Brenner & Rector's
THE
KIDNEY

Brenner & Rector's
THE
KIDNEY

8TH EDITION

Barry M. Brenner, MD, AM (Hon), DSc (Hon),
DMSc (Hon), MD (Hon), Dipl (Hon),
FRCP (London, Hon)
Samuel A. Levine Professor of Medicine
Harvard Medical School
Director Emeritus, Renal Division, and Senior Physician
Department of Medicine
Brigham and Women's Hospital
Boston, Massachusetts

VOLUME 1

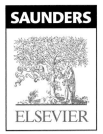

SAUNDERS

ELSEVIER

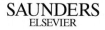

1600 John F. Kennedy Blvd.
Ste 1800
Philadelphia, PA 19103-2899

BRENNER & RECTOR'S THE KIDNEY

ISBN: 978-1-4160-3105-5
E-dition: 978-1-4160-3110-9
Two volume set: 978-1-4160-3105-5
Vol. 1: 9996014460
Vol. 2: 9996014525

Notice

Knowledge and best practice in this field are constantly changing. As new research and experience broaden our knowledge, changes in practice, treatment and drug therapy may become necessary or appropriate. Readers are advised to check the most current information provided (i) on procedures featured or (ii) by the manufacturer of each product to be administered, to verify the recommended dose or formula, the method and duration of administration, and contraindications. It is the responsibility of the practitioner, relying on their own experience and knowledge of the patient, to make diagnoses, to determine dosages and the best treatment for each individual patient, and to take all appropriate safety precautions. To the fullest extent of the law, neither the Publisher nor the Editor assumes any liability for any injury and/or damage to persons or property arising out or related to any use of the material contained in this book.

The Publisher

Previous editions copyrighted 2004, 2000, 1996, 1991, 1986, 1981, 1976 by Elsevier Inc.

Front Cover

Magnetic resonance images of human kidneys. Reproduced with permission from L Hofmann, S Simon-Zoula, A Nowak et al. BOLD-MRI for the assessment of renal oxygenation in humans: Acute effect of nephrotoxic xenobiotics. Nature Publishing Group: Kidney International, Volume 70, Issue 1, July 1, 2006.

Back Cover

Top Left. Two color image of renal tubules and contiguous dendritic cells. Reprinted with permission from T J Soos, T N Sims, L Barisoni et al. CX3CR1 interstitial dendritic cells form a contiguous network throughout the entire kidney. Nature Publishing Group: Kidney International, Volume 70, Issue 3, August 1, 2006.

Top Right. Arrow diagram of transtubular chloride transport. From Chapter 5.

Bottom Left. Hemisection of rodent kidney stained to reveal cortical glomeruli. From Chapter 1.

Bottom Right. Scanning electron photomicrograph of abnormal human glomerulus. Reprinted with permission from A-M Kuusniemi, J Merenmies, A-T Lahdenkari et al. Glomerular sclerosis in kidneys with congenital nephrotic syndrome (NPHS1). Nature Publishing Group: Kidney International, Volume 70, Issue 8, October 1, 2006.

Library of Congress Cataloging-in-Publication Data
Brenner & Rector's The Kidney / [edited by] Barry M. Brenner—8th ed.
    p. ; cm.
  Includes bibliographical references and index.
  ISBN 978-1-4160-3105-5
  1. Kidneys—Diseases. 2. Kidneys. I. Brenner, Barry M., 1937- II. Rector, Floyd C. III. Title: Brenner and Rector's The Kidney. IV. Title: Kidney.
  [DNLM: 1. Kidney Diseases. 2. Kidney—physiology. 3. Kidney—physiopathology. WJ 300 B8375 2008]
RC902.K53 2008
616.6′1—dc22

2006033461

Acquisitions Editor: Susan Pioli
Developmental Editor: Arlene Chappelle
Project Manager: Mary B. Stermel
Design Direction: Steven Stave

Printed in China
Last digit is the print number: 9 8 7 6 5 4 3 2 1

Dedicated to
Jane
Our Parents
Louis and Sally and Murray and Beatrice
Our Children
Rob and Molly and Jen and Ron
And Our Grandchildren
Sam, Max, and Elliott

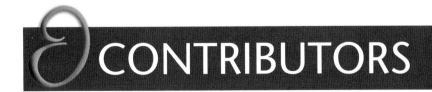

Zaid A. Abassi, DSc
Associate Professor, Department of Physiology and
Biophysics, Faculty of Medicine, Technion—Israel
Institute of Technology; Principal Investigator,
Department of Vascular Surgery, Rambam Medical
Center, Haifa, Israel
Extracellular Fluid and Edema Formation

Nada M. Abou Hassan, MD
Medicine Chief Resident, American University of
Beirut, Beirut, Lebanon
Microvascular and Macrovascular Diseases of the Kidney

Michael Allon, MD
Professor of Medicine, University of Alabama at
Birmingham, Birmingham, Alabama
Interventional Nephrology

Sharon Anderson, MD
Professor of Medicine, Division of Nephrology and
Hypertension, Oregon Health and Science
University, Portland, Oregon
*Renal and Systemic Manifestations of Glomerular
Disease*

Mohammed Javeed Ansari, MBBS, MRCP(UK)
Instructor in Medicine, Harvard Medical School;
Staff Physician, Brigham and Women's Hospital,
Boston, Massachusetts
Clinical Management

Gerald B. Appel, MD
Professor of Clinical Medicine, Columbia University
College of Physicians and Surgeons; Director,
Clinical Nephrology, Columbia University Medical
Center, New York, New York
Secondary Glomerular Disease

Allen I. Arieff, MS, MD
Professor of Medicine Emeritus, University of
California School of Medicine, San Francisco;
Attending Physician, Cedars-Sinai Medical Center,
Los Angeles, California
Neurologic Aspects of Kidney Disease

Michael B. Atkins, MD
Professor of Medicine, Harvard Medical School;
Deputy Director, Division of Hematology/Oncology,
and Director, Cutaneous Oncology and Biologic
Therapy Programs, Beth Israel Deaconess Medical
Center, Boston, Massachusetts
Renal Neoplasia

Kamal F. Badr, MD
Founding Dean, Lebanese American University,
Beirut, Lebanon
*Microvascular and Macrovascular Diseases of the
Kidney*

Tomas Berl, MD
Professor of Medicine and Head of Renal Diseases
and Hypertension, University of Colorado School of
Medicine, Denver, Colorado
Disorders of Water Balance

Daniel G. Bichet, MD, MSc
Professor of Medicine and Physiology, and Canada
Research Chair in Genetics of Renal Diseases,
Université de Montréal; Nephrologist, Hôpital du
Sacré-Coeur de Montréal, Montréal, Québec, Canada
Inherited Disorders of the Renal Tubule

Peter G. Blake, MB, MSc, FRCPC, FRCPI
Professor of Medicine and Chair of Nephrology,
University of Western Ontario; Staff Nephrologist,
London Health Sciences Centre, London, Ontario,
Canada
Peritoneal Dialysis

Jon D. Blumenfeld, MD
Professor of Clinical Medicine, Weill Medical College
of Cornell University; Director, Hypertension
Section and The Susan R. Knafel Polycystic
Kidney Disease Center of The Rogosin Institute,
New York-Presbyterian Hospital; Attending
Physician, Department of Medicine, The Rockefeller
University Hospital, New York, New York
Primary and Secondary Hypertension

Alain Bonnardeaux, MD
Associate Professor of Medicine, Université de
Montréal; Nephrologist, Hôpital Maisonneuve-
Rosemont, Montréal, Québec, Canada
Inherited Disorders of the Renal Tubule

Joseph V. Bonventre, MD, PhD
Robert H. Ebert Professor of Medicine, Harvard
Medical School; Director, Renal Division, Brigham
and Women's Hospital, Boston, Massachusetts
Genomics and Proteomics in Nephrology

William D. Boswell, Jr., MD
Associate Professor of Radiology, and Associate
Chairman, Department of Radiology, Keck School
of Medicine, University of Southern California;
Chief of Radiology, USC/Norris Cancer Center,
Los Angeles, California
Diagnostic Kidney Imaging

Barry M. Brenner, MD
Samuel A. Levine Professor of Medicine, Harvard
Medical School; Director Emeritus, Renal Division,
and Senior Physician, Department of Medicine,
Brigham and Women's Hospital, Boston,
Massachusetts
*The Renal Circulations and Glomerular Ultrafiltration;
Nephron Endowment; Adaptation to Nephron Loss;
Renal and Systemic Manifestations of Glomerular
Disease*

Matthew D. Breyer, MD
Professor of Medicine, Division of Nephrology,
Vanderbilt University, Nashville, Tennessee; Senior
Medical Fellow II, Biotherapeutics Discovery
Research, Eli Lilly and Company Corporate Center,
Indianapolis, Indiana
Arachidonic Acid Metabolites and the Kidney

Dennis Brown, PhD
Professor of Medicine, Harvard Medical School;
Director, Massachusetts General Hospital Program
in Membrane Biology, Massachusetts General
Hospital, Boston, Massachusetts
Cell Biology of Vasopressin Action

Louise M. Burrell, MB, ChB, MRCP, MD, FRACP, FAHA
Professor of Medicine, University of Melbourne,
Melbourne; Senior Clinician, Austin Health,
Victoria, Australia
Vasoactive Peptides and the Kidney

David A. Bushinsky, MD
Professor of Medicine and of Pharmacology and
Physiology, University of Rochester School of
Medicine; Chief, Nephrology Division, University of
Rochester Medical Center, Rochester, New York
Nephrolithiasis

Riccardo Candido, MD, PhD
Diabetic Centre, Azienda per i Servizi Sanitari n. 1
Triestina, Trieste, Italy
Vasoactive Peptides and the Kidney

Anil Chandraker, MB, ChB, FRCP
Assistant Professor of Medicine, Harvard Medical
School; Associate Physician, Brigham and Women's
Hospital; Research Associate, Children's Hospital
Boston, Boston, Massachusetts
Transplantation Immunobiology

Ingrid J. Chang, MD
Instructor of Medicine, Division of Nephrology and
Hypertension, Vanderbilt University Medical
Center, Nashville, Tennessee
Extracorporeal Treatment of Poisoning

Devasmita Choudhury, MD
Associate Professor, Department of Medicine,
University of Texas Southwestern Medical School;
Director of In-center and Home Dialysis, VA North
Texas Health Care Systems, Dallas VA Medical
Center, Dallas, Texas
Aging and Kidney Disease

Peale Chuang, MD
Fellow, Vanderbilt University Medical Center,
Nashville, Tennessee
Hemodialysis

Michael R. Clarkson, MD, MRCPI
Senior Lecturer in Clinical Nephrology, University
College Cork School of Medicine; Consultant
Nephrologist, Cork University Hospital, Wilton,
Cork, Ireland
Acute Kidney Injury

Fredric L. Coe, MD
Professor of Medicine and Physiology, and Director,
Kidney Stone Prevention Program, Pritzker School
of Medicine, University of Chicago, Chicago,
Illinois
Nephrolithiasis

Mark E. Cooper, MB, PhD, FRACP, FAHA, FASN
Professor of Medicine (Eastern Clinical School),
Monash University; Senior Endocrinologist,
Alfred Hospital; Head, Diabetes and Metabolism
Division, Baker Heart Research Institute,
Melbourne, Victoria, Australia
Vasoactive Peptides and the Kidney

Josef Coresh, MD, PhD, MHS
Professor of Epidemiology, Biostatistics and
Medicine, Johns Hopkins University Bloomberg
School of Public Health, Johns Hopkins University
School of Medicine, Baltimore, Maryland
Epidemiology of Kidney Disease

Ramzi S. Cotran, MD*
Former Frank B. Mallory Professor of Pathology,
Harvard Medical School; Former Chair, Department
of Pathology, Brigham and Women's Hospital and
Children's Hospital Boston, Boston, Massachusetts
*Urinary Tract Infection, Pyelonephritis, and Reflux
Nephropathy*

Gary C. Curhan, MD, ScD
Associate Professor of Medicine, Harvard Medical
School; Associate Professor of Epidemiology,
Harvard School of Public Health; Physician, Renal
Division, Department of Medicine, Brigham and
Women's Hospital, Boston, Massachusetts
Diet and Kidney Disease

Vivette D'Agati, MD
Professor of Pathology, Department of Pathology,
Columbia University College of Physicians and
Surgeons; Chief, Renal Pathology, Columbia
University Medical Center, New York, New York
Secondary Glomerular Disease

M.R. Davids, MD
Professor of Medicine, and Chief of Nephrology,
Stellenbosch University School of Medicine,
Cape Town, South Africa
*Interpretation of Electrolyte and Acid-Base Parameters in
Blood and Urine*

Marc E. De Broe, MD
Professor in Nephrology, University of Antwerp,
Wilrijk/Antwerpen, Belgium
Tubulointerstitial Diseases

Paul E. De Jong, MD
Professor of Nephrology, Nephrologist, and Chief,
Division of Nephrology, Department of Medicine,
University Medical Center Groningen, Groningen,
The Netherlands
*Specific Pharmacologic Approaches to Clinical
Renoprotection*

*Deceased

Dick de Zeeuw, MD
Professor of Clinical Pharmacology, University Medical Center Groningen, Groningen, The Netherlands
Specific Pharmacologic Approaches to Clinical Renoprotection

Bradley M. Denker, MD
Associate Professor of Medicine, Harvard Medical School; Physician, Brigham and Women's Hospital; Chief of Nephrology, Harvard Vanguard Medical Associates, Boston, Massachusetts
Plasmapheresis

Matthew Dollins, MD
Assistant Professor of Clinical Medicine, Indiana University, Indianapolis, Indiana
Intensive Care Nephrology

Thomas D. DuBose, Jr., MD
Tinsley R. Harrison Professor and Chair of Internal Medicine, and Professor of Physiology and Pharmacology, Wake Forest University School of Medicine; Chief of Internal Medicine Service, North Carolina Baptist Hospital, Winston-Salem, North Carolina
Disorders of Acid-Base Balance

Lance D. Dworkin, MD
Professor of Medicine, Vice Chairman for Research and Academic Affairs, and Director, Division of Kidney Diseases and Hypertension, Warren Alpert Medical School of Brown University; Director, Division of Kidney Diseases and Hypertension, Rhode Island and The Miriam Hospitals, Providence, Rhode Island
The Renal Circulations and Glomerular Ultrafiltration

David H. Ellison, MD
Professor of Medicine, and Head, Division of Nephrology and Hypertension, Oregon Health and Science University; Oregon Health and Science University Hospital; Portland VA Medical Center, Portland, Oregon
Diuretics

Joseph A. Eustace, MB, MRCPI, MHS
Senior Lecturer in Clinical Nephrology, University College Cork School of Medicine; Consultant Nephrologist, Cork University Hospital, Wilton, Cork, Ireland
Epidemiology of Kidney Disease; Acute Kidney Injury

Ronald J. Falk, MD
Doc J. Thurston Distinguished Professor of Medicine, University of North Carolina; Chief, Division of Nephrology, UNC Health Care, Chapel Hill, North Carolina
Primary Glomerular Disease

Robert A. Fenton, PhD
Assistant Professor, University of Aarhus, Aarhus, Denmark
Urine Concentration and Dilution

Steven Fishbane, MD
Professor of Medicine, SUNY Stony Brook School of Medicine, Stony Brook; Chief, Division of Nephrology, Winthrop-University Hospital, Mineola, New York
Hematologic Aspects of Kidney Disease; Erythropoietin Therapy in Renal Disease and Renal Failure

Jay A. Fishman, MD
Associate Professor of Medicine, Harvard Medical School; Associate Director, Transplantation Center, and Director, Massachusetts General Hospital Transplant Infectious Disease and Compromised Host Program, Massachusetts General Hospital, Boston, Massachusetts
Xenotransplantation

John J. Friedewald, MD
Assistant Professor, Division of Nephrology/Hypertension, Northwestern University Medical School, Chicago, Illinois
Acute Kidney Injury

Jørgen Frøkiaer, MD, DMSc
Professor of Medicine, Faculty of Health Sciences, University of Aarhus; Chief Consultant, Aarhus University Hospital—Skejby, Aarhus, Denmark
Urinary Tract Obstruction

Ladan Golestaneh, MD, MS
Assistant Professor of Medicine, Albert Einstein College of Medicine; Medical Director of Inpatient Dialysis and CRRT, Montefiore Medical Center, Bronx, New York
Gender and Kidney Disease

Rujun Gong, MD, PhD
Assistant Professor of Medicine, Division of Kidney Diseases and Hypertension, Warren Alpert Medical School of Brown University; Medical Research Scientist, Division of Kidney Diseases and Hypertension, Rhode Island Hospital, Providence, Rhode Island
The Renal Circulations and Glomerular Ultrafiltration

William G. Goodman, MD
Medical Affairs Director, Nephrology Therapeutic Area, Amgen Inc., Thousand Oaks, California
Vitamin D, Calcimimetics, and Phosphate-Binders

Jared J. Grantham, MD
Harry Statland Professor of Nephrology, Associate Dean for Medical Graduate Studies, and Consultant, The Kidney Institute, University of Kansas Medical Center, Kansas City, Kansas
Cystic Diseases of the Kidney

M.L. Halperin, MD, FRCPC, FRS
Emeritus Professor, University of Toronto School of Medicine; Attending Physician, St. Michael's Hospital, Toronto, Ontario, Canada
Interpretation of Electrolyte and Acid-Base Parameters in Blood and Urine

x L. Lee Hamm, MD
Chair, Department of Internal Medicine, Tulane
  University School of Medicine, New Orleans,
  Louisiana
  Renal Acidification

Marc R. Hammerman, AB, MD
Chromalloy Professor of Renal Diseases in Medicine,
  Washington University School of Medicine;
  Physician, Barnes-Jewish Hospital, St. Louis,
  Missouri
  Tissue Engineering and Regeneration

Donna S. Hanes, MD
Associate Professor of Medicine, University of
  Maryland School of Medicine, Baltimore,
  Maryland
  Antihypertensive Drugs

Raymond C. Harris, Jr., MD
Ann and Roscoe R. Robinson Professor of Medicine,
  Director, Vanderbilt Division of Nephrology and
  Hypertension, and Director, Vanderbilt O'Brien
  Center for the Study of Renal Disease, Vanderbilt
  University School of Medicine; Staff Physician/
  Nephrologist, Veterans Administration Hospital,
  Nashville, Tennessee
  Arachidonic Acid Metabolites and the Kidney

Jonathan Himmelfarb, MD
Clinical Professor of Medicine, University of Vermont
  College of Medicine, Burlington, Vermont; Director,
  Division of Nephrology and Transplantation, Maine
  Medical Center, Portland, Maine
  Hemodialysis

Jason D. Hoffert, PhD
Physiologist, National Heart, Lung, and Blood
  Institute, Bethesda, Maryland
  Urine Concentration and Dilution

Thomas H. Hostetter, MD
Professor of Medicine, Albert Einstein College of
  Medicine, New York, New York
  Pathophysiology of Uremia

Stephen I-Hong Hsu, MD, PhD
R. Glenn Davis Associate Professor in Clinical and
  Translational Medicine, Division of Nephrology,
  Hypertension and Dialysis, Department of
  Medicine, University of Florida College of
  Medicine; Nephrologist, Division of Nephrology,
  Hypertension and Dialysis, Department of
  Medicine, Shands Healthcare at the University of
  Florida, Gainesville, Florida
  Genomics and Proteomics in Nephrology

John J. Iacomini, PhD
Associate Professor of Medicine, Harvard Medical
  School; Associate Biologist, Brigham and Women's
  Hospital; Associate Scientist, Children's Hospital
  Boston, Boston, Massachusetts
  Transplantation Immunobiology

Hassan N. Ibrahim, MD, MS
Assistant Professor of Medicine, and Director, Renal
  Fellowship Program, University of Minnesota,
  Minneapolis, Minnesota
  Donor and Recipient Issues

Ajay K. Israni, MD, MS
Assistant Professor of Medicine, University of
  Minnesota School of Medicine; Adjunct Assistant
  Professor of Epidemiology and Community Health,
  University of Minnesota School of Public Health;
  Attending Nephrologist, Hennepin County Medical
  Center, Minneapolis, Minnesota
  *Laboratory Assessment of Kidney Disease: Clearance,
    Urinalysis, and Kidney Biopsy*

Hossein Jadvar, MD, PhD, MPH, MBA
Associate Professor of Radiology and Biomedical
  Engineering, and Director of Research, Department
  of Radiology, Keck School of Medicine, University
  of Southern California, Los Angeles, California
  Diagnostic Kidney Imaging

Karin A.M. Jandeleit-Dahm, MD, PhD, FRACP
Associate Professor of Medicine (Eastern Clinical
  School), Monash University, Melbourne, Victoria,
  Australia
  Vasoactive Peptides and the Kidney

J. Charles Jennette, MD
Kenneth M. Brinkhous Distinguished Professor,
  University of North Carolina; Chair, UNC Health
  Care, Chapel Hill, North Carolina
  Primary Glomerular Disease

Eric Jonasch, MD
Assistant Professor, Genitourinary Medical Oncology,
  University of Texas M.D. Anderson Cancer Center,
  Houston, Texas
  Renal Neoplasia

K.S. Kamel, MD, FRCPC
Professor, University of Toronto School of Medicine;
  Chief, Nephrology, St. Michael's Hospital, Toronto,
  Ontario, Canada
  *Interpretation of Electrolyte and Acid-Base Parameters in
    Blood and Urine*

Abbas A. Kanso, MD
Nephrology Fellow, Division of Nephrology, Metro
  Health Medical Center, Case Western Reserve
  University, Cleveland, Ohio
  *Microvascular and Macrovascular Diseases of the
    Kidney*

S. Ananth Karumanchi, MD
Associate Professor of Medicine, Obstetrics and
  Gynecology, Harvard Medical School; Attending
  Physician, Nephrology, Beth Israel Deaconess
  Medical Center, Boston, Massachusetts
  Hypertension and Kidney Disease in Pregnancy

Bertram L. Kasiske, MD
Professor, University of Minnesota School of
  Medicine; Director, Division of Nephrology, and
  Medical Director, Kidney Transplant, Hennepin
  County Medical Center; Medical Director, Kidney
  Transplant and Pancreas Transplant, University of
  Minnesota Medical Center-Fairview, Minneapolis,
  Minnesota
*Laboratory Assessment of Kidney Disease: Clearance,
  Urinalysis, and Kidney Biopsy; Donor and Recipient
  Issues*

David K. Klassen, MD
Professor of Medicine, University of Maryland School
  of Medicine, Baltimore, Maryland
Antihypertensive Drugs

Mark A. Knepper, MD, PhD
Senior Investigator, National Heart, Lung, and Blood
  Institute, Bethesda, Maryland
Urine Concentration and Dilution

Radko Komers, MD, PhD
Research Assistant Professor of Medicine, Division of
  Nephrology and Hypertension, Oregon Health and
  Science University, Portland, Oregon
*Renal and Systemic Manifestations of Glomerular
  Disease*

Bruce C. Kone, MD
Dean and Folke H. Peterson Dean's Distinguished
  Professor, University of Florida College of
  Medicine, Gainesville, Florida
Metabolic Basis of Solute Transport

Michael A. Kraus, MD
Clinical Chief of Nephrology, Indiana University
  School of Medicine; Medical Director, Home
  Dialysis and Acute Dialysis, and Co-Chief of
  Nephrology, Clarion Health Partners, Indianapolis,
  Indiana
Intensive Care Nephrology

Jordan Kreidberg, MD, PhD
Associate Professor of Pediatrics, Department of
  Nephrology, Children's Hospital Boston, Boston,
  Massachusetts
Embryology of the Kidney

John H. Laragh, MD
Professor of Clinical Medicine in Cardiothoracic
  Surgery, Weill Medical College of Cornell
  University; Director, Cardiovascular Center,
  Department of Cardiothoracic Surgery, New York-
  Presbyterian Hospital, New York, New York
Primary and Secondary Hypertension

Andrew S. Levey, MD
Dr. Gerald J. and Dorothy R. Friedman Professor of
  Medicine, Tufts University School of Medicine;
  Chief, Division of Nephrology, Tufts-New England
  Medical Center, Boston, Massachusetts
Risk Factors and Kidney Disease

Moshe Levi, MD
Professor of Medicine, Physiology and Biophysics,
  and Vice Chair of Medicine for Research, University
  of Colorado Health Sciences Center, Denver,
  Colorado
Aging and Kidney Disease

S.H. Lin, MD
Professor, Tri-Services General Medical School;
  Director, Dialysis Service, Division of Nephrology,
  Tri-Services General Hospital, Taipei, Taiwan
*Interpretation of Electrolyte and Acid-Base Parameters in
  Blood and Urine*

Valerie A. Luyckx, MD
Assistant Professor, Division of Nephrology and
  Immunology, Department of Medicine, University
  of Alberta, Edmonton, Alberta, Canada
Nephron Endowment

David A. Maddox, PhD
Professor of Internal Medicine, University of South
  Dakota Sanford School of Medicine; Coordinator of
  Research and Development, VA Medical Center;
  Director of Basic Research, Avera Research Institute,
  Sioux Falls, South Dakota
The Renal Circulations and Glomerular Ultrafiltration

Kirsten M. Madsen, MD, DMSc
Associate Professor of Medicine, University of Florida
  College of Medicine, Gainesville, Florida
Anatomy of the Kidney

Colm C. Magee, MD, MPH, MRCPI
Assistant Professor of Medicine, Harvard Medical
  School; Staff Physician, Brigham and Women's
  Hospital, Boston, Massachusetts
Clinical Management

Daniella Magen, MD
Lecturer, Faculty of Medicine, Technion—Israel
  Institute of Technology; Senior Physician, Pediatric
  Nephrology Unit, Meyer Children's Hospital,
  Rambam Health Care Campus, Haifa, Israel
Stem Cells in Renal Biology and Medicine

Michael Mauer, MD
Department of Pediatric Nephrology, University of
  Minnesota Hospital and Clinic, Minneapolis,
  Minnesota
Diabetic Nephropathy

Ivan D. Maya, MD, FACP
Assistant Professor of Medicine and Radiology,
  University of Alabama at Birmingham; Associate
  Director of Interventional Nephrology, University of
  Alabama Hospitals, Birmingham, Alabama
Interventional Nephrology

Sharon E. Maynard, MD
Assistant Professor of Medicine, Division of Renal
  Diseases and Hypertension, George Washington
  University Medical School, and George Washington
  University Hospital, Washington, D.C.
Hypertension and Kidney Disease in Pregnancy

xii Christopher W. McIntyre, MBBS, MD
Associate Professor and Reader in Vascular Medicine,
School of Graduate Entry Medicine and Healthcare,
University of Nottingham Medical School at Derby;
Honorary Consultant Nephrologist, Derby City
General Hospital, Derby, United Kingdom
Prescribing Drugs in Kidney Disease

Lawrence P. McMahon, MD, FRACP
Director of Nephrology, Western Hospital, Melbourne,
Victoria, Australia
Cardiovascular Aspects of Chronic Kidney Disease

Vandana Menon, MD, PhD, MPH
Assistant Professor of Medicine, Tufts University
School of Medicine, and Tufts-New England
Medical Center, Boston, Massachusetts
Risk Factors and Kidney Disease

Timothy W. Meyer, MD
Professor of Medicine, Stanford University, Stanford;
VA Palo Alto Health Care System, Palo Alto,
California
Pathophysiology of Uremia

Edgar L. Milford, MD
Associate Professor of Medicine, Harvard Medical
School; Staff Physician, Brigham and Women's
Hospital, Boston, Massachusetts
Clinical Management

William E. Mitch, MD
Gordon A. Cain Professor of Medicine, and Director,
Division of Nephrology, Baylor College of Medicine,
Houston, Texas
Diet and Kidney Disease

Orson W. Moe, MD
Director, Charles and Jane Pak Center for Mineral
Metabolism and Clinical Research, University of
Texas Southwestern Medical Center at Dallas;
Professor, Internal Medicine, Parkland Memorial
Hospital, and St. Paul Hospital, Dallas, Texas
Renal Handling of Organic Solutes; Nephrolithiasis

Sharon M. Moe, MD
Professor of Medicine, and Vice Chair for Research,
Department of Medicine, Indiana University School
of Medicine, and Roudebush VA Medical Center,
Indianapolis, Indiana
Mineral Bone Disorders in Chronic Kidney Disease

Bruce A. Molitoris, MD
Director of Nephrology, Indiana University School of
Medicine, and Roudebush VA Medical Center;
Indiana University Hospital; Clarion Hospital;
Veterans Affairs Hospital, Indianapolis, Indiana
Intensive Care Nephrology

David B. Mount, MD
Assistant Professor, Harvard Medical School;
Attending Physician, Renal Division, Brigham and
Women's Hospital, and Division of General Internal
Medicine, VA Boston Health Care System, Boston,
Massachusetts
*Transport of Inorganic Solutes: Sodium, Chloride,
Potassium, Magnesium, Calcium, and Phosphate;
Disorders of Potassium Balance*

Jean Mulder, MD
Instructor in Medicine, Harvard Medical School;
Brigham and Women's Hospital, Boston,
Massachusetts
Endocrine Aspects of Kidney Disease

Patrick H. Nachman, MD
Associate Professor of Medicine, UNC Kidney Center,
University of North Carolina, and UNC Health Care,
Chapel Hill, North Carolina
Primary Glomerular Disease

Nazih L. Nakhoul, PhD
Research Associate Professor, Department of Internal
Medicine, Tulane University School of Medicine,
New Orleans, Louisiana
Renal Acidification

Gerjan Navis, MD
Professor of Experimental Nephrology, and
Nephrologist, Division of Nephrology, Department
of Medicine, University Medical Center Groningen,
Groningen, The Netherlands
*Specific Pharmacologic Approaches to Clinical
Renoprotection*

Joel Neugarten, MD
Professor of Medicine, Albert Einstein College of
Medicine; Site Director, Renal Division, Montefiore
Medical Center, Bronx, New York
Gender and Kidney Disease

Søren Nielsen, MD, PhD, DMSc
Professor of Cell Biology and Pathophysiology, and
Director, The Water and Salt Research Center,
Institute of Anatomy, University of Aarhus, Aarhus,
Denmark
*Anatomy of the Kidney; Cell Biology of Vasopressin
Action*

Allen R. Nissenson, MD
Professor of Medicine, Associate Dean, and Director,
Dialysis Program, David Geffen School of Medicine
at UCLA, Los Angeles, California
*Erythropoietin Therapy in Renal Disease and Renal
Failure*

Paul J. Owen, MBBS
Research Fellow in Renal Medicine, School of
Graduate Entry Medicine and Healthcare,
University of Nottingham Medical School at Derby,
Derby, United Kingdom
Prescribing Drugs in Kidney Disease

Randall K. Packer, PhD
Professor of Biology and Deputy Chair of Biology
Department, George Washington University,
Washington, D.C.
Urine Concentration and Dilution

Manuel Palacín, DSc
Full Professor of Biochemistry and Molecular Biology,
Department of Biochemistry and Molecular Biology,
Faculty of Biology, University of Barcelona; Group
Leader, Molecular Medicine Program, Institute for
Research in Biomedicine (IRB), Barcelona, Spain
Renal Handling of Organic Solutes

Biff F. Palmer, MD
Professor of Internal Medicine, University of Texas
  Southwestern Medical Center at Dallas; Physician,
  Parkland Health and Human Services, Dallas,
  Texas
Endocrine Aspects of Kidney Disease

Suzanne L. Palmer, MD
Associate Professor of Clinical Radiology, and Chief,
  Body Imaging Division, Keck School of Medicine,
  University of Southern California, Los Angeles,
  California
Diagnostic Kidney Imaging

Patrick S. Parfrey, MD, FRCP(C)
University Research Professor, Memorial University;
  Research Chief, and Staff Nephrologist, Eastern
  Health, St. John's, Newfoundland, Canada
Cardiovascular Aspects of Chronic Kidney Disease

Hans-Henrik Parving, MD, DMSc
Professor and Chief Physician, Rigshospitalet,
  Copenhagen, Denmark
Diabetic Nephropathy

Norberto Perico, MD
Head, Laboratory of Drug Development, Clinical
  Research Center for Rare Diseases "Aldo e Cele
  Daccò", Mario Negri Institute for Pharmacological
  Research, Bergamo, Italy
Tubulointerstitial Diseases

Martin R. Pollak, MD
Associate Professor of Medicine, Harvard Medical
  School; Physician, Brigham and Women's Hospital,
  Boston, Massachusetts
*Disorders of Calcium, Magnesium, and Phosphate
  Balance; Inherited Disorders of Podocyte Function*

Susan E. Quaggin, MD
Canada Research Chair in Vascular Biology,
  The Samuel Lunnenfeld Research Institute,
  University of Toronto, Toronto, Ontario, Canada
Embryology of the Kidney

L. Darryl Quarles, MD
Summerfield Endowed Professor of Nephrology, Vice
  Chairman, Department of Internal Medicine, and
  Director, The Kidney Institute and Division of
  Nephrology, University of Kansas Medical Center,
  Kansas City, Kansas
Vitamin D, Calcimimetics, and Phosphate-Binders

Hamid Rabb, MD, FACP
Associate Professor of Medicine, and Physician
  Director, Kidney Transplant Program, Johns
  Hopkins University School of Medicine, Baltimore,
  Maryland
Acute Kidney Injury

Jai Radhakrishnan, MD
Associate Professor of Clinical Medicine, Columbia
  University College of Physicians and Surgeons;
  Director, Renal Fellowship Program, Columbia
  University Medical Center, New York, New York
Secondary Glomerular Disease

Jochen Reiser, MD, PhD
Assistant Professor of Medicine, Harvard Medical
  School; Associate Physician, Massachusetts General
  Hospital, Boston, Massachusetts
Inherited Disorders of Podocyte Function

Giuseppe Remuzzi, MD
Professor in Nephrology, and Director of Division of
  Nephrology and Dialysis, Azienda Ospedaliera
  Ospedali Riuniti di Bergamo; Director of Mario
  Negri Institute for Pharmacological Research, Negri
  Bergamo Laboratories, Bergamo, Italy
Tubulointerstitial Diseases

Eberhard Ritz, MD
Professor of Nephrology, Dialysis, and
  Transplantation, Sektion Nephrologie, Med.
  Universitätsklinik, Heidelberg, Germany
Diabetic Nephropathy

Robert H. Rubin, MD
Professor of Medicine, Harvard Medical School;
  Associate Director, Division of Infectious Diseases,
  Brigham and Women's Hospital, Boston,
  Massachusetts
*Urinary Tract Infection, Pyelonephritis, and Reflux
  Nephropathy*

Ernesto Sabath, MD
Physician, Universidad Autonoma de Queretaro,
  Queretaro, Mexico
Plasmapheresis

David H. Sachs, MD, AB, DES
Professor of Surgery and Immunology, Harvard
  Medical School, Boston; Director of the
  Transplantation Biology Research Center,
  Massachusetts General Hospital, Charlestown,
  Massachusetts
Xenotransplantation

Souheil Saddekni, MD
Professor of Radiology, University of Alabama at
  Birmingham, Birmingham, Alabama
Interventional Nephrology

Alan D. Salama, MBBS, MA, PhD, FRCP
Senior Lecturer and Honorary Consultant Physician,
  Imperial College London; Honorary Consultant
  Physician, Hammersmith Hospital, London,
  United Kingdom
Attaining Immunologic Tolerance in the Clinic

Mark J. Sarnak, MD, MS
Associate Director, Research Training Program,
  Division of Nephrology, Tufts-New England Medical
  Center; Associate Professor of Medicine, Tufts
  University School of Medicine, Boston,
  Massachusetts
Risk Factors and Kidney Disease

Ramesh Saxena, MD, PhD
Associate Professor of Medicine, Department
  of Internal Medicine, University of Texas
  Southwestern Medical Center at Dallas,
  Dallas, Texas
Approach to the Patient with Kidney Disease

xiv Mohamed H. Sayegh, MD
Professor of Medicine and Pediatrics, Harvard
   Medical School; Director, Transplantation
   Research Center, Brigham and Women's Hospital,
   and Children's Hospital Boston,
   Boston, Massachusetts
   *Transplantation Immunobiology; Attaining Immunologic
      Tolerance in the Clinic*

Asher D. Schachter, MD, MMSc, MS
Assistant Professor of Pediatrics, Harvard Medical
   School; Division of Nephrology, Children's Hospital
   Boston, Boston, Massachusetts
   Genomics and Proteomics in Nephrology

Gerald Schulman, MD
Professor of Medicine, Vanderbilt University School
   of Medicine; Professor of Medicine, Director of
   Hemodialysis, and Co-Director of Clinical Trials
   Center in Nephrology, Vanderbilt University
   Medical Center, Nashville, Tennessee
   Hemodialysis

Ajay Sharma, MD
Assistant Professor of Pediatrics, University of
   Western Ontario; Pediatric Nephrologist, London
   Health Sciences Centre, London, Ontario, Canada
   Peritoneal Dialysis

Sharon R. Silbiger, MD
Professor of Clinical Medicine, Albert Einstein
   College of Medicine; Director, Internal Medicine
   Residency Program (AECOM/Montefiore),
   Montefiore Medical Center, Bronx, New York
   Gender and Kidney Disease

Ajay K. Singh, MB, MRCP
Associate Professor of Medicine, Harvard Medical
   School; Clinical Director, Renal Division, and
   Director of Dialysis Services, Brigham and Women's
   Hospital, Boston, Massachusetts
   Endocrine Aspects of Kidney Disease

Karl L. Skorecki, MD
Annie Chutick Professor and Chair in Medicine
   (Nephrology), Technion—Israel Institute of
   Technology; Director of Medical and Research
   Development, Rambam Health Care Campus,
   Haifa, Israel
   *Extracellular Fluid and Edema Formation; Stem Cells in
      Renal Biology and Medicine*

James P. Smith, MD
Clinical Fellow, Nephrology, Vanderbilt University
   Medical Center, Nashville, Tennessee
   Extracorporeal Treatment of Poisoning

Stuart M. Sprague, DO
Professor of Medicine, Northwestern University
   Feinberg School of Medicine, Chicago; Chief,
   Division of Nephrology and Hypertension, Evanston
   Northwestern Healthcare, Evanston, Illinois
   Mineral Bone Disorders in Chronic Kidney Disease

John C. Stivelman, AB, MD
Associate Professor of Medicine, Division of
   Nephrology, Department of Medicine,
   University of Washington School of Medicine;
   Chief Medical Officer, Northwest Kidney Centers,
   Seattle, Washington
   *Erythropoietin Therapy in Renal Disease and Renal
      Failure*

Maarten W. Taal, MB, ChB, MMed, MD,
FCP(SA), FRCP
Special Lecturer, University of Nottingham Medical
   School at Derby; Consultant Renal Physician, Derby
   City General Hospital, Derby, United Kingdom
   Adaptation to Nephron Loss

Eric N. Taylor, MD, MSc
Instructor in Medicine, Harvard Medical School;
   Associate Physician, Renal Division, Brigham and
   Women's Hospital, Boston, Massachusetts
   *Disorders of Calcium, Magnesium, and Phosphate
      Balance*

Stephen C. Textor, MD
Professor of Medicine, Mayo Clinic College of
   Medicine; Vice-Chair, Nephrology and Hypertension
   Division, Mayo Clinic, Rochester, Minnesota
   Renovascular Hypertension and Ischemic Nephropathy

Ravi Thadhani, MD, MPH
Associate Professor of Medicine, Harvard Medical
   School; Director of Clinical Research in
   Nephrology, Massachusetts General Hospital,
   Boston, Massachusetts
   Hypertension and Kidney Disease in Pregnancy

C. Craig Tisher, MD
Professor, Departments of Medicine, Pathology, and
   Anatomy and Cell Biology, and Dean Emeritus,
   University of Florida College of Medicine;
   Attending Physician, Shands Hospital, University
   of Florida, Gainesville, Florida
   Anatomy of the Kidney

Nina E. Tolkoff-Rubin, MD
Associate Professor of Medicine, Harvard Medical
   School; Director, Hemodialysis and Continuous
   Ambulatory Peritoneal Dialysis Units,
   Massachusetts General Hospital, Boston,
   Massachusetts
   *Urinary Tract Infection, Pyelonephritis, and Reflux
      Nephropathy*

Vicente E. Torres, MD, PhD
Professor of Medicine, Mayo Clinic College of
   Medicine; Chair, Division of Nephrology and
   Hypertension, Mayo Clinic and Mayo Foundation,
   Rochester, Minnesota
   Cystic Diseases of the Kidney

Robert D. Toto, MD
Mary M. Conroy Professorship in Kidney Disease,
   Department of Internal Medicine, and Director,
   Patient Oriented Research in Nephrology,
   University of Texas Southwestern Medical Center at
   Dallas, Dallas, Texas
   Approach to the Patient with Kidney Disease

Joseph G. Verbalis, MD
Professor of Medicine and Physiology, and Interim
  Chair of Medicine, Georgetown University,
  Washington, D.C.
Disorders of Water Balance

Bernardo C. Vidal, Jr., MSc
Research Assistant, Population Genetics Group,
  Genome Institute of Singapore, Singapore,
  Singapore
Genomics and Proteomics in Nephrology

David G. Warnock, MD
Marie K. Ingaus Professor of Medicine, Director,
  Division of Nephrology, and Director, Office of
  Human Research, University of Alabama at
  Birmingham, Birmingham, Alabama
Interventional Nephrology

Matthew R. Weir, MD
Professor of Medicine, and Director, Division of
  Nephrology, University of Maryland School of
  Medicine, Baltimore, Maryland
Antihypertensive Drugs

Christopher S. Wilcox, MD, PhD
George E. Schreiner Chair of Nephrology, and
  Professor of Medicine, Georgetown University,
  Washington, D.C.
Diuretics

Joseph Winaver, MD
Professor, Department of Physiology and Biophysics,
  Faculty of Medicine, Technion—Israel Institute of
  Technology, Haifa, Israel
Extracellular Fluid and Edema Formation

Christopher G. Wood, MD
Associate Professor, University of Texas M.D.
  Anderson Cancer Center, Houston, Texas
Renal Neoplasia

Stephen H. Wright, PhD
Professor of Physiology, University of Arizona College
  of Medicine, Tucson, Arizona
Renal Handling of Organic Solutes

Alan S. L. Yu, MB, BChir
Associate Professor of Medicine, Keck School of
  Medicine, University of Southern California;
  Attending Nephrologist, Los Angeles County-USC
  Medical Center, Los Angeles, California
*Transport of Inorganic Solutes: Sodium, Chloride,
  Potassium, Magnesium, Calcium, and Phosphate;
  Disorders of Calcium, Magnesium, and Phosphate
  Balance*

Kambiz Zandi-Nejad, MD
Instructor in Medicine, Harvard Medical School;
  Attending Physician, Renal Division, Brigham and
  Women's Hospital, Boston, Massachusetts
Disorders of Potassium Balance

Mark L. Zeidel, MD
Herrman L. Blumgart Professor of Medicine, Harvard
  Medical School; Chair, Department of Medicine,
  Beth Israel Deaconess Medical Center, Boston,
  Massachusetts
Urinary Tract Obstruction

Israel Zelikovic, MD
Associate Professor of Pediatrics/Nephrology and
  Physiology, Faculty of Medicine, Technion—Israel
  Institute of Technology; Director, Pediatric
  Nephrology Unit, Meyer Children's Hospital,
  Rambam Health Care Campus, Haifa, Israel
Stem Cells in Renal Biology and Medicine

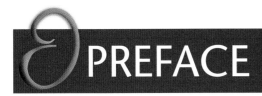

PREFACE

For the past 35 years, one of my main professional activities has been devoted to the formidable task of editing the serial editions of *Brenner and Rector's The Kidney,* initially with my colleague Dr. Floyd C. Rector, Jr., and for the past four editions as sole editor. The greatest challenge has been to recognize and incorporate an ever-increasing body of new knowledge that has spurred enormous progress in nephrology. As the treadmill spins faster and faster, the task for each edition has been to meet this challenge for our readership in ways that ensure clarity, accuracy and extensive documentation.

As readers approach this *Eighth* edition, they will immediately appreciate our radical change in book design, with vibrant cover art and pages in full color to enhance visual appeal and illustration clarity. Despite growth in knowledge, we have beseeched authors to adhere to strictly assigned length limitations and to emphasize literature published since 1990, since older references are readily available in cited reviews and previous editions. As a result, overall book length is less than the previous edition, despite growing from *66 to 70 chapters.* To more effectively integrate the ever-enlarging knowledge base in renal physiology, pathophysiology, clinical diagnosis and therapeutics, we have also initiated a radical reorganization of the textbook into *12 sections,* each distinguished by separate color code. This is the first such reorganization since publication of the First edition in 1976. Of the *70* chapters, one-fourth are *entirely new titles,* one-fourth have been *completely revised by newly invited authors* and for the remaining half each chapter has undergone *major updates and revisions,* often with addition of new co-authors. Through the collective efforts of our very able contributors, the intellectual and practical value of this new edition of *Brenner and Rector's The Kidney* has not only been continued but further strengthened. There are now 161 contributors to the Eighth Edition (compared to 151 in the Seventh Edition), and 73 of these 161 (over 40%) are new to this edition.

The new organization in *12 sections* proceeds as follows:

Section I: Normal Renal Function: Molecular, Cellular, Structural and Physiological Principles. This section devoted to basic renal structure and function is made up of *nine chapters*, dealing in detail with embryology, anatomy and topography, hemodynamics, tubule solute transport, urinary acidification, concentration and dilution, and the cellular actions of vasopressin. The principles outlined enable the reader to approach subsequent considerations of pathogenesis, pathophysiology and clinical nephrology in the most rational way possible.

Section II: Integrated Control of Body Fluid Volume and Composition. Of the *seven chapters* in this section, two deal with vasoactive peptides and arachidonate metabolites, molecules that greatly influence renal function. These are followed by in-depth discussions of disorders of sodium and water, acid-base, potassium, calcium, magnesium and phosphate homeostasis.

Section III: Epidemiology and Risk Factors in Kidney Disease. This novel section contains *five chapters* dealing with epidemiology, risk factor assessment, and the increasingly recognized roles of nephron endowment, gender and aging on renal disease risk and outcomes.

Section IV: Pathogenesis of Renal Disease. In this section of *seven chapters,* experienced clinicians describe the approach to the patient with known or suspected kidney disease, and how to apply the most cost-effective diagnostic assessments by laboratory evaluation and radiologic and other new imaging procedures. This very extensive imaging library is in itself a comprehensive primer for the nephrologist. Also reviewed in this section are the growing number of interventional approaches made possible by these ingenious new imaging procedures. Finally, this section includes two chapters dealing with the fundamental renal and systemic adaptations to nephron injury and chronic loss of renal function, providing insight into the mechanisms that ultimately contribute to the progression of renal disease and its attendant systemic complications.

Section V: Disorders of Kidney Function. The *ten chapters* in this section deal with the major clinical entities that constitute the full spectrum of acute and chronic kidney disease. Pathogenesis, diagnosis and therapy of acute kidney injury, primary and secondary glomerulopathies, micro- and macrovascular disorders of the kidney, tubulo-interstitial disease, diabetic nephropathy, urinary tract infection, obstruction, nephrolithiasis, and renal neoplasia are extensively reviewed by authors with vast clinical experience in each of their assigned areas.

Section VI: Genetic Basis of Kidney Disease. The *three chapters* devoted to this very active area of renal research address the inherited podocytopathies and tubule transport disorders as well as the various cystic diseases of the kidney, with thorough discussions of relevant genetic abnormalities and current understanding of how mutational events lead to clinical manifestations of disordered renal structure and function.

Section VII: Hypertension and the Kidney. This section of *five chapters* deals with the important clinical entities of primary and secondary hypertension, renovascular disease and ischemic nephropathy, and hypertension and kidney disease in pregnancy. Treatment for these conditions has evolved considerably, and these advances are thoroughly reviewed in two relevant chapters on antihypertensive drugs and diuretics, again by recognized experts.

Section VIII: The Consequences of Renal Failure. The *six chapters* in this section examine the biochemical and pathophysiological consequences of advancing renal insufficiency on cardiovascular, hematologic, endocrine, neurologic and musculoskeletal systems, areas in which new research findings have shed considerable light on causes and management of these systemic manifestations of the uremic state.

Section IX: Conservative and Pharmacological Management of Kidney Disease. This section of *five chapters* reviews in detail the best available dietary and pharmacologic therapies for patients with progressive kidney disease, including specific pharmacologic approaches to renoprotection, and the rational uses of erythropoietic stimulating proteins, vitamin D analogs and calcimimetic and phosphate binding agents. The final chapter in this section updates our knowledge of faulty drug metabolism in the patient with advancing renal disease and the necessary precautions that must be applied to drug use in this at-risk population.

Section X: Invasive Therapy of Renal Failure. In *five chapters* in this section the major treatment modalities of hemodialysis, peritoneal dialysis, and plasmapheresis are reviewed, along with the special challenges that increasingly confront nephrologists in the setting of the intensive care unit and in the patient in whom intentional or accidental poisoning necessitates extracorporeal treatment for toxin-removal and life support.

Section XI: Renal Transplantation. The *three chapters* in this penultimate section deal with the still-challenging treatment modality of renal transplantation, with extensive reviews of relevant basic immunology, specific issues related to both the organ donor and recipient, and principles of management of the early and later phases of the post-transplant clinical response.

Section XII: Frontiers in Nephrology. In these final *five chapters*, experts working at the cutting edge of the frontiers that hold great promise for nephrology are asked to foresee the future from their unique vantage points. Can we ultimately attain immunologic tolerance, achieve success with xenotransplantation, engineer the regrowth of normal renal parenchyma, and utilize stem cells and the promise of genomics and proteomics to advance our diagnostic and therapeutic horizons in nephrology? The answers to these provocative challenges will hopefully spur dramatic improvements in the care of our deserving patients with end stage renal disease.

As was the case with previous editions of *Brenner and Rector's The Kidney,* our goal for the *Eighth* edition is to educate and update all those concerned with the workings of the kidney in health and disease, i.e., medical and graduate students, internists, pediatricians, urologists and of course nephrologists, from trainees to highly experienced clinicians and scientists.

But even a two-volume, extensively illustrated, updated and abundantly referenced tome cannot by itself encompass the full universe of nephrology of 2008 and beyond. In recognition of this limitation, we have systematically labored to construct a formidable *Library of Nephrology* consisting of several regularly revised and updated *Companion Volumes,* including *Therapy in Nephrology and Hypertension,* second edition, edited by Hugh Brady and Christopher Wilcox, *Hypertension,* second edition, edited by Suzanne Oparil and Michael Weber, *Chronic Kidney Disease, Dialysis, and Transplantation,* second edition, edited by Brian Pereira, Mohamed Sayegh, and Peter Blake, *Acute Renal Failure,* edited by Bruce Molitoris and William Finn, *Acid-Base and Electrolyte Disorders,* edited by Thomas DuBose and Lee Hamm, *Diagnostic Atlas of Renal Pathology,* edited by Agnes Fogo and Michael Kashgarian and *Pocket Companion,* edited by Michael Clarkson and Barry Brenner. The aim of these, and several additional volumes now in preparation or planned, is to assist the active and often time-constrained renal physician and scientist in acquiring familiarity with the latest advances in contemporary nephrology.

Keeping pace can also be achieved by utilizing the **e-dition** of the *Eighth* edition, which provides immediate *electronic access* to the entire text and its myriad of tables and figures, all of which can be readily downloaded in PowerPoint format for individual use. Moreover, since our four year cycle for new editions still leaves time gaps for those most in immediate need of new information, I now routinely scan dozens of relevant journals each month and prepare abstracts of articles that I believe contain important new information. These abstracts are posted at frequent intervals directly into the page of the electronic text dealing with the exact topic so as to create a constantly updated ***e-dition,*** in effect *a living textbook.*

My goal for the *Eighth* edition is the most user-friendly informational resource possible in nephrology via print and electronic formats. I am particularly indebted to our many renowned and devoted authors whose scholarly and practical contributions constitute the essence of this enterprise. For their adherence to deadlines, page and content constraints, I am in their debt. Nor could my goal have been accomplished without the extraordinary efforts of my local editorial associates, Gabriela Salomé Álvarez and Anna Elizabeth Besch, and the highly professional and devoted staff of Elsevier. I especially thank Susan Pioli, Publishing Director, Arlene Chappelle, Senior Developmental Editor, and Mary B. Stermel, Senior Project Manager, for their guidance, technical excellence, and unrelenting support. I also thank Berta Steiner for overseeing the production of the edition and Steven Stave for his innovative book design.

My appreciation also extends to our many devoted readers who have reacted so favorably to previous editions and offered encouragement and sound advice over the years. It is to them and the betterment of their patients that our efforts are ultimately directed.

Finally, to my family and friends, for their continued acceptance of my benign neglect due to the assumption of this and all too many other time-consuming projects, I express my heartfelt gratitude and unbounded love. And soon their patience will be rewarded. Just as blazing embers eventually grow dimmer, I recognize that now is the appropriate time to begin the orderly transition of responsibility for future editions of *Brenner and Rector's The Kidney,* as well as the other components of our *Library of Nephrology,* to a new generation of editors. An international team consisting of Drs. Glenn M. Chertow (San Francisco, California, USA), Philip A. Marsden (Toronto, Canada), Karl L. Skorecki (Haifa, Israel), Maarten W. Taal (Derby, United Kingdom) and Alan S. L. Yu (Los Angeles, California, USA) will join me in developing the *Ninth* edition and I am certain that with their exceptional abilities and dedication to task the future excellence of *Brenner and Rector's The Kidney,* and indeed our entire *Library* will be assured.

Barry M. Brenner, M.D.
Boston, 2007

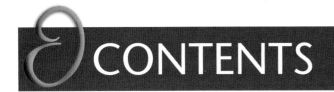

CONTENTS

SECTION I

Normal Renal Function: Molecular, Cellular, Structural and Physiological Principles

CHAPTER 1

Embryology of the Kidney

Susan E. Quaggin • Jordan Kreidberg

Over the past several decades, the identification of genes and molecular pathways required for normal renal development have provided insight into our understanding of obvious developmental diseases such as renal agenesis and renal dysplasia. However, many of the genes identified have also been shown to play roles in adult-onset and acquired renal diseases such as focal segmental glomerulosclerosis. The number of nephrons present in the kidney at birth, which is determined during fetal life, predicts the risk of renal disease and hypertension later in life; a reduced number is associated with greater risk.[1-3] Discovery of novel therapeutic targets and strategies to slow and reverse kidney disease, requires an understanding of the molecular mechanisms that underlie kidney development.

MAMMALIAN KIDNEY DEVELOPMENT: EMBRYOLOGY

Development of the Urogenital System

The vertebrate kidney derives from the intermediate mesoderm of the urogenital ridge, a structure found along the posterior wall of the abdomen in the developing fetus.[7] It develops in three successive stages known as the pronephros, the mesonephros, and the metanephros (Fig. 1–1), although only the metanephros gives rise to the definitive adult kidney. However, earlier stages are required for development of other organs, such as the adrenal gland and gonad that also develop within the urogenital ridge. Furthermore, many of the signaling pathways and genes that play important roles in the metanephric kidney appear to play parallel roles during earlier stages of renal development, in the pronephros and mesonephros. The pronephros consists of pronephric tubules and the pronephric duct (also known as the precursor to the Wolffian duct) and develops from the rostral-most region of the urogenital ridge at 22 days of gestation (humans) and 8 days post coitum (d.p.c.; mouse). It functions in the larval stages of amphibians and fish, but not in mammals. The mesonephros develops caudal to the pronephric tubules in the mid-section of the urogenital ridge. The mesonephros becomes the functional excretory apparatus in lower vertebrates and may perform a filtering function during embryonic life in mammals. However, it largely degenerates before birth. Prior to its degeneration, endothelial, peritubular myoid, and steroidogenic cells from the mesonephros migrate into the adjacent adrenogonadal primordia, which ultimately form the adrenal gland and gonads.[10] Abnormal mesonephric migration leads to gonadal dysgenesis, a fact that emphasizes the intricate association between these organ systems during development and explains the common association of gonadal and renal defects in congenital syndromes.[11,12] In males, production of testosterone also induces the formation of seminal vesicles, tubules of the epididymis, and portions of the vas deferens from the Wolffian duct.

Development of the Metanephros

The metanephros is the third and final stage, and gives rise to the definitive adult kidney of higher vertebrates; it results from a series of inductive interactions that occur between the metanephric mesenchyme and the epithelial ureteric bud at the caudal end of the urogenital ridge. The ureteric bud (UB) is first visible as an outgrowth at the distal end of the Wolffian duct at approximately 5 weeks of gestation in humans or 10.5 days post coitus (d.p.c.) in mice. The metanephric mesenchyme (MM) becomes histologically distinct from the surrounding mesenchyme and is found adjacent to the UB. Upon invasion of UB into the MM at 11.5 d.p.c. in mice and 5 weeks in humans, signals from the MM cause the UB to branch into a T-tubule and then to undergo dichotomous branching, giving rise to the urinary collecting system and all of the collecting ducts (Fig. 1–2). Simultaneously, the UB sends reciprocal signals to the MM, which is induced to condense along the surface of the bud. Following condensation, a subset of MM aggregates adjacent and inferior to the tips of the branching ureteric bud. These collections of cells are known as pre-tubular aggregates, which undergo mesenchymal-to-epithelial conversion to become the renal vesicle (Fig. 1–3).

The renal vesicle segments and proceeds through a series of morphological changes to form the glomerulus and components of the tubular nephron from the proximal convoluted tubule to the distal nephron. These stages are known as comma shape, S-shape, capillary loop, and mature stage and require precise proximal-to-distal patterning and structural transformation (see Fig. 1–3). Remarkably, this process is repeated 600,000 to 1 million times in each developing human kidney as new nephrons are sequentially born at the tips of the UB throughout fetal life.

The glomerulus develops from the most proximal end of the renal vesicle that is furthest from the UB tip.[13,14] Distinct cell types of the glomerulus can first be identified in the S-shape stage, where presumptive podocytes appear as a columnar-shaped epithelial cell layer. A vascular cleft develops and separates the presumptive podocyte layer from more distal cells that will form the proximal tubule. Parietal epithelial cells differentiate and flatten becoming Bowman's capsule, a structure that surrounds the urinary space and is continuous with the proximal tubular epithelium. Concurrently, endothelial cells migrate into the vascular cleft. Together with the glomerular visceral epithelial cells, the endothelial cells produce the glomerular basement membrane, a major component of the mature filtration barrier. Initially the podocytes are connected by intercellular tight-junctions at their apical surface.[15] As glomerulogenesis proceeds, the podocytes revert to a mesenchymal-type phenotype, flatten and spread out to cover the increased surface area of the growing glomerular capillary bed. They develop microtubular-based primary processes and actin-based secondary foot processes. During this time, the intercellular junctions become restricted to the basal aspect of the podocyte and eventually are replaced by a modified adherens-like structure known as the slit diaphragm (SD).[15] At the same time, the podocyte foot processes of adjacent cells become highly inter-digitated. The slit diaphragms function as signaling centers as well as structural components of the renal filtration apparatus that connect foot processes of adjacent podocytes and link the SD to the specialized cytoskeleton that supports foot process structure.[17–19] Mesangial cell ingrowth follows the migration of endothelial cells and is required for development and patterning of the capillary loops that are found in normal glomeruli. The endothelial cells also flatten considerably and capillary lumens are formed due to apoptosis of a subset of endothelial cells.[20] At the capillary loop stage, glomerular endothelial cells develop fenestrae, transmembrane pores that are found in semi-permeable capillary beds exposed to high flux. Positioning of the foot processes on the glomerular basement membrane and

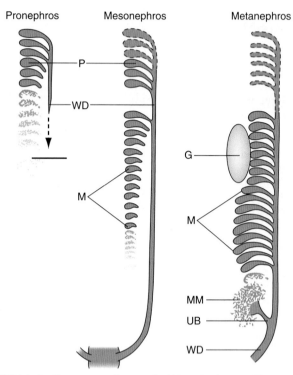

FIGURE 1–1 Three stages of mammalian kidney development. The pronephros (P) and mesonephros (M) develop in a rostral-to-caudal direction and the tubules are aligned adjacent to the Wolffian or nephric duct (WD). The metanephros develops from an outgrowth of the distal end of the Wolffian duct known as the ureteric bud epithelium (UB) and a cluster of cells known as the metanephric mesenchyme (MM). Cells migrate from the mesonephros (M) into the developing gonad (G), which develop in close association with one another. (Adapted from Saxen L: Organogenesis of the Kidney. Cambridge, Cambridge University Press, 1987.)

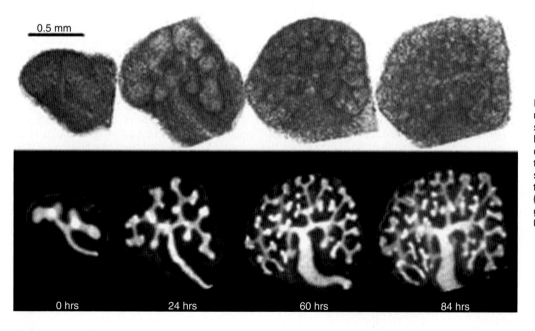

0.5 mm

0 hrs   24 hrs   60 hrs   84 hrs

FIGURE 1–2 Organ culture of rat metanephroi dissected at T-tubule stage. Within 84 hours, dichotomous branching of the ureteric bud has occurred to provide basic architecture of the kidney. Bottom panel is stained with dolichos biflorus agglutin—a lectin specific for the UB. (Adapted from Saxen L: Organogenesis of the Kidney. Cambridge, Cambridge University Press, 1987.)

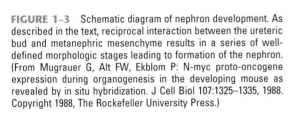

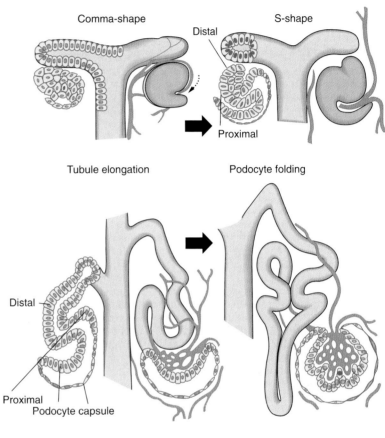

Loose mesenchyme

Condensation

Epithelial ureter bud — Mesenchyme

Comma-shape

S-shape

Distal

Proximal

Tubule elongation

Podocyte folding

Distal

Proximal
Podocyte capsule

FIGURE 1–3 Schematic diagram of nephron development. As described in the text, reciprocal interaction between the ureteric bud and metanephric mesenchyme results in a series of well-defined morphologic stages leading to formation of the nephron. (From Mugrauer G, Alt FW, Ekblom P: N-myc proto-oncogene expression during organogenesis in the developing mouse as revealed by in situ hybridization. J Cell Biol 107:1325–1335, 1988. Copyright 1988, The Rockefeller University Press.)

spreading of podocyte cell bodies are still incompletely understood, but share many features of synapse formation and neuronal migration.[21,22]

In the mature stage glomerulus, the podocytes, fenestrated endothelial cells, and intervening glomerular basement membrane (GBM) comprise the filtration barrier that separates the urinary from the blood space. Together, these components provide a size- and charge-selective barrier that permits free passage of small solutes and water but prevents the loss of larger molecules such as proteins. The mesangial cells are found between the capillary loops (approximately 3 per loop); they are required to provide ongoing structural support to the capillaries and possess smooth-muscle cell-like characteristics that have the capacity to contract, which may account for the dynamic properties of the glomerulus.

The tubular portion of the nephron becomes segmented in a proximal-distal order, into the proximal convoluted tubule, the descending and ascending loops of Henle, and distal convoluted tubule. The latter portion connects to the collecting ducts, which are derived from the ureteric bud derivatives and not from the original mesenchymal component of the metanephric rudiment. Fusion events between the MM- and UB-derived portions of the nephron are required, although are poorly understood at present.

Although all segments of the nephron are present at birth and filtration occurs prior to birth, maturation of the tubule continues in the postnatal period. Increased levels of transporters, switch in transporter isoforms, alterations in paracellular transport mechanisms, and permeability and biophysical properties of tubular membranes have all been observed to occur postnatally.[23] Although additional studies are needed, these observations emphasize the importance of considering developmental stage of the nephron in interpretation of renal transport and may explain the age of onset of symptoms in inherited transport disorders; some of these issues may be recapitulated in acute renal injury.

The Nephrogenic Zone

After the first few rounds of branching of the ureteric bud derivatives, and the concomitant induction of nephrons from the mesenchyme, the kidney begins to become divided between an outer cortical region where nephrons are being induced, and an inner medullary region where the collecting system will form. As growth continues, successive groups of nephrons are induced at the peripheral regions of the kidney, known as the nephrogenic zone (Fig. 1–4). Thus, within the developing kidney, the most mature nephrons are found in

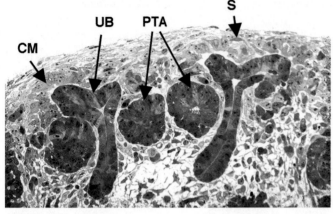

FIGURE 1–4 The nephrogenic zone. As described in the text, nephrons are continually produced in the nephrogenic zone throughout fetal life. CM, condensing mesenchyme; UB, ureteric bud; PTA, pretubular aggregate; S, stromal cell lineage (spindle-shaped cells).

the innermost layers of the cortex, and the most immature nephrons in the most peripheral regions. At the extreme peripheral lining, under the renal capsule, a process that appears to nearly exactly recapitulate the induction of the original nephrons can be observed, where numerous ureteric bud-like structures are inducing areas of condensed mesenchyme. Indeed, whether there are significant molecular differences between the induction of the original nephrons and these subsequent inductive events is not known. Also unknown is whether there exists a stem-like population of cells within or adjacent to the nephrogenic zone. It is apparent from the histology of the nephrogenic zone that the mesenchyme condensed around these derivatives of the ureteric bud must continually replenish itself, as well as provide a substrate for the induction of successive rounds of nephrons. However, it is not known whether there is a small subset of cells that have the stem-like properties of self-renewal and differentiation, or whether these properties apply to the whole population of condensed mesenchyme present in the nephrogenic zone.

Branching Morphogenesis— Development of the Collecting System

The collecting system is composed of hundreds of tubules through which the filtrate produced by the nephrons is conducted out of the kidney and to the ureter and then the bladder. Water and salt absorption and excretion, NH3 transport and H+ ion secretion required for acid-base homeostasis also occur in the collecting ducts, under different regulatory mechanisms, and using different transporters and channels than are active in the tubular portions of the nephron. The collecting ducts are all derived from the original ureteric bud. So, whereas each nephron is an individual unit separately induced and originating from a distinct pretubular aggregate, the collecting ducts are the product of branching morphogenesis from the ureteric bud. Considerable remodeling is involved in forming collecting ducts from branches of ureteric bud, and how this occurs remains incompletely understood.[24] The branching is highly patterned, with the first several rounds of branching being somewhat symmetrical, followed by additional rounds of asymmetric branching, in which a main trunk of the collecting duct continues to extend towards the nephrogenic zone, while smaller buds branch as they induce new nephrons

within the nephrogenic zone. Originally, the ureteric bud derivatives are branching within a surrounding mesenchyme. Ultimately, they form a funnel-shaped structure in which a cone-shaped grouping of ducts or papilla sits within a funnel or calyce that drains into the ureter. The mouse kidney has a single papilla and calyce, whereas a human kidney has 8 to 10 papillae, each of which drains into a minor calyce, with several minor calyces draining into a smaller number of major calyces.

Renal Stroma and Interstitial Populations

For decades in classic embryologic studies of kidney development, emphasis has been placed on the reciprocal inductive signals between MM and UB. However, in recent years, interest in the stromal cell as a key regulator of nephrogenesis has arisen.[14,25–27] Stromal cells also derive from the metanephric mesenchyme, but are not induced to condense by the UB. Two distinct populations of stromal cells have been described: cortical stromal cells exist as a thin layer beneath the renal capsule while medullary stromal cells populate the interstitial space between the collecting ducts and tubules (see Fig. 1–8). Cortical stromal cells also surround the condensates and provide signals required for ureteric bud branching and patterning of the developing kidney. Disruption or loss of these stromal cells leads to failure of UB branching, a reduction in nephron number, and disrupted patterning of nephric units with failure of cortical-medullary boundary formation. A reciprocal signaling loop from the UB exists to properly pattern stromal cell populations. Loss of these UB-derived signals leads to a buildup of stromal cells beneath the capsule that are several layers thick. As nephrogenesis proceeds, stromal cells differentiate into peritubular interstitial cells and pericytes that are required for vascular remodeling, and production of extracellular matrix responsible for proper nephric formation. These cells migrate from their position around the condensates to areas between the developing nephrons within the medulla. Although stromal cells derive from MM, it is not yet clear if MM that give rise to stromal cell and nephric lineages derive from the same progenitor cell or a different cell.

Development of the Vasculature

The microcirculations of the kidney include the specialized glomerular capillary system responsible for production of the ultrafiltrate and the vasa rectae, peritubular capillaries involved in the countercurrent mechanism. In the adult, each kidney receives 10% of the cardiac output.

Vasculogenesis and angiogenesis have been described as two distinct processes in blood vessel formation. The first refers to de novo differentiation of previously nonvascular cells into structures that resemble capillary beds, whereas angiogenesis refers to sprouting from these early beds to form mature vessel structures including arteries, veins, and capillaries. Both processes are involved in development of the renal vasculature. At the time of UB invasion (11 d.p.c.; all timing given is for mice), the MM is avascular but by 12 d.p.c. a rich capillary network is present and by 14 d.p.c. vascularized glomeruli are present. Transplantation experiments support a model whereby endothelial progenitors within the MM give rise to renal vessels in situ,[28] although the origin of large blood vessels is still debated. At 13 d.p.c., capillaries form networks around the developing nephric tubules and by 14 d.p.c., the hilar artery and first-order interlobar renal artery branches can be identified. These branches

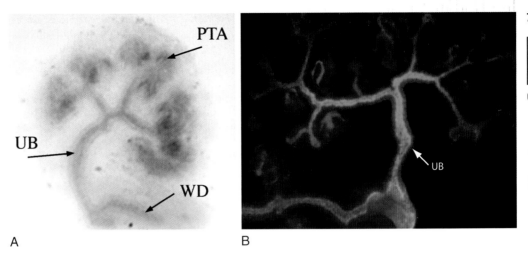

FIGURE 1-5 Metanephric organ explants. **A,** In situ analysis for Pax2 that marks pretubular aggregates (PTA) and the ureteric (UB) and Wolffian duct (WD). **B,** Immunohistochemical stain for proximal tubular cell brush border (red) and pan cytokeratin (green) marks the developing nephrons and ureteric bud, respectively.

will form the cortico-medullary arcades; and interlobular arteries that branch from these arcades. Further branching produces the glomerular afferent arterioles. From 13.5 d.p.c. onward, endothelial cells migrate into the vascular cleft of developing glomeruli, where they undergo differentiation to form the glomerular capillary loops. The efferent arterioles carry blood away from the glomerulus to a system of fenestrated peritubular capillaries that are in close contact with the adjacent tubules and receive filtered water and solutes reabsorbed from the filtrate. These capillaries have few pericytes. In comparison, the vasa recta, which surround the medullary tubules and are involved in urinary concentration are also fenestrated but have more pericytes. They arise from the efferent arterioles of deep glomeruli. The peritubular capillary system surrounding the proximal tubules is well developed in the late fetal period, whereas the vasa rectae mature 1 to 3 weeks postnatally.

MODEL SYSTEMS TO STUDY KIDNEY DEVELOPMENT

Organ Culture

The Kidney Organ Culture System: Classical Studies
Metanephric kidney organ culture (Fig. 1–5) formed the basis for extensive classical studies of embryonic induction. Parameters of induction such as the temporal and physical constraints on exposure of the inductive tissue to the mesenchyme were determined, as were the time periods during which various tubular elements of the nephron were first observed in culture.

Mutant Phenotypic Analyses
As originally shown by Grobstein, Saxen, and colleagues in classical studies of embryonic induction, the two major components of the metanephric kidney, the mesenchyme and the ureteric bud, could be separated from each other, and the isolated mesenchyme could be induced to form nephron-like tubules by a selected set of other embryonic tissues, the best example of which is embryonic neural tube.[7,29] This phenomenon can be distinguished from placing the whole metanephric rudiment, including the ureteric bud, in culture, in that when the whole rudiment is placed in culture, there is induction of nephrons, branching of the ureteric bud, and continued growth of the rudiment. In contrast, when neural tube is used to induce the separated mesenchyme, there is terminal

differentiation of the mesenchyme into tubules, but not significant tissue expansion. The isolated mesenchyme experiment has proven useful in the analysis of renal agenesis phenotypes, where there is no outgrowth of the ureteric bud. In these cases the mesenchyme can be placed in contact with neural tube to determine whether it has the intrinsic ability to differentiate. Most often, when the renal agenesis is due to the mutation of a transcription factor, tubular induction is not rescued by neural tube, as could be predicted for transcription factors, which would be expected to act in a cell-autonomous fashion.[6] In the converse situation, in which renal agenesis is caused by loss of a gene function in the ureteric bud, such as EMX-2, it is usually possible for embryonic neural tube to induce tubule formation in isolated mesenchymes.[30] Therefore the organ culture induction assay can be used to test hypotheses concerning whether a particular gene is required in the mesenchyme or ureteric bud. Recently, as chemical inhibitors specific for various signal transduction pathways have been synthesized and become available, it has been possible to add these to organ cultures and observe effects that are informative about the roles of specific pathways in development of the kidney. Examples are the use of MAP kinase inhibitors and inhibitors of the Notch signaling pathway.

Anti-Sense Oligonucleotides and siRNA in Organ Culture
Several studies have described the use of antisense oligonucleotides and more recently, siRNA molecules, to inhibit gene expression in kidney organ culture. Among the earliest of these was the inhibition of the low affinity nerve growth factor receptor, p75 or NGFR, by anti-sense oligonucleotides,[31] a treatment that decreased the growth of the organ culture. A subsequent study could not duplicate this phenotype,[32] though there were possible differences in experimental techniques.[33] An additional study using anti-sense oligonucleotides to Pax2 also showed this gene to be crucial in the mesenchymal to epithelial transformation.[8,9] More recently, one report has demonstrated that siRNA to the WT1 and Pax2 genes can inhibit early nephron differentiation.[34]

Organ Culture Microinjection
A novel approach to the organ culture system has also yielded insights as to a possible function of the WT1 gene in early kidney development. A system was established to microinject and electroporate DNA plasmid expression constructs into the condensed mesenchyme of organ cultures.[35]

The results with this system are described in the section on Wt1.

Transgenic and Knockout Mouse Models

Over the past two decades, the generation and analysis of knockout and transgenic mice have provided tremendous insight into kidney development (Table 1–1).[36,37] Although homologous recombination to delete genes within the germline also known as standard "knockout" technology has provided information about the biological functions of many genes in kidney development, several disadvantages exist. Disruption of gene function in embryonic stem (ES) cells may result in embryonic or perinatal lethality, precluding the functional analysis of the gene in the kidney that develops relatively late in fetal life. Additionally, many genes are expressed in multiple cell types, and the resulting knockout phenotypes can be complex and difficult or impossible to dissect. The ability to limit gene targeting to specific renal cell types overcomes some of these problems and the temporal control of gene expression permits more precise dissection of a gene's function. A number of mouse lines exist that may be used to target specific kidney cell lineages (Table 1–2; Fig. 1–6). As with any experimental procedure, numerous caveats exist that the investigator must take into account in interpretation of data (reviewed in Refs 38, 39); these include determining the completeness of excision at the locus of interest, the timing and extrarenal expression of the promoters, and general toxicity of expressed proteins to the cell of interest. In spite of these caveats, they remain a powerful tool. The next generation of targeting includes improved efficiency using BAC targeting approaches, siRNA and microRNA approaches, and large genome-wide targeting efforts already underway at many academic and pharmaceutical institutions.

In contrast to gene targeting experiments where the gene is known at the beginning of the experiment (reverse genetics), random mutagenesis represents a complimentary phenotype-driven approach (forward genetics). Random mutations are introduced into the genome at high efficiency by chemical or "gene-trap" mutagenesis. Consecutively, large numbers of animals are screened systematically for specific phenotypes of interest. As soon as a phenotype is identified, test breeding is used to confirm the genetic nature of the trait. The mutated gene is then identified by chromosomal mapping and positional cloning. There are two major advantages to genome-wide based approaches compared to reverse genetics: (1) most knockouts lead to major gene disruptions, which may not be relevant to the subtle gene alterations that underlie human renal disease; (2) many of the complex traits underlying congenital anomalies and acquired diseases of the kidney are unknown, making predictions about the nature of the genes that are involved in these diseases difficult.

One of the most powerful and well-characterized mutagens in the mouse is the chemical mutagen, N-ethyl-N-nitrosourea (ENU). It acts through random alkylation of nucleic acids inducing point mutations in spermatogonial stem cells of injected male mice.[40,41] This results in multiple point mutations within the spermatogonia of the male, who is then bred to a female mouse of different genetic background. Resulting F1 offspring are screened for renal phenotypes of interest (e.g., dysplastic, cystic) and heritability. Mutations may be complete or partial loss-of-function, gain-of-function, or altered function and can be dominant or recessive. The specific locus mutation frequency of ENU is 1 in 1000. Assuming a total number of 25,000 to 40,000 genes in the mouse genome, a single treated male mouse should have between 25 and 40

different heterozygous mutagenized genes. In the case of multigenic phenotypes, segregation of the mutations in the next generation allows the researcher to focus on monogenic traits. In each generation, 50% of the mutations are lost, and only the mutation underlying the selected phenotype is maintained in the colony. A breeding strategy that includes backcrossing to the female genetic strain enables rapid mapping of the ENU mutation that occurred on the male genetic background.

The screening in ENU-mutagenesis experiments can focus on dominant or recessive renal mutations. Screening for dominant phenotypes is popular as breeding schemes are simple and a great amount of mutants can be recovered through this approach. About 2% of all F1 mice display a heritable phenotypic abnormality.[42,43] A number of large ENU mutagenesis projects are now underway, with mutant strains available to interested researchers. It is possible to design "sensitized screens" on a smaller scale, which increases the ability to identify genes in a pathway of interest. For example, in renal glomerular development, the phenotype of a genetic mouse strain with a tendency to develop congenital nephrosis (e.g., CD2AP haploinsufficiency[44]) may be enhanced or suppressed by breeding to a mutagenized male. The modifier gene may then be mapped using the approach outlined earlier. This approach has been successfully used to identify genes involved in neural development,[45,46] but has not yet been exploited to full potential by the renal community.

Other genome-wide approaches that have led to the discovery of novel genes in kidney development and disease include gene trap consortia,[47,48] and transcriptome/proteome projects.[49] The interested reader is referred to the following web site: www.cmhd.on.ca.

Non-mammalian Model Systems for Kidney Development

Organisms separated by millions of years of evolution from humans, still provide useful models to study the genetic basis and function of mammalian kidney development. This stems from the fact that all of these organisms possess excretory organs designed to remove metabolic wastes from the body, and that genetic pathways involved in other aspects of invertebrate development may serve as templates to dissect pathways in mammalian kidney development. In support of the latter argument, elucidation of the genetic interactions and molecular mechanism of the Neph1 ortholog and nephrin-like molecule—SYG1 and SYG2—in synapse formation in C. Elegans is providing major clues to the function of these genes in glomerular and slit diaphragm formation and function in mammals.[50]

The excretory organs of invertebrates differ greatly in their structure and complexity and range in size from a few cells in C. elegans, to several hundred cells in the Malpighian tubules of Drosophila, to the more recognizable kidneys in amphibians, birds, and mammals. In the soil nematode, C. elegans, the excretory system consists of a single large H-shaped excretory cell, a pore cell, a duct cell, and a gland cell.[51,52] C. elegans provides many benefits as a model system: the availability of powerful genetic tools including "mutants by mail", a short life and reproductive cycle, a publicly available genome sequence and resource database (www.wormbase.org), the ease of performing genetic enhancer-suppressor screens in worms and the fact that they share many genetic pathways with mammals. Major contributions in our understanding of the function of polycystic and cilia-related genes have been made from studying C. elegans. The PKD1 and PKD2 homologs, LOV1 and LOV2, are involved in cilia development and function of the mating organ required for mating behavior.[53,54] Strides in understanding the function

TABLE 1–1	Summary of Knockout and Transgenic Models for Kidney Development		
Kidney Phenotype	**Mouse (Knockout or Mutation) Other Affected Organs**	**Human (Naturally Occurring Mutation)**	**References**
Aplasia (Variable)			
WT-1	Gonad, mesothelium, heart, lung	Wilms tumor, WAGR, Denys-Drash	4–6
Pax-2	Genital tract, gonad	Renal hypoplasia, VUR, and optic nerve colobomas	8, 9
Pax-2/Pax-8	Defect in intermediate mesoderm transition, failure of pronephric duct formation		
Emx-2	Genital tract, gonad		30
Lim-1	Genital tract, gonads, anterior head		66
Hox-A11/D11	Distal limbs, vas deferens		217
Retinoic acid receptor $\alpha\gamma/\alpha\beta2$	Skeleton, many visceral abnormalities including renal hypoplasia, dysplasia		12, 14, 16
GDNF, c-ret, GRFα1	UB failure, enteric neurons	Hirschsprung disease	67–69, 173–177
Integrin-α8	Reduced UB branching		87
Danforth Short Tail	Short tail, UB failure		218
KAL mutation		Kallman syndrome (olfactory bulb agenesis)	
Heparan sulfate 2-sulfotransferase	Lack of UB branching and mesenchymal condensation		219
EYA-1 (Eyes absent-1)		Branchio-oto-renal syndrome (branchial fistulae, deafness)	62, 74
Six1		Branchio-oto-renal syndrome	64
Gremlin			71
Sal1	Severe renal dysplasia/renal agenesis	Townes-Brock syndrome (anal, renal, limb, ear anomalies)	65, 178
Dysplasia/Hypoplasia/Low Nephron Mass			
FoxD1 (BF-2)	Reduced UB branching/stromal patterning defects		26
BMP-7	Reduced MM survival		86
Wnt-4	Failure of MM induction		84, 179
AP-2	MM failure, craniofacial and skeletal defects		220
Cyclooxygenase-2	Oligonephronia		221
Lmx-1b	Renal dysplasia, skeletal abnormalities	Nail-patella syndrome	160, 180
FGF-7	Small kidneys, reduction in nephron number		91
Increased Branching			
Slit2/robo2	Increased branching of UB		102
Cysts			
KIF3A	Polycystic kidney disease (tubular-selective)		181
HNF1β			182
VHL	Renal cysts (tubular-selective)		183
Peroxisomal assembly factor-1		Zellweger syndrome	OMIM*214100
Bcl-2	Renal hypoplasia and cysts		
MKS1		Meckel syndrome (multicystic dysplasia, neural tube defect)	222
PKD1, PKD2	Renal cysts	AD PKD	184
Later phenotypes (Glomerular, vascular, glomerular basement membrane)			
PDGFB/PDGFR-β	Lack of mesangial cells, ballooned glomerular capillary loop		157, 158
MPV-17	Nephrotic syndrome		223
Integrin-α3	Reduced UB branching, glomerular defects, poor foot process formation, lung		98
CD151	Focal segmental glomerulosclerosis, massive proteinuria, disorganized GBM, tubular cystic dilation	End stage kidney failure, regional skin blistering, sensorineural deafness	228
Col4a3	Alport syndrome		185, 186
Col4a3/a4			187
Col4a5			188
Col4a1		Intracerebral hemorrhage and strokes	189
Lamb2	Proteinuria prior to the onset of foot process effacement		190, 191
Lama5	Defective glomerulogenesis, abnormal GBM, poor podocyte adhesion, loss of mesangial cells		192
Lama5;Mr51	Ballooned capillary loop, proteinuria		193
Lama5;Mr5G2	Nephrotic syndrome		194

Continued

TABLE 1–1	Summary of Knockout and Transgenic Models for Kidney Development—cont'd		
Kidney Phenotype	**Mouse (Knockout or Mutation) Other Affected Organs**	**Human (Naturally Occurring Mutation)**	**References**
Agrin	No glomerular permeability defect (podocyte-selective)		224
Perlecan heparan sulfated sites	No baseline defects; proteinuria with albumin loading		195
Entactin-1	Abnormal GBM		196
Angiotensin II type-2 receptor	Various collecting system defects	CAKUT syndrome	143, 144, 147
Eagle-Barrett (prune belly) syndrome		(–) Abdominal wall musculature, VUR, cryptorchidism	
BMP-4 (heterozygous)	Renal hypoplasia/dysplasia, hydroureter, ectopic uterovesical junction		89
Foxc1 (Mfl)	Renal duplication, multiple ureters, hydroureter/hydronephrosis		101
Mf2	Small kidneys with few nephrons		197
Glypican-3	Disorganized tubules and medullary cysts	Simpson-Golabi-Behmel syndrome	198–201
Notch2	Lack of glomerular endothelial and mesangial cells		103, 104
Pod1/tcf21	Lung and cardiac defects, sex reversal and gonadal dysgenesis, vascular defects, disruption in UB branching, impaired podocyte differentiation, dilated glomerular capillary, poor mesangial migration		11, 111
FoxC2	Impaired podocyte differentiation, dilated glomerular capillary loop, poor mesangial migration		49
Kreisler (maf-1)	Abnormal podocyte differentiation		159
Nephrin	Absent slit diaphragms	Congenital nephrosis of the Finnish variety	162
Neph 1	Abnormal slit diaphragm function, FSGS		48
Podocin	Congenital nephrosis, FSGS, vascular defects	Steroid-resistant FSGS	166, 202
PLCε1		Diffuse mesangial sclerosis; FSGS	225
GNE/MNK (M712T)	Hyposialation defect, foot process effacement, GBM splitting, proteinuria and hematuria	Hereditary inclusion body myopathy	226
FAT1	Foot process fusion, failure of foot process formation		203
NCK1/2	Failure of foot process formation (podocyte-selective)		17
CD2AP	FSGS, immunotactoid nephropathy		169
Alpha-actinin 4	Glomerular developmental defects, FSGS	AD FSGS	167, 168
VEGF-A	Endotheliosis, disruption of glomerular filtration barrier formation, nephrotic syndrome (podocyte-selective)		118, 119
Angiopoietin2	Cortical peritubular capillary abnormalities		131
ILK1	Nephrotic syndrome (podocyte-selective)		204
VHL	RPGN (podocyte-selective)		137

VUR, vesicoureteral reflux; UB, ureter bud; MM, metanephric mesenchyme; AD, autosomal dominant; PKD, polycystic kidney disease; VHL, von Hippel-Lindau; GBM, glomerular basement membrane; FSGS, focal segmental glomerulosclerosis; RPGN, rapidly progressive glomerulonephritis.

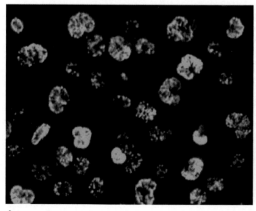
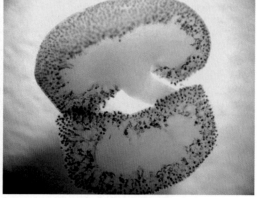

FIGURE 1–6 Glomeruli expressing cyan fluorescent protein (**A**) or beta galactosidase (**B**). Transgenic mice were generated using the nephrin-promoter to direct expression of either CFP or beta-galactosidase specifically to developing and mature podocytes.

A

B

Promoter	Renal Expression	Extrarenal Expression	Reference
Kidney androgen promoter 2	Proximal tubules	Brain	205
γ-Glutamyl transpeptidase	Cortical tubules	None	206
Na/glucose cotransporter (SGLT2)	Proximal tubules	None	207
PEPCK	Proximal tubules	Liver	183
Aquaporin-2	Principal cells of collecting duct	Testis, vas deferens	208
Hox-B7	Collecting ducts, Ureteric bud, Wolffian bud, ureter	Spinal cord, dorsal root ganglia	209
Ksp-cadherin	Renal tubules, collecting ducts, ureteric bud, Wolffian duct, mesonephros	Müllerian duct	210
Tamm-Horsfall protein	Thick ascending limbs of loops of Henle	Testis, brain	211
Nephrin	Podocytes	Brain	212, 213
Podocin	Podocytes	None	214
Renin	Juxtaglomerular cells, afferent arterioles	Adrenal gland, testis, sympathetic ganglia, etc.	141
FoxD1/BF2	Stromal cells	?	
Six2	Metanephric mesenchyme	?	
Pax3	Metanephric mesenchyme	Neural tube, neural crest	215, 216

TABLE 1–2 Conditional Mouse Lines for the Kidney

of the slit diaphragm have also been made from C. elegans as described earlier.

In Drosophila, the "kidney" consists of Malpighian tubules that develop from the hindgut and perform a secretion reabsorption filtering function.[55] They express a number of mammalian gene homologues (e.g., Cut, members of the Wingless pathway) that have subsequently been shown to play major roles in mammalian kidney development. Furthermore, studies on myoblast fusion and neural development in Drosophila—two processes that may not appear to be related to kidney development at first glance—have provided major clues into development and function of slit diaphragms.[56] Mutations in the Neph ortholog Irregular chiasm C-roughest (IrreC-rst) are associated with neuronal defects and abnormal patterning of the eye.[57,58]

The pronephros, which is only the first of three stages of kidney development in mammals, is the final and only kidney of jawless fish, whereas the mesonephros is the definitive kidney in amphibians. The pronephros found in larval stage zebra fish consists of two tubules connected to a fused, single, midline glomerulus. The zebrafish pronephric glomerulus expresses many of the same genes found in mammalian glomeruli including VEGFA, NPHS1, NPHS2, Wt1 and contain podocytes and fenestrated endothelial cells.[59] Advantages to the zebra fish as a model system include its short reproductive cycle, transparency of the larvae with easy visualization of defects in pronephric development without sacrificing the organism, availability of the genome sequence, the ability to rapidly knockdown gene function using morpholino oligonucleotides, and the ability to perform functional studies of filtration using fluorescently tagged labels of varying sizes.[60] These features lend the zebra fish to both forward and reverse

genetic screens and currently, there are several labs performing knockdown screens of mammalian homologues in zebra fish and genome-wide mutagenesis screens to study renal function.

The pronephros of Xenopus has also been used as a simple model to study early events in nephrogenesis. Similar to the fish, the pronephros consists of a single glomus, paired tubules, and a duct. The fact that Xenopus embryos develop rapidly outside the body (all major organ systems are formed by 6 days of age), the ease of injecting DNA, mRNA, and protein and ability to perform grafting and in vitro culture experiments establish the frog as a valuable model system to dissect early inductive and patterning cues.[61]

GENETIC ANALYSIS OF MAMMALIAN KIDNEY DEVELOPMENT

Much has been learned about the molecular genetic basis of kidney development over the past 15 years. This understanding has primarily been gained through the phenotypic analysis of mice carrying targeted mutations that affect kidney development. Additional information has been gained by identification and study of genes that are expressed in the developing kidney, even though the targeted mutation, or "knockout", either has not yet been done, or the knockout has not affected kidney development or function. In this section, we categorize the genetic defects based on the major phenotype and stage of disrupted development. It must be emphasized that many genes are expressed at multiple time stages of renal development and may play pleiotropic roles that are not yet entirely clear.

The molecular analysis of the initiation of metanephric kidney development has included a series of classical experiments using organ culture systems that allow separation of the ureteric bud and metanephric mesenchyme, and more recently, the analysis of many gene targeted mice whose phenotypes have included various degrees of renal agenesis. The organ culture system has been in use since the seminal experiments, beginning in the 1950s, of Grobstein, Saxen, and colleagues. These experiments showed that the induction of the mesenchymal to epithelial transformation within the mesenchyme required the presence of an inducing agent, provided by the ureteric bud. The embryonic neural tube was found to be able to substitute for the epithelial bud, and experiments involving the placement of the inducing agent on the opposite side of a porous filter from the mesenchyme provided information about the degree of contact required between them. A large series of experiments using the organ culture provided information about the timing of appearance of different proteins normally observed during the induction of nephrons, and the time intervals that were crucial in maintaining contact between the inducing agent and the mesenchyme to obtain induction of tubules.

The work with the organ culture system provided an extensive framework on which to base further studies of organ development, and remains in extensive use to this day. However, the modern era of studies on the early development of the kidney began with the observation of renal agenesis phenotypes in gene targeted or knockout mice, the earliest among these, the knockout of several transcription factors including the Wilms' Tumor-1 gene, also known as WT-1,[6] Pax-2,[9] Eya-1,[62] Six-1,[63,64] Sall-1,[65] Lim-1,[66] and Emx-2.[30] The knockout of several secreted signaling molecules such as GDNF,[67–69] GDF-11,[70] Gremlin[71] or their receptors, including c-Ret[72] and GFRα-1[73] also resulted in renal agenesis, at least in the majority of embryos.

Renal Agenesis Phenotypes from Transcription Factor Mutations

In embryos with the phenotype of renal agenesis, the most common observation is for there to be a histologically distinct patch of mesenchyme located in the normal location of the metanephric mesenchyme, but for there to be no outgrowth of the ureteric bud. An exception is the Eya-1 mutant embryo, where this distinct patch of mesenchyme is not found, suggesting that Eya-1 expression may indeed be the earliest determinant of the metanephric mesenchyme yet identified (Fig. 1–7). Together, the phenotypes of these knockout mice have provided an initial molecular hierarchy of early kidney development. There is evidence for at least three major pathways involved in determining the appearance and early function of the metanephric mesenchyme. One is the Eya-1/Six-1 pathway, which has also been implicated in kidney development through the study of humans with urogenital defects. Eya1 and Six1 mutations are found in humans with branchio-oto-renal (BOR) syndrome.[74] It is now known, through in vitro experiments, that Eya1 and Six1 form a regulatory complex that appears to be involved in transcriptional regulation.[75,76] Interestingly, a phosphatase activity is associated with this complex.[76] Moreover, Eya and Six family genes are co-expressed in several tissues in mammals, Xenopus and Drosophila, further supporting a functional interaction of these genes.[62–64,77,78] Direct transcriptional targets of this complex appear to include the pro-proliferative factor c-Myc.[76] In the Eya1-deficient urogenital ridge, it has recently been demonstrated that, unlike with some other renal agenesis phenotypes, there is no histologically distinct group of

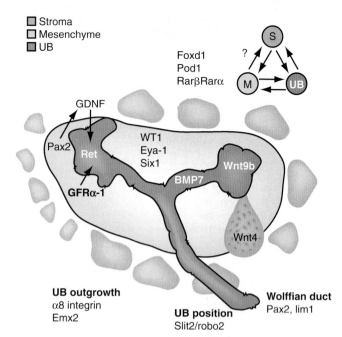

☐ Stroma
☐ Mesenchyme
☐ UB

FIGURE 1–7 Reciprocal interactions occur between all three major compartments of the metanephros (stroma, mesenchyme, and ureteric bud (UB)). Pretubular aggregate is shown on right side. Selected molecules that play key roles in these interactions are shown for simplicity. The Pax2/GDNF loop underlies a push to UB branching whereas the Wnt side represents induction of nephrons.

cells in the normal location of the metanephric mesenchyme.[79] Consistent with this finding, Six1 is either not expressed or highly diminished in expression in the location of the metanephric mesenchyme of Eya1 –/– embryos.[76–79] These findings may identify Eya1 as a gene involved in early commitment of this group of cells to the metanephric lineage. Although Six1 and Eya1 may act in a complex together, the Six1 phenotype is somewhat different, in that a histologically distinct mesenchyme is present at E11.5, without an invading ureteric bud, similar to the other renal agenesis phenotypes.[63,64] Eya1 is expressed in the Six1–/– mesenchyme, suggesting that Eya1 is upstream of Six1. Additionally, Sal1 and Pax2 are not expressed in the Six1 mutant mesenchyme, though Wt1 is expressed.[63,64,79] (There are discrepancies in the literature about Pax2 expression in Six1 mutant embryos, which may reflect the exact position along the anterior-posterior axis of the urogenital ridge of Six1 mutant embryos from which sections are obtained.)

A second pathway in the metanephric mesenchyme involves Pax-2 and GDNF. In Pax2 –/– embryos, Eya1, Six1 and Sal1 are expressed,[79] suggesting that the Eya-1/Six-1 pathway is not downstream, but may be upstream of Pax-2. Through a combination of molecular and in vivo studies, it has been demonstrated that Pax2 appears to act as a transcriptional activator of GDNF,[80] the major growth factor attracting and maintaining outgrowth of the ureteric bud and its derivative branches.

The third major pathway involves WT-1 and VEGF-A.[35] A novel approach to the organ culture system involving microinjection and electroporation has also yielded insights as to a possible function of the WT1 gene in early kidney development. Over-expression of WT1 from an expression construct led to high-level expression of vascular endothelial growth factor-A (VEGF-A). The target of VEGF-A appeared to be Flk-1 (VEGFR-2) expressing angioblasts at the periphery of the mesenchyme. Blocking signaling through Flk-1, if done when the metanephric rudiment was placed in culture, blocked expression of Pax2 and GDNF, and consequently the continued branching of the ureteric bud and induction of nephrons by the bud. Addition of the Flk-1 blockade after the organ had been in culture for 48 hours had no effect, indicating that the angioblast-derived signal was required to initiate kidney development, but not to maintain continued development. The signal provided by the angioblasts is not yet known, nor is it known whether WT1 is a direct transcriptional activator of VEGF-A. Flk-1 signaling is also known to be required to initiate hepatocyte differentiation during liver development.

Genes Required by the Ureteric Bud in Early Kidney Development

Genes expressed by the ureteric bud are also crucially involved in the inductive events of early kidney development. Examples include the transcription factor Emx-2 and c-Ret, the receptor for GDNF. C-Ret is a receptor tyrosine kinase, and presumably transduces signals to the epithelial cells of the bud that result in continued branching and proliferation. Interestingly, the failure of ureteric bud growth and branching of the GDNF homozygous mutant embryos can be rescued in situations in which the embryo also carries a transgene that specifically directs GDNF expression in the ureteric bud, and not in the mesenchyme. This autocrine-like rescue of ureteric bud growth and branching indicates that the pattern of branching is not determined by a specific pattern of GDNF expression in the mesenchyme; rather, any local source of GDNF elicits the usual pattern of branching.

Signaling Factors in Early Kidney Development

The signaling pathways described in the metanephric mesenchyme were identified by mutation of transcription factors. Presumably these transcription factors direct the expression of genes that encode proteins that act within the cell, in addition to genes encoding secreted molecules that act to convey signals from one group of cells to an adjacent or nearby group of cells. As previously mentioned, it has been demonstrated that Pax2 regulates the expression of GDNF, and WT1 regulates VEGF-A. In the case of other signaling molecules, it has yet to be determined what transcription factors control their expression in different cell types within the early kidney. Nevertheless, several groups of signaling molecules have been identified to be of great importance in early kidney development.

Fibroblast growth factors (FGFs) have been implicated in the very early stages of differentiation of the nephron. Conditional mutation of fibroblast growth factor receptors in the mesenchyme results in renal agenesis with a ureteric bud, with expression of early markers such as Eya1 and Six1 in the vicinity of the ureteric bud, but without expression of slightly later markers such as Six2 or Pax2, and no branching of the bud or induction of nephrons.[81] Two groups have published conditional mutations in the FGF8 gene, which eliminate expression of FGF8 in the mesenchyme of the early kidney.[82,83] Failure to properly express FGF8 did not block formation of a WT1 and Pax2-expressing condensed mesenchyme, but Wnt4-expressing pretubular aggregates were not present, and consequently S-shaped bodies, the precursor of the nephron, never developed.[82,83] Interestingly, these conditionally mutant kidneys were smaller with fewer branches of the collecting ducts, suggesting that nephron differentiation may have a role in driving continued branching morphogenesis of the collecting system.

Two members of the Wnt family of signaling molecules are expressed by the ureteric bud, Wnt 11 and Wnt 9b. The Wnt

family was originally discovered as the Wingless mutation in Drosophila, and in mammals as genes found at retroviral integration sites in mammary tumors in mice. Wnt11 is expressed at the tips of the buds, and decreased branching is observed in its absence, though there is no specific effect on the induction of the mesenchymal to epithelial transformation. In contrast, Wnt9b, which is expressed in the entire ureteric bud except the very tips, appears to be the vital molecule expressed by the bud that induces the mesenchyme. In the absence of Wnt 9b, the bud merges from the Wolffian duct and invades the mesenchyme, which condenses around the bud, but pretubular aggregates do not form, and there is no mesenchymal to epithelial transformation. No further branching of the bud is observed. Thus, Wnt 9b is the closest candidate identified to date, which is likely to be the crucial molecule produced by the bud that stimulates induction of the nephrons.

A third member of the Wnt family, Wnt 4, is expressed in the pretubular aggregate, and is required for the mesenchymal to epithelial transformation.[84] In Wnt4 mutant embryos, pretubular aggregates are present but they fail to undergo the mesenchymal to epithelial transformation into the tubular precursor of the mature nephron, indicating a role for Wnt4 in the formation of epithelial cells from mesenchyme.[84] The role of Wnt signaling has been studied in vitro, by exposing isolated metanephric mesenchymes to fibroblast cultures transfected with Wnt-expressing DNA vectors. Several Wnt's were found to be able to induce the mesenchymal to epithelial transformation, similar to that observed using embryonic neural tube. In considering these experiments in light of the more recently published Wnt 9b phenotype, it is worth considering whether the neural tube induction experiment can be viewed as a recapitulation of the Wnt 4 or Wnt 9b function, or both. As previously noted, a distinction between the induction by the ureteric bud versus neural tube, is that the bud stimulates both proliferation and mesenchymal to epithelial transformation, whereas the neural tube, or Wnt 4 expression by fibroblasts, only stimulates differentiation, without significant proliferation. On the other hand, both the classical neural tube experiment and the Wnt-expressing fibroblast experiment seemingly bypass a step normally observed in kidney development, that of formation of the pretubular aggregate inferior to the tips of the bud. Instead, aggregates form randomly within the isolated mesenchyme. Therefore, the neural tube rescue experiments are more consistent with a Wnt 4 rather than a Wnt 9b function. Further experimentation will be needed, however, to determine whether Wnt 9b, in the absence of the bud, can stimulate proliferation in addition to differentiation, in order to determine whether the expression of Wnt 9b is the major criterion that distinguishes the induction by the bud from induction by neural tube.

The bone morphogenetic protein (BMP) family of proteins is an additional family of secreted signaling proteins that plays a crucial role in the developing kidney.

Bmp-7 is first expressed in the ureteric bud, and then in the condensed mesenchyme.[85,86] In the absence of Bmp7, the first round of nephrons are induced, but there is no further kidney development.[85,86] It has been suggested that this first round of nephrons might result from maternal contribution of Bmp7 across the placenta, and it is not known whether Bmp7 is absolutely required for the induction of nephrons.

Adhesion Proteins in Early Kidney Development

A current theme in cell biology is that growth factor signaling often occurs coordinately with signals from the extracellular matrix transduced by adhesion receptors such as members of the integrin family. α8β1 integrin is expressed by cells of the metanephric mesenchyme,[87] which binds a novel molecule named nephronectin,[88] expressed on the ureteric bud. In most α8 integrin mutant embryos, the ureteric bud arrests its outgrowth upon contact with the metanephric mesenchyme.[87] In a small portion of embryos, this block is overcome, and a single, usually hypoplastic, kidney develops. Thus, the interaction of α8β1 integrin with nephronectin must have an important role in the continued growth of the ureteric bud into the mesenchyme. This phenotype also implies that there is something about the interaction of ureteric bud cells with the metanephric mesenchyme, which distinguishes it from the interaction of the ureteric bud with the undifferentiated mesenchyme of the urogenital ridge, through which it must briefly pass before encountering the metanephric mesenchyme. Whether α8β1 integrin:nephronectin signaling occurs in concert with growth factor signaling is not yet known.

Formation of the Collecting System

Formation of the collecting system is the result of the branching morphogenesis of the ureteric bud and its derivative branches, followed by extensive remodeling of those initial branches, to finally form the papillary region of the medulla, as well as the collecting ducts within the cortex and outer medulla. The overall structure of the kidney is largely patterned by the collecting system, and understanding the pathways that drive the formation of the collecting system will be an essential component of understanding how the kidney derives its overall structure.

The molecular events crucial to the development of the collecting system occur largely as interactions between the mesenchymal cells and the epithelial derivatives of the ureteric bud. This is especially true in the early phases of kidney development, when the epithelial branches of the bud are surrounded by mesenchyme. At later stages of development, when the cortex and medulla form distinct areas of the kidney, and nephrons and stromal cells compose much of the cortex, it is presently much less clear what the important cellular interactions are, even when it is known what molecules are important.

Several families of secreted growth factors have been demonstrated to be important in the patterning of the collecting system, including members of the BMP,[89] sonic hedgehog,[90] and FGF families.[91] The role of GDNF, required for initial outgrowth of the bud and to drive continued branching, was previously discussed. Conditional gene targeting of FGF receptor 2 (but not of FGFR1) in the ureteric bud results in greatly decreased branching of the bud.[92] Mice carrying a mutation of FGF7 have smaller collecting systems,[91] though this phenotype is not as severe as the conditional mutation of FGFR2, implying that additional FGFs are probably involved in branching of the ureteric bud. The role of FGF8 in the mesenchyme, with regard to nephron development, was previously discussed. Whether FGF8 or another FGF is also driving development of the collecting system is not clear, but it is interesting to note that mutations that block induction of nephrons also tend to eliminate further branching and growth of the derivative branches of the ureteric bud.

The role of BMP7 in early kidney development has been discussed in a previous section. Two other prominent members of the BMP family, BMP2 and 4, also have significant roles in formation of the collecting system,[89] which were more difficult to decipher, as mouse embryos carrying mutations in these factors undergo embryonic demise too early to identify an effect on kidney development. In organ culture, BMP7 stimulates branching, whereas BMP2 was found to inhibit branching of the derivatives of the ureteric bud.[93,94] Further study of the role of BMP2 utilized a constitutively

active form of the BMP2 receptor, ALK3, specifically expressed in the derivatives of the ureteric bud. This resulted in medullary dysplasia, resembling medullary cystic disease observed in humans.[95] It appears that BMP2 signaling normally acts to suppress a proliferation signal mediated by smad signaling and β-catenin, which acts to stimulate expression of the pro-proliferative transcription factor c-Myc.[96]

Diminished branching is also observed in kidneys of sonic hedgehog (shh)-deficient embryos.[90] This phenotype bears resemblance to the renal dysplasia observed in humans with mutations of the Gli3 gene, which encodes an effector of the Shh signaling pathway.[97] Increased expression of Pax2 and Sal1, required for normal kidney development, as well as cell cycle regulatory genes N-myc and cyclin D1, were observed in Shh-deficient kidneys.[97] Interestingly, the Shh-deficient kidney phenotype was rescued by inhibiting signaling through Gli3, providing genetic confirmation that Gli3 is a regulator of the Shh pathway.[97]

Targeted mutation in mice of the α3 integrin gene, discussed later in regard to its role in glomerular development, also results in a poorly formed papilla, with fewer collecting ducts and increased interstitium.[98] α3β1 integrin is expressed in the ureteric bud and collecting ducts.[99] In vitro, α3β1 integrin appears to have a role both in cell-matrix and cell-cell interaction,[100] but the latter role has not been verified in vivo, though α3β1 integrin is expressed basolaterally in developing tubules, consistent with both roles. As integrins are known to signal in coordination with growth factor receptors, it will be of interest to determine if α3β1 integrin is involved in any of the signaling pathways discussed previously in this section.

Positioning of the Ureteric Bud

A final aspect of kidney development that is of great relevance to renal and urological congenital defects in humans relates to the positioning of the ureteric bud. Incorrect position of the bud, or duplication of the bud, results in abnormally shaped kidneys, and/or incorrect insertion of the ureter into the bladder, and resultant ureteral reflux that can pre-dispose to infection and scarring of the kidneys and urological tract.

FoxC1 is a transcription factor of the Forkhead family, expressed in the intermediate mesoderm and the metanephric mesenchyme adjacent to the Wolffian duct. In the absence of Foxc1, the expression of GDNF adjacent to the Wolffian duct is less restricted than in wild-type embryos, and there are resultant ectopic ureteric buds, giving rise to duplex ureters, one of which is a hydroureter, and to hypoplastic kidneys.[101] Additional molecules that regulate the location of ureteric bud outgrowth are slit2 and ROBO2, signaling molecules best known for their role in axon guidance in the developing nervous system. Slit is a secreted factor, and ROBO is its receptor. Slit2 is mainly expressed in the Wolffian duct, whereas Robo2 is expressed in the mesenchyme.[102] In embryos deficient in either Slit2 or ROBO2, there are ectopic ureteric buds, similar to the Foxc1 mutant. (Dissimilar to the Foxc1 phenotype was the observation that none of the ureters in Slit2/ROBO2 mutants failed to undergo the normal remodeling that results in insertion in the bladder; instead, the ureters remained connected to the nephric duct.[102]) The domain of GDNF expression is expanded anteriorly in the absence of either Slit2 or ROBO2. The expression of Pax2, Eya1, and Foxc1, all thought to regulate GDNF expression, was not dramatically different in the absence of Slit2 or ROBO2, suggesting that Slit/ROBO signaling was not upstream of these genes. It is possible that Slit/ROBO signaling is regulating the point of ureteric bud outgrowth, by regulating the GDNF expression domain downstream of Pax2 or Eya1. An alternative explanation is that Slit/ROBO are acting independently of GDNF, and that the expanded GDNF domain is a response to, rather than a cause of, ectopic ureteric buds.

Molecular Biology of Nephron Development: Tubulogenesis

While gene targeting and other analyses have identified many genes involved in the initial induction of the metanephric kidney and the formation of the pre-tubular aggregate, much less is presently known about how the pre-tubular aggregate develops into the mature nephron, a process through which a simple tubule elongates, convolutes, and differentiates into multiple distinct segments with different functions. In considering how this segmentation occurs, it has been considered whether there will be similarities to other aspects of development, such as the limb or neural tube, where there is segmentation along various axes.

The Notch group of signaling molecules has been implicated in directing segmentation of the nephron. Notch family members are transmembrane proteins whose cytoplasmic domains are cleaved by the γ-secretase enzyme, upon the interaction of the extracellular domain with transmembrane ligand proteins of the delta and jagged families, found on adjacent cells.[103] Thus, Notch signaling occurs between adjacent cells, in contrast to signaling by secreted growth factors, which may occur at a distance from the growth factor-expressing cells. The cleaved portion of the Notch cytoplasmic domain translocates to the nucleus, where it has a role in directing gene expression. Mice homozygous for a hypomorphic allele of Notch2 have abnormal glomeruli, with a failure to form a mature capillary tuft.[104,105] Because null mutants of notch family members usually result in early embryonic lethality, further analysis of Notch family function in kidney development has made use of the organ culture model. When metanephric rudiments are cultured in the presence of a γ-secretase inhibitor,[106,107] there is diminished expression of podocyte and proximal tubule markers, in comparison with distal tubule markers and branching of the ureteric bud. When the γ-secretase inhibitor is removed, there seems to be a better recovery of expression of proximal tubule markers, in comparison with markers of podocyte differentiation. Similar results were observed in mice carrying targeted mutation of the PSEN1 and PSEN2 genes that encode a component of the γ-secretase complex.[108] These results, while requiring confirmation from mice carrying conditional mutations in notch genes themselves, suggest that Notch signaling is involved in patterning the proximal tubule and glomerulus. Similar results were obtained from mice with mutations in the gene encoding γ-secretase.

There is one example so far of a transcription factor being involved in the differentiation of a specific cell type in the kidney. The phenotype is actually found in the collecting ducts, rather than in the nephron itself, but is discussed in this section as it is demonstrative of the types of phenotypes it is expected will be found as additional mutant mice are examined. Two cell types are normally found in the collecting ducts— principal cells, which mediate water and salt reabsorption, and intercalated cells that mediate acid-base transport. In the absence of the Foxi1 transcription factor, there is only one cell type present in collecting ducts, and many acid-base-transport proteins normally expressed by intercalated cells are absent.[109]

Molecular Analysis of the Nephrogenic Zone

The molecular biology of the nephrogenic zone remains largely to be explored, especially that pertaining to whether there exists a population of kidney stem cells. As noted, the histology of this zone resembles the early developing kidney, with condensed mesenchyme, which expresses Pax2 and low levels of Wt1, surrounding ureteric bud-like structures. Unknown is how this population of condensed mesenchyme is maintained; whether it self-replenishes, such that it could be regarded as a stem-like population, or whether there is a subset of cells within the condensed mesenchyme that are the stem-like cells. Alternatively, there may be a population of cells, not within the condensed mesenchyme itself, which both self-replenishes and gives rise to successive populations of condensed mesenchyme in each successive layer of the nephrogenic zone. At present, no molecular markers have been identified that distinguish a subset of cells that might be a stem-like population, apart from the condensed mesenchyme as a whole.

Molecular Genetics of the Stromal Cell Lineage

In recent years, a key role for the stromal cell lineage in kidney development was discovered largely through the analysis of knockout mice. FoxD1 (formerly BF2) is a winged helix transcription factor; in the kidney it is only expressed in stromal cells that are found in a rim beneath the renal capsule and as a layer of cells surrounding the mesenchymal condensates.[26] Despite the restricted distribution of FoxD1-positive cells, major defects in the development of adjacent renal tubules and glomeruli were observed in FoxD1 KO mice. These results demonstrate that stromal cells are required for nephrogenesis and furthermore that the model of reciprocal signaling between the UB and condensates must be extended to include the stromal cell compartment[14] (Fig. 1–8).

Pod1 (tcf21/capsulin/epicardin), a member of the basic-helix-loop-helix family of transcription factors, is also expressed in the stromal cell lineage, as well as in condensing MM.[110,111] Pod1 is also expressed in a number of differentiated renal cell types that derive from these mesenchymal cells and include developing and mature podocytes of the renal glomerulus, cortical and medullary peritubular interstitial cells, pericytes surrounding small renal vessels, and adventitial cells surrounding larger blood vessels. The defect in nephrogenesis observed in Pod1 KO mice is similar to the defect seen in BF2 knockout mice, with disruption of branching morphogenesis and an arrest and delay in glomerulogenesis and tubulogenesis. Analysis of chimeric mice that are derived from Pod1 KO embryonic stem cells and GFP-expressing embryos, demonstrated both cell autonomous and non-cell-autonomous roles for Pod1 in nephrogenesis.[112] Most strikingly, the glomerulogenesis defect is rescued by the presence of wild-type stromal cells (i.e., mutant cells will epithelialize and form nephrons normally as long as they are surrounded by wild-type stromal cells in keeping with the model outlined in Figs. 1–7 and 1–8). In addition, there is a cell autonomous requirement for Pod1 in stromal mesenchymal cells to allow differentiation into interstitial cell and pericyte cell lineages of the cortex and medulla as Pod1 null ES cells were unable to contribute to these populations.

Although many of the defects in the Pod1 mutant kidneys phenocopy those seen in the BF2 mutant kidneys, there are important differences. In the kidneys of Pod1 KO mice, there are vascular anomalies and absence of pericyte differentiation that were not reported in FoxD1 mutant mice. These differences might result from the broader domain of Pod1 expression, which also includes the condensing mesenchyme, podocytes and medullary stromal cells, in addition to the stromal cells that surround the condensates. In contrast to FoxD1, Pod1 is not highly expressed in the thin rim of stromal cells found immediately beneath the capsule, suggesting that FoxD1 and Pod1 might mark early and late stromal cell lineages, respectively, with overlap in the stroma that surrounds the condensates.[27] However, definitive co-labeling studies to address this issue have not been performed. As both Pod1 and FoxD1 are transcription factors it is interesting to speculate that they might interact or regulate the expression of a common stromal "inducing factor".

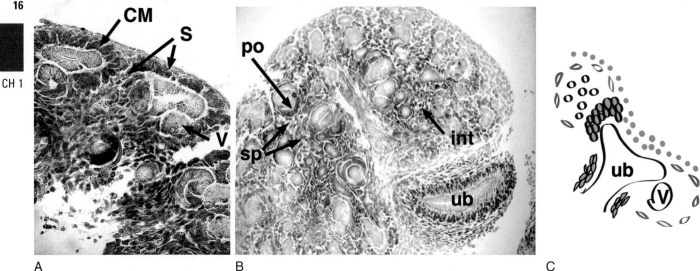

FIGURE 1-8 Populations of cells within the metanephric mesenchyme. As described in the text, these populations are defined by morphologic and molecular characteristics. Metanephroi from a 14.5 d.p.c (**A**) and 15.5 d.p.c. (**B**) Pod1/lacZ mouse are stained with lacZ. Pod1-expressing cells stain blue. Stromal cells (S; pink in **C**) are seen surrounding condensing mesenchyme (CM). Metanephrogenic population (green in **C**) remain unstained. By 15.5 d.p.c. a well-developed interstitial compartment is seen and consists of peritubular fibroblasts, medullary fibroblasts, and pericytes. Loose and condensed mesenchymal cells are also observed around the stalk of the ureteric bud in **B**. v, renal vesicle; po, podocyte precursors; sp, stromal pericytes; int, interstitium. **C**, Schematic diagram of mesenchymal populations include the metanephrogenic precursors (in green), uninduced mesenchyme (white), condensing mesenchyme around the UB tips and stalk (blue) and stromal cell lineage (pink). (Reproduced with permission from Developmental Dynamics.)

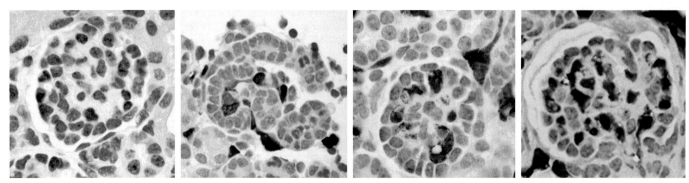

FIGURE 1-9 Developing glomeruli stained with an antibody to the GFP (green fluorescent protein). Control glomerulus from a wild-type mouse. S-shape, capillary and mature glomeruli in an 18.5 d.p.c. metanephros from a Flk1-GFP mouse strain. All endothelial cells express the GFP protein that is expressed under control of the endogenous Flk1/VEGFR-2 promoter. (Reproduced with permission from the Journal of American Society of Nephrology.)

Vitamin A deficiency has been associated with a variety of birth defects, including renal dysplasia; vitamin A is the ligand for retinoic acid receptors (RARs) including RARA and RARB2, both of which are expressed in the stromal cell lineage. Mice that lack both of these receptors and thus have decreased vitamin A signaling, demonstrate decreased branching of the UB, patterning defects in the stromal cell lineage with a buildup of stromal cell layers beneath the capsule and defects in nephron patterning.[14,27,113] Transgenic overexpression of the tyrosine kinase receptor, c-ret, under the regulation of a ureteric bud-specific promoter from the Hoxb7 gene rescued the observed defects although retinoic acid treatment alone could not. Taken together, these results show that a vitamin A dependent signal is required in stromal cells for UB branching and that UB branching is required to pattern the stroma.

Molecular Genetics of Vascular Formation

Vasculogenesis and angiogenesis both contribute to vascular development within the kidney. Endothelial cells may be identified through the expression of the tyrosine kinase signaling receptor, VEGFR −2 (flk1/KDR).[114] Reporter mouse strains that carry lacZ or GFP cDNA cassettes "knocked into" the VEGFR-2 locus, permit precise snapshots of vessel development, as all the vascular progenitor and differentiated cells in these organs express a blue or green color (Fig. 1–9). Use of other knock-in strains allows identification of endothelial cells lining arteriolar or venous vessels.[115]

Over the past decade, a number of growth factors and their receptors have been identified that are required for vasculogenesis and angiogenesis. Gene deletion studies in mice have shown that VEGF-A and its cognate receptor VEGFR-2 are essential for vasculogenesis.[114,116] Mice that are null for the VEGF-A gene die at 9.5 days post coitum (d.p.c.) due to a failure of vasculogenesis while mice lacking a single VEGF-A allele (i.e., they are heterozygotes for the VEGF-A gene) die at 11.5 d.p.c. also from vascular defects.[116] These data demonstrate gene dosage sensitivity to VEGF-A during development. In the developing kidney, podocytes and renal tubular epithelial cells express VEGF-A[117] and continue to express it constitutively in the adult kidney, while the cognate tyrosine-kinase receptors for VEGF-A, VEGFR-1 (Flt1), and

VEGFR-2 (Flk1/KDR) are predominantly expressed by all endothelial cells. Which non-endothelial cells might also express the VEGF receptors in the kidney in vivo is still debated, although renal cell lines clearly do and metanephric mesenchymal cells express VEGFR-2 in organ culture as outlined earlier.

Conditional gene targeting experiments and cell-selective deletion of VEGF-A from podocytes demonstrates that VEGF-A signaling is required for formation and maintenance of the glomerular filtration barrier.[118,119] Glomerular endothelial cells express VEGFR-2 as they migrate into the vascular cleft. Although a few endothelia migrate into the developing glomeruli of VEGF[lox/lox]/Pod-Cre mice (mice with selective deletion of VEGF from podocytes), likely due to a small amount of VEGF-A produced by presumptive podocytes at the S-shaped stage of glomerular development prior to Cre-mediated genetic deletion, the endothelia failed to develop fenestrations and rapidly disappeared leaving capillary "ghosts" (Fig. 1–10). Similar to the dosage sensitivity observed in the whole embryo, deletion of a single VEGF-A allele from podocytes also led to glomerular endothelial defects known as endotheliosis that progressed to end-stage kidney failure at 3 months of age; as the dose of VEGF-A decreased, the associated endothelial phenotypes became more severe (Fig. 1–11). Upregulation of the major 164 angiogenic VEGF-A isoform in developing podocytes of transgenic mice led to massive proteinuria and collapse of the glomerular tuft by 5 days of age. Taken together, these results show a requirement for VEGF-A

for development and maintenance of the specialized glomerular endothelia and demonstrate a major paracrine signaling function for VEGF-A in the glomerulus. Furthermore, tight regulation of the dose of VEGF-A is essential for proper formation of the glomerular capillary system; the molecular basis and mechanism of dosage sensitivity is unclear at present and is particularly intriguing given the documented inducible regulation of VEGF-A by hypoxia inducible factors (HIFs) at a transcriptional level. Despite this, it is clear that in vivo, a single VEGF-A allele is unable to compensate for loss of the other. Immortalized podocyte cell lines express a variety of VEGF receptors opening up the possibility that VEGF-A also plays an autocrine role in the developing glomerulus[120–122]; however, the functional relevance of these findings for the glomerulus in vivo is unclear at present.

A second major receptor tyrosine kinase (RTK) signaling pathway required for maturation of developing blood vessels is the Angiopoietin-Tie signaling system. Angiopoietin 1 stabilizes newly formed blood vessels and is associated with loss of vessel plasticity and concurrent recruitment of pericytes or vascular support cells to the vascular wall.[123] The molecular switch or pathway leading to vessel maturation through activation of Tie2 (previously known as Tek), the major receptor for Ang1 is not known and appears to be independent of the PDGF signaling system that is also required for pericyte recruitment. Ang1 knockout mice die at 12.5 d.p.c precluding analysis of its role in glomerular development. In contrast, it is proposed that Ang2 functions as a natural

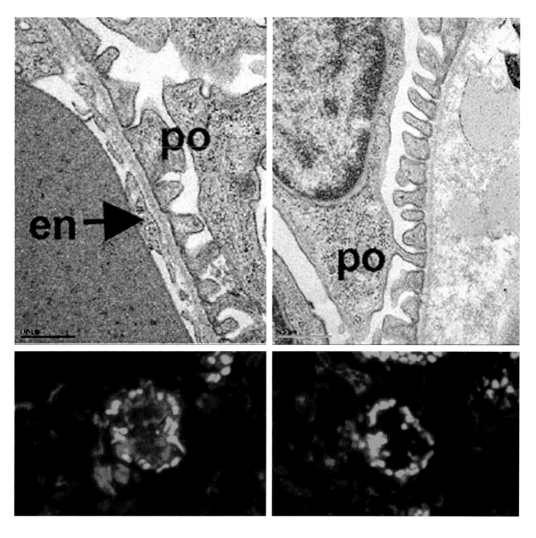

FIGURE 1–10 Transmission electron micrographs of the glomerular filtration barrier from a wild-type (left) or transgenic mouse with selective knockout of VEGF from the podocytes. Podocytes (po) are seen in both but the endothelial layer (en) is entirely missing from the knockout mouse leaving a "capillary ghost." Immunostaining for WT1 (podocytes/green) and PECAM (endothelial cells/red) confirms the absence of capillary wall in VEGF knockouts. (Adapted from Eremina V, Sood M, Haigh J, et al: Glomerular-specific alterations of VEGF-A expression lead to distinct congenital and acquired renal diseases. J Clin Invest 111:707–716, 2003.)

CH 1

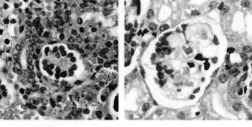
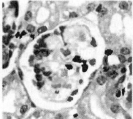
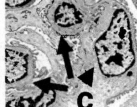
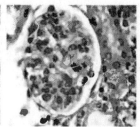
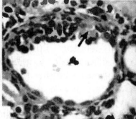

| −/− | hypo/− | +/− | +/+ | ++++ |
| Perinatal death | Mesangiolysis | Endotheliosis | Wildtype | Collapsing glomerulopathy |

FIGURE 1–11 Vascular endothelial growth factor dose and glomerular development: Photomicrographs of glomeruli from mice carrying different copy numbers of the VEGF gene within podocytes. A total knockout (loss of both alleles;−/−) results in failure of glomerular filtration barrier formation and perinatal death; a single hypomorphic allele (hypo/−) leads to massive mesangiolysis in the first weeks of life and death at 3 weeks of age; loss of one copy (+/−) results in endotheliosis (swelling of the endothelium) and death at 12 weeks of age. Overexpression (20-fold increase in VEGF;++++) results in collapsing glomerulopathy. (Adapted from Eremina V, Baeld HJ, Quaggin SE: Role of the VEGF-A signaling pathway in the glomerulus: evidence for crosstalk between components of the glomerular filtration barrier. Nephron Physiol 106:32–37, 2007.)

antagonist of the Tie2 receptor, as Ang2 can bind to this receptor but fails to phosphorylate it in endothelial cultures.[124,125] Consistent with this hypothesis is the fact that overexpression of Ang2 in transgenic mice results in a phenotype similar to the Ang1 or Tie2 KO mice. Ang1, Ang2, Tie2, and Tie1 (an orphan receptor for this system) are all expressed in the developing kidney.[126–130] Whereas Ang1 is quite broadly expressed in condensing mesenchyme, podocytes, and tubular epithelial cells, Ang2 is more restricted to pericytes and smooth muscle cells surrounding cortical and large vessels as well as in the mesangium. Angiopoietin 2 KO mice are viable but exhibit defects in peritubular cortical capillary development; the mice died prior to differentiation of vasa rectae precluding analysis of the role of Ang2 in these other capillary beds.[131] Both angiopoietin ligands function in concert with VEGF, although precise degree of crosstalk between these pathways is still under investigation. (VEGF and Ang1 work together to promote sprouting.) Chimeric studies showed that the orphan receptor Tie1 is required for development of the glomerular capillary system, because Tie1 null cells are not able to contribute to glomerular capillary endothelium.[132]

The Ephrin-Eph family is a third tyrosine kinase dependent growth factor signaling system that is expressed in the developing kidney; in the whole embryo, it is involved in neural sprouting and axon finding as well as in arterial/venous specification of arterial and venous components of the vasculature.[133,134] Ephrins and their cognate receptors are expressed widely during renal development. Overexpression of EPH4 leads to defects in glomerular arteriolar formation whereas conditional deletion of EphrinB2 from perivascular smooth muscle cells and mesangial cells leads to glomerular vascular abnormalities.[135,136] How this occurs is not entirely clear as Ephrin B2 has a dynamic pattern of expression in the developing glomerulus, beginning in podocyte precursors and rapidly switching to glomerular endothelial cells and mesangial cells.[115]

An additional pathway that is likely to play a role in glomerular endothelial development and perhaps of the entire vasculature of the kidney, is the CXCR4-SDF1 axis. CXCR4, a chemokine receptor is expressed by bone marrow derived cells, but is also expressed in endothelial cells. SDF-1 (Cxcl12), the only known ligand for CXCR4 is expressed in a dynamic segmental pattern in the podocyte-endothelial compartment and later in the mesangial cells of the glomerulus.[137] Embryonic deletion of CXCR4 results in glomerular developmental defects with a dilated capillary network (presented at American Society of Nephrology, 2005).

Mice carrying a hypomorphic allele of Notch 2, which is missing 2 epidermal growth factor (EGF) motifs are born with a reduced number of glomeruli that lack both endothelial and mesangial cells as discussed in the section on nephron segmentation.[103,104]

There is evidence from other model systems that vascular development is required for patterning and terminal differentiation of adjacent tissues. For example, vascular signals and basement membrane produced by adjacent endothelial cells are required for differentiation of the islet cells of the pancreas.[138,139] In the kidney, it is possible that vascular signals are required for branching morphogenesis, and patterning of the nephron and may explain some of the defects observed in KO mice such as Pod1 (Tcf21) mutants. Given the complex reciprocal interactions between tissue types, these signals will be a challenge to sort out, but with the increasing arsenal of genetic tools, should be possible.

The Juxta-Glomerular Apparatus and the Renin-Angiotensin System

The juxtaglomerular apparatus consists of juxtaglomerular cells that line the afferent arteriole, the macula densa cells of the distal tubule, and the extraglomerular mesangial cells that are in contact with intraglomerular mesangium.[140] Renin-expressing cells may be seen in arterioles in early mesonephric kidneys in 5-week human fetus and in metanephric kidney by week 8, at a stage prior to hemodynamic flow changes within the kidney. Recently, Gomez and colleagues generated a Renin-knockin mouse that expresses Cre recombinase in the renin locus.[141] Offspring of matings between the renin-Cre and a reporter strain that expresses beta-galactosidase or GFP upon Cre-mediated DNA excision showed that renin-expressing cells may be found within MM and give rise not only to JG cells, but also to mesangial cells, epithelial cells, and extrarenal cells including interstitial Leydig cells of the XY gonad and cells within the adrenal gland. Although most of these cells cease to express renin in the adult, they appear to re-express renin in stress conditions and are recruited to the afferent arteriole.

The only known substrate for renin, angiotensinogen, is converted to angiotensin I and angiotensin II by angiotensin converting enzyme.[142] The renin-angiotensin-aldosterone axis is required for normal renal development. In humans, the use of angiotensin-converting enzyme inhibitors in early or late pregnancy have been associated with congenital defects including renal anomalies.[143,144] Two subtypes of angiotensin receptors exist[145]: AT1 receptors are responsible for most of the classically recognized functions of the RAS including pressor effects and aldosterone release mediated through angiotensin; functions of the type 2 receptors have been more difficult to characterize, but generally seem to oppose the actions of the AT1 receptors. Genetic deletion of angiotensinogen[146,147] or the ACE[148,149] result in hypotension, and defects in formation of the renal papilla and pelvis. Humans have one AT1 gene while mice have two: AT1a and AT1b. Mice carrying a knockout for either AT1 receptor alone exhibit no major defects,[150,151] while combined deficiency phenocopies the angiotensinogen and ACE phenotypes.[152,153] While AT2 receptor expression is markedly up-regulated in the embryonic kidney, genetic deletion of the AT2 receptor does not cause major impairment of renal development.[154,155] However, an association between AT2 receptor-deficiency and malformations of the collecting system, including VUR (vesicoureteral reflux) and ureteropelvic junction obstruction, has been reported.[156]

Nephron Development and Glomerulogenesis

Mesangial Cell Ingrowth

Mesangial cells grow into the developing glomerulus and come to sit between the capillary loops. Gene deletion studies have demonstrated a critical role for PDGF-B/beta receptor signaling in this process. Deletion of PDGF-B, which is expressed by glomerular endothelia, or the PDGF beta receptor that is expressed by mesangial cells, results in glomeruli with a single balloon-like capillary loop, instead of the intricately folded glomerular endothelial capillaries of wild-type kidneys. Furthermore, the glomeruli contain no mesangial cells.[157] Endothelial-cell specific deletion of PDGF-B results in the same glomerular phenotype and show that production of PDGF-B by the endothelium is required for mesangial migration.[158] In turn, mesangial cells and the matrix they produce are required to pattern the glomerular capillary system. Loss of podocyte-derived factors such as VEGF-A also lead to failure of mesangial cell ingrowth, likely through primary loss of endothelial cells and failure of PDGF-B signaling.

A number of other knockouts demonstrate defects in both vascular/capillary development and mesangial cell ingrowth. Transcription factors expressed by podocytes including Pod1 and Foxc2 show defects in mesangial cell migration (Fig. 1–12).[49,111] What factors are disrupted in these mutant mice to result in the phenotype are not yet known but emphasize the importance of "crosstalk" between cell compartments within the glomerulus.

Glomerular Epithelial Development

Presumptive podocytes are observed at the most proximal end of the S-shape body at the furthest point away from the ureteric bud tip. They form as columnar epithelial cells in apposition to the developing vascular cleft. A number of transcription factors have been identified that are expressed within developing and mature podocytes including: Wilms tumor suppressor 1, Pod1 (tcf21), Kreisler (maf1), Foxc2, and lmx1b (Fig. 1–13).[6,49,110,111,159,160] Genetic deletion studies have shown that Pod1, Foxc2, lmx1b, and Kreisler are all required for elaboration of podocyte foot processes and spreading of podocytes around the glomerular capillary beds. Pod1 appears to function upstream of Kreisler, as the latter factor is down-regulated in glomeruli from Pod1 KO mice.[159] Transcriptional programs regulated by these factors are incompletely known, however, Pod1, Foxc2, and lmx1b knockout mice all display remarkably similar glomerular phenotypes with major podocyte developmental/maturation defects together with capillary loop, glomerular basement membrane, and mesangial ingrowth abnormalities. It is believed that loss of podocyte-expressed factors regulated by these proteins leads to the dramatic arrest in development resulting in abnormal capillary loop stage glomeruli. Immunostaining and gene expression profiling performed in glomeruli from each of these mutant mice have identified reduced expression of some common downstream effector molecules including collagen alpha 4. In turn, a podocyte-specific protein, podocin (NPHS2) is reduced in the glomeruli of Foxc2, lmx1b, and Pod1 KO mice.[49,161] Mutations in lmx1b are associated with nail patellar syndrome in humans, a disease characterized by absent patellae and nephrotic syndrome in a subset of patients. All of these genes are expressed from the S-shape stage onward and remain constitutively expressed in adult glomeruli.

WT1 is also expressed in presumptive and mature podocytes. As WT1 knockout mice fail to develop any kidneys, the role of WT1 in the developing and mature podocyte is not entirely clear. However, a series of experimental models support an important role for WT1 in the podocyte. The null phenotype was largely rescued using a yeast artificial chromosome (YAC) containing the human WT1 gene[5]; depending on the level of WT1 expression, these mice developed crescentic glomerulonephritis or mesangial sclerosis, defects in the glomerulus reminiscent of some of the human phenotypes observed with Denys Drash syndrome resulting from mutations in the KTS isoform of WT1.[5] Transgenic mice expressing a Denys-Drash mutant WT1 allele under the regulation of a podocyte-specific promoter also developed glomerular disease with abnormalities observed in the adjacent endothelium.[4]

Alpha 3 integrin KO mice also demonstrate defects in glomerular development with specific abnormalities in podocyte maturation.[98] Alpha 3 integrin forms a heterodimer with β1 integrin and is expressed by podocytes. Loss of this integrin results in poorly formed foot processes and abnormalities in adjacent glomerular basement membrane. Elaboration of foot processes during development requires the interaction of an

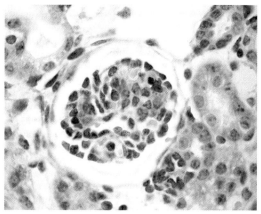 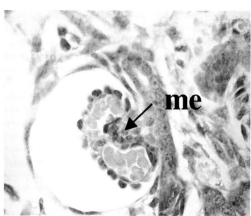

FIGURE 1–12 Glomeruli from wild-type (**A**) or Pod1 knockout mice (**B**). Note dilated capillary loop and poor ingrowth of mesangial cells (me).

A B

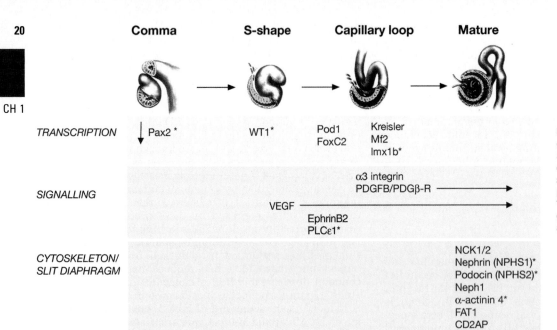

	Comma	S-shape	Capillary loop	Mature
TRANSCRIPTION	↓ Pax2 *	WT1*	Pod1 FoxC2	Kreisler Mf2 lmx1b*
SIGNALLING		VEGF	EphrinB2 PLCε1*	α3 integrin PDGFB/PDGβ-R
CYTOSKELETON/ SLIT DIAPHRAGM				NCK1/2 Nephrin (NPHS1)* Podocin (NPHS2)* Neph1 α-actinin 4* FAT1 CD2AP

FIGURE 1–13 Molecular basis of glomerular development. Key factors are shown; time point of major effect observed in knockout or transgenic studies is identified. Many factors play roles at more than one time point. *Mutations identified in patients with glomerular disease. (Top panel adapted from Saxen.)

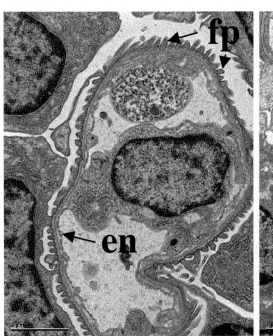
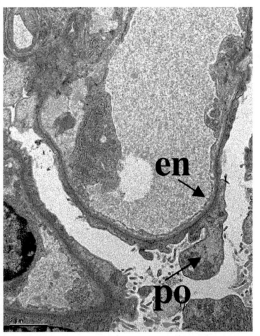

FIGURE 1–14 Foot processes (fp) are seen surrounding a capillary loop of a newborn wild-type mouse. In the right panel, a capillary loop from a NCK1/2 knockout mouse shows complete lack of foot process formation. En, glomerular endothelial cell. (Adapted from Jones N, Blasutig IM, Eremina V, et al: Nck adaptor proteins link nephrin to the actin cytoskeleton of kidney podocytes. Nature 440:818–823, 2006.)

adaptor signaling molecule, NCK, with slit diaphragm proteins. The slit diaphragm is a specialized intercellular junction that connects foot processes of adjacent podocytes. In mature glomeruli, the slit diaphragm appears as a dense band on transmission electron micrographs. In 1998, Karl Tryggvason's group identified the nephrin (NPHS1) gene and showed that mutations in this gene cause congenital nephrosis of the Finnish (CNF) variety.[162] Glomeruli from infants with CNF, lack slit diaphragms and die from renal failure and nephrotic syndrome unless they receive renal replacement therapy. Nephrin is a member of the immunoglobulin superfamily and makes up a major structural component of the slit diaphragm. Recently, it was shown that the nephrin molecule contains 3 intracellular tyrosine residues (1176, 1193, 1217) that can be phosphorylated leading to recruitment of the SH2 adaptor proteins, NCK 1 and 2.[17,18] In vitro, this association leads to reorganization of the actin cytoskeleton, the backbone of foot

process structure. Mice born with podocyte-selective deletion of the NCK1 and 2 genes exhibit congenital nephrosis and fail to form any foot processes (Fig. 1–14), emphasizing the biologic link between the slit diaphragm and cytoskeleton in vivo. The phenotype observed in Nck-deficient mice is similar to that of FAT1 KO mice, with complete absence of foot process formation and podocyte effacement. FAT1 is a large protocadherin expressed in podocytes. In contrast, Nephrin KO mice exhibit narrowed slits with loss of the diaphragm but the degree of foot process effacement or fusion varies and may be dependent on mouse strain. Additional proteins of the slit diaphragm and cytoskeleton have been identified that play major roles in glomerulogenesis and in human disease. Three Nephrin-like molecules exist (neph1–3) that are also expressed in podocytes and interact with other slit diaphragm proteins.[163,164] Mice generated through a gene-trap screen with loss of Neph1 function develop focal segmental glomerulosclerosis (FSGS), suggesting that these molecules are also important for function of the slit diaphragm.[48] NPHS2 (podocin) is a homologue of the Caenorhabditis elegans mechanosensory channel (MEC), MEC2, and co-localizes with nephrin at the slit diaphragm. Mutations in NPHS2 have been identified in patients with steroid-resistant congenital autosomal recessive FSGS.[165] Although foot process effacement is a feature of the NPHS2 KO mice, vascular defects are also observed and suggest that podocin or the slit diaphragm (or both) may regulate components of the crosstalk between podocytes and endothelium.[166] Mutations in alpha actinin 4, a component of the actin cytoskeleton, were identified in autosomal dominant FSGS, a disease with its onset in adulthood.[167] Pollak and colleagues hypothesized that the mutant actinin functions in a dominant negative manner to cause the phenotype. Interestingly, ACTN4 KO mice also develop glomerular disease, despite the proteins rather ubiquitous expression.[168] Clearly, elucidation of the mechanism(s) is important, and will provide exciting insights into glomerular biology.

CD2AP (CD2-associated protein), is an SH3 domain containing protein in lymphoid cells and podocytes that interacts with the cytoplasmic tail of nephrin and with the actin cytoskeleton.[169] Null CD2AP mice rapidly develop massive proteinuria and mesangial sclerosis, a finding that highlights the interplay of all of these molecules in the glomerulus. CD2AP heterozygous mice are susceptible to glomerular disease and exhibit glomerular lesions at 12 to 18 months that are similar to immunotactoid glomerulopathy in humans.[44,170] CD2AP has been implicated in endocytosis and lysosomal sorting and may be required to clear immunoglobulins that are normally filtered at the glomerulus. Consistent with this hypothesis, the investigators showed that a large proportion of CD2AP heterozygous mice develop FSGS-like lesions when injected with a nephrotoxic antibody.[170] Mutations in TRPC6 channel underlie another inherited form of AD-FSGS in patients. Some, but not all, of the identified mutations lead to activation of the channel and increased influx of calcium inside the cell.[171,172] TRPC6 is expressed in podocytes but also other glomerular cell types. Elucidation of the mechanism whereby TRPC6 leads to glomerular disease is exciting and may provide a mechanism that is amenable to pharmacologic intervention.

From all of these studies, it follows that intrinsic proteins and functions of podocytes play a key role in the development and maintenance of the permselective properties of the glomerular filtration barrier; however, as outlined earlier in the section on vascular development, podocytes also function as vasculature supporting cells producing VEGF and other angiogenic growth factors. It is likely that endothelial cells also produce factors required for terminal differentiation of podocytes, although these factors are currently unknown.

Maturation of Glomerular Endothelial Cells and Glomerular Basement Membrane

Following migration into the glomerular vascular cleft, endothelial cells are rounded and capillaries do not possess a lumen. During glomerulogenesis, lumens form through apoptosis of a subset of endothelial cells and the endothelial cells flatten considerably and develop fenestrations and a complex glycocalyx. This process is believed to be dependent on a TGFβ1-dependent signal.[227] Loss of these specialized features of the glomerular endothelium as in endotheliosis, leads to disruption of the filtration barrier and protein loss, emphasizing that this layer of the GFB plays a major role in permselectivity.

Another chapter in the book deals with properties and development of the glomerular basement membrane although informative knockouts are included in Table 1–1 for completeness. It is important to note that components are produced by both podocytes and glomerular endothelium and that a number of vital growth factors, such as VEGF-A are stored and processed in the GBM.

References

1. Zandi-Nejad K, Luyckx VA, Brenner BM: Adult hypertension and kidney disease: The role of fetal programming. Hypertension 47:502–508, 2006.
2. Luyckx VA, Brenner BM: Low birth weight, nephron number, and kidney disease. Kidney Int Suppl:S68–77, 2005.
3. Rossing P, Tarnow L, Nielsen FS, et al: Low birth weight. A risk factor for development of diabetic nephropathy? Diabetes 44:1405–1407, 1995.
4. Natoli TA, Liu J, Eremina V, et al: A mutant form of the Wilms' tumor suppressor gene WT1 observed in Denys-Drash Syndrome interferes with glomerular capillary development. J Am Soc Nephrol 13:2058–2067, 2002.
5. Moore AW, McInnes L, Kreidberg J, et al: YAC complementation shows a requirement for Wt1 in the development of epicardium, adrenal gland and throughout nephrogenesis. Development 126:1845–1857, 1999.
6. Kreidberg JA, Sariola H, Loring JM, et al: WT-1 is required for early kidney development. Cell 74:679–691, 1993.
7. Saxen L: Organogenesis of the Kidney. Cambridge, Cambridge University Press, 1987.
8. Rothenpieler UW, Dressler GR: Pax-2 is required for mesenchyme-to-epithelium conversion during kidney development. Development 119:711–720, 1993.
9. Torres M, Gomez-Pardo E, Dressler GR, Gruss P: Pax-2 controls multiple steps of urogenital development. Development 121:4057–4065, 1995.
10. Capel B, Albrecht KH, Washburn LL, Eicher EM: Migration of mesonephric cells into the mammalian gonad depends on Sry. Mech Dev 84:127–131, 1999.
11. Cui S, Ross A, Stallings N, et al: Disrupted gonadogenesis and male-to-female sex reversal in Pod1 knockout mice. Development 131:4095–4105, 2004.
12. Mendelsohn C, Lohnes D, Decimo D, et al: Function of the retinoic acid receptors (RARs) during development (II. Multiple abnormalities at various stages of organogenesis in RAR double mutants). Development 120:2749–2771, 1994.
13. Kreidberg JA: Podocyte differentiation and glomerulogenesis. J Am Soc Nephrol 14:806–814, 2003.
14. Batourina E, Gim S, Bello N, et al: Vitamin A controls epithelial/mesenchymal interactions through Ret expression. Nat Genet 27:74–78, 2001.
15. Reeves W, Caulfield JP, Farquhar MG: Differentiation of epithelial foot processes and filtration slits: Sequential appearance of occluding junctions, epithelial polyanion, and slit membranes in developing glomeruli. Lab Invest 39:90–100, 1978.
16. Batourina E, Tsai S, Lambert S, et al: Apoptosis induced by vitamin A signaling is crucial for connecting the ureters to the bladder. Nat Genet 37:1082–1089, 2005.
17. Jones N, Blasutig IM, Eremina V, et al: Nck adaptor proteins link nephrin to the actin cytoskeleton of kidney podocytes. Nature 440:818–823, 2006.
18. Verma R, Kovari I, Soofi A, et al: Nephrin ectodomain engagement results in Src kinase activation, nephrin phosphorylation, Nck recruitment, and actin polymerization. J Clin Invest 116:1346–1359, 2006.
19. Tryggvason K, Pikkarainen T, Patrakka J: Nck links nephrin to actin in kidney podocytes. Cell 125:221–224, 2006.
20. Fierlbeck W, Liu A, Coyle R, Ballermann BJ: Endothelial cell apoptosis during glomerular capillary lumen formation in vivo. J Am Soc Nephrol 14:1349–1354, 2003.
21. Rastaldi MP, Armelloni S, Berra S, et al: Glomerular podocytes possess the synaptic vesicle molecule Rab3A and its specific effector rabphilin-3a. Am J Pathol 163:889–899, 2003.
22. Kobayashi N, Gao SY, Chen J, et al: Process formation of the renal glomerular podocyte: Is there common molecular machinery for processes of podocytes and neurons? Anat Sci Int 79:1–10, 2004.
23. Baum M, Quigley R, Satlin L: Maturational changes in renal tubular transport. Curr Opin Nephrol Hypertens 12:521–526, 2003.
24. Osathanondh V, Potter EL: Development of human kidney as shown by microdissection. iii. Formation and interrelationship of collecting tubules and nephrons. Arch Pathol 76:290–302, 1963.
25. Bard J: A new role for the stromal cells in kidney development. Bioessays 18:705–707, 1996.
26. Hatini V, Huh SO, Herzlinger D, et al: Essential role of stromal mesenchyme in kidney morphogenesis revealed by targeted disruption of Winged Helix transcription factor BF-2. Genes Dev 10:1467–1478, 1996.
27. Levinson R, Mendelsohn C: Stromal progenitors are important for patterning epithelial and mesenchymal cell types in the embryonic kidney. Semin Cell Dev Biol 14:225–231, 2003.
28. Robert B, St. John PL, Hyink DP, Abrahamson DR: Evidence that embryonic kidney cells expressing flk-1 are intrinsic, vasculogenic angioblasts. Am J Physiol 271:F744–F753, 1996.
29. Grobstein C: Inductive epitheliomesenchymal interaction in cultured organ rudiments of the mouse. Science 118:52–55, 1953.
30. Miyamoto N, Yoshida M, Kuratani S, et al: Defects of urogenital development in mice lacking Emx2. Development 124:1653–1664, 1997.
31. Sariola H, Saarma M, Sainio K, et al: Dependence of kidney morphogenesis on the expression of nerve growth factor receptor. Science 254:571–573, 1991.
32. Durbeej M, Soderstrom S, Ebendal T, et al: Differential expression of neurotrophin receptors during renal development. Development 119:977–989, 1993.
33. Sainio K, Saarma M, Nonclercq D, et al: Antisense inhibition of low-affinity nerve growth factor receptor in kidney cultures: Power and pitfalls. Cell Mol Neurobiol 14:439–457, 1994.

34. Davies JA, Ladomery M, Hohenstein P, et al: Development of an siRNA-based method for repressing specific genes in renal organ culture and its use to show that the Wt1 tumour suppressor is required for nephron differentiation. Hum Mol Genet 13:235–246, 2004.

35. Gao X, Chen X, Taglienti M, et al: Angioblast-mesenchyme induction of early kidney development is mediated by Wt1 and Vegfa. Development 132:5437–5449, 2005.

36. Vainio S, Lin Y: Coordinating early kidney development: Lessons from gene targeting. Nat Rev Genet 3:533–543, 2002.

37. Dressler GR: Kidney development branches out. Dev Genet 24:189–193, 1999.

38. Gawlik A, Quaggin SE: Conditional gene targeting in the kidney. Curr Mol Med 5:527–536, 2005.

39. Gawlik A, Quaggin SE: Deciphering the renal code; advances in conditional gene targeting in the kidney. Physiology (Bethesda) 19:245–252, 2004.

40. Justice M: Capitalizing on large-scale mouse mutagenesis screens. Nat Rev Genet 2:109–115, 2000.

41. Justice M, Carpenter D, Favor J, et al: Effects of ENU dosage on mouse strains. Mamm Genome 11:484–488, 2000.

42. Hrabe de Angelis MH, Flaswinkel H, Fuchs H, et al: Genome-wide, large-scale production of mutant mice by ENU mutagenesis. Nat Genet 25:444–447, 2000.

43. Nolan PM, Peters J, Strivens M, et al: A systematic, genome-wide, phenotype-driven mutagenesis programme for gene function studies in the mouse. Nat Genet 25:440–443, 2000.

44. Huber TB, Kwoh C, Wu H, et al: Bigenic mouse models of focal segmental glomerulosclerosis involving pairwise interaction of CD2AP, Fyn, and synaptopodin. J Clin Invest 116:1337–1345, 2006.

45. Beier DR, Herron BJ: Genetic mapping and ENU mutagenesis. Genetica 122:65–69, 2004.

46. Cordes SP: N-ethyl-N-nitrosourea mutagenesis: Boarding the mouse mutant express. Microbiol Mol Biol Rev 69:426–439, 2005.

47. Stanford WL, Cohn JB, Cordes SP: Gene-trap mutagenesis: past, present and beyond. Nat Rev Genet 2:756–768, 2001.

48. Donoviel DB, Freed DD, Vogel H, et al: Proteinuria and parinatal lethality in mice lacking NEPH1, a novel protein with homology to NEPHRIN. Mol Cell Biol 21:4829–4836, 2001.

49. Takemoto M, He L, Norlin J, et al: Large-scale identification of genes implicated in kidney glomerulus development and function. EMBO J 25:1160–1174, 2006.

50. Shen K, Fetter RD, Bargmann CI: Synaptic specificity is generated by the synaptic guidepost protein SYG-2 and its receptor, SYG-1. Cell 116:868–881, 2004.

51. Nelson FK, Albert PS, Riddle DL: Fine structure of the Caenorhabditis elegans secretory-excretory system. J Ultrastruct Res 82:156–171, 1983.

52. Barr MM: Caenorhabditis elegans as a model to study renal development and disease: Sexy cilia. J Am Soc Nephrol 16:305–312, 2005.

53. Barr MM, DeModena J, Braun D, et al: The Caenorhabditis elegans autosomal dominant polycystic kidney disease gene homologs lov-1 and pkd-2 act in the same pathway. Curr Biol 11:1341–1346, 2001.

54. Simon JM, Sternberg PW: Evidence of a mate-finding cue in the hermaphrodite nematode Caenorhabditis elegans. Proc Natl Acad Sci U S A 99:1598–1603, 2002.

55. Jung AC, Denholm B, Skaer H, Affolter M: Renal tubule development in Drosophila: A closer look at the cellular level. J Am Soc Nephrol 16:322–328, 2005.

56. Dworak HA, Charles MA, Pellerano LB, Sink H: Characterization of Drosophila hibris, a gene related to human nephrin. Development 128:4265–4276, 2001.

57. Schneider T, Reiter C, Eule E, et al: Restricted expression of the irreC-rst protein is required for normal axonal projections of columnar visual neurons. Neuron 15:259–271, 1995.

58. Venugopala Reddy G, Reiter C, Shanbhag S, et al: Irregular chiasm-C-roughest, a member of the immunoglobulin superfamily, affects sense organ spacing on the Drosophila antenna by influencing the positioning of founder cells on the disc ectoderm. Dev Genes Evol 209:581–591, 1999.

59. Majumdar A, Drummond IA: Podocyte differentiation in the absence of endothelial cells as revealed in the zebrafish avascular mutant, cloche. Dev Genet 24:220–229, 1999.

60. Drummond IA: Kidney development and disease in the zebrafish. J Am Soc Nephrol 16:299–304, 2005.

61. Jones EA: Xenopus: a prince among models for pronephric kidney development. J Am Soc Nephrol 16:313–321, 2005.

62. Xu PX, Adams J, Peters H, et al: Eya1-deficient mice lack ears and kidneys and show abnormal apoptosis of organ primordia. Nat Genet 23:113–117, 1999.

63. Laclef C, Souil E, Demignon J, Maire P: Thymus, kidney and craniofacial abnormalities in Six 1 deficient mice. Mech Dev 120:669–679, 2003.

64. Xu PX, Zheng W, Huang L, et al: Six1 is required for the early organogenesis of mammalian kidney. Development 130:3085–3094, 2003.

65. Nishinakamura R, Matsumoto Y, Nakao K, et al: Murine homolog of SALL1 is essential for ureteric bud invasion in kidney development. Development 128:3105–3115, 2001.

66. Shawlot W, Behringer RR: Requirement for Lim1 in head-organizer function. Nature 374:425–430, 1995.

67. Moore MW, Klein RD, Farinas I, et al: Renal and neuronal abnormalities in mice lacking GDNF. Nature 382:76–79, 1996.

68. Pichel JG, Shen L, Sheng HZ, et al: Defects in enteric innervation and kidney development in mice lacking GDNF. Nature 382:73–76, 1996.

69. Sanchez MP, Silos-Santiago I, Frisen J, et al: Renal agenesis and the absence of enteric neurons in mice lacking GDNF. Nature 382:70–73, 1996.

70. Esquela AF, Lee SJ: Regulation of metanephric kidney development by growth/differentiation factor 11. Dev Biol 257:356–370, 2003.

71. Michos O, Panman L, Vintersten K, et al: Gremlin-mediated BMP antagonism induces the epithelial-mesenchymal feedback signaling controlling metanephric kidney and limb organogenesis. Development 131:3401–3410, 2004.

72. Schuchardt A, D'Agati V, Larsson-Blomberg L, et al: RET-deficient mice: An animal model for Hirschsprung's disease and renal agenesis. J Intern Med 238:327–332, 1995.

73. Cacalano G, Farinas I, Wang LC, et al: GFRalpha1 is an essential receptor component for GDNF in the developing nervous system and kidney. Neuron 21:53–62, 1998.

74. Buller C, Xu X, Marquis V, et al: Molecular effects of Eya1 domain mutations causing organ defects in BOR syndrome. Hum Mol Genet 10:2775–2781, 2001.

75. Ikeda K, Watanabe Y, Ohto H, Kawakami K: Molecular interaction and synergistic activation of a promoter by Six, Eya, and Dach proteins mediated through CREB binding protein. Mol Cell Biol 22:6759–6766, 2002.

76. Li X, Oghi KA, Zhang J, et al: Eya protein phosphatase activity regulates Six1-Dach-Eya transcriptional effects in mammalian organogenesis. Nature 426:247–254, 2003.

77. Fougerousse F, Durand M, Lopez S, et al: Six and Eya expression during human somitogenesis and MyoD gene family activation. J Muscle Res Cell Motil 23:255–264, 2002.

78. Pandur PD, Moody SA: Xenopus Six1 gene is expressed in neurogenic cranial placodes and maintained in the differentiating lateral lines. Mech Dev 96:253–257, 2000.

79. Sajithlal G, Zou D, Silvius D, Xu PX: Eya 1 acts as a critical regulator for specifying the metanephric mesenchyme. Dev Biol 284:323–336, 2005.

80. Brophy PD, Ostrom L, Lang KM, Dressler GR: Regulation of ureteric bud outgrowth by Pax2-dependent activation of the glial derived neurotrophic factor gene. Development 128:4747–4756, 2001.

81. Poladia DP, Kish K, Kutay B, et al: Role of fibroblast growth factor receptors 1 and 2 in the metanephric mesenchyme. Dev Biol 291:325–339, 2006.

82. Grieshammer U, Cebrian C, Ilagan R, et al: FGF8 is required for cell survival at distinct stages of nephrogenesis and for regulation of gene expression in nascent nephrons. Development 132:3847–3857, 2005.

83. Perantoni AO, Timofeeva O, Naillat F, et al: Inactivation of FGF8 in early mesoderm reveals an essential role in kidney development. Development 132:3859–3871, 2005.

84. Stark K, Vainio S, Vassileva G, McMahon AP: Epithelial transformation of metanephric mesenchyme in the developing kidney regulated by Wnt-4. Nature 372:679–683, 1994.

85. Luo G, Hofmann C, Bronckers AL, et al: BMP-7 is an inducer of nephrogenesis, and is also required for eye development and skeletal patterning. Genes Dev 9:2808–2820, 1995.

86. Dudley AT, Lyons KM, Robertson EJ: A requirement for bone morphogenetic protein-7 during development of the mammalian kidney and eye. Genes Dev 9:2795–2807, 1995.

87. Muller U, Wang D, Denda S, et al: Integrin alpha8beta1 is critically important for epithelial-mesenchymal interactions during kidney morphogenesis. Cell 88:603–613, 1997.

88. Brandenberger R, Schmidt A, Linton J, et al: Identification and characterization of a novel extracellular matrix protein nephronectin that is associated with integrin alpha-8beta1 in the embryonic kidney. J Cell Biol 154:447–458, 2001.

89. Miyazaki Y, Oshima K, Fogo A, et al: Bone morphogenetic protein 4 regulates the budding site and elongation of the mouse ureter. J Clin Invest 105:863–873, 2000.

90. Chiang C, Litingtung Y, Lee E, et al: Cyclopia and defective axial patterning in mice lacking Sonic hedgehog gene function. Nature 383:407–413, 1996.

91. Qiao J, Uzzo R, Obara-Ishihara T, et al: FGF-7 modulates ureteric bud growth and nephron number in the developing kidney. Development 126:547–554, 1999.

92. Zhao H, Kegg H, Grady S, et al: Role of fibroblast growth factor receptors 1 and 2 in the ureteric bud. Dev Biol 276:403–415, 2004.

93. Gupta IR, Macias-Silva M, Kim S, et al: BMP-2/ALK3 and HGF signal in parallel to regulate renal collecting duct morphogenesis. J Cell Sci 113 Pt 2:269–278, 2000.

94. Piscione TD, Yager TD, Gupta IR, et al: BMP-2 and OP-1 exert direct and opposite effects on renal branching morphogenesis. Am J Physiol 273:F961–F975, 1997.

95. Hu MC, Piscione TD, Rosenblum ND: Elevated SMAD1/beta-catenin molecular complexes and renal medullary cystic dysplasia in ALK3 transgenic mice. Development 130:2753–2766, 2003.

96. Hu MC, Rosenblum ND: Smad1, beta-catenin and Tcf4 associate in a molecular complex with the Myc promoter in dysplastic renal tissue and cooperate to control Myc transcription. Development 132:215–225, 2005.

97. Hu MC, Mo R, Bhella S, et al: GLI3-dependent transcriptional repression of Gli1, Gli2 and kidney patterning genes disrupts renal morphogenesis. Development 133:569–578, 2006.

98. Kreidberg JA, Donovan MJ, Goldstein SL, et al: Alpha 3 beta 1 integrin has a crucial role in kidney and lung organogenesis. Development 122:3537–3547, 1996.

99. Korhonen M, Ylanne J, Laitinen L, Virtanen I: The alpha 1-alpha 6 subunits of integrins are characteristically expressed in distinct segments of developing and adult human nephron. J Cell Biol 111:1245–1254, 1990.

100. Chattopadhyay N, Wang Z, Ashman LK, et al: alpha3beta1 integrin-CD151, a component of the cadherin-catenin complex, regulates PTPmu expression and cell-cell adhesion. J Cell Biol 163:1351–1362, 2003.

101. Kume T, Deng K, Hogan BL: Murine forkhead/winged helix genes Foxc1 (Mf1) and Foxc2 (Mfh1) are required for the early organogenesis of the kidney and urinary tract. Development 127:1387–1395, 2000.

102. Grieshammer U, Le M, Plump AS, et al: SLIT2-mediated ROBO2 signaling restricts kidney induction to a single site. Dev Cell 6:709–717, 2004.

103. McCright B: Notch signaling in kidney development. Curr Opin Nephrol Hypertens 12:5–10, 2003.

104. McCright B, Gao X, Shen L, et al: Defects in development of the kidney, heart and eye vasculature in mice homozygous for a hypomorphic Notch2 mutation. Development 128:491–502, 2001.

105. McCright B, Lozier J, Gridley T: A mouse model of Alagille syndrome: Notch2 as a genetic modifier of Jag1 haploinsufficiency. Development 129:1075–1082, 2002.

106. Cheng HT, Kopan R: The role of Notch signaling in specification of podocyte and proximal tubules within the developing mouse kidney. Kidney Int 68:1951–1952, 2005.
107. Cheng HT, Miner JH, Lin M, et al: Gamma-secretase activity is dispensable for mesenchyme-to-epithelium transition but required for podocyte and proximal tubule formation in developing mouse kidney. Development 130:5031–5042, 2003.
108. Wang P, Pereira FA, Beasley D, Zheng H: Presenilins are required for the formation of comma- and S-shaped bodies during nephrogenesis. Development 130:5019–5029, 2003.
109. Blomqvist SR, Vidarsson H, Fitzgerald S, et al: Distal renal tubular acidosis in mice that lack the forkhead transcription factor Foxi1. J Clin Invest 113:1560–1570, 2004.
110. Quaggin SE, Vanden Heuvel GB, Igarashi P: Pod-1, a mesoderm-specific basic-helix-loop-helix protein expressed in mesenchymal and glomerular epithelial cells in the developing kidney. Mech Dev 71:37–48, 1998.
111. Quaggin SE, Schwartz L, Post M, Rossant J: The basic-helix-loop-helix protein Pod-1 is critically important for kidney and lung organogenesis. Development 126:5771–5783, 1999.
112. Cui S, Schwartz L, Quaggin SE: Pod1 is required in stromal cells for glomerulogenesis. Dev Dyn 226:512–522, 2003.
113. Mendelsohn C, Batourina E, Fung S, et al: Stromal cells mediate retinoid-dependent functions essential for renal development. Development 126:1139–1148, 1999.
114. Shalaby F, Rossant J, Yamaguchi TP, et al: Failure of blood-island formation and vasculogenesis in Flk-1-deficient mice. Nature 376:62–66, 1995.
115. Takahashi T, Takahashi K, Gerety S, et al: Temporally compartmentalized expression of ephrin-B2 during renal glomerular development. J Am Soc Nephrol 12:2673–2682, 2001.
116. Carmeliet P, Ferreira V, Breier G, et al: Abnormal blood vessel development and lethality in embryos lacking a single VEGF allele. Nature 380:435–439, 1996.
117. Villegas G, Lange-Sperandio B, Tufro A: Autocrine and paracrine functions of vascular endothelial growth factor (VEGF) in renal tubular epithelial cells. Kidney Int 67:449–457, 2005.
118. Eremina V, Sood M, Haigh J, et al: Glomerular-specific alterations of VEGF-A expression lead to distinct congenital and acquired renal diseases. J Clin Invest 111:707–716, 2003.
119. Eremina V, Cui S, Gerber H, et al: VEGF-A signaling in the podocyte-endothelial compartment is required for mesangial cell migration and survival. J Am Soc Nephrol 17:724–735, 2006.
120. Foster RR, Hole R, Anderson K, et al: Functional evidence that vascular endothelial growth factor may act as an autocrine factor on human podocytes. Am J Physiol Renal Physiol 284:F1263–F1273, 2003.
121. Foster RR, Saleem MA, Mathieson PW, et al: Vascular endothelial growth factor and nephrin interact and reduce apoptosis in human podocytes. Am J Physiol Renal Physiol 288:F48–F57, 2005.
122. Guan F, Villegas G, Teichman J, et al: Autocrine VEGF-A system in podocytes regulates podocin and its interaction with CD2AP. Am J Physiol Renal Physiol 291: F422–428, 2006.
123. Suri C, Jones PF, Patan S, et al: Requisite role of angiopoietin-1, a ligand for the TIE2 receptor, during embryonic angiogenesis [see comments]. Cell 87:1171–1180, 1996.
124. Maisonpierre PC, Suri C, Jones PF, et al: Angiopoietin-2, a natural antagonist for Tie2 that disrupts in vivo angiogenesis [see comments]. Science 277:55–60, 1997.
125. Augustin HG, Breier G: Angiogenesis: Molecular mechanisms and functional interactions. Thromb Haemost 89:190–197, 2003.
126. Yuan HT, Suri C, Yancopoulos GD, Woolf AS: Expression of angiopoietin-1, angiopoietin-2, and the Tie-2 receptor tyrosine kinase during mouse kidney maturation. J Am Soc Nephrol 10:1722–1736, 1999.
127. Woolf AS, Yuan HT: Angiopoietin growth factors and Tie receptor tyrosine kinases in renal vascular development. Pediatr Nephrol 16:177–184, 2001.
128. Yuan HT, Suri C, Landon DN, et al: Angiopoietin-2 is a site-specific factor in differentiation of mouse renal vasculature. J Am Soc Nephrol 11:1055–1066, 2000.
129. Satchell SC, Harper SJ, Mathieson PW: Angiopoietin-1 is normally expressed by periendothelial cells. Thromb Haemost 86:1597–1598, 2001.
130. Satchell SC, Harper SJ, Tooke JE, et al: Human podocytes express angiopoietin 1, a potential regulator of glomerular vascular endothelial growth factor. J Am Soc Nephrol 13:544–550, 2002.
131. Pitera JE, Woolf AS, Gale NW, et al: Dysmorphogenesis of kidney cortical peritubular capillaries in angiopoietin-2-deficient mice. Am J Pathol 165:1895–1906, 2004.
132. Partanen J, Puri MC, Schwartz L, et al: Cell autonomous functions of the receptor tyrosine kinase TIE in a late phase of angiogenic capillary growth and endothelial cell survival during murine development. Development 122:3013–3021, 1996.
133. Gerety SS, Anderson DJ: Cardiovascular ephrinB2 function is essential for embryonic angiogenesis. Development 129:1397–1410, 2002.
134. Wang HU, Anderson DJ: Eph family transmembrane ligands can mediate repulsive guidance of trunk neural crest migration and motor axon outgrowth. Neuron 18:383–396, 1997.
135. Andres AC, Munarini N, Djonov V, et al: EphB4 receptor tyrosine kinase transgenic mice develop glomerulopathies reminiscent of aglomerular vascular shunt. Mech Dev 120:511–516, 2003.
136. Foo SS, Turner CJ, Adams S, et al: Ephrin-B2 controls cell motility and adhesion during blood-vessel-wall assembly. Cell 124:161–173, 2006.
137. Ding M, Cui S, Li C, et al: Loss of the tumor suppressor Vhlh leads to upregulation of Cxcr4 and rapidly progressive glomerulonephritis in mice. Nature Medicine 12:1081–1087, 2006.
138. Nikolova G, Jabs N, Konstantinova I, et al: The vascular basement membrane: A niche for insulin gene expression and Beta cell proliferation. Dev Cell 10:397–405, 2006.
139. Lammert E, Cleaver O, Melton D: Induction of pancreatic differentiation by signals from blood vessels. Science 294:564–567, 2001.
140. Schnermann J: Homer W. Smith Award lecture. The juxtaglomerular apparatus: from anatomical peculiarity to physiological relevance. J Am Soc Nephrol 14:1681–1694, 2003.
141. Sequeira Lopez ML, Pentz ES, Nomasa T, et al: Renin cells are precursors for multiple cell types that switch to the renin phenotype when homeostasis is threatened. Dev Cell 6:719–728, 2004.
142. Husain A, Graham R: Enzymes and Receptors of the Renin-Angiotensin System: Celebrating a Century of Discovery. Sidney, Harwood Academic, 2000.
143. Cooper WO, Hernandez-Diaz S, Arbogast PG, et al: Major congenital malformations after first-trimester exposure to ACE inhibitors. N Engl J Med 354:2443–2451, 2006.
144. Friberg P, Sundelin B, Bohman SO, et al: Renin-angiotensin system in neonatal rats: induction of a renal abnormality in response to ACE inhibition or angiotensin II antagonism. Kidney Int 45:485–492, 1994.
145. Timmermans PB, Wong PC, Chiu AT, et al: Angiotensin II receptors and angiotensin II receptor antagonists. Pharmacol Rev 45:205–251, 1993.
146. Kim HS, Krege JH, Kluckman KD, et al: Genetic control of blood pressure and the angiotensinogen locus. Proc Natl Acad Sci U S A 92:2735–2739, 1995.
147. Niimura F, Labosky PA, Kakuchi J, et al: Gene targeting in mice reveals a requirement for angiotensin in the development and maintenance of kidney morphology and growth factor regulation. J Clin Invest 96:2947–2954, 1995.
148. Krege JH, John SW, Langenbach LL, et al: Male-female differences in fertility and blood pressure in ACE-deficient mice. Nature 375:146–148, 1995.
149. Esther CR, Jr, Howard TE, Marino EM, et al: Mice lacking angiotensin-converting enzyme have low blood pressure, renal pathology, and reduced male fertility. Lab Invest 74:953–965, 1996.
150. Ito M, Oliverio MI, Mannon PJ, et al: Regulation of blood pressure by the type 1A angiotensin II receptor gene. Proc Natl Acad Sci U S A 92:3521–3525, 1995.
151. Sugaya T, Nishimatsu S, Tanimoto K, et al: Angiotensin II type 1a receptor-deficient mice with hypotension and hyperreninemia. J Biol Chem 270:18719–18722, 1995.
152. Tsuchida S, Matsusaka T, Chen X, et al: Murine double nullizygotes of the angiotensin type 1A and 1B receptor genes duplicate severe abnormal phenotypes of angiotensinogen nullizygotes. J Clin Invest 101:755–760, 1998.
153. Oliverio MI, Kim HS, Ito M, et al: Reduced growth, abnormal kidney structure, and type 2 (AT2) angiotensin receptor-mediated blood pressure regulation in mice lacking both AT1A and AT1B receptors for angiotensin II. Proc Natl Acad Sci U S A 95:15496–15501, 1998.
154. Ichiki T, Labosky PA, Shiota C, et al: Effects on blood pressure and exploratory behaviour of mice lacking angiotensin II type-2 receptor. Nature 377:748–750, 1995.
155. Hein L, Barsh GS, Pratt RE, et al: Behavioural and cardiovascular effects of disrupting the angiotensin II type-2 receptor in mice. Nature 377:744–747, 1995.
156. Nishimura H, Yerkes E, Hohenfellner K, et al: Role of the angiotensin type 2 receptor gene in congenital anomalies of the kidney and urinary tract, CAKUT, of mice and men. Mol Cell 3:1–10, 1999.
157. Lindahl P, Hellstrom M, Kalen M, et al: Paracrine PDGF-B/PDGF-Rbeta signaling controls mesangial cell development in kidney glomeruli. Development 125:3313–3322, 1998.
158. Bjarnegard M, Enge M, Norlin J, et al: Endothelium-specific ablation of PDGFB leads to pericyte loss and glomerular, cardiac and placental abnormalities. Development 131:1847–1857, 2004.
159. Sadl V, Jin F, Yu J, et al: The mouse Kreisler (Krml1/MafB) segmentation gene is required for differentiation of glomerular visceral epithelial cells. Dev Biol 249:16–29, 2002.
160. Chen H, Lun Y, Ovchinnikov D, et al: Limb and kidney defects in Lmx1b mutant mice suggest an involvement of LMX1B in human nail patella syndrome. Nat Genet 19:51–55, 1998.
161. Cui S, Li C, Ema M, et al: Rapid isolation of glomeruli coupled with gene expression profiling identifies downstream targets in pod1 knockout mice. J Am Soc Nephrol 16:3247–3255, 2005.
162. Kestila M, Lenkkeri U, Mannikko M, et al: Positionally cloned gene for a novel glomerular protein—nephrin—is mutated in congenital nephrotic syndrome. Mol Cell 1:575–582, 1998.
163. Sellin L, Huber TB, Gerke P, et al: NEPH1 defines a novel family of podocin interacting proteins. FASEB J 17:115–117, 2003.
164. Huber TB, Hartleben B, Kim J, et al: Nephrin and CD2AP associate with phosphoinositide 3-OH kinase and stimulate AKT-dependent signaling. Mol Cell Biol 23:4917–4928, 2003.
165. Lenkkeri U, Mannikko M, McCready P, et al: Structure of the gene for congenital nephrotic syndrome of the Finnish type (NPHS1) and characterization of mutations. Am J Hum Genet 64:51–61, 1999.
166. Roselli S, Heidet L, Sich M, et al: Early glomerular filtration defect and severe renal disease in podocin-deficient mice. Mol Cell Biol 24:550–560, 2004.
167. Kaplan JM, Kim SH, North KN, et al: Mutations in ACTN4, encoding alpha-actinin-4, cause familial focal segmental glomerulosclerosis. Nat Genet 24:251–256, 2000.
168. Kos CH, Le TC, Sinha S, et al: Mice deficient in alpha-actinin-4 have severe glomerular disease. J Clin Invest 111:1683–1690, 2003.
169. Shih NY, Li J, Karpitskii V, et al: Congenital nephrotic syndrome in mice lacking CD2-associated protein [see comments]. Science 286:312–315, 1999.
170. Kim JM, Wu H, Green G, et al: CD2-associated protein haploinsufficiency is linked to glomerular disease susceptibility. Science 300:1298–1300, 2003.
171. Winn MP, Conlon PJ, Lynn KL, et al: A mutation in the TRPC6 cation channel causes familial focal segmental glomerulosclerosis. Science 308:1801–1804, 2005.
172. Reiser J, Polu KR, Moller CC, et al: TRPC6 is a glomerular slit diaphragm-associated channel required for normal renal function. Nat Genet 37:739–744, 2005.
173. Srinivas S, Wu Z, Chen C-M, et al: Dominant effects of RET receptor misexpression and ligand-independent RET signaling on ureteric bud development. Development 126:1375–1386, 1999.
174. Vega QC, Worby CA, Lechner MS, et al: Glial cell line-derived neurotrophic factor activates the receptor tyrosine kinase RET and promotes kidney morphogenesis. Proc Natl Acad Sci U S A 93:10657–10661, 1996.

175. Jing S, Wen D, Yu Y, et al: GDNF-induced activation of the ret protein tyrosine kinase is mediated by GDNFR-alpha, a novel receptor for GDNF. Cell 85:1113–1124, 1996.

176. Schuchardt A, D'Agati V, Larsson-Blomberg L, et al: Defects in the kidney and enteric nervous system of mice lacking the tyrosine kinase receptor Ret. Nature 367:380–383, 1994.

177. Schuchardt A, D'Agati V, Pachnis V, Costantini F: Renal agenesis and hypodysplasia in ret-k- mutant mice result from defects in ureteric bud development. Development 122:1919–1929, 1996.

178. Sato A, Kishida S, Tanaka T, et al: Sall1, a causative gene for Townes-Brocks syndrome, enhances the canonical Wnt signaling by localizing to heterochromatin. Biochem Biophys Res Commun 319:103–113, 2004.

179. Kispert A, Vainio S, McMahon AP: Wnt-4 is a mesenchymal signal for epithelial transformation of metanephric mesenchyme in the developing kidney. Development 125:4225–4234, 1998.

180. Dreyer SD, Zhou G, Baldini A, et al: Mutations in *LMX1B* cause abnormal skeletal patterning and renal dysplasia in nail patella syndrome. Nat Genet 19:47–50, 1998.

181. Lin F, Hiesberger T, Cordes K, et al: Kidney-specific inactivation of the KIF3A subunit of kinesin-II inhibits renal ciliogenesis and produces polycystic kidney disease. Proc Natl Acad Sci U S A 100:5286–5291, 2003.

182. Gresh L, Fischer E, Reimann A, et al: A transcriptional network in polycystic kidney disease. EMBO J 23:1657–1668, 2004.

183. Rankin EB, Tomaszewski JE, Haase VH: Renal cyst development in mice with conditional inactivation of the von Hippel-Lindau tumor suppressor. Cancer Res 66:2576–2583, 2006.

184. Lu W, Peissel B, Babakhanlou H, et al: Perinatal lethality with kidney and pancreas defects in mice with a targeted Pkd1 mutation. Nat Genet 17:179–181, 1997.

185. Miner JH, Sanes JR: Molecular and functional defects in kidneys of mice lacking collagen alpha 3(IV): Implications for Alport syndrome. J Cell Biol 135:1403–1413, 1996.

186. Cosgrove D, Meehan DT, Grunkemeyer JA, et al: Collagen COL4A3 knockout: A mouse model for autosomal Alport syndrome. Genes Dev 10:2981–2992, 1996.

187. Lu W, Phillips CL, Killen PD, et al: Insertional mutation of the collagen genes Col4a3 and Col4a4 in a mouse model of Alport syndrome. Genomics 61:113–124, 1999.

188. Rheault MN, Kren SM, Thielen BK, et al: Mouse model of X-linked Alport syndrome. J Am Soc Nephrol 15:1466–1474, 2004.

189. Gould DB, Phalan FC, van Mil SE, et al: Role of COL4A1 in small-vessel disease and hemorrhagic stroke. N Engl J Med 354:1489–1496, 2006.

190. Noakes PG, Miner JH, Gautam M, et al: The renal glomerulus of mice lacking s-laminin/laminin beta 2: Nephrosis despite molecular compensation by laminin beta 1. Nat Genet 10:400–406, 1995.

191. Jarad G, Cunningham J, Shaw AS, Miner JH: Proteinuria precedes podocyte abnormalities in Lamb2-/- mice, implicating the glomerular basement membrane as an albumin barrier. J Clin Invest 116:2272–2279, 2006.

192. Miner JH, Li C: Defective glomerulogenesis in the absence of laminin alpha5 demonstrates a developmental role for the kidney glomerular basement membrane. Dev Biol 217:278–289, 2000.

193. Kikkawa Y, Virtanen I, Miner JH: Mesangial cells organize the glomerular capillaries by adhering to the G domain of laminin alpha5 in the glomerular basement membrane. J Cell Biol 161:187–196, 2003.

194. Kikkawa Y, Miner JH: Molecular dissection of laminin alpha5 in vivo reveals separable domain-specific roles in embryonic development and kidney function. Dev Biol 296:265–277, 2006.

195. Morita H, Yoshimura A, Inui K, et al: Heparan sulfate of perlecan is involved in glomerular filtration. J Am Soc Nephrol 16:1703–1710, 2005.

196. Lebel SP, Chen Y, Gingras D, et al: Morphofunctional studies of the glomerular wall in mice lacking entactin-1. J Histochem Cytochem 51:1467–1478, 2003.

197. Kume T, Deng K, Hogan BL: Minimal phenotype of mice homozygous for a null mutation in the forkhead/winged helix gene, Mf2. Mol Cell Biol 20:1419–1425, 2000.

198. Cano-Gauci DF, Song HH, Yang H, et al: Glypican-3-deficient mice exhibit developmental overgrowth and some of the abnormalities typical of Simpson-Golabi-Behmel syndrome. J Cell Biol 146:255–264, 1999.

199. Grisaru S, Rosenblum ND: Glypicans and the biology of renal malformations. Pediatr Nephrol 16:302–306, 2001.

200. Grisaru S, Cano-Gauci D, Tee J, et al: Glypican-3 modulates BMP- and FGF-mediated effects during renal branching morphogenesis. Dev Biol 231:31–46, 2001.

201. Hartwig S, Hu MC, Cella C, et al: Glypican-3 modulates inhibitory Bmp2-Smad signaling to control renal development in vivo. Mech Dev 122:928–938, 2005.

202. Boute N, Gribouval O, Roselli S, et al: NPHS2, encoding the glomerular protein podocin, is mutated in autosomal recessive steroid-resistant nephrotic syndrome [In Process Citation]. Nat Genet 24:349–354, 2000.

203. Ciani L, Patel A, Allen ND, French-Constant C: Mice lacking the giant protocadherin mFAT1 exhibit renal slit junction abnormalities and a partially penetrant cyclopia and anophthalmia phenotype. Mol Cell Biol 23:3575–3582, 2003.

204. El-Aouni C, Herbach N, Blattner SM, et al: Podocyte-specific deletion of integrin-linked kinase results in severe glomerular basement membrane alterations and progressive glomerulosclerosis. J Am Soc Nephrol 17:1334–1344, 2006.

205. Lavoie JL, Lake-Bruse KD, Sigmund CD: Increased blood pressure in transgenic mice expressing both human renin and angiotensinogen in the renal proximal tubule. Am J Physiol Renal Physiol 286:F965–F971, 2004.

206. Sepulveda AR, Huang SL, Lebovitz RM, Lieberman MW: A 346-base pair region of the mouse gamma-glutamyl transpeptidase type II promoter contains sufficient cis-acting elements for kidney-restricted expression in transgenic mice. J Biol Chem 272:11959–11967, 1997.

207. Rubera I, Poujeol C, Bertin G, et al: Specific cre/lox recombination in the mouse proximal tubule. J Am Soc Nephrol 15:2050–2056, 2004.

208. Nelson RD, Stricklett P, Gustafson C, et al: Expression of an AQP2 Cre recombinase transgene in kidney and male reproductive system of transgenic mice. Am J Physiol 275:C216–226, 1998.

209. Srinivas S, Goldberg MR, Watanabe T, et al: Expression of green fluorescent protein in the ureteric bud of transgenic mice: A new tool for the analysis of ureteric bud morphogenesis. Dev Genet 24:241–251, 1999.

210. Shao X, Somlo S, Igarashi P: Epithelial-specific Cre/lox recombination in the developing kidney and genitourinary tract. J Am Soc Nephrol 13:1837–1846, 2002.

211. Zhu X, Cheng J, Gao J, et al: Isolation of mouse THP gene promoter and demonstration of its kidney-specific activity in transgenic mice. Am J Physiol Renal Physiol 282: F608–F617, 2002.

212. Moeller MJ, Kovari IA, Holzman LB: Evaluation of a new tool for exploring podocyte biology: Mouse Nphs1 5' flanking region drives LacZ expression in podocytes. J Am Soc Nephrol 11:2306–2314, 2000.

213. Wong MA, Cui S, Quaggin SE: Identification and characterization of a glomerular-specific promoter from the human nephrin gene. Am J Physiol Renal Physiology 279: F1027–F1032, 2000.

214. Moeller MJ, Sanden SK, Soofi A, et al: Two gene fragments that direct podocyte-specific expression in transgenic mice. J Am Soc Nephrol 13:1561–1567, 2002.

215. Engleka KA, Gitler AD, Zhang M, et al: Insertion of Cre into the Pax3 locus creates a new allele of Splotch and identifies unexpected Pax3 derivatives. Dev Biol 280:396–406, 2005.

216. Li J, Chen F, Epstein JA: Neural crest expression of Cre recombinase directed by the proximal Pax3 promoter in transgenic mice. Genesis 26:162–164, 2000.

217. Patterson LT, Pembaur M, Potter SS: Hoxa11 and Hoxd11 regulate branching morphogenesis of the ureteric bud in the developing kidney. Development 128:2153–2161, 2001.

218. Mesrobian HG, Sulik KK: Characterization of the upper urinary tract anatomy in the Danforth spontaneous murine mutation. J Urol 148:752–755, 1992.

219. Bullock SL, Fletcher JM, Beddington RS, Wilson VA: Renal agenesis in mice homozygous for a gene trap mutation in the gene encoding heparan sulfate 2-sulfotransferase. Genes Dev 12:1894–1906, 1998.

220. Moser M, Pscherer A, Roth C, et al: Enhanced apoptotic cell death of renal epithelial cells in mice lacking transcription factor AP-2beta. Genes Dev 11:1938–1948, 1997.

221. Norwood VF, Morham SG, Smithies O: Postnatal development and progression of renal dysplasia in cyclooxygenase-2 null mice. Kidney Int 58:2291–2300, 2000.

222. Kyttala M, Tallila J, Salonen R, et al: MKS1, encoding a component of the flagellar apparatus basal body proteome, is mutated in Meckel syndrome. Nat Genet 38:155–157, 2006.

223. Weiher H, Noda T, Gray DA, et al: Transgenic mouse model of kidney disease: insertional inactivation of ubiquitously expressed gene leads to nephrotic syndrome. Cell 62:425–434, 1990.

224. Harvey SJ, Jarad G, Gunningham J, et al: Disruption of glomerular basement membrane charge through podocyte-specific mutation of agrin does not alter glomerular permselectivity. Am J Pathol 171:139–152, 2007.

225. Hinkes B, Wiggins RC, Gbadegesin R, et al: Positional cloning uncovers mutations in PLCE1 responsible for a nephrotic syndrome variant that may be reversible. Nat Genet 38:1397–1405, 2006.

226. Galeano B, Klootwijk R, Manoli I, et al: Mutation in the key enzyme of sialic acid biosynthesis causes severe glomerular proteinuria and is rescued by N-acetylmannosamine. J Clin Invest 117:1585–1594, 2007.

227. Fierlbeck W, Liu A, Coyle R, Ballermann BJ: Endothelial cell apoptosis during glomerular capillary lumen formation in vivo. J Am Soc Nephrol 14:1349–1354, 2003.

228. Sachs N, Kreft M, van den Bergh Weerman MA, et al: Kidney failure in mice lacking the tetraspanin CD151. Cell Biol 175:33–39, 2006.

CHAPTER 2

Anatomy of the Kidney

Kirsten M. Madsen • Søren Nielsen • C. Craig Tisher

Knowledge of the complex structure of the mammalian kidney provides a basis for understanding the multitude of functional characteristics of this organ in both healthy and diseased states. In this chapter, gross observations coupled with light microscopic and ultrastructural information and examples of immunohistochemical localization of selected channels, transporters, and regulatory proteins are presented using illustrative material derived from a variety of laboratory animals and humans.

GROSS FEATURES

Kidneys are paired retroperitoneal organs situated in the posterior part of the abdomen on each side of the vertebral column. In the human, the upper pole of each kidney lies opposite the twelfth thoracic vertebra, and the lower pole lies opposite the third lumbar vertebra. The right kidney is usually slightly more caudal in position. The weight of each kidney ranges from 125 g to 170 g in the adult male and from 115 g to 155 g in the adult female. The human kidney is approximately 11 cm to 12 cm in length, 5.0 cm to 7.5 cm in width, and 2.5 cm to 3.0 cm in thickness. Located on the medial or concave surface of each kidney is a slit, called the hilus, through which the renal pelvis, the renal artery and vein, the lymphatics, and a nerve plexus pass into the sinus of the kidney. The organ is surrounded by a tough fibrous capsule, which is smooth and easily removable under normal conditions.

In the human, as in most mammals, each kidney is supplied normally by a single renal artery, although the presence of one or more accessory renal arteries is not uncommon. The renal artery enters the hilar region and usually divides to form an anterior and a posterior branch. Three segmental or lobar arteries arise from the anterior branch and supply the upper, middle, and lower thirds of the anterior surface of the kidney (Fig. 2–1). The posterior branch supplies more than half of the posterior surface and occasionally gives rise to a small apical segmental branch. However, the apical segmental or lobar branch arises most commonly from the anterior division. No collateral circulation has been demonstrated between individual segmental or lobar arteries or their subdivisions. Not uncommonly, the kidneys receive aberrant arteries from the superior mesenteric, suprarenal, testicular, or ovarian arteries. True accessory arteries that arise from the abdominal aorta usually supply the lower pole of the kidney. The arterial and venous circulations in the kidney are described in detail in Chapter 3 and are not discussed further in this chapter.

Two distinct regions can be identified on the cut surface of a bisected kidney: a pale outer region, the cortex, and a darker inner region, the medulla (Fig. 2–2). In humans, the medulla is divided into 8 to 18 striated conical masses, the renal pyramids. The base of each pyramid is positioned at the corticomedullary boundary, and the apex extends toward the renal pelvis to form a papilla. On the tip of each papilla are 10 to 25 small openings that represent the distal ends of the collecting ducts (of Bellini). These openings form the area cribrosa (Fig. 2–3). In contrast to the human kidney, the kidney of the rat and of many other laboratory animals has a single renal pyramid and is therefore termed "unipapillate." Otherwise, these kidneys resemble the human kidney in their gross appearance. In humans, the renal cortex is about 1 cm in

thickness, forms a cap over the base of each renal pyramid, and extends downward between the individual pyramids to form the renal columns of Bertin (Fig. 2–4; see Fig. 2–2). From the base of the renal pyramid, at the corticomedullary junction, longitudinal elements termed the "medullary rays of Ferrein" extend into the cortex. Despite their name, the medullary rays are actually considered a part of the cortex and are formed by the collecting ducts and the straight segments of the proximal and distal tubules.

The renal pelvis is lined by transitional epithelium and represents the expanded portion of the upper urinary tract. In humans, two and sometimes three outpouchings, the major calyces, extend outward from the upper dilated end of the renal pelvis. From each of the major calyces, several minor calyces extend toward the papillae of the pyramids and drain the urine formed by each pyramidal unit. In mammals possessing a unipapillate kidney, the papilla is directly surrounded by the renal pelvis. The ureters originate from the lower portion of the renal pelvis at the ureteropelvic junction, and in humans they descend a distance of approximately 28 cm to 34 cm to open into the fundus of the bladder. The walls of the calyces, pelvis, and ureters contain smooth muscle that contracts rhythmically to propel the urine to the bladder.

THE NEPHRON

The functional unit of the kidney is the nephron. Each human kidney contains about 0.6×10^6 to 1.4×10^6 nephrons,[1-3] which contrasts with the approximately 30,000 nephrons in each adult rat kidney.[4,5] The essential components of the nephron include the renal or malpighian corpuscle (glomerulus and Bowman's capsule), the proximal tubule, the thin limbs, the distal tubule, and the connecting tubule. The origin of the nephron is the metanephric blastema. Although there has not been universal agreement on the origin of the connecting tubule, it is now generally believed to derive from the metanephric blastema.[6] The collecting duct system, which includes the initial collecting tubule, the cortical collecting duct (CCD) in the medullary ray, the outer medullary collecting duct (OMCD), and the inner medullary collecting duct

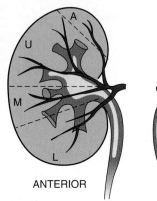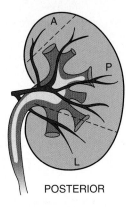

ANTERIOR   POSTERIOR

FIGURE 2–1 Diagram of the vascular supply of the human kidney. The anterior half of the kidney can be divided into upper (U), middle (M), and lower (L) segments, each supplied by a segmental branch of the anterior division of the renal artery. A small apical segment (A) is usually supplied by a division from the anterior segmental branch. The posterior half of the kidney is divided into apical (A), posterior (P), and lower (L) segments, each supplied by branches of the posterior division of the renal artery. (Modified from Graves FT: The anatomy of the intrarenal arteries and its application to segmental resection of the kidney. Br J Surg 42:132, 1954.)

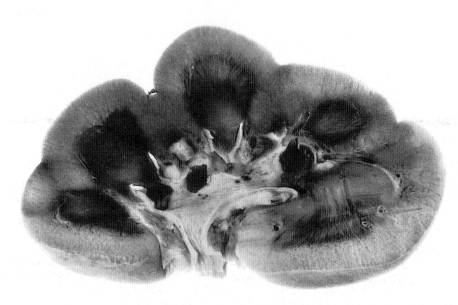

FIGURE 2–2 Bisected kidney from a 4-year-old child, demonstrating the difference in appearance between the light-staining cortex and the dark-staining outer medulla. The inner medulla and papillae are less dense than the outer medulla. The columns of Bertin can be seen extending downward to separate the papillae.

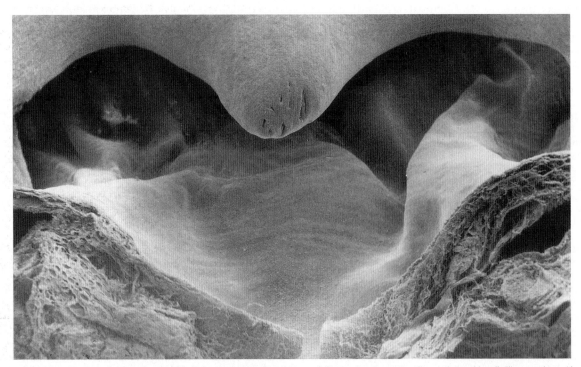

FIGURE 2–3 Scanning electron micrograph of papilla from a rat kidney (upper center), illustrating the area cribrosa formed by slit-like openings where the ducts of Bellini terminate. The renal pelvis (below) surrounds the papilla. (Magnification, ×24.)

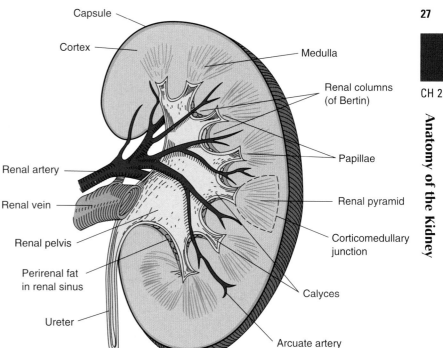

FIGURE 2–4 Diagram of the cut surface of a bisected kidney, depicting important anatomic structures.

(IMCD), is not, strictly speaking, considered part of the nephron because embryologically it arises from the ureteric bud. However, all of the components of the nephron and the collecting duct system are interrelated functionally.

Two main populations of nephrons are recognizable in the kidney: those possessing a short loop of Henle and those with a long loop of Henle (Fig. 2–5). The loop of Henle is composed of the straight portion of the proximal tubule (pars recta), the thin limb segments, and the straight portion of the distal tubule (thick ascending limb, or pars recta). The length of the loop of Henle is generally related to the position of its parent glomerulus in the cortex. Most nephrons originating from superficial and midcortical locations have short loops of Henle that bend within the inner stripe of the outer medulla close to the inner medulla. A few species, including humans, also possess cortical nephrons with extremely short loops that never enter the medulla but turn back within the cortex. Nephrons originating from the juxtamedullary region near the corticomedullary boundary have long loops of Henle with long descending and ascending thin limb segments that enter the inner medulla. Many variations exist, however, between the two basic types of nephrons, depending on their relative position in the cortex. The ratio between long and short loops varies among species. Humans and most rodents have a larger number of short-looped than long-looped nephrons.

On the basis of the segmentation of the renal tubule, the medulla can be divided into an inner and an outer zone, with the outer zone further subdivided into an inner and an outer stripe (see Fig. 2–5). The inner medulla contains both descending and ascending thin limbs and large collecting ducts, including the ducts of Bellini. In the inner stripe of the outer medulla, thick ascending limbs are present in addition to descending thin limbs and collecting ducts. The outer stripe of the outer medulla contains the terminal segments of the pars recta of the proximal tubule, the thick ascending limbs (partes rectae of the distal tubule), and collecting ducts. The division of the kidney into cortical and medullary zones and the further subdivision of the medulla into inner and outer zones are of considerable importance in relating renal structure to the ability of an animal to form a maximally concentrated urine.

Renal Corpuscle (Glomerulus)

The renal corpuscle is composed of a capillary network lined by a thin layer of endothelial cells; a central region of mesangial cells with surrounding mesangial matrix material; the visceral epithelial cells and the associated basement membrane; and the parietal layer of Bowman's capsule with its basement membrane (Figs. 2–6 through 2–8). Between the two epithelial layers is a narrow cavity called Bowman's space, or the urinary space. Although the term renal corpuscle is more precise anatomically than the term glomerulus when referring to that portion of the nephron composed of the glomerular tuft and Bowman's capsule, the term glomerulus is employed throughout this chapter because of its common use. The visceral epithelium is continuous with the parietal epithelium at the vascular pole, where the afferent arteriole enters and the efferent arteriole exits the glomerulus. The parietal layer of Bowman's capsule continues into the epithelium of the proximal tubule at the so-called urinary pole. The average diameter of the glomerulus is approximately 200 μm in the human kidney and 120 μm in the rat kidney. However, glomerular number and size vary significantly with age and gender as well as birth weight. The average glomerular volume has been reported to be 3 to 7 million μm^3 in humans[1–3] and 0.6 to 1 million μm^3 in the rat.[4,5] In the rat, juxtamedullary glomeruli are larger than glomeruli in the superficial cortex. However, this is not the case in the human kidney.[7]

The glomerulus is responsible for the production of an ultrafiltrate of plasma. The filtration barrier between the blood and the urinary space is composed of a fenestrated endothelium, the peripheral glomerular basement membrane (GBM), and the slit pores between the foot processes of the visceral epithelial cells (Fig. 2–9). The mean area of filtration surface per glomerulus has been reported to be 0.203 mm^2 in the human kidney[8] and 0.184 mm^2 in the rat kidney.[9]

Endothelial Cells

The glomerular capillaries are lined by a thin fenestrated endothelium (Fig. 2–10; see Fig. 2–9). The endothelial cell nucleus usually lies adjacent to the mesangium, away from

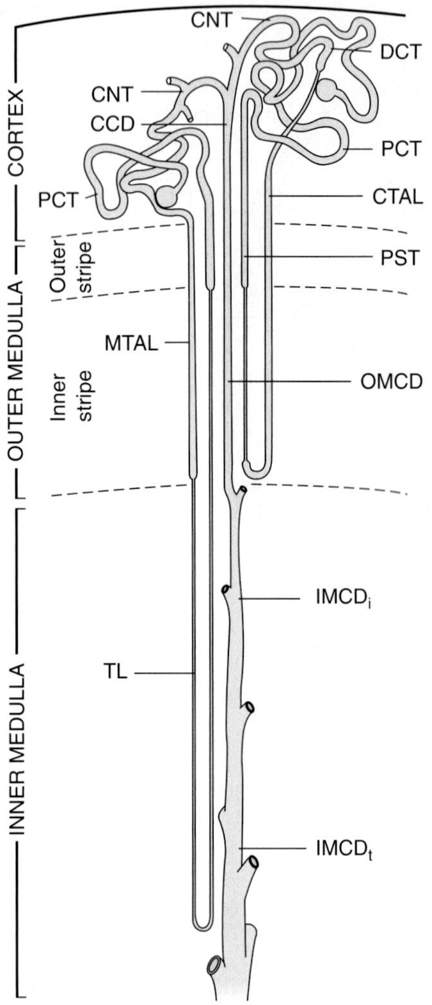

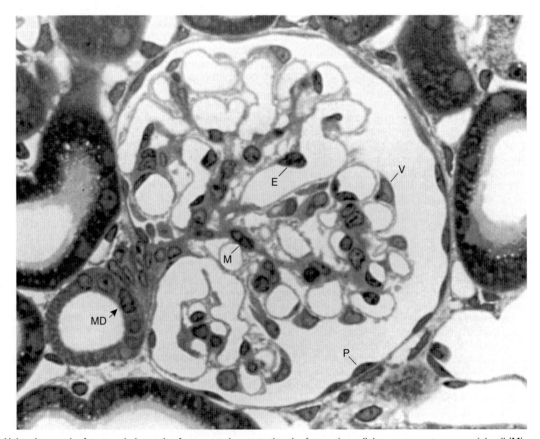

CORTEX

OUTER MEDULLA

INNER MEDULLA

CNT

DCT

CNT

CCD

PCT

PCT

CTAL

Outer stripe

PST

Inner stripe

MTAL

OMCD

IMCD$_i$

TL

IMCD$_t$

FIGURE 2–5 Diagram illustrating superficial and juxtamedullary nephron. CCD, cortical collecting duct; CNT, connecting tubule; CTAL, cortical thick ascending limb; DCT, distal convoluted tubule; IMCD$_i$, initial inner medullary collecting duct; IMCD$_t$, terminal inner medullary collecting duct; MTAL, medullary thick ascending limb; OMCD, outer medullary collecting duct; PCT, proximal convoluted tubule; PST, proximal straight tubule; TL, thin limb of loop of Henle. (Modified from Madsen KM, Tisher CC: Structural-functional relationship along the distal nephron. Am J Physiol 250:F1, 1986.)

FIGURE 2–6 Light micrograph of a normal glomerulus from a rat, demonstrating the four major cellular components: mesangial cell (M), endothelial cell (E), visceral epithelial cell (V), and parietal epithelial cell (P). MD, macula densa. (Magnification, ×750.)

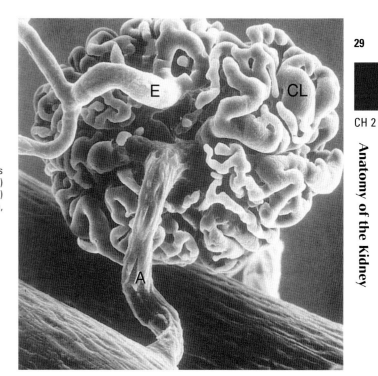

FIGURE 2–7 Scanning electron micrograph of a cast of a glomerulus with its many capillary loops (CL) and adjacent renal vessels. The afferent arteriole (A) takes its origin from an interlobular artery at lower left. The efferent arteriole (E) branches to form the peritubular capillary plexus (upper left). (Magnification, ×300.) (Courtesy of Waykin Nopanitaya, PhD.)

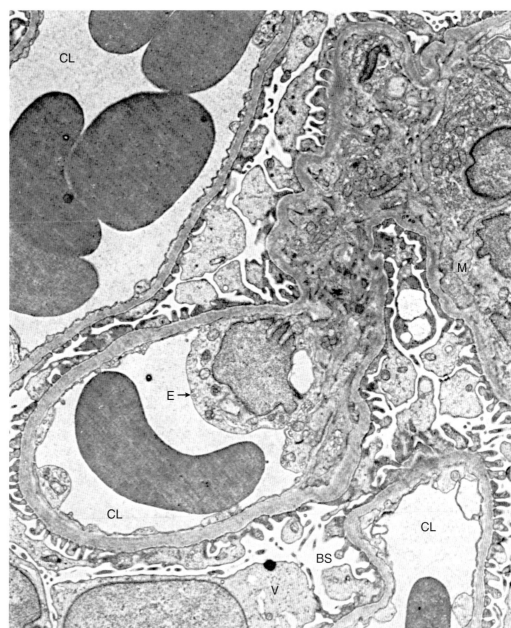

FIGURE 2–8 Electron micrograph of a portion of a glomerulus from normal human kidney in which segments of three capillary loops (CL) are evident. The relationship between mesangial cells (M), endothelial cells (E), and visceral epithelial cells (V) is demonstrated. Several electron-dense erythrocytes lie in the capillary lumens. BS, Bowman's space. (Magnification, ×6700.)

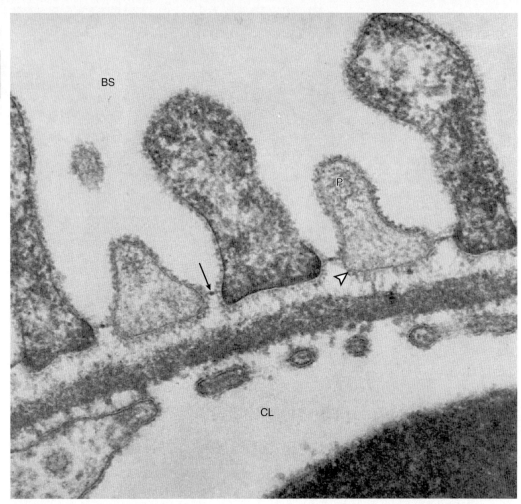

FIGURE 2–9 Electron micrograph of normal rat glomerulus fixed in a 1% glutaraldehyde solution containing tannic acid. Note the relationship among the three layers of the glomerular basement membrane and the presence of the pedicels (P) embedded in the lamina rara externa (arrowhead). The filtration slit diaphragm with the central dense spot (arrow) is especially evident between the individual pedicels. The fenestrated endothelial lining of the capillary loop is shown below the basement membrane. A portion of an erythrocyte is located in the extreme lower right corner. BS, Bowman's space; CL, capillary lumen. (Magnification, ×120,000.)

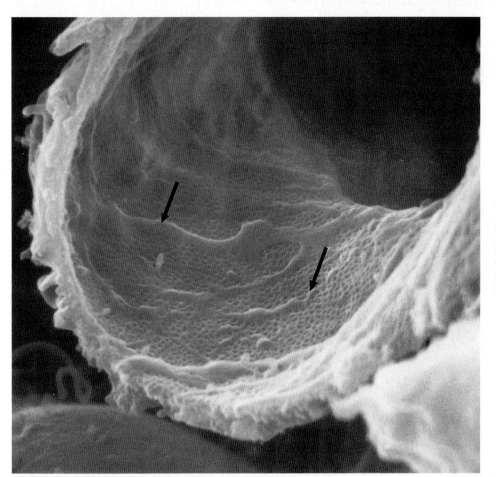

FIGURE 2–10 Scanning electron micrograph demonstrating the endothelial surface of a glomerular capillary from the kidney of a normal rat. Numerous endothelial pores, or fenestrae, are evident. The ridge-like structures (arrows) represent localized thickenings of the endothelial cells. (Magnification, ×21,400.)

the urinary space, and the remainder of the cell is irregularly attenuated around the capillary lumen (see Fig. 2–8). The endothelium is perforated by pores or fenestrae, which in the human kidney range from 70 nm to 100 nm in diameter (see Fig. 2–10).[10] Thin diaphragms have been observed extending across these fenestrae and electron microscopic studies using a modified fixation method reported the presence of filamentous sieve plugs in the fenestrae.[11] The function of these plugs remains to be established and it is not known whether they represent a significant barrier to the passage of macromolecules. Recent studies have confirmed the presence of electron-dense filamentous material in the fenestrae and also demonstrated a thick filamentous surface layer on the endothelial cells.[12] Nonfenestrated, ridge-like structures termed cytofolds are found near the cell borders.

In both human and rat kidney, an extensive network of intermediate filaments and microtubules is present in the endothelial cells, and microfilaments surround the endothelial fenestrations.[13] Knowledge of the exact functions of the cytoskeleton in these cells is incomplete. The surface of the glomerular endothelial cells is negatively charged because of the presence of a surface coat or glycocalyx rich in polyanionic glycosaminoglycans and glycoproteins that are synthesized by the endothelial cells.[14] Recent studies have suggested that the endothelial cell glycocalyx contributes to the charge-selective properties of the glomerular capillary wall and thus may constitute an important part of the filtration barrier.[15] The glomerular endothelial cells synthesize both nitric oxide (NO), previously called endothelium-derived relaxing factor, and endothelin-1, a vasoconstrictor.[16] The synthesis of NO is catalyzed by endothelial nitric oxide synthase (eNOS), which is expressed in glomerular endothelial cells.[17]

Receptors for vascular endothelial growth factor (VEGF) are expressed on the surface of the glomerular endothelial cells.[18] VEGF is produced by the glomerular visceral epithelial cells and is an important regulator of microvascular permeability.[18,19] In vitro studies in endothelial cells of different origins have demonstrated that VEGF increases endothelial cell permeability and induces the formation of endothelial fenestrations,[20,21] and VEGF-induced formation of fenestrae has also been demonstrated in renal microvascular endothelial cells.[22] Gene deletion studies in mice have demonstrated that VEGF is required for normal differentiation of glomerular endothelial cells[23,24] and there is evidence that VEGF is important for endothelial cell survival and repair in glomerular diseases characterized by endothelial cell damage.[25] Thus, VEGF produced by the visceral epithelial cells plays a critical role in the differentiation and maintenance of glomerular endothelial cells and is an important regulator of endothelial cell permeability.

The endothelial cells form the initial barrier to the passage of blood constituents from the capillary lumen to Bowman space and they contribute to the charge-selective properties of the glomerular capillary wall through their negatively charged glycocalyx. Under normal conditions, the formed elements of the blood, including erythrocytes, leukocytes, and platelets, do not gain access to the subendothelial space.

Visceral Epithelial Cells

The visceral epithelial cells, also called podocytes, are the largest cells in the glomerulus (see Fig. 2–6). They have long cytoplasmic processes, or trabeculae, that extend from the main cell body and divide into individual foot processes, or pedicels, that come into direct contact with the lamina rara externa of the GBM (see Figs. 2–8 and 2–9). By scanning electron microscopy, it is apparent that adjacent foot processes are derived from different podocytes (Fig. 2–11). The podocytes contain a well-developed Golgi complex, and lysosomes are often observed. Large numbers of microtubules,

microfilaments, and intermediate filaments are present in the cytoplasm[13] and actin filaments are especially abundant in the foot processes[26] where they connect the slit membrane with the GBM.

In the normal glomerulus, the distance between adjacent foot processes near the GBM varies from 25 nm to 60 nm (see Fig. 2–9). This gap, referred to as the filtration slit or slit pore, is bridged by a thin membrane called the filtration slit membrane[27,28] or slit diaphragm,[29] which is located approximately 60 nm from the GBM. A continuous central filament with a diameter of approximately 11 nm can be seen in the filtration slit diaphragm.[27] Detailed studies of the slit diaphragm in the rat, mouse, and human glomerulus have revealed that the 11-nm-wide central filament is connected to the cell membrane of the adjacent foot processes by regularly spaced cross bridges approximately 7 nm in diameter and 14 nm in length, giving the slit diaphragm a zipper-like configuration (Fig. 2–12).[29,30] The dimensions of the pores between the cross bridges are approximately 4×14 nm. The slit diaphragm has the morphologic features of an adherens junction[31] and the ZO-1 protein that is specific to tight junctions has been localized to the sites where the slit diaphragm is connected to the plasma membrane of the foot processes.[32]

The molecular structure of the slit diaphragm has long escaped identification, and its role in establishing the perm-selective properties of the filtration barrier has been a matter of dispute. However, there is evidence that a newly identified protein, nephrin, may constitute a key component of the filtration barrier.[33] Nephrin is the product of the gene that is mutated in congenital nephrotic syndrome of the Finnish type (NPHS1).[34,35] Based on the deduced amino acid sequence, nephrin is a transmembrane protein that belongs to the immunoglobulin family of adhesion molecules.[35] Nephrin is expressed in the visceral epithelial cells in the glomerulus, where it is located exclusively in the slit diaphragm.[36,37] This suggests that nephrin and the slit diaphragm are essential components of the glomerular filtration barrier, as illustrated in the hypothetical model of the filter in Figure 2–13. A second protein, CD2-associated protein (CD2AP) has recently been identified in the slit diaphragm.[38] CD2AP is an adapter molecule that binds to the cytoplasmic domain of nephrin and is believed to connect nephrin to the cytoskeleton.[39,40] Deletion of CD2AP is also associated with congenital nephrotic syndrome and morphologically with effacement and fusion of foot processes.[39] Therefore, both nephrin and CD2AP appear to be required for normal filtration to occur. The gene responsible for familial steroid-resistant nephrotic syndrome has also been identified.[41] Its product, podocin, is an integral membrane protein that is expressed in the foot process membrane at the site of insertion of the slit diaphragm.[42,43] Podocin is connected to both nephrin and CD2AP.

Various membrane components have been identified on the surface of the visceral epithelial cells. Kerjaschki and co-workers[44] identified and characterized the principal sialoprotein on the urinary surface of the podocytes and termed it "podocalyxin." The human glomerular C3b receptor[45] and the Heymann nephritis antigen (gp330 or megalin)[46] have also been identified in the plasma membrane of the visceral epithelial cell. In Heymann nephritis induced in the Lewis rat, this antigen reacts with an antibody directed against a constituent of the microvilli that form the brush border of the proximal tubule.[46] The visceral epithelial cells then undergo capping on their surface and the antigen-antibody complex is shed into the subepithelial space adjacent to the GBM. There is evidence that pathogenic epitopes are present in all four clusters of ligand-binding repeats in megalin. Injection of domain-specific antibodies against each of the four megalin fragments produced glomerular immune deposits indicative of passive Heymann nephritis in rats.[47]

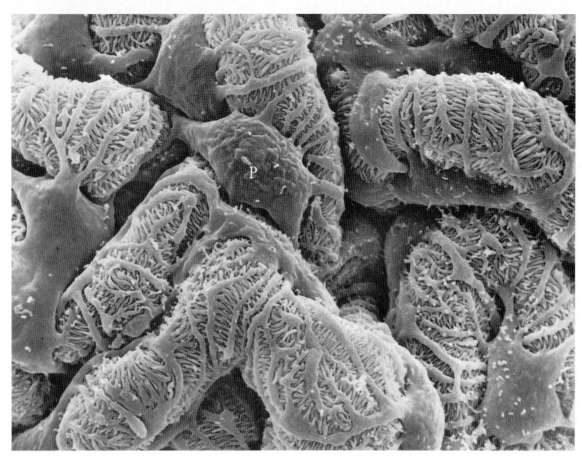

FIGURE 2–11 Scanning electron micrograph of a glomerulus from the kidney of a normal rat. The visceral epithelial cells, or podocytes (P), extend multiple processes outward from the main cell body to wrap around individual capillary loops. Immediately adjacent pedicels, or foot processes, arise from different podocytes. (Magnification, ×6000.)

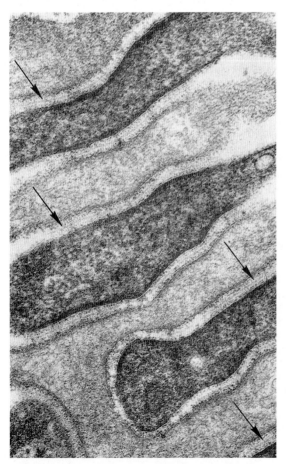

FIGURE 2–12 Electron micrograph showing the epithelial foot processes of normal rat glomerulus preserved in a 1% glutaraldehyde solution containing tannic acid. In several areas, the slit diaphragm has been sectioned parallel to the plane of the basement membrane, revealing a highly organized substructure. The thin central filament corresponding to the central dot observed on cross section (see Fig. 2–9) is indicated by the arrows. (Magnification, ×52,000.)

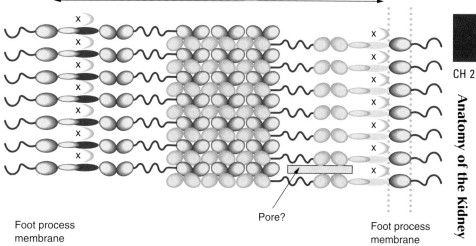

FIGURE 2–13 Diagram illustrating hypothetical assembly of nephrin forming the filter of the podocyte slit diaphragm. Nephrin molecules from adjacent interdigitating foot processes are shown in different shades of purple. X indicates proteins interacting with nephrin and connecting with the plasma membrane. (From Tryggvason K: Unraveling the mechanisms of glomerular ultrafiltration: Nephrin, a key component of the slit diaphragm. J Am Soc Nephrol 10:2440, 1999.)

In many diseases associated with proteinuria, the foot processes are replaced by a continuous cytoplasmic band along the GBM. This process is commonly referred to as foot process fusion or effacement. Similar ultrastructural changes have been described in the rat kidney after intra-arterial infusion of protamine sulfate, a polycationic substance that interacts with anionic sites on the cell membrane.[48] Furthermore, perfusion of rat kidneys with neuraminidase, which removes sialic acid, causes a detachment of both endothelial and epithelial cells from the GBM,[49] suggesting that negatively charged sites on these cells are important for the maintenance of normal structure and function of the filtration barrier. More recent evidence has assigned a possible role for the plasma membrane protein, podoplanin, in the maintenance of podocyte shape. A single intravenous injection of antipodoplanin immunoglobulin G antibodies into rats induced rapid and reversible flattening of foot processes and heavy albeit transient proteinuria.[50] It has also been demonstrated that podoplanin is transcriptionally down-regulated in puromycin aminonucleoside nephrosis, in which there is flattening of foot processes and proteinuria.[51] Therefore, anionic sites on the podocytes as well as the presence of an intact slit diaphragm are important in establishing the permselective properties of the filtration barrier. The visceral epithelial cells are capable of endocytosis, and the heterogeneous content of their lysosomes most likely reflects the uptake of proteins and other components from the ultrafiltrate. In conditions associated with heavy proteinuria, an increase occurs in the number of protein droplets in the cytoplasm of the podocytes.

For a detailed discussion of the structure, cell biology, and function of the glomerular podocyte, the reader is referred to a recent review article by Pavenstadt and colleagues.[52]

Mesangial Cells

The mesangial cells and their surrounding matrix material constitute the mesangium, which is separated from the capillary lumen by the endothelium (see Figs. 2–6 and 2–8). Zimmermann provided the first detailed description of the mesangium by light microscopy in 1933 and proposed the current nomenclature based on his theory of the development of the glomerulus by invagination.[10] It was not until the advent of the electron microscope, however, that the mesangial cell was distinguished clearly from the endothelial cell and described in detail.[53,54] The mesangial cell is irregular in shape, with a dense nucleus and elongated cytoplasmic processes that can extend around the capillary lumen and insinuate themselves between the GBM and the overlying endothelium (see Fig. 2–8). In addition to the usual complement of subcellular organelles, mesangial cells possess an extensive array of microfilaments composed at least in part of actin, α-actinin, and myosin.[55] There is an especially heavy concentration of microfilaments situated along the paramesangial region and within the mesangial cell processes adjacent to the glomerular capillaries.[56] The contractile mesangial cell processes appear to bridge the gap in the GBM encircling the capillary, and bundles of microfilaments interconnect opposing parts of the GBM, an arrangement that is believed to prevent capillary wall distention secondary to elevation of the intracapillary hydraulic pressure.[55,56]

The mesangial cell is surrounded by a matrix material that is similar to but not identical with the GBM; the mesangial matrix is more coarsely fibrillar and slightly less electron dense. The mesangial matrix contains sulfated glycosaminoglycans[57] as well as large amounts of fibronectin, laminin, and various collagens.[58,59] Several cell surface receptors of the β-integrin family have been identified on the mesangial cells, including α1β1, α3β1, and the fibronectin receptor, α5β1.[60–62] An additional α-chain, α8, has been identified on mesangial cells in human as well as rat and mouse kidneys.[63] The α8β1 integrin receptor can also serve as a receptor for fibronectin. The integrin receptors mediate attachment of the mesangial cells to specific molecules in the extracellular mesangial matrix and link the matrix to the cytoskeleton. The attachment to the mesangial matrix is important for cell anchorage, contraction, and migration, and ligand-integrin binding also serves as a signal transduction mechanism that regulates the production of extracellular matrix as well as the synthesis of various vasoactive mediators, growth factors, and cytokines.[64]

As reviewed by Schlondorff,[65] the mesangial cell in all likelihood represents a specialized pericyte and possesses many of the functional properties of smooth muscle cells. In addition to providing structural support for the glomerular capillary loops, the mesangial cell has contractile properties and is believed to play a role in the regulation of glomerular filtration. Mesangial cells also exhibit phagocytic properties and participate in the clearance or disposal of macromolecules from the mesangium.[65,66] Finally, mesangial cells are involved in the generation and metabolism of the extracellular mesangial matrix and participate in various forms of glomerular injury.[64,65]

The contractile properties of cultured mesangial cells are well established. Studies employing antibodies against actin, α-actinin, and myosin documented their colocalization with microfilaments in the rat mesangial cell.[55] Cell contraction is stimulated by a variety of vasoactive agents, including angiotensin II, vasopressin, norepinephrine, thromboxane, leukotrienes, and platelet-activating factor.[65,67,68] In contrast, such agents as PGE$_2$, atrial peptides, and dopamine cause relaxation of cultured mesangial cells, in most instances by increasing intracellular levels of cyclic guanosine monophosphate (cGMP).[65] Furthermore, receptors for angiotensin II, vasopressin, and platelet-activating factor have been demonstrated on the mesangial cell.[65,67] The location of the mesangial cell in the intercapillary or centrilobular stalk region, combined with its contractile and relaxant properties, makes this cell an ideal candidate to participate in the control of glomerular filtration. It is possible that mesangial cell contraction decreases glomerular filtration by reducing blood flow through selected capillary loops, thereby eliminating their contribution to the process of filtration.[65] The local generation of autacoids, such as PGE$_2$, by the mesangial cell, may provide a counterregulatory mechanism to oppose the effect of the vasoconstrictors.

Morphologic aspects of the phagocytic properties of the mesangial cells are well documented.[66] Uptake of tracers such as ferritin,[53] colloidal carbon,[69] aggregated proteins,[70] and immune complexes has been described, and investigators have suggested that phagocytosed material may be cleared from the mesangium by cell-to-cell transport to the extraglomerular mesangial region at the vascular pole of the glomerular tuft.[69] Although some have reported that much of the phagocytic capability of the mesangium resides in the bone marrow–derived resident monocyte-macrophages, a population of cells possessing immune region–associated antigens (Ia),[71,72] there is evidence that the mesangial cell is also capable of phagocytosis. Studies in cultured mesangial cells have demonstrated phagocytosis of opsonized zymosan, which was associated with the production of prostaglandins, reactive oxygen species, and lipoxygenase products.[73] Endocytosis of immune complexes by mesangial cells was found to be associated with stimulation of PGE$_2$ and platelet-activating factor and was dependent on Fc receptor activity.[74] Thus, there is evidence that both the Ia-bearing cell and the mesangial cell possess phagocytic capability.

Mesangial cells produce prostaglandins, and several vasoactive substances are known to influence this production.[65] In addition to their proposed role in counter-regulating the effect of vasoconstrictors, prostaglandins can influence local cell proliferation and the production of cytokines, including platelet-derived growth factor, interleukin-1, and epithelial growth factor. This interaction among cytokines, mesangial cells, and prostaglandins may be important for understanding the mechanisms of the glomerular injury that is associated with mesangial cell proliferation and mesangial expansion in a host of kidney diseases.

Glomerular Basement Membrane

The GBM is composed of a central dense layer, the lamina densa, and two thinner, more electron-lucent layers, the lamina rara externa and the lamina rara interna (see Fig. 2–9). The latter two layers measure approximately 20 nm to 40 nm in thickness.[10] The layered configuration of the GBM results in part from the fusion of endothelial and epithelial basement membranes during development.[75]

Several investigators have provided estimates of the width of the GBM of peripheral glomerular capillary loops. Jørgensen and Bentzon[76] reported a geometric mean of 329 nm in 24 patients who showed no clinical evidence of renal disease. In a quantitative study of the GBM in five healthy individuals, Østerby[77] calculated a mean width of 310 nm. Steffes and co-workers[78] determined the GBM width in a large group of donor kidneys for transplantation and found a significantly thicker basement membrane in men (373 nm) than in women (326 nm). For the purpose of comparison with the

human, the thickness of the GBM in the rat was found to be 132 nm.[79]

Like other basement membranes in the body, the GBM is composed primarily of collagen IV, laminin, entactin/nidogen, and sulfated proteoglycans.[58,59,80–82] In addition, the GBM contains specific components, such as laminin 11, distinct collagen IV α chains, and the proteoglycans agrin and perlecan,[57,82,83] that most likely reflect its specialized function as part of the glomerular filtration barrier. Collagen IV is the major constituent of the GBM.[84] As reviewed by Kashtan,[85] six isomeric chains, designated α1 through α6 (IV), comprise the type IV collagen family of proteins.[86] Of these six chains, α1 through α5 have been identified in the normal GBM.[85] The six chains, α1 through α6 (IV), are encoded by genes located on human chromosomes 2, 13, and X. There is evidence that distinct networks of type IV collagen exist in different basement membranes. Although networks of α1/α2 (IV) chains are ubiquitous in all basement membranes, the GBM also contains networks of α3/α4/α5 (IV) chains, which are restricted in distribution. The exact significance of the restricted networks remains unclear, but they may reflect specialization of function.[85] Mutations in the genes encoding α3, α4, and α5 (IV) chains are known to cause Alport syndrome, a hereditary basement membrane disorder associated with progressive glomerulopathy.[84,85]

The GBM possesses fixed, negatively charged sites that may influence the filtration of macromolecules. Caulfield and Farquhar[87] demonstrated the existence of anionic sites in all three layers of the GBM with use of the cationic protein lysozyme. Additional studies employing cationic ferritin and ruthenium red, a cationic dye, revealed a lattice of anionic sites with a spacing of approximately 60 nm (Fig. 2–14) throughout the lamina rara interna and lamina rara externa, which might contribute to the formation of the charge barrier.[88] Kanwar and Farquhar[89,90] demonstrated that the anionic sites in the GBM consist of glycosaminoglycans rich in heparan sulfate. Their removal by enzymatic digestion resulted in an increase in permeability of the GBM to ferritin[91] and to bovine serum albumin,[92] suggesting that glycosaminoglycans play a role in establishing the permeability properties of the GBM to plasma proteins (see Fig. 2–14). It has also been suggested that the glycosaminoglycans might serve as anticlogging agents in the GBM.[93]

The glomerular capillary wall functions as a sieve or filter that allows the passage of small molecules but almost completely restricts the passage of molecules the size of albumin or larger. Physiologic studies have established that the glomerular capillary wall possesses both size-selective and charge-selective properties.[94] To cross the capillary wall, a molecule must pass sequentially through the fenestrated endothelium, the GBM, and the epithelial slit diaphragm. The fenestrated endothelium, with its negatively charged glycocalyx, excludes formed elements of the blood and probably plays a role in determining the access of proteins to the GBM.

The exact role of the GBM in establishing the glomerular filtration barrier remains somewhat controversial. Ultrastructural tracer studies have provided evidence that the GBM constitutes both a size-selective and a charge-selective barrier. Caulfield and Farquhar[95] infused dextrans of different molecular weights into rats and demonstrated that filtration depended on the size of the molecule and that the GBM was the main barrier to filtration. Rennke and co-workers[96,97] used ultrastructural tracers such as ferritin and horseradish peroxidase with isoelectric points varying from 4.5 to 11.5 to examine the effect of molecular charge on the filtration of macromolecules. These studies demonstrated that the clearance of cationic molecules greatly exceeded that of neutral and anionic molecules. Furthermore, the electrostatic barrier appeared to be located mainly in the GBM. Subsequent

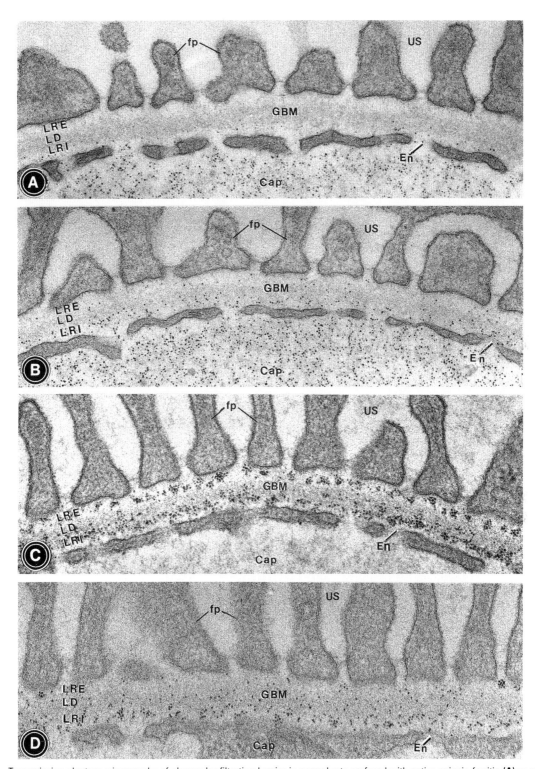

FIGURE 2–14 Transmission electron micrographs of glomerular filtration barrier in normal rats perfused with native anionic ferritin **(A)** or cationic ferritin **(C)** and in rats treated with heparitinase before perfusion with anionic **(B)** or cationic **(D)** ferritin. In normal animals, anionic ferritin is present in the capillary (Cap) but does not enter the glomerular basement membrane (GBM), as shown in **A**. In contrast, cationic ferritin binds to the negatively charged sites in the lamina rara interna (LRI) and lamina rara externa (LRE) of the GBM (see **C**). After treatment with heparitinase, both anionic **(B)** and cationic **(D)** ferritin penetrates into the GBM, but there is no labeling of negatively charged sites by cationic ferritin. En, endothelial fenestrae; fp, foot processes; LD, lamina densa; US, urinary space. (Magnification, ×80,000.) (From Kanwar YS: Biophysiology of glomerular filtration and proteinuria. Lab Invest 51:7, 1984.)

studies reported that removal of negatively charged glycosaminoglycans resulted in increased permeability of the GBM to ferritin and albumin.[91,92] Taken together these studies provided convincing experimental evidence that the GBM plays a major role in establishing a charge-selective filter in the glomerulus. However, the role of the GBM as the main determinant of charge selectivity was challenged subsequently because studies in the isolated GBM failed to demonstrate charge selectivity in vitro.[98]

Because of the unique structure of the negatively charged filtration slit diaphragm and recent advances in its molecular characterization demonstrating that lack of distinct proteins associated with the slit diaphragm leads to massive proteinuria, it is now generally accepted that this structure plays a major role in establishing the ultrafiltration characteristics of the glomerular capillary wall. Most investigators, however, believe that the existence of all of the three structural components of the filtration barrier placed in series is important for the normal permeability properties of the glomerulus. A detailed discussion of glomerular permeability and the filtration barrier is provided in a recent review article by Deen and colleagues.[98]

Parietal Epithelial Cells

The parietal epithelium, which forms the outer wall of Bowman's capsule, is continuous with the visceral epithelium at the vascular pole. The parietal epithelial cells are squamous in character, but at the urinary pole there is an abrupt transition to the taller cuboidal cells of the proximal tubule, which have a well-developed brush border (Figs. 2–15 and 2–16). The parietal epithelium of the capsule was described in detail by Jørgensen.[10] The cells are 0.1 μm to 0.3 μm in height, except at the nucleus, where they increase to 2.0 μm to 3.5 μm. Each cell has a long cilium and occasional microvilli up to 600 nm in length. Cell organelles are generally sparse and include small mitochondria, numerous vesicles that are 40 nm to 90 nm in diameter, and the Golgi apparatus. Large vacuoles and multivesicular bodies are rarely, if ever, seen. The thickness of the basement membrane of Bowman's capsule is variable but has been found to range from 1200 nm to 1500 nm.[10] The basement membrane is composed of multiple layers, or lamellae, which increase in thickness with many disease processes. At both the vascular pole and the urinary pole, the thickness of Bowman's capsule decreases markedly. In certain disease processes, such as rapidly progressive glomerulonephritis, the parietal epithelial cells proliferate to contribute to the formation of crescents.

Peripolar Cells

Ryan and colleagues[99] have described a peripolar cell that they believe is a component of the juxtaglomerular apparatus. It is located at the origin of the glomerular tuft in Bowman's

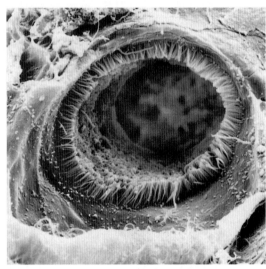

FIGURE 2–15 Scanning electron micrograph depicting the transition from the parietal epithelial cells of Bowman's capsule (foreground) to the proximal tubule cells, with their well-developed brush border, in the kidney of a rat. (Magnification, ×3200.)

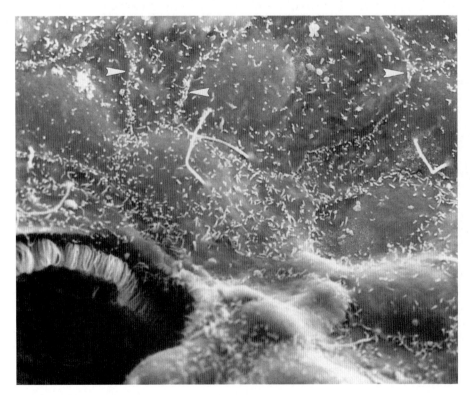

FIGURE 2–16 Scanning electron micrograph illustrating the appearance of the surface of the parietal epithelial cells adjacent to the early proximal tubule at the urinary pole (lower left). Parietal epithelial cells possess a single cilium, and their lateral cell margins are accentuated by short microvilli (arrowheads). (Magnification, ×12,500.) (Courtesy of Jill W. Verlander, DVM.)

space and is interposed between the visceral and parietal epithelial cells. The base of these cells rests on the basement membrane of Bowman's capsule, and the opposite surface is exposed to the urinary space. They contain multiple membrane-bound electron-dense granules and are separated from the afferent arteriole only by the basement membrane of Bowman's capsule.[99] The peripolar cells are especially prominent in sheep, but they have also been identified in other species, including humans, and have been localized predominantly in glomeruli in the outer cortex.[100]

Juxtaglomerular Apparatus

The juxtaglomerular apparatus is located at the vascular pole of the glomerulus, where a portion of the distal nephron comes into contact with its parent glomerulus. It has a vascular and a tubule component. The vascular component is composed of the terminal portion of the afferent arteriole, the initial portion of the efferent arteriole, and the extraglomerular mesangial region. The tubule component is the macula densa, which is that portion of the thick ascending limb that is in contact with the vascular component.[101–103] The extraglomerular mesangial region, which has also been referred to as the polar cushion (polkissen) or the lacis, is bounded by the cells of the macula densa, the specialized regions of the afferent and efferent glomerular arterioles, and

the mesangial cells of the glomerular tuft (the intraglomerular mesangial cells). Within the vascular component of the juxtaglomerular apparatus, two distinct cell types can be distinguished: the juxtaglomerular granular cells, also called epithelioid or the myoepithelial cells, and the agranular extraglomerular mesangial cells, which are also referred to as the lacis cells or pseudo-meissnerian cells of Goormaghtigh.

Juxtaglomerular Granular Cells

The granular cells are located primarily in the walls of the afferent and efferent arterioles, but they are also present in the extraglomerular mesangial region.[101,103–105] They exhibit features of both smooth muscle cells and secretory epithelial cells and therefore have been called myoepithelial cells.[101] The juxtaglomerular granular cells are believed to represent modified smooth muscle cells. They contain myofilaments in the cytoplasm and, except for the presence of granules, are indistinguishable from the neighboring arteriolar smooth muscle cells. They also exhibit features suggestive of secretory activity, including a well-developed endoplasmic reticulum and a Golgi complex containing small granules with a crystalline substructure.[101,106]

The juxtaglomerular granular cells are characterized by the presence of numerous membrane-bound granules of variable size and shape (Fig. 2–17).[105] Some of these granules, termed

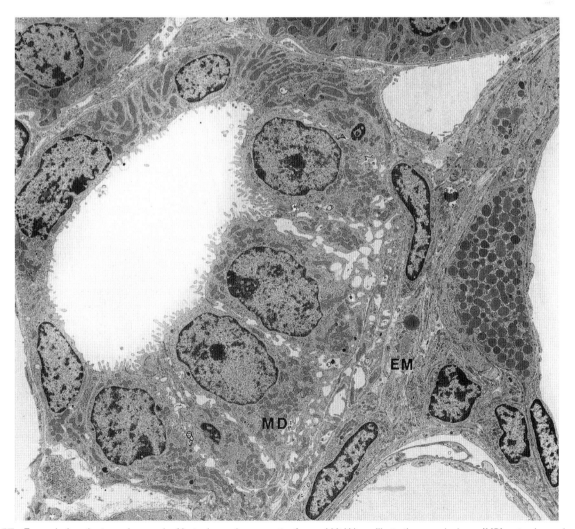

FIGURE 2–17 Transmission electron micrograph of juxtaglomerular apparatus from rabbit kidney, illustrating macula densa (MD), extraglomerular mesangium (EM), and a portion of an arteriole (on the right), containing numerous electron-dense granules. (Magnification, ×3700.)

protogranules, have a crystalline substructure and are believed to represent precursors that fuse to form the larger mature granules.[105,107] In addition to these so-called specific granules, lipofuscin-like granules are commonly observed in the human kidney.[104,106]

There is convincing evidence that the specific granules represent renin or its precursor. As early as 1945, Goormaghtigh proposed that the granular cells were the source of renin. That hypothesis was later proven correct by immunohistochemical and in situ hybridization studies as well as biochemical studies demonstrating renin enzyme activity in the juxtaglomerular apparatus.[103,105] Immunohistochemical studies demonstrated the presence of both renin and angiotensin II in the juxtaglomerular granular cells, with activities being highest in the afferent arteriole.[108] Through use of the immunogold technique in combination with electron microscopy, renin and angiotensin II were found to coexist in the same granules.[105] Studies using in situ hybridization techniques demonstrated renin messenger RNA (mRNA) in the juxtaglomerular cells in normal kidneys, thus providing evidence that these cells produce renin.[109] Histochemical and immunocytochemical studies also have demonstrated the presence of lysosomal enzymes, including acid phosphatase and cathepsin B, in renin-containing granules of the juxtaglomerular epithelioid cells, suggesting that these granules may represent modified lysosomes.[105]

Extraglomerular Mesangium

The extraglomerular mesangium is also called the lacis or the cells of Goormaghtigh. It is located between the afferent and efferent arterioles in close contact with the macula densa (see Fig. 2–17). The extraglomerular mesangium is continuous with the intraglomerular mesangium and is composed of cells that are similar in ultrastructure to the mesangial cells.[101,103] The extraglomerular mesangial cells possess long, thin cytoplasmic processes that are separated by basement membrane material. Under normal conditions, these cells do not contain granules; however, juxtaglomerular granular cells are occasionally observed in the extraglomerular mesangium. The extraglomerular mesangial cells are in contact with the arterioles and the macula densa, and gap junctions are commonly observed between the various cells of the vascular portion of the juxtaglomerular apparatus.[110,111] Gap junctions have also been described between extraglomerular and intraglomerular mesangial cells, suggesting that the extraglomerular mesangium may serve as a functional link between the macula densa and the glomerular arterioles and mesangium.[111] Moreover, there is evidence that mesangial cell damage and selective disruption of gap junctions eliminate the tubuloglomerular feedback response.[112]

Macula Densa

The macula densa is a specialized region of the thick ascending limb adjacent to the hilus of the glomerulus (see Fig. 2–17). Only those cells immediately adjacent to the hilus are morphologically distinctive and form the macula densa. They are low columnar cells and exhibit an apically placed nucleus. With electron microscopy,[101,102] the cell base is seen to interdigitate with the adjacent extraglomerular mesangial cells to form a complex relationship. Although mitochondria are numerous, their orientation is not perpendicular to the base of the cell, and they are rarely enclosed within plications of the basolateral plasma membrane. The position of the Golgi apparatus is lateral to and beneath the cell nucleus. In addition, other cell organelles, including lysosomes, autophagic vacuoles, ribosomes, and profiles of smooth and granular endoplasmic reticulum, are located principally beneath the cell nucleus. The basement membrane of the macula densa is continuous with that surrounding the granular and agranular cells of the extraglomerular mesangial region, which in turn is continuous with the matrix material surrounding the mesangial cells within the glomerular tuft. The macula densa cells lack the lateral cell processes and interdigitations that are characteristic of the thick ascending limb. Ultrastructural studies have provided evidence that the widths of the lateral intercellular spaces in the macula densa vary, depending on the physiologic status of the animal.[113] This finding, coupled with the demonstrated absence of Tamm-Horsfall protein in the macula densa,[114] has prompted some investigators to suggest that, in contrast to the thick ascending limb, where the presence of this glycoprotein may contribute to the water impermeability, the macula densa may be relatively permeable to water.[103] Furthermore, direct visualization of the isolated perfused macula densa by use of differential interference contrast microscopy has revealed reversible dilatation of the lateral intercellular spaces between the macula densa cells with reduction of luminal osmolality.[115]

Morphologic evidence suggests that the autonomic nervous system is involved in the regulation of the function of the juxtaglomerular apparatus. Electron microscopic studies have demonstrated the existence of synapses between granular and agranular cells of the juxtaglomerular apparatus and autonomic nerve endings.[116] On serial sections of the rat juxtaglomerular apparatus, Barajas and Müller[117] analyzed the frequency of contacts between axons and the various cellular components of the juxtaglomerular apparatus. Nerve endings, principally adrenergic in type, were observed to be in contact with approximately one third of the cells of the efferent arteriole and with somewhat less than one third of the cells of the afferent arteriole in the region of the juxtaglomerular apparatus. The frequency of innervation of the tubule component of the juxtaglomerular apparatus was far less. Electron microscopic autoradiography demonstrated uptake of tritiated norepinephrine in axons in contact with afferent and efferent arterioles, which suggests that the nerves are adrenergic in character.[118] Extensive studies by Kopp and DiBona[119] provided convincing evidence that renin secretion is modulated by renal sympathetic nerve activity, which is consistent with the existence of neuroeffector junctions on renin-positive granular cells of the juxtaglomerular apparatus.

The juxtaglomerular apparatus represents a major structural component of the renin-angiotensin system. The role of the juxtaglomerular apparatus is to regulate glomerular arteriolar resistance and glomerular filtration and to control the synthesis and secretion of renin.[120,121] The cells of the macula densa sense changes in the luminal concentrations of sodium and chloride, presumably via absorption of these ions across the luminal membrane by the Na^+-K^+-$2Cl$ cotransporter,[122,123] which is expressed in the macula densa.[124] This initiates the tubuloglomerular feedback response by which signals generated by acute changes in sodium chloride concentration are transferred via the macula densa cells to the glomerular arterioles to control the glomerular filtration rate. Signals from the macula densa, in response to changes in luminal sodium and chloride, are also transmitted to the renin-secreting cells in the afferent arteriole.[121]

Renin synthesis and secretion by the juxtaglomerular granular cells are controlled by several factors, including neurotransmitters of the sympathetic nervous system, glomerular perfusion pressure (presumably through arteriolar baroreceptors), and mediators in the macula densa.[121,125,126] There is increasing evidence that the macula densa control of renin secretion is mediated by NO, cyclooxygenase products such as PGE_2, and adenosine.[121,126,127]

At least two immunologically distinct isoforms of nitric oxide synthase (NOS) are present in the juxtaglomerular apparatus, a fact that, when coupled with complementary physiologic observations, indicates that NO may be an important regulator of the functions of the juxtaglomerular apparatus. Several investigators have demonstrated immunostaining of macula densa cells with antibodies directed against the neuronal isoform of nitric oxide synthase (nNOS),[17,128-130] and the mRNA for nNOS has also been demonstrated in macula densa cells by in situ hybridization.[17,129] In addition, the endothelial isoform of nitric oxide synthase (eNOS) is expressed in endothelial cells of both the glomerular arterioles and the glomerular capillary tuft.[17] The localization of NOS in the macula densa and glomerular endothelial cells was confirmed by use of an independent histochemical technique to detect reduced nicotinamide adenine dinucleotide phosphate (NADPH)–dependent diaphorase activity, which has served as a marker for NOS.[17,130] In functional studies, it has been reported that NO regulates renin release both in vivo and in vitro.[131-133]

Macula densa–controlled renin secretion plays an important role in the adaptation of tubuloglomerular feedback that occurs during long-term perturbations of macula densa sodium chloride concentration.[121] Several investigators have provided evidence that NO modulates the tubuloglomerular feedback response.[128,134-136] NO is believed to cause a resetting of the feedback mechanism, probably via its effect on renin secretion and by reducing ecto-5′-nucleotidase (CD73) activity (discussed later), but it is not a mediator of the response.[121,126,136,137] Therefore, although NO blunts glomerular arteriolar constriction and is important for regulation of the feedback mechanism, it is not required for the feedback response to occur.[136] In contrast, there is evidence that adenosine may play a role as a mediator of the tubuloglomerular feedback response, as discussed in detail by Schnermann and Levine.[138] Mice lacking the type 1 adenosine receptor had a completely abolished feedback response, supporting a role for adenosine as a physiological mediator in this process.[139] Moreover, mice with a genetic deletion of the ecto-5′-nucleotidase (CD73), an enzyme converting extracellular AMP to adenosine, has a markedly impaired tubuloglomerular feedback response.[140]

The stimulation of renin secretion in response to a decrease in macula densa sodium chloride concentration is abolished by inhibition of NOS, indicating that NO produced in the macula densa stimulates renin secretion.[132,133] There is also evidence that prostaglandins generated by the cyclooxygenase (COX) enzymes are involved in macula densa–controlled renin secretion.[141] Harris and co-workers[142] using both in situ hybridization and immunohistochemical techniques, have demonstrated that COX-2 is expressed in the macula densa and that its expression is up-regulated in animals receiving a low-salt diet. Inhibition of COX-2 prevents macula densa–mediated stimulation of renin secretion[143] and causes a decrease in the expression of renin in the kidney.[144] Studies in COX-2 knockout mice demonstrated a significant decrease in renin expression and activity compared with wild-type animals, and the increase in renin mRNA expression observed in wild-type mice in response to a low-salt diet was abolished in COX-2 knockout animals.[145] These studies indicate that COX-2 products such as PGE_2 are involved in the regulation of renin production and secretion. Therefore, there is both structural and functional evidence that both NO and COX-2–generated prostaglandins participate in the signaling pathway between the macula densa and the renin-producing cells in the afferent arteriole. The exact relationship between the two mediators remains to be established. However, studies suggest that the increase in COX-2 expression in the macula densa in response to a low-salt diet is mediated by

NO.[144,146] In addition to serving as a mediator of the tubuloglomerular feedback response, adenosine appears to be required for the inhibition of renin secretion that occurs in response to an increased NaCl concentration at the macula densa.[127]

Proximal Tubule

The proximal tubule begins abruptly at the urinary pole of the glomerulus (see Fig. 2–15). It consists of an initial convoluted portion, the pars convoluta, which is a direct continuation of the parietal epithelium of Bowman's capsule, and a straight portion, the pars recta, which is located in the medullary ray (see Fig. 2–5). The length of the proximal tubule is approximately 10 mm in the rabbit,[147] 8 mm in the rat, and 4 nm to 5 mm in the mouse,[148] compared with approximately 14 mm in the human. The outside diameter of the proximal tubule is about 40 µm. In the rat, three morphologically distinct segments—S1, S2, and S3— have been identified.[149] The S1 segment is the initial portion of the proximal tubule; it begins at the glomerulus and constitutes approximately two thirds of the pars convoluta. The S2 segment consists of the remainder of the pars convoluta and the initial portion of the pars recta. The S3 segment represents the remainder of the proximal tubule, located in the deep inner cortex and the outer stripe of the outer medulla.

The structural features that distinguish the cells in the three segments in the rat have been described in detail by Maunsbach[149] and are illustrated in Figures 2–18 through 2–20. The S1 segment has a tall brush border and a well-developed vacuolar-lysosomal system. The basolateral plasma membrane forms extensive lateral invaginations, and lateral cell processes extending from the apical to the basal surface interdigitate with similar processes from adjacent cells. Elongated mitochondria are located in the lateral cell processes in proximity to the plasma membrane. The ultrastructure of the S2 segment is similar to that of the S1 segment; however, the brush border is shorter, the basolateral invaginations are less prominent, and the mitochondria are smaller. Numerous small lateral processes are located close to the base of the cell. The endocytic compartment is less prominent than in the S1 segment. However, the number and size of the lysosomes vary among species and between males and females, and numerous large lysosomes are often observed in the S2 segment of the male rat.[147,149] In the S3 segment, lateral cell processes and invaginations are essentially absent, and mitochondria are small and randomly distributed within the cell. The length of the brush border in the S3 segment varies among species. It is tall in the rat, fairly short in the rabbit, and intermediate in length in the human kidney. Considerable species variation is also observed in the vacuolar-lysosomal compartment in the S3 segment. In the rat[149] and the human,[150] endocytic vacuoles and lysosomes are small and sparse, whereas in the rabbit, large endocytic vacuoles and numerous small lysosomes are present in the S3 segment.[147] Peroxisomes are present throughout the proximal tubule. They increase in number along the length of the proximal tubule and are most prominent in the S3 segment.

Three segments have also been described in the proximal tubule of the rabbit[151,152] and the rhesus monkey.[153] However, according to Kaissling and Kriz,[151] in the rabbit the S2 segment is not clearly demarcated morphologically and represents a transition between the S1 and S3 segments. Interestingly, a recent ultrastructural study found no evidence of structural segmentation along the proximal tubule of the mouse.[148] Only the pars convoluta and the pars recta have been positively identified and described in the nondiseased human kidney.[150] Because most functional studies have

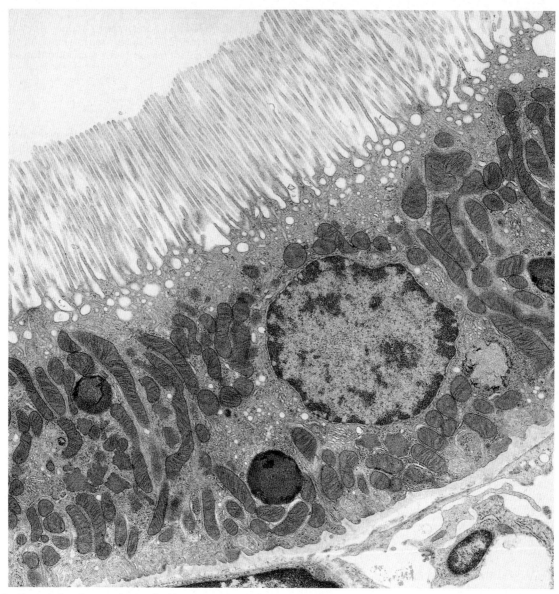

FIGURE 2–18 Transmission electron micrograph of S1 segment of rat proximal tubule. The cells are characterized by a tall brush border, a prominent endocytic-lysosomal apparatus, and extensive invaginations of the basolateral plasma membrane. (Magnification, ×10,600.)

distinguished between the convoluted and the straight portions of the proximal tubule rather than the S1, S2, and S3 segments, the former distinction is used in the following description.

Pars Convoluta

The individual cells of the pars convoluta are extremely complex in shape as described for the S1 segment of the rat proximal tubule (Fig. 2–21).[154] From the main cell body, large primary ridges extend laterally from the apical to the basal surface of the cells. Lateral processes large enough to contain mitochondria extend outward from the primary ridges and interdigitate with similar processes from adjacent cells. These lateral processes can be demonstrated by scanning electron microscopy (Fig. 2–22). At the luminal surface of the cells, smaller apical lateral processes extend outward from the primary ridges to interdigitate with those of adjacent cells. Small basal villi that do not contain mitochondria are found along the basal cell surface (see Fig. 2–21).

As a result of the extensive interdigitations of lateral and basal processes between adjacent cells, a complex extracellular compartment is formed. It is referred to as the basolateral intercellular space (Fig. 2–23; see Fig. 2–22). This space is separated from the tubule lumen by a specialization of the plasma membrane called the zonula occludens, or tight junction.[155] The zonula occludens forms a continuous band around the luminal surface of each cell, where the outer leaflets of the plasma membrane of adjacent cells appear to be fused, resulting in a pentilaminar appearance of the tight junction. Early tracer studies employing high-molecular-weight substances such as ferritin,[156] peroxidase,[157] and hemoglobin[155] failed to provide morphologic evidence of a pathway between proximal tubule cells. However, physiologic and electrophysiologic studies have revealed the presence of a low-resistance shunt pathway in parallel with a high-resistance pathway across the apical and basal plasma membranes of the proximal tubule cell.[158–160] The low-resistance pathway is believed to be formed by the tight junction and the lateral intercellular space. In ultrastructural studies of in vivo perfused rat proxi-

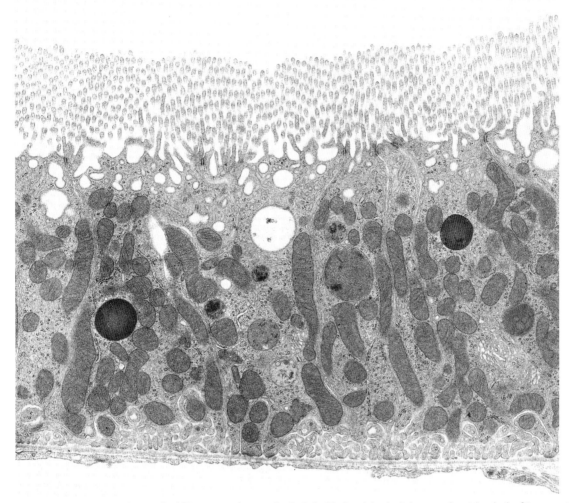

FIGURE 2–19   Transmission electron micrograph of S2 segment of rat proximal tubule. The brush border is less prominent than in the S1 segment. Note numerous small lateral processes at the base of the cell. (Magnification, ×10,600.)

mal tubules, Tisher and Yarger[161] demonstrated that both ionic and colloidal lanthanum were capable of penetrating the entire region of the tight junction from either the luminal or the peritubular surface of the cell. These results were confirmed by Martinez-Palomo and Erlij[162] thus providing further support for the existence of a paracellular pathway in the proximal tubule.

Freeze-fracture electron microscopy of proximal convoluted tubules of mouse,[163] several other species of animals including rat and rabbit,[164] and human kidney[165] has revealed that the tight junction is formed by one or two strands. These strands are equivalent to ridges on the P face (that half of the plasma membrane adjacent to the cytoplasm of the cell) and grooves on the E face (that half of the plasma membrane adjacent to the intercellular space). In the proximal convoluted tubule of the rat, up to 10% of the strands forming the tight junction are discontinuous,[164] which may explain the ability of lanthanum to penetrate the tight junction of the proximal convoluted tubule. Thus, morphologic as well as physiologic data provide evidence for the presence of a paracellular shunt pathway between cells of the mammalian proximal convoluted tubule.

Immediately beneath the tight junction is a second specialized region of the plasma membrane, termed the intermediate junction or zonula adherens.[155] It is a seven-layered structure formed by the two adjacent, triple-layered plasma membranes separated by a narrow upper extension of the intercellular space. Dense condensations of cytoplasm are located adjacent to the regions of the plasma membranes that form the intermediate junction. Desmosomes, or maculae adherentes, are also found in the proximal convoluted tubule, distributed randomly at variable distances beneath the intermediate junction. These seven-layered structures are also formed by the two adjacent plasma membranes and the intervening intercellular space. However, they are disk-shaped rather than belt-like in configuration and they are responsible for cell-cell adhesion. Gap junctions are present in small numbers in mammalian and invertebrate renal proximal tubules.[166] They are specialized connections between adjacent cells where the plasma membranes are separated by a 2-nm gap that contains characteristic subunits. The gap junction is believed to provide a pathway for the movement of ions between cells.

The intercellular space is open toward the basement membrane, which separates it from the peritubular interstitium and capillaries. The thickness of the basement membrane gradually decreases along the proximal tubule. In the rhesus monkey, it decreases in thickness from approximately 250 nm in the S1 segment to 145 nm in the S2 segment and to only 70 nm in the S3 segment.[153] In the rat, the basement membrane of the proximal convoluted tubule was found to be 143 nm in thickness.[167]

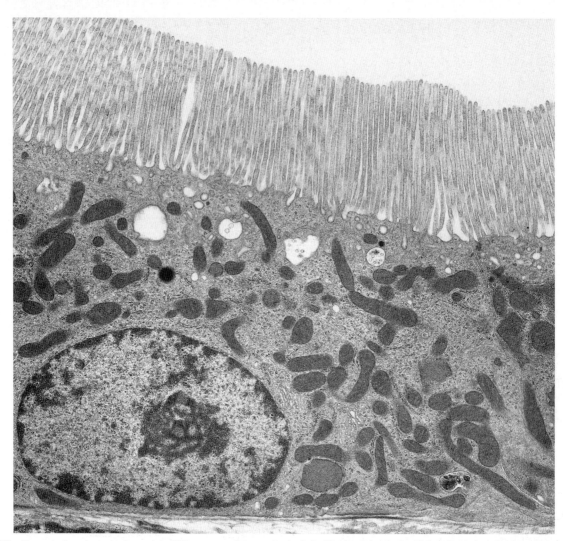

FIGURE 2–20   Transmission electron micrograph of S3 segment of rat proximal tubule. The brush border is tall, but the endocytic-lysosomal apparatus is less prominent than in the S1 and S2 segments. Basolateral invaginations are sparse, and mitochondria are scattered randomly throughout the cytoplasm. (Magnification, ×10,600.)

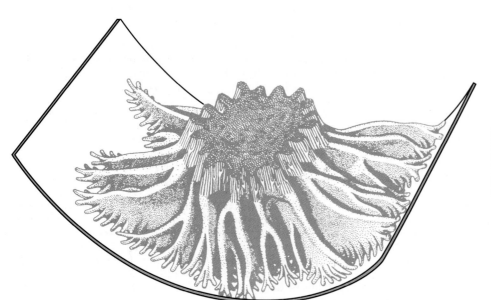

FIGURE 2–21   Schematic drawing illustrating three-dimensional configuration of proximal convoluted tubule cell. (From Welling LW, Welling DJ: Shape of epithelial cells and intercellular channels in the rabbit proximal nephron. Kidney Int 9:385, 1976.)

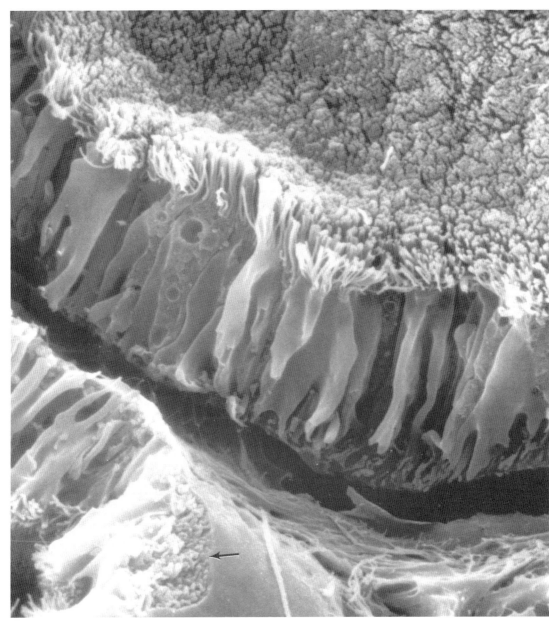

FIGURE 2–22   Scanning electron micrograph of proximal convoluted tubule illustrating prominent lateral cell processes. Arrow on adjacent proximal convoluted tubule denotes small basal processes. (Magnification, ×8200.) (From Madsen KM, Brenner BM: Structure and function of the renal tubule and interstitium. *In* Tisher CC, Brenner BM (eds): Renal Pathology with Clinical and Functional Correlations. Philadelphia, JB Lippincott, 1989, p 606.)

The lateral cell processes and invaginations of the plasma membrane serve to increase the intercellular space and the area of the basolateral plasma membrane, where the sodium-potassium adenosine triphosphatase (Na$^+$,K$^+$-ATPase) or Na$^+$ pump is located.[168,169] Morphometric studies of the proximal convoluted tubule in the rabbit have demonstrated that the area of the lateral surface equals that of the luminal surface and amounts to 2.9 mm^2/mm tubule.[170] Elongated mitochondria are located in the lateral cell processes in close proximity to the plasma membrane (see Fig. 2–23), an arrangement that is characteristic of epithelia involved in active ion transport. With standard transmission electron microscopy, these organelles appear rod-shaped and tortuous; however, studies using high-voltage electron microscopy of 0.5- to 1.0-μm-thick sections have revealed that many mitochondria in the proximal tubule are branched and anastomose with one another.[171] A system of smooth membranes, called the paramembranous

cisternal system, is often observed between the plasma membrane and the mitochondria. The function of the paramembranous cisternal system is not known, but studies suggest that it is in continuity with the smooth endoplasmic reticulum.[172]

The cells throughout the proximal tubule contain large quantities of smooth and rough endoplasmic reticulum, and free ribosomes are also abundant in the cytoplasm. A well-developed Golgi apparatus is located above and lateral to the nucleus in the midregion of the cell. It is composed of four basic elements: smooth-surfaced sacs or cisternae, coated vesicles, uncoated vesicles, and larger vacuoles. The cisternae form parallel stacks that possess a convex surface, the cis side, and a concave surface, the trans side, from which small, coated vesicles appear to bud off (Fig. 2–24). An extensive system of microtubules is located throughout the cytoplasm of the proximal tubule cells.

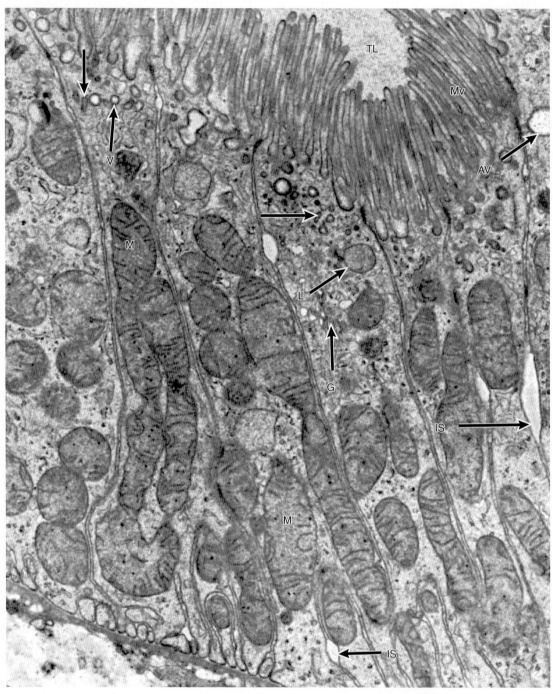

FIGURE 2–23 Electron micrograph of the pars convoluta of the proximal tubule from a normal human kidney. The mitochondria (M) are elongated and tortuous, occasionally doubling back on themselves. The endocytic apparatus, composed of apical vacuoles (AV), apical vesicles (V), and apical dense tubules (arrows), is well developed. G, Golgi apparatus; IS, intercellular space; L, lysosome; Mv, microvilli forming the brush border; TL, tubule lumen. (Magnification, ×15,000.)

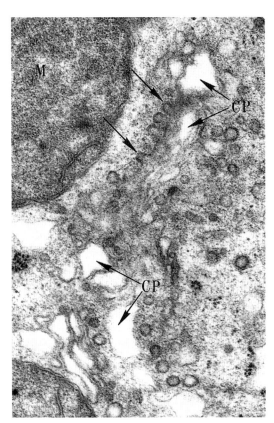

FIGURE 2–24 Electron micrograph of a Golgi apparatus from a normal human proximal tubule. Small vesicles (arrows) consistent with the appearance of primary lysosomes are seen budding from the larger cisternal profiles (CP). M, mitochondrion. (Magnification, ×32,900.) (From Tisher CC, Bulger RE, Trump BF: Human renal ultrastructure. I. Proximal tubule of healthy individuals. Lab Invest 15:1357, 1966.)

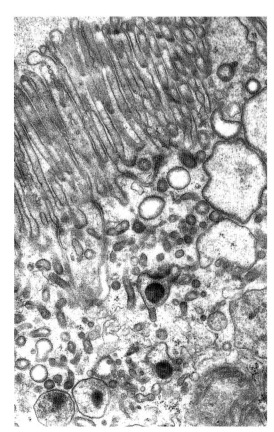

FIGURE 2–25 Transmission electron micrograph of the apical region of a human proximal tubule, illustrating the endocytic apparatus, including coated pits, coated vesicles, apical dense tubules, and endosomes. (Magnification, ×18,500.)

A well-developed brush border forms the apical or luminal surface of the proximal convoluted tubule. It is formed by numerous finger-like projections of the apical plasma membrane, the microvilli (see Figs. 2–18 through 2–20). Morphometric studies performed on isolated segments of rabbit proximal convoluted tubules found that the brush border increases the apical cell surface 36-fold.[170] On cross section, 6 to 10 filaments, approximately 6 nm in diameter, can be seen within individual microvilli, often extending downward into the apical region of the cell for considerable distances. A network of filaments, called the terminal web, is located in the apical cytoplasm just beneath and perpendicular to the microvilli.[173] The filaments of the microvilli are actin filaments. Immunocytochemical studies have demonstrated the presence of the cytoskeletal proteins, villin and fimbrin, in the microvillar core, whereas myosin and spectrin were found in the terminal web.[174] It is well established that the protein composition of the brush border membrane is different from that of the basolateral membrane.[175] Biochemical studies have reported the presence of alkaline phosphatase, aminopeptidase, 5′-nucleotidase, and Mg^{2+}-ATPase activity within brush border membranes from the kidney cortex while Na^+-K^+-ATPase is present in the basolateral plasma membrane.[175] Furthermore, immunocytochemical studies have demonstrated microdomains with different glycoproteins in brush border membranes. The Heymann nephritis antigen (gp330 or megalin) is located mainly in the apical invaginations between the microvilli, whereas maltase, a disaccharidase, is concentrated on the microvilli.[176] Ecto-5′-

nucleotidase, which is involved in the generation of adenosine, is also expressed in the brush border of the proximal tubule.[177]

The pars convoluta of the proximal tubule contains a well-developed endocytic-lysosomal apparatus that is involved in the reabsorption and degradation of macromolecules from the ultrafiltrate.[178] The endocytic compartment consists of an extensive system of coated pits, small coated vesicles, apical dense tubules, and larger endocytic vacuoles without a cytoplasmic coat (Fig. 2–25). The coated pits are invaginations of the apical plasma membrane at the base of the microvilli that form the brush border. The cytoplasmic coat of the small vesicles is similar in ultrastructure to the coat that is present on the cytoplasmic side of the coated pits. Immunocytochemical studies have demonstrated that this coat contains clathrin,[179] a protein believed to play a role in receptor-mediated endocytosis. The Heymann nephritis antigen demonstrated in brush border membranes from the proximal tubule is also located mainly in the clathrin-coated pits and clathrin-coated vesicles.[176,180]

A large number of lysosomes are present in the proximal convoluted tubule. Lysosomes are membrane-bound, heterogeneous organelles that contain a variety of acid hydrolases, including acid phosphatase, and various proteases, lipases, and glycosidases (Fig. 2–26).[178,181] They vary considerably in size, shape, and ultrastructural appearance. Lysosomes are involved in the degradation of material absorbed by endocytosis (heterophagocytosis), and they often contain multiple electron-dense deposits that are believed to

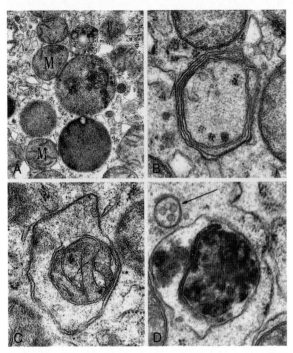

FIGURE 2–26 Electron micrographs illustrating the appearance of different types of lysosomes from human proximal tubules. **A,** Lysosomes. Several mitochondria (M) are also shown. (Magnification, ×15,500.) **B,** Early stage of formation of an autophagic vacuole. (Magnification, ×23,500.) **C,** Fully formed autolysosome containing a mitochondrion undergoing digestion. (Magnification, ×28,500.) **D,** Autolysosome, containing a microbody undergoing digestion. A multivesicular body (arrow) is also shown. (Magnification, ×29,250.) (From Tisher CC, Bulger RE, Trump BF: Human renal ultrastructure. I. Proximal tubule of healthy individuals. Lab Invest 15:1357, 1966.)

represent reabsorbed substances such as proteins (see Fig. 2–26). Lysosomes also play a role in the normal turnover of intracellular constituents by autophagocytosis, and autophagic vacuoles containing fragments of cell organelles are often seen in the proximal tubule (see Fig. 2–26).[181] Lysosomes containing nondigestible residues are called residual bodies, and they can empty their contents into the tubule lumen by exocytosis. Multivesicular bodies that are part of the vacuolar-lysosomal system are often observed in the cytoplasm of the proximal convoluted tubule. They are believed to be involved in membrane retrieval or membrane disposal (or both).

Studies using the weak base N-(3-((2,4-dinitrophenyl)amino) propyl)-N-(3-aminopropyl) methylamine dihydrochloride (DAMP), in combination with immunocytochemical techniques at the ultrastructural level, to identify intracellular acidic compartments in the proximal tubule of the rat and rabbit found that lysosomes and a population of endosomes were acidic.[182,183] In agreement with these observations, biochemical studies demonstrated the presence of an electrogenic H+ pump in endosomes isolated from the kidney cortex.[184] Furthermore, immunocytochemical studies using antibodies to the vacuolar H+ pump demonstrated labeling of both endosomes and the apical plasma membrane at the base of the microvilli, thus confirming that an H+-ATPase exists in these structures.[185] Polybasic cationic drugs, such as aminoglycoside antibiotics, are absorbed and accumulate in acidic organelles in the proximal tubule.[186] Certain heavy metals also accumulate in renal lysosomes, probably because they are bound to protein in the tubule fluid and undergo endocytosis.[187] Long-term exposure to mercuric chloride was found to cause both structural and functional changes in the lysosomal system of the proximal tubule of the rat.[188,189]

The vacuolar-lysosomal system plays an important role in the reabsorption and degradation of albumin and low-molecular-weight plasma proteins from the glomerular filtrate.[178,190,191] Proteins are absorbed from the tubule lumen by endocytosis or pinocytosis (Fig. 2–27). By this process, the protein becomes located in invaginations of the apical plasma membrane—the so-called coated pits—which pinch off to form small coated vesicles. The coated vesicles fuse with endosomes and the absorbed protein is transferred through the endosomal compartment to the lysosomes, where it is catabolized by proteolytic enzymes. The apical dense tubules are part of the vacuolar system and are believed to be involved in the recycling of membrane back to the apical plasma membrane.[192] Interestingly, binding sites for insulin are present on both the apical and basolateral plasma membrane. However, the uptake of insulin is much greater from the luminal side than from the peritubular side.[193]

Under normal conditions, the vacuolar-lysosomal system is most prominent in the S1 segment.[147,149] In proteinuric states, however, with large amounts of protein being presented to the proximal tubule cells, large vacuoles—the so-called protein droplets—and lysosomes can be observed in the proximal tubule, especially in the S2 segment. In agreement with these ultrastructural observations, biochemical studies on individual tubule segments have demonstrated that under normal nonproteinuric conditions, the activity of the lysosomal proteolytic enzymes, cathepsins B and L, is significantly higher in the S1 segment than in the S2 and S3 segments of the proximal tubule.[147,194] In proteinuric conditions, the activity of cathepsins B and L in the proximal tubule is increased, and activity is highest in the S2 segment.[194]

Studies in the isolated perfused rat kidney,[195] in vivo micropuncture studies,[196] and studies using isolated perfused rabbit proximal tubule,[197,198] have provided evidence that the absorption of protein by the proximal tubule is a selective process determined by the net charge, size, and configuration of the protein molecule and possibly by the presence of preferential endocytic sites on the apical plasma membrane. Based on studies by Farquhar and co-workers[199] and by Christensen and Birn,[200] it is now generally accepted that the reabsorption of numerous proteins and polypeptides by the proximal tubule is mediated by megalin, a multiligand endocytic receptor. Kerjaschki and Farquhar[180] purified megalin (gp330) from rat kidney brush border membrane and demonstrated that it represents the antigen for rat Heymann nephritis. Megalin was subsequently cloned and found to be a 600-kD glycoprotein belonging to the low-density-lipoprotein receptor gene family.[201] The receptor-associated protein, RAP, which binds to megalin, is also an antigen for Heymann nephritis. RAP is believed to function as a chaperone for megalin.[199] Immunocytochemical studies have demonstrated that megalin is located in the brush border, coated pits, endocytic vesicles, and apical dense tubules in the proximal tubule, particularly in the S2 segment (Fig. 2–28).[176,202,203]

As reviewed in detail by Christensen and Birn,[200] megalin serves as a receptor for numerous ligands, including low-molecular-weight proteins,[204] polypeptide hormones,[204] albumin,[205] vitamin-binding proteins,[206–208] and polybasic drugs such as aminoglycosides.[209] Orlando and co-workers[204] demonstrated that megalin binds and internalizes insulin, and evidence was also provided from ligand blotting assays that megalin serves as a receptor for various low-molecular-weight polypeptides including β2-microglobulin, lysozyme, prolactin, cytochrome C, and epidermal growth factor. Moestrup, Christensen, Nykjaer, and their co-workers[206–208] demonstrated that megalin serves as the principal receptor for the

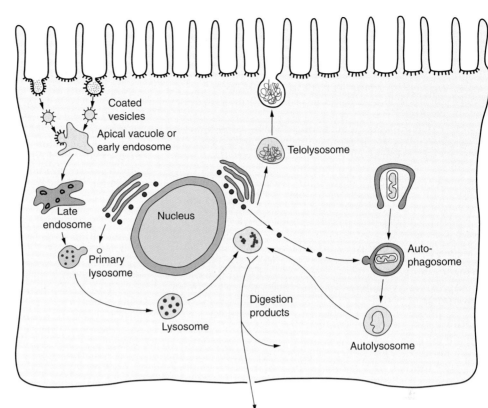

FIGURE 2–27 Schematic drawing of the endocytic-lysosomal system in a proximal tubule cell.

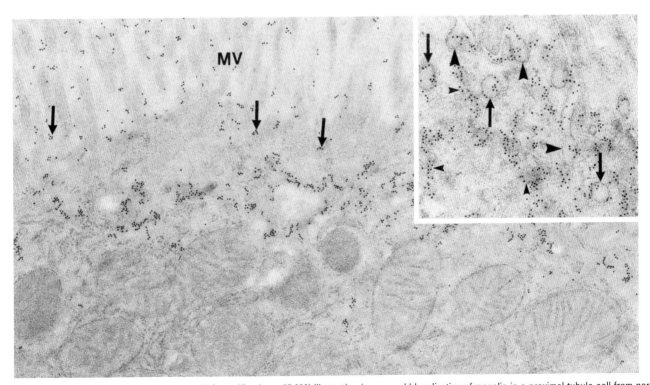

FIGURE 2–28 Transmission electron micrograph (magnification, ×35,000) illustrating immunogold localization of megalin in a proximal tubule cell from normal mouse kidney. Labeling of megalin is seen on microvilli (MV), coated pits (arrows), and the apical endocytic apparatus. Inset is a higher-magnification (×53,000) micrograph illustrating the labeling of coated pits (large arrowheads), apical endosomes (arrows), and apical dense tubules (small arrowheads). (From Christensen EI, Willnow TE: Essential role of megalin in renal proximal tubule for vitamin homeostasis. J Am Soc Nephrol 10:2224, 1999.)

carrier proteins of various vitamins, including vitamin B_{12}, vitamin D, and retinol, suggesting that megalin may play a role in vitamin metabolism and homeostasis.[210] Other studies demonstrated a loss of components of the endocytic apparatus and increased excretion of low-molecular-weight proteins in the urine of megalin-deficient mice, providing further support for the role of megalin in proximal tubule reabsorption of protein.[210,211]

A second multiligand endocytic receptor, cubilin, which is identical to the intestinal intrinsic factor–cobalamin receptor, has been identified in the proximal tubule.[200,212] Cubilin is a 460 kD glycoprotein that binds to megalin. It is expressed in the brush border and in the endocytic compartment in a pattern similar to that of megalin.[200] Studies by Christensen, Birn, and their co-workers[212,213] demonstrated that cubilin binds several ligands present in the glomerular ultrafiltrate, including albumin and various vitamin-binding proteins, and that both megalin and cubilin are essential for the reabsorption of these proteins in the proximal tubule.

The proximal convoluted tubule plays a major role in the reabsorption of Na^+, HCO_3^-, Cl^-, K^+, Ca^{2+}, PO_4^{3-}, water, and organic solutes such as glucose and amino acids. Approximately half of the ultrafiltrate is reabsorbed in the proximal tubule. Fluid reabsorption is coupled to the active transport of Na^+, and little change occurs in the osmolality or in the Na^+ concentration of the tubule fluid along the proximal tubule, indicating that fluid reabsorption in this segment is almost isosmotic.[214] The rate of fluid absorption from the proximal tubule to the peritubular capillaries is influenced by the hydraulic and oncotic pressures across the tubule and capillary wall. Changes in these parameters cause significant ultrastructural changes in the proximal tubule, especially in the configuration of the lateral intercellular spaces.[215,216]

In the early 1990s Preston and co-workers cloned a water channel protein, CHIP28 or aquaporin-1 (AQP1), from human erythrocytes.[217,218] AQP1 is believed to mediate osmotic water permeability in red blood cells as well as in renal tubule cells. Immunocytochemical studies[219–221] using antibodies to AQP1 demonstrated the presence of this water channel protein in both the proximal tubule (Fig. 2–29) and the descending thin limb, segments known to have high osmotic water permeability. Labeling was observed in both the apical and the basolateral plasma membrane, which indicates that water is reabsorbed across the epithelium through these channels in response to the existent osmotic gradient. AQP8[222,223] is also expressed in the renal proximal tubule where it is located mainly in intracellular structures with little or no expression at the plasma membrane.[224] Biophysical studies in Xenopus oocytes and yeast have revealed that AQP8 conducts water as well as ammonia/ammonium and formamide.[225,226] AQP8 gene knockout mice have no major phenotype. Thus, the role of AQP8 remains to be established.

Aquaporin-11 (AQP11) is a channel protein with unusual pore-forming NPA (asparagine-proline-alanine) boxes.[227] Immunocytochemical studies have demonstrated intracellular expression of AQP11 in the proximal tubule[228] as well as in AQP11-transfected CHO-K1 cells. A predominantly intracellular expression has also been reported in other cell types including cells in the brain.[229] AQP11-null mice exhibit vacuolization and cyst formation of the proximal tubule.[228] The mice appeared normal at birth, but developed polycystic kidneys and died before weaning due to advanced renal failure. Interestingly, primary cultured proximal tubule cells from AQP11-null mice exhibited an endosomal acidification defect. However, the physiologic role of AQP11 in the proximal tubule remains to be identified.

Sodium reabsorption by the proximal tubule is an active process driven by Na^+,K^+-ATPase, which is located in the basolateral plasma membrane, as demonstrated by both histochemical[230] and immunocytochemical[169] studies. The active transport of Na^+ out of the cell across the basolateral membrane creates a lumen-to-cell concentration gradient for Na^+. The transport of various anions and organic solutes is coupled with the transport of Na^+ down its concentration gradient.[231] The main anions transported together with Na^+ are HCO_3^- and Cl^-. HCO_3^- reabsorption takes place primarily in the early proximal tubule and is secondary to H^+ secretion, which is mediated predominantly by an Na^+/H^+ exchange mechanism located in the brush border membrane.[232,233] Studies in several laboratories have demonstrated expression of the Na^+/H^+ exchanger isoform, NHE3, in the brush border of the proximal tubule.[234,235] In addition, there is evidence that active H^+ secretion mediated by an H^+-ATPase occurs in the proximal tubule.[236] An H^+-ATPase has been demonstrated in brush border membrane vesicles[237] as well as in endosome vesicles isolated from the kidney cortex.[184] Immunocytochemical studies using antibodies to a renal H^+-ATPase have revealed labeling of both endosomes and coated pits at the base of the brush border microvilli, which supports the presence of H^+-ATPase at both sites.[185] Studies in mice lacking the NHE3 have confirmed the importance of NHE3 for bicarbonate and fluid reabsorption in the proximal convoluted tubule.[238,239] The expression and activity of NHE3 is regulated by various hormones, including angiotensin II and aldosterone.[240,241] The regulation involves multiple signaling pathways and molecules such as PKA/cAMP and EPAC,[242] NHERF-1,[243,244] and Rho GTPases.[245] It has also been suggested that mechanosensory pathways involving the microvilli may play a role in the regulation of NHE3 in the proximal tubule.[246]

Bicarbonate reabsorption in the proximal tubule is mediated by an electrogenic Na^+/HCO_3^- co-transporter, NBC1, with a stoichiometry of 3 HCO_3^- for each Na^+.[247,248] NBC1 belongs to a superfamily of bicarbonate transporters that includes the anion exchangers (AE) and the sodium bicarbonate co-transporters (NBC).[249] NBC1 in the proximal tubule was the first sodium bicarbonate co-transporter to be identified. It was cloned initially from Ambystoma[250] and later from both human[251] and rat kidney.[252] In situ hybridization studies in the rabbit kidney demonstrated that NBC1 mRNA was present only in the renal cortex where it was localized to the proximal tubule.[253] Subsequent immunofluorescence studies in rat and rabbit[254] and high-resolution electron microscopic studies in the rat kidney[255] revealed that NBC1 was expressed exclusively in the basolateral plasma membrane of the S1 and S2 segments of the proximal tubule (Fig. 2–30). This is in agreement with the results of physiologic studies demonstrating that bicarbonate is reabsorbed primarily in the initial part of the proximal tubule.[233] Humans with mutations in NBC1 develop permanent proximal renal tubular acidosis with associated ocular abnormalities consistent with NBC1 being the primary pathway for basolateral bicarbonate transport.[256]

The proximal tubule is a major site of ammonia production in the kidney.[257–259] Ammonia is produced in the mitochondria from the metabolism of glutamine. At the pH that exists in the proximal tubule cells, ammonia combines with H^+ to form NH_4^+, which is secreted into the tubule lumen.[260]

Pars Recta

The pars recta of the proximal tubule consists of the terminal portion of the S2 segment and the entire S3 segment. The epithelium of the S3 segment is simpler than that of the S1 and S2 segments.[149,151] Basolateral invaginations of the plasma membrane are virtually absent, mitochondria are small and randomly scattered throughout the cytoplasm, and the intercellular spaces are smaller and less complex (Fig. 2–31;

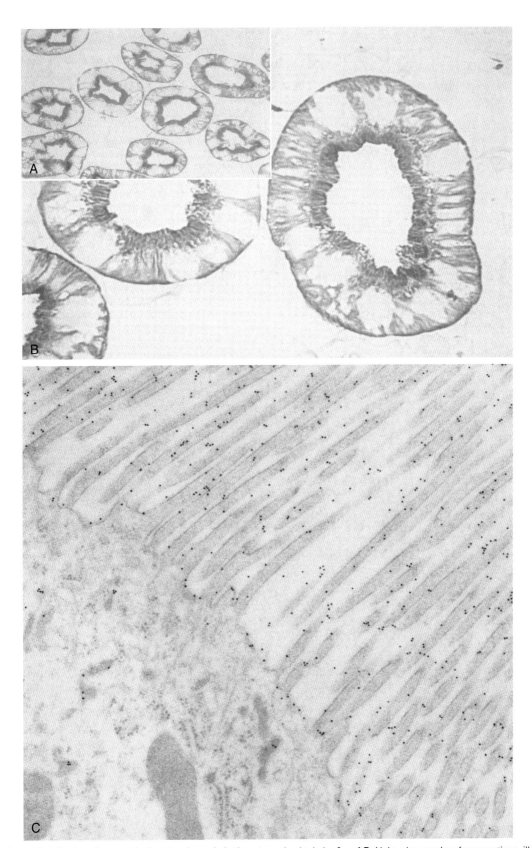

FIGURE 2–29 Immunolocalization of aquaporin-1 water channels in the rat proximal tubule. **A and B,** Light micrographs of cryosections, illustrating immuno-staining of the apical and basolateral plasma membrane of the S3 segment of the proximal tubule with use of a horseradish peroxidase technique. (Magnification: A, ×670; B, ×800.) **C,** Electron micrograph of cryosubstituted Lowicryl section, illustrating immunogold labeling of microvilli and apical invaginations of the S3 segment of the proximal tubule. (Magnification, ×48,000.)

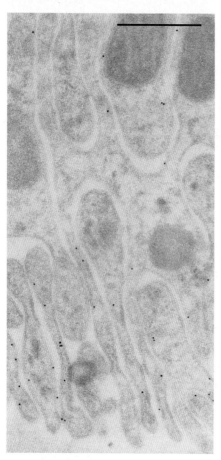

FIGURE 2–30 Transmission electron micrograph illustrating immunogold localization of NBC1 in the basal part of a proximal convoluted tubule cell from normal rat kidney. Labeling of NBC1 is seen on the cytoplasmic side of the basolateral plasma membrane. (Magnification, ×68,000.) (From Maunsbach AB, Vorum H, Kwon TH, et al: Immunoelectron microscopic localization of the electrogenic Na/HCO(3) cotransporter in rat and ambystoma kidney. J Am Soc Nephrol 11:2179, 2000.)

see Fig. 2–20). These morphologic characteristics are in agreement with results of biochemical studies demonstrating that Na+,K+-ATPase activity is significantly lower in the pars recta than in the pars convoluta.[261] In addition, studies examining transport parameters in individual segments of the proximal tubule have demonstrated that fluid reabsorption in the S3 segment is significantly less than in the S1 and S2 segments.[262]

The morphologic appearance of the pars recta varies considerably among species. In the rat, the microvilli of the brush border measure up to 4 μm in length, whereas in the rabbit and human kidney they are much shorter. The vacuolar-lysosomal system is less prominent in the S3 segment of the proximal tubule. However, in both rabbit and human, many small lysosomes with electron-dense membrane-like material are common in the S3 segment.[147,150] The specific role of lysosomes in this segment is not known.

Peroxisomes are common in the pars recta. In contrast to lysosomes, the peroxisomes are surrounded by a 6.5-nm-thick membrane and do not contain acid hydrolases.[181] Peroxisomes are irregular in shape and vary considerably in appearance among species. In the rat, small, circular profiles can be observed just inside the limiting membrane, and rod-shaped structures often project outward from the organelle. In addition, a small nucleoid is often present in peroxi-somes in the rat proximal tubule. In the proximal tubule of both rabbit and human, electron-dense structures called marginal plates are located at the periphery of the organelle (see Fig. 2–31). The functional significance of the peroxisomes in the kidney is not known with certainty; however, they are believed to be involved in lipid metabolism and to play a role in fatty acid oxidation. They have a high content of catalase, which is involved in the degradation of hydrogen peroxide, and of various oxidative enzymes, including L-α-hydroxy-acid oxidase and D-amino acid oxidase.[263,264]

The pars recta of the proximal tubule is involved in the secretion of organic anions and cations and it is a portion of the nephron that is often damaged by nephrotoxic compounds, including various drugs and heavy metals. Woodhall and colleagues[152] examined the secretion of p-aminohippuric acid, an organic anion, in individual S1, S2, and S3 segments of superficial and juxtamedullary proximal tubules of the rabbit and found that secretion was significantly higher in the S2 segment of both nephron populations. In similar studies of organic cation transport, McKinney[265] demonstrated that the secretion of procainamide was greatest in S1 segments of superficial nephrons and in S1 and S2 segments of juxtamedullary nephrons.

Recent studies from several laboratories have identified a family of transporters involved in the uptake of organic anions and cations across the basolateral membrane into the cells of the proximal tubule.[266] The organic ion transporters play an important role in the excretion of numerous commonly used drugs, including various antibiotics, nonsteroidal anti-inflammatory drugs, loop diuretics, and the immunosuppressive drug cyclosporine.[266] The uptake of organic anions, including p-aminohippuric acid, from the blood into the proximal tubule cells is mediated by an organic anion transporter, OAT1, which has been cloned[267–269] and found to be expressed in the proximal tubule by both in situ hybridization[267,268] and immunohistochemistry.[270,271] In the kidney, OAT1 is present only in the basolateral plasma membrane of the proximal tubule, and studies in the rat have demonstrated that OAT1 is expressed predominantly in the S2 segment of the proximal tubule.[271] Organic cation transporters, OCT1 and OCT2, have also been demonstrated in the proximal tubule of the rat.[272] By in situ hybridization, expression of both OCT1 and OCT2 was detected in all three segments of the proximal tubule. By immunohistochemistry, OCT1 was observed mainly in S1 and S2 segments, whereas OCT2 was expressed in S2 and S3 segments.[272]

The aquaglyceroporin AQP7, which is abundantly expressed in the testis[273] has also been demonstrated in the proximal tubule brush border[274,275] but exclusively in the part recta. AQP7 knockout mice fail to reabsorb glycerol and exhibit marked glyceroluria[276] indicating a role for AQP7 in glycerol metabolism.

Thin Limbs of the Loop of Henle

The transition from the proximal tubule to the descending thin limb of the loop of Henle is abrupt (Figs. 2–32 and 2–33) and marks the boundary between the outer and inner stripes of the outer medulla. Short-looped nephrons originating from superficial and midcortical glomeruli have a short descending thin limb located in the inner stripe of the outer medulla. Close to the hairpin turn of the short loops of Henle, the thin limb continues into the thick ascending limb. Long-looped nephrons originating from juxtamedullary glomeruli have a long descending thin limb that extends into the inner medulla and a long ascending thin limb that continues into the thick

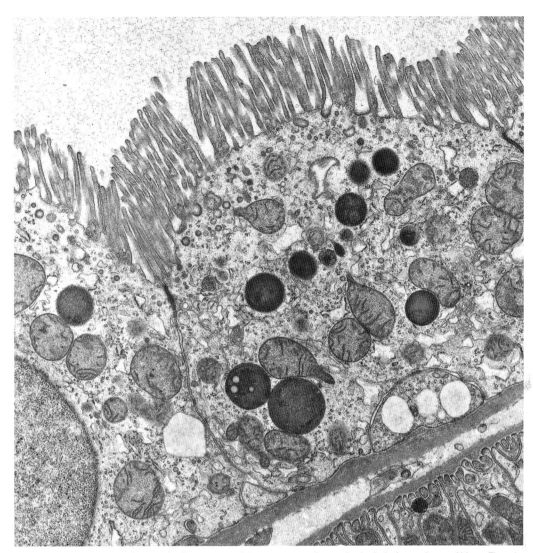

FIGURE 2-31   Low-magnification electron micrograph of a segment of the pars recta of a proximal tubule from a human kidney. The microvilli on the convex apical cell surface are not as long as those from the pars recta of the rat. The lysosomes are extremely electron-dense. The clear, single- membrane-limited structures at the base of the cell to the right represent lipid droplets. (Magnification, ×10,400.) (Courtesy of R.E. Bulger, PhD.)

ascending limb. The transition from the thin to the thick ascending limb forms the boundary between the outer and inner medulla (see Fig. 2-5). Nephrons arising in the extreme outer cortex may possess short cortical loops that do not extend into the medulla.

Considerable effort has been expended toward identification of the histotopographic organization of the renal medulla in several laboratory animals. Most mammals, including rabbits, guinea pigs, prairie dogs, cats, dogs, pigs, and humans, have a simple medulla in which the vascular bundles contain only descending and ascending vasa recta. The thin limb segments of both short- and long-looped nephrons are located outside the vascular bundles.[277] In contrast, most animals with a high urine concentrating ability, such as the rat,[278] mouse,[279] and desert sand rat (Psammomys obesus),[280] have a complex medulla in which the descending thin limbs of the short-looped nephrons are incorporated into the vascular bundles in the outer medulla together with the vasa recta. Descending thin limbs from long-looped nephrons descend through the outer medulla outside the vascular bundles, in the so-called interbundle regions. In

most species studied thus far, the inner medulla appears to lack the discrete compartmentalization that is characteristic of the outer medulla.[281] Recent 3-D reconstruction studies of the mouse nephron indicate that a highly complex structural relationship exists between the thin limb segments and the thick ascending limbs in the outer medulla of the mouse.[282]

Early ultrastructural studies demonstrated that the cells of the initial part of the descending thin limb of Henle were complex because of extensive interdigitation with one another, whereas the cells of the ascending thin limb near the transition with the thick ascending limb, and thin limb cells in the inner medulla, were less complex in configuration. Dieterich and associates[283] later described the presence of four types of epithelia (types I through IV) in the thin limbs of the mouse kidney and devised a classification based on the ultrastructural characteristics of the cells and their location within the different regions of the medulla. Subsequent studies in other species, including rat,[277] rabbit,[151] hamster,[284] and P. obesus,[280,281] confirmed the existence of four morphologically distinct segments in the thin limb of Henle

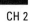

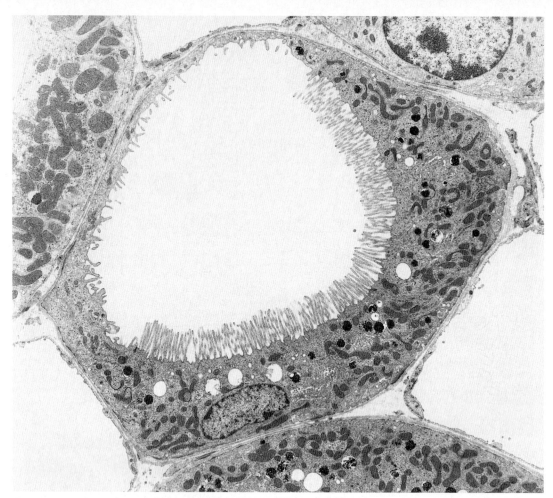

FIGURE 2–32 Transmission electron micrograph from rabbit kidney, illustrating the transition from the pars recta of the proximal tubule to the descending thin limb of the loop of Henle. (Magnification, ×4500.) (From Madsen KM, Park CH: Lysosome distribution and cathepsin B and L activity along the rabbit proximal tubule. Am J Physiol 253:F1290, 1987.)

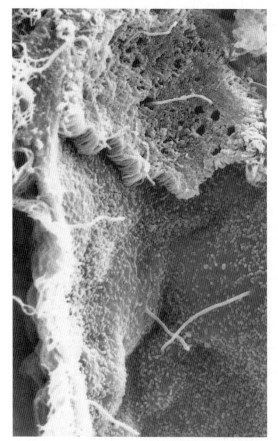

FIGURE 2–33 Scanning electron micrograph from a normal rat kidney depicting the transition from the terminal S3 segment of the proximal tubule (above) to the early descending thin limb of Henle (below). Note the elongated cilia projecting into the lumen from cells of the proximal tubule and the thin limb of Henle. (Magnification, ×4500.)

(Fig. 2–34). In these animals, type I epithelium is found exclusively in the descending thin limb of short-looped nephrons. Type II epithelium forms the descending thin limb of long-looped nephrons in the outer medulla. This epithelium gives way to type III epithelium in the inner medulla. Type IV epithelium forms the bends of the long loops and the entire ascending thin limb to the transition into the thick ascending limb at the boundary between the inner and outer medulla.

In all animals studied thus far, type I epithelium is extremely thin and has few basal or luminal surface specializations, the latter in the form of microvilli (see Fig. 2–34). There is a virtual absence of lateral interdigitations with adjacent cells, and cellular organelles are relatively sparse. Microbodies have not been identified in the thin limbs of the loop of Henle. Tight junctions between cells are intermediate in depth with several junctional strands, which suggests a tight epithelium.[285-287] Type II epithelium is taller and exhibits considerable species differences. In the rat,[278] mouse,[283] P. obesus,[281] and hamster,[284] the type II epithelium is complex and characterized by extensive lateral and basal interdigitations and a well-developed paracellular pathway (Fig. 2–35). The tight junctions are extremely shallow and contain a single junctional strand, which is characteristic of a leaky epithelium. The luminal surface is covered by short blunt microvilli, and cell organelles, including mitochondria, are more prominent than in other segments of the thin limb. In the rabbit,[151] the type II epithelium is less complex. Lateral interdigitations and paracellular pathways are less prominent, and tight junctions are deeper.[286] As in the rat and mouse, the luminal surface is covered with short microvilli, and many small mitochondria are present in the cytoplasm. In comparison with type II epithelium, type III epithelium is lower and has a simpler structure. The cells do not interdigitate, the tight junctions are intermediate in depth, and fewer microvilli cover the luminal surface. Type IV epithelium (see Fig. 2–34) is generally low and flattened and possesses relatively few organelles. It is characterized by an absence of surface microvilli but has an abundance of lateral cell processes and interdigitations as well as prominent paracellular pathways. The tight junctions are shallow and are characteristic of a leaky epithelium. The basement membrane of the thin limb segments varies greatly in thickness from species to species and in many animals is multilayered. A secreted phosphoprotein, osteopontin, is constitutively expressed in the type I and especially the type II epithelium of the descending thin limb in the inner stripe of the outer medulla.[288,289] The function of osteopontin in the descending thin limb is unknown.

Freeze-fracture studies have confirmed the structural heterogeneity along the thin limb of the loop of Henle in the rat,[287] rabbit,[286] and P. obesus.[285] Segmental as well as species

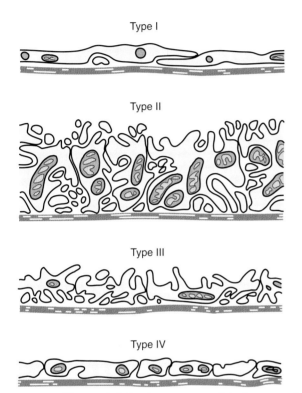

FIGURE 2–34 Diagram depicting the appearance of the four types of thin limb segments in rat kidney. (See text for explanation.)

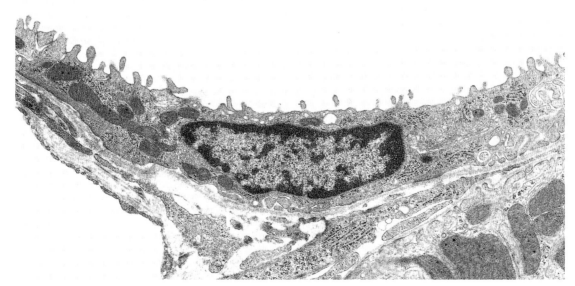

FIGURE 2–35 Transmission electron micrograph of type II epithelium of the thin limb of the loop of Henle in the inner stripe of the outer medulla of rat kidney. (Magnification, ×11,800.)

differences were found in the number of strands and the depth of the tight junctions. The most striking finding in these studies was an extremely high density of intramembrane particles in both the luminal and the basolateral membrane of type II epithelium in all animals studied. Biochemical studies in isolated nephron segments,[290] as well as histochemical studies,[230] demonstrated significant levels of Na$^+$,K$^+$-ATPase activity in type II epithelium of the thin limb in the rat. Little or no activity was present in other segments of the rat thin limb or in any segment of the rabbit thin limb.[291] The functional significance of these observations is not known. However, physiologic studies determining the permeability properties of isolated perfused segments of descending thin limbs from different species have demonstrated that the permeability of the type II epithelium to Na$^+$ and K$^+$ is higher in the rat and hamster than in the rabbit,[292] supporting the described ultrastructural and biochemical differences among species in this epithelium.

Studies of salt and water permeability in descending thin limb segments from the hamster have demonstrated that both type I and type II epithelia are highly permeable to water, whereas the permeability to Na$^+$ and Cl$^-$ is significantly higher in type II than in type I epithelium.[293] In contrast, urea permeability is higher in the type I epithelium.[293] No evidence has been found for active transport of Na$^+$ or Cl$^-$ in the thin limb of the loop of Henle. In support of the reported permeability characteristics of the different thin limb segments, immunohistochemical studies have demonstrated high levels of expression of the water channel protein, AQP1, in the descending thin limb and especially in the type II epithelium of long-looped nephrons in the outer medulla (Fig. 2–36).[219,294] There is no AQP1 immunoreactivity in the ascending thin limb and AQP1 is not expressed in the innermost part of the type I epithelium of short-looped nephrons. Detailed studies by Pannabecker and Dantzler have described the heterogeneity in the expression of AQP1 in descending thin limbs in the inner medulla. Those investigators reported that descending thin limbs that form loops more than 1 mm below the base of the inner medulla express AQP1 only in the initial portion of the segment, leaving almost 60% of the inner medullary segment of long-looped thin descending limbs with no detectable AQP1 expression.[295] Moreover, AQP1 stainable descending thin limbs and collecting ducts were separated into two distinct lateral compartments, suggesting that water transport may occur between these compartments.[296]

Interestingly, the innermost part of the thin descending limb of short-looped nephrons that lacks AQP1 does express high levels of the urea transporter, UT-A2, as demonstrated at both the mRNA[297] and protein level (Fig. 2–37).[298–302] There is also weak expression of UT-A2 mRNA and protein in the type III epithelium of the descending thin limb of long-looped nephrons in the outer portion of the inner medulla.[297,298,300–302] The expression of UT-A2 in the descending thin limb is upregulated by vasopressin,[301,302] although specific receptors for vasopressin have not been detected in this segment. The urea transporter is believed to be involved in urea recycling in the renal medulla, a process that is important for the maintenance of medullary hypertonicity.[303]

The thin limbs of the loop of Henle play an important role in the countercurrent multiplication process that is responsible for the maintenance of a hypertonic medullary interstitium and for the dilution and concentration of the urine.[303] According to the passive model of the countercurrent multiplier mechanism described by Kokko and Rector,[304] the descending thin limb epithelium is permeable to water but has a low permeability to Na$^+$ and Cl$^-$; this allows water to be extracted from the tubule fluid as the thin limb descends through the hypertonic interstitium of the medulla. In contrast, the ascending thin limb is largely impermeable to water but highly permeable to Na$^+$ and Cl$^-$, which causes salt to diffuse out of the tubule. A kidney-specific chloride channel, ClC-K1, was cloned from rat kidney and was found to be expressed in the ascending thin limb.[305] Immunohistochemical studies revealed that ClC-K1 is expressed exclusively in

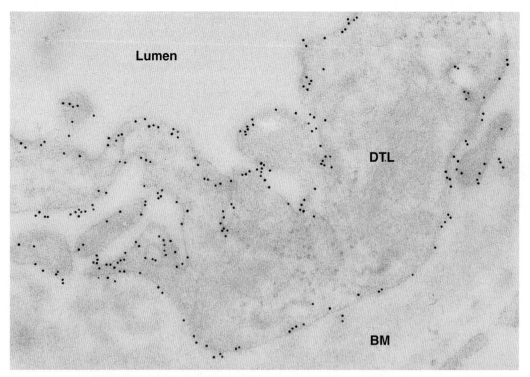

FIGURE 2–36 Transmission electron micrograph illustrating immunogold labeling of aquaporin-1 in the descending thin limb (DTL) of a long-looped nephron from rat kidney. Labeling of aquaporin-1 is seen in both the apical and basolateral plasma membrane. BM, basement membrane. (Magnification, ×120,000.) (From Nielsen S, Kwon TH, Christensen BM, et al: Physiology and pathophysiology of renal aquaporins. J Am Soc Nephrol 10:647, 1999.)

important for the maintenance of a hypertonic interstitium **55**
and for the urine concentration mechanism.

CH 2

Anatomy of the Kidney

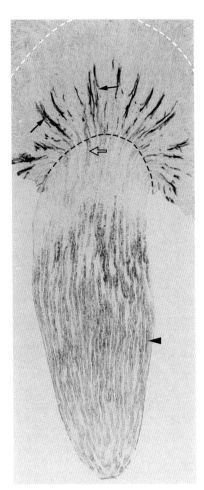

FIGURE 2–37 Light micrograph illustrating immunoperoxidase staining of the urea transporters UT-A2 in the descending thin limb of short-looped nephrons (closed arrows) and UT-A1 in the inner medullary collecting duct (arrowhead) in normal rat kidney. Open arrow indicates weak UT-A2 immunolabeling in descending thin limb segments of long-looped nephrons in the outer part of the inner medulla. (Magnification, ×20.) (Courtesy of Young-Hee Kim, PhD.)

The cells in the renal medulla are exposed to a hypertonic environment. To protect the cells against extreme changes in tonicity and allow them to maintain cell volume, intracellular organic osmolytes, including sorbitol, myoinositol, glycerophosphorylcholine, and betaine, are generated and accumulate in the cells in the renal medulla.[313,314] Several genes are known to be regulated in response to hyperosmotic stimuli. Some of these osmoprotective genes include the sodium/myo-inositol cotransporter, aldose reductase (catalyzes the enzymatic conversion of glucose to sorbitol), and heat shock protein 70.[315] The regulation of the osmoprotective genes appears to be mediated via the tonicity-responsive element (TonE)/TonE-binding protein (TonEBP) pathway,[316,317] which is activated during hyperosmotic stimuli.[318] Mice lacking the TonEBP gene suffer from increased mortality and exhibit an altered medullary morphology with atrophy of the renal medulla.[319] Consistently, mice lacking the TonEBP gene have a reduced renal expression of osmoprotective genes.[319]

Distal Tubule

The distal tubule is composed of three morphologically distinct segments: the thick ascending limb of the loop of Henle (pars recta), the macula densa, and the distal convoluted tubule (pars convoluta). Studies of rat kidney[320] and rabbit kidney[151] revealed that the cortical thick ascending limb extends beyond the vicinity of the macula densa and forms an abrupt transition with the distal convoluted tubule. Therefore, the macula densa is a specialized region of the thick ascending limb.

Thick Ascending Limb

The thick ascending limb, or pars recta, represents the initial portion of the distal tubule and can be divided into a medullary and a cortical segment (see Fig. 2–5). In long-looped nephrons, there is an abrupt transition from the thin ascending limb to the thick ascending limb, which marks the boundary between the inner medulla and the inner stripe of the outer medulla. In short-looped nephrons, the transition to the thick ascending limb occurs shortly before the hairpin turn. From its transition with the thin limb, the thick ascending limb extends upward through the outer medulla and the cortex to the glomerulus of the nephron of origin, where the macula densa is formed. At the point of contact with the extraglomerular mesangial region, only the immediately contiguous portion of the wall of the tubule actually forms the macula densa. The transition to the distal convoluted tubule occurs shortly after the macula densa. The cells forming the medullary segment in the inner stripe of the outer medulla measure approximately 7 μm to 8 μm in height.[151,321] As the tubule ascends toward the cortex, cell height gradually decreases to approximately 5 μm in the cortical thick ascending limb of the rat[321] and to 2 μm in the terminal part of the cortical thick ascending limb of the rabbit. Welling and coworkers[322] reported an average cell height of 4.5 μm in the cortical thick ascending limb of the rabbit kidney.

The cells of the thick ascending limb are characterized by extensive invaginations of the basolateral plasma membrane and interdigitations between adjacent cells. The lateral invaginations often extend a distance of two thirds or more from the base to the luminal border of the cell. This arrangement is most prominent in the thick ascending limb of the inner stripe of the outer medulla (Fig. 2–38). Numerous elongated mitochondria are located in lateral cell processes, and their orientation is perpendicular to the basement membrane. The mitochondria resemble those in the proximal tubule but contain very prominent granules in the matrix. Other subcellular organelles in this segment of the nephron include a

this segment, where it is located in both the apical and basolateral plasma membrane.[306] Expression of ClC-K1 in the ascending thin limb has also been demonstrated in the human kidney.[307] The presence of ClC-K1 in the ascending thin limb is in agreement with results of physiologic studies demonstrating that this segment is highly permeable to chloride.[308,309] Mice lacking ClC-K1 became dehydrated after water deprivation and were not able to concentrate their urine in response to vasopressin, indicating that ClC-K1 is essential for the urinary concentrating mechanism.[310]

The passive model for the countercurrent multiplier system is supported by both functional and immunohistochemical studies. However, for this model to work the permeability of the ascending thin limb to outward movement of Na⁺ and Cl⁻ must be considerably higher than the permeability to inward movement of urea from the interstitium. Evidence from studies in isolated thin limb segments from hamster[311] and chinchilla[312] suggests that the difference between the permeabilities of Na⁺ and urea in the ascending thin limb may not be sufficient to account for the osmolality gradient in the inner medulla. Various mathematical models (reviewed by Knepper and Rector[303]) have also failed to explain the countercurrent multiplication process and the concentration of solutes in the inner medulla on the basis of purely passive mechanisms. However, it is generally accepted that the permeability properties of the thin limb epithelium are extremely

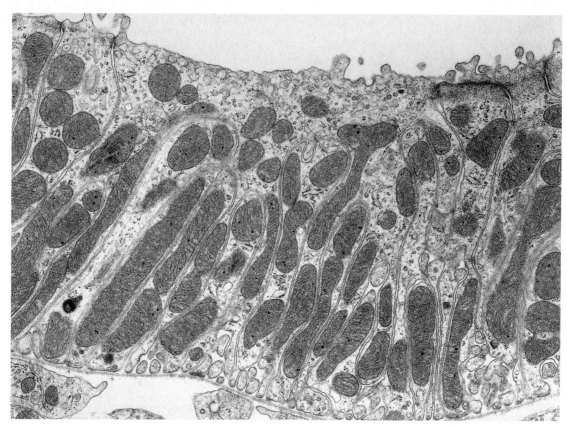

FIGURE 2–38 Transmission electron micrograph from a thick ascending limb in the outer stripe of the outer medulla of the rat. Note the deep, complex invaginations of the basal plasma membrane, which enclose elongated mitochondrial profiles and extend into the apical region of the cell. (Magnification, ×13,000.)

well-developed Golgi complex, multivesicular bodies and lysosomes, and abundant quantities of smooth- and rough-surfaced endoplasmic reticulum. Numerous small vesicles are commonly observed in the apical portion of the cytoplasm. The cells are attached to one another via tight junctions that are 0.1 μm to 0.2 μm in depth in the rat.[155] Intermediate junctions are also present, but desmosomes appear to be lacking. In the rat, ultrastructural tracer studies using colloidal lanthanum have demonstrated that the tracer readily penetrates the tight junction, which suggests the presence of a potential paracellular shunt pathway for movement of solute and fluid.[323]

Scanning electron microscopy of the thick ascending limb of the rat kidney has revealed the existence of two distinct surface configurations of the luminal membrane.[320] Some cells have a rough surface because of the presence of numerous small microprojections, whereas others have a smooth surface that is largely devoid of microprojections except along the apical cell margins (Fig. 2–39). Most cells possess one cilium; some have two cilia. The rough-surfaced cells possess more extensive lateral processes radiating from the main cell body than do the smooth-surfaced cells. In contrast, small vesicles and tubulovesicular profiles are more numerous in the apical region of the smooth-surfaced cells. A predominance of cells with the smooth-surface pattern is observed in the medullary segment. As the thick limb ascends toward the cortex, the number of cells with a rough surface pattern increases, and luminal microprojections and apical lateral invaginations become more prominent. Consequently, the surface area of the luminal plasma membrane is significantly greater in the cortical than in the medullary thick ascending limb.[321] The functional significance of the two surface configurations is not known; however, physiologic studies have provided evidence for the presence of two func-

tionally distinct cell types in the medullary thick ascending limb of the hamster.[324] One cell type has a low Cl⁻ conductance in the basolateral membrane, and the other has a high basolateral Cl⁻ conductance. Immunohistochemical studies of the localization of ROMK channels in the rat kidney have also demonstrated cellular heterogeneity along the thick ascending limb.[325,326] Some cells exhibited strong ROMK immunoreactivity in the apical plasma membrane, whereas other cells showed little or no labeling for ROMK. Tamm-Horsfall protein is a glycoprotein that is produced and secreted by the thick ascending limb. It has been demonstrated along the luminal membrane of the thick ascending limb of both the rat[114] and human[327] kidney, and by use of the immunogold technique, labeling was found mainly over apical vesicles.[328] The functional significance of Tamm-Horsfall protein in the distal tubule is not known.

The thick ascending limb is involved in active transport of NaCl from the lumen to the surrounding interstitium. Because this epithelium is almost impermeable to water, the reabsorption of salt contributes to the formation of a hypertonic medullary interstitium and the delivery of a dilute tubule fluid to the distal convoluted tubule. The reabsorption of NaCl in both the medullary and the cortical segments of the thick ascending limb is mediated by a Na⁺-K⁺-2Cl⁻ cotransport mechanism,[329–332] which is inhibited by loop diuretics such as furosemide and bumetanide.[332] The cDNA sequences for a kidney-specific bumetanide-sensitive Na⁺-K⁺-2Cl⁻ cotransporter (BSC-1 or NKCC2) have been cloned from rat,[333] rabbit,[334] and mouse.[335] The expression of the transporter in the cortical and medullary thick ascending limb was subsequently confirmed by reverse transcription polymerase chain reaction on microdissected tubule segments[336] as well as by in situ hybridization.[124,337] Immunohistochemical studies using antibodies against a fusion protein or peptides based

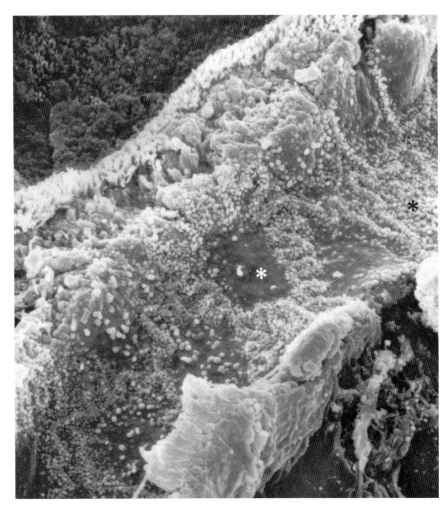

FIGURE 2–39 Scanning electron micrograph illustrating the luminal surface of rat medullary thick ascending limb. The white asterisk denotes smooth-surfaced cells; the black asterisk identifies rough-surfaced cells. (Magnification, ×4300.) (From Madsen KM, Verlander JW, Tisher CC: Relationship between structure and function in distal tubule and collecting duct. J Electron Microsc Tech 9:187, 1988.)

on the sequence of the cloned cDNAs demonstrated the presence of BSC-1 in the apical plasma membrane of the thick ascending limb in the rat.[337–339]

Different splice variants of NKCC2 have been located in rat kidney. They are distributed spatially throughout the thick ascending limb. In situ hybridization revealed that the F isoform was most highly expressed in the inner stripe of the outer medulla, isoform A was mostly expressed in the outer stripe of the outer medulla and cortex, and isoform B was expressed mainly in the macula densa.[335,340,341] An AF splice variant has also been detected in the thick ascending limb. Flux studies investigating three of the splice variants (A, B, and F) have demonstrated marked differences in their kinetics, especially in their affinity for Na+, K+, and Cl−.[342] The function of the AF splice variant remains obscure and it does not appear to be functional when expressed in *Xenopus oocytes*.[343] Moreover, it exerts a dominant-negative effect on the A or F splice variants by forming nonfunctional heterodimers when expressed together in *Xenopus oocytes*.[340] In addition, the A, F, and AF variants are regulated differently in response to water loading and furosemide administration.[340]

Three phosphorylation sites have been described in NKCC2 corresponding to Thr[99], Thr[104], and Thr[117] in rabbit NKCC2.[344] Gimenez and Forbush have provided evidence for the involvement of these phospho-sites in the regulation of NKCC2 cotransport activity in the oocyte expression system. They found that deletion of all three phosphorylation sites abolished the increase in NKCC2 transport normally observed during exposure to hypertonic media and that the phospho-sites worked in concert to increase transport during hyper-

tonic stimulation.[344] Moreover, the A, B, and F splice variants all experienced the same amount of activation when expressed in *Xenopus oocytes* and exposed to hypertonic media.[344]

Chronic vasopressin administration strongly up-regulates the expression of the Na+-K+-2Cl− cotransporter in the thick ascending limb.[345] The energy for the reabsorptive process is provided by the Na+,K+-ATPase that is located in the basolateral plasma membrane. Biochemical[346] and histochemical[230] studies have demonstrated that Na+,K+-ATPase activity is greatest in that segment of the thick ascending limb that is located in the inner stripe of the outer medulla, which also has a larger basolateral membrane area and more mitochondria than does the remainder of the thick ascending limb.[321] In agreement with these observations, physiologic studies using the isolated perfused tubule technique have demonstrated that NaCl transport is greater in the medullary segment than in the cortical segment of the thick ascending limb.[347] However, the cortical segment can create a steeper concentration gradient and therefore can achieve a lower NaCl concentration and a lower osmolality in the tubule fluid.[348] Thus, an excellent correlation exists between the structural and functional properties of the thick ascending limb.

Studies by Good and colleagues[349,350] provided evidence that the thick ascending limb is involved in HCO3− reabsorption in the rat. The reabsorption of HCO3− is Na+ dependent and is inhibited by amiloride, which indicates that it is mediated by an Na+/H+ exchanger.[349] The identity of the Na+/H+ exchanger isoform responsible for HCO3− reabsorption in the thick ascending limb was established by immunohistochemical studies demonstrating strong expression of NHE3 in the apical plasma membrane.[235] Immunohistochemical studies[351] also demonstrated labeling for carbonic anhydrase IV in the rat thick ascending limb, thus providing additional support for a role of this part of the nephron in acid-base transport in the rat. Activation of adenylate cyclase by various peptide hormones was shown to inhibit HCO_3^- reabsorption in the thick ascending limb.[352] There is no evidence for HCO_3^- reabsorption or carbonic anhydrase activity in the thick ascending limb of the rabbit,[233] and NHE3 is not expressed in this segment in the rabbit.[234]

The mechanism of base exit across the basolateral plasma membrane is not known with certainty. However, studies in rat, mouse, and human kidneys have demonstrated that a Cl^-/HCO_3^- exchanger, AE2, is expressed in the thick ascending limb, suggesting that this transporter may be, at least in part, responsible for HCO_3^- exit from the cells.[353-355] Moreover, a recent immunohistochemical study revealed that an electroneutral sodium bicarbonate cotransporter, NBCn1, is also expressed in the basolateral membrane of the medullary thick ascending limb in the rat.[356] NBCn1 was expressed only in the renal medulla, and there was no labeling of the cortical thick ascending limb.[356]

In addition to its role in producing a dilute tubule fluid and a hypertonic interstitium and in the reabsorption of bicarbonate, the thick ascending limb is involved in the transport of divalent cations such as Ca^{2+}[357] and Mg^{2+}[358] The extracellular Ca^{2+}/polyvalent cation-sensing receptor, which was originally cloned from bovine parathyroid gland[359] and subsequently from rat kidney,[360] is strongly expressed in the distal tubule, particularly in the cortical thick ascending limb.[361,362] It modulates various cellular functions in response to changes in extracellular Ca^{2+} and other polyvalent cations and is believed to play a central role in mineral ion homeostasis.[363,364]

The function of the thick ascending limb is regulated by a variety of hormones, including vasopressin, parathyroid hormone, and calcitonin, which exert their effects through activation of the adenylate cyclase system. However, significant differences exist between segments, as well as between species, in the response to these hormones.[365] Vasopressin stimulates adenylate cyclase activity[365] and NaCl reabsorption[366,367] in the medullary thick ascending limb of both the rat and the mouse but has little or no effect on this segment in the rabbit.[365,367] In contrast, vasopressin has less effect on adenylate cyclase activity in the cortical thick ascending limb[365] and does not stimulate NaCl transport in this segment.[366] In mice, acute vasopressin administration increases the phosphorylation of the Na^+K^+-$2Cl^-$ co-transporter (BSC-1/NKCC2) in the thick ascending limb in the inner stripe of the outer medulla, whereas the cortical thick ascending limb appears unresponsive.[368] Recent data has provided direct evidence for shuttling of NKCC2 in response to cAMP administration. Addition of dibutyryl cAMP to rat medullary thick ascending limb suspensions increases surface expression of NKCC2, whereas preincubation of suspensions with tetanus toxin (which inactivates VAMP-2 and VAMP-3), blocks the effect of dibutyryl cAMP on NKCC2 surface expression and transport.[369] Prolonged administration of vasopressin to Brattleboro rats with hereditary diabetes insipidus was found to cause hypertrophy of the cells of the medullary thick ascending limb.[370] Furthermore, vasopressin stimulated Cl^- reabsorption in the isolated perfused medullary thick ascending limb from Brattleboro rats,[371] providing further support for the role of vasopressin in the regulation of ion transport in this segment. Drug-induced hypothyroidism in rats is associated with a decrease in cell height and basolateral membrane area in the medullary thick ascending limb.[372,373] Given that a decrease in vasopressin-stimulated adenylate cyclase activity has been reported in the medullary thick ascending limb in a similar model of hypothyroidism,[374] it is conceivable that the reduction in cell size observed in

this segment was caused by an impairment of vasopressin-stimulated ion transport.

Segmental differences in the response of the thick ascending limb to parathyroid hormone have also been demonstrated. Whereas parathyroid hormone stimulates adenylate cyclase activity in the cortical thick ascending limb of all species studied, it has no effect in the medullary segment.[365] In agreement with these findings, physiologic studies demonstrated that parathyroid hormone stimulates the reabsorption of Ca^{2+}[357] and Mg^{2+}[358] in the cortical thick ascending limb but has no effect on ion transport in the medullary segment. In contrast, calcitonin and glucagon stimulate adenylate cyclase activity and ion transport in both the cortical and the medullary segments of the thick ascending limb.[375]

Distal Convoluted Tubule

The distal convoluted tubule, or pars convoluta, measures approximately 1 mm in length.[151,376] It begins at a variable distance beyond the macula densa and extends to the connecting tubule that connects the nephron with the collecting duct. The transition from the thick ascending limb is abrupt (Fig. 2-40). The cells of the distal convoluted tubule resemble those of the thick ascending limb but are considerably taller. By light microscopy, the cells appear tall and cuboid, and they contain numerous mitochondria. The cell nuclei occupy a middle to apical position. The distal convoluted tubule lacks the well-developed brush border and the extensive endocytic apparatus that are characteristic of the pars convoluta of the proximal tubule.

Scanning electron microscopy has demonstrated that the luminal surface of the distal convoluted tubule differs substantially from that of the thick ascending limb (Fig. 2-41; compare with Fig. 2-39). The distal convoluted tubule is covered with numerous small microprojections, and the lateral cell margins are straight, without the apical interdigitations that are characteristic of the thick ascending limb. The individual cells possess one centrally placed cilium, and occasionally two cilia are observed. The epithelium of the distal convoluted tubule is characterized by extensive invaginations of the basolateral plasma membrane and by interdigitations between adjacent cells similar to the arrangement in the thick ascending limb. Transmission electron microscopy reveals numerous elongated mitochondria that are located in lateral cell processes and are closely aligned with the plasma membrane. They are oriented perpendicular to the basement membrane and often extend from the basal to the apical cell surface (Fig. 2-42). The junctional complex in this segment of the nephron is composed of a tight junction, or zonula occludens, which is approximately 0.3 μm in depth, and an intermediate junction, or zonula adherens.[155] Tracer studies have demonstrated that the tight junction is freely permeable to both colloidal and ionic lanthanum.[161,162] These observations, together with the demonstration of a relatively low transepithelial electrical resistance,[377] suggest the existence of a potential paracellular shunt pathway for solute and water movement in this segment of the nephron.

Lysosomes and multivesicular bodies are common in the cells of the distal convoluted tubule, but microbodies are absent. The Golgi complex is well developed, and its location is lateral to the cell nucleus. The cells contain numerous microtubules and abundant quantities of rough- and smooth-surfaced endoplasmic reticulum and free ribosomes. The basement membrane is complex, often multilayered, and frequently irregular in configuration. Numerous small vesicles are located in the apical region of the cells. Electron microscopic studies examining the uptake of electron-dense tracer from the luminal side showed no uptake of anionic ferritin in the distal convoluted tubule. However, cationic ferritin was absorbed into small apical vesicles and multivesicular bodies, suggesting that these vesicles may be involved in

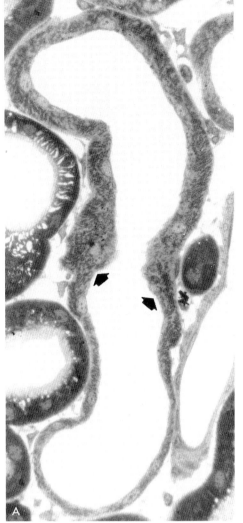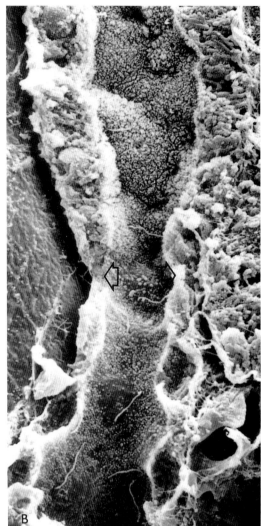

FIGURE 2–40 Micrographs depicting the abrupt transition (arrows) from the thick ascending limb of Henle (below) to the distal convoluted tubule (above). **A,** Light micrograph of normal rat kidney. (Magnification, ×775.) **B,** Scanning electron micrograph of normal rabbit kidney. (Magnification, ×2700.) (B, Courtesy of Ann LeFurgey, PhD.)

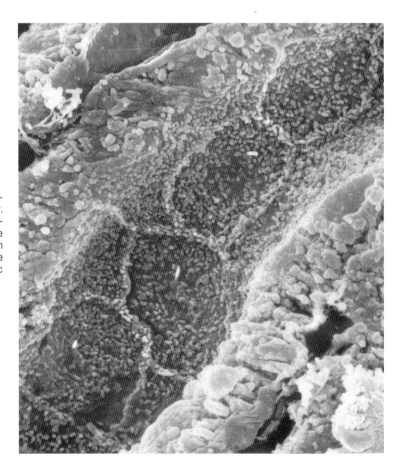

FIGURE 2–41 Scanning electron micrograph illustrating the appearance of the luminal surface of a distal convoluted tubule from rat kidney. Microvilli are prominent, but there is a marked absence of lateral interdigitations in the apical region of the cells. The cell boundaries are accentuated by taller microvilli. (Magnification, ×3000.) (Modified from Madsen KM, Verlander JW, Tisher CC: Relationship between structure and function in distal tubule and collecting duct. J Electron Microsc Tech 9:187, 1988.)

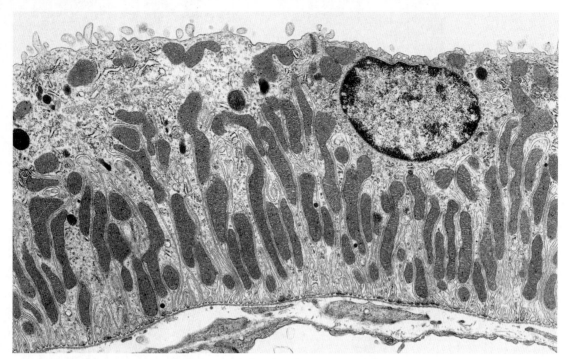

FIGURE 2–42 Transmission electron micrograph illustrating a typical portion of the pars convoluta segment of the distal tubule of a rat. The ultrastructural features closely resemble those of the pars recta of the distal tubule (see Fig. 2–38). (Magnification, ×10,000.)

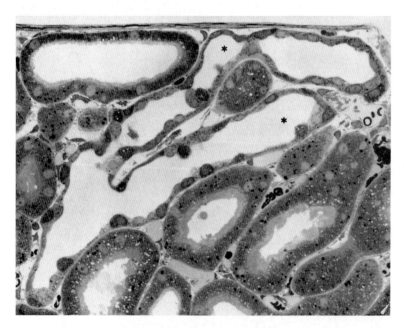

FIGURE 2–43 Light micrograph of initial collecting tubules (asterisks) of a cortical collecting duct in a rat kidney. One tubule is situated just beneath the surface of the capsule (top of picture) and hence is easily accessible to micropuncture. This segment of the cortical collecting duct corresponds to the so-called late distal tubule as defined at the micropuncture table. (Magnification, ×360.)

some form of transport or in membrane recycling in the distal convoluted tubule.[378]

Investigators working with micropuncture techniques arbitrarily defined the distal tubule as that region of the nephron that begins just after the macula densa and extends to the first junction with another renal tubule. With that definition, however, the distal tubule can be formed by as many as four different types of epithelia. In general, the "early" distal tubule corresponds largely to the distal convoluted tubule and the short segment of the thick ascending limb that extends beyond the macula densa, whereas the "late" distal tubule actually represents the connecting tubule and the first portion of the collecting duct, which is usually referred to as the initial collecting tubule (Fig. 2–43).[376,379] (A more detailed discussion of the anatomy of this region of the renal tubule can be found in the next section, which describes the connecting segment or connecting tubule.)

Micropuncture studies in the rat have demonstrated net NaCl reabsorption and K+ secretion in the distal tubule.[377] Because the microscopic anatomy of the segments under study was not carefully defined at the time, it was not possible to state with certainty whether these functional properties were limited to the early distal tubule or whether they occurred along the entire "distal tubule." Stanton and Giebisch,[380] using in vivo microperfusion, succeeded in perfusing short segments of the rat distal tubule. They demonstrated that Na+ is reabsorbed in both early and late segments, whereas K+ is secreted only in the late segment of the distal tubule, corresponding to the connecting segment and the initial collecting tubule. These findings agree with the results of a combined structural-functional study from the same laboratory, which demonstrated significant morphologic changes in the connecting segment and initial collecting tubule of the rat during K^+ loading but no changes in the distal convoluted tubule.[381] Ultrastructural changes were also seen in the connecting tubule and cortical collecting duct of the rabbit after ingestion of a high-potassium, low-sodium diet, whereas no changes occurred in the distal convoluted tubule.[382] After ingestion of a high-sodium, low-potassium diet, an increase occurred in cell height and in basolateral membrane area in the rabbit distal convoluted tubule.[382]

The distal convoluted tubule has a higher Na^+,K^+-ATPase activity than any other segment of the nephron.[261,291] As in the thick ascending limb, Na^+,K^+-ATPase is located in the basolateral membrane and provides the driving force for ion transport in this segment. Reabsorption of sodium and chloride is a main function of the distal convoluted tubule. It is mediated by a thiazide-sensitive Na^+/Cl^- cotransporter, TSC or NCC, that is distinct from the Na^+ K^+ $2Cl^-$ co-transporter, BSC-1, present in the thick ascending limb.[377] The TSC mRNA and protein are expressed exclusively in the distal convoluted tubule, as revealed by in situ hybridization[383] and immunohistochemistry.[384,385] By immunoelectron microscopy, TSC was localized to the apical plasma membrane and apical cytoplasmic vesicles.[385,386]

The expression of the thiazide-sensitive cotransporter in the rat distal convoluted tubule is up-regulated by the mineralocorticoid, aldosterone.[387] In agreement with this observation, immunohistochemical and in situ hybridization studies demonstrated that the mineralocorticoid receptor as well as the enzyme that confers mineralocorticoid specificity, 11-β-hydroxysteroid dehydrogenase 2, are expressed in the distal convoluted tubule of the rat.[388,389] Studies in the rat have distinguished between the early segment, DCT1, and the late segment, DCT2, of the distal convoluted tubule.[388,389] The thiazide-sensitive cotransporter was expressed throughout the distal convoluted tubule, whereas a Na^+/Ca^{2+} exchanger and a calcium-binding protein, calbindin—proteins normally expressed only in the connecting segment—were found in DCT2 but not in DCT1. A similar distinction between DCT1 and DCT2 could not be established in the mouse kidney, where both the Na^+/Ca^{2+} exchanger and calbindin were expressed in most of the distal convoluted tubule.[390] The sodium transport–related proteins in the distal tubule have been reviewed in detail by Bachmann and colleagues.[389]

Detailed studies by Kaissling and colleagues[391-393] demonstrated that the ultrastructure and the functional capacity of the distal convoluted tubule and connecting tubule are highly dependent on the delivery and uptake of sodium. Animals treated with a loop diuretic, furosemide, and given sodium chloride in their drinking water exhibited a striking increase in epithelial cell volume and in basolateral membrane area in the distal convoluted tubule and connecting tubule, and in vivo microperfusion studies demonstrated increased rates of sodium reabsorption in these nephron segments. The observed structural and functional changes were independent of changes in extracellular fluid volume and levels of aldosterone and vasopressin.[391-393]

Gitelman syndrome, an autosomal recessive renal tubulopathy caused by loss-of-function mutations in NCC/TSC, is characterized by mild renal sodium wasting, hypocalciuria, hypomagnesemia, and hypokalemic alkalosis. Studies in NCC-deficient mice[394] demonstrated that these animals have significantly elevated plasma aldosterone levels and exhibit hypocalciuria, hypomagnesemia, and compensated alkalosis. Immunofluorescent detection of distal tubule marker proteins and ultrastructural analysis revealed that the early DCT, which physiologically lacks epithelial Na^+ (ENaC) and Ca^{2+}

(TRPV5) channels, was virtually absent in NCC-deficient mice. In contrast, the late DCT appeared intact with normal expression of ENaC, TRPV5, and the Na^+-Ca^{2+} exchanger. The connecting tubule exhibited a marked epithelial hypertrophy accompanied by an increased apical abundance of ENaC. Reduced glomerular filtration and enhanced fractional reabsorption of Na^+ and Ca^{2+} upstream and of Na^+ downstream of the DCT provided some compensation for the Na^+ transport defect in the DCT. Thus, loss of NCC leads to major structural remodeling of the renal distal tubule that goes along with marked changes in glomerular and tubular function, which may explain some of the clinical features of Gitelman syndrome. A modest reduction of dietary potassium induced a marked reduction in plasma potassium and elevated renal potassium excretion in NCC null mice, which was associated with a pronounced polydipsia and polyuria of central origin.[395]

The distal convoluted tubule is also involved in the reabsorption of Ca^{2+} and has a higher Ca^{2+}, Mg^{2+}-ATPase activity than any other segment of the nephron.[396] Immunohistochemical studies using antibodies to the erythrocyte Ca^{2+}, Mg^{2+}-ATPase demonstrated labeling of the basolateral plasma membrane of the distal convoluted tubule cells,[397] and immunoreactivity for a vitamin D–dependent Ca^{2+}-binding protein has also been observed in this segment.[398]

Because of the heterogeneity of the distal tubule, there has been some confusion regarding the functional properties of this segment of the nephron.[377] Early micropuncture studies in the rat demonstrated that a hypotonic tubule fluid was delivered to the early distal tubule. In the presence of vasopressin, the tubule fluid approached isotonicity somewhere beyond the midportion of the distal tubule. From these data, investigators concluded that vasopressin-induced osmotic water flow occurs along the entire length of the distal tubule that is accessible to micropuncture. In a combined morphologic-physiologic study performed in rats with hereditary hypothalamic diabetes insipidus, Woodhall and Tisher[379] could not find morphologic evidence, in the form of cell swelling and intercellular space dilatation, of transepithelial water flow in the early distal tubule (distal convoluted tubule). Vasopressin-induced osmotic water flow was evident, however, in the late distal tubule (connecting segment and initial collecting tubule). Subsequently, studies using the isolated perfused tubule technique demonstrated that osmotic water permeability in the distal convoluted tubule of the rabbit was low and unaffected by exposure of the tubule to exogenous vasopressin.[399] These data agree with the demonstration that adenylate cyclase activity in the distal convoluted tubule is not increased after vasopressin stimulation.[365] The combined data suggest that the distal convoluted tubule, like the thick ascending limb, is relatively impermeable to water.

Connecting Tubule

The connecting tubule (or connecting segment) represents a transitional region between the distal nephron and the collecting duct, and it constitutes the main portion of the late distal tubule as defined in the micropuncture literature. The connecting tubules of superficial nephrons continue directly into initial collecting tubules, whereas connecting tubules from midcortical and juxtamedullary nephrons join to form arcades that ascend in the cortex and continue into initial collecting tubules (Fig. 2–44; see Fig. 2–43).[151,400] In the rabbit, the connecting tubule is a well-defined segment composed of two cell types: the connecting tubule cell and the intercalated cell.[151,382] In most other species, however, including rat,[376,379] mouse,[382] and human,[401] there is a gradual transition from the distal convoluted tubule to the cortical collecting duct, and the connecting tubule is not clearly

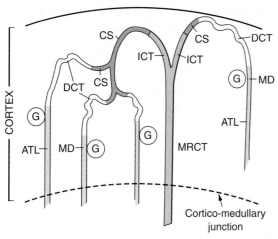

FIGURE 2–44 Diagram of the various anatomic arrangements of the distal tubule and cortical collecting duct in superficial and juxtamedullary nephrons. (See text for detailed explanation.) ATL, ascending thick limb (of Henle); CS, connecting segment; DCT, distal convoluted tubule; G, glomerulus; ICT, initial collecting tubule; MD, macula densa; MRCT, medullary ray collecting tubule.

demarcated because of intermingling of cells from neighboring segments.

The connecting tubule in the rat measures 150 μm to 200 μm in length.[379] It is composed of four different cell types: connecting tubule cells, intercalated cells, distal convoluted tubule cells, and principal cells, which are similar to principal cells in the cortical collecting duct. The connecting tubule cell is characteristic of this segment. It is intermediate in ultrastructure between the distal convoluted tubule cell and the principal cell and exhibits a mixture of lateral invaginations and basal infoldings of the plasma membrane.[402] Connecting tubule cells are taller than principal cells and have an apically located nucleus. Mitochondria are fewer and more randomly distributed than in the distal tubule. A main function of the connecting tubule cells is potassium secretion (see later discussion).

At least two configurations of intercalated cells are present in the connecting tubule. In the rabbit, a "black" form and a "gray" form have been described.[151] Investigators found both configurations to be rich in mitochondria, but the flat and spherical vesicles characteristic of intercalated cells were much more common in the gray cell. In the rat, variations were also reported in the density of the cytoplasm of intercalated cells in the connecting tubule.[376] Two configurations of intercalated cells, type A and type B, were described in both the connecting tubule and the cortical collecting duct of the rat.[403] In the connecting tubule, type A cells were more numerous than type B cells, and they resembled the gray cells described in the rabbit. More recently, a third type of intercalated cell was identified in the connecting tubule of both rat and mouse.[404,405] This cell has been referred to as the nonA-nonB type of intercalated cell. In the mouse, this is the most prevalent form of intercalated cell in the connecting tubule.[404] The function of the intercalated cells in the connecting tubule is not known with certainty. However, ultrastructural changes have been demonstrated in the type A intercalated cells in both the connecting tubule and the cortical collecting duct of rats with acute respiratory acidosis, indicating that these cells may be involved in acid secretion, as are the intercalated cells in the outer medullary collecting duct. The functional properties and immunohistochemical features of the intercalated cells have been studied extensively and are described later.

Both morphologic and physiologic studies have provided evidence that the connecting tubule plays an important role

in K+ secretion, which is at least in part regulated by mineralocorticoids.[377] Free-flow micropuncture studies in rats demonstrated high levels of K+ secretion in the superficial distal tubule.[406] In a combined structural-functional study, Stanton and co-workers[381] demonstrated that chronic K+ loading, which stimulates aldosterone secretion, caused an increase in K+ secretion by the late distal tubule and a simultaneous increase in the surface area of the basolateral plasma membrane of connecting tubule cells and principal cells of both the connecting tubule and the initial collecting tubule, which indicates that these cells are responsible for K+ secretion. No changes were observed, however, in the cells of the distal convoluted tubule. Studies in the rabbit revealed a similar increase in the basolateral membrane area of the connecting tubule cells after ingestion of a high-potassium, low-sodium diet.[382] Studies in adrenalectomized rats demonstrated a decrease in K+ secretion in the superficial distal tubule[407] as well as a decrease in the surface area of the basolateral membrane of the principal cells in the initial collecting tubule.[408] Both structural and functional changes could be prevented by aldosterone treatment, which indicates that K+ secretion in the connecting tubule and initial collecting tubule is regulated by mineralocorticoids.

Immunocytochemical studies have demonstrated staining for kallikrein in the connecting tubule cells in the vicinity of the juxtaglomerular apparatus at the vascular pole of the glomerulus.[409,410] Immunostaining was observed in the endoplasmic reticulum, the Golgi apparatus, the cytoplasmic vesicles, and the plasma membrane, suggesting that kallikrein may be both produced and secreted by the connecting tubule cells.[409]

The connecting tubule is an important site of calcium reabsorption in the kidney. Immunohistochemical studies have demonstrated the presence of an Na+/Ca2+ exchanger,[383,411] as well as a Ca2+-ATPase,[397,412] in the basolateral plasma membrane of the connecting tubule cells. Strong expression of a vitamin D–dependent calcium-binding protein, calbindin D28K, has also been demonstrated in the connecting tubule cells.[398,412,413] The exact role of calbindin in these cells is not known. Interestingly, treatment with cyclosporine is associated with a striking decrease in calbindin expression in the connecting tubule and with increased excretion of calcium in the urine.[413]

Immunohistochemical studies in rats[388,411] revealed that a subpopulation of cells in the late part of the distal convoluted tubule, at the transition to the connecting tubule, expresses both the thiazide-sensitive cotransporter, TSC, and the Na+/Ca2+ exchanger, which are traditionally considered specific for distal convoluted tubule cells and connecting tubule cells, respectively. In the rat kidney, the vasopressin V2 receptor and the vasopressin-regulated water channel, AQP2, are also expressed in the connecting tubule,[414] and AQP2 immunoreactivity has been demonstrated in connecting tubule cells in both rats and mice.[404] In the rabbit the connecting tubule constitutes a distinct segment with respect to both structure and function, and there is no co-expression of TSC and the Na+/Ca2+ exchanger in any cells in the distal convoluted tubule or connecting tubule.[384] Furthermore, vasopressin has no effect on either adenylate cyclase activity or water permeability in the connecting tubule of the rabbit.[415] Biochemical studies on isolated nephron segments have demonstrated that parathyroid hormone and isoproterenol stimulate adenylate cyclase activity in this segment.[365]

Subunits of the amiloride-sensitive sodium channel, ENaC, which are responsible for sodium absorption in the collecting duct, are also highly expressed in the connecting tubule as well as in DCT2.[416] Studies in collecting duct-selective gene knockout mice generated by exploiting the CRE/LoxP approach revealed that selective deletion of alpha ENaC in the collecting duct system with retained expression in the

DCT2 and connecting tubule failed to produce major phenotypic changes.[417] In contrast, global gene knockout of the alpha subunit was postnatally lethal.[418] Thus, the DCT2 and connecting tubule represent the major aldosterone-sensitive pathway for sodium reabsorption. In contrast to these observations, collecting duct specific AQP2 gene-knock out animals developed using the same CRE/LoxP approach exhibited a dramatic phenotype with severe polyuria.[419] Mice with global AQP2 gene knockout died postnatally within 2 weeks with severe hydronephrosis.[419] Thus, in contrast to ENaC (with regard to sodium reabsorption), expression of AQP2 in the entire connecting tubule and collecting duct is essential for water balance regulation.[419]

Recent studies have reported that in experimental forms of diabetes insipidus (either in vasopressin-deficient Brattleboro rats or in rats with lithium-induced nephrogenic DI), exogenous aldosterone markedly reduced remnant apical AQP2 with increased basolateral AQP2 targeting. This was paralleled by a marked further increase in urine production. Conversely, increased apical AQP2 and reduced urine output were seen in response to treatment with spironolactone, a mineralocorticoid receptor antagonist.[420]

COLLECTING DUCT

The collecting duct extends from the connecting tubule in the cortex through the outer and inner medulla to the tip of the papilla. It can be divided into at least three regions, based primarily on their location in the kidney. These include the cortical collecting duct, the outer medullary collecting duct, and the inner medullary collecting duct. The inner medullary segments terminate as the papillary collecting ducts, or ducts of Bellini, which open on the surface of the papilla to form the area cribrosa (see Fig. 2–3). Traditionally, two types of cells have been described in the mammalian collecting duct: principal or light cells, and intercalated or dark cells.

Principal cells are the major cell type; they were originally believed to be present in the entire collecting duct, whereas intercalated cells disappear in the inner medulla. However, there is both structural and functional evidence that the cells in the terminal portion of the inner medullary collecting duct constitute a distinct cell population.[421] Furthermore, at least two, and in certain species three, configurations of intercalated cells have been described in the cortical collecting duct.[403,404] Therefore, significant structural axial heterogeneity exists along the collecting duct.

Cortical Collecting Duct

The cortical collecting duct can be further subdivided into two parts: the initial collecting tubule and the medullary ray portion (see Fig. 2–5). The cells of the initial collecting tubule are taller than those of the medullary ray segment, but otherwise no major morphologic differences exist between the two subsegments. The cortical collecting duct is composed of principal cells and intercalated cells, the latter constituting approximately one third of the cells in this segment in the rat,[404,422] the mouse,[404,405] and the rabbit.[423] Principal cells have a light-staining cytoplasm and relatively few cell organelles (Fig. 2–45). They are characterized by numerous infoldings of the basal plasma membrane that are restricted to the basal region of the cell below the nucleus. The infoldings do not enclose mitochondria or other cell organelles, which causes the basal region to appear as a light rim by light microscopy. Lateral cell processes and interdigitations are virtually absent.[424] Mitochondria are small and scattered randomly in the cytoplasm. A few lysosomes, autophagic vacuoles, and multivesicular bodies are also present, as are rough- and smooth-surfaced endoplasmic reticulum and free ribosomes. Scanning electron microscopy of the luminal surface of the principal cells reveals a relatively smooth membrane covered with short, stubby microvilli and a single cilium (Fig. 2–46).

Intercalated cells in the cortical collecting duct have a dense-staining cytoplasm and therefore have been called dark cells (Fig. 2–47). They are characterized by the presence of various tubulovesicular membrane structures in the

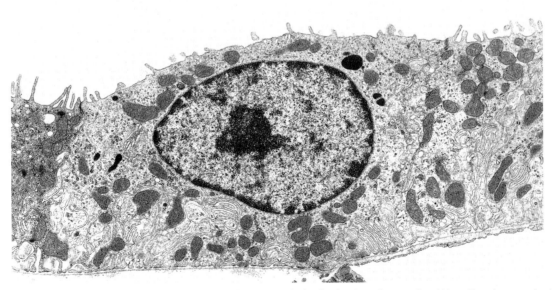

FIGURE 2–45 Transmission electron micrograph of a principal cell from the cortical collecting duct of a normal rat kidney. Note the extensive infoldings of the basal plasma membrane. (Magnification, ×11,000.) (From Madsen KM, Tisher CC: Structural-functional relationship along the distal nephron. Am J Physiol 250:F1, 1986.)

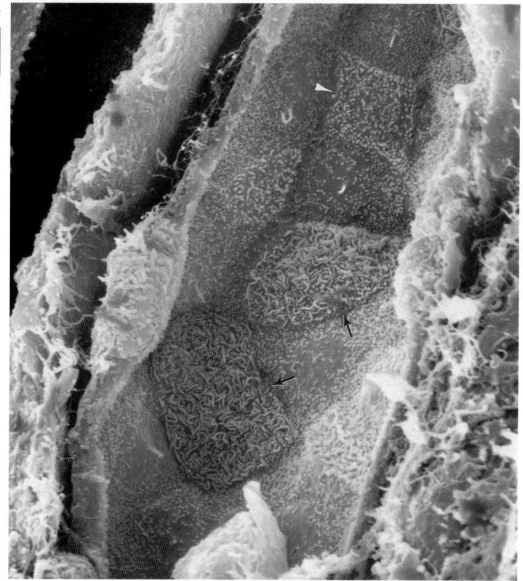

FIGURE 2–46 Scanning electron micrograph illustrating the luminal surface of a rat cortical collecting duct. The principal cells possess small, stubby microprojections and a single cilium. Two configurations of intercalated cells are present: type A (arrows), with a large luminal surface covered mostly with microplicae, and type B (arrowhead), with a more angular outline and a surface covered mostly with small microvilli. (Magnification, ×5900.) (From Madsen KM, Verlander JW, Tisher CC: Relationship between structure and function in distal tubule and collecting duct. J Electron Microsc Tech 9:187, 1988.)

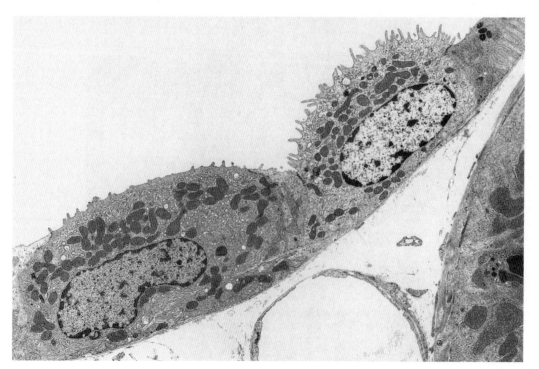

FIGURE 2–47 Transmission electron micrograph from rat cortical collecting duct illustrating type A (right) and type B (left) intercalated cells. Note differences in density of cytoplasm and in apical microprojections. (Magnification, ×5300.) (From Madsen KM, Verlander JW, Tisher CC: Relationship between structure and function in distal tubule and collecting duct. J Electron Microsc Tech 9:187, 1988.)

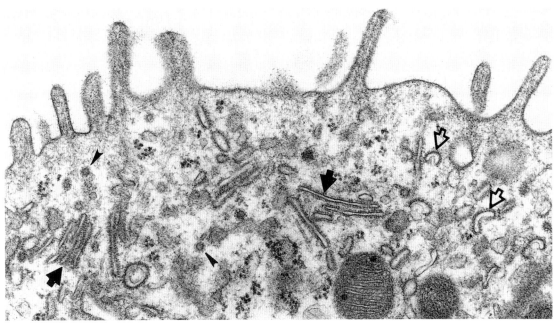

FIGURE 2–48   Higher-magnification transmission electron micrograph illustrating the apical region of an intercalated cell from rat kidney. Note especially the large number of tubulocisternal profiles (solid arrows), invaginated vesicles (open arrows), and small coated vesicles with the appearance of clathrin vesicles (arrowheads). (Magnification, ×38,000.)

cytoplasm and prominent microprojections on the luminal surface. In addition, numerous mitochondria and polyribosomes are located throughout the cells, which also contain a well-developed Golgi apparatus. Previous studies have described two distinct populations of intercalated cells, type A and type B, in the cortical collecting duct of the rat,[403,425] each constituting approximately 50% of the intercalated cells in this segment (see Fig. 2–47). Type A intercalated cells are similar in ultrastructure to intercalated cells in the outer medullary collecting duct. They have a prominent tubulovesicular membrane compartment that includes both spherical and invaginated vesicles and flat saccules or cisternae that appear as tubular profiles on section (Fig. 2–48). The cytoplasmic face of these membrane structures is coated with characteristic club-shaped particles or studs, similar to the coat that lines the cytoplasmic face of the apical plasma membrane.[426] The ultrastructural appearance of the apical region of type A intercalated cells can vary considerably, depending on the physiologic state. Some cells have numerous tubulovesicular structures and few microprojections on the luminal surface, whereas other cells have extensive microprojections on the surface but only a few tubulovesicular structures in the apical cytoplasm.

The type B intercalated cell has a denser cytoplasm and more mitochondria than the type A cell, which gives it a darker appearance (see Fig. 2–47). Numerous vesicles are present throughout the cytoplasm, but tubular profiles and studded membrane structures are rare in the cytoplasm of type B cells. The apical membrane exhibits small, blunt microprojections, and often a band of dense cytoplasm without organelles is present just beneath the apical membrane. Morphometric analysis in the rat has demonstrated that type B intercalated cells have a smaller apical membrane area but a larger basolateral membrane area when compared with type A cells.[403] By scanning electron microscopy, two different surface configurations have been described in the rat.[403] Type A cells have a large luminal surface covered with microplicae or a mixture of microplicae and microvilli; type B cells have a smaller, angular surface with a few microprojections, mostly in the form of small microvilli (see Fig. 2–46).

Both type A and type B intercalated cells are present in the cortical collecting duct of the mouse.[405] However, the type B cells are less common than in the rat. More recent studies have identified and characterized a third type of intercalated cell in both rat[404] and mouse.[404,405] This so-called nonA-nonB type of intercalated cell constitutes approximately 40% to 50% percent of the intercalated cells in the connecting tubule and initial collecting duct of the mouse but is fairly rare in the rat.[404]

Kaissling and Kriz[151] described both light and dark manifestations of intercalated cells in the collecting duct of the rabbit. The light form was most commonly observed in the outer medulla, whereas the dark form was observed mainly in the cortex. Flat and invaginated vesicles were present in both cell configurations. The two manifestations of intercalated cells in the rabbit possibly correspond to type A and type B intercalated cells in the rat. Scanning electron microscopy has also revealed different surface configurations of intercalated cells in the collecting duct of the rabbit.[423] Cells with either microplicae or microvilli, or both, have been described, but their relationship to the two cell types has not been investigated. Cells with microvilli are prevalent in the cortex, however. Most intercalated cells in the cortical collecting duct of the rabbit bind peanut lectin on the luminal surface[427] and are believed to correspond to the type B intercalated cells. In the rat, the binding of various lectins to intercalated cells varies between the cortical collecting duct and outer medullary collecting duct,[428] and peanut lectin labels all cells in the collecting duct of the rat.[429] Histochemical and immunocytochemical studies have demonstrated high levels of carbonic anhydrase in intercalated cells,[430–432] which suggests that these cells are involved in tubule fluid acidification in the collecting duct. The cortical collecting duct is capable of both reabsorption and secretion of HCO_3^-. Studies using the isolated perfused tubule technique have demonstrated that cortical collecting tubules from acid-loaded rats[433] and rabbits[434,435] reabsorb HCO_3^- (i.e., secrete H^+), whereas tubules from HCO_3^--loaded or deoxycorticosterone-treated rats[433,436] and rabbits[434,437,438] secrete HCO_3^-.

Both morphologic and immunocytochemical studies have provided evidence that the type A intercalated cells are involved in H[+] secretion in the cortical collecting duct of the rat.[439] In a study of the effect of acute respiratory acidosis on the cortical collecting duct of the rat, Verlander and colleagues[403] demonstrated a significant increase in the surface area of the apical plasma membrane of type A intercalated cells. No ultrastructural changes were observed in type B intercalated cells. Similar ultrastructural findings were reported in intercalated cells in the outer cortex of rats with acute metabolic acidosis; however, no distinction was made between type A and type B cells.[440] Immunocytochemical studies using antibodies to the vacuolar H[+]-ATPase and the erythrocyte anion exchanger, band 3 protein, (now known as AE1) have confirmed the presence of two types of intercalated cells in the cortical collecting duct of both mouse and rat. Type A intercalated cells have an apical H[+]-ATPase (Fig. 2–49)[404,405,441–445] and a basolateral band 3–like Cl[-]/HCO_3[-] exchanger, AE1,[404,405,441,446,447] which indicates that they are involved in H[+] secretion. In contrast, type B intercalated cells have the H[+]-ATPase in the basolateral plasma membrane and in cytoplasmic vesicles throughout the cell (see Fig. 2–49A), and they do not express AE1.[404,405,441,447]

There is convincing evidence that type B cells secrete HCO_3[-] by an apical Cl[-]/HCO_3[-] exchanger that is distinct from AE1, the anion exchanger in the type A cells. Recent studies have demonstrated that a novel anion exchanger, pendrin, is expressed in a subpopulation of cells in the renal cortex.[448,449] Pendrin is structurally unrelated to AE1, and mutations in the gene encoding pendrin causes Pendred syndrome, a genetic disorder associated with deafness and goiter.[450] Immu-

nohistochemical studies revealed that pendrin expression is restricted to the apical region of AE1–negative intercalated cells (see Fig. 2–49B), suggesting that pendrin might represent the long sought-after apical Cl[-]/HCO_3[-] exchanger of type B intercalated cells.[448,451] Immunogold electron microscopy confirmed that pendrin is located in the apical plasma membrane and apical cytoplasmic vesicles of type B (Fig. 2–50) as well as in nonA-nonB intercalated cells in the connecting tubule and cortical collecting duct of both mouse and rat.[451] Elegant microperfusion studies in isolated cortical collecting duct segments from alkali-loaded mice deficient in pendrin demonstrated a failure to secrete HCO_3[-], compared with tubules from wild-type mice,[448] indicating that pendrin is important for HCO_3[-] secretion in the cortical collecting duct. This conclusion is also supported by studies in the rat demonstrating that the expression of pendrin in the renal cortex is significantly increased in chronic metabolic alkalosis and decreased in chronic metabolic acidosis.[452] In addition, ultrastructural studies have demonstrated changes in type B intercalated cells during experimental conditions designed to stimulate HCO_3[-] secretion in the collecting duct.[443,444] Recent studies have focused on the possible role of pendrin in hypertension. Deoxycorticosterone induces hypertension and metabolic alkalosis in mice. However, pendrin-deficient mice appear resistant to deoxycorticosterone-induced hypertension and more sensitive to deoxycorticosterone induced metabolic alkalosis.[453] In addition, Wall and co-workers[454] found that during NaCl restriction, Cl[-] excretion and urinary volume were increased in pendrin-deficient mice compared with wild-type animals, suggesting that pendrin may play a role in renal Cl[-] conservation. Recent studies examining pendrin

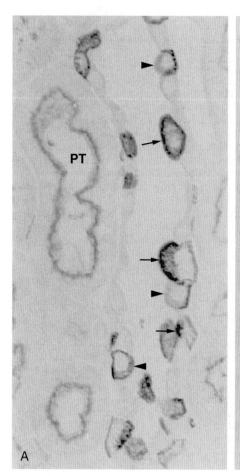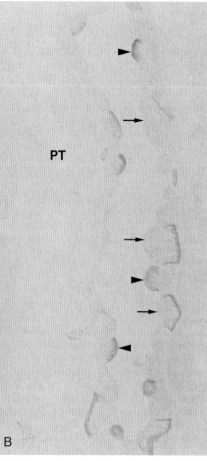

FIGURE 2–49 Light micrograph illustrating immunostaining for (**A**) the vacuolar H[+]-ATPase and the anion exchanger, AE1, and (**B**) pendrin and AE1 in serial sections of the mouse cortical collecting duct with use of a horseradish peroxidase technique. In **A**, type A intercalated cells (arrows) have strong apical labeling for H[+]-ATPase and basolateral labeling for AE1, whereas type B intercalated cells (arrowheads) have basolateral and diffuse labeling for H[+]-ATPase and no AE1. In contrast, type B intercalated cells have apical labeling for pendrin (**B**). PT, proximal tubule. (Differential interference microscopy; magnification, ×800.) (Courtesy of Jin Kim, MD, Catholic University, Seoul, Korea.)

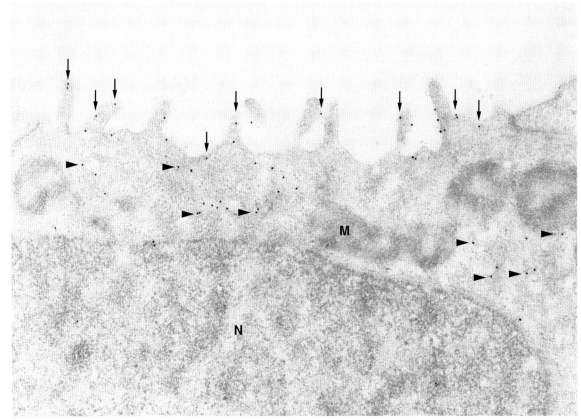

FIGURE 2–50 Transmission electron micrograph illustrating immunogold localization of pendrin in a type B intercalated cell from rat kidney. Labeling of pendrin is seen in the apical plasma membrane (arrows) and in small vesicles (arrowheads) in the apical cytoplasm. M, mitochondrion; N, nucleus. (Magnification, ×46,000.) (Courtesy of Tae-Hwan Kwon, MD, University of Aarhus, Denmark.)

regulation in response to changes in chloride balance have demonstrated an inverse relationship between pendrin expression and the level of chloride loading and provided evidence that distal chloride delivery may be the chief regulator of pendrin expression.[455,456] Taken together, these findings suggest a prominent role for pendrin in chloride transport in the connecting tubule and cortical collecting duct.

Recently researchers cloned the cDNA of a member of the AE family of anion exchangers, AE4, from rabbit collecting duct cells and demonstrated that the AE4 protein is expressed in the apical membrane of type B intercalated cells in the rabbit kidney.[457] Whether AE4 is expressed in intercalated cells in rodents remains to be established.

In the rabbit cortical collecting duct, about 70% of the intercalated cells bind peanut lectin, which has been considered a marker of HCO_3-secreting cells in the rabbit, and originally it was reported that the remainder of the intercalated cells were labeled with antibodies to band 3 protein.[427] However, subsequent studies[458] reported immunostaining for band 3 protein in about 40% of the intercalated cells, including some of the peanut lectin–positive cells, indicating that binding of peanut lectin may not be specific for type B intercalated cells. Finally, studies by Verlander and colleagues[459] revealed that in the rabbit approximately 50% of the intercalated cells in the connecting tubule and 30% to 40% of the intercalated cells in the cortical collecting duct were band 3 positive. These investigators also demonstrated staining for peanut lectin in band 3–positive intercalated cells in the outer medulla of acidotic rabbits, thus raising further doubt about the specificity of peanut lectin as a marker of type B intercalated cells.

Interestingly, in the cortical collecting duct of the rabbit, band 3 immunoreactivity is located mainly in intracellular vesicles and multivesicular bodies in a subpopulation of intercalated cells, and there is little labeling of the basolateral plasma membrane.[460] Moreover, immunocytochemical studies have demonstrated that H^+-ATPase is located in intracellular vesicles in most intercalated cells in the rabbit cortical collecting duct, and only a minority of intercalated cells have H^+-ATPase immunoreactivity in the apical plasma membrane characteristic of type A intercalated cells.[461] These observations suggest that, under normal conditions, most type A intercalated cells in the rabbit cortical collecting duct are not functionally active. However, after chronic ammonium chloride loading there is increased band 3 immunolabeling in the basolateral plasma membrane and increased labeling for H^+-ATPase in the apical plasma membrane of intercalated cells in the cortical collecting duct of the rabbit.[462]

A subpopulation of intercalated cells in the rabbit cortical collecting duct exhibits H^+-ATPase immunolabeling in the basolateral plasma membrane, which is characteristic of type B intercalated cells.[461] Physiologic studies using pH-sensitive dyes to monitor changes in intracellular pH have provided evidence for HCO_3^- secretion by an apical Cl^-/HCO_3^- exchange mechanism in peanut lectin–positive intercalated cells in the rabbit cortical collecting duct.[463,464] Because these cells are more prevalent than cells with basolateral H^+-ATPase, it is likely that some of the cells with diffuse labeling for H^+-ATPase also represent HCO_3^--secreting cells.

It has been suggested that the type A and type B configurations of intercalated cells could represent different functional states of the same cell population and that these cells may change polarity in response to changes in the acid-base status of the animal.[465] Support for this hypothesis was provided by the presence of H[+]-ATPase in the apical membrane of the acid-secreting type A cell and in the basolateral membrane of the type B cell, which might suggest a reversed polarity.[442] However, there is no evidence that a reversal of intercalated cell polarity occurs in vivo, and AE1 and pendrin have never been observed in the same cell in the kidney. The observation that AE1 is expressed only in type A intercalated cells,[447] whereas pendrin is expressed only in type B and nonA-nonB intercalated cells,[451] is more consistent with the concept that type A and type B cells represent structurally and functionally distinct cell types. This concept is also supported by studies demonstrating that distinct members of the chloride channel gene family are expressed in the two types of intercalated cells. ClC-3 mRNA is present only in type B intercalated cells, whereas ClC-5 mRNA is expressed in type A intercalated cells.[466]

A major function of the cortical collecting duct is the secretion of K[+]. This process is, at least in part, regulated by mineralocorticoids, which stimulate K[+] secretion and Na[+] reabsorption in the isolated perfused cortical collecting duct of the rabbit.[467,468] Treatment with mineralocorticoids has also been shown to stimulate Na[+],K[+]-ATPase activity in individual segments of the cortical collecting duct of both rat[469] and rabbit.[291,470] Morphologic studies of the collecting duct of rabbits given a low-sodium, high-potassium diet[382] and of rabbits treated with deoxycorticosterone[471] demonstrated a significant increase in the surface area of the basolateral plasma membrane of the principal cells. The observed changes were similar to those reported in principal cells in the connecting segment and in the initial collecting duct of rats on a high-potassium diet,[381] indicating that these cells are responsible for K[+] secretion in the connecting tubule and cortical collecting duct.

Sodium is absorbed through an amiloride-sensitive sodium channel, ENaC, which is located in the apical plasma membrane of connecting tubule cells and in principal cells along the entire collecting duct.[472,473] The amiloride-sensitive sodium channel is composed of three homologous ENaC subunits, α, β, and γ, which together constitute the functional channel.[474] Immunohistochemical[472,473] and in situ hybridization studies[472] have demonstrated that all three subunits are expressed in connecting tubule cells and principal cells in the collecting duct. However, high-resolution immunohistochemistry and immunogold electron microscopy revealed that α-ENaC was expressed in both the apical plasma membrane and apical cytoplasmic vesicles, whereas β-ENaC and γ-ENaC appeared to be located in small vesicles throughout the cytoplasm.[473]

The activity of ENaC in the collecting duct is regulated by aldosterone and vasopressin as well as other hormonal systems via mechanisms that involve complex signaling pathways and incorporate changes in expression and subcellular trafficking of ENac subunits. In mice receiving a high sodium diet, which is associated with a low plasma aldosterone level, α-ENaC was not detectable and β- and γ-ENaC were distributed throughout the cytoplasm.[475] In mice given a low-sodium diet, which is associated with high plasma aldosterone levels, all three subunits of ENaC were expressed in the apical and subapical region of the connecting tubule cells and in principal cells of the cortical collecting duct. In the medullary collecting duct, however, cytoplasmic staining for β- and γ-ENaC was still observed.[475] Vasopressin increases the abundance of all three ENaC subunits in the rat kidney[476] and angiotensin II also plays a role in the regulation of ENaC.[477,478]

Epithelial Na[+] transport is regulated in large part through trafficking mechanisms that control ENaC expression at the apical cell surface. Delivery of ENaC to the cell surface is regulated by aldosterone (and corticosteroids) and vasopressin, which increase ENaC synthesis and exocytosis. Endocytosis and degradation is at least in part controlled by a PPPXYXXL motif in the C terminus of alpha, beta, and gamma ENaC that serves as a binding site for Nedd4-2, an E3 ubiquitin protein ligase that targets ENaC for degradation.[479] Mutations that delete or disrupt this so-called PY motif cause accumulation of channels at the cell surface, resulting in Liddle syndrome.[480,481] Nedd4-2 is central for ENaC regulation by aldosterone and vasopressin; both induce phosphorylation of Nedd4-2 residues, which blocks Nedd4-2 binding to ENaC. Thus, aldosterone and vasopressin regulate epithelial Na[+] transport in part by altering ENaC trafficking to and from the cell surface (for recent review see Ref 479). An essential role of serum- and glucocorticoid-regulated kinase (sgk1) in the regulation of ENaC has also been established.[482] A series of studies have also underscored a role of proteolytic processing in the activation and regulation of ENaC.[483–485]

Recent immunohistochemical studies also provide evidence that aldosterone-mediated ENaC targeting may (at least in certain experimental conditions) occur via mineralocorticoid receptor-independent mechanisms. This conclusion is based on the observation that targeting of ENaC subunits is maintained in the presence of spironolactone,[486] a mineralocorticoid receptor blocker, and it is consistent with previous findings regarding non-genomic effects of aldosterone.[487] Abnormal regulation of ENaC is associated with salt retention or wasting by the collecting duct (reviewed by Shaefer[488]). Certain single-gene defects affecting ENaC or its regulation by aldosterone cause severe hypertension, whereas others cause sodium wasting and hypotension. Such gene defects underscore the role of the collecting duct in maintaining normal extracellular volume and blood pressure. Changes in the regulatory actions of other hormones, such as vasopressin, and various autocrine and paracrine regulators, such as norepinephrine, dopamine, and prostaglandin E2, which inhibit the antinatriuretic effects of vasopressin, may also be associated with abnormal regulation of sodium reabsorption and lead to sodium retention or wasting, as seen in hypertension, congestive heart failure, or cirrhosis. Recent studies have provided evidence for dysregulation of ENaC via enhanced apical targeting in experimental conditions with severe sodium retention such as in various forms of nephrotic syndrome[489,490] and in CCl4-induced liver cirrhosis.[491] However, ENaC dysregulation in such conditions is only one of several factors because adrenalectomized animals also have sodium retention, suggesting that dysregulation of the alpha-1 subunit of the Na[+],K[+]-ATPase may also play a significant role.[492,493]

Outer Medullary Collecting Duct

The collecting duct segments in the outer and inner stripe of the outer medulla are abbreviated OMCD$_o$ and OMCD$_i$, respectively. The outer medullary collecting duct is composed of principal cells and intercalated cells. In the rat[422] and mouse,[405] intercalated cells constitute approximately one third of the cells in both the OMCD$_o$ and the OMCD$_i$, and a similar ratio between the two cell types is found in the OMCD$_o$ of the rabbit. In the rabbit OMCD$_i$, however, the number of intercalated cells varies between animals. In some animals intercalated cells are present only in the outer half, where they represent 10% to 15% of the total cell population.

Principal cells in the outer medullary collecting duct are similar in ultrastructure to those in the cortical collecting duct. The cells become slightly taller, however, and the number of organelles and basal infoldings decreases as the collecting duct descends through the outer medulla. Whether principal cells in the outer medullary collecting duct are

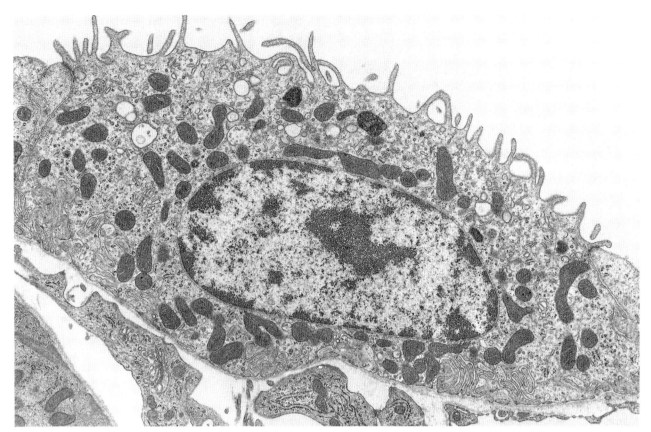

FIGURE 2–51 Transmission electron micrograph of an intercalated cell in the outer medullary collecting duct of a normal rat kidney. The cell has a prominent tubulovesicular membrane compartment and many microprojections on the apical surface. (Magnification, ×10,000.) (From Madsen KM, Tisher CC: Response of intercalated cells of rat outer medullary collecting duct to chronic metabolic acidosis. Lab Invest 51:268, 1984.)

functionally similar to those in the cortical collecting duct is not known with certainty. They express Na^+,K^+-ATPase in the basolateral plasma membrane[169] and the amiloride-sensitive sodium channel in the apical plasma membrane,[472,473] and they are believed to be involved in Na^+ reabsorption; however, there is no evidence that they secrete K^+ as in the cortical collecting duct. In fact, the $OMCD_i$ is a site of K^+ reabsorption, at least in the rabbit.[494] In the rat, intercalated cells in the outer medullary collecting duct are similar in ultrastructure to type A intercalated cells in the cortical collecting duct (Fig. 2–51).

In the $OMCD_i$, the cells become taller and less electron-dense, and little or no difference in the density of the cytoplasm exists between intercalated cells and principal cells in this segment. The main characteristics of the intercalated cells in the outer medulla include numerous tubulovesicular structures in the apical cytoplasm and prominent microprojections on the luminal surface. Scanning electron microscopy has revealed that intercalated cells are covered with microplicae and often bulge into the tubule lumen.

The outer medullary collecting duct plays an important role in urine acidification,[435] which is believed to be a primary function of this segment. There is evidence that H^+ secretion in the $OMCD_i$ is an Na^+-independent electrogenic process,[495] similar to that described in the turtle urinary bladder.[496] In the turtle bladder, H^+ secretion is mediated by an N-ethylmaleimide-sensitive H^+-translocating ATPase that has been isolated in a microsomal fraction from bladder epithelial cells.[497,498] A similar H^+-ATPase has been isolated from bovine[499] and rat[500] renal medulla. Furthermore, biochemical studies on isolated tubule segments have demonstrated the presence of N-ethylmaleimide-sensitive H^+-ATPase

activity in both the cortical collecting duct and the outer medullary collecting duct. The activity varies with the acid-base status of the animal,[501,502] and it is stimulated by mineralocorticoids.[503,504]

Morphologic studies have demonstrated characteristic ultrastructural changes in intercalated cells in the collecting duct after stimulation of H^+ secretion. In rats with acute respiratory acidosis[426] or chronic metabolic acidosis,[505] an increase occurred in the surface area of the apical plasma membrane concomitant with a decrease in the number of tubulovesicular structures in the apical cytoplasm. These findings are similar to those reported in the carbonic anhydrase-rich cells in the turtle urinary bladder after stimulation of H^+ secretion.[506] On the basis of these observations, it was suggested that membrane containing the H^+-ATPase is transferred from the tubulovesicular structures to the luminal membrane in intercalated cells in response to stimulation of H^+ secretion. Subsequent immunocytochemical studies using antibodies against the H^+-ATPase from bovine renal medulla confirmed the presence of an H^+-ATPase in the tubulovesicular structures and apical membrane of intercalated cells.[507] These studies, together with the demonstration that antibodies against band 3 protein (AE1) label the basolateral membrane of intercalated cells, provided convincing evidence that these cells are involved in acid secretion in the collecting duct. Finally, there is now convincing evidence that mutations in the human H^+-ATPase gene lead to renal tubular acidosis (extensively reviewed by Wagner and co-workers[508]).

There is evidence that an H^+,K^+-ATPase is present in the collecting duct, where it plays an important role in K^+ reabsorption as well as H^+ secretion.[509] Biochemical studies have demonstrated H⁺,K⁺-ATPase activity in individual segments of both the cortical collecting duct and the outer medullary collecting duct of the rat[510] and the rabbit.[510,511] The activity was inhibited by omeprazole and Sch-28080, both of which are potent inhibitors of the gastric H⁺,K⁺-ATPase. In addition, H⁺,K⁺-ATPase activity was found to increase in rats receiving a potassium-deficient diet,[510] which suggests that the transporter may be involved in K⁺ reabsorption. Transport studies in the isolated perfused OMCD$_i$ of rabbits receiving a potassium-deficient diet demonstrated K⁺ reabsorption and H⁺ secretion that were inhibited by omeprazole.[512]

Immunohistochemical studies have revealed that antibodies to the gastric H⁺,K⁺-ATPase label the intercalated cells in the collecting duct of both the rat and the rabbit.[513] Subsequent in situ hybridization studies confirmed the expression of the gastric isoform of H⁺,K⁺-ATPase in intercalated cells of rat and rabbit collecting duct.[514,515] Therefore, intercalated cells are capable of both electrogenic H⁺ secretion, mediated by a vacuolar-type H⁺-ATPase, and electroneutral H⁺ secretion in exchange for K⁺, mediated by an H⁺,K⁺-ATPase. However, the two processes seem to be regulated differently. A study examining the role of aldosterone and dietary potassium in the regulation of ATPase activity in the collecting duct reported that H⁺-ATPase activity is dependent on plasma aldosterone levels, whereas H⁺,K⁺-ATPase activity varies with changes in dietary potassium.[516] An isoform of the α-subunit of the colonic H⁺-K⁺-ATPase, encoded by the HK-alpha 2 gene has been shown to be expressed in the kidney, where it mainly localizes to the outer medullary collecting duct principal cells.[517,518] Additionally, transgenic mice expressing green fluorescent protein after the H⁺,K⁺-alpha 2 promoter, show fluorescence in the collecting duct system.[519] The colonic H⁺-K⁺-ATPase isoform has been shown to be regulated by chronic Na⁺ and K⁺ depletion[517,518] and in IMCD-3 cells vasopressin and forskolin stimulates H⁺,K⁺-Alpha 2 mRNA abundance as does overexpression of cAMP/Ca²⁺-responsive elements binding protein.[520] Immunohistochemical studies have also demonstrated that a splice variant of the colonic isoform of the H⁺,K⁺-ATPase is expressed in the apical domain of both intercalated cells and principal cells in the rabbit collecting duct.[521] Generation of colonic H⁺,K⁺-ATPase deficient mice showed no apparent renal phenotype in either normal or K⁺-depleted mice.[522]

Secretion of ammonia/ammonium by the collecting duct is an important component of net acid secretion. However, NH₄⁺-specific transporters have not been identified with certainty in the kidney. Recent studies have reported that members of the Rhesus protein superfamily are expressed in the kidney and, based on sequence homology and structural similarities between the human Rhesus associated glycoprotein (RhAG) and the methylammonium and ammonium permease/ammonium transporters in yeast and bacteria,[523] it was suggested that these proteins may function as NH₄⁺ transporters in the kidney.[524,525] Recently two nonerythroid Rhesus glycoprotein homologs, RhBG[526] and RhCG,[527] were cloned from both mouse and human. Determination of their tissue-specific expression demonstrated high abundance in the kidney, adding further attention to their role in ammonium transport.[526,527] Indeed, subsequent studies revealed that these proteins, when expressed in yeast or in Xenopus oocytes, were capable of ammonium transport,[528–530] suggesting that they could play a major role in renal ammonium transport. Immunohistochemical analysis revealed that RhBG and RhCG are coexpressed in cells along the connecting tubule and collecting duct[531–533] with strong immunoreactivity in intercalated cells.[531,533] The RhCG protein is predominantly expressed in the apical plasma membrane whereas RhBG is expressed in the basolateral membrane.[532,533] Moreover, RhCG appears to be regulated in response to chronic metabolic acidosis, whereas RhBG remained unchanged.[534,535] The generation and detailed phenotyping of a RhBG deficient mice, did not reveal any phenotypical changes, suggesting that RhBG my not contribute significantly to distal tubular ammonium excretion.[536] Further studies are needed to establish the exact role of these proteins in renal ammonium transport.

Inner Medullary Collecting Duct

The inner medullary collecting duct extends from the boundary between the outer and inner medulla to the tip of the papilla. As the collecting ducts descend through the inner medulla, they undergo successive fusions, which result in fewer tubules that have larger diameters (Fig. 2–52). The final ducts, the ducts of Bellini, open on the tip of the papilla to form the area cribrosa (see Fig. 2–3).

The epithelium of the ducts of Bellini is tall, columnar, and similar to that covering the tip of the papilla.[151,537] There are considerable species differences regarding the length of the papilla, the number of fusions of the collecting ducts, and the height of the cells.[277,537] In the rabbit, the height of the cells gradually increases from approximately 10 μm in the initial portion to approximately 50 μm close to the papillary tip, where the tubules form the ducts of Bellini. In the rat the epithelium is considerably lower, and the increase in height occurs mainly in the inner half, from approximately 6 μm to 15 μm at the papillary tip.[421,537]

The inner medullary collecting duct has been subdivided arbitrarily into three portions: the outer third (IMCD₁), middle third (IMCD₂), and inner third (IMCD₃).[421,538,539] The IMCD₁ is similar in ultrastructure to the OMCD$_i$, but most of the IMCD₂ and the IMCD₃ appear to represent a distinct segment.[539] The inner medullary collecting duct was originally believed to be a functionally homogeneous segment. However, transport studies have provided evidence that two functionally distinct segments exist in the inner medulla: an initial portion, the IMCD$_i$, which corresponds to the IMCD₁, and a terminal portion, the IMCD$_t$, which includes most of the IMCD₂ and the IMCD₃. In the following text, the terminology IMCD$_i$ and IMCD$_t$ is used to distinguish these two functionally distinct segments of the inner medullary collecting duct.

In both rat[538] and mouse,[405] the IMCD$_i$ consists of principal cells (Fig. 2–53) and intercalated cells, the latter constituting approximately 10% of the total cell population.[538] Both cell types are similar in ultrastructure to the cells in the OMCD$_i$ and are believed to have the same functional properties. In the rabbit, the IMCD$_i$ is often composed of only one cell type, similar in ultrastructure to the predominant cell type in the OMCD$_i$.[151] However, in some rabbits, intercalated cells can be found in this segment.

In the rat, the transition from the IMCD$_i$ to the IMCD$_t$ is gradual and occurs in the outer part of the IMCD₂.[421,539] The IMCD$_t$ consists mainly of one cell type, the inner medullary collecting duct cell. It is cuboid to columnar with a light-staining cytoplasm and few cell organelles (Fig. 2–54). It contains numerous ribosomes and many small, coated vesicles resembling clathrin-coated vesicles. Small, electron-dense bodies representing lysosomes or lipid droplets are present in the cytoplasm, often located beneath the nucleus. The luminal membrane has short, stubby microvilli that are more numerous than on principal cells, and they are covered with an extensive glycocalyx. Infoldings of the basal plasma membrane are sparse. By scanning electron microscopy, the luminal surface of inner medullary collecting duct cells is

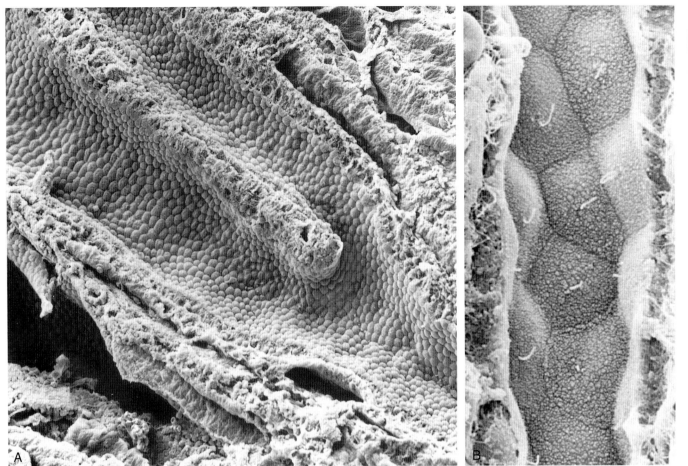

FIGURE 2–52 Scanning electron micrographs of normal papillary collecting duct of a rabbit. **A,** The junction between two subdivisions at low magnification (×600). **B,** Higher magnification view (×4250), illustrating the luminal surface of individual cells with prominent microvilli and a single cilium. (A, Courtesy of Ann LeFurgey, PhD. B, From LeFurgey A, Tisher CC: Morphology of rabbit collecting duct. Am J Anat 155:111, 1979.)

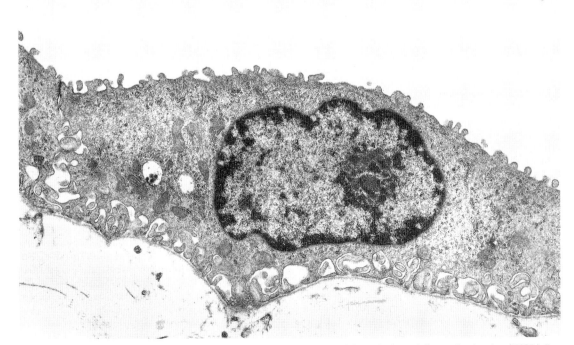

FIGURE 2–53 Transmission electron micrograph of a principal cell from the initial portion of the rat inner medullary collecting duct (IMCD$_i$). Few organelles are present in the cytoplasm, and apical microprojections are sparse. (Magnification, ×11,750.) (From Madsen KM, Clapp WL, Verlander JW: Structure and function of the inner medullary collecting duct. Kidney Int 34:441, 1988.)

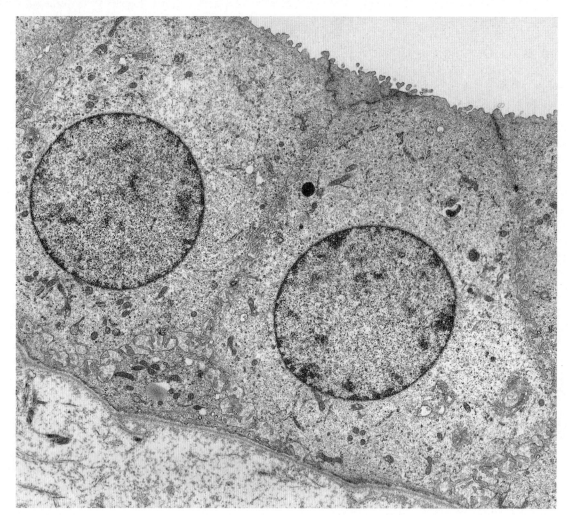

FIGURE 2–54 Transmission electron micrograph of cells from the terminal portion of rabbit inner medullary collecting duct (IMCD$_t$). The cells are tall, possess few organelles, and exhibit small microprojections on the apical surface. Ribosomes and small coated vesicles are scattered throughout the cytoplasm. (Magnification, ×7000.)

covered with numerous small microvilli (Figs. 2–55 and 2–56). However, these cells lack the central cilium that is characteristic of principal cells.[539]

The functional properties of the inner medullary collecting duct have been studied mainly by in vivo micropuncture of the exposed rat papilla or by microcatheterization through a duct of Bellini.[277,421] Use of these techniques has established that the inner medullary collecting duct is involved in the reabsorption of Na$^+$, Cl$^-$, K$^+$, and urea and water. Only a few studies using the isolated perfused tubule technique had been performed until recently[540] because of difficulties in dissection of this segment of the collecting duct. Sands and Knepper[541] described an improved method of microdissection and perfusion of segments of the inner medullary collecting duct from both rat and rabbit. Use of this technique has revealed significant functional differences between the IMCD$_i$ and the IMCD$_t$.[541,542] In the absence of the antidiuretic hormone, vasopressin, the IMCD$_i$ is impermeable to both urea and water, whereas significant permeabilities for both urea and water were demonstrated in the IMCD$_t$. Vasopressin stimulated water permeability in both segments of the inner medullary collecting duct, but urea permeability was stimulated only in the IMCD$_t$. There is evidence that salt and water transport in the inner medullary collecting duct is regulated by atrial natriuretic peptides.

Studies in the isolated perfused IMCD$_t$ have demonstrated that atrial natriuretic peptides cause a significant decrease in vasopressin-stimulated osmotic water permeability but have no effect on urea permeability.[543] Furthermore, evidence indicates that cGMP is the second messenger mediating the effect of atrial natriuretic peptides on the collecting duct.[544,545]

Urea transport in the IMCD$_t$ is a facilitated process that is mediated by specific transport proteins located in the plasma membrane of the inner medullary collecting duct cells.[300] The renal urea transporters, UTA, belong to a large family of urea transporters that also include the erythrocyte urea transporter, UT-B, which is expressed in the descending vasa recta.[298,300] The UT-A1 and UT-A2 isoforms were first cloned from rabbit inner medulla[546] and subsequently also from rat inner medulla.[547] Studies of the segmental distribution of these transporters by in situ hybridization and immunohistochemistry revealed that UT-A1 was expressed exclusively in the IMCD$_t$, whereas UT-A2 was expressed in the descending thin limb of Henle's loop (see Fig. 2–37).[297-299] A third isoform, UT-A3, has also been identified in the IMCD$_t$.[548] UT-A1 and UT-A3 are expressed exclusively in IMCD cells and immunocytochemistry has revealed that UT-A1 is present in the apical region of the IMCD,[299,549] whereas UT-A3 is localized both intracellularly and in the basolateral membrane.[548,550] To

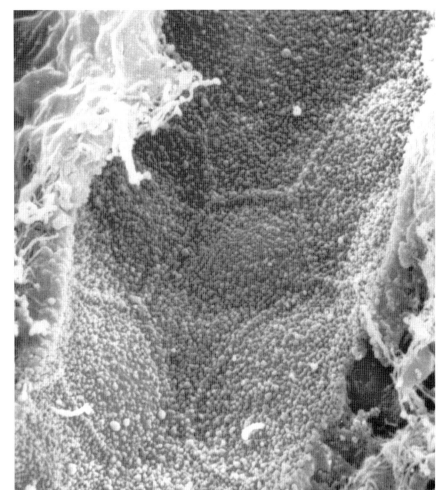

FIGURE 2–55 Scanning electron micrograph from the middle portion of the rat inner medullary collecting duct. The luminal surface is covered with small microvilli, and some cells possess a single cilium. (Magnification, ×10,500.) (From Madsen KM, Clapp WL, Verlander JW: Structure and function of the inner medullary collecting duct. Kidney Int 34:441, 1988.)

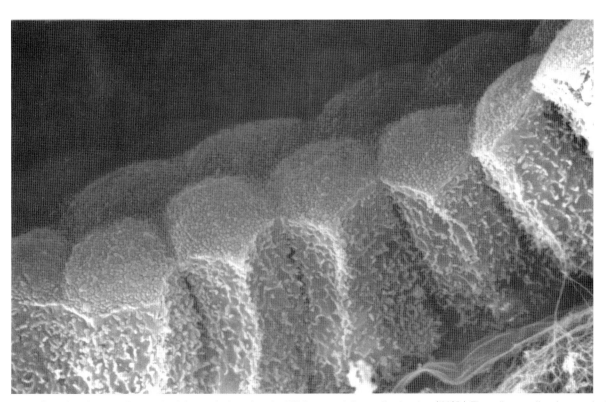

FIGURE 2–56 Scanning electron micrograph of the terminal portion of rabbit inner medullary collecting duct (IMCD$_t$). The cells are tall and covered with small microvilli on the luminal surface. Small lateral cell processes project into the lateral intercellular spaces. (Magnification, ×6000.) (From Madsen KM, Clapp WL, Verlander JW: Structure and function of the inner medullary collecting duct. Kidney Int 34:441, 1988.)

assess the role of inner medullary urea transport in kidney function, Fenton and colleagues developed a mouse model by deleting both UT-A1 and UT-A3 using standard gene targeting techniques (*UT-A1/3–/–* mice) and found that the animals exhibited a urinary concentrating defect.[551] However, there were no differences in inner medullary Na$^+$ and Cl$^-$ concentrations between *UT-A1/3–/–* mice and wild-type control mice indicating that NaCl accumulation in the inner medulla was not dependent on either IMCD urea transport or accumulation of urea in the inner medullary interstitium. Thus, the passive countercurrent multiplier mechanism in the form originally proposed by Stephenson (see review in Ref 303) and by Kokko and Rector[304] where NaCl reabsorption from Henle's loop depends on a high IMCD urea permeability, cannot completely explain how NaCl is concentrated in the inner medulla.

Physiologic studies have provided evidence that the inner medullary collecting duct is involved in urine acidification. Microcatheterization experiments estimating in situ pH demonstrated a decrease in pH along the inner medullary collecting duct,[552] and micropuncture of the papillary collecting duct revealed reabsorption of bicarbonate, which could be inhibited with acetazolamide.[553,554] In addition, microcatheterization studies demonstrated an increase in net acid secretion in the inner medullary collecting duct of rats with acute and chronic metabolic acidosis.[555,556] The mechanism of H$^+$ secretion in this segment of the collecting duct is not known. In the rat, intercalated cells are present in the IMCD$_i$. They are similar in ultrastructure to intercalated cells in the outer medullary collecting duct, and they exhibit immunostaining for both H$^+$-ATPase and AE1, which suggests that they are involved in H$^+$ secretion.

Urine acidification has been demonstrated along the papillary portion of the collecting duct, where there are no intercalated cells, which indicates that the inner medullary collecting duct cells must also be involved in H$^+$ secretion; however, carbonic anhydrase has not been demonstrated in inner medullary collecting duct cells of adult animals, and these cells are also negative for AE1. An H$^+$-ATPase has been isolated from both bovine[499] and rat[500] renal medulla, but the exact cellular origin of this ATPase is not known. Although there is no immunoreactivity for either H$^+$-ATPase or H$^+$,K$^+$-ATPase in inner medullary collecting duct cells in vivo, studies in cultured inner medullary collecting duct cells have demonstrated acid secretion mediated by H$^+$-ATPase[557] as well as H$^+$,K$^+$-ATPase.[558] Moreover, acid secretion mediated by an H$^+$,K$^+$-ATPase was demonstrated in isolated perfused IMCD$_t$ segments from the rat kidney.[559] Interestingly, studies in AQP1-deficient mice revealed strong H$^+$ATPase immunoreactivity in the apical plasma membrane of IMCD cells and increased H$^+$ATPase protein expression in the inner medulla of AQP1 null mice compared with wild-type mice.[560] Recently studies have also demonstrated the presence of NBCn1 in IMCD cells implicating a role of this transporter in regulation of urinary acidification.[561,562]

The epithelium of the collecting duct is tight and relatively impermeable to water in the absence of the antidiuretic hormone, vasopressin. Freeze-fracture examination of the cortical collecting duct and outer medullary collecting duct has revealed relatively complex tight junctions with 6 to 10 individual strands or ridges that form an anastomosing network in all species studied.[163,563] As the medullary collecting duct descends toward the papillary tip, both the depth and the number of strands that form the tight junction gradually decrease.[564] This observation is in agreement with the studies of Tisher and Yarger,[161,565] who demonstrated that the tight junctions of the cortical and outer medullary segments of the collecting duct resist penetration by the extracellular tracer lanthanum, whereas those

of the inner medullary collecting duct are permeable to lanthanum.

In the presence of vasopressin, all segments of the collecting duct become permeable to water. Morphologic changes, including cell swelling, dilatation of intercellular spaces, and an increased number of intracellular vacuoles, have been demonstrated along the entire collecting duct in association with vasopressin-induced osmotic water reabsorption (Fig. 2–57).[379,566–568] Vasopressin binds to specific receptors on the surface of the basolateral plasma membrane, which stimulates adenylate cyclase to generate cyclic adenosine monophosphate (cAMP), the second messenger for activation of the water transport system in the apical membrane. Freeze-fracture studies have demonstrated characteristic intramembrane particle aggregates in the apical membrane of vasopressin-responsive cells in the collecting duct.[569,570] Demonstration of a correlation between the frequency of particle aggregates in the apical membrane and water permeability of the epithelium suggested that these aggregates represent water channels. Subsequent studies demonstrated that similar particle aggregates exist in the membrane of tubulovesicles, the so-called aggrephores, in the apical cytoplasm, and it was hypothesized that vasopressin increases water permeability by stimulating the fusion of vesicles containing water channels with the apical membrane.[571]

In the collecting duct the intramembrane particle clusters are present in the principal cells and in the inner medullary collecting duct cells. Furthermore, specific vasopressin receptors have been demonstrated on the basolateral membrane of the principal cells.[572] Transmission electron microscopy revealed the presence of coated pits in the luminal plasma membrane of principal cells; these coated pits correspond to the location of intramembrane particle clusters, which suggests that endocytosis plays a role in the regulation of water permeability.[573] Studies using horseradish peroxidase as a marker of endocytosis demonstrated that removal of vasopressin stimulates endocytosis in principal cells of the collecting duct in the rabbit,[574] which suggests that water channels are internalized from the luminal membrane. Similar studies in Brattleboro rats with hereditary diabetes insipidus also indirectly suggested that insertion and retrieval of water channels in the principal cells are regulated by vasopressin.[575]

Since the cloning and characterization of AQP1, the water channel protein in the proximal tubule and descending thin limb, an entire family of aquaporins has been cloned and sequenced. The complementary DNA for the vasopressin-regulated water channel, AQP2, was cloned from a rat kidney library by polymerase chain reaction amplification using degenerate oligonucleotide probes based on the published sequence of AQP1.[217,576] Using antibodies generated to synthetic peptides based on the sequence for AQP2, Nielsen and co-workers[577] demonstrated selective labeling of principal cells and inner medullary collecting duct cells along the entire collecting duct of the rat (Fig. 2–58). Immunolabeling was localized to the apical plasma membrane and small subapical vesicles. There was no labeling of other cells in the kidney. Subsequent immunohistochemical studies demonstrated that AQP3 and AQP4 are expressed in the basolateral plasma membrane representing exit pathways for water reabsorbed through AQP2 channels.[578–580] Thus, the water channels demonstrated in the collecting duct are distinct from the water channel responsible for the high water permeability in the proximal tubule and descending thin limb of the loop of Henle. The regulation of AQP2 involves both short-term and long-term mechanisms and is described in detail in this volume (see Chapter 8). Briefly, studies in isolated perfused tubules[581] and in whole animals[582–584]

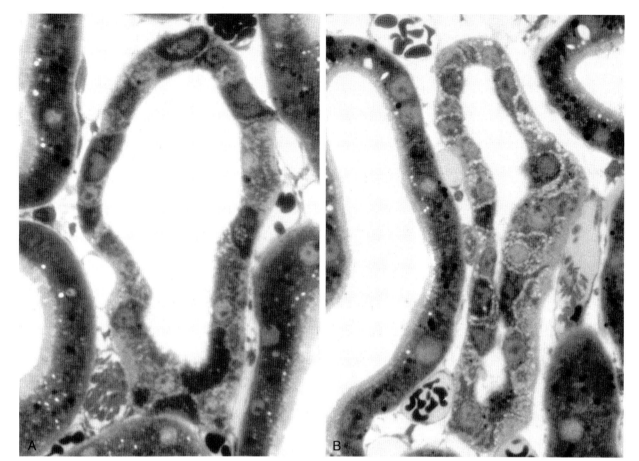

FIGURE 2–57 Light micrographs of cortical collecting ducts of rats with hypothalamic diabetes insipidus. **A,** Tissue preserved during water diuresis in the absence of exogenous vasopressin. **B,** Tissue preserved after the water diuresis was interrupted by intravenous administration of exogenous vasopressin. Note the presence of cell swelling and marked dilatation of the intercellular spaces. (Magnification: A, ×960; B, ×960.)

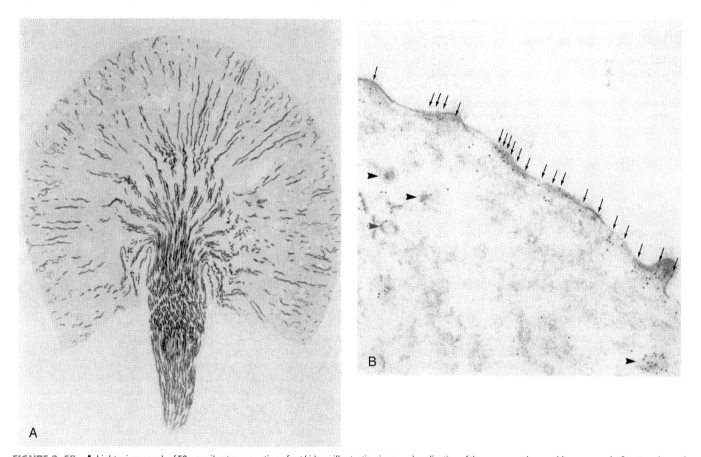

FIGURE 2–58 **A,** Light micrograph of 50-μm vibratome section of rat kidney illustrating immunolocalization of the vasopressin-sensitive aquaporin-2 water channel in the collecting duct using a horseradish peroxidase procedure. **B,** Immunoelectron microscopy of the vasopressin-sensitive aquaporin-2 water channel in the collecting duct using an immunogold procedure. The labeling of aquaporin-2 is seen in the apical plasma membrane of principal cells in the inner medullary collecting duct and the labeling is associated with the apical plasma membrane and intracellular vesicles (×20,000). (A, Courtesy of Jin Kim, MD, Catholic University, Seoul, Korea.)

revealed that vasopressin acutely regulates collecting duct water permeability, and hence body water balance, by inducing a translocation of AQP2 from vesicles to the apical plasma membrane. On a longer-term basis vasopressin regulates the expression of AQP2.[577,585] A series of detailed studies have been devoted to elucidate and characterize the regulation of AQP2, including signaling pathways, cytoskeletal elements, targeting receptors, and associated regulatory proteins (see Chapter 8). Mutations in AQP2 or in vasopressin V2-receptors lead to very severe forms of nephrogenic diabetes insipidus.[586] Dysregulation of AQP2 expression, as well as of AQP3 expression is associated with a number of acquired forms of nephrogenic diabetes insipidus such as lithium-induced polyuria, hypokalemia, hypercalcemia, and post-obstructive polyuria.[586–588] Conversely up-regulation of AQP2 expression has been seen in conditions with water and sodium retention such as congestive heart failure[589,590] and CCl$_4$-induced liver cirrhosis.[491]

INTERSTITIUM

The renal interstitium is composed of interstitial cells and a loose, flocculent extracellular matrix material consisting of sulfated and nonsulfated glucosaminoglycans.[591,592] The amount of interstitial tissue in the cortex is limited, and the tubules and capillaries are often directly opposed to each other. The interstitium constitutes 7% to 9% of the cortical volume in the rat.[593,594] Three percent of the 7% represents the interstitial cells, and the remaining 4% represents the extracellular space.[591] In humans, the relative volume of cortical interstitial tissue has been found to be 11.7% ± 5.5% in kidneys from patients younger than 36 years of age and 15.7% ± 3.0% in older patients.[595] Bohle and associates[596] reported a mean cortical interstitial volume of 9% with a range of 5% to 11% in 20 kidneys, but the age of the patients was not given. Hestbech and co-workers[597] reported similar values, with a mean of 13.6% and a range of 6.3% to 21.3%, in 13 kidneys from patients 33 to 65 years of age. Kappel and Olsen[598] evaluated 54 donor kidneys that were unsuitable for transplantation and reported a range of 7.1% to 37.1%, with values dependent on age.

In the medulla, a gradual increase occurs in interstitial volume, from 10% to 20% in the outer medulla to approximately 30% to 40% at the papillary tip in both the rat and the rabbit.[537,594] In a study using the volume of distribution of inulin and similar extracellular markers, the interstitial volume in the rat kidney was found to constitute approximately 13% of the total kidney volume; in the rabbit kidney, the value was 17.5%.[599]

Cortical Interstitium

The cortical interstitium can be divided into a wide interstitial space, located between two or more adjacent renal tubules, and a narrow or slit-like interstitial space, located between the basement membrane of a single tubule and the adjacent peritubular capillary.[600,601] Whether such a division has any functional significance is unknown; however, it is of interest that approximately two thirds of the total peritubular capillary wall faces the narrow compartment and that this portion of the vessel wall is fenestrated.[593] This relationship might facilitate the control of fluid reabsorption across the basolateral membrane of the proximal tubule by Starling forces.

There are two types of interstitial cells in the cortex: one that resembles a fibroblast (type 1 cortical interstitial cell) (Fig. 2–59) and another, less common mononuclear or lymphocyte-like cell (type 2 cortical interstitial cell).[591,600] Type 1 cells are positioned between the basement membranes of adjacent tubules and peritubular capillaries. They have a stellate appearance and contain an irregularly shaped nucleus and a well-developed rough- and smooth-surfaced endoplasmic reticulum. Type 2 cells are usually round, with sparse cytoplasm and few cell organelles. Studies by Kaissling and Le Hir[602] demonstrated antigen-presenting dendritic cells among the fibroblasts in the peritubular interstitium in both cortex and outer medulla of the normal rat kidney. The interstitial space contains a loose, flocculent material of low density and small bundles of collagen fibrils. Immunocytochemical staining of immature and mature human kidney has revealed types I and III collagen and fibronectin in the interstitium of the cortex.[603] Type V collagen has been described in the cortical interstitium of the rat.[604]

There is evidence that the peritubular, fibroblast-like interstitial cells are the site of erythropoietin production in the kidney. In situ hybridization studies using sulfur 35–labeled probes detected erythropoietin mRNA in peritubular cells in the kidney cortex of anemic mice.[605] This localization was confirmed by Bachmann and co-workers,[606] who demonstrated colocalization of erythropoietin mRNA and immunoreactivity for ecto-5′-nucleotidase, a marker of the fibroblast-like interstitial cells in the renal cortex,[607] thus identifying the erythropoietin-producing cells in the renal cortex as being interstitial cells. The lymphocyte-like interstitial cells in the cortex are believed to represent bone marrow-derived cells.

Medullary Interstitium

Bohman[601] described three types of interstitial cells in the rat renal medulla. Type 1 cells are the prominent, lipid-containing interstitial cells and resemble the type 1 cells in the cortex. However, they do not express erythropoietin mRNA and do not contain ecto-5′-nucleotidase.[606,607] They are present throughout the inner medulla and are also found in the inner stripe of the outer medulla. The type 2 medullary interstitial cell is a lymphocyte-like cell that is virtually identical to the mononuclear cell (type 2 interstitial cell) described previously in the cortex. It is present in the outer medulla and in the outer part of the inner medulla. It is free of lipid droplets, but lysosome-like bodies are often observed. Type 2 cells are sometimes found together with type 1 cells. The type 3 cell is a pericyte that is located in the outer medulla and the outer portion of the inner medulla. It is closely related to the descending vasa recta, where it is found between two leaflets of the basement membrane. These three types of interstitial cells are also found in the rabbit.[600]

Most interstitial cells in the inner medulla are the lipid-containing type 1 interstitial cells,[608] which are often referred to as the renomedullary interstitial cells. They have long cytoplasmic projections that give them an irregular, star-shaped appearance. The cells are often arranged in rows between the loops of Henle and vasa recta, with their long axes perpendicular to those of adjacent tubules and vessels, thus resembling the rungs of a ladder (Fig. 2–60). The elongated cell processes are in close contact with the thin limbs of Henle and the vasa recta, but direct contact with collecting ducts is observed only rarely. Often, a single cell is in contact with several vessels and thin limbs.[601] The long cytoplasmic processes from different cells are often connected by specialized cell junctions that vary in both size and shape and contain elements of tight junctions, intermediate junctions, and gap junctions.[609,610]

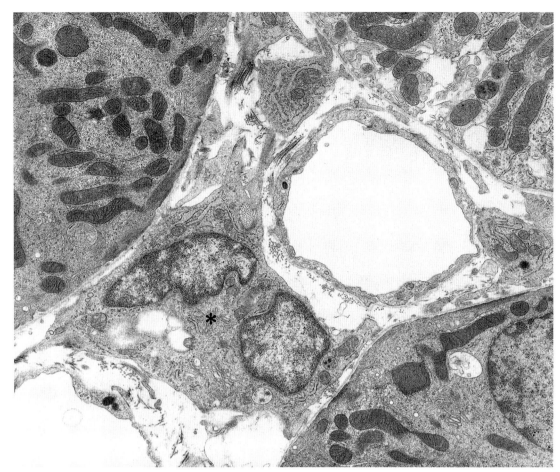

FIGURE 2–59 Transmission electron micrograph of type 1 cortical interstitial cell (asterisk) from rat. A peritubular capillary is located at right center. (Magnification, ×9300.)

Several investigators have described the ultrastructure of the type 1 medullary interstitial cells in rat,[601] rabbit,[600,608] and human kidney. They contain numerous lipid inclusions or droplets in the cytoplasm that vary considerably in both size and number (Fig. 2–61). An average diameter of 0.4 μm to 0.5 μm has been reported in the rat, but profiles of up to 1 μm in diameter were also observed.[611] The droplets have a homogeneous content, but they have no limiting membrane; however, they are often surrounded by whorls of smooth cytomembranes with a thickness of 6 nm to 7 nm. The cells contain large amounts of rough endoplasmic reticulum that often is continuous with elements of the smooth cytoplasmic membranes. Mitochondria are sparse and scattered randomly in the cytoplasm. A small number of lysosomes are present, but endocytic vacuoles are sparse, although interstitial cells are capable of endocytosis of particulate material. Cavallo[612] reported that the type 1 interstitial cells in the inner medulla of the rat kidney contain endogenous peroxidase activity in the endoplasmic reticulum, in the perinuclear cisterna, and in small cytoplasmic vesicles. In contrast, no activity was observed in interstitial cells in the outer medulla or the cortex.

An unusual type of cylindrical body, measuring 0.1 μm to 0.2 μm in diameter and up to 11 mm in length and believed to be derived from the endoplasmic reticulum, has been described in the type 1 interstitial cells.[591,613–615] These structures were observed originally in dehydrated rats and were believed to represent a response to severe dehydration,[613] but subsequent studies demonstrated their presence under normal conditions.[614] The wall of the cylinders consists of two triple-layered membranes, each measuring 6 nm in thickness, and connections between the walls and the membranes of the endoplasmic reticulum have been observed.[613] The functional significance of these cylindrical structures remains unknown.

The number and size of the lipid inclusions in the type 1 medullary interstitial cells vary considerably, depending on the physiologic state of the animal[616,617] and on the species.[608] In the rat, lipid droplets constitute 2% to 4% of the interstitial cell volume, and the volume depends largely on the physiologic state of the animal.[611] The lipid droplets were originally reported to decrease in both size and number after 24 hours of dehydration,[617] but in a later study Bohman and Jensen[611] were unable to confirm these findings. However, an increase occurred in both the size and the number of lipid droplets in water-loaded rats, whereas the interstitial cells were almost depleted of lipid inclusions in water-loaded rabbits.[608] Although the lipid droplets and the diuretic state of an animal seem to be related, the exact nature of this relationship remains to be established.

The function of type 1 interstitial cells (renomedullary interstitial cells) is not known. They probably provide structural support in the medulla because of their special arrangement that is perpendicular to the tubules and vessels. The close relationship between these cells and the thin limbs and capillaries also suggests a possible interaction with these structures. Because of the presence of a well-developed endoplasmic reticulum and prominent lipid droplets, researchers

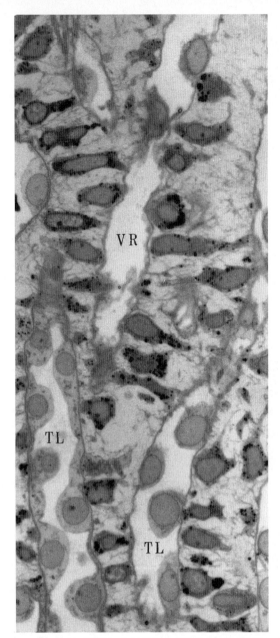

FIGURE 2–60 Light micrograph of the renal medullary interstitium from a normal rat. The lipid-laden type 1 interstitial cells bridge the interstitial space between adjacent thin limbs of Henle (TL) and vasa recta (VR). (Magnification, ×830.)

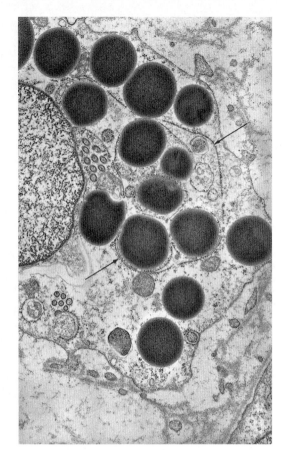

FIGURE 2–61 Higher-magnification electron micrograph illustrating the relationship between the electron-dense lipid droplets, which almost fill the type 1 interstitial cells, and the granular endoplasmic reticulum (arrows). Wisps of basement membrane–like material adjacent to the surface of the cells are contiguous with the basement membrane of the adjacent tubules (lower right). (Magnification, ×12,000.)

have suggested that the type 1 interstitial cells may also be secretory in nature.[618] The lipid droplets are not secretory granules in the usual sense, however, because they have no limiting membrane and there is no evidence that they are secreted by the cell. The droplets have been isolated from homogenates of the renal medulla of both rat[619,620] and rabbit.[621] They consist mainly of triglycerides and small amounts of cholesterol esters and phospholipids.[620] The triglycerides are rich in unsaturated fatty acids, including arachidonic acid.[619,621] The renomedullary interstitial cells are a major site of prostaglandin synthesis. Studies using tissue cultures of renal medullary interstitial cells demonstrated synthesis of prostaglandins by these cells,[622,623] with the major product being PGE_2.[624] However, prostaglandin synthetase activity has been found in rabbit collecting duct cells, which suggests

that prostaglandin synthesis is not limited to the interstitial cells.[625]

Prostaglandin synthesis in the renomedullary interstitial cells is mediated by COX-2.[626] The expression of COX-2 in these cells increases in response to water deprivation and hypertonicity.[144,626] Binding sites for several vasoactive peptides, including angiotensin II, are present in renomedullary interstitial cells,[627,628] and there is evidence that angiotensin may be involved in the regulation of prostaglandin production in the renal medulla.[629] Using histochemical techniques, Kugler[630] demonstrated aminopeptidase A (EC 3.4.11.7), an angiotensinase that is capable of degrading angiotensin, in the type 1 renomedullary interstitial cells of rat, rabbit, golden hamster, and guinea pig. Therefore, another possible mechanism to control angiotensin stimulation of prostaglandin production seems to be present in the medulla.

The type 1 renomedullary interstitial cells may have an endocrine antihypertensive function.[622] Muirhead and coworkers demonstrated that transplantation of renal papillary tissue[631,632] and cultured renomedullary interstitial cells[622] into hypertensive animals was followed by a decrease in blood pressure. The lipid droplets may be related to the antihypertensive function of the interstitial cells, but the precise mechanism has yet to be established. Finally, the interstitial cells are responsible for the synthesis of the glycosaminoglycans, in particular hyaluronic acid, which are present in the matrix material of the interstitium.[633]

Little is known about the function of the type 2 and type 3 medullary interstitial cells. Bohman[591] suggested that the type 2 cells are probably phagocytic, but the function of type 3 cells remains unknown.

LYMPHATICS

Interstitial fluid can leave the kidney by two different lymphatic networks, a superficial capsular system and a deeper hilar system.[634,635] Our knowledge of the distribution of lymphatics within the kidney, however, is restricted. Intrarenal lymphatics are embedded in the periarterial loose connective tissue around the renal arteries and are distributed primarily along the interlobular and arcuate arteries in the cortex.[634–636] Kriz and Dieterich[636] believed that the cortical lymphatics begin as lymphatic capillaries in the area of the interlobular arteries and that these capillaries drain into the arcuate lymphatic vessels at the region of the corticomedullary junction (Fig. 2–62). The arcuate lymphatic vessels drain to hilar lymphatic vessels through interlobar lymphatics. Numerous valves have been described within the interlobar and hilar lymphatic channels.[636] Similar findings were reported by Bell and associates[635] in both calves and dogs. In the horse, glomeruli are often completely surrounded by lymphatic channels, whereas in the dog, only a portion of the glomerulus is surrounded by lymphatics.[635] Electron microscopic studies in the dog kidney after injection of India ink into capsular lymphatic vessels revealed the presence of small lymphatic channels, in close apposition to both proximal and distal tubules, in addition to the interlobular arteries.[637] An electron microscopic study of the lymphatic system in the dog kidney demonstrated the existence of cortical intralobular lymphatics

closely associated with terminal arteries, arterioles, renal corpuscles, and tubule elements.[638] Morphometric analysis revealed that the cross-sectional area of interlobular lymphatics was almost twice that of intralobular lymphatics in the cortex. The volume density of renal cortical lymphatics was 0.17%.[638] Similar morphometric studies in the rat, hamster, and rabbit revealed volume densities of cortical lymphatics of 0.11%, 0.37%, and 0.02%, respectively.[639]

A less extensive system of lymphatic vessels is present within and immediately beneath the renal capsule.[635,636] The lymphatic vessels of the renal capsule drain into subcapsular lymphatic channels that lie adjacent to interlobular arteries located just beneath the renal capsule. These lymphatic vessels appear to provide continuity between the major intrarenal lymphatic vessels within the cortex (interlobular and arcuate lymphatic vessels) and the capsular lymphatic vessels; thus, in some animals, a continuous system of lymphatic drainage has been observed from the renal capsule, through the cortex, and into the hilar region (Fig. 2–63). In the dog kidney, two types of tributaries have been described in association with the surface lymphatics.[640] So-called communicating lymphatic channels were found in small numbers, usually in association with an interlobular artery and vein; these lymphatics penetrated the capsule and appeared to represent a connection between the hilar and capsular systems. The second type of vessel, the so-called perforating lymphatic channel, penetrated the capsule alone or in association with a small vein; these channels appeared to repre-

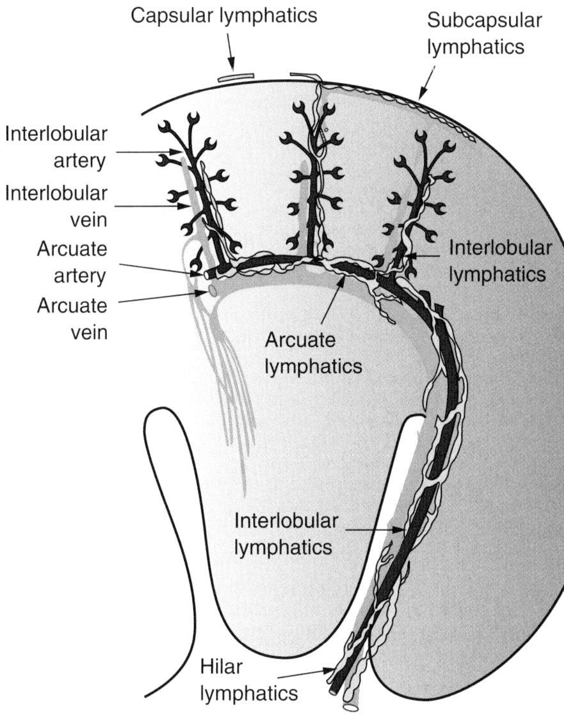

FIGURE 2–62 Diagram of the lymphatic circulation in the mammalian kidney. (Modified from Kriz W, Dieterich HJ: [The lymphatic system of the kidney in some mammals. Light and electron microscopic investigations]. Z Anat Entwicklungsgesch 131:111, 1970.)

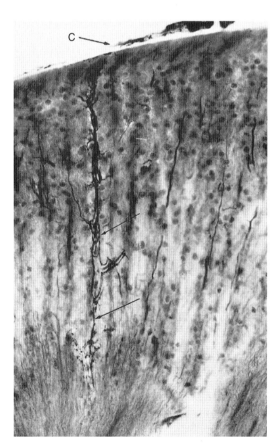

FIGURE 2–63 Light micrograph of a sagittal section through the cortex and outer medulla of a dog kidney. A capsular lymphatic (C) was injected with India ink. Intrarenal lymphatics (arrows) follow the distribution of the interlobular arteries in the cortex. (Magnification, ×10.) (From Bell RD, Keyl MJ, Shrader FR, et al: Renal lymphatics: The internal distribution. Nephron 5:454, 1968.)

sent a primary pathway for lymph drainage from the superficial cortex. From a study in the dog kidney, investigators concluded that intramedullary lymphatics do not exist in this species, and they suggested that interstitial fluid from the medulla may drain to the arcuate or interlobar lymphatics.[641] It has also been suggested that plasma proteins are cleared from the medullary interstitium through the ascending vasa recta.[642-644]

On microscopic examination, the wall of the interlobular lymphatic vessel is formed by a single endothelial layer and does not have the support of a basement membrane.[636] The arcuate and interlobar lymphatic vessels are similar in appearance, although the latter possess valves.

INNERVATION

The efferent nerve supply to the kidney arises largely from the celiac plexus, with additional contributions originating from the greater splanchnic nerve, the intermesenteric plexus, and the superior hypogastric plexus.[645] The postganglionic sympathetic nerve fiber distribution generally follows the arterial vessels throughout the cortex and outer stripe of the outer medulla.[646] Adrenergic fibers have been observed lying adjacent to smooth muscle cells of arcuate and interlobular arteries and afferent arterioles.[647-649] An extensive innervation of the efferent arteriolar vessels of the juxtamedullary glomeruli, which eventually divide to form the afferent vasa recta, has been described.[648,650] However, quantitation of monoaminergic innervation by autoradiography revealed a higher density of norepinephrine-containing nerves associated with the afferent rather than the efferent arteriole.[649] Newstead and Munkacsi[650] reported the existence of large bundles of unmyelinated nerve fibers that accompanied the efferent arterioles from the region of the juxtamedullary glomeruli to the level of the inner stripe of the outer medulla. Nerve fibers and nerve endings were no longer present at the site at which the smooth muscle layer of the efferent arterioles and arteriolae rectae gave way to the pericytes surrounding the arterial vasa recta, which begin in the deep inner stripe of the outer medulla. There is also evidence for the presence of transitory adrenergic fibers in the inner medulla of the cat kidney.[651]

For some time, controversy has existed regarding the presence of direct tubule innervation in the renal cortex. Nerve bundles arising from perivascular nerves have been described in proximity to both proximal and distal tubules.[652] Structures termed varicosities, which are believed to represent nerve endings, have been described as being in close contact with proximal and distal tubules, often in the vicinity of the hilus of the glomerulus and the juxtaglomerular apparatus,[117,652,653] and in the connecting segment and the cortical collecting duct.[654] Autoradiographic studies have also revealed that injected tritiated norepinephrine is associated with both proximal and distal convoluted tubules, which indicates monoaminergic innervation of these tubules.[655] The thick ascending limb of Henle receives the largest nerve supply.[655] Both myelinated and unmyelinated nerve fibers have been demonstrated in the corticomedullary region and in perivascular connective tissue.[656] Electron microscopic autoradiography revealed that tritiated norepinephrine is concentrated mainly on unmyelinated fibers, suggesting that these fibers are adrenergic in nature.[656] There is evidence that renal nerves possess fibers containing neuropeptide Y, a potent vasoconstrictor,[657,658] as well as immunoreactive somatostatin and neurotensin.[658] Vasoactive intestinal polypeptide immunoreactive nerve fibers are also well documented in the kidney.[658] Earlier studies describing cholinergic nerve fibers within the renal parenchyma have fallen into disrepute because the conclusions were based largely on the presence of acetylcholinesterase.[647]

The afferent renal nerves are found principally in the pelvic region, the major vessels, and the corticomedullary connective tissue.[653] Most, although not all, afferent renal nerves are unmyelinated.[659] Largely on the basis of immunocytochemical localization of calcitonin gene–related peptide, a marker of afferent nerve fibers, Barajas and co-workers[653] suggested that these immunoreactive nerve fibers may be involved in baroreceptor and afferent nerve responses to changes in arterial, venous, interstitial, or intrapelvic pressure.

References

1. Hughson M, Farris AB, III, Douglas-Denton R, et al: Glomerular number and size in autopsy kidneys: The relationship to birth weight. Kidney Int 63:2113, 2003.
2. Keller G, Zimmer G, Mall G, et al: Nephron number in patients with primary hypertension. N Engl J Med 348:101, 2003.
3. Nyengaard JR, Bendtsen TF: Glomerular number and size in relation to age, kidney weight, and body surface in normal man. Anat Rec 232:194, 1992.
4. Bertram JF, Soosaipillai MC, Ricardo SD, Ryan GB: Total numbers of glomeruli and individual glomerular cell types in the normal rat kidney. Cell Tissue Res 270:37, 1992.
5. Nyengaard JR: The quantitative development of glomerular capillaries in rats with special reference to unbiased stereological estimates of their number and sizes. Microvasc Res 45:243, 1993.
6. Neiss WF: Morphogenesis and histogenesis of the connecting tubule in the rat kidney. Anat Embryol (Berl) 165:81, 1982.
7. Samuel T, Hoy WE, Douglas-Denton R, et al: Determinants of glomerular volume in different cortical zones of the human kidney. J Am Soc Nephrol 16:3102, 2005.
8. Guasch A, Myers BD: Determinants of glomerular hypofiltration in nephrotic patients with minimal change nephropathy. J Am Soc Nephrol 4:1571, 1994.
9. Shea SM, Morrison AB: A stereological study of the glomerular filter in the rat. Morphometry of the slit diaphragm and basement membrane. J Cell Biol 67:436, 1975.
10. Jørgensen F: The Ultrastructure of the Normal Human Glomerulus. Copenhagen, Ejnar Munksgaard, 1966.
11. Rostgaard J, Thuneberg L: Electron microscopical observations on the brush border of proximal tubule cells of mammalian kidney. Z Zellforsch Mikrosk Anat 132:473, 1972.
12. Hjalmarsson C, Johansson BR, Haraldsson B: Electron microscopic evaluation of the endothelial surface layer of glomerular capillaries. Microvasc Res 67:9, 2004.
13. Vasmant D, Maurice M, Feldmann G: Cytoskeleton ultrastructure of podocytes and glomerular endothelial cells in man and in the rat. Anat Rec 210:17, 1984.
14. Sorensson J, Bjornson A, Ohlson M, et al: Synthesis of sulfated proteoglycans by bovine glomerular endothelial cells in culture. Am J Physiol Renal Physiol 284:F373, 2003.
15. Jeansson M, Haraldsson B: Morphological and functional evidence for an important role of the endothelial cell glycocalyx in the glomerular barrier. Am J Physiol Renal Physiol 290:F111, 2006.
16. Ballermann BJ, Marsden PA: Endothelium-derived vasoactive mediators and renal glomerular function. Clin Invest Med 14:508, 1991.
17. Bachmann S, Bosse HM, Mundel P: Topography of nitric oxide synthesis by localizing constitutive NO synthases in mammalian kidney. Am J Physiol 268:F885, 1995.
18. Simon M, Grone HJ, Johren O, et al: Expression of vascular endothelial growth factor and its receptors in human renal ontogenesis and in adult kidney. Am J Physiol 268:F240, 1995.
19. Brown LF, Berse B, Tognazzi K, et al: Vascular permeability factor mRNA and protein expression in human kidney. Kidney Int 42:1457, 1992.
20. Esser S, Wolburg K, Wolburg H, et al: Vascular endothelial growth factor induces endothelial fenestrations in vitro. J Cell Biol 140:947, 1998.
21. Roberts WG, Palade GE: Increased microvascular permeability and endothelial fenestration induced by vascular endothelial growth factor. J Cell Sci 108 (Pt 6):2369, 1995.
22. Chen J, Braet F, Brodsky S, et al: VEGF-induced mobilization of caveolae and increase in permeability of endothelial cells. Am J Physiol Cell Physiol 282:C1053, 2002.
23. Ballermann BJ: Glomerular endothelial cell differentiation. Kidney Int 67:1668, 2005.
24. Eremina V, Sood M, Haigh J, et al: Glomerular-specific alterations of VEGF-A expression lead to distinct congenital and acquired renal diseases. J Clin Invest 111:707, 2003.
25. Ostendorf T, Kunter U, Eitner F, et al: VEGF(165) mediates glomerular endothelial repair. J Clin Invest 104:913, 1999.
26. Andrews PM, Bates SB: Filamentous actin bundles in the kidney. Anat Rec 210:1, 1984.
27. Farquhar MG, Wissig SL, Palade GE: Glomerular permeability. I. Ferritin transfer across the normal glomerular capillary wall. J Exp Med 113:47, 1961.
28. Latta H: The glomerular capillary wall. J Ultrastruct Res 32:526, 1970.

29. Rodewald R, Karnovsky MJ: Porous substructure of the glomerular slit diaphragm in the rat and mouse. J Cell Biol 60:423, 1974.

30. Schneeberger EE, Levey RH, McCluskey RT, Karnovsky MJ: The isoporous substructure of the human glomerular slit diaphragm. Kidney Int 8:48, 1975.

31. Reiser J, Kriz W, Kretzler M, Mundel P: The glomerular slit diaphragm is a modified adherens junction. J Am Soc Nephrol 11:1, 2000.

32. Schnabel E, Anderson JM, Farquhar MG: The tight junction protein ZO-1 is concentrated along slit diaphragms of the glomerular epithelium. J Cell Biol 111:1255, 1990.

33. Tryggvason K: Unraveling the mechanisms of glomerular ultrafiltration: Nephrin, a key component of the slit diaphragm. J Am Soc Nephrol 10:2440, 1999.

34. Kestila M, Lenkkeri U, Mannikko M, et al: Positionally cloned gene for a novel glomerular protein—nephrin—is mutated in congenital nephrotic syndrome. Mol Cell 1:575, 1998.

35. Lenkkeri U, Mannikko M, McCready P, et al: Structure of the gene for congenital nephrotic syndrome of the Finnish type (NPHS1) and characterization of mutations. Am J Hum Genet 64:51, 1999.

36. Holzman LB, St John PL, Kovari IA, et al: Nephrin localizes to the slit pore of the glomerular epithelial cell. Kidney Int 56:1481, 1999.

37. Ruotsalainen V, Ljungberg P, Wartiovaara J, et al: Nephrin is specifically located at the slit diaphragm of glomerular podocytes. Proc Natl Acad Sci U S A 96:7962, 1999.

38. Shih NY, Li J, Cotran R, et al: CD2AP localizes to the slit diaphragm and binds to nephrin via a novel C-terminal domain. Am J Pathol 159:2303, 2001.

39. Li C, Ruotsalainen V, Tryggvason K, et al: CD2AP is expressed with nephrin in developing podocytes and is found widely in mature kidney and elsewhere. Am J Physiol Renal Physiol 279:F785, 2000.

40. Yuan H, Takeuchi E, Salant DJ: Podocyte slit-diaphragm protein nephrin is linked to the actin cytoskeleton. Am J Physiol Renal Physiol 282:F585, 2002.

41. Boute N, Gribouval O, Roselli S, et al: NPHS2, encoding the glomerular protein podocin, is mutated in autosomal recessive steroid-resistant nephrotic syndrome. Nat Genet 24:349, 2000.

42. Roselli S, Gribouval O, Boute N, et al: Podocin localizes in the kidney to the slit diaphragm area. Am J Pathol 160:131, 2002.

43. Schwarz K, Simons M, Reiser J, et al: Podocin, a raft-associated component of the glomerular slit diaphragm, interacts with CD2AP and nephrin. J Clin Invest 108:1621, 2001.

44. Kerjaschki D, Sharkey DJ, Farquhar MG: Identification and characterization of podocalyxin—the major sialoprotein of the renal glomerular epithelial cell. J Cell Biol 98:1591, 1984.

45. Kazatchkine MD, Fearon DT, Appay MD, et al: Immunohistochemical study of the human glomerular C3b receptor in normal kidney and in seventy-five cases of renal diseases: Loss of C3b receptor antigen in focal hyalinosis and in proliferative nephritis of systemic lupus erythematosus. J Clin Invest 69:900, 1982.

46. Kerjaschki D, Farquhar MG: Immunocytochemical localization of the Heymann nephritis antigen (GP330) in glomerular epithelial cells of normal Lewis rats. J Exp Med 157:667, 1983.

47. Yamazaki H, Ullrich R, Exner M, et al: All four putative ligand-binding domains in megalin contain pathogenic epitopes capable of inducing passive Heymann nephritis. J Am Soc Nephrol 9:1638, 1998.

48. Seiler MW, Venkatachalam MA, Cotran RS: Glomerular epithelium: Structural alterations induced by polycations. Science 189:390, 1975.

49. Kanwar YS, Farquhar MG: Detachment of endothelium and epithelium from the glomerular basement membrane produced by kidney perfusion with neuraminidase. Lab Invest 42:375, 1980.

50. Matsui K, Breiteneder-Geleff S, Kerjaschki D: Epitope-specific antibodies to the 43-kD glomerular membrane protein podoplanin cause proteinuria and rapid flattening of podocytes. J Am Soc Nephrol 9:2013, 1998.

51. Breiteneder-Geleff S, Matsui K, Soleiman A, et al: Podoplanin, novel 43-kd membrane protein of glomerular epithelial cells, is down-regulated in puromycin nephrosis. Am J Pathol 151:1141, 1997.

52. Pavenstadt H, Kriz W, Kretzler M: Cell biology of the glomerular podocyte. Physiol Rev 83:253, 2003.

53. Farquhar MG, Palade GE: Functional evidence for the existence of a third cell type in the renal glomerulus. J Cell Biol 13:55, 1962.

54. Latta H, Maunsbach AB, Madden SC: The centrolobular region of the renal glomerulus studied by electron microscopy. J Ultrastruct Res 4:455, 1960.

55. Drenckhahn D, Schnittler H, Nobiling R, Kriz W: Ultrastructural organization of contractile proteins in rat glomerular mesangial cells. Am J Pathol 137:1343, 1990.

56. Kriz W, Elger M, Mundel P, Lemley KV: Structure-stabilizing forces in the glomerular tuft. J Am Soc Nephrol 5:1731, 1995.

57. Groffen AJ, Hop FW, Tryggvason K, et al: Evidence for the existence of multiple heparan sulfate proteoglycans in the human glomerular basement membrane and mesangial matrix. Eur J Biochem 247:175, 1997.

58. Courtoy PJ, Kanwar YS, Hynes RO, Farquhar MG: Fibronectin localization in the rat glomerulus. J Cell Biol 87:691, 1980.

59. Courtoy PJ, Timpl R, Farquhar MG: Comparative distribution of laminin, type IV collagen, and fibronectin in the rat glomerulus. J Histochem Cytochem 30:874, 1982.

60. Kerjaschki D, Ojha PP, Susani M, et al: A beta 1-integrin receptor for fibronectin in human kidney glomeruli. Am J Pathol 134:481, 1989.

61. Cosio FG, Sedmak DD, Nahman NS, Jr: Cellular receptors for matrix proteins in normal human kidney and human mesangial cells. Kidney Int 38:886, 1990.

62. Petermann A, Fees H, Grenz H, et al: Polymerase chain reaction and focal contact formation indicate integrin expression in mesangial cells. Kidney Int 44:997, 1993.

63. Hartner A, Schocklmann H, Prols F, et al: Alpha8 integrin in glomerular mesangial cells and in experimental glomerulonephritis. Kidney Int 56:1468, 1999.

64. Rupprecht HD, Schocklmann HO, Sterzel RB: Cell-matrix interactions in the glomerular mesangium. Kidney Int 49:1575, 1996.

65. Schlondorff D: The glomerular mesangial cell: an expanding role for a specialized pericyte. FASEB J 1:272, 1987.

66. Michael AF, Keane WF, Raij L, et al: The glomerular mesangium. Kidney Int 17:141, 1980.

67. Ausiello DA, Kreisberg JI, Roy C, Karnovsky MJ: Contraction of cultured rat glomerular cells of apparent mesangial origin after stimulation with angiotensin II and arginine vasopressin. J Clin Invest 65:754, 1980.

68. Kreisberg JI, Venkatachalam M, Troyer D: Contractile properties of cultured glomerular mesangial cells. Am J Physiol 249:F457, 1985.

69. Elema JD, Hoyer JR, Vernier RL: The glomerular mesangium: Uptake and transport of intravenously injected colloidal carbon in rats. Kidney Int 9:395, 1976.

70. Mauer SM, Fish AJ, Blau EB, Michael AF: The glomerular mesangium. I. Kinetic studies of macromolecular uptake in normal and nephrotic rats. J Clin Invest 51:1092, 1972.

71. Schreiner GF, Cotran RS: Localization of an Ia-bearing glomerular cell in the mesangium. J Cell Biol 94:483, 1982.

72. Schreiner GF, Kiely JM, Cotran RS, Unanue ER: Characterization of resident glomerular cells in the rat expressing Ia determinants and manifesting genetically restricted interactions with lymphocytes. J Clin Invest 68:920, 1981.

73. Baud L, Hagege J, Sraer J, et al: Reactive oxygen production by cultured rat glomerular mesangial cells during phagocytosis is associated with stimulation of lipoxygenase activity. J Exp Med 158:1836, 1983.

74. Singhal PC, Ding GH, DeCandido S, et al: Endocytosis by cultured mesangial cells and associated changes in prostaglandin E2 synthesis. Am J Physiol 252:F627, 1987.

75. Abrahamson DR: Structure and development of the glomerular capillary wall and basement membrane. Am J Physiol 253:F783, 1987.

76. Jorgensen F, Bentzon MW: The ultastructure of the normal human glomerulus. Thickness of glomerular basement membrane. Lab Invest 18:42, 1968.

77. Osterby R: Morphometric studies of the peripheral glomerular basement membrane in early juvenile diabetes. I. Development of initial basement membrane thickening. Diabetologia 8:84, 1972.

78. Steffes MW, Barbosa J, Basgen JM, et al: Quantitative glomerular morphology of the normal human kidney. Lab Invest 49:82, 1983.

79. Rasch R: Prevention of diabetic glomerulopathy in streptozotocin diabetic rats by insulin treatment. Diabetologia 16:319, 1979.

80. Dean DC, Barr JF, Freytag JW, Hudson BG: Isolation of type IV procollagen-like polypeptides from glomerular basement membrane. Characterization of pro-alpha 1(IV). J Biol Chem 258:590, 1983.

81. Katz A, Fish AJ, Kleppel MM, et al: Renal entactin (nidogen): Isolation, characterization and tissue distribution. Kidney Int 40:643, 1991.

82. Miner JH: Renal basement membrane components. Kidney Int 56:2016, 1999.

83. Groffen AJ, Ruegg MA, Dijkman H, et al: Agrin is a major heparan sulfate proteoglycan in the human glomerular basement membrane. J Histochem Cytochem 46:19, 1998.

84. Hudson BG, Tryggvason K, Sundaramoorthy M, Neilson EG: Alport's syndrome, Goodpasture's syndrome, and type IV collagen. N Engl J Med 348:2543, 2003.

85. Kashtan CE: Alport syndrome and thin glomerular basement membrane disease. J Am Soc Nephrol 9:1736, 1998.

86. Zhou J, Reeders ST: The alpha chains of type IV collagen. Contrib Nephrol 117:80, 1996.

87. Caulfield JP, Farquhar MG: Distribution of anionic sites in glomerular basement membranes: Their possible role in filtration and attachment. Proc Natl Acad Sci U S A 73:1646, 1976.

88. Kanwar YS, Farquhar MG: Anionic sites in the glomerular basement membrane. In vivo and in vitro localization to the laminae rarae by cationic probes. J Cell Biol 81:137, 1979.

89. Kanwar YS, Farquhar MG: Isolation of glycosaminoglycans (heparan sulfate) from glomerular basement membranes. Proc Natl Acad Sci U S A 76:4493, 1979.

90. Kanwar YS, Farquhar MG: Presence of heparan sulfate in the glomerular basement membrane. Proc Natl Acad Sci U S A 76:1303, 1979.

91. Kanwar YS, Linker A, Farquhar MG: Increased permeability of the glomerular basement membrane to ferritin after removal of glycosaminoglycans (heparan sulfate) by enzyme digestion. J Cell Biol 86:688, 1980.

92. Rosenzweig LJ, Kanwar YS: Removal of sulfated (heparan sulfate) or nonsulfated (hyaluronic acid) glycosaminoglycans results in increased permeability of the glomerular basement membrane to 125I-bovine serum albumin. Lab Invest 47:177, 1982.

93. Kanwar YS, Rosenzweig LJ: Clogging of the glomerular basement membrane. J Cell Biol 93:489, 1982.

94. Brenner BM, Bohrer MP, Baylis C, Deen WM: Determinants of glomerular permselectivity: Insights derived from observations in vivo. Kidney Int 12:229, 1977.

95. Caulfield JP, Farquhar MG: The permeability of glomerular capillaries to graded dextrans. Identification of the basement membrane as the primary filtration barrier. J Cell Biol 63:883, 1974.

96. Rennke HG, Venkatachalam MA: Glomerular permeability: in vivo tracer studies with polyanionic and polycationic ferritins. Kidney Int 11:44, 1977.

97. Rennke HG, Patel Y, Venkatachalam MA: Glomerular filtration of proteins: clearance of anionic, neutral, and cationic horseradish peroxidase in the rat. Kidney Int 13:278, 1978.

98. Deen WM, Lazzara MJ, Myers BD: Structural determinants of glomerular permeability. Am J Physiol Renal Physiol 281:F579, 2001.

99. Ryan GB, Coghlan JP, Scoggins BA: The granulated peripolar epithelial cell: A potential secretory component of the renal juxtaglomerular complex. Nature 277:655, 1979.

100. Gall JA, Alcorn D, Butkus A, et al: Distribution of glomerular peripolar cells in different mammalian species. Cell Tissue Res 244:203, 1986.

101. Barajas L: Anatomy of the juxtaglomerular apparatus. Am J Physiol 237:F333, 1979.

102. Barajas L: The ultrastructure of the juxtaglomerular apparatus as disclosed by three-dimensional reconstructions from serial sections. The anatomical relationship between the tubular and vascular components. J Ultrastruct Res 33:116, 1970.

103. Barajas L, Salido E: Pathology of the juxtaglomerular apparatus. In Tisher CC, Brenner BM (eds): Renal Pathology with Clinical and Functional Correlations, 2nd ed. Philadelphia, JB Lippincott, 1994, p 948.

104. Tisher CC, Bulger RE, Trump BF: Human renal ultrastructure. 3. The distal tubule in healthy individuals. Lab Invest 18:655, 1968.

105. Hackenthal E, Paul M, Ganten D, Taugner R: Morphology, physiology, and molecular biology of renin secretion. Physiol Rev 70:1067, 1990.

106. Biava CG, West M: Fine structure of normal human juxtaglomerular cells. II. Specific and nonspecific cytoplasmic granules. Am J Pathol 49:955, 1966.

107. Barajas L: The development and ultrastructure of the juxtaglomerular cell granule. J Ultrastruct Res 15:400, 1966.

108. Celio MR, Inagami T: Angiotensin II immunoreactivity coexists with renin in the juxtaglomerular granular cells of the kidney. Proc Natl Acad Sci U S A 78:3897, 1981.

109. Deschepper CF, Mellon SH, Cumin F, et al: Analysis by immunocytochemistry and in situ hybridization of renin and its mRNA in kidney, testis, adrenal, and pituitary of the rat. Proc Natl Acad Sci U S A 83:7552, 1986.

110. Pricam C, Humbert F, Perrelet A, Orci L: Gap junctions in mesangial and lacis cells. J Cell Biol 63:349, 1974.

111. Taugner R, Schiller A, Kaissling B, Kriz W: Gap junctional coupling between the JGA and the glomerular tuft. Cell Tissue Res 186:279, 1978.

112. Ren Y, Carretero OA, Garvin JL: Role of mesangial cells and gap junctions in tubuloglomerular feedback. Kidney Int 62:525, 2002.

113. Kaissling B, Kriz W: Variability of intercellular spaces between macula densa cells: A transmission electron microscopic study in rabbits and rats. Kidney Int Suppl 12: S9, 1982.

114. Hoyer JR, Sisson SP, Vernier RL: Tamm-Horsfall glycoprotein: Ultrastructural immunoperoxidase localization in rat kidney. Lab Invest 41:168, 1979.

115. Kirk KL, Bell PD, Barfuss DW, Ribadeneira M: Direct visualization of the isolated and perfused macula densa. Am J Physiol 248:F890-F894, 1985.

116. Barajas L: The innervation of the juxtaglomerular apparatus. An electron microscopic study of the innervation of the glomerular arterioles. Lab Invest 13:916, 1964.

117. Barajas L, Muller J: The innervation of the juxtaglomerular apparatus and surrounding tubules: A quantitative analysis by serial section electron microscopy. J Ultrastruct Res 43:107, 1973.

118. Barajas L, Wang P: Localization of tritiated norepinephrine in the renal arteriolar nerves. Anat Rec 195:525, 1979.

119. Kopp UC, DiBona GF: Neural regulation of renin secretion. Semin Nephrol 13:543, 1993.

120. Schnermann J, Briggs JP: The function of the juxtaglomerular apparatus: Control of glomerular hemodynamics and renin secretion. In Seldin DW, Giebisch G (eds): The Kidney: Physiology and Pathophysiology, 2nd ed. New York, Raven Press, 1992, p 1249.

121. Schnermann J: Juxtaglomerular cell complex in the regulation of renal salt excretion. Am J Physiol 274:R263-R279, 1998.

122. Schlatter E, Salomonsson M, Persson AE, Greger R: Macula densa cells sense luminal NaCl concentration via furosemide sensitive Na$^+$2Cl$^-$-K$^+$ cotransport. Pflugers Arch 414:286, 1989.

123. Lapointe JY, Laamarti A, Hurst AM, et al: Activation of Na:2Cl:K cotransport by luminal chloride in macula densa cells. Kidney Int 47:752, 1995.

124. Obermuller N, Kunchaparty S, Ellison DH, Bachmann S: Expression of the Na-K-2Cl cotransporter by macula densa and thick ascending limb cells of rat and rabbit nephron. J Clin Invest 98:635, 1996.

125. Kurtz A, Wagner C: Cellular control of renin secretion. J Exp Biol 202:219, 1999.

126. Persson AE, Bachmann S: Constitutive nitric oxide synthesis in the kidney—functions at the juxtaglomerular apparatus. Acta Physiol Scand 169:317, 2000.

127. Kim SM, Mizel D, Huang YG, et al: Adenosine as a mediator of macula densa-dependent inhibition of renin secretion. Am J Physiol Renal Physiol 290:F1016, 2006.

128. Wilcox CS, Welch WJ, Murad F, et al: Nitric oxide synthase in macula densa regulates glomerular capillary pressure. Proc Natl Acad Sci U S A 89:11993, 1992.

129. Mundel P, Bachmann S, Bader M, et al: Expression of nitric oxide synthase in kidney macula densa cells. Kidney Int 42:1017, 1992.

130. Tojo A, Gross SS, Zhang L, et al: Immunocytochemical localization of distinct isoforms of nitric oxide synthase in the juxtaglomerular apparatus of normal rat kidney. J Am Soc Nephrol 4:1438, 1994.

131. Sigmon DH, Carretero OA, Beierwaltes WH: Endothelium-derived relaxing factor regulates renin release in vivo. Am J Physiol 263:F256, 1992.

132. Beierwaltes WH: Selective neuronal nitric oxide synthase inhibition blocks furosemide-stimulated renin secretion in vivo. Am J Physiol Renal Physiol 269:F134, 1995.

133. He XR, Greenberg SG, Briggs JP, Schnermann JB: Effect of nitric oxide on renin secretion. II. Studies in the perfused juxtaglomerular apparatus. Am J Physiol 268:F953, 1995.

134. Ito S, Ren Y: Evidence for the role of nitric oxide in macula densa control of glomerular hemodynamics. J Clin Invest 92:1093, 1993.

135. Thorup C, Persson AE: Inhibition of locally produced nitric oxide resets tubuloglomerular feedback mechanism. Am J Physiol 267:F606, 1994.

136. Welch WJ, Wilcox CS, Thomson SC: Nitric oxide and tubuloglomerular feedback. Semin Nephrol 19:251, 1999.

137. Satriano J, Wead L, Cardus A, et al: Regulation of ecto-5'-nucleotidase by NaCl and nitric oxide: Potential roles in tubuloglomerular feedback and adaptation. Am J Physiol Renal Physiol 291:F1078-1082, 2006.

138. Schnermann J, Levine DZ: Paracrine factors in tubuloglomerular feedback: Adenosine, ATP, and nitric oxide*. Ann Rev Physiol 65:501, 2003.

139. Sun D, Samuelson LC, Yang T, et al: Mediation of tubuloglomerular feedback by adenosine: Evidence from mice lacking adenosine 1 receptors. Proc Natl Acad Sci U S A 98:9983, 2001.

140. Castrop H, Huang Y, Hashimoto S, et al: Impairment of tubuloglomerular feedback regulation of GFR in ecto-5'-nucleotidase/CD73-deficient mice. J Clin Invest 114:634, 2004.

141. Harris RC, Zhang MZ, Cheng HF: Cyclooxygenase-2 and the renal renin-angiotensin system. Acta Physiol Scand 181:543, 2004.

142. Harris RC, McKanna JA, Akai Y, et al: Cyclooxygenase-2 is associated with the macula densa of rat kidney and increases with salt restriction. J Clin Invest 94:2504, 1994.

143. Traynor TR, Smart A, Briggs JP, Schnermann J: Inhibition of macula densa-stimulated renin secretion by pharmacological blockade of cyclooxygenase-2. Am J Physiol 277: F706, 1999.

144. Harris RC, Breyer MD: Physiological regulation of cyclooxygenase-2 in the kidney. Am J Physiol Renal Physiol 281:F1, 2001.

145. Yang T, Endo Y, Huang YG, et al: Renin expression in COX-2-knockout mice on normal or low-salt diets. Am J Physiol Renal Physiol 279:F819, 2000.

146. Cheng HF, Wang JL, Zhang MZ, et al: Nitric oxide regulates renal cortical cyclooxygenase-2 expression. Am J Physiol Renal Physiol 279:F122, 2000.

147. Madsen KM, Park CH: Lysosome distribution and cathepsin B and L activity along the rabbit proximal tubule. Am J Physiol 253:F1290, 1987.

148. Zhai XY, Birn H, Jensen KB, et al: Digital three-dimensional reconstruction and ultrastructure of the mouse proximal tubule. J Am Soc Nephrol 14:611, 2003.

149. Maunsbach AB: Observations on the segmentation of the proximal tubule in the rat kidney. Comparison of results from phase contrast, fluorescence and electron microscopy. J Ultrastruct Res 16:239, 1966.

150. Tisher CC, Bulger RE, Trump BF: Human renal ultrastructure. I. Proximal tubule of healthy individuals. Lab Invest 15:1357, 1966.

151. Kaissling B, Kriz W: Structural analysis of the rabbit kidney. Adv Anat Embryol Cell Biol 56:1, 1979.

152. Woodhall PB, Tisher CC, Simonton CA, Robinson RR: Relationship between para-aminohippurate secretion and cellular morphology in rabbit proximal tubules. J Clin Invest 61:1320, 1978.

153. Tisher CC, Rosen S, Osborne GB: Ultrastructure of the proximal tubule of the rhesus monkey kidney. Am J Pathol 56:469, 1969.

154. Welling LW, Welling DJ: Shape of epithelial cells and intercellular channels in the rabbit proximal nephron. Kidney Int 9:385, 1976.

155. Farquhar MG, Palade GE: Junctional complexes in various epithelia. J Cell Biol 17:375, 1963.

156. Maunsbach AB: Absorption of ferritin by rat kidney proximal tubule cells. Electron microscopic observations of the initial uptake phase in cells of microperfused single proximal tubules. J Ultrastruct Res 16:1, 1966.

157. Graham RC, Jr, Karnovsky MJ: The early stages of absorption of injected horseradish peroxidase in the proximal tubules of mouse kidney: ultrastructural cytochemistry by a new technique. J Histochem Cytochem 14:291, 1966.

158. Grandchamp A, Boulpaep EL: Pressure control of sodium reabsorption and intercellular backflux across proximal kidney tubule. J Clin Invest 54:69, 1974.

159. Schultz SG: The role of paracellular pathways in isotonic fluid transport. Yale J Biol Med 50:99, 1977.

160. Lutz MD, Cardinal J, Burg MB: Electrical resistance of renal proximal tubule perfused in vitro. Am J Physiol 225:729, 1973.

161. Tisher CC, Yarger WE: Lanthanum permeability of the tight junction (zonula occludens) in the renal tubule of the rat. Kidney Int 3:238, 1973.

162. Martinez-Palomo A, Erlij D: The distribution of lanthanum in tight junctions of the kidney tubule. Pflugers Arch 343:267, 1973.

163. Claude P, Goodenough DA: Fracture faces of zonulae occludentes from "tight" and "leaky" epithelia. J Cell Biol 58:390, 1973.

164. Roesinger B, Schiller A, Taugner R: A freeze-fracture study of tight junctions in the pars convoluta and pars recta of the renal proximal tubule. Cell Tissue Res 186:121, 1978.

165. Kuhn K, Reale E: Junctional complexes of the tubular cells in the human kidney as revealed with freeze-fracture. Cell Tissue Res 160:193, 1975.

166. Silverblatt FJ, Bulger RE: Gap junctions occur in vertebrate renal proximal tubule cells. J Cell Biol 47:513, 1970.

167. Christensen EI, Madsen KM: Renal age changes: Observations of the rat kidney cortex with special reference to structure and function of the lysosomal system in the proximal tubule. Lab Invest 39:289, 1978.

168. Ernst SA: Transport ATPase cytochemistry: Ultrastructural localization of potassium-dependent and potassium-independent phosphatase activities in rat kidney cortex. J Cell Biol 66:586, 1975.

169. Kashgarian M, Biemesderfer D, Caplan M, Forbush B, III: Monoclonal antibody to Na,K-ATPase: Immunocytochemical localization along nephron segments. Kidney Int 28:899, 1985.

170. Welling LW, Welling DJ: Surface areas of brush border and lateral cell walls in the rabbit proximal nephron. Kidney Int 8:343, 1975.

171. Bergeron M, Guerette D, Forget J, Thiery G: Three-dimensional characteristics of the mitochondria of the rat nephron. Kidney Int 17:175, 1980.

172. Bergeron M, Thiery G: Three-dimensional characteristics of the endoplasmic reticulum of rat renal tubule cells: An electron microscopy study in thick sections. Biol Cell 43:1981.

173. Coudrier E, Kerjaschki D, Louvard D: Cytoskeleton organization and submembranous interactions in intestinal and renal brush borders. Kidney Int 34:309, 1988.

174. Rodman JS, Mooseker M, Farquhar MG: Cytoskeletal proteins of the rat kidney proximal tubule brush border. Eur J Cell Biol 42:319, 1986.

175. Heidrich HG, Kinne R, Kinne-Saffran E, Hannig K: The polarity of the proximal tubule cell in rat kidney. Different surface charges for the brush-border microvilli and plasma membranes from the basal infoldings. J Cell Biol 54:232, 1972.

176. Kerjaschki D, Noronha Blob L, Sacktor B, Farquhar MG: Microdomains of distinctive glycoprotein composition in the kidney proximal tubule brush border. J Cell Biol 98:1505, 1984.

177. Le Hir M, Kaissling B: Distribution and regulation of renal ecto-5′-nucleotidase: Implications for physiological functions of adenosine [editorial]. Am J Physiol 264:F377, 1993.

178. Christensen EI, Nielsen S: Structural and functional features of protein handling in the kidney proximal tubule. Semin Nephrol 11:414, 1991.

179. Rodman JS, Kerjaschki D, Merisko E, Farquhar MG: Presence of an extensive clathrin coat on the apical plasmalemma of the rat kidney proximal tubule cell. J Cell Biol 98:1630, 1984.

180. Kerjaschki D, Farquhar MG: The pathogenic antigen of Heymann nephritis is a membrane glycoprotein of the renal proximal tubule brush border. Proc Natl Acad Sci U S A 79:5557, 1982.

181. Maunsbach AB: Observations on the ultrastructure and acid phosphatase activity of the cytoplasmic bodies in rat kidney proximal tubule cells. With a comment on their classification. J Ultrastruct Res 16:197, 1966.

182. Larsson L, Clapp WL, Park CH, et al: Ultrastructural localization of acidic compartments in cells of isolated rabbit PCT. Am J Physiol 253:F95, 1987.

183. Verlander JW, Madsen KM, Larsson L, et al: Immunocytochemical localization of intracellular acidic compartments: Rat proximal nephron. Am J Physiol 257:F454, 1989.

184. Sabolic I, Burckhardt G: Characteristics of the proton pump in rat renal cortical endocytotic vesicles. Am J Physiol 250:F817, 1986.

185. Brown D, Hirsch S, Gluck S: Localization of a proton-pumping ATPase in rat kidney. J Clin Invest 82:2114, 1988.

186. Morin JP, Viotte G, Vandewalle A, et al: Gentamicin-induced nephrotoxicity: a cell biology approach. Kidney Int 18:583, 1980.

187. Madsen KM: Mercury accumulation in kidney lysosomes or proteinuric rats. Kidney Int 18:445, 1980.

188. Madsen KM, Christensen EI: Effects of mercury on lysosomal protein digestion in the kidney proximal tubule. Lab Invest 38:165, 1978.

189. Madsen KM, Maunsbach AB: Effects of chronic mercury exposure on the rat kidney cortex a studied morphometrically by light and electron microscopy. Virchows Arch B 37:137, 1981.

190. Maunsbach AB: Absorption of I^{125}-labeled homologous albumin by rat kidney proximal tubule cells. A study of microperfused single proximal tubules by electron microscopic autoradiography and histochemistry. 1966 [classical article]. J Am Soc Nephrol 8:323, 1997.

191. Maack T, Johnson V, Kau ST, et al: Renal filtration, transport, and metabolism of low-molecular-weight proteins: A review. Kidney Int 16:251, 1979.

192. Christensen EI: Rapid membrane recycling in renal proximal tubule cells. Eur J Cell Biol 29:43, 1982.

193. Nielsen S, Nielsen JT, Christensen EI: Luminal and basolateral uptake of insulin in isolated, perfused, proximal tubules. Am J Physiol 253:F857, 1987.

194. Olbricht CJ, Cannon JK, Garg LC, Tisher CC: Activities of cathepsins B and L in isolated nephron segments from proteinuric and nonproteinuric rats. Am J Physiol 250:F1055, 1986.

195. Sumpio BE, Maack T: Kinetics, competition, and selectivity of tubular absorption of proteins. Am J Physiol 243:F379, 1982.

196. Christensen EI, Rennke HG, Carone FA: Renal tubular uptake of protein: Effect of molecular charge. Am J Physiol 244:F436, 1983.

197. Park CH, Maack T: Albumin absorption and catabolism by isolated perfused proximal convoluted tubules of the rabbit. J Clin Invest 73:767, 1984.

198. Park CH: Time course and vectorial nature of albumin metabolism in isolated perfused rabbit PCT. Am J Physiol 255:F520, 1988.

199. Farquhar MG, Saito A, Kerjaschki D, Orlando RA: The Heymann nephritis antigenic complex: megalin (gp330) and RAP. J Am Soc Nephrol 6:35, 1995.

200. Christensen EI, Birn H: Megalin and cubilin: Synergistic endocytic receptors in renal proximal tubule. Am J Physiol Renal Physiol 280:F562, 2001.

201. Saito A, Pietromonaco S, Loo AK, Farquhar MG: Complete cloning and sequencing of rat gp330/"megalin," a distinctive member of the low density lipoprotein receptor gene family. Proc Natl Acad Sci U S A 91:9725, 1994.

202. Abbate M, Bachinsky D, Zheng G, et al: Location of gp330/α_2-m recptor-associated protein (α_2-MRAP) and its binding sites in kidney: Distribution of endogenous α_2-MRAP is modified by tissue processing. Eur J Cell Biol 61:139, 1993.

203. Christensen EI, Nielsen S, Moestrup SK, et al: Segmental distribution of the endocytosis receptor gp330 in renal proximal tubules. Eur J Cell Biol 66:349, 1995.

204. Orlando RA, Rader K, Authier F, et al: Megalin is an endocytic receptor for insulin. J Am Soc Nephrol 9:1759, 1998.

205. Cui S, Verroust PJ, Moestrup SK, Christensen EI: Megalin/gp330 mediates uptake of albumin in renal proximal tubule. Am J Physiol 271:F900, 1996.

206. Christensen EI, Moskaug JO, Vorum H, et al: Evidence for an essential role of megalin in transepithelial transport of retinol. J Am Soc Nephrol 10:685, 1999.

207. Moestrup SK, Birn H, Fischer PB, et al: Megalin-mediated endocytosis of transcobalamin-vitamin-B12 complexes suggests a role of the receptor in vitamin-B12 homeostasis. Proc Natl Acad Sci U S A 93:8612, 1996.

208. Nykjaer A, Dragun D, Walther D, et al: An endocytic pathway essential for renal uptake and activation of the steroid 25-(OH) vitamin D3. Cell 96:507, 1999.

209. Moestrup SK, Cui S, Vorum H, et al: Evidence that epithelial glycoprotein 330/megalin mediates uptake of polybasic drugs. J Clin Invest 96:1404, 1995.

210. Christensen EI, Willnow TE: Essential role of megalin in renal proximal tubule for vitamin homeostasis. J Am Soc Nephrol 10:2224, 1999.

211. Leheste JR, Rolinski B, Vorum H, et al: Megalin knockout mice as an animal model of low molecular weight proteinuria. Am J Pathol 155:1361, 1999.

212. Christensen EI, Birn H: Megalin and cubilin: multifunctional endocytic receptors. Nat Rev Mol Cell Biol 3:256, 2002.

213. Birn H, Fyfe JC, Jacobsen C, et al: Cubilin is an albumin binding protein important for renal tubular albumin reabsorption. J Clin Invest 105:1353, 2000.

214. Burg MB: Renal handling of sodium, chloride, water, amino acids, and glucose. In Brenner BM, Rector FC Jr (eds): The Kidney. Philadelphia, WB Saunders, 1986, p 145.

215. Maunsbach AB, Tripathi S, Boulpaep EL: Ultrastructural changes in isolated perfused proximal tubules during osmotic water flow. Am J Physiol 253:F1091, 1987.

216. Tripathi S, Boulpaep EL, Maunsbach AB: Isolated perfused Ambystoma proximal tubule: Hydrodynamics modulates ultrastructure. Am J Physiol 252:F1129, 1987.

217. Agre P, Preston GM, Smith BL, et al: Aquaporin CHIP: The archetypal molecular water channel. Am J Physiol 265:F463, 1993.

218. Preston GM, Agre P: Isolation of the cDNA for erythrocyte integral membrane protein of 28 kilodaltons: Member of an ancient channel family. Proc Natl Acad Sci U S A 88:11110, 1991.

219. Nielsen S, Smith B, Christensen EI, et al: CHIP28 water channels are localized in constitutively water-permeable segments of the nephron. J Cell Biol 120:371, 1993.

220. Sabolic I, Valenti G, Verbavatz JM, et al: Localization of the CHIP28 water channel in rat kidney. Am J Physiol 263:C1225, 1992.

221. Maunsbach AB, Marples D, Chin E, et al: Aquaporin-1 water channel expression in human kidney. J Am Soc Nephrol 8:1, 1997.

222. Ishibashi K, Kuwahara M, Kageyama Y, et al: Cloning and functional expression of a second new aquaporin abundantly expressed in testis. Biochem Biophys Res Commun 237:714, 1997.

223. Ma T, Yang B, Verkman AS: Cloning of a novel water and urea-permeable aquaporin from mouse expressed strongly in colon, placenta, liver, and heart. Biochem Biophys Res Commun 240:324, 1997.

224. Elkjar ML, Nejsum LN, Gresz V, et al: Immunolocalization of aquaporin-8 in rat kidney, gastrointestinal tract, testis, and airways. Am J Physiol Renal Physiol 281: F1047, 2001.

225. Liu KF, Nagase HF, Huang CG, et al: Purification and functional characterization of aquaporin-8. Biol Cell 98:153–161, 2006.

226. Holm LM, Jahn TP, Moller AL, et al: NH3 and NH4+ permeability in aquaporin-expressing Xenopus oocytes. Pflugers Arch 450:415, 2005.

227. Ishibashi K, Kuwahara M, Kageyama Y, et al: Molecular cloning of a new aquaporin superfamily in mammals: AQPX1 and AQPX2. In Hohmann S, Nielsen S (eds): Molecular Biology and Physiology of Water and Solute Transport. New York, Kluwer Academic/Plenum Publishers, 2006, p 123.

228. Morishita Y, Matsuzaki T, Hara-chikuma M, et al: Disruption of aquaporin-11 produces polycystic kidneys following vacuolization of the proximal tubule. Mol Cell Biol 25:7770, 2005.

229. Gorelick D, Praetorius J, Tsunenari T, et al: Aquaporin-11: A channel protein lacking apparent transport function expressed in brain. BMC Biochemistry 7:14, 2006.

230. Ernst SA, Schreiber JH: Ultrastructural localization of Na+,K+-ATPase in rat and rabbit kidney medulla. J Cell Biol 91:803, 1981.

231. Rector FC, Jr: Sodium, bicarbonate, and chloride absorption by the proximal tubule. Am J Physiol 244:F461, 1983.

232. Aronson PS: Mechanisms of active H+ secretion in the proximal tubule. Am J Physiol 245:F647, 1983.

233. Alpern RJ, Stone DK, Rector FC Jr: Renal acidification mechanisms. In Brenner BM, Rector FC Jr (eds): The Kidney. Volume I. Philadelphia and London, WB Saunders, 1991, p 318.

234. Biemesderfer D, Pizzonia J, Abu-Alfa A, et al: NHE3: A Na+/H+ exchanger isoform of renal brush border. Am J Physiol 265:F736, 1993.

235. Amemiya M, Loffing J, Lotscher M, et al: Expression of NHE-3 in the apical membrane of rat renal proximal tubule and thick ascending limb. Kidney Int 48:1206, 1995.

236. Preisig PA, Ives HE, Cragoe EJ, Jr, et al: Role of the Na+/H+ antiporter in rat proximal tubule bicarbonate absorption. J Clin Invest 80:970, 1987.

237. Kinne-Saffran E, Beauwens R, Kinne R: An ATP-driven proton pump in brush-border membranes from rat renal cortex. J Membr Biol 64:67, 1982.

238. Lorenz JN, Schultheis PJ, Traynor T, et al: Micropuncture analysis of single-nephron function in NHE3-deficient mice. Am J Physiol 277:F447, 1999.

239. Schultheis PJ, Clarke LL, Meneton P, et al: Renal and intestinal absorptive defects in mice lacking the NHE3 Na+/H+ exchanger. Nat Genet 19:282, 1998.

240. Hayashi H, Szaszi K, Grinstein S: Multiple modes of regulation of Na+/H+ exchangers. Ann N Y Acad Sci 976:248, 2002.

241. Good DW, George T, Watts BA, III: Nongenomic regulation by aldosterone of the epithelial NHE3 Na+/H+ exchanger. Am J Physiol Cell Physiol 290:C757, 2006.

242. Honegger KJ, Capuano P, Winter C, et al: Regulation of sodium-proton exchanger isoform 3 (NHE3) by PKA and exchange protein directly activated by cAMP (EPAC). Proc Natl Acad Sci 103:803, 2006.

243. Weinman EJ, Steplock D, Shenolikar S: NHERF-1 uniquely transduces the cAMP signals that inhibit sodium-hydrogen exchange in mouse renal apical membranes. FEBS Lett 536:141, 2003.

244. Huang P, Steplock D, Weinman EJ, et al: κ Opioid receptor interacts with Na+/H+-exchanger regulatory factor-1/ezrin-radixin-moesin-binding phosphoprotein-50 (NHERF-1/EBP50) to stimulate Na$^+$/H$^+$ exchange independent of Gi/Go proteins. J Biol Chem 279:25002, 2004.

245. Alexander RT, Furuya W, Szaszi K, et al: Rho GTPases dictate the mobility of the Na/H exchanger NHE3 in epithelia: Role in apical retention and targeting. Proc Natl Acad Sci 102:12253, 2005.

246. Du Z, Duan Y, Yan Q, et al: Mechanosensory function of microvilli of the kidney proximal tubule. Proc Natl Acad Sci 101:13068, 2004.

247. Alpern RJ: Mechanism of basolateral membrane H+/OH-/HCO-3 transport in the rat proximal convoluted tubule. A sodium-coupled electrogenic process. J Gen Physiol 86:613, 1985.

248. Soleimani M, Grassi SM, Aronson PS: Stoichiometry of Na+-HCO-3 cotransport in basolateral membrane vesicles isolated from rabbit renal cortex. J Clin Invest 79:1276, 1987.

249. Soleimani M, Burnham CE: Na+:HCO(3−) cotransporters (NBC): Cloning and characterization. J Membr Biol 183:71, 2001.

250. Romero MF, Hediger MA, Boulpaep EL, Boron WF: Expression cloning and characterization of a renal electrogenic Na+/HCO3− cotransporter. Nature 387:409, 1997.

251. Burnham CE, Amlal H, Wang Z, et al: Cloning and functional expression of a human kidney Na+:HCO3- cotransporter. J Biol Chem 272:19111, 1997.

252. Romero MF, Fong P, Berger UV, et al: Cloning and functional expression of rNBC, an electrogenic Na(+)-HCO3- cotransporter from rat kidney. Am J Physiol 274:F425, 1998.

253. Abuladze N, Lee I, Newman D, et al: Axial heterogeneity of sodium-bicarbonate cotransporter expression in the rabbit proximal tubule. Am J Physiol Renal Physiol 274:F628, 1998.

254. Schmitt BM, Biemesderfer D, Romero MF, et al: Immunolocalization of the electrogenic Na+-HCO-3 cotransporter in mammalian and amphibian kidney. Am J Physiol 276:F27, 1999.

255. Maunsbach AB, Vorum H, Kwon TH, et al: Immunoelectron microscopic localization of the electrogenic Na/HCO(3) cotransporter in rat and ambystoma kidney. J Am Soc Nephrol 11:2179, 2000.

256. Igarashi T, Inatomi J, Sekine T, et al: Mutations in SLC4A4 cause permanent isolated proximal renal tubular acidosis with ocular abnormalities. Nat Genet 23:264, 1999.

257. Good DW, Burg MB: Ammonia production by individual segments of the rat nephron. J Clin Invest 73:602, 1984.

258. Good DW, DuBose TD, Jr: Ammonia transport by early and late proximal convoluted tubule of the rat. J Clin Invest 79:684, 1987.

259. Nagami GT, Kurokawa K: Regulation of ammonia production by mouse proximal tubules perfused in vitro. Effect of luminal perfusion. J Clin Invest 75:844, 1985.

260. Knepper MA, Packer R, Good DW: Ammonium transport in the kidney. Physiol Rev 69:179, 1989.

261. Katz AI, Doucet A, Morel F: Na-K-ATPase activity along the rabbit, rat, and mouse nephron. Am J Physiol 237:F114, 1979.

262. Clapp WL, Park CH, Madsen KM, Tisher CC: Axial heterogeneity in the handling of albumin by the rabbit proximal tubule. Lab Invest 58:549, 1988.

263. Ohno S: Peroxisomes of the kidney. Int Rev Cytol 95:131, 1985.

264. Angermuller S, Leupold C, Zaar K, Fahimi HD: Electron microscopic cytochemical localization of alpha-hydroxyacid oxidase in rat kidney cortex. Heterogeneous staining of peroxisomes. Histochemistry 85:411, 1986.

265. McKinney TD: Heterogeneity of organic base secretion by proximal tubules. Am J Physiol 243:F404, 1982.

266. Burckhardt G, Wolff NA: Structure of renal organic anion and cation transporters. Am J Physiol Renal Physiol 278:F853, 2000.

267. Lopez-Nieto CE, You G, Bush KT, et al: Molecular cloning and characterization of NKT, a gene product related to the organic cation transporter family that is almost exclusively expressed in the kidney. J Biol Chem 272:6471, 1997.

268. Sekine T, Watanabe N, Hosoyamada M, et al: Expression cloning and characterization of a novel multispecific organic anion transporter. J Biol Chem 272:18526, 1997.

269. Sweet DH, Wolff NA, Pritchard JB: Expression cloning and characterization of ROAT1. The basolateral organic anion transporter in rat kidney. J Biol Chem 272:30088, 1997.

270. Hosoyamada M, Sekine T, Kanai Y, Endou H: Molecular cloning and functional expression of a multispecific organic anion transporter from human kidney. Am J Physiol 276:F122–F128, 1999.

271. Tojo A, Sekine T, Nakajima N, et al: Immunohistochemical localization of multispecific renal organic anion transporter 1 in rat kidney. J Am Soc Nephrol 10:464, 1999.

272. Karbach U, Kricke J, Meyer-Wentrup F, et al: Localization of organic cation transporters OCT1 and OCT2 in rat kidney. Am J Physiol Renal Physiol 279:F679, 2000.

273. Ishibashi K, Kuwahara M, Gu Y, et al: Cloning and functional expression of a new water channel abundantly expressed in the testis permeable to water, glycerol, and urea. J Biol Chem 272:20782, 1997.

274. Nejsum LN, Elkjaer M-L, Hager H, et al: Localization of aquaporin-7 in rat and mouse kidney using RT-PCR, immunoblotting, and immunocytochemistry. Biochem Biophys Res Commun 277:164, 2000.

275. Ishibashi K, Imai M, Sasaki S: Cellular localization of aquaporin 7 in the rat kidney. Nephron Exp Nephrol 8:252, 2000.

276. Sohara E, Rai T, Miyazaki Ji, et al: Defective water and glycerol transport in the proximal tubules of AQP7 knockout mice. Am J Physiol Renal Physiol 289:F1195, 2005.

277. Jamison RL, Kriz W: Urinary Concentrating Mechanism: Structure and Function. New York, Oxford University Press, 1982.

278. Schwartz MM, Venkatachalam MA: Structural differences in thin limbs of Henle: Physiological implications. Kidney Int 6:193, 1974.

279. Kriz W, Koepsell H: The structural organization of the mouse kidney. Z Anat Entwicklungsgesch 144:137, 1974.

280. Barrett JM, Kriz W, Kaissling B, de-Rouffignac C: The ultrastructure of the nephrons of the desert rodent (Psammomys obesus) kidney. I. Thin limb of Henle of short-looped nephrons. Am J Anat 151:487, 1978.

281. Barrett JM, Kriz W, Kaissling B, de-Rouffignac C: The ultrastructure of the nephrons of the desert rodent (Psammomys obesus) kidney. II. Thin limbs of Henle of long-looped nephrons. Am J Anat 151:499, 1978.

282. Zhai XY, Thomsen JS, Birn H, et al: Three-dimensional reconstruction of the mouse nephron. J Am Soc Nephrol 17:77, 2006.

283. Dieterich HJ, Barrett JM, Kriz W, Bulhoff JP: The ultrastructure of the thin loop limbs of the mouse kidney. Anat Embryol Berl 147:1, 1975.

284. Bachmann S, Kriz W: Histotopography and ultrastructure of the thin limbs of the loop of Henle in the hamster. Cell Tissue Res 225:111, 1982.

285. Kriz W, Schiller A, Taugner R: Freeze-fracture studies on the thin limbs of Henle's loop in Psammomys obesus. Am J Anat 162:23, 1981.

286. Schiller A, Taugner R, Kriz W: The thin limbs of Henle's loop in the rabbit. A freeze fracture study. Cell Tissue Res 207:249, 1980.

287. Schwartz MM, Karnovsky MJ, Venkatachalam MA: Regional membrane specialization in the thin limbs of Henle's loops as seen by freeze-fracture electron microscopy. Kidney Int 16:577, 1979.

288. Kleinman JG, Beshensky A, Worcester EM, Brown D: Expression of osteopontin, a urinary inhibitor of stone mineral crystal growth, in rat kidney. Kidney Int 47:1585, 1995.

289. Madsen KM, Zhang L, bu Shamat AR, et al: Ultrastructural localization of osteopontin in the kidney: Induction by lipopolysaccharide. J Am Soc Nephrol 8:1043, 1997.

290. Garg LC, Tisher CC: Na-K-ATPase activity in thin limbs of rat nephron. Abstract. Kidney Int 23:255, 1983.

291. Garg LC, Knepper MA, Burg MB: Mineralocorticoid effects on Na-K-ATPase in individual nephron segments. Am J Physiol 240:F536-F544, 1981.

292. Imai M: Functional heterogeneity of the descending limbs of Henle's loop. II. Interspecies differences among rabbits, rats, and hamsters. Pflugers Arch 402:393, 1984.

293. Imai M, Hayashi M, Araki M: Functional heterogeneity of the descending limbs of Henle's loop. I. Internephron heterogeneity in the hamster kidney. Pflugers Arch 402:385, 1984.

294. Nielsen S, Pallone TL, Smith BL, et al: Aquaporin-1 water channels in short and long loop descending thin limbs and in descending vasa recta in rat kidney. Am J Physiol 268:F1023, 1995.

295. Pannabecker TL, Abbott DE, Dantzler WH: Three-dimensional functional reconstruction of inner medullary thin limbs of Henle's loop. Am J Physiol Renal Physiol 286: F38, 2004.

296. Pannabecker TL, Dantzler WH: Three-dimensional lateral and vertical relationships of inner medullary loops of Henle and collecting ducts. Am J Physiol Renal Physiol 287:F767, 2004.

297. Shayakul C, Knepper MA, Smith CP, et al: Segmental localization of urea transporter mRNAs in rat kidney. Am J Physiol 272:F654, 1997.

298. Kim YH, Kim DU, Han KH, et al: Expression of urea transporters in the developing rat kidney. Am J Physiol Renal Physiol 282:F530, 2002.

299. Nielsen S, Terris J, Smith CP, et al: Cellular and subcellular localization of the vasopressin-regulated urea transporter in rat kidney. Proc Natl Acad Sci U S A 93:5495, 1996.

300. Sands JM, Timmer RT, Gunn RB: Urea transporters in kidney and erythrocytes. Am J Physiol 273:F321, 1997.

301. Shayakul C, Smith CP, Mackenzie HS, et al: Long-term regulation of urea transporter expression by vasopressin in Brattleboro rats. Am J Physiol Renal Physiol 278:F620, 2000.

302. Wade JB, Lee AJ, Liu J, et al: UT-A2: A 55-kDa urea transporter in thin descending limb whose abundance is regulated by vasopressin. Am J Physiol Renal Physiol 278: F52, 2000.

303. Knepper MA, Rector FC Jr: Urinary concentration and dilution. In Brenner BM, Rector FC Jr. (eds) The Kidney. Volume I. Philadelphia, London, WB Saunders, 1991, p 445.

304. Kokko JP, Rector FC, Jr: Countercurrent multiplication system without active transport in inner medulla. Kidney Int 2:214, 1972.

305. Uchida S, Sasaki S, Furukawa T, et al: Molecular cloning of a chloride channel that is regulated by dehydration and expressed predominantly in kidney medulla. J Biol Chem 268:3821, 1993.

306. Uchida S, Sasaki S, Nitta K, et al: Localization and functional characterization of rat kidney-specific chloride channel, ClC-K1. J Clin Invest 95:104, 1995.

307. Takeuchi Y, Uchida S, Marumo F, Sasaki S: Cloning, tissue distribution, and intrarenal localization of ClC chloride channels in human kidney. Kidney Int 48:1497, 1995.

308. Imai M, Kokko JP: Mechanism of sodium and chloride transport in the thin ascending limb of Henle. J Clin Invest 58:1054, 1976.

309. Yoshitomi K, Kondo Y, Imai M: Evidence for conductive Cl- pathways across the cell membranes of the thin ascending limb of Henle's loop. J Clin Invest 82:866, 1988.

310. Matsumura Y, Uchida S, Kondo Y, et al: Overt nephrogenic diabetes insipidus in mice lacking the CLC-K1 chloride channel. Nat Genet 21:95, 1999.

311. Imai M: Function of the thin ascending limbs of Henle of rats and hamsters perfused in vitro. Am J Physiol 232:F201, 1977.

312. Chou CL, Knepper MA: In vitro perfusion of chinchilla thin limb segments: urea and NaCl permeabilities. Am J Physiol 1993.

313. Bagnasco S, Balaban R, Fales HM, et al: Predominant osmotically active organic solutes in rat and rabbit renal medullas. J Biol Chem 261:5872, 1986.

314. Garcia-Perez A, Burg MB: Renal medullary organic osmolytes. Physiol Rev 71:1081, 1991.

315. Burg MB, Kwon AE, Kultz D: Regulation of gene expression by hypertonicity. Ann Rev Physiol 59:437, 1997.

316. Na KY, Woo SK, Lee SD, Kwon HM: Silencing of TonEBP/NFAT5 transcriptional activator by RNA interference. J Am Soc Nephrol 14:283, 2003.

317. Woo SK, Lee SD, Na KY, et al: TonEBP/NFAT5 stimulates transcription of HSP70 in response to hypertonicity. Mol Cell Biol 22:5753, 2002.

318. Miyakawa H, Woo SK, Dahl SC, et al: Tonicity-responsive enhancer binding protein, a Rel-like protein that stimulates transcription in response to hypertonicity. Proc Natl Acad Sci 96:2538, 1999.

319. Lopez-Rodriguez C, Antos CL, Shelton JM, et al: Loss of NFAT5 results in renal atrophy and lack of tonicity-responsive gene expression. Proc Natl Acad Sci 101:2392, 2004.

320. Allen F, Tisher CC: Morphology of the ascending thick limb of Henle. Kidney Int 9:8, 1976.

321. Kone BC, Madsen KM, Tisher CC: Ultrastructure of the thick ascending limb of Henle in the rat kidney. Am J Anat 171:217, 1984.

322. Welling LW, Welling DJ, Hill JJ: Shape of cells and intercellular channels in rabbit thick ascending limb of Henle. Kidney Int 13:144, 1978.

323. Kokko JP, Tisher CC: Water movement across nephron segments involved with the countercurrent multiplication system. Kidney Int 10:64, 1976.

324. Yoshitomi K, Koseki C, Taniguchi J, Imai M: Functional heterogeneity in the hamster medullary thick ascending limb of Henle's loop. Pflugers Arch 408:600, 1987.

325. Mennitt PA, Wade JB, Ecelbarger CA, et al: Localization of ROMK channels in the rat kidney. J Am Soc Nephrol 8:1823, 1997.

326. Xu JZ, Hall AE, Peterson LN, et al: Localization of the ROMK protein on apical membranes of rat kidney nephron segments. Am J Physiol 273:F739, 1997.

327. Sikri KL, Foster CL, MacHugh N, Marshall RD: Localization of Tamm-Horsfall glyco-protein in the human kidney using immuno-fluorescence and immuno-electron microscopical techniques. J Anat 132:597, 1981.

328. Bachmann S, Koeppen-Hagemann I, Kriz W: Ultrastructural localization of Tamm-Horsfall glycoprotein (THP) in rat kidney as revealed by protein A-gold immunocy-tochemistry. Histochemistry 83:531, 1985.

329. Greger R, Schlatter E: Presence of luminal K+, a prerequisite for active NaCl transport in the cortical thick ascending limb of Henle's loop of rabbit kidney. Pflugers Arch 392:92, 1981.

330. Hebert SC, Andreoli TE: Control of NaCl transport in the thick ascending limb. Am J Physiol 246:F745, 1984.

331. Greger R, Schlatter E, Lang F: Evidence for electroneutral sodium chloride cotransport in the cortical thick ascending limb of Henle's loop of rabbit kidney. Pflugers Arch 396:308, 1983.

332. Schlatter E, Greger R, Weidtke C: Effect of "high ceiling" diuretics on active salt transport in the cortical thick ascending limb of Henle's loop of rabbit kidney. Correlation of chemical structure and inhibitory potency. Pflugers Arch 396:210, 1983.

333. Gamba G, Miyanoshita A, Lombardi M, et al: Molecular cloning, primary structure, and characterization of two members of the mammalian electroneutral sodium-(potas-sium)-chloride cotransporter family expressed in kidney. J Biol Chem 269:17713, 1994.

334. Xu JC, Lytle C, Zhu TT, et al: Molecular cloning and functional expression of the bumetanide-sensitive Na-K-Cl cotransporter. Proc Natl Acad Sci U S A 91:2201, 1994.

335. Igarashi P, Vanden Heuvel GB, Payne JA, Forbush B, III: Cloning, embryonic expres-sion, and alternative splicing of a murine kidney-specific Na-K-Cl cotransporter. Am J Physiol 269:F405, 1995.

336. Yang T, Huang YG, Singh I, et al: Localization of bumetanide- and thiazide-sensitive Na-K-Cl cotransporters along the rat nephron. Am J Physiol 271:F931, 1996.

337. Kaplan MR, Plotkin MD, Lee WS, et al: Apical localization of the Na-K-Cl cotrans-porter, rBSC1, on rat thick ascending limbs. Kidney Int 49:40, 1996.

338. Ecelbarger CA, Terris J, Hoyer JR, et al: Localization and regulation of the rat renal Na(+)-K(+)-2Cl– cotransporter, BSC-1. Am J Physiol 271:F619, 1996.

339. Nielsen S, Maunsbach AB, Ecelbarger CA, Knepper MA: Ultrastructural localization of Na-K-2Cl cotransporter in thick ascending limb and macula densa of rat kidney. Am J Physiol 275:F885, 1998.

340. Brunet GM, Gagnon E, Simard CF, et al: Novel insights regarding the operational characteristics and teleological purpose of the renal Na+-K+-2Cl cotransporter (NKCC2s) splice variants. J Gen Physiol 126:325, 2005.

341. Yang T, Huang YG, Singh I, et al: Localization of bumetanide- and thiazide-sensitive Na-K-Cl cotransporters along the rat nephron. Am J Physiol Renal Physiol 271:F931-F939, 1996.

342. Gimenez I, Isenring P, Forbush B: Spatially distributed alternative splice variants of the renal Na-K-Cl cotransport exhibit dramatically different affinities for the trans-ported ions. J Biol Chem 277:8767, 2002.

343. Gagnon E, Bergeron MJ, Daigle ND, et al: Molecular mechanisms of cation transport by the renal Na+-K+-Cl– cotransporter: Structural insight into the operating charac-teristics of the ion transport sites. J Biol Chem 280:32555, 2005.

344. Gimenez I, Forbush B: Regulatory phosphorylation sites in the NH2 terminus of the renal Na-K-Cl cotransporter (NKCC2). Am J Physiol Renal Physiol 289:F1341, 2005.

345. Kim GH, Ecelbarger CA, Mitchell C, et al: Vasopressin increases Na-K-2Cl cotrans-porter expression in thick ascending limb of Henle's loop. Am J Physiol 276:F96, 1999.

346. Garg LC, Mackie S, Tisher CC: Effect of low potassium-diet on Na-K-ATPase in rat nephron segments. Pflugers Arch 394:113, 1982.

347. Rocha AS, Kokko JP: Sodium chloride and water transport in the medullary thick ascending limb of Henle. Evidence for active chloride transport. J Clin Invest 52:612, 1973.

348. Burg MB, Green N: Function of the thick ascending limb of Henle's loop. Am J Physiol 224:659, 1973.

349. Good DW: Sodium-dependent bicarbonate absorption by cortical thick ascending limb of rat kidney. Am J Physiol 248:F821, 1985.

350. Good DW, Knepper MA, Burg MB: Ammonia and bicarbonate transport by thick ascending limb of rat kidney. Am J Physiol 247:F35, 1984.

351. Brown D, Zhu XL, Sly WS: Localization of membrane-associated carbonic anhydrase type IV in kidney epithelial cells. Proc Natl Acad Sci U S A 87:7457, 1990.

352. Good DW: Inhibition of bicarbonate absorption by peptide hormones and cyclic ade-nosine monophosphate in rat medullary thick ascending limb. J Clin Invest 85:1006, 1990.

353. Alper SL, Stuart-Tilley AK, Biemesderfer D, et al: Immunolocalization of AE2 anion exchanger in rat kidney. Am J Physiol 273:F601, 1997.

354. Stuart-Tilley AK, Shmukler BE, Brown D, Alper SL: Immunolocalization and tissue-specific splicing of AE2 anion exchanger in mouse kidney. J Am Soc Nephrol 9:946, 1998.

355. Castillo JE, Martinez-Anso E, Malumbres R, et al: In situ localization of anion exchanger-2 in the human kidney. Cell Tissue Res 299:281, 2000.

356. Vorum H, Kwon TH, Fulton C, et al: Immunolocalization of electroneutral Na-HCO(3)(-) cotransporter in rat kidney. Am J Physiol Renal Physiol 279:F901, 2000.

357. Suki WN, Rouse D, Ng RC, Kokko JP: Calcium transport in the thick ascending limb of Henle. Heterogeneity of function in the medullary and cortical segments. J Clin Invest 66:1004, 1980.

358. Shareghi GR, Agus ZS: Magnesium transport in the cortical thick ascending limb of Henle's loop of the rabbit. J Clin Invest 69:759, 1982.

359. Brown EM, Pollak M, Chou YH, et al: Cloning and functional characterization of extracellular Ca(2+)-sensing receptors from parathyroid and kidney. Bone 17:7S, 1995.

360. Riccardi D, Park J, Lee WS, et al: Cloning and functional expression of a rat kidney extracellular calcium/polyvalent cation-sensing receptor. Proc Natl Acad Sci U S A 92:131, 1995.

361. Riccardi D, Lee WS, Lee K, et al: Localization of the extracellular Ca(2+)-sensing receptor and PTH/PTHrP receptor in rat kidney. Am J Physiol 271:F951, 1996.

362. Riccardi D, Hall AE, Chattopadhyay N, et al: Localization of the extracellular Ca2+/polyvalent cation-sensing protein in rat kidney. Am J Physiol 274:F611, 1998.

363. Brown EM, Pollak M, Hebert SC: The extracellular calcium-sensing receptor: Its role in health and disease. Annu Rev Med 49:15, 1998.

364. Brown EM, Hebert SC: A cloned Ca(2+)-sensing receptor: A mediator of direct effects of extracellular Ca2+ on renal function? J Am Soc Nephrol 6:1530, 1995.

365. Morel F: Sites of hormone action in the mammalian nephron. Am J Physiol 240:F159–F164, 1981.

366. Hebert SC, Culpepper RM, Andreoli TE: NaCl transport in mouse medullary thick ascending limbs. I. Functional nephron heterogeneity and ADH-stimulated NaCl cotransport. Am J Physiol 241:F412, 1981.

367. Sasaki S, Imai M: Effects of vasopressin on water and NaCl transport across the in vitro perfused medullary thick ascending limb of Henle's loop of mouse, rat, and rabbit kidneys. Pflugers Arch 383:215, 1980.

368. Wittner M, Stefano A, Wangemann P, et al: Differential effects of ADH on sodium, chloride, potassium, calcium and magnesium transport in cortical and medullary thick ascending limbs of mouse nephron. Pflugers Archiv Eur J Physiol 412:516, 1988.

369. Ortiz PA: cAMP increases surface expression of NKCC2 in rat thick ascending limbs: role of VAMP. Am J Physiol Renal Physiol 290:F608, 2006.

370. Bouby N, Bankir L, Trinh-Trang-Tan MM, et al: Selective ADH-induced hypertrophy of the medullary thick ascending limb in Brattleboro rats. Kidney Int 28:456, 1985.

371. Work J, Galla JH, Booker BB, et al: Effect of ADH on chloride reabsorption in the loop of Henle of the Brattleboro rat. Am J Physiol 249:F698, 1985.

372. Davis RG, Madsen KM, Fregly MJ, Tisher CC: Kidney structure in hypothyroidism. Am J Pathol 113:41, 1983.

373. Bentley AG, Madsen KM, Davis RG, Tisher CC: Response of the medullary thick ascending limb to hypothyroidism in the rat. Am J Pathol 120:215, 1985.

374. Kim JK, Summer SN, Schrier RW: Cellular action of arginine vasopressin in the iso-lated renal tubules of hypothyroid rats. Am J Physiol 253:F104, 1987.

375. De Rouffignac C, Di Stefano A, Wittner M, et al: Consequences of differential effects of ADH and other peptide hormones on thick ascending limb of mammalian kidney. Am J Physiol Regul Integr Comp Physiol 260:R1023, 1991.

376. Crayen ML, Thoenes W: Architecture and cell structures in the distal nephron of the rat kidney. Cytobiologie 17:197, 1978.

377. Reilly RF, Ellison DH: Mammalian distal tubule: physiology, pathophysiology, and molecular anatomy. Physiol Rev 80:277, 2000.

378. Madsen KM, Harris RH, Tisher CC: Uptake and intracellular distribution of ferritin in the rat distal convoluted tubule. Kidney Int 21:354, 1982.

379. Woodhall PB, Tisher CC: Response of the distal tubule and cortical collecting duct to vasopressin in the rat. J Clin Invest 52:3095, 1973.

380. Stanton BA, Giebisch GH: Potassium transport by the renal distal tubule: effects of potassium loading. Am J Physiol 243:F487, 1982.

381. Stanton BA, Biemesderfer D, Wade JB, Giebisch G: Structural and functional study of the rat distal nephron: Effects of potassium adaptation and depletion. Kidney Int 19:36, 1981.

382. Kaissling B: Structural aspects of adaptive changes in renal electrolyte excretion. Am J Physiol 243:F211, 1982.

383. Obermuller N, Bernstein P, Velazquez H, et al: Expression of the thiazide-sensitive Na-Cl cotransporter in rat and human kidney. Am J Physiol 269:F900, 1995.

384. Bachmann S, Velazquez H, Obermuller N, et al: Expression of the thiazide-sensitive Na-Cl cotransporter by rabbit distal convoluted tubule cells. J Clin Invest 96:2510, 1995.

385. Plotkin MD, Kaplan MR, Verlander JW, et al: Localization of the thiazide sensitive Na-Cl cotransporter, rTSC1 in the rat kidney. Kidney Int 50:174, 1996.

386. Verlander JW, Tran TM, Zhang L, et al: Estradiol enhances thiazide-sensitive NaCl cotransporter density in the apical plasma membrane of the distal convoluted tubule in ovariectomized rats. J Clin Invest 101:1661, 1998.

387. Kim GH, Masilamani S, Turner R, et al: The thiazide-sensitive Na-Cl cotransporter is an aldosterone-induced protein. Proc Natl Acad Sci U S A 95:14552, 1998.

388. Bostanjoglo M, Reeves WB, Reilly RF, et al: 11Beta-hydroxysteroid dehydrogenase, mineralocorticoid receptor, and thiazide-sensitive Na-Cl cotransporter expression by distal tubules. J Am Soc Nephrol 9:1347, 1998.

389. Bachmann S, Bostanjoglo M, Schmitt R, Ellison DH: Sodium transport-related proteins in the mammalian distal nephron—distribution, ontogeny and functional aspects. Anat Embryol (Berl) 200:447, 1999.

390. Campean V, Kricke J, Ellison D, et al: Localization of thiazide-sensitive Na(+)-Cl(−) cotransport and associated gene products in mouse DCT. Am J Physiol Renal Physiol 281:F1028, 2001.

391. Kaissling B, Bachmann S, Kriz W: Structural adaptation of the distal convoluted tubule to prolonged furosemide treatment. Am J Physiol 248:F374, 1985.

392. Kaissling B, Stanton BA: Adaptation of distal tubule and collecting duct to increased sodium delivery. I. Ultrastructure. Am J Physiol 255:F1256, 1988.

393. Stanton BA, Kaissling B: Adaptation of distal tubule and collecting duct to increased Na delivery. II. Na$^+$ and K$^+$ transport. Am J Physiol 255:F1269, 1988.

394. Loffing J, Vallon V, Loffing-Cueni D, et al: Altered renal distal tubule structure and renal Na$^+$ and Ca^{2+} handling in a mouse model for Gitelman's syndrome. J Am Soc Nephrol 15:2276, 2004.

395. Morris RG, Hoorn EJ, Knepper MA: Hypokalemia in a mouse model of Gitelman syndrome. Am J Physiol Renal Physiol 290:F1416–1420, 2006.

396. Doucet A, Katz AI: High-affinity Ca-Mg-ATPase along the rabbit nephron. Am J Physiol 242:F346, 1982.

397. Borke JL, Minami J, Verma A, et al: Monoclonal antibodies to human erythrocyte membrane Ca++-Mg++ adenosine triphosphatase pump recognize an epitope in the basolateral membrane of human kidney distal tubule cells. J Clin Invest 80:1225, 1987.

398. Roth J, Brown D, Norman AW, Orci L: Localization of the vitamin D-dependent calcium-binding protein in mammalian kidney. Am J Physiol 243:F243, 1982.

399. Gross JB, Imai M, Kokko JP: A functional comparison of the cortical collecting tubule and the distal convoluted tubule. J Clin Invest 55:1284, 1975.

400. Morel F, Chabardes D, Imbert M: Functional segmentation of the rabbit distal tubule by microdetermination of hormone-dependent adenylate cyclase activity. Kidney Int 9:264, 1976.

401. Myers CE, Bulger RE, Tisher CC, Trump BF: Human renal ultrastructure. IV. Collecting duct of healthy individuals. Lab Invest 16:655, 1966.

402. Welling LW, Evan AP, Welling DJ, Gattone VH, III: Morphometric comparison of rabbit cortical connecting tubules and collecting ducts. Kidney Int 23:358, 1983.

403. Verlander JW, Madsen KM, Tisher CC: Effect of acute respiratory acidosis on two populations of intercalated cells in rat cortical collecting duct. Am J Physiol 253:F1142, 1987.

404. Kim J, Kim YH, Cha JH, et al: Intercalated cell subtypes in connecting tubule and cortical collecting duct of rat and mouse. J Am Soc Nephrol 10:1, 1999.

405. Teng-umnuay P, Verlander JW, Yuan W, et al: Identification of distinct subpopulations of intercalated cells in the mouse collecting duct. J Am Soc Nephrol 7:260, 1996.

406. Wright FS, Giebisch G: Renal potassium transport: Contributions of individual nephron segments and populations. Am J Physiol 235:F515, 1978.

407. Field MJ, Stanton BA, Giebisch GH: Differential acute effects of aldosterone, dexamethasone, and hyperkalemia on distal tubular potassium secretion in the rat kidney. J Clin Invest 74:1792, 1984.

408. Stanton B, Janzen A, Klein-Robbenhaar G, DeFronzo R, et al: Ultrastructure of rat initial collecting tubule. Effect of adrenal corticosteroid treatment. J Clin Invest 75:1327, 1985.

409. Vio CP, Figueroa CD: Subcellular localization of renal kallikrein by ultrastructural immunocytochemistry. Kidney Int 28:36, 1985.

410. Barajas L, Powers K, Carretero O, et al: Immunocytochemical localization of renin and kallikrein in the rat renal cortex. Kidney Int 29:965, 1986.

411. Reilly RF, Shugrue CA, Lattanzi D, Biemesderfer D: Immunolocalization of the Na$^+$/Ca^{2+} exchanger in rabbit kidney. Am J Physiol 265:F327, 1993.

412. Borke JL, Caride A, Verma AK, et al: Plasma membrane calcium pump and 28-kDa calcium binding protein in cells of rat kidney distal tubules. Am J Physiol 257:F842, 1989.

413. Yang CW, Kim J, Kim YH, et al: Inhibition of calbindin D28K expression by cyclosporin A in rat kidney: The possible pathogenesis of cyclosporin A-induced hypercalciuria. J Am Soc Nephrol 9:1416, 1998.

414. Kishore BK, Mandon B, Oza NB, et al: Rat renal arcade segment expresses vasopressin-regulated water channel and vasopressin V2 receptor. J Clin Invest 97:2763, 1996.

415. Imai M: The connecting tubule: A functional subdivision of the rabbit distal nephron segments. Kidney Int 15:346, 1979.

416. Loffing J, Loffing-Cueni D, Valderrabano V, et al: Distribution of transcellular calcium and sodium transport pathways along mouse distal nephron. Am J Physiol Renal Physiol 281:F1021, 2001.

417. Rubera I, Loffing J, Palmer LG, et al: Collecting duct-specific gene inactivation of αENaC in the mouse kidney does not impair sodium and potassium balance. J Clin Invest 112:554, 2003.

418. Hummler E, Barker P, Gatzy J, et al: Early death due to defective neonatal lung liquid clearance in [alpha]ENaC-deficient mice. Nat Genet 12:325, 1996.

419. Rojek A, Fuchtbauer EM, Kwon TH, et al: Severe urinary concentrating defect in renal collecting duct-selective AQP2 conditional-knockout mice. Proc Natl Acad Sci U S A 103:6037–6042, 2006.

420. Nielsen J, Kwon TH, Praetorius J, et al: Aldosterone increases urine production and decreases apical AQP2 expression in rats with diabetes insipidus. Am J Physiol Renal Physiol 290:F438, 2006.

421. Madsen KM, Clapp WL, Verlander JW: Structure and function of the inner medullary collecting duct. Kidney Int 34:441, 1988.

422. Hansen GP, Tisher CC, Robinson RR: Response of the collecting duct to disturbances of acid-base and potassium balance. Kidney Int 17:326, 1980.

423. LeFurgey A, Tisher CC: Morphology of rabbit collecting duct. Am J Anat 155:111, 1979.

424. Welling LW, Evan AP, Welling DJ: Shape of cells and extracellular channels in rabbit cortical collecting ducts. Kidney Int 20:211, 1981.

425. Madsen KM, Tisher CC: Structural-functional relationship along the distal nephron. Am J Physiol 250:F1, 1986.

426. Madsen KM, Tisher CC: Cellular response to acute respiratory acidosis in rat medullary collecting duct. Am J Physiol 245:F670, 1983.

427. Schuster VL, Bonsib SM, Jennings ML: Two types of collecting duct mitochondria-rich (intercalated) cells: Lectin and band 3 cytochemistry. Am J Physiol 251:C347, 1986.

428. Brown D, Roth J, Orci L: Lectin-gold cytochemistry reveals intercalated cell heterogeneity along rat kidney collecting ducts. Am J Physiol 248:C348, 1985.

429. Le Hir M, Dubach UC: The cellular specificity of lectin binding in the kidney. I. A light microscopical study in the rat. Histochemistry 74:521, 1982.

430. Holthofer H, Schulte BA, Pasternack G, et al: Immunocytochemical characterization of carbonic anhydrase-rich cells in the rat kidney collecting duct. Lab Invest 57:150, 1987.

431. Kim J, Tisher CC, Linser PJ, Madsen KM: Ultrastructural localization of carbonic anhydrase II in subpopulations of intercalated cells of the rat kidney. J Am Soc Nephrol 1:245, 1990.

432. Lonnerholm G, Ridderstrale Y: Intracellular distribution of carbonic anhydrase in the rat kidney. Kidney Int 17:162, 1980.

433. Atkins JL, Burg MB: Bicarbonate transport by isolated perfused rat collecting ducts. Am J Physiol 249:F485, 1985.

434. McKinney TD, Burg MB: Bicarbonate transport by rabbit cortical collecting tubules. Effect of acid and alkali loads in vivo on transport in vitro. J Clin Invest 60:766, 1977.

435. Lombard WE, Kokko JP, Jacobson HR: Bicarbonate transport in cortical and outer medullary collecting tubules. Am J Physiol 244:F289, 1983.

436. Knepper MA, Good DW, Burg MB: Ammonia and bicarbonate transport by rat cortical collecting ducts perfused in vitro. Am J Physiol 249:F870, 1985.

437. Garcia-Austt J, Good DW, Burg MB, Knepper MA: Deoxycorticosterone-stimulated bicarbonate secretion in rabbit cortical collecting ducts: Effects of luminal chloride removal and in vivo acid loading. Am J Physiol 249:F205, 1985.

438. Star RA, Burg MB, Knepper MA: Bicarbonate secretion and chloride absorption by rabbit cortical collecting ducts. Role of chloride/bicarbonate exchange. J Clin Invest 76:1123, 1985.

439. Verlander JW, Madsen KM, Tisher CC: Structural and functional features of proton and bicarbonate transport in the rat collecting duct. Semin Nephrol 11:465, 1991.

440. Dorup J: Structural adaptation of intercalated cells in rat renal cortex to acute metabolic acidosis and alkalosis. J Ultrastruct Res 92:119, 1985.

441. Alper SL, Natale J, Gluck S, et al: Subtypes of intercalated cells in rat kidney collecting duct defined by antibodies against erythroid band 3 and renal vacuolar H+-ATPase. Proc Natl Acad Sci 86:5429, 1989.

442. Brown D, Hirsch S, Gluck S: An H+-ATPase in opposite plasma membrane domains in kidney epithelial cell subpopulations. Nature 331:622, 1988.

443. Kim J, Welch WJ, Cannon JK, et al: Immunocytochemical response of type A and type B intercalated cells to increased sodium chloride delivery. Am J Physiol 262:F288, 1992.

444. Verlander JW, Madsen KM, Galla JH, et al: Response of intercalated cells to chloride depletion metabolic alkalosis. Am J Physiol 262:F309, 1992.

445. Bastani B, Purcell H, Hemken P, et al: Expression and distribution of renal vacuolar proton-translocating adenosine triphosphatase in response to chronic acid and alkali loads in the rat. J Clin Invest 88:126, 1991.

446. Drenckhahn D, Schluter K, Allen DP, Bennett V: Colocalization of band 3 with ankyrin and spectrin at the basal membrane of intercalated cells in the rat kidney. Science 230:1287, 1985.

447. Verlander JW, Madsen KM, Low PS, et al: Immunocytochemical localization of band 3 protein in the rat collecting duct. Am J Physiol 255:F115, 1988.

448. Royaux IE, Wall SM, Karniski LP, et al: Pendrin, encoded by the Pendred syndrome gene, resides in the apical region of renal intercalated cells and mediates bicarbonate secretion. Proc Natl Acad Sci U S A 98:4221, 2001.

449. Soleimani M, Greeley T, Petrovic S, et al: Pendrin: An apical Cl-OH/HCO₃⁻ exchanger in the kidney cortex. Am J Physiol Renal Physiol 280:F356, 2001.

450. Everett LA, Glaser B, Beck JC, et al: Pendred syndrome is caused by mutations in a putative sulphate transporter gene (PDS). Nat Genet 17:411, 1997.

451. Kim YH, Kwon TH, Frische S, et al: Immunocytochemical localization of pendrin in intercalated cell subtypes in rat and mouse kidney. Am J Physiol Renal Physiol 283:F744, 2002.

452. Frische S, Kwon TH, Frokiaer J, et al: Regulated expression of pendrin in rat kidney in response to chronic NH4Cl or NaHCO3 loading. Am J Physiol Renal Physiol 284:F584, 2003.

453. Verlander JW, Hassell KA, Royaux IE, et al: Deoxycorticosterone upregulates PDS (Slc26a4) in mouse kidney: Role of pendrin in mineralocorticoid-induced hypertension. Hypertension 42:356, 2003.

454. Wall SM, Kim YH, Stanley L, et al: NaCl restriction upregulates renal Slc26a4 through subcellular redistribution: Role in Cl- conservation. Hypertension 44:982, 2004.

455. Vallet M, Picard N, Loffing-Cueni D, et al: Pendrin regulation in mouse kidney primarily is chloride-dependent. J Am Soc Nephrol 17:2153, 2006.

456. Quentin F, Chambrey R, Trinh-Trang-Tan MM, et al: The Cl–/HCO3– exchanger pendrin in the rat kidney is regulated in response to chronic alterations in chloride balance. Am J Physiol Renal Physiol 287:F1179, 2004.

457. Tsuganezawa H, Kobayashi K, Iyori M, et al: A new member of the HCO3(–) transporter superfamily is an apical anion exchanger of beta-intercalated cells in the kidney. J Biol Chem 276:8180, 2001.

458. Schuster VL, Fejes-Toth G, Naray-Fejes-Toth A, Gluck S: Colocalization of H(+)-ATPase and band 3 anion exchanger in rabbit collecting duct intercalated cells. Am J Physiol 260:F506, 1991.

459. Verlander JW, Madsen KM, Tisher CC: Axial distribution of band 3-positive intercalated cells in the collecting duct of control and ammonium chloride-loaded rabbits. Kidney Int Suppl 57:S137, 1996.

460. Madsen KM, Kim J, Tisher CC: Intracellular band 3 immunostaining in type A intercalated cells of rabbit kidney. Am J Physiol 262:F1015, 1992.

461. Verlander JW, Madsen KM, Stone DK, Tisher CC: Ultrastructural localization of H+ATPase in rabbit cortical collecting duct. J Am Soc Nephrol 4:1546, 1994.

462. Verlander JW, Madsen KM, Cannon JK, Tisher CC: Activation of acid-secreting intercalated cells in rabbit collecting duct with ammonium chloride loading. Am J Physiol 266:F633, 1994.

463. Weiner ID, Hamm LL: Regulation of intracellular pH in the rabbit cortical collecting tubule. J Clin Invest 85:274, 1990.

464. Weiner ID, Hamm LL: Use of fluorescent dye BCECF to measure intracellular pH in cortical collecting tubule. Am J Physiol 256:F957, 1989.

465. Schwartz GJ, Barasch J, Al-Awqati Q: Plasticity of functional epithelial polarity. Nature 318:368, 1985.

466. Obermuller N, Gretz N, Kriz W, et al: The swelling-activated chloride channel ClC-2, the chloride channel ClC-3, and ClC-5, a chloride channel mutated in kidney stone disease, are expressed in distinct subpopulations of renal epithelial cells. J Clin Invest 101:635, 1998.

467. O'Neil RG, Helman SI: Transport characteristics of renal collecting tubules: influences of DOCA and diet. Am J Physiol 233:F544, 1977.

468. Schwartz GJ, Burg MB: Mineralocorticoid effects on cation transport by cortical collecting tubules in vitro. Am J Physiol 235:F576, 1978.

469. Mujais SK, Chekal MA, Jones WJ, et al: Regulation of renal Na-K-ATPase in the rat. Role of the natural mineralo- and glucocorticoid hormones. J Clin Invest 73:13, 1984.

470. Petty KJ, Kokko JP, Marver D: Secondary effect of aldosterone on Na-KATPase activity in the rabbit cortical collecting tubule. J Clin Invest 68:1514, 1981.

471. Wade JB, O'Neil RG, Pryor JL, Boulpaep EL: Modulation of cell membrane area in renal collecting tubules by corticosteroid hormones. J Cell Biol 81:439, 1979.

472. Duc C, Farman N, Canessa CM, et al: Cell-specific expression of epithelial sodium channel alpha, beta, and gamma subunits in aldosterone-responsive epithelia from the rat: Localization by in situ hybridization and immunocytochemistry. J Cell Biol 127:1907, 1994.

473. Hager H, Kwon TH, Vinnikova AK, et al: Immunocytochemical and immunoelectron microscopic localization of alpha-, beta-, and gamma-ENaC in rat kidney. Am J Physiol Renal Physiol 280:F1093, 2001.

474. Canessa CM, Schild L, Buell G, et al: Amiloride-sensitive epithelial Na+ channel is made of three homologous subunits. Nature 367:463, 1994.

475. Loffing J, Pietri L, Aregger F, et al: Differential subcellular localization of ENaC subunits in mouse kidney in response to high- and low-Na diets. Am J Physiol Renal Physiol 279:F252, 2000.

476. Ecelbarger CA, Kim GH, Terris J, et al: Vasopressin-mediated regulation of epithelial sodium channel abundance in rat kidney. Am J Physiol Renal Physiol 279:F46, 2000.

477. Peti-Peterdi J, Warnock DG, Bell PD: Angiotensin II directly stimulates ENaC activity in the cortical collecting duct via AT1 receptors. J Am Soc Nephrol 13:1131, 2002.

478. Beutler KT, Masilamani S, Turban S, et al: Long-term regulation of ENaC expression in kidney by angiotensin II. Hypertension 41:1143, 2003.

479. Snyder PM: Minireview: Regulation of epithelial Na+ channel trafficking. Endocrinology 146:5079, 2005.

480. Schild L, Lu Y, Gautschi I, et al: Identification of a PY motif in the epithelial Na channel subunits as a target sequence for mutations causing channel activation found in Liddle syndrome. EMBO J 15:2381, 1996.

481. Kamynina E, Debonneville C, Bens M, et al: A novel mouse Nedd4 protein suppresses the activity of the epithelial Na+ channel. FASEB J 15:204, 2001.

482. Vallon V, Wulff P, Huang DY, et al: Role of Sgk1 in salt and potassium homeostasis. Am J Physiol Regul Integr Comp Physiol 288:R4, 2005.

483. Rossier BC: The epithelial sodium channel: Activation by membrane-bound serine proteases. Proc Am Thorac Soc 1:4, 2004.

484. Adebamiro A, Cheng Y, Johnson JP, Bridges RJ: Endogenous protease activation of enac: effect of serine protease inhibition on ENaC single channel properties. J Gen Physiol 126:339, 2005.

485. Hughey RP, Mueller GM, Bruns JB, et al: Maturation of the epithelial Na+ channel involves proteolytic processing of the α- and γ-subunits. J Biol Chem 278:37073, 2003.

486. Nielsen J, Kwon TH, Masilamani S, et al: Sodium transporter abundance profiling in kidney: effect of spironolactone. Am J Physiol Renal Physiol 283:F923, 2002.

487. Zhou ZH, Bubien JK: Nongenomic regulation of ENaC by aldosterone. Am J Physiol Cell Physiol 281:C1118, 2001.

488. Schafer JA: Abnormal regulation of ENaC: syndromes of salt retention and salt wasting by the collecting duct. Am J Physiol Renal Physiol 283:F221, 2002.

489. Sassen MC, Kim SW, Kwon TH, et al: Dysregulation of renal sodium transporters in gentamicin-treated rats. Kidney Int 2006.

490. Kim SW, de Seigneux S, Sassen MC, et al: Increased apical targeting of renal ENaC subunits and decreased expression of 11betaHSD2 in HgCl2-induced nephrotic syndrome in rats. Am J Physiol Renal Physiol 290:F674, 2006.

491. Kim SW, Schou UK, Peters CD, et al: Increased apical targeting of renal epithelial sodium channel subunits and decreased expression of type 2 11β-hydroxysteroid dehydrogenase in rats with ccl4-induced decompensated liver cirrhosis. J Am Soc Nephrol 16:3196, 2005.

492. de Seigneux S, Kim SW, Hemmingsen SC, et al: Increased expression but not targeting of ENaC in adrenalectomized rats with PAN-induced nephrotic syndrome. Am J Physiol Renal Physiol 291:F208, 2006.

493. Lourdel S, Loffing J, Favre G, et al: Hyperaldosteronemia and activation of the epithelial sodium channel are not required for sodium retention in puromycin-induced nephrosis. J Am Soc Nephrol 16:3642, 2005.

494. Wingo CS: Potassium transport by medullary collecting tubule of rabbit: Effects of variation in K intake. Am J Physiol 253:F1136, 1987.

495. Stone DK, Seldin DW, Kokko JP, Jacobson HR: Mineralocorticoid modulation of rabbit medullary collecting duct acidification. A sodium-independent effect. J Clin Invest 72:77, 1983.

496. Steinmetz PR: Cellular organization of urinary acidification. Am J Physiol 251:F173, 1986.

497. Gluck S, Cannon C, Al-Awqati Q: Exocytosis regulates urinary acidification in turtle bladder by rapid insertion of H+ pumps into the luminal membrane. Proc Natl Acad Sci U S A 79:4327, 1982.

498. Gluck S, Kelly S, Al-Awqati Q: The proton translocating ATPase responsible for urinary acidification. J Biol Chem 257:9230, 1982.

499. Gluck S, Al-Awqati Q: An electrogenic proton-translocating adenosine triphosphatase from bovine kidney medulla. J Clin Invest 73:1704, 1984.

500. Kaunitz JD, Gunther RD, Sachs G: Characterization of an electrogenic ATP and chloride-dependent proton translocating pump from rat renal medulla. J Biol Chem 260:11567, 1985.

501. Sabatini S, Laski ME, Kurtzman NA: NEM-sensitive ATPase activity in rat nephron: Effect of metabolic acidosis and alkalosis. Am J Physiol 258:F297, 1990.

502. Khadouri C, Marsy S, Barlet-Bas C, et al: Effect of metabolic acidosis and alkalosis on NEM-sensitive ATPase in rat nephron segments. Am J Physiol 262:F583, 1992.

503. Garg LC, Narang N: Effects of aldosterone on NEM-sensitive ATPase in rabbit nephron segments. Kidney Int 34:13, 1988.

504. Khadouri C, Marsy S, Barlet-Bas C, Doucet A: Short-term effect of aldosterone on NEM-sensitive ATPase in rat collecting tubule. Am J Physiol 257:F177, 1989.

505. Madsen KM, Tisher CC: Response of intercalated cells of rat outer medullary collecting duct to chronic metabolic acidosis. Lab Invest 51:268, 1984.

506. Stetson DL, Steinmetz PR: Role of membrane fusion in CO₂ stimulation of proton secretion by turtle bladder. Am J Physiol 245:C113, 1983.

507. Brown D, Gluck S, Hartwig J: Structure of the novel membrane-coating material in proton- secreting epithelial cells and identification as an H+ATPase. J Cell Biol 105:1637, 1987.

508. Wagner CA, Finberg KE, Breton S, et al: Renal Vacuolar H+-ATPase. Physiol Rev 84:1263, 2004.

509. Wingo CS, Cain BD: The renal H-K-ATPase: Physiological significance and role in potassium homeostasis. Annu Rev Physiol 55:323, 1993.

510. Doucet A, Marsy S: Characterization of K-ATPase activity in distal nephron: stimulation by potassium depletion. Am J Physiol 253:F418, 1987.

511. Garg LC, Narang N: Ouabain-insensitive K-adenosine triphosphatase in distal nephron segments of the rabbit. J Clin Invest 81:1204, 1988.

512. Wingo CS: Active proton secretion and potassium absorption in the rabbit outer medullary collecting duct. Functional evidence for proton-potassium-activated adenosine triphosphatase. J Clin Invest 84:361, 1989.

513. Wingo CS, Madsen KM, Smolka A, Tisher CC: H-K-ATPase immunoreactivity in cortical and outer medullary collecting duct. Kidney Int 38:985, 1990.

514. Ahn KY, Kone BC: Expression and cellular localization of mRNA encoding the "gastric" isoform of H(+)-K(+)-ATPase alpha-subunit in rat kidney. Am J Physiol Renal Physiol 268:F99, 1995.

515. Campbell-Thompson ML, Verlander JW, Curran KA, et al: In situ hybridization of H-K-ATPase beta-subunit mRNA in rat and rabbit kidney. Am J Physiol 269:F345, 1995.

516. Eiam-Ong S, Kurtzman NA, Sabatini S: Regulation of collecting tubule adenosine triphosphatases by aldosterone and potassium. J Clin Invest 91:2385, 1993.

517. Sangan P, Rajendran VM, Mann AS, et al: Regulation of colonic H-K-ATPase in large intestine and kidney by dietary Na depletion and dietary K depletion. Am J Physiol Cell Physiol 272:C685, 1997.

518. Ahn KY, Park KY, Kim KK, Kone BC: Chronic hypokalemia enhances expression of the H(+)-K(+)-ATPase alpha 2-subunit gene in renal medulla. Am J Physiol Renal Physiol 271:F314, 1996.

519. Zhang W, Xia X, Zou L, et al: In vivo expression profile of a H+-K+-ATPase α2-subunit promoter-reporter transgene. Am J Physiol Renal Physiol 286:F1171, 2004.

520. Xu X, Zhang W, Kone BC: CREB trans-activates the murine H+-K+-ATPase α 2-subunit gene. Am J Physiol Cell Physiol 287:C903, 2004.

521. Verlander JW, Moudy RM, Campbell WG, et al: Immunohistochemical localization of H-K-ATPase alpha(2c)-subunit in rabbit kidney. Am J Physiol Renal Physiol 281:F357, 2001.

522. Meneton P, Schultheis PJ, Greeb J, et al: Increased sensitivity to K+ deprivation in colonic H,K-ATPase-deficient mice. J Clin Invest 101:536, 1998.

523. Marini AM, Urrestarazu A, Beauwens R, Andre B: The Rh (rhesus) blood group polypeptides are related to NH4+ transporters. Trends Biochem Sci 22:460, 1997.

524. Nakhoul N, Hamm LL: Non-erythroid Rh glycoproteins: A putative new family of mammalian ammonium transporters. Pflugers Archiv Eur J Physiol 447:807, 2004.

525. Weiner ID: The Rh gene family and renal ammonium transport. Curr Opin Nephrol Hypertens 13:533, 2004.

526. Liu Z, Peng J, Mo R, et al: Rh type B glycoprotein is a new member of the rh super-family and a putative ammonia transporter in mammals. J Biol Chem 276:1424, 2001.

527. Liu Z, Chen Y, Mo R, et al: Characterization of human RhCG and mouse Rhcg as novel nonerythroid rh glycoprotein homologues predominantly expressed in kidney and testis. J Biol Chem 275:25641, 2000.

528. Marini AM, Matassi G, Raynal V, et al: The human Rhesus-associated RhAG protein and a kidney homologue promote ammonium transport in yeast. Nat Genet 26:341, 2000.

529. Westhoff CM, Ferreri-Jacobia M, Mak D-OD, Foskett JK: Identification of the erythrocyte rh blood group glycoprotein as a mammalian ammonium transporter. J Biol Chem 277:12499, 2002.

530. Mak DO, Dang B, Weiner ID, et al: Characterization of ammonia transport by the kidney Rh glycoproteins RhBG and RhCG. Am J Physiol Renal Physiol 290:F297-F305, 2006.

531. Eladari D, Cheval L, Quentin F, et al: Expression of RhCG, a new putative NH3/NH4+ transporter, along the rat nephron. J Am Soc Nephrol 13:1999, 2002.

532. Quentin F, Eladari D, Cheval L, et al: RhBG and RhCG, the putative ammonia transporters, are expressed in the same cells in the distal nephron. J Am Soc Nephrol 14:545, 2003.

533. Verlander JW, Miller RT, Frank AE, et al: Localization of the ammonium transporter proteins RhBG and RhCG in mouse kidney. Am J Physiol Renal Physiol 284:F323, 2003.

534. Seshadri RM, Klein JD, Kozlowski S, et al: Renal expression of the ammonia transporters, Rhbg and Rhcg, in response to chronic metabolic acidosis. Am J Physiol Renal Physiol 290:F397, 2006.

535. Seshadri RM, Klein JD, Smith T, et al: Changes in subcellular distribution of the ammonia transporter, Rhcg, in response to chronic metabolic acidosis. Am J Physiol Renal Physiol 290:F1443, 2006.

536. Chambrey R, Goossens D, Bourgeois S, et al: Genetic ablation of Rhbg in the mouse does not impair renal ammonium excretion. Am J Physiol Renal Physiol 289:F1281, 2005.

537. Knepper MA, Danielson RA, Saidel GM, Post RS: Quantitative analysis of renal medullary anatomy in rats and rabbits. Kidney Int 12:313, 1977.

538. Clapp WL, Madsen KM, Verlander JW, Tisher CC: Intercalated cells of the rat inner medullary collecting duct. Kidney Int 31:1080, 1987.

539. Clapp WL, Madsen KM, Verlander JW, Tisher CC: Morphologic heterogeneity along the rat inner medullary collecting duct. Lab Invest 60:219, 1989.

540. Rocha AS, Kudo LH: Water, urea, sodium, chloride, and potassium transport in the in vitro isolated perfused papillary collecting duct. Kidney Int 22:485, 1982.

541. Sands JM, Knepper MA: Urea permeability of mammalian inner medullary collecting duct system and papillary surface epithelium. J Clin Invest 79:138, 1987.

542. Sands JM, Nonoguchi H, Knepper MA: Vasopressin effects on urea and H2O transport in inner medullary collecting duct subsegments. Am J Physiol 253:F823, 1987.

543. Nonoguchi H, Sands JM, Knepper MA: Atrial natriuretic factor inhibits vasopressin-stimulated osmotic water permeability in rat inner medullary collecting duct. J Clin Invest 82:1383, 1988.

544. Nonoguchi H, Knepper MA, Manganiello VC: Effects of atrial natriuretic factor on cyclic guanosine monophosphate and cyclic adenosine monophosphate accumulation in microdissected nephron segments from rats. J Clin Invest 79:500, 1987.

545. Zeidel ML, Silva P, Brenner BM, Seifter JL: cGMP mediates effects of atrial peptides on medullary collecting duct cells. Am J Physiol 252:F551, 1987.

546. You G, Smith CP, Kanai Y, et al: Cloning and characterization of the vasopressin-regulated urea transporter. Nature 365:844, 1993.

547. Smith CP, Lee WS, Martial S, et al: Cloning and regulation of expression of the rat kidney urea transporter (rUT2). J Clin Invest 96:1556, 1995.

548. Terris JM, Knepper MA, Wade JB: UT-A3: Localization and characterization of an additional urea transporter isoform in the IMCD. Am J Physiol Renal Physiol 280: F325, 2001.

549. Fenton RA, Stewart GS, Carpenter B, et al: Characterization of mouse urea transporters UT-A1 and UT-A2. Am J Physiol Renal Physiol 283:F817, 2002.

550. Stewart GS, Fenton RA, Wang W, et al: The basolateral expression of mUT-A3 in the mouse kidney. Am J Physiol 286:F979–F987, 2004.

551. Fenton RA, Chou CL, Stewart GS, et al: Urinary concentrating defect in mice with selective deletion of phloretin-sensitive urea transporters in the renal collecting duct. Proc Natl Acad Sci 101:7469, 2004.

552. Graber ML, Bengele HH, Schwartz JH, Alexander EA: pH and PCO2 profiles of the rat inner medullary collecting duct. Am J Physiol 241:F659, 1981.

553. Richardson RM, Kunau RT, Jr: Bicarbonate reabsorption in the papillary collecting duct: effect of acetazolamide. Am J Physiol 243:F74, 1982.

554. Ullrich KJ, Papavassiliou F: Bicarbonate reabsorption in the papillary collecting duct of rats. Pflugers Arch 389:271, 1981.

555. Bengele HH, Schwartz JH, McNamara ER, Alexander EA: Chronic metabolic acidosis augments acidification along the inner medullary collecting duct. Am J Physiol 250: F690, 1986.

556. Graber ML, Bengele HH, Mroz E, et al: Acute metabolic acidosis augments collecting duct acidification rate in the rat. Am J Physiol 241:F669, 1981.

557. Schwartz JH, Masino SA, Nichols RD, Alexander EA: Intracellular modulation of acid secretion in rat inner medullary collecting duct cells. Am J Physiol 266:F94, 1994.

558. Ono S, Guntupalli J, DuBose TD, Jr: Role of H(+)-K(+)-ATPase in pHi regulation in inner medullary collecting duct cells in culture. Am J Physiol 270:F852, 1996.

559. Wall SM, Truong AV, DuBose TD, Jr: H(+)-K(+)-ATPase mediates net acid secretion in rat terminal inner medullary collecting duct. Am J Physiol 271:F1037, 1996.

560. Kim YH, Kim J, Verkman AS, Madsen KM: Increased expression of H+-ATPase in inner medullary collecting duct of aquaporin-1-deficient mice. Am J Physiol Renal Physiol 285:F550, 2003.

561. Damkier HH, Nielsen S, Praetorius J: An anti-NH2-terminal antibody localizes NBCn1 to heart endothelia and skeletal and vascular smooth muscle cells. Am J Physiol Heart Circ Physiol 290:H172, 2006.

562. Praetorius J, Kim YH, Bouzinova EV, et al: NBCn1 is a basolateral Na+-HCO3 cotransporter in rat kidney inner medullary collecting ducts. Am J Physiol Renal Physiol 286:F903, 2004.

563. Schiller A, Forssmann WG, Taugner R: The tight junctions of renal tubules in the cortex and outer medulla. A quantitative study of the kidneys of six species. Cell Tissue Res 212:395, 1980.

564. Schiller A, Taugner R: Heterogeneity of tight junctions along the collecting duct in the renal medulla. A freeze-fracture study in rat and rabbit. Cell Tissue Res 223:603, 1982.

565. Tisher CC, Yarger WE: Lanthanum permeability of tight junctions along the collecting duct of the rat. Kidney Int 7:35, 1975.

566. Ganote CE, Grantham JJ, Moses HL, et al: Ultrastructural studies of vasopressin effect on isolated perfused renal collecting tubules of the rabbit. J Cell Biol 36:355, 1968.

567. Grantham JJ, Ganote CE, Burg MB, Orloff J: Paths of transtubular water flow in isolated renal collecting tubules. J Cell Biol 41:562, 1969.

568. Tisher CC, Bulger RE, Valtin H: Morphology of renal medulla in water diuresis and vasopressin-induced antidiuresis. Am J Physiol 220:87, 1971.

569. Harmanci MC, Kachadorian WA, Valtin H, DiScala VA: Antidiuretic hormone-induced intramembranous alterations in mammalian collecting ducts. Am J Physiol 235:440, 1978.

570. Harmanci MC, Stern P, Kachadorian WA, et al: Vasopressin and collecting duct intramembranous particle clusters: A dose-response relationship. Am J Physiol 239:F560, 1980.

571. Wade JB, Stetson DL, Lewis SA: ADH action: evidence for a membrane shuttle mechanism. Ann N Y Acad Sci 372:106, 1981.

572. Kirk KL, Buku A, Eggena P: Cell specificity of vasopressin binding in renal collecting duct: Computer-enhanced imaging of a fluorescent hormone analog. Proc Natl Acad Sci 84:6000, 1987.

573. Brown D, Orci L: Vasopressin stimulates formation of coated pits in rat kidney collecting ducts. Nature 302:253, 1983.

574. Strange K, Willingham MC, Handler JS, Harris HW, Jr: Apical membrane endocytosis via coated pits is stimulated by removal of antidiuretic hormone from isolated, perfused rabbit cortical collecting tubule. J Membr Biol 103:17, 1988.

575. Brown D, Weyer P, Orci L: Vasopressin stimulates endocytosis in kidney collecting duct principal cells. Eur J Cell Biol 46:336, 1988.

576. Fushimi K, Uchida S, Hara Y, et al: Cloning and expression of apical membrane water channel of rat kidney collecting tubule. Nature 361:549, 1993.

577. Nielsen S, DiGiovanni SR, Christensen EI, et al: Cellular and subcellular immunolocalization of vasopressin-regulated water channel in rat kidney. Proc Natl Acad Sci U S A 90:11663, 1993.

578. Ecelbarger CA, Terris J, Frindt G, et al: Aquaporin-3 water channel localization and regulation in rat kidney. Am J Physiol 269:F663, 1995.

579. Terris J, Ecelbarger CA, Marples D, et al: Distribution of aquaporin-4 water channel expression within rat kidney. Am J Physiol 269:F775, 1995.

580. Frigeri A, Gropper MA, Turck CW, Verkman AS: Immunolocalization of the mercurial-insensitive water channel and glycerol intrinsic protein in epithelial cell plasma membranes. Proc Natl Acad Sci U S A 92:4328, 1995.

581. Nielsen S, Chou CL, Marples D, et al: Vasopressin increases water permeability of kidney collecting duct by inducing translocation of aquaporin-CD water channels to plasma membrane. Proc Natl Acad Sci U S A 92:1013, 1995.

582. Marples D, Knepper MA, Christensen EI, Nielsen S: Redistribution of aquaporin-2 water channels induced by vasopressin in rat kidney inner medullary collecting duct. Am J Physiol 269:C655, 1995.

583. Yamamoto T, Sasaki S, Fushimi K, et al: Vasopressin increases AQP-CD water channel in apical membrane of collecting duct cells in Brattleboro rats. Am J Physiol Cell Physiol 268:C1546, 1995.

584. Sabolic I, Katsura T, Verbavatz JM, Brown D: The AQP2 water channel: Effect of vasopressin treatment, microtubule disruption, and distribution in neonatal rats. J Membr Biol 143:165, 1995.

585. DiGiovanni SR, Nielsen S, Christensen EI, Knepper MA: Regulation of collecting duct water channel expression by vasopressin in Brattleboro rat. Proc Natl Acad Sci U S A 91:8984, 1994.

586. Robben JH, Knoers N, Deen PMT: Cell biological aspects of the vasopressin type-2 receptor and aquaporin 2 water channel in nephrogenic diabetes insipidus. Am J Physiol Renal Physiol 291:F257, 2006.

587. Marples D, Christensen S, Christensen EI, et al: Lithium-induced downregulation of aquaporin-2 water channel expression in rat kidney medulla. J Clin Invest 95:1838, 1995.

588. Li C, Shi Y, Wang W, et al: α-MSH prevents impairment in renal function and dysregulation of AQPs and Na-K-ATPase in rats with bilateral ureteral obstruction. Am J Physiol Renal Physiol 290:F384, 2006.

589. Nielsen S, Terris J, Andersen D, et al: Congestive heart failure in rats is associated with increased expression and targeting of aquaporin-2 water channel in collecting duct. Proc Natl Acad Sci U S A 94:5450, 1997.

590. Xu DL, Martin PY, Ohara M, et al: Upregulation of aquaporin-2 water channel expression in chronic heart failure rat. J Clin Invest 99:1500, 1997.

591. Bohman SO: The ultrastructure of the renal medulla and the interstitial cells. In Mandal AK (ed): The Renal Papilla and Hypertension. New York, Plenum, 1980, p 7.

592. Lemley KV, Kriz W: Anatomy of the renal interstitium. Kidney Int 39:370, 1991.

593. Pedersen JC, Persson AE, Maunsbach AB: Ultrastructure and quantitative characterization of the cortical interstitium in the rat kidney. In Maunsbach AB, Olsen TS, Christensen EI (eds): Functional Ultrastructure of the Kidney. London, Academic Press, 1980, p 443.

594. Pfaller W: Structure function correlation on rat kidney. Quantitative correlation of structure and function in the normal and injured rat kidney. Berlin, Springer-Verlag, 70:1, 1982.

595. Dunnill MS, Halley W: Some observations on the quantitative anatomy of the kidney. J Pathol 110:113, 1973.

596. Bohle A, Grund KE, Mackensen S, Tolon M: Correlations between renal interstitium and level of serum creatinine. Morphometric investigations of biopsies in perimembranous glomerulonephritis. Virchows Arch A Pathol Anat Histol 373:15, 1977.

597. Hestbech J, Hansen HE, Amdisen A, Olsen S: Chronic renal lesions following long-term treatment with lithium. Kidney Int 12:205, 1977.

598. Kappel B, Olsen S: Cortical interstitial tissue and sclerosed glomeruli in the normal human kidney, related to age and sex. A quantitative study. Virchows Arch A Pathol Anat Histol 387:271, 1980.

599. Wolgast M, Larson M, Nygren K: Functional characteristics of the renal interstitium. Am J Physiol 241:F105, 1981.

600. Bulger RE, Nagle RB: Ultrastructure of the interstitium in the rabbit kidney. Am J Anat 136:183, 1973.

601. Bohman SO: The ultrastructure of the rat renal medulla as observed after improved fixation methods. J Ultrastruct Res 47:329, 1974.

602. Kaissling B, Le Hir M: Characterization and distribution of interstitial cell types in the renal cortex of rats. Kidney Int 45:709, 1994.

603. Mounier F, Foidart JM, Gubler MC: Distribution of extracellular matrix glycoproteins during normal development of human kidney. An immunohistochemical study. Lab Invest 54:394, 1986.

604. Martinez-Hernandez A, Gay S, Miller EJ: Ultrastructural localization of type V collagen in rat kidney. J Cell Biol 92:343, 1982.

605. Lacombe C, Da Silva JL, Bruneval P, et al: Peritubular cells are the site of erythropoietin synthesis in the murine hypoxic kidney. J Clin Invest 81:620, 1988.

606. Bachmann S, Le HM, Eckardt KU: Co-localization of erythropoietin mRNA and ecto-5′-nucleotidase immunoreactivity in peritubular cells of rat renal cortex indicates that fibroblasts produce erythropoietin. J Histochem Cytochem 41:335, 1993.

607. Le Hir M, Kaissling B: Distribution of 5′-nucleotidase in the renal interstitium of the rat. Cell Tissue Res 258:177, 1989.

608. Bohman SO, Jensen PK: The interstitial cells in the renal medulla of rat, rabbit, and gerbil in different states of diuresis. Cell Tissue Res 189:1, 1978.

609. Schiller A, Taugner R: Junctions between interstitial cells of the renal medulla: a freeze-fracture study. Cell Tissue Res 203:231, 1979.

610. Majack RA, Larsen WJ: The bicellular and reflexive membrane junctions of renomedullary interstitial cells: Functional implications of reflexive gap junctions. Am J Anat 157:181, 1980.

611. Bohman SO, Jensen PK: Morphometric studies on the lipid droplets of the interstitial cells of the renal medulla in different states of diuresis. J Ultrastruct Res 55:182, 1976.

612. Cavallo T: Fine structural localization of endogenous peroxidase activity in inner medullary interstitial cells of the rat kidney. Lab Invest 31:458, 1974.

613. Bulger RE, Griffith LD, Trump BF: Endoplasmic reticulum in rat renal interstitial cells: molecular rearrangement after water deprivation. Science 151:83, 1966.

614. Ledingham JM, Simpson FO: Bundles of intracellular tubules in renal medullary interstitial cells. J Cell Biol 57:594, 1973.

615. Moffat DB: A new type of cell inclusion in the interstitial cells of the medulla of the rat kidney. J Microsc 6:1073, 1967.

616. Nissen HM: On lipid droplets in renal interstitial cells. II. A histological study on the number of droplets in salt depletion and acute salt repletion. Z Zellforsch Mikrosk Anat 85:483, 1968.

617. Nissen HM: On lipid droplets in renal interstitial cells. 3. A histological study on the number of droplets during hydration and dehydration. Z Zellforsch Mikrosk Anat 92:52, 1968.

618. Mandal AK, Frolich ED, Claude P: A morphologic study of the renal papillary granule: Analysis in the interstitial cell and in the interstitium. J Lab Clin Med 85:120, 1975.

619. Nissen HM, Bojesen I: On lipid droplets in renal interstitial cells. IV. Isolation and identification. Z Zellforsch Mikrosk Anat 97:274, 1969.

620. Bohman SO, Maunsbach AB: Ultrastructure and biochemical properties of subcellular fractions from rat renal medulla. J Ultrastruct Res 38:225, 1972.

621. Anggard E, Bohman SO, Griffin JE, et al: Subcellular localization of the prostaglandin system in the rabbit renal papilla. Acta Physiol Scand 84:231, 1972.

622. Muirhead EE, Germain GS, Armstrong FB, et al: Endocrine-type antihypertensive function of renomedullary interstitial cells. Kidney Int Suppl S271, 1975.

623. Dunn MJ, Staley RS, Harrison M: Characterization of prostaglandin production in tissue culture of rabbit renal medulla. Prostaglandins 12:37, 1976.

624. Zusman RM, Keiser HR: Prostaglandin biosynthesis by rabbit renomedullary interstitial cells in tissue culture. Stimulation by angiotensin II, bradykinin, and arginine vasopressin. J Clin Invest 60:215, 1977.

625. Bohman SO: Demonstration of prostaglandin synthesis in collecting duct cells and other cell types of the rabbit renal medulla. Prostaglandins 14:729, 1977.

626. Guan Y, Chang M, Cho W, et al: Cloning, expression, and regulation of rabbit cyclooxygenase-2 in renal medullary interstitial cells. Am J Physiol 273:F18, 1997.

627. Maric C, Aldred GP, Antoine AM, et al: Effects of angiotensin II on cultured rat renomedullary interstitial cells are mediated by AT1A receptors. Am J Physiol 271:F1020, 1996.

628. Zhuo J, Dean R, Maric C, et al: Localization and interactions of vasoactive peptide receptors in renomedullary interstitial cells of the kidney. Kidney Int Suppl 67:S22, 1998.

629. Brown CA, Zusman RM, Haber E: Identification of an angiotensin receptor in rabbit renomedullary interstitial cells in tissue culture. Correlation with prostaglandin biosynthesis. Circ Res 46:802, 1980.

630. Kugler P: Angiotensinase A in the renomedullary interstitial cells. Histochemistry 77:105, 1983.

631. Muirhead EE, Brooks B, Pitcock JA, Stephenson P: Renomedullary antihypertensive function in accelerated (malignant) hypertension. Observations on renomedullary interstitial cells. J Clin Invest 51:181, 1972.

632. Muirhead EE, Brooks B, Pitcock JA, et al: Role of the renal medulla in the sodium-sensitive component of renoprival hypertension. Lab Invest 27:192, 1972.

633. Pitcock JA, Lyons H, Brown PS, et al: Glycosaminoglycans of the rat renomedullary interstitium: Ultrastructural and biochemical observations. Exp Mol Pathol 49:373, 1988.

634. Peirce EC: Renal lymphatics. Anat Rec 90:315, 1944.

635. Bell RD, Keyl MJ, Shrader FR, et al: Renal lymphatics: The internal distribution. Nephron 5:454, 1968.

636. Kriz W, Dieterich HJ: [The lymphatic system of the kidney in some mammals. Light and electron microscopic investigations]. Z Anat Entwicklungsgesch 131:111, 1970.

637. Nordquist RE, Bell RD, Sinclair RJ, Keyl MJ: The distribution and ultrastructural morphology of lymphatic vessels in the canine renal cortex. Lymphology 6:13, 1973.

638. Albertine KH, O'Morchoe CC: Distribution and density of the canine renal cortical lymphatic system. Kidney Int 16:470, 1979.

639. Niiro GK, Jarosz HM, O'Morchoe PJ, O'Morchoe CC: The renal cortical lymphatic system in the rat, hamster, and rabbit. Am J Anat 177:21, 1986.

640. Holmes MJ, O'Morchoe PJ, O'Morchoe CC: Morphology of the intrarenal lymphatic system. Capsular and hilar communications. Am J Anat 149:333, 1977.

641. Albertine KH, O'Morchoe CC: An integrated light and electron microscopic study on the existence of intramedullary lymphatics in the dog kidney. Lymphology 13:100, 1080.

642. Michel CC: Renal medullary microcirculation: Architecture and exchange. Microcirculation 2:125, 1995.

643. Tenstad O, Heyeraas KJ, Wiig H, Aukland K: Drainage of plasma proteins from the renal medullary interstitium in rats. J Physiol 536:533, 2001.

644. Wang W, Michel CC: Modeling exchange of plasma proteins between microcirculation and interstitium of the renal medulla. Am J Physiol Renal Physiol 279:F334, 2000.

645. Mitchell GA: The nerve supply of the kidneys. Acta Anat (Basel) 10:1, 1950.

646. Gosling JA: Observations on the distribution of intrarenal nervous tissue. Anat Rec 163:81, 1969.

647. McKenna OC, Angelakos ET: Acetylcholinesterase-containing nerve fibers in the canine kidney. Circ Res 23:645, 1968.

648. McKenna OC, Angelakos ET: Adrenergic innervation of the canine kidney. Circ Res 22:345, 1968.

649. Barajas L, Powers K: Monoaminergic innervation of the rat kidney: A quantitative study. Am J Physiol 259:F503, 1990.

650. Newstead J, Munkacsi I: Electron microscope observations on the juxtamedullary efferent arterioles and Arteriolae rectae in kidneys of rats. Z Zellforsch Mikrosk Anat 97:465, 1969.

651. Knight DS, Russell HW, Cicero SR, Beal JA: Transitory inner medullary nerve terminals in the cat kidney. Neurosci Lett 114:173, 1990.

652. Barajas L: Innervation of the renal cortex. Fed Proc 37:1192, 1978.

653. Barajas L, Liu L, Powers K: Anatomy of the renal innervation: intrarenal aspects and ganglia of origin. Can J Physiol Pharmacol 70:735, 1992.

654. Barajas L, Powers K, Wang P: Innervation of the late distal nephron: an autoradiographic and ultrastructural study. J Ultrastruct Res 92:146, 1985.

655. Barajas L, Powers K, Wang P: Innervation of the renal cortical tubules: A quantitative study. Am J Physiol 247:F50, 1984.

656. Barajas L, Wang P: Myelinated nerves of the rat kidney. A light and electron microscopic autoradiographic study. J Ultrastruct Res 65:148, 1978.

657. Ballesta J, Polak JM, Allen JM, Bloom SR: The nerves of the juxtaglomerular apparatus of man and other mammals contain the potent peptide NPY. Histochemistry 80:483, 1984.

658. Reinecke M, Forssmann WG: Neuropeptide (neuropeptide Y, neurotensin, vasoactive intestinal polypeptide, substance P, calcitonin gene-related peptide, somatostatin)

immunohistochemistry and ultrastructure of renal nerves. Histochemistry 89:1, 1988.

659. Knuepfer MM, Schramm LP: The conduction velocities and spinal projections of single renal afferent fibers in the rat. Brain Res 435:167, 1987.

660. Graves FT: The anatomy of the intrarenal arteries and its application to segmental resection of the kidney. Br J Surg 42:132, 1954.

661. Kanwar YS: Biophysiology of glomerular filtration and proteinuria. Lab Invest 51:7, 1984.

662. Madsen KM, Brenner BM: Structure and function of the renal tubule and interstitium. *In* Tisher CC, Brenner BM (eds): Renal Pathology with Clinical and Functional Correlations. Philadelphia, JB Lippincott, 1989, p.606.

663. Nielsen S, Kwon TH, Christensen BM, et al: Physiology and pathophysiology of renal aquaporins. J Am Soc Nephrol 10:647, 1999.

664. Madsen KM, Verlander JW, Tisher CC: Relationship between structure and function in distal tubule and collecting duct. J Electron Microsc Tech 9:187, 1988.

CHAPTER 3

The Renal Circulations and Glomerular Ultrafiltration

Rujun Gong • Lance D. Dworkin • Barry M. Brenner •
David A. Maddox

Under resting conditions, about 20% of the cardiac output in humans perfuses the kidneys, organs that constitute only about 0.5% of the human body mass. This rate of blood flow, approximately 400 mL/100 g of tissue per minute, is much greater than that observed in other vascular beds ordinarily considered to be well perfused, such as heart, liver, and brain.[1] From this enormous blood flow (about 1 L/minute) only a small quantity of urine is formed (about 1 mL/minute). Although the metabolic energy requirement of urine production is great— about 10% of basal O_2 consumption— examination of the renal arteriovenous O_2 difference reveals that blood flow far exceeds metabolic demands. In fact, the high rate of blood flow is essential to the process of urine formation.

Traditionally, reviews of the renal circulation have focused on whole-organ blood flow, as measured by arterial flowmeters or by clearance techniques, and on the variations in this flow induced by pharmacologic agents. Technologic advances, however, now permit both a more precise definition of renal vascular anatomy and direct measurements of microvascular pressures, flows, resistances, and permeabilities in regions of mammalian kidneys previously considered inaccessible. The results obtained make it clear that the kidney contains several distinct microvascular networks, including the glomerular microcirculation, the cortical peritubular microcirculation, and the unique microcirculations that nourish and drain the inner and outer medulla. In this chapter, we consider (1) the intrarenal organization of these discrete microcirculatory networks, (2) the total and regional renal blood flows, and (3) the physiologic factors that regulate these flows. For detailed discussions of the effects of pharmacologic agents on renal blood flow and intrarenal blood flow distribution, the reader is referred to Chapters 45 and 46.

MAJOR ARTERIES AND VEINS

The human renal artery usually divides just before entry into the renal parenchyma. The anterior main branch further divides into four segmental arteries, which supply the apex of the kidney, the upper and middle segments of the anterior surface, and the entire lower pole, respectively. The posterior main branch supplies the remainder of the kidney; an occasional branch from this trunk supplies blood to the apex. These segmental arteries are end arteries, there being no anastomoses between their branches at any level of division.[2] Therefore, obstruction of an arterial vessel should lead to complete ischemia and infarction of the tissue in its area of distribution. In fact, ligation of individual segmental arteries has frequently been performed in the rat to reduce renal mass and produce the remnant kidney model of chronic renal failure. Morphologic studies in this model reveal the presence of ischemic zones adjacent to the totally infarcted areas. These regions contain viable glomeruli that appear shrunken and crowded together, demonstrating that some portions of the renal cortex may have partial dual perfusion.[3]

The anatomic distribution of segmental arteries just described is most common; however, other patterns may occur.[4,5] Not infrequently, "accessory" renal arteries may result from precocious division of the renal artery at the aorta. These vessels, which most often supply the lower pole,[6] are not in fact accessory because each is the sole arterial supply of some part of the organ.[2] Such additional arteries are found in 20% to 30% of normal individuals.

Within the renal sinus of the human kidney, division of the segmental arteries gives rise to the interlobar arteries, which extend toward the cortex along the columns of Bertin located between adjacent medullary pyramids. These vessels, in turn, give rise to the arcuate arteries, whose several divisions tend to lie in a plane parallel to the kidney surface at the border between the cortex and outer medulla. From the arcuate arteries, the interlobular arteries branch more or less sharply, most often as a common

CH 3

trunk that divides two to five times as it extends toward the kidney surface[7-10] (Fig. 3–1). Afferent arterioles leading to glomeruli arise from the smaller branches of the interlobular arteries (Fig. 3–2). Except for the terminal portion of the afferent arteriole, the wall structure of the intrarenal arteries and the afferent arterioles resembles that of vessels of similar size in other locations.

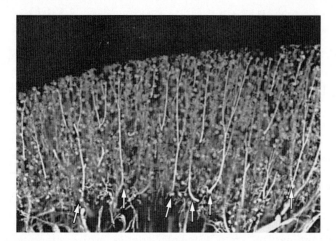

FIGURE 3–1 Low-power photomicrograph of silicone-injected vascular structures in human renal cortex. The tissue has been made transparent by dehydration and clearing procedures after injection. Interlobular arteries (some indicated by arrows) arise from arcuate arteries (not seen) and extend toward the kidney surface. The glomeruli, visible as small round objects, arise from the interlobular vessels at all cortical levels. (Magnification ×5.) (Courtesy of R Beeuwkes, Ph.D.)

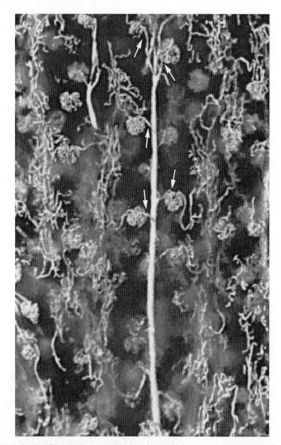

FIGURE 3–2 Photomicrograph of a single interlobular artery and glomeruli arising from it as seen in a cleared section of a silicone rubber–injected human kidney. Afferent arterioles (arrows) extend to glomeruli. Efferent vessels emerging from glomeruli branch to form the cortical postglomerular capillary network. The photomicrograph is oriented so that the outer cortex is at the top and the inner cortex is at the bottom. (Magnification ×25.) (Courtesy of R Beeuwkes, Ph.D.)

The capillary network of each glomerulus is connected to the postglomerular (peritubular) capillary circulation by way of efferent arterioles. Venous connections between peritubular capillaries and veins are made at every cortical level. Superficial veins drain the region near the kidney surface. These lie within the cortex and may run parallel to the capsule before descending along the interlobular axes.[10] Interlobular veins, close to the corresponding arteries, drain the bulk of the cortex. As these converge they are joined by vessels from the medullary rays and veins returning from the medulla in vascular bundles. Unlike the arterial system, which has no collateral pathways, the venous vessels anastomose at several levels.[2,8] Convergence at the arcuate and interlobar veins gives rise to several main trunks that join to form the renal vein. The large veins of the renal hilum have no clear segmental organization, and because of the earlier anastomoses, obstruction of one large venous channel usually leads to diversion of blood flow to the others.

The pattern of the renal arterial system is similar in most of the mammals commonly used experimentally. Nomenclature is also similar. For example, the main arterial branches that lie beside the medullary pyramid are called interlobar, even in animals that have but a single lobe. The absence of arterial anastomoses seems to be a general finding.[10] In contrast to the similarity in arterial vessels, the venous pattern shows more marked species differences. The canine kidney has a major outer cortical venous system that is drained by way of the interlobular axes.[9,10] Superficial cortical veins are also a feature of the feline kidney, but in this species these vessels are subcapsular and extend around the surface of the kidney to join with the renal vein at the hilum.[8,11] This arrangement has permitted experiments involving separate collection of the venous drainage from the superficial and deep cortex.[12] In the ringed seal, the subcapsular system is so developed that virtually the entire venous outflow of the kidney is directed to the peripheral plexuses. This species differs from most other mammals in that no arcuate venous system exists and no major vein of consequence emerges from the renal hilum.[13] In the hamster, rat, and mouse, superficial veins are absent and blood leaves the cortex entirely by way of interlobular veins descending in a direction perpendicular to the capsule.[8,14] Such veins can also be seen in photographs of injected rabbit kidneys.[15] Anastomoses between the arcuate vessels of the venous system appear to be a consistent finding in all species except the seal.

ORGANIZATION AND FUNCTION OF THE INTRARENAL MICROCIRCULATIONS

Hydraulic Pressure Profile of the Renal Circulation

Based on studies of the vasculature of a unique set of juxtamedullary nephrons[16,17] most of the preglomerular pressure drop between the arcuate artery and the glomerulus occurs along the afferent arteriole (Fig. 3–3). The pressure drop between the systemic vasculature and the end of the interlobular artery in both the superficial and juxtamedullary microvasculature, however, can be as much as 25 mm Hg at normal perfusion pressures, with the majority of that pressure drop occurring along the interlobular arteries (see Fig. 3–3 and Refs 17, 18). Approximately 70% of the postglomerular hydraulic pressure drop takes place along the efferent arterioles with approximately 40% of the total postglomerular resistance accounted for by the early efferent arteriole (see

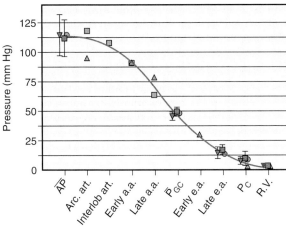

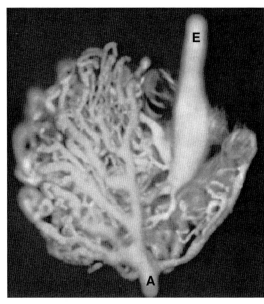

FIGURE 3-3 Hydraulic pressure profile in the renal vasculature. Filled squares and triangles denote values (mean± 2 SD) obtained from a variety of micropuncture studies in euvolemic and hydropenic rats, respectively. Values obtained from studies of the squirrel monkey are shown as open diamonds. Values shown by open inverted triangles and open squares were obtained by micropunture of juxtamedullary nephrons in the Sprague-Dawley rat. In these studies the arcuate artery (Arc.art.) was perfused with whole blood (at the perfusion pressures shown) and hydraulic pressures measured at downstream sites including the interlobular artery (Interlob. art.), the proximal (Early a.a.) and distal (Late a.a.) portions of the afferent arteriole, the glomerular capillaries ($\bar{P}_{GC}$), the proximal (Early e.a.) and late (Late e.a.) segments of the efferent arteriole, the peritubular capillaries (P_C), and the renal vein (R.V.). (See Refs 18 and 551 for sources of data.)

FIGURE 3-4 Photomicrograph of a silicone-injected and cleared canine glomerulus. The afferent arteriole (A) enters at the bottom of the photograph. The efferent arteriole (E) extends upward. The vascular tuft has been teased apart slightly to reveal the distinctive dilation in the early part of the efferent vessel. (Magnification ×360.) (Reprinted with permission from Barger AC, Herd JA: The renal circulation. N Engl J Med 284:482, 1971.)

Fig. 3–3). Of note, studies using this preparation now demonstrate that the very late portion of the afferent arteriole (last 50 μm–150 μm) and the very early portion of the efferent arteriole (first 50 μm–150 μm) provide a large portion of the total pre- and postglomerular resistance (see Fig. 3–3).

Structure of the Glomerular Microcirculation

The glomerulus and glomerular filtration are discussed in detail in a later part of this chapter. Structurally, the glomerulus consists of an enlargement of the proximal end of the tubule to incorporate a vascular tuft. The vascular structure of the tuft is strikingly similar in different species and appears to be genetically defined, at least in its major divisions. For example, vascular pathways of the injected canine glomerulus, shown in Figure 3–4, are similar to those of a human glomerulus drawn from a reconstruction by Elias (Fig. 3–5).[19,20] The efferent vessel is formed by an abrupt and distinctive convergence of the glomerular capillary pathways (see Figs. 3–4 and 3–5).

Elger and co-workers[21] provided a detailed ultrastructural analysis of the vascular pole of the renal glomerulus. They described significant differences in the structure and branching patterns of the afferent and efferent arterioles as they enter and exit the tuft. Afferent arterioles lose their internal elastic layer and smooth muscle cell layer prior to entering the glomerular tuft. Smooth muscle cells are replaced by granular cells that are in close contact with the extraglomerular mesangium. Upon entering, afferent arterioles branch immediately and are distributed along the surface of the glomerular tuft. These primary branches have wide lumens and immediately acquire features of glomerular capillaries, including a fenestrated endothelium, characteristic glomerular basement membrane, and epithelial foot processes. In contrast, the efferent arteriole arises deep within the tuft, from the convergence of capillaries arising from multiple lobules. Additional tributar-

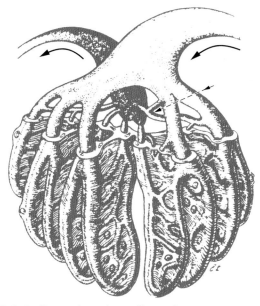

FIGURE 3-5 Human glomerular capillary pathways, as reconstructed by Elias. This drawing shows the abrupt connections of capillary pathways to the efferent arteriole. Such connections are apparent in the dog glomerulus (see Fig. 3–4). This diagram does not indicate the details of the capillary walls or membranes. The dashed arrow indicates a short pathway between afferent and efferent arterioles. (From Elias H, Hossmann A, Barth IB, Solmor A: Blood flow in the renal glomerulus. J Urol 83:790–798, 1960.)

ies join the arteriole as it travels toward the vascular pole. The structure of the capillary wall begins to change even before the vessels coalesce to form the efferent arteriole, losing fenestrae progressively until a smooth epithelial lining is formed. At its terminal portion within the tuft, endothelial cells may bulge into the lumen, reducing its internal diameter. Typically, the diameter of the efferent arteriole within the tuft is significantly less than that of the afferent arteriole.

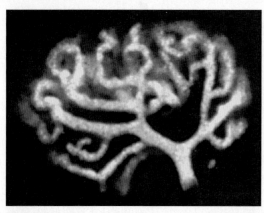

FIGURE 3–6 Photomicrograph of a silicone-injected and cleared glomerulus from a dog in which only relatively large-diameter channels have filled. In contrast with the glomerulus shown in Figure 3–4, with its myriad of small pathways, the simple structure of this capillary tuft is striking. Such variability of intraglomerular perfusion may play a role in regulating filtration rate in mammals (see text). (Reprinted with permission from Barger AC, Herd JA: The renal circulation. N Engl J Med 284:482, 1971.)

Depending on the location of the final confluence of capillaries, efferent arterioles may acquire a smooth muscle cell layer, which is observed distal to the entry point of the final capillary. The efferent arteriole is also in close contact with the glomerular mesangium as it forms inside the tuft and with the extraglomerular mesangium as it exits the tuft. This precise and close anatomic relationship between the afferent and efferent arterioles and mesangium is of uncertain physiologic significance, but is consistent with the presence of an intraglomerular signaling system that may participate in the regulation of blood flow and filtration rate.

The appearance of the vascular pathways within the glomerulus may change under different physiologic conditions. In injection studies, some glomeruli show only simple, large-diameter paths (Fig. 3–6), whereas other glomeruli nearby may show a myriad of small pathways, as in Figure 3–4. This may result from variability in the degree of filling of available intraglomerular pathways.[21] Intermittent flow within glomeruli has been reported in amphibian species,[22] and Hall[23] has suggested that variation in filling of different intraglomerular pathways is a means of regulating filtration by altering the filtration surface area and axial resistance to blood flow. For a given cross-sectional area, small channels have much higher resistance than large channels.

Some insight into the mechanism by which intraglomerular flow patterns might be changed has been obtained. The glomerular mesangium has been shown to contain contractile elements[24] and exhibit contractile activity when exposed to angiotensin II (AII).[25] Mesangial cells, which possess specific receptors for angiotensin II, undergo contraction when exposed to this peptide in vitro.[26] Three-dimensional reconstruction of the entire mesangium in the rat suggests that approximately 15% of capillary loops may be entirely enclosed within armlike extensions of mesangial cells that, together with the body of the mesangial cell, are anchored to the extracellular matrix.[27] Contraction of these cells might alter local blood flow and filtration rate as well as alter the intraglomerular distribution of blood flow and total filtration surface area. Many hormones and other vasoactive substances capable of altering the glomerular ultrafiltration coefficient bring about this adjustment by altering the state of contraction of mesangial cells.

Recent studies have employed newer imaging techniques to more accurately assess the three-dimensional structure of the glomerular tuft. Yu and co-workers[28] applied scanning electron microscopy to mouse glomeruli that were fixed by an in vivo cryotechnique with freeze substitution, as opposed to more conventional methods. This technique maintained open capillary lumens and may preserve the ultrastructure of the glomerulus closer to the living state. Kaczmarek[29] applied confocal microscopy of normal rats to more precisely reveal the lobular structure of glomeruli and to estimate the average length of the capillary network. He proposed that three-dimensional models based on confocal data were much easier to generate than reconstructions based on serial sections. In addition, Antiga and colleagues[30] developed an automated method to produce a three-dimensional model of the glomerular capillary network using digitized images of serial sections of a tuft. This method was used to produce a topographic map of the glomerulus and to derive data on the length, radius, and spatial configuration of capillary segments. More recently, a novel technology, termed two-photon microscopy, has been applied to optimize three-dimensional, multicolor imaging and single-cell segmentation of glomerular components in either biopsy or intravital kidney tissue.[31]

A detailed discussion of the various driving forces and physiologic modulators of the glomerular ultrafiltration process are provided later. The sieving characteristics of the glomerular capillary wall for macromolecules are considered in Chapter 26.

Cortical Postglomerular Microcirculation

Vascular Patterns

The precise description of efferent vascular patterns in each cortical region has been achieved through careful microscopic examination of kidneys after vascular injection with appropriate media, usually silicone rubber.[11,32–35] More recently, microcomputed tomography has allowed visualization of injected renal microvessels without sectioning the kidney.[36] From these studies, it has become clear that the appearance of efferent arterioles, and of the peritubular capillary networks arising from them, varies markedly from one cortical region to another[37] (see Fig. 3–8). This intracortical heterogeneity may have important physiologic consequences. Indeed, some functional characteristics of the cortical circulation suggest that at least three different circulations exist in parallel within the cortex (see "Intrarenal Blood Flow Distribution").

In the outermost, or subcapsular, region of the cortex, the efferent arterioles give rise to a dense capillary network that surrounds the convoluted tubule segments arising from the superficial glomeruli (rectangle 1 in Fig. 3–7). There is evidence suggesting that this arrangement is of great importance for reabsorption of water and electrolytes in proximal tubule segments of superficial nephrons (see Chapter 9). In contrast, the efferent arterioles originating from the comparatively fewer juxtamedullary glomeruli (rectangle 4 in Fig. 3–7) extend into the medulla and give rise to the medullary microcirculatory patterns: an intricate capillary network in the outer medulla and long, unbranched capillary loops, the so-called vasa recta, in the inner medulla. More localized, inner cortical capillary networks may also arise from juxtamedullary glomeruli (rectangle 4 in Fig. 3–4). The arrangement of the medullary microcirculation plays an important role in the process of concentration of urine (see Chapter 9).

Differences in wall structure are also observed when one compares the efferent arterioles of juxtamedullary glomeruli with those of other nephrons. Superficial and midcortical efferent arterioles are smaller in diameter than juxtamedullary

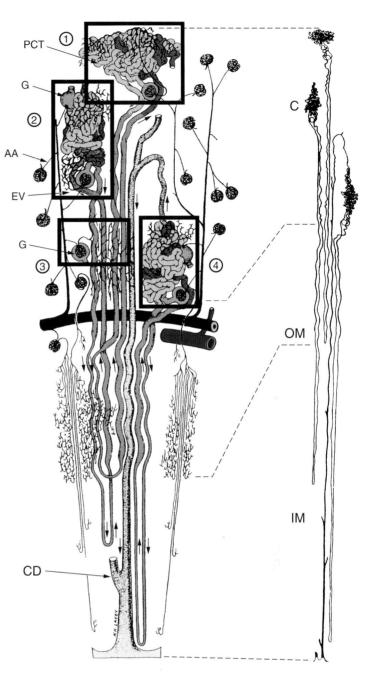

FIGURE 3–7 Diagram showing the vascular and tubule organization of the kidney in the dog. In the right-hand portion of the figure, nephrons arising from glomeruli in outer, middle, and inner cortex are shown to scale. Cortex (C), outer medulla (OM), and inner medulla (IM) are indicated. The left portion of the figure illustrates the pattern of glomeruli (G) arising from afferent arterioles (AA). The efferent vessels (EV) from these glomeruli divide to form the peritubular capillaries. At the kidney surface, proximal convoluted tubules (PCT) are associated with a dense capillary network arising from division of superficial efferent arterioles (rectangle 1). In the middle and inner cortex, convoluted tubule segments are located close to interlobular arteries and are perfused by a complex peritubular capillary network, usually derived from the efferent vessels of many glomeruli (rectangles 2 and 4). Midway between interlobular vessels, loops of Henle are grouped together with collecting ducts (CD). The peritubular capillary network of this region, derived from midcortical efferent arterioles, is largely oriented parallel to the tubular structures of the medullary ray (rectangle 3). In the inner or juxtamedullary cortex, glomeruli have efferent arterioles that extend downward and divide to form outer medullary vascular bundles (rectangle 4). A dense outer medullary capillary network arises from these bundles. Only thin limbs of Henle extend with collecting ducts to the papillary tip. These are accompanied by vasa recta extending from the cores of the vascular bundles. For simplicity, venous vessels have not been shown. (Modified from Beeuwkes R III, Bonventre JV: Tubular organization and vascular tubular relations in the dog kidney. Am J Physiol 229:F695, 1975.)

vessels,[10,15,38,39] and usually possess only one layer of smooth muscle cells (Fig. 3–8A). The larger juxtamedullary efferent arterioles (see Fig. 3–8B) characteristically display two to four layers of smooth muscle cells. The endothelial layer consists of a large number of longitudinally arranged cells.[39,40] Kriz and Kaissling[41] have described basal lamina material filling irregular, wide spaces between the smooth muscle and endothelial cell layers in efferent arterioles of both superficial and deep nephrons.

The complex microcirculatory architecture described, with its striking "vertical" heterogeneity, is further complicated by the existence of a "horizontal" heterogeneity: near the interlobular arteries, a dense capillary network, with no definable orientation, is formed by efferent arterioles and enmeshes both proximal and distal convoluted segments (see rectangles 2 and 4 in Fig. 3–7). However, when one examines the central portion of the lobule, in the region of the medullary rays (see Chapter 2), less dense capillary networks are found, most of them oriented parallel to the tubule structures with which

they are associated, namely cortical segments of loops of Henle and collecting ducts (see rectangle 3 in Fig. 3–7). This variability in cortical efferent arteriolar branching patterns, whose physiologic significance is unknown, is further illustrated in Fig. 3–9.

The cortical venous circulation also shows a high degree of regional variability. The most superficial cortex is drained, at least in humans, dogs, and cats, by way of the superficial cortical veins.[8,10,12] In middle and inner cortex, venous drainage is achieved mainly by the interlobular veins. The dense peritubular capillary network surrounding the interlobular vessels (see rectangles 2 and 4 in Fig. 3–7) drains directly into the interlobular veins through multiple connections, whereas the less dense, long-meshed network of the medullary rays (see rectangle 3 in Fig. 3–7) appears to anastomose with the interlobular network and thus drain laterally. The medullary circulation also shows two different types of drainage: the outer medullary networks typically extend into the medullary rays before joining interlobular veins, whereas

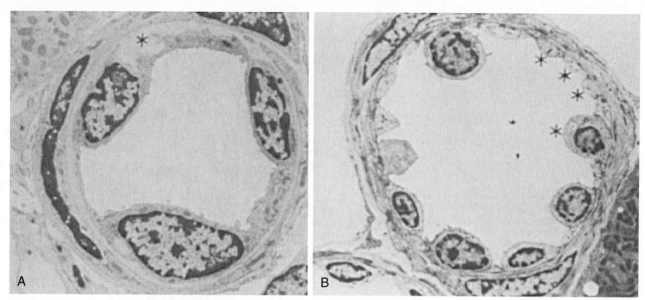

FIGURE 3–8 Transmission electron micrographs of efferent arterioles. **A,** A vessel arising from a superficial glomerulus of a rabbit. The thick basal lamina frequently broadens to lakelike structures (∗) underneath the endothelium. (Magnification ×2400.) **B,** A vessel derived from a juxtamedullary glomerulus in the rat. Note the many profiles of endothelial cells (∗). (Magnification ×1800.) (Adapted from Kriz W, Kaissling B: Structural organization of the mammalian kidney. *In* Seldin DW, Giebisch G (eds): The Kidney: Physiology and Pathophysiology. New York, Raven Press, 1985, p 281.)

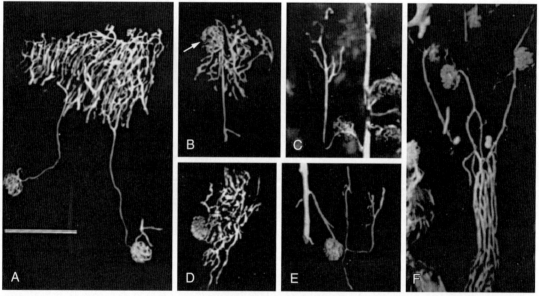

FIGURE 3–9 Photomicrographs of glomeruli and efferent vessels as observed in silicone-injected and cleared canine kidneys. **A and B,** Superficial cortex. Near the kidney surface, many glomeruli have long efferent arterioles that extend to, or nearly to, the surface before dividing **(A)**. Other glomeruli located at the same cortical level are nearly obscured by the surrounding dense peritubular capillary network **(B)**. The glomerulus is indicated by an arrow. **C, D, and E,** Midcortex. In the midcortex, most glomeruli are located near the interlobular arterioles. Although the peritubular capillary network often remains close to its parent glomerulus **(C)**, many midcortical glomeruli have efferent arterioles that extend to perfuse the tubule structures of many nephrons in the medullary ray. Such efferent arterioles are long and simply branched **(D and E)**. **F,** Inner cortex. In the inner, or juxtamedullary cortex, many glomeruli are associated with long efferent arterioles that divide in the outer medulla to form characteristic vascular bundles. Here, the contribution of two such efferent vessels to a vascular bundle is shown. Typically, such bundles are formed from efferent arterioles of 10 or more glomeruli. All panels are shown at approximately the same magnification. Scale bar in A equals 0.5 mm. (Modified from Beeuwkes R: Efferent vascular patterns and early vascular-tubular relations in the dog kidney. Am J Physiol 221:1361, 1971.)

the long vascular bundles of the inner medulla (vasa recta) converge abruptly and join the arcuate veins (see later section on medullary circulation).

Vascular-Tubule Relations

Diagrams of renal vascular and tubule organization in earlier textbooks often showed nephrons that were associated throughout their entire length with the postglomerular network arising from the same glomerulus. However, given the limited spatial extent and local venous drainage of cortical efferent networks, this description is now recognized as incorrect. The development of suitable double-injection techniques permitted vascular-tubule relationships to be defined in detail.[10,35,42,43] In such studies, the blood vessels are injected with a colored silicone rubber. Then, after the tissue is cleared, selected nephrons in all cortical regions are injected with silicone materials of contrasting color. Because only single nephrons are made visible, their relationships to nearby peritubular capillaries can be evaluated. Vascular-tubule relationships on the kidney surface have also been defined by techniques based on conventional micropuncture, and such studies have yielded additional valuable information.[33,44]

Cortical vascular-tubule relations have been described most completely in the canine kidney.[10,35,45] These studies show that, except for convoluted tubule segments in the outermost region of the cortex, the efferent peritubular capillary network and the nephron arising from each glomerulus are dissociated. In addition, even though many superficial proximal and distal convoluted tubules are perfused, at least in part, by pertitubular capillaries arising from the parent glomerulus of the same nephron, the loops of Henle of such nephrons, descending in the medullary ray, are perfused successively by blood emerging from many midcortical glomeruli through efferent arterioles that extend directly into the ray (see Fig. 3–7). The early divisions of such efferent arterioles probably supply only a small region of tubule, because typical networks extend only about 1 mm. Nephrons originating from midcortical glomeruli have proximal and distal convoluted tubule segments lying close to the interlobular axis in the region above the glomerulus of origin. This region is perfused by capillary networks arising from the efferents of more superficial glomeruli (see Fig. 3–7). It is in the inner cortex, however, that this dissociation between individual tubules and the corresponding postglomerular capillary network is most apparent (see Fig. 3–7). The convoluted tubule segments of these nephrons lie above the glomeruli, surrounded either by the dense network close to the interlobular vessels or by capillary networks arising from other inner cortical glomeruli.

In the human kidney, efferent vessel patterns and vascular-tubule relationships are similar to those of the dog.[42,43] Vascular-tubule relationships in the superficial cortex of the rat have also been defined in micropuncture studies. In general, a close association between the initial portions of peritubular capillaries and early and late proximal tubule segments of the same glomerulus has been shown.[34,46,47] However, this close association does not mean that each vessel adjacent to a given tubule necessarily arises from the same glomerulus. In fact, Briggs and Wright[44] have found that, although superficial nephron segments and stellate vessels arising from the same glomerulus are closely associated, each stellate vessel may serve segments of more than one nephron. Thus, of 142 stellate vessels studied, only one third were entirely surrounded by convoluted tubule segments arising from a single nephron.

Peritubular Capillary Dynamics

The same Starling forces that control fluid movement across all capillary beds govern the rate of fluid movement across peritubular capillary walls. Because of a large drop in hydraulic pressure along the efferent arteriole, the oncotic pressure difference across the walls of peritubular capillaries exceeds the hydraulic pressure difference, thereby favoring fluid movement into the capillaries. The absolute amount of movement resulting from this driving force also depends on the peritubular capillary surface area available for fluid uptake and the hydraulic conductivity of the capillary wall. Values for the hydraulic conductivity of the glomerular capillaries far exceed those of all other microvascular beds measured thus far, including the peritubular capillaries. This difference is offset by the much larger total surface area of the peritubular capillary network. For detailed values, the reader is referred to Chapter 7 of the 7th Edition of this book.

The electron microscope shows that the endothelium of the peritubular capillary is fenestrated. In the rat, it has been estimated that approximately 50% of the capillary surface is composed of fenestrated areas.[38] Unlike the glomerular

capillaries, peritubular capillary fenestrations are bridged by a thin diaphragm[38] that is negatively charged.[48] Beneath the fenestrae of the endothelial cells lies a basement membrane that completely surrounds the capillary. Glomerular and peritubular capillaries are distinguished, however, by the absence in the latter of an epithelial structure comparable to the glomerular podocyte. For the most part, peritubular capillaries are closely apposed to cortical tubules so that the extracellular space between the tubules and capillaries constitutes only about 5% of the cortical volume.[49] The tubular epithelial cells are surrounded by the tubular basement membrane, which is distinct from and wider than the capillary basement membrane. Numerous microfibrils connect the tubular and capillary basement membranes.[50] The function of these fibrils is uncertain, but as reviewed elsewhere,[51] they may help limit expansion of the interstitium and maintain close contact between the tubular epithelial cells and peritubular capillaries during periods of high fluid flux. Thus, the pathway for fluid reabsorption from the tubular lumen to the peritubular capillary is composed in series of the epithelial cell, tubular basement membrane, a narrow interstitial region containing microfibrils, the capillary basement membrane, and the thin membrane closing the endothelial fenestrae.[51]

Like the endothelial cells, the basement membrane of the peritubular capillaries possesses anionic sites.[48] The electronegative charge density of the peritubular capillary basement membrane is significantly greater than that observed in the unfenestrated capillaries of skeletal muscle and similar to that observed in the glomerular capillary bed. Although the function of the anionic sites in the peritubular capillaries is uncertain, by analogy to the glomerulus, it is likely that they are an adaptation to compensate for the greater permeability of fenestrated capillaries, allowing free exchange of water and small molecules while restricting anionic plasma proteins to the circulation. In fact, some workers have reported that the renal peritubular capillaries are more permeable to both small and large molecules than are other beds.[52] This conclusion is based on tracer studies in which the renal artery was clamped or the kidney removed before fixation. Because normal plasma flow conditions appear necessary for the maintenance of the glomerular permeability barrier,[53] it is likely that these high stop-flow peritubular permeabilities are also due to the unfavorable experimental conditions employed. Indeed, studies by Deen and associates[54] indicate that, at least under free-flow conditions, the permeability of these vessels to dextrans and albumin is extremely low.

Because the peritubular capillary uptake process is in series with all cellular mechanisms for tubule fluid reabsorption, it is ideally situated to modulate the rate of tubule fluid reabsorption. In fact, even the diameter or total number of functioning peritubular capillaries may be important in the regulation of proximal fluid reabsorption.[55] Typically, however, alterations in peritubular capillary hydraulic pressure or intracapillary oncotic pressure lead to major alterations in proximal tubule reabsorption. During volume expansion, the correlation between physical factors and proximal tubule fluid reabsorption is sufficiently strong that it is possible to model the reabsorptive mechanism as if transcapillary exchange were the only regulatory process involved, implying that peritubular capillary uptake is rate-limiting for reabsorption. However, a number of micropuncture and microperfusion studies indicate that alterations in peritubular capillary oncotic or hydraulic pressure do not always result in parallel changes in proximal tubule fluid transfer.[56] Furthermore, significant changes in proximal reabsorption may occur in the absence of detectable variations in Starling forces (i.e., direct inhibition of ion pumps in epithelia).

In actuality, the interaction between blood vessel and tubule is undoubtedly quite complex. Ott and colleagues[57] determined that the state of hydration affected the ability of peritubular capillary oncotic pressure to alter proximal reabsorption. They found that increasing oncotic pressure increased proximal reabsorption in volume-expanded animals but not in hydropenic animals. This finding is consistent with a model of proximal tubule function that envisions the magnitude of back-leakage, into the tubule lumen, of fluid originally transported into the intercellular spaces as an important factor in the control of net proximal reabsorption.[58] During volume expansion, decreasing capillary uptake leads to increased hydraulic pressure in the interstitial space between the tubules and the peritubular capillaries. Increased renal interstitial pressure would, in turn, reduce fluid flux out of the lateral intercellular spaces. In contrast, during hydropenia, transport of solute into the lateral intercellular spaces might be reduced to the point at which changes in oncotic pressure would have little effect on proximal reabsorption. In fact, a variety of studies support an association between renal interstitial pressure and Na excretion,[59] although some investigators have suggested that the augmenting effect of increased interstitial pressure on Na excretion depends on sites distal to the proximal tubule. Haas and colleagues[60] reported that only proximal tubules of deep nephrons were sensitive to changes in renal perfusion pressure, suggesting that these nephrons may be more responsive to changes in interstitial pressure.

More recently, Granger and co-workers[61] suggested that alterations in cortical interstitial pressure may be a major determinant of capillary uptake in settings where the oncotic pressure gradient across the capillary wall is absent or low. This occurs experimentally in isolated kidneys perfused with colloid-free solutions[62] or when interstitial pressure is artificially reduced by exposing the kidney to subatmospheric pressure,[63] and in vivo in older animals in which interstitial protein concentration and oncotic pressures approach plasma levels.[64] In these settings, peritubular capillary uptake of fluid persists despite the absence of a significant oncotic pressure gradient. Evidence suggests[61] that the interstitial hydrostatic pressure rises in this setting, possibly as a result of ongoing transport of solute into the peritubular interstitium, which has limited ability to expand due to the presence of the microfilaments described above that bridge that space. Increased interstitial pressure creates a favorable hydrostatic pressure gradient for fluid movement into the capillary, which also does not collapse due to the same cytoskeletal support system.

Because the peritubular capillaries that surround a given nephron are derived from many efferent vessels, regulatory processes related to capillary factors need not be viewed as a mechanism only for balancing filtration and reabsorption in a single nephron. Instead, assuming that capillary dynamics throughout the cortex are the same as has thus far been defined for the microcirculation of the superficial cortex, we may consider that, within broad regions of the cortex, all tubule segments are surrounded by capillary vessels that are operating in a similar reabsorptive mode. Thus, the function of the cortex as a whole may reflect the average reabsorptive capacity of all cortical peritubular vessels. This is obviously a first approximation. For further discussion of the factors that regulate proximal tubule fluid reabsorption, the reader is referred to Chapter 5.

Medullary Microcirculation

Vascular Patterns

The precise location of the boundary between the renal cortex and medulla is difficult to discern because the medullary rays of the cortex merge imperceptibly with the medulla. In general, the sites at which the interlobular arteries branch into arcuate arteries, or the arcuate arteries themselves, mark this boundary. When considering the medullary circulation,

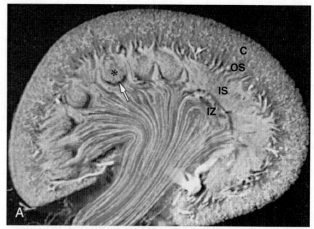
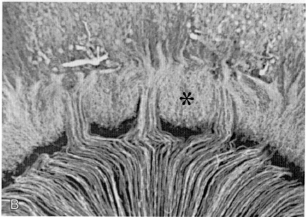

FIGURE 3–10 Longitudinal section of kidney of the sand rat (Psammomys obesus) after arterial injection of Microfil silicone rubber and clearing. **A,** The low-power magnification reveals distinct zonation of the kidney (c, cortex; OS and IS, outer and inner stripes of the outer medulla, respectively; IZ, inner medulla). The inner medulla is long and extends a short distance below the bottom of the picture. Giant vascular bundles, including a mixture of descending and ascending vasa recta, traverse the outer medulla to supply blood to the inner medulla. **B,** The outer medulla at a higher magnification. Between the vascular bundles (three are visible), a rich capillary plexus (asterisk) supplies the tubule segments present in this zone. (From Bankir L, Kaissling B, de Rouffignac C, Kriz W: The vascular organization of the kidney of Psammomys obesus. Anat Embryol 155:149, 1979.)

most focus on its relation to the countercurrent mechanism as facilitated by the parallel array of descending and ascending vasa recta. However, although this configuration is characteristic of the inner medulla, the medulla also contains an outer zone, which contains two morphologically distinct regions, the outer and inner stripes (Figs. 3–10 and 3–11). The boundary between the outer and inner medullary zones is defined by the beginning of the thick ascending limbs of Henle.[65] In addition to the thick ascending limbs, the outer medulla contains descending straight segments of proximal tubules (pars recta), descending thin limbs, and collecting ducts (see Fig. 3–11). The inner stripe of the outer medulla is the region in which thick ascending limbs overlap with thin descending limbs. Each of these morphologically distinct medullary regions is supplied and drained by an independent, specific vascular system.

The blood supply of the medulla is entirely derived from the efferent arterioles of the juxtamedullary glomeruli.[8,14,35,66] Infrequent aglomerular vessels mark sites where corresponding glomeruli have degenerated.[67] Depending on the species and the method of evaluation, it has been estimated that from 7% to 18% of glomeruli give rise to efferents that ultimately supply the medulla.[66,68] As already discussed, efferent

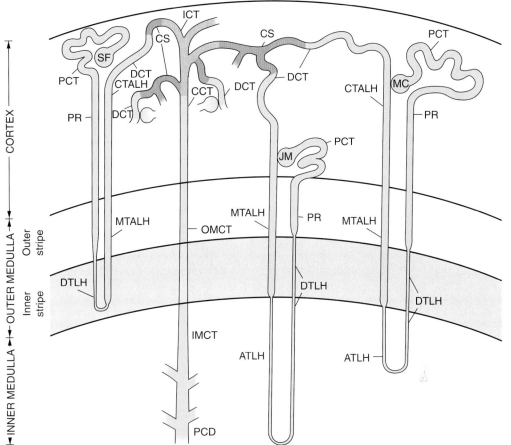

FIGURE 3–11 Three populations of nephrons based on location of their glomeruli are depicted schematically: superficial (SF), midcortical (MC), and juxtamedullary (JM) nephrons. The major nephron segments are labeled as follows: ATLH, ascending thin limb of Henle; CCT, cortical collecting tubule; CS, connecting segment; CTALH, cortical thick ascending limb of Henle; DCT, distal convoluted tubule; DTLH, descending thin limb of Henle; ICT, initial collecting tubule; IMCT, inner medullary collecting tubule; MTALH, medullary thick ascending limb of Henle; OMCT, outer medullary collecting tubule; PCD, papillary collecting duct; PCT, proximal convoluted tubule; PR, pars recta. Transport characteristics of these segments are discussed in the text. (From Jacobson HR: Functional segmentation of the mammalian nephron. Am J Physiol 241:F203, 1981.)

arterioles of juxtamedullary nephrons are larger in diameter and possess a thicker endothelium and more prominent smooth muscle layer than arterioles originating from superficial glomeruli.[39–41] In the rat, cat, and dog, afferent arterioles supplying juxtamedullary glomeruli also differ and are distinguished by the presence, at their origins from the interlobular arteries, of intra-arterial "cushions," smooth muscle cell–like structures that protrude into the lumen of the vessel.[69] These structures are not found in a variety of other mammalian species, including humans.[8] Although their function is unknown, these cushions are ideally located to regulate blood flow to the deeper medullary structures.

Although the vasculature of the outer medulla displays both vertical and lateral heterogeneity, in general, both the outer and inner stripes contain two distinct circulatory regions. These are the vascular bundles, formed by the coalescence of the descending and ascending vasa recta, and the interbundle capillary plexus. The descending vasa recta arise from the efferent arterioles and descend through the outer stripe of the outer medulla to supply the inner stripe of the outer medulla and the inner medulla (see Fig. 3–10). Within the outer stripe, the descending vasa recta also give rise, via small side branches, to a complex capillary plexus. Early studies suggested that this capillary network was limited and, therefore, not the main blood supply to this region. Instead, it was thought that nutrient flow was provided by the ascending vasa recta rising from the inner medulla and the inner stripe. This was further suggested by the large area of contact between ascending vasa recta and the descending proximal straight tubules within this zone (Fig. 3–12).[38,68,70] Using resin casting and scanning electron microscopy, Yamamoto and co-workers[71] visualized a dense capillary network perfusing the entire outer medulla.

Within the inner stripe, the two vascular regions are even more easily identified (see Figs. 3–11 and 3–13). The exact organization of the ascending and descending vasa recta within the vascular bundles displays significant interspecies variation (discussed later). The interbundle region contains the tubules, including the metabolically active thick ascending limbs. Nutrient and O_2 supply to this energy-demanding tissue is by a dense capillary plexus arising from a few descending vasa recta at the periphery of the bundles. Approximately 10% to 15% of total renal blood flow is directed to the medulla, and of this probably the largest portion perfuses this inner stripe capillary plexus. Ultrastructurally, medullary capillaries resemble their counterparts within the cortex and consist of a flattened endothelium encased in a thin basal lamina. Fenestrations, which are bridged by a thin diaphragm, are regularly and densely distributed throughout the non-nuclear regions of the endothelial cells.[41]

The rich capillary network of the inner stripe drains into numerous veins, which, for the most part, do not join the vascular bundles but ascend directly to the outer stripe. These veins subsequently rise to the cortical-medullary junction as wide, wavy channels and the majority joins with cortical veins at the level of the inner cortex. A minority of the wavy veins may extend within the medullary rays to regions near the kidney surface.[8,10] Thus, the capillary network of the inner stripe makes no contact with the vessels draining the inner medulla.

The inner medulla contains thin descending and thin ascending limbs of Henle, together with collecting ducts (see Fig. 3–11). Within this region, the straight, unbranching vasa recta descend in bundles, with individual vessels leaving at every level to divide into a simple capillary network

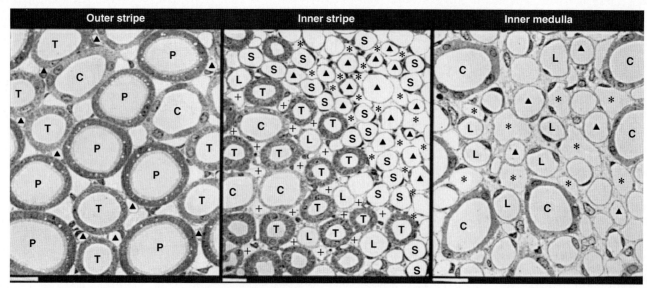

Outer stripe	Inner stripe	Inner medulla

FIGURE 3–12 Electron micrograph showing cross sections of both outer stripe and inner stripe of outer medulla and a cross section of inner medulla. C, collecting duct; P, pars recta; S and L, thin descending limbs of short and long loops, respectively; T, thick ascending limb. Triangles indicate arterial descending vasa recta; asterisks indicate venous ascending vasa recta. In the outer stripe, note the large area of contact between ascending vasa recta and pars recta and the paucity of interstitial space. In the inner stripe, part of a vascular bundle is shown in the upper right half of the photograph, and the interbundle region is shown in the lower half. Note that the thin descending limbs of short loops are surrounded by venous vasa recta ascending from the inner medulla. The wall of these vessels adapts to available space between the descending vasa recta and the thin limbs, offering a large area of contact with these descending structures. Thin limbs of long loops lie in the interbundle region and are surrounded by vessels belonging to the interbundle capillary plexus. In the inner medulla, note abundant interstitium surrounding all tubule and vascular structures. Walls of tubules and vessels are not in direct contact. (Outer stripe is from rabbit kidney; inner stripe and inner medulla are from rat kidney.) Bar is approximately 30 (μm). (Adapted from Bankir L, de Rouffignac C: Urinary concentration ability: Insights derived from comparative anatomy. Am J Physiol 249:R643, 1985.)

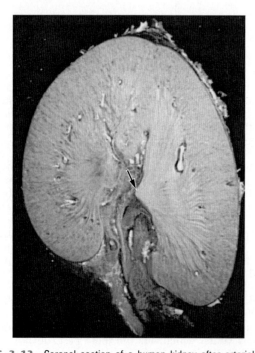

FIGURE 3–13 Coronal section of a human kidney after arterial silicone injection and clearing. Complete injection of the renal vascular system enables the intense vascularity of the organ to be visualized. Although the renal papilla (arrow) has often been considered to be relatively poorly vascularized, this injection study shows that capillary density of the papilla is at least as great as that found in the cortex. (Actual size.)

characterized by elongated links.[68] These capillaries converge to form the venous vasa recta. Within the inner medulla the descending and ascending vascular pathways remain in close apposition, although distinct vascular regions can no longer be clearly discerned. The venous vasa recta rise toward the outer medulla in parallel with the supply vessels to join the vascular bundles. Thus, the outer medullary vascular bundles include both supplying and draining vessels of the inner medulla.[40] Within the outer stripe of the outer medulla, the vascular bundles spread out and traverse the outer stripe as wide, tortuous channels that lie in close apposition to the tubules, eventually emptying into arcuate or deep intertubular veins.[68] The venous pathways within the bundles are both larger and more numerous than the arterial vessels, suggesting lower flow velocities in the ascending (venous) than in the descending (arterial) direction.[72,73] The importance of the close apposition of the arterial and venous pathways within the vascular bundles for maintaining the hypertonicity of the inner medulla is discussed in Chapter 9.

The number of inner medullary vessels is large; studies show that the capillary volume fraction of the inner medulla is nearly twice that of the cortex.[9,74] However, because of the long lengths and narrow diameters of these vessels, they can be filled by arterial injection only with great difficulty. If an injection is continued long enough, the intense vascularity of the inner medulla becomes apparent, as shown in Figure 3–14.

Morphologists have recognized important differences in the structure of the ascending and descending vasa recta. The descending vasa recta possess a contractile layer composed of smooth muscle cells in the early segments that evolve into pericytes by the more distal portions of the vessels. Immunohistochemical studies demonstrate that these pericytes contain smooth muscle alpha-actin, suggesting that they may serve as contractile elements and participate in the regulation of medullary blood flow.[75] These vessels also display a continuous endothelium that persists until the hairpin turn is reached and the vessels divide to form the medullary capillaries. In contrast, ascending vasa recta, like true capillaries, lack a contractile layer and are characterized by a highly fenestrated endothelium.[76,77] Although the precise functional role of these anatomic differences is not known, it is of interest that essentially identical morphologic patterns are found in the rete mirabile of the swim bladder of fishes, a structure

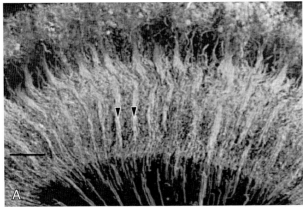

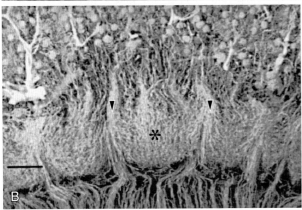

FIGURE 3–14 Sagittal section of rat (**A**) and Mongolian gerbil (Meriones shawii) (**B**) kidneys after arterial injection with Microfil silicone rubber, showing deep cortex, outer and inner stripes of the outer medulla, and early inner medulla (from top to bottom of each micrograph, respectively). In the inner stripe, vascular bundles (arrowheads) alternate with interbundle capillary plexuses (asterisk). The functional separation between the two adjacent compartments is present in both species but is amplified in the desert-adapted Mongolian gerbil. Bar=600 (µm) (A) and 350 (µm) (B). (From Bankir L, Bouby N, Trinh-Trang-Tan MM: Organization of the medullary circulation: Functional implications. *In* Robinson RR (ed): Nephrology: Proceedings of the IXth International Congress of Nephrology. New York, Springer-Verlag, 1984, pp 84–106.)

that serves a countercurrent exchange function (gas exchange) quite independent of urine concentration.[78,79]

Vascular-Tubule Relations

The mechanism of urine concentration requires coordinated function of the vascular and tubule components of the medulla (see Chapter 9). In species capable of marked concentrating ability, medullary vascular-tubule relations show a high degree of organization with at least three functionally distinct compartments, each favoring particular exchange processes by the juxtaposition of specific tubule segments and blood vessels. In addition to anatomic proximity, the absolute magnitude of these exchanges is greatly influenced by the permeability characteristics of the structures involved, which may vary significantly among species.[80] For a further discussion of the anatomic relations and permeability characteristics of various medullary structures as they relate to mechanisms of urine concentration, the reader is referred to Chapter 9.

Most of our detailed knowledge of vascular-tubule relations within the medulla is based on histologic studies of rodent s pecies.[14,40,41,70,71,75,81] In the inner medulla, descending and ascending vasa recta are interspersed with thin limbs of the loops of Henle in a homogeneous and apparently random manner (see Fig. 3–12). Although the relative number of these structures varies considerably among species, this overall

organization of the inner medulla is well conserved. As already discussed, the inner stripe of the outer medulla contains two distinct territories, the vascular bundles and the interbundle regions (see Figs. 3–10, 3–12, and 3–14). In most mammals, the vascular bundles contain only closely juxtaposed descending and ascending vasa recta running in parallel. The tubule structures of the inner stripe, including thin descending limbs, thick ascending limbs, and collecting ducts, are found in the interbundle regions and are supplied by the dense capillary bed described earlier.[40] Commonly, the interbundle territory is organized with the long loops of the juxtamedullary nephrons lying closest to the vascular bundles. The shorter loops arising from superficial glomeruli are more peripheral and, therefore, closer to the collecting ducts. The vascular bundles themselves contain no tubule structures.

Medullary Capillary Dynamics

The functional role of the medullary peritubular vasculature is basically the same as that of cortical peritubular vessels. These capillaries supply the metabolic needs of the tissues near them and are responsible for the uptake and removal of water extracted from collecting ducts during the process of urine concentration. However, because the concentration process is based on the maintenance of a hypertonic interstitium, medullary blood flow must not only avoid washing out the solute gradient but also assist in its formation. These processes are discussed in detail in Chapter 9.

TOTAL RENAL BLOOD FLOW

Total renal blood flow in humans typically exceeds 20% of the cardiac output. For detailed discussion of methods of measurements, the reader is referred to Chapter 7 of the previous, 7th Edition of this book. Renal blood flow in women is slightly lower than in men, even when normalized to body surface area. Early clearance measurements by Smith[82] revealed that renal blood flow in women averaged 982 ± 184 (SD) mL/minute/1.73 m^2 of body surface area. The wide range of normal in these subjects is illustrated by 95% confidence intervals encompassing a range between 614 and 1350 mL/minute/1.73 m^2. In men, Smith found that normalized renal blood flow averaged 1209 ± 256 (SD) mL/minute/1.73 m^2. Later studies using other methods have consistently yielded measurements with similar means and wide ranges.[82] Amith found renal plasma flow averaged 592 ± 153 mL/minute/1.73 m^2 in women and 654 ± 163 mL/minute/1.73 m^2 in men.[83] In children between 6 months and 1 year of age, normalized renal plasma flow is approximately half that of adults, but it increases progressively and reaches the adult level at about 3 years of age.[84] After age 30, renal blood flow decreases progressively with age; at 90 years it is about half that at 20 years.[85]

INTRARENAL BLOOD FLOW DISTRIBUTION

Cortical Blood Flow

It has long been recognized that the perfusion rate in different regions of the kidney is not uniform, especially after trauma or hemorrhage.[86] Experimentally, the existence of several compartments having different flow rates has been recognized from the dispersion of transit times and uptake rates of injected indicators and the presence of multiple components in the washout curves of radioactive tracers. Accordingly, there has been much interest in determining whether differences in flow rate are associated with definable anatomic regions and whether correlations exist between renal blood flow distribution and renal function. Because the regions of interest lie within the interior of the organ, considerable experimental ingenuity has been required, and no single technique for estimating regional flow has yet become generally accepted. Furthermore, because of differences in observations made with different methods and under different experimental conditions, results have often been difficult to interpret. To date, no clear correlation between intrarenal blood flow distribution and renal function has been established. For a detailed discussion of methods of measurements, the reader is referred to Chapter 7 of the 7th Edition of this book.

Redistribution of Cortical Blood Flow

The redistribution of renal cortical blood flow has been extensively investigated using numerous different animal models. Studies of renal blood flow distribution after hemorrhage were among the first performed. They were provoked by the report of Trueta and colleagues[11]that, in shock states, renal blood flow appeared to be shunted through the medulla. This phenomenon, observed in qualitative studies of the distribution of India ink and radiographic contrast media, was subsequently termed "cortical ischemia with maintained blood flow through the medulla."[87] Trueta's observations suggested a medullary bypass or shunt during hemorrhage or shock, including the rapid appearance of arterially injected contrast medium in the renal vein during systemic hypotension and the visible pallor of the superficial cortex at a time when radiographs showed considerable amounts of contrast medium in the outer medullary area.[11] Although 60 years have passed since Trueta's original proposal, only the qualitative observation of relative outer cortical ischemia with hemorrhage is accepted; neither the quantitative magnitude nor the mechanism of the flow redistribution associated with hemorrhage has been established.

Medullary Blood Flow

Medullary blood flow constitutes about 10% to 15% of total renal blood flow.[86] For detailed methods of measurements, the reader is again referred to the 7th Edition of this book. In terms of flow per unit tissue mass, estimates of outer medullary flow range from 1.3 to 2.3 mL/minute/g of kidney, inner medullary flow between 0.23 and 0.7 mL/minute/g, and papillary flow between 0.22 and 0.42 mL/minute/g. Although these medullary flows are less than one fourth as high as cortical flows, medullary flow is still substantial. Thus, per gram of tissue, outer medullary flow exceeds that of liver, and inner medullary flow is comparable to that of resting muscle or brain.[83] The fact that such large flows are compatible with the existence and maintenance of the inner medullary solute concentration gradient attests to the efficiency of countercurrent mechanisms in this region. Besides, the hematocrit in the vasa recta is approximately one half that of arterial blood.[88] Autoregulatory ability has been observed[89] and is discussed in more detail later. Medullary blood flow is highest under conditions of water diuresis and declines during antidiuresis.[90] This decrease depends, at least in part, on a direct vasoconstrictive action of vasopressin on the medullary microcirculation.[91] Acetylcholine,[92] Lameire,[88] vasodilator prostaglandins,[93,94] kinins,[95] adenosine,[96,97] atrial peptides,[98,99] and nitric oxide[100] may increase, and angiotensin II,[101] vasopressin,[91,102] endothelin,[103] and increased renal nerve activity[104] may decrease, medullary flow. The role of these hormones in normal physiology is still uncertain; however, alterations in medullary blood flow may be a key determinant of medullary tonicity and, thereby, solute transport in the loops of Henle. In addition, and reviewed by Mattson,[105]

the medullary circulation may play an important role in the control of sodium excretion and blood pressure.

∎ REGULATION OF RENAL CIRCULATION AND GLOMERULAR FILTRATION

Vasomotor Properties of the Renal Microcirculations

Whether mediated by neural, humoral, or intrarenal physical factors, the regulation of the renal circulation ultimately depends on resistance changes resulting from the constriction or relaxation of vascular smooth muscle. The vessels up to and including the interlobular arteries contain smooth muscle in many layers, enclosed within elastic intimal and advential sheaths. Afferent arterioles contain less smooth muscle—only one or two layers—and lack intimal and adventitial laminae.[40] Near the glomerular pole, smooth muscle cells around the entire circumference of the arteriole are modified to form the granular cells of the juxtaglomerular apparatus.[106,107] The hydraulic pressure within glomerular capillaries depends on afferent and efferent arteriolar resistances, increasing with selective efferent constriction or afferent dilation. Flow within the glomerular capillaries, on the other hand, is reduced by an increase in resistance of either vessel. As early as 1924, Richards and Schmidt[22] recognized the potential role of contractile elements in the control of glomerular capillary flow and pressure.

Functional proof of afferent and efferent vascular reactivity has come from micropuncture studies of glomerular dynamics. Click and colleagues[108] grafted renal tissue from neonatal hamsters into the cheek pouch of adult hamsters. Such grafts developed primitive glomerular circulations with visible afferent and efferent vessels. Local application of norepinephrine or angiotensin II by means of micropipettes resulted in clearly visible constriction of both vessel types. Afferent vessels responded more strongly to norepinephrine, whereas efferent vessels were more sensitive to angiotensin II.[108] This technique has also been used to demonstrate the presence of myogenic responses to alterations in extravascular pressure in afferent arterioles whereas efferent arterioles responded passively to changes in applied pressure.[109]

Steinhausen and co-workers[110] applied epi- and transillumination microscopic techniques to the split, hydronephrotic rat kidney. At 6 to 8 weeks after unilateral ureteral ligation, the tubule system had undergone atrophy; however, the vascular system remained relatively intact. The kidney was split at its large curvature, immobilized, and placed in a tissue bath. This preparation permits the arcuate artery, interlobular artery, afferent arteriole, and efferent arteriole to be visualized and studied in situ during perfusion with systemic blood. Changes in the diameter of these vessels have been measured in response to systemically or locally applied vasoactive substance. The effect of acute, intravenous infusion of angiotensin II on the pre- and postglomerular circulation was assessed. The diameter of the large, preglomerular vessels decreased in a dose-dependent fashion, with the interlobular artery displaying the greatest percent reduction. Significant but less constriction was observed in efferent arterioles. Studies in which perfusion pressure was held constant indicated that preglomerular constriction resulted primarily from receptor-mediated effects of angiotensin II on these vessels. When angiotensin II was infused chronically, an attenuated vascular response was observed. In other studies using this technique, dilation of the preglomerular vasculature has been observed during infusion of low doses of dopamine[111] and after administration of a Ca^{2+} channel blocker.[112,113] Atrial peptide infused intravenously dilated the preglomerular vessels but caused postglomerular vasoconstriction.[104] Subsequently, Gabriels and co-workers[114] examined the effects of diadenosine phosphates, which bind to A_1 and P_2 purinoceptors, on afferent and efferent vessels using this technique. These agents induced transient constrictions that were more prominent in intralobular arteries and afferent arterioles than in efferent arterioles.

Loutzenhiser and co-workers[112,113,115] employed a modification of the hydronephrotic kidney technique in which the kidney is mounted and perfused in vitro to examine the response of the afferent arteriole to various stimuli. They[112] found that low concentrations of adenosine produced a vasodilation in afferent arterioles that had been previously constricted by exposure to pressure. They[115] also observed complex responses to prostaglandin E_2 in this preparation, which elicited both vasodilator and vasoconstrictor responses in the afferent arteriole via different receptors. More recently, Loutzenhiser and co-workers[113] examined the kinetic aspects of the myogenic response in afferent arterioles by examining pressure-dependent vasoconstriction and vasodilation in this model. They found that high systolic pressures elicited a contractile response even when mean arterial pressure was reduced. These data suggest that the main role of the afferent

arteriolar constriction is to protect the glomerular capillary bed from increases in pulse pressure, rather than autoregulation per se.

In vitro perfusion of rat kidney has also been utilized to assess segmental vascular reactivity directly in the juxtamedullary nephrons that lie in apposition to the pelvic cavity.[116] To expose these nephrons, the perfused kidney is removed and bisected along its longitudinal axis. The intact papilla, left on one half of the kidney, is lifted back, exposing the pelvic mucosa, which is then removed to reveal the underlying vessels. Applying epifluorescence videomicroscopy to these structures, the inside diameters of the various renal vascular segments can be determined.[116] The effects of angiotensin II on segmental diameters as measured by this technique are shown in Figure 3–15 (*Top*). Angiotensin II reversibly decreased the diameters of both pre- and postglomerular vessels. The estimated effects of the alterations in vessel caliber on segmental resistance are summarized in Figure 3–15 (*Bottom*). This analysis suggests that despite the large changes in arcuate and interlobular artery diameter, the majority of the increase in resistance occurs near the glomerulus. This is due to the fact that equivalent changes in

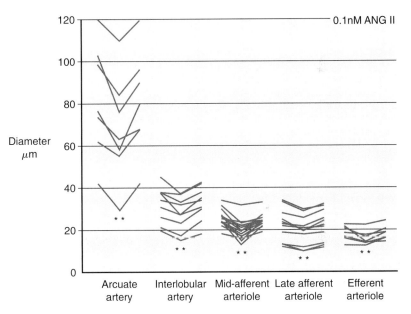

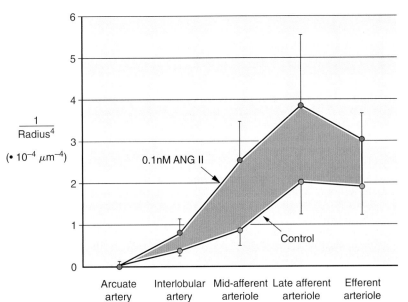

FIGURE 3–15 Effect of angiotensin II on the blood-perfused juxtamedullary nephron microvasculature. Top, Vessel inside-diameter responses to angiotensin II (AII). Each line denotes observations of a single vessel segment during control, angiotensin II, and recovery periods. Bottom, Estimation of angiotensin II–induced changes in segmental vascular resistance, calculated from data in upper panel. **P<.01. (From Navar LG, Gilmore JP, Joyner WL, et al: Direct assessment of renal microcirculatory dynamics. Fed Proc 45:2851, 1986.)

diameter elicit greater effects on resistance in smaller than in larger vessels.[117]

In fact, the exact anatomic distribution of preglomerular vascular resistance has been a matter of debate. Initially, it was assumed that resistance at the level of the afferent arteriole was responsible for the entire pressure drop from the aorta to the glomerular capillaries. However, subsequent data obtained using a variety of other techniques suggests that this is not correct. Interlobular arteries respond to changes in perfusion pressure[118] and to a broad spectrum of vasoactive substances in vivo[110,111] and in vitro.[119–122] Examination of vascular casts suggests that even interlobar arteries may be involved.[123] Direct measurements of interlobular artery pressure indicate that the afferent arteriole accounts for approximately 50% of preglomerular vascular resistance.[124] In fact, hydraulic pressure has been observed to decline in a continuous manner from the arcuate artery to the distal afferent arteriole in the split hydronephrotic kidney preparation,[125] which allows visualization and direct puncture of the entire renal vascular tree. These data are also consistent with findings in other vascular beds.[126]

Edwards developed an in vitro technique to study the reactivity of isolated segments of interlobular arteries and superficial afferent and efferent arterioles dissected from rabbit kidneys.[119] All three types of vessels responded with a dose-dependent decrease in luminal diameter when norepinephrine was added to the system. In contrast, only efferent arteriolar segments showed a similar dose-dependent vasoconstriction in response to angiotensin II. The reasons for the differences between the sites of action of angiotensin II shown by this technique and those shown by the techniques described earlier are uncertain. The isolated vessel technique has also been utilized to assess the renal vascular reactivity to a variety of vasodilator substances.[120,121] As shown in Figure 3–16, dopamine, acetylcholine, and prostaglandins E_2 and I_2 (prostacyclin) all dilate the afferent arteriole of the rabbit, whereas bradykinin, adenosine, and prostaglandins D_2 and $F_{2\alpha}$ do not. The efferent arteriole dilated in response not only to dopamine, acetylcholine, and prostacyclin but also to bradykinin and adenosine. Prostaglandins E_2, D_2, and $F_{2\alpha}$ had no effect on this vessel.

Ito and colleagues[127] developed an in vitro approach to study changes in preglomerular resistance using the isolated perfused afferent arteriole with its glomerulus attached. Angiotensin II and endothelin produce afferent arteriolar constriction in this preparation that is modulated by nitric oxide.[128] The afferent arteriolar response to angiotensin II was also enhanced when the NaCl concentration at the macula densa was raised.[129] In contrast to angiotensin II, Ren and co-workers[101] found that angiotensin 1–7 induced dilation in afferent arterioles that was not mediated by either angiotensin II AT_1 or AT_2 receptors.

Numerous studies indicate that preglomerular vessels including the arcuate artery, interlobular artery, and afferent arteriole do constrict in response to exogenous and endogenous AII.[127,130–134] The efferent arteriole, however, has a 10-fold to 100-fold greater sensitivity to AII.[130,131,133] The vasoconstrictor effects of AII are blunted by the endogenous production of vasodilators including the endothelium-derived relaxing factor nitric oxide as well as cyclooxygenase and cytochrome P450 epoxygenase metabolites in the afferent but not the efferent arteriole.[115,127,130,135–138] AII-simulated release of NO in the afferent arteriole occurs through activation of the AT_1 receptors.[139] AII increases the production of prostaglandins in afferent arteriolar smooth muscle cells (both PGE_2 and PGI_2) and PGE_2, PGI_2, and cAMP all blunt AII-induced calcium entry into these cells[138] potentially explaining, at least in part, the different effects of AII on vasoconstriction of the afferent and efferent arteriole.[137,138] PGE_2 was without effect on AII-induced vasoconstriction of the efferent

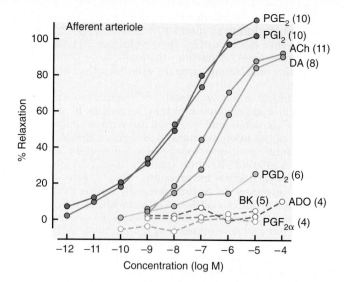

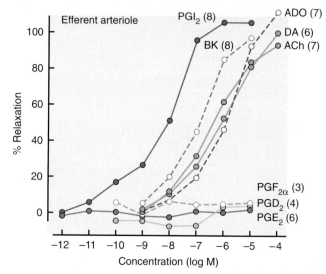

FIGURE 3–16 Relaxation response of afferent (top) and efferent (bottom) arterioles to acetylcholine (ACh), dopamine (DA), bradykinin (BK), adenosine (ADO), and prostaglandins (PGE_2, PGI_2, PGD_2, and $PGF_{2\alpha}$). Tone was induced with 3×10^7 M norepinephrine. Numbers in parentheses represent numbers of arterioles. (From Navar LG, Gilmore JP, Joyner WL, et al: Direct assessment of renal microcirculatory dynamics. Fed Proc 45:2851, 1986.)

arteriole.[115] The effects of PGE_2 on AII-induced vasoconstriction of the afferent arteriole are concentration-dependent with low concentrations acting as a vasodilator via interaction with prostaglandin EP_4 receptors whereas high concentrations of PGE_2 act on prostaglandin EP_3 receptors to restore the AII effects in that segment.[115] While AII infusion alone has little effect on single nephron glomerular filtration rate (SNGFR) when combined with cyclooxygenase inhibition AII causes marked reductions in SNGFR as well as glomerular plasma flow rate (Q_A) suggesting an important role for endogenous vasodilatory prostaglandins in ameliorating the vasoconstrictor effects of AII.[140] Because AII increases renal production of vasodilatory prostaglandin production this may serve as a feedback loop to modulate the vasoconstrictor effects on AII under chronic conditions when the renin angiotensin system is stimulated.[18]

In addition to causing renal vasoconstriction, reduced blood flow, and glomerular capillary hypertension, AII causes a decrease in the glomerular ultrafiltration coefficient (K_f).[18,140,141] As discussed later in "Determinants of Glomerular Ultrafiltration" K_f is the product of the surface area available for filtration (S) and hydraulic conductivity of the filtration barrier (k) and is one of the primary determinants of SNGFR. A decrease in K_f induced by AII could be the result of either a decrease in S or k. As noted earlier, glomerular AII receptors are found on the mesangial cells, glomerular capillary endothelial cells, and podocytes. Because AII causes contraction of mesangial cells[142] one possibility is that contraction of the mesangial cells reduces effective filtration area by blocking flow through some glomerular capillaries but no direct evidence has been obtained that would support this hypothesis. Alternatively the AII-induced decrease in K_f could be the result of a decrease in hydraulic conductivity rather than a reduction in the surface area available for filtration.[141] A role for glomerular epithelial cells in the effects of AII on K_f is suggested by the fact that they possess both AT_1 and AT_2 receptors and respond to AII by increasing cAMP production.[143] Alterations in epithelial structure or the size of the filtration slits were not detected, however, following infusion of AII at a dose sufficient to decrease glomerular filtration rate (GFR) and K_f and increase blood pressure[144] and the mechanisms by which AII causes a reduction in K_f have not yet been determined.

Just as the renal vascular effects of AII are moderated by production of vasodilator prostaglandins and nitric oxide, AII-induced changes in K_f are also be affected by such substances. Endogenous prostaglandins help to prevent the reduction in K_f caused by AII.[140] The vasoconstrictive effect of AII on glomerular mesangial cells is markedly reduced by endothelial derived relaxing factor (EDRF, now known to be nitric oxide, NO—see later).[145] Mesangial cells co-incubated with endothelial cells have increased cGMP production induced by NO release from the endothelial cells resulting in decreased vasoconstrictive effects of AII, indicating that local NO production can modify the effects of agents such as AII.[145] Whether a similar effect would be observed for glomerular epithelial cells co-incubated with endothelial cells and whether either would translate into protection from AII-induced alterations on glomerular capillary surface area or hydraulic conductivity is not known but inhibition of NO production in the normal rat does produce a marked decrease in K_f.[145–147]

Arima and co-workers[148] examined angiotensin II AT_2 receptor–mediated effects on afferent arteriolar tone. When the AT_1 receptor was blocked, angiotension II caused a dose-dependent dilation of the afferent arteriole that could be blocked by disruption of the endothelium or by simultaneous inhibition of the cytochrome P-450 pathway. These data suggest that AT_2 receptor vasodilation in efferent arterioles is endothelium-dependent, possibly via the synthesis of epoxyeicosatrienoic acids via a cytochrome P450 pathway, partially blocking the vasoconstrictor effects of AII.[148,149]

Role of Endothelial Factors in the Control of Renal Circulation and Glomerular Filtration

Endothelial cells were once considered to be simple cells that passively lined the vascular tree. We now recognize that these cells produce a number of substances that can profoundly alter vascular tone, including vasodilator substances such as prostacyclin and the endothelium-derived relaxing factor, NO, as well as vasoconstrictor substances such as the endothelins. These factors play an important role in the minute-to-minute regulation of renal vascular flow and resistance.

Nitric Oxide

In 1980, Furchgott and Zawadzki[150] demonstrated that the action of the vasodilator acetylcholine required the presence of an intact endothelium to be vasorelaxant. The binding of

acetylcholine and many other vasodilator substances to receptors on endothelial cells leads to the formation and release of an endothelial relaxing factor subsequently determined to be NO.[151,152] NO is formed from L-arginine[153] by a family of enzymes that are encoded by separate genes called nitric oxide synthases (NOSs) that are present in many cells, including vascular endothelial cells, macrophages, neurons,[154] glomerular mesangial cells,[155] macula densa,[156] and renal tubular cells. Once released by the endothelium, NO diffuses into adjacent and downstream vascular smooth muscle cells,[157] where it activates soluble guanylate cyclase leading to cyclic guanosine monophosphate (cGMP) accumulation.[145,158–162] Cyclic GMP reduces phosphatidyl inositol hydrolysis and calcium influx and intracellular calcium release, thereby reducing the amount of calcium available for contraction hence promoting relaxation.[163] In addition to stimulation by acetylcholine, NO formation in the vascular endothelium increases in response to bradykinin,[145,164–167] thrombin,[168] platelet activating factor,[169] endothelin,[170] and calcitonin gene-related peptide.[165,171–173] Increased flow through blood vessels with intact endothelium or across cultured endothelial cells resulting in increased shear stress, also increases NO release[159,164,167,174–178] and elevated perfusion pressure/shear stress increased NO release from afferent arterioles.[179] Both pulse frequency and amplitude modulate flow-induced NO release.[174]

In the kidney nitric oxide (NO) has numerous important functions including the regulation of renal hemodynamics, maintenance of medullary perfusion, mediation of pressure-natriuresis, blunting of tubuloglomerular feedback, inhibition of tubular sodium reabsorption, and modulation of renal sympathetic neural activity. The net effect of NO in the kidney is to promote natriuresis and diuresis.[180] Experimental studies also support the presence of an important interaction between NO, angiotensin II, and renal nerves in the control of renal function.[181] Renal hemodynamics are continuously affected by endogenous NO production as evidenced by the fact that nonselective NOS inhibition results in marked decreases in renal plasma flow rate (RPF), an increase in mean arterial blood pressure (AP), and generally a reduction in GFR.[182–184] These effects are largely prevented by the simultaneous administration of excess L arginine.[182] Selective inhibition of neuronal NOS (nNOS or type I NOS), which is found in the thick ascending limb of the loop of Henle, the macula densa, and efferent arterioles,[156,185] decreases GFR without affecting blood pressure or renal blood flow (RBF).[186] Because eNOS (endothelial NOS or type II NOS) is found in the endothelium of renal blood vessels including the afferent and efferent arterioles and glomerular capillary endothelial cells,[156] differences in the effects of inhibition of NO formation on RBF from generalized NOS inhibition versus specific inhibition of nNOS appear to be related to the distinct distribution of eNOS versus nNOS in the kidney. Both acute and chronic inhibition of NO production results in systemic and glomerular capillary hypertension, an increase in preglomerular (R_A) and efferent arteriolar (R_E) resistance, a decrease in K_f, and decreases in both Q_A and SNGFR.[146,147,187–189] These responses to NO inhibition are largely mediated through the actions of AII and endothelin.[127,128,187,190] Administration of nonpressor doses of an inhibitor of NO formation through the renal artery yielded an increase in preglomerular resistance and a decrease in SNGFR and K_f but no effect on efferent resistance was observed unless systemic blood pressure increased.[147] These studies suggested that the cortical afferent, but not efferent, arterioles were under tonic control by NO. However, others have found that the renal artery, arcuate and interlobular arteries and the afferent and efferent arterioles have all been shown to produce NO and constrict in response to inhibition of endogenous NO production.[17,127,128,130,157,191,192] In agreement with this finding, other investigators[193,194] have reported that

NO dilates both efferent and afferent arterioles in the perfused juxtamedullary nephron.

Controversy exists regarding the role of the renin-angiotensin system in the genesis of the increase in vascular resistance that follows blockade of NOS. Studies of in vitro perfused nephrons[191] and of anesthetized rats in vivo[195] suggest that the increase in renal vascular resistance that follows NOS blockade is blunted when angiotensin II formation or binding is blocked. NO inhibits renin release while acute AII infusion increases cortical NOS activity and protein expression and chronic AII infusion increases mRNA levels for both eNOS and nNOS.[196,197] AII increases NO production in isolated perfused afferent arterioles via activation of the AT1 AII receptors.[198] On the other hand, Baylis and colleagues[199] reported that inhibition of NOS in the conscious rats had similar effects on renal hemodynamics in the intact and angiotensin II–blocked state. This suggests that the vasoconstrictor response of NOS blockade is not mediated by angiotensin II. In a later study, workers in this laboratory[200] showed that when the angiotensin II level was acutely raised by infusion of exogenous peptide, acute NO blockade amplified the renal vascoconstrictor actions of angiotensin II. In agreement with this finding, Ito and co-workers[127] showed that intrarenal inhibition of NO enhanced angiotensin II–induced afferent, but not efferent, arteriolar vasoconstriction in the rabbit. Similar results have also been obtained in dogs.[135] These data suggest that NO modulates the vasoconstrictor effects of angiotensin II on glomerular arterioles in vivo in settings where angiotensin II levels are elevated.

Endothelin

Endothelin, a potent vasoconstrictor derived primarily from vascular endothelial cells, was first described by Yanagisawa and colleagues.[201] There are three distinct genes for endothelin, each encoding distinct 21 amino acid isopeptides termed ET-1, ET-2, ET-3.[201–203] Endothelin is produced following cleavage by endothelin converting enzyme of the 38–40 amino acid proendothelin which, in turn, is produced from proteolytic cleavage of prepro-endothelin (~212 amino acids) by furin.[204,205] ET-1 is the primary endothelin produced in the kidney including arcuate arteries and veins, interlobular arteries, afferent and efferent arterioles, glomerular capillary endothelial cells, glomerular epithelial cells, and glomerular mesangial cells of both rat and human[206–216] and acts in an autocrine or paracrine fashion or both[217] to alter a variety of biologic processes in these cells. Endothelins are extremely potent vasoconstrictors and the renal vasculature is highly sensitive to these agents.[218] Once released from endothelial cells, endothelins bind to specific receptors on vascular smooth muscle, the ET_A receptors, that bind both ET-1 and ET-2.[217,219–222] ET_B receptors are expressed in the glomerulus on mesangial cells and podocytes with equal affinity for ET-1, ET-2, or ET-3.[217,219,220,223–225] There are two subtypes of ET_B receptors, the ET_{B1} linked to vasodilation and the ET_{B2} linked to vasoconstriction.[226] An endothelin-specific protease modulates endothelin levels in the kidney.[227]

Endothelin production is stimulated by physical factors including increased shear stress and vascular stretch.[228,229] In addition a variety of hormones, growth factors, and vasoactive peptides increase endothelin production including transforming growth factor-β, platelet-derived growth factor, tumor necrosis factor-α, angiotensin II, arginine vasopressin, insulin, bradykinin, thromboxane A_2, and thrombin.[206,207,211,213,216,230–233] Endothelin production is inhibited by atrial and brain natriuretic peptides acting through a cyclic GMP-dependent process[227] and by factors that increase intracellular cyclic AMP and protein kinase A activation such as β-adrenergic agonists.[211]

Typically, intravenous infusion of ET-1 induces a marked, prolonged pressor response[201,234] accompanied by increases in preglomerular and efferent arteriolar resistances and a decrease in renal blood flow and GFR.[234] Infusion of subpressor doses of ET-1 also decreases whole kidney and single nephron GFR and blood flow,[235–239] again accompanied by increases in both preglomerular and postglomerular resistances and filtration fraction.[235,239,240] Vasoconstriction of afferent and efferent arterioles by endothelin has been confirmed in the split, hydronephrotic rat kidney preparation[241,242] and in isolated perfused arterioles.[128,131,243] In both micropuncture[239] and isolated arteriole[131] studies, the sensitivity and response of the efferent arteriole exceeded those of the afferent vessel. Endothelin also causes mesangial cell contraction.[244,245] Finally, other studies have suggested that the vasoconstrictor effects of the endothelins can be modulated by a number of factors[221,246] including endothelium-derived relaxing factor,[128] bradykinin,[247] and prostaglandin E_2[248] and prostacyclin.[248,249]

There are multiple endothelin receptors; most is known about the ET_A and ET_B receptors, which have been cloned and characterized.[220,250,251] According to the traditional view, ET_A receptors, abundant on vascular smooth muscle, have a high affinity for ET-1 and play a prominent role in the pressor response to endothelin.[252] ET_B receptors are present on endothelial cells where they may mediate NO release and endothelial-dependent relaxation.[251] However, the distribution and function of ET_A and ET_B receptors vary greatly among species and, in the rat, even according to strain. In the normal rat, both ET_A and ET_B receptors are expressed in the media of interlobular arteries, afferent and efferent arterioles. In interlobar and arcuate arteries only ET_A receptors were present on vascular smooth muscle cells.[253] ET_B receptor immunoreactivity is sparse on endothelial cells of renal arteries, while there is strong labeling of peritubular and glomerular capillaries as well as vasa recta endothelium.[253] ET_A receptors are evident on glomerular mesangial cells and pericytes of descending vasa recta bundles.[253] In the rat, endogenous endothelin may actually tonically dilate the afferent arteriole and lower K_f via ET_B receptors.[254] However, ET_B receptors on vascular smooth muscle also mediate vasoconstriction in the rat and this is potentiated in hypertensive animals.[255]

Endothelin stimulates the production of vasodilatory prostaglandins[238,249,256–258] yielding a feedback loop to modify the vasoconstrictor effects of endothelin. ET-1, ET-2, and ET-3 also stimulate NO production in the arteriole and glomerular mesangium via activation of the ET_B receptor.[128,168,170,257,259] Resistance in the renal and systemic vasculature are markedly increased during inhibition of nitric oxide production and these effects can be partially reversed by ET_A blockade or inhibition of endothelin-converting enzyme, indicating the dynamic interrelationship between nitric oxide and endothelin effects.[260,261] The vasoconstrictive effects of AII may be mediated, in part, by a stimulation of endothelin-1 production that acts on endothelin type A (ET_A) receptors to produce vasoconstriction.[231,232] Indeed chronic administration reduces renal blood flow, an effect prevented by administration of a mixed ET_A/ET_B receptor antagonist suggesting that endothelin contributes importantly to the renal vasoconstrictive effects of AII.[232]

Tubuloglomerular Feedback Control of Renal Blood Flow and Glomerular Filtration

The nephron is organized in a manner such that each tubule that leaves the glomerulus returns again to come in contact with it in a specialized nephron segment lying between the end of the thick ascending limb of the loop of Henle and the distal convoluted tubule. The specialized cells in this region are the known as the macula densa cells and they sit adjacent to the cells of the extraglomerular mesangium, which fill the space in the angle formed by the afferent and efferent arterioles of the glomerulus of the same nephron. This anatomical arrangement of macula densa cells, extraglomerular mesangial cells, vascular smooth muscle cells, and renin-secreting cells of the afferent arteriole, is known as the juxtaglomerular apparatus (JGA). The JGA is ideally suited for a feedback system whereby a stimulus received at the macula densa might be transmitted to the arterioles of the same nephron to alter renal blood flow and glomerular filtration rate. Changes in the delivery and composition of the fluid flowing past the macula densa have now been shown to elicit rapid changes in glomerular filtration of the same nephron with increases in delivery of fluid out of the proximal tubule resulting in decreases in SNGFR and glomerular capillary hydraulic pressure (P_{GC}) of the same nephron.[262,263] This feedback between delivery of fluid to the macula densa and filtration rate, termed tubuloglomerular feedback, provides a powerful mechanism to regulate the pressures and flows that govern glomerular filtration rate in response to acute perturbations in delivery of fluid out of the proximal tubule.

Changes in delivery of Na^+, Cl^-, and K^+ are thought to be sensed by the macula densa through the $Na^+/2Cl^-/K^+$ cotransporter on the luminal cell membrane of the macula densa cells.[263] Alterations in Na^+, K^+, and Cl^- reabsorption result in inverse changes in SNGFR and renal vascular resistance, primarily in the preglomerular vessels.[263] Agents such as furosemide that interfere with the $Na^+/2Cl^-/K^+$ cotransporter in the macula densa cells inhibit the feedback response.[262] Evidence now indicates that adenosine and possibly ATP play a central role in mediating the relationship between Na^+, Cl^-, K^+ transport at the luminal cell membrane of the macula densa and glomerular filtration rate of the same nephron. This is illustrated in Figure 3–17 adapted from Vallon.[264] According to this scheme increased delivery of solute to the macula densa results in concentration-dependent increases in solute uptake by the $Na^+/2Cl^-/K^+$ cotransporter. This, in turn, stimulates Na^+/K^+-ATPase activity on the basolateral side of the cells leading to the formation of ADP and subsequent formation of adenosine monophosphate (AMP). Dephosphorylation of AMP by cytosolic 5′ nucleotidase or endo-5′ nucleotidase bound to the cell membrane yields the formation of adenosine.[264] AMP might also be extruded into the interstitum where it is converted to adenosine by ecto-5′ nucleotidases. According to the scheme shown in Figure 3–17 once adenosine leaves the macula densa cells or is formed in the adjacent interstitum it interacts with adenosine A_1 receptors on the extraglomerular mesangial cells resulting in an increase in $[Ca^{2+}]_i$.[265] The increase in $[Ca^{2+}]_i$ may occur via in part basolateral membrane depolarization through Cl^- channel followed by Ca^{2+} entry into the cells via voltage-gated Ca^{2+} channels.[266] As indicated in Figure 3–17 gap junctions then transmit the calcium transient to the adjacent afferent arteriole leading to vasoconstriction and renin release.[264] Macula densa cells respond to an increase in luminal [NaCl] by releasing ATP at the basolateral cell membrane through ATP-permeable large conductance anion channels, possibly providing a communication link between macula densa cells and adjacent mesangial cells via purinoceptors receptors on the latter.[267]

Several lines of evidence support the role for adenosine in mediating tubuloglomerular feedback. Intraluminal administration of an adenosine A_1 receptor agonist enhances the TGF response.[268] In addition tubuloglomerular feedback is completely absent in adenosine A_1 receptor-deficient mice despite the fact that the animals had plasma renin activities that were twice normal.[269,270] Blocking adenosine A_1 receptors or by inhibition of 5′-nucleotidase reduce tubuloglomerular feedback efficiency and combining the two inhibitors nearly completely blocked tubuloglomerular feedback.[271] Addition of

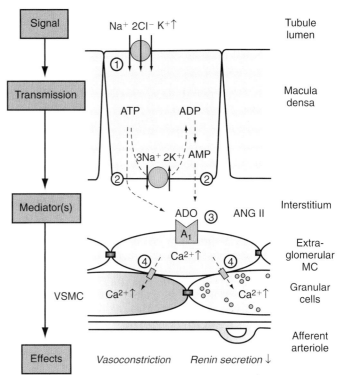

FIGURE 3–17 Proposed mechanism of tubuloglomerular feedback (TGF). The sequence of events (numbers in circles) are (1) uptake of Na^+, Cl^-, and K^+ by the $Na^+/2Cl^-/K^+$ cotransporter on the luminal cell membrane of the macula densa cells; (2) intracellular or extracellular production of adenosine (ADO); (3) ADO activation of adenosine A_1 receptors triggering an increase in cytosolic Ca^{2+} in extraglomerular mesangial cells (MC); (4) coupling between extraglomerular MC and granular cells (containing renin) and smooth muscle cells of the afferent arteriole (VSMC) by gap junctions allowing propagation of the increased $[Ca^{2+}]_i$ resulting in afferent arteriolar vasoconstriction and inhibition of renin release. Local angiotensin II and nNOS activity modulate the response. (Figure reproduced by permission from Vallon V: Tubuloglomerular feedback and the control of glomerular filtration rate. News Physiol Sci 18:169–174, 2003.)

adenosine to the afferent arteriole causes vasoconstriction via activation of the adenosine A_1 receptor and addition of an A_1 receptor antagonist blocked both the effects of adenosine and of high macula densa [NaCl].[272] Of note, the effects only occur when adenosine is added to the extravascular space and do not occur when adenosine is added to the lumen of the macula densa.[272] These results are consistent with the proposed scheme in Figure 3–17, which suggests that an increase in [NaCl] to the macula densa stimulates Na^+/K^+-ATPase activity leading to increased adenosine synthesis followed by constriction of the afferent arterioles via A_1 receptor activation.[272]

Efferent arterioles preconstricted with norepinephrine vasodilate in response to an increase in [NaCl] at the macula densa, an effect blocked with adenosine A_2 receptor antagonists but not by blocking the A_1 receptor.[273] The changes in efferent arteriolar resistance are in opposite direction to that of the afferent arterioles, which vasoconstrict in response to increased [NaCl] at the macula densa.[272,274] The net result would be decreased glomerular blood flow, decreased glomerular hydraulic pressure, and a reduction in SNGFR. Extracellular ATP attenuates the TGF system.[275]

The tubuloglomerular feedback (TGF) response is blunted by AII antagonists and AII synthesis inhibitors and is absent in knockout mice lacking either the AT_{1A} angiotensin II receptor or angiotensin converting enzyme (ACE) and systemic infusion of AII in ACE knockout mice restores

108

tubuloglomerular feedback.[276–280] AII enhances tubuloglomerular feedback via activation of AT_1 receptors on the luminal membrane of the macula densa.[281] Acute inhibition of the AT_1 receptor in normal mice blocked tubuloglomerular feedback and reduced autoregulatory efficiency.[278] These results indicate that AII plays a central role in modulating tubuloglomerular feedback and that this response is mediated through the AT_1 receptor.

The macula densa is a site of immunocytochemical localization of neuronal nitric oxide synthase (nNOS or NOS 1).[282] Nitric oxide derived from nNOS in the macula densa provides a vasodilatory influence on tubuloglomerular feedback, decreasing the amount of vasoconstriction of the afferent arteriole than otherwise would occur.[282,283] Increased distal sodium chloride delivery to the macula densa stimulates nNOS activity and also increases activity of the inducible form of cyclooxygenase (COX-2) to generate metabolites that also participate in counteracting TGF-mediated constriction of the afferent arteriole.[282,284] Macula densa cell pH increases in response to increased luminal sodium concentration and may be related to the stimulation of nNOS.[285] Inhibition of macula densa guanylate cyclase increases the TGF response to high luminal [NaCl] further indicating the importance of NO in modulating TGF.[274] Ito and Ren, using an isolated perfused complete JGA preparation, found that microperfusion of the macula densa with an inhibitor of nitric oxide production led to constriction of the adjacent afferent arteriole.[286] When the macula densa was perfused with a low sodium solution, however, the response was blocked, indicating that solute reabsorption is required.[286] Microperfusion of the macula densa with the precursor of nitric oxide, L-arginine, blunts tubuloglomerular feedback, especially in salt depleted animals.[287–289] Thus it appears that the afferent arteriole acutely vasodilates in response to NO, blunting TGF. An increase in NO production may also inhibit renin release by increasing cGMP in the granular cells of the afferent arteriole,[290] thereby accentuating its vasodilatory effects. Of note, however, Schnermann and co-workers reported that when nitric oxide production is chronically blocked in knockout mice lacking nNOS tubuloglomerular feedback in response to acute perturbations in distal sodium delivery is normal.[276] They did observe, however, that the presence of intact nNOS in the JGA is required for sodium chloride-dependent renin secretion.[276] The tubuloglomerular feedback system, which elicits vasoconstriction and a reduction in SNGFR in response to acute increases in delivery to the macula densa, appears to secondarily activate a vasodilatory response. Stimulation of NO production in response to increased distal salt delivery under conditions of volume expansion would be advantageous by resetting tubuloglomerular feedback and limiting TGF-mediated vasoconstrictor responses.

Tubuloglomerular feedback responses might be temporally divided into two opposing events. The initial, rapid (seconds) tubuloglomerular feedback response would yield vasoconstriction and a decrease in GFR and P_{GC} when sodium delivery out of the proximal tubule is acutely increased. The same increase in delivery would be expected with time (minutes) to decrease renin secretion, which in the face of a continued stimulus such as volume expansion, would reduce AII production and allow filtration rate to increase, thereby helping to increase urinary excretion rates. The rapid tubuloglomerular feedback system would prevent large changes in GFR under such conditions as spontaneous fluctuations in blood pressure that might otherwise occur, thereby maintaining tight control of distal sodium delivery in the short term.[276] Schnermann and co-workers hypothesized that the juxtaglomerular apparatus functions to maintain tight control of distal sodium delivery only for the short term.[276] Over the long term, renin secretion is controlled by the JGA in accordance with the requirements for sodium balance and the TGF system resets at a new sodium delivery rate.[276] The TGF system then continues to operate around this new setpoint. The resetting of the TGF system may thus be the result of sustained increases in GFR and distal delivery rather than the cause of the resetting.[276,291,292]

Renal Autoregulation

Many organs are capable of maintaining relative constancy of blood flow in the face of major changes in perfusion pressure. Although the efficiency with which blood flow is maintained differs from organ to organ (being most efficient in brain and kidney), virtually all organs and tissues, including skeletal muscle and intestine, exhibit this property, termed autoregulation. The ability of the kidney to autoregulate renal blood flow and glomerular filtration rate over a wide range of renal perfusion pressures was first demonstrated by Forster and Maes[293] and subsequently confirmed by others.[294,295] Figure 3–18 shows typical patterns of autoregulation for the dog and rat kidney.

Autoregulation of blood flow requires parallel changes in resistance with changes in perfusion pressure. However, if efferent arteriolar resistance declined significantly when perfusion pressure was reduced, glomerular capillary pressure and GFR would also fall. Therefore, the finding that both renal plasma flow and GFR are autoregulated suggests that the principal resistance change is in the preglomerular vasculature. In support of this hypothesis, early micropuncture studies in the rat indicate that pressures in postglomerular surface microvessels remain relatively constant despite variations in perfusion pressure throughout the autoregulatory range.[296–299] Subsequent studies using the Munich-Wistar rat, which has glomeruli on the renal cortical surface that are readily accessible to micropuncture, afforded an opportunity to observe the renal cortical microvascular adjustments that take place in response to variations in renal arterial perfusion pressure. Figure 3–19 summarizes the effects in the normal hydropenic rat of graded reductions in renal perfusion pressure on glomerular capillary blood flow rate, mean glomerular capillary hydraulic pressure (P_{GC}), and preglomerular (R_A) and efferent arteriolar (R_E) resistance.[300] As shown in Figure 3–19, graded reduction in renal perfusion pressure from 120 mm Hg to 80 mm Hg resulted in only a modest decline in glomerular capillary blood flow, whereas further reduction in perfusion pressure to 60 mm Hg led to a more pronounced decline. Despite the decline in perfusion pressure from 120 mm Hg to 80 mm Hg, values of P_{GC} fell

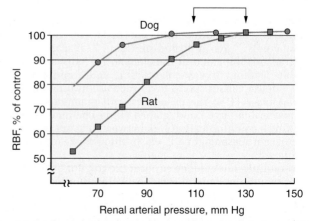

FIGURE 3–18 Autoregulatory response of total renal blood flow to changes in renal perfusion pressure in the dog and rat. In general, the normal anesthetized dog exhibits greater autoregulatory capability to lower arterial pressure than does the rat. (From Navar LG, Bell PD, Burke TJ: Role of a macula densa feedback mechanism as a mediator of renal autoregulation. Kidney Int 22:S157, 1982.)

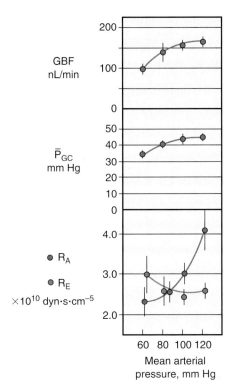

FIGURE 3-19 Glomerular dynamics in response to reduction of renal arterial perfusion pressure in the normal hydropenic rat. As can be seen, glomerular blood flow (GBF) and glomerular capillary hydraulic pressure ($\bar{P}_{GC}$) remained relatively constant over the range of perfusion pressure examined, primarily as a result of a marked decrease in afferent arteriolar resistance (R_A). R_E, efferent arteriolar resistance. (Adapted from Robertson CR, Deen WM, Troy JL, Brenner BM: Dynamics of glomerular ultrafiltration in the rat. III. Hemodynamics and autoregulation. Am J Physiol 223:1191, 1972.)

nephrons to changes in perfusion pressure might account for this difference.

Preglomerular vessels including the afferent arterioles and vessels as large as the arcuate and interlobular arteries participate in the autoregulatory response. In the split, hydronephrotic rat kidney preparation, Steinhausen and co-workers[118] observed dilation of all preglomerular vessels from the arcuate to interlobular arteries in response to reductions in perfusion pressure from 120 mm Hg to 95 mm Hg. The proximal afferent arteriole did not respond to pressure changes in this range but did dilate when perfusion pressure was reduced to 70 mm Hg. The diameter of the distal afferent arteriole did not change at any pressure. Also consistent with an important role of large, preglomerular vessels in the autoregulatory response, Heyeraas and Aukland[304] reported that interlobular arterial pressure remained constant when renal perfusion pressure was reduced by 20 mm Hg, again suggesting that these vessels contribute importantly to the constancy of outer cortical blood flow in the upper autoregulatory range. A number of observations suggest that the major preglomerular resistor is located close to the glomerulus, at the level of the afferent arteriole.[99,305-307] As in superficial nephrons, direct observations of perfused juxtamedullary nephrons revealed parallel reductions in the luminal diameters of arcuate, interlobular, and afferent arterioles in response to elevation in perfusion pressure. However, because quantitatively similar reductions in vessel diameter produce much greater elevations in resistance in small than in large vessels, the predominant effect of these changes is an increase in afferent arteriolar resistance.[308]

Renal Autoregulatory Mechanisms
Cellular Mechanisms Involved in Renal Autoregulation
Autoregulation of the afferent arteriole and interlobular artery is blocked by administration of L-type calcium channel blockers, inhibition of mechanosensitive cation channels, and a calcium-free perfusate.[309-312] The autoregulatory response thus involves gating of mechanosensitive channels producing membrane depolarization and activation of voltage-dependent calcium channels leading to an increase in intracellular calcium concentration and vasoconstriction.[309,313,314] Indeed calcium channel blockade almost completely blocks autoregulation of renal blood flow.[315,316] The autoregulatory capacity of the afferent arteriole is attenuated by intrinsic metabolites of the cytochrome P450 epoxygenase pathway while metabolites of the cytochrome P450 hydroxylase pathway enhance autoregulatory responsiveness.[317]

Autoregulation of both GFR and RBF occur in the presence of inhibition of nitric oxide but values for RBF were reduced at any given renal perfusion pressure as compared with control values.[183,318-320] In the isolated perfused juxtamedullary afferent arteriole the initial vasodilatation observed when pressure was increased was of shorter duration when endogenous nitric oxide formation was blocked but the autoregulatory response was unaffected.[313] Cortical and juxtamedullary preglomerular vessels in the split hydronephrotic kidney also autoregulate in the presence of NO inhibition.[192] The majority of evidence therefore suggests that NO is not essential at least for the myogenic component of renal autoregulation, though nitric oxide may play a role in tubuloglomerular feedback (see later discussion).[193]

Several other vasoactive substances have been implicated in the autoregulation of renal blood flow, including various vasoactive eicosanoids,[321-323] kinins,[324] and the renin-angiotensin system[323,325] but definitive evidence in favor of any of these is lacking. Kaloyanides and co-workers[326] found that autoregulation of renal blood flow and GFR persists when prostaglandin synthesis is inhibited. On the other hand, Schnermann and co-workers[323] have shown renal autoregulatory ability to be severely impaired by indomethacin

only modestly on average, from 45 mm Hg to 40 mm Hg. Further reduction in perfusion pressure from 80 mm Hg to 60 mm Hg resulted in a further fall in P_{GC} (from 40 mm Hg to 35 mm Hg). Calculated values for R_A and R_E are shown in Figure 3-19. The better autoregulation of glomerular capillary blood flow in the perfusion pressure range 80 mm Hg to 120 mm Hg was due to the more pronounced fall in R_A than occurred in the lower range of perfusion pressure. Over the range of renal perfusion pressure from 120 mm Hg to 60 mm Hg, R_E tended to increase slightly. In that study when plasma volume was expanded, R_A declined while R_E increased as renal perfusion pressure was lowered so that P_{GC} and ΔP were virtually unchanged over the entire range of renal perfusion pressures.[300] In plasma-expanded animals, the mean glomerular transcapillary hydraulic pressure difference (ΔP) exhibited nearly perfect autoregulation over the entire range of perfusion pressures because of concomitant increases in R_E as R_A fell.[300] These results indicate that autoregulation of GFR is the consequence of the autoregulation of both glomerular blood flow and glomerular capillary pressure.

The medullary circulation has also been shown to possess autoregulatory capacity.[301,302] Cohen and co-workers[89] demonstrated that vasa recta blood flow remained relatively constant for the pressure range 85 mm Hg to 125 mm Hg. Mattson and associates[303] reported that outer and inner medullary blood flow in rats decreased when perfusion pressure was reduced below 100 mm Hg. In contrast, simultaneously measured superficial and deep cortical blood flows were well autoregulated in this range. Thus, the autoregulatory range of the medulla may be narrower than that of the cortex and altered responses of the postglomerular circulation of deep infusion. Suppression of renin release by high-salt diets and administration of desoxycorticosterone also yielded conflicting results.[327] Although many studies have shown that angiotensin II plays an important role in regulating TGF mechanism,[280,322,328] intrarenal administration of angiotensin II antagonists has not been associated with impairment of renal blood flow autoregulation.[329-333]

As noted previously, autoregulation of renal blood flow is demonstrable in denervated and isolated organ preparations and is therefore thought to be independent of circulating humoral or neurogenic factors but governed instead by a mechanism or mechanisms intrinsic to the kidney.[299,334] Several hypotheses have been proposed to account for this phenomenon including (1) a role for an intrinsic myogenic mechanism first proposed by Bayliss,[335] (2) a role for the tubuloglomerular feedback system, and (3) a role for a metabolic mechanism.

The Myogenic Mechanism for Autoregulation

According to the myogenic theory arterial smooth muscle contracts and relaxes in response to increases and decreases in vascular wall tension.[335] Thus, an increase in perfusion pressure, which initially distends the vascular wall, is followed by a contraction of resistance vessels, resulting in a recovery of blood flow from an initial elevation to a value comparable to the control level. Renal blood flow thus tends to remain relatively constant. This autoregulatory mechanism has also been proposed for other organs.[336,337] Lush and co-workers[338,339] presented a model of myogenic control of renal blood flow based on the assumption that flow remains constant when the distending force and the constricting forces, determined by the properties of the vessel wall, are equal. The constricting force is envisioned to have both a passive and an active component, the latter sensitive to stretch in the vessel.

Several lines of evidence indicate that such a myogenic mechanism is important in renal autoregulation. Autoregulation of renal blood flow is observed even when tubuloglomerular feedback is inhibited by furosemide suggesting an important role for a myogenic mechanism.[134] This myogenic mechanism of autoregulation occurs very rapidly, reaching a full response in 3 to 10 seconds.[134] Autoregulation occurs in all of the preglomerular resistance vessels of the in vitro blood-perfused juxtamedullary nephron preparation.[317,340-343] Of note the afferent arteriole in this preparation was able to constrict in response to rapid changes in perfusion pressure even when all flow to the macula densa was stopped by resection of the papilla indicating an important role for a myogenic mechanism in autoregulation.[340] Isolated perfused rabbit afferent arterioles respond to step increases of intraluminal pressure with a decrease in luminal diameter.[119] In contrast, efferent arteriolar segments showed vasodilation when submitted to the same procedure, probably reflecting simple passive physical properties. Autoregulation is also observed in the afferent arteriole and arcuate and interlobular artery of the split hydronephrotic kidney,[192,309-322,344] but again the efferent arteriole did not autoregulate in this model.[192] Further evidence that the renal vasculature is indeed intrinsically responsive to variations in the transmural hydraulic pressure difference was obtained by Gilmore and co-workers[109] who provided direct evidence for myogenic autoregulation in renal vessels transplanted into a cheek pouch of the hamster. In this nonfiltering system, contraction of afferent but not efferent arterioles was observed in response to increased interstitial pressure in the pouch. However, it should be noted that, in vivo, efferent arteriolar resistance may increase in response to decreases in arterial pressure,[300,345] and this may result from increased activity of the renin-angiotensin system. These data may also explain why autoregulation of GFR is more efficient than autoregulation of renal blood flow.

The autoregulatory threshold can be reset in response to a variety of perturbations. Autoregulation in the afferent arteriole is greatly attenuated in diabetic kidneys and may contribute to the hyperfiltration seen in this disease.[344] Autoregulation is partially restored by insulin treatment or by inhibition of endogenous prostaglandin production (or both).[344] Autoregulation in the remnant kidney is markedly attenuated 24 hours after the reduction in renal mass and is again restored by cyclooxygenase inhibition, suggesting that release of vasodilatory prostaglandins may be involved in the initial response to increase SNGFR in the remaining nephrons after acute partial nephrectomy.[346] Much higher pressures than normal are required to evoke a vasoconstrictor response in the afferent arteriole during the development of spontaneous hypertension.[347] The intermediate portion of the interlobular artery of the spontaneously hypertensive rat exhibits an enhanced myogenic response, with a lower threshold pressure and a greater maximal response.[310] Both the afferent arterioles and the interlobular arteries of the Dahl salt-sensitive hypertensive rat exhibit a reduced myogenic responsiveness to increases in perfusion pressure in rats fed a high-salt diet.[348] Thus, alterations in autoregulatory responses of the renal vasculature occur in a variety of disease states for the control of renal blood flow and glomerular ultrafiltration.

Autoregulation Mediated by Tubuloglomerular Feedback

The tubuloglomerular feedback (TGF) mechanism has been suggested as an alternative to the myogenic response to explain the autoregulation of renal blood flow and GFR. This system is envisioned to operate through the following sequence as described in detail later. Increased arterial pressure augments renal blood flow and glomerular capillary hydraulic pressure. These alterations cause GFR and therefore delivery of solute to the distal tubule to rise. Increased distal delivery is sensed by the macula densa, which activates effector mechanisms that increase preglomerular resistance, reducing renal blood flow, glomerular pressure, and GFR. A number of observations support this hypothesis. Perfusion of the renal distal tubule at increasing flows causes reduction in glomerular blood flow and GFR.[349] Furthermore, as reviewed by Navar and colleagues,[193,307] a variety of experimental maneuvers that cause distal tubule fluid flow to decline or cease induce afferent arteriolar vasodilation and interfere with the normal autoregulatory response. In addition, Moore and Casellas[350] found that infusion of furosemide into the macula densa segment of juxtamedullary nephrons significantly abrogated the normal constrictor response of afferent arterioles to increased perfusion pressure. A similar observation was made by Takenaka and co-workers.[343] These studies suggested that the autoregulatory response in juxtamedullary nephrons was mainly dependent on the TGF mechanism.

To examine the mechanisms responsible for autoregulation, investigators have studied spontaneous oscillations in proximal tubule pressure and renal blood flow and the response of the renal circulation to high-frequency oscillations in tubule flow rates or renal perfusion pressure.[351] Oscillations in tubule pressure have been observed in anesthetized rats at a rate of about three cycles per minute.[352] These spontaneous oscillations do not correlate with changes in blood pressure,[352] can be induced by maneuvers that alter NaCl delivery to the macula densa,[352] vary from nephron to nephron,[353,354] and are eliminated by loop diuretics,[355] findings consistent with the hypothesis that they are mediated by the TGF response. To examine this hypothesis, Holstein-Rathlou[351] induced sinusoidal oscillations in distal tubule flow in rats at a frequency similar to that of the spontaneous fluctuations in tubule pressure. Varying distal delivery at this rate caused parallel fluctuations in stop-flow pressure (an index of glomerular capillary pressure), probably mediated by alterations in afferent resistance, again consistent with dynamic regulation of glomerular blood flow by the TGF system. To investigate the role of this system in autoregulation, Holstein-Rathlou and colleagues[356] examined the effects of sinusoidal variations in arterial pressure at varying frequencies on renal blood flow in rats. Two separate components of autoregulation were identified, one operating at about the same frequency as the spontaneous fluctuations in tubule pressure (the TGF component) and one operating at a much higher frequency consistent with spontaneous fluctuations in vascular smooth muscle tone (the myogenic component). Subsequently, Flemming and co-workers[357] reported that renal vascular responses to alterations in renal perfusion pressure varied considerably depending on the dynamics of the change and that rapid and slow changes in perfusion pressure could have opposite effects. They suggested that slow pressure changes elicited a predominant TGF response, whereas rapid changes invoked the myogenic mechanism. Despite these observations, the conclusion that the TGF system plays a central role in autoregulation is complicated by several factors. First, there is the process of glomerulotubular balance, by which proximal tubule reabsorption increases as GFR rises. This mechanism would tend to blunt the effects of alterations in GFR on distal delivery. In addition, the persistence of autoregulatory behavior in nonfiltering kidneys[358] and in isolated blood vessels suggests that the delivery of filtrate to the distal tubule is not absolutely required for constancy of blood flow, at least in superficial nephrons. Consistent with this view, Just and colleagues[134,359] demonstrated in the conscious dog that although TGF contributes to maximum autoregulatory capacity of renal blood flow, autoregulation is observed even when tubuloglomerular feedback is inhibited by furosemide suggesting an important role for a myogenic mechanism. Finally, it should be noted that the myogenic and TGF mechanisms are not mutually exclusive and Aukland and Hien[360] have proposed a model of renal autoregulation that incorporates both systems. Because the myogenic and TGF responses share the same effector site, the afferent arteriole, interactions between these two systems are unavoidable and each response is capable of modulating the other. The prevailing view is that these two mechanisms act in concert to accomplish the same end, a stabilization of renal function when blood pressure is altered.[361]

Autoregulation Mediated by Metabolic Mechanisms

The metabolic theory predicts that, given the relative constancy of tissue metabolism, a decrease in organ blood flow leads to local accumulation of a vasodilator metabolite, maintaining blood flow at or near its previous level.[360–364] Some investigators believe this mechanism is valid for the kidney as well.[362] A strong objection to this theory is related to the unique relationship between renal blood flow and renal metabolism.[365] The latter is determined mainly by Na reabsorption (see Chapter 4), which in turn is roughly proportional to GFR (glomerulotubular balance). Because it has been demonstrated in many species that GFR varies in proportion to renal blood flow under physiologic conditions, it follows that renal metabolism should also vary directly with renal blood flow. If it is true that some vasodilator metabolite plays a major role in the autoregulation of renal blood flow, then elevation in the latter would increase the production of the putative vasodilator, leading to further elevation in renal blood flow and rendering autoregulation of this parameter impossible.[365] Recent evidence indicates, however, that adenosine triphosphate (ATP) and its metabolites adenosine diphosphate (ADP) and adenosine have important effects on renal vascular smooth muscle and thus may provide a metabolic link to autoregulation.

Role of Purine Nucleotides in Autoregulation and Renal Hemodynamics
Adenosine Triphosphate

Navar[193] proposed that adenosine triphosphate (ATP) may function as a metabolic regulator tubuloglomerular feedback and autoregulation of renal blood flow. ATP is present in and required for the function of all cells. ATP is released from vascular smooth muscle cells and endothelial cells[366] as well as from ATP-releasing nerve fibers or "purinergic" nerve fibers.[366–368] When ATP is released from the nerves or other types of cells into the extracellular space it activates two types of purinoceptors, the P_{2X} and the P_{2Y} receptors, resulting in vasoconstriction.[322,369–372] Activation of P_{2X} purinoceptors by ATP leads to increases in intracellular calcium concentration ($[Ca^{2+}]_i$) through an initial rapid influx through nonselective ligand-gated cation channels followed by sustained entry through opening of voltage-dependent L-type calcium channels.[369,370,373,374] ATP also activates P_{2Y} receptors leading to activation of phospholipase C, formation of 1,4,5-trisphosphate, and mobilization of intracellular calcium stores promoting vasoconstriction.[369,370,373,375] Superfusion with ATP leads to vasoconstriction of arcuate arteries, interlobular arteries, and the afferent arteriole with effects on the afferent arteriole being stronger and lasting longer than in the other vessels, but ATP does not constrict the efferent arteriole.[369,371,372,374,376] ATP promotes a transient vasoconstriction in the arcuate and interlobular arteries followed by a gradual return to control diameter.[374] In the afferent arteriole ATP induces a rapid initial vasoconstriction (vessel diameter ~70% smaller than control) followed by a gradual relaxation to a final diameter still at least 10% smaller than control.[374] This suggests that the vasoconstrictor effects of ATP may be more prolonged in the afferent arteriole than in other preglomerular vessels. These results indicate a unique role for ATP in the selective control of preglomerular resistance.

Despite the ability of ATP to promote vasoconstriction when applied from the extravascular side of the blood vessel,[369,371,372,374,376] intrarenal infusion of ATP leads to renal vasodilatation rather than vasoconstriction.[162,319] ATP from the luminal side of the blood vessel activates P_{2Y} purinoceptors on vascular endothelial cells leading to increased synthesis and release of nitric oxide as well as stimulation of the production of prostacyclin resulting in vasodilatation.[162,319] The net effect of ATP on renal vascular resistance in vivo may depend on whether the ATP is delivered from the blood side or the interstitial side, and NO and prostacyclin production stimulated by ATP in the endothelium may modulate any direct vasoconstrictive effects of this compound on the renal circulation.[369,371,372,374,376] Thus ATP serves as a metabolic regulator of renal blood flow and glomerular filtration rate. Majid and co-workers[318] found that infusion of ATP in large enough amounts to saturate the P_2 purinergic receptors completely blocked autoregulation that was then fully restored adjustments in renal blood flow. Interstitial levels of ATP decrease with reductions in perfusion pressure, which would decrease ATP-induced preglomerular vasoconstriction.[377] These results thus suggest that ATP-mediated effects on autoregulation are significant.

Adenosine Diphosphate

Adenosine diphosphate (ADP) acts as a vasodilator by activating ATP-sensitive potassium (K_{ATP}) channels resulting in membrane hyperpolarization whereas ATP closes the channel leading to membrane depolarization.[378–380] When intracellular ATP levels are decreased and ADP concentrations are increased (such as inhibition of glycolysis) vasodilatation occurs[380,381] suggesting that [ADP] and/or the ATP/ADP ratio plays a significant role in regulating renal vascular tone. Exogenous ADP does not affect the renal vasculature[380] but alterations in intracellular ADP concentrations may play an important role in modulating renal vascular resistance and glomerular ultrafiltration by its effects on the K_{ATP} channel. The vasodilatation induced by ADP is, at least in part, endothelium-dependent.[379] These data suggest a potential role for ADP in the metabolic control of renal hemodynamics and autoregulation but further studies are needed.

Adenosine

The metabolism of ATP generates the purinergic agonist adenosine, which binds to the P_1 class of purinergic receptors that preferentially bind adenosine over ATP, ADP, or AMP.[366,382] Four subtypes of membrane bound G protein-coupled adenosine receptors of the P_1 class have been identified; the A_1, the A_{2a}, the A_{2b}, and the A_3 receptor.[366,383,384] Low levels of adenosine (nanomolar concentrations) activate A_1 receptors resulting in inhibition of adenylate cyclase activity, mobilization of intracellular Ca^{2+}, and vasoconstriction whereas activation of either type of A_2 receptors by higher adenosine levels (micromolar concentrations) stimulates adenylate cyclase activity and promotes vasorelaxation.[384–387] Adenosine-induced vasodilation of afferent arterioles occurs via activation of adenosine A_{2A} receptors.[387] Intracellular adenosine formation is an important component in the macula densa cells for tubuloglomerular feedback control of glomerular filtration rate (see later) and thus is involved in that component of autoregulation. Delivery of solute to the macula densa cells increases $Na^+/2Cl^-/K^+$ transport at the luminal cell membrane leading to increased basolateral Na^+/K^+-ATPase activity and the formation of ADP. Conversion of ADP to AMP by intracellular phosphodiesterase and subsequently to adenosine by intracellular 5′nucleotidase results in adenosine formation with subsequent effects on vascular tone and renin production of the adjacent arterioles as presented in the earlier discussion of tubuloglomerular feedback. An additional pathway leading to adenosine production is the transport of intracellular cAMP to the extracellular compartment leading to the production of adenosine by membrane bound ectophosphodiesterase and ecto-5′-nucleotidase.[384,388] This extracellular adenosine may directly regulate vascular tone through interaction with vascular adenosine receptors and indirectly affect tone by inhibition of renin release from juxtaglomerular cells via activation of A_1 receptors,[389] the adenosine brake hypothesis, to block production of the vasoconstrictor AII.[384,388,390]

Intravenous infusion of adenosine results in a transient renal vasoconstriction followed by vasodilatation and an increase in RBF.[391,392] The initial vasoconstriction is potentiated and the duration of the contraction prolonged by NO inhibition suggesting that at least a portion of the recovery from adenosine-induced renal vasoconstriction is mediated by increases in NO production[392] and indeed adenosine stimulates NO production in vascular endothelial cells.[386] Both A_1 and A_{2b} adenosine receptors are present in afferent and efferent arterioles and activation of the A_1 receptor by low concentrations of adenosine results in vasoconstriction of these vessels whereas activation of the A_{2b} receptors by high concentrations of adenosine results in vasodilatation.[112,376,393,394] Selective blockade of the A_{2a} receptors significantly augmented the vasoconstrictor response of the arterioles to adenosine indicating that adenosine-mediated vasoconstriction is modified by vasodilatory influences of adenosine A_{2a} receptor activation.[393]

A_1 adenosine receptors in the afferent arteriole are selectively activated from the interstitial side resulting in vasoconstriction suggesting a paracrine role for adenosine in the control of GFR.[391] Vasoconstriction of the afferent and efferent arterioles in response to addition of adenosine to the bathing solution is prevented by adenosine receptor blockade.[395] Adenosine concentrations in cortical and medullary interstitial fluid averaged 23 nM and 55 nM, respectively, in animals on a low (0.15%) sodium diet and increased markedly to 418 nM and 1040 nM in the cortex and medulla, respectively for rats on a high-salt (4%) diet.[396] High adenosine levels under conditions of a high-salt diet may contribute to a decrease in macula densa-mediated reductions in renin secretion.[397] Intravenous infusion of adenosine in conscious, healthy humans results in a decrease in GFR with only slight (nonsignificant) declines in renal plasma flow[398] whereas administration of a selective A_1 antagonist produces increases in GFR[399] suggesting that under normal circumstances adenosine concentrations are low enough to activate the vasoconstrictor response via A_1 receptors but activation of A_{2A} receptors provides counteracting vasodilatation. Glomerular mesangial cells constrict in response to adenosine via A_1 receptors.[265] Based on the effects of adenosine on the mesangial cell, an adenosine-induced decrease in GFR may be related, in part, to a decrease in the glomerular ultrafiltration coefficient (K_f). Specific adenosine A_1 receptor antagonists block tubuloglomerular feedback-mediated reductions in glomerular pressure in response to increases in delivery of fluid out of the proximal tubule suggesting that at least part of the vasoconstrictor effect of adenosine is mediated through the tubuloglomerular feedback loop and thus might affect autoregulation.[400] Because of the link between local adenosine concentrations and the divergent hemodynamic responses that can result, adenosine plays an important role in the control of renal blood flow and glomerular filtration rate.

Other Factors Involved in Autoregulation

Studies have shown that endothelium-dependent factors might play a role in the myogenic response of renal arteries and arterioles to changes in perfusion pressure. For example, in 1992 Hishikawa and co-workers[401] reported that increased transmural pressure increased NO release by cultured endothelial cells. In addition, Tojo and co-workers[402] used histochemical techniques to demonstrate the presence of NOS in the macula densa, suggesting that NO also participates in the TGF response. More recent studies suggest that NO produced by the macula densa can dampen the TGF response.[287] In fact, studies have examined the role of this endothelial factor in the autoregulatory response. In dogs, inhibition of production of endothelium-dependent relaxing factor leads to an increase in blood pressure and a decline in basal renal vascular resistance; however, autoregulatory ability is unimpaired.[183] On the other hand, Salom and co-workers[403] reported that inhibition of NO production causes a greater decline in renal blood flow in the kidneys of rats perfused at hypertensive compared with normotensive pressure. This suggests that increased NO production might modulate the vasoconstrictor response to an increase in perfusion pressure. Consistent with this view are the data of Imig and co-workers,[404] who utilized the isolated perfused juxtamedullary nephron technique to examine the response of the preglomerular circulation to an increase in perfusion pressure in the presence and absence of NOS blockade. They found that pressure-induced contraction of the interlobular artery and afferent arteriole was enhanced when NO production was inhibited.

Elevations in transmural pressure also increase endothelin release by cultured endothelial cells and this was not altered by the presence of a calcium channel blocker, nifedipine, or a channel activator, gadolinium.[405] These findings suggest that endothelin, via a mechanism other than extracellular Ca^2 influx, may play a role in pressure-induced control of renal blood flow. Of note, endothelin production is also stimulated by a rise in sheer stress.[229] However, infusions of endothelin produce a prolonged constrictor response that is ill suited to an autoregulatory role,[224,225,239] and there is little or no evidence linking this factor to the minute-to-minute control of renal vascular resistance in normal animals.

Other Hormones and Vasoactive Substances Controlling Renal Blood Flow and Glomerular Filtration

Prostaglandins

Processing of linoleic acid (an essential polyunsaturated fatty acid in the diet) by the liver yields arachidonic acid (AA) that is then stored in membrane phospholipids. Following interaction of a variety of hormones and vasoactive substances with their membrane receptors phospholipase A_2 (PLA_2) is activated resulting in the release of AA from the cell membranes, allowing the enzymatic action of cyclooxygenase to process arachidonic acid into prostaglandins (PG) PGG_2 and subsequently PGH_2. PGH_2 is then converted into a number of biologically active prostaglandins including PGE_2, prostacyclin (PGI_2), $PGF_{2\alpha}$, PGE_1, PGD_2, and thromboxane (TxA_2) (see Chapter 11).

PGE_1, PGE_2, and PGI_2 are vasodilator prostaglandins that generally increase renal plasma flow yet produce little or no increase in GFR and SNGFR, in part due to a large decline in K_f.[406–408] PGE_1 infusion yields little or no increase in SNGFR despite an increase in Q_A due to a large decline in K_f, with little or no change in $\overline{\Delta P}$ or π_A.[408] During blockade of endogenous prostaglandin production infusion of PGE_2 or PGI_2 induce large declines in SNGFR and Q_A accompanied by an increase in renal vascular resistance (particularly R_E), increases in $\overline{P}_{GC}$ and $\overline{\Delta P}$, and a decline in K_f.[409] Additional blockade of AII recep- tors during cyclooxygenase inhibition yielded marked vasodilation in response to PGE_2 or PGI_2 resulting in a return of SNGFR and Q_A equal to or greater than control values, a fall in P_{GC} below control values, and a return of K_f to normal.[409] Thus, the renal vasoconstriction induced by exogenous PGE_2 or PGI_2 appears to be mediated by induction of renin and AII production. Vasodilatation at the whole kidney level resulting from PGI_2 infusion during cyclooxygenase and AII inhibition has not always been observed.[410] Topical application (but not luminal) of PGE_2 to the afferent arteriole increased the vasoconstrictive effect of AII and norepinephrine whereas PGI_2 only attenuated norepinephrine-induced vasoconstriction.[411] PGE_2 also constricted interlobular arteries but neither prostaglandin produced vasodilatation of vessels preconstricted by AII.[411] Indomethacin alone induced vasoconstriction of all pre- and postglomerular resistance vessels of superficial and juxtamedullary nephrons suggesting that vasodilatory prostaglandins normally modulate endogenous vasoconstrictors.[412] The combination of cyclooxygenase inhibition with an ACE inhibitor caused vasodilatation of pre- but not postglomerular vessels of the cortical nephrons due to the effects of continued NO production on preglomerular vessels.[412] These data taken together indicate that there could indeed be differences in the response to vasoactive prostaglandins between superficial and deep nephrons.

Norepinephrine

Systemic infusion of norepinephrine increases arterial blood pressure and induces vasoconstriction of the preglomerular vessels and the efferent arteriole, resulting in a decrease in Q_A but with unknown effects on K_f.[413] $\overline{P}_{GC}$ and $\overline{\Delta P}$ increase with norepinephrine infusion, however, so that SNGFR is relatively unchanged.[413] Like angiotensin II, norepinephrine constricts the arcuate artery, the interlobular arteries, and the afferent and efferent arterioles as well as mesangial cells.[130,133,313,411,423,414] Vasoconstriction of the afferent and efferent arterioles occurs via activation of α_1 receptors.[415] This is partially counterbalanced, however, by activation of cycloxygensase-2 (COX-2) to increase production of the prostaglandins PGE_2 and $PGF_{2\alpha}$.[414]

Antidiuretic Hormone

Antidiuretic hormone (ADH or arginine vasopressin, AVP) at low doses causes renal vasodilatation in the dog[416] whereas acute intravenous infusion of AVP in Munich-Wistar rats undergoing a chronic water diuresis does not change SNGFR or Q_A but markedly decreases K_f.[417] SNGFR was maintained despite the fall in K_f because of a decline in proximal tubule hydraulic pressure that resulted in a rise in ΔP. By contrast chronic administration of AVP or the V2 agonist dDAVP causes a large increase in GFR in the conscious rat in direct relationship with increases in urine osmolality suggesting possible renal vasodilatation, but glomerular dynamics were not studied in this model.[418–420] AVP-induced renal vasodilatation appears to be mediated by increased nitric oxide production[421,422] and vasodilatory prostaglandins and a vasoconstrictor effect is unmasked when prostaglandin production is blocked.[423]

Arginine vasopressin has been shown to constrict afferent and efferent arterioles and mesangial cells by activating V_1 subtype vasopressin receptors.[424–426] However, when afferent arterioles were pretreated with a V_1 receptor antagonist and constricted with norepinephrine, AVP caused vasodilatation, an effect blocked by a V_2 receptor antagonist.[426] This suggests that AVP causes vasoconstriction through interaction with V_1 receptors and causes vasodilatation through interaction with V_2 receptors and both are present on the same vessel.[426]

Leukotrienes and Lipoxins

Leukotrienes are a class of lipid products formed from arachidonic acid following activation of the 5-lipoxygenase enzymes glutathione-S-alkyl-transferase and glutamyl transpeptidase.[427] Leukotrienes known to affect glomerular filtration and renal blood flow are leukotrienes C_4 (LTC_4), leukotriene D_4 (LTD_4), and leukotriene B_4 (LTB_4). LTC_4 and LTD_4 are potent vasoconstrictors[428] whereas LTB_4 produces moderate renal vasodilatation and an increase in renal blood flow with no change in GFR in the normal rat.[429] Intravenous infusion of LTC_4 increases renal vascular resistance leading to a fall in renal blood flow and GFR as well as a decrease in plasma volume and cardiac output.[430,431] The decline in renal blood flow is partially but not completely reversed by saralasin (AII receptor antagonist) and indomethacin (inhibitor of cyclooxygenase), indicating (1) involvement of angiotensin II and cyclooxygenase products in the response to LTC_4 and (2) an additional direct effect of LTC_4 on the renal resistance vessels.[431] Similarly LTD_4 induced a marked decrease in K_f, a rise in renal vascular resistance, particularly in R_E, a fall in Q_A and SNGFR, and a rise in $\overline{P}_{GC}$ and $\overline{\Delta P}$ during blockade of AII and control of renal perfusion pressure demonstrating a direct effect of this leukotriene on renal hemodynamics.[432]

Inflammatory injury also activates the 5-, 12-, and 15-lipoxygenase pathways in neutorphils and platelets to form acyclic eicosanoids called lipoxins (LX) of which there are two main types, LXA_4 and LXB_4.[433] The lipoxins produce diverse effects on renal hemodynamics. LXB_4 and 7-cis-11-trans-LXA_4 produce renal vasoconstriction.[434] By contrast intrarenal infusion of LXA_4 induces a marked reduction in preglomerular hydraulic resistance (R_A) without affecting R_E, thereby resulting in an increase in $\overline{P}_{GC}$ and $\overline{\Delta P}$.[435] The specific vasodilatation of the preglomerular vessels by LXA_4 was blocked by cyclooxygenase inhibition indicating that vasodilatory prostaglandins were responsible for this effect.[434,435] Unique to this compound, LXA_4 produced vasodilatation while simultaneously causing a reduction in K_f.[434] Because $\overline{P}_{GC}$, $\overline{\Delta P}$, and Q_A were increased, however, SNGFR also increased.[435]

Platelet-Activating Factor

Platelet-activating factor (PAF) (1-O-alkyl-2-acetyl-sn-glycero-3-phosphorylcholine) is a phospholipid involved in allergic reactions and inflammatory processes.[436] In the kidney PAF is both produced and metabolized by glomerular mesangial cells.[437] Intrarenal infusion of low dose PAF results in renal vasodilatation and an increase in renal blood flow mediated through enhanced nitric oxide production.[169,438] Higher intrarenal doses of PAF, by contrast, result in AII-independent renal vasoconstriction and a decrease in K_f resulting in declines in both SNGFR and Q_A.[437,439,440] These effects were blocked by inhibition of cyclooxygenase suggesting that PAF stimulates production of vasoconstrictor cyclooxygenase products such as thromboxane A_2. Indeed concomitant administration of a thromboxane A_2 receptor antagonist resulted in a PAF-induced increase in renal plasma flow and GFR.[439] PAF in picomolar concentrations causes vasodilatation of afferent arteriole through stimulation of NO production whereas nanomolar doses result in vasoconstriction.[440] PAF in nanomolar concentrations also constricts the efferent arteriole, an effect that is attenuated by pretreatment with indomethecin.[441] Possibly related to the PAF-induced decrease in K_f, PAF constricts mesangial cells, probably through increased production of thromboxane A_2.[439] Endothelin increases PAF production by isolated glomeruli and blockade of PAF receptor binding prevents endothelin-induced renal vasoconstriction as well as endothelin-induced contraction of isolated glomeruli and mesangial cells, suggesting that PAF may be a mediator of the effects of endothelin.[442]

Acetylcholine

Acetylcholine is a potent vasodilator that increases renal blood flow without changing SNGFR.[403,408,443] The interlobular arteries and afferent and efferent arterioles vasodilate in response to acetylcholine and the effects can be prevented by muscarinic receptor antagonists.[120,408,443] As a consequence of the decrease in renal vascular resistance Q_A increased in response to acetylcholine in the rat as did ΔP (R_A decreased more than R_E so that $\overline{P}_{GC}$ and $\overline{\Delta P}$ increased), yet SNGFR remained unchanged because of a marked decline in K_f.[408]

Acetylcholine-induced renal and systemic vasodilatation is mediated in part through the stimulation of NO production,[150,172,191,313,403,444–446] enhanced production of vasodilatory prostaglandins,[166,403,447] and production of a putative endothelium-derived hyperpolarizing factor (EDHF) that hyperpolarizes adjacent vascular smooth muscle.[447–453] Figure 3–20 summarizes the mechanisms by which a number of vasodilators including acetylcholine and bradykinin might lead to vasodilatation. Acetylcholine acts on muscarinic receptors of the endothelium to increase endothelial intracellular $[Ca^{2+}]_i$ leading to opening of Ca^{2+}-activated K^+ channels and endothelial membrane hyperpolarization.[453] By way of myoendothelial gap junctions hyperpolarization of adjacent smooth muscle cells results in closure of voltage-gated Ca^{2+} channels, a decrease in $[Ca^{2+}]_i$, and vasodilatation.[452,453] The increase in endothelial $[Ca^{2+}]_i$ following stimulation of the muscarinic receptors also triggers the production of nitric oxide and prostanoids in the endothelium, which hyperpolarize the underlying smooth muscle by activation of ATP-sensitive K^+ channels.[451] Thus acetylcholine can stimulate three endothelium-dependent vasodilatation pathways, the production of vasodilatory prostaglandins, the production of nitric oxide, and the production of EDHF.[454]

Bradykinin

Bradykinin is a potent vasodilator that produces large increases in renal blood flow due to dilation of both the preglomerular blood vessels and the efferent arteriole mediated through the bradykinin B_2 receptor.[408,455–457] Although in the rat bradykinin had no significant effects on $\overline{\Delta P}$, the increase in Q_A that might be expected to increase SNGFR failed to do so because K_f fell to levels half of those seen in normal rats.[408] Figure 3–20 summarizes potential mechanisms of bradykinin-induced vasodilatation. Bradykinin stimulates inositol (1,4,5)-trisphosphate production and increased cytosolic free $[Ca^{2+}]$ in cultured mesangial cells, glomerular epithelial cells, and vascular endothelial cells.[314,412,458,459] Subsequent activation

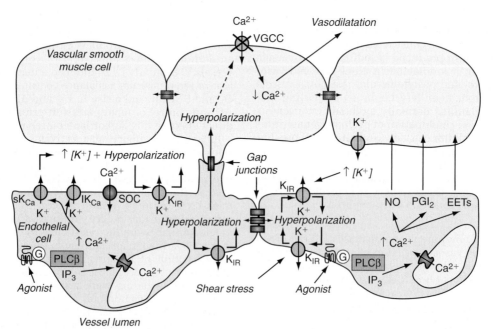

FIGURE 3–20 Potential mechanisms involved in endothelium-dependent vasodilatation in response to agonists such as acetylcholine, bradykinin, or ATP. Coupling of agonists to G-protein coupled receptors activates the beta isoform of protein kinase C (PKC-β) leading to the production of inositol 3,4,5, trisphosphate (IP_3) with subsequent rapid release of intracellular calcium stores followed by increased calcium influx through store-operated calcium channels (SOC). Increased $[Ca^{2+}]_i$ opens intermediate or small Ca^{2+}-activated K^+ channels (IK_{Ca} and/or sK_{Ca}, respectively) leading to endothelial cell membrane hyperpolarization. The hyperpolarization may activate K^+_{IR} channels, contributing to the hyperpolarization. Endothlieal shear stress may also active these channels. Coupling of endothelial cell hyperpolarization to adjacent vascular smooth muscle cells through gap junctions may then close voltage-gated calcium channels (VGCC) leading to a fall in smooth muscle intracellular calcium concentration and vasodilatation. Agonist-induced increases in endothelial cell $[Ca^{2+}]_i$ also increases production of NO and cyclooxygenase and epoxygenase-derived vasodilator compounds, which when combined with hyperpolarization, yields smooth muscle vasodilatation. (Figure reproduced by permission from Jackson WF: Silent inward rectifier K^+ channels in hypercholesterolemia. Circ Res 98:982–984, 2006.)

of Ca^{2+}-dependent potassium channels and activation of chloride channels leads to membrane depolarization and relaxation.[166,460-462] Low concentrations of bradykinin induce vasodilatation of isolated afferent and efferent arterioles in the rat[120] mediated via bradykinin B_2 receptors.[412] In the rabbit low concentrations of bradykinin (10^{-12} mol/L to 10^{-10} mol/L) dilate the afferent arteriole via B_2 receptor activation while high concentrations (10^{-9} mol/L to 10^{-8} mol/L) result in vasoconstriction.[456] By contrast, high concentrations of bradykinin cause vasodilatation of the efferent arteriole in that species.[456] Vasoconstriction of the afferent arteriole to high concentrations of bradykinin appears to be mediated through vasoconstrictor prostanoids.[463] Bradykinin-induced vasodilatation of the afferent arteriole is mediated by cyclooxygenase vasodilator products including PGE_2 and epoxyeicosatrienoic acids (EETs) via increased epoxygenase activity.[464] When the efferent arteriole is perfused in a retrograde fashion with bradykinin the response, acting through B_2 receptors, is a dose-dependent vasodilatation that is independent of either NO or cyclooxygenase metabolites.[463] Instead the vasodilator effects in that segment under such conditions are mediated by cytochrome P450 metabolites, probably EETs.[463] In the absence of cyclooxygenase inhibitors bradykinin infused orthograde through the afferent arteriole induces the glomerular release of a vasoconstrictor (20-hydroxyeicosatetraenoic acid, 20-HETE) that blunts the vasodilator effects of bradykinin-induced release of EETs from the efferent arteriole and glomerulus.[465]

Glucocorticoids

Chronic administration of glucocorticoid hormones increases glomerular filtration rate as a direct consequence of an increase in plasma flow since K_f, π_A, and $\overline{\Delta P}$ are unaffected.[466,467] For cortisol renal vasodilatation involves stimulation of NO production.[467] Volume retention, tubuloglomerular feedback, and alterations in eicosanoid production do not appear to be involved in the renal response to glucocorticoids.[466]

Insulin

Insulin, necessary for tissue glucose metabolism, is also a vasoactive hormone important in the regulation of blood pressure and glomerular filtration rate.[468] Insulin is a vasodilator in the systemic and renal vasculature, acting in part through a stimulation of nitric oxide formation.[469-472] Vasodilatation in response to insulin can still take place during inhibition of nitric oxide synthesis, however and this effect is mediated in part through increased production of the metabolite adenosine.[473] In normal rats acute insulin infusion (during euglycoemic clamp) decreases preglomerular and efferent arteriolar resistance resulting in increases in Q_A, SNGFR, and $\overline{\Delta P}$.[474]

Early insulin-dependent diabetes is characterized by high rates of renal blood flow and glomerular filtration due, in part, to elevations in atrial natriuretic peptide and vasodilatory prostaglandins.[474,475] Insulin administration in diabetic animals produces preglomerular vasoconstriction rather than the vasodilatation seen in normal animals resulting in decreases in Q_A, $\overline{P}_{GC}$ and $\overline{\Delta P}$, and SNGFR.[474] The increase in preglomerular resistance observed following insulin infusion in the diabetic animal could be related to a stimulation of vasoconstrictor prostaglandin (thromboxane A_2) and endothelin production that might obviate any vasodilatory effects of insulin.[206,474]

Insulin-Like Growth Factor

Insulin-like growth factor (IGF) is produced as two peptides hormones, IGF-I and IGF-II, which upon secretion, are >99% bound to IGF-binding proteins that regulate the bioavailability of IGFs.[476] IGF-1 is produced in several portions of the nephron including mesangial cells that also contain IGF-1 receptors.[476,477] High dietary protein intake (which increases GFR) increases IGF-1 production and increases the bioavail-

ability of the peptide, whereas decreased protein intake or fasting decrease IGF-1 production and increase binding protein levels.[476] The response to acute IGF-1 administration is vasodilatation of preglomerular blood vessels and the efferent arteriole leading to increases in GFR and RPF.[478-483] Administration of IGF-1 to either non-starved (12h food restriction) or in rats with short-term starvation (60–72 h food restriction), which would have low levels of circulating IGF-1, resulted in increases in SNGFR and Q_A.[478] The increase in SNGFR was a consequence of the large increases in Q_A and a near doubling of K_f because $\overline{P}_{GC}$ and $\overline{\Delta P}$ were unaffected by IGF-1.[478] Increases in vasodilatory prostaglandins and nitric oxide production combined with stimulation of the renal kalikrein/kinin system are largely responsible for the renal vasodilatation induced by IGF-1.[479,481,484] Inhibition of the effects of AII by IGF-1[149] may be responsible for the increase in K_f observed with IGF-I infusions.[478]

Calcitonin Gene-Related Peptide (CGRP)

Calcitonin-gene related peptide (CGRP) is a 37-amino acid peptide that is an important cardiovascular vasodilator that also causes renal vasodilatation yielding an increase in renal blood flow and GFR while decreasing systemic blood pressure.[485] Atrial natriuretic peptide (ANP) and two other peptides, long-acting natriuretic peptide and vessel dilator, all increase circulating CGRP threefold to fourfold with the effects of ANP on CGRP being of shorter duration than with the other two peptides.[486] Immunohistochemical staining of CGRP-containing nerves and nerve terminals are observed in the main renal artery, arcuate arteries, interlobular arteries, afferent arterioles including the juxtaglomerular apparatus, and the veins, with some staining of the efferent arterioles.[487] CGRP by itself does not affect the diameter of isolated afferent or efferent arterioles,[488] but CGRP produced a dose-dependent inhibition of myogenic reactivity in the afferent arteriole and vasodilatation of both afferent and efferent arterioles preconstricted by AII.[488-490] CGRP can also induce vasodilatation in norepinephrine-contracted afferent, but not efferent, arterioles.[488,489] CGRP reverses renal vasoconstriction and the accompanying reduction in GFR in the kidney induced by endothelin[485] as well as norepinephrine-induced constriction in the isolated perfused kidney.[491] Calcitonin, by contrast, had no vasodilatory effects on either the afferent or efferent arteriole.[489]

The renal vasodilatory effects of CGRP are mediated at least in part through stimulation of the production of NO.[171-173,485,492] CGRP also increases the production of cAMP in isolated glomeruli[489] as well as in the whole kidney[493] suggesting a role for cAMP in the vasodilatation produced by CGRP. Pretreatment with indomethacin does not block the renal vasodilatation and increase in GFR observed with CGRP administration indicating that prostaglandins are not involved in the response to CGRP.[485]

Relaxin

Relaxin, an ovarian hormone secreted by the corpus luteum in pregnancy, appears to be involved in the endothelin-nitric oxide-cGMP pathway responsible for the renal vasodilatation seen in the first two trimesters.[494-496] Relaxin is a potent vasodilator and chronic administration of relaxin to virgin females increases in GFR and RPF and produces a decrease in plasma osmolality and hematocrit suggesting plasma volume expansion[494,496] similar to that seen in pregnancy.[497] Relaxin antibodies block the gestational elevation of GFR and RPF and prevent the reduction in myogenic activity of small renal arteries.[498] In addition chronic administration of relaxin to either overiectomized rats or to male rats results in an increase in GFR and RPF indicating that estrogen and progesterone are not necessary for the vasodilatory effects of relaxin.[494,496] Acute blockade of NO production completely reverses chronic relaxin-induced hyperfiltration and hyperperfusion indicating that relaxin stimulates NO production.[496] The vasodilatory effects of chronic relaxin administration are completely reversed by a specific ET_B receptor antagonist or a NOS inhibitor.[494,498] Pressure-induced myogenic reactivity is reduced in small renal and mesenteric arteries isolated from midgestational rats leading to a greater increase in diameter in response to a greater increase in pressure than normal.[499] Myogenic reactivity of these vessels was restored to levels seen in vessels obtained from virgin rats when the vessels from the pregnant animals were incubated with NOS inhibitors, a selective ET_B receptor antagonist, or had the endothelium removed.[499] Thus plasma volume expansion and the renal vasodilatation and glomerular hyperfiltration observed in pregnancy appear to be largely mediated through the release of relaxin leading to activation of ET_B receptors, increased NO production, and increased GFR and RPF.

Natriuretic Peptides

Increased left atrial pressure such as that induced by blood volume expansion leads to natriuresis and diuresis[500,501] caused by release of an atrial natriuretic peptide (ANP).[502] ANP is synthesized as part of a larger (151 amino acid) preprohormone (preproANP) and is stored in the atria as a high molecular weight 126 amino acid precursor, proANP.[503] Upon release from the atria proANP is cleaved yielding two polypeptides including the 28 amino acid active form of the peptide, ANP.[503] Other ANP-like natriuretic compounds include brain natriuretic peptide (BNP) and two ANP-like natriuretic peptides produced by the kidney, one a natriuretic peptide containing 32 amino acids known as urodilatin (URO)[460,504,505] and a C-type natriuretic peptide (C-ANP).[506,507] Receptors for ANP have been identified in the glomerulus,[508] the arcuate and interlobular arteries, and the afferent and efferent arterioles.[509] ANP A-Type receptors mediate the vascular response to ANP in the afferent and efferent arterioles but ANP binds to both ANP Type-A and ANP Type-C receptors.[509] The biological effects of URO are mediated by cGMP following interaction with an ANP A-type receptor whereas C-ANP binds to both C-ANP type and B-ANP type receptors but only exerts its effects through the ANP B-Type receptor located primarily in the glomerulus, the afferent arteriole, and distal portions of the nephron.[149,506,507,509,510] The C-ANP dilates afferent arterioles via a prostaglandin/nitric oxide pathway. A third type of ANP receptor, the ANP C-type receptor, serves to clear natriuretic peptides with no vasoactive effects.[509] ANP stimulates secretion of URO resulting in large increases in circulating URO.[511] Glomerular ANP receptor density is down-regulated in rats on a high-salt diet and upregulated in rats on a low-salt diet.[508,512] ANP stimulates NO production and increases guanylate cyclase activity and cyclic GMP production in the kidney.[446]

Acute and chronic blood volume expansion and increased atrial pressure increase plasma levels of ANP and BNP.[513–516] Systemic blood pressure decreases and GFR, filtration fraction, and salt and water excretion increase in response to exogenous ANP.[98,513,516,517] Studies in the hydronephrotic kidney preparation demonstrated increased glomerular blood flow in a dose-dependent manner in response to both ANP and urodilantin.[412] In the euvolemic rat, pretreatment with an ANP receptor antagonist resulted in a significantly lower GFR during subsequent ANP infusion than was observed in control rats receiving vehicle prior to the ANP infusion,[475,518] again suggesting a role for ANP in the control of GFR in the normal rat. Renal hemodynamics are not altered by ANP antibody administration or ANP receptor antagonists in rats with myocardial infarction or congestive heart failure.[516,519] ANP receptor antagonists decreased GFR in DOCA-salt hypertension, a model associated with elevated ANP and BNP levels.[515] Infusion of ANP antibodies into diabetic animals that already had elevated baseline values of GFR and RPF reduced GFR toward normal animal levels, indicating that high endogenous ANP contributes to hyperfiltration in early diabetes.[475,514] The effect of natriuretic peptide inhibition on GFR and RPF is greatest under conditions of high levels of endogenous natriuretic peptides such as chronic high sodium intake.[520] Elevated prostacyclin and PGE_2 production also contribute to the hyperfiltration seen in diabetes.[514,521]

Atrial natriuretic peptide increases SNGFR without altering Q_A in the rat resulting in an increase in filtration fraction.[98] Unique among vasoactive agents, ANP induces preglomerular vasodilatation (arcuate arteries, interlobular arteries, and afferent aterioles) but efferent arteriolar vasoconstriction.[98,412,506,509] As a consequence $\overline{P}_{GC}$ and $\overline{\Delta P}$ increased with little effect on K_f indicating that the increase in SNGFR was almost entirely the consequence of the increase in ΔP.[98] The preglomerular vasodilatation and efferent arteriolar constriction occurred even when AII receptors were blocked or renal perfusion pressure was controlled.[98]

Similar to the effects of ANP, urodilatin also produces dose-dependent vasodilatation of the arcuate and interlobular arteries and afferent arteriole, vasoconstriction of the efferent arteriole, and a net increase in glomerular blood flow in both cortical and juxtamedullary nephrons.[412] Low-dose URO inhibits the renin-angiotensin system whereas high concentrations of URO activate it leading to variable effects on RPF and GFR depending on the dose used.[412,518,522,523] Angiotensin converting enzyme inhibition (ACEI) combined ACEI and cyclooxygenase inhibition (CYOI), and endothelin receptor blockade reduced the URO-induced vasodilatation of the preglomerular vessels.[412] URO-induced vasoconstriction of the efferent arteriole is exaggerated by NO blockade and was completely blocked by combined AII and cyclooxygenase inhibition, by bradykinin receptor blockade, and by endothelin blockade.[412] C-ANP induces dose-dependent vasodilatation of both the preglomerular and postglomerular vessels and a large increase in renal blood flow.[509]

Parathyroid Hormone

Parathyroid hormone (PTH) has renal hemodynamic effects in addition to regulating calcium and phosphate transport in the kidney. Intrarenal infusion of PTH (1–34) produces a dose-dependent increase in RBF when given at low enough doses to prevent a fall in blood pressure.[524] Low-dose PTH administered intravenously to thyroparathyroidectomized (TPTX) animals or high-dose PTH to normal animals causes a marked reduction in K_f.[525] PTH in the rat caused a decline in SNGFR without affecting Q_A, $\overline{P}_{GC}$, or $\overline{\Delta P}$ owing to the reduction in K_f.[525] In the dog SNGFR did not decrease despite the decline in K_f because of a small increase in $\overline{\Delta P}$.[526] Intravenous administration of PTH in some studies increases renal blood flow in the intact animal.[527] Trizna and Edwards observed relaxation of isolated norepinephrine-contracted afferent and efferent arterioles in response to PTH that was completely blocked by a specific PTH antagonist.[528] These data indicate that PTH is a vasodilator, but in vivo administration of PTH can secondarily lead to the release of counteracting vasoconstrictor substances.

Parathyroid hormone increases cAMP production in glomeruli, vascular endothelial cells, mesangial cells, and proximal tubules.[528–531] If prostaglandin synthesis is inhibited, subsequent administration of PTH results in reductions in both SNGFR and Q_A and a decrease in K_f.[409] When prostaglandin synthesis inhibition and AII receptor blockade are combined, the effects of PTH on glomerular hemodynamics are completely abolished and K_f returns to normal.[409] PTH also stimulates NO and cGMP production.[531] Thus the effects of PTH appear to be mediated through stimulation of cAMP production leading to enhanced renin/AII production[532] and a reduction in K_f. The hemodynamic effects of AII, in turn, are modulated by enhanced production of nitric oxide and vasodilatory prostaglandins.

Parathyroid Hormone-Related Protein (PTHrP)

PTH-related protein (PTHrP) has an amino acid sequence at the N-terminus that is similar to PTH and binds to and acts through a common PTH/PTHrP receptor.[533] PTHrP is found in the media of smooth muscle cells and in endothelial cells of all renal microvessels including the afferent and efferent arterioles, the interlobular and arcuate arteries, and the macula densa as well as in the visceral and parietal cells of the glomerulus and the tubules.[534] Intrarenal infusion of PTHrP in the rat at low doses increased RBF and GFR in the absence of changes in heart rate or mean arterial pressure similar to effects seen with PTH.[524,535] Both PTH and PTHrP cause renal vasodilatation in the isolated kidney ruling out a role for the renal nerves or stimulation of other extrarenal hormones in producing the effects.[536] Preglomerular vessels vasodilate in response to either PTH or PTHrP in almost an identical fashion[535] and both PTH and PTHrP stimulate renin release.[531] This may account for the failure of the efferent arteriole in the intact animal to vasodilate in response to PTH or PTHrP in the absence of angiotensin II inhibition[535] because that segment is more sensitive to AII. In accord with that hypothesis isolated perfused afferent and efferent arterioles both vasodilate in response to PTHrP as well as PTH.[528] PTHrP as well as PTH stimulates adenylate cyclase activity and cAMP formation in isolated glomeruli, vascular endothelial cells, and cultured mesangial cells as well as in the isolated kidney.[529-531] Both PTH and PTHrP stimulate activation of endothelial-derived NO production via PTH/PTHrP receptors and mediated by the calcium/calmodulin pathway,[530] and inhibition of NOS markedly reduces PTHrP-induced vasorelaxation.[534,537] PTHrP also inhibits endothelin-1 production in cultured endothelial cells, possibly mediated through increased NO and cGMP production.[537,538] Thus PTHrP may play an important role in the local regulation of renal blood flow and glomerular filtration rate.

Adrenomedullin

Adrenomedullin (ADM) is a 52 amino acid peptide that was isolated from human pheochromocytoma in the adrenal medulla that induces hypotension.[539] Messenger RNA for ADM is found in a number of organs including the kidney.[540,541] ADM induces arterial vasodilatation via interaction with $CGRP_1$ receptors[542] and both ADM and CGRP stimulate cAMP formation in glomeruli and glomerular mesangial cells, but ADM is more potent.[543,544] Intrarenal administration of ADM increases renal blood flow and GFR whereas intravenous infusion decreases RBF in the absence of changes in GFR.[543,545-547] The increase in RBF induced by ADM occurs even in the presence of a CGRP antagonist and both the renal artery and outer cortical glomeruli have high affinity ADM binding sites specific to ADM and have a very low or no affinity for CGRP.[543,547] ADM inhibits PDGF-induced ET-1 production in mesangial cells suggesting that its vasodilatory capability is mediated, in part, through reduced vasoconstrictor production.[544] This peptide may therefore play a role, indirectly or directly, in the control of glomerular filtration rate and renal blood flow.

Neural Regulation of Glomerular Filtration Rate

The renal vasculature including the afferent arteriole and the efferent arteriole, the macula densa cells of the distal tubule, and the glomerular mesangium are richly innervated.[18,548] Innervation includes renal efferent sympathetic adrenergic nerves[548,549] and renal afferent sensory fibers containing

peptides such as calcitonin gene-related peptide (CGRP) and substance P.[18,548] Acetylcholine is a potent vasodilator of the renal vasculature (discussed previously), suggesting a role for this neurotransmitter in the control of the renal circulation. Sympathetic efferent nerves are found in all segments of the vascular tree from the main renal artery to the afferent arteriole (including the renin-containing juxtaglomerular cells) and the efferent arteriole[548,549] and play an important role in the regulation of renal hemodynamics, sodium transport, and renin secretion.[550] Afferent nerves containing CGRP and substance P are localized primarily in the main renal artery and interlobar arteries, with some innervation also observed in the arcuate artery, the interlobular artery, and the afferent arteriole including the juxtaglomerular apparatus.[548,549] Peptidergic nerve fibers immunoreactive for neuropeptide Y (NPY), neurotensin, vasoactive intestinal polypeptide, and somatostatin are also found in the kidney.[551] Neuronal nitric oxide synthase-immunoreactive neurons have now been identified in the kidney.[548,552] The NOS-containing neuronal somata are seen in the wall of the renal pelvis, at the renal hilus close to the renal artery, along the interlobar arteries, the arcuate arteries, and extending to the afferent arteriole suggesting they have a role in the control of renal blood flow.[548,552] They were also present in nerve bundles having vasomotor and sensory fibers suggesting they might modulate renal neural function.[548,552]

In micropuncture studies of the effects of renal nerve stimulation (RNS), RNS alone increased R_A and R_E resulting in a fall in Q_A and SNGFR without any effect on K_f.[553] When prostaglandin production was inhibited by indomethacin, however, the same level of RNS produced even greater increases in R_A and R_E accompanied by very large declines in Q_A and SNGFR and decreases in K_f, $\overline{P}_{GC}$, and $\overline{\Delta P}$.[553] When saralasin was administered as a competitive inhibitor of endogenous AII in conjunction with indomethacin, RNS had no effect on K_f, but both R_A and R_E were still increased, and $\overline{\Delta P}$ was slightly reduced.[553] The release of norepinephrine by RNS enhances AII production to yield arteriolar vasoconstriction and reduction in K_f. The increase in AII production may then enhance vasodilator prostaglandin production,[553,554] which partially ameliorates the constriction. Continued vasoconstriction by RNS during blockade of endogenous prostaglandins and AII suggests that norepinephrine has separate vasoconstrictive properties by itself. In agreement with this suggestion are the findings that norepinephrine causes constriction of preglomerular vessels.[137] Inhibition of nitric oxide synthase results in a decline in SNGFR in normal rats but not in rats with surgical renal denervation suggesting that nitric oxide normally modulates the effects of renal adrenergic activity.[555] This modulation does not appear, however, to be related to sympathetic modulation of renin secretion.[556]

Renal denervation in animals undergoing acute water deprivation (48 h duration) or with congestive heart failure produces increases in SNGFR, Q_A, and K_f.[557] This suggests that the natural activity of the renal nerves in these settings plays an important role in the constriction of the arterioles and reduction in K_f that were observed.[557] The vasoconstrictive effects of the renal nerves in both settings were mediated in part by a stimulatory effect on AII release, together with a direct vasoconstrictive effect on the preglomerular and postglomerular blood vessels.[557] These studies demonstrate the important role of the renal nerves in pathophysiological settings.

DETERMINANTS OF GLOMERULAR ULTRAFILTRATION

The filtration of a nearly protein-free fluid from the glomerular capillaries into Bowman space represents the first step in the process of urine formation. Electrolytes, amino acids, glucose, and other endogenous or exogenous compounds with molecular radii smaller than 20 Å are freely filtered while molecules larger than ~50 Å are virtually excluded from filtration.[551,558-562] This process of ultrafiltration of fluid is governed by the net balance between the transcapillary hydraulic pressure gradient (ΔP), the transcapillary colloid osmotic pressure gradient ($\Delta \pi$), and the hydraulic permeability of the filtration barrier (k), which determine the rate of fluid movement (J_v) across any given point of a capillary wall based on the expression:

$$J_V = k(\Delta P - \Delta \pi)$$
$$= k[(P_{GC} - P_T) - (\pi_{GC} - \pi_T)] \quad (1)$$

where P_{GC} and P_T are the hydraulic pressures in the glomerular capillaries and Bowman space, respectively, and π_{GC} and π_T are the corresponding colloid osmotic pressures. The protein concentration of the fluid in Bowman space is essentially zero and thus π_T is also zero. Total glomerular filtration rate for a single nephron (SNGFR) is equal to the product of the surface area for filtration (S) and average values along the length of the glomerular capillaries of the right-hand terms in Equation 1, yielding the expression:

$$SNGFR = kS \times (\Delta P - \Delta \pi)$$
$$= K_f \bar{P}_{UF} \quad (2)$$

K_f, the glomerular ultrafiltration coefficient, is the product of S and k while $\bar{P}_{UF}$, the mean net ultrafiltration pressure, is the difference between the mean transcapillary and colloid osmotic pressure differences, $\overline{\Delta P}$ and $\overline{\Delta \pi}$, respectively.

The barrier for ultrafiltration consists of the glomerular capillary endothelium with its fenestrations, the glomerular basement membrane, the filtration slits between glomerular epithelial cell foot processes, and ultimately the filtration slit diaphragm within the filtration slits. Mathematical modeling based on known ultrastructural detail and the hydrodynamic properties of the individual components of the filtration barrier

suggests that only ~2% of the total hydraulic resistance is accounted for by the fenestrated capillary endothelium whereas the basement membrane accounts for nearly 50%.[563-565] The filtration slits between the glomerular epithelial foot processes account for the remaining hydraulic resistance with the majority of that resistance residing in the filtration slit diaphragm.[563,564] A reduction in the frequency of the filtration slits is an important factor in controlling filtration in some disease states.[564,566]

Hydraulic Pressures in the Glomerular Capillaries and Bowman Space

The first direct measurements of P_{GC} in the Munich-Wistar rat were obtained 36 years ago by Brenner and co-workers[560] who found that $\bar{P}_{GC}$* averaged 46 mm Hg. Many studies subsequently confirmed the original observations demonstrating that values for $\bar{P}_{GC}$ average 43 mm Hg to 49 mm Hg (Fig. 3–21) with similar values found in the squirrel monkey.[567] Because P_{GC} is nearly constant along the length of the capillary bed the transcapillary hydraulic pressure difference averages 34 mm Hg in the hydropenic Munich-Wistar rat (see Fig. 3–21). Coupling these hydraulic pressure measurements with direct determinations of efferent arteriolar protein concentrations of superficial nephrons[568] permits direct determination of all of hydraulic and oncotic pressures that govern glomerular ultrafiltration at the beginning and end of the capillary network.

The early direct measurements of $\bar{P}_{GC}$ were obtained in the hydropenic rats that exhibit a surgically induced reduction in plasma volume and glomerular filtration rate.[569] As shown in Figure 3–21, following restoration of plasma volume to the

*$\bar{P}_{GC}$ represents the average value for the mean pulsatile glomerular capillary hydraulic pressure as measured along the whole glomerulus.[551]

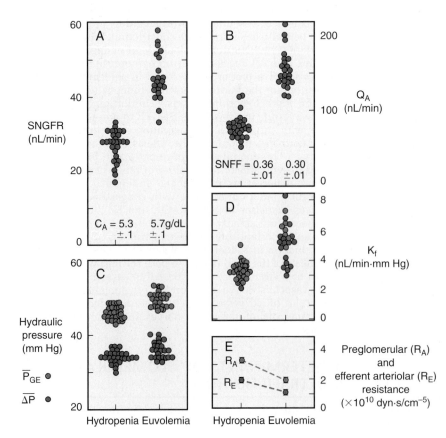

FIGURE 3–21 Glomerular ultrafiltration in the Munich-Wistar rat. Each point represents the mean value reported for studies in hydropenic and euvolemic rats provided food and water ad libitum until the time of study. Only studies using male or a mix of male and female rats are shown. Values of the ultrafiltration coefficient, K_f, shown by filled circles in panel D denote minimum values because the animals were in filtration pressure equilibrium. Open circles represent unique values of K_f calculated under conditions of filtration pressure disequilibrium $\pi_E/\overline{\Delta P} \leq 0.95$. (See Refs 18 and 551 for data sources.)

"euvolemic" state by infusion of isooncotic plasma yields single nephron glomerular filtration rates (SNGFR) substantially higher in euvolemic animals than in hydropenic rats primarily as a consequence of a marked increase in glomerular plasma flow (Q_A) associated with a fall in preglomerular (R_A) and efferent arteriolar (R_E) resistance values. Because surface glomeruli are not available in most experimental animals the stop-flow technique has been used by a number of investigators to estimate $\bar{P}_{GC}$ and comparisons of glomerular capillary pressure calculated using the stop-flow technique (P_{GCSF}) with direct determinations of $\bar{P}_{GC}$ generally indicate that P_{GCSF} provides a reasonable estimate of $\bar{P}_{GC}$ with P_{GCSF} generally being ~2 mm Hg greater than that for $\bar{P}_{GC}$ measured directly.[18]

Glomerular Capillary Hydraulic and Colloid Osmotic Pressure Profiles

Figure 3–22 depicts the glomerular capillary hydraulic and oncotic pressure profiles for hydropenic and euvolemic Munich-Wistar rats using the mean values determined from the studies shown in Figure 3–21. Plasma oncotic pressure at the efferent end of the glomerular capillary (π_E) rises to a value that, on average, equals ΔP yielding a reduction in net local ultrafiltration pressure, P_{UF}, [$P_{GC} - (P_T + \pi_{GC})$] from approximately 17 mm Hg at the afferent end of the glomerular capillary network to essentially zero by the efferent end in hydropenic animals. The equality between π_E and $\overline{\Delta P}$ is referred to as filtration pressure equilibrium. As seen in Figure 3–21, panel D, filtration pressure equilibrium (π_E/ $\Delta P \cong 1.00$) is almost always observed in the hydropenic Munich-Wistar but is present in only ~40% of the studies in the euvolemic Munich-Wistar rat, suggesting that the normal condition in the glomerulus of the conscious animal is poised on the verge of disequilibrium.

P_{UF} declines between the afferent end and efferent ends of the glomerular capillary network in the hydropenic animal primarily due to the rise in π_{GC} because ΔP remains nearly constant along the glomerular capillaries (see Fig. 3–22). The decline in P_{UF} depicted by Curve A in Figure 3–22 shows that

this decline in P_{UF} (the difference between ΔP and $\Delta \pi$ curves) is nonlinear. This is because (1) filtration is more rapid at the afferent end where P_{UF} is greatest, and (2) the relationship between plasma protein concentration and colloid osmotic pressure is nonlinear (see refs 18, 551). The exact profile of $\Delta \pi$ along the capillary network cannot be determined under conditions of filtration pressure disequilibrium and Curves A and B in Figure 3–22 are only two of many possibilities.

Determination of the Ultrafiltration Coefficient

Single nephron glomerular filtration rates equals the ultrafiltration coefficient (K_f) times the net driving force for ultrafiltration averaged over the length of the glomerular capillaries ($\bar{P}_{UF}$) (Equation 2). Under conditions of filtration pressure equilibrium determination of a unique value of $\bar{P}_{UF}$ is not possible because an exact $\Delta \pi$ profile cannot be defined but if a linear rise in $\Delta \pi$ between the afferent and efferent ends of the glomerular capillaries is assumed a maximum value for $\bar{P}_{UF}$ can be determined (curve C, dashed line in Fig. 3–22). Using this maximum value for P_{UF} and measured values of SNGFR, a minimum estimate of K_f can be obtained. This minimum estimate of K_f in the hydropenic Munich-Wistar rat averages 3.5 ± 0.2 nl/(min·mm Hg) (Fig. 3–21, panel D). In the euvolemic Munich-Wistar rat K_f increases with age with little differences noted between sexes when body mass is taken into account (Fig. 3–23).

Under conditions of filtration pressure equilibrium changes in glomerular plasma flow rate (Q_A) (in the absence of significant changes in π_A or ΔP) are predicted to result in proportional changes in SNGFR.[570] This occurs because in the absence of changes in any other determinants of SNGFR an increase in Q_A slows the rate of increase of plasma protein concentration and therefore $\Delta \pi$ along the glomerular capillary network. This shifts the point at which filtration equilibrium is achieved toward the efferent end of the glomerular capillary network, effectively increasing the total capillary surface area exposed to a positive net ultrafiltration pressure and increases the magnitude of the local P_{UF} at any point along

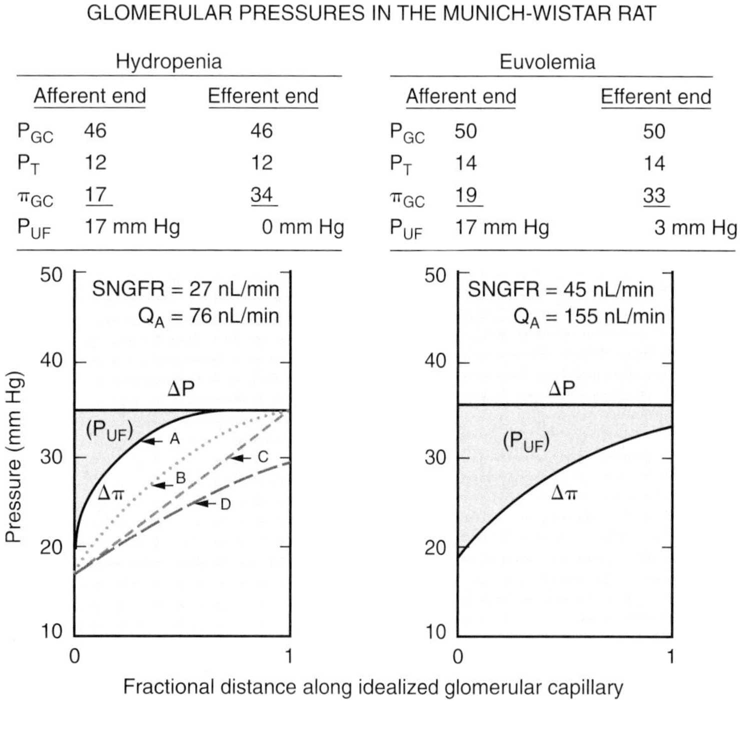

GLOMERULAR PRESSURES IN THE MUNICH-WISTAR RAT

	Hydropenia		Euvolemia	
	Afferent end	Efferent end	Afferent end	Efferent end
P_{GC}	46	46	50	50
P_T	12	12	14	14
π_{GC}	17	34	19	33
P_{UF}	17 mm Hg	0 mm Hg	17 mm Hg	3 mm Hg

FIGURE 3–22 Hydraulic and colloid osmotic pressure profiles along idealized glomerular capillaries in hydropenic and euvolemic rats. Values shown are mean values derived from the studies shown in Figure 3–21. $\Delta P = P_{GC} - P_T$ and $\Delta \pi = \pi_{GC} - \pi_T$, where P_{GC} and P_T are the hydraulic pressures in the glomerular capillary and Bowman space, respectively, and π_{GC} and π_T are the corresponding colloid osmotic pressures. Because the value of π_T is negligible, $\Delta \pi$ essentially equals π_{GC}. P_{UF} is the ultrafiltration pressure at any point. The area between the ΔP and $\Delta \pi$ curves represents the net ultrafiltration pressure, P_{UF}. Curves A and B in the left panel represent two of the many possible profiles under conditions of filtration pressure equilibrium whereas Line D represents disequilibrium. Line C represents the hypothetical linear $\Delta \pi$ profile.

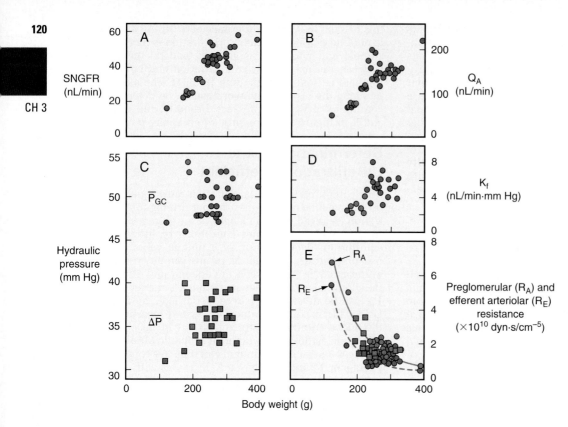

FIGURE 3-23 Maturational alterations in the determinants of glomerular ultrafiltration in the euvolemic Munich-Wister rat. In panels A, B, C, and D filled symbols denote values obtained from female rats whereas open symbols were from studies of male or male plus female rats. In panel E the filled symbols denote values of R_A whereas open symbols are values of R_E. In panel E the circles were from studies of male or male plus female rats whereas squares were from studies of female animals. Each point represents the mean value for a given study. (See Refs 18 and 551 for sources of data.)

the glomerular capillary network. This is illustrated in Figure 3-22, which shows that even in the absence of changes in $\overline{\Delta P}$ or plasma protein concentration an increase in Q_A can result in a change in the profile from that seen with curve A to that of curve B while still achieving filtration pressure equilibrium. For curve B, however, $\overline{P}_{UF}$ is significantly greater than with curve A, and hence SNGFR will increase proportionately.

If Q_A increases enough, $\Delta\pi$ no longer rises to an extent that π_E equals $\overline{\Delta P}$, and filtration pressure disequilibrium is obtained.[570] Under these conditions a unique profile of $\Delta\pi$ can be derived, $\overline{P}_{UF}$ can be accurately determined, and a unique value of K_f can be calculated.[570] The first unique determinations of K_f in the Munich-Wistar rat were obtained by Deen and colleagues using iso-oncotic plasma volume expansion to increase Q_A sufficiently to produce filtration pressure disequilibrium.[570] Under these conditions K_f was found to exceed the minimum estimate obtained in hydropenic rats by 37%, averaging 4.8 nl/(min·mmHg). This value remained essentially unchanged over a twofold range of changes in Q_A, however, suggesting that changes in Q_A per se did not affect K_f.[570]

Filtration pressure equilibrium is generally achieved when Q_A is less than 130 nl/min whereas Q_A values greater than 130 nl/min generally yield filtration pressure disequilibrium.[18] The values of K_f for all of the studies in euvolemic Munich-Wistar rats shown in Figure 3-21 averaged 5.0 ± 0.3 nl/(min·mm Hg) and are similar to those obtained in plasma expanded Munich Wistar rats in which only unique values of K_f were obtained (4.8 ± 0.3 nl/(min·mm Hg)).[551,570] Measured values of $\overline{\Delta P}$ are slightly higher in euvolemic rats than in hydropenic animals (see Fig. 3-21), but this is offset by higher plasma protein concentrations (C_A and hence π_A), so that P_{UF} at the afferent end of the glomerular capillary network is nearly identical in euvolemia versus hydropenia. Thus SNGFR euvolemic rats is higher primarily as a result of increases in Q_A (see Fig. 3-21), yielding a greater value of $\overline{P}_{UF}$ (see Fig. 3-22).

K_f is the product of the total surface area available for filtration and the hydraulic conductivity of the filtration barrier (k). Total capillary basement membrane area per glomerulus (A_s) in the rat has been determined to be equal to ~0.003 cm^2 in superficial nephrons and 0.004 cm^2 in the deep nephrons.[571] Only the peripheral area of the capillaries surrounded by podocytes participates in filtration and that peripheral area available for filtration (A_p) has been estimated to be 0.0016–0.0018 and 0.0019–0.0022 cm^2 in the superficial and deep glomeruli, respectively, or about half that of the total.[571] Using these estimates of A_p and a value of K_f of ~5 nl/(min·mm Hg) as determined by micropuncture techniques, then k=45–48 nl/(s·mm Hg·cm^2). These estimates of k for the rat glomerulus are all 1 to 2 orders in magnitude higher than those reported for capillary networks in mesentery, skeletal muscle, omentum, or in peritubular capillaries of the kidney.[18,551] This very high glomerular hydraulic permeability permits very rapid rates of filtration across glomerular capillaries despite mean net ultrafiltration pressures (P_{UF}) of only 5 mm Hg to 6 mm Hg in hydropenia and 8 mm Hg to 9 mm Hg in euvolemia.

Selective Alterations in the Primary Determinants of Glomerular Ultrafiltration

Alterations in any of the four primary determinants of ultrafiltration, Q_A, $\overline{\Delta P}$, K_f, and π_A, will affect glomerular filtration rate. The degree to which selective alterations will modify SNGFR has been examined by mathematical modeling[570] and compared with values obtained experimentally.[18]

Glomerular Plasma Flow Rate (Q_A)

Because protein is normally excluded from the glomerular ultrafiltrate, conservation of mass dictates that the total amount of protein entering the the glomerular capillary network from the afferent arteriole equals the total amount leaving at the efferent arteriole:

$$Q_A C_A = Q_E C_E \quad (3)$$

For Equation 3, Q_E = efferent arteriolar plasma flow rate, and C_A and C_E are the afferent and efferent arteriolar plasma concentrations of protein, respectively. This can be expressed as:

$$Q_A C_A = (Q_A - SNGFR) C_E \quad (4)$$

Rearranging Equation 4 yields

$$SNGFR = (1 - (C_A/C_E)) \times Q_A \quad (5)$$

$$\text{with } SNFF = 1 - (C_A/C_E) \quad (6)$$

where SNFF is the single nephron filtration fraction. Although the relationship between colloid osmotic pressure (π) and protein concentration deviates from linearity,[572] Equation 4 can be approximated as:

$$SNGFR \cong (1 - (\pi_A/\pi_E)) * Q_A \quad (7)$$

Because at filtration pressure equilibrium $\pi_E = \Delta P$,

$$SNGFR \cong (1 - (\pi_A/\Delta P)) * Q_A \quad (8)$$

Under conditions of filtration pressure equilibrium, filtration fraction $[\cong (1 - (\pi_A/\Delta P))]$ is constant if π_A and ΔP are unchanged. SNGFR will then vary directly with changes in Q_A (Equation 8). Increases in Q_A great enough to produce disequilibrium (π_E less than $\overline{\Delta P}$) yields a fall in C_E, a decrease in SNFF (Equation 5), and SNGFR no longer varies linearly with Q_A. Brenner and colleagues first demonstrated the plasma flow dependence of GFR[573] and as shown in Figure 3–24 increases in glomerular plasma flow are associated with increases in SNGFR in studies of rats, dogs, nonhuman primates, and humans. Because filtration pressure equilibrium occurs in most studies at plasma flow rates less than 100 nl/min to 150 nl/min, increases in Q_A result in proportional increases in SNGFR, and SNFF remains constant. Further increases in Q_A are associated with proportionately lower increases in SNGFR resulting in decreased SNFF as filtration pressure disequilibrium is achieved.

Transcapillary Hydraulic Pressure Difference (ΔP)

Isolated changes in the glomerular transcapillary hydraulic pressure gradient are also predicted to affect SNGFR.[570] Until ΔP exceeds the colloid osmotic pressure at the afferent end of the glomerular capillary there is no filtration. Once that point is reached SNGFR increases as ΔP increases, but the rate of increase is nonlinear because the rise in SNGFR at any given fixed value of Q_A results in a concurrent (but smaller) increase in $\Delta \pi$. Because $\overline{\Delta P}$ is normally 30 mm Hg to 40 mm Hg (see Fig. 3–21), changes in $\overline{\Delta P}$ generally result in relatively minor variations in SNGFR.

Glomerular Capillary Ultrafiltration Coefficient (K_f)

The glomerular ultrafiltration coefficient is reduced in a variety of kidney diseases, in part as a consequence of a reduction in surface area available for filtration as glomerulosclerosis progresses. In addition, the hydraulic permeability of the glomerular basement membrane is inversely related to $\overline{\Delta P}$, indicating that K_f, the product of surface area and hydraulic conductivity, may be directly affected by $\overline{\Delta P}$.[574] The hydraulic conductivity of the GBM and K_f, are also affected by the plasma protein concentration (see later discussion). Because filtration pressure equilibrium is generally observed at low values of Q_A, reductions in K_f do not affect SNGFR until K_f is reduced enough to produce filtration pressure disequilibrium. At low Q_A values increases in K_f above normal values move the point of equilibrium closer to the afferent end of the capillaries but have little affect on SNGFR.[18,570] For high Q_A values filtration pressure disequilibrium occurs and there is a more direct relationship between K_f and SNGFR.[570]

Colloid Osmotic Pressure (π_A)

Single nephron glomerular filtration rate and SNFF are predicted to vary reciprocally as a function of π_A.[570] This is because changes in π_A are associated with alterations in K_f, thereby offsetting variations in P_{UF} that occur with changes in π_A.[18] These divergent results can be partially explained by the results from studies of isolated glomerular basement membranes by Daniels and co-workers, who observed a biphasic relationship between albumin concentration and hydraulic permeability.[574] They observed lower values of hydraulic permeability at albumin concentrations of 4 g/dl than at either 0 or 8 g/dl, but they did not study the effects of extremely high protein concentrations (e.g., 11 g/dl).[574] Their studies suggest a primary effect on hydraulic conductivity,[574] but the mechanism is unknown.

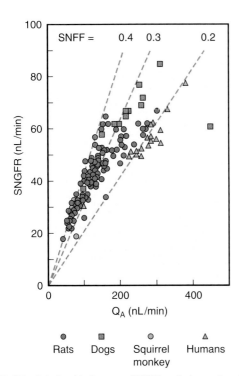

FIGURE 3–24 Relationship between SNGFR and glomerular plasma flow rate. Values from studies in rats are denoted by open circles whereas data from dogs are presented as filled squares. Also shown are values from primates including the squirrel monkey (filled circle) and humans (filled triangles). The values for SNGFR and Q_A for humans were calculated by dividing whole kidney GFR and renal plasma flow by the estimated total number of nephrons/kidney (one million). Each point represents the mean value for a given study. (See Refs 18 and 551 for sources of data.)

References

1. Stein JH, Fadem SZ: The renal circulation. JAMA 239(13):1308–1312, 1978.
2. Graves F: The Arterial Anatomy of the Kidney. Philadelphia, Williams & Wilkins, 1971.
3. Correa-Rotter R, Hostetter TH, Manivel JC, Rosenberg ME: Renin expression in renal ablation. Hypertension 20(4):483–490, 1992.
4. Sykes D: The arterial supply of the human kidney, with special reference to accessory renal arteries. Br J Urol 50:68, 1963.
5. Sykes D: The correlation between renal vascularization and lobulation of the kidney. Br J Urol 36:549, 1964.
6. Boijsen E: Angiographic studies of the anatomy of single and multiple renal arteries. Acta Radiol Suppl 183:1–135, 1959.
7. Kosinski H: Variation of the structure and course of the interlobular arteries in human kidney. Folia Morphol (Warsz) 56(4):249–252, 1997.

8. Fourman J: The Blood Vessels of the Kidney. Oxford, Blackwell Scientific Publications, 1971.

9. von Kogelgen A: Die Gefassarchitektur der Niere. Untersuchungen an der Hundeiere. Stuttgart, Georg Thieme, 1959.

10. Beeuwkes R, 3rd: Efferent vascular patterns and early vascular-tubular relations in the dog kidney. Am J Physiol 221(5):1361–1374, 1971.

11. Trueta J: Studies on the Renal Circulation. Oxford, Blackwell Scientific Publications, 1947.

12. Rasmussen SN, Nissen OI: Effects of saline on continuously recorded filtration fractions in cat kidney. Am J Physiol 243(1):F96–101, 1982.

13. Munkacsi IM, Newstead JD: The intrarenal and pericapsular venous systems of kidneys of the ringed seal, Phoca hispida. J Morphol 184(3):361–373, 1985.

14. Kriz W, Koepsell H: The structural organization of the mouse kidney. Z Anat Entwicklungsgesch 144(2):137–163, 1974.

15. Bankir L, Farman N: [Heterogeneity of the glomeruli in the rabbit]. Arch Anat Microsc Morphol Exp 62(3):281–291, 1973.

16. Casellas D, Navar LG: In vitro perfusion of juxtamedullary nephrons in rats. Am J Physiol 246(3 Pt 2):F349–F358, 1984.

17. Imig JD, Roman RJ: Nitric oxide modulates vascular tone in preglomerular arterioles. Hypertension 19(6 Pt 2):770–774, 1992.

18. Maddox DA, Brenner BM: Glomerular ultrafiltration. In Brenner BM (ed): The Kidney. Philadelphia, WB Saunders, 2004.

19. Elias H: De structura glomeruli renalis. Acta Anat (Basel) 104:26, 1957.

20. Barger AC, Herd JA: The renal circulation. N Engl J Med 284(9):482–490, 1971.

21. Elger M, Sakai T, Kriz W: The vascular pole of the renal glomerulus of rat. Adv Anat Embryol Cell Biol 139:1–98, 1998.

22. Richards A, Schmidt C: A description of the glomerular circulation in the frog's kidney and observations concerning the action of adrenalin and various other substances upon it. Am J Physiol 71:178, 1924.

23. Hall V: The protoplasmic basis of glomerular ultrafiltration. Am Heart J 54(1):1–9, 1957.

24. Scheinman JI, Fish AJ, Brown DM, Michael AJ: Human glomerular smooth muscle (mesangial) cells in culture. Lab Invest 34(2):150–158, 1976.

25. Sraer JD, Adida C, Peraldi MN, Rondeau E, et al: Species-specific properties of the glomerular mesangium. J Am Soc Nephrol 3(7):1342–1350, 1993.

26. Feng Z, Wei C, Chen X, et al: Essential role of Ca^{2+} release channels in angiotensin II-induced Ca^{2+} oscillations and mesangial cell contraction. Kidney Int 70(1):130–138, 2006.

27. Inkyo-Hayasaka K, Sakai T, Kobayashi N, et al: Three-dimensional analysis of the whole mesangium in the rat. Kidney Int 50(2):672–683, 1996.

28. Yu Y, Leng CJ, Terada N, Ohno S: Scanning electron microscopic study of the renal glomerulus by an in vivo cryotechnique combined with freeze-substitution. J Anat 192 (Pt 4):595–603, 1998.

29. Kaczmarek E: Visualisation and modelling of renal capillaries from confocal images. Med Biol Eng Comput 37(3):273–277, 1999.

30. Antiga L, Ene-Iordache B, Remuzzi G, Remuzzi A: Automatic generation of glomerular capillary topological organization. Microvasc Res 62(3):346–354, 2001.

31. Phillips CL, Gattone VH, 2nd, Bonsib SM: Imaging glomeruli in renal biopsy specimens. Nephron Physiol 103(2):75–81, 2006.

32. Sobin SS, Frasher, Jr, WG, Tremer HM: Vasa vasorum of the pulmonary artery of the rabbit. Circ Res 11:257–263, 1962.

33. Birch AG, Zakheim RM, Jones LG, Barger AC: Redistribution of renal blood flow produced by furosemide and ethacrynic acid. Circ Res 21(6):869–878, 1967.

34. Weinstein SW, Szyjewicz J: Superficial nephron tubular-vascular relationships in the rat kidney. Am J Physiol 234(3):F207–214, 1978.

35. Beeuwkes R, III, Bonventre JV: Tubular organization and vascular-tubular relations in the dog kidney. Am J Physiol 229(3):695–713, 1975.

36. Garcia-Sanz A, Rodriguez-Barbero A, Bentley MD, et al: Three-dimensional micro-computed tomography of renal vasculature in rats. Hypertension 31(1 Pt 2):440–444, 1998.

37. Evan AP, Dail, Jr, WG: Efferent arterioles in the cortex of the rat kidney. Anat Rec 187(2):135–145, 1977.

38. Edwards JG: Efferent arterioles of glomeruli in the juxtamedullary zone of the human kidney. Anat Rec 125(3):521–529, 1956.

39. Dieterich HJ: Structure of blood vessels in the kidney. Norm Pathol Anat (Stuttg), 35:1–108, 1978.

40. Kriz W, Dieterich H: The supplying and draining vessels of the renal medulla in mammals. Proceed of the Fourth Int Cong Nephrol, 1970(138).

41. Kriz W, Kaissling B: Structural organization of the mammalian kidney. In Seldin DW, Giebeisch G (eds): The Kidney: Physiology and Pathophysiology, New York, Raven Press, 1985, p 268.

42. Beeuwkes R, 3rd: Vascular-tubular relationships in the human kidney. Renal Pathophysiol: Recent Advances:155, 1979.

43. Beeuwkes R, 3rd: Dissociation of proximal tubule and efferent peritubular capillaries in the same glomerulus. Physiologist 13:146, 1970.

44. Briggs JP, Wright FS: Feedback control of glomerular filtration rate: Site of the effector mechanism. Am J Physiol 236(1):F40–47, 1979.

45. Beeuwkes R, 3rd, Bonventre J: The organization and vascular perfusion of canine renal tubules. Physiologist 16:264, 1973.

46. Steinhausen M, Eisenbach GM, Galaske R: Countercurrent system in the renal cortex of rats. Science 167(925):1631–1633, 1970.

47. Steinhausen M: Further information on the cortical countercurrent system in rat kidney. Yale J Biol Med 45(3):451–456, 1972.

48. Charonis AS, Wissig SL: Anionic sites in basement membranes. Differences in their electrostatic properties in continuous and fenestrated capillaries. Microvasc Res 25(3):265–285, 1983.

49. Kriz W, Napiwotzky P: Structural and functional aspects of the renal interstitium. Contrib Nephrol 16:104–108, 1979.

50. Langer K: Niereninterstitium-Feinstruckturen und Kapillarpermeabilitat I. Feinstruckturen der zellularen und extrazellularen Komponenten des peritubularen Niereninterstitiums. Cytobiology 10:161–184, 1975.

51. Aukland K, Bogusky RT, Renkin EM: Renal cortical interstitium and fluid absorption by peritubular capillaries. Am J Physiol 266(2 Pt 2):F175–184, 1994.

52. Venkatachalam MA, Karnovsky MJ: Extravascular protein in the kidney. An ultrastructural study of its relation to renal peritubular capillary permeability using protein tracers. Lab Invest 27(5):435–444, 1972.

53. Ryan GB, Karnovsky MJ: Distribution of endogenous albumin in the rat glomerulus: role of hemodynamic factors in glomerular barrier function. Kidney Int 9(1):36–45, 1976.

54. Deen WM, Ueki IF, Brenner BM: Permeability of renal peritubular capillaries to neutral dextrans dextrans and endogenous albumin. Am J Physiol 231(2):283–291, 1976.

55. Kon V, Hughes ML, Ichikawa I: Blood flow dependence of postglomerular fluid transfer and glomerulotubular balance. J Clin Invest 72(5):1716–1728, 1983.

56. Bank N, Aynedjian HS: Failure of changes in intracapillary pressures to alter proximal fluid reabsorption. Kidney Int 26(3):275–282, 1984.

57. Ott CE, Haas JA, Cuche JL, Knox FG: Effect of increased peritubule protein concentration on proximal tubule reabsorption in the presence and absence of extracellular volume expansion. J Clin Invest 55(3):612–620, 1975.

58. Knox FG, Mertz JI, Burnett JC Jr, Haramati A: Role of hydrostatic and oncotic pressures in renal sodium reabsorption. Circ Res 52(5):491–500, 1983.

59. Granger JP: Regulation of sodium excretion by renal interstitial hydrostatic pressure. Fed Proc 45(13):2892–2896, 1986.

60. Haas JA, Granger JP, Knox FG: Effect of renal perfusion pressure on sodium reabsorption from proximal tubules of superficial and deep nephrons. Am J Physiol 250(3 Pt 2):F425–429, 1986.

61. Granger JP: Pressure natriuresis. Role of renal interstitial hydrostatic pressure. Hypertension 19(1 Suppl):I9–17, 1992.

62. Schurek HJ, Alt JM: Effect of albumin on the function of perfused rat kidney. Am J Physiol 240(6):F569–576, 1981.

63. Clausen G, Oien AH, Aukland K: Myogenic vasoconstriction in the rat kidney elicited by reducing perirenal pressure. Acta Physiol Scand 144(3):277–290, 1992.

64. Pinter G: Renal lymph: Vital for the kidney, and valuable for the physiologist. News Physiol Sci 3:183–193, 1988.

65. Beeuwkes R, 3rd: Functional anatomy of the medullary vasculature of the dog kidney. In Wirz H, Spinelli F (eds). Recent Advances in Renal Physiology, 1972, p. 184.

66. Moffat DB, Fourman J: The vascular pattern of the rat kidney. J Anat 97:543–553, 1963.

67. Moffat D: The Mammalian Kidney. Cambridge, Cambridge University Press, 1975.

68. Kriz W: Structural organization of renal medullary circulation. Nephron 31(4):290–295, 1982.

69. Moffat DB, Creasey M: The fine structure of the intra-arterial cushions at the origins of the juxtamedullary afferent arterioles in the rat kidney. J Anat 110(Pt 3):409–419, 1971.

70. Kriz W, Schnermann J, Koepsell H: The position of short and long loops of Henle in the rat kidney. Z Anat Entwicklungsgesch 138(3):301–319, 1972.

71. Yamamoto K, Wilson DR, Baumal R: Blood supply and drainage of the outer medulla of the rat kidney: Scanning electron microscopy of microvascular casts. Anat Rec 210(2):273–277, 1984.

72. Kaissling B, de Rouffignac C, Barrett JM, Kriz W: The structural organization of the kidney of the desert rodent Psammomys obesus. Anat Embryol (Berl) 148(2):121–143, 1975.

73. Marsh DJ, Segel LA: Analysis of countercurrent diffusion exchange in blood vessels of the renal medulla. Am J Physiol 221(3):817–828, 1971.

74. Pfaller V, Rittinger M: Quantitative morphologie der niere. Mikroskopie 33:74, 1977.

75. Park F, Mattson DL, Roberts LA, Cowley AW Jr: Evidence for the presence of smooth muscle alpha-actin within pericytes of the renal medulla. Am J Physiol 273(5 Pt 2):R1742–1748, 1997.

76. Kriz W, Barrett JM, Potor S: The renal vasculature: Anatomical-functional aspects. Int Rev Physiol 11:1–21, 1976.

77. Schwartz MM, Karnovsky MJ, Vehkatachalam MA: Ultrastructural differences between rat inner medullary descending and ascending vasa recta. Lab Invest 35(2):161–170, 1976.

78. Fawcett D: The fine structure of capillaries in the rete mirabile of the swim bladder of Opsanus tau. Anat Rec 13:274, 1959.

79. Longley JB, Banfield WG, Brindley DC: Structure of the rete mirabile in the kidney of the rat as seen with the electron microscope. J Biophys Biochem Cytol 7:103–106, 1960.

80. Imai M: Functional heterogeneity of the descending limbs of Henle's loop. II. Interspecies differences among rabbits, rats, and hamsters. Pflugers Arch 402(4):393–401, 1984.

81. Valtin H: Structural and functional heterogeneity of mammalian nephrons. Am J Physiol 233(6):F491–501, 1977.

82. Smith H: Lectures on the Kidney. University Extension Division of University of Kansas, 1943:97.

83. Altman P: Respiration and circulation. Fed Am Soc Exp Biol, p. 427, 1971.

84. McCrory W: Developmental Nephrology. Cambridge, Harvard Univ Press, 1972.

85. Davies DF, Shock NW: Age changes in glomerular filtration rate, effective renal plasma flow, and tubular excretory capacity in adult males. J Clin Invest 29(5):496–507, 1950.

86. Barger AC, Herd JA: Renal vascular anatomy and distribution of blood flow. In Orloff J, Berliner RW (eds): Handbook of Physiology, Sec 8, Renal Physiology. Washington, DC, American Physiological Society, 1973, p 249.

87. Daniel PM, Peabody CN, Prichard MM: Cortical ischaemia of the kidney with maintained blood flow through the medulla. Q J Exp Physiol Cogn Med Sci 37(1):11–18, 1952.

88. Zimmerhackl B, Dussel R, Steinhausen M: Erythrocyte flow and dynamic hematocrit in the renal papilla of the rat. Am J Physiol 249(6 Pt 2):F898–902, 1985.
89. Cohen HJ, Marsh DJ, Kayser B: Autoregulation in vasa recta of the rat kidney. Am J Physiol 245(1):F32–40, 1983.
90. Zimmerhackl B, Robertson CR, Jamison RL: The microcirculation of the renal medulla. Circ Res 57(5):657–667, 1985.
91. Zimmerhackl B, Robertson CR, Jamison RL: Effect of arginine vasopressin on renal medullary blood flow. A videomicroscopic study in the rat. J Clin Invest 76(2):770–778, 1985.
92. Fadem SZ, Hernandez-Llamas G, Patak RV, et al: Studies on the mechanism of sodium excretion during drug-induced vasodilatation in the dog. J Clin Invest 69(3):604–610, 1982.
93. Ganguli M, Tobian L, Azar S, O'Donnell M: Evidence that prostaglandin synthesis inhibitors increase the concentration of sodium and chloride in rat renal medulla. Circ Res 40(5 Suppl 1):I135–139, 1977.
94. Solez K, Kramer EC, Fox JA, Heptinstall RH: Medullary plasma flow and intravascular leukocyte accumulation in acute renal failure. Kidney Int 6(1):24–37, 1974.
95. Nafz B, Berger K, Rosler C, Persson PB: Kinins modulate the sodium-dependent autoregulation of renal medullary blood flow. Cardiovasc Res 40(3):573–579, 1998.
96. Miyamoto M, Yagil Y, Larson T, et al: Effects of intrarenal adenosine on renal function and medullary blood flow in the rat. Am J Physiol 255(6 Pt 2):F1230–1234, 1988.
97. Zou AP, Nithipatikom K, Li PL, Cowlet AW Jr: Role of renal medullary adenosine in the control of blood flow and sodium excretion. Am J Physiol 276(3 Pt 2):R790–798, 1999.
98. Dunn BR, Ichikawa I, Pfeffer JM, et al: Renal and systemic hemodynamic effects of synthetic atrial natriuretic peptide in the anesthetized rat. Circ Res 59(3):237–246, 1986.
99. Hansell P, Ulfendahl HR: Atriopeptins and renal cortical and papillary blood flow. Acta Physiol Scand 127(3):349–357, 1986.
100. Pallone TL, Mattson DL: Role of nitric oxide in regulation of the renal medulla in normal and hypertensive kidneys. Curr Opin Nephrol Hypertens 11(1):93–98, 2002.
101. Ren Y, Garvin JL, Carretero OA: Vasodilator action of angiotensin-(1–7) on isolated rabbit afferent arterioles. Hypertension 39(3):799–802, 2002.
102. Kiberd B, Robertson CR, Larson T, Jamison RL: Effect of V2-receptor-mediated changes on inner medullary blood flow induced by AVP. Am J Physiol 253(3 Pt 2):F576–581, 1987.
103. Abassi Z, Gurbanov K, Rubinstein I, et al: Regulation of intrarenal blood flow in experimental heart failure: Role of endothelin and nitric oxide. Am J Physiol 274(4 Pt 2):F766–774, 1998.
104. Hermansson K, Ojteg G, Wolgast M: The cortical and medullary blood flow at different levels of renal nerve activity. Acta Physiol Scand 120(2):161–169, 1984.
105. Mattson DL: Importance of the renal medullary circulation in the control of sodium excretion and blood pressure. Am J Physiol Regul Integr Comp Physiol 284(1):R13–27, 2003.
106. Cantin M, Araujo-Nascimente MD, Benchimol S, Desormeaux Y: Metaplasia of smooth muscle cells into juxtaglomerular cells in the juxtaglomerular apparatus, arteries, and arterioles of the ischemic (endocrine) kidney. An ultrastructural-cytochemical and autoradiographic study. Am J Pathol 87(3):581–602, 1977.
107. Gorgas K: [Structure and innervation of the juxtaglomerular apparatus of the rat (author's transl)]. Adv Anat Embryol Cell Biol 54(2):3–83, 1978.
108. Click RL, Joyner WL, Gilmore JP: Reactivity of gomerular afferent and efferent arterioles in renal hypertension. Kidney Int 15(2):109–115, 1979.
109. Gilmore JP, Cornish KG, Rogers SD, Joyner WL: Direct evidence for myogenic autoregulation of the renal microcirculation in the hamster. Circ Res 47(2):226–230, 1980.
110. Steinhausen M, Sterzel RB, Fleming JT, et al: Acute and chronic effects of angiotensin II on the vessels of the split hydronephrotic kidney. Kidney Int Suppl 20:S64–73, 1987.
111. Steinhausen M, Weis S, Fleming J, et al: Responses of in vivo renal microvessels to dopamine. Kidney Int 30(3):361–370, 1986.
112. Tang L, Parker M, Fei Q, Loutzenhiser R: Afferent arteriolar adenosine A2a receptors are coupled to KATP in in vitro perfused hydronephrotic rat kidney. Am J Physiol 277(6 Pt 2):F926–933, 1999.
113. Loutzenhiser R, Bidani A, Chilton L: Renal myogenic response: Kinetic attributes and physiological role. Circ Res 90(12):1316–1324, 2002.
114. Gabriels G, Endlich K, Rahn KH, et al: In vivo effects of diadenosine polyphosphates on rat renal microcirculation. Kidney Int 57(6):2476–2484, 2000.
115. Tang L, Loutzenhiser K, Loutzenhiser R: Biphasic actions of prostaglandin E(2) on the renal afferent arteriole: Role of EP(3) and EP(4) receptors. Circ Res 86(6):663–670, 2000.
116. Carmines PK, Morrison TK, Navar LG: Angiotensin II effects on microvascular diameters of in vitro blood-perfused juxtamedullary nephrons. Am J Physiol 251(4 Pt 2):F610–618, 1986.
117. Navar LG, Gilmore JP, Joyner WL, et al: Direct assessment of renal microcirculatory dynamics. Fed Proc 45(13):2851–2861, 1986.
118. Steinhausen M, Blum M, Fleming JT, et al: Visualization of renal autoregulation in the split hydronephrotic kidney of rats. Kidney Int 35(5):1151–1160, 1989.
119. Edwards RM: Segmental effects of norepinephrine and angiotensin II on isolated renal microvessels. Am J Physiol 244(5):F526–534, 1983.
120. Edwards RM: Response of isolated renal arterioles to acetylcholine, dopamine, and bradykinin. Am J Physiol 248(2 Pt 2):F183–189, 1985.
121. Edwards RM: Effects of prostaglandins on vasoconstrictor action in isolated renal arterioles. Am J Physiol 248(6 Pt 2):F779–784, 1985.
122. Edwards RM, Trizna W, Kinter LB: Renal microvascular effects of vasopressin and vasopressin antagonists. Am J Physiol 256(2 Pt 2):F274–278, 1989.
123. Endlich K, Kuhn R, Steinhausen M: Visualization of serotonin effects on renal vessels of rats. Kidney Int 43(2):314–323, 1993.
124. Boknam L, Ericson AC, Aberg B, Ulfendahl HR: Flow resistance of the interlobular artery in the rat kidney. Acta Physiol Scand 111(2):159–163, 1981.
125. Fretschner M, Endlich K, Fester C, et al: A narrow segment of the efferent arteriole controls efferent resistance in the hydronephrotic rat kidney. Kidney Int 37(5):1227–1239, 1990.
126. Mulvaney M, Aalkjaer C: Structure and function of small arteries. Physiol Rev 70:921–961, 1990.
127. Ito S, Johnson CS, Carretero OA: Modulation of angiotensin II-induced vasoconstriction by endothelium-derived relaxing factor in the isolated microperfused rabbit afferent arteriole. J Clin Invest 87(5):1656–1663, 1991.
128. Ito S, Juncos LA, Nushiro N, et al: Endothelium-derived relaxing factor modulates endothelin action in afferent arterioles. Hypertension 17(6 Pt 2):1052–1056, 1991.
129. Ren YL, Carretero OA, Ito S: Influence of NaCl concentration at the macula densa on angiotensin II-induced constriction of the afferent arteriole. Hypertension 27(3 Pt 2):649–652, 1996.
130. Ito S, Arima S, Ren YL, et al: Endothelium-derived relaxing factor/nitric oxide modulates angiotensin II action in the isolated microperfused rabbit afferent but not efferent arteriole. J Clin Invest 91(5):2012–2019, 1993.
131. Lanese DM, Yuan BH, McMurtry IF, Conger JD: Comparative sensitivities of isolated rat renal arterioles to endothelin. Am J Physiol 263(5 Pt 2):F894–899, 1992.
132. Denton KM, Anderson WP, Sinniah R: Effects of angiotensin II on regional afferent and efferent arteriole dimensions and the glomerular pole. Am J Physiol Regul Integr Comp Physiol 279(2):R629–R638, 2000.
133. Uan BH, Robinette J, Conger JD: Effect of angiotensin II and norepinephrine on isolated rat afferent and efferent arterioles. Am J Physiol 258:F741–F750, 1990.
134. Just A, Ehmke H, Toktomambetova L, Kirchheim HR: Dynamic characteristics and underlying mechanisms of renal blood flow autoregulation in the conscious dog. Am J Physiol Renal Physiol 280(6):F1062–F1071, 2001.
135. Schnackenberg CG, Wilkins FC, Granger JP: Role of nitric oxide in modulating the vasoconstrictor actions of angiotensin II in preglomerular and postglomerular vessels in dogs. Hypertension 26(6 Pt 2):1024–1029, 1995.
136. Kohagura K, Endo Y, Ito O, et al: Endogenous nitric oxide and epoxyeicosatrienoic acids modulate angiotensin II-induced constriction in the rabbit afferent arteriole. Acta Physiol Scand 168(1):107–112, 2000.
137. Juncos LA, Ren Y, Arima S, et al: Angiotensin II action in isolated microperfused rabbit afferent arterioles is modulated by flow. Kidney Int 49(2):374–381, 1996.
138. Purdy KE, Arendshorst WJ: Prostaglandins buffer ANG II-mediated increases in cytosolic calcium in preglomerular VSMC. Am J Physiol 277(6 Pt 2):F850–F858, 1999.
139. Patzak A, Lai E, Persson PB, Persson AE: Angiotensin II-nitric oxide interaction in glomerular arterioles. Clin Exp Pharmacol Physiol 32(5–6):410–414, 2005.
140. Baylis C, Brenner BM: Modulation by prostaglandin synthesis inhibitors of the action of exogenous angiotensin II on glomerular ultrafiltration in the rat. Circ Res 43(6):889–898, 1978.
141. Wiegmann TB, MacDougall ML, Savin VJ: Glomerular effects of angiotensin II require intrarenal factors. Am J Physiol 258(3 Pt 2):F717–F721, 1990.
142. Takeda K, Meyer-Lehnert H, Kim JK, Schrier W: Effect of angiotensin II on Ca^{2+} kinetics and contraction in cultured rat glomerular mesangial cells. Am J Physiol 254(2 Pt 2):F254–F266, 1988.
143. Sharma M, Sharma R, Greene AS, et al: Documentation of angiotensin II receptors in glomerular epithelial cells. Am J Physiol 274(3 Pt 2):F623–F627, 1998.
144. Pagtalunan ME, Rasch R, Rennke HG, Meyer TW: Morphometric analysis of effects of angiotensin II on glomerular structure in rats. Am J Physiol 268(1 Pt 2):F82–F88, 1995.
145. Schultz PJ, Schorer AE, Raij L: Effects of endothelium-derived relaxing factor and nitric oxide on rat mesangial cells. Am J Physiol 258:F162–F167, 1990.
146. Baylis C, Mitruka B, Deng A: Chronic blockade of nitric oxide synthesis in the rat produces systemic hypertension and glomerular damage. J Clin Invest 90(1):278–281, 1992.
147. Deng A, Baylis C: Locally produced EDRF controls preglomerular resistance and ultrafiltration coefficient. Am J Physiol 264(2 Pt 2):F212–215, 1993.
148. Arima S, Endo Y, Yaoita H, et al: Possible role of P-450 metabolite of arachidonic acid in vasodilator mechanism of angiotensin II type 2 receptor in the isolated microperfused rabbit afferent arteriole. J Clin Invest 100(11):2816–2823, 1997.
149. Inishi Y, Okuda T, Arakawa T, Kurokawa K: Insulin attenuates intracellular calcium responses and cell contraction caused by vasoactive agents. Kidney Int 45(5):1318–1325, 1994.
150. Furchgott RF, Zawadzki JV: The obligatory role of endothelial cells in the relaxation of arterial smooth muscle by acetylcholine. Nature 288(5789):373–376, 1980.
151. Ignarro LJ, Buga GM, Wood KS, et al: Endothelium-derived relaxing factor produced and released from artery and vein is nitric oxide. Proc Natl Acad Sci U S A 84(24):9265–9269, 1987.
152. Palmer RM, Ferrige AG, Moncada S: Nitric oxide release accounts for the biological activity of endothelium-derived relaxing factor. Nature 327(6122):524–526, 1987.
153. Ignarro LJ: Biosynthesis and metabolism of endothelium-derived nitric oxide. Annu Rev Pharmacol Toxicol 30:535–560, 1990.
154. Romero JC, Lahera V, Salom MG, Biondi ML: Role of the endothelium-dependent relaxing factor nitric oxide on renal function. J Am Soc Nephrol 2(9):1371–1387, 1992.
155. Shultz PJ, Tayeh MA, Marletta MA, Raij L: Synthesis and action of nitric oxide in rat glomerular mesangial cells. Am J Physiol 261(4 Pt 2):F600–606, 1991.
156. Bachmann S, Bosse HM, Mundel P: Topography of nitric oxide synthesis by localizing constitutive NO synthases in mammalian kidney. Am J Physiol 268(5 Pt 2):F885–898, 1995.
157. Kon V, Harris RC, Ichikawa I: A regulatory role for large vessels in organ circulation. Endothelial cells of the main renal artery modulate intrarenal hemodynamics in the rat. J Clin Invest 85(6):1728–1733, 1990.

158. Tolins JP, Palmer RM, Moncada S, Raij L: Role of endothelium-derived relaxing factor in regulation of renal hemodynamic responses. Am J Physiol 258(3 Pt 2):H655–H662, 1990.

159. Lamontagne D, Pohl U, Busse R: Mechanical deformation of vessel wall and shear stress determine the basal release of endothelium-derived relaxing factor in the intact rabbit coronary vascular bed. Circ Res 70(1):123–130, 1992.

160. Murphy RA: What is special about smooth muscle? The significance of covalent crossbridge regulation. FASEB J 8(3):311–318, 1994.

161. Greenberg SG, He XR, Schnermann B, Briggs JP: Effect of nitric oxide on renin secretion. I. Studies in isolated juxtaglomerular granular cells. Am J Physiol 268(5 Pt 2):F948–F952, 1995.

162. Radermacher J, Forstermann U, Frolich JC: Endothelium-derived relaxing factor influences renal vascular resistance. Am J Physiol 259(1 Pt 2):F9–17, 1990.

163. Rapoport RM: Cyclic guanosine monophosphate inhibition of contraction may be mediated through inhibition of phosphatidylinositol hydrolysis in rat aorta. Circ Res 58:407–410, 1986.

164. Buga GM, Gold ME, Fukuto JM, Ignarro LJ: Shear stress-induced release of nitric oxide from endothelial cells grown on beads. Hypertension 17(2):187–193, 1991.

165. Chin JH, Azhar S, Hoffman BB: Inactivation of endothelial derived relaxing factor by oxidized lipoproteins. J Clin Invest 89(1):10–18, 1992.

166. Luckhoff A, Busse R: Calcium influx into endothelial cells and formation of endothelium-derived relaxing factor is controlled by the membrane potential. Pflugers Arch 416(3):305–311, 1990.

167. Cooke JP, Rossitch E Jr, Andon NA, et al: Flow activates an endothelial potassium channel to release an endogenous nitrovasodilator. J Clin Invest 88(5):1663–1671, 1991.

168. Marsden PA, Brock TA, Ballermann BJ: Glomerular endothelial cells respond to calcium-mobilizing agonists with release of EDRF. Am J Physiol 258(5 Pt 2):F1295–F1303, 1990.

169. Handa RK, Strandhoy JW: Nitric oxide mediates the inhibitory action of platelet-activating factor on angiotensin II-induced renal vasoconstriction, in vivo. J Pharmacol Exp Ther 277(3):1486–1491, 1996.

170. Edwards RM, Pullen M, Nambi P: Activation of endothelin ETB receptors increases glomerular cGMP via an L-arginine-dependent pathway. Am J Physiol 263(6 Pt 2):F1020–F1025, 1992.

171. Samuelson UE, Jernbeck J: Calcitonin gene-related peptide relaxes porcine arteries via one endothelium-dependent and one endothelium-independent mechanism. Acta Physiol Scand 141(2):281–282, 1991.

172. Gray DW, Marshall I: Nitric oxide synthesis inhibitors attenuate calcitonin gene-related peptide endothelium-dependent vasorelaxation in rat aorta. Eur J Pharmacol 212(1):37–42, 1992.

173. Fiscus RR, Zhou HL, Wang X, et al: Calcitonin gene-related peptide (CGRP)-induced cyclic AMP, cyclic GMP and vasorelaxant responses in rat thoracic aorta are antagonized by blockers of endothelium-derived relaxant factor (EDRF). Neuropeptides 20(2):133–143, 1991.

174. Hutcheson IR, Griffith TM: Release of endothelium-derived relaxing factor is modulated both by frequency and amplitude of pulsatile flow. Am J Physiol 261(1 Pt 2):H257–H262, 1991.

175. Koller A, Kaley G: Endothelial regulation of wall shear stress and blood flow in skeletal muscle microcirculation. Am J Physiol 260(3 Pt 2):H862–H868, 1991.

176. Pohl U, Herlan K, Huang A, Bassenge E: EDRF-mediated shear-induced dilation opposes myogenic vasoconstriction in small rabbit arteries. Am J Physiol 261(6 Pt 2):H2016–H2023, 1991.

177. Nollert MU, Eskin SG, McIntire LV: Shear stress increases inositol trisphosphate levels in human endothelial cells. Biochem Biophys Res Commun 170(1):281–287, 1990.

178. O'Neill WC: Flow-mediated NO release from endothelial cells is independent of K+ channel activation or intracellular Ca2+. Am J Physiol 269(4 Pt 1):C863–C869, 1995.

179. Pittner J, Wolgast M, Casellas D, Persson AE: Increased shear stress-released NO and decreased endothelial calcium in rat isolated perfused juxtamedullary nephrons. Kidney Int 67(1):227–236, 2005.

180. Mount PF, Power DA: Nitric oxide in the kidney: Functions and regulation of synthesis. Acta Physiol (Oxf) 187(4):433–446, 2006.

181. Gabbai FB, Blantz RC: Role of nitric oxide in renal hemodynamics. Semin Nephrol 19(3):242–250, 1999.

182. Baylis C, Harton P, Engels K: Endothelial derived relaxing factor controls renal hemodynamics in the normal rat kidney. J Am Soc Nephrol 1(6):875–881, 1990.

183. Baumann JE, Persson PB, Emke H, et al: Role of endothelium-derived relaxing factor in renal autoregulation in conscious dogs. Am J Physiol 263(2 Pt 2):F208–213, 1992.

184. Treeck B, Aukland K: Effect of L-NAME on glomerular filtration rate in deep and superficial layers of rat kidneys. Am J Physiol 272(3 Pt 2):F312–F318, 1997.

185. Welch WJ, Tojo A, Lee JU, et al: Nitric oxide synthase in the JGA of the SHR: Expression and role in tubuloglomerular feedback. Am J Physiol 277(1 Pt 2):F130–F138, 1999.

186. Sigmon DH, Bierwaltes WH: Influence of nitric oxide derived from neuronal nitric oxide synthase on glomerular function. Gen Pharmacol 34:95–100, 2000.

187. Qiu C, Baylis C: Endothelin and angiotensin mediate most glomerular responses to nitric oxide inhibition. Kidney Int 55(6):2390–2396, 1999.

188. Zatz R, de Nucci G: Effects of acute nitric oxide inhibition on rat glomerular microcirculation. Am J Physiol 261(2 Pt 2):F360–F363, 1991.

189. Gonzalez JD, Llinas MT, Nava E, et al: Role of nitric oxide and prostaglandins in the long-term control of renal function. Hypertension 32(1):33–38, 1998.

190. Qiu C, Engels K, Baylis C: Endothelin modulates the pressor actions of acute systemic nitric oxide blockade. J Am Soc Nephrol 6(5):1476–1481, 1995.

191. Ohishi K, Carmines PK, Inscho EW, Navar LG, et al: EDRF-angiotensin II interactions in rat juxtamedullary afferent and efferent arterioles. Am J Physiol 263(5 Pt 2):F900–906, 1992.

192. Hoffend J, Cavarape A, Endlich K, Steinhausen M: Influence of endothelium-derived relaxing factor on renal microvessels and pressure-dependent vasodilation. Am J Physiol 265(2 Pt 2):F285–F292, 1993.

193. Navar LG: Integrating multiple paracrine regulators of renal microvascular dynamics. Am J Physiol 274(3 Pt 2):F433–444, 1998.

194. Raij L, Baylis C: Glomerular actions of nitric oxide. Kidney Int 48(1):20–32, 1995.

195. Sigmon DH, Carretero OA, Beierwaltes WH: Angiotensin dependence of endothelium-mediated renal hemodynamics. Hypertension 20(5):643–650, 1992.

196. Sigmon DH, Carretero OA, Beierwaltes WH: Endothelium-derived relaxing factor regulates renin release in vivo. Am J Physiol 263(2 Pt 2):F256–F261, 1992.

197. Moreno C, Lopez A, Llinas MT, et al: Changes in NOS activity and protein expression during acute and prolonged ANG II administration. Am J Physiol Regul Integr Comp Physiol 282(1):R31–R37, 2002.

198. Patzak A, Lai EY, Mrowka R, et al: AT1 receptors mediate angiotensin II-induced release of nitric oxide in afferent arterioles. Kidney Int 66(5):1949–1958, 2004.

199. Baylis C, Engels K, Samsell L, Harton P: Renal effects of acute endothelial-derived relaxing factor blockade are not mediated by angiotensin II. Am J Physiol 264(1 Pt 2):F74–78, 1993.

200. Baylis C, Harvey J, Engels K: Acute nitric oxide blockade amplifies the renal vasoconstrictor actions of angiotension II. J Am Soc Nephrol 5(2):211–214, 1994.

201. Yanagisawa M, Kurihara H, Kimura S, et al: A novel potent vasoconstrictor peptide produced by vascular endothelial cells. Nature 332(6163):411–415, 1988.

202. Inoue A, Yanagisawa M, Kimura S, et al: The human endothelin family: Three structurally and pharmacologically distinct isopeptides predicted by three separate genes. Proc Natl Acad Sci U S A 86(8):2863–2867, 1989.

203. Simonson MS, Dunn MJ: Ca2+ signaling by distinct endothelin peptides in glomerular mesangial cells. Exp Cell Res 192(1):148–156, 1991.

204. Barnes K, Murphy LJ, Takahashi M, et al: Localization and biochemical characterization of endothelin-converting enzyme. J Cardiovasc Pharmacol 26 Suppl 3:S37–S39, 1995.

205. Barnes K, Brown C, Turner AJ: Endothelin-converting enzyme: Ultrastructural localization and its recycling from the cell surface. Hypertension 31(1):3–9, 1998.

206. Bakris GL, Fairbanks R, Traish AM: Arginine vasopressin stimulates human mesangial cell production of endothelin. J Clin Invest 87(4):1158–1164, 1991.

207. Kohan DE: Production of endothelin-1 by rat mesangial cells: Regulation by tumor necrosis factor. J Lab Clin Med 119(5):477–484, 1992.

208. Karet FE, Davenport AP: Localization of endothelin peptides in human kidney. Kidney Int 49(2):382–387, 1996.

209. Marsden PA, Dorfman DM, Collins T, et al: Regulated expression of endothelin 1 in glomerular capillary endothelial cells. Am J Physiol 261(1 Pt 2):F117–F125, 1991.

210. Sakamoto H, Sasaki S, Hirata Y, et al: Production of endothelin-1 by rat cultured mesangial cells. Biochem Biophys Res Commun 169(2):462–468, 1990.

211. Sakamoto H, Asak S, Nakamura Y, et al: Regulation of endothelin-1 production in cultured rat mesangial cells. Kidney Int 41(2):350–355, 1992.

212. Herman WH, Emancipator SN, Rhoten RL, Simonson MS: Vascular and glomerular expression of endothelin-1 in normal human kidney. Am J Physiol 275(1 Pt 2):F8–F17, 1998.

213. Kasinath BS, Fried TA, Davalath S, Marsden PA: Glomerular epithelial cells synthesize endothelin peptides. Am J Pathol 141(2):279–283, 1992.

214. Ujiie K, Terada Y, Nonoguchi H, et al: Messenger RNA expression and synthesis of endothelin-1 along rat nephron segments. J Clin Invest 90(3):1043–1048, 1992.

215. Wilkes BM, Susin M, Mento PF, et al: Localization of endothelin-like immunoreactivity in rat kidneys. Am J Physiol 260(6 Pt 2):F913–F920, 1991.

216. Zoja C, Orisio S, Perico N, et al: Constitutive expression of endothelin gene in cultured human mesangial cells and its modulation by transforming growth factor-beta, thrombin, and a thromboxane A2 analogue. Lab Invest 64(1):16–20, 1991.

217. Kohan DE: Endothelins in the normal and diseased kidney. Am J Kidney Dis 29(1):2–26, 1997.

218. Madeddu P, Troffa C, Glorioso N, et al: Effect of endothelin on regional hemodynamics and renal function in awake normotensive rats. J Cardiovasc Pharmacol 14(6):818–825, 1989.

219. Martin ER, Brenner BM, Ballermann BJ: Heterogeneity of cell surface endothelin receptors. J Biol Chem 265(23):14044–14049, 1990.

220. Sakurai T, Yanagisawa M, Masaki T: Molecular characterization of endothelin receptors. Trends Pharmacol Sci 13(3):103–108, 1992.

221. Marsden PA, Danthuluri NR, Brenner BM, et al: Endothelin action on vascular smooth muscle involves inositol trisphosphate and calcium mobilization. Biochem Biophys Res Commun 158(1):86–93, 1989.

222. Clozel M, Fischli W, Guilly C: Specific binding of endothelin on human vascular smooth muscle cells in culture. J Clin Invest 83(5):1758–1761, 1989.

223. Kohzuki M, Johnston CI, Chai SY, et al: Localization of endothelin receptors in rat kidney. Eur J Pharmacol 160(1):193–194, 1989.

224. Gauquelin G, Thibault G, Garcia R: Characterization of renal glomerular endothelin receptors in the rat. Biochem Biophys Res Commun 164(1):54–57, 1989.

225. Orita Y, Fujiwara Y, Ochi S, et al: Endothelin-1 receptors in rat renal glomeruli. J Cardiovasc Pharmacol 13 Suppl 5:S159–161, 1989.

226. Pollock DM, Keith TL, Highsmith RF: Endothelin receptors and calcium signaling. FASEB J 9(12):1196–1204, 1995.

227. Deng Y, et al: A soluble protease identified from rat kidney degrades endothelin-1 but not proendothelin-1. J Biochem (Tokyo) 112(1):168–172, 1992.

228. Katusic ZS, Shepherd JT, Vanhoutte PM: Endothelium-dependent contraction to stretch in canine basilar arteries. Am J Physiol 252(3 Pt 2):H671–H673, 1987.

229. Yoshizumi M, Kurihara H, Sugiyama T, et al: Hemodynamic shear stress stimulates endothelin production by cultured endothelial cells. Biochem Biophys Res Commun 161(2):859–864, 1989.

230. Kohno M, Horio T, Ikeda M, et al: Angiotensin II stimulates endothelin-1 secretion in cultured rat mesangial cells. Kidney Int 42(4):860–866, 1992.

231. Rajagopalan S, Laursen JB, Borthayre A, et al: Role for endothelin-1 in angiotensin II–mediated hypertension. Hypertension 30(1 Pt 1):29–34, 1997.

232. Herizi A, Jover B, Bouriquet N, Mimran A: Prevention of the cardiovascular and renal effects of angiotensin II by endothelin blockade. Hypertension 31(1):10–14, 1998.

233. Marsden PA, Brenner BM: Transcriptional regulation of the endothelin-1 gene by TNF-alphA Am J Physiol 262(4 Pt 1):C854–C861, 1992.

234. King AJ, Brenner BM, Anderson S: Endothelin: A potent renal and systemic vasoconstrictor peptide. Am J Physiol 256(6 Pt 2):F1051–1058, 1989.

235. Heller J, Kramer HJ, Horacek V: Action of endothelin-1 on glomerular haemodynamics in the dog: Lack of direct effects on glomerular ultrafiltration coefficient. Clin Sci (Lond) 90(5):385–391, 1996.

236. Stacy DL, Scott JW, Granger JP: Control of renal function during intrarenal infusion of endothelin. Am J Physiol 258(5 Pt 2):F1232–F1236, 1990.

237. Clavell AL, Stingo AJ, Margulies KB, et al: Role of endothelin receptor subtypes in the in vivo regulation of renal function. Am J Physiol 268(3 Pt 2):F455–F460, 1995.

238. Perico N, Dadan J, Gabanelli M, et al: Cyclooxygenase products and atrial natriuretic peptide modulate renal response to endothelin. J Pharmacol Exp Ther 252(3):1213–1220, 1990.

239. Badr KF, Murray JJ, Breyer MD, et al: Mesangial cell, glomerular and renal vascular responses to endothelin in the rat kidney. Elucidation of signal transduction pathways. J Clin Invest 83(1):336–342, 1989.

240. Kon V, Yoshioka T, Fogo A, Ichikawa I: Glomerular actions of endothelin in vivo. J Clin Invest 83(5):1762–1767, 1989.

241. Loutzenhiser R, Epstein M, Hayashi K, Horton C: Direct visualization of effects of endothelin on the renal microvasculature. Am J Physiol 258(1 Pt 2):F61–F68, 1990.

242. Fretschner M, Endlich K, Gulbins E, et al: Effects of endothelin on the renal microcirculation of the split hydronephrotic rat kidney. Ren Physiol Biochem 14(3):112–127, 1991.

243. Edwards RM, Trizna W, Ohlstein EH: Renal microvascular effects of endothelin. Am J Physiol 259(2 Pt 2):F217–F221, 1990.

244. Dlugosz JA, Munk S, Zhou X, Whiteside CI: Endothelin-1-induced mesangial cell contraction involves activation of protein kinase C-alpha, -delta, and -epsilon. Am J Physiol 275(3 Pt 2):F423–F432, 1998.

245. Simonson MS, Dunn MJ: Endothelin-1 stimulates contraction of rat glomerular mesangial cells and potentiates beta-adrenergic-mediated cyclic adenosine monophosphate accumulation. J Clin Invest 85(3):790–797, 1990.

246. Noll G, Wenzel RR, Luscher TF: Endothelin and endothelin antagonists: Potential role in cardiovascular and renal disease. Mol Cell Biochem 157(1–2):259–267, 1996.

247. Momose N, Fukuo K, Morimoto S, Ogihara T: Captopril inhibits endothelin-1 secretion from endothelial cells through bradykinin. Hypertension 21(6 Pt 2):921–924, 1993.

248. Prins BA, Hu RM, Nazario B, et al: Prostaglandin E2 and prostacyclin inhibit the production and secretion of endothelin from cultured endothelial cells. J Biol Chem 269(16):11938–11944, 1994.

249. Chou SY, Dahhan A, Porush JG: Renal actions of endothelin: Interaction with prostacyclin. Am J Physiol 259(4 Pt 2):F645–652, 1990.

250. Arai H, Hori S, Aramori I, et al: Cloning and expression of a cDNA encoding an endothelin receptor. Nature 348(6303):730–732, 1990.

251. Sakurai T, Yanagisawa M, Takuwa Y, et al: Cloning of a cDNA encoding a non-isopeptide-selective subtype of the endothelin receptor. Nature 348(6303):732–735, 1990.

252. Ihara M, Noguchi K, Saeki T, et al: Biological profiles of highly potent novel endothelin antagonists selective for the ETA receptor. Life Sci 50(4):247–255, 1992.

253. Wendel M, Knels L, Kummer W, Koch T: Distribution of endothelin receptor subtypes ETA and ETB in the rat kidney. J Histochem Cytochem 54:1193–1203, 2006.

254. Qiu C, Samsell L, Baylis C: Actions of endogenous endothelin on glomerular hemodynamics in the rat. Am J Physiol 269(2 Pt 2):R469–473, 1995.

255. Gellai M, DeWolf R, Pullen M, Nambi P: Distribution and functional role of renal ET receptor subtypes in normotensive and hypertensive rats. Kidney Int 46(5):1287–1294, 1994.

256. Stier CT, Jr, Quilley CP, McGiff JC: Endothelin-3 effects on renal function and prostanoid release in the rat isolated kidney. J Pharmacol Exp Ther 262(1):252–256, 1992.

257. Lin H, Smith MJ Jr, Young DB: Roles of prostaglandins and nitric oxide in the effect of endothelin-1 on renal hemodynamics. Hypertension 28(3):372–378, 1996.

258. Oyekan AO, McGiff JC: Cytochrome P-450-derived eicosanoids participate in the renal functional effects of ET-1 in the anesthetized rat. Am J Physiol 274:R52–R61, 1998.

259. Owada A, Tomita K, Terada Y, et al: Endothelin (ET)-3 stimulates cyclic guanosine 3',5'-monophosphate production via ETB receptor by producing nitric oxide in isolated rat glomerulus, and in cultured rat mesangial cells. J Clin Invest 93(2):556–563, 1994.

260. Filep JG: Endogenous endothelin modulates blood pressure, plasma volume, and albumin escape after systemic nitric oxide blockade. Hypertension 30(1 Pt 1):22–28, 1997.

261. Thompson A, Valeri CR, Lieberthal W: Endothelin receptor A blockade alters hemodynamic response to nitric oxide inhibition in rats. Am J Physiol 269(2 Pt 2):H743–H748, 1995.

262. Schnermann J, et al: Tubuloglomerular feedback control of renal vascular resistance. In Windhager EE, Giebisch G (eds): Handbook of Physiology: Renal Physiology. Baltimore: American Physiological Society, Williams and Wilkins, 1992.

263. Schnermann J, Briggs J: Function of the juxtaglomerular apparatus: Control of glomerular hemodynamics and renin secretion. 3rd ed. In Seldin DW, Giebisch G (eds). The Kidney: Physiology and Pathophysiology. Philadelphia: Lippincott, Williams, and Wilkins, 2000.

264. Vallon V: Tubuloglomerular feedback and the control of glomerular filtration rate. News Physiol Sci 18:169–174, 2003.

265. Olivera A, Lamas S, Rodriguez-Puyol D, Lopez-Novoa JM: Adenosine induces mesangial cell contraction by an A1-type receptor. Kidney Int 35(6):1300–1305, 1989.

266. Peti-Peterdi J, Bell PD: Cytosolic [Ca^{2+}] signaling pathway in macula densa cells. Am J Physiol 277(3 Pt 2):F472–F476, 1999.

267. Bell PD, Lapointe JY, Sabirov R, et al: Macula densa cell signaling involves ATP release through a maxi anion channel. Proc Natl Acad Sci U S A 100(7):4322–4327, 2003.

268. Franco M, Bell PD, Navar LG: Effect of adenosine A1 analogue on tubuloglomerular feedback mechanism. Am J Physiol 257(2 Pt 2):F231–F236, 1989.

269. Brown R, Ollerstam A, Johansson B, et al: Abolished tubuloglomerular feedback and increased plasma renin in adenosine A1 receptor-deficient mice. Am J Physiol Regul Integr Comp Physiol 281(5):R1362–1367, 2001.

270. Sun D, Samuelson LC, Yang T, et al: Mediation of tubuloglomerular feedback by adenosine: Evidence from mice lacking adenosine 1 receptors. Proc Natl Acad Sci U S A 98(17):9983–9988, 2001.

271. Thomson S, Bao D, Deng A, Vallon V: Adenosine formed by 5'-nucleotidase mediates tubuloglomerular feedback. J Clin Invest 106(2):289–298, 2000.

272. Ren Y, Arima S, Carretero OA, Ito S: Possible role of adenosine in macula densa control of glomerular hemodynamics. Kidney Int 61(1):169–176, 2002.

273. Ren Y, Garvin JL, Carretero OA: Efferent arteriole tubuloglomerular feedback in the renal nephron. Kidney Int 59(1):222–229, 2001.

274. Ren YL, Garvin JL, Carretero OA: Role of macula densa nitric oxide and cGMP in the regulation of tubuloglomerular feedback. Kidney Int 58(5):2053–2060, 2000.

275. Mitchell KD, Navar LG: Modulation of tubuloglomerular feedback responsiveness by extracellular ATP. Am J Physiol 264(3 Pt 2):F458–F466, 1993.

276. Schnermann J, Traynor T, Yang T, et al: Tubuloglomerular feedback: New concepts and developments. Kidney Int Suppl 67:S40–S45, 1998.

277. Welch WJ, Wilcox CS: Feedback responses during sequential inhibition of angiotensin and thromboxane. Am J Physiol 258(3 Pt 2):F457–F466, 1990.

278. Traynor TR, Schnermann J: Renin-angiotensin system dependence of renal hemodynamics in mice. J Am Soc Nephrol 10 Suppl 11:S184–S188, 1999.

279. Vallon V: Tubuloglomerular feedback in the kidney: Insights from gene-targeted mice. Pflugers Arch 445(4):470–476, 2003.

280. Schnermann JB, Traynor T, Yang T, et al: Absence of tubuloglomerular feedback responses in AT1A receptor-deficient mice. Am J Physiol 273(2 Pt 2):F315–320, 1997.

281. Wang H, Garvin JL, Carretero OA: Angiotensin II enhances tubuloglomerular feedback via luminal AT(1) receptors on the macula densA Kidney Int 60(5):1851–1857, 2001.

282. Wilcox CS, Welch WJ, Murad F, et al: Nitric oxide synthase in macula densa regulates glomerular capillary pressure. Proc Natl Acad Sci U S A 89(24):11993–11997, 1992.

283. Ichihara A, Imig JD, Inscho EW, Navar LG: Cyclooxygenase-2 participates in tubular flow-dependent afferent arteriolar tone: Interaction with neuronal NOS. Am J Physiol 275(4 Pt 2):F605–F612, 1998.

284. Ichihara A, Imig JD, Navar LG: Neuronal nitric oxide synthase-dependent afferent arteriolar function in angiotensin II-induced hypertension. Hypertension 33(1 Pt 2):462–466, 1999.

285. Liu R, Carretero OA, Ren Y, Garvin JL: Increased intracellular pH at the macula densa activates nNOS during tubuloglomerular feedback. Kidney Int 67(5):1837–1843, 2005.

286. Ito S, Ren Y: Evidence for the role of nitric oxide in macula densa control of glomerular hemodynamics. J Clin Invest 92(2):1093–1098, 1993.

287. Thorup C, Erik A, Persson G: Macula densa derived nitric oxide in regulation of glomerular capillary pressure. Kidney Int 49(2):430–436, 1996.

288. Wilcox CS, Welch WJ: Macula densa nitric oxide synthase: Expression, regulation, and function. Kidney Int Suppl 67:S53–S57, 1998.

289. Welch WJ, Wilcox CS: Macula densa arginine delivery and uptake in the rat regulates glomerular capillary pressure. Effects of salt intake. J Clin Invest 100(9):2235–2242, 1997.

290. Vidal MJ, Romero JC, Vanhoutte PM: Endothelium-derived relaxing factor inhibits renin release. Eur J Pharmacol 149(3):401–402, 1988.

291. Thomson SC, Blantz RC, Vallon V: Increased tubular flow induces resetting of tubuloglomerular feedback in euvolemic rats. Am J Physiol 270(3 Pt 2):F461–F468, 1996.

292. Thomson SC, Vallon V, Blantz RC: Resetting protects efficiency of tubuloglomerular feedback. Kidney Int Suppl 67:S65–S70, 1998.

293. Forster R, Maes J: Effect of experimental neurogenic hypertension on renal blood flow and glomerular filtration rate in intact denervated kidneys of unanesthetized rabbits with adrenal glands demedullated. Am J Physiol 150:534–540, 1947.

294. Jones RD, Berne RM: Intrinsic regulation of skeletal muscle blood flow. Circ Res 14:126–138, 1964.

295. Selkurt EE, Hall PW, Spencer MP: Influence of graded arterial pressure decrement on renal clearance of creatinine, p-aminohippurate and sodium. Am J Physiol 159(2):369–378, 1949.

296. Shipley RE, Study RS: Changes in renal blood flow, extraction of inulin, glomerular filtration rate, tissue pressure and urine flow with acute alterations of renal artery blood pressure. Am J Physiol 167(3):676–688, 1951.

297. Gertz KH, Mangos JA, Braun G, Pagel HD: Pressure in the glomerular capillaries of the rat kidney and its relation to arterial blood pressure. Pflugers Arch Gesamte Physiol Menschen Tiere 288(4):369–374, 1966.

298. Navar LG: Minimal preglomerular resistance and calculation of normal glomerular pressure. Am J Physiol 219(6):1658–1664, 1970.

299. Gottschalk CW, Mylle M: Micropuncture study of pressures in proximal tubules and peritubular capillaries of the rat kidney and their relation to ureteral and renal venous pressures. Am J Physiol 185(2):430–439, 1956.

300. Robertson CR, Deen WM, Troy JL, Brenner BM: Dynamics of glomerular ultrafiltration in the rat. 3. Hemodynamics and autoregulation. Am J Physiol 223(5):1191–1200, 1972.

126
CH 3

301. Loyning EW: Effect of reduced perfusion pressure on intrarenal distribution of blood flow in dogs. Acta Physiol Scand 83(2):191–202, 1971.
302. Grangsjo G, Wolgast M: The pressure-flow relationship in renal cortical and medullary circulation. Acta Physiol Scand 85(2):228–36, 1972.
303. Mattson D, Lu S, Roman RJ, Cowley AW Jr: Relationship between renal perfusion pressure and blood flow in different regions of the kidney. Am J Physiol 264:R578, 1993.
304. Heyeraas KJ, Aukland K: Interlobular arterial resistance: Influence of renal arterial pressure and angiotensin II. Kidney Int 31(6):1291–1298, 1987.
305. Ofstad J, Iversen BM, Morkrid L, Sekse I: Autoregulation of renal blood flow (RBF) with and without participation of afferent arterioles. Acta Physiol Scand 130(1):25–32, 1987.
306. Sossenheimer M, Fleming JT, Steinhausen M: Passage of microspheres through vessels of normal and split hydronephrotic rat kidneys. Am J Anat 180(2):185–194, 1987.
307. Navar LG, Bell PD, Burke TJ: Role of a macula densa feedback mechanism as a mediator of renal autoregulation. Kidney Int Suppl 12:S157–164, 1982.
308. Carmines PK, Inscho EW, Gensure RC: Arterial pressure effects on preglomerular microvasculature of juxtamedullary nephrons. Am J Physiol 258(1 Pt 2):F94–102, 1990.
309. Takenaka T, Suzuki H, Okada H, et al: Mechanosensitive cation channels mediate afferent arteriolar myogenic constriction in the isolated rat kidney. J Physiol 511 (Pt 1):245–253, 1998.
310. Hayashi K, Epstein M, Loutzenhiser R: Enhanced myogenic responsiveness of renal interlobular arteries in spontaneously hypertensive rats. Hypertension 19(2):153–160, 1992.
311. Hayashi K, Epstein M, Loutzenhiser R: Determinants of renal actions of atrial natriuretic peptide. Lack of effect of atrial natriuretic peptide on pressure-induced vasoconstriction. Circ Res 67(1):1–10, 1990.
312. Davis MJ, Hill MA: Signaling mechanisms underlying the vascular myogenic response. Physiol Rev 79(2):387–423, 1999.
313. Yip KP, Marsh DJ: $[Ca^{2+}]_i$ in rat afferent arteriole during constriction measured with confocal fluorescence microscopy. Am J Physiol 271(5 Pt 2):F1004–F1011, 1996.
314. Wagner AJ, Holstein-Rathlou NH, Marsh DJ: Endothelial Ca^{2+} in afferent arterioles during myogenic activity. Am J Physiol 270(1 Pt 2):F170–F178, 1996.
315. Navar LG, Inscho EW, Imig JD, Mitchell KD: Heterogeneous activation mechanisms in the renal microvasculature. Kidney Int Suppl 67:S17–S21, 1998.
316. Griffin KA, Hacioglu R, Abu-Amarah I, et al: Effects of calcium channel blockers on "dynamic" and "steady-state step" renal autoregulation. Am J Physiol Renal Physiol 286(6):F1136–1143, 2004.
317. Imig JD, Falck JR, Inscho EW: Contribution of cytochrome P450 epoxygenase and hydroxylase pathways to afferent arteriolar autoregulatory responsiveness. Br J Pharmacol 127(6):1399–1405, 1999.
318. Majid DS, Inscho EW, Navar LG: P2 purinoceptor saturation by adenosine triphosphate impairs renal autoregulation in dogs. J Am Soc Nephrol 10(3):492–498, 1999.
319. Majid DS, Navar LG: Suppression of blood flow autoregulation plateau during nitric oxide blockade in canine kidney. Am J Physiol 262(1 Pt 2):F40–F46, 1992.
320. Beierwaltes WH, Sigmon DH, Carretero OA: Endothelium modulates renal blood flow but not autoregulation. Am J Physiol 262(6 Pt 2):F943–F949, 1992.
321. Katoh T, Chang H, Uchida S, et al: Direct effects of endothelin in the rat kidney. Am J Physiol 258(2 Pt 2):F397–402, 1990.
322. Navar LG, Inscho EW, Majid SA, et al: Paracrine regulation of the renal microcirculation. Physiol Rev 76(2):425–536, 1996.
323. Schnermann J, Briggs JP, Weber PC: Tubuloglomerular feedback, prostaglandins, and angiotensin in the autoregulation of glomerular filtration rate. Kidney Int 25(1):53–64, 1984.
324. Maier M, Starlinger M, Wagner M, et al: The effect of hemorrhagic hypotension on urinary kallikrein excretion, renin activity, and renal cortical blood flow in the pig. Circ Res 48(3):386–392, 1981.
325. Levens NR, Peach MJ, Carey RM: Role of the intrarenal renin-angiotensin system in the control of renal function. Circ Res 48(2):157–167, 1981.
326. Kaloyanides GJ, Ahrens RE, Shepherd JA, DiBona GF: Inhibition of prostaglandin E2 secretion. Failure to abolish autoregulation in the isolated dog kidney. Circ Res 38(2):67–73, 1976.
327. Brech WJ, Sigmund E, Kadatz R, et al: The influence of renin on the intrarenal distribution of blood flow and autoregulation. Nephron 12(1):44–58, 1974.
328. Schnermann J, Briggs JP: Restoration of tubuloglomerular feedback in volume-expanded rats by angiotensin II. Am J Physiol 259(4 Pt 2):F565–572, 1990.
329. Kaloyanides GJ, DiBona GF: Effect of an angiotensin II antagonist on autoregulation in the isolated dog kidney. Am J Physiol 230(4):1078–1083, 1976.
330. Arendshorst WJ, Finn WF: Renal hemodynamics in the rat before and during inhibition of angiotensin II. Am J Physiol 233(4):F290–297, 1977.
331. Zimmerman BG, Wong PC, Kounenis GK, Kraft EJ: No effect of intrarenal converting enzyme inhibition on canine renal blood flow. Am J Physiol 243(2):H277–283, 1982.
332. Hall JE, Coleman TG, Guyton AC, et al: Intrarenal role of angiotensin II and [des-Asp1]angiotensin II. Am J Physiol 236(3):F252–259, 1979.
333. Macias JF, Fiksen-Olsen M, Romero JC, Knox FG: Intrarenal blood flow distribution during adenosine-mediated vasoconstriction. Am J Physiol 244(1):H138–141, 1983.
334. Arendshorst WJ, Beierwaltes WH: Renal tubular reabsorption in spontaneously hypertensive rats. Am J Physiol 237(1):F38–47, 1979.
335. Bayliss W: On the local reactions of the arterial wall to changes in internal pressure. J Physiol (London) 28:220, 1902.
336. Thurau KW: Autoregulation of renal blood flow and glomerular filtration rate, including data on tubular and peritubular capillary pressures and vessel wall tension. Circ Res 15:suppl:132–141, 1964.
337. Johnson P: The myogenic response. Handbook of Physiol, The Cardiovascular System, Am Physiol Soc 2(2):409, 1980.
338. Lush DJ, Fray JC: Steady-state autoregulation of renal blood flow: A myogenic model. Am J Physiol 247(1 Pt 2):R89–99, 1984.
339. Fray JC, Lush DJ, Park CS: Interrelationship of blood flow, juxtaglomerular cells, and hypertension: Role of physical equilibrium and CA. Am J Physiol 251(4 Pt 2):R643–662, 1986.
340. Walker M, III, Harris-Bernard LM, Cook AK, Navar LG: Dynamic interaction between myogenic and TGF mechanisms in afferent arteriolar blood flow autoregulation. Am J Physiol Renal Physiol 279(5):F858–F865, 2000.
341. Casellas D, Bouriquet N, Moore LC: Branching patterns and autoregulatory responses of juxtamedullary afferent arterioles. Am J Physiol 272(3 Pt 2):F416–F421, 1997.
342. Casellas D, Moore LC: Autoregulation of intravascular pressure in preglomerular juxtamedullary vessels. Am J Physiol 264(2 Pt 2):F315–F321, 1993.
343. Takenaka T, Harris-Bernard LM, Inscho EW, et al: Autoregulation of afferent arteriolar blood flow in juxtamedullary nephrons. Am J Physiol 267(5 Pt 2):F879–887, 1994.
344. Hayashi K, Epstein M, Loutzenhiser R, Forster H: Impaired myogenic responsiveness of the afferent arteriole in streptozotocin-induced diabetic rats: Role of eicosanoid derangements. J Am Soc Nephrol 2(11):1578–1586, 1992.
345. Heller J, Horacek V: Autoregulation of superficial nephron function in the alloperfused dog kidney. Pflugers Arch 382(1):99–104, 1979.
346. Pelayo JC, Westcott JY: Impaired autoregulation of glomerular capillary hydrostatic pressure in the rat remnant nephron. J Clin Invest 88(1):101–105, 1991.
347. Hayashi K, Epstein M, Loutzenhiser R: Pressure-induced vasoconstriction of renal microvessels in normotensive and hypertensive rats. Studies in the isolated perfused hydronephrotic kidney. Circ Res 65(6):1475–1484, 1989.
348. Takenaka T, Forster H, De Micheli A, Epstein M: Impaired myogenic responsiveness of renal microvessels in Dahl salt-sensitive rats. Circ Res 71(2):471, 1992.
349. Schnermann J: Localization, mediation and function of the glomerular vascular response to alterations of distal fluid delivery. Fed Proc 40(1):109–115, 1981.
350. Moore LC, Casellas D: Tubuloglomerular feedback dependence of autoregulation in rat juxtamedullary afferent arterioles. Kidney Int 37(6):1402–8, 1990.
351. Holstein-Rathlou NH: Oscillations and chaos in renal blood flow control. J Am Soc Nephrol 4(6):1275–1287, 1993.
352. Leyssac PP, Baumbach L: An oscillating intratubular pressure response to alterations in Henle loop flow in the rat kidney. Acta Physiol Scand 117(3):415–419, 1983.
353. Holstein-Rathlou NH: Synchronization of proximal intratubular pressure oscillations: Evidence for interaction between nephrons. Pflugers Arch 408(5):438–443, 1987.
354. Leyssac PP: Further studies on oscillating tubulo-glomerular feedback responses in the rat kidney. Acta Physiol Scand 126(2):271–277, 1986.
355. Leyssac PP, Holstein-Rathlou NH: Effects of various transport inhibitors on oscillating TGF pressure responses in the rat. Pflugers Arch 407(3):285–291, 1986.
356. Holstein-Rathlou NH, Wagner AJ, Marsh DJ: Dynamics of renal blood flow autoregulation in rats. Kidney Int Suppl 32:S98–101, 1991.
357. Flemming B, Arenz N, Seeliger E, et al: Time-dependent autoregulation of renal blood flow in conscious rats. J Am Soc Nephrol 12(11):2253–2262, 2001.
358. Gotshall R, Hess T, Mills T: Efficiency of canine renal blood flow autoregulation in kidneys with or without glomerular filtration. Blood Vessels 22(1):25–31, 1985.
359. Just A, Wittmann U, Ehmke H, Kirchheim R: Autoregulation of renal blood flow in the conscious dog and the contribution of the tubuloglomerular feedback. J Physiol 506 (Pt 1):275–290, 1998.
360. Aukland K, Oien AH: Renal autoregulation: Models combining tubuloglomerular feedback and myogenic response. Am J Physiol 252(4 Pt 2):F768–783, 1987.
361. Loutzenhiser R, Griffin K, Williamson G, Bidani A: Renal autoregulation: new perspectives regarding the protective and regulatory roles of the underlying mechanisms. Am J Physiol Regul Integr Comp Physiol 290(5):R1153–1167, 2006.
362. Haddy FJ, Scott JB: Metabolically linked vasoactive chemicals in local regulation of blood flow. Physiol Rev 48(4):688–707, 1968.
363. Tabaie HM, Scott JB, Haddy FJ: Reduction of exercise dilation by theophylline. Proc Soc Exp Biol Med 154(1):93–97, 1977.
364. Berne RM: Metabolic regulation of blood flow. Circ Res 15:suppl:261–268, 1964.
365. Spielman WS, Thompson CI: A proposed role for adenosine in the regulation of renal hemodynamics and renin release. Am J Physiol 242(5):F423–435, 1982.
366. Olsson RA, Pearson JD: Cardiovascular purinoceptors. Physiol Rev 70(3):761–845, 1990.
367. Katsuragi T, Tokunaga T, Ogawa S, et al: Existence of ATP-evoked ATP release system in smooth muscles. J Pharmacol Exp Ther 259(2):513–518, 1991.
368. Inscho EW, Mitchell KD, Navar LG: Extracellular ATP in the regulation of renal microvascular function. FASEB J 8(3):319–328, 1994.
369. Inscho EW, Cook AK: P2 receptor-mediated afferent arteriolar vasoconstriction during calcium blockade. Am J Physiol Renal Physiol 282(2):F245–F255, 2002.
370. Inscho EW: P2 receptors in regulation of renal microvascular function. Am J Physiol Renal Physiol 280(6):F927–F944, 2001.
371. Inscho EW, Cook AK, Mui V, Miller J: Direct assessment of renal microvascular responses to P2-purinoceptor agonists. Am J Physiol 274(4 Pt 2):F718–F727, 1998.
372. Inscho EW, Ohishi K, Navar LG: Effects of ATP on pre- and postglomerular juxtamedullary microvasculature. Am J Physiol 263(5 Pt 2):F886–893, 1992.
373. Inscho EW, Schroeder AC, Deichmann PC, Imig JD: ATP-mediated Ca2+ signaling in preglomerular smooth muscle cells. Am J Physiol 276(3 Pt 2):F450–F456, 1999.
374. Inscho EW, Ohishi K, Cook AK, et al: Calcium activation mechanisms in the renal microvascular response to extracellular ATP. Am J Physiol 268(5 Pt 2):F876–F884, 1995.
375. Pfeilschifter J: Extracellular ATP stimulates polyphosphoinositide hydrolysis and prostaglandin synthesis in rat renal mesangial cells. Involvement of a pertussis toxin-sensitive guanine nucleotide binding protein and feedback inhibition by protein kinase C. Cell Signal 2(2):129–138, 1990.

376. Inscho EW, Carmines PK, Navar LG: Juxtamedullary afferent arteriolar responses to P1 and P2 purinergic stimulation. Hypertension 17(6 Pt 2):1033–1037, 1991.
377. Nishiyama A, Majid DS, Walker M 3rd, et al: Renal interstitial atp responses to changes in arterial pressure during alterations in tubuloglomerular feedback activity. Hypertension 37(2 Part 2):753–759, 2001.
378. Brayden JE, Nelson MT: Regulation of arterial tone by activation of calcium-dependent potassium channels. Science 256(5056):532–535, 1992.
379. Brayden JE: Hyperpolarization and relaxation of resistance arteries in response to adenosine diphosphate. Distribution and mechanism of action. Circ Res 69(5):1415–1420, 1991.
380. Lorenz JN, Schnermann J, Brosius FC, et al: Intracellular ATP can regulate afferent arteriolar tone via ATP-sensitive K^+ channels in the rabbit. J Clin Invest 90(3):733–740, 1992.
381. Gaposchkin CG, Tornheim K, Sussman I, et al: Glucose is required to maintain ATP/ADP ratio of isolated bovine cerebral microvessels. Am J Physiol 258(3 Pt 1):E543–E547, 1990.
382. Le Hir M, Kaissling B: Distribution and regulation of renal ecto-5′-nucleotidase: implications for physiological functions of adenosine. Am J Physiol 264(3 Pt 2):F377–F387, 1993.
383. Stehle JH, Rivkees SA, Lee JJ, et al: Molecular cloning and expression of the cDNA for a novel A2-adenosine receptor subtype. Mol Endocrinol 6(3):384–393, 1992.
384. Jackson EK, Dubey RK: Role of the extracellular cAMP-adenosine pathway in renal physiology. Am J Physiol Renal Physiol 281(4):F597–F612, 2001.
385. Spielman WS, Arend LJ: Adenosine receptors and signaling in the kidney. Hypertension 17(2):117–130, 1991.
386. Li JM, Fenton RA, Cutler BS, Dobson JG Jr: Adenosine enhances nitric oxide production by vascular endothelial cells. Am J Physiol 269(2 Pt 1):C519–C523, 1995.
387. Lai EY, Patzak A, Steege A, et al: Contribution of adenosine receptors in the control of arteriolar tone and adenosine-angiotensin II interaction. Kidney Int 70(4):690–698, 2006.
388. Jackson EK, Mi Z: Preglomerular microcirculation expresses the cAMP-adenosine pathway. J Pharmacol Exp Ther 295(1):23–28, 2000.
389. Weaver DR, Reppert SM: Adenosine receptor gene expression in rat kidney. Am.J.Physiol 263(6 Pt 2):F991–F995, 1992.
390. Jackson EK: Adenosine: A physiological brake on renin release. Annu Rev Pharmacol Toxicol 31:1–35, 1991.
391. Hansen PB, Schnermann J: Vasoconstrictor and vasodilator effects of adenosine in the kidney. Am J Physiol Renal Physiol 285(4):F590–F599, 2003.
392. Okumura M, Miura K, Yamashita Y, et al: Role of endothelium-derived relaxing factor in the in vivo renal vascular action of adenosine in dogs. J Pharmacol Exp Ther 260(3):1262–1267, 1992.
393. Nishiyama A, Inscho EW, Navar LG: Interactions of adenosine A1 and A2a receptors on renal microvascular reactivity. Am J Physiol Renal Physiol 280(3):F406–F414, 2001.
394. Weihprecht H, Lorenz JN, Briggs JP, Schnermann J: Vasomotor effects of purinergic agonists in isolated rabbit afferent arterioles. Am J Physiol 263(6 Pt 2):F1026–F1033, 1992.
395. Carmines PK, Inscho EW: Renal arteriolar angiotensin responses during varied adenosine receptor activation. Hypertension 23(1 Suppl):I114–I119, 1994.
396. Siragy HM, Linden J: Sodium intake markedly alters renal interstitial fluid adenosine. Hypertension 27(3 Pt 1):404–407, 1996.
397. Lorenz JN, Weihprecht H, He XR, et al: Effects of adenosine and angiotensin on macula densa-stimulated renin secretion. Am J Physiol 265(2 Pt 2):F187–F194, 1993.
398. Balakrishnan VS, Coles GA, Williams JD: Effects of intravenous adenosine on renal function in healthy human subjects. Am J Physiol 271(2 Pt 2):F374–F381, 1996.
399. Balakrishnan VS, Coles GA, Williams JD: A potential role for endogenous adenosine in control of human glomerular and tubular function. Am J Physiol 265(4 Pt 2):F504–F510, 1993.
400. Kawabata M, Ogawa T, Takabatake T: Control of rat glomerular microcirculation by juxtaglomerular adenosine A1 receptors. Kidney Int Suppl 67:S228–S230, 1998.
401. Hishikawa K, Nakaki T, Suzuki H, et al: Transmural pressure inhibits nitric oxide release from human endothelial cells. Eur J Pharmacol 215(2–3):329–331, 1992.
402. Tojo A, Gross SS, Zhang L, et al: Immunocytochemical localization of distinct isoforms of nitric oxide synthase in the juxtaglomerular apparatus of normal rat kidney. J Am Soc Nephrol 4(7):1438–1447, 1994.
403. Salom MG, Lahera V, Romero JC: Role of prostaglandins and endothelium-derived relaxing factor on the renal response to acetylcholine. Am J Physiol 260(1 Pt 2):F145–149, 1991.
404. Imig JD, Gebremehdin D, Harder DR, Roman RJ: Modulation of vascular tone in renal microcirculation by erythrocytes: Role of EDRF. Am J Physiol 264(1 Pt 2):H190–195, 1993.
405. Hishikawa K, Nakaki T, Marumo T, et al: Pressure enhances endothelin-1 release from cultured human endothelial cells. Hypertension 25(3):449–452, 1995.
406. Nielsen CB, Bech JN, Pedersen EB: Effects of prostacyclin on renal haemodynamics, renal tubular function and vasoactive hormones in healthy humans. A placebo-controlled dose-response study. Br J Clin Pharmacol 44(5):471–476, 1997.
407. Villa E, Garcia-Robles R, Haas J, Romero JC: Comparative effect of PGE2 and PGI2 on renal function. Hypertension 30(3 Pt 2):664–666, 1997.
408. Baylis C, Deen WM, Myers BD, Brenner BM: Effects of some vasodilator drugs on transcapillary fluid exchange in renal cortex. Am J Physiol 230(4):1148–1158, 1976.
409. Schor N, Ichikawa I, Brenner BM: Mechanisms of action of various hormones and vasoactive substances on glomerular ultrafiltration in the rat. Kidney Int 20(4):442–451, 1981.
410. Yoshioka T, Yared A, Miyazawa H, Ichikawa I: In vivo influence of prostaglandin I2 on systemic and renal circulation in the rat. Hypertension 7(6 Pt 1):867–872, 1985.
411. Inscho EW, Carmines PK, Navar LG: Prostaglandin influences on afferent arteriolar responses to vasoconstrictor agonists. Am J Physiol 259(1 Pt 2):F157–F163, 1990.
412. Endlich K, Forssmann WG, Steinhausen M: Effects of urodilatin in the rat kidney: Comparison with ANF and interaction with vasoactive substances. Kidney Int 47(6):1558–1568, 1995.
413. Myers BD, Deen WM, Brenner BM: Effects of norepinephrine and angiotensin II on the determinants of glomerular ultrafiltration and proximal tubule fluid reabsorption in the rat. Circ Res 37(1):101–110, 1975.
414. Llinas MT, Lopez R, Rodriguez F, et al: Role of COX-2-derived metabolites in regulation of the renal hemodynamic response to norepinephrine. Am J Physiol Renal Physiol 281(5):F975–F982, 2001.
415. Edwards RM, Trizna W: Characterization of alpha-adrenoceptors on isolated rabbit renal arterioles. Am J Physiol 254(2 Pt 2):F178–F183, 1988.
416. Naitoh M, Suzuki H, Murakami M, et al: Arginine vasopressin produces renal vasodilation via V2 receptors in conscious dogs. Am J Physiol 265(4 Pt 2):R934–R942, 1993.
417. Ichikawa I, Brenner BM: Evidence for glomerular actions of ADH and dibutyryl cyclic AMP in the rat. Am J Physiol 233(2):F102–F117, 1977.
418. Bouby N, Ahloulay M, Ngsebe E, et al: Vasopressin increases glomerular filtration rate in conscious rats through its antidiuretic action. J Am Soc Nephrol 7(6):842–851, 1996.
419. Bankir L, Ahloulay M, Bouby N: Direct and indirect effects of vasopressin on renal hemodynamics. *In* Gross P, Richter D, Robinson GL (eds): Vasopressin. Paris: John Libby Eurotext, 1993.
420. Bankir L, Ahloulay M, Bouby N, et al: Is the process of urinary urea concentration responsible for a high glomerular filtration rate? J Am Soc Nephrol 4(5):1091–1103, 1993.
421. Aki Y, Tamaki T, Kiyomoto H, et al: Nitric oxide may participate in V2 vasopressin-receptor-mediated renal vasodilation. J Cardiovasc Pharmacol 23(2):331–336, 1994.
422. Rudichenko VM, Beierwaltes WH: Arginine vasopressin-induced renal vasodilation mediated by nitric oxide. J Vasc Res 32(2):100–105, 1995.
423. Yared A, Kon V, Ichikawa I: Mechanism of preservation of glomerular perfusion and filtration during acute extracellular fluid volume depletion. Importance of intrarenal vasopressin-prostaglandin interaction for protecting kidneys from constrictor action of vasopressin. J Clin Invest 75(5):1477–1487, 1985.
424. Weihprecht H, Lorenz JN, Briggs JP, Schnermann J: Vasoconstrictor effect of angiotensin and vasopressin in isolated rabbit afferent arterioles. Am J Physiol 261(2 Pt 2):F273–F282, 1991.
425. Briner VA, Tsai P, Choong HL, Schrier RW: Comparative effects of arginine vasopressin and oxytocin in cell culture systems. Am J Physiol 263(2 Pt 2):F222–F227, 1992.
426. Tamaki T, Kiyomoto K, He H, et al: Vasodilation induced by vasopressin V2 receptor stimulation in afferent arterioles. Kidney Int 49(3):722–729, 1996.
427. Gunning ME, et al: Vasoactive peptides and the kidney. *In* Brenner BM (ed): The Kidney. Philadelphia: WB Saunders, 1996.
428. Dahlen SE, Bjork J, Hedqvist P, et al: Leukotrienes promote plasma leakage and leukocyte adhesion in postcapillary venules: In vivo effects with relevance to the acute inflammatory response. Proc Natl Acad Sci U S A 78(6):3887–3891, 1981.
429. Yared A, Albrightson-Winslow C, Griswold D, et al: Functional significance of leukotriene B4 in normal and glomerulonephritic kidneys. J Am Soc Nephrol 2(1):45–56, 1991.
430. Filep J, Rigter B, Frolich JC: Vascular and renal effects of leukotriene C4 in conscious rats. Am J Physiol 249(5 Pt 2):F739–F744, 1985.
431. Badr KF, Baylis C, Pfeffer JM, et al: Renal and systemic hemodynamic responses to intravenous infusion of leukotriene C4 in the rat. Circ Res 54(5):492–499, 1984.
432. Badr KF, Brenner BM, Ichikawa I: Effects of leukotriene D4 on glomerular dynamics in the rat. Am J Physiol 253(2 Pt 2):F239–F243, 1987.
433. Serhan CN, Sheppard KA: Lipoxin formation during human neutrophil-platelet interactions. Evidence for the transformation of leukotriene A4 by platelet 12-lipoxygenase in vitro. J Clin Invest 85(3):772–780, 1990.
434. Katoh T, Takahashi K, DeBoer DK, et al: Renal hemodynamic actions of lipoxins in rats: A comparative physiological study. Am J Physiol 263(3 Pt 2):F436–F442, 1992.
435. Badr KF, Serhan CN, Nicolaou KC, Samuelsson B: The action of lipoxin-A on glomerular microcirculatory dynamics in the rat. Biochem Biophys Res Commun 145(1):662–670, 1987.
436. Braquet P, Touqui L, Shen TY, Vargaftig BB: Perspectives in platelet-activating factor research. Pharmacol Rev 39(2):97–145, 1987.
437. Lianos EA, Zanglis A: Biosynthesis and metabolism of 1-O-alkyl-2-acetyl-sn-glycero-3-phosphocholine in rat glomerular mesangial cells. J Biol Chem 262(19):8990–8993, 1987.
438. Handa RK, Strandhoy JW, Buckalew, Jr VM: Platelet-activating factor is a renal vasodilator in the anesthetized rat. Am J Physiol 258(6 Pt 2):F1504–F1509, 1990.
439. Badr KF, DeBoer DK, Takahashi K, et al: Glomerular responses to platelet-activating factor in the rat: Role of thromboxane A2. Am J Physiol 256(1 Pt 2):F35–F43, 1989.
440. Juncos LA, Ren YL, Arima S, Ito S: Vasodilator and constrictor actions of platelet-activating factor in the isolated microperfused afferent arteriole of the rabbit kidney. Role of endothelium-derived relaxing factor/nitric oxide and cyclooxygenase products. J Clin Invest 91(4):1374–1379, 1993.
441. Arima S, Ren Y, Juncos LA, Ito S: Platelet-activating factor dilates efferent arterioles through glomerulus-derived nitric oxide. J Am Soc Nephrol 7(1):90–96, 1996.
442. Lopez-Farre A, Gomez-Garre D, Bernabeu F, et al: Renal effects and mesangial cell contraction induced by endothelin are mediated by PAF. Kidney Int 39(4):624–630, 1991.
443. Thomas CE, Ott CE, Bell PD, et al: Glomerular filtration dynamics during renal vasodilation with acetylcholine in the dog. Am J Physiol 244(6):F606–F611, 1983.
444. Mugge A, Elwell JH, Peterson TE, Harrison DG: Release of intact endothelium-derived relaxing factor depends on endothelial superoxide dismutase activity. Am J Physiol 260(2 Pt 1):C219–C225, 1991.

445. Jacobs M, Plane F, Bruckdorfer KR: Native and oxidized low-density lipoproteins have different inhibitory effects on endothelium-derived relaxing factor in the rabbit aorta. Br J Pharmacol 100(1):21–26, 1990.

446. Burton GA, MacNeil S, de Jonge A, Haylor J: Cyclic GMP release and vasodilatation induced by EDRF and atrial natriuretic factor in the isolated perfused kidney of the rat. Br J Pharmacol 99(2):364–368, 1990.

447. Urakami-Harasawa L, Shimokawa H, Nakashima M, et al: Importance of endothelium-derived hyperpolarizing factor in human arteries. J Clin Invest 100(11):2793–2799, 1997.

448. Brayden JE: Membrane hyperpolarization is a mechanism of endothelium-dependent cerebral vasodilation. Am J Physiol 259(3 Pt 2):H668–H673, 1990.

449. Kamori K, Vanhoutte PM: Endothelium-derived hyperpolarizing factor. Blood Vessels 272:238–245, 1990.

450. Najibi S, Cowan CL, Palacino JJ, Cohen RA: Enhanced role of potassium channels in relaxations to acetylcholine in hypercholesterolemic rabbit carotid artery. Am J Physiol 266(5 Pt 2):H2061–H2067, 1994.

451. Murphy ME, Brayden JE: Apamin-sensitive K+ channels mediate an endothelium-dependent hyperpolarization in rabbit mesenteric arteries. J Physiol 489 (Pt 3):723–734, 1995.

452. Jackson WF: Potassium channels in the peripheral microcirculation. Microcirculation 12:113–127, 2005.

453. Jackson WF: Silent inward rectifier K+ channels in hypercholesterolemia. Circ Res 98(8):982–984, 2006.

454. Hayashi K, Loutzenhiser R, Epstein M, et al: Multiple factors contribute to acetylcholine-induced renal afferent arteriolar vasodilation during myogenic and norepinephrine- and KCl-induced vasoconstriction. Studies in the isolated perfused hydronephrotic kidney. Circ Res 75(5):821–828, 1994.

455. Siragy HM, Jaffa AA, Margolius HS: Bradykinin B2 receptor modulates renal prostaglandin E2 and nitric oxide. Hypertension 29(3):757–762, 1997.

456. Yu H, Carretero OA, Juncos LA, Garvin JL: Biphasic effect of bradykinin on rabbit afferent arterioles. Hypertension 32(2):287–292, 1998.

457. Hoagland KM, Maddox DA, Martin DS: Bradykinin B2-receptors mediate the pressor and renal hemodynamic effects of intravenous bradykinin in conscious rats. J Auton Nerv Syst 75(1):7–15, 1999.

458. Bascands JL, Emond C, Pecher C, et al: Bradykinin stimulates production of inositol (1,4,5) trisphosphate in cultured mesangial cells of the rat via a BK2-kinin receptor. Br J Pharmacol 102(4):962–966, 1991.

459. Pavenstadt H, Sapth M, Fiedler C, et al: Effect of bradykinin on the cytosolic free calcium activity and phosphoinositol turnover in human glomerular epithelial cells. Ren Physiol Biochem 15(6):277–288, 1992.

460. Greenwald JE, Needleman P, Wilkins MR, Schreiner GF: Renal synthesis of atriopeptin-like protein in physiology and pathophysiology. Am J Physiol 260(4 Pt 2):F602–F607, 1991.

461. Mehrke G, Pohl U, Daut J: Effects of vasoactive agonists on the membrane potential of cultured bovine aortic and guinea-pig coronary endothelium. J Physiol 439:277–299, 1991.

462. Pavenstadt H, Bengen F, Spath M, et al: Effect of bradykinin and histamine on the membrane voltage, ion conductances and ion channels of human glomerular epithelial cells (hGEC) in culture. Pflugers Arch 424(2):137–144, 1993.

463. Ren Y, Garvin J, Carretero OA: Mechanism involved in bradykinin-induced efferent arteriole dilation. Kidney Int 62(2):544–549, 2002.

464. Imig JD, Falck JR, Wei S, Capdevila JH: Epoxygenase metabolites contribute to nitric oxide-independent afferent arteriolar vasodilation in response to bradykinin. J Vasc Res 38(3):247–255, 2001.

465. Wang H, Garvin JL, Falck JR, et al: Glomerular cytochrome P-450 and cyclooxygenase metabolites regulate efferent arteriole resistance. Hypertension 46(5):1175–1179, 2005.

466. Baylis C, Handa RK, Sorkin M: Glucocorticoids and control of glomerular filtration rate. Semin Nephrol 10(4):320–329, 1990.

467. De Matteo R, May CN: Glucocorticoid-induced renal vasodilatation is mediated by a direct renal action involving nitric oxide. Am J Physiol 273(6 Pt 2):R1972–R1979, 1997.

468. Kotchen TA: Attenuation of hypertension by insulin-sensitizing agents. Hypertension 28(2):219–223, 1996.

469. Hayashi K, Fujiwara K, Oka K, et al: Effects of insulin on rat renal microvessels: Studies in the isolated perfused hydronephrotic kidney. Kidney Int 51(5):1507–1513, 1997.

470. Schroeder CA, Jr, Chen YL, Messina EJ: Inhibition of NO synthesis or endothelium removal reveals a vasoconstrictor effect of insulin on isolated arterioles. Am J Physiol 276(3 Pt 2):H815–H820, 1999.

471. Steinberg HO, Brechtel G, Johnson A, et al: Insulin-mediated skeletal muscle vasodilation is nitric oxide dependent. A novel action of insulin to increase nitric oxide release. J Clin Invest 94(3):1172–1179, 1994.

472. Scherrer U, Randin D, Vollenweider P, et al: Nitric oxide release accounts for insulin's vascular effects in humans. J Clin Invest 94(6):2511–2515, 1994.

473. McKay MK, Hester RL: Role of nitric oxide, adenosine, and ATP-sensitive potassium channels in insulin-induced vasodilation. Hypertension 28(2):202–208, 1996.

474. Tucker BJ, Anderson CM, Thies RS, et al: Glomerular hemodynamic alterations during acute hyperinsulinemia in normal and diabetic rats. Kidney Int 42(5):1160–1168, 1992.

475. Zhang PL, Mackenzie HS, Troy JL, Brenner BM: Effects of an atrial natriuretic peptide receptor antagonist on glomerular hyperfiltration in diabetic rats. J Am Soc Nephrol 4(8):1564–1570, 1994.

476. Hirschberg R, Adler S: Insulin-like growth factor system and the kidney: Physiology, pathophysiology, and therapeutic implications. Am J Kidney Dis 31(6):901–919, 1998.

477. Aron DC, Rosenzweig JL, Abboud HE: Synthesis and binding of insulin-like growth factor I by human glomerular mesangial cells. J Clin Endocrinol Metab 68(3):564–571, 1989.

478. Hirschberg R, Kopple JD, Blantz RC, Tucker BJ: Effects of recombinant human insulin-like growth factor I on glomerular dynamics in the rat. J Clin Invest 87(4):1200–1206, 1991.

479. Jaffa AA, LeRoith D, Roberts CT Jr, et al: Insulin-like growth factor I produces renal hyperfiltration by a kinin-mediated mechanism. Am J Physiol 266(1 Pt 2):F102–F107, 1994.

480. Hirschberg R, Brunori G, Kopple JD, Guler HP: Effects of insulin-like growth factor I on renal function in normal men. Kidney Int 43(2):387–397, 1993.

481. Hirschberg R, Kopple JD: Evidence that insulin-like growth factor I increases renal plasma flow and glomerular filtration rate in fasted rats. J Clin Invest 83(1):326–330, 1989.

482. Baumann U, Eisenhauer T, Hartmann H: Increase of glomerular filtration rate and renal plasma flow by insulin-like growth factor-I during euglycaemic clamping in anaesthetized rats. Eur J Clin Invest 22(3):204–209, 1992.

483. Giordano M, DeFronzo RA: Acute effect of human recombinant insulin-like growth factor I on renal function in humans. Nephron 71(1):10–15, 1995.

484. Tsukahara H, Gordienko DV, Tonshoff B, et al: Direct demonstration of insulin-like growth factor-I-induced nitric oxide production by endothelial cells. Kidney Int 45(2):598–604, 1994.

485. Amuchastegui CS, Remuzzi G, Perico N: Calcitonin gene-related peptide reduces renal vascular resistance and modulates ET-1-induced vasoconstriction. Am J Physiol 267(5 Pt 2):F839–F844, 1994.

486. Vesely DL, Overton RM, McCormick MT, Schocken DD: Atrial natriuretic peptides increase calcitonin gene-related peptide within human circulation. Metabolism 46(7):818–825, 1997.

487. Knight DS, Cicero S, Beal JA: Calcitonin gene-related peptide-immunoreactive nerves in the rat kidney. Am J Anat 190(1):31–40, 1991.

488. Reslerova M, Loutzenhiser R: Renal microvascular actions of calcitonin gene-related peptide. Am J Physiol 274(6 Pt 2):F1078–F1085, 1998.

489. Edwards RM, Trizna W: Calcitonin gene-related peptide: Effects on renal arteriolar tone and tubular cAMP levels. Am J Physiol 258(1 Pt 2):F121–F125, 1990.

490. Bankir L, Martin H, Dechaux M, Ahloulay M: Plasma cAMP: A hepatorenal link influencing proximal reabsorption and renal hemodynamics? Kidney Int Suppl 59: S50–S56, 1997.

491. Castellucci A, Maggi CA, Evangelista S: Calcitonin gene-related peptide (CGRP)1 receptor mediates vasodilation in the rat isolated and perfused kidney. Life Sci 53(9): L153–L158, 1993.

492. Gray DW, Marshall I: Human alpha-calcitonin gene-related peptide stimulates adenylate cyclase and guanylate cyclase and relaxes rat thoracic aorta by releasing nitric oxide. Br J Pharmacol 107(3):691–696, 1992.

493. Zaidi M, Datta H, Bevis PJ: Kidney: A target organ for calcitonin gene-related peptide. Exp Physiol 75(1):27–32, 1990.

494. Danielson LA, Kercher LJ, Conrad KP: Impact of gender and endothelin on renal vasodilation and hyperfiltration induced by relaxin in conscious rats. Am J Physiol Regul Integr Comp Physiol 279(4):R1298–R1304, 2000.

495. Novak J, Danielson LA, Kerchner LJ, et al: Relaxin is essential for renal vasodilation during pregnancy in conscious rats. J Clin Invest 107(11):1469–1475, 2001.

496. Danielson LA, Sherwood OD, Conrad KP: Relaxin is a potent renal vasodilator in conscious rats. J Clin Invest 103(4):525–533, 1999.

497. Cadnapaphornchai MA, Ohara M, Morris KG Jr, et al: Chronic NOS inhibition reverses systemic vasodilation and glomerular hyperfiltration in pregnancy. Am J Physiol Renal Physiol 280(4):F592–F598, 2001.

498. Novak J, Ramirez RJ, Gandley RE, et al: Myogenic reactivity is reduced in small renal arteries isolated from relaxin-treated rats. Am J Physiol Regul Integr Comp Physiol 283(2):R349–R355, 2002.

499. Gandley RE, Conrad KP, McLaughlin MK: Endothelin and nitric oxide mediate reduced myogenic reactivity of small renal arteries from pregnant rats. Am J Physiol Regul Integr Comp Physiol 280(1):R1–R7, 2001.

500. Henry JP, Gauer OH, Reeves JL: Evidence of the atrial location of receptors influencing urine flow. Circ Res 4(1):85–90, 1956.

501. Henry JP, Gauer OH, Sieker HO: The effect of moderate changes in blood volume on left and right atrial pressures. Circ Res 4(1):91–94, 1956.

502. de Bold AJ, Borenstein HB, Veress AT, Sonnenberg H: A rapid and potent natriuretic response to intravenous injection of atrial myocardial extract in rats. Life Sci 28(1):89–94, 1981.

503. Brenner BM, Ballermann BJ, Gunning ME, Seidel ML: Diverse biological actions of atrial natriuretic peptide. Physiol Rev 70(3):665–699, 1990.

504. Saxenhofer H, Raselli A, Weidmann P, et al: Urodilatin, a natriuretic factor from kidneys, can modify renal and cardiovascular function in men. Am J Physiol 259(5 Pt 2):F832–F838, 1990.

505. Goetz KL: Renal natriuretic peptide (urodilatin?) and atriopeptin: Evolving concepts. Am J Physiol 261(6 Pt 2):F921–F932, 1991.

506. Amin J, Carretero OA, Ito S: Mechanisms of action of atrial natriuretic factor and C-type natriuretic peptide. Hypertension 27(3 Pt 2):684–687, 1996.

507. Lohe A, Yeh I, Hyver T, et al: Natriuretic peptide B receptor and C-type natriuretic peptide in the rat kidney. J Am Soc Nephrol 6(6):1552–1558, 1995.

508. Michel H, Meyer-Lehnert H, Backer A, et al: Regulation of atrial natriuretic peptide receptors in glomeruli during chronic salt loading. Kidney Int 38(1):73–79, 1990.

509. Endlich K, Steinhausen M: Natriuretic peptide receptors mediate different responses in rat renal microvessels. Kidney Int 52(1):202–207, 1997.

510. Maack T: Receptors of atrial natriuretic factor. Annu Rev Physiol 54:11–27, 1992.

511. Maack T: Role of atrial natriuretic factor in volume control. Kidney Int 49(6):1732–1737, 1996.

512. Ballermann BJ, Hoover RL, Karnovsky MJ, Brenner BM: Physiologic regulation of atrial natriuretic peptide receptors in rat renal glomeruli. J Clin Invest 76(6):2049–2056, 1985.

513. Lee RW, Raya TE, Michael U, et al: Captopril and ANP: Changes in renal hemodynamics, glomerular-ANP receptors and guanylate cyclase activity in rats with heart failure. J Pharmacol Exp Ther 260(1):349–354, 1992.

514. Perico N, Benigni A, Gabanelli M, et al: Atrial natriuretic peptide and prostacyclin synergistically mediate hyperfiltration and hyperperfusion of diabetic rats. Diabetes 41(4):533–538, 1992.

515. Hirata Y, Matsuoka H, Suzuki E, et al: Role of endogenous atrial natriuretic peptide in DOCA-salt hypertensive rats. Effects of a novel nonpeptide antagonist for atrial natriuretic peptide receptor. Circulation 87(2):554–561, 1993.

516. Abassi Z, Haramati A, Hoffman A, et al: Effect of converting-enzyme inhibition on renal response to ANF in rats with experimental heart failure. Am J Physiol 259(1 Pt 2):R84–R89, 1990.

517. Genovesi S, Protasoni G, Assi C, et al: Interactions between the sympathetic nervous system and atrial natriuretic factor in the control of renal functions. J Hypertens 8(8):703–710, 1990.

518. Zhang PL, Jimenez W, Mackenzie HS, et al: HS-142–1, a potent antagonist of natriuretic peptides in vitro and in vivo. J Am Soc Nephrol 5(4):1099–1105, 1994.

519. Nishikimi T, Miura K, Minamino M, et al: Role of endogenous atrial natriuretic peptide on systemic and renal hemodynamics in heart failure rats. Am J Physiol 267(1 Pt 2):H182–H186, 1994.

520. Zhang PL, Mackenzie HS, Troy JL, Brenner BM: Effects of natriuretic peptide receptor inhibition on remnant kidney function in rats. Kidney Int 46(2):414–420, 1994.

521. Pomeranz A, Podjamy E, Rathaus M, et al: Atrial natriuretic peptide-induced increase of glomerular filtration rate, but not of natriuresis, is mediated by prostaglandins in the rat. Miner Electrolyte Metab 16(1):30–33, 1990.

522. Bestle MH, Olsen NV, Christensen P, et al: Cardiovascular, endocrine, and renal effects of urodilatin in normal humans. Am J Physiol 276(3 Pt 2):R684–R695, 1999.

523. Carstens J, Jensen KT, Pedersen EB: Effect of urodilatin infusion on renal haemodynamics, tubular function and vasoactive hormones. Clin Sci (Lond) 92(4):397–407, 1997.

524. Massfelder T, Parekh N, Endlich K, et al: Effect of intrarenally infused parathyroid hormone-related protein on renal blood flow and glomerular filtration rate in the anaesthetized rat. Br J Pharmacol 118(8):1995–2000, 1996.

525. Ichikawa I, Humes HD, Dousa TP, Brenner BM: Influence of parathyroid hormone on glomerular ultrafiltration in the rat. Am J Physiol 234(5):F393–F401, 1978.

526. Marchand GR: Effect of parathyroid hormone on the determinants of glomerular filtration in dogs. Am J Physiol 248(4 Pt 2):F482–F486, 1985.

527. Pang PK, Janssen HF, Yee JA: Effects of synthetic parathyroid hormone on vascular beds of dogs. Pharmacology 21(3):213–222, 1980.

528. Trizna W, Edwards RM: Relaxation of renal arterioles by parathyroid hormone and parathyroid hormone-related protein. Pharmacology 42(2):91–96, 1991.

529. Massfelder T, Saussine C, Simeoni U, et al: Evidence for adenylyl cyclase-dependent receptors for parathyroid hormone (PTH)-related protein in rabbit kidney glomeruli. Life Sci 53(11):875–881, 1993.

530. Kalinowski L, Dobrucki LW, Malinski T: Nitric oxide as a second messenger in parathyroid hormone-related protein signaling. J Endocrinol 170(2):433–440, 2001.

531. Bosch RJ, Rojo-Linares P, Torrecillas-Casamayor G, et al: Effects of parathyroid hormone-related protein on human mesangial cells in culture. Am J Physiol 277(6 Pt 1):E990–E995, 1999.

532. Saussine C, Massfelder T, Parnin F, et al: Renin stimulating properties of parathyroid hormone-related peptide in the isolated perfused rat kidney. Kidney Int 44(4):764–773, 1993.

533. Philbrick WM, Wysolmerski JJ, Galbraith S, et al: Defining the roles of parathyroid hormone-related protein in normal physiology. Physiol Rev 76(1):127–173, 1996.

534. Massfelder T, Stewart AF, Endlich K, et al: Parathyroid hormone-related protein detection and interaction with NO and cyclic AMP in the renovascular system. Kidney Int 50(5):1591–1603, 1996.

535. Endlich K, Massfelder T, Helwig JJ, Steinhausen M: Vascular effects of parathyroid hormone and parathyroid hormone-related protein in the split hydronephrotic rat kidney. J Physiol 483 (Pt 2):481–490, 1995.

536. Musso MJ, Plante M, Judes C, et al: Renal vasodilatation and microvessel adenylate cyclase stimulation by synthetic parathyroid hormone-like protein fragments. Eur J Pharmacol 174(2–3):139–151, 1989.

537. Simeoni U, Massfelder T, Saussine C, et al: Involvement of nitric oxide in the vasodilatory response to parathyroid hormone-related peptide in the isolated rabbit kidney. Clin Sci (Lond) 86(3):245–249, 1994.

538. Jiang B, Morimoto S, Fukuo K, et al: Parathyroid hormone-related protein inhibits indothelin-1 production. Hypertension 27(3 Pt 1):360–363, 1996.

539. Kitamura K, Matsui E, Kato J, et al: Adrenomedullin: A novel hypotensive peptide isolated from human pheochromocytoma. Biochem Biophys Res Commun 192(2):553–560, 1993.

540. Chini EN, Chini CC, Bolliger C, et al: Cytoprotective effects of adrenomedullin in glomerular cell injury: Central role of cAMP signaling pathway. Kidney Int 52(4):917–925, 1997.

541. Sakata J, Shimokubo T, Kitamura K, et al: Molecular cloning and biological activities of rat adrenomedullin, a hypotensive peptide. Biochem Biophys Res Commun 195(2):921–927, 1993.

542. Berthiaume N, Claing A, Lippton H, et al: Rat adrenomedullin induces a selective arterial vasodilation via CGRP1 receptors in the double-perfused mesenteric bed of the rat. Can J Physiol Pharmacol 73(7):1080–1083, 1995.

543. Edwards RM, Trizna W, Stack E, Aiyar N: Effect of adrenomedullin on cAMP levels along the rat nephron: Comparison with CGRP. Am J Physiol 271(4 Pt 2):F895–F899, 1996.

544. Kohno M, Yasunari K, Yokokawa K, et al: Interaction of adrenomedullin and platelet-derived growth factor on rat mesangial cell production of endothelin. Hypertension 27(3 Pt 2):663–667, 1996.

545. Ebara T, Miura K, Okumura M, et al: Effect of adrenomedullin on renal hemodynamics and functions in dogs. Eur J Pharmacol 263(1–2):69–73, 1994.

546. Jougasaki M, Wei CM, Aarhus LL, et al: Renal localization and actions of adrenomedullin: A natriuretic peptide. Am J Physiol 268(4 Pt 2):F657–F663, 1995.

547. Hjelmqvist H, Keil R, Mathai M, et al: Vasodilation and glomerular binding of adrenomedullin in rabbit kidney are not CGRP receptor mediated. Am J Physiol 273(2 Pt 2):R716–R724, 1997.

548. Liu L, Liu GL, Barajas L: Distribution of nitric oxide synthase-containing ganglionic neuronal somata and postganglionic fibers in the rat kidney. J Comp Neurol 369(1):16–30, 1996.

549. Barajas L, Liu L, Powers K: Anatomy of the renal innervation: intrarenal aspects and ganglia of origin. Can J Physiol Pharmacol 70(5):735–749, 1992.

550. DiBona GF: Neural control of renal function in health and disease. Clin Auton Res 4(1–2):69–74, 1994.

551. Maddox DA, Deen WM, Brenner BM: Glomerular Filtration. Handbook of Physiology: Renal Physiology. In Windhager EE, Giebisch G (eds): Handbook of Physiology Renal Physiology. Baltimore: American Physiological Society, Williams and Wilkins, 1992.

552. Liu GL, Liu L, Barajas L: Development of NOS-containing neuronal somata in the rat kidney. J Auton Nerv Syst 58(1–2):81–88, 1996.

553. Pelayo JC: Renal adrenergic effector mechanisms: Glomerular sites for prostaglandin interaction. Am J Physiol 254(2 Pt 2):F184–F190, 1988.

554. Pelayo JC, Ziegler MG, Blantz RC: Angiotensin II in adrenergic-induced alterations in glomerular hemodynamics. Am J Physiol 247(5 Pt 2):F799–F807, 1984.

555. Gabbai FB, Thomson SC, Peterson O, et al: Glomerular and tubular interactions between renal adrenergic activity and nitric oxide. Am J Physiol 268(6 Pt 2):F1004–F1008, 1995.

556. Beierwaltes WH: Sympathetic stimulation of renin is independent of direct regulation by renal nitric oxide. Vascul Pharmacol 40(1):43–49, 2003.

557. Kon V, Yared A, Ichikawa I: Role of renal sympathetic nerves in mediating hypoperfusion of renal cortical microcirculation in experimental congestive heart failure and acute extracellular fluid volume depletion. J Clin Invest 76(5):1913–1920, 1985.

558. Wearn JT, Richards AN: Observations on the composition of glomerular urine, with particular reference to the problem of reabsorption in the renal tubule. Am J Physiol 71:209–227, 1924.

559. Walker AM, et al: The collection and analysis of fluid from single nephrons, of the mammalian kidney. Am J Physiol 134:580–595, 1941.

560. Brenner BM, Troy JL, Daugharty TM: The dynamics of glomerular ultrafiltration in the rat. J Clin Invest 50(8):1776–1780, 1971.

561. Oliver JD, III, Anderson S, Troy JL, et al: Determination of glomerular size-selectivity in the normal rat with Ficoll. J Am Soc Nephrol 3(2):214–228, 1992.

562. Scandling JD, Myers BD: Glomerular size-selectivity and microalbuminuria in early diabetic glomerular disease. Kidney Int 41(4):840–846, 1992.

563. Drumond MC, Deen WM: Structural determinants of glomerular hydraulic permeability. Am J Physiol 266(1 Pt 2):F1–F12, 1994.

564. Deen WM, Lazzara MJ, Myers BD: Structural determinants of glomerular permeability. Am J Physiol Renal Physiol 281(4):F579–F596, 2001.

565. Deen WM: What determines glomerular capillary permeability? J Clin Invest 114(10):1475–1483, 2004.

566. Drumond MC, Kristal B, Myers BD, Deen WM: Structural basis for reduced glomerular filtration capacity in nephrotic humans. J Clin Invest 94(3):1187–1195, 1994.

567. Maddox DA, Deen WM, Brenner BM: Dynamics of glomerular ultrafiltration. VI. Studies in the primate. Kidney Int 5(4):271–278, 1974.

568. Brenner BM, Falchuk KH, Keimowitz RI, Berliner RW: The relationship between peritubular capillary protein concentration and fluid reabsorption by the renal proximal tubule. J Clin Invest 48(8):1519–1531, 1969.

569. Maddox DA, Price DC, Rector FC Jr: Effects of surgery on plasma volume and salt and water excretion in rats. Am J Physiol 233(6):F600–F606, 1977.

570. Deen WM, Robertson CR, Brenner BM: A model of glomerular ultrafiltration in the rat. Am J Physiol 223(5):1178–1183, 1972.

571. Pinnick RV, Savin VJ: Filtration by superficial and deep glomeruli of normovolemic and volume-depleted rats. Am J Physiol 250(1 Pt 2):F86–F91, 1986.

572. Brenner BM, Ueki IF, Daugharty TM: On estimating colloid osmotic pressure in pre- and postglomerular plasma in the rat. Kidney Int 2(1):51–53, 1972.

573. Brenner BM, Troy JL, Daugharty TM, et al: Dynamics of glomerular ultrafiltration in the rat. II. Plasma-flow dependence of GFR. Am J Physiol 223(5):1184–1190, 1972.

574. Daniels BS, Hauser EB, Deen WM, Hostetter TH: Glomerular basement membrane: In vitro studies of water and protein permeability. Am J Physiol 262(6 Pt 2):F919–F926, 1992.

CHAPTER 4

Metabolic Basis of Solute Transport

Bruce C. Kone

The normal kidney encounters extreme metabolic demands even under physiologic conditions. The reabsorption of 99% of the 180 L of glomerular ultrafiltrate each day expends considerable metabolic energy and requires commensurate levels of energy production. Accordingly, though contributing less than 1% of the total body mass, the kidney basally consumes 10% of the total body oxygen, a value surpassed only by the heart among parenchymal organs. The functional capacity of the kidney to perform active transport and biosynthetic processes is dependent on its energy supply. The energy needed to perform such work is chiefly derived from biologic oxidation (O_2-requiring) reactions that convert metabolic substrates into high-energy compounds such as ATP. These oxidative processes, in particular mitochondrial oxidative phosphorylation, account for roughly 95% of total renal ATP production, although nonoxidative ATP generation, principally glycolysis (lactate generation from glucose), generates a greater share of ATP to support active solute transport in certain nephron segments.

Through their direct or indirect influence on electrochemical gradients, membrane ionic conductances, membrane permeability, and ion pump activity, metabolic components exert considerable control over transepithelial solute transport. Given this level of importance to renal function, the relationship between renal solute transport and metabolism has been the subject of extensive study over the past century. This chapter reviews the elements that couple ATP synthesis to solute transport, the preferred metabolic substrates for these processes, and the integration of individual nephron segments in generating and consuming energy to conduct solute transport.

ATP AND ACTIVE TRANSPORT

Since membranes are generally impermeable to ions distributed across them, ion-motive pumps are used to interconvert chemical energy derived from the hydrolysis of ATP ($ATP \rightarrow ADP + P_i$) or other high-energy phosphate molecules into an electrochemical gradient to drive transport against a concentration gradient. This process is termed *primary active transport* (Fig. 4–1). In the kidney, the principal mechanism for primary active transport is the Na+,K+-ATPase, an enzyme that serves to maintain the low concentration of Na+ and high concentration of K+ in the intracellular environment. *Secondary active transport* refers to transport that allows solutes to move along an electrochemical gradient, without chemical modification or direct consumption of energy (see Fig. 4–1). Thus, the energy stored in the steep Na+ gradient generated by the Na+,K+-ATPase can be used to direct Na+-coupled transport of sugars, amino acids, and a variety of other solutes along the nephron. H+-ATPases and Ca2+-ATPases in the plasma membranes of specific renal tubular epithelial cells can also generate ion gradients that can fuel Na+-independent secondary active transport. Indeed the H+-ATPase in the brush border membrane of the proximal tubule appears to be a significant energy-consuming process in certain species. Finally, the energy stored in the Na+ gradient generated by the Na+,K+-ATPase can be indirectly used to drive the transport of other ions and organic molecules. As one example, peptide transport in the proximal tubule is driven by a H+ gradient across the brush border membrane. As another example, the Na+/H+ exchanger, a secondary active transport system located in the brush border membrane, couples the influx of Na+ into the cell with the efflux of H+ from the cell and is thus principally responsible for the existence of this H+ gradient (see Fig. 4–1). The driving force for the Na+/H+ exchanger, a transmembrane Na+ gradient, is in turn generated and maintained by the Na+,K+-ATPase, a primary active transport system in the basolateral membrane of these cells. In tertiary active transport, the H+ gradient generated by the operation of the Na+,K+-ATPase and Na+/H+ exchanger is used to drive the tertiary active transport of Cl– across the brush border membrane via a Cl–/HCO3– exchanger (see Fig. 4–1).

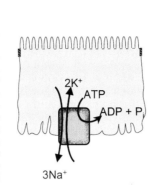 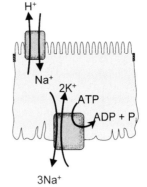 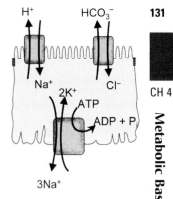

PRIMARY ACTIVE TRANSPORT   **SECONDARY ACTIVE TRANSPORT**   **TERTIARY ACTIVE TRANSPORT**

FIGURE 4–1 Active transport processes in renal epithelial cells. Models of three epithelial cells are shown to illustrate the different modes of active transport. Primary active transporters (in this example, the Na^+,K^+-ATPase) use the energy derived from ATP hydrolysis to power the transport of solutes across the plasma membrane against their electrochemical gradients. Secondary active transporters utilize the energy in the electrochemical gradient (in this example, Na^+) generated by the primary active transport process to drive the influx of efflux of a coupled solute. Tertiary active transport links the transport of a solute (in this example, Cl^-) to the gradient (in this case, H^+) created by the secondary active transport process.

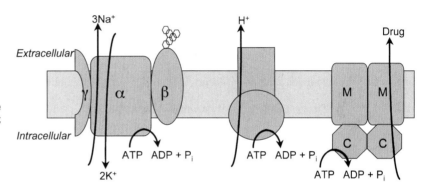

FIGURE 4–2 Major classes of transport ATPases in the kidney. M=membrane-spanning domain; C=catalytic domain; MDR1=multi-drug resistance protein 1.

P-type ATPase (example: Na^+,K^+-ATPase)   **V-ATPase** (example: H^+-ATPase)   **ABC superfamily** (example: MDR1)

ENERGY CONSUMPTION TO CONDUCT SOLUTE TRANSPORT

The intracellular ionic composition differs markedly from that of the extracellular fluid, and maintenance or restoration of this condition requires the input of energy. As previously emphasized, primary active transport processes make direct use of ATP, whereas secondary active transport makes use of the potential energy stored in transmembrane ion gradients. Various classes of ATP-driven solute pumps perform primary active transport. Many schemes exist to classify these pumps, but for simplicity, three broad classes important for renal transport are considered here (Fig. 4–2 and Table 4–1). These energy-requiring pumps provide for all solute transport along the nephron either by conducting the transport themselves or by establishing electrochemical gradients that allow the solute transport by secondary or tertiary active transport processes. In general, the distribution and level of expression of specific ATPases along the nephron correlates with the demands for solute transport and the required metabolic machinery (e.g., mitochondria, enzymes for ATP synthetic pathways) to support the transport. Numerous studies have also established that the activities and level of expression of these active transporters in specific nephron segments respond to changes in overall ion balance, hormones, and autocoids.

P-type ATPases are an evolutionarily conserved family of over 300 ATP hydrolysis-driven ion pumps that form an acyl-

TABLE 4–1	Major Classes of Inorganic Ion-Translocating ATPases Active in Kdney and Their Structural and Functional Characteristics		
Ion Pump	**Class**	**Subunit Structure**	**Ionic Stoichiometry**
Na^+,K^+-ATPase	P-type	$\alpha\beta$	$3Na^+:2K^+:ATP$
H^+,K^+-ATPase	P-type	$\alpha\beta$	$H^+:K^+:ATP$
Ca^{2+}-ATPase	P-type	α	$Ca^{2+}: (H^+):ATP$
Cu^{2+}-ATPase	P-type	α	$Cu^{2+}:ATP$
H^+-ATPase	V-type	F_1F_0 12 subunits	$H^+:ATP$

phosphate intermediate as part of the reaction mechanism and bear a seven amino acid signature motif, beginning with the aspartate to which the terminal phosphate of ATP is attached during the enzymatic cycle. These enzymes share four highly conserved protein domains ten transmembrane domains, as well as highly conserved phosphorylation and ATP-binding sites. The activity of most P-type ATPases is tightly controlled by extraregulatory domains or protein subunits. The Na^+,K^+-ATPase and the closely related gastric H^+,K^+-ATPase (H^+,K^+-ATPase $\alpha1$ subunit) are the only members of the P-type ATPase family comprising more than one subunit. On the basis of sequence similarities, phylogenetic analyses, and substrate specificities, Axelsen and Palmgren[1] classified this superfamily into 5 families and 11 subfamilies. The type Ia ATPases include the B subunit of the bacterial Kdp K^+-ATPase. Type Ib ATPases transport heavy metals such as Cu^{2+}, Cd^{2+}, and Zn^{2+}. Mutations in the ATP7A and ATP7B genes encoding Cu^{2+}-ATPases are responsible for Menkes disease and Wilson's disease, respectively. The type II subfamily transports non–heavy metal cations and includes the sarcoplasmic-endoplasmic reticulum Ca^{2+}-ATPases (SERCA; group IIa; three SERCA genes in humans); the secretory pathway Ca^{2+}-ATPases (SPCA; two genes in humans), which transport both Ca^{2+} and Mn^{2+} in the Golgi lumen and therefore play an important role in the cytosolic and intra-Golgi Ca^{2+} and Mn^{2+} homeostasis; the plasma membrane Ca^{2+}-ATPases (PMCA; group IIb, four genes in humans); and type IIc with the four isoforms of the Na^+,K^+-ATPase α-subunit and the gastric and "nongastric" H^+,K^+-ATPase α -subunits. The type III family is expressed only in plants and fungi and includes ATPases involved in the transport of Mg^{2+} and H^+. Type IV subfamily members are exclusively expressed in eukaryotic cells and translocate phospholipids, rather than cations, from the outer and inner leaflet of membrane bilayers,[2] and may play a role in vesicular (protein) trafficking in yeast. Finally, the recently identified type V subfamily, which is also exclusively expressed in eukaryotic cells, has been implicated in cellular Ca^{2+} homeostasis and endoplasmic reticulum function in yeast.

Vacuolar H^+-ATPases (V-ATPases) are a family of multisubunit ATP-dependent H^+ pumps responsible for acidification of intracellular organelles, including endosomes, lysomes, secretory vesicles, Golgi, and clathrin-coated vesicles, and of luminal or interstitial spaces. The V-ATPases are large multimeric complexes and differ from P-type ATPases in that they do not form a phosphoenzyme intermediate and are resistant to vanadate inhibition.

ATP-binding–cassette (ABC) transporters are a superfamily of proteins that couple ATP hydrolysis to the transport of a wide array of molecules across biologic membranes. Forty-nine ABC protein genes exist on human chromosomes. Eukaryotic ABC proteins were originally recognized as drug efflux pumps involved in the multidrug resistance of cancer cells, but it is now appreciated that they have multiple physiologic roles and their dysfunction can be often associated with human diseases. Collectively, they are known to transport a diverse array of drugs and toxins, conjugated organic anions comprising dietary and environmental carcinogens, pesticides, metals, metalloids, and lipid peroxidation products. They are recognized by their shared modular organization and by two sequence motifs that make up a nucleotide-binding fold. The functional protein generally contains two nuclear-binding folds and two transmembrane domains, typically consisting of six membrane-spanning α-helices.[3] ABC proteins that confer drug resistance include (but are not limited to) P-glycoprotein (ABCB1), the multidrug resistance protein 1 (MDR1, gene symbol ABCC1), MDR2 (gene symbol ABCC2), and the breast cancer resistance protein (BCRP, gene symbol ABCG2). Proteins of the ABC transporter superfamily have been implicated in the outward transport, or "flopping," of choline-containing phospholipids.[2] Multidrug resistance protein (MDR) 3 (ABCB4) specifically translocates phosphatidylcholine from the inner to the outer leaflet of the bilayer when expressed in LLC-PK1 cells.[4] MDR1 (ABCB1) protein, a broad-range xenobiotic transporter, translocates choline-containing lipids, including short-chain analogs of phosphatidylcholine, glucosylceramide, and platelet-activating factor. Studies of extracellular acidification rates in MDR1-transfected and null cells indicate that P-glycoprotein is tightly coupled to the metabolic state of the cell. The energy required for P-glycoprotein activation relative to the basal metabolic energy in glucose-deficient cells

was double that of glucose-fed cells, suggesting cellular protection by P-glycoprotein even under conditions of starvation.[5] Unlike P-glycoptorein and MDR1, ABCG2 is a half-transporter that must homodimerize to acquire transport activity. ABCG2 is found in a variety of stem cells and may protect them from exogenous and endogenous toxins. Its expression is upregulated under low-oxygen conditions, consistent with its high expression in tissues exposed to low-oxygen environments. ABCG2 interacts with heme and other porphyrins and protects cells and/or tissues from protoporphyrin accumulation under hypoxic conditions.[6]

P-type ATPases

Na^+,K^+-ATPASE. The Na^+,K^+-ATPase is an oligomeric membrane protein that couples the hydrolysis of one ATP molecule to the translocation of three Na^+ and two K^+ ions against their electrochemical gradients to maintain or restore the normally high K^+ and low Na^+ concentrations inside mammalian cells. The Na^+,K^+-ATPase plays a central role in the regulation of the membrane potential, cell ion content, and cell volume. In renal tubular epithelial cells, this enzyme is distributed in the basolateral membrane, and it provides the principal driving force for net Na^+ reabsorption and the secondary active transport of other ions and organic solutes. The specific activity of the purified Na^+,K^+-ATPase from renal medulla, approximately 10,000 ATP/min/enzyme molecule, is among the highest of any tissue.[7,8] Studies in the isolated perfused rat kidney suggest that the Na^+,K^+-ATPase directly accounts for about half of the total Na^+ reabsorbed by the kidney.[9]

Structurally, the minimal functional unit of the enzyme is a heterodimer of α and β subunits. The ~100-kD α-subunit is responsible for ATP hydrolysis, cation transport, and ouabain binding, whereas the ~40- to 60-kD (depending on the degree of glycosylation) β-subunit appears to play a role in the occlusion of K^+, the modulation of the K^+ and Na^+ affinity of the enzyme, and directing the holoenzyme to the plasma membrane. The $K_{0.5}$ for ATP of the enzyme is between 5 and 400 µM,[7,8] so that the ATP concentration in most cells is saturating for the enzyme. Four α- and three β-subunit isoforms have been identified, and these exhibit different tissue distributions and produce Na^+,K^+-ATPase isozymes with different transport properties.[7,8]

The α1β1 enzyme is found in nearly every tissue and is the principal isozyme of the kidney. The renal expression of the other Na^+,K^+-ATPase isoforms has been debated.[10-12] The α2 and α3 isoforms have been detected in renal cortex, medulla, and papilla and using RT-PCR,[11] in situ hybridization,[10] and differential [^{3}H]ouabain titration analysis.[12] Measurement of mRNA and protein levels together with [^{3}H]ouabain titration data, however, indicates that the α2- and α3-isoforms constitute less than or equal to 0.1% of the α1β1 enzyme of the kidney.[12] In contrast to the widespread expression of α1 and β1, the other α- and β-isoforms exhibit more restricted patterns of expression. The α2-isoform is expressed principally in adipocytes, skeletal and cardiac muscle, and brain. The α3-isoform is abundant in nervous tissues, whereas the α4-isoform is a testis-specific isoform.[7,8] The β2-isoform is present primarily in skeletal muscle, pineal gland, and neural tissues. Estimates of mRNA abundance by RNase protection assay showed that β2 constituted only 5% of the total β subunit mRNA.[11] β3 is present in testis, retina, liver, and lung.[13] The expression pattern of the Na^+,K^+-ATPase isoforms is under developmental and hormonal controls and may vary in pathologic states. However, no consistent data have emerged to indicate significant changes in the α1β1 enzyme predominance in the kidney under such transitions.

The distribution of the Na^+,K^+-ATPase α-subunit in the kidney has been extensively examined, using immunohistochemistry, Western blots, in situ hybridization, and RT-PCR

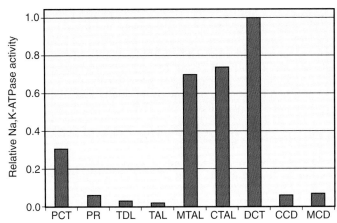

FIGURE 4–3 Relative levels of Na⁺,K⁺-ATPase activity measured in individual segments of the rat nephron. CCD, cortical collecting duct; CTAL, cortical thick ascending limb of Henle's loop; DCT, distal convoluted tubule; MCD, outer medullary collecting duct; MTAL, medullary thick ascending limb of Henle's loop; PCT, proximal convoluted tubule; PR, pars recta (proximal straight tubule); TAL, thin ascending limb of Henle's loop; TDL, thin descending limb of Henle's loop. (Data are normalized to that of the DCT and are redrawn from Katz AI, Doucet A, Morel F: Na⁺-K⁺-ATPase activity along the rabbit, rat, and mouse nephron. Am J Physiol 237:F114–F120, 1979.)

analysis of mRNA levels in microdissected nephron segments. In the aggregate, these studies indicate that the highest levels of Na⁺,K⁺-ATPase expression are in the medullary thick ascending limb of Henle's loop (MTAL), cortical thick ascending limb of Henle's loop (CTAL), and the distal convoluted tubule (DCT). Lower levels are evident in the proximal convoluted tubule (PCT) and cortical collecting duct (CCD), and very low levels are expressed in glomeruli, descending and ascending thin limbs of Henle (DTL and ATL, respectively), outer medullary collecting duct (OMCD), and inner medullary collecting duct (IMCD). These data correlate with studies in rabbit, rat, and mouse that have examined the amount of Na⁺,K⁺-ATPase hydrolytic activity and specific binding of [³H]ouabain in isolated nephron segments, indicating that the highest activity is in the MTAL, CTAL, and DCT, intermediate activity is in the PCT and CCD, and very low activity is in the proximal straight tubule (PST), DTL, and ATL[14,15] (Fig. 4–3). The distribution and relative abundance of the Na⁺,K⁺-ATPase along the nephron are generally comparable among these three species. Moreover, the differences in activity from different segments of the nephron appear to be the result of differences in pump number rather than differences in enzyme turnover rates or ATP dependence. El-Mernissi and Doucet[15] found that Na⁺,K⁺-ATPase hydrolytic activity and specific binding of [³H]ouabain to its single site on the Na⁺,K⁺-ATPase α-subunit were similar along the nephron.

In addition, the Na⁺,K⁺-ATPase has been shown to be regulated in a tissue-specific and isoform-specific fashion by direct interaction with at least five of the seven members of the FXYD family, including FXYD1 (phospholemman), FXYD2 (the γ-subunit), FXYD3 (Mat-8), FXYD4 (corticosteroid hormone–induced factor [CHIF]), and FXYD7, all members of the FXYD family of type II transmembrane proteins.[16] In addition, a dominant-negative mutation in FXYD2 has been linked to cases of autosomal dominant renal magnesium wasting.[17] A signature FXYD motif in the N-terminus and conserved glycine and serine residues in the transmembrane domain characterizes the FXYD proteins. The γ-subunit is expressed principally in the kidney, and CHIF is expressed in the medullary collecting duct and in the epithelium of the distal colon.[16] Two principal subtypes of the 8- to 14-kD hydrophobic polypeptide, termed "γₐ" and "γᵦ," have been

characterized in rat kidney. Both isoforms are highly expressed with the Na⁺,K⁺-ATPase α1-subunit in the MTAL, whereas γₐ is specific for cells in the macula densa and principal cells of the CCD but is not expressed in the CTAL. In contrast, γᵦ is present in the CTAL.[16] It is becoming increasingly apparent that the γ-subunit is a component of the renal Na⁺,K⁺-ATPase and that this subunit may influence kinetic properties of the holoenzyme. The γ-subunit decreases the apparent Na⁺ affinity of the Na⁺,K⁺-ATPase, increases the apparent affinity for ATP, and increases the K⁺ antagonism of cytoplasmic Na⁺ activation.[16] In contrast, CHIF increases the apparent Na⁺ affinity of the Na⁺,K⁺-ATPase.[16] CHIF knockout mice exhibit twofold higher urine volumes and an increased glomerular filtration rate under K-loaded conditions. In addition, treatment of K⁺-loaded mice for 10 days with furosemide resulted in increased mortality in the knockout mice but not in the wild-type group. These findings are consistent with an effect of CHIF on the Na⁺,K⁺-ATPase of the OMCD and IMCD.[18]

H⁺,K⁺-ATPASES. The H⁺,K⁺-ATPases are a family of integral membrane proteins closely related to the Na⁺,K⁺-ATPase. The H⁺,K⁺-ATPase in vertebrates exists as an α/β heterodimer and is encoded by at least two distinct genes. The H⁺,K⁺-ATPase α1-subunit (HKα1, also termed the *"gastric" H⁺,K⁺-ATPase*) was originally cloned from rat stomach,[19] and cDNAs encoding the HKα1-subunit have since been cloned from a wide range of species, including humans. The H⁺,K⁺-ATPase α2-subunit (HKα2, also termed the *"colonic"* or *"non-gastric" H⁺,K⁺-ATPase*) was first cloned from rat colon,[20] and an orthologous gene product ATP1AL1 has been characterized in humans.[21] Alternative splicing gives rise to HKα2 N-terminal splice variants in rabbit[22] and rat,[23] but these are not encoded by the mouse or human genes.[24] The members of the H⁺,K⁺-ATPase gene family appear to participate in the control of body K⁺ balance, renal HCO₃⁻ absorption, the enhanced ammonium secretion in the IMCD during chronic hypokalemia, and intracellular Na⁺ regulation in the macula densa.[25] The two isoforms differ in their tissue distribution, response to chronic K⁺ depletion, and inhibitor sensitivity. The HKα1-subunit is expressed in stomach and the medullary collecting ducts,[26] but not distal colon, and is inhibited by low concentrations of Sch-28080 but not by ouabain,[27] and its expression in the collecting duct is not affected by chronic hypokalemia.[26] In contrast, the HKα2-subunit is expressed in the medullary collecting ducts[28] and distal colon, but not stomach,[20] is Sch-28080–resistant and partially ouabain-sensitive,[27] and its expression in the collecting duct is upregulated by chronic hypokalemia.[28] From an energetics standpoint, both H⁺,K⁺-ATPase isoforms are believed to have identical stoichiometries for ATP.

Ca²⁺-ATPASE. The human plasma membrane Ca²⁺-ATPase (PMCA) isoforms are encoded by at least four separate genes. The diversity of these enzymes is further amplified by tissue-specific alternative splicing within regulatory sites, which generate multiple subtypes of each isoform. The functional enzyme is thought to consist an ~115-kD monomer. The enzyme isolated from kidney is calmodulin-dependent and has a $K_{0.5}$ for Ca²⁺ of approximately 0.7 µM, which correlates with the value obtained for ATP-dependent Ca²⁺ uptake in basolateral membrane vesicles from kidney cortex.[29]

Differences in the structure and localization of PMCA splice variants confer specific regulatory properties that may have consequences for proper cellular Ca²⁺ signaling. The isoforms are expressed in a tissue-dependent manner, with PMCA1 and PMCA4 widely expressed among tissues, whereas PMCA2 and PMCA3 are expressed predominantly in brain and skeletal muscle.[30] PMCA in concert with the NCX1 Na⁺/Ca²⁺ exchanger regulates intracellular Ca²⁺ concentrations and mediates both basal and hormone-stimulated Ca²⁺ efflux by distal tubules. Among nephron segments, the DCT possesses the highest Ca²⁺-ATPase activity[31] and exhibits the strongest immunocytochemical reactivity for PMCA protein expression.[32] Magocsi and colleagues[33] reported the presence of multiple PMCA isoform mRNAs detected by RT-PCR in the kidney. PMCA1 was found in cortex, outer medulla, and inner medulla, PMCA2 in cortex and outer medulla, and PMCA3 in outer medulla (the PMCA4 cDNA sequence was unknown at that time). RT-PCR of cDNA generated from microdissected rat tubules demonstrated PMCA2 expression exclusively in proximal tubules, CTALs, and distal tubules.[33] In a subsequent RT-PCR analysis by another laboratory, mRNAs for PMCA1 and PMCA2 were discovered to be abundant in the glomerulus, PCT, DTL, DCT, and CCD. PMCA3 mRNA was identified in the DTL and CTAL, and PMCA4 was found throughout the nephron.[34] The concordance of data obtained in human, rat, and mouse indicates that PMCA1 and PMCA4 are the principal transcripts and protein expressed in kidney,[32] whereas PMCA2 mRNA constitutes less than 2% of the total PMCA mRNA in the kidney and PMCA3 could not be detected. Molecular studies in immortalized mouse DCT cells (mDCT) demonstrated that PMCA1 and PMCA4 are the isoforms in these cells.[32] Transcripts of the SERCA3 isoforms, which like the other SERCA members is inhibited by thapsigargin but unlike the others does not appear to be regulated by phospholamban, have also been detected in kidney.[35] However, the physiologic role of this pump in the kidney is unknown.

Cu²⁺-ATPASES. The Menkes protein ATP7A and the Wilson's disease protein ATP7B are monomeric proteins with eight predicted transmembrane domains that export Cu^{2+}, and possibly other metals, from the cytoplasm to an intracellular organelle. The Menkes protein is essential for efficient dietary Cu^{2+} uptake in the small intestine but also in the delivery of Cu^{2+} to the brain across the blood-brain barrier and recovery of Cu^{2+} from the proximal tubules of the kidney. Patients with Menkes disease exhibit defective Cu^{2+} efflux. Under normal Cu^{2+} conditions, both ATP7A and ATP7B are located in the trans-Golgi network where they provide Cu^{2+} to secreted cuproenzymes.[36] When intracellular Cu^{2+} levels rise, ATP7A traffics to the plasma membrane to export the excess Cu^{2+}. Patients with Menkes disease and Wilson's disease both suffer Cu^{2+} accumulation in proximal tubules. In some Wilson's disease patients this Cu^{2+} accumulation causes tubular dysfunction, resulting in the increased urinary amino acid and Ca^{2+} excretion. In situ hybridization and immunolocalization studies have demonstrated that both Atp7a and Atp7b are expressed in glomeruli; however, Atp7b is also seen in the kidney medulla.[37]

Vacuolar H⁺-ATPases

In the kidney, V-ATPases play an important role in H⁺ secretion in the proximal tubule and along the length of the distal tubule and collecting duct. Immunohistochemical, biochemical, and physiologic studies demonstrated that the V-ATPase is present in proximal tubules, TALs, DCT, and intercalated cells of the collecting duct.[38] Several heritable diseases have been attributed to defects in genes that encode V-ATPase subunits, including renal tubular acidosis and osteopetrosis.[39] The renal V-ATPases can be inhibited by N,N'-dicyclohexyl carbodiimide (DCCD), the sulfhydryl reagent N-ethylmaleimide, and more specifically, by the macrolide antibiotic bafilomycin A. The H⁺:ATP stoichiometry of the V-ATPase has been suggested to be up to 3:1, and the K_m for ATP of the purified V-ATPases is roughly 150 µM. V-ATPases are composed of a cytoplasmic catalytic domain (V_1), responsible for ATP hydrolysis, and a transmembrane domain (V_0), responsible for H⁺ translocation. The V_1 domain consists of eight distinct subunits (A–H), with an aggregate molecular mass of ~570 kD. The 260-kDa V_0 domain complex is composed of 5 subunits (subunits a-d).[38] The V-ATPase in kidney

is regulated at multiple levels from changes in gene transcription and protein synthesis, to alterations in membrane insertion and interaction with heterologous proteins. Monogenic defects in two subunits (ATP6V0A4, ATP6V1B1) of the V-ATPase have been observed in patients with distal renal tubular acidosis.[38] As discussed later, recent work suggests that the V-ATPase may also be functionally coupled to ATP production from glycolysis.

ATP-Binding-Cassette Transporters

P-GLYCOPROTEINS. P-glycoproteins are ABC transporters originally discovered as drug pumps in multidrug-resistant cancer cells, but have since been found in many normal tissues. The 170-kD multidrug resistance transporter (MDR) confers resistance by active, ATP-dependent extrusion of a broad range of drugs that do not share obvious structural characteristics. These include anticancer drugs, immunosuppressive agents such as cyclosporine and FK506, cardiac glycosides, and antibiotics.[3] Humans have two known P-glycoprotein genes, ABCB1 and ABCB4 (formerly known as MDR1 and MDR3), whereas rodents have three genes, termed mdr1a, mdr1b, and mdr2. The human MDR1 and mouse mdr1a and mdr1b encode an ~170-kD plasma membrane ATPase (K_m ~ 38 µM ATP) that transports a wide range of structurally unrelated drugs, steroids, and phospholipids, and thereby confers multidrug resistance. In contrast, MDR3 and its ortholog mouse mdr2 encode P-glycoproteins that are phosphatidylcholine translocases and that have limited ability to transport numerous drugs, although they may transport some drugs in cell culture systems.[40] In the kidney, the MDR1 mRNA and protein are expressed in mesangial cells, proximal tubule, TAL, and collecting duct.[41] In mesangial[42] and proximal tubule cells, P-glycoprotein has been shown to transport xenobiotics. Human MDR2 was localized to the of proximal tubules by double and triple immunofluorescence microscopy.[43]

CYSTIC FIBROSIS TRANSMEMBRANE REGULATOR. Cystic fibrosis transmembrane regulator (CFTR), another member of the ABC transporter family, couples ATP signaling with ion transport. CFTR is regulated by phosphorylation of its regulatory R domain and ATP hydrolysis at two nucleotide-binding domains, but it is unique among the ABC transporter family in that it functions as a Cl⁻ channel. Mutations of this transporter lead to a defect of epithelial Cl⁻ secretion causing the disease cystic fibrosis. CFTR transcripts have been identified in all nephron segments, and the encoded protein participates in Cl⁻ secretion in the distal tubule and the principal cells of the CCD and IMCD.[44] Although patients with cystic fibrosis do not manifest serious renal dysfunction, they do have impaired ability to concentrate and dilute the urine and to excrete certain drugs.[44] In addition to Cl⁻ secretion, CFTR has also been shown to secrete ATP directly[45] or to modulate other ATP release channels.[46] In this manner, CFTR may regulate other ionic conductances, such as the epithelial Na⁺ channel (ENaC)[47] and ATP-regulated K⁺ channels (Kir 1.1., also known as ROMK)[48] in the collecting duct. The effect of CFTR on the renal K⁺ secretory channel is mediated by protein kinase A, which may provide a functional switch designating the distribution of open and ATP-inhibited K⁺ channels in apical membranes. Recent studies also revealed that overexpression of CFTR promotes cell volume recovery from swelling or a regulatory volume decrease, enhances both constitutive and volume-sensitive ATP release, and through purinergic receptors, facilitates autocrine control of cell volume.[49] CFTR requires the hydrolysis of ATP for activity and has been shown to interact physically with AMP-activated protein kinase (AMPK), with activation of AMPK resulting in an inhibition of CFTR in epithelial cells colonic and pulmonary epithelial cells (detailed later).[50]

ENERGY PRODUCTION TO FUEL SOLUTE TRANSPORT

The various metabolic pathways that support and regulate solute transport along the nephron are highly integrated and interdependent. The oxidation of carbohydrate, lipid, and protein is tightly coupled to the generation and utilization of energy. The tricarboxylic acid (TCA) cycle and β oxidation of fatty acids are tightly linked to mitochondrial electron transport via the supply and demand of nicotinamide and flavin nucleotides. Similarly, electron transport is tightly coupled to oxidative phosphorylation and the supply and demand for ADP and ATP. Given its high transport demands, the kidney favors the more efficient ATP generation of aerobic metabolism (36 ATP produced per glucose consumed) over anaerobic metabolism (e.g., 6 ATP per glucose consumed in anaerobic glycolysis). Studies using diverse experimental methods in a variety of species, including humans, have provided a model of the relative contributions and intrarenal localization of specific metabolic pathways that fuel renal solute transport under physiologic and pathophysiologic conditions. These methods have included studies in the intact organism, isolated perfused kidney, renal tissue slices, tubule suspensions, and isolated nephron segments. Techniques applied to these studies have included measurements of $^{14}CO_2$ production from ^{14}C-labeled substrates, oxygen consumption (QO_2), ATP contents, and NADH fluorescence, ^{31}P nuclear magnetic resonance (NMR) spectroscopy, blood oxygen level–dependent (BOLD)-MRI, and others.

Mitochondrial ATP Production

Oxidative Phosphorylation

In 1924, Otto Warburg characterized the O_2 transferring component of the "respiratory enzyme" and established the phenomenon of cellular respiration. A few years later, Lohmann, Fiske, and Subbarow isolated ATP from muscle extract, and in 1937, Kaclkar reported the link between cellular respiration and ATP synthesis. In 1961, Mitchell proposed the chemiosmotic theory, which states that the energy stored in an electrochemical gradient across the inner mitochondrial membrane could be coupled to ATP synthesis. Although this theory met with controversy until the mid-1970s, it has now gained widespread acceptance.

Oxidative phosphorylation occurs in the mitochondrial inner membrane and includes the oxidation of metabolic fuels by O_2 and the associated transduction of energy into ATP. The electron transport chain, or respiratory chain, is a system of mitochondrial enzymes and redox carrier molecules that transfer reducing equivalents (electrons), obtained from the oxidation of respiratory substrates, to O_2 (Fig. 4–4). It comprises five enzyme complexes (complexes I–V), ubiquinone (or coenzyme Q), and cytochrome c. This set of enzymes consists of NADH:ubiquinone oxidoreductase (complex I), succinate:ubiquinone oxidoreductase (complex II), ubiquinone:cytochrome c oxidoreductase (complex III, cytochrome reductase, cytochrome $bc1$), cytochrome c oxidase (complex IV, cytochrome oxidase), and ATP synthase (complex V, F_1F_0-ATPase). Other membrane-bound enzymes, such as the energy linked transhydrogenase, fulfill ancillary roles. The crystal structures of the major complexes of the electron transport chain (except complex I) have been established, permitting detailed analyses of the mechanism of H^+ pumping coupled to electron transport in the mitochondria.

The first step in the oxidation process involves transfer of electrons from NADH to complex I. Alternatively, electrons can transfer from $FADH_2$ to complex II. Because the latter complex does not move H^+, oxidation of $FADH_2$ results in the movement of fewer H^+ across the membrane and the production of less ATP. Hence, NAD-linked substrates give consistently higher ADP:O ratios (~2.5) compared with FAD-linked substrates, such as succinate (ADP:O ratio ~1.5). Variability of coupling may occur under some conditions but is generally not significant. The fractional values result from the coupling ratios of proton transport. An additional revision of ADP:O ratio may be required because a recent report of the structure of ATP synthase suggests that the H^+:ATP ratio is 10:3, rather than 3, consistent with ADP:O ratios of 2.3 with NADH and 1.4 with succinate.[51]

After entry into the respiratory chain, electrons are transferred sequentially to coenzyme Q, complex III), cytochrome c, complex IV, and finally to O_2, which is reduced to H_2O (see Fig. 4–4). The free energy released by the fall in redox potential of the passing electrons during electron transfer drives the translocation of H^+ via complexes I, II, and IV from the mitochondrial matrix to the inner mitochondrial space. This process generates a H^+ electrochemical potential gradient across the inner mitochondrial membrane of 200 to 230 mV,[52] which is known as the *proton-motive force*. The H^+ then

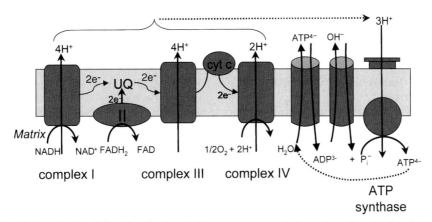

FIGURE 4–4 Mitochondrial oxidative phosphorylation. The mitochondrial electron transport chain conducts the oxidation of NADH or $FADH_2$, generates an H^+ gradient across the inner mitochondrial membrane to drive ATP synthesis, and consumes O_2. The proteins that make up the electron transport chain are integral membrane proteins of the inner mitochondrial membrane. Substrate-level dehydrogenase reactions within the mitochondrial space generate NADH, which contributes 2 electrons (e^{-1}) to complex I. These electrons are sequentially transferred to complexes III and IV, with O_2 as the final acceptor. Ubiquinone (UQ) and cytochrome c (cyt c) function as mobile carriers of electrons between complexes. The flow of electrons from higher to lower redox potentials generates energy that is used to extrude 10 to 12 H^+ from the matrix space. The H^+ gradient across the inner mitochondrial membrane is used to drive ATP synthesis by the ATP synthase (F_1F_0-ATPase, complex V). An adenine nucleotide translocase, which exchanges ATP^{4-} for ADP^{3-}, and a PO_4^-/OH^- exchanger in the inner mitochondrial membrane function to deliver and extrude ADP, P_i, and ATP.

reenters the matrix via the F_1F_0-ATPase of complex V (ATP synthase), driving ATP synthesis. The F_1F_0-ATPase complex (Mr ~500,000) contains at least 12 distinct subunits, several of which are present in multiple copies. The catalytic F_1 head group, which contains three nucleotide binding sites, is connected by an oligomycin-sensitive stalk to a H^+-conducting F_0 baseplate embedded in the mitochondrial inner membrane. Three H^+ are thought to pass through the membrane for each molecule of ATP manufactured by the complex. An increase in Na^+,K^+-ATPase activity, therefore, decreases the intramitochondrial phosphorylation potential ($[ATP]/[ADP][P_i]$), which results in more rapid H^+ entry via the F_1F_0-ATPase, a dissipation of the H^+ gradient, and more rapid electron transfer along the electron transport chain to extrude H^+ and increase QO_2.

The proton-motive force arises both from the change in membrane potential from the net movement of positive charge across the inner mitochondrial membrane and the pH gradient. Of these two components, the membrane potential contributes most of the energy stored in the gradient. The H^+ gradient can also be dissipated by the presence of the uncoupling proteins UCP1, UCP2, UCP3, or by other transport processes for various ions and small molecules. Additional transporters influence the membrane potential of the inner mitochondrial membrane, and thereby the proton-motive force. The adenosine nucleotide translocator, which conducts the electrogenic 1:1 exchange of ADP^{3-} for ATP^{4-}, a phosphate transporter, which imports PO_4^- in exchange for OH^-, and a constitutive proton H^+ leak reside in the inner mitochondrial membrane protein (see Fig. 4–4). The voltage-dependent anion channel localizes to the outer mitochondrial membrane. In addition to the proteins involved in the TCA cycle, the electron transport chain, and ATP synthesis, a number of other factors, including shuttles and transporters, are required for oxidative phosphorylation. Mitochondrial carrier proteins, integral membrane proteins that transport metabolites and cofactors across the inner membrane of mitochondria, are also required for ATP synthesis, the TCA cycle, fatty acid β-oxidation, and the malate shuttle.

Under certain stresses, such as free radical–mediated damage, mitochondria experience an irreversible autocatalytic collapse, with a loss of the normal membrane potential and a failure of ATP production, termed the *mitochondrial permeability transition*. The transition involves the integration of adenine nucleotide transporter subunits and other outer membrane proteins into a large pore, which allows free entrance of small ions to the mitochondrial interior. Atractyloside inactivates the ATP/ADP antiporter and favors pore formation, whereas bongkrekic acid and cyclosporine inhibit the process. Mitochondria that undergo the permeability transition release pro-apoptotic molecules.

Oxygen Consumption, Respiratory Control, and Coupled Respiration

Much of our understanding of mitochondrial respiration has come from studies of QO_2 in cells and isolated mitochondria. When normal mitochondria are incubated in an isotonic medium containing substrate and phosphate, ADP addition promotes a sudden increase in QO_2 as the ADP is converted into ATP. This active state of respiration, termed *"state 3" respiration*, distinguishes the maximal QO_2 that is coupled to ATP production. In permeabilized proximal tubules for example, ADP stimulates QO_2 by four- to fivefold over baseline.[53] The subsequent slower rate of QO_2 after all the ADP has been phosphorylated to form ATP is referred to as *state 4*. The ratio of QO_2 in state 3 to that in state 4 is termed the *respiratory control index,* and it reflects the O_2 uptake (oxidation of NADH and/or $FADH_2$) by intact mitochondria and the simultaneous conversion of ADP and inorganic phosphate into ATP. Because the catalytic site for ATP synthesis by the

F_1F_0-ATPase is in the mitochondrial matrix, respiratory control is likely related to the availability of ADP and the kinetics of its transport by the adenine nucleotide translocase, a hypothesis first proposed by Chance and Williams in the 1950s.[54] *Coupled respiration* refers to O_2 uptake dependent on the presence of ADP and P_i. Respiratory control reflects the fact that the oxidation of NADH and $FADH_2$ is coupled to the H^+ transport across the mitochondrial inner membrane. If the movement of H^+ through the F_1F_0-ATPase to drive ATP synthesis does not dissipate the H^+ gradient, the energy required for H^+ translocation would exceed that derived from electron transfer and thus inhibit further electron transport. Competing hypotheses have been proposed to explain the factor(s) responsible for respiratory control. Lemasters and Sowers[55] proposed that the kinetics of the adenine nucleotide translocase, an inner mitochondrial membrane protein that exchanges cytosolic ADP^{3-} for intramitochondrial ATP^4, governs the rate of ATP synthesis. The adenine nucleotide translocase operates in parallel with a P_i/OH^- exchanger in the inner mitochondrial membrane that uses the H^+ gradient to drive P_i entry (see Fig. 4–4). Inhibitors of the adenine nucleotide translocase, such as atractyloside, caused inhibition of ADP influx, respiration, and ATP synthesis.[55] However, it is unclear whether [ADP] itself or the [ATP]/[ADP] ratio preferentially regulates the translocase.

The near-equilibrium hypothesis of Erecinska and Wilson[56] proposed that respiration and ATP synthesis are mainly regulated by the phosphorylation potential and the $NADH/NAD^+$ ratio. However, oxidative phosphorylation may not always be near equilibrium, and relative proximity to equilibrium does not necessarily exclude the contributions of the electron transport chain, H^+ leak, F_1F_0-ATPase, or adenine nucleotide translocase to regulation of essential fluxes. In some instances, for example, respiration rate may correlate better with [ADP] than with phosphorylation potential, and may be relatively insensitive to mitochondrial $NADH/NAD^+$ ratio. Although it is clear from these considerations that mitochondrial respiratory control is a complex process potentially involving ATP, ADP, P_i, the NAD redox state, cytochrome c, O_2, and other factors as signals, there is compelling evidence to support the concept that the dynamics of cytosolic ATP, ADP, and P_i participate in the coupling between mitochondrial respiration and active transport.

QO_2 measurements also provide important insights into the coupling of active Na^+ transport and cellular respiration (Table 4–2). As noted earlier, the state 3 rate of respiration provides an index of the maximal rate at which mitochondrial oxygen consumption is coupled to ATP production. Because tubule cells are impermeable to ADP, the tubules are first permeabilized by additions of low concentrations of digitonin, before addition of ADP. Assays of carbonylcyanide-m-chlorophenylhydrazone (CCCP)–uncoupled QO_2, provide similar information about mitochondrial respiratory capacity in the intact cell. The oligomycin-sensitive component of basal QO_2 represents that directly related to ATP synthesis. In proximal tubules, oligomycin inhibits at least 80% of basal QO_2.[57] The ouabain-sensitive rate of respiration indicates that proportion of respiration devoted to the operation of the Na^+,K^+-ATPase and of secondary active transport coupled to the Na^+,K^+-ATPase. The value of ouabain-sensitive QO_2 varies among nephron segments ranging from 8% in the OMCD to 60% of total QO_2 in the PCT, according to the proportionate needs of active Na^+ transport (see Fig. 4–8). The basal, ouabain-insensitive respiration reflects mitochondrial respiration devoted to Na^+-independent processes, such as the operation of other primary and secondary active transport processes (e.g., H^+-ATPase, Ca^{2+}-ATPase), synthesis of DNA, RNA, protein, lipids, and glucose (gluconeogenesis), mitochondrial H^+ leak, and substrate interconversions. For unclear reasons, the basal, ouabain-insensitive QO_2 is considerably

TABLE 4-2	Components of QO₂
QO₂ Parameter	**Interpretation**
Ouabain-insensitive	Basal rate, composed of Primary and secondary active transport not coupled to the Na⁺,K⁺-ATPase (e.g., H⁺-ATPase) Biosynthetic functions (lipids, glucose) Cell growth and repair Substrate interconversions and transformations
Ouabain-sensitive	Na⁺,K⁺-ATPase and secondary active transport coupled to the Na⁺,K⁺-ATPase
Nystatin-simulated	Maximal activation of the Na⁺,K⁺-ATPase; should be completely inhibited by ouabain
CCCP uncoupled	Maximal mitochondrial respiratory capacity
Oligomycin-sensitive	QO₂ coupled to ATP synthesis from mitochondrial oxidative phosphorylation

QO₂ can be used to dissect mechanisms that couple active Na⁺ transport and mitochondrial oxidative phosphorylation. The ouabain-insensitive QO₂ provides a measurement of basal QO₂ that is independent of Na⁺ transport. The ouabain-sensitive rate is related to active Na⁺ transport mediated by the Na⁺,K⁺-ATPase. The nystatin-stimulated QO₂ tests the integrity of the functions of and links between Na⁺ entry, Na⁺,K⁺-ATPase, and mitochondrial respiration. The carbonylcyanide-m-chlorophenylhydrazone (CCCP)-uncoupled QO₂ and the oligomycin-sensitive of QO₂ provide information regarding mitochondrial integrity and function.

higher in isolated renal cells and tubules (40%–90%), compared with measurements in whole kidney (<20%). Addition of cationophores, such as nystatin or monensin, allows the Na⁺ concentration to equilibrate across the membrane and provides maximal stimulation of the Na⁺,K⁺-ATPase without adversely affecting mitochondrial function. Thus, the effects of the maximal stimulation, with nystatin, and maximal inhibition, with ouabain, of Na⁺,K⁺-ATPase activity on QO₂ provide an assessment of the integrity of this ion pump and its coupling to Na⁺ entry and to mitochondrial respiration. Elegant studies in suspensions of cortical tubules by Mandel's laboratory, for example, found that nystatin stimulated QO₂ by nearly 60% above its spontaneous rate and to the respiratory capacity of the tubules as defined by the state 3 rate. In contrast, ouabain inhibited spontaneous QO₂ by about 50%.[58] In these same studies, ATP contents were found to change little during these maneuvers: ATP declined by 15% during nystatin stimulation and increased by 6% during ouabain inhibition.[59]

Mitochondrial Substrate Entry

Many important metabolites show an asymmetrical distribution across the mitochondrial inner membrane. Therefore, normal operation of the respiratory chain requires highly specific transporters to control the movement of substrates across the membrane. These include electroneutral uptake mechanisms for phosphate, malate, succinate, 2-oxoglutarate, and citrate, as well as several exchangers for organic solutes (Fig. 4–5). In general, these transporters exploit directly or

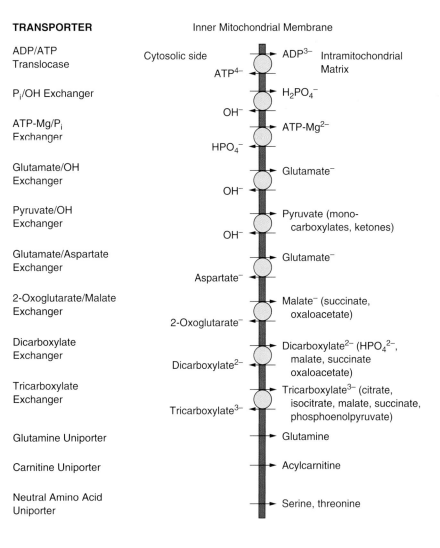

FIGURE 4-5 Major metabolite transporters in the mitochondrial inner membrane. These transporters permit the selective accumulation of organic solutes in the mitochondrial matrix that can be metabolized by the TCA cycle and other mitochondrial enzymes, as well as ADP and Pᵢ needed for ATP synthesis. These pathways are driven directly or indirectly by the H⁺ gradient (matrix side alkaline), membrane potential (matrix side negative), and/or solute gradients.

indirectly the H^+ gradient generated by the electron transport chain. Consequently, conditions that alter the mitochondrial pH gradient, such as intracellular acidosis or certain drugs, can change the concentrations of metabolites within the mitochondria and thereby influence oxidative metabolism. The transporter expression and specificity governs the ability of various tissues to conduct substrate oxidations (see Fig. 4–5). Although many of these transporters have been identified in the kidney, the intrarenal distribution of specific transporters has not yet been defined. Moreover, the role of these transporters has largely been studied in mitochondria from heart or liver, so that there is little information regarding the specific properties of these transporters in renal cells.

Three of the most important metabolite carriers are the energy-driven aspartate/glutamate exchange (aspartate exchanges for glutamate plus a H^+), the aspartate carrier, and the carnitine palmitoyltransferase (CPT) system. The aspartate/glutamate exchange plays an important role in maintaining the cytosolic compartment in a relatively "oxidizing" state (with a low $NADH/NAD^+$ ratio), while keeping the mitochondrial space correspondingly reduced and suppressing the aerobic synthesis of lactic acid. The aspartate carrier plays a central role in the reoxidation of glycolytic NADH by the malate-aspartate cycle, involving malate dehydrogenase and glutamate oxaloacetate transaminase. This cycle overcomes the fact that the inner membrane is impermeable to NAD^+ and NADH. The carnitine palmitoyltransferase (CPT) system (CPTI and CPTII) mediates the transport of long-chain fatty acids into the mitochondria for oxidation. CPTI exchanges carnitine for the CoA attached to long-chain fatty acids to create a fatty acid–carnitine conjugate. This conjugate is transported into the matrix by a transporter protein in the inner mitochondrial membrane. Once the fatty acid–carnitine conjugate is inside the matrix, CPTII exchanges CoA for carnitine to produce new fatty acid–CoA again, which is ready to enter fatty acid oxidation in the matrix. The liberated carnitine is exported to renew the cytoplasmic pool of carnitine and allow the transfer process to continue.

Inhibitors of Mitochondrial Function

Much of our knowledge of mitochondrial function has resulted from the use of specific inhibitors to probe discrete mechanisms. These compounds have been used to distinguish the electron transport system from the phosphorylation system and to establish the sequence of redox carriers along the respiratory chain (Fig. 4–6). In addition, they have been used to probe the contributions of specific metabolic pathways to solute transport along the nephron. Several categories of mitochondrial inhibitors can be distinguished. *Respiratory chain inhibitors* (e.g., antimycin and rotenone) block mitochondrial respiration, even in the presence of either ADP or uncoupling agents. Rotenone inhibits complex I, and

antimycin A inhibits cytochrome *c. Phosphorylation inhibitors,* such as oligomycin, block the burst of QO_2 and ATP manufacture after ADP addition, but only if the respiratory coupling is intact. *Uncoupling agents* (e.g., dinitrophenol, CCCP) inhibit the coupling between the respiratory chain and the phosphorylation system. By shuttling H^+ across the inner mitochondrial membrane, uncoupling agents dissipate the H^+ gradient, uncouple the processes of oxidation and phosphorylation, and block ATP synthesis. This results in a high rate of QO_2 in the absence of ADP until all O_2 is consumed. *Transport inhibitors* (e.g., atractyloside, bongkrekic acid, *N*-ethylmaleimide) prevent either ATP export or substrate import across the mitochondrial inner membrane. *Ionophores* (e.g., valinomycin, nigericin) render the inner membrane leaky to ions to which the membrane is usually impermeable.

Renal Transport Defects Associated with Mitochondrial Genetic Disorders

Genetic mutations in components of the electron transport chain or ATP synthase that affect renal solute transport have been described. In general, renal manifestations of these disorders tend to be more commonly observed in children than in adults. Most of these diseases affect other organ systems as well, particularly the central nervous system and muscle. Of the renal manifestations, the most common defect reported is a proximal tubulopathy resulting in a form of the Fanconi syndrome, but other patients developed tubulointerstitial nephritis, renal failure, or nephrotic syndrome.[60] Because the Na^+,K^+-ATPase drives the secondary active transport of glucose, phosphate, and amino acids, insufficient ATP supply to this pump results in impaired reabsorption of these solutes. Renal biopsy often shows giant mitochondria and nonspecific abnormalities of the tubules, including tubular atrophy and casts.[60] Diagnosis rests on establishing proper oxidoreduction status and activity of enzymatic complexes of the respiratory chain. For most patients—especially those presenting with tubulopathy—plasma lactate, pyruvate, ß-OH butyrate, acetoacetate, and their molar ratios were within the normal ranges. This could be ascribed to renal leakage, which contributes to lowering blood lactate. Thus, normal lactatemia does not rule out the hypothesis of a mitochondrial disorder in patients with renal involvement. However, urinary organic acids chromatography revealed high lactate and Krebs cycle intermediates, which are highly suggestive of mitochondrial disorder. Treatment is generally unsatisfactory. However, patients with complex I deficiency may be treated with riboflavin and ubidecarone (coenzyme Q10),[61] and patients with complex III deficiency may benefit from menadione (vitamin K_3) or ubidecarone. Patients with secondary carnitine deficiency may benefit from carnitine supplementation.

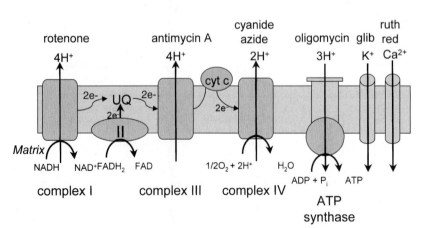

FIGURE 4–6 Inhibitors of mitochondrial respiration. Representative inhibitors of mitochondrial oxidative phosphorylation and their sites of action in the inner mitochondrial membrane are shown. Glib, glibenclamide; Ruth red, ruthenium red.

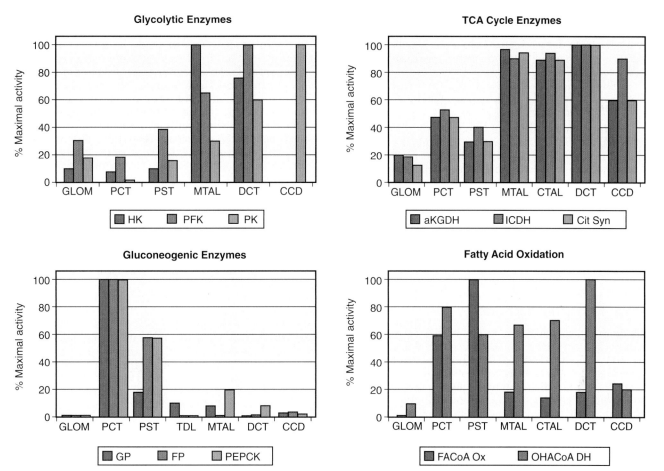

FIGURE 4–7 Intrarenal distribution of enzymes involved in four major metabolic pathways. Assays of enzymatic activity for each of the indicated enzymes were performed on microdissected nephron segments. The data represent the percent of maximal activity for each enzyme. α-KGDH, α-ketoglutarate dehydrogenase; FACoA Ox, fatty acyl-CoA oxidase; FP, fructose bisphosphatase; GP, glucose-6-phosphatase; HK, hexokinase; ICDH, isocitrate dehydrogenase; OHACoA DH, 3-hydroxyacyl-CoA dehydrogenase; PEPCK, phosphoenolpyruvate carboxykinase; PFK, phosphofructokinase; PK, pyruvate kinase. (Data from references 62, 63, 66, 68, 169, 199.)

Glycolysis

Glycolysis, the formation of lactate from glucose or glycogen, is accomplished by the actions of 11 cytoplasmic enzymes. In the kidney, glycolysis derives principally from glucose because glycogen stores are minimal. Glycolysis can occur under anaerobic or aerobic conditions, in which case mitochondria can continue the oxidation of glucose by converting lactate or pyruvate to CO_2. Glycolysis may be particularly important in the renal medulla and papilla where O_2 concentrations are low and aerobic metabolism is not effectively supported. The key regulatory enzymes—hexokinase, phosphofructokinase, and pyruvate kinase—are most active in the renal medulla. The distribution of these enzymes along the rodent and rabbit nephron has been examined[62,63] (Fig. 4–7). In the rat, hexokinase and pyruvate kinase activities were relatively low in the proximal tubule but are at least 10-fold greater in the MTAL and about 8-fold greater in the DCT. In the rabbit, the activity of the hexokinase is lowest in the PCT and progressively increases in parallel with pyruvate kinase and phosphofructokinase along the distal nephron, including the MTAL, CTAL, DCT, and the entire collecting duct, with highest values in the connecting tubule. In addition, superficial nephrons exhibited lower activities of pyruvate kinase and phosphofructokinase compared with juxtamedullary nephrons.[64] RT-PCR analysis of rat nephron segments demonstrated the expression of aldolase A and pyruvate kinase in the thin limb and collecting ducts of the medulla and in the distal tubules and glomeruli of the cortex.[65]

Tricarboxylic Acid Cycle

The enzymes for the TCA cycle are located in the matrix of the mitochondria. Acetyl coenzyme A is the major substrate entering the TCA cycle, and three products are generated: (1) H^+, for oxidative phosphorylation, (2) CO_2 from the metabolism of carbohydrate, fat, and proteins, and (3) ATP, synthesized by a substrate phosphorylation step in the TCA cycle. The activity of the TCA cycle enzymes oxoglutarate dehydrogenase, citrate synthase, isocitrate dehydrogenase, and α-ketoglutarate dehydrogenase, and isocitrate dehydrogenase are particularly high in the CTAL, MTAL, and DCT, and very low in the TDL and the medullary collecting duct (see Fig. 4–7). Oxoglutarate dehydrogenase shows the lowest activities along the whole nephron and appears to catalyze the rate-limiting step of the TCA cycle.[66]

Ketone Body Metabolism

The kidney can utilize ketone bodies as an energy source. In studies of cortical tissue slices, for example, acetoacetate met the majority of energy demands.[67] Guder and colleagues[68] described the distribution of two enzymes of ketone body metabolism, 3-oxoacid CoA-transferase and 3-hydroxybutyrate dehydrogenase in dissected segments of the mouse nephron. Both enzymes were found in all nephron segments, and their distribution generally paralleled the distribution of mitochondria along the nephron. The highest activities of the enzymes were observed in the TAL and DCT and decreased to only 20% of these values in the collecting duct. The proximal tubule exhibited heterogeneity, with uniform activity of 3-hydroxybutyrate dehydrogenase along its length, whereas the activity of 3-oxoacid CoA-transferase increased fivefold from PCT to PST (see Fig. 4–7).

Fatty Acid Oxidation

The oxidation of fatty acids is an important source of energy for ATP production in mitochondria through the entry of acetyl-CoA into the TCA cycle. Fatty acids can be oxidized in all nephron segments, with their rates of oxidation mirroring the mitochondrial mass of the nephron segments.[69] Fatty acyl-CoA oxidase activity is greatest in the proximal tubule, increasing along its length, whereas there is little activity in more distal structures (see Fig. 4–7). The mitochondrial enzyme 3-hydroxyacyl-CoA dehydrogenase generally followed the distribution of mitochondrial density along the nephron, with highest activities in the PCT and DCT.[66]

Pentose-Phosphate Shunt

The pentose-phosphate cycle yields the reducing energy needed for the biosynthesis of fatty acids, steroids, and nucleotides. It completely oxidizes glucose under anaerobic conditions. Glucose 6-phosphate dehydrogenase, the first enzyme in the pentose phosphate shunt, is found throughout the nephron, with highest catalytic activities in the proximal tubules and the DCT (see Fig. 4–7). Pentose-phosphate shunt activity has been demonstrated using radiolabeled glucose consumption in tissue slices and nephron segments.[70] Based on these studies, this pathway is estimated to account for about 10% of total glucose utilization in the kidney.

GLUCONEOGENESIS AND ITS ROLE IN SOLUTE TRANSPORT

In 1937, Benoy and Elliott[71] demonstrated the capacity of the kidney to perform gluconeogenesis, the de novo formation of glucose from noncarbohydrate precursors. Gram-for-gram, the kidney exhibits glucose synthetic rates several times higher than that observed in the liver.[72] However, because arteriovenous difference measurements revealed that the kidneys of postabsorptive subjects show little or no net take-up or release of glucose, renal gluconeogenesis in humans under normal or pathologic conditions was believed to be of little consequence compared with that of the liver until the mid-1990s. Then, the combination of arteriovenous difference measurements with tracer techniques demonstrated that, in healthy postabsorptive humans, the renal glucose release approaches 20% of all glucose released in the circulation.[73] The kidney has minimal glycogen stores, and its cells that are capable of storing glycogen lack glucose-6-phosphatase. Thus, renal glucose release occurs almost exclusively from gluconeogenesis. Renal glucose release is of the same order of magnitude as splanchnic glucose release during the postabsorptive period in humans, appears to be more sensitive to hormone action than hepatic glucose release, and may have a more important role during the adaptation to various physiologic and pathologic conditions. The kidney is now recognized as playing a key role in interorgan glucose metabolism, and particularly in the Cori cycle and glutamine-glucose cycle.

Compared with liver, renal gluconeogenesis has different substrate requirements and responds to different regulatory stimuli. The preferred gluconeogenic precursors in the kidney are lactate, glutamine, glycerol, α-ketoglutarate, and citrate.

Of these, lactate is the predominant precursor for both renal and systemic gluconeogenesis in humans. Renal gluconeogenesis from lactate was shown to be 3.5-, 2.5-, and 9.6-fold greater than that from glycerol, glutamine, and alanine, respectively. These four substrates accounted for ~90% of renal gluconeogenesis in humans.[73] In vitro studies of microdissected S1, S2, and S3 human proximal tubules incubated with physiologic concentrations of glutamine or lactate revealed that the three successive segments have roughly the same capacity to synthesize glucose from glutamine, whereas the S2 and S3 segments synthesize more glucose from lactate than the S1 segment.[74] Studies in multiple species indicate that it is difficult to extrapolate results concerning the metabolic heterogeneity of the nephron obtained in a given animal species to humans. In humans, renal gluconeogenesis is altered under physiologic and pathophysiologic states, including fasting, hypoglycemia, and diabetes mellitus. cAMP was a potent agonist of gluconeogenesis from lactate and glutamine by human proximal tubules, whereas adrenaline and noradrenaline were ineffective, suggesting that the stimulation of renal gluconeogenesis observed in vivo with adrenaline infusion may result from an indirect action on the renal proximal tubule.[74]

Studies in animals and humans indicated that only the proximal tubule is capable of synthesizing glucose, and the only nephron segment that contains the key gluconeogenic enzymes glucose 6-phosphatase, fructose 1,6-diphosphatase, and phoshoenolpyruvate carboxykinase (PEPCK)[69] (see Fig. 4–7). mRNA transcripts encoding fructose-1,6-bisphosphatase aldolase B and PEPCK have been detected in rat proximal cells.[65] Aldolase B was found to be bound specifically to fructose 1,6-diphosphatase in these cells. In the absence of glutamine and lactate, glucose synthesis from endogenous substrates is negligible[74] and consistent with the very low glycogen content of the proximal tubule in normal subjects. The proximal tubule is metabolically heterogeneous along its course, however, and species differences exist. Microdissected S1, S2, and S3 segments of the human proximal tubule synthesize glucose from lactate and glutamine at physiologic concentrations, with the S2 and S3 segments capable of more glucose from a physiologic concentration of lactate than the S1 segment. Similar heterogeneity was observed in the proximal tubule, in which the pars recta was shown to generate more glucose from lactate or pyruvate than the pars convoluta.[75]

Studies in cortical tubule suspensions and the isolated perfused kidney revealed a reciprocal relationship between Na$^+$ transport and gluconeogenesis. In some experiments, inhibition of Na$^+$,K$^+$-ATPase activity, and thereby, active Na$^+$ reabsorption, stimulated gluconeogenesis in the kidney. Conversely, stimulation of Na$^+$,K$^+$-ATPase activity by nystatin[76] or monensin inhibited gluconeogenesis in proximal tubules. Nagami and Lee[77] demonstrated that increased Na$^+$ transport in isolated proximal tubules was associated with a fall in glucose production and that inhibition of secondary active Na$^+$ transport with amiloride increased glucose production. In agreement with this work, furosemide, ethacrynic acid, and chlorthiazide, all inhibitors of secondary active Na$^+$ transport pathways, stimulated gluconeogenesis in kidney cortex slices.[78] Because both gluconeogenesis and the Na$^+$,K$^+$-ATPase are ATP-consuming processes, it was proposed that they might compete for energy availability in the proximal tubule. However, ouabain inhibition of Na$^+$,K$^+$-ATPase does not always stimulate gluconeogenesis. In the isolated perfused kidneys of rat, for example, ouabain inhibited gluconeogenesis from lactate.[79] In the aggregate, the studies suggested that under normal circumstances, the renal proximal tubule can meet the energetic demands of both gluconeogenesis and active Na$^+$ transport and that these processes are subject to complex control.

Whole Kidney Studies

Given the high rates of active Na[+] transport in the kidney and the high mitochondrial densities in many portions of the nephron, it is not surprising that there is a linear correlation between the rate of Na[+] reabsorption (T$_{Na+}$) and the QO$_2$ over a wide range of Na[+] transport rates. The relationship of T$_{Na+}$/QO$_2$ has been reported to be in the range of 26 to 30.[80] Several investigators challenged the legitimacy of using T$_{Na+}$ as an accurate measure of active Na[+] reabsorption. For example, various provocative maneuvers, such as water deprivation or administration of mannitol,[80] loop diuretics, or dopamine, resulted in a higher T$_{Na+}$/QO$_2$ coupling ratio than was predicted. In contrast, studies in tight epithelia such as frog skin or toad urinary bladder, revealed lower than predicted T$_{Na+}$/QO$_2$ coupling ratios, in the range of 16 to 20 and in closer agreement to the predicted value of 18.[81] The greater T$_{Na+}$/QO$_2$ coupling efficiency in the kidney compared with other systems was attributed to a significant (~30%) proportion of passive Na[+] transport. Studies subsequently designed to minimize passive transport obtained lower values for the coupling ratio, in the range of 12.5 to 20.[82] Ostensen and colleagues[83] used transport inhibitors to quantify the relative proportions of NaHCO$_3$ and NaCl transport that were actively and passively transported in the proximal and distal tubule of dogs. Under conditions of saturated distal NaCl reabsorption, acetazolamide, an inhibitor of carbonic anhydrase–dependent HCO$_3^-$ and Na[+] reabsorption in the proximal tubule, reduced HCO$_3^-$ reabsorption, Na[+] reabsorption, and QO$_2$, whereas mannitol reduced NaCl reabsorption without significantly affecting NaHCO$_3$ reabsorption or QO$_2$. The investigators concluded that proximal NaHCO$_3$ reabsorption is the only important active Na[+] transport process that is sensitive to inhibition of carbonic anhydrase and that NaCl transport is passive in this segment. In addition, they concluded that the distal nephron exhibits a T$_{Na+}$/QO$_2$ of 18 when proximal Na[+] reabsorption is blocked with acetazolamide and ouabain is added. These whole kidney studies, however, suffered from major limitations related to the numerous assumptions made and the inability to determine Na[+] transport in specific nephron segments.

Correlation Between Na[+] Transport and QO$_2$ Along the Nephron

The heterogeneity of oxidative metabolism and active Na[+] transport along the nephron has been studied extensively in isolated cell or tubule suspensions from selected nephron segments using measurements of ouabain-sensitive QO$_2$, Na[+],K[+]-ATPase activity, cellular ATP content, and mitochondrial density. In general, there is a strong correlation between active Na[+] transport and these parameters along the nephron (Fig. 4–8). Segments with high rates of active Na[+] transport, such as the MTAL, exhibit high rates of ouabain-sensitive QO$_2$ and Na[+],K[+]-ATPase activity, abundant cellular ATP, and many mitochondria (see Fig. 4–8). At the other end of the spectrum, the IMCD conducts lower amounts of active Na[+] transport, has fewer mitochondria, and accordingly, has lower rates of ouabain-sensitive QO$_2$ and Na[+],K[+]-ATPase activity.

In addition, the coupling efficiency of transepithelial Na[+] transport and mitochondrial ATP generation differs considerably among nephron segments. In the proximal tubule, the T$_{Na+}$/QO$_2$ has been reported to be in the range of 24 to 30, indicating a Na[+]/ATP ratio of about 4 to 5 (assuming that six ATP are produced per O$_2$ consumed). Because the proximal tubule is a leaky epithelium, minor osmotic and electrochemical gradients are able to drive passive NaCl transport across the epithelium. Fromter and colleagues[84] calculated that as much as 50% of net Na[+] reabsorption in the proximal tubule is passively mediated, whereas Kiil and coworkers[85] suggested that this number was 30%. Because ATP hydrolysis is not directly coupled to passive transepithelial Na[+] transport, passive transport increases the T$_{Na+}$/QO$_2$ and Na[+]/ATP ratios. In addition, apical Na[+] influx is coupled to H[+] efflux by the Na[+]/H[+] exchanger NHE3, a process that generates intracellular HCO$_3^-$ (Fig. 4–9). This HCO$_3^-$ is then extruded across the basolateral membrane by an electrogenic Na[+]/HCO$_3^-$ cotransporter kNCB1. The ionic stoichiometry of this transporter in the proximal tubule has been reported to be 3Na[+]:1HCO$_3^-$, although it may be 2Na[+]:1HCO$_3^-$ in other cell types.[86] Therefore, with these stoichiometries, one third of the Na[+] transported into the cell by the apical Na[+]/H[+] exchanger could be transported across the epithelium and extruded by the basolateral 3Na[+]:1HCO$_3^-$ exchanger without the need for ATP hydrolysis. Thus, the Na[+]:ATP would be 4.5 (one third greater than the 3Na[+]:1ATP stoichiometry of the Na[+],

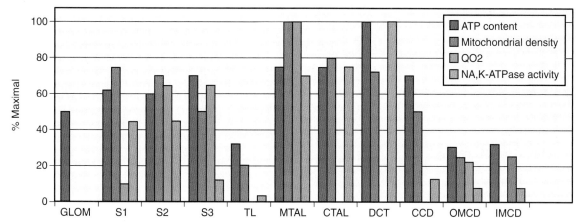

FIGURE 4–8 Relative distributions of QO$_2$, mitochondrial density, ATP content, and Na[+],K[+]-ATPase activity along the mammalian nephron. For each item, the results were normalized to the maximal value in the nephron. QO$_2$ data obtained from references 76, 157, 158, 171, 200–202 with the maximal value for total QO$_2$ in the MTAL (2000 ng/mg protein/h). The percentages indicated in the unshaded portion of the bars represent the ouabain-sensitive component of QO$_2$. Mitochondrial density data from reference 100 with a maximal value of 44% in the MAL. ATP content from reference 154 with a maximal value of 16.8 mmol/kg dry wt reported in DCT. Na[+],K[+]-ATPase activities from reference 203 with the DCT value of 6679 pmol/mm tubule/h being maximal. CCD, cortical collecting duct; CTAL, cortical thick ascending limb of Henle's loop; GLOM, glomerulus; IMCD, inner medullary collecting duct; MTAL, medullary thick ascending limb of Henle's loop; OMCD, outer medullary collecting duct; S1, S1 segment of proximal tubule; S2, S2 segment of proximal tubule; S3, S3 segment of proximal tubule; TL, thin limbs of Henle's loop; (Adapted from Soltoff SP: ATP and the regulation of renal cell function. Annu Rev Physiol 48:9–31, 1986.)

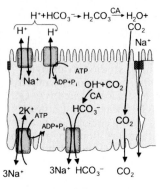
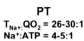
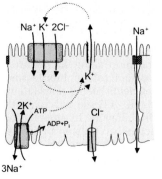
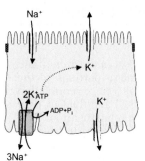

PT
$T_{Na+}:QO_2 = 26\text{-}30:1$
$Na^+:ATP = 4\text{-}5:1$

TAL
$T_{Na+}:QO_2 = 36:1$
$Na^+:ATP = \sim6:1$

CCD principal cell
$T_{Na+}:QO_2 = 18:1$
$Na^+:ATP = 3:1$

FIGURE 4–9 Cellular models characterizing the stoichiometric relationships between transepithelial sodium reabsorption (T_{Na+}) and QO_2 or ATP utilization (ATP) for the proximal tubule (PT), medullary thick ascending limb of Henle's loop (TAL), and cortical collecting duct (CCD) principal cell. See text for discussion.

K^+-ATPase), with a T_{Na+}/QO_2 ratio of 27:1. However, HCO_3^- absorption in the proximal tubule is also mediated by an apical H^+-ATPase working in tandem with the apical Na^+/H^+ exchanger. The H^+-ATPase has been estimated to mediate between 10% and 50% of the total apical H^+ transport.[57] Therefore, this transporter would contribute to HCO_3^- absorption at the expense of the Na^+/H^+ exchanger, which would reduce the Na^+/ATP ratio toward 3:1, depending on the $H^+:ATP$ stoichiometry of the apical H^+-ATPase. Thus, through the contributions of passive paracellular Na^+ transport and of Na^+-HCO_3^- coupled transport, the proximal tubule operates a highly efficient mechanism for transepithelial Na^+ transport.

The coupling efficiency of transepithelial Na^+ transport and mitochondrial ATP generation in the MTAL is believed to be greater than that observed in other nephron segments, although this has not been directly established. Studies in model epithelia such as the shark rectal gland[87] and tracheal epithelium[88] suggest that the T_{Na+}/QO_2 of the MTAL is 36:1 and the Na^+/ATP ratio is 6:1 (see Fig. 4–9). The high coupling efficiency in this epithelium is the result of the stoichiometry of the $Na^+/K^+/2Cl^-$ transporter of the apical membrane, which allows the energy derived from the Na^+ pump to drive the secretion of 2Cl^- molecules per Na^+. The resulting Cl^- electrochemical gradient drives passive transepithelial Na^+ transport via paracellular pathways. Like other high-resistance Na^+-transporting epithelia, the CCD is thought to have a relatively low efficiency of Na^+ to ATP coupling. Because the apical entry of Na^+ via the Na^+ channels is not linked to the transport of other solutes, and the basolateral Na^+,K^+-ATPase represents the only significant pathway for Na^+ exit, the Na^+/ATP relationship is the same 3:1 ratio as that of the Na^+,K^+-ATPase (see Fig. 4–9).

Coupling of Na+,K+-ATPase and Mitochondrial Oxidative Phosphorylation

Na+/K+/O2/ATP Stoichiometry
In the early 1960s, Whittam's laboratory[89] provided experimental evidence for a functional coupling between active Na^+ and K^+ transport and respiration in renal cortical slices. In this classic model, ATP hydrolysis by the Na^+,K^+-ATPase produces ADP+P_i, which acts as a feedback signal to the mitochondrial for the regulation of ATP synthesis (Fig. 4–10). In cells that rely exclusively on mitochondrial oxidative phosphorylation to support transport, activation of Na^+ would be exactly coupled to coordinate increases in QO_2 and ATP generation. There is no direct experimental proof that adenine nucleotides are the coupling signal between Na^+,K^+-ATPase and mitochondrial oxidative phosphorylation, but there is

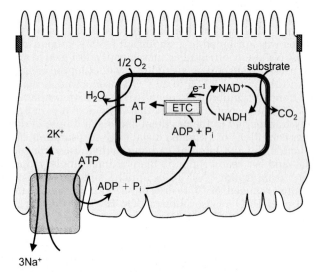

FIGURE 4–10 Whittam model for the coupling of ATP production by mitochondrial oxidative phosphorylation and ATP utilization by the Na^+,K^+-ATPase. ATP hydrolysis by the Na^+,K^+-ATPase produces ADP+P_i, which serve as a feedback regulator of mitochondrial ATP synthesis, and consequently, QO_2. This model suggests a direct relationship between Na^+,K^+-ATPase turnover, mitochondrial ATP synthesis, and QO_2 in cells that rely on mitochondrial ATP production. e^{-1}, electron; ETC, electron transport chain.

compelling correlative evidence in the renal tubules. Balaban and colleagues[59] made simultaneous measurements of the redox state of mitochondrial NAD fluorescence, cellular ATP and ADP concentrations, and QO_2 in renal cortical tubule suspensions (see Fig. 4–10). Ouabain caused a net reduction of NAD, a 30% increase in the ATP/ADP ratio, and a 54% inhibition of QO_2. Conversely, activation of Na^+,K^+-ATPase by addition of K^+ to K^+-depleted tubules promoted a 127% stimulation of QO_2, a large oxidation of NAD, and a 47% decrease in the cellular ATP/ADP ratio. These results suggested that the intracellular concentrations of ATP and ADP represented a cytoplasmic coupling signal in a feedback loop between ATP utilization by the Na^+,K^+-ATPase and ATP production by mitochondrial oxidative phosphorylation.

Additional studies examined the $Na^+/K^+/O_2$ stoichiometry in proximal tubule suspensions and their correlation with the known stoichiometries of the Na^+,K^+-ATPase and mitochondrial oxidative phosphorylation. Reintroducing K^+ into a K^+-depleted suspension of renal proximal tubules to activate the Na^+,K^+-ATPase resulted in an initial net K^+ influx and simultaneous increase in QO_2.[53,90] In two studies, the K^+ transport/QO_2 ratios were reported as 10.4 and 11.8,[53,90] near the expected theoretical value of 12 (two K^+ transported per ATP hydrolyzed by the Na^+,K^+-ATPase and six ATP molecules produced per O_2 by mitochondrial oxidative phosphorylation). Extensions of these studies by different methods, including ^{23}Na NMR spectroscopy coupled with extracellular K^+ electrodes[91] and direct measurements of net Na^+ and K^+ fluxes by extracellular ion-sensitive electrodes,[92] have largely concluded that the $Na^+/K^+/O_2$ in the intact proximal tubule is 18:12:1 as predicted.[93]

ATP Dependence of Na^+,K^+-ATPase Activity

Given the coupling of Na^+,K^+-ATPase activity to ATP production, much attention has been directed at determining the ATP dependence of the Na^+,K^+-ATPase in the intact kidney, isolated tubules and cells under physiologic and provocative conditions. Different interpretations have arisen depending on whether the studies were performed in intact or permeabilized tubules. In permeabilized proximal tubules, with Na^+,K^+-ATPase activity studied under V_{max} conditions for Na^+ and K^+, Soltoff and Mandel[94] reported that plots of Na^+,K^+-ATPase activity as a function of ATP concentration were hyperbolic, with $K_{0.5}$ of roughly 0.4 mM for ATP, in the range of values later obtained by others (Fig. 4–11). In contrast, studies in the intact in vitro microperfused proximal tubule showed that a decrement in intracellular ATP content, achieved by pharmacologic inhibition of mitochondrial oxidative phosphorylation, resulted in coordinate reductions in Na^+-dependent transport of fluid, phosphate, and glucose.[95] Soltoff and Mandel[94] extended these studies by examining the ATP dependence of Na^+,K^+-ATPase activity, indexed by the initial rate of K^+ uptake in intact, K^+-depleted proximal tubules, following graded reductions in intracellular ATP content achieved by serial reductions in the dose of rotenone. Because the Na^+,K^+-ATPase turnover is reduced in the K^+-depleted tubules, the intracellular Na^+ concentration is elevated and not limiting for subsequent activation of Na^+,K^+-ATPase turnover by reintroduction of K^+. These investigators found that the relationship of Na^+,K^+-ATPase activity to ATP concentration was linear, even at ATP concentrations known to saturate the enzyme in in vitro enzymatic assays (see Fig. 4–11). The authors postulated that the differences in the data obtained in the permeabilized versus the intact proximal tubule might reflect differences in the local concentrations of ATP, ADP, and P_i in the vicinity for the Na^+,K^+-ATPase in the intact tubule compared with permeabilized preparations. In permeabilized tubules, respiration measured in the presence of excess extramitochondrial P_i is dependent on the extramitochondrial concentration of ADP, a relationship with saturable kinetics. The K_m for ADP has been reported to be 15 to 50 µM.[54] Extrapolated to the intact proximal tubule, these values would saturate the ATP-ADP translocase of the mitochondria and maximally stimulate respiration. Most likely, differences in the measurements of the total cellular concentration of ADP in the cellular extract and the actual free ADP in the cytoplasm likely accounts for this discrepancy.

Similarly, Amman and colleagues[96] studying dog cortical tubules observed a fixed increment of ouabain-sensitive QO_2 upon stimulation of Na^+,K^+-ATPase activity at ATP concentrations ranging from 2 to 7 mM, and phosphorylation potential ($[ATP]/[ADP][P_i]$) ranging from 1.5 to 7.5 mM⁻¹. They concluded that the Na^+/ATP stoichiometry of the Na^+,K^+-ATPase remains unmodified by intracellular ATP concentrations in these tubules even when the ATP content equals or exceeds the physiologic value. Taken together, these results suggest a complex coupling between the supply of ATP generated by mitochondrial oxidative phosphorylation and the energetic demands of the Na^+,K^+-ATPase and further suggest that the stoichiometry of the Na^+,K^+-ATPase is unaltered when ATP concentration or the phosphorylation potential is changed to values greater than or equal to normal. Furthermore, although neither ATP nor phosphorylation potential appears to be rate-limiting for the Na^+,K^+-ATPase in the proximal tubule under physiologic conditions, small reductions in these parameters lessen the activity of the Na^+,K^+-ATPase.

NAD Redox State

NADH fluorescence can be used to monitor the redox state of the cytoplasm. The ratio $[NADH]/[NAD^+]$ provides an index of the redox state within the cytoplasm. Inhibition of active transport causes reduction of NAD^+, whereas increased transport work elicits oxidation of NAD^+, both occurring as expected from mitochondrial transitions to a lesser or more active state, respectively (Fig. 4–12). Another use of this method is the determination of the relative effectiveness of metabolic substrates to deliver reducing equivalents to the respiratory chain in a particular tissue. Combining QO_2 measurements with optical determinations of the redox level of the mitochondrial respiratory chain permits the distinction between energy utilization by primary transport processes, primary metabolic processes, or both (see Fig. 4–12). Balaban and coworkers[97] applied this method coupled with measurements of QO_2 to study substrate utilization in suspensions of proximal tubules. Short-chain fatty acids increased NADH fluorescence and QO_2 to a greater extent than did carboxylic acids and amino acids. Because NADH fluorescence increased proportionally with QO_2, it was concluded that the substrates increase QO_2 by increasing the delivery of reducing equivalents to NAD and not by direct stimulation of ATP hydrolysis. In another example, glucose removal caused a decrease in QO_2 in proximal tubules in the presence or absence of butyrate, a readily oxidizable fatty acid. This result suggested that these QO_2 changes were related to the transport and not the metabolism of glucose.[76] The nystatin-stimulated QO_2 was the same in the presence and absence of glucose, and NADH fluorescence showed that glucose addition to tubules suspended in glucose-free medium caused NAD oxidation. Thus, glucose increases respiration by stimulating Na^+ entry followed by increased Na^+ pump activity and its associated increase in mitochondrial respiration.

High-Resolution Nuclear Magnetic Resonance Spectroscopy

^{31}P, ^{14}N, and ^{1}H NMR spectroscopy are noninvasive means to measure in real-time renal metabolic pathways and the structure, dynamics, and interactions of biochemical compounds of the nephron in vivo and in vitro.[98] An important strength

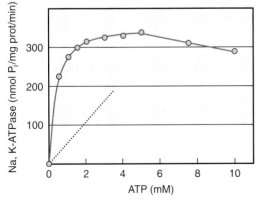

FIGURE 4–11 ATP dependence of the Na^+,K^+-ATPase in permeabilized (solid line) and intact (dashed line) rabbit proximal tubules. See text for discussion. (From Soltoff SP, Mandel LJ: Active ion transport in the renal proximal tubule. III. The ATP dependence of the Na^+ pump. J Gen Physiol 84:643–662, 1984.)

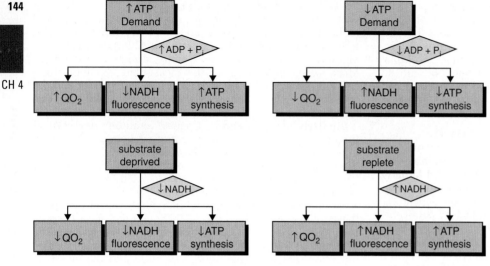

FIGURE 4–12 Mitochondrial responses to physiologic changes. QO_2, oxygen consumption. The indicator in the diamond represents the controlling factor for the mitochondrial response.

of this method is that prior selection of metabolites or substrates is not required. The data obtained are determined principally by the nucleus used for detection (e.g., ^{31}P, ^{14}N, ^{13}C, and ^{1}H). With ^{31}P NMR, all manner of inorganic phosphate and high-energy phosphate compounds can be analyzed, including but not limited to ATP, ADP, P_i, and phosphocreatine. Studies of renal metabolism with ^{31}P NMR measurements have been applied to the intact kidney in vivo and in vitro, extracts of kidney tissue, and isolated tubules. ^{31}P spectra of kidney show strong signals for ATP, P_i, 2-3-diphosphoglycerate (from erythrocytes) but lack an appreciable phosphocreatine signal evident in the heart, brain, and other metabolically active tissues. In addition, ^{31}P spectra show relatively little ADP or P_i in the intact kidney. Compared with enzymatic analysis, 100% of ATP, but only 25% of ADP and 27% of P_i, are visible to NMR in the intact kidney.[99] These results suggest that most of the ADP and P_i is bound within the cell, likely unavailable for biochemical reactions, and invisible by NMR. Thus, of the estimated 0.5 to 1.0 mM ADP and 0.7 mM P_i in the cell, only about 25% of these compounds may be free in the cytoplasm. Consequently, the intracellular phosphorylation potential (i.e., [ATP]/[ADP][Pi]), as judged by ^{31}P NMR, is some 10-fold greater than that assayed by biochemical techniques. Biochemical studies estimated a higher total of free cytosolic ADP concentration in the cytosol. Pfaller and colleagues[100] isolated mitochondrial and cytosolic fractions from proximal tubular suspensions by the digitonin method and analyzed the amount of ATP for each compartment. In parallel experiments, they measured the absolute volumes of mitochondrial and extramitochondrial spaces in similar suspensions utilizing electron microscopic morphometry. When ATP content was related to the morphometrically determined absolute volumes, the ATP concentrations were calculated to be 4.33 mmol/L for the cytosolic and 2.62 mmol/L for the mitochondrial space. Thus, cytosolic and mitochondrial ATP represent 70% and 30% of the total cellular ATP, respectively, in these studies.

Saturation transfer NMR studies in the intact kidney revealed a ADP:O ratio of 2.45 and that the energy cost of Na^+ transport, calculated from the theoretical Na:ATP of 3.0, exceeded the measured rate of ATP synthesis. Instead, Na:ATP for active transport in the perfused kidney was 12.[99] ^{13}C NMR spectroscopy using ^{13}C-labelled substrates has also been used to examine substrate utilization and metabolic fluxes simultaneously through glycolysis, gluconeogenesis, and other cycles. For example, Kinne and coworkers[101] used ^{13}C NMR analysis of IMCD cell extracts to examine carbohydrate biochemistry with this nonradioactive isotope. The advent of magic-angle spinning (MAS) ^{1}H NMR technology has allowed the analysis of a wider range of biochemical processes in intact tissue samples, without the need for conventional acetonitrile extraction. However, this promising methodology has not been extensively applied to studies of renal transport and metabolism.

ATP-Sensitive Ion Channels and Coupling to Cation Transport

Several laboratories have identified ATP-sensitive K^+ channels (K-ATP) in renal epithelial cells. These K^+ channels are defined by their inhibition in response to increased cytosolic ATP concentrations. They couple the metabolic demands of the cell, including those imposed by the demands of the Na^+,K^+-ATPase, with the macroscopic K^+ conductance of the plasma membrane. K-ATP channels are found in a variety of cell types, and their regulation by ATP, other nucleotides, and other molecular mediators varies depending on the roles these channels fulfill. Along the nephron, K-ATP channels are found in the proximal tubule, the TAL, and the CCD.[102] Structurally, the K-ATP channels in the principal cell of the CCD are heteromultimers composed of an inwardly rectifying K^+ channel and a sulphonylurea-binding subunit(s). Under basal conditions, these channels exhibit a high open probability and contribute to solute reabsorption and whole body K^+ homeostasis. Elegant studies in the proximal tubule by Welling and coworkers[103] found that the macroscopic K^+ conductance of the basolateral membrane increased upon stimulation of Na^+,K^+-ATPase activity and that these responses were accompanied by a fall in intracellular ATP levels (see Fig. 4–9). Conversely, intracellular ATP loading uncoupled this response. It has been postulated that this pump-leak coupling via the nucleotide sensitivity of the K-ATP channel ensures that cell membrane potential, intracellular K^+ activity, and cell volume are defended during physiologic variations in transepithelial ion transport.

The K-ATP channel plays an important role in K^+ recycling in the TAL and in K^+ secretion in the collecting duct (see Fig. 4–9). A cDNA encoding an inwardly rectifying K-ATP channel (ROMK1, Kir1.1a) was initially isolated from outer medulla of rat kidney by expression cloning.[104] Since then, multiple alternative splice variants of ROMK have been characterized. In the rat, alternative splicing at the 5′-end gives rise to channel proteins differing at their amino-termini: ROMK2 (Kir1.1b) lacks the first 19 amino acids of ROMK1, and

ROMK3 (Kir1.1c) contains a 7-amino acid extension.[105] These splice variants are differentially expressed along the distal nephron, ROMK1 transcripts are expressed in the CCD and the OMCD, ROMK2 mRNA is highly expressed from the MTAL to the CCD and connecting tubule (CNT), and ROMK3 is expressed in the MTAL, macula densa, and DCT.[106] ROMK protein has also been immunolocalized to the apical border of the TAL, macula densa, DCT, CNT, CCD principal cells, and OMCD principal cells.[107] This localization is in agreement with the known distribution of low-conductance K⁺ channels identified in the apical membrane of the distal nephron segments.

More recently, a stretch-activated nonselective cation channel that is inhibited by intracellular ATP ($K_i = 0.48$ mM) has been discovered in the basolateral membrane of the proximal tubule. The channel allows permeation of Ca^{2+} and other cations, and its activity in cell-attached patches is completely inhibited by the venom of the common Chilean tarantula, *Grammosola spatulata*. The investigators postulated that the channel may be involved in cell volume regulation, intracellular Ca^{2+} homeostasis, and may have increased importance during states of ATP depletion.[108] Finally, a small-conductance K⁺ channel, with properties similar to those of the K-ATP channel from the plasma membrane, has been characterized in the inner membrane of rat liver and beef heart mitochondria and designated the *mitochondrial ATP-regulated K⁺ channel*.[109] The mitochondrial K-ATP channel is inhibited not only by ATP but also, like the plasma membrane K-ATP channel, by sulfonylureas. This channel, which is also expressed in kidney mitochondria, may play an important role in mitochondrial ATP production during physiologic and hypoxic states.[110] K⁺ transport by this channel results in increased respiration and decreased in the inner mitochondrial membrane potential. Furthermore, diazoxide-triggered activation of ATP-sensitive K⁺ uptake results in decreased ATP hydrolysis through the reverse activity of the F_1F_0-ATPase when respiration is inhibited. Thus, this pathway may have a role in the prevention of mitochondrial ATP hydrolysis.[111]

ATP (Purinergic) Receptors Modulating Active Na⁺ Transport

In addition to its role as a metabolic fuel, ATP and its metabolites play important roles in autocrine and/or paracrine processes through activation of P2 purinergic receptors in the kidney and most other tissues. Many of these local regulatory functions modulate solute transport in the kidney. P2 receptors are specific membrane–bound receptors sensitive to ATP and uridine triphosphate. Two major subtypes of P2 receptors—ionotropic P2X and metabotropic P2Y receptors—have been characterized. P2X receptors are ligand-gated channels, whereas the P2Y receptors are linked by G proteins to second-messenger systems. RT-PCR studies revealed more intense expression of P2Y(6) receptor mRNA in the proximal tubule and the TAL, less intense expression in the thin descending limb and the CCD and OMCD, and no detectable expression in either the thin ascending limb or the IMCD.[112] Functional studies revealed luminal P2Y receptors in principal cells of mouse CCD but not in rabbit CCD.[113] Patch-clamp studies demonstrated that extracellular ATP inhibits the small-conductance K⁺ channel on the apical membrane of the mouse CCD.[114] Luminal ATP and UTP, presumably acting through P2Y2 receptors, inhibit amiloride-sensitive short-circuit current in perfused mouse CCD.[115] Activation of P2 receptors also attenuates the inhibitory effect of PTH on Na⁺-dependent phosphate uptake,[116] Ca^{2+} and Na⁺ absorption, as well as K⁺ secretion. ATP release from epithelial cells onto their luminal aspect, where ecto-nucleotidases promote their metabolism,

results in adenosine generation, which may elicit further effects on ion transport, often opposite those of ATP. Moreover, ATP and adenosine may be important autocrine/paracrine mediators of cellular protection and regeneration after ischemic cell damage.[117] ATP stimulation of purinergic P2Y receptors hydrolyzes anionic phospholipids of the inner leaflet of the plasma membrane, such as phosphatidylinositol-bisphosphates (PIP2), resulting in inhibition of ENaC activity.[118] Recent studies have also demonstrated that aldosterone promotes ATP release from the basolateral side of target kidney cells, which then acts via a purinergic mechanism to produce contraction of small groups of neighboring epithelial cells and increased transepithelial electrical conductance in a process that involves phosphatidylinositol 3-kinase. It has been hypothesized that this lateral contaction redistributes cell volume resulting in apical swelling, which, in turn, disrupts the interaction of ENaC with the F-actin cytoskeleton, opening the channel for increased sodium transport.[119]

Purinergic P2Y(2) receptors are also expressed in mesangial cells and play an important role in the coupling of macular densa signaling to the mesangial cell-afferent arteriolar complex and thus the tubuloglomerular feedback response. Macula densa cells serve as biosensors, detecting changes in luminal NaCl concentration and relaying signals to the mesangial cell-afferent arteriolar complex. Patch-clamp and ATP bioassay studies of macula densa cells revealed a NaCl concentration-sensitive, ATP-permeable large-conductance (380 pS) anion channel that mediated release of ATP (up to 10 mM) across the basolateral membrane. Moreover, ATP released from macula densa cells via this maxi-anion channel acted at mesangial cell purinergic P2Y(2) receptors to provoke increased in intracellular Ca^{2+} concentration.[120] In vivo studies demonstrated that ATP release occurs over the same range of NaCl concentrations known to effect the tubuloglomerular feedback response and, like the tubuloglomerular feedback response, was increased by dietary salt restriction, suggesting that macula densa ATP release is a signaling component of the tubuloglomerular feedback pathway.[121]

AMP-activated Protein Kinase Coupling Ion Transport and Metabolism

AMP-activated protein kinase (AMPK) is a heterotrimeric serine/threonine kinase that functions as a sensor of intracellular energy stores, increasing its activity during conditions of metabolic stress as a result of an elevated intracellular AMP/ATP ratio. AMPK responds to alterations in cellular energy stores by adjusting both ATP-consuming and ATP-generating pathways. AMPK activation has been shown to inhibit fatty acid, triglyceride, and sterol synthesis and to stimulate glucose uptake, glycolysis, and fatty acid oxidation in various cell types.[122] Recent studies indicate that as a metabolic sensor in cells, AMPK may be important in tuning transepithelial transport by CFTR and ENaC to cellular metabolism.[123]

CFTR is unique among ion channels in requiring ATP hydrolysis for its gating, suggesting the coupling of CFTR activity with cellular energetics. Recent studies by Hallows and associates[50,124,125] have shown that AMPK colocalizes with, binds to, and phosphorylates CFTR in colonic and lung epithelial cells and that AMPK phosphorylation of CFTR in vitro inhibits cAMP-activated CFTR conductance in *Xenopus* oocytes and T84 cells. AMPK has also been shown to inhibit ENaC activity in microinjected *Xenopus* oocytes expressing mouse ENaC and cultured cortical collecting duct mpkCCD(c14) cells. In contrast to CFTR, the AMPK-ENaC interaction effect appears to be indirect, because AMPK did not bind ENaC by in vivo pull-down assays, nor did it phosphorylate ENaC in vitro.[126] Moreover, the AMPK-dependent ENaC inhibition appears to be mediated through a decrease in the number of active channels at the plasma membrane rather than a change in open probability of the channel.[126] AMPK inhibition of ENaC may limit excessive Na$^+$ influx under conditions of metabolic stress, thereby limiting Na$^+$,K$^+$-ATPase turnover and ATP utilization by this pump. It is intriguing to speculate that AMPK may serve to functionally couple the activities of CFTR and ENaC to coordinate transepithelial NaCl transport during states of metabolic stress.

Functional Coupling of Glycolysis with Ion Pumps

Several studies in different renal cell types have suggested a functional coupling of a primary active transport process with ATP generated locally from glycolysis. Paul and coworkers[127] demonstrated a link between increases in activity of the Na$^+$,K$^+$-ATPase, consumption of ATP, and stimulation of aerobic glycolysis in vascular smooth muscle and suggested that carbohydrate metabolism is compartmentalized in these cells.[128] Such coupling was also reported in the renal cell lines A6 and MDCK.[129] Similarly, functional coupling of glycolytic ATP production to the energy requirements of the Ca^{2+}-ATPase of the sarcoplasmic reticulum of skeletal and cardiac muscle[130] and to the renal V-ATPase[131] has been reported. Lu and colleagues[131] established that the glycolytic enzyme aldolase directly binds the V-ATPase E subunit. The two proteins colocalized in the brush border of the proximal tubule, but not in the intercalated cells of the collecting duct. Expression studies in yeast indicated that the interaction with aldolase was necessary for proper association of the V$_1$ and V$_0$ domains of the V-ATPase. Further studies demonstrated that aldolase interacts with three different subunits of V-ATPase on distinct interfaces of the glycolytic enzyme and that this interaction increases dramatically in the presence of glucose, suggesting that aldolase may act as a glucose sensor for V-ATPase regulation.[131] The effects of glucose on V-ATPase–dependent acidification of intracellular compartments and V-ATPase assembly and trafficking are mediated through a phosphatidylinositol 3-kinase–dependent pathway in renal epithelial cells.[132] The authors postulated that the specific binding of aldolase to the V-ATPase provides a means for the generation of local ATP pools by glycolysis while at the same time regulating the local pH by excreting the H$^+$ generated by glycolysis (glycolysis generates two H$^+$ for every glucose molecule oxidized and one H$^+$ for every ATP molecule produced).[131] In addition to aldolase, phosphofructokinase-1, the rate-limiting step in glycolysis, has been shown to interact with the C-terminus of the a4 subunit of the V-ATPase and to colocalize in α-intercalated cells, providing another link between the pump and glycolysis.[133]

RENAL SUBSTRATE PREFERENCES

Whole Kidney and Regional Profiles of Metabolism

By the early 1900s, it was established that the kidney exhibited a high QO$_2$ compared with other organs and that this was related in large part to Na$^+$ reabsorption. In 1928, Gyoergy and coworkers[134] reported metabolic differences between cortex and medulla. Studies in renal tissue slices later provided evidence for regional differences in intrarenal metabolism and suggested that this distinction may reflect the varying metabolic demands of different nephron segments. In vivo studies measuring carbon-labeled substrate consumption

demonstrated the capacity of the kidney to oxidize numerous metabolic substrates. Of these fuels, lactate, glutamine, glucose, free fatty acids, citrate, and ketone bodies are most readily utilized.[135,136] Cellular respiration provides the majority of ATP needed for energy-dependent transport processes. A smaller proportion of ATP arises from glycolysis and substrate-level oxidation.[137] These studies, in conjunction with studies in the isolated perfused rat kidney, provided considerable information about the integration of renal metabolism and ion transport. For example, glucose metabolism was found to be intimately involved in several overall transport processes in the isolated perfused kidney, including K$^+$ secretion,[138] HCO$_3^-$ transport, H$^+$ secretion,[139] and active Na$^+$ transport.[137] However, because of the complex distribution of metabolic enzymes along the nephron, disparate metabolic needs and environments of various nephron segments, dicarboxylation reactions unrelated to oxidative metabolism, and methodologic factors, the relative contributions of individual substrates to overall renal metabolism have been difficult to assay.

Studies in renal tissue slices provided important early observations about renal metabolism. The cortex was shown to exhibit a high rate of aerobic metabolism, a low respiratory quotient (CO$_2$ generated per O$_2$ consumed), which is indicative of fatty acid oxidation,[140] gluconeogenesis,[71] and low glycogen content. In contrast, the medulla is characterized by a high rate of anaerobic or aerobic glycolysis, a respiratory quotient of unity,[141] which is indicative of glucose oxidation,[140] glucose consumption resulting in lactate accumulation in the medulla, and a high glycogen content.[142] However, these studies were limited by the fact that the tissue preparation, with its collapsed tubules and prominent diffusion barriers to O$_2$ and solutes, did not reflect renal metabolism that occurs in the actively transporting nephron in vivo. Moreover, tissue slices did not allow investigators to attribute specific metabolic pathways to distinct nephron segments. With the development in the 1970s of microprocedures to analyze substrate utilization and enzymatic activities in single microdissected segments of rodents and rabbits, the heterogeneity of renal metabolism among nephron structures was appreciated.

Segmental Profiles of Nephron Metabolism

Substrate Preferences and Dominant Metabolic Pathways

PROXIMAL TUBULE. Proximal tubules have relatively little glycolytic capacity and are thus dependent on aerobic mitochondrial metabolism for ATP synthesis. The intact proximal tubule normally conducts transport work at 50% to 60% of its maximal respiratory capacity, so that substantial reserve capacity is available under physiologic conditions to meet increased ATP utilization. This segment has the ability to oxidize a variety of metabolic substrates, and its preferences for a given substrate are dictated by substrate availability and physiologic state. Experiments using QO$_2$, ^{14}CO$_2$ production from radiolabeled substrates and ATP content in cortical tubule suspensions and microdissected proximal tubule segments revealed that lactate, glutamine, fatty acids, ketone bodies, and triglycerides are avidly oxidized, whereas glucose is poorly oxidized by the proximal tubule.[97,143–146] In the rat proximal tubule, the rank order of preferred substrates is ketone bodies>fatty acids>lactate>glutamine (Fig. 4–13). However, some variability in this hierarchy exists among species. The proximal tubule has also significant endogenous fuels, likely neutral lipids, that support about half of the respiratory energy in the absence of exogenous substrates.

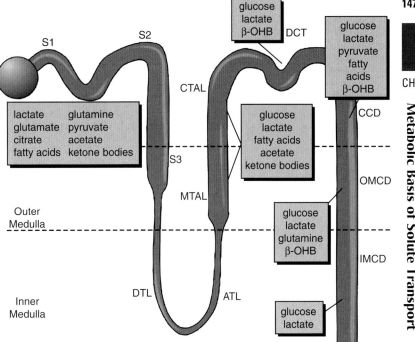

FIGURE 4-13 Substrate preferences along the nephron. Summary of preferred substrates to fuel active transport in nephron segments as gleaned primarily from studies using QO_2, ion fluxes, $^{14}CO_2$ generation from ^{14}C-labeled substrates, ATP contents, and NADH fluorescence. β-OHB, β-hydroxybutyrate.

Uchida and Endou[146] analyzed the ability of exogenous substrates to support ATP content in individual mouse proximal tubules. ATP production by glucose alone was minimal in the early proximal tubule (S1) but was significant in the late proximal tubule (S3). Based on the support of ATP content, these investigators concluded that glutamine and lactate were the preferred substrates in proximal tubules. Similarly, studies in rabbit cortical tubule suspensions enriched for PST and PCT showed differences in the metabolic responses to glucose. In glucose-containing buffer, PST segments were able to maintain QO_2 and ATP contents at levels significantly higher than PCT segments.[147] These differential responses between PST and PCT were glucose-dependent and suggested that the PCT cannot utilize glucose to support oxidative metabolism, whereas PST segments can oxidatively metabolize this substrate. Because these differences in glucose utilization do not correlate with the distribution of glycolytic enzyme activities, differential metabolic regulation of these enzymes may determine the ability of each segment to utilize glucose. Glucose cotransported with Na^+ stimulated ouabain-sensitive QO_2 and NADH oxidation, indicating that it preferentially stimulated ATP utilization.[148] In contrast, lactate maintains normal ATP content, stimulates QO_2, and increases NADH content in both the PCT and the PST.[97,146] Substrate-starved proximal tubules demonstrate an increased QO_2 and/or NADH fluorescence when provided TCA cycle intermediates, such as succinate, citrate, and malate, as well as glutamine and acetate.[97,146] β-hydroxybutyrate and glutamine supported ATP content in all proximal tubule segments.[146]

Of the various substrates studied, the short-chain fatty acids butyrate, valerate, and heptanoate most dramatically stimulated QO_2 and NADH fluorescence.[97] Harris and coworkers[90] demonstrated that butyrate supported, to a greater extent than lactate, glucose, or alanine, the high rates of mitochondrial oxidative phosphorylation needed to sustain maximal rates of Na^+,K^+-ATPase activity, provoked by nystatin addition. In another study, addition of fatty acids (butyrate or valerate) or TCA intermediates (succinate or malate) to proxi-

mal tubules incubated in lactate, alanine, and glucose resulted in enhanced Na^+-dependent phosphate transport in the absence of net fluid flux or ATP content.[149] Butyrate was also shown to enhance the capacity of isolated, nonperfused PSTs to regulate volume under hypo-osmotic conditions by promoting NaCl transport.[150] Gullans and coworkers[76,144] showed that succinate stimulated gluconeogenesis, hyperpolarized the plasma membrane potential, and promoted intracellular K^+ accumulation without altering Na^+,K^+-ATPase activity. Thus, the proximal tubule responds to a variety of substrates to support ion transport but has varied metabolic capabilities and substrate preferences along its length.

THIN LIMBS OF HENLE. Relatively few studies have investigated the metabolic profile of the thin ascending limb of Henle or TDL. These segments have few mitochondria and limited oxidative metabolism. In studies of microdissected TDLs from short- and long-looped nephrons, ATP was depleted when the tubules were incubated in the absence of exogenous substrate at 37°C,[151] indicating limited endogenous fuel stores. In the presence of exogenous substrates, however, TDLs from long-loop nephrons exhibited two to three times greater ATP contents per mm tubule length than did TDLs from short-loop nephrons. Glucose and pyruvate were the preferred substrates to sustain cellular ATP in TDLs from both short- and long-loop nephrons. ATP production from glutamine, β-hydroxybutyrate, and lactate was significant in TDLs from long-loop nephrons, whereas in TDLs from short-loop nephrons, glutamine was the preferred substrate, and β-hydroxybutyrate and lactate provided minimal metabolic support.[151] The tubules exhibited a tight coupling of ATP production and active Na^+ transport. When active Na^+ transport was stimulated by the ionophore monensin, ATP levels were depleted, and conversely, ouabain inhibition of Na^+ transport resulted in increased ATP levels.[151] There have been no published studies profiling the metabolic pathways of the thin ascending limbs of Henle.

CTAL. ^{14}C-labeled substrate studies demonstrated that glucose and lactate both efficiently generated $^{14}CO_2$ in the CTAL.[70] Glutamine, glutamate, malate, 2-oxoglutarate, and palmitate were also oxidized, but to a lesser degree.[152] The ATP content of CTALs was maintained in the presence of glucose, β-hydroxybutyrate, or lactate, but glutamine was ineffective.[146] The isolated perfused CTAL of the rabbit nephron utilizes glucose and/or pyruvate, acetate, β-hydroxybutyrate, acetoacetate, and butyrate to energize active Na^+ transport as measured by short-circuit current.[153] Glutamine, glutamate, citrate, 2-oxoglutarate, and succinate were less effective in supporting maximal rates of transepithelial Na^+ transport. Substrate removal resulted in a substantial decrease in I_{sc} over 10 minutes, indicating limited endogenous energy stores. Lactate was produced from glucose under aerobic conditions, and lactate synthesis was greatly enhanced when antimycin A was used to inhibit mitochondrial oxidative phosphorylation.[154] The CTAL exhibits a tight coupling of active Na^+ transport and QO_2. Ouabain inhibits about 40% to 50% of the QO_2 in CTALs in the presence of glucose, lactate, and alanine.

Inhibition of active Na^+ transport with ouabain or furosemide abrogated $^{14}CO_2$ production with ^{14}C-labeled lactate as substrate, indicating a tight coupling of active Na^+ transport and lactate oxidation.[152] In addition, some studies indicate that enzymes active in fatty acid oxidation are active in the CTAL and that CO_2 can be formed from palmitate. Other work, however, demonstrated that proprionate, caprylate, and oleate did not support active Na^+ transport in this segment, suggesting an inability of the CTAL to metabolize odd-chain or long-chain fatty acids.[155] In the aggregate, these studies indicate that the preferred exogenous substrates to fuel active Na^+ transport in the CTAL are glucose, lactate, pyruvate, ketone bodies, and fatty acids.

MTAL. The TAL exhibits the highest rates of active Na^+ transport among nephron segments, and possesses abundant mitochondria[156] and a high QO_2 to meet these energy demands.[157,158] In fact, the QO_2 in the MTAL is nearly 50% greater than that of the proximal tubule.[159] The MTAL has substantial endogenous energy reserves. In the absence of exogenous substrates, QO_2 is 85% of that achieved in the presence of substrate.[158] Studies by Eveloff and coworkers,[157] using pharmacologic inhibitors to block glycolysis, fatty acid oxidation, and amino acid transferase, showed that the endogenous fuels included glycogen, fatty acids, and amino acids. These endogenous fuels were inadequate to support fully nystatin-stimulated Na^+,K^+-ATPase activity, but addition of exogenous glucose stimulated QO_2 by nearly 20% and sustained higher rates of nystatin-stimulated QO_2. In the presence of glucose, inhibition of fatty acid oxidation had less inhibitory effect on QO_2. The short-chain fatty acid butyrate as well as acetoacetate and acetate but not lactate, further augmented QO_2 in the presence of glucose. These results suggested that the tubules were substrate-limited in the absence of fatty acids or ketone bodies. Glucose, acetate, malate, and succinate fully supported QO_2 in the MTAL.[157] Inhibition of salt transport by furosemide or ouabain markedly decreased glucose oxidation.[160]

Substrate oxidation assessed by measuring $^{14}CO_2$ production from tracer amounts of ^{14}C-labeled substrates in microdissected MTALs showed that glucose, 2-oxoglutarate, palmitate, lactate, glutamate, and glutamine were utilized as fuels, whereas the TCA cycle intermediates succinate, citrate, and malate were not significantly oxidized.[70] Leucine, a branched-chain amino acid, is also used as metabolic fuel by this nephron segment, although to a fivefold lower extent than glucose.[160] In a separate study, glucose, β-hydroxybutyrate, and lactate supported normal ATP content, whereas glutamine was only partially effective in restoring ATP content.

Compared with the proximal tubule, TAL segments exhibit a greater capacity for anaerobic metabolism to support cellular functions but still require mitochondrial respiration for maintenance of active Na^+ transport. In in vitro microperfusion studies of isolated rabbit CTALs, removal of substrates led to a rapid decline in transepithelial Na^+ transport, measured as short-circuit current. Addition of glucose from the basolateral side sustained short-circuit current, indicating that the CTAL of rabbit utilizes glucose to energize Na^+ reabsorption. However, when mitochondrial oxidative phosphorylation was poisoned with cyanide, glucose was only minimally superior to lactate in supporting transport. Studies in both rat[154] and mice[146] CTALs demonstrated that inhibition of mitochondrial oxidative phosphorylation resulted in activation of glycolysis, but this was insufficient to maintain normal rates of NaCl transport. The MTAL exhibits a greater capacity for anaerobic glycolysis but, like the CTAL, requires ATP production from mitochondrial oxidative phosphorylation to maintain active Na^+ transport. In the rat MTAL, lactate generation from glucose is greatly enhanced after chemical inhibition of cellular respiration,[154] but insufficient to support normal ATP levels.[146] Chamberlin and Mandel[158] tested the effects of anoxia on Na^+,K^+-ATPase activity, ATP content, extracellular K^+ release, and QO_2 in suspensions of rabbit MTALs. Under oxygenated conditions, the tubules exhibited efficient coupling between oxidative metabolism (six ATP/ O_2) and Na^+,K^+-ATPase (two K^+/ATP). When anoxic, the tubules released K^+, indicating substrate limitation of Na^+,K^+-ATPase activity. However, this rate was accelerated with complete Na^+,K^+-ATPase blockade by ouabain, indicating a reserve of Na^+,K^+-ATPase activity even in anoxia. Anaerobic metabolism maintained 73% of cellular ATP during 10 min of anoxia, and iodoacetate, an inhibitor of glycolysis, produced a 57% decline in ATP levels and a 33% decline in K^+ content during anoxia. Thus, glycolysis contributes significant energy during anoxia but is insufficient to maintain the high rates of active transport conducted by this segment.

DISTAL CONVOLUTED TUBULE. The metabolic profile and substrate preferences of the DCT are not as clearly described as for other nephron segments. Vinay and coworkers[161] established that this segment is glycolytic. The DCT contains abundant mitochondria, Na^+,K^+-ATPase activity,[162] high ATP levels (as compared with the proximal tubule),[163] and contains enzymatic activities that would support utilization of glucose, fatty acids, and ketone bodies.[68,135] In isolated DCTs from the mouse provided glucose, lactate, β-hydroxybutyrate, or L-glutamine as single substrates, lactate and β-hydroxybutyrate were preferred substrates for ATP maintenance. ATP contents were supported at somewhat lower levels by glucose alone, and glutamine did not increase ATP levels over basal conditions.[146] Bagnasco and coworkers[154] found that microdissected DCTs produced lactate with glucose as the only substrate and that inhibition of respiration with antimycin A increased lactate production by 98%. A single report of CO_2 production from ^{14}C-labeled substrates demonstrated glucose oxidation in isolated DCT,[164] but no data are published concerning QO_2 in this segment.

CORTICAL COLLECTING DUCT. Oxidative metabolism provides the majority of the support of cellular ATP content and active Na^+ transport in this nephron segment. In measurements of metabolic CO_2 production from ^{14}C-labelled lactate or glucose in microdissected nonperfused tubules, ouabain decreased by more than 50% the CO_2 production by CCD, indicating tight coupling of oxidative metabolism to active Na^+ transport. Similarly, blockade of Na^+ entry steps with amiloride reduced the rate of CO_2 production to an extent almost similar to that obtained with ouabain.[165] Substrate deprivation for 30 min at 37°C produced no change in ATP content of the isolated rat CCD, indicating significant endogenous fuels.[166] ATP production was greater from glucose than from lactate, β-hydroxybutyrate, or glutamine.[146] Likewise, in the isolated perfused rabbit CCD, endogenous substrates supported a small component of Na^+ transport.[167] Inhibition of mitochondrial respiration in the isolated rat CCD with antimycin A caused a significant decrement in cell ATP level within 5 min. Rabbit nonperfused CCDs subjected to hyperosmotic challenge undergo a regulatory volume increase in the presence of extracellular Na^+ that is supported by butyrate,[168] suggesting a role for fatty acids in this process, despite the relative low activity of enzymes for fatty acid oxidation present in the rat CCD.[169]

Nonaka and Stokes[170] examined the role of metabolism in the support of CCD ion transport using transepithelial electrical measurements and concurrent determination of lumen-to-bath Na^+ flux. Glucose provided the better support of Na^+ transport than lactate, pyruvate, glutamine, glutamate, alanine, and several short-chain fatty acids. With glucose absent, near-maximal support of Na^+ transport was provided by lactate, butyrate hexanoate, or acetate. Hering-Smith and Hamm[167] assayed lumen-to-bath $^{22}Na^+$ flux and HCO_3^- in microperfused rabbit CCDs before and after metabolic substrate changes or application of metabolic inhibitors. Both Na^+ reabsorption, predominantly a principal cell function in the CCD, and HCO_3^- secretion, predominantly an intercalated cell process, were inhibited by antimycin A but were not significantly affected by inhibitors of glycolysis or the hexosemonophosphate shunt pathway.[167] Basolateral perfusion of glucose and acetate best supported Na^+ reabsorption, whereas either glucose or acetate fully maintained HCO_3^- secretion. In addition, luminal glucose to some degree supported HCO_3^- secretion, but not Na^+ transport. The investigators concluded that principal cells and intercalated cells differ not only in their morphology and function but also in their metabolic support of transport.[167]

OMCD. The OMCD is a major site of H^+ secretion along the nephron and is largely responsible for the final acidification of the urine. The OMCD appears to have appreciable endogenous fuels, presumably glycogen, as evidenced by the fact that substrate deprivation for 30 min at 37°C resulted in no change in ATP content of the isolated, nonperfused rat OMCD.[166] Likewise, HCO_3^- secretion in the isolated perfused rabbit OMCD was fully supported by endogenous substrates.[167] The segment exhibits has considerable reliance on oxidative metabolism. Addition of cyanide to inhibit mitochondrial oxidative phosphorylation depleted greater than 95% of the ATP content of isolated rabbit OMCD cells in the absence of glucose fuels.[166] Anaerobic glycolysis can also contribute significantly to cellular energetics. Inhibition of oxidative phosphorylation with antimycin A resulted in an ~350% increase in lactate production from the isolated rat OMCD.[154] The OMCD has relatively low rates of active Na^+ transport and, in the rabbit, exhibits a relatively low level of ouabain-sensitive QO_2. Active Na^+ transport appears to be tightly coupled to oxidative metabolism. Ouabain decreased by more than 50% the CO_2 production from radiolabeled glucose in isolated, nonperfused rat OMCD, indicating that oxidative metabolism was substantially coupled to active Na^+ transport.[165]

IMCD. A major function of the IMCD is the final absorption of about 5% of filtered Na^+. Studies in isolated rat IMCD cells showed that ouabain-sensitive QO_2 is only 25% to 35%,[171] and accordingly, ATP turnover is relatively low.[172] Cellular energetics are largely dependent upon glucose availability under aerobic or anaerobic conditions,[172] although these cells appear to have considerable endogenous substrates. Stokes and colleagues[171] found that, in the absence of any exogenous substrate, respiration and ATP contents were near-normal, but lactate production was markedly decreased. Based on ^{13}C-NMR analysis of IMCD cell suspensions, enzyme assays on cell homogenates, and enzymatic determination of metabolites and cofactors, the major pathways of glucose metabolism in the IMCD are aerobic and anaerobic glycolysis, the pentose-phosphate shunt, and gluconeogenesis, although the latter two pathways represent minor ones for glucose metabolism in this tissue.[101] Studies of suspensions of dog IMCDs incubated under aerobic and anaerobic conditions demonstrated that glucose is the preferred substrate for this segment, even if lactate can be oxidized under aerobic conditions.[172] Glycogen consumption also occurs and to a greater extent during anoxia.[172]

Under aerobic conditions, the net oxidation of glucose to CO_2 contributes significantly to the cellular energetics. In studies of isolated rat IMCDs, lactate production was at least three times greater than other distal nephron segments.[154] In another study, aerobic glycolysis accounted for more than 20% of the ATP production in the IMCD.[171] Cohen postulated that that the high rate of aerobic glycolysis in the presence of an adequate O_2 supply stems from the small mass of mitochondria in relation to the amount of work done by the papillary tissue. The limited ATP synthesis from mitochondrial oxidative phosphorylation shifts both the phosphorylation state ($[ATP]/[ADP][P_i]$) and the cytoplasmic redox state ($[NAD^+]/[NADH]$) of the IMCD cells to a more reduced state, enhancing glycolytic rates and enabling these cells with few mitochondria to sustain substantial active transport in a low O_2 environment.

Given the low density of mitochondria in the IMCD and the low PO_2 it encounters, the IMCD relies to a greater degree on anaerobic glycolysis to sustain normal ion transport rates. Stokes and colleagues[171] reported that glycolysis increased by 56% and was able to maintain the cellular ATP level at 65% of control values when mitochondrial oxidative phosphorylation was inhibited with rotenone. Similarly, Bagnasco and colleagues[154] found that antimycin A treatment resulted in a 28% increase in lactate production from glucose. In studies that examined the metabolic determinants of K^+ transport in the rabbit IMCD, glucose as sole substrate augmented basal QO_2 and cell K^+ content by about 12% each, whereas iodoacetic acid, an inhibitor of glycolysis, or rotenone, an inhibitor of mitochondrial oxidative phosphorylation, promoted a release of cell K^+, indicative of substrate limitation of the Na^+,K^+-ATPase.[173] Similarly, in dog IMCD, anoxia resulted in a shift to glycolytic production of ATP, but both the apparent ATP turnover and the activity of the Na^+, K^+-ATPase were reduced.[172] Collectively, these data indicate that both glycolysis and oxidative phosphorylation are required to maintain optimal cellular K^+ gradients and ATP levels in the IMCD. In addition, Kinne and coworkers[101] posit that substrate recycling helps to conserve carbohydrate. Based on IMCD cell isolation studies, they propose that sorbitol, taken up by neighboring interstitial cells, is converted into fructose and then recycled to the collecting duct cells. This cycle might represent a beneficial adaptation to low O_2 tension, low substrate supply, and extreme changes in extracellular osmolality in this region.

In summary, a variety of methodologies, both to examine specific metabolic pathways and to define intrarenal heterogeneity of metabolism, have been applied to the study of renal metabolism along the nephron. Differences are evident among cell types and are in large part dictated by the local environment and the requirements of the specific cell type to perform active Na^+ transport. Though differences in mechanisms for substrate uptake differ among nephron cell populations, substrate availability is not generally rate-limiting under physiologic conditions in the kidney. To date, work has principally focused on the proximal tubule and the IMCD, so much is to be learned about the metabolism in other segments of the nephron. Because most studies have sought to isolate single metabolic pathways and used single substrates to analyze substrate preferences in substrate-starved cells, little is known about true preferences when multiple substrates are present and what factors may govern such preferences. There also appears to be considerable interspecies differences in metabolic profile among nephron segments, and very little is known about nephron heterogeneity of metabolism in humans.

SOLUTE TRANSPORT AND ENERGY AVAILABILITY DURING HYPOXIC OR ISCHEMIC CONDITIONS

Several investigators have explored the ability of isolated nephron segments supplied selected substrates to maintain active transport and ATP levels in the face of environmental or chemical inhibitors of mitochondrial oxidative phosphorylation. These studies sought to determine whether endogenous fuel reserves were sufficient to maintain active transport and ATP content, whether ATP-generation derived from anaerobic glycolysis was enhanced, and whether ATP from glycolytic metabolism could support cellular functions when mitochondrial oxidative respiration was limited. In the rabbit proximal tubule, disparate results have been obtained depending on the experimental model. Glycolysis, measured as lactate production from glucose, was not appreciably evident under aerobic conditions or when mitochondrial respiration was inhibited with antimycin A.[154] In contrast, Dickman and Mandel,[174] using different means to inhibit oxidative, namely hypoxia (1% O_2) or inhibition of the respiratory chain with rotenone, showed that suspensions of rabbit proximal tubules can generate lactate and ATP through anaerobic glycolysis to maintain 90% of basal ATP levels. In addition, a differential susceptibility of proximal tubule segments to hypoxia, related at least in part to differences in glycolytic capacity, was discovered: The PCT, with its more limited glycolytic capacity, was more vulnerable to hypoxia than the PST.[175] Finally, in ischemia, the reduced ATP/ADP ratio would be predicted to increase the open probability of the K-ATP channels independently from pump activity, leading to detrimental imbalance of pump and K^+ leak.

Weinberg and coworkers[176,177] conducted a comprehensive analysis of proximal tubule metabolism following hypoxia/reoxygenation. During hypoxia/reoxygenation, the cells developed severe energy deficits, respiratory inhibition, and diminished mitochondrial membrane potential. The decreased respiration persists for substantial periods of time before onset of the mitochondrial permeability transition and/or loss of cytochrome *c*. Interestingly, there is a high level of resistance to development of complex I dysfunction during hypoxia-reoxygenation in these cells, implicating events upstream of complex I to be important for the energetic deficit.[177] The function of both the F_1F_0-ATPase and the adenine nucleotide translocase are largely intact, and uncoupling appears to play the principal role in the mitochondrial dysfunction.[176] Provision of supplements, as substrates for anaerobic ATP generation, during either hypoxia or only during reoxygenation abrogated these abnormalities. Provision of the citric acid cycle metabolites α-ketoglutarate plus malate during either hypoxia or reoxygenation promotes mitochondrial anaerobic metabolism to increase ATP production by substrate-level phosphorylation and energization by anaerobic respiration in electron transport complexes I and II and provide succinate to bypass the complex I block when aerobic metabolism resumes. Accumulation of nonesterified fatty acids appears to underlie the energetic failure of reoxygenated proximal tubules. Moreover, lowering levels of nonesterified fatty acids is a major contributor to the benefit from supplementation with α-ketoglutarate and malate.[176]

Compared with the proximal tubule, TAL segments exhibit a greater capacity for anaerobic metabolism to support cellular functions but still require mitochondrial respiration for maintenance of active Na^+ transport. In in vitro microperfusion studies of isolated rabbit CTALs, removal of substrates led to a rapid decline in transepithelial Na^+ transport, measured as I_{sc}. Addition of glucose from the basolateral side sustained the I_{sc}, indicating that the CTAL of rabbit utilizes glucose to energize salt reabsorption. However, when mitochondrial oxidative phosphorylation was poisoned with cyanide, glucose was only minimally superior to lactate in supporting transport.[153] In studies in both rat[154] and mice[146] CTALs, inhibition of mitochondrial oxidative phosphorylation resulted in activation of glycolysis, but this was insufficient to maintain normal rates of NaCl transport. The MTAL exhibits a greater capacity for anaerobic glycolysis but, like the CTAL, requires ATP production from mitochondrial oxidative phosphorylation to maintain active Na^+ transport. In the rat MTAL, lactate generation from glucose is greatly enhanced after chemical inhibition of cellular respiration[154] but insufficient to support normal ATP levels.[146] Chamberlin and Mandel[158] tested the effects of anoxia on Na^+,K^+-ATPase activity, ATP content, extracellular K^+ release, and QO_2 in suspensions of rabbit MTALs. Under oxygenated conditions, the tubules exhibited efficient coupling between oxidative metabolism (six ATP/O_2) and Na^+,K^+-ATPase (two K^+/ATP). When anoxic, the tubules released K^+, indicating insufficient Na^+,K^+-ATPase activity. However, this rate was accelerated with complete Na^+,K^+-ATPase blockade by ouabain, indicating a reserve of Na^+,K^+-ATPase activity even in anoxia. Anaerobic metabolism maintained 73% of cellular ATP during 10 min of anoxia, and iodoacetate, an inhibitor of glycolysis, produced a 57% decline in ATP levels and a 33% decline in potassium content during anoxia. Thus, glycolysis contributes significant energy during anoxia but is insufficient to maintain the high rates of active transport conducted by this segment.

Given the fact that requirement the MTAL in vitro requires mitochondrial respiration to maintain normal ATP contents and transport rates, it is somewhat surprising that the MTAL in vivo sustains high active transport rates despite the low O_2 tension of this region. The countercurrent flow of the vasa recta, coupled with the high rates of active solute transport and gradient generation by the MTAL, results in a steep corticomedullary gradient of oxygen, ranging from a PO_2 of 50 mm Hg in the cortex to 10 to 20 mm Hg in the medulla.[178] The tenuous balance of oxygen supply and demand in the relatively hypoxic renal medulla places this nephron segment at high risk for hypoxic cellular dysfunction and injury. Prasad and coworkers[179] used the noninvasive technique blood oxygenation level–dependent (BOLD) MRI, a method that exploits deoxygenated blood as an endogenous source of contrast, to demonstrate the dynamics of intrarenal oxygenation in humans. Furosemide, which inhibits active Na^+ reabsorption and QO_2 in the MTAL, increased medullary PO_2 in healthy young adults, whereas acetazolamide, which principally inhibits solute reabsorption in the proximal tubules, had no effect on medullary PO_2.[179] Indeed, Brezis and coworkers[180] suggested that decreased transport workload in the MTAL may help to spare it from injury. In the isolated rat kidney perfused with hypoxic solutions, furosemide-treated kidneys exhibited 86% lower fraction of MTALs showing severe damage compared with vehicle-treated kidneys.

Given the low density of mitochondria in the IMCD and the low PO_2 it encounters, the IMCD relies to a greater degree on anaerobic glycolysis to sustain normal ion transport rates. In IMCD cell suspension from rabbit, glucose augmented basal QO_2 and cell K^+ content by about 12% each, and iodoacetic acid, an inhibitor of glycolysis, promoted a release of cell K^+. However, inhibition of mitochondrial oxidative phosphorylation with rotenone demonstrated that glycolysis alone could not maintain cell K^+ content.[173] In dog IMCD, anoxia resulted in a shift to glycolytic production of ATP, but both the apparent ATP turnover and the activity of the Na^+, K^+-ATPase were reduced.[172] Thus, both glycolysis and oxidative phosphorylation are required to maintain optimal cellular K^+

gradients and ATP levels in the IMCD. In addition, Kinne and coworkers[101] postulated that substrate recycling helps to conserve carbohydrate. Based on IMCD cell isolation studies, they propose that sorbitol, taken up by neighboring interstitial cells, is converted into fructose and then recycled to the collecting duct cells. This cycle might represent a beneficial adaptation to low oxygen tension, low substrate supply, and extreme changes in extracellular osmolality in this region.

EFFECTS OF L-ARGININE METABOLISM ON SOLUTE TRANSPORT AND CELLULAR ENERGETICS

L-arginine is a semi-essential amino acid that is metabolized to several molecules that influence renal function, including NO, L-proline, or polyamines. L-Arginine is the only known substrate for all NO synthase isoforms and, as such, helps to regulate the potent effects of NO on solute transport and metabolism in the kidney.

L-Arginine Metabolism

The uptake, recycling, and degradation of L-arginine modulate NO production. The amino acid is transported into renal tubular epithelial cells by the cationic amino acid transporter (CAT) family of system y(+), proteins. In some cell types, CAT-2 activity is coordinately induced with NO synthase activity to support higher substrate demands of the enzyme. CAT-1 mRNA is expressed predominantly in the collecting ducts and vasa recta in the inner medulla, where L-arginine uptake by this transporter is important in the production of NO and maintenance of blood flow in the renal medulla.[181] In addition to the importance of L-arginine uptake for NO generation, L-citrulline, which is formed as a byproduct of the NO synthase reaction, can be recycled to L-arginine by consecutive actions of argininosuccinate synthetase and argininosuccinate lyase. Immunolocalization studies in mouse kidney determined that both enzymes are expressed predominantly in the proximal tubule.[182] In agreement with this work, studies examining the fate of radiolabeled L-citrulline documented substantial generation of radiolabeled L-arginine in the proximal tubule, predominantly in the proximal convoluted tubule.[183]

In addition to its metabolism via NO synthases, L-arginine can be metabolized by arginase to ornithine and then via ornithine decarboxylase to growth stimulatory polyamines, and by arginine decarboxylase to agmatine following the action of arginine decarboxylase (Fig. 4–14).[184] These latter pathways effectively decrease intracellular arginine available for NO production. There is likely competition for substrate among the various arginine metabolic pathways, and the products of these enzymes appear to have a regulatory role on the various pathways.[184] Immunolocalization studies have shown that the arginase II isoenzyme is strongly expressed in the outer stripe of the outer medulla, presumably in the proximal straight tubules, and in a subpopulation of the proximal convoluted tubules in the cortex.[185] Similarly, within the mouse and rat nephron, ornithine decarboxylase activity is found exclusively in the proximal tubule, primarily in the proximal convoluted tubule.[186] Filtered ornithine reabsorbed along the PCT may be a major source of ornithine for ornithine decarboxylase.

Effects of NO on Renal Solute Transport

In the proximal tubule, NO has been reported to both stimulate and inhibit net fluid and HCO_3^- flux, but only inhibitory effects of NO have been found on the Na^+/H^+ exchanger and Na^+,K^+-ATPase activity in this segment.[187] In the MTAL, NO inhibits net Cl^- and HCO_3^- absorption, effects in part mediated by a direct inhibitory action of NO on the Na^+-K^+-$2Cl^-$ cotransporter and the Na^+/H^+ exchanger.[187] In contrast, NO stimulates the activity of apical K^+ channels in this segment.[188] In the collecting duct, NO inhibits Na^+ absorption and vasopressin-stimulated osmotic water permeability.[187] In addition, Lu and coworkers[189] demonstrated that NO inhibits apical Na^+ channels in the CCD and linked this mechanism to the inhibition of the basolateral small-conductance K^+ channel. NO has also been reported to inhibit the H^+-ATPase of intercalated cells of the collecting duct.[190] In the dog, nonselective NO synthase inhibitors renal increase QO_2 and T_{Na+}/QO_2. Rats treated with nonselective NO synthase inhibitors exhibited increased T_{Na+}/QO_2, and these inhibitors also increased QO_2 in proximal tubules in vitro at presumed lower levels of vectorial NaCl transport, suggesting that this effect was not mediated by influences on sodium transport alone. Thus, nonselective NO synthase inhibition increases the oxygen costs of kidney function via angiotensin II–independent mechanisms.[191]

Effects of NO on Mitochondrial Respiration

Experiments on isolated mitochondria and intact cells have shown that NO plays important roles in regulating mitochondrial QO_2, membrane potential, ATP production, and free radical generation.[192] Several groups demonstrated that NO potently and reversibly inhibits cytochrome oxidase through interactions with complex IV and S-nitrosation of complex I[193] with very rapid binding and dissociation kinetics and reduces the affinity of the enzyme for O_2.[194] In addition, mounting evidence indicates that an NO synthase, recently identified as the full-length neuronal NO synthase isoform with unique post-translational modifications, is expressed in mitochondria and produces NO under physiologic conditions.[195] Transcripts for this mitochondrial NO synthase were detected in kidney.[195] Although mitochondria cannot release physiologically relevant levels of NO, they produce biologically active nitrates through arginine-independent mechanisms, which raises the possibility that modulating mitochondrial functions can alter nitrate metabolism. In the aggregate, these findings suggested that NO might serve as a physiologic regulator of cellular respiration. Studies in renal tubules and isolated mitochondria indicated that NO could potently and reversibly inhibit respiration at nanomolar concentrations. There were no differences in sensitivity to NO-mediated inhibition between outer medullary and cortical tubules. The result suggested that, because of its low PO_2, the renal outer medulla may be more vulnerable to hypoxia, not simply because of the low PO_2 as such, but more likely because of the competition between NO and O_2 to control respiration.[196]

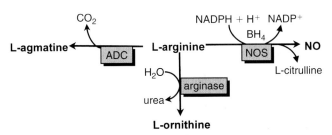

FIGURE 4–14 Pathways of L-arginine metabolism. ADC, arginine decarboxylase; BH_4, tetrahydrobiopterin, a necessary cofactor for NOS activity; NO, nitric oxide; NOS, NO synthase.

In addition to limiting cellular respiration, the inhibition of cytochrome oxidase by NO also shifts the electron transport chain to a more reduced state, favoring the formation of superoxide anions (O_2^-) at the level of complexes I and III of the electron transport chain. The O_2^- can then be converted by superoxide dismutase into hydrogen peroxide or, depending on intracellular redox conditions, react with NO to form peroxynitrite ($ONOO^-$).[197] Both reactive species can produce alteration of solute transport pathways, cell damage, and apoptosis. The attendant depletion of the glutathione pool and enhanced production of $ONOO^-$ in the mitochondria promotes the induction of the permeability transition pore, which collapses the membrane potential and leads to mitochondrial swelling, rupture of the outer mitochondrial membrane, release of pro-apoptotic factors, and apoptosis.[198]

SUMMARY AND CONCLUSIONS

The heterogeneity of renal transport systems to maintain cellular homeostasis is coupled in a dynamic and interactive manner to a diverse, but highly integrated system of metabolic pathways that effect or influence energy production. A family of ion-translocating ATPases mediates the primary active transport of Na^+, K^+, Ca^{2+}, and perhaps Cl^-, drives the secondary active transport of other ions and solutes, and consumes the majority of the renal energy supply. To address these demands, kidney epithelial cells have a high capacity for mitochondrial oxidative phosphorylation to generate ATP. Studies in whole kidney, isolated tubules, and renal cells have demonstrated that the energy demands of active Na^+ transport are coupled to the availability and synthesis of ATP, often indexed by QO_2. The coupling factors between these processes appear to be the cytosolic concentrations of ATP, ADP, and P_i. These adenine nucleotides also influence ATP-sensitive K^+ channels and link the activity of the Na^+ pump with the K^+ leak in at least some nephron segments. There is considerable variability along the nephron among ion transport demand, specific ion transport pathways, metabolic substrate preferences to fuel ion transport, and biochemical pathways and mitochondrial density used to generate ATP and reducing equivalents. In addition to its role as a metabolic fuel, ATP and its metabolites serve as autocrine and/or paracrine regulators of solute transport via activation of P2 purinergic receptors in the kidney. Similarly, the generation of NO from L-arginine affects both specific ion transport mechanisms and mitochondrial respiration. Finally, a wealth of data indicate that the ion transport mechanisms and metabolic processes that support and regulate them along the nephron are subject to complex control by changes in local and systemic environmental conditions (e.g., diet, hormones, drugs, dysfunction of other organs). The extent to which the responses of ion transport and metabolism remain coordinated is largely predictive of successful adaptation to the environmental challenge.

References

1. Axelsen KB, Palmgren MG: Evolution of substrate specificities in the P-type ATPase superfamily. J Mol Evol 46:84–101, 1998.
2. Paulusma CC, Oude Elferink RP: The type 4 subfamily of P-type ATPases, putative aminophospholipid translocases with a role in human disease. Biochim Biophys Acta 1741:11–24, 2005.
3. Gottesman MM, Fojo T, Bates SE: Multidrug resistance in cancer: Role of ATP-dependent transporters. Nat Rev Cancer 2:48–58, 2002.
4. van Helvoort A, Smith AJ, Sprong H, et al: MDR1 P-glycoprotein is a lipid translocase of broad specificity, while MDR3 P-glycoprotein specifically translocates phosphatidylcholine. Cell 87:507–517, 1996.
5. Gatlik-Landwojtowicz E, Aanismaa P, Seelig A: The rate of P-glycoprotein activation depends on the metabolic state of the cell. Biochemistry 43:14840–14851, 2004.
6. Krishnamurthy P, Schuetz JD: Role of ABCG2/BCRP in biology and medicine. Annu Rev Pharmacol Toxicol 46:381–410, 2006.
7. Horisberger JD: Recent insights into the structure and mechanism of the sodium pump. Physiology (Bethesda) 19:377–387, 2004.
8. Jorgensen PL, Hakansson KO, Karlish SJ: Structure and mechanism of Na,K-ATPase: Functional sites and their interactions. Annu Rev Physiol 65:817–849, 2003.
9. Ross B, Leaf A, Silva P, Epstein FH: Na-K-ATPase in sodium transport by the perfused rat kidney. Am J Physiol 226:624–629, 1974.
10. Ahn KY, Madsen KM, Tisher CC, Kone BC: Differential expression and cellular distribution of a- and b-isoforms of Na^+-K^+-ATPase in rat kidney. Am J Physiol 265:F792–F801, 1993.
11. Clapp WL, Bowman P, Shaw GS, et al: Segmental localization of mRNAs encoding Na+-K+-ATPase a- and b-subunit isoforms in rat kidney using RT-PCR. Kidney Int 46:627–638, 1994.
12. Lucking K, Nielsen JM, Pedersen PA, Jorgensen PL: Na-K-ATPase isoform (a3, a2, a1) abundance in rat kidney estimated by competitive RT-PCR and ouabain binding. Am J Physiol 271:F253–260, 1996.
13. Arystarkhova E, Sweadner KJ: Tissue-specific expression of the Na,K-ATPase b3 subunit. The presence of b3 in lung and liver addresses the problem of the missing subunit. J Biol Chem 272:22405–22408, 1997.
14. Katz AI: Distribution and function of classes of ATPases along the nephron. Kidney Int 29:21–31, 1986.
15. El Mernissi G, Doucet A: Quantitation of [³H]ouabain binding and turnover of Na-K-ATPase along the rabbit nephron. Am J Physiol 247:F158–F167, 1984.
16. Geering K: FXYD proteins: New regulators of Na-K-ATPase. Am J Physiol Renal Physiol 290:F241–F250, 2006.
17. Meij IC, Koenderink JB, van Bokhoven H, et al: Dominant isolated renal magnesium loss is caused by misrouting of the Na+,K+-ATPase g-subunit. Nat Genet 26:265–266, 2000.
18. Aizman R, Asher C, Fuzesi M, et al: Generation and phenotypic analysis of CHIF knockout mice. Am J Physiol Renal Physiol 283:F569–F277, 2002.
19. Shull GE, Lingrel JB: Molecular cloning of the rat stomach (H++K+)-ATPase. J Biol Chem 261:16788–16791, 1986.
20. Crowson MS, Shull GE: Isolation and characterization of a cDNA encoding the putative distal colon H+,K+-ATPase. Similarity of deduced amino acid sequence to gastric H+,K+-ATPase and Na+,K+-ATPase and mRNA expression in distal colon, kidney, and uterus. J Biol Chem 267:13740–13748, 1992.
21. Grishin AV, Sverdlov VE, Kostina MB, Modyanov NN: Cloning and characterization of the entire cDNA encoded by ATP1AL1—A member of the human Na,K/H,K-ATPase gene family. FEBS Lett 349:144–150, 1994.
22. Campbell WG, Weiner ID, Wingo CS, Cain BD: H-K-ATPase in the RCCT-28A rabbit cortical collecting duct cell line. Am J Physiol 276:F237–F245, 1999.
23. Kone BC, Higham SC: A novel N-terminal splice variant of the rat H+-K+-ATPase α2 subunit. Cloning, functional expression, and renal adaptive response to chronic hypokalemia. J Biol Chem 273:2543–2552, 1998.
24. Zhang W, Kuncewicz T, Higham SC, Kone BC: Structure, promoter analysis, and chromosomal localization of the murine H+/K+-ATPase α2 subunit gene. J Am Soc Nephrol 12:2554–2564, 2001.
25. Kone BC: Renal H,K-ATPase: Structure, function and regulation. Miner Electrolyte Metab 22:349–365, 1996.
26. Ahn KY, Turner PB, Madsen KM, Kone BC: Effects of chronic hypokalemia on renal expression of the "gastric" H+-K+-ATPase α-subunit gene. Am J Physiol 270:F557–F566, 1996.
27. Codina J, Kone BC, Delmas-Mata JT, DuBose TD Jr: Functional expression of the colonic H+,K+-ATPase α-subunit. Pharmacologic properties and assembly with X+,K+-ATPase β-subunits. J Biol Chem 271:29759–29763, 1996.
28. Ahn KY, Park KY, Kim KK, Kone BC: Chronic hypokalemia enhances expression of the H+-K+-ATPase α2-subunit gene in renal medulla. Am J Physiol 271:F314–F321, 1996.
29. Ramachandran C, Chan M, Brunette MG: Characterization of ATP-dependent Ca^{2+} transport in the basolateral membrane vesicles from proximal and distal tubules of the rabbit kidney. Biochem Cell Biol 69:109–114, 1991.
30. Strehler EE, Zacharias DA: Role of alternative splicing in generating isoform diversity among plasma membrane calcium pumps. Physiol Rev 81:21–50, 2001.
31. Doucet A, Katz AI: High-affinity Ca-Mg-ATPase along the rabbit nephron. Am J Physiol 242:F346–F352, 1982.
32. Magyar CE, White KE, Rojas R, et al: Plasma membrane Ca^{2+}-ATPase and NCX1 Na+/Ca^{2+} exchanger expression in distal convoluted tubule cells. Am J Physiol Renal Physiol 283:F29–F40, 2002.
33. Magosci M, Yamaki M, Penniston JT, Dousa TP: Localization of mRNAs coding for isozymes of plasma membrane Ca^{2+}-ATPase pump in rat kidney. Am J Physiol 263:F7–F14, 1992.
34. Caride AJ, Chini EN, Homma S, et al: mRNA encoding four isoforms of the plasma membrane calcium pump and their variants in rat kidney and nephron segments. J Lab Clin Med 132:149–156, 1998.
35. Martin V, Bredoux R, Corvazier E, et al: Three novel sarco/endoplasmic reticulum Ca2+-ATPase (SERCA) 3 isoforms. Expression, regulation, and function of the membranes of the SERCA3 family. J Biol Chem 277:24442–24452, 2002.
36. Greenough M, Pase L, Voskoboinik I, et al: Signals regulating trafficking of Menkes (MNK; ATP7A) copper-translocating P-type ATPase in polarized MDCK cells. Am J Physiol Cell Physiol 287:C1463–C1471, 2004.
37. Moore SD, Cox DW: Expression in mouse kidney of membrane copper transporters ATP7a and ATP7b. Nephron 92:629–634, 2002.
38. Wagner CA, Finberg KE, Breton S, et al: Renal vacuolar H+-ATPase. Physiol Rev 84:1263–1314, 2004.
39. Borthwick KJ, Karet FE: Inherited disorders of the H+-ATPase. Curr Opin Nephrol Hypertens 11:563–568, 2002.
40. Smith AJ, van Helvoort A, van Meer G, et al: MDR3 P-glycoprotein, a phosphatidylcholine translocase, transports several cytotoxic drugs and directly interacts with

drugs as judged by interference with nucleotide trapping. J Biol Chem 275:23530–23539, 2000.

41. Ernest S, Rajaraman S, Megyesi J, Bello-Reuss EN: Expression of MDR1 (multidrug resistance) gene and its protein in normal human kidney. Nephron 77:284–289, 1997.

42. Bello-Reuss E, Ernest S: Expression and function of P-glycoprotein in human mesangial cells. Am J Physiol 267:C1351–C1358, 1994.

43. Schaub TP, Kartenbeck J, Konig J, et al: Expression of the MRP2 gene-encoded conjugate export pump in human kidney proximal tubules and in renal cell carcinoma. J Am Soc Nephrol 10:1159–1169, 1999.

44. Stanton BA: Cystic fibrosis transmembrane conductance regulator (CFTR) and renal function. Wien Klin Wochenschr 109:457–464, 1997.

45. Cantiello HF: Electrodiffusional ATP movement through CFTR and other ABC transporters. Pflugers Arch 443(suppl 1):S22–S27, 2001.

46. Sugita M, Yue Y, Foskett JK: CFTR Cl⁻ channel and CFTR-associated ATP channel: Distinct pores regulated by common gates. Embo J 17:898–908, 1998.

47. Ismailov II, Awayda MS, Jovov B, et al: Regulation of epithelial sodium channels by the cystic fibrosis transmembrane conductance regulator. J Biol Chem 271:4725–4732, 1996.

48. Ruknudin A, Schulze DH, Sullivan SK, et al: Novel subunit composition of a renal epithelial KATP channel. J Biol Chem 273:14165–14171, 1998.

49. Braunstein GM, Roman RM, Clancy JP, et al: Cystic fibrosis transmembrane conductance regulator facilitates ATP release by stimulating a separate ATP release channel for autocrine control of cell volume regulation. J Biol Chem 276:6621–6630, 2001.

50. Hallows KR, Raghuram V, Kemp BE, et al: Inhibition of cystic fibrosis transmembrane conductance regulator by novel interaction with the metabolic sensor AMP-activated protein kinase. J Clin Invest 105:1711–1721, 2000.

51. Hinkle PC: P/O ratios of mitochondrial oxidative phosphorylation. Biochim Biophys Acta 1706:1–11, 2005.

52. Mitchell P, Moyle J: Estimation of membrane potential and pH difference across the cristae membrane of rat liver mitochondria. Eur J Biochem 7:471–484, 1969.

53. Harris SI, Balaban RS, Mandel LJ: Oxygen consumption and cellular ion transport: Evidence for adenosine triphosphate to O₂ ratio near 6 in intact cell. Science 208:1148–1150, 1980.

54. Jacobus WE, Moreadith RW, Vandegaer KM: Mitochondrial respiratory control. Evidence against the regulation of respiration by extramitochondrial phosphorylation potentials or by [ATP]/[ADP] ratios. J Biol Chem 257:2397–2402, 1982.

55. Lemasters JJ, Sowers AE: Phosphate dependence and atractyloside inhibition of mitochondrial oxidative phosphorylation. The ADP-ATP carrier is rate-limiting. J Biol Chem 254:1248–1251, 1979.

56. Erecinska M, Wilson DF: Regulation of cellular energy metabolism. J Membr Biol 70:1–14, 1982.

57. Noel J, Vinay P, Tejedor A, et al: Metabolic cost of bafilomycin-sensitive H⁺ pump in intact dog, rabbit, and hamster proximal tubules. Am J Physiol 264:F655–F661, 1993.

58. Harris SI, Balaban RS, Barrett L, Mandel LJ: Mitochondrial respiratory capacity and Na⁺- and K⁺-dependent adenosine triphosphatase-mediated ion transport in the intact renal cell. J Biol Chem 256:10319–10328, 1981.

59. Balaban RS, Mandel LJ, Soltoff SP, Storey JM: Coupling of active ion transport and aerobic respiratory rate in isolated renal tubules. Proc Natl Acad Sci U S A 77:447–451, 1980.

60. Niaudet P: Mitochondrial disorders and the kidney. Arch Dis Child 78:387–390, 1998.

61. Rotig A, Appelkvist EL, Geromel V, et al: Quinone-responsive multiple respiratory-chain dysfunction due to widespread coenzyme Q10 deficiency. Lancet 356:391–395, 2000.

62. Guder WG, Schmidt U: The localization of gluconeogenesis in rat nephron. Determination of phosphoenolpyruvate carboxykinase in microdissected tubules. Hoppe Seylers Z Physiol Chem 355:273–278, 1974.

63. Burch HB, Narins RG, Chu C, et al: Distribution along the rat nephron of three enzymes of gluconeogenesis in acidosis and starvation. Am J Physiol 235:F246–F253, 1978.

64. Vandewalle A, Wirthensohn G, Heidrich HG, Guder WG: Distribution of hexokinase and phosphoenolpyruvate carboxykinase along the rabbit nephron. Am J Physiol 240: F492–F500, 1981.

65. Yanez AJ, Ludwig HC, Bertinat R, et al: Different involvement for aldolase isoenzymes in kidney glucose metabolism: Aldolase B but not aldolase A colocalizes and forms a complex with FBPase. J Cell Physiol 220:743–753, 2005.

66. Le Hir M, Dubach UC: Activities of enzymes of the tricarboxylic acid cycle in segments of the rat nephron. Pflugers Arch 395:239–243, 1982.

67. Weidemann MJ, Krebs HA: The fuel of respiration of rat kidney cortex. Biochem J 112:149–166, 1969.

68. Guder WG, Purschel S, Wirthensohn G: Renal ketone body metabolism. Distribution of 3-oxoacid CoA-transferase and 3-hydroxybutyrate dehydrogenase along the mouse nephron. Hoppe Seylers Z Physiol Chem 364:1727–1737, 1983.

69. Guder WG, Ross BD: Enzyme distribution along the nephron. Kidney Int 26:101–111, 1984.

70. Klein KI, Wang MS, Torikai S, et al: Substrate oxidation by defined single nephron segments of rat kidney. Int J Biochem 12:53–54, 1980.

71. Benoy MP, Elliot KAC: The metabolism of lactic and pyruvic acids in normal and tumble tissue. V. Synthesis of carbohydrate. Biochem J 31:1268–1275, 1937.

72. Krebs HA: Renal gluconeogenesis. Adv Enzyme Regul 1:385–400, 1963.

73. Meyer C, Stumvoll M, Dostou J, et al: Renal substrate exchange and gluconeogenesis in normal postabsorptive humans. Am J Physiol Endocrinol Metab 282:E428–E434, 2002.

74. Conjard A, Martin M, Guitton J, et al: Gluconeogenesis from glutamine and lactate in the isolated human renal proximal tubule: Longitudinal heterogeneity and lack of response to adrenaline. Biochem J 360:371–377, 2001.

75. Maleque A, Endou H, Koseki C, Sakai F: Nephron heterogeneity: Gluconeogenesis from pyruvate in rabbit nephron. FEBS Lett 116:154–156, 1980.

76. Gullans SR, Brazy PC, Dennis VW, Mandel LJ: Interactions between gluconeogenesis and sodium transport in rabbit proximal tubule. Am J Physiol 246:F859–F869, 1984.

77. Nagami GT, Lee P: Effect of luminal perfusion on glucose production by isolated proximal tubules. Am J Physiol 256:F120–F127, 1989.

78. Fulgraff G, Nunemann H, Sudhoff DE Effects of the diuretics furosemide, ethacrynic acid, and chlorothiazide on gluconeogenesis from various substrates in rat kidney cortex slices. Naunyn Schmiedebergs Arch Pharmacol 273:86–98, 1972.

79. Silva P, Hallac R, Spokes K, Epstein FH: Relationship among gluconeogenesis, QO₂, and Na⁺ transport in the perfused rat kidney. Am J Physiol 242:F508–F513, 1982.

80. Kiil F, Aukland K, Refsum HE: Renal sodium transport and oxygen consumption. Am J Physiol 201:511–526, 1961.

81. Sen AK, Post RL: Stoichiometry and localization of adenosine triphosphate-dependent sodium and potassium transport in the erythrocyte. J Biol Chem 239:345–352, 1964.

82. Mathisen O, Monclair T, Kiil F: Oxygen requirement of bicarbonate-dependent sodium reabsorption in the dog kidney. Am J Physiol 238:F175–F180, 1980.

83. Ostensen J, Stokke ES, Hartmann A, et al: Low oxygen cost of carbonic anhydrase-dependent sodium reabsorption in the dog kidney. Acta Physiol Scand 137:189–198, 1989.

84. Fromter E, Rumrich G, Ullrich KJ: Phenomenologic description of Na⁺, Cl⁻, and HCO₃⁻ absorption from proximal tubules of the rat kidney. Pflugers Arch 343:189–220, 1973.

85. Kiil F, Sejersted OM, Steen PA: Energetics and specificity of transcellular NaCl transport in the dog kidney. Int J Biochem 12:245–250, 1980.

86. Gross E, Hawkins K, Abuladze N, et al: The stoichiometry of the electrogenic sodium bicarbonate cotransporter NBC1 is cell-type dependent. J Physiol 531:597–603, 2001.

87. Silva P, Myers MA: Stoichiometry of sodium chloride transport by rectal gland of *Squalus acanthias*. Am J Physiol 250:F516–F519, 1986.

88. Welsh MJ: Energetics of chloride secretion in canine tracheal epithelium. Comparison of the metabolic cost of chloride transport with the metabolic cost of sodium transport. J Clin Invest 74:262–268, 1984.

89. Whittam R: Active cation transport as a pacemaker of respiration. Nature 191:603–604, 1961.

90. Harris SI, Patton L, Barrett L, Mandel LJ: (Na⁺,K⁺)-ATPase kinetics within the intact renal cell. The role of oxidative metabolism. J Biol Chem 257:6996–7002, 1982.

91. Avison MJ, Gullans SR, Ogino T, et al: Measurement of Na⁺-K⁺ coupling ratio of Na⁺-K⁺-ATPase in rabbit proximal tubules. Am J Physiol 253:C126–C136, 1987.

92. Brady HR, Kone BC, Gullans SR: Extracellular Na⁺ electrode for monitoring net Na⁺ flux in cell suspensions. Am J Physiol 256:C1105–C1110, 1989.

93. Blostein R, Harvey WJ: Na⁺, K⁺-pump stoichiometry and coupling in inside-out vesicles from red blood cell membranes. Methods Enzymol 173:377–380, 1989.

94. Soltoff SP, Mandel LJ: Active ion transport in the renal proximal tubule. III. The ATP dependence of the Na pump. J Gen Physiol 84:643–662, 1984.

95. Gullans SR, Brazy PC, Soltoff SP, et al: Metabolic inhibitors: Effects on metabolism and transport in the proximal tubule. Am J Physiol 243:F133–F140, 1982.

96. Ammann H, Noel J, Boulanger Y, Vinay P: Relationship between intracellular ATP and the sodium pump activity in dog renal tubules. Can J Physiol Pharmacol 68:57–67, 1990.

97. Balaban RS, Mandel LJ: Metabolic substrate utilization by rabbit proximal tubule. An NADH fluorescence study. Am J Physiol 254:F407–F416, 1988.

98. Foxall PJ, Nicholson JK: Nuclear magnetic resonance spectroscopy: A non-invasive probe of kidney metabolism and function. Exp Nephrol 6:409–414, 1998.

99. Freeman D, Bartlett S, Radda G, Ross B: Energetics of sodium transport in the kidney. Saturation transfer ³¹P-NMR. Biochim Biophys Acta 762:325–336, 1983.

100. Pfaller W, Guder WG, Gstraunthaler G, et al: Compartmentation of ATP within renal proximal tubular cells. Biochim Biophys Acta 805:152–157, 1984.

101. Kinne RK, Grunewald RW, Ruhfus B, Kinne-Saffran E: Biochemistry and physiology of carbohydrates in the renal collecting duct. J Exp Zool 279:436–442, 1997.

102. Quast U: ATP-sensitive K+ channels in the kidney. Naunyn Schmiedebergs Arch Pharmacol 354:213–225, 1996.

103. Tsuchiya K, Wang W, Giebisch G, Welling PA: ATP is a coupling modulator of parallel Na,K-ATPase-K-channel activity in the renal proximal tubule. Proc Natl Acad Sci U S A 89:6418–6422, 1992.

104. Ho K, Nichols CG, Lederer WJ, et al: Cloning and expression of an inwardly rectifying ATP-regulated potassium channel. Nature 362:31–38, 1993.

105. Boim MA, Ho K, Shuck ME, et al: ROMK inwardly rectifying ATP-sensitive K⁺ channel. II. Cloning and distribution of alternative forms. Am J Physiol 268:F1132–F1140, 1995.

106. Lee WS, Hebert SC: ROMK inwardly rectifying ATP-sensitive K⁺ channel. I. Expression in rat distal nephron segments. Am J Physiol 268:F1124–F1131, 1995.

107. Kohda Y, Ding W, Phan E, et al: Localization of the ROMK potassium channel to the apical membrane of distal nephron in rat kidney. Kidney Int 54:1214–1223, 1998.

108. Hurwitz CG, Hu VY, Segal AS: A mechanogated nonselective cation channel in proximal tubule that is ATP sensitive. Am J Physiol Renal Physiol 283:F93–F104, 2002.

109. Paucek P, Mironova G, Mahdi F, et al: Reconstitution and partial purification of the glibenclamide-sensitive, ATP-dependent K⁺ channel from rat liver and beef heart mitochondria. J Biol Chem 267:26062–26069, 1992.

110. Garlid KD, Paucek P: The mitochondrial potassium cycle. IUBMB Life 52:153–158, 2001.

111. Cancherini DV, Trabuco LG, Reboucas NA, Kowaltowski AJ: ATP-sensitive K+ channels in renal mitochondria. Am J Physiol Renal Physiol 285:F1291–F1296, 2003.

112. Bailey MA, Imbert-Teboul M, Turner C, et al: Evidence for basolateral P2Y(6) receptors along the rat proximal tubule: Functional and molecular characterization. J Am Soc Nephrol 12:1640–1647, 2001.

113. Deetjen P, Thomas J, Lehrmann H, et al: The luminal P2Y receptor in the isolated perfused mouse cortical collecting duct. J Am Soc Nephrol 11:1798–1806, 2000.

114. Lu M, MacGregor GG, Wang W, Giebisch G: Extracellular ATP inhibits the small-conductance K channel on the apical membrane of the cortical collecting duct from mouse kidney. J Gen Physiol 116:299–310, 2000.

115. Lehrmann H, Thomas J, Kim SJ, et al: Luminal P2Y2 receptor-mediated inhibition of Na+ absorption in isolated perfused mouse CCD. J Am Soc Nephrol 13:10–18, 2002.

116. Lederer ED, McLeish KR: P2 purinoceptor stimulation attenuates PTH inhibition of phosphate uptake by a G protein-dependent mechanism. Am J Physiol 269:F309–F316, 1995.

117. Leipziger J: Control of epithelial transport via luminal P2 receptors. Am J Physiol 284:F419–F432, 2003.

118. Ishikawa T, Jiang C, Stutts MJ, et al: Regulation of the epithelial Na+ channel by cytosolic ATP. J Biol Chem 278:38276–38286, 2003.

119. Gorelik J, Zhang Y, Sanchez D, et al: Aldosterone acts via an ATP autocrine/paracrine system: The Edelman ATP hypothesis revisited. Proc Natl Acad Sci U S A 102:15000–15005, 2005.

120. Bell PD, Lapointe JY, Sabirov R, et al: Macula densa cell signaling involves ATP release through a maxi anion channel. Proc Natl Acad Sci U S A 100:4322–4327, 2003.

121. Komlosi P, Peti-Peterdi J, Fuson AL, et al: Macula densa basolateral ATP release is regulated by luminal [NaCl] and dietary salt intake. Am J Physiol Renal Physiol 286:F1054–F1058, 2004.

122. Carling D: AMP-activated protein kinase: Balancing the scales. Biochimie 87:87–91, 2005.

123. Hallows KR: Emerging role of AMP-activated protein kinase in coupling membrane transport to cellular metabolism. Curr Opin Nephrol Hypertens 14:464–471, 2005.

124. Hallows KR, Kobinger GP, Wilson JM, et al: Physiological modulation of CFTR activity by AMP-activated protein kinase in polarized T84 cells. Am J Physiol Cell Physiol 284:C1297–C1308, 2003.

125. Hallows KR, McCane JE, Kemp BE, et al: Regulation of channel gating by AMP-activated protein kinase modulates cystic fibrosis transmembrane conductance regulator activity in lung submucosal cells. J Biol Chem 278:998–1004, 2003.

126. Carattino MD, Edinger RS, Grieser HJ, et al: Epithelial sodium channel inhibition by AMP-activated protein kinase in oocytes and polarized renal epithelial cells. J Biol Chem 280:17608–17616, 2005.

127. Paul RJ, Bauer M, Pease W: Vascular smooth muscle: Aerobic glycolysis linked to sodium and potassium transport processes. Science 206:1414–1416, 1979.

128. Lynch RM, Paul RJ: Compartmentation of glycolytic and glycogenolytic metabolism in vascular smooth muscle. Science 222:1344–1346, 1983.

129. Lynch RM, Balaban RS: Coupling of aerobic glycolysis and Na+-K+-ATPase in renal cell line MDCK. Am J Physiol 253:C269–C276, 1987.

130. Xu KY, Zweier JL, Becker LC: Functional coupling between glycolysis and sarcoplasmic reticulum Ca²⁺ transport. Circ Res 77:88–97, 1995.

131. Lu M, Sautin YY, Holliday LS, Gluck S: The glycolytic enzyme aldolase mediates assembly, expression, and activity of vacuolar H+-ATPase. J Biol Chem 279:8732–8739, 2004.

132. Sautin YY, Lu M, Gaugler A, et al: Phosphatidylinositol 3-kinase-mediated effects of glucose on vacuolar H+-ATPase assembly, translocation, and acidification of intracellular compartments in renal epithelial cells. Mol Cell Biol 25:575–589, 2005.

133. Su Y, Zhou A, Al-Lamki RS, Karet FE: The α-subunit of the V-type H+-ATPase interacts with phosphofructokinase-1 in humans. J Biol Chem 278:20013–20018, 2003.

134. Gyoergy P, Keller W, Brehme TH: Nierenstoffwechsel und Nierenentwicklung. Biochem Zeitschr 200:356–366, 1928.

135. Wirthensohn G, Guder WG: Renal substrate metabolism. Physiol Rev 66:469–497, 1986.

136. Guder WG, Wagner S, Wirthensohn G: Metabolic fuels along the nephron: Pathways and intracellular mechanisms of interaction. Kidney Int 29:41–45, 1986.

137. Ross BD, Epstein FH, Leaf A: Sodium reabsorption in the perfused rat kidney. Am J Physiol 225:1165–1171, 1973.

138. Silva P, Ross BD, Charney AN, et al: Potassium transport by the isolated perfused kidney. J Clin Invest 56:862–869, 1975.

139. Besarab A, Silva P, Ross B, Epstein FH: Bicarbonate and sodium reabsorption by the isolated perfused kidney. Am J Physiol 228:1525–1530, 1975.

140. Dickens F, Simer F: The respiratory quotient and the relationship of respiration to glycolysis. Biochem J 24:1301–1326, 1930.

141. Lee JB, Peter HM: Effect of oxygen tension on glucose metabolism in rabbit kidney cortex and medulla. Am J Physiol 217:1464–1471, 1969.

142. Cohen JJ: Is the function of the renal papilla coupled exclusively to an anaerobic pattern of metabolism? Am J Physiol 236:F423–F433, 1979.

143. Gullans SR, Brazy PC, Mandel LJ, Dennis VW: Stimulation of phosphate transport in the proximal tubule by metabolic substrates. Am J Physiol 247:F582–F587, 1984.

144. Gullans SR, Kone BC, Avison MJ, Giebisch G: Succinate alters respiration, membrane potential, and intracellular K⁺ in proximal tubule. Am J Physiol 255:F1170–F1177, 1988.

145. Soltoff SP, Mandel LJ: Active ion transport in the renal proximal tubule. I. Transport and metabolic studies. J Gen Physiol 84:601–622, 1984.

146. Uchida S, Endou H: Substrate specificity to maintain cellular ATP along the mouse nephron. Am J Physiol 255:F977–F983, 1988.

147. Ruegg CE, Mandel LJ: Bulk isolation of renal PCT and PST. I. Glucose-dependent metabolic differences. Am J Physiol 259:F164–F175, 1990.

148. Gullans SR, Harris SI, Mandel LJ: Glucose-dependent respiration in suspensions of rabbit cortical tubules. J Membr Biol 78:257–262, 1984.

149. Mandel LJ: Use of noninvasive fluorometry and spectrophotometry to study epithelial metabolism and transport. Fed Proc 41:36–41, 1982.

150. Rome L, Grantham J, Savin V, et al: Proximal tubule volume regulation in hyperosmotic media: Intracellular K⁺, Na⁺, and Cl. Am J Physiol 257:C1093–C1100, 1989.

151. Jung KY, Endou H: Cellular adenosine triphosphate production and consumption in the descending thin limb of Henle's loop in the rat. Ren Physiol Biochem 13:248–258, 1990.

152. LeBouffant F, Hus-Citharel A, Morel F: In vitro ¹⁴CO₂ production by single pieces of cortical thick ascending limbs and its coupling to active salt transport. In Morel F (ed): Biochemistry of Kidney Functions. INSERM Symposium 21. Amsterdam, Elsevier Biomedical Press, 1982, pp 363–370.

153. Wittner M, Weidtke C, Schlatter E, et al: Substrate utilization in the isolated perfused cortical thick ascending limb of rabbit nephron. Pflugers Arch 402:52–62, 1984.

154. Bagnasco S, Good D, Balaban R, Burg M: Lactate production in isolated segments of the rat nephron. Am J Physiol 254:F522–F526, 1985.

155. Guder WG, Wirthensohn G: Metabolism of isolated kidney tubules. Interactions between lactate, glutamine and oleate metabolism. Eur J Biochem 99:577–584, 1979.

156. Kone BC, Madsen KM, Tisher CC: Ultrastructure of the thick ascending limb of Henle in the rat kidney. Am J Anat 171:217–226, 1984.

157. Eveloff J, Bayerdorffer E, Silva P, Kinne R: Sodium-chloride transport in the thick ascending limb of Henle's loop. Oxygen consumption studies in isolated cells. Pflugers Arch 389:263–270, 1981.

158. Chamberlin ME, Mandel LJ: Na+-K+-ATPase activity in medullary thick ascending limb during short-term anoxia. Am J Physiol 252:F838–F843, 1987.

159. Mandel LJ: Primary active sodium transport, oxygen consumption, and ATP: Coupling and regulation. Kidney Int 29:3–9, 1986.

160. Trinh-Trang-Tan MM, Levillain O, Bankir L: Contribution of leucine to oxidative metabolism of the rat medullary thick ascending limb. Pflugers Arch 411:676–680, 1988.

161. Vinay P, Gougoux A, Lemieux G: Isolation of a pure suspension of rat proximal tubules. Am J Physiol 241:F403–F411, 1981.

162. Katz AI, Doucet A, Morel F: Na-K-ATPase activity along the rabbit, rat, and mouse nephron. Am J Physiol 237:F114–F120, 1979.

163. Kiebzak GM, Yusufi AN, Kusano E, et al: ATP and cAMP system in the in vitro response of microdissected cortical tubules to PTH. Am J Physiol 248:F152–F159, 1985.

164. Le Bouffant F, Hus-Citharel A, Morel F: Metabolic CO₂ production by isolated single pieces of rat distal nephron segments. Pflugers Arch 401:346–353, 1984.

165. Hus-Citharel A, Morel F: Coupling of metabolic CO₂ production to ion transport in isolated rat thick ascending limbs and collecting tubules. Pflugers Arch 407:421–427, 1986.

166. Torikai S: Dependency of microdissected nephron segments upon oxidative phosphorylation and exogenous substrates: A relationship between tubular anatomical location in the kidney and metabolic activity. Clin Sci (Lond) 77:287–295, 1989.

167. Hering-Smith KS, Hamm LL: Metabolic support of collecting duct transport. Kidney Int 53:408–415, 1998.

168. Natke E Jr: Cell volume regulation of rabbit cortical collecting tubule in anisotonic media. Am J Physiol 258:F1657–F1665, 1990.

169. Le Hir M, Dubach UC: Peroxisomal and mitochondrial beta-oxidation in the rat kidney: Distribution of fatty acyl-coenzyme A oxidase and 3-hydroxyacyl-coenzyme A dehydrogenase activities along the nephron. J Histochem Cytochem 30:441–444, 1982.

170. Nonaka T, Stokes JB: Metabolic support of Na⁺ transport by the rabbit CCD: Analysis of the use of equivalent current. Kidney Int 45:743–752, 1994.

171. Stokes JB, Grupp C, Kinne RK: Purification of rat papillary collecting duct cells: Functional and metabolic assessment. Am J Physiol 253:F251–F262, 1987.

172. Meury L, Noel J, Tejedor A, et al: Glucose metabolism in dog inner medullary collecting ducts. Ren Physiol Biochem 17:246–266, 1994.

173. Kone BC, Kikeri D, Zeidel ML, Gullans SR: Cellular pathways of potassium transport in renal inner medullary collecting duct. Am J Physiol 256:C823–C830, 1989.

174. Dickman KG, Mandel LJ: Differential effects of respiratory inhibitors on glycolysis in proximal tubules. Am J Physiol 258:F1608–F1615, 1990.

175. Ruegg CE, Mandel LJ: Bulk isolation of renal PCT and PST. II. Differential responses to anoxia or hypoxia. Am J Physiol 259:F176–F185, 1990.

176. Feldkamp T, Kribben A, Roeser NF, et al: Accumulation of nonesterified fatty acids causes the sustained energetic deficit in kidney proximal tubules after hypoxia-reoxygenation. Am J Physiol 288:F1092–F1102, 2005.

177. Feldkamp T, Kribben A, Roeser NF, et al: Preservation of complex I function during hypoxia-reoxygenation-induced mitochondrial injury in proximal tubules. Am J Physiol 286:F749–F759, 2004;.

178. Leichtweiss HP, Lubbers DW, Weiss C, et al: The oxygen supply of the rat kidney: Measurements of intrarenal pO₂. Pflugers Arch 309:328–349, 1969.

179. Prasad PV, Edelman RR, Epstein FH: Noninvasive evaluation of intrarenal oxygenation with BOLD-MRI. Circulation 94:3271–3275, 1996.

180. Brezis M, Rosen S, Silva P, Epstein FH: Transport activity modifies thick ascending limb damage in the isolated perfused kidney. Kidney Int 25:65–72, 1984.

181. Kakoki M, Kim HS, Arendshorst WJ, Mattson DL: L-Arginine uptake affects nitric oxide production and blood flow in the renal medulla. Am J Physiol Regul Integr Comp Physiol 2004;287:R1478–85.

182. Morris SM Jr, Sweeney WE Jr, Kepka DM, et al: Localization of arginine biosynthetic enzymes in renal proximal tubules and abundance of mRNA during development. Pediatr Res 29:151–154, 1991.

183. Levillain O, Hus-Citharel A, Morel F, Bankir L: Localization of arginine synthesis along rat nephron. Am J Physiol 259:F916–F923, 1990.

184. Blantz RC, Satriano J, Gabbai F, Kelly C: Biological effects of arginine metabolites. Acta Physiol Scand 168:21–25, 2000.

185. Miyanaka K, Gotoh T, Nagasaki A, et al: Immunohistochemical localization of arginase II and other enzymes of arginine metabolism in rat kidney and liver. Histochem J 30:741–751, 1998.

186. Levillain O, Hus-Citharel A, Morel F, Bankir L: Arginine synthesis in mouse and rabbit nephron: Localization and functional significance. Am J Physiol 264:F1038–F1045, 1993.

187. Ortiz PA, Garvin JL: Role of nitric oxide in the regulation of nephron transport. Am J Physiol Renal Physiol 282:F777–F784, 2002.

188. Lu M, Wang X, Wang W: Nitric oxide increases the activity of the apical 70-pS K^+ channel in TAL of rat kidney. Am J Physiol 274:F946–F950, 1998.

189. Lu M, Giebisch G, Wang W: Nitric oxide links the apical Na^+ transport to the basolateral K^+ conductance in the rat cortical collecting duct. J Gen Physiol 110:717–726, 1997.

190. Tojo A, Guzman NJ, Garg LC, et al: Nitric oxide inhibits bafilomycin-sensitive H^+-ATPase activity in rat cortical collecting duct. Am J Physiol 267:F509–F515, 1994.

191. Deng A, Miracle CM, Suarez JM, et al: Oxygen consumption in the kidney: Effects of nitric oxide synthase isoforms and angiotensin II. Kidney Int 68:723–730, 2005.

192. Moncada S, Erusalimsky JD: Does nitric oxide modulate mitochondrial energy generation and apoptosis? Nat Rev Mol Cell Biol 3:214–220, 2002.

193. Burwell LS, Nadtochiv SM, Tompkins AJ, et al: Direct evidence for S-nitrosation of mitochondrial complex I. Biochem J 15:627–634, 2006.

194. Loke KE, McConnell PI, Tuzman JM, et al: Endogenous endothelial nitric oxide synthase-derived nitric oxide is a physiological regulator of myocardial oxygen consumption. Circ Res 84:840–845, 1999.

195. Elfering SL, Sarkela TM, Giulivi C: Biochemistry of mitochondrial nitric-oxide synthase. J Biol Chem 277:38079–38086, 2002.

196. Garvin JL, Hong NJ: Nitric oxide inhibits sodium/hydrogen exchange activity in the thick ascending limb. Am J Physiol 277:F377–F382, 1999.

197. Packer MA, Porteous CM, Murphy MP: Superoxide production by mitochondria in the presence of nitric oxide forms peroxynitrite. Biochem Mol Biol Int 40:527–534, 1996.

198. Halestrap AP, Doran E, Gillespie JP, O'Toole A: Mitochondria and cell death. Biochem Soc Trans 28:170–177, 2000.

199. Schmid H, Scholz M, Mall A, et al: Carbohydrate metabolism in rat kidney: Heterogeneous distribution of glycolytic and gluconeogenic key enzymes. Curr Probl Clin Biochem 8:282–289, 1977.

200. Zeidel ML, Seifter JL, Lear S, et al: Atrial peptides inhibit oxygen consumption in kidney medullary collecting duct cells. Am J Physiol 251:F379–F383, 1986.

201. Grunewald RW, Kinne RK: Sugar transport in isolated rat kidney papillary collecting duct cells. Pflugers Arch 413:32–37, 1988.

202. Chamberlin ME, Mandel LJ: Substrate support of medullary thick ascending limb oxygen consumption. Am J Physiol 251:F758–F763, 1986.

203. Terada Y, Knepper MA: Na^+-K^+-ATPase activities in renal tubule segments of rat inner medulla. Am J Physiol 256:F218–F223, 1989.

CHAPTER 5

Transport of Inorganic Solutes: Sodium, Chloride, Potassium, Magnesium, Calcium, and Phosphate

David B. Mount • Alan S. L. Yu

SODIUM AND CHLORIDE TRANSPORT

Sodium (Na^+) is the principal osmole in extracellular fluid; as such, the total body content of Na^+ and Cl^-, its primary anion, determine the extracellular fluid volume. Renal excretion or retention of salt (Na^+-Cl^-) is thus the major determinant of the extracellular fluid volume, such that genetic loss-in-function or gains-in-function in renal Na^+-Cl^- transport can be associated with relative hypotension or hypertension, respectively. On a quantitative level, at a glomerular filtration rate of 180 liters/day and serum Na^+ of ~140 mM, the kidney filters some 25,200 millimoles per day of Na^+; this is equivalent to ~1.5 kilograms of salt, which would occupy roughly ten times the extracellular space.[1] Minute changes in renal Na^+-Cl^- excretion can thus have profound effects on the extracellular fluid volume; furthermore, 99.6% of this filtered Na^+-Cl^- must be reabsorbed to excrete 100 millimoles per day. Energetically, this renal absorption of Na^+ consumes one molecule of ATP per 5 molecules of Na^+.[1] This is gratifyingly economical, given that the absorption of Na^+-Cl^- is driven by basolateral Na^+/K^+-ATPase, which has a stoichiometry of three molecules of transported Na^+ per molecule of ATP. This estimate reflects a net expenditure, however, because the cost of transepithelial Na^+-Cl^- transport varies considerably along the nephron, from a predominance of passive transport by thin ascending limbs to the purely active transport mediated by the aldosterone-sensitive distal nephron (distal convoluted tubule, connecting tubule, and collecting duct). The bulk of filtered Na^+-Cl^- transport is reabsorbed by the proximal tubule and thick ascending limb (Fig. 5–1), nephron segments which utilize their own peculiar combinations of paracellular and transcellular Na^+-Cl^- transport; whereas the proximal tubule can theoretically absorb as much as 9 Na^+ molecules for each hydrolyzed ATP,[1] paracellular Na^+ transport by the thick ascending limb doubles the efficiency of transepithelial Na^+-Cl^- transport (6 Na^+ per ATP).[2] Finally, the "fine-tuning" of renal Na^+-Cl^- absorption occurs at full cost[1] (3 Na^+ per ATP) in the aldosterone-sensitive distal nephron, while affording the generation of considerable transepithelial gradients.

The nephron thus constitutes a serial arrangement of tubule segments with considerable heterogeneity in the physiological consequences, mechanisms, and regulation of transepithelial Na^+-Cl^- transport. These issues will be reviewed in this section, in anatomical order, with an emphasis on particularly recent developments.

Proximal Tubule

A primary function of the renal proximal tubule is the near-isosomotic reabsorption of two thirds to three quarters of the glomerular ultrafiltrate. This encompasses the reabsorption of approximately 60% of filtered Na^+-Cl^- (see Fig. 5–1), such that this nephron segment plays a critical role in the maintenance of extracellular fluid volume. Although all segments of the proximal tubule share the ability to transport a variety of inorganic and organic solutes, there are considerable differences in the transport characteristics and capacity of early, mid, and late segments of the proximal tubule. There is thus is a gradual reduction in the volume of transported fluid and solutes as one proceeds along the proximal nephron. This corresponds to distinct ultrastructural characteristics in the tubular epithelium, moving from the S1 segment (early proximal convoluted tubule), to the S2 segment (late proximal convoluted tubule and beginning of the proximal straight tubule), and the S3 segment (remainder of the proximal straight tubule) (Fig. 5–2). Cells of the S1 segment are thus characterized by a tall brush border, with extensive lateral invaginations of the basolateral membrane.[3] Numerous elongated mitochondria are located in lateral cell processes, with a proximity to the plasma membrane that is characteristic of epithelial cells involved in active transport. Ultrastructure of the S2 segment is similar, albeit with a shorter brush border, fewer lateral invaginations, and less prominent mitochondria. In epithelial cells of the S3 segment, lateral cell processes and invaginations are essentially absent, with small mitochondria that are randomly distributed within the cell.[3] The extensive brush border of proximal tubular cells serves to amplify the apical cell surface that is available for reabsorption; again, this amplification is axially distributed, increasing apical area 36-fold in S1 and 15-fold in S3.[4] At the functional

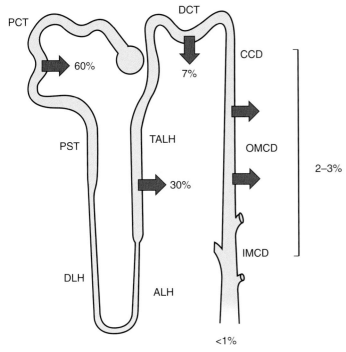

FIGURE 5–1 Percentage reabsorption of filtered Na⁺-Cl⁻ along the euvolemic nephron. ALH, thin ascending limb of the loop of Henle; CCD, cortical collecting duct: DCT, distal convoluted tubule; DLH, descending thin limb of the loop of Henle; PCT, proximal convoluted tubule; PST, proximal straight tubule; TAL, thick ascending limb; IMCD, inner medullary collecting duct; OMCD, outer medullary collecting duct.

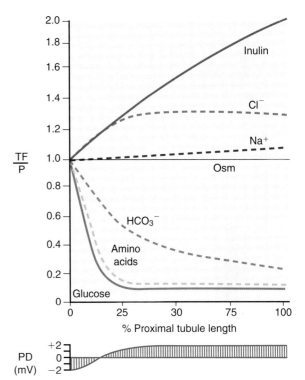

FIGURE 5–3 Reabsorption of solutes along the proximal tubule, in relation to transepithelial potential difference (PD). TF/P represents to ratio of tubule fluid to plasma concentration. OSM, osmolality. (From Rector FC, Jr: Sodium, bicarbonate, and chloride absorption by the proximal tubule. Am J Physiol 244: F461–71, 1983.)

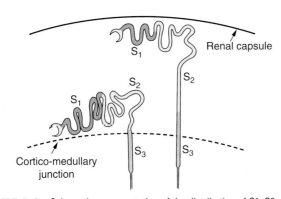

FIGURE 5–2 Schematic representation of the distribution of S1, S2, and S3 segments in the proximal tubules of superficial (SF) and juxtamedullary (JM) nephrons. (Redrawn from Woodhall PB, Tisher CC, Simonton CA, Robinson RR: Relationship between para-aminohippurate secretion and cellular morphology in rabbit proximal tubules. J Clin Invest 61:1320–1329, 1978.)

level, there is a rapid drop in the absorption of bicarbonate and Cl⁻ after the first millimeter of perfused proximal tubule, consistent with a much greater reabsorptive capacity in S1 segments.[5]

There is also considerable axial heterogeneity in the quantitative capacity of the proximal nephron for organic solutes such as glucose and amino acids, with predominant reabsorption of these substrates in S1 segments.[6] The Na⁺-dependent reabsorption of glucose, amino acids, and other solutes in S1 segments results in a transepithelial potential difference (PD) that is initially lumen-negative, due to electrogenic removal of Na⁺ from the lumen[7] (Fig. 5–3). This is classically considered the first phase of volume reabsorption by the proximal tubule.[8,9] The lumen-negative PD serves to drive both paracellular Cl⁻ absorption and a "backleak" of Na⁺ from the peritu-

bular space to the lumen. Paracellular Cl⁻ absorption in this setting accomplishes the net transepithelial absorption of a solute such as glucose, along with equal amounts of Na⁺ and Cl⁻; in contrast, backleak of Na⁺ leads only to reabsorption of the organic solute, with no net transepithelial transport of Na⁺ or Cl⁻. The amount of Cl⁻ reabsorption that is driven by this lumen-negative PD thus depends on the relative permeability of the paracellular pathway to Na⁺ and Cl⁻. There appears to be considerable heterogeneity in the relative paracellular permeability to Na⁺ and Cl⁻; for example, whereas superficial proximal convoluted tubules and proximal straight tubules in the rabbit are Cl⁻-selective, juxtamedullary proximal tubules in this species are reportedly Na⁺-selective.[10,11] Regardless, the component of paracellular Cl⁻ transport that is driven by this lumen-negative PD is restricted to the very early proximal tubule.

The second phase of volume reabsorption by the proximal tubule is dominated by Na⁺-Cl⁻ reabsorption, via both paracellular and transcellular pathways.[9] In addition to the Na⁺-dependent reabsorption of organic solutes, the early proximal tubule has a much higher capacity for HCO₃⁻ absorption,[6] via the coupling of apical Na⁺-H⁺ exchange, carbonic anhydrase, and basolateral Na⁺-HCO₃⁻ cotransport. As the luminal concentrations of HCO₃⁻ and other solutes begin to drop, the concentration of Na⁺-Cl⁻ rises to a value greater than that of the peritubular space.[8] This is accompanied by a reversal of the lumen-negative PD, to a lumen-*positive* value generated by passive Cl⁻ diffusion[12] (see Fig. 5–3). This lumen-positive PD serves to drive paracellular Na⁺ transport, whereas the *chemical* gradient between the lumen and peritubular space provides the driving force for paracellular reabsorption of Cl⁻. This passive, paracellular pathway is thought to mediate ~40% of transepithelial Na⁺-Cl⁻ reabsorption by the mid-to-late proximal tubule.[11] Of note, however, there may be heterogeneity in the relative importance of this paracellular pathway, with evidence that active (i.e., transcellular)

158

CH 5

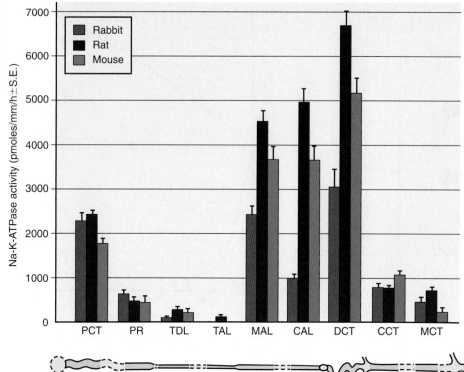

FIGURE 5–4 *Distribution of Na$^+$/K$^+$-ATPase activity along the nephron. CAL, cortical thick ascending limb; CCT, cortical collecting duct; DCT, distal convoluted tubule; MAL, medullary thick ascending limb; MCT, medullary collecting duct; PCT, proximal convoluted tubule; PR, pars recta; TAL, thin ascending limb of the loop of Henle; TDL, descending thin limb of the loop of Henle. (From Katz AI, Doucet A, Morel F: Na-K-ATPase activity along the rabbit, rat, and mouse nephron. Am J Physiol 237:F114–120, 1979.)*

reabsorption predominates in proximal convoluted tubules from juxtamedullary versus superficial nephrons.[13] Regardless, the combination of both passive and active transport of Na$^+$-Cl$^-$ explains how the proximal tubule is able to reabsorb ~60% of filtered Na$^+$-Cl$^-$ despite Na$^+$/K$^+$-ATPase activity that is considerably lower than that of distal segments of the nephron[14] (Fig. 5–4).

The transcellular component of Na$^+$-Cl$^-$ reabsorption initially emerged from studies of the effect of cyanide, ouabain, luminal anion transport inhibitors, cooling, and luminal/peritubular K$^+$ removal.[9] For example, the luminal addition of SITS, an inhibitor of anion transporters, reduces volume reabsorption of proximal convoluted tubules perfused with a high Cl$^-$, low HCO$_3^-$ solution that mimics the luminal composition of the late proximal tubule; this occurs in the absence of an effect on carbonic anhydrase.[15] This transcellular component of Na$^+$-Cl$^-$ reabsorption is clearly electroneutral. For example, in the absence of anion gradients across the perfused proximal tubule there is no change in transepithelial PD after the inhibition of active transport by ouabain, despite a marked reduction in volume reabsorption.[16] Transcellular Na$^+$-Cl$^-$ reabsorption is accomplished by the coupling of luminal Na$^+$-H$^+$ exchange or Na$^+$-SO$_4^{2-}$ cotransport with a heterogeneous population of anion exchangers, as reviewed later.

Paracellular Na$^+$-Cl$^-$ Transport

A number of factors serve to optimize the conditions for paracellular Na$^+$-Cl$^-$ transport by the mid-to-late proximal tubule. First, the proximal tubule is a low-resistance, "leaky" epithelium,[11] with tight junctions that are highly permeable to both Na$^+$ and Cl$^-$.[10] Second, these tight junctions are preferentially permeable to Cl$^-$ over HCO$_3^-$,[17] a feature that helps generate the lumen-positive PD in the mid-to-late proximal tubule. Third, the increase in luminal Na$^+$-Cl$^-$ concentrations in the mid-to-late proximal tubule generates the electrical and chemical driving forces for paracellular transport. Diffusion of Cl$^-$ thus generates a lumen-positive PD,[12] which drives paracellular Na$^+$ transport; the *chemical* gradient between the

lumen and peritubular space provides the driving force for paracellular reabsorption of Cl$^-$. This rise in luminal Na$^+$-Cl$^-$ is the direct result of the robust reabsorption of HCO$_3^-$ and other solutes by the early S1 segment,[6,8] combined with the iso-osmotic reabsorption of filtered water.[18]

A highly permeable paracellular pathway is a consistent feature of epithelia that function in the near-isosmolar reabsorption of Na$^+$-Cl$^-$, including small intestine, proximal tubule, and gallbladder. Morphologically, the apical tight junction of proximal tubular cells and other "leaky" epithelia is considerably less complex than that of "tight" epithelia. Freeze-fracture microscopy thus reveals that the tight junction of proximal tubular cells is comparatively shallow, with as few as one junctional strand (Fig. 5–5); in contrast, high-resistance epithelia have deeper tight junctions with a complex, extensive network of junctional strands.[19] At the functional level, tight junctions of epithelia function as charge- and size-selective "paracellular tight-junction channels",[20] physiological characteristics that are thought to be conferred by integral membrane proteins that cluster together at the tight junction[21]; changes in the expression of these proteins can have marked effects on permeability, without affecting the number of junctional strands.[22] In particular, the charge[23] and size[24] selectivity of tight junctions appears to be conferred in large part by the claudins, a large (>20) gene family of tetraspan transmembrane proteins. The repertoire of claudins expressed by proximal tubular epithelial cells may thus determine the high paracellular permeability of this nephron segment. At a minimum, proximal tubular cells co-express claudin-2, -10, and -11.[25,26] The robust expression of claudin-2 in proximal tubule is of particular interest because this claudin can dramatically decrease the resistance of transfected epithelial cells.[22] Consistent with this cellular phenotype, targeted deletion of claudin-2 in knockout mice generates a "tight" epithelium in the proximal tubule, with a reduction in Na$^+$-Cl$^-$ reabsorption.[27]

The reabsorption of HCO$_3^-$ and other solutes from the glomerular ultrafiltrate would be expected to generate an osmotic

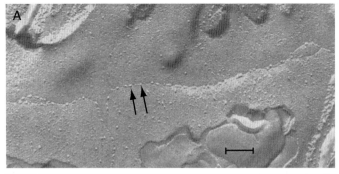

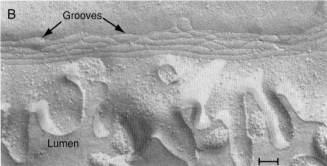

FIGURE 5–5 Freeze fracture electron microscopy of tight junctions in mouse proximal and distal nephron. **A,** Proximal convoluted tubule, a "leaky" epithelium; the tight junction contains only one junctional strand, seen as a groove in the fracture face (arrows). **B,** Distal convoluted tubule, a "tight" epithelium. The tight junction is deeper and contains several anastamosing strands, seen as grooves in the fracture face. (From Claude P, Goodenough DA: Fracture faces of zonulae occludentes from "tight" and "leaky" epithelia. J Cell Biol 58:390–400, 1973.)

gradient across the epithelium, resulting in a hypotonic lumen. This appears to be the case, although the absolute difference in osmolality between lumen and peri-tubular space has been a source of considerable controversy.[18] Another controversial issue has been the relative importance of paracellular versus transcellular water transport from this hypotonic lumen. These issues have both been elegantly addressed through characterization of knockout mice with a targeted deletion of Aquaporin-1, a water channel protein expressed at the apical and basolateral membranes of the proximal tubule. Mice deficient in Aquaporin-1 have an 80% reduction in water permeability in perfused S2 segments, with a 50% reduction in transepithelial fluid transport.[28] Aquaporin-1 deficiency also results in a marked increase in luminal hypotonicity, providing definitive proof that near-isosmotic reabsorption by the proximal tubule requires transepithelial water transport via Aquaporin-1.[18] The residual water transport in the proximal tubules of Aquaporin-1 knockout mice is mediated in part by Aquaporin-7.[29] Alternative pathways for water reabsorption may include "co-transport" of H_2O via the multiple Na^+-dependent solute transporters in the early proximal tubule[30]; this novel hypothesis is, however, a source of considerable controversy.[31] A related issue is the relative importance of diffusional versus convective transport of Na^+-Cl^-, also known as "solvent drag", across the paracellular tight junction[11]; convective transport of Na^+-Cl^- with water would seem to play a lesser role than diffusion, given the evidence that the transcellular pathway is the dominant transepithelial pathway for water in the proximal tubule.[18,28,29]

Transcellular Na^+-Cl^- transport
Apical Mechanisms
Apical Na^+-H^+ exchange plays a critical role in both transcellular and paracellular reabsorption of Na^+-Cl^- by the proximal

tubule. In addition to providing an entry site in the transcellular transport of Na^+, Na^+-H^+ exchange plays a dominant role in the robust absorption of HCO_3^- by the early proximal tubule[32]; this absorption of HCO_3^- serves to increase the luminal concentration of Cl^-, which in turn increases the driving forces for the passive paracellular transport of both Na^+ and Cl^-. Increases in luminal Cl^- also help drive the apical uptake of Cl^- during transcellular transport. Not surprisingly, there is a considerable reduction in fluid transport of perfused proximal tubules exposed to concentrations of amiloride that are sufficient to inhibit proximal tubular Na^+-H^+ exchange.[33]

Na^+-H^+ exchange is predominantly mediated by the NHE proteins, encoded by the nine members of the SLC9 gene family; NHE3 in particular plays an important role in proximal tubular physiology. The NH3 protein is expressed at the apical membrane of S1, S2, and S3 segments.[34] The apical membrane of the proximal tubule also expresses alternative Na^+-dependent H^+ transporters,[35] including NHE8.[36] Regardless, the primacy of NHE3 in proximal Na^+-Cl^- reabsorption is illustrated by the renal phenotype of *NHE3*-null knockout mice, which have a 62% reduction in proximal fluid absorption[37] and a 54% reduction in baseline chloride absorption.[38]

Much as amiloride and other inhibitors of Na^+-H^+ exchange revealed an important role for this transporter in transepithelial salt transport by the proximal tubule,[33] evidence for the involvement of an apical anion exchanger first came from the use of anion transport inhibitors; DIDS, furosemide, and SITS all reduce fluid absorption from the lumen of PT segments perfused with solutions containing Na^+-Cl^-.[15,33] In the simplest arrangement for the coupling of Na^+-H^+ exchange to Cl^- exchange, Cl^- would be exchanged with the OH^- ion during Na^+-Cl^- transport (Fig. 5–6). Evidence for such a Cl^--OH^- exchanger was reported by a number of groups in the early 1980's, using membrane vesicles isolated from the proximal tubule (reviewed in Ref 39). These findings could not however be replicated in similar studies from other groups.[39,40] Moreover, experimental evidence was provided for the existence of a dominant Cl^--formate exchange activity in brush border vesicles, in the absence of significant Cl^--OH^- exchange.[40] It was postulated that recycling of formate by the back-diffusion of formic acid would sustain the net transport of Na^+-Cl^- across the apical membrane. Vesicle formate transport stimulated by a pH gradient (H^+-formate cotransport or formate-OH^- exchange) is saturable, consistent with a carrier-mediated process rather than diffusion of formic acid across the apical membrane of the proximal tubule.[41] Transport studies using brush border vesicles have also detected the presence of Cl^--*oxalate* exchange mechanisms in the apical membrane of the PT,[42] in addition to SO_4^{2-}-oxalate exchange.[43] Based on differences in the affinities and inhibitor sensitivity of the Cl^--oxalate and Cl^--formate exchange activities, it was suggested that there are two separate apical exchangers in the proximal nephron, a Cl^--formate exchanger and a Cl^--formate/oxalate exchanger capable of transporting both formate and oxalate (see Fig. 5–6).

The physiological relevance of apical Cl-formate and Cl-oxalate exchange has been addressed by perfusing individual proximal tubule segments with solutions containing Na^+-Cl^- and either formate or oxalate. Both formate and oxalate significantly increased fluid transport under these conditions, in rabbit, rat, and mouse proximal tubule.[38] This increase in fluid transport was inhibited by DIDS, suggesting involvement of the DIDS-sensitive anion exchanger(s) detected in brush border vesicle studies. A similar mechanism for Na^+-Cl^- transport in the distal convoluted tubule (DCT) has also been detected, independent of thiazide-sensitive Na^+-Cl^- cotransport.[44] Further experiments indicated that the oxalate- and formate-dependent anion transporters in the PT are

A

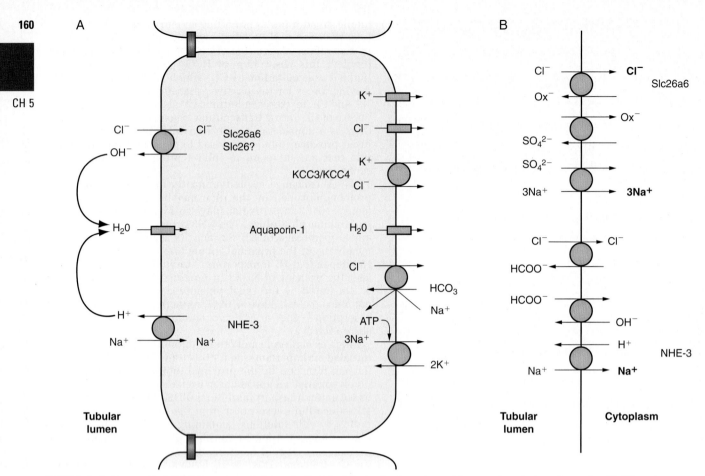

B

FIGURE 5–6 Transepithelial Na$^+$-Cl$^-$ transport in the proximal tubule. **A,** In the simplest scheme, Cl$^-$ enters the apical membrane via a Cl$^-$-OH$^-$ exchanger, coupled to Na$^+$ entry via NHE-3. **B,** Alternative apical anion exchange activities that couple to Na$^+$-H$^+$ exchange and Na$^+$-SO$_4$$^{2-}$ cotransport; see text for details.

coupled to distinct Na$^+$ entry pathways, to Na$^+$-SO$_4$$^{2-}$ cotransport and Na$^+$-H$^+$ exchange, respectively.[45] The coupling of Cl$^-$-oxalate transport to Na$^+$-SO$_4$$^{2-}$ cotransport requires the additional presence of SO$_4$$^{2-}$-oxalate exchange, which has been demonstrated in brush border membrane vesicle studies.[43] The obligatory role for NHE3 in formate stimulated Cl$^-$ transport was illustrated using *NHE3*-null mice, in which the formate effect is abolished[38]; of note, oxalate stimulation of Cl$^-$ transport is preserved in the *NHE3*-null mice. Finally, tubular perfusion data from superficial and juxtamedullary proximal convoluted tubules suggest that there is heterogeneity in the dominant mode of anion exchange along the PT, such that Cl$^-$-formate exchange is absent in juxtamedullary PCTs, in which Cl$^-$-OH$^-$ exchange may instead be dominant.[46]

The molecular identity of the apical anion exchanger(s) involved in transepithelial Na$^+$-Cl$^-$ by the proximal tubule has been the object of more than two decades of investigation. A key breakthrough was the observation that the SLC26A4 anion exchanger, also known as pendrin, is capable of Cl$^-$-formate exchange when expressed in *Xenopus laevis* oocytes.[47] However, expression of SLC26A4 in the proximal tubule is minimal or absent in several species, and murine Slc26a4 is quite clearly not involved in formate-stimulated Na$^+$-Cl$^-$ transport in this nephron segment.[48] There is however robust expression of SLC26A4 in distal type B intercalated cells[49]; the role of this exchanger in Cl$^-$ transport by the distal nephron is reviewed elsewhere in this chapter (see Na$^+$-Cl$^-$ transport in the CNT and CCD; Cl$^-$ transport). Regardless, this data for

SLC26A4 led to the identification and characterization of SLC26A6, a widely expressed member of the SLC26 family that is expressed at the apical membrane of proximal tubular cells. Murine Slc26a6, when expressed in *Xenopus* oocytes, mediates the multiple modes of anion exchange that have been implicated in transepithelial Na$^+$-Cl$^-$ by the proximal tubule, including Cl$^-$-formate exchange, Cl$^-$-OH$^-$ exchange, Cl$^-$-SO$_4$$^{2-}$, and SO$_4$$^{2-}$-oxalate exchange.[50] However, tubule perfusion experiments in mice deficient in Slc26a6 do not reveal a reduction in baseline Cl$^-$ or fluid transport, indicative of considerable heterogeneity in apical Cl$^-$ transport by the proximal tubule.[51] Candidates for the residual Cl$^-$ transport in Slc26a6-deficient mice include Slc26a7, which is expressed at the apical membrane of proximal tubule[52]; however, this member of the SLC26 family appears to function as a Cl$^-$ channel rather than as an exchanger.[53] It does however appear that Slc26a6 is the dominant Cl$^-$-oxalate exchanger of the proximal brush border. The usual increase in tubular fluid transport induced by oxalate is thus abolished in Slc26a6-knockout mice,[51] with an attendant loss of Cl$^-$-oxalate exchange in brush border membrane vesicles.[54]

Somewhat surprisingly, Slc26a6 mediates electrogenic Cl$^-$-OH$^-$ and Cl$^-$-HCO$_3$$^-$ exchange,[50] and most if not all the members of this family are electrogenic in at least one mode of anion transport.[55] This begs the question of how the electroneutrality of transcellular Na$^+$-Cl$^-$ transport is preserved. Notably, however, the stoichiometry and electrophysiology of Cl$^-$-base exchange differ for individual members of the family; for example, Slc26a6 exchanges one Cl$^-$ for two HCO$_3$$^-$ anions, whereas SLC26A3 exchanges two Cl^- anions for one HCO_3^- anion.[55] Co-expression of two or more electrogenic SLC26 exchangers in the same membrane may thus yield a net electroneutrality of apical Cl^- exchange. Alternatively, apical K^+ channels in the proximal tubule may function to stabilize membrane potential during Na^+-Cl^- absorption.[56]

Another puzzle is why Cl^--formate exchange preferentially couples to Na^+-H^+ exchange mediated by NH3 38 (see Fig. 5–6), without evident coupling of Cl^--oxalate exchange to Na^+-H^+ exchange or Cl^--formate exchange to Na^+-SO_4^{2-} cotransport; it is evident that Slc26a6 is capable of mediating SO_4^{2-}-formate exchange,[50] which would be necessary to support coupling between Na^+-SO_4^{2-} cotransport and formate. Scaffolding proteins may serve to cluster these different transporters together in separate "micro-domains", leading to preferential coupling. Notably, whereas both Slc26a6 and NHE have been reported to bind to the scaffolding protein PDZK1, distribution of Slc26a6 is selectively impaired in PDZK1 knockout mice.[57] Petrovic and colleagues[58] have also reported a novel activation of proximal Na^+-H^+ exchange by luminal formate, suggesting a direct effect of formate *per se* on NHE3; this may in part explain the preferential coupling of Cl^--formate exchange to NHE3.

Basolateral Mechanisms

As in other absorptive epithelia, basolateral Na^+/K^+-ATPase activity establishes the Na^+ gradient for transcellular Na^+-Cl^- transport by the proximal tubule and provides a major exit pathway for Na^+. To preserve the electroneutrality of transcellular Na^+-Cl^- transport[16] this exit of Na^+ across the basolateral membrane must be balanced by an equal exit of Cl^-. Several exit pathways for Cl^- have been identified in proximal tubular cells, including K^+-Cl^- cotransport, Cl^- channels, and various modalities of Cl^--HCO_3^- exchange (see Fig. 5–6).

Several lines of evidence support the existence of a swelling-activated basolateral K^+-Cl^- cotransporter (KCC) in the proximal tubule.[59] The KCC proteins are encoded by four members of the cation-chloride cotransporter gene family; KCC1, KCC3, and KCC4 are all expressed in kidney. In particular, there is very heavy co-expression of KCC3 and KCC4 at the basolateral membrane of the proximal tubule, from S1 to S3.[60] At the functional level, basolateral membrane vesicles from renal cortex reportedly contain K^+-Cl^- cotransport activity.[59] The use of ion-sensitive microelectrodes, combined with luminal charge injection and manipulation of bath K^+ and Cl^-, suggest the presence of an electroneutral K^+-Cl^- cotransporter at the basolateral membrane proximal straight tubules. Increases or decreases in basolateral K^+ increase or decrease intracellular Cl^- activity, respectively, with reciprocal effects of basolateral Cl^- on K^+ activity; these data are consistent with coupled K^+-Cl^- transport.[61,62] Notably, a 1 mM concentration of furosemide, sufficient to inhibit all four of the KCCs, does not inhibit this K^+-Cl^- cotransport under baseline conditions.[61] However, only 10% of baseline K^+ efflux in the proximal tubule is mediated by furosemide-sensitive K^+-Cl^- cotransport, which is likely quiescent in the absence of cell swelling. Thus the activation of apical Na^+-glucose transport in proximal tubular cells strongly activates a barium-resistant (Ba^{2+}) K^+ efflux pathway that is 75% inhibited by 1 mM furosemide.[63] In addition, volume regulatory decrease (VRD) in Ba^{2+}-blocked proximal tubules swollen by hypotonic conditions is blocked by 1 mM furosemide.[59] Cell swelling in response to apical Na^+ absorption[64] is postulated to activate a volume-sensitive basolateral K^+-Cl^- cotransporter, which participates in transepithelial absorption of Na^+-Cl^-. Notably, targeted deletion of KCC3 and KCC4 in the respective knockout mice reduces VRD in the proximal tubule.[65] Furthermore, perfused proximal tubules from KCC3-deficient mice have a considerable reduction in transepithelial fluid transport,[66]

suggesting an important role for basolateral K^+-Cl^- cotransport in transcellular Na^+-Cl^- reabsorption.

The basolateral chloride conductance of mammalian proximal tubular cells is relatively low, suggesting a lesser role for Cl^- channels in transepithelial Na^+-Cl^- transport. Basolateral anion substitutions have minimal effect on the membrane potential, despite considerable effects on intracellular Cl^- activity,[67] nor for that matter do changes in basolateral membrane potential affect intracellular Cl^-.[61,62] However, as with basolateral K^+-Cl^- cotransport, basolateral Cl^- channels in the proximal tubule may be relatively inactive in the absence of cell swelling. Cell swelling thus activates both K^+ and Cl^- channels at the basolateral membranes of proximal tubular cells.[68–70] Seki and colleagues[71] have reported the presence of a basolateral Cl^- channel within S3 segments of the rabbit nephron, wherein they did not seen affect of the KCC inhibitor H74 on intracellular Cl^- activity. The molecular identity of these and other basolateral Cl^- channels in the proximal nephron is not known with certainty, although S3 segments have been shown to exclusively express mRNA for the swelling-activated CLC-2 Cl^- channel[72]; the role of this channel in transcellular Na^+-Cl^- reabsorption is not known.

Finally, there is functional evidence for both Na^+-dependent and Na^+-independent Cl^--HCO_3^- exchange at the basolateral membrane of proximal tubular cells.[10,67,73] The impact of Na^+-independent Cl^--HCO_3^- exchange on basolateral exit is thought to be minimal.[67] For one, this exchanger is expected to mediate Cl^- *entry* under physiological conditions.[73] Second, there is only a modest difference between the rate of decrease in intracellular Cl^- activity between the combined removal of Na^+ and Cl^- versus Cl^- and HCO_3^- removal, suggesting that pure Cl^--HCO_3^- exchange does not contribute significantly to Cl^- exit. In contrast, there is a 75% decrease rate of decrease in intracellular Cl^- activity after the removal of basolateral Na^+.[67] The Na^+-dependent Cl^--HCO_3^- exchanger may thus play a considerable role in basolateral Cl^- exit, with recycled exit of Na^+ and HCO_3^- via the basolateral Na^+-HCO_3^- cotransporter NBC1 (see Fig. 5–6). Molecular candidates for this Na^+-dependent Cl^--HCO_3^- exchanger have emerged from the human, squid, and *Drosophila* genomes[74]; however, immunolocalization in mammalian proximal tubule has not as yet been reported.

Regulation of Proximal Tubular Na⁺-Cl⁻ Transport

Glomerulotubular Balance

A fundamental property of the kidney is the phenomenon of glomerulotubular balance, wherein changes in glomerular filtration rate (GFR) are balanced by equivalent changes in tubular reabsorption, thus maintaining a constant *fractional* reabsorption of fluid and Na^+-Cl^- (Fig. 5–7). Although the distal nephron is capable of adjusting reabsorption in response to changes in tubular flow,[75] the impact of GFR on Na^+-Cl^- reabsorption by the proximal tubule is particularly pronounced (Fig. 5–8). Glomerulotubular balance is independent of direct neurohumoral control, and thought to be mediated by the additive effects of luminal and peri-tubular factors.[76]

At the luminal side, changes in GFR increase the filtered load of HCO_3^-, glucose, and other solutes, increasing their reabsorption by the load-responsive proximal tubule[6] and thus preserving a constant fractional reabsorption. Changes in tubular flow rate have additional stimulatory effects on luminal transport, in both the proximal and distal nephron.[75] In the proximal tubule, increases in tubular perfusion clearly increase the rate of both Na^+ and HCO_3^- absorption, due to increases in luminal Na^+-H^+ exchange.[75] Increases in GFR during volume expansion are also accompanied by a modest increase in the capacity of Na^+-H^+ exchange, as measured in brush-border membrane vesicles, with the opposite effect in volume contraction.[75]

Notably, influential experiments from almost four decades ago, performed in rabbit proximal tubules, failed to demonstrate a significant effect of tubular flow on fluid absorption.[77] This issue has been revisited by Du and co-workers, who

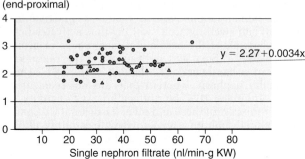

TF/p Inulin (end-proximal)

$y = 2.27 + 0.0034x$

Single nephron filtrate (nl/min-g KW)

FIGURE 5-7 Glomerulotubular balance; fractional water absorption by the proximal tubule does not change as a function of single nephron GFR. (From Schnermann J, Wahl M, Liebau G, Fischbach H: Balance between tubular flow rate and net fluid reabsorption in the proximal convolution of the rat kidney. I. Dependency of reabsorptive net fluid flux upon proximal tubular surface area at spontaneous variations of filtration rate. Pflugers Arch 304:90–103, 1968.)

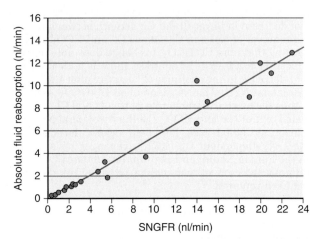

Absolute fluid reabsorption (nl/min)

SNGFR (nl/min)

FIGURE 5-8 Glomerulotubular balance; linear increase in absolute fluid reabsorption by the late proximal tubule as a functional of single nephron GFR (SNGFR). (From Spitzer A, Brandis M: Functional and morphologic maturation of the superficial nephrons. Relationship to total kidney function. J Clin Invest 53:279–287, 1974.)

recently reported a considerable flow-dependence of fluid and HCO_3^- transport in perfused murine proximal tubules[76,78] (Fig. 5–9). These data were analyzed using a mathematical model that estimated microvillus torque as a function of tubular flow[78]; accounting for increases in tubular diameter, which reduce torque, there is a linear relationship between calculated torque and both fluid and HCO_3^- absorption.[76,78] Consistent with an effect of torque rather than flow *per se,* increasing viscosity of the perfusate by the addition of dextran increases the effect on fluid transport; the extra viscosity increases the hydrodynamic effect of flow and thus increases torque. The mathematical analysis of Du and assoicates provide an excellent explanation of the discrepancy between their results and those of Burg and co-workers.[77] Whereas Burg and colleagues performed their experiments in rabbit,[77] the more recent report utilized mice[76,78]; other studies that had found an effect of flow utilized perfusion of rat proximal tubules, presumably more similar to mouse than rabbit.[75] Increased flow has a considerably greater effect on tubular diameter in rabbit proximal tubule, thus reducing the increase in torque. Mathematical analysis of the rabbit data[77] thus predicts a 43% increase in torque, due to a 41% increase in tubule diameter at a threefold increase in flow; this corresponds to the statistically insignificant 36% increase in volume reabsorption reported by Burg and colleagues (Table 2 in Ref 77).

Pharmacological inhibition reveals that tubular flow activates proximal HCO_3^- reabsorption mediated by both NHE3 and apical H^+-ATPase.[76] The flow-dependent increase in proximal fluid and HCO_3^- reabsorption is also attenuated in NHE3-deficient knockout mice.[76,78] Inhibition of the actin cytoskeleton with cytochalasin-D reduces the effect of flow on fluid and HCO_3^- transport, suggesting that flow-dependent movement of microvilli serves to activate NHE3 and H^+-ATPase via their linkage to the cytoskeleton (see Fig. 5–13 for NHE3).

Peritubular factors also play an important, additive role in glomerulotubular balance. Specifically, increases in GFR result in an increase in filtration fraction and an attendant increase in postglomerular protein and peritubular oncotic pressure. It has long been appreciated that changes in peritubular protein concentration have important effects on proximal tubular Na^+-Cl^- reabsorption[79]; these effects are also seen in combined capillary and tubular perfusion experiments (reviewed in Ref 76). Peritubular protein also has an effect in isolated perfused proximal tubule segments, where the effect of hydrostatic pressure is abolished.[76] Increases in peritubular protein concentration have an additive effect on flow-dependent activation of proximal fluid and HCO_3^- absorption (see Fig. 5–9). The effect of peritubular protein on HCO_3^- absorption, which is a predominantly transcellular phenom-

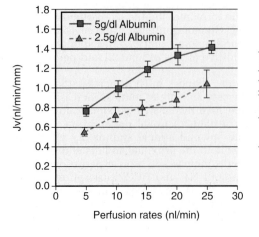

Jv (nl/min/mm)

Perfusion rates (nl/min)

— ■ — 5g/dl Albumin
‑ ▲ ‑ 2.5g/dl Albumin

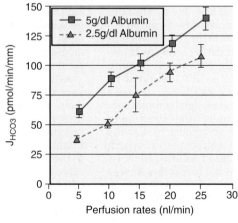

J_{HCO3} (pmol/min/mm)

Perfusion rates (nl/min)

— ■ — 5g/dl Albumin
‑ ▲ ‑ 2.5g/dl Albumin

FIGURE 5-9 Glomerulotubular balance; flow dependent increases in fluid (J_v) and HCO_3^- (J_{HCO3}) absorption by perfused mouse proximal tubules. Absorption increases when bath albumin concentration increases from 2.5 g/dl to 5 g/dl. (From Du Z, Yan Q, Duan Y, et al: Axial flow modulates proximal tubule NHE3 and H-ATPase activities by changing microvillus bending moments. Am J Physiol Renal Physiol 290:F289–96, 2006.)

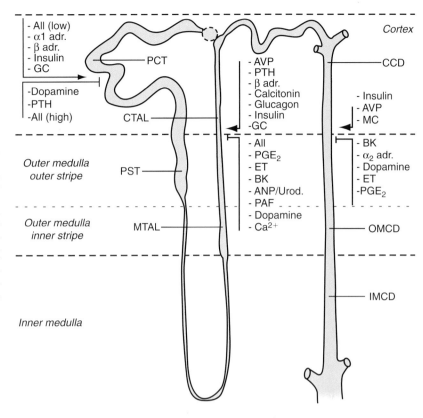

FIGURE 5–10 Neurohumoral influences on Na⁺-Cl⁻ absorption by the proximal tubule, thick ascending limb, and collecting duct. Factors that stimulate (→) and inhibit (⊢) sodium reabsorption are as follows: ANGII, angiotensin II (low and high referring to pico- and micromolar concentrations); adr, adrenergic agonists; AVP, arginine vasopressin; PTH, parathyroid hormone; GC, glucocorticoids; MC, mineralocorticoids; PGE₂, prostaglandin E₂; ET, endothelin; ANP/Urod, atrial natriuretic peptide and urodilatin; PAF, platelet-activating factor; BK, bradykinin. PCT, proximal convoluted tubule; PST, proximal straight tubule; MTAL, medullary thick ascending limb of loop of Henle; CTAL, cortical thick ascending limb; CCD, cortical collecting duct; OMCD, outer medullary collecting duct; IMCD, inner medullary collecting duct. (Redrawn from Feraille E, Doucet A: Sodium-potassium-adenosinetriphosphatase-dependent sodium transport in the kidney: hormonal control. Physiol Rev 81:345–418, 2001.)

enon,[17] suggests that changes in peritubular oncotic pressure do not affect transport via the paracellular pathway. However, the mechanism of the stimulatory effect of peritubular protein on transcellular transport is still not completely clear.[76]

Neurohumoral Influences

Fluid and Na⁺-Cl⁻ reabsorption by the proximal tubule is affected by a number of hormones and neurotransmitters. The major hormonal influences on renal Na⁺-Cl⁻ transport are shown in Figure 5–10. Renal sympathetic tone exerts a particularly important stimulatory influence, as does angiotensin II (AII); dopamine is a major inhibitor of proximal tubular Na⁺-Cl⁻ reabsorption.

Unilateral denervation of the rat kidney causes a marked natriuresis and a 40% reduction in proximal Na⁺-Cl⁻ reabsorption, without effects on single nephron GFR or on the contralateral innervated kidney.[80] In contrast, low-frequency electrical stimulation of renal sympathetic nerves reduces proximal tubular fluid absorption, with a 32% drop in natriuresis and no change in GFR.[81] Basolateral epinephrine and/or nor-epinephrine stimulate proximal Na⁺-Cl⁻ reabsorption via both α- and β-adrenergic receptors. Several lines of evidence suggest that α_1-adrenergic receptors exert a stimulatory effect on proximal Na⁺-Cl⁻ transport, via activation of basolateral Na⁺/K⁺-ATPase and apical Na⁺-H⁺ exchange; the role of α_2-adrenergic receptors is more controversial.[82] Ligand-dependent recruitment of the scaffolding protein NHERF-1 by β_2-adrenergic receptors resorts in direct activation of apical NHE3,[83] bypassing the otherwise negative effect of downstream cyclic AMP (cAMP—see later).

Angiotensin II (ANGII) has potent, complex effects on proximal Na⁺-Cl⁻ reabsorption. Several issues unique to ANGII deserve emphasis. First, it has been appreciated for three decades that this hormone has a biphasic effect on the proximal tubule[84]; stimulation of Na⁺-Cl⁻ reabsorption occurs at low doses (10^{-12} to 10^{-10} M), whereas concentrations greater than 10^{-7} M are inhibitory (Fig. 5–11). Further complexity arises from the presence of AT1 receptors for ANGII at both

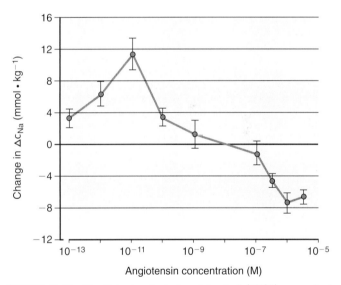

FIGURE 5–11 The biphasic effect of angiotensin II (ANGII) on proximal tubular Na⁺-Cl⁻ absorption. The steady-state Na⁺ concentration gradient (Δc_{Na}) is plotted as a function of peritubular ANGII concentration; low concentrations activate Na⁺-Cl⁻ absorption by the proximal tubule, whereas higher concentrations inhibit. (From Harris PJ, Navar LG: Tubular transport responses to angiotensin. Am J Physiol 248:F621–630, 1985.)

luminal and basolateral membranes in the proximal tubule.[85] ANGII application to either the luminal or peritubular side of perfused tubules has a similar biphasic effect on fluid transport, albeit with more potent effects at the luminal side.[86] Experiments using both receptor antagonists and knockout mice have indicated that the stimulatory and inhibitory effects of ANGII are both mediated via AT1 receptors, due to signaling at both the luminal and basolateral membrane.[87] Finally, ANGII is also synthesized and secreted by the proximal tubule, exerting a potent autocrine effect on proximal tubular Na$^+$-Cl$^-$ reabsorption.[88] Proximal tubular cells thus express mRNA for angiotensinogen, renin, and angiotensin-converting enzyme,[82] allowing for autocrine generation of ANGII. Indeed, luminal concentrations of ANGII can be 100–1000-fold higher than circulating levels of the hormone.[82] Proximal tubular and systemic synthesis of ANGII may be subject to different control. In particular, Thomson and co-workers have recently demonstrated that proximal tubular ANGII is increased considerably after high-salt diet, with a preserved inhibitory effect of losartan on proximal fluid reabsorption.[89] These authors have argued that the increase in proximal tubular ANGII after a high-salt diet contributes to a more stable distal salt delivery.[89]

The proximal tubule is also a target for natriuretic hormones; in particular, dopamine synthesized in the proximal tubule has negative autocrine effects on proximal Na$^+$-Cl$^-$ reabsorption.[82] Proximal tubular cells have the requisite enzymatic machinery for the synthesis of dopamine, using L-dopa reabsorbed from the glomerular ultrafiltrate. Dopamine synthesis by proximal tubular cells and release into the tubular lumen is increased after volume expansion or high-salt diet, resulting in a considerable natriuresis.[90,91] Luminal dopamine antagonizes the stimulatory effect of epinephrine on volume absorption in perfused proximal convoluted tubules,[92] consistent with an autocrine effect of dopamine released into the tubular lumen.[90] Dopamine primarily exerts its natriuretic effect via D$_1$-like dopamine receptors (D1 and D5 in human); as is the case for the AT1 receptors for ANGII,[85] D1 receptors are expressed at both the apical and luminal membranes of proximal tubule.[93] Targeted deletion of the D1A[94] and D5 receptors[95] in mice leads to hypertension, by mechanisms that include reduced proximal tubular natriuresis.[94]

The natriuretic effect of dopamine in the proximal tubule is modulated by atrial natriuretic peptide (ANP), which inhibits apical Na$^+$-H$^+$ exchange via a dopamine-dependent mechanism.[96] ANP appears to induce recruitment of the D1 dopamine receptor to the plasma membrane of proximal tubular cells, thus sensitizing the tubule to the effect of dopamine.[97] The inhibitory effect of ANP on basolateral Na$^+$/K$^+$-ATPase occurs via a D1-dependent mechanism, with a synergistic inhibition of Na$^+$/K$^+$-ATPase by the two hormones.[97] Furthermore, dopamine and D1 receptors appear to play critical permissive roles in the *in vivo* natriuretic effect of ANP.[98,99]

Finally, there is considerable crosstalk between the major anti-natriuretic and natriuretic influences on the proximal tubule. For example, ANP inhibits ANGII dependent stimulation of proximal tubular fluid absorption,[100] presumably via the dopamine-dependent mechanisms discussed earlier.[96] Dopamine also decreases the expression of AT1 receptors for ANGII in cultured proximal tubular cells.[101] Furthermore, the provision of L-dopa in the drinking water of rats decreases AT1 receptor expression in the proximal tubule, suggesting that dopamine synthesis in the proximal tubule "resets" the sensitivity to ANGII.[101] ANGII signaling through AT1 receptors decreases expression of the D5 dopamine receptor, whereas renal cortical expression of AT1 receptors is in turn increased in knockout mice deficient in the D5 receptor.[102] Similar interactions have been found between proximal tubular AT1 receptors and the D$_2$-like D3 receptor.[103]

Regulation of Proximal Tubule Transporters

The apical Na$^+$-H$^+$ exchanger NHE3 and the basolateral Na$^+$/K$^+$-ATPase are primary targets for signaling pathways elicited by the various anti-natriuretic and natriuretic stimuli discussed earlier; NHE3 mediates the rate-limiting step in transepithelial Na$^+$-Cl$^-$ absorption,[78] and as such is perhaps the dominant target for regulatory pathways. NHE3 is regulated by the combined effects of direct phosphorylation and interaction with scaffolding proteins, which primarily regulate transport via changes in trafficking of the exchanger protein to and from the brush border membrane (see Fig. 5–2).[34,104,105] Increases in cyclic AMP (cAMP) have a profound inhibitory effect on apical Na$^+$-H$^+$ exchange in the proximal tubule. Intracellular cAMP is increased in response to dopamine signaling via D$_1$-like receptors and/or PTH-dependent signaling via the PTH receptor, whereas ANGII-dependent activation of NHE3 is associated with a reduction in cAMP.[106] PTH is a potent inhibitor of NHE3, presumably so as to promote distal delivery of Na$^+$-HCO$_3^-$ and an attendant stimulation of distal calcium reabsorption.[105] The activation of protein kinase A (PKA) by increased cAMP results in direct phosphorylation of NHE3; although several sites in NHE3 are phosphorylated by PKA, the phosphorylation of serine 552 (S552) and 605 (S605) been specifically implicated in the inhibitory effect of cAMP on Na$^+$-H$^+$ exchange.[107] "Phospho-specific" antibodies that specifically recognize the phosphorylated forms of S552 and S605 were recently utilized to demonstrate dopamine-dependent increases in the phosphorylation of both these serines.[108] Moreover, immunostaining of rat kidney revealed that S552-phosphorylated NHE3 localizes at the coated pit region of the coated pit region of the brush border membrane,[108] where the oligomerized inactive form of NHE3 predominates.[109] The cAMP-stimulated phosphorylation of NHE3 by PKA thus results in a redistribution of the transporter from the microvillar membrane to an inactive, sub-microvillar population (Fig. 5–12).

The regulation of NHE3 by cAMP also requires the participation of homologous scaffolding proteins that contain protein-protein interaction motifs known as PDZ domains (named for the **P**SD95, **D**iscs large (Drosophila), and **Z**O-1 proteins in which these domains were first discovered) (Fig. 5–13). The first of these proteins, NHE Regulatory Factor-1 (NHERF-1), was purified as a cellular factor required for the inhibition of NHE3 by PKA.[104] NHERF-2 was in turn cloned by yeast two-hybrid screens as a protein that interacts with the C-terminus of NHE3; NHERF-1 and NHERF-2 have very similar effects on the regulation of NHE3 in cultured cells. The related protein PDZK1 interacts with NHE3 and a number of other epithelial transporters, and is required for expression of the anion exchanger Slc26a6 at brush border membranes of the proximal tubule.[57]

NHERF-1 and NHERF-2 are both expressed in human and mouse proximal tubule cells; NHERF-1 colocalizes with NHE3 in microvilli of the brush border, whereas NHERF-2 is predominantly expressed at the base of microvilli in the vesicle-rich domain.[104] The NHERFs assemble a multi-protein signaling complex in association with NHE3 and other epithelial transporters and channels. In addition to NHE3 they bind to the actin-associated protein ezrin, thus linking NHE3 to the cytoskeleton[104]; this linkage to the cytoskeleton may be particularly important for the mechanical activation of NHE3 by microvillar bending, as has been implicated in glomerulo-tubular balance (see earlier).[76,78] Ezrin also functions as an anchoring protein for PKA, bringing PKA into close proximity with NHE3 and facilitating its phosphorylation (see Fig. 5–13).[104] Analysis of knockout mice for NHERF-1 has revealed that it is not required for baseline activity of NHE3; as expected, however, it is required for cAMP-dependent regulation of the exchanger by PTH.[104] One longstanding paradox has been that β-adrenergic receptors, which increase cAMP in the proximal tubule, cause an activation of apical Na$^+$-H$^+$ exchange.[82] This has been resolved by the observation that the first PDZ domain of NHERF-1 interacts with the β$_2$-adrenergic receptor in an agonist-dependent fashion; this interaction serves to disrupt the interaction between the second PDZ domain and NHE3, resulting in a stimulation of the exchanger despite the catecholamine-dependent increase in cAMP.[104]

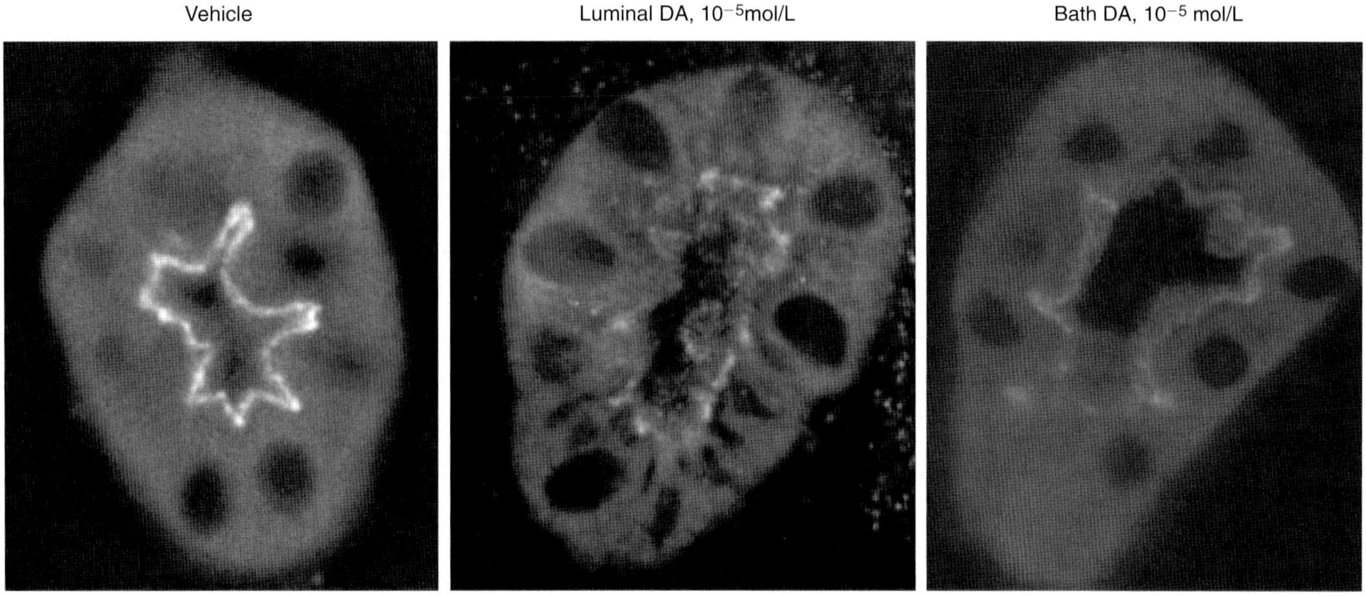

Transport of Inorganic Solutes: Sodium, Chloride, Potassium, Magnesium, Calcium, and Phosphate

FIGURE 5–12 The effect of dopamine on trafficking of the Na^+-H^+ exchanger NHE3 in the proximal tubule. Microdissected proximal convoluted tubules were perfused for 30 minutes with 10^{-5} mol/L dopamine (DA) in the lumen or the bath, as noted, inducing a retraction of immunoreactive NHE3 protein from the apical membrane. (From Bacic D, Kaissling B, McLeroy P, et al: Dopamine acutely decreases apical membrane Na/H exchanger NHE3 protein in mouse renal proximal tubule. Kidney Int 64:2133–2141, 2003.)

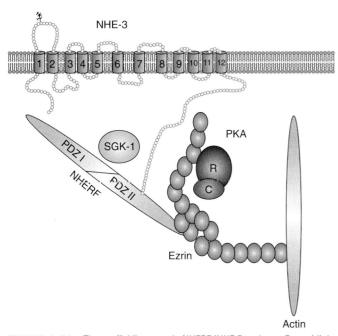

FIGURE 5–13 The scaffolding protein NHERF (NHE Regulatory Factor) links the Na^+-H^+ exchanger NHE3 to the cytoskeleton and signaling proteins. NHERF binds to ezrin, which in turn links to protein kinase A (PKA) and the actin cytoskeleton. NHERF also binds to the SGK-1 protein kinase, which activates NHE-3. PDZ, **P**SD95, **D**iscs large (Drosophila), and **Z**O-1 domain; SGK-1, serum and glucocorticoid-induced kinase-1. (Redrawn from Weinman EJ, Cunningham R, Shenolikar S: NHERF and regulation of the renal sodium-hydrogen exchanger NHE3. Pflugers Arch 450:137–144, 2005.)

As discussed earlier, at concentrations greater than 10^{-7} M (see Fig. 5–11) ANGII has an inhibitory effect on proximal tubular Na^+-Cl^- absorption.[84] This inhibition is dependent on the activation of brush border phospholipase A_2, which results in the liberation of arachidonic acid.[86] Metabolism of arachidonic acid by cytochrome P450 mono-oxygenases in turn generates 20-hydroxyeicosatetraenoic acid (20-HETE)

and epoxyeicosatrioenoic acids (EETs), compounds that inhibit NHE3 and the basolateral Na^+/K^+-ATPase.[82,110] EETs and 20-HETE have also been implicated in the reduction in proximal Na^+-Cl^- absorption that occurs during pressure natriuresis, inhibiting Na^+/K^+-ATPase and retracting NHE3 from the brush border membrane.[111]

Anti-natriuretic stimuli such as ANGII acutely increase expression of NHE3 at the apical membrane, at least in part by inhibiting the generation of cAMP.[106] "Low-dose" ANGII (10^{-10} M) also increases exocytic insertion of NHE3 into the plasma membrane, via a mechanism that is dependent on phosphatidylinositol 3-kinase (PI 3-kinase).[112] Treatment of rats with captopril thus results in a retraction of NHE3 and associated proteins from the brush border of proximal tubule cells.[113] Glucocorticoids also increase NHE3 activity, due to both transcriptional induction of the NHE3 gene and an acute stimulation of exocytosis of the exchanger to the plasma membrane.[114] Glucorticoid-dependent exocytosis of NHE3 appears to require NHERF-2, which acts in this context as a scaffolding protein for the glucocorticoid-induced serine-threonine kinase SGK1 (see also Regulation of Na^+-Cl^- transport in the CNT and CCD; aldosterone).[115] The acute effect of dexamethasone has thus been shown to require direct phosphorylation of serine 663 in the NHE3 protein by SGK1.[116]

Finally, many of the natriuretic and anti-natriuretic pathways that influence NHE3 have parallel effects on the basolateral Na^+/K^+-ATPase (see Ref 82 for a detailed review). The molecular mechanisms underlying inhibition of Na^+/K^+-ATPase by dopamine have been particularly well characterized. Inhibition by dopamine is associated with removal of active Na^+/K^+-ATPase units from the basolateral membrane,[117] analogous somewhat to the effect on NHE3 expression at the apical membrane. This inhibitory effect is primarily mediated by protein kinase C (PKC), which directly phosphorylates the α_1 subunit of Na^+/K^+-ATPase, the predominant α subunit in the kidney.[82] The effect of dopamine requires phosphorylation of serine 18 of the α_1 subunit by PKC; this phosphorylation event does not affect enzymatic activity of the Na^+/K^+-ATPase, but rather induces a conformational change that enhances the binding of PI 3-kinase to an adjacent proline-rich domain. The PI-3 kinase recruited by this phosphorylated α_1 subunit then stimulates the dyamin-dependent endocytosis of the Na$^+$/K$^+$-ATPase complex via clathrin-coated pits.[117]

Loop of Henle and Thick Ascending Limb

The loop of Henle encompasses the thin descending limb, the thin ascending limb, and the thick ascending limb (TAL). The descending and ascending thin limbs function in passive absorption of water [118] and Na$^+$-Cl$^-$,[119–121] respectively, whereas the TAL reabsorbs ~30% of filtered Na$^+$-Cl$^-$ via active transport. There is considerable cellular and functional heterogeneity along the entire length of the loop of Henle, with consequences for the transport of water, Na$^+$-Cl$^-$, and other solutes. The thin descending limb begins in the outer medulla after an abrupt transition from S3 segments of the proximal tubule, marking the boundary between the outer and inner stripes of the outer medulla. Thin descending limbs end at a hairpin turn at the end of the loop of Henle. Short-looped nephrons that originate from superficial and midcortical nephrons have a short descending limb within the inner stripe of the outer medulla; close to the hairpin turn of the loop these tubules merge abruptly into the TAL (see also later). Long-looped nephrons originating from juxtamedullary glomeruli have a long ascending thin limb that then merges with the TAL. The TALs of long-looped nephrons begin at the boundary between the inner and outer medulla, whereas the TALs of short-looped nephrons may be entirely cortical. The ratio of medullary to cortical TAL for a given nephron is a function of the depth of its origin, such that superficial nephrons are primarily composed of cortical TALs whereas juxtamedullary nephrons primarily possess medullary TALs.

Transport Characteristics of the Descending Thin Limb

It has long been appreciated that the osmolality of tubular fluid increases progressively between the corticomedullary junction and the papillary tip, due to either active secretion of solutes or passive absorption of water along the descending thin limb.[122] Subsequent reports revealed a very high water permeability of perfused outer medullary thin descending limbs, in the absence of significant permeability to Na$^+$-Cl$^-$.[123] Notably, however, the permeability properties of descending thin limbs vary as a function of depth in the inner medulla and inclusion in short-versus long-looped nephrons.[124,125] Descending thin limbs from short-looped nephrons contain "type I" cells—very flat, endothelial-like cells with intermediate-depth tight junctions suggesting a relative tight epithelium (reviewed in 124, 125). The epithelium of descending limbs from long-looped nephrons is initially more complex, with taller type II cells possessing more elaborate apical microvilli and more prominent mitochondria. In the lower medullary portion of long-looped nephrons these cells change into a type III morphology, endothelial-like cells similar to the type I cells from short-looped nephrons.[124] The permeability properties appear to change as a function of cell type, with a progressive axial drop in water permeability of long-looped descending limbs; the water permeability of descending thin limbs in the middle part of the inner medulla is thus ~42% that of outer medullary thin descending limbs.[126] Furthermore, the distal 20% of descending thin limbs have a very low water permeability.[126] These changes in water permeability along the descending thin limb are accompanied by a progressive increase in Na$^+$-Cl$^-$ permeability, although the ionic permeability remains considerably less than that of the ascending thin limb.[125]

Consistent with a primary role in passive water and solute absorption, Na$^+$/K$^+$-ATPase activity in the descending thin limb is almost undetectable,[14] suggesting that these cells do not actively transport Na$^+$-Cl$^-$; those ion transport pathways that have been identified in descending thin limb cells are thought to primarily contribute to cellular volume regulation.[127] In contrast to the relative lack of Na$^+$-Cl$^-$ transport, transcellular water reabsorption by the thin descending limb is a critical component of the renal countercurrent concentrating mechanism.[118,123] Consistent with this role, epithelial cells of the descending thin limbs express very high levels of the Aquaporin-1 water channel, at both apical and basolateral membranes.[128] The expression is highest in type II cells of descending thin limbs in the outer medulla,[128] which have the highest Aquaporin-1 content of all the tubule segments along the nephron.[129] Aquaporin-1 is also expressed in type I cells of short-looped nephrons[128]; notably, however, Aquaporin-1-expressing cells in descending limbs from short-looped nephrons extend into segments that do not express Aquaporin-1, just prior to the juncture with thick ascending limbs.[128] In addition, the terminal sections of deep descending limbs of long-looped nephrons, which do not exhibit appreciable water permeability,[126] do not express Aquaporin-1.[130] The analysis of knockout mice with targeted deletion of Aquaporin-1 has dramatically proven the primary role of water absorption, as opposed to solute secretion, in the progressive increase in osmolality along the descending thin limb.[122] Homozygous Aquaporin-1 knockout mice thus have a marked reduction in water permeability of perfused descending thin limbs, resulting in a vasopressin-resistant concentrating defect.[118]

Na$^+$-Cl$^-$ Transport by the Thin Ascending Limb

Fluid entering the thin ascending limb has a very high concentration of Na$^+$-Cl$^-$, due to osmotic equilibration by the water-permeable descending limbs. The passive reabsorption of this delivered Na$^+$-Cl$^-$ by the thin ascending limb is a critical component of the passive equilibration model of the renal countercurrent multiplication system.[119,120] Consistent with this role, the permeability properties of the thin ascending limb are dramatically different from those of the descending thin limb, with a much higher permeability to Na$^+$-Cl$^-$[125] and vanishingly-low water permeability.[131] Passive Na$^+$-Cl$^-$ reabsorption by thin ascending limbs occurs via a combination of paracellular Na$^+$ transport[121,132,133] and transcellular Cl$^-$ transport.[134–136] The inhibition of paracellular conductance by protamine thus selectively inhibits Na$^+$ transport across perfused thin ascending limbs, consistent with paracellular transport of Na$^+$.[132] As in the descending limb, thin ascending limbs have a modest Na$^+$/K$^+$-ATPase activity (see Fig. 5–4); however, the active transport of Na$^+$ across thin ascending limbs for only an estimated 2% of Na$^+$ reabsorption by this nephron segment.[137] Anion transport inhibitors[134] and chloride channel blockers[135] reduce Cl$^-$ permeability of the thin ascending limb, consistent with passive transcellular Cl$^-$ transport. Direct measurement of the membrane potential of impaled hamster thin ascending limbs has also yielded evidence for apical and basolateral Cl$^-$ channel activity.[136] This transepithelial transport of Cl$^-$, but not Na$^+$, is activated by vasopressin, with a pharmacology that is consistent with direct activation of thin ascending limb Cl$^-$ channels.[138]

Both apical and basolateral Cl$^-$ transport in the thin ascending limb appears to be mediated by the CLC-K1 Cl$^-$ channel, in co-operation with the Barttin subunit (see also Na$^+$-Cl$^-$ transport in the thick ascending limb; basolateral mechanisms). Immunofluorescence[139] and in situ hybridization[140] indicate a selective expression of CLC-K1 in thin ascending limbs, although single-tubule RT-PCR studies have suggested additional expression in the thick ascending limb, distal convoluted tubule, and cortical collecting duct.[141] Notably, immunofluorescence and immunogold labeling indicate that

CLC-K1 is expressed exclusively at both the apical and basolateral membrane of thin ascending limbs,[139] such that both the luminal and basolateral Cl⁻ channels of this nephron segment[136] are encoded by the same gene. Homozygous knockout mice with a targeted deletion of CLC-K1 have a vasopressin-resistant nephrogenic diabetes insipidus,[142] reminiscent of the phenotype of Aquaporin-1 knockout mice.[118] Given that CLC-K1 is potentially expressed in the thick ascending limb (TAL),[141] dysfunction of this nephron segment might also contribute to the renal phenotype of CLC-K1 knockout mice; however, the closely homologous channel CLC-K2 (CLC-NKB) is clearly expressed in TAL,[141] where it can likely substitute for CLC-K1. Furthermore, loss-of-function mutations in CLC-NKB are an important cause of Bartter syndrome,[143] indicating that CLC-K2, rather than CLC-K1, is critical for transport function of the TAL.

Detailed characterization of CLC-K1 knockout mice has revealed a selective impairment in Cl⁻ transport by the thin ascending limb.[121] Whereas Cl⁻ absorption is profoundly reduced, Na⁺ absorption by thin ascending limbs is not significantly impaired (Fig. 5–14). The diffusion voltage induced by a transepithelial Na⁺-Cl⁻ gradient is reversed by the absence of CLC-K1, from +15.5 mV in homozygous wild-type controls (+/+) to −7.6 mV in homozygous knockout mice (−/−). This change in diffusion voltage is due to the dominance of paracellular Na⁺ transport in the CLC-K1 deficient −/− mice, leading to a lumen-negative potential; this corresponds to a marked reduction in the relative permeability of Cl⁻ to that of Na⁺ (P_{Cl}/P_{Na}), from 4.02 to 0.63 (see Fig. 5–14). The inhibition of paracellular transport by protamine has a comparable effect on the diffusion voltage in −/− mice versus +/− and +/+ mice that have been treated with NPPB to inhibit CLC-K1; the respective diffusion voltages are 7.9 mV (−/− plus protamine), 8.6 mV (+/− plus protamine and NPPB), and 9.8 (+/+ plus protamine and NPPB). Therefore, the paracellular Na⁺ conductance is unimpaired and essentially the same in CLC-K1 mice, when compared to littermate controls. This study thus provides elegant proof for the relative independence of para-

cellular and transcellular conductances for Na⁺ and Cl⁻, respectively, in thin ascending limbs.

Finally, CLC-K1 associates with "Barttin", a novel accessory subunit identified via positional cloning of the gene for Bartter syndrome with sensorineural deafness[144] (see also Na⁺-Cl⁻ transport in thick ascending limb: basolateral mechanisms). Barttin is expressed with CLC-K1 in thin ascending limbs, in addition to TAL, distal convoluted tubule, and α-intercalated cells.[141,144] Rat CLC-K1 is unique among the CLC-K orthologs and paralogs (CLC-K1/2 in rodent, CLC-NKB/NKA in humans) in that it can generate Cl⁻ channel activity in the absence of co-expression with Barttin[139,145]; however, its human ortholog CLC-NKA is non-functional in the absence of Barttin.[144] Regardless, Barttin co-immunoprecipitates with CLC-K1,[141] and increases expression of the channel protein at the cell membrane.[141,145] This "chaperone" function seems to involve the transmembrane core of Barttin, whereas domains within the cytoplasmic carboxy terminus modulate channel properties (open probability and unitary conductance).[145]

Thick Ascending Limb
Apical Na⁺-Cl⁻ Transport

The thick ascending limb (TAL) reabsorbs ~30% of filtered Na⁺-Cl⁻ (see Fig. 5–1). In addition to an important role in the defense of the extracellular fluid volume, Na⁺-Cl⁻ reabsorption by the water-impermeable TAL is a critical component of the renal countercurrent multiplication system. The separation of Na⁺-Cl⁻ and water in the TAL is thus responsible for the capacity of the kidney to either dilute or concentrate the urine. In collaboration with the countercurrent mechanism, Na⁺-Cl⁻ reabsorption by the thin and thick ascending limb increases medullary tonicity, facilitating water absorption by the collecting duct.

The TAL begins abruptly after the thin ascending limb of long-looped nephrons and after the Aquaporin-negative segment of short-limbed nephrons.[128] The TAL extends into the renal cortex, where it meets its parent glomerulus at the

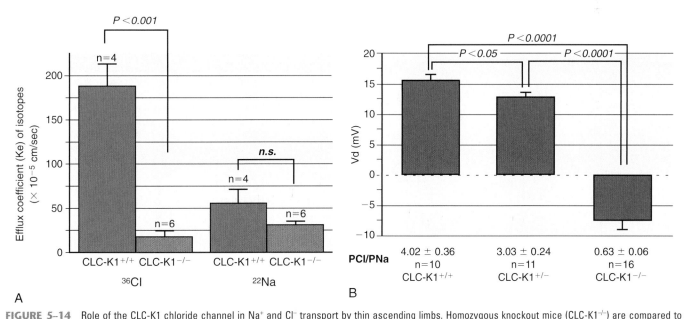

FIGURE 5–14 Role of the CLC-K1 chloride channel in Na⁺ and Cl⁻ transport by thin ascending limbs. Homozygous knockout mice (CLC-K1⁻/⁻) are compared to their littermate controls (CLC-K1⁺/⁺). **A,** Efflux coefficients for ³⁶Cl⁻ and ²²Na⁺ in the thin ascending limbs; Cl⁻ absorption is essentially abolished in the knockout mice, whereas there is no significant effect of CLC-K1 deficiency on Na⁺ transport. **B,** The diffusion voltage induced by a transepithelial Na⁺-Cl⁻ gradient is reversed by the absence of CLC-K1, from +15.5 mV in controls to −7.6 mV in homozygous knockout mice. This change in diffusion voltage is due to the dominance of paracellular Na⁺ transport in the CLC-K1 deficient −/− mice, leading to a lumen-negative potential; this corresponds to a marked reduction in the relative permeability of Cl⁻ to that of Na⁺ (P_{Cl}/P_{Na}), from 4.02 to 0.63. (From Liu W, Morimoto T, Kondo Y, et al: Analysis of NaCl transport in thin ascending limb of the loop of Henle in CLC-K1 null mice. Am J Physiol Renal Physiol 282:F451–457, 2002.)

vascular pole; the plaque of cells at this junction form the macula densa, which function as the tubular sensor for both tubuloglomerular feedback and tubular regulation of renin release by the juxtaglomerular apparatus. Cells in the medullary TAL are 7 μM to 8 μM in height, with extensive invaginations of the basolateral plasma membrane and interdigitations between adjacent cells.[3] As in the proximal tubule, these lateral cell processes contain numerous elongated mitochondria, perpendicular to the basement membrane. Cells in the cortical TAL are considerably shorter, 2 μM in height at the end of the cortical TAL in rabbit, with less mitochondria and a simpler basolateral membrane.[3] Macula densa cells also lack the lateral cell processes and interdigitations that are characteristic of medullar TAL cells.[3] However, scanning electron microscopy has revealed that the TAL of both rat[146] and hamster[147] contains two morphological subtypes, a rough-surfaced cell type (R cells) with prominent apical microvilli and a smooth-surfaced cell type (S cells) with an abundance of sub-apical vesicles.[3,148] In the hamster TAL, cells can also be separated into those with high apical and low basolateral K^+ conductance and a weak basolateral Cl^- conductance (LBC cells), versus a second population with low apical and high basolateral K^+ conductance, combined with high basolateral Cl^- conductance (HBC).[136,147] The relative frequency of the morphological and functional subtypes in the cortical and medullary TAL suggests that HBC cells correspond to S cells and LBC cells to R cells.[147]

Morphological heterogeneity notwithstanding, the cells of the medullary TAL, cortical TAL, and macula densa share the same basic transport mechanisms (Fig. 5–15). Na^+-Cl^- reabsorption by the TAL is thus a secondarily active process, driven by the favorable electrochemical gradient for Na^+ established by the basolateral Na^+/K^+-ATPase.[149,150] Na^+, K^+, and Cl^- are co-transported across by the apical membrane by an electroneutral Na^+-K^+-$2Cl^-$ cotransporter; this transporter generally requires the simultaneous presence of all three ions, such that the transport of Na^+ and Cl^- across the epithelium is mutually co-dependent and dependent on the luminal presence of K^+.[151–153] Of note, under certain circumstances apical Na^+-Cl^- transport in the TAL appears to be K^+-

independent; this issue is reviewed below (see Regulation of Na^+-Cl^- transport in the TAL). Regardless, this transporter is universally sensitive to furosemide, which has been known for more than three decades to inhibit transepithelial Cl^- transport by the TAL.[154] Apical Na^+-K^+-$2Cl^-$ cotransport is mediated by the cation-chloride cotransporter NKCC2, encoded by the SLC12A1 gene.[155] Functional expression of NKCC2 in Xenopus laevis oocytes yields Cl^-- and Na^+-dependent uptake of $^{86}Rb^+$ (a radioactive substitute for K^+) and Cl^-- and K^+-dependent uptake of $^{22}Na^+$.[155–157] As expected, NKCC2 is sensitive to micromolar concentrations of furosemide, bumetanide, and other loop diuretics.[155]

Immunofluorescence indicates expression of NKCC2 protein along the entire length of the TAL.[155] In particular, immunoelectron microscopy reveals expression in both rough (R—see earlier) and smooth (S) cells of the TAL (also see earlier).[148] NKCC2 expression in subapical vesicles is particularly prominent in smooth cells,[148] suggesting a role for vesicular trafficking in the regulation of NKCC2 (see Regulation of Na^+-Cl^- transport in the TAL). NKCC2 is also expressed in macula densa cells,[148] which have been shown to possess apical Na^+-K^+-$2Cl^-$ cotransport activity.[158] This latter observation is of considerable significance, given the role of the macula densa in tubuloglomerular feedback and renal renin secretion; luminal loop diuretics block both tubuloglomerular feedback[159] and the suppression of renin release by luminal Cl^-.[160]

Alternative splicing of exon 4 of the SLC12A1 gene yields NKCC2 proteins that differ within transmembrane domain 2 and the adjacent intracellular loop. There are thus three different variants of exon 4, denoted "A", "B", and "F"; the variable inclusion of these cassette exons yields the NKCC2-A, NKCC2-B, and NKCC2-F proteins.[155,157] Kinetic characterization reveals that these isoforms differ dramatically in ion affinities.[155,157] In particular, NKCC2-F has a very low affinity for Cl^- (K_m of 113 mM) and NKCC2-B has a very high affinity (K_m of 8.9 mM); NKCC2-A has an intermediate affinity for Cl^- (K_m of 44.7 mM).[157] These isoforms differ in axial distribution along the tubule, with the F cassette expressed in inner stripe of the outer medulla, the A cassette in outer stripe, and the B cassette in cortical TAL.[161] There is thus an axial distribution of the anion affinity of NKCC2 along the TAL, from a low-affinity, high-capacity transporter (NKCC2-F) to a high-affinity, low-capacity transporter (NKCC2-B). Although technically compromised by the considerable homology between the 3′ end of these 96 base-pair exons, in situ hybridization has suggested that rabbit macula densa exclusively expresses the NKCC2-B isoform.[162] Notably, however, selective knockout of the B cassette exon 4 does not eliminate NKCC2 expression in the murine macula densa, which also seems to express NKCC2-A by in situ hybridization.[163] These NKCC2-B knockout mice do however have a shift in the sensitivity of both tubuloglomerular feedback and tubular regulation of renin release.[163]

It should be mentioned in this context that the Na^+-H^+ exchanger NHE3 functions as an alternative mechanism for apical Na^+ absorption by the TAL. There is also evidence in mouse cortical TAL for Na^+-Cl^- transport via parallel Na^+-H^+ and Cl^--HCO_3^- exchange,[164] although the role of this mechanism in transepithelial Na^+-Cl^- transport seems less prominent than in the proximal tubule. Indeed, apical Na^+-H^+ exchange mediated by NHE3 appears to function primarily in HCO_3^- absorption by the TAL.[165] There is thus a considerable upregulation of both apical Na^+-H^+ exchange and NHE3 protein in the TAL of acidotic animals,[166] paired with an induction of AE2, a basolateral Cl^--HCO_3^- exchanger.[167]

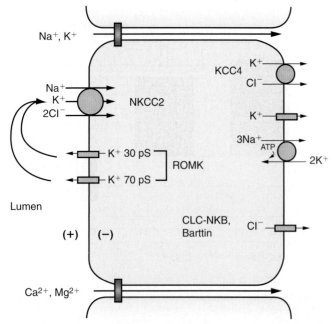

FIGURE 5–15 Transepithelial Na^+-Cl^- transport pathways in the thick ascending limb (TAL). NKCC2, Na^+-K^+-$2Cl^-$ cotransporter-2; ROMK, renal outer medullary K^+ channel; CLC-NKB, human Cl^- channel; Barttin, Cl^- channel subunit; KCC4, K^+-Cl^- cotransporter-4.

Apical K^+ Channels

Microperfused TALs develop a lumen-positive potential difference (PD) during perfusion with Na^+-Cl^-.[168,169] This lumen-negative PD plays a critical role in physiology of the TAL, driving the paracellular transport of Na^+, Ca^{2+}, and Mg^{2+} (see Fig. 5–15). Originally attributed to electrogenic Cl^- transport,[169] the lumen-positive, transepithelial PD in the TAL is generated by the combination of apical K^+ channels and basolateral Cl^- channels.[149,150,170] The conductivity of the apical membrane of TAL cells is predominantly, if not exclusively, K^+ selective. Luminal recycling of K^+ via Na^+-K^+-$2Cl^-$ cotransport and apical K^+ channels, along with basolateral depolarization due to Cl^- exit through Cl^- channels, results in the lumen-negative transepithelial PD.[149,150]

Several lines of evidence indicate that apical K^+ channels are required for transepithelial Na^+-Cl^- transport by the TAL.[149,150] First, the removal of K^+ from luminal perfusate results in a marked decrease in Na^+-Cl^- reabsorption by the TAL, as measured by short circuit current; the residual Na^+-Cl^- transport in the absence of luminal K^+ is sustained by the exit of K^+ via apical K^+ channels, since the combination of K^+ removal and a luminal K^+ channel inhibitor (barium) almost abolishes the short-circuit current.[151] Apical K^+ channels are thus required for continued functioning of NKCC2, the apical Na^+-K^+-$2Cl^-$ cotransporter; the low luminal concentration of K^+ in this nephron segment would otherwise become limiting for transepithelial Na^+-Cl^- transport. Second, the net transport of K^+ across perfused TAL is <10% that of Na^+ and Cl^-[171]; ~90% of the K^+ transported by NKCC2 is recycled across the apical membrane via K^+ channels, resulting in minimal net K^+ absorption by the TAL.[150] Third, the intracellular K^+ activity of perfused TAL cells is ~15 mV to 20 mV above equilibrium, due to furosemide-sensitive entry of K^+ via NKCC2.[170] Given an estimated apical K^+ conductivity of ~12 m/cm², this intracellular K^+ activity yields a calculated K^+ current of ~200 µA/cm²; this corresponds quantitatively to the uptake of K^+ by the apical Na^+-K^+-$2Cl^-$ cotransporter.[149] Finally, the observation that Bartter syndrome can be caused by mutations in ROMK[172] provides genetic proof for the importance of K^+ channels in Na^+-Cl^- absorption by the TAL (see later).

Three types of apical K^+ channels have been identified in the TAL, a 30 pS channel, a 70 pS channel, and a high-conductance, calcium-activated maxi K^+ channel[173–175] (see Fig. 5–15). The higher open probability and greater density of the 30 pS and 70 pS channels, versus the maxi K^+ channel, suggest that these are the primary route for K^+ recycling across the apical membrane; the 70 pS channel in turn appears to mediate ~80% of the apical K^+ conductance of TAL cells.[176] The low conductance 30 pS channel shares several electrophysiological and regulatory characteristics with ROMK, the cardinal inward-rectifying K^+ channel that was initially cloned from renal outer medulla.[177] ROMK protein has been identified at the apical membrane of medullary TAL, cortical TAL, and macula densa.[178] Furthermore, the 30 pS channel is absent from the apical membrane of mice with homozygous deletion of the gene encoding ROMK.[179] Notably, not all cells in the TAL are labeled with ROMK antibody, suggesting that ROMK might be absent in the co-called HBC cells with high basolateral Cl^- conductance and low apical/high basolateral K^+ conductance (see also earlier).[136,147] HBC cells are thought to correspond to the smooth-surfaced morphological subtype of TAL cells (S cells)[147]; however, distribution of ROMK protein by immunoelectron microscopy has not as yet been published.

ROMK clearly plays a critical role in Na^+-Cl^- absorption by the TAL, given that loss-of-function mutations in this gene are associated with Bartter syndrome.[172] The role of ROMK in Bartter syndrome was initially discordant with the data suggesting that the 70 pS K^+ channel is the dominant conductance at the apical membrane of TAL cells[176]; heterologous expression of the ROMK protein in *Xenopus* oocytes had yielded a channel with a conductance of ~30 pS,[177] suggesting

that the 70 pS channel was distinct from ROMK. This paradox has been resolved by the observation that the 70 pS channel is absent from the TAL of ROMK knockout mice, indicating that ROMK proteins form a subunit of the 70 pS channel.[180] ROMK activity in the TAL is clearly modulated by association with other proteins, such that co-association with other subunits to generate the 70 pS channel is perfectly compatible with the known physiology of this protein. ROMK thus associates with scaffolding proteins NHERF-1 and NHERF-2 (see Proximal tubule, neurohumoral influences), via the C-terminal PDZ-binding motif of ROMK; NHERF-2 is co-expressed with ROMK in the TAL.[181] The association of ROMK with NHERFs serves to bring ROMK into closer proximity to the cystic fibrosis transmembrane regulator protein (CFTR).[181] This ROMK-CFTR interaction is in turn required for the native ATP and glybenclamide sensitivity of apical K^+ channels in the TAL.[182]

Paracellular Transport

Microperfused TALs perfused with Na^+-Cl^- develop a lumen-positive transepithelial potential difference (PD)[168,169] generated by the combination of apical K^+ secretion and basolateral Cl^- efflux.[149,150,170] This lumen-positive PD plays a critical role in the paracellular reabsorption of Na^+, Ca^{2+}, and Mg^{2+} by the TAL (see Fig. 5–15). In the transepithelial transport of Na^+, the stoichiometry of NKCC2 ($1Na^+$:$1K^+$:$2Cl^-$) is such that other mechanisms are necessary to balance the exit of Cl^- at the basolateral membrane; consistent with this requirement, data from mouse TAL indicate that ~50% of transepithelial Na^+ transport occurs via the paracellular pathway.[2,183] For example, the ratio of net Cl^- transepithelial absorption to net Na^+ absorption through the paracellular pathway is 2.4 +/– 0.3 in microperfused mouse medullary TAL segments,[183] the expected ratio if 50% of Na^+ transport occurs via the paracellular pathway. In the absence of vasopressin, apical Na^+-Cl^- cotransport is not K^+-dependent (see Regulation of Na^+-Cl^- transport in the TAL), reducing the lumen-positive PD; switching to K^+-dependent Na^+-K^+-$2Cl^-$ cotransport in the presence of vasopressin results in a doubling of Na^+-Cl^- reabsorption, without an effect on oxygen consumption.[2] Therefore, the combination of a cation-permeable paracellular pathway and an "active transport" lumen-positive PD,[149] generated indirectly by the basolateral Na^+/K^+-ATPase,[184] results in a doubling of active Na^+-Cl^- transport for a given level of oxygen consumption.[2]

Unlike the proximal tubule,[12] the voltage-positive PD in the TAL is generated almost entirely by transcellular transport, rather than diffusion across the lateral tight junction. In vasopressin-stimulated mouse TAL segments, with a lumen-positive PD of 10 mV, the maximal increase in Na^+-Cl^- in the lateral interspace is ~10 mM.[183] Tight junctions in the TAL are cation-selective, with P_{Na}/P_{Cl} ratios of 2 to 5.[149,183] Notably, however, P_{Na}/P_{Cl} ratios can be highly variable in individual tubules, ranging from 2 to 5 in a single study of perfused mouse TAL.[183] Regardless, assuming a P_{Na}/P_{Cl} ratio of ~3, the maximal dilution potential in the mouse TAL is between 0.7 mV to 1.1 mV, consistent with a dominant effect of transcellular processes on the lumen-positive PD.[183]

The reported transepithelial resistance in the TAL is between 10 and 50 Ω-cm²; although this resistance is higher than that of the proximal tubule, the TAL is not considered a "tight" epithelium.[149,184] Notably, however, water permeability of the TAL is extremely low, <1% that of the proximal tubule.[149] These "hybrid" characteristics[184]—relatively low resistance and very low water permeability—allow the TAL to generate and sustain Na^+-Cl^- gradients of up to 120 mM.[149] Not unexpectedly, given its lack of water permeability, the TAL does not express aquaporin water channels; as in the proximal tubule, the particular repertoire of claudins expressed in the TAL determines the resistance and

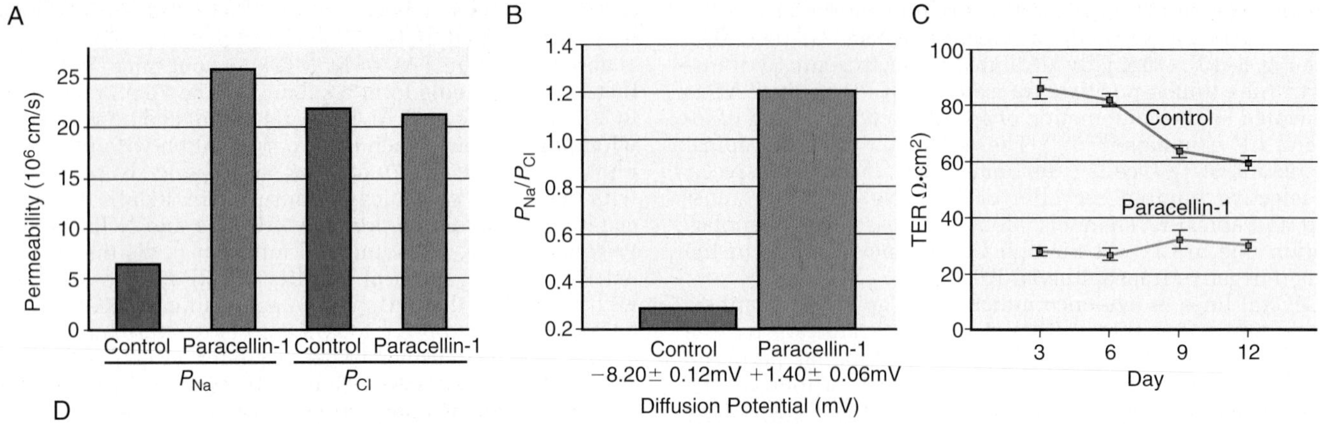

A

B

C

D

	P_{Li} (10^{-6}cm/s)	P_{Na} (10^{-6}cm/s)	P_K (10^{-6}cm/s)	P_{Rb} (10^{-6}cm/s)	P_{Cs} (10^{-6}cm/s)	P_{Mg} (10^{-6}cm/s)
Control	9.101 ± 0.107	6.381 ± 0.107	5.753 ± 0.099	5.370 ± 0.205	5.175 ± 0.104	6.564 ± 0.023
Paracellin-1	28.810 ± 0.180	25.750 ± 0.092	29.630 ± 0.270	26.577 ± 0.057	25.083 ± 0.055	10.740 ± 0.059

FIGURE 5–16 The effect of claudin-16 (paracellin-1) overexpression in LLC-PK1 cells. **A,** Effects of paracellin-1 on the permeability of Na^+ and Cl^- in LLC-PK1 cells. **B,** Ratio of P_{Na} to P_{Cl} and diffusion potential (bottom) across a LLC-PK1 cell monolayer. **C,** Transepithelial resistance across an LLC-PK1 cell monolayer over a period of 12 days in cells expressing paracellin-1 and control cells. **D,** Summary of the effects of paracellin-1 upon permeability of various cations in LLC-PK1 cells. (From Hou J, Paul DL, Goodenough DA: Paracellin-1 and the modulation of ion selectivity of tight junctions. J Cell Sci 118:5109–5118, 2005.)

ion-selectivity of this nephron segment. Mouse TAL segments co-express claudin-3, -10, -11, -16, and -19.[26,185,186] Of particular significance, mutations in human claudin-16 (paracellin-1)[185] and claudin-19[186] are associated with hereditary hypomagnesemia, suggesting that these claudins are particularly critical for the cation-selectivity of TAL tight junctions. Heterologous expression of claudin-16 (paracellin-1) in the anion-selective LLC-PK1 cell line markedly increases Na^+ permeability, without affecting Cl^- permeability; this yields a marked increase in the P_{Na}/P_{Cl} ratio (Fig. 5–16).[187] LLC-PK1 cells expressing claudin-16 also have increased permeability to other monovalent cations. There is however only a modest increase in Mg^{2+} permeability, suggesting that claudin-16 does not form a Mg^{2+}-specific pathway in the tight junction; rather, it may serve to increase the overall cation selectivity of the tight junction. Notably, no such effects on P_{Na}/P_{Cl} ratio or Mg^{2+} permeability were seen in cation-selective MDCK-II cells[187]; Kausalya and colleagues also report minimal effect of claudin-16 on P_{Na}/P_{Cl} ratio in MCDK-C7 cells, although they did detect a modest increase in Mg^{2+} permeability.[188] Regardless, the functional[187] and genetic[185] data suggest that claudin-16 expression is critical for the cation-selectivity of tight junctions in the TAL.

Basolateral Mechanisms

The basolateral Na^+/K^+-ATPase is the primary exit pathway for Na^+ at the basolateral membrane of TAL cells. The Na^+ gradient generated by Na^+/K^+-ATPase activity is also thought to drive the apical entry of Na^+, K^+, and Cl^- via NKCC2, the furosemide-sensitive Na^+-K^+-$2Cl^-$ cotransporter.[150] Inhibition of Na^+/K^+-ATPase with ouabain thus collapses the lumen-positive PD and abolishes transepithelial Na^+-Cl^- transport in the TAL.[168,169,184] Basolateral exit of Cl^- from TAL cells is primarily but not exclusively[189] electrogenic, mediated by Cl^- channel activity.[149,150] Reductions in basolateral Cl^- depolarize the basolateral membrane, whereas increases in intracellular Cl^- induced by luminal furosemide have a hyperpolarizing effect.[189] Intracellular Cl^- activity during transepithelial Na^+-Cl^- transport is above its electrochemical equilibrium,[190] with an intracellular-negative voltage of −40 to −70 mV that drives basolateral Cl^- exit.[149,150,189]

There has been considerable recent progress in the molecular physiology of basolateral Cl^- channels in the TAL. At least two CLC channels, CLC-K1 and CLC-K2 (CLC-NKA and CLC-NKB in humans), are co-expressed in this nephron segment.[141,144] However, an increasing body of evidence indicates that the dominant Cl^- channel in the TAL is encoded by CLC-K2. First, CLC-K1 is heavily expressed at both apical and basolateral membranes of the thin ascending limb,[139] and the phenotype of the corresponding knockout mouse is consistent with primary dysfunction of thin ascending limbs, rather than the TAL[121,142] (see Na^+-Cl^- transport in the thin ascending limb). Second, loss-of-function mutations in CLC-NKB are associated with Bartter syndrome,[143] genetic evidence for a dominant role of this channel in Na^+-Cl^- transport in the TAL. More recently, a very common T481S polymorphism in human CLC-NKB was shown to increase channel activity by a factor of 20[191]; preliminary data indicate an association with hypertension,[192] suggesting that this gain-of-function in CLC-NKB increases Na^+-Cl^- transport by the TAL and/or other segments of the distal nephron. Finally, CLC-K2 protein is heavily expressed at the basolateral membrane of the mouse TAL, with additional expression in the DCT, CNT, and α-intercalated cells.[193]

A key advance was the characterization of the "Barttin" subunit of CLC-K channels, which is co-expressed with CLC-K1 and CLC-K2 in several nephron segments, including TAL (see also Na^+-Cl^- transport in the thin ascending limb).[141,144] Unlike rat CLC-K1, the rat CLC-K2, human CLC-NKA, and human CLC-NKB paralogs are not functional in the absence of Barttin co-expression.[144,145] CLC-NKB co-expressed with Barttin is highly selective for Cl^-, with a permeability series of $Cl^->>Br^-=NO_3^->I^-$.[141,144,191] CLC-NKB/Barttin channels are activated by increases in extracellular Ca^{2+} and are pH-sensitive, with activation at alkaline extracellular pH and marked inhibition at acidic pH.[144] CLC-NKA/Barttin channels have similar pH and calcium sensitivities, but exhibit higher permeability to Br^-.[144] Strikingly, despite the considerable homology between the CLC-NKA/NKB proteins, these channels also differ considerably in pharmacological sensitivity to various Cl^- channel blockers, potential lead compounds for the development of paralog-specific inhibitors.[194]

Correlation between functional characteristics of CLC-K proteins with native Cl^- channels in TAL has been problematic. In particular, a wide variation in single channel conductance has been reported for basolateral Cl^- channels in this nephron segment (reviewed in Ref 195). This is perhaps due to the use of collagenase and other conditions for the preparation of tubule fragments and/or basolateral vesicles, manipulations that potentially affect channel characteristics.[195] There may also be considerable molecular heterogeneity of Cl^- channels in the TAL, although the genetic evidence would seem to suggest a functional dominance of CLC-NKB.[143] Notably, single channel conductance has not been reported for CLC-NKB/Barttin channels, due to the difficulty in expressing the channel in heterologous systems; this complicates the comparison of CLC-NKB/Barttin to native Cl^- channels. Single channel conductance has however been reported for the V166E mutant of rat CLC-K1, which alters gating of the channel without expected effects on single channel amplitude; co-expression with Barttin increases the single channel conductance of V166E CLC-K1 from ~7 pS to ~20 pS.[145] Therefore, part of the reported variability in native single channel conductance may reflect heterogeneity in the interaction between CLC-NKB and/or CLC-NKA with Barttin. Regardless, a recent study using whole-cell recording techniques suggests that CLC-K2 (CLC-NKB in humans) is the dominant Cl^- channel in TAL and other segments of the rat distal nephron.[195] Like CLC-NKB/Barttin[141,144,191] this native channel is highly Cl^--selective, with considerably weaker conductance for Br^- and I^-[195]; CLC-NKA/Barttin channels exhibit higher permeability to Br^-.[144] This renal channel is also inhibited by acidic extracellular pH,[195] but seems to lack the activation by alkaline pH seen in CLC-NKB/Barttin-expressing cells.[144]

Electroneutral K^+-Cl^- cotransport has also been implicated in transepithelial Na^+-Cl^- transport in the TAL (see Figure 5–15), functioning in K^+-dependent Cl^- exit at the basolateral membrane.[189] The K^+-Cl^- cotransporter KCC4 is thus expressed at the basolateral membrane of medullary and cortical TAL, in addition to macula densa.[196,197] There is also functional evidence for K^+-Cl^- cotransport at the basolateral membrane of this section of the nephron. First, TAL cells contain a Cl^--dependent NH_4^+ transport mechanism that is sensitive to 1.5 mM furosemide and 10 mM barium (Ba^{2+}).[198] NH_4^+ ions have the same ionic radius as K^+ and are transported by KCC4 and other K^+-Cl^- cotransporters[199]; KCC4 is also sensitive to Ba^{2+} and millimolar furosemide[200], consistent with the pharmacology of NH_4^+-Cl^- cotransport in the TAL.[198] Second, to account for the effects on transmembrane potential difference of basolateral Ba^{2+} and/or increased K^+, it has been suggested that the basolateral membrane of TAL contains a Ba^{2+}-sensitive K^+-Cl^- transporter[189,201]; this is also consistent with the known expression of Ba^{2+}-sensitive[200] KCC4 at the basolateral membrane.[196,197] Third, increases in basolateral K^+ cause Cl^--dependent cell swelling in *Amphiuma* early distal tubule, an anolog of the mammalian TAL; in *Amphiuma* LBC cells with low basolateral conductance, analogous to mammalian LBC cells[136,147] (see Na^+-Cl^- transport in the TAL: Apical Na^+-Cl^- transport), this cell swelling was not accompanied by changes in basolateral membrane voltage or resistance,[202] consistent with K^+-Cl^- transport.

There is thus considerable evidence for basolateral K^+-Cl^- cotransport in the TAL, mediated by KCC4.[196,197] However, direct confirmation of a role for basolateral K^+-Cl^- cotransport in transepithelial transepithelial Na^+-Cl^- transport is lacking. Indeed, KCC4-deficient mice do not have a prominent defect in function of the TAL, but exibit instead a renal tubular acidosis.[197] The renal tubular acidosis in these mice has been attributed to defects in acid extrusion by H^+-ATPase in α-intercalated cells[197]; however, this phenotype is conceivably due to reduction in medullary NH_4^+ reabsorption by the TAL,[203] due to the loss of basolateral NH_4^+ exit mediated by KCC4.[199]

Finally, there is also evidence for the existence of Ba^{2+}-sensitive K^+ channel activity at the basolateral membrane of TAL,[204–206] providing an alternative exit pathway for K^+ to that mediated by KCC4. These channels may function in transepithelial transport of K^+, which is however only <10% that of Na^+ and Cl^- transport by the TAL.[171] Basolateral K^+ channels may also attenuate the increases in intracellular K^+ that are generated by the basolateral Na^+/K^+-ATPase, thus maintaining transepithelial Na^+-Cl^- transport.[204–206] In addition, basolateral K^+ channel activity may help stabilize the basolateral membrane potential above the equilibrium potential for Cl^-,[206] thus maintaining a continuous driving force for Cl^- exit via CLC-NKB/Barttin Cl^- channels.

Regulation of Na^+-Cl^- Transport by the Thick Ascending Limb
Activating Influences

Transepithelial Na^+-Cl^- transport by the TAL is regulated by a complex blend of competing neurohumoral influences. In particular, increases in intracellular cAMP tonically stimulate ion transport in the TAL; the list of stimulatory hormones and mediators that increase cAMP in this nephron segment includes vasopressin, PTH, glucagon, calcitonin, and β-adrenergic activation (see Fig. 5–10). These overlapping cAMP-dependent stimuli are thought to result in maximal baseline stimulation of transepithelial Na^+-Cl^- transport.[82] For example, characterization of the *in vivo* effect of these hormones requires the prior simultaneous suppression or absence of circulating vasopressin, PTH, calcitonin, and glucagon.[82] This baseline activation is in turn modulated by a number of negative influences; most prominently PGE_2 and extracellular Ca^{2+} (see Fig. 5–10).

Vasopressin is perhaps the most extensively studied positive modulator of transepithelial Na^+-Cl^- transport in the TAL. The TAL expresses V2 vasopressin receptors at both the mRNA and protein level, and micro-dissected TALs respond to the hormone with an increase in intracellular cAMP.[207] Vasopressin activates apical Na^+-K^+-$2Cl^-$ cotransport within minutes in perfused mouse TAL segments, and also exerts longer term influence on NKCC2 expression and function. The acute activation of apical Na^+-K^+-$2Cl^-$ cotransport is achieved at least in part by the stimulated exocytosis of NKCC2 proteins, from subapical vesicles to the plasma membrane.[208] This trafficking-dependent activation is abrogated by treatment of perfused tubules with tetanus toxin, which cleaves the vesicle-associated membrane proteins VAMP-2 and VAMP-3.[208] Activation of NKCC2 is also associated with the phosphorylation of a cluster of N-terminal threonines in the transporter protein; treatment of rats with the V2 agonist dDAVP induces phosphorylation of these residues *in vivo*, as measured with a potent phospho-specific antibody.[208] These threonine residues are thought to be substrates for the SPAK and OSR1 kinases, recently identified by Delpire and colleagues as key regulatory kinases for NKCC1 and other cation-chloride cotransporters.[209] SPAK and OSR1 are in turn activated by upstream WNK (With No Lysine (K)) kinases (see also Regulation of Na^+-Cl^- transport in the DCT), such that SPAK or OSR1 require co-expression with WNK4 to fully activate NKCC1.[209] WNK kinases can however influence transport when co-expressed alone in *Xenopus* oocytes with cation-chloride cotransporters, in the absence of exogenous SPAK/OSR1, reflective perhaps of the activation of endogenous *Xenopus laevis* orthologs of SPAK and/or OSR1.

Regardless, co-expression with WNK3 in *Xenopus* oocytes results in activatory phosphorylation of the N-terminal threonines in NKCC2 that are phosphorylated in TAL cells after treatment with dDAVP.[208,210] The WNK3 protein is also expressed in TAL cells,[210] although the link(s) between activation of the V2 receptor and this particular kinase are as yet uncharacterized.

Vasopressin has also been shown to alter the stoichiometry of furosemide-sensitive apical Cl^- transport in the TAL, from a K^+-independent Na^+-Cl^- mode to the classical Na^+-K^+-2Cl^- cotransport stoichiometry.[2] In the absence of vasopressin, $^{22}Na^+$ uptake by mouse medullary TAL cells is not dependent on the presence of extracellular K^+, whereas the addition of the hormone induces a switch to K^+-dependent $^{22}Na^+$ uptake. Underscoring the metabolic advantages of paracellular Na^+ transport, which is critically dependent on the apical entry of K^+ via Na^+-K^+-2Cl^- cotransport (see earlier), vasopressin accomplishes a doubling of transepithelial Na^+-Cl^- transport without affecting $^{22}Na^+$ uptake (an indicator of transcellular Na^+-Cl^- transport); this doubling in transepithelial absorption occurs without an increase in O_2 consumption,[2] highlighting the energy efficiency of ion transport by the TAL. The mechanism of this shift in the apparent stoichiometry of NKCC2 is not completely clear. However, splice variants of mouse NKCC2 with a novel, shorter C-terminus have been found to confer sensitivity to cAMP when co-expressed with full-length NKCC2.[211] Notably, these shorter splice variants appear to encode furosemide-sensitive, K^+-independent Na^+-Cl^- cotransporters when expressed alone in *Xenopus* oocytes.[212] The *in vivo* relevance of these phenomena is not clear, however, nor is it known whether similar splice variants exist in species other than mouse.

In addition to its acute effects on NKCC2, the apical Na^+-K^+-2Cl^- cotransporter, vasopressin increases transepithelial Na^+-Cl^- transport by activating apical K^+ channels and basolateral Cl^- channels in the TAL.[82,207] Details have yet to emerge of the regulation of the basolateral CLC-NKB/Barttin Cl^- channel complex by vasopressin, cAMP, and related pathways. However, the apical K^+ channel ROMK is directly phosphorylated by protein kinase A on three serine residues (S25, S200, and S294 in the ROMK2 isoform). Phosphorylation of at least two of these three serines is required for detectable K^+ channel activity in *Xenopus* oocytes; mutation of all three serines to alanine abolishes phosphorylation and transport activity, and all three serines are required for full channel activity.[213] These three phospho-acceptor sites have distinct effects on ROMK activity and expression.[214] Phosphorylation of the N-terminal S25 residue appears to regulate trafficking of the channel to the cell membrane, without affects on channel gating; this serine is also a substrate for the SGK1 kinase, which activates the channel via an increase in expression at the membrane.[214] In contrast, phosphorylation of the two C-terminal serines modulates open channel probability, via effects on pH-dependent gating[215] and on activation by the binding of phosphatidyl 4,5-biphosphate (PIP2) to the C-terminal domain of the channel.[216]

Vasopressin also has considerable long-term effects on transepithelial Na^+-Cl^- transport by the TAL. Sustained increases in circulating vasopressin result in marked hypertrophy of medullary TAL cells, accompanied by a doubling in baseline active Na^+-Cl^- transport.[207] Water restriction or treatment with dDAVP also results in an increase in abundance of the NKCC2 protein in rat TAL cells. Consistent with a direct effect of vasopressin-dependent signaling, expression of NKCC2 is reduced in mice with a heterozygous deletion of the G_s stimulatory G protein, through which the V2 receptor activates cAMP generation.[207] Increases in cAMP are thought to directly induce transcription of the *SLC12A1* gene that encodes NKCC2, given the presence of a cAMP-response element in the 5′ promoter.[207,208] Abrogation of the tonic nega-

tive effect of PGE_2 on cAMP generation with indomethacin also results in a considerable increase in abundance of the NKCC2 protein.[207] Finally, in addition to these effects on NKCC2 expression, water restriction or dDAVP treatment increases abundance of the ROMK protein at the apical membrane of TAL cells.[217]

Inhibitory Influences

The tonic stimulation of transepithelial Na^+-Cl^- transport by cAMP-generating hormones (e.g., vasopressin, PTH) is modulated by a number of negative neurohumoral influences (see Fig. 5–10 and Ref 82). In particular, extracellular Ca^{2+} and PGE_2 exert dramatic inhibitory effects on ion transport by this and other segments of the distal nephron, through a plethora of synergistic mechanisms. Both extracellular Ca^{2+} and PGE_2 activate the G_i inhibitory G protein in TAL cells, opposing the stimulatory, G_s-dependent effects of vasopressin on intracellular levels of cAMP.[218,219] Extracellular Ca^{2+} exerts its effect through the calcium-sensing receptor (CaSR), which is heavily expressed at the basolateral membrane of TAL cells[219,220]; PGE_2 primarily signals through EP_3 prostaglandin receptors.[82] The increases in intracellular Ca^{2+} due to the activation of the CaSR and other receptors directly inhibits cAMP generation by a Ca^{2+}-inhibitable adenylate cyclase that is expressed in the TAL, accompanied by an increase in phosphodiesterase-dependent degradation of cAMP[219,221] (Fig. 5–17).

Activation of the CaSR and other receptors in the TAL also results in the downstream generation of arachidonic acid metabolites with potent negative effects on Na^+-Cl^- transport (see Fig. 5–17). Extracellular Ca^{2+} thus activates phospholipase A_2 in TAL cells, leading to the liberation of arachidonic acid. This arachidonic acid is in turn metabolized by P450 ω-hydroxylase to 20-HETE (20-hydroxyeicosatetraenoic acid), or by cyclooxygenase-2 (COX-2) to PGE_2; P450 ω-hydroxylation generally predominates in response to activation of the CaSR in TAL.[219] 20-HETE has very potent negative effects on apical Na^+-K^+-2Cl^- cotransport, apical K^+ channels, and the basolateral Na^+/K^+-ATPase.[82,219] PLA_2-dependent generation of 20-HETE also underlies in part the negative effect of bradykinin and angiotensin-II on Na^+-Cl^- transport.[82,219] Activation of the CaSR also induces TNFα expression in the TAL, which activates COX-2 and thus generation of PGE_2 (see Fig. 5–17); this PGE_2 in turn results in additional inhibition of Na^+-Cl^- transport.[219]

The relative importance of the CaSR in the regulation of Na^+-Cl^- transport by the TAL is dramatically illustrated by the phenotype of a handful of patients with gain-of-function mutations in this receptor. In addition to suppressed PTH and hypocalcemia, the usual phenotype caused by gain-of-function mutations in the CaSR (autosomal dominant hypoparathyroidism), these patients manifest a hypokalemic alkalosis, polyuria, and increases in circulating renin and aldosterone.[222,223] Therefore, the persistent inhibition of Na^+-Cl^- transport in the TAL by these over-active mutants of the CaSR causes a rare subtype of Bartter syndrome, type V in the genetic classification of this disease.[219]

Distal Convoluted Tubule, Connecting Tubule, and Collecting Duct

The distal nephron that extends beyond the thick ascending limb is the final arbiter of urinary Na^+-Cl^- excretion, and a critical target for both natriuretic and anti-natriuretic stimuli. The understanding of the cellular organization and molecular phenotype of the distal nephron continues to evolve, and merits a brief review in this context. The distal convoluted tubule (DCT) begins at a variable distance after the macula densa, with an abrupt transition between NKCC2-positive cortical TAL cells and DCT cells that express the

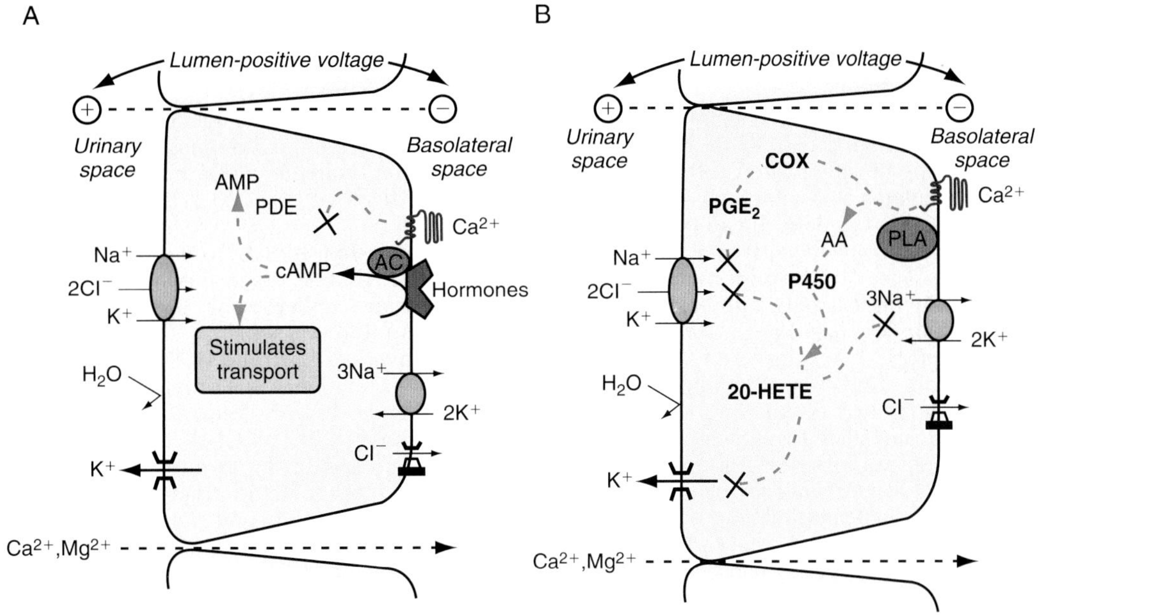

FIGURE 5–17 Inhibitory effects of the calcium-sensing receptor (CaSR) on transepithelial Na$^+$-Cl$^-$ transport in the TAL. **A,** Activation of the basolateral CaSR inhibits the generation of cyclic AMP (cAMP) in response to vasopressin and other hormones (see text for details). **B,** Stimulation of phospholipase A2 by the CaSR leads to liberation of arachidonic acid, which is in turn metabolized by P450 ω-hydroxylase to 20-HETE (20-hydroxyeicosatetraenoic acid), or by cyclooxygenase-2 (COX-2) to PGE$_2$. 20-HETE is a potent natriuretic factor, inhibiting apical Na$^+$-K$^+$-2Cl$^-$ cotransport, apical K$^+$ channels, and the basolateral Na$^+$/K$^+$-ATPase. Activation of the CaSR also induces TNFα expression in the TAL, which activates COX-2 and thus generation of PGE$_2$, leading to additional inhibition of Na$^+$-Cl$^-$ transport. (Redrawn from Hebert SC: Calcium and salinity sensing by the thick ascending limb: A journey from mammals to fish and back again. Kidney Int Suppl: S28–33, 2004.)

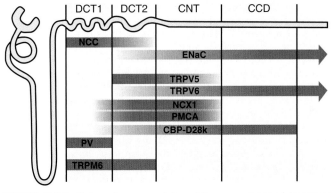

FIGURE 5–18 Schematic representation of the segmentation of the mouse distal nephron and of the distribution and abundance of Na$^+$-, Ca^{2+}- and Mg^{2+}-transporting proteins. ENaC, epithelial Na$^+$ channel; NCC, thiazide-sensitive Na$^+$-Cl$^-$ cotransporter; CB, calbindin D$_{28K}$; PV, paravalbumin. TRPV5 and TRPV6, apical Ca^{2+} entry channels; NCX1, Na$^+$-Ca^{2+} exchanger; PMCA, plasma membrane Ca^{2+}-ATPase; CBP-D28k, calbindin D28k; TRPM6, apical Mg^{2+} entry channel. Data compiled from Refs 225, 522, 661.

thiazide-sensitive Na$^+$-Cl$^-$ cotransporter NCC. Considerable progress has been made in the phenotypic classification of cell types in the DCT and adjacent nephron segments, based on the expression of an expanding list of transport proteins and other markers[224] (Fig. 5–18). This analysis has revealed considerable differences in the organization of the DCT, connecting segment (CNT), and cortical collecting duct (CCD) in rodent, rabbit, and human kidneys. In general, rabbit kidneys are unique in the axial demarcation of DCT, CNT, and CCD segments, at both a molecular and morphological level; the organization of the DCT to CCD is considerably more complex in other species, with boundaries that are much less absolute.[224] Notably, however, the overall repertoire of transport proteins expressed does not vary between these species; what differs is the specific cellular and molecular organization of this segment of the nephron.

The early DCT (DCT1) of mouse kidney expresses NCC and a specific marker, parvalbumin, which also distinguishes the DCT1 from the adjacent cortical TAL[225] (see Fig. 5–18). Mouse DCT2 cells co-express NCC with proteins involved in transcellular Ca^{2+} transport, including the apical calcium channel ECaC1 (TRPV5), the cytosolic calcium-binding protein calbindin D$_{28K}$, and the basolateral Na$^+$-Ca^{2+} exchanger NCX1.[225] NCC is co-expressed with the amiloride-sensitive Na$^+$ channel (ENaC) in the late DCT2 of mouse, with robust expression of ENaC continuing in the downstream CNT and CCD.[225] In contrast, rabbit kidney does not have a DCT1 or DCT2, and exhibits abrupt transitions between NCC- and ENaC-positive DCT and CNT segments, respectively.[224] Human kidneys that have been studied thus far exhibit expression of calbindin D$_{28K}$ all along the DCT and CNT, extending into the CCD; however, the intensity of expression varies at these sites. Approximately 30% of cells in the distal convolution of human kidney express NCC, with 70% expressing ENaC (CNT cells); ENaC and NCC overlap in expression at the end of the human DCT segment. Finally, cells of the early CNT of human kidneys express ENaC in the absence of Aquaporin-2, the apical vasopressin-sensitive water channel.[224]

Although primarily contiguous with the DCT, CNT cells share several traits with principal cells of the CCD, including apical expression of ENaC and ROMK, the K$^+$ secretory channel; the capacity for Na$^+$-Cl$^-$ reabsorption and K$^+$ secretion in this nephron segment is as much as 10 times higher than that of the CCD[226] (see also Na$^+$-Cl$^-$ transport in the CNT and CCD; Apical Na$^+$ transport). Intercalated cells are the minority cell type within the distal nephron, emerging within the DCT and CNT and extending into the early inner medullary collecting duct (IMCD).[227] Three subtypes of intercalated cells have been defined, based on differences in the subcellular distribution of the H$^+$-ATPase and the presence or absence of the basolateral AE1 Cl$^-$-HCO$_3^-$ exchanger. Type A intercalated cells extrude protons via an apical H$^+$-ATPase in series with basolateral AE1; type B intercalated cells secrete HCO$_3^-$ and OH$^-$ via an apical anion exchanger (SLC26A4 or pendrin) in series with basolateral H$^+$-ATPase.[227] In rodents, the most prevalent subtype of intercalated cells in the CNT is the non-A, non-B intercalated cell, which possess an apical Cl$^-$-HCO$_3^-$ exchanger (SLC26A4 or pendrin) along with apical H$^+$-ATPase.[227] Although intercalated cells play a dominant role in acid-base homeostasis, Cl$^-$ transport by type B intercalated cells performs an increasingly appreciated role in distal nephron Na$^+$-Cl$^-$ transport (see Na$^+$-Cl$^-$ transport in the CNT and CCD; Cl$^-$ transport).

The outer medullary collecting duct encompasses two separate subsegments, corresponding to the outer and stripes of the inner medulla, OMCDo and OMCDi, respectively. OMCDo and OMCDi contain principal cells with apical amiloride-sensitive Na$^+$ channels (ENaC)[228]; however, the primary role of this nephron segment is renal acidification, with a particular dominance of Type A intercalated cells in OMCDi.[3] The OMCD also plays a critical role in K$^+$ reabsorption, via the activity of apical H$^+$/K$^+$-ATPase pumps.[229-231]

Finally, the inner medullary collecting duct begins at the boundary between the outer and inner medulla, and extends to the tip of the papilla. The IMCD is arbitrarily separated into three equal zones, denoted IMCD1, IMCD2, and IMCD3; at the functional level, an early IMCD (IMCDi) and a terminal portion (IMCDt) can be appreciated.[3] The IMCD plays particularly prominent roles in vasopressin-sensitive water and urea transport.[3] The early IMCD contains both principal cells and intercalated cells; all three subsegments (IMCD1-3) express apical ENaC protein, albeit considerably weaker expression than in the CNT and CCD.[232] The roles of the IMCD and OMCD in Na$^+$-Cl$^-$ homeostasis have been more elusive than that of the CNT and CCD; however, to the extent that ENaC is expressed in the IMCD and OMCD, homologous mechanisms are expected to function in Na$^+$-Cl$^-$ reabsorption by CNT, CCD, OMCD, and IMCD segments.

Distal Convoluted Tubule
Mechanisms of Na$^+$-Cl$^-$ Transport in the Distal Convoluted Tubule

Earlier micropuncture studies that did not distinguish between early and late DCT indicate that this nephron segment reabsorbs ~10% of filtered Na$^+$-Cl$^-$.[233,234] The apical absorption of Na$^+$ and Cl$^-$ by the DCT is mutually dependent; ion substitution does not affect transepithelial voltage, suggesting electroneutral transport.[235] The absorption of Na$^+$ by perfused DCT segments is also inhibited by chlorothiazide, localized proof that this nephron segment is the target for thiazide diuretics.[236] Similar thiazide-sensitive Na$^+$-Cl$^-$ cotransport exists in the urinary blander of winter flounder, the species in which the thiazide-sensitive Na$^+$-Cl$^-$ cotransporter (NCC) was first identified by expression cloning.[237] Functional characterization of rat NCC indicates very high affinities for both Na$^+$ and Cl$^-$ (Michaelis-Menten constants of 7.6 ± 1.6 and 6.3 ± 1.1 mM, respectively)[238]; equally high affinities had previously been obtained by Velazquez and co-workers in perfused rat DCT.[235] The measured Hill coefficients of rat NCC are ~1 for each ion, consistent with electroneutral co-transport.[238]

NCC expression is the defining characteristic of the DCT[224] (see Figs. 5–18 and 5–19). There is also evidence for expression of this transporter in osteoblasts, peripheral blood mononuclear cells, and intestinal epithelium[239]; however, kidney is the dominant expression site.[155] Loss-of-function mutations in the SLC12A2 gene encoding human NCC cause Gitelman syndrome, familial hypokalemic alkalosis with hypomagnesemia, and hypocalciuria (see also Chapter 15). Mice with

homozygous deletion of the Slc12a2 gene encoding NCC exhibit marked morphological defects in the early DCT,[240,241] with both a reduction in the absolute number of DCT cells and changes in ultrastructural appearance. Similarly, thiazide treatment promotes marked apoptosis of the DCT,[242] suggesting that thiazide-sensitive Na$^+$-Cl$^-$ cotransport plays an important role in modulating growth and regression of this nephron segment (see also Regulation of Na$^+$-Cl$^-$ transport in the DCT).

Co-expression of NCC and the amiloride-sensitive Na$^+$ channel (ENaC) occurs in the late DCT and CNT segments of many species, either in the same cells or in adjacent cells in the same tubule.[224] Notably, ENaC is the primary Na$^+$ transport pathway of CNT and CCD cells, rather than DCT. There is however evidence for other Na$^+$ and Cl$^-$ entry pathways in DCT cells. In particular, the Na$^+$-H$^+$ exchanger NHE2 is co-expressed with NCC at the apical membrane of rat DCT cells.[243] As in the proximal tubule, perfusion of distal convoluted tubule with formate and oxalate stimulates DIDS-sensitive Na$^+$-Cl$^-$ transport that is distinct from the thiazide-sensitive transport mediated by NCC.[44] Therefore, a parallel arrangement of Na$^+$-H$^+$ exchange and Cl$^-$-anion exchangers may play an important role in electroneutral Na$^+$-Cl$^-$ absorption by the DCT (see Fig. 5–19). Of note, the anion exchanger SLC26A6 is evidently expressed in the human distal nephron, including perhaps in DCT cells[244]; NHE2[243] and SLC26A6 are thus candidates mechanisms for this alternative pathway of DCT Na$^+$-Cl$^-$ absorption.

At the basolateral membrane, as in other nephron segments, Na$^+$ exits via Na$^+$/K$^+$-ATPase; bearing in mind the considerable caveats in morphological identification of the DCT,[224] this nephron segment appears to have the highest Na$^+$/K$^+$-ATPase activity of the entire nephron[14] (see Fig. 5–4). Basolateral membranes of DCT cells in both rabbit[245] and mouse[196] express the K$^+$-Cl$^-$ cotransporter KCC4, a potential exit pathway for Cl$^-$. However, several lines of evidence indicate that Cl$^-$ primarily exits DCT cells via basolateral Cl$^-$ channels. First, the basolateral membrane of rabbit DCT contains Cl$^-$ channel activity, with functional characteristics that are similar to those of CLC-K2.[195,246] Second, CLC-K2 protein is expressed at the basolateral membrane of DCT and CNT cells[193]; mRNA for CLC-K1 can also be detected by RT-PCR of microdissected DCT segments.[141] Third, loss-of-function mutations in CLC-NKB, the human ortholog of CLC-K2, typically cause Bartter syndrome (dysfunction of the TAL)[143]; however, in some of these patients, mutations in CLC-NKB lead to more of a Gitelman syndrome phenotype, consistent with loss-of-function of DCT segments.[247]

Regulation of Na$^+$-Cl$^-$ Transport in the Distal Convoluted Tubule

Considerable hypertrophy of the DCT occurs in response to chronic increases in delivery of Na$^+$-Cl$^-$ to the DCT, typically induced by furosemide treatment with dietary Na$^+$-Cl$^-$ supplementation.[224,233] These morphological changes are reportedly independent of changes in aldosterone or glucocorticoid, suggesting that increased Na$^+$-Cl$^-$ entry via NCC promotes hypertrophy of the DCT[224]; this is the inverse of the hypomorphic changes seen in NCC-deficiency[240,241] or thiazide treatment.[224] Notably, however, changes in aldosterone do have dramatic effects on both the morphology of the DCT[248] and expression of NCC.[224,249,250] The DCT is thus an aldosterone-sensitive epithelium, expressing both mineralocorticoid receptor and the 11β-hydroxysteroid dehydrogenase-2 (11β-HSD2) enzyme that confers specificity for aldosterone over glucocorticoids.[224] Mice with a targeted deletion of 11β-HSD2, with activation of the mineralocorticoid receptor by circulating gluocorticoid, exhibit massive hypertrophy of what appear to be DCT cells[248]; this suggests an important role for mineralocorticoid activity in shaping this nephron segment.

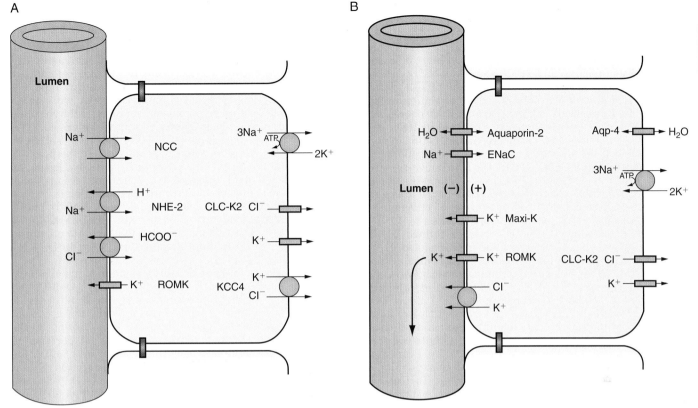

FIGURE 5–19 Transport pathways for Na⁺-Cl⁻ and K⁺ in **(A)** DCT cells and **(B)** principal cells of the CNT and CCD. ENaC, epithelial Na⁺ channel; NCC, thiazide-sensitive Na⁺-Cl⁻ cotransporter; ROMK, renal outer medullary K⁺ channel; KCC4, K⁺-Cl⁻ cotransporter-4; NHE-2, Na⁺-H⁺ exchanger-2.

Furthermore, NCC expression is dramatically increased by treatment of normal rats with fludrocortisone or aldosterone[249]; adrenalectomized rats also show an increase in NCC expression after rescue with aldosterone, and treatment with spironolactone reduces expression of NCC in salt-restricted rats.[230]

Considerable insight into the role of NCC in the pathobiology of the DCT has recently emerged from the study of the WNK4 kinase.[251] WNK1 and WNK4 were initially identified as causative genes for pseudohypopaldosteronism type II (PHA-II) (also known as Gordon syndrome or "hereditary hypertension with hyperkalemia"). PHA-II is in every respect the "mirror image" of Gitelman syndrome, encompassing hypertension, hyperkalemia, hyperchloremic metabolic acidosis, suppressed PRA and aldosterone, and hypercalciuria.[252] Furthermore, PHA-II behaves like a gain-of-function in NCC and/or the DCT, in that treatment with thiazides typically results in resolution of the entire syndrome.[252] Intronic mutations in WNK1 have been detected in patients with PHA-II, leading to increased abundance of WNK1 mRNA in patient leukocytes; WNK4-associated disease is due to clustered point mutations in an acidic-rich, conserved region of the protein.[253] The WNK1 and WNK4 proteins are co-expressed within the distal nephron, in both DCT and CCD cells; whereas WNK1 localizes to the cytoplasm and basolateral membrane, WNK4 protein is found at the apical tight junctions.[253]

Consistent with the physiological gain-of-function in NCC associated with PHA-II,[252] WNK4 co-expression with NCC in Xenopus oocytes inhibits transport, and both kinase-dead and disease-associated mutations abolish the effect.[254,255] WNK1 in turn has no effect on NCC, but abrogates the inhibitory effect of WNK4.[256] WNK4 reportedly interacts directly with the NCC protein[254]; however, the WNK kinases appear to exert their effect on NCC and other cation-chloride cotransporters via the phosphorylation and activation of the SPAK and OSR1 serine/threonine kinases, which in turn phosphorylate the transporter proteins.[209,257,258] Notably, however, the in vivo relevance of these cell culture experiments is not entirely clear, particularly because the WNK1 and WNK4 kinases appear to regulate a number of other transport pathways in the distal nephron.[259–261]

To develop in vivo models relevant to both PHA-II and the physiological role of WNK4 in the distal nephron, Lalioti and colleagues generated two strains of BAC-transgenic mice that overexpress wild-type WNK4 (TgWnk4ᵂᵀ) or a PHA-II mutant of WNK4 (TgWnk4ᴾᴴᴬᴵᴵ, bearing a Q562E mutation associated with the disease).[251] Consistent with the inhibitory effect of WNK4 on NCC,[254,255] the blood pressure of TgWnk4ᵂᵀ is less than that of wild-type littermate controls; in contrast, TgWnk4ᴾᴴᴬᴵᴵ mice are hypertensive. The biochemical phenotype of TgWnk4ᴾᴴᴬᴵᴵ is also similar to that of PHA-II (i.e., hyperkalemia, acidosis, and hypercalciuria, with a suppressed expression of renal renin). TgWnk4ᴾᴴᴬᴵᴵ mice also exhibit marked hyperplasia of the DCT, compared to a relative hypoplasia in the TgWnk4ᵂᵀ mice; morphology and phenotype of the CCD was not particularly affected. Of particular significance, the DCT hyperplasia of TgWnk4ᴾᴴᴬᴵᴵ mice was completely suppressed on an NCC-deficient background, generated by mating TgWnk4ᴾᴴᴬᴵᴵ mice with NCC knockout mice.[240,241] Therefore, the DCT is the primary target for PHA-II associated mutations in WNK4. In addition, as suggested by prior studies[224,240,241] changes in Na⁺-Cl⁻ entry via NCC can evidently modulate hyperplasia or regression of the DCT.[251] Furthermore, the results obtained with transgenic mice[251] provide a dramatic validation of the selective use of Xenopus oocytes for the analysis of regulatory interactions with ion transport proteins such as NCC.[254–256]

Connecting Tubules and Cortical Collecting Duct

Apical Na⁺ Transport

The apical membrane of CNT cells and principal cells contain prominent Na⁺ and K⁺ conductances,[226,262] without a measurable apical conductance for Cl⁻.[195] The entry of Na⁺ occurs via the highly selective epithelial Na⁺ channel (ENaC), which is sensitive to micromolar concentrations of amiloride (see Fig. 5–19).[263] This selective absorption of positive charge generates a lumen-negative potential difference (PD), the magnitude of which varies considerably as a function of mineralocorticoid status and other factors (see also Regulation of Na⁺-Cl⁻ transport in the CNT and CCD). This lumen-negative PD serves to drive the following critical processes: (1) K⁺ secretion via apical K⁺ channels; (2) paracellular Cl⁻ transport through the adjacent tight junctions; or (3) electrogenic H⁺ secretion via adjacent Type A intercalated cells.

ENaC is a heteromeric channel complex formed by the assembly of separate, homologous subunits, denoted α-, β-, and γ-ENaC.[264] These channel subunits share a common structure, with intracellular N- and C-terminal domains, two transmembrane segments, and a large glycosylated extracellular loop.[265] Xenopus oocytes expressing α-ENaC alone have detectable Na⁺ channel activity (Fig. 5–20), which facilitated the initial identification of this subunit by expression cloning; functional complementation of this modest activity was then utilized to clone the other two subunits by expression cloning.[264] Full channel activity requires the co-expression of all three subunits, which causes a dramatic increase in expression of the channel complex at the plasma membrane[266] (see Fig. 5–20). The subunit stoichiometry has been a source of considerable controversy, with some reports favoring a tetramer with ratios of two α-ENaC proteins to one each of β-, and γ-ENaC (2α:1β:1γ), and others favoring a higher-order assembly with a stoichiometry of 3α:3β:3γ.[267] Regardless, the single channel characteristics of heterologously expressed ENaC are essentially identical to the amiloride-sensitive channel detectable at the apical membrane of CCD cells.[263,264]

ENaC plays a critical role in renal Na⁺-Cl⁻ reabsorption and maintenance of the extracellular fluid volume (see also Regulation of Na⁺-Cl⁻ transport in the CNT and CCD). In particular, recessive loss-of-function mutations in the three subunits of ENaC are a cause of pseudohypoaldosteronism type I.[268] Patients with this syndrome typically present with severe neonatal salt wasting, hypotension, acidosis, and hyperkalemia; this dramatic phenotype underscores the critical roles of ENaC activity in renal Na⁺-Cl⁻ reabsorption, K⁺ secretion, and H⁺ secretion. Gain-of-function mutations in the β- and γ-ENaC subunits are in turn a cause of Liddle syndrome, an autosomal-dominant hypertensive syndrome accompanied by suppressed aldosterone and variable hypokalemia.[269] With one exception,[270] ENaC mutations associated with Liddle syndrome disrupt interactions between a PPxY motif in the C-terminus of channel subunits with the Nedd4-2 ubiquitin-ligase (see also Regulation of Na⁺-Cl⁻ transport in the CNT and CCD).

The ENaC protein is detectable at the apical membrane of CNT cells and principal cells within the CCD, OMCD, and IMCD.[228,232] Notably, however, several lines of evidence support the hypothesis that the CNT makes the dominant contribution to amiloride-sensitive Na⁺ reabsorption by the distal nephron. First, amiloride-sensitive Na⁺ currents in the CNT are twofold to fourfold higher than in the CCD; the maximal capacity of the CNT for Na⁺ reabsorption is estimated to be ~10 times higher than that of the CCD.[226] Second, targeted deletion of α-ENaC in the collecting duct abolishes amiloride-sensitive currents in CCD principal cells, but does not affect Na⁺ or K⁺ homeostasis; the residual ENaC expression in the late DCT and CNT of these knockout mice easily compensates for the loss of the channel in CCD cells.[271] Third, Na⁺/K⁺-ATPase activity in the CCD is considerably less than that of the DCT[14] (see also Fig. 5–4); this speaks to a greater capacity for transepithelial Na⁺-Cl⁻ absorption by the DCT

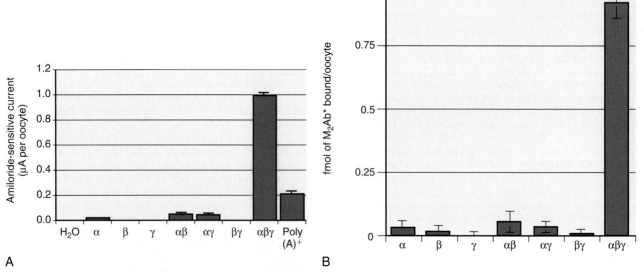

A

B

FIGURE 5–20 Maximal expression of the amiloride-sensitive epithelial Na⁺ channel (ENaC) at the plasma membrane requires the co-expression of all three subunits (α-, β-, and γ-ENaC). **A,** Amiloride-sensitive current in *Xenopus* oocytes expressing the individual subunits and various combinations thereof; channel activity is considerably enhanced in cells expressing all three subunits ("αβγ"). (From Canessa CM, Schild L, Buell G, et al: Amiloride-sensitive epithelial Na⁺ channel is made of three homologous subunits. Nature 367:463–467, 1994.) **B,** Surface expression is markedly enhanced in *Xenopus* oocytes that co-express all three subunits. The individual cDNAs were engineered with an external epitope tag; expression of the channel proteins at the cell surface is measured by binding of a monoclonal antibody to the tag. (From Firsov D, Schild L, Gautschi I, et al: Cell surface expression of the epithelial Na channel and a mutant causing Liddle syndrome: A quantitative approach. Proc Natl Acad Sci U S A 93:15370–15375, 1996.)

and CNT. Fourth, the apical recruitment of ENaC subunits in response to dietary Na^+ restriction begins in the CNT, with progressive recruitment of subunits in the downstream CCD at lower levels of dietary Na^{+272}; under conditions of high Na^+-Cl^- and low K^+ intake, the bulk of aldosterone-stimulated Na^+ transport likely occurs prior to the entry of tubular fluid into the CCD.[273]

Cl^- Transport

There are two major pathways for Cl^- absorption in the CNT and CCD; paracellular transport across the tight junction, and transcellular transport across type B intercalated cells (Fig. 5–21).[227,274] The CNT and CCD are "tight" epithelia, with comparatively low paracellular permeability that is not selective for Cl^- over Na^+; however, voltage-driven paracellular Cl^- transport in the CCD may play a considerable role in transepithelial Na^+-Cl^- absorption.[275] The CNT, DCT, and collecting duct co-express claudin-3, -4, and -8[26,276]; claudin-8 in particular may function as a paracellular cation barrier that prevents backleak of Na^+, K^+, and H^+ in this segment of the nephron.[276] Regulated changes in paracellular permeability may also contribute to Cl^- absorption by the CNT and CCD.

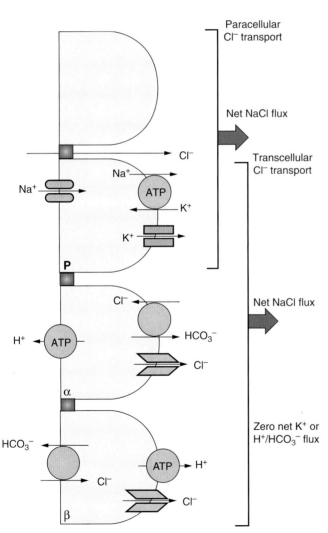

In particular, wild-type WNK4 appears to increase paracellular Cl^- permeability in transfected MDCK II cell lines; a WNK4 PHA-II mutant has a much larger effect, with no effect seen in cells expressing kinase-dead WNK4 constructs.[261] Yamauchi and co-workers have also reported that PHA-II–associated WNK4 increases paracellular permeability, due perhaps to an associated hyper-phosphorylation of claudin proteins.[277]

Transcellular Cl^- absorption across intercalated cells is thought to play a quantitatively greater role in the CNT and CCD than that of paracellular transport.[274] In the simplest scheme, this process requires the concerted function of both type A and type B intercalated cells, achieving net electrogenic Cl^- absorption without affecting HCO_3^- or H^+ excretion[274] (see also Fig. 5–21). Chloride thus enters type B intercalated cells via apical Cl^--HCO_3^- exchange, followed by exit from the cell via basolateral Cl^- channels. Recycling of Cl^- at the basolateral membrane of adjacent type A intercalated cells results in HCO_3^- absorption and extrusion of H^+ at the apical membrane. The net effect of apical Cl^--HCO_3^- exchange in type B intercalated cells, leading to apical secretion of HCO_3^-, and recycling of Cl^- at the basolateral membrane type A intercalated cells, leading to apical secretion of H^+, is electrogenic Cl^- absorption across type B intercalated cells (see Fig. 5–21).

At the basolateral membrane, intercalated cells have a very robust Cl^- conductance with transport characteristics similar to those of CLC-K2/Barttin.[195] CLC-K2 protein is also detected at the basolateral membrane of type A intercalated cells, although expression in type B cells was not clarified.[193] At the apical membrane, the SLC26A4 exchanger (also known as pendrin), has been conclusively identified as the elusive Cl^--HCO_3^- exchanger of type B and non-A, non-B intercalated cells[227]; this exchanger functions as the apical entry site during transepithelial Cl^- transport by the distal nephron. Human SLC26A4 is mutated in Pendred syndrome, which encompasses sensorineural hearing loss and goiter; these patients do not have an appreciable renal phenotype.[227] However, Slc26a4-deficient knockout mice are sensitive to restriction of dietary Na^+-Cl^-, developing hypotension during severe restriction.[278] Slc26a4 knockout mice are also resistant to mineralocorticoid-induced hypertension.[370] Finally, dietary Cl^- restriction with provision of Na^+-HCO_3^- results in Cl^- wasting in Slc26a4 knockout mice and increased apical expression of Slc26a4 protein in the type B intercalated cells of normal littermate controls.[280] Therefore, Slc26a4 plays a critical role in distal nephron Cl^- absorption, underlining the particular importance of transcellular Cl^- transport in this process.

Regulation of Na^+-Cl^- Transport in the Connecting Tubule and Cortical Collecting Duct
Aldosterone
The DCT, CNT, and collecting ducts collectively constitute the aldosterone-sensitive distal nephron, expressing both the mineralocorticoid receptor and the 11β-hydroxysteroid dehydrogenase-2 (11β-HSD2) enzyme that protects against illicit activation by glucocorticoids.[224] Aldosterone plays perhaps the dominant positive role in the regulation of distal nephron Na^+-Cl^- transport, with a plethora of mechanisms and transcriptional targets.[281] For example, aldosterone increases expression of the Na^+/K^+-ATPase α-1 and β-1 subunits in the CCD,[282] in addition to inducing Slc26a4, the apical Cl^--HCO_3^- exchanger of intercalated cells.[279] Adosterone may also affect paracellular permeability of the distal nephron, via posttranscriptional modification of claudins and other components of the tight junction.[283] However, particularly impressive progress has been made in the understanding of the downstream

FIGURE 5–21 Transepithelial Cl^- transport by principal and intercalated cells. The lumen-negative PD generated by principal cells drives paracellular Cl^- absorption. Alternatively, transepithelial transport occurs in type B intercalated cells, via apical Cl^--HCO_3^- exchange (SLC26A4/pendrin) and basolateral Cl^- exit via CLC-K2.

effects of aldosterone on synthesis, trafficking, and membrane-associated activity of ENaC subunits.

Aldosterone increases abundance of α-ENaC, via a glucocorticoid-response element in promoter of the SCNN1A gene that encodes this subunit.[284] This transcriptional activation results in an increased abundance of α-ENaC protein in response to either exogenous aldosterone or dietary Na+-Cl− restriction[285,286] (Fig. 5–22); the response to Na+-Cl− restriction is blunted by spironolactone, indicating involvement of the mineralocorticoid receptor.[250] At baseline, α-ENaC transcripts in the kidney are less abundant than those encoding β- and γ-ENaC[287] (see Fig. 5–22). All three subunits are required for efficient processing of heteromeric channels in the endoplasmic reticulum and trafficking to the plasma membrane (see Fig. 5–20), such that the induction of α-ENaC is thought to relieve a major "bottleneck" in the processing and trafficking of active ENaC complexes.[287]

Aldosterone also plays an indirect role in the regulated trafficking of ENaC subunits to the plasma membrane, via the regulation of accessory proteins that interact with pre-existing ENaC subunits. Aldosterone rapidly induces expression of a serine-threonine kinase denoted SGK-1 (serum and glucocorticoid-induced kinase-1)[288,289]; co-expression of SGK-1 with ENaC subunits in *Xenopus* oocytes results in a dramatic activation of the channel, due to increased expression at the plasma membrane.[286] Notably, an analogous redistribution of ENaC subunits occurs in the CNT and early CCD, from a largely cytoplasmic location during dietary Na+-Cl− excess to a purely apical distribution after aldosterone or Na+-Cl− restriction (see Fig. 5–22).[250,272,286] Furthermore, there is a temporal correlation between the appearance of induced SGK-1 protein in the CNT and the redistribution of ENaC protein to the plasma membrane.[286]

SGK-1 modulates membrane expression of ENaC by interfering with regulated endocytosis of its channel subunits. Specifically, the kinase interferes with interactions between ENaC subunits and the ubiquitin-ligase Nedd4-2.[287] PPxY domains in the C-termini of all three ENaC subunits bind to WW domains of Nedd4-2[290]; these PPxY domains are deleted, truncated, or mutated in patients with Liddle syndrome,[269] leading to a gain-of-function in channel activity.[266] Co-expression of Nedd4-2 with wild-type ENaC channel results in a marked inhibition of channel activity due to retrieval from the cell membrane, whereas channels bearing Liddle

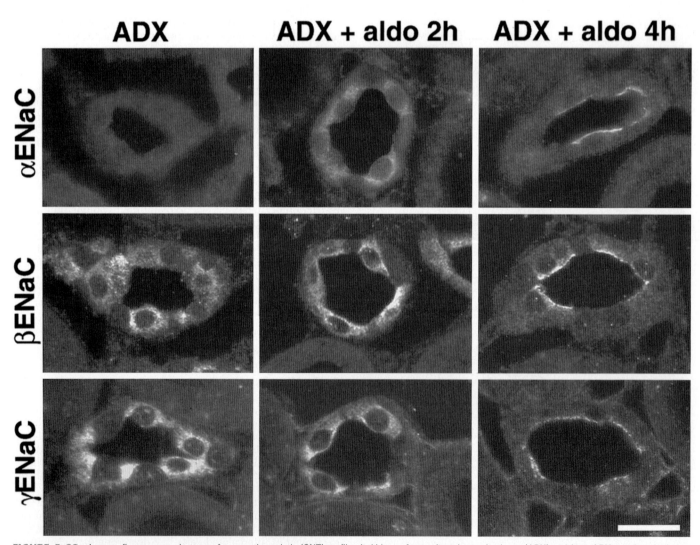

FIGURE 5–22 Immunofluorescence images of connecting tubule (CNT) profiles in kidneys from adrenalectomized rats (ADX) and from ADX rats 2 and 4 hours after aldosterone injection. Antibodies against the α-, β-, and γ-subunits of ENaC reveal absent expression of the former in ADX rats, with progressive induction by aldosterone. All three subunits traffic to the apical membrane in response to aldosterone. This coincides with rapid aldosterone induction of the SGK kinase in the same cells; SGK is known to increase the expression of ENaC at the plasma membrane (see text for details). Bar ~ 15 μm. (From Loffing J, Zecevic M, Feraille E, et al. Aldosterone induces rapid apical translocation of ENaC in early portion of renal collecting system: Possible role of SGK. Am J Physiol Renal Physiol 280:F675–682, 2001.)

syndrome mutations are resistant; Nedd4-2 is thought to ubiquitinate ENaC subunits, resulting in the removal of channel subunits from the cell membrane and degradation in lysosomes and the proteosome.[287] A PPxY domain in SGK-1 also binds to Nedd4-2, which is a phosphorylation substrate for the kinase; phosphorylation of Nedd4-2 by SGK-1 abrogates its inhibitory effect on ENaC subunits.[291,292] Aldosterone also stimulates Nedd4-2 phosphorylation in vivo.[293] Nedd4-2 phosphorylation in turn results in ubiquitin-mediated degradation of SGK-1,[294] suggest that there is considerable feedback regulation in this system. Furthermore, the hormone reduces Nedd4-2 protein expression in cultured CCD cells,[295] suggesting additional levels of in vivo regulation.

The induction of SGK-1 by aldosterone thus appears to stimulate the redistribution of ENaC subunits from the cytoplasm to the apical membrane of CNT and CCD cells. This phenomenon involves SGK-1-dependent phosphorylation of the Nedd4-2 ubiquitin ligase, which is co-expressed with ENaC and SGK-1 in the distal nephron.[295] Of note, there is considerable axial heterogeneity in the recruitment and redistribution of ENaC to the plasma membrane, which begins in the CNT and only extends into the CCD and OMCD in Na$^+$-Cl$^-$ restricted or aldosterone-treated animals.[224,286] The underlying causes of this progressive axial recruitment are not as yet clear.[224] However, Nedd4-2 expression is inversely related to the apical distribution of ENaC, with low expression in the CNT and increased expression levels in the CCD[295]; in all likelihood, the relative balance between SGK-1, ENaC, and Nedd4-2 figures prominently in the recruitment of the channel subunits to the apical membrane.

Finally, aldosterone indirectly activates ENaC channels through the induction of "channel activating proteases", which increase open channel probability by cleavage of the extracellular domain of α- and γ-ENaC. Western blotting of renal tissue from rats subjected to Na$^+$-Cl$^-$ restriction or treatment with aldosterone reveals α- and γ-ENaC subunits of lower molecular mass than those detected in control animals, indicating that aldosterone induces proteolytic cleavage.[285,296] Proteases that have been implicated in the processing of ENaC include furin, elastase, and three novel, membrane-associated proteases denoted CAP1-3 (channel activating proteases-1/2/3).[297,298] CAP1 was initially identified from Xenopus A6 cells as an ENaC activating protease[299]; the mammalian ortholog is an aldosterone-induced protein in principal cells.[300] Urinary excretion of CAP1, also known as prostasin, is increased in hyperaldosteronism, with a reduction after adrenalectomy.[300] CAP1 is tethered to the plasma membrane by a glycosylphosphatidylinositol (GPI) linkage,[299] whereas CAP2 and CAP3 are transmembrane proteases.[298] All three of these proteases activate ENaC by increasing the open probability of the channel, without increasing expression at the cell surface.[298] Proteolytic cleavage of ENaC appears to activate the channel by removing the "self-inhibitory" effect of external Na$^+$[297]; in the case of furin-mediated proteolysis of αENaC, this appears to involve the removal of an inhibitory domain from within the extracellular loop.[301] Unprocessed channels at the plasma membrane are thought to function as a "reserve pool", capable of rapid activation by membrane-associated luminal proteases.[297]

One would expect synergistic activation by co-expressed CAP1-3 and SGK-1, given that this kinase increases channel expression at the cell surface[286]; this is indeed the case.[298] Notably, the C-terminal mutations that cause Liddle syndrome, which abrogate interaction with Nedd4-2, appear to have a greater relative effect on channel activity than on surface expression[266]; this observation led to a longstanding controversy as to whether the gain-of-function in these mutant channels is partially due to an increase in channel activity at the membrane.[302] This issue has been dramatically resolved by the observation that Liddle syndrome mutations result in an increased proportion of cleaved channels at the plasma membrane; dominant-negative inhibition of Nedd4-2 leads to a similar increased in processing at the cell membrane, whereas over-expression of wild-type Nedd4-2 has the opposite effect.[302] Therefore, aldosterone-dependent induction of SGK-1 also affects protease-dependent cleavage and activation of ENaC at the cell membrane, in addition to reducing Nedd4-2-dependent degradation of the channel.

Vasopressin and Other Factors

Although not classically considered an anti-natriuretic hormone, vasopressin has well-characterized stimulatory effects on Na$^+$-Cl$^-$ transport by the CCD.[82,303] In perfused rat CCD segments, vasopressin and aldosterone can have synergistic effects on Na$^+$ transport, with a combined effect that exceeds that of the individual hormones.[303] Prostaglandins inhibit this effect of vasopressin, particularly in the rabbit CCD; this inhibition occurs at least in part through reductions in vasopressin-generated cAMP.[82,303] There are however considerable species-dependent differences in the interactions between vasopressin and negative modulators of Na$^+$-Cl$^-$ transport in the CCD, which include prostaglandins, bradykinin, endothelin, and α$_2$-adrenergic tone.[82,303] Regardless, cyclic-AMP causes a rapid increase in the Na$^+$ conductance of apical membranes in the CCD; this effect appears to be due to increases in surface expression of ENaC subunits at the plasma membrane,[304] in addition to effects on open channel probability (reviewed in Ref 305). Notably, cyclic-AMP inhibits retrieval of ENaC subunits from the plasma membrane, via PKA-dependent phosphorylation of the phosphoacceptor sites in Nedd4-2 that are targeted by SGK-1[306]; therefore, both aldosterone and vasopressin converge on Nedd4-2 in the regulation of ENaC activity in the distal nephron. Analogous to the effect on trafficking of aquaporin-2 in principal cells, cAMP also seems to stimulate exocytosis of ENaC subunits to the plasma membrane.[305] Finally, similar to the long-term effects of vasopressin on aquaporin-2 expression and NKCC2 expression,[207] chronic treatment with dDAVP results in an increase in abundance of the β- and γ-ENaC subunits.[307]

Systemic generation of circulating angiotensin II (ANGII) induces aldosterone release by the adrenal gland, with downstream activation of ENaC. However, ANGII also activates amiloride-sensitive Na$^+$ transport directly in perfused CCDs; blockade by losartan or candesartan suggests that this activation is mediated by AT$_1$ receptors.[308] Of particular significance, the effect of luminal ANGII (10^{-9}) was greater than that of bath ANGII, suggesting that intra-tubular ANGII may regulate ENaC in the distal nephron. Similar stimulation of ENaC is seen when tubules are perfused with ANGI; this effect is blocked by ACE-inhibition with captopril, indicating that intraluminal conversion of ANGI to ANGII can occur in the CCD.[309] Notably, CNT cells express considerable amounts of immunoreactive renin, versus the vanishingly low expression of renin mRNA in the proximal tubule.[310] Angiotensinogen secreted into the tubule by proximal tubule cells[310] may thus be converted to ANGII in the CNT via locally generated renin and angiotensin converting enzyme, and/or related proteases.

As in other segments of the nephron, Na$^+$-Cl$^-$ transport by the CNT and CCD is modulated by metabolites of arachidonic acid generated by cytochrome P450 mono-oxygenases. In particular, arachidonic acid inhibits ENaC channel activity in the rat CCD, via generation of the epoxygenase product 11,12-EET (epoxyeicosatreinoic acid) by the CYP2C23 enzyme expressed in principal cells.[311] Targeted deletion of the murine Cyp4a10 enzyme, another P450 mono-oxygenase, results in salt-sensitive hypertension; urinary excretion of 11,12-EET is reduced in these knockout mice, with a blunted effect of arachidonic acid on ENaC channel activity in the CCD.[312] These mice also became normotensive after treatment with amiloride, indicative of *in vivo* activation of ENaC. It appears that deletion of Cyp4a10 reduces activity of the murine ortholog of rat CYPC23 (Cyp2c44 in mouse), and/or related expoxygenases, via reduced generation of a ligand for PPARα (peroxisome proliferator-activated receptor-α) that induces expoxygenase activity.[312] The mechanism(s) whereby 11,12-EET inhibits ENaC are unknown as of yet. However, renal 11,12-EET production is known to be salt-sensitive, suggesting that generation of this mediator may serve to reduce ENaC activity during high dietary Na^+-Cl^- intake.[311]

Finally, activation of PPARγ by thiazolidinediones results in amiloride-sensitive hypertension, suggesting *in vivo* activation of ENaC.[313,314] Thiazolidinediones (TZDs—rosiglitazone, pioglitazone, and troglitazone) are insulin-sensitizing drugs utilized for the management of type II diabetes. Treatment with these agents is frequently associated with fluid retention, suggesting an effect on renal Na^+-Cl^- transport. Given robust expression of PPARγ in the collecting duct, activation of ENaC was an attractive hypothesis for this TZD-associated edema syndrome.[313,314] This appears to be the case, in that selective deletion of the murine PPARγ gene in principal cells abrogates the increase in amiloride-sensitive transport seen in response to TZDs.[313,314] TZDs appear to induce transcription of the Sccn1g gene encoding γENaC,[313] in addition to inducing SGK-1.[315] However, the mechanism(s) of this intriguing stimulation of ENaC activity are not completely clear, nor is the physiological renal ligand for PPARγ known. Regardless, the beneficial effect of spironolactone in type II diabetics with TZD-associated volume expansion is consistent with *in vivo* activation of ENaC in the aldosterone-responsive distal nephron.[316] In addition, the risk of peripheral edema is increased considerably in patients treated with both TZDs and insulin therapy.[316] Notably, insulin appears to activate ENaC via SGK1-dependent mechanisms,[317,318] such that this clinical observation may be a consequence of the synergistic activation of ENaC by insulin and TZDs.

POTASSIUM TRANSPORT

Maintenance of K^+ balance is important for a multitude of physiological processes. Changes in intracellular K^+ impact on cell volume regulation, regulation of intracellular pH, enzymatic function, protein synthesis,[319] DNA synthesis,[320] and apoptosis.[321] Changes in the ratio of intracellular to extracellular K^+ affect the resting membrane potential, leading to depolarization in hyperkalemia and hyperpolarization in hypokalemia. In consequence, disorders of extracellular K^+ have a dominant effect on excitable tissues, chiefly heart and muscle. In addition, a growing body of evidence implicates hypokalemia or reduced dietary K^+ (or both) in the pathobiology of hypertension, heart failure, and stroke[322]; these and other clinical consequences of K^+ disorders are reviewed in Chapter 15.

Potassium is predominantly an intracellular cation, with only 2% of total body K^+ residing in the extracellular fluid. Extracellular K^+ is maintained within a very narrow range by three primary mechanisms. First, the distribution of K^+ between the intracellular and extracellular space is determined by the activity of a number of transport pathways, namely Na^+/K^+-ATPase, the Na^+-K^+-$2Cl^-$ cotransporter NKCC1, the four K^+-Cl^- cotransporters, and a plethora of K^+ channels. In particular, skeletal muscle contains as much as 75% of body potassium (see Fig. 15–1), and exerts considerable influence on extracellular K^+. Short-term and long-term regulation of muscle Na^+/K^+-ATPase plays a dominant role in determining the distribution of K^+ between the intracellular and extracellular space; the various hormones and physiological conditions that affect the uptake of K^+ by skeletal muscle are reviewed in Chapter 15 (see Table 15–1). Second, the colon

has the ability to absorb and secrete K^+, with considerable mechanistic[323] and regulatory[324] similarities to renal K^+ secretion. K^+ secretion in the distal colon is increased after dietary loading[324] and in end-stage renal disease.[325] However, the colon has a relatively limited capacity for K^+ excretion, such that changes in renal K^+ excretion play the dominant role in responding to changes in K^+ intake. In particular, regulated K^+ secretion by the CNT and CCD play a critical role in the response to hyperkalemia and K^+ loading; increases in the reabsorption of K^+ by the CCD and OMCD function in the response to hypokalemia or K^+ deprivation.

This section will review the mechanisms and regulation of transepithelial K^+ transport along the nephron. As in other sections of this chapter, the emphasis will be on particularly recent developments in the molecular physiology of renal K^+ transport. Of note, transport pathways for K^+ play important roles in renal Na^+-Cl^- transport, particularly within the TAL; furthermore, Na^+ absorption via ENaC in the aldosterone-sensitive distal nephron generates a lumen-negative potential difference that drives distal K^+ excretion. These pathways are primarily discussed in the section on renal Na^+-Cl^- transport; related issues relevant to K^+ homeostasis *per se* will be specifically addressed in this section.

Proximal Tubule

The proximal tubule reabsorbs some 50% to 70% of filtered K^+ (Fig. 5–23). Proximal tubules generate minimal transepithelial K^+ gradients, and fractional reabsorption of K^+ is similar to that of Na^+.[229] K^+ absorption follows that of fluid, Na^+, and other solutes,[326,327] such that this nephron segment does not play a direct role in regulated renal excretion. Notably, however, changes in Na^+-Cl^- reabsorption by the proximal tubule have considerable effects on distal tubular flow and distal tubular Na^+ delivery, with attendant effects on the excretory capacity for K^+ (see K^+ secretion by the DCT, CNT, and CCD).

The mechanisms involved in transepithelial K^+ transport by the proximal tubule are not completely clear, although active

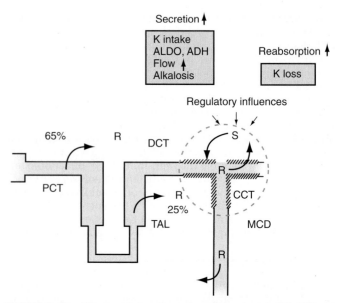

FIGURE 5–23 K^+ transport along the nephron. Approximately 90% of filtered K^+ is reabsorbed by the proximal tubule and the loop of Henle. K^+ is secreted along the initial and cortical collecting tubule; net reabsorption occurs in response to K^+ depletion, primarily within the medullary collecting duct. PCT, proximal tubule; TAL, thick ascending limb; CCT, cortical collecting tubule; DCT, distal convoluted tubule; S, secretion; R, reabsorption; ALDO, aldosterone; ADH, antidiuretic hormone; MCD, medullary collecting duct; ICT, initial connecting tubule.

transport does not appear to play a major role.[327,328] Luminal barium has modest effects on transepithelial K⁺ transport by the proximal tubule, suggesting a component of transcellular transport via barium-sensitive K⁺ channels.[329] However, the bulk of K⁺ transport is thought to occur via the paracellular pathway,[329,330] driven by the lumen-positive potential difference in the mid-to-late proximal tubule (see Fig. 5–3). The total K⁺ permeability of the proximal tubule is thus rather high, apparently due to characteristics of the paracellular pathway.[329,330] The combination of luminal K⁺ concentrations that are ~10% higher than that of plasma, a lumen-positive PD of ~2 mV (see Fig. 5–3), and high paracellular permeability leads to considerable paracellular absorption in the proximal tubule. This absorption is thought to primarily proceed via convective transport—"solvent drag" due to frictional interactions between water and K⁺—rather than diffusional transport.[331] Notably, however, the primary pathway for water movement in the proximal tubule is quite conclusively transcellular, via Aquaporin-1 and Aquaporin-7 water channels in the apical and basolateral membrane.[18,28,29] Therefore, the apparent convective transport of K⁺ would have to constitute "pseudo-solvent drag", with hypothetical, uncharacterized interactions between water traversing the transcellular route and diffusion of K⁺ along the paracellular pathway.[331]

The Loop of Henle and Medullary K⁺ Recycling

Transport by the loop of Henle plays a critical role in medullary K⁺ recycling (Fig. 5–24). Several lines of evidence indicate that a considerable fraction of K⁺ secreted by the CCD is reabsorbed by the medullary collecting ducts and then secreted into the late proximal tubule or descending thin limbs of long-looped nephrons (or both).[332] In potassium-loaded rats there is thus a doubling of luminal K⁺ in terminal thin descending limbs, with a sharp drop after inhibition of CCD K⁺ secretion by amiloride.[333] Enhancement of CCD K⁺ secretion by treatment with dDAVP also results in an increase in luminal K⁺ in descending thin limbs.[334] This recycling pathway (secretion in CCD, absorption in OMCD and IMCD,

secretion in descending thin limb) is associated with a marked increase in medullary interstitial K⁺. Passive transepithelial K⁺ absorption by the thin ascending limb and active absorption by the thick ascending limb (TAL)[171] also contribute to this increase in interstitial K⁺ (see Fig. 5–24). Specifically, the absorption of K⁺ by ascending thin limb, TAL, and OMCD exceeds the secretion by descending thin limbs, thus trapping K⁺ in the interstitium.

The physiological significance of medullary K⁺ recycling is not completely clear. However, an increase in interstitial K⁺ from 5 mM to 25 mM dramatically inhibits Cl⁻ transport by perfused thick ascending limbs.[171] By inhibiting Na⁺-Cl⁻ absorption by the TAL, increases in interstitial K⁺ would increase Na⁺ delivery to the CNT and CCD, thus enhancing the lumen-negative PD in these tubules and increasing K⁺ secretion.[171] Alternatively, the marked increase in medullary interstitial K⁺ after dietary K⁺ loading serves to limit the difference between luminal and peritubular K⁺ in the collecting duct, thus minimizing passive K⁺ loss from the collecting duct.

K⁺ is secreted into descending thin limbs by passive diffusion, driven by the high medullary interstitial K⁺ concentration. Descending thin limbs thus have a very high K⁺ permeability, without evidence for active transepithelial K⁺ transport.[335] Transepithelial K⁺ transport by ascending thin limbs has not to our knowledge been measured; however, as is the case for Na⁺-Cl⁻ transport (see Na⁺-Cl⁻ transport in the thin ascending limb), the absorption of K⁺ by thin ascending limbs is presumably passive. Active transepithelial K⁺ transport across the TAL includes both a transcellular component, via apical Na⁺-K⁺-2Cl⁻ cotransport mediated by NKCC2, and a paracellular pathway (see Fig. 5–15). Luminal K⁺ channels play a critical role in generating the lumen-positive PD in the TAL, as summarized in the section on Na⁺-Cl⁻ transport (see Na⁺-Cl⁻ transport in the TAL; apical K⁺ channels).

K⁺ Secretion by the Distal Convoluted Tubule, Connecting Tubule, and Cortical Collecting Duct

Approximately 90% of filtered K⁺ is reabsorbed by the proximal tubule and loop of Henle (see Fig. 5–23); the "fine tuning" of renal K⁺ excretion occurs in the remaining distal nephron. The bulk of regulated secretion occurs in principal cells within the CNT and CCD, whereas K⁺ reabsorption primarily occurs in the OMCD (see later). K⁺ secretion is initially detectable in the early DCT,[336] where NCC-positive cells express ROMK, the apical K⁺ secretory channel.[178] Classically, the CCD is considered the primary site for distal K⁺ secretion, partially due to the greater ease with which this segment is perfused and studied. However, as is the case for Na⁺-Cl⁻ absorption (see Na⁺-Cl⁻ transport in the CNT and CCD; apical Na⁺ transport), the bulk of distal K⁺ secretion appears to occur prior to the CCD,[229] within the CNT.[337]

In principal cells, apical Na⁺ entry via ENaC generates a lumen-negative potential difference, which drives passive K⁺ exit through apical K⁺ channels. Distal K⁺ secretion is therefore dependent on delivery of adequate luminal Na⁺ to the CNT and CCD,[338,339] essentially ceasing when luminal Na⁺ drops below 8 mmol/L.[340] Dietary Na⁺ intake also influences K⁺ excretion, such that excretion is enhanced by excess Na⁺ intake and reduced by Na⁺ restriction (see Fig. 15–4).[338,339] Secreted K⁺ enters principal cells via the basolateral Na⁺/K⁺-ATPase, which also generates the gradient that drives apical Na⁺ entry via ENaC (see Fig. 5–23).

Two major subtypes of apical K⁺ channels function in secretion by the CNT and CCD, +/– DCT; a small-conductance (SK) 30 pS channel[337,341] and a large-conductance, Ca²⁺-activated 150 pS ("maxi-K") channel.[179,226] The density and high open

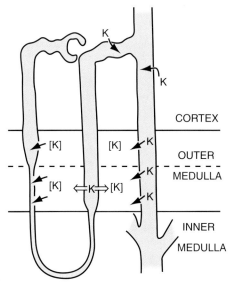

FIGURE 5–24 Schematic representation of medullary K⁺ recycling. Medullary interstitial K⁺ increases considerably after dietary K⁺ loading, due to the combined effects of secretion in the CCD, absorption in OMCD, TAL, and IMCD, and secretion in descending thin limb (see text for details). (Redrawn from Stokes JB: Consequences of potassium recycling in the renal medulla. Effects of ion transport by the medullary thick ascending limb of Henle's loop. J Clin Invest 70:219–229, 1982.)

probability of the SK channel indicates that this pathway alone is sufficient to mediate the bulk of K^+ secretion in the CCD under baseline conditions,[342] hence its designation as the "secretory" K^+ channel. Notably, SK channel density is considerably higher in the CNT than in the CCD,[337] consistent with the greater capacity for Na^+ absorption and K^+ secretion in the CNT. The characteristics of the SK channel are similar to those of the ROMK K^+ channel,[343] and ROMK protein has been localized at the apical membrane of principal cells.[178] SK channel activity is absent from apical membranes of the CCD in homozygous knockout mice with a targeted deletion of the Kcnj1 gene that encodes ROMK, definitive proof that ROMK is the SK channel.[179] The observation that these knock-out mice are normokalemic with an increased excretion of K^+ illustrates the considerable redundancy in distal K^+ secretory pathways[179]; distal K^+ secretion in these mice is mediated by apical maxi-K channels[344] (see later). Of interest, loss-of-function mutations in human KCNJ1 are associated with Bartter syndrome; ROMK expression is critical for the 30 pS and 70 pS channels that generate the lumen-positive PD in the TAL[179,180] (see Fig. 5–15). These patients typically have slightly higher serum K^+ than the other genetic forms of Bartter syndrome,[172] and affected patients with severe neonatal hyperkalemia have also been described[345]; this neonatal hyperkalemia is presumably the result of a transient developmental deficit in apical maxi-K channel activity.

The apical Ca^{2+}-activated maxi-K channel plays a critical role in flow-dependent K^+ secretion by the CNT and CCD.[341] Maxi-K channels have a heteromeric structure, with α-subunits that form the ion channel pore and modulatory β-subunits that affect the biophysical, regulatory, and pharmacological characteristics of the channel complex.[341] Maxi-K α-subunit transcripts are expressed in multiple nephron segments, and channel protein is detectable at the apical membrane of principal and intercalated cells in the CCD and CNT.[341] Increased distal flow has a well-established stimulatory effect on K^+ secretion, due in part to both enhanced delivery and absorption of Na^+ and to increased removal of secreted K^+,[338,339] but also due to the activation of apical K^+ conductance. The pharmacology of flow-dependent K^+ secretion in the CCD is consistent with dominant involvement of maxi-K channels,[346] and flow-dependent K^+ secretion is reduced in mice with targeted deletion of the α1 and β1 subunits.[341] The physiological rationale for the presence of two apical secretory K^+ channels—ROMK/SK and maxiK channels—is not completely clear. However, the high density and higher open probability of SK/ROMK channels is perhaps better suited for a role in basal K^+ secretion, with additional recruitment of the higher capacity, flow-activated maxi-K channels when additional K^+ secretion is required.[341]

Other K^+ channels reportedly expressed at the luminal membranes of the CNT and CCD include voltage-sensitive channels such as Kv1.3,[347,348] double-pore K^+ channels such as TWIK-1,[349] and KCNQ1.[350] KCNQ1 mediates K^+ secretion in the inner ear and is expressed at the apical membrane of principal cells in the CCD,[350] whereas TWIK-1 is expressed at the apical membrane of intercalated cells.[349] The role of these channels in renal K^+ secretion or absorption is not as yet known.

K^+ channels present at the basolateral membrane of principal cells appear to set the resting potential of the basolateral membrane, and function in K^+ secretion and Na^+ absorption at the apical membrane, the latter via K^+ recycling at the basolateral membrane to maintain activity of the Na^+/K^+-ATPase. A variety of different K^+ channels have been described in the electrophysiological characterization of the basolateral membrane of principal cells, which has a number of technical barriers to overcome (reviewed in Ref 351). However, a singe predominant activity can be identified in principal cells from the rat CCD, using whole-cell recording techniques

under conditions in which ROMK is inhibited (low intracellular pH or presence of the ROMK inhibitor tertiapin-Q).[351] This basolateral current is TEA-insensitive, barium-sensitive, and acid-sensitive (pKa ~ 6.5), with a conductance of ~17 pS and weak inward-rectification. These properties do not correspond exactly to specific characterized K^+ channels, or combinations thereof. However, candidate inward-rectifying K^+ channel subunits that have been localized at the basolateral membrane of the CCD include Kir4.1, Kir5.1, Kir7.1, and Kir 2.3.[351] Notably, basolateral K^+ channel activity increases on a high-K^+ diet, suggesting a role in transepithelial K^+ secretion.[351]

In addition to apical K^+ channels, considerable evidence implicates apical K^+-Cl^- cotransport (or functionally equivalent pathways[352]) in distal K^+ secretion.[59,338,353] Thus in rat distal tubules, a reduction in luminal Cl^- markedly increases K^+ secretion[354]; the replacement of luminal Cl^- with SO_4^- or gluconate has an equivalent stimulatory effect on K^+ secretion. This anion-dependent component of K^+ secretion is not influenced by luminal Ba^{2+},[354] suggesting that it does not involve apical K^+ channel activity. Perfused surface distal tubules are a mixture of distal convoluted tubule (DCT), connecting segment, and initial collecting duct (see Fig. 5–18); however, Cl^--coupled K^+ secretion is detectable in both the DCT and in early CNT.[355] In addition, similar pathways are detectable in rabbit CCD, where a decrease in luminal Cl^- from 112 mmol/L to 5 mmol/L increases K^+ secretion by 48%.[356] A reduction in basolateral Cl^- also decreases K^+ secretion without an effect on transepithelial voltage or Na^+ transport, and the direction of K^+ flux can be reversed by a lumen-to-bath Cl^- gradient, resulting in K^+ absorption.[356] In perfused CCDs from rats treated with mineralocorticoid, vasopressin increases K^+ secretion[357]; because this increase in K^+ secretion is resistant to luminal Ba^{2+} (2 mmol/L), vasopressin may stimulate Cl^--dependent K^+ secretion.[356] Recent pharmacological studies of perfused tubules are consistent with K^+-Cl^- cotransport mediated by the KCCs[59,353]; however, of the three renal KCCs, only KCC1 is apically expressed along the nephron (D.B.M., unpublished observations). Other functional possibilities for Cl^--dependent K^+ secretion include parallel operation of apical H^+-K^+-exchange and Cl^--HCO_3^- exchange in type B intercalated cells.[352]

K^+ Reabsorption by the Collecting Duct

In addition to K^+ secretion, the distal nephron is capable of considerable reabsorption, primarily during restriction of dietary K^+.[229–231] This reabsorption is accomplished in large part by intercalated cells in the outer medullary collecting duct (OMCD), via the activity of apical H^+/K^+-ATPase pumps. Under K^+-replete conditions, apical H^+/K^+-ATPase activity recycles K^+ with an apical K^+ channel, without effect on transepithelial K^+ absorption. Under K^+-restricted conditions, K^+ absorbed via apical H^+/K^+-ATPase appears to exit intercalated cells via a basolateral K^+ channel, thus achieving the transepithelial transport of K^+.[358]

H^+-K^+-ATPase holoenzymes are members of the P-type family of ion transport ATPases, which also includes subunits of the basolateral Na^+-K^+-ATPase.[359] HKα-1 and HKα-2 are also referred to as the "gastric" and "colonic" subunits, respectively; humans also have an HKα-4 subunit.[359,360] A specific HKβ subunit interacts with the HKα subunits to ensure delivery to the cell surface and complete expression of H^+-K^+-ATPase activity[361]; HKα-2 and HKα-4 subunits are also capable of interaction with Na^+-K^+-ATPase β subunits.[362,363] The pharmacology of H^+-K^+-ATPase holoenzymes differs considerably, such that the gastric HKα-1 is classically sensitive to the H^+-K^+-ATPase inhibitors SCH-28080 and omeprazole and resistant to ouabain; the colonic HKα-2 subunit is usually sensitive to ouabain and resistant to SCH-28080.[361] Within the kidney, the HKα-1 subunit is expressed at the apical membrane of at least a subset of type A intercalated cells in the distal nephron.[360] HKα-2 distribution in the distal nephron is more diffuse,[364] with robust expression at the apical membrane of type A and B intercalated cells and connecting segment cells and lesser expression in principal cells.[365,366] The human HKα-4 subunit is reportedly expressed in intercalated cells.[360]

HKα-1 and HKα-2 are both constitutively expressed in the distal nephron. However, tubule perfusion of K+-replete animals suggests a functional dominance of omeprazole/SCH-28080-sensitive, oubain-resistant H+-K+-ATPase activity, consistent with holoenzymes containing HKα-1.[367] K+ deprivation increases the overall activity of H+-K+-ATPase in the collecting duct, with the emergence of a oubain-sensitive H+-K+-ATPase activity[368,369]; this is consistent with a relative dominance of HKα-2 during K+-restricted conditions. K+-restriction also induces a dramatic up-regulation of HKα-2 transcript and protein in the outer and inner medulla during K+ depletion[370,371]; HKα-1 expression is unaffected.[370,371] Mice with a targeted deletion of HKα-2 exhibit lower plasma and muscle K+ than wild-type littermates when maintained on a K+-deficient diet. However, this appears to be due to marked loss of K+ in the colon rather than kidney because renal K+ excretion is appropriately reduced in the K+-depleted knockout mice.[372] Presumably the lack of an obvious renal phenotype in either HKα-1[373] or HKα-2[372] knockout mice reflects the marked redundancy in the expression of HKα subunits in the distal nephron. Indeed, collecting ducts from the HKα-1 knockout mice have significant residual oubain-resistant and SCH-28080-sensitive H+-K+-ATPase activities, consistent with the expression of other HKα subunits that confer characteristics similar to the "gastric" H+-K+-ATPase.[374] However, more recent data from HKα-1 and HKα-2 knockout mice suggest that compensatory mechanisms in these mice are not accounted for by ATPase-type mechanisms.[375]

The importance of K+ reabsorption mediated by the collecting duct is dramatically illustrated by the phenotype of transgenic mice with generalized over-expression of a gain-of-function mutation in H+-K+-ATPase, effectively bypassing the redundancy and complexity of this reabsorptive pathway. This transgene expresses a mutant form of the HKβ subunit, in which a tyrosine-to-alanine mutation within the C-terminal tail abrogates regulated endocytosis from the plasma membrane; these mice have higher plasma K+ than their wild-type littermates, with approximately half the fractional excretion of K+.[376]

Regulation of Distal K+ Transport

Aldosterone and K+ Loading

Aldosterone has a potent kaliuretic effect,[377] with important inter-relationships between circulating K+ and aldosterone. Aldosterone release by the adrenal is thus induced by hyperkalemia or a high K+ diet (or both), suggesting an important "feedback" effect of aldosterone on K+ homeostasis.[378] Aldosterone also has clinically relevant effects on K+ homeostasis, with a clear relationship at all levels of serum K+ between circulating levels of the hormone and the ability to excrete K+ (see Chapter 15 and Fig. 15–4).

Aldosterone has no effect on the density of apical SK channels in the CCD[379]; it does however induce a marked increase in the density of apical Na+ channels in the CNT and CCD.[379] This hormone activates ENaC via inter-related effects on the synthesis, trafficking, and membrane-associated activity of the subunits encoding the channel (see Regulation of Na+-Cl− transport in the CNT and CCD). Aldosterone is thus induced by high K+ diet (see Table 5–1), and strongly stimulates apical ENaC activity, which provides the lumen-negative PD that stimulates K+ secretion by principal cells.

The important relationships between K+ and aldosterone notwithstanding, it is increasingly clear that much of the adaptation to high K+ intake is aldosterone-independent. For example, a high K+ diet in adrenalectomized animals increases apical Na+ reabsorption and K+ secretion in the CCD.[380] At the tubular level, when basolateral K+ is increased there is a significant activation of the Na+/K+-ATPase, accompanied by a secondary activation of apical Na+ and K+ channels.[381] Increased dietary K+ also markedly increases the density of SK channels in the CCD, along with a modest increase in Na+ channel (ENaC) density[379]; this is associated with changes in the subcellular distribution of the ROMK protein, with an increase in apical expression.[382] Notably, this increase in ENaC and SK density in the CCD occurs within hours of assuming a high K+ diet, with a minimal associated increase in circulating aldosterone[383] (Fig. 5–25 and Table 5–1). In

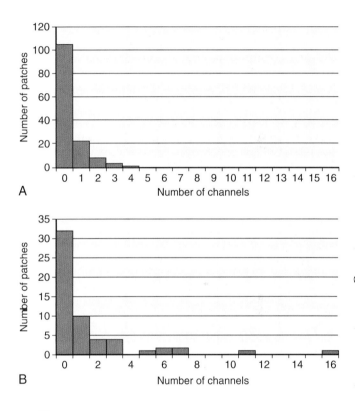

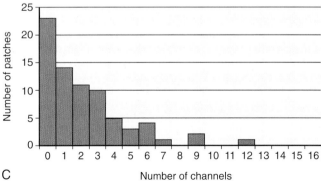

FIGURE 5–25 High K+ diet rapidly activates SK channels in the CCD, mediated by the ROMK (Kir 1.1) K+ channel. Histograms of *N* (channels/patch) are shown for rats on control diet (**A**), on a high-K diet for 6 hours (**B**), and on a high-K diet for 48 hours (**C**). Each determination of *N* represents a single cell-attached patch. High K+ diet results in a progressive recruitment of SK channels at the apical membrane. (From Palmer LG, Frindt G: Regulation of apical K channels in rat cortical collecting tubule during changes in dietary K intake. Am J Physiol 277:F805–812, 1999.)

TABLE 5–1	Effect of High K⁺ Diet, Aldosterone, and/or Na⁺-Cl⁻ Restriction on SK Channel Density in the Rat Cortical Collecting Duct		
Condition	K Channel Density/μm^2	Plasma aldo (ng/dL)	Plasma K (mM)
Control	0.41	15	3.68
High K diet, 6 h	1.51	36	NM
High K diet, 48 h	2.13	98	4.37
Low Na diet, 7 days	0.48	1260	NM
Aldo infusion, 48 h	0.44	550	2.44
Aldo + High K diet	0.32	521	3.80

Modified from Palmer LG, Frindt G: Regulation of apical K channels in rat cortical collecting tubule during changes in dietary K intake. Am J Physiol 277:F805–812, 1999.

contrast, a week of low Na⁺-Cl⁻ intake, with almost a thousand-fold increase in aldosterone, has no effect on SK channel density; nor for that matter does 2 days of aldosterone infusion, despite the development of hypokalemia[383] (Table 5–1). Of note, unlike the marked increase seen in the CCD,[379,383] the density of SK channels in the CNT is not increased by high dietary K⁺[337]; this suggests that SK channels in the CNT are already maximally active, consistent with a progressive, axial recruitment of transport capacity for Na⁺ and K⁺ along the distal nephron (see Na⁺-Cl⁻ transport in the CNT and CCD; apical Na⁺ transport).

Maxi-K channels in the CNT and CCD play an important role in the flow-activated component of distal K⁺ excretion[341]; these channels are also activated by dietary K⁺ loading. Flow-stimulated K⁺ secretion by the CCD of both mice[344] and rats[384] is thus enhanced on a high-K⁺ diet, with an absence of flow-dependent K⁺ secretion in rats on a low-K⁺ diet.[384] This is accompanied by the appropriate changes in transcript levels for α- and β₂₋₄-subunits of the maxi-K channel proteins in micro-dissected CCDs (β₁ subunits are restricted to the CNT[341]). Trafficking of maxi-K subunits is also affected by dietary K⁺, with largely intracellular distribution of α-subunits in K⁺-restricted rats and prominent apical expression in K⁺-loaded rats.[384]

The changes in trafficking and/or activity of the ROMK channel that are induced by dietary K⁺ appear in large part to involve tyrosine phosphorylation/dephosphorylation of the ROMK protein (see later). However, a recent series of reports have linked changes in expression of WNK1 kinase subunits in the response to high K⁺ diet. WNK1 and WNK4 were initially identified as causative genes for pseudohypoaldosteronism type II (PHA-II), also known as Gordon syndrome or "hereditary hypertension with hyperkalemia" (see also Regulation of Na⁺-Cl⁻ transport in the DCT). ROMK expression at the membrane of Xenopus oocytes is dramatically reduced by co-expression of WNK4; PHA-II–associated mutations dramatically increase this effect, suggesting a direction inhibition of SK channels in PHA-II.[260] The study of WNK1 is further complicated by the transcriptional complexity of its gene, which has at least three separate promoters and a number of alternative splice forms. In particular, the predominant intra-renal WNK1 isoform is generated by a distal nephron transcriptional site that bypasses the N-terminal exons that encode the kinase domain, yielding a kinase-deficient "short" isoform[385] ("WNK1-S"). Full-length WNK1 (WNK1-L) inhibits ROMK activity by inducing endocytosis of the channel protein[259,386,387]; kinase activity or the N-terminal kinase domain of WNK1 (or both) appear to be required for this effect,[259,387] although Cope and colleagues

have reported that a kinase-dead mutant of WNK1 is unimpaired.[386] The shorter WNK1-S isoform, which lacks the kinase domain, appears to inhibit the effect of WNK1-L.[259,387] The ratio of WNK1-S to WNK1-L transcripts is reduced by K⁺ restriction (greater endocytosis of ROMK)[259,388] and increased by K⁺ loading (reduced endocytosis of ROMK),[387,388] suggesting that this ratio between WNK1-S and WNK1-L functions as a "switch" to regulate distal K⁺ secretion. Notably, in contrast to the prior data in Xenopus oocytes,[260] changes in the apical distribution of ROMK protein in CNT or CCD segments were reportedly not detected in BAC-transgenic mice overexpressing wild-type WNK4 or a PHA-II mutant (see Regulation of Na⁺-Cl⁻ transport in the DCT)[251]; this does not, however, rule out a more direct role for WNK1 in trafficking of ROMK and/or the maxi-K channel.

K⁺ Deprivation

A reduction in dietary K⁺ leads within 24 hours to a dramatic drop in urinary K⁺ excretion.[388,389] This drop in excretion is due to both an induction of reabsorption by intercalated cells in the OMCD[230,231] and to a reduction in SK channel activity in principal cells.[390] The mechanisms involved in K⁺ reabsorption by intercalated cells are discussed earlier; notably, H⁺/K⁺-ATPase activity in the collecting duct does not appear to be regulated by aldosterone.[391]

Considerable progress has recently been made in defining the signaling pathways that regulate the activity of the SK channel (ROMK) in response to changes in dietary K⁺. Dietary K⁺ intake modulates trafficking of the ROMK channel protein to the plasma membrane of principal cells, with a marked increase in the relative proportion of intracellular channel protein in K⁺-depleted animals[382,392] and clearly defined expression at the plasma membrane of CCD cells from animals on a high K⁺ diet.[382] The membrane insertion and activity of ROMK is modulated by tyrosine phosphorylation of the channel protein, such that phosphorylation of tyrosine residue[337] stimulates endocytosis and dephosphorylation induces exocytosis[393,394]; this tyrosine phosphorylation appears to play a dominant role in the regulation of ROMK by dietary K⁺.[395] Whereas the levels of protein tyrosine phosphatase-1D do not vary with K⁺ intake, intra-renal activity of the cytoplasmic tyrosine kinases c-src and c-yes are inversely related to dietary K⁺ intake, with a decrease under high K⁺ conditions and a marked increase after several days of K⁺ restriction.[390,396] Localization studies indicate co-expression of c-src with ROMK in thick ascending limb and principal cells of the CCD.[382] Moreover, inhibition of protein tyrosine phosphatase activity, leading to a dominance of tyrosine phosphorylation, dramatically increases the proportion of intracellular ROMK in the CCD of animals on a high-K⁺ diet.[382]

The neurohumoral factors that induce the K⁺-dependent trafficking and expression of apical ROMK[382,392] and maxi-K channels[384] are not as yet known. However, a landmark study recently implicated the intra-renal generation of superoxide anions in the activation of cytoplasmic tyrosine kinases and downstream phosphorylation of the ROMK channel protein by K⁺ depletion.[397] Potential candidates for the upstream kaliuretic factor include angiotensin II and growth factors such as IGF-1.[397] Regardless, reports of a marked post-prandial kaliuresis in sheep, independent of changes in plasma K⁺ or aldosterone, have led to the suggestion that an enteric or hepatoportal K⁺ "sensor" controls kaliuresis via a sympathetic reflex.[398] Changes in dietary K⁺ absorption may thus have a direct "anticipatory" effect on K⁺ homeostasis, in the absence of changes in plasma K⁺. Such a "feedfoward" control has the theoretical advantage of greater stability because it operates prior to changes in plasma K⁺.[399] Notably, changes in ROMK phosphorylation status and insulin-sensitive muscle uptake can be seen in K⁺-deficient animals in the absence of a change in plasma K^+,[400] suggesting that upstream activation of the major mechanisms that serve to reduce K^+ excretion (reduced K^+ secretion in the CNT/CCD, decreased peripheral uptake, and increased K^+ reabsorption in the OMCD) does not require changes in plasma K^+.

Vasopressin

Vasopressin has a well-characterized stimulatory effect on K^+ secretion by the distal nephron.[334,401] Teleologically, this vasopressin-dependent activation serves to preserve K^+ secretion during dehydration and extracellular volume depletion, when circulating levels of vasopressin are high and tubular delivery of Na^+ and fluid is reduced. The stimulation of basolateral V2 receptors results in an activation of ENaC, which increases the driving force for K^+ secretion by principal cells; the relevant mechanisms are discussed earlier in this chapter (see Regulation of Na^+-Cl^- transport in the CNT and cortical collecting duct; vasopressin). In addition, vasopressin activates SK channels directly in the CCD,[402] as does cAMP.[342] The ROMK protein is directly phosphorylated by protein kinase A on three serine residues (S25, S200, and S294 in the ROMK2 isoform), with phosphorylation of all three sites required for full activity in *Xenopus* oocytes (see Regulation of Na^+-Cl^- transport in TAL; activating influences). Finally, the stimulation of luminal V1 receptors also stimulate K^+ secretion in the CCD, apparently via activation of maxi-K channels.[403]

CALCIUM TRANSPORT

Calcium Homeostasis

Total body Calcium

Calcium, which exists in the body as a divalent cation (Ca^{2+}), plays an important structural role as a key component of the bony skeleton, and acts as an extracellular and intracellular signal. A total of 1 kg to 2 kg of Ca^{2+} is present in the body of an average adult, of which approximately 99% is in bone and teeth, and most of the remaining 1% is in soft tissues and the extracellular space. The normal total plasma Ca^{2+} concentration is 8.8 to 10.3 mg/dL (2.2 to 2.6 mM). (The atomic mass of calcium is 40.1. Thus, 1 mmol Ca^{2+} ≡ 2 mEq = 40 mg; and 1 mM Ca^{2+} concentration ≡ 2 mEq/L ≡ 4 mg/dL.) Normally, approximately 40% of plasma Ca^{2+} is bound to plasma proteins, predominantly albumin. The remaining 60%, which is filterable through artificial and biological membranes (ultrafilterable Ca^{2+} or UF_{Ca}), consists of Ca^{2+} in complex with various anions, 10%, and free Ca^{2+} ions (ionized Ca^{2+} or iCa), 50%. The ionized Ca^{2+} is the fraction of plasma Ca^{2+} that is physiologically important and its concentration (1.05 mM to 1.23 mM) is tightly regulated by the hormones, parathyroid hormone (PTH), 1, 25-dihydroxyvitamin D (1,25(OH)$_2$D, the active metabolite of vitamin D), calcitonin, and iCa itself, acting on three major organs, the kidneys, intestinal tract, and bone. The relative distribution of Ca^{2+} in plasma may be altered by changes in plasma protein concentration and pH. For example, the proportion of total plasma Ca^{2+} that is ionized is increased in hypoalbuminemia and acidemia. Under such circumstances, the total plasma Ca^{2+} concentration may not accurately reflect the status of physiologically relevant ionized Ca^{2+} in the extracellular fluid.

Within cells, Ca^{2+} is sequestered in the endoplasmic reticulum and mitochondria, or bound to cytoplasmic proteins and ligands, so that the basal intracellular iCa concentration is maintained at a very low level (0.1 μM to 1 μM). The steep gradient between the extracellular and intracellular iCa is maintained by active extrusion of Ca^{2+} across the plasma membrane mediated by a Ca^{2+}-ATPase pump present in all cells, and also by a sodium-calcium exchanger in certain tissues.

Intake and Output

The daily dietary intake of Ca^{2+}, of which the majority is obtained from milk and other dairy products, is 600 mg to 800 mg for adults in the United States. Many adults also take Ca^{2+} supplements, so that the average total intake of Ca^{2+} is approximately 1000 mg (Fig. 5–26). Approximately 20% to 25% of dietary Ca^{2+} is absorbed by the intestine. In addition, the intestine also reabsorbs approximately 200 mg of Ca^{2+} from luminal secretions in the distal small intestine and colon. The efficiency of Ca^{2+} absorption is increased when dietary Ca^{2+} is reduced, as well as during periods of rapid growth in children, during pregnancy, and during lactation. Once absorbed, Ca^{2+} in the extracellular fluid may exchange with the pool in bone, with 300 mg of Ca^{2+} typically entering and leaving the skeleton daily as it is continuously remodeled. Ultimately, the kidneys are responsible for the excretion of about 200 mg of Ca^{2+} per day. More importantly, regulation of renal Ca^{2+} excretion is one of the principal ways in which the body regulates extracellular Ca^{2+} balance.

Overview of Calcium Regulation

The plasma concentration of iCa is meticulously maintained within a narrow range. This is accomplished by PTH, 1,25(OH)$_2$D, calcitonin, and extracellular Ca^{2+} itself, acting on three major target organs, the kidneys, intestinal tract and bone (Fig. 5–27). A fall in plasma iCa acutely stimulates secretion of PTH from the parathyroid gland, increases PTH gene expression, and chronically leads to parathyroid gland hyperplasia. These effects are thought to be mediated by the calcium-sensing receptor (CaSR),[404] a G-protein-coupled receptor located on the cell membrane of parathyroid glands. Extracellular Ca^{2+} acts as an agonist of the CaSR, thereby

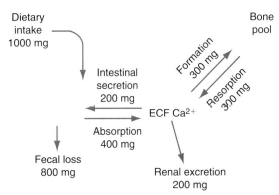

FIGURE 5–26 Typical daily Ca^{2+} intake and output for a normal adult in neutral Ca^{2+} balance (see text for details).

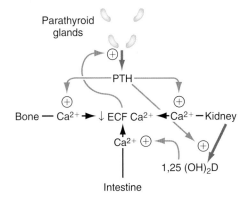

FIGURE 5–27 Summary of overall Ca^{2+} homeostasis. The primary homeostatic mechanisms activated in response to a fall in extracellular fluid (ECF) ionized Ca^{2+} concentration are shown.

activating phospholipase C, generating inositol 1,4,5-triphosphate, and releasing intracellular Ca^{2+} stores, as well as inhibiting adenylate cyclase and reducing intracellular cyclic AMP levels.[404] Reduction in extracellular iCa leads to the opposite effects and thereby stimulates release of PTH. PTH acts to increase iCa and return it to normal by mobilizing Ca^{2+} from bone stores, and by stimulating renal Ca^{2+} reabsorption in the distal tubule (see later). In addition, PTH stimulates 25-hydroxyvitamin D-1α-hydroxylase, the enzyme in the proximal renal tubule that converts 25-hydroxyvitamin D to its active metabolite, $1,25(OH)_2D$, which in turn promotes intestinal absorption of Ca^{2+}. An abnormal rise in iCa has the opposite effects on PTH and vitamin D metabolism. Hypercalcemia also activates the secretion from thyroid C-cells of calcitonin, a hormone that inhibits osteoclast-mediated bone resorption. However, calcitonin is not thought to play an important role in normal Ca^{2+} homeostasis in humans. In addition to its effects on the parathyroid gland, extracellular Ca^{2+} itself has hormone-like actions on other organs, which are mediated by the CaSR. For example, hypercalcemia is thought to directly inhibit renal tubule Ca^{2+} reabsorption, likely via engagement of the CaSR on the basolateral membrane of the thick ascending limb of Henle (see later).

Renal Handling of Calcium

Only the ionized and complexed forms of plasma Ca^{2+} are ultrafiltered at the glomerulus. The Ca^{2+} concentration of fluid in Bowman space, determined by micropuncture in rodents, has generally been found to be 60% to 70% of the total plasma Ca^{2+} concentration,[405] consistent with the values for UF_{Ca} determined with artificial membranes. Renal clearance studies have demonstrated that 98% to 99% of the filtered load of Ca^{2+} is reabsorbed by the renal tubules, so that only about 200 mg/d is ultimately excreted. The contribution of individual nephron segments is summarized in Table 5–2.

Calcium Handling by individual Nephron Segments
Proximal Convoluted Tubule (PCT) Segments, S1 and S2

Most of the filtered load of Ca^{2+} (50% to 60%) is reabsorbed in the PCT. The ratio of the concentration of Ca^{2+} in tubule fluid to its concentration in the glomerular ultrafiltrate (TF/UF_{Ca}), as determined by micropuncture, is 1.0 in the early convolutions of the superficial PCT, rising to 1.1 to 1.2 in the later convolutions.[405] The finding that the proximal tubule fluid Ca^{2+} concentration is close to UF_{Ca} suggests that Ca^{2+} is absorbed in parallel with Na^+ and water. The modest increase

in the later convolutions could be attributed either to a lag in the reabsorption of Ca^{2+} relative to water, creating a favorable concentration gradient for diffusive reabsorption downstream, or to a rising concentration of nonabsorbable complexed Ca^{2+}.

The passive permeability of the PCT to Ca^{2+} is high, as demonstrated by a large backflux component in *in vivo* microperfusion experiments.[406] *In vitro* microperfusion studies of PCT S2 segments confirmed the high Ca^{2+} permeability, and also showed that there was no net flux of Ca^{2+} in the absence of a transtubular electrochemical gradient.[407] These findings suggest that Ca^{2+} reabsorption in the PCT is primarily passive in nature. The observation that PCT Ca^{2+} reabsorption parallels closely that of Na^+ and water not only under normal basal conditions, but also following maneuvers that change urinary Ca^{2+} excretion[405] such as administration of saline, diuretics, PTH, and acid-base disturbances, is also consistent with a passive mechanism. Passive reabsorption could potentially occur either by solvent drag or by diffusion. The reflection coefficient for Ca^{2+} in this segment is 0.9,[407] arguing against a major component of convective transport. Furthermore, recent evidence indicates that the majority of water reabsorption in the proximal tubule is transcellular and mediated by aquaporin-1 water channels. Given that transcellular transport would require uphill transport of Ca^{2+} against a steep, unfavorable electrochemical gradient at the basolateral membrane, and that aquaporin-1 channels are impermeable to cations, solvent drag is an unlikely mechanism for Ca^{2+} reabsorption in this segment.

By contrast, diffusion is thought to play the major role in Ca^{2+} reabsorption, particularly in the S2 and later segments of the proximal tubule where the TF/UF_{Ca} rises above 1.0 and the transepithelial electrical potential difference (PD) becomes lumen-positive, so that a favorable electrochemical gradient exists to drive vectorial transport (Fig. 5–28). The unfavorable electrochemical gradient across the basolateral membrane precludes simple transcellular diffusion, so passive Ca^{2+} reabsorption by diffusion must occur via the paracellular route. The rate-limiting barrier in paracellular transport is the tight junction, and recent evidence suggests that a family of integral membrane tight junction proteins, the claudins, regulate paracellular permeability, possibly by constituting the pore of a paracellular channel. One of the members of this family, claudin-2, forms paracellular cation pores[408] and is strongly expressed in the tight junctions of the proximal nephron.[25] Claudin-2 is therefore a strong candidate for the paracellular Ca^{2+} channel.

The question of if, and how Ca^{2+} is reabsorbed in the earliest (S1) segment of the PCT remains open, as there are no direct studies of this segment. The TF/UF_{Ca} initially approximates 1.0 and the transepithelial electrical potential difference (PD) is lumen-negative due to the reabsorption of Na^+ with uncharged organic solutes, so there is no driving force for Ca^{2+} diffusion. In certain situations, Ca^{2+} is apparently reabsorbed against an uphill electrochemical gradient in the PCT, suggesting that it may be actively transported in the PCT. However, the observation that TF/UF_{Ca} rises progressively to 1.1 to 1.2 along the length of this segment, and does so seemingly in parallel with an initially proportionate rise in the TF/UF of inulin, a nonreabsorbable filtration marker, suggests that more likely there is simply no Ca^{2+} reabsorption in the S1 segment.

In summary, the bulk of Ca^{2+} reabsorption in the PCT, probably mainly mediated by the S2 segment, is passive and diffusive, driven by a modest concentration gradient and lumen-positive PD.

Proximal Straight Tubule Segments, S2 and S3

Whereas the TF/UF_{Ca} is similar to TF/UF_{Na} at the end of the PCT, tubular fluid obtained by micropuncture from the

TABLE 5–2	Segmental Handling of Ca^{2+} Along the Renal Tubule	
Nephron Segment	**Fractional Reabsorption (%)**	**Cellular Transport Mechanism**
Proximal tubule	50–60	Passive, paracellular
Thin descending and ascending limbs	0	
TAL	15	Passive, paracellular Active component stimulated by PTH
DCT/CNT	10–15	Active, transcellular
Collecting duct	+/–	Unknown

TAL, thick ascending limb; DCT, distal convoluted tubule; CNT, connecting tubule.

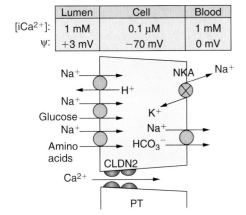
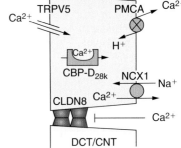

FIGURE 5–28 Models depicting the putative cellular mechanism of Ca^{2+} reabsorption in different nephron segments. In the proximal tubule S2 segment (PT), transcellular Na^+ and water generate a concentration gradient that drives passive paracellular Ca^{2+} reabsorption, likely through the tight junction channel protein, claudin-2 (CLDN2). In the thick ascending limb (TAL), transcellular Na^+ reabsorption through the apical electroneutral Na-K-2Cl cotransporter (NKCC2), coupled to apical K^+ recycling through the ATP-sensitive K^+ channel, ROMK, generates a lumen-positive voltage that drives passive paracellular Ca^{2+} reabsorption through claudin-16/paracellin (CLDN16). In the distal convoluted tubule and connecting tubule (DCT/CNT), Ca^{2+} is reabsorbed transcellularly. Ca^{2+} enters apically through an epithelial Ca^{2+} channel (TRPV5), diffuses across the cytosol bound to calbindin-D28k (CBP-D$_{28k}$), and exits basolaterally through a plasma membrane Ca^{2+} pump (PMCA), or Na-Ca exchanger (NCX1). Ca^{2+} backflux is blocked by a paracellular Ca^{2+} barrier constituted in part by claudin-8 (CLDN8). Other abbreviations: [iCa^{2+}], ionized Ca^{2+} concentration; ψ, electrical potential; NKA, Na-K-ATPase; CLC-Kb, basolateral Cl^- channel.

hairpin bend of the loop of Henle has a TF/UF$_{Ca}$ that is 35% less than TF/UF$_{Na}$, suggesting that there is disproportionate reabsorption of Ca^{2+}, dissociated from that of Na^+, in either the PST or the thin descending limb (TDL).[405] As the TDL has been found to be impermeable to Ca^{2+},[409] this implicates the PST as a site of Na^+-independent Ca^{2+} reabsorption.

The S2 segment of the PST exhibits passive Ca^{2+} reabsorption driven by a lumen-positive PD and favorable concentration gradient,[410] identical to the S2 segment of the PCT. The S3 segment of the PST, when perfused *in vitro* with symmetrical solutions, reabsorbs Ca^{2+} despite the absence of a concentration gradient, and a lumen-negative PD,[411] indicating the active transport of Ca^{2+}. Furthermore, this reabsorption is not affected by ouabain, confirming its dissociation from Na^+ movement, and excluding any involvement of a Na-Ca exchanger. The molecular mechanisms for active Ca^{2+} reabsorption in this segment are currently unknown.

Thin Descending And Ascending Limbs of the Loop of Henle
The permeability of the thin limbs to Ca^{2+} is very low and no significant net transport of Ca^{2+} is believed to take place in these segments.[405]

Thick Ascending Limb of the Loop of Henle
Approximately 15% of the filtered load of Ca^{2+} is reabsorbed in the TAL. In this segment, active reabsorption of NaCl and luminal membrane recycling of K^+ generate a lumen-positive PD (see Fig. 5–28). *In vitro* tubule perfusion studies have demonstrated that this segment has a significant permeability to Ca^{2+} and that the direction of net Ca^{2+} transport is voltage-dependent, consistent with passive, and presumably paracellular, diffusion.[405] Indeed, Bourdeau and Burg found no net flux of Ca^{2+} when the cortical TAL was perfused with symmetrical salt solutions and the transepithelial PD was abolished by administration of the loop diuretic, furosemide, which inhibits the apical Na-K-2Cl cotransporter and thereby establishes a chemical voltage clamp.[412] This suggests that transport of Ca^{2+} in this segment is entirely passive. Furthermore, they found that the Ussing flux ratio varied linearly with voltage, in a manner consistent with a model of single-file ionic diffusion. Mg^{2+} transport in the TAL is also thought to be primarily mediated by passive paracellular diffusion (see later). Such a model nicely explains why both hypercalciuria and hypermagnesuria occur in situations in which the

ability to generate the TAL transepithelial PD is compromised, such as pharmacological inhibition of the Na-K-2Cl cotransporter with loop diuretics, and inherited loss-of-function mutations in either the Na-K-2Cl cotransporter, the ROMK K^+ channel, or the ClC-Kb Cl^- channel, as in Bartter syndrome.

Another disorder with both renal Ca^{2+} and Mg^{2+} wasting, familial hypomagnesemic hypercalcuria, has recently been found to be caused by mutations in claudin-16 (also known as paracellin), a member of the claudin family of integral membrane tight junction proteins that is expressed in the tight junctions of the TAL.[185] This suggests that claudin-16 plays an important role in the paracellular transport of divalent cations. Furthermore, careful analysis of the claudin-16 amino-acid sequence revealed a cluster of negatively charged residues in one of the two putative extracellular loops of the protein, which is not found in other homologous members of the claudin family. The extracellular domains of the protein would be predicted to protrude into the lateral intercellular space, potentially in directly contact with ions traversing the paracellular pathway. It is therefore tempting to speculate that claudin-16 may in fact constitute part of a paracellular Ca^{2+} and Mg^{2+} channel, with the negatively charged residues forming the mouth of the pore, as found in other transmembrane Ca^{2+} channels.

Controversy exists over whether there is an additional component of Ca^{2+} reabsorption in the TAL that is active. Suki and co-workers found that although furosemide decreased the tubular efflux of Ca^{2+} in the medullary TAL concomitant with abolition of the transepithelial PD, it actually increased Ca^{2+} efflux in the cortical TAL.[413] Imai varied the transepithelial PD of cortical TAL by perfusion with solutions of varying Na^+ concentrations and showed that net reabsorption of Ca^{2+} occurred even when the transepithelial PD was zero.[414] Friedman demonstrated significant Ca^{2+} reabsorption in the cortical TAL but not in medullary TAL under furosemide voltage-clamp conditions.[415] Furthermore, the residual, presumably active, component of net Ca^{2+} flux in the cortical TAL under these conditions was increased almost threefold by PTH.

Distal Convoluted Tubule and Connecting Tubule
Approximately 10% to 15% of filtered Ca^{2+} is reabsorbed in the distal tubule, which includes the DCT, CNT, and collecting tubule. The PD in the distal tubule is lumen-negative

throughout, and the Ca^{2+} concentration below that of plasma, so any Ca^{2+} reabsorption must be active. By micropuncture, only the early and late convolutions of the superficial DCT are accessible. It is well established that there is Ca^{2+} reabsorption in the superficial DCT.[405] Costanzo and Windhager demonstrated that this reabsorption is active, and that back-flux of Ca^{2+} is negligible, precluding a component of passive transport.[416] However, the fractional delivery of Ca^{2+} to the final urine is less than that to the late distal tubule, indicating that there must be further reabsorption of Ca^{2+} after the DCT. Indeed both Shareghi and Stoner,[417] and Imai[418] have perfused isolated segments of CNT and demonstrated active Ca^{2+} reabsorption in these segments (as well as in the DCT). Importantly, Ca^{2+} reabsorption in both the DCT and CNT are stimulated by PTH and by cyclic AMP. Thus, these are the major segments for the anti-calciuric action of PTH, working through adenylate cyclase. The molecular mechanisms of distal tubule Ca^{2+} transport are discussed in the subsequent section and summarized in Figure 5–28. It is important to note that although the absolute amount of Ca^{2+} reabsorbed in these segments is quite modest, the fraction excretion of Ca^{2+} into the final urine is only about 1% to 2%. Thus, even very small changes in DCT/CNT fractional reabsorption can have a large effect on the final amount excreted. This underscores the importance of the DCT and CNT for the hormonal regulation of renal Ca^{2+} excretion.

Collecting Duct

The collecting duct likely plays a minor role in renal Ca^{2+} reabsorption. In isolated perfused cortical collecting ducts (CCD), a small net reabsorption of Ca^{2+} has been observed by some, but not by others.[405] If there is indeed Ca^{2+} reabsorption in this segment, it would occur against a negative luminal voltage and uphill transepithelial Ca^{2+} concentration gradient, and would therefore have to be active and transcellular. Consistent with this, some of the components that could potentially mediate transcellular Ca^{2+} transport (see later) are also expressed in the CCD, including TRPV6[419] and calbindin-D28k in mice,[225] and NCX1, calbindin-D28k and the plasma membrane Ca-ATPase in humans.[420] Ca^{2+} reabsorption may also occur in the medullary collecting ducts.

Molecular Mechanisms of Transcellular Ca^{2+} Reabsorption

Transcellular Ca^{2+} reabsorption occurs primarily in the DCT and CNT, with perhaps minor components in the cortical TAL (when activated by PTH) and CCD. This process can be divided into three key steps: apical entry, cytosolic diffusion, and basolateral efflux (see Fig. 5–28). The intracellular free Ca^{2+} level in most cells is several orders of magnitude below that of extracellular fluid, and the membrane potential inside-negative. Thus, the basolateral efflux step must necessarily be active, whereas the apical entry step would rationally be expected to be passive.

Apical Ca^{2+} entry

The apical entry step is likely to be the rate-limiting step in vectorial Ca^{2+} transport. In rabbit CNT/CCD cells, apical Ca^{2+} entry and basolateral Ca^{2+} exit are closely coupled.[421,422] Stimulation of adenylyl cyclase with forskolin increases intracellular Ca^{2+} levels and transcellular Ca^{2+} transport, suggesting that this occurs through stimulation of apical Ca^{2+} entry.[421] Conversely, inhibition of Ca^{2+} influx by apical acidification causes a decrease in intracellular Ca^{2+} and subsequent down-regulation of transcellular Ca^{2+} transport.[422]

The apical entry step is mediated by a Ca^{2+} channel. Numerous groups have reported voltage-dependent Ca^{2+} channels with varying properties in the distal tubule by patch clamp study.[405] Bacskai and Friedman observed Ca^{2+} entry into DCT/

cortical TAL cells that was regulated by dihydropyridines, which are ligands of L-type voltage-dependent Ca^{2+} channels, and upregulated by PTH.[423] Expression of various L-type voltage-dependent Ca^{2+} channels has been found in distal renal tubule segments or cultured distal convoluted tubule cells.[424–426] However, the role of voltage-dependent Ca^{2+} channels in vectorial transepithelial Ca^{2+} transport remains unproven.

It is now clear that the principal apical epithelial Ca^{2+} channel in the distal tubule is TRPV5 (also known as ECaC1) a member of the TRP superfamily of cation channels. TRPV5 was identified by an expression cloning strategy[427] and found to be expressed on the apical membrane of CNT principal cells in the rabbit,[428] and in both the late distal convoluted tubule (DCT2) and the CNT in the mouse[225] and rat (see Fig. 5–18).[429] Toward the more distal segments, its location becomes intracellular, suggesting that its surface abundance may be regulated by vesicle trafficking.[225] Its functional properties are also consistent with a role in apical Ca^{2+} entry. When expressed in *Xenopus* oocytes or in human embryonic kidney cells, TRPV5 is highly selective for Ca^{2+} (P_{Ca}/P_{Na} 100:1) and exhibits inwardly rectifying currents that would be expected to be constitutively activated at physiological membrane potentials.[430] Furthermore, entry of Ca^{2+} into the cell leads to inactivation of the channel.[431] This negative feedback mechanism may account in part for the tight coupling between apical Ca^{2+} entry and basolateral efflux that has been observed.[421] TRPV5 currents are also inhibited by reduction in extracellular pH.[432] This may account for the hypercalciuria observed in association with acidosis. There are no specific ligands of TRPV5, but it is blocked by ruthenium red, econazole, and inorganic polycations such as Gd^{3+} and Cd^{2+}.[433]

TRPV6 (also referred to as CaT1 or ECaC2)[434] is a homolog of TRPV5 with similar functional properties.[435,436] TRPV6 is the predominant apical Ca^{2+} entry channel in the duodenum, where it likely mediates transepithelial Ca^{2+} absorption. TRPV6 is also expressed in the kidney, specifically in DCT2, CNT, cortical and medullary collecting ducts (see Fig. 5–18).[419] When expressed in HEK293 cells, TRPV6 can assemble with TRPV5 into functional heterotetrameric Ca^{2+} channels.[437] However, the role of TRPV6 in the kidney *in vivo* remains undefined.

The critical role of TRPV5 in distal tubule Ca^{2+} reabsorption was demonstrated by the finding that TRPV5 knockout mice are hypercalciuric.[438] In these mice, renal TRPV6 expression is preserved. Fractional delivery of Ca^{2+} to the earliest segments of the distal convolution was found to be normal, but as more distal puncture sites were sampled, fractional delivery of Ca^{2+} appeared to rise, indicating not only the absence of reabsorption, but also significant secretion of Ca^{2+} into the tubule lumen. The latter is presumably due to passive back-leak of Ca^{2+} via the paracellular pathway. These findings indicate that TRPV6 cannot compensate for absence of TRPV5 in the kidney.

TRPV5, particularly its C-terminus, participates in interactions with numerous proteins that may be important in its regulation, including S100A10, 80K-H, BSPRY, and calmodulin. S100A10 is a member of the S100 protein superfamily that forms a heterotetrameric complex with annexin-2, and serves to stabilize plasma membrane domains and provide a link to the actin cytoskeleton. This interaction is required for TRPV5 trafficking to the plasma membrane.[439] 80K-H is a protein with two EF hands that binds Ca^{2+} and appears to function as an intracellular Ca^{2+} sensor for TRPV5. Inactivation of the EF-hand pair reduces the TRPV5-mediated Ca^{2+} current and increases the TRPV5 sensitivity to intracellular Ca^{2+}, accelerating feedback inhibition of the channel.[440] BSPRY (B-box and SPRY domain-containing protein) is a protein of unknown function that appears to inhibit Ca^{2+}

influx in MDCK cells expressing TRPV5.[441] Both S100A10 and 80K-H mRNA are up-regulated by vitamin D, whereas BSPRY is down-regulated, suggesting these as possible modes of vitamin D regulation of TRPV5. Both TRPV5 and TRPV6 also bind calmodulin.[442] In TRPV6, calmodulin acts as a Ca^{2+} sensor and is responsible for slow inactivation of the channel by high levels of intracellular Ca^{2+}.[443] The role of calmodulin in TRPV5 function has not been studied.

Cytosolic Diffusion of Ca^{2+}

The baseline cytosolic free Ca^{2+} concentration in all cells is maintained at a very low level (submicromolar range). Against this low background, acute spikes in intracellular Ca^{2+} level can thereby be detected for signalling purposes. This poses a unique problem for Ca^{2+}-transporting epithelia such as the distal renal tubule and the duodenum: at such low concentrations, the theoretical rate of diffusive flux of Ca^{2+} across the cytosol is insufficient to support the observed rates of transcellular Ca^{2+} transport.[444]

Both the distal tubule and duodenal epithelium contain the cytosolic calcium-binding protein, calbindin. Two isoforms exist, calbindin-D28k, which is predominantly expressed in the mammalian kidney (except in birds where it is also in the intestine), and calbindin-D9k, which is primarily in the intestine (but also in the kidney in the mouse).[405] The importance of calbindin-D28k for renal Ca^{2+} reabsorption is supported by three lines of evidence. First, it colocalizes to the exact same nephron segments as other Ca^{2+}-transporting proteins (see Fig. 5–18). Calbindin-D28k is found in the DCT, particularly in the late DCT, and in principal cells of the CNT and CCD,[225,420] coinciding with the localization of TRPV5 and NCX1 (see later). Second, its level of expression is induced by 1,25(OH)$_2$D,[445] thus correlating with the increase in Ca^{2+} reabsorption stimulated by this hormone.[446] Finally, calbindin-D28k knockout mice [447] have a twofold to threefold increase in urinary Ca^{2+}-creatinine ratio,[448] suggestive of a defect in renal tubule Ca^{2+} reabsorption.

It has been postulated that the role of calbindin is to buffer cytosolic Ca^{2+}, so that a high total intracellular Ca^{2+} concentration may exist despite a very low free Ca^{2+} concentration. Bronner and Stein calculated that the predicted maximum transcellular flux across the distal tubule in the absence of calbindin is less than 2% of the actual transcellular flux observed experimentally. In the presence of calbindin, even though Ca^{2+} bound to it diffuses more slowly than unbound Ca^{2+}, there is more total Ca^{2+} to diffuse, so that the predicted maximum transcellular flux is similar to the observed value.[444] Feher has performed *in vitro* studies using the intestinal isoform, calbindin-D9k, which confirm the predicted effect of Ca^{2+}-binding protein to increase Ca^{2+} flux.[449] Calbindin may augment transcellular Ca^{2+} flux by an additional mechanism: by buffering intracellular Ca^{2+}, it would prevent feedback inhibition of TRPV5 by high intracellular free Ca^{2+} concentrations and thereby increase apical Ca^{2+} entry. Finally it has been proposed, by analogy to calmodulin that calbindins may also act as Ca^{2+} sensors that directly bind to, and regulate, membrane transport proteins. Although there is no direct evidence for this hypothesis at this time, there are reports indicating that calbindin-D28k is not only in the cytosol but can be associated with the membrane fraction as well.[450,451]

Basolateral Ca^{2+} Exit

Two classes of transport protein could potentially mediate active extrusion of Ca^{2+} at the basolateral membrane, plasma membrane Ca-ATPases (PMCA), and Na-Ca exchangers (NCX). Na-Ca exchange appears to be the major Ca extrusion mechanism in primary cultured CNT/CCD cells, with PMCA playing a minor role.[445,452]

The Na-Ca exchanger is a secondary active transporter that utilizes the inwardly directed transmembrane Na^+ gradient generated by the Na-K-ATPase to drive Ca^{2+} countertransport. Na^+ gradient-dependent Ca^{2+} transport activity can be detected in renal cortical basolateral membranes,[453] and in liposomes reconstituted with partially purified protein.[454] Furthermore, it has been observed in isolated perfused tubules of the rabbit DCT and CNT,[455] and in membrane vesicles derived from the rat distal tubule but not from the proximal tubule,[456] consistent with a role in distal tubule transcellular Ca^{2+} reabsorption. The renal NCX shares similar properties to the NCX of excitable tissues; it is reversible, electrogenic with a stoichiometry of 3 to 4 Na^+ ions per 1 Ca^{2+} ion, and the K_m for Ca^{2+} is in the micromolar range.[454]

Three NCX genes have been identified. NCX1 is the gene expressed in the kidney.[457,458] Alternative splicing within a large intracellular loop further increases the complexity of NCX1. Six small exons are used in different combinations in different tissues, giving rise to heart (NCX1.1), brain (NCX1.4), and kidney (NCX1.3) splice variants.[459] This has functional importance because the large intracellular loop is the site responsible for two regulatory mechanisms, Ca^{2+} activation, and Na^+-dependent inactivation.[460] Intracellular Ca^{2+}-activation is likely to be a mechanism to match exchanger activity with Ca^{2+} transport requirements. Specifically in the distal tubule, increased apical Ca^{2+} entry would increase intracellular Ca^{2+} levels, and thereby stimulate exchange activity to facilitate basolateral Ca^{2+} efflux. The physiological role of Na^+-dependent inactivation is unclear.

NCX1 is expressed most strongly in the DCT2 with lesser expression in the CNT and late DCT1 in the mouse (see Fig. 5–4),[225] and most strongly in the CNT with lesser expression in the late DCT and CCD in humans.[420]

The other potential route for basolateral efflux of Ca^{2+} is via the PMCA. PMCA are primary active pumps of the P-type ATPase family. They are ubiquitous in eukaryotic cells where they serve to maintain low levels of intracellular free Ca^{2+}. Biochemical evidence of Ca^{2+}-dependent ATPase activity can be detected along the entire length of the nephron,[461] and ATP-dependent Ca^{2+} transport can be detected in membrane vesicles derived from both proximal and distal tubules.[456] If PMCA play an additional, more specialized role in transcellular Ca^{2+} reabsorption, one might expect that they would either be more strongly expressed, or a unique isoform would be expressed at the basolateral membrane of the DCT and CNT. Indeed early studies using a monoclonal antibody, raised against purified erythrocyte PMCA, stained exclusively the basolateral membrane of the DCT.[462] Four genes encode for the PMCA (named PMCA 1-4), and multiple alternatively spliced mRNA variants exist (denoted by a letter, *a–d*, after the gene number).[463]

So far, the distal tubule basolateral PMCA has not been identified. PMCA1 and PMCA4 are widely expressed throughout the body and are thought to play a housekeeping role. Consistent with this, PMCA1b and 4b are found ubiquitously within the kidney.[464,465] By reverse-transcription polymerase chain reaction (RT-PCR) amplification of mRNA from individually microdissected nephron segments, PMCA2b was found to be most highly expressed in the DCT and cTAL.[464,465] It is therefore the strongest candidate for the basolateral Ca^{2+} pump. However, a study using isoform-specific antibodies found that PMCA2 was confined to the brain.[466] Furthermore, in the distal tubule cell lines, mDCT[467] and MDCK,[467] the only PMCA transcripts and protein that have been detected are PMCA1b and 4b.

Paracellular Cation Barrier

In contrast to the proximal tubule and TAL, the distal nephron segments have a very low passive permeability to Ca^{2+}

TABLE 5–3	Summary of Factors Affecting Ca^{2+} Reabsorption		
	Nephron Location		
Factor	**Proximal**	**TAL**	**Distal**
Volume expansion	↓		↓
Calcium			
Hypercalcemia	↓	↓	↓ (PTH)
Hypocalcemia	↑	↑	
Phosphate			
Loading			↑ (PTH)
Depletion	↓		↓ (PTH)
Acid-base status			
Acidosis	↓		↓
Alkalosis	↑		
Hormones			
PTH	↓	↑	↑
Vitamin D			↑
Calcitonin		↑	↑
Insulin/glucose	↓		↓
Diuretics			
Loop diuretics		↓	
Thiazides	↑		↑
Amiloride			↑

PTH, indirect effect mediated by parathyroid hormone.

backflux,[416] and likewise to other cations including H^+, K^+, and Na^+. This indicates that the paracellular pathway must be relatively impermeable to Ca^{2+}, and indeed this would be expected to be a prerequisite for active transcellular reabsorption to proceed efficiently in these segments. Claudin-8, a tight junction membrane protein expressed in the distal renal tubule, can markedly impede paracellular permeability to cations, including Ca^{2+}, implicating it as a key component of the paracellular Ca^{2+} barrier.[468]

Regulation of Renal Calcium Handling

Many factors influence renal Ca^{2+} handling. These are summarized in Table 5–3, and only the most important are discussed here.

Glomerular Filtration Rate

Increasing GFR with protein feeding, dexamethasone, or dopamine is associated with minimal change in renal Ca^{2+} excretion, presumably due to a compensatory increase in tubule reabsorption.[405] This demonstrates that glomerulotubular balance for Ca^{2+} is well maintained. A modest reduction in GFR, as in early renal failure, is associated with a decrease in the fractional excretion of Ca^{2+}, perhaps in part due to secondary hyperparathyroidism. In advanced renal failure, however, although absolute Ca^{2+} excretion is low, fractional excretion increases, due to a reduction in Ca^{2+} reabsorption in the proximal tubule and TAL segments of the remaining intact nephrons.[469] This explains in part why serum Ca^{2+} does not normally rise during advanced renal failure.

Sodium and Extracellular Fluid Volume

Upon volume expansion with saline, the fractional excretion of Ca^{2+} increases in parallel with that of Na^+. This is hardly surprising because Ca^{2+} reabsorption is dependent on Na^+ reabsorption in the PCT and the TAL. However, Agus and co-workers observed that fractional delivery of Ca^{2+} to the late DCT was not increased with saline loading.[470] This seems to suggest that any effects in the proximal nephron are irrelevant

and that the increased Ca^{2+} excretion is actually due to decreased reabsorption in a segment downstream of the DCT, presumably either the CNT or CCD.

Hypercalcemia

Hypercalcemia reduces the GFR and can cause a prerenal syndrome, as well as acute renal failure. In mild hypercalcemia the ultrafiltration coefficient, K_f, is reduced,[471] whereas more severe hypercalcemia causes renal arteriolar vasoconstriction and reduced renal plasma flow.[472]

Hypercalcemia also reduces renal tubule Ca^{2+} reabsorption, an adaptive response that presumably serves to rid the body of the excess Ca^{2+}.[405] In the PCT, hypercalcemia reduces reabsorption of Ca^{2+}, presumably by increasing the peritubular Ca^{2+} concentration and thereby reducing the concentration gradient driving paracellular transport. Hypercalcemia also inhibits Ca^{2+} reabsorption in the TAL,[473] likely by activating the CaSR, which is located on the basolateral membrane.[220] One postulated mechanism is through activation of phospholipase A_2, generating arachidonic acid metabolites, such as 20-hydroxyeicosatetraenoic acid (20-HETE), which inhibit the apical Na-K-2Cl cotransporter[474] and the apical K^+ channel.[475] In this scheme, the generation of the normal lumen-positive voltage, which is the driving force for paracellular Ca^{2+} reabsorption, is impaired, and hence Ca^{2+} reabsorption inhibited. However, in a recent study in isolated, perfused cortical thick ascending limbs, activation of the CaSR with the agonists, Gd^{3+} or NPS R-467, did not seem to affect either active Na^+ reabsorption or the transepithelial voltage generated by it, but rather inhibited PTH-stimulated transcellular Ca^{2+} reabsorption by an unexplained mechanism.[476]

Finally, hypercalcemia induced by Ca^{2+} infusion also inhibits Ca^{2+} reabsorption in the DCT/CNT.[477] This is probably not a direct effect of Ca^{2+}, but is likely secondary to the suppression of PTH. In the in vitro perfused DCT that is not subjected to PTH, increased luminal Ca^{2+} delivery actually leads to increased Ca^{2+} reabsorption.[473]

Acidosis and Alkalosis

Acute and chronic metabolic acidosis cause hypercalciuria, primarily due to a decrease in distal tubule Ca^{2+} reabsorption.[478] Conversely, induction of metabolic alkalosis enhances tubule Ca^{2+} reabsorption and leads to hypocalciuria.[405] Furthermore, in the isolated perfused DCT, Ca^{2+} reabsorption is increased by a high perfusate pH and decreased by a low perfusate pH, suggesting that in metabolic acid-base disturbances it is the luminal pH of the distal tubule that is sensed.[479] The conductance of TRPV5, the apical Ca^{2+} entry channel in the distal tubule, is increased by an acute decrease in apical extracellular pH and decreased by a high pH.[432] Furthermore, chronic metabolic acidosis decreases renal TRPV5 and calbindin-D28k mRNA and protein abundance in wild-type mice, whereas chronic metabolic alkalosis has the opposite effect.[480] Thus, pH-regulation of TRPV5 expression and activity could potentially explain the effects of chronic and acute acidosis and alkalosis.

Hormones

Parathyroid Hormone and Parathyroid Hormone-Related Peptide

Parathyroid hormone is secreted by the parathyroid gland and is one of the most important regulators of body Ca^{2+} homeostasis. Parathyroid hormone-related peptide (PTHrP) is a paracrine factor with PTH-like effects on Ca^{2+} handling. Two types of PTH receptors have been identified, PTH1R, which binds both PTH and PTHrP, and PTH2R, which binds only to PTH. In the kidney, PTH1R mRNA is expressed in glomerular podocytes, PCT, PST, cortical TAL, and DCT.[481] By immunohistochemistry, it is expressed more strongly at the basolateral membrane of proximal tubules than at the apical

TABLE 5–4	Parathyroid Effects on Renal Ca²⁺ Handling	
Segment	Effect	Putative Mechanism
Glomerulus	↓ Filtered Ca²⁺ load	↓ K_f
Proximal tubule	↓ Ca²⁺ reabsorption	↓ Apical Na-H exchanger
Cortical TAL	↑ Ca²⁺ reabsorption	↑ Paracellular permeability
DCT/CNT	↑ Ca²⁺ reabsorption	↑ Apical Ca²⁺ channels ↑ Luminal NaHCO₃ delivery

DCT, distal convoluted tubule; CNT, connecting tubule.

membrane.[482] PTH2R is expressed in vascular endothelium and smooth muscle, and in lung and pancreas.[483] In the kidney, it is expressed only at the vascular pole of the glomerulus. For this reason, PTH1R is considered to be the receptor primarily responsible for the effects of PTH and PTHrP on renal tubule Ca²⁺ (and phosphate) transport.

Parathyroid hormone and PTHrP stimulation of PTH1R can activate at least two second messenger signaling systems: the classical adenylyl cyclase/protein kinase A (PKA) pathway and the phospholipase C/protein kinase C pathway (PKC). Chabardés and colleagues have shown that PTH-stimulated adenylyl cyclase is present in the PCT, PST, cortical TAL, CNT, and early CCD in rabbits.[405] There is some species variation, so that in mice it is also present in the DCT, but is absent from the CCD, whereas in humans it is primarily in the early DCT rather than the CNT, and is found in medullary as well as cortical TAL. The precise roles of the different signalling pathways in mediating the physiological effects of PTH and PTHrP are not well defined at present.

Parathyroid hormone has multiple different effects on the kidney (Table 5–4). It directly decreases K_f,[471] thereby reducing GFR and the filtered load of Ca²⁺. PTH also stimulates tubular Ca²⁺ reabsorption, so that its overall effect is to reduce renal Ca²⁺ excretion.

In the proximal tubule, the primary action of PTH is to inhibit NaHCO₃ reabsorption via PKA-dependent phosphorylation and endocytosis of the Na-H exchanger, NHE3.[105] The reduced proximal tubule Na⁺ and water reabsorption is accompanied by a proportionate decrease in passive Ca²⁺ reabsorption in this segment.[484] However, this is counteracted by increased Ca²⁺ reabsorption in more distal segments.

In the TAL, PTH increases Ca²⁺ reabsorption. In mice, this effect has been shown to be confined to the cortical segment,[415] consistent with the known tubular distribution of PTH1R[481] and adenylyl cyclase. The mechanism of this effect is controversial. Several studies using isolated perfused tubules suggest that PTH affects the passive permeability of the cortical TAL. Bourdeau and Burg,[485] and Imai[418] both found that PTH increased Ca²⁺ reabsorption without increasing the transepithelial voltage. Wittner showed that the effect of PTH disappeared when the transepithelial voltage was abolished by administration of furosemide and perfusion of both tubule surfaces with symmetrical solutions (in effect, the imposition of a chemical voltage clamp).[486] Because the transepithelial voltage provides the driving force for passive paracellular Ca²⁺ reabsorption in this segment,[412] these studies suggest that the paracellular permeability of the cortical TAL can be regulated by PTH, perhaps via an effect on claudin-16. By contrast, Friedman found that PTH stimulated net Ca²⁺ reabsorption in cortical TAL tubules even when they were chemically voltage-clamped, suggesting that there may be a PTH-dependent component of active, transcellular Ca²⁺ transport in this segment.[415]

The primary site for PTH action is thought to be the DCT/CNT.[487] PTH increases Ca²⁺ reabsorption in these segments without affecting transepithelial voltage,[418] and its effects can be mimicked by cyclic AMP analogs,[487] suggesting that they are mediated by PKA. In the rabbit, Shimizu and co-workers[488] and Imai[418] observed that PTH-responsiveness was confined to the CNT, which would be consistent with the known distribution of adenylyl cyclase in this species, whereas Shareghi and Stoner found that both DCT and CNT were responsive to PTH.[417]

Because Ca²⁺ reabsorption in these segments is active and transcellular, PTH presumably regulates one or more of the steps involved in transcellular transport. In microdissected rabbit CNT,[489] and in isolated mouse cortical TAL/DCT cells,[423] PTH induces a sustained increase in intracellular Ca²⁺ within minutes that is due to extracellular Ca²⁺ entry, suggesting that PTH may regulate TRPV5. However, the mechanism of these acute effects is unknown. Chronic reduction in PTH in mice or rats, by parathyroidectomy or administration of a calcimimetic, reduces expression of TRPV5, calbindin-D28k and NCX1 over a period of 1 week, whereas PTH supplementation restores their expression. Furthermore, inhibition of Ca²⁺ entry by the TRPV5-specific inhibitor, ruthenium red, blocks the PTH-stimulated expression of calbindin-D28k and NCX1.[490] This suggests that PTH exerts its effects primarily on gene expression of TRPV5 and that the increased intracellular Ca²⁺ secondarily up-regulates expression of other components of transcellular Ca²⁺ reabsorption in a coordinated manner.

Vitamin D

Vitamin D metabolites play a minor role in regulating renal Ca²⁺ handling. The overall effect of vitamin D on renal Ca²⁺ clearance in parathyroidectomized animals is small and variable. However, there does appear to be good evidence for an effect of vitamin D metabolites to selectively increase Ca²⁺ reabsorption in the distal tubule. In primary cultures of rabbit CNT/CCD cells, 1,25(OH)₂D significantly increases transepithelial Ca²⁺ reabsorption.[446] This is in part due to increased gene expression of Ca²⁺ transport proteins. In vitamin D-deficient knockout mouse models, there was downregulation of TRPV5, NCX1, and calbindin D28 mRNA that could be normalized by 1,25(OH)₂-D supplementation.[491]

In addition, vitamin D appears to regulate TRPV5 activity through interaction with other proteins. The TRPV5-binding proteins, S100A10 and 80K-H are positive regulators of its activity, whereas BSPRY is a negative regulator of TRPV5 activity. Consistent with this, vitamin D up-regulates S100A10 and 80K-H, and down-regulates BSPRY.[439–441] Klotho is a newly described type I membrane protein of the β-glycosidase family that is expressed principally in distal tubule cells of the kidney. It hydrolyzes extracellular N-linked oligosaccharides on TRPV5 and stabilizes it at the plasma membrane, facilitating Ca²⁺ reabsorption.[492] Interestingly, Klotho is upregulated by 1,25(OH)₂-D, which may be a novel mechanism by which vitamin D regulates Ca²⁺ metabolism.

Calcitonin

Supraphysiologic doses of calcitonin are hypercalciuric. By contrast, at physiologic doses, calcitonin has been observed to decrease renal Ca²⁺ excretion.[405] Part of this effect is simply due to concomitant hypocalcemia, but there is also a direct effect of calcitonin to increase distal tubule Ca²⁺ reabsorption. Calcitonin receptors were detected in the TAL and DCT by ligand binding,[493] and in the TAL and CCD by RT-PCR,[494] whereas calcitonin-sensitive adenylyl cyclase has been demonstrated in the cortical and medullary TAL of rabbit, rat, and human, and in the DCT of mouse, rat, and human.[495] By isolated perfused tubule studies, calcitonin and cyclic AMP analogs enhance Ca^{2+} reabsorption in the rabbit medullary TAL[496] and DCT.[488]

Tissue Kallikrein
Kallikrein is a serine protease that cleaves kinninogens to activate kinins. Tissue kallikrein (TK) is expressed in the late DCT and CNT and is up-regulated on a low Ca^{2+} diet. TK knockout mice are hypercalciuric.[497] However, abolition of signalling by the two kinin receptors, B1 (by a receptor blocker) and B2 (by gene targeting), did not affect urine Ca^{2+} excretion. Thus, TK likely stimulates renal Ca^{2+} reabsorption by a kinin-independent mechanism.

Diuretics
Loop Diuretics
Loop diuretics inhibit the TAL apical Na-K-2Cl cotransporter, NKCC2. They cause profound natriuresis and calciuresis. The effect of loop diuretics on Ca^{2+} excretion is clearly a consequence of inhibition of NKCC2, because hypercalciuria is also seen in patients with type I Bartter syndrome, who have inactivating mutations in NKCC2.[498] Entry of Na^+, K^+, and Cl^- through NKCC2 in a 1:1:2 ratio, in concert with apical K^+ recycling through the K^+ channel, ROMK, generates the lumen-positive electrical potential that drives paracellular Ca^{2+} reabsorption in this segment (see Fig. 5–28). The effect of loop diuretics is due to dissipation of this electrical potential.[412]

Thiazide Diuretics
Acute administration of thiazides causes marked natriuresis due to inhibition of the thiazide-sensitive NaCl cotransporter, NCC, in the DCT. At the same time, urinary Ca^{2+} excretion changes minimally.[499] This is likely because thiazides acutely stimulate Ca^{2+} reabsorption in the DCT, leading to a dissociation between Na^+ and Ca^{2+} handling in this segment.[416]

Chronic administration of thiazides causes frank hypocalciuria. This effect is dependent on inhibition of NCC because hypocalciuria is also seen in patients with Gitelman syndrome. Several lines of evidence suggest that the likely mechanism is extracellular fluid volume contraction leading to increased proximal tubule reabsorption of Na^+, and hence Ca^{2+}. First, micropuncture experiments in mice demonstrated increased reabsorption of Na^+ and Ca^{2+} in the proximal tubule during chronic thiazide treatment, whereas Ca^{2+} reabsorption in the DCT was not affected.[500] Second, thiazides induce hypocalciuria in TRPV5 knockout mice, which have no active distal Ca^{2+} reabsorption.[500] Third, increased reabsorption of Ca^{2+} in the proximal tubule is also observed in NCC knockout mice.[241] Finally, the hypocalciuria in humans can be reversed by salt replacement.[501]

MAGNESIUM TRANSPORT

Magnesium Homeostasis

Total Body Magnesium
Magnesium, which exists in the body as a divalent cation (Mg^{2+}), is the second most abundant intracellular cation.[405] It is a component of the bony skeleton, an essential cofactor for many metabolic enzymes, and a key regulator of ion channels and transporters in excitable tissues. The normal body content of Mg^{2+} is approximately 24 g (2000 mEq), of which 50% to 60% resides in mineralized bone, and 40 to 50% is in the intracellular compartment. (The atomic mass of Mg is 24.3. Thus, 1 mmol $Mg^{2+} \equiv 2$ mEq $\equiv 24.3$ mg; and 1 mM Mg^{2+} concentration $\equiv 2$ mEq/L $\equiv 2.43$ mg/dL.) Only about 1% of total body Mg^{2+} is present in extracellular fluid. The total concentration of Mg^{2+} in serum is normally 1.8 to 2.3 mg/dL (1.5 to 1.9 mEq/L). Approximately 70% to 80% is ultrafilter-

able, of which 90% is in an ionized form, and the rest is complexed to citrate, bicarbonate, and phosphate. Twenty percent to 30% of serum Mg^{2+} is bound to proteins, chiefly albumin. The ionized fraction of total Mg^{2+} is considered to be the physiologically important moiety. Unlike Ca^{2+}, the relative distribution of Mg^{2+} in plasma does not vary much with pH.

Within cells, greater than 90% of Mg^{2+} is bound to anions such as ATP, ADP, citrate, proteins, RNA, and DNA, or is sequestered in subcellular compartments, chiefly mitochondria and the endoplasmic reticulum. Measurements of intracellular ionized Mg^{2+} by nuclear magnetic resonance or ion-sensitive fluorescent dyes in a variety of mammalian tissues have generally been found to be in the range of 0.25 to 1 mM.[405] No direct measurements have been performed in renal tubule epithelial cells, but in MDCK cells[502] and in immortalized mouse DCT cells,[503] intracellular free Mg^{2+} is approximately 0.5 mM. Thus, the intracellular free Mg^{2+} concentration is not substantially different from that of the extracellular fluid. However, most cells have an inside-negative resting membrane potential, so that the intracellular free Mg^{2+} concentration is actually maintained below its electrochemical equilibrium. Although most plasma membranes are relatively impermeable to Mg^{2+}, there must exist active transport mechanisms to extrude excess Mg^{2+} that leaks into the cell. In heart and erthyrocytes, there is some evidence that this role is undertaken by a Na-Mg exchanger.

Intake and Output
The average daily dietary intake of Mg^{2+} in North America is 300 mg (Fig. 5–29), the main sources of which are green vegetables, soybeans, nuts, whole grain cereals, and seafood. The minimum daily dietary Mg^{2+} intake needed to maintain Mg^{2+} balance in the average person is controversial, with estimates ranging from 12 mg up to 100 mg. Mg^{2+} is absorbed in the small intestine, primarily the jejunum and ileum. Of the dietary Mg^{2+} intake, 30% to 50% is normally absorbed, but this can increase to 75% on a low Mg^{2+} diet, and decrease to 24% on a high Mg^{2+} diet. Lower intestinal secretions can contain up to 16 mg/dL of Mg^{2+}. Under normal circumstances, their contribution to overall Mg^{2+} elimination is minimal (about 20 mg/day), but these losses can become quite significant in diarrheal states. Urinary excretion normally accounts for about 100 mg of Mg^{2+} output per day.

Overview of Magnesium Regulation
Extracellular Mg^{2+} levels are regulated by three effector organs: intestine, bone, and kidney. Although several hormones have effects on Mg^{2+} homeostasis, none are specific for Mg^{2+}, and no single hormone appears to play a very important role. For example, in contrast to their effects on Ca^{2+}, the active metabolites of vitamin D have a slight, but probably physiologically

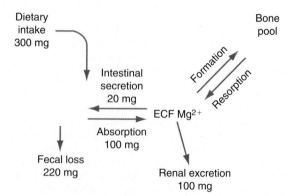

FIGURE 5–29 Typical daily Mg^{2+} intake and output for a normal adult in neutral Mg^{2+} balance (see text for details).

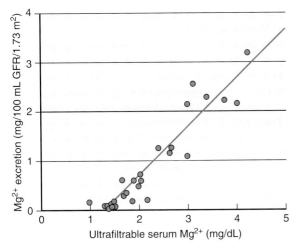

FIGURE 5–30 Relationship of urinary Mg^{2+} excretion to serum ultrafiltrable Mg^{2+} in normal human subjects before and during Mg^{2+} infusion. The apparent threshold for appearance of urinary Mg^{2+} is a serum ultrafiltrable Mg^{2+} concentration of 1.4 mg/dL. (From Rude RK, Bethune JE, Singer FR: Renal tubular maximum for magnesium in normal, hyperparathyroid, and hypoparathyroid man. J Clin Endocrinol Metabol 51:1425–1431, 1980.)

TABLE 5–5	Segmental Handling of Mg^{2+} Along the Renal Tubule	
Nephron Segment	**Fractional Reabsorption (%)**	**Cellular Transport Mechanism**
Proximal tubule	5–15	Unknown
Thin descending and ascending limbs	0	
TAL	60–70	Passive, paracellular
DCT/CNT	5–10	Active, transcellular
Collecting duct	0	

TAL, thick ascending limb; DCT, distal convoluted tubule; CNT, connecting tubule.

insignificant, stimulatory effect on intestinal Mg^{2+} absorption. PTH induces a modest decrease in urinary Mg^{2+} excretion.[504] Mg^{2+} is also an agonist at the CaSR, but its affinity is relatively weak. In sharks and teleost fish, the CaSR senses Mg^{2+} at concentrations found in seawater in order to osmoregulate in response to environmental salinity.[505] Whether CaSR sensing of extracellular Mg^{2+} in mammals has any physiological significance is unknown.

Renal Magnesium Handling

Seventy percent to 80% of serum Mg^{2+} is freely filtered at the glomerulus, of which most is reabsorbed along the length of the nephron. Only about 3% of filtered Mg^{2+} normally appears in the final urine.[405] During severe dietary Mg^{2+} deprivation, the kidney avidly retains Mg^{2+}. Under these circumstances, urinary Mg^{2+} excretion may be reduced to less than 24 mg/day (and often less than 12 mg/day), and the fractional excretion of filtered Mg^{2+} (F_eMg) to less than 1%.[506] Conversely, with Mg^{2+} loading a threshold effect is observed[507]: when the threshold serum Mg^{2+} concentration (1.8 mg/dL in humans[507]) is exceeded, increasing Mg^{2+} spills into the urine in an amount equivalent to the excess filtered load (Fig. 5–30). This observation of an apparent transport maximum (T_m) in such clearance studies initially suggested the existence of a saturable reabsorptive pathway. However, careful *in vivo* tubule perfusion studies have shown that Mg^{2+} reabsorption is not, in fact, saturable with respect to luminal Mg^{2+} concentration in any segment of the nephron, but is inhibited in a concentration-dependent manner by increasing peritubular Mg^{2+} levels in the TAL, giving rise to an apparent T_m effect in studies of whole kidney clearance.[508] The contribution of individual nephron segments is summarized in Table 5–5.

Magnesium Handling by Individual Nephron Segments

Proximal Convoluted Tubule

Only 5% to 15% of filtered Mg^{2+} is reabsorbed in the PCT. Free-flow micropuncture studies have shown that the TF/UF_{Mg} is greater than 1, rises progressively along the length of the PCT, but is always less than the TF/UF for inulin.[405] This indicates that Mg^{2+} is reabsorbed in the PCT, but at a lower rate than that of Na^+ and water. The cellular mechanism of Mg^{2+} reabsorption is unknown. *In vivo* tubule microperfusion

studies showed that PCT Mg^{2+} reabsorption is not saturable, but increases linearly in response to increasing luminal Mg^{2+} conentrations even up to ten times that of plasma UF_{Mg}.[508] Conversely, increasing basolateral Mg^{2+} by induction of hypermagnesemia inhibited Mg^{2+} reabsorption. These findings are consistent with passive Mg^{2+} transport. Furthermore, Mg^{2+} reabsorption in the PCT is inhibited by volume expansion, in parallel with changes in Na^+ and water reabsorption in this segment. The model that best explains Mg^{2+} reabsorption in this segment is one in which the rise in luminal Mg^{2+} concentration due to water reabsorption provides a concentration gradient that drives diffusive paracellular flux. However, two studies have shown very little backflux of peritubular Mg^{2+} into the lumen, suggesting that the passive permeability of this segment is in fact very low.[406,508] Thus, the mechanism for PCT Mg^{2+} reabsorption remains controversial.

In immature animals, the PCT plays a more important role, reabsorbing 60% to 70% of the filtered load.[509] The mechanism for this is unknown.

Proximal Straight Tubule

The only direct data on PST function come from a single study of isolated perfused PST segments, showing that they behave similarly to the PCT.[510] In this study, PST segments reabsorbed Mg^{2+} concomitant with, but at a lower fractional rate than, the reabsorption of Na^+ and water.

Thin Descending and Ascending Limbs of the Loop of Henle

Mg^{2+} transport has not been studied directly in either the thin descending or ascending limbs. It is unlikely that there is any significant net reabsorption in these segments.

Thick Ascending Limb of the Loop of Henle

The TAL is the major site for tubular Mg^{2+} reabsorption and accounts for 60% to 70% of reabsorption along the nephron.[405] The TF/P_{Mg} decreases from 1.5 at the end of the PCT to 0.5 to 0.6 at the beginning of the DCT, indicating that there is net Mg^{2+} reabsorption without water reabsorption and that it can proceed against an uphill concentration gradient. The site of Mg^{2+} reabsorption is species-specific: in the mouse, it occurs in the cortical TAL only, whereas in the rabbit it has been found in both cortical and medullary segments.[405] Quamme and Dirks have shown by *in vivo* microperfusion that Mg^{2+} reabsorption in this segment increases linearly with luminal Mg^{2+} concentration and is unsaturable.[508] When plasma Mg^{2+} and hence peritubular Mg^{2+} concentration is increased while luminal Mg^{2+} is held constant, Mg^{2+} reabsorption is inhibited. Similar results were obtained in *in vitro* perfused TAL segments.[511] These observations probably explain the apparent T_m observed in clearance studies (see Fig. 5–30).

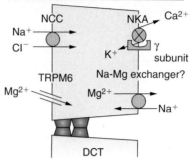

Lumen	Cell	Blood
0.25 mM	~0.5 mM	0.75 mM
+10 mV	−70 mV	0 mV

Lumen	Cell	Blood
0.25 mM	~0.5 mM	0.75 mM
−10 mV	−70 mV	0 mV

FIGURE 5–31 Models depicting the putative cellular mechanism of Mg^{2+} reabsorption in different nephron segments.

The mechanism of Mg^{2+} transport in the TAL is primarily passive and driven by the transepithelial voltage.[486,511] Under normal circumstances, there is a lumen-positive transepithelial potential difference that is generated by apical Na^+, K^+, and Cl^- entry via NKCC2, concomitant with apical K^+ recycling via ROMK (Fig. 5–31).[486] This transepithelial voltage would be expected to drive passive reabsorption of Mg^{2+} even against an uphill concentration gradient. Loop diuretics, such as furosemide and bumetanide, inhibit the Na-K-2Cl cotransporter, and prevent the establishment of a transepithelial potential difference, thereby abolishing Mg^{2+} reabsorption.[486,512] Similarly, extracellular volume expansion decreases Na^+ reabsorption, transepithelial voltage, and hence Mg^{2+} reabsorption in this segment.[513] The route of transport is likely to be a paracellular pathway that is shared with Ca^{2+}. Claudin-16, the tight junction protein mutated in familial hypercalciuric hypomagenesemia, is postulated to be the paracellular Mg^{2+} and Ca^{2+} pore.[185]

Most hormones regulate Mg^{2+} transport in the TAL by altering the transepithelial voltage, or the paracellular permeability (see later). However, glucagon and ADH appear to enchance Mg^{2+} reabsorption in the mouse cortical TAL with little or no change in the transepithelial voltage,[514,515] suggesting the possibility of an additional, transcellular component.

The CaSR is present on the basolateral membrane in this segment[220] and when stimulated, inhibits Na^+ reabsorption,[474] reduces the lumen-positive voltage, and hence inhibits Mg^{2+} reabsorption. This is presumably the mechanism by which hypercalcemia induces magnesuria.[473] The CaSR could also provide a convenient feedback loop for regulating hypermagnesemia. However, the affinity of the CaSR for Mg^{2+} is quite low (EC_{50} of 10 mM when expressed in *Xenopus* oocytes), so it is unlikely to play such a regulatory role under normal circumstances.

Distal Convoluted Tubule and Connecting Tubule

The DCT/CNT reabsorbs 5% to 10% of filtered Mg^{2+}.[405] TF/P_{Mg} increases along the distal tubule, though to a lesser extent than that of inulin, indicating that there is net reabsorption at a lower rate than that of Na^+ and water. Because Mg^{2+} transport in this segment normally operates close to maximum capacity, whereas fractional excretion of Mg^{2+} can vary over a very wide range, the DCT/CNT is unlikely to play a very important regulatory role in Mg^{2+} homeostasis. There are no direct studies to indicate whether reabsorption occurs in the DCT or the CNT, nor is the cellular mechanism known.

Quamme and colleagues have addressed the mechanisms of Mg^{2+} transport in a series of studies in the MDCT cell line. They found that Mg^{2+} entry is stimulated by hyperpolarization, amiloride, and PTH, and inhibited by dihydropyridine Ca^{2+} channel blockers (reviewed in Ref 516). Although these studies have yielded potentially interesting insights into the biology of Mg^{2+} transport, these cells have never been demonstrated to mediate vectorial transepithelial Mg^{2+} transport, nor have the observations ever been corroborated in the DCT itself. Thus, it is unclear at this point whether data obtained from the MDCT cell line have any direct relevance to the situation in the *in vivo* distal tubule.

Collecting Duct

Micropuncture studies comparing the Mg^{2+} content of late superficial distal tubule fluid to the final urine suggested that 1% to 3% of the filtered load may be reabsorbed in the collecting duct.[405] However, this interpretation is flawed because it does not account for the possibility of heterogeneity in handling of Mg^{2+} between superficial and juxtamedullary nephrons. There have been three direct studies of collecting tubule Mg^{2+} transport. Brunette and colleagues micropunctured early and late collecting tubule sites,[517] Shareghi and Agus isolated and perfused CCD segments,[518] and Bengele and co-workers microcatheterized the IMCD *in vivo*.[519] No significant Mg^{2+} reabsorption was observed in any of these studies, indicating that the collecting duct system does not contribute to renal tubule Mg^{2+} handling.

Molecular Mechanisms of Transcellular Mg^{2+} Reabsorption

Apical Mg^{2+} Entry

The apical entry step is primarily mediated by the epithelial Mg^{2+} channel, TRPM6 (see Fig. 5–31). TRPM6, which is also a member of the TRP family, was first identified as the culprit gene for familial hypomagnesemia with secondary hypocalcemia, an autosomal recessive disease characterized by intestinal malabsorption of Mg^{2+} associated with renal Mg^{2+} wasting.[520,521] TRPM6 is expressed at the apical membrane of DCT1 and DCT2 (see Fig. 5–18),[522] and also at the brush border of intestinal absorptive epithelial cells in the colon and cecum. When expressed in HEK cells, TRPM6 forms cation channels that permeate both Ca^{2+} and Mg^{2+}. However, the affinity of the channel is much higher for Mg^{2+} than for Ca^{2+} suggesting that under physiological conditions, it primarily conducts Mg^{2+}.[522]

TRPM7, a close homolog of TRPM6, is ubiquitously expressed, and also encodes divalent cation channels.[523] Interestingly, TRPM6 and TRPM7 are distinct from all other ion channels in that they are composed of a channel linked to an atypical protein α-kinase domain whose function is so far undefined.[523] TRPM6 associates with TRPM7. In *Xenopus* oocytes and in HEK cells, this appears to be necessary for trafficking of TRPM6 to the cell surface.[524] Thus, TRPM6/TRPM7 heteromultimers may represent the functional unit of the Mg^{2+} channel in the DCT.

Basolateral Mg^{2+} Exit

The identity of the basolateral Mg^{2+} transport protein(s) remains unknown. One hypothesis is that this step is mediated by a Na-Mg exchanger, such as has been observed in a variety of other tissues, including squid axon, myocardium, and erythrocytes. However, the molecular identity of such a Na-Mg exchanger has yet to be elucidated.

Interestingly, mutations in FXYD2,[525] which encodes a Na-K-ATPase γ-subunit, have been found in autosomal dominant isolated familial hypomagnesemia, which is characterized by hypomagnesemia with renal Mg^{2+} wasting.[526] Mutation of the γ-subunit was shown to abolish its ability to facilitate trafficking of the α- and β-subunits of the Na-K-ATPase to the cell surface.[525] A plausible explanation is that active, transcellular Mg^{2+} reabsorption in the distal tubule requires a secondary active transport step (i.e., Na-Mg exchange) that is energetically dependent on the Na^+ gradient across the basolateral membrane, and hence on Na-K-ATPase activity (see Fig. 5–31). Mutation of the γ-subunit impairs Na-K-ATPase surface trafficking leading to loss of the basolateral Na^+ gradient and therefore defective Na-Mg exchange.

Regulation of Renal Magnesium Handling

Many factors influence renal Mg^{2+} handling. These are summarized in Table 5–6, and only the most important are discussed here.

Sodium and Extracellular Fluid Volume
Saline expansion increases the excretion of Mg^{2+}, concomitant with that of Na^+ and water. This occurs even when the renal artery perfusion pressure is reduced to decrease the GFR, and is associated with an increase in the fractional excretion, indicating that tubule Mg^{2+} reabsorption is inhibited. In the PCT, Wen and colleagues showed that fractional reabsorption of Mg^{2+} declined from 30% to 15%.[527] This is consistent with the observation that Mg^{2+} handling in this segment generally parallels that of Na^+ and water. There was also a substantial reduction in TAL fractional reabsorption so that the bulk of the increased load of Mg^{2+} delivered to the loop of Henle appeared in the urine.

Hypermagnesemia and Hypomagnesemia
Hypermagnesemia increases renal Mg^{2+} excretion, not only due to an increased filtered load, but also due to inhibition

of tubule reabsorption. In the proximal tubule, absolute reabsorption increases, due to increased delivery, but fractional reabsorption decreases, in parallel with a decrease in Na^+ and water reabsorption of unknown cause.[527] In the TAL, Mg^{2+} reabsorption is specifically inhibited by the high peritubular Mg^{2+} concentration.[508] Several possible mechanisms could explain this. First, the concentration gradient for passive diffusion of Mg^{2+} would be reduced if basolateral Mg^{2+} concentrations were high. However, in hypermagnesemia luminal Mg^{2+} concentrations would also be expected to be high, yet this does not seem to be sufficient to overcome the inhibition. Second, basolateral Mg^{2+} may direct inhibit Mg^{2+} transport, perhaps by binding to the basolateral opening of a paracellular Mg^{2+} channel such as claudin-16, in the same way that Mg^{2+} blocks other cation channels. Third, basolateral Mg^{2+} may, like Ca^{2+}, stimulate the TAL CaSR,[220] thereby triggering the generation of arachidonic acid metabolites that inhibit NKCC2 and ROMK and abolishing the transepithelial voltage that drives Mg^{2+} reabsorption.

During profound Mg^{2+} depletion, fractional excretion of Mg^{2+} falls markedly, usually to below 1% in humans.[506,528] Studies of Mg^{2+} depletion in rats demonstrated that proximal tubule fractional reabsorption did not change; because the delivered load was less, though, the absolute reabsorption of Mg^{2+} in this segment was reduced.[529] The major site of adaptive change is the TAL, where fractional reabsorption was increased by 12%, so that only 3% of the filtered load exited the TAL.[529] The mechanism by which the TAL can conserve Mg^{2+} under these circumstances is not well understood. A recent study found that dietary Mg^{2+} restriction caused upregulation of TRPM6 mRNA in the kidney.[530] This could also increase Mg^{2+} reabsorption in the DCT.

Hypercalcemia and Hypocalcemia
Hypercalcemia causes an increase in renal excretion of Mg^{2+}, concomitant with, but exceeding, the increase in excretion of Ca^{2+}. In the proximal tubule, hypercalcemia reduces Na^+ and water reabsorption, which is presumably the mechanism that then reduces reabsorption of Ca^{2+} and Mg^{2+}.[473] In the TAL, both Ca^{2+} and Mg^{2+} reabsorption are inhibited by hypercalcemia, most likely due to stimulation of the basolateral CaSR. The DCT increases reabsorption of Ca^{2+} and Mg^{2+} in response to the increased delivered load.[473] In hypocalcemia, the opposite effects may be observed. Mg^{2+} excretion is reduced, consistent with an increase in reabsorption primarily in the TAL.[508]

Acid-Base Status
In most studies, metabolic acidosis has been found to increase Mg^{2+} excretion. This has been attributed to a decrease in TAL Mg^{2+} reabsorption.[506] However, chronic metabolic acidosis also decreases TRPM6 mRNA expression, suggesting an effect in the DCT.[480]

Metabolic alkalosis causes a consistent decrease in Mg^{2+} excretion. Mg^{2+} reabsorption is increased in the juxtamedullary loop and persists despite the administration of furosemide, excluding an effect in the TAL. Micropuncture studies suggested that the site of increased Mg^{2+} reabsorption is between the late PCT and the early DCT. However, TRPM6 mRNA expression is also increased, suggesting that alkalosis may also stimulate DCT Mg^{2+} reabsorption.[480]

Hormones
No single hormone plays a primary role in regulating Mg^{2+} homeostasis.

Parathyroid Hormone
Parathyroid hormone enhances the reabsorption of Mg^{2+}, as it does for Ca^{2+}, in hypoparathyroid humans and in experimental animals.[405] This appears to be due to increased reabsorption in the TAL.[508] In the in vitro perfused cortical TAL,

TABLE 5–6	Summary of Factors Affecting Mg^{2+} Reabsorption		
	Nephron Location		
Factor	**Proximal**	**TAL**	**Distal**
Volume expansion	↓	↓	?
Magnesium			
Hypermagnesemia	↑	↓	No Δ
Hypomagnesemia	↓	↑	No Δ
Hypercalcemia	↓	↓	No Δ
Phosphate depletion	No Δ	↓	↓
Acid-base status			
Acidosis		↓	↓
Alkalosis			↑
Hormones			
PTH	No Δ	↑	↑?
Calcitonin	No Δ	↑?	No Δ
Estrogens			↑
Diuretics			
Loop diuretics	No Δ	↓	No Δ
Calcineurin inhibitors			↓

TAL, thick ascending limb; PTH, parathyroid hormone.
No Δ, no change.

PTH stimulates Mg^{2+} and Ca^{2+} reabsorption in parallel, both by increasing NaCl reabsorption and therefore the generation of a transepithelial potential difference, and by increasing the passive permeability of the TAL to paracellular transport.[486]

Estrogens

Menopausal women are magnesuric and estrogen replacement therapy decreases urinary Mg^{2+} excretion.[405] In rats, TRPM6 mRNA was downregulated by ovariectomy and restored to normal levels by estrogen administration, suggesting that estrogen effects on the DCT are responsible.[530]

Diuretics
Thiazide Diuretics

The administration of thiazide diuretics causes a very small and variable increase in Mg^{2+} excretion in animals and humans.[405] Thiazides primarily act on the NaCl cotransporter, NCC, which is located in the DCT. However, micropuncture studies in the hamster found that Mg^{2+} reabsorption in this segment was unchanged by chlorothiazide.[531] These findings are at odds with the observation that patients with Gitelman syndrome, who have inactivating mutations in NCC, universally have renal Mg^{2+} wasting.[498]

Loop Diuretics

Loop diuretics increase Mg^{2+} excretion by abolishing the lumen-positive voltage in the TAL (see Fig. 5–31).[499] Interestingly, the increase in Mg^{2+} excretion with furosemide is greater than that of Na^+ or Ca^{2+}.[512] The reasons for this are unknown, but it is possible that furosemide inhibits other aspects of Mg^{2+} transport, or that, unlike with Na^+ or Ca^{2+}, the distal nephron is unable to compensate for the increased Mg^{2+} delivered from the TAL.

Calcineurin Inhibitors

Transplant patients on calcineurin inhibitors such as cyclosporine and tacrolimus are frequently hypomagnesemic due to renal Mg^{2+} wasting.[532] One potential mechanism may be by downregulation of TRPM6 mRNA.[419]

PHOSPHATE TRANSPORT

Phosphate Homeostasis

Total Body Phosphate

Phosphate has multiple functions in the body. Like Ca^{2+}, it is a key component of the bony skeleton. Phosphate is important for metabolic processes, including the formation of high energy phosphate bonds such as those in ATP. It is also an important component of nucleic acids. Phosphorylation of cellular proteins is an important mechanism for regulation of cellular function. Finally, phosphate is an important blood and urinary pH buffer.

The total body content of phosphorus is 700 g in an average adult, of which 85% is in bone and teeth, 14% in soft tissues, and only 1% in extracellular fluid. The normal concentration of phosphorus in plasma is 3 mg/dL to 4.5 mg/dL (1 to 1.5 mM). Phosphorus is present in plasma primarily as HPO_4^{-2} and $H_2PO_4^{-1}$, which exist in a pH-dependent equilibrium (pK_a 6.8). Thus, at pH 7.4, the ratio of HPO_4^{-2} to $H_2PO_4^{-1}$ is $4:1$ and the average valence is 1.8. (The atomic mass of phosphorus is 31. Thus, 1 mmol plasma phosphate $\equiv$ 1.8 mEq $\equiv$ 31 mg; and 1 mM phosphate $\equiv$ 1.8 mEq/L $\equiv$ 3.1 mg/dL.)

Plasma phosphate exists in ionized, complexed, and protein-bound forms. If phosphate were totally filterable through artificial and glomerular membranes, its concentration in the ultrafiltrate would be 1.18 times that of plasma (corrected for plasma water and the Gibbs-Donnan factor). Measured ultrafilterable phosphate to plasma phosphate ratios have been found to range from 0.89 to 0.96, indicating that about 25% of plasma phosphate is bound to protein.

Of ultrafilterable phosphate, approximately 60% is ionized and 40% is complexed to the major plasma cations, chiefly Ca^{2+}, Mg^{2+}, and Na^+. The fraction of total phosphate that is ultrafilterable declines with hypercalcemia, probably due to the formation of calcium-phosphate-proteinate complexes.

Intracellular phosphate is primarily sequestered in intracellular organelles, or incorporated into organic compounds such as creatine phosphate, adenosine phosphates and, in erythrocytes, 2,3-diphosphoglycerate. The cytosolic free inorganic phosphate concentration is only about 1 mM. Nevertheless, this is above its electrochemical equilibrium value as predicted from the membrane potential, suggesting that there must be active transport of phosphate into cells. The regulation of intracellular phosphate levels is closely linked to cellular metabolic activity. Inhibition of phosphate uptake impairs cellular metabolic function, whereas increasing extracellular phosphate concentration stimulates mitochondrial respiration. Conversely, bathing cells in glucose reduces phosphate uptake and in conditions of limited phosphate availability reduces mitochondrial respiration, oxidative phosphorylation, and ATP content, a phenomenon called the Crabtree effect.

Intake and Output

The daily dietary intake of phosphate is 800 mg to 1500 mg (Fig. 5–32). Phosphate is found in many foods, including dairy products, meat, and cereal grains, so that dietary deficiency is rare. Approximately 65% of ingested phosphate is absorbed, primarily by the duodenum and jejunum. This varies proportionally with dietary intake. Dietary polyvalent cations such as Ca^{2+}, Mg^{2+}, and Al^{3+} bind to intestinal luminal phosphate and decrease its absorption. Secreted digestive juices contain about 3 mg/kg/day of phosphate. Once absorbed, phosphate in the extracellular fluid may exchange with the pool in bone, with 200 mg of phosphate typically entering and leaving the skeleton daily as it is continuously remodeled. Ultimately, the kidneys are responsible for the excretion of a substantial excess of phosphate, about 900 mg per day. During periods of growth, a greater proportion of phosphate is retained for bone deposition, but this still constitutes a small percentage of dietary intake. Thus, renal phosphate excretion is the principal mechanism by which the body regulates extracellular phosphate balance.

Overview of Phosphate Regulation

The plasma concentration of phosphate is maintained by $1,25(OH)_2D$, PTH and phosphatonins (Fig. 5–33). The phosphatonins refer to a group of humoral phosphaturic factors, of which the most well characterized is fibroblast growth factor 23 (FGF-23),[533] which were first isolated from tumors of patients with tumor-induced osteomalacia,[534] and are produced primarily in bone. A rise in plasma phosphate stimulates the release of PTH in three ways. First, phosphate

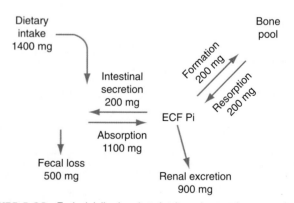

FIGURE 5–32 Typical daily phosphate intake and output for a normal adult in neutral phosphate balance (see text for details).

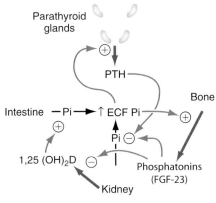

FIGURE 5–33 Summary of overall phosphate homeostasis. The primary homeostatic mechanisms activated in response to a rise in extracellular fluid (ECF) phosphate concentration are shown.

TABLE 5–7	Segmental Handling of Phosphate Along the Renal Tubule	
Nephron Segment	**Fractional Reabsorption (%)**	**Cellular Transport Mechanism**
Proximal tubule	80	Active, transcellular
Thin descending and ascending limbs	0	
TAL	0	
DCT/CNT	5	Active, transcellular
Collecting duct	+/–	Unknown

TAL, thick ascending limb; DCT, distal convoluted tubule; CNT, connecting tubule.

directly stimulates PTH synthesis and release from the parathyroid gland, as well as parathyroid cell growth.[535,536] Second, a rise in serum phosphate causes a fall in serum free Ca^{2+}, which stimulates PTH release via activation of the CaSR. Third, hyperphosphatemia decreases circulating 1,25(OH)$_2$D, alleviating its inhibition of PTH secretion.[535] Hyperphosphatemia also stimulates FGF-23 expression and release.[537] Both PTH and FGF-23 (and perhaps other phosphatonins) then inhibit renal tubular phosphate reabsorption and hence increase phosphate excretion. In addition, hyperphosphatemia also inhibits expression of the enzyme, 25-hydroxyvitamin D 1α-hydroxylase, in the proximal tubule, perhaps mediated by FGF-23.[537] This decreases 1,25(OH)$_2$D, a hormone that normally stimulates intestinal phosphate absorption. Decreased intestinal phosphate absorption then contributes to the restoration of normal plasma phosphate levels. A fall in plasma phosphate would trigger the opposite effects.

Renal Handling of Phosphate

Only the ionized and complexed forms of plasma phosphate are ultrafiltered at the glomerulus, so that the phosphate concentration of fluid in Bowman space is approximately 90% of the total plasma phosphate concentration.[405] Renal clearance studies have demonstrated that 80% to 97% of the filtered load of phosphate is reabsorbed by the renal tubules, so that only 3% to 20% is ultimately excreted. The contribution of individual nephron segments is summarized in Table 5–7.

The relationship between plasma phosphate and phosphate excretion is shown in Figure 5–34. Initially as the plasma

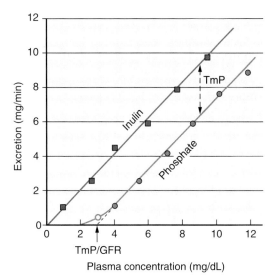

FIGURE 5–34 Relationship between urinary excretion rate and plasma concentration of phosphate in a normal human subject during fasting (open circle) and phosphate infusion (solid circles). Also shown is the excretion-concentration relationship for inulin (squares). The slope of both lines is the same and equal to the GFR. The vertical distance between the two lines represents the maximum tubular reabsorption rate of phosphate (TmP). The x-intercept, extrapolated from the line connecting the solid circles, represents the theoretical renal phosphate threshold (TmP/GFR). (From Bijvoet OL: Relation of plasma phosphate concentration to renal tubular reabsorption of phosphate. Clin Sci 37:23–36, 1969.)

phosphate, and hence filtered load, increases, there is a commensurate increase in the reabsorption of phosphate, so that minimal phosphate appears in the urine. When the plasma phosphate exceeds a certain level, the renal threshold, phosphate begins to appear in the urine, increasing in proportion to the filtered load. This indicates that tubular reabsorption of phosphate is saturable. In humans, with a GFR above 40 ml/min, the maximum tubular reabsorption rate of phosphate, TmP, varies proportionately with GFR. Thus, TmP/GFR, which is the theoretical renal threshold, is kept constant and is a reliable index of tubule reabsorptive capacity.

With advanced renal insufficiency (GFR <40 ml/min), TmP is further decreased (in part due to secondary hyperparathyroidism) and the fractional excretion of phosphate further increased. However, the decrease in TmP is less than the decrease in GFR, so that TmP/GFR rises and hyperphosphatemia ensues.

Phosphate Handling by individual Nephron Segments
Proximal Tubule
About 80% of filtered phosphate is reabsorbed in the proximal tubule. There is marked axial heterogeneity in reabsorptive activity. Micropuncture studies show that 60% to 70% of filtered phosphate is reabsorbed within the PCT itself.[538] Of this, most is reabsorbed in the S1 segment. The net reabsorptive rate has been estimated to be 11 to 14 pmol/min/mm in the S1 segment, 3 pmol/min/mm in the S2 segment, and 2 pmol/min/mm in the S3 segment.[538,539] In thyroparathyroidectomized animals, the later convolutions become capable of higher reabsorptive rates, suggesting that the S2 segment may be more sensitive to suppression by PTH.[540]

These findings have been confirmed in primary cultured cell lines and in isolated membrane vesicles. Primary cell cultures derived from the S1 segments had higher reabsorptive rates than those from S3 segments.[541] Furthermore, PTH and cyclic AMP analogs suppressed phosphate reabsorption in S3 cells but not in S1 cells. Two studies have compared brush border membrane vesicles (BBMV) derived from the superficial cortex (primarily PCT segments), and those derived from the juxtamedullary cortex and/or outer stripe of outer medulla (primarily PST segments).[542,543] These showed that the V_{max} for Na-phosphate cotransport was four times higher in the superficial cortex BBMV than those from the juxtamedullary cortex, whereas the K_m for phosphate was slightly lower. Furthermore, the density of Na-Pi transporters, as estimated by binding studies with phosphonoformic acid, was also higher in the superficial cortex.[543] These findings indicate that the earliest convolutions of the PCT have the highest density of phosphate transporters and the highest capacity to reabsorb phosphate. The PST has a lower reabsorptive capacity but higher affinity for phosphate. These are appropriate characteristics for a downstream segment that sees less delivered phosphate load and lower luminal concentrations than the PCT.

There is also some evidence for internephron heterogeneity in reabsorptive activity. The fractional delivery of phosphate to the micropuncture-accessible DCT, which is derived from superficial nephrons, is consistently greater than that delivered to the bend of the loop of Henle of juxtamedullary nephrons.[544] This suggests that the proximal reabsorptive capacity of juxtamedullary nephrons is greater than that of superficial nephrons. In rats, this discrepancy is observed only when they are thyroparathyroidectomized, but not when PTH is repleted, suggesting that juxtamedullary nephrons are more sensitive to the inhibitory effect of PTH.[544] In rats loaded with excess phosphate, the superficial nephrons reabsorb more than the juxtamedullary nephrons, suggesting that superficial nephrons adapt more effectively to increased filtered phosphate load than do juxtamedullary nephrons.[545] Conversely, in a study of isolated perfused tubule segments, no difference was found between the reabsorptive rates of superficial and juxtamedullary nephrons.[539]

Loop of Henle

There is likely no reabsorption of phosphate in the loop of Henle, other than the PST. In parathyroid-intact animals, micropuncture studies show no phosphate reabsorption between the late PCT and early DCT. In thyroparathyroidecomized animals there is some phosphate reabsorption in this region, but it could all be attributable to the transport occurring in the PST.[405] Consistent with this, the phosphate permeability measured in isolated perfused thin descending and ascending limbs, and cortical thick ascending limbs is extremely low.[409]

Distal Convoluted Tubule and Connecting Tubule

Micropuncture studies have observed reabsorption of phosphate between the early DCT and the final urine.[405] In the interpretation of these early micropuncture studies, one potential source of artifact that must be considered is the heterogeneity in proximal transport between nephrons. As mentioned previously, the proximal tubules of juxtamedullary nephrons reabsorb more phosphate than their superficial counterparts. Because the micropuncture fluid from the superficial DCT reflects delivery only from superficial nephrons while the final urine reflects delivery from both superficial and juxtamedullary nephrons, the phosphate concentration in the urine may be less than that in the early DCT, even when there is no distal tubule reabsorption.

Several lines of evidence suggest there may be true distal tubule phosphate reabsorption, at least under conditions of phosphate deprivation, and that this is not simply an artifact of nephron heterogeneity. First, micropuncture studies that have sampled fluid from both the early DCT (derived from superficial nephrons) and the papillary loop of Henle (derived from juxtamedullary nephrons) find that the fractional delivery of phosphate to *both* sites is similar and 6% to 8% greater than in the final urine, but only when the animal is on a low phosphate diet.[546] Second, micropuncture studies that have sampled fluid directly from both early and late convolutions of the DCT show that approximately 5% of filtered phosphate is reabsorbed between these two sites.[547] Third, in stop-flow studies of the DCT, the $TF/UF_{phosphate}$ concentration ratio, corrected for water absorption, doubled after PTH administration, consistent with a reduction in the normal phosphate reabsorption rate in this segment.[548]

Several studies have failed to find phosphate transport in the distal tubules from animals on a normal diet.[405] Because distal tubule phosphate transport is enhanced by low phosphate diet, it is possible that reabsorption in this segment is difficult to detect in animals on a normal phosphate diet.

The cellular mechanism for DCT phosphate reabsorption is unknown, but on thermodynamic grounds luminal uptake must occur by active transport. Whether transport occurs in both the DCT and CNT or in the DCT alone is also unclear.

Collecting Duct

The collecting duct accounts for very little, if any, phosphate reabsorption. In isolated perfused CCD, a small amount of phosphate reabsorption was found by some investigators but not by others.[405] One study found phosphate reabsorption by microcatheterization of the IMCD but only in thyroparathyroidectomized animals. In another study, no phosphate transport was found in the papillary collecting duct.

Molecular Mechanisms of Transcellular Phosphate Reabsorption

Transcellular phosphate reabsorption occurs primarily in the proximal tubule, where its mechanism has been studied in detail (Fig. 5–35). Intracellular phosphate levels are higher than the level expected for electrochemical equilibrium with luminal fluid, so apical entry must occur by active transport, while basolateral exit may occur by diffusion.

Apical Phosphate Entry

The apical entry of phosphate is the rate-limiting step in transcellular phosphate transport, and the target for virtually all physiological mechanisms that alter tubule phosphate reabsorption. Hoffmann and colleagues[549] were the first to show that kidney cortex BBMV exhibit Na^+-dependent phosphate cotransport. Some of the key features of the apical Na-phosphate cotransporter have emerged from this and subsequent vesicle studies. The coupling ratio of Na^+ to phosphate is greater than unity. Both HPO_4^{-2} and $H_2PO_4^{-1}$ are transported, so transport is partly electrogenic (net positive charge movement with phosphate entry); however, transport of the divalent form is preferred. There is normally a steep inward concentration gradient for Na^+ across the plasma membrane that is maintained by the basolateral Na-K-ATPase, and an inside-negative membrane potential. Thus, the high

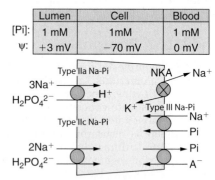

FIGURE 5–35 Model depicting the putative cellular mechanisms of phosphate transport in the proximal tubule. Pi, phosphate; A^-, inorganic anion.

TABLE 5–8	The Three Families of Na-Pi Cotransporters				
	Type I	Type II			Type III
		Type IIa	Type IIb	Type IIc	
Protein name	NaPi-1	NaPi-2/3/4/6/7	NaPi-5		PiT-1 (Glvr-1) PiT-2 (Ram-1)
Gene name	*SLC17*	*SLC34A1*	*SLC34A2*	*SLC34A3*	*SLC20*
Tissue expression	Kidney cortex/PT, liver, brain	Kidney cortex/PT	Small intestine, lung	Kidney cortex/PT	Ubiquitous
Substrates	Phosphate, Cl$^-$, organic anions	Phosphate	Phosphate	Phosphate	Phosphate
Affinity for phosphate	~1 mM	0.1–0.2 mM	0.05 mM	0.07 mM	0.025 mM
Affinity for Na$^+$	50–60 mM	50–70 mM	33 mM	48 mM	40–50 mM
Na$^+$-phosphate coupling ratio	>1	3	3	2	3
pH dependence	None	Stimulated at high pH	Inhibited at high pH	Stimulated at high pH	Inhibited at high pH
Regulation by PTH or dietary phosphate	No	PTH and diet	Diet	Diet	?Diet

PT, proximal tubule.
Modified from Murer H, Hernando N, Forster I, Biber J: Proximal tubular phosphate reabsorption: molecular mechanisms. Physiol Rev 80:1373–1409, 2000.

coupling ratio and electrogenicity are both thermodynamically important for the secondary active transport of phosphate against its steep electrochemical gradient at the apical membrane, particularly in the late proximal tubule, where luminal phosphate levels are low. The transporter is stimulated by increasing extravesicular pH, which not only increases the proportion of phosphate in the preferred, divalent form, but also increases the affinity of the transporter for Na$^+$, either by a competitive or allosteric effect. Extravesicular Na$^+$ enhances the transporter's affinity for phosphate. Thus, there may be allosteric sites for modulation both by Na$^+$ and by H$^+$. Additionally, an inwardly directed H$^+$ gradient stimulates transport, probably by trapping intravesicular phosphate in the monovalent (non-preferred) form and thereby impeding its efflux. Finally, transport is competitively inhibited by arsenate and foscarnet (phosphonoformic acid).

Three subclasses of the Na-phosphate (Na-Pi) cotransporters have now been identified at the molecular level, and named type I, II, and III (Table 5–8). The type I Na-Pi cotransporter[550] is expressed on the brush border of the proximal tubule,[551,552] as well as in liver and brain. However, the characteristics of the type I Na-Pi transporter do not resemble renal brush border Na-phosphate cotransport[553,554] making it unlikely that the type I transporter plays an important role in transcellular phosphate transport. The type III Na-Pi cotransporters are ubiquitously expressed, including at the basolateral membrane of the proximal tubule,[555] and are probably housekeeping proteins required for phosphate uptake for cellular metabolic needs.

The type II Na-Pi cotransporters include three homologous isoforms, type IIa,[556] and IIc,[557] which are expressed at the proximal tubule brush border, and type IIb, which in mammals is expressed in the small intestine and in pneumocytes.[558,559] The type IIa Na-Pi cotransporter is probably the predominant apical phosphate entry transporter in the proximal tubule. When expressed in *Xenopus* oocytes and studied by radioisotope uptake or by electrophysiology under whole cell voltage clamp, its functional characteristics match well those of the BBMV transport system (see Table 5–8).[556] Like the BBMV Na$^+$-phosphate transport system, it is electrogenic.[560]

By simultaneous measurement of substrate flux and charge movement under voltage-clamp conditions, the stoichiometry was determined to be 3 Na$^+$:1 phosphate.[560] Furthermore, the dependence on external pH was confirmed, and shown to be due both to a competitive interaction of H$^+$ with the Na$^+$-binding site,[561] and to an additional effect on reorientation of the empty transporter.[562]

The role of the type IIa cotransporter is also supported by gene knockout studies. Mice with targeted inactivation of the Npt2 gene exhibited phosphaturia, hypophosphatemia, and an appropriate elevation in the serum concentration of 1,25(OH)$_2$D with attendant hypercalcemia, hypercalciuria, and decreased serum PTH levels.[563] Na$^+$-phosphate cotransport in BBMV derived from the knockout mice was reduced by 85% compared to wild-type controls, indicating that the cause of the phosphaturia was loss of the major brush border Na$^+$-phosphate transport system.[564] Furthermore, two patients have now been described that have heterozygous inactivating mutations in this the type IIa cotransporter. Both have idiopathic hypophosphatemia with renal Pi wasting, associated in one case with recurrent nephrolithiasis and in the other with osteoporosis.[565]

The type IIa cotransporter participates in multiple protein interactions via a PDZ-binding motif on its C-terminal tail.[566] This is a peptide motif that binds to the PDZ domains on PDZ-containing proteins, including PDZK1 (NaPi-Cap1) and Na-H exchanger-regulatory factor 1 (NHERF1),[567] both of which are also located on the brush border membrane of the proximal tubule.[568] Disruption of these interactions by competition with PDZ domain peptides prevent normal trafficking of the type IIa cotransporter to the apical membrane.[569] The importance of NHERF1 is demonstrated by the finding that in knockout mice that lack NHERF1, the proximal tubule type IIa Na-Pi cotransporter is aberrantly localized intracellularly, and the mice are overtly phosphaturic.[570] Thus NHERF1 is required for normal trafficking of the type IIa cotransporter to the cell surface. By contrast, PDZK1-knockout mice had very little phenotype. When chronically fed a high-phosphate diet, the type IIa cotransporter expression at the brush border was decreased, and urinary excretion of phosphate was slightly elevated.[571] Thus the physiological role of PDZK1 is unclear.

The type IIc Na-Pi cotransporter is likely to be important in renal phosphate reabsorption primarily in early life. It exhibits Na-dependent phosphate cotransport that is electroneutral, with a stoichiometry of 2 Na^+:1 phosphate, and is stimulated by alkaline extracellular pH.[557,572] The type IIc cotransporter is expressed primarily in the kidney at the apical membrane of the proximal tubule, and at significantly higher levels in weaning animals than adults. mRNA hybrid depletion experiments suggest that both the type IIa and type IIc proteins function as Na-phosphate cotransporters in weaning animals, but only type IIa in adults.[557] The 2:1 stoichiometry, as well as the lack of coupled movement of net charge, would be expected to reduce the thermodynamic ability of the transporter to concentrate phosphate within the proximal tubule epithelial cell. However, weaning animals have substantially lower renal intracellular phosphate concentrations.[573] Thus, the type IIc cotransporter may be expressed in weaning animals to take advantage of the increased phosphate gradient and thereby transport phosphate more efficiently.

The physiological importance of the type IIc Na-Pi cotransporter has now been confirmed by the demonstration that inactivating mutations in its gene, SLC34A3, cause the autosomal recessive renal phosphate wasting disorder, hereditary hypophosphatemic rickets with hypercalciuria.[574,575]

Basolateral Phosphate Exit

Transport of phosphate at the basolateral membrane in the proximal tubule must be sufficiently flexible to mediate two different functions. First, to mediate transcellular phosphate reabsorption it must be able to efflux some or all of the phosphate that enters from the luminal membrane. Second, it must be able to mediate influx of phosphate for intracellular metabolic processes, if apical phosphate entry is insufficient to meet cellular requirements.

The precise mechanisms for basolateral phosphate exit are poorly understood. Several studies have found evidence for Na^+-independent phosphate uptake in basolateral membrane vesicles that is driven by an intravesicular-positive membrane potential, *trans*-stimulated by intravesicular loading with phosphate or other inorganic anions, and insensitive to distilbenes.[405] Thus, the evidence supports the existence of an electrogenic phosphate-anion exchanger as the probable basolateral phosphate efflux system.

In addition, Na^+-phosphate cotransport has been found in basolateral membranes from dog kidney, but not from the rat. It has been suggested that such conflicting results may be caused by variable contamination of basolateral vesicle preparations with brush border membranes. If basolateral Na^+-phosphate cotransport does occur, it would likely serve as the "housekeeping" phosphate influx system. As mentioned earlier, the most likely molecular candidate for such a transporter is the type III Na-Pi cotransporter.

Regulation of Renal Phosphate Handling

Many factors influence renal phosphate handling. These are summarized in Table 5–9, and only the most important are discussed here.

Dietary Phosphate

Clearance studies have demonstrated that phosphate excretion is remarkably responsive to antecedent phosphate intake. Fractional excretion of phosphate increases with a high phosphate diet and decreases with a low phosphate diet, independent of any effect on plasma phosphate, Ca^{2+}, or PTH concentration.[405] By micropuncture, the major site of adapta-

tion is the proximal tubule, though the distal tubule also shows upregulation of phosphate reabsorption during phosphate deprivation. Superficial nephrons demonstrate a greater suppression of phosphate reabsorption on a high phosphate diet than do juxtamedullary nephrons. BBMV transport studies demonstrate that this adaptation is due to changes in the V_{max} of the apical Na^+-phosphate cotransporter.

The acute adaptive changes in response to dietary phosphate are due to trafficking of the type IIa and type IIc Na-phosphate cotransporters, whereas chronic adaptive changes are mediated by changes in transcription and translation. In animals chronically fed a high phosphate diet, the type IIa transporter mRNA and protein abundance are low. By immunofluorescence the transporter is mostly found in juxtamedullary nephrons; within the proximal tubule it is largely localized to intracellular vesicles.[576] Upon acutely switching to a low phosphate diet, brush border membrane transporter protein is increased,[577] but without any change in mRNA abundance.[576] The transporter is recruited to more superficial nephrons and redistributed within the proximal tubule to the brush border.[576] This redistribution is due to microtubule-dependent insertion of membrane vesicles into the apical membrane.[578] These changes are not inhibited by actinomycin D nor by cycloheximide, confirming that new RNA and protein synthesis are not required.[578] With chronic feeding of a low phosphate diet, the type IIa transporter mRNA also increases. Refeeding a high phosphate diet to animals chronically adapted to a low phosphate diet reverses all these changes.[579,580] Acutely after switching to a high phosphate diet, the type IIa transporter is internalized by membrane retrieval from the apical surface and sequestration in the subapical vacuolar network. This process was found to be dependent on microtubules in one study,[581] but not in another.[578] The endocytosed transporter is subsequently trafficked to lysosomes for degradation.[582] Chronic high phosphate diet also down-regulates transporter mRNA and protein. The effects of dietary phosphate are not mediated by PTH because they could be observed even in parathyroidectomized animals.[580]

Similarly a high phosphate diet causes acute internalization of type IIc transporter but, unlike type IIa Na-Pi cotransporters that are trafficked to lysosomes, type IIc transporters are trafficked to an intracellular, subapical pool and are not degraded.[583] Similar to type IIa cotransporters, type IIc cotransporter protein abundance was decreased in mice fed a chronic high-phosphate diet.[584]

The upstream signals that mediate the acute and chronic effects of dietary phosphate are not well understood. Dietary phosphate affects the concentrations of phosphate in plasma and in tubular fluid, so it is possible that that proximal tubule cells sense phosphate directly. In this regard, it is interesting to note that type IIa cotransporter adaptation can also be observed in opposum kidney (OK) cells simply by culturing in low or high phosphate media.[585] The basis of transcriptional activation of the NPT2 gene in response to chronic low phosphate diet has been investigated by two groups. Kido and colleagues used DNA footprinting analysis to identify a putative phosphate response element in the NPT2 promoter that binds to mouse transcription factor µE3 (TFE3).[586] TFE3 was found to be upregulated by a low phosphate diet, and stimulated transcription from the NPT2 promoter. Custer and colleagues[587] used differential display-PCR to identify PDZ1 as an mRNA upregulated by low phosphate diet. When PDZ1 was coexpressed with NaPi-2 cRNA in *Xenopus* oocytes, it stimulated Na^+-phosphate cotransport, suggesting that PDZ1 may have a post-transcriptional regulatory role.

Calcium

Acute hypercalcemia, especially when severe, decreases phosphate excretion by several mechanisms. Hypercalcemia

TABLE 5–9 Summary of Factors Affecting Phosphate Reabsorption

Factor	Proximal Tubule Reabsorption	Effect on Type IIa Na-Pi Cotransporter	Putative Mechanism Acute/Chronic
Volume expansion	↓		
Hypercalcemia Acute Chronic	↑ ↓		Activation of CaSR
Phosphate Loading Depletion	↓ ↑	↓ ↑	Endocytosis/↓ mRNA Exocytosis/↑ mRNA
Metabolic acidosis Acute Chronic	No Δ ↓	↓	Endocytosis/↓ mRNA
Metabolic alkalosis Acute Chronic	↓ ↑	↑	?Inhibition of basolateral Pi transport Exocytosis/↑ mRNA
Respiratory acidosis	↓	?↓	?↓ mRNA
Respiratory alkalosis	↑	?↑	↓ filtered load/↑ mRNA
Hormones PTH	↓	↓	Endocytosis/↓ mRNA
Vitamin D Acute Chronic	↑ ↓	↑ ↓	↑ mRNA ↓ mRNA
Dopamine	↓		Endocytosis of Na-K-ATPase α_1 subunit
Insulin	↑		
Stanniocalcin-1	↑	↑	
FGF-23	↓	↓	↓ mRNA
Diuretics Acetazolamide Thiazides Mannitol	↓ ↓ ↓		

PTH, parathyroid hormone.

decreases the plasma concentration of ultrafilterable phosphate because of the formation Ca²⁺-phosphate-proteinate complexes. Hypercalcemia also decreases renal blood flow and GFR. As a consequence, filtered load of phosphate falls. In most studies, tubule reabsorption of phosphate is increased with acute hypercalcemia. This is in part due to the decreased filtered phosphate load, and partly due to a reduction in circulating PTH.

Whether acute hypercalcemia also directly affects tubule phosphate reabsorption is controversial.[405] Micropuncture studies generally agree that hypercalcemia increases distal tubule reabsorption, but there are conflicting results regarding its effect on the proximal tubule. *In vitro* microperfused proximal tubule S2 segments showed increased phosphate reabsorption in response to increased luminal Ca²⁺, whereas S3 segments did not. Of note, the CaSR is expressed at the brush border of the proximal tubule, predominantly in S1 and S2 segments,[220] raising the possibility that it might mediate the effects of luminal Ca²⁺ on phosphate transport.

In contrast to its acute effects, chronic hypercalcemia decreases tubule phosphate reabsorption whereas chronic hypocalcemia increases phosphate reabsorption, independent of the effects of PTH, vitamin D, or serum Ca²⁺. The mechanism is unknown.

Sodium and Extracellular Volume

Extracellular volume expansion increases (and volume contraction decreases) phosphate excretion by several mechanisms.[405] First, volume expansion increases GFR and the filtered load of phosphate. Second, volume expansion inhibits proximal tubule Na⁺ and water reabsorption, diluting the concentration of luminal phosphate available for reabsorption. Third, volume expansion decreases plasma Ca²⁺ and increases PTH, which inhibits proximal tubule phosphate reabsorption (see later). Finally, there is probably a direct effect of volume expansion to inhibit tubule phosphate reabsorption, which is independent of filtered load, plasma Ca²⁺, or PTH.

Acid-Base Status

Acute metabolic acidosis (3 hours) has minimal effect on phosphate excretion but blunts the phosphaturic effect of PTH.[405] Acute metabolic alkalosis causes an increase in phosphate excretion. Paradoxically, alkalinization of proximal tubule luminal fluid would be expected to stimulate the type IIa and IIc Na-Pi cotransporters and increase phosphate reabsorption. Conversely, alkalinization of peritubular fluid has been shown to inhibit phosphate reabsorption in perfused PCT segments. Thus, the effects of acute metabolic alkalosis are best explained by regulation of basolateral rather than apical phosphate transport in the proximal tubule.

In contrast to the effects of acute acid-base disturbances, chronic metabolic acidosis decreases and chronic metabolic alkalosis increases renal tubule phosphate reabsorption. In early chronic metabolic acidosis (6 hours), the type IIa Na-Pi cotransporter protein expression at the brush border is decreased, but the protein abundance in total cortical homogenate, and the mRNA abundance are unchanged, suggesting that there is retrieval of transporters from the apical membrane.[588] Late chronic metabolic acidosis (12 hours to 10 days) is associated with progressive decrease in type IIa Na-Pi cotransporter mRNA abundance as well.[588]

Respiratory acidosis and alkalosis are associated with an increase and decrease in phosphate excretion, respectively. Acute respiratory alkalosis causes a redistribution of phosphate into cells, resulting in hypophosphatemia, so the effects on renal excretion may be attibutable to alterations in filtered load. Indeed in rats fed a high phosphate diet, which would be expected to induce saturating phosphate concentrations, the effect of acute respiratory alkalosis on fractional excretion of phosphate was abolished. By contrast, chronic respiratory alkalosis also causes reduced phosphate excretion, but is accompanied by hyperphosphatemia. In OK cells, decreasing the HCO_3^-/CO_2 concentration of the media without changing the pH caused an increase in type IIa Na-Pi cotransporter expression due to transcriptional activation.[589] This suggests that the effects of respiratory acid-base status may be mediated by a direct effect of CO_2 on proximal tubule cells.

Hormones

Parathyroid Hormone

Parathyroid hormone is the major hormonal regulator of renal phosphate handling. It inhibits tubule phosphate reabsorption, primarily in the PCT.[405] The juxtamedullary nephrons are more sensitive to PTH than superficial nephrons,[544] and the S2 segment of the PCT may be more sensitive than the S1 segment.[540] PTH also inhibits phosphate transport in the PST, DCT, and the CCD.

The effects of PTH on phosphate reabsorption in proximal tubule, as well as in OK cells, are primarily mediated by its effects on the type IIa Na-Pi cotransporter. Acutely, PTH causes endocytosis of type IIa cotransporters from the apical surface in a microtubule-dependent manner.[590] Endocytosis occurs at the intermicrovillar clefts. There, the transporter is internalized into clathrin- and adapter protein-2 (AP2)-coated vesicles, where it colocalizes with endocytosed fluid-phase markers such as horseradish peroxidase, and is transiently trafficked to the subapical region.[591] Unlike other membrane transport proteins, type IIa cotransporters are not routed to a recycling compartment from which they can be recruited back to the surface. Instead, they are trafficked directly to the lysosomes and irreversibly degraded.[591,592] The recognition signal for PTH-mediated endocytosis is a dibasic peptide "KR" motif located in the last intracellular loop of the type IIa Na-Pi cotransporter.[593] This KR motif interacts with PEX19, a protein normally involved in the binding and trafficking of peroxisomal proteins that stimulates endocytosis of the type IIa Na-Pi cotransporter.[594]

Chronic administration of PTH additionally causes a small decrease in type IIa cotransporter mRNA.[595] Withdrawal of PTH, or parathyroidectomy, reverses these changes and up-regulates brush border type IIa cotransporters, a process that requires *de novo* protein synthesis.[596] In knockout mice that lack the type IIa Na-Pi cotransporter, PTH has no effect on serum phosphate, fractional excretion of phosphate, or Na+-dependent phosphate transport in BBMV.[597]

Parathyroid hormone can signal in proximal tubules via several different signalling pathways, including the classical adenylate cyclase/PKA pathway, phospholipase C/PKC, and the extracellular signal-regulated kinase (ERK). PTH can inhibit Na+-phosphate cotransport via activation of either the PKA or PKC pathway alone.[598] In OK cells, the reduction in type IIa cotransporter expression by PTH has been shown to be mediated by PKA.[599] The type IIa cotransporter has now been shown to physically associate with PKA through an A kinase anchoring protein (AKAP) that is required for the regulation of phosphate transport by PTH.[600]

It has recently been recognized that proximal tubules have PTH receptors not only on their basolateral membrane, but also on their brush border membrane.[601] By perfusing either luminal or peritubular compartments of proximal tubules with PTH analogs, Traebert and colleagues[598] showed that activation of the PTH receptors at either surface was sufficient to cause Na+-phosphate cotransporter internalization. The luminal receptors signalled preferentially via PKC, while the basolateral receptors required activation of both PKA and PKC. As PTH is a small polypeptide that is probably freely filtered at the glomerulus, a sufficiently high concentration is likely to normally be present in the lumen of the proximal tubule to be sensed by these brush border receptors. The importance of luminal signaling is indicated by studies in mice with targeted inactivation of CLC5, the Dent disease gene.[602] These mice, which have defective endocytosis of luminal PTH and therefore high concentrations of PTH in proximal tubule luminal fluid, exhibit abnormal internalization of the type IIa Na+-phosphate cotransporter, and hence phosphaturia.

In addition to its effects on the type IIa Na+-phosphate cotransporter, PTH inhibits phosphate reabsorption by several other mechanisms. PTH inhibits the basolateral Na-K-ATPase, thereby indirectly preventing secondary active Na+-gradient dependent phosphate transport at the apical membrane. The signal transduction pathway for this is complex, and involves an early phase that depends on PKC, phospholipase A_2, and ERK, and a late phase dependent on PKA, phospholipase A_2, and ERK.[603,604] ERK activation alone also inhibits phosphate transport.[605] It does not affect Na+-phosphate cotransporter expression, but its downstream target has not been defined. PTH-stimulated cyclic AMP generation can also inhibit phosphate transport via another pathway. It has been postulated that the cyclic AMP generated can be exported to the tubule lumen, where it is metabolized by 5'-ectonucleotidase to adenosine, re-enters the cell, and inhibits phosphate transport.[606] PTH-activated PKC acts synergistically by inhibiting phosphodiesterase,[607] the enzyme that degrades intracellular cyclic AMP, and also by activating the 5'-ectonucleotidase.[608]

Vitamin D

The effects of vitamin D metabolites on renal phosphate handling are complex. Chronic administration of vitamin D causes phosphaturia, a reduction in renal cortical BBMV phosphate transport, and reduced renal cortical expression of type IIa Na-Pi cotransporter mRNA and protein.[609] Because chronic vitamin D administration increases intestinal phosphate absorption, it is possible that the adaptive mechanism is the same as that of high dietary phosphate intake. The phosphaturic response to chronic vitamin D requires the presence of PTH,[609] whereas the downregulation of BBMV transport and cotransporter expression do not. This suggests that the vitamin D-induced decrease in proximal tubule phosphate reabsorption can be compensated by increased reabsorption at downstream nephron sites that are PTH-responsive.

Acute administration of vitamin D metabolites reduces renal phosphate excretion. This effect requires the presence of PTH, is associated with a decrease in urinary cyclic AMP and renal tubular adenylate cyclase activity, and can be inhibited by cycloheximide, which blocks *de novo* protein synthesis.[610] 1,25(OH)$_2$D stimulated Na+-phosphate cotransport in a subclone of OK cells,[611] and phosphate uptake in isolated renal cells from vitamin D-deficient chicks,[612] both of which could be inhibited by actinomycin D and cycloheximide. In vitamin D-deficient rats, Taketani and colleagues showed that type IIa Na-Pi cotransporter mRNA and protein is downregulated in the juxtamedullary cortex, but somewhat up-regulated in the superficial cortex.[613] Administration of

1,25(OH)$_2$D caused upregulation of its mRNA and protein expression in the juxtamedullary cortex within 12 hours. Thus, the evidence suggests that vitamin D acts acutely by antagonizing the actions of PTH on adenylate cyclase, and thereby induces de novo synthesis of type IIa Na-Pi cotransporter, perhaps in the PST.

Dopamine

Dopamine is a renal paracrine phosphaturic hormone. Renal dopamine is produced in the proximal tubule from its precursor, L-dopa; a small amount is also released from nerve endings. Dopamine production is stimulated by a high phosphate diet and suppressed by a low phosphate diet. Exogenous dopamine inhibits phosphate transport in isolated perfused proximal tubule S3 segments,[614] and Na$^+$-phosphate cotransport in BBMV.[615] Inhibition of endogenous dopamine production with carbidopa decreased renal phosphate excretion[616] and increased Na$^+$-phosphate cotransport in BBMV.[616] Carbidopa also decreased Na$^+$-gradient-dependent phosphate uptake into OK cells.[617] A synthetic L-dopa analog that is selectively activated in the proximal tubules was shown to inhibit BBMV Na$^+$-phosphate cotransport and to cause phosphaturia.[618]

The action of dopamine is primarily mediated by DA1 receptors.[619] It is now clear that the primary action of dopamine in the proximal tubule is to inhibit the basolateral Na-K-ATPase, a process dependent on both PKA and PKC.[604] Activation of PKC causes phosphorylation of, and thereby induces endocytosis of the α_1-subunit of the Na-K-ATPase. This would indirectly inhibit phosphate reabsorption because the apical Na$^+$-phosphate transport step depends on the extracellular-to-intracellular Na$^+$ gradient generated by the Na-K-ATPase. Whether dopamine also directly affects the type IIa Na-Pi cotransporter is unclear.

Insulin, Glucose, and Glucagon

Insulin reduces renal phosphate excretion,[620] independently of its effects on glucose. It increases phosphate uptake into cells, causing hypophosphatemia, a reduced filtered load, and hence increased proximal tubule reabsorption. Insulin has also been shown to directly stimulate phosphate uptake in BBMV[621] and in OK cells.[622] The effects of insulin may in part be explained by inhibition of gluconeogenesis, which causes intracellular phosphate depletion. Glucagon, which stimulates gluconeogenesis and increases cytosolic phosphate, is phosphaturic,[623] probably due to inhibition of phosphate reabsorption in the PST.[624] Glucose infusion is also phosphaturic.[620] It acts in part as an osmotic diuretic. Glucose also inhibits luminal phosphate uptake, probably because Na$^+$-glucose cotransport depolarizes the apical membrane and dissipates the Na$^+$ gradient, thereby inhibiting electrogenic Na$^+$-phosphate cotransport.[625]

Stanniocalcin-1

The mammalian stanniocalcins, STC1 and STC2, are homologs of a fish anticalcemic hormone. STC1 is ubiquitously expressed. The intrarenal sites of STC1 expression are controversial. In humans, STC1 protein appears to be expressed in the "distal tubule" and collecting duct.[626,627] In rodents, STC1 mRNA has been detected in collecting ducts only, whereas STC1 protein is found in almost all tubule segments.[628,629] STC1 mRNA expression in cortical and outer medullary collecting ducts was reduced by a low phosphate diet and increased on a high phosphate diet.[629] Expression of STC1 mRNA in the kidney is also increased by 1,25(OH)$_2$D, whereas that of STC2 is decreased.[630] STC1 has a very short plasma half-life and circulating levels are not normally detectable, so it probably acts as a local paracrine factor.[631]

STC1 is an antiphosphaturic hormone. Recombinant human STC1, when injected into rats, caused a decrease in fractional excretion of phosphate,[626,632] and an increase in

Na$^+$-phosphate cotransport in BBMV.[632] However, STC1-knockout mice have normal serum Ca^{2+} and phosphate and respond normally to acute injections of vitamin D, raising doubt as to the physiological significance of STC1.[633] No physiologic role has been proposed for STC2.

Phosphatonins

Phosphatonins are humoral factors, secreted by tumors of patients with tumor-induced osteomalacia, which have phosphaturic activity. Several proteins have now been found to be overexpressed by such tumors: FGF-23,[533] matrix extracellular phosphoglycoprotein (MEPE),[534] secreted frizzled related protein-4 (FRP-4),[634] and fibroblast growth factor-7 (FGF-7).[635]

The evidence for a role in regulating renal phosphate excretion is strongest for FGF-23. Mutations in FGF-23 that prevent its cleavage (and presumably increase functional levels) cause autosomal dominant hypophosphatemic rickets/osteomalacia,[636–640] whereas missense mutations in FGF-23 that presumably abolish its function have been identified in familial tumoral calcinosis, which is characterized by decreased urinary excretion of phosphorus, hyperphosphatemia, and ectopic calcification.[641,642] Inactivating mutations in a metalloproteinase, PHEX, which inhibits FGF-23 expression and release,[643,644] cause X-linked hypophosphatemic rickets.[645] Finally, targeted ablation of FGF-23 in mice causes hyperphosphatemia.[646]

FGF-23 is expressed in osteoblasts. Its expression is upregulated by hyperphosphatemia[537,647] and also perhaps by 1,25-vit D[648] either directly, or via downregulation of PHEX gene transcription.[649] FGF-23[533] inhibits Na$^+$-dependent phosphate transport in kidneys[650] and in OK cells.[651,652] In FGF-23 transgenic mice, reduction in mRNA expression of both the type IIa and IIc Na-Pi cotransporters is the cause of phosphaturia.[653] In contrast, sFRP-4 increases renal phosphate excretion by inducing internalization of the type IIa Na-Pi cotransporter from the brush border of the proximal tubule.[654]

Diuretics

Most diuretics are somewhat phosphaturic.[405] Mannitol modestly increases phosphate excretion by decreasing Na$^+$ and water reabsorption in the proximal tubule, and hence diluting luminal phosphate. Acetazolamide, which inhibits carbonic anhydrase, is quite phosphaturic, probably by setting up an acidic disequilibrium pH in the proximal tubule lumen that inhibits the type IIa Na-Pi cotransporter. Thiazides and fursosemide in high doses have a small phosphaturic effect, attributable to inhibition of carbonic anhydrase.

Ontogeny

In contrast to other tubule transport processes, phosphate reabsorption is highest in infants, and declines with age.[405] This is important to maintain positive phosphate balance in the immature animal during active growth and development. The increased phosphate reabsorption in newborns is observed in both proximal and distal tubules. Furthermore, newborn animals exhibit a greater increase in phosphate reabsorption in response to a dietary phosphate deprivation, and a lesser decrease in response to high phosphate diet, or PTH. BBMV from neonates show a greater V_{max} for Na$^+$-phosphate transport than those of adults.[655] Type IIa Na-Pi cotransporter protein is concomitantly increased.[656–658] Early in development, the type IIa Na-Pi cotransporter is expressed in the brush borders of all proximal tubules, whereas in adulthood it is primarily expressed at the brush borders of juxtamedullary nephrons.[657] Furthermore, the type IIc Na-Pi cotransporter is expressed in weaning animals but not in adults, suggesting that it may supply added capacity for phosphate reabsorption just during development.[557] The mechanisms for regulating these developmental changes are unknown, but growth hormone[659] and triiodothyronine appear to play a role.[660]

References

1. Greger R: Physiology of renal sodium transport. Am J Med Sci 319:51–62, 2000.
2. Sun A, Grossman EB, Lombardi M, Hebert SC: Vasopressin alters the mechanism of apical Cl– entry from Na+:Cl– to Na+:K+:2Cl– cotransport in mouse medullary thick ascending limb. J Membr Biol 120:83–94, 1991.
3. Madsen KM, Tishler CC: Anatomy of the Kidney. In Brenner BM (ed): Brenner and Rector's The Kidney. Philadelphia, WB Saunders, 2004, pp 3–72.
4. Welling LW, Welling DJ: Surface areas of brush border and lateral cell walls in the rabbit proximal nephron. Kidney Int 8:343–348, 1975.
5. Liu FY, Cogan MG: Axial heterogeneity of bicarbonate, chloride, and water transport in the rat proximal convoluted tubule. Effects of change in luminal flow rate and of alkalemia. J Clin Invest 78:1547–1557, 1986.
6. Maddox DA, Gennari FJ: The early proximal tubule: A high-capacity delivery-responsive reabsorptive site. Am J Physiol 252:F573–84, 1987.
7. Kokko JP: Proximal tubule potential difference. Dependence on glucose on glucose, HCO 3, and amino acids. J Clin Invest 52:1362–1367, 1973.
8. Neumann KH, Rector FC, Jr: Mechanism of NaCl and water reabsorption in the proximal convoluted tubule of rat kidney. J Clin Invest 58:1110–1111, 1976.
9. Alpern RJ, Howlin KJ, Preisig PA: Active and passive components of chloride transport in the rat proximal convoluted tubule. J Clin Invest 76:1360–1366, 1985.
10. Moe OW, Baum M, Berry CA, Rector FC, Jr: Renal transport of glucose, amino acids, sodium, chloride, and water. In Brenner BM (ed): Brenner and Rector's The Kidney. Philadelphia, WB Saunders, 2004, pp 413–452.
11. Schild L, Giebisch G, Green R: Chloride transport in the proximal renal tubule. Annu Rev Physiol 50:97–110, 1988.
12. Barratt LJ, Rector FC, Jr, Kokko JP, Seldin DW: Factors governing the transepithelial potential difference across the proximal tubule of the rat kidney. J Clin Invest 53:454–464, 1974.
13. Jacobson HR: Characteristics of volume reabsorption in rabbit superficial and juxtamedullary proximal convoluted tubules. J Clin Invest 63:410–418, 1979.
14. Katz AI, Doucet A, Morel F: Na-K-ATPase activity along the rabbit, rat, and mouse nephron. Am J Physiol 237:F114–120, 1979.
15. Lucci MS, Warnock DG: Effects of anion-transport inhibitors on NaCl reabsorption in the rat superficial proximal convoluted tubule. J Clin Invest 64:570–579, 1979.
16. Baum M, Berry CA: Evidence for neutral transcellular NaCl transport and neutral basolateral chloride exit in the rabbit proximal convoluted tubule. J Clin Invest 74:205–211, 1984.
17. Green R, Giebisch G: Reflection coefficients and water permeability in rat proximal tubule. Am J Physiol 257:F658–668, 1989.
18. Vallon V, Verkman AS, Schnermann J: Luminal hypotonicity in proximal tubules of aquaporin-1-knockout mice. Am J Physiol Renal Physiol 278:F1030–1033, 2000.
19. Claude P, Goodenough DA: Fracture faces of zonulae occludentes from "tight" and "leaky" epithelia. J Cell Biol 58:390–400, 1973.
20. Tang VW, Goodenough DA: Paracellular ion channel at the tight junction. Biophys J 84:1660–1673, 2003.
21. Yu AS: Paracellular solute transport: more than just a leak? Curr Opin Nephrol Hypertens 9:513–515, 2000.
22. Furuse M, Furuse K, Sasaki H, Tsukita S: Conversion of zonulae occludentes from tight to leaky strand type by introducing claudin-2 into Madin-Darby canine kidney I cells. J Cell Biol 153:263–272, 2001.
23. Yu AS, Enck AH, Lencer WI, Schneeberger EE: Claudin-8 expression in Madin-Darby canine kidney cells augments the paracellular barrier to cation permeation. J Biol Chem 278:17350–17359, 2003.
24. Nitta T, Hata M, Gotoh S, et al: Size-selective loosening of the blood-brain barrier in claudin-5-deficient mice. J Cell Biol 161:653–660, 2003.
25. Enck AH, Berger UV, Yu AS: Claudin-2 is selectively expressed in proximal nephron in mouse kidney. Am J Physiol Renal Physiol 281:F966–974, 2001.
26. Kiuchi-Saishin Y, Gotoh S, Furuse M, et al: Differential expression patterns of claudins, tight junction membrane proteins, in mouse nephron segments. J Am Soc Nephrol 13:875–886, 2002.
27. Muto S, et al: Disruption of claudin-2 gene converts from a leaky to a tight epithelium in mouse proximal tubule, leading to an inhibition of NaCl reabsorption (abstract). J Am Soc Nephrol 15:4A, 2004.
28. Schnermann J, Chou CL, Ma T, et al: Defective proximal tubular fluid reabsorption in transgenic aquaporin-1 null mice. Proc Natl Acad Sci U S A 95:9660–9664, 1998.
29. Sohara E, Rai T, Miyazaki J, et al: Defective water and glycerol transport in the proximal tubules of AQP7 knockout mice. Am J Physiol Renal Physiol 289:F1195–1200, 2005.
30. Zeuthen T, Meinild AK, Loo DD, et al: Isotonic transport by the Na+-glucose cotransporter SGLT1 from humans and rabbit. J Physiol 531:631–644, 2001.
31. Charron FM, Blanchard MG, Lapointe JY: Intracellular hypertonicity is responsible for water flux associated with Na+/glucose cotransport. Biophys J 90:3546–3554, 2006.
32. Maddox DA, Gennari FJ: Load dependence of HCO3 and H2O reabsorption in the early proximal tubule of the Munich-Wistar rat. Am J Physiol 248:F113–121, 1985.
33. Baum M: Evidence that parallel Na+-H+ and Cl(–)-HCO3-(OH–) antiporters transport NaCl in the proximal tubule. Am J Physiol 252:F338–345, 1987.
34. Bacic D, Kaissling B, McLeroy P, et al: Dopamine acutely decreases apical membrane Na/H exchanger NHE3 protein in mouse renal proximal tubule. Kidney Int 64:2133–2141, 2003.
35. Choi JY, Shah M, Lee MG, et al: Novel amiloride-sensitive sodium-dependent proton secretion in the mouse proximal convoluted tubule. J Clin Invest 105:1141–1146, 2000.
36. Goyal S, Vanden Heuvel G, Aronson PS: Renal expression of novel Na+/H+ exchanger isoform NHE8. Am J Physiol Renal Physiol 284:F467–473, 2003.
37. Schultheis PJ, Clarke LL, Meneton P, et al: Renal and intestinal absorptive defects in mice lacking the NHE3 Na+/H+ exchanger. Nat Genet 19:282–285, 1998.
38. Wang T, Yang CL, Abbiati T, et al: Essential role of NHE3 in facilitating formate-dependent NaCl absorption in the proximal tubule. Am J Physiol Renal Physiol 281:F288–292, 2001.
39. Kurtz I, Nagami G, Yanagawa N, et al: Mechanism of apical and basolateral Na(+)-independent Cl–/base exchange in the rabbit superficial proximal straight tubule. J Clin Invest 94:173–183, 1994.
40. Karniski LP, Aronson PS: Chloride/formate exchange with formic acid recycling: A mechanism of active chloride transport across epithelial membranes. Proc Natl Acad Sci U S A 82:6362–6365, 1985.
41. Saleh AM, Rudnick H, Aronson PS: Mechanism of H(+)-coupled formate transport in rabbit renal microvillus membranes. Am J Physiol 271:F401–407, 1996.
42. Karniski LP, Aronson PS: Anion exchange pathways for Cl– transport in rabbit renal microvillus membranes. Am J Physiol 253:F513–521, 1987.
43. Kuo SM, Aronson PS: Pathways for oxalate transport in rabbit renal microvillus membrane vesicles. J Biol Chem 271:15491–15497, 1996.
44. Wang T, Agulian SK, Giebisch G, Aronson PS: Effects of formate and oxalate on chloride absorption in rat distal tubule. Am J Physiol 264:F730–736, 1993.
45. Wang T, Egbert AL, Jr, Abbiati T, et al: Mechanisms of stimulation of proximal tubule chloride transport by formate and oxalate. Am J Physiol 271:F446–450, 1996.
46. Sheu JN, Quigley R, Baum M: Heterogeneity of chloride/base exchange in rabbit superficial and juxtamedullary proximal convoluted tubules. Am J Physiol 268:F847–853, 1995.
47. Scott DA, Karniski LP: Human pendrin expressed in Xenopus laevis oocytes mediates chloride/formate exchange. Am J Physiol Cell Physiol 278:C207–211, 2000.
48. Karniski LP, Wang T, Everett LA, et al: Formate-stimulated NaCl absorption in the proximal tubule is independent of the pendrin protein. Am J Physiol Renal Physiol 283:F952–956, 2002.
49. Royaux IE, Wall SM, Karniski LP, et al: Pendrin, encoded by the Pendred syndrome gene, resides in the apical region of renal intercalated cells and mediates bicarbonate secretion. Proc Natl Acad Sci U S A 98:4221–4226, 2001.
50. Xie Q, Welch R, Mercado A, et al: Molecular characterization of the murine Slc26a6 anion exchanger, functional comparison to Slc26a1. Am J Physiol 283:F826–F838, 2002.
51. Wang Z, Wang T, Petrovic S, et al: Renal and intestinal transport defects in Slc26a6-null mice. Am J Physiol Cell Physiol 288:C957–965, 2005.
52. Dudas PL, Greineder CF, Mentone SA, Aronson PS: Immunolocalization of anion exchanger Slc26a7 in mouse kidney. J Am Soc Nephrol 14:313A, 2003.
53. Kim KH, Shcheynikov N, Wang Y, Muallem S: SLC26A7 is a Cl– channel regulated by intracellular pH. J Biol Chem 280:6463–6470, 2005.
54. Jiang Z, Asplin JR, Evan AP, et al: Calcium oxalate urolithiasis in mice lacking anion transporter Slc26a6. Nat Genet 38: 403–404, 2006.
55. Shcheynikov N, Wang Y, Park M, et al: Coupling modes and stoichiometry of Cl–/HCO3– exchange by slc26a3 and slc26a6. J Gen Physiol 127:511–524, 2006.
56. Vallon V, Grahammer F, Volkl H, et al: KCNQ1-dependent transport in renal and gastrointestinal epithelia. Proc Natl Acad Sci U S A 102:17864–17869, 2005.
57. Thomson RB, Wang T, Tomson BR, et al: Role of PDZK1 in membrane expression of renal brush border ion exchangers. Proc Natl Acad Sci U S A 102:13331–13336, 2005.
58. Petrovic S, Barone S, Weinstein AM, Soleimani M: Activation of the apical Na+/H+ exchanger NHE3 by formate: A basis of enhanced fluid and electrolyte reabsorption by formate in the kidney. Am J Physiol Renal Physiol 287:F336–346, 2004.
59. Mount DB, Gamba G: Renal potassium-chloride cotransporters. Curr Opin Nephrol Hypertens 10:685–691, 2001.
60. Mercado A, Vazquez N, Song L, et al: NH2-terminal heterogeneity in the KCC3 K+-Cl– cotransporter. Am J Physiol Renal Physiol 289:F1246–1261, 2005.
61. Ishibashi K, Rector FC, Jr, Berry CA: Chloride transport across the basolateral membrane of rabbit proximal convoluted tubules. Am J Physiol 258:F1569–1578, 1990.
62. Sasaki S, Ishibashi K, Yoshiyama N, Shiigai T: KCl co-transport across the basolateral membrane of rabbit renal proximal straight tubules. J Clin Invest 81:194–199, 1988.
63. Avison MJ, Gullans SR, Ogino T, Giebisch G: Na+ and K+ fluxes stimulated by Na+-coupled glucose transport: evidence for a Ba2+-insensitive K+ efflux pathway in rabbit proximal tubules. J Membr Biol 105:197–205, 1988.
64. Schild L, Aronson PS, Giebisch G: Effects of apical membrane Cl(–)-formate exchange on cell volume in rabbit proximal tubule. Am J Physiol 258:F530–536, 1990.
65. Boettger T, Rust MB, Maier H, et al: Loss of K-Cl co-transporter KCC3 causes deafness, neurodegeneration and reduced seizure threshold. EMBO J 22:5422–5434, 2003.
66. Wang T, Delpire E, Giebisch G, et al: Impaired fluid and bicarbonate absorption in proximal tubules (PT) of KCC3 knockout mice. FASEB J 17:A464, 2003.
67. Ishibashi K, Rector FC, Jr, Berry CA: Role of Na-dependent Cl/HCO3 exchange in basolateral Cl transport of rabbit proximal tubules. Am J Physiol 264:F251–258, 1993.
68. Macri P, Breton S, Beck JS, et al: Basolateral K+, Cl–, and HCO3– conductances and cell volume regulation in rabbit PCT Am J Physiol 264:F365–376, 1993.
69. Schild L, Aronson PS, Giebisch G: Basolateral transport pathways for K+ and Cl– in rabbit proximal tubule: Effects on cell volume. Am J Physiol 260:F101–109, 1991.
70. Welling PA, O'Neil RG: Ionic conductive properties of rabbit proximal straight tubule basolateral membrane. Am J Physiol 258:F940–950, 1990.

71. Seki G, Taniguchi S, Uwatoko S, et al: Evidence for conductive Cl– pathway in the basolateral membrane of rabbit renal proximal tubule S3 segment. J Clin Invest 92:1229–1235, 1993.

72. Obermuller N, Gretz N, Kriz W, et al: The swelling-activated chloride channel ClC-2, the chloride channel ClC-3, and ClC-5, a chloride channel mutated in kidney stone disease, are expressed in distinct subpopulations of renal epithelial cells. J Clin Invest 101:635–642, 1998.

73. Alpern RJ, Chambers M: Basolateral membrane Cl/HCO3 exchange in the rat proximal convoluted tubule. Na-dependent and -independent modes. J Gen Physiol 89:581–598, 1987.

74. Virkki LV, Choi I, Davis BA, Boron WF: Cloning of a Na+-driven Cl/HCO3 exchanger from squid giant fiber lobe. Am J Physiol Cell Physiol 285:C771–780, 2003.

75. Wang T: Flow-activated transport events along the nephron. Curr Opin Nephrol Hypertens 15:530–536, 2006.

76. Du Z, Yan Q, Duan Y, et al: Axial flow modulates proximal tubule NHE3 and H-ATPase activities by changing microvillus bending moments. Am J Physiol Renal Physiol 290:F289–296, 2006.

77. Burg MB, Orloff J: Control of fluid absorption in the renal proximal tubule. J Clin Invest 47:2016–2024, 1968.

78. Du Z, Duan Y, Yan Q, et al: Mechanosensory function of microvilli of the kidney proximal tubule. Proc Natl Acad Sci U S A 101:13068–13073, 2004.

79. Brenner BM, Troy JL: Postglomerular vascular protein concentration: evidence for a causal role in governing fluid reabsorption and glomerulotublar balance by the renal proximal tubule. J Clin Invest 50:336–349, 1971.

80. Bello-Reuss E, Colindres RE, Pastoriza-Munoz E, et al: Effects of acute unilateral renal denervation in the rat. J Clin Invest 56:208–217, 1975.

81. Bell-Reuss E, Trevino DL, Gottschalk CW: Effect of renal sympathetic nerve stimulation on proximal water and sodium reabsorption. J Clin Invest 57:1104–1107, 1976.

82. Feraille E, Doucet A: Sodium-potassium-adenosinetriphosphatase-dependent sodium transport in the kidney: Hormonal control. Physiol Rev 81:345–418, 2001.

83. Hall RA, Premont RT, Chaw CW, et al: The beta2-adrenergic receptor interacts with the Na+/H+-exchanger regulatory factor to control Na+/H+ exchange. Nature 392:626–630, 1998.

84. Harris PJ, Young JA: Dose-dependent stimulation and inhibition of proximal tubular sodium reabsorption by angiotensin II in the rat kidney. Pflugers Arch 367:295–297, 1977.

85. Harrison-Bernard LM, Navar LG, Ho MM, et al: Immunohistochemical localization of ANG II AT1 receptor in adult rat kidney using a monoclonal antibody. Am J Physiol 273:F170–177, 1997.

86. Li L, Wang YP, Capparelli AW, et al: Effect of luminal angiotensin II on proximal tubule fluid transport: Role of apical phospholipase A2. Am J Physiol 266:F202–209, 1994.

87. Zheng Y, Horita S, Hara C, et al: Biphasic regulation of renal proximal bicarbonate absorption by luminal (AT1A) receptor. J Am Soc Nephrol 14:1116–1122, 2003.

88. Quan A, Baum M: Endogenous production of angiotensin II modulates rat proximal tubule transport. J Clin Invest 97:2878–2882, 1996.

89. Thomson SC, Deng A, Wead L, et al: An unexpected role for angiotensin II in the link between dietary salt and proximal reabsorption. J Clin Invest 116:1110–1116, 2006.

90. Wang ZQ, Siragy HM, Felder RA, Carey RM: Intrarenal dopamine production and distribution in the rat. Physiological control of sodium excretion. Hypertension 29:228–234, 1997.

91. Hegde SS, Jadhav AL, Lokhandwala MF: Role of kidney dopamine in the natriuretic response to volume expansion in rats. Hypertension 13:828–834, 1989.

92. Baum M, Quigley R: Inhibition of proximal convoluted tubule transport by dopamine. Kidney Int 54:1593–1600, 1998.

93. Yu P, Asico LD, Luo Y, et al: D1 dopamine receptor hyperphosphorylation in renal proximal tubules in hypertension. Kidney Int 70:1072–1079, 2006.

94. Albrecht FE, Drago J, Felder RA, et al: Role of the D1A dopamine receptor in the pathogenesis of genetic hypertension. J Clin Invest 97:2283–2288, 1996.

95. Hollon TR, Bek MJ, Lachowicz JE, et al: Mice lacking D5 dopamine receptors have increased sympathetic tone and are hypertensive. J Neurosci 22:10801–1010, 2002.

96. Winaver J, Burnett JC, Tyce GM, Dousa TP: ANP inhibits Na(+)-H+ antiport in proximal tubular brush border membrane: Role of dopamine. Kidney Int 38:1133–1140, 1990.

97. Holtback U, Brismar H, Dibona GF, et al: Receptor recruitment: A mechanism for interactions between G protein-coupled receptors. Proc Natl Acad Sci U S A 96:7271–7275, 1999.

98. Katoh T, Sophasan S, Kurokawa K: Permissive role of dopamine in renal action of ANP in volume-expanded rats. Am J Physiol 257:F300–309, 1989.

99. Hegde SS, Chen CJ, Lokhandwala MF: Involvement of endogenous dopamine and DA-1 receptors in the renal effects of atrial natriuretic factor in rats. Clin Exp Hypertens A 13:357–369, 1991.

100. Harris PJ, Thomas D, Morgan TO: Atrial natriuretic peptide inhibits angiotensin-stimulated proximal tubular sodium and water reabsorption. Nature 326:697–698, 1987.

101. Cheng HF, Becker BN, Harris RC: Dopamine decreases expression of type-1 angiotensin II receptors in renal proximal tubule. J Clin Invest 97:2745–2752, 1996.

102. Zeng C, Yang Z, Wang Z, et al: Interaction of angiotensin II type 1 and D5 dopamine receptors in renal proximal tubule cells. Hypertension 45:804–810, 2005.

103. Zeng C, Liu Y, Wang Z, et al: Activation of D3 dopamine receptor decreases angiotensin II type 1 receptor expression in rat renal proximal tubule cells. Circ Res 99:494–500, 2006.

104. Weinman EJ, Cunningham R, Shenolikar S: NHERF and regulation of the renal sodium-hydrogen exchanger NHE3. Pflugers Arch 450:137–144, 2005.

105. Collazo R, Fan L, Hu MC, et al: Acute regulation of Na+/H+ exchanger NHE3 by parathyroid hormone via NHE3 phosphorylation and dynamin-dependent endocytosis. J Biol Chem 275:31601–31608, 2000.

106. Liu FY, Cogan MG: Angiotensin II stimulates early proximal bicarbonate absorption in the rat by decreasing cyclic adenosine monophosphate. J Clin Invest 84:83–91, 1989.

107. Zhao H, Wiederkehr MR, Fan L, et al. Acute inhibition of Na/H exchanger NHE-3 by cAMP Role of protein kinase a and NHE-3 phosphoserines 552 and 605. J Biol Chem 274:3978–3987, 1999.

108. Kocinsky HS, Girardi AC, Biemesderfer D, et al: Use of phospho-specific antibodies to determine the phosphorylation of endogenous Na+/H+ exchanger NHE3 at PKA consensus sites. Am J Physiol Renal Physiol 289:F249–258, 2005.

109. Biemesderfer D, DeGray B, Aronson PS: Active (9.6 s) and inactive 21 s) oligomers of NHE3 in microdomains of the renal brush border. J Biol Chem 276:10161–10167, 2001.

110. Sanchez-Mendoza A, Lopez-Sanchez P, Vazquez-Cruz B, et al: Angiotensin II modulates ion transport in rat proximal tubules through CYP metabolites. Biochem Biophys Res Commun 272:423–430, 2000.

111. Dos Santos EA, Dahly-Vernon AJ, Hoagland KM, Roman RJ: Inhibition of the formation of EETs and 20-HETE with 1-aminobenzotriazole attenuates pressure natriuresis. Am J Physiol Regul Integr Comp Physiol 287:R58–68, 2004.

112. du Cheyron D, Chalumeau C, Defontaine N, et al: Angiotensin II stimulates NHE3 activity by exocytic insertion of the transporter: Role of PI 3-kinase. Kidney Int 64:939–949, 2003.

113. Leong PK, Devillez A, Sandberg MB, et al: Effects of ACE inhibition on proximal tubule sodium transport. Am J Physiol Renal Physiol 290:F854–863, 2006.

114. Bobulescu IA, Dwarakanath V, Zou L, et al: Glucocorticoids acutely increase cell surface Na+/H+ exchange activity (NHE3) by activation of NHE3 exocytosis. Am J Physiol Renal Physiol 289:F685–691, 2005.

115. Yun CC, Chen Y, Lang F: Glucocorticoid activation of Na(+)/H(+) exchanger isoform 3 revisited. The roles of SGK1 and NHERF2. J Biol Chem 277:7676–7683, 2002.

116. Wang D, Sun H, Lang F, Yun CC: Activation of NHE3 by dexamethasone requires phosphorylation of NHE3 at Ser663 by SGK1. Am J Physiol Cell Physiol 289:C802–810, 2005.

117. Pedemonte CH, Efendiev R, Bertorello AM: Inhibition of Na,K-ATPase by dopamine in proximal tubule epithelial cells. Semin Nephrol 25:322–327, 2005.

118. Chou CL, Knepper MA, Hoek AN: Reduced water permeability and altered ultrastructure in thin descending limb of Henle in aquaporin-1 null mice. J Clin Invest 103:491–496, 1999.

119. Imai M, Kokko JP: Sodium chloride, urea, and water transport in the thin ascending limb of Henle. Generation of osmotic gradients by passive diffusion of solutes. J Clin Invest 53:393–402, 1974.

120. Stephenson JL: Concentration of urine in a central core model of the renal counterflow system. Kidney Int 2:85–94, 1972.

121. Liu W, Morimoto T, Kondo Y, et al: Analysis of NaCl transport in thin ascending limb of Henle's loop in CLC-K1 null mice. Am J Physiol Renal Physiol 282:F451–457, 2002.

122. Gottschalk CW, Lassiter WE, Mylle M, et al: Micropuncture study of composition of loop of Henle fluid in desert rodents. Am J Physiol 204:532–535, 1963.

123. Kokko JP: Sodium chloride and water transport in the descending limb of Henle. J Clin Invest 49:1838–1846, 1970.

124. Imai M, Taniguchi J, Yoshitomi K: Transition of permeability properties along the descending limb of long-loop nephron. Am J Physiol 254:F323–328, 1988.

125. Chou CL, Knepper MA: In vitro perfusion of chinchilla thin limb segments: Urea and NaCl permeabilities Am J Physiol 264:F337–343, 1993.

126. Chou CL, Knepper MA: In vitro perfusion of chinchilla thin limb segments: Segmentation and osmotic water permeability. Am J Physiol 263:F417–426, 1992.

127. Lopes AG, Amzel LM, Markakis D, Guggino WB: Cell volume regulation by the thin descending limb of Henle's loop. Proc Natl Acad Sci U S A 85:2873–2877, 1988.

128. Nielsen S, Pallone T, Smith BL, et al: Aquaporin-1 water channels in short and long loop descending thin limbs and in descending vasa recta in rat kidney. Am J Physiol 268:F1023–1037, 1995.

129. Maeda Y, Smith BL, Agre P, Knepper MA: Quantification of Aquaporin-CHIP water channel protein in microdissected renal tubules by fluorescence-based ELISA. J Clin Invest 95:422–428, 1995.

130. Chou CL, Nielsen S, Knepper MA: Structural-functional correlation in chinchilla long loop of Henle thin limbs: A novel papillary subsegment. Am J Physiol 265:F863–874, 1993.

131. Imai M: Function of the thin ascending limb of Henle of rats and hamsters perfused in vitro. Am J Physiol 232:F201–209, 1977.

132. Koyama S, Yoshitomi K, Imai M: Effect of protamine on ion conductance of ascending thin limb of Henle's loop from hamsters. Am J Physiol 261:F593–599, 1991.

133. Takahashi N, Kondo Y, Fukiwara I, et al: Characterization of Na+ transport across the cell membranes of the ascending thin limb of Henle's loop. Kidney Int 47:789–794, 1995.

134. Kondo Y, Yoshitomi K, Imai M: Effects of anion transport inhibitors and ion substitution on Cl– transport in TAL of Henle's loop. Am J Physiol 253:F1206–1215, 1987.

135. Isozaki T, Yoshitomi K, Imai M: Effects of Cl– transport inhibitors on Cl– permeability across hamster ascending thin limb. Am J Physiol 257:F92–98, 1989.

136. Yoshitomi K, Kondo Y, Imai M: Evidence for conductive Cl– pathways across the cell membranes of the thin ascending limb of Henle's loop. J Clin Invest 82:866–871, 1988.

137. Kondo Y, Abe K, Igarashi Y, et al: Direct evidence for the absence of active Na+ reabsorption in hamster ascending thin limb of Henle's loop. J Clin Invest 91:5–11, 1993.

138. Takahashi N, Kondo Y, Ito O, et al: Vasopressin stimulates Cl– transport in ascending thin limb of Henle's loop in hamster. J Clin Invest 95:1623–1627, 1995.

139. Uchida S, Sasaki S, Nitta K, et al: Localization and functional characterization of rat kidney-specific chloride channel, ClC-K1. J Clin Invest 95:104–113, 1995.

140. Wolf K, Meier-Meitinger M, Bergler T, et al: Parallel down-regulation of chloride channel CLC-K1 and barttin mRNA in the thin ascending limb of the rat nephron by furosemide. Pflugers Arch 446:665–671, 2003.
141. Waldegger S, Jeck N, Barth P, et al: Barttin increases surface expression and changes current properties of ClC-K channels. Pflugers Arch 444:411–418, 2002.
142. Matsumura Y, Uchida S, Kondo Y, et al: Overt nephrogenic diabetes insipidus in mice lacking the CLC-K1 chloride channel. Nat Genet 21:95–98, 1999.
143. Simon DB, Bindra RS, Mansfield TA, et al: Mutations in the chloride channel gene, CLCNKB, cause Bartter's syndrome type III. Nat Genet 17:171–178, 1997.
144. Estevez R, et al: Barttin is a Cl− channel beta-subunit crucial for renal Cl− reabsorption and inner ear K+ secretion. Nature 414:558–561, 2001.
145. Scholl U, Hebeisen S, Janssen AG, et al: Barttin modulates trafficking and function of ClC-K channels. Proc Natl Acad Sci U S A 103:11411–11416, 2006.
146. Allen F, Tisher CC: Morphology of the ascending thick limb of Henle. Kidney Int 9:8–22, 1976.
147. Tsuruoka S, Koseki C, Muto S, et al: Axial heterogeneity of potassium transport across hamster thick ascending limb of Henle's loop. Am J Physiol 267:F121–129, 1994.
148. Nielsen S, Maunsbach AB, Ecelbarger CA, Knepper MA: Ultrastructural localization of Na-K-2Cl cotransporter in thick ascending limb and macula densa of rat kidney. Am J Physiol 275: F885–893, 1998.
149. Greger R: Ion transport mechanisms in thick ascending limb of Henle's loop of mammalian nephron. Physiol Rev 65:760–797, 1985.
150. Hebert SC, Andreoli TE: Control of NaCl transport in the thick ascending limb. Am J Physiol 246:F745–756, 1984.
151. Greger R, Schlatter E: Presence of luminal K+, a prerequisite for active NaCl transport in the cortical thick ascending limb of Henle's loop of rabbit kidney. Pflugers Arch 392:92–94, 1981.
152. Hebert SC, Culpepper RM, Andreoli TE: NaCl transport in mouse medullary thick ascending limbs. I. Functional nephron heterogeneity and ADH-stimulated NaCl cotransport. Am J Physiol 241:F412–431, 1981.
153. Hebert SC, Andreoli TE: Effects of antidiuretic hormone on cellular conductive pathways in mouse medullary thick ascending limbs of Henle: II. Determinants of the ADH-mediated increases in transepithelial voltage and in net Cl− absorption. J Membr Biol 80:221–233, 1984.
154. Burg M, Stoner L, Cardinal J, Green N: Furosemide effect on isolated perfused tubules. Am J Physiol 225:119–124, 1973.
155. Hebert SC, Mount DB, Gamba G: Molecular physiology of cation-coupled Cl− cotransport: The SLC12 family. Pflugers Arch 447:580–593, 2004.
156. Plata C, Mount DB, Rubio V, et al: Isoforms of the apical Na-K-2Cl transporter in murine thick ascending limb. II: Functional characterization and mechanism of activation by cyclic-AMP. Am J Physiol 276:F359–F366, 1999.
157. Gimenez I, Isenring P, Forbush B: Spatially distributed alternative splice variants of the renal Na-K-Cl cotransporter exhibit dramatically different affinities for the transported ions. J Biol Chem 277:8767–8770, 2002.
158. Lapointe JY, Laamarti A, Bell PD: Ionic transport in macula densa cells. Kidney Int Suppl 67:S58–64, 1998.
159. Ito S, Carretero OA: In in vitro approach to the study of macula densa-mediated glomerular hemodynamics. Kidney Int 38:1206–1210, 1990.
160. He XR, Greenberg SG, Briggs JP, Schnermann J: Effects of furosemide and verapamil on the NaCl dependency of macula densa-mediated renin secretion. Hypertension 26:137–142, 1995.
161. Igarashi P, Vanden Heuvel GB, Payne JA, Forbush B, 3rd: Cloning, embryonic expression, and alternative splicing of a murine kidney-specific Na-K-Cl cotransporter. Am J Physiol 269:F405–418:1995.
162. Flemmer AW, Gimenez I, Dowd BF, et al: Activation of the Na-K-Cl otransporter NKCC1 detected with a phospho-specific antibody. J Biol Chem 277:37551–37558, 2002.
163. Oppermann M, Mizel D, Huang G, et al: Macula densa control of renin secretion and preglomerular resistance in mice with selective deletion of the B isoform of the Na,K,2Cl Co-transporter. J Am Soc Nephrol 17:2143–2152, 2006.
164. Friedman PA, Andreoli TE: CO2-stimulated NaCl absorption in the mouse renal cortical thick ascending limb of Henle. Evidence for synchronous Na +/H+ and Cl−/HCO3− exchange in apical plasma membranes. J Gen Physiol 80:683–711, 1982.
165. Good DW, Watts BA, 3rd: Functional roles of apical membrane Na+/H+ exchange in rat medullary thick ascending limb. Am J Physiol 270:F691–699, 1996.
166. Laghmani K, Borensztein P, Ambuhl P, et al: Chronic metabolic acidosis enhances NHE-3 protein abundance and transport activity in the rat thick ascending limb by increasing NHE-3 mRNA. J Clin Invest 99:24–30, 1997.
167. Quentin F, et al: Regulation of the Cl−/HCO3− exchanger AE2 in rat thick ascending limb of Henle's loop in response to changes in acid-base and sodium balance. J Am Soc Nephrol 15:2988–2997, 2004.
168. Burg MB, Green N: Function of the thick ascending limb of Henle's loop. Am J Physiol 224:659–668, 1973.
169. Rocha AS, Kokko JP: Sodium chloride and water transport in the medullary thick ascending limb of Henle. Evidence for active chloride transport. J Clin Invest 52:612–623, 1973.
170. Greger R, Weidtke C, Schlatter E, et al: Potassium activity in cells of isolated perfused cortical thick ascending limbs of rabbit kidney. Pflugers Arch 401:52–57, 1984.
171. Stokes JB: Consequences of potassium recycling in the renal medulla. Effects of ion transport by the medullary thick ascending limb of Henle's loop. J Clin Invest 70:219–229, 1982.
172. Simon DB, Karet FE, Rodriguez-Soriano J, et al: Genetic heterogeneity of Bartter's syndrome revealed by mutations in the K+ channel, ROMK. Nat Genet 14:152–156, 1996.
173. Taniguchi J, Guggino WB: Membrane stretch: A physiological stimulator of Ca^{2+}-activated K+ channels in thick ascending limb. Am J Physiol 257:F347–352, 1989.
174. Bleich M, Schlatter E, Greger R: The luminal K+ channel of the thick ascending limb of Henle's loop. Pflugers Arch 415:449–460, 1990.
175. Wang WH: Two types of K+ channel in thick ascending limb of rat kidney. Am J Physiol 267:F599–605, 1994.
176. Wang W, Lu M: Effect of arachidonic acid on activity of the apical K+ channel in the thick ascending limb of the rat kidney. J Gen Physiol 106:727–743, 1995.
177. Ho K, Nichols CJ, Lederer WJ, et al: Cloning and expression of an inwardly rectifying ATP-regulated potassium channel. Nature 362:31–38, 1993.
178. Xu JZ, Hall AE, Peterson LN, et al: Localization of the ROMK protein on apical membranes of rat kidney nephron segments. Am J Physiol 273:F739–F748, 1997.
179. Lu M, Wang T, Yan Q, et al: Absence of small conductance K+ channel (SK) activity in apical membranes of thick ascending limb and cortical collecting duct in ROMK (Bartter's) knockout mice. J Biol Chem 277:37881–37887, 2002.
180. Lu M, Wang T, Yan Q, et al: ROMK is required for expression of the 70-pS K channel in the thick ascending limb. Am J Physiol Renal Physiol 286:F490–495, 2004.
181. Yoo D, Flagg TP, Olsen O, et al: Assembly and trafficking of a multiprotein ROMK (Kir 1.1) channel complex by PDZ interactions. J Biol Chem 279:6863–6873, 2004.
182. Lu M, Leng Q, Egan ME, et al: CFTR is required for PKA-regulated ATP sensitivity of Kir1.1 potassium channels in mouse kidney. J Clin Invest 116:797–807, 2006.
183. Hebert SC, Andreoli TE: Ionic conductance pathways in the mouse medullary thick ascending limb of Henle. The paracellular pathway and electrogenic Cl− absorption. J Gen Physiol 87:567–590, 1986.
184. Hebert SC, Culpepper RM, Andreoli TE: NaCl transport in mouse medullary thick ascending limbs. II. ADH enhancement of transcellular NaCl cotransport; origin of transepithelial voltage. Am J Physiol 241:F432–442, 1981.
185. Simon DB, Lu Y, Choate KA, et al: Paracellin-1, a renal tight junction protein required for paracellular Mg^{2+} resorption. Science 285:103–106, 1999.
186. Konrad M, Schaller A, Seelow D, et al: Mutations in the tight-junction gene Claudin 19 (CLDN19) are associated with renal magnesium wasting, renal failure, and severe ocular involvement. Am J Hum Genet 79:949–957, 2006.
187. Hou J, Paul DL, Goodenough DA: Paracellin-1 and the modulation of ion selectivity of tight junctions. J Cell Sci 118:5109–5118, 2005.
188. Kausalya PJ, Amashesh S, Gunzel D, et al: Disease-associated mutations affect intracellular traffic and paracellular Mg^{2+} transport function of Claudin-16. J Clin Invest 116:878–891, 2006.
189. Greger R, Schlatter E: Properties of the basolateral membrane of the cortical thick ascending limb of Henle's loop of rabbit kidney. A model for secondary active chloride transport. Pflugers Arch 396:325–334, 1983.
190. Greger R, Oberleithner H, Schlatter E, et al: Chloride activity in cells of isolated perfused cortical thick ascending limbs of rabbit kidney. Pflugers Arch 399:29–34, 1983.
191. Jeck N, Waldegger P, Doroszewicz J, et al: A common sequence variation of the CLCNKB gene strongly activates ClC-Kb chloride channel activity. Kidney Int 65:190–197, 2004.
192. Geller DS: A genetic predisposition to hypertension? Hypertension 44:27–28, 2004.
193. Kobayashi K, Uchida S, Mizutani S, et al: Intrarenal and cellular localization of CLC-K2 protein in the mouse kidney. J Am Soc Nephrol 12:1327–1334, 2001.
194. Picollo A, Liantonio A, Didonna MP, et al: Molecular determinants of differential pore blocking of kidney CLC-K chloride channels. EMBO Rep 5:584–589, 2004.
195. Palmer LG, Frindt G: Cl− channels of the distal nephron. Am J Physiol Renal Physiol 291:F1157–1168, 2006.
196. Song L, Delpire E, Gamba G, Mount DB: Localization of the K-Cl Cotransporters KCC3 and KCC4 in Mouse Kidney. FASEB J A341, 2000.
197. Boettger T, Hubner CA, Maier H, et al: Deafness and renal tubular acidosis in mice lacking the K-Cl co-transporter Kcc4. Nature 416:874–878, 2002.
198. Amlal H, Paillard M, Bichara M: Cl(−)-dependent NH4+ transport mechanisms in medullary thick ascending limb cells. Am J Physiol 267:C1607–1615, 1994.
199. Bergeron MJ, Gagnon E, Wallendorff B, et al: Ammonium transport and pH regulation by K(+)-Cl(−) cotransporters. Am J Physiol Renal Physiol 285:F68–78, 2003.
200. Mercado A, Song L, Vazquez N, et al: Functional comparison of the K+-Cl− cotransporters KCC1 and KCC4. J Biol Chem 275:30326–30334, 2000.
201. Di Stefano A, Greger R, Desfleurs E, et al: Ba($^{2+}$)-insensitive K+ conductance in the basolateral membrane of rabbit cortical thick ascending limb cells. Cell Physiol Biochem 8:89–105, 1998.
202. Guggino WB: Functional heterogeneity in the early distal tubule of the Amphiuma kidney: Evidence for two modes of Cl− and K+ transport across the basolateral cell membrane. Am J Physiol 250:F430–440, 1986.
203. Good DW: Ammonium transport by the thick ascending limb of Henle's loop. Annu Rev Physiol 56:623–647, 1994.
204. Hurst AM, Duplain M, Lapointe JY: Basolateral membrane potassium channels in rabbit cortical thick ascending limb. Am J Physiol 263:F262–267, 1992.
205. Paulais M, Lachheb S, Teulon J: A Na+- and Cl−-activated K+ channel in the thick ascending limb of mouse kidney. J Gen Physiol 127:205–215, 2006.
206. Paulais M, Lourdel S, Teulon J: Properties of an inwardly rectifying K(+) channel in the basolateral membrane of mouse TAL. Am J Physiol Renal Physiol 282:F866–876, 2002.
207. Knepper MA, Kim GH, Fernandez-Llama P, Ecelbarger CA: Regulation of thick ascending limb transport by vasopressin. J Am Soc Nephrol 10:628–634, 1999.
208. Mount DB: Membrane trafficking and the regulation of NKCC2. Am J Physiol Renal Physiol 290:F606–607, 2006.
209. Gagnon KB, England R, Delpire E: Volume sensitivity of cation-Cl− cotransporters is modulated by the interaction of two kinases: Ste20-related proline-alanine-rich kinase and WNK4. Am J Physiol Cell Physiol 290:C134–142, 2006.
210. Rinehart J, Kahle KT, de Los Heros JP, et al: WNK3 kinase is a positive regulator of NKCC2 and NCC, renal cation-Cl− cotransporters required for normal blood pressure homeostasis. Proc Natl Acad Sci U S A 102:16777–16782, 2005.
211. Mount DB, Baekgaard A, Hall AE, et al: Isoforms of the apical Na-K-2Cl transporter in murine thick ascending limb. I: Molecular characterization and intra-renal localization. Am J Physiol 276:F347–F358, 1999.

212. Plata C, Meade P, Hall A, et al: Alternatively spliced isoform of apical Na(+)-K(+)-Cl(−) cotransporter gene encodes a furosemide-sensitive Na(+)-Cl(−)cotransporter. Am J Physiol Renal Physiol 280:F574–582, 2001.
213. Xu ZC, Yang Y, Hebert SC: Phosphorylation of the ATP-sensitive, inwardly rectifying K+ channel, ROMK, by cyclic AMP-dependent protein kinase. J Biol Chem 271:9313–9319, 1996.
214. Yoo D, Kim BY, Campo C, et al: Cell surface expression of the ROMK (Kir 1.1) channel is regulated by the aldosterone-induced kinase, SGK-1, and protein kinase A. J Biol Chem 278:23066–23075, 2003.
215. Leipziger J, MacGregor GG, Cooper GJ, et al: PKA site mutations of ROMK2 channels shift the pH dependence to more alkaline values. Am J Physiol Renal Physiol 279: F919–926, 2000.
216. Liou HH, Zhou SS, Huang CL: Regulation of ROMK1 channel by protein kinase A via a phosphatidylinositol 4,5-bisphosphate-dependent mechanism. Proc Natl Acad Sci U S A 96:5820–5825, 1999.
217. Ecelbarger CA, Kim GH, Knepper MA, et al: Regulation of potassium channel Kir 1.1 (ROMK) abundance in the thick ascending limb of Henle's loop. J Am Soc Nephrol 12:10–18, 2001.
218. Takaichi K, Kurokawa K: Inhibitory guanosine triphosphate-binding protein-mediated regulation of vasopressin action in isolated single medullary tubules of mouse kidney. J Clin Invest 82:1437–1444, 1988.
219. Hebert SC: Calcium and salinity sensing by the thick ascending limb: A journey from mammals to fish and back again. Kidney Int Suppl:S28–33, 2004.
220. Riccardi D, Hall AE, Chattopadhyay N, et al: Localization of the extracellular Ca^{2+}/(polyvalent cation)-sensing protein in rat kidney. Am J Physiol 274:F611–F622, 1998.
221. de Jesus Ferreira MC, Helies-Toussaint C, Imbert-Teboul M, et al: Co-expression of a Ca^{2+}-inhibitable adenylyl cyclase and of a Ca^{2+}-sensing receptor in the cortical thick ascending limb cell of the rat kidney. Inhibition of hormone-dependent cAMP accumulation by extracellular Ca^{2+}. J Biol Chem 273:15192–15202, 1998.
222. Watanabe S, Fukumoto S, Chang H, et al: Association between activating mutations of calcium-sensing receptor and Bartter's syndrome. Lancet 360:692–694, 2002.
223. Vargas-Poussou R, Huang C, Hulin P, et al: Functional characterization of a calcium-sensing receptor mutation in severe autosomal dominant hypocalcemia with a Bartter-like syndrome. J Am Soc Nephrol 13:2259–2266, 2002.
224. Loffing J, Kaissling B: Sodium and calcium transport pathways along the mammalian distal nephron: from rabbit to human. Am J Physiol Renal Physiol 284:F628–643, 2003.
225. Loffing J, Loffing-Cueni D, Valderrabano D, et al: Distribution of transcellular calcium and sodium transport pathways along mouse distal nephron. Am J Physiol Renal Physiol 281:F1021–1027, 2001.
226. Frindt G, Palmer LG: Na channels in the rat connecting tubule. Am J Physiol Renal Physiol 286:F669–674, 2004.
227. Wall SM: Recent advances in our understanding of intercalated cells. Curr Opin Nephrol Hypertens 14:480–484, 2005.
228. Duc C, Farman N, Canessa CM, et al: Cell-specific expression of epithelial sodium channel alpha, beta, and gamma subunits in aldosterone-responsive epithelia from the rat: Localization by in situ hybridization and immunocytochemistry. J Cell Biol 127:1907–1921, 1994.
229. Malnic G, Klose RM, Giebisch G: Micropuncture study of renal potassium excretion in the rat. Am J Physiol 206:674–686, 1964.
230. Wingo CS, Armitage FE: Rubidium absorption and proton secretion by rabbit outer medullary collecting duct via H-K-ATPase. Am J Physiol 263:F849–857, 1992.
231. Okusa MD, Unwin RJ, Velazquez H, et al: Active potassium absorption by the renal distal tubule. Am J Physiol 262:F488–493, 1992.
232. Hager H, Kwon TH, Vinnikova AK, et al: Immunocytochemical and immunoelectron microscopic localization of alpha-, beta-, and gamma-ENaC in rat kidney. Am J Physiol Renal Physiol 280:F1093–1106, 2001.
233. Ellison DH, Velazquez H, Wright FS: Adaptation of the distal convoluted tubule of the rat. Structural and functional effects of dietary salt intake and chronic diuretic infusion. J Clin Invest 83:113–126, 1989.
234. Khuri RN, Strieder N, Wiederholt M, Giebisch G: Effects of graded solute diuresis on renal tubular sodium transport in the rat. Am J Physiol 228:1262–1268, 1975.
235. Velazquez H, Good DW, Wright FS: Mutual dependence of sodium and chloride absorption by renal distal tubule. Am J Physiol 247:F904–911, 1984.
236. Costanzo LS: Localization of diuretic action in microperfused rat distal tubules: Ca and Na transport. Am J Physiol 248:F527–535, 1985.
237. Gamba G, Saltzberg SN, Lombardi M, et al: Primary structure and functional expression of a cDNA encoding the thiazide-sensitive, electroneutral sodium-chloride cotransporter. Proc Natl Acad Sci U S A 90:2749–2753 1993.
238. Monroy A, Plata C, Hebert SC, Gamba G: Characterization of the thiazide-sensitive Na(+)-Cl(−) cotransporter: A new model for ions and diuretics interaction. Am J Physiol Renal Physiol 279:F161–169, 2000.
239. Bazzini C, Vezzoli V, Sironi C, et al: Thiazide-sensitive NaCl-cotransporter in the intestine: Possible role of hydrochlorothiazide in the intestinal Ca^{2+} uptake. J Biol Chem 280:19902–19910, 2005.
240. Schultheis PJ, Lorenz JN, Meneton P, et al: Phenotype resembling Gitelman's syndrome in mice lacking the apical Na+-Cl− cotransporter of the distal convoluted tubule. J Biol Chem 273:29150–29155, 1998.
241. Loffing J, Vallon V, Loffing-Cueni D, et al: Altered renal distal tubule structure and renal Na(+) and Ca($^{2+}$) handling in a mouse model for Gitelman's syndrome. J Am Soc Nephrol 15:2276–2288, 2004.
242. Loffing J, Loffing-Cueni D, Hegyi I, et al: Thiazide treatment of rats provokes apoptosis in distal tubule cells. Kidney Int 50:1180–1190, 1996.
243. Chambrey R, Warnock DG, Podevin RA, et al: Immunolocalization of the Na+/H+ exchanger isoform NHE2 in rat kidney. Am J Physiol 275:F379–386, 1998.
244. Kujala M, Tienari J, Lohi H, et al: SLC26A6 and SLC26A7 anion exchangers have a distinct distribution in human kidney. Nephron Exp Nephrol 101:e50–58, 2005.
245. Velazquez H, Silva T: Cloning and localization of KCC4 in rabbit kidney: expression in distal convoluted tubule. Am J Physiol Renal Physiol 285:F49–58, 2003.
246. Lourdel S, Paulais M, Marvao P, et al: A chloride channel at the basolateral membrane of the distal-convoluted tubule: A candidate ClC-K channel. J Gen Physiol 121:287–300, 2003.
247. Jeck N, Konrad M, Peters M, et al: Mutations in the chloride channel gene, CLCNKB, leading to a mixed Bartter-Gitelman phenotype. Pediatr Res 48:754–758, 2000.
248. Kotelevtsev Y, Brown RW, Fleming S, et al: Hypertension in mice lacking 11beta-hydroxysteroid dehydrogenase type 2. J Clin Invest 103:683–689, 1999.
249. Kim GH, Masilamani S, Turner R, et al: The thiazide-sensitive Na-Cl cotransporter is an aldosterone-induced protein. Proc Natl Acad Sci U S A 95:14552–14557, 1998.
250. Nielsen J, Kwon TH, Masilamani S, et al: Sodium transporter abundance profiling in kidney: Effect of spironolactone. Am J Physiol Renal Physiol 283:F923–933, 2002.
251. Lalioti MD, Zhang J, Volkman HM, et al: Wnk4 controls blood pressure and potassium homeostasis via regulation of mass and activity of the distal convoluted tubule. Nat Genet 38:1124–1132, 2006.
252. Mayan H, Vered I, Mouallem M, et al: Pseudohypoaldosteronism type II: Marked sensitivity to thiazides, hypercalciuria, normomagnesemia, and low bone mineral density. J Clin Endocrinol Metab 87:3248–3254, 2002.
253. Wilson FH, Disse-Nicodeme S, Choate KA, et al: Human hypertension caused by mutations in WNK kinases. Science 293:1107–1112, 2001.
254. Wilson FH, Kahle KT, Sabath E, et al: Molecular pathogenesis of inherited hypertension with hyperkalemia: The Na-Cl cotransporter is inhibited by wild-type but not mutant WNK4. Proc Natl Acad Sci U S A 100:680–684 2003.
255. Golbang AP, Cope G, Hamad A, et al: Regulation of the expression of the Na/Cl cotransporter (NCCT) by WNK4 and WNK1: Evidence that accelerated dynamin-dependent endocytosis is not involved. Am J Physiol Renal Physiol 291:F139–1376, 2006.
256. Yang CL, Angell J, Mitchell R, Ellison DH: WNK kinases regulate thiazide-sensitive Na-Cl cotransport. J Clin Invest 111:1039–1045, 2003.
257. Vitari AC, Deak M, Morrice NA, Alessi DR: The WNK1 and WNK4 protein kinases that are mutated in Gordon's hypertension syndrome phosphorylate and activate SPAK and OSR1 protein kinases. Biochem J 391:17–24, 2005.
258. Moriguchi T, Urushiyama S, Hisamoto N, et al: WNK1 regulates phosphorylation of cation-chloride-coupled cotransporters via the STE20-related kinases, SPAK and OSR1. J Biol Chem 280, 42685–42693, 2005.
259. Lazrak A, Liu Z, Huang CL: Antagonistic regulation of ROMK by long and kidney-specific WNK1 isoforms. Proc Natl Acad Sci U S A 103:1615–1620, 2006.
260. Kahle KT, Wilson FH, Leng Q, et al: WNK4 regulates the balance between renal NaCl reabsorption and K+ secretion. Nat Genet 35:372–376, 2003.
261. Kahle KT, Macgregor GG, Wilson FH, et al: Paracellular Cl− permeability is regulated by WNK4 kinase: Insight into normal physiology and hypertension. Proc Natl Acad Sci U S A 101:14877–14882, 2004.
262. Frindt G, Palmer LG: Low-conductance K channels in apical membrane of rat cortical collecting tubule. Am J Physiol 256:F143–151, 1989.
263. Palmer LG, Frindt G: Amiloride-sensitive Na channels from the apical membrane of the rat cortical collecting tubule. Proc Natl Acad Sci U S A 83:2767–2770, 1986.
264. Canessa CM, Schild L, Buell G, et al: The amiloride-sensitive epithelial sodium channel is made of three homologous subunits. Nature 367:463–467, 1994.
265. Canessa CM, Morillat AM, Rossier BC: Membrane topology of the epithelial sodium channel in intact cells. Am J Physiol 267:C1682–1690 1994.
266. Firsov D, Schild L, Gautschi I, et al: Cell surface expression of the epithelial Na channel and a mutant causing Liddle syndrome: A quantitative approach. Proc Natl Acad Sci U S A 93:15370–15375 1996.
267. Staruschenko A, Adams E, Booth RE, Stockand JD: Epithelial Na+ channel subunit stoichiometry. Biophys J 88:3966–3975, 2005.
268. Lifton RP, Gharavi AG, Geller DS: Molecular mechanisms of human hypertension. Cell 104:545–556, 2001.
269. Findling JW, Raff H, Hansson JH, Lifton RP: Liddle's syndrome: prospective genetic screening and suppressed aldosterone secretion in an extended kindred. J Clin Endocrinol Metab 82:1071–1074, 1997.
270. Hiltunen TP, Hamila-Handelberg T, Petajaniemi N, et al: Liddle's syndrome associated with a point mutation in the extracellular domain of the epithelial sodium channel gamma subunit. J Hypertens 20:2383–2390, 2002.
271. Rubera I, Loffing J, Palmer LG, et al: Collecting duct-specific gene inactivation of alphaENaC in the mouse kidney does not impair sodium and potassium balance. J Clin Invest 112:554–565, 2003.
272. Loffing J, Pietri L, Agregger F, et al: Differential subcellular localization of ENaC subunits in mouse kidney in response to high- and low-Na diets. Am J Physiol Renal Physiol 279:F252–258, 2000.
273. Meneton P, Loffing J, Warnock DG: Sodium and potassium handling by the aldosterone-sensitive distal nephron: The pivotal role of the distal and connecting tubule. Am J Physiol Renal Physiol 287:F593–601, 2004.
274. Schuster VL, Stokes JB: Chloride transport by the cortical and outer medullary collecting duct. Am J Physiol 253:F203–212, 1987.
275. Warden DH, Schuster VL, Stokes JB: Characteristics of the paracellular pathway of rabbit cortical collecting duct. Am J Physiol 255:F720–727, 1988.
276. Li WY, Huey CL, Yu AS: Expression of claudin-7 and -8 along the mouse nephron. Am J Physiol Renal Physiol 286:F1063–1071, 2004.
277. Yamauchi K, Rai T, Kobayashi K, et al: Disease-causing mutant WNK4 increases paracellular chloride permeability and phosphorylates claudins. Proc Natl Acad Sci U S A 101:4690–4694, 2004.
278. Wall SM, Kim YH, Stanley L, et al: NaCl restriction upregulates renal Slc26a4 through subcellular redistribution. role in Cl− Conservation. Hypertension 44:982–987, 2004.

208

CH 5

279. Verlander JW, Hassell KA, Royaux IE, et al: Deoxycorticosterone upregulates PDS (Slc26a4) in mouse kidney: Role of pendrin in mineralocorticoid-induced hypertension. Hypertension 42:356–362, 2003.

280. Verlander JW, Kim YH, Shin W, et al: Dietary Cl(–) restriction upregulates pendrin expression within the apical plasma membrane of type B intercalated cells. Am J Physiol Renal Physiol 291:F833–839, 2006.

281. Fuller PJ, Young MJ: Mechanisms of mineralocorticoid action. Hypertension 46:1227–1235, 2005.

282. Welling PA, Caplan M, Sutters M, Giebisch G: Aldosterone-mediated Na/K-ATPase expression is alpha 1 isoform specific in the renal cortical collecting duct. J Biol Chem 268:23469–23476, 1993.

283. Le Moellic C, Boulkroun S, Gonzalez-Nunez D, et al: Aldosterone and tight junctions: Modulation of claudin-4 phosphorylation in renal collecting duct cells. Am J Physiol Cell Physiol 289:C1513–1521, 2005.

284. Mick VE, Itani OA, Loftus RW, et al: The alpha-subunit of the epithelial sodium channel is an aldosterone-induced transcript in mammalian collecting ducts, and this transcriptional response is mediated by distinct cis-elements in the 5′-flanking region of the gene. Mol Endocrinol 15:575–588, 2001.

285. Masilamani S, Kim GH, Mitchell C, et al: Aldosterone-mediated regulation of ENaC alpha, beta, and gamma subunit proteins in rat kidney. J Clin Invest 104:R19–23, 1999.

286. Loffing J, Zecevic M, Feraille E, et al: Aldosterone induces rapid apical translocation of ENaC in early portion of renal collecting system: Possible role of SGK Am J Physiol Renal Physiol 280:F675–682, 2001.

287. Snyder PM: Minireview: Regulation of epithelial Na+ channel trafficking. Endocrinology 146:5079–5085, 2005.

288. Chen SY, Bhargava A, Mastroberardino L, et al: Epithelial sodium channel regulated by aldosterone-induced protein sgk. Proc Natl Acad Sci U S A 96:2514–2519, 1999.

289. Naray-Fejes-Toth A, Canessa C, Cleaveland ES, et al: sgk is an aldosterone-induced kinase in the renal collecting duct. Effects on epithelial na+ channels. J Biol Chem 274:16973–16978, 1999.

290. Kamynina E, Tauxe C, Staub O: Distinct characteristics of two human Nedd4 proteins with respect to epithelial Na(+) channel regulation. Am J Physiol Renal Physiol 281: F469–477, 2001.

291. Snyder PM, Olson DR, Thomas BC: Serum and glucocorticoid-regulated kinase modulates Nedd4-2-mediated inhibition of the epithelial Na+ channel. J Biol Chem 277:5–8, 2002.

292. Debonneville C, Flores SY, Kamynina E, et al: Phosphorylation of Nedd4-2 by Sgk1 regulates epithelial Na(+) channel cell surface expression. EMBO J 20:7052–7059, 2001.

293. Flores SY, Loffing-Cueni D, Kamynina E, et al: Aldosterone-induced serum and glucocorticoid-induced kinase 1 expression is accompanied by Nedd4-2 phosphorylation and increased Na+ transport in cortical collecting duct cells. J Am Soc Nephrol 16:2279–2287, 2005.

294. Zhou R, Snyder PM: Nedd4-2 phosphorylation induces serum and glucocorticoid-regulated kinase (SGK) ubiquitination and degradation. J Biol Chem 280:4518–4523, 2005.

295. Loffing-Cueni D, Flores SY, Sauter D, et al: Dietary sodium intake regulates the ubiquitin-protein ligase nedd4-2 in the renal collecting system. J Am Soc Nephrol 17:1264–1274, 2006.

296. Ergonul Z, Frindt G, Palmer LG: Regulation of maturation and processing of ENaC subunits in the rat kidney. Am J Physiol Renal Physiol 291:F683–693, 2006.

297. Kleyman TR, Myerburg MM, Hughey RP: Regulation of ENaCs by proteases: An increasingly complex story. Kidney Int 70:1391–1392, 2006.

298. Vuagniaux G, Vallet V, Jaeger NF, et al: Synergistic activation of ENaC by three membrane-bound channel-activating serine proteases (mCAP1, mCAP2, and mCAP3) and serum- and glucocorticoid-regulated kinase (Sgk1) in Xenopus Oocytes. J Gen Physiol 120:191–201, 2002.

299. Vallet V, Chraibi A, Gaeggeler HP, et al: An epithelial serine protease activates the amiloride-sensitive sodium channel. Nature 389:607–610, 1997.

300. Narikiyo T, Kitamura K, Adachi M, et al: Regulation of prostasin by aldosterone in the kidney. J Clin Invest 109:401–408 2002.

301. Carattino MD, Sheng S, Bruns JB, et al: The epithelial Na+ channel is inhibited by a peptide derived from proteolytic processing of its alpha subunit. J Biol Chem 281:18901–18907, 2006.

302. Knight KK, Olson DR, Zhou R, Snyder PM: Liddle's syndrome mutations increase Na+ transport through dual effects on epithelial Na+ channel surface expression and proteolytic cleavage. Proc Natl Acad Sci U S A 103:2805–2808, 2006.

303. Schafer JA: Abnormal regulation of ENaC: Syndromes of salt retention and salt wasting by the collecting duct. Am J Physiol Renal Physiol 283:F221–235, 2002.

304. Morris RG, Schafer JA: cAMP increases density of ENaC subunits in the apical membrane of MDCK cells in direct proportion to amiloride-sensitive Na(+) transport. J Gen Physiol 120, 71–85 2002.

305. Butterworth MB, Edinger RS, Johnson JP, Frizzell RA: Acute ENaC stimulation by cAMP in a kidney cell line is mediated by exocytic insertion from a recycling channel pool. J Gen Physiol 125:81–101, 2005.

306. Snyder PM, Olson DR, Kabra R, et al: cAMP and serum and glucocorticoid-inducible kinase (SGK) regulate the epithelial Na(+) channel through convergent phosphorylation of Nedd4-2. J Biol Chem 279:45753–45758, 2004.

307. Ecelbarger CA, Kim GH, Terris J, et al: Vasopressin-mediated regulation of epithelial sodium channel abundance in rat kidney. Am J Physiol Renal Physiol 279:F46–53, 2000.

308. Peti-Peterdi J, Warnock DG, Bell PD: Angiotensin II directly stimulates ENaC activity in the cortical collecting duct via AT1) receptors. J Am Soc Nephrol 13:1131–1135, 2002.

309. Komlosi P, Fuson AL, Fintha A, et al: Angiotensin I conversion to angiotensin II stimulates cortical collecting duct sodium transport. Hypertension 42:195–199, 2003.

310. Rohrwasser A, Morgan T, Dillon HF, et al: Elements of a paracrine tubular renin-angiotensin system along the entire nephron. Hypertension 34:1265–1274, 1999.

311. Wei Y, Lin DH, Kemp R, et al: Arachidonic acid inhibits epithelial Na channel via cytochrome P450 (CYP) epoxygenase-dependent metabolic pathways. J Gen Physiol 124:719–727, 2004.

312. Nakagawa K, Holla VR, Wei Y, et al: Salt-sensitive hypertension is associated with dysfunctional Cyp4a10 gene and kidney epithelial sodium channel. J Clin Invest 116:1696–1702, 2006.

313. Guan Y, Hao C, Cha DR, et al: Thiazolidinediones expand body fluid volume through PPARgamma stimulation of ENaC-mediated renal salt absorption. Nat Med 11:861–866, 2005.

314. Zhang H, Zhang A, Kohan DE, et al: Collecting duct-specific deletion of peroxisome proliferator-activated receptor gamma blocks thiazolidinedione-induced fluid retention. Proc Natl Acad Sci U S A 102:9406–9411, 2005.

315. Hong G, Lockhart A, Davis B, et al: PPARgamma activation enhances cell surface ENaCalpha via up-regulation of SGK1 in human collecting duct cells. FASEB J 17:1966–1968, 2003.

316. Karalliedde J, Buckingham R, Starkie M, et al: Effect of various diuretic treatments on rosiglitazone-induced fluid retention. J Am Soc Nephrol 17:3482–3490, 2006.

317. Alvarez de la Rosa D, Canessa CM: Role of SGK in hormonal regulation of epithelial sodium channel in A6 cells. Am J Physiol Cell Physiol 284:C404–414, 2003.

318. Wang J, Barbry P, Maiyar AC, et al: SGK integrates insulin and mineralocorticoid regulation of epithelial sodium transport. Am J Physiol Renal Physiol 280:F303–313, 2001.

319. Ledbetter ML, Lubin M: Control of protein synthesis in human fibroblasts by intracellular potassium. Exp Cell Res 105:223–236, 1977.

320. Lopez-Rivas A, Adelberg EA, Rozengurt E: Intracellular K+ and the mitogenic response of 3T3 cells to peptide factors in serum-free medium. Proc Natl Acad Sci U S A 79:6275–6279, 1982.

321. Bortner CD, Hughes FMJ, Cidlowski JA: A primary role for K+ and Na+ efflux in the activation of apoptosis. J Biol Chem 272:32436–32442, 1997.

322. Coca SG, Perazella MA, Buller GK: The cardiovascular implications of hypokalemia. Am J Kidney Dis 45:233–247, 2005.

323. Sausbier M, Matos JE, Sausbier U, et al: Distal colonic K(+) secretion occurs via BK channels. J Am Soc Nephrol 17:1275–1282, 2006.

324. Foster ES, Jones WJ, Hayslett JP, Binder HJ: Role of aldosterone and dietary potassium in potassium adaptation in the distal colon of the rat. Gastroenterology 88:41–46, 1985.

325. Bastl C, Hayslett JP, Binder HJ: Increased large intestinal secretion of potassium in renal insufficiency. Kidney Int 12:9–16, 1977.

326. Bomsztyk K, Wright FS: Dependence of ion fluxes on fluid transport by rat proximal tubule. Am J Physiol 250:F680–689, 1986.

327. Kaufman JS, Hamburger RJ: Passive potassium transport in the proximal convoluted tubule. Am J Physiol 248:F228–232, 1985.

328. Wilson RW, Wareing M, Green R: The role of active transport in potassium reabsorption in the proximal convoluted tubule of the anaesthetized rat. J Physiol 500 (Pt 1):155–164, 1997.

329. Kibble JD, Wareing, M, Wilson RW, Green R: Effect of barium on potassium diffusion across the proximal convoluted tubule of the anesthetized rat. Am J Physiol 268: F778–783, 1995.

330. Wilson RW, Wareing M, Kibble J, Green R: Potassium permeability in the absence of fluid reabsorption in proximal tubule of the anesthetized rat. Am J Physiol 274: F1109–1112, 1998.

331. Wareing M, Wilson RW, Kibble JD, Green R: Estimated potassium reflection coefficient in perfused proximal convoluted tubules of the anaesthetized rat in vivo. J Physiol 488 (Pt 1):153–161, 1995.

332. Johnston PA, Battilana CA, Lacy FB, Jamison RL: Evidence for a concentration gradient favoring outward movement of sodium from the thin loop of Henle. J Clin Invest 59:234–240, 1977.

333. Battilana CA, Dobyan DC, Lacy FB, et al: Effect of chronic potassium loading on potassium secretion by the pars recta or descending limb of the juxtamedullary nephron in the rat. J Clin Invest 62:1093–1103, 1978.

334. Elalouf JM, Roinel N, de Rouffignac C: Effects of dDAVP on rat juxtamedullary nephrons: stimulation of medullary K recycling. Am J Physiol 249:F291–298, 1985.

335. Tabei K, Imai MK: transport in upper portion of descending limbs of long-loop nephron from hamster. Am J Physiol 252:F387–392, 1987.

336. Schnermann J, Steipe B, Briggs JP: In situ studies of distal convoluted tubule in rat. II. K secretion. Am J Physiol 252:F970–976, 1987.

337. Frindt G, Palmer LG: Apical potassium channels in the rat connecting tubule. Am J Physiol Renal Physiol 287:F1030–1037, 2004.

338. Giebisch G: Renal potassium transport: Mechanisms and regulation. Am J Physiol 274:F817–833, 1998.

339. Muto S: Potassium transport in the mammalian collecting duct. Physiol Rev 81:85–116, 2001.

340. Stokes JB: Potassium secretion by cortical collecting tubule: Relation to sodium absorption, luminal sodium concentration, and transepithelial voltage. Am J Physiol 241:F395–402, 1981.

341. Pluznick JL, Sansom SC: BK channels in the kidney: Role in K(+) secretion and localization of molecular components. Am J Physiol Renal Physiol 291:F517–529, 2006.

342. Gray DA, Frindt G, Palmer LG: Quantification of K+ secretion through apical low-conductance K channels in the CCD Am J Physiol Renal Physiol 289:F117–126, 2005.

343. Palmer LG, Choe H, Frindt G: Is the secretory K channel in the rat CCT ROMK? Am J Physiol 273:F404–410, 1997.

344. Bailey MA, Cantone A, Yan Q, et al: Maxi-K channels contribute to urinary potassium excretion in the ROMK-deficient mouse model of Type II Bartter's syndrome and in adaptation to a high-K diet. Kidney Int 70:51–59, 2006.

345. Finer G, Shalev H, Birk OS, et al: Transient neonatal hyperkalemia in the antenatal (ROMK defective) Bartter syndrome. J Pediatr 142:318–323, 2003.

346. Woda CB, Bragin A, Kleyman TR, Satlin LM: Flow-dependent K+ secretion in the cortical collecting duct is mediated by a maxi-K channel. Am J Physiol Renal Physiol 280:F786–793, 2001.

347. Giebisch GH: A trail of research on potassium. Kidney Int 62:1498–1512, 2002.

348. Giebisch G: Renal potassium channels: Function, regulation, and structure. Kidney Int 60:436–445, 2001.

349. Lesage F, Lazdunski M: Molecular and functional properties of two-pore-domain potassium channels. Am J Physiol Renal Physiol 279:F793–7801, 2000.

350. Zheng W, Verlander JW, Lynch IJ, et al: Cellular distribution of the potassium channel, KCNQ1, in normal mouse kidney. Am J Physiol Renal Physiol 292:456–466, 2006.

351. Gray DA, Frindt G, Zhang YY, Palmer LG: Basolateral K+ conductance in principal cells of rat CCD. Am J Physiol Renal Physiol 288:F493–504, 2005.

352. Zhou X, Xia SL, Wingo CS: Chloride transport by the rabbit cortical collecting duct: dependence on H,K-ATPase. J Am Soc Nephrol 9:2194–2202, 1998.

353. Amorim JB, Bailey MA, Musa-Aziz R, et al: Role of luminal anion and pH in distal tubule potassium secretion. Am J Physiol Renal Physiol 284:F381–388, 2003.

354. Ellison DH, Velazquez H, Wright FS: Unidirectional potassium fluxes in renal distal tubule: effects of chloride and barium. Am J Physiol 250:F885–894, 1986.

355. Velazquez H, Ellison DH, Wright FS: Chloride-dependent potassium secretion in early and late renal distal tubules. Am J Physiol 253:F555–562, 1987.

356. Wingo CS: Reversible chloride-dependent potassium flux across the rabbit cortical collecting tubule. Am J Physiol 256:F697–7704, 1989.

357. Schafer JA, Troutman SL: Potassium transport in cortical collecting tubules from mineralocorticoid-treated rat. Am J Physiol 253:F76–88, 1987.

358. Zhou X, Lynch IJ, Xia SL, Wingo CS: Activation of H(+)-K(+)-ATPase by CO2) requires a basolateral Ba^{2+})-sensitive pathway during K restriction. Am J Physiol Renal Physiol 279:F153–160, 2000.

359. Jaisser F, Beggah AT: The nongastric H+-K+-ATPases: Molecular and functional properties. Am J Physiol 276:F812–824, 1999.

360. Kraut JA, Helander KG, Helander HF, et al: Detection and localization of H+-K+-ATPase isoforms in human kidney. Am J Physiol Renal Physiol 281:F763–768, 2001.

361. Sangan P, Thevananther, S, Sangan S, et al: Colonic H-K-ATPase alpha- and beta-subunits express ouabain-insensitive H-K-ATPase. Am J Physiol Cell Physiol 278:C182–189, 2000.

362. Codina J, Delmas-Mata JT, DuBose, TD, Jr: The alpha-subunit of the colonic H+,K+-ATPase assembles with beta1-Na+,K+-ATPase in kidney and distal colon. J Biol Chem 273:7894–7899, 1998.

363. Kraut JA, Hiura J, Shin JM, et al: The Na(+)-K(+)-ATPase beta 1 subunit is associated with the HK alpha 2 protein in the rat kidney. Kidney Int 53:958–962, 1998.

364. Fejes-Toth G, Naray-Fejes-Toth A, Velazquez H: Intrarenal distribution of the colonic H,K-ATPase mRNA in rabbit. Kidney Int 56:1029–1036, 1999.

365. Verlander JW, Moudy RM, Campbell WG, et al: Immunohistochemical localization of H-K-ATPase alpha2c)-subunit in rabbit kidney. Am J Physiol Renal Physiol 281:F357–365, 2001.

366. Fejes-Toth G, Naray Fejes-Toth A: Immunohistochemical localization of colonic H-K-ATPase to the apical membrane of connecting tubule cells. Am J Physiol Renal Physiol 281:F318–325, 2001.

367. Silver RB, Soleimani M: H+-K+-ATPases: regulation and role in pathophysiological states. Am J Physiol 276:F799–811, 1999.

368. Buffin-Meyer B, Younes-Ibrahim M, Barlet-Bas C, et al: K depletion modifies the properties of Sch-28080-sensitive K-ATPase in rat collecting duct. Am J Physiol 272:F124–131, 1997.

369. Nakamura S, Wang Z, Galla JH, Soleimani M: K+ depletion increases HCO3– reabsorption in OMCD by activation of colonic H(+)-K(+)-ATPase. Am J Physiol 274:F687–692, 1998.

370. Kraut JA, Hiura J, Besancon M, et al: Effect of hypokalemia on the abundance of HK alpha 1 and HK alpha 2 protein in the rat kidney. Am J Physiol 272:F744–750, 1997.

371. Codina J, Delmas-Mata JT, DuBose TD, Jr: Expression of HKalpha2 protein is increased selectively in renal medulla by chronic hypokalemia. Am J Physiol 275:F433–440, 1998.

372. Meneton P, Schultheis PJ, Greeb J, et al: Increased sensitivity to K+ deprivation in colonic H,K-ATPase-deficient mice. J Clin Invest 101:536–542, 1998.

373. Spicer Z, Miller ML, Andringa A, et al: Stomachs of mice lacking the gastric H,K-ATPase alpha-subunit have achlorhydria, abnormal parietal cells, and ciliated metaplasia. J Biol Chem 275:21555–21565, 2000.

374. Petrovic S, Spicer Z, Greeley T, et al: Novel Schering and ouabain-insensitive potassium-dependent proton secretion in the mouse cortical collecting duct. Am J Physiol Renal Physiol 282:F133–143, 2002.

375. Dherbecourt O, Cheval L, Bloch-Faure M, et al: Molecular identification of Sch28080-sensitive K-ATPase activities in the mouse kidney. Pflugers Arch 451:769–775, 2006.

376. Abuladze N, Lee I, Newman D, et al: Axial heterogeneity of sodium-bicarbonate cotransporter expression in the rabbit proximal tubule. Am J Physiol 274:F628–633, 1998.

377. August JT, Nelson DH, Thorn GW: Response of normal subjects to large amounts of aldosterone. J Clin Invest 37:1549–1555, 1958.

378. Palmer LG, Frindt G: Aldosterone and potassium secretion by the cortical collecting duct. Kidney Int 57:1324–1328, 2000.

379. Palmer LG, Antonian L, Frindt G: Regulation of apical K and Na channels and Na/K pumps in rat cortical collecting tubule by dietary K. J Gen Physiol 104:693–710, 1994.

380. Muto S, Sansom S, Giebisch G: Effects of a high potassium diet on electrical properties of cortical collecting ducts from adrenalectomized rabbits. J Clin Invest 81:376–380, 1988.

381. Muto S, Asano Y, Seldin D, Giebisch G: Basolateral Na+ pump modulates apical Na+ and K+ conductances in rabbit cortical collecting ducts. Am J Physiol 276:F143–158, 1999.

382. Lin DH, Sterling H, Yang B, et al: Protein tyrosine kinase is expressed and regulates ROMK1 location in the cortical collecting duct. Am J Physiol Renal Physiol 286:F881–892, 2004.

383. Palmer LG, Frindt G: Regulation of apical K channels in rat cortical collecting tubule during changes in dietary K intake. Am J Physiol 277:F805–812, 1999.

384. Najjar F, Zhou H, Morimoto T, et al: Dietary K+ regulates apical membrane expression of maxi-K channels in rabbit cortical collecting duct. Am J Physiol Renal Physiol 289:F922–932, 2005.

385. Delaloy C, Lu J, Houot AM, et al: Multiple promoters in the WNK1 gene: One controls expression of a kidney-specific kinase-defective isoform. Mol Cell Biol 23:9208–9221, 2003.

386. Cope G, Murthy M, Golbang AP, et al: WNK1 affects surface expression of the ROMK potassium channel independent of WNK4. J Am Soc Nephrol 17:1867–1874, 2006.

387. Wade JB, Fang L, Liu J, et al: WNK1 kinase isoform switch regulates renal potassium excretion. Proc Natl Acad Sci U S A 103:8558–8563, 2006.

388. O'Reilly M, Marshall E, Macgillivray T, et al: Dietary electrolyte-driven responses in the renal WNK kinase pathway in vivo. J Am Soc Nephrol 17:2402–2413, 2006.

389. Ornt DB, Tannen RL: Demonstration of an intrinsic renal adaptation for K+ conservation in short-term K+ depletion. Am J Physiol 245:F329–338, 1983.

390. Wang W, Lerea KM, Chan M, Giebisch G: Protein tyrosine kinase regulates the number of renal secretory K channels. Am J Physiol Renal Physiol 278:F165–171, 2000.

391. Eiam-Ong S, Kurtzman NA, Sabatini S: Regulation of collecting tubule adenosine triphosphatases by aldosterone and potassium. J Clin Invest 91:2385–2392, 1993.

392. Mennitt PA, Frindt G, Silver RB, Palmer LG: Potassium restriction downregulates ROMK expression in rat kidney. Am J Physiol Renal Physiol 278:F916–924, 2000.

393. Lin DH, Sterling H, Lerea KM, et al: K depletion increases protein tyrosine kinase-mediated phosphorylation of ROMK. Am J Physiol Renal Physiol 283:F671–677, 2002.

394. Sterling H, Lin DH, Gu RM, et al: Inhibition of protein-tyrosine phosphatase stimulates the dynamin-dependent endocytosis of ROMK1. J Biol Chem 277:4317–4323, 2002.

395. Lin DH, Sterling H, Wang WH: The protein tyrosine kinase-dependent pathway mediates the effect of K intake on renal K secretion. Physiology (Bethesda) 20:140–146, 2005.

396. Wei Y, Bloom P, Lin D, et al: Effect of dietary K intake on apical small-conductance K channel in CCD: Role of protein tyrosine kinase. Am J Physiol Renal Physiol 281:F206–212, 2001.

397. Babilonia E, Wei Y, Sterling H, et al: Superoxide anions are involved in mediating the effect of low K intake on c-Src expression and renal K secretion in the cortical collecting duct. J Biol Chem 280:10790–10796, 2005.

398. Rabinowitz L: Aldosterone and potassium homeostasis. Kidney Int 49:1738–1742, 1996.

399. McDonough AA, Youn JH: Role of muscle in regulating extracellular [K+]. Semin Nephrol 25:335–342, 2005.

400. Chen P, Guzman JP, Leong PK, et al: Modest dietary K+ restriction provokes insulin resistance of cellular K+ uptake and phosphorylation of renal outer medulla K+ channel without fall in plasma K+ concentration. Am J Physiol Cell Physiol 290:C1355–1363, 2006.

401. Field MJ, Stanton BA, Giebisch GH: Influence of ADH on renal potassium handling: A micropuncture and microperfusion study. Kidney Int 25:502–511, 1984.

402. Cassola AC, Giebisch G, Wang W: Vasopressin increases density of apical low-conductance K+ channels in rat CCD. Am J Physiol 264:F502–509, 1993.

403. Amorim JB, Musa-Aziz R, Mello-Aires M, Malnic G: Signaling path of the action of AVP on distal K+ secretion. Kidney Int 66:696–704, 2004.

404. Brown EM: Extracellular Ca^{2+} sensing, regulation of parathyroid cell function, and role of Ca^{2+} and other ions as extracellular (first) messengers. Physiol Rev 71:371–411, 1991.

405. Yu AS: Renal transport of calcium, magnesium, and phosphate. In Brenner BM (ed): Brenner and Rector's The Kidney, Vol. 1. Saunders, Philadelphia, 2004, pp 535–572.

406. Brunette M, Aras M: A microinjection study of nephron permeability to calcium and magnesium. Am J Physiol 221:1442–1448, 1971.

407. Ng RC, Rouse D, Suki WN: Calcium transport in the rabbit superficial proximal convoluted tubule. J Clin Invest 74:834–842, 1984.

408. Amasheh S, Meiri N, Gitter AH, et al: Claudin-2 expression induces cation-selective channels in tight junctions of epithelial cells. J Cell Sci 115:4969–4976, 2002.

409. Rocha AS, Magaldi JB, Kokko JP: Calcium and phosphate transport in isolated segments of rabbit Henle's loop. J Clin Invest 59:975–983, 1977.

410. Bourdeau JE: Calcium transport across the pars recta of cortical segment 2 proximal tubules. Am J Physiol 251:F718–724, 1986.

411. Rouse D, Ng RCK, Suki WN: Calcium transport in the pars recta and thin descending limb of Henle of the rabbit, perfused in vitro. J Clin Invest 65:37–42, 1980.

412. Bourdeau JE, Burg MB: Voltage dependence of calcium transport in the thick ascending limb of Henle's loop. Am J Physiol 236:F357–F364, 1979.

413. Suki WN, Rouse D, Ng RCK, Kokko JP: Calcium transport in the thick ascending limb of Henle. Heterogeneity of function in the medullary and cortical segments. J Clin Invest 66:1004–1009, 1980.

414. Imai M: Calcium transport across the rabbit thick ascending limb of Henle's loop perfused in vitro. Pflugers Arch 374:255–263, 1978.

415. Friedman PA: Basal and hormone-activated calcium absorption in mouse renal thick ascending limbs. Am J Physiol 254:F62–F70, 1988.

416. Costanzo LS, Windhager EE: Calcium and sodium transport by the distal convoluted tubule of the rat. Am J Physiol (Renal Fluid Electrolyte Physiol.) 235:F492–F506, 1978.

417. Shareghi GR, Stoner LC: Calcium transport across segments of the rabbit distal nephron in vitro. Am J Physiol 235:F367–F375, 1978.

418. Imai M: Effects of parathyroid hormone and N^6, $O^{2'}$-dibutyryl cyclic AMP on Ca^{2+} transport across the rabbit distal nephron segments perfused in vitro. Pflügers Arch 390:145–151, 1981.

419. Nijenhuis T, Hoenderop JG, Bindels RJ: Downregulation of $Ca^{(2+)}$ and $Mg^{(2+)}$ transport proteins in the kidney explains tacrolimus (FK506)-induced hypercalciuria and hypomagnesemia. J Am Soc Nephrol 15:549–557, 2004.

420. Biner HL, Arpin-Bott MP, Loffing J, et al: Human cortical distal nephron: Distribution of electrolyte and water transport pathways. J Am Soc Nephrol 13:836–847, 2002.

421. Raber G, Willems PH, Lang F, et al: Co-ordinated control of apical calcium influx and basolateral calcium efflux in rabbit cortical collecting system. Cell Calcium 22:157–166, 1997.

422. Bindels RJM, Hartog A, Abrahamse SL, van Os CH: Effects of pH and calcium channel blockers on apical calcium entry and active calcium transport in rabbit cortical collecting system. Am J Physiol 266:F620–F627, 1994.

423. Bacskai BJ, Friedman PA: Activation of latent Ca^{2+} channels in renal epithelial cells by parathyroid hormone. Nature (London) 347:388–391, 1990.

424. Yu ASL, Hebert SC, Brenner BM, Lytton J: Molecular characterization and nephron distribution of a family of transcripts encoding the pore-forming subunit of Ca^{2+} channels in the kidney. Proc Natl Acad Sci U S A 89:10494–10498, 1992.

425. Barry EL, Gesek FA, Yu AS, et al: Distinct calcium channel isoforms mediate parathyroid hormone and chlorothiazide-stimulated calcium entry in transporting epithelial cells. J Membr Biol 161:55–64, 1998.

426. Zhao PL, Wang XT, Zhang XM, et al: Tubular and cellular localization of the cardiac L-type calcium channel in rat kidney. Kidney Int 61:1393–1406, 2002.

427. Hoenderop JG, van der Kemp AW, Hartog A, et al: Molecular identification of the apical Ca^{2+} channel in 1,25-dihydroxyvitamin D3-responsive epithelia. J Biol Chem 274:8375–8378, 1999.

428. Hoenderop JG, Hartog A, Stuiver M, et al: Localization of the epithelial $Ca^{(2+)}$ channel in rabbit kidney and intestine. J Am Soc Nephrol 11:1171–1178, 2000.

429. Hoenderop JG, Muller D, van der Kemp AW, et al: Calcitriol controls the epithelial calcium channel in kidney. J Am Soc Nephrol 12:1342–1349, 2001.

430. Vennekens R, Hoenderop JG, Prenen J, et al: Permeation and gating properties of the novel epithelial $Ca^{(2+)}$ channel. J Biol Chem 275:3963–3969, 2000.

431. Nilius B, Vennekens R, Prenens J, et al: Whole-cell and single channel monovalent cation currents through the novel rabbit epithelial Ca^{2+} channel ECaC. J Physiol 527 Pt 2:239–248, 2000.

432. Vennekens R, Prenen J, Hoenderop JG, et al: Modulation of the epithelial Ca^{2+} channel ECaC by extracellular pH. Pflugers Arch 442:237–242, 2001.

433. Nilius B, Prenen J, Vennekens R, et al: Pharmacological modulation of monovalent cation currents through the epithelial Ca^{2+} channel ECaC1. Br J Pharmacol 134:453–462, 2001.

434. Peng J-B, Chen XZ, Berger UV, et al: Molecular cloning and characterization of a channel-like transporter mediating intestinal calcium absorption. J Biol Chem 274:22739–22746, 1999.

435. Hoenderop JG, Vennekns R, Muller D, et al: Function and expression of the epithelial $Ca^{(2+)}$ channel family: Comparison of mammalian ECaC1 and 2. J Physiol 537:747–761, 2001.

436. Vassilev PM, Peng JB, Hediger, MA, Brown EM: Single-channel activities of the human epithelial Ca^{2+} transport proteins CaT1 and CaT2. J Membr Biol 184:113–120, 2001.

437. Hoenderop JG, Voets T, Hoefs S, et al: Homo- and heterotetrameric architecture of the epithelial Ca^{2+} channels TRPV5 and TRPV6. EMBO J 22:776–785, 2003.

438. Hoenderop JG, van Leeuwen JB, van der Eerden BC, et al: Renal Ca^{2+} wasting, hyperabsorption, and reduced bone thickness in mice lacking TRPV5. J Clin Invest 112:1906–1914, 2003.

439. van de Graaf SF, Hoenderop JG, Gkika D, et al: Functional expression of the epithelial $Ca^{(2+)}$ channels (TRPV5 and TRPV6) requires association of the S100A10-annexin 2 complex. EMBO J 22:1478–1487, 2003.

440. Gkika D, Mahieu F, Nilius B, et al: 80K-H as a new Ca^{2+} sensor regulating the activity of the epithelial Ca^{2+} channel transient receptor potential cation channel V5 (TRPV5). J Biol Chem 279:26351–26357, 2004.

441. van de Graaf SF, et al: Identification of BSPRY as a novel auxiliary protein inhibiting TRPV5 activity. J Am Soc Nephrol 17:26–30, 2006.

442. Lambers TT, Weidema AF, Nilius B, et al: Regulation of the mouse epithelial Ca2(+) channel TRPV6 by the $Ca^{(2+)}$-sensor calmodulin. J Biol Chem 279:28855–28861, 2004.

443. Niemeyer BA, Bergs C, Wissenbach U, et al: Competitive regulation of CaT-like-mediated Ca^{2+} entry by protein kinase C and calmodulin. Proc Natl Acad Sci U S A 98:3600–3605, 2001.

444. Bronner F, Stein WD: CaBPr facilitates intracellular diffusion for Ca pumping in distal convoluted tubule. Am J Physiol 255:F558–562, 1988.

445. Van Baal J, Yu A, Hartog A, et al: Localization and regulation by vitamin D of calcium transport proteins in rabbit cortical collecting system. Am. J Physiol 271:F985–993, 1996.

446. Bindels RJM, Hartog A, Timmermans J, Van Os CH: Active Ca^{2+} transport in primary cultures of rabbit kidney CCD: stimulation by 1,25-dihydroxyvitamin D_3 and PTH. Am J Physiol 261:F799–F807, 1991.

447. Airaksinen MS, Eilers J, Garaschuk O, et al: Ataxia and altered dendritic calcium signaling in mice carrying a targeted null mutation of the calbindin D28k gene. Proc Natl Acad Sci U S A 94:1488–1493, 1997.

448. Sooy K, Kohut J, Christakos S: The role of calbindin and 1,25dihydroxyvitamin D3 in the kidney. Curr Opin Nephrol Hypertens 9:341–347, 2000.

449. Feher JJ: Facilitated calcium diffusion by intestinal calcium-binding protein. Am J Physiol 244:C303–307, 1983.

450. Shimura F, Wasserman RH: Membrane-associated vitamin D-induced calcium-binding protein (CaBP): Quantification by a radioimmunoassay and evidence for a specific CaBP in purified intestinal brush borders. Endocrinology 115:1964–1972, 1984.

451. Freud TS, Christakos S: Enzyme modification by renal calcium-binding proteins. In Norman AW, Schaefer K, Gringoleit H-G, Herrath DV (eds): Vitamin D, Chemical, Biochemical and Clinical Endocrinology of Calcium Metabolism. Berlin, DeGruyter, 1985, 369–370.

452. Bindels RJ, Ramakers PL, Dempster JA, et al: Role of Na+/Ca^{2+} exchange in transcellular Ca^{2+} transport across primary cultures of rabbit kidney collecting system. Pflugers Arch 420:566–572, 1992.

453. Gmaj P, Murer H, Kinne R: Calcium ion transport across plasma membranes isolated from rat kidney cortex. Biochem J 178:549–557, 1979.

454. Talor Z, Arruda JAL: Partial purification and reconstitution of renal basolateral Na+-Ca^{2+} exchanger into liposomes. J Biol Chem 260:15473–15476, 1985.

455. Bourdeau JE, Lau K: Basolateral cell membrane Ca-Na exchange in single rabbit connecting tubules. Am J Physiol 258:F1497–1503, 1990.

456. Ramachandran C, Brunette MG: The renal Na+/Ca^{2+} exchange system is located exclusively in the distal tubule. Biochem J 257:259–264, 1989.

457. Yu, ASL, Hebert SC, Lee S-L, et al: Identification and localization of the renal Na+-Ca^{2+} exchanger by the polymerase chain reaction. Am J Physiol 263:F680–F685, 1992.

458. Reilly RF, Shugrue CA: cDNA cloning of a renal Na+-Ca^{2+} exchanger. Am J Physiol 262:F1105–F1109, 1992.

459. Lee S-L, Yu ASL, Lytton J: Tissue-specific expression of Na+-Ca^{2+} exchanger isoforms. J Biol Chem 269:14849–14852, 1994.

460. Hilgemann DW, Collins A, Matsuoka S: Steady-state and dynamic properties of cardiac sodium-calcium exchange. Secondary modulation by cytoplasmic calcium and ATP J Gen Physiol 100, 933–961, 1992.

461. Doucet A, Katz AI: High-affinity Ca-Mg-ATPase along the rabbit nephron. Am J Physiol 242:F346–F352, 1982.

462. Borke JL, Caride A, Verma A, et al: Plasma membrane calcium pump and 28-kDa calcium binding protein in cells of rat kidney distal tubules. Am J Physiol 257: F842–F849, 1989.

463. Strehler EE, Zacharias DA: Role of alternative splicing in generating isoform diversity among plasma membrane calcium pumps. Physiol Rev 81:21–50, 2001.

464. Caride AJ, Chini EN, Homma S, et al: mRNA encoding four isoforms of the plasma membrane calcium pump and their variants in rat kidney and nephron segments. J Lab Clin Med 132:149–156, 1998.

465. Magocsi M, Yamaki M, Penniston JT, Dousa TP: Localization of mRNA coding isozymes of plasma membrane Ca^{2+}-ATPase pump in rat kidney. Am J Physiol 263:F7–F14, 1992.

466. Stauffer TP, Guerini D, Carafoli E: Tissue distribution of the four gene products of the plasma membrane Ca^{2+} pump. A study using specific antibodies. J Biol Chem 270:12184–12190, 1995.

467. Magyar CE, White KE, Rojas R, et al: Plasma membrane Ca^{2+}-ATPase and NCX1 Na+/Ca^{2+} exchanger expression in distal convoluted tubule cells. Am J Physiol Renal Physiol 283:F29–40, 2002.

468. Yu AS, Enck AH, Lencer WI, Schneeberger EE: Claudin-8 expression in MDCK cells augments the paracellular barrier to cation permeation. J Biol Chem 278:17350–17359, 2003.

469. Wong NL, Quamme GA, Dirks JH, Sutton RA: Divalent ion transport in dogs with experimental chronic renal failure. Can J Physiol Pharmacol 60:1296–1302, 1982.

470. Agus ZS, Chiu PJ, Goldberg M: Regulation of urinary calcium excretion in the rat. Am J Physiol 232:F545–549, 1977.

471. Humes HD, Ichikawa I, Troy JL, Brenner BM: Evidence for a parathyroid hormone-dependent influence of calcium on the glomerular ultrafiltration coefficient. J Clin Invest 61:32–40, 1978.

472. Castelli I, Steiner LA, Kaufmann MA, Drop LJ: Renovascular responses to high and low perfusate calcium steady-state experiments in the isolated perfused rat kidney with baseline vascular tone. J Surg Res 61:51–57, 1996.

473. Quamme GA: Effect of hypercalcemia on renal tubular handling of calcium and magnesium. Can J Physiol Pharmacol 60:1275–1280, 1982.

474. Amlal H, Legoff C, Vernimmen C, et al: Na(+)-K+(NH4+)-2Cl− cotransport in medullary thick ascending limb: Control by PKA, PKC, and 20-HETE. Am J Physiol 271: C455–63 1996.

475. Wang WH, Lu M, Hebert SC: Cytochrome P-450 metabolites mediate extracellular $Ca^{(2+)}$-induced inhibition of apical K+ channels in the TAL Am J Physiol 271:C103–111, 1996.

476. Motoyama HI, Friedman PA: Calcium-sensing receptor regulation of PTH-dependent calcium absorption by mouse cortical ascending limbs. Am J Physiol Renal Physiol 283:F399–406, 2002.

477. Edwards BR, Sutton RA, Dirks JH: Effect of calcium infusion on renal tubular reabsorption in the dog. Am J Physiol 227:13–18, 1974.

478. Sutton RA, Wong NL, Dirks JH: Effects of metabolic acidosis and alkalosis on sodium and calcium transport in the dog kidney. Kidney Int 15:520–533, 1979.

479. Mori Y, Machida T, Miyakawa S, Bomsztyk K: Effects of amiloride on distal renal tubule sodium and calcium absorption: Dependence on luminal pH. Pharmacol Toxicol 70:201–204, 1992.

480. Nijenhuis T, Renkema KY, Hoenderop JG, Bindels RJ: Acid-base status determines the renal expression of Ca^{2+} and mg^{2+} transport proteins. J Am Soc Nephrol 17:617–626, 2006.

481. Lee K, Brown D, Urena P, et al: Localization of parathyroid hormone/parathyroid hormone-related peptide receptor mRNA in kidney. Am J Physiol 270:F186–191, 1996.

482. Amizuka N, Lee HS, Kwan MY, et al: Cell-specific expression of the parathyroid hormone (PTH)/PTH-related peptide receptor gene in kidney from kidney-specific and ubiquitous promoters. Endocrinology 138:469–481, 1997.
483. Usdin TB, Bonner TI, Harta G, Mezey E: Distribution of parathyroid hormone-2 receptor messenger ribonucleic acid in rat. Endocrinology 137:4285–4297, 1996.
484. Agus ZS, Gardner LB, Beck LH, Goldberg M: Effects of parathyroid hormone on renal tubular reabsorption of calcium, sodium, and phosphate. Am J Physiol 224:1143–1148, 1973.
485. Bourdeau JE, Burg MB: Effect of PTH on calcium transport across the cortical thick ascending limb of Henle's loop. Am J Physiol 239:F121–126, 1980.
486. Wittner M, Mandon B, Roinel N, et al: Hormonal stimulation of Ca^{2+} and Mg^{2+} transport in the cortical thick ascending limb of Henle's loop of the mouse: Evidence for a change in the paracellular pathway permeability. Pflügers Arch 423:387–396, 1993.
487. Costanzo LS, Windhager EE: Effects of PTH, ADH, and cyclic AMP on distal tubular Ca and Na reabsorption. Am J Physiol 239:F478–F485, 1980.
488. Shimizu, T, Yoshitomi K, Nakamura M, Imai M: Effects of PTH, calcitonin, and cAMP on calcium transport in rabbit distal nephron segments. Am J Physiol 259:F408–414, 1990.
489. Bourdeau JE, Lau K: Effects of parathyroid hormone on cytosolic free calcium concentration in individual rabbit connecting tubules. J Clin Invest 83:373–379, 1989.
490. van Abel M, Hoenderop JG, van der Kemp AW, et al: Coordinated control of renal $Ca(^{2+})$ transport proteins by parathyroid hormone. Kidney Int 68:1708–1721, 2005.
491. Hoenderop JG, Dardenne O, Van Abel M, et al: Modulation of renal Ca^{2+} transport protein genes by dietary Ca^{2+} and 1,25-dihydroxyvitamin D3 in 25-hydroxyvitamin D3–1alpha-hydroxylase knockout mice. FASEB J 16:1398–1406, 2002.
492. Chang Q, Hoefs S, van der Kemp AW, et al: The beta-glucuronidase klotho hydrolyzes and activates the TRPV5 channel. Science 310:490–493, 2005.
493. Sexton PM, Adam WR, Moseley JM, et al: Localization and characterization of renal calcitonin receptors by in vitro autoradiography. Kidney Int 32:862–868, 1987.
494. Firsov D, Bellanger AC, Marsy S, Elalouf JM: Quantitative RT-PCR analysis of calcitonin receptor mRNAs in the rat nephron. Am J Physiol 269:F702–709, 1995.
495. Morel F, Doucet A: Hormonal control of kidney functions at the cell level. Physiol Rev 66:377–468, 1986.
496. Suki WN, Rouse D: Hormonal regulation of calcium transport in thick ascending limb renal tubules. Am J Physiol 241:F171–174, 1981.
497. Picard N, Van Abel M, Campone C, et al: Tissue kallikrein-deficient mice display a defect in renal tubular calcium absorption. J Am Soc Nephrol 16:3602–3610, 2005.
498. Peters M, Jeck N, Reinalter S, et al: Clinical presentation of genetically defined patients with hypokalemic salt-losing tubulopathies. Am J Med 112:183–190, 2002.
499. Eknoyan G, Suki WN, Martinez-Maldonado M: Effect of diuretics on urinary excretion of phosphate, calcium, and magnesium in thyroparathyroidectomized dogs. J Lab Clin Med 76:257–266, 1970.
500. Nijenhuis T, Vallon V, van der Kemp AW, et al: Enhanced passive Ca^{2+} reabsorption and reduced Mg^{2+} channel abundance explains thiazide-induced hypocalciuria and hypomagnesemia. J Clin Invest 115:1651–1658, 2005.
501. Brickman AS, Massry SG, Coburn JW: Changes in serum and urinary calcium during treatment with hydrochlorothiazide: Studies on mechanisms. J Clin Invest 51:945–954, 1972.
502. Quamme GA, Dai LJ: Presence of a novel influx pathway for Mg^{2+} in MDCK cells. Am J Physiol 259:C521–525, 1990.
503. Dai LJ, Raymond L, Friedman PA, Quamme GA: Mechanisms of amiloride stimulation of Mg^{2+} uptake in immortalized mouse distal convoluted tubule cells. Am J Physiol 272:F249–256, 1997.
504. Harris CA, Burnatowska MA, Seely JF, et al: Effects of parathyroid hormone on electrolyte transport in the hamster nephron. Am J Physiol 236:F342–348, 1979.
505. Nearing J, Betka M, Quinn S, et al: Polyvalent cation receptor proteins (CaRs) are salinity sensors in fish. Proc Natl Acad Sci U S A 99:9231–9236, 2002.
506. Barnes BA, Cope O, Gordon EB: Magnesium requirements and deficits: An evaluation of two surgical patients. Ann Surg 152:518–533, 1960.
507. Rude RK, Bethune JE, Singer FR: Renal tubular maximum for magnesium in normal, hyperparathyroid, and hypoparathyroid man. J Clin Endocrinol Metabol 51:1425–1431, 1980.
508. Quamme GA, Dirks JH: Intraluminal and contraluminal magnesium on magnesium and calcium transfer in the rat nephron. Am J Physiol 238:F187–198, 1980.
509. Lelievre-Pegorier M, Merlet-Benichou C, Roinel N, de Rouffignac C: Developmental pattern of water and electrolyte transport in rat superficial nephrons. Am J Physiol 245:F15–21, 1983.
510. Quamme GA, Smith CM: Magnesium transport in the proximal straight tubule of the rabbit. Am J Physiol 246:F544–50, 1984.
511. Shareghi GR, Agus ZS: Magnesium transport in the cortical thick ascending limb of Henle's loop of the rabbit. J Clin Invest 69:759–769, 1982.
512. Quamme GA: Effect of furosemide on calcium and magnesium transport in the rat nephron. Am J Physiol 241:F340–347, 1981.
513. Poujeol P, Chabardes D, Roinel N, De Rouffignac C: Influence of extracellular fluid volume expansion on magnesium, calcium and phosphate handling along the rat nephron. Pflugers Arch 365:203–211, 1976.
514. Wittner M, di Stefano A, Wangemann P, et al: Differential effects of ADH on sodium, chloride, potassium, calcium and magnesium transport in cortical and medullary thick ascending limbs of mouse nephron. Pflugers Arch 412:516–523, 1988.
515. Di Stefano A, Wittner M, Nitschke R, et al: Effects of glucagon on Na^+, Cl–, K^+, Mg^{2+} and Ca^{2+} transports in cortical and medullary thick ascending limbs of mouse kidney. Pflugers Arch 414:640–646, 1989.
516. Dai LJ, Ritchie G, Kerstan D, et al: Magnesium transport in the renal distal convoluted tubule. Physiol Rev 81:51–84, 2001.
517. Brunette MG, Vigneault N, Carriere S: Magnesium handling by the papilla of the young rat. Pflugers Arch 373:229–235, 1978.
518. Shareghi GR, Agus ZS: Phosphate transport in the light segment of the rabbit cortical collecting tubule. Am J Physiol 242:F379–384, 1982.
519. Bengele HH, Alexander EA, Lechene CP: Calcium and magnesium transport along the inner medullary collecting duct of the rat. Am J Physiol 239:F24–29, 1980.
520. Schlingmann KP, Weber S, Peters M, et al: Hypomagnesemia with secondary hypocalcemia is caused by mutations in TRPM6, a new member of the TRPM gene family. Nat Genet 31:166–170, 2002.
521. Walder RY, Landau D, Meyer P, et al: Mutation of TRPM6 causes familial hypomagnesemia with secondary hypocalcemia. Nat Genet 31:171–174, 2002.
522. Voets T, Nilius B, Hoefs S, et al: TRPM6 forms the Mg^{2+} influx channel involved in intestinal and renal Mg^{2+} absorption. J Biol Chem 279:19–25, 2004.
523. Montell C: Mg^{2+} homeostasis: The Mg^{2+}nificent TRPM chanzymes. Curr Biol 13: R799–801 2003.
524. Chubanov V, Waldegger S, Mederos Y, Schnitzler M, et al: Disruption of TRPM6/TRPM7 complex formation by a mutation in the TRPM6 gene causes hypomagnesemia with secondary hypocalcemia. Proc Natl Acad Sci U S A 101:2894–2899, 2004.
525. Meij IC, Koenderink JB, De Jong JC, et al: Dominant isolated renal magnesium loss is caused by misrouting of the Na(+),K(+)-ATPase gamma-subunit. Nat Genet 26:265–266, 2000.
526. Geven WB, Monnens LA, Willems HL, et al: Renal magnesium wasting in two families with autosomal dominant inheritance. Kidney Int 31:1140–1144, 1987.
527. Wen SF, Evanson RL, Dirks JH: Micropuncture study of renal magnesium transport in proximal and distal tubule of the dog. Am J Physiol 219:570–576, 1970.
528. Barnes BA, Cope O, Harrison T: Magnesium conservation in the human being on a low magnesium diet. J Clin Invest 37:430–440, 1958.
529. Carney SL, Wong NL, Quamme GA, Dirks JH: Effect of magnesium deficiency on renal magnesium and calcium transport in the rat. J Clin Invest 65:180–188, 1980.
530. Groenestege WM, Hoenderop JG, van den Heuvel L, et al: The epithelial mg^{2+} channel transient receptor potential melastatin 6 is regulated by dietary Mg^{2+} content and estrogens. J Am Soc Nephrol 174:1035–1043, 2006.
531. Wong NL, Quamme GA, Dirks JH: Effect of chlorothiazide on renal calcium and magnesium handling in the hamster. Can J Physiol Pharmacol 60:1160–1165, 1982.
532. Barton CH, Vaziri ND, Martin DC, et al: Hypomagnesemia and renal magnesium wasting in renal transplant recipients receiving cyclosporine. Am J Med 83:693–699, 1987.
533. Shimada T, Mizutani S, Muto T, et al: Cloning and characterization of FGF23 as a causative factor of tumor-induced osteomalacia. Proc Natl Acad Sci U S A 98:6500–6505, 2001.
534. De Beur SM, Finnegan RB, Vassiliadis J, et al: Tumors associated with oncogenic osteomalacia express genes important in bone and mineral metabolism. J Bone Miner Res 17:1102–1110, 2002.
535. Naveh-Many T, Rahamimov R, Livni N, Silver J: Parathyroid cell proliferation in normal and chronic renal failure rats. The effects of calcium, phosphate, and vitamin D. J Clin Invest 96:1786–1793, 1995.
536. Slatopolsky E, Finch J, Denda M, et al: Phosphorus restriction prevents parathyroid gland growth. High phosphorus directly stimulates PTH secretion in vitro. J Clin Invest 97:2534–2540, 1996.
537. Perwad F, Azam N, Zhang MY, et al: Dietary and serum phosphorus regulate fibroblast growth factor 23 expression and 1,25-dihydroxyvitamin D metabolism in mice. Endocrinology 146:5358–5364, 2005.
538. Ullrich KJ, Rumrich G, Kloss S: Phosphate transport in the proximal convolution of the rat kidney. I. Tubular heterogeneity, effect of parathyroid hormone in acute and chronic parathyroidectomized animals and effect of phosphate diet. Pflugers Arch 372:269–274, 1977.
539. McKeown JW, Brazy PC, Dennis VW: Intrarenal heterogeneity for fluid, phosphate, and glucose absorption in the rabbit. Am J Physiol 237:F312–8 1979.
540. Agus ZS, Puschett JB, Senesky D, Goldberg M: Mode of action of parathyroid hormone and cyclic adenosine 3′,5′-monophosphate on renal tubular phosphate reabsorption in the dog. J Clin Invest 50:617–626, 1971.
541. Suzuki M, Capparelli A, Jo OD, et al: Phosphate transport in the in vitro cultured rabbit proximal convoluted and straight tubules. Kidney Int 34:268–272, 1988.
542. Turner ST, Dousa TP: Phosphate transport by brushborder membranes from superficial and juxtamedullary cortex. Kidney Int 27:879–885, 1985.
543. Levi M: Heterogeneity of Pi transport by BBM from superficial and juxtamedullary cortex of rat. Am J Physiol 258:F1616–1624, 1990.
544. Haramati A, Haas JA, Knox FG: Nephron heterogeneity of phosphate reabsorption: Effect of parathyroid hormone. Am J Physiol 246:F155–158, 1984.
545. Knox FG, Haas JA, Berndt T, et al: Phosphate transport in superficial and deep nephrons in phosphate-loaded rats. Am J Physiol 233:F150–153, 1977.
546. Haramati A, Haas JA, Knox FG: Adaptation of deep and superficial nephrons to changes in dietary phosphate intake. Am J Physiol 244:F265–269, 1983.
547. Bailly C, Roinel N, Amiel C: Stimulation by glucagon and PTH of Ca and Mg reabsorption in the superficial distal tubule of the rat kidney. Pflugers Arch 403:28–34, 1985.
548. Knox FG, Lechene C: Distal site of action of parathyroid hormone on phosphate reabsorption. Am J Physiol 229:1556–1560, 1975.
549. Hoffmann N, Thees M, Kinne R: Phosphate transport by isolated renal brush border vesicles. Pflugers Arch 362:147–156, 1976.
550. Werner A, Moore ML, Mantei N, et al: Cloning and expression of cDNA for a Na/Pi cotransport system of kidney cortex. Proc Natl Acad Sci U S A 88:9608–9612, 1991.
551. Custer M, Meier F, Schlatter E, et al: Localization of NaPi-1, a Na-Pi cotransporter, in rabbit kidney proximal tubules. I. mRNA localization by reverse transcription/polymerase chain reaction. Pflugers Arch 424:203–209, 1993.
552. Biber J, Custer M, Werner A, et al: Localization of NaPi-1, a Na/Pi cotransporter, in rabbit kidney proximal tubules. II. Localization by immunohistochemistry. Pflugers Arch 424:210–215, 1993.
553. Quabius ES, Murer H, Biber J: Expression of a renal Na/Pi cotransporter (NaPi-1) in MDCK and LLC-PK1 cells. Pflugers Arch 430:132–136, 1995.

554. Busch AE, Biber J, Murer H, Lang F: Electrophysiological insights of type I and II Na/Pi transporters. Kidney Int 49:986–987, 1996.

555. Murer H, Hernando N, Forster I, Biber J: Proximal tubular phosphate reabsorption: molecular mechanisms. Physiol Rev 80:1373–1409, 2000.

556. Magagnin S, Werner A, Markovich D, et al: Expression cloning of human and rat renal cortex Na/Pi cotransport. Proc Natl Acad Sci U S A 90:5979–5983, 1993.

557. Segawa H, Kaneko I, Takahashi A, et al: Growth-related renal type II Na/Pi cotransporter. J Biol Chem 277:19665–19672, 2002.

558. Traebert M, Hattenhauer O, Murer H, et al: Expression of type II Na-P(i) cotransporter in alveolar type II cells. Am J Physiol 277:L868–873, 1999.

559. Hilfiker H, Hattenhauer O, Traebert M, et al: Characterization of a murine type II sodium-phosphate cotransporter expressed in mammalian small intestine. Proc Natl Acad Sci U S A 95:14564–14569, 1998.

560. Forster IC, Loo DD, Eskandari S: Stoichiometry and Na+ binding cooperativity of rat and flounder renal type II Na+-Pi cotransporters. Am J Physiol 276:F644–649, 1999.

561. Busch A, Waldegger S, Herzer T, et al: Electrophysiological analysis of Na+/Pi cotransport mediated by a transporter cloned from rat kidney and expressed in Xenopus oocytes. Proc Natl Acad Sci U S A 91:8205–8208, 1994.

562. Forster IC, Biber J, Murer H: Proton-sensitive transitions of renal type II Na(+)-coupled phosphate cotransporter kinetics. Biophys J 79:215–230, 2000.

563. Beck L, Karaplis AC, Amizuka N, et al: Targeted inactivation of Npt2 in mice leads to severe renal phosphate wasting, hypercalciuria and skeletal abnormalities. Proc Natl Acad Sci U S A 95:5372–5377, 1998.

564. Hoag HM, Martel J, Gauthier C, Tenenhouse HS: Effects of Npt2 gene ablation and low-phosphate diet on renal Na(+)/phosphate cotransport and cotransporter gene expression. J Clin Invest 104:679–686, 1999.

565. Prie D, Huart V, Bakouh N, et al: Nephrolithiasis and osteoporosis associated with hypophosphatemia caused by mutations in the type 2a sodium-phosphate cotransporter. N Engl J Med 347:983–991, 2002.

566. Karim-Jimenez Z, Hernando N, Biber J, Murer H: Molecular determinants for apical expression of the renal type IIa Na+/Pi-cotransporter. Pflugers Arch 442:782–790, 2001.

567. Gisler SM, Stagljar I, Traebert M, et al: Interaction of the type IIa Na/Pi cotransporter with PDZ proteins. J Biol Chem 276:9206–9213, 2001.

568. Wade JB, Welling PA, Donowitz M, et al: Differential renal distribution of NHERF isoforms and their colocalization with NHE3, ezrin, and ROMK Am J Physiol Cell Physiol 280:C192–198, 2001.

569. Hernando N, Deliot N, Gisler SM, et al: PDZ-domain interactions and apical expression of type IIa Na/P(i) cotransporters. Proc Natl Acad Sci U S A 99:11957–11962, 2002.

570. Shenolikar S, Voltz JW, Minkoff CM, et al: Targeted disruption of the mouse NHERF-1 gene promotes internalization of proximal tubule sodium-phosphate cotransporter type IIa and renal phosphate wasting. Proc Natl Acad Sci U S A 99:11470–11475, 2002.

571. Capuano P, Bacic D, Stange G, et al: Expression and regulation of the renal Na/phosphate cotransporter NaPi-IIa in a mouse model deficient for the PDZ protein PDZK1. Pflugers Arch 449:392–402, 2005.

572. Bacconi A, Virkki LV, Biber J, et al: Renouncing electroneutrality is not free of charge: Switching on electrogenicity in a Na+-coupled phosphate cotransporter. Proc Natl Acad Sci U S A 102:12606–12611, 2005.

573. Barac-Nieto M, Dowd TL, Gupta RK, Spitzer A: Changes in NMR-visible kidney cell phosphate with age and diet: relationship to phosphate transport. Am J Physiol 261: F153–62 1991.

574. Bergwitz C, Roslin NM, Tieder M, et al: SLC34A3 mutations in patients with hereditary hypophosphatemic rickets with hypercalciuria predict a key role for the sodium-phosphate cotransporter NaPi-IIc in maintaining phosphate homeostasis. Am J Hum Genet 78:179–192, 2006.

575. Lorenz-Depiereux B, Benet-Pages A, Eckstein G, et al: Hereditary hypophosphatemic rickets with hypercalciuria is caused by mutations in the sodium-phosphate cotransporter gene SLC34A3. Am J Hum Genet 78:193–201, 2006.

576. Ritthaler T, Traebert M, Lotscher M, et al: Effects of phosphate intake on distribution of type II Na/Pi cotransporter mRNA in rat kidney. Kidney Int 55:976–983, 1999.

577. Levi M, Lotscher M, Sorribas V, et al: Cellular mechanisms of acute and chronic adaptation of rat renal Pi transporter to alterations in dietary Pi. Am J Physiol 267: F900–F908, 1994.

578. Lotscher M, Kaissling B, Biber J, et al: Role of microtubules in the rapid regulation of renal phosphate transport in response to acute alterations in dietary phosphate content. J Clin Invest 99:1302–1312, 1997.

579. Werner A, Kempson SA, Biber J, Murer H: Increase of Na/Pi-cotransport encoding mRNA in response to low Pi diet in rat kidney cortex. J Biol Chem 269:6637–6639, 1994.

580. Takahashi F, Morita K, Katai K, et al: Effects of dietary Pi on the renal Na+-dependent Pi transporter NaPi-2 in thyroparathyroidectomized rats. Biochem J 333:175–181, 1998.

581. Katai K, Segawa H, Haga H, et al: Acute regulation by dietary phosphate of the sodium-dependent phosphate transporter (NaP(i)-2) in rat kidney. J Biochem (Tokyo) 121:50–55, 1997.

582. Keusch I, Traebert M, Lotscher M, et al: Parathyroid hormone and dietary phosphate provoke a lysosomal routing of the proximal tubular Na/Pi-cotransporter type II. Kidney Int 54:1224–1232, 1998.

583. Segawa H, Yamanaka S, Ito M, et al: Internalization of renal type IIc Na-Pi cotransporter in response to a high-phosphate diet. Am J Physiol Renal Physiol 288:F587–596, 2005.

584. Ohkido I, Segawa H, Yanagida R, et al: Cloning, gene structure and dietary regulation of the type-IIc Na/Pi cotransporter in the mouse kidney. Pflugers Arch 446:106–115, 2003.

585. Pfister MF, Hilfiker H, Forgo J, et al: Cellular mechanisms involved in the acute adaptation of OK cell Na/Pi-cotransport to high- or low-Pi medium. Pflugers Arch 435:713–719, 1998.

586. Kido S, Miyamoto K, Mizobuchi H, et al: Identification of regulatory sequences and binding proteins in the type II sodium/phosphate cotransporter NPT2 gene responsive to dietary phosphate. J Biol Chem 274:28256–28263, 1999.

587. Custer M, Spindler B, Verrey F, et al: Identification of a new gene product (diphor-1) regulated by dietary phosphate. Am J Physiol 273:F801–806, 1997.

588. Ambuhl PM, Zajicek HK, Wang H, et al: Regulation of renal phosphate transport by acute and chronic metabolic acidosis in the rat. Kidney Int 53:1288–1298, 1998.

589. Jehle AW, Hilfiker H, Pfister MF, et al: Type II Na-Pi cotransport is regulated transcriptionally by ambient bicarbonate/carbon dioxide tension in OK cells. Am J Physiol 276:F46–53, 1999.

590. Lotscher M, Scarpetta Y, Levi M, et al: Rapid downregulation of rat renal Na/P(i) cotransporter in response to parathyroid hormone involves microtubule rearrangement. J Clin Invest 104:483–494, 1999.

591. Traebert M, Roth J, Biber J, et al: Internalization of proximal tubular type II Na-P(i) cotransporter by PTH: Immunogold electron microscopy. Am J Physiol Renal Physiol 278:F148–154, 2000.

592. Pfister MF, Ruf I, Stange G, et al: Parathyroid hormone leads to the lysosomal degradation of the renal type II Na/Pi cotransporter. Proc Natl Acad Sci U S A 95:1909–1914, 1998.

593. Karim-Jimenez Z, Hernando N, Biber J, Murer H: A dibasic motif involved in parathyroid hormone-induced down-regulation of the type IIa NaPi cotransporter. Proc Natl Acad Sci U S A 97:12896–12901, 2000.

594. Ito M, Iidawa S, Izuka M, et al: Interaction of a farnesylated protein with renal type IIa Na/Pi co-transporter in response to parathyroid hormone and dietary phosphate. Biochem J 377:607–616, 2004.

595. Kempson SA, Lotscher M, Kaissling B, et al: Parathyroid hormone action on phosphate transporter mRNA and protein in rat renal proximal tubules. Am J Physiol 268: F784–791, 1995.

596. Malmstrom K, Murer H: Parathyroid hormone regulates phosphate transport in OK cells via an irreversible inactivation of a membrane protein. FEBS Lett 216:257–260, 1987.

597. Zhao N, Tenenhouse HS: Npt2 gene disruption confers resistance to the inhibitory action of parathyroid hormone on renal sodium-phosphate cotransport. Endocrinology 141:2159–2165, 2000.

598. Traebert M, Volkl H, Biber J, et al: Luminal and contraluminal action of 1–34 and 3–34 PTH peptides on renal type IIa Na-P(i) cotransporter. Am J Physiol Renal Physiol 278: F792–798, 2000.

599. Lederer ED, Sohi SS, Mathiesen JM, Klein JB: Regulation of expression of type II sodium-phosphate cotransporters by protein kinases A and C. Am J Physiol 275: F270–277, 1998.

600. Khundmiri SJ, Rane, MJ, Lederer, ED: Parathyroid hormone regulation of type II sodium-phosphate cotransporters is dependent on an a kinase anchoring protein. J Biol Chem 20:20, 2002.

601. Kaufmann M, Muff R, Stieger B, et al: Apical and basolateral parathyroid hormone receptors in rat renal cortical membranes. Endocrinology 134:1173–1178, 1994.

602. Piwon N, Gunther W, Schwake M, et al: ClC-5 Cl−-channel disruption impairs endocytosis in a mouse model for Dent's disease. Nature 408:369–373, 2000.

603. Derrickson BH, Mandel LJ: Parathyroid hormone inhibits Na(+)-K(+)-ATPase through Gq/G11 and the calcium-independent phospholipase A2. Am J Physiol 272:F781–788, 1997.

604. Khundmiri SJ, Lederer E: PTH and DA regulate Na-K ATPase through divergent pathways. Am J Physiol Renal Physiol 282:F512–522, 2002.

605. Lederer ED, Sohi SS, McLeish KR: Parathyroid hormone stimulates extracellular signal-regulated kinase (ERK) activity through two independent signal transduction pathways: Role of ERK in sodium-phosphate cotransport. J Am Soc Nephrol 11:222–231, 2000.

606. Friedlander G, Couette S, Coureau C, Amiel C: Mechanisms whereby extracellular adenosine 3′,5′-monophosphate inhibits phosphate transport in cultured opossum kidney cells and in rat kidney. Physiological implication. J Clin Invest 90:848–858, 1992.

607. Le Goas F, Amiel C, Friedlander G: Protein kinase C modulates cAMP content in proximal tubular cells: Role of phosphodiesterase inhibition. Am J Physiol 261: F587–592, 1991.

608. Siegfried G, Vrtovsnik F, Prie D, et al: Parathyroid hormone stimulates ecto-5′-nucleotidase activity in renal epithelial cells: Role of protein kinase-C. Endocrinology 136:1267–1275, 1995.

609. Friedlaender MM, Wald H, Dranitzki-Elhalel M, et al: Vitamin D reduces renal NaPi-2 in PTH-infused rats: Complexity of vitamin D action on renal P(i) handling. Am J Physiol Renal Physiol 281:F428–433, 2001.

610. Brezis M, Wald H, Shilo R, Popovtzer, MM: Blockade of the renal tubular effects of vitamin D by cycloheximide in the rat. Pflugers Arch 398:247–252, 1983.

611. Allon M, Parris M: Calcitriol stimulates Na(+)-Pi cotransport in a subclone of opossum kidney cells (OK-7A) by a genomic mechanism. Am J Physiol 264:F404–410, 1993.

612. Liang CT, Barnes J, Balakir R, et al: In vitro stimulation of phosphate uptake in isolated chick renal cells by 1,25-dihydroxycholecalciferol. Proc Natl Acad Sci U S A 79:3532–3536, 1982.

613. Taketani Y, Segawa H, Chikamori M, et al: Regulation of type II renal Na+-dependent inorganic phosphate transporters by 1,25-dihydroxyvitamin D3. Identification of a vitamin D-responsive element in the human NAPi-3 gene. J Biol Chem 273:14575–14581, 1998.

614. Kaneda Y, Bello-Reuss E: Effect of dopamine on phosphate reabsorption in isolated perfused rabbit proximal tubules. Miner Electrolyte Metab 9:147–150, 1983.

615. Isaac J, Glahn RP, Appel MM, et al: Mechanism of dopamine inhibition of renal phosphate transport. J Am Soc Nephrol 2:1601–1607, 1992.

616. Debska-Slizien A, Ho P, Drangova R, Baines AD: Endogenous renal dopamine production regulates phosphate excretion. Am J Physiol 266:F858–867, 1994.

617. Glahn RP, Onsgard MJ, Tyce GM, et al: Autocrine/paracrine regulation of renal Na(+)-phosphate cotransport by dopamine. Am J Physiol 264:F618–622, 1993.

618. de Toledo FG, Thompson MA, Bolliger C, et al: gamma-L-glutamyl-L-DOPA inhibits Na(+)-phosphate cotransport across renal brush border membranes and increases renal excretion of phosphate. Kidney Int 55:1832–1842, 1999.

619. Perrichot R, Garcia-Ocana A, Couette S, et al: Locally formed dopamine modulates renal Na-Pi co-transport through DA1 and DA2 receptors. Biochem J 312 (Pt 2):433–437, 1995.

620. DeFronzo RA, Goldberg M, Agus ZS: The effects of glucose and insulin on renal electrolyte transport. J Clin Invest 58:83–90, 1976.

621. Hammerman MR, Rogers S, Hansen VA, Gavin JR, 3rd: Insulin stimulates Pi transport in brush border vesicles from proximal tubular segments. Am J Physiol 247:E616–624, 1984.

622. Abraham MI, McAteer JA, Kempson SA: Insulin stimulates phosphate transport in opossum kidney epithelial cells. Am J Physiol 258:F1592–1598, 1990.

623. Rubinger D, Wald H, Friedlaender MM, et al: Effect of intravenous glucagon on the urinary excretion of adenosine 3′,5′-monophosphate in man and in rats. Evidence for activation of renal adenylate cyclase and formation of nephrogenous cAMP. Miner Electrolyte Metab 14:211–220, 1988.

624. de Rouffignac C, Elalouf JM, Roinel N: Glucagon inhibits water and NaCl transports in the proximal convoluted tubule of the rat kidney. Pflugers Arch 419:472–477, 1991.

625. Dennis VW, Brazy PC: Sodium phosphate, glucose, bicarbonate, and alanine interactions in the isolated proximal convoluted tubule of the rabbit kidney. J Clin Invest 62:387–397, 1978.

626. Olsen HS, Cepeda MA, Zhang QQ, et al: Human stanniocalcin: A possible hormonal regulator of mineral metabolism. Proc Natl Acad Sci U S A 93:1792–1796, 1996.

627. De Niu P, Olsen HS, Gentz R, Wagner GF: Immunolocalization of stanniocalcin in human kidney. Mol Cell Endocrinol 137:155–159, 1998.

628. Wong CK, Ho MA, Wagner GF: The co-localization of stanniocalcin protein, mRNA and kidney cell markers in the rat kidney. J Endocrinol 158:183–189, 1998.

629. Deol H, Stasko SE, De Niu P, et al: Post-natal ontogeny of stanniocalcin gene expression in rodent kidney and regulation by dietary calcium and phosphate. Kidney Int 60:2142–2152, 2001.

630. Honda S, Kashiwagi M, Ookata K, et al: Regulation by 1alpha,25-dihydroxyvitamin D(3) of expression of stanniocalcin messages in the rat kidney and ovary. FEBS Lett 459:119–122, 1999.

631. De Niu P, Radman DP, Jaworski EM, et al: Development of a human stanniocalcin radioimmunoassay: Serum and tissue hormone levels and pharmacokinetics in the rat. Mol Cell Endocrinol 162:131–144, 2000.

632. Wagner GF, Vozzolo BL, Jaworski E, et al: Human stanniocalcin inhibits renal phosphate excretion in the rat. J Bone Miner Res 12:165–171, 1997.

633. Chang AC, Cha J, Koentgen F, Reddel RR: The murine stanniocalcin 1 gene is not essential for growth and development. Mol Cell Biol 25:10604–10610, 2005.

634. Kumar R: New insights into phosphate homeostasis: Fibroblast growth factor 23 and frizzled-related protein-4 are phosphaturic factors derived from tumors associated with osteomalacia. Curr Opin Nephrol Hypertens 11:547–553, 2002.

635. Carpenter TO, Ellis BK, Insogna KL, et al: Fibroblast growth factor 7: An inhibitor of phosphate transport derived from oncogenic osteomalacia-causing tumors. J Clin Endocrinol Metab 90:1012–1020, 2005.

636. The ADHR Consortium: Autosomal dominant hypophosphataemic rickets is associated with mutations in FGF23. Nat Genet 26:345–348, 2000.

637. Shimada T, Muto T, Urakawa I, et al: Mutant FGF-23 responsible for autosomal dominant hypophosphatemic rickets is resistant to proteolytic cleavage and causes hypophosphatemia in vivo. Endocrinology 143:3179–3182, 2002.

638. White KE, Carn G, Lorenz-Depiereux B, et al: Autosomal-dominant hypophosphatemic rickets (ADHR) mutations stabilize FGF-23. Kidney Int 60:2079–2086, 2001.

639. Yamazaki Y, Okazaki R, Shibata M, et al: Increased circulatory level of biologically active full-length FGF-23 in patients with hypophosphatemic rickets/osteomalacia. J Clin Endocrinol Metab 87:4957–4960, 2002.

640. White KE, Jonsson KB, Carn G, et al: The autosomal dominant hypophosphatemic rickets (ADHR) gene is a secreted polypeptide overexpressed by tumors that cause phosphate wasting. J Clin Endocrinol Metab 86:497–500, 2001.

641. Larsson T, Yu X, Davis SI, et al: A novel recessive mutation in fibroblast growth factor-23 causes familial tumoral calcinosis. J Clin Endocrinol Metab 90:2424–2427, 2005.

642. Benet-Pages A, Orlik P, Strom TM, Lorenz-Depiereux B: An FGF23 missense mutation causes familial tumoral calcinosis with hyperphosphatemia. Hum Mol Genet 14:385–390, 2005.

643. Liu S, Guo R, Simpson LG, et al: Regulation of fibroblastic growth factor 23 expression but not degradation by PHEX. J Biol Chem 278:37419–37426, 2003.

644. Liu S, Zhou J, Tang W, et al: Pathogenic role of FGF23 in Hyp Mice. Am J Physiol Endocrinol Metab 291:E38–49, 2006.

645. The HYP Consortium: A gene (PEX) with homologies to endopeptidases is mutated in patients with X-linked hypophosphatemic rickets. Nat Genet 11:130–136, 1995.

646. Shimada T, Lakitani M, Yamazaki Y, et al: Targeted ablation of Fgf23 demonstrates an essential physiological role of FGF23 in phosphate and vitamin D metabolism. J Clin Invest 113:561–568, 2004.

647. Mirams M, Robinson BG, Mason RS, Nelson AE: Bone as a source of FGF23: Regulation by phosphate? Bone 35:1192–1199, 2004.

648. Collins MT, Lindsay JR, Jain A, et al: Fibroblast growth factor-23 is regulated by 1alpha,25-dihydroxyvitamin D J Bone Miner Res 20:1944–1950, 2005.

649. Hines ER, Kolek OI, Jones MD, et al: 1,25-dihydroxyvitamin D3 down-regulation of PHEX gene expression is mediated by apparent repression of a 110 kDa transfactor that binds to a polyadenine element in the promoter. J Biol Chem 279:46406–46414, 2004.

650. Saito H, Kusano K, Kinosaki M, et al: Human fibroblast growth factor-23 mutants suppress Na+-dependent phosphate Co-transport activity and 1alpha,25-dihydroxyvitamin D3 production. J Biol Chem 278:2206–2211, 2003.

651. Bowe AE, Finnegan R, Jan de Beur SM, et al: FGF-23 inhibits renal tubular phosphate transport and is a PHEX substrate. Biochem Biophys Res Commun 284:977–981, 2001.

652. Yamashita T, Konishi M, Miyake A, et al: Fibroblast growth factor (FGF)-23 inhibits renal phosphate reabsorption by activation of the mitogen-activated protein kinase pathway. J Biol Chem 277:28265–28270, 2002.

653. Larsson T, Marsell R, Schipani E, et al: Transgenic mice expressing fibroblast growth factor 23 under the control of the alpha1(I) collagen promoter exhibit growth retardation, osteomalacia, and disturbed phosphate homeostasis. Endocrinology 145:3087–3094, 2004.

654. Berndt TJ, Bielesz B, Craig TA, et al: Secreted frizzled-related protein-4 reduces sodium-phosphate co-transporter abundance and activity in proximal tubule cells. Pflugers Arch 451:579–587, 2006.

655. Neiberger RE, Barac-Nieto M, Spitzer A: Renal reabsorption of phosphate during development: Transport kinetics in BBMV. Am J Physiol 257:F268–274, 1989.

656. Taufiq S, Collins JF, Ghishan FK: Posttranscriptional mechanisms regulate ontogenic changes in rat renal sodium-phosphate transporter. Am J Physiol 272:R134–141, 1997.

657. Traebert M, Lotscher M, Aschwanden R, et al: Distribution of the sodium/phosphate transporter during postnatal ontogeny of the rat kidney. J Am Soc Nephrol 10:1407–1415, 1999.

658. Woda C, Mulroney SE, Halaihel N, et al: Renal tubular sites of increased phosphate transport and NaPi-2 expression in the juvenile rat. Am J Physiol Regul Integr Comp Physiol 280:R1524–1533, 2001.

659. Haramati A, Mulroney SE, Lumpkin MD: Regulation of renal phosphate reabsorption during development: Implications from a new model of growth hormone deficiency. Pediatr Nephrol 4:387–391, 1990.

660. Euzet S, Lelievre-Pegorier M, Merlet-Benichou C: Effect of 3,5,3′-triiodothyronine on maturation of rat renal phosphate transport: Kinetic characteristics and phosphate transporter messenger ribonucleic acid and protein abundance. Endocrinology 137:3522–3530, 1996.

661. Nijenhuis T, Hoenderop JG, van der Kemp AW, Bindels RJ: Localization and regulation of the epithelial Ca2+ channel TRPV6 in the kidney. J Am Soc Nephrol 14:2731–27340, 2003.

662. Bijvoet OL: Relation of plasma phosphate concentration to renal tubular reabsorption of phosphate. Clin Sci 37:23–36, 1969.

CHAPTER 6

Renal Handling of Organic Solutes

Orson W. Moe • Stephen H. Wright • Manuel Palacín

Archaic nephrons in lower life forms are largely secretory in nature. Kidneys in higher vertebrates handle solutes by the processes of filtration, reabsorption, and secretion. The handling of organic solutes involves all three of these means. The human kidney produces approximately 150 L to 170 L of low protein cell-free ultrafiltrate per day. The renal tubules processes this large volume of fluid to conserve the essential nutrients (glucose, amino acids, Krebs cycle intermediates, vitamins), to eliminate potentially toxic substances (organic acids and bases), and to reduce the quantity of salt and water excreted in the final urine. The handling of organic solutes spans a wide range from a clearance that exceeds glomerular filtration rate (GFR) in the form of filtration followed by secretion (fractional excretion > 1) to filtration followed by complete reabsorption (fractional excretion ~0), and everything in between (Fig. 6–1).

The kidney participates in homeostasis by adjusting the body content of specific solutes in the body as well as concentration of specific solutes in certain body fluid compartments; usually in the plasma. To achieve these regulatory functions, there must be sensing mechanisms for both the pool size and the concentration of the solute. Unlike inorganic solutes such as sodium or potassium, with organic solutes, the total pool is difficult to define as these solutes are constantly being synthesized and metabolized. For glucose, the maintenance of a discrete plasma concentration is clearly important. For amino acids and organic cation and anions, it is less clear whether plasma levels are as tightly regulated. The renal regulation of this latter group of organic solutes is more concerned with external balance and adjustment of urinary concentrations.

A filtration-reabsorption design is absolutely critical to maintain a high GFR, which is required for the complex metabolism and homeothermy of terrestrial mammals as tubular reabsorption salvages all the valuable solutes (e.g., sodium, bicarbonate, glucose) that would have otherwise been lost in the urine (see Fig. 6–1). In addition to allowance of high GFR, filtration-reabsorption commences by disposing everything and then selectively reclaims and retains substances the organism desires to keep in the appropriate amount. All that is not reclaimed is excreted. This mechanism economizes on genes and gene products required to identify and excrete the myriad of undesirable substances. In the filtration-secretion or secretion mode, the burden is on the kidney to recognize the substrates to be secreted. Therefore, in contrast to glucose transport (reabsorption), which is highly specific to certain hexose structures, organic anion and cation transport (secretion) can engage hundreds of structurally distinct substrates.

Unlike the handling of a lot of other solutes described in this textbook, the reabsorption and secretion of organic solutes are primarily performed by the proximal tubule with little or no contribution past the pars recta. This chapter summarizes the physiology, cell, and molecular biology of organic solute transport in the kidney, and highlights certain aspects of clinical relevance. Although only renal mechanisms will be covered in this chapter, it is important to note that homeostasis of organic solutes involves the concerted action of multiple organs.

GLUCOSE

Physiology of Renal Glucose Transport

Overview

Plasma glucose concentration is regulated at about 5 mM with balanced actions of glucose ingestion, glycogenolysis, and gluconeogenesis against glucose utilization and in some circumstances renal glucose excretion. Although transient increments and decrements of plasma glucose is tolerated in post-prandial and fasting states, neither hypoglycemia nor hyperglycemia is desirable for the organism. The robust metabolic rate of mammals mandates a high glomerular filtration rate (GFR) so the loss of glucose through the ultrafiltrate will be colossal if not reclaimed. Therefore the main physiologic task of the kidney is to retrieve as much glucose as possible so the normal urine is glucose-free. This was described by Cushny as early as 1917.[5]

Renal Glucose Handling

Plasma glucose is neither protein-bound nor complexed with macromolecules and is filtered freely at the glomerulus. Glucose reabsorption by the proximal tubule increases as the filtered load increases (Plasma [glucose] × GFR) until it reaches a threshold ($Tm_{Glucose}$) that represents the maximal reabsorptive capacity of the proximal tubule, then glycosuria ensues (Fig. 6–2). This concept was first inducted by the classic studies of Shannon and is still quite valid today.[6] With normal GFR, the value of plasma glucose for glycosuria to occur is about 11 mM or 200 mg/dl. One can predict that glycosuria will occur at lower plasma glucose concentrations in physiologic states of hyperfiltration such as pregnancy or a unilateral kidney (e.g., nephrectomy, transplant allograft, etc.). In these circumstances, glycosuria may not indicate significant hyperglycemia. Conversely, in patients with renal insufficiency, it will take a plasma glucose concentration of more than 11 mM

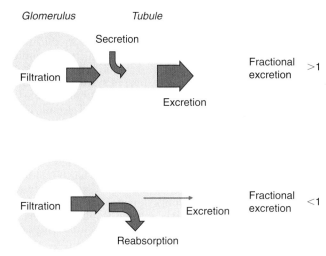

FIGURE 6–1 Secretory and reabsorptive modes of the mammalian nephron.

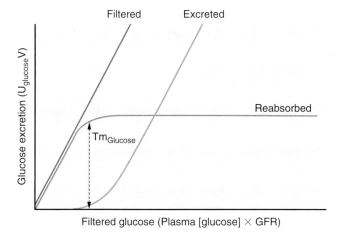

FIGURE 6–2 Urinary glucose excretion and tubular reabsorption as a function of filtered load. Tubular reabsorption increases linearly with filtered load as a part of glomerulotubular balance. When reabsorption reaches the tubular capacity (Tm$_{glucose}$), glucose starts appearing in the urine. The plasma glucose concentration for the given GFR is the glycosuric threshold.

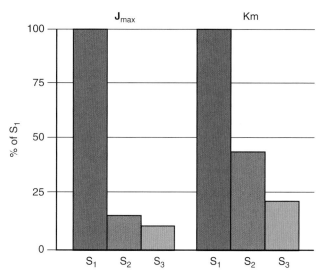

FIGURE 6–3 Relative magnitude of glucose transport characteristics in different segments of the proximal tubule. Jmax, maximal glucose transport rate; Km, affinity constant for glucose. (Data from Barfuss DW, Schafer JA: Differences in active and passive glucose transport along the proximal nephron. Am J Physiol 241:F322, 1981.)

TABLE 6–1	Renal Glucose Handing in Humans under Physiologic States
Excretion rate	2.7 µmoles/min (3.4 mmoles/day)
Urinary concentration	0.50 mM–0.65 mM
Reabsorptive capacity	1.85–2.17 mmoles/min
Tm$_{Glucose}$	(2664–3125 mmoles/day)

(200 mg/dl) for glycosuria to occur. The reduced filtered load for a given plasma glucose concentration is partially counterbalanced by lower Tm$_{Glucose}$ (see Fig. 6–2) but glycosuria still occurs at a higher plasma glucose concentration. Some of the whole organism values for renal glucose handling in humans are summarized in Table 6–1.[7]

Microperfusion data for rabbit proximal tubules indicate that the maximal rate of glucose transport slows as one progresses from S_1 to S_3 (Fig. 6–3).[1] However, the affinity for glucose rises, with a Michaelis constant (Km; concentration of substrate where half maximal rates of transport is attained) of approximately 2 mM in S_1 to 0.4 mM in S_3.[1] The net result of different Na$^+$-glucose carrier kinetics along the length of the proximal tubule is that S_1 can reabsorb glucose with higher capacity but the S_3 can decrease the tubule fluid glucose concentration to a much lower level. Theoretically, a single uniform segment cannot perform both high-capacity and high-gradient glucose absorption. Transport studies with brush border membrane vesicles and molecular cloning methods have now firmly established the existence of two Na$^+$-glucose transport systems with kinetic characteristics consistent with earlier microperfusion findings.

When Na$^+$ and glucose move as a net positive charge into the negatively charged cell interior, it partially depolarizes the cell interior. Consequently, when glucose is removed from the luminal solution, the PD becomes more negative (i.e., it hyperpolarizes).[8,9] Using microelectrodes from the basolateral membrane to measure cell hyperpolarization, Biagi and coworkers found that elimination of Na$^+$-glucose cotransport results in 14 mV of hyperpolarization in S_1 and early S_2 and about 4 mV in late S_2.[10] Na$^+$-glucose transport accounts for approximately 15% of the apical membrane current and for about half of the luminal negative PD in the early PCT.

Aronson and Sacktor first described Na$^+$-dependent glucose transport in renal brush border vesicles in 1974.[11,12] The two major Na$^+$-glucose transporters are distinguished by their glucose transport capacity; their affinities for glucose, Na$^+$, and phlorhizin; and their location within the kidney. In the outer cortex, where the S_1 and S_2 segments of the proximal tubule are located, there is predominantly a high-capacity, low-affinity glucose transport system.[13-15] The low-affinity system has a Km for glucose of approximately 6 mM. The transporter carries one Na$^+$ per glucose with a Km for Na$^+$ of 228 mM.[14] Phlorhizin binds and inhibits the transporter with a dissociation constant (Kd) of 1 mM to 2 mM.[14]

In the outer medulla, where S_3 is located, there is a high-affinity system with a Km for glucose of approximately 0.3 mM, carrying two Na$^+$ per glucose.[13,14,16] The coupling of two Na$^+$ to one glucose allows the cotransporter to utilize the square of the electrochemical driving force of Na$^+$ to energize glucose uptake. The S_3 transporter has a K$_{0.5}$ for Na$^+$ of approximately 50 mM. Although the S_3 transporter binds phlorhizin with a Kd of 1 mM to 2 mM, it inhibits glucose transport with a Kd of 50 mM. The S_3 transporter has an affinity for D-galactose that is more than 10-fold higher than that of the S1 transporter.[13]

Molecular Biology of Renal Glucose Transport Proteins

Cell Model of Proximal Tubule Glucose Transport

Glucose reabsorption in the proximal tubule cell occurs in two steps: (1) carrier-mediated, Na^+-glucose cotransport across the apical membrane, followed by (2) facilitated glucose transport and active Na^+ extrusion across the basolateral membrane (see Fig. 6–2). Electroneutrality is maintained by either paracellular Cl^- diffusion or Na^+ back-diffusion, depending on the relative permeabilities of the intercellular tight junction to Na^+ and Cl^- (Fig. 6–4). Two specific Na^+-coupled carriers (sodium glucose cotransporter SGLT-1 and SGLT-2) have been identified in the proximal tubule cell apical membrane that bind Na^+ and glucose in the tubule fluid. A third gene SGLT-3 has been cloned from a porcine kidney cell line and is transcribed in kidney.[17] SGLT3 has been studied in heterologously expressed system but its localization and functional role in the kidney is undetermined so the current paradigm still contains only SGLT-1 and -2 (see Fig. 6–4). The translocation of the Na^+ and glucose across the apical cell membrane is driven by the electrochemical driving force for Na^+ from tubule fluid to cell and is therefore termed "secondary active transport." Exit of glucose across the basolateral membrane does not consume energy but is mediated by specific carriers belonging to the GLUT gene family (see Fig. 6–4). SGLT-1 and -2 belongs to a broader group of solute carriers called SLC5, which currently encompasses 11 members in the human genome of which 6 are Na^+-glucose cotransporters.[18]

Transporter Proteins
Apical Entry

Molecular studies have confirmed with striking fidelity the physiologic data on glucose transport obtained in perfused tubules and membrane vesicles. It has been known since the 1960s that patients with the rare congenital disorder of glucose-galactose malabsorption have a partial defect in renal absorption of glucose,[19–24] but patients with renal glycosuria have normal intestinal glucose transport.[20] This finding led to the conjecture that one of the two renal glucose transporters may also be found in the intestine. Hediger and co-workers cloned the intestinal Na^+-glucose transporter and found expression in both intestine and kidney.[23,24] Within the kidney, it was later shown to be expressed almost exclusively in the S_3 segment of the proximal tubule.[25] Sequence comparison showed similarity to the proline transporter of *Escherichia coli,* the Na^+-dependent neutral amino acid transporter, and the Na^+-dependent *myo*-inositol transporter. This transporter, termed SGLT-1, has a Km for glucose of 0.4 mM, is inhibited by 5 mM to 10 mM of phlorhizin, and binds two Na^+ with a Km for Na^+ of 32 mM (Table 6–2).[24] The high affinity allows SGLT-1 to reclaim even low concentrations glucose from the urinary lumen. The 2Na^+: 1 glucose stoichiometry squares the electrochemical driving force of the lumen-to-cell Na^+ gradient. These properties are virtually identical to those of the S_3 glucose transport system determined from earlier microperfusion studies and transport studies in membrane vesicles.

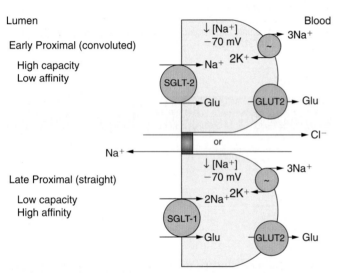

FIGURE 6–4 Model of proximal tubule glucose absorption. The Na^+-K^+-ATPase lowers cell [Na^+] and generates a negative interior voltage. This drives the uphill Na^+-coupled glucose entry from the apical membrane via the SGLT transporters 1 and 2. Glucose leaves the basolateral membrane via the facilitative glucose transporters GLUT1 and GLUT down its electrochemical gradient.

TABLE 6–2	Na⁺-coupled Glucose Transporter Family		
	SGLT1	**SGLT2**	**SGLT3**
Gene name	*SLC5A1*	*SLC5A2*	*SLC5A4*
Human chromosome	22p13.1	16p11.2	22p12.1
OMIM	182380	233100	—
Genetic disease	Intestinal glucose galactose malabsorption	Familial renal glycosuria	—
Amino acids	664	672	659
Tissue distribution	Kidney, intestine	Kidney	Kidney, intestine, liver spleen
Renal expression	Proximal straight tubule	Proximal convoluted tubule	Unknown
Affinity glucose ($K_{0.5}$, mM)	0.4	2	6
Hexose selectivity	Gluc = Gal	Gluc >> Gal	Gluc >> Gal
Affinity sodium ($K_{0.5}$, mM)	32	100	1.5
Substrate stoichiometry	2Na^+: glucose	Na^+: glucose	2Na^+: glucose

Gluc, Glucose; Gal, Galactose.

Hediger and colleagues cloned a second glucose transporter termed SGLT-2.[26,27] This clone exhibits 59% homology to SGLT-1 and is expressed in kidney, but not intestine.[28] SGLT-2 confers phlorhizin-sensitive (1 mM to 5 mM) glucose transport with a Km for glucose of approximately 1.6 mM. One Na^+ is bound per glucose with a Km for Na^+ of 200 mM to 300 mM (see Table 6–2). *In situ* hybridization localized SGLT-2 to the cortex in S1 proximal tubule segments. SGLT-2 is most likely the previously described "low-affinity" glucose transporter.

SGLT-1 and SGLT-2 are responsible for bringing glucose into the proximal tubule cell via secondary active transport, but clearly a different system is needed to return this glucose from the cell to the blood. The transporter was found to be inhibited by phloretin and cytochalasin B, but not phlorhizin.[29,30] Although stereospecific for D-glucose, it also transports 2-deoxy-D-glucose and 3-O-methyl-D-glucose, but not α-methyl-D-glucoside.[31] These characteristics are similar to those of proteins found in polarized intestinal and liver cells and to those of the insulin-sensitive D-glucose transporters in red blood cells, muscle cells, and adipocytes.[32] Another cDNA from the SGLT family was cloned from a pig kidney cell line and then subsequently human now termed SGLT-3.[33-35] SGLT-3 resembles SGLT-2 in terms of its low affinity for glucose and high specificity for glucose over other hexose substrates, but it functions more like SGLT-1 in terms of its tissue distribution and 2:1 Na^+: glucose stoichiometry (see Table 6–2).[36-38] The SGLT-3 transcript is present in the kidney but in low levels[39]; nephron segmental distribution is not yet available. At present, SGLT-3 has been characterized in expression systems but its role in the kidney is unclear.

Basolateral Exit

The relationships between glucose transport in the proximal tubule basolateral membrane and glucose transport in other tissues has been clarified with the discovery of a large gene family termed the GLUT genes. There are now 17 known members of the GLUT gene family (Table 6–3).[40] One classi-

fication based on sequence dendrograms has been proposed (see Table 6–3). A thorough discussion is beyond the scope of this book. Several excellent reviews are available.[40-42] At present, the two isoforms that are believed to be important for transepithelial glucose transport are GLUT1 and GLUT2 (see Fig. 6–4). The first member of the GLUT family to be discovered was GLUT-1, cloned via an antibody to the red blood cell glucose transporter. The carrier has a high affinity for glucose (1 mM to 2 mM) and is found at variable levels in virtually all nephron segments.[43,44] Its expression may correlate with nutritive requirements of the cell,[45] and it is probably also the mechanism for glucose exit in S_3.[46] GLUT-2 is a high-capacity, low-affinity (15 mM to 20 mM) basolateral transporter found in tissues with large glucose fluxes, such as intestine, liver, and pancreas, and the S_1 segment of the PCT.[47,48] GLUT-4 is the insulin-responsive glucose transporter found almost exclusively in fat and muscle.[49,50] This transporter has also been found in glomeruli and renal microvessels.[51] The regulation of this and other glucose transporters in diabetes is discussed elsewhere.[40,52] The role of GLUT-2 in renal glucose transport has been demonstrated by the presence of renal glycosuria in mice with GLUT-2 deletion[53] as well as in humans with GLUT-2 mutations who present interestingly with Fanconi syndrome, which is glycosuria with generalized proximal tubule dysfunction.[54,55] Transcripts of some of the other GLUT transporters have been detected in the kidney but their roles are unclear.

Renal Glucose Transport in Diseases States

Monogenic Defects of Glucose Transport
SGLT-1
The best characterized monogenic disease in the SGLT family is glucose-galactose malabsorption due to inactivating mutation of SGLT1 gene (OMIM 182380).[56-60] This rare autosomal recessive disease presents in infancy with an intestinal

TABLE 6–3	Facilitative Sugar Transporters		
Protein	**Gene**	**Glut Class**	**Renal Expression**
GLUT1	SLC2A1	I	All nephron segments Proximal tubule basolateral membrane S_2
GLUT2	SLC2A2	I	Proximal tubule basolateral membrane S_1
GLUT3	SLC2A3	I	Absent
GLUT4	SLC2A4	I	mRNA *in situ* in thick ascending limb
GLUT5	SLC2A5	II	mRNA *in situ* in proximal straight tubule
GLUT6	SLC2A6	III	Absent
GLUT7	SLC2A7	II	Unknown
GLUT8	SLC2A8	III	Absent
GLUT9	SLC2A9	II	mRNA present
GLUT10	SLC2A10	III	mRNA present
GLUT11	SLC2A11	II	Absent
GLUT12	SLC2A12	III	Unknown
HMIT	SLC2A13	III	Unknown
No gene product	SLC2A3P1	—	
No gene product	SLC2A3P2	—	
No gene product	SLC2A3P3	—	
No gene product	SLC2AXP1	—	

phenotype. The osmotic diarrhea resolves upon cessation of dietary glucose, galactose, and lactose; substrates of SGLT-1. The diarrhea returns when rechallenged with one of more these substrates. The diagnosis of the disease can be readily confirmed by oral administration of glucose or galactose (2 g/ kg) followed by lactic acid determination in breath. Patients with inactivating mutations of SGLT-1 exhibit some degree of renal glycosuria.[19,22,61] In general the severity is very mild and reduction of tubular maximal absorptive capacity was not always demonstrable.[62] This is in keeping though with the low capacity late proximal tubule SGLT-1 transport system.

Renal Glycosuria

There is considerable controversy as to the inheritance pattern (autosomal dominant versus recessive), clinical classification of the reabsorptive defect (glucose threshold versus maximal absorptive capacity, versus both), and associated overlapping defects with aminoaciduria in this syndrome.[63,64] Due to the lack of intestinal defect and the renal-restricted distribution of SGLT-2, the SGLT-2 gene has been repeatedly proposed as the candidate for renal glycosuria. To date, the strongest evidence that SGLT2 is the major transporter involved in the reabsorption of glucose from the glomerular filtrate comes from the analysis of one patient with autosomal recessive renal glycosuria with a homozygous nonsense mutation in exon 11 of SGLT2, and a heterozygous mutation at the same position in both parents and a younger brother.[65] In contrast, the linkage of the autosomal dominant form of renal glycosuria to the HLA complex on chromosome 6 are not supportive of the SGLT transporters being causative.[66] Based on circumstantial evidence, an autoimmune mechanism has been proposed for this disease.[67] It is possible that this entity represents a heterogeneous group of disorders.

Diseases of GLUTs

The first patient with Fanconi–Bickel syndrome[68] had hepatorenal glycogenosis and renal Fanconi syndrome.[69] This child presented at age 6 months with failure to thrive, polydipsia, and constipation followed later in childhood by osteopenia, short stature, hepatomegaly, and a proximal tubulopathy consisting of glycosuria, phosphaturia, aminoaciduria, proteinuria, and hyperuricemia. The liver was infiltrated with glycogen and fat. Disturbance of glucose homeostasis includes fasting hypoglycemia and ketosis and postprandially hyperglycemia. A mutation in the GLUT2 gene was demonstrated by Santer and co-workers.[70] Most patients with the Fanconi–Bickel syndrome are homozygous for the disease-related mutations consistent with an autosomal recessive pattern of inheritance. Some patients have been shown to be compound heterozygotes.[71] The mechanism by which GLUT2 mutation cause the proximal tubulopathy is unclear. It is conceivable that impaired basolateral exit of glucose in the proximal convoluted tubule can lead to glucose accumulation and glycotoxicity. GLUT2 gene deletion in rodents leads to glucose-insensitive islet cells but proximal tubulopathy was not described.[72] GLUT1 mutations presents with primarily a neurologic syndrome with no documented renal involvement.[68,73,74]

Pharmacologic Manipulation of SGLT

Antidiabetic therapy traditionally targets several broad levels: gut glucose absorption, insulin release, and insulin sensitivity. One additional strategy is providing a glucose sink to alleviate hyperglycemia and the ravages of glycotoxicity without actual direct manipulation of insulin secretion or sensitivity. If one decreases the capacity of proximal absorption, the same filtered load will lead to higher glycosuria resulting in lower plasma glucose concentration (Fig. 6–5). In addition to providing a glucose sink, the proximal osmotic diuresis can potentially act via tubuloglomerular feedback and reduce GFR, especially in the setting of diabetic hyper-

filtration. One advantage of this approach is the self-limiting effect. Increased filtered load from hyperglycemia in the presence of reduced proximal reabsorption increases glycosuria (see Fig. 6–5). Once hyperglycemia is corrected and filtered load is reduced, the renal glucose leak ceases even if the drug is still on board (see Fig. 6–5). This approach is receiving increasing attention[75] with new technical advances in high through-put screening.[76] A variety compounds with widely divergent structures has been shown to inhibit SGLT function.[77–83] Glycemic control with these agents has been shown in animal models.[84–86] The long-term consequence of escalated glycosylation of epithelial proteins exposed to the urinary lumen has not been examined. Because hyperglycemia fluctuates, so does osmotic diuresis. The staccato natriuresis may present a challenge in control of extracellular fluid volume.

■ ORGANIC CATIONS

Physiology of Renal Organic Cation Transport

Overview

The kidney is capable of clearing the plasma of a vast array of compounds that share little in common other than possessing a net positive charge at physiological pH. These "organic cations" (OCs) include a structurally diverse array of primary, secondary, tertiary, or quaternary amines, although compounds that have non-nitrogen cationic moieties (e.g., phosphoniums[87]) can also interact effectively with what is frequently referred to as the "classical organic cation secretory pathway".[88] Studies employing the techniques of stop flow, micropuncture, and microperfusion identified the renal proximal tubule (RPT) as the principal site of renal OC secretion.[89–91] Although a number of endogenous OCs are actively secreted by the proximal tubule (e.g., N^1-methylnicotinamide (NMN), choline, epinephrine, and dopamine; see Ref 90), an equally, if not more important function of this process is clearing the body of xenobiotic compounds,[18,89] including a wide range of alkaloids and other positively charged, heterocyclic dietary constituents; cationic drugs of therapeutic or recreational use; or other cationic toxins of environmental origin (e.g., nicotine). Importantly, the secretory process is also a site of clinically significant interactions between OCs in humans. For example, therapeutic doses of cimetidine retard the renal elimination of procainamide[2,92] and nicotine.[93]

The Cellular Basis of Renal Organic Cation Secretion

Renal OC secretion involves the concerted activity of a suite of distinct transport processes arranged in series (i.e., in the basolateral [peritubular] and apical [luminal] poles of RPT cells); or in parallel (i.e., within the same pole of RPT cells). In developing a model for the functional basis of this complexity, it is useful to consider the "Type I" and "Type II" classifications for different structural classes of organic cations developed to describe OC secretion in the liver.[94] In general, Type I OCs are comparatively small (generally <400 Da) monovalent compounds, such as tetraethylammonium (TEA), tributylmethylammonium, and procainamide ethobromide. Importantly, the majority of cationic drugs from a wide array of clinical classes, including antihistamines, skeletal muscle relaxants, antiarrhythmics, and β-adrenoceptor blocking agents, are adequately described as being Type I OCs. Type II OCs are usually bulkier (generally >500 Da) and frequently polyvalent, including d-tubocurarine, vecuronium, and hexafluorenium. Although the kidney plays a quantitatively significant role in the secretion of selected Type II OCs, the liver plays the predominant role in

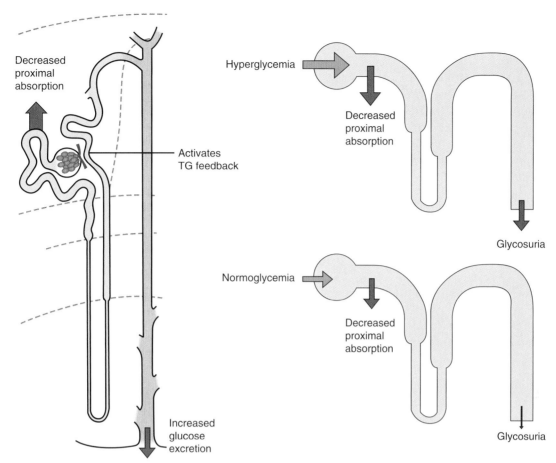

FIGURE 6–5 Effect of SGLT inhibition. Inhibition of proximal absorption leads to increased glucose excretion. Proximal osmotic diuresis activates tubuloglomerular (TG) feedback and reduces hyperfiltration. Right panel shows self-adjusting features of the renal glucose sink. As plasma glucose level falls, so does filtered load and glycosuria ceases even proximal absorption is still inhibited.

excretion (into the bile) of large hydrophobic cations (e.g., see Ref 95). In contrast, renal excretion is a predominant avenue for clearance of Type I OCs. Thus, although the processes associated with the renal handling of Type II OCs will be briefly described as currently understood, the renal transport of Type I OCs of substrates will be the central focus of this discussion. The reader is directed to recent reviews that consider the molecular biology and physiology of MDR1 (P-gp) in more depth.[96–98]

Basolateral Organic Cation Entry

Figure 6–6 shows a model for transcellular OC transport by RPT that is consistent with studies employing isolated renal plasma membranes and intact proximal tubules[89,99] and supported by recent molecular data. The first step in transcellular OC secretion involves OC entry into RPT cells from the blood across the peritubular membrane. For Type I OCs this entry step involves either an electrogenic uniport (facilitated diffusion), driven by the inside-negative electrical potential difference (PD),[100] or an electroneutral antiport (exchange) of OCs[100,101] (it is likely that these two mechanisms represent alternative modes of action of the same transporter(s)[102]. The PD across the basolateral membrane of RPT cells is in the order of 50 mV to 60 mV (inside negative[103,104]), which is sufficient to account for an accumulation of OCs within proximal cells to levels approximately 10 times that in the blood. A hallmark of peritubular OC uptake is its broad selectivity, frequently termed "multispecificity".[105] Studies by Ullrich and colleagues on the structural specificity of peritubular OC transport in microperfused rat proximal tubules in vivo indi-

cated a clear correlation between an increase in substrate hydrophobicity and an increase in interaction with basolateral OC transporters,[105,106] although it is also clear that steric factors influence this interaction.[107–109]

The molecular identity of the transport processes responsible for basolateral entry of Type I OCs is relatively clear. OCT1 (organic cation transporter 1; SLC22A1), OCT2 (SLC22A2), and OCT3 (SLC22A3) are electrogenic uniporters that are expressed in the basolateral membrane of renal proximal tubule cells (although their individual levels of expression display marked species differences). Significantly, elimination of OCT1 and OCT2 activity (in OCT1/OCT2 null mice) completely eliminates active secretion of TEA.[3] The molecular biology of each of these processes is discussed in more detail in an upcoming section.

The process(es) responsible for basolateral entry of Type II OCs into RPT cells is(are) not clear. The bulky ring structures that characterize Type II OCs generally render them substantially more hydrophobic than Type I OCs and, in the liver, generally makes Type II OCs (e.g., rocuronium) substrates for one or more homologues of the organic anion transporting polypeptide (OATPs) family of transporters.[110] However, (in the rat) renal OATP expression is typically low, compared to the liver (the sole exception being Oatp5, the function and location of which in rat kidney is unknown, and for which no human ortholog has been identified[111]). It is likely that the marked hydrophobicity of most Type II OCs results in a substantial diffusive flux across the peritubular membrane that provides Type II OCs with a passive, electrically conductive avenue for entry into proximal cells.

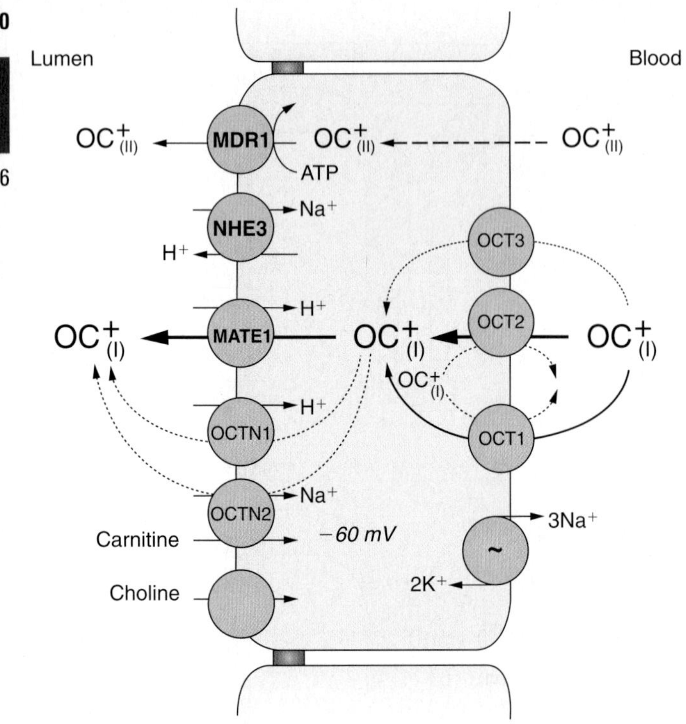

220

CH 6

Lumen   Blood

FIGURE 6–6 Schematic model of the transport processes associated with the secretion of organic cations (OCs) by renal proximal tubule cells. Circles depict carrier mediated transport processes. Arrows indicate the direction of net substrate transport. Solid lines depict the principal pathways of OC transport; dotted lines indicate pathways that are believed to be of secondary importance; dashed line indicates diffusive movement. Na$^+$-K$^+$-ATPase; maintains the K$^+$ gradient associated with the inside negative membrane potential and the inwardly directed Na$^+$ gradient, both of which represent driving forces associated with active OC secretion. OCT1, OCT2, and OCT3; support electrogenic facilitated diffusion associated with basolateral uptake of Type I OCs (these processes are also believed to support electroneutral OC/OC exchange, as indicated by the outwardly directed arrows). MDR1; supports the ATP dependent, active luminal export of Type II OCs. NHE3; the Na$^+$/H$^+$ exchanger that plays a principal role in sustaining the inwardly directed hydrogen electrochemical gradient that, in turn, supports activity of transport processes mediated by physiologically characterized Type I OC/H$^+$ exchanger, which includes MATE1 (the broadly specific process that accepts TEA as a prototypic substrate) and the narrowly specific process that accepts guanidine as a substrate, and OCTN1; supports electroneutral OC/H$^+$ exchange but with selectivity properties that make it distinct from process 7. OCTN2 supports Na$^+$-carnitine cotransport and the electrogenic flux of TEA and selected Type I substrates, as well as mediated exchange of TEA for Na$^+$-carnitine. Finally, there is a physiologically characterized electrogenic choline reabsorption pathway.

Apical Organic Cation Exit

Exit of Type I OCs across the luminal membrane involves carrier-mediated antiport of OC for H$^+$ (see Fig. 6–6), a process observed in brush border membrane vesicles (BBMV) isolated from human, rabbit, rat, dog, chicken, and snake kidneys.[89] Luminal OC efflux is the rate-limiting step in trans-tubular OC secretion.[112] It is unlikely that net OC secretion requires a transluminal H$^+$-gradient. Indeed, in the early proximal tubule, where the pH of the tubular filtrate is on the order of 7.4 (i.e., the same as plasma), tubular secretion exceeds that of later segments[112] even though it is in these latter regions where an inwardly directed H$^+$ gradient is most likely to develop.[113] Instead, it is the electrically silent nature of the exchanger (which involves the obligatory 1:1 exchange of monovalent cations[114]) that, even in the absence of an inwardly directed H$^+$ gradient, will permit OCs to exit the electrically negative cytoplasm of RPT cells and develop a luminal concentration as large as (or larger than, if there is an inwardly

directed H$^+$ gradient) that in the cytoplasm. Net transepithelial secretion, therefore, is a consequence of combining luminal OC/H$^+$ exchange with the electrically driven flux of OCs across the basolateral membrane. From an energetic perspective, OC/H$^+$ antiport is the active step in the earlier outlined scenario because it depends on the displacement of H$^+$ away from electrochemical equilibrium, a state maintained through the activity in the luminal membrane of the Na$^+$/H$^+$ exchanger[115,116] and, to a lesser extent, a V-type H-ATPase (not shown in figure).[117] The basolateral Na,K-ATPase, ultimately, drives OC secretion by (1) maintaining the inside negative membrane potential that supports concentrative uptake of OCs across the basolateral membrane (the result of the developed K$^+$ gradient); and (2) sustaining the inwardly directed Na gradient that drives the aforementioned luminal Na$^+$/H$^+$ exchange. Evidence on the structural specificity of luminal OC transport indicates that, as with the peritubular transport process, binding of substrate to the OC/H$^+$ exchanger is profoundly influenced by substrate hydrophobicity and, to a lesser extent, the 3D structure of the substrate.[118] At least two distinct OC/H$^+$ exchangers, distinguished by their substrate selectivities, have been described in renal cortical BBMV. One, which is regarded as being the principal avenue for luminal OC secretion, displays a very broad selectivity and accepts TEA as a substrate.[118] The second displays mechanistically similar characteristics to this former process, but displays a narrower selectivity and accepts guanidine as a substrate.[119]

Two members of the SLC22A family are suspected to play a role in mediating apical efflux of (at least) selected OC substrates. OCTN1 (organic cation transporter-novel 1; SLC22A4) supports mediated exchange of TEA and H$^+$ and, consequently, it has been suggested to contribute to luminal OC/H$^+$ exchange activity.[120] However, the kinetics, selectivity, and tissue distribution of OCTN1 do not fit the physiological profile of the OC/H$^+$ exchanger of renal BBMV,[18] making it unlikely that OCTN1 is a major contributor to renal secretion of Type I OCs. OCTN2 (SLC22A5) is unique in displaying both Na$^+$ coupled transport of carnitine (and structurally related zwitterions[121]) and the electrogenic uniport of TEA and selected Type I OCs.[122] The potential significance of OCTN2 in mediating apical OC export is evident in the observation that a genetic defect in Octn2 in the jvs mouse is associated with a marked decrease in renal clearance of TEA.[3]

The recent cloning from human and mouse kidney of a member of the MOP (Multidrug/Oligosaccharidyl-lipid/Polysaccharide) superfamily of multidrug/H$^+$ exchangers[123] offers the promise of identifying the principal elements in luminal OC/H$^+$ exchange. The multidrug and toxicant extruder, MATE1, supports TEA/H$^+$ exchange and in the human is expressed in the apical membrane of renal proximal tubules and in the canalicular membrane of hepatic cells[123] (i.e., locations known to contains OC/H$^+$ exchange activity). Moreover, the kinetics and selectivity of the process[123,124] are consistent with those of OC/H$^+$ exchange characterized in isolated renal BBMV, further supporting the contention that MATE1 may comprise a quantitatively significant element in luminal OC secretion.

The apical export of Type II OCs is likely to involve the multidrug resistance transporter, MDR1 (ABCB1), which is expressed in the apical membrane of RPT cells and has been implicated in the apical efflux of Type II OCs (and other bulky hydrophobic substrates) in in vitro studies.[125-127] However, whereas the influence of MDR1 in biliary excretion of Type II OCs is evident (e.g., in studies employing Mdr1 knockout mice)[128]; the quantitative influence of MDR1 on renal secretion is less clear. For example, whereas biliary excretion of doxorubicin is markedly decreased in Mdr1 knockout mice, urinary clearance increases.[129] Similarly, elimination of Mdr1 activity in knockout mice is associated with marked changes in the distribution of Type II OCs across brain, intestinal, and hepatic barriers, whereas the renal phenotype in these animals is modest.[128]

Axial Distribution of Organic Cation Transport in the Renal Proximal Tubule

Renal secretion of TEA and procainamide by isolated perfused rabbit RPT shows a marked axial heterogeneity that differs from that of secretion of PAH[130,131] with a profile of TEA secretion of S1 > S2 > S3,[112] and a profile of procainamide secretion of $S_1 = S_2 > S_3$.[132] This axial distribution of secretory function is correlated (in rat and rabbit) with a marked difference in the distribution of distinct basolateral transporters, with OCT1 expression dominating in the early proximal tubule and OCT2 expression dominating in the mid and later portions of the proximal tubule.[133,134] Despite these differences, the kinetics of basolateral TEA uptake, as determined in isolated, non-perfused tubules, is effectively the same in all three segments,[133] suggesting that the apical exit step for OCs is both rate limiting and the source of the axial heterogeneity observed for TEA secretion.[112] Consistent with this conclusion is the observation that the maximal rate of TEA/H^+ exchange is significantly higher in rabbit renal BBMV isolated from outer cortex (enriched in membranes from S1/S2 segments) than from outer medulla (enriched in S_3 segments[135]).

We can summarize the current, overall understanding of the cellular processes associated with secretion of organic cations as follows: Type I OCs enter RPT cells across the peritubular membrane via electrogenic facilitated diffusion (mediated by one or more OCT transporters) and leave cells across the luminal membrane via electroneutral exchange for H^+ (possibly by means of one or more MATE and/or OCTN transporters). Type II OCs diffuse into proximal cells across the peritubular membrane and are exported into the tubule filtrate via the primary active MDR1 transporter. Importantly, considerable overlap appears to exist in the selectivity of these parallel transport pathways.[110,136]

Organic Cation Reabsorption

Whereas secretion dominates the net flux of OCs transported by the proximal tubule, net reabsorption has been reported for a few cationic substrates, most notably choline.[89,90,137,138] The apical membrane of renal proximal tubule cells expresses an electrogenic uniporter that accepts choline and structurally similar compounds with relatively high affinity.[139,140] In contrast, the apical OC/H^+ exchanger has a low affinity (but high capacity) for choline.[139] Consequently, choline is effectively reabsorbed when plasma concentration do not exceed the comparatively low, physiological concentrations (10 μM to 20 μM), and is secreted when concentrations are raised to levels >100 μM.[138]

Substrate Interactions and Renal Clearance of Organic Cations

The renal OC secretory process has sufficient transport capacity to extract >90% of many OCs, when present in low (clinically relevant) concentrations, during a single passage of blood through the kidney.[141] The presence of multiple OCs in the blood can result in competition between these compounds for one or more common elements in the OC secretory pathway, leading to decreased rates of elimination of one or more of these compounds with resultant elevation(s) in their blood levels (see Fig. 6–6). This has been shown to occur when the antiarrhythmic, procainamide, is administered with either cimetidine or ranitidine (Fig. 6–7).[2,92,142,143] The clinical impact of such interactions will depend on the therapeutic index of the drugs in question.

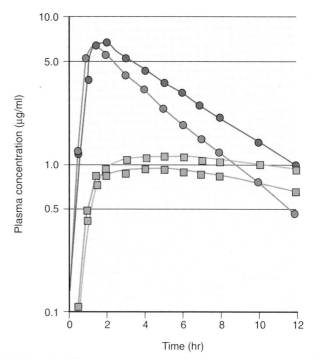

FIGURE 6–7 Effect of drug-drug competition at the level of renal organic cation secretion on mean plasma concentration-time profiles of procainamide (–■–) and n—acetylprocainamide (–●–) in six subjects with (–●–) or without (–■–) co-administration of cimetidine. (From Somogyi A, McLean A, Heinzow B: Cimetidine-procainamide pharmacokinetic interaction in man: Evidence of competition for tubular secretion of basic drugs. Eur J Clin Pharmacol 25:339, 1983.)

Molecular Biology of Renal Organic Cation Transport

The cloning in 1994 of OCT1[144] by Gründemann and Koepsell resulted in a rapid increase in understanding of the molecular and cellular basis of renal OC transport. As outlined earlier, strong evidence supports the conclusion that basolateral entry of Type I OCs into RPT cells occurs by a (species specific) combination of the activities of OCT1, OCT2, and OCT3; and that apical exit of Type I OCs includes a combination of the activities of MATE1, MATE2, OCTN1, and OCTN2. The OCTs and OCTNs are all found within the SLC22A family of solute carriers and share a common set of structural features that place them within the Major Facilitator Superfamily (MFS) of transport proteins,[145] whereas the MATEs are members of the Multidrug/Oligosaccharidyl-lipid/Polysaccharide (MOP) superfamily.[146] Renal secretion of Type II OCs involves MDR1 in the luminal membranes of proximal tubular cells, although the role its activity plays in clearance of these compounds from the body is currently the subject of speculation. Following is a discussion of the molecular characteristics of the earlier listed transport proteins.

Basolateral Organic Cation Transporters
Organic Cation Transporters

Basolateral OC transport is dominated by the combined activity of three members of the SLC22A family of transport proteins, OCT1 (SLC22A1), OCT2 (SLC22A2), and OCT3 (SLC22A3).[18] As MFS transporters, they share several structural characteristics including 12 transmembrane spanning helices (TMHs), cytoplasmic N- and C-termini, a long cytoplasmic loop between TMHs 6 and 7, and several conserved sequence motifs.[18,147] Several additional features are unique to the OCT members of SLC22A, including a long (~110 amino acid residues) extracellular loop between TMHs 1 and 2, as well as a distinguishing sequence motif.[148] The human orthologs of OCT1, OCT2, and OCT3 contain 554, 555, and 556 amino acid residues, respectively, and several consensus sites for PKC-, PKA-, PKG-, CKII-, and/or CaMII-mediated phosphorylation located within or near the long cytoplasmic loop between TMHs 6 and 7, or in the cytoplasmic C-terminal sequence.[147,149] The long extracellular loop between TMHs 1 and 2 contains three N-linked glycosylation sites in all three homologs. Elimination of these sites is associated with both decreased trafficking of protein to the membrane and with changes in apparent affinity for substrate,[150] the latter observation suggesting that the configuration of the long extracellular loop influences the position of TMHs 1 and 2, which are elements of the hydrophilic "binding cleft" common to the OCTs and in which substrate is suspected to bind ([4,151]; and discussed later).

The human genes for OCT1, OCT2, and OCT3 have 11 coding exons.[152] Several alternatively spliced variants of OCT1 have been described. rOCT1A lacks putative TMHs 1 and 2 and the large extracellular loop that separates those two TMHs, yet supports mediated transport of TEA.[153] In the human, four alternatively spliced isoforms of OCT1 are present in human glioma cells,[154] a long (full-length) form and three shorter forms. Only the long form (hOCT1G/L554) supports transport when expressed in HEK293 cells.[154] Human kidney expresses at least one splice variant of OCT2. Designated hOCT2-A, it is characterized by the insertion of a 1169 bp sequence arising from the intron found between exons 7 and 8 of hOCT2[155] resulting in a truncated protein that is missing the last three putative TMHs (i.e., 10, 11, 12). Despite the absence of the last three TMHs, hOCT2-A retains the capacity to transport TEA and cimetidine, though guanidine transport is lost.

In the rat and rabbit, OCT1 expression appears to dominate basolateral OC entry in the early (S_1 segment) of renal proximal tubule, whereas OCT2 expression appears to dominate the mid and late (S_2 and S_3) segments of RPT.[133,134] In the human kidney it is likely that basolateral OC transport is dominated by activity of OCT2. OCT2 is heavily expressed in the human kidney, and the relative expression profile of mRNAs coding for OCT1, OCT2, and OCT3 in human renal cortex is 1:100:10.[156] However, the observation that, in the rabbit, OCT1 activity dominates OC transport in the early proximal tubule, despite the fact that OCT2 mRNA expression is >10 times larger,[133] suggests that it would be premature to conclude that OCT1 (and OCT3) have no influence on renal clearance of selected compounds by human kidney.

The relative role of OCTs expressed in the proximal tubule may also be influenced by their site of expression. In the rodent, as in the rabbit, OCT expression in the early proximal tubule is dominated by OCT1, whereas OCT2 expression is restricted to the later portions of the RPT.[3,134] Jonker and colleagues[3] found that targeted elimination of OCT1 actually resulted in an increase in renal clearance of TEA (presumably reflecting the increase in plasma TEA levels that resulted from the elimination of OCT1-mediated hepatic clearance of TEA), and elimination of OCT2 had no effect on renal clearance of TEA (Fig. 6–8). In other words, the level of *functional* expression of each transporter was sufficient to maintain fractional clearance of TEA at control levels in the absence of the other. Importantly, the elimination of both OCT1 and OCT2 completely eliminated active clearance of TEA (see Fig. 6–3),[3] indicating that (in the mouse) OCT3 plays no significant role in renal clearance of TEA. Indeed, mice in which OCT3 has been eliminated display no apparent renal phenotype[157] (although OCT3 may still play a role in the renal elimination of substrates for which it displays a particularly high affinity[133]). Thus, under normal conditions, transporters restricted to later portions of the RPT may see little or no substrate if

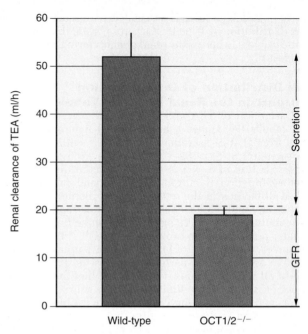

FIGURE 6–8 Renal clearance of TEA in wild-type and Oct1/2–/– mice. Renal clearance was calculated by dividing the amount of TEA excreted in the urine over 60 minutes by the plasma AUC(0–60). The estimated GFR was approximately 21 ml/h for both genotypes and is indicated with a dashed line. (From Jonker JW, Wagenaar E, Van Eijl S, et al: Deficiency in the organic cation transporters 1 and 2 (Oct1/Oct2 [Slc22a1/Slc22a2]) in mice abolishes renal secretion of organic cations. Mol Cell Biol 23:7902, 2003.)

that compound is effectively cleared by transporters located in "upstream" portions of the tubule. Transport capacity in later portions of the tubule may only come into play when the activity in the early RPT is saturated or inhibited, as may occur in the event of a drug-drug interaction.

All the OCTs share a common transport mechanism (i.e., electrogenic uniport). Transport is independent of extracellular Na^+ and H^+, with membrane potential providing the driving force for transport of cationic substrates.[102,158] The transport of positively charged substrates is electrogenic, as shown directly in studies characterizing the saturable inward currents that result from exposing *Xenopus* oocytes injected with the cRNA for OCT1,[102] OCT2,[158] or OCT3[159] to increasing concentrations of substrate. Koepsell and colleagues[102] showed that membrane potential provides the driving force for OCT1-mediated TEA, NMN, and choline uptake, and that OCT1 can also support the electrogenic efflux of substrate in the presence of energetically favorable outwardly directed substrate gradients, as well as electroneutral OC/OC exchange.

Although the three OCTs display marked overlap in substrate selectivity, they are also distinguished by their selectivities for specific compounds. For example, OCT1 and OCT2 generally have a similar affinity for TEA (20 μM–200 μM)[133] whereas OCT3 has a very low affinity for TEA (~2 mM[160]); Cimetidine has a much higher (50-fold) affinity for OCT2 than OCT1,[161] whereas tyramine has a higher affinity (20-fold) for OCT1 than OCT2[161]; and all three homologs display a similar, comparatively high affinity for MPP.[162] In general, the three homologs all support transport of a structurally diverse array of Type I OCs,[133] and interact with a limited number of neutral and even anionic substrates.[163] With respect to the latter observation that OCTs can interact with (selected) neutral or anionic substrates, Ullrich and colleagues observed "cross-over" interactions of a number of what they referred to as "bisubstrates" with both cation and anion transport pathways in rat kidney.[164,165] Nevertheless, despite the (generally weak) interaction of neutral and anionic substrates with OCTs, the presence of a charged moiety clearly enhances interaction with these transporters, as shown in studies demonstrating more efficient interaction of the weak base, cimetidine (pK_a = 6.9), with OCT2 when the substrate is protonated.[166] OCTs also typically interact with Type II OCs, though this interaction generally appears to be restricted to binding with modest or no translocation of substrate.[110]

It is likely that the kinetics of binding of the OCTs with many, if not most, substrates is asymmetric (i.e., differs when the interaction occurs at the extracellular versus cytoplasmic face of the membrane). Koepsell and colleagues,[167] using giant excised patches of *Xenopus* oocyte membrane, determined that the binding of corticosterone and tetrabutylammonium to the extracellular face of rat OCT2 is 20-fold lower versus 4-fold higher, respectively, than that measured for binding to the intracellular face of the transporter. This is not a surprising observation when considered in the light of information concerning the probable 3D structure of OCTs and the likelihood that binding regions will have (at least) modestly different 3D configurations when exposed to the inside versus the outside of cells. This issue is discussed in more detail in an upcoming section.

In addition to operating as electrogenic uniporters, the OCTs also support OC/OC exchange.[102,168-172] Preloading *Xenopus* oocytes with unlabeled TEA, for example, stimulates the uptake of [³H]MPP by human, rabbit, mouse, and rat OCT1.[168] The symmetry of this type of trans-effect is apparent in observations of accelerated efflux of preloaded [3H]MPP from rOCT1-expressing oocytes in the presence of inwardly-directed gradients of unlabeled TEA[102] or MPP.[169] Human OCT1 also supports trans-stimulation of both influx and efflux (of TEA), but quantitative differences in the extent of these stimulated fluxes produced by some substrates (e.g., tributylmethylammonium) support the suggestion, as dis-

cussed earlier, of asymmetrical binding properties on the extracellular versus intracellular face of the transporter.[170]

Organic Cation Transporter Structure

The elucidation of the crystal structure of two MFS transporters, LacY,[173] and GlpT,[174] and the discovery that these two proteins share a marked structural homology (i.e., a common helical fold) despite having a low sequence homology (<15%), paved the way for efforts to use homology modeling as a means to develop structural models for other MFS transporters.[175] LacY and GlpT have served as "templates" for the modeling of OCT1[151] and OCT2,[4] respectively, and the resulting models share a number of common structural features (owing, in part, to shared structural features of the templates), including a large hydrophilic "cleft" formed by the juxtaposition of the N- and C-terminal halves of the proteins that is comprised of the amino acid residues of the "pore forming" helices: TMHs 1, 2, 4, 5, 7, 8, 10, and 11 (Fig. 6–9). Significantly, amino acid residues that have been independently shown in site-directed studies to influence substrate binding are found, in both models, at locations consistent with roles in stabilizing substrate-transporter interactions. In particular, an aspartate residue in TMH 11 that is conserved in all OCT homologues (i.e., D475 in hOCT2) and that markedly influences substrate binding in rOCT1[176] and in rOCT2,[177] is directed toward the hydrophilic pore at a position within the protein that coincides closely to the binding site identified in both GlpT[174] and in LacY[173] (see Fig. 6–9). Similarly, residues within TMHs 4 and 10 that influence substrate binding are also directed toward the pore region of OCT1[151] and OCT2,[4] including three residues in TMH10 that play a key role in defining the selectivity differences that distinguish OCT1 and OCT2.[4,151,178] The comparatively large extent of the pore or cleft region of OCTs (20 Å × 60 Å × 80 Å[151]), is consistent with the suggestion that the broad substrate selectivity these proteins reflects binding

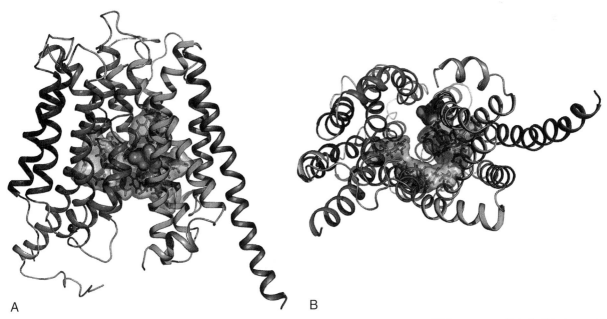

FIGURE 6–9 Model of the 3D structure of the rabbit ortholog of OCT2, based on structural homology with the MFS transporter, GlpT. **A,** Side view of OCT2, with the cytoplasmic face directed downward. The helices (TMHs 1–6) comprising the N-terminal half of the protein are colored blue; the helices comprising the C-terminal half of the protein are colored cyan. The lighter colored helices (1, 2, 4, 5, 7, 8, 10, and 11) border the hydrophilic cleft region formed by the juxtaposition of the N- and C-terminal halves of the protein. The amino acid residues that comprise the postulated substrate-binding region within the cleft are rendered as sticks with a pink colored van der Waals surface. D475 is rendered as a space-filling reside in orange. Note: residues from the long extracellular loop (between TMHs 1 and 2) and the cytoplasmic loop (between TMHs 6 and 7) were eliminated to facilitate homology modeling with the GlpT template. **B,** An end-on view of the cleft and postulated binding region from the cytoplasmic aspect of the protein. (From Zhang X, Shirahatti NV, Mahadevan D, et al: A conserved glutamate residue in transmembrane helix 10 influences substrate specificity of rabbit OCT2 (SLC22A2). J Biol Chem 280:34813, 2005.)

interactions over a large surface that contains several distinct sites or regions.[4,178]

The recent discovery of altered transport function of hOCT1 and hOCT2 that contain single nucleotide polymorphisms present in different ethnic populations[179–181] has underscored the importance of understanding structure-activity relationships for these processes. For example, 28 variable sites in the hOCT2 gene were discovered in a collection of 247 ethnically diverse DNA samples (White, African American, Asian American, Mexican American, and Pacific Islander). Eight of these polymorphisms caused non-synonymous amino acid changes, of which four were present in at least 1% of an ethnic population. These four displayed altered transporter function, including up to a threefold change in K_t values for MPP and TBA, changes that could result in differences in the pharmacokinetics of renal drug excretion between individuals expressing different variants of hOCT2. However, population-genetic analysis suggests that selection has acted against amino acid changes to hOCT2, which may reflect a necessary role of OCT2 in the renal elimination of endogenous amines or xenobiotics.[179]

Regulation of Organic Cation Transporter-Mediated Transport

Organic cation transporter activity responds to both short- and long-term regulation, although there appear to be significant species differences in the extent of such responses.[149] For example, when expressed heterologously, activation of protein kinase A acutely up-regulates rat OCT1-mediated transport,[182] but down-regulates human OCT1-mediated transport.[183] Of particular significance to the issue of short-term regulation of renal OC transport in humans is the observation that basolateral uptake of the fluorescent cation 4-[4-(dimethylamino)-styryl]-N-methylpyridinium into isolated single non-perfused proximal tubules from human kidney, is acutely down-regulated following activation of PKC,[184] and this presumably reflects acute regulation of OCT2 activity. In fact, hOCT2 (expressed heterologously) is acutely down-regulated following activation of PKA, PKC, Ca^{2+}/CaM, or PI3-kinase.[185] The decrease in transport associated with acute activation of these kinases appears to reflect a decrease in the maximal rate of transport (i.e., K_t is not affected[186]), consistent with the hypothesis that acute down-regulation of OCT2 activity reflects the rapid sequestration of transporters into a cytoplasmic vesicular compartment, a mechanism that has been shown to account for the acute down-regulation of the closely related OAT transporters.[187]

Sex steroids have been shown to regulate the long-term activity of OCT2. TEA uptake is greater in renal cortical slices of male rats than female rats, and this is correlated with a higher level of expression (mRNA and protein) of OCT2 in kidneys of male rats, with no sex-linked differences in either OCT1 or rOCT3.[188] Moreover, treatment of male and female rats with testosterone significantly increases OCT2 expression in the kidney,[189] via the androgen receptor mediated transcriptional pathway,[190] suggesting that testosterone plays a significant role in the transcriptional regulation of the OCT2 gene in rats. A similar profile is not, however, evident in all species. Although OCT2 mRNA expression is higher in kidneys from male rabbits than female rabbits, this difference does not extend to either protein expression or in rates of TEA transport in renal tubules isolated from male and female rabbit kidneys.[191] On the other hand, humans, like rats, exhibit a significant sex difference in the renal excretion of the OC substrate, amantadine (which is a substrate for OCT1, OCT2, and OCT3[192,193]). It is noteworthy that renal clearance involves transport across both basolateral and apical membranes. Thus, sex differences in renal clearance may involve apical transporters either in addition to or rather than basolateral transporters.

Apical Organic Cation Transporters

Although the physiological characteristics of apical OC transport have been studied extensively using isolated BBMV (see Refs 89, 133), the molecular identity of the processes that mediate the exit step in renal secretion of Type I OCs, particularly the identity of the "OC/H$^+$ exchanger," is still unclear. The OCTNs (i.e., OCTN1 and OCTN2) have been implicated and may well play a role in the mediating transport of at least some OCs. Perhaps more attractive, though still in a very early state of study, are the MATEs, which have a physiological profile consistent that of apical OC transport observed in isolated renal membranes and intact renal tubules.

OCTN

OCTN1 (SLC22A4) and OCTN2 (SLC22A5) are 551–557 amino acid peptides with ~30% to 33% sequence identity with hOCT1. As with other members of the OCT family, the OCTNs have 12 putative TMHs and, consistent with the OCTs, 3 N-linked glycosylation sites and a number of consensus sites for phosphorylation mediated by PKA, PKC, and CKII. OCTN1, although widely expressed in human tissues, is weakly expressed in the kidney.[156] OCTN2, in contrast, is most heavily expressed in kidney, heart, placenta, skeletal muscle and pancreas.[194]

OCTN1 supports electroneutral transport of TEA, and flux of TEA across Xenopus oocyte membrane is trans-stimulated by oppositely oriented H$^+$ gradients.[120] It is this latter observation that led to speculation that OCTN1 may play a role in the OC/H$^+$ exchange observed in isolated renal BBMV preparations. However, TEA/H$^+$ exchange has been noted in very few tissues, most notably in isolated membranes from kidney (apical BBMV[133]) and liver (canalicular BBMV[195]). OCTN1, however, is expressed in many tissues, including the placenta and intestine,[196] neither of which support TEA/H$^+$ exchange. The comparatively low level of expression of OCTN1 in human kidney[156] also appears to be inconsistent with the observation that OC/H$^+$ exchange is the dominant mechanism for OC flux across isolated human renal brush border membrane vesicles.[197] In addition, the kinetic/selectivity characteristics of OCTN1 are inconsistent with this process playing a major role in luminal OC transport. As noted earlier, a transporter with even modest levels of expression may play a quantitatively significant role in renal secretion of selected substrates, so OCTN1 could influence the secretion of some OCs. However, the paucity of data on the selectivity characteristics of OCTN1 makes it difficult to draw conclusions concerning its potential role in renal OC transport.

OCTN2 appears to be unique in that it supports both Na-dependent transport of the zwitterion, carnitine (and related compounds), and Na-independent, electrogenic facilitated diffusion of Type I OCs. Importantly, lesions in OCTN2 result in primary carnitine deficiency in humans[198,199] and mice,[200] and the Na-dependent interaction of OCTN2 with carnitine and its role in supporting the reabsorption of this important metabolite is discussed extensively elsewhere.[201,202] The Na-independent transport of TEA, MPP, and a wide range of other Type I OCs[122,194] occurs electrogenically,[122] and operating in this mode OCTN2 would be expected to support OC reabsorption, rather than secretion. Significantly, however, jvs mice, which express an inoperative OCTN2 (and display primary carnitine deficiency), show a 50% reduction in TEA clearance and a 2.5-fold increase in the kidney-plasma ratio of TEA,[203] both of which implicate OCTN2 in the apical efflux step of TEA secretion. A possible, and intriguing, explanation for these results may be found in the observation that outwardly directed TEA gradients trans-stimulate OCTN2-mediated carnitine-Na cotransport.[203] Thus, OCTN2-mediated reabsorption of carnitine could serve as a driving force to support electroneutral luminal efflux of TEA (and selected Type I OCs); under normal physiological conditions, the comparatively high concentrations of Na$^+$ and carnitine in the plasma (and filtrate) should maximize the operation of OCTN2 as a reabsorptive pathway for carnitine, rather than as an electrogenic pathway for Type I OC reabsorption, and in the presence of elevated cytoplasmic levels of a suitable Type I substrate (e.g., TEA), OCTN2 would mediate the secretory efflux of that molecule (e.g., Na-carnitine/TEA exchange) (see Fig. 6–6).

MATE

Two members of the MOP family of transport proteins, MATE1 and MATE2, were recently cloned in the human and mouse.[123,124] A splice variant of MATE2 (MATE2-K) was also identified in human kidney.[204] The human ortholog of MATE1 is a 570 aa protein with 12 putative TMHs, no N-linked glycosylation sites (in extracellular loops), and 3 consensus PKG phosphorylation sites (and no PKC, PKA, CKII, or CaMII sites). In the human, MATE1 is expressed in the kidney and liver (and, less so, in the heart), where it is found in the apical and canalicular membranes, respectively, of renal proximal tubules and hepatocytes.[123] Importantly, MATE1-mediated transport of TEA is electroneutral, pH sensitive, and markedly *trans*-stimulated by oppositely-oriented H$^+$ gradients. TEA transport is *cis*-inhibited by Type I OCs, including cimetidine, quinidine, and MPP, only weakly inhibited by NMN and choline, and is refractory to guanidine, PAH and probenecid.[124] Thus, the (1) profile of expression, (2) energetic mechanism, and (3) selectivity characteristics of MATE1 are reasonably comparable to those of the apical OC/H$^+$ exchanger as expressed in renal BBMV, making MATE1 a strong candidate for the molecular identity of this process. MATE2 is also expressed in the kidney, but not in the liver, and its physiological characteristics remain undetermined; its role in mediating renal OC transport is, therefore, unclear. However, its splice variant, MATE2-K, displays characteristics similar to those of MATE1, and its kidney-specific expression suggests that it, too, may play a role in the luminal export of OCs.

Multidrug Resistance

The multidrug resistance transporter (MDR1; ABCB1; also called the P-glycoprotein, or p-GP) was first characterized within the context of its role in the development of cross-resistance of cancer cells to a structurally diverse range of chemotherapeutic agents. The human ortholog of MDR1 is a protein of 1279 amino acids (141 kDa) and is composed of two homologous halves, each containing six TMDs and an ATP-binding domain, separated by a linker polypeptide. The normal expression of MDR1 in barrier epithelia, including the intestine, liver, and kidney, supports the conclusion that it plays a role in limiting absorption (in the intestine) and facilitating excretion (by the liver and kidney) of xenobiotic compounds. In the kidney, MDR1 is expressed in the apical membrane of proximal tubule cells in human[205] and mouse kidneys.[206] MDR1 is also expressed, albeit at apparently lower levels, in the mesangium, thick ascending limb of Henle's loop, and collecting tubule of the normal human kidney[207] MDR1 supports ATP-dependent export of a structurally diverse range of comparatively bulky, hydrophobic cationic substrates that, in general, fall within the Type II OC classification. These traditional MDR1 substrates include the vinca alkaloids (e.g., vinblastine, vincristine), cyclosporine, anthracyclines (e.g., daunorubicin, doxorubicin), and verapamil. In addition, MDR1 mediates the transport of a number of relatively hydrophobic compounds that are either uncharged or are neutral at physiological pH, including digoxin, colchicine, propafenone, and selected corticosteroids. Although substantial evidence supports the conclusion that MDR1 is involved in the luminal secretion of at least Type II OCs, its quantitative significance is not known.

Clinical Diseases from Genetic Defects of Organic Cation Transporters

Lesions in OCTN2 have been clearly linked to systemic carnitine deficiency, owing to the central role this transporter plays in reabsorption of carnitine from the tubular filtrate.[200,208,209] In addition, single nucleotide polymorphisms (SNPs) in the genes coding for OCTN1 and OCTN2 have been linked to increased incidence of inflammatory bowel diseases, including Crohn disease.[210] There is not, however, a clear disease phenotype associated with the failure of renal OC secretion, as shown by the normal phenotypes of mice in which OCT1, OCT2, and/or OCT3 have been eliminated.[3,133] Instead, the focus has been on the influence of naturally occurring genetic variation in human populations for the OCTs and OCTNs and the influence such variation may have on the pharmacokinetics of drug elimination (see Ref 180, 211). For example, a study of six monozygotic twin pairs showed that genetic factors contribute substantially to the renal clearance of metformin, a drug that is a substrate of OCT2 and eliminated exclusively by the kidney. Indeed, the genetic component contributing to variation in the renal clearance of metformin, which undergoes transporter-mediated secretion, is suspected of being particularly high (>90%),[181] suggest that variation in the renal clearance of metformin has a strong genetic component, and that genetic variation in OCT2 may explain a large part of this pharmacokinetic variability. Common variants of OCT2, as well as genetic variants of OCT1, OCTN1, and OCTN2, may alter protein function and could cause inter-individual differences in the renal handling of organic cation drugs. Genetic variants of all these processes have been identified in human populations[179–181,212–214] and studies in heterologous expressions systems have confirmed that common (typically, with occurrences in specific population groups of >1%) SNPs result in substantial changes in transporter activity. Further studies examining the pharmacokinetic phenotypes of individuals harboring genetic variants that change transport function should help to define the roles of each transporter in renal elimination.[211] Furthermore, such studies may help identify particular genetic variants that lead to susceptibility to drug toxicities resulting from drug-drug interactions.

ORGANIC ANIONS

Organic Anion Physiology

Organic anions represent an immensely broad group of solutes being transported by the kidney, which renders it barely justifiable to be discussed in a single section. An organic anion can be loosely defined as any organic compound that bears a net negative charge at the pH of the fluid in which the compound resides. These can be endogenous substances, or exogenously acquired toxins or drugs. The physiology can be poised for conservation with extremely low fractional excretion similar to glucose. Such is the case with metabolic intermediates like mono- and di-carboxylates (Fig. 6–1; fractional excretion ≈ 0). On the other end, the system can gear itself for elimination utilizing combined glomerular filtration and secretion (Fig. 6–1; fractional excretion >>1). In addition to the large range of fractional excretion, this group of transporters also has the broadest array of substrates that spans compounds with completely disparate chemical structures. Multi-specificity in substrate recognition is a prevalent feature within each gene family and across different families of organic anion transporters.

The precise analysis of the field of renal anion excretion was ushered by the seminal work of Marshall and co-workers who studied the elimination of dyes and arrived at the conclusion that mammalian renal tubules possess high capacity secretory function.[215,216] This was followed by the classical studies of Smith and associates who described the tubular secretion of *p*-aminohippurate (PAH) and provided a marker for estimating renal blood flow (RPF) by PAH clearance for decades that followed.[217] Reabsorptive physiology was illustrated in the previous section on glucose. Figure 6–5 illustrates the secretory nature of the proximal tubule using PAH as a surrogate. In low plasma concentrations, PAH has a fractional excretion of $\gg$1 and PAH clearance (C_{PAH}) approaches renal plasma flow (RPF) as most of the PAH is removed from the plasma in a single pass. As plasma PAH increases, both filtered and secreted PAH increases and C_{PAH} remains a good estimate of RPF. When the secretory maximal is reached and subsequently exceeded, the commensurate increment in excretion is contributed solely by increasing filtered load. At this stage, C_{PAH} starts to gradually drift further below RPF toward the value of GFR (Fig. 6–10).

Classic studies using stop-flow, micropuncture, and microperfusion[218–220] in multiple species have demonstrated that organic anions are secreted in the proximal tubule. The study of Tune and co-workers definitely demonstrated uphill transport from peritubular fluid into urinary lumen.[220] As noted earlier, the secretory mode mandates broad substrate recognition and one simply cannot afford to devote one gene per compound that the organism wishes to excrete. Table 6–4 is

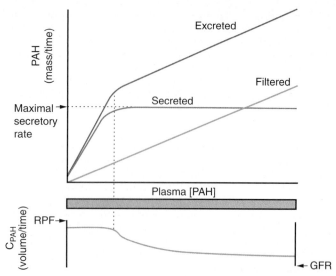

FIGURE 6–10 Illustration of filtration-secretion using PAH clearance (C_{PAH}). PAH clearance = GFR + PAH secretion. For a given GFR, both secreted and filtered PAH increases with increasing plasma [PAH]. At this point, C_{PAH} approximates renal plasma flow (RPF). With increasing plasma [PAH], maximal secretion is reached and any further increase in C_{PAH} is due to increasing filtered PAH. At high plasma [PAH], C_{PAH} numerically drifts towards GFR.

TABLE 6–4	Classes of Organic Anions Transported by the Proximal Tubule
Endogenous	
Metabolic intermediates	α-ketoglutarate, succinate, citrate
Eicosanoids	PGE1, PGE2, PGD2, PGF2a, PGI2, TxB2
Cyclic nucleotides	cAMP, cGMP
Others	Urate, folate, bile acids, oxalate, 5-HIA, HVA
Metabolic Conjugates	
Sulfate	Estrone sulfate, DHEAS,
Glucuronide	Estradiol glucuronide, salicylglucuronide
Acetyl	Acetylated sulphonamide
Glycine	PAH, *o*-hydroxyhippurate
Cysteine	CTFC, DCVC, N-acetyl-S-farnesyl–cysteine
Drugs	
Antibiotics	β-lactam, cepham, tetracycline, sulphonamide
Antiviral	Acyclovir, amantadine, adefovir
Anti-inflammatory	Salicylates, indomethacin,
Diuretics	Loop diuretics, thiazides, acetazolamide
Antihypertensive	ACE inhibitors, ARB
Chemotherapeutic	Methotrexate, azathioprine, cyclophosphamide, 5-FU
Antiepileptic	Vaproate
Uricosuric	Probenicid
Environmental Toxins	
Fungal products	Ochratoxin A & B, aflatoxin G1, patulin
Herbicides	2,4-dichlorophenoxyacetic acid

PG, prostaglandins; Tx, thromboxane; 5-HIA, 5-Hydroxyindoleacetate; HVA, homovanillic acid; DHEAS, dihydroxyepiandronesterone sulfate; PAH, p-amino hippurate; CTFC, S-(2-chloro-1,1,2-trifluoroethyl)-L-cysteine; DCVC, S-(1,2-dichlorovinyl)-L-cysteine; ACE inhibitors, angiotensin converting enzyme inhibitor; ARB, angiotensin receptor blockers; 5-FU, 5-fluorouracil.

an illustrative but incomplete inventory that demonstrates the extremely broad substrate spectra of organic anion handling by the kidney. It is impossible to fathom any structural similarities among these compounds. In addition, the number of substances transported far exceeds the number of proteins required to excrete these substance. This is not unlike proteins such as P-glycoprotein (ATP-binding cassette multidrug resistance protein) or the multi-ligand receptor megalin where the ability to engage with multiple compounds is intrinsic to their biologic function.[221,222] The classical microperfusion study from Fritzch and co-workers proposed a minimal requirement of a hydropic region in the anion to be a substrate.[223] The protein structure that permits this broad range of substrate to be bound and transported is unknown but undoubtedly fascinating.

Molecular Biology of Organic Anion Transporters

Several families of solute transporters can be included in this discussion. Three will be mentioned: the dicarboxylate-sulphate transporters (NaDC/NaS SLC13 family), the organic anion transporters (OAT SLC22 family), and the organic anion transporting polypeptides (OATP SLC21 family). A

detail account is beyond the scope of this chapter. The reader is referred to several excellent recent reviews.[224-231]

NaDC (*SLC13A*) Family
These transporters function to reclaim filtered solutes and are functionally directly opposite to the next group of secretory proteins. This family is related by similarities in primary sequences but the isoforms are quite distinct in their function. The nomenclature is still in a state of evolution and five genes are identified to date (Table 6–5).[229,230] NaS1 is a low-affinity sulfate transporter[232] expressed at the proximal tubule apical membrane (see Table 6–5)[233] but does not take organic anions. NaS2 and NaCT are not expressed in the kidney (see Table 6–5). These proteins will not be discussed. NaDC1 and NaDC3 are the main transporters of interest in this discussion.

NaDC1
NaDC1 was first cloned by Pajor's group[234-237] and subsequently by others.[238,239] NaDC1 is found on apical membranes of both the renal proximal tubule and small intestine where it mediates absorption of tricarboxylic acid cycle intermediates from the glomerular filtrate or the intestinal lumen. The preferred substrates of NaDC1 are 4-carbon dicarboxylates such as succinate, fumarate, and α-ketoglutarate. Citrate

TABLE 6–5	Organic Anion Transporters			
NaDC Family				
Name	Gene Name	Human Chromosome	Renal Proximal Tubule Localization	Transport Mode/substrate (All Na$^+$-dependent)
NaS1	*SLC13A1*	7q31-32	Apical	Sulphate, thiosulfate selenate
NaDC1	*SLC13A2*	17p11.1-q11.1	Apical	Succinate, citrate, α-ketoglutarate
NaDC3	*SLC13A3*	20q12-13.1	Basolateral	Succinate, citrate, α-ketoglutarate
NaS2	*SLC13A4*	7q33	Absent	Sulphate
NaCT	*SLC13A5*	12q12-13	Absent	Citrate, succinate, pyruvate

OAT Family				
Name	Gene Name	Human Chromosome	Renal Proximal Tubule Localization	Transport Mode/substrate (Na$^+$-independent)
OAT1	*SLC22A6*	11q12.3	Basolateral	OA dicarboxylate exchange
OAT2	*SLC22A7*	6q21.1-2	Basolateral	OA dicarboxylate exchange
OAT3	*SLC22A8*	11q12.3	Basolateral	OA dicarboxylate exchange
OAT4	*SLC22A11*	11q13.1	Apical	OA dicarboxylate exchange
URAT1	*SLC22A12*	11q13.1	Apical	Urate OA exchange
OAT5	*Slc22a19*	(murine)		

OA, organic anion (broad substrate specificity).

OATP				
Name	Gene Name	Human Chromosome	Renal Tubule Localization	Transport Mode/substrate (Na$^+$-independent)
OATP4C1	*SLCO4C1*	5q21	PT: basolateral	Digoxin, ouabain, T3
OATP1A2	*SLCO1A2*	12p12	CCD: basolateral	Bile salts, estrogen conjugates PG's, T3, T4, antibiotics ouabain, ochratoxin A
OATP2A1	*SLCO2A1*	3q21	mRNA+	PG's
OATP2B1	*SLCO2B1*	11q13	mRNA+	Estrogen conjugates, antibiotics
OATP3A1	*SLCO3A1*	15q26	mRNA+	Estrogen conjugates, antibiotics
OATP4A1	*SLCO4A1*	20q13.1	mRNA+	Bile salts, estrogen conjugates, PG's, T3, T4, antibiotics

PT, proximal tubule; CCD, cortical collecting duct; T3, thyroid hormone; PGs, prostaglandin.

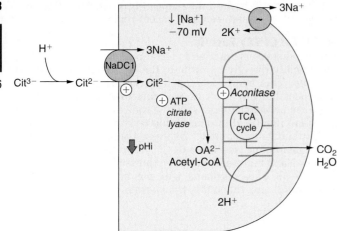

FIGURE 6–11 Proximal tubule citrate absorption and metabolism. The Na⁺-K⁺-ATPase generates the low cell [Na⁺]. As a secondary active transporter NaDC1 uses the electrochemical gradient to pick up filtered citrate, which metabolized in the cytoplasm or the mitochondria. Ambient and cytoplasmic pH increase citrate uptake and metabolism. (1) Acidification of urinary lumen titrates citrate to the divalent transported species; (2) NaDC1 is directly activated by pH and chronic low pH increases expression of NaDC1 (circled arrow); (3) Intracellular acidification increases the expression of ATP citrate lyase and aconitase (circled arrows).

exists mostly as a tricarboxylate at plasma pH, but in the proximal tubule lumen, because of apical H⁺ transport, citrate³⁻ is titrated (citrate³⁻/citrate²⁻ pK 5.7–6.0) and is taken up in protonated form as citrate²⁻. The Km for dicarboxylates ranges between 0.3 mM and 1 mM. Transport of one divalent anion substrate is coupled to three Na⁺ ions.

Once absorbed across the apical membrane, cytosolic citrate is either metabolized through ATP citrate lyase, which cleaves citrate to oxaloacetate and acetyl CoA, or transported into the mitochondria where it can be metabolized in the tricarboxylic acid cycle to neutral end products such as carbon dioxide (Fig. 6–11).[240,241] When a divalent organic anion is converted to neutral products, two H⁺ are consumed, which renders citrate²⁻ an important urinary base.

NaDC3

NaDC3 has a wider tissue distribution and much broader substrate specificity than NaDC1. NaDC3 is expressed on basolateral membranes in renal proximal tubule cells,[242] as well as liver, brain, and placenta. The basolateral location of NaDC3 was mapped to a motif in its amino-terminal cytoplasmic domain.[243–246] The K_m for succinate in NaDC3 is lower than NaDC1 (10 μM-100 μM).[246] Similarly, NADC3 displays a much higher affinity for α-ketoglutarate[247] than does NaDC1.[248] Like NaDC1, NaDC3 is sodium-coupled and electrogenic so it is very unlikely that NaDC3 will mediate citrate efflux from the proximal tubule into the peritubular space. It is more likely that the NaDC3 helps support the outwardly directed α-ketoglutarate gradient required for OAT transporters to perform organic anion exchange (see later). In fact, the activity of NaDC3 has been shown to support approximately 50% of the OAT-mediated uptake of the organic anion fluorescein across the basolateral membrane in isolated rabbit renal tubules[249] with half of this effect reflecting the accumulation of exogenous α-ketoglutarate from the blood, and the other half arising from "recycling" endogenous α-ketoglutarate that exited the cell in OAT-mediated exchange for the organic anion substrate.

OAT (*SLC22A*) Family

Two features of these transporters should once again be emphasized—their high capacity for substrate and tremen-

dously diverse substrate selectivity (see Table 6–4). The importance of these proteins in rescuing the organism from succumbing to toxins cannot be over-emphasized. The uptake of substrates from the basolateral membrane of the proximal tubule is a thermodynamically uphill process utilizing tertiary active transport (Fig. 6–12). The Na⁺ and voltage gradient generated by the Na⁺-K⁺-ATPase drives the accumulation of the dicarboxylate α-ketoglutarate in the proximal tubule via NaDC3, which in a tertiary fashion (thrice removed from ATP hydrolysis) energizes uptake of organic anions into the proximal tubule (see Fig. 6–12). Endogenously produced α-ketoglutarate from deamination and deamidation of glutamine (ammoniagenesis) may also participate in the exchange process. Some of the organic anions transported may be endogenous or relatively innocuous exogenous compounds but many of the substrates (see Table 6–4) are toxins. Although its function is in defending the body, the proximal tubule cells cannot afford a self-sacrificial approach as the end result can be destruction of the very mechanism that secretes these toxins. There exists detoxifying mechanism in the proximal tubule cell that protects the cell while the toxins are en route to the apical membrane to be disposed. The details of these mechanisms are still elusive but current data in isolated proximal tubules and cell culture models suggests compartmentalization that may serve to sequester the toxins from imparting their harmful effects.[250]

Basolateral Transporters

More than half a century after the seminal paper from Homer Smith's laboratory[251] that described PAH secretion into the urine, the "PAH transporter" was cloned by several laboratories almost contemporaneously.[252–254] The OAT members OAT1 and OAT3 are present in the basolateral membrane of the proximal tubule (see Fig. 6–12, Table 6–5). OAT1-mediated uptake of PAH is stimulated by an outwardly directed gradient of dicarboxylates such as α-ketoglutarate, indicating that OAT1 is an organic anion-dicarboxylate exchanger.[255] The substrate selectivity of OAT1 is extremely broad with affinities for substrate that are comparable to that reported for the functional PAH transport system. OAT3 is localized in the basolateral membrane of the kidney and, like OAT1, has a broad extra-renal expression.[256] OAT3 also has a promiscuous substrate list comparable to that of OAT1.[231] The purpose for the OAT1/3 redundancy in the kidney is unclear. OAT2 was originally identified from the liver and its expression in the kidney appears to be weaker than OAT1 and OAT3.[257] It transports PAH, dicarboxylates, prostaglandins, salicylate, acetylsalicylate, and tetracycline.[231]

Apical Transporters

There is no overlap of polarized expression of OATs in the proximal tubule. OAT4 was cloned from the kidney and is expressed in the apical membrane of the proximal tubule.[258] When characterized in oocytes, it transports PAH, conjugated sex hormones, prostaglandins, and mycotoxins in an organic anion/dicarboxylate exchange mode and is capable of bi-directional movement of organic anions.[259] It is not known whether OAT4 represents an exceptional OAT-mediated luminal uptake, although it is hard to fathom from the list of candidate substrates why OAT will participate in absorption. The other apical transporter is URAT1, which is renal-specific in its expression.[260] The human URAT1 appears to be quite specific for urate transport.[260] As discussed later, the role of URAT1 as a urate transporter was proven at the whole organism levels from an experiment of nature in humans with renal hypouricemia.

OATP (*SLCO*) Family

This family of organic anion transporting polypeptides is expressed widely in the brain, choroid plexus, liver, heart, heart, intestine, kidney, placenta, and testis[261] and, like the

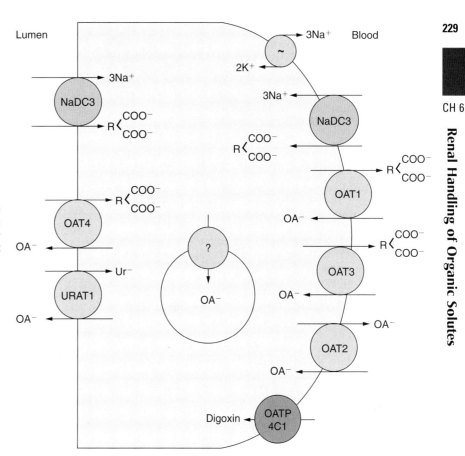

FIGURE 6–12 NaDC (green), OAT (blue), and OATP (black) families of anionic transporters in the proximal tubule. OA⁻, organic anion; Ur⁻, urate. The intracellular transport and sequestration of organic anions are not understood.

OATs, they also have a wide spectrum of substrates.[262] The first member oatp1 was cloned from rat liver by Meier's group as a sodium-independent bile acid transporter.[263] Eleven human isoforms and even more rodent isoforms have been appended to the OATP family.[224,264] In place of the older nomenclature of SLC21A, a new nomenclature has recently been assigned to the OATP family of solute transporters,[226,231] which subdivides the OATP superfamily into multiple subfamilies (reviewed in Ref 226). A comprehensive discussion of this complex classification is beyond the scope of this chapter. One noteworthy point is that there are considerable inter-species differences that engender difficulties in extrapolating rodent data to humans. Among human OATPs, only OATP4C1 is predominantly and definitively expressed in the kidney. The myriad of rodent isoforms that have not been confirmed in humans will not be discussed in this section (an excellent account can be found in two recent reviews).[226,231] One important compound carried by OATP2C1 is the cardiac glycoside digoxin.[264] OATP4C1 is expressed exclusively in the basolateral membrane of proximal tubular cells and mediates the high-affinity transport of digoxin (K_m: 7.8 μM) and ouabain (K_m: 0.38 μM), as well as thyroid hormones such as triiodothyronine (K_m: 5.9 μM). The apical pathway for digoxin has been presumed to be an ATP-dependent efflux pump such as P-glycoprotein.

Clinical Relevance of Organic Anion Transporters

NaDC1
The role of NaDC1 in physiology and pathophysiology has been well studied. Citrate has multiple functions in mam-

malian urine and the two most important ones are as a chelator for urinary calcium, and as a physiologic urinary base.[265] It is a tricarboxylic acid cycle intermediate, and the majority of citrate reabsorbed by the proximal tubule is oxidized to electroneutral end products so H⁺ is consumed in the process rendering citrate a major urinary base (see Fig. 6–11). Calcium associates in a one-to-one stoichiometry. The highest affinity and solubility is a monovalent anionic ($Ca^{2+}Citrate^{3-})^-$ complex.[265]

The final urinary excretion of citrate is determined by reabsorption in the proximal tubule and the most important regulator of citrate reabsorption is proximal tubule cell pH. Acid loading increases citrate absorption by four mechanisms (see Fig. 6–11): (1) Low luminal pH titrates citrate³⁻ to citrate²⁻ which is the preferred transported species[266]; (2) NaDC1 is also gated by pH such that low pH acutely stimulates its activity[267]; (3) Intracellular acidosis increases expression of the NaDC1 transporter[268] and insertion of NaDC1 into the apical membrane; (4) Intracellular acidosis stimulates enzymes that metabolize citrate in the cytoplasm and mitochondria.[268,270] This is a well concerted response and an appropriate response of the proximal tubule to cellular acidification is hypocitraturia. Although perfectly adaptive from an acid-base point of view, this response is detrimental to prevention of calcium chelation. All conditions that lead to proximal tubular cellular acidification (e.g., distal renal tubular acidosis, high-protein diet, potassium deficiency) are clinical risk factors for calcareous nephrolithiasis. Hypocitraturia can cause kidney stones by itself or by acting with other risk factors such as hypercalciuria, and therapy with potassium citrate has been shown to reverse the biochemical defect and reduce stone recurrence.[271]

URAT1 and Hyperuricosuria

The model for renal handling of uric acid has been rather controversial with a popular but yet unproven paradigm of tandem filtration-reabsorption-secretion-reabsorption. Molecular identity and functional evidence of the proteins involved are just beginning to emerge. The current model suggest that apical urate absorption is mediated by URAT1,[260,272–274] whereas apical secretion is mediated the ATP-binding cassette protein MRP4[273,274] and the galectin-9/uric acid transporter (UAT).[275–277]

A host of uricosuric substances such as probenecid, phenylbutazone, sulfinpyrazone, benzbromarone, and some nonsteroidal anti-inflammatory agents inhibits URAT1 from the luminal side.[278] The angiotensin II receptor losartan, which lowers blood uric acid via its uricosuric actions[279] also inhibits URAT1.

Mutations of URAT1 (*SLC22A12*) cause idiopathic renal hypouricemia.[260,280] This is a rare autosomal recessive disorder seen in Japanese and Iraqi Jews. The lack of functional URAT1 transporter leads to hypouricemia and hyperuricosuria resulting in crystalluria and kidney stones. Some patients can get exercise-induced acute renal failure from likely a combination of rhabdomyolysis and acute urate nephropathy.[281] Sequencing of *SLC22A12* in Japanese cohorts with idiopathic renal hypouricemia revealed two patients who did not have missense mutations in this gene.[280] This suggests that non-coding sequences or additional loci related to urate transport or metabolism could be involved in renal hypouricemia.

AMINO ACIDS

Physiology of Renal Amino Acid Transport

Overview

The amino acid, cystine, was discovered in the urine of a patient suffering from urolithiasis in 1810.[282] We know now that the presence of this amino acid in the urine reflected the failure of this patient to reabsorb cystine properly. In fact, the filtered load of amino acids is comparatively large: with a total concentration of free amino acids in the plasma on the order of 2.5 mM,[283] the result is a daily filtered load at the glomerulus of some 400+ mmoles. Indeed, Cushny recognized in 1917[284] that potent reabsorptive mechanisms must be found in the tubular walls of the nephron to recover amino acids because almost none of the filtered load is actually lost in the urine.

As with the other substrates discussed in this chapter, the powerful techniques of stop flow, micropuncture, and microperfusion identified the renal proximal tubule (RPT) as the principal site of renal amino acid reabsorption.[283] However, although net transepithelial reabsorption typically predominates, there is also a physiologically important influx of many amino acids from the blood into renal cells across the basolateral membrane. The situation is further complicated by tubular amino acid metabolism. Renal glutamine breakdown, for example, plays a key role in acid-base balance by yielding NH3 for urinary acid excretion, and renal conversion of citrulline to arginine is the most important source of this dibasic amino acid in the whole body.[284,285] Finally, unlike the other transport processes highlighted in this chapter that are generally restricted in their distribution to cells of the proximal tubule, all cells of the renal nephron express an array of distinct amino acid transporters that play important roles in supporting the metabolic needs of the cells. In addition, amino acid transporters distributed in cells of Henle's loop play critical roles in generating large medullary concentrations of amino acid that serve a protective role against the

high ionic strength associated the urine concentrating mechanism.[286–289] These latter process are, however, beyond the scope of the present discussion and the reader is directed to reviews that consider them in detail.[288,289] The detailed discussion of the tubular and organ physiology of renal amino acid transport, as deduced from classical studies employing intact single renal tubules and perfused organs, is also beyond the scope of the present treatment, and the reader is directed to the discussion of these data by Silbernagl.[283] Here we focus our attention on the molecular and cellular physiology of the multiple amino acid transport processes of the proximal tubule.

Molecular Biology of Amino Acid Transport

Overview

The renal reabsorption of amino acids occurs mainly in the proximal convoluted tubule (S_1-S_2 segments),[283] and the absorption of these compounds occurs in the small intestine.[290] The plasma membrane of epithelial cells in these two locations has a similar set of amino acid transporters (Fig. 6–13). Trans-epithelial flux of amino acids from the intestinal or renal tubular lumen to the intercellular space requires transport through apical and basolateral plasma membranes. Several amino acid transporters have been identified in the apical domain: (1) for neutral amino acids B^0AT1 (system B^0), ASCT2 (system ASC), SIT (system Imino), and PAT1 (also representing system Imino; reviewed in Ref 291); (2) for dibasic amino acids, the heterodimer complex rBAT/$b^{0,+}$AT (system $b^{0,+}$); and (3) for dicarboxylic amino acids, EAAC1 (system X_{AG}^-). Transporters localized in the basolateral domain of these cells are the heterodimers 4F2hc/y^+LAT1 (system y^+L) and 4F2hc/LAT2 (exchanger L for all neutral amino acids), and TAT1 (*SLC16A10;* aromatic amino acid (Trp) transporter). Several of these transporters present higher expression in the renal proximal convoluted (S_1 and S_2 segments) than in the straight tubule (S3 segment): rBAT/$b^{0,+}$AT,[292] 4F2hc/y^+LAT1,[293] and 4F2hc/LAT2,[293,294] B^0AT1,[295,296] ASCT2,[297] and SIT.[298,299] PAT1 is expressed in kidney, but its expression pattern along the nephron has not been studied.[300] Transporter ATB$^{0,+}$ (*SLC6A14;* system B$^{0,+}$: Na$^+$ and Cl– dependent co-transporter for neutral and dibasic amino acids), which is not shown in Figure 6–13, is expressed in distal ileum and colon but not in kidney, indicating a role for this transporter in the absorption of amino acids produced by bacterial metabolism.[301]

Neutral amino acids are mainly absorbed in the small intestine and reabsorbed in the proximal convoluted tubule by system B^0. B^0AT1 accounts for system B^0 activity (electrogenic Na$^+$ co-transport of neutral amino acids) (see Fig. 6–13). Two additional B^0-like activities are expressed in the proximal straight tubule; the molecular identity of these transporters is unknown (reviewed in Ref 291). Mutations in B^0AT1 cause Hartnup disease, characterized by wastage of all neutral amino acids in urine, with the exception of proline, hydroxyproline, glycine, and cystine.[302] This observation suggests that other transporters also mediate the reabsorption of proline. Indeed, renal iminoglycinuria, characterized by aminoaciduria of proline and glycine, also indicates that specific transporters contribute to the reabsorption of these amino acids. PAT1 and SIT are candidate transporters underlying the molecular bases of this disorder. PAT1 is a H$^+$ co-transporter of proline, glycine and alanine[303] whereas SIT is Na$^+$ co-transporter of proline and hydroxyproline (see Fig. 6–13).[298,299] Although PAT1 is proton-dependent, sustained uptake in epithelial cells appears to be Na$^+$-dependent because removal of H$^+$ is coupled to the Na$^+$-gradient via the Na$^+$/H$^+$ exchanger.[300] Recently, Broer and co-workers[291] proposed a model for renal reabsorption of proline and glycine. PAT1, SIT, and B^0AT1

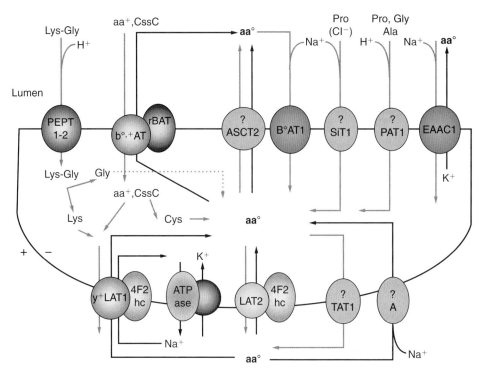

FIGURE 6-13 Proximal tubule model for amino acid transporters involved in renal and intestinal reabsorption of amino acids. Transporters with a proven role in renal reabsorption or intestinal absorption of amino acids are colored, whereas those expressed in the plasma membrane of epithelial cells of the proximal convoluted tubule (or of the small intestine) but with no direct experimental evidence supporting their role in reabsorption, are shown in light blue. Amino acid fluxes in the reabsorption direction are in red. PEPT1 and PEPT2 are expressed in the small intestine and kidney, respectively.

together will reabsorb proline at the convoluted tubule with a capacity exceeding normal kidney load. In contrast, reabsorption of glycine will approach the capacity of two transporters (glycine is not a substrate for SIT): PAT1 and B^0AT1. SIT would be the major player for intestinal reabsorption of proline in the small intestine. This model predicts that PAT1 mutations would result in iminoglycinuria: iminoglycinuria without intestinal phenotype may be caused by two mutated alleles in PAT1, whereas one mutated PAT1 allele would lead to isolated glycinuria. In contrast, iminoglycinuria with a defect in intestinal proline transport may be due to mutations in SIT. The possibility that a third gene is involved in renal iminoglycinuria cannot be ruled out. Indeed, the murine *Slc6a18*-knockout model presents with hyperglycinuria.[304] *SLC6A18* codes for the orphan transporter XT2, which is expressed in the proximal straight tubule.[305]

System $b^{0,+}$ mediates the influx of cystine and dibasic amino acids in exchange with neutral amino acids efflux (see Fig. 6-13). The high intracellular concentration of neutral amino acids drives the direction of this exchange. The membrane potential (negative inside) favors the influx of dibasic amino acids (i.e., with a net positive charge at neutral pH) and the intracellular reduction of cystine to cysteine favors the influx of cystine. As a result, patients with cystinuria presents with urinary hyperexcretion of cystine and dibasic amino acids but not other neutral amino acids. Interestingly, the mean and range (i.e., 5th-95th centile limits) of cystine, lysine, arginine, and ornithine in the urine of patients with mutations rBAT and in $b^{0,+}AT$ are almost identical (see patients AA with phenotype I and patients BB with non-I phenotype in Table 6-6). This result is expected because all $b^{0,+}AT$ heterodimerizes with rBAT in renal brush-border membranes, constituting the holotransporter $b^{0,+}$.[292] Cystinuric patients may show almost no cystine reabsorption in kidney, whereas dibasic amino acid reabsorption in this organ remains intact (reviewed in Ref 292). This observation indicates that $b^{0,+}$ is the main reabsorption system for cystine, but other transporters also participate in the reabsorption of dibasic amino acids. The

molecular identity of these transporters is currently unknown.

The intracellular concentration of neutral amino acids is a major determinant of the active uptake of cystine and dibasic amino acids via system $b^{0,+}$. Apical (e.g., B^0AT1) and basolateral (e.g., system A) co-transporters of Na^+ and neutral amino acids should contribute to the high intracellular concentration of neutral amino acids (see Fig. 6-13). Moderate hyperexcretion of dibasic amino acids occurs in Hartnup disorder,[306] suggesting coordinated function between systems B^0 and $b^{0,+}$: a defective system B^0 will reduce the intracellular concentration of neutral amino acids, which drives the influx of dibasic amino acids via system $b^{0,+}$. In contrast, the impact of system A on renal reabsorption is unknown. The electrochemical gradient of Na^+ drives the active transport of the Na^+ co-transporters of neutral amino acids B^0 and A. Thus, system $b^{0,+}$ mediates active transport of cystine and dibasic amino acids with a tertiary active mechanism of transport.

Apical PEPT1 (*SLC15A1*) and PEPT2 (*SLC15A1*) are expressed in the small intestine and in kidney, respectively.[307] These transporters co-transport H^+ with di- and tripeptides. The physiological role of PEPT2 in kidney is largely unknown.[308] The contribution of PEPT1 to the assimilation of amino acids has not been properly evaluated in mammals or humans, but it is assumed that absorption of di- and tripeptides accounts for a significant proportion of the intestinal absorption of amino acids.[307] A deeper study of the phenotype of the *Slc15A2*-knockout mouse[308] and generation and study of the PEPT1 model may answer these questions. Meanwhile, the role of PEPT1 in amino acid nutrition is supported by observations of the lack of pathology associated with amino acid malabsorption in cystinuria and in many patients with Hartnup disorder. Patients with cystinuria do not show pathology, with the exception of cystine urolithiasis. It is believed that absorption of di- and tri-peptides via PEPT1 compensate for the defective absorption of cystine and dibasic amino acids via system $b^{0,+}$. Similarly, phenotype severity in Hartnup disorder is reduced in well-nourished patients.

TABLE 6–6 Urine Amino Acid Excretion in Patients Classified by Genotype and Clinical Type of Cystinuria

Genotype	Cystinuria Type	n	Urine Amino Acid Excreted (mmol/g creatinine)			
			Cystine	Lysine	Arginine	Ornithine
AA	I	34	1.66 [0.65–3.40]	6.58 [2.65–11.6]	3.14 [0.23–8.37]	1.74 [0.59–3.44]
AA	Mixed	3	0.78, 2.12, 5.56	3.31, 5.72, 11.4	1.23, 2.82, 7.03	0.72, 1.64, 1.92
AA(B)	Mixed	1	2.57	9.84	2.95	5.17
BB	I	1	2.69	2.28	1.11	0.30
BB	Non-I	37	1.62 [0.50–3.30]	6.51 [1.72–14.7]	3.45 [0.50–6.15]	2.20 [0.30–4.77]
B+	Non-I carriers	3	0.26*, 0.44*, 0.80	1.64*, 2.45, 3.88	0.02*, 0.12*, 0.15*	0.04*, 0.27*, 0.29*
BB	Mixed	11	1.82 [0.43–3.18]	4.58 [1.57–8.72]	1.54 [0.21–3.51]	1.33 [0.47–2.45]
BB(A)	Mixed	1	0.43	3.27	0.489	0.603

The mean of the amino acid levels for each group is indicated, with the exception of categories with less than 11 patients, where individual data points are shown.
  When applicable, the 5th and 95th percentile limits are in square brackets.
*Excretion values below fifth percentile of homozygotes of cystinuria Type non-I (BB) in carriers of cystinuria Type non-I.
A, allele *SLC3A1* mutated; B, allele *SLC7A9* mutated; +, normal allele.
N, number of patients.
Extracted from Font-Llitjos M, Jimenez-Vidal M, Bisceglia L, et al: New insights into cystinuria: 40 new mutations, genotype-phenotype correlation, and digenic
  inheritance causing partial phenotype. J Med Genet 42:58, 2005.

The heterodimer 4F2hc/y⁺LAT1 has a basolateral location and accounts for system y⁺L activity (the electroneutral efflux of dibasic amino acids in exchange with neutral amino acids plus sodium) (see Fig. 6–13). Mutations in y⁺LAT1 cause lysinuric protein intolerance (LPI), which is characterized by hyperdibasic aminoaciduria and malabsorption of dibasic amino acids. On the one hand, wastage of lysine in urine in LPI and cystinuria are similar, whereas that of arginine and ornithine are less severe in LPI than in cystinuria (see Table 6–6). Regarding the renal reabsorption of dibasic amino acids, these findings indicate that: (1) lysine appears to be a preferred substrate for basolateral efflux via 4F2hc/y⁺LAT1, and (2) other basolateral transporters mediate efflux of arginine and ornithine. The molecular identity of these transporters is unknown. On the other hand, LPI produces a larger depletion of the three dibasic amino acids in plasma than cystinuria (see Table 6–6). All these observations suggest that malabsorption of dibasic amino acids is more severe in LPI than in cystinuria. Two reasons may account for this: (1) the contribution of the apical peptide transporter PEPT1 cannot compensate for the basolateral defect associated with LPI (see Fig. 6–13); and (2) 4F2hc/y⁺LAT1 is probably the main basolateral system for intestinal absorption of dibasic amino acids.

The basolateral 4F2hc-LAT2 heterodimer is an exchanger with broad specificity for small and large neutral amino acids with characteristics of system L (see Fig. 6–13).[294] This transporter may be involved in intestinal absorption and renal reabsorption of neutral amino acids. Indeed, LAT2 knockdown experiments in the polarized opossum kidney cell line OK, derived from proximal tubule epithelial cells, demonstrated that LAT2 participates in the transepithelial flux of cystine, and the basolateral efflux of cysteine and influx of alanine, serine, and threonine.[309] To our knowledge, no inherited human disease has yet been related to LAT2 mutations. Therefore, a final demonstration of the role of LAT2 in reabsorption requires the generation of LAT2-knockout mouse models.

The model proposed in Figure 6–13 for renal reabsorption of amino acids requires a basolateral efflux system for neutral amino acids. A defective amino acid transport system for this efflux would increase the intracellular concentration of these compounds, resulting in their hyperexcretion in urine and intestinal malabsorption. Candidate transporters for this function may be found within transporter families SLC16 and SLC43. Amino acid transporters in these families mediate facilitated diffusion and may therefore mediate the efflux of neutral amino acids from the high intracellular concentration to the interstitial space. T-type amino acid transporter 1 (TAT1; *SLC16A10*) transports aromatic amino acids in a Na⁺- and H⁺-independent manner.[310,311] TAT1 is expressed in human kidney and small intestine with a basolateral location and can function as a net efflux pathway for aromatic amino acids.[312] Thus, TAT1 may supply parallel exchangers (systems y⁺L and L) with recycling uptake substrates that could drive the efflux of other amino acids. The SLC16 family (also named MCT for monocarboxylate transporters) holds members that transport monocarboxylates and also thyroid hormones. Several members within this family are orphan transporters.[313] Knockout murine models for TAT1, and their related orphan transporters expressed in kidney cortex and small intestine, may help to identify the basolateral transporters involved in reabsorption of neutral amino acids. LAT3[314] and LAT4[315] within family SLC43 mediate the facilitated diffusion of neutral amino acids with characteristics of system L. Neither of these two transporters is expressed in epithelial cells of the renal proximal convoluted tubule or the small intestine. Interestingly, the SLC43 family has a third member with no identified transport function (EEG1[316]). Functional and tissue-expression studies are required to ascertain the role of EEG1 in the reabsorption of amino acids.

The bulk (>90%) of filtered acidic amino acids is reabsorbed within segment S_1 (i.e., the first part of the proximal convoluted tubule).[317,318] Two apical acidic transport systems have been described in the proximal tubule: one of high capacity and low affinity and the other of low capacity and high affinity.[319] The Na⁺/K⁺-dependent acidic amino acid transporter EAAC1 (also named EAAT3), which localized to chromosome 9p24[320] (system X_{AG}^-) is expressed mainly in the brush-border membranes of segments S2 and S3 of the nephron (see Fig. 6–13).[321] The transport characteristics of *SLC1A1* correspond to the high-affinity system.[322] The *Slc1a1*-knockout mouse develops dicarboxylic aminoaciduria,[323] demonstrating the role of this transporter in renal reabsorption of dibarboxylic amino acids. Mutational analysis of *SLC1A1* in patients with dicarboxylic aminoaciduria has not been performed. The apical low-affinity transport system for acidic amino acids in kidney has been characterized in brush-border membrane preparations,[324] but its molecular entity remains elusive. At renal basolateral plasma membranes, a high-affinity Na⁺/K⁺-dependent trans-

TABLE 6–7 Primary Inherited Aminoacidurias

	Prevalence	Inheritance	Gene	Chromosome	Mutations	Transport System
Cystinuria*	1:7000	AR/ADIP	SLC3A1	2p16.3	112	
			SLC7A9	19q13.1	73	$b^{0,+}$
Isolated cystinuria	Very rare	AR?	?	?	?	?
Lysine Protein Intolerance	~200 cases	AR	SLC7A7	14q11	26	y^+L
Hyperdibasic aminoaciduria Type 1	Very rare	AD	?	?	?	?
Isolated lysinuria	Very rare	AR?	?	?	?	?
Hartnup disorder	1:26000	AR	SLC6A19	5p15	10	B^0
Renal familial iminoglycinuria	1:15000	AR	?	?	?	Imino(?)[†]
Dicarboxylic amino aciduria	Very rare	AR?	SLC1A1 (?)	9p24	KO null[‡]	X_{AG}^-

AR, autosomal recessive; ADIP, autosomal dominant with incomplete penetrance; AD, autosomal dominant; AR?, familial studies in the very few cases described for these diseases suggest an autosomal recessive mode of inheritance.
*Three phenotypes of cystinuria, depending on the obligate heterozygotes, are considered: Type I (with AR inheritance), Type non-I (ADIP inheritance), and Mixed Type (combination of both).
[†]The amino acids hyperexcreted in patients with renal familial iminoglycinuria (glycine and proline) suggest defects in Imino system.
[‡]Slc1a1-null knockout mice present dicarboxylic aminoaciduria, pointing to this gene as a candidate for the human disease.

port system for acidic amino acids has been reported,[325] but its molecular structure has not been identified. GLT1 (i.e., the glial high-affinity glutamate transporter,[326,327] also named EAAT2; SLC1A2) may be responsible for this activity. GLT1 mRNA is expressed in rat kidney cortex and porcine small intestine[328,329] but the expression of GLT1 protein has not been studied in kidney or intestine. Slc1a2-knockout mice show lethal spontaneous epileptic seizures[330] but the renal phenotype in these mice has not been examined.

Inherited Aminoacidurias in Humans

Overview
Primary inherited aminoacidurias (PIA) are caused by defective amino acid transport, which affect renal reabsorption of these compounds and may also affect intestinal absorption as well. Several PIA have been described (Table 6–7). Inherited disorders of renal tubule like the renal Fanconi syndrome (MIM: 134600), which is a generalized dysfunction of the proximal tubule that results in wasting of phosphate, glucose, amino acid and bicarbonate, or cystinosis (MIM: 219800; 219900), affecting lysosomal efflux of cystine are not discussed in this chapter. Neither are the inherited defects of amino acid metabolism resulting in aminoaciduria (e.g., homocystinuria, MIM 236200) described in this chapter.

Plasma membrane transport of dibasic amino acids (i.e., basic amino acids) is abnormal in four inherited diseases:

1. Cystinuria (MIM 220100; 600918), in which patients present hyperexcretion of cystine and dibasic amino acids (first described by Sir Archibald Garrod in 1908).[331] There is phenotypic variability in obligate heterozygotes (i.e., silent or hyperexcretors of amino acids).[332]
2. Lysinuric protein intolerance (LPI) (also named hyperdibasic aminoaciduria type 2, or familial protein intolerance; MIM 222700) (first described in Finland).[333]
3. Autosomal dominant hyperdibasic aminoaciduria type I (MIM 222690).[334]
4. Isolated lysinuria described in one Japanese patient.[335]

Cystinuria and LPI are caused by defective amino acid transporter systems $b^{0,+}$ and y^+L respectively. These two transporters belong to the family of heteromeric amino acid transporters (HAT).[336,337] Mutations in the two subunits of system $b^{0,+}$ (rBAT and $b^{0,+}$AT) causes cystinuria.[338,339] whereas mutations in one of the two subunits of system y^+L (y^+LAT1), but

not in the other subunit (4F2hc), produce LPI.[340,341] At the molecular level, the relationship between LPI, and the very rare autosomal dominant hyperdibasic aminoaciduria type I, and isolated lysinuria is unknown.

Plasma membrane transport of zwitterionic amino acids (i.e., neutral amino acids at physiological pH) is defective in three inherited diseases:

1. Hartnup disorder (MIM 234500), in which patients present hyperexcretion of neutral amino acids (first described in two siblings of the Hartnup family).[342]
2. Renal familial iminoglycinuria (MIM 242600) is an autosomal recessive benign disorder in which individuals present hyperexcretion of proline and glycine (first described in the sixties).[313,314] There is phenotypic complexity in this disorder[345,346]; (1) renal iminoglycinuria with defective intestinal absorption and normal heterozygotes; (2) renal iminoglycinuria without intestinal phenotype and normal heterozygotes; and (3) renal iminoglycinuria without intestinal phenotype and isolated glycinuria in heterozygotes.
3. Isolated cystinuria (MIM 238200), in which patients present hyperexcretion of cystine but not dibasic amino acids.[347]

Hartnup disorder is due to a defective amino acid transport system B^0 (also named neutral brush border) caused by mutations in B^0AT1 (SLC6A19).[296,348] The relationship between isolated cystinuria and cystinuria at the molecular level is unknown. The molecular basis of iminoglycinuria is unknown but candidate genes are[291]: SLC36A1 (coding for transporter PAT1),[300] SLC6A20 (coding for transporter SIT [also called IMINO]),[298,299] and SLC6A18 (coding for the orphan transporter XT2).

Plasma membrane transport of dicarboxylic amino acids is defective in Dicarboxylic aminoaciduria (MIM 222730).[349,350] The molecular basis of this disease is unknown but the glutamate transporter EAAC1 (SLC1A1[351]) is an obvious candidate because the murine knockout of Slc1a1 presents dicarboxylic aminoaciduria.[323]

Defects Associated with Heteromeric Amino Acid Transporters
Heteromeric amino acid transporters (HATs) are composed of a heavy subunit and a light subunit (see Table 6–2).[337,352,353] These are unique features among mammalian plasma membrane amino acid transporters. Two homologous heavy

subunits from the SLC3 family have been cloned, rBAT (i.e., related to b[0,+] amino acid transport) and 4F2hc (i.e., heavy chain of the surface antigen 4F2hc, also named CD98 or fusion regulatory protein 1 [FRP1]).[354] Ten light subunits (SLC7 family members from *SLC7A5* to *SLC7A14*) have been identified. Six of these are partners of 4F2hc (LAT1, LAT2, y[+]LAT1, y[+]LAT2, asc1, and xCT); one forms a heterodimer with rBAT (b[0,+]AT); two (asc2 and AGT-1) appear to interact with as yet unknown heavy subunits[355,356]; and the last one (arpAT) may interact with rBAT, 4F2hc, or an unidentified heavy subunit.[357] Two light subunits are not present in humans: asc2 is not found in the genome sequence and arpAT is heavily inactivated in this genome.[357] Members *SLC7A1-4* of family SLC7 correspond to system y[+] isoforms (i.e., cationic amino acid transporters; CATs) and related proteins, which on average show <25% amino acid identity with the light subunits of HATs.

The general features of HATs are as follows[352,353]:

1. The heavy subunits (molecular mass of ~90 and ~80 kDa for rBAT and 4F2hc, respectively) are type II membrane N-glycoproteins with a single transmembrane domain, an intracellular N-terminus, and an extracellular C-terminus significantly homologous to insect and bacterial glucosidases (Fig. 6–14). X-ray diffraction of the extracellular domain of human 4F2hc revealed a three-dimensional structure similar to that of bacterial glucosidases (a triose phosphate isomerase (TIM) barrel [(αβ)8] and eight antiparallel β-strands); Fig. 6–14 (unpublished results).

2. The light subunits (~50 kDa) are highly hydrophobic and not glycosylated. This results in anomalously high mobility in SDS-PAGE (35 kDa-40 kDa). Cysteine-scanning mutagenesis studies of xCT, as a model for the

light subunits of HATs, support a 12-transmembrane-domain topology, with the N- and C- terminals located inside the cell and with a reentrant-like structure in the intracellular loop IL2-3 (see Fig. 6–14).[358]

3. The light and the corresponding heavy subunit are linked by a disulfide bridge (see Fig. 6–14). For this reason, HATs are also named glycoprotein-associated amino acid transporters. The intervening cysteine residues are located in the putative extracellular loop EL3-4 of the light subunit and a few residues away from the transmembrane domain of the heavy subunit (see Fig. 6–14).

4. The light subunit cannot reach the plasma membrane unless it interacts with the heavy subunit.

5. The light subunit confers specific amino acid transport activity to the heteromeric complex (LAT1 and LAT2 for system L isoforms, y[+]LAT1 and y[+]LAT2 for system y[+]L isoforms, asc1 and asc2 for system asc isoforms, xCT for system x[-]_c, b[0,+]AT for system b[0,+], AGT-1 for a system serving aspartate and glutamate transport, and arpAT for a transport system with aromatic amino acids as preferred substrates). Moreover, reconstitution in liposomes showed that the light subunit b[0,+]AT is fully functional in the absence of the heavy subunit rBAT.[382]

6. The light subunit b[0,+]AT stabilizes the heavy subunit rBAT. No data are available as to whether this also holds for 4F2hc and associated light subunits.

7. HAT are, with the exception of system asc isoforms, tightly coupled amino acid antiporters.[359]

The transport characteristics of two HAT-associated transport systems are relevant to cystinuria and LPI (see Table 6–6): system b[0,+] [due to the rBAT (*SLC3A1*) and b[0,+]AT (*SLC7A9*)

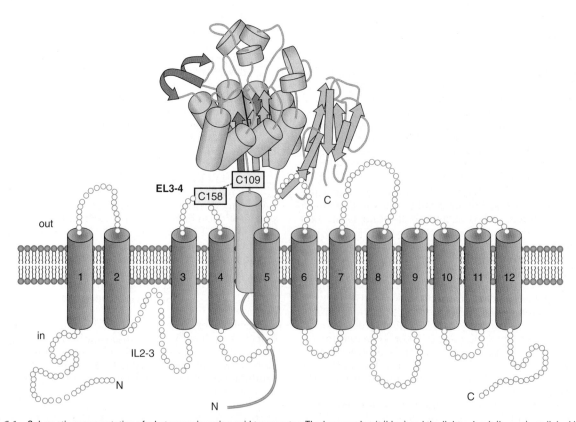

FIGURE 6–14 Schematic representation of a heteromeric amino acid transporter. The heavy subunit (blue) and the light subunit (brown) are linked by a disulfide bridge with conserved cysteine residues (cysteine 158 for the human xCT and cysteine 109 for human 4F2hc). The heavy subunits (4F2hc or rBAT) are type II membrane glycoproteins with an intracellular NH2 terminus, a single transmembrane domain, and a bulky COOH terminal domain (~50 kDa without glycosylation; i.e., similar to the size of the light subunits). This part of the protein shows homology with bacterial glycosidases (a schematic representation of the TIM barrel and the all-β domain is shown). The light subunits are polytopic proteins with 12 transmembrane domains, with the NH2 and COOH terminals located intracellularly and with a reentrant loop-like structure in the intracellular loop IL2-3 (on the basis of studies on xCT[358]).

heterodimer] is a tertiary active mechanism of renal reabsorption and intestinal absorption of dibasic amino acid and cystine in the apical plasma membrane. It mediates the electrogenic exchange of dibasic amino acids (influx) for neutral amino acids (efflux) (see Fig. 6–13). System y⁺L (4F2hc/y⁺LAT1 heterodimer) mediates the electroneutral exchange of dibasic amino acids (efflux) for neutral amino acids plus sodium (influx).[361–363] This transport system allows the efflux of dibasic amino acids against the membrane potential at the basolateral domain of epithelial cells (see Fig. 6–13). The 4F2hc/y⁺LAT2 heterodimer also mediates system y⁺L in many other cell types (see Ref 353 for review).

Cystinuria: Overview

Cystinuria is an autosomal inherited disorder, characterized by impaired transport of cystine and dibasic amino acids in the proximal renal tubule and the gastrointestinal tract. The overall prevalence of the disease is 1 in 7000 neonates, ranging from 1 in 2500 neonates in Libyan Jews to 1 in 100,000 among Swedes. Patients present with normal to low-normal levels in blood (Table 6–8), hyperexcretion in urine, and intestinal malabsorption of these amino acids. High cystine concentration in the urinary tract most often causes the formation of recurring cystine stones as a result of the low solubility of this amino acid. This is the only symptom associated with the disease. Therefore, treatment attempts to increase cystine solubility in urine (increased hydration, urine alkalinization, and formation of soluble cystine adducts with thiol drugs). Cystinuria is not accompanied by malnutrition, suggesting that intestinal malabsorption is not severe. The transport defect occurs in the apical plasma membrane of renal and intestinal epithelial cells. Absorption of di- and tripeptides via PEPT1 (SLC15A1) may prevent malnutrition in cystinuria (see Fig. 6–13).[307]

Traditionally, three types of cystinuria have been recognized in humans: type I, type II, and type III.[364] This classification correlates poorly with molecular findings, and it has recently been revised to type I (MIM 220100) and non-type I (MIM 600918) cystinuria (with the latter corresponding to old types II and III). These two are distinguished on the basis of the cystine and dibasic aminoaciduria of the obligate heterozygotes[332]: type I heterozygotes are silent, whereas non-type I heterozygotes present a variable degree of urinary hyperexcretion of cystine and dibasic amino acids that is higher in type II than in type III. This indicates that type I cystinuria is transmitted as an autosomal recessive trait, whereas non-type I is transmitted dominantly, with incomplete penetrance. Not surprisingly, urolithiasis has been reported in a minority of non-type I heterozygotes. Thus, in the cohort of patients of the International Cystinuria Consortium (ICC) three type non-I heterozygotes with cystine urolithiasis have been identified from 164 cystinuria probands (Table 6–9).[365] Patients with a mixed type, inheriting type I and non-type I alleles from either parent, have also been described.[366] Data on the relative proportion of the two types in specific populations are scarce. In 97 well-characterized families of the ICC cohort of patients, mainly from Italy, Spain, and Israel, 38%, 47%, and 14% transmitted type I, non-type I, and mixed cystinuria, respectively (see Table 6–9).[365] This cohort is not a registry, and therefore it may not be representative of the whole population within these countries.[367]

The characteristics of rBAT expression in the plasma membrane of the epithelial cells of kidney proximal tubule and small intestine, and induction of system b⁰,⁺ in oocytes (for review see Ref 352) pointed to this gene as a candidate for

TABLE 6–8	Plasma and Urine Amino Acids in Lysine Protein Intolerance and Cystinuria				
Plasma Amino Acids (µM)					
Amino Acid	Range in Normal Children	Patients with LPI		Controls Cystinuria (mean ± SD)	Patients with Cystinuria (mean ± SD)
		Mean	Range		
Lysine	71–151	70	32–179	171 ± 26	121 ± 30
Arginine	23–86	27	12–58	82 ± 16	46 ± 12
Ornithine	27–86	21	2–83	58 ± 11	36 ± 11
Cystine	48–140	80	57–105	79 ± 12	43 ± 12
Glutamine	57–467	5583	3644–7161	n.d.	n.d.
Alanine	173–305	772	417–1017	n.d.	n.d.
Amino Acids in Urine					
Amino Acid	Range in Controls (mmol/g creatinine)		Patients with LPI (mmol/1.73 m²/24 h)		Patients with Cystinuria Type B (mmol/g creatinine)
	Mean	Range*	Mean	Range	Mean	Range*
Lysine	0.18	0.04–0.50	4.13	1.02–7.00	6.51	1.72–14.7
Arginine	0.02	0.00–0.05	0.36	0.08–0.69	3.45	0.50–6.15
Ornithine	0.03	0.01–0.07	0.11	0.09–0.13	2.20	0.30–4.77
Cystine	0.05	0.02–0.11	0.12	0.06–0.21	1.62	0.50–3.30

Plasma amino acids are expressed in µM. Data for normal children, and patients with LPI (n = 20) are from (Simell, 2001). Plasma glutamine data also include asparagine concentration. Plasma amino acids from controls (n = 12) and patients with cystinuria (n = 8) are from Morin CL, Thompson MW, Jackson SH, et al: Biochemical and genetic studies in cystinuria: Observations on double heterozygotes of genotype I–II. J Clin Invest 50:1961, 1971. In patients with LPI, urinary excretion is expressed in mmol/1.73 m²/24 h (n = 4) (Simell, 2001), whereas in controls (n = 83) (Dello SL, Pras E, Pontesilli C, et al: Comparison between SLC3A1 and SLC7A9 cystinuria patients and carriers: A need for a new classification. J Am Soc Nephrol 13:2547, 2002) and patients with cystinuria type B (i.e., due to mutations in SLC7A9) (n = 37) (Font-Llitjos M, Jimenez-Vidal M, Bisceglia L, et al: New insights into cystinuria: 40 new mutations, genotype-phenotype correlation, and digenic inheritance causing partial phenotype. J Med Genet 42:58, 2005.) it is expressed in mmol/g creatinine.
*Fifth-95th centile range.
SD, standard deviation. n.d., not determined.

TABLE 6–9 Cystinuria Type and Genetic Frequencies of the Probands from the International Cystinuria Consortium

Genotype	Cystinuria Phenotype						
	I	Non-I	Non-I Carriers*	Mixed	Untyped	Total Probands (%)	
AA	29			2	25	56 (34.1)	
AA(B)				1		1 (0.6)	
BB	1	34		7	23	65 (39.6)	
B+			3			3 (1.8)	
BB(A)				1		1 (0.6)	126 (76.8)
A?	5			1	5	11 (6.7)	
B?	2	7		2	11	22 (13.3)	33 (20.1)
??		2			3	5 (3.0)	5 (3.0)
Total probands (%)	37 (22.6)	43 (26.2)	3 (1.8)	14 (8.5)	67 (40.9)	164 (100)	
Total alleles	74	89	3	28	134		
Explained alleles (%)	67 (90.5)	78 (87.6)	3 (100)	25 (89.3)	112 (83.6)		

A total of 164 probands have been studied. In 126 probands (76.8%) the alleles causing the disease have been identified. In 33 probands (20.1%) one of the two mutated alleles has been identified. In five probands (3.0%) no mutated alleles have been identified.
*Heterozygote probands with cystine lithiasis. For patients AA(B) and BB(A), two alleles causing the disease and two explained alleles in each case have been taken into account in the calculations.
A, allele *SLC3A1* mutated; B, allele *SLC7A9* mutated; +, normal allele; ?, unknown allele.
Extracted from Font-Llitjos M, Jimenez-Vidal M, Bisceglia L, et al: New insights into cystinuria: 40 new mutations, genotype-phenotype correlation, and digenic inheritance causing partial phenotype. J Med Genet 42:58, 2005.

cystinuria. In 1994 it was demonstrated that mutations in *SLC3A1* cause type I cystinuria.[338] Since then 112 distinct rBAT mutations have been described, including nonsense, missense, splice-site, and frameshift mutations, as well as large deletions and chromosome rearrangements (mutations are listed in Ref 365; for more recently described mutations, see Refs 368–370). Cystinuria resembling type I caused by mutations in canine *Slc3a1* has been reported in Newfoundland dogs.[371] Similarly, *Pebbels* mice (homozygous for the rBAT mutation D140G) develop type I cystinuria with urolithiasis.[372]

Most of the cystinuria-associated rBAT missense mutations occur in the ectodomain.[365] Unfortunately, amino acid sequence identity of the ectodomains of rBAT and 4F2hc is very low. This precludes the generation of a structural model of the ectodomain of rBAT using the crystal structure of that of 4F2hc. Therefore, at present, functional analysis is the easiest study available for missense rBAT mutations. The most common *SLC3A1* mutation, M467T, showed a trafficking defect, with the protein reaching the plasma membrane inefficiently.[373] A trafficking defect, also suggested for other *SLC3A1* mutations,[359,373,374] is consistent with the proposed role of rBAT as an ancillary subunit of b$^{0,+}$AT. *SLC3A1* mutations may also affect transport properties of the holo-transporter b$^{0,+}$: the cystinuria-specific mutation R365W, in addition to temperature-sensitive protein stability and trafficking defect, shows a defect in the efflux of arginine but not in its influx.[359] This observation indicates two pathways for the transport unit of system b$^{0,+}$, one for influx and the other for efflux. This scenario is consistent with two additional sets of results: (1) the intestinal system b$^{0,+}$ of the chicken has a sequential mechanism of exchange, compatible with the formation of a ternary complex (i.e., the transporter bound to its intracellular and extracellular amino acid substrates)[375]; and (2) the analog amino isobutyrate (AIB) induces an unequal exchange with other substrates through the rBAT-induced system b$^{0,+}$ in oocytes (i.e., using the endogenous b$^{0,+}$AT subunit). The oligomeric structure of system b$^{0,+}$ (i.e., rBAT-b$^{0,+}$AT heteromer) is unknown. Functional coordination of

two rBAT-b$^{0,+}$AT heterodimers in a heterotetrameric structure would explain these results. If this is not the case, the transport defect associated with mutation R365W would suggest that a single b$^{0,+}$AT subunit contains two translocation pathways.

The gene causing non-type I cystinuria was assigned to 19q12-13.1 by linkage analysis.[376–378] *SLC7A9* was a positional and functional candidate gene for non-type I cystinuria (i.e., appropriate chromosomal location, rBAT-associated amino acid transport activity (system b$^{0,+}$), and proper tissue expression in kidney and small intestine (reviewed in Ref 379). In 1999 the non-type I cystinuria gene was identified as *SLC7A9*.[339] The protein product encoded by *SLC7A9* was termed b$^{0,+}$AT for b$^{0,+}$ amino acid transporter. Seventy-three *SLC7A9* mutations causing cystinuria have been described (mutations are listed in Ref 365; for more recently described mutations see Refs 368–370). Mutation G105R is the most frequent *SLC7A9* mutation in the ICC cohort of patients (~27% of the *SLC7A9* alleles identified). Similarly to the human disease, the *Slc7a9*-knockout mouse presents with non-type I cystinuria with urolithiasis.[380] Several cystinuria-specific *SLC7A9* missense mutations have been reported to lead to a defect in transport function.[381] Reconstitution in proteoliposomes showed that A182T-mutated b$^{0,+}$AT is active, whereas mutation A354T renders the transporter inactive.[382]

Very recently, the ICC performed an exhaustive mutational analysis of 164 probands[365]: ~87% of the independent alleles were identified. The coverage of identified alleles was similar in all cystinuria types (see Table 6–9). The unidentified alleles (~13%) may be due to mutations in intronic or promoter regions, to *SLC3A1* or *SLC7A9* polymorphisms in combination with cystinuria-specific mutations in the other allele,[383] or to unidentified genes. These three possibilities have not been confirmed or ruled out. Of particular interest is the possibility of a third cystinuria gene. In this regard, Goodyer's group proposed *SLC7A10* as a candidate.[384] This gene is located near the cystinuria gene *SLC7A9* on chromosome 19q13.1 and codes for asc1, a 4F2hc-associated renal light subunit with substrate specificity for cysteine and other small neutral amino acids. Moreover, these authors identified the missense mutation E112D associated with cystinuria. In contrast, recent studies have ruled out this hypothesis[359]: (1) cystinuria-specific mutations are not found in patients with alleles not explained by mutations in the two cystinuria genes; (2) the conservative mutation E112D does not affect transport of 4F2hc-asc1; and (3) asc1 mRNA is expressed in the distal tubule where renal reabsorption of amino acids is not relevant but where asc1 may have a role in osmoregulation. The possibility of a third cystinuria gene cannot be discarded, but it would be relegated to a very small proportion of patients (only 3% of the probands of the ICC show no mutation in either of the two cystinuria genes) (see Table 6–9).

Genotype/Phenotype Correlations in Cystinuria

Initial data suggested a close correlation between the phenotype and the mutated gene (mutations in SLC3A1 resulted in type I, and mutations in SLC7A9 resulted in non-type I).[385,386] In contrast to this simple view, recent data show a more complex scenario. On the one hand, all SLC3A1 mutations in well-characterized families cause type I cystinuria, with the exception of mutation dupE5–E9, which shows the non-type I phenotype in four of six heterozygotes studied.[365] This mutation consists of a gene rearrangement c.(891+1524_1618-1600)dup, which results in the duplication of exons 5–9 and the corresponding in-frame duplication of amino acid residues E298–D539 of rBAT, as shown by RNA studies.[365,387] Functional studies are required to explain the dominant negative effect of dup E5–E9 mutation on the rBAT/b$^{0,+}$AT heteromeric complex. On the other hand, most of the heterozygotes carrying a SLC7A9 mutation have a phenotype of non-I (i.e., hyperexcretion of dibasic amino acids and cystine), but may also have a phenotype of I (i.e., silent heterozygotes). Approximately 14% of the SLC7A9 heterozygotes have phenotype I.[367] SLC7A9 mutations associated with phenotype I in some families are I44T, G63R, G105R, T123M, A126T, V170M (the Libyan Jewish mutation), A182T, G195R, Y232C, P261L, W69X, and c.614dupA.[365,388] There is no clear explanation of why these mutations associate with phenotype I because some proteins show residual transport activity when expressed in heterologous expression systems whereas others do not. A182T is the most frequent SLC7A9 mutation associated with phenotype I (i.e., 6 of 11 A182T heterozygotes in the ICC cohort), and this mutation leads to a protein with 50% residual transport activity at the plasma membrane. Moreover, in the ICC cohort the 11 mixed cystinuria patients and the single patient with cystinuria type I, which all carry two mutations in SLC7A9 presented aminoaciduria in the lower range of non-type I patients with two mutations in this gene.[365] This suggests that, in addition to individual and population variability, mild SLC7A9 mutations may be more prone to associate with silent phenotype in heterozygotes (i.e., phenotype I).

The lack of a direct relationship between the mutated cystinuria gene and the type of cystinuria led the ICC to propose a parallel classification to describe cystinuria on the basis of the genotype of the patients (type A due to mutations in SLC3A1, type B due to mutations in SLC7A9, and type AB to define a possible digenic cystinuria).[367] Table 6–8 summarizes the double classification for 78 cystinuria probands by the ICC as follows: (1) most type I patients have two mutations in SLC3A1 (i.e., individuals AA); (2) all non-type I patients (including type non-type I heterozygotes with urolithiasis) have mutations in SLC7A9 (i.e., individuals BB and B+); (3) patients with mixed cystinuria carry mutations in SLC3A1 (2 probands AA) or in SLC7A9 (7 probands BB); and (4) 2 of 126 fully genotyped probands carry mutations in both genes.

To our knowledge, only four patients with mutations in both cystinuria genes have been described.[365,389] There is no report of the urine phenotype of the Swedish patient AA(B). Two sisters AA(B) and one male BB(A) from 2 families of 126 fully genotyped families in the ICC cohort have been identified and classified as mixed cystinuria patients (i.e., each of the two mutated alleles in the same gene is associated with phenotype I or non-phenotype I in the obligate heterozygotes). The aminoaciduria levels of these patients and their double-heterozygote (i.e., AB) relatives indicate that digenic inheritance in cystinuria has only a partial effect on the phenotype, restricted to a variable impact on the aminoaciduria. Indeed, none of the individuals AB presented urolithiasis. Given that the frequencies of type A and B alleles are similar in this cohort, if digenic inheritance was the rule in cystinuria, we would expect a quarter of patients to be AA, a quarter to be BB, and half to be AB. This indicates that digenic inheritance affecting phenotype is an exception in cystinuria. However, the possibility that some combinations of mutations A and B produce enough cystine hyperexcretion to cause urolithiasis cannot be ruled out.

A working hypothesis on the biogenesis of the rBAT/b$^{0,+}$AT heterodimer may explain the urine phenotypes and the apparent lack of full digenic inheritance in cystinuria: b$^{0,+}$AT controls the amount of active holotransporter at the plasma membrane. Thus, the rBAT protein would be produced in excess in kidney, and therefore an rBAT mutation in heterozygosis in humans and in mice does not lead to hyperexcretion of amino acids (phenotype I). The only exception to this rule that has been identified to date is the human rBAT mutation dupE5–E9, thereby indicating a dominant effect for this mutation. b$^{0,+}$AT controls the expression of the functional rBAT/b$^{0,+}$AT heterodimeric complex: interaction with b$^{0,+}$AT stabilizes rBAT, and the excess of rBAT is degraded, as shown in transfected cells.[382,390] As a result, a half dose of b$^{0,+}$AT (i.e., heterozygotes of severe human SLC7A9 mutations or of the Slc7a9-knockout mice) causes hyperexcretion of cystine and dibasic amino acids (i.e., phenotype non-I) as a result of a significant decrease in the expression of functional rBAT/b$^{0,+}$AT (system b$^{0,+}$). In this scenario, the lack of a full cystinuria phenotype because of digenic inheritance indicates that in double heterozygotes (AB), the mutated rBAT does not compromise the heterodimerization and trafficking to the plasma membrane of the half dose of wild-type b$^{0,+}$AT with the half dose of wild-type rBAT. Thus individuals AB behave as heterozygotes B with a variable degree of aminoaciduria, which could be greater than that of single heterozygotes within the family, depending on the particular combination of mutations. Demonstration of this hypothesis requires an in-depth study of the effect of cystinuria-specific rBAT and b$^{0,+}$AT mutations on the biogenesis of the heteromeric complex rBAT/b$^{0,+}$AT both in cell culture studies and in vivo, using double heterozygote mice (Slc3a1 D140G/+, Slc7a9 –/–).

Urolithiasis shows a clear gender and individual variability among cystinuria patients.[367] In the ICC cohort, the age of onset of lithiasis ranges from 2 to 40 years with a median of 12 and 15 years for males and females, respectively. Similarly, the number of total stone events (i.e., spontaneously emitted stones plus those surgically removed) is higher in males than females (0.42 and 0.21 events per year in males and females, respectively). Of the 224 patients studied, ten with full genetic confirmation of the disease and presenting aminoaciduria did not develop renal stones, and two of these patients were over 40 years of age. In contrast, clinical symptoms (i.e., urolithiasis and its consequences) are almost identically represented in the two cystinuria types when either the clinical or the genetic classification is considered. The differences in severity between the genders and marked differences between siblings sharing the same mutations[367] suggest that other lithogenic factors, genetic or environmental, contribute to the urolithiasis phenotype. Indeed, only about half of the Slc7a9-knockout mice, in a mixed genetic background, develop urolithiasis.[380] Moreover, lithiasic and non lithiasic *Slc7a9*-knockout mice hyperexcrete similar levels of cystine. Studies in *Slc7a9*-knockout mice with distinct genetic backgrounds may unravel the genetic factors, in addition to mutations in *Slc7a9* and the cystine levels in urine, which contribute to urolithiasis.

Lysinuric Protein Intolerance: Overview

Lysinuric protein intolerance is a primary inherited aminoaciduria with an autosomal recessive mode of inheritance predominantly reported in Finland where the prevalence of the disorder is 1 in 60,000. Two other geographic locations with a relatively high prevalence are Southern Italy and Japan,[332] with the northern part of Iwate (Japan) registering a prevalence of 1 in 50,000.[391] The diagnosis of LPI is often difficult because of an unspecific clinical presentation. Therefore it is not surprising that LPI is mainly known in Finland, Italy, and Japan (~200 patients described) where clinicians are accustomed to diagnose this disorder.[332]

In LPI there is massive urinary excretion of dibasic amino acids, especially lysine, and the intestinal absorption of these amino acids is poor; therefore the concentration of dibasic amino acids in plasma is low (see Table 6–8).[392,393] Arginine and ornithine are intermediates of the urea cycle that provide the carbon skeleton to the cycle. Their reduced availability results in a functional deficiency of the urea cycle.[394] Other characteristics of the LPI phenotype are as follows. Protein malnutrition and deficiency of the essential amino acid lysine contribute to the patient's failure to thrive. Patients with LPI are usually asymptomatic while breast-feeding, and symptoms (e.g., vomiting, diarrhea, and hyperammonemic coma when force-fed high-protein food) appear only after weaning. After infancy, patients with LPI reject high-protein diets, and show a delay in bone growth and prominent osteoporosis, hepatosplenomegaly, muscle hypotonia, and sparse hair. Most patients have a normal mental development, but some may show moderate retardation. Low-protein diet and citrulline, a urea cycle intermediate, are used to correct the functional deficiency of intermediates of the urea cycle. The final height in treated patients is slightly subnormal or low normal. This treatment does not correct all symptoms such as poor growth, hepatosplenomegaly, delayed bone age, and osteoporosis, which are all probably due to the lysine deficiency. Recently, Simell's group reported recovery of plasma lysine by oral supplementation with the amino acid.[395]

About two thirds of patients with LPI have interstitial changes in chest radiographs, and some develop acute or chronic respiratory insufficiency[396] that can lead to fatal pulmonary alveolar proteinosis and to multiple organ dysfunction syndrome. Further symptoms suggesting that the immune system is affected are glomerulonephritis and erythroblastophagia.[397,398]

System y⁺L transports dibasic amino acids with high affinity (Km in the micromolar range) in a sodium-independent way, but requires sodium to transport neutral amino acids with high affinity[399]: (1) in the absence of sodium, the transport of neutral amino acids through system y⁺L is of very low affinity; and (2) system y⁺L catalyzes the electroneutral efflux of cationic amino acids in exchange for neutral amino acids plus sodium, using the driving force of the sodium concentration gradient. In the early 1990s, two groups described the expression of a system y⁺-like transport activity in *Xenopus* oocytes after injection of 4F2hc cRNA.[400,401] Two closely related proteins (y⁺LAT-1 and y⁺LAT-2) that induce y⁺L transport activity when expressed together with 4F2hc were identified by homology screening,[402] using the light subunit of HAT LAT-1.[403,404] The transport characteristics of 4F2hc/y⁺LAT-1 have been studied in heterologous expression systems, where co-immunoprecipitation of these two proteins has been substantiated.[363,402,405] The transport activity elicited matches the characteristics of system y⁺L;

electroneutral exchange of dibasic amino acids for neutral amino acids plus sodium with a 1:1:1 stoichiometry. y⁺LAT-1 is expressed in the basolateral plasma membrane in the epithelial cells of kidney tubules and polarized cellular models (see Fig. 6–13).[293]

The gene responsible for LPI was localized to 14q11.2 in Finnish and non-Finnish populations.[406,407] The cloning of y⁺LAT-1, encoded by *SLC7A7*, revealed characteristics that made this gene an excellent candidate for LPI (i.e., appropriate chromosome location, co-expression of system y⁺L with 4F2hc, and proper expression in LPI affected tissues).

In 1999 two consortiums[340,341] independently reported the first mutational analysis of *SLC7A7* in patients with LPI. A single Finnish mutant allele (1181-2A>T) was found with an A>T transversion at position -2 of the acceptor splice site in intron 6 of *SLC7A7*. This inactivates the normal splice site acceptor and activates a cryptic acceptor 10 bp downstream with the result that 10 bp of the ORF are deleted and the reading frame is shifted. This mutation has been found in all Finnish LPI patients (i.e., "the Finnish mutation").[408] These two seminal studies also identified LPI-specific *SLC7A7* mutations in Spanish and Italian patients, and established that mutations in *SLC7A7* cause LPI. The fact that system y⁺L activity is present in LPI erythrocytes or fibroblasts[409,410] indicates the expression of a distinct y⁺L transporter isoform in these cells, most probably y⁺LAT-2. Additional studies showed the nonsense mutation W242X and the insertion 1625insATAC as the most prevalent mutations in the south of Italy[411] and the nonsense mutation R410X as the most prevalent in Japan. A total of 26 *SLC7A7* mutations of any kind (large genomic rearrangements, missense and nonsense mutations, splicing mutations, insertions and deletions) has been described in 106 patients with LPI (>90% allele explained).[412] No LPI-associated mutations have been reported in *SLC3A2*, coding for the heavy subunit of y⁺LAT-1 (4F2hc). This strongly suggests that *SLC7A7* is the only gene involved in the primary cause of LPI. It is believed that mutations in *SLC3A2* would be deleterious. 4F2hc serves as the heavy subunit of six other HAT (see earlier). Therefore, a defect in 4F2hc will result in six defective amino acid transport activities expressed in many cell types and tissues. Indeed, the murine *Slc3a2* knockout is lethal.[413]

Functional studies in oocytes and transfected cells showed that frameshift mutations (e.g., 1291delCTTT, 1548delC, and the Finnish mutation) produce a severe trafficking defect (e.g., the mutated proteins do not localize to the plasma membrane when co-expressed with 4F2hc).[408,414] In contrast, the missense mutations G54V and L334R inactivate the transporter (e.g., the mutated proteins reach the plasma membrane when co-expressed with 4F2hc but no transport activity is elicited).[408,414] Mutation E36del showed a dominant negative effect when expressed in *Xenopus* oocytes.[415] The molecular basis for this effect is not yet fully understood.

Pathophysiology of Lysinuric Protein Intolerance

Lysinuric protein intolerance is a multisystemic disease. Some of the symptoms of this disease, like the renal and intestinal phenotypes, are easily explained by a defect in the basolateral amino acid transport system y⁺L. Urea cycle malfunction is a characteristic of patients with LPI after weaning. Patients with LPI have a decreased tolerance for nitrogen and present with hyperammonemia after ingestion of even moderate amounts of protein. The malfunction of the urea cycle in LPI is less severe than that caused by defects in the enzymes of the cycle. y⁺LAT1 is not expressed in hepatoytes.[402,405] It is believed that urea cycle malfunction is due to diminished availability of the intermediates of this cycle because of their low concentration in plasma ("intermediate functional deficiency hypothesis"). The mechanisms underlying the LPI-associated immune-related disorders (e.g., alveolar proteinosis, erythroblastophagia, and glomerulonephritis) are unknown. In addition, individual phenotypic variability precluded establishment of genotype/phenotype correlations.[408,411] Thus, Finnish patients with LPI, all with the same Finnish mutation in homozygosis, show a wide range of phenotypic severity ranging from nearly normal growth with minimal protein intolerance to severe cases with hepatosplenomegaly, osteoporosis, alveolar proteinosis, and severe protein intolerance. In the following part of this section, the mechanisms that explain the renal and intestinal pathophysiology in LPI are discussed.

Table 6–9 compares plasma and urine levels for several amino acids in patients with LPI and cystinuria. Plasma concentrations of the dibasic amino acids (i.e., lysine, arginine, and ornithine) are usually subnormal (one third to one half of the normal values), but occasionally may fall within the normal range. Similarly, but to a lesser extent, plasma dibasic and cystine concentrations are lower in patients with cystinuria.[416] This observation indicates that the defects in renal reabsorption and intestinal absorption of dibasic amino acids may have a greater impact in LPI than in cystinuria, and therefore produce a larger depletion of these amino acids in plasma. In contrast to dibasic amino acids, the plasma concentrations of the neutral amino acids glutamine and alanine are increased in patients with LPI (see Table 6–9), and to a lesser extent serine, glycine, citrulline, and proline. The considerable increase in plasma glutamine and alanine in LPI is believed to be the result of the large amount of waste nitrogen not incorporated into urea as a result of urea cycle malfunction.

In LPI, urinary excretion and renal clearance of lysine is massively increased, whereas that of arginine and ornithine is moderately augmented[417]: lysine excretion is 10-fold and 30-fold that of arginine and ornithine in LPI patients, respectively (see Table 6–8). In contrast, lysine excretion is only twofold to threefold higher than that of arginine and ornithine in patients with cystinuria. Renal reabsorption of lysine is comparable in LPI and cystinuria, whereas hyperexcretion of arginine and ornithine are lower in LPI than in cystinuria (see Table 6–8). These observations indicate that the LPI-defective transporter (y+LAT-1/4F2hc) may have a more pronounced role in the reabsorption of lysine than of the other dibasic amino acids. In contrast to cystinuria, where cystine excretion in urine is four times lower than that of lysine, in LPI there is only a slight increase of renal cystine excretion (see Table 6–8). This may be explained by the large tubular lysine load (i.e., caused by the reabsorption defect of lysine) that competes for absorption through the apical system b0,+, and shares uptake of cystine and dibasic amino acids in exchange with other neutral amino acids. The increased plasma concentration of serine, glycine, citrulline, proline, alanine, and glutamine in LPI explains hyperexcretion of these amino acids, and their renal clearance is within the normal range.

The defect in kidney and intestine in LPI is located in the basolateral membrane and thus affects the basolateral efflux of dibasic amino acids.[418,419] An oral load with the dipeptide lysyl-glycine increased glycine plasma concentrations, but plasma lysine remained almost unchanged in patients with LPI, whereas both amino acids increased in plasma of control subjects or in patients with cystinuria.[420,421] Figure 6–13 shows the present knowledge on the molecular bases of the intestinal absorption of dibasic amino acids. At the luminal membrane of the enterocyte, the transport of oligopeptides (not shared with amino acids) is mediated by PEPT1.[422] A major route for dibasic amino acids across the apical membrane is system b0,+ (i.e., the transporter defective in cystinuria). The absorbed peptides are hydrolyzed to release amino acids in the cytoplasm of the enterocyte[423–425] and are able to cross the basolateral membrane only as free amino acids. The lack of increased plasma lysine after the lysyl-glycine load,

but normal increase in plasma glycine, shows that the basolateral efflux of the intracellularly delivered lysine is defective in LPI. In patients with cystinuria, the cleaved glycine and lysine cross the epithelial cell normally because the defect is apical (i.e., system b0,+) (see Fig. 6–13). The defect in the basolateral system y+L explains the renal and the intestinal phenotypes in LPI. The protein y+LAT-1 has a basolateral location in epithelial cells. System y+L (i.e., the 4F2hc/y+LAT-1 heteromeric complex) mediates the efflux of cationic amino acids by exchange with extracellular neutral amino acids and sodium (see Fig. 6–13). Thus, the loss of transport function of the LPI-associated y+LAT-1 mutations results in a defective basolateral efflux of dibasic amino acids in the intestinal absorptive and renal reabsorptive epithelial cells.

Hartnup Disorder

The original patients with Hartnup disorder presented cerebellar ataxia, tremor, nystagmus, pellagra-like photosensitive skin rash, and delayed intellectual development. Hartnup disorder affects the renal reabsorption and intestinal absorption of neutral amino acids with the exception of proline, hydroxyproline, glycine, and cystine. Pellagra-like symptoms (i.e., niacin deficiency) are frequent in patients with this disorder. Low tryptophan availability (i.e., defective renal and intestinal reabsorption of the amino acids) appears to be at the basis of the niacin deficiency: tryptophan and niacin deficiencies are thought to generate similar symptoms because this amino acid is a major source of NAD(P)H in humans. In this regard, pellagra-like symptoms respond to nicotinic acid supplementation.

The incidence of Hartnup disorder has been estimated at 1 in 26,000 in newborn screening programs.[306] The trait is transmitted in autosomal recessive fashion, but clinical manifestations are probably modulated by environmental and genetic factors.[426]

System B0 neutral amino acid transporter has been considered the defective transporter in Hartnup disorder. Large neutral amino acids are mainly absorbed in the small intestine and reabsorbed in the proximal convoluted tubule (i.e., S1-S2 segments) by the apical system B0 (reviewed in Ref 291). Functional studies in renal and intestinal brush-border membrane vesicles and derived cell models defined system B0 (B for broad and 0 for neutral charge[427]) as a transporter serving a broad spectrum of neutral amino acids. System B0 mediates co-transport of Na+ and neutral amino acids with 1:1 stoichiometry, where Na+ and amino acid affects each other's kinetic parameters (reviewed in Ref 291).

Broer's group demonstrated that mouse B0AT1 (previously the orphan XTR2-related transporter) when expressed in Xenopus oocytes induces Na+-dependent and Cl-independent transport of neutral amino acids with broad specificity, matching the characteristic of system B0.[295,428] Apparent Km for neutral amino acids ranges from 1 mM to 10 mM with the following substrate specificity (one letter code for amino acids): M=L=I=V > Q=N=C=F=A > S=G=Y=T=H=P > W.[428] The human ortholog showed similar transport characterisics.[296,348] Human B0AT1 mRNA is expressed mainly in kidney and small intestine, and to a lesser extent in colon, pancreas, and prostate.[296,348] Mouse B0AT1 was localized to the brush-border membrane of the epithelial cells of the renal proximal convoluted tubule (S1-S2 segments) and of the small intestine with a gradient of expression from the crypts toward the tip of the microvilli.[295,296] Human B0AT1 gene (SLC6A19) localized to chromosome 5p15.33,[348] and Hartnup disorder to chromosome 5p15 in Japanese families transmitting the disease.[429] Thus, SLC6A19 was an obvious functional and positional candidate gene for Hartnup disorder.

In 2004, two independent studies demonstrated that mutations in SLC6A19 are associated with Hartnup disorder and confirmed the recessive mode of inheritance.[296,348] Patients

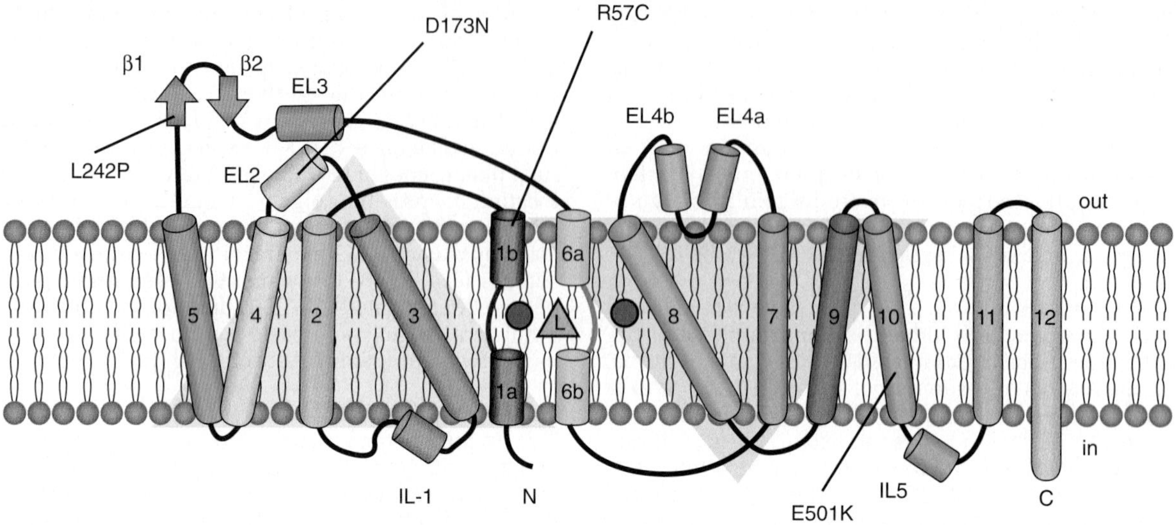

FIGURE 6–15 The predicted topology is based on the crystal structure of LeuT$_{Aa}$ from bacteria *Aquifex aeolicus*.[409] There is a structural repeat, not based on amino acid sequence, in the first ten transmembrane (TM) helices of LeuT$_{Aa}$, relating TM1–TM5 (pink triangle) and TM6–TM10 (blue triangle) by a pseudo-twofold axis located in the plane of the membrane. LeuT$_{Aa}$ is a bacterial homolog of Na$^+$/Cl$^-$-dependent neurotransmitter transporters (family SLC6), to which the defective Hartnup disorder transporter (B^{0}AT1) belongs. Amino acid sequence homology of B^{0}AT1 and LeuT$_{Aa}$ is ~20% and covers the whole sequences (CLUSTAL alignment; data not shown). Major amino acid sequence differences between LeuT$_{Aa}$ and the eukaryotic SLC6 transporters are located at the N- and C termini, between TM3 and TM4, and between extracellular α-helices EL4a and EL4b (these segments are longer in B^{0}AT1 and in other SLC6 eukaryotic transporters). The positions of the substrate leucine and the two sodium ions are shown as a yellow triangle and two blue circles, respectively. Residues interacting with the substrate and ions are located within and surrounding the unwound regions between TM1a and TM1b, and TM6a and TM6b, as well as in TM3 and TM8. Hartnup disorder-specific missense B^{0}AT1 mutations are indicated within the LeuT$_{Aa}$ topology. Rectangle, α-helix. Arrow, β-sheet. (Figure modified from Smith DW, Scriver CR, Simell O: Lysinuric protein intolerance mutation is not expressed in the plasma membrane of erythrocytes. Hum Genet 80:395, 1988.) Location of mutations within the topology of SLC6 transporters. R57C destroys a saline bridge with Asp486 holding the position of TM1b, which interacts with the amino acid substrate and the two Na$^+$ ions. Leu242 involves the extracellular β1 sheet, and L242P, most probably, disrupt this structure. Glu501 in TM10 interacts with one of two water molecules that hold the structure of the unwound residues between TM6a and TM6b, which interact with the amino acid substrate and one of the Na$^+$ ions. Mutation E501K most probably affects the folding of this unwound region. Finally, mutation D173N is a conservative amino acid substitution affecting a residue not conserved among the SLC6 transporters in the extracellular α–helix EL2.

from the Hartnup family were homozygotes for mutation IVS8+2T>G affecting the donor splice consensus sequence of exon 8.[296] In seven Australian pedigrees, six distinct mutations that cosegregated with the disorder were identified (three missense, one nonsense, and two splice site mutations), including one Australian family transmitting the Hartnup family mutation in one allele. In the Australian population, D173N and R240X mutations occur at a frequency of 1 in 140 and 1 in 1000 people, respectively. Four further mutations were identified in three Japanese families (one missense, one nonsense, and two small deletions causing frameshift).[296] In total, 10 Hartnup disorder-specific *SLC6A19* mutations have been identified in 13 independent pedigrees. This implies that ~73% of the independently studied alleles have been identified (19 of 26 alleles).

Recently the crystal structure of a prokaryotic homolog (LeuT$_{Aa}$ from *Aquifex aeolicus*) of the SLC6 family has been reported.[430] This structure will be very useful to ascertain the molecular events underlining the defects associated with Hartnup disorder mutations. The four Hartnup disorder-specific *SLC6A19* missense mutations (R57C, D173N, L242P, E501K) were checked for function in oocytes.[296,348] These mutations showed no transport function, with the exception of the most common mutation D173N, which has residual transport activity (~50%). Figure 6–15 shows the location of these mutations within the topology of SLC6 transporters. R57C destroys a saline bridge with residue Asp486. This bond helps to hold the position of TM1b, which interacts with the amino acid substrate and the two Na$^+$ ions. Leu242 involves the first of two residues constituting the extracellular β1 sheet, and mutation L242P, most likely, disrupt this structure. Glu501 in TM10 interacts with one of two water molecules that holds the structure of the unwound residues

between TM6a and TM6b, which interact with the amino acid substrate and one of the Na$^+$ ions. Then, mutation E501K most probably affects the folding of this unwound region. Finally, mutation D173N is a conservative amino acid substitution affecting a residue not conserved among the SLC6 transporters in the extracellular α–helix EL2. Then, not surprisingly, this mutation retains significant transport activity.[348]

Genetic Heterogeneity and Phenotype Variability

Taken together, these results demonstrated that mutations in *SLC6A19* cause Hartnup disorder. However, individuals that display Hartnup-like aminoaciduria without apparent mutations in *SLC6A19* (in two American pedigrees[296]) have been reported; similar results have been described by the Australian Hartnup Consortium.[291] Indeed, genetic linkage of Hartnup disorder with the 5p15 region has been excluded in an American family.[296] This finding indicates that additional Hartnup disorder genes may be involved and remain to be identified. Five candidate neutral amino acid transporters have been excluded (genetic linkage exclusion and/or lack of co-segregating mutations) as causative genes of the disorder[348]: *SLC3A2* (4F2hc), *SLC7A8* (LAT2), *SLC1A5* (ASCT2 or ATB0), *SLC6A18* (orphan Xtrp2), and *SLCA20* (orphan XT3). A system B^0-like activity in the proximal straight tubule (S3 segment), which has not yet been identified, is an obvious candidate for Hartnup disorder.[291]

Patients with Hartnup disorder display a wide phenotype range. This was described in the original report of the Hartnup family: of the four siblings with clear aminoaciduria, two presented severe clinical symptoms, one had mild symptoms, and one was asymptomatic. Symptoms most likely appear in individuals with subnormal plasma amino acid levels (reviewed in Ref 426). Intestinal absorption of peptides, via

PEPT1, is thought to compensate for the lack of amino acid transport in Hartnup disorder (see Fig. 6–13).[307] This compensation has two consequences. On the one hand, in developed societies, characterized by high protein intake, most patients will remain asymptomatic. Only a limited number of patients will display symptoms (e.g., subnormal body weight, episodes of diarrhea, pellagra-like rash, etc.).[431] On the other hand, genetic factors may predispose individuals to a more severe deficiency in amino acid uptake. The phenotype of Hartnup disorder could be influenced by the amino acid transporters, which participate in the renal reabsorption and intestinal absorption of amino acids: other apical transporters for neutral amino acids (e.g., the B⁰-like activity in the proximal straight tubule) and basolateral transporters. Polymorphisms in these transporters may contribute to heterogeneity in the phenotype of Hartnup disorder.

References

1. Barfuss DW, Schafer JA: Differences in active and passive glucose transport along the proximal nephron. Am J Physiol 241:F322, 1981.
2. Somogyi A, McLean A, Heinzow B: Cimetidine-procainamide pharmacokinetic interaction in man: Evidence of competition for tubular secretion of basic drugs. Eur J Clin Pharmacol 25:339, 1983.
3. Jonker JW, Wagenaar E, Van Eijl S, et al: Deficiency in the organic cation transporters 1 and 2 (Oct1/Oct2 [Slc22a1/Slc22a2]) in mice abolishes renal secretion of organic cations. Mol Cell Biol 23:7902, 2003.
4. Zhang X, Shirahatti NV, Mahadevan D, et al: A conserved glutamate residue in transmembrane helix 10 influences substrate specificity of rabbit OCT2 (SLC22A2). J Biol Chem 280:34813, 2005.
5. Cushny AR: The secretion of the urine. 1917.
6. Shannon JA, Fisher S: The renal tubular reabsorption of glucose in the normal dog. Am J Physiol 133:752, 1938.
7. Brod J: Investigation of tubular function. Techniques based on clearance methods. In The Kidney. London, Butterworth, 1973, p 98.
8. Aronson PS, Sacktor B: Transport of D-glucose by brush border membranes isolated from the renal cortex. Biochim Biophys Acta 356:231, 1974.
9. Lapointe JY, Laprade R, Cardinal J: Characterization of the apical membrane ionic permeability of the rabbit proximal convoluted tubule. Am J Physiol 250:F339, 1986.
10. Biagi B, Kubota T, Sohtell M, et al: Intracellular potentials in rabbit proximal tubules perfused in vitro. Am J Physiol 240:F200, 1981.
11. Aronson PS, Sacktor B: Transport of D glucose by brush border membranes isolated from the renal cortex. Biochim Biophys Acta 356:231, 1974.
12. Aronson PS, Sacktor B: The Na⁺ gradient-dependent transport of D-glucose in renal brush border membranes. J Biol Chem 250:6032, 1975.
13. Turner RJ, Moran A: Heterogeneity of sodium-dependent D-glucose transport sites along the proximal tubule: Evidence from vesicle studies. Am J Physiol 242:F406, 1982.
14. Turner RJ, Moran A: Further studies of proximal tubular brush border membrane D-glucose transport heterogeneity. J Membr Biol 70:37, 1982.
15. Quamme GA, Freeman HJ: Evidence for a high-affinity sodium-dependent D-glucose transport system in the kidney. Am J Physiol 253:F151, 1987.
16. Turner RJ, Moran A: Stoichiometric studies of the renal outer cortical brush border membrane D-glucose transporter. J Membr Biol 67:73, 1982.
17. Kong CT, Yet SF, Lever JE: Cloning and expression of a mammalian Na⁺/amino acid cotransporter with sequence similarity to Na⁺/glucose cotransporters. J Biol Chem 268:1509, 1993.
18. Wright SH, Dantzler WH: Molecular and cellular physiology of renal organic cation and anion transport. Physiol Rev 84:987, 2004.
19. Lindquist B, Meeuwisse G, Melin K: Glucose-galactose malabsorption. Lancet 2:666, 1962.
20. Elsas LJ, Rosenberg LE: Familial renal glycosuria: A genetic reappraisal of hexose transport by kidney and intestine. J Clin Invest 48:1845, 1969.
21. Elsas LJ, Hillman RE, Patterson JH, et al: Renal and intestinal hexose transport in familial glucose-galactose malabsorption. J Clin Invest 49:576, 1970.
22. Melin K, Meeuwisse GW: Glucose-galactose malabsorption. A genetic study. Acta Paediatr Scand :Suppl 188:19+:Suppl, 1969.
23. Hediger MA, Coady MJ, Ikeda TS, et al: Expression cloning and cDNA sequencing of the Na⁺/glucose co-transporter. Nature 330:379, 1987.
24. Ikeda TS, Hwang ES, Coady MJ, et al: Characterization of a Na⁺/glucose cotransporter cloned from rabbit small intestine. J Membr Biol 110:87, 1989.
25. Lee WS, Kanai Y, Wells RG, et al: The high affinity Na+/glucose cotransporter. Re-evaluation of function and distribution of expression. J Biol Chem 269:12032, 1994.
26. Wells RG, Pajor AM, Kanai Y, et al: Cloning of a human kidney cDNA with similarity to the sodium-glucose cotransporter. Am J Physiol 254:F711, 1992.
27. Kanai Y, Lee WS, You G, et al: The human kidney low affinity Na+/glucose cotransporter SGLT2. Delineation of the major renal reabsorptive mechanism for D-glucose. J Clin Invest 93:397, 1994.
28. Wells RG, Pajor AM, Kanai Y, et al: Cloning of a human kidney cDNA with similarity to the sodium-glucose cotransporter. Am J Physiol 263:F459, 1992.
29. Ling KY, Im WB, Faust RG: Na⁺-independent sugar uptake by rat intestinal and renal brush border and basolateral membrane vesicles. Int J Biochem 13:693, 1981.
30. Cheung PT, Hammerman MR: Na⁺-independent D-glucose transport in rabbit renal basolateral membranes. Am J Physiol 254:F711, 1988.
31. Cheung PT, Hammerman MR: Na⁺-independent D-glucose transport in rabbit renal basolateral membranes. Am J Physiol 254:F711, 1988.
32. Gliemann J, Rees WD: The insulin-sensitive hexose transport system in adipocytes. Curr Top Member Transp 18:339, 1983.
33. Kong CT, Yet SF, Lever JE: Cloning and expression of a mammalian Na⁺/amino acid cotransporter with sequence similarity to Na⁺/glucose cotransporters. J Biol Chem 268:1509, 1993.
34. Diez-Sampedro A, Lostao MP, Wright EM, et al: Glycoside binding and translocation in Na(+)-dependent glucose cotransporters: Comparison of SGLT1 and SGLT3. J Membr Biol 176:111, 2000.
35. Dunham I, Shimizu N, Roe BA, et al: The DNA sequence of human chromosome 22. Nature 402:489, 1999.
36. Mackenzie B, Panayotova-Heiermann M, Loo DD, et al: SAAT1 is a low affinity Na+/glucose cotransporter and not an amino acid transporter. A reinterpretation. J Biol Chem 269:22488, 1994.
37. Mackenzie B, Loo DD, Panayotova-Heiermann M, et al: Biophysical characteristics of the pig kidney Na⁺/glucose cotransporter SGLT2 reveal a common mechanism for SGLT1 and SGLT2. J Biol Chem 20;271:32678, 1996.
38. Diez-Sampedro A, Eskandari S, Wright EM, et al: Na⁺-to-sugar stoichiometry of SGLT3. Am J Physiol Renal Physiol 280:F278, 2001.
39. Mackenzie B, Panayotova-Heiermann M, Loo DD, et al: SAAT1 is a low affinity Na+/glucose cotransporter and not an amino acid transporter. A reinterpretation. J Biol Chem 269:22488, 1994.
40. Joost HG, Thorens B: The extended GLUT-family of sugar/polyol transport facilitators: nomenclature, sequence characteristics, and potential function of its novel members (review). Mol Membr Biol 18:247, 2001.
41. Uldry M, Thorens B: The SLC2 family of facilitated hexose and polyol transporters. Pflugers Arch 447:480–489, 2004.
42. Thorens B: Glucose transporters in the regulation of intestinal, renal, and liver glucose fluxes. Am J Physiol 270:G541, 1996.
43. Takata K, Kasahara T, Kasahara M, et al: Localization of Na(+)-dependent active type and erythrocyte/HepG2-type glucose transporters in rat kidney: Immunofluorescence and immunogold study. J Histochem Cytochem 39:287, 1991.
44. Thorens B, Lodish HF, Brown D: Differential localization of two glucose transporter isoforms in rat kidney. Am J Physiol 259:C286, 1990.
45. Thorens B, Lodish HF, Brown D: Differential localization of two glucose transporter isoforms in rat kidney. Am J Physiol 259:C286, 1990.
46. Dominguez JH, Camp K, Maianu L, et al: Glucose transporters of rat proximal tubule: differential expression and subcellular distribution. Am J Physiol 262:F807, 1992.
47. Thorens B, Lodish HF, Brown D: Differential localization of two glucose transporter isoforms in rat kidney. Am J Physiol 259:C286, 1990.
48. Dominguez JH, Camp K, Maianu L, et al: Glucose transporters of rat proximal tubule: Differential expression and subcellular distribution. Am J Physiol 262:F807, 1992.
49. James DE, Strube M, Mueckler M: Molecular cloning and characterization of an insulin-regulatable glucose transporter. Nature 338:83, 1989.
50. Birnbaum MJ: Identification of a novel gene encoding an insulin-responsive glucose transporter protein. Cell 57:305, 1989.
51. Brosius FC, III, Briggs JP, Marcus RG, et al: Insulin-responsive glucose transporter expression in renal microvessels and glomeruli. Kidney Int 42:1086, 1992.
52. Dominguez JH, Camp K, Maianu L, et al: Molecular adaptations of GLUT1 and GLUT2 in renal proximal tubules of diabetic rats. Am J Physiol 266:F283, 1994.
53. Guillam MT, Hummler E, Schaerer E, et al: Early diabetes and abnormal postnatal pancreatic islet development in mice lacking Glut-2. Nat Genet 17:327, 1997.
54. Santer R, Schneppenheim R, Dombrowski A, et al: Mutations in GLUT2, the gene for the liver-type glucose transporter, in patients with Fanconi-Bickel syndrome. Nat Genet 17:324, 1997.
55. Sakamoto O, Ogawa E, Ohura T, et al: Mutation analysis of the GLUT2 gene in patients with Fanconi-Bickel syndrome. Pediatr Res 48:586, 2000.
56. Turk E, Zabel B, Mundlos S, et al: Glucose/galactose malabsorption caused by a defect in the Na⁺/glucose cotransporter. Nature 350:354, 1991.
57. Martin MG, Turk E, Lostao MP, et al: Defects in Na⁺/glucose cotransporter (SGLT1) trafficking and function cause glucose-galactose malabsorption. Nat Genet 12:216, 1996.
58. Martin MG, Lostao MP, Turk E, et al: Compound missense mutations in the sodium/D-glucose cotransporter result in trafficking defects. Gastroenterology 112:1206, 1997.
59. Lam JT, Martin MG, Turk E, et al: Missense mutations in SGLT1 cause glucose-galactose malabsorption by trafficking defects. Biochim Biophys Acta 1453:297, 1999.
60. Kasahara M, Maeda M, Hayashi S, et al: A missense mutation in the Na(+)/glucose cotransporter gene SGLT1 in a patient with congenital glucose-galactose malabsorption: Normal trafficking but inactivation of the mutant protein. Biochim Biophys Acta 1536:141, 2001.
61. Elsas LJ, Hillman RE, Patterson JH, et al: Renal and intestinal hexose transport in familial glucose-galactose malabsorption. J Clin Invest 49:576, 1970.
62. Meeuwisse GW: Glucose-galactose malabsorption. Studies on renal glucosuria. Helv Paediatr Acta 25:13, 1970.
63. Desjeux JF, Turk E, Wright E: Congenital selective Na⁺ D-glucose cotransport defects leading to renal glycosuria and congenital selective intestinal malabsorption of glucose and galactose. In Scriver CR, Beaudet AL, Sly WS, Valle D (eds): The

Metabolic and Molecular Basis of Inherited Disease. New York, McGraw-Hill, 1995, p 3563.

64. Brodehl J, Oemar BS, Hoyer PF: Renal glucosuria. Pediatr Nephrol 1:502, 1987.

65. Wright EM, Turk E: The sodium/glucose cotransport family SLC5. Pflugers Arch 447:510, 2004.

66. De Marchi S, Cecchin E, Basile A, et al: Close genetic linkage between HLA and renal glycosuria. Am J Nephrol 4:280, 1984.

67. De Paoli P, Battistin S, Jus A, et al: Immunological characterization of renal glycosuria patients. Clin Exp Immunol 56:289, 1984.

68. Pascual JM, Wang D, Lecumberri B, et al: GLUT1 deficiency and other glucose transporter diseases. Eur J Endocrinol 150:627, 2004.

69. Fanconi G, Bickel H: Die chronische aminoacidurie (aminosaeurediabetes oder nephrotisch-glukosurisscher zwergwuchs) ber der glykogenose und cystinkrankheit. Helv Paediatr Acta 4:359, 1949.

70. Santer R, Schneppenheim R, Dombrowski A, et al: Mutations in GLUT2, the gene for the liver-type glucose transporter, in patients with Fanconi-Bickel syndrome. Nat Genet 17:324, 1997.

71. Santer R, Groth S, Kinner M, et al: The mutation spectrum of the facilitative glucose transporter gene SLC2A2 (GLUT2) in patients with Fanconi-Bickel syndrome. Hum Genet 110:21, 2002.

72. Guillam MT, Hummler E, Schaerer E, et al: Early diabetes and abnormal postnatal pancreatic islet development in mice lacking Glut-2. Nat Genet 17:327, 1997.

73. De Vivo DC, Trifiletti RR, Jacobson RI, et al: Defective glucose transport across the blood-brain barrier as a cause of persistent hypoglycorrhachia, seizures, and developmental delay. N Engl J Med 325:703, 1991.

74. Seidner G, Alvarez MG, Yeh JI, et al: GLUT-1 deficiency syndrome caused by haploinsufficiency of the blood-brain barrier hexose carrier. Nat Genet 18:188, 1998.

75. Asano T, Ogihara T, Katagiri H, et al: Glucose transporter and Na+/glucose cotransporter as molecular targets of anti-diabetic drugs. Curr Med Chem 11:2717, 2004.

76. Castaneda F, Kinne RK: A 96-well automated method to study inhibitors of human sodium-dependent D-glucose transport. Mol Cell Biochem 280:91, 2005.

77. Tsujihara K, Hongu M, Saito K, et al: Na(+)-glucose cotransporter inhibitors as antidiabetics. I. Synthesis and pharmacological properties of 4'-dehydroxyphlorizin derivatives based on a new concept. Chem Pharm Bull (Tokyo) 44:1174, 1996.

78. Tsujihara K, Hongu M, Saito K, et al: Na(+)-glucose cotransporter (SGLT) inhibitors as antidiabetic agents. 4. Synthesis and pharmacological properties of 4'-dehydroxyphlorizin derivatives substituted on the B ring. J Med Chem 42:5311, 1999.

79. Oku A, Ueta K, Arakawa K, et al: Antihyperglycemic effect of T-1095 via inhibition of renal Na+-glucose cotransporters in streptozotocin-induced diabetic rats. Biol Pharm Bull 23:1434, 2000.

80. Ader P, Block M, Pietzsch S, et al: Interaction of quercetin glucosides with the intestinal sodium/glucose co-transporter (SGLT-1). Cancer Lett 162:175, 2001.

81. Ohsumi K, Matsueda H, Hatanaka T, et al: Pyrazole-O-glucosides as novel Na(+)-glucose cotransporter (SGLT) inhibitors. Bioorg Med Chem Lett 13:2269, 2003.

82. Yoo O, Son JH, Lee DH: 4-acetoxyscirpendiol of Paecilomyces tenuipes inhibits Na(+)/D-glucose cotransporter expressed in Xenopus laevis oocytes. J Biochem Mol Biol 38:211, 2005.

83. Yoo O, Lee DH: Inhibition of sodium glucose cotransporter-I expressed in Xenopus laevis oocytes by 4-acetoxyscirpendiol from Cordyceps takaomantana (anamorph = Paecilomyces tenuipes). Med Mycol 44:79, 2006.

84. Arakawa K, Ishihara T, Oku A, et al: Improved diabetic syndrome in C57BL/KsJ-db/db mice by oral administration of the Na(+)-glucose cotransporter inhibitor T-1095. Br J Pharmacol 132:578, 2001.

85. Ueta K, Ishihara T, Matsumoto Y, et al: Long-term treatment with the Na+-glucose cotransporter inhibitor T-1095 causes sustained improvement in hyperglycemia and prevents diabetic neuropathy in Goto-Kakizaki Rats. Life Sci 76:2655, 2005.

86. Ueta K, Yoneda H, Oku A, et al: Reduction of renal transport maximum for glucose by inhibition of NA(+)-glucose cotransporter suppresses blood glucose elevation in dogs. Biol Pharm Bull 29:114, 2006.

87. Wright SH, Wunz TM: Influence of substrate structure on turnover of the organic cation/H+ exchanger of the renal luminal membrane. Pflugers Arch 436:469, 1998.

88. Clark BA, Shannon RP, Rosa RM, et al: Increased susceptibility to thiazide-induced hyponatremia in the elderly. J Am Soc Nephrol 5:1106, 1994.

89. Pritchard JB, Miller DS: Mechanisms mediating renal secretion of organic anions and cations. Physiol Rev 73:765, 1993.

90. Roch-Ramel F, Besseghir K, Murer H: Renal physiology. Section 8:2189, 1992.

91. Rennick BR, Moe GK: Stop-flow localization of renal tubular excretion of tetraethylammonium. Am J Physiol 198:1267–70:1267, 1960.

92. Somogyi A, Heinzow B: Cimetidine reduces procainamide elimination. N Engl J Med 307:1080, 1982.

93. Bendayan R, Sullivan JT, Shaw C, et al: Effect of cimetidine and ranitidine on the hepatic and renal elimination of nicotine in humans. Eur J Clin Pharmacol 38:165, 1990.

94. Meijer DK, Mol WE, Muller M, et al: Carrier-mediated transport in the hepatic distribution and elimination of drugs, with special reference to the category of organic cations. J Pharmacokinet Biopharm 18:35, 1990.

95. Chandra P, Brouwer KL: The complexities of hepatic drug transport: Current knowledge and emerging concepts. Pharm Res 21:719, 2004.

96. Blackmore CG, McNaughton PA, van Veen HW: Multidrug transporters in prokaryotic and eukaryotic cells: Physiological functions and transport mechanisms. Mol Membr Biol 18:97, 2001.

97. Ambudkar SV, Dey S, Hrycyna CA, et al: Biochemical, cellular, and pharmacological aspects of the multidrug transporter. Annu Rev Pharmacol Toxicol 39:361–98:361, 1999.

98. Higgins CF, Callaghan R, Linton KJ, et al: Structure of the multidrug resistance P-glycoprotein. Semin Cancer Biol 8:135, 1997.

99. Pritchard JB, Miller DS: Renal secretion of organic anions and cations. Kidney Int 49:1649, 1996.

100. Sokol PP, McKinney TD: Mechanism of organic cation transport in rabbit renal basolateral membrane vesicles. Am J Physiol 258:F1599, 1990.

101. Dantzler WH, Wright SH, Chatsudthipong V, et al: Basolateral tetraethylammonium transport in intact tubules: Specificity and trans-stimulation. Am J Physiol 261:F386, 1991.

102. Busch AE, Quester S, Ulzheimer JC, et al: Electrogenic properties and substrate specificity of the polyspecific rat cation transporter rOCT1. J Biol Chem 271:32599, 1996.

103. Cardinal J, Lapointe JY, Laprade R: Luminal and peritubular ionic substitutions and intracellular potential of the rabbit proximal convoluted tubule. Am J Physiol 247:F352, 1984.

104. Bello-Reuss E: Electrical properties of the basolateral membrane of the straight portion of the rabbit proximal renal tubule. J Physiol 326:49–63:49, 1982.

105. Ullrich KJ, Rumrich G, Neiteler K, et al: Contraluminal transport of organic cations in the proximal tubule of the rat kidney. II. Specificity: anilines, phenylalkylamines (catecholamines), heterocyclic compounds (pyridines, quinolines, acridines). Pflugers Arch 420:29, 1992.

106. Ullrich KJ, Papavassiliou F, David C, et al: Contraluminal transport of organic cations in the proximal tubule of the rat kidney. I. Kinetics of N1-methylnicotinamide and tetraethylammonium, influence of K+, HCO3, pH; inhibition by aliphatic primary, secondary and tertiary amines, and mono- and bisquaternary compounds. Pflugers Arch 419:84, 1991.

107. Bednarczyk D, Ekins S, Wikel JH, et al: Influence of molecular structure on substrate binding to the human organic cation transporter, hOCT1. Mol Pharmacol 63:489, 2003.

108. Ullrich KJ, Rumrich G: Morphine analogues: Relationship between chemical structure and interaction with proximal tubular transporters-contraluminal organic cation and anion transporter, luminal H+/organic cation exchanger, and luminal choline transporter. Cell Physiol Biochem 5:290, 1995.

109. Suhre WM, Ekins S, Chang C, et al: Molecular determinants of substrate/inhibitor binding to the human and rabbit renal organic cation transporters hOCT2 and rbOCT2. Mol Pharmacol 67:1067, 2005.

110. van Montfoort JE, Muller M, Groothuis GM, et al: Comparison of "type I" and "type II" organic cation transport by organic cation transporters and organic anion-transporting polypeptides. J Pharmacol Exp Ther 298:110, 2001.

111. Li N, Hartley DP, Cherrington NJ, et al: Tissue expression, ontogeny, and inducibility of rat organic anion transporting polypeptide 4. J Pharmacol Exp Ther 301:551, 2002.

112. Schali C, Schild L, Overney J, et al: Secretion of tetraethylammonium by proximal tubules of rabbit kidneys. Am J Physiol 245:F238, 1983.

113. Yoshitomi K, Fromter E: Cell pH of rat renal proximal tubule in vivo and the conductive nature of peritubular HCO3– (OH–) exit. Pflugers Arch 402:300, 1984.

114. Wright SH, Wunz TM: Transport of tetraethylammonium by rabbit renal brush-border and basolateral membrane vesicles. Am J Physiol 253:F1040, 1987.

115. Wright SH: Transport of N1-methylnicotinamide across brush border membrane vesicles from rabbit kidney. Am J Physiol 249:F903, 1985.

116. Holohan PD, Ross CR: Mechanisms of organic cation transport in kidney plasma membrane vesicles: 2. delta pH studies. J Pharmacol Exp Ther 216:294, 1981.

117. Gluck S, Nelson R: The role of the V-ATPase in renal epithelial H+ transport. J Exp Biol 172:205, 1992.

118. Wright SH, Wunz TM, Wunz TP: Structure and interaction of inhibitors with the TEA/H+ exchanger of rabbit renal brush border membranes. Pflugers Arch 429:313, 1995.

119. Miyamoto Y, Tiruppathi C, Ganapathy V, et al: Multiple transport systems for organic cations in renal brush-border membrane vesicles. Am J Physiol 256:F540, 1989.

120. Yabuuchi H, Tamai I, Nezu J, et al: Novel membrane transporter OCTN1 mediates multispecific, bidirectional, and pH-dependent transport of organic cations. J Pharmacol Exp Ther 289:768, 1999.

121. Ohashi R, Tamai I, Yabuuchi H, et al: Na(+)-dependent carnitine transport by organic cation transporter (OCTN2): its pharmacological and toxicological relevance. J Pharmacol Exp Ther 291:778, 1999.

122. Wagner CA, Lukewille U, Kaltenbach S, et al: Functional and pharmacological characterization of human Na(+)-carnitine cotransporter hOCTN2. Am J Physiol Renal Physiol 279:F584, 2000.

123. Otsuka M, Matsumoto T, Morimoto R, et al: A human transporter protein that mediates the final excretion step for toxic organic cations. Proc Natl Acad Sci U S A 102:17923, 2005.

124. Haisa M, Matsumoto T, Komatsu T, et al: Wide variety of locations for rodent MATE1, a transporter protein that mediates the final excretion step for toxic organic cations. Am J Physiol Cell Physiol 2006.

125. Gutmann H, Miller DS, Droulle A, et al: P-glycoprotein- and mrp2-mediated octreotide transport in renal proximal tubule. Br J Pharmacol 129:251, 2000.

126. Miller DS, Sussman CR, Renfro JL: Protein kinase C regulation of p-glycoprotein-mediated xenobiotic secretion in renal proximal tubule. Am J Physiol 275:F785, 1998.

127. Miller DS, Fricker G, Drewe J: p-Glycoprotein-mediated transport of a fluorescent rapamycin derivative in renal proximal tubule. J Pharmacol Exp Ther 282:440, 1997.

128. Chen C, Liu X, Smith BJ: Utility of Mdr1-gene deficient mice in assessing the impact of P-glycoprotein on pharmacokinetics and pharmacodynamics in drug discovery and development. Curr Drug Metab 4:272, 2003.

129. Hartmann G, Vassileva V, Piquette-Miller M: Impact of endotoxin-induced changes in P-glycoprotein expression on disposition of doxorubicin in mice. Drug Metab Dispos 33:820, 2005.

130. Shimomura A, Chonko AM, Grantham JJ: Basis for heterogeneity of para-aminohippurate secretion in rabbit proximal tubules. Am J Physiol 240:F430, 1981.

131. Woodhall PB, Tisher CC, Simonton CA, et al: Relationship between para-aminohippurate secretion and cellular morphology in rabbit proximal tubules. J Clin Invest 61:1320, 1978.

132. McKinney TD: Heterogeneity of organic base secretion by proximal tubules. Am J Physiol 243:F404, 1982.

133. Wright SH, Evans KK, Zhang X, et al: Functional map of TEA transport activity in isolated rabbit renal proximal tubules. Am J Physiol Renal Physiol 287:F442, 2004.

134. Karbach U, Kricke J, Meyer-Wentrup F, et al: Localization of organic cation transporters OCT1 and OCT2 in rat kidney. Am J Physiol Renal Physiol 279:F679, 2000.

135. Montrose-Rafizadeh C, Roch-Ramel F, Schali C: Axial heterogeneity of organic cation transport along the rabbit renal proximal tubule: Studies with brush-border membrane vesicles. Biochim Biophys Acta 904:175, 1987.

136. Smit JW, Duin E, Steen H, et al: Interactions between P-glycoprotein substrates and other cationic drugs at the hepatic excretory level. Br J Pharmacol 123:361, 1998.

137. Acara M, Roch-Ramel F, Rennick B: Bidirectional renal tubular transport of free choline: A micropuncture study. Am J Physiol 236:F112, 1979.

138. Acara M, Rennick B: Regulation of plasma choline by the renal tubule: Bidirectional transport of choline. Am J Physiol 225:1123, 1973.

139. Wright SH, Wunz TM, Wunz TP: A choline transporter in renal brush-border membrane vesicles: Energetics and structural specificity. J Membr Biol 126:51, 1992.

140. Ullrich KJ, Rumrich G: Luminal transport system for choline+ in relation to the other organic cation transport systems in the rat proximal tubule. Kinetics, specificity: alkyl/arylamines, alkylamines with OH, O, SH, NH2, ROCO, RSCO and H2PO4-groups, methylaminostyryl, rhodamine, acridine, phenanthrene and cyanine compounds. Pflugers Arch 432:471, 1996.

141. Besseghir K, Pearce LB, Rennick B: Renal tubular transport and metabolism of organic cations by the rabbit. Am J Physiol 241:F308, 1981.

142. Christian CD, Jr., Meredith CG, Speeg KV, Jr: Cimetidine inhibits renal procainamide clearance. Clin Pharmacol Ther 36:221, 1984.

143. Rodvold KA, Paloucek FP, Jung D, et al: Interaction of steady-state procainamide with H2-receptor antagonists cimetidine and ranitidine. Ther Drug Monit 9:378, 1987.

144. Grundemann D, Gorboulev V, Gambaryan S, et al: Drug excretion mediated by a new prototype of polyspecific transporter. Nature 372:549, 1994.

145. Pao SS, Paulsen IT, Saier MH, Jr: Major facilitator superfamily. Microbiol Mol Biol Rev 62:1, 1998.

146. Hvorup RN, Winnen B, Chang AB, et al: The multidrug/oligosaccharidyl-lipid/polysaccharide (MOP) exporter superfamily. Eur J Biochem 270:799, 2003.

147. Burckhardt G, Wolff NA: Structure of renal organic anion and cation transporters. Am J Physiol Renal Physiol 278:F853, 2000.

148. Schomig E, Spitzenberger F, Engelhardt M, et al: Molecular cloning and characterization of two novel transport proteins from rat kidney. FEBS Lett 425:79, 1998.

149. Ciarimboli G, Schlatter E: Regulation of organic cation transport. Pflugers Arch 449:423, 2005.

150. Pelis RM, Suhre WM, Wright SH: Functional influence of N-glycosylation in OCT2-mediated tetraethylammonium transport. Am J Physiol Renal Physiol 290:F1118, 2006.

151. Popp C, Gorboulev V, Muller TD, et al: Amino acids critical for substrate affinity of rat organic cation transporter 1 line the substrate binding region in a model derived from the tertiary structure of lactose permease. Mol Pharmacol 67:1600, 2005.

152. Eraly SA, Monte JC, Nigam SK: Novel slc22 transporter homologs in fly, worm, and human clarify the phylogeny of organic anion and cation transporters. Physiol Genomics 18:12, 2004.

153. Zhang L, Dresser MJ, Chun JK, et al: Cloning and functional characterization of a rat renal organic cation transporter isoform (rOCT1A). J Biol Chem 272:16548, 1997.

154. Hayer M, Bonisch H, Bruss M: Molecular cloning, functional characterization and genomic organization of four alternatively spliced isoforms of the human organic cation transporter 1 (hOCT1/SLC22A1). Ann Hum Genet 63:473, 1999.

155. Urakami Y, Akazawa M, Saito H, et al: cDNA cloning, functional characterization, and tissue distribution of an alternatively spliced variant of organic cation transporter hOCT2 predominantly expressed in the human kidney. J Am Soc Nephrol 13:1703, 2002.

156. Motohashi H, Sakurai Y, Saito H, et al: Gene expression levels and immunolocalization of organic ion transporters in the human kidney. J Am Soc Nephrol 13:866, 2002.

157. Zwart R, Verhaagh S, Buitelaar M, et al: Impaired activity of the extraneuronal monoamine transporter system known as uptake-2 in Orct3/Slc22a3-deficient mice. Mol Cell Biol 21:4188, 2001.

158. Budiman T, Bamberg E, Koepsell H, et al: Mechanism of electrogenic cation transport by the cloned organic cation transporter 2 from rat. J Biol Chem 275:29413, 2000.

159. Kekuda R, Prasad PD, Wu X, et al: Cloning and functional characterization of a potential-sensitive, polyspecific organic cation transporter (OCT3) most abundantly expressed in placenta. J Biol Chem 273:15971, 1998.

160. Wu X, Huang W, Ganapathy ME, et al: Structure, function, and regional distribution of the organic cation transporter OCT3 in the kidney. Am J Physiol Renal Physiol 279:F449, 2000.

161. Kaewmokul S, Chatsudthipong V, Evans KK, et al: Functional mapping of rbOCT1 and rbOCT2 activity in the S2 segment of rabbit proximal tubule. Am J Physiol Renal Physiol 285:F1149, 2003.

162. Sata R, Ohtani H, Tsujimoto M, et al: Functional analysis of organic cation transporter 3 expressed in human placenta. J Pharmacol Exp Ther 315:888, 2005.

163. Arndt P, Volk C, Gorboulev V, et al: Interaction of cations, anions, and weak base quinine with rat renal cation transporter rOCT2 compared with rOCT1. Am J Physiol Renal Physiol 281:F454, 2001.

164. Ullrich KJ, Rumrich G, David C, et al: Bisubstrates: Substances that interact with both, renal contraluminal organic anion and organic cation transport systems. II. Zwitterionic substrates: dipeptides, cephalosporins, quinolone-carboxylate gyrase inhibitors and phosphamide thiazine carboxylates; nonionizable substrates: steroid hormones and cyclophosphamides. Pflugers Arch 425:300, 1993.

165. Ullrich KJ, Rumrich G, David C, et al: Bisubstrates: Substances that interact with renal contraluminal organic anion and organic cation transport systems. I. Amines, piperidines, piperazines, azepines, pyridines, quinolines, imidazoles, thiazoles, guanidines and hydrazines. Pflugers Arch 425:280, 1993.

166. Barendt WM, Wright SH: The human organic cation transporter (hOCT2) recognizes the degree of substrate ionization. J Biol Chem 277:22491, 2002.

167. Volk C, Gorboulev V, Budiman T, et al: Different affinities of inhibitors to the outwardly and inwardly directed substrate binding site of organic cation transporter 2. Mol Pharmacol 64:1037, 2003.

168. Dresser MJ, Gray AT, Giacomini KM: Kinetic and selectivity differences between rodent, rabbit, and human organic cation transporters (OCT1). J Pharmacol Exp Ther 292:1146, 2000.

169. Nagel G, Volk C, Friedrich T, et al: A reevaluation of substrate specificity of the rat cation transporter rOCT1. J Biol Chem 272:31953, 1997.

170. Zhang L, Gorset W, Dresser MJ, et al: The interaction of n-tetraalkylammonium compounds with a human organic cation transporter, hOCT1. J Pharmacol Exp Ther 288:1192, 1999.

171. Zhang L, Gorset W, Washington CB, et al: Interactions of HIV protease inhibitors with a human organic cation transporter in a mammalian expression system. Drug Metab Dispos 28:329, 2000.

172. Zhang L, Schaner ME, Giacomini KM: Functional characterization of an organic cation transporter (hOCT1) in a transiently transfected human cell line (HeLa). J Pharmacol Exp Ther 286:354, 1998.

173. Abramson J, Smirnova I, Kasho V, et al: Structure and mechanism of the lactose permease of Escherichia coli. Science 301:610, 2003.

174. Huang Y, Lemieux MJ, Song J, et al: Structure and mechanism of the glycerol-3-phosphate transporter from Escherichia coli. Science 301:616, 2003.

175. Vardy E, Arkin IT, Gottschalk KE, et al: Structural conservation in the major facilitator superfamily as revealed by comparative modeling. Protein Sci 13:1832, 2004.

176. Gorboulev V, Volk C, Arndt P, et al: Selectivity of the polyspecific cation transporter rOCT1 is changed by mutation of aspartate 475 to glutamate. Mol Pharmacol 56:1254, 1999.

177. Bahn A, Hagos Y, Rudolph T, et al: Mutation of amino acid 475 of rat organic cation transporter 2 (rOCT2) impairs organic cation transport. Biochimie 86:133, 2004.

178. Gorboulev V, Shatskaya N, Volk C, et al: Subtype-specific affinity for corticosterone of rat organic cation transporters rOCT1 and rOCT2 depends on three amino acids within the substrate binding region. Mol Pharmacol 67:1612, 2005.

179. Leabman MK, Huang CC, Kawamoto M, et al: Polymorphisms in a human kidney xenobiotic transporter, OCT2, exhibit altered function. Pharmacogenetics 12:395, 2002.

180. Leabman MK, Huang CC, DeYoung J, et al: Natural variation in human membrane transporter genes reveals evolutionary and functional constraints. Proc Natl Acad Sci U S A 100:5896, 2003.

181. Shu Y, Leabman MK, Feng B, et al: Evolutionary conservation predicts function of variants of the human organic cation transporter, OCT1. Proc Natl Acad Sci U S A 100:5902, 2003.

182. Mehrens T, Lelleck S, Cetinkaya I, et al: The affinity of the organic cation transporter rOCT1 is increased by protein kinase C-dependent phosphorylation. J Am Soc Nephrol 11:1216, 2000.

183. Ciarimboli G, Struwe K, Arndt P, et al: Regulation of the human organic cation transporter hOCT1. J Cell Physiol 201:420, 2004.

184. Pietig G, Mehrens T, Hirsch JR: Properties and regulation of organic cation transport in freshly isolated human proximal tubules. J Biol Chem 276:33741, 2001.

185. Cetinkaya I, Ciarimboli G, Yalcinkaya G, et al: Regulation of human organic cation transporter hOCT2 by PKA, PI3K, and calmodulin-dependent kinases. Am J Physiol Renal Physiol 284:F293, 2003.

186. Biermann J, Lang D, Gorboulev V, et al: Characterization of regulatory mechanisms and states of human organic cation transporter 2. Am J Physiol Cell Physiol 290: C1521, 2006.

187. Wolff NA, Thies K, Kuhnke N, et al: Protein kinase C activation downregulates human organic anion transporter 1-mediated transport through carrier internalization. J Am Soc Nephrol 14:1959, 2003.

188. Urakami Y, Nakamura N, Takahashi K, et al: Gender differences in expression of organic cation transporter OCT2 in rat kidney. FEBS Lett 461:339, 1999.

189. Urakami Y, Okuda M, Saito H, et al: Hormonal regulation of organic cation transporter OCT2 expression in rat kidney. FEBS Lett 473:173, 2000.

190. Asaka J, Terada T, Okuda M, et al: Androgen receptor is responsible for rat organic cation transporter 2 gene regulation but not for rOCT1 and rOCT3. Pharm Res 23:697, 2006.

191. Groves CE, Suhre WB, Cherrington NJ, et al: Sex differences in the mRNA, protein, and functional expression of organic anion transporter (Oat) 1, Oat3, and organic cation transporter (Oct) 2 in rabbit renal proximal tubules. J Pharmacol Exp Ther 316:743, 2006.

192. Goralski KB, Lou G, Prowse MT, et al: The cation transporters rOCT1 and rOCT2 interact with bicarbonate but play only a minor role for amantadine uptake into rat renal proximal tubules. J Pharmacol Exp Ther 303:959, 2002.

193. Kristufek D, Rudorfer W, Pifl C, et al: Organic cation transporter mRNA and function in the rat superior cervical ganglion. J Physiol 543:117, 2002.

194. Wu X, Prasad PD, Leibach FH, et al: cDNA sequence, transport function, and genomic organization of human OCTN2, a new member of the organic cation transporter family. Biochem Biophys Res Commun 246:589, 1998.

195. Moseley RH, Jarose SM, Permoad P: Organic cation transport by rat liver plasma membrane vesicles: Studies with tetraethylammonium. Am J Physiol 263:G775, 1992.

196. Wu X, George RL, Huang W, et al: Structural and functional characteristics and tissue distribution pattern of rat OCTN1, an organic cation transporter, cloned from placenta. Biochim Biophys Acta 1466:315, 2000.

197. Ott RJ, Hui AC, Yuan G, et al: Organic cation transport in human renal brush-border membrane vesicles. Am J Physiol 261:F443, 1991.

198. Wang Y, Ye J, Ganapathy V, et al: Mutations in the organic cation/carnitine transporter OCTN2 in primary carnitine deficiency. Proc Natl Acad Sci U S A 96:2356, 1999.

199. Tang NL, Ganapathy V, Wu X, et al: Mutations of OCTN2, an organic cation/carnitine transporter, lead to deficient cellular carnitine uptake in primary carnitine deficiency. Hum Mol Genet 8:655, 1999.

200. Lu K, Nishimori H, Nakamura Y, et al: A missense mutation of mouse OCTN2, a sodium-dependent carnitine cotransporter, in the juvenile visceral steatosis mouse. Biochem Biophys Res Commun 252:590, 1998.

201. Tein I: Carnitine transport: Pathophysiology and metabolism of known molecular defects. J Inherit Metab Dis 26:147, 2003.

202. Lahjouji K, Mitchell GA, Qureshi IA: Carnitine transport by organic cation transporters and systemic carnitine deficiency. Mol Genet Metab 73:287, 2001.

203. Ohashi R, Tamai I, Nezu JJ, et al: Molecular and physiological evidence for multifunctionality of carnitine/organic cation transporter OCTN2. Mol Pharmacol 59:358, 2001.

204. Masuda S, Terada T, Yonezawa A, et al: Identification and functional characterization of a new human kidney-specific h+/organic cation antiporter, kidney-specific multidrug and toxin extrusion 2. J Am Soc Nephrol 17:2127–2135, 2006.

205. Thiebaut F, Tsuruo T, Hamada H, et al: Cellular localization of the multidrug-resistance gene product P-glycoprotein in normal human tissues. Proc Natl Acad Sci U S A 84:7735, 1987.

206. Ernest S, Bello-Reuss E: Expression and function of P-glycoprotein in a mouse kidney cell line. Am J Physiol 269:C323, 1995.

207. Ernest S, Rajaraman S, Megyesi J, et al: Expression of MDR1 (multidrug resistance) gene and its protein in normal human kidney. Nephron 77:284, 1997.

208. Lahjouji K, Mitchell GA, Qureshi IA: Carnitine transport by organic cation transporters and systemic carnitine deficiency. Mol Genet Metab 73:287, 2001.

209. Tamai I, Ohashi R, Nezu J, et al: Molecular and functional identification of sodium ion-dependent, high affinity human carnitine transporter OCTN2. J Biol Chem 273:20378, 1998.

210. Peltekova VD, Wintle RF, Rubin LA, et al: Functional variants of OCTN cation transporter genes are associated with Crohn disease. Nat Genet 36:471, 2004.

211. Fujita T, Urban TJ, Leabman MK, et al: Transport of drugs in the kidney by the human organic cation transporter, OCT2 and its genetic variants. J Pharm Sci 95:25, 2006.

212. Fukushima-Uesaka H, Maekawa K, Ozawa S, et al: Fourteen novel single nucleotide polymorphisms in the SLC22A2 gene encoding human organic cation transporter (OCT2). Drug Metab Pharmacokinet 19:239, 2004.

213. Sakata T, Anzai N, Shin HJ, et al: Novel single nucleotide polymorphisms of organic cation transporter 1 (SLC22A1) affecting transport functions. Biochem Biophys Res Commun 313:789, 2004.

214. Itoda M, Saito Y, Maekawa K, et al: Seven novel single nucleotide polymorphisms in the human SLC22A1 gene encoding organic cation transporter 1 (OCT1). Drug Metab Pharmacokinet 19:308, 2004.

215. Marshall EK Jr, Vickers JL: The mechanism of elimination of phenolsulphonepthalein by the kidney- a proof of secretion by the convoluted tubules. Johns Hopkins Hops (Bull) 34:1, 1923.

216. Marshall EK Jr: The secretion of phenol red by the mammalian kidney. Am J Physiol 24:99, 1931.

217. Smith HW, Finkelstein N, Aliminosa L, et al: The renal clearances of substituted hippuric acid derivatives and other aromatic acids in dog and man. J Clin Invest 24:388, 1945.

218. Malvin RL, Wilde WS, Sullivan LP: Localization of nephron transport by stop flow analysis. Am J Physiol 194:135, 1958.

219. Cortney MA, Mylle M, Lassiter WE, et al: Renal tubular transport of water, solute, and PAH in rats loaded with isotonic saline. Am J Physiol 209:1199, 1965.

220. Tune BM, Burg MB, Patlak CS: Characteristics of p-aminohippurate transport in proximal renal tubules. Am J Physiol 217:1057, 1969.

221. Deeley RG, Cole SP: Substrate recognition and transport by multidrug resistance protein 1 (ABCC1). FEBS Lett 580:1103, 2006.

222. Christensen EI, Birn H: Megalin and cubilin: Multifunctional endocytic receptors. Nat Rev Mol Cell Biol 3:256, 2002.

223. Fritzsch G, Rumrich G, Ullrich KJ: Anion transport through the contraluminal cell membrane of renal proximal tubule. The influence of hydrophobicity and molecular charge distribution on the inhibitory activity of organic anions. Biochim Biophys Acta 978:249, 1989.

224. Hagenbuch B, Meier PJ: The superfamily of organic anion transporting polypeptides. Biochim Biophys Acta 1609:1, 2003.

225. You G: Towards an understanding of organic anion transporters: Structure-function relationships. Med Res Rev 24:762, 2004.

226. Hagenbuch B, Meier PJ: Organic anion transporting polypeptides of the OATP/SLC21 family: Phylogenetic classification as OATP/SLCO superfamily, new nomenclature and molecular/functional properties. Pflugers Arch 447:653, 2004.

227. Mikkaichi T, Suzuki T, Abe T, et al: The organic anion transporter (OATP) family. Drug Metab Pharmacokinet 19:171, 2004.

228. Anzai N, Jutabha P, Kanai Y, et al: Integrated physiology of proximal tubular organic anion transport. Curr Opin Nephrol Hypertens 14:472, 2005.

229. Markovich D, Murer H: The SLC13 gene family of sodium sulphate/carboxylate cotransporters. Pflugers Arch 447:594, 2004.

230. Pajor AM: Molecular properties of the SLC13 family of dicarboxylate and sulfate transporters. Pflugers Arch 451:597, 2006.

231. Sekine T, Miyazaki H, Endou H: Molecular physiology of renal organic anion transporters. Am J Physiol Renal Physiol 290:F251, 2006.

232. Markovich D, Forgo J, Stange G, et al: Expression cloning of rat renal Na+/SO4(2−) cotransport. Proc Natl Acad Sci U S A 90:8073, 1993.

233. Lotscher M, Custer M, Quabius ES, et al: Immunolocalization of Na/SO4-cotransport (NaSi-1) in rat kidney. Pflugers Arch 432:373, 1996.

234. Pajor AM: Sequence and functional characterization of a renal sodium/dicarboxylate cotransporter. J Biol Chem 270:5779, 1995.

235. Pajor AM: Molecular cloning and functional expression of a sodium-dicarboxylate cotransporter from human kidney. Am J Physiol 270:F642, 1996.

236. Bai L, Pajor AM: Expression cloning of NaDC-2, an intestinal Na(+)- or Li(+)-dependent dicarboxylate transporter. Am J Physiol 273:G267, 1997.

237. Pajor AM, Sun NN: Molecular cloning, chromosomal organization, and functional characterization of a sodium-dicarboxylate cotransporter from mouse kidney. Am J Physiol Renal Physiol 279:F482, 2000.

238. Sekine T, Cha SH, Hosoyamada M, et al: Cloning, functional characterization, and localization of a rat renal Na+-dicarboxylate transporter. Am J Physiol 275:F298, 1998.

239. Chen XZ, Shayakul C, Berger UV, et al: Characterization of a rat Na+-dicarboxylate cotransporter. J Biol Chem 273:20972, 1998.

240. Srere PA: The molecular physiology of citrate. Curr Top Cell Regul 33:261–75:261, 1992.

241. Simpson DP: Citrate excretion: a window on renal metabolism. Am J Physiol 244: F223, 1983.

242. Hentschel H, Burckhardt BC, Scholermann B, et al: Basolateral localization of flounder Na+-dicarboxylate cotransport (fNaDC-3) in the kidney of Pleuronectes americanus. Pflugers Arch 446:578, 2003.

243. Bai X, Chen X, Feng Z, et al: Identification of basolateral membrane targeting signal of human sodium-dependent dicarboxylate transporter 3. J Cell Physiol 206:821, 2006.

244. Chen X, Tsukaguchi H, Chen XZ, et al: Molecular and functional analysis of SDCT2, a novel rat sodium-dependent dicarboxylate transporter. J Clin Invest 103:1159, 1999.

245. Kekuda R, Wang H, Huang W, et al: Primary structure and functional characteristics of a mammalian sodium-coupled high affinity dicarboxylate transporter. J Biol Chem 274:3422, 1999.

246. Pajor AM, Gangula R, Yao X: Cloning and functional characterization of a high-affinity Na(+)/dicarboxylate cotransporter from mouse brain. Am J Physiol Cell Physiol 280: C1215, 2001.

247. Chen X, Tsukaguchi H, Chen XZ, et al: Molecular and functional analysis of SDCT2, a novel rat sodium-dependent dicarboxylate transporter. J Clin Invest 103:1159, 1999.

248. Pajor AM, Sun N: Functional differences between rabbit and human Na(+)-dicarboxylate cotransporters, NaDC-1 and hNaDC-1. Am J Physiol 271:F1093, 1996.

249. Welborn JR, Shpun S, Dantzler WH, et al: Effect of alpha-ketoglutarate on organic anion transport in single rabbit renal proximal tubules. Am J Physiol 274:F165, 1998.

250. Miller DS, Stewart DE, Pritchard JB: Intracellular compartmentation of organic anions within renal cells. Am J Physiol 264:R882, 1993.

251. Smith HW, Finkelstein N, Aliminosa L, et al: The renal clearances of substituted hippuric acid derivatives and other aromatic acids in dog and man. J Clin Invest 24:388, 1945.

252. Sekine T, Watanabe N, Hosoyamada M, et al: Expression cloning and characterization of a novel multispecific organic anion transporter. J Biol Chem 272:18526, 1997.

253. Sweet DH, Wolff NA, Pritchard JB: Expression cloning and characterization of ROAT1. The basolateral organic anion transporter in rat kidney. J Biol Chem 272:30088, 1997.

254. Wolff NA, Werner A, Burkhardt S, et al: Expression cloning and characterization of a renal organic anion transporter from winter flounder. FEBS Lett 417:287, 1997.

255. Shimada H, Moewes B, Burckhardt G: Indirect coupling to Na+ of p-aminohippuric acid uptake into rat renal basolateral membrane vesicles. Am J Physiol 253:F795, 1987.

256. Kusuhara H, Sekine T, Utsunomiya-Tate N, et al: Molecular cloning and characterization of a new multispecific organic anion transporter from rat brain. J Biol Chem 274:13675, 1999.

257. Sekine T, Cha SH, Tsuda M, et al: Identification of multispecific organic anion transporter 2 expressed predominantly in the liver. FEBS Lett 429:179, 1998.

258. Cha SH, Sekine T, Kusuhara H, et al: Molecular cloning and characterization of multispecific organic anion transporter 4 expressed in the placenta. J Biol Chem 275:4507, 2000.

259. Ekaratanawong S, Anzai N, Jutabha P, et al: Human organic anion transporter 4 is a renal apical organic anion/dicarboxylate exchanger in the proximal tubules. J Pharmacol Sci 94:297, 2004.

260. Enomoto A, Kimura H, Chairoungdua A, et al: Molecular identification of a renal urate anion exchanger that regulates blood urate levels. Nature 417:447, 2002.

261. Tamai I, Nezu J, Uchino H, et al: Molecular identification and characterization of novel members of the human organic anion transporter (OATP) family. Biochem Biophys Res Commun 273:251, 2000.

262. Meier PJ, Eckhardt U, Schroeder A, et al: Substrate specificity of sinusoidal bile acid and organic anion uptake systems in rat and human liver. Hepatology 26:1667, 1997.

263. Jacquemin E, Hagenbuch B, Stieger B, et al: Expression cloning of a rat liver Na(+)-independent organic anion transporter. Proc Natl Acad Sci U S A 91:133, 1994.

264. Mikkaichi T, Suzuki T, Onogawa T, et al: Isolation and characterization of a digoxin transporter and its rat homologue expressed in the kidney. Proc Natl Acad Sci U S A 101:3569, 2004.

265. Moe OW, Preisig PA: Dual role of citrate in mammalian urine. Curr Opin Nephrol Hypertens 15:419, 2006.

266. Brennan S, Hering-Smith K, Hamm LL: Effect of pH on citrate reabsorption in the proximal convoluted tubule. Am J Physiol 255:F301, 1988.

267. Wright SH, Kippen I, Wright EM: Effect of pH on the transport of Krebs cycle intermediates in renal brush border membranes. Biochim Biophys Acta 684:287, 1982.

268. Aruga S, Wehrli S, Kaissling B, et al: Chronic metabolic acidosis increases NaDC-1 mRNA and protein abundance in rat kidney. Kidney Int 58:206, 2000.

269. Melnick JZ, Srere PA, Elshourbagy NA, et al: Adenosine triphosphate citrate lyase mediates hypocitraturia in rats. J Clin Invest 98:2381, 1996.

270. Melnick JZ, Preisig PA, Moe OW, et al: Renal cortical mitochondrial aconitase is regulated in hypo- and hypercitraturia. Kidney Intern 54:160, 1998.

271. Moe OW: Kidney stones: Pathophysiology and medical management. Lancet 367:333, 2006.

272. Enomoto A, Endou H: Roles of organic anion transporters (OATs) and a urate transporter (URAT1) in the pathophysiology of human disease. Clin Exp Nephrol 9:195, 2005.

273. Anzai N, Enomoto A, Endou H: Renal urate handling: Clinical relevance of recent advances. Curr Rheumatol Rep 7:227, 2005.

274. Hediger MA, Johnson RJ, Miyazaki H, et al: Molecular physiology of urate transport. Physiology (Bethesda) 20:125–33:125, 2005.

275. Leal-Pinto E, Cohen BE, Abramson RG: Functional analysis and molecular modeling of a cloned urate transporter/channel. J Membr Biol 169:13, 1999.

276. Rappoport JZ, Lipkowitz MS, Abramson RG: Localization and topology of a urate transporter/channel, a galectin, in epithelium-derived cells. Am J Physiol Cell Physiol 281:C1926, 2001.

277. Lipkowitz MS, Leal-Pinto E, Cohen BE, et al: Galectin 9 is the sugar-regulated urate transporter/channel UAT. Glycoconj J 19:491, 2004.

278. Sekine T, Cha SH, Endou H: The multispecific organic anion transporter (OAT) family. Pflugers Arch 440:337, 2000.

279. Nakashima M, Uematsu T, Kosuge K, et al: Pilot study of the uricosuric effect of DuP-753, a new angiotensin II receptor antagonist, in healthy subjects. Eur J Clin Pharmacol 42:333, 1992.

280. Ichida K, Hosoyamada M, Hisatome I, et al: Clinical and molecular analysis of patients with renal hypouricemia in Japan-influence of URAT1 gene on urinary urate excretion. J Am Soc Nephrol 15:164, 2004.

281. Kikuchi Y, Koga H, Yasutomo Y, et al: Patients with renal hypouricemia with exercise-induced acute renal failure and chronic renal dysfunction. Clin Nephrol 53:467, 2000.

282. Wollaston WH: On cystic oxide: a new species of urinary calculus. Trans R Soc Edinb 100:223, 1810.

283. Silbernagl S: The renal handling of amino acids and oligopeptides. Physiol Rev 68:911, 1988.

284. Featherston WR, Rogers QR, Freedland RA: Relative importance of kidney and liver in synthesis of arginine by the rat. Am J Physiol 224:127, 1973.

285. Windmueller HG, Spaeth AE: Source and fate of circulating citrulline. Am J Physiol 241:E473, 1981.

286. Silbernagl S, Volker K, Dantzler WH: Cationic amino acid fluxes beyond the proximal convoluted tubule of rat kidney. Pflugers Arch 429:210, 1994.

287. Dantzler WH, Silbernagl S: Basic amino acid transport in renal papilla: Microinfusion of Henle's loops and vasa recta. Am J Physiol 265:F830, 1993.

288. Handler JS, Kwon HM: Kidney cell survival in high tonicity. Comp Biochem Physiol A Physiol 117:301, 1997.

289. Kwon HM, Handler JS: Cell volume regulated transporters of compatible osmolytes. Curr Opin Cell Biol 7:465, 1995.

290. Mariotti F, Huneau JF, Mahe S, et al: Protein metabolism and the gut. Curr Opin Clin Nutr Metab Care 3:45, 2000.

291. Broer A, Cavanaugh JA, Rasko JE, et al: The molecular basis of neutral aminoacidurias. Pflugers Arch 451:511, 2006.

292. Fernandez E, Carrascal M, Rousaud F, et al: rBAT-b(0,+)AT heterodimer is the main apical reabsorption system for cystine in the kidney. Am J Physiol Renal Physiol 283:F540, 2002.

293. Bauch C, Forster N, Loffing-Cueni D, et al: Functional cooperation of epithelial heteromeric amino acid transporters expressed in madin-darby canine kidney cells. J Biol Chem 278:1316, 2003.

294. Pineda M, Fernandez E, Torrents D, et al: Identification of a membrane protein, LAT-2, that Co-expresses with 4F2 heavy chain, an L-type amino acid transport activity with broad specificity for small and large zwitterionic amino acids. J Biol Chem 274:19738, 1999.

295. Broer A, Klingel K, Kowalczuk S, et al: Molecular cloning of mouse amino acid transport system B0, a neutral amino acid transporter related to Hartnup disorder. J Biol Chem 279:24467, 2004.

296. Kleta R, Romeo E, Ristic Z, et al: Mutations in SLC6A19, encoding B0AT1, cause Hartnup disorder. Nat Genet 36:999, 2004.

297. Avissar NE, Ryan CK, Ganapathy V, et al: Na(+)-dependent neutral amino acid transporter ATB(0) is a rabbit epithelial cell brush-border protein. Am J Physiol Cell Physiol 281:C963, 2001.

298. Kowalczuk S, Broer A, Munzinger M, et al: Molecular cloning of the mouse IMINO system: An Na+- and Cl--dependent proline transporter. Biochem J 386:417, 2005.

299. Takanaga H, Mackenzie B, Suzuki Y, et al: Identification of mammalian proline transporter SIT1 (SLC6A20) with characteristics of classical system imino. J Biol Chem 280:8974, 2005.

300. Anderson CM, Grenade DS, Boll M, et al: H+/amino acid transporter 1 (PAT1) is the imino acid carrier: An intestinal nutrient/drug transporter in human and rat. Gastroenterology 127:1410, 2004.

301. Nakanishi T, Hatanaka T, Huang W, et al: Na+- and Cl--coupled active transport of carnitine by the amino acid transporter ATB(0,+) from mouse colon expressed in HRPE cells and Xenopus oocytes. J Physiol 532:297, 2001.

302. Levy LL: Hartnup disorder. In Scriver CS, Beaudet AL, Sly WS, Valle D (eds): The Metabolic and Molecular Basis of Inherited Diseases, 8th ed. New York, McGraw-Hill, 2001, p 4957.

303. Boll M, Foltz M, Rubio-Aliaga I, et al: Functional characterization of two novel mammalian electrogenic proton-dependent amino acid cotransporters. J Biol Chem 277:22966, 2002.

304. Quan H, Athirakul K, Wetsel WC, et al: Hypertension and impaired glycine handling in mice lacking the orphan transporter XT2. Mol Cell Biol 24:4166, 2004.

305. Obermuller N, Kranzlin B, Verma R, et al: Renal osmotic stress-induced cotransporter: Expression in the newborn, adult and post-ischemic rat kidney. Kidney Int 52:1584, 1997.

306. Levy HL: Genetic screening. Adv Hum Genet 4:1–104:1, 1973.

307. Daniel H: Molecular and integrative physiology of intestinal peptide transport. Annu Rev Physiol 66:361–384, 2004.

308. Rubio-Aliaga I, Frey I, Boll M, et al: Targeted disruption of the peptide transporter Pept2 gene in mice defines its physiological role in the kidney. Mol Cell Biol 23:3247, 2003.

309. Fernandez E, Torrents D, Chillaron J, et al: Basolateral LAT-2 has a major role in the transepithelial flux of L-cystine in the renal proximal tubule cell line OK. J Am Soc Nephrol 14:837, 2003.

310. Kim DK, Kanai Y, Chairoungdua A, et al: Expression cloning of a Na+-independent aromatic amino acid transporter with structural similarity to H+/monocarboxylate transporters. J Biol Chem 276:17221, 2001.

311. Kim dK, Kanai Y, Matsuo H, et al: The human T-type amino acid transporter-1: Characterization, gene organization, and chromosomal location. Genomics 79:95, 2002.

312. Ramadan T, Camargo SM, Summa V, et al: Basolateral aromatic amino acid transporter TAT1 (Slc16a10) functions as an efflux pathway. J Cell Physiol 206:771, 2006.

313. Halestrap AP, Meredith D: The SLC16 gene family-from monocarboxylate transporters (MCTs) to aromatic amino acid transporters and beyond. Pflugers Arch 447:619, 2004.

314. Babu E, Kanai Y, Chairoungdua A, et al: Identification of a novel system L amino acid transporter structurally distinct from heterodimeric amino acid transporters. J Biol Chem 278:43838, 2003.

315. Bodoy S, Martin L, Zorzano A, et al: Identification of LAT4, a novel amino acid transporter with system L activity. J Biol Chem 280:12002, 2005.

316. Stuart RO, Pavlova A, Beier D, et al: EEG1, a putative transporter expressed during epithelial organogenesis: Comparison with embryonic transporter expression during nephrogenesis. Am J Physiol Renal Physiol 281:F1148, 2001.

317. Silbernagl S, Volkl H: Molecular specificity of the tubular resorption of "acidic" amino acids. A continuous microperfusion study in rat kidney in vivo. Pflugers Arch 396:225, 1983.

318. Silbernagl S: Kinetics and localization of tubular resorption of "acidic" amino acids. A microperfusion and free flow micropuncture study in rat kidney. Pflugers Arch 396:218, 1983.

319. Hediger MA: Glutamate transporters in kidney and brain. Am J Physiol 277:F487, 1999.

320. Smith CP, Weremowicz S, Kanai Y, et al: Assignment of the gene coding for the human high-affinity glutamate transporter EAAC1 to 9p24: Potential role in dicarboxylic aminoaciduria and neurodegenerative disorders. Genomics 20:335, 1994.

321. Shayakul C, Kanai Y, Lee WS, et al: Localization of the high-affinity glutamate transporter EAAC1 in rat kidney. Am J Physiol 273:F1023, 1997.

322. Kanai Y, Hediger MA: Primary structure and functional characterization of a high-affinity glutamate transporter. Nature 360:467, 1992.

323. Peghini P, Janzen J, Stoffel W: Glutamate transporter EAAC-1-deficient mice develop dicarboxylic aminoaciduria and behavioral abnormalities but no neurodegeneration. EMBO J 16:3822, 1997.

324. Weiss SD, McNamara PD, Pepe LM, et al: Glutamine and glutamic acid uptake by rat renal brushborder membrane vesicles. J Membr Biol 43:91, 1978.

325. Sacktor B, Rosenbloom IL, Liang CT, et al: Sodium gradient- and sodium plus potassium gradient-dependent L-glutamate uptake in renal basolateral membrane vesicles. J Membr Biol 60:63, 1981.

326. Pines G, Danbolt NC, Bjoras M, et al: Cloning and expression of a rat brain L-glutamate transporter. Nature 360:464, 1992.

327. Shashidharan P, Wittenberg I, Plaitakis A: Molecular cloning of human brain glutamate/aspartate transporter II. Biochim Biophys Acta 1191:393, 1994.

328. Fan MZ, Matthews JC, Etienne NM, et al: Expression of apical membrane L-glutamate transporters in neonatal porcine epithelial cells along the small intestinal crypt-villus axis. Am J Physiol Gastrointest Liver Physiol 287:G385, 2004.

329. Welbourne TC, Matthews JC: Glutamate transport and renal function. Am J Physiol 277:F501, 1999.

330. Tanaka K, Watase K, Manabe T, et al: Epilepsy and exacerbation of brain injury in mice lacking the glutamate transporter GLT-1. Science 276:1699, 1997.

331. Garrod AE: Inborn errors of metabolism (lectures I-IV). Lancet 2:1, 1908.

332. Palacin M, Fernandez E, Chillaron J, et al: The amino acid transport system b(o,+) and cystinuria. Mol Membr Biol 18:21, 2001.

333. Perheentupa J, Visakorpi JK: Protein intolerance with deficient transport of basic aminoacids. Another inborn error of metabolism. Lancet 2:813, 1965.

334. Whelan DT, Scriver CR: Hyperdibasicaminoaciduria: An inherited disorder of amino acid transport. Pediatr Res 2:525, 1968.

335. Omura K, Yamanaka N, Higami S, et al: Lysine malabsorption syndrome: A new type of transport defect. Pediatrics 57:102, 1976.

336. Palacin M, Estevez R, Bertran J, et al: Molecular biology of mammalian plasma membrane amino acid transporters. Physiol Rev 78:969, 1998.

337. Chillaron J, Roca R, Valencia A, et al: Heteromeric amino acid transporters: Biochemistry, genetics, and physiology. Am J Physiol Renal Physiol 281:F995, 2001.

338. Calonge MJ, Gasparini P, Chillaron J, et al: Cystinuria caused by mutations in rBAT, a gene involved in the transport of cystine. Nat Genet 6:420, 1994.

339. Feliubadalo L, Font M, Purroy J, et al: Non-type I cystinuria caused by mutations in SLC7A9, encoding a subunit (bo,+AT) of rBAT. Nat Genet 23:52, 1999.

340. Borsani G, Bassi MT, Sperandeo MP, et al: SLC7A7, encoding a putative permease-related protein, is mutated in patients with lysinuric protein intolerance. Nat Genet 21:297, 1999.

341. Torrents D, Mykkanen J, Pineda M, et al: Identification of SLC7A7, encoding y+LAT-1, as the lysinuric protein intolerance gene. Nat Genet 21:293, 1999.

342. Baron DN, Dent CE, Harris H, et al: Hereditary pellagra-like skin rash with temporary cerebellar ataxia, constant renal amino-aciduria, and other bizarre biochemical features. Lancet 271:421, 1956.

343. Scriver CR, Efron ML, Schafer IA: Renal tubular transport of proline, hydroxyproline, and glycine in health and in familial hyperprolinemia. J Clin Invest 43:374–85:374, 1964.

344. Rosenberg LE, Durant JL, Elsas LJ: Familial iminoglycinuria. An inborn error of renal tubular transport. N Engl J Med 278:1407, 1968.

345. Scriver CR: Renal tubular transport of proline, hydroxyproline, and glycine. 3. Genetic basis for more than one mode of transport in human kidney. J Clin Invest 47:823, 1968.

346. Chesney RW: Iminoglycinuria. In Scriver CR, Beaudet AL, Sly WS, Valle D (eds): The Metabolic and Molecular Basis of Inherited Disease, 8th ed. New York, McGraw-Hill, 2001, p 4971.

347. Brodehl J, Gellissen K, Kowalewski S: [An isolated defect of the tubular cystine reabsorption in a family with idiopathic hypoparathyroidism]. Klin Wochenschr 45:38, 1967.

348. Seow HF, Broer S, Broer A, et al: Hartnup disorder is caused by mutations in the gene encoding the neutral amino acid transporter SLC6A19. Nat Genet 36:1003, 2004.

349. Teijema HL, van Gelderen HH, Giesberts MA, et al: Dicarboxylic aminoaciduria: An inborn error of glutamate and aspartate transport with metabolic implications, in combination with a hyperprolinemia. Metabolism 23:115, 1974.

350. Melancon SB, Dallaire L, Lemieux B, et al: Dicarboxylic aminoaciduria: An inborn error of amino acid conservation. J Pediatr 91:422, 1977.

351. Kanai Y, Stelzner M, Nussberger S, et al: The neuronal and epithelial human high affinity glutamate transporter. Insights into structure and mechanism of transport. J Biol Chem 269:20599, 1994.

352. Palacin M, Kanai Y: The ancillary proteins of HATs: SLC3 family of amino acid transporters. Pflugers Arch 447:490, 2004.

353. Verrey F, Closs EI, Wagner CA, et al: CATs and HATs: the SLC7 family of amino acid transporters. Pflugers Arch 447:532, 2004.

354. Ohgimoto S, Tabata N, Suga S, et al: Molecular characterization of fusion regulatory protein-1 (FRP-1) that induces multinucleated giant cell formation of monocytes and HIV gp160-mediated cell fusion. FRP-1 and 4F2/CD98 are identical molecules. J Immunol 155:3585, 1995.

355. Chairoungdua A, Kanai Y, Matsuo H, et al: Identification and characterization of a novel member of the heterodimeric amino acid transporter family presumed to be associated with an unknown heavy chain. J Biol Chem 276:49390, 2001.

356. Matsuo H, Kanai Y, Kim JY, et al: Identification of a novel Na+-independent acidic amino acid transporter with structural similarity to the member of a heterodimeric amino acid transporter family associated with unknown heavy chains. J Biol Chem 277:21017, 2002.

357. Fornandez E, Torrents D, Zorzano A, et al: Identification and functional characterization of a novel low affinity aromatic-preferring amino acid transporter (arpAT). One of the few proteins silenced during primate evolution. J Biol Chem 280:19364, 2005.

358. Gasol E, Jimenez-Vidal M, Chillaron J, et al: Membrane topology of system xc light subunit reveals a re-entrant loop with substrate-restricted accessibility. J Biol Chem 279:31228, 2004.

359. Pineda M, Wagner CA, Broer A, et al: Cystinuria-specific rBAT(R365W) mutation reveals two translocation pathways in the amino acid transporter rBAT-b0,+AT. Biochem J 377:665, 2004.

360. Palacin M, Estevez R, Zorzano A: Cystinuria calls for heteromultimeric amino acid transporters. Curr Opin Cell Biol 10:455, 1998.

361. Chillaron J, Estevez R, Mora C, et al: Obligatory amino acid exchange via systems bo,+-like and y+L-like. A tertiary active transport mechanism for renal reabsorption of cystine and dibasic amino acids. J Biol Chem 271:17761, 1996.

362. Broer A, Wagner CA, Lang F, et al: The heterodimeric amino acid transporter 4F2hc/y+LAT2 mediates arginine efflux in exchange with glutamine. Biochem J 349 Pt 3:787–95:787, 2000.

363. Kanai Y, Fukasawa Y, Cha SH, et al: Transport properties of a system y+L neutral and basic amino acid transporter. Insights into the mechanisms of substrate recognition. J Biol Chem 275:20787, 2000.

364. Segal S, Thier SO: Cystinuria. In Scriver CS, Beaudet AL, Sly WS, Valle D (eds): The Metabolic and Molecular Basis of Inherited Disease. New York, McGraw-Hill, 1995, p 3581.

365. Font-Llitjos M, Jimenez-Vidal M, Bisceglia L, et al: New insights into cystinuria: 40 new mutations, genotype-phenotype correlation, and digenic inheritance causing partial phenotype. J Med Genet 42:58, 2005.

366. Goodyer PR, Clow C, Reade T, et al: Prospective analysis and classification of patients with cystinuria identified in a newborn screening program. J Pediatr 122:568, 1993.

367. Dello SL, Pras E, Pontesilli C, et al: Comparison between SLC3A1 and SLC7A9 cystinuria patients and carriers: A need for a new classification. J Am Soc Nephrol 13:2547, 2002.

368. Skopkova Z, Hrabincova E, Stastna S, et al: Molecular genetic analysis of SLC3A1 and SLC7A9 genes in Czech and Slovak cystinuric patients. Ann Hum Genet 69:501, 2005.

369. Jaeken J, Martens K, Francois I, et al: Deletion of PREPL, a gene encoding a putative serine oligopeptidase, in patients with hypotonia-cystinuria syndrome. Am J Hum Genet 78:38, 2006.

370. Yuen YP, Lam CW, Lai CK, et al: Heterogeneous mutations in the SLC3A1 and SLC7A9 genes in Chinese patients with cystinuria. Kidney Int 69:123, 2006.

371. Henthorn PS, Liu J, Gidalevich T, et al: Canine cystinuria: Polymorphism in the canine SLC3A1 gene and identification of a nonsense mutation in cystinuric Newfoundland dogs. Hum Genet 107:295, 2000.

372. Peters T, Thaete C, Wolf S, et al: A mouse model for cystinuria type I. Hum Mol Genet 12:2109, 2003.

373. Chillaron J, Estevez R, Samarzija I, et al: An intracellular trafficking defect in type I cystinuria rBAT mutants M467T and M467K. J Biol Chem 272:9543, 1997.

374. Saadi I, Chen XZ, Hediger M, et al: Molecular genetics of cystinuria: mutation analysis of SLC3A1 and evidence for another gene in type I (silent) phenotype. Kidney Int 54:48, 1998.

375. Torras-Llort M, Torrents D, Soriano-Garcia JF, et al: Sequential amino acid exchange across b(0,+)-like system in chicken brush border jejunum. J Membr Biol 180:213, 2001.

376. Bisceglia L, Calonge MJ, Totaro A, et al: Localization, by linkage analysis, of the cystinuria type III gene to chromosome 19q13.1. Am J Hum Genet 60:611, 1997.

377. Wartenfeld R, Golomb E, Katz G, et al: Molecular analysis of cystinuria in Libyan Jews: Exclusion of the SLC3A1 gene and mapping of a new locus on 19q. Am J Hum Genet 60:617, 1997.

378. Stoller ML, Bruce JE, Bruce CA, et al: Linkage of type II and type III cystinuria to 19q13.1: Codominant inheritance of two cystinuric alleles at 19q13.1 produces an extreme stone-forming phenotype. Am J Med Genet 86:134, 1999.

379. Palacin M, Nunes V, Font-Llitjos M, et al: The genetics of heteromeric amino acid transporters. Physiology (Bethesda) 20:112–24:112, 2005.

380. Feliubadalo L, Arbones ML, Manas S, et al: Slc7a9-deficient mice develop cystinuria non-I and cystine urolithiasis. Hum Mol Genet 12:2097, 2003.

381. Font MA, Feliubadalo L, Estivill X, et al: Functional analysis of mutations in SLC7A9, and genotype-phenotype correlation in non-Type I cystinuria. Hum Mol Genet 10:305, 2001.

382. Reig N, Chillaron J, Bartoccioni P, et al: The light subunit of system b(o,+) is fully functional in the absence of the heavy subunit. EMBO J 21:4906, 2002.

383. Schmidt C, Tomiuk J, Botzenhart E, et al: Genetic variations of the SLC7A9 gene: allele distribution of 13 polymorphic sites in German cystinuria patients and controls. Clin Nephrol 59:353, 2003.

384. Leclerc D, Wu Q, Ellis JR, et al: Is the SLC7A10 gene on chromosome 19 a candidate locus for cystinuria? Mol Genet Metab 73:333, 2001.

385. Calonge MJ, Volpini V, Bisceglia L, et al: Genetic heterogeneity in cystinuria: The SLC3A1 gene is linked to type I but not to type III cystinuria. Proc Natl Acad Sci U S A 92:9667, 1995.

386. Gasparini P, Calonge MJ, Bisceglia L, et al: Molecular genetics of cystinuria: Identification of four new mutations and seven polymorphisms, and evidence for genetic heterogeneity. Am J Hum Genet 57:781, 1995.

387. Schmidt C, Vester U, Wagner CA, et al: Significant contribution of genomic rearrangements in SLC3A1 and SLC7A9 to the etiology of cystinuria. Kidney Int 64:1564, 2003.

388. Leclerc D, Boutros M, Suh D, et al: SLC7A9 mutations in all three cystinuria subtypes. Kidney Int 62:1550, 2002.

389. Harnevik L, Fjellstedt E, Molbaek A, et al: Mutation analysis of SLC7A9 in cystinuria patients in Sweden. Genet Test 7:13, 2003.

390. Bauch C, Verrey F: Apical heterodimeric cystine and cationic amino acid transporter expressed in MDCK cells. Am J Physiol Renal Physiol 283:F181, 2002.

391. Koizumi A, Matsuura N, Inoue S, et al: Evaluation of a mass screening program for lysinuric protein intolerance in the northern part of Japan. Genet Test 7:29, 2003.

392. Kekomaki M, Visakorpi JK, Perheentupa J, et al: Familial protein intolerance with deficient transport of basic amino acids. An analysis of 10 patients. Acta Paediatr Scand 56:617, 1967.

393. Oyanagi K, Miura R, Yamanouchi T: Congenital lysinuria: A new inherited transport disorder of dibasic amino acids. J Pediatr 77:259, 1970.

394. Pineda M, Font M, Bassi MT, et al: The amino acid transporter asc-1 is not involved in cystinuria. Kidney Int 66:1453, 2004.

395. Lukkarinen M, Nanto-Salonen K, Pulkki K, et al: Oral supplementation corrects plasma lysine concentrations in lysinuric protein intolerance. Metabolism 52:935, 2003.

396. Parto K, Svedstrom E, Majurin ML, et al: Pulmonary manifestations in lysinuric protein intolerance. Chest 104:1176, 1993.

397. DiRocco M, Garibotto G, Rossi GA, et al: Role of haematological, pulmonary and renal complications in the long-term prognosis of patients with lysinuric protein intolerance. Eur J Pediatr 152:437, 1993.

398. Nagata M, Suzuki M, Kawamura G, et al: Immunological abnormalities in a patient with lysinuric protein intolerance. Eur J Pediatr 146:427, 1987.

399. Deves R, Boyd CA: Transporters for cationic amino acids in animal cells: Discovery, structure, and function. Physiol Rev 78:487, 1998.

400. Bertran J, Magagnin S, Werner A, et al: Stimulation of system y(+)-like amino acid transport by the heavy chain of human 4F2 surface antigen in Xenopus laevis oocytes. Proc Natl Acad Sci U S A 89:5606, 1992.

401. Wells RG, Lee WS, Kanai Y, et al: The 4F2 antigen heavy chain induces uptake of neutral and dibasic amino acids in Xenopus oocytes. J Biol Chem 267:15285, 1992.

402. Torrents D, Estevez R, Pineda M, et al: Identification and characterization of a membrane protein (y+L amino acid transporter-1) that associates with 4F2hc to encode the amino acid transport activity y+L. A candidate gene for lysinuric protein intolerance. J Biol Chem 273:32437, 1998.

403. Mastroberardino L, Spindler B, Pfeiffer R, et al: Amino-acid transport by heterodimers of 4F2hc/CD98 and members of a permease family. Nature 395:288, 1998.

404. Kanai Y, Segawa H, Miyamoto K, et al: Expression cloning and characterization of a transporter for large neutral amino acids activated by the heavy chain of 4F2 antigen (CD98). J Biol Chem 273:23629, 1998.

405. Pfeiffer R, Rossier G, Spindler B, et al: Amino acid transport of y+L-type by heterodimers of 4F2hc/CD98 and members of the glycoprotein-associated amino acid transporter family. EMBO J 18:49, 1999.

406. Lauteala T, Sistonen P, Savontaus ML, et al: Lysinuric protein intolerance (LPI) gene maps to the long arm of chromosome 14. Am J Hum Genet 60:1479, 1997.

407. Lauteala T, Mykkanen J, Sperandeo MP, et al: Genetic homogeneity of lysinuric protein intolerance. Eur J Hum Genet 6:612, 1998.

408. Mykkanen J, Torrents D, Pineda M, et al: Functional analysis of novel mutations in y(+)LAT-1 amino acid transporter gene causing lysinuric protein intolerance (LPI). Hum Mol Genet 9:431, 2000.

409. Smith DW, Scriver CR, Simell O: Lysinuric protein intolerance mutation is not expressed in the plasma membrane of erythrocytes. Hum Genet 80:395, 1988.

410. Dall'Asta V, Bussolati O, Sala R, et al: Arginine transport through system y(+)L in cultured human fibroblasts: Normal phenotype of cells from LPI subjects. Am J Physiol Cell Physiol 279:C1829, 2000.

411. Sperandeo MP, Bassi MT, Riboni M, et al: Structure of the SLC7A7 gene and mutational analysis of patients affected by lysinuric protein intolerance. Am J Hum Genet 66:92, 2000.

412. Sperandeo MP, Annunziata P, Ammendola V, et al: Lysinuric protein intolerance: Identification and functional analysis of mutations of the SLC7A7 gene. Hum Mutat 25:410, 2005.

413. Tsumura H, Suzuki N, Saito H, et al: The targeted disruption of the CD98 gene results in embryonic lethality. Biochem Biophys Res Commun 308:847, 2003.

414. Toivonen M, Mykkanen J, Aula P, et al: Expression of normal and mutant GFP-tagged y(+)L amino acid transporter-1 in mammalian cells. Biochem Biophys Res Commun 291:1173, 2002.

415. Sperandeo MP, Paladino S, Maiuri L, et al: A y(+)LAT-1 mutant protein interferes with y(+)LAT-2 activity: Implications for the molecular pathogenesis of lysinuric protein intolerance. Eur J Hum Genet 13:628, 2005.

416. Morin CL, Thompson MW, Jackson SH, et al: Biochemical and genetic studies in cystinuria: Observations on double heterozygotes of genotype I-II. J Clin Invest 50:1961, 1971.

417. Simell O, Perheentupa J: Renal handling of diamino acids in lysinuric protein intolerance. J Clin Invest 54:9, 1974.

418. Desjeux JF, Simell RO, Dumontier AM, et al: Lysine fluxes across the jejunal epithelium in lysinuric protein intolerance. J Clin Invest 65:1382, 1980.

419. Rajantie J, Simell O, Perheentupa J: Lysinuric protein intolerance. Basolateral transport defect in renal tubuli. J Clin Invest 67:1078, 1981.

420. Rajantie J, Simell O, Perheentupa J: Basolateral-membrane transport defect for lysine in lysinuric protein intolerance. Lancet 1:1219, 1980.

421. Rajantie J, Simell O, Perheentupa J: Intestinal absorption in lysinuric protein intolerance: Impaired for diamino acids, normal for citrulline. Gut 21:519, 1980.

422. Groneberg DA, Doring F, Eynott PR, et al: Intestinal peptide transport: Ex vivo uptake studies and localization of peptide carrier PEPT1. Am J Physiol Gastrointest Liver Physiol 281:G697, 2001.

423. Adibi SA: Intestinal transport of dipeptides in man: Relative importance of hydrolysis and intact absorption. J Clin Invest 50:2266, 1971.

424. Asatoor AM, Crouchman MR, Harrison AR, et al: Intestinal absorption of oligopeptides in cystinuria. Clin Sci 41:23, 1971.

425. Mathews DM, Adibi SA: Peptide absorption. Gastroenterology 71:151, 1976.

426. Scriver CR, Mahon B, Levy HL, et al: The Hartnup phenotype: Mendelian transport disorder, multifactorial disease. Am J Hum Genet 40:401, 1987.

427. Mailliard ME, Stevens BR, Mann GE: Amino acid transport by small intestinal, hepatic, and pancreatic epithelia. Gastroenterology 108:888, 1995.

428. Bohmer C, Broer A, Munzinger M, et al: Characterization of mouse amino acid transporter B0AT1 (slc6a19). Biochem J 389:745, 2005.

429. Nozaki J, Dakeishi M, Ohura T, et al: Homozygosity mapping to chromosome 5p15 of a gene responsible for Hartnup disorder. Biochem Biophys Res Commun 284:255, 2001.

430. Yamashita A, Singh SK, Kawate T, et al: Crystal structure of a bacterial homologue of Na$^+$/Cl$^-$-dependent neurotransmitters. Nature 437:215, 2005.

431. Wilcken B, Yu JS, Brown DA: Natural history of Hartnup disease. Arch Dis Child 52:38, 1977.

CHAPTER 7

Renal Acidification

L. Lee Hamm • Nazih L. Nakhoul

The kidneys have two major roles in acid-base homeostasis: (1) reabsorption of the bicarbonate (HCO_3^-) filtered at the glomerulus (~4000 mmoles to 4500 mmoles per day depending on glomerular filtration rate (GFR) and plasma bicarbonate); and (2) excretion of acid and ammonium (NH_4^+) to accomplish production of "new" bicarbonate to replace that consumed by dietary or endogenous metabolic acids. As will be discussed, both functions rely on H^+ secretion in the various segments of the nephron. Dietary and endogenous acids usually amount to about 1 mEq/Kg body weight per day on a typical Western diet.[1] Regarding the reabsorption of filtered HCO_3^-, the proximal tubule accounts for the majority (~75% to 80%) of this reabsorption as illustrated in Figure 7–1. Without this reabsorption, as in proximal renal tubular acidosis, HCO_3^- spills into the urine, lowering plasma HCO_3^- and causing metabolic acidosis. However, normally almost all of the filtered HCO_3^- is reabsorbed.

The second function of the kidneys is to generate "new" HCO_3^-; "new" HCO_3^- refers to HCO_3^- that is produced by the kidneys, but that was not filtered at the glomerulus. Production of new HCO_3^- is also critical in regulating plasma HCO_3^- concentration and hence acid-base balance. This is accomplished in two ways: excretion of titratable acid (TA) and excretion of NH_4^+. Titratable acid refers to acid excreted that has titrated urinary buffers. Titratable acid equals the amount of acid (H^+) that is added to tubular fluid along the nephron, thus titrating urinary buffers. Titratable acid is a function of both urine pH and buffering capacity.[2] Excretion of H^+ (or the equivalent) produces HCO_3^- in a HCO_3^-/CO_2 buffered physiologic system in which pCO_2 is in essence fixed by pulmonary excretion. Although HCO_3^-/CO_2 is not the only physiologic buffer system, it reflects the status of all the physiologic buffers. Phosphate is the principal urinary buffer, but creatinine, citrate, and a variety of organic solutes also function as urinary buffers to some extent.[2]

Urinary NH_4^+ accomplishes production of "new" HCO_3^- and excretion of acid indirectly; in contrast to prior concepts this does not occur directly via NH_3 acting as a proton acceptor ($NH_3 + H^+ \leftrightarrow NH_4^+$). Total ammonia, $NH_3 + NH_4^+$, is predominantly NH_4^+ at physiologic pH (because the pKa of NH_4^+ is ~9) as discussed subsequently. Excretion of NH_4^+ produces "new" bicarbonate from the metabolism of glutamine to HCO_3^- and NH_4^+.[3] Addition of HCO_3^- to plasma is the physiologic equivalent of acid excretion.

The production of new HCO_3^-, or equivalently excretion of acid, is quantified as net acid excretion (NAE). Urinary NAE is usually calculated as

$$NAE = NH_4^+ + TA - HCO_3^-$$

Urinary HCO_3^- is subtracted because the loss of a HCO_3^- in the urine is equivalent to the gain of acid. Urinary HCO_3^- is usually small. The urine also contains a variety of organic anions such as citrate, which if retained, rather than excreted, could be metabolized to HCO_3^-. However, this loss of organic anions has not traditionally been thought to contribute to overall acid-base balance in humans (see discussion of organic acids).

This chapter will cover carbonic anhydrase, then the mechanisms of acid-base transport along the nephron and separately the generation and excretion of NH_4^+. Carbonic anhydrase is important in most nephron segments for acid-base transport and will be covered initially. The prior editions of this text have thoroughly reviewed the development of current concepts of acid-base transport and therefore some aspects that were covered extensively before will be abbreviated. References are selective with emphasis on more recent work. More extensive historical references have been provided in earlier editions.[4]

Prior decades of study of acid-base physiology focused on identifying mechanisms of acid-base transport along the nephron. After clearance studies that relied on indirect inferences about specific nephron segment transport properties, initial studies of proximal tubule transport beginning in the 1960s used in vivo micropuncture of rat superficial proximal tubules.[5] Beginning in the late 1970s, in vitro microperfusion studies, using rabbit and later rat and mouse, expanded the types of studies that could be performed[6,7]; in vivo microperfusion of rat proximal tubules later accomplished similar control of both luminal and basolateral composition. In a similar time frame, studies of transport by membrane vesicles, particularly from the apical and basolateral membranes of the proximal tubule, were extremely valuable in identifying and characterizing mechanisms of acid-base transport. The past decade has been noted for the molecular identification and understanding of acid-base transporters, and the signaling that regulates them; emphasis will be placed on these aspects.

CARBONIC ANHYDRASE AND CO₂ TRANSPORT

Carbonic Anhydrase

Carbonic anhydrase (CA) is an important aspect of HCO_3^- transport all along the nephron. This zinc metalloenzyme catalyzes the reversible reaction[8–11]:

$$CO_2 + OH^- \leftrightarrow HCO_3^-$$

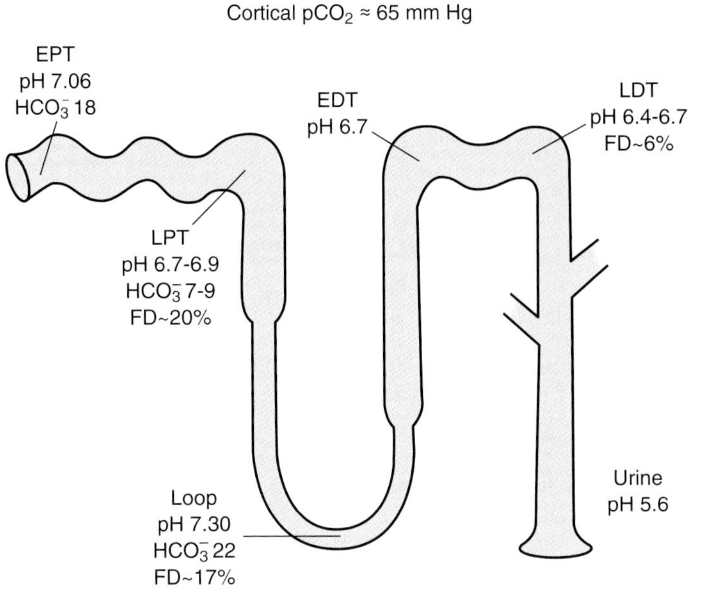

Cortical $pCO_2 \approx 65$ mm Hg

EPT
pH 7.06
HCO_3^- 18

EDT
pH 6.7

LDT
pH 6.4-6.7
FD~6%

LPT
pH 6.7-6.9
HCO_3^- 7-9
FD~20%

Loop
pH 7.30
HCO_3^- 22
FD~17%

Urine
pH 5.6

FIGURE 7-1 Model of over-all bicarbonate reabsorption and lumen pH profile along the nephron. Derived from data in control rats in references 162 and 163. pH and HCO_3^- concentration values are shown for the following sequential nephron segments: early superficial proximal tubule (EPT), late superficial proximal tubule (LPT), bend of Henle's loop (loop), early superficial distal tubule (EDT), and late superficial distal tubule(LDT). FD is fractional delivery of HCO_3^- to those sites where measured. The pCO_2 in the renal cortex has been determined to be ~65 mm Hg.[48-51] See text for additional details.

In physiologic solutions this is equivalent to the more commonly written equation:

$$CO_2 + H_2O \leftrightarrow H_2CO_3 \leftrightarrow HCO_3^- + H^+$$

The uncatalyzed rate of this reaction is very slow, but the catalyzed rate with carbonic anhydrase is accelerated by several orders of magnitude. The presence of CA both inside cells and on the apical and basolateral membrane of tubular epithelial cells greatly accelerates acid-base transport, particularly HCO_3^- reabsorption. In the absence of CA, H^+ secretion into the tubule lumen will result in an H^+ concentration significantly above equilibrium values (a lower pH-H^+ higher-than equilibrium due to the slow equilibration of the previous equation going from right to left). This is a so-called acid disequilibrium pH. A higher H^+ concentration (lower pH) will impede further H^+ secretion whether via Na-H exchange or H^+ ATPase, the two main mechanisms of H^+ secretion (discussed later). The mammalian isoenzymes appear to share three zinc binding histidine residues[8]; the bound zinc metal is crucial for the functional activity of CA.[8,10]

Because of the importance of CA for acid-base transport, the distribution of CA in the kidney has been studied for many years. Initially these studies used histochemical approaches (Hanson's cobalt-phosphate) to detect hydratase activity in tissue sections.[12] Later studies used functional approaches with CA inhibitors. More recent studies have used immuncytochemical methods and molecular methods to detect mRNA for specific isoforms of CA. A great difficulty in integrating these studies is the apparent differences among experimental species and humans. An additional difficulty has been differences between varying techniques and even different antibodies in the same species. These differences have been well reviewed earlier.[4,8,13]

Although there are more than a dozen isoforms of mammalian CA, two isoforms of carbonic anhydrase have been best studied in the kidney, cytosolic CA II and membrane bound CA IV.[8] CA II is present in most cells along the nephron

involved in acid-base transport. CA II is quite sensitive to inhibition by a variety of sulfonamides. In the proximal tubule, cytosolic CA functions to continuously provide both cellular H^+ for luminal secretion and HCO_3^- for extrusion across the basolateral membrane (see model figures in later sections); both H^+ and HCO_3^- derive from H_2O and CO_2 as in the earlier equation. Similar functions pertain to both H^+ secretion and HCO_3^- secretion in more distal nephron segments. An important, but still not completely defined, aspect of CA function now appears to be direct binding and interaction with HCO_3^- transporters such as AE1 and NBC1[14,15]; such interactions may also extend both to other CA, such as CA IV, and to other acid-base transporters such as NHE1.[16-18] CA II also appears to be important in the development of intercalated cells of the collecting duct.[19]

CA IV is less abundant but critically important in several nephron segments, particularly the proximal tubule where large amounts of HCO_3^- are reabsorbed.[20,21] The apical distribution of CA IV is shown in Figure 7-2. CA IV is bound to the apical membrane by a glycosylphosphatidylinositol (GPI) moiety. The presence of functional luminal CA prevents a spontaneous acid disequilibrium pH that would inhibit significant HCO_3^- reabsorption (see later discussion of proximal tubule).[22] Usually a GPI linkage is only associated with apical localization of a membrane protein, but CA IV is also found in the basolateral membranes of some nephron segments (not shown well in Figure 7-2, but well documented). The mechanism of basolateral localization (such as alternately spliced isoform of CA IV or immunologically overlapping isoform) is unknown. CA IV is present on the basolateral membrane of the proximal tubule, probably facilitating HCO_3^- efflux from the cell.[21,23,24] CA IV is also present on the apical and basolateral membranes of the thick ascending limb (TAL).[21]

The importance of membrane bound CA, as distinct from cytosolic CA, has been studied using relatively impermeant CA inhibitors such as benzolamide and also CA inhibitors chemically bound to polymers such as dextran. Such inhibitors can block activity of extracellular CA, but presumably not cytosolic CA. These studies have demonstrated a critical role of both luminal and basolateral membrane bound CA in the proximal tubule.[25-27] Similar studies have also demonstrated the importance of luminal carbonic anhydrous in some distal nephron segments such as the inner stripe portion of outer medullary collecting duct.[28] Direct studies of luminal pH have also been used to establish the presence or absence of functional luminal CA. These studies suggest that most segments of the collecting duct and the final portion of the proximal tubule, the S3 segment, do not have luminal CA.[29-33] However, some segments of the distal tubule and collecting duct (inner stripe portion of the outer medullary collecting duct in rabbit and initial inner medullary collecting duct of rat) have functional luminal CA.[30,31] Those nephron segments without luminal CA are expected to secrete H^+ or reabsorb HCO_3^- at lower rates and luminal pH will be lower (for the same rate of H^+ secretion). The lower luminal pH particularly in the distal collecting duct may augment NH_4^+ secretion by keeping NH_3 concentration lower (see later discussion).

Recent studies demonstrate that both CA II and CA IV increase with metabolic acidosis, facilitating increased rates of acid-base transport.[34-36]

Two other isozymes of membrane bound CA have been recently found in kidney, CA XII and CA XIV.[37-39] CA XII is in the basolateral membranes of the TAL, the distal tubule, and principal cells of the collecting duct.[37,40] CA XII is also present in the proximal tubule and collecting tubules of some species.[41] CA XIV is present in the proximal tubule and thin descending limb.[38] Identifying the functional roles of these enzymes and integration of these findings with prior studies of CA activity will be important in the future.

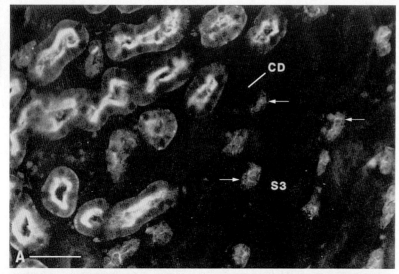

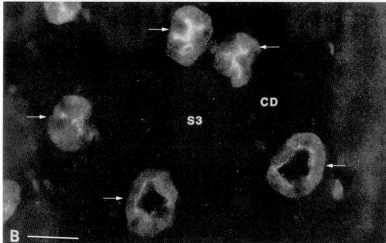

FIGURE 7–2 CA IV staining distribution. **A,** Corticomedullary boundary of a rat kidney. On left, apical aspects of S2 segments of the proximal tubule within the cortex are heavily stained for CA IV. On right, proximal S3 segments in the outer stripe of the outer medulla are negative. With other methods basolateral membranes were also stained. Thick ascending limbs (arrows) are positive, but collecting ducts (CD) are unstained. **B,** Outer stripe of the outer medulla. The CA IV-positive tubules are thick ascending limbs of Henle (arrows). The proximal S3 segments are unstained, and both intercalated and principal cells in collecting ducts (CD) are negative. (From Brown D, Zhu XL, Sly WS: Localization of membrane-associated carbonic anhydrase type IV in kidney epithelial cells. Proc Natl Acad Sci U S A 87:7457–7461, 1990.)

Despite the importance of CA, complete inhibition of CA activity in vivo only reduces whole kidney HCO_3^- reabsorption by 30% to 40%.[42] In vivo, the proximal tubule continues to reabsorb 20% of the filtered load,[42] and the loop of Henle and distal nephron reabsorb significant HCO_3^-.[20,43] The mechanism of the residual HCO_3^- reabsorption in vivo appears to be HCO_3^- gradients from tubule lumen to interstitium during luminal volume absorption.[4,20] Consistent with this mechanism, little if any HCO_3^- reabsorption occurs in nephron segments perfused in vitro during CA inhibition; in this case there are only small transepithelial HCO_3^- gradients.

CO₂ Transport

CO_2 diffusion across cell membranes is critical for HCO_3^- transport, as discussed in the section on the proximal tubule in particular. For instance, CO_2, with H_2O, provides for the cellular H^+ to be secreted across the apical membrane and HCO_3^- to be transported across the basolateral membrane. Rapid CO_2 diffusion across cell membranes is predictable based on high lipid solubility of CO_2.[44] And in fact, very high CO_2 permeability has been measured in intact proximal tubules.[45,46] However, CO_2 diffusion through aqueous solutions is facilitated by CA.[45,47]

Surprisingly, measurements of pCO_2 in most structures of the renal cortex reveal levels higher than arterial pCO_2 (or renal venous blood) by as much as 25 mm Hg.[48–51] This has been attributed to the process of H^+/HCO_3^- transport in the proximal tubule, but more importantly to metabolic CO_2 production, coupled with a counter-current type vascular exchange of CO_2 in the cortex.[4,52–54]

The urine pCO_2 is also significantly greater than arterial pCO_2 during bicarbonaturia; in fact, the urine minus blood pCO_2 gradient has been used to index distal nephron H^+ secretion. The origin of the elevated urine pCO_2 derives from H^+ secretion into the collecting duct lumen, combining with HCO_3^-.[55,56] In this setting two factors contribute to the high CO_2: first, slow uncatalyzed rate of CO_2 formation in the absence of luminal CA in the collecting duct lumen, and second, the countercurrent system in the medulla and low surface area:volume ratio in the renal pelvis and remaining urinary tract, slowing diffusion of CO_2.[4,55,56]

PROXIMAL TUBULE

The proximal tubule reabsorbs 75% to 80% of the filtered bicarbonate. The general features of HCO_3^- reabsorption are shown in Figure 7–3: apical H^+ secretion, basolateral Na^+ coupled HCO_3^- exit from the cell, and facilitation by both membrane bound and cellular carbonic anhydrase. Apical H^+ secretion occurs by both an apical Na-H exchanger and a H^+-ATPase. The apically secreted H^+ reacts with luminal HCO_3^- to form CO_2 and H_2O that are readily permeable across all membranes of the proximal tubule. This initial process removes luminal HCO_3^-. To complete the process of net transepithelial HCO_3^- reabsorption, cellular HCO_3^- derived from $CO_2 + H_2O$ is transported across the basolateral membrane.

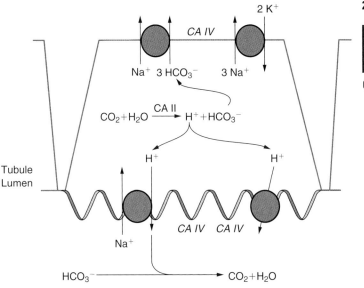

FIGURE 7–3 Model of HCO_3^- reabsorption in the proximal tubule. See text for details.

Mechanisms of H^+ and HCO_3^- Transport

Both the apically secreted H^+ and the basolaterally transported HCO_3^- derive from $CO_2 + H_2O \rightarrow HCO_3^- + H^+$; the CO_2 can be conceptualized as derived from luminal $HCO_3^- \rightarrow CO_2$. Each of the reactions of $HCO_3^- + H^+ \leftrightarrow CO_2 + H_2O$ (in the lumen net $HCO_3^- + H^+ \rightarrow CO_2 + H_2O$; in the cell, net $CO_2 + H_2O \rightarrow HCO_3^- + H^+$) is catalyzed (accelerated) by carbonic anhydrase, both cytoplasmic and membrane bound on the apical and basolateral membranes; in the absence or inhibition of carbonic anhydrase, net transepithelial HCO_3^- reabsorption is markedly inhibited.[42]

The proximal tubule is composed of three specific subsegments (S1, S2, and S3) and differs between juxtamedullary and superficial nephrons[57–59]; the acid-base transport in these subsegments differ both quantitatively (e.g., S1 higher rates of transport than S3) and qualitatively to some extent as will be discussed in more detail later.[60,61] However, many of the mechanisms and regulation of acid-base transport are similar among these areas. The main differences appear to be lower rates of HCO_3^- reabsorption and some different mechanisms in the late proximal tubule (identified as the terminal proximal straight tubule).

Mechanisms of H^+ and HCO_3^- Transport

Conceptually, HCO_3^- reabsorption could occur by either direct HCO_3^- (or base) reabsorption, or secretion of acid (or H^+). The mechanism of HCO_3^- reabsorption was determined to be H^+ secretion rather than direct HCO_3^- reabsorption more than three decades ago.[5] Investigators demonstrated an acid disequilibrium pH using microelectrodes in the proximal tubule lumen during carbonic anhydrase inhibition.[5,62] An acid disequilibrium pH (explained earlier) implies H^+ secretion, rather than base absorption.[4] The acid disequilibrium pH was only seen with inhibition of luminal CA because normally membrane bound CA is active in the proximal tubule.

HCO_3^- reabsorption across the luminal membrane was also found to be sodium dependent, chloride independent, and electroneutral.[7,63,64] Subsequently, studies demonstrated that the mechanism of H^+ secretion involves a Na-H exchanger that exchanges one luminal Na^+ for one cellular H^+; this was shown first using brush border membrane vesicles and later with intact tubules.[65–67] Membrane vesicle experiments demonstrated acid transport with an imposed sodium gradient, and sodium transport with an imposed pH gradient. Additional vesicle experiments demonstrated that the Km for Na^+

is ~5 mM to 15 mM and that the exchanger is sensitive to amiloride and its analogs.[66,68,69] Similar features were subsequently found in intact tubules.[70–73] The high affinity (low Km) for sodium implies that the exchanger will always be maximally saturated for sodium in the proximal tubule in vivo. The competitive inhibition by amiloride and its analogs has been a key feature in identifying Na-H exchangers experimentally.[68,74] This exchange process is responsible for ~2/3 of proximal HCO_3^- reabsorption and is also the major mode of Na^+ reabsorption in the proximal tubule. The driving force for transport is the Na^+ concentration gradient from lumen to cell (~140 mM and ~10–20 mM in lumen and cell, respectively) maintained by basolateral Na-K ATPase. The luminal Na^+ concentration is constant ~140 mEq/L along the length of the proximal tubule due to the near equivalent reabsorption of Na^+ and water.

The apical membrane Na-H exchanger has now been determined to be NHE-3 (Na-H Exchanger 3), a member of the ubiquitous family of Na-H exchangers that regulate intracellular pH and volume, and respond to growth factors, in many cell types.[75] NHE-3 is a 93 kD molecule with 10–13 transmembrane domains and consensus phosphorylation sites for PKA and PKC.[75–77] NHE-3 is distinct from NHE-1, the first cloned and more ubiquitous Na-H exchanger, particularly in tissue distribution and regulation. In contrast to the presence of NHE-1 in most cell types and on the basolateral aspect of many epithelial cells, NHE-3 is restricted to the kidney (predominantly cortex) and intestine, and in these cell types is located on the apical membrane. The regulatory mechanisms are also quite distinct.[75] Many of the molecular features of NHE-3 have been determined and are discussed elsewhere in this volume and also recently reviewed.[75,78] Immunohistochemical studies and studies of NHE-3 knockout animals are the most definitive in indicating a predominant role for NHE-3 in mediating most of proximal HCO_3^- reabsorption.[78–86] In NHE-3 knockout mice, proximal tubule HCO_3^- and volume reabsorption is significantly reduced (leaving most remaining HCO_3^- reabsorption mediated by a bafilomycin sensitive mechanism); a mild acidosis is present, partially compensated by increased distal tubule acid secretion.[81,82,84] This is illustrated in Figure 7–4, which shows the overall reduction of HCO_3^- and fluid reabsorption in NHE-3 knock-out animals, the lack of response to the amiloride analog EIPA, and the bafilomycin sensitive HCO_3^- reabsorption (related to H^+-ATPase discussed later) in both control and knock-out animals. Immunohistochemical studies have demonstrated NHE-3 appropriately localized to the apical membranes of proximal tubules (and thick ascending limbs) (Fig. 7–5).[79,80] Some evidence has supported the possible role of other (possibly unidentified) NHE isoforms in proximal tubule apical transport,[86,87] but this remains controversial. Some studies have suggested a possible role for NHE-2, but most immunohistochemical studies and knock-out mice do not suggest a proximal tubule location or function.[88–90] Similarly, NHE-1 deficient animals do not have systemic acid-base abnormalities.[91] However, Na-H exchange in the late proximal tubule may not be NHE-3.[79] Recently NHE-8 has been localized to the proximal tubule and may play a role in acid excretion.[92] The exchanger in the proximal tubule also transports other cations such as lithium and

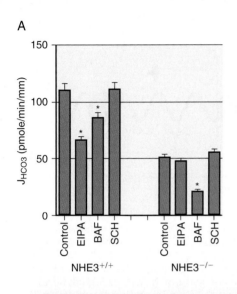

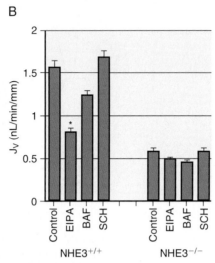

FIGURE 7–4 HCO_3^- and fluid reabsorptive rates (JHCO3 and Jv, respectively) in wild-type and NHE3 null mice. Effects of inhibitors: EIPA, ethylisopropylamiloride to inhibit Na-H exchange; BAF, bafilomycin to inhibit H^+-ATPase; SCH, Sch-28080 to inhibit H-K-ATPase. *Significant difference from control ($P < 0.05$). (From Wang T, Yang CL, Abbiati T, et al: Mechanism of proximal tubule bicarbonate absorption in NHE3 null mice. Am J Physiol 277:F298–F302, 1999.)

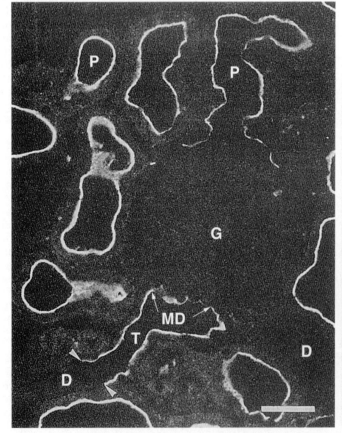

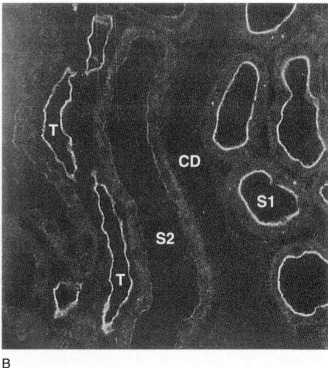

FIGURE 7–5 Immunohistochemical demonstration of NHE-3 distribution in the rat kidney. Shown are staining in the apical membranes of proximal tubules (P) and thick ascending limb (T), but no staining in the distal tubule (D) or glomerulus (G). **A,** *Cortical labyrinth, Immunostaining fro NHE-3.* The proximal brush border is stained from the beginning of the proximal tubule (P). The luminal membranes of the macula densa cells (MD) are weaker stained than those of thick ascending limb cells. NHE-3 protein staining ceases at the transition (arrow heads) of the thick ascending limb (T) to the dista convoluted tubule (D). **B,** *Medullary ray.* Immunostaining for NHE-3 showing that the luminal membranes of thick ascending limbs (T) are heavily stained, collecting ducts (CD) are unstained; weak staining of S2 segments of the proximal tubules in the medullary ray compared to strong staining of S1 in the cortex. (From Amemiya M, Loffing J, Lotscher M, et al: Expression of NHE-3 in the apical membrane of rat renal proximal tubule and thick ascending limb. Kidney Int 48:1206–1215, 1995.)

NH$_4^{+93,94}$ (see later discussion). An important physiologic feature is that the transport rate of the apical Na-H exchanger is augmented by intracellular acidosis via both kinetic and allosteric mechanisms[95] (see later discussion).

The proximal tubule also has a second mechanism of H$^+$ secretion, a Na$^+$ independent electrogenic ATPase that was first identified in membrane vesicles.[96] Subsequent work has identified this as an apical membrane, multi-subunit vacuolar type H$^+$ATPase like that in the distal nephron, discussed later.[97–101] In addition to the vesicle studies, experiments in intact tubules have also been consistent with an apical H$^+$ATPase: electrophysiologic studies showing a lumen positive voltage in the appropriate setting, cell pH measurements demonstrating Na$^+$ independent intracellular pH recovery from acid loads, and response of HCO$_3^-$ reabsorption and cell pH to inhibitors of H$^+$ATPase.[102–105] The vacuolar H$^+$ATPases are blocked by DCCD (N,N′-dicyclohexylcarbodiimide), NEM (N-ethylmaleimide), and more specifically by bafilomycin A1.[105,106] The most convincing evidence has been the immunocytochemical staining for subunits of the vacuolar H$^+$-ATPase.[107] The H$^+$ATPase mechanism accounts for much, if not all, of the remaining $\frac{1}{3}$ of HCO$_3^-$ reabsorption in the proximal tubule not mediated by Na-H exchange. This is illustrated by the knock-out of NHE-3 experiments in Figure 7–4.

The proximal tubule apical membrane also exhibits Cl$^-$/base (OH$^-$ or HCO$_3^-$) exchange,[108–112] but the role in acid-base transport is doubtful because net HCO$_3^-$ reabsorption is independent of Cl$^-$.[113,114] The predominant role of Cl$^-$/base exchange is in fluid reabsorption. Cl$^-$/base exchange in parallel with Na-H exchange (Na and Cl$^-$ moving into the cell, and H$^+$ and base moving into the lumen) will result in no net effect on acid-base transport but result in NaCl absorption. The apical membrane also has other Cl$^-$/anion exchangers (the anions formate and oxalate in particular) that can augment net NaCl reabsorption, but these are probably not involved in HCO$_3^-$ reabsorption[115,116]; the transporter SLC26A6 (CFEX, PAT1) is probably at least one of the responsible transport proteins.[117–119]

Basolateral HCO$_3^-$ extrusion from the proximal tubule cell is also necessary to accomplish net transepithelial HCO$_3^-$ reabsorption (see Fig. 7–3). HCO$_3^-$, derived from CO$_2$ and H$_2$O in the presence of cytoplasmic CA, is transported into the basolateral interstitium and capillary blood. The major mechanism of this was first suggested from experiments on salamander proximal tubules; these experiments demonstrate that changes in basolateral HCO$_3^-$ or sodium concentration simultaneously altered intracellular pH and sodium concentration, and altered basolateral membrane voltage (Fig. 7–6).[120] These changes were independent of Cl– and sensitive to 4-acetamido-4-isothiocyanostilbene-2,2′-disulfonate (SITS).[120] Subsequent experiments using mammalian tubules[121–124] and basolateral membrane vesicles[125,126] demonstrated results consistent with coupled Na and HCO$_3^-$ co-transport, carrying negative charge (more HCO$_3^-$ than Na transported). The driving force for basolateral Na-HCO$_3^-$ co-transport is the cell negative transmembrane voltage, maintained by the high cell-to-interstitium K$^+$ gradient. To achieve basolateral HCO$_3^-$ extrusion based on the known ionic content and voltage of the proximal tubule, the stoichiometry should be three HCO$_3^-$ per Na$^{+127,128}$; this has been demonstrated both in tubules and in membrane vesicles.[123,129] Several studies demonstrated that the transported base is HCO$_3^-$ and not OH$^-$.[23,125,126] Carbonate (CO$_3^{-2}$) has been suggested by one study to be a transported species[130]; it would be the electrical and acid-base transport equivalent of two HCO$_3^-$. This has not been confirmed with the cloned transporter, discussed later.

The basolateral Na-HCO$_3^-$ co-transporter has now been cloned (named NBC transporter for <u>N</u>a <u>b</u>icarbonate <u>c</u>otransporter) and found to be distantly related to the red cell Cl$^-$/HCO$_3^-$ exchanger AE1.[131,132] The basolateral NBC in the

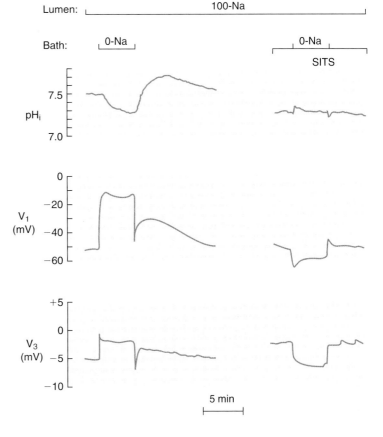

FIGURE 7–6 Electrogenic Na-HCO$_3^-$ co-transport in the basolateral membrane of the Ambystoma proximal tubule. VI and *V3* represent basolateral membrane potential and transepithelial potential, respectively. Basolateral Na$^+$ removal causes both cell acidification and basolateral depolarization. Basolateral SITS (4-acetamido-4-isothiocyanostilbene-2,2′-disulfonate, 0.5 mM) blocks these changes. (From Boron WF, Boulpaep EL: Intracellular pH regulation in the renal proximal tubule of the salamander. Basolateral HCO$_3^-$ transport. J Gen Physiol 81:53–94, 1983.)

proximal tubule is the NBC1 isoform first cloned from the sala-mander Ambystoma[131] and later from human.[132] The human gene is designated SLC4A4. NBC1 (also called kNBC for kidney NBC) encodes a 1035 amino acids protein with pre-dicted size of 116 kDa several potential phosphorylation sites, and 12 predicted membrane spanning segments.[133] The NBC transporter in the late proximal tubule may not be NBC1.[134] Other isoforms are known to be electroneutral.[15,133,135] All of the NBC are sensitive to inhibition by DIDS (4,4'-Diisothiocyanostilbene-2,2'-Disulfonic Acid), SITS, and other disulfonic stilbenes. The large family of HCO_3^- transporters also includes a K^+/HCO_3^- cotransporter and a Na^+-dependent Cl^-/HCO_3^- exchanger. These features are discussed in more detail in another chapter.

Although the physiologic studies discussed earlier suggest that NBC-1 functions in a $3:1$ $HCO_3^-:Na^+$ mode, some experi-ments support that it can also operate in a $2:1$ mode in certain circumstances.[136–140] These recent experiments suggest that cAMP through PKA phosphorylates the C-terminus of NBC1 and changes the stoichiometry to $2:1$.[138–140] There may also be some interaction in this process with CA.[141]

For the basolateral membrane, both Na^+ dependent Cl^-/HCO_3^- exchange[142–145] and Na^+ independent Cl^-/HCO_3^- exchange (in the S3 segment)[126,146,147] have also been found, but the role in transepithelial acid-base has not been estab-lished. Variable evidence exists for basolateral Na-H exchange in some proximal segments of some species[147–149]; when present basolateral Na-H exchange would not function in transepithelial HCO_3^- reabsorption, but to regulate cell volume and pH as in other cells.

Citrate and other organic anions are also reabsorbed in the proximal tubule. Changes in their reabsorption and urinary excretion could alter acid-base balance in that these organics anions can be metabolized to HCO_3^- if reabsorbed. Thus, this reabsorption prevents the loss of excess "potential base" into the urine. In fact, in the rat, urinary excretion of citrate and other organic anions contributes substantially to the excre-tion of alkali, for instance in the recovery from metabolic alkalosis.[150–153] And urinary citrate and other organic anions increase in the urine with alkalosis, and decrease with aci-dosis.[2] In humans, urinary citrate does change in the ap-propriate direction with acid-base changes—a decrease in excretion with acidosis or acid loads, and an increase in excretion with alkalosis or alkali loads, but the magnitude is usually sufficiently small (usually ~5–10 mEq/day) that major influences on systemic acid-base balance are limited.[154] Other organic acids and their anions, in particular lactate and acetate, have been shown to modulate intracellular pH, at least in salamander proximal tubules, and probably only in the absence of CO_2 and HCO_3^-.[155–157]

The proximal tubule has high ionic permeabilities for H^+ and HCO_3^-, and also for CO_2 discussed earlier.[45,158,159] The high H^+ permeability results in little H^+ transport because of the low concentrations of free H^+. The high CO_2 permeability does allow rapid equilibration of CO_2 in the adjacent struc-tures of the kidney (e.g., tubule lumen, cell, and interstitium); see earlier discussion. The large paracellular HCO_3^- permea-bility limits net HCO_3^- reabsorption in the late proximal tubule (where luminal HCO_3^- concentration is low compared with peritubular concentrations) and hence allows greater delivery of HCO_3^- out of the proximal tubule.[160] Therefore, because of this relatively large permeability of the proximal tubule to HCO_3^-[159] and the thermodynamics of Na-H exchange,[161] the proximal tubule is only able to lower the luminal pH to ~6.7 and the luminal HCO_3^- to ~7 mM to 8 mM.[162,163] (Regarding the thermodynamics, because the Na-H exchanger is a neutral exchanger driven by the Na gradient, which is ~140 mM lumen: ~10 mM to 20 mM cytoplasm or $10:1$, the induced H^+ gradient can theoretically only be ~$10:1$ H^+ concentration or 1 pH unit.) Therefore, the proximal tubule

is a "high capacity, low gradient" system for H^+/HCO_3^- trans-port in contrast to the distal nephron discussed later. Contin-ued Na-H exchange, even when the luminal fluid has reached a plateau phase HCO_3^- level, is important however for net NaCl reabsorption.

Regulation of Proximal Tubule Acid-Base Transport

Acid-base transport in the proximal tubule is a complex process, responding in most circumstances to maintain acid-base homeostasis, but also responding to a variety of hor-mones that are not necessarily homeostatic for acid-base balance. For instance, in some disease states, these hormones may actually cause or perpetuate acid-base disorders. Meta-bolic alkalosis for example is often perpetuated by renal retention of HCO_3^- and urinary acid excretion; and the proxi-mal tubule participates in this process. In the proximal tubule, HCO_3^- reabsorption may increase secondary to angiotensin II, increased filtered load of bicarbonate, decreased HCO_3^- back-leak across the paracellular pathway, and potassium dele-tion—each discussed later.

Acid-Base Balance and Peritubular pH
In general, the proximal tubule responds to systemic acid-base changes (either frank acid-base disorders or acid or base loads) in a direction to restore acid-base balance. So, acidosis or acid loads increase proximal tubule H^+ secretion and HCO_3^- reabsorption, and alkalosis or base loads decrease H^+ secretion and HCO_3^- reabsorption. The responses to acidosis or decreases in peritubular pH are complex, apparently involving a variety of both intrinsic mechanisms and sys-temic hormonal mechanisms. In addition, there are different mechanisms for acute and chronic responses to acid or base loads.

With decreases in peritubular pH (either increased pCO_2 or decreased HCO_3^- concentration), proximal tubule HCO_3^- reab-sorption increases; and the opposite occurs with increases in peritubular pH.[57,164–170] (There are some conflicting data on acute increases in CO_2.[168,171] Also, the amount of HCO_3^- reab-sorption in vivo will also depend on the filtered load and concentration of HCO_3^-, which may be reduced in metabolic acidosis.[172]) Decreases in cell pH, which result from HCO_3^- exit on the Na-HCO_3^- cotransporter with decreases in baso-lateral HCO_3^-,[73] stimulate apical H^+ secretion via the apical Na-H exchanger. This will occur via kinetic effects with increased cell H^+ concentrations, but intracellular acidosis also has an allosteric stimulation of the Na-H exchanger.[95] This is illustrated in Figure 7–7. An allosteric activation of Na-H exchange is a feature of most isoforms of NHE, and appears to depend on amino acid residues in the C terminus portion of the molecules.[173] These changes occur immedi-ately. There is also acute exocytic insertion of vesicles (prob-ably containing both H^+-ATPase and NHE-3) into the brush border apical membrane, at least with acidosis caused by increased CO_2.[174] As discussed later, NHE-3 exists associated with other proteins and in different domains of the apical region of the cell; the precise steps of exocytic insertion and retrieval are not known, but are being actively investigated.

Boron and colleagues have also demonstrated that H^+ secre-tion in the proximal tubule is directly stimulated in response to basolateral CO_2, apparently independent of pH; they have postulated that there is a "CO_2 sensor" in the proximal tubule.[175–178] This CO_2 sensor mechanism appears to interact with angiotensin II and to involve a tyrosine kinase.[179,180]

Over a more prolonged period of acidosis (days), a variety of other adaptive changes occur to increase HCO_3^- reabsorp-tion even more.[181,182] With chronic acidosis, Na-H exchange in the brush border increases and Na-HCO_3^- co-transport in basolateral membranes increases, whether studied in cells

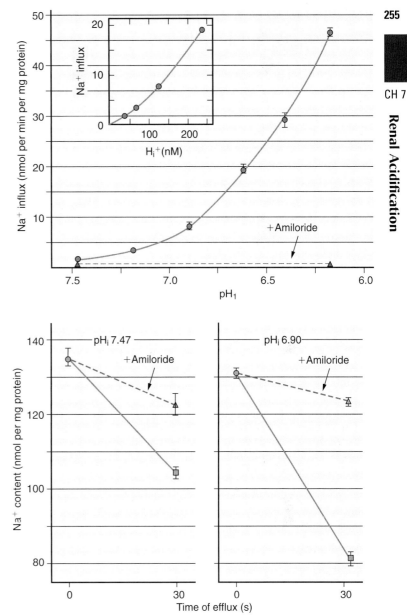

FIGURE 7–7 Allosteric regulation of Na-H exchange in proximal tubule brush border membrane vesicles. Upper panel. Sodium influx as a function of intravesicular pH. The insert shows the same data expressed as a function of intravesicular H^+ concentration, showing a non-linear (sloping upward) increase of Na transport with decreasing pH, increasing H^+. Lower panel. Sodium efflux from vesicles at two intravesicular pH values. The remaining sodium content is plotted as a function of time in the presence and absence of amiloride at intravesicular pH values of 7.47 and 6.90. At the lower intravesicular pH, there is a greater rate of amiloride-sensitive sodium efflux. The effect of pH in this case can not be a substrate effect of more H^+ for exchange with Na^+. (From Aronson PS, Nee J, Suhm MA: Modifier role of internal H^+ in activating the Na^+-H^+ exchanger in renal microvillus membrane vesicles. Nature 299:161–163, 1982.)

or membrane vesicles.[183–188] The increase in basolateral Na-HCO_3^- co-transport with metabolic acidosis may result from post-translational modifications of NBC-1 because protein levels do not change.[189] Some of the effects of acidosis (perhaps exocytic insertion) can occur in vitro, in as little time as two hours.[190] Similar types of changes are seen with respiratory acidosis, and opposite changes with alkalosis[186,191–193]; however, some investigators have not found the same results with respiratory acidosis.[194,195] With acidosis, there is an increase in NHE3 protein in the apical membrane brush border, but not an increase in NHE3 mRNA in vivo; there is, however, an increase in NHE-3 mRNA in the OKP cell culture model.[196] The increase in NHE-3 protein in the apical membrane results predominantly from increased exocytic insertion from subapical membrane vesicles, but there may be increased protein translation as well.[197–199]

Hormones also play a critical role in the response to acidosis. These include endothelin-1 (ET-1), glucocorticoids, and possibly PTH. With acidosis, increases in renal endothelin-1[200,201] and cortisol from the adrenal[202] occur and may play significant roles (see later discussion). Alpern and colleagues have proposed and experimentally supported the elegant

scheme illustrated in Figure 7–8 whereby endothelin is an integral autocrine or paracrine component of the mechanism whereby acidosis causes adaptation in NHE-3. These aspects are presented later in the section on endothelin. In sum, the response to acidosis is complex, involving multiple steps and separate mechanisms. Key elements are turning out to be intrinsic allosteric responses of NHE-3, hormonal responses that secondarily up-regulate Na-H exchange, and exocytic insertion of NHE-3.

Potassium Depletion

Potassium depletion also increases proximal tubule HCO_3^- reabsorption.[167] There is an increase in both the apical Na-H exchanger and the basolateral Na-HCO_3^- co-transporter.[203] These changes may result in large part from low potassium inducing an intracellular acidosis and resulting adaptive changes in the transporters.[204,205]

Extracellular Volume, luminal Flow Rate, and Delivery of HCO_3^-

Increases in luminal HCO_3^- concentration, usually accompanied by increased luminal pH, increase proximal HCO_3^-

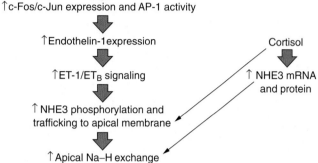

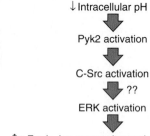

FIGURE 7–8 Signal transduction mechanism of acidosis-induced adaptation of Na-H exchange proposed by Alpern and colleagues. (Adapted from Laghmani K, Preisig PA, Alpern RJ: The role of endothelin in proximal tubule proton secretion and the adaptation to a chronic metabolic acidosis. J Nephrol 15 Suppl 5:S75–S87, 2002.)

reabsorption.[160,166] This increased reabsorption is due to an increased rate of H^+ secretion by the apical Na-H exchanger, probably due to positive kinetic effects of decreases in the luminal H^+ concentration.[160,166,206,207] As Na-H exchange increases, cell pH will rise and stimulate basolateral Na-HCO_3^- co-transport out of the cell. Alpern[4,208] has noted that this HCO_3^- concentration effect will attenuate the effects of other influences on HCO_3^- reabsorption. For instance, if a hormone stimulates HCO_3^- reabsorption, this will decrease luminal HCO_3^- concentration, which will in turn secondarily decrease HCO_3^- reabsorption, attenuating the original change.

Increasing luminal flow also increases proximal tubule HCO_3^- reabsorption. This occurs both by increases in mean luminal HCO_3^- concentration, which will have effects as discussed earlier and by a direct effect of flow rate on Na-H exchange.[167,209,210] This effect of flow rate on the apical Na-H exchanger appears to be a direct effect, possibly on an apical diffusion barrier.[211] Chronic changes in luminal flow rate in vivo (induced experimentally by hyperfiltration from uninephrectomy, renal mass reduction, or high protein diets) cause additional long-term adaptive increases in both the apical Na-H exchanger and the basolateral Na-HCO_3^- co-transporter.[212–215] An important consequence of increasing proximal HCO_3^- reabsorption with increasing delivery (glomerulotubular balance for HCO_3^-) is prevention of excessive delivery downstream and urinary excretion.

Volume expansion usually leads to a reduction in proximal HCO_3^- reabsorption.[165,216–218] This is in spite of the fact that extracellular volume expansion may increase GFR, filtered HCO_3^-, and luminal flow, factors discussed earlier that could increase proximal HCO_3^- reabsorption. Part of the effect of volume expansion to decrease HCO_3^- reabsorption is via increased HCO_3^- permeability,[165] but part is due to an effect on H^+ secretion.[219] PTH may also be involved in this process.[220] Hypertension, and the often associated natriuresis, has been associated with a redistribution of NHE-3 in the proximal tubule also.[221–223] In contrast, volume contraction or low dietary sodium is often accompanied by increased proximal tubule HCO_3^- reabsorption. This may be secondary to angio-tensin II, catecholamines, or dopamine causing changes in Na-H exchange.[224]

Hormones

A variety of hormones modulate proximal tubule acid-base transport. Some of these effects are involved in the response to acidosis and alkalosis as discussed earlier, but others are not involved in acid-base homeostasis, and the acid-base effects appear collateral.

Endothelin-1

Endothelin-1 (ET-1), acting on the ET_B receptor in proximal tubules, may be a critical factor in the response to acidosis as discussed above and illustrated in Figure 7–8.[201,225] Renal ET-1 is produced in response to acidosis,[201,226,227] and its effects on the ET_B receptor are critical in the NHE-3 response to acidosis.[225] Acidosis, and decreases in intracellular pH, increase ET-1 synthesis in the kidney, specifically by microvascular endothelial cells and proximal tubule cells.[225–227] ET-1 in low concentrations (10^{-13} M) increases proximal tubule reabsorption[228]; high concentrations inhibit reabsorption. Both apical Na-H exchange as well as basolateral Na-HCO_3^- cotransport increase with low concentrations of ET-1.[229,230] The ET_B receptor is responsible for these acid-base effects.[201,231] ET_B activation leads to phosphorylation of NHE-3 and its insertion in the apical membrane.[199–201,225,232] In ET_B receptor deficient mice, acid ingestion does not lead to normal apical insertion of NHE-3 and ET-1 does not lead to increased Na-H exchange activity; however, there is normal urinary excretion of titratable acid and NH_4^+.[201] Distal tubule effects of ET-1 are discussed later. The signal transduction mechanisms whereby acidosis and/or low intracellular pH stimulate ET-1 synthesis has been extensively studied by Alpern's group in cultured proximal tubule cells (OKP), and to a lesser extent in vivo; the mechanism appears to involve sequential activation of Pyk2 (a non-receptor tyrosine kinase), c-Src (another non-receptor tyrosine kinase), followed by ERK activation, and c-fos/c-jun (immediate early genes) activating the AP-1 promoter site of the ET-1 gene.[225,233–236] ET-1 stimulation leads to a calcium and tyrosine kinase dependent phosphorylation, membrane insertion, and hence activation of NHE-3; other proteins such as paxillin and p125FAK are phosphorylated in this process as well.[199,200,231–233] Similar signaling pathways have been implicated in the stimulation of basolateral Na-HCO_3^- co-transport.[237,238]

Glucocorticoids

Glucocorticoids also are an important component of the response to metabolic acidosis.[187,202] Metabolic acidosis increases cortisol,[239] which is necessary for the increase in Na-H exchange activity in response to metabolic acidosis.[187] Glucocorticoids increase Na-H exchange by multiple steps, but importantly include an increased translation and insertion of NHE-3 protein into the apical membrane.[202,240–242] Cortisol may also increase NHE-3 mRNA.[243] Glucocorticoids increase NBC1 mRNA levels and activity in the proximal tubule.[244,245] Therefore, glucocorticoids appear to be a parallel and perhaps synergistic pathway with ET-1/ET_B in the response to acidosis. Glucocorticoids also stimulate ammonium excretion, discussed later. Thus, glucocorticoids represent one of the hormone systems that integrate the response to acidosis.[246] Glucocorticoids are also important in the development and maturation of proximal tubule transport.[247]

Parathyroid Hormone

Parathyroid hormone (PTH) acutely decreases proximal HCO_3^- reabsorption via increases in cAMP.[248–250] PTH increases cAMP, which activates PKA. PTH via PKA immediately phosphorylates NHE-3 and inhibits activity, and over a slightly longer time frame NHE-3 undergoes phosphorylation-dependent endocytosis.[251–254] This endocytosis is microtubule and dynamin dependent. NHERF, Na-H exchange regulatory factor discussed later, may also be involved. PTH also inhibits basolateral Na-HCO$_3^-$ co-transport.[255,256] NHERF is necessary for this inhibition of Na-HCO$_3^-$ co-transport.[257,258]

The chronic effects of PTH may differ substantially. PTH levels rise in metabolic acidosis and may be important in the ultimate adaptive *increase* in net acid excretion (both TA and ammonium). Although there may be a transient increase in urinary HCO$_3^-$, PTH effects on the loop of Henle and distal nephron are to increase acid excretion.[259-261] Consistent with an adaptive chronic role of PTH via stimulating cAMP, on a chronic basis cAMP (and hormones that stimulate cAMP) may actually increase Na-H exchange.[262] The acute hormonal regulation of NHE-3 is a complex mechanism that is an intense area of investigation; this area is discussed more later and has recently been reviewed thoroughly.[263]

Angiotensin II
Angiotensin II increases HCO$_3^-$ reabsorption by increases in apical H$^+$ secretion and basolateral HCO$_3^-$ transport.[264] Angiotensin II produced by the proximal tubule may stimulate luminal receptors to stimulate HCO$_3^-$ reabsorption.[265] Angiotensin II increases exocytic insertion and activity of NHE3.[266-268] Basolateral Na-HCO$_3^-$ transport is also directly stimulated.[269,270] The mechanisms of these responses include decreased cAMP, activation of protein kinase C, and activation of tyrosine kinase (src)/MAPK pathways.[271-274]

Other Hormones
Other hormones also can regulate proximal tubule acid-base transport, but in some cases the physiologic and pathophysiologic implications are not well understood. Insulin,[275] dopamine,[276-278] thyroid hormone,[279] glucagon,[280] adenosine,[281,282] cholinergic agents,[283,284] and others modulate proximal tubule HCO$_3^-$ transport. For instance, dopamine modulates apical Na-H exchange and this has anticipated effects on sodium balance, but particular systemic acid-base changes are not known. Catecholamines stimulate HCO$_3^-$ reabsorption.[285,286] α-2 receptors activate NHE-3 by interacting with NHERF (Na-H exchanger regulatory factor)[287] discussed later. Activation of adenosine A1 receptor inhibits NHE-3 via a PKC and phospholipase C mechanism involving calcineurin homologous protein interaction.[288] Neuronal and inducible nitricoxide synthase also modulate HCO$_3^-$ reabsorption.[289,290]

Common Acute Signal Transduction Mechanisms
Several hormones and perhaps other signals share some common acute signal transduction mechanisms in the proximal tubule.[263] A number of hormones such as PTH and catecholamines (in addition to angiotensin II discussed earlier) function at least in large part via changes in cAMP and protein kinase A (PKA). As recently reviewed thoroughly by Moe,[263] phosphorylation of the carboxy-terminal domain of NHE-3 and endocytosis of NHE-3 appear to be key events. The exact mechanism whereby phosphorylation leads to decreased activity is still being investigated; both endocytosis and intrinsic changes in NHE-3 may be involved, and co-factors discussed later are likely necessary.[263] Trafficking of NHE-3 between the apical membrane and other compartments is also a common theme (see discussion of acidosis, PTH, endothelin). In addition to NHE-3 phosphorylation by PKA, endocytosis can also be regulated by a phosphatidylinositol 3' kinase-dependent pathways.[291]

NHERF (also known as EBP50) is a protein cofactor that is important for cAMP mediated regulation of NHE-3 activity.[292-294] NHERF, a 55 kD phosphoprotein with two PDZ domains, links ezrin, NHE-3, and PKA to the actin cytoskeleton.[292,293] This linkage allows NHE-3 phosphorylation and inactivation.[295-298] NHERF may also regulate basolateral Na-HCO$_3^-$ co-transport.[257,258] The α2-adrenergic receptor can

directly associate with NHERF through its PDZ domain, providing a mechanism of regulation of NHE-3 activity.[287] Reorganization of the cytoskeleton may also be involved in inactivation of NHE-3 by cAMP.[299] The PDZ-based adaptor Shank2 is another protein likely involved in trafficking of NHE-3.[300]

Linkage of NHE-3 to megalin may also be important. Recent studies demonstrated that NHE-3 exists as both 9.6 and 21 S oligomers in the renal brush border.[301,302] The lighter fraction localizes to the microvilli, not associated with megalin, and is functionally active. The denser fraction contains NHE-3 associated with megalin in the intermicrovillar region of the brush border and is not active. Shifting of NHE-3 between these two fractions and domains may be an important mechanism of acute regulation.[301,302]

LOOP OF HENLE AND THICK ASCENDING LIMB

The loop of Henle (including the thick ascending limb, TAL) reabsorbs much of the HCO$_3^-$ that leaves the proximal tubule (see Fig. 7–1); this represents 10% to 20% of the total filtered HCO$_3^-$.[303-305] The amount of HCO$_3^-$ reabsorbed in vivo in the loop of Henle has been determined using micropuncture to measure the HCO$_3^-$ delivery to the end of the superficial proximal tubule and to the early distal tubule, see Figure 7–1. Between these two sites, several distinct nephron segments exist: the late proximal tubule, the thin descending and ascending limbs, and the medullary and cortical TAL. Probably only the late proximal tubule and the thick ascending limbs account for the active HCO$_3^-$ reabsorption and most of this HCO$_3^-$ reabsorption probably occurs in the TAL as discussed in detail later.[306,307] The amount of HCO$_3^-$ reabsorbed by the late proximal tubule in vivo is relatively small. This is probably due to limited amount of delivered HCO$_3^-$ from the early proximal tubule and a limited intrinsic capacity of this segment to reabsorb HCO$_3^-$. This is supported by in vivo studies, which indicate that fractional delivery (FD) of HCO$_3^-$ at the late superficial proximal tubule is minimally different from that at the bend of the loop of Henle (see Fig. 7–1). However these data are complicated by the fact that measurements in the loop of Henle are derived from deep (or juxtamedullary nephrons) whereas measurements in the late proximal tubule are drawn from outer cortical nephrons. Importantly, in the descending loop of Henle, the luminal HCO$_3^-$ concentration rises toward the bend of the loop of Henle as water is abstracted with minimal HCO$_3^-$ reabsorption (see Fig. 7–1). Subsequently, reabsorption of HCO$_3^-$ in the TAL is resumed, which lowers luminal HCO$_3^-$ before the start of the distal tubule. As will be discussed, HCO$_3^-$ reabsorption in the TAL is concentration dependent and therefore the rise in luminal HCO$_3^-$ concentration before this segment is physiologically important.

The general features of HCO$_3^-$ reabsorption in the thick ascending limb are shown in Figure 7–9. Although specific properties may differ between cortical and medullary TAL (and among experimental species) HCO$_3^-$ reabsorption, like in other segments, is dependent on luminal H$^+$ secretion and basolateral efflux of HCO$_3^-$. As expected, HCO$_3^-$ reabsorption in the TAL can be inhibited by CA inhibitors.[303,308] Apical Na-H exchange mediates most, if not all, of H$^+$ secretion in the TAL.[308] This has been demonstrated by in vitro and in vivo inhibitor and ion substition experiments.[303,308,309] NHE-3 is likely the dominant isoform; NHE-3 has been demonstrated by immunohistochemical studies and specific functional inhibitor studies.[79,310-312] NHE-2 is present in the apical membrane,[89] and could be functionally active.[313] Na-H exchange in the TAL is usually relatively pH independent and is inhibited by hyperosmolality in contrast to other epithelia.[312,314]

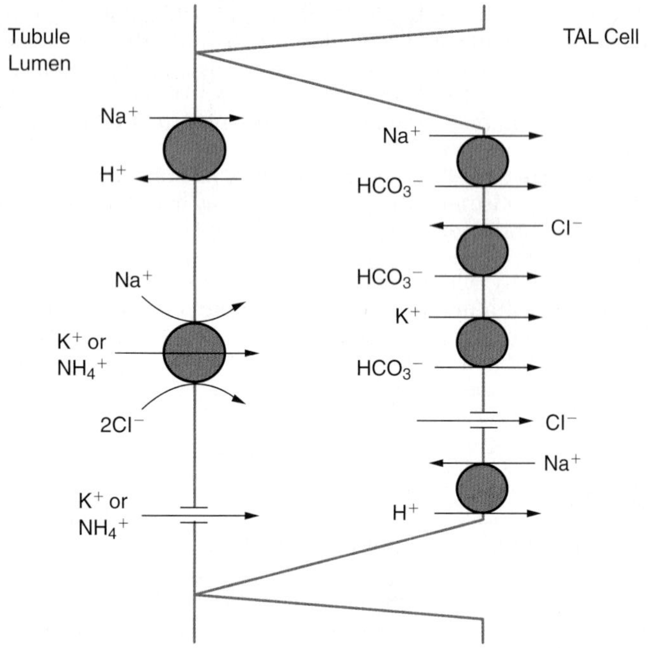

Tubule
Lumen

TAL Cell

FIGURE 7–9 Model of acid-base transporters in the thick ascending limb. See text for details. (Adapted from Hamm LL, Alpern RJ: Cellular mechanisms of renal tubular acidification. *In* Seldin DW, Giebisch G (eds): The Kidney: Physiology and Pathophysiology. Philadelphia, Lippincott Williams & Wilkins, 2000, pp 1935–1979.)

H-ATPase is present in the apical membrane of the TAL,[107] and some HCO_3^- reabsorption in the loop is sensitive to bafilomycin, although some of this could be late proximal tubule sensitivity.[303] Because HCO_3^- reabsorption in the TAL in vitro is predominantly Na dependent, a major role for H^+-ATPase in HCO_3^- reabsorption is unlikely.[312] A K^+-dependent HCO_3^- transport pathway, possibly a K^+-HCO_3^- cotransporter was also identified in the apical membrane of medullary TAL.[315] This mechanism, driven by a large cell to lumen K^+ concentration gradient, opposes transepithelial HCO_3^- reabsorption. The molecular identity and physiological role of this mechanism are not yet clear.

Renal excretion of NH_4^+ plays a very important role in renal acid base transport. In the TAL, NH_4^+ is predominantly reabsorbed, which is counter to what is expected if acid is to be excreted. Yet reabsorption of NH_4^+ by the TAL is necessary for establishing a medullary high concentration of NH_4^+ that is needed for regulating acid secretion into the collecting duct. In general, NH_4^+ is transported in the TAL by substituting for K^+, which it resembles in size and charge. The apical mechanisms responsible for reabsorbing NH_4^+ include $Na^+/K/2Cl^-$ and K^+ channels. Other mechanisms include a K/H exchanger and Na^+-H exchange.[316] Transport of NH_4^+ is discussed in details in a later section.

Na-HCO_3^- co-transport at the basolateral membrane may mediate HCO_3^- transport into the peritubular fluid from the TAL cell.[317] Electroneutral NBC 2 (also known as NBCn1) is thought to be the predominate isoform, at least in the medullary portion of the TAL.[318,319] But, basolateral Cl^-/HCO_3^- exchange and K-HCO_3^- transport are present and may be important mediators of transepithelial HCO_3^- transport.[320–324] AE2 (anion exchanger 2) is present in abundance in the TAL[325,326] and may mediate some of the adaptive changes that occur in acid-base transport.[327,328] A basolateral Na-H exchanger, NHE-1 and probably NHE-4, is also present and likely functions in part to regulate apical Na-H exchange, as discussed later.[148,329,330] The specific role of each of these multiple transporters is not clear, but might be important in independently regulating the transport of specific solutes (and simultaneously cell pH and volume) in a segment in which Na^+, Cl^-, HCO_3^-, and ammonium are reabsorbed in single cell types.

Regulation of HCO_3^- Transport in the Thick Ascending Limb

Systemic acid-base balance, particularly metabolic acidosis, regulates HCO_3^- reabsorption in the loop of Henle and thick ascending limb.[331,332] NHE-3 and basolateral Na-HCO_3^- co-transport increase in response to acidosis.[319,333] Similar adaptations occur for NH_4^+ transport as discussed later. In contrast, as metabolic alkalosis and respiratory acid base disturbances do not cause major changes in HCO_3^- transport in the TAL.[304,334] This apparent lack of adaptation may result from opposing influences of the acid-base status and sodium delivery (discussed later) in the experimental models studied. NHE-3 does change with metabolic alkalosis.[335]

Thick ascending limb HCO_3^- reabsorption increases as luminal HCO_3^- concentration increases.[303,308] Therefore, the increasing concentration of HCO_3^- in the descending loop of Henle as H_2O is reabsorbed is physiologically important for TAL HCO_3^- reabsorption. As shown in Figure 7–1, the concentration of HCO_3^- delivered to the TAL is above 20 mM, significantly greater than the ~7 mM to 10 mM concentration at the end of the proximal tubule.[336]

Changes in dietary sodium and a variety of hormones also modulate loop and TAL HCO_3^- transport. Increases in dietary sodium increase loop and TAL HCO_3^- reabsorption measured in vivo and in vitro respectively.[331,332] Although prior studies had suggested that aldosterone might increase TAL HCO_3^- transport,[304] recent studies reported that aldosterone inhibits TAL HCO_3^- reabsorption by a non-genomic mechanism inhibition of NHE3 action.[337,338] Therefore, the effects of dietary sodium could be secondary to changes in aldosterone because aldosterone would be suppressed with high dietary sodium. In contrast, physiologic doses of glucocorticoids, or supraphysiologic doses of aldosterone, restore loop of Henle HCO_3^- reabsorption after adrenalectomy.[339] Changes in NHE-3 expression do not appear to be responsible for the effects of dietary sodium.[335]

A variety of other hormones alter TAL HCO_3^- transport: angiotensin II, nerve growth factor, prostaglandin PGE2, PTH, and glucagon. Angiotensin II inhibits TAL HCO_3^- reabsorption in contrast to its effects in the proximal tubule.[340] The physiologic importance of these hormonal effects has not been clearly delineated yet. PTH increases loop acid secretion, which has been proposed to be an important component of the response to acidosis.[260,261] The role of changes in HCO_3^- transport in the TAL are difficult to determine in vivo because of the large amount of bicarbonate reabsorption upstream in the proximal nephron and the final regulation of urine acidification in the collecting duct. The signaling pathways for regulation of TAL HCO_3^- transport are diverse: extracellular signal-regulated kinase (ERK), cytochrome P-450, and phosphatidylinositol 3-kinase (PI3-K), and the cAMP pathway.[340–345]

A novel mechanism of regulation of TAL HCO_3^- transport is regulation of apical Na-H exchange by basolateral Na-H exchange.[329,346] NHE1 is proposed to control activity of NHE3, and consequently HCO_3^- reabsorption, by a mechanism involving a change in cellular polymerized actin.[347] Both NHE-1 and NHE-4 are likely present in the basolateral membrane of the TAL.[148,329,330]

Hyper- and hypo-osmolality also affect HCO_3^- transport in the TAL.[343,348–350] Hypertonicity inhibits HCO_3^- reabsorption and hypotonicity stimulates HCO_3^- reabsorption. These actions depend on a tyrosine kinase dependent pathway.[349]

ADH, which will lead to medullary hypertonicity, also directly reduces TAL HCO$_3^-$ reabsorption.[345,351,352] Loop diuretics stimulate TAL HCO$_3^-$ reabsorption, possibly via increases in cell sodium, but also possibly secondary to medullary hypotonicity.[304,353]

DISTAL NEPHRON

The distal nephron is responsible for the final regulation of acid excretion. To accomplish this, the distal nephron reabsorbs the remaining filtered bicarbonate, generates titratable acid, and "traps" NH$_4^+$ for excretion into the final urine.[162,163] All of these functions result from H$^+$ secretion just as in the preceding nephron segments. The distal nephron does have a limited capacity for H$^+$ secretion and normally reabsorbs only ~5% to 10% of the filtered HCO$_3^-$.

The distal nephron is composed of several distinct segments including the distal convoluted tubule, the connecting segment, the cortical collecting duct, the medullary collecting duct (outer and inner stripe portions), and the inner medullary collecting duct (with initial and terminal portions). Some of these segments also have multiple cell types. Despite these different cell types, several segments share features of acid secretion, depicted in Figure 7–10. The differences between segments will be detailed later. The cell model in Figure 7–10 is derived mostly from work in the type A or α intercalated cells (IC) in the cortical collecting duct (CCD), and from prior studies in the turtle bladder model epithelium,[354,355] but similar mechanisms exist in most acid secreting cells of the distal nephron. (Types A and B IC are sometimes used to only indicate rat cells, whereas α and β are used for rabbit IC cells; here, A and B refer to any experimental species.) The turtle bladder, an ancestral and embryologic relative of the collecting tubule, was used extensively in the past as an in vitro model of distal nephron acid-base transport and established many of the mechanisms now accepted in mammalian distal nephron.[354,356] These studies established that active, electro-genic H$^+$ secretion, independent of other ions and HCO$_3^-$, mediates apical acidification. (One study suggested primary base absorption in the turtle bladder, but this has not been confirmed.[357]) In the CCD, type A IC are the prototypical acid secreting cells interspersed among more numerous principal cells. The principal cells are responsible for most of Na$^+$, K$^+$, and H$_2$O transport. A vacuolar-type H$^+$ ATPase mediates much of the H$^+$ secretion by the type A IC. A Cl$^-$/HCO$_3^-$ exchanger, anion exchanger 1 or AE1 (also called band 3 protein), on the basolateral membrane mediates HCO$_3^-$ extrusion into the interstitium and peritubular blood. Another H$^+$ pump, H-K-ATPase (probably of at least two types discussed later), is also important for H$^+$ secretion, at least with some conditions such as K$^+$ deficiency. An apical Na-H exchanger (NHE-2) also secretes H$^+$ in the distal convoluted tubule and connecting segment.[88,310,358]

A unique feature of acid-base transport in the distal nephron is HCO$_3^-$ secretion; this occurs by type B or β intercalated cells in the CCD and connecting tubule, discussed later. The general mechanism of HCO$_3^-$ secretion is modeled in Figure 7–11 and discussed in detail later. HCO$_3^-$ secretion is electroneutral, independent of Na$^+$, and coupled to Cl$^-$ reabsorption. The driving force for HCO$_3^-$ secretion is likely basolateral H$^+$ATPase as discussed later, with apical HCO$_3^-$ transport occurring via an apical chloride bicarbonate exchanger. This apical exchanger is likely pendrin, discussed later. Bicarbonate secretion was originally described in CCD from alkali loaded rabbits, but was subsequently shown in the superficial distal nephron and CCD of rats, and in CCD of mice.[359-362] Metabolic alkalosis (and recovery from metabolic alkalosis), mineralocorticoids (possibly via metabolic alkalosis), and isoproterenol stimulate HCO$_3^-$ secretion[363-367]; and acid loads inhibit HCO$_3^-$ secretion.[365,368] (The time frame over which HCO$_3^-$ secretion is stimulated in metabolic alkalosis has not been studied in detail and may depend on the experimental model used.) The process of HCO$_3^-$ secretion occurs simultaneously with H$^+$ secretion by a separate cell type (see discussion of interconversion of cell types later)[369-371]; whether net

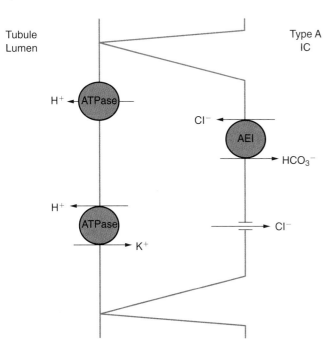

FIGURE 7–10 Model of acid-base transport in the H$^+$ secreting type A intercalated cells of the cortical collecting duct. See text for details. (Adapted from Hamm LL, Alpern RJ: Cellular mechanisms of renal tubular acidification. *In* Seldin DW, Giebisch G (eds): The Kidney: Physiology and Pathophysiology. Philadelphia, Lippincott Williams & Wilkins, 2000, pp 1935–1979.)

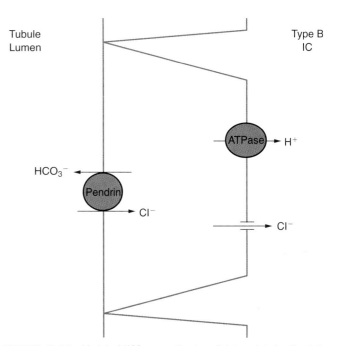

FIGURE 7–11 Model of HCO$_3^-$ secreting type B intercalated cells of the cortical collecting duct. See text for details. (Adapted from Hamm LL, Alpern RJ: Cellular mechanisms of renal tubular acidification. *In* Seldin DW, Giebisch G (eds): The Kidney: Physiology and Pathophysiology. Philadelphia, Lippincott Williams & Wilkins, 2000, pp 1935–1979.)

HCO$_3^-$ reabsorption or secretion occurs depends on the relative magnitude of the two processes in the CCD and distal tubule.

Both type A and B IC cells in the distal nephron have abundant cytoplasmic carbonic anhydrase as discussed earlier. In contrast, functional luminal membrane bound carbonic anhydrase is present in only a minority of cells along the distal nephron.

Although these general models of acid-base transport pertain to several acid-base transporting cells along the distal nephron, there are differences among the various segments and between experimental species. These differences will be discussed later. The unique characteristics of each segment have been studied with different techniques (e.g., in vivo micropuncture, microperfusion, cell culture) because of the relative inaccessibility of each segment.

Distinct Features of Specific Distal Tubule Segments

Distal Tubule

Micropuncture studies of rats usually define the distal tubule as beginning after the macula densa and extending to the first junction with another tubule. Defined this way, the distal tubule includes four distinct morphologic segments: a short segment of the TAL, the distal convoluted tubule, the connecting segment, and the initial collecting tubule (see Chapter 1). However, the exact morphology depends on species; and function has essentially only been examined in rats, with few exceptions. Micropuncture studies in rats have clearly shown H$^+$ secretion (or HCO$_3^-$ reabsorption) in the superficial distal tubule of the rat.[170,372-378] Although both the early and late distal tubule secrete H$^+$, only the more distal aspects of the superficial distal nephron (connecting tubule) have intercalated cells. The early superficial distal nephron (predominantly distal convoluted tubule) secretes H$^+$ via both an apical Na-H exchanger (likely NHE-2) and H$^+$ ATP.[310,358,379] The late superficial distal tubule (connecting segment and initial collecting duct) secretes H$^+$ via a H$^+$ ATPase, and probably H$^+$-K$^+$-ATPase.[380] The colonic isoform of H-K-ATPase is particularly prominent in the apical membranes of some cells of the connecting segment and early CCD.[381,382]

The late superficial distal tubule (and connecting segment specifically) also secretes HCO$_3^-$ with alkali loading.[352,361,383-385] Net HCO$_3^-$ transport (the sum of secretion and reabsorption) varies with diet, acid loading, and other conditioning in vivo and also with luminal flow rate.[386] Studies using variations in luminal Cl$^-$ demonstrate that both HCO$_3^-$ reabsorption and HCO$_3^-$ secretion are present in the late distal tubule, just as in the cortical collecting duct described in the next section.[358,387]

Cortical Collecting Duct (CCD)

The CCD has been the most studied of the distal nephron segments in vitro, and findings in these cells have been used to extrapolate to other distal nephron segments. In a pivotal group of studies, McKinney, Burg, and colleagues demonstrated that the rabbit CCD in vitro can either reabsorb or secrete HCO$_3^-$, depending on the acid-base conditioning of the animals.[359,388,389] These studies were later extended to the rat CCD.[360,390,391] As implied earlier, many studies suggest that HCO$_3^-$ reabsorption (H$^+$ secretion) and HCO$_3^-$ secretion are separate processes mediated by distinct cell types, type A and B IC as in Figures 7-10 and 7-11.[392]

Most CCD from untreated normal rabbits secrete HCO$_3^-$ when studied in vitro[332,359,393-395]; in contrast, most CCD from untreated rats reabsorb HCO$_3^-$.[390,391] Simultaneous processes of HCO$_3^-$ secretion and reabsorption are probably occurring in separate IC types in both species. The existence of two distinct, opposing processes has been inferred from HCO$_3^-$

flux studies that selectively inhibit HCO$_3^-$ reabsorption (with removal of luminal HCO$_3^-$ or peritubular Cl$^-$) or alternatively inhibit HCO$_3^-$ secretion (with removal of luminal Cl$^-$ or basolateral HCO$_3^-$).[365,368,391] HCO$_3^-$ reabsorption is also blocked by disulfonic stilbenes such as SITS and DIDS added to the basolateral aspect.[394,396] HCO$_3^-$ secretion is not inhibited by luminal addition of stilbenes as discussed later. Simultaneous HCO$_3^-$ secretion and H$^+$ secretion was also demonstrated in rabbit CCD by measuring an acid disequilibrium pH in CCD with net HCO$_3^-$ secretion.[32]

H$^+$ secretion (often measured as HCO$_3^-$ reabsorption) has actually been studied most clearly in outer medullary collecting ducts in which no HCO$_3^-$ secretion occurs; H$^+$ secretion in the CCD is thought to have the same mechanisms.[32] H$^+$ secretion in both outer medullary collecting duct (OMCD) and CCD is electrogenic (lumen-positive transepithelial voltage with inhibition of Na$^+$ transport) and sodium-independent.[388,396] CCD HCO$_3^-$ secretion is electroneutral, Na$^+$-independent, and coupled to Cl$^-$ absorption.[389,394,395,397] Both reabsorption and secretion of HCO$_3^-$ are inhibited by acetazolamide. Acid loads in vivo increase net HCO$_3^-$ reabsorption in the CCD. However, the predominant effect of acid loads is inhibition of unidirectional HCO$_3^-$ secretion, with a smaller effect of stimulation of unidirectional HCO$_3^-$ reabsorption.[365,368,384,398-400] HCO$_3^-$ secretion is increased by mineralocorticoids given in vivo (at least in alkalotic animals).[365] CCD H$^+$ secretion may also be increased by mineralocorticoids, both by direct stimulation and by stimulation of Na$^+$ transport and a lumen negative transepithelial voltage.[396]

The existence of separate functional and morphologic IC types is again analogous to findings in the turtle urinary bladder. The rat CCD has at least two distinct morphologic types of IC, both containing carbonic anhydrase.[401-403] The type A cell has a mixture of apical microplicae and microvilli, apical intramembranous rod-shaped particles (which are associated with H-ATPase as described later), apical immunoreactivity for H-ATPase, and basolateral AE-1 (or band 3 protein).[107,402,404,405] In contrast, type B IC have few apical microvilli, H-ATPase, and rod-shaped particles on the basolateral membrane, but no AE1.[402,404-407] Pendrin is also located on the apical membranes of rat (and mouse) type B IC[408,409] (see Figs. 7-10 to 7-13). In the rabbit CCD, which has been studied more functionally, IC do not separate as clearly into types based on morphology.[410] All rabbit CCD ICs contain both apical and basolateral rod-shaped particles, although to varying extent.[410] Rabbit ICs, however, are functionally distinct and have distinct polarization of certain transport proteins. Type A IC from rabbit CCD have apical H-ATPase and basolateral AE-1.[411,412] As expected with basolateral Cl$^-$/HCO$_3^-$ exchange, type A IC alkalinize on removal of basolateral Cl$^-$.[413,414] These cells also exhibit endocytosis of luminal fluorescent macromolecules, presumably reflecting in part recycling of apical membrane H-ATPase as discussed later.[174,413,414] type A IC in the rabbit CCD are relatively infrequent in the outer cortex, but become more abundant toward the medulla.[415,416] Type B (or HCO$_3^-$ secreting) IC from rabbit, the predominant IC type in the outer cortex, have expected rapid changes in intracellular pH (pHi) with changes in luminal Cl$^-$ or HCO$_3^-$, and cell acidification on removal of basolateral Cl$^-$. These cells can be identified by apical labeling with peanut lectin.[369,370,411,414] Rabbit B IC (peanut lectin positive) usually have diffuse staining for H-ATPase, rather than basolateral staining as in the rat type B IC.[412] ICs also express H,K-ATPase as discussed later.[382,417,418] Both A and B ICs have basolateral Cl$^-$ channels and basolateral Na-H exchange to regulate intracellular pH.[370,419,420]

Besides type A and B IC, other types or intermediate phenotypes have been demonstrated. Some H$^+$ secreting IC do not exhibit luminal endocytosis, a property of prototypical type A IC.[416] Also, other ICs, sometimes referred to as rat G

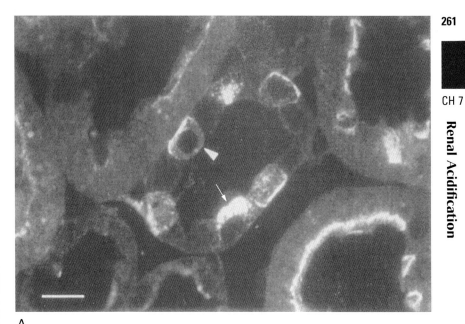

A

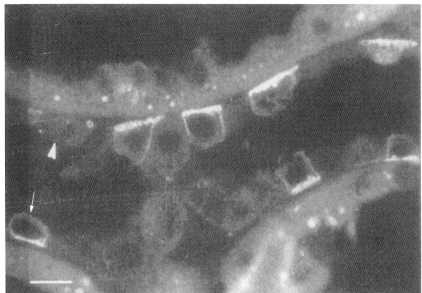

B

FIGURE 7-12 Illustration of AE-1 and H-ATPase distribution in cells of the CCD. **A,** Cryostained section showing CCD from rat with acute metabolic alkalosis immunostained with monoclonal antibody to H^+-ATPase. Basolateral H^+-ATPase staining of type B IC is shown by arrowhead. Closed arrow indicates type A with apical H^+-ATPase. **B,** CCD taken from rat with acute metabolic acidosis, immunostained with polyclonal antibody to AE1. Basolateral AE1 staining of type A IC is shown with closed arrow. Arrowhead indicates type B IC with no AE1 staining. (From Sabolic I, Brown D, Gluck SL, Alper SL: Regulation of AE1 anion exchanger and H(+)-ATPase in rat cortex by acute metabolic acidosis and alkalosis. Kidney Int 51:125–137, 1997.)

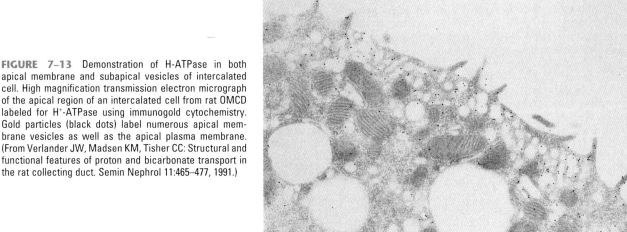

FIGURE 7-13 Demonstration of H-ATPase in both apical membrane and subapical vesicles of intercalated cell. High magnification transmission electron micrograph of the apical region of an intercalated cell from rat OMCD labeled for H^+-ATPase using immunogold cytochemistry. Gold particles (black dots) label numerous apical membrane vesicles as well as the apical plasma membrane. (From Verlander JW, Madsen KM, Tisher CC: Structural and functional features of proton and bicarbonate transport in the rat collecting duct. Semin Nephrol 11:465–477, 1991.)

or rabbit γ or also as "non-A, non-B" IC, have been defined by studies of intracellular pH or atypical labeling by various antibodies.[421,422] Non-A, non-B IC are also seen in the mouse.[423] In the studies of intracellular pH, these cells are typically identified by both apical and basolateral Cl^-/HCO_3^- exchange; these cells typically bind peanut lectin on the apical membrane. Other cells have apical H-ATPase, but no basolateral AE1.[423] The exact morphologic characteristics, functional features, and adaptive responses for these atypical cells have not been clarified. The conjecture that these cells represent a versatile cell type, able to respond to acid or base loads, remains unproved, but as discussed later there is growing evidence for significant functional modification of some CCD ICs with acid loads.[414,424,425] Perhaps corresponding to the diversity and spectrum of cell types, studies of the cellular distribution of H-ATPase in rat CCD and OMCD show a range of staining patterns: from predominantly apical location, to predominantly cytoplasmic, to predominantly basolateral, depending on the acid-base status of the animal.[426]

The IC are interspersed between more numerous principal cells (PC, ~⅓ of CCD cells) which mediate sodium, water, and most of potassium transport under normal conditions.[427] Although PC have several acid-base transporters on the basolateral membrane: Na-H exchanger, Na^+- independent Cl^-/HCO_3^- exchanger, and Na/HCO_3^- cotransporter,[370,428,429] these cells are not likely involved in transepithelial acid-base transport under normal conditions. As in many cells, these transporters in PC probably function to regulate pHi. No apical membrane acid-base transporters have been shown in PC.[370,429] Also, immunocytochemical and electron microscopy studies do not show H-ATPase, AE-1, pendrin, or significant H-K-ATPase.[107,409–411,417] Therefore PC (and the analogous granular cells of the turtle bladder) are not normally involved in transepithelial acid-base transport.[430]

Therefore, different types of ICs mediate acid-base transport in the CCD, with separate processes of HCO_3^- reabsorption and HCO_3^- secretion, occurring in separate cell types. The specific transporters mediating these processes and the regulation are discussed later.

Outer Medullary Collecting Duct (OMCD)

The OMCD differs from the CCD in that this segment only reabsorbs HCO_3^-; HCO_3^- secretion has not been found.[390,393,431] For this reason, many studies have used this segment to better identify mechanisms of H^+ secretion. OMCD HCO_3^- reabsorption is Na independent and coupled to basolateral Cl^-/HCO_3^- exchange.[431–433] In contrast to the CCD, HCO_3^- reabsorption is relatively insensitive to inhibition by carbonic anhydrase.[431] ICs constitute ⅓ of the OMCD cells in the rat.[403] In the rabbit, the outer most part, the "outer stripe" (OMCDos), has ICs, but the inner stripe portion (OMCDis) has predominantly cells that differ morphologically from both PCs and ICs and have been termed "inner stripe cells".[410,434] Although, only some OMCDis cells stain for apical H-ATPase and basolateral AE-1, all have at least some apical intramembranous rod-shaped particles associated with H-ATPase.[107,410,412] The OMCDis does not reabsorb Na^+, and has a lumen positive transepithelial voltage from H^+ secretion.

The H^+ secreting ICs of the OMCD are similar in almost all respects to the type A ICs of the CCD described earlier and represented in Figure 7–10: apical or cytoplasmic H-ATPase, Na-independent H^+ extrusion sensitive to NEM, basolateral AE-1, basolateral Cl^-/HCO_3^- exchange, H-K-ATPase, and no peanut lectin binding.[411,412,416,417,419,435–438] H-K-ATPase mediates significant HCO_3^- reabsorption in the OMCDis, particularly in potassium depleted rabbits.[439–441] OMCDis intercalated cells also have an apical electroneutral EIPA-sensitive, DIDS-insensitive $Na-HCO_3^-$ cotransporter (NBC3) that functions predominantly in intracellular pH homeostasis.[442] As with many epithelial cells, these cells express basolateral Na-H

exchange, probably functioning to regulate intracellular pH rather than to participate in transepithelial acid-base transport.[419] The electrophysiologic properties of both PCs and ICs have been characterized. ICs have a Cl^- selective basolateral membrane, and virtually no measurable ionic conductance across the apical membrane.[443]

In contrast to the most segments of the distal nephron, the rabbit OMCDis has functional luminal carbonic anhydrase, indicated by the lack of an acid luminal disequilibrium pH.[30] This may facilitate a higher rate of HCO_3^- reabsorption.

Inner Medullary Collecting Duct (IMCD)

Morphologically and functionally, the IMCD has initial (first ~⅓ of IMCD) and terminal segments, IMCDi and IMCDt respectively (see Chapter 1).[444,445] The rat IMCDi contains ~10% ICs; but in the rabbit, the cells of the IMCDi are more homogeneous and resemble the inner stripe cells discussed earlier.[445] The IMCDt cells are homogeneous without ICs and are referred to as IMCD cells.[410,445] The IC of the IMCD are similar to the IC of prior segments. Although the cells of the IMCDi have apical rod-shaped particles and membrane-associated CA, the IMCDt does not have these characteristics and yet secretes H^+.[410,445] Immunoreactivity for H-ATPase, AE1, and H-K-ATPase has usually been demonstrated in only IC of the IMCD, but may be present in lower density in other cells based on functional studies discussed later.

The IMCD has been studied in the rat in vivo with micropuncture and micro-catheterization techniques.[446,447] The IMCD has luminal acidification, sodium-independent HCO_3^- reabsorption, and an acid disequilibrium pH (at least during systemic bicarbonate infusion).[56,448–455] Limited in vitro microperfusion studies of acid-base transport in the IMCD have been reported. Although, earlier studies found no luminal acidification in the rabbit IMCD,[456] Wall and colleagues found low rates of H^+ secretion and HCO_3^- reabsorption in the rat IMCD (both IMCDi and IMCDt) perfused in vitro.[457,458] Similar to the OMCDis, the IMCDi has functional luminal CA; this is not found in IMCDt.[31]

However, there have been a relatively large number of cell culture and cell suspension studies of IMCD cells. These studies demonstrate both Na^+-dependent and Na^+-independent H^+ transport.[446,459–467] H-ATPase clearly mediates H^+ secretion in cultured IMCD cells.[446,468] NEM-sensitive ATPase activity (ascribed to H-ATPase) is found in the IMCDi.[469,470] However, as discussed later, H-K-ATPase also participates in H^+ secretion as demonstrated by both cell culture and intact tubule studies.[458,471] As discussed for other collecting duct cells, a basolateral Na-H exchanger functions in pHi regulation, not likely in transepithelial transport.[460,472] Basolateral Cl^-/HCO_3^- in the IMCD is likely mediated by AE1 and AE2.[473–475] Basolateral Na-coupled HCO_3^- transport has also been found in IMCD cells.[476] In sum, the IMCD clearly secretes acid and participates in the regulation of final acidification, but the exact cellular localization of many key acid-base transport proteins has not been well defined except in IC.

Cellular Mechanisms of H^+ Secretion and HCO_3^- Reabsorption

H^+ ATPase

Primary H^+ secretion as the mechanism of acid secretion in the distal nephron has been demonstrated by studies showing an acid luminal disequilibrium pH in the superficial distal tubule, in the cortical and outer medullary collecting tubules, and in papillary collecting tubules.[22,30,32,56,396,453,477] An apical membrane H^+-ATPase is thought to be responsible for most of the H^+ secretion along the collecting duct,[98,478] but H-K-ATPase discussed below likely contributes, particularly in certain conditions (see later discussion). This H^+ ATPase is a member of the "vacuolar-type" H^+ translocating ATPase that acidifies many intracellular organelles such as lysosomes, clathrin-coated vesicles, endosomes, Golgi-derived vesicles, endoplasmic reticulum, and chromaffin granules.[97,98,479] The H-ATPase is related by sequence and structure to the F_1F_0 H-ATPases, which includes mitochondrial ATP synthetase.[100,480] The vacuolar H-ATPases contain 8–10 subunits with a total molecular weight of 500 kD to 700 kD. This class of H-ATPases is inhibited by NEM, 7-chloro-4-nitrobenz-2-oxa-1, 3-diazole (NBD-Cl), DCCD, omeprazole, and bafilomycin, but resistant to vanadate, azide, and oligomycin.[106,480]

The initial evidence for H-ATPase mediating urine acidification derived from turtle bladder experiments.[354,481,482] The evidence that H-ATPase mediates urine acidification is considerable. First, the physiology of distal tubule H^+ secretion correlates well with an electrogenic, sodium-independent ATP-requiring process.[356,396,433] Second, antibodies against H-ATPase stain the apical plasma membranes of ICs.[107,404,406] Third, OMCDis have H^+ secretion that is sensitive to luminal NEM.[437] Also purified H-ATPase forms arrays of stud-like structures in liposomes that are identical to structures found in apical membranes of H^+ secreting cells.[483] And, finally as described in other chapters, mutations in subunits of H-ATPase cause distal renal tubular acidosis.[484,485]

Regulation of H^+ ATPase occurs predominantly via recycling between the apical membrane and subapical vesicles, reviewed in Ref. 98. Insertion occurs in response to intracellular acidification or increased pCO_2; these cause an increase in cell calcium that may be crucial.[413,468,486,487] This process is also microtubule/microfilament dependent and similar to mechanisms of neurosecretory exocytosis, involving SNARE and SNAP proteins.[487,488]

H^+ATPase is electrogenic and therefore influenced by the effects of electrogenic Na^+ reabsorption in Na^+ transporting segments. (Parallel anion channels are present to shunt current in intracellular organelles, but not in most distal nephron H^+ secreting cells; the superficial distal tubule may be an exception.[489])

An additional mechanism of regulation may be regulated assembly and disassembly of the H-ATPase subunits.[490,491] Also, cytosolic regulatory proteins of H^+-ATPase have been identified, although the role remains uncertain.[492,493] An intriguing possible aspect of regulation is interaction with several glycolytic enzymes.[494,495] Transcriptional and translational regulation appears to be a less important mechanism of regulation, although the 31 kD subunit increases in IC with acidosis.[426,496] NEM sensitive ATPase increases with acidosis, but the mechanism is not clarified.[469,497]

Basolateral H^+-ATPase likely mediates HCO_3^- secretion from type B IC; see later discussion. The distal tubule H^+-ATPase shares most subunits with the proximal tubule H^+-ATPase, except that the 56 kD subunit in the distal nephron is the B1 or "kidney isoform" and that in the proximal tubule is a distinct B2 subunit or "brain isoform".[498] Other subunits also differ.[499]

H-K-ATPase

H-K-ATPases also probably have a significant role in distal nephron acid secretion, especially with potassium deficiency.[418,440,500,501] These were first identified as K-ATPase activity in distal tubules that is insensitive to sodium and ouabain, but sensitive to inhibitors of the gastric H,K-ATPase.[502,503] Importantly, functional evidence for a role in H^+ secretion was then found in perfused rabbit collecting ducts.[440,504] Functionally, H^+ secretion by H,K-ATPase has usually been identified by inhibition with K^+ removal or by the use of inhibitors such as omeprazole or SCH28080 (Schering-Plough, Kenilworth, NJ).[440]

H-K-ATPases exchange H^+ and K^+ in an electroneutral manner. At least two isoforms of H-K-ATPase, gastric and colonic, are in the kidney; and strong evidence supports at

least one additional type of H-K-ATPase in the distal nephron. These pumps are K-dependent ATPases of the E1,E2 class (P-type ATPase) Each have a unique α subunit (α1 for gastric and α2 for the colonic isoform) and a β subunit (a unique isoform for the gastric or the β subunit of Na-K-ATPase for the colonic pump).[440,500,501,505–507] The human ortholog of the α2 gene is probably ATP1AL1, also known as α4.[508,509] The colonic α2 subunit has at least two molecular variants.[382,510,511] The gastric isoform is sensitive to omeprazole and SCH28080, but not to ouabain; and the colonic isoform is sensitive to ouabain, but not SCH28080. Another isoform α3 has been found in toad bladder but not in mammals.[512] At least three distinct types of H-K-ATPases have been determined in studies of the enzyme activities,[500] but the correlation with transport studies is not totally clarified. The identity of a third isoform in mammals (in addition to gastric and colonic) has not been established. The isoforms of H-K-ATPase, which mediate acid-base and potassium transport in the collecting duct during various conditions has remained uncertain. Heterologous expression studies in Xenopus oocytes do not correspond well with functional studies in perfused kidney tubules. For instance, colonic H-K-ATPase expressed in oocytes is sensitive to ouabain, but not to SCH28080; however, in the distal tubule, studies have identified acid secretion sensitive to SCH28080, simultaneous with up-regulation of colonic H-K-ATPase, and down-regulation of gastric H-K-ATPase.[500] Studies are on-going to identify additional isoforms, particularly ones up-regulated with potassium deficiency.[513–515]

Although animals with knockouts for either gastric or colonic H^+-K^+-ATPase have normal acid-base status,[516,517] compensatory adaptations may occur. New evidence for a novel form of H-K-ATPase comes from mice with no gastric isoform; CCD from these animals during potassium depletion have a ouabain and SCH28080 insensitive, K^+ dependent H^+ secretion.[515]

Potassium deficiency stimulates omeprazole and SCH28080 sensitive HCO_3^- absorption and colonic H-K-ATPase mRNA, particularly in the medullary collecting duct.[358,439,518–524] Gastric H-K-ATPase may be stimulated in the CCD with potassium depletion.

Metabolic acidosis also stimulates H-K-ATPase activity.[520,525] In the OMCDis, 35% to 70% of HCO_3^- reabsorption is via H-K-ATPase under normal conditions,[441,518] but increased HCO_3^- reabsorption in response to metabolic acidosis is from increased H-ATPase.[398,441,519] The acute response to respiratory acidosis may be H,K-ATPase, at least in the CCD.[526] The role of H-K-ATPase in bicarbonate secretion is not clear; although there is functional and mRNA expression data suggesting a role,[363,527] H-K-ATPase in the type B IC is at the apical membrane.[381,528,529] A role in sodium transport has been proposed because sodium can substitute for potassium to accomplish sodium absorption and low Na diets up-regulate H-K-ATPase activity.[530–532] NH_4^+ may also substitute for H^+ and then H-K-ATPase secrete NH_4^+.[533–535]

The cellular distribution of H-K-ATPase in the distal nephron is complex, with differences found with various species, with technique (e.g., immunocytochemistry versus in situ hybridization studies), and even with different antibodies.[381,382,418,536] Both colonic and gastric isoforms are clearly located in ICs, but may also be present in certain principal cells (connecting segment cells) and even in some aspects of the TAL and macula densa.[381,382,536] As mentioned earlier, colonic type H-K-ATPase and H-K-ATPase activity has been found on the apical membrane of type B IC; the function there is uncertain.[382,418,520,537]

Basolateral Chloride-Bicarbonate Exchange

The basolateral HCO_3^- transport step in the H^+ secreting cells of the distal nephron is Cl^-/HCO_3^- exchange. Inhibition of basolateral Cl^-/HCO_3^- exchange inhibits acid secretion and HCO_3^- reabsorption in the collecting duct.[431,432,455] Studies of pHi in IC of rabbit are also consistent with basolateral Na-independent Cl^-/HCO_3^- exchange.[414,416,419,438] Conductive pathways or significant sodium-coupled pathways for HCO_3^- transport are not present in most distal tubule H^+ secreting cells.[419,438,474] In the rat IMCDi, a basolateral HCO_3^- conductance has been found, without a basolateral Cl^- channel.[538]

This Cl^-/HCO_3^- exchanger is a kidney form of AE1, also known as band 3 protein, the red blood cell exchanger involved in CO_2 transport. Although a single gene encodes both the red cell and the kidney AE1, an alternate start site leads to an mRNA in the kidney, which has exons 1 through 3 deleted.[326,539,540] Therefore, the kidney AE 1 protein has a truncated N-terminus. The truncated part of the cytoplasmic domain is not directly involved in Cl^-/HCO_3^- exchange.[541,542] Antibodies to AE1 stain the basolateral membranes of H^+ secreting mitochondria rich cells of the turtle bladder and type A ICs of rat, rabbit, and human collecting ducts.[404,405,411,542,543]

AE1 (both renal and red blood cell forms) exchanges one chloride for one bicarbonate ion in an electroneutral fashion. The interstitium-to-cell chloride concentration gradient will therefore drive HCO_3^- extrusion from the cell. The driving force for basolateral Cl^-/HCO_3^- exchange is the interstitium-to-cell Cl^- concentration gradient because most studies of pHi in the collecting tubule suggest that the intracellular HCO_3^- is close to or below plasma HCO_3^-.[414,416,419,438] Cell Cl^- will be low due to basolateral Cl^- channels and the cell negative voltage. The basolateral membranes of H^+ secreting cells are predominantly Cl^- conductive.[443,544-547] At least one study has reported that the Km for Cl^- in the OMCDis is in a range such that physiologic changes in extracellular $[Cl^-]$ could alter H^+ secretion.[438] In contrast, another study suggests that the exchanger is always saturated with Cl^-.[419] Basolateral AE1 in the collecting duct does adapt to acid-base conditions.[548,549]

AE2 is also on the basolateral membrane of collecting duct cells, particularly in the inner medulla.[325,473,550,551] AE4 discussed later may also mediate some of basolateral HCO_3^- extrusion.[552] SLC26A7 may also be another mechanism of basolateral Cl^-/HCO_3^- exchange in the OMCD.[553,554]

Cellular Mechanisms of HCO_3^- Secretion

Apical Chloride-Bicarbonate Exchange

HCO_3^- secretion from the type B IC occurs via an electroneutral, DIDS insensitive Cl^-/HCO_3^- exchange process now thought to be pendrin (discussed later). The transport properties were demonstrated by transepithelial flux studies and directly demonstrated by studies of pHi in rabbit ICs.[370,389,394,395,414,416,420,555] The exchanger also mediates Cl^- self-exchange (at a rate greater than Cl^-/HCO_3^- exchange) and is activated by cAMP.[364,394,420,556-558] The relative DIDS resistance in vivo is an unusual feature of HCO_3^- transporters that is not shared by many transporters in heterologous expression systems. The apical Cl^-/HCO_3^- exchanger in type B ICs is not likely the same protein as the basolateral $Cl^-HCO_3^-$ exchanger in type A IC. In addition to functional differences, the apical membranes of type B IC do not stain with antibodies to AE1, in contrast to the basolateral membranes of type A IC.[404,405,411,543] However, some investigators have suggested that AE1 could be responsible, just exhibiting different properties in the type B IC.[559-563]

Pendrin (SLC26A4), the gene product previously cloned as responsible for Pendred Syndrome, an autosomal recessive deafness and goiter, localizes to the apical membrane of HCO_3^- secreting type B IC and non-A, non-B IC. (Pendrin was originally identified as an iodine transporter.) CCD from mice deficit in pendrin do not secrete HCO_3^-.[362,408,564] Pendrin expression and distribution appears to be regulated as expected for a HCO_3^- secretory process, increasing with alkali loads and mineralocorticoids and decreasing with acid loads.[408,565-568] Pendrin expression appears to respond particularly to chloride balance and may participate in blood pressure regulation.[568-571]

A novel anion exchanger AE4 has been proposed to account for apical Cl^-/HCO_3^- exchange, at least in the rabbit.[572] However, recent studies have shown characteristics of AE4 that do not seem compatible with a general role in CCD HCO_3^- secretion: DIDS sensitive, basolateral membrane distribution in type A IC in rats, and lack of change with acid-base perturbations.[552] In rabbits, AE4 is present on the apical membranes of type B IC.

Although an electroneutral apical Cl^-/HCO_3^- exchanger clearly mediates mammalian HCO_3^- secretion, the situation is more complex in the turtle bladder, involving both electroneutral Cl^-/HCO_3^- exchange and a separate electrogenic component during stimulation with alkaline loads, cAMP, or vasoactive intestinal peptide.[573-576] This process has not been demonstrated in mammalian distal tubules.

Basolateral H^+ Extrusion

HCO_3^- secretion in the CCD is active and acetazolamide sensitive.[389] The active driving force for HCO_3^- secretion is basolateral H extrusion and most evidence supports predominantly H-ATPase. Again, key findings were first identified in turtle bladder.[577,578] HCO_3^- secretion is insensitive to ouabain, peritubular amiloride, and removal of sodium.[389,395,411] (One study did show a decrease in HCO_3^- secretion with removal of sodium.[389]) In the rat, H-ATPase antibodies stain the basolateral membrane of a portion of the IC in the CCD.[107,404,406,426] In rabbit CCD however, diffuse cytoplasmic staining, rather than basolateral staining, for H-ATPase, is seen in most lectin positive cells (type B ICs).[412] However, H-ATPase is clearly seen in the basolateral membrane of some IC.[579] Rod-shaped particles associated with H-ATPase are present in both membranes of rabbit CCD ICs and in the basolateral membrane of some rat ICs.[407,410] Although Na-H exchange is present on the basolateral membranes of type B ICs, no evidence supports a role in HCO_3^- secretion.[370] There also appears to be a basolateral Na dependent Cl^-/HCO_3^- exchange mechanism in type B IC.[580] The possible role of H-K-ATPase is discussed earlier.

Other Transporters

Basolateral Cl^- channels are present in both type A and type B ICs. In type A IC, Cl^- channels presumably recycle Cl^- across the basolateral membrane, extruding Cl^-, which enters the cells on the basolateral Cl^-/HCO_3^- exchanger. A predominant basolateral Cl^- conductance has been clearly demonstrated by electrophysiologic techniques in some H^+ secreting cell types.[443,544,545] The apical membranes of H^+ secreting cells from intact tubules do not appear to possess functional Cl^- channels, despite the usual association of vacuolar H-ATPase with Cl^- channels.[443,544,545] In contrast some cultured collecting duct cells do have apical Cl^- channels.[581] The chloride channel ClC-5 has been found to colocalize with H-ATPase in type A ICs, but its function there is unknown.[582] ClC-5, which also is located in the proximal tubule, may function in endocytosis rather than in transepithelial transport.[582]

Cl^- channels are also present in the basolateral membranes of type B ICs.[547] cAMP appears to activate basolateral Cl^- channels in type B ICs in conjunction with acceleration of apical Cl^-/HCO_3^- exchange.[556,558] Also, low concentrations of intracellular HCO_3^- activate these channels.[7,557,583] Recently, the chloride channel ClC-3 has been localized to type B ICs.[584]

A basolateral Na-H exchanger (NHE-1) is present in most cells of the distal nephron.[370,437] This basolateral NHE-1 probably regulates intracellular pH and volume, but not transepithelial acid-base transport.

Electroneutral NBC-3 (or NBCn1) is present in the apical membrane of type A IC and OMCD cells, and in the basolateral membranes of type B IC and IMCD cells.[585–587] Little, if any, function in transepithelial acid-base transport is known.[139,442]

Cystic fibrosis transmembrane conductance regulator (CFTR) is also located in the collecting duct and could regulate other transporters, but its function in the collecting duct is unknown.[588]

Regulation of Distal Nephron Acid-Base Transport

Acid-Base Balance and pH

The distal nephron usually responds appropriately to systemic acid-base changes (e.g., increasing HCO_3^- reabsorption and H^+ secretion with acidosis). However, a number of factors also regulate distal nephron acid-base transport.

Acute or chronic acidosis stimulate distal nephron acid-base transport in several distal segments (reviewed extensively in Refs. 4, 386, 397, 589). In vivo, systemic acid-base changes alter U-B pCO_2 (an index of distal nephron H secretion,[56,590,591] HCO_3^- transport in the superficial distal tubule,[380,384,399] and inner medullary H^+ secretion.[452] In vitro, acutely lowering basolateral pH by either lowering peritubular HCO_3^- or raising pCO_2 increases collecting duct luminal acidification and bicarbonate reabsorption.[592–594] Acute reductions in peritubular HCO_3^- will stimulate basolateral Cl^-/HCO_3^- exchange, and the reduction in intracellular pH will stimulate insertion of H^+ ATPase into the apical membrane from subapical vesicles.[486,549] As discussed earlier, this insertion process is calcium and microtubule/microfilament dependent, similar to mechanisms of neurosecretory exocytosis.[488,593,595] A similar process may occur for basolateral AE1.[549] Some, but not all, studies demonstrate that increased peritubular pCO_2 increases HCO_3^- reabsorption in the OMCDos and OMCDis.[592,593]

Acute changes in peritubular Cl^- will also alter HCO_3^- transport due to effects on the basolateral Cl^-/HCO_3^- exchanger in type A IC; peritubular Cl^- will also alter transport in type B IC.[370,371,596] With low luminal Cl^-, the HCO_3^- secretory process will be inhibited. This may be relevant to the maintenance and recovery from metabolic alkalosis.

Luminal pH also acutely alters H^+ secretion. Decreasing luminal pH will inhibit the H-ATPase due to increased lumen to cell H^+ gradient.[597] However, luminal pH has minimal effects on cell pH or passive fluxes of HCO_3^- or H^+, because the distal nephron has low apical membrane and paracellular permeabilities.[371,374,438,474,592] However, luminal HCO_3^- and pH do influence the pH of type B ICs based on the apical Cl^-/HCO_3^- exchanger.[371]

Chronic changes in acid-base balance in vivo induce more persistent adaptations in the distal nephron. With acid loading in vivo, HCO_3^- secretion decreases and the type B IC undergo morphologic and functional changes.[30,359,368,389,400,414,598] Similar persistent changes in transport are seen in superficial distal tubules and IMCD.[361,383,457] Some of these effects can occur rapidly with in vivo treatment.[391] In segments such as the distal tubule and the CCD that can reabsorb or secrete HCO_3^-, changes in HCO_3^- secretion appear to be predominant over changes in HCO_3^- reabsorption,[365,368,399] although some data in the rat CCD show significant changes in both processes.[391]

In the CCD, interconversion between type B and type A intercalated cells has been proposed as a major mechanism of adaptation.[414,563] In further studies, Schwartz, Al-Awqati, and colleagues have demonstrated possible reversal of polarity of Cl^-/HCO_3^- exchange. Although this was initially

shown only in cultured cells,[559,561,599] more recent studies in freshly isolated CCD demonstrate similar findings. With acid media incubation, some type B IC not only lost apical Cl^-/HCO_3^- exchange, but acquired basolateral Cl^-/HCO_3^- exchange, an effect mediated in part by the extracellular protein hensin.[400,424,563,600,601] In fact, recent studies suggest that cyclosporine may cause distal renal tubular acidosis by intefering with hensin's function.[602] However, total interconversion of cell type remains controversial. Immunocytochemical studies do show changes in the distributions of intercalated cells with particular patterns of staining for H^+-ATPase with acid or alkali loads.[426] Respiratory acidosis induces distinct changes in type A cells but no clear evidence of interconversion of cell types.[402] The presence of numerous "atypical" cells in the CCD, discussed earlier, which are neither classic type A IC or classic type B IC, raises the issue of whether there are "hybrid cells," which can modulate transport phenotype within some spectrum.

Regulation of H^+-ATPase at the mRNA level is not thought to be a major mechanism of the response to acidosis,[426] but there is some evidence of increases in at least the 31 kD subunit of H^+-ATPase in acidosis.[496] With acidosis, AE1 mRNA and protein increase.[548,603] Regulation of pendrin expression and localization may mediate changes in HCO_3^- secretion.[565,566]

The "signal" for these adaptive changes might not be pH per se because systemic pH is not necessarily changed; endothelin discussed later has been proposed to be such a signal.[226] Renal cortical acid content may be altered even when systemic pH is normal.[604] Acid loads in the form of protein induce distal tubule transport adaptations without major changes in systemic pH.[361,375,605]

Sodium delivery, Transepithelial Voltage, Angiotensin, and Mineralocorticoids

Classic studies demonstrated that sodium delivery and the accompanying anion have marked influences on distal nephron acidification.[606–608] Increasing sodium delivery, especially with non-reabsorbable anions, increases H^+ secretion, particularly with volume depletion or increased mineralocorticoids.[607] Because almost all of the mechanisms of H^+ secretion in the distal nephron are Na^+ independent, an indirect mechanism must be invoked: electrogenic H^+ secretion responding to transepithelial voltage.[356,609] Increasing sodium delivery, poorly reabsorbable anions (anions other than chloride), and mineralocorticoids will increase the lumen negative transepithelial voltage and secondarily H^+ secretion. This electrogenic response has been shown directly in CCD and OMCDis.[396,433,610] Chloride concentration gradients may also alter H^+ secretion by altering transepithelial voltage.[596,610]

Changes in luminal Cl^- and peritubular Cl^- will alter HCO_3^- reabsorption and secretion by effects on the apical and basolateral Cl^-/HCO_3^- transporters; low luminal Cl^- will limit HCO_3^- secretion in the collecting duct.[387,395,596] Cl^- delivery in vivo will be important because the Km for luminal Cl^-/HCO_3^- exchange in B IC is approximately 5 mM to 10 mM.[558] Luminal flow rate and HCO_3^- delivery also influence HCO_3^- transport in the rat superficial distal tubule.[372,374,383]

Mineralocorticoids are important determinants of net acid excretion.[611,612] In addition to the indirect voltage effects described earlier, mineralocorticoids directly stimulate H^+ATPase.[396,433] This effect is directly seen in the OMCDis, which has no sodium reabsorption.[433] A rapid nongenomic stimulation of H^+ATPase has recently been reported in OMCD.[613] Mineralocorticoids also stimulate IMCD H^+ secretion.[614] In contrast to the effects on H^+ secretion, mineralocorticoids also stimulate bicarbonate secretion by type B IC, an effect that may be secondary to metabolic alkalosis.[360,365,615]

Angiotensin II has been reported to have a variety of direct effects on distal nephron acid-base transport.[616] Angiotensin II increases HCO_3^- reabsorption in the superficial distal tubule.[617,618] However, it increases HCO_3^- secretion in the CCD and decreases HCO_3^- reabsorption in the OMCD.[619,620]

Potassium

Hypokalemia or potassium depletion increases HCO_3^- reabsorption in the superficial distal tubule.[372,373] Similar findings have been made in the collecting duct.[621] These findings parallel the increased ammonium production and enhanced proximal tubule HCO_3^- reabsorption with potassium depletion. Increased membrane insertion of H-ATPase in K depletion is a possible mechanism of the distal effects because an increased number of rod-shaped particles is found in ICs.[622]

However, stimulation of distal nephron H-K-ATPase activity is likely very important as discussed previously.[439,500,502,623] Increased H-K-ATPase will cause both increased potassium reabsorption and increased H^+ secretion. As reviewed, the mRNA of the colonic isoform of H-K-ATPase increases with potassium depletion, but the functional activity is sensitive to SCH28080, which should not affect the colonic isoform.[500,523,524,624] Another, so far unidentified, H-K-ATPase isoform may be induced by hypokalemia.[500,515] Alternatively, the properties of existing isoforms may be altered in potassium depletion.

Endothelin

Endothelin may be particularly important in the distal nephron, just as in the proximal tubule.[625] Endothelin-1 levels in the renal interstitium increase with acidosis and stimulate superficial distal tubule H^+ secretion via the ET_B receptor.[226,626] Endothelin-1 is released from microvascular endothelia cells.[626] The increased HCO_3^- reabsorption may be due to increased Na-H exchange and decreased HCO_3^- secretion.[380,626] Recent in vitro studies indicate that the ETB receptor regulates the adaptation of the cortical collecting duct to metabolic acidosis, and that the NO-guanylate cyclase component of ETB receptor signaling mediates down-regulation of HCO_3^- secretion.[627]

Other Hormones

A variety of other hormones also modulate distal nephron acid-base transport, but the physiologic significance is not as certain. PTH stimulates distal nephron acidification,[259,261,449,628] and PTH increases with acidosis.[261] A significant part of the effect of PTH may be from increased distal delivery of phosphate.[628] Vasopressin also increases distal nephron acidification.[352,617,629] In contrast, angiotensin II increases CCD HCO_3^- secretion[619] but increases HCO_3^- reabsorption in rat distal tubule.[617] Prostaglandin E2 inhibits and indomethacin stimulates HCO_3^- reabsorption in the OMCDis to some extent.[630] Prostacyclin (PGI2) increases rat distal tubule HCO_3^- secretion and alkali loads increase urinary metabolites of PGI2.[631] Isoproterenol increases HCO_3^- secretion in the CCD via a cAMP-dependent mechanism.[394] In contrast, HCO_3^- reabsorption increase in response to isoproterenol in the rat distal tubule[617] and cAMP in the rabbit OMCDis.[630] Glucagon stimulates HCO_3^- secretion in the rat superficial distal tubule in vivo.[632]

▮ AMMONIUM EXCRETION

Urinary excretion of ammonium (NH_4^+) accounts for approximately two thirds of net acid excretion usually, but can represent an even larger proportion of net acid excretion with acid loads. Production of NH_4^+ occurs predominantly from the metabolism of glutamine in the proximal tubule. NH_4^+ is a weak acid with a pKa of approximately 9.0:

$$NH_4^+ \rightarrow NH_3 + H^+$$

At physiologic pH, most of total ammonia (NH_4^+ and NH_3) is in the form of NH_4^+. Based on this pKa, at pH 7 the ratio of NH_4^+ to NH_3 is approximately 100:1. Therefore in contrast

to historical concepts, physiologically NH_3 is not an effective buffer because most is already protonated as NH_4^+. The manner in which NH_4^+ excretion in the urine represents acid excretion depends on the metabolism of glutamine. Complete deamidation of glutamine yields two NH_4^+ ions, and complete metabolism of the carbon skeleton of glutamine yields two HCO_3^-. (The carbon skeleton can alternatively be converted to glucose, as indicated in Figure 7–14, which is ultimately metabolized elsewhere to HCO_3^-.) Therefore, glutamine metabolism produces both NH_4^+, which is excreted into the urine and HCO_3^-, which is returned to the blood.[3] Because the excretion of NH_4^+ is linked quantitatively to the production of HCO_3^- conceptually (just as urinary H^+ excretion as titratable acid is linked to production of HCO_3^-), excretion of NH_4^+ represents acid excretion. NH_4^+ that is not excreted in the urine will be metabolized in the liver to produce urea, a process consuming HCO_3^-, with no overall effect on acid-base balance. Therefore, only the NH_4^+ excreted into the urine is linked to the production of HCO_3^- and is the equivalent of acid excretion.

NH_4^+ production results predominantly from the metabolism of glutamine (see Fig. 7–14).[4,633,634] Although all nephron segments appear to be capable of producing NH_4^+, the proximal tubule is quantitatively the most important and also the segment where there is adaptation to acidosis, in terms of both NH_4^+ production and key ammoniagenesis enzymes.[635-638] Many of the steps of NH_4^+ production and secretion into the urine are regulated by acid-base and potassium balance, as discussed later.

Ammoniagenesis

Ammoniagenesis and the response to acidosis have been extensively reviewed,[634,634,639] and will only be briefly

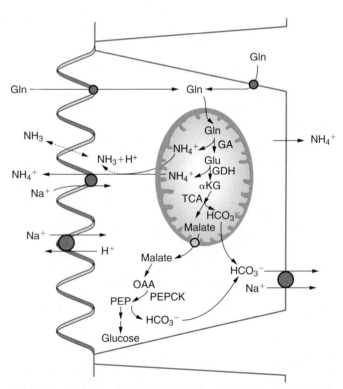

FIGURE 7–14 Major pathway of ammoniagenesis in the proximal tubule (with a cartoon of one large mitochondria). Gln, glutamine; glu, glutamate; αKG, alpha-ketoglutarate; GA, glutaminase I; GDH, glutamate dehydrogenase; PEPCK, phospho*enol*pyruvate carboxykinase; PEP, phosphoenolpyruvate; TCA, tricarboxylic acid cycle enzymes; OAA, oxaloacetate. (Adapted from Curthoys NP, Gstraunthaler G: Mechanism of increased renal gene expression during metabolic acidosis. Am J Physiol Renal Physiol 281:F381–F390, 2001.)

described (see Fig. 7–14). Ammoniagenesis is increased by both acute and chronic acidosis.[633] Several enzymes involved in ammoniagenesis appear to be most important in this regulation: glutaminase I, glutamate dehydrogenase, and PEPCK. However, multiple steps are involved. Release of glutamine from muscles and glutamine uptake into proximal tubule cells from both the luminal fluid and from the basolateral aspect of the cells is stimulated by acidosis.[640,641] Uptake of glutamine from the cytoplasm into mitochondria then occurs via a specific transporter that is stimulated by acidosis.[642] Mitochondrial glutaminase I (also called phosphate-dependent glutaminase) then initiates the most important pathway of ammoniagenesis. Glutaminase is present in other nephron segments, but in these locations is not regulated by acid-base balance nor is quantitatively as significant.[637] Glutaminase I deamidates glutamine to yield glutamate and one NH_4^+. When ammoniagenesis is stimulated, an additional NH_4^+ results from the oxidative deamination of glutamate (also yielding alpha ketoglutarate) by glutamate dehydrogenase (GDH) in the mitochodria. Glutaminase I and GDH are both up-regulated by acid loads, predominantly by an increase in mRNA stability of these enzymes.[643–646] With glutaminase, the increase in mRNA stability may result from a pH responsive binding of zeta-crystallin/NADPH:quinone reductase to an eight-base AU sequence in the 3′-untranslated region of the mRNA. Metabolism of alpha-ketoglutarate by alpha-ketoglutarate dehydrogenase and Krebs cycle enzymes results in malate, which is then transported from the mitochondria to the cytoplasm. Alpha-ketoglutarate dehydrogenase is also stimulated by acidosis. Malate is converted to oxaloacetate and finally to phosphoenolpyruvate by phospho*enol*pyruvate carboxykinase (PEPCK). PEPCK, in addition to glutaminase and GDH, is also importantly regulated by acid-base homeostasis. PEPCK is induced by mRNA transcription.[639] Increased transcription of PEPCK occurs via an acidosis induced phosphorylation of p38 MAPK and activating transcription factor-2 (ATF-2) acting via the cAMP-response element-1 site of the PEPCK promoter.[647] The phosphoenolpyruvate can be metabolized to either produce glucose or further metabolized to yield HCO_3^-. NH_4^+ can be produced by other metabolic pathways (such as gamma-glutamyltranspeptidase) but these are thought to be less important.[634]

Chronic hypokalemia, probably via an intracellular acidosis, also stimulates ammoniagenesis.[205,648,649] In contrast, hyperkalemia reduces both ammoniagenesis and NH_4^+ transport in the TAL and consequent transfer into the collecting duct.[634,650–652]

Angiotensin II increases ammoniagenesis and transport of ammonia from the proximal tubule cell into the lumen.[653,654] Other hormones such as insulin, PTH, dopamine, and alpha adrenergic agonists also increase ammoniagenesis.[633,655] As discussed earlier, glucocorticoids increase with acidosis, and in turn glucocorticoids also stimulate ammoniagenesis.[239,656,657] Prostaglandins inhibit ammoniagenesis.[658]

NH_4^+ and NH_3 Transport

Total ammonia transport has often been considered to occur by free lipophilic diffusion of NH_3 across all cell membranes and trapping of NH_4^+ in the acidic tubular lumen. This simple concept has gradually been replaced over the past several years with information that NH_4^+ transport occurs on a variety of membrane transporters and that NH_3 diffusion does not occur across all tubule segments with equally high permeability.[659–663] Although permeabilities to NH_3 are high, particularly in the proximal tubule, NH_3 concentrations are not in equilibrium,[659,664–667] as expected for CO_2.

As discussed earlier, total ammonia is produced predominantly in the proximal tubule and NH_4^+ produced there is preferentially secreted into the tubule lumen. However, a

substantial portion of NH_4^+ produced in the kidneys exits via the renal veins, instead of being excreted into the urine.[668] Secretion of ammonia in the proximal tubule occurs by both NH_3 diffusion and by NH_4^+ transport on the apical Na-H exchanger.[93,94] NH_4^+ transport on the Na-H exchanger was first demonstrated in membrane vesicles, but later also demonstrated to occur in intact mouse proximal tubules in vitro.[93,94] However, studies using rat proximal tubules in vivo demonstrated that total ammonia transport probably occurs nearly equally by NH_3 diffusion and NH_4^+ movement on the Na-H exchanger.[669–671] (Experimentally, NH_4^+ transport is difficult to separate from parallel NH_3 and H^+ transport.) NH_3 diffusion is facilitated by a low luminal pH created by H^+ secretion; this keeps the luminal NH_3 concentration low. And NH_4^+ secretion will be accelerated by stimuli that increase Na-H exchanger activity. Therefore, both NH_3 transport and NH_4^+ transport on the Na-H exchanger will be accelerated by increased activity of the Na-H exchanger. NH_4^+ transport in the proximal tubule may also occur via a barium-sensitive K^+ pathway.[672] NH_4^+ may substitute for K^+ on the basolateral Na-K-ATPase[673,674] and there may also be a basolateral K^+/NH_4^+ exchanger.[675] Angiotensin II and increasing luminal flow rate stimulate NH_4^+ production and secretion into the proximal tubule lumen.[654,676] In normal conditions, total ammonia is secreted by the early proximal tubule and is reabsorbed to some extent late in the proximal tubule; with chronic acidosis, ammonia secretion also occurs in the late proximal tubule, stimulated by angiotensin II.[665,677] More than 20% of ammonia produced in the proximal tubule is released across the basolateral membrane and reaches the renal venous blood.[634,665]

Although NH_4^+ is produced and secreted in the proximal tubule, much of the NH_4^+ does not simply traverse down the tubule lumen. Total ammonia delivered to the loop of Henle is higher than that at the end of the superficial proximal tubule, but is considerably less at the beginning of the superficial distal tubule. Therefore, total ammonia is lost or reabsorbed in the ascending loop of Henle and/or thick ascending limb.[163,666,678,679] Ammonia may be secreted into the descending limb of Henle (and perhaps late proximal straight tubule) but is then reabsorbed in the thick ascending limb.[306] The total ammonia lost in the loop of Henle, however, is eventually secreted into the collecting duct for excretion into the urine. The reabsorption and concentration of total ammonia by the loop of Henle and thick ascending limb indicates recycling and countercurrent concentration for total ammonia, creating high concentrations in the deep medulla.[660] Total ammonia concentrations in the renal interstitium increase from the outer medullary region to higher concentrations in the deep papilla as illustrated in Figure 7–15. This creates a concentration driving force for secretion into the late collecting duct. NH_3 concentrations in the loop of Henle will be increased by the high luminal pH values (see earlier discussion of medullary concentration of HCO_3^- in the loop as water is extracted); and NH_3 concentrations in the collecting duct will be decreased by H^+ secretion.

NH_4^+ reabsorption in the thick ascending limb is the driving force for medullary concentration of total ammonia. NH_4^+ is absorbed despite the simultaneous reabsorption of HCO_3^-; therefore NH_4^+ transport in the TAL occurs in a direction opposite to that expected for non-ionic diffusion of NH_3 and "trapping" of NH_4^+.[306] In fact, non-ionic diffusion of NH_3 is limited in the TAL because of an apical membrane that has a low permeability to NH_3.[661,680] (Initially the low NH_3 permeability, relative to NH_4^+ entry in TAL, was interpreted as an impermeable apical membrane[661]; later analysis has suggested that the NH_3 permeability is only relatively low compared to NH_4^+ entry, probably due to a small surface area compared to the basolateral membrane.[681–683])

NH_4^+ is transported from the lumen of the thick ascending limb by several mechanisms: substitution for K^+ on both the

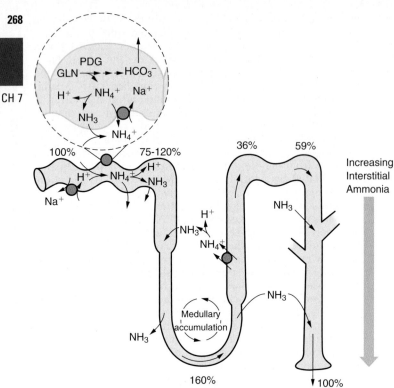

FIGURE 7–15 Overall scheme of ammonia transport along the nephron. Numbers (%) refer to percentage of delivery to each site compared to final urine; data from 2, 163, 665, 666, 678, 679. These numbers are shown to illustrate the large addition of ammonia in the proximal tubule, the high concentrations in the loop of Henle, and the loss of ammonia before the distal tubule. (Adapted from Hamm LL, Alpern RJ: Cellular mechanisms of renal tubular acidification. *In* Seldin DW, Giebisch G (eds): The Kidney: Physiology and Pathophysiology. Philadelphia, Lippincott Williams & Wilkins, 2000, pp 1935–1979.)

Na-K-2Cl transporter (also known as BSC1 or NKCC2) and the apical membrane K^+ channel.[680,684] The Na-K-2Cl transporter in the TAL is enhanced in metabolic acidosis and by the increase in glucocorticoids that occurs with acidosis.[685,686] In addition, there is a separate NH_4^+ conductance (amiloride sensitive) and an electroneutral K^+/NH_4^+ (or H^+) exchanger (verapamil and barium sensitive).[315,675,687,688] NH_4^+ can also be transported on Na-H exchangers and Na-K-ATPase as discussed earlier. Also some NH_4^+ may be driven through the paracellular pathway by the lumen positive voltage; this has been estimated to account for some 35% of TAL NH_4^+ transport.[684,689] Consistent with the physiologic importance of the TAL for NH_4^+ transport, NH_4^+ transport in the TAL is increased by acidosis and decreased by increasing potassium concentration.[332,650,684] However, NH_4^+ and HCO_3^- reabsorption are also increased with metabolic alkalosis induced by $NaHCO_3$ loading (a response inappropriate for correction of the alkalosis), probably secondary to the increased delivery of NaCl to this segment in vivo.[332]

Ammonia secretion along the collecting duct is critical for urinary excretion. Total ammonia secretion in the collecting duct occurs in large part by non-ionic diffusion of NH_3, driven by the concentration gradient for NH_3, which is maintained by high medullary interstitial concentrations of NH_3.[33,457,679,690] As discussed earlier, NH_3 concentrations increase deeper in the medulla. This secretion is abetted by H^+ secretion and an acid luminal disequilibrium pH in most segments of the collecting duct[615,659]; without H^+ secretion, collecting duct luminal pH and NH_3 concentrations would rise concurrently as NH_3 entered. Although non-ionic diffusion of NH_3 has been presumed (with some experimental verification) to account for much of total ammonia transport in the collecting duct, recent evidence suggests that facilitated transport, perhaps via Rh proteins discussed later, may account for a significant portion of this transport across both apical and basolateral membranes.[691,692]

In the collecting duct, total ammonia may be transported across the basolateral membrane by NH_4^+ substitution for potassium on the Na-K-ATPase.[693–695] NH_4^+ may serve as a proton source for acid secretion.[696] There is competition between K^+ and NH_4^+, so that NH_4^+ uptake increases with lower interstitial K^+ concentrations.[697] NH_4^+ transport across the apical membrane may occur on H-K-ATPase, by substitution for potassium, particularly in states of potassium deficiency.[533–535] Recent studies have shown that NH_3 can be transported by water channels (AQP1),[698,699] but the physiologic importance of this has not been established. Although, NH_4^+ can be transported on the Na-K-2Cl co-transporter (BSC2) in the inner medullary collecting duct and is upregulated by acidosis, this transporter does not greatly alter acid-base transport.[700–703] An $NH_4^+/K+$ exchanger that is sensitive to verapamil and SCH28080 has also been described in cultured inner medullary collecting duct cells.[704]

Recently, two new described membrane proteins belonging to the erythrocyte Rh family have been proposed to be involved in NH_3 and/or NH_4^+ transport (for a review see Refs. 663, 705). In the kidney, RhCG and RhBG are respectively expressed in the apical and basolateral membranes of the intercalated cells of the distal nephron including the connecting tubule and the cortical and medullary collecting ducts.[706,711] However, localization in CCD principal cells is also found and RhCG is also found on the basolateral membranes depending on species.[712–714] Metabolic acidosis causes increased RhCG protein and redistribution within cells, whereas no changes in RhBG are found.[713,714] Several studies indicate that these membrane proteins act as carriers of NH_4^+ transport. RhCG and RhBG were reported to be electroneutral NH_4^+-H^+ exchangers.[715,716] Other studies proposed that RhCG actually transports NH_3[717] and possibly CO_2.[718] When expressed in oocytes, Rhbg was reported to be an electrogenic NH_4^+ transporter.[719] Based on recently resolved crystallographic structure of bacterial Amt-B (a related protein), Rh glycoproteins were proposed to act as gas channels through a unique mechanism involving recruitment of NH_4^+ and passage of NH_3 through a hydrophobic core.[720] Increasingly, evidence is accumulating to indicate that renal NH_4^+-specific transporters may actually be the Rh glycoproteins. Of note however, animals with knock out of Rhbg do not have acid-base abnormalities or detectable defects in ammonia transport[721]; whether this represents redundancy of transporters or other adaptation has not been determined.

In sum, NH_4^+ excretion into the urine is regulated by three processes: ammoniagenesis, specific transport of NH_4^+, and by H^+ secretion.[2,633,662] Regulation of NH_4^+ transport occurs in the proximal tubule, in the TAL (and resulting medullary concentration of total ammonia), and in the collecting duct.

References

1. Sebastian A, Frassetto LA, Sellmeyer DE, et al: Estimation of the net acid load of the diet of ancestral preagricultural Homo sapiens and their hominid ancestors. Am J Clin Nutr 76:1308–1316, 2002.
2. Hamm LL, Simon EE: Roles and mechanisms of urinary buffer excretion. Am J Physiol 253:F595–F605, 1987.
3. Alpern RJ, Star R, Seldin DW: Hepatic renal interrelations in acid-base regulation. Am J Physiol 255:F807–F809, 1988.
4. Alpern RJ: Renal acidification mechanisms. In Brenner B (ed): The Kidney. Philadelphia, W.B. Saunders Company, 2000, pp 455–519.
5. Rector FC Jr., Carter NW, Seldin DW: The mechanism of bicarbonate reabsorption in the proximal and distal tubules of the kidney. J Clin Invest 44:278–290, 1965.
6. Warnock DG, Burg MB: Urinary acidification: CO_2 transport by the rabbit proximal straight tubule. Am J Physiol 232:F20–F25, 1977.
7. McKinney TD, Burg MB: Bicarbonate and fluid absorption by renal proximal straight tubules. Kidney Int 12:1–8, 1977.
8. Schwartz GJ: Physiology and molecular biology of renal carbonic anhydrase. J Nephrol 15 Suppl 5:S61–S74, 2002.
9. Sly WS, Hu PY: Human carbonic anhydrases and carbonic anhydrase deficiencies. Annu Rev Biochem 64:375–401, 1995.
10. Lindskog S: Structure and mechanism of carbonic anhydrase. Pharmacol Ther 74:1–20, 1997.
11. Maren TH: Carbonic anhydrase: Chemistry, physiology, and inhibition. Physiol Rev 47:595–781, 1967.
12. Hansson HP: Histochemical demonstration of carbonic anhydrase activity. Histochemie 11:112–128, 1967.
13. Dobyan DC, Bulger RE: Renal carbonic anhydrase. Am J Physiol 243:F311–F324, 1982.
14. Sterling D, Reithmeier RA, Casey JR: A transport metabolon. Functional interaction of carbonic anhydrase II and chloride/bicarbonate exchangers. J Biol Chem 276:47886–47894, 2001.
15. Soleimani M: Na^+:HCO_3^- cotransporters (NBC): Expression and regulation in the kidney. J Nephrol 15 Suppl 5:S32–S40, 2002.
16. Sterling D, Alvarez BV, Casey JR: The extracellular component of a transport metabolon. Extracellular loop 4 of the human AE1 Cl^-/HCO_3^- exchanger binds carbonic anhydrase IV. J Biol Chem 277:25239–25246, 2002.
17. Li X, Alvarez B, Casey JR, et al: Carbonic anhydrase II binds to and enhances activity of the Na^+/H^+ exchanger. J Biol Chem 277:36085–36091, 2002.
18. Alvarez BV, Loiselle FB, Supuran CT, et al: Direct extracellular interaction between carbonic anhydrase IV and the human NBC1 sodium/bicarbonate co-transporter. Biochemistry 42:12321–12329, 2003.
19. Breton S, Alper SL, Gluck SL, et al: Depletion of intercalated cells from collecting ducts of carbonic anhydrase II-deficient (CAR2 null) mice. Am J Physiol 269:t–74, 1995.
20. DuBose TD, Jr, Lucci MS: Effect of carbonic anhydrase inhibition on superficial and deep nephron bicarbonate reabsorption in the rat. J Clin Invest 71:55–65, 1983.
21. Brown D, Zhu XL, Sly WS: Localization of membrane-associated carbonic anhydrase type IV in kidney epithelial cells. Proc Natl Acad Sci U S A 87:7457–7461, 1990.
22. DuBose TD, Jr: Application of the disequilibrium pH method to investigate the mechanism of urinary acidification [review] [55 refs]. Am J Physiol 245:F535–F544, 1983.
23. Krapf R, Alpern RJ, Rector FC, Jr, Berry CA: Basolateral membrane Na/base cotransport is dependent on CO_2/HCO_3 in the proximal convoluted tubule. J Gen Physiol 90:833–853, 1987.
24. Schwartz GJ, Kittelberger AM, Barnhart DA, Vijayakumar S: Carbonic anhydrase IV is expressed in H(+)-secreting cells of rabbit kidney. Am J Physiol Renal Physiol 278:F894–F904, 2000.
25. Lucci MS, Pucacco LR, DuBose TD, Jr, et al: Direct evaluation of acidification by rat proximal tubule: Role of carbonic anhydrase. Am J Physiol 238:F372–F379, 1980.
26. Lucci MS, Tinker JP, Weiner IM, DuBose TD, Jr: Function of proximal tubule carbonic anhydrase defined by selective inhibition. Am J Physiol 245:F443–F449, 1983.
27. Tsuruoka S, Swenson ER, Petrovic S, et al: Role of basolateral carbonic anhydrase in proximal tubular fluid and bicarbonate absorption. Am J Physiol Renal Physiol 280:F146–F154, 2001.
28. Tsuruoka S, Schwartz GJ: HCO_3^- absorption in rabbit outer medullary collecting duct: Role of luminal carbonic anhydrase. Am J Physiol 274:F139–F147, 1998.
29. Kurtz I, Star R, Balaban RS, et al: Spontaneous luminal disequilibrium pH in S3 proximal tubules. Role in ammonia and bicarbonate transport. J Clin Invest 78:989–996, 1986.
30. Star RA, Burg MB, Knepper MA: Luminal disequilibrium pH and ammonia transport in outer medullary collecting duct [corrected and issued with original paging in Am J Physiol 1987;253(2 Pt 2)]. Am J Physiol 252:F1148–F1157, 1987.
31. Wall SM, Flessner MF, Knepper MA: Distribution of luminal carbonic anhydrase activity along rat inner medullary collecting duct. Am J Physiol 260:F738–F748, 1991.
32. Star RA, Kurtz I, Mejia R, et al: Disequilibrium pH and ammonia transport in isolated perfused cortical collecting ducts. Am J Physiol 253:F1232–F1242, 1987.
33. Flessner MF, Wall SM, Knepper MA: Ammonium and bicarbonate transport in rat outer medullary collecting duct. Am J Physiol 262:F1–F7, 1992.
34. Brion LP, Zavilowitz BJ, Rosen O, Schwartz GJ: Changes in soluble carbonic anhydrase activity in response to maturation and NH4Cl loading in the rabbit. Am J Physiol 261:R1204–R1213, 1991.
35. Brion LP, Zavilowitz BJ, Suarez C, Schwartz GJ: Metabolic acidosis stimulates carbonic anhydrase activity in rabbit proximal tubule and medullary collecting duct. Am J Physiol 266:F185–F195, 1994.
36. Tsuruoka S, Kittelberger AM, Schwartz GJ: Carbonic anhydrase II and IV mRNA in rabbit nephron segments: Stimulation during metabolic acidosis. Am J Physiol 274:F259–F267, 1998.
37. Tureci O, Sahin U, Vollmer E, et al: Human carbonic anhydrase XII: cDNA cloning, expression, and chromosomal localization of a carbonic anhydrase gene that is overexpressed in some renal cell cancers. Proc Natl Acad Sci U S A 95:7608–7613, 1998.
38. Mori K, Ogawa Y, Ebihara K, et al: Isolation and characterization of CA XIV, a novel membrane-bound carbonic anhydrase from mouse kidney. J Biol Chem 274:15701–15705, 1999.
39. Purkerson JM, Schwartz GJ: Expression of membrane-associated carbonic anhydrase isoforms IV, IX, XII, and XIV in the rabbit: Induction of CA IV and IX during maturation. Am J Physiol Regul Integr Comp Physiol 288:R1256–R1263, 2005.
40. Parkkila S, Parkkila AK, Saarnio J, et al: Expression of the membrane-associated carbonic anhydrase isozyme XII in the human kidney and renal tumors. J Histochem Cytochem 48:1601–1608, 2000.
41. Schwartz GJ, Kittelberger AM, Watkins RH, O'Reilly MA: Carbonic anhydrase XII mRNA encodes a hydratase that is differentially expressed along the rabbit nephron. Am J Physiol Renal Physiol 284:F399–F410, 2003.
42. Cogan MG, Maddox DA, Warnock DG, et al: Effect of acetazolamide on bicarbonate reabsorption in the proximal tubule of the rat. Am J Physiol 237:F447–F454, 1979.
43. Frommer JP, Laski ME, Wesson DE, Kurtzman NA: Internephron heterogeneity for carbonic anhydrase-independent bicarbonate reabsorption in the rat. J Clin Invest 73:1034–1045, 1984.
44. Gutknecht J, Bisson MA, Tosteson DC: Diffusion of carbon dioxide through lipid bilayer membranes: Effects of carbonic anhydrase, bicarbonate, and unstirred layers. J Gen Physiol 69:779–794, 1977.
45. Schwartz GJ, Weinstein AM, Steele RE, et al: Carbon dioxide permeability of rabbit proximal convoluted tubules. Am J Physiol 240:F231–F244, 1981.
46. Lucci MS, Pucacco LR, Carter NW, DuBose TD, Jr: Direct evaluation of the permeability of the rat proximal convoluted tubule to CO_2. Am J Physiol 242:F470–F476, 1982.
47. Gros G, Moll W: Facilitated diffusion of CO_2 across albumin solutions. J Gen Physiol 64:356–371, 1974.
48. Sohtell M: CO_2 along the proximal tubules in the rat kidney. Acta Physiol Scand 105:146–155, 1979.
49. Sohtell M: PCO_2 of the proximal tubular fluid and the efferent arteriolar blood in the rat kidney. Acta Physiol Scand 105:137–145, 1979.
50. DuBose TD, Jr, Pucacco LR, Seldin DW, Carter NW: Direct determination of PCO2 in the rat renal cortex. J Clin Invest 62:338–348, 1978.
51. DuBose TD, Jr., Caflisch CR, Bidani A: Role of metabolic CO_2 production in the generation of elevated renal cortical PCO2. Am J Physiol 246:F592–F599, 1984.
52. Gennari FJ, Caflisch CR, Johns C, et al: PCO2 measurements in surface proximal tubules and peritubular capillaries of the rat kidney. Am J Physiol 242:F78–F85, 1982.
53. Maddox DA, Atherton LJ, Deen WM, Gennari FJ: Proximal HCO_3^- reabsorption and the determinants of tubular and capillary PCO2 in the rat. Am J Physiol 247:F73–F81, 1984.
54. Atherton LJ, Deen WM, Maddox DA, Gennari FJ: Analysis of the factors influencing peritubular PCO2 in the rat. Am J Physiol 247:F61–F72, 1984.
55. Graber ML, Bengele HH, Alexander EA: Elevated urinary PCO2 in the rat: An intrarenal event. Kidney Int 21:795–799, 1982.
56. DuBose TD, Jr: Hydrogen ion secretion by the collecting duct as a determinant of the urine to blood PCO2 gradient in alkaline urine. J Clin Invest 69:145–156, 1982.
57. Jacobson HR: Effects of CO_2 and acetazolamide on bicarbonate and fluid transport in rabbit proximal tubules. Am J Physiol 240:F54–F62, 1981.
58. Jacobson HR: Functional segmentation of the mammalian nephron [review] [153 refs]. Am J Physiol 241:F203–F218, 1981.
59. Holmberg C, Kokko JP, Jacobson HR: Determination of chloride and bicarbonate permeabilities in proximal convoluted tubules. Am J Physiol 241:F386–F394, 1981.
60. Sheu JN, Quigley R, Baum M: Heterogeneity of chloride/base exchange in rabbit superficial and juxtamedullary proximal convoluted tubules. Am J Physiol 268:F847–F853, 1995.
61. Liu FY, Cogan MG: Axial heterogeneity in the rat proximal convoluted tubule. I. Bicarbonate, chloride, and water transport. Am J Physiol 247:F816–F821, 1984.
62. Vieira FL, Malnic G: Hydrogen ion secretion by rat renal cortical tubules as studied by an antimony microelectrode. Am J Physiol 214:710–718, 1968.

63. Chantrelle B, Cogan MG, Rector FC, Jr: Evidence for coupled sodium/hydrogen exchange in the rat superficial proximal convoluted tubule. Pflugers Arch 395:186–189, 1982.

64. Chan YL, Giebisch G: Relationship between sodium and bicarbonate transport in the rat proximal convoluted tubule. Am J Physiol 240:F222–F230, 1981.

65. Murer H, Hopfer U, Kinne R: Sodium/proton antiport in brush-border-membrane vesicles isolated from rat small intestine and kidney. Biochem J 154:597–604, 1976.

66. Kinsella JL, Aronson PS: Properties of the Na⁺-H⁺ exchanger in renal microvillus membrane vesicles. Am J Physiol 238:F461–F469, 1980.

67. Warnock DG, Reenstra WW, Yee VJ: Na⁺/H⁺ antiporter of brush border vesicles: Studies with acridine orange uptake. Am J Physiol 242:F733–F739, 1982.

68. Kinsella JL, Aronson PS: Amiloride inhibition of the Na⁺-H⁺ exchanger in renal microvillus membrane vesicles. Am J Physiol 241:F374–F379, 1981.

69. Ives HE, Yee VJ, Warnock DG: Mixed type inhibition of the renal Na⁺/H⁺ antiporter by Li+ and amiloride. Evidence for a modifier site. J Biol Chem 258:9710–9716, 1983.

70. Boron WF, Boulpaep EL: Intracellular pH regulation in the renal proximal tubule of the salamander. Na-H exchange. J Gen Physiol 81:29–52, 1983.

71. Sasaki S, Shigai T, Takeuchi J: Intracellular pH in the isolated perfused rabbit proximal straight tubule. Am J Physiol 249:F417–F423, 1985.

72. Preisig PA, Ives HE, Cragoe EJ, Jr, et al: Role of the Na⁺/H⁺ antiporter in rat proximal tubule bicarbonate absorption. J Clin Invest 80:970–978, 1987.

73. Alpern RJ, Chambers M: Cell pH in the rat proximal convoluted tubule. Regulation by luminal and peritubular pH and sodium concentration. J Clin Invest 78:502–510, 1986.

74. Kleyman TR, Cragoe EJ, Jr: Amiloride and its analogs as tools in the study of ion transport. J Membr Biol 105:1–21, 1988.

75. Counillon L, Pouyssegur J: The expanding family of eucaryotic Na(+)/H(+) exchangers. J Biol Chem 275:1–4, 2000.

76. Tse CM, Brant SR, Walker MS, et al: Cloning and sequencing of a rabbit cDNA encoding an intestinal and kidney-specific Na⁺/H⁺ exchanger isoform (NHE-3). J Biol Chem 267:9340–9346, 1992.

77. Orlowski J, Kandasamy RA, Shull GE: Molecular cloning of putative members of the Na/H exchanger gene family. cDNA cloning, deduced amino acid sequence, and mRNA tissue expression of the rat Na/H exchanger NHE-1 and two structurally related proteins. J Biol Chem 267:9331–9339, 1992.

78. Burckhardt G, Di Sole F, Helmle-Kolb C: The Na⁺/H⁺ exchanger gene family. J Nephrol 15 Suppl 5:S3–21, 2002.

79. Amemiya M, Loffing J, Lotscher M, et al: Expression of NHE-3 in the apical membrane of rat renal proximal tubule and thick ascending limb. Kidney Int 48:1206–1215, 1995.

80. Biemesderfer D, Pizzonia J, Abu-Alfa A, et al: NHE3: A Na⁺/H⁺ exchanger isoform of renal brush border. Am J Physiol 265:F736–F742, 1993.

81. Nakamura S, Amlal H, Schultheis PJ, et al: HCO-3 reabsorption in renal collecting duct of NHE-3-deficient mouse: A compensatory response. Am J Physiol 276:F914–F921, 1999.

82. Wang T, Yang CL, Abbiati T, et al: Mechanism of proximal tubule bicarbonate absorption in NHE3 null mice. Am J Physiol 277:F298–F302, 1999.

83. Ledoussal C, Lorenz JN, Nieman ML, et al: Renal salt wasting in mice lacking NHE3 Na⁺/H⁺ exchanger but not in mice lacking NHE2. Am J Physiol Renal Physiol 281:F718–F727, 2001.

84. Schultheis PJ, Clarke LL, Meneton P, et al: Renal and intestinal absorptive defects in mice lacking the NHE3 Na⁺/H⁺ exchanger. Nat Genet 19:282–285, 1998.

85. Lorenz JN, Schultheis PJ, Traynor T, et al: Micropuncture analysis of single-nephron function in NHE3-deficient mice. Am J Physiol 277:F447–F453, 1999.

86. Choi JY, Shah M, Lee MG, et al: Novel amiloride-sensitive sodium-dependent proton secretion in the mouse proximal convoluted tubule. J Clin Invest 105:1141–1146, 2000.

87. Weinman EJ, Steplock D, Corry D, Shenolikar S: Identification of the human NHE-1 form of Na(+)-H⁺ exchanger in rabbit renal brush border membranes. J Clin Invest 91:2097–2102, 1993.

88. Chambrey R, Warnock DG, Podevin RA, et al: Immunolocalization of the Na⁺/H⁺ exchanger isoform NHE2 in rat kidney. Am J Physiol 275:F379–F386, 1998.

89. Sun AM, Liu Y, Dworkin LD, et al: Na⁺/H⁺ exchanger isoform 2 (NHE2) is expressed in the apical membrane of the medullary thick ascending limb. J Membr Biol 160:85–90, 1997.

90. Schultheis PJ, Clarke LL, Meneton P, et al: Targeted disruption of the murine Na⁺/H⁺ exchanger isoform 2 gene causes reduced viability of gastric parietal cells and loss of net acid secretion. J Clin Invest 101:1243–1253, 1998.

91. Cox GA, Lutz CM, Yang CL, et al: Sodium/hydrogen exchanger gene defect in slow-wave epilepsy mutant mice [erratum appears in Cell 91:861, 1997]. Cell 91:139–148, 1997.

92. Goyal S, Mentone S, Aronson PS: Immunolocalization of NHE8 in rat kidney. Am J Physiol Renal Physiol 288:F530–F538, 2005.

93. Kinsella JL, Aronson PS: Interaction of NH4+ and Li+ with the renal microvillus membrane Na⁺-H⁺ exchanger. Am J Physiol 241:C220–C226, 1981.

94. Nagami GT: Luminal secretion of ammonia in the mouse proximal tubule perfused in vitro. J Clin Invest 81:159–164, 1988.

95. Aronson PS, Nee J, Suhm MA: Modifier role of internal H⁺ in activating the Na⁺-H⁺ exchanger in renal microvillus membrane vesicles. Nature 299:161–163, 1982.

96. Kinne-Saffran E, Beauwens R, Kinne R: An ATP-driven proton pump in brush-border membranes from rat renal cortex. J Membr Biol 64:67–76, 1982.

97. Nakhoul NL, Hamm LL: Vacuolar H(+)-ATPase in the kidney. J Nephrol 15 Suppl 5:S22–S31, 2002.

98. Brown D, Breton S: Structure, function, and cellular distribution of the vacuolar H⁺ATPase (H⁺V-ATPase/proton pump). In Seldin DW, Giebisch G (eds): The Kidney:

Physiology and Pathophysiology. Philadelphia, Lippincott Williams & Wilkins, 2000, pp 171–191.

99. Forgac M: Structure, function and regulation of the vacuolar (H⁺)-ATPases. FEBS Lett 440:258–63, 1998.

100. Stone DK, Crider BP, Xie XS: Structural properties of vacuolar proton pumps. Kidney Int 38:649–653, 1990.

101. Gluck SL, Lee BS, Wang SP, et al: Plasma membrane V-ATPases in proton-transporting cells of the mammalian kidney and osteoclast [review] [84 refs]. Acta Physiol Scand Suppl 643:203–212, 1998.

102. Kurtz I: Apical Na⁺/H⁺ antiporter and glycolysis-dependent H⁺-ATPase regulate intracellular pH in the rabbit S3 proximal tubule. J Clin Invest 80:928–935, 1987.

103. Fromter E, Gessner K: Active transport potentials, membrane diffusion potentials and streaming potentials across rat kidney proximal tubule. Pflugers Arch 351:85–98, 1974.

104. Fromter E, Gessner K: Effect of inhibitors and diuretics on electrical potential differences in rat kidney proximal tubule. Pflugers Arch 357:209–224, 1975.

105. Bank N, Aynedjian HS, Mutz BF: Evidence for a DCCD-sensitive component of proximal bicarbonate reabsorption. Am J Physiol 249:F636–F644, 1985.

106. Bowman EJ, Siebers A, Altendorf K: Bafilomycins: A class of inhibitors of membrane ATPases from microorganisms, animal cells, and plant cells. Proc Natl Acad Sci U S A 85:7972–7976, 1988.

107. Brown D, Hirsch S, Gluck S: Localization of a proton-pumping ATPase in rat kidney. J Clin Invest 82:2114–2126, 1988.

108. Baum M: Evidence that parallel Na⁺-H⁺ and Cl(–)-HCO₃⁻(OH–) antiporters transport NaCl in the proximal tubule. Am J Physiol 252:F338–F345, 1987.

109. Lucci MS, Warnock DG: Effects of anion-transport inhibitors on NaCl reabsorption in the rat superficial proximal convoluted tubule. J Clin Invest 64:570–579, 1979.

110. Warnock DG, Yee VJ: Chloride uptake by brush border membrane vesicles isolated from rabbit renal cortex. Coupling to proton gradients and K⁺ diffusion potentials. J Clin Invest 67:103–115, 1981.

111. Shiuan D, Weinstein SW: Evidence for electroneutral chloride transport in rabbit renal cortical brush border membrane vesicles. Am J Physiol 247:F837–F847, 1984.

112. Chen PY, Illsley NP, Verkman AS: Renal brush-border chloride transport mechanisms characterized using a fluorescent indicator. Am J Physiol 254:F114–F120, 1988.

113. Burg M, Green N: Bicarbonate transport by isolated perfused rabbit proximal convoluted tubules. Am J Physiol 233:F307–F314, 1977.

114. Sasaki S, Berry CA: Mechanism of bicarbonate exit across basolateral membrane of the rabbit proximal convoluted tubule. Am J Physiol 246:F889–F896, 1984.

115. Aronson PS, Giebisch G: Mechanisms of chloride transport in the proximal tubule. Am J Physiol 273:F179–F192, 1997.

116. Knauf F, Yang CL, Thomson RB, et al: Identification of a chloride-formate exchanger expressed on the brush border membrane of renal proximal tubule cells. Proc Natl Acad Sci U S A 98:9425–9430, 2001.

117. Aronson PS: Ion exchangers mediating Na⁺, HCO₃⁻ and Cl⁻ transport in the renal proximal tubule. J Nephrol 19 Suppl 9:S3-S10:S3–S10, 2006.

118. Wang Z, Wang T, Petrovic S, et al: Renal and intestinal transport defects in Slc26a6-null mice. Am J Physiol Cell Physiol 288:C957–C965, 2005.

119. Chernova MN, Jiang L, Friedman DJ, et al: Functional comparison of mouse slc26a6 anion exchanger with human SLC26A6 polypeptide variants: Differences in anion selectivity, regulation, and electrogenicity. J Biol Chem 280:8564–8580, 2005.

120. Boron WF, Boulpaep EL: Intracellular pH regulation in the renal proximal tubule of the salamander. Basolateral HCO₃⁻ transport. J Gen Physiol 81:53–94, 1983.

121. Alpern RJ: Mechanism of basolateral membrane H⁺/OH⁻/HCO₃ transport in the rat proximal convoluted tubule. A sodium-coupled electrogenic process. J Gen Physiol 86:613–636, 1985.

122. Biagi BA, Sohtell M: Electrophysiology of basolateral bicarbonate transport in the rabbit proximal tubule. Am J Physiol 250:F267–F272, 1986.

123. Yoshitomi K, Burckhardt BC, Fromter E: Rheogenic sodium-bicarbonate cotransport in the peritubular cell membrane of rat renal proximal tubule. Pflugers Arch 405:360–366, 1985.

124. Biagi BA: Effects of the anion transport inhibitor, SITS, on the proximal straight tubule of the rabbit perfused in vitro. J Membr Biol 88:25–31, 1985.

125. Akiba T, Alpern RJ, Eveloff J, et al: Electrogenic sodium/bicarbonate cotransport in rabbit renal cortical basolateral membrane vesicles. J Clin Invest 78:1472–1478, 1986.

126. Grassl SM, Aronson PS: Na⁺/HCO₃⁻co-transport in basolateral membrane vesicles isolated from rabbit renal cortex. J Biol Chem 261:8778–8783, 1986.

127. Preisig PA, Alpern RJ: Basolateral membrane H-OH-HCO3 transport in the proximal tubule [review]. Am J Physiol 256:F751–F765, 1989.

128. Alpern RJ: Cell mechanisms of proximal tubule acidification [review]. Phys Rev 70:79–114, 1990.

129. Soleimani M, Grassi SM, Aronson PS: Stoichiometry of Na⁺-HCO-3 cotransport in basolateral membrane vesicles isolated from rabbit renal cortex. J Clin Invest 79:1276–1280, 1987.

130. Soleimani M, Aronson PS: Ionic mechanism of Na⁺-HCO₃⁻ cotransport in rabbit renal basolateral membrane vesicles. J Biol Chem 264:18302–18308, 1989.

131. Romero MF, Hediger MA, Boulpaep EL, Boron WF: Expression cloning and characterization of a renal electrogenic Na⁺/HCO₃⁻ cotransporter. Nature 387:409–413, 1997.

132. Burnham CE, Amlal H, Wang Z, et al: Cloning and functional expression of a human kidney Na⁺:HCO₃⁻ cotransporter. J Biol Chem 272:19111–19114, 1997.

133. Romero MF: The electrogenic Na⁺/HCO₃⁻ cotransporter, NBC. JOP 2:182–191, 2001.

134. Maunsbach AB, Vorum H, Kwon TH, et al: Immunoelectron microscopic localization of the electrogenic Na/HCO(3) cotransporter in rat and ambystoma kidney. J Am Soc Nephrol 11:2179–2189, 2000.

135. Romero MF, Boron WF: Electrogenic Na⁺/HCO₃⁻ cotransporters: Cloning and physiology. Annu Rev Physiol 61:699–723, 1999.
136. Seki G, Coppola S, Fromter E: The Na(+)-HCO3⁻ cotransporter operates with a coupling ratio of 2 HCO₃⁻ to 1 Na⁺ in isolated rabbit renal proximal tubule. Pflugers Arch 425:409–416, 1993.
137. Planelles G, Thomas SR, Anagnostopoulos T: Change of apparent stoichiometry of proximal-tubule Na(+)-HCO₃⁻ cotransport upon experimental reversal of its orientation. Proc Natl Acad Sci U S A 90:7406–7410, 1993.
138. Gross E, Hawkins K, Abuladze N, et al: The stoichiometry of the electrogenic sodium bicarbonate cotransporter NBC1 is cell-type dependent. J Physiol 531:597–603, 2001.
139. Gross E, Kurtz I: Structural determinants and significance of regulation of electrogenic Na(+)-HCO(3)(–) cotransporter stoichiometry. Am J Physiol Renal Physiol 283:F876–F887, 2002.
140. Gross E, Hawkins K, Pushkin A, et al: Phosphorylation of Ser(982) in the sodium bicarbonate cotransporter kNBC1 shifts the HCO(3)(–):Na(+) stoichiometry from 3:1 to 2:1 in murine proximal tubule cells. J Physiol 537:659–665, 2001.
141. Gross E, Pushkin A, Abuladze N, et al: Regulation of the sodium bicarbonate cotransporter kNBC1 function: Role of Asp(986), Asp(988) and kNBC1-carbonic anhydrase II binding. J Physiol 544:679–685, 2002.
142. Guggino WB, London R, Boulpaep EL, Giebisch G: Chloride transport across the basolateral cell membrane of the Necturus proximal tubule: Dependence on bicarbonate and sodium. J Membr Biol 71:227–240, 1983.
143. Alpern RJ, Chambers M: Basolateral membrane Cl/HCO₃ exchange in the rat proximal convoluted tubule. Na-dependent and -independent modes. J Gen Physiol 89:581–598, 1987.
144. Sasaki S, Yoshiyama N: Interaction of chloride and bicarbonate transport across the basolateral membrane of rabbit proximal straight tubule. Evidence for sodium coupled chloride/bicarbonate exchange. J Clin Invest 81:1004–1011, 1988.
145. Chen PY, Verkman AS: Sodium-dependent chloride transport in basolateral membrane vesicles isolated from rabbit proximal tubule. Biochemistry 27:655–660, 1988.
146. Nakhoul NL, Chen LK, Boron WF: Intracellular pH regulation in rabbit S3 proximal tubule: Basolateral Cl·HCO₃ exchange and Na-HCO₃ cotransport. Am J Physiol 258:F371–F381, 1990.
147. Kurtz I: Basolateral membrane Na⁺/H⁺ antiport, Na⁺/base cotransport, and Na⁺-independent Cl⁻/base exchange in the rabbit S3 proximal tubule. J Clin Invest 83:616–622, 1989.
148. Biemesderfer D, Reilly RF, Exner M, et al: Immunocytochemical characterization of Na(+)-H⁺ exchanger isoform NHE-1 in rabbit kidney. Am J Physiol 263:F833–F840, 1992.
149. Geibel J, Giebisch G, Boron WF: Basolateral sodium-coupled acid-base transport mechanisms of the rabbit proximal tubule. Am J Physiol 257:F790–F797, 1989.
150. Kaufman AM, Brod-Miller C, Kahn T: Role of citrate excretion in acid-base balance in diuretic-induced alkalosis in the rat. Am J Physiol 248:F796–F803, 1985.
151. Kaufman AM, Kahn T: Complementary role of citrate and bicarbonate excretion in acid-base balance in the rat. Am J Physiol 255:F182–F187, 1988.
152. Brown JC, Packer RK, Knepper MA: Role of organic anions in renal response to dietary acid and base loads. Am J Physiol 257:F170–F176, 1989.
153. Cheema-Dhadli S, Lin SH, Halperin ML: Mechanisms used to dispose of progressively increasing alkali load in rats. Am J Physiol Renal Physiol 282:F1049–F1055, 2002.
154. Hamm LL, Hering-Smith KS: Pathophysiology of hypocitraturic nephrolithiasis. Endocrinol Metab Clin North Am 31:885–893, viii, 2002.
155. Siebens AW, Boron WF: Effect of electroneutral luminal and basolateral lactate transport on intracellular pH in salamander proximal tubules. J Gen Physiol 90:799–831, 1987.
156. Nakhoul NL, Lopes AG, Chaillet JR, Boron WF: Intracellular pH regulation in the S3 segment of the rabbit proximal tubule in HCO₃⁻-free solutions. J Gen Physiol 92:369–393, 1988.
157. Nakhoul NL, Boron WF: Acetate transport in the S3 segment of the rabbit proximal tubule and its effect on intracellular pH. J Gen Physiol 92:395–412, 1988.
158. Hamm LL, Pucacco LR, Kokko JP, Jacobson HR: Hydrogen ion permeability of the rabbit proximal convoluted tubule. Am J Physiol 246:F3–F11, 1984.
159. Preisig PA, Alpern RJ: Contributions of cellular leak pathways to net NaHCO₃ and NaCl absorption. J Clin Invest 83:1859–1867, 1989.
160. Alpern RJ, Cogan MG, Rector FC, Jr: Effect of luminal bicarbonate concentration on proximal acidification in the rat. Am J Physiol 243:F53–F59, 1982.
161. Aronson PS: Kinetic properties of the plasma membrane Na⁺-H⁺ exchanger. Ann Rev Physiol 47:545–560, 1985.
162. DuBose TD, Jr, Pucacco LR, Lucci MS, Carter NW: Micropuncture determination of pH, PCO₂, and total CO₂ concentration in accessible structures of the rat renal cortex. J Clin Invest 64:476–482, 1979.
163. Buerkert J, Martin D, Trigg D: Segmental analysis of the renal tubule in buffer production and net acid formation. Am J Physiol 244:F442–F454, 1983.
164. Cogan MG, Maddox DA, Lucci MS, Rector FC: Control of proximal bicarbonate reabsorption in normal and acidotic rats. J Clin Invest 64:1168–1180, 1979.
165. Alpern RJ, Cogan MG, Rector FC, Jr: Effects of extracellular fluid volume and plasma bicarbonate concentration on proximal acidification in the rat. J Clin Invest 71:736–746, 1983.
166. Sasaki S, Berry CA, Rector FC, Jr: Effect of luminal and peritubular HCO3(–) concentrations and PCO₂ on HCO3(–) reabsorption in rabbit proximal convoluted tubules perfused in vitro. J Clin Invest 70:639–649, 1982.
167. Chan YL, Biagi B, Giebisch G: Control mechanisms of bicarbonate transport across the rat proximal convoluted tubule. Am J Physiol 242:F532–F543, 1982.
168. Cogan MG: Effects of acute alterations in PCO₂ on proximal HCO-3, Cl⁻, and H₂O reabsorption. Am J Physiol 246:F21–F26, 1984.
169. Mello AM, Malnic G: Peritubular pH and PCO'2 in renal tubular acidification. Am J Physiol 228:1766–1774, 1975.
170. Giebisch G, Malnic G, De Mello GB, de Mello AM: Kinetics of luminal acidification in cortical tubules of the rat kidney. J Physiol 267:571–599, 1977.
171. Levine DZ: Effect of acute hypercapnia on proximal tubular water and bicarbonate reabsorption. Am J Physiol 221:1164–1170, 1971.
172. Cogan MG, Rector FC, Jr: Proximal reabsorption during metabolic acidosis in the rat. Am J Physiol 242:F499–F507, 1982.
173. Wakabayashi S, Bertrand B, Shigekawa M, et al: Growth factor activation and "H(+)-sensing" of the Na⁺/H⁺ exchanger isoform 1 (NHE1). Evidence for an additional mechanism not requiring direct phosphorylation. J Biol Chem 269:5583–5588, 1994.
174. Schwartz GJ, Al Awqati Q: Carbon dioxide causes exocytosis of vesicles containing H⁺ pumps in isolated perfused proximal and collecting tubules. J Clin Invest 75:1638–1644, 1985.
175. Nakhoul NL, Chen LK, Boron WF: Effect of basolateral CO₂/HCO₃⁻ on intracellular pH regulation in the rabbit S3 proximal tubule. J Gen Physiol 102:1171–1205, 1993.
176. Chen LK, Boron WF: Acid extrusion in S3 segment of rabbit proximal tubule. II. Effect of basolateral CO₂/HCO₃⁻. Am J Physiol 268:F193–F203, 1995.
177. Zhao J, Zhou Y, Boron WF: Effect of isolated removal of either basolateral HCO-3 or basolateral CO₂ on HCO-3 reabsorption by rabbit S2 proximal tubule. Am J Physiol Renal Physiol 285:F359–F369, 2003.
178. Zhou Y, Zhao J, Bouyer P, Boron WF: Evidence from renal proximal tubules that HCO3⁻ and solute reabsorption are acutely regulated not by pH but by basolateral HCO3⁻ and CO₂. Proc Natl Acad Sci U S A 102:3875–3880, 2005.
179. Zhou Y, Bouyer P, Boron WF: Role of a tyrosine kinase in the CO₂-induced stimulation of HCO3⁻ reabsorption by rabbit S2 proximal tubules. Am J Physiol Renal Physiol 291:F358–F367, 2006.
180. Zhou Y, Bouyer P, Boron WF: Effects of angiotensin II on the CO₂ dependence of HCO3⁻ reabsorption by the rabbit S2 renal proximal tubule. Am J Physiol Renal Physiol 290: F666–F673, 2006.
181. Kunau RT, Jr., Hart JI, Walker KA: Effect of metabolic acidosis on proximal tubular total CO₂ absorption. Am J Physiol 249:F62–F68, 1985.
182. Cogan MG: Chronic hypercapnia stimulates proximal bicarbonate reabsorption in the rat. J Clin Invest 74:1942–1947, 1984.
183. Cohn DE, Klahr S, Hammerman MR: Metabolic acidosis and parathyroidectomy increase Na⁺-H⁺ exchange in brush border vesicles. Am J Physiol 245:F217–F222, 1983.
184. Tsai CJ, Ives HE, Alpern RJ, et al: Increased Vmax for Na⁺/H⁺ antiporter activity in proximal tubule brush border vesicles from rabbits with metabolic acidosis. Am J Physiol 247:F339–F343, 1984.
185. Preisig PA, Alpern RJ: Chronic metabolic acidosis causes an adaptation in the apical membrane Na/H antiporter and basolateral membrane Na(HCO3)3 symporter in the rat proximal convoluted tubule. J Clin Invest 82:1445–1453, 1988.
186. Akiba T, Rocco VK, Warnock DG: Parallel adaptation of the rabbit renal cortical sodium/proton antiporter and sodium/bicarbonate cotransporter in metabolic acidosis and alkalosis. J Clin Invest 80:308–315, 1987.
187. Kinsella J, Cujdik T, Sacktor B: Na⁺-H⁺ exchange activity in renal brush border membrane vesicles in response to metabolic acidosis: The role of glucocorticoids. Proc Natl Acad Sci U S A 81:630–634, 1984.
188. Kinsella J, Cujdik T, Sacktor B: Na⁺-H⁺ exchange in isolated renal brush-border membrane vesicles in response to metabolic acidosis. Kinetic effects. J Biol Chem 259:13224–13227, 1984.
189. Amlal H, Chen Q, Greeley T, et al: Coordinated down-regulation of NBC-1 and NHE-3 in sodium and bicarbonate loading. Kidney Int 60:1824–1836, 2001.
190. Soleimani M, Bizal GL, McKinney YJ: Effect of in vitro metabolic acidosis on luminal Na⁺/H⁺ exchange and basolateral Na⁺:HCO₃⁻ cotransport in rabbit kidney proximal tubules. J Clin Invest 90:211–218, 1992.
191. Chang CS, Talor Z, Arruda JA: Effect of metabolic or respiratory acidosis on rabbit renal medullary proton-ATPase. Biochem Cell Biol 66:20–24, 1988.
192. Ruiz OS, Arruda JA, Talor Z: Na-HCO3 cotransport and Na-H antiporter in chronic respiratory acidosis and alkalosis. Am J Physiol 256:F414–F420, 1989.
193. Krapf R: Mechanisms of adaptation to chronic respiratory acidosis in the rabbit proximal tubule. J Clin Invest 83:890–896, 1989.
194. Zeidel ML, Seifter JL: Regulation of Na/H exchange in renal microvillus vesicles in chronic hypercapnia. Kidney Int 34:60–66, 1988.
195. Northrup TE, Garella S, Perticucci E, Cohen JJ: Acidemia alone does not stimulate rat renal Na⁺-H⁺ antiporter activity. Am J Physiol 255:F237–F243, 1988.
196. Amemiya M, Yamaji Y, Cano A, et al: Acid incubation increases NHE-3 mRNA abundance in OKP cells. Am J Physiol 269:C126–C133, 1995.
197. Wu MS, Biemesderfer D, Giebisch G, Aronson PS: Role of NHE3 in mediating renal brush border Na⁺-H⁺ exchange. Adaptation to metabolic acidosis. J Biol Chem 271:32749–32752, 1996.
198. Ambuhl PM, Amemiya M, Danczkay M, et al: Chronic metabolic acidosis increases NHE3 protein abundance in rat kidney. Am J Physiol 271:F917–F925, 1996.
199. Yang X, Amemiya M, Peng Y, et al: Acid incubation causes exocytic insertion of NHE3 in OKP cells. Am J Physiol Cell Physiol 279:C410–C419, 2000.
200. Peng Y, Amemiya M, Yang X, et al: ET(B) receptor activation causes exocytic insertion of NHE3 in OKP cells. Am J Physiol Renal Physiol 280:F34–F42, 2001.
201. Laghmani K, Preisig PA, Moe OW, et al: Endothelin-1/endothelin-B receptor-mediated increases in NHE3 activity in chronic metabolic acidosis. J Clin Invest 107:1563–1569, 2001.
202. Ambuhl PM, Yang X, Peng Y, et al: Glucocorticoids enhance acid activation of the Na⁺/H⁺ exchanger 3 (NHE3). J Clin Invest 103:429–435, 1999.
203. Soleimani M, Bergman JA, Hosford MA, McKinney TD: Potassium depletion increases luminal Na⁺/H⁺ exchange and basolateral Na⁺:CO3=:HCO₃⁻ cotransport in rat renal cortex. J Clin Invest 86:1076–1083, 1990.

204. Amemiya M, Tabei K, Kusano E, et al: Incubation of OKP cells in low-K+ media increases NHE3 activity after early decrease in intracellular pH. Am J Physiol 276: C711–C716, 1999.

205. Adam WR, Koretsky AP, Weiner MW: 31P-NMR in vivo measurement of renal intracellular pH: Effects of acidosis and K+ depletion in rats. Am J Physiol 251:F904–F910, 1986.

206. Malnic G, Mello-Aires M: Kinetic study of bicarbonate reabsorption in proximal tubule of the rat. Am J Physiol 220:1759–1767, 1971.

207. Aronson PS, Suhm MA, Nee J: Interaction of external H+ with the Na+-H+ exchanger in renal microvillus membrane vesicles. J Biol Chem 258:6767–6771, 1983.

208. Alpern RJ, Rector FC, Jr: A model of proximal tubular bicarbonate absorption. Am J Physiol 248:F272–F281, 1985.

209. Alpern RJ, Cogan MG, Rector FC, Jr: Flow dependence of proximal tubular bicarbonate absorption. Am J Physiol 245:F478–F484, 1983.

210. Maddox DA, Gennari FJ: Load dependence of HCO3 and H2O reabsorption in the early proximal tubule of the Munich-Wistar rat. Am J Physiol 248:F113–F121, 1985.

211. Preisig PA: Luminal flow rate regulates proximal tubule H-HCO3 transporters. Am J Physiol 262:F47–F54, 1992.

212. Preisig PA, Alpern RJ: Increased Na/H antiporter and Na/3HCO3 symporter activities in chronic hyperfiltration. A model of cell hypertrophy. J Gen Physiol 97:195–217, 1991.

213. Harris RC, Seifter JL, Brenner BM: Adaptation of Na+-H+ exchange in renal microvillus membrane vesicles. Role of dietary protein and uninephrectomy. J Clin Invest 74:1979–1987, 1984.

214. Nord EP, Hafezi A, Kaunitz JD, et al: pH gradient-dependent increased Na+-H+ antiport capacity of the rabbit remnant kidney. Am J Physiol 249:F90–F98, 1985.

215. Cohn DE, Hruska KA, Klahr S, Hammerman MR: Increased Na+-H+ exchange in brush border vesicles from dogs with renal failure. Am J Physiol 243:F293–F299, 1982.

216. Cogan MG: Volume expansion predominantly inhibits proximal reabsorption of NaCl rather than NaHCO3. Am J Physiol 245:F272–F275, 1983.

217. Bichara M, Paillard M, Corman B, et al: Volume expansion modulates NaHCO3 and NaCl transport in the proximal tubule and Henle's loop. Am J Physiol 247: F140–F150, 1984.

218. Chan YL, Malnic G, Giebisch G: Passive driving forces of proximal tubular fluid and bicarbonate transport: Gradient dependence of H+ secretion. Am J Physiol 245:F622–F633, 1983.

219. Alpern RJ: Bicarbonate-water interactions in the rat proximal convoluted tubule. An effect of volume flux on active proton secretion. J Gen Physiol 84:753–770, 1984.

220. Mercier O, Bichara M, Paillard M: Parathyroid hormone contributes to volume expansion-induced inhibition of proximal reabsorption. Am J Physiol 248:F100–F103, 1985.

221. Zhang Y, Mircheff AK, Hensley CB, et al: Rapid redistribution and inhibition of renal sodium transporters during acute pressure natriuresis. Am J Physiol 270:F1004–F1014, 1996.

222. Yip KP, Tse CM, McDonough AA, Marsh DJ: Redistribution of Na+/H+ exchanger isoform NHE3 in proximal tubules induced by acute and chronic hypertension. Am J Physiol 275:F565–F575, 1998.

223. Yang L, Leong PK, Chen JO, et al: Acute hypertension provokes internalization of proximal tubule NHE3 without inhibition of transport activity. Am J Physiol Renal Physiol 282:F730–F740, 2002.

224. Moe OW, Tejedor A, Levi M, et al: Dietary NaCl modulates Na(+)-H+ antiporter activity in renal cortical apical membrane vesicles. Am J Physiol 260:F130–F137, 1991.

225. Laghmani K, Preisig PA, Alpern RJ: The role of endothelin in proximal tubule proton secretion and the adaptation to a chronic metabolic acidosis. J Nephrol 15 Suppl 5: S75–S87, 2002.

226. Wesson DE: Endogenous endothelins mediate increased distal tubule acidification induced by dietary acid in rats. J Clin Invest 99:2203–2211, 1997.

227. Wesson DE, Simoni J, Green DF: Reduced extracellular pH increases endothelin-1 secretion by human renal microvascular endothelial cells. J Clin Invest 101:578–583, 1998.

228. Garcia NH, Garvin JL: Endothelin's biphasic effect on fluid absorption in the proximal straight tubule and its inhibitory cascade. J Clin Invest 93:2572–2577, 1994.

229. Guntupalli J, DuBose TD, Jr: Effects of endothelin on rat renal proximal tubule Na(+)-Pi cotransport and Na+/H+ exchange. Am J Physiol 266:F658–F666, 1994.

230. Eiam-Ong S, Hilden SA, King AJ, et al: Endothelin-1 stimulates the Na+/H+ and Na+/HCO3− transporters in rabbit renal cortex. Kidney Int 42:18–24, 1992.

231. Chu TS, Peng Y, Cano A, et al: Endothelin(B) receptor activates NHE-3 by a Ca2+-dependent pathway in OKP cells. J Clin Invest 97:1454–1462, 1996.

232. Peng Y, Moe OW, Chu T, et al: ETB receptor activation leads to activation and phosphorylation of NHE3. Am J Physiol 276:C938–C945, 1999.

233. Chu TS, Tsuganezawa H, Peng Y, et al: Role of tyrosine kinase pathways in ETB receptor activation of NHE3. Am J Physiol 271:C763–C771, 1996.

234. Yamaji Y, Tsuganezawa H, Moe OW, Alpern RJ: Intracellular acidosis activates c-Src. Am J Physiol 272:C886–C893, 1997.

235. Tsuganezawa H, Sato S, Yamaji Y, et al: Role of c-SRC and ERK in acid-induced activation of NHE3. Kidney Int 62:41–50, 2002.

236. Li S, Sato S, Yang X, et al: Pyk2 activation is integral to acid stimulation of sodium/hydrogen exchanger 3. J Clin Invest 114:1782–1789, 2004.

237. Ruiz OS, Robey RB, Qiu YY, et al: Regulation of the renal Na-HCO(3) cotransporter. XI. Signal transduction underlying CO(2) stimulation. Am J Physiol 277:F580–F586, 1999.

238. Espiritu DJ, Bernardo AA, Robey RB, Arruda JA: A central role for Pyk2-Src interaction in coupling diverse stimuli to increased epithelial NBC activity. Am J Physiol Renal Physiol 283:F663–F670, 2002.

239. Welbourne TC: Acidosis activation of the pituitary-adrenal-renal glutaminase I axis. Endocrinology 99:1071–1079, 1976.

240. Freiberg JM, Kinsella J, Sacktor B: Glucocorticoids increase the Na+-H+ exchange and decrease the Na+ gradient-dependent phosphate-uptake systems in renal brush border membrane vesicles. Proc Natl Acad Sci U S A 79:4932–4936, 1982.

241. Loffing J, Lotscher M, Kaissling B, et al: Renal Na/H exchanger NHE-3 and Na-PO4 cotransporter NaPi-2 protein expression in glucocorticoid excess and deficient states. J Am Soc Nephrol 9:1560–1567, 1998.

242. Bobulescu IA, Dwarakanath V, Zou L, et al: Glucocorticoids acutely increase cell surface Na+/H+ exchanger-3 (NHE3) by activation of NHE3 exocytosis. Am J Physiol Renal Physiol 289:F685–F691, 2005.

243. Baum M, Amemiya M, Dwarakanath V, et al: Glucocorticoids regulate NHE-3 transcription in OKP cells. Am J Physiol 270:F164–F169, 1996.

244. Ali R, Amlal H, Burnham CE, Soleimani M: Glucocorticoids enhance the expression of the basolateral Na+:HCO3− cotransporter in renal proximal tubules. Kidney Int 57:1063–1071, 2000.

245. Ruiz OS, Wang LJ, Pahlavan P, Arruda JA: Regulation of renal Na-HCO3 cotransporter: III. Presence and modulation by glucocorticoids in primary cultures of the proximal tubule. Kidney Int 47:1669–1676, 1995.

246. Hamm LL, Hering-Smith KS, Alpern RJ: Role of glucocorticoids in acidosis. Am J Kidney Dis 34:960–965, 1999.

247. Gupta N, Tarif SR, Seikaly M, Baum M: Role of glucocorticoids in the maturation of the rat renal Na+/H+ antiporter (NHE3). Kidney Int 60:173–181, 2001.

248. McKinney TD, Myers P: PTH inhibition of bicarbonate transport by proximal convoluted tubules. Am J Physiol 239:F127–F134, 1980.

249. Puschett JB, Zurbach P, Sylk D: Acute effects of parathyroid hormone on proximal bicarbonate transport in the dog. Kidney Int 9:501–510, 1976.

250. Bank N, Aynedjian HS: A micropuncture study of the effect of parathyroid hormone on renal bicarbonate reabsorption. J Clin Invest 58:336–344, 1976.

251. Moe OW, Amemiya M, Yamaji Y: Activation of protein kinase A acutely inhibits and phosphorylates Na/H exchanger NHE-3. J Clin Invest 96:2187–2194, 1995.

252. Fan L, Wiederkehr MR, Collazo R, et al: Dual mechanisms of regulation of Na/H exchanger NHE-3 by parathyroid hormone in rat kidney. J Biol Chem 274:11289–11295, 1999.

253. Collazo R, Fan L, Hu MC, et al: Acute regulation of Na+/H+ exchanger NHE3 by parathyroid hormone via NHE3 phosphorylation and dynamin-dependent endocytosis. J Biol Chem 275:31601–31608, 2000.

254. Zhao H, Wiederkehr MR, Fan L, et al: Acute inhibition of Na/H exchanger NHE-3 by cAMP. Role of protein kinase a and NHE-3 phosphoserines 552 and 605. J Biol Chem 274:3978–3987, 1999.

255. Pastoriza-Munoz E, Harrington RM, Graber ML: Parathyroid hormone decreases HCO3 reabsorption in the rat proximal tubule by stimulating phosphatidylinositol metabolism and inhibiting base exit. J Clin Invest 89:1485–1495, 1992.

256. Ruiz OS, Qiu YY, Wang LJ, Arruda JA: Regulation of the renal Na-HCO3 cotransporter: V. Mechanism of the inhibitory effect of parathyroid hormone. Kidney Int 49:396–402, 1996.

257. Weinman EJ, Evangelista CM, Steplock D, et al: Essential role for NHERF in cAMP-mediated inhibition of the Na+-HCO3− co-transporter in BSC-1 cells. J Biol Chem 276:42339–42346, 2001.

258. Bernardo AA, Kear FT, Santos AV, et al: Basolateral Na(+)/HCO(3)(−) cotransport activity is regulated by the dissociable Na(+)/H(+) exchanger regulatory factor. J Clin Invest 104:195–201, 1999.

259. Bichara M, Mercier O, Paillard M, Leviel F: Effects of parathyroid hormone on urinary acidification. Am J Physiol 251:F444–F453, 1986.

260. Paillard M, Bichara M: Peptide hormone effects on urinary acidification and acid-base balance: PTH, ADH, and glucagon. Am J Physiol 256:F973–F985, 1989.

261. Bichara M, Mercier O, Borensztein P, Paillard M: Acute metabolic acidosis enhances circulating parathyroid hormone, which contributes to the renal response against acidosis in the rat. J Clin Invest 86:430–443, 1990.

262. Cano A, Preisig P, Alpern RJ: Cyclic adenosine monophosphate acutely inhibits and chronically stimulates Na/H antiporter in OKP cells. J Clin Invest 92:1632–1638, 1993.

263. Moe OW: Acute regulation of proximal tubule apical membrane Na/H exchanger NHE-3: Role of phosphorylation, protein trafficking, and regulatory factors. J Am Soc Nephrol 10:2412–2425, 1999.

264. Geibel J, Giebisch G, Boron WF: Angiotensin II stimulates both Na(+)-H+ exchange and Na+/HCO3− cotransport in the rabbit proximal tubule. Proc Natl Acad Sci U S A 87:7917–7920, 1990.

265. Baum M, Quigley R, Quan A: Effect of luminal angiotensin II on rabbit proximal convoluted tubule bicarbonate absorption. Am J Physiol 273:F595–F600, 1997.

266. Bloch RD, Zikos D, Fisher KA, et al: Activation of proximal tubular Na(+)-H+ exchange by angiotensin II. Am J Physiol 263:F135–F143, 1992.

267. Liu FY, Cogan MG: Angiotensin II: A potent regulator of acidification in the rat early proximal convoluted tubule. J Clin Invest 80:272–275, 1987.

268. Liu FY, Cogan MG: Angiotensin II stimulation of hydrogen ion secretion in the rat early proximal tubule. Modes of action, mechanism, and kinetics. J Clin Invest 82:601–607, 1988.

269. Eiam-Ong S, Hilden SA, Johns CA, Madias NE: Stimulation of basolateral Na(+)-HCO3− cotransporter by angiotensin II in rabbit renal cortex. Am J Physiol 265: F195–F203, 1993.

270. Ruiz OS, Qiu YY, Wang LJ, Arruda JA: Regulation of the renal Na-HCO3 cotransporter: IV. Mechanisms of the stimulatory effect of angiotensin II. J Am Soc Nephrol 6:1202–1208, 1995.

271. Liu FY, Cogan MG: Angiotensin II stimulates early proximal bicarbonate absorption in the rat by decreasing cyclic adenosine monophosphate. J Clin Invest 84:83–91, 1989.

272. Liu FY, Cogan MG: Role of protein kinase C in proximal bicarbonate absorption and angiotensin signaling. Am J Physiol 258:F927–F933, 1990.

273. Tsuganezawa H, Preisig PA, Alpern RJ: Dominant negative c-Src inhibits angiotensin II induced activation of NHE3 in OKP cells. Kidney Int 54:394–398, 1998.

274. Robey RB, Ruiz OS, Espiritu DJ, et al: Angiotensin II stimulation of renal epithelial cell Na/HCO3 cotransport activity: A central role for Src family kinase/classic MAPK pathway coupling. J Membr Biol 187:135–145, 2002.

275. Klisic J, Hu MC, Nief V, et al: Insulin activates Na(+)/H(+) exchanger 3: Biphasic response and glucocorticoid dependence. Am J Physiol Renal Physiol 283:F532–F539, 2002.

276. Felder CC, Campbell T, Albrecht F, Jose PA: Dopamine inhibits Na(+)-H+ exchanger activity in renal BBMV by stimulation of adenylate cyclase. Am J Physiol 259:F297–F303, 1990.

277. Wiederkehr MR, Di Sole F, Collazo R, et al: Characterization of acute inhibition of Na/H exchanger NHE-3 by dopamine in opossum kidney cells. Kidney Int 59:197–209, 2001.

278. Hu MC, Fan L, Crowder LA, Karim-Jimenez Z, et al: Dopamine acutely stimulates Na(+)/H+ exchanger (NHE3) endocytosis via clathrin-coated vesicles: Dependence on protein kinase A-mediated NHE3 phosphorylation. J Biol Chem 276:26906–26915, 2001.

279. Cano A, Baum M, Moe OW: Thyroid hormone stimulates the renal Na/H exchanger NHE3 by transcriptional activation. Am J Physiol 276:C102–C108, 1999.

280. Amemiya M, Kusano E, Muto S, et al: Glucagon acutely inhibits but chronically activates Na(+)/H(+) antiporter 3 activity in OKP cells. Exp Nephrol 10:26–33, 2002.

281. Di Sole F, Casavola V, Mastroberardino L, et al: Adenosine inhibits the transfected Na+-H+ exchanger NHE3 in Xenopus laevis renal epithelial cells (A6/C1). J Physiol 515:829–842, 1999.

282. Di Sole F, Cerull R, Casavola V, et al: Molecular aspects of acute inhibition of Na(+)-H(+) exchanger NHE3 by A(2)-adenosine receptor agonists. J Physiol 541:529–543, 2002.

283. Ruiz OS, Qiu YY, Cardoso LR, Arruda JA: Regulation of the renal Na-HCO3 cotransporter: VII. Mechanism of the cholinergic stimulation. Kidney Int 51:1069–1077, 1997.

284. Robey RB, Ruiz OS, Baniqued J, et al: SFKs, Ras, and the classic MAPK pathway couple muscarinic receptor activation to increased Na-HCO(3) cotransport activity in renal epithelial cells. Am J Physiol Renal Physiol 280:F844–F850, 2001.

285. Chan YL: Adrenergic control of bicarbonate absorption in the proximal convoluted tubule of the rat kidney. Pflugers Arch 388:159–164, 1980.

286. Nord EP, Howard MJ, Hafezi A, et al: Alpha 2 adrenergic agonists stimulate Na+-H+ antiport activity in the rabbit renal proximal tubule. J Clin Invest 80:1755–1762, 1987.

287. Hall RA, Premont RT, Chow CW, et al: The beta2-adrenergic receptor interacts with the Na+/H+-exchanger regulatory factor to control Na+/H+ exchange. Nature 392:626–630, 1998.

288. Di SF, Cerull R, Babich V, et al: Acute regulation of Na/H exchanger NHE3 by adenosine A(1) receptors is mediated by calcineurin homologous protein. J Biol Chem 279:2962–2974, 2004.

289. Wang T: Role of iNOS and eNOS in modulating proximal tubule transport and acid-base balance. Am J Physiol Renal Physiol 283:F658–F662, 2002.

290. Wang T, Inglis FM, Kalb RG: Defective fluid and HCO(3)(–) absorption in proximal tubule of neuronal nitric oxide synthase-knockout mice. Am J Physiol Renal Physiol 279:F518–F524, 2000.

291. Kurashima K, Szabo EZ, Lukacs G, et al: Endosomal recycling of the Na+/H+ exchanger NHE3 isoform is regulated by the phosphatidylinositol 3-kinase pathway. J Biol Chem 273:20828–20836, 1998.

292. Shenolikar S, Weinman EJ: NHERF: Targeting and trafficking membrane proteins [review]. Am J Physiol Renal Physiol 280:F389–F395, 2001.

293. Weinman EJ: New functions for the NHERF family of proteins [letter; comment]. J Clin Invest 108:185–186, 2001.

294. Weinman EJ, Steplock D, Shenolikar S: CAMP-mediated inhibition of the renal brush border membrane Na+-H+ exchanger requires a dissociable phosphoprotein cofactor. J Clin Invest 92:1781–1786, 1993.

295. Lamprecht G, Weinman EJ, Yun CH: The role of NHERF and E3KARP in the cAMP-mediated inhibition of NHE3. J Biol Chem 273:29972–29978, 1998.

296. Weinman EJ, Steplock D, Wade JB, Shenolikar S: Ezrin binding domain-deficient NHERF attenuates cAMP-mediated inhibition of Na(+)/H(+) exchange in OK cells. Am J Physiol Renal Physiol 281:F374–F380, 2001.

297. Weinman EJ, Steplock D, Donowitz M, Shenolikar S: NHERF associations with sodium-hydrogen exchanger isoform 3 (NHE3) and ezrin are essential for cAMP-mediated phosphorylation and inhibition of NHE3. Biochemistry 39:6123–6129, 2000.

298. Zizak M, Lamprecht G, Steplock D, et al: cAMP-induced phosphorylation and inhibition of Na(+)/H(+) exchanger 3 (NHE3) are dependent on the presence but not the phosphorylation of NHE regulatory factor. J Biol Chem 274:24753–24758, 1999.

299. Szaszi K, Kurashima K, Kaibuchi K, et al: Role of the cytoskeleton in mediating cAMP-dependent protein kinase inhibition of the epithelial Na+/H+ exchanger NHE3. J Biol Chem 276:40761–40768, 2001.

300. Han W, Kim KH, Jo MJ, et al: Shank2 associates with and regulates Na+/H+ exchanger 3. J Biol Chem 281:1461–1469, 2006.

301. Biemesderfer D, Nagy T, DeGray B, Aronson PS: Specific association of megalin and the Na+/H+ exchanger isoform NHE3 in the proximal tubule. J Biol Chem 274:17518–17524, 1999.

302. Biemesderfer D, DeGray B, Aronson PS: Active (9.6 s) and inactive (21 s) oligomers of NHE3 in microdomains of the renal brush border. J Biol Chem 276:10161–10167, 2001.

303. Capasso G, Unwin R, Agulian S, Giebisch G: Bicarbonate transport along the loop of Henle. I. Microperfusion studies of load and inhibitor sensitivity. J Clin Invest 88:430–437, 1991.

304. Capasso G, Unwin R, Rizzo M, et al: Bicarbonate transport along the loop of Henle: Molecular mechanisms and regulation. J Nephrol 15 Suppl 5:S88–S96, 2002.

305. Capasso G, Evangelista C, Zacchia M, et al: Acid-base transport in Henle's loop: the effects of reduced renal mass and diabetes. J Nephrol 19 Suppl 9:S11–S17, 2006.

306. Good DW, Knepper MA, Burg MB: Ammonia and bicarbonate transport by thick ascending limb of rat kidney. Am J Physiol 247:F35–F44, 1984.

307. Good DW: The thick ascending limb as a site of renal bicarbonate reabsorption. Semin Nephrol 13:225–235, 1993.

308. Good DW: Sodium-dependent bicarbonate absorption by cortical thick ascending limb of rat kidney. Am J Physiol 248:F821–F829, 1985.

309. Kikeri D, Azar S, Sun A, et al: Na(+)-H+ antiporter and Na(+)-(HCO3–)n symporter regulate intracellular pH in mouse medullary thick limbs of Henle. Am J Physiol 258:F445–F456, 1990.

310. Wang T, Hropot M, Aronson PS, Giebisch G: Role of NHE isoforms in mediating bicarbonate reabsorption along the nephron. Am J Physiol Renal Physiol 281:F1117–F1122, 2001.

311. Biemesderfer D, Rutherford PA, Nagy T, et al: Monoclonal antibodies for high-resolution localization of NHE3 in adult and neonatal rat kidney. Am J Physiol 273:F289–F299, 1997.

312. Good DW, Watts BA, III: Functional roles of apical membrane Na+/H+ exchange in rat medullary thick ascending limb. Am J Physiol 270:F691–F699, 1996.

313. Vallon V, Schwark JR, Richter K, Hropot M: Role of Na(+)/H(+) exchanger NHE3 in nephron function: Micropuncture studies with S3226, an inhibitor of NHE3. Am J Physiol Renal Physiol 278:F375–F379, 2000.

314. Watts BA, III, Good DW: Apical membrane Na+/H+ exchange in rat medullary thick ascending limb. pH-dependence and inhibition by hyperosmolality. J Biol Chem 269:20250–20255, 1994.

315. Watts BA, III, Good DW: An apical K(+)-dependent HCO(3)- transport pathway opposes transepithelial HCO(3)- absorption in rat medullary thick ascending limb. Am J Physiol Renal Physiol 287:F57–F63, 2004.

316. Attmane-Elakeb A, Amlal H, Bichara M: Ammonium carriers in medullary thick ascending limb. Am J Physiol Renal Physiol 280:F1–F9, 2001.

317. Krapf R: Basolateral membrane H/OH/HCO3 transport in the rat cortical thick ascending limb. Evidence for an electrogenic Na/HCO3 cotransporter in parallel with a Na/H antiporter. J Clin Invest 82:234–241, 1988.

318. Vorum H, Kwon TH, Fulton C, et al: Immunolocalization of electroneutral Na-HCO(3)(–) cotransporter in rat kidney. Am J Physiol Renal Physiol 279:F901–F909, 2000.

319. Kwon TH, Fulton C, Wang W, et al: Chronic metabolic acidosis upregulates rat kidney Na-HCO cotransporters NBCn1 and NBC3 but not NBC1. Am J Physiol Renal Physiol 282:F341–F351, 2002.

320. Hebert SC: Hypertonic cell volume regulation in mouse thick limbs. II. Na+-H+ and Cl(–)-HCO3– exchange in basolateral membranes. Am J Physiol 250:C920–C931, 1986.

321. Blanchard A, Leviel F, Bichara M, et al: Interactions of external and internal K+ with K(+)-HCO3– cotransporter of rat medullary thick ascending limb. Am J Physiol 271:C218–C225, 1996.

322. Leviel F, Eladari D, Blanchard A, et al: Pathways for HCO-3 exit across the basolateral membrane in rat thick limbs. Am J Physiol 276:F847–F856, 1999.

323. Bourgeois S, Masse S, Paillard M, Houillier P: Basolateral membrane Cl(–)-, Na(+)-, and K(+)-coupled base transport mechanisms in rat MTALH. Am J Physiol Renal Physiol 282:F655–F668, 2002.

324. Eladari D, Blanchard A, Leviel F, et al: Functional and molecular characterization of luminal and basolateral Cl-/HCO-3 exchangers of rat thick limbs. Am J Physiol 275:F334–F342, 1998.

325. Alper SL, Stuart-Tilley AK, Biemesderfer D, et al: Immunolocalization of AE2 anion exchanger in rat kidney. Am J Physiol 273:F601–F614, 1997.

326. Alper SL, Darman RB, Chernova MN, Dahl NK: The AE gene family of Cl/HCO3– exchangers. J Nephrol 15 Suppl 5:S41–S53, 2002.

327. Quentin F, Eladari D, Frische S, et al: Regulation of the Cl-/HCO3– exchanger AE2 in rat thick ascending limb of Henle's loop in response to changes in acid-base and sodium balance. J Am Soc Nephrol 15:2988–2997, 2004.

328. Frische S, Zolotarev AS, Kim YH, et al: AE2 isoforms in rat kidney: Immunohistochemical localization and regulation in response to chronic NH4Cl loading. Am J Physiol Renal Physiol 286:F1163–F1170, 2004.

329. Good DW, George T, Watts BA, III: Basolateral membrane Na+/H+ exchange enhances HCO3– absorption in rat medullary thick ascending limb: Evidence for functional coupling between basolateral and apical membrane Na+/H+ exchangers. Proc Natl Acad Sci U S A 92:12525–12529, 1995.

330. Chambrey R, St John PL, Eladari D, et al: Localization and functional characterization of Na+/H+ exchanger isoform NHE4 in rat thick ascending limbs. Am J Physiol Renal Physiol 281:F707–F717, 2001.

331. Capasso G, Unwin R, Ciani F, et al: Bicarbonate transport along the loop of Henle. II. Effects of acid-base, dietary, and neurohumoral determinants. J Clin Invest 94:830–838, 1994.

332. Good DW: Adaptation of HCO-3 and NH+4 transport in rat MTAL: Effects of chronic metabolic acidosis and Na+ intake. Am J Physiol 258:F1345–F1353, 1990.

333. Laghmani K, Borensztein P, Ambuhl P, et al: Chronic metabolic acidosis enhances NHE-3 protein abundance and transport activity in the rat thick ascending limb by increasing NHE-3 mRNA. J Clin Invest 99:24–30, 1997.

334. Unwin R, Stidwell R, Taylor S, Capasso G: The effects of respiratory alkalosis and acidosis on net bicarbonate flux along the rat loop of Henle in vivo. Am J Physiol 273:F698–F705, 1997.

335. Laghmani K, Chambrey R, Froissart M, et al: Adaptation of NHE-3 in the rat thick ascending limb: Effects of high sodium intake and metabolic alkalosis. Am J Physiol 276:F18–F26, 1999.

336. DuBose TD, Jr., Lucci MS, Hogg RJ, et al: Comparison of acidification parameters in superficial and deep nephrons of the rat. Am J Physiol 244:F497–F503, 1983.

337. Good DW, George T, Watts BA, III: Aldosterone inhibits HCO absorption via a nongenomic pathway in medullary thick ascending limb. Am J Physiol Renal Physiol 283: F699–F706, 2002.

338. Good DW, George T, Watts BA, III: Nongenomic regulation by aldosterone of the epithelial NHE3 Na(+)/H(+) exchanger. Am J Physiol Cell Physiol 290:C757–C763, 2006.

339. Unwin R, Capasso G, Giebisch G: Bicarbonate transport along the loop of Henle effects of adrenal steroids. Am J Physiol 268:F234–F239, 1995.

340. Good DW, George T, Wang DH: Angiotensin II inhibits HCO-3 absorption via a cytochrome P-450-dependent pathway in MTAL. Am J Physiol 276:F726–F736, 1999.

341. Good DW: Nerve growth factor regulates HCO3− absorption in thick ascending limb: Modifying effects of vasopressin. Am J Physiol 274:C931–C939, 1998.

342. Watts BA, III, Di Mari JF, Davis RJ, Good DW: Hypertonicity activates MAP kinases and inhibits HCO-3 absorption via distinct pathways in thick ascending limb. Am J Physiol 275:F478–F486, 1998.

343. Good DW, Di Mari JF, Watts BA, III: Hyposmolality stimulates Na(+)/H(+) exchange and HCO(3)(–) absorption in thick ascending limb via PI 3-kinase. Am J Physiol Cell Physiol 279:C1443–C1454, 2000.

344. Watts BA, III, Good DW: ERK mediates inhibition of Na(+)/H(+) exchange and HCO(3)(–) absorption by nerve growth factor in MTAL. Am J Physiol Renal Physiol 282:F1056–F1063, 2002.

345. Borensztein P, Juvin P, Vernimmen C, et al: cAMP-dependent control of Na+/H+ antiport by AVP, PTH, and PGE2 in rat medullary thick ascending limb cells. Am J Physiol 264:F354–F364, 1993.

346. Watts BA, III, George T, Good DW: Nerve growth factor inhibits HCO3− absorption in renal thick ascending limb through inhibition of basolateral membrane Na+/H+ exchange. J Biol Chem 274:7841–7847, 1999.

347. Watts BA, III, George T, Good DW: The basolateral NHE1 Na+/H+ exchanger regulates transepithelial HCO3− absorption through actin cytoskeleton remodeling in renal thick ascending limb. J Biol Chem 280:11439–11447, 2005.

348. Good DW: Effects of osmolality on bicarbonate absorption by medullary thick ascending limb of the rat. J Clin Invest 89:184–190, 1992.

349. Good DW: Hyperosmolality inhibits bicarbonate absorption in rat medullary thick ascending limb via a protein-tyrosine kinase-dependent pathway. J Biol Chem 270:9883–9889, 1995.

350. Watts BA, III, Good DW: Hyposmolality stimulates apical membrane Na(+)/H(+) exchange and HCO(3)(–) absorption in renal thick ascending limb. J Clin Invest 104:1593–1602, 1999.

351. Good DW: Inhibition of bicarbonate absorption by peptide hormones and cyclic adenosine monophosphate in rat medullary thick ascending limb. J Clin Invest 85:1006–1013, 1990.

352. Bichara M, Mercier O, Houillier P, et al: Effects of antidiuretic hormone on urinary acidification and on tubular handling of bicarbonate in the rat. J Clin Invest 80:621–630, 1987.

353. DuBose TD, Jr, Good DW: Effects of diuretics on renal acid-base transport. Semin Nephrol 8:282–294, 1988.

354. Steinmetz PR: Cellular organization of urinary acidification. Am J Physiol 251: F173–F187, 1986.

355. Steinmetz PR: Characteristics of hydrogen ion transport in urinary bladder of water turtle. J Am Soc Nephrol 11:1160–1169, 2000.

356. Al Awqati Q: H + transport in urinary epithelia. Am J Physiol 235:F77–F88, 1978.

357. Schilb TP, Durham JH, Brodsky WA: In vivo environmental temperature and the in vitro pattern of luminal acidification in turtle bladders. Evidence for HCO3 ion reabsorption. J Gen Physiol 92:613–642, 1988.

358. Wang T, Malnic G, Giebisch G, Chan YL: Renal bicarbonate reabsorption in the rat. IV. Bicarbonate transport mechanisms in the early and late distal tubule. J Clin Invest 91:2776–2784, 1993.

359. McKinney TD, Burg MB: Bicarbonate transport by rabbit cortical collecting tubules. Effect of acid and alkali loads in vivo on transport in vitro. J Clin Invest 60:766–768, 1977.

360. Knepper MA, Good DW, Burg MB. Ammonia and bicarbonate transport by rat cortical collecting ducts perfused in vitro. Am J Physiol 247:F870–F877, 1985.

361. Levine DZ, Iacovitti M, Nash L, Vandorpe D: Secretion of bicarbonate by rat distal tubules in vivo. Modulation by overnight fasting. J Clin Invest 81:1873–1878, 1988.

362. Royaux IE, Wall SM, Karniski LP, et al: Pendrin, encoded by the Pendred syndrome gene, resides in the apical region of renal intercalated cells and mediates bicarbonate secretion. Proc Natl Acad Sci U S A 98:4221–4226, 2001.

363. Gifford JD, Rome L, Galla JH: H(+)-K(+)-ATPase activity in rat collecting duct segments. Am J Physiol 262:F692–F695, 1992.

364. Hayashi M, Yamaji Y, Iyori M, et al: Effect of isoproterenol on intracellular pH of the intercalated cells in the rabbit cortical collecting ducts. J Clin Invest 87:1153–1157, 1991.

365. Garcia-Austt J, Good DW, Burg MB, Knepper MA: Deoxycorticosterone-stimulated bicarbonate secretion in rabbit cortical collecting ducts: Effects of luminal chloride removal and in vivo acid loading. Am J Physiol 249:F205–F212, 1985.

366. Wesson DE, Dolson GM: Enhanced HCO3 secretion by distal tubule contributes to NaCl-induced correction of chronic alkalosis. Am J Physiol 264:F899–F906, 1993.

367. Galla JH, Gifford JD, Luke RG, Rome L: Adaptations to chloride-depletion alkalosis. Am J Physiol 261:R771–R781, 1991.

368. Hamm LL, Hering-Smith KS, Vehaskari VM: Control of bicarbonate transport in collecting tubules from normal and remnant kidneys. Am J Physiol 256:F680–F687, 1989.

369. Weiner ID, Hamm LL: Use of fluorescent dye BCECF to measure intracellular pH in cortical collecting tubule. Am J Physiol 256:F957–F964, 1989.

370. Weiner ID, Hamm LL: Regulation of intracellular pH in the rabbit cortical collecting tubule. J Clin Invest 85:274–281, 1990.

371. Weiner ID, Hamm LL: Regulation of Cl−/HCO3− exchange in the rabbit cortical collecting tubule. J Clin Invest 87:1553–1558, 1991.

372. Capasso G, Jaeger P, Giebisch G, et al: Renal bicarbonate reabsorption in the rat. II. Distal tubule load dependence and effect of hypokalemia. J Clin Invest 80:409–414, 1987.

373. Capasso G, Kinne R, Malnic G, Giebisch G: Renal bicarbonate reabsorption in the rat. I. Effects of hypokalemia and carbonic anhydrase. J Clin Invest 78:1558–1567, 1986.

374. Chan YL, Malnic G, Giebisch G: Renal bicarbonate reabsorption in the rat. III. Distal tubule perfusion study of load dependence and bicarbonate permeability 2639. J Clin Invest 84:931–938, 1989.

375. Kunau RT, Jr, Walker KA: Total CO2 absorption in the distal tubule of the rat 1591. Am J Physiol 252:F468–F473, 1987.

376. Levine DZ: An in vivo microperfusion study of distal tubule bicarbonate reabsorption in normal and ammonium chloride rats. J Clin Invest 75:588–595, 1985.

377. Lucci MS, Pucacco LR, Carter NW, DuBose TD, Jr: Evaluation of bicarbonate transport in rat distal tubule: Effects of acid-base status. Am J Physiol 243:F335–F341, 1982.

378. Malnic G, de Mello AM, Giebisch G: Micropuncture study of renal tubular hydrogen ion transport in the rat. Am J Physiol 222:147–158, 1972.

379. Bailey MA, Giebisch G, Abbiati T, et al: NHE2-mediated bicarbonate reabsorption in the distal tubule of NHE3 null mice. J Physiol 561:765–775, 2004.

380. Wesson DE: Na/H exchange and H-K ATPase increase distal tubule acidification in chronic alkalosis. Kidney Int 53:945–951, 1998.

381. Fejes-Toth G, Naray-Fejes-Toth A: Immunohistochemical localization of colonic H-K-ATPase to the apical membrane of connecting tubule cells. Am J Physiol Renal Physiol 281:F318–F325, 2001.

382. Verlander JW, Moudy RM, Campbell WG, et al: Immunohistochemical localization of H-K-ATPase alpha(2c)-subunit in rabbit kidney. Am J Physiol Renal Physiol 281: F357–F365, 2001.

383. Iacovitti M, Nash L, Peterson LN, et al: Distal tubule bicarbonate accumulation in vivo. Effect of flow and transtubular bicarbonate gradients. J Clin Invest 78:1658–1665, 1986.

384. Wesson DE: Dietary HCO3 reduces distal tubule acidification by increasing cellular HCO3 secretion. Am J Physiol 271:F132–F142, 1996.

385. Tsuruoka S, Schwartz GJ: Mechanisms of HCO(−)(3) secretion in the rabbit connecting segment. Am J Physiol 277:t–74, 1999.

386. Levine DZ: Single-nephron studies: Implications for acid-base regulation. Kidney Int 38:744–761, 1990.

387. Levine DZ, Vandorpe D, Iacovitti M: Luminal chloride modulates rat distal tubule bidirectional bicarbonate flux in vivo. J Clin Invest 85:1793–1798, 1990.

388. McKinney TD, Burg MB: Bicarbonate absorption by rabbit cortical collecting tubules in vitro 3199. Am J Physiol 234:F141–F145, 1978.

389. McKinney TD, Burg MB: Bicarbonate secretion by rabbit cortical collecting tubules in vitro 3198. J Clin Invest 61:1421–1427, 1978.

390. Atkins JL, Burg MB: Bicarbonate transport by isolated perfused rat collecting ducts. Am J Physiol 249:F485–F489, 1985.

391. Gifford JD, Sharkins K, Work J, et al: Total CO2 transport in rat cortical collecting duct in chloride-depletion alkalosis. Am J Physiol 258:F848–F853, 1990.

392. Schuster VL: Bicarbonate reabsorption and secretion in the cortical and outer medullary collecting tubule. Semin Nephrol 10:139–147, 1990.

393. Lombard WE, Kokko JP, Jacobson HR: Bicarbonate transport in cortical and outer medullary collecting tubules. Am J Physiol 244:F289–F296, 1983.

394. Schuster VL: Cyclic adenosine monophosphate-stimulated bicarbonate secretion in rabbit cortical collecting tubules. J Clin Invest 75:2056–2064, 1985.

395. Star RA, Burg MB, Knepper MA: Bicarbonate secretion and chloride absorption by rabbit cortical collecting ducts. Role of chloride/bicarbonate exchange. J Clin Invest 76:1123–1130, 1985.

396. Koeppen BM, Helman SI: Acidification of luminal fluid by the rabbit cortical collecting tubule perfused in vitro. Am J Physiol 242:F521–F531, 1982.

397. Levine DZ, Jacobson HR: The regulation of renal acid secretion: New observations from studies of distal nephron segments. Kidney Int 29:1099–1109, 1986.

398. Tsuruoka S, Schwartz GJ: Adaptation of rabbit cortical collecting duct HCO3− transport to metabolic acidosis in vitro 194. J Clin Invest 97:1076–1084, 1996.

399. Wesson DE: Reduced bicarbonate secretion mediates increased distal tubule acidification induced by dietary acid. Am J Physiol 271:F670–F678, 1996.

400. Satlin LM, Schwartz GJ: Cellular remodeling of HCO3(−)-secreting cells in rabbit renal collecting duct in response to an acidic environment. J Cell Biol 109:1279–1288, 1989.

401. Madsen KM, Tisher CC: Structural-functional relationship along the distal nephron. Am J Physiol 250:F1–15, 1986.

402. Verlander JW, Madsen KM, Tisher CC: Effect of acute respiratory acidosis on two populations of intercalated cells in rat cortical collecting duct. Am J Physiol 253: F1142–F1156, 1987.

403. Verlander JW, Madsen KM, Tisher CC: Structural and functional features of proton and bicarbonate transport in the rat collecting duct. Semin Nephrol 11:465–477, 1991.

404. Alper SL, Natale J, Gluck S, et al: Subtypes of intercalated cells in rat kidney collecting duct defined by antibodies against erythroid band 3 and renal vacuolar H+-ATPase. Proc Natl Acad Sci U S A 86:5429–5433, 1989.

405. Verlander JW, Madsen KM, Low PS, et al: Immunocytochemical localization of band 3 protein in the rat collecting duct. Am J Physiol 255:F115–F125, 1988.

406. Brown D, Hirsch S, Gluck S: An H+-ATPase in opposite plasma membrane domains in kidney epithelial cell subpopulations. Nature 331:622–624, 1988.

407. Brown D, Orci L: Junctional complexes and cell polarity in the urinary tubule. J Electron Microsc Tech 9:145–170, 1988.

408. Kim YH, Kwon TH, Frische S, et al: Immunocytochemical localization of pendrin in intercalated cell subtypes in rat and mouse kidney. Am J Physiol Renal Physiol 283: F744–F754, 2002.

409. Wall SM, Hassell KA, Royaux IE, et al: Localization of pendrin in mouse kidney. Am J Physiol Renal Physiol 284:F229–F241, 2003.

410. Ridderstrale Y, Kashgarian M, Koeppen B, et al: Morphological heterogeneity of the rabbit collecting duct. Kidney Int 34:655–670, 1988.

411. Schuster VL, Bonsib SM, Jennings ML: Two types of collecting duct mitochondria-rich (intercalated) cells: Lectin and band 3 cytochemistry. Am J Physiol 251:C347–C355, 1986.

412. Schuster VL, Fejes-Toth G, Naray-Fejes-Toth A, Gluck S: Colocalization of H(+)-ATPase and band 3 anion exchanger in rabbit collecting duct intercalated cells. Am J Physiol 260:F506–F517, 1991.

413. Schwartz GJ, Al Awqati Q: Regulation of transepithelial H+ transport by exocytosis and endocytosis. Annu Rev Physiol 48:153–161, 1986.

414. Schwartz GJ, Barasch J, Al Awqati Q: Plasticity of functional epithelial polarity. Nature 318:368–371, 1985.

415. Emmons CL, Matsuzaki K, Stokes JB, Schuster VL: Axial heterogeneity of rabbit cortical collecting duct. Am J Physiol 260:F498–F505, 1991.

416. Schwartz GJ, Satlin LM, Bergmann JE: Fluorescent characterization of collecting duct cells: A second H+-secreting type. Am J Physiol 255:F1003–F1014, 1988.

417. Wingo CS, Madsen KM, Smolka A, Tisher CC: H-K-ATPase immunoreactivity in cortical and outer medullary collecting duct. Kidney Int 38:985–990, 1990.

418. Silver RB, Soleimani M: H+-K+-ATPases: Regulation and role in pathophysiological states. Am J Physiol 276:F799–F811, 1999.

419. Breyer MD, Jacobson HR: Regulation of rabbit medullary collecting duct cell pH by basolateral Na+/H+ and Cl−/base exchange. J Clin Invest 84:996–1004, 1989.

420. Schuster VL, Stokes JB: Chloride transport by the cortical and outer medullary collecting duct. Am J Physiol 253:F203–F212, 1987.

421. Emmons C, Kurtz I: Functional characterization of three intercalated cell subtypes in the rabbit outer cortical collecting duct. J Clin Invest 93:417–423, 1994.

422. Weiner ID, Weill AE, New AR: Distribution of Cl−/HCO3− exchange and intercalated cells in rabbit cortical collecting duct. Am J Physiol 267:F952–F964, 1994.

423. Teng-umnuay P, Verlander JW, Yuan W, et al: Identification of distinct subpopulations of intercalated cells in the mouse collecting duct. J Am Soc Nephrol 7:260–274, 1996.

424. Schwartz GJ, Tsuruoka S, Vijayakumar S, et al: Acid incubation reverses the polarity of intercalated cell transporters, an effect mediated by hensin. J Clin Invest 109:89–99, 2002.

425. Al Awqati Q, Vijayakumar S, Takito J, et al: Phenotypic plasticity and terminal differentiation of the intercalated cell: The hensin pathway [Review] [32 refs]. Exp Nephrol 8:66–71, 2000.

426. Bastani B, Purcell H, Hemken P, et al: Expression and distribution of renal vacuolar proton-translocating adenosine triphosphatase in response to chronic acid and alkali loads in the rat. J Clin Invest 88:126–136, 1991.

427. O'Neil RG, Hayhurst RA: Functional differentiation of cell types in cortical collecting duct. Am J Physiol 248:F449–F453, 1985.

428. Chaillet JR, Lopes AG, Boron WF: Basolateral Na-H exchange in the rabbit cortical collecting tubule. J Gen Physiol 86:795–812, 1985.

429. Wang X, Kurtz I: H+/base transport in principal cells characterized by confocal fluorescence imaging. Am J Physiol 259:C365–C373, 1990.

430. Schwartz JH, Bethencourt D, Rosen S: Specialized function of carbonic anhydrase-rich and granular cells of turtle bladder. Am J Physiol 242:F627–F633, 1982.

431. McKinney TD, Davidson KK: Bicarbonate transport in collecting tubules from outer stripe of outer medulla of rabbit kidneys. Am J Physiol 253:F816–F822, 1987.

432. Stone DK, Seldin DW, Kokko JP, Jacobson HR: Anion dependence of rabbit medullary collecting duct acidification. J Clin Invest 71:1505–1508, 1983.

433. Stone DK, Seldin DW, Kokko JP, Jacobson HR: Mineralocorticoid modulation of rabbit medullary collecting duct acidification. A sodium-independent effect. J Clin Invest 72:77–83, 1983.

434. Hamm LL, Hering-Smith KS: Acid-base transport in the collecting duct. Semin Nephrol 13:246–255, 1993.

435. Kuwahara M, Sasaki S, Marumo F: Cell pH regulation in rabbit outer medullary collecting duct cells: mechanisms of HCO3(−)-independent processes. Am J Physiol 259:F902–F909, 1990.

436. Weiner ID, Wingo CS, Hamm LL: Regulation of intracellular pH in two cell populations of inner stripe of rabbit outer medullary collecting duct. Am J Physiol 265:F406–F415, 1993.

437. Hays SR, Alpern RJ: Apical and basolateral membrane H+ extrusion mechanisms in inner stripe of rabbit outer medullary collecting duct. Am J Physiol 259:F628–F635, 1990.

438. Hays SR, Alpern RJ: Basolateral membrane Na(+)-independent Cl−/HCO3− exchange in the inner stripe of the rabbit outer medullary collecting tubule. J Gen Physiol 95:347–367, 1990.

439. Wingo CS: Active proton secretion and potassium absorption in the rabbit outer medullary collecting duct. Functional evidence for proton-potassium-activated adenosine triphosphatase. J Clin Invest 84:361–365, 1989.

440. Wingo CS, Smolka AJ: Function and structure of H-K-ATPase in the kidney. Am J Physiol 269:F1–16, 1995.

441. Tsuruoka S, Schwartz GJ: Metabolic acidosis stimulates H+ secretion in the rabbit outer medullary collecting duct (inner stripe) of the kidney. J Clin Invest 99:1420–1431, 1997.

442. Yip KP, Tsuruoka S, Schwartz GJ, Kurtz I: Apical H(+)/base transporters mediating bicarbonate absorption and pH(i) regulation in the OMCD. Am J Physiol Renal Physiol 283:F1098–F1104, 2002.

443. Koeppen BM: Conductive properties of the rabbit outer medullary collecting duct: outer stripe. Am J Physiol 250:F70–F76, 1986.

444. Clapp WL, Madsen KM, Verlander JW, Tisher CC: Morphologic heterogeneity along the rat inner medullary collecting duct. Lab Invest 60:219–230, 1989.

445. Madsen KM, Clapp WL, Verlander JW: Structure and function of the inner medullary collecting duct. Kidney Int 34:441–454, 1988.

446. Schwartz JH: Renal acid-base transport: the regulatory role of the inner medullary collecting duct. Kidney Int 47:333–341, 1995.

447. Wall SM, Knepper MA: Acid-base transport in the inner medullary collecting duct. Semin Nephrol 10:148–158, 1990.

448. Bengele HH, Graber ML, Alexander EA: Effect of respiratory acidosis on acidification by the medullary collecting duct. Am J Physiol 244:F89–F94, 1983.

449. Bengele HH, McNamara ER, Alexander EA: Effect of acute thyroparathyroidectomy on nephron acidification. Am J Physiol 246:F569–F574, 1984.

450. Bengele HH, Schwartz JH, McNamara ER, Alexander EA: Chronic metabolic acidosis augments acidification along the inner medullary collecting duct. Am J Physiol 250:F690–F694, 1986.

451. Bengele HH, McNamara ER, Schwartz JH, Alexander EA: Acidification adaptation along the inner medullary collecting duct. Am J Physiol 255:F1155–F1159, 1988.

452. Graber ML, Bengele HH, Mroz E, et al: Acute metabolic acidosis augments collecting duct acidification rate in the rat. Am J Physiol 241:F669–F676, 1981.

453. Graber ML, Bengele HH, Schwartz JH, Alexander EA: pH and PCO2 profiles of the rat inner medullary collecting duct. Am J Physiol 241:F659–F668, 1981.

454. Richardson RM, Kunau RT, Jr: Bicarbonate reabsorption in the papillary collecting duct: Effect of acetazolamide. Am J Physiol 243:F74–F80, 1982.

455. Ullrich KJ, Papavassiliou F: Bicarbonate reabsorption in the papillary collecting duct of rats. Pflugers Arch 389:271–275, 1981.

456. Ishibashi K, Sasaki S, Yoshiyama N, et al: Generation of pH gradient across the rabbit collecting duct segments perfused in vitro. Kidney Int 31:930–936, 1987.

457. Wall SM, Sands JM, Flessner MF, et al: Net acid transport by isolated perfused inner medullary collecting ducts. Am J Physiol 258:F75–F84, 1990.

458. Wall SM, Truong AV, DuBose TD, Jr: H(+)-K(+)-ATPase mediates net acid secretion in rat terminal inner medullary collecting duct. Am J Physiol 271:F1037–F1044, 1996.

459. Brion LP, Schwartz JH, Lachman HM, et al: Development of H+ secretion by cultured renal inner medullary collecting duct cells. Am J Physiol 257:F486–F501, 1989.

460. Hering-Smith KS, Cragoe EJ, Jr, Weiner D, Hamm LL: Inner medullary collecting duct Na(+)-H+ exchanger. Am J Physiol 260:C1300–C1307, 1991.

461. Kikeri D, Zeidel ML: Intracellular pH regulation in freshly isolated suspensions of rabbit inner medullary collecting duct cells: Role of Na+:H+ antiporter and H(+)-ATPase. J Am Soc Nephrol 1:890–901, 1990.

462. Kleinman JG, Blumenthal SS, Wiessner JH, et al: Regulation of pH in rat papillary tubule cells in primary culture. J Clin Invest 80:1660–1669, 1987.

463. Ono S, Guntupalli J, DuBose TD, Jr: Role of H(+)-K(+)-ATPase in pHi regulation in inner medullary collecting duct cells in culture. Am J Physiol 270:F852–F861, 1996.

464. Prigent A, Bichara M, Paillard M: Hydrogen transport in papillary collecting duct of rabbit kidney. Am J Physiol 248:C241–C246, 1985.

465. Selvaggio AM, Schwartz JH, Bengele HH, et al: Mechanisms of H+ secretion by inner medullary collecting duct cells. Am J Physiol 254:F391–F400, 1988.

466. Wall SM, Kraut JA, Muallem S: Modulation of Na+-H+ exchange activity by intracellular Na+, H+, and Li+ in IMCD cells. Am J Physiol 255:F331–F339, 1988.

467. Wall SM, Muallem S, Kraut JA: Detection of a Na+-H+ antiporter in cultured rat renal papillary collecting duct cells. Am J Physiol 253:F889–F895, 1987.

468. Schwartz JH, Masino SA, Nichols RD, Alexander EA: Intracellular modulation of acid secretion in rat inner medullary collecting duct cells. Am J Physiol 266:F94–101, 1994.

469. Garg LC, Narang N: Stimulation of an N-ethylmaleimide-sensitive ATPase in the collecting duct segments of the rat nephron by metabolic acidosis. Can J Physiol Pharmacol 63:1291–1296, 1985.

470. Garg LC, Narang N: Effects of aldosterone on NEM-sensitive ATPase in rabbit nephron segments. Kidney Int 34:13–17, 1988.

471. DuBose TD, Jr, Codina J: H,K-ATPase. Curr Opin Nephrol Hypertens 5:411–416, 1996.

472. Hart D, Nord EP: Polarized distribution of Na+/H+ antiport and Na+/HCO3− cotransport in primary cultures of renal inner medullary collecting duct cells. J Biol Chem 266:2374–2382, 1991.

473. Obrador G, Yuan H, Shih TM, et al: Characterization of anion exchangers in an inner medullary collecting duct cell line. J Am Soc Nephrol 9:746–754, 1998.

474. Star RA: Basolateral membrane sodium-independent Cl−/HCO3− exchanger in rat inner medullary collecting duct cell. J Clin Invest 85:1959–1966, 1990.

475. Weill AE, Tisher CC, Conde MF, Weiner ID: Mechanisms of bicarbonate transport by cultured rabbit inner medullary collecting duct cells. Am J Physiol 266:F466–F476, 1994.

476. Kraut JA, Hart D, Nord EP: Basolateral Na(+)-independent Cl(−)-HCO3− exchange in primary cultures of rat IMCD cells. Am J Physiol 263:F401–F410, 1992.

477. DuBose TD, Jr, Pucacco LR, Carter NW: Determination of disequilibrium pH in the rat kidney in vivo: Evidence of hydrogen secretion. Am J Physiol 240:F138–F146, 1981.

478. Breton S, Brown D: New insights into the regulation of V-ATPase-dependent proton secretion. Am J Physiol 292:F1–10, 2007.

479. Wagner CA, Finberg KE, Breton S, et al: Renal vacuolar H+-ATPase. Physiol Rev 84:1263–1314, 2004.

480. Forgac M: Structure and function of vacuolar class of ATP-driven proton pumps. Physiol Rev 69:765–96, 1989.

481. Dixon TE, Al Awqati Q: Urinary acidification in turtle bladder is due to a reversible proton-translocating ATPase. Proc Natl Acad Sci U S A 76:3135–3138, 1979.

482. Gluck S, Kelly S, Al Awqati Q: The proton translocating ATPase responsible for urinary acidification. J Biol Chem 257:9230–9233, 1982.

483. Brown D, Gluck S, Hartwig J: Structure of the novel membrane-coating material in proton-secreting epithelial cells and identification as an H⁺ATPase 78. J Cell Biol 105:1637–1648, 1987.

484. Alper SL: Genetic diseases of acid-base transporters. Annu Rev Physiol 64:899–923, 2002.

485. Borthwick KJ, Karet FE: Inherited disorders of the H⁺-ATPase. Curr Opin Nephrol Hypertens 11:563–568, 2002.

486. Gluck S, Cannon C, Al Awqati Q: Exocytosis regulates urinary acidification in turtle bladder by rapid insertion of H⁺ pumps into the luminal membrane. Proc Natl Acad Sci U S A 79:4327–4331, 1982.

487. Alexander EA, Brown D, Shih T, et al: Effect of acidification on the location of H⁺-ATPase in cultured inner medullary collecting duct cells. Am J Physiol 276:t–63, 1999.

488. Banerjee A, Li G, Alexander EA, Schwartz JH: Role of SNAP-23 in trafficking of H⁺-ATPase in cultured inner medullary collecting duct cells. Am J Physiol Cell Physiol 280:C775–C781, 2001.

489. Fernandez R, Bosqueiro JR, Cassola AC, Malnic G: Role of Cl⁻ in electrogenic H⁺ secretion by cortical distal tubule. J Membr Biol 157:193–201, 1997.

490. Gluck SL, Iyori M, Holliday LS, et al: Distal urinary acidification from Homer Smith to the present. Kidney Int 49:1660–1664, 1996.

491. Gluck SL, Underhill DM, Iyori M, et al: Physiology and biochemistry of the kidney vacuolar H⁺-ATPase. Annu Rev Physiol 58:427–445, 1996.

492. Zhang K, Wang ZQ, Gluck S: Identification and partial purification of a cytosolic activator of vacuolar H(+)-ATPases from mammalian kidney. J Biol Chem 267:9701–9705, 1992.

493. Zhang K, Wang ZQ, Gluck S: A cytosolic inhibitor of vacuolar H(+)-ATPases from mammalian kidney. J Biol Chem 267:14539–14542, 1992.

494. Su Y, Zhou A, Al Lamki RS, Karet FE: The "a" subunit of the V-type H⁺-ATPase interacts with phosphofructokinase-1 in humans. J Biol Chem 278:20013–20018, 2003.

495. Lu M, Holliday LS, Zhang L, et al: Interaction between aldolase and vacuolar H⁺-ATPase: evidence for direct coupling of glycolysis to the ATP-hydrolyzing proton pump. J Biol Chem 276:30407–30413, 2001.

496. Fejes-Toth G, Naray-Fejes-Toth A: Effect of acid/base balance on H-ATPase 31 kD subunit mRNA levels in collecting duct cells. Kidney Int 48:1420–1426, 1995.

497. Sabatini S, Laski ME, Kurtzman NA: NEM-sensitive ATPase activity in rat nephron: effect of metabolic acidosis and alkalosis. Am J Physiol 258:F297–F304, 1990.

498. Nelson RD, Guo XL, Masood K, et al: Selectively amplified expression of an isoform of the vacuolar H(+)-ATPase 56-kilodalton subunit in renal intercalated cells. Proc Natl Acad Sci U S A 89:3541–3545, 1992.

499. Hemken P, Guo XL, Wang ZQ, et al: Immunologic evidence that vacuolar H⁺ ATPases with heterogeneous forms of Mr = 31,000 subunit have different membrane distributions in mammalian kidney. J Biol Chem 267:9948–9957, 1992.

500. Doucet A, Horisberger J: Renal ion-translocating ATPases: The p-type family. In Seldin D, Giebisch G (eds): The Kidney: Physiology and Pathophysiology. Philadelphia: Lippincott Williams & Wilkins, 2000, pp 140–170.

501. Caviston TL, Campbell WG, Wingo CS, Cain BD: Molecular identification of the renal H⁺,K⁺-ATPases. Semin Nephrol 19:431–437, 1999.

502. Doucet A, Marsy S: Characterization of K-ATPase activity in distal nephron: stimulation by potassium depletion. Am J Physiol 253:F418–F423, 1987.

503. Garg LC, Narang N: Ouabain-insensitive K-adenosine triphosphatase in distal nephron segments of the rabbit. J Clin Invest 81:1204–1208, 1988.

504. Wingo CS, Cain BD: The renal H-K-ATPase: Physiological significance and role in potassium homeostasis. Annu Rev Physiol 55:323–347, 1993.

505. Kraut JA, Hiura J, Shin JM, et al: The Na(+)-K(+)-ATPase beta 1 subunit is associated with the HK alpha 2 protein in the rat kidney. Kidney Int 53:958–962, 1998.

506. Codina J, Delmas-Mata JT, DuBose TD, Jr: The alpha-subunit of the colonic H⁺, K⁺-ATPase assembles with beta1-Na⁺,K⁺-ATPase in kidney and distal colon. J Biol Chem 273:7894–7899, 1998.

507. Sangan P, Kolla SS, Rajendran VM, et al: Colonic H-K-ATPase beta-subunit: identification in apical membranes and regulation by dietary K depletion. Am J Physiol 276:C350–C360, 1999.

508. Grishin AV, Bevensee MO, Modyanov NN, et al: Functional expression of the cDNA encoded by the human ATP1AL1 gene. Am J Physiol 271:F539–F551, 1996.

509. Kraut JA, Helander KG, Helander HF, et al: Detection and localization of H⁺-K⁺-ATPase isoforms in human kidney. Am J Physiol Renal Physiol 281:F763–F768, 2001.

510. Kone BC, Higham SC: A novel N-terminal splice variant of the rat H⁺-K⁺-ATPase alpha2 subunit. Cloning, functional expression, and renal adaptive response to chronic hypokalemia. J Biol Chem 273:2543–2552, 1998.

511. Zies DL, Wingo CS, Cain BD: Molecular regulation of the HKalpha2 subunit of the H⁺,K(+)-ATPases. J Nephrol 15 Suppl 5:S54–S60, 2002.

512. Jaisser F, Horisberger JD, Geering K, Rossier BC: Mechanisms of urinary K⁺ and H⁺ excretion: Primary structure and functional expression of a novel H,K-ATPase. J Cell Biol 123:1421–1429, 1993.

513. Laroche-Joubert N, Marsy S, Doucet A: Cellular origin and hormonal regulation of K(+)-ATPase activities sensitive to Sch-28080 in rat collecting duct. Am J Physiol Renal Physiol 279:F1053–F1059, 2000.

514. Jaisser F, Beggah AT: The nongastric H⁺-K⁺-ATPases: molecular and functional properties. Am J Physiol 276:F812–F824, 1999.

515. Petrovic S, Spicer Z, Greeley T, et al: Novel Schering and ouabain-insensitive potassium-dependent proton secretion in the mouse cortical collecting duct. Am J Physiol Renal Physiol 282:F133–F143, 2002.

516. Spicer Z, Miller ML, Andringa A, et al: Stomachs of mice lacking the gastric H,K-ATPase alpha-subunit have achlorhydria, abnormal parietal cells, and ciliated metaplasia. J Biol Chem 275:21555–21565, 2000.

517. Meneton P, Schultheis PJ, Greeb J, et al: Increased sensitivity to K⁺ deprivation in colonic H,K-ATPase-deficient mice. J Clin Invest 101:536–542, 1998.

518. Armitage FE, Wingo CS: Luminal acidification in K-replete OMCDi: contributions of H-K-ATPase and bafilomycin-A1-sensitive H-ATPase. Am J Physiol 267:F450–F458, 1994.

519. Guntupalli J, Onuigbo M, Wall S, et al: Adaptation to low-K⁺ media increases H(+)-K(+)-ATPase but not H(+)-ATPase-mediated pHi recovery in OMCD1 cells. Am J Physiol 273:t–71, 1997.

520. Silver RB, Mennitt PA, Satlin LM: Stimulation of apical H-K-ATPase in intercalated cells of cortical collecting duct with chronic metabolic acidosis. Am J Physiol 270:F539–F547, 1996.

521. Ahn KY, Park KY, Kim KK, Kone BC: Chronic hypokalemia enhances expression of the H(+)-K(+)-ATPase alpha 2-subunit gene in renal medulla. Am J Physiol 271:F314–F321, 1996.

522. Marsy S, Elalouf JM, Doucet A: Quantitative RT-PCR analysis of mRNAs encoding a colonic putative H,K-ATPase alpha subunit along the rat nephron: effect of K⁺ depletion. Pflugers Arch 432:494–500, 1996.

523. Nakamura S, Wang Z, Galla JH, Soleimani M: K⁺ depletion increases HCO3⁻ reabsorption in OMCD by activation of colonic H(+)-K(+)-ATPase. Am J Physiol 274:F687–F692, 1998.

524. Kraut JA, Hiura J, Besancon M, et al: Effect of hypokalemia on the abundance of HK alpha 1 and HK alpha 2 protein in the rat kidney. Am J Physiol 272:F744–F750, 1997.

525. Silver RB, Frindt G, Mennitt P, Satlin LM: Characterization and regulation of H-K-ATPase in intercalated cells of rabbit cortical collecting duct. J Exp Zool 279:443–455, 1997.

526. Zhou X, Wingo CS: Stimulation of total CO₂ flux by 10% CO₂ in rabbit CCD: role of an apical Sch-28080- and Ba-sensitive mechanism. Am J Physiol 267:F114–F120, 1994.

527. Fejes-Toth G, Rusvai E, Longo KA, Naray-Fejes-Toth A: Expression of colonic H-K-ATPase mRNA in cortical collecting duct: Regulation by acid/base balance. Am J Physiol 269:F551–F557, 1995.

528. Weiner ID, Milton AE: H(+)-K(+)-ATPase in rabbit cortical collecting duct B-type intercalated cell. Am J Physiol 270:F518–F530, 1996.

529. Silver RB, Frindt G: Functional identification of H-K-ATPase in intercalated cells of cortical collecting tubule. Am J Physiol 264:F259–F266, 1993.

530. Cougnon M, Bouyer P, Planelles G, Jaisser F: Does the colonic H,K-ATPase also act as an Na,K-ATPase? Proc Natl Acad Sci U S A 95:6516–6520, 1998.

531. Zhou X, Wingo CS: H-K-ATPase enhancement of Rb efflux by cortical collecting duct. Am J Physiol 263: F43–F48, 1992.

532. Silver RB, Choe H, Frindt G: Low-NaCl diet increases H-K-ATPase in intercalated cells from rat cortical collecting duct. Am J Physiol 275:F94–102, 1998.

533. Cougnon M, Bouyer P, Jaisser F, et al: Ammonium transport by the colonic H(+)-K(+)-ATPase expressed in Xenopus oocytes. Am J Physiol 277:C280–C287, 1999.

534. Codina J, Pressley TA, DuBose TD, Jr: The colonic H⁺,K⁺-ATPase functions as a Na⁺-dependent K⁺(NH4+) ATPase in apical membranes from rat distal colon. J Biol Chem 274:19693–19698, 1999.

535. Nakamura S, Amlal H, Galla JH, Soleimani M: NH4+ secretion in inner medullary collecting duct in potassium deprivation: Role of colonic H⁺-K⁺-ATPase. Kidney Int 56:2160–2167, 1999.

536. Ahn KY, Kone BC: Expression and cellular localization of mRNA encoding the "gastric" isoform of H(+)-K(+)-ATPase alpha-subunit in rat kidney. Am J Physiol 268:F99–109, 1995.

537. Constantinescu A, Silver RB, Satlin LM: H-K-ATPase activity in PNA-binding intercalated cells of newborn rabbit cortical collecting duct. Am J Physiol 272:F167–F177, 1997.

538. Stanton BA: Characterization of apical and basolateral membrane conductances of rat inner medullary collecting duct. Am J Physiol 256:F862–F868, 1989.

539. Brosius FC, III, Alper SL, Garcia AM, Lodish HF: The major kidney band 3 gene transcript predicts an amino-terminal truncated band 3 polypeptide. J Biol Chem 264:7784–7787, 1989.

540. Kudrycki KE, Shull GE: Primary structure of the rat kidney band 3 anion exchange protein deduced from a cDNA. J Biol Chem 264:8185–8192, 1989.

541. Janoshazi A, Ojcius DM, Kone B, et al: Relation between the anion exchange protein in kidney medullary collecting duct cells and red cell band 3. J Membr Biol 103:181–189, 1988.

542. Wagner S, Vogel R, Lietzke R, et al: Immunochemical characterization of a band 3-like anion exchanger in collecting duct of human kidney. Am J Physiol 253:F213–F221, 1987.

543. Drenckhahn D, Schluter K, Allen DP, Bennett V: Colocalization of band 3 with ankyrin and spectrin at the basal membrane of intercalated cells in the rat kidney. Science 230:1287–1289, 1985.

544. Koeppen BM: Conductive properties of the rabbit outer medullary collecting duct: Inner stripe. Am J Physiol 500:F500–F506, 1985.

545. Koeppen BM: Electrophysiological identification of principal and intercalated cells in the rabbit outer medullary collecting duct. Pflugers Arch 409:138–141, 1987.

546. Koeppen BM: Electrophysiology of collecting duct H⁺ secretion: Effect of inhibitors. Am J Physiol 256:F79–F84, 1989.

547. Muto S, Yasoshima K, Yoshitomi K, et al: Electrophysiological identification of alpha- and beta-intercalated cells and their distribution along the rabbit distal nephron segments. J Clin Invest 86:1829–1839, 1990.

548. Sabolic I, Brown D, Gluck SL, Alper SL: Regulation of AE1 anion exchanger and H(+)-ATPase in rat cortex by acute metabolic acidosis and alkalosis. Kidney Int 51:125–137, 1997.

549. Verlander JW, Madsen KM, Cannon JK, Tisher CC: Activation of acid-secreting intercalated cells in rabbit collecting duct with ammonium chloride loading. Am J Physiol 266:F633–F645, 1994.

550. Fejes-Toth G, Rusvai E, Cleaveland ES, Naray-Fejes-Toth A: Regulation of AE2 mRNA expression in the cortical collecting duct by acid/base balance. Am J Physiol 274:F596–F601, 1998.

551. Stuart-Tilley AK, Shmukler BE, Brown D, Alper SL: Immunolocalization and tissue-specific splicing of AE2 anion exchanger in mouse kidney. J Am Soc Nephrol 9:946–959, 1998.
552. Ko SB, Luo X, Hager H, et al: AE4 is a DIDS-sensitive Cl(–)/HCO(–)(3) exchanger in the basolateral membrane of the renal CCD and the SMG duct. Am J Physiol Cell Physiol 283:C1206–C1218, 2002.
553. Petrovic S, Barone S, Xu J, et al: SLC26A7: a basolateral $Cl^-/HCO3^-$ exchanger specific to intercalated cells of the outer medullary collecting duct. Am J Physiol Renal Physiol 286:F161–F169, 2004.
554. Xu J, Worrell RT, Li HC, et al: Chloride/bicarbonate exchanger SLC26A7 is localized in endosomes in medullary collecting duct cells and is targeted to the basolateral membrane in hypertonicity and potassium depletion. J Am Soc Nephrol 17:956–967, 2006.
555. Emmons C: Transport characteristics of the apical anion exchanger of rabbit cortical collecting duct beta-cells. Am J Physiol 276:F635–F643, 1999.
556. Tago K, Schuster VL, Stokes JB: Regulation of chloride self exchange by cAMP in cortical collecting tubule. Am J Physiol 251:F40–F48, 1986.
557. Tago K, Schuster VL, Stokes JB: Stimulation of chloride transport by $HCO3^-CO2$ in rabbit cortical collecting tubule. Am J Physiol 251:F49–F56, 1986.
558. Schuster VL: Cyclic adenosine monophosphate-stimulated anion transport in rabbit cortical collecting duct. Kinetics, stoichiometry, and conductive pathways. J Clin Invest 78:1621–1630, 1986.
559. Al Awqati Q, Vijayakumar S, Hikita C, et al: Phenotypic plasticity in the intercalated cell: the hensin pathway. Am J Physiol 275:F183–F190, 1998.
560. van't Hof W, Malik A, Vijayakumar S, et al: The effect of apical and basolateral lipids on the function of the band 3 anion exchange protein. J Cell Biol 139:941–949, 1997.
561. van Adelsberg J, Edwards JC, Takito J, et al: An induced extracellular matrix protein reverses the polarity of band 3 in intercalated epithelial cells. Cell 76:1053–1061, 1994.
562. van Adelsberg JS, Edwards JC, Al Awqati Q: The apical Cl/HCO3 exchanger of beta intercalated cells. J Biol Chem 268:11283–11289, 1993.
563. Al Awqati Q: Terminal differentiation of intercalated cells: The role of hensin. Annu Rev Physiol 65:567–583, 2003.
564. Soleimani M, Greeley T, Petrovic S, et al: Pendrin: An apical $Cl^-/OH^-/$ $HCO3^-$ exchanger in the kidney cortex. Am J Physiol Renal Physiol 280:F356–F364, 2001.
565. Wagner CA, Finberg KE, Stehberger PA, et al: Regulation of the expression of the $Cl^-/$ anion exchanger pendrin in mouse kidney by acid-base status. Kidney Int 62:2109–2117, 2002.
566. Petrovic S, Wang Z, Ma L, Soleimani M: Regulation of the apical Cl^-/HCO-3 exchanger pendrin in rat cortical collecting duct in metabolic acidosis. Am J Physiol Renal Physiol 284:F103–F112, 2003.
567. Frische S, Kwon TH, Frokiaer J, et al: Regulated expression of pendrin in rat kidney in response to chronic NH4Cl or NaHCO3 loading. Am J Physiol Renal Physiol 284: F584–F593, 2003.
568. Verlander JW, Hassell KA, Royaux IE, et al: Deoxycorticosterone upregulates PDS (Slc26a4) in mouse kidney: Role of pendrin in mineralocorticoid-induced hypertension. Hypertension 42:356–362, 2003.
569. Quentin F, Chambrey R, Trinh-Trang-Tan MM, et al: The $Cl^-/HCO3^-$ exchanger pendrin in the rat kidney is regulated in response to chronic alterations in chloride balance. Am J Physiol Renal Physiol 287:F1179–F1188, 2004.
570. Wall SM, Kim YH, Stanley L, et al: NaCl restriction upregulates renal Slc26a4 through subcellular redistribution: Role in Cl^- conservation. Hypertension 44:982–987, 2004.
571. Verlander JW, Kim YH, Shin W, et al: Dietary Cl^- restriction upregulates pendrin expression within the apical plasma membrane of type B intercalated cells. Am J Physiol Renal Physiol 291:F833–F839, 2006.
572. Tsuganezawa H, Kobayashi K, Iyori M, et al: A new member of the HCO3(–) transporter superfamily is an apical anion exchanger of beta-intercalated cells in the kidney. J Biol Chem 276:8180–8189, 2001.
573. Satake N, Durham JH, Ehrenspeck G, Brodsky WA: Active electrogenic mechanisms for alkali and acid transport in turtle bladders. Am J Physiol 244:C259–C269, 1983.
574. Durham JH, Matons C: Chloride-induced increment in short-circuiting current of the turtle bladder. Effects of in-vivo acid-base state. Biochim Biophys Acta 769:297–310, 1984.
575. Durham JH, Matons C, Brodsky WA: Vasoactive intestinal peptide stimulates alkali excretion in turtle urinary bladder. Am J Physiol 252:C428–C435, 1987.
576. Stetson DL, Beauwens R, Palmisano J, et al: A double-membrane model for urinary bicarbonate secretion. Am J Physiol 249:F546–F552, 1985.
577. Fritsche C, Schwartz JH, Heinen RR, et al: HCO_3^- secretion in mitochondria-rich cells is linked to an H^+-ATPase. Am J Physiol 256:F869–F874, 1989.
578. Stetson DL, Steinmetz PR: Alpha and beta types of carbonic anhydrase-rich cells in turtle bladder. Am J Physiol 249:F553–F565, 1985.
579. Verlander JW, Madsen KM, Stone DK, Tisher CC: Ultrastructural localization of H^+ATPase in rabbit cortical collecting duct. J Am Soc Nephrol 4:1546–1557, 1994.
580. Emmons C, Stokes JB: Cellular actions of cAMP on HCO3(–)-secreting cells of rabbit CCD: Dependence on in vivo acid-base status. Am J Physiol 266:F528–F535, 1994.
581. Light DB, Schwiebert EM, Fejes-Toth G, et al: Chloride channels in the apical membrane of cortical collecting duct cells. Am J Physiol 258:F273–F280, 1990.
582. Gunther W, Luchow A, Cluzeaud F, et al: ClC-5, the chloride channel mutated in Dent's disease, colocalizes with the proton pump in endocytotically active kidney cells. Proc Natl Acad Sci U S A 95:8075–8080, 1998.
583. Matsuzaki K, Schuster VL, Stokes JB: Reduction in sensitivity to Cl^- channel blockers by $HCO3^-$ –CO2 in rabbit cortical collecting duct. Am J Physiol 257:C102–C109, 1989.
584. Obermuller N, Gretz N, Kriz W, et al: The swelling-activated chloride channel ClC-2, the chloride channel ClC-3, and ClC-5, a chloride channel mutated in kidney stone disease, are expressed in distinct subpopulations of renal epithelial cells. J Clin Invest 101:635–642, 1998.
585. Kwon TH, Pushkin A, Abuladze N, et al: Immunoelectron microscopic localization of NBC3 sodium-bicarbonate cotransporter in rat kidney. Am J Physiol Renal Physiol 278:F327–F336, 2000.
586. Pushkin A, Abuladze N, Lee I, et al: Cloning, tissue distribution, genomic organization, and functional characterization of NBC3, a new member of the sodium bicarbonate cotransporter family. J Biol Chem 274:16569–16575, 1999.
587. Praetorius J, Kim YH, Bouzinova EV, et al: NBCn1 is a basolateral Na^+-$HCO3^-$ cotransporter in rat kidney inner medullary collecting ducts. Am J Physiol Renal Physiol 286:F903–F912, 2004.
588. Todd-Turla KM, Rusvai E, Naray-Fejes-Toth A, Fejes-Toth G: CFTR expression in cortical collecting duct cells. Am J Physiol 270:F237–F244, 1996.
589. Hamm LL, Alpern RJ: Cellular mechanisms of renal tubular acidification. *In* Seldin DW, Giebisch G (eds): The Kidney: Physiology and Pathophysiology. Philadelphia, Lippincott Williams & Wilkins, 2000, pp 1935–1979.
590. Gougoux A, Vinay P, Lemieux G, et al: Studies on the mechanism whereby acidemia stimulates collecting duct hydrogen ion secretion in vivo 1483. Kidney Int 20:643–648, 1981.
591. Gougoux A, Vinay P, Lemieux G, et al: Effect of blood pH on distal nephron hydrogen ion secretion. Kidney Int 17:615–621, 1980.
592. Breyer MD, Kokko JP, Jacobson HR: Regulation of net bicarbonate transport in rabbit cortical collecting tubule by peritubular pH, carbon dioxide tension, and bicarbonate concentration. J Clin Invest 77:1650–1660, 1986.
593. McKinney TD, Davidson KK: Effects of respiratory acidosis on $HCO3^-$ transport by rabbit collecting tubules. Am J Physiol 255:F656–F665, 1988.
594. Jacobson HR: Medullary collecting duct acidification. Effects of potassium, HCO_3 concentration, and pCO_2. J Clin Invest 74:2107–2114, 1984.
595. Banerjee A, Shih T, Alexander EA, Schwartz JH: SNARE proteins regulate H(+)-ATPase redistribution to the apical membrane in rat renal inner medullary collecting duct cells. J Biol Chem 274:26518–26522, 1999.
596. Laski ME, Warnock DG, Rector FC, Jr: Effects of chloride gradients on total CO_2 flux in the rabbit cortical collecting tubule. Am J Physiol 244:F112–F121, 1983.
597. Steinmetz PR, Lawson LR: Effect of luminal pH on ion permeability and flows of $Na^+$and H^+ in turtle bladder. Am J Physiol 220:1573–1580, 1971.
598. Madsen KM, Verlander JW, Kim J, Tisher CC: Morphological adaptation of the collecting duct to acid-base disturbances. Kidney Int Suppl 33:S57–S63, 1991.
599. Takito J, Hikita C, Al Awqati Q: Hensin, a new collecting duct protein involved in the in vitro plasticity of intercalated cell polarity. J Clin Invest 98:2324–2331, 1996.
600. Yasoshima K, Satlin LM, Schwartz GJ: Adaptation of rabbit cortical collecting duct to in vitro acid incubation. Am J Physiol 263:F749–F756, 1992.
601. Schwartz GJ, Al-Awqati Q: Role of hensin in mediating the adaptation of the cortical collecting duct to metabolic acidosis. Curr Opin Nephrol Hypertens 14:383–388, 2005.
602. Watanabe S, Tsuruoka S, Vijayakumar S, et al: Cyclosporin A produces distal renal tubular acidosis by blocking peptidyl prolyl cis-trans isomerase activity of cyclophilin. Am J Physiol Renal Physiol 288:F40–F47, 2005.
603. Silva Junior JC, Perrone RD, Johns CA, Madias NE: Rat kidney band 3 mRNA modulation in chronic respiratory acidosis. Am J Physiol 260:F204–F209, 1991.
604. Wesson DE: Dietary acid increases blood and renal cortical acid content in rats. Am J Physiol 274:F97–103, 1998.
605. McKinney TD, Davidson KK: Effect of potassium depletion and protein intake in vivo on renal tubular bicarbonate transport in vitro. Am J Physiol 252:F509–F516, 1987.
606. Bank N, Schwartz WB: The influence of anion penetrating ability on urinary acidification and the excretion of titratable acid. J Clin Invest 39:1516–1525, 1960.
607. Schwartz WB JRRA: Acidification of the urine and increased ammonium excretion without change in acid-base equilibrium: Sodium reabsorption as a stimulus to the acidifying process. J Clin Invest 34:673–680, 1955.
608. Tam SC, Goldstein MB, Stinebaugh BJ, et al: Studies on the regulation of hydrogen ion secretion in the collecting duct in vivo: Evaluation of factors that influence the urine minus blood PCO_2 difference. Kidney Int 20:636–642, 1981.
609. Al Awqati Q, Mueller A, Steinmetz PR: Transport of H^+ against electrochemical gradients in turtle urinary bladder. Am J Physiol 233:F502–F508, 1977.
610. Laski ME, Kurtzman NA: Characterization of acidification in the cortical and medullary collecting tubule of the rabbit. J Clin Invest 72:2050–2059, 1983.
611. Hulter HN, Ilnicki LP, Harbottle JA, Sebastian A: Impaired renal H^+ secretion and NH3 production in mineralocorticoid-deficient glucocorticoid-replete dogs. Am J Physiol 232:F136–F146, 1977.
612. Hulter HN, Licht JH, Glynn RD, Sebastian A: Renal acidosis in mineralocorticoid deficiency is not dependent on NaCl depletion or hyperkalemia. Am J Physiol 236: F283–F294, 1979.
613. Winter C, Schulz N, Giebisch G, et al: Nongenomic stimulation of vacuolar H^+-ATPases in intercalated renal tubule cells by aldosterone. Proc Natl Acad Sci U S A 101:2636–2641, 2004.
614. DuBose TD, Jr, Caflisch CR: Effect of selective aldosterone deficiency on acidification in nephron segments of the rat inner medulla. J Clin Invest 82:1624–1632, 1988.
615. Knepper MA, Good DW, Burg MB: Mechanism of ammonia secretion by cortical collecting ducts of rabbits. Am J Physiol 247:F729–F738, 1984.
616. Geibel JP: Distal tubule acidification. J Nephrol 19 Suppl 9:S18–S26, 2006.
617. Levine DZ, Iacovitti M, Buckman S, Harrison V: In vivo modulation of rat distal tubule net HCO_3 flux by VIP, isoproterenol, angiotensin II, and ADH. Am J Physiol 266: F878–F883, 1994.
618. Wang T, Giebisch G: Effects of angiotensin II on electrolyte transport in the early and late distal tubule in rat kidney. Am J Physiol 271:F143–F149, 1996.

619. Weiner ID, New AR, Milton AE, Tisher CC: Regulation of luminal alkalinization and acidification in the cortical collecting duct by angiotensin II. Am J Physiol 269: F730–F738, 1995.

620. Wall SM, Fischer MP, Glapion DM, De La Calzada M: ANG II reduces net acid secretion in rat outer medullary collecting duct. Am J Physiol Renal Physiol 285:F930–F937, 2003.

621. Hays SR, Seldin DW, Kokko JP, et al: Effect of K depletion on HCO₃ transport across rabbit collecting duct segments [abstract]. Kidney Int 29, 368A. 1986.

622. Stetson DL, Wade JB, Giebisch G: Morphologic alterations in the rat medullary collecting duct following potassium depletion. Kidney Int 17:45–56, 1980.

623. Buffin-Meyer B, Younes-Ibrahim M, Barlet-Bas C, et al: K depletion modifies the properties of Sch-28080-sensitive K-ATPase in rat collecting duct. Am J Physiol 272: F124–F131, 1997.

624. Nakamura S, Amlal H, Galla JH, Soleimani M: Colonic H⁺-K⁺-ATPase is induced and mediates increased HCO₃⁻ reabsorption in inner medullary collecting duct in potassium depletion. Kidney Int 54:1233–1239, 1998.

625. Wesson DE: Physiologic and pathophysiologic renal consequences of H(+)-stimulated endothelin secretion. Am J Kidney Dis 35:LII–LIV, 2000.

626. Wesson DE, Dolson GM: Endothelin-1 increases rat distal tubule acidification in vivo. Am J Physiol 273:F586–F594, 1997.

627. Tsuruoka S, Watanabe S, Purkerson JM, et al: Endothelin and nitric oxide mediate the adaptation of the cortical collecting duct to metabolic acidosis. Am J Physiol Renal Physiol 291:F866–F873, 2006.

628. Mercier O, Bichara M, Paillard M, Prigent A: Effects of parathyroid hormone and urinary phosphate on collecting duct hydrogen secretion. Am J Physiol 251:F802–F809, 1986.

629. Tomita K, Pisano JJ, Burg MB, Knepper MA: Effects of vasopressin and bradykinin on anion transport by the rat cortical collecting duct. Evidence for an electroneutral sodium chloride transport pathway. J Clin Invest 77:136–141, 1986.

630. Hays S, Kokko JP, Jacobson HR: Hormonal regulation of proton secretion in rabbit medullary collecting duct. J Clin Invest 78:1279–1286, 1986.

631. Wesson DE: Prostacyclin increases distal tubule HCO₃ secretion in the rat 1636. Am J Physiol 271:F1183–F1192, 1996.

632. Mercier O, Bichara M, Delahousse M, et al: Effects of glucagon on H(+)-HCO₃⁻ transport in Henle's loop, distal tubule, and collecting ducts in the rat. Am J Physiol 257: F1003–F1014, 1989.

633. Nagami GT: Renal ammonia production and excretion. *In* Seldin D, Giebisch G (eds): The Kidney: Physiology and Pathophysiology. Philadelphia, Lippincott Williams & Wilkins, 2000, pp 1996–2013.

634. Tannen RL: Renal ammonia production and excretion. *In* Windhager EE (ed): Handbook of Physiology: Renal Physiology. New York, Oxford University Press, 1992, pp 1017–1059.

635. Good DW, Burg MB: Ammonia production by individual segments of the rat nephron. J Clin Invest 73:602–610, 1984.

636. Wright PA, Knepper MA: Glutamate dehydrogenase activities in microdissected rat nephron segments: Effects of acid-base loading. Am J Physiol 259:F53–F59, 1990.

637. Wright PA, Knepper MA: Phosphate-dependent glutaminase activity in rat renal cortical and medullary tubule segments. Am J Physiol 259:F961–F970, 1990.

638. Curthoys NP, Lowry OH: The distribution of glutaminase isoenzymes in the various structures of the nephron in normal, acidotic, and alkalotic rat kidney. J Biol Chem 248:162–168, 1973.

639. Curthoys NP, Gstraunthaler G: Mechanism of increased renal gene expression during metabolic acidosis. Am J Physiol Renal Physiol 281:F381–F390, 2001.

640. Hughey RP, Rankin BB, Curthoys NP: Acute acidosis and renal arteriovenous differences of glutamine in normal and adrenalectomized rats. Am J Physiol 238:F199–F204, 1980.

641. Curthoys NP, Tang A, Gstraunthaler G: pH regulation of renal gene expression. Novartis Found Symp 240:100–111, 2001.

642. Sastrasinh S, Sastrasinh M: Glutamine transport in submitochondrial particles. Am J Physiol 257:F1050–F1058, 1989.

643. Laterza OF, Curthoys NP: Effect of acidosis on the properties of the glutaminase mRNA pH-response element binding protein. J Am Soc Nephrol 11:1583–1588, 2000.

644. Laterza OF, Hansen WR, Taylor L, Curthoys NP: Identification of an mRNA-binding protein and the specific elements that may mediate the pH-responsive induction of renal glutaminase mRNA. J Biol Chem 272:22481–22488, 1997.

645. Wright PA, Packer RK, Garcia-Perez A, Knepper MA: Time course of renal glutamate dehydrogenase induction during NH4Cl loading in rats. Am J Physiol 262: F999–1006, 1992.

646. Kaiser S, Hwang JJ, Smith H, et al: Effect of altered acid-base balance and of various agonists on levels of renal glutamate dehydrogenase mRNA. Am J Physiol 262:F507–F512, 1992.

647. Feifel E, Obexer P, Andratsch M, et al: p38 MAPK mediates acid-induced transcription of PEPCK in LLC-PK(1)-FBPase(+) cells. Am J Physiol Renal Physiol 283:F678–F688, 2002.

648. Tannen RL: Effect of potassium on renal acidification and acid-base homeostasis. Semin Nephrol 7:263–273, 1987.

649. Tannen RL, Sahai A: Biochemical pathways and modulators of renal ammoniagenesis. Miner Electrolyte Metab 16:249–258, 1990.

650. Good DW: Effects of potassium on ammonia transport by medullary thick ascending limb of the rat. J Clin Invest 80:1358–1365, 1987.

651. DuBose TD, Jr, Good DW: Effects of chronic hyperkalemia on renal production and proximal tubule transport of ammonium in rats. Am J Physiol 260:F680–F687, 1991.

652. DuBose TD, Jr, Good DW: Chronic hyperkalemia impairs ammonium transport and accumulation in the inner medulla of the rat. J Clin Invest 90:1443–1449, 1992.

653. Nagami GT: Effect of angiotensin II on ammonia production and secretion by mouse proximal tubules perfused in vitro. J Clin Invest 89:925–931, 1992.

654. Nagami GT: Effect of luminal angiotensin II on ammonia production and secretion by mouse proximal tubules. Am J Physiol 269:F86–F92, 1995.

655. Schoolwerth AC: Regulation of renal ammoniagenesis in metabolic acidosis. Kidney Int 40:961–973, 1991.

656. Welbourne TC: Influence of adrenal glands on pathways of renal glutamine utilization and ammonia production. Am J Physiol 226:535–539, 1974.

657. Welbourne TC: Glucocorticoid control of ammoniagenesis in the proximal tubule. Semin Nephrol 10:339–349, 1990.

658. Jones ER, Beck TR, Kapoor S, et al: Prostaglandins inhibit renal ammoniagenesis in the rat. J Clin Invest 74:992–1002, 1984.

659. Hamm LL, Trigg D, Martin D, et al: Transport of ammonia in the rabbit cortical collecting tubule. J Clin Invest 75:478–485, 1985.

660. Knepper MA, Packer R, Good DW: Ammonium transport in the kidney. Physiol Rev 69:179–249, 1989.

661. Kikeri D, Sun A, Zeidel ML, Hebert SC: Cell membranes impermeable to NH3. Nature 339:478–480, 1989.

662. DuBose TD, Jr, Good DW, Hamm LL, Wall SM: Ammonium transport in the kidney: New physiological concepts and their clinical implications [review]. J Am Soc Nephrol 1:1193–1203, 1991.

663. Weiner ID, Hamm LL: Molecular mechanisms of renal ammonia transport. Annu Rev Physiol 69:317–340, 2007.

664. Garvin JL, Burg MB, Knepper MA: NH3 and NH4+ transport by rabbit renal proximal straight tubules. Am J Physiol 252:F232–F239, 1987.

665. Good DW, DuBose TD, Jr: Ammonia transport by early and late proximal convoluted tubule of the rat. J Clin Invest 79:684–691, 1987.

666. Simon E, Martin D, Buerkert J: Contribution of individual superficial nephron segments to ammonium handling in chronic metabolic acidosis in the rat. Evidence for ammonia disequilibrium in the renal cortex. J Clin Invest 76:855–864, 1985.

667. Preisig PA, Alpern RJ: Pathways for apical and basolateral membrane NH3 and NH4+ movement in rat proximal tubule. Am J Physiol 259:F587–F593, 1990.

668. Tizianello A, Deferrari G, Garibotto G, et al: Renal ammoniagenesis during the adaptation to metabolic acidosis in man. Contrib Nephrol 31:40–46, 1982.

669. Simon EE, Hamm LL: Ammonia entry along rat proximal tubule in vivo: Effects of luminal pH and flow rate. Am J Physiol 253:F760–F766, 1987.

670. Simon EE, Fry B, Hering-Smith K, Hamm LL: Ammonia loss from rat proximal tubule in vivo: Effects of luminal pH and flow rate. Am J Physiol 255:F861–F867, 1988.

671. Simon EE, Merli C, Herndon J, et al: Determinants of ammonia entry along the rat proximal tubule during chronic metabolic acidosis. Am J Physiol 256:F1104–F1110, 1989.

672. Simon EE, Merli C, Herndon J, et al: Effects of barium and 5-(N-ethyl-N-isopropyl)-amiloride on proximal tubule ammonia transport. Am J Physiol 262:F36–F39, 1992.

673. Garvin JL, Burg MB, Knepper MA: Ammonium replaces potassium in supporting sodium transport by the Na-K-ATPase of renal proximal straight tubules. Am J Physiol 249:F785–F788, 1985.

674. Kurtz I, Balaban RS: Ammonium as a substrate for Na⁺-K⁺-ATPase in rabbit proximal tubules. Am J Physiol 250:F497–F502, 1986.

675. Karim Z, Attmane-Elakeb A, Bichara M: Renal handling of NH4+ in relation to the control of acid-base balance by the kidney. J Nephrol 15 Suppl 5:S128–S134, 2002.

676. Nagami GT, Kurokawa K: Regulation of ammonia production by mouse proximal tubules perfused in vitro. Effect of luminal perfusion. J Clin Invest 75:844–849, 1985.

677. Nagami GT: Ammonia production and secretion by S3 proximal tubule segments from acidotic mice: role of ANG II. Am J Physiol Renal Physiol 287:F707–F712, 2004.

678. Buerkert J, Martin D, Trigg D: Ammonium handling by superficial and juxtamedullary nephrons in the rat. Evidence for an ammonia shunt between the loop of Henle and the collecting duct. J Clin Invest 70:1–12, 1982.

679. Good DW, Caflisch CR, DuBose TD, Jr: Transepithelial ammonia concentration gradients in inner medulla of the rat. Am J Physiol 252:F491–F500, 1987.

680. Kikeri D, Sun A, Zeidel ML, Hebert SC: Cellular NH4+/K⁺ transport pathways in mouse medullary thick limb of Henle. Regulation by intracellular pH. J Gen Physiol 99:435–461, 1992.

681. Rivers R, Blanchard A, Eladari D, et al: Water and solute permeabilities of medullary thick ascending limb apical and basolateral membranes. Am J Physiol 274:F453–F462, 1998.

682. Hering-Smith KS, Kovach K, Hamm LL: Ammonia transport across distal tubule cells. Contrib Nephrol 110:60–66, 1994.

683. Laamarti MA, Lapointe JY: Determination of NH4+/NH3 fluxes across apical membrane of macula densa cells: A quantitative analysis. Am J Physiol 273:F817–F824, 1997.

684. Good DW: Active absorption of NH4+ by rat medullary thick ascending limb: Inhibition by potassium. Am J Physiol 255:F78–F87, 1988.

685. Attmane-Elakeb A, Mount DB, Sibella V, et al: Stimulation by in vivo and in vitro metabolic acidosis of expression of rBSC-1, the Na⁺-K⁺(NH4+)-2Cl⁻ cotransporter of the rat medullary thick ascending limb. J Biol Chem 273:33681–33691, 1998.

686. Attmane-Elakeb A, Sibella V, Vernimmen C, et al: Regulation by glucocorticoids of expression and activity of rBSC1, the Na⁺-K⁺(NH4+)-2Cl⁻ cotransporter of medullary thick ascending limb. J Biol Chem 275:33548–33553, 2000.

687. Amlal H, Paillard M, Bichara M: NH4+ transport pathways in cells of medullary thick ascending limb of rat kidney. NH4+ conductance and K⁺/NH4+(H⁺) antiport. J Biol Chem 269:21962–21971, 1994.

688. Attmane-Elakeb A, Boulanger H, Vernimmen C, Bichara M: Apical location and inhibition by arginine vasopressin of K⁺/H⁺ antiport of the medullary thick ascending limb of rat kidney. J Biol Chem 272:25668–25677, 1997.

689. Garvin JL, Burg MB, Knepper MA: Active NH4+ absorption by the thick ascending limb. Am J Physiol 255:F57–F65, 1988.

690. Sajo IM, Goldstein MB, Sonnenberg H, et al: Sites of ammonia addition to tubular fluid in rats with chronic metabolic acidosis. Kidney Int 20:353–358, 1981.

691. Handlogten ME, Hong SP, Westhoff CM, Weiner ID: Basolateral ammonium transport by the mouse inner medullary collecting duct cell (mIMCD-3). Am J Physiol Renal Physiol 287:F628–F638, 2004.

692. Handlogten ME, Hong SP, Westhoff CM, Weiner ID: Apical ammonia transport by the mouse inner medullary collecting duct cell (mIMCD-3). Am J Physiol Renal Physiol 289:F347–F358, 2005.

693. Wall SM, Koger LM: NH$^+$4 transport mediated by Na(+)-K(+)-ATPase in rat inner medullary collecting duct. Am J Physiol 267:F660–F670, 1994.

694. Wall SM: Ouabain reduces net acid secretion and increases pHi by inhibiting NH4+ uptake on rat tIMCD Na(+)-K(+)-ATPase. Am J Physiol 273:F857–F868, 1997.

695. Wall SM, Davis BS, Hassell KA, et al: In rat tIMCD, NH4+ uptake by Na$^+$-K$^+$-ATPase is critical to net acid secretion during chronic hypokalemia. Am J Physiol 277:F866–F874, 1999.

696. Wall SM: NH$^+$4 augments net acid secretion by a ouabain-sensitive mechanism in isolated perfused inner medullary collecting ducts. Am J Physiol 270:F432–F439, 1996.

697. Wall SM, Fischer MP, Kim GH, et al: In rat inner medullary collecting duct, NH uptake by the Na,K-ATPase is increased during hypokalemia. Am J Physiol Renal Physiol 282:F91–102, 2002.

698. Nakhoul NL, Hering-Smith KS, Abdulnour-Nakhoul SM, Hamm LL: Transport of NH(3)/NH in oocytes expressing aquaporin-1. Am J Physiol Renal Physiol 281:F255–F263, 2001.

699. Holm LM, Jahn TP, Moller AL, et al: NH3 and NH4+ permeability in aquaporin-expressing Xenopus oocytes. Pflugers Arch 450:415–428, 2005.

700. Wall SM, Trinh HN, Woodward KE: Heterogeneity of NH$^+$4 transport in mouse inner medullary collecting duct cells. Am J Physiol 269:F536–F544, 1995.

701. Wall SM, Fischer MP: Contribution of the Na(+)-K(+)-2Cl(–) cotransporter (NKCC1) to transepithelial transport of H(+), NH(4)(+), K(+), and Na(+) in rat outer medullary collecting duct. J Am Soc Nephrol 13:827–835, 2002.

702. Kaplan MR, Plotkin MD, Brown D, et al: Expression of the mouse Na-K-2Cl cotransporter, mBSC2, in the terminal inner medullary collecting duct, the glomerular and extraglomerular mesangium, and the glomerular afferent arteriole. J Clin Invest 98:723–730, 1996.

703. Ikebe M, Nonoguchi H, Nakayama Y, et al: Upregulation of the secretory-type Na(+)/K(+)/2Cl(–)-cotransporter in the kidney by metabolic acidosis and dehydration in rats. J Am Soc Nephrol 12:423–430, 2001.

704. Amlal H, Soleimani M: K$^+$/NH4+ antiporter: a unique ammonium carrying transporter in the kidney inner medulla. Biochim Biophys Acta 1323:319–333, 1997.

705. Nakhoul NL, Hamm LL: Non-erythroid Rh glycoproteins: A putative new family of mammalian ammonium transporters. Pflugers Arch 447:807–812, 2004.

706. Eladari D, Cheval L, Quentin F, et al: Expression of RhCG, a new putative NH(3)/NH(4)(+) transporter, along the rat nephron. J Am Soc Nephrol 13:1999–2008, 2002.

707. Verlander JW, Miller RT, Frank AE, et al: Localization of the ammonium transporter proteins RhBG and RhCG in mouse kidney. Am J Physiol Renal Physiol 284:F323–F337, 2003.

708. Quentin F, Eladari D, Cheval L, et al: RhBG and RhCG, the putative ammonia transporters, are expressed in the same cells in the distal nephron. J Am Soc Nephrol 14:545–554, 2003.

709. Huang CH, Liu PZ: New insights into the Rh superfamily of genes and proteins in erythroid cells and nonerythroid tissues. Blood Cells Mol Dis 27:90–101, 2001.

710. Heitman J, Agre P: A new face of the Rhesus antigen. Nat Genet 26:258–259, 2000.

711. Liu Z, Peng J, Mo R, et al: Rh type B glycoprotein is a new member of the Rh superfamily and a putative ammonia transporter in mammals. J Biol Chem 276:1424–1433, 2001.

712. Verlander JW, Miller RT, Frank AE, et al: Localization of the ammonium transporter proteins RhBG and RhCG in mouse kidney. Am J Physiol Renal Physiol 284:F323–F337, 2003.

713. Seshadri RM, Klein JD, Kozlowski S, et al: Renal expression of the ammonia transporters, Rhbg and Rhcg, in response to chronic metabolic acidosis. Am J Physiol Renal Physiol 290:F397–F408, 2006.

714. Seshadri RM, Klein JD, Smith T, et al: Changes in subcellular distribution of the ammonia transporter, Rhcg, in response to chronic metabolic acidosis. Am J Physiol Renal Physiol 290:F1443–F1452, 2006.

715. Ludewig U: Electroneutral ammonium transport by basolateral rhesus B glycoprotein. J Physiol 559:751–759, 2004.

716. Mak DO, Dang B, Weiner ID, et al: Characterization of ammonia transport by the kidney Rh glycoproteins RhBG and RhCG. Am J Physiol Renal Physiol 290:F297–F305, 2006.

717. Bakouh N, Benjelloun F, Cherif-Zahar B, Planelles G: The challenge of understanding ammonium homeostasis and the role of the Rh glycoproteins. Transfus Clin Biol 13:139–146, 2006.

718. Kustu S, Inwood W: Biological gas channels for NH3 and CO2: Evidence that Rh (Rhesus) proteins are CO$_2$ channels. Transfus Clin Biol 13:103–110, 2006.

719. Nakhoul NL, Dejong H, Abdulnour-Nakhoul SM, et al: Characteristics of renal Rhbg as an NH4(+) transporter. Am J Physiol Renal Physiol 288:F170–F181, 2005.

720. Khademi S, O'Connell J, III, Remis J, et al: Mechanism of ammonia transport by Amt/MEP/Rh: structure of AmtB at 1.35 A. Science 305:1587–1594, 2004.

721. Chambrey R, Goossens D, Bourgeois S, et al: Genetic ablation of Rhbg in the mouse does not impair renal ammonium excretion. Am J Physiol Renal Physiol 289:F1281–F1290, 2005.

722. Sabolic I, Brown D, Gluck SL, Alper SL: Regulation of AE1 anion exchanger and H(+)-ATPase in rat cortex by acute metabolic acidosis and alkalosis. Kidney Int 51:125–137, 1997.

CHAPTER 8

Cell Biology of Vasopressin Action

Dennis Brown • Søren Nielsen

The antidiuretic hormone, vasopressin (VP) plays a multifaceted role in urinary concentration in mammals via activation of a G-protein coupled receptor (GPCR), the vasopressin receptor (V2R). VP increases the water permeability of renal collecting ducts by stimulating the plasma membrane accumulation of a water channel, aquaporin 2 (AQP2); it stimulates NaCl reabsorption by thick ascending limbs of Henle to increase the osmolality of the medullary interstitium; it facilitates the transepithelial movement of urea along its concentration gradient in terminal portions of the collecting duct, an important facet of the renal concentrating mechanism that allows high levels of urea to be excreted without reducing urinary concentrating ability. Many of the proteins that are involved in fluid and electrolyte transport in the kidney have now been identified and in several cases their function has been verified in animal models, providing a critical link between molecular function and animal physiology. This chapter will focus on two of the major protein elements that constitute the vasopressin-activated renal concentrating mechanism, the V2R and AQP2. Other critical channels and transporters that contribute to urinary concentration are dealt with elsewhere in this volume.

We will address functionally relevant properties of the V2R and AQP2 proteins that have emerged over the past few years, and we will update our understanding of signaling cascades, protein–protein interactions, membrane transport, intracellular trafficking, and synthesis and degradation pathways—areas that continue to evolve rapidly as the powerful new tools of genomics and proteomics are applied to renal physiology. However, in the face of an explosion of information related to the genetic and protein components that interact in these pathways, it becomes even more critical to integrate this information into whole organ and whole animal physiology in order to fulfill the promise of the emerging "Systems Biology" revolution as it applies to the renal concentrating mechanism.

VASOPRESSIN—THE ANTIDIURETIC HORMONE

Arginine vasopressin, a nine amino acid peptide, is the antidiuretic hormone of most mammals, although members of the pig family have a slightly different peptide known as lysine vasopressin (LVP) in which a lysine replaces the arginine in position 8 of the molecule. VP is synthesized in cells of the supraoptic and paraventricular nuclei of the hypothalamus, and the hormone is transported to nerve terminals in the posterior pituitary where it is stored in secretory granules. Secretion of VP is stimulated by a variety of factors, most notably an increase in plasma osmolality, but also by plasma volume.[1] A recent study indicates that vasopressin gene transcription is activated by decreased plasma volume, but not by increased plasma osmolality,[2] whereas another report shows increased VP heteronuclear RNA (hnRNA) levels in the hypothalamus after acute salt loading of rats.[3] The secretion of vasopressin in response to plasma osmolality is very sensitive, and a change in osmolality as small as 1% can cause a significant rise in plasma VP levels, which then activates regulatory systems necessary to retain water and restore osmolality to normal. Although the physiological response of VP to volume is less sensitive, with a 5% to 10% decrease in volume required to stimulate VP secretion, VP has important clinical applications in the control of vasodilatory shock.[4,5] Finally, the usual mammalian form of VP, arginine VP (AVP), is an effective agonist for all vasopressin receptor isoforms—the V1a and V1b/V3 forms that are located mainly in blood vessels and hepatocytes,[6] and the pituitary,[7–9] respectively—as well as the V2R that is expressed in the kidney[10] and in some other tissues, including the inner ear.[11,12] A modified form of AVP, known as desamino d-arginine[8] vasopressin (dDAVP), is specific for the V2R and has little or no V1-related pressor effect. It is, therefore, commonly used in studies (or in the clinical situation) when V2R activation is required in the absence of the V1 effect.

THE VASOPRESSIN V2 RECEPTOR (V2R)— A G-PROTEIN COUPLED RECEPTOR

The V2R is a 371 amino acid protein[10,13]—a member of the family of seven membrane-spanning domain receptors that couple to heterotrimeric G-proteins.[14] In the kidney, it is expressed on the plasma membrane of collecting duct principal cells and epithelial cells of the thick ascending limb of Henle. The V2R is also expressed in the endolymphatic sac in the inner ear,[11,12,15,16] and on endothelial cells in a variety of tissues, where it may be involved in a vasodilatory response that includes NO generation and Von Willebrand factor secretion.[17-19] The presence of vasopressin receptors on these cell types has been demonstrated by a variety of techniques, including functional and morphological assays of vasopressin action both *in situ* and in isolated tubule and cellular preparations from the kidney.[20-25] Attempts to localize the V2R using specific antibodies have met with variable success, and some studies have even reported a significant apical staining for the V2R in renal tubules, in addition to the expected basolateral staining and staining inside the cell.[26,27] Considerable use has also been made of cell culture systems, especially LLC-PK1 cells from porcine kidney, to evaluate ligand receptor interactions and signal transduction mechanisms via stimulatory and inhibitory heterotrimeric GTP-binding proteins.[28] A variety of transfected cell systems, both epithelial and non-epithelial, have proven valuable in elucidating several aspects of the V2R signaling cascade following ligand binding, as well as intracellular pathways of V2R recycling, down-regulation, and desensitization.

In target cells, the V2R is activated by the binding of its ligand, AVP, which stimulates adenylyl cyclase activity and increases cytosolic cAMP levels.[29] The increase in cAMP activates protein kinase A (PKA) and results in the PKA-mediated phosphorylation of several proteins. As will be discussed in more detail later, the vasopressin-sensitive water channel AQP2 is itself phosphorylated under these conditions and accumulates in the apical plasma membrane of collecting duct principal cells, thus increasing transepithelial water permeability and facilitating osmotically driven water reabsorption from the tubule lumen into the renal interstitium (Fig. 8–1). In addition, intracellular calcium is also increased by VP via a mechanism involving interaction with calmodulin,[30] a phenomenon that is also involved in the regulated trafficking of AQP2.[31,32]

Structure of the V2R

Homologs of the V2R have been cloned from several mammalian species including human, pig, and rat, and the receptor sequences are more than 90% identical. The membrane topology of the receptor and several functionally important features are illustrated in Figure 8–2. These include (1) an extracellular N-terminus with a consensus site for N-linked glycosylation (N22), (2) a cytoplasmic carboxy terminus and large intracellular loop that contain multiple sites for serine and threonine phosphorylation, and probably play a role in receptor desensitization, internalization, sequestration, and recycling,[33,34,36,37] (3) conserved sites for fatty acylation (palmitoylation), which may serve as an additional membrane anchor in the C-terminal tail, and be involved in membrane accumulation or in endocytosis and MAPK signaling,[38,39] (4) two highly conserved cysteine residues in the second and third extracellular loops, which may form a disulfide bridge that is important for correct folding of the molecule and stabilization of the ligand binding site, (5) hydrophobic residues at the C-terminus, including a dileucine motif, which are involved in ER to Golgi transfer, and in receptor folding that is required for receptor transport from the ER.[40]

Interaction of V2R with Heterotrimeric G-Proteins

Upon binding of VP, the V2R assumes an active configuration and promotes the disassembly of the bound heterotrimeric G-protein, Gs, into Gα and Gβγ subunits.[29] GDP-GTP exchange occurs on the alpha subunit. This G-protein is located on the basolateral plasma membrane of TAL and principal cells.[41,42] The activated Gsα then stimulates adenylate cyclase (AC), resulting in an increase in cAMP levels in the cell. In the rat kidney, several AC isoforms are expressed, but AC-6 is the predominant isoform in the adult rat kidney, and AC-4, -5, and -9 have lower expression levels.[43] The calmodulin-sensitive AC-3 is also expressed in the collecting duct, however, and the vasopressin-induced increase in cAMP and AQP2 trafficking in principal cells has been reported to be calmodulin-dependent.[31,32] The liganded V2R interacts with Gs via its cytosolic domain, and the third intracellular loop of the V2R is involved in this interaction.[44,45] A peptide corresponding to this loop inhibits V2R signaling though Gs when introduced into cells expressing the V2R.[46] Interestingly, this same peptide also reduces VP binding to the V2R by converting the receptor from a high to a low affinity state.

A complex cross-talk mechanism also results in activation of an inhibitory GTP-binding protein, which down-regulates the vasopressin response.[28,29] Other factors involved in a blunting of the vasopressin response are receptor down-regulation and desensitization. This results at least in part from a decreased number of receptors at the cell surface as receptors are internalized via clathrin-coated pits.[47,48] The level of V2R mRNA also decreases rapidly after an elevation of plasma AVP.[49] Many additional mechanisms that down-regulate the vasopressin response have been described. These include destruction of cAMP by cytosolic phosphodiesterases[50] and inhibition of the vasopressin response by prostaglandins,[51] dopamine,[52,53] adenosine receptor stimulation,[54] adrenergic agonists,[55,56] endothelin-1,[57] and bradykinin.[58]

The V2R Enters a Lysosomal Degradative Pathway after Internalization

G-protein coupled receptors (GPCR) are constitutively expressed on the plasma membrane and are down-regulated following ligand binding. Ligand-induced changes in receptor conformation are followed by receptor phosphorylation, desensitization, internalization, and sequestration. Phosphorylation triggers the binding of β-arrestin to the V2R.[33,59] Arrestins uncouple GPCRs from heterotrimeric G-proteins, effectively producing a desensitized receptor.[60] Arrestin-receptor complexes are also capable of recruiting the clathrin adaptor protein AP-2, an important component of the endocytotic mechanism,[61] and the complex is then internalized via clathrin-mediated endocytosis.[47,48] In most cases, hormone ligands dissociate from their receptors in acidic endosomes, and the receptors subsequently reappear at the cell surface in a process known as receptor recycling. However, different GPCRs recycle back to the cell surface at different rates. The β2-adrenergic receptor (β2AR) is a so-called "rapid recycler", and pre-stimulation levels of the β2AR are restored on the cell surface within an hour of ligand-induced internalization.[33] In contrast, the same process requires several hours in the case of the V2R.[33,34,62]

An earlier study[35] showed that the vasopressin ligand is delivered to lysosomes after binding to the V2R, as are many other ligands that are internalized by receptor-mediated endocytosis, but the fate of the actual vasopressin receptor was not followed in this report. It is known that the V2R forms a stable complex with β-arrestin throughout the

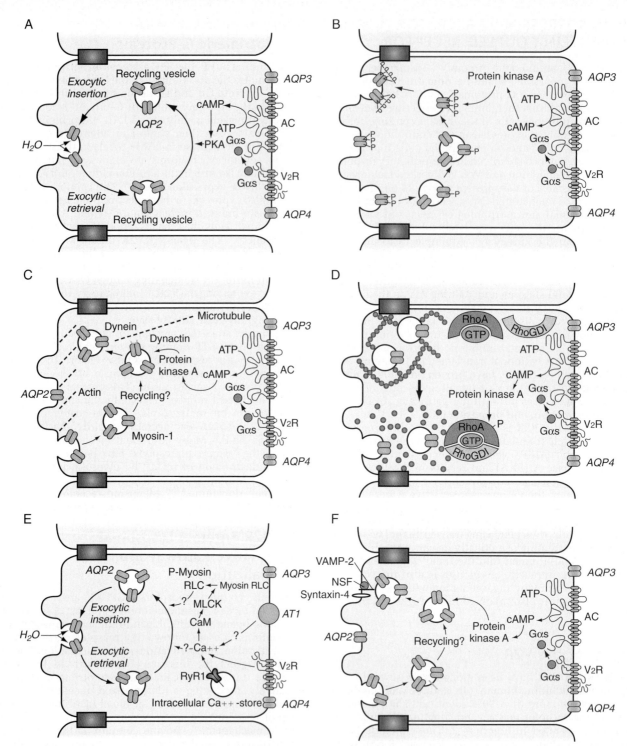

FIGURE 8–1 Overview of vasopressin-controlled short-term regulation of AQP2 trafficking in AQP2-containing collecting duct cell. Signaling cascades and molecular apparatus involved in vasopressin regulation of AQP2 trafficking are shown. **A,** Vasopressin binding to the G-protein-linked V2-receptor stimulates adenylyl cyclase leading to elevated cAMP levels and activation of protein kinase A. AQP2 is subsequently translocated to the apical plasma membrane. **B,** Role of AQP2-phosphorylation in AQP2 recruitment to the plasma-membrane. Protein kinase A phosphorylates AQP2-monomers and phosphorylation of at least three of four AQP2 monomers in an AQP2-tetramer is associated with translocation to the plasma membrane. It is currently unknown if dephosphorylation of AQP2 is necessary for endocytosis of AQP2. **C,** Overview of cytoskeletal elements, which may be involved in AQP2-trafficking. AQP2 containing vesicles may be transported along microtubules by dynein/dynactin. The cortical actin web may act as a barrier to fusion with the plasma-membrane. **D,** Changes in the actin cytoskeleton associated with AQP2-trafficking to the plasma membrane. Inactivation of RhoA by phosphorylation and increased formation of RhoARhoGDI complexes seem to control the dissociation of actin fibers seen after vasopressin stimulation. **E,** Intracellular calcium signaling and AQP2-trafficking. Increases in intracellular Ca^{2+} concentration may arise from stimulation of the V2 receptor. The existence and potential role of other receptors and pathways affecting Ca^{2+} mobilization is still uncertain but may potentially include AT1 receptors. The downstream targets of the calcium signal are unknown. **F,** Vesicle targeting receptors and AQP2-trafficking. A number of vesicle targeting receptors, for example, SNARE-proteins have been localized to the AQP2-containing collecting duct cells and cultured cells. The exact role of these remains to be established. V2R, vasopressin-V2-receptors; AC, adenylyl cyclase, PKA, cAMP and protein kinase A (PKA).

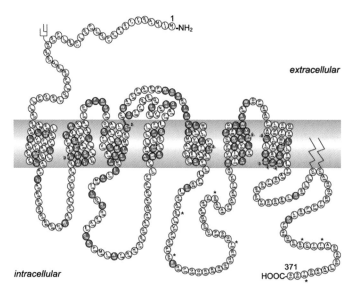

FIGURE 8–2 Membrane topology of the vasopressin receptor (V2R). The 371 amino acid protein has seven membrane spanning domains, an extracellular N-terminus, and a cytoplasmic C-terminus. Several features of the molecule are illustrated. Residue N22 is a putative N-glycosylation site; a functionally important disulfide bridge occurs between cysteines 112 and 192; the dileucine motif LL339–340 is an endocytotic signaling motif; C341/342 are sites of palmitoylation; phosphorylation sites (serine and threonine residues) between T347 and S364 play a critical role in V2R internalization and recycling. Potential sites of phosphorylation by GRK are indicated with asterisks. (Figure slightly modified from an original kindly provided by Dr. Daniel Bichet, University of Montreal.)

internalization pathway[33,63] and this prolonged association of β-arrestin with the V2R could be responsible for the intracellular retention, but not the final destination of the receptor.[37]

Recent immunofluorescence, biochemical, and ligand binding data have now clearly shown that much of the V2R that is internalized after vasopressin addition to cells enters a lysosomal degradation compartment, and that re-establishment of baseline levels of vasopressin binding sites (V2R) at the cell surface requires *de novo* protein synthesis.[64,65] Furthermore, VP stimulation leads to rapid, β-arrestin–dependent ubiquitination of the V2R and increased degradation.[66]

The process of internalization and delivery to lysosomes can be followed using transfected cells expressing the V2R coupled to green fluorescent protein (GFP). Real-time spinning disk confocal microscopy shows that after ligand binding, the V2R-GFP moves from a predominant plasma membrane location to a perinuclear vesicular compartment (Fig. 8–3).[67] Colocalization of the V2R-GFP construct with Lysotracker, a marker of acidic late endosomes and lysosomes, after VP-induced internalization of V2R-GFP is shown in Figure 8–4, indicating that the perinuclear vesicles are predominantly lysosomes.[64] Western blotting also reveals a time-dependent degradation of the V2R after internalization that is completely inhibited by chloroquine (a lysosome inhibitor) but not by lactacystin (a proteasome inhibitor). Furthermore, re-establishment of pre-stimulation levels of the V2R at the cell surface is significantly inhibited by cycloheximide, illustrating the requirement for new protein synthesis in this process.[64]

In summary, the V2R—classified as a "slow-recycling" GPCR—appears to be mainly degraded in lysosomes after ligand-induced internalization. This pathway may have evolved to allow the V2R to function in the harsh environment of the renal medulla, which can be acidic and of high osmolality.[68] Normally, receptors and ligands dissociate in the acidic endosomal environment, but the V2R must actually

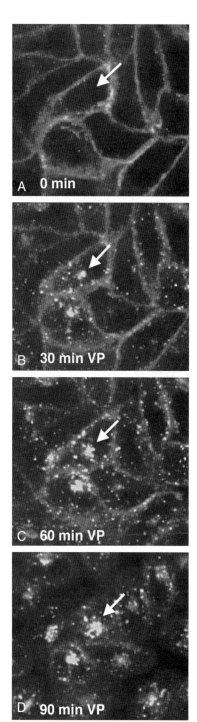

FIGURE 8–3 Spinning disk confocal microscopy (live cell imaging) of LLC-PK1 cells stably expressing V2R-GFP seen at various times (0–90 min) after addition of the ligand, vasopressin (VP). Initially, most of the V2R-GFP is located on the plasma membrane **(A)**. After VP treatment, the V2R-GFP is down-regulated from the cell surface and is progressively internalized **(B, C)** into a perinuclear compartment that is seen as a bright fluorescent patch (indicated with an arrow in each panel). The degree of internalization can be easily followed in the same cells using this technique. After VP treatment for 90 minutes, virtually no plasma membrane V2R-GFP is detectable—it is all concentrated in an area close to the nucleus **(D)**. (Figure adapted from a review by Brown D: Imaging protein trafficking. Nephron Exp Nephrol 103:e55–61, 2006.)

associate with VP in the acidic renal medulla. Thus, the V2R-VP pair should be resistant to pH-induced dissociation, and the delivery of both the ligand and receptor to lysosomes may be required in order to terminate the physiological response to VP.

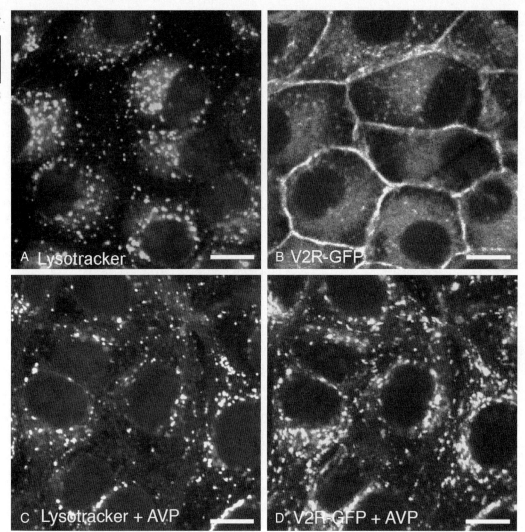

FIGURE 8–4 In non-stimulated LLC-PK1 cells expressing V2R-GFP, the patterns of staining for Lysotracker (**A**)—a marker of acidic lysosomes and late endosomes—and the V2R-GFP (**B**) are distinct, with most of the V2R-GFP at the plasma membrane (although some intracellular V2R is also present). After VP-induced down-regulation, the V2R-GFP is internalized as shown in Fig. 8–3, and accumulates in vesicles, many of which are also stained with Lysotracker (**C, D**). These data indicate that internalized V2R is mainly trafficked to lysosomes for degradation. (Figure adapted from Bouley R, Lin HY, Raychowdhury MK, et al: Down-regulation of the vasopressin type 2 receptor after vasopressin-induced internalization: Involvement of a lysosomal degradation pathway. Am J Physiol Cell Physiol 288:C1390–1401, 2005.)

Diabetes Insipidus (Central and Nephrogenic)

Diabetes insipidus is the generic name for conditions affecting the VP, V2R, AQP2 axis that result in a failure to maximally concentrate the urine. Patients with this disease produce large amounts of dilute urine—up to 20 L per day in extreme cases.[69,70] Clinically, this condition is recognizable soon after birth, and if not corrected can result in severe dehydration, hypernatremia, and damage to the central nervous system. The molecular basis for many of these related disorders has been examined and elucidated thanks to the cloning and sequencing of the key proteins involved, the V2R[13] and the vasopressin-sensitive collecting duct water channel, AQP2,[71] as well as the gene coding for the vasopressin/neurophysin/glycopeptide precursor protein from which active vasopressin is derived by further processing.[72,73]

Congenital Central Diabetes Insipidus

The autosomal dominant form of familial neurohypophyseal (central) diabetes insipidus (adFNDI) has been linked to over 40 different mutations of the gene encoding the vasopressin-neurophysin II (AVP-NPII) precursor. Most of these mutations have been located in either the signal peptide or the neurophysin II moiety, but a mutation in the portion of the gene coding for the VP protein has also been identified.[74] A three-generation kindred with severe adFNDI was found to cosegregate with a novel missense mutation in the part of the AVP-NPII gene encoding the AVP moiety.[75] Normally, newly synthesized pre-pro-AVP-NPII is translocated into the endoplasmic reticulum, where the signal peptide is removed, enabling the prohormone to fold, form the appropriate intrachain disulfide bonds, and dimerize. This conformation permits the prohormone to move to the Golgi where it is packaged into neurosecretory granules, cleaved into its individual moieties (AVP, NPII, and copeptin), and transported along the axon to be stored in nerve terminals until release. Many studies over the past several years have documented that mutations leading to adFNDI result in impaired folding or dimerization of the mutant precursor (or both). This interferes with normal intracellular trafficking and processing of the prohormone through the regulated secretory pathway.[75,76]

The congenital (or acquired) absence of a functional vasopressin hormone can be generally treated by administration of vasopressin or dDAVP, usually via nasal aerosol. In this form of the disease, the V2R and the AQP2 genes and proteins are unaffected, and VP administration leads to the reestablishment of urine concentration.[77–80] An animal model of CDI, the Brattleboro rat, has proven to be an invaluable system in which many of the consequences of defective urinary concentration resulting from an absence of functional VP have been elucidated.[81,82] A single base pair deletion in the neurophysin domain of the vasopressin gene was identified in these animals.[83] This frameshift mutation results in the loss of a stop codon and abnormal processing of the neurophysin/vasopressin/glycopeptide precursor, leading to a failure in the production, storage, and secretion of vasopressin.[72] The ability to convert these rats from non-concentrators to concentrators simply by administering exogenous VP has resulted in many important discoveries on the vasopressin signaling cascade that will be alluded to later.

Nephrogenic Diabetes Insipidus

Nephrogenic diabetes insipidus (NDI) on the other hand, results from a loss of an appropriate response of the kidneys to circulating vasopressin, and in most cases cannot be treated simply by administering vasopressin. As for central DI, NDI can be congenital/hereditary or acquired.[69,77,84,85] CNDI was first described over 50 years ago[86] and genetic linkage studies in several families established that the predominant form is an X-linked trait.[87,88] Acquired disease is more frequent than hereditary NDI, and of all causes, lithium-induced NDI is the most common.[84,89] This will be addressed in more detail in a later section of this chapter, along with other acquired forms of the disease. Distinct forms of nephrogenic diabetes insipidus are produced by a variety of gene mutations that result in defective targeting and/or function of the V2R or the AQP2 water channel.[69,85,90–93]

Type I CNDI (congenital nephrogenic DI), the more frequent X-linked form, is a recessive disease caused by mutations in the vasopressin receptor.[93] Type II CNDI is an autosomal recessive disease resulting from mutations in the AQP2 water channel[91–94] although an autosomal dominant form of CNDI has also been described.[95,96]

Mutations in the V2R

Close to 200 disease-causing mutations have been identified in the V2R[97] (see Fig. 8–2), many of which result in the production of a non-functional receptor by target cells in the kidney.[98] While this is predominantly an X-linked disease (the V2R gene is located on the X-chromosome), some very rare female cases have been described, which are believed to be associated with aberrant X-chromosome inactivation.[99] Some of the mutations result in the appearance of premature stop codons, others result in frame shifts that result in nonsense protein sequences, whereas others are single point mutations that cause an amino acid replacement at critical locations in the receptor. Mutations in the V2R sequence that allow the production of a full-length or near full-length protein could result in CNDI by interfering with different aspects of the receptor-ligand signal transduction cascade. For example (1) the receptor could be expressed normally at the cell surface, but not bind vasopressin, (2) the receptor could bind its ligand normally at the cell surface, but fail to couple to its stimulatory GTP-binding protein, so that adenylyl cyclase is not activated, (3) the mutated receptor may be incorrectly folded and might be retained for degradation in the rough endoplasmic reticulum (RER), and may never reach the cell surface—this is an example of a targeting mutation, (4) changes in the ability of the receptor to be phosphorylated may affect several aspects of function, including trafficking and desensitization.[91,100] The R137H mutation produces NDI because it is constitutively desensitized via an arrestin-mediated mechanism—the mutant V2R is phosphorylated and sequestered in arrestin-containing vesicles even in the absence of agonist.[101] Interestingly, this mutation can result in either severe or mild NDI, indicating that genetic or environmental modifiers (or both) may affect the final phenotype within affected members of the same family.[102]

Some mutations in the V2R have been associated with specific functional defects that are believed to explain the loss of receptor function. For example, many of the missense mutations that have been described (R181C, G185C, and Y205C) result in the addition of cysteine residues in the extracellular loops, and this is believe to interfere with the disulfide bond formation that connects the first and second loops in the wild-type receptor. However, a newly discovered Y205H mutation also abolishes receptor function and leads to NDI, suggesting that loss of the tyrosine is the cause of dysfunction, rather than the addition of a cysteine at least at residue 205.[103]

Many mutations cause folding defects that are recognized by cellular quality control mechanisms, leading to retention and degradation in intracellular compartments. However, different mutations are handled in different ways, and some temporarily escape from the ER before being rerouted back to this compartment for degradation. Cell transfection experiments have shown that whereas the L62P, DeltaL62-R64, and S167L mutants are trapped in the ER, the R143P, Y205C, InsQ292, V226E, and R337X mutant receptors actually reach the ER/Golgi intermediate compartment (ERGIC) before being rerouted to the ER. Differences in the folding characteristics of these receptors that allow interactions with different sets of accessory proteins are thought to explain these differences.[94]

Correcting the Defect: Approaches to Nephrogenic Diabetes Insipidus Therapy Involving the V2R

Several approaches have been considered as potential therapeutic strategies in X-linked forms of NDI that involve V2R mutations. These have developed from our increased understanding of the cell biology and signaling pathways that are involved in the response to VP. If the mutated V2R is mistrafficked in cells but is otherwise functional, then persuading the mutant receptor to move to the cell surface would be therapeutically beneficial. This strategy is also being explored for other diseases of protein trafficking, including cystic fibrosis, in which a single point mutation prevents efficient delivery of the CFTR protein to the cell surface. Instead, it is retained intracellularly and degraded. A variety of approaches including the use of chemical-induced or drug-induced rescue of cell surface expression have been attempted. Among the first chemical chaperones to be tested for the V2R were substances such as glycerol and dimethylsulfoxide. Additional reagents (thapsigargin/curcumin and ionomycin) that modify calcium levels in cellular compartments were also tested.[105] However, their reported efficacy in partially restoring transport activity to cells and tissues expressing the ΔF508 CFTR mutation that leads to cystic fibrosis[106,107] has subsequently been contested in an independent study.[108] Furthermore, of 9 V2R mutants tested, the surface expression of only one of them—V2R-V206D—was increased using these reagents.[105]

However, the use of V2R antagonists to increase cell surface expression and functionality of mutant V2R protein seems more promising.[109] Small, cell permeant non-peptidic antagonists were shown to rescue the cell surface appearance of 8 mutant receptors that were tested, whereas a non-permeable antagonist had no positive effect.[110,111] Importantly, the antagonist SR49059, which was shown to be effective in three patients harboring the R137H V2R mutation, acts by improving the maturation and cell surface targeting of the mutant receptor.[112] Furthermore, the pharmacological V2R antagonist SR121463B resulted in greater maturation and surface expression of the V2R mutations V206D and S167T than chemical chaperones.[105]

Finally, aminoglycoside antibiotics are known to suppress premature stop codons in some cases. In the case of the V2R, an E242X mutation produces a premature stop codon in humans, and when introduced into mice, this mutation causes NDI. However, urine concentrating ability can be restored by administering the antibiotic Geneticin (G418) to mice, and the AVP-mediated cAMP response is increased by G418 in cultured cells expressing this V2R mutation.[113] This provides a potential means of suppressing NDI that is caused by a premature stop codon in the V2R.

THE AQUAPORINS—A FAMILY OF WATER CHANNEL PROTEINS

The first water channel (aquaporin) was identified and characterized as a Nobel Prize winning discovery by Peter Agre and his associates in 1988.[114] This protein—originally known as CHIP28—is now known as aquaporin 1 (AQP1).[115–117] Functional studies in Xenopus oocytes (injected with AQP1 mRNA) and liposomes (reconstituted with purified AQP1 protein)[117–119] confirmed its role as the long-sought erythrocyte transmembrane water channel protein whose existence had been proposed for many years prior to its ultimate identification. The AQP1 protein is homologous to the lens fiber channel-forming protein MIP26 (Major Intrinsic Protein of 26 kDa, now renamed AQP0), which was cloned several years earlier[120] but whose physiological function was a matter of speculation. AQP1 is expressed in many cells and tissues with high constitutive water permeability, in addition to erythrocytes, including proximal tubules and thin descending limbs of Henle in the kidney,[121,122] the choroid plexus,[123] reabsorptive portions of the male reproductive tract that are embryologically related to renal tubules,[124] parts of the inner ear,[125] and many others.[126,127]

AQP2, the collecting duct vasopressin-sensitive water channel was then discovered by homology cloning from the renal medulla,[71] and a variety of studies that are described in more detail later confirmed that it is the principal cell water channel that is involved in distal urinary concentration ion the kidney.[128–132] Other aquaporins were subsequently discovered in rapid succession, and at the time of writing,12 mammalian homologs are known. Although aquaporins show considerable homology among different mammalian species,[133] homology among the different aquaporins from the same species may be as little as 35%. Aquaporins have also been found in virtually all species examined, including bacteria and plants. The membrane topography and some key features (e.g., phosphorylation sites) of the aquaporins (AQP2) are illustrated in Figure 8–5.

Other Permeability Properties of Aquaporins

Aquaporins were so named because they function as transmembrane water channels. However, the single channel water permeability of different aquaporins varies greatly. AQP1, AQP2, and AQP4 have high permeabilities whereas and AQP0 and AQP3 have much lower permeabilities.[134] Furthermore, some aquaporins including AQP3, AQP8, and AQP9 also allow the passage of other molecules, including urea, glycerol, ammonia, and other small solutes.[134–141] Based on

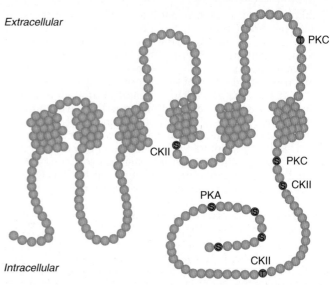

FIGURE 8–5 Membrane topology of the aquaporin 2 (AQP2) water channel. This 271 amino acid protein spans the lipid bilayer six times. Both N- and C-termini are in the cytoplasm. Phosphorylation sites for PKC, PKA, and casein kinase II (CKII) are shown.

such properties and phylogenetic considerations, aquaporins were divided into one of two groups, the "orthodox set" (aquaporins) and the "cocktail set" (aquaglyceroporins).[142] Distinct physiological functions for aquaporins in the transport of non-water molecules, including glycerol, are beginning to emerge.[143]

Remarkably, water channels do not allow the passage of protons, a property that was first shown using isolated apical endosomes from rat kidney papilla.[144,145] Crystallographic evidence has provided a structural explanation for their ability to prevent proton conductance.[146] This and other structural features of the aquaporins that contribute to their remarkable specificity will be described in more detail later. However, some results in oocytes and liposomes indicate that AQP1 serves as a CO_2 channel,[147–150] (reviewed in Ref 151) whereas whole animal studies using AQP1-deficient mice have refuted this claim.[152] Other groups examining the potential role of erythrocyte AQP1 in CO_2 transport have produced data in favor[147] or against[153,154] a role of AQP1 in this process. Recent developments have not reached a final consensus, and the role of AQP1 in transmembrane CO_2 permeability in mammalian cells remains controversial.[155] Support of this idea, however, comes from plant systems in which aquaporin-mediated CO_2 permeability is reported to be an important step in the photosynthetic process.[156–158]

Although some aquaporins including AQP1[159] and AQP8 have been reported to allow passage of ammonia in some expression systems, including yeast and oocytes,[135,138] the physiological relevance of this has been questioned in AQP8 knockout mice.[160] AQPs 7 and 9 have both been implicated in arsenite transport in mammalian cells.[161]

Aquaporin 2: The Vasopressin-Sensitive, Collecting Duct Water Channel

Many studies have localized aquaporin mRNA or protein (or both) in a wide range of cell types, and aquaporins have been attributed a wide range of functions in the normal physiology of many tissues and organ systems. This section will focus on aquaporin 2 (AQP2), which was identified as the VP-regulated water channel in kidney collecting duct principal cells.[71] VP stimulation of the kidney collecting duct results

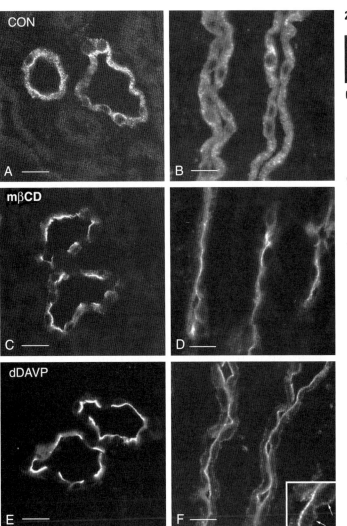

FIGURE 8–6 Increased plasma membrane expression of AQP2 in principal cells of Sprague Dawley kidney perfused in the presence of 5 mM mβCD (an endocytosis inhibitor) or 4 nM dDAVP for 60 minutes. Kidneys were then fixed, sectioned, and immunostained using anti-AQP2 antibodies. Examples of tubules sectioned transversely from the inner stripe of the outer medulla (**A, C, E**) and longitudinally in the inner medulla/papilla (**B, D, F**) are illustrated. Under control conditions (**A, B**), AQP2 has a cytosolic distribution in principal cells. After perfusion with 5 mM mβCD (**C, D**), AQP2 shows an increased apical localization in principal cells of the inner stripe and inner medulla. After perfusion with 4 nM dDAVP, a similar and expected increased apical localization of AQP2 in medullary collecting ducts is seen in the isolated perfused kidney preparation. dDAVP also induced a basolateral localization of AQP2 in the inner medulla (**F** and arrows, inset) but not in the inner stripe (**E**) principal cells. Bar = 40 μm.

in the accumulation of AQP2 on the plasma membrane of principal cells via a membrane trafficking mechanism that involves the recycling of AQP2 between intracellular vesicles and the cell surface (Fig. 8–6).[94,128–130,134,162,163] However, it should be mentioned that AQP3, present in the basolateral membrane of principal cells,[137] is also regulated at the expression level by vasopressin or dehydration (or both),[164] although no evidence for an acute regulation of this basolateral channel has been forthcoming. Hormonal (VP) stimulation of the collecting duct epithelium increases its plasma membrane water permeability, which in turn allows the luminal fluid to equilibrate osmotically with the surrounding interstitium. The osmolality in the renal inner medulla reaches about 1200 mOsm/kg in humans, and thus the urine can reach the same concentration in the presence of vasopressin. The mechanism by which the apical plasma membrane of collecting duct principal cells shifts from a low-to-high permeability state upon vasopressin action is the subject of much of the remainder of this chapter, and involves the redistribution of AQP2 from cytoplasmic vesicles to the plasma membrane under the influence of a signaling cascade that is triggered by the binding of VP to the V2R in these cells.

Although AQP2 was discovered in the kidney, it is also expressed in a limited number of non-renal epithelia. These are the vas deferens of the male reproductive tract,[165,166] the inner ear in which its expression is regulated by vasopres-

sin,[15,16] and the colon.[167] Interestingly, AQP2 in the vas deferens is inserted into the apical plasma membrane in a non-regulated, constitutive pathway, implying that the same aquaporin can be regulated in different ways depending on the cell type in which it is expressed.[166]

Intramembranous Particle Aggregates— An Early Morphological Hallmark of Membrane Water Permeability

The "cell biological" era of vasopressin action can be considered to have begun in 1974, when Chevalier and colleagues described an alteration in the appearance of frog urinary bladder plasma membranes in parallel with an increase in epithelial water permeability induced by another neurohypophyseal hormone, oxytocin.[168] Freeze-fracture electron microscopy revealed numerous small aggregates of intramembranous particles (IMPs), which represent integral membrane proteins, on the apical plasma membranes of frog bladder epithelial cells under these conditions. The correlation between this membrane structural change and hormonally induced transepithelial water flow was strengthened by a large body of subsequent work from several groups.[169–173] The data suggested that the IMP aggregates were water-permeable patches, and that the individual IMPs in each aggregate were the morphological correlate of a putative (but not yet identified at that time) water channel protein that spanned the lipid bilayer.

In support of this idea, apical plasma membrane IMP aggregates or IMP clusters were induced by VP administration in both amphibian epidermis and the mammalian collecting duct.[174,175] IMP clusters were not present in mice with hereditary diabetes insipidus that cannot concentrate their urine.[176] In the amphibian epidermis, both ADH and isoproterenol stimulate water flow, and both caused IMP aggregates to appear.[177] In all three target epithelia (amphibian urinary bladder and skin, and mammalian collecting duct), there was a dose response relationship between the number of IMP aggregates in the membrane, and the magnitude of the water permeability response.

AQP4 Splice Variants and Orthogonal Arrays of Intramembranous Particles

The IMP aggregates seen by freeze-fracture EM in toad epidermis are virtually identical to the characteristic orthogonal arrays of IMPs (OAPs) that have now been identified as AQP4.[178–180] These AQP4 arrays are present on the basolateral plasma membrane of collecting duct principal cells where AQP4 is located,[181–183] as well as on other cell types that express AQP4 including gastric parietal cells[184,185] and astroglial cells.[178] AQP4 is an unusual water channel in that two splice variants are expressed—known as M1 and M23—due to the presence of alternative transcription initiation sites in the AQP4 gene.[186,187] Two recent reports have shown that M23 is more abundant in most cells, and that this variant arranges into typical orthogonal arrays when expressed in cultured cells.[188,189] M1 expression does not result in orthogonal arrays but interestingly, M1 co-expression in cells along with M23 actually is disruptive to OAP formation. Furthermore, the single channel water permeability of M23 when arranged into OAPs is significantly greater than that of M1, which does not form OAPs. These data raise the intriguing possibility that OAP formation enhances membrane water permeability due to AQP4, and that M1 expression and incorporation into the membrane disrupts OAPs and may decrease membrane water permeability. Interestingly, the water permeability of AQP4 expressed in LLC-PK1 cells and oocytes was reported to be gated (decreased) by PKC phosphorylation of residue S180, without any apparent change in membrane distribution of this protein,[190,191] but the expression of OAPs in these cells was not examined. Thus, it is possible that the basolateral membrane permeability of collecting duct principal cells may be modulated by AQP4 phosphorylation. Indeed there is one report showing that the basolateral membrane permeability of collecting ducts from the outer and inner medulla increases after dehydration and/or vasopressin (desmopressin) action, but the aquaporin responsible for this was not clearly identified.[192] However, it is unlikely to be AQP4 because the cell swelling effect was abolished by mercuric chloride, and AQP4 is known to be insensitive to this inhibitor.[193] Another basolateral aquaporin, AQP3, is up-regulated at the transcriptional level by VP[164] and could be responsible for the increased basolateral permeability. Furthermore, AQP2 can also be inserted into basolateral membranes of principal cells under some conditions, and thereby increase the permeability of this membrane domain.[194–196]

Aquaporin 2 Recycling: The "Shuttle Hypothesis" of Vasopressin Action

Based on many studies using vasopressin-sensitive amphibian epithelia, it was proposed that "water channels" are located on intracellular vesicles that fuse with the apical plasma membrane upon vasopressin stimulation, and then are retrieved back into the cell by endocytosis after vasopressin washout. The internalized water channels can then be re-inserted back into the plasma membrane upon subsequent re-stimulation by vasopressin. This so-called "shuttle hypothesis" of vasopressin action, proposed by Wade and associates in 1981,[173] was an elegant idea that has guided studies on the cell biology of vasopressin action for the past two decades. Developments in aquaporin cloning and expression in various cell systems, as well as in vivo studies, over the past decade have allowed a direct examination of many of the subcellular mechanisms underlying vasopressin regulation of collecting duct water permeability. The basic principles of the shuttle hypothesis (i.e., that water channels [AQP2] recycle between an intracellular vesicle pool and the plasma membrane [Fig. 8–1]) have withstood the test of time, but the details of this process remain to be fully elucidated at the cellular and mechanistic level. The following sections will provide an update on specific parts of the recycling itinerary of AQP2, and will outline the current state of our understanding of the regulation of the complex pathways that lead to a VP-induced increase in collecting duct water permeability.

Vasopressin-Regulated Trafficking of AQP2 in Collecting Duct Principal Cells

AQP2 was first identified by Fushimi and colleagues and sequencing of this protein from rat allowed several groups to develop antibodies against AQP2.[71,195,196] These reagents were used to show that AQP2 is abundantly expressed in the apical plasma membrane of collecting duct principal cells, as well as in numerous intracellular vesicles.[195] This distribution was consistent with the shuttle hypothesis of VP action (see Fig. 8–1). The onset and offset phase of VP action were then examined in vitro and in vivo, and the immunocytochemical data showed clearly that VP induced a striking and reversible redistribution of AQP2 from intracellular vesicles to the apical plasma membrane of principal cells (see Fig. 8–6).[197–200] Rapid internalization of AQP2 was induced by VP washout in isolated perfused collecting ducts, and in whole animals infused with a V2R antagonist or water loading.[201–203] These studies, taken together, provided strong evidence that vasopressin acutely regulates the osmotic water permeability of collecting duct principal cells by inducing exocytosis of AQP2 from intracellular vesicles to the apical plasma membrane, and that AQP2 removal from the membrane by endocytosis restores the low baseline water permeability of the apical plasma membrane of principal cells.

The internalized AQP2 that accumulates in endosomes after VP withdrawal follows a complex intracellular pathway prior to re-insertion into the plasma membrane. Studies in cells stably transfected with AQP2 have shown that recycling of AQP2 can occur in conditions in which protein synthesis is inhibited (see later), indicating that de novo protein synthesis is not required for this process to occur.[204] However, not all AQP2 is recycled. There is significant accumulation of AQP2 in larger cellular structures including multivesicular endosomes (MVEs) in response to treatment of rats with a VP antagonist.[201] Late endosomes often have the appearance of MVBs, and proteins in this compartment could be moved to lysosomes for degradation, be transferred to a recycling compartment via vesicular carriers that bud from the MVB, or be directly transported to the cell surface via other distinct transport vesicles that derive from the MVBs. It has been shown that AQP2 is "secreted" into the tubule lumen, where it can be found partially associated with small vesicles called exosomes in the urine.[205,206] The amount of AQP2 in the urine increases in conditions of antidiuresis when more AQP2 is present in the apical membrane of principal cells. The physiological relevance of this urinary excretion of AQP2 is unknown but interestingly, urinary AQP2 correlates with the severity of nocturnal enuresis in children, and lowering urinary calcium levels (by low calcium diet) has a beneficial effect in reducing the severity of the enuresis and reducing AQP2 secretion in hypercalcemic children treated with dDAVP.[207]

Reconstitution of Aquaporin Expression in Non-Polarized Cells

Expression of Aquaporins in Xenopus Oocytes

Xenopus oocytes were the first expression system that was used to demonstrate that aquaporin 1 (CHIP28) was a functional transmembrane water channel.[117] This system has been used in many subsequent studies to assess the water (and solute) permeability of virtually all mammalian aquaporins. Membrane permeability resulting from injection of an appropriate mRNA is measured by computer-assisted analysis of oocyte swelling in response to a hypotonic buffer, as initially described by Verkman and colleagues.[208] This system has also proven useful in assessing the function of mutated aquaporins including those that are known to cause NDI in humans, posttranslational modifications (phosphorylation, glycosylation), as well as potential modifiers of aquaporin permeability by co-expressing proteins such as CFTR.[209] Many of the mutant AQP2 proteins are not expressed at the cell surface of oocytes, probably due to folding defects that cause retention and ultimate degradation in the rough endoplasmic reticulum or retention (or both) in the Golgi apparatus.[96,210,211] Oocytes have also been useful for dissection of the role of aquaporin oligomerization in cell surface expression.[212]

Expression of Aquaporins in Non-Epithelial Cells

Expression systems such as CHO cells have been extremely useful for morphological and functional studies on the different aquaporins. However, by definition, they cannot be used for studies on factors that regulate the polarized expression of aquaporins in renal epithelia. Freeze-fracture studies on transfected CHO cells revealed that the AQP1 protein assembles as a tetramer in the lipid bilayer,[213,214] a result in agreement with biochemical cross-linking data[215] and with data from cryo- and atomic force microscopy of 2D crystals of AQP1.[216–218] Transfection of CHO cells with AQP4 cDNA showed that this protein forms a characteristic pattern of orthogonal IMP arrays (OAPs) that are found in several cell types, including collecting duct principal cells (on the basolateral plasma membrane).[180,182] A comparison of membrane IMP organization in CHO cells expressing AQPs 1–5 showed that only AQP4 forms OAPs, that AQP2 does not spontaneously form IMP aggregates, and that AQP3 has a limited tendency to form small, densely packed clusters of IMPs.[219]

When various AQP2 mutations were expressed in CHO cells, important information was gathered concerning the abnormal intracellular location and the defective functional activity of these proteins.[210] CHO cells were also used to demonstrate that chemical chaperones could increase the delivery of misfolded AQP2 protein to the cell surface, a potentially important observation in terms of managing autosomal CNDI.[220,221]

Expression of AQP2 in Polarized Epithelial Cells

Transfected Cells Expressing Exogenous AQP2

Early observations revealed that renal epithelial cell lines that are commonly used for cell biological studies (LLC-PK1, MDCK, OMCD, IMCD, OK) showed little or no endogenous expression of AQP2. Cultures of cells from the inner medullary collecting duct (IMCD) showed a progressive loss of AQP2 mRNA expression over the first 4 days of culture.[222] Transcription of the AQP2 gene appears to be rapidly inactivated in these cells cultures and was shown, at least in part, to be mediated by repressors present in its 5'-flanking region.[222] Several laboratories, therefore, developed stably transfected cells and used them to dissect intracellular processes related to AQP2 trafficking and V2R signaling. cAMP-dependent translocation of AQP2 was first reconstituted in LLC-PK1 cells (Fig. 8–7),[223] and subsequently in transfected rabbit collecting duct epithelial cells,[224] MDCK cells,[225] and primary cultures of inner medullary collecting duct cells.[226] Two lines of stably transfected LLC-PK1 and MDCK renal epithelial cells were produced that retained constitutive (AQP1) and vasopressin-regulated (AQP2) membrane localization of these aquaporins.[204,223,225,227] AQP1-transfected LLC-PK1 and MDCK cells showed constitutive plasma membrane expression of the protein, whereas AQP2-transfected LLC-PK1 cells had a baseline intracellular vesicular labeling that relocated to the plasma membrane only after increasing cytosolic cAMP levels with forskolin or vasopressin stimulation (see Fig. 8–7). Interestingly, transfected MDCK cells also show constitutive membrane AQP2 expression under baseline conditions unless they are pre-treated with indomethacin, which is presumed to reduce cAMP levels and induce AQP2 internalization in these cells.[225] After indomethacin treatment, AQP2 can then be returned to the cell surface by vasopressin/forskolin exposure of the cells. Functional studies showed that AQP1-transfected cells had a high constitutive water permeability, whereas AQP2- transfected cells acquired the same degree of permeability only after stimulation.[223] Similar data were obtained using transformed rabbit collecting duct epithelial cells.[224]

Tissue slices[228,229] and isolated papillary collecting ducts[230] have also been used to dissect vasopressin and forskolin-stimulated AQP2 trafficking events. These systems more closely mimic the in vivo situation than pure cell culture models, and may be very useful to elucidate many of the signaling cascades that are involved in regulating AQP2 trafficking or that are involved in modulating the vasopressin response.

Cells Expressing Endogenous AQP2

Endogenous expression of AQP2 has been reported in a collecting duct cell line known as mpkCCD(cl4).[231,232] These cells have the advantage that factors regulating AQP2 expression at the transcriptional levels can be addressed because endogenous flanking regions that contain promoter, repressor, and enhancer elements are presumably present. The involvement of the tonicity-responsive enhancer binding protein (TonEBP) in regulating AQP2 gene transcription in response to hypertonicity was demonstrated using mpkCCD(cl4) cells.[233] These cells have not yet been used extensively to address questions related to VP-induced AQP2 trafficking, however.

Expression of Multiple Basolateral Aquaporins (AQP2, AQP3, and/or AQP4) in Principal Cells

Although VP regulates collecting duct water permeability by modulating the amount of AQP2 in the apical plasma membrane of principal cells, AQP2 is also localized in the basolateral plasma membrane of these cells in some regions of the collecting duct. The bipolar expression of AQP2 is most evident in the inner medulla (see Fig. 8–6F) and the cortical connecting segment.[195,198,234,235] In the inner medulla, basolateral expression of AQP2 is increased by VP and oxytocin.[194,196]

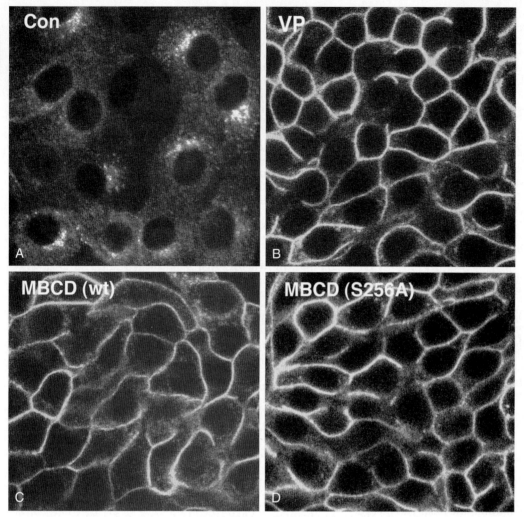

FIGURE 8–7 Immunofluorescence staining for AQP2 in LLC-PK1 cells expressing wild-type AQP2 **(A–C)** or a mutant in which the S256 residue has been replaced by alanine (S256A) **(D)**. Under baseline conditions, both wild-type **(A)** and the S256A mutation (not shown) are mainly located on intracellular vesicles, with very little plasma membrane staining. After vasopressin (VP) treatment, the wild-type AQP2 relocates to the plasma membrane **(B)**, whereas the S256A mutation remains on intracellular vesicles (not shown). However, when endocytosis is inhibited in these cells by application of the cholesterol-depleting drug methyl-β-cyclodextrin (MBCD), both wild-type and S256A AQP2 accumulate at the cell surface **(C, D)**. This result shows that both wt AQP2 and S256A AQP2 are constitutively recycling between intracellular vesicles and the plasma membrane, and that inhibiting endocytosis (using MBCD) is sufficient to cause membrane accumulation, even in the absence of S256 phosphorylation of AQP2.

Intriguingly, the basolateral membrane of principal cells contains two other aquaporins—AQP3 and AQP4—although their relative abundance varies in different regions of the collecting duct, with AQP3 expression being predominant in the cortex and decreasing toward the inner medulla, with the reverse pattern for AQP4, which is most abundant in the inner medulla.[164,183] No AQP4 expression could be detected in the connecting segment.[236] In view of this apparent redundancy of basolateral aquaporin expression in some principal cells, the physiological role of basolateral AQP2 is unclear. Whether all three of these aquaporins are ever co-expressed in the same basolateral membrane has not been definitively examined, but clearly the following AQP pairs can be present in the basolateral membrane of the same principal cell: AQP2/AQP3 (connecting segments), AQP2/AQP4 (inner medulla), and AQP3/AQP4 (outer medulla). Although AQP2 and AQP3 have similar water permeabilities, AQP3 may also function as a solute channel under normal circumstances. However, AQP3 knockout mice have a severe concentrating defect, indicating an important role in the urinary concentrating mechanism.[237] In addition, AQP3 message and protein are both up-regulated by VP,[164] although trafficking to the membrane appears not to be acutely regulated by VP.

AQP4 on the other hand has a much greater single channel water permeability than AQP2 and AQP3; this may be due to the arrangement of the M23 AQP4 variant into tightly packed OAPs within the plasma membrane.[189] Interestingly, the involvement of AQP4 in urine concentration is less clear cut than that of AQP2 and AQP3. First, AQP4 knockout mice have only a minor concentrating defect that becomes detectable only after water deprivation,[238] although the water permeability of isolated collecting ducts from these animals is reduced to about 25% of that measured in wild-type tubules.[239] Second, kangaroo rats that can concentrate their urine to more than 5000 mOsm/kg do not express AQP4 in any cell type in their kidneys, indicating that AQP4 is not necessary for the extreme concentrating ability of these rodents.[240] Indeed, the complete absence of AQP4 from kangaroo rat kidneys suggests that expression of this channel might even be detrimental in some way to maximal urinary concentration.

As mentioned earlier, the amount of AQP2 at the basolateral membrane of principal cells in some collecting duct regions appears to be regulated. Both VP and oxytocin have been reported to cause basolateral AQP2 insertion in the inner medullary collecting duct,[194,195] and one report has shown that basolateral membrane water permeability in this region is increased after VP treatment in a mercurial-sensitive manner, ruling out the contribution of the mercurial-insensitive AQP4 to this process.[192] Recent data indicate that interstitial osmolality may be at least partially responsible for the basolateral targeting of AQP2 in the inner medulla and in MDCK cells.[196] However, hypertonicity cannot be the only factor involved in this change in polarity of AQP2 insertion because cortical connecting segments in an isotonic environment also show an abundant basolateral insertion of AQP2.[234,235] Furthermore, a recent study found basolateral AQP2 in IMCD cells in vasopressin-deficient Brattleboro rats in vivo.[234] The physiological role of basolateral AQP2 and the signaling events that lead to basolateral delivery are the subject of ongoing research in several laboratories.

The apical to basolateral distribution of AQP2 in connecting segments and cortical collecting ducts can also be modified by aldosterone in rats with two types of diabetes insipidus. In lithium-treated rats, aldosterone treatment increases urine output even more than lithium alone, and causes a significant redistribution of AQP2 to the basolateral plasma membrane in these cortical segments.[241] A similar effect is seen in aldosterone treated Brattleboro rats that lack endogenous vasopressin. Although the mechanism for this profound effect on AQP2 polarity is unknown, it is clearly independent of VP action. However, in humans, a frameshift mutation in AQP2 that results in basolateral targeting when expressed in polarized MDCK cells causes NDI.[242] This shows that, as expected, increased basolateral expression of AQP2 is not sufficient to increase transepithelial water permeability in the collecting duct. Whether basolateral AQP2 represents a mechanism to further increase the water permeability of the basolateral membrane under some conditions (despite the presence of other water channels in the same membrane), or whether it represents a transient step in an indirect apical targeting pathway for the AQP2 protein remains uncertain.

Apical and Basolateral Expression of AQP2 in Cell Cultures

In the original study describing trafficking of AQP2 expressed exogenously in transfected cells,[223] AQP2 was inserted into the basolateral plasma membrane of LLC-PK1 cells after vasopressin stimulation (see Fig. 8–7). In MDCK and rabbit collecting duct cells, a predominant apical insertion of exogenous AQP2 was described.[224,225] However, in primary cultures of IMCD cells, AQP2 is inserted both apically and basolaterally, but the predominant pattern in vitro reflects basolateral insertion.[31,226] This pattern is reminiscent of the basolateral expression of AQP2 that is seen in IMCD cells in the renal inner medulla in situ.[195] Thus, regulated trafficking of AQP2 occurs in a variety of transfected cell lines, and these unique targeting properties can be used to examine how polarity signals on proteins are interpreted by different cell types, and how they are translated by the intracellular transport machinery.

Studies on transfected epithelial cells have also shown that motifs in the sixth transmembrane domain of AQP2, including a dileucine motif, are involved in regulated trafficking of this water channel.[243] Domain-swap experiments however, show that while the cytoplasmic C-terminus of AQP2 is necessary for regulated insertion of AQP2, it is not sufficient, implying that other domains of the protein play a role in this process.[244] One study has identified an AQP2 mutation causing NDI in humans that adds a C-terminal extension containing both a tyrosine- and a leucine-based basolateral targeting motif to the AQP2 protein.[242] Presumably, if active in humans, this would lead to basolateral insertion of AQP2 in the collecting duct and would prevent the VP-induced increase in epithelial permeability.

INTRACELLULAR PATHWAYS OF AQP2 TRAFFICKING

As discussed earlier, early studies using model amphibian epithelia led to the shuttle hypothesis of water channel trafficking, according to which water channels were stored in intracellular vesicles before insertion into the apical plasma membrane following VP stimulation of target cells. Thus, the water channels were said to be part of a "regulated" membrane recycling pathway. More recent data have shown that

in fact, AQP2 is recycled continually between intracellular vesicles and the cell surface. This section will describe the known pathways that AQP2 passes through during its recycling itinerary. The potential mechanisms by which this pathway is regulated will be discussed in a later section.

Role of Clathrin-Coated Pits in Water Channel Recycling

Clathrin-coated pits concentrate and internalize selected populations of many plasma membrane proteins, including receptors (with or without their cognate ligands), transporters, and channels. The role of clathrin-coated pits in V2R internalization has been shown previously.[47,63] Based on morphological studies on collecting duct principal cells in situ, it was proposed that coated pits were also involved in the endocytotic step of water channel recycling long before aquaporins were identified.[245] IMP clusters believed to represent water channels were shown to correspond to sites of clathrin-coated pit formation at the cell surface.[245] Studies using horseradish peroxidase to follow apical membrane endocytosis during vasopressin stimulation of principal cells supported a role of clathrin-mediated endocytosis in water channel retrieval from the plasma membrane, and the rate of endocytosis was increased by VP washout to terminate the permeability response.[246,247]

These early studies were confirmed by direct visualization of AQP2 in clathrin-coated pits by immunogold electron microscopy (Fig. 8–8).[250] A relationship between IMP clusters first described more than two decades earlier[174,175] and AQP2 endocytosis was shown using a technique known as fracture-labeling. In a transfected cell culture system (LLC-PK1 cells), AQP2 is concentrated in these coated-pit related IMP clusters after stimulation of the cells with forskolin followed by a 10-minute washout period (see Fig. 8–8).[250] Thus, IMP clusters in principal cells are markers of endocytotic, but probably not exocytotic events, and may result from a concentration of AQP2 protein into clathrin-coated membrane domains during the internalization phase of the vasopressin-induced recycling process. Whether exocytosis of AQP2 from intracellular stores results in the immediate formation of detectable membrane IMP clusters (representing patches of AQP2) at the sites of vesicle fusion with the plasma membrane remains uncertain.

Finally, when clathrin-mediated endocytosis was inhibited by the expression of a dominant negative form of the protein dynamin in LLC-PK1 cells, AQP2 accumulated on the plasma membrane and was depleted from cytoplasmic vesicles.[250] Dynamin is a GTPase that is involved in the formation and pinching off of clathrin-coated pits to form clathrin-coated vesicles.[248,249] The dominant negative form has a single point mutation K44A that renders the protein GTPase-deficient, and arrests clathrin-mediated endocytosis.

AQP2 Localization in Intracellular Compartments during Recycling

Observations on the complex recycling pathways followed by AQP2 have been greatly facilitated by studies on transfected cells. Recycling of the AQP2 protein was directly demonstrated in cycloheximide-treated, AQP2-transfected LLC-PK1 cells, in which several rounds of exo- and endocytosis of AQP2 could be followed despite the complete inhibition of de novo AQP2 synthesis.[204] Several studies have been carried out to identify the intracellular compartments in which AQP2 resides during this recycling process. After internalization from the plasma membrane via clathrin-coated pits, AQP2 enters an early endosomal compartment that can be identified using antibodies against EEA1 (early endosomal antigen 1).[252]

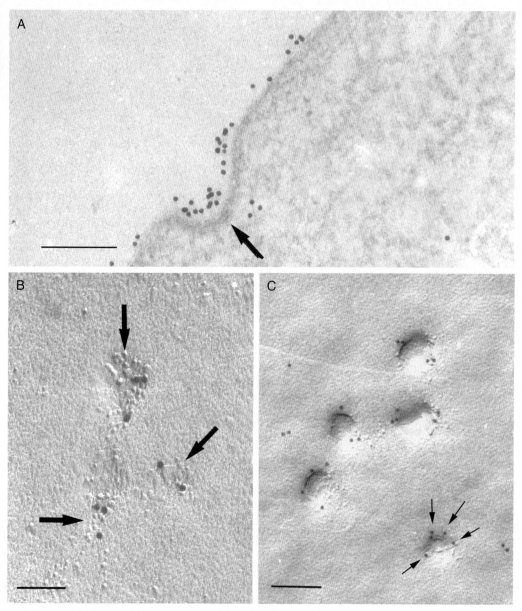

FIGURE 8–8 Aquaporin 2 is internalized by clathrin-coated pits. **A,** immunogold labeling of AQP2 in clathrin-coated pit (arrow) at the apical plasma membrane of collecting duct principal cells. An antibody against an external epitope of AQP2 was used. Panels B and C show label-fracture images of LLC-PK1 cells expressing AQP2. Immunogold label for AQP2 is located in IMP clusters on the membrane (**B,** arrows) and is associated with membrane invaginations that resemble clathrin-coated pits (**C,** arrows). Bars = 0.25 μm.

However, in collecting duct principal cells in situ, the endosomes that are formed during water channel recycling are highly specialized because they are non-acidic, and lack important functional subunits of the vacuolar H⁺ATPase.[144,145] It has been reported that after forskolin washout from transfected MDCK cells, AQP2 enters an apical storage compartment that is sensitive to wortmannin and LY294002, which are phosphatidylinositol 3-kinase inhibitors. In the same cells, AQP2 is localized in a subapical recycling compartment that is distinct from organelles such as the Golgi, the TGN (trans-Golgi network), and lysosomes.[252] Furthermore, this AQP2 compartment does not contain transferrin receptor, and it is distinct from vesicles that contain Glut4 (another recycling protein) in adipocytes that co-express AQP2 and Glut4.[253] Stimulation of these coexpressing cells with forskolin results in the membrane accumulation of AQP2, but not of Glut4. Similarly, stimulation of cells with insulin causes membrane accumulation of Glut4 but not AQP2.[253] Together, these data suggest that prior to insertion into the cell surface, AQP2—like Glut4 in smooth muscle cells and adipocytes—is located in specialized vesicles that are not

easily identified using markers of known intracellular compartments, although in the adipocyte system AQP2 showed significant overlap with the distribution of vesicle associated membrane protein (VAMP) 2. Whether these vesicles represent a novel organelle that appears in cells transfected with AQP2, or whether AQP2 usurps an already existing pathway and modifies it based on intrinsic signals within the AQP2 sequence, remains unclear. It is likely that as newly synthesized AQP2 is loaded into transporting vesicles as it exits the TGN, the fate of the vesicles is indeed determined by signals on the AQP2 protein itself that will be discussed in more detail later.

However, experiments in which the recycling of AQP2 has been artificially interrupted show that in transfected LLC-PK1 cells, AQP2 can be concentrated in a clathrin-positive, Golgi-associated compartment by lowering the incubation temperature of the cells to 20°C, or by incubating cells with bafilomycin, an inhibitor of the vacuolar H⁺ATPase.[254] This accumulation occurs even in the presence of cycloheximide, an inhibitor of protein synthesis, indicating that recycling AQP2 is also accumulating in this juxta-nuclear compartment. It is known that the 20°C block prevents exit of proteins from the trans Golgi,[255] and that clathrin-coated vesicles are enriched in this cellular compartment.[256] However, some portions of the so-called "recycling endosome", which is located in a similar juxtanuclear region of the cells, also have clathrin-coated domains.[257] Therefore, the AQP2 could be recycling either via the trans Golgi, via a specialized clathrin-coated recycling endosome, or both. Indeed recycling AQP2 is at least partially colocalized with internalized transferrin in recycling endosomes in LLC-PK1 cells[258] and is partially colocalized with rab11, a marker of the recycling endosomal compartment, in subapical vesicles.[259]

AQP2 is a Constitutively Recycling Membrane Protein

Whereas AQP2 was originally believed to be present in subapical vesicles awaiting a signal (VP stimulation) to move to the cell surface, it is now clear that AQP2 in fact recycles continually between intracellular vesicles and the cell surface, both in transfected cells in culture and in principal cells in situ. In this respect, AQP2 resembles the glucose transporter, Glut4, which also recycles constitutively, but whose plasma membrane accumulation is increased by insulin.[260-262] This provides the opportunity to modulate the plasma membrane content of AQP2 by increasing the rate of exocytosis, decreasing endocytosis, or both. Indeed such a dual action of VP was predicted by Knepper and Nielsen[263] by comparing mathematical models of VP-induced permeability changes to actual experimental data from isolated perfused collecting ducts.

Data showing that AQP2 recycles constitutively have been obtained by blocking the AQP2 recycling pathway either in an intracellular perinuclear compartment identified as the TGN as discussed earlier,[254] or at the cell surface.[250,264] When cells are infected with a dynamin K44A virus, clathrin-mediated endocytosis is arrested, and in parallel, AQP2 accumulates at the plasma membrane in a VP-independent manner.[250] This process takes several hours as the mutant dynamin is expressed in cultured cells and the endogenous wild-type dynamin is overwhelmed. A more rapid means of preventing clathrin-mediated endocytosis is to treat cells with the cholesterol-depleting drug, methyl-β-cyclodextrin.[265,266] When this was done in LLC-PK1 cells expressing AQP2, the water channel accumulated at the plasma membrane in a matter of minutes, indicating that it is recycling rapidly through the plasma membrane and that inhibition of endocytosis is sufficient to cause membrane accumulation of AQP2 (Fig. 8-7C).[264] Importantly, this drug also causes a significant accumulation of AQP2 in the apical membrane of collecting duct principal cells in situ (Fig. 8-6C),[267] confirming the relevance of the cell culture studies to the intact organ. This observation raises the exciting possibility that inhibition of endocytosis is a potential pathway by which AQP2 can be accumulated at the cell surface of collecting duct principal cells in patients with X-linked NDI. How recent insights into AQP2 trafficking and signaling might provide novel strategies to alleviate the symptoms of NDI will be discussed in more detail later.

▌ REGULATION OF AQP2 TRAFFICKING

Our understanding of AQP2 recycling continues to evolve in parallel with new discoveries related to the targeting and trafficking of membrane proteins in general. These include the discovery of alternative signaling pathways for AQP2 trafficking in addition to the "conventional" cAMP pathway, the role of phosphorylation by various kinases, the involvement of the actin cytoskeleton, and the gradual discovery of accessory interacting proteins. However, as will be pointed out, several fundamental questions related to the cell biology of VP action remain unanswered, the most important of which is precisely how phosphorylation of AQP2 on residue S256 induces membrane accumulation of this water channel.

Role of Phosphorylation in AQP2 Trafficking

The AQP2 sequence contains several putative phosphorylation sites for kinases including protein kinase A (PKA) and protein kinase G (PKG), protein kinase C (PKC), Golgi casein kinase, and casein kinase II (see Fig. 8-5). A recent study using phosphoproteomics on inner medullary protein samples identified an additional site at S261 on AQP2 that may be a MAP kinase site.[268] Most work has focused on the role of PKA-induced phosphorylation of S256 in the vasopressin-induced signaling cascade because this site appears to be critical to the vasopressin-induced membrane accumulation of AQP2.[269,270] Upon VP binding to the V2R, activation of protein kinase A by increased levels of cytosolic cAMP leads to phosphorylation of S256 on the cytoplasmic C-terminus (see Fig. 8-1). This S256 residue is required for a cAMP-induced increase in water permeability of oocytes expressing AQP2.[271]

Phosphorylation could in theory modulate the water permeability of AQP2 already in the plasma membrane, or it could be involved in the regulated trafficking of vesicles containing AQP2 and insertion of AQP2 into the plasma membrane. The permeability of AQP4[190,191] and of several plant water channels is regulated by phosphorylation,[272,273] and some structural features of the phosphorylation-dependent gating mechanism were recently elucidated for SoPIP2, a spinach plasma membrane aquaporin.[274] In addition, the ion channel properties of AQP0 (MIP26) are modulated by a calcium/calmodulin-mediated event.[275] Some reports have suggested that PKA-induced phosphorylation may increase the permeability of AQP1 to cations,[276-278] but this result is controversial and has not been repeated in other laboratories.[279] However, evidence against a role of phosphorylation in gating AQP2 was obtained by Lande and colleagues[280] who showed that the water permeability of isolated kidney papillary vesicles containing AQP2 was not modified significantly by PKA or phosphatase treatment of the AQP2-containing vesicles. However, a more direct assessment of the effect of phosphorylation on AQP2 permeability in systems overexpressing AQP2 or using purified protein in liposomes has not been performed to date.

In contrast, regulation of membrane permeability by AQP2 trafficking has been established in a variety of experimental systems. Using a point mutation of AQP2, serine 256 to alanine (S256A) expressed in LLC-PK1 cells, it was clearly shown that phosphorylation of the S256 residue by PKA is required for the VP-induced accumulation of AQP2 in the plasma membrane.[269,270] VP also stimulates S256 phosphorylation of native AQP2 in collecting duct principal cells in situ.[281,282] The in vivo importance of S256 phosphorylation was shown by the identification of a mutant AQP2 in a patient with NDI that destroys the consensus PKA phosphorylation site. This S254L mutation, when expressed in epithelial cells, is retained in intracellular vesicles and is not phosphorylated upon forskolin addition.[283] Furthermore, PKA and several protein kinase A anchoring proteins (AKAPs) are enriched in AQP2-immunopurified vesicles from IMCD cells. Inhibition of forskolin-induced AQP2 translocation with a peptide that prevents PKA-AKAP interaction demonstrated that, besides its enzymatic activity, tethering of PKA to subcellular compartments is essential for AQP2 translocation.[284,285] Of particular interest and importance is the finding that the rat AKAP Ht31 directly interacts with the actin modifying GTPase RhoA, which plays a crucial role in modulating AQP2 trafficking (see later). Most recently, an AKAP18 splice variant—AKAP18δ—was shown to colocalize with AQP2 in IMCD cells. Elevation of cAMP caused the dissociation of AKAP18δ and PKA suggesting a role for this novel AKAP in the VP response.[286]

However, more recent data have shown that phosphorylation of AQP2 at S256 is not necessary for its exocytotic insertion into the plasma membrane. As indicated earlier, AQP2 follows a constitutive recycling pathway and the S256A mutant, from which the PKA phosphorylation site is absent, also accumulates on the plasma membrane upon inhibition of endocytosis with either K44A dynamin or methyl-β-cyclodextrin (Fig. 8–7D).[264] Thus, while VP-induced *accumulation* of AQP2 at the cell surface requires S256 phosphorylation, exocytotic *insertion* of AQP2 into the plasma membrane is independent of this phosphorylation event.

However, dephosphorylation of AQP2 at S256 is not necessary for its internalization. Prostaglandin E2 stimulates removal of AQP2 from the surface of principal cells when added after AVP treatment, but does not alter the phosphorylated state of AQP2.[282] In support of this, it was shown in cell cultures that PKC-mediated endocytosis of AQP2 is also independent of the phosphorylation state of this water channel and in addition, the AQP2 mutant S256D—which mimics the phosphorylated state of the channel—is constitutively expressed mainly at the cell surface in overexpressing cells.[287] However, internalization of S256D AQP2 can be induced by treating cells with either PGE2 or dopamine, but only after pre-exposing the cells to forskolin.[288] The authors concluded that PGE2 and dopamine induce internalization of AQP2 independently of AQP2 dephosphorylation, and that preceding activation of cAMP production is necessary for PGE2 and dopamine to cause AQP2 internalization. These data imply that phosphorylation of another intracellular target or targets (presumably by forskolin-stimulated elevation of cAMP) is necessary for AQP2 endocytosis to occur, but these proteins remain to be identified.

Preventing dephosphorylation of AQP2 with the phosphatase inhibitor okadaic acid also has the expected effect of increasing cell surface accumulation of AQP2 in cultured cells but surprisingly, the same effect of okadaic acid was observed in the presence of the PKA inhibitor H-89. The authors concluded that okadaic acid stimulates the membrane translocation of AQP2 in a phosphorylation-independent manner.[289] The transduction mechanism responsible for this effect remains to be determined, but these data support the idea that AQP2 can accumulate on the plasma membrane in an S256 phosphorylation-independent manner.

The mechanism by which phosphorylation of AQP2 on residue S256 affects the steady-state redistribution of AQP2 is unknown. No other phosphorylation sites on AQP2 have yet been shown to be involved in its VP-induced membrane accumulation, although one report has suggested that a Golgi casein kinase mediated phosphorylation of S256 is involved in the passage of AQP2 through the Golgi apparatus in its biosynthetic pathway.[290] One possibility is that phosphorylation results in a modified interaction of vesicles with the cytoskeleton, via microtubule or microtubule motors (or both). These proteins are a driving force for intracellular vesicle movement, and must be brought into play in order for vesicles to be transported through the cytosol in the direction of the plasma membrane. Alternatively, phosphorylation could inhibit the endocytotic step of AQP2 recycling, leading to accumulation at the cell surface, although results

discussed earlier show that phosphorylated AQP2 can still be internalized.

Actin, Actin-Associated Proteins, and AQP2 Trafficking

The literature on the role of actin in water channel trafficking dates back over three decades, but its role in this process still remains unclear. Actin has been shown to associate directly with AQP2,[291,292] implying a functional relationship that remains to be clearly demonstrated. VP exposure was reported to depolymerize actin in the toad bladder and collecting duct principal cells,[169,293,294] allowing water channel containing vesicles to break through the "actin barrier" and fuse with the plasma membrane. However, actin depolymerization resulting from the inactivation of RhoA, a GTPase that regulates the actin cytoskeleton, increases the membrane accumulation of AQP2 and membrane water permeability in cultured cells even in the absence of VP.[295,296] Cytochalasins, which disrupt actin filaments, markedly inhibit the vasopressin response in target epithelia,[297–300] but such treatment increases AQP2 membrane accumulation in cultured renal epithelial cells in some studies.[295,296] Although actin depolymerization was originally believed to simply remove a physical barrier that prevented vesicles fusion with the plasma membrane, it is now clear that the role of actin in vesicle trafficking and vesicle endo- and exocytosis is much more complex.

Role of Actin Polymerization in AQP2 Trafficking

The potential role of actin in AQP2 membrane insertion was directly examined in transfected CDB cells in culture. Exposure of these cells to Clostridium toxin B, which inhibits RhoGTPases that are involved in regulating the actin cytoskeleton,[301] caused actin depolymerization and an accumulation of AQP2 in the plasma membrane.[296] A similar AQP2 translocation was seen in cells treated with the downstream Rho kinase inhibitor, Y-27632.[295] This occurred in the absence of any detectable elevation of intracellular cAMP. Conversely, expression of constitutively active RhoA in these cells induced stress fiber formation, indicating actin polymerization, and inhibited the normal AQP2 translocation response to forskolin. Although these data provide strong evidence for a major regulatory role of the actin cytoskeleton in the vasopressin-induced trafficking of AQP2 from intracellular vesicles to the cell surface, it remains unclear whether the net accumulation of AQP2 under these conditions is due to increased exocytosis or decreased endocytosis. There is a considerable body of evidence showing that actin depolymerization inhibits endocytosis, although whether apical and/or basolateral endocytosis is most affected remains a matter of debate.[302–304] Interestingly, actin depolymerization was sufficient to provoke membrane accumulation of AQP2 in either the apical or the basolateral plasma membrane, depending on the transfected cell type that was examined.[295,296] In contrast to the data discussed earlier, showing membrane accumulation of AQP2 after actin depolymerization, a more recent study using transfected MDCK cells reported that AQP2 was concentrated in an EEA1-positive early endosomal compartment upon actin filament disruption by either cytochalasin D or latrunculin.[259] These contrasting effects may reflect the use of different model systems, and the physiological role played by actin on AQP2 trafficking in renal principal cells *in situ* remains to be determined.

Identification of Actin-Associated Proteins Potentially Involved in AQP2 Trafficking

Many studies in other systems have implicated actin and associated proteins such as the myosins, as well as microtubules (see later), in sequential transport steps of vesicle trafficking.[305,306] Several actin-associated proteins appear to be involved in AQP2 trafficking, and in some cases have been localized on or close to vesicles that contain AQP2 by immunocytochemistry or immuno-isolation of vesicles coupled to mass spectrometry/proteomic analysis.[307] Immunogold localization showed that myosin I, an actin-associated motor protein is associated with AQP2 containing vesicles.[308] Various myosin isoforms including myosin 1C, non-muscle myosins IIA and IIB, myosin VI, and myosin IXB were associated with vesicles prepared for the proteomic analysis by immunoprecipitation with AQP2 antibodies, although the profile of identified proteins indicates that virtually all compartments in the secretory and recycling pathways were represented in the immunoprecipitated material.[307] Myosin light chain kinase, the myosin regulatory light chain (MLC), and the IIA and IIB isoforms of the non-muscle myosin heavy were also found in rat IMCD cells and were implicated in a calcium/calmodulin regulated pathway leading to AQP2 membrane accumulation.[309] These data supported previous work from the same group that Ca^{2+} release from ryanodine-sensitive stores plays an essential role in vasopressin-mediated aquaporin-2 trafficking via a calmodulin-dependent mechanism.[31] A role of Epac (exchange protein directly activated by cAMP) in VP-induced calcium mobilization and AQP2 exocytosis in perfused collecting ducts has also been shown.[310] However, the role of calcium in the vasopressin response was questioned by another group who provided capacitance data in support of a cAMP-dependent, but calcium-independent exocytotic process after VP stimulation.[311]

In another study, AQP2-interacting proteins were identified by mass spectrometry in a complex containing ionized calcium binding adapter molecule 2, myosin regulatory light chain smooth muscle isoforms 2-A and 2-B, alpha-tropomyosin 5b, annexin A2 and A6, scinderin, gelsolin, alpha-actinin 4, alpha-II spectrin, and myosin heavy chain nonmuscle type A.[312] The proteins were suggested to comprise a multiprotein motor complex involved in AQP2 trafficking. Interestingly, the gelsolin-like protein adseverin is much more highly expressed in collecting duct principal cells than gelsolin (which is abundant in intercalated cells), indicating that it might be a physiologically important player in calcium-activated actin remodeling in these cells.[313] In addition to myosins, moesin, a member of the ERM (ezrin-radixin-moesin) family of scaffolding proteins, has also been implicated in the apical trafficking process.[314] The GTPase Rap1 and the signal-induced proliferation-associated gene-1 (SPA-1) may also have a role in regulating AQP2 trafficking.[315] Activation of Rap1 was found to inhibit AQP2 plasma membrane targeting, possibly by increasing actin polymerization. This effect is most likely mediated by SPA-1.

Based on these studies, it is clear that actin and its complex array of regulatory proteins play critical roles in the membrane accumulation and recycling of AQP2. However, the precise steps in the pathway, and how these processes are regulated by vasopressin have not been established in any detail, other than to show that disruption of the cytoskeleton has end results compatible with a perturbation of the physiologically regulated process. How AQP2 interaction with the cytoskeleton is affected by phosphorylation, for example, is completely unknown.

Microtubules and AQP2 Trafficking

Many studies have shown that vesicles can move along microtubules and that such transport may be driven by microtubule mechanoenzymes or motors.[316–318] It is, therefore, not surprising that microtubule-depolymerizing agents such as colchicine and nocodazole have long been known to partially inhibit the VP-induced water permeability increase in target epithelia.[298–300,319–322] Colchicine treatment disrupts the apical localization of AQP2 in rat kidney principal cells, and causes it to be scattered on vesicles throughout the cytoplasm.[197] Furthermore, cold treatment, which depolymerizes microtubules, also inhibits the vasopressin response, indicating that caution must be exercised in the interpretation of data from cell or tissue preparations that involve a cold incubation step as part of the experimental procedure.[229] However, relatively little insight is available concerning the mechanism(s) by which AQP2-containing vesicles interact with the microtubule network in a regulated manner.

As is the case for the actin cytoskeleton, microtubules have an array of accessory proteins that are necessary for their biological activity. Two large protein families are of particular importance for microtubule-based vesicle movement—these are ATPases known as motor proteins, the dyneins,[323] and the kinesins.[324] The ones with minus end-directed motors such as dynein will transport vesicles toward the microtubule-organizing center whereas plus end-directed motors (such as kinesin) will transport vesicles in the opposite direction.[325–327] Both immunoblotting using immunoisolated vesicles and double-immunogold microscopy revealed that dynein and dynactin, a protein complex thought to link dynein to microtubules and vesicles, are associated with AQP2-bearing vesicles,[328] consistent with the view that microtubule motor proteins are involved in the vasopressin-regulated trafficking of AQP2-bearing vesicles. Furthermore, early studies had shown that an inhibitor of the dynein ATPase, erythro-9-[3-(2-hydroxynonyl)] adenine (EHNA), significantly reduced the effect of VP on water flow in the amphibian urinary bladder model system.[329] However, although treatment of transfected epithelial cells with nocodazole or colchicine to depolymerize microtubules resulted in a dispersion of AQP2 vesicles throughout the cytoplasm, forskolin-induced membrane accumulation was apparently not inhibited in these cells as judged by immunofluorescence staining.[259] Even in earlier work using toad bladder and collecting duct epithelia, the effect of VP on transepithelial water flow was only partially inhibited by microtubule disruption (about 65% in collecting ducts)[320]; this could be accounted for by a reduction in aquaporin delivery that might not be detectable without careful quantification. This also supports the idea that microtubules are involved in the long-range trafficking of vesicles toward the plasma membrane, but that the final step of approach and fusion involves a cooperative interaction between the microtubule and actin-based cytoskeleton.[306,326,330,331] Thus, in cells in which AQP2 containing vesicles are already quite close to the cell surface, AQP2 delivery to the membrane might be less dependent on intact microtubules. Furthermore, recent studies have shown that a protein complex exists at the plus ends of microtubules that is involved in cellular processes involving force generation at the interface between microtubule ends and the actin-rich cortical cytoskeleton.[332] Thus, the delivery of AQP2 vesicles to the sub-plasma membrane region probably involves both microtubules and the actin cytoskeleton, as well as their respective cohorts of accessory and motor proteins that are also involved in membrane trafficking processes in most cell types. Most of the specific protein–protein interactions, as well as their regulation, which render the process VP-sensitive in the case of AQP2 trafficking in the collecting duct remain to be elucidated.

SNARE Proteins and AQP2 Trafficking

As for most if not all membrane fusion events, it has been postulated that the docking step for vasopressin-induced exocytosis of AQP2-bearing vesicles could be mediated by vesicle targeting proteins.[333–336] The final delivery steps of vesicle tethering, docking, and fusion involve a complex series of protein–protein interactions that are combined under the name "the SNARE hypothesis".[337-341] This process requires a complex interaction between integral membrane proteins, the "SNAREs", present in the vesicle (v-SNAREs) and the target membrane (t-SNAREs) as has been suggested for docking of synaptic vesicles to the presynaptic plasma membrane in the central nervous system. In the synapse, this core complex consists of a v-SNARE (VAMP-2) and two t-SNAREs (syntaxin-1 and SNAP-25),[342] which form a 7S core complex that binds the ATPase NSF ("N-ethylmaleimide sensitive factor") via an intervening soluble NSF attachment protein (a-SNAP) to form a larger 20S complex. The formation of this complex is thought to be vital to the eventual vesicle fusion process. In the collecting duct principal cell, several proteins of the SNARE complex are associated with AQP2-containing vesicles or the apical plasma membrane (or both) of principal cell cells. These include VAMP-2,[336] the t-SNAREs syntaxin-4[334] and SNAP23,[343] and Hrs-2, an ATPase that may regulate exocytosis via interaction with SNAP25.[344] Other proteins that are involved in exocytotic processes in other cell types, such as rab3, rab5a, and a synaptobrevin II-like protein,[345] as well as cellubrevin[346] have also been identified in isolated vesicles containing AQP2. Several additional SNARE proteins, including syntaxin-7, syntaxin-12, syntaxin-13 were identified in a proteomic screen using vesicles immunoisolated with anti AQP2 antibodies.[307] However, as mentioned earlier, such isolated vesicles represent a mixed population that contain AQP2, but are not all in the exocytotic pathway. While a role of some of these proteins in exocytosis is likely by analogy with other secretory pathways, the functions of most of these SNARE proteins in AQP2 trafficking have not been formally examined. One exception is VAMP 2/synaptobrevin. Studies on collecting duct cells in culture have shown that treatment with tetanus toxin, which cleaves VAMP2, abolishes vasopressin-induced AQP2 translocation to the plasma membrane.[347] Interestingly, the related protein cellubrevin, also present in principal cells,[346] is involved in the exocytosis of the vacuolar ATPase in proton secreting cells of the epididymis,[348] which closely resemble intercalated cells of the collecting duct. Thus, SNARE proteins are part of a ubiquitous fusion machinery that is required for vesicle exocytosis. Whether they have any specific features in principal cells that allow them to be specifically regulated upon vasopressin action to modulate AQP2 insertion into the plasma membrane is unknown and requires additional studies.

cAMP-Independent Membrane Insertion of AQP2—Potential Strategies for Treating Nephrogenic Diabetes Insipidus

Important progress has been made in the past 3 or 4 years in our understanding of intracellular signaling or alternative trafficking pathways that bypass the V2R, cAMP, PKA cascade and that allow membrane accumulation of AQP2 even in the absence of a functional V2R. This is especially important for the generation of novel strategies to alleviate the symptoms of X-linked NDI, in which a mutated V2R is defective for a number of reasons, as described earlier. Principal cells in these patients still produce AQP2, but the defective V2R signaling mechanism means that it does not accumulate at the cell surface in order to increase urine concentration upon an increase in circulating VP levels. Recent developments in understanding the cell biology of AQP2 trafficking have provided some hope that AQP2 can in fact accumulate at the cell surface independently of VP signaling in collecting ducts of these patients. Two promising approaches will be discussed below.

Activation of a cGMP Signaling Pathway

In both cell cultures (Fig. 8–9) and principal cells in kidney slices in vitro (Fig. 8–10), several hormones and drugs that increase cGMP levels also induce AQP2 accumulation at the cell surface. These include sodium nitroprusside (a nitric oxide donor), L-arginine (which stimulates nitric oxide synthase), and atrial natriuretic peptide.[228] Similar data showing that ANP increases AQP2 surface expression in vivo after 90 minutes of infusion have also been reported.[349] This effect was paralleled by an increased apical expression of EnaC, and may represent a direct or a compensatory effect to increase sodium and water reabsorption, which would prevent volume depletion in response to prolonged ANP infusion. Importantly, it has also been shown that elevation of intracellular

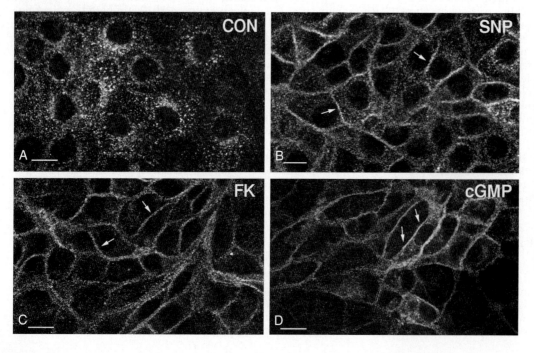

FIGURE 8–9 Effect of activation of the cGMP pathway on AQP2 membrane accumulation in cells and tissues. Immunofluorescence staining of an AQP2-c-myc construct expressed in LLC-PK1 epithelial cells. Under basal conditions, the AQP2 is located on intracellular, perinuclear vesicles (**A,** CON). After 10 minutes stimulation with the nitric oxide donor sodium nitroprusside (SNP) to increase cGMP (**B**), forskolin (FK) to increase cAMP (**C**), or with a permeant cGMP analog (**D**), AQP2 is relocated to the plasma membrane. Bar = 10 μm.

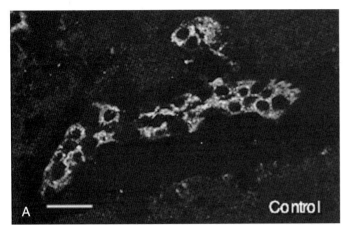

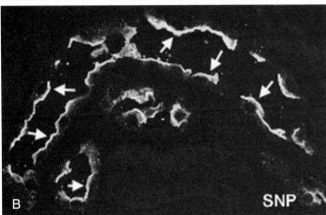

FIGURE 8–10 The nitric oxide donor, sodium nitroprusside (SNP), has a vasopressin-like effect on AQP2 distribution in principal cells. Rat kidney slices were incubated *in vitro* without (**A**) or with SNP for 15 minutes. A marked redistribution of AQP2 to the apical plasma membrane is induced by SNP treatment (**B**, arrows) compared to the scattered intracellular location of AQP2 under non-stimulated conditions (**A**). See Ref 284 for more details. Bar = 20 μm.

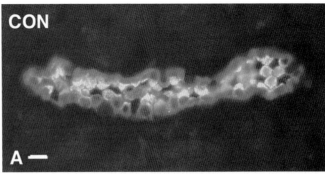

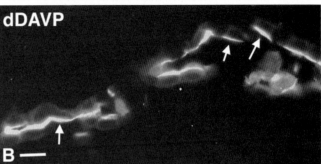

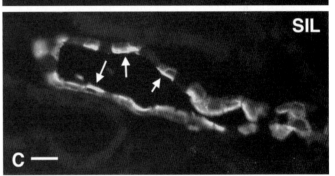

FIGURE 8–11 Viagra stimulates membrane accumulation of AQP2 in rat kidney inner stripe collecting duct principal cells after acute *in vivo* treatment of Brattleboro rats. Animals were injected with saline, dDAVP, or sildenafil through the jugular vein. Injection of saline was used as a control (**A**) and compared to 25 mg/kg dDAVP (**B**) and (**C**) 4 mg/kg of sildenafil. In controls (**A**), AQP2 is diffusely located throughout the subapical cytoplasm of principal cells. dDAVP (**B**) and sildenafil (**C**) both induce a marked redistribution of AQP2, which appears as a narrow, brightly stained band at the apical pole of principal cells, consistent with plasma membrane staining (arrows). Bar = 10 μm.

cGMP using the phosphodiesterase (PDE5) inhibitor sildenafil citrate (Viagra) also increases cell surface expression of AQP2 both in vitro and in vivo (Fig. 8–11).[350] Although no significant increase in urinary concentration was detectable in rats treated with Viagra for 90 minutes, possibly due to increased renal blood flow as a result of vasodilatation, this observation nevertheless provides a strategy to induce the VP-independent cell surface accumulation of AQP2. Adaptation of this approach to the human condition will require further dose-response studies, as well as the potential development of PDE5 inhibitors that may be more selective for tubular epithelial cells, or that may be delivered more specifically to these cells at an appropriate concentration to elicit the required response.

Inhibition of AQP2 Endocytosis

As discussed earlier, it is now evident that AQP2 recycles constitutively between the cell surface and intracellular vesicles. It has been shown using dominant negative dynamin (K44A dynamin) and methyl-β-cyclodextrin treatment that AQP2 accumulation at the cell surface can be achieved simply by blocking endocytosis[250,264] (Figs. 8–6C, D and 8–7C, D). It has also been shown that endocytosis of AQP2 is stimulated by PGE2 (or dopamine) under some conditions[288] and that activation of PKC by PMA treatment of cells also stimulates AQP2 endocytosis, independently of its S256 phosphorylation state.[287] Thus, an attractive possibility is to modulate the endocytotic pathway in X-linked NDI as a means of

increasing its cell surface expression. Potential approaches are to decrease prostaglandin production using specific COX2 inhibitors, or to use a discovery approach to screen small chemical libraries for specific inhibitors of endocytosis that might be applied in vivo. For example, such a strategy was recently used to identify a small chemical named "dynasore" that is a specific inhibitor of the dynein GTPase, a protein critically involved in clathrin and caveolin-mediated endocytosis.[351]

LONG-TERM REGULATION OF WATER BALANCE (see also Chapter 13)

In addition to the acute regulation of collecting duct water permeability and body water balance, long-term regulation of water balance also plays an important role in the homeostatic response. De Wardener and colleagues showed several decades ago that prolonged dehydration is as potent as acute vasopressin treatment in increasing urinary concentration, while water loading efficiently reduced the urinary concentrating capacity.[352] Although multiple nephron segments are involved in these effects, Lankford and colleagues[353] demonstrated that part of this long-term adaptational regulation occurs in the kidney collecting duct; isolated perfused collecting tubules dissected from thirsted rats displayed much higher osmotic water permeability than tubules from water-loaded rats. It was later shown that AQP2 expression levels markedly increase in response to dehydration with an increased abundance of AQP2 in the apical plasma membrane.[195] Both vasopressin-dependent and -independent signal transduction pathways are involved in this process.[198,354–357] Thus, collecting duct water permeability and body water balance are regulated in a concerted fashion by short-term and long-term mechanisms, both critically involving AQP2.

Other studies have also documented that the expression of AQP3, a water channel that is abundantly expressed in the basolateral plasma membranes of collecting duct principal cells, is also regulated by vasopressin[358] suggesting that adaptational regulation of AQP3 may also be involved. DDAVP treatment of vasopressin-deficient Brattleboro rats results in a significant increase in AQP3 expression (in addition to AQP2), whereas AQP1 and AQP4 remain unchanged.[358] The key role of AQP3 in urinary concentration was demonstrated in transgenic mice lacking AQP3, which had a very severe urinary concentrating defect.[237] One complicating factor is that the expression of AQP2 was (surprisingly) markedly down-regulated in the cortex and outer medulla but not in the inner medulla of these knockout mice. The mechanisms responsible for this segment-specific down-regulation of AQP2 remain unknown. There are major differences in the different segments also with regard to the expression and localization of AQP2.[234] Because most water is reabsorbed in the proximal regions (i.e., the connecting tubule and cortical collecting duct) reduced expression of AQP2 in the renal cortex could contribute to the development of severe polyuria in AQP3 knockout mice. Because AQP4 is not present or only present at low levels in the CNT and CCD,[163,235,236] it would not be able to provide a compensatory exit route for basolateral water flow, which it may accomplish in the IMCD where AQP4 is abundantly expressed. Moreover AQP2 is normally present in the basolateral plasma membrane in the CNT (at least in the rat) and could therefore also potentially be involved in basolateral exit of water.[234,235] Thus, the absence of AQP4 and reduced levels of both apical and basolateral AQP2 may participate in the polyuria in AQP3-deficient mice. However, the precise role of basolateral AQP4 in urinary concentration is also unclear, because (1) AQP4 knockout mice have only a slight impairment of concentrating ability,[238] and (2) AQP4 is completely absent from kidneys of the desert rodent, which can concentrate urine up to 5000 to 6000 mOsm/kg.[240] Clearly, further studies are needed to provide a better understanding of the functional interactions among the different collecting duct aquaporins.

AQP2 and Nephrogenic Diabetes Insipidus

Hereditary nephrogenic diabetes insipidus, resulting in the inability to produce a concentrated urine, can be a result of mutations in the V2R, as described earlier, or can be a result of mutations in the AQP2 water channel. The latter form is characterized mainly as an autosomal recessive disorder,[359] although some mutations causing a dominant phenotype have been described.[95] In addition, there are several known forms of acquired NDI that also lead to a concentrating defect, and these are much more common than the hereditary forms of the disease. Many of these disorders have now been associated with alterations in the expression of AQP2 in principal cells. This section will summarize both hereditary and acquired NDI with emphasis on the role of AQP2 in these pathological conditions.

Autosomal Recessive Nephrogenic Diabetes Insipidus and Mutations in AQP2

Important data on the role of AQP2 in non X-linked NDI was obtained by examining the AQP2 molecule in human disease.[360] In the first patient studied[211] two distinct point mutations were found that resulted in a substitution of Cys for Arg[187], and Pro for Ser[216]. The R187C mutation occurs in a region of the third extracellular loop that is strongly conserved in members of the aquaporin family. The S216P mutation is located in the last transmembrane domain of AQP2. When mRNAs coding for these mutated proteins (which had the predicted size of 29 kD) were expressed in Xenopus oocytes, no increase in membrane osmotic water permeability was detected above that seen in water-injected controls.[211]

Mutations in the AQP2 gene that result in production of a full-length protein could have at least two consequences that would result in a loss of principal cell vasopressin-sensitivity; (1) the production of an AQP2 channel that is still vasopressin-sensitive, and is inserted into the plasma membrane after vasopressin action, but has lost the capacity to function as a water channel; (2) the production of a water channel that is still functional, but that is no longer targeted to the plasma membrane after vasopressin action. Oocyte expression studies have shown that the missense mutations R187C and S216P are impaired in their delivery to the cell surface.[361] The trapped form of these AQP2 mutants is a 32 kD high mannose form, indicating that the protein is blocked in the RER[361] in much the same way as the ΔF508 CFTR mutation is trapped inside the RER. Recent data indicate that some point mutations, including mutations in asparagine residue 123, significantly affect AQP2 water permeability.[362] The plasma membrane expression of this mutation was only slightly decreased from that shown by the wild-type protein in oocytes. Most recently, an additional AQP2 mutation has been found that causes the protein to be blocked at the level of the Golgi apparatus.[96]

An unusual dominant form of autosomal NDI due to a single nucleotide deletion (727ΔG) was ascribed to the ability of the mutated AQP2 monomers to form tetramers with normal protein in heterozygotes, and to block the delivery of the entire tetramer to the plasma membrane. The AQP2 tetramers were retained in late endosomes and lysosomes.[95] In addition, a frameshift mutation in the AQP2 molecule has been identified in some patients that causes basolateral targeting of AQP2 in epithelial cells in culture.[242] This mutation results in the addition of both a leucine- and a tyrosine-based basolateral targeting motif to the AQP2 COOH terminus.

Acquired Water Balance Disorders

Acquired forms of NDI are much more common than the hereditary forms described earlier, and they arise as a consequence of drug treatments, electrolyte disturbances, following urinary tract obstruction, as well as a variety of other causes that are listed in Table 8–1. There is considerable experimental support for the view that dysregulation of AQP2 plays a fundamental role in the development of polyuria associated with multiple acquired forms of nephrogenic diabetes insipidus,[357] and some quantitative data on AQP2 levels in various experimental conditions is summarized in Figure 8–12. Dysregulation of AQP3 often accompanies AQP2 down-regulation and may also participate in the development of

TABLE 8–1	Physiologic or Pathophysiologic Conditions Associated with Altered Abundance or Targeting (or Both) of Aquaporin-2	
Reduced Abundance of AQP2		**Increased Abundance of AQP2**

Reduced Abundance of AQP2

With Polyuria

Genetic defects
   Brattleboro rats (central DI)
   DI +/+ Severe mice (low cAMP)

   AQP2 mutants (human)
   V2 receptor variants (human)*
Acquired NDI (rat models)
   Lithium treatment
   Hypokalemia
   Hypercalcemia
   Postobstructive NDI
     Bilateral
     Unilateral
Low-protein diet (urinary concentrating defect
   without polyuria)
Water loading (compulsive water drinking)
Chronic renal failure (5/6 nephrectomy model)
Ischemia-induced acute renal failure
   (polyuric phase in rat model)
Cisplatin-induced acute renal failure
Calcium channel blocker (nifedipine) treatment
   (rat model)
Age-induced NDI

With Altered Urinary Concentration without Polyuria

Nephrotic syndrome models (rat models)
   PAN-induced
   Adriamycin-induced
Hepatic cirrhosis (CBL, compensated)
Ischemia-induced acute renal failure
   (oliguric phase in rat model)

Increased Abundance of AQP2

With Expansion of Extracellular Fluid Volume
   Vasopressin infusion (SIADH)
   Congestive heart failure
   Hepatic cirrhosis (CCI4-induced
     noncompensated)?
   Pregnancy

With Polyuria
   Osmotic diuresis (DM model in rat)

cAMP, cyclic adenosine monophosphate; CBL, common bile duct ligation; CCI4, carbon tetrachloride; DI, diabetes insipidus; DM, diabetes mellitus; NDI, nephrogenic diabetes insipidus; PAN, puromycin aminonucleoside; SIADH, syndrome of inappropriate secretion of antidiuretic hormone.
*Reduced V2-receptor density has a profound effect on AQP2 targeting and expression.

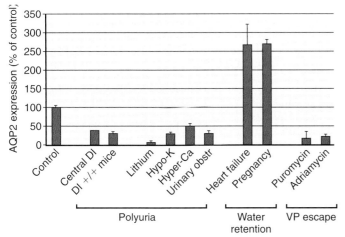

FIGURE 8–12 Quantitation of AQP2 levels in various conditions of fluid and electrolyte imbalance, including acquired NDI.

polyuria, but this has not been examined in as great a depth as the AQP2 contribution. Moreover, in some forms of acquired NDI, defects in the expression of important renal sodium transporters that participate in the urinary concentrating ability have also been encountered.

Lithium Treatment

One per thousand of the population is on lithium treatment in the Western world, and of these 20% to 30% develop clini-

cally significant polyuria. Rats treated with lithium for 1 month showed a dramatic decrease in AQP2 expression both in the inner medulla as well as in cortical and outer medullary parts of the collecting duct.[363,364] This down-regulation was paralleled by the progressive development of severe polyuria with a daily urinary output matching their own weight. The reduction in AQP2 expression was originally believed to result from an impairment in the production of cAMP in collecting duct principal cells, consistent with the presence of a cAMP-responsive element in the 5′ untranslated region of the AQP2 gene[365,366] and with the recent demonstration that mice with inherently low cAMP levels also have low expression of AQP2.[367] However, recent data have shown that the reduction in AQP2 levels is independent of adenylyl cyclase activity and cytosolic cAMP concentration.[368] Blood dDAVP levels were clamped in Brattleboro lacks lacking endogenous VP, and these animals showed no difference in dDAVP-induced cAMP generation between kidneys of rats with lithium-induced NDI and control rats. These data were supported by in vitro experiments using the collecting duct cell line mpkCCD(c14)—lithium did not alter VP-stimulated cAMP elevation in these cells, but it did decrease AQP2 mRNA levels.[368] Thus, the mechanism by which lithium reduces AQP2 expression remains unknown.

There was a very slow recovery in AQP2 expression and restoration of urinary concentration after cessation of lithium treatment[364] consistent with clinical findings. Kwon and colleagues[363] used two different treatment protocols—one leading to moderate lithium-induced NDI and one leading to severe lithium-induced NDI. In both protocols there was a dramatic down-regulation of AQP2 expression and a comparable down-regulation also of the basolateral AQP3 to less than 10% of control levels. Thus, down-regulation of AQP3 may also play a significant role. Interestingly, lithium treatment also caused a marked decrease in the fraction of principal cells in collecting duct in cortex and inner medulla[369] with a parallel increase in the population of intercalated cells. This architectural restructuring of the collecting duct, together with down-regulation of collecting duct aquaporins, is likely to be important in lithium-induced NDI. After a 4-week recovery period (cessation of lithium treatment), urine production, AQP2 protein levels, as well as the fraction of principal cells returned completely to control levels.[369] The mechanism underlying the change in principal/intercalated cell ratio after lithium treatment remains unclear, but other procedures such as chronic carbonic anhydrase inhibition by acetazolamide also increase the intercalated cell population in the medulla, implying a phenotypic plasticity of collecting duct epithelial cells.[370]

In addition to the large increase in urinary water excretion, lithium-induced NDI is also associated with significant sodium wasting.[371] The molecular explanation for this has been investigated by functional and biochemical analysis. Kwon and colleagues did not find changes in the expression levels of proximal tubule and thick ascending limb sodium transporters that could be ascribed any role in the sodium wasting or in the reduced urinary concentrating ability.[363] However, amiloride had a lower effect on sodium excretion in rats with lithium-induced NDI than in controls, suggesting that potential changes in the epithelial sodium channel ENaC function could be involved in the sodium wasting.[372] Immunoblotting and immunocytochemical analysis demonstrated a marked reduction in protein expression levels of alpha, beta, and gamma subunits in the cortical and outer medullary collecting duct principal cells in rats with lithium-induced NDI,[373] but there were no changes in proximal tubule and thick ascending limb sodium transporters, consistent with the data of Kwon and colleagues.[363] Thus reduction in ENaC subunits appears to represent the molecular background for the sodium wasting observed in lithium treatment.

Interestingly, treatment of rats with amiloride attenuates the severity of lithium-induced NDI in rats,[374] and in humans,[375,376] presumably due to an inhibition of lithium uptake into principal cells via the ENaC channel.

Hypokalemia and Hypercalcemia

Hypokalemia and hypercalcemia are both associated with significant vasopressin-resistant polyuria, and both were associated with a reduced expression of AQP2 levels and polyuria in rats.[377,378] The polyuria associated with these conditions is less severe than that seen in lithium-induced NDI and consistent with this, a less marked reduction in AQP2 was observed. In addition, expression of AQP2 is reduced in hypercalcemic rats contributing to the development of polyuria.[379] With regard to hypercalcemia, it was found that in addition to down-regulation of AQP2, the expression levels of AQP1 and AQP3 protein were also reduced.[379] Hypercalcemia is known to be associated with sodium absorption defects in the thick ascending limb, which would affect the counter current multiplication system. Wang and associates examined the protein expression levels of several key sodium transporters, including the vasopressin-regulated bumetanide-sensitive sodium potassium 2 chloride co-transporter BSC-1 or NKCC-2.[380] BSC-1 expression was markedly reduced both in cortex and in the inner stripe of the outer medulla (ISOM). Also ROMK protein expression was reduced. In contrast there was no reduction in NHE3 and Na, K-ATPase (alpha subunit) in ISOM. Thus reduced TAL BSC-1 and ROMK in hypercalcemia is likely to participate in the known defect in TAL sodium reabsorption and hence in the impaired urinary concentration together with reduced AQP2 and AQP3 expression in the collecting duct.

Ureteral Obstruction

Chronic urinary outflow obstruction with impaired ability of the kidney to concentrate urine is a common condition amongst elderly men, whereas acute obstruction can also cause a similar concentrating defect at all ages. Rat models in which one or both ureters were reversibly obstructed[381,382] showed that after 24 hours, AQP2 expression was markedly reduced, even before release of the obstruction. Following release of the obstruction, there was a vasopressin-resistant and persistent polyuria, and an increase in solute-free water clearance. Although urine output was almost normalized after a week, the animals still had a concentrating defect. Consistent with this, AQP2 expression levels were significantly reduced to about 25% of control levels 2 days after release of obstruction and remained at about 50% of controls at 7 days. Thus, the persisting concentrating defect is likely to be related to the continued depression in AQP2 levels.[381] Interestingly, unilateral ureteral obstruction also showed significantly reduced renal AQP2 levels indicating that local intrarenal factors are involved in the signaling pathways resulting in reduced expression. Thus there is increasing evidence that down-regulation of AQP2 expression plays a major role for the development of polyuria associated with acquired forms of NDI. This has been further supported by additional studies showing a marked down-regulation of collecting duct aquaporins (AQP2–4) as well as proximal tubule AQP1.[383] Moreover ureteral obstruction and release of ureteral obstruction is also associated with a marked down-regulation of key renal sodium transporters including the TAL transporters involved in countercurrent multiplication.[384] Thus there is growing evidence that many of the energy-consuming processes involved in urinary concentration are dramatically down-regulated in conditions that result in obstruction of the urinary tract. However, there is very little information regarding the signaling processes that are responsible for this down-regulation. In support of a role of inflammatory processes, alpha-MSH treatment of rats with ureteral obstruction or release of obstruction markedly prevented the down-regulation of several key aquaporins and sodium transporters. In particular, the down-regulation of AQP1 and Na,K-ATPase was significantly inhibited.[385] Importantly, it has been found that acute ureteral obstruction leads to marked upregulation of COX-2 in the inner medulla and that selective COX-2 inhibition prevents the observed dysregulation of AQP2, BSC-1, and NHE3.[386] These data indicate that COX-2 may be an important factor contributing to the impaired renal water and sodium handling in response to bilateral ureteral obstruction.

Cirrhosis and Congestive Heart Failure

In some conditions with extracellular fluid expansion such as hepatic cirrhosis and congestive heart failure, which are known to be associated with hyponatremia and a defect in urinary dilution, an increase in AQP2 expression has been found, for example in rats with severe CCl4-induced hepatic cirrhosis.[387,388] In contrast, conditions with compensated biliary hepatic cirrhosis showed a reduction in AQP2 expression.[389] In experimental congestive heart failure, a marked increase in AQP2 expression and apical targeting was observed,[251,390] but no change in AQP2 expression was noted in rats with compensatory heart failure.[251] Vasopressin-V2-receptor antagonist treatment of rats with severe congestive heart failure normalized AQP2 expression and eliminated sodium and water retention.[390] Both observations support the view that dysregulation of AQP2 may play a significant role in the development of water retention and hyponatremia. A baroreceptor-mediated increase in circulating vasopressin is likely to play a key role in the increase in AQP2 expression and targeting. It remains to be established why vasopressin-escape does not take place in rats with congestive heart failure in contrast to what is seen in normal experimental SIADH rats.[391]

It should be emphasized that other mechanisms including changes in NaCl transporter expression are also likely to play a major role in the development of sodium and water retention. Recently, it was demonstrated that the expression of BSC-1 (or NKCC2) in the thick ascending limb of the loop of Henle was increased in rats with mild congestive heart failure.[392] Moreover, vasopressin-mediated renal water reabsorption (evaluated by the aquaretic response to selective V(2)-receptor blockade) was significantly increased. Losartan treatment normalized expression of BSC-1 and decreased the protein expression levels of AQP2. This was associated with normalization of daily sodium excretion and normalization of the aquaretic response to V(2)-receptor blockade. Together, these results indicate that, in rats with congestive heart failure, losartan treatment inhibits increased sodium reabsorption through BSC-1 in the thick ascending limb of the loop of Henle and water reabsorption through AQP2 in the collecting ducts, which in part may result in an improved renal function.

Dysregulation of AQP2 (as well as AQP3 and AQP1) is also associated with multiple other water balance disorders including experimental nephrotic syndrome,[393,394] low-protein feeding,[395] experimentally induced chronic renal failure,[396] and experimental ischemic renal failure.[363,397] There is substantial evidence that the down-regulation of AQP2 in many pathological conditions is a primary event in acquired NDI. The changes in AQP2 expression in kidney cortex are identical with those seen in the inner medulla[377] indicating that a local effect of interstitial tonicity is not a major factor. Moreover, treatment with the loop diuretic furosemide causes the washout of the medullary osmotic gradient by blocking salt reabsorption in the loop of Henle, but resulted in no significant change in AQP2 expression after either 1 or 5 days treatment.[357,377] This also indicates that the high urine flow itself is not responsible for the decrease in AQP2 expression in experimental NDI. Indeed homozygous Brattleboro rats express substantial levels of intracellular AQP2 in principal cells (although less than in normal rats), despite high urine volume. This is further supported by the observation that AQP2 expression was increased in polyuric, glycosuric streptozotocin-diabetic rats that had a raised AQP2 level,[398] probably as a consequence of increased circulating vasopressin. These results strengthen the view that the decrease in AQP2 is, at least in part, a cause rather than a consequence of the polyuria.

Thus, dysregulation of aquaporins is likely to play a significant role in a variety of water balance disorders associated with common and often severe kidney, liver, and heart diseases. Studies are underway in many laboratories to fully examine the signal transduction pathways, and to define the exact role of dysregulated expression and targeting in the development of these conditions. Further analysis of aquaporins and aquaporin cell biology, in combination with our increasing understanding of ion channel and transporter expression and function in the kidney, is expected to provide further insights into the molecular understanding of water balance and its disorders.

ACKNOWLEDGMENT

Work from the laboratories of the authors was carried out with the support of National Institutes of Health (NIH) Grant DK38452 (DB) and a grant from the National Danish Research Foundation (Grundforskningsfonden; SN) and the Danish Medical Research Council (SN). We thank our many excellent colleagues for their invaluable contributions to our research endeavors over the past several years.

References

1. Robertson GL: Vasopressin. In Seldin DW, Giebisch G (eds): The Kidney. Physiology and Pathophysiology. Philadelphia, Lippincott Williams and Wilkins, 2000, pp 1133–1151.
2. Hayashi M, Arima H, Goto M, et al: Vasopressin gene transcription increases in response to decreases in plasma volume, but not to increases in plasma osmolality, in chronically dehydrated rats. Am J Physiol Endocrinol Metab 290:E213–E217, 2006.
3. Yue C, Mutsuga N, Scordalakes EM, et al: Studies of oxytocin and vasopressin gene expression in the rat hypothalamus using exon- and intron-specific probes. Am J Physiol Regul Integr Comp Physiol 290:R1233–R1241, 2006.
4. Argenziano M, Choudhri AF, Oz MC, et al: A prospective randomized trial of arginine vasopressin in the treatment of vasodilatory shock after left ventricular assist device placement. Circulation 96:II-286–290, 1997.
5. Landry DW, Oliver JA: The pathogenesis of vasodilatory shock. N Engl J Med 345:588–595, 2001.
6. Morel A, O'Carroll AM, Brownstein MJ, et al: Molecular cloning and expression of a rat V1a arginine vasopressin receptor. Nature 356:523–526, 1992.
7. Baertschi AJ, Friedli M: A novel type of vasopressin receptor on anterior pituitary corticotrophs? Endocrinology 116:499–502, 1985.
8. de Keyzer Y, Auzan C, Lenne F, et al: Cloning and characterization of the human V3 pituitary vasopressin receptor. FEBS Lett 356:215–220, 1994.
9. Sugimoto T, Saito M, Mochizuki S, et al: Molecular cloning and functional expression of a cDNA encoding the human V1b vasopressin receptor. J Biol Chem 269:27088–27092, 1994.
10. Lolait SJ, O'Carroll AM, Konig M, et al: Cloning and characterization of a vasopressin V2 receptor and possible link to nephrogenic diabetes insipidus. Nature 357:336–339, 1992.
11. Kitano H, Suzuki M, Kitanishi T, et al: Regulation of inner ear fluid in the rat by vasopressin. Neuroreport 10:1205–1207, 1999.
12. Zenner HP, Zenner B: Vasopressin and isoproterenol activate adenylate cyclase in the guinea pig inner ear. Arch Otorhinolaryngol 222:275–283, 1979.
13. Birnbaumer M, Seibold A, Gilbert S: Molecular cloning of the receptor for human antidiuretic hormone. Nature 357:333–335, 1992.
14. Dohlman HG, Thorner J, Caron MG, et al: Model systems for the study of seven-transmembrane segment receptors. Ann Rev Biochem 60:653–688, 1991.
15. Kumagami H, Loewenheim H, Beitz E, et al: The effect of anti-diuretic hormone on the endolymphatic sac of the inner ear. Pflugers Arch 436:970–975, 1998.
16. Sawada S, Takeda T, Kitano H, et al: Aquaporin-2 regulation by vasopressin in the rat inner ear. Neuroreport 13:1127–1129, 2002.
17. Kaufmann JE, Iezzi M, Vischer UM: Desmopressin (DDAVP) induces NO production in human endothelial cells via V2 receptor- and cAMP-mediated signaling. J Thromb Haemost 1:821–828, 2003.
18. Kaufmann JE, Oksche A, Wollheim CB, et al: Vasopressin-induced von Willebrand factor secretion from endothelial cells involves V2 receptors and cAMP. J Clin Invest 106:107–116, 2000.
19. Liard JF: L-NAME antagonizes vasopressin V2-induced vasodilatation in dogs. Am J Physiol 266:H99–H106, 1994.
20. Fejes-Toth G, Naray-Fejes-Toth A: Isolated principal and intercalated cells: Hormone responsiveness and Na⁺-K⁺-ATPase activity. Am J Physiol 256:F742–F750, 1989.
21. Ganote CE, Grantham JJ, Moses HL, et al: Ultrastructural studies of vasopressin effect on isolated perfused renal collecting tubules of the rabbit. J Cell Biol 36:355–367, 1968.
22. Grantham JJ, Burg MB: Effect of vasopressin and cyclic AMP on permeability of isolated collecting tubules. Am J Physiol 211:255–259, 1966.
23. Kirk K: Binding and internalization of a fluorescent vasopressin analogue by collecting duct cells. Am J Physiol 255:C622–C632, 1988.
24. Morel F, Imbert-Teboul M, Chabardes D: Distribution of hormone-dependent adenylate cyclase in the nephron and its physiological significance. Ann Rev Physiol 43:569–581, 1981.
25. Woodhall PB, Tisher CC: Response of the distal tubule and cortical collecting duct to vasopressin in the rat. J Clin Invest 52:3095–3108, 1973.
26. Nonoguchi H, Owada A, Kobayashi N, et al: Immunohistochemical localization of V2 vasopressin receptor along the nephron and functional role of luminal V2 receptor in terminal inner medullary collecting ducts. J Clin Invest 96:1768–1778, 1995.
27. Sarmiento JM, Ehrenfeld P, Anazco CC, et al: Differential distribution of the vasopressin V receptor along the rat nephron during renal ontogeny and maturation. Kidney Int 68:487–496, 2005.
28. Ausiello DA, Holtzman EJ, Gronich JH, et al: Cell signalling. In Seldin DW, Giebisch G (eds): The Kidney: Physiology and Pathophysiology. New York, Raven Press, 1992, pp 645–692.
29. Skorecki KL, Brown D, Ercolani L, et al:. Molecular mechanisms of vasopressin action in the kidney. In Windhager EE (ed): Handbook of Physiology: Section 8, Renal Physiology. New York, Oxford University Press, 1992, pp 1185–1218.
30. Nickols HH, Shah VN, Chazin WJ, et al: Calmodulin interacts with the V2 vasopressin receptor: Elimination of binding to the C terminus also eliminates arginine vasopressin-stimulated elevation of intracellular calcium. J Biol Chem 279:46969–46980, 2004.
31. Chou CL, Yip KP, Michea L, et al: Regulation of aquaporin-2 trafficking by vasopressin in the renal collecting duct. Roles of ryanodine-sensitive Ca²⁺ stores and calmodulin. J Biol Chem 275:36839–36846, 2000.

32. Hoffert JD, Chou CL, Fenton RA, et al: Calmodulin is required for vasopressin-stimulated increase in cyclic AMP production in inner medullary collecting duct. J Biol Chem 280:13624–13630, 2005.

33. Innamorati G, Le Gouill C, Balamotis M, et al: The long and the short cycle. Alternative intracellular routes for trafficking of G-protein-coupled receptors. J Biol Chem 276:13096–13103, 2001.

34. Innamorati G, Sadeghi H Birnbaumer M: Phosphorylation and recycling kinetics of G protein-coupled receptors. J Recept Signal Transduct Res 19:315–326, 1999.

35. Lutz W, Sanders M, Salisbury J, et al: Internalization of vasopressin analogs in kidney and smooth muscle cells: Evidence for receptor-mediated endocytosis in cells with V2 or V1 receptors. Proc Natl Acad Sci U S A 87:6507–6511, 1990.

36. Innamorati G, Sadeghi H, Eberle AN, et al: Phosphorylation of the V2 vasopressin receptor. J Biol Chem 272:2486–2492, 1997.

37. Innamorati G, Sadeghi HM, Tran NT, et al: A serine cluster prevents recycling of the V2 vasopressin receptor. Proc Natl Acad Sci U S A 95:2222–2226, 1998.

38. Charest PG, Bouvier M: Palmitoylation of the V2 vasopressin receptor carboxyl tail enhances beta-arrestin recruitment leading to efficient receptor endocytosis and ERK1/2 activation. J Biol Chem 278:41541–41551, 2003.

39. Sadeghi HM, Innamorati G, Dagarag M, et al: Palmitoylation of the V2 vasopressin receptor. Mol Pharmacol 52:21–29, 1997.

40. Thielen A, Oueslati M, Hermosilla R, et al: The hydrophobic amino acid residues in the membrane-proximal C tail of the G protein-coupled vasopressin V2 receptor are necessary for transport-competent receptor folding. FEBS Lett 579:5227–5235, 2005.

41. Brunskill N, Bastani B, Hayes C, et al: Localization and polar distribution of several G-protein subunits along nephron segments. Kidney Int 40:997–1006, 1991.

42. Stow JL, Sabolic I, Brown D: Heterogenous localization of G protein a-subunits in rat kidney. Am J Physiol 261:F831–F840, 1991.

43. Shen T, Suzuki Y, Poyard M, et al: Expression of adenylyl cyclase mRNAs in the adult, in developing, and in the Brattleboro rat kidney. Am J Physiol 273:C323–C330, 1997.

44. Postina R, Kojro E, Fahrenholz F: Identification of neurohypophysial hormone receptor domains involved in ligand binding and G protein coupling. Adv Exp Med Biol 449:371–385, 1998.

45. Schoneberg T, Kostenis E, Liu J, et al: Molecular aspects of vasopressin receptor function. Adv Exp Med Biol 449:347–358, 1998.

46. Granier S, Terrillon S, Pascal R, et al: A cyclic peptide mimicking the third intracellular loop of the V2 vasopressin receptor inhibits signaling through its interaction with receptor dimer and G protein coupling. J Biol Chem 279:50904–50914, 2004.

47. Bouley R, Sun TX, Chenard M, et al: Functional role of the NPxxY motif in internalization of the type 2 vasopressin receptor in LLC-PK1 cells. Am J Physiol Cell Physiol 285:C750–C762, 2003.

48. Oakley RH, Laporte SA, Holt JA, et al: Differential affinities of visual arrestin, beta arrestin1, and beta arrestin2 for G protein-coupled receptors delineate two major classes of receptors. J Biol Chem 275:17201–17210, 2000.

49. Terashima Y, Kondo K, Mizuno Y, et al: Influence of acute elevation of plasma AVP level on rat vasopressin V2 receptor and aquaporin-2 mRNA expression. J Mol Endocrinol 20:281–285, 1998.

50. Dousa TP: Cyclic-3′, 5′-nucleotide phosphodiesterases in the cyclic adenosine monophosphate (cAMP)-mediated actions of vasopressin. Semin Nephrol 14:333–340, 1994.

51. Stokes JB: Modulation of vasopressin-induced water permeability of the cortical collecting tubule by endogenous and exogenous prostaglandins. Miner Electrolyte Metab 11:240–248, 1985.

52. Li L, Schafer JA: Dopamine inhibits vasopressin-dependent cAMP production in the rat cortical collecting duct. Am J Physiol 275:F62–F67, 1998.

53. Muto S, Tabei K, Asano Y, et al: Dopaminergic inhibition of the action of vasopressin on the cortical collecting tubule. Eur J Pharmacol 114:393–397, 1985.

54. Edwards RM, Spielman WS: Adenosine A1 receptor-mediated inhibition of vasopressin action in inner medullary collecting tubule. Am J Physiol 266:F791–F796, 1994.

55. Hawk CT, Kudo LH, Rouch AJ, et al: Inhibition by epinephrine of AVP- and cAMP-stimulated Na+ and water transport in Dahl rat CCD. Am J Physiol 265:F449–F460, 1993.

56. Rouch AJ, Kudo LH: Alpha 2-adrenergic-mediated inhibition of water and urea permeability in the rat IMCD. Am J Physiol 271:F150–F157, 1996.

57. Oishi R, Nonoguchi H, Tomita K, et al: Endothelin-1 inhibits AVP-stimulated osmotic water permeability in rat inner medullary collecting duct. Am J Physiol 261:F951–F956, 1991.

58. Tamma G, Carmosino M, Svelto M, et al: Bradykinin signaling counteracts cAMP-elicited aquaporin 2 translocation in renal cells. J Am Soc Nephrol 16:2881–2889, 2005.

59. Shenoy SK, Lefkowitz RJ: Receptor regulation: beta-arrestin moves up a notch. Nat Cell Biol 7:1159–1161, 2005.

60. Perry SJ, Lefkowitz RJ: Arresting developments in heptahelical receptor signaling and regulation. Trends Cell Biol 12:130–138, 2002.

61. Laporte SA, Oakley RH, Zhang J, et al: The beta2-adrenergic receptor/betaarrestin complex recruits the clathrin adaptor AP-2 during endocytosis. Proc Natl Acad Sci U S A 96:3712–3717, 1999.

62. Bowen-Pidgeon D, Innamorati G, Sadeghi HM, et al: Arrestin effects on internalization of vasopressin receptors. Mol Pharmacol 59:1395–1401, 2001.

63. Oakley RH, Laporte SA, Holt JA, et al: Association of beta-arrestin with G protein-coupled receptors during clathrin-mediated endocytosis dictates the profile of receptor resensitization. J Biol Chem 274:32248–32257, 1999.

64. Bouley R, Lin HY, Raychowdhury MK, et al: Downregulation of the vasopressin type 2 receptor after vasopressin-induced internalization: Involvement of a lysosomal degradation pathway. Am J Physiol Cell Physiol 288:C1390–C1401, 2005.

65. Robben JH, Knoers NV, Deen PM: Regulation of the vasopressin V2 receptor by vasopressin in polarized renal collecting duct cells. Mol Biol Cell 15:5693–5699, 2004.

66. Martin NP, Lefkowitz RJ, Shenoy SK: Regulation of V2 vasopressin receptor degradation by agonist-promoted ubiquitination. J Biol Chem 278:45954–45959, 2003.

67. Bouley R, Hawthorn G, Russo LM, et al: Aquaporin 2 (AQP2) and vasopressin type 2 receptor (V2R) endocytosis in kidney epithelial cells: AQP2 is located in 'endocytosis-resistant' membrane domains after vasopressin treatment. Biol Cell 98:215–232, 2006.

68. Kersting U, Dantzler DW, Oberleithner H, et al: Evidence for an acid pH in rat renal inner medulla: Paired measurements with liquid ion-exchange microelectrodes on collecting ducts and vasa recta. Pflugers Arch 426:354–356, 1994.

69. Bichet DG: Hereditary polyuric disorders: New concepts and differential diagnosis. Semin Nephrol 26:224–233, 2006.

70. Sands JM, Bichet DG: Nephrogenic diabetes insipidus. Ann Intern Med 144:186–194, 2006.

71. Fushimi K, Uchida S, Hara Y, et al: Cloning and expression of apical membrane water channel of rat kidney collecting tubule. Nature 361:549–552, 1993.

72. Kim JK, Summer SN, Wood WM, et al: Arginine vasopressin secretion with mutants of wild-type and Brattleboro rats AVP gene. J Am Soc Nephrol 8:1863–1869, 1997.

73. Schmale H, Heinsohn S, Richter D: Structural organization of the rat gene for the arginine vasopressin-neurophysin precursor. EMBO J 2:763–767, 1983.

74. Wahlstrom JT, Fowler MJ, Nicholson WE, et al: A novel mutation in the preprovasopressin gene identified in a kindred with autosomal dominant neurohypophyseal diabetes insipidus. J Clin Endocrinol Metab 89:1963–1968, 2004.

75. Rittig S, Siggaard C, Ozata M, et al: Autosomal dominant neurohypophyseal diabetes insipidus due to substitution of histidine for tyrosine(2) in the vasopressin moiety of the hormone precursor. J Clin Endocrinol Metab 87:3351–3355, 2002.

76. Siggaard C, Rittig S, Corydon TJ, et al: Clinical and molecular evidence of abnormal processing and trafficking of the vasopressin preprohormone in a large kindred with familial neurohypophyseal diabetes insipidus due to a signal peptide mutation. J Clin Endocrinol Metab 84:2933–2941, 1999.

77. Khanna A: Acquired nephrogenic diabetes insipidus. Semin Nephrol 26:244–248, 2006.

78. Makaryus AN, McFarlane SI: Diabetes insipidus: Diagnosis and treatment of a complex disease. Cleve Clin J Med 73:65–71, 2006.

79. Moses AM, Miller M, Streeten DH: Pathophysiologic and pharmacologic alterations in the release and action of ADH. Metabolism 25:697–721, 1976.

80. Moses AM, Scheinman SJ, Schroeder ET: Antidiuretic and PGE2 responses to AVP and dDAVP in subjects with central and nephrogenic diabetes insipidus. Am J Physiol 248:F354–F359, 1985.

81. Valtin H: The discovery of the Brattleboro rat, recommended nomenclature and the question of proper controls. Ann N Y Acad Sci 394:1–9, 1982.

82. Valtin H, Schroeder HA: Familial hypothalamic diabetes insipidus in rats (Brattleboro Strain). Am J Physiol 206:425–430, 1964.

83. Schmale H, Richter D: Single base deletion in the vasopressin gene is the cause of diabetes insipidus in Brattleboro rats. Nature 308:705–709, 1984.

84. Garofeanu CG, Weir M, Rosas-Arellano MP, et al: Causes of reversible nephrogenic diabetes insipidus: A systematic review. Am J Kidney Dis 45:626–637, 2005.

85. Holtzman EJ, Kolakowski LF, Ausiello DA: The molecular biology of congenital nephrogenic diabetes insipidus. In Schlondorff D, Bonventre JV (eds): Molecular Nephrology. New York, Marcel Dekker, 1995, pp 887–910.

86. Forssmann H: On hereditary diabetes insipidus. Acta Med Scand 121 (Suppl. 159):9–46, 1945.

87. Robinson MG, Kaplan SA: Inheritance of vasopressin-resistant nephrogenic diabetes insipidus. Am J Dis Child 99:164–171, 1960.

88. Williams RH, Henry C: Nephrogenic diabetes insipidus transmitted by females and appearing during infancy in males. Ann Int Med 27:84–95, 1947.

89. Livingstone C, Rampes H: Lithium: A review of its metabolic adverse effects. J Psychopharmacol 20:347–355, 2006.

90. Deen PM, Knoers NV: Physiology and pathophysiology of the aquaporin-2 water channel. Curr Opin Nephrol Hypertens 7:37–42, 1998.

91. Oksche A, Rosenthal W: The molecular basis of nephrogenic diabetes insipidus. J Mol Med 76:326–337, 1998.

92. Robben JH, Knoers NV, Deen PM: Cell biological aspects of the vasopressin type-2 receptor and aquaporin 2 water channel in nephrogenic diabetes insipidus. Am J Physiol Renal Physiol 291:F257–F270, 2006.

93. Rosenthal WA, Seibold A, Antaramian A, et al: Molecular identification of the gene responsible for congenital nephrogenic diabetes insipidus. Nature 359:233–235, 1992.

94. Deen PMT, Brown D: Trafficking of native and mutant mammalian MIP proteins. In Hohmann S, Nielsen S, Agre P (eds): Aquaporins: Current Topics in Membranes. New York, Academic Press, 2001, pp 235–276.

95. Marr N, Bichet DG, Lonergan M, et al: Heteroligomerization of an Aquaporin-2 mutant with wild-type Aquaporin-2 and their misrouting to late endosomes/lysosomes explains dominant nephrogenic diabetes insipidus. Hum Mol Genet 11:779–789, 2002.

96. Mulders SM, Bichet DG, Rijss JP, et al: An aquaporin-2 water channel mutant which causes autosomal dominant nephrogenic diabetes insipidus is retained in the Golgi complex. J Clin Invest 102:57–66, 1998.

97. Arthus MF, Lonergan M, Crumley MJ, et al: Report of 33 novel AVPR2 mutations and analysis of 117 families with X-linked nephrogenic diabetes insipidus. J Am Soc Nephrol 11:1044–1054, 2000.

98. Knoers NV, Deen PM: Molecular and cellular defects in nephrogenic diabetes insipidus. Pediatr Nephrol 16:1146–1152, 2001.

99. Kinoshita K, Miura Y, Nagasaki H, et al: A novel deletion mutation in the arginine vasopressin receptor 2 gene and skewed X chromosome inactivation in a female patient with congenital nephrogenic diabetes insipidus. J Endocrinol Invest 27:167–170, 2004.

100. Morello JP, Bichet DG: Nephrogenic diabetes insipidus. Annu Rev Physiol 63:607–630, 2001.

101. Barak LS, Oakley RH, Laporte SA, et al: Constitutive arrestin-mediated desensitization of a human vasopressin receptor mutant associated with nephrogenic diabetes insipidus. Proc Natl Acad Sci U S A 98:93–98, 2001.

102. Kalenga K, Persu A, Goffin E, et al: Intrafamilial phenotype variability in nephrogenic diabetes insipidus. Am J Kidney Dis 39:737–743, 2002.

103. Sangkuhl K, Rompler H, Busch W, et al: Nephrogenic diabetes insipidus caused by mutation of Tyr205: A key residue of V2 vasopressin receptor function. Hum Mutat 25:505, 2005.

104. Hermosilla R, Oueslati M, Donalies U, et al: Disease-causing V(2) vasopressin receptors are retained in different compartments of the early secretory pathway. Traffic 5:993–1005, 2004.

105. Robben JH, Sze M, Knoers NV, et al: Rescue of vasopressin V2 receptor mutants by chemical chaperones: specificity and mechanism. Mol Biol Cell 17:379–386, 2006.

106. Egan ME, Glockner-Pagel J, Ambrose C, et al: Calcium-pump inhibitors induce functional surface expression of Delta F508-CFTR protein in cystic fibrosis epithelial cells. Nat Med 8:485–492, 2002.

107. Egan ME, Pearson M, Weiner SA, et al: Curcumin, a major constituent of turmeric, corrects cystic fibrosis defects. Science 304:600–602, 2004.

108. Song Y, Sonawane ND, Salinas D, et al: Evidence against the rescue of defective DeltaF508-CFTR cellular processing by curcumin in cell culture and mouse models. J Biol Chem 279:40629–40633, 2004.

109. Thibonnier M: Genetics of vasopressin receptors. Curr Hypertens Rep 6:21–26, 2004.

110. Morello JP, Petaja-Repo UE, Bichet DG, et al: Pharmacological chaperones: A new twist on receptor folding. Trends Pharmacol Sci 21:466–469, 2000.

111. Morello JP, Salahpour A, Laperriere A, et al: Pharmacological chaperones rescue cell-surface expression and function of misfolded V2 vasopressin receptor mutants. J Clin Invest 105:887–895, 2000.

112. Bernier V, Lagace M, Lonergan M, et al: Functional rescue of the constitutively internalized V2 vasopressin receptor mutant R137H by the pharmacological chaperone action of SR49059. Mol Endocrinol 18:2074–2084, 2004.

113. Sangkuhl K, Schulz A, Rompler H, et al: Aminoglycoside-mediated rescue of a disease-causing nonsense mutation in the V2 vasopressin receptor gene in vitro and in vivo. Hum Mol Genet 13:893–903, 2004.

114. Knepper MA, Nielsen S: Peter Agre, 2003 Nobel Prize winner in chemistry. J Am Soc Nephrol 15:1093–1095, 2004.

115. Denker BM, Smith BL, Kuhajda FP, et al: Identification, purification and partial characterization of a novel Mr 28,000 integral membrane protein from erythrocytes and renal tubules. J Biol Chem 263:15634–15642, 1988.

116. Preston GM, Agre P: Isolation of the cDNA for erythrocyte integral membrane protein of 28 kilodaltons: Member of an ancient channel family. Proc Natl Acad Sci U S A 88:11110–11114, 1991.

117. Preston GM, Carroll TP, Guggino WB, et al: Appearance of water channels in Xenopus oocytes expressing red cell CHIP28 protein. Science 256:385–387, 1992.

118. Van Hoek AN, Verkman AS: Functional reconstitution of the isolated erythrocyte water channel CHIP28. J Biol Chem 267:18267–18269, 1992.

119. Zeidel ML, Ambudkar SV, Smith BL, et al: Reconstitution of functional water channels in liposomes containing purified red cell CHIP28 protein. Biochemistry Biochemistry 31:7436–7440, 1992.

120. Gorin MB, Yancey SB, Cline J, et al: The major intrinsic protein (MIP) of the bovine lens fiber membrane: Characterization and structure based on cDNA cloning. Cell 39:49–59, 1984.

121. Nielsen S, Smith BL, Christensen EI, et al: CHIP28 water channels are localized in constitutively water-permeable segments of the nephron. J Cell Biol 120:371–383, 1993.

122. Sabolic I, Valenti G, Verbavatz J-M, et al: Localization of the CHIP28 water channel in rat kidney. Am J Physiol 263:C1225–C1233, 1992.

123. Nielsen S, Smith BL, Christensen EI, et al: Distribution of the aquaporin CHIP in secretory and resorptive epithelia and capillary endothelia. Proc Natl Acad Sci U S A 90:7275–7279, 1993.

124. Brown D, Verbavatz JM, Valenti G, et al: Localization of the CHIP28 water channel in reabsorptive segments of the rat male reproductive tract. Eur J Cell Biol 61:264–273, 1993.

125. Stankovic KM, Adams JC, Brown D: Immunolocalization of aquaporin CHIP in the guinea pig inner ear. Am J Physiol 269:C1450–C1456, 1995.

126. Borgnia M, Nielsen S, Engel A, et al: Cellular and molecular biology of the aquaporin water channels. Annu Rev Biochem 68:425–458, 1999.

127. Verkman AS: Novel roles of aquaporins revealed by phenotype analysis of knockout mice. Rev Physiol Biochem Pharmacol 155:31–55, 2005.

128. Agre P, Kozono D: Aquaporin water channels: Molecular mechanisms for human diseases. FEBS Lett 555:72–78, 2003.

129. Brown D: The ins and outs of aquaporin-2 trafficking. Am J Physiol Renal Physiol 284:F893–F901, 2003.

130. Frokiaer J, Nielsen S, Knepper MA: Molecular physiology of renal aquaporins and sodium transporters: Exciting approaches to understand regulation of renal water handling. J Am Soc Nephrol 16:2827–2829, 2005.

131. Ishikawa SE, Schrier RW: Pathophysiological roles of arginine vasopressin and aquaporin-2 in impaired water excretion. Clin Endocrinol (Oxf) 58:1–17, 2003.

132. Valenti G, Procino G, Tamma G, et al: Minireview: aquaporin 2 trafficking. Endocrinology 146:5063–5070, 2005.

133. Madsen O, Deen PM, Pesole G, et al: Molecular evolution of mammalian aquaporin-2: Further evidence that elephant shrew and aardvark join the paenungulate clade. Mol Biol Evol 14:363–371, 1997.

134. Yang B, Verkman AS: Water and glycerol permeabilities of aquaporins 1–5 and MIP determined quantitatively by expression of epitope-tagged constructs in Xenopus oocytes. J Biol Chem 272:16140–16146, 1997.

135. Holm LM, Jahn TP, Moller AL, et al: NH3 and NH4+ permeability in aquaporin-expressing Xenopus oocytes. Pflugers Arch 450:415–428, 2005.

136. Ishibashi K, Kuwahara M, Gu Y, et al: Cloning and functional expression of a new aquaporin (AQP9) abundantly expressed in the peripheral leukocytes permeable to water and urea but not to glycerol. Biochem Biophys Res Commun 244:268–274, 1998.

137. Ishibashi K, Sasaki S, Fushimi K, et al: Molecular cloning and expression of a member of the aquaporin family with permeability to glycerol and urea in addition to water expressed at the basolateral membrane of kidney collecting duct cells [see comments]. Proc Natl Acad Sci U S A 91:6269–6273, 1994.

138. Jahn TP, Moller AL, Zeuthen T, et al: Aquaporin homologues in plants and mammals transport ammonia. FEBS Lett 574:31–36, 2004.

139. Tsukaguchi H, Shayakul C, Berger UV, et al: Molecular characterization of a broad selectivity neutral solute channel. J Biol Chem 273:24737–24743, 1998.

140. Verkman AS, Shi LB, Frigeri A, et al: Structure and function of kidney water channels. Kidney Int 48:1069–1081, 1995.

141. Wintour EM: Water channels and urea transporters. Clin Exp Pharmacol Physiol 24:1–9, 1997.

142. Agre P, Bonhivers M, Borgnia MJ: The aquaporins, blueprints for cellular plumbing systems. J Biol Chem 273:14659–14662, 1998.

143. Hara-Chikuma M, Verkman AS: Physiological roles of glycerol-transporting aquaporins: The aquaglyceroporins. Cell Mol Life Sci 63:1386–1392, 2006.

144. Lencer WI, Verkman AS, Arnaout MA, et al: Endocytic vesicles from renal papilla which retrieve the vasopressin-sensitive water channel do not contain a functional H+ ATPase. J Cell Biol 111:379–389, 1990.

145. Sabolic I, Wuarin F, Shi LB, et al: Apical endosomes isolated from kidney collecting duct principal cells lack subunits of the proton pumping ATPase. J Cell Biol 119:111–122, 1992.

146. Murata K, Mitsuoka K, Hirai T, et al: Structural determinants of water permeation through aquaporin-1. Nature 407:599–605, 2000.

147. Blank ME, Ehmke H: Aquaporin-1 and HCO3(-)-Cl- transporter-mediated transport of CO2 across the human erythrocyte membrane. J Physiol 550:419–429, 2003.

148. Cooper GJ, Boron WF: Effect of PCMBS on CO2 permeability of Xenopus oocytes expressing aquaporin 1 or its C189S mutant. Am J Physiol 275:C1481–1486, 1998.

149. Nakhoul NL, Davis BA, Romero MF, et al: Effect of expressing the water channel aquaporin-1 on the CO2 permeability of Xenopus oocytes. Am J Physiol 274:C543–C548, 1998.

150. Prasad GV, Coury LA, Finn F, et al: Reconstituted aquaporin 1 water channels transport CO2 across membranes. J Biol Chem 273:33123–33126, 1998.

151. Cooper GJ, Zhou Y, Bouyer P, et al: Transport of volatile solutes through AQP1. J Physiol 542:17–29, 2002.

152. Fang X, Yang B, Matthay MA, et al: Evidence against aquaporin-1-dependent CO(2) permeability in lung and kidney. J Physiol 542:63–69, 2002.

153. Ripoche P, Goossens D, Devuyst O, et al: Role of RhAG and AQP1 in NH3 and CO2 gas transport in red cell ghosts: A stopped-flow analysis. Transfus Clin Biol 13:117–122, 2006.

154. Swenson ER, Deem S, Kerr ME, et al: Inhibition of aquaporin-mediated CO2 diffusion and voltage-gated H+ channels by zinc does not alter rabbit lung CO2 and NO excretion. Clin Sci (Lond) 103:567–575, 2002.

155. Verkman AS: Does aquaporin-1 pass gas? An opposing view. J Physiol 542:31, 2002.

156. Kaldenhoff R, Fischer M: Functional aquaporin diversity in plants. Biochim Biophys Acta 1758:1134–1141, 2006.

157. Terashima I, Ono K: Effects of HgCl(2) on CO(2) dependence of leaf photosynthesis: Evidence indicating involvement of aquaporins in CO(2) diffusion across the plasma membrane. Plant Cell Physiol 43:70–78, 2002.

158. Uehlein N, Lovisolo C, Siefritz F, et al: The tobacco aquaporin NtAQP1 is a membrane CO2 pore with physiological functions. Nature 425:734–737, 2003.

159. Nakhoul NL, Hering-Smith KS, Abdulnour-Nakhoul SM, et al: Transport of NH(3)/NH in oocytes expressing aquaporin-1. Am J Physiol Renal Physiol 281:F255–F263, 2001.

160. Yang B, Zhao D, Solenov E, et al: Evidence from knockout mice against physiologically significant aquaporin-8 facilitated ammonia transport. Am J Physiol Cell Physiol 291:C417–423, 2006.

161. Liu Z, Shen J, Carbrey JM, et al: Arsenite transport by mammalian aquaglyceroporins AQP7 and AQP9. Proc Natl Acad Sci U S A 99:6053–6058, 2002.

162. Ishibashi K, Kuwahara M, Sasaki S: Molecular biology of aquaporins. Rev Physiol Biochem Pharmacol 141:1–32, 2000.

163. Nielsen S, Frokiaer J, Marples D, et al: Aquaporins in the kidney: From molecules to medicine. Physiol Rev 82:205–244, 2002.

164. Ishibashi K, Sasaki S, Fushimi K, et al: Immunolocalization and effect of dehydration on AQP3, a basolateral water channel of kidney collecting ducts. Am J Physiol 272:F235–F241, 1997.

165. Nelson RD, Stricklett P, Gustafson C, et al: Expression of an AQP2 cre recombinase transgene in kidney and male reproductive system of transgenic mice. Am J Physiol Cell Physiol 275:C216–C226, 1998.

166. Stevens AL, Breton S, Gustafson CE, et al: Aquaporin 2 is a vasopressin-independent, constitutive apical membrane protein in rat vas deferens. Am J Physiol Cell Physiol 278:C791–C802, 2000.

167. Gallardo P, Cid LP, Vio CP, et al: Aquaporin-2, a regulated water channel, is expressed in apical membranes of rat distal colon epithelium. Am J Physiol Gastrointest Liver Physiol 281:G856–G863, 2001.

168. Chevalier J, Bourguet J, Hugon JS: Membrane-associated particles: Distribution in frog urinary bladder epithelium at rest and after oxytocin treatment. Cell Tissue Res 152:129–140, 1974.

169. Hays RM: Alteration of luminal membrane structure by antidiuretic hormone. Am J Physiol 245:C289–C296, 1983.

170. Kachadorian WA, Wade JB, DiScala VA: Vasopressin: Induced structural changes in toad bladder luminal membrane. Science 190:67–69, 1975.

171. Kachadorian WA, Wade JB, Uiterwyk CC, et al: Membrane structural and functional responses to vasopressin in toad bladder. J Membrane Biol 30:381–401, 1977.

172. Wade JB: Membrane structural specialization of the toad urinary bladder revealed by the freeze-fracture technique. III. Location, structure and vasopressin dependence of intramembranous particle arrays. J Membr Biol 40 (Special Issue):281–296, 1978.

173. Wade JB, Stetson DL, Lewis SA: ADH action: Evidence for a membrane shuttle mechanism. Ann N Y Acad Sci 372:106–117, 1981.

174. Harmanci MC, Stern P, Kachadorian WA, et al: Antidiuretic hormone-induced intramembranous alteration in mammalian collecting ducts. Am J Physiol 235:F440–F443, 1978.

175. Harmanci MC, Stern P, Kachadorian WA, et al: Vasopressin and collecting duct intramembranous particle clusters: A dose-response relationship. Am J Physiol 239:F560–F564, 1980.

176. Brown D, Shields GI, Valtin H, et al: Lack of intramembranous particle clusters in collecting ducts of mice with nephrogenic diabetes insipidus. Am J Physiol 249:F582–F589, 1985.

177. Brown D, Grosso A, DeSousa RC: Correlation between water flow and intramembrane particle aggregates in toad epidermis. Am J Physiol 245:C334–C342, 1983.

178. Rash JE, Yasumura T, Hudson CS, et al: Direct immunogold labeling of aquaporin-4 in square arrays of astrocyte and ependymocyte plasma membranes in rat brain and spinal cord. Proc Natl Acad Sci U S A 95:11981–11986, 1998.

179. Verbavatz JM, Ma T, Gobin R, et al: Absence of orthogonal arrays in kidney, brain and muscle from transgenic knockout mice lacking water channel aquaporin-4. J Cell Sci 110: 2855–2860, 1997.

180. Yang B, Brown D, Verkman AS: The mercurial insensitive water channel (AQP-4) forms orthogonal arrays in stably transfected Chinese hamster ovary cells. J Biol Chem 271:4577–4580, 1996.

181. Humbert F, Pricam C, Perrelet A, et al: Specific plasma membrane differentiations in the cells of the kidney collecting tubule. J Ultrastr Res 52: 13–20, 1975.

182. Orci L, Humbert F, Brown D, et al: Membrane ultrastructure in urinary tubules. Int Rev Cytol 73:183–242, 1981.

183. Terris J, Ecelbarger CA, Marples D, et al: Distribution of aquaporin-4 water channel expression within rat kidney. Am J Physiol 269:F775–F785, 1995.

184. Bordi C, Perrelet A: Orthogonal arrays of particles in plasma membranes of the gastric parietal cell. Anat Rec 192:297–303, 1978.

185. Misaka T, Abe K, Iwabuchi K, et al: A water channel closely related to rat brain aquaporin 4 is expressed in acid- and pepsinogen-secretory cells of human stomach. FEBS Lett 381:208–212, 1996.

186. Jung JS, Bhat RV, Preston GM, et al: Molecular characterization of an aquaporin cDNA from brain: Candidate osmoreceptor and regulator of water balance. Proc Natl Acad Sci U S A 91:13052–13056, 1994.

187. Lu M, Lee MD, Smith BL, et al: The human AQP4 gene: Definition of the locus encoding two water channel polypeptides in brain. Proc Natl Acad Sci U S A 93:10908–10912, 1996.

188. Furman CS, Gorelick-Feldman DA, Davidson KG, et al: Aquaporin-4 square array assembly: Opposing actions of M1 and M23 isoforms. Proc Natl Acad Sci U S A 100:13609–13614, 2003.

189. Silberstein C, Bouley R, Huang Y, et al: Membrane organization and function of M1 and M23 isoforms of aquaporin-4 in epithelial cells. Am J Physiol Renal Physiol 287:F501–F511, 2004.

190. Han Z, Wax MB, Patil RV: Regulation of aquaporin-4 water channels by phorbol ester-dependent protein phosphorylation. J Biol Chem 273:6001–6004, 1998.

191. Zelenina M, Zelenin S, Bondar AA, et al: Water permeability of aquaporin-4 is decreased by protein kinase C and dopamine. Am J Physiol Renal Physiol 283:F309–318, 2002.

192. Baturina GS, Isaeva LE, Khodus GR, et al: [Water permeability of the OMCD and IMCD cells' basolateral membrane under the conditions of dehydration and dDAVP action]. Ross Fiziol Zh Im I M Sechenova 90:865–873, 2004.

193. Shi LB, Verkman AS: Selected cysteine point mutations confer mercurial sensitivity to the mercurial-insensitive water channel MIWC/AQP-4. Biochemistry 35:538–544, 1996.

194. Jeon US, Joo KW, Na KY, et al: Oxytocin induces apical and basolateral redistribution of aquaporin-2 in rat kidney. Nephron 93:E36–E45, 2003.

195. Nielsen S, DiGiovanni SR, Christensen EI, et al: Cellular and subcellular immunolocalization of vasopressin-regulated water channel in rat kidney. Proc Natl Acad Sci U S A 90:11663–11667, 1993.

196. van Balkom BW, van Raak M, Breton S, et al: Hypertonicity is involved in redirecting the aquaporin-2 water channel into the basolateral, instead of the apical, plasma membrane of renal epithelial cells. J Biol Chem 278:1101–1107, 2003.

197. Sabolic I, Katsura T, Verbavatz JM, et al: The AQP2 water channel: Effect of vasopressin treatment, microtubule disruption, and distribution in neonatal rats. J Membr Biol 143:165–175, 1995.

198. Marples D, Knepper MA, Christensen EI, et al: Redistribution of aquaporin-2 water channels induced by vasopressin in rat kidney inner medullary collecting duct. Am J Physiol 269:C655–664, 1995.

199. Nielsen S, Chou CL, Marples D, et al: Vasopressin increases water permeability of kidney collecting duct by inducing translocation of aquaporin-CD water channels to plasma membrane. Proc Natl Acad Sci U S A 92:1013–1017, 1995.

200. Yamamoto T, Sasaki S, Fushimi K, et al: Localization and expression of a collecting duct water channel, aquaporin, in hydrated and dehydrated rats. Exp Nephrol 3:193–201, 1995.

201. Christensen BM, Marples D, Jensen UB, et al: Acute effects of vasopressin V2-receptor antagonist on kidney AQP2 expression and subcellular distribution. Am J Physiol 275:F285–F297, 1998.

202. Hayashi M, Sasaki S, Tsuganezawa H, et al: Expression and distribution of aquaporin of collecting duct are regulated by vasopressin V2 receptor in rat kidney. J Clin Invest 94:1778–1783, 1994.

203. Saito T, Ishikawa SE, Sasaki S, et al: Alteration in water channel AQP-2 by removal of AVP stimulation in collecting duct cells of dehydrated rats. Am J Physiol 272:F183–F191, 1997.

204. Katsura T, Ausiello DA, Brown D: Direct demonstration of aquaporin-2 water channel recycling in stably transfected LLC-PK1 epithelial cells. Am J Physiol 270:F548–F553, 1996.

205. Pisitkun T, Shen RF, Knepper MA: Identification and proteomic profiling of exosomes in human urine. Proc Natl Acad Sci U S A 101:13368–13373, 2004.

206. Wen H, Frokiaer J, Kwon TH, et al: Urinary excretion of aquaporin-2 in rat is mediated by a vasopressin-dependent apical pathway. J Am Soc Nephrol 10:1416–1429, 1999.

207. Valenti G, Laera A, Gouraud S, et al: Low-calcium diet in hypercalciuric enuretic children restores AQP2 excretion and improves clinical symptoms. Am J Physiol Renal Physiol 283:F895–F903, 2002.

208. Zhang R, Logee K, Verkman AS: Expression of mRNA coding for kidney and red cell water channels in Xenopus oocytes. J Biol Chem 265:15375–15378, 1990.

209. Cheung KH, Leung CT, Leung GP, et al: Synergistic effects of cystic fibrosis transmembrane conductance regulator and aquaporin-9 in the rat epididymis. Biol Reprod 68:1505–1510, 2003.

210. Canfield MC, Tamarappoo BK, Moses AM, et al: Identification and characterization of aquaporin-2 water channel mutations causing nephrogenic diabetes insipidus with partial vasopressin response. Hum Mol Genet 6:1865–1871, 1997.

211. Deen PM, Verdijk MA, Knoers NV, et al: Requirement of human renal water channel aquaporin-2 for vasopressin- dependent concentration of urine. Science 264:92–95, 1994.

212. Kamsteeg EJ, Wormhoudt TA, Rijss JP, et al: An impaired routing of wild-type aquaporin-2 after tetramerization with an aquaporin-2 mutant explains dominant nephrogenic diabetes insipidus. EMBO J 18:2394–2400, 1999.

213. Verbavatz J-M, Brown D, Sabolic I, et al: Tetrameric assembly of CHIP28 water channels in liposomes and cell membranes: A freeze-fracture study. J Cell Biol 123:605–618, 1993.

214. Zeidel ML, Nielsen S, Smith BL, et al: Ultrastructure, pharmacologic inhibition, and transport selectivity of aquaporin channel-forming integral protein in proteoliposomes. Biochemistry 33:1606–1615, 1994.

215. Smith BL, Agre P: Erythrocyte Mr 28,000 transmembrane protein exists as a multisubunit oligomer similar to channel proteins. J Biol Chem 266:6407–6415, 1991.

216. de Groot BL, Heymann JB, Engel A, et al: The fold of human aquaporin 1. J Mol Biol 300:987–994, 2000.

217. Moller C, Fotiadis D, Suda K, et al: Determining molecular forces that stabilize human aquaporin-1. J Struct Biol 142:369–378, 2003.

218. Walz T, Tittmann P, Fuchs KH, et al: Surface topographies at subnanometer-resolution reveal asymmetry and sidedness of aquaporin-1. J Mol Biol 264:907–918, 1996.

219. Van Hoek AN, Yang B, Kirmiz S, et al: Freeze-fracture analysis of plasma membranes of CHO cells stably expressing aquaporins 1–5. J Membrane Biol 165:243–254, 1998.

220. Tamarappoo BK, Verkman AS: Defective aquaporin-2 trafficking in nephrogenic diabetes insipidus and correction by chemical chaperones. J Clin Invest 101:2257–2267, 1998.

221. Tamarappoo BK, Yang B, Verkman AS: Misfolding of mutant aquaporin-2 water channels in nephrogenic diabetes insipidus. J Biol Chem 274:34825–34831, 1999.

222. Furuno M, Uchida S, Marumo F, et al: Repressive regulation of the aquaporin-2 gene. Am J Physiol 271:F854–F860, 1996.

223. Katsura T, Verbavatz JM, Farinas J, et al: Constitutive and regulated membrane expression of aquaporin 1 and aquaporin 2 water channels in stably transfected LLC-PK1 epithelial cells. Proc Natl Acad Sci U S A 92:7212–7216, 1995.

224. Valenti G, Frigeri A, Ronco PM, et al: Expression and functional analysis of water channels in a stably AQP2- transfected human collecting duct cell line. J Biol Chem 271:24365–24370, 1996.

225. Deen PM, Rijss JP, Mulders SM, et al: Aquaporin-2 transfection of Madin-Darby canine kidney cells reconstitutes vasopressin-regulated transcellular osmotic water transport. J Am Soc Nephrol 8:1493–1501, 1997.

226. Maric K, Oksche A, Rosenthal W: Aquaporin-2 expression in primary cultured rat inner medullary collecting duct cells. Am J Physiol 275:F796–F801, 1998.

227. Deen PM, Nielsen S, Bindels RJ, et al: Apical and basolateral expression of aquaporin-1 in transfected MDCK and LLC-PK cells and functional evaluation of their transcellular osmotic water permeabilities. Pflugers Arch 433:780–787, 1997.

228. Bouley R, Breton S, Sun T, et al: Nitric oxide and atrial natriuretic factor stimulate cGMP-dependent membrane insertion of aquaporin 2 in renal epithelial cells. J Clin Invest 106:1115–1126, 2000.

229. Breton S, Brown D: Cold-induced microtubule disruption and relocalization of membrane proteins in kidney epithelial cells. J Am Soc Nephrol 9:155–166, 1998.

230. Shaw S, Marples D: A rat kidney tubule suspension for the study of vasopressin-induced shuttling of AQP2 water channels. Am J Physiol Renal Physiol 283:F1160–F1166, 2002.

231. Bens M, Vallet V, Cluzeaud F, et al: Corticosteroid-dependent sodium transport in a novel immortalized mouse collecting duct principal cell line. J Am Soc Nephrol 10:923–934, 1999.

232. Hasler U, Mordasini D, Bens M, et al: Long term regulation of aquaporin-2 expression in vasopressin-responsive renal collecting duct principal cells. J Biol Chem 277:10379–10386, 2002.

233. Hasler U, Jeon US, Kim JA, et al: Tonicity-responsive enhancer binding protein is an essential regulator of aquaporin-2 expression in renal collecting duct principal cells. J Am Soc Nephrol 17:1521–1531, 2006.

234. Christensen BM, Wang W, Frokiaer J, et al: Axial heterogeneity in basolateral AQP2 localization in rat kidney: Effect of vasopressin V2-receptor activation and deactivation. Am J Physiol Renal Physiol 284:F701–F717, 2003.

235. Coleman RA, Wu DC, Liu J, et al: Expression of aquaporins in the renal connecting tubule. Am J Physiol Renal Physiol 279:F874–F883, 2000.

236. Kim YH, Earm JH, Ma T, et al: Aquaporin-4 expression in adult and developing mouse and rat kidney. J Am Soc Nephrol 12:1795–1804, 2001.

237. Ma T, Song Y, Yang B, et al: Nephrogenic diabetes insipidus in mice lacking aquaporin-3 water channels. Proc Natl Acad Sci U S A 97:4386–4391, 2000.

238. Ma T, Yang B, Gillespie A, et al: Generation and phenotype of a transgenic knockout mouse lacking the mercurial-insensitive water channel aquaporin-4. J Clin Invest 100:957–962, 1997.

239. Chou CL, Ma T, Yang B, et al: Fourfold reduction of water permeability in inner medullary collecting duct of aquaporin-4 knockout mice. Am J Physiol 274:C549–C554, 1998.

240. Huang Y, Tracy R, Walsberg GE, et al: Absence of aquaporin-4 water channels from kidneys of the desert rodent Dipodomys merriami merriami. Am J Physiol Renal Physiol 280:F794–F802, 2001.

241. Nielsen J, Kwon TH, Praetorius J, et al: Aldosterone increases urine production and decreases apical AQP2 expression in rats with diabetes insipidus. Am J Physiol Renal Physiol 290:F438–F449, 2006.

242. Kamsteeg EJ, Bichet DG, Konings IB, et al: Reversed polarized delivery of an aquaporin-2 mutant causes dominant nephrogenic diabetes insipidus. J Cell Biol 163:1099–1109, 2003.

243. Yamashita Y, Hirai K, Katayama Y, et al: Mutations in sixth transmembrane domain of AQP2 inhibit its translocation induced by vasopression. Am J Physiol Renal Physiol 278:F395–F405, 2000.

244. Deen PM, Van Balkom BW, Savelkoul PJ, et al: Aquaporin-2: COOH terminus is necessary but not sufficient for routing to the apical membrane. Am J Physiol Renal Physiol 282:F330–F340, 2002.

245. Brown D, Orci L: Vasopressin stimulates formation of coated pits in rat kidney collecting ducts. Nature 302:253–255, 1983.

246. Brown D, Weyer P, Orci L: Vasopressin stimulates endocytosis in kidney collecting duct epithelial cells. Eur J Cell Biol 46:336–340, 1988.

247. Strange K, Willingham MC, Handler JS, et al: Apical membrane endocytosis via coated pits is stimulated by removal of antidiuretic hormone from isolated, perfused rabbit cortical collecting tubule. J Membr Biol 103:17–28, 1988.

248. Hinshaw JE: Dynamin and its role in membrane fission. Annu Rev Cell Dev Biol 16:483–519, 2000.

249. McNiven MA, Cao H, Pitts KR, et al: The dynamin family of mechanoenzymes: Pinching in new places. Trends Biochem Sci 25:115–120, 2000.

250. Sun TX, Van Hoek A, Huang Y, et al: Aquaporin-2 localization in clathrin-coated pits: Inhibition of endocytosis by dominant-negative dynamin. Am J Physiol Renal Physiol 282:F998–F1011, 2002.

251. Nielsen S, Terris J, Andersen D, et al: Congestive heart failure in rats is associated with increased expression and targeting of aquaporin-2 water channel in collecting duct. Proc Natl Acad Sci U S A 94:5450–5455, 1997.

252. Tajika Y, Matsuzaki T, Suzuki T, et al: Aquaporin-2 is retrieved to the apical storage compartment via early endosomes and phosphatidylinositol 3-kinase-dependent pathway. Endocrinology 145:4375–4383, 2004.

253. Procino G, Caces DB, Valenti G, et al: Adipocytes support cAMP-dependent translocation of aquaporin-2 from intracellular sites distinct from the insulin-responsive GLUT4 storage compartment. Am J Physiol Renal Physiol 290:F985–F994, 2006.

254. Gustafson CE, Katsura T, McKee M, et al: Recycling of aquaporin 2 occurs through a temperature- and bafilomycin-sensitive trans-Golgi-associated compartment in LLC-PK1 cells. Am J Physiol (Renal Physiology) 278:F317–F326, 1999.

255. Matlin KS, Simons K: Reduced temperature prevents transfer of a membrane glycoprotein to the cell surface but does not prevent terminal glycosylation. Cell 34:233–243, 1983.

256. Griffiths G, Simons K: The trans Golgi network: Sorting at the exit site of the Golgi complex. Science 234:438–443, 1986.

257. Futter CE, Gibson A, Allchin EH, et al: In polarized MDCK cells basolateral vesicles arise from clathrin-gamma- adaptin-coated domains on endosomal tubules. J Cell Biol 141:611–623, 1998.

258. Yamauchi K, Fushimi K, Yamashita Y, et al: Effects of missense mutations on rat aquaporin-2 in LLC-PK1 porcine kidney cells. Kidney Int 56:164–171, 1999.

259. Tajika Y, Matsuzaki T, Suzuki T, et al: Differential regulation of AQP2 trafficking in endosomes by microtubules and actin filaments. Histochem Cell Biol 124:1–12, 2005.

260. Bryant NJ, Govers R, James DE: Regulated transport of the glucose transporter GLUT4. Nat Rev Mol Cell Biol 3:267–277, 2002.

261. Jhun BH, Rampal AL, Liu H, et al: Effects of insulin on steady state kinetics of GLUT4 subcellular distribution in rat adipocytes. Evidence of constitutive GLUT4 recycling. J Biol Chem 267:17710–17715, 1992.

262. Martin S, Slot JW, James DE: GLUT4 trafficking in insulin-sensitive cells. A morphological review. Cell Biochem Biophys 30:89–113, 1999.

263. Knepper MA, Nielsen S: Kinetic model of water and urea permeability regulation by vasopressin in collecting duct. Am J Physiol 265:F214–F224, 1993.

264. Lu H, Sun TX, Bouley R, et al: Inhibition of endocytosis causes phosphorylation (S256)-independent plasma membrane accumulation of AQP2. Am J Physiol Renal Physiol 286:F233–F243, 2004.

265. Rodal SK, Skretting G, Garred O, et al: Extraction of cholesterol with methyl-beta-cyclodextrin perturbs formation of clathrin-coated endocytic vesicles. Mol Biol Cell 10:961–974, 1999.

266. Subtil A, Gaidarov I, Kobylarz K, et al: Acute cholesterol depletion inhibits clathrin-coated pit budding. Proc Natl Acad Sci U S A 96:6775–6780, 1999.

267. Russo LM, McKee M, Brown D: Methyl-beta-cyclodextrin induces vasopressin-independent apical accumulation of aquaporin-2 in the isolated, perfused rat kidney. Am J Physiol Renal Physiol 291:F246–F253, 2006.

268. Hoffert JD, Pisitkun T, Wang G, et al: Quantitative phosphoproteomics of vasopressin-sensitive renal cells: Regulation of aquaporin-2 phosphorylation at two sites. Proc Natl Acad Sci U S A 103:7159–7164, 2006.

269. Fushimi K, Sasaki S, Marumo F: Phosphorylation of serine 256 is required for cAMP-dependent regulatory exocytosis of the aquaporin-2 water channel. J Biol Chem 272:14800–14804, 1997.

270. Katsura T, Gustafson CE, Ausiello DA, et al: Protein kinase A phosphorylation is involved in regulated exocytosis of aquaporin-2 in transfected LLC-PK1 cells. Am J Physiol 272:F817–822, 1997.

271. Kuwahara M, Fushimi K, Terada Y, et al: cAMP-dependent phosphorylation stimulates water permeability of aquaporin-collecting duct water channel protein expressed in Xenopus oocytes. J Biol Chem 270:10384–10387, 1995.

272. Chaumont F, Moshelion M, Daniels MJ: Regulation of plant aquaporin activity. Biol Cell 97:749–764, 2005.

273. Maurel C, Javot H, Lauvergeat V, et al: Molecular physiology of aquaporins in plants. Int Rev Cytol 215:105–148, 2002.

274. Tornroth-Horsefield S, Wang Y, Hedfalk K, et al: Structural mechanism of plant aquaporin gating. Nature 439:688–694, 2006.

275. Peracchia C, Girsch SJ: Calmodulin site at the C-terminus of the putative lens gap junction protein MIP26. Lens Eye Toxic Res 6:613–621, 1989.

276. Anthony TL, Brooks HL, Boassa D, et al: Cloned human aquaporin-1 is a cyclic GMP-gated ion channel. Mol Pharmacol 57:576–588, 2000.

277. Han Z, Patil RV: Protein kinase A-dependent phosphorylation of aquaporin-1. Biochem Biophys Res Commun 273:328–332, 2000.

278. Yool AJ, Stamer WD, Regan JW: Forskolin stimulation of water and cation permeability in aquaporin 1 water channels. Science 273:1216–1218, 1996.

279. Agre P, Lee MD, Devidas S, et al: Aquaporins and ion conductance. Science 275:1490; discussion 1492, 1997.

280. Lande MB, Jo I, Zeidel ML, et al: Phosphorylation of aquaporin-2 does not alter the membrane water permeability of rat papillary water channel-containing vesicles. J Biol Chem 271:5552–5557, 1996.

281. Nishimoto G, Zelenina M, Li D, et al: Arginine vasopressin stimulates phosphorylation of aquaporin-2 in rat renal tissue. Am J Physiol 276:F254–F259, 1999.

282. Zelenina M, Christensen BM, Palmer J, et al: Prostaglandin E(2) interaction with AVP: Effects on AQP2 phosphorylation and distribution. Am J Physiol Renal Physiol 278:F388–F394, 2000.

283. de Mattia F, Savelkoul PJ, Kamsteeg EJ, et al: Lack of arginine vasopressin-induced phosphorylation of aquaporin-2 mutant AQP2-R254L explains dominant nephrogenic diabetes insipidus. J Am Soc Nephrol 16:2872–2880, 2005.

284. Klussmann E, Maric K, Wiesner B, et al: Protein kinase A anchoring proteins are required for vasopressin-mediated translocation of aquaporin-2 into cell membranes of renal principal cells. J Biol Chem 274:4934–4938, 1999.

285. Klussmann E, Rosenthal W: Role and identification of protein kinase A anchoring proteins in vasopressin-mediated aquaporin-2 translocation. Kidney Int 60:446–449, 2001.

286. Henn V, Edemir B, Stefan E, et al: Identification of a novel A-kinase anchoring protein 18 isoform and evidence for its role in the vasopressin-induced aquaporin-2 shuttle in renal principal cells. J Biol Chem 279:26654–26665, 2004.

287. Van Balkom BW, Savelkoul PJ, Markovich D, et al: The role of putative phosphorylation sites in the targeting and shuttling of the Aquaporin-2 water channel. J Biol Chem 277:41473–41479, 2002.

288. Nejsum LN, Zelenina M, Aperia A, et al: Bidirectional regulation of AQP2 trafficking and recycling: Involvement of AQP2-S256 phosphorylation. Am J Physiol Renal Physiol 288:F930–F938, 2005.

289. Valenti G, Procino G, Carmosino M, et al: The phosphatase inhibitor okadaic acid induces AQP2 translocation independently from AQP2 phosphorylation in renal collecting duct cells. J Cell Sci 113:1985–1992, 2000.

290. Procino G, Carmosino M, Marin O, et al: Ser-256 phosphorylation dynamics of Aquaporin 2 during maturation from the ER to the vesicular compartment in renal cells. FASEB J 17:1886–1888, 2003.

291. Brown D, Cunningham C, Hartwig J, et al: Association of AQP2 with actin in transfected LLC-PK1 cells and rat papilla. J Am Soc Nephrol 7:1265a, 1996.

292. Noda Y, Horikawa S, Katayama Y, et al: Water channel aquaporin-2 directly binds to actin. Biochem Biophys Res Commun 322:740–745, 2004.

293. Hays RM, Condeelis J, Gao Y, et al: The effect of vasopressin on the cytoskeleton of the epithelial cell. Pediatr Nephrol 7:672–679, 1993.

294. Hays RM, Ding GH, Franki N: Morphological aspects of the action of ADH. Kidney Int Suppl 21:S51–S55, 1987.

295. Klussmann E, Tamma G, Lorenz D, et al: An inhibitory role of Rho in the vasopressin-mediated translocation of aquaporin-2 into cell membranes of renal principal cells. J Biol Chem 276:20451–20457, 2001.

296. Tamma G, Klussmann E, Maric K, et al: Rho inhibits cAMP-induced translocation of aquaporin-2 into the apical membrane of renal cells. Am J Physiol Renal Physiol 281:F1092–F1101, 2001.

297. DeSousa RC, Grosso A, Rufener C: Blockade of the hydrosmotic effect of vasopressin by cytochalasin B. Experientia 30:175–177, 1974.

298. Iyengar R, Lepper KG, Mailman DS: Involvement of microtubules and microfilaments in the action of vasopressing in canine renal medulla. J Supramol Struct 5:521(373)–530(382), 1976.

299. Kachadorian WA, Ellis SJ, Muller J: Possible roles for microtubules and microfilaments in ADH action on toad urinary bladder. Am J Physiol 236:F14–F20, 1979.

300. Taylor A, Mamelak M, Reaven E, et al: Vasopressin: Possible role of microtubules and microfilaments in its action. Science 181:347–350, 1973.

301. Ridley AJ: Rho proteins: Linking signaling with membrane trafficking. Traffic 2:303–310, 2001.

302. Gottlieb TA, Ivanov IE, Adesnik M, et al: Actin microfilaments play a critical role in endocytosis at the apical but not the basolateral surface of polarized epithelial cells. J Cell Biol 120:695–710, 1993.

303. Hyman T, Shmuel M, Altschuler Y: Actin is required for endocytosis at the apical surface of Madin-Darby canine kidney cells where ARF6 and clathrin regulate the actin cytoskeleton. Mol Biol Cell 17:427–437, 2006.

304. Leung SM, Rojas R, Maples C, et al: Modulation of endocytic traffic in polarized Madin-Darby canine kidney cells by the small GTPase RhoA. Mol Biol Cell 10:4369–4384, 1999.

305. Bi GQ, Morris RL, Liao G, et al: Kinesin- and myosin-driven steps of vesicle recruitment for Ca²⁺-regulated exocytosis. J Cell Biol 138:999–1008, 1997.

306. Rogers SL, Gelfand VI: Myosin cooperates with microtubule motors during organelle transport in melanophores. Curr Biol 8:161–164, 1998.

307. Barile M, Pisitkun T, Yu MJ, et al: Large scale protein identification in intracellular aquaporin-2 vesicles from renal inner medullary collecting duct. Mol Cell Proteomics 4:1095–1106, 2005.

308. Marples D, Smith J, Nielsen S: Myosin-I is associated with AQP-2 water channel bearing vesicles in rat kidney and may be involved in the antidiuretic response to vasopressin. J Am Soc Nephrol 8:62a, 1997.

309. Chou CL, Christensen BM, Frische S, et al: Non-muscle myosin II and myosin light chain kinase are downstream targets for vasopressin signaling in the renal collecting duct. J Biol Chem 279:49026–49035, 2004.

310. Yip KP: Epac mediated Ca²⁺ mobilization and exocytosis in inner medullary collecting duct. Am J Physiol Renal Physiol, 2006.

311. Lorenz D, Krylov A, Hahm D, et al: Cyclic AMP is sufficient for triggering the exocytic recruitment of aquaporin-2 in renal epithelial cells. EMBO Rep 4:88–93, 2003.

312. Noda Y, Horikawa S, Katayama Y, et al: Identification of a multiprotein "motor" complex binding to water channel aquaporin-2. Biochem Biophys Res Commun 330:1041–1047, 2005.

313. Lueck A, Brown D, Kwiatkowski DJ: The actin-binding proteins adseverin and gelsolin are both highly expressed but differentially localized in kidney and intestine. J Cell Sci 111:3633–3643, 1998.

314. Tamma G, Klussmann E, Oehlke J, et al: Actin remodeling requires ERM function to facilitate AQP2 apical targeting. J Cell Sci 118:3623–3630, 2005.

315. Noda Y, Horikawa S, Furukawa T, et al: Aquaporin-2 trafficking is regulated by PDZ-domain containing protein SPA-1. FEBS Lett 568:139–145, 2004.

316. Allan VJ, Schroer TA: Membrane motors. Curr Opin Cell Biol 11:476–482, 1999.

317. Schroer TA, Sheetz MP: Functions of microtubule-based motors. Annu Rev Physiol 53:629–652, 1991.

318. Vale RD: Intracellular transport using microtubule-based motors. Annu Rev Cell Biol 3:347–378, 1987.

319. Dousa TP, Barnes LD: Effects of colchicine and vinblastine on the cellular action of vasopressin in mammalian kidney. A possible role of microtubules. J Clin Invest 54:252–262, 1974.

320. Phillips ME, Taylor A: Effect of nocodazole on the water permeability response to vasopressin in rabbit collecting tubules perfused in vitro. J Physiol (Lond) 411:529–544, 1989.

321. Taylor A, Mamelak M, Golbetz H, et al: Evidence for involvement of microtubules in the action of vasopressin in toad urinary bladder. I. Functional studies on the effects of antimitotic agents on the response to vasopressin. J Membr Biol 40:213–235, 1978.

322. Valenti G, Hugon JS, Bourguet J: To what extent is microtubular network involved in antidiuretic response? Am J Physiol 255:F1098–F1106, 1988.

323. Pfister KK, Fisher EM, Gibbons IR, et al: Cytoplasmic dynein nomenclature. J Cell Biol 171:411–413, 2005.

324. Lawrence CJ, Dawe RK, Christie KR, et al: A standardized kinesin nomenclature. J Cell Biol 167:19–22, 2004.

325. Brown CL, Maier KC, Stauber T, et al: Kinesin-2 is a motor for late endosomes and lysosomes. Traffic 6:1114–1124, 2005.

326. Levi V, Serpinskaya AS, Gratton E, et al: Organelle transport along microtubules in Xenopus melanophores: Evidence for cooperation between multiple motors. Biophys J 90:318–327, 2006.

327. Reilein AR, Rogers SL, Tuma MC, et al: Regulation of molecular motor proteins. Int Rev Cytol 204:179–238, 2001.

328. Marples D, Schroer TA, Ahrens N, et al: Dynein and dynactin colocalize with AQP2 water channels in intracellular vesicles from kidney collecting duct. Am J Physiol 274:F384–F394, 1998.

329. Marples D, Barber B, Taylor A: Effect of a dynein inhibitor on vasopressin action in toad urinary bladder. J Physiol 490 (Pt 3):767–774, 1996.

330. Rogers SL, Gelfand VI: Membrane trafficking, organelle transport, and the cytoskeleton. Curr Opin Cell Biol 12:57–62, 2000.

331. Vale RD, Milligan RA: The way things move: Looking under the hood of molecular motor proteins. Science 288:88–95, 2000.

332. Wu X, Xiang X, Hammer JA, 3rd: Motor proteins at the microtubule plus-end. Trends Cell Biol 16:135–143, 2006.

333. Hays RM, Franki N, Simon H, et al: Antidiuretic hormone and exocytosis: lessons from neurosecretion. Am J Physiol 267:C1507–C1524, 1994.

334. Mandon B, Chou CL, Nielsen S, et al: Syntaxin-4 is localized to the apical plasma membrane of rat renal collecting duct cells: possible role in aquaporin-2 trafficking. J Clin Invest 98:906–913, 1996.

335. Mandon B, Nielsen S, Kishore BK, et al: Expression of syntaxins in rat kidney. Am J Physiol 273:F718–F730, 1997.

336. Nielsen S, Marples D, Birn H, et al: Expression of VAMP-2-like protein in kidney collecting duct intracellular vesicles. Colocalization with Aquaporin-2 water channels. J Clin Invest 96:1834–1844, 1995.

337. Mayer A: Intracellular membrane fusion: SNAREs only? Curr Opin Cell Biol 11:447–452, 1999.

338. Rothman JE, Sollner TH: Throttles and dampers: Controlling the engine of membrane fusion. Science 276:1212–1213, 1997.

339. Rothman JE, Warren G: Implications of the SNARE hypothesis for intracellular membrane topology and dynamics. Curr Biol 4:220–233, 1994.

340. Scheller RH: Membrane trafficking in the presynaptic nerve terminal. Neuron 14:893–897, 1995.

341. Weber T, Zemelman BV, McNew JA, et al: SNAREpins: Minimal machinery for membrane fusion. Cell 92:759–772, 1998.

342. Sollner T, Whiteheart SW, Brunner M, et al: SNAP receptors implicated in vesicle targeting and fusion. Nature 362:318–324, 1993.

343. Inoue T, Nielsen S, Mandon B, et al: SNAP-23 in rat kidney: Colocalization with aquaporin-2 in collecting duct vesicles. Am J Physiol 275:F752–F760, 1998.

344. Shukla A, Hager H, Corydon TJ, et al: SNAP-25-associated Hrs-2 protein colocalizes with AQP2 in rat kidney collecting duct principal cells. Am J Physiol Renal Physiol 281:F546–F556, 2001.

345. Liebenhoff U, Rosenthal W: Identification of Rab3-, Rab5a- and synaptobrevin II-like proteins in a preparation of rat kidney vesicles containing the vasopressin-regulated water channel. FEBS Lett 365:209–213, 1995.

346. Franki N, Macaluso F, Schubert W, et al: Water channel-carrying vesicles in the rat IMCD contain cellubrevin. Am J Physiol 269:C797–C801, 1995.

347. Gouraud S, Laera A, Calamita G, et al: Functional involvement of VAMP/synaptobrevin-2 in cAMP-stimulated aquaporin 2 translocation in renal collecting duct cells. J Cell Sci 115:3667–3674, 2002.

348. Breton S, Nsumu NN, Galli T, et al: Tetanus toxin-mediated cleavage of cellubrevin inhibits proton secretion in the male reproductive tract. Am J Physiol Renal Physiol 278:F717–F725, 2000.

349. Wang W, Li C, Nejsum LN, et al: Biphasic effects of ANP infusion in conscious, euvolumic rats: Roles of AQP2 and ENaC trafficking. Am J Physiol Renal Physiol 290:F530–F541, 2006.

350. Bouley R, Pastor-Soler N, Cohen O, et al: Stimulation of AQP2 membrane insertion in renal epithelial cells in vitro and in vivo by the cGMP phosphodiesterase inhibitor sildenafil citrate (Viagra). Am J Physiol Renal Physiol 288:F1103–F1112, 2005.

351. Macia E, Ehrlich M, Massol R, et al: Dynasore, a cell-permeable inhibitor of dynamin. Dev Cell 10:839–850, 2006.

352. Jones RVH, DeWardener HF: Urine concentration after fluid deprivation or pitressin tannate in oil. Brit Med J 1:271–274, 1956.

353. Lankford SP, Chou CL, Terada Y, et al: Regulation of collecting duct water permeability independent of cAMP-mediated AVP response. Am J Physiol 261:F554–F566, 1991.

354. DiGiovanni SR, Nielsen S, Christensen EI, et al: Regulation of collecting duct water channel expression by vasopressin in Brattleboro rat. Proc Natl Acad Sci U S A 91:8984–8988, 1994.

355. Ecelbarger CA, Chou CL, Lolait SJ, et al: Evidence for dual signaling pathways for V2 vasopressin receptor in rat inner medullary collecting duct. Am J Physiol 270:F623–F633, 1996.

356. Hayashi M, Sasaki S, Tsuganezawa H, et al: Role of vasopressin V2 receptor in acute regulation of aquaporin-2. Kidney Blood Press Res 19:32–37, 1996.

357. Marples D, Christensen BM, Frokiaer J, et al: Dehydration reverses vasopressin antagonist-induced diuresis and aquaporin-2 downregulation in rats. Am J Physiol 275:F400–F409, 1998.

358. Terris J, Ecelbarger CA, Nielsen S, et al: Long-term regulation of four renal aquaporins in rats. Am J Physiol 271:F414–F422, 1996.

359. Marr N, Kamsteeg EJ, van Raak M, et al: Functionality of aquaporin-2 missense mutants in recessive nephrogenic diabetes insipidus. Pflugers Arch 442:73–77, 2001.

360. van Lieburg AF, Verdijk MA, Knoers VV, et al: Patients with autosomal nephrogenic diabetes insipidus homozygous for mutations in the aquaporin 2 water-channel gene. Am J Hum Genet 55:648–652, 1994.

361. Deen PM, Croes H, van Aubel RA, et al: Water channels encoded by mutant aquaporin-2 genes in nephrogenic diabetes insipidus are impaired in their cellular routing. J Clin Invest 95:2291–2296, 1995.

362. Bai L, Fushimi K, Sasaki S, et al: Structure of aquaporin-2 vasopressin water channel. J Biol Chem 271:5171–5176, 1996.

363. Kwon TH, Laursen UH, Marples D, et al: Altered expression of renal AQPs and Na(+) transporters in rats with lithium-induced NDI. Am J Physiol Renal Physiol 279:F552–F564, 2000.

364. Marples D, Christensen S, Christensen EI, et al: Lithium-induced downregulation of aquaporin-2 water channel expression in rat kidney medulla. J Clin Invest 95:1838–1845, 1995.

365. Hozawa S, Holtzman EJ, Ausiello DA: cAMP motifs regulating transcription in the aquaporin 2 gene. Am J Physiol 270:C1695–C1702, 1996.

366. Matsumura Y, Uchida S, Rai T, et al: Transcriptional regulation of aquaporin-2 water channel gene by cAMP. J Am Soc Nephrol 8:861–867, 1997.

367. Frokiaer J, Marples D, Valtin H, et al: Low aquaporin-2 levels in polyuric DI +/+ severe mice with constitutively high cAMP-phosphodiesterase activity. Am J Physiol 276:F179–F190, 1999.

368. Li Y, Shaw S, Kamsteeg EJ, et al: Development of lithium-induced nephrogenic diabetes insipidus is dissociated from adenylyl cyclase activity. J Am Soc Nephrol 17:1063–1072, 2006.

369. Christensen BM, Marples D, Wang W, et al: Decreased fraction of principal cells in parallel with increased fraction of intercalated cells in rats with lithium-induced NDI. J Am Soc Nephrol 13:270A, 2002.

370. Bagnis C, Marshansky V, Breton S, et al: Remodeling the cellular profile of collecting ducts by chronic carbonic anhydrase inhibition. Am J Physiol Renal Physiol 280:F437–F448, 2001.

371. Timmer RT, Sands JM: Lithium intoxication. J Am Soc Nephrol 10:666–674, 1999.

372. Thomsen K, Bak M, Shirley DG: Chronic lithium treatment inhibits amiloride-sensitive sodium transport in the rat distal nephron. J Pharmacol Exp Ther 289:443–447, 1999.

373. Nielsen J, Kwon TH, Toftgaard A, et al: Regulation of ENaC in Rats with Lithium Induced Nephrogenic Diabetes Insipidus. J Am Soc Nephrol 13:278A, 2002.

374. Feuerstein G, Zilberman Y, Hemmendinger R, et al: Attenuation of the lithium-induced diabetes-insipidus-like syndrome by amiloride in rats. Neuropsychobiology 7:67–73, 1981.

375. Batlle DC, von Riotte AB, Gaviria M, et al: Amelioration of polyuria by amiloride in patients receiving long-term lithium therapy. N Engl J Med 312:408–414, 1985.

376. Kosten TR, Forrest JN: Treatment of severe lithium-induced polyuria with amiloride. Am J Psychiatry 143:1563–1568, 1986.

377. Marples D, Frokiaer J, Dorup J, et al: Hypokalemia-induced downregulation of aquaporin-2 water channel expression in rat kidney medulla and cortex. J Clin Invest 97:1960–1968, 1996.

378. Sands JM, Flores FX, Kato A, et al: Vasopressin-elicited water and urea permeabilities are altered in IMCD in hypercalcemic rats. Am J Physiol 274:F978–F985, 1998.

379. Wang W, Li C, Kwon TH, et al: AQP3, p-AQP2, and AQP2 expression is reduced in polyuric rats with hypercalcemia: Prevention by cAMP-PDE inhibitors. Am J Physiol Renal Physiol 283:F1313–F1325, 2002.

380. Wang XY, Beutler K, Nielsen J, et al: Decreased abundance of collecting duct urea transporters UT-A1 and UT-A3 with ECF volume expansion. Am J Physiol Renal Physiol 282:F577–F584, 2002.

381. Frokiaer J, Christensen BM, Marples D, et al: Downregulation of aquaporin-2 parallels changes in renal water excretion in unilateral ureteral obstruction. Am J Physiol 273:F213–F223, 1997.

382. Frokiaer J, Marples D, Knepper MA, et al: Bilateral ureteral obstruction downregulates expression of vasopressin- sensitive AQP-2 water channel in rat kidney. Am J Physiol 270:F657–F668, 1996.

383. Li C, Wang W, Kwon TH, et al: Downregulation of AQP1, -2, and -3 after ureteral obstruction is associated with a long-term urine-concentrating defect. Am J Physiol Renal Physiol 281:F163–F171, 2001.

384. Li C, Wang W, Kwon TH, et al: Altered expression of major renal Na transporters in rats with unilateral ureteral obstruction. Am J Physiol Renal Physiol 284:F155–F166, 2003.

385. Li C, Wang W, Kwon TH, et al: Alpha-MSH treatment prevents downregulation of AQP1, AQP2 and AQP3 expression in rats with bilateral ureteral obstruction. J Am Soc Nephrol 13:272A, 2002.

386. Norregaard R, Jensen BL, Li C, et al: COX-2 inhibition prevents downregulation of key renal water and sodium transport proteins in response to bilateral ureteral obstruction. Am J Physiol Renal Physiol 289:F322–F333, 2005.

387. Fujita N, Ishikawa SE, Sasaki S, et al: Role of water channel AQP-CD in water retention in SIADH and cirrhotic rats. Am J Physiol 269:F926–F931, 1995.

388. Ishikawa SE, Schrier RW: Pathophysiological roles of arginine vasopressin and aquaporin-2 in impaired water excretion. Clin Endocrinol (Oxf) 58:1–17, 2003.

389. Johansson I, Karlsson M, Shukla VK, et al: Water transport activity of the plasma membrane aquaporin PM28A is regulated by phosphorylation. Plant Cell 10:451–459, 1998.

390. Xu DL, Martin PY, Ohara M, et al: Upregulation of aquaporin-2 water channel expression in chronic heart failure rat. J Clin Invest 99:1500–1505, 1997.

391. Ecelbarger CA, Nielsen S, Olson BR, et al: Role of renal aquaporins in escape from vasopressin-induced antidiuresis in rat. J Clin Invest 99:1852–1863, 1997.

392. Staahltoft D, Nielsen S, Janjua NR, et al: Losartan treatment normalizes renal sodium and water handling in rats with mild congestive heart failure. Am J Physiol Renal Physiol 282:F307–F315, 2002.

393. Apostol E, Ecelbarger CA, Terris J, et al: Reduced renal medullary water channel expression in puromycin aminonucleoside–induced nephrotic syndrome. J Am Soc Nephrol 8:15–24, 1997.

394. Fernandez-Llama P, Andrews P, Nielsen S, et al: Impaired aquaporin and urea transporter expression in rats with adriamycin-induced nephrotic syndrome. Kidney Int 53:1244–1253, 1998.

395. Sands JM, Naruse M, Jacobs JD, et al: Changes in aquaporin-2 protein contribute to the urine concentrating defect in rats fed a low-protein diet. J Clin Invest 97:2807–2814, 1996.

396. Kwon TH, Frokiaer J, Knepper MA, et al: Reduced AQP1, -2, and -3 levels in kidneys of rats with CRF induced by surgical reduction in renal mass. Am J Physiol 275:F724–F741, 1998.

397. Kwon TH, Frokiaer J, Fernandez-Llama P, et al: Reduced abundance of aquaporins in rats with bilateral ischemia-induced acute renal failure: prevention by alpha-MSH. Am J Physiol 277:F413–F427, 1999.

398. Nejsum LN, Kwon TH, Marples D, et al: Compensatory increase in AQP2, p-AQP2, and AQP3 expression in rats with diabetes mellitus. Am J Physiol Renal Physiol 280:F715–F726, 2001.

399. Brown D: Imaging protein trafficking. Nephron Exp Nephrol 103:e55–e61, 2006.

CHAPTER 9

Urine Concentration and Dilution

Mark A. Knepper • Jason D. Hoffert • Randall K. Packer • Robert A. Fenton

THE KIDNEY CAN REGULATE WATER EXCRETION WITHOUT LARGE CHANGES IN SOLUTE EXCRETION

The tonicity of body fluids is controlled predominantly through the regulation of renal water excretion. The kidney also carries out several other homeostatic functions, including regulation of extracellular fluid volume (through control of NaCl excretion), regulation of systemic acid-base balance (through control of net acid excretion), regulation of systemic K balance (through the control of K^+ excretion), and maintenance of nitrogen balance (through excretion of urea). Water excretion and the excretion of individual solutes must be regulated independently to allow all of the homeostatic functions of the kidney to be performed simultaneously. Thus, when water intake changes in the absence of changes in solute intake or of changes in metabolic production of waste solutes, the kidney can excrete the appropriate amount of water without marked perturbations in solute excretion (i.e., without disturbing the other homeostatic functions of the kidney). This phenomenon, shown in Figure 9–1, occurs as a result of operation of the renal concentrating and diluting mechanism, the focus of this chapter.

Figure 9–1 highlights several important features of the concentrating and diluting mechanism viewed from the perspective of whole-kidney function. The major effector in the regulation of renal water excretion is the antidiuretic hormone vasopressin. Vasopressin is a peptide hormone secreted into the peripheral plasma by the posterior pituitary gland (see Chapter 8). As shown in the upper panel of Figure 9–1, the kidney is capable of wide variations in water excretion (i.e., urine flow) in response to changing levels of vasopressin in the peripheral plasma. Water excretion is typically more than 100-fold lower in extreme antidiuresis (high vasopressin level) than in extreme water diuresis (low vasopressin level). These large changes in water excretion are achieved without substantial changes in the steady-state rate of total solute excretion (measured as osmolar clearance). As shown in the bottom panel of Figure 9–1, this behavior is dependent on the ability of the kidney to concentrate and dilute the urine. When water excretion is rapid because of a low circulating vasopressin level, the urine is diluted to an osmolality less than that of plasma (290 mOsm/kg H_2O). When water excretion is low because of a high circulating vasopressin level, the urine is concentrated to an osmolality much higher than that of plasma.

Under normal circumstances, the circulating vasopressin level is determined by osmoreceptors in the hypothalamus that trigger increases in vasopressin secretion (by the posterior pituitary gland) when the osmolality of the blood rises above a threshold value, about 292 mOsm/kg H_2O. This mechanism can be subverted when other inputs to the hypothalamus (e.g., associated with arterial underfilling, severe fatigue, or physical stress) override this osmotic mechanism. Such non-osmotic stimuli, coupled with continued water intake, explain the hyponatremia that occurs in severe congestive heart failure and cirrhosis.[1] Similar circumstances (stress induced vasopressin secretion coupled with continued water intake) are believed to be responsible for the hyponatremia seen in marathon runners[2] and for the high incidence of hyponatremia seen in Coalition troops during the 2003 invasion of Iraq.[3]

A PARALLEL ORGANIZATION OF STRUCTURES IN THE RENAL MEDULLA IS CRITICAL TO URINARY CONCENTRATING AND DILUTING PROCESS

The ability of the kidney to vary water excretion over a broad range, without altering steady-state solute excretion, would not be predicted from simple consideration of sequential transport processes along the nephron.[4] Urine concentration and dilution cannot be explained by simple models based on the sequential action of several nephron segments. Instead, it is necessary to consider the parallel interactions between nephron segments that result from its folded or looped structure (see Chapter 2). An understanding of these interactions depends on knowledge of the regional architecture of the renal medulla and medullary rays illustrated in Figure 9–2. The nomenclature used for the various renal tubule segments is summarized in Table 9–1. Except where indicated, we follow the terminology recommended by Kriz and Bankir[5] on behalf of the Renal Commission of the International Union of Physiological Sciences.

Renal Tubules

Loops of Henle

Two populations of nephrons merge to form a common collecting duct system (see Fig. 9–2). One population (short-looped

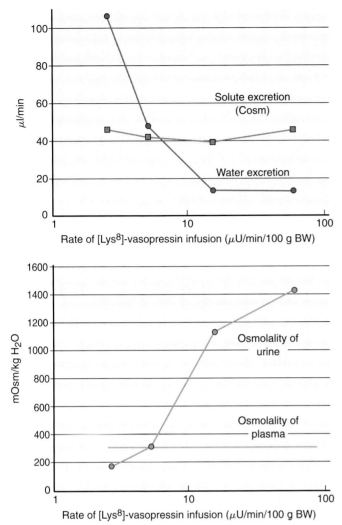

FIGURE 9–1 Steady-state renal response to varying rates of vasopressin infusion in conscious rats.[212] A water load (4% of body weight) was maintained throughout the experiments to suppress endogenous vasopressin secretion. Although the urine flow rate was markedly reduced at higher vasopressin infusion rates, the osmolar clearance changed little. (Data from Atherton JC, Green R, Thomas S: Influence of lysine-vasopressin dosage on the time course of changes in renal tissue and urinary composition in the conscious rat. J Physiol 213:291–309, 1971.)

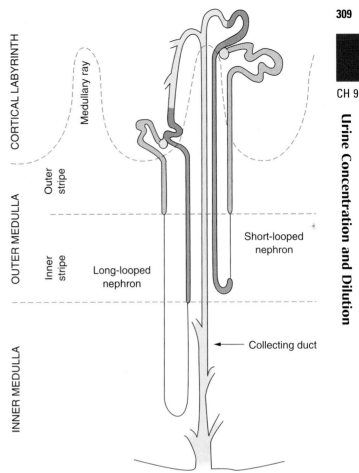

FIGURE 9–2 Mammalian renal structure.[81] Major regions of the kidney are shown on the left. Configurations of a long-looped and a short-looped nephron are depicted. The major portions of the nephron are proximal tubules (medium blue), thin limbs of loops of Henle (single line), thick ascending limbs of loops of Henle (green), distal convoluted tubules (lavender), and the collecting duct system (yellow). (Modified from Knepper MA, Stephenson JL: Urinary concentrating and diluting processes. In Andreoli TE, Fanestil DD, Hoffman JF, Schultz SG (eds): Physiology of Membrane Disorders, 2nd ed. New York, Plenum, 1986, pp 713–726.)

nephrons) has loops that bend in the outer medulla. The other population (long-looped nephrons) has loops that bend at various levels of the inner medulla. Figure 9–3 shows three examples of long loops of Henle in mouse as traced using computer reconstruction techniques from serial histological sections through the kidney, providing a realistic view of the course of individual tubules. In rats, more than 70% of long loops of Henle bend in the outer half of the inner medulla, and progressively fewer loops extend to deeper levels of the inner medulla. The loops of Henle receive the effluent from the proximal convoluted tubules. They carry tubule fluid into and out of the renal medulla, establishing countercurrent flow between the two limbs of the hairpin loop as emphasized in Figure 9–3.

Several discrete nephron segments compose the loop of Henle (see Figs. 9–2 and 9–3, and Table 9–1). In Figure 9–3, proximal tubule segments are depicted as blue-green and thin limbs of Henle are depicted as green. The descending part of the loop consists of the S_2 proximal straight tubules in the medullary rays, the S_3 proximal straight tubule in the outer

stripe of the outer medulla, and the thin descending limbs in the inner stripe of the outer medulla and the inner medulla. The descending thin limbs of short loops of Henle (SDL) differ structurally and functionally from the descending thin limbs of long loops of Henle (LDL).[6] The SDLs are not depicted in Figure 9–3 but their arrangement in the renal outer medulla is illustrated in Figure 9–4 (labeled in green). As can be seen, the SDLs tend to be organized in a ring-like pattern surrounding the vascular bundles of the outer medulla (Fig. 9–4, inset). Long-looped descending limbs in the outer medulla (LDL$_{OM}$) differ morphologically and functionally from long-looped descending limbs in the inner medulla (LDL$_{IM}$).[7-10] The transition from the LDL$_{OM}$ to the LDL$_{IM}$ is gradual; it often occurs a considerable distance into the inner medulla. Figure 9–5 shows a computerized reconstruction of the inner medullary portions of several long loops of Henle from rats featuring labeling with antibodies to aquaporin-1 (AQP1) and the ClC-K1 chloride channel.[11] AQP1, a marker of the LDL$_{OM}$ in the outer medulla, is present in LDLs for a variable distance into the inner medulla. ClC-K1 labeling, marking the thin ascending limb-type epithelium, is first seen at variable distances before the loop bends, consistent with many morphological studies that have demonstrated that the DL-to-AL transition

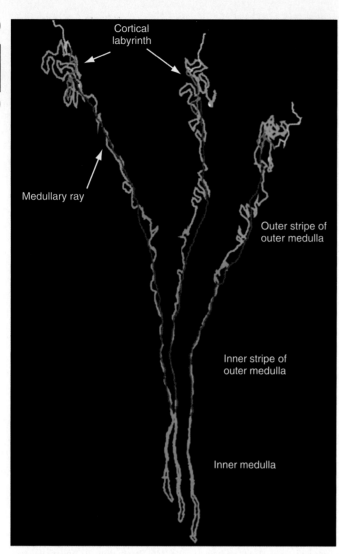

FIGURE 9–3 The courses of three long-loop nephrons from mouse as determined by computer reconstruction from histological images. Color codes: proximal tubule segments, blue-green; thin limbs segments, green; thick ascending limb segments, red; distal convoluted tubule, purple; connecting tubules, yellow. (From Zhai XY, Thomsen JS, Birn H, et al: Three-dimensional reconstruction of the mouse nephron. J Am Soc Nephrol 17:77–88, 2006.)

TABLE 9–1	Nomenclature for Renal Tubule Segments*		
Major Segment	**Subsegment**	**Abbreviation**	**Region of Kidney**
Proximal convoluted tubule	Early proximal convolution Cortical labyrinth	PCT(S$_1$)	Cortical labyrinth Late proximal convolution PCT(S$_2$)
Loop of Henle	Early proximal straight	PST(S$_2$)	Medullary rays
	Late proximal straight	PST(S$_3$)	Outer medulla (outer stripe)
	Descending thin limb of short loops	SDL	Outer medulla (inner stripe)
	Descending thin limb of long loops, outer medulla	LDL$_{OM}$	Outer medulla (inner stripe)
	Descending thin limb of long loops, inner medulla	LDL$_{IM}$	Inner medulla
	Ascending thin limb	ATL	Inner medulla
	Medullary thick ascending limb	MTAL	Outer medulla
	Cortical thick ascending limb	CTAL	Medullary rays
Distal	Distal convoluted tubule	DCT	Cortical labyrinth
	Connecting tubule	CNT	Cortical labyrinth
Collecting ducts	Initial collecting tubule	ICT	Cortical labyrinth
	Cortical collecting duct	CCD	Medullary rays
	Outer medullary collecting duct, outer stripe	OMCD-OS	Outer medulla
	Outer medullary collecting duct, inner stripe	OMCD-IS	Outer medulla
	Inner medullary collecting duct, initial part	IMCD$_i$	Inner medulla (base)
	Inner medullary collecting duct, terminal part	IMCD$_t$	Inner medulla (papilla)

*Terminology is based on that proposed by the Renal Commission of the International Union of Physiological Sciences[5] with two exceptions: (1) Terminology for descending thin limb subsegments based on that proposed by Imai and colleagues[6] is used because it is more literally descriptive of the locations and topography of the segments; (2) Expanded terminology for the inner medullary collecting duct is based on studies[53,218] demonstrating two distinct inner medullary collecting duct subsegments.

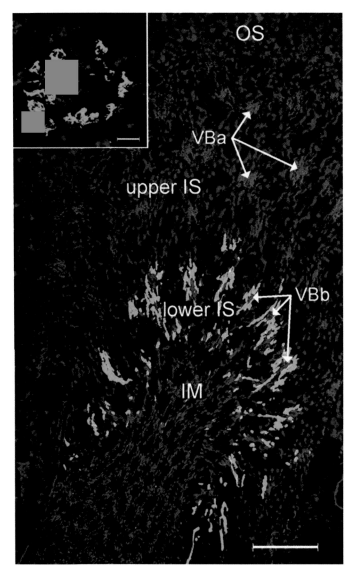

FIGURE 9–4 Triple immunolabeling of rat renal medulla showing localization of UT-A2 (green) marking late SDL segments, von Willebrand factor (blue) marking endothelial cells of vasa recta, and aquaporin-1 (red) marking LDL_{OM} segments and early SDL segments. Inset shows a cross section of a vascular bundle demonstrating that UT-A2 positive SDL segments surround the vascular bundles in the deep part of the outer medulla. Labels in this diagram: IM, inner medulla; IS, inner stripe of outer medulla; OS, outer stripe of outer medulla; VBa, vascular bundles in outer part of inner stripe; VBb, vascular bundles in inner part of inner stripe. (From Wade JB, Lee AJ, Liu J, et al: UTA-2: A 55 kDa urea transporter in thin descending limb whose abundance is regulated by vasopressin. Am J Physiol 278:F52–F62, 2000.)

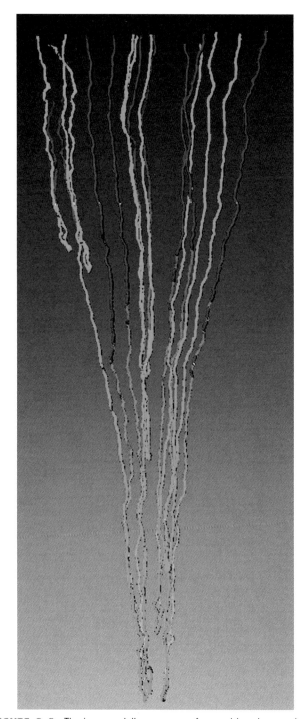

FIGURE 9–5 The inner medullary courses of several long-loop nephrons from rat as determined by computer reconstruction from immunolabeled histological sections. Colors: aquaporin-1, red; ClC-K1, green; no labeling, light blue. (From Pannabecker TL, Abbott DE, Dantzler WH: Three-dimensional functional reconstruction of inner medullary thin limbs of Henle's loop. Am J Physiol Renal Physiol 286:F38–F45, 2004 and Zhai XY, Thomsen JS, Birn H, et al: Three-dimensional reconstruction of the mouse nephron. J Am Soc Nephrol 17:77–88, 2006.)

occurs before the loop bend. A substantial portion of the inner medullary LDL (presumably the LDL_{IM}) did not express either AQP1 or ClC-K1. Overall, the ascending part of the loop of Henle consists of the ascending thin limbs (which are present only in long loops), the medullary thick ascending limbs in the inner stripe of the outer medulla, and the cortical thick ascending limbs in the medullary rays. (Medullary and cortical thick ascending limbs are shown in red in Figure 9–3.)

Distal Tubule Segments in the Cortical Labyrinth

After exiting the loop of Henle, tubule fluid enters the distal convoluted tubules in the cortical labyrinth (violet tubules in Fig. 9–3). Several distal tubules merge to form a connecting tubule arcade in most mammalian species. (Connecting tubules are depicted as yellow in Figure 9–3.) The arcades ascend upward through the cortical labyrinth in association with the interlobular arteries and veins.[12] The connecting tubule cells of the arcades express both aquaporin-2 (the vasopressin-regulated water channel) and the vasopressin V_2-subtype receptor,[13] suggesting that, like the collecting ducts, the arcades are sites of regulated water absorption (see later). The arcades deliver their tubule fluid to initial collecting tubules in the superficial cortex and finally to the cortical collecting ducts. In rats and rabbits, five or six nephrons combine to form a single cortical collecting duct.[14] In mice, six to seven nephrons merge to form a single collecting duct.[15]

Collecting Duct System

The collecting duct system spans all the regions of the kidney between the superficial cortex and the tip of the inner medulla (see Fig. 9–2). The collecting ducts are arrayed parallel to the loops of Henle in the medulla and medullary rays. Like the loop of Henle, the collecting duct system is composed of several morphologically and functionally discrete tubule segments (see Table 9–1). In general, the collecting ducts descend straight through the medullary rays and outer medulla without joining other collecting ducts. However, repeated joinings occur in the inner medulla, which results in a progressive reduction in the number of inner medullary collecting ducts (IMCDs) toward the renal papillary tip.[14] This reduction in the number of collecting ducts, combined with the progressive reduction in the number of loops of Henle reaching successive levels of the inner medulla, accounts for the tapered structure of the renal papilla.

Vasculature

The major blood vessels that carry blood into and out of the renal medulla are called the vasa recta. The descending vasa recta receive blood from efferent arterioles of juxtamedullary nephrons and supply blood to the capillary plexuses at each level of the medulla. The capillary plexus in the outer medulla is considerably more dense and much better perfused than the plexus in the inner medulla.[16] Blood from the capillary plexus of the inner medulla feeds into ascending vasa recta. (Ascending vasa recta are never formed directly from descending vasa recta in a loop-like structure.) Ascending vasa recta from the inner medulla traverse the inner stripe of the outer medulla in close physical association with the descending vasa recta in vascular bundles.[17] In many animal species, the vascular bundles are surrounded by the thin limbs of short loops of Henle (SDLs) as shown in Figure 9–4. Here the SDL segments are labeled with an antibody to the UT-A2 urea transporter, suggesting a route for urea recycling from the vasa recta to the short loops of Henle. The capillary plexus of the outer medulla is drained by vasa recta that ascend through the outer stripe of the outer medulla separate from the descending vasa recta.[18]

The counterflow arrangement of vasa recta in the medulla promotes countercurrent exchange of solutes and water. This exchange is abetted by the presence of aquaporin-1 water channels[19,20] and the UT-B urea transporters[21,22] in the endothelial cells of the descending portion of the vasa recta. Countercurrent exchange provides a means of reducing the effective blood flow to the medulla while maintaining a high absolute perfusion rate.[23] The low effective blood flow that results from countercurrent exchange is thought to be important to the preservation of solute concentration gradients in the medullary tissue (see later).

In contrast to the medulla, the cortical labyrinth has a high effective blood flow. The rapid vascular perfusion to this region promotes the rapid return of solutes and water absorbed from the nephron to the general circulation. The rapid perfusion is thought to maintain the interstitial concentrations of most solutes at levels close to those in the peripheral plasma. The medullary rays of the cortex have a capillary plexus that is considerably sparser than that of the cortical labyrinth. Consequently, the effective blood flow to the medullary

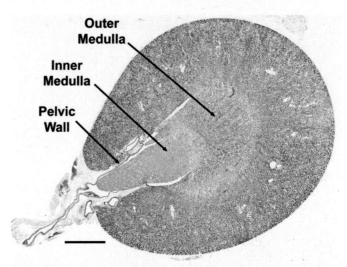

FIGURE 9–6 Alcian blue staining of normal rat kidney showing distribution of hyaluronic acid with high levels in inner medulla. Bar is 2 mm. (From Knepper MA, Saidel GM, Hascall VC, Dwyer T: Concentration of solutes in the renal inner medulla: Interstitial hyaluronan as a mechano-osmotic transducer. Am J Physiol Renal Physiol 284:F433–F446, 2003.)

rays has been postulated to be lower than that of the cortical labyrinth.[4]

Medullary Interstitium

The renal medullary interstitium is a complex space that contains fluid, microfibrils, extracellular matrix, and interstitial cells.[24] In the outer medulla and the outer portion of the inner medulla, the interstitium is relatively small in volume,[4] which may be important in limiting diffusion of solutes upward along the medullary axis. The interstitial space is much larger in the inner half of the inner medulla.[4] A gelatinous matrix found in this region contains large amounts of highly polymerized hyaluronic acid (HA), consisting of alternating D-glucuronate and N-acetyl-D-glucosamine moieties.[25] Figure 9–6 shows a rat kidney labeled with a dye (Alcian Blue) that binds selectively to HA showing its distribution in the kidney. The inner medullary HA interstitial matrix (stained blue in Fig. 9–6) has recently been proposed to play a direct role in generation of an inner medullary osmotic gradient through its ability to store and transduce energy from the smooth muscle contractions of the renal pelvis[25] (see later).

Renal Pelvis

Urine exits the collecting duct system and enters the renal pelvis at the tip of the renal papilla (Fig. 9–7; compare with Fig. 9–6). The renal pelvis (or the calyx in multipapillate kidneys) is a complex intrarenal urinary space surrounding the renal papilla. The renal pelvis (calyx) has extensions called fornices and secondary pouches whose lumens contact portions of the renal outer medulla. Although a transitional epithelium lines most of the pelvic space, a simple cuboidal epithelium separates the pelvic space from the renal parenchyma.[26] It has been proposed that solute and water transport could occur across this epithelium, modifying the composition of the renal medullary interstitial fluid.[27]

The renal pelvic (calyceal) wall (see Fig. 9–6) contains two smooth muscle layers.[28] Contractions of these smooth muscle layers are responsible for powerful peristaltic waves that appear to displace the renal papilla downward with a "milking" action.[29] The peristaltic waves have been reported

Urine Concentration and Dilution

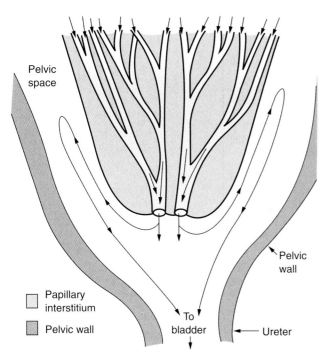

FIGURE 9–7 Pattern of urine flow in papillary collecting ducts and renal pelvis. Urine exits the papillary collecting ducts (ducts of Bellini) at the tip of the renal papilla and is carried to the urinary bladder by the ureter. (Compare with Figure 9–6.) Under some circumstances, a fraction of the urine may reflux backward in the pelvic space and contact the outer surface of the renal papilla. Solute and water exchange across the papillary surface epithelium has been postulated (see text).

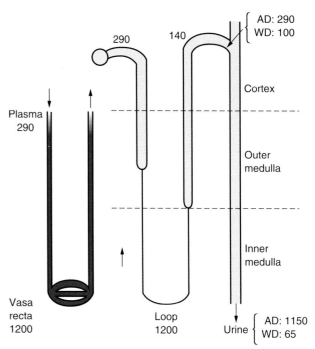

FIGURE 9–8 Typical osmolalities (in mOsm/kg H_2O) found in various vascular (left) and renal tubule (right) sites in rat kidneys. AD, antidiuresis (i.e., high vasopressin); WD, water diuresis (i.e., low vasopressin). Fluid in the proximal tubule is always isosmotic with plasma (290 mOsm/kg H_2O). Fluid emerging from the loop of Henle (entering the early distal tubule) is always hypotonic. Osmolality in the late distal tubule increases to plasma level only during antidiuresis. Final urine is hypertonic when the circulating vasopressin level is high, and hypotonic when the vasopressin level is low. A high osmolality is always maintained in the loop of Henle and vasa recta. During antidiuresis, osmolalities in all inner medullary structures are nearly equal. Osmolalities are somewhat attenuated in the loop and vasa recta during water diuresis (not shown). (Based on micropuncture studies; see text.)

to intermittently propel the urine along the collecting ducts. The contractions compress all structures in the renal inner medulla including the collecting ducts, the loops of Henle, and the interstitium.[30] The contractions have been proposed to furnish part of the energy for concentrating solutes in the inner medulla,[25] as discussed subsequently.

GENERAL FEATURES OF THE URINE CONCENTRATION AND DILUTION PROCESS

Sites of Urine Concentration and Dilution

The sites of tubule fluid concentration and dilution along the mammalian nephron have been investigated by micropuncture studies in rats and other rodents. These results are summarized in Figure 9–8. The tubule fluid in the proximal convoluted tubule is always approximately isosmotic with plasma, regardless of whether the kidney is concentrating or diluting the urine.[31,32] In contrast, the fluid in the early distal convoluted tubule is always hypotonic, regardless of the osmolality of the urine. The earliest site along the nephron where differences in tubule fluid osmolality between antidiuresis and water diuresis can be detected is the late distal tubule. At this site, the tubule fluid becomes isosmotic with plasma during antidiuresis, but remains hypotonic during water diuresis. Between the late distal tubule and the final urine, the tubule fluid osmolality rises to a level greater than that of plasma during antidiuresis but remains hypotonic during water diuresis. On the basis of the foregoing observations, it has been concluded that the chief site of dilution of tubule fluid is the loop of Henle and that the dilution process

in the loop occurs regardless of whether the final urine is dilute or concentrated. During water diuresis, further dilution occurs in the collecting ducts.[33] The chief site of urine concentration is beyond the distal tubule (i.e., in the collecting duct system). The following sections consider in turn the mechanism of urinary dilution and of urinary concentration.

Mechanism of Tubule Fluid Dilution

Micropuncture measurements in rats have revealed that the hypotonicity of the fluid in the early distal tubule is due chiefly to a reduction in luminal NaCl concentration relative to the proximal tubule.[34] In principle, a low luminal NaCl concentration could result from active NaCl absorption from the loop of Henle or water secretion into the loop. However, micropuncture studies, using inulin as a volume marker, demonstrated net water absorption from the superficial loop of Henle during antidiuresis,[35] which rules out the possibility of water secretion as a mechanism of tubule fluid dilution. Thus, we can conclude that luminal dilution occurs because of NaCl reabsorption in the loop of Henle in excess of water absorption. The mechanism of dilution has been demonstrated in classic studies of isolated perfused rabbit thick ascending limbs of loops of Henle.[36,37] NaCl is rapidly absorbed by active transport, which lowers the luminal NaCl concentration and osmolality to levels below those in the peritubular fluid. The osmotic water permeability is low, which prevents dissipation of the transepithelial osmolality gradient by water fluxes. Details of the active NaCl transport process at a cellular level are discussed later in the section "Molecular Physiology of Urinary Concentrating and Diluting Processes."

The hypotonicity of tubule fluid is maintained throughout the distal tubule and collecting duct system during water diuresis, abetted by the low osmotic water permeability of the collecting ducts when circulating levels of vasopressin are low (see Chapter 8). Although the dilute state is sustained in the collecting ducts, the solute composition of the tubule fluid is modified in the collecting duct system, chiefly by Na absorption and K secretion. Active NaCl reabsorption by the collecting ducts is responsible for the further dilution of the collecting duct fluid beyond that achieved in the thick ascending limbs.[33]

Mechanism of Tubule Fluid Concentration

When circulating vasopressin levels are high, extensive net water absorption occurs at sites between the late distal tubule and the final urine (i.e., in the collecting ducts).[35] Measurements along the IMCDs of antidiuretic hamsters demonstrated directly that water is absorbed in excess of solutes, with a resulting rise in osmolality along the collecting ducts toward the papillary tip.[38] Thus, the collecting duct fluid is concentrated chiefly by water absorption, rather than by solute addition.

The osmotic driving force for water absorption along the collecting ducts is present because of the existence of an axial osmolality gradient in the renal medullary tissue, with the highest degree of hypertonicity at the papillary tip. Such an osmolality gradient was initially demonstrated by Wirz and colleagues[39] in a classic study that used an ingenious microcryoscopic method to measure the osmolality in the lumens of individual renal tubules in tissue slices from quick-frozen rat kidneys. The measurements revealed that in antidiuretic rats, there was a continuous osmolality gradient throughout the medullary axis, including both the outer medulla and inner medulla, with the highest osmolality in the deepest part of the inner medulla, the papillary tip. Furthermore, in the medulla, the osmolality was about as high in the large tubules (presumably collecting ducts) as in the small tubules (presumably loops of Henle); this demonstrates that the high tissue osmolality was not simply a manifestation of a high osmolality in a single structure, namely, the collecting duct. Consistent with this view, Wirz demonstrated by micropuncture that the osmolality of vasa recta blood, sampled from near the papillary tip in antidiuretic hamsters, was virtually equal to that of the final urine.[31] Subsequently, Gottschalk and Mylle,[32] using micropuncture in antidiuretic hamsters, confirmed that the osmolality of the fluid in the loops of Henle, the vasa recta, and the collecting ducts was approximately the same (see Fig. 9–8), in support of the view that the collecting duct fluid is concentrated by osmotic equilibration with a hypertonic medullary interstitium. Furthermore, *in vitro* studies demonstrated that collecting ducts have a high water permeability in the presence of vasopressin[40,41] as is required for osmotic equilibration. The mechanism by which the corticomedullary osmolality gradient is generated is considered later.

The overall axial osmolality gradient in the renal medulla is composed of gradients of several individual solutes. However, the principal solutes responsible for the osmolality gradient are NaCl and urea, as demonstrated initially in dog kidneys by Ullrich and Jarausch[42] by use of the tissue slice analysis technique. These data are summarized in Figure 9–9. The increase in NaCl concentration along the corticomedullary axis occurs predominantly in the outer medulla, with only a small increase in the inner medulla. In contrast,

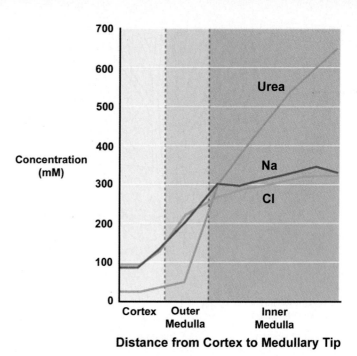

FIGURE 9–9 Cortico-medullary gradients of urea, sodium, and chloride in kidneys of antidiuretic dogs. Summary of data from Ullrich and Jarausch.[42] (From Giebisch G, Windhager EE: Urine concentration and dilution. *In* Boron WF, Boulpaep EL (eds): Medical Physiology. Philadelphia, Saunders, 2006, pp 828–844.)

the increase in urea concentration along the corticomedullary axis occurs predominantly in the inner medulla, with little or no increase in the outer medulla. Although some aspects of the process that generates the renal medullary solute gradient are in doubt, the major aspects are well understood, viz. the mechanism of generation of the NaCl gradient in the outer medulla and the mechanism of urea accumulation in the inner medulla. In the following, we will emphasize these well understood aspects first and then briefly address the frontiers of our knowledge.

Generation of An Axial NaCl Gradient in the Renal Outer Medulla: Countercurrent Multiplication

The concept of countercurrent multiplication originally evolved from a consideration of industrial processes that separate and concentrate economically useful products (e.g., countercurrent extraction and distillation). In these processes, a single stage (given the appropriate energy input) is capable of modest concentration of one component. However, the effect of a single stage ("single effect") can be multiplied by successive applications of the effect. Werner Kuhn, a Swiss applied physical chemist, and his colleagues used this concept to provide an explanation for the corticomedullary osmolality gradient in the renal medulla.[43–45] They showed, using mathematical techniques, that a small concentration difference (single effect) between the ascending and descending limbs of a hairpin counterflow system could be multiplied by the countercurrent flow to obtain an axial gradient much larger than the transverse concentration difference between the limbs. They demonstrated the feasibility of such a concept by constructing physical counterflow models that developed axial solute concentration gradients. In the following paragraphs, we develop in greater detail the conceptual basis of the countercurrent multiplier model.

Figure 9–10A shows a hypothetical single-stage process that provides a starting point for consideration of the

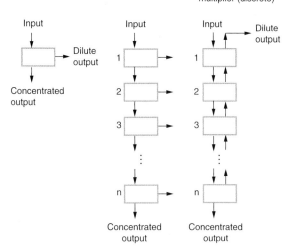
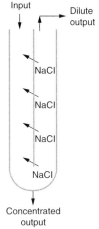
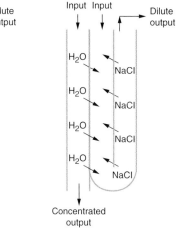

FIGURE 9–10 Conceptual development of the countercurrent multiplier hypothesis based on the work of Kuhn and associates.[43–45] See text for explanation.

countercurrent multiplication concept. We assume that a volume of fluid containing a dissolved solute can be added to such a single stage and, with an appropriate energy input, can be divided into two smaller volumes, one slightly more concentrated than the input, one slightly less concentrated. If the more concentrated output were reintroduced into the same single stage and similarly divided into two smaller volumes, the overall action would be to concentrate a fraction of the original starting fluid more than could have been achieved by a single stage applied only once. If the concentrated output of a single stage is "y" times more concentrated than the input, then the two steps would concentrate the output $R = y^2$ times more than the original input. That is, the single effect y is <u>multiplied</u> to obtain the overall concentration ratio R. Similarly, if there are "n" successive applications of a single stage, the single effect will be multiplied n times, and the overall concentration ratio R will be y^n. It is evident that by such a scheme, the action of a single stage with a modest single-stage concentration ratio can be multiplied to yield any arbitrary overall concentration ratio R.

Instead of successive applications of a single stage, it is theoretically feasible to stack several such stages in a cascade so that all can operate simultaneously in a steady-state operation (Fig. 9–10B). In this configuration, the concentrated output from a given stage is passed downward to the next stage to be further concentrated. As with the sequential operation of a single stage, this scheme can multiply the single effect of an individual stage to yield any arbitrary overall concentration ratio, given enough stages. The disadvantage of such a scheme is that the volume of fluid reaching each successive stage will be progressively smaller, and the volume of the overall effluent at the bottom of the stack would approach zero as the number of stages n became large. This drawback is avoided, however, if the more dilute output from each stage is passed upward to the next stage, allowing recycling of the fluid (Fig. 9–10C). This change results in a countercurrent arrangement, with the upward-flowing fluid interacting with the downward-flowing fluid at each stage. This countercurrent multiplication scheme allows several concentrating stages to interact to produce a relatively large volume of concentrated fluid at the bottom of the stack.

Kuhn and colleagues recognized that it was a simple matter to extend the countercurrent multiplier scheme involving several discrete stages shown in Figure 9–10C to a continuous-flow scheme in which discrete stages are replaced by ascending and descending streams whose interaction is distributed uniformly throughout their lengths, as would have to exist in the loop of Henle (Fig. 9–10D). A small concentration difference between the counterflowing descending and ascending streams could result in a large axial concentration gradient. The development of the concept by Kuhn and colleagues[43–45] that such a continuous countercurrent scheme could explain urine concentration was a landmark event in renal physiology. The terminology derived from the stagewise process was retained in the description of renal countercurrent multiplication. Thus, the term "single effect" (Einzeleffekt, individual effect), which referred to the action of an individual stage, was retained to denote a small solute concentration difference between ascending and descending limbs, although in fact discrete individual stages do not exist.

Hydrostatic pressure was initially considered a possible energy source for creation of a single effect in the loop of Henle.[43] High pressure on the descending limb side of the loop could theoretically force water to exit the lumen, thus concentrating the descending limb luminal fluid relative to the ascending limb fluid. The realization that hydrostatic pressures in the descending limb lumen were not likely to be high enough to provide a substantial osmolality difference between the two limbs led Kuhn and Ramel[45] to describe a model in which *active NaCl transport* out of the ascending limb lowered its concentration with respect to that of the descending limb (see Fig. 9–10D). Later studies in isolated perfused thick ascending limbs demonstrated that this renal tubule segment indeed has the capability of generating a transepithelial osmotic gradient as required.[36,37]

A continuous countercurrent multiplier is capable of producing a small volume of concentrated output, which in theory could be withdrawn from the bend of the hairpin loop (see Fig. 9–10D). However, Hargitay and Kuhn[44] recognized that a more realistic scheme would include a third tube (a "collecting duct") that equilibrates osmotically with the loop fluid to produce a concentrated output (Fig. 9–10E). Such a scheme has the advantage that it can concentrate solutes in the collecting ducts other than those responsible for the axial osmolality gradient in the loop. The volume flow into the collecting duct must be considerably less than in the loop for a significant overall concentrating effect to be maintained.

Figure 9–10 depicts a countercurrent multiplier that works strictly by recycling NaCl between ascending and descending limbs of the loop of Henle, thus increasing the

316

mean residence time of Na and Cl ions in the renal medulla. Subsequent work has revealed that early portions of the descending limbs of long-loop nephrons are highly permeable to water[7,8,10] due to the expression of high levels of aquaporin-1 in the apical and basolateral plasma membrane of descending limb cells.[19,46–48] Thus, as shown in Figure 9–11, countercurrent multiplication works not only by *NaCl recycling* into the descending limb, but also by *water short-circuiting* from the descending limb.[49] The water reabsorbed from the descending limb is rapidly returned to the general circulation by the vasa recta, thus reducing the *mean residence time* for water molecules in the renal medulla. Either an increase in residence time of solute particles or a decrease

in residence time of water molecules serves to concentrate the renal medulla.

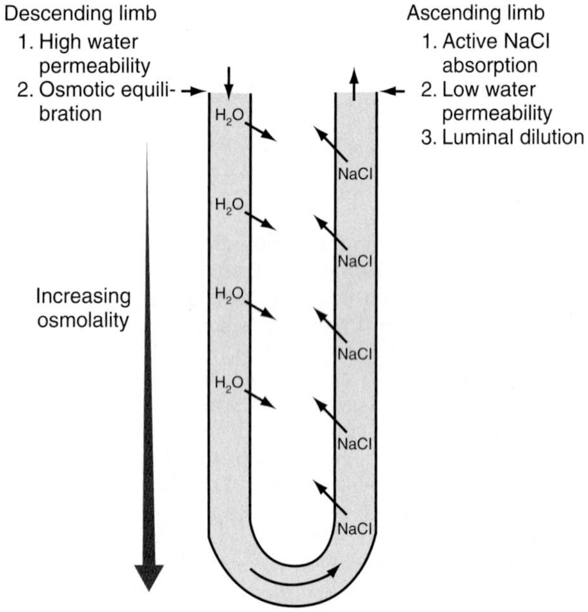

It is now generally accepted that the axial osmolality gradient in the outer medulla is generated by countercurrent multiplication driven by active NaCl transport in the thick ascending limbs. However, as discussed in greater detail subsequently, this basic mechanism does not exist in the inner medulla of the kidney. Indeed, the ascending limb of Henle's loop in the inner medulla has thin limb morphology and little or no capacity for active NaCl transport.[41,50–52] The solute responsible for most of the inner medullary osmolality gradient is urea (see Fig. 9–9). Mechanisms responsible for urea accumulation in the inner medulla are discussed next.

Accumulation of Urea in Renal Inner Medulla: Facilitated Urea Transport, Diffusion Trapping, and Urea Recycling

Urea accumulation in the inner medulla is dependent on differential urea permeability along the collecting duct system (Fig. 9–12). The pattern of urea permeability differences among tubule segments has been defined chiefly using the isolated, perfused tubule technique. Figure 9–12 shows a long loop of Henle, a short loop of Henle, and the collecting ducts with each segment distorted so that its width is proportional to the urea permeability coefficient in that segment. Among collecting duct segments, a high urea permeability has been found only in the terminal part of the IMCD.[53] The urea permeability of the terminal IMCD is regulated by vasopressin, increasing to extremely high values within minutes of vasopressin exposure.[41,54,55] This action of vasopressin is mediated by cyclic adenosine monophosphate (cyclic AMP).[56] As discussed subsequently, the high urea permeability of the terminal part of the IMCD is due to the presence of specialized phloretin-sensitive urea transporters in the apical and basolateral plasma membranes of the IMCD cells. The low urea permeability of the collecting duct system proximal to the terminal IMCD is due to a lack of urea transporter expression.

The mechanism of urea accumulation in the renal medulla is shown in Figure 9–13.[57] The accumulation process is a result of passive urea absorption from the IMCDs. The tubule fluid entering the collecting duct system in the renal cortex has a relatively low urea concentration. During antidiuresis, water is osmotically absorbed from the urea-impermeable parts of the collecting duct system in the cortex and outer medulla. This causes a progressive increase in luminal urea concentration along the connecting tubules, cortical

FIGURE 9–11 Countercurrent multiplication in the renal outer medulla. The thick ascending limb actively reabsorbs NaCl, but because of low water permeability, water is not reabsorbed, resulting in luminal dilution necessary for 'single effect'. The descending limb is highly permeable to water due to high levels of expression of aquaporin-1. Hypertonic NaCl reabsorbed from ascending limb drives osmotic water reabsorption from descending limb, resulting in short-circuiting of water back to the general circulation (see text). (From Knepper MA, Nielsen S, Chou C-L: Physiological roles of aquaporins in the kidney. Curr Top Membr 51:121–153, 2001.)

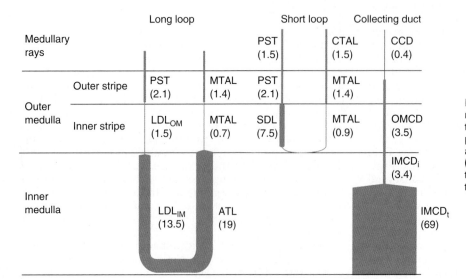

FIGURE 9–12 Urea permeabilities of mammalian renal tubule segments. The width of each segment in the diagram is distorted to be proportional to the urea permeability of that segment. Numbers in parentheses are measured values for the permeability coefficient ($\times 10^{-5}$ cm/sec). Values are from isolated perfused tubules studies.[54,68,70,71,214–216] Abbreviations for renal tubule segments are the same as in Table 9–1.

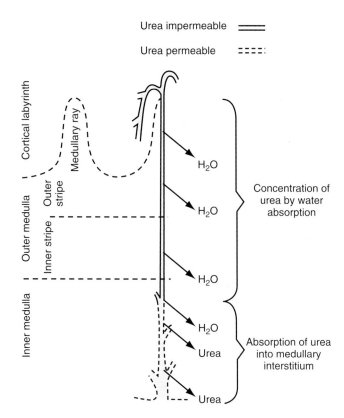

FIGURE 9–13 Diagram of mammalian collecting duct system showing principal sites of water absorption and urea absorption. Water is absorbed in early part of the collecting duct system, driven by an osmotic gradient. Because urea permeabilities of cortical collecting duct, outer medullary collecting duct and initial IMCD are very low, the water absorption concentrates urea in the lumen of these segments. When the tubule fluid reaches the terminal IMCD, which is highly permeable to urea, urea rapidly exits from the lumen. This urea is trapped in the inner medulla as a result of countercurrent exchange.

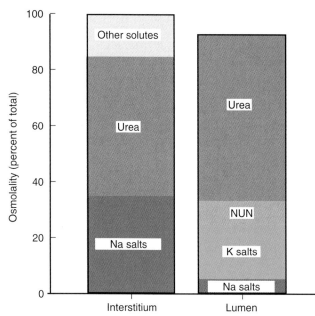

FIGURE 9–14 Solutes that account for osmolality of medullary interstitium and tubule fluid in the inner medullary collecting duct during antidiuresis in rats. Urea nearly equilibrates across the IMCD epithelium as a result of rapid facilitated urea transport. Although the osmolalities of the fluid in the two spaces are nearly equal, the non-urea solutes can differ considerably between the two compartments. Typical values in untreated rats are presented. Values can differ considerably in other species and in the same species with different diets. NUN, non-urea nitrogen.

collecting ducts, and outer medullary collecting ducts. Then, when the tubule fluid reaches the terminal IMCD, which is highly permeable to urea, urea can exit rapidly from the lumen to the inner medullary interstitium. The urea is trapped in the inner medullary interstitium because the effective blood flow is low owing to countercurrent exchange by the vasa recta (see later). Because the urea permeability of the terminal IMCD is extremely high, particularly in the presence of vasopressin, urea nearly equilibrates across the IMCD epithelium under steady-state conditions. This allows urea in the intersititum to almost completely balance osmotically the high urea concentration in the collecting duct lumen, preventing the osmotic diuresis that would otherwise occur (Fig. 9–14).

Close association of descending and ascending vasa recta facilitates countercurrent exchange of urea between the two structures.[23] The concentration of urea in the ascending vasa recta exiting the inner medulla approaches the concentration in the descending vasa recta entering the inner medulla, which minimizes the washout of urea from the inner medulla. The permeability of the vasa recta to urea is extremely high (>40 × 10⁻⁵ cm/sec),[21,41] which abets the countercurrent exchange process. Countercurrent exchange cannot completely eliminate loss of urea from the inner medullary interstitium because the volume flow rate of blood in the ascending vasa recta normally exceeds that in the descending vasa recta.[58] The water added to the vasa recta derives from the IMCDs and descending limbs, both of which reabsorb water during antidiuresis. Because the mass flow rate of urea is the product of the urea concentration and the volume flow rate,

the higher volume flow rate in the ascending vasa recta will ensure that the inner medullary vasculature continually removes urea from the inner medulla. Quantitatively, the most important loss of urea from the inner medullary interstitium is thought to occur via the vasa recta.[59]

Recycling pathways limit the loss of urea from the inner medulla. Flow in the ascending vasa recta and ascending limb of the loop of Henle tends to carry urea out of the inner medulla. These losses are minimized by urea recycling pathways, which return to the inner medulla much of the urea that leaves through the vasa recta or ascending limbs. Three major urea recycling pathways are described in Figure 9–15.[59]

Recycling of Urea through the Ascending Limbs, Distal Tubules, and Collecting Ducts
Urea exiting the inner medulla in the ascending limbs of the long loops of Henle is carried through the thick ascending limbs, the distal convoluted tubules, and the early part of the collecting duct system by the flow of tubule fluid[35] (Fig. 9–15A). When it reaches the urea-permeable part of the collecting duct in the inner medulla, it passively exits into the inner medullary interstitium, completing the cycle.

Recycling of Urea through the Vasa Recta, Short Loops of Henle, and Collecting Ducts
Micropuncture studies of non diuretic rats have revealed that the delivery of urea to the superficial distal tubule exceeds the delivery out of the superficial proximal tubule.[35,60,61] This implies that, in addition to urea recycling via the long loops as described in Figure 9–15A, net urea addition occurs along the short loops of Henle. To explain this finding, it has been proposed[60,62] that urea leaving the inner medulla in the vasa recta is transferred to the descending limbs of the short loops of Henle (Fig. 9–15B). The urea that enters the short loops can then be carried through the superficial distal tubules and back to the inner medulla by the collecting ducts where it is

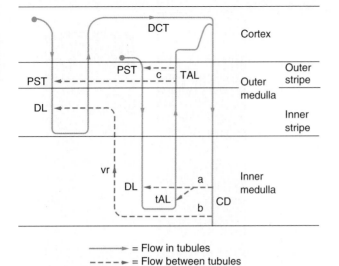

= Flow in tubules

---- = Flow between tubules

FIGURE 9–15 Pathways of urea recycling in the mammalian kidney. Solid lines represent a short-looped nephron (left) and a long-looped nephron (right). Transfer of urea between nephron segments is indicated by dashed arrows labeled a, b, and c corresponding to recycling pathways described in the text. tAL, thin ascending limb; CD, collecting duct; DCT, distal convoluted tubule; DL, descending limb; PST, proximal straight tubule; TAL, thick ascending limb; vr, vasa recta. (From Knepper MA, Roch-Ramel F: Pathways of urea transport in the mammalian kidney. Kidney Int 31:629–633, 1987.)

reabsorbed, completing the recycling pathway. Transfer of urea from the vasa recta to the short loops of Henle is facilitated by a close physical association between the vasa recta and the descending limbs of the short loops in the vascular bundles of the inner stripe of the outer medulla.[18,63] The recent finding that the urea transporter UT-A2 is selectively expressed in the thin descending limb of short loops of Henle[64,65] provides support for this hypothesis. However, recent research using mathematical modeling[66] and UT-A2 knockout mice[67] (see later) has raised doubts about the importance of this pathway.

Recycling of Urea between Ascending Limb and Descending Limb

Studies in isolated perfused thick ascending limbs have revealed that the urea permeability of thick ascending limbs from the inner stripe of the outer medulla is too low to permit a substantial amount of urea absorption.[68,69] However, similar studies in segments from the outer stripe and medullary rays have demonstrated a higher urea permeability.[68,70] It has been proposed that urea reabsorbed from these thick ascending limbs enters neighboring proximal straight tubules, completing a recycling pathway between the ascending limb and descending limbs of the loop[4] (Fig. 9–15C). The urea transfer between thick ascending limbs and proximal straight tubules is facilitated by the parallel relationship between these two structures in the outer stripe and in the medullary rays. The transfer may also depend on a relatively attenuated effective blood flow in these regions. Urea secretion into the proximal straight tubules can occur by active transport,[71] by passive diffusion,[70] or by a combination of both. Urea presumably enters the proximal straight tubules of both short and long loops of Henle. The urea that enters the short-looped nephrons will be carried back to the inner medulla by the flow of tubule fluid through the superficial distal tubules and collecting ducts, reentering the inner medullary interstitium by reabsorption from the terminal IMCD. The urea that enters proximal straight tubules of long loops returns to the inner medulla directly through the descending limbs.

Collecting Duct Water Absorption

The process of urine concentration consists of two relatively independent components: (1) countercurrent processes that generate a hypertonic medullary interstitium by concentrating NaCl and urea (discussed earlier); and (2) osmotic equilibration of the tubule fluid in the medullary collecting ducts with the hypertonic medullary interstitium to form a hypertonic final urine. In this section, we discuss the mechanism of the latter.

Water excretion is regulated by vasopressin (see Fig. 9–1) largely as a result of its effect on the water permeability of the collecting ducts. The cellular mechanism of this response is discussed in considerable detail elsewhere (see Chapter 8). When the water permeability is low in collecting ducts because of a low circulating level of vasopressin, relatively little water is absorbed in the collecting ducts. The dilute fluid exiting the loops of Henle remains dilute as it passes through the collecting duct system, yielding a large volume of hypotonic urine. When the water permeability of the collecting ducts is high because of a high circulating level of vasopressin, water is rapidly reabsorbed along the collecting duct system by osmosis, drawn by the osmolality gradient between the lumen and the peritubular interstitium. The osmolality of the final urine approaches that of the inner medullary interstitium, which results in formation of a small volume of hypertonic urine.

Micropuncture studies have demonstrated that the late distal tubule is the earliest site along the renal tubule where water absorption increases during antidiuresis.[31] The "distal tubule", as defined by micropuncturists, is made up of three segments, the distal convoluted tubule, the connecting tubule, and the initial collecting tubule. Osmotic water permeability is difficult to measure in these segments owing to their short length. The evidence available indicates that the distal convoluted tubule has a low water permeability and does not express any of the known water channels. In contrast, the connecting tubule expresses both the type 2 vasopressin receptor (V_2R) and the vasopressin-regulated water channel aquaporin-2 (AQP2) and is presumably the segment responsible for distal tubular osmotic equilibration in micropuncture studies.[13] In addition, AQP2 is expressed in the initial collecting tubule as well as the cortical collecting duct.[72] Thus, among the segments making up the portion of the distal tubule accessible by cortical micropuncture (distal convoluted tubule, connecting segment, and initial collecting tubule), only the connecting segment and the initial collecting tubule appear to exhibit vasopressin-regulated water transport.

The amount of water absorption in the connecting segment and initial collecting tubule required to raise tubule fluid to isotonicity is considerably greater than the additional amount required to concentrate the urine above the osmolality of plasma in the medullary portion of the collecting duct system.[4] Consequently, most of the water reabsorbed from the collecting duct system during antidiuresis enters the cortical labyrinth, where the effective blood flow is high enough to return the reabsorbed water to the general circulation without diluting the interstitium. If such a large amount of water were absorbed along the medullary collecting ducts, it would be expected to have a significant dilutional effect on the medullary interstitium and impair concentrating ability.[73,74]

During water diuresis, a corticomedullary osmolality gradient persists, although it is attenuated.[75–77] In the absence of vasopressin, the water permeability of the collecting ducts is low but not zero.[54,78] Consequently, some water is absorbed by the collecting ducts during water diuresis. Most of the water absorption occurs from the terminal part of IMCDs, where the transepithelial osmolality gradient is highest and the basal water permeability is also highest. In fact, more water is absorbed from the terminal collecting ducts during water diuresis than during antidiuresis owing to a much larger transepithelial osmolality gradient.[73] A high rate of water absorption from the IMCDs is thought to contribute to the reduction of the medullary interstitial osmolality during water diuresis by its dilutional effect. The fall in inner medullary tissue osmolality during water diuresis results largely from an increase in tissue water content[74,79] associated with the higher rate of water absorption from the collecting ducts, although reductions in the quantities of urea and NaCl in the medullary tissue have also been documented.

Determinants of Concentrating Ability

Figure 9–16 summarizes the major determinants of urinary concentrating ability based on the classical theoretical analysis of Stephenson.[80] We present this here because it provides a basis for understanding the effects of vasopressin and specific gene knockouts on the concentrating process discussed later (in section titled "Molecular Physiology of Urinary Concentrating and Diluting Processes"). Obviously, active transport of NaCl from the thick ascending limb (factor 2) and collecting duct water permeability (factor 4) are two determinants that are self evident from the foregoing description of the urinary concentrating mechanism. In addition, the "distal delivery" of NaCl and water to the loop of Henle (factor 1) is an important determinant because it places an upper bound on the amount of NaCl actively absorbed by the thick ascend-

ing limb to drive the countercurrent multiplier mechanism. Finally, the fluid delivery to the medullary collecting duct (factor 3) has an underappreciated effect on the concentrating process. Too much delivery saturates the water absorption process along the medullary collecting ducts and is associated with interstitial dilution owing to rapid osmotic water transport. Too little fluid delivery to the medullary collecting ducts, even in the absence of vasopressin, results in sustained osmotic equilibration across the collecting duct epithelium owing to the non-zero osmotic water permeability of the IMCD.[54,73,78]

An Unanswered Question: Concentration of NaCl in the Renal Inner Medulla

As described in Figure 9–9, tissue slice studies have demonstrated that the corticomedullary osmolality gradient is made up largely of a NaCl gradient in the outer medulla and a urea gradient in the inner medulla. Accordingly, in the foregoing we have emphasized the process that concentrates NaCl in the outer medulla (classic countercurrent multiplication) and the process responsible for urea accumulation in the inner medulla (passive urea absorption from the inner medullary collecting duct plus diffusion trapping). Not addressed was the origin of the small NaCl gradient in the renal inner medulla (see Fig. 9–9), as well as the energy source for concentration of non-urea solutes in the inner medullary interstitium. These remain unanswered questions.

Presumably a countercurrent multiplication process is responsible for the inner medullary NaCl and osmolality gradient, but what is the single effect? As discussed earlier, the single-effect mechanism in the outer medulla is active NaCl transport out of the water-impermeable thick ascending limb, diluting the luminal fluid relative to the interstitium. However, repeated studies of thin ascending limbs[41,50–52] have failed to show evidence for such an active transport process in the inner medulla. General analysis of inner medullary concentrating processes indicates that, to satisfy mass balance requirements, either an ascending stream (thin ascending limbs or ascending vasa recta) must be diluted relative to the inner medullary interstitium, or a descending stream (descending thin limbs, descending vasa recta, or collecting ducts) must be concentrated locally relative to the inner medulla.[25,81,82] In previous versions of this chapter (in earlier editions) and in published review papers,[25,82,83] we have categorized possible single effect mechanisms for inner medullary concentrating processes. In the following, we summarize the three mechanisms that garnered the greatest interest in the current literature.

The Kokko-Rector Stephenson Model: The "Passive Mechanism"

Kokko and Rector[84] and Stephenson[85] simultaneously proposed a model by which the osmolality in the ascending thin limb could be lowered below that of the interstitium entirely by passive transport processes in the inner medulla. This formulation is generally referred to as the "passive model" or the "passive countercurrent multiplier mechanism". In this model, rapid efflux of urea from the inner medullary collecting duct causes osmotic withdrawal of water from the thin descending limb, concentrating NaCl in the lumen. The highly concentrated NaCl is then proposed to exit passively from the thin ascending limb, thus diluting the luminal fluid, providing a single effect for countercurrent multiplication. This model requires that the thin descending limb be highly permeable to water but not NaCl or urea, whereas the thin ascending limb would have to be permeable to NaCl but not water or urea. Previously objections to the model have been made largely on the basis of the high urea permeabilities that have been measured in the thin descending limb[86] and thin ascending limb.[25] Recent studies in mice[87,88] in which

Determinants of Concentrating Ability

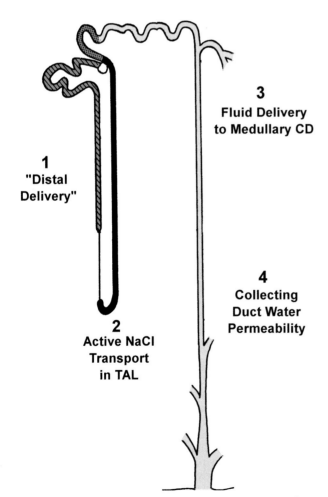

1 "Distal Delivery"

2 Active NaCl Transport in TAL

3 Fluid Delivery to Medullary CD

4 Collecting Duct Water Permeability

FIGURE 9–16 Major determinants of urinary concentrating ability. See text for details.

facilitated urea transport from the inner medullary collecting duct was eliminated via a gene knockout strategy provided strong evidence that seemingly rules out the passive model (see later). Specifically, when the UT-A1 and UT-A3 urea transporter genes were deleted, urea accumulation in the inner medulla was largely eliminated, but inner medullary NaCl accumulation was not affected in contradiction to the passive model (see "UT-A1/3 knockout" later).

A more thorough discussion of the Kokko-Rector-Stephenson passive countercurrent multiplier model may be found in the corresponding chapter on urinary concentration and dilution in previous editions of this book.

Lactate-Driven Concentrating Mechanism

Because of a failure of models accounting only for urea, NaCl, and water to explain solute gradients in the inner medullary interstitium, consideration has been given to possible other solutes that could play a role.[89] In such a model, an unspecified solute may be assumed to be added continuously to the inner medullary interstitium. Such a solute would have to be generated *de novo* via a chemical reaction that generates more osmotically active particles than it consumes. In a subsequent mathematical modeling study, Thomas and Wexler[90] confirmed that addition of such a solute to the inner medullary interstitium could theoretically explain the concentration gradient along the inner medullary axis by driving water absorption from the thin descending limb. This action would concentrate NaCl in the descending limb, establishing a gradient for NaCl efflux from the ascending limb and dilution of the ascending limb lumen relative to the interstitium. This model is like the Kokko-Rector-Stephenson passive model discussed earlier except that the external solute substitutes for urea.

Thomas[91,92] has proposed that the "external solute" is lactate, generated by anaerobic glycolysis (the predominant means of ATP generation in the inner medulla) in the proportion of two lactate ions per glucose molecule consumed:

$$\text{glucose} \rightarrow 2 \text{ lactate} + 2 \text{ H}^+$$

The success of the proposed model in generating a medullary osmotic gradient depends on the fate of the H generated. If the H ions titrate bicarbonate, they will remove two osmotically active particles (HCO_3 ions) causing net disappearance of osmotically active particles:

$$\text{glucose} + 2 \text{ HCO}_3 \rightarrow \text{lactate} + 2 \text{ CO}_2$$

Because CO_2 readily permeates lipid bilayers, it is unlikely to be osmotically effective. Alternatively, if the H ions titrate buffers other than bicarbonate, such as phosphate or NH_3, net generation of osmotically active particles can occur. Thus far, this hypothesis has not been pursued experimentally. Recent mathematical modeling studies re-evaluating factors involved in inner medullary lactate accumulation suggest that countercurrent exchange of glucose from descending (DVR) to ascending vasa recta (AVR) in the outer medulla (OM) and upper inner medulla (IM) may severely limit lactate generation in the deepest part of the inner medulla,[93] raising doubts about the feasibility of the lactate generation model.

Hyaluronan as a Mechano-Osmotic Transducer

As proposed by Schmidt-Nielsen,[94] the contractions of the smooth muscle of the pelvic wall may provide energy for the inner medullary concentrating mechanism by compressing the spongelike interstitial hyaluronan matrix. Following this proposal, Knepper and collaborators[25] have described a periodic (non–steady state) concentrating model of the inner medulla (summarized later in this section) based on the assumption that the inner medullary interstitium consists of a semisolid viscoelastic hyaluronan gel rather than being a freely flowing aqueous medium.

Hyaluronan (or "hyaluronic acid") is a glycosaminoglycan (GAG). GAGs consist of unbranched polysaccharide chains composed of repeating disaccharide units. Aside from hyaluronan, the family of mammalian GAGs include dermatan sulfate, chondroitin sulfates, keratan sulfate, heparan sulfate, and heparin. Hyaluronan differs from the other GAGs because it is not covalently linked to proteins to form proteoglycans and is not sulfated.[95] In contrast to the other GAGs, which are produced in the Golgi apparatus, hyaluronan is synthesized at the plasma membrane by an integral membrane protein, hyaluronan synthase (HAS).[96,97] Three mammalian HAS genes are recognized, namely, HAS1, HAS2, and HAS3. All three HAS proteins produce hyaluronan on the cytoplasmic side of the plasma membrane and transport it across the plasma membrane to the extracellular space. Therefore, hyaluronan secretion is not dependent on vesicular trafficking. Because of the importance of GAGs in the structure of connective tissues such as cartilage, tendon, bone, synovial fluid, intervertebral disks, and skin, the physico chemical properties of these substances have been thoroughly investigated.[98]

As shown in Figure 9–6, hyaluronan is extremely abundant in the renal inner medullary interstitium.[99,100] Other GAGs are present in the inner medulla, but in much lower amounts. The hyaluronan in the inner medulla is produced by a specialized interstitial cell (the type 1 interstitial cell) that forms characteristic "bridges" between the thin limbs of Henle and vasa recta.[101] Thus, the inner medullary interstitium can be visualized as being composed of a compressible, viscoelastic hyaluronan matrix.

The compression of hyaluronan in the medullary interstitium by the peristaltic contractions of the pelvic wall can hypothetically serve to generate a single effect for inner medullary concentration without measurable changes in hydrostatic pressure.[25] During inner medullary compression due to the contraction of the pelvic wall, the compression of the hyaluronan matrix stores some of the mechanical energy generated from the smooth muscle contraction. This compression does not require a generalized increase in hydrostatic pressure, but simply involves a direct mechanical compression of the hyaluronan matrix as one would compress a steel spring. After passage of a peristaltic wave, the compressed hyaluronan springs back from its compressed state, exerting an elastic force that can theoretically drive water efflux from the descending limb of the loop of Henle and other water-permeable structures. This water efflux would concentrate solutes in the tubule lumens. In the descending limb, the total solute concentration would thereby rise above that of the surrounding interstitium, satisfying the requirement for an inner medullary single effect, which could be multiplied by the counterflow between ascending and descending limbs. Thus, hyaluronan compression and relaxation would facilitate an energy conversion starting with ATP hydrolysis in the smooth muscle cells of the pelvic wall, leading to an increase in electrochemical potential due to concentration of solutes in the tubule lumen.

Hyaluronan has other properties that would enhance the concentrating process.[102] It is a large (1000 kD to 10000 kD) polyanion. Its charge is due to the COO (carboxylate) groups of the glucuronic acid subunits. It is strongly hydrophilic and adopts a highly expanded, stiffened random-coil conformation that occupies a huge volume relative to its mass. The extended state of hyaluronan owes partly to repulsive electrostatic forces exerted by neighboring carboxylate groups, which maximize the distance between neighboring negative charges, and partly by the constraints of the glycosidic bonds that prefer somewhat extended conformations. This creates a swelling pressure (turgor) that allows the hyaluronan matrix to generate the elastic-like force (resilience) that resists compression. When hyaluronan is compressed, as occurs in a meniscus in the knee joint in response to load bearing, the repulsive force of neighboring carboxylate groups is overcome in part by condensation of cations (chiefly Na) forming a localized crystalloid structure. Thus, compression of a hyaluronan gel results in a decrease of the local sodium ion activity in the gel.[25] In aqueous solutions in equilibrium with the gel, the NaCl concentration will be decreased secondary to the compression-induced reduction in Na activity within the gel. Therefore, the free fluid that is expressed from the hyaluronan matrix during the contraction phase would have a lower total solute concentration than that of the gel as a whole. The slightly hypotonic fluid expressed from the interstitial matrix is likely to escape the inner medulla via the ascending vasa recta, the only structure that remains open during the compressive phase of the contraction cycle.[103] As a consequence, an ascending stream (the ascending vasa recta) would have a lower total solute concentration than the interstitium as a whole, creating a single effect for medullary concentration during the compression phase of the pelvic contraction cycle.

The *HAS2* gene has been knocked out in mice.[104] However, the mice die during fetal development due to cardiac developmental abnormalities, preventing the evaluation of the inner medullary concentrating process in these mice. Thus, either a targeted deletion in the inner medullary interstitial cells or an inducible knockout of *HAS2* would be needed for the studies to address a role for hyaluronan in the inner medullary concentrating mechanism.

MOLECULAR PHYSIOLOGY OF URINARY CONCENTRATING AND DILUTING PROCESSES

Transport Proteins Involved in Urinary Concentration and Dilution

Figure 9–17 summarizes the renal tubule sites of expression of water channels (aquaporins), urea transporters, and ion transporters important to the urinary concentrating process. In the following, we summarize the roles of these transport proteins in urinary concentrating and diluting mechanisms. We emphasize these proteins as molecular targets for vasopressin action.

Aquaporins

Abundant expression of aquaporin-1 in the LDL-OM, LDL-IM, and the early part of the SDL accounts for the high water permeability in these segments.[19,46–48] In contrast, the ascending limb segments (ATL, MTAL, and CTAL) do not express any known water channel, accounting for the low osmotic water permeability measured in these segments.[36,37,51] Aquaporin-2 is a major target for vasopressin action in the CNT and throughout the collecting duct system.[105] Aquaporin-2 is regulated in two ways by vasopressin: (1) short-term regulation of aquaporin-2 trafficking to and from the apical plasma membrane[106]; and (2) long-term regulation of aquaporin-2 abundance,[107] chiefly through transcriptional mechanisms.[108] Aquaporin-2 is chiefly expressed apically throughout the collecting duct system. The basolateral component of water transport across CNT cells and collecting duct principal cells is mediated by aquaporin-3[109] and aquaporin-4.[110] Aquaporin-3 is the dominant basolateral water channel in the CNT and early parts of the collecting duct system, whereas aquaporin-4 predominates in the outer medullary and inner medullary collecting ducts.[110] The abundance of aquaporin-3, but not that of aquaporin-4 is regulated by the long-term effect of vasopressin.[109–111] The regulation of aquaporin-3 occurs via changes in aquaporin-3 mRNA levels.[108]

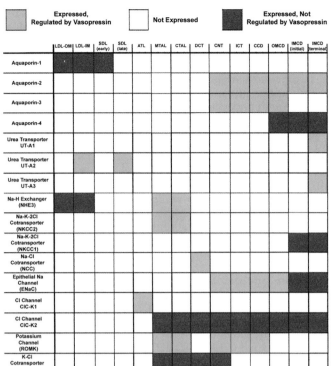

FIGURE 9–17 Grid showing sites of expression of water channels, urea transporters, and ion transporters important to the urinary concentrating process. See text for details.

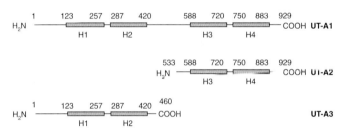

FIGURE 9–18 Urea transporters derived from UT-A gene. UT-A1 and UT-A3 are driven by the same promotor and are identical through amino acid 459. Use of an alternative exon inserts a stop codon that terminates UT-A3 after amino acid 460 (an aspartic acid). UT-A2 is identical to the terminal 397 amino acids of UT-A1 and is driven by an alternative promotor in intron 13 of the mouse gene.[117] Numbers indicate amino acid sequence number.

Urea Transporters

The three urea transporters shown in Figure 9–17 are derived from the same gene, UT-A (Fig. 9–18). The transcription of UT-A1 and UT-A3 is driven by the same promotor and are expressed in the terminal part of the IMCD.[64,87,112–116] In contrast, transcription of UT-A2 is driven by a downstream promotor present in an intron[117] and is expressed in the late portion of the SDL (see Fig. 9–4).[64,65] The presence of UT-A2 is presumably responsible for the high urea permeability of the LDL-IM and the SDL (see Fig. 9–12) but the high urea permeability of the ATL is not attributable to any known urea transporter. We speculate that the high urea permeability of the ATL is due to paracellular urea movement. The extremely high urea permeability of the terminal IMCD corresponds to the localization of UT-A1 and UT-A3 (see also "Knockout Mice", later).

All three of the UT-A urea transporters expressed in the kidney are regulated by vasopressin. UT-A2 protein abundance has been shown to be increased in the LDL-IM and SDL in response to long-term treatment with vasopressin.[65] This may be an indirect effect of vasopressin because V2 receptors have not been demonstrated in the LDL or SDL. Isolated perfused terminal IMCD segments exhibit a rapid increase in urea permeability in response to vasopressin.[54,118] This may be in part due to direct phosphorylation of UT-A1[119] although the phosphorylation site has not yet been identified. Exposure of *Xenopus* oocytes injected with UT-A1 or UT-A3 cRNA to PKA agonists (cAMP/forskolin/IBMX) caused a significant increase in passive urea transport, whereas these agents had no effect in UT-A2 injected oocytes.[117] These results suggest that both UT-A1 and UT-A3 are targets for the short-term action of vasopressin working though cyclic AMP. New studies have demonstrated that UT-A2 activity can also be acutely regulated by both vasopressin and its second messengers in cultured MDCK cells.[120]

Long-term vasopressin stimulation or water deprivation has resulted in a *decrease* in UT-A1 protein abundance in the IMCD.[121,122] Changes in osmolality could be responsible.

Na Transporters and Channels
NHE3
The Na-H exchanger, NHE3, is the major absorptive pathway for Na in the proximal tubule. Immunocytochemical studies have demonstrated that it is also expressed in the thin descending limb of Henle (LDL-OM) and the thick ascending limb (MTAL and CTAL)[123] (Fig. 9–19). NHE3 activity in the MTAL is increased by hypotonicity through activation of a PI 3-K-dependent pathway, which is inhibited by vasopressin working through cAMP.[124] Thus, vasopressin has the net effect to inhibit NHE3 activity in the thick ascending limb of Henle.

Na-K-2Cl Cotransporters
Both of the known Na-K-2Cl cotransporters are expressed in the kidney. The ubiquitous form, NKCC1, is expressed in the basolateral plasma membrane of the inner medullary collecting duct,[125] where it is thought to play a role in NaCl secretion.[55] It is also present in the basolateral plasma membrane of outer medullary alpha-intercalated cells.[126]

The "renal" Na-K-Cl cotransporter isoform, NKCC2, is expressed in the apical plasma membrane of the cells of the MTAL (see Fig. 9–19) and the CTAL[127–129] as well as the macula densa.[129] NKCC2 is regulated on a long-term basis by vasopressin, which increases the abundance of NKCC2 protein in the thick ascending limb.[130] This effect is associ-

ated with an increase in maximal urinary concentrating capacity.[131] Vasopressin also acutely increases NaCl absorption in the MTAL,[132,133] in part by regulating trafficking of NKCC2 to the apical plasma membrane[134,135] in association with phosphorylation of the N-terminal tail of NKCC2.[134]

NCC and ENaC
The thiazide-sensitive Na-Cl cotransporter NCC and the amiloride-sensitive sodium channel ENaC are important targets for the action of aldosterone in the regulation of sodium excretion.[136,137] NCC is expressed in distal convoluted tubule cells,[136,138–140] whereas ENaC is expressed predominantly in the connecting tubule, initial collecting tubule, and cortical collecting duct.[141,142] Both NCC[143] and the beta- and gamma- subunits of ENaC[143,144] are increased in abundance by the long-term action of vasopressin. Furthermore, vasopressin acutely increases Na absorption in the rat cortical collecting duct[145,146] by increasing apical Na entry via the amiloride-sensitive Na channel ENaC.[147] The increase in apical ENaC activity has been proposed to be due to vasopressin-induced trafficking of ENaC-containing vesicles from intracellular stores to the apical plasma membrane.[148]

Increasing NaCl absorption via the action of vasopressin on NCC in the distal convoluted tubule and ENaC activity in the connecting tubule and cortical collecting duct can have an important positive effect on urinary concentrating ability by reducing fluid delivery to the medullary collecting ducts (see Fig. 9–16).

Chloride Channels
Two closely related chloride channel (ClC) paralogs, ClC-K1 and ClC-K2 are expressed in renal tubule segments. Strong expression of ClC-K1 is found in both the apical and basolateral plasma membrane of the thin ascending limb of Henle.[149] Although generally viewed as being predominantly or exclusively expressed in the thin ascending limb, there is evidence from RT-PCR studies in microdissected tubules that ClC-K1 is expressed in the thick ascending limb and distal convoluted tubule as well.[150] In contrast, there is general agreement that the chloride channel ClC-K2 is broadly expressed basolaterally along the nephron from the thick ascending limb (see Fig. 9–19) through the collecting ducts.[150–152] Isolated perfused tubule studies have demonstrated that vasopressin increases chloride conductance in the thin ascending limb of hamster,[153] presumably by affecting unit conductance or localization of ClC-K1 chloride channels.

ROMK Potassium Channel
The ROMK potassium channel, an ATP-sensitive inwardly rectifier potassium channel, has been localized to the thick ascending limb, distal convoluted tubule, connecting tubule, and collecting duct system by *in situ* hybridization[154] and immunocytochemistry.[155,156] ROMK is expressed predominantly or entirely in the apical plasma membrane in these segments.[155–157]

ROMK is critical in the active NaCl transport process in the thick ascending limb of Henle (see Fig. 9–19) and consequently plays an important role in urinary concentration and dilution. Vasopressin has a long-term effect to increase the abundance of ROMK protein in thick ascending limb cells,[158] thus contributing to the long-term effect of vasopressin to increase NaCl transport in this segment.[159]

In the connecting tubule and collecting duct, ROMK is responsible for the potassium secretion process that regulates urinary potassium excretion and systemic potassium balance. The later process is strongly regulated by vasopressin.[145] This secretory process may be an indirect consequence of vasopressin's action to increase Na entry via ENaC, which results in apical plasma membrane depolarization and an increase in the electrochemical driving force for K movement through

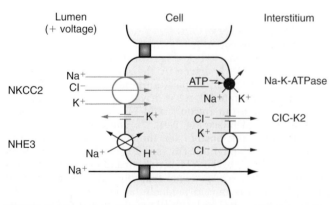

FIGURE 9–19 Ion transporters in thick ascending limb cell. Ion transporters and channels that account for net NaCl transport across the thick ascending limb epithelium. Transporters regulated by vasopressin indicated in green. Transporters not known to be regulated by vasopressin in red. Tight junctional pathway for cations is via a junctional protein called paracellin or claudin-16.[217]

ROMK.[160] An alternative view is that the open probability of the ROMK channel may be regulated by vasopressin in a process that is mediated by CFTR, a cAMP responsive protein.[161,162]

K-Cl cotransporter, KCC4

K-Cl cotransport was first detected in the basolateral plasma membranes of isolated, perfused thick ascending limbs by Greger and Schlatter.[163] Molecular cloning[164] followed by immunohistochemical studies[165] demonstrated that KCC4 is likely to be the basolateral K-Cl cotransporter in the thick ascending limb (see Fig. 9–19). This cotransporter also appears to be expressed in the distal convoluted tubule and the connecting tubule.[165]

Use of Knockout Mice to Study the Urinary Concentrating Mechanism and Vasopressin Action

Expression of a number of the transporters depicted in Figures 9–17, 9–18, and 9–19 as well as the vasopressin V2 receptor have been deleted in mice using targeted gene deletion approaches. The phenotypes of these mice have been informative with regard to the role of these gene products in the urinary concentrating mechanism. This section summarizes the key studies.

Aquaporin-1 Knockout (AQP1 KO) Mice

Verkman and colleagues developed a mouse model in which aquaporin-1 expression was deleted in all tissues.[166] In comparison with wild-type littermates, AQP1 knockout mice had reduced urinary osmolality that was not increased in response to water deprivation. Indeed, the urinary concentrating defect was so severe that after 36 hours of water deprivation, the average body weight decreased by 35% and serum osmolality increased to greater than 500 mOsm/kg H$_2$O. Although proximal tubule fluid absorption is markedly impaired in these mice, distal delivery of NaCl and water was not impaired, owing to a TGF-mediated reduction in glomerular filtration rate.[167] However, the function of the thin descending limb (LDL-OM and LDL-IM), normally a site of aquaporin-1 expression, was markedly impaired. The osmotic water permeability of isolated perfused LDL segments from AQP1 KO mice was markedly reduced compared to control animals.[168] As discussed earlier (see Fig. 9–11), rapid water absorption from the thin descending limbs has been found to be a key component of the countercurrent multiplication process, and presumably impairment of LDL water absorption is largely responsible for the concentrating defect in AQP1 KO mice. In addition, descending vasa recta, a second renal medullary site of aquaporin-1 expression[19] also displayed a marked reduction in osmotic water permeability in AQP1 KO mice compared to controls.[20] Hence, countercurrent exchange processes involving the descending vasa recta are likely to be impaired in AQP1 KO mice. Thus, the concentrating defect in AQP1 KO mice is likely to be due to impairment of both countercurrent multiplication and countercurrent exchange in the renal medulla.

Aquaporin-2 Knockout (AQP2 KO) Mice

Despite the strong evidence implicating an essential role of AQP2 in the urinary concentrating mechanism, a suitable mouse model to examine its function has only recently been developed. In 2001, a mouse knock-in model of AQP2 dependent nephrogenic diabetes insipidus (NDI) was generated by inserting a T126M mutation into the mouse AQP2 gene.[169] This mutation results in a mouse equivalent of humans with a form of autosomal NDI. Although the mutant mice appeared normal at birth, they failed to thrive and generally died within 1 week. Analysis of the urine and serum revealed serum

hyperosmolality and low urine osmolality, typical characteristics of a defective urinary concentrating mechanism. Forward genetic screening of ethylnitrosourea-mutagenized mice isolated another mouse model of NDI with a F204V mutation in AQP2. These mice survived beyond the neonatal period and had a much milder form of NDI.[170]

Recently, two other mouse models have been developed that allow the role of AQP2 in the adult mouse to be examined. One model, developed by Nielsen and colleagues, makes use of the Cre-loxP system of gene disruption to create a collecting duct specific deletion of AQP2.[171] Another model with complete AQP2 protein deletion in the CD was accomplished by tamoxifen-inducible Cre-recombinase expression in homozygous mice in which loxP sites were introduced in introns of the mouse AQP2 gene.[172] The major phenotype in both of these mouse lines is severe polyuria, with average basal urine volumes approximately equivalent to bodyweight. However, despite the polyuria, with free access to water, plasma concentrations of electrolytes, urea, and creatinine are not different in knockout mice compared to controls, and neither was the estimated GFR. Thus, despite having normal renal function (presumably normal active Na$^+$ transport along the nephron), there is a major defect in the urinary concentrating mechanism in these mice. This defect confirms that AQP2 is responsible for the majority of transcellular water reabsorption in the collecting duct system.

Aquaporin-3 Knockout (AQP3 KO) Mice

AQP3 knockout mice have been generated by targeted gene deletion and found to have a greater than threefold reduced osmotic water permeability of the basolateral membrane of the cortical collecting duct compared to wild-type control mice.[173] AQP3 null mice are markedly polyuric (10-fold greater daily urine volume than controls), with an average urine osmolality of less than 300 mOsm/kg H$_2$O. However, unlike AQP1 or AQP2 null mice, AQP3 KO mice are able to raise their urine osmolalities to a modest degree after either water deprivation or the administration of the vasopressin analog dDAVP. It is likely that when AQP3 is deleted, the reduced osmotic water permeability of the basolateral membrane results in a decrease in transepithelial water transport in the connecting tubule, initial collecting tubule and cortical collecting duct, where AQP3 is normally the predominant basolateral water channel. The relatively severe polyuria in this model is consistent with the view from micropuncture data that the majority of post-macula densa fluid reabsorption in the normal kidney is from the cortical portion of the collecting duct system.[4]

Aquaporin-4 Knockout (AQP4 KO) Mice

AQP4 null mice have been generated by standard gene deletion methods.[174] Isolated perfused tubule studies demonstrated a fourfold decrease in IMCD osmotic water permeability, indicating that AQP4 is responsible for most of the water movement across the basolateral membrane in this segment.[175] Despite this reduced water permeability in the IMCD, in hydrated mice, there was no difference in urine osmolality compared to controls and no difference in serum electrolyte concentrations. However, there was a small (15%–20%) but significant reduction in maximal urine osmolality in AQP4 null mice after 36 hours of water deprivation, and this reduced urine osmolality could not be further increased by vasopressin administration, indicating a mild urinary concentrating defect. Why does deletion of AQP4 manifest a modest decrease in urinary concentrating ability while another basolateral water channel AQP3 manifests a profound concentrating defect? The answer to this is based on the normal distribution of water transport along the collecting duct (discussed earlier).[4] The amount of water reabsorbed osmotically in the cortical portion of the collecting duct system (where AQP3 is predominant) is much greater than that absorbed in the medullary collecting ducts (where AQP4 is the predominant basolateral water channel).

UT-A1/3 Urea Transporter Knockout Mice

In 2004, a mouse model was reported in which the two collecting duct urea transporters, UT-A1 and UT-A3, were deleted by standard gene targeting techniques (UT-A1/3[-/-] mice).[87] Isolated perfused tubule studies demonstrated a complete absence of phloretin-sensitive and vasopressin-regulated urea transport in IMCD segments from UT-A1/3[-/-] mice. UT-A1/3[-/-] mice on either a normal protein (20% protein by weight) or high-protein (40%) diet had a significantly greater fluid intake and urine flow, resulting in a decreased urine osmolality, than wild-type animals. However, UT-A1/3[-/-] mice on a low-protein diet did not show a substantial degree of polyuria. In this latter condition, hepatic urea production is low and urea delivery to the IMCD is predicted to be low, thus rendering collecting duct urea transport largely immaterial to water balance. Studies investigating the maximal urinary concentrating capacity of UT-A1/3[-/-] mice showed that after an 18-hour water restriction, mice on a 20% or 40% protein intake are unable to reduce their urine flow to levels below those observed under basal conditions, resulting in volume depletion and loss of body weight. In contrast, UT-A1/3[-/-] mice on a 4% protein diet were able to maintain fluid balance. Thus, the concentrating defect in UT-A1/3[-/-] mice is caused by a urea-dependent osmotic diuresis; greater urea delivery to the IMCD results in greater levels of water excretion. These results are compatible with a model for the role of urea in the urinary concentrating mechanism proposed in the 1950s by Berliner and colleagues.[23] They hypothesized that luminal urea in the IMCD is normally osmotically ineffective because of the high concentrations of urea in the inner medullary interstitium, which balance osmotically the luminal urea and thus prevent the osmotic diuresis that would otherwise occur.

UT-A1/3[-/-] mice have been exploited to study the mechanism responsible for Na and Cl accumulation in the inner medulla. For many years, a model independently proposed by Stephenson and by Kokko and Rector in 1972[84,85] has been the chief paradigm for concentration of Na and Cl in the inner medulla (see earlier). In this mechanism, known colloquially as the 'Passive Mechanism', the generation of a passive electrochemical gradient that drives Na and Cl exit from the thin ascending limb is indirectly dependent on rapid absorption of urea from the IMCD (see earlier for full description). This model would predict that UT-A1/3[-/-] mice, which lack facilitated urea transport in the IMCD would fail to accumulate Na and Cl to a normal degree. However, two independent studies in UT-A1/3[-/-] mice failed to demonstrate the predicted decline in inner medullary Na and Cl concentration, despite a profound decrease in urea accumulation in the renal inner medulla.[87,88] Thus, the passive\pard\plain concentrating model in the form originally proposed by Stephenson and by Kokko and Rector, where NaCl reabsorption from Henle's loop depends on a high IMCD urea permeability, is not the mechanism by which NaCl is concentrated in the inner medulla. Overall, the results with UT-A1/3[-/-] mice demonstrate that the primary role of IMCD urea transporters in the urinary concentrating mechanism is in their ability to prevent a urea-induced osmotic diuresis when urea excretion rates are high.[87,88,176]

UT-A2 and UT-B Urea Transporter Knockout Mice

UT-A2 knockout mice have recently been developed and some aspects of their renal phenotype have been described.[67] On a normal level of protein intake (20% protein), the UT-A2 null mice do not have significant differences in daily urine output compared to control mice and even after a 36-hour period of water deprivation, differences in urine output and urine osmolality are not observed. Furthermore, UT-A2 knockout mice do not have an impairment of urea or chloride accumulation in the inner medulla. Only on a low-protein diet (4% protein), did the UT-A2 knockout mice have a somewhat reduced maximal urinary concentrating capacity compared to wild-type controls, associated with a reduction in urea accumulation in the inner medulla. These results are surprising, considering the role that UT-A2 has been proposed to play in urea recycling in the renal medulla,[65] a process postulated to play a key role in maintenance of a high inner medullary urea concentration. Therefore, they call into question either the importance of UT-A2 in urea recycling or the importance of urea recycling in the concentrating mechanism.

In contrast, mice in which UT-B, the erythrocyte and vasa recta urea transporter, was deleted demonstrated a moderate decrease in maximal urinary osmolality (averaging 2403 mOsmol/kg H_2O in UT-B null mice and 3438 mOsmol/kg H_2O in wild-type mice). These findings suggest that urea transport by UT-B in the erythrocyte or vasa recta is important for the urinary concentrating process.[177,178] In addition, a selective defect in urea accumulation is observed in the renal medullae of the UT-B knockout mice, compatible with the idea that UT-B is important for countercurrent exchange of urea in the renal medulla.

NHE3 and NKCC2 Knockout Mice

Both of the major apical Na transporters mediating Na entry in the thick ascending limb (see Fig. 9–19) have been knocked out in mice, namely NHE3[179] and NKCC2.[180] From the perspective of the urinary concentrating mechanism, the renal phenotypes are much different and a comparison is informative.

The NHE3 knockout mice are viable and the chief elements of the renal phenotype are associated with the fact that NHE3 is the major Na entry pathway in proximal tubule cells. These animals manifest a marked reduction in proximal tubule fluid absorption and a compensatory decrease in glomerular filtration rate owing to an intact tubulo-glomerular feedback mechanism.[181] On ad libitum water intake, they manifest a moderate increase in water intake associated with lower urinary osmolalities,[182] although urinary osmolality in the NHE3 knockout mice still averaged 1737 mOsmol/kg H_2O and maximal urinary osmolality was not evaluated. The NHE3 knockout mice exhibited a marked decrease in renal NKCC2 expression[182,183] despite elevated circulating levels of vasopressin. Thus, NHE3 mice retain the ability to concentrate the urine although they may exhibit a concentrating defect associated with a reduction in NKCC2 expression.

In contrast, NKCC2 knockout mice were not viable because of perinatal renal fluid wasting and dehydration resulting in death prior to weaning.[180] Although these mice could be induced to survive by treatment with indomethacin and fluid administration, extreme polyuria, hydronephrosis, and growth retardation could not be abrogated.

Why does deletion of NKCC2 result in such a severe phenotype, when deletion of NHE3, a transporter responsible for reabsorption of far more Na, results in a viable mouse capable of maintaining extracellular fluid volume? The answer appears to be in the special role that NKCC2 plays in the macula densa in the mediation of tubulo-glomerular feedback. Tubulo-glomerular feedback allows NHE3 knockout mice to maintain a relatively normal distal delivery through a decrease in glomerular filtration rate, whereas NKCC2 mice cannot compensate in this manner because the transporter is necessary for the feedback to occur.

NKCC1 Knockout Mice

NKCC1, expressed in the basolateral plasma membrane of the IMCD cells and intercalated cells, has also been knocked out in mice.[184] NKCC1 null mice had a reduced capacity to excrete free water relative to wild-type mice, and also had a blunted increase in urinary osmolality following vasopressin administration, suggesting abnormalities in vasopressin signaling in the collecting duct.[185]

NCC and ENaC Knockout Mice

Both of the major apical Na transporters mediating Na entry beyond the macula densa have been knocked out in mice, namely NCC[186] and ENaC.[187–189] The renal phenotypes are much different and a comparison is informative.

The NCC knockout mice appear to have a mildly altered phenotype with only a small decrease in blood pressure. On a normal diet they are not polyuric, but with restriction of potassium intake they develop hypokalemia and consequent polyuria, associated with an apparent central defect in the regulation of vasopressin secretion.[190] Only after prolonged hypokalemia do these animals develop evidence of NDI with suppressed aquaporin-2 expression in the kidney.[190]

In contrast to the NCC knockouts, knockout of any of the ENaC subunits results in a severe phenotype with neonatal death. In the alpha ENaC knockouts, early death appears to be due to failure to adequately clear fluid from the pulmonary alveoli after birth,[187] whereas the beta and gamma ENaC knockout mice appear to die of hyperkalemia and sodium chloride wasting.[188,189] When alpha ENaC expression was deleted selectively from the renal collecting ducts, leaving intact ENaC expression in the renal connecting tubule and non-renal tissues, the mice were viable and exhibited only a very mild phenotype with little or no difficulty in maintaining homeostasis in the face of salt or water restriction.[191] Urinary osmolality after a 23-hour period of water restriction was not different from wild-type mice. Thus, Na absorption from the renal collecting duct via ENaC does not appear to be necessary for urinary concentration.

Thus, NCC deleted only from the distal convoluted tubule or ENaC deleted only from the collecting duct results in a very mild phenotype, presumably because one can compensate for the other with regard to sodium balance. It remains unclear whether the severity of the phenotype seen when any ENaC subunit is deleted globally is chiefly because of the importance of ENaC in non-renal tissues or is related to the role of ENaC in the connecting tubule, which is conserved in the collecting duct-only alpha ENaC deletion mice.

ClC-K1 Knockout Mice

In 1999, Matsumura and colleagues generated CLC-K1 null mice (Clcnk1⁻/⁻) and have made use of this model to examine the role of CLC-K1 in the urinary concentrating mechanism.[192] Microperfusion studies determined that there was drastically reduced transepithelial chloride transport in the tAL of knockout mice. Physiological studies revealed that Clcnk1⁻/⁻ mice had significantly greater urine volume and lower urine osmolality compared to controls. Even after a 24-hour period of water deprivation knockout mice were unable to concentrate their urine. This observed polyuria was insensitive to dDAVP administration. The studies demonstrated that the polyuria observed in CLC-K1 null mice is due to water diuresis and not osmotic diuresis such as would be expected with NaCl wasting. Solute analysis of the inner medulla of Clcnk1⁻/⁻ mice determined that the concentrations of urea, Na, and Cl were approximately half those of controls, resulting in a significantly reduced osmolality of the papilla. These studies demonstrate that the ClC-K1 chloride channel, expressed chiefly in the thin ascending limb, is necessary for maintenance of a maximal osmolality in the inner medullary tissue. The findings in the Clcnk1⁻/⁻ mice, therefore emphasize the importance of rapid chloride exit (and presumably Na exit) from the thin ascending limb to the inner medullary concentrating process. As discussed earlier, all inner medul-

lary models not including active NaCl transport from the thin ascending limb must include rapid NaCl (and urea) exit from the thin ascending limb as a component of the model.

ROMK Knockout Mice

Expression of the ROMK potassium channel (Kir1.1) has been deleted in mice by Lorenz and colleagues.[193] These mice manifest early death associated with hydronephrosis and severe dehydration, consistent with the known role of ROMK in active NaCl absorption in the thick ascending limb (see Fig. 9–19). About 5% of these mice survived the perinatal period, but surviving adults still manifested polydipsia, polyuria, impaired urinary concentrating ability, hypernatremia, and reduced blood pressure. From these animals, a line of mice has been derived that has a greater survival rate and no hydronephrosis in adults, albeit possessing higher water excretion rates.[194] Interestingly, these mice do not exhibit hyperkalemia, indicating that the connecting tubule or collecting duct principal cells (or both) must be capable of secreting K via some other pathway, presumably flow-dependent, Ca^{2+}-activated K channels referred to as "Maxi-K" channels.[195]

Vasopressin V2 Receptor Knockout Mice

In 2000, Yun and colleagues created a mouse model of X-linked NDI (XNDI), by introducing a nonsense mutation (Glu-242stop) into the mouse V2 receptor gene.[196] This mutation is known to cause XNDI in humans. This particular mutation was chosen as it has been shown that the encoded mutant receptor is retained intracellularly and completely lacks functional activity, thus mimicking the functional properties of many other disease-causing V2R mutants.

Male V2R mutant mice (V2R⁻/y) died within 7 days after birth. Urine osmolalities, collected from the bladders of 3-day-old pups, were significantly lower than controls. Serum electrolyte analysis revealed that V2R⁻/y pups have increased Na^+ and Cl^- levels, indicative of a severe state of hypernatremia. In control mice, an intraperitoneal injection of the V2R agonist dDAVP resulted in a significant increase in urine osmolality, whereas there was no effect in V2R⁻/y mice. Analysis of adult female V2R⁺/⁻ mice revealed that the mice have polyuria, polydipsia, and a reduced urinary concentrating ability; consistent with NDI. Furthermore, they have an approximate 50% decrease in total AVP binding capacity, resulting in an approximately 50% decrease in dDAVP-induced intracellular cAMP levels. Taken together, the results obtained from this loss-of-function mutation in the V2R are consistent with the general view that the antidiuretic effects of AVP result from an initial interaction between AVP and the V2R, resulting in increased intracellular cAMP and eventually promoting water reabsorption in the kidney collecting duct via aquaporins. The implication is that there is no other significant compensatory event that can generate cAMP and increase water permeability in the renal collecting duct.

AMMONIUM ACCUMULATES IN THE RENAL MEDULLA

Ammonium can be concentrated in urine to concentrations of several hundred millimolar.[197] Production of a final urine with a high NH_4^+ concentration depends on two processes: (1) trapping of NH_4^+ in the renal medulla, which raises the medullary interstitial NH_4^+ concentration to well above that present in the cortex; and (2) diffusion trapping in the collecting ducts (i.e., parallel H^+ and NH_3 transport), which raises the luminal concentration of NH_4^+ above that present in the medullary interstitium.

A substantial corticomedullary NH_4^+ gradient develops in antidiuretic rats and is regulated according to the acid-base state of rats, such that the gradient is markedly increased by

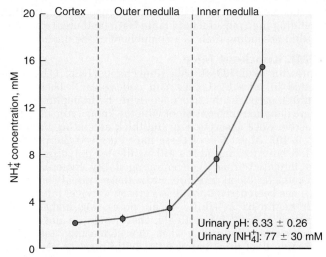

FIGURE 9–20 Corticomedullary NH_4 gradient in canine renal medulla. NH_4 concentrations were measured in tissue water from slices from cortex and medulla of untreated dogs. (Plotted from data of Robinson RR, Owen EE: Intrarenal distribution of ammonia during diuresis and antidiuresis. Am J Physiol 208:1129–1134, 1965.)

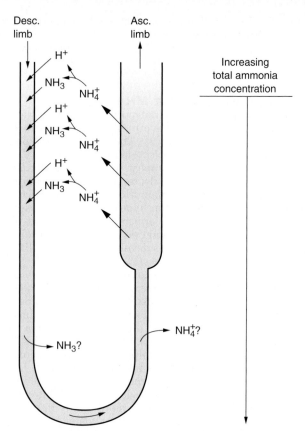

FIGURE 9–21 Countercurrent multiplier for NH_4 in renal medulla. Active absorption of NH_4 from thick ascending limb of loop of Henle provides a single effect for countercurrent multiplication (see text). (Modified from Good DW, Knepper MA: Ammonia transport in the mammalian kidney. Am J Physiol 248: F459–F471, 1985.)

systemic acid loading.[198] Similar medullary NH_4^+ gradients have been found in dogs (Fig. 9–20).[199] Micropuncture studies have shown that NH_4^+ concentrations in the inner medullary vasa recta of rats (and presumably in the medullary interstitium) greatly exceed values in the cortex or peripheral plasma.[200]

NH_4^+ is produced in the mammalian proximal tubule as part of the overall renal process that regulates systemic acid-base balance. The increased NH_4^+ production in the proximal tubule in response to acid loading in rats is associated with increased activity of several ammoniagenic enzymes. Acid loading in rats increases glutaminase, glutamate dehydrogenase, and phosphoenolpyruvate carboxykinase mRNA levels,[201,202] contributing to increased NH_4^+ production and secretion in the proximal tubule.[203]

The trapping of NH_4^+ in the medullary interstitium is thought to occur by a countercurrent multiplication process analogous to the countercurrent multiplication of Na^+ (Fig. 9–21). Studies in isolated perfused tubules have demonstrated NH_4^+ absorption from the thick ascending limb of the loop of Henle against an NH_4^+ concentration gradient,[204,205] which identifies a single effect for the countercurrent NH_4^+ multiplier. The NH_4^+ absorption from the thick ascending limb occurs by direct NH_4^+ transport. Most of the NH_4^+ absorption is active, resulting from coupled Na^+-NH_4^+-Cl^- transport in the apical membranes of the thick ascending limb cells. NH_4^+ absorbed from the thick ascending limb is presumably secreted into the proximal straight tubule and thin descending limb, which creates a recycling pathway around the loop of Henle (see Fig. 9–21). Studies by Flessner and colleagues[206] have demonstrated that the long-looped thin descending limb in the outer medulla is permeable to both NH_4^+ and NH_3, providing a pathway for passive secretion of NH_4^+ actively absorbed from the thick ascending limb. For a high concentration of NH_4^+ to be delivered to the interstitium of the inner medulla, some of the NH_4^+ recycled around the loop must be reabsorbed by either the thin ascending limb or the inner medullary part of the descending limb. Studies of isolated perfused thin ascending limbs[207] from the inner medullae of chinchillas and rats suggest that direct passive NH_4^+ efflux from this segment is the most likely pathway of NH_4^+ delivery to the inner medullary interstitium.

The ammonium that accumulates in the medullary interstitium is then transported from the medullary interstitium into collecting duct cells and is subsequently secreted into the collecting duct lumen, where NH_4^+ can be concentrated to levels much higher than in the interstitium.[200] A number of specific mechanisms for transport of NH_4^+ across the collecting duct epithelium have been proposed. Wall and co-workers[208] demonstrated active NH_4^+ transport across basolateral membranes by substitution for K^+ on the Na^+,K^+-ATPase. Recent studies by Weiner and associates[209,210] suggest that both apical and basolateral transport of NH_4^+ into medullary collecting duct cells of rats is mediated in part by the putative NH_4^+ transporter RhB-glycoprotein. However, in mice, elimination of RhBG expression by genetic inactivation did not disrupt urinary NH_4^+ excretion nor did it inhibit NH_4^+ uptake across the basolateral membrane of cortical collecting duct cells in microperfused tubules,[211] raising doubts about the role of RhBG in renal ammonia transport. In order for NH_4^+ to accumulate in urine to concentrations as high as several hundred millimolar,[197] the most likely mechanism appears to be parallel H^+ and lipid phase NH_3 diffusion (diffusion trapping) across the plasma membranes of collecting duct cells.

References

1. Schrier RW, Gurevich AK, Cadnapaphornchai MA: Pathogenesis and management of sodium and water retention in cardiac failure and cirrhosis. Semin Nephrol 21:157–172, 2001.

2. Almond CS, Shin AY, Fortescue EB, et al: Hyponatremia among runners in the Boston Marathon. N Engl J Med 352:1550–1556, 2005.

3. Bricknell M: Prevention of heat illness in Iraq. *In* Proceedings of NATO Research and Technology Agency Specialists Meeting, Boston, Massachusetts, NATO, 2006.

4. Knepper M, Burg M: Organization of nephron function. Am J Physiol 244:F579–F589, 1983.

5. Kriz W, Bankir L: A standard nomenclature for structures of the kidney. Am J Physiol 254:F1–F8, 1988.

6. Imai M, Taniguchi J, Tabei K: Function of thin loops of Henle. Kidney Int 31:565–579, 1987.

7. Imai M, Taniguchi J, Yoshitomi K: Transition of permeability properties along the descending limb of long-looped nephron. Am J Physiol 254:F323–F328, 1988.

8. Chou CL, Knepper MA: In vitro perfusion of chinchilla thin limb segments: Segmentation and osmotic water permeability. Am J Physiol 263:F417–F426, 1992.

9. Chou CL, Knepper MA: In vitro perfusion of chinchilla thin limb segments: Urea and NaCl permeabilities. Am J Physiol 264:F337–F343, 1993.

10. Chou CL, Nielsen S, Knepper MA: Structural-functional correlation in thin limbs of the chinchilla long-loop of Henle: Evidence for a novel papillary subsegment. Am J Physiol 265:F863–F874, 1993.

11. Pannabecker TL, Abbott DE, Dantzler WH: Three-dimensional functional reconstruction of inner medullary thin limbs of Henle's loop. Am J Physiol Renal Physiol 286: F38–F45, 2004.

12. Kaissling B, Kriz W: Structural analysis of the rabbit kidney. Adv Anat Embryol Cell Biol 56:1–123, 1979.

13. Kishore BK, Mandon B, Oza NB, et al: Rat renal arcade segment expresses vasopressin-regulated water channel and vasopressin V₂ receptor. J Clin Invest 97:2763–2771, 1996.

14. Knepper MA, Danielson RA, Saidel GM, Post RS: Quantitative analysis of renal medullary anatomy in rats and rabbits. Kidney Int 12:313–323, 1977.

15. Zhai XY, Thomsen JS, Birn H, et al: Three-dimensional reconstruction of the mouse nephron. J Am Soc Nephrol 17:77–88, 2006.

16. Rollhuser H, Kriz W, Heinke W: Das Gefs system der Rattenniere. Z Zellforsch 64:381–403, 1964.

17. Kriz W: Der architektonische und funktionelle Aufbau der Rattenniere. Z Zellforsch 82:495–535, 1967.

18. Lemley KV, Kriz W: Cycles and separations: The histopathology of the urinary concentrating process. Kidney Int 31:538–548, 1987.

19. Nielsen S, Pallone T, Smith BL, et al: Aquaporin-1 water channels in short and long loop descending thin limbs and in descending vasa recta in rat kidney. Am J Physiol 268:F1023–F1037, 1995.

20. Pallone TL, Kishore BK, Nielsen S, et al: Evidence that aquaporin-1 mediates NaCl-induced water flux across descending vasa recta. Am J Physiol 272:F587–F596, 1997.

21. Pallone TL: Characterization of the urea transporter in outer medullary descending vasa recta. Am J Physiol 267:R260–R267, 1994.

22. Xu Y, Olives B, Bailly P, et al: Endothelial cells of the kidney vasa recta express the urea transporter HUT11. J Am Soc Nephrol 51:138–146, 1997.

23. Berliner RW, Levinsky NG, Davidson DG, Eden M: Dilution and concentration of the urine and the action of antidiuretic hormone. Am J Med 27:730–744, 1958.

24. Bulger RE, Nagle RB: Ultrastructure of the interstitium in the rabbit kidney. Am J Anat 136:183–204, 1973.

25. Knepper MA, Saidel GM, Hascall VC, Dwyer T: Concentration of solutes in the renal inner medulla: Interstitial hyaluronan as a mechano-osmotic transducer. Am J Physiol: Renal Physiol 284:F433–F446, 2003.

26. Lacy ER, Schmidt-Nielsen B: Ultrastructural organization of the hamster renal pelvis. Am J Anat 155:403–424, 1979.

27. Schmidt-Nielsen B: Excretion in mammals: Role of the renal pelvis in the modification of the urinary concentration and composition. Fed Proc 36:2493–2503, 1977.

28. Sheehan HL, Davis JC: Anatomy of the pelvis in the rabbit kidney. J Anat 93:499–502, 1959.

29. Reinking LN, Schmidt-Nielsen B: Peristaltic flow of urine in the renal papillary collecting ducts of hamsters. Kidney Int 20:55060, 1981.

30. Schmidt-Nielsen B, Graves B: Changes in fluid compartments in hamster renal papilla due to peristalsis in the pelvic wall. Kidney Int 22:613–625, 1982.

31. Wirz H: Der osmotische Druck in den corticalin Tubuli der Rattenniere. Helv Physiol Pharmacol Acta 14:353–362, 1956.

32. Gottschalk CW, Mylle M: Micropuncture study of the mammalian urinary concentrating mechanism: Evidence for the countercurrent hypothesis. Am J Physiol 196:927–936, 1959.

33. Jamison RL, Lacy FB: Evidence for urinary dilution by the collecting tubule. Am J Physiol 223:898–902, 1972.

34. Giebisch G, Windhager EE: Renal tubular transfer of sodium chloride and potassium. Am J Med 36:643–669, 1964.

35. Lassiter WE, Gottschalk CW, Mylle M: Micropuncture study of net transtubular movement of water and urea in nondiuretic mammalian kidney. Am J Physiol 200:1139–1146, 1961.

36. Burg MB, Green N: Function of the thick ascending limb of Henle's loop. Am J Physiol 224:659–668, 1973.

37. Rocha AS, Kokko JP: Sodium chloride and water transport in the medullary thick ascending limb of Henle. J Clin Invest 52:612–624, 1973.

38. Ullrich KJ: Function of the collecting ducts. Circulation 21:869–874, 1960.

39. Wirz H, Hargitay B, Kuhn W: Lokalisation des Konzentrierungsprozesses in der Niere durch direkte Kryoskopie. Helv Physiol Acta 9:196–207, 1951.

40. Grantham JJ, Burg MB: Effect of vasopressin and cyclic AMP on permeability of isolated collecting tubules. Am J Physiol 211:255–259, 1966.

41. Morgan T, Berliner RW: Permeability of the loop of Henle, vasa recta, and collecting duct to water, urea, and sodium. Am J Physiol 215:108–115, 1968.

42. Ullrich KJ, Jarausch KH: Untersuchungen zum Problem der Harnkonzentrierung und Harnverd nnung. Pflugers Archiv 262:S537–S550, 1956.

43. Kuhn W, Ryffel K: Herstellung konzentrierter Lösungen aus verdünnten durch blosse Membranwirkung. Ein Modellversuch zur Funktion der Niere. Hoppe-Seylers Z. Physiol Chemie 276:145–178, 1942.

44. Hargitay B, Kuhn W: Das Multiplikationsprinzip als Grundlage der Harnkonzentrierung in der Niere. Z Elektrochem angew phys Chemie 55:539–558, 1951.

45. Kuhn W, Ramel A: Activer Salztransport als moeglicher (und wahrscheinlicher) Einzeleffekt bei der Harnkonzentrierung in der Niere. Helv Chim Acta 42:628–660, 1959.

46. Sabolic I, Valenti G, Verbabatz JM, et al: Localization of the CHIP28 water channel in rat kidney. Am J Physiol 263:C1225–C1233, 1992.

47. Nielsen S, Smith BL, Christensen EI, et al: CHIP28 water channels are localized in constitutively water-permeable segments of the nephron. J Cell Biol 120:371–383, 1993.

48. Maeda Y, Smith BL, Agre P, Knepper MA: Quantification of Aquaporin-CHIP water channel protein in microdissected renal tubules by fluorescence-based ELISA. J Clin Invest 95:422–428, 1995.

49. Knepper MA, Nielsen S, Chou C-L: Physiological roles of aquaporins in the kidney. Current Topics in Membranes 251:121–153, 2001.

50. Marsh DJ, Solomon S: Analysis of electrolyte movement in thin Henle's loops of hamster papilla. Am J Physiol 208:1119–1128, 1965.

51. Imai M, Kokko JP: Sodium chloride, urea, and water transport in the thin ascending limb of Henle. Generation of osmotic gradients by passive diffusion of solutes. J Clin Invest 53:393–402, 1974.

52. Imai M, Kusano E: Effects of arginine vasopressin on the thin ascending limb of Henle's loop of hamsters. Am J Physiol 243:F167–F172, 1982.

53. Sands JM, Knepper MA: Urea permeability of mammalian inner medullary collecting duct system and papillary surface epithelium. J Clin Invest 79:138–147, 1987.

54. Sands JM, Nonoguchi H, Knepper MA: Vasopressin effects on urea and H₂O transport in inner medullary collecting duct subsegments. Am J Physiol 253:F823–F832, 1987.

55. Rocha AS, Kudo LH: Water, urea, sodium, chloride, and potassium transport in the in vitro isolated perfused papillary collecting duct. Kidney Int 22:485–491, 1982.

56. Star RA, Nonoguchi H, Balaban R, Knepper MA: Calcium and cyclic adenosine monophosphate as second messengers for vasopressin in the rat inner medullary collecting duct. J Clin Invest 81:1879–1888, 1988.

57. Knepper MA, Star RA: The vasopressin-regulated urea transporter in renal inner medullary collecting duct. Am J Physiol 259:F393–F401, 1990.

58. Zimmerhackl BL, Robertson CR, Jamison RL: The medullary microcirculation. Kidney Int 31:641–647, 1987.

59. Knepper MA, Roch-Ramel F: Pathways of urea transport in the mammalian kidney. Kidney Int 31:629–633, 1987.

60. DeRouffignac C, Morel F: Micropuncture study of water, electrolytes, and urea along the loops of Henle in Psammomys. J Clin Invest 48:474–486, 1969.

61. DeRouffignac C, Bankir L, Roinel N: Renal function and concentrating ability in a desert rodent: the gundi (Ctenodactylus vali). Pflugers Arch 390:138–144, 1981.

62. Valtin H: Structural and functional heterogeneity of mammalian nephrons. Am J Physiol 233:F491–F501, 1977.

63. Kriz W: Structural organization of the renal medulla: Comparative and functional aspects. Am J Physiol 241:R3–R16, 1981.

64. Nielsen S, Terris J, Smith CP, et al: Cellular and subcellular localization of the vasopressin-regulated urea transporter in rat kidney. Proc Natl Acad Sci U S A 93:5495–5500, 1996.

65. Wade JB, Lee AJ, Liu J, et al: UTA-2: A 55 kDa urea transporter in thin descending limb whose abundance is regulated by vasopressin. Am J Physiol 278:F52–F62, 2000.

66. Layton AT, Layton HE: A region-based mathematical model of the urine concentrating mechanism in the rat outer medulla. II. Parameter sensitivity and tubular inhomogeneity. Am J Physiol Renal Physiol 289:F1367–F1381, 2005.

67. Uchida S, Sohara E, Rai T, et al: Impaired urea accumulation in the inner medulla of mice lacking the urea transporter UT-A2. Mol Cell Biol 25:7357–7363, 2005.

68. Knepper MA: Urea transport in isolated thick ascending limbs and collecting ducts from rats. Am J Physiol 245:F634–F639, 1983.

69. Rocha AS, Kokko JP: Permeability of medullary nephron segments to urea and water: Effect of vasopressin. Kidney Int 6:379–387, 1974.

70. Knepper MA: Urea transport in nephron segments from medullary rays of rabbits. Am J Physiol 244:F622–F627, 1983.

71. Kawamura S, Kokko JP: Urea secretion by the straight segment of the proximal tubule. J Clin Invest 58:604–612, 1976.

72. Nielsen S, DiGiovanni SR, Christensen EI, et al: Cellular and subcellular immunolocalization of vasopressin-regulated water channel in rat kidney. Proc Natl Acad Sci U S A 90:11663–11667, 1993.

73. Jamison RL, Buerkert J, Lacy F: A micropuncture study of collecting tubule function in rats with hereditary diabetes insipidus. J Clin Invest 50:2444–2452, 1971.

74. Schmidt-Nielsen B, Graves B, Roth J: Water removal and solute additions determining increases in renal medullary osmolality. Am J Physiol 244:F472–F482, 1983.

75. Hai MA, Thomas S: The time-course of changes in renal composition during lysine vasopressin infusion in the rat. Pflugers Arch 310:297–319, 1969.

76. Bray GA: Freezing point depression of rat kidney slices during water diuresis and antidiuresis. Am J Physiol 199:915–918, 1960.

77. Saikia TC: Composition of the renal cortex and medulla of rats during water diuresis and antidiuresis. Quart J Exp Physiol 50:146–157, 1965.

78. Lankford SP, Chou CL, Terada Y, et al: Regulation of collecting duct water permeability independent of cAMP-mediated AVP response. Am J Physiol 261:F554–F566, 1991.

79. Atherton JC, Hai MA, Thomas S: The time course of changes in renal tissue composition during water diuresis in the rat. J Physiol (London) 197:429–443, 1968.

80. Stephenson JL: Countercurrent transport in the kidney. Annu Rev Biophys Bioeng 7:15–39, 1978.

81. Knepper MA, Stephenson JL: Urinary concentrating and diluting processes. In Andreoli TE (ed): Physiology of Membrane Disorders. 2nd ed. New York, Plenum, 1986, pp 713–726.

82. Knepper MA, Chou CL, Layton HE: How is urine concentrated by the renal inner medulla? Contrib Nephrol 102:144–160, 1993.

83. Chou CL, Knepper MA, Layton HE: Urinary concentrating mechanism: The role of the inner medulla. Semin Nephrol 13:168–181, 1993.

84. Kokko JP, Rector FC, Jr: Countercurrent multiplication system without active transport in inner medulla. Kidney Int 2:214–223, 1972.

85. Stephenson JL: Concentration of urine in a central core model of the renal counterflow system. Kidney Int 2:85–94, 1972.

86. Layton HE, Knepper MA, Chou CL: Permeability criteria for effective function of passive countercurrent multiplier. Am J Physiol 270:F9–F20, 1996.

87. Fenton RA, Chou CL, Stewart GS, et al: Urinary concentrating defect in mice with selective deletion of phloretin-sensitive urea transporters in the renal collecting duct. Proc Natl Acad Sci U S A 101:7469–7474, 2004.

88. Fenton RA, Flynn A, Shodeinde A, et al: Renal phenotype of UT-A urea transporter knockout mice. J Am Soc Nephrol 16:1583–1592, 2005.

89. Jen JF, Stephenson JL: Externally driven countercurrent multiplication in a mathematical model of the urinary concentrating mechanism of the renal inner medulla. Bull Math Biol 56:491–514, 1994.

90. Thomas SR, Wexler AS: Inner medullary external osmotic driving force in a 3-D model of the renal concentrating mechanism. Am J Physiol 269:F159–F171, 1995.

91. Thomas SR: Inner medullary lactate production and accumulation: A vasa recta model. Am J Physiol: Renal Physiol 279:F468–F481, 2000.

92. Hervy S, Thomas SR: Inner medullary lactate production and urine-concentrating mechanism: A flat medullary model. Am J Physiol Renal Physiol 284:F65–F81, 2003.

93. Zhang W, Edwards A: A model of glucose transport and conversion to lactate in the renal medullary microcirculation. Am J Physiol Renal Physiol 290:F87–102, 2006.

94. Schmidt-Nielsen B: The renal concentrating mechanism in insects and mammals: A new hypothesis involving hydrostatic pressures. Am J Physiol 268:R1087–R1100, 1995.

95. Hascall VC, Heinegaard DK, Wight TN: Proteoglycans: Metabolism and pathology. In Hay ED (ed): Cell Biology of Extracellular Matrix. New York, Plenum, 1991, pp 149–175.

96. Weigel PH, Hascall VC, Tammi M: Hyaluronan synthases. J Biol Chem 272:13997–14000, 1997.

97. Toole BP: Hyaluronan is not just goo! J Clin Invest 106:335–336, 2000.

98. Comper WD, Laurent TC: Physiological function of connective tissue polysaccharides. Physiol Rev 58:255–315, 1978.

99. Castor CW, Greene JA: Regional distribution of acid mucopolysaccharides in the kidney. J Clin Invest 47:2125–2132, 1968.

100. Dwyer TM, Banks SA, Alonso-Galicia M, et al: Distribution of renal medullary hyaluronan in lean and obese rabbits. Kidney Int 58:721–729, 2000.

101. Pitcock JA, Lyons H, Brown PS, et al: Glycosaminoglycans of the rat renomedullary interstitium: Ultrastructural and biochemical observations. Exp Mol Pathol 49:373–387, 1988.

102. Laurent TC: The Chemistry, Biology and Medical Applications of Hyaluronan and its Derivatives. London, Portland Press, 1998.

103. MacPhee PJ, Michel CC: Subatmospheric closing pressures in individual microvessels of rats and frogs. J Physiol (London) 484:183–187, 1995.

104. Camenisch TD, Spicer AP, Brehm-Gibson T, et al: Disruption of hyaluronan synthase-2 abrogates normal cardiac morphogenesis and hyaluronan-mediated transformation of epithelium to mesenchyme. J Clin Invest 106:349–360, 2000.

105. Nielsen S, Frokiaer J, Marples D, et al: Aquaporins in the kidney: From molecules to medicine. Physiol Rev 82:205–244, 2002.

106. Nielsen S, Chou CL, Marples D, et al: Vasopressin increases water permeability of kidney collecting duct by inducing translocation of aquaporin-CD water channels to plasma membrane. Proc Natl Acad Sci U S A 92:1013–1017, 1995.

107. DiGiovanni SR, Nielsen S, Christensen EI, Knepper MA: Regulation of collecting duct water channel expression by vasopressin in Brattleboro rat. Proc Natl Acad Sci U S A 91:8984–8988, 1994.

108. Ecelbarger CA, Nielsen S, Olson BR, et al: Role of renal aquaporins in escape from vasopressin-induced antidiuresis in rat. J Clin Invest 99:1852–1863, 1997.

109. Ecelbarger CA, Terris J, Frindt G, et al: Aquaporin-3 water channel localization and regulation in rat kidney. Am J Physiol: Renal Physiol 269:F663–F672, 1995.

110. Terris J, Ecelbarger CA, Marples D, et al: Distribution of aquaporin-4 water channel expression within rat kidney. Am J Physiol: Renal Physiol 269:F775–F785, 1995.

111. Terris J, Ecelbarger CA, Nielsen S, Knepper MA: Long-term regulation of four renal aquaporins in rat. Am J Physiol 271:F414–F422, 1996.

112. Fenton RA, Shodeinde A, Knepper MA: UT-A urea transporter promoter, UT-Aalpha, targets principal cells of the renal inner medullary collecting duct. Am J Physiol Renal Physiol 290:F188–F195, 2006.

113. Karakashian A, Timmer RT, Klein JD, et al: Cloning and characterization of two new isoforms of the rat kidney urea transporter: UT-A3 and UT-A4. J Am Soc Nephrol 10:230–237, 1999.

114. Bagnasco SM, Peng T, Nakayama Y, Sands JM: Differential expression of individual UT-A urea transporter isoforms in rat kidney. J Am Soc Nephrol 11:1980–1986, 2000.

115. Terris JM, Knepper MA, Wade JB: UT-A3: Localization and characterization of an additional urea transporter isoform in the IMCD. Am J Physiol: Renal Physiol 280:F325–F332, 2001.

116. Shayakul C, Tsukaguchi H, Berger UV, Hediger MA: Molecular characterization of a novel urea transporter from kidney inner medullary collecting ducts. Am J Physiol Renal Physiol 280:F487–F494, 2001.

117. Fenton RA, Cooper GJ, Morris ID, Smith CP: Coordinated expression of UT-A and UT-B urea transporters in rat testis. Am J Physiol Cell Physiol 282:C1492–C1501, 2002.

118. Chou CL, Knepper MA: Inhibition of urea transport in inner medullary collecting duct by phloretin and urea analogues. Am J Physiol 257:F359–F365, 1989.

119. Zhang C, Sands JM, Klein JD: Vasopressin rapidly increases the phosphorylation of the UT-A1 urea transporter in rat IMCDs through PKA. Am J Physiol: Renal Physiol 282:F85–F90, 2002.

120. Potter EA, Stewert G, Smith CP: Urea flux across MDCK-mUT-A2 monolayers is acutely sensitive to AVP, cAMP and [Ca²⁺]i. Am J Physiol Renal Physiol 291:F122–128, 2006.

121. Terris J, Ecelbarger CA, Sands JM, Knepper MA: Long-term regulation of renal urea transporter protein expression in rat. J Am Soc Nephrol 9:729–736, 1998.

122. Lim SW, Han KH, Jung JY, et al: Ultrastructural localization of UT-A and UT-B in rat kidneys with different hydration status. Am J Physiol Regul Integr Comp Physiol 290:R479–R492, 2006.

123. Biemesderfer D, Rutherford PA, Nagy T, et al: Monoclonal antibodies for high-resolution localization of NHE3 in adult and neonatal rat kidney. Am J Physiol 273:F289–F299, 1997.

124. Good DW, Di Mari JF, Watts BA, III: Hyposmolality stimulates Na⁺/H⁺ exchange and HCO₃⁻ absorption in thick ascending limb via PI 3-kinase. Am J Physiol Cell Physiol 279:C1443–C1454, 2000.

125. Kaplan MR, Plotkin MD, Brown D, et al: Expression of the mouse Na-K-2Cl cotransporter, mBSC2, in the terminal inner medullary collecting duct, the glomerular and extraglomerular mesangium, and the glomerular afferent arteriole. J Clin Invest 98:723–730, 1996.

126. Ginns SM, Knepper MA, Ecelbarger CA, et al: Immunolocalization of the secretory isoform of Na-K-Cl contransporter in rat renal intercalated cells. J Am Soc Nephrol 7:2533–2542, 1996.

127. Kaplan MR, Plotkin MD, Lee WS, et al: Apical localization of the Na-K-Cl cotransporter, rBSC1, on membranes of thick ascending limbs. Kidney Int 49:40–47, 1996.

128. Ecelbarger CA, Terris J, Hoyer JR, et al: Localization and regulation of the rat renal Na⁺-K⁺-2Cl⁻ cotransporter, BSC-1. Am J Physiol 271:F619–F628, 1996.

129. Nielsen S, Maunsbach AB, Ecelbarger CA, Knepper MA: Ultrastructural localizatioon of Na-K-2Cl cotransporter in thick ascending limb and macula densa of rat kidney. Am J Physiol 275:F885–F893, 1998.

130. Kim GH, Ecelbarger CA, Mitchell C, et al: Vasopressin increases Na-K-2Cl cotransporter expression in thick ascending limb of Henle's loop. Am J Physiol 276:F96–F103, 1999.

131. Kim JK, Summer SN, Erickson AE, Schrier RW: Role of arginine vasopressin in medullary thick ascending limb on maximal urinary concentration. Am J Physiol 251:F266–F270, 1986.

132. Hall DA, Varney DW: Effect of vasopressin on electrical potential difference and chloride transport in mouse medullary thick ascending limb of Henle's loop. J Clin Invest 66:792–802, 1980.

133. Sasaki S, Imai M: Effects of vasopressin on water and NaCl transport across the in vitro perfused medullary thick ascending limb of Henle's loop of mouse, rat and rabbit kidneys. Pflugers Archiv 383:215–221, 1980.

134. Gimenez I, Forbush B: Short-term stimulation of the renal Na-K-Cl cotransporter (NKCC2) by vasopressin involves phosphorylation and membrane translocation of the protein. J Biol Chem 278:26946–26951, 2003.

135. Ortiz PA: cAMP increases surface expression of NKCC2 in rat thick ascending limbs: Role of VAMP. Am J Physiol Renal Physiol 290:F608–F616, 2006.

136. Kim GH, Masilamani S, Turner R, et al: The thiazide-sensitive Na-Cl cotransporter is an aldosterone-induced protein. Proc Natl Acad Sci U S A 95:14552–14557, 1998.

137. Masilamani S, Kim GH, Mitchell C, et al: Aldosterone-mediated regulation of ENaC α, β, and γ subunit proteins in rat kidney. J Clin Invest 104:R19–R23, 1999.

138. Ellison DH, Biemesderfer D, Morrisey J, et al: Immunocytochemical characterization of the high-affinity thiazide diuretic receptor in rabbit renal cortex. Am J Physiol 264:F141–F148, 1993.

139. Plotkin MD, Kaplan MR, Verlander JW, et al: Localization of the thiazide sensitive Na-Cl cotransporter, rTSC1 in the rat kidney. Kidney Int 50:174–183, 1996.

140. Yang T, Huang YG, Singh I, et al: Localization of bumetanide- and thiazide-sensitve Na-K-Cl cotransporters along the rat nephron. Am J Physiol 271:F931–F939, 1996.

141. Hager H, Kwon TH, Vinnikova AK, et al: Immunocytochemical and immunoelectron microscopic localization of α-, β- and γ-ENaC in rat kidney. Am J Physiol: Renal Physiol 280:F1093–F1106, 2001.

142. Loffing J, Loffing-Cueni D, Macher A, et al: Localization of epithelial sodium channel and aquaporin-2 in rabbit kidney cortex. Am J Physiol 278:F530–F539, 2000.

143. Ecelbarger CA, Kim GH, Terris J, et al: Vasopressin-mediated regulation of ENaC abundance in rat kidney. Am J Physiol: Renal Physiol 279:F46–F53, 2000.

144. Nicco C, Wittner M, DiStefano A, et al: Chronic exposure to vasopressin upregulates ENaC and sodium transport in the rat renal collecting duct and lung. Hypertension 38:1143–1149, 2001.

145. Tomita K, Pisano JJ, Knepper MA: Control of sodium and potassium transport in the cortical collecting duct of the rat. Effects of bradykinin, vasopressin, and deoxycorticosterone. J Clin Invest 76:132–136, 1985.

146. Reif MC, Troutman SL, Schafer JA: Sodium transport by rat cortical collecting tubule: Effects of vasopressin and desoxycorticosterone. J Clin Invest 77:1291–1298, 1986.

147. Schlatter E, Schafer JA: Electrophysiological studies in principal cells of rat cortical collecting tubules: ADH increases the apical membrane Na⁺-conductance. Pflugers Archiv 409:81–92, 1987.

148. Snyder PM: Minireview: Regulation of epithelial Na+ channel trafficking. Endocrinology 146:5079–5085, 2005.

149. Uchida S, Sasaki S, Nitta K, et al: Localization and functional characterization of rat kidney-specific chloride channel, ClC-K1. J Clin Invest 95:104–113, 1995.

150. Vandewalle A, Cluzeaud F, Bens M, et al: Localization and induction by dehydration of ClC-K chloride channels in the rat kidney. Am J Physiol 272:F678–F688, 1997.

151. Yoshikawa M, Uchida S, Yamauchi A, et al: Localization of rat CLC-K2 chloride channel mRNA in the kidney. Am J Physiol 276:F552–F558, 1999.

152. Kobayashi K, Uchida S, Mizutani S, et al: Intrarenal and cellular localization of CLC-K2 protein in the mouse kidney. J Am Soc Nephrol 12:1327–1334, 2001.

153. Takahashi N, Kondo Y, Ito O, et al: Vasopressin stimulates Cl⁻ transport in ascending thin limb of Henle's loop in hamster. J Clin Invest 95:1623–1627, 1995.

154. Lee WS, Hebert SC: ROMK inwardly rectifying ATP-sensitive K⁺ channel. I. Expression in rat distal nephron segments. Am J Physiol 268:F1124–F1131, 1995.

155. Xu JZ, Hall AE, Peterson LN, et al: Localization of the ROMK protein on apical membranes of rat kidney nephron segments. Am J Physiol 273:F739–F748, 1997.

156. Mennitt PA, Wade JB, Ecelbarger CA, et al: Localization of ROMK channels in the rat kidney. J Am Soc Nephrol 8:1823–1830, 1997.

157. Kohda Y, Ding W, Phan E, et al: Localization of the ROMK potassium channel to the apical membrane of distal nephron in rat kidney. Kidney Int 54:1214–1223, 1998.

158. Ecelbarger CA, Kim GH, Knepper MA, et al: Regulation of potassium channel Kir 1.1 (ROMK) abundance in the thick ascending limb of Henle's loop. J Am Soc Nephrol 12:10–18, 2001.

159. Besseghir K, Trimble ME, Stoner L: Action of ADH on isolated medullary thick ascending limb of the Brattleboro rat. Am J Physiol 251:F271–F277, 1986.

160. Schafer JA, Troutman SL, Schlatter E: Vasopressin and mineralocorticoid increase apical membrane driving force for K⁺ secretion in rat CCD. Am J Physiol 258:F199–F210, 1990.

161. Konstas AA, Koch JP, Tucker SJ, Korbmacher C: Cystic fibrosis transmembrane conductance regulator-dependent up-regulation of Kir1.1 (ROMK) renal K⁺ channels by the epithelial sodium channel. J Biol Chem 277:25377–25384, 2002.

162. Lu M, Leng Q, Egan ME, et al: CFTR is required for PKA-regulated ATP sensitivity of Kir1.1 potassium channels in mouse kidney. J Clin Invest 116:797–807, 2006.

163. Greger R, Schlatter E: Properties of the basolateral membrane of the cortical thick ascending limb of Henle's loop of rabbit kidney. Pflugers Archiv 1983:325–334, 1983.

164. Mount DB, Mercado A, Song L, et al: Cloning and characterization of KCC3 and KCC4, new members of the cation-chloride cotransporter gene family. J Biol Chem 274:16355–16362, 1999.

165. Velazquez H, Silva T: Cloning and localization of KCC4 in rabbit kidney: Expression in distal convoluted tubule. Am J Physiol Renal Physiol 285:F49–F58, 2003.

166. Ma T, Yang B, Gillespie A, et al: Severely impaired urinary concentrating ability in transgenic mice lacking aquaporin-1 water channels. J Biol Chem 273:4296–4299, 1998.

167. Schnermann J, Chou CL, Ma T, et al: Defective proximal tubular fluid reabsorption in transgenic aquaporin-1 null mice. Proc Natl Acad Sci U S A 95:9660–9664, 1998.

168. Chou CL, Knepper MA, van Hoek AN, et al: Reduced water permeability and altered ultrastructure in thin descending limb of Henle in aquaporin-1 null mice. J Clin Invest 103:491–496, 1999.

169. Yang B, Gillespie A, Carlson EJ, et al: Neonatal mortality in an aquaporin-2 knock-in mouse model of recessive nephrogenic diabetes insipidus. J Biol Chem 276:2775–2779, 2001.

170. Lloyd DJ, Hall FW, Tarantino LM, Gekakis N: Diabetes insipidus in mice with a mutation in aquaporin-2. PLoS Genet 1:e20, 2005.

171. Rojek A, Fuchtbauer EM, Kwon TH, et al: Severe urinary concentrating defect in renal collecting duct-selective AQP2 conditional-knockout mice. Proc Natl Acad Sci U S A 10315:6037–6042, 2006.

172. Yang B, Zhao D, Qian L, Verkman AS: Mouse model of inducible nephrogenic diabetes insipidus produced by floxed aquaporin-2 gene deletion. Am J Physiol Renal Physiol 291:F465–472, 2006.

173. Ma T, Song Y, Yang B, et al: Nephrogenic diabetes insipidus in mice lacking aquaporin-3 water channels. Proc Natl Acad Sci U S A 97:4386–4391, 2000.

174. Ma T, Yang B, Gillespie A, et al: Generation and phenotype of a transgenic knockout mouse lacking the mercurial-insensitive water channel aquaporin-4. J Clin Invest 100:957–962, 1997.

175. Chou CL, Ma T, Yang B, et al: Fourfold reduction in water permeability in inner medullary collecting duct of aquaporin-4 knockout mice. Am J Physiol 274:C549–C554, 1998.

176. Fenton RA, Chou CL, Sowersby H, et al: Gamble's 'Economy of Water' revisited: Studies in urea transporter knockout mice. Am J Physiol Renal Physiol 291:F148–154, 2006.

177. Yang B, Bankir L, Gillespie A, et al: Urea-selective concentrating defect in transgenic mice lacking urea transporter UT-B. J Biol Chem 277:10633–10637, 2002.

178. Bankir L, Chen K, Yang B: Lack of UT-B in vasa recta and red blood cells prevents urea-induced improvement of urinary concentrating ability. Am J Physiol Renal Physiol 286:F144–F151, 2004.

179. Schultheis P, Clarke LL, Meneton P, et al: Renal and intestinal absorptive defects in mice lacking the NHE3 Na⁺/H⁺ exchanger. Nat Genet 19:282–285, 1998.

180. Takahashi N, Chernavvsky DR, Gomez RA, et al: Uncompensated polyuria in a mouse model of Bartter's syndrome. Proc Natl Acad Sci U S A 97:5434–5439, 2000.

181. Lorenz JN, Schultheis PJ, Traynor T, et al: Micropuncture analysis of single-nephron function in NHE3-deficient mice. Am J Physiol 277:F447–F453, 1999.

182. Amlal H, Ledoussal C, Sheriff S, et al: Downregulation of renal AQP2 water channel and NKCC2 in mice lacking the apical Na⁺-H⁺ exchanger NHE3. J Physiol 553:511–522, 2003.

183. Brooks HL, Sorensen AM, Terris J, et al: Profiling of renal tubule Na⁺ transporter abundances in NHE3 and NCC null mice using targeted proteomics. J Physiol (London) 530:359–366, 2001.

184. Flagella M, Clarke LL, Miller ML, et al: Mice lacking the basolateral Na-K-2Cl cotransporter have impaired epithelial chloride secretion and are profoundly deaf. J Biol Chem 274:26946–26955, 1999.

185. Wall SM, Knepper MA, Hassell KA, et al: Hypotension in NKCC1 null mice: Role of the kidneys. Am J Physiol Renal Physiol 290:F409–F416, 2006.

186. Schultheis PJ, Lorenz JN, Meneton P, et al: Phenotype resembling Gitelman's syndrome in mice lacking the apical Na⁺-Cl⁻ cotransporter of the distal convoluted tubule. J Biol Chem 273:29150–29155, 1998.

187. Hummler E, Barker P, Gatzy J, et al: Early death due to defective neonatal lung liquid clearance in alpha-ENaC-deficient mice. Nat Genet 12:325–328, 1996.

188. Barker PM, Nguyen MS, Gatzy JT, et al: Role of gammaENaC subunit in lung liquid clearance and electrolyte balance in newborn mice. Insights into perinatal adaptation and pseudohypoaldosteronism. J Clin Invest 102:1634–1640, 1998.

189. McDonald FJ, Yang B, Hrstka RF, et al: Disruption of the beta subunit of the epithelial Na⁺ channel in mice: Hyperkalemia and neonatal death associated with a pseudohypoaldosteronism phenotype. Proc Natl Acad Sci U S A 96:1727–1731, 1999.

190. Morris RG, Hoorn EJ, Knepper MA: Hypokalemia in a mouse model of Gitelman syndrome. Am J Physiol Renal Physiol 290:F1416–1420, 2006.

191. Rubera I, Loffing J, Palmer LG, et al: Collecting duct-specific gene inactivation of alphaENaC in the mouse kidney does not impair sodium and potassium balance. J Clin Invest 112:554–565, 2003.

192. Matsumura Y, Uchida S, Kondo Y, et al: Overt nephrogenic diabetes insipidus in mice lacking the CLC-K1 chloride channel. Nat Genet 21:67–68, 1999.

193. Lorenz JN, Baird NR, Judd LM, et al: Impaired renal NaCl absorption in mice lacking the ROMK potassium channel, a model for type II Bartter's syndrome. J Biol Chem 277:37871–37880, 2002.

194. Lu M, Wang T, Yan Q, et al: Absence of small conductance K⁺ channel (SK) activity in apical membranes of thick ascending limb and cortical collecting duct in ROMK (Bartter's) knockout mice. J Biol Chem 277:37881–37887, 2002.

195. Woda CB, Bragin A, Kleyman TR, Satlin LM: Flow-dependent K⁺ secretion in the cortical collecting duct is mediated by a maxi-K channel. Am J Physiol Renal Physiol 280:F786–F793, 2001.

196. Yun J, Schoneberg T, Liu J, et al: Generation and phenotype of mice harboring a nonsense mutation in the V2 vasopressin receptor gene. J Clin Invest 106:1361–1371, 2000.

197. Kim GH, Martin SW, Fernandez-Llama P, et al: Long-term regulation of renal Na-dependent cotransporters and ENaC: Response to altered acid-base intake. Am J Physiol: Renal Physiol 279:F459–F467, 2000.

198. Packer RK, Desai SS, Hornbuckle K, Knepper MA: Role of countercurrent multiplication in renal ammonium handling—Regulation of medullary ammonium accumulation. J Am Soc Nephrol 2:77–83, 1991.

199. Robinson RR, Owen EE: Intrarenal distribution of ammonia during diuresis and antidiuresis. Am J Physiol 208:1129–1134, 1965.

200. DuBose TD, Jr, Good DW: Chronic hyperkalemia impairs ammonium transport and accumulation in the inner medulla of the rat. J Clin Invest 90:1443–1449, 1992.

201. Wright PA, Packer RK, Garcia-Perez A, Knepper MA: Time course of renal glutamate dehydrogenase induction during NH4Cl loading in rats. Am J Physiol 262:F999–F1006, 1992.

202. Curthoys NP, Gstraunthaler G: Mechanism of increased renal gene expression during metabolic acidosis. Am J Physiol Renal Physiol 281:F381–F390, 2001.

203. Nagami GT: Ammonia production and secretion by S₃ proximal tubulo oogmonts from acidotic mice: Role of ANG II. Am J Physiol Renal Physiol 287:F707–F712, 2004.

204. Good DW: Active absorption of NH4⁺ by rat medullary thick ascending limb: Inhibition by potassium. Am J Physiol 255:F78–F87, 1988.

205. Garvin JL, Burg MB, Knepper MA: Active NH4⁺ absorption by the thick ascending limb. Am J Physiol 255:F57–F65, 1988.

206. Flessner MF, Mejia R, Knepper MA: Ammonium and bicarbonate transport in isolated perfused rodent long-loop thin descending limbs. Am J Physiol 264:F388–F396, 1993.

207. Flessner MF, Knepper MA: Ammonium and bicarbonate transport in isolated perfused rodent ascending limbs of the loop of Henle. Am J Physiol 264:F837–F844, 1993.

208. Wall SM, Davis BS, Hassell KA, et al: In rat tIMCD, NH4⁺ uptake by Na⁺-K⁺-ATPase is critical to net acid secretion during chronic hypokalemia. Am J Physiol 277:F866–F874, 1999.

209. Verlander JW, Miller RT, Frank AE, et al: Localization of the ammonium transporter proteins RhBG and RhCG in mouse kidney. Am J Physiol Renal Physiol 284:F323–F337, 2003.

210. Weiner ID: The Rh gene family and renal ammonium transport. Curr Opin Nephrol Hypertens 13:533–540, 2004.

211. Chambrey R, Goossens D, Bourgeois S, et al: Genetic ablation of Rhbg in the mouse does not impair renal ammonium excretion. Am J Physiol Renal Physiol 289:F1281–F1290, 2005.

212. Atherton JC, Green R, Thomas S: Influence of lysine-vasopressin dosage on the time course of changes in renal tissue and urinary composition in the conscious rat. J Physiol (London) 213:291–309, 1971.

213. Giebisch G, Windhager EE: Urine concentration and dilution. Ch. 37. In Boron WF, Boulpaep EL (eds): Medical Physiology, 1st ed. Philadelphia, Saunders, 2006, pp 828–844.

214. Imai M, Taniguchi J, Yoshitomi K: Osmotic work across inner medullary collecting duct accomplished by difference in reflection coefficients for urea and NaCl. Pflugers Archiv 412:557–567, 1988.

215. Imai M: Function of the thin ascending limb of Henle of rats and hamsters perfused in vitro. Am J Physiol 232:F201–F209, 1977.

216. Imai M, Hayashi M, Araki M: Functional heterogeneity of the descending limbs of Henle's loops. I. Internephron heterogeneity in the hamster kidney. Pflugers Archiv 402:385–392, 1984.

217. Simon DB, Lu Y, Choate KA, et al: Paracellin-1, a renal tight junction protein required for paracellular Mg²⁺ resorption. Science 285:103–106, 1999.

218. Madsen KM, Clapp WL, Verlander JW: Structure and function of the inner medullary collecting duct. Kidney Int 34:441–454, 1988.

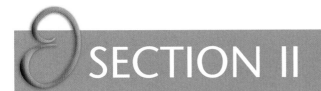

SECTION II

Integrated Control of Body Fluid Volume and Composition

CHAPTER 10

Vasoactive Peptides and the Kidney

Riccardo Candido • Louise M. Burrell • Karin A. M. Jandeleit-Dahm • Mark E. Cooper

RENIN-ANGIOTENSIN SYSTEM

The renin-angiotensin system (RAS) cascade has been viewed historically as an integral component of cardiovascular and renal regulation primarily to maintain and modulate blood pressure and water and sodium balance. Recently, the RAS has proved to be an important regulator of cardiovascular and renal structure and function, in addition to salt and water balance.

The RAS has been implicated in the pathophysiology of various diseases including hypertension, cardiac hypertrophy, and myocardial infarction as well as various progressive renal diseases.[1–3] Of particular interest are newly described roles for the RAS in other situations such as retinal neovascularization[4] and hepatic fibrosis.[5] For this reason, there has been a major effort in the past several years to understand the molecular and cellular mechanisms governing the biosynthesis and the activity of the RAS components, so that novel means might be developed to control their activities. In the classic view of the RAS (Fig. 10–1), the glycoprotein angiotensinogen is secreted into the circulation by the liver, where it is cleaved by renin, an aspartyl protease produced by the juxtaglomerular (JG) cells, to release the decapeptide angiotensin (Ang) I. This peptide is an inactive intermediate, and it is further processed by angiotensin-converting enzyme (ACE), a metalloprotease, into the eight–amino acid peptide Ang II. Ang II binds to high-affinity cell surface receptors, the most well known are the Ang II subtype 1 (AT_1) and Ang II subtype 2 (AT_2) receptors, which cause a remarkably diverse range of physiologic effects.[6] In addition, Ang II can be formed via non-ACE and nonrenin enzymes including chymase, cathepsin G, cathepsin A, chymostatin-sensitive Ang II-generated enzyme (CAGE), tissue plasminogen activator, and tonin.[7] Ang II induces vascular smooth muscle constriction and raises peripheral vascular resistance. In response to Ang II, renal proximal tubular epithelium increases absorption of salt and water. Within the adrenal gland, zona glomerulosa cells are stimulated to produce aldosterone, which in turn regulates sodium reabsorption from the distal tubule. Ang II elevates the resistance of both efferent and afferent arterioles in the kidney and increases filtration fraction. In the heart, Ang II is associated with positive inotropy and in the brain, it induces a variety of responses including the onset of thirst and increased vasopressin release.[8] These and other actions of Ang II act to increase intracellular volume, peripheral vascular resistance, and blood pressure. In addition to its effects on fluid homeostasis, Ang II has been found to have a myriad of local tissue influences, ranging from growth and repair to a role in ovulation.[9]

Given the physiologic diversity of Ang II, it is not surprising that pharmaceutical companies sought inhibitors of this vasoactive peptide at the level of synthesis and action. Three strategies have already been developed: inhibition of the enzymatic action of renin, inhibition of the enzymatic action of ACE, and competitive inhibition of the binding of Ang II to cell surface receptors. ACE inhibitors and, increasingly, Ang II receptor antagonists are now widely prescribed for the treatment of hypertension, heart failure, myocardial infarction, diabetic nephropathy, and other proteinuric renal diseases.

During the development of angiotensin II receptor antagonists, peptidic and nonpeptidic inhibitors were developed that discriminate between the two major classes of angiotensin II receptors (AT_1 and AT_2).[10] Whereas the AT_2 inhibitors are still under experimental investigation, the AT_1 receptor blockers have been extensively evaluated in large clinical trials and have been shown to demonstrate significant beneficial end-organ effects not only in hypertension but also in both cardiac[11] and renal diseases.

In addition to the circulating RAS, there are complete RASs within a variety of tissues and organs, the functions of which are quite varied. Local synthesis of all the components of the RAS has been demonstrated within the kidney. Messenger RNA (mRNA) for both angiotensinogen and renin is found in the JG cells and renal tubular

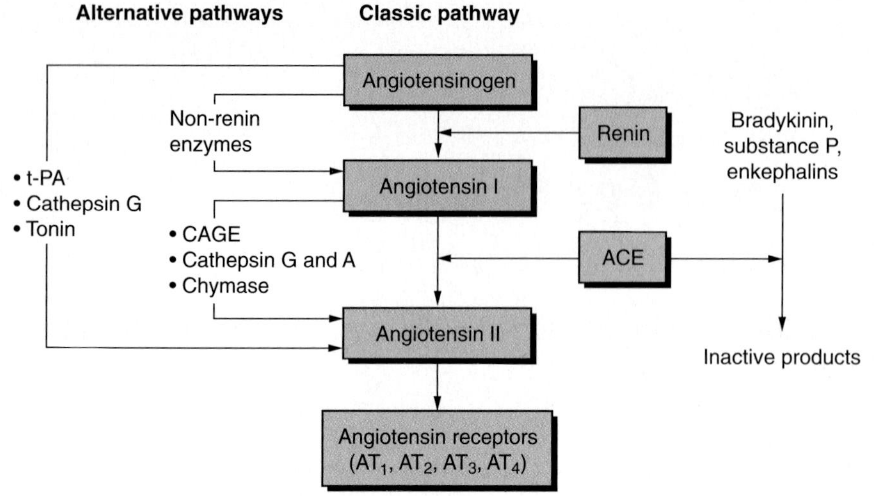

Alternative pathways   **Classic pathway**

FIGURE 10–1 Enzymatic cascade of the RAS: classic and alternative pathways. CAGE, chymostatin-sensitive angiotensin II–generated enzyme; t-PA, tissue plasminogen activator.

cells.[12] AT_1 receptors are found on the efferent and afferent arterioles of the glomerulus as well as in mesangial and tubular epithelial cells. Expression of AT_2 receptor mRNA is highly localized to interlobular arteries. However, emulsion autoradiography and immunohistochemical staining have recently localized AT_2 receptors in the glomeruli and proximal tubules,[13,14] albeit at much lower levels. Multiple functions have been proposed for the intrarenal RAS.[15] Ang II constriction of the afferent arteriole would have the effect of reducing glomerular flow and glomerular capillary pressure, with a corresponding decrease in glomerular filtration rate (GFR). Conversely, constriction of the efferent arteriole, while also reducing flow, would increase glomerular pressure and GFR. The action of Ang II on mesangial cells results in a morphologic appearance of contraction with a corresponding decrease in the glomerular capillary ultrafiltration coefficient. In the proximal tubule, Ang II regulates sodium and pH balance through modulation of the activity of the sodium/hydrogen (Na^+/H^+) antiporter. Indeed, there is much compelling evidence that locally produced components of the RAS may play an important role in both the physiology and the pathophysiology of renal function.

This chapter discusses each component of the RAS and its physiologic and pathophysiologic roles in the kidney.

Angiotensinogen

Plasma angiotensinogen is the source of Ang I in all animal species. Physical isolation of this protein has shown that it is heterogeneous in molecular weight (52–60 kDa). The variance in molecular size appears to stem from a difference in glycosylation.

The human angiotensinogen gene is 12 kilobases long, consisting of five exons and four introns, and is present as a single copy in the human genome.[16] Human angiotensinogen has 452 and rat has 453 predicted amino acids.

The liver is the primary site of angiotensinogen mRNA and protein synthesis. Angiotensinogen mRNA expression has also been demonstrated in the central nervous system, kidney, heart, vascular tissues, adrenal glands, fat, and leukocytes.

In the kidney, both in situ studies and reverse transcription–polymerase chain reaction (RT-PCR) reveal that angiotensinogen gene expression is most abundant in the cortex, primarily within the proximal tubule, with smaller amounts in the glomerulus and even less in the outer and inner medulla.[12,17]

Adrenal angiotensinogen mRNA is most abundant in the zona glomerulosa, consistent with local angiotensin II production being involved in the regulation of aldosterone production.

In the heart, both atria and ventricles have lower levels of angiotensinogen mRNA.[18] Angiotensinogen is found in cerebrospinal fluid, and this is the source of locally produced cerebrospinal fluid Ang II, which appears to be involved in the regulation of thirst and blood pressure through effects on paraventricular structures.

Like α_1-antitrypsin, angiotensinogen is an acute-phase reactant and production by the liver is markedly elevated in response to stresses such as bacterial infection and tissue injury. Finally, Ang II, the final active product of the RAS, participates in a positive feedback loop that stimulates the hepatic production of angiotensinogen. This feedback loop would have the effect that during periods of high Ang II production, the peptide stimulates production of its own precursor protein to ensure constant availability of Ang II. Ang II also increases angiotensinogen mRNA production in the kidney and liver,[19] whereas renin appears to inhibit angiotensinogen release.

Renin

Renin is produced and stored in granular JG cells, which are modified smooth muscle cells found in the media of afferent arterioles.[2,20] Renin is synthesized as an inactive precursor form, preprorenin. Cleavage of the signal peptide from the carboxyl terminus of preprorenin results in prorenin, which is also considered to be biologically inactive. Subsequent glycosylation and proteolytic cleavage leads to the formation of renin, a 37- to 40-kDa proteolytic enzyme. Both prorenin and renin are secreted from JG cells. Because prorenin is the major circulating form, it is postulated that significant conversion of prorenin to renin follows secretion. Prorenin-activating enzymes have been localized to neutrophils, endothelial cells, and the kidney.[2] In addition to JG cells, renin production has also been detected in the submandibular gland, liver, brain, prostate, testis, ovary, spleen, pituitary, thymus, and lung.[2] Circulating renin, however, appears to be derived almost entirely from the kidney.

Within the circulation in humans, active renin cleaves a leucine-valine bond within angiotensinogen (Fig. 10–2) to form the decapeptide Ang I. Based on measurements of the enzymatic activity of renin, several investigators have sug-

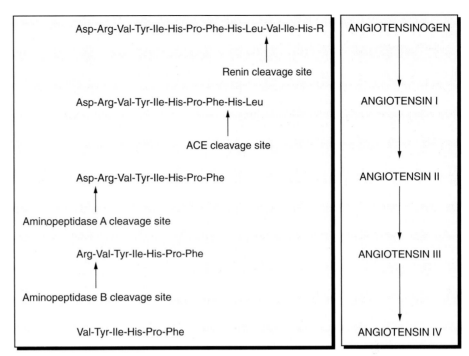

FIGURE 10–2 Comparison of the structure of the RAS components and sites of enzymic cleavage.

gested that inhibitors of renin are present in plasma. Indeed, a number of renin-inhibiting substances such as phospholipids, neutral lipids, unsaturated fatty acids, and synthetic analogs of natural renin substrate have been identified.[21] Recently, Nguyen and colleagues have reported, for the first time, the existence of a functional receptor of renin that was localized to the mesangium of glomeruli.[22] The renin receptor is able to trigger intracellular signalling by activating the mitogen-activated protein (MAP) kinase (ERK1 and ERK2) pathway. It also acts as a cofactor by increasing the efficiency of angiotensinogen cleavage by receptor-bound renin, thereby facilitating Ang II generation and action on a cell surface.[22] These findings emphasize the role of the cell surface in Ang II generation and open a new perspective on renin effects, independent of Ang II.

Renin Secretion

The majority of renin production occurs in the JG apparatus, where these specialized smooth muscle cells of afferent arterioles contain electron-dense granules that are the major storage sites for renin.[2] Renin-containing cells are found throughout the afferent glomerular arteriole, with greatly increased density near the glomerular hilum, hence the term JG cells.[2] Direct secretion of renin into the afferent arteriolar plasma appears to be facilitated by the fenestrated endothelium overlying JG cells. Such fenestrations are a feature commonly observed in endocrine organs, supporting the concept of the JG apparatus as an endocrine structure. Between the afferent and the efferent glomerular arterioles at the glomerular hilum lies a region containing lacelike (lacis) cells (also termed Goormaghtigh cells or extraglomerular mesangium), the so-called polkisen. The extraglomerular mesangium is in direct contact with both the macula densa region of the ascending limb of the loop of Henle and the intraglomerular mesangium. Lacis cells have numerous cell processes extending from their ends and have connecting gap junctions suggesting electrical coupling to each other and to cells of the glomerular mesangium and glomerular arterioles. The region of the macula densa of the thick ascend-

TABLE 10–1	Mechanisms Regulating Renin Secretion
Renal baroreceptors	
Mechanisms involving the macula densa	
Neural mechanisms	
Endocrine and paracrine mechanisms	
Intracellular mechanisms	

ing limb of Henle (so named because of its appearance of tightly packed nuclei) is in close apposition with the lacis cells as well as the cells of afferent and efferent glomerular arterioles. However, macula densa cells and lacis cells are not joined by gap junctions, despite their close relationship. Rather, the intercellular matrix between macula densa and lacis cells appears continuous, and the basolateral surface of macula densa cells is irregular, with spaces between the cells varying in size, depending on the rate of fluid reabsorption at this site. The renal vasculature and tubules are richly innervated, yet nerve endings do not seem to make direct contact with macula densa or lacis cells. The possible role of innervation to the adjacent vascular or ascending limb cells in the function of the JG apparatus remains to be fully elucidated.

Several mechanisms are involved in the control of renin secretion (Table 10–1).

RENAL BARORECEPTORS. In the kidney, renin secretion is controlled by at least two independent mechanisms: a renal baroreceptor and the macula densa. Renin secretion is inhibited by increased pressure or stretch within the afferent arteriole. By contrast, renin secretion increases in response to decreased stretch. In support of this concept, alterations in renal perfusion pressure were shown to result in changes in renal renin release, even when the confounding influences of the macula densa mechanism and renal innervation were eliminated. It is thought that diminished JG cell stretch hyperpolarizes the cells, resulting in a fall in intracellular calcium concentration and increase renin release.

MECHANISMS INVOLVING THE MACULA DENSA. Renin secretion is also related to the composition of tubule fluid at the macula densa.[23] Renal arterial infusions of sodium chloride inhibit renin secretion. Volume expansion with sodium chloride has a more profound inhibitory effect on renin secretion than comparable expansion with dextran, presumably because of an effect of sodium chloride at the macula densa. Initial studies assumed sodium dependence of renin secretion, but later observations have suggested that suppression of plasma renin activity (PRA) by administration of sodium is dependent upon the concomitant administration of chloride (Cl⁻). In fact, sodium fails to suppress PRA when administered with other anions. Similarly, PRA is suppressed by potassium chloride and choline chloride but not by potassium bicarbonate or lysine glutamate. Sodium chloride transport, rather than load, appears to be the important signal. Macula densa cells do not have direct contact with the renin-secreting granular cells in the afferent arteriolar wall. Thus, ion transport plus subsequent second-messenger signaling is necessary. In addition, it has been proposed that adenosine released from adenosine triphosphate (ATP) hydrolysis in macula densa cells serves as the chemical signal that inhibits renin release. Another influence may be the fluid resorption into the lacis cells leading to a stretch receptor mechanism controlling renin release. Mesangial cells appear to contain voltage-activated calcium (Ca^{2+}) channels, as well as Ca^{2+}-activated Cl^- channels, so that changes in extracellular Cl^- concentration might directly affect granular cells. Indeed, whole cell patch-clamp studies have shown a large Ca^{2+}-activated Cl^- conductance in plasma membrane JG granular cells. Arachidonic acid metabolites may also be important in renin release, and arachidonic acid infusion increases PRA (see later). It also appears that nitric oxide (NO) may modulate renin release from the macula densa.[23]

NEURAL MECHANISMS. Renin release is modulated by the central nervous system, primarily via the sympathetic nervous system. Nerve terminals are present on the JG apparatus, and renin secretion is stimulated by electrical stimulation of the renal nerves, by infusion of catecholamines, and by increasing sympathetic nervous system activity. Based primarily on experiments with adrenergic antagonists and agonists, the neural component of renin secretion appears to be mediated by beta-adrenergic receptors, specifically beta₁-receptors.[21] Beta-adrenergic stimulation of renin release appears to involve activation of adenylate cyclase and the formation of cyclic adenosine monophosphate (cAMP).

ENDOCRINE AND PARACRINE MECHANISMS. Several endocrine and paracrine hormones regulate renin secretion by the kidney. Arachidonic acid, prostaglandin E_2 (PGE₂), 13,14-dihydro-PGE₂ (a metabolite of PGE₂) and prostacyclin stimulate renin secretion from renal cortical slices in vitro and from both filtering and nonfiltering denervated kidneys in vivo.[21]

Renin release is also stimulated by other agonists that act through cAMP, namely histamine, parathyroid hormone, glucagon, and dopamine.[21] Whether or how these agonists play a role in the day-to-day physiologic control of renin release is still not fully understood.

Atrial natriuretic peptide (ANP) has been shown to inhibit renin release from isolated JG cells (see later). Other inhibitory hormones include vasopressin, endothelin, and adenosine.[20,23] It has been postulated that adenosine may serve as the macula densa–derived signal that suppresses renin release in response to enhanced solute transport by ascending limb cells. Inhibition of renin release by endothelin suggests a possible paracrine regulation of renin release.[20]

Regulation of renin secretion by Ang II is probably the most physiologically relevant.[24] Ang II inhibits renin secretion and renin gene expression in a negative feedback loop. Treatment of transgenic mice bearing the human renin gene with an ACE inhibitor increases renin expression in the kidney by 5- to 10-fold.[25] Similarly, ACE inhibition in rats augments renal renin mRNA expression, an effect that is reversed by infusion of Ang II.[26] Indeed, ACE inhibition has been shown to be associated with a marked increase in cells with a JG phenotype expressing renin protein.[27] The effects of Ang II on renin are believed to be direct and not dependent on changes in renal hemodynamics or tubular transport.

INTRACELLULAR MECHANISMS. Most investigators have shown that increased extracellular Ca^{2+} concentrations inhibit renin secretion both in vitro and in vivo and attenuate stimulation of renin release by catecholamines. As previously reported, ANP inhibits renin release. The mechanisms whereby ANP and NO, and thus cyclic guanosine monophosphate (cGMP), inhibit renin release need further clarification. The sum effect of ANP on renin release probably depends on the integration between a variety of concomitant stimuli that either augment or inhibit renin release.

Renin secretion is invariably augmented by agonists that stimulate adenylate cyclase activity in JG cells. The finding of a cAMP-responsive element in the renin gene and the finding that forskolin, a diterpene that directly activates adenylate cyclase activity, markedly enhances renin release further indicate that cAMP is an important second messenger in renin release. Renin release in vitro is increased by direct exposure of renal cortical slices to dibutyryl cAMP, with in vivo infusion of dibutyryl cAMP also augmenting renin release. The phosphodiesterase inhibitor theophylline, which increases cAMP levels, enhances the actions of PGE₂ on renin release, providing further evidence that cAMP acts as the second messenger for renin release. cGMP has an important function in the regulation of vascular tone, and an increase in intracellular cGMP induces a vasorelant action. However, no consistent link between glomerular cGMP and renin release has been identified.[28]

Angiotensin-Converting Enzyme

ACE is a zinc-containing dipeptidyl carboxypeptidase that is responsible for the cleavage of the dipeptide His-Leu from the carboxyl end of Ang I to form the octapeptide Ang II (see Fig. 10–2). The main site of synthesis of ACE is in the pulmonary vasculature and, it has a molecular weight of approximately 200 kDa. The structure of ACE has now been determined with the recent crystallization of this enzyme.[29] The analysis of the three-dimensional structure of ACE by Natesh and colleagues[29] shows that it bears little similarity to that of carboxypeptidase A. This new finding provides the opportunity to design domain-selective ACE inhibitors that may exhibit new pharmacologic profiles. Whereas renin is extraordinarily precise in its substrate specificity, ACE is enzymatically far more promiscuous. Indeed, many other small peptides (enkephalins, substance P, luteinizing hormone-releasing hormone) can be cleaved by this enzyme. Moreover, ACE cleaves bradykinin into inactive fragments (see later) and thus functionally degrades this potent vasodilator. The same enzyme produces the pressor substance Ang II and inactivates the vasodepressor kinins. It is perhaps because of this wide diversity of substrates that inhibitors of ACE are so effective in the treatment of hypertension and other cardiovascular and renal diseases.

ACE is also located in plasma and in endothelium of pulmonary and other vascular beds, including the kidney. This enzyme is ubiquitous and has an enormous capacity to convert Ang I to Ang II. Thus, the conversion step has not been regarded as rate limiting for Ang II production. Many tissues produce ACE, but it is the production of the enzyme by vascular endothelial cells that is thought to be most important for the regulation of blood pressure. Nascent ACE protein contains a 29–amino acid signal sequence, and its NH$_2$ terminus is extruded from the cell. A COOH-terminal hydrophobic anchor sequence secures the protein to the luminal face of the endothelial cell membrane. Thus, Ang II is formed at the luminal surface of endothelial cells in close proximity to vascular smooth muscle, a critical target organ for this vasoconstrictor. Studies have examined the ACE levels in human sera, and although levels vary by up to fourfold among individuals, no significant association with clinical hypertension has been identified.[30,31] ACE exists as two isozymes transcribed from a single gene by the differential utilization of two different promoters. In addition, a soluble form of ACE exists that is presumably derived from the vascular endothelium. The larger isozyme, termed somatic ACE, is present as an ectoenzyme in vascular endothelial cells and other somatic tissues including the renal proximal tubule. Analysis of the cDNA shows that somatic ACE contains 1306 amino acids.

A striking feature of the ACE sequence is the presence of two internal homologous domains, each of which in now known to be catalytic. Each domain is composed of 357 amino acids, and overall the two domains are 68% identical in amino acid sequence.

Human ACE in encoded by a single gene located on chromosome 17.[31] It spans 21 kilobases and is made up of 25 exons.[32] Each of the two homologous domains of the enzyme is encoded by a cluster of eight exons (exons 4 to 11 and exons 16 to 23). The similarity of the exon-intron organization of the two clusters strongly suggests that the mammalian ACE gene is the result of an ancestral gene duplication event.

The testis has a distinct form of ACE that is shorter and has only one catalytic site. Whereas the testicular form of ACE seems to be under the control of androgens, DNA elements possibly responsive to glucocorticoids and cAMP have been found in the upstream region of the endothelial promoter.[33] Also, it has been shown that the gene expression of the endothelial ACE is down-regulated by plasma Ang II levels[34] and upregulated by ACE inhibitors[35] and dexamethasone.[36]

Within the kidney, ACE has been localized to glomerular endothelial cells and the proximal tubule brush border.[21] Several potential roles for proximal tubule brush border ACE have been considered. It has been postulated that ACE may play a role in the cleavage of dipeptides from filtered proteins for subsequent uptake and processing by epithelial cells, a role suggested by localization of ACE in intestinal microvilli, a site without Ang II receptors. ACE probably also serves to form Ang II within proximal tubule fluid, thereby affecting reabsorption. In blood vessels, ACE may be located in vascular cells other than the endothelium.[37] In most cells, ACE appears to be located on the external surface of the cell membrane, although there is some evidence that it may also be located intracellularly. It has been demonstrated by Diet and coworkers[38] that ACE is expressed in lipid-laden macrophages within the atherosclerotic plaques in humans. Recently, our group has confirmed and extended these observations to diabetes-induced atherosclerotic lesions. We observed that ACE gene expression was significantly increased in diabetic vessels and that ACE protein expression was consistently found to be at the site of macrophage accumulation within the atherosclerotic plaques.[39] Moreover, recently, our group has demonstrated that ACE is highly expressed in areas of active fibrogenesis in bile duct–ligated livers in the rat suggesting a key role for the RAS in the pathogenesis of liver fibrosis.[5]

The role of plasma ACE is still unknown. Interestingly, studies have shown that a deletion polymorphism of the ACE gene is associated with an increase in plasma ACE levels and with target organ damage in hypertension. Specifically, the D allele of the ACE gene has been associated with microalbu-

minuria, left ventricular hypertrophy, and coronary artery disease, as well as with renal complications in diabetes.[40,41] In addition, we recently demonstrated that the D allele of the ACE gene was associated with renal failure in patients with essential hypertension.[42] Further observations suggest that the ACE genotype may influence the response to ACE inhibitor therapy. In particular, it has been observed that the beneficial short- and long-term renoprotective effects of ACE inhibition are lower in albuminuric diabetic patients homozygous for the deletion compared with the insertion polymorphism of the ACE gene.[43,44] By contrast, Parving's group[45] has demonstrated that treatment with the AT$_1$ receptor blocker losartan offers similar short-term renoprotective and blood pressure–lowering effects in albuminuric hypertensive type 1 diabetic patients with the ACE II and DD genotype, indicating that there is no evidence for an interaction between ACE genotype and blockade of the AT$_1$ receptor. However, this finding remains to be confirmed.

Recently, the classical view of the RAS has been challenged by the discovery of the enzyme ACE2. In addition, there is increasing awareness that many agiotensin peptides other than Ang II have biologic activity and physiologic importance.[46] Two separate groups have described the first human homolog of ACE.[47,48] ACE-related carboxypeptidase (ACE2), like ACE, is a membrane-associated and -secreted enzyme. The ACE2 and ACE catalytic domains are 42% identical in amino acid sequence, and conservation of exon-intron organization further indicates that the two genes evolved from a common ancestor.[47] In contrast to ACE, however, ACE2 is highly tissue specific. Whereas ACE is expressed ubiquitously in the vasculature, human ACE2 is restricted to the heart, kidney, and testis.[47] In addition to endothelial expression, ACE2 is present in smooth muscle in some coronary vessels and focally in tubular epithelium of the kidney. Both ACE and ACE2 cleave Ang I, but their activities are distinct. Whereas ACE is a dipeptidase, ACE2 removes the single C-terminal Leu residue to generate Ang 1-9 (Fig. 10–3). Ang 1-9 has been identified in vivo in rat and human plasma, but its function is unknown.[49] Ang 1-9 is then subjected to further cleavage by ACE to yield Ang 1-7, a vasodilator.[46,50] In addition, Ang II can be degraded by ACE2 to also yield Ang 1-7 (see Fig. 10–3). Thus, ACE2 may function to limit the vasoconstrictor action of Ang II not only by its inactivation but also by the formation of a counteracting vasodilatory angiotensin, Ang 1-7. Although Ang II is considered to be the main effector of the RAS, the reported vasodilatory actions of Ang 1-7,[46,50] taken together with the discovery of ACE2 and its potential involvement in both Ang II degradation and Ang 1-7 production, adds another level of complexity to the RAS. Thus, the identification and characterization of ACE2 has uncovered an exciting new area of cardiovascular and renal physiology as well as providing possible novel therapeutic targets. In addition, an unexpected function of ACE2 has recently been identified and characterized. Specifically, ACE2 is a functional receptor for coronaviruses, including the coronavirus that cause severe acute respiratory syndrome, and is involved in mediating virus entry and cell fusion.[51] Although not directly relevant to cardiovascular function, this would indicate that the RAS including ACE2 has multiple roles in physiology and various pathophysiologic states.[52]

Indeed, a recent study[53] has shown that ACE2 mRNA levels are reduced in animal models of hypertension and ACE2 knockout mice exhibit severe defects in cardiac contractility that are restored by concomitant ACE ablation. These findings support the concept that ACE2 acts in a counter-regulatory manner to ACE and may play an important role to modulate the balance between vasoconstrictors and vasodilators in the heart and kidney. Recent immunohistochemical studies have shown that in the kidney, both ACE2 and ACE protein

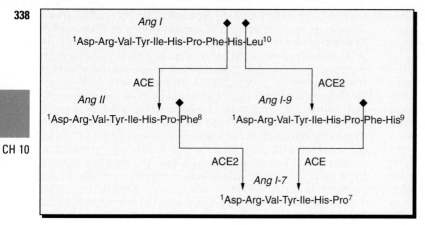

FIGURE 10–3 A schema showing where ACE and ACE2 cleave angiotensin (Ang) I as well as how the cleavage products are processed by the two peptidases.

are localized to tubular epithelial cells.[54] Furthermore, we have reported that ACE2 protein expression is reduced in the diabetic kidney and that this reduction is prevented by ACE inhibitor therapy, suggesting that ACE2 might have a reno-protective role in diabetes.[54] Given the findings of altered expression levels of ACE2 in the diseased kidney, it is postulated that there is an important role for ACE2 in angiotensin metabolism, renal physiology, and potentially, a variety of renal diseases.[55]

Angiotensins and Angiotensinases

Ang II has a very short biologic half-life. After intravenous injection, the pressor response in animals lasts only 1 to 3 minutes. This very rapid effect would suggest rapid uptake from the circulation and/or degradation. Seventy percent or more of Ang II is removed in one circulation, through the liver or the femoral or vascular beds. However, Ang II passes undestroyed through the pulmonary circulation.

AMINOPEPTIDASES. Ang II, with aspartic acid in position 1, is most susceptible to cleavage by an acid aminopeptidase, known as aminopeptidase A, angiotensinase A, or more precisely, glutamyl aminopeptidase. Glutamyl aminopeptidase is a metalloprotease containing zinc. In vivo, cleavage by glutamyl aminopeptidase is the step that usually begins the degradation of Ang II.[56] Removal of aspartic acid from Ang II forms the heptapeptide Ang 2-8, also called Ang III (see Fig. 10–2). This heptapeptide is a less potent vaso-constrictor than Ang II, but it is at least as potent as the octapeptide in the adrenal zona glomerulosa and central nervous system. Indeed, it has been postulated that Ang III is the principal effector of the RAS in the brain. Ang III is even more rapidly hydrolyzed than Ang II in vivo. Like Ang II, the heptapeptide is first cleaved by aminopeptidase action into the hexapeptide Ang 3-8 or Ang IV (see Fig. 10–2). The enzyme most active in its further cleavage is arginyl aminopeptidase (angiotensinase B or aminopeptidase B). Another enzyme, aminopeptidase N, can convert Ang III into the hexapeptide Ang IV. Other aminopeptidases that cleave angiotensins include leucyl aminopeptidase, alanyl aminopeptidase, and dipeptidyl peptidase I (also known as cathepsin C).

Ang IV, another breakdown product once thought to be a virtually inactive peptide, has been demonstrated by Kerins and colleagues[57] to be the form of angiotensin that stimulates endothelial expression of plasminogen inactivator inhibitor (PAI)-1. This effect appears to be mediated via the stimulation of an endothelial AT$_4$ receptor because neither AT$_1$ nor AT$_2$ receptor antagonists could inhibit the Ang IV-induced PAI-1

gene expression.[57,58] There is also some evidence that Ang IV is involved in the pathogenesis of some renal diseases.

ENDOPEPTIDASES. Angiotensins are susceptible to hydroly-sis by several classical endopeptidases, including trypsin and chymotrypsin, which probably never gain access to these peptides either at their origin in the circulation or at their targets outside of the gut. The endopeptidase most likely to be involved in limiting the duration of action of angiotensin is neutral endopeptidase (NEP), also called enkephalinase. This enzyme has also been throughly studied for its action on ANP (see later). NEP can directly convert Ang I to Ang 1-7.[59] Whereas Ang I is the primary substrate for the formation of Ang 1-7, the heptapeptide may be formed also from Ang II by the cleavage of the Pro^7-Phe^8 bond by prolyl-endopeptidase and a prolyl carboxypeptidase.[60] Formerly considered physi-ologically inactive, Ang 1-7 has been recently demonstrated to have effects on the vasculature and on kidney function. In the vasculature, it produces opposite effects to the growth promoting and constrictor actions of Ang II. In the kidney, Ang 1-7 exerts important regulatory effects on the long-term control of arterial pressure, particularly to counterbalance the actions of Ang II. Infusion of Ang 1-7 into the renal artery stimulates marked diuresis and natriuresis.[61–63] Ang 1-7 is hydrolyzed at the Ile^5-His^6 bond to form Ang 1-5 and the dipeptide His-Pro by ACE.[64,65] This observation suggests that chronic treatment with ACE inhibitors is able to prolong the half-life of Ang 1-7.[66] Thus, ACE constitutes a critical conver-gence point between the pressor and proliferative properties of Ang II and the depressor and antiproliferative actions of Ang 1-7, similarly to that observed for bradykinin (see later).

Angiotensin II Receptors

Ang II is known to interact with at least two distinct Ang II receptor subtypes, designated AT$_1$ and AT$_2$.[67] The character-ization of Ang II receptor subtypes was made possible by the discovery and development of selective nonpeptide Ang II receptor antagonists, namely losartan (AT$_1$-selective) and PD123319 (AT$_2$-selective).[68] Virtually all the known biologic actions of Ang II, including vasoconstriction, release of aldosterone, stimulation of sympathetic transmission, and cellular growth, are mediated by the AT$_1$ receptor.[68,69] The functional role of the AT$_2$ receptor is not fully understood. Recent studies have described a possible role for AT$_2$ recep-tors in mediating antiproliferation, apoptosis, differentia-tion, and possibly vasodilation.[70,71] However, recent evidence indicates that proinflammatory, growth stimulatory, and pro-fibrogenic effects of Ang II may not be solely transduced through AT_1 receptors, but also involve activation of AT_2 receptors.

AT_1 Receptors

AT_1 receptors selectively bind biphenylimidazoles, including losartan, candesartan, and irbesartan, with high affinity and are rather insensitive to tetrahydroimidazolpyridines, such as PD123319 and PD123177.[68]

The gene for the AT_1 receptor was first cloned from rat vascular smooth muscle cells[72] and bovine adrenal gland.[73] The AT_1 receptor gene product consists of 359 amino acids and has a molecular mass of 41 kDa. The human genome contains a unique gene coding for the AT_1 receptor, which is localized on chromosome 3.[74]

The AT_1 receptor belongs to the seven transmembrane class of G-protein–coupled receptors.[75] The transmembrane domain and the extracellular loop play an important role in Ang II binding.[76] The binding site for Ang II is different from the binding site for AT_1 receptor antagonists, which interact only with the transmembrane domain of the receptor.[77] Like most G-protein–coupled receptors, the AT_1 receptor is also subject to internalization when stimulated by Ang II, a process dependent on specific residues on the cytoplasmic tail.[78]

There are five classical signal transduction mechanisms for the AT_1 receptor: activation of phospholipase A_2, phospholipase C, phospholipase D, and L-type Ca^{2+} channels and inhibition of adenylate cyclase.

It has been observed that activation of the AT_1 receptor stimulates growth factor pathways, such as tyrosine phosphorylation and phospholipase C-gamma, leading to activation of downstream proteins, including MAP kinases, janus kinases (JAK), and the signal transducers and activators of transcription (STAT) proteins.[79,80] Ang II–stimulated cellular proliferation and growth has been defined in adrenal medulla and vascular smooth muscle cells. These growth-like effects have been linked to cardiovascular and kidney diseases.

The tissue distribution of AT_1 receptors has been studied extensively in humans and animals. AT_1 receptors are found primarily in the brain, adrenal glands, heart, vasculature, and kidney, serving to regulate blood pressure and fluid and electrolyte balance. AT_1 receptors have been demonstrated in the central nervous system of the rat,[81] rabbit,[82] and human.[83,84] AT_1 receptors are localized to areas of the brain that are exposed to blood-borne Ang II, such as the circumventricular organs, including the subfornical organ, median eminence, vascular organ of the lamina terminalis, anterior pituitary, and the area postrema in the hindbrain.[81] Furthermore, other regions of the hypothalamus, nucleus of the solitary tract, and ventrolateral medulla in the hindbrain also contain a high density of AT_1 receptors.[81]

AT_1 receptors have also been identified in the adrenal gland of rodents, primates, and humans,[6] where they are localized mainly to the zona glomerulosa of the cortex and chromaffin cells of the medulla. In the heart, the highest density of AT_1 receptors is found in the conducting system.[85] Punctate AT_1 receptor binding is found in the epicardium surrounding the atria, with low binding seen throughout the atrial and ventricular myocardium.[86] Moreover, AT_1 receptors in the vasculature, including the aorta, pulmonary, and mesenteric arteries, are present at high levels on smooth muscle cells and at low levels in the adventitia.[87]

The anatomic distribution of the AT_1 receptor in the kidney has been mapped in various species.[87] High levels of AT_1 receptor binding occur in glomerular mesangial cells and renal interstitial cells located between the tubules and the vasa recta bundles within the inner stripe of the outer medulla.[88] Moreover, moderate binding is localized to proximal convoluted tubular epithelia.

Ang II stimulation of AT_1 receptors in blood vessels causes vasoconstriction, leading to an increase in peripheral vascular tone and systemic blood pressure. AT_1 receptors in the heart are known to mediate the positive inotropic and chronotropic effects of Ang II on cardiomyocytes.[89] Ang II is also known to mediate cell growth and proliferation in cardiac myocytes and fibroblasts, as well as in vascular smooth muscle cells.[90,91] Ang II induces the expression and release of various endogenous growth factors, including basic fibroblast growth factor (bFGF), transforming growth factor (TGF)-β1 and platelet-derived growth factor (PDGF).[90,91] It is now clear that these long-term trophic effects of Ang II occur as a result of activation of AT_1 receptors.[92] It is well documented that AT_1 receptor activation mediates the Ang II–induced release of catecholamines from the adrenal medulla and aldosterone from the adrenal cortex.[93] Finally, in the kidney Ang II influences sodium and water reabsorption from the proximal tubules and inhibits renin secretion from the macula densa cells via the AT_1 receptor.[94]

AT_2 Receptors

The AT_2 receptor is characterized by its high affinity for PD123319, PD123177, and CGP42112 and its very low affinity for losartan and candesartan.[68] Ang II binds to the AT_2 receptor with similar affinity as to the AT_1 receptor.[67]

The AT_2 receptor has been cloned in a variety of species, including human,[95,96] rat,[97] and mouse.[98,99] The AT_2 receptor is also a seven transmembrane domain receptor, encoded by a 363–amino acid protein with a molecular mass of 41 kDa, and shares only 34% sequence identity with the AT_1 receptor.[100] The AT_2 receptor gene has been mapped in humans to chromosome X.[95]

Previously, various second messengers coupled to the AT_2 receptor have been described and include indirect negative coupling to guanylate cyclase (inhibition of cGMP production)[100] and activation of potassium channels.[101] There have been new insights into AT_2 receptor signalling pathways, including activation of protein phosphatases and protein dephosphorylation, the NO-cGMP system, and phospholipase A_2 (release of arachidonic acid). In particular, stimulation of AT_2 receptors leads to activation of various phosphatases, such as protein tyrosine phosphatase, MAP kinase phosphatase 1 (MKP-1),[102,103] SH2-domain–containing phosphatase 1 (SHP-1)[104] and serine/threonine phosphatase 2A,[105] resulting in the inactivation of extracellular signal-regulated kinase (ERK), opening of potassium channels and inhibition of T-type Ca^{2+} channels.[106] It has been confirmed that the AT_2 receptor is a G-protein–coupled receptor[13] and that an inhibitory G-protein (G_i) is linked to the AT_2 receptor signalling mechanism.[107]

In the human heart, the AT_2 receptor is localized mainly to fibroblasts in interstitial regions, with a lower degree of binding seen in the surrounding myocardium.[108,109] Moreover, AT_2 receptors are highly expressed in the adrenal medulla of most species, but expression is much lower in humans.[6,110] In human kidneys, the AT_2 receptor is localized to glomeruli, tubules, and renal blood vessels.[14]

Using emulsion autoradiography, our group demonstrated the presence of AT_2 receptors in the glomeruli and proximal tubules of adult rat kidney.[13] These findings are similar to those reported by Ozono and coworkers[14] who demonstrated, using immunohistochemistry and Western blot analysis, that the AT_2 receptor is localized mainly to glomeruli, but it is also found at low levels in cortical tubules and interstitial cells.

Because the AT_2 receptor is highly abundant in fetal tissues, it is believed to play an important role in fetal development. However, AT_2 receptor knockout mice appear to develop and grow normally (see later), suggesting that AT_2 receptors may not be as crucial as previously thought for fetal development.[111,112] In mice lacking the AT_2 receptor, the drinking response is impaired and locomotion is reduced. In addition, the animals exhibit an increase in the vasopressor response to Ang II.

It has been demonstrated that the AT_2 receptor is involved in the production of cGMP,[113] NO,[114] and prostaglandin F2α[115] in the kidney, suggesting an important role in renal function, including vasodilatation and blood pressure regulation. In addition, evidence suggests that, in the kidney, AT_2 receptor stimulation induces the bradykinin/NO pathway.[116]

Our group has explored the renal expression of the AT_2 receptor in subtotally nephrectomized rats and the effects of AT_2 receptor blockade on renal injury.[117] In that study, we observed increased gene expression of the AT_2 receptor in the kidney, whereas no global differences in AT_2 receptor protein expression and binding were found between remnant and control kidneys. However, the AT_2 receptor protein was identified specifically in the injured tubules after renal mass reduction. Treatment with the AT_2 receptor blocker PD123319 significantly reduced tubulointerstitial injury, tubular cell proliferation, renal inflammatory cell infiltration, and proteinuria.[117] These findings suggest a key role for the AT_2 receptor in mediating kidney damage in certain contexts.

Other Angiotensin Receptors

There is mounting evidence for the existence of additional angiotensin receptors, which are pharmacologically distinct from AT_1 and AT_2 receptors. The angiotensin AT_4 receptor is a novel binding site that displays high specificity and affinity for the hexapeptide fragment Ang IV, but with low affinity for Ang II.[118] The binding of Ang IV to the AT_4 receptor is insensitive to both losartan and PD123319 but is selectively blocked by the peptide antagonist divalinal-Ang IV.[119] Although it is not clear yet whether the AT_4 receptor belongs to the G-protein–coupled receptor superfamily as reported for the AT_1 and AT_2 receptor subtypes, it has been demonstrated that this transmembrane protein is distributed in many tissues, and in particular, in the brain and kidney. Harding and colleagues[120] have shown that the AT_4 receptor is preferentially concentrated in the outer stripe of the medulla. Moreover, using autoradiography Handa and coworkers[121] localized AT_4 receptors to the cell body and apical membrane of convoluted and straight proximal tubules not only in the outer medulla but also in the cortex of rat kidney. The same authors demonstrated that human proximal tubular epithelial cells contain functional AT_4 receptors that are pharmacologically similar to the AT_4 receptor described in more distal segments of the nephron and other renal cells.[122,123] The functional role of this receptor remains to be fully clarified, but it has been suggested that it may play an important role in mediating cerebral and renal blood flow, memory retention, and neuronal development.[118]

Studies using the selective Ang 1-7 antagonist A-779 provide evidence for an Ang 1-7 receptor distinct from the classical Ang II receptors AT_1 and AT_2.[124,125] Recent studies by Santos and colleagues[126] have identified the G protein–coupled receptor Mas as a functional receptor for Ang 1-7 because it binds Ang 1-7 and is involved in mediating biologic actions of this angiotensin peptide. Because Ang 1-7 counteracts Ang II, these findings clearly widen the possibilities for treating cardiovascular diseases using agonists for the Ang 1-7-Mas axis.

Another atypical angiotensin binding site, loosely termed the AT_3 receptor, has also been identified in cultured mouse neuroblastoma cells and binds Ang II with high affinity, but has low affinity for Ang III and no affinity for losartan or PD123319.[127]

Renin-Angiotensin System Knockout or Transgenic Models

Targeted gene manipulation has provided significant insights into the physiologic and pathologic roles of the RAS in regulating blood pressure, cardiovascular homeostasis, renal function, and development (Table 10–2). In angiotensinogen-deficient mice, who have complete loss of plasma immunoreactive Ang I,[128] the systolic blood pressure was approximately 20 to 30 mmHg lower than in wild-type mice.[128] Similarly, in ACE-deficient mice, markedly reduced blood pressure was observed, and interestingly, there was also severe renal disease.[129,130] The renal papilla in these mice was markedly reduced, and the intrarenal arteries exhibited vascular hyperplasia associated with a perivascular inflammatory infiltrate. Moreover, these animals could not effectively concentrate urine and had an abnormally low urinary sodium–to-potassium ratio despite reduced levels of aldosterone.

Deletion of the gene encoding the AT_{1A} receptor subtype in mice is associated with a significant reduction in blood pressure and an attenuated pressor response to infused Ang II.[131,132] Conversely, in AT_{1B} receptor knockout mice, systemic blood pressure is normal, suggesting that the AT_{1A} receptor subtype is the major receptor involved in blood pressure regulation.[133] Deletion of either the AT_{1A} or the AT_{1B} receptor in mice is not associated with impaired development, survival, or tissue abnormalities.[131,132,134] However, deletion of both receptor subtypes results in decreased blood pressure, impaired growth, and renal abnormalities, a phenotype similar to that seen with deletion of angiotensinogen or ACE.[134,135] Thus, the AT_{1B} receptor, although considered to be of less importance, may compensate for the effects seen in AT_{1A} knockout mice.

In contrast to AT_1 receptor gene deletion, targeted deletion of the AT_2 receptor gene in mice results in raised blood pressure and enhanced sensitivity to the pressor effects of Ang II.[111,112] This suggests that the AT_2 receptor mediates a vasodepressor effect and may functionally oppose the effects mediated by the AT_1 receptor, possibly via bradykinin and NO.[136] Although AT_2 receptors are abundant in fetal tissues, such as the heart, kidney, and brain, AT_2 receptor knockout mice apparently develop and grow normally.[111,112] However, these mice have impaired drinking responses to water deprivation and reduced exploratory behavior.[111,112] More recently, it has been reported that mice lacking the AT_2 receptor exhibit anxiety-like behavior[137] and have increased sensitivity to pain.[138] Thus, the AT_2 receptor may also play a role in modulating behavioral effects, mood, and the threshold for pain.

The RAS has been the focus of the largest number of transgenic studies reported in the renal literature using animal models overexpressing various components of the RAS.[139] Rats transgenic for either the human renin or the human angiotensin gene have normal plasma Ang II levels despite high circulating levels of renin or angiotensinogen.[140,141] These negative findings can be explained by the species specificity of the renin-angiotensinogen interaction. Human renin does not act on rat angiotensinogen, and human angiotensinogen does not serve as a substrate for rat renin.[140] However, transgenic mice expressing both human angiotensinogen and human renin genes under the control of the appropriate human promoter[142] develop hypertension and renal fibrosis. Administration of the ACE inhibitor lisinopril to these mice significantly decreased the glomerulosclerosis index without decreasing systolic blood pressure. These results suggest that activation of the renal RAS induces renal sclerosis independently of systemic hypertension. Findings from other animal models support the hypothesis that endogenous Ang II produced locally plays a role in the formation of renal

Model	Systolic Blood Pressure	Fetal Kidney Development	Postnatal Kidney Development
AGT −/−	Very low (reduction of 20 mm Hg)	Normal	Hypertrophy of renal arteries and arterioles, atrophy of the papilla, focal areas of tubular dropout, interstitial inflammation and fibrosis
Renin −/−	Very low (reduction of 20 mm Hg)	Normal	Similar to that observed in AGT −/− model
ACE −/−	Very low (reduction of 20 mm Hg)	Normal	Similar to that observed in AGT −/− model
AT_{1A}/AT_{1B} −/−	Very low (reduction of 20 mm Hg)	Normal	Similar to that observed in AGT −/− model
AT_{1A} −/−	Moderately low (reduction of 12 mm Hg)	Normal	Normal or slight dilatation of the renal pelvis, mild compression of the papilla, shortening of the renal papilla, and reduction in the area of the inner medulla
AT_{1B} −/−	Normal	Normal	Normal
AT_2 −/−	High (increase of 13 mm Hg)	Normal	Normal

TABLE 10–2 Differential Phenotypes Among Various Renin-Angiotensin System Knockout Models

ACE −/−, ACE knockout model; AGT −/−, angiotensinogen knockout model; AT_{1A} −/−, angiotensin II subtype 1A receptor knockout model; AT_{1B} −/−, angiotensin II subtype 1B receptor knockout model; AT_{1A}/AT_{1B} −/−, angiotensin II subtype 1A and 1B receptors knockout model; AT_2 −/−, angiotensin II subtype 2 receptor knockout model; Renin −/−, renin knockout model.

fibrosis, independent of alterations in systemic vascular resistance.[143]

Mullins and coworkers[140,144] introduced the mouse Ren-2 gene into normotensive rats, thus creating a transgenic strain that expresses high levels of Ren-2 mRNA in many sites including the adrenal gland and to a much lesser extent the kidney. In these rats, fulminant hypertension develops between 5 and 10 weeks of age. Treatment with low-dose ACE inhibitors or Ang II antagonists normalized blood pressure.[145] Despite severe hypertension in Ren-2 transgenic rats, the systemic RAS was not stimulated and plasma levels of active renin, angiotensinogen, Ang I, and Ang II were lower than those seen in control animals.[144] By contrast, the plasma concentration of prorenin was dramatically elevated. This increase in prorenin originated mainly from the adrenal glands with adrenalectomy normalizing blood pressure in these rats.[140] Because the activation of the RAS has been implicated in the progression of chronic renal disease, Ganten and colleagues[140] studied progression of glomerular sclerosis after subtotal nephrectomy in Ren-2 transgenic rats. Compared with blood pressure–matched spontaneously hypertensive rats, the transgenic animals had significant acceleration of glomerulosclerosis, consistent with a pathogenetic role for the intrarenal RAS in the progression to renal failure. Similarly, it has been observed that induction of diabetes in Ren-2 transgenic rats was associated with glomerulosclerosis, tubulointerstitial fibrosis, and decline in renal function, features not observed in other rodent models of diabetes.[146] Moreover, blocking the RAS with either an ACE inhibitor or an AT_1 receptor blocker preserves renal function and attenuates renal structural damage in this model. These effects on renal disease progression appear to be due to attenuation of expression and activation of the local RAS and not solely the result of reducing systemic blood pressure because an equihypotensive dose of an endothelin antagonist

failed to confer a similar degree of renoprotection in this model.

Physiologic Effects of the Renin-Angiotensin System

The predominant function of the RAS is regulation of vascular tone and renal salt excretion in response to changes in extracellular fluid volume or blood pressure. Ang II represents the effector limb of this hormonal system, acting on several organs, including the vascular system, heart, adrenal glands, central nervous system, and kidney. We focus on the renal effects of Ang II.

Effects of Angiotensin II on Renal Hemodynamics

In the kidney, the primary action of Ang II is on the small-diameter resistance arterioles supplying the glomeruli. It is well established that both endogenous and exogenous Ang II affect preglomerular (afferent) as well as efferent arteriolar tone. The tendency of the filtration fraction to rise is due to smaller reductions in GFR relative to a larger decrease in renal blood flow. This is interpreted as consistent with a predominant action of Ang II on the postglomerular (efferent) arterioles. Micropuncture studies indicate that Ang II usually decreases the filtration coefficient and increases permeability to macromolecules.[147] The precise in vivo role of the contractile mesangial cells in producing changes in capillary hydraulic conductivity and/or capillary surface area is not fully known.[147]

SEGMENTAL VASCULAR RESISTANCE. Early studies on single nephron function demonstrated that Ang II increases total resistance as a result of contraction of preglomerular arteries and afferent and efferent arterioles.[147,148] The most convincing in vivo evidence for direct actions of Ang II on the afferent arteriole was obtained during infusion of Ang I or Ang II into the renal artery. Several studies using direct microscopic visualization and calcium-sensitive dye fluorescence provide convincing evidence that Ang II constricts both afferent and efferent arterioles, with similar potency or slightly greater effects on the efferent arteriole.[149,150] There are high concentrations of Ang II in the vicinity of the JG apparatus and glomerular arterioles with at least a hundredfold increase in intrarenal versus systemic Ang II concentrations (nM versus pM).[151]

PARACRINE/AUTOCRINE AGENTS. In addition to direct effects on vascular smooth muscle cells, Ang II can stimulate release of other vasoactive factors from endothelial cells. Accordingly, the vascular actions of Ang II can be modulated by paracrine and autocrine agents produced in response to Ang II, with either buffering or amplifying effects. The most common integrated response to Ang II is net vasoconstriction. Within the kidney, these secondary vasoactive agents may originate from endothelial, vascular smooth muscle, or mesangial cells (and perhaps reno medullary interstitial cells). Most widely known are the protective or opposing effects provided by NO and vasodilator products of arachidonic acid metabolism, notably PGE_2, PGI_2, and possibly epoxyeicosatrienoic acid.

Endothelin-1 may be another endothelial factor that regulates Ang II–induced vasoconstriction.[152] Ang II can increase gene expression and synthesis of endothelin-1 in vascular smooth muscle cells.[153] Blockade of both endothelin A and endothelin B receptors with bosentan attenuates the vasoconstrictor and proteinuric effects of chronic Ang II infusion.[154] Other modulatory factors include adenosine and ATP, dopamine, and lipoxygenase and cytochrome P-450 metabolites derived from arachidonic acid.[148]

Effects of Angiotensin II on Renal Autoregulatory Mechanisms

The renal vasculature plays an important role in protecting the glomerulus and tubules from large changes in arterial pressure that occur during normal daily activity as well as during stress. These autoregulatory mechanisms continually adjust renal vasomotor tone to counterbalance fluctuations in arterial pressure to maintain renal blood flow and GFR constant, thereby blunting the natriuretic effects of increases in arterial pressure.[147] Whole kidney blood flow studies show that renal blood flow is regulated near constancy during acute changes in systolic arterial pressure between 90 and 180 mmHg. Such renal autoregulation is thought to be mediated by two basic mechanisms, both of which involve the afferent arteriole. One is a pressure-induced myogenic response of vascular smooth muscle cells in the interlobular arteries and afferent arterioles. The other is a tubuloglomerular feedback (TGF) loop involving the JG apparatus. This TGF system functions as a negative feedback system, regulating afferent arteriolar tone as a function of solute delivery and transport by macula densa cells at the start of the distal tubule.

Effects of Angiotensin II on Tubular Transport

Direct actions of Ang II on tubular transport function have been suggested for more than 2 decades. In sodium-depleted dogs, chronic blockade of Ang II formation decreased blood pressure and increased urinary sodium excretion, independent of any changes in circulating aldosterone levels. Similarly, it has been observed that in sodium-depleted dogs with activation of the RAS, increases in sodium excretion in response to increases in arterial pressure were attenuated, compared with dogs maintained on normal sodium diets. Furthermore, with administration of the ACE inhibitor captopril, absolute and fractional sodium excretion increased at all levels of arterial pressure, an effect that could not be explained by changes in the filtered load of sodium. These studies and others provide compelling evidence that increases in fractional sodium excretion in response to RAS blockade are greater than can be accounted for by associated changes in GFR or renal blood flow. Accordingly, it is suggested that Ang II exerts direct stimulatory effects on tubular transport.

In the proximal tubule, Ang II plays a central role in promoting the reabsorption of sodium, fluid, and bicarbonate (HCO_3^-). A luminal Na^+/H^+ exchanger is activated by Ang II, resulting in sodium uptake from the lumen into the cells.[155,156] The increased activity of the Na^+/H^+ exchanger promotes HCO_3^- transport by the basolateral Na^+/HCO_3^- cotransporter, which may be directly affected by Ang II.[157,158] Ang II also increases basolateral Na^+-K^+-ATPase activity in the proximal tubule, thereby contributing to sodium transport.[155] In addition, Ang II can modify sodium-independent H^+ secretion by insertion of H^+-ATPase–containing vesicles into the brush border membrane.[159] Finally, Garvin[160] has investigated the effect of Ang II on glucose and fluid absorption in isolated, perfused rat proximal tubules and determined that Ang II stimulates Na^+/glucose cotransport in this nephron segment.

There is a well-characterized biphasic effect of Ang II on transport activities in the proximal tubule. Low concentrations of Ang II ($<10^{-9}$ M) appear to stimulate fluid reabsorption whereas high concentrations of Ang II ($>10^{-9}$ M) inhibit transport.

Most studies suggest that both inhibitory and stimulatory effects of Ang II are mediated by the AT_1 receptor subtype.[68,69] This notion is supported by the use of specific antagonists against AT_1 and AT_2 receptors in a number of studies.[161,162] For example, Quan and Baum[163] demonstrated that luminally applied AT_1 or AT_2 receptor antagonists decreased endogenous Ang II–stimulated proximal tubule volume reabsorption. Clearly, studies assessing transport in tubules isolated from both AT_1 and AT_2 receptor-deficient mice may clarify the role of these receptor subtypes on proximal tubule transport.

Some studies suggest that the inhibitory effects of high-dose Ang II on transport may be mediated via AT_2 receptors in the proximal tubule. Jacobs and Douglas[164] have localized AT_2 receptor function to apical membranes of rabbit proximal tubule cells, associated with stimulation of arachidonic acid release through phospholipase A_2. It has been suggested that the effect described previously appears to be mediated by a novel mechanism involving the AT_2 receptor, with coupling to the G protein β-γ subunit and stimulation of phospholipase A_2 activity, arachidonate release, p21ras, and MAP kinase.[165] Effects of Ang II on other sites within the nephron have also been reported, including stimulation of bicarbonate transport in the superficial loop of Henle and stimulation of apical Na^+/H^+ exchange in the early distal tubule. In the late distal tubule, Ang II activates apical amiloride-sensitive sodium channels on principal cells and also potently stimulates bicarbonate reabsorption at this site in an AT_1 receptor–dependent manner. The effects of Ang II on the collecting duct have been less well studied, with lower concentrations of Ang II having no effect on bicarbonate transport.[166] Ang II appears to directly modulate water transport in the inner medulla, with AT_1 receptors having been identified in these inner medullary collecting ducts.[167] Finally, there is indirect evidence for interactions of Ang II and AT_1 receptors in renomedullary interstitial cells, which may be important in the regulation of the renal medullary microcirculation. These cells are situated in the medullary interstitium between and anchored closely into the basement membranes of the loop of Henle and vasa recta blood vessels.[168] These cells are distinct from two other cell types, macrophages and dendritic cells, which are also present in the renal medullary interstitium.[169] A number of studies have been performed exploring the effects of Ang II in inducing vasoconstriction of medullary blood vessels. These effects are considered partly to occur via paracrine actions on renomedullary interstitial cells in addition to direct actions on these vessels.

Intrarenal Renin-Angiotensin System

Although traditionally the RAS has been thought primarily as an endocrine system that delivers circulating Ang II to target tissues, significant insights have been generated during the past 20 years regarding the capacity of kidney tissue to directly synthesize Ang II. It has now been convincingly shown that the major components of the RAS (angiotensinogen, renin, ACE, and AT_1 and AT_2 receptors) are synthesized within the kidney, in both glomeruli and tubules.[24,170,171]

Renin production and secretion from the JG apparatus are controlled by intrarenal as well as by systemic factors. Ang II is clearly produced within the kidney, and ACE, which is found on peritubular and capillary endothelial cells, plays a role in its production. It has been demonstrated that intrarenal Ang II production occurs within the kidney in the interstitium, within JG cells, and within tubular cells.[24,170,171]

The interstitium has long been considered to be an important site for the RAS within the kidney. Renin, angiotensinogen, Ang I, and Ang II are present not only in the intravascular compartment of the kidney but also in renal lymph with the interstitium containing high levels of Ang II.[172]

The colocalization of renin and Ang II in JG cell granules originally led to the concept that Ang II may also be synthesized in JG cells. Indeed, it has been shown that Ang II peptides are generated within JG cells, presumably by a mechanism which involves the action of endogenous renin on internalized, exogenous angiotensinogen.[173]

mRNAs for angiotensinogen, renin, ACE, and AT_1 and AT_2 receptors have been localized to proximal tubule cells, and the corresponding proteins have also been identified in this segment by immunohistochemistry.[24,170,171] In studies performed by Seikaly and coworkers[174] and Braam and colleagues,[175] the lumen of the proximal tubule was shown to contain concentrations of Ang II ranging from 100- to 1000-fold higher than the concentrations normally present in plasma. It appears that Ang II may be formed within proximal tubule cells, and secreted into the tubular lumen, or converted from intraluminal Ang I by the presence of apical membrane–bound ACE.[176] Interestingly, in rats maintained on salt-restricted diets, Tank and coworkers[177] reported a significant increase in proximal tubule renin mRNA expression, suggesting an enhanced capacity for local Ang II generation. Several studies by our group reported similar findings of proximal tubular renin expression in association with immunoreactive Ang II in two different models of progressive renal injury, subtotal nephrectomy,[178] and diabetes in transgenic Ren-2 rats.[146] Together, these data indicate that the proximal tubule has an endogenous RAS and that locally generated Ang II could exert autocrine and/or paracrine effects in this segment.

Advances have also been made in our understanding of the distribution of Ang II receptors along the nephron. Radioligand binding studies demonstrated that Ang II binding sites were present in discrete nephron segments in the rat, including the proximal convoluted tubule (where the density of receptors is highest), pars recta, loop of Henle, distal convoluted tubule, and cortical and medullary collecting ducts. It appears that the majority of tubular Ang II receptors are of the AT_1 subtype. Immunohistochemical studies have revealed the presence of AT_1 receptors along the entire nephron, on apical and basolateral membranes of proximal tubule cells, but also in other segments including the macula densa, distal tubule, and inner medullary collecting ducts.[167] There is evidence that AT_1 receptors are also expressed on renomedullary

interstitial cells and that these receptors are regulated in a manner similar to those in glomerular mesangial cells during alterations in the activity of the RAS.

In contrast, it is estimated that up to 10% to 15% of intrarenal Ang II receptors in the adult may be of the AT_2 subtype. AT_2 receptors are abundant in the fetal kidney, with diminished expression immediately after birth. In the adult rat kidney, these receptors have been localized to cortical and medullary tubular segments, with up-regulation following sodium depletion.[14]

Pathophysiologic Effects of the Renin-Angiotensin System in the Kidney

Most forms of progressive renal disease lead to a common histologic end point: the end-stage kidney, which is usually fibrotic and reduced in mass. In both humans and animals with chronic renal disease, the evolution of glomerulosclerosis is characterized by progressive involvement of segments within individual glomeruli, eventual global sclerosis and a decrease in the number of glomeruli, and obliteration of tubular structures.[21] Impairment of glomerular and tubular function correlates to a certain extent with histologic changes.[21] Tubular atrophy is manifested by a progressive impairment of the kidney's capacity to concentrate the urine or excrete acid.[21] A number of kidney diseases, and their progression to end-stage renal failure, are driven by the autocrine, paracrine, and endocrine effects of Ang II. Moreover, despite the beneficial effects of ACE inhibitors,[179,180] the findings that the systemic RAS is not activated in most types of chronic renal disease has led to the suggestion that it is the local intrarenal RAS that may be a particularly important determinant in the progression of renal disease (Fig. 10–4).

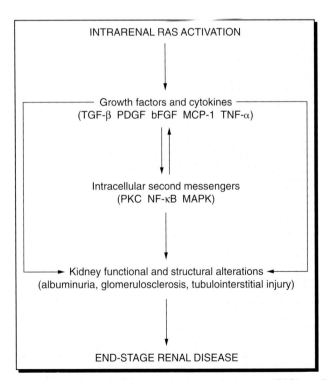

FIGURE 10–4 Pathophysiologic mechanisms for the intrarenal RAS in mediating renal injury. bFGF, basic fibroblast growth factor; MAPK, mitogen-activated protein kinase; MCP-1, monocyte chemoattractant protein-1; NF-κB, nuclear factor-κB; PDGF, platelet-derived growth factor; PKC, protein kinase C; TGF-β, transforming growth factor-β; TNF, tumor necrosis factor.

Effects of Angiotensin II on the Kidney

In Vitro Studies

Diabetes mellitus, systemic hypertension, and inflammatory disease are important causes of chronic progressive renal disease.[181–183] The glomerular findings in these diseases include mesangial expansion and excessive accumulation of extracellular matrix proteins.[181–183] This leads to glomerular capillary obliteration and decline in the GFR, ultimately leading to renal failure.[184] The three major cell types in the glomerulus, mesangial, endothelial, and epithelial are all implicated in progressive renal diseases and respond to Ang II.

Besides its hemodynamic effects in the kidney, Ang II has been shown to have various important direct actions on mesangial cells. Indeed, these nonhemodynamic effects of Ang II may play a crucial role in Ang II–mediated glomerular injury. In cultured murine mesangial cells, Ang II stimulates cellular hypertrophy, and this effect is blocked by AT_1 receptor antagonism.[185] On the other hand, other investigators[186,187] have shown that Ang II causes not only cellular hypertrophy but also proliferation in mesangial cells.

Accumulating evidence supports the notion that TGF-β1 plays a key role in progression of glomerulosclerosis by directly enhancing mesangial hypertrophy and extracellular matrix production.[188,189] The treatment of rat mesangial cells with Ang II increased mRNA and protein levels for TGF-β1 and extracellular matrix components including biglycan, fibronectin, and collagen type I. Furthermore, a neutralizing antibody to TGF-β1 blocked Ang II–induced mesangial cell hypertrophy. A wide range of other in vitro findings, including assessment of PAI-1 and fibronectin expression, supports the notion that TGF-β1 is a key mediator in Ang II–induced glomerulosclerosis. A range of inflammatory pathways is also activated by Ang II in cultured mesangial cells. This includes activation of nuclear factor-κB (NF-κB) and increased expression of the NF-κB–dependent chemokine, monocyte chemoattractant protein (MCP)-1.[190] An inhibitor of NF-κB activation, the antioxidant, pyrrolidine dithiocarbamate, inhibited not only Ang II–induced NF-κB activation but also MCP-1 gene expression.[190]

Cultured rat glomerular endothelial cells have been found to possess not only AT_1 receptors but also AT_2 receptors. Ang II treatment stimulated mRNA and protein synthesis of RANTES, a chemokine with chemoattractant properties for macrophages/monocytes.[191] This effect was blocked by the AT_2 receptor ligands PD123177 and CGP-42112, but not by the AT_1 receptor antagonist losartan, suggesting a possible role for the endothelial AT_2 receptor in Ang II–induced RANTES expression and the subsequent development of glomerular inflammation.[191] Glomerular epithelial cells, which play an important role in the glomerular filtration barrier, have both AT_1 and AT_2 receptors. Ang II has been shown to increase cAMP accumulation in these cells via the AT_1 but not the AT_2 receptor.[192] However, the significance of this observation is as yet unknown.

Studies on cultured renomedullary interstitial cells have suggested that interactions between Ang II and these cells may exert several important influences in the kidney in a manner similar to that seen with respect to Ang II and mesangial cells.[193] Like mesangial cells, in which AT_{1A} receptors are expressed and Ang II stimulates protein synthesis,[194] Ang II also acts in these cells on AT_{1A} receptors to increase [3H]-thymidine incorporation and induces extracellular matrix accumulation.[195] The proliferative effects of Ang II on renomedullary interstitial cells in vitro may be physiologically important both in maintaining normal structural arrangements in the renal medulla and in the pathogenesis of progressive renal disease.[196]

In Vivo Studies

Ang II infusion in vivo in rats leads to glomerulosclerosis.[197] A range of cellular and molecular mechanisms linking glomerular injury to Ang II have been identified in these studies.[198] Continuous Ang II infusion in rats led to dramatic up-regulation of alpha-smooth muscle actin in glomerular mesangial cells and desmin in epithelial cells.[199] Continuous administration of Ang II in rats for 7 days caused increases in glomerular expression of TGF-β1 and collagen type I.[200] Moreover, infusion of Ang II in rats for 4 days significantly stimulated glomerular expression of chemokine RANTES and increased glomerular macrophage/monocyte influx. Notably, oral treatment with the AT_2 receptor antagonist PD123177 did not affect blood pressure but did attenuate glomerular RANTES expression and glomerular macrophage/monocyte influx.[191]

Our group[13] has demonstrated that subcutaneous infusion of Ang II for 14 days in normotensive rats induced proliferation and apoptosis of proximal tubular epithelial cells. The administration of the AT_2 receptor antagonist PD123319 or the AT_1 receptor antagonist valsartan was associated with a reduction in renal injury and attenuation of cell proliferation and apoptosis following Ang II infusion.[13] Furthermore, in that study, Ang II infusion was associated with increased osteopontin gene and protein expression, which could be reduced by treatment with either AT_1 or AT_2 receptor blockers. These findings on the matrix protein osteopontin should be interpreted in the light of recent findings from microarray studies in vascular smooth muscle cells in which osteopontin was shown to be a gene that is highly responsive to exogenous Ang II.[201] Interestingly, our findings indicated that not only the AT_1 but also the AT_2 receptor have a role in mediating Ang II–induced proliferation and apoptosis in proximal tubular cells and expression of osteopontin. These observations are in agreement with other studies previously mentioned, which suggest a role for the AT_2 receptor in mediating cellular processes, including cell recruitment in the kidney.[191]

Role of the Renin-Angiotensin System in the Pathophysiology of Kidney Diseases

Studies by Hostetter and Brenner[21] first suggested that increases in capillary pressure and/or flow cause glomerular injury. Furthermore, Anderson and colleagues[21] showed in the subtotally nephrectomized rat model that chronic ACE inhibition normalized both systemic and glomerular capillary pressure. These striking hemodynamic effects were associated with prevention of glomerular injury in the remnant kidney. More recent studies, in the same experimental model (remnant kidney model), demonstrated that the Ang II antagonist candesartan significantly reduced the expression of glomerular alpha-smooth muscle actin and desmin, while decreasing urinary albumin excretion and attenuating glomerulosclerosis.[202]

Although the glomerulus is often the primary site of injury in renal disease, it is the extent of tubulointerstitial rather than glomerular injury that correlates most closely with and predicts future loss of renal function in patients with primary glomerular disease. Following subtotal nephrectomy, our group demonstrated that renin synthesis is suppressed at the JG apparatus but appears de novo in the tubular epithelium. Furthemore, we observed in the same study that the JG apparatus and tubule responded in a divergent manner to ACE inhibition with regard to renin synthesis. As seen in an intact kidney, ACE inhibition led to increased JG apparatus renin expression with proximal extension into the afferent arteriole, whereas in the tubule, this intervention led to suppression of renin production.[203] These findings provide evidence that within the kidney, the regulation of the RAS differs between the JG apparatus and the tubules. The relevance of this altered pattern of renin synthesis is confirmed by concomitant de novo appearance of the effector molecule of the RAS, Ang II in the renal tubule in response to subtotal nephrectomy. The expression of renin by tubular epithelial cells described in this study may reflect a phenotypic change that occurs as a nonspecific response to injury.[178] Activation in this model of the tubular RAS was associated with an increased expression of TGF-β1 within the tubular epithelium and an increase in collagen IV expression. Interruption of the RAS by ACE inhibition was associated with disappearance of aberrant tubular expression of renin and Ang II in association with the restoration of high levels of renin expression in the JG apparatus. Furthermore, ACE inhibition significantly reduced expression of the Ang II–induced mediator of renal fibrosis, TGF-β1 in association with amelioration of the functional and structural manifestations of renal injury.[178]

It has been recently demonstrated that the integrity of the podocyte and specifically the slit diaphragm is crucial to the process of glomerular filtration.[204] The recently discovered protein nephrin is a major constituent of the molecular structure of the slit pore, and its absence has been implicated in the pathogenesis of the congenital nephrotic syndrome of the Finnish type.[205] Down-regulation of nephrin has been implicated in various models of proteinuria including puromycin aminonucleoside nephrosis,[206] mercuric-chloride–treated rat,[207] and more recently, in the diabetic rat and subtotal nephrectomy model.[117] In the subtotal nephrectomy model, it was observed that increased proteinuria was associated with reduced gene and protein expression of this slit diaphragm protein. This alteration in nephrin expression was prevented by both the AT₁ receptor blocker valsartan and the AT₂ receptor antagonist PD123319, suggesting a role for the RAS in influencing expression of nephrin. In addition, both antagonists were antiproteinuric in association with reduced cellular proliferation. Moreover, it seems that the combination of the AT₁ and the AT₂ receptor antagonists may confer additive renoprotective effects.

Although not extensively reviewed here, a role for Ang II per se in a range of other renal diseases has been described including cyclosporine nephrotoxicity, deoxycortocosterone acetate (DOCA)-salt hypertension, and ureteral obstruction.

Unlike the role of Ang II in the progression of chronic renal failure, there is less direct evidence that the RAS is involved in the mediation of acute kidney injury (AKI). However, PRA and renal renin content increase in experimental ischemic renal failure.[208] An important pathogenic role for the RAS in the development of AKI during hypertensive crises in scleroderma has long been recognized, and this was one of the first conditions in which ACE inhibitors were considered appropriate therapy.[209]

Role of the Renin-Angiotensin System in the Pathophysiology of Diabetic Nephropathy

Diabetic nephropathy is the leading cause of end-stage renal disease in the Western world. Measurements of circulating components of the RAS in experimental or human diabetes mellitus do not appear to accurately predict the state of activation of the RAS or its response to blockade at the kidney level.[210] Although measurements of components of the RAS in plasma have, in general, suggested suppression of this system in diabetes, there is increasing evidence for activation of the local intrarenal RAS in the diabetic kidney. Indeed, in the proximal tubule, there is evidence for up-regulation of renin and angiotensinogen expression.[211,212] An increase in ACE levels within the glomerulus has been reported in diabetes, as have direct effects of high extracellular glucose levels on mesangial cell expression of RAS components. Despite the possibility of increased local production of Ang II, several studies have described suppression of AT₁ and AT₂ receptor mRNA and protein expression in the diabetic kidney.[213] It remains to be determined whether the balance of intrarenal AT₁ and AT₂ receptors is important in determining the cellular responses to Ang II in diabetic nephropathy.

The importance of the RAS in mediating the kidney damage in diabetes has been demostrated by a large number of clinical and experimental studies showing that ACE inhibitors as well as AT₁ receptor antagonists decrease proteinuria and slow the progression of diabetic nephropathy in both type 1 and type 2 diabetes.[214–217] Studies by Hostetter and Brenner[21] first showed that increases in glomerular capillary pressure and flow were responsible for the above-normal elevation of GFR in diabetic rats. The hemodynamic abnormalities in rats with diabetes were different from those observed in rats with renal insufficiency, as a result of subtotal nephrectomy. Specifically, diabetic rats exhibited an increase in glomerular capillary pressure without any increase in systemic blood pressure. Chronic Ang II blockade, however, was found to reduce glomerular pressure in diabetes as well as in experimental renal insufficiency. These hemodynamic changes were associated with protection of the glomerulus from accelerated renal sclerotic injury that was seen in experimental diabetes.

Increased TGF-β and type IV collagen expression have been demonstrated in experimental diabetic nephropathy[218,219] as well as in human diabetic nephropathy.[220] Although most studies of diabetic nephropathy have addressed the glomerular changes, there is increasing interest in the tubulointerstitial abnormalities in this disease. Indeed, tubulointerstitial changes in diabetic nephopathy are closely related to declining renal function.

In a series of studies in diabetic rodents, investigators have explored the effects of agents that interrupt the RAS on growth factors and extracellular matrix protein expression. These studies have demonstrated renoprotective effects of these agents in both hypertensive and normotensive models of diabetic nephropathy. In particular, the tubulointerstitial lesions observed in experimental diabetes were attenuated by ACE inhibition in association with reduced proximal tubular TGF-β expression.[221] A range of other Ang II–mediated effects that are relevant to diabetic kidney disease include stimulation of proliferative cytokines such as PDGF, induction of oxidative stress, activation of NF-κB, and enhancement of expression of chemokines and cytokines that are proinflammatory such as RANTES and MCP-1.[221]

Future Perspectives of the Renin-Angiotensin System

Twenty years ago, it was assumed that Ang II, the main effector of the RAS, was a systemic circulating hormone that was considered primarily to be a peripheral vasoconstrictor involved in blood pressure regulation, a regulator of glomerular filtration, and a secretagog for aldosterone. Major scientific advances in this area have changed this simple view of Ang II, and it is increasingly recognized that specific organs exhibit their own local RASs, which act independently from their systemic counterparts interacting with specific Ang II receptors. In parallel with these findings, it became clear that Ang II has many additional properties above and beyond being a simple vasoconstrictor. In fact, it has been clearly demonstrated that Ang II is directly involved in the control of tubular transport and cell growth and that it has profibrogenic and proinflammatory effects. In addition, it has gradually become clear that not only Ang II but also related peptides such as Ang III, Ang IV, and Ang 1-7 have specific effects independent of the parent peptide. Among the local RASs, the renal RAS has been particularly characterized. It is now known that specific cell populations such as renal proximal tubular cells exhibit all components of the RAS. The RAS plays a major role in the pathogenesis of hypertension, cardiovascular, and renal diseases. Moreover, the RAS has been demonstrated to mediate the progression of glomerular and tubulointerstitial injury in numerous experimental and clinical conditions. These observations provide a clear explanation for the beneficial effects observed for the ACE inhibitors and AT_1 receptor blockers in renal diseases. The future elucidation of the increasing complexity of this system will greatly assist in the rational use of agents that interrupt the RAS in chronic progressive renal injury.

ENDOTHELIN

Structure

Endothelins (ETs) are potent endothelium-derived vasoconstrictor peptides first described by Yanagisawa and coworkers in 1988. Three structurally and pharmacologically distinct ET isoforms (endothelin-1, -2, and -3 [ET-1, -2, and -3]) have been described. All three isoforms consist of 21 amino acids, are highly homologous, and share a common structure. ET-1 is considered to be the most dominant isoform in the cardiovascular system.

Synthesis and Secretion

ETs are synthesized via posttranslational proteolytic cleavage of specific prohormones. Dibasic pair specific processing endopeptidases, which recognize Arg-Arg or Lys-Arg paired amino acids, cleave prepro ETs and reduce their size from approximately 203 to 39 amino acids. These proETs are subsequently proteolytically cleaved by ET-converting enzymes, yielding mature ETs. These endothelin-converting enzymes (ECEs) are the key enzymes in the endothelin biosynthetic pathways that catalyze the conversion of big ET, the biologically inactive precursor of mature ET. ECEs are type II membrane bound metalloproteases and share significant amino acid sequence identity with neutral endopeptidase 24.11. Therefore, it is not surprising that the majority of ECE inhibitors also possess potent NEP inhibitory activity.

Polarized endothelial cells secrete the majority of the ET-1 into the basolateral compartment.[222] Secretion occurs at a constant level, suggesting constitutive pathways. However, a variety of triggers stimulate ET synthesis via transcriptional regulation (Table 10–3).

ET stimulation is endothelium dependent and requires de novo protein synthesis because protein synthesis inhibitors such as cycloheximide prevent the release of the mature peptide. However, ET production is not exclusively released by the endothelium but also by nonvascular tissues, albeit at much lower levels than by endothelial cells.

Numerous cells in the kidney produce ETs, including glomerular endothelial cells,[223] glomerular epithelial cells,[224] mesangial cells,[225] and tubular epithelial cells.[226] The kidney synthesizes ET-3 as well as ET-1.[226] In microdissected rat kidney nephron segments, ET-1 mRNA was reported to be in glomeruli and innermedullary collecting ducts but was undetectable in other nephron segments.[227,228]

ECE mRNA has been found to be more abundant in the renal medulla than in the cortex. However, in disease states such as chronic heart failure, there is up-regulation of ECE mRNA expression, predominantly in the renal cortex.[229] In human kidney, ECE-1 was localized to endothelial and tubular epithelial cells in the cortex and medulla of kidneys.[230]

ETs bind to two G-protein–coupled receptors, the ET(A) and ET(B) receptors.[231,232] The specific distribution of the two distinct ET receptors has been determined using RT-PCR in microdissected rat nephrons. ET(A) receptors are found in the proximal straight tubule, and both ET receptor subtypes are

TABLE 10–3	Endothelin Gene and Protein Expression
Stimulation	
Vasoactive Peptides	**Growth Factors**
Angiotensin II	Epidermal growth factor
Bradykinin	Insulin-like growth factor
Vasopressin	Transforming growth factor-β (TGF-β)
Endothelin-1	
Epinephrine	**Coagulation**
Insulin	Thrombin
Glucocorticoids	Thromboxane A_2
Prolactin	Tissue plasminogen-activating factor
Inflammatory Mediators	**Other**
Endotoxin	Calcium
Interleukin-1	Hypoxia
Tumor necrosis factor-α (TNF-α)	Shear stress
	Phorbol esters
Interferon-β	Oxidized low-density lipoproteins
Inhibition	
ANP	
BNP	
Bradykinin	
Heparin	
Prostacyclin	
Protein kinase A activators	
Nitric oxide	
ACE inhibitors	

found in glomeruli and in the afferent and efferent arterioles. The ET(B) receptor has been demonstrated in the proximal convoluted tubule, cortical inner and outer medullary collecting duct, and medullary thick ascending limb. ET(B) receptors have also been identified on podocytes.[233]

Physiologic Actions of Endothelin on the Kidney

The kidney is both the source and an important target for ETs. The effects of ETs include regulation of vascular and mesangial tone, regulation of sodium and water excretion, and cell proliferation and matrix formation. The highest concentrations of ET are found in the renal medulla, where it mediates natriuretic and diuretic effects through the ET(B) receptor and is regulated by sodium intake.[234] The ET(B) receptor is considered to exert predominantly renoprotective effects such as natriuresis and vasodilation via NO and prostaglandins.

ET exerts its hemodynamic effects in almost all vessels, but the sensitivity of the different vascular beds to this peptide varies considerably. The renal and the mesenteric vasculatures have the greatest susceptibility to the actions of endothelins. ET-1 increases renal vascular resistance via contraction of the glomerular arterioles and arcuate and interlobular arteries and decreases blood flow.[235] Long-lasting vasoconstriction that is mediated by the ET(A) receptor is temporarily preceded by transient vasodilation. Vasodilation results from ET(B) receptor mediated release of NO but possibly also involves PGE_2 synthesis and cAMP release from mesangial cells.[235] ET(B) receptors may also be involved in the clearance of ET-1 from the plasma.[236] Micropuncture techniques have demonstrated that ET-1 results in a decline in net filtration pressure and a reduction in the glomerular ultrafiltration coefficient, as a result of constriction of pre- and postglomerular arterioles, reduction of blood flow, and mesangial contraction. ET also influences tubular reabsorption and secretion.

In the glomerular tuft, mesangial cells are important targets for ETs. ET-1 induces mesangial cell contraction and mitogenesis. Contraction of the mesangium by ET-1 may reduce glomerular ultrafiltration in vivo, as is the case in post-ischemic renal failure (see later).

ET synthesis in endothelial and mesangial cells is increased after exposure to proinflammatory agents and shear stress (see Table 10–3), supporting the view that ET-1 serves as a biologic signal in glomerular injury and inflammation. A large number of proinflammatory stimuli induce ET-1 synthesis, including Ang II, TGF-β, thromboxane A_2, thrombin, hypoxia, and shear stress. In glomerular injury, infiltrating inflammatory cells such as macrophages, neutrophils, and mast cells may also become important sources of ET-1. Receptor interactions with ET trigger cell contraction, proliferation, and matrix synthesis. In vitro, ET-1 stimulates proliferation of human renal interstitial fibroblasts and gene expression of collagen I, TGF-β, matrix metalloproteinase (MMP)-1, tissue inhibitor of metalloproteinase (TIMP)-1, and TIMP-2. All these effects are blocked by ET(A) receptor blockade.[237] In response to injury, stimulation of ET isopeptide synthesis may cause complex rearrangement of actin microfilament bundles and transform mesangial cells from a quiescent to an activated status. The resulting long-term changes in glomerular cell phenotype would then contribute to progressive renal disease and, ultimately, glomerulosclerosis and tubulointerstitial injury.

Endothelin and Renal Pathophysiology

The kidney is an important source and target for ETs. ET has been implicated in several disorders associated with the renal endothelium including cyclosporine toxicity, vascular rejection of kidney transplants, various forms of AKI and chronic renal failure, and hepatorenal syndrome (Table 10–4). Renal vasoconstriction and reductions in GFR are characteristic of these disorders. In chronic progressive renal injury of diverse etiologies, the promitogenic and proinflammatory actions of ET may be even more important.

Acute Renal Ischemia

The role of ET has been extensively investigated in a range of renal disorders including acute renal ischemia, cyclosporine-induced nephrotoxicity, and renal allograft rejection. In these experimental models, ET(A) and dual ET(A)/ET(B) antagonists have, in general, demonstrated a degree of renoprotection, although this has not been a universal finding.[238–241]

Chronic Renal Disease/Fibrosis

The renal ET system appears to be involved in the pathogenesis of kidney fibrosis as well as blood pressure regulation by regulating tubular sodium excretion. It has been demonstrated that renal tubular cells synthesize ETs and that protein overload of these cells induces a dose-dependent increase in the synthesis and release of ET-1.[242,243] This peptide accumulates in the interstitium and participates in the activation of a sequence of events that leads to interstitial inflammation and, ultimately, renal scarring. In several animal models of proteinuric progressive nephropathies, the enhanced renal ET-1 expression as well as the excretion of the peptide in the urine correlated with urinary protein excretion. Similarly, in patients with chronic renal disease an association has been found between increased urinary ET-1 excretion and renal damage. In nephrotic patients, not only is ET-1 localized to endothelial cells but de novo expression of ET-1 also occurs in tubular cells, suggesting a possible relationship between proteinuria and renal ET-1 production.[244] In patients with remission of proteinuria, urinary ET-1 levels decreased, whereas in patients with persistent proteinuria, ET-1 levels remained elevated.

Transgenic mice models selectively overexpressing the ET gene represent an opportunity to investigate directly the mechanisms of ET-mediated vascular and renal changes. Human ET-1 transgenic mice demonstrate heightened expression of ET-1 in the kidney.[245] Although blood pressure was similar to that in control animals, the kidneys of these animals demonstrated interstitial fibrosis and glomerulosclerosis in association with increased extracellular matrix protein expression both in the glomeruli and in the interstitium. From studies in mice with overexpression of ET-1, it was observed that ET did not directly cause hypertension but triggered renal injury that led to increased susceptibility to salt-induced hypertension.[246] Indeed, the ET antagonist bosentan was effective in reducing renal fibrosis in this model independent of effects on blood pressure.[247,248]

A strong argument in favor of ET-1 as a mediator of renal injury derives from preclinical studies with selective and nonselective ET receptor antagonists that have become available over the last decade. These studies, performed in Ren-2 transgenic animals and in the subtotal nephrectomy model, have demonstrated variable findings on renal protection and suggest that ET antagonists are not as effective as agents that interrupt the RAS.

Diabetic Nephropathy

ETs may contribute to both the pathogenesis and the progression of diabetic nephropathy by at least two separate mechanisms. First, ET acts as a vasoconstrictor with subsequent cortical and inner medullary hypoperfusion. Second, as a trophic agent, ET causes extracellular matrix deposition, a prominent pathologic feature of diabetic nephropathy. Nevertheless, compared with the role of the RAS in the development and progression of diabetic nephropathy, the effects of the ET system remain less clear.

In diabetic population studies, measuring plasma and urine ET levels have been conflicting. In general, in uncomplicated type 1 or 2 diabetes, plasma ET-1 levels are usually not elevated. If albuminuria is present, plasma ET-1 levels may be elevated and could reflect generalized endothelial dysfunction and damage. Furthermore, correlations between plasma ET-1 levels and the degree of albuminuria have been demonstrated. In the presence of diabetic macrovascular complications, plasma ET-1 levels are consistently elevated. There is now accumulating evidence that smoking aggravates and accelerates diabetic and nondiabetic nephropathies by increasing the renal ET-system and impairing endothelial vasodilation.[249]

The effect of glucose per se on ET production remains controversial.[250–253] In high glucose conditions, mesangial cells lose their contractile response to ET-1 in association with filamentous F-actin disassembly and a reduction in cell size. Loss of the contractile response of mesangial cells to ET-1 occurs in the presence of normal Ca^{2+} signalling and normal myosin light chain phosphorylation. Recently, it has been shown that these changes are mediated by protein kinase C-ζ.[254–256] In contrast, if mesangial cells are exposed to high glucose, mesangial cell p38 responsiveness to ET-1, Ang II, and PDGF, and consequent CREB (cAMP responsive element binding) phosphorylation are enhanced through a PKC-independent pathway.[256]

Insulin itself has been shown to stimulate ET-1 release and ET- receptor gene expression.[250] Rats on a high-fructose diet develop hyperinsulinemia, hypertriglyceridemia, and hypertension and subsequently develop renal and cardiac injury. A novel dual ET(A/B) inhibitor, enrasentan, has been reported to prevent the rise in blood pressure as well as renal and cardiac injury in this model.[257]

In several different animal models of type 1 and 2 diabetes, plasma ET-1 levels were increased. However, most of these studies were unable to detect any change at the receptor level.[258,259] Studies performed by our group using in vitro autoradiographic techniques did not show a significant

TABLE 10–4 Endothelin and Renal Pathophysiology

Model	ET Antagonists	Renal Effect	BP Effect	Reference
Renal ablation	ET(A) FR139317	Proteinuria ↓ Renal injury ↓		242
	Bosentan	Proteinuria ↓ Renal injury ↓, survival ↑	↓	388
	Bosentan, ET(A) blocker BMS 193884	No beneficial effect on fibrosis, renal injury, proteinuria	↓	389
	Bosentan+AT₁ blocker	Combination no additional effect to AT₁ blocker		
	ACEi vs ET(A) and combination	GSI all treatments ↓ Better on GSI and TI, not on albumin excretion		390
	ET(A) 127722	Response to exogenous big ET ↓	No effect	391
	ET(A) PD 155080	No adverse effect on creatinine clearance or proteinuria	↓	392
	ET(A) BMS 182874 or ET(A/B) Ro 46-2005	GSI ↓ Only ET(A) TI ↓ No effect on glomerular hypertrophy	No effect	393
	ET(A) LU 135252	Serum creatinine and proteinuria, plasma and urinary ET-1 ↓	↓	394
Transgenic ET-1 mice	Bosentan	Renal fibrosis ↓	No effect	247
SHR+salt	ET(A) blocker LU 135252	Albuminuria ↓ vascular hypertrophy ↓	No effect	395
PA nephrosis	NEP/ECE inhibitor CGS 26302	Renal injury ↓		396
PHN nephritis	ET(A) LU 135252 and trandolapril	Both proteinuria ↓ GSI and TI ↓ Combination superior		397
Diabetes	ET(A) blocker FR 139317	Matrix proteins↓, chemokines and cytokines ↓		398 262
	ET(B) blocker	No effect on ECM or growth factors		262
	ET(A/B) PD 142893 and ET(A) blocker	Proteinuria ↓, glomerular damage ↓	↓	243
	ET(A) 135252 or ET(A/B) 224332	Both: ECM ↓ Fibronectin ↓ Collgen IV ↓ Proteinuria ↓ 50%		264
6 months diabetes	ET(A) LU135252 or trandolapril	Thickening of glomerular basement membrane ↓ matrix deposition ↓ fibronectin and collagen ↓		399
Diabetic Ren2	Bosentan versus valsartan	No effect on glomerulosclerosis index, tubulointerstitial injury TGF-β and collagen IV	↓	267
Diabetic SHR	Bosentan+amlodipine	Similar to cilazapril TGF-β, collagen and fibrosis ↓ Renal injury ↓		269
	NEP/ECE and NEP/ACE	Renal injury ↓	↓	270
Galactose feeding	bosentan	Renal injury ↓		266
DOCA salt renal fibrosis	ET(A) A 127722 AT₁ (candesartan) and combination	Improved hemodynamics but no effect on renal injury in all treatment groups		400
Radiocontrast nephropathy	ET(A) 127722	Plasma creatinine ↓ Proteinuria ↓		401
Stroke prone SHR	ET(A) BMS 182874	Survival ↑, renal injury ↓	No effect	271
	ET(A) BMS 182874	TGF-β, bFGF, MMP-2, procollagen I ↓		402
Chronic renal allograft rejection	Bosentan	No prevention of rejection, no improvement of survival		403
	ET(A)	Prevention of rejection		404
Proliferative nephritis	Bosentan	Proteinuria and injury ↓, renal function↑, urinary ET-1 excretion ↓	BP normal	405

ACEi, ACE inhibitor; BP, blood pressure; ECE, endothelin-converting enzyme; ECM, extracellular matrix; ET, endothelin; GSI, glomerulosclerotic index; MMP-2, matrix metalloproteinase-2; NEP, neutral endopeptidase; TI, tubulointerstitial injury.

difference in renal ET receptor distribution between control and streptozotocin-diabetic rats.[260]

In various animal models of diabetes, there have been reports showing renoprotection by treatment with ET(A) blockade. For example, the renoprotective effect of ET(A) blockade with FR 139317 was associated with a reduction in the mRNA levels of various extracellular matrix proteins including type IV collagen and laminin as well as a reduction in cytokines and growth factors including TNF-α, PDGF-B, TGF-β, and bFGF.[261,262]

Blockade of the ET(B) receptor alone by selective ET(B) blockers has not proven to be beneficial in diabetic nephropathy and had no effect on extracelluar matrix deposition or growth factor expression.[261] The ET(B) receptor is now thought to confer renoprotection by increasing natriuresis and diuresis as well as by promoting vasodilation. Indeed, diabetic ET(B) receptor–deficient rats develop severe low-renin hypertension and progressive renal failure. These mice have high ET-1 plasma levels, suggesting a clearance role for the ET(B) receptor. This study supports a protective role for the ET(B) receptor in the progression of diabetic nephropathy.[263]

Further studies exploring nonselective ET(A/B) receptor blockers or ET(A) antagonists in diabetes have not led to consistent findings. These studies performed in animal models of type 1 and type 2 diabetes have demonstrated variable findings on the development and progression of diabetic nephropathy and have confirmed that the RAS plays a more critical role in the physiopathology of experimental diabetic nephropathy than does the ET pathway.[264–268]

Rather than considering approaches blocking ET-dependent events as monotherapy, it may be worth considering these agents as part of a combination regimen. For example, the combination of bosentan and amlodipine conferred similar renoprotection to a treatment with the ACE inhibitor cilazapril as monotherapy in diabetic SHR. These effects occurred in association with reduced urinary excretion of TGF-β, renal fibrosis, and collagen accumulation. However, that study did not include control groups treated with bosentan or amlodipine alone.[269] In another study, a novel treatment strategy was employed including a dual inhibitor CGS 26303 that blocked both NEP and ECE (NEP/ECE). This treatment was shown to be effective in reducing renal injury and blood pressure in diabetic SHR and was similar in efficacy to a dual NEP/ACE inhibitor.[270]

Human Studies

ET antagonism in experimental hypertension may result in regression of vascular damage, prevention of stroke and renal failure, and improvement of heart failure. Whether the same is true in human hypertension remains to be established.[271,272] In humans, moderate to severe hypertension was associated with enhanced expression of pre-pro ET1 mRNA in the endothelium of subcutaneous resistance arteries.[273] Severity of blood pressure, salt-sensitivity, and insulin resistance may be common denominators of involvement of the ET system in hypertension. In essential hypertension, bosentan reduced blood pressure to a similar extent to enalapril without reflex neurohumoral activation.[274] In 47 patients with essential hypertension, salt-depleted–salt-sensitive hypertensive patients exhibited enhanced catecholamine-stimulated ET-1 release. This response pattern was associated with a better response to ET blocker treatment than in nonselected patients.[275]

Summary

ETs are important at several stages in embryonic development, in normal postnatal growth, and in cardiovascular and renal homeostasis under healthy conditions. In addition, there is now overwhelming evidence that ET-1 plays an important pathophysiologic role in conditions of decompensated vascular homeostasis.

ET receptor antagonists hold the potential to improve the outcome in patients with various cardiovascular disorders. Most of the progress has been achieved in heart failure and pulmonary hypertension with some exciting preliminary data in the field of atherosclerosis.

With respect to renal disease, inhibitors of the RAS appear to be superior to inhibition of the ET system. Thus, if there is a role for ET antagonists in renal disease, it is likely to be in the context of concomitant RAS blockade.

▌UROTENSIN II

Urotensin II (U-II) was initially isolated from the goby urophysis, a neurosecretory system in the caudal portion of the spinal cord of fish that is functionally similar to the human hypothalamic-pituitary system.[276] Named urotensin for its smooth muscle–stimulating activity, it has notably hemodynamic, gastrointestinal, reproductive, osmoregulatory, and metabolic functions in fish. Subsequntly, homologs of U-II were identified in tissues of many other animals such as rat and ultimately man.[277,278]

Human U-II, cloned in 1998, is a cyclic dodecapeptide that is derived from post-translational processing of two distinct precursors (Fig. 10–5), which are alternate splice variants.[279,280]

In 1999, Ames and colleagues demonstrated that U-II was the ligand for the rat orphan receptor known as GPR14/SENR, which had been cloned by two independent groups.[279] The U-II receptor, known as UT, is a seven transmembrane, G-protein–coupled receptor encoded on chromosome 17q25.3.[281] It shares significant structural similarity with somastatin receptor subtype 4 and the opioid receptors. It has been demonstrated, ex vivo, that vessels taken from UT receptor knockout mice fail to vasoconstrict in the presence of U-II, demonstrating that this receptor is required for U-II–mediated vasoconstriction.[282]

Binding of U-II to UT leads to activation of the G protein, leading to activation of protein kinase C, calmodulin, and phospholipase C, as evidenced by inhibition of vasoconstriction by specific inhibitors to these enzymes.[281,283]

U-II has also been demonstrated to be a vascular smooth muscle mitogen. Further studies have linked U-II to the ERK/MAP and RhoA/Rho kinase pathways.[284,285]

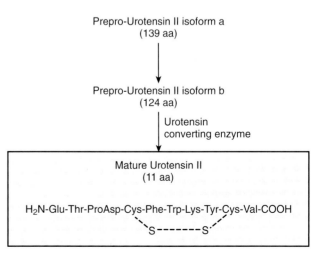

FIGURE 10–5 Comparison of the structure of urotensin II and its precursors and sites of enzymic cleavage.

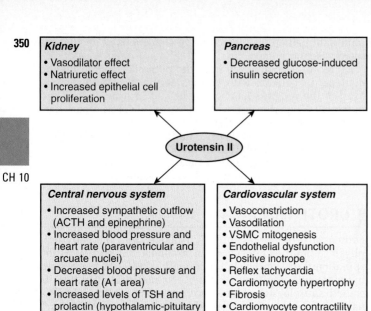

Kidney
- Vasodilator effect
- Natriuretic effect
- Increased epithelial cell proliferation

Pancreas
- Decreased glucose-induced insulin secretion

Urotensin II

Central nervous system
- Increased sympathetic outflow (ACTH and epinephrine)
- Increased blood pressure and heart rate (paraventricular and arcuate nuclei)
- Decreased blood pressure and heart rate (A1 area)
- Increased levels of TSH and prolactin (hypothalamic-pituitary axis)

Cardiovascular system
- Vasoconstriction
- Vasodilation
- VSMC mitogenesis
- Endothelial dysfunction
- Positive inotrope
- Reflex tachycardia
- Cardiomyocyte hypertrophy
- Fibrosis
- Cardiomyocyte contractility

FIGURE 10–6 Biologic actions of urotensin II in several major organ systems in humans. ACTH, adrenocorticotropic hormone; VSMC, vascular smooth muscle cells.

Role in the Kidney

In fish, U-II affects sodium transport, lipid, and glucose metabolism.[276] The urinary human U-II (hU-II) concentration is about three orders of magnitude greater than the plasma concentration.[286] U-II may play a role in the regulation of GFR via tubuloglomerular feedback and reflex control of GFR (Fig. 10–6).[287] In the kidney, U-II has vasodilator and natriuretic effects (see Fig. 10–6). Increases in renal blood flow and GFR were observed after the infusion of synthetic human U-II into the renal artery of anesthetized rats, and this can be completely inhibited by an NO synthase inhibitor.[288]

The plasma U-II concentration is twofold higher in patients with renal dysfunction not on hemodialysis and threefold higher in patients on hemodialysis compared with healthy individuals.[289] Although there is no correlation between blood pressure and urinary U-II levels, a higher urinary U-II level was observed in patients with essential hypertension, patients with both glomerular disease and hypertension, and patients with renal tubular disorders but not in normotensive patients with glomerular disease.[286] Abundant U-II–like immunoactivity is observed in tubular epithelial cells and collecting ducts with lower expression in capillaries and glomerular endothelium in the normal kidney as well as renal clear-cell carcinoma.[278,287]

In type 2 diabetic patients, plasma and urinary U-II levels are higher in those with renal dysfunction than in those with normal renal function.[290] This may be due to increased production of U-II by various organs as well as by renal tubular cells as a result of renal damage.[286] In diabetic nephropathy, there are dramatic increases in the expression of U-II and the UT receptor in tubular epithelial cells.[291]

U-II and its receptor have been extensively investigated in various nonrenal contexts including cardiovascular disease, the nervous system, and diabetes and the metabolic syndrome. U-II appears to have a powerful vasoconstrictor action, promotes fatty acid release, and appears to be highly expressed in certain sites within the peripheral and central nervous systems (see Fig. 10–6).[280,281,292,293] There are only very limited renal data including two studies using the specific nonpeptide U-II receptor antagonist palosuran. Intravenous administration of palosuran protected against renal ischemia in a rat

model,[294] perhaps by inhibiting U-II–mediated renal vasoconstriction. Furthermore, palosuran has been reported to decrease albuminuria in a diabetic rat model.[295] Clinical studies of palosuran are now in progress to examine its effect on diabetic nephropathy.

Summary

U-II is the most potent vasoconstrictor known, causing endothelium-independent vasoconstriction and endothelium-dependent vasodilation. There is increasing evidence that U-II is associated with renal dysfunction, various cardiovascular diseases, atherosclerosis, diabetes, and hypertension, although the results of some studies are ambiguous. More research is needed to elucidate the physiology and pathophysiology of U-II and its receptor. Plasma and urinary concentrations of U-II are elevated in several cardiorenal and metabolic disease states in humans, including hypertension, heart failure, renal disease, and diabetes. The rapid development of research tools, such as knockout mice and novel UT receptor antagonists, will advance our understanding of the physiology and pharmacology of U-II and the UT receptor and may provide a novel treatment for cardiorenal diseases.

KALLIKREIN-KININ SYSTEM

The kallikrein-kinin system (KKS) is a complex multienzymatic system, the main components of which are the enzyme kallikrein, the substrate kininogen, effector hormones or kinins (lysyl-bradykinin, bradykinin), and metabolizing enzymes (several kininases, the most relevant being kininase I and II and NEP) (Fig. 10–7). The kinins were discovered in 1909 when Abelous reported an acute fall in blood pressure induced by experimental injection of urine. Kinins are formed from partial hydrolysis of kininogens by a family of kininogenases called kallikreins. Kinins produce their effects by the binding and activation of specific cell surface receptors. At least two types of kinin receptors have been described, B_1 and B_2. The B_1 receptor is activated predominantly by desArg[9]-bradykinin, a natural degradation product of bradykinin produced by the enzyme kininase I. Although it is generally agreed that B_1 receptors are inducible by tissue injury,[296] it has been suggested that B_1 receptors may also be functionally expressed under normal conditions in the vasculature and the kidney.[297,298] The B_2 receptor is activated by lys-bradykinin and bradykinin and mediates all the known physiologic actions of kinins, including the regulation of organ blood flow, systemic blood pressure, transepithelial water and electrolyte transport, cellular growth, capillary permeability, and the inflammatory response.[299]

Kinins have a very short half-life (<30 sec) and are degraded by a number of peptidases. Kininase II, which is the same as ACE, is the predominant kinin-degrading enzyme.[300] Other important enzymes in the degradation pathway include NEP and kininase.[300] Because of their short half-life, kinins are paracrine rather than true endocrine hormones.

The discovery of specific and potent kinin receptor antagonists, such as Hoe 140,[301,302] and the availability of animal models with defined genetic modifications of the KKS have facilitated the efforts to uncover the functional relevance of endogenous kinins. In the kidney, kinins play a significant role in the modulation of renal hemodynamics and sodium excretion and therefore participate in the regulation of blood volume.[303,304] Kinins have bifunctional effects on cell growth. Bradykinin increases IP_3 and intracellular calcium and stimulates the proliferation of a variety of mesenchymal cells, including fibroblasts, vascular smooth muscle cells, and glomerular mesangial cells.[305–308] Conversely, in the injured vascular wall, kinins may be responsible for the antiproliferative

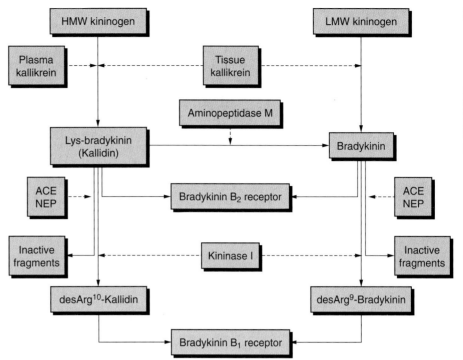

FIGURE 10–7 Enzymatic cascade of the KKS. ACE, angiotensin-converting enzyme; HMW, high molecular weight; LMW, low molecular weight; NEP, neutral endopeptidase.

action of ACE inhibitors by stimulating the production of NO.[309]

Kininogens

The single human kininogen gene is localized to chromosome 3q26-qter and is close to two closely related genes, the α-2-HS-glycoprotein and the histidine-rich glycoprotein.[310,311] It codes for the production of both high-molecular-weight (HMW) kininogen (626 amino acids and 88–120 kDa) and low-molecular-weight (LMW) kininogen (409 amino acids and 50–68 kDa) via alternative splicing from 11 exons spread over a 27-kilobase pair span.

In the human kidney, kallikrein has been demonstrated in connecting tubule cells (see later) and kininogen in the principal cells of the same tubule just preceding the collecting duct. The site is juxtaposed to the afferent arteriole, where synthesized kallikrein (known to traffic to basolateral membranes of these epithelial cells) might affect interstitial cell or vascular wall function via local kinin formation. Alternatively, the known kallikrein trafficking to the apical membranes of these epithelial cells, with subsequent tubular secretion, might result in kininogen being present in the adjacent principal cells to generate kinin locally, thereby modulating tubular ion and water transport.

Kallikreins and Kallikrein Inhibitors

Kallikrein exists in two major forms, plasma and tissue or glandular kallikrein. Renal kallikrein is the so-called true tissue kallikrein, a serine protease. The human genes are clustered on chromosome 19 at q13.2-13.2 and the enzyme is expressed in the epithelial or secretory cells of various ducts, including salivary, sweat, pancreatic, prostatic, intestinal, and distal nephron.[312] Some studies suggest that renal kallikrein mRNA is also detectable by in situ hybridization at the glomerular vascular pole.

The tissue kallikreins are acid glycoproteins, variably and extensively glycosylated.[312] The purified human renal enzyme is synthesized as a zymogen (prokallikrein) with an attached 17–amino acid signal peptide preceding a 7–amino acid activation sequence, which must be cleaved to activate the enzyme.

In the human kidney, kallikrein is localized to tubular segments that, according to cytologic criteria, correspond to the connecting tubule. Close anatomic contact between the kallikrein-containing tubules and the afferent arteriole of the JG apparatus is consistently observed. The close anatomic association of the kallikrein-containing cells with the renin-containing cells at the afferent arteriole close to the JG apparatus suggest a physiologic function and is consistent with a paracrine function for the KKS in the regulation of renal blood flow, GFR, and renin release.

Kallikrein, which is not filtered under normal conditions, crosses the glomerular basement membrane in pathologic conditions such as chronic renal failure. In the rat remnant kidney model, kallikrein is consistently observed in reabsorption droplets of the proximal tubule and is almost certainly secondary to an alteration in glomerular permeability, grossly manifested as proteinuria.[313]

Once activated, renal kallikrein cleaves both HMW and LMW kininogens to release Lys-bradykinin (kallidin). In most mammals including humans, tissue kallikrein cleaves Lys-bradykinin from kininogens, whereas plasma kallikrein releases bradykinin.

Renal kallikrein gene expression is modulated by physiologic factors such as development, thyroid hormones, glucocorticoids, and salt intake.[314–317] Interestingly, high dietary salt intake down-regulates renal kallikrein synthesis and enzymatic activity in both newborn and adult rats.[316]

Kinin Generation

Two independent KKSs can be distinguished in humans that involve specific subtypes of both kallikreins and kininogens.[299] The circulating plasma KKS consists of the HMW kininogen and plasma prekallikrein, both of which are synthesized in the liver and secreted as plasma proteins. Plasma kallikrein is proteolytically cleaved by the activity of an endothelial cell-borne prekallikrein activator. Previous investigation has identified Ang II and bradykinin as substrates of the same processing enzyme. As reported previously in the RAS section of this chapter, prolylcarboxypeptidase can activate the biologically inert Ang I or the vasoconstrictor Ang II to form Ang 1-7, a biologically active peptide that induces vasodilation by stimulating NO formation.[50,318] Interestingly, the finding that prolylcarboxypeptidase also activates prekallikrein indicates that it can produce two biologically active peptides, bradykinin and Ang 1-7, each of which could potentially reduce blood pressure, counterbalancing the vasoconstrictor effects of Ang II.

Apart from the plasma KKS, there are also tissue-specific systems consisting of locally synthesized or liver-derived LMW kininogen and tissue kallikrein, a serine protease that has been demonstrated in various glands, as previously described.[299] Unlike the plasma KKS, a continuous synthesis and secretion of kallikrein can occur in these organ-specific tissue systems so that kallidin can be produced physiologically from local and plasma-derived LMW kininogen. Some of these tissue KKSs have been shown to express LMW-kininogen. This applies expecially to the kidney, where large quantities of kininogen and kallikrein are synthesized by the tubular epithelium and are secreted in the urine. Kinin formed within the kidney is detectable in urine, renal interstitial fluid, and even in renal venous blood. However, both the local and the systemic half-life of kinins is widely considered to be very short, in the order of 10 to 30 seconds. Owing to the fact that kinins are produced continuously and that there is a clear evidence for powerful effects of kinins on renal vasculature resistance, electrolyte and water excretion, and renal function modulators (such as renin and angiotensin, eicosanoids, cathecholamines, NO, vasopressin, and ET), it is presumed that the renal KKS contributes to physiologic regulatory processes within the mammalian kidney.[299]

The activity of the renal KKS is usually inferred from measurements of urinary kallikrein. However, the activity of this system could be regulated not only by the amount of kallikrein secreted in the tubular fluid but also by the substrate concentration, the presence of kallikrein inhibitors, the pH and ionic composition of the tubular fluid, the presence of kininases, and the sensitivity of the target organs. In most studies, urinary kallikrein excretion has been the only parameter measured. The activity of the renal KKS can also be assessed by measuring kinins formed in the renal vascular compartment or by determining urinary kinin excretion, because kinins are the biologically active component of this system. However, kinins are rapidly catabolized in the kidney and blood, and in urine while in the bladder. Thus, renal vein kinins and urinary excretion of kinins may not reflect the intrarenal activity of the system. Campbell and colleagues[319] have developed high-performance liquid chromatography–based radioimmunoassays for the specific measurement of hydroxylated and nonhydroxylated bradykinin and kallidin peptides and their metabolites. Using this technique, it was observed that the levels of kinin peptides in urine were several orders of magnitude higher than in plasma or tissue, and kallidin peptides were more abundant than bradykinin peptides in urine.[320]

Kinin Receptors

The most prominent effects of kinins are mediated via the B_2 kinin–receptor subtype. This receptor is a constitutively expressed G-protein–coupled receptor that is present in a large number of organs and tissues (e.g., endothelium, fibroblasts, glandular epithelium, kidney, heart, skeletal muscle, central nervous system, as well as in the smooth muscle of blood vessels, vas deferens, trachea, intestine, uterus, and bladder). The B_2 receptor is stimulated by both bradykinin and kallidin. By contrast, bradykinin has hardly any effect on the B_1 receptor subtype.

The signal transduction mechanisms of the kinin receptors are well characterized only for the B_2 subtype. This receptor is responsible for the vasodilatatory activity of kinins at its location on endothelial cells. B_2 receptors stimulate phospholipase C and intracellular production of both IP_3 and diacylglycerol via activation of certain G-proteins such as $G\alpha_q$ and $G\alpha_i$.

Substantially less information exists about the functionality and signal transduction mechanisms of the B_1 receptor subtype. The amino acid sequence is 36% identical with that of the B_2 receptor. The B_1 receptors, which are physiologically present in only a few tissues, are also associated with vasoactive and inflammatory effects. This receptor subtype does not appear to play a major role in the kidney.

Kininases

Kinins are cleaved by a number of peptidases that have been described as kininases (Fig. 10–8). Apart from the metabolites desArg[9]-bradykinin and desArg[10]-kallidin, all kinin cleavage products are biologically inactive, and thus, kininase activities can significantly influence kinin effectiveness. These include various carboxypeptidases, ACE, and NEP. ACE, which has been described in detail in the RAS section of this chapter, truncates its own reaction product, 1-7 bradykinin, further to 1-5 bradykinin.

NEP is a membrane enzyme that, like ACE, cleaves bradykinin at the 7-8 position, but without breaking down the resulting 1-7 bradykinin peptide any farther. NEP has been demonstrated in renal tubules, intestinal epithelium, the central nervous system, the prostate, the heart, and the epididymis. It has also been localized to fibroblasts, endothelial cells, and granulocytes.[321,322] Most of the kininase activity present in urine and seminal fluid is derived from NEP. Like ACE, NEP also has a broad substrate specificity for a variety of the other substances, including substance P, Ang II, ANP, brain natriuretic peptide (BNP), ET-11, big-ET, enkephalins, oxytocin, and gastrin.[321]

At the NH_2-terminal end of bradykinin, only a proline-specific exopeptidase, aminopeptidase P, is able to attack the molecule owing to the presence of two proline residues. After bradykinin breakdown by aminopeptidase P, the resulting peptide 2-9-bradykinin is susceptible to other proteases including the endothelial enzyme dipeptidyl-aminopeptidase IV that reduces this metabolite to 4-9-bradykinin. A variety of other peptidases are also known to be capable of breaking down kinins, including a range of rarely discussed enzymes such as aminopeptidase M.

Physiologic Functions of the Kallikrein-Kinin System: Focus on the Kidney

Kinins can provoke a variety of biologic effects including effects on inflammation, coagulation, and vascular permeability.

Concerning the importance of kinins in the control of blood pressure and organ perfusion, the local KKSs in the myocardium, vascular system, and kidney are the most important. The vasodilatatory effects of kinins are related to an increased release of the mediators NO, PGI_2, and endothelium-derived hyperpolarizing factor (EDHF) from the endothelium.[323] Whereas the increase in kidney perfusion is primarily mediated by prostaglandins, NO appears to be essential for the anti-ischemic effect of kinins on the isolated heart.[324] Many of the beneficial effects of kinins can be explained by their ability to stimulate endothelial mediators. Regarding NO and prostacyclin, in addition to their vasodilatory activity, they can also inhibit platelet aggregation and granulocyte adhesion and reduce the release of cardiac catecholamines. The ability of NO to act as a free radical scavenger can also be considered as a further beneficial effect.[325]

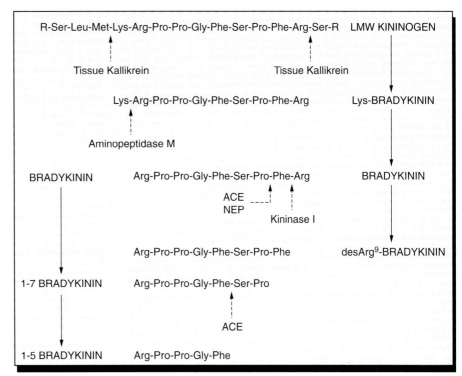

R-Ser-Leu-Met-Lys-Arg-Pro-Pro-Gly-Phe-Ser-Pro-Phe-Arg-Ser-R   LMW KININOGEN

Tissue Kallikrein   Tissue Kallikrein

Lys-Arg-Pro-Pro-Gly-Phe-Ser-Pro-Phe-Arg   Lys-BRADYKININ

Aminopeptidase M

BRADYKININ   Arg-Pro-Pro-Gly-Phe-Ser-Pro-Phe-Arg   BRADYKININ

ACE
NEP
Kininase I

Arg-Pro-Pro-Gly-Phe-Ser-Pro-Phe   desArg⁹-BRADYKININ

1-7 BRADYKININ   Arg-Pro-Pro-Gly-Phe-Ser-Pro

ACE

1-5 BRADYKININ   Arg-Pro-Pro-Gly-Phe

FIGURE 10–8 Comparison of the structure of tissue KKS components and sites of enzymic cleavage. ACE, angiotensin-converting enzyme; LMW, low molecular weight; NEP, neutral endopeptidase.

Recent studies using animal models with defined genetic modifications have helped to demonstrate the role of the KKS in normal physiology and in disease states. The kininogen-deficient Brown-Norway Katholiek strain of rat shows increased sensitivity to the pressor effects of increased dietary salt, mineralocorticoid administration and Ang II infusion, and an impairment of the cardioprotective effects of preconditioning.[326]

The B₂ receptor gene knockout mouse is reported to have elevated blood pressure, increased heart weight–to–body weight ratio, and an exaggerated pressor response to Ang II infusion and chronic dietary salt loading.[327] In addition to various cardiac defects, bradykinin B₂ receptor gene knockout mice also demonstrate increased urinary concentration in response to vasopressin, indicating that endogenous kinins acting through the B₂ receptor oppose the antidiuretic effect of vasopressin.[328]

Wang and coworkers[329] have observed that two transgenic mouse lines expressing the human B₂ receptor showed a significant reduction in blood pressure. Furthermore, administration of Hoe 140, a bradykinin B₂ receptor antagonist, restored the blood pressure of the transgenic mice to normal levels within 1 hour, the effect diminishing within 4 hours. The transgenic mice displayed an enhanced blood pressure–lowering effect induced by a bolus intra-aortic injection of kinin and showed an increased response in kinin-induced uterine smooth muscle contractility compared with control littermates. These observations suggest that overexpression of the human bradykinin B₂ receptor causes a sustained reduction in blood pressure in transgenic mice, confirming an important physiologic role for the KKS in the control of systemic blood pressure. Moreover, it has recently been demonstrated that transgenic mice overexpressing human tissue kallikrein showed a sustained reduction in blood pressure throughout their life span, indicating the lack of sufficient compensatory mechanisms to reverse the hypotensive effect of kallikrein.[330]

In the kidney, kinins have been reported to increase renal blood flow and papillary blood flow and mediate the hyper-filtration induced by high-protein diet. Furthermore, kinins inhibit in cortical collecting ducts the osmotic response to antidiuretic hormone and reduce net sodium reabsorption. Kinins also inhibit conductive sodium entry in inner medullary collecting duct cells and induce the release of renin in isolated glomeruli.[331]

There are observations that bradykinin can reset tubuloglomerular feedback.[332] In particular, it has been suggested that endogenously produced kinins in the normal rat may, via effects upon prostaglandin production, lower tubuloglomerular feedback sensitivity.

The natriuretic effect of kinins is either due to inhibition of sodium reabsorption in the distal part of the nephron or to changes in deep nephron reabsorption. Kinins may affect sodium reabsorption as a result of a direct effect on the transport of sodium along the nephron, a vasodilator effect, changes in the osmotic gradient of the renal medulla, or a combination of all three effects. These findings imply that the renal KKS is involved in the physiologic regulation of blood pressure, body fluid, and sodium balance. Further experimental studies, both in vitro and in vivo, predominantly using Hoe 140, suggest that bradykinin is antihypertrophic and antiproliferative. This has been reported in mesangial cells, fibroblasts, and renomedullary interstitial cells.

Kallikrein-Kinin System Function in Renal Diseases

Role of the Kallikrein-Kinin System in the Pathogenesis of Hypertension

Based on findings from gene knockout animals, it is hypothesised that impaired kinin levels/action may be involved in the pathogenesis of primary or secondary hypertension. Considering the genetically determined causes of hypertension, the kidney in particular may play an important role. A reduced activity of kallikrein has been observed in the urine of hypertensive patients and rats. Furthermore, epidemiologic studies have shown that a genetically determined impairment of renal kallikrein excretion is associated with the development of high blood pressure and is apparent even prior to the manifestation of clinical hypertension. However, the interpretation of such results is limited by the fact that any preexisting or hypertension-induced kidney disease might also be the underlying cause for a reduction in renal kallikrein excretion. Therefore, the epidemiologic association cannot conclusively be considered to indicate a causal role of reduced renal kallikrein in the pathogenesis of hypertension. Other associations between renal kallikrein excretion and hypertension-related factors, such as age, race, and dietary sodium and potassium intake of the patients, have also been reported.[333] Hence, the fact that reduced renal kallikrein activity is associated with hypertension remains to be explained fully at a mechanistic level.

Role of the Kallikrein-Kinin System in the Pathogenesis of Renal Diseases: Focus on Diabetes

Rats with streptozotocin-induced diabetes mellitus have markedly altered KKS function.[334] Early in the course of the diabetic state, these animals, if treated with insulin, show glomerular hyperfiltration along with increased renal kallikrein synthesis levels and urinary excretion.[334] Treatment of such animals with aprotinin or a B_2 receptor antagonist reduces renal blood flow and GFR.[334] These studies have been confirmed in patients with type 1 diabetes.[335] Diabetic subjects with glomerular hyperfiltration showed greater active kallikrein and PGE_2 excretion than diabetic patients with normal GFR or control nondiabetic subjects. Kallikrein levels correlated directly with GFR and distal tubular sodium reabsorption. These findings in diabetic rat models and patients provide evidence that the renal KKS is a contributor to the renal adaptation to diabetes and may play a role in diabetic nephropathy. Our own group[336] has explored the possible role of the bradykinin in mediating the renoprotective effects of ACE inhibitors in experimental diabetic nephropathy. In that study, the administration of the bradykinin B_2 receptor antagonist Hoe 140 to diabetic rats did not attenuate the antialbuminuric effects of the ACE inhibitor, nor did it have any effect itself. Moreover, treatment with Hoe 140 did not attenuate the beneficial effect of ACE inhibition on glomerular morphology.[336] These findings demonstrate that blockade of Ang II is the major pathway responsible for renoprotection afforded by ACE inhibition and implies that there is no or only a minor involvement of the KKS to the long-term changes of the kidney in diabetes. However, the importance of the KKS in diabetic renal disease has recently been reconsidered with a study in Akita diabetic B2 receptor knockout mice demonstrating accelerated renal injury.[337]

In patients with chronic renal failure, kallikrein excretion has been reported to be greatly increased, and it has been postulated that an increase in kallikrein activity per nephron may play a role in the maintenance of high sodium excretion and blood flow in the surviving nephrons.

In patients with both renal parenchymal disease and hypertension, kallikrein excretion is conspicuously decreased, and the severity of hypertension inversely correlates with kallikrein excretion. Kallikrein excretion in these patients was lower than in patients with essential hypertension of comparable severity without renal failure.[21]

Summary

In the last decade, our knowledge of the KKS, in particular the renal KKS, has been significantly advanced. There are two main classes of KKSs: the plasma KKS and the tissue KKS. Studies involving receptors antagonists, kininogen-deficient animals, B_2 receptor knockout mice, and genetic activation of the KKS have suggested a physiologic role for this system

in the regulation of blood pressure, blood flow distribution, coagulation, and sodium and water excretion. Moreover, recent observations suggest a crucial role for the KKS and, in particular, for the B_2 receptor in mediating renal growth and development. Data are available that indicate that the KKS interacts with other renal hormonal systems such as the prostaglandins and the RAS. Indeed, the KKS may participate in mediating some of the effects of treatment with ACE inhibitors. Abnormalities of the KKS have been found in hypertension, diabetes mellitus, and chronic renal failure, and it has been postulated that this system may participate in the pathogenesis and pathophysiology of these diseases. Future studies are needed to assess whether new therapeutic strategies based on stimulation or interruption of KKS actions will be important to the treatment or perhaps even the prevention of some of these common disorders.

THE NATRIURETIC PEPTIDES

The natriuretic peptides are a well characterized family of hormones that play a major role in salt and water homeostasis.[338] The first member of the family to be described was ANP, but at least five structurally similar but genetically distinct peptides including BNP, C-type natriuretic peptide (CNP),[339] dendroaspis natriuretic peptide,[340] and urodilantin[341,342] also exist. There are other peptides involved in salt and water balance including adrenomedullin, guanylin, uroguanylin,[343] and oubain-like factor, but these are not discussed further in this review.

ANP and BNP are similar in their ability to act as endogenous antagonists of the RAS to cause natriuresis and diuresis, vasodilation, and suppression of the sympathetic nervous system, as well as inhibiting cell growth and reducing secretion of aldosterone and renin.[338,344,345]

The natriuretic peptides (NPs) play an important role in the regulation of cardiovascular, renal, and endocrine function,[344] but their therapeutic potential is limited by their peptide nature and the need for intravenous administration. Despite this, several studies have used intravenous administration of the NPs to treat heart failure and AKI in humans, with limited success. An alternative approach is to increase endogenous NP levels by inhibition of the enzymatic degradation by NEP EC 3.4.24.11 (NEP).[321,346–348] Selective orally active NEP inhibitors have been demonstrated to protect the NPs from inactivation in vivo and to potentiate their biologic actions. Novel compounds that simultaneously inhibit both NEP and ACE have been developed and are known as vasopepeptidase inhibitors (VPIs).[349,350] Although these agents have been successful in various animal models of disease, the first of these compounds, omapatrilat, that was used in large clinical trials in hypertension (OCTAVE) and in heart failure (OVERTURE), showed adverse effects that slowed the further development of these VPIs.[351,352]

Atrial Natriuretic Peptide—Structure, Processing, and Synthesis

The main site of synthesis of ANP is the cardiac atria, and the main stimulus to release is wall tension secondary to increased intravascular volume. In the adult heart, ANP mRNA levels are approximately 30- to 50-fold higher in the atria than observed in the ventricle. However, ventricular expression is dramatically increased in the developing heart[338] and during hemodynamic overload such as heart failure and hypertension.[353] There are also extracardiac sites of ANP gene expression including the kidney, lung, brain, adrenal gland, and liver.[21,354,355] In the kidney, alternate processing of proANP adds four amino acids to the N-terminus of ANP to generate a 32–amino acid peptide, proANP 95-126 or urodilatin.[356]

Brain Natriuretic Peptide

BNP is synthesised predominantly from the heart.[338] BNP is found in the highest concentrations in the cardiac ventricles, where it is constitutively expressed. Like ANP, the expression of BNP is regulated by changes in intracardiac pressure and/or stretch.[357,358] Cardiac BNP gene expression and plasma levels increase in heart failure,[359] hypertension,[360,361] and renal failure.[362–364] The physiologic actions of BNP are qualitatively similar to those of ANP and include effects on the kidney (natriuresis and diuresis), the vasculature (decrease in blood pressure and intravascular fluid volume), endocrine systems (inhibition of plasma renin and aldosterone secretion), and the brain (central vasodepressor activity).[338] In pathophysiologic states such as heart failure and renal failure, the levels of BNP often exceed those of ANP, which may reflect slower clearance of BNP by the degradation system and suggests differences in the regulation of BNP compared with that of ANP.

Natriuretic Peptide Receptors

NPs mediate their effects through binding to high-affinity receptors on the cell surface with subsequent intracellular generation of cGMP.[338] Only two of these receptors, NPR-A and NPR-B, exhibit the intracellular guanylyl cyclase (GC) catalytic domain.[365] Upon ligand binding, a change in receptor conformation allows cytosolic factors to interact with the kinase-like domain, leading to activation of GC and the consequent generation of cGMP, the second messenger of the NPs.

NPR-A mRNA is expressed mainly in the kidney, in the glomeruli, in the renal vasculature, and in the proximal tubules and is highest in the innermedullary collecting duct (IMCD),[366,367] consistent with the known physiologic actions of ANP on these structures.[368]

Clearance Receptor

The inactivation of the NPs occurs via two pathways, binding to the clearance receptor NPR-C and enzymatic degradation. This results in a half-life of the NPs in the range of minutes. The NPR-C clears the NPs through receptor-mediated uptake, internalization, and lysosomal hydrolysis of the NPs, with rapid and efficient recycling of internalized receptors to the cell surface. NPR-C is the most abundant of the receptors, accounting for more than 95% of the total receptor population, and is expressed at high density in kidney, vascular endothelium, smooth muscle cell, and the heart.[369] The NPR-C binds all members of the NP family with high affinity.

Neutral Endopeptidase

Enzymatic degradation of the NPs takes place in the lung, liver, and kidney, and the main enzyme responsible for this degradation is NEP.[321,346,348] NEP, originally referred to as enkephalinase because of its ability to degrade opioid peptides within the brain, was subsequently shown to be identical to an already well-characterized zinc metallopeptidase present in the kidney. NEP has a ubiquitous tissue distribution and multiple functions, sharing structural similarities with various metallopeptidases including aminopeptidase (APN), ACE, ECE, and carboxypeptidases A, B, and E.[321] NEP is most abundant in the brush borders of the proximal tubules of the kidney, where it rapidly degrades filtered ANP, thus preventing the peptide from reaching more distal luminal receptors. Despite its lack of substrate specificity in vitro, the primary function of NEP in vivo is to metabolize the NPs.

Renal Actions of the Natriuretic Peptides

The NPs are endogenous antagonists of the RAS. Levels of ANP and BNP rise in response to volume expansion and pressure overload and have actions to antagonize the effects of Ang II on blood pressure, renal tubular reabsorption, vascular tone and growth, and aldosterone secretion.[370]

The glomerulus and the IMCD are the two regions of the nephron at which most NP receptors have been identified. Not surprisingly, the natriuretic and diuretic actions of the NPs result from both hemodynamic effects and direct tubular actions.[371] The most notable hemodynamic action is to increase GFR by enhancing glomerular hydrostatic pressure as a result of afferent arteriolar dilation and efferent arteriolar constriction. The contrasting effects of the NPs on the afferent and efferent arterioles differ from the actions of classical vasodilators such as BK. The NPs also increase accumulation of cGMP in mesangial cells to cause relaxation of these cells and increase the effective surface area for filtration.[372] The NPs are considered to have direct tubular actions. ANP inhibits Ang II–induced sodium and water transport in the proximal tubule, tubular water transport through vasopressin antagonism in the cortical collecting duct, and the distal tubular actions of aldosterone.[21] In addition, NPs induce increases in sodium delivery to the macula densa, thereby indirectly inhibiting renin secretion and subsequent secretion of Ang II and aldosterone.

The NPs decrease blood pressure by a number of pathways. ANP reduces cardiac preload by shifting intravascular fluid into the extravascular compartment through increases in capillary hydrostatic permeability. ANP also increases venous capacitance and reduces extracellular fluid volume,[370] as well as reduces peripheral vascular resistance. ANP also reduces sympathetic tone, suppresses the release of catecholamines, and reduces central sympathetic outflow. BNP has cardiovascular effects similar to those of ANP, whereas CNP is a more potent dilator than either ANP or BNP.

Therapeutic Uses of the Natriuretic Peptides

Given the properties of the NPs, their efficacy in the treatment of diseases such as hypertension, heart failure, and renal insufficiency has been examined in both experimental models and humans. The following section focuses on the therapeutic uses of the NPs in humans. In essential hypertension, ANP infusion lowers blood pressure and increases urinary sodium excretion.[338] In heart failure, ANP decreases systemic vascular resistance, increases natriuresis and diuresis,[338] and is registered for the treatment of pulmonary edema in Japan, under the name Carperitide (Fujisawa, Japan).[373] Although experimental studies in acute renal dysfunction had encouraging results in terms of improvement in renal function, studies in humans have been disappointing.[374] Anaritide is a 25–amino acid synthetic form of ANP (102-106) and was used in a multicenter, randomized, double-blind, placebo-controlled clinical trial in 504 critically ill patients with acute tubular necrosis.[375] Anaritide did not improve the overall rate of dialysis-free survival, and although it may have improved dialysis-free survival in patients with oliguria, it actually worsened survival in patients without oliguria with acute tubular necrosis. In a larger study of 1222 patients with oliguric AKI, a 24-hour infusion of anaritide (0.2 μg/kg/min) had similar effects on the primary end-point of dialysis-free survival (21%) to placebo (15%, $p=.22$).[376] Thus, ANP is not considered to be of use in the treatment of AKI.[377]

With regard to BNP, an infusion increases sodium excretion and lowers blood pressure in mild to moderate hypertension.[378] As the natriuretic and blood pressure-lowering effects of BNP are two- to threefold greater than ANP,[379] BNP may represents a more beneficial therapeutic modality than ANP. Indeed, BNP or nesiritide (Scios, Sunnyvale, CA, USA), gained U.S. Food and Drug Administration approval as the first new parenteral agent approved for heart failure therapy in more than a decade.[380] Nesiritide is identical to endogenous BNP and has been evaluated in clinical trials involving more than 700 subjects. The rapid and sustained beneficial hemodynamic effects of nesiritide supports its use as a first-line intravenous therapy for patients with symptomatic decompensated CHF.[381] However, a recent meta-analysis of the clinical trials of BNP in acutely decompensated heart failure and data from the company suggest that the risk of worsening renal dysfunction increases with its use in heart failure.[382] To date, there are no data as to the efficacy of BNP in renal failure per se in humans.

Neural Endopeptidase Inhibition

Although there has been some success with ANP and BNP infusions, such a mode of administration is not suitable for the long-term treatment of chronic diseases in humans. As there has been little success with orally active analogs or alternative routes of peptide administration, efforts to use the biologic actions of the NPs as a therapy have centered on NEP inhibitors. Although NEP inhibitors do elevate plasma levels of the NPs and under certain experimental conditions cause the expected responses such as diuresis and natriuresis and peripheral vasodilatation, clinical trials in hypertension and heart failure have, in general, had disappointing results. This may relate to the biologic activity of the compounds themselves, but is probably also due to the fact that a fall in blood pressure activates the RAS. Therefore, any increase in the NPs, be it from infusions or inhibition of breakdown, is unable to overcome an activated RAS. The biologic actions of the NPs are restored in the presence of an inhibited RAS, which has led to the development of compounds that simultaneously inhibit NEP and ACE, known as VPIs. These compounds may offer advantages in the treatment of hypertension, heart failure, and renal disease.

Dual Inhibition of Neural Endopeptidase and Angiotensin-Converting Enzyme

The VPIs have been rationally designed, taking into account the similar structural characteristics of the catalytic site of both peptidases, NEP and ACE.[350] Several such inhibitors are available including mixanpril (S21402), CGS30440, aladotril, MDL 100173, sampatrilat, and omapatrilat. All these compounds show potent activity to inhibit ACE and NEP, although the degree of potency against the individual enzymes does vary among compounds. Omapatrilat, the most clinically advanced VPI, has similar potency against both NEP and ACE (NEP K_i = 9 nmol/L; ACE K_i = 6 nmol/L).[383] Unfortunately, in initial clinical studies focused on hypertension and heart failure, a high incidence of angioedema, a potentially life-threatening complication, occurred with omapatrilat. It is not clear that this represents a side effect of all VPIs, especially given the differences in potencies for ACE versus NEP that exist. However, this life-threatening side effect has significant impaired development of this new class of agents for the time being.

VASOPEPTIDASE INHIBITORS AND RENAL DISEASE. In experimental models of renal disease, the VPIs offer some hope in terms of achieving more aggressive blood pressure targets. In the diabetic hypertensive rat, the VPI S21402 had increased efficacy on blood pressure in diabetic SHR, compared with ACE or NEP inhibition alone over a 4-week period.[384] Urinary albumin excretion rate was lower in both diabetic and non-diabetic SHR treated with the dual NEP/ACE inhibitor. In a long-term study in diabetic SHR, another VPI, omapatrilat, conferred renoprotection in a dose-dependent manner, in association with a reduction in expression of TGF-β and β-inducible gene-H3, a TGF-β–dependent matrix protein.[385]

This dual ACE/NEP inhibition has also been reported by several groups to attenuate the progression of renal injury in the model of subtotal nephrectomy (STNx).[386,387] Overall, these findings suggest that vasopeptidase inhibition may be a therapeutic approach for retarding progression of renal injury, in which reducing both blood pressure and proteinuria are considered important targets.

There are no clinical studies that have specifically assessed VPIs in diabetic or nondiabetic renal disease. However, if clinical studies produce results similar to those in animal models, this new class of drugs may have a major effect in reducing the number of patients that progresses to end-stage renal failure.

Summary

The NP system includes ANP, BNP, CNP, and dendroaspis natriuretic peptide. ANP and BNP are similar in their ability to act as endogenous antagonists of the RAS to cause natriuresis and diuresis, vasodilation, and suppression of the sympathetic nervous system, as well as inhibiting cell growth and reducing secretion of aldosterone and renin. Although less is known about the actions of the other NPs, CNP has been demonstrated to be a potent vasodilator in arteries and veins and to inhibit mitogenesis, migration, and growth of vascular smooth muscle cells. NPs mediate their effects through binding to high-affinity receptors, NPR-A, B, and C. The NPs play an important role in the regulation of cardiovascular, renal, and endocrine function. Therapeutic approach to increase endogenous NP levels by inhibition of the enzymatic degradation by NEP has been proposed, and novel compounds that simultaneously inhibit both NEP and ACE, the VPIs, were developed. Unfortunately, preclinical and early clinical trials with omapatrilat in hypertension and heart failure were disappointing, partly because of the potentially life-threatening side effect, angioedema, with this agent.

References

1. Lindpaintner K, Ganten D: Tissue renin-angiotensin systems and their modulation: The heart as a paradigm for new aspects of converting enzyme inhibition. Cardiology 79(suppl 1):32–44, 1991.
2. Griendling KK, Murphy TJ, Alexander RW: Molecular biology of the renin-angiotensin system. Circulation 87:1810–1828, 1993.
3. Neuringer JR, Brenner BM: Hemodynamic theory of progressive renal disease: A 10-year update in brief review. Am J Kidney Dis 22:98–104, 1993.
4. Moravski CJ, Kelly DJ, Cooper ME, et al: Retinal neovascularization is prevented by blockade of the renin-angiotensin system. Hypertension 36:1099–1104, 2000.
5. Paizis G, Cooper ME, Schembri JM, et al: Up-regulation of components of the renin-angiotensin system in the bile duct-ligated rat liver. Gastroenterology 123:1667–1676, 2002.
6. Allen AM, Zhuo J, Mendelsohn FA: Localization of angiotensin AT1 and AT2 receptors. J Am Soc Nephrol 10(suppl 11):S23–S29, 1999.
7. Urata H, Nishimura H, Ganten D: Mechanisms of angiotensin II formation in humans. Eur Heart J 16 (suppl N):79–85, 1995.
8. Saavedra JM: Brain and pituitary angiotensin. Endocr Rev 13:329–380, 1992.
9. Taubman MB: Angiotensin II: A vasoactive hormone with ever-increasing biological roles. Circ Res 92:9–11, 2003.
10. Timmermans PB, Wong PC, Chiu AT, et al: Nonpeptide angiotensin II receptor antagonists. Trends Pharmacol Sci 12:55–62, 1991.
11. Dahlof B, Devereux RB, Kjeldsen SE, et al: Cardiovascular morbidity and mortality in the Losartan Intervention For Endpoint reduction in hypertension study (LIFE): A randomised trial against atenolol. Lancet 359:995–1003, 2002.
12. Ingelfinger JR, Zuo WM, Fon EA, et al: In situ hybridization evidence for angiotensinogen messenger RNA in the rat proximal tubule. An hypothesis for the intrarenal renin angiotensin system. J Clin Invest 85:417–423, 1990.
13. Cao Z, Kelly DJ, Cox A, et al: Angiotensin type 2 receptor is expressed in the adult rat kidney and promotes cellular proliferation and apoptosis. Kidney Int 58:2437–2451, 2000.
14. Ozono R, Wang ZQ, Moore AF, et al: Expression of the subtype 2 angiotensin (AT2) receptor protein in rat kidney. Hypertension 30:1238–1246, 1997.

15. Ichikawi I, Harris RC: Angiotensin actions in the kidney: Renewed insight into the old hormone. Kidney Int 40:583–596, 1991.

16. Fukamizu A, Takahashi S, Seo MS, et al: Structure and expression of the human angiotensinogen gene. Identification of a unique and highly active promoter. J Biol Chem 265:7576–7582, 1990.

17. Terada Y, Tomita K, Nonoguchi H, et al: PCR localization of angiotensin II receptor and angiotensinogen mRNAs in rat kidney. Kidney Int 43:1251–1259, 1993.

18. Sawa H, Tokuchi F, Mochizuki N, et al: Expression of the angiotensinogen gene and localization of its protein in the human heart. Circulation 86:138–146, 1992.

19. Schunkert H, Ingelfinger JR, Jacob H, et al: Reciprocal feedback regulation of kidney angiotensinogen and renin mRNA expressions by angiotensin II. Am J Physiol 263: E863–E869, 1992.

20. Hackenthal E, Paul M, Ganten D, et al: Morphology, physiology, and molecular biology of renin secretion. Physiol Rev 70:1067–1116, 1990.

21. Candido R, Burrell LM, Jandeleit-Dahm KA, et al: Vasoactive peptides and the kidney. In Brenner BM (ed): The Kidney, 7th ed. Philadelphia, WB Saunders, 2003.

22. Nguyen G, Delarue F, Burckle C, et al: Pivotal role of the renin/prorenin receptor in angiotensin II production and cellular responses to renin. J Clin Invest 109:1417–1427, 2002.

23. Lorenz JN, Greenberg SG, Briggs JP: The macula densa mechanism for control of renin secretion. Semin Nephrol 13:531–542, 1993.

24. Burns KD, Homma T, Harris RC: The intrarenal renin-angiotensin system. Semin Nephrol 13:13–30, 1993.

25. Sigmund CD, Jones CA, Kane CM, et al: Regulated tissue- and cell-specific expression of the human renin gene in transgenic mice. Circ Res 70:1070–1079, 1992.

26. Johns DW, Peach MJ, Gomez RA, et al: Angiotensin II regulates renin gene expression. Am J Physiol 259:F882–F887, 1990.

27. Berka JL, Alcorn D, Ryan GB, et al: Renin processing studied by immunogold localization of prorenin and renin in granular juxtaglomerular cells in mice treated with enalapril. Cell Tissue Res 268:141–148, 1992.

28. Sigmon DH, Carretero OA, Beierwaltes WH: Endothelium-derived relaxing factor regulates renin release in vivo. Am J Physiol 263:F256–F261, 1992.

29. Natesh R, Schwager SL, Sturrock ED, et al: Crystal structure of the human angiotensin-converting enzyme-lisinopril complex. Nature 421:551–554, 2003.

30. Rigat B, Hubert C, Alhenc-Gelas F, et al: An insertion/deletion polymorphism in the angiotensin I-converting enzyme gene accounting for half the variance of serum enzyme levels. J Clin Invest 86:1343–1346, 1990.

31. Jeunemaitre X, Lifton RP, Hunt SC, et al: Absence of linkage between the angiotensin converting enzyme locus and human essential hypertension. Nat Genet 1:72–75, 1992.

32. Hubert C, Houot AM, Corvol P, et al: Structure of the angiotensin I-converting enzyme gene. Two alternate promoters correspond to evolutionary steps of a duplicated gene. J Biol Chem 266:15377–15383, 1991.

33. Shai SY, Langford KG, Martin BM, et al: Genomic DNA 5′ to the mouse and human angiotensin-converting enzyme genes contains two distinct regions of conserved sequence. Biochem Biophys Res Commun 167:1128–1133, 1990.

34. Schunkert H, Ingelfinger JR, Hirsch AT, et al: Feedback regulation of angiotensin converting enzyme activity and mRNA levels by angiotensin II. Circ Res 72:312–318, 1993.

35. King SJ, Oparil S: Converting-enzyme inhibitors increase converting-enzyme mRNA and activity in endothelial cells. Am J Physiol 263:C743–C749, 1992.

36. Dasarathy Y, Lanzillo JJ, Fanburg BL: Stimulation of bovine pulmonary artery endothelial cell ACE by dexamethasone: Involvement of steroid receptors. Am J Physiol 263:L645–L649, 1992.

37. Okamura T, Okunishi H, Ayajiki K, et al: Conversion of angiotensin I to angiotensin II in dog isolated renal artery: Role of two different angiotensin II-generating enzymes. J Cardiovasc Pharmacol 15:353–359, 1990.

38. Diet F, Pratt RE, Berry GJ, et al: Increased accumulation of tissue ACE in human atherosclerotic coronary artery disease. Circulation 94:2756–2767, 1996.

39. Candido R, Jandeleit-Dahm KA, Cao Z, et al: Prevention of accelerated atherosclerosis by angiotensin-converting enzyme inhibition in diabetic apolipoprotein E-deficient mice. Circulation 106:246–253, 2002.

40. Pontremoli R, Sofia A, Tirotta A, et al: The deletion polymorphism of the angiotensin I-converting enzyme gene is associated with target organ damage in essential hypertension. J Am Soc Nephrol 7:2550–2558, 1996.

41. Marre M, Jeunemaitre X, Gallois Y, et al: Contribution of genetic polymorphism in the renin-angiotensin system to the development of renal complications in insulin-dependent diabetes: Genetique de la Nephropathie Diabetique (GENEDIAB) study group. J Clin Invest 99:1585–1595, 1997.

42. Fabris B, Bortoletto M, Candido R, et al: Genetic polymorphisms of the renin-angiotensin-aldosterone system and renal insufficiency in essential hypertension. J Hypertens 23:309–316, 2005.

43. Tarnow L, Cambien F, Rossing P, et al: Lack of relationship between an insertion/deletion polymorphism in the angiotensin I-converting enzyme gene and diabetic nephropathy and proliferative retinopathy in IDDM patients. Diabetes 44:489–494, 1995.

44. Parving HH, Jacobsen P, Tarnow L, et al: Effect of deletion polymorphism of angiotensin converting enzyme gene on progression of diabetic nephropathy during inhibition of angiotensin converting enzyme: Observational follow up study. BMJ 313:591–594, 1996.

45. Andersen S, Tarnow L, Cambien F, et al: Renoprotective effects of losartan in diabetic nephropathy: Interaction with ACE insertion/deletion genotype? Kidney Int 62:192–198, 2002.

46. Burrell LH, Johnston CI, Tikellis C, Cooper ME: ACE2, a new regulator of the renin angiotensin system. Trends Endocrinol Metab 15:166–169, 2004.

47. Donoghue M, Hsieh F, Baronas E, et al: A novel angiotensin-converting enzyme-related carboxypeptidase (ACE2) converts angiotensin I to angiotensin 1–9. Circ Res 87:E1–E9, 2000.

48. Tipnis SR, Hooper NM, Hyde R, et al: A human homolog of angiotensin-converting enzyme. Cloning and functional expression as a captopril-insensitive carboxypeptidase. J Biol Chem 275:33238–33243, 2000.

49. Vickers C, Hales P, Kaushik V, et al: Hydrolysis of biological peptides by human angiotensin-converting enzyme-related carboxypeptidase. J Biol Chem 277:14838–14843, 2002.

50. Ren Y, Garvin JL, Carretero OA: Vasodilator action of angiotensin-(1–7) on isolated rabbit afferent arterioles. Hypertension 39:799–802, 2002.

51. Li W, Moore MJ, Vasilieva N, et al: Angiotensin-converting enzyme 2 is a functional receptor for the SARS coronavirus. Nature 426:450–454, 2003.

52. Dimitrov DS: The secret life of ACE2 as a receptor for the SARS virus. Cell 115:652–653, 2003.

53. Crackower MA, Sarao R, Oudit GY, et al: Angiotensin-converting enzyme 2 is an essential regulator of heart function. Nature 417:822–828, 2002.

54. Tikellis C, Johnston CI, Forbes JM, et al: Characterization of renal angiotensin-converting enzyme 2 in diabetic nephropathy. Hypertension 41:392–397, 2003.

55. Dean RG, Burrell LH: ACE2 and diabetic complications. Curr Pharm Des 2007 (in press).

56. Ahmad S, Ward PE: Role of aminopeptidase activity in the regulation of the pressor activity of circulating angiotensins. J Pharmacol Exp Ther 252:643–650, 1990.

57. Kerins DM, Hao Q, Vaughan DE: Angiotensin induction of PAI-1 expression in endothelial cells is mediated by the hexapeptide angiotensin IV. J Clin Invest 96:2515–2520, 1995.

58. Nishimura H, Tsuji H, Masuda H, et al: The effects of angiotensin metabolites on the regulation of coagulation and fibrinolysis in cultured rat aortic endothelial cells. Thromb Haemost 82:1510–1521, 1999.

59. Yamamoto K, Chappell MC, Brosnihan KB, et al: In vivo metabolism of angiotensin I by neutral endopeptidase (EC 3.4.24.11) in spontaneously hypertensive rats. Hypertension 19:692–696, 1992.

60. Welches WR, Santos RA, Chappell MC, et al: Evidence that prolyl endopeptidase participates in the processing of brain angiotensin. J Hypertens 9:631–638, 1991.

61. Hilchey SD, Bell-Quilley CP: Association between the natriuretic action of angiotensin-(1–7) and selective stimulation of renal prostaglandin I2 release. Hypertension 25:1238–1244, 1995.

62. Handa RK, Ferrario CM, Strandhoy JW: Renal actions of angiotensin-(1–7): in vivo and in vitro studies. Am J Physiol 270:F141–F147, 1996.

63. Vallon V, Heyne N, Richter K, et al: [7-D-ALA]-angiotensin 1–7 blocks renal actions of angiotensin 1–7 in the anesthetized rat. J Cardiovasc Pharmacol 32:164–167, 1998.

64. Chappell MC, Pirro NT, Sykes A, et al: Metabolism of angiotensin-(1–7) by angiotensin-converting enzyme. Hypertension 31:362–367, 1998.

65. Deddish PA, Marcic B, Jackman HL, et al:. N-domain-specific substrate and C-domain inhibitors of angiotensin-converting enzyme: angiotensin-(1–7) and keto-ACE. Hypertension 31:912–917, 1998.

66. Yamada K, Iyer SN, Chappell MC, et al: Converting enzyme determines plasma clearance of angiotensin-(1–7). Hypertension 32:496–502, 1998.

67. de Gasparo M, Husain A, Alexander W, et al: Proposed update of angiotensin receptor nomenclature. Hypertension 25:924–927, 1995.

68. Timmermans PB, Wong PC, Chiu AT, et al:. Angiotensin II receptors and angiotensin II receptor antagonists. Pharmacol Rev 45:205–251, 1993.

69. Timmermans PB, Benfield P, Chiu AT, et al: Angiotensin II receptors and functional correlates. Am J Hypertens 5:221S–235S, 1992.

70. Horiuchi M: Functional aspects of angiotensin type 2 receptor. Adv Exp Med Biol 396:217–24, 1996.

71. Csikos T, Chung O, Unger T: Receptors and their classification: Focus on angiotensin II and the AT2 receptor. J Hum Hypertens 12:311–318, 1998.

72. Murphy TJ, Alexander RW, Griendling KK, et al: Isolation of a cDNA encoding the vascular type-1 angiotensin II receptor. Nature 351:233–236, 1991.

73. Sasaki K, Yamano Y, Bardhan S, et al: Cloning and expression of a complementary DNA encoding a bovine adrenal angiotensin II type-1 receptor. Nature 351:230–233, 1991.

74. Guo DF, Furuta H, Mizukoshi M, et al: The genomic organization of human angiotensin II type 1 receptor. Biochem Biophys Res Commun 200:313–319, 1994.

75. Griendling KK, Alexander RW: The angiotensin (AT1) receptor. Semin Nephrol 13:558–66, 1993.

76. Hunyady L, Balla T, Catt KJ: The ligand binding site of the angiotensin AT1 receptor. Trends Pharmacol Sci 17:135–140, 1996.

77. Groblewski T, Maigret B, Nouet S, et al: Amino acids of the third transmembrane domain of the AT1A angiotensin II receptor are involved in the differential recognition of peptide and nonpeptide ligands. Biochem Biophys Res Commun 209:153–160, 1995.

78. Thomas WG, Thekkumkara TJ, Baker KM: Molecular mechanisms of angiotensin II (AT1A) receptor endocytosis. Clin Exp Pharmacol Physiol Suppl 3:S74–S80, 1996.

79. Schieffer B, Paxton WG, Marrero MB, et al: Importance of tyrosine phosphorylation in angiotensin II type 1 receptor signaling. Hypertension 27:476–480, 1996.

80. Marrero MB, Schieffer B, Paxton WG, et al: Direct stimulation of Jak/STAT pathway by the angiotensin II AT1 receptor. Nature 375:247–250, 1995.

81. Song K, Allen AM, Paxinos G, et al: Mapping of angiotensin II receptor subtype heterogeneity in rat brain. J Comp Neurol 316:467–484, 1992.

82. Aldred GP, Chai SY, Song K, et al: Distribution of angiotensin II receptor subtypes in the rabbit brain. Regul Pept 44:119–130, 1993.

83. Barnes JM, Steward LJ, Barber PC, et al: Identification and characterisation of angiotensin II receptor subtypes in human brain. Eur J Pharmacol 230:251–258, 1993.

84. MacGregor DP, Murone C, Song K, et al: Angiotensin II receptor subtypes in the human central nervous system. Brain Res 675:231–240, 1995.

85. Allen AM, Yamada H, Mendelsohn FA: In vitro autoradiographic localization of binding to angiotensin receptors in the rat heart. Int J Cardiol 28:25–33, 1990.

86. Sechi LA, Griffin CA, Grady EF, et al: Characterization of angiotensin II receptor subtypes in rat heart. Circ Res 71:1482–1489, 1992.

87. Zhuo J, Allen AM, Alcorn D, et al: The distribution of angiotensin II receptors. In Laragh JH, Brenner BM (eds): Hypertension: Pathophysiology, Diagnosis, and Management. New York: Raven Press, 1995, pp 1739–1762.

88. Zhuo J, Alcorn D, Allen AM, et al: High resolution localization of angiotensin II receptors in rat renal medulla. Kidney Int 42:1372–1380, 1992.

89. Moravec CS, Schluchter MD, Paranandi L, et al: Inotropic effects of angiotensin II on human cardiac muscle in vitro. Circulation 82:1973–1984, 1990.

90. Rosendorff C: The renin-angiotensin system and vascular hypertrophy. J Am Coll Cardiol 28:803–812, 1996.

91. Dzau VJ: Cell biology and genetics of angiotensin in cardiovascular disease. J Hypertens Suppl 12:S3–S10, 1994.

92. Paradis P, Dali-Youcef N, Paradis FW, et al: Overexpression of angiotensin II type I receptor in cardiomyocytes induces cardiac hypertrophy and remodeling. Proc Natl Acad Sci U S A 97:931–936, 2000.

93. Giacchetti G, Opocher G, Sarzani R, et al: Angiotensin II and the adrenal. Clin Exp Pharmacol Physiol Suppl 3:S119–S124, 1996.

94. Bell PD, Peti-Peterdi J: Angiotensin II stimulates macula densa basolateral sodium/hydrogen exchange via type 1 angiotensin II receptors. J Am Soc Nephrol 10(suppl 11):S225–S259, 1999.

95. Koike G, Horiuchi M, Yamada T, et al: Human type 2 angiotensin II receptor gene: Cloned, mapped to the X chromosome, and its mRNA is expressed in the human lung. Biochem Biophys Res Commun 203:1842–1850, 1994.

96. Martin MM, Elton TS: The sequence and genomic organization of the human type 2 angiotensin II receptor. Biochem Biophys Res Commun 209:554–562, 1995.

97. Koike G, Winer ES, Horiuchi M, et al: Cloning, characterization, and genetic mapping of the rat type 2 angiotensin II receptor gene. Hypertension 26:998–1002, 1995.

98. Nakajima M, Mukoyama M, Pratt RE, et al: Cloning of cDNA and analysis of the gene for mouse angiotensin II type 2 receptor. Biochem Biophys Res Commun 197:393–399, 1993.

99. Ichiki T, Herold CL, Kambayashi Y, et al: Cloning of the cDNA and the genomic DNA of the mouse angiotensin II type 2 receptor. Biochim Biophys Acta 1189:247–250, 1994.

100. Bottari SP, King IN, Reichlin S, et al: The angiotensin AT2 receptor stimulates protein tyrosine phosphatase activity and mediates inhibition of particulate guanylate cyclase. Biochem Biophys Res Commun 183:206–211, 1992.

101. Kang J, Posner P, Sumners C: Angiotensin II type 2 receptor stimulation of neuronal K+ currents involves an inhibitory GTP binding protein. Am J Physiol 267:C1389–C1397, 1994.

102. Horiuchi M, Hayashida W, Kambe T, et al: Angiotensin type 2 receptor dephosphorylates Bcl-2 by activating mitogen-activated protein kinase phosphatase-1 and induces apoptosis. J Biol Chem 272:19022–19026, 1997.

103. Fischer TA, Singh K, O'Hara DS, et al: Role of AT1 and AT2 receptors in regulation of MAPKs and MKP-1 by ANG II in adult cardiac myocytes. Am J Physiol 275:H906–H916, 1998.

104. Bedecs K, Elbaz N, Sutren M, et al: Angiotensin II type 2 receptors mediate inhibition of mitogen-activated protein kinase cascade and functional activation of SHP-1 tyrosine phosphatase. Biochem J 325(pt 2):449–454, 1997.

105. Huang XC, Richards EM, Sumners C: Mitogen-activated protein kinases in rat brain neuronal cultures are activated by angiotensin II type 1 receptors and inhibited by angiotensin II type 2 receptors. J Biol Chem 271:15635–15641, 1996.

106. Nouet S, Nahmias C: Signal transduction from the angiotensin II AT2 receptor. Trends Endocrinol Metab 11:1–6, 2000.

107. Zhang J, Pratt RE: The AT2 receptor selectively associates with Gialpha2 and Gialpha3 in the rat fetus. J Biol Chem 271:15026–15033, 1996.

108. Tsutsumi Y, Matsubara H, Ohkubo N, et al: Angiotensin II type 2 receptor is upregulated in human heart with interstitial fibrosis, and cardiac fibroblasts are the major cell type for its expression. Circ Res 83:1035–1046, 1998.

109. Wharton J, Morgan K, Rutherford RA, et al: Differential distribution of angiotensin AT2 receptors in the normal and failing human heart. J Pharmacol Exp Ther 284:323–336, 1998.

110. Breault L, Lehoux JG, Gallo-Payet N: Angiotensin II receptors in the human adrenal gland. Endocr Res 22:355–361, 1996.

111. Hein L, Barsh GS, Pratt RE, et al: Behavioural and cardiovascular effects of disrupting the angiotensin II type-2 receptor in mice. Nature 377:744–747, 1995.

112. Ichiki T, Labosky PA, Shiota C, et al: Effects on blood pressure and exploratory behaviour of mice lacking angiotensin II type-2 receptor. Nature 377:748–750, 1995.

113. Siragy HM, Carey RM: The subtype-2 (AT2) angiotensin receptor regulates renal cyclic guanosine 3′,5′-monophosphate and AT1 receptor-mediated prostaglandin E2 production in conscious rats. J Clin Invest 97:1978–1982, 1996.

114. Siragy HM, Carey RM: The subtype 2 (AT2) angiotensin receptor mediates renal production of nitric oxide in conscious rats. J Clin Invest 100:264–269, 1997.

115. Siragy HM, Carey RM: The subtype 2 angiotensin receptor regulates renal prostaglandin F2 alpha formation in conscious rats. Am J Physiol 273:R1103–R1107, 1997.

116. Carey RM, Wang ZQ, Siragy HM: Role of the angiotensin type 2 receptor in the regulation of blood pressure and renal function. Hypertension 35:155–163, 2000.

117. Cao Z, Bonnet F, Candido R, et al: Angiotensin type 2 receptor antagonism confers renal protection in a rat model of progressive renal injury. J Am Soc Nephrol 13:1773–1787, 2002.

118. Wright JW, Harding JW: Important role for angiotensin III and IV in the brain renin-angiotensin system. Brain Res Brain Res Rev 25:96–124, 1997.

119. Krebs LT, Kramar EA, Hanesworth JM, et al: Characterization of the binding properties and physiological action of divalinal-angiotensin IV, a putative AT4 receptor antagonist. Regul Pept 67:123–130, 1996.

120. Harding JW, Wright JW, Swanson GN, et al: AT4 receptors: Specificity and distribution. Kidney Int 46:1510–1512, 1994.

121. Handa RK, Krebs LT, Harding JW, et al: Angiotensin IV AT4-receptor system in the rat kidney. Am J Physiol 274:F290–F299, 1998.

122. Handa RK: Characterization and signaling of the AT(4) receptor in human proximal tubule epithelial (HK-2) cells. J Am Soc Nephrol 12:440–449, 2001.

123. Chansel D, Czekalski S, Vandermeersch S, et al: Characterization of angiotensin IV-degrading enzymes and receptors on rat mesangial cells. Am J Physiol 275:F535–F542, 1998.

124. Tallant EA, Lu X, Weiss RB, et al: Bovine aortic endothelial cells contain an angiotensin-(1–7) receptor. Hypertension 29:388–393, 1997.

125. Santos RA, Campagnole-Santos MJ: Central and peripheral actions of angiotensin-(1–7). Braz J Med Biol Res 27:1033–1047, 1994.

126. Santos RA, Simoes e Silva AC, Maric C, et al: Angiotensin-(1–7) is an endogenous ligand for the G protein-coupled receptor Mas. Proc Natl Acad Sci U S A 100:8258–8263, 2003.

127. Chaki S, Inagami T: Identification and characterization of a new binding site for angiotensin II in mouse neuroblastoma neuro-2A cells. Biochem Biophys Res Commun 182:388–394, 1992.

128. Tanimoto K, Sugiyama F, Goto Y, et al: Angiotensinogen-deficient mice with hypotension. J Biol Chem 269:31334–31337, 1994.

129. Esther CR, Jr., Howard TE, Marino EM, et al: Mice lacking angiotensin-converting enzyme have low blood pressure, renal pathology, and reduced male fertility. Lab Invest 74:953–965, 1996.

130. de Gasparo M, Catt KJ, Inagami T, et al: International union of pharmacology. XXIII. The angiotensin II receptors. Pharmacol Rev 52:415–472, 2000.

131. Ito M, Oliverio MI, Mannon PJ, et al: Regulation of blood pressure by the type 1A angiotensin II receptor gene. Proc Natl Acad Sci U S A 92:3521–3525, 1995.

132. Sugaya T, Nishimatsu S, Tanimoto K, et al: Angiotensin II type 1a receptor-deficient mice with hypotension and hyperreninemia. J Biol Chem 270:18719–18722, 1995.

133. Chen X, Li W, Yoshida H, et al: Targeting deletion of angiotensin type 1B receptor gene in the mouse. Am J Physiol 272:F299–F304, 1997.

134. Oliverio MI, Kim HS, Ito M, et al: Reduced growth, abnormal kidney structure, and type 2 (AT2) angiotensin receptor-mediated blood pressure regulation in mice lacking both AT1A and AT1B receptors for angiotensin II. Proc Natl Acad Sci U S A 95:15496–15501, 1998.

135. Tsuchida S, Matsusaka T, Chen X, et al: Murine double nullizygotes of the angiotensin type 1A and 1B receptor genes duplicate severe abnormal phenotypes of angiotensinogen nullizygotes. J Clin Invest 101:755–760, 1998.

136. Siragy HM, Inagami T, Ichiki T, et al: Sustained hypersensitivity to angiotensin II and its mechanism in mice lacking the subtype-2 (AT2) angiotensin receptor. Proc Natl Acad Sci U S A 96:6506–6510, 1999.

137. Okuyama S, Sakagawa T, Chaki S, et al: Anxiety-like behavior in mice lacking the angiotensin II type-2 receptor. Brain Res 821:150–159, 1999.

138. Sakagawa T, Okuyama S, Kawashima N, et al: Pain threshold, learning and formation of brain edema in mice lacking the angiotensin II type 2 receptor. Life Sci 67:2577–2585, 2000.

139. Kopp JB, Klotman PE: Transgenic animal models of renal development and pathogenesis. Am J Physiol 269:F601–F620, 1995.

140. Wagner J, Ganten D: The renin-angiotensin system in transgenic rats: Characteristics and functional studies. Semin Nephrol 13:586–592, 1993.

141. Ganten D, Wagner J, Zeh K, et al: Species specificity of renin kinetics in transgenic rats harboring the human renin and angiotensinogen genes. Proc Natl Acad Sci U S A 89:7806–7810, 1992.

142. Kai T, Kino H, Sugimura K, et al: Significant role of the increase in renin-angiotensin system in cardiac hypertrophy and renal glomerular sclerosis in double transgenic tsukuba hypertensive mice carrying both human renin and angiotensinogen genes. Clin Exp Hypertens 20:439–449, 1998.

143. Fern RJ, Yesko CM, Thornhill BA, et al: Reduced angiotensinogen expression attenuates renal interstitial fibrosis in obstructive nephropathy in mice. J Clin Invest 103:39–46, 1999.

144. Mullins JJ, Peters J, Ganten D: Fulminant hypertension in transgenic rats harbouring the mouse Ren-2 gene. Nature 344:541–544, 1990.

145. Bader M, Zhao Y, Sander M, et al: Role of tissue renin in the pathophysiology of hypertension in TGR(mREN2)27 rats. Hypertension 19:681–686, 1992.

146. Kelly DJ, Wilkinson-Berka JL, Allen TJ, et al: A new model of diabetic nephropathy with progressive renal impairment in the transgenic (mRen-2)27 rat (TGR). Kidney Int 54:343–352, 1998.

147. Arendshorst WJ, Brannstrom K, Ruan X: Actions of angiotensin II on the renal microvasculature. J Am Soc Nephrol 10(suppl 11):S149–S161, 1999.

148. Navar LG, Inscho EW, Majid SA, et al: Paracrine regulation of the renal microcirculation. Physiol Rev 76:425–536, 1996.

149. Takenaka T, Forster H, Epstein M: Protein kinase C and calcium channel activation as determinants of renal vasoconstriction by angiotensin II and endothelin. Circ Res 73:743–750, 1993.

150. Tolins JP, Shultz PJ, Raij L, et al: Abnormal renal hemodynamic response to reduced renal perfusion pressure in diabetic rats: Role of NO. Am J Physiol 265:F886–F895, 1993.

151. Ito S, Amin J, Ren Y, et al: Heterogeneity of angiotensin action in renal circulation. Kidney Int Suppl 63:S128–S131, 1997.

152. Dohi Y, Hahn AW, Boulanger CM, et al: Endothelin stimulated by angiotensin II augments contractility of spontaneously hypertensive rat resistance arteries. Hypertension 19:131–137, 1992.

153. Rossi GP, Sacchetto A, Cesari M, et al: Interactions between endothelin-1 and the renin-angiotensin-aldosterone system. Cardiovasc Res 43:300–307, 1999.

154. Herizi A, Jover B, Bouriquet N, et al: Prevention of the cardiovascular and renal effects of angiotensin II by endothelin blockade. Hypertension 31:10–14, 1998.

155. Wang T, Chan YL: Mechanism of angiotensin II action on proximal tubular transport. J Pharmacol Exp Ther 252:689–695, 1990.

156. Wu MS, Biemesderfer D, Giebisch G, et al: Role of NHE3 in mediating renal brush border Na+-H+ exchange. Adaptation to metabolic acidosis. J Biol Chem 271:32749–32752, 1996.

157. Romero MF, Fong P, Berger UV, et al: Cloning and functional expression of rNBC, an electrogenic Na(+)-HCO3- cotransporter from rat kidney. Am J Physiol 274:F425–F432, 1998.

158. Ruiz OS, Qiu YY, Wang LJ, et al: Regulation of the renal Na-HCO3 cotransporter: IV. Mechanisms of the stimulatory effect of angiotensin II. J Am Soc Nephrol 6:1202–1208, 1995.

159. Wagner CA, Giebisch G, Lang F, et al: Angiotensin II stimulates vesicular H+-ATPase in rat proximal tubular cells. Proc Natl Acad Sci U S A 95:9665–9668, 1998.

160. Garvin JL: Angiotensin stimulates glucose and fluid absorption by rat proximal straight tubules. J Am Soc Nephrol 1:272–277, 1990.

161. Han HJ, Park SH, Koh HJ, et al: Mechanism of regulation of Na+ transport by angiotensin II in primary renal cells. Kidney Int 57:2457–2467, 2000.

162. Wong PS, Johns EJ: The receptor subtype mediating the action of angiotensin II on intracellular sodium in rat proximal tubules. Br J Pharmacol 124:41–46, 1998.

163. Quan A, Baum M: Effect of luminal angiotensin II receptor antagonists on proximal tubule transport. Am J Hypertens 12:499–503, 1999.

164. Jacobs LS, Douglas JG: Angiotensin II type 2 receptor subtype mediates phospholipase A2-dependent signaling in rabbit proximal tubular epithelial cells. Hypertension 28:663–668, 1996.

165. Haithcock D, Jiao H, Cui XL, et al: Renal proximal tubular AT2 receptor: Signaling and transport. J Am Soc Nephrol 10(suppl 11):S69–S74, 1999.

166. Kennedy CR, Burns KD: Angiotensin II as a mediator of renal tubular transport. Contrib Nephrol 135:47–62, 2001.

167. Harrison-Bernard LM, Navar LG, Ho MM, et al: Immunohistochemical localization of ANG II AT1 receptor in adult rat kidney using a monoclonal antibody. Am J Physiol 273:F170–F177, 1997.

168. Lemley KV, Kriz W: Anatomy of the renal interstitium. Kidney Int 39:370–381, 1991.

169. Kaissling B, Hegyi I, Loffing J, et al: Morphology of interstitial cells in the healthy kidney. Anat Embryol (Berl) 193:303–318, 1996.

170. Johnston CI, Fabris B, Jandeleit K: Intrarenal renin-angiotensin system in renal physiology and pathophysiology. Kidney Int Suppl 42:S59–S63, 1993.

171. Kakinuma Y, Fogo A, Inagami T, et al: Intrarenal localization of angiotensin II type 1 receptor mRNA in the rat. Kidney Int 43:1229–1235, 1993.

172. Lindop GB, Lever AF: Anatomy of the renin-angiotensin system in the normal and pathological kidney. Histopathology 10:335–362, 1986.

173. Mercure C, Ramla D, Garcia R, et al: Evidence for intracellular generation of angiotensin II in rat juxtaglomerular cells. FEBS Lett 422:395–399, 1998.

174. Seikaly MG, Arant BS, Jr., Seney FD, Jr: Endogenous angiotensin concentrations in specific intrarenal fluid compartments of the rat. J Clin Invest 86:1352–1357, 1990.

175. Braam B, Mitchell KD, Fox J, et al: Proximal tubular secretion of angiotensin II in rats. Am J Physiol 264:F891–F898, 1993.

176. Navar LG, Harrison-Bernard LM, Wang CT, et al: Concentrations and actions of intraluminal angiotensin II. J Am Soc Nephrol 10(suppl 11):S189–S195, 1999.

177. Tank JE, Henrich WL, Moe OW: Regulation of glomerular and proximal tubule renin mRNA by chronic changes in dietary NaCl. Am J Physiol 273:F892–F898, 1997.

178. Gilbert RE, Wu LL, Kelly DJ, et al: Pathological expression of renin and angiotensin II in the renal tubule after subtotal nephrectomy. Implications for the pathogenesis of tubulointerstitial fibrosis. Am J Pathol 155:429–440, 1999.

179. The GISEN Group: Randomised placebo-controlled trial of effect of ramipril on decline in glomerular filtration rate and risk of terminal renal failure in proteinuric, non-diabetic nephropathy. Lancet 349:1857–1863, 1997.

180. Lewis EJ, Hunsicker LG, Bain RP, et al: The effect of angiotensin-converting-enzyme inhibition on diabetic nephropathy. The Collaborative Study Group. N Engl J Med 329:1456–1462, 1993.

181. Marinides GN: Progression of chronic renal disease and diabetic nephropathy: A review of clinical studies and current therapy. J Med 24:266–288, 1993.

182. Maschio G, Oldrizzi L, Marcantoni C, et al: Hypertension and progression of renal disease. J Nephrol 13:225–227, 2000.

183. Remuzzi G, Ruggenenti P, Benigni A: Understanding the nature of renal disease progression. Kidney Int 51:2–15, 1997.

184. Wesson LG: Physical factors and glomerulosclerosis. Cause or coincidence? Nephron 78:125–130, 1998.

185. Anderson PW, Do YS, Hsueh WA: Angiotensin II causes mesangial cell hypertrophy. Hypertension 21:29–35, 1993.

186. Wolf G, Haberstroh U, Neilson EG: Angiotensin II stimulates the proliferation and biosynthesis of type I collagen in cultured murine mesangial cells. Am J Pathol 140:95–107, 1992.

187. Gomez-Garre D, Ruiz-Ortega M, Ortego M, et al: Effects and interactions of endothelin-1 and angiotensin II on matrix protein expression and synthesis and mesangial cell growth. Hypertension 27:885–892, 1996.

188. Border WA, Ruoslahti E: Transforming growth factor-beta in disease: The dark side of tissue repair. J Clin Invest 90:1–7, 1992.

189. Border WA, Noble NA: Transforming growth factor beta in tissue fibrosis. N Engl J Med 331:1286–1292, 1994.

190. Ruiz-Ortega M, Bustos C, Hernandez-Presa MA, et al: Angiotensin II participates in mononuclear cell recruitment in experimental immune complex nephritis through nuclear factor-kappa B activation and monocyte chemoattractant protein-1 synthesis. J Immunol 161:430–439, 1998.

191. Wolf G, Ziyadeh FN, Thaiss F, et al: Angiotensin II stimulates expression of the chemokine RANTES in rat glomerular endothelial cells. Role of the angiotensin type 2 receptor. J Clin Invest 100:1047–1058, 1997.

192. Sharma M, Sharma R, Greene AS, et al: Documentation of angiotensin II receptors in glomerular epithelial cells. Am J Physiol 274:F623–F627, 1998.

193. Zhuo J, Maric C, Harris PJ, et al: Localization and functional properties of angiotensin II AT1 receptors in the kidney: Focus on renomedullary interstitial cells. Hypertens Res 20:233–250, 1997.

194. Chansel D, Llorens-Cortes C, Vandermeersch S, et al: Regulation of angiotensin II receptor subtypes by dexamethasone in rat mesangial cells. Hypertension 27:867–874, 1996.

195. Maric C, Aldred GP, Antoine AM, et al: Effects of angiotensin II on cultured rat renomedullary interstitial cells are mediated by AT1A receptors. Am J Physiol 271:F1020–F1028, 1996.

196. Zhuo JL: Renomedullary interstitial cells: A target for endocrine and paracrine actions of vasoactive peptides in the renal medulla. Clin Exp Pharmacol Physiol 27:465–473, 2000.

197. Miller PL, Rennke HG, Meyer TW: Glomerular hypertrophy accelerates hypertensive glomerular injury in rats. Am J Physiol 261:F459–F465, 1991.

198. Kim S, Iwao H: Molecular and cellular mechanisms of angiotensin II-mediated cardiovascular and renal diseases. Pharmacol Rev 52:11–34, 2000.

199. Johnson RJ, Alpers CE, Yoshimura A, et al: Renal injury from angiotensin II-mediated hypertension. Hypertension 19:464–474, 1992.

200. Kagami S, Border WA, Miller DE, et al: Angiotensin II stimulates extracellular matrix protein synthesis through induction of transforming growth factor-beta expression in rat glomerular mesangial cells. J Clin Invest 93:2431–2437, 1994.

201. Campos AH, Zhao Y, Pollman MJ, et al: DNA microarray profiling to identify angiotensin-responsive genes in vascular smooth muscle cells: potential mediators of vascular disease. Circ Res 92:111–118, 2003.

202. Hamaguchi A, Kim S, Wanibuchi H, et al: Angiotensin II and calcium blockers prevent glomerular phenotypic changes in remnant kidney model. J Am Soc Nephrol 7:687–693, 1996.

203. Berka JL, Alcorn D, Coghlan JP, et al: Granular juxtaglomerular cells and prorenin synthesis in mice treated with enalapril. J Hypertens 8:229–238, 1990.

204. Tryggvason K, Wartiovaara J: Molecular basis of glomerular permselectivity. Curr Opin Nephrol Hypertens 10:543–549, 2001.

205. Kestila M, Lenkkeri U, Mannikko M, et al: Positionally cloned gene for a novel glomerular protein—nephrin—is mutated in congenital nephrotic syndrome. Mol Cell 1:575–582, 1998.

206. Kawachi H, Koike H, Kurihara H, et al: Cloning of rat nephrin: Expression in developing glomeruli and in proteinuric states. Kidney Int 57:1949–1961, 2000.

207. Luimula P, Ahola H, Wang SX, et al: Nephrin in experimental glomerular disease. Kidney Int 58:1461–1468, 2000.

208. Honda N, Hishida A, Kato A: Factors affecting severity of renal injury and recovery of function in acute renal failure. Ren Fail 14:337–340, 1992.

209. Torres MA, Furst DE: Treatment of generalized systemic sclerosis. Rheum Dis Clin North Am 16:217–241, 1990.

210. Burns KD: Angiotensin II and its receptors in the diabetic kidney. Am J Kidney Dis 36:449–467, 2000.

211. Anderson S, Jung FF, Ingelfinger JR: Renal renin-angiotensin system in diabetes: Functional, immunohistochemical, and molecular biological correlations. Am J Physiol 265:F477–F486, 1993.

212. Correa-Rotter R, Hostetter TH, Rosenberg ME: Renin and angiotensinogen gene expression in experimental diabetes mellitus. Kidney Int 41:796–804, 1992.

213. Bonnet F, Candido R, Carey RM, et al: Renal expression of angiotensin receptors in long-term diabetes and the effects of angiotensin type 1 receptor blockade. J Hypertens 20:1615–1624, 2002.

214. Wolf G, Ziyadeh FN: The role of angiotensin II in diabetic nephropathy: Emphasis on nonhemodynamic mechanisms. Am J Kidney Dis 29:153–163, 1997.

215. Bonnet F, Cooper ME, Kawachi H, et al: Irbesartan normalises the deficiency in glomerular nephrin expression in a model of diabetes and hypertension. Diabetologia 44:874–877, 2001.

216. Jandeleit-Dahm K, Cooper ME: Hypertension and diabetes: role of the renin-angiotensin syndrome. Endocrinol Metab Clin North Am 35:469–490, 2006.

217. Kim S, Wanibuchi H, Hamaguchi A, et al: Angiotensin blockade improves cardiac and renal complications of type II diabetic rats. Hypertension 30:1054–1061, 1997.

218. Gilbert RE, Cox A, Wu LL, et al: Expression of transforming growth factor-beta1 and type IV collagen in the renal tubulointerstitium in experimental diabetes: Effects of ACE inhibition. Diabetes 47:414–422, 1998.

219. Gilbert RE, Cooper ME: The tubulointerstitium in progressive diabetic kidney disease: More than an aftermath of glomerular injury? Kidney Int 56:1627–1637, 1999.

220. Yamamoto T, Nakamura T, Noble NA, et al: Expression of transforming growth factor beta is elevated in human and experimental diabetic nephropathy. Proc Natl Acad Sci U S A 90:1814–1818, 1993.

221. Cao Z, Cooper ME: Role of angiotensin II in tubulointerstitial injury. Semin Nephrol 21:554–562, 2001.

222. Wagner OF, Christ G, Wojta J, et al: Polar secretion of endothelin-1 by cultured endothelial cells. J Biol Chem 267:16066–16068, 1992.

223. Marsden PA, Dorfman DM, Collins T, et al: Regulated expression of endothelin 1 in glomerular capillary endothelial cells. Am J Physiol 261:F117–F125, 1991.

224. Ohta K, Hirata Y, Imai T, et al: Cytokine-induced release of endothelin-1 from porcine renal epithelial cell line. Biochem Biophys Res Commun 169:578–584, 1990.

225. Sakamoto H, Sasaki S, Hirata Y, et al: Production of endothelin-1 by rat cultured mesangial cells. Biochem Biophys Res Commun 169:462–468, 1990.

226. Kohan DE: Endothelin synthesis by rabbit renal tubule cells. Am J Physiol 261:F221–F226, 1991.

227. Uchida S, Takemoto F, Ogata E, et al: Detection of endothelin-1 mRNA by RT-PCR in isolated rat renal tubules. Biochem Biophys Res Commun 188:108–113 1992.

228. Ujiie K, Terada Y, Nonoguchi H, et al: Messenger RNA expression and synthesis of endothelin-1 along rat nephron segments. J Clin Invest 90:1043–1048, 1992.

229. Abassi Z, Winaver J, Rubinstein I, et al: Renal endothelin-converting enzyme in rats with congestive heart failure. J Cardiovasc Pharmacol 31:S31–S34, 1998.

230. Pupilli C, Romagnani P, Lasagni L, et al: Localization of endothelin-converting enzyme-1 in human kidney. Am J Physiol 273:F749–F756, 1997.

231. Arai H, Hori S, Aramori I, et al: Cloning and expression of a cDNA encoding an endothelin receptor. Nature 348:730–732, 1990.

232. Sakurai T, Yanagisawa M, Takuwa Y, et al: Cloning of a cDNA encoding a non-iso-peptide-selective subtype of the endothelin receptor. Nature 348:732–735, 1990.

233. Yamamoto T, Hirohama T, Uemura H: Endothelin B receptor-like immunoreactivity in podocytes of the rat kidney. Arch Histol Cytol 65:245–250, 2002.

234. Vanni S, Polidori G, Cecioni I, et al: ET(B) receptor in renal medulla is enhanced by local sodium during low salt intake. Hypertension 40:179–185, 2002.

235. Hirata Y, Emori T, Eguchi S, et al: Endothelin receptor subtype B mediates synthesis of nitric oxide by cultured bovine endothelial cells. J Clin Invest 91:1367–1373, 1993.

236. Spieker LE, Noll G, Luscher TF: Therapeutic potential for endothelin receptor antagonists in cardiovascular disorders. Am J Cardiovasc Drugs 1:293–303, 2001.

237. Tian X, Tang G, Chen Y: [The effects of endothelin-1 and selective endothelin receptor-type A antagonist on human renal interstitial fibroblasts in vitro]. Zhonghua Yi Xue Za Zhi 82:5–9, 2002.

238. Forbes JM, Jandeleit-Dahm K, Allen TJ, et al: Endothelin and endothelin A/B receptors are increased after ischaemic acute renal failure. Exp Nephrol 9:309–316, 2001.

239. Forbes JM, Leaker B, Hewitson TD, et al: Macrophage and myofibroblast involvement in ischemic acute renal failure is attenuated by endothelin receptor antagonists. Kidney Int 55:198–208, 1999.

240. Forbes JM, Hewitson TD, Becker GJ, et al: Simultaneous blockade of endothelin A and B receptors in ischemic acute renal failure is detrimental to long-term kidney function. Kidney Int 59:1333–1341, 2001.

241. Gottmann U, van der Woude FJ, Braun C: Endothelin receptor antagonists: A new therapeutic option for improving the outcome after solid organ transplantation? Curr Vasc Pharmacol 1:281–299, 2003.

242. Benigni A, Zoja C, Corna D, et al: A specific endothelin subtype A receptor antagonist protects against injury in renal disease progression. Kidney Int 44:440–444, 1993.

243. Benigni A, Colosio V, Brena C, et al: Unselective inhibition of endothelin receptors reduces renal dysfunction in experimental diabetes. Diabetes 47:450–456, 1998.

244. Vlachojannis JG, Tsakas S, Petropoulou C, et al: Endothelin-1 in the kidney and urine of patients with glomerular disease and proteinuria. Clin Nephrol 58:337–343, 2002.

245. Schwarz A, Godes M, Thone-Reineke C, et al: Tissue-dependent expression of matrix proteins in human endothelin-1 transgenic mice. Clin Sci (Lond) 103(suppl 48):39S–43S, 2002.

246. Shindo T, Kurihara H, Maemura K, et al: Renal damage and salt-dependent hypertension in aged transgenic mice overexpressing endothelin-1. J Mol Med 80:105–116, 2002.

247. Dussaule JC, Tharaux PL, Boffa JJ, et al: Mechanisms mediating the renal profibrotic actions of vasoactive peptides in transgenic mice. J Am Soc Nephrol 11(suppl 16):S124–S128, 2000.

248. Chatziantoniou C, Dussaule JC: Endothelin and renal vascular fibrosis: Of mice and men. Curr Opin Nephrol Hypertens 9:31–36, 2000.

249. Ritz E, Ogata H, Orth SR: Smoking: A factor promoting onset and progression of diabetic nephropathy. Diabetes Metab 26(suppl 4):54–63, 2000.

250. Frank HJ, Levin ER, Hu RM, et al: Insulin stimulates endothelin binding and action on cultured vascular smooth muscle cells. Endocrinology 133:1092–1097, 1993.

251. Hu RM, Levin ER, Pedram A, et al: Insulin stimulates production and secretion of endothelin from bovine endothelial cells. Diabetes 42:351–358, 1993.

252. Yamauchi T, Ohnaka K, Takayanagi R, et al: Enhanced secretion of endothelin-1 by elevated glucose levels from cultured bovine aortic endothelial cells. FEBS Lett 267:10–18, 1990.

253. Ferri C, De Mattia G: The effect of insulin on endothelin-1 (ET-1) secretion in human cultured endothelial cell. Metabolism 44:689–690, 1995.

254. Whiteside CI, Dlugosz JA: Mesangial cell protein kinase C isozyme activation in the diabetic milieu. Am J Physiol Renal Physiol 282:F975–F980, 2002.

255. Dlugosz JA, Munk S, Ispanovic E, et al: Mesangial cell filamentous actin disassembly and hypocontractility in high glucose are mediated by PKC-zeta. Am J Physiol Renal Physiol 282:F151–F163, 2002.

256. Tsiani E, Lekas P, Fantus IG, et al: High glucose-enhanced activation of mesangial cell p38 MAPK by ET-1, ANG II, and platelet-derived growth factor. Am J Physiol Endocrinol Metab 282:E161–E169, 2002.

257. Cosenzi A, Bernobich E, Bonavita M, et al: Antihypertensive treatment with enrasentan (SB217242) in an animal model of hypertension and hyperinsulinemia. J Cardiovasc Pharmacol 39:488–495, 2002.

258. Fukui M, Nakamura T, Ebihara I, et al: Gene expression for endothelins and their receptors in glomeruli of diabetic rats. J Lab Clin Med 122:149–156, 1993.

259. Turner NC, Morgan PJ, Haynes AC, et al: Elevated renal endothelin-I clearance and mRNA levels associated with albuminuria and nephropathy in non-insulin-dependent diabetes mellitus: Studies in obese fa/fa Zucker rats. Clin Sci (Lond) 93:565–571, 1997.

260. Jandeleit-Dahm K, Allen TJ, Youssef S, et al: Is there a role for endothelin antagonists in diabetic renal disease? Diabetes Obes Metab 2:15–24, 2000.

261. Nakamura T, Ebihara I, Tomino Y, et al: Effect of a specific endothelin A receptor antagonist on murine lupus nephritis. Kidney Int 47:481–489, 1995.

262. Koide H, Nakamura T, Ebihara I, et al: Endothelins in diabetic kidneys. Kidney Int Suppl 51:S45–S49, 1995.

263. Pfab T, Thone-Reineke C, Theilig F, et al: Diabetic endothelin B receptor-deficient rats develop severe hypertension and progressive renal failure. J Am Soc Nephrol 17:1082–1089, 2006.

264. Hocher B, Schwarz A, Reinbacher D, et al: Effects of endothelin receptor antagonists on the progression of diabetic nephropathy. Nephron 87:161–169, 2001.

265. Gu Y, Chen J, Yang H, et al: [The effects of endothelin blockade on renal expression of angiotensin II type 1 receptor in diabetic hypertensive rats]. Zhonghua Yi Xue Za Zhi 82:10–13, 2002.

266. Chen S, Evans T, Deng D, et al: Hyperhexosemia induced functional and structural changes in the kidneys: Role of endothelins. Nephron 90:86–94, 2002.

267. Kelly DJ, Skinner SL, Gilbert RE, et al: Effects of endothelin or angiotensin II receptor blockade on diabetes in the transgenic (mRen-2)27 rat. Kidney Int 57:1882–1894, 2000.

268. Gross ML, Ritz E, Schoof A, et al: Renal damage in the SHR/N-cp type 2 diabetes model: Comparison of an angiotensin-converting enzyme inhibitor and endothelin receptor blocker. Lab Invest 83:1267–1277, 2003.

269. Chen J, Gu Y, Lin F, et al: Endothelin receptor antagonist combined with a calcium channel blocker attenuates renal injury in spontaneous hypertensive rats with diabetes. Chin Med J (Engl) 115:972–978, 2002.

270. Tikkanen I, Tikkanen T, Cao Z, et al: Combined inhibition of neutral endopeptidase with angiotensin converting enzyme or endothelin converting enzyme in experimental diabetes. J Hypertens 20:707–714, 2002.

271. Touyz RM, Turgeon A, Schiffrin EL: Endothelin-A-receptor blockade improves renal function and doubles the lifespan of stroke-prone spontaneously hypertensive rats. J Cardiovasc Pharmacol 36:S300–S304, 2000.

272. Schiffrin EL: Endothelin: Role in experimental hypertension. J Cardiovasc Pharmacol 35:S33–S35, 2000.

273. Schiffrin EL, Deng LY, Sventek P, et al: Enhanced expression of endothelin-1 gene in resistance arteries in severe human essential hypertension. J Hypertens 15:57–63, 1997.

274. Krum H, Viskoper RJ, Lacourciere Y, et al: The effect of an endothelin-receptor antagonist, bosentan, on blood pressure in patients with essential hypertension. Bosentan Hypertension Investigators. N Engl J Med 338:784–790, 1998.

275. Elijovich F, Laffer CL, Amador E, et al: Regulation of plasma endothelin by salt in salt-sensitive hypertension. Circulation 103:263–268, 2001.

276. Ong KL, Lam KS, Cheung BM: Urotensin II: Its function in health and its role in disease. Cardiovasc Drugs Ther 19:65–75, 2005.

277. Conlon JM, Yano K, Waugh D, et al: Distribution and molecular forms of urotensin II and its role in cardiovascular regulation in vertebrates. J Exp Zool 275:226–238, 1996.

278. Conlon JM, Tostivint H, Vaudry H: Somatostatin- and urotensin II-related peptides: Molecular diversity and evolutionary perspectives. Regul Pept 69:95–103, 1997.

279. Ames RS, Sarau HM, Chambers JK, et al: Human urotensin-II is a potent vasoconstrictor and agonist for the orphan receptor GPR14. Nature 401:282–286, 1999.

280. Coulouarn Y, Lihrmann I, Jegou S, et al: Cloning of the cDNA encoding the urotensin II precursor in frog and human reveals intense expression of the urotensin II gene in motoneurons of the spinal cord. Proc Natl Acad Sci U S A 95:15803–15808, 1998.

281. Thanassoulis G, Huyhn T, Giaid A: Urotensin II and cardiovascular diseases. Peptides 25:1789–1794, 2004.

282. Behm DJ, Harrison SM, Ao Z, et al: Deletion of the UT receptor gene results in the selective loss of urotensin-II contractile activity in aortae isolated from UT receptor knockout mice. Br J Pharmacol 139:464–472, 2003.

283. Wang YX, Ding YJ, Zhu YZ, et al: Role of PKC in the novel synergistic action of urotensin II and angiotensin II and in urotensin II-induced vasoconstriction. Am J Physiol Heart Circ Physiol 292:H348–H353, 2007.

284. Tamura K, Okazaki M, Tamura M, et al: Urotensin II-induced activation of extracellular signal-regulated kinase in cultured vascular smooth muscle cells: Involvement of cell adhesion-mediated integrin signaling. Life Sci 72:1049–1060, 2003.

285. Sauzeau V, Le Mellionnec E, Bertoglio J, et al: Human urotensin II-induced contraction and arterial smooth muscle cell proliferation are mediated by RhoA and Rho-kinase. Circ Res 88:1102–1104, 2001.

286. Matsushita M, Shichiri M, Imai T, et al: Co-expression of urotensin II and its receptor (GPR14) in human cardiovascular and renal tissues. J Hypertens 19:2185–2190, 2001.

287. Shenouda A, Douglas SA, Ohlstein EH, et al: Localization of urotensin-II immunoreactivity in normal human kidneys and renal carcinoma. J Histochem Cytochem 50:885–889, 2002.

288. Zhang AY, Chen YF, Zhang DX, et al: Urotensin II is a nitric oxide-dependent vasodilator and natriuretic peptide in the rat kidney. Am J Physiol Renal Physiol 285:F792–F798, 2003.

289. Totsune K, Takahashi K, Arihara Z, et al: Role of urotensin II in patients on dialysis. Lancet 358:810–811, 2001.

290. Totsune K, Takahashi K, Arihara Z, et al: Elevated plasma levels of immunoreactive urotensin II and its increased urinary excretion in patients with Type 2 diabetes mellitus: Association with progress of diabetic nephropathy. Peptides 25:1809–1814, 2004.

291. Langham RG, Kelly DJ, Gow RM, et al: Increased expression of urotensin II and urotensin II receptor in human diabetic nephropathy. Am J Kidney Dis 44:826–831, 2004.

292. Maguire JJ, Kuc RE, Davenport AP: Orphan-receptor ligand human urotensin II: Receptor localization in human tissues and comparison of vasoconstrictor responses with endothelin-1. Br J Pharmacol 131:441–446, 2000.

293. Silvestre RA, Rodriguez-Gallardo J, Egido EM, et al: Inhibition of insulin release by urotensin II—A study on the perfused rat pancreas. Horm Metab Res 33:379–381, 2001.

294. Clozel M, Binkert C, Birker-Robaczewska M, et al: Pharmacology of the urotensin-II receptor antagonist palosuran (ACT-058362; 1-[2-(4-benzyl-4-hydroxy-piperidin-1-yl)-ethyl]-3-(2-methyl-quinolin-4-yl)-urea sulfate salt): First demonstration of a patho-

physiological role of the urotensin system. J Pharmacol Exp Ther 311:204–212, 2004.

295. Clozel M, Hess P, Qiu C, et al: The urotensin-II receptor antagonist palosuran improves pancreatic and renal function in diabetic rats. J Pharmacol Exp Ther 316:1115–1121, 2006.

296. Pruneau D, Luccarini JM, Robert C, et al: Induction of kinin B1 receptor-dependent vasoconstriction following balloon catheter injury to the rabbit carotid artery. Br J Pharmacol 111:1029–1034, 1994.

297. Lortie M, Regoli D, Rhaleb NE, et al: The role of B1- and B2-kinin receptors in the renal tubular and hemodynamic response to bradykinin. Am J Physiol 262:R72–R76, 1992.

298. Nakhostine N, Ribuot C, Lamontagne D, et al: Mediation by B1 and B2 receptors of vasodepressor responses to intravenously administered kinins in anaesthetized dogs. Br J Pharmacol 110:71–76, 1993.

299. Bhoola KD, Figueroa CD, Worthy K: Bioregulation of kinins: Kallikreins, kininogens, and kininases. Pharmacol Rev 44:1–80, 1992.

300. Skidgel RA: Bradykinin-degrading enzymes: Structure, function, distribution, and potential roles in cardiovascular pharmacology. J Cardiovasc Pharmacol 20(suppl 9): S4–S9, 1992.

301. Hock FJ, Wirth K, Albus U, et al: Hoe 140 A new potent and long acting bradykinin-antagonist: In vitro studies. Br J Pharmacol 102:769–773, 1991.

302. Lembeck F, Griesbacher T, Eckhardt M, et al: New, long-acting, potent bradykinin antagonists. Br J Pharmacol 102:297–304, 1991.

303. Fenoy FJ, Roman RJ: Effect of kinin receptor antagonists on renal hemodynamic and natriuretic responses to volume expansion. Am J Physiol 263:R1136–R1140, 1992.

304. Madeddu P, Anania V, Parpaglia PP, et al: Effects of Hoe 140, a bradykinin B2-receptor antagonist, on renal function in conscious normotensive rats. Br J Pharmacol 106:380–386, 1992.

305. Bascands JL, Pecher C, Rouaud S, et al: Evidence for existence of two distinct brady-kinin receptors on rat mesangial cells. Am J Physiol 264:F548–F556, 1993.

306. Dixon BS, Breckon R, Fortune J, et al: Effects of kinins on cultured arterial smooth muscle. Am J Physiol 258:C299–308, 1990.

307. Godin C, Smith AD, Riley PA: Bradykinin stimulates DNA synthesis in competent Balb/c 3T3 cells and enhances inositol phosphate formation induced by platelet-derived growth factor. Biochem Pharmacol 42:117–122, 1991.

308. Van Zoelen EJ, Peters PH, Afink GB, et al: Bradykinin-induced growth inhibition of normal rat kidney (NRK) cells is paralleled by a decrease in epidermal-growth-factor receptor expression. Biochem J 298(pt 2):335–340, 1994.

309. Farhy RD, Carretero OA, Ho KL, et al: Role of kinins and nitric oxide in the effects of angiotensin converting enzyme inhibitors on neointima formation. Circ Res 72:1202–1210, 1993.

310. Fong D, Smith DI, Hsieh WT: The human kininogen gene (KNG) mapped to chromosome 3q26-qter by analysis of somatic cell hybrids using the polymerase chain reaction. Hum Genet 87:189–192, 1991.

311. Cheung PP, Cannizzaro LA, Colman RW: Chromosomal mapping of human kininogen gene (KNG) to 3q26-qter. Cytogenet Cell Genet 59:24–26, 1992.

312. Margolius HS: Kallikreins and kinins. Some unanswered questions about system characteristics and roles in human disease. Hypertension 26:221–229 1995;.

313. Vio CP, Loyola S, Velarde V: Localization of components of the kallikrein-kinin system in the kidney: Relation to renal function. State of the art lecture. Hypertension 19: II10–II16, 1992.

314. Madeddu P, Glorioso N, Maioli M, et al: Regulation of rat renal kallikrein expression by estrogen and progesterone. J Hypertens Suppl 9:S244–S245, 1991.

315. el-Dahr SS, Yosipiv I: Developmentally regulated kallikrein enzymatic activity and gene transcription rate in maturing rat kidneys. Am J Physiol 265:F146–F150, 1993.

316. el-Dahr SS, Yosipiv IV, Muchant DG, et al: Salt intake modulates the developmental expression of renal kallikrein and bradykinin B2 receptors. Am J Physiol 270:F425–F431, 1996.

317. el-Dahr SS, Chao J: Spatial and temporal expression of kallikrein and its mRNA during nephron maturation. Am J Physiol 262:F705–F711, 1992.

318. Santos RA, Brosnihan KB, Jacobsen DW, et al: Production of angiotensin-(1–7) by human vascular endothelium. Hypertension 19:II56–II61, 1992.

319. Duncan AM, Kladis A, Jennings GL, et al: Kinins in humans. Am J Physiol Regul Integr Comp Physiol 278:R897–R904, 2000.

320. Rosamilia A, Clements JA, Dwyer PL, et al: Activation of the kallikrein kinin system in interstitial cystitis. J Urol 162:129–134, 1999.

321. Roques BP, Noble F, Dauge V, et al: Neutral endopeptidase 24.11: Structure, inhibition, and experimental and clinical pharmacology. Pharmacol Rev 45:87–146, 1993.

322. Dendorfer A, Wolfrum S, Wellhoner P, et al: Intravascular and interstitial degradation of bradykinin in isolated perfused rat heart. Br J Pharmacol 122:1179–1187, 1997.

323. Dendorfer A, Wolfrum S, Dominiak P: Pharmacology and cardiovascular implications of the kinin-kallikrein system. Jpn J Pharmacol 79:403–426, 1999.

324. Linz W, Wiemer G, Gohlke P, et al: Contribution of kinins to the cardiovascular actions of angiotensin-converting enzyme inhibitors. Pharmacol Rev 47:25–49, 1995.

325. Massoudy P, Becker BF, Gerlach E: Nitric oxide accounts for postischemic cardioprotection resulting from angiotensin-converting enzyme inhibition: Indirect evidence for a radical scavenger effect in isolated guinea pig heart. J Cardiovasc Pharmacol 25:440–447, 1995.

326. Yang XP, Liu YH, Scicli GM, et al: Role of kinins in the cardioprotective effect of preconditioning: Study of myocardial ischemia/reperfusion injury in B2 kinin receptor knockout mice and kininogen-deficient rats. Hypertension 30:735–740, 1997.

327. Madeddu P, Varoni MV, Palomba D, et al: Cardiovascular phenotype of a mouse strain with disruption of bradykinin B2-receptor gene. Circulation 96:3570–3578, 1997.

328. Alfie ME, Alim S, Mehta D, et al: An enhanced effect of arginine vasopressin in bradykinin B2 receptor null mutant mice. Hypertension 33:1436–1440, 1999.

329. Wang DZ, Chao L, Chao J: Hypotension in transgenic mice overexpressing human bradykinin B2 receptor. Hypertension 29:488–493, 1997.

330. Chao J, Chao L: Functional analysis of human tissue kallikrein in transgenic mouse models. Hypertension 27:491–494, 1996.

331. Zeidel ML, Jabs K, Kikeri D, et al: Kinins inhibit conductive Na+ uptake by rabbit inner medullary collecting duct cells. Am J Physiol 258:F1584–F1591, 1990.

332. Morsing P, Persson AE: Kinin and tubuloglomerular feedback in normal and hydronephrotic rats. Am J Physiol 260:F868–F873, 1991.

333. Madeddy P, Emanueli C, el-Dahr SS: Mechanisms of disease: the tissue Kallikrein-Kinin system in hypertension and vascular remodeling. Nat Clin Pract Nephrol 3:208–221, 2007.

334. Harvey JN, Jaffa AA, Margolius HS, et al: Renal kallikrein and hemodynamic abnormalities of diabetic kidney. Diabetes 39:299–304, 1990.

335. Harvey JN, Edmundson AW, Jaffa AA, et al: Renal excretion of kallikrein and eicosanoids in patients with type 1 (insulin-dependent) diabetes mellitus. Relationship to glomerular and tubular function. Diabetologia 35:857–862, 1992.

336. Allen TJ, Cao Z, Youssef S, et al: Role of angiotensin II and bradykinin in experimental diabetic nephropathy. Functional and structural studies. Diabetes 46:1612–1618, 1997.

337. Kakoki M, Takahashi N, Jennette JC, et al: Diabetic nephropathy is markedly enhanced in mice lacking the bradykinin B2 receptor. Proc Natl Acad Sci U S A 101:13302–13305, 2004.

338. Levin ER, Gardner DG, Samson WK: Natriuretic peptides. N Engl J Med 339:321–328, 1998.

339. Sudoh T, Minamino N, Kangawa K, et al: C-type natriuretic peptide (NP): A new member of natriuretic peptide family identified in porcine brain. Biochem Biophys Res Commun 168:863–870, 1990.

340. Schweitz H, Vigne P, Moinier D, et al: A new member of the natriuretic peptide family is present in the venom of the Green Mamba (Dendroaspis angusticeps). J Biol Chem 267:13928–13932, 1992.

341. Hirsch JR, Meyer M, Forssmann WG: ANP and urodilatin: who is who in the kidney. Eur J Med Res 11:447–454, 2006.

342. Forssmann W, Meyer M, Forssmann K: The renal urodilatin system: Clinical implications. Cardiovasc Res 51:450–462, 2001.

343. Sindic A, Schlatter E: Cellular effects of guanylin and uroguanylin. J Am Soc Nephrol 17:607–616, 2006.

344. Brenner BM, Ballermann BJ, Gunning ME, et al: Diverse biological actions of atrial natriuretic peptide. Physiol Rev 70:665–699, 1990.

345. Vesely DL: Atrial natriuretic peptides in pathophysiological diseases. Cardiovasc Res 51:647–658, 2001.

346. Turner AJ, Brown CD, Carson JA, et al: The neprilysin family in health and disease. Adv Exp Med Biol 477:229–240, 2000.

347. Turner AJ: Exploring the structure and function of zinc metallopeptidases: Old enzymes and new discoveries. Biochem Soc Trans 31:723–727, 2003.

348. Skidgel RA, Erdos EG: Angiotensin converting enzyme (ACE) and neprilysin hydrolyze neuropeptides: A brief history, the beginning and follow-ups to early studies. Peptides 25:521–525, 2004.

349. Kubota E, Dean RG, Hubner RA, et al: Evidence for cardioprotective, renoprotective, and vasculoprotective effects of vasopeptidase inhibitors in disease. Curr Hypertens Rep 3(suppl 2):S31–S33, 2001.

350. Corti R, Burnett JC Jr, Rouleau JL, et al: Vasopeptidase inhibitors: A new therapeutic concept in cardiovascular disease? Circulation 104:1856–1862, 2001.

351. Coats AJ: Omapatrilat—The story of Overture and Octave. Int J Cardiol 86:1–4, 2002.

352. Zanchi A, Maillard M, Burnier M: Recent clinical trials with omapatrilat: New developments. Curr Hypertens Rep 5:346–352, 2003.

353. Poulos JE, Gower WR, Sullebarger JT, et al: Congestive heart failure: Increased cardiac and extra-cardiac atrial natriuretic peptide gene expression. Cardiovasc Res 32:909–919, 1996.

354. Greenwald JE, Ritter D, Tetens E, et al: Renal expression of the gene for atrial natriuretic factor. Am J Physiol 263:F974–F978, 1992.

355. Vollmar AM, Paumgartner G, Gerbes AL: Differential gene expression of the three natriuretic peptides and natriuretic peptide receptor subtypes in human liver. Gut 40:145–150, 1997.

356. Forssmann WG, Richter R, Meyer M: The endocrine heart and natriuretic peptides: Histochemistry, cell biology, and functional aspects of the renal urodilatin system. Histochem Cell Biol 110:335–357, 1998.

357. Kinnunen P, Vuolteenaho O, Ruskoaho H: Mechanisms of atrial and brain natriuretic peptide release from rat ventricular myocardium: Effect of stretching. Endocrinology 132:1961–1970, 1993.

358. Gerbes AL, Dagnino L, Nguyen T, et al: Transcription of brain natriuretic peptide and atrial natriuretic peptide genes in human tissues. J Clin Endocrinol Metab 78:1307–1311, 1994.

359. Troughton RW, Frampton CM, Yandle TG, et al: Treatment of heart failure guided by plasma aminoterminal brain natriuretic peptide (N-BNP) concentrations. Lancet 355:1126–1130, 2000.

360. Kohno M, Horio T, Yoshiyama M, et al: Accelerated secretion of brain natriuretic peptide from the hypertrophied ventricles in experimental malignant hypertension. Hypertension 19:206–211, 1992.

361. Dagnino L, Lavigne JP, Nemer M: Increased transcripts for B-type natriuretic peptide in spontaneously hypertensive rats. Quantitative polymerase chain reaction for atrial and brain natriuretic peptide transcripts. Hypertension 20:690–700, 1992.

362. Cataliotti A, Malatino LS, Jougasaki M, et al: Circulating natriuretic peptide concentrations in patients with end-stage renal disease: Role of brain natriuretic peptide as a biomarker for ventricular remodeling. Mayo Clin Proc 76:1111–1119, 2001.

363. Zoccali C, Mallamaci F, Benedetto FA, et al: Cardiac natriuretic peptides are related to left ventricular mass and function and predict mortality in dialysis patients. J Am Soc Nephrol 12:1508–1515, 2001.

CH 10

364. Nishikimi T, Futoo Y, Tamano K, et al: Plasma brain natriuretic peptide levels in chronic hemodialysis patients: Influence of coronary artery disease. Am J Kidney Dis 37:1201–1208, 2001.

365. Koller KJ, Goeddel DV: Molecular biology of the natriuretic peptides and their receptors. Circulation 86:1081–1088, 1992.

366. Figueroa CD, Lewis HM, MacIver AG, et al: Cellular localisation of atrial natriuretic factor in the human kidney. Nephrol Dial Transplant 5:25–31, 1990.

367. Terada Y, Tomita K, Nonoguchi H, et al: PCR localization of C-type natriuretic peptide and B-type receptor mRNAs in rat nephron segments. Am J Physiol 267:F215–222, 1994.

368. Gunning ME, Brady HR, Otuechere G, et al: Atrial natriuretic peptide(31–67) inhibits Na+ transport in rabbit inner medullary collecting duct cells. Role of prostaglandin E2. J Clin Invest 89:1411–1417, 1992.

369. Maack T: Receptors of atrial natriuretic factor. Annu Rev Physiol 54:11–27, 1992.

370. Hunt PJ, Espiner EA, Nicholls MG, et al: Differing biological effects of equimolar atrial and brain natriuretic peptide infusions in normal man. J Clin Endocrinol Metab 81:3871–3876, 1996.

371. Zeidel ML: Renal actions of atrial natriuretic peptide: Regulation of collecting duct sodium and water transport. Annu Rev Physiol 52:747–759, 1990.

372. Stockand JD, Sansom SC: Glomerular mesangial cells: Electrophysiology and regulation of contraction. Physiol Rev 78:723–744, 1998.

373. Kitashiro S, Sugiura T, Takayama Y, et al: Long-term administration of atrial natriuretic peptide in patients with acute heart failure. J Cardiovasc Pharmacol 33:948–952, 1999.

374. Brusq JM, Mayoux E, Guigui L, et al: Effects of C-type natriuretic peptide on rat cardiac contractility. Br J Pharmacol 128:206–212, 1999.

375. Allgren RL, Marbury TC, Rahman SN, et al: Anaritide in acute tubular necrosis. Auriculin Anaritide Acute Renal Failure Study Group. N Engl J Med 336:828–834, 1997.

376. Lewis J, Salem MM, Chertow GM, et al: Atrial natriuretic factor in oliguric acute renal failure. Anaritide Acute Renal Failure Study Group. Am J Kidney Dis 36:767–774, 2000.

377. Brenner RM, Chertow GM: The rise and fall of atrial natriuretic peptide for acute renal failure. Curr Opin Nephrol Hypertens 6:474–476, 1997.

378. Richards AM, Crozier IG, Holmes SJ, et al: Brain natriuretic peptide: Natriuretic and endocrine effects in essential hypertension. J Hypertens 11:163–170, 1993.

379. Pidgeon GB, Richards AM, Nicholls MG, et al: Differing metabolism and bioactivity of atrial and brain natriuretic peptides in essential hypertension. Hypertension 27:906–913, 1996.

380. Elkayam U, Akhter MW, Tummala P, et al: Nesiritide: A new drug for the treatment of decompensated heart failure. J Cardiovasc Pharmacol Ther 7:181–194, 2002.

381. Mills RM, LeJemtel TH, Horton DP, et al: Sustained hemodynamic effects of an infusion of nesiritide (human b-type natriuretic peptide) in heart failure: A randomized, double-blind, placebo-controlled clinical trial. Natrecor Study Group. J Am Coll Cardiol 34:155–162, 1999.

382. Sackner-Bernstein JD, Kowalski M, Fox M, et al: Short-term risk of death after treatment with nesiritide for decompensated heart failure: A pooled analysis of randomized controlled trials. JAMA 293:1900–1905, 2005.

383. Trippodo NC, Robl JA, Asaad MM, et al: Effects of omapatrilat in low, normal, and high renin experimental hypertension. Am J Hypertens 11:363–372, 1998.

384. Tikkanen T, Tikkanen I, Rockell MD, et al: Dual inhibition of neutral endopeptidase and angiotensin-converting enzyme in rats with hypertension and diabetes mellitus. Hypertension 32:778–785, 1998.

385. Davis BJ, Johnston CI, Burrell LM, et al: Renoprotective effects of vasopeptidase inhibition in an experimental model of diabetic nephropathy. Diabetologia 46:961–971, 2003.

386. Cao ZM, Burrell LM, Tikkanen I, et al: Vasopeptidase inhibition attenuates the progression of renal injury in subtotal nephrectomized rats. Kidney Int 60:715–721, 2001.

387. Taal MW, Nenov VD, Wong W, et al: Vasopeptidase inhibition affords greater renoprotection than angiotensin-converting enzyme inhibition alone. J Am Soc Nephrol 12:2051–2059, 2001.

388. Benigni A, Zola C, Corna D, et al: Blocking both type A and B endothelin receptors in the kidney attenuates renal injury and prolongs survival in rats with remnant kidney. Am J Kidney Dis 27:410–423, 1996.

389. Cao Z, Cooper ME, Wu LL, et al: Blockade of the renin-angiotensin and endothelin systems on progressive renal injury. Hypertension 36:561–568, 2000.

390. Amann K, Simonaviciene A, Medwedewa T, et al: Blood pressure-independent additive effects of pharmacologic blockade of the renin-angiotensin and endothelin systems on progression in a low-renin model of renal damage. J Am Soc Nephrol 12:2572–2584, 2001.

391. Pollock DM, Polakowski JS: ETA receptor blockade prevents hypertension associated with exogenous endothelin-1 but not renal mass reduction in the rat. J Am Soc Nephrol 8:1054–1060, 1997.

392. Potter GS, Johnson RJ, Fink GD: Role of endothelin in hypertension of experimental chronic renal failure. Hypertension 30:1578–1584, 1997.

393. Nabokov A, Amann K, Wagner J, et al: Influence of specific and non-specific endothelin receptor antagonists on renal morphology in rats with surgical renal ablation. Nephrol Dial Transplant 11:514–520, 1996.

394. Brochu E, Lacasse S, Moreau C, et al: Endothelin ET(A) receptor blockade prevents the progression of renal failure and hypertension in uraemic rats. Nephrol Dial Transplant 14:1881–1888, 1999.

395. Trenkner J, Priem F, Bauer C, et al: Endothelin receptor A blockade reduces proteinuria and vascular hypertrophy in spontaneously hypertensive rats on high-salt diet in a blood-pressure-independent manner. Clin Sci (Lond) 103(suppl 48):385S–388S, 2002.

396. Feldman DL, Mogelesky TC, Chou M, et al: Attenuation of puromycin aminonucleoside-induced glomerular lesions in rats by CGS 26303, a dual neutral endopeptidase/endothelin-converting enzyme inhibitor. J Cardiovasc Pharmacol 36:S342–S345, 2000.

397. Benigni A, Corna D, Maffi R, et al: Renoprotective effect of contemporary blocking of angiotensin II and endothelin-1 in rats with membranous nephropathy. Kidney Int 54:353–359, 1998.

398. Nakamura T, Ebihara I, Fukui M, et al: Effect of a specific endothelin receptor A antagonist on mRNA levels for extracellular matrix components and growth factors in diabetic glomeruli. Diabetes 44:895–899, 1995.

399. Dhein S, Hochreuther S, Aus Dem Spring C, et al: Long-term effects of the endothelin(A) receptor antagonist LU 135252 and the angiotensin-converting enzyme inhibitor trandolapril on diabetic angiopathy and nephropathy in a chronic type I diabetes mellitus rat model. J Pharmacol Exp Ther 293:351–359, 2000.

400. Pollock DM, Derebail VK, Yamamoto T, et al: Combined effects of AT(1) and ET(A) receptor antagonists, candesartan, and A-127722 in DOCA-salt hypertensive rats. Gen Pharmacol 34:337–342, 2000.

401. Pollock DM, Polakowski JS, Wegner CD, et a: Beneficial effect of ETA receptor blockade in a rat model of radiocontrast-induced nephropathy. Ren Fail 19:753–761, 1997.

402. Tostes RC, Touyz RM, He G, et al: Endothelin A receptor blockade decreases expression of growth factors and collagen and improves matrix metalloproteinase-2 activity in kidneys from stroke-prone spontaneously hypertensive rats. J Cardiovasc Pharmacol 39:892–900, 2002.

403. Braun C, Conzelmann T, Vetter S, et al: Treatment with a combined endothelin A/B-receptor antagonist does not prevent chronic renal allograft rejection in rats. J Cardiovasc Pharmacol 36:428–437, 2000.

404. Braun C, Conzelmann T, Vetter S, et al: Prevention of chronic renal allograft rejection in rats with an oral endothelin A receptor antagonist. Transplantation 68:739–746, 1999.

405. Gomez-Garre D, Largo R, Liu XH, et al: An orally active ETA/ETB receptor antagonist ameliorates proteinuria and glomerular lesions in rats with proliferative nephritis. Kidney Int 50:962–972, 1996.

CHAPTER 11

Arachidonic Acid Metabolites and the Kidney

Raymond C. Harris, Jr • Matthew D. Breyer

CELLULAR ORIGIN OF EICOSANOIDS

Eicosanoids comprise a family of biologically active, oxygenated arachidonic acid (AA) metabolites. Arachidonic acid is a polyunsaturated fatty acid possessing 20 carbon atoms and 4 double bonds (C20:4) and is formed from linoleic acid (C18:2) by addition of two carbons to the chain and further desaturation. In mammals, linoleic acid is derived strictly from dietary sources. Essential fatty acid (EFA) deficiency occurs when dietary fatty acid precursors, including linoleic acid, are omitted, thereby depleting the hormone-responsive pool of AA. EFA deficiency thereby reduces the intracellular availability of AA in response to hormonal stimulation and abrogates many biological actions of hormone-induced eicosanoid release.[1]

Of an approximate 10 gm of linoleic acid ingested per day, only about 1 mg/day is eliminated as end products of AA metabolism. Following its formation, AA is esterified into cell membrane phospholipids, principally at the 2 position of the phosphatidylinositol fraction (i.e., sn-2 esterified AA), the major hormone-sensitive pool of AA that is susceptible to release by phospholipases.

Multiple stimuli lead to release of membrane-bound AA, via activation of cellular phospholipases, principally phospholipase A2's (PLA$_2$).[2] This cleavage step is rate limiting in the production of biologically relevant arachidonate metabolites. In the case of PLA2 activation, membrane receptors activate guanine nucleotide-binding (G) proteins, leading to release of AA directly from membrane phospholipids. Activation of phospholipase C or PLD, on the other hand, releases AA via the sequential action of the phospholipase-mediated production of diacylglycerol (DAG) with subsequent release of AA from DAG by DAG lipase.[3] When considering eicosanoid formation, the physiological significance of AA release by these other phospholipases remains uncertain because at least in the setting of inflammation, phospholipase A$_2$ action appears essential for the generation of biologically active AA metabolites.[4]

More than 15 proteins with PLA$_2$ activity are known to exist, including secreted (sPLA$_2$) and cytoplasmic PLA$_2$ (cPLA$_2$) isoforms.[5,6] A mitogen activated cytoplasmic PLA$_2$ has been found to mediate AA release in a calcium/calmodulin-dependent manner. Other hormones and growth factors, including epidermal growth factor (EGF) and platelet derived growth factors, activate PLA$_2$ directly through tyrosine residue kinase activity, allowing the recruitment of co-activators to the enzyme without an absolute requirement for the intermediate action of Ca^{++}/calmodulin or other cellular kinases.

Following de-esterification, AA is rapidly re-esterified into membrane lipids or avidly bound by intracellular proteins in which case it becomes unavailable to further metabolism. Should it escape re-esterification and protein binding, free AA becomes available as a substrate for one of three major enzymatic transformations, the common result of which is the incorporation of oxygen atoms at various sites of the fatty acid backbone, with accompanying changes in its molecular structure (such as ring formation).[7,8] This results in the formation of biologically active molecules, referred to as "eicosanoids". The specific nature of the products generated is a function of the initial stimuli for AA release, as well as the metabolic enzyme available, which is determined in part by the cell type involved.[8,9]

These products, in turn, either mediate or modulate the biologic actions of the agonist in question. AA release may also result from non-specific stimuli, such as cellular trauma including ischemia and hypoxia,[10] oxygen free radicals,[11] or osmotic stress.[12] The identity of the specific AA metabolite generated in a particular cell system depends on both the proximate stimulus and the availability of the down stream AA metabolizing enzymes present in that cell.

Three major enzymatic pathways of AA metabolism are present in the kidney: cyclooxygenases, lipoxygenases, and cytochrome P450s (Fig. 11–1). The cyclooxygenase pathway mediates the formation of prostaglandins (PGs) and thromboxanes, the lipoxygenase pathway mediates the formation of mono-, di-, and

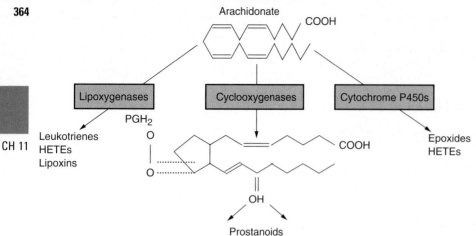

FIGURE 11-1 Pathways of enzymatically mediated arachidonic acid metabolism. Arachidonic acid can be converted into biologically active compounds by cyclooxygenase- (COX), lipoxygenase- (LO), or cytochrome P450- (CYP450) mediated metabolism.

trihydroxyeicosatetraenoic acids (HETEs) leukotrienes (LTs), and lipoxins (LXs) and the cytochrome P-450-dependent oxygenation of AA mediates the formation of epoxyeicosatrienoic acids (EETs), their corresponding diols, HETEs, and monooxygenated AA derivatives. Fish oil diets, rich in ω-3 polyunsaturated fatty acids[13] interfere with metabolism via all three pathways by competing with AA oxygenation, resulting in the formation of biologically inactive end products.[14] Interference with the production of pro-inflammatory lipids has been hypothesized to underlie the beneficial effects of fish-oil in IgA nephropathy and other cardiovascular diseases.[15] The following sections deal with the current understanding of the chemistry, biosynthesis, renal metabolism, mechanisms of release, receptor biology, signal transduction pathways, biologic activities, and functional significance of each of the metabolites generated by the three major routes of AA metabolism in the kidney.

THE CYCLOOXYGENASE (COX) PATHWAY

Molecular Biology

The cyclooxygenase enzyme system is the major pathway for AA metabolism in the kidney (Fig. 11–2). Cyclooxygenase (prostaglandin synthase G_2/H_2) is the enzyme responsible for the initial conversion of arachidonic acid to prostaglandin G_2 and subsequently to prostaglandin H_2. Cyclooxygenase was first purified from ram seminal vesicles and cloned in 1988. The protein was found to be widely expressed and the level of activity not dynamically regulated. Other studies supported the presence of a cyclooxygenase that was dynamically regulated and responsible for increased prostanoid production in inflammation. This second, inducible cyclooxygenase isoform was identified shortly after the cloning of the initial enzyme and designated cyclooxygenase-2 (COX-2), whereas the initially isolated isoform is now designated COX-1.[7,16,17] COX-1 and COX-2 are encoded by distinct genes located on different chromosomes. The human COX-1 gene (PTGS1=prostaglandin synthase 1) is distributed over 40 kB on 11 exons on chromosome 9, whereas COX-2 is localized on chromosome 1 and spans approximately 9 kB. The genes are also subject to dramatically different regulatory signals.

Regulation of Cyclooxygenase Gene Expression

At the cellular level, COX-2 expression is highly regulated by several processes that alter its transcription rate, message export from the nucleus, message stability, and efficiency of

message translation.[18,19] These processes tightly control the expression of COX-2 in response to many of the same cellular stresses that activate arachidonate release (e.g., cell volume changes, shear stress, hypoxia),[10,20] as well as a variety of cytokines and growth factors, including tumor necrosis factor (TNF) interleukin 1β, epidermal growth factor, and platelet derived growth factor (PDGF). Activation of COX-2 gene transcription is mediated via the coordinated activation of several transcription factors that bind to and activate consensus sequences in the 5′ flanking region of the COX-2 gene for NF-κB, and NF-IL6/C-EBP, and a cyclic AMP response element (CRE).[21] Induction of COX-2 mRNA transcription by endotoxin (lipopolysaccharide) may also involve CRE sites[22] and NF-κB sites.[23]

Regulation of Cyclooxygenase Expression by Anti-inflammatory Steroids

A molecular basis linking the anti-inflammatory effects of cyclooxygenase inhibiting nonsteroidal anti-inflammatory drugs (NSAIDs) and anti-inflammatory glucocorticoids has long been sought. A novel mechanism for the suppression of arachidonate metabolism by corticosteroids involving translational inhibition of COX formation had been suggested prior to the molecular recognition of COX-2. With the cloning of COX-2 it became well established that glucocorticoids suppress COX-2 expression and prostaglandin synthesis, an effect now viewed as central to the anti-inflammatory effects of glucocorticoids. Post-transcriptional control of COX-2 expression represents another robust mechanism by which adrenal steroids regulate COX-2 expression.[24] Accumulating evidence suggests COX-2 is modulated at multiple steps in addition to transcription rate, including stabilization of the mRNA and enhanced translation.[18,25] Glucocorticoids, including dexamethasone, down regulate COX-2 mRNA in part by destabilizing the mRNA.[25] The 3′untranslated region of COX-2 mRNA contains 22 copies of an AUUUA motif, which are important in destabilizing COX-2 message in response to dexamethasone, whereas other 3′ sequences appear important for COX-2 mRNA stabilization in response to interleukin-1β.[25] Effects of the 3′UTR as well as other factors regulating efficiency of COX-2 translation have also been suggested.[18] The factors determining the expression of COX1 are more obscure.

Enzymatic Chemistry

Despite these differences, both prostaglandin (PG) synthases catalyze a similar reaction, resulting in cyclization of C-8 to

Arachidonic Acid Metabolites and the Kidney

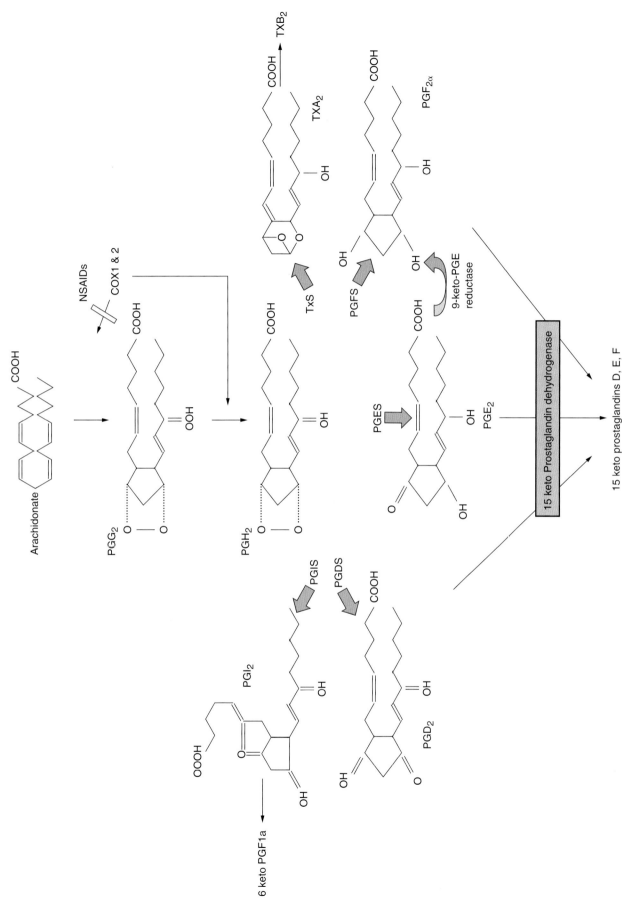

FIGURE 11–2 Cyclooxygenase metabolism of arachidonic acid. Both COX-1 and COX-2 convert AA to PGH₂ which is then acted upon by specific synthases to produce prostanoids that act at G-protein coupled receptors that either increase or decrease cAMP or increase intracellular calcium.

C-12 of the AA backbone forming cyclic endoperoxide, accompanied by the concomitant insertion of two oxygen atoms at C-15 to form PGG$_2$ (a 15-hydroperoxide). In the presence of a reduced glutathione-dependent peroxidase, PGG$_2$ is converted to the 15-hydroxy derivative, PGH$_2$. The endoperoxides (PGG$_2$ and PGH$_2$) have very short half lives of about 5 minutes and are biologically active in inducing aortic contraction and platelet aggregation.[26] However under some circumstances, the formation of these endoperoxides may be strictly limited, via the self-deactivating properties of the enzyme.

Expression of recombinant enzymes and determination of the crystal structure of COX-2 have provided further insight into the observed physiologic and pharmacologic similarities to, and differences from, COX-1. It is now clear that cyclooxygenase inhibiting NSAIDs work by sterically blocking access of AA to the heme containing, active enzymatic site.[27] Particularly well conserved are sequences surrounding the aspirin-sensitive serine residues, at which acetylation by aspirin irreversibly inhibits activity.[28] More recent evidence has developed showing that COX-1 and COX-2 are capable of forming heterodimers and sterically modulating each other's function.[29] The substrate binding pocket of COX-2 is larger and therefore accepting of bulkier inhibitors and substrates. This difference has allowed the development and marketing of both relatively and highly selective COX-2 inhibitors for clinical use as analgesics,[30] antipyretics,[31] and anti-inflammatory agents.[30] In addition to its central role in

inflammation, aberrantly up-regulated COX-2 expression has been implicated in the pathogenesis of a number of epithelial cell carcinomas[32] and in Alzheimer disease and other degenerative neurologic conditions.[33]

RENAL COX-1 AND COX-2 EXPRESSION

COX-2 Expression in the Kidney

There is now definitive evidence for significant COX-2 expression in the mammalian kidney (Fig. 11–3). COX-2 mRNA and immunoreactive COX-2 are present at low but detectable levels in normal adult mammalian kidney, where in situ hybridization and immunolocalization demonstrated localized expression of COX-2 mRNA and immunoreactive protein in the cells of the macula densa and a few cells in the cortical thick ascending limb cells immediately adjacent to the macula densa.[34] COX-2 expression is also abundant in the lipid-laden medullary interstitial cells in the tip of the papilla.[34–36] Some investigators have reported that COX-2 may be expressed in inner medullary collecting duct cells or intercalated cells in the renal cortex.[37] Nevertheless COX-1 expression is constitutive and clearly the most abundant isoform in the collecting duct, so potential existence and physiological significance of COX-2 co-expression in this segment remains uncertain.

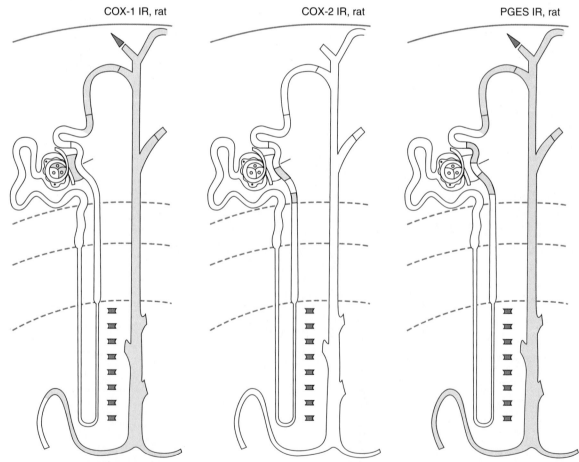

FIGURE 11–3 Localization (indicated in shaded areas) of immunoreactive COX-1, COX-2, and microsomal prostaglandin E synthase along the rat nephron. (Reproduced with permission from S. Bachmann.)

COX-2 Expression in the Renal Cortex

It is now well documented that COX-2 is expressed in macula densa/cTALH and in kidney of mouse, rat, rabbit, and dog. Furthermore, despite initial controversy regarding COX-2 localization in primate and human kidney, more recent studies confirm a similar distribution of COX-2 in macula densa (as well as medullary interstitial cells) especially in kidneys of the elderly,[38,39] patients with diabetes mellitus, congestive heart failure,[40] and Bartter-like Syndrome.[41]

The presence of COX-2 in the unique group of cells comprising the macula densa, points to a potential role for COX-2 derived prostanoids in regulating glomerular function. Studies of the prostanoid-dependent control of glomerular filtration rate by the macula densa suggest effects via both dilator and constrictor effects of prostanoids contributing to tubuloglomerular feedback (TGF).[42,43] Some studies suggest that COX-2 derived prostanoids are predominantly vasodilators.[44,45] By inhibiting production of dilator prostanoids contributing to the patency of adjacent afferent arteriole, COX-2 inhibition may contribute to the decline in GFR observed in patients taking NSAIDs or selective COX-2 inhibitors[46] (see later discussion). The identity of the specific prostanoids elaborated by the COX-2 expressing macula densa cells remains uncertain.

The volume-depleted state is typified by low NaCl delivery to the macula densa, and COX-2 expression in the macula densa is also increased in states associated with volume depletion (Fig. 11–4).[34] Of note, COX-2 expression in cultured macula densa cells and cTAL cells is also increased in vitro by reducing extracellular Cl^- concentration. Studies in which cortical thick limbs and associated glomeruli were removed and perfused from rabbits pretreated with a low salt diet to upregulate macula densa COX-2 demonstrated COX-2-dependent release of PGE2 from the macula densae in response to decreased chloride perfusate.[47] Furthermore the induction of

COX2 by low Cl^- can be blocked by a specific p38 MAP kinase inhibitor.[48,49] Finally, in vivo, renal cortical immunoreactive pp38 expression (the active form of p38) predominantly localized to the macula densa and cTALH and increases in response to a low salt diet.[48] These findings point to a molecular pathway whereby enhanced COX-2 expression occurring in circumstances associated with intracellular volume depletion could result from decreased luminal chloride delivery. Recent studies have also indicated that the carbonic anhydrase inhibitor, acetazolamide, and dopamine may both indirectly regulate macula densa COX-2 expression by inhibiting proximal reabsorption and thereby increasing luminal macula densa chloride delivery.[50]

In the mammalian kidney, the macula densa is involved in regulating renin release by sensing alterations in luminal chloride via changes in the rate of $Na^+/K^+/2Cl^-$ cotransport (Fig. 11–5).[51] Measurements in vivo, in isolated perfused kidney and in isolated perfused juxtaglomerular preparation all indicated that that administration of non-specific cyclooxygenase inhibitors prevented the increases in renin release mediated by macula densa sensing of decreases in luminal NaCl.[51] Induction of a high renin state by imposition of a salt deficient diet, ACE inhibition, diuretic administration, or experimental renovascular hypertension all significantly increase macula densa/cTALH COX-2 mRNA, and immunoreactive protein. COX-2 selective inhibitors blocked elevations in plasma renin activity, renal renin activity, and renal cortical renin mRNA in response to loop diuretics, ACE inhibitors, or a low salt diet,[52–55] and in an isolated perfused juxtaglomerular preparation, increased renin release in response to lowering the perfusate NaCl concentration was blocked by COX-2 inhibition.[56] In COX-2 knockout mice, increases in renin in response to low salt or ACE inhibitors were significantly blunted[57,58] but were unaffected in COX-1 knockout mice.[59,60] COX-2 inhibitors have also been shown to decrease renin production in models of renovascular hypertension[61] and recent studies in mice with targeted

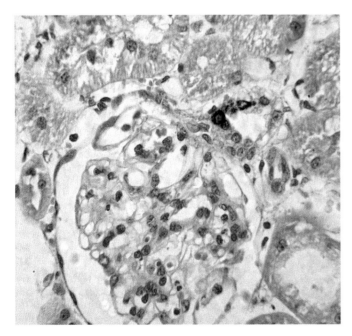

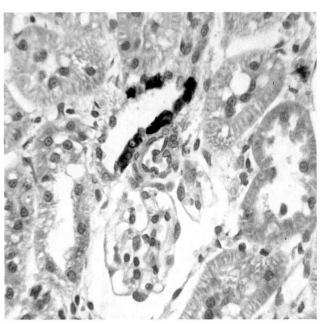

Control

Low salt

FIGURE 11–4 COX-2 expression is regulated in renal cortex in rats. *Left*, Under basal conditions, sparse immunoreactive COX-2 is localized to the macula densa and surrounding cortical thick ascending limb. *Right*, Following chronic administration of a sodium deficient diet, macula densa/cTAL COX-2 expression increases markedly.

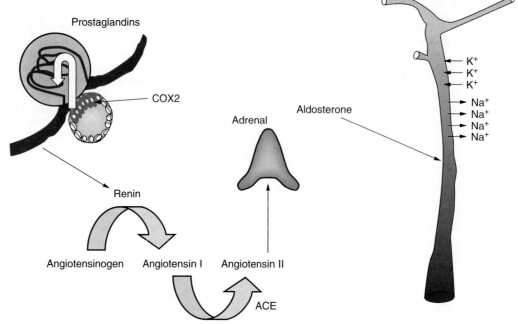

FIGURE 11–5 Proposed intrarenal roles for vasodilatory prostaglandins to regulate renal function and blood pressure control. Prostaglandins released from the macula densa and/or the afferent arteriole can both vasodilate the afferent arteriole and modulate renin release from juxtaglomerular cells.

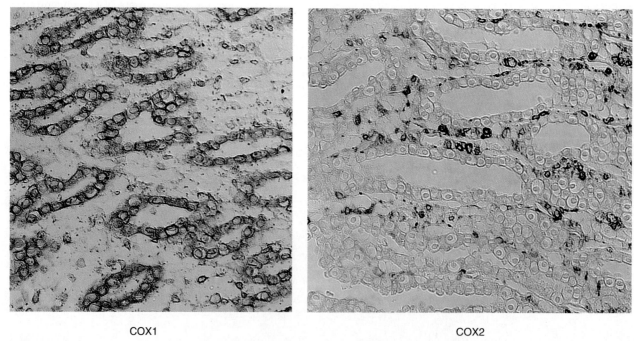

COX1   COX2

FIGURE 11–6 Differential immunolocalization of COX-1 *(left)* and COX-2 *(right)* in the renal medulla of rodents. COX-1 is predominantly localized to the collecting duct and is also found in a subset of medullary interstitial cells, whereas COX-2 is predominantly localized to a subset of interstitial cells.

deletion of the prostacyclin receptor suggest a predominant role for prostacyclin in mediating renin production and release in these models.[62]

COX-2 Expression in the Renal Medulla

The renal medulla is a major site of prostaglandin synthesis and abundant COX-1 and COX-2 expression (Fig. 11–6).[63] COX-1 and COX-2 exhibit differential compartmentalization within the medulla, with COX-1 predominating in the medullary collecting ducts and COX-2 predominating in medullary interstitial cells. COX-2 may also be expressed in endothelial cells of the vasa recta supplying the inner medulla.

The factors determining this differential tissue expression of COX-2 remain uncertain but likely include distinct upstream promoter elements and gene organization. In the collecting duct or human ureter and bladder epithelium, which are also derived from ureteric bud, COX-2 expression

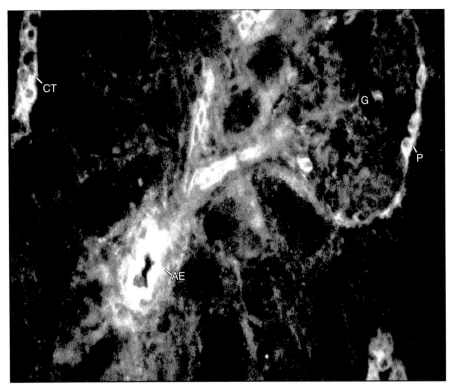

FIGURE 11–7 Renal cortical COX-1 expression. Immunoreactive COX-1 is predominantly localized to the afferent arteriole, glomerular mesangial cells and parietal glomerular epithelial cells, and the cortical collecting duct. (From Hirata M, Hayashi Y, Ushikubi F, et al: Cloning and expression of cDNA for a human thromboxane A2 receptor. Nature 349:617–620, 1991.)

is only detected in the setting of malignant transformation.[64] Because of the potential chemopreventive and therapeutic effects of NSAIDs in epithelial cancers[65] the factors contributing to the aberrant expression of COX-2 in malignant epithelia is an area of intense investigation.[32] Aberrant methylation of COX-2 DNA has been associated with silencing of COX-2 expression in some colon cancers,[66] but whether differential methylation contributes to the cellular compartmentalization of COX-2 in the normal kidney is unknown.

In those cells normally expressing COX-2, dynamic regulation of its expression appears to be an important adaptive response to physiological stresses, including water deprivation and exposure to endotoxin.[37,63,67] Following dehydration renal medullary COX-2 mRNA and protein expression are significantly induced,[37,63] primarily in medullary interstitial cells.[63] In contrast, COX-1 expression is unaffected by water deprivation. Although hormonal factors could also contribute to COX-2 induction, shifting cultured renal medullary interstitial cells to hypertonic media (using either NaCl or mannitol) is sufficient to induce COX-2 expression directly. Because prostaglandins play an important role in maintaining renal function during volume depletion or water deprivation, induction of COX-2 by hypertonicity provides an important adaptive response.

As is the case for the macula densa, medullary interstitial cell COX-2 expression is transcriptionally regulated in response to renal extracellular salt and tonicity. Water deprivation activates COX-2 expression in medullary interstitial cells by activating the NF-κB pathway.[63] Other studies suggest roles for MAP kinase/JNK in COX-2 induction following hypertonicity.[68]

COX-1 Expression in the Kidney

Whereas well-defined factors regulating COX-2 and determining the role of COX-2 expression in the kidney are coming to light, the role of renal COX-1 remains more obscure. COX-1

is constitutively expressed in platelets[69] in renal microvasculature, and glomerular parietal epithelial cells (Fig. 11–7). In addition COX-1 is abundantly expressed in the collecting duct, but there is little COX-1 expressed in the proximal tubule or thick ascending limb.[44] COX-1 expression levels do not appear to be dynamically regulated, and consistent with this observation, the COX-1 promoter does not possess a TATA box. The factors accounting for the tissue specific expression of COX-1 are uncertain but may involve histone acetylation and the presence of two tandem Sp1 sites in the upstream region of the gene.[70]

RENAL COMPLICATIONS OF NSAIDs

Na+ Retention, Edema, and Hypertension

Use of non-selective NSAIDs may be complicated by the development of significant Na+ retention, edema, congestive heart failure, and hypertension.[71] These complications are also apparent in patients using COX-2 selective NSAIDs. Studies with celecoxib and rofecoxib demonstrate that like non-selective NSAIDs, these COX-2 selective NSAIDs reduce urinary Na+ excretion, and are associated with modest Na+ retention in otherwise healthy subjects.[72,73] COX-2 inhibition likely promotes salt retention via multiple mechanisms (Fig. 11–8). Reduced glomerular filtration rate may limit the filtered Na+ load and salt excretion.[74,75] In addition, PGE_2 directly inhibits Na+ absorption in the thick ascending limb and collecting duct.[76] The relative abundance of COX-2 in medullary interstitial cells places this enzyme adjacent to both these nephron segments, allowing for COX-2 derived PGE_2 to modulate salt absorption. COX-2 inhibitors decrease renal PGE_2 production[72,77] and thereby may enhance renal sodium retention. Finally, reduction in renal medullary blood flow by inhibition of vasodilator prostanoids may significantly reduce

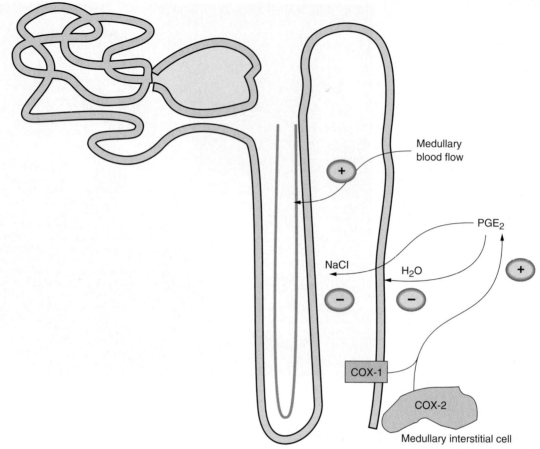

FIGURE 11–8 Integrated role of PGE$_2$ on regulation of salt and water excretion. PGE$_2$ can both increase medullary blood flow and directly inhibit NaCl reabsorption in mTAL and water reabsorption in collecting duct.

renal salt excretion and promote the development of edema and hypertension. COX-2 selective NSAIDs have been demonstrated to exacerbate salt dependent hypertension in rats.[78] Similarly, patients with pre-existing treated hypertension commonly experience hypertensive exacerbations with COX-2 selective NSAIDs.[73] Taken together these data suggest that COX-2 selective NSAIDs have similar effects as non-selective NSAIDs with respect to salt excretion.

Hyperkalemia

Non-selective NSAIDs cause hyperkalemia due to suppression of the renin/aldosterone axis. Both decreased GFR and inhibition of renal renin release may compromise renal K$^+$ excretion. Two recent studies in patients on a salt-restricted diet demonstrated that a COX-2 selective inhibitor (either rofecoxib or celecoxib) decreased urinary potassium excretion.[74,75] In sub-populations of patients at risk, development of overt hyperkalemia with COX-2 selective inhibitors seems likely.

Papillary Necrosis

Both acute and sub-acute forms of papillary necrosis have been observed with NSAID use.[79–81] Acute NSAID-associated renal papillary injury is more likely to occur in the setting of dehydration, suggesting a critical dependence of renal function upon COX metabolism in this setting.[63] Long-term use of COX-inhibiting NSAIDs has been associated with papillary

necrosis and progressive renal structural and functional deterioration much like the syndrome of analgesic nephropathy observed with acetaminophen, aspirin, and caffeine combinations.[80] Experimental studies suggest that renal medullary interstitial cells are an early target of injury in analgesic nephropathy.[82] COX-2 has been shown to be an important survival factor for cells exposed to a hypertonic medium.[36,63,83] The coincident localized expression of COX-2 in these interstitial cells[36,63] raises the possibility that, like non-selective NSAIDs, long-term use of COX-2 selective NSAIDs may contribute to development of papillary necrosis and analgesic nephropathy.[84] Because the development of analgesic nephropathy requires the regular ingestion of NSAIDs or analgesics over years, this possibility remains to be verified.

Acute Renal Insufficiency

Acute renal failure is a well-described complication of NSAID use.[71] This is generally considered to be a result of altered intra-renal microcirculation and glomerular filtration secondary to the inability to produce beneficial endogenous prostanoids when the kidney is dependent on them for normal function. Recent reports suggest that like the traditional, non-selective NSAIDs, COX-2 selective NSAIDs will also reduce glomerular filtration in susceptible patients.[71] Although rare overall, NSAID-associated renal insufficiency occurs in a significant proportion of patients with underlying volume depletion, renal insufficiency, congestive heart failure, diabetes, and old age.[71] These risk factors are additive and rarely are present in patients included in study cohorts used for safety assessment of these drugs. It is therefore relevant that both celecoxib and rofecoxib caused a slight but significant fall in glomerular filtration rate in salt depleted but otherwise healthy subjects.[74,75] More than 200 cases of acute renal insufficiency due to COX-2 selective NSAIDs have now been reported.[46,85] Pre-clinical studies support the concept that inhibition of COX-2 derived prostanoids generated in the macula densa contributes to a fall in GFR by reducing the diameter of the afferent arteriole. In vivo video microscopy studies document reduced afferent arteriolar diameter following administration of a COX-2 inhibitor.[45] Taken together these animal data not only support the concept that COX-2 plays an important role regulating glomerular filtration rate but also the clinical observations that COX-2 selective inhibitors can cause renal insufficiency similar to that reported with non-selective NSAIDs.

Interstitial Nephritis

The gradual development of renal insufficiency characterized by a subacute inflammatory interstitial infiltrate may occur after several months of continuous NSAID ingestion. Less commonly, the interstitial nephritis and renal failure may be fulminant. The infiltrate is typically accompanied by eosinophils; however, the clinical picture is typically much less dramatic than the allergic interstitial nephritis associated with β-lactam antibiotics, lacking fever or rash.[86] This syndrome has also been reported with the COX-2 selective drug, celecoxib.[87,88] Dysregulation of the immune system is thought to play an important role in the syndrome, which typically abates rapidly following discontinuation of the NSAID or COX-2 inhibitor.

Nephrotic Syndrome

Like interstitial nephritis, nephrotic syndrome typically occurs in patients chronically ingesting any one of a myriad of NSAIDs over course of months.[86,89] The renal pathology is usually consistent with minimal change disease with foot process fusion of glomerular podocytes observed on EM, but membranous nephropathy has also been reported.[90] Typically, the nephrotic syndrome occurs together with the interstitial nephritis.[86] Nephrotic syndrome without interstitial nephritis may occur, as well as immune-complex glomerulopathy, in a small subset of patients receiving NSAIDs. It remains uncertain whether this syndrome results from mechanism-based cyclooxygenase inhibition by these drugs, an idiosyncratic immune drug reaction, or a combination of both.

Renal Dysgenesis

Reports of renal dysgenesis and oligohydramnios in offspring of women administered non-selective NSAIDs during the third trimester of pregnancy[91] have implicated prostaglandins in the process of normal renal development. A similar syndrome of renal dysgenesis has been reported in mice with targeted disruption of the COX-2 gene, as well as mice treated with the specific COX-2 inhibitor SC58236.[92] Since neither COX-1−/− mice or mice treated with the COX-1 selective inhibitor SC58560 exhibited altered renal development, a specific role for COX-2 in nephrogenesis is suggested.[93–95] A report of renal dysgenesis in the infant of a woman exposed to the COX-2 selective inhibitor nimesulide suggests COX-2 also plays a role in renal development in humans.[91]

The intra-renal expression of COX-2 in the developing kidney peaks in mouse at post-natal day 4 and in the rat in the second post-natal week.[92,96] It has not yet been determined if a similar pattern of COX-2 is seen in humans. Although the most intense staining is observed in a small subset of cells in the nascent macula densa and cortical thick ascending limb, expression in the papilla is also observed.[92,96] Considering the similar glomerular developmental defects observed in rodents treated with the COX-2 inhibitor and in mice with targeted disruption of the COX-2 gene, it seems likely that prostanoids or other products resulting from COX-2 activity in cortical thick limb (and macula densa) act in a paracrine manner to influence glomerular development. The identity of the COX-2 derived prostanoids that promote glomerulogenesis, remains uncertain. In vitro studies show that exogenous PGE_1 promotes renal metanephric development,[97] and is a critical growth factor for renal epithelia cells. Nevertheless, none of the prostaglandin receptor knockout mice recapitulate the phenotype of the COX-2 knockout mouse.[98]

CARDIOVASCULAR EFFECTS OF COX-2 INHIBITORS

Effects of COX-2 Inhibition on Vascular Tone

In addition to their propensity to reduce renal salt excretion and decrease medullary blood flow, NSAIDs and selective COX-2 inhibitors have been shown to exert direct effects on systemic resistance vessels. The acute pressor effect of angiotensin infusion in human subjects was significantly increased by pretreatment with the non-selective NSAID, indomethacin, at all angiotensin II doses studied. More recently, administration of selective COX-2 inhibitors or COX-2 gene knockout has been shown to accentuate the pressor effects of angiotensin II in mice.[44] These studies also demonstrated that Ang II-mediated blood pressure increases were markedly reduced by administration of a selective COX-1 inhibitor or in COX-1 gene knockout mice.[44] These findings support the conclusion that COX-1 derived prostaglandins participate in, and are integral to the pressor activity of angiotensin II, whereas COX-2 derived prostaglandins are vasodilators that oppose and mitigate the pressor activity of angiotensin II. Other animal studies more directly show that that both NSAIDs and COX-2 inhibitors blunt arteriolar dilation and decrease flow through resistance vessels.[99]

Increased Cardiovascular Thrombotic Events

COX-2 is known to be induced in vascular endothelial cells in response to shear stress, and selective COX-2 inhibition reduces circulating prostacyclin levels in normal human subjects.[100] Therefore, increasing evidence indicates that COX-2 selective antagonism may carry increased thrombogenic risks due to selective inhibition of the endothelial-derived anti-thrombogenic prostacyclin without any inhibition of the prothrombotic platelet-derived thromboxane generated by COX-1.[101] Although animal studies have provided conflicting results about the role of COX-2 inhibition on development of atherosclerosis,[102–106] there are recent indications that COX-2 inhibition may destabilize atherosclerotic plaques,[107] as suggested by studies indicating increased COX-2 expression and colocalization with microsomal PGE synthase-1 and metalloproteinases-2 and -9 in carotid plaques from individuals with symptomatic disease before endarterectomy.[108] Because of the concerns about increased cardiovascular risk, two selective COX-2 inhibitors, rofecoxib and valdecoxib, have been withdrawn from the market, and remaining coxibs and other NSAIDs have been relabeled to highlight the increased risk for cardiovascular events.

Once PGH_2 is formed in the cell, it can undergo a number of possible transformations, yielding biologically active prostaglandins and thromboxane A2. As seen in Figure 11–9, in the presence of isomerase and reductase enzymes, PGH_2 is converted to PGE_2 and $PGF_{2\alpha}$, respectively. Thromboxane synthase converts PGH_2 into a bicyclic oxetane-oxane ring metabolite, thromboxane A_2 (TxA_2), a prominent reaction product in the platelet and an established synthetic pathway in the glomerulus. Prostacyclin synthase, a 50 kD protein located in plasma and nuclear membranes and found mostly in vascular endothelial cells, catalyzes the biosynthesis of prostacyclin (PGI_2). PGD_2, the major prostaglandin product in mast cells, is also derived directly from PGH_2, but its role in the kidney is uncertain. The enzymatic machinery and their localization in the kidney are discussed in detail later.

Sources and Nephronal Distribution of Cyclooxygenase Products

COX activity is present in arterial and arteriolar endothelial cells, including glomerular afferent and efferent arterioles. The predominant metabolite from these vascular endothelial cells is PGI_2.[109] Whole glomeruli generate PGE_2, PGI_2, $PGF_{2\alpha}$, and TxA_2. The predominant products in rat and rabbit glomeruli are PGE_2, followed by PGI2 and $PGF_{2\alpha}$ and finally TxA_2.

Analysis of individual cultured glomerular cell subpopulations has also provided insight into the localization of prostanoid synthesis. Cultured mesangial cells are capable of generating PGE_2, and in some cases $PGF_{2\alpha}$ and PGI_2 have also been detected.[110] Other studies suggest mesangial cells may produce the endoperoxide PGH_2 as a major cyclooxygenase product.[111] Glomerular epithelial cells also appear to participate in prostaglandin synthesis, but the profile of COX products generated in these cells remains controversial. Immunocytochemical studies of rabbit kidney demonstrate intense staining for COX-1 predominantly in the parietal epithelial cells. Glomerular capillary endothelial cell PG generation profiles remain undefined but may well include prostacyclin.

The predominant synthetic site of prostaglandin synthesis along the nephron is the collecting duct (CD), particularly its medullary portion (MCT).[112] In the presence of exogenous arachidonic acid, PGE_2 is the predominant PG formed in collecting duct, the variations among the other products being insignificant. PGE_2 is also the major COX metabolite generated in medullary interstitial cells.[113] The role that specific prostanoid synthases may play in the generation of these products is outlined later.

Thromboxane Synthase

Thromboxane A_2 (TxA_2) is produced from PGH_2 by thromboxane synthase (TxAS), a microsomal protein of 533 amino acids with a predicted molecular weight of ~60 kDa. The amino acid of sequence of the enzyme exhibits homology to the cytochrome P450s and is now classified as CYP5A1.[114] The human gene is localized on Chromosome 7q and spans 180 kB. TxAS mRNA is highly expressed in hematopoietic cells, including platelets, macrophages, and leukocytes. TxAS mRNA is expressed in thymus, kidney, lung, spleen, prostate, and placenta. Immunolocalization of TxA synthase demonstrates high expression in the dendritic cells of the interstitium, with lower expression in glomerular podocytes of human kidney.[115] TxA_2 synthase expression is regulated by dietary salt intake.[116] Furthermore experimental use of ridogrel, a specific thromboxane synthase inhibitor, reduced

blood pressure in spontaneously hypertensive rats.[117] The clinical use of TxA_2 synthase inhibitors is complicated by the fact that its endoperoxide precursors (PGG_2/PGH_2) are also capable of activating its downstream target, the TP receptor.[26]

Prostacyclin Synthase

The biological effects of prostacyclin are numerous and include nociception, anti-thrombosis, and vasodilator actions, which have been targeted therapeutically to manage pulmonary hypertension.

Prostacyclin (PGI_2) is derived by the enzymatic conversion of PGH_2 via prostacyclin synthase (PGIS). The cloned cDNA contains a 1500 base pair open reading frame that encodes a 500 amino acid protein of approximately 56 kDa. The human prostacyclin synthase gene is present as a single copy per haploid genome and is localized on chromosome 20q. Northern blot analysis shows prostacyclin synthase mRNA is widely expressed in human tissues and is particularly abundant in ovary, heart, skeletal muscle, lung, and prostate. PGI synthase expression exhibits segmental expression in the kidney especially in kidney inner medulla tubules and interstitial cells.

Recently, PGI_2 synthase-null mice were generated.[118] PGI_2 levels in the plasma, kidneys, and lungs, were reduced, documenting the role of this enzyme as an in vivo source of PGI_2. Blood pressure and blood urea nitrogen and creatinine in the PGIS knockout mice were significantly increased and renal pathological findings included surface irregularity, fibrosis, cysts, arterial sclerosis, and hypertrophy of vessel walls. Thickening of the thoracic aortic media and adventitia were observed in aged PGI null mice.[118] Interestingly this is a phenotype different from that reported for the IP receptor knockout mouse.[119] These differences points to the presence of additional IP independent PGI_2 activated signaling pathways. Regardless, these findings demonstrate the importance of PGI_2 to maintenance of blood vessels and to the kidney.

Prostaglandin Synthase

Prostaglandin D_2 is derived from PGH_2 via the action of specific enzymes designated PGD synthases. Two major enzymes are capable of transforming PGH_2 to PGD_2 including a lipocalin type PGD synthase and a hematopoietic type PGDS.[120,121] Mice lacking the lipocalin D synthase gene exhibit altered sleep and pain sensation.[122] PGD_2 is the major prostanoid released from mast cells following challenge with IgE. The kidney also appears capable of synthesizing PGD_2. RNA for the lipocalin type PGD synthase has been reported to be widely expressed along the rat nephron, whereas the hematopoietic type PGD synthase is restricted to the collecting duct.[123] Urinary excretion of lipocalin D synthase has recently been proposed as a biomarker predictive of renal injury[124] and lipocalin D synthase knockout mice appear to be more prone to diabetic nephropathy.[125] However the physiologic roles of these enzymes in the kidney remain less certain. Once synthesized, PGD_2 is available to interact with the either the DP or CRTH2 receptors (see later discussion) or undergo further metabolism to a PGF_2 like compound.

Prostaglandin F Synthesis

Prostaglandin $F_{2\alpha}$ is a major urinary cyclooxygenase product. Its synthesis may derive either directly from PGH_2 via a PGF synthase[126] or indirectly by metabolism of PGE_2 via a 9-keto-reductase.[126] Another more obscure pathway for PGF formation is by the action of a PGD_2 ketoreductase, yielding a stereoisomer of PGF_2, 9α, 11β-PGF_2 (11epi-$PGF_{2\alpha}$).[126] This reaction, and conversion of PGD_2 into an apparently

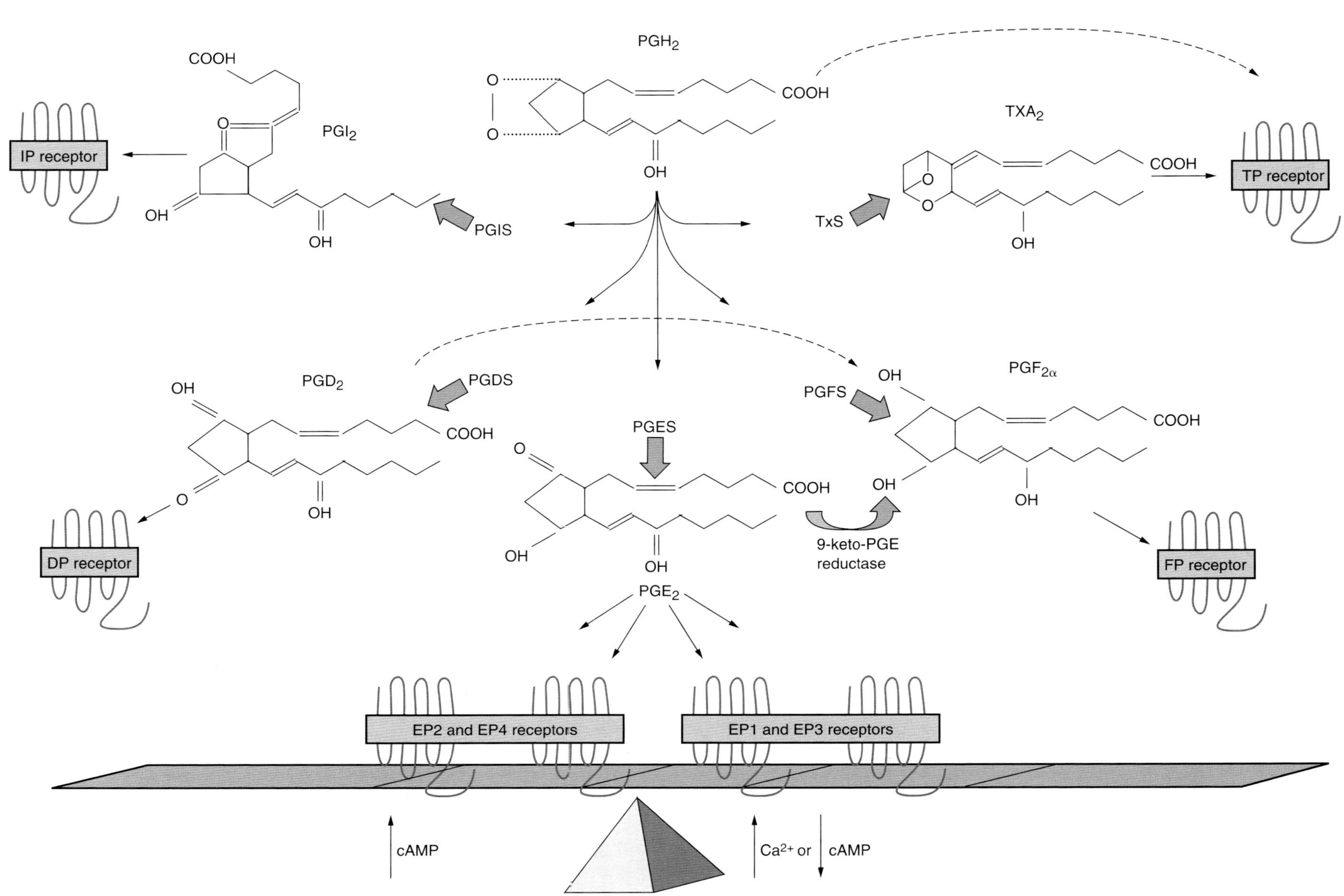

FIGURE 11-9 Prostaglandin synthases.

biologically active metabolite (9a,11b-PGF$_{2\alpha}$) has been documented in vivo.[127] Interestingly this isomer can also ligate and activate the FP receptor.[128] The physiologically relevant enzymes responsible for renal PGF$_{2\alpha}$ formation remain incompletely characterized.

Prostaglandin 9 Ketoreductase

Physiologically relevant transformations of COX products occur in the kidney via a NADPH-dependent 9-ketoreductase, which converts PGE$_2$ into PGF$_{2a}$. This enzymatic activity is typically cytosolic[126] and may be detected in homogenates from renal cortex, medulla, or papilla. The activity appears to be particularly robust in suspensions from the thick ascending limb of Henle (TALH). Renal PGE$_2$ 9 keto-reductase also exhibits 20α hydroxysteroid reductase activity that could affect steroid metabolism.[126] This enzyme appears to be a member of the aldo-keto reductase family 1C.[129]

Interestingly, some studies suggest activity of a 9-ketoreductase may be modulated by salt intake and AT$_2$ receptor activation, and may play an important role in hypertension.[130] Mice deficient in the AT$_2$ receptor exhibit salt sensitive hypertension, increased PGE$_2$ production, and reduced production of PGF$_{2\alpha}$,[131] consistent with reduced 9-ketoreductase activity. Other studies suggest dietary potassium intake may also enhance the activity of conversion from PGE$_2$ to PGF$_{2\alpha}$.[132] The intra-renal sites of expression of this enzymatic activity remain to be characterized.

Prostaglandin E Synthases

PGE$_2$ is the other major product of cyclooxygenase-initiated arachidonic acid metabolism in the kidney and is synthesized at high rates along the nephron, particularly in the collecting duct. Two membrane associated PGE$_2$ synthases have been identified: a 33 kDa and a 16 kDa membrane associated enzyme.[133,134] The initial report describing the cloning of a glutathione dependent microsomal enzyme (the 16 kDa form) that specifically converts PGH$_2$ to PGE$_2$[134] showed mRNA for this enzyme is highly expressed in reproductive tissues as well as in kidney. Genetic disruption confirms that mPGES1−/− mice exhibit a marked reduction in inflammatory responses compared with mPGES1+/+[135] and indicate that mPGES1 is also critical for the induction of inflammatory fever.[136]

Intra-renal expression of mPGES1 has been demonstrated and mapped to collecting duct with lower expression in the medullary interstitial cells and macula densa (see Fig. 11–3).[112,137] Thus in the kidney this isoform co-localizes with both cyclooxygenase 1 and -2. In contrast, in inflammatory cells, this PGE synthase is co-induced with COX-2 and appears to be functionally coupled to it.[138] Notably, the kidneys of mPGES1−/− mice are normal and do not exhibit the renal dysgenesis observed in COX2−/− mice.[94,139] Nor do these mice exhibit perinatal death from patent ductus arteriosus observed with the prostaglandin EP4 receptor knockout mouse.[140]

More recently another membrane associated PGE synthase with a relative mass of ~33 kDa was purified from heart. The recombinant enzyme was activated by several SH-reducing reagents, including dithiothreitol, glutathione (GSH), and beta-mercaptoethanol. Moreover, the mRNA distribution was high in the heart and brain, and was also expressed in the kidney, but the mRNA was not expressed in the seminal vesicles. The intra-renal distribution of this enzyme is, at present, uncharacterized.[133]

Other cytosolic proteins exhibit lower prostaglandin E synthase activity, including a 23 kDa GST requiring cytoplasmic PGES[141] that is expressed in the kidney and lower genitourinary tract.[142] Some evidence suggests this isozyme may constitutively couple to COX-1 in inflammatory cells. In addition several cytosolic glutathione-S-transferases have the capability to convert PGH$_2$ to PGE$_2$; however their physiologic role in this process remains uncertain.[143]

CELLULAR ORIGIN OF EICOSANOIDS PROSTANOID RECEPTORS

TP Receptors

The TP receptor was originally purified by chromatography using a high affinity ligand to capture the receptor (Figs. 11–10 and 11–11).[144] This was the first eicosanoid receptor cloned and is a G-protein coupled transmembrane receptor capable of activating a calcium coupled signaling mechanism (Fig. 11–12). The cloning of other prostanoid receptors was achieved by finding cDNAs homologous to this TP receptor cDNA. Two alternatively spliced variants of the human thromboxane receptor have been described[145] that differ in their carboxyl-terminal tail distal to Arg^{328}. Similar patterns of alternative splicing have been described for both the EP$_3$ receptor and the FP receptor.[146] Heterologous cAMP mediated signaling of the thromboxane receptor may occur via its heterodimerization with the prostacyclin (IP) receptor.[147]

Either the endoperoxide, PGH$_2$ or its metabolite, TxA2 can activate the TP receptor.[26] Competition radioligand binding studies have demonstrated a rank order of potency on human platelet TP receptor of the ligands I-BOP, S145>SQ29-48>STA$_2$>U-46619.[148,149] Whereas I-BOP, STA$_2$, and U-46619 are agonists, SQ29548 and S145, are potent TP receptor antagonists.[150] Studies have suggested that the TP receptor may mediate some of the biological effects of the non-enzymatically derived isoprostanes,[151] including modulation of tubuloglomerular feedback.[152] This latter finding may have significance in pathophysiological conditions associated with increased oxidative stress.[153] Signal transduction studies show the TP receptor activates phosphatidylinositol hydrolysis (PIP$_2$) dependent Ca^{++} influx.[144,154] Northern analysis of mouse tissues revealed that the highest level of TP mRNA expression is in the thymus followed by spleen, lung, and kidney, with lower levels of expression in heart, uterus, and brain.[155]

Thromboxane is a potent modulator of platelet shape change and aggregation as well as smooth muscle contraction and proliferation. Moreover, a point mutation (Arg^{60} to Leu) in the first cytoplasmic loop of the TXA$_2$ receptor was identified in a dominantly inherited bleeding disorder in humans, characterized by defective platelet response to TXA$_2$.[156] Targeted gene disruption of the murine TP receptor also resulted in prolonged bleeding times and reduction in collagen stimulated platelet aggregation (Table 11–1). Conversely, overexpression of the TP receptor in vascular tissue increases the severity of vascular pathology following injury. Increased thromboxane synthesis has been linked to cardiovascular diseases, including acute myocardial ischemia, heart failure, and inflammatory renal diseases.

In the kidney, TP receptor mRNA has been reported in glomeruli and vasculature. Radioligand autoradiography using ^{125}I-BOP suggests a similar distribution of binding sites in mouse renal cortex, but additional renal medullary binding sites were observed.[157] These medullary TxA$_2$ binding sites are absent following disruption of the TP receptor gene, suggesting they also represent authentic TP receptors.[158] Glomerular TP receptors may participate in potent vasoconstrictor effects of TxA$_2$ analogs on the glomerular microcirculation associated with reduced glomerular filtration rate. Mesangial TP receptors coupled to phosphatidylinositol hydrolysis, protein kinase C activation, and glomerular mesangial cell contraction may contribute to these effects.[159]

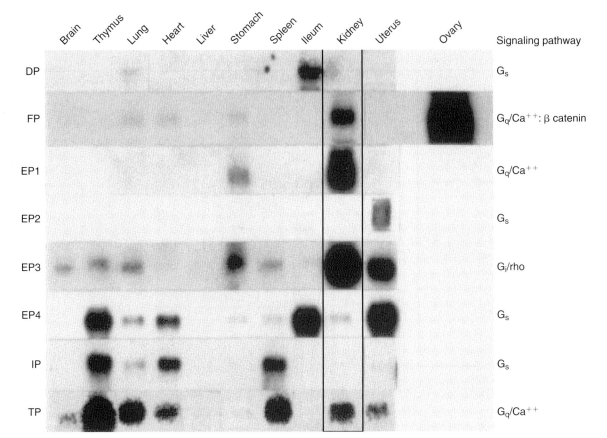

FIGURE 11–10 Tissue distribution of prostanoid receptor mRNA. (Adapted from Bek M, Nusing R, Kowark P, et al: Characterization of prostanoid receptors in podocytes. J Am Soc Nephrol 10:2084–2093, 1999.)

An important role for TP receptors in regulating renal hemodynamics and systemic blood pressure has also been suggested. Administration of a TP receptor antagonist reduces blood pressure in spontaneously hypertensive rats (SHRs)[117] and in angiotensin-dependent hypertension.[160] The TP receptor also appears to modulate renal blood flow in AngII dependent hypertension[161] and in endotoxemia-induced renal failure.[162] Modulation of renal TP receptor mRNA expression and function by dietary salt intake has also been reported.[163] These studies also suggested an important role for luminal TP receptors in the distal tubule to enhance glomerular vasoconstriction indirectly via effects on the macula densa and tubuloglomerular feedback (TGF).[164] However, recent studies reveal no significant difference in tubuloglomerular feedback between wild type and TP receptor knockout mice.[43]

Despite the renal effects of thromboxane mimetics, the major phenotype of TP receptor disruption in mice and humans appears to be reduced platelet aggregation and prolonged bleeding time.[158] Thromboxane may also modulate the glomerular fibrinolytic system by increasing the production of an inhibitor of plasminogen activator (PAI-1) in mesangial cells.[165] Although a specific renal phenotype in the TP receptor knockout mouse has not yet been reported, important pathogenic roles for TxA$_2$ and glomerular TP receptors in mediating renal dysfunction in glomerulonephritis, diabetes mellitus, and sepsis seem likely.

Prostacyclin Receptors

The cDNA for the IP receptor encodes a transmembrane protein of approximately 41 kDa. The IP receptor is selectively activated by the analog cicaprost.[166] Iloprost and carbaprostacyclin potently activate the IP receptor but also activate the EP$_1$ receptor. Most evidence suggests the PGI$_2$ receptor signals via stimulation of cAMP generation; however at 1000 fold higher concentrations the cloned mouse PGI$_2$ receptor also signaled via PIP$_2$.[167] It remains unclear whether PIP$_2$ hydrolysis plays any significant role in the physiologic action of PGI$_2$.

IP receptor mRNA is highly expressed in mouse thymus, heart, and spleen[167] and in human kidney, liver, and lung.[168] In situ hybridization shows IP receptor mRNA predominantly in neurons of the dorsal root ganglia and vascular tissue including aorta, pulmonary artery, and renal interlobular and glomerular afferent arterioles.[169] The expression of IP receptor mRNA in the dorsal root ganglia is consistent with a role for prostacyclin in pain sensation. Mice with IP receptor gene disruption exhibit a predisposition to arterial thrombosis, diminished pain perception, and inflammatory responses.[119]

PGI$_2$ has been demonstrated to play an important vasodilator role in the kidney[170] including in the glomerular microvasculature[171] as well as regulating renin release.[172,173] The capacity of PGI$_2$ and PGE$_2$ to stimulate cAMP generation in the glomerular microvasculature is distinct and additive,[174] demonstrating the effects of these two prostanoids are mediated via separate receptors. IP receptor knockout mice also exhibit salt sensitive hypertension.[175] Prostacyclin is a potent stimulus of renal renin release, and studies using IP–/– mice confirm an important role for the IP receptor in the development of renin dependent hypertension of renal artery stenosis.[62]

Renal epithelial effects of PGI$_2$ in the thick ascending limb have also been suggested[176] and IP receptors have been reported in the collecting duct[177] but the potential expression and role of prostacyclin in these segments are less well established. Of interest, in situ hybridization also demonstrated

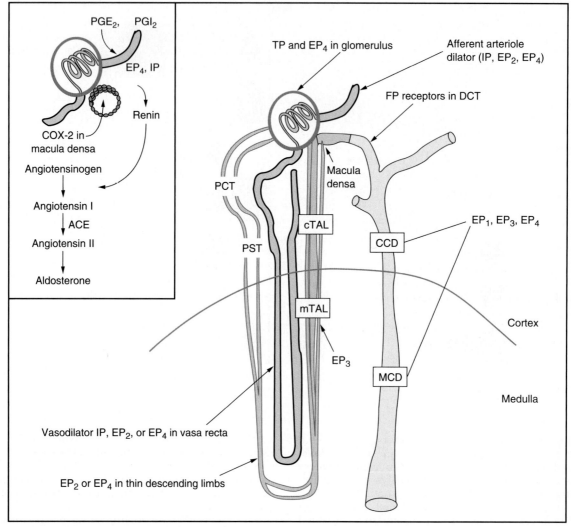

FIGURE 11–11 Intrarenal localization of prostanoid receptors.

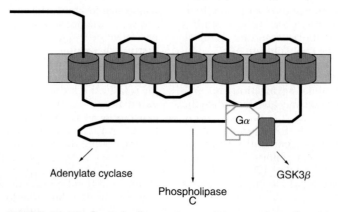

FIGURE 11–12 Prostaglandin receptors are 7-transmembrane G-protein coupled receptors.

TABLE 11–1	Published Phenotypes of Prostanoid Receptor Knockout Mice		
	Renal Expression	Knockout Phenotype	References
DP	Minimal?	No Reduced allergic asthma	185
IP	++ Afferent arteriole	± Reduced inflammation, pain; increased thrombosis	119
TP	+ Glomerulus, tubules?	No Prolonged bleeding time, platelet defect	158
FP	+++ Distal tubules	No Failure of parturition	193
EP1	++++ MCD	No Decreased pain, sensation	K. Watanabe et al, 1997
EP2	++ Interstitial, stromal	Impaired ovulation, salt sensitive hypertension (?)	Hizaki et al, 1999; 215, 217, 253
EP3	++++ TAL, MCD	± Impaired febrile response, Mild diluting defect	140, 236
EP4	+++ Glomerulus, + distal tubules	± Perinatal death from persistent patent ductus arteriosus	140, 236

significant expression of prostacyclin synthase in medullary collecting ducts,[178] consistent with a role for this metabolite in this region of the kidney. In summary, whereas IP receptors appear to play an important role regulating renin release and a vasodilator in the kidney, their role in regulating renal epithelial function remains to be firmly established.

DP Receptors

The DP receptor has been cloned and like the IP and EP2/4 receptors, the DP receptor predominantly signals by increasing cAMP generation. The human DP receptor binds PGD_2 with a high affinity binding of 300 pM, and a lower affinity site of 13.4 nM.[179] DP selective PGD_2 analogs, include the agonist BW 245C.[180] DP receptor mRNA is highly expressed in leptomeninges, retina, and ileum but was not detected in the kidney.[181] Northern blot analysis of the human DP receptor demonstrated mRNA expression in the small intestine and retina,[182] whereas in the mouse the DP receptor mRNA was detected in the ileum and lung.[179] PGD_2 has also been shown to affect the sleep-wake cycle,[183] pain sensation,[122] and body temperature.[184] Peripherally, PGD_2 has been shown to mediate vasodilation as well as possibly inhibiting platelet aggregation. Consistent with this latter finding, the DP receptor knockout displayed reduced inflammation in the ovalbumin model of allergic asthma.[185] Although the kidney appears capable of synthesizing PGD_2, its role in the kidney remains

poorly defined. Intra-renal infusion of PGD_2 resulted in dose-dependent increase in renal artery flow, urine output, creatinine clearance, and sodium and potassium excretion.[186]

Recently, another G-protein coupled receptor capable of binding and being activated by PGD_2 was cloned from eosinophils and T-cells (TH2 subset) and designated the CRTH2 receptor.[187] This receptor, also referred to by some as the DP2 receptor, bears no significant sequence homology to the family of prostanoid receptors discussed earlier, and couples to increased cell calcium rather than increased cAMP. The use of DP selective agonists should help clarify whether renal effects of PGD_2 are mediated by authentic DP receptors or the CRTH2 receptor. The recognition of this molecularly unrelated receptor allows for the possibility of existence of a distinct and new family of prostanoid activated membrane receptors.

FP Receptors

The cDNA encoding the $PGF_{2\alpha}$ receptor (FP receptor) was cloned from a human kidney cDNA library and encodes a protein of 359 amino acid residues. The bovine and murine FP receptors, cloned from corpora lutea similarly encode proteins of 362 and 366 amino acid residues, respectively. Transfection of HEK293 cells with the human FP receptor cDNA, conferred preferential ^3H-$PGF_{2\alpha}$ binding with a KD of 4.3 ± 1.0 nM.[150,188] Selective activation of the FP receptor may be achieved using fluprostenol or latanoprost.[150] ^3H-$PGF_{2\alpha}$ binding was displaced by a panel of ligands with a rank order potency of: $PGF_{2\alpha}$=fluprostenol>PGD_2>PGE_2>U466-9>iloprost.[166] When expressed in oocytes, $PGF_{2\alpha}$ or fluprostenol induced a Ca^{++} dependent Cl^- current. Increased cell calcium has been observed in fibroblasts expressing an endogenous FP receptor.[189] Recent studies suggest FP receptors may also activate protein kinase C dependent and Rho mediated/PKC independent signaling pathways.[190] An alternatively spliced isoform with a shorter carboxy-terminal tail, has been identified that appears to signal via a similar manner as the originally described FP receptor.[191] More recent studies suggest these two isoforms may exhibit differential desensitization and may also activate a glycogen synthase kinase/β-catenin coupled signaling pathway.[192]

Tissue distribution of FP receptor mRNA shows highest expression in ovarian corpus luteum followed by kidney, with lower expression in lung, stomach, and heart.[193] Expression of the FP receptor in corpora lutea is critical for normal birth, and homozygous disruption of the murine FP receptor gene results in failure of parturition in females apparently due to failure of the normal pre-term decline in progesterone levels.[194] $PGF_{2\alpha}$ is a potent constrictor of smooth muscle in the uterus, bronchi, and blood vessels; however an endothelial FP receptor may also play a dilator role.[195] The FP receptor is also highly expressed in skin, where it may play an important role in carcinogenesis.[196] A clinically important role for the FP receptor in the eye has been demonstrated to increase uveoscleral outflow and reduce ocular pressure. The FP selective agonist latanoprost has been used clinically as an effective treatment for glaucoma.[197]

The role of FP receptors in regulating renal function is only partially defined. FP receptor expression has been mapped to the cortical collecting duct in mouse and rabbit kidney.[198] FP receptor activation in the collecting duct inhibits vasopressin-stimulated water absorption via a pertussis toxin sensitive (presumably Gi) dependent mechanism. Although $PGF_{2\alpha}$ increases cell Ca^{++} in cortical collecting duct, the FP selective agonists latanoprost and fluprostenol did not increase calcium.[199] Because $PGF_{2\alpha}$ can also bind to EP1 and EP3 receptors[166,200,201] these data suggest that the calcium increase activated by $PGF_{2\alpha}$ in the collecting duct may be mediated via an EP receptor. $PGF_{2\alpha}$ also increases Ca^{++} in cultured glomerular mesangial cells and podocytes,[202,203] suggesting an FP receptor may modulate glomerular contraction. In contrast to these findings, demonstration of glomerular FP receptors at the molecular level has not been forthcoming. Other vascular effects of $PGF_{2\alpha}$ have been described, including selective modulation of renal production of $PGF_{2\alpha}$ by sodium or potassium loading and AT_2 receptor activation.[130]

Multiple EP Receptors

Four EP receptor subtypes have been identified.[204] Although these four receptors uniformly bind PGE_2 with a higher affinity than other endogenous prostanoids, the amino-acid homology of each is more closely related to other prostanoid receptors that signal through similar mechanisms.[149] Thus the relaxant/cAMP coupled EP_2 receptor is more closely related to other relaxant prostanoid receptors such as the IP and DP receptors, whereas the constrictor/Ca^{++} coupled EP_1 receptor is more closely related to the other Ca^{++} coupled prostanoid receptors such as the TP and FP receptors.[205] These receptors may also be selectively activated or antagonized by different analogs. EP receptor subtypes also exhibit differential expression along the nephron, suggesting distinct functional consequences of activating each EP receptor subtype in the kidney.[204]

EP₁ Receptors

The human EP1 receptor cDNA encodes a 402 amino acid polypeptide that signals via IP_3 generation and increased cell Ca^{++} with IP_3 generation. Studies of EP1 receptors may utilize one of several relatively selective antagonists including SC51089, SC19220, or SC53122. EP_1 receptor mRNA predominates in the kidney>>gastric muscularis mucosae>adrenal.[206] Renal EP_1 mRNA expression determined by in situ hybridization is expressed primarily in the collecting duct, and increases from the cortex to the papillae.[206] Activation of the EP_1 receptor increases intracellular calcium and inhibits Na^+ and water reabsorption absorption in the collecting duct,[206] suggesting renal EP_1 receptor activation might contribute to the natriuretic and diuretic effects of PGE_2.

Hemodynamic, microvascular effects of EP_1 receptors have also been supported. The EP_1 receptor was originally described as a smooth muscle constrictor.[207] A recent report suggests the EP_1 receptor may also be present in cultured glomerular mesangial cells[208] where it could play a role as a vasoconstrictor and a stimulus for mesangial cell proliferation. Although a constrictor PGE_2 effect has been reported in the afferent arteriole of rat,[209] it remains unclear whether this is mediated by an EP_1 or EP_3 receptor. There does not appear to be very high expression of the EP_1 receptor mRNA in preglomerular vasculature or other arterial resistance vessels in either mice or rabbits.[210] Other reports suggest EP_1 receptor knockout mice exhibit hypotension and hyperreninemia, supporting a role for this receptor in maintaining blood pressure.[211]

EP₂ Receptors

Two cAMP stimulating EP receptors, designated EP_2 and EP_4 have been identified. The EP_2 receptor can be pharmacologically distinguished from the EP_4 receptor by its sensitivity to butaprost.[212] Prior to 1995 literature the cloned EP_4 receptor was designated the EP_2 receptor, but then a butaprost sensitive EP receptor was cloned,[213] and the original receptor reclassified as the EP_4 receptor and the newer butaprost sensitive protein designated the EP_2 receptor.[214] A pharmacologically defined EP_2 receptor has now also been cloned for the mouse, rat, rabbit, dog, and cow.[215] The human EP_2 receptor cDNA encodes a 358 amino acid polypeptide, which signals through increased cAMP. The EP_2 receptor may also be distinguished from the EP_4 receptor, the other major relaxant EP receptor, by its relative insensitivity to the EP_4 agonist

PGE_1-OH and insensitivity to the weak EP4 antagonist AH23848.[212]

The precise distribution of the EP_2 receptor mRNA has been partially characterized. This reveals a major mRNA species of ~3.1 kb, which is most abundant in the uterus, lung, and spleen, exhibiting only low levels of expression in the kidney.[215] EP_2 mRNA is expressed at much lower levels than EP_4 mRNA in most tissues.[216] There is scant evidence to suggest segmental distribution of the EP_2 receptor along the nephron.[215] Interestingly it is expressed in cultured renal interstitial cells, supporting the possibility that the EP_2 receptor is predominantly expressed in this portion of the nephron.[215] Studies in knockout mice demonstrate a critical role for the EP_2 receptor role in ovulation and fertilization.[217] In addition these studies suggest a potential role for the EP_2 receptor in salt sensitive hypertension.[217] This latter finding supports an important role for the EP_2 receptor in protecting systemic blood pressure, perhaps via its vasodilator effect or effects on renal salt excretion.

EP₃ Receptors

The EP_3 receptor generally acts as a constrictor of smooth muscle.[218] Nuclease protection and northern analysis demonstrate relatively high levels of EP_3 receptor expression in several tissues including kidney, uterus, adrenal, and stomach, with riboprobes hybridizing to major mRNA species at ~2.4 and ~7.0 kb.[219] This receptor is unique in that multiple (more than eight) alternatively spliced variants differing only in their C-terminal cytoplasmic tails, exist.[220-222] The EP3 splice variants bind PGE_2, and the EP_3 agonists MB28767 and sulprostone with similar affinity, and although they exhibit common inhibition of cAMP generation via a pertussis toxin sensitive Gi-coupled mechanism, the tails may recruit different signaling pathways, including Ca^{++} dependent signaling[149,212] and the small G-protein, rho.[223] Differences in agonist independent activity have been observed for several of the splice variants, suggesting that they may play a role in constitutive regulation of cellular events.[224] The physiologic roles of these different C-terminal splice variants and sites of expression within the kidney remains uncertain.

In situ hybridization demonstrates EP_3 receptor mRNA is abundant in the thick ascending limb and collecting duct.[225] This distribution has been confirmed by RT-PCR on microdissected rat and mouse collecting ducts and corresponds to the major binding sites for radioactive PGE_2 in the kidney.[226] An important role for a G_i coupled prostaglandin E receptor in regulating water and salt transport along the nephron has been recognized for many years. PGE_2 directly inhibits salt and water absorption in both microperfused thick ascending limbs (TAL) and collecting ducts (CD). PGE_2 directly inhibits Cl^- absorption in the mouse or rabbit medullary TAL from either the luminal or basolateral surfaces.[227] PGE_2 also inhibits hormone stimulated cAMP generation in TAL. Good demonstrated that PGE_2 modulates ion transport in the rat TAL by a pertussis toxin sensitive mechanism.[227] Interestingly these effects also appear to involve protein kinase C activation,[228] possibly reflecting activation of a novel EP_3 receptor signaling pathway, possibly corresponding to alternative signaling pathways as described earlier.[223] Taken together, these data support a role for the EP3 receptor in regulating transport in both the collecting duct and TAL.

Blockade of endogenous PGE_2 synthesis by NSAIDs enhances urinary concentration. It is likely PGE_2 mediated antagonism of vasopressin-stimulated salt absorption in the TAL and water absorption in the collecting duct contributes to its diuretic effect. In the in vitro microperfused collecting duct, PGE_2 inhibits both vasopressin-stimulated osmotic water absorption and vasopressin-stimulated cAMP generation.[199] Furthermore PGE_2 inhibition of water absorption and cAMP generation are both blocked by pertussis toxin, suggesting effects mediated by the inhibitory G protein, G_i.[199] When administered in the absence of vasopressin, PGE_2 actually stimulates water absorption in the collecting duct from either the luminal or the basolateral side.[229] These stimulatory effects of PGE_2 on transport in the collecting duct appear to be related to activation of the EP_4 receptor.[229] Despite the presence of this absorption enhancing EP receptor, in vivo studies suggest that, in the presence of vasopressin, the predominant effects of endogenous PGE_2 on water transport are diuretic.

Based on the preceding functional considerations, one would expect $EP_3-/-$ mice to exhibit inappropriately enhanced urinary concentration. Surprisingly $EP_3-/-$ mice exhibited a comparable urinary concentration following dDAVP, similar 24 hour water intake, and similar maximal and minimal urinary osmolality.[230] The only clear difference was that in mice allowed free access to water, indomethacin increased urinary osmolality in normal mice but not in the knockout animals. These findings raise the possibility that some of the renal actions of PGE_2 normally mediated by the EP_3 receptor have been co-opted by other receptors (such as the EP_1 or FP receptor) in the EP_3 knockout mouse. This remains to be formally tested.

The significance of EP_3 receptor activation to animal physiology has been significantly advanced by the availability of mice with targeted disruption of this gene.[230,231] Mice with targeted deletion of the EP_3 receptor exhibit an impaired febrile response, suggesting that EP_3 receptor antagonists could be effective antipyretic agents.[231] Other studies suggest the EP_3 receptor plays an important vasopressor role in the peripheral circulation of mice.[210] Studies in knockout mice also support a potential role for the EP_3 receptor as an important systemic vasopressor.[210,232]

The EP_4 Receptor

Like the EP_2 receptor, the EP_4 receptor signals through increased cAMP.[233] The human EP_4 receptor cDNA encodes a 488 amino acid polypeptide with a predicted molecular mass of ~53 kDa.[234] Note, care must be taken in reviewing the literature prior to 1995, when this receptor was generally referred to as the EP_2 receptor.[214] In addition to the human receptor, EP_4 receptors for the mouse, rat, rabbit, and dog have been cloned. EP_4 receptors can be pharmacologically distinguished from the EP_1 and EP_3 receptors by insensitivity to sulprostone and from EP_2 receptors by its insensitivity to butaprost and relatively selective activation by PGE_1-OH.[150] Recently an EP_4 selective agonist (ONO-AE1-329) and antagonist have been generated[212]; however, to date, their use has not been widely reported.

EP_4 receptor mRNA is highly expressed relative to the EP_2 receptor and widely distributed, with a major species of ~3.8 kb detected by northern analysis in thymus, ileum, lung, spleen, adrenal, and kidney.[216,235] Dominant vasodilator effects of EP_4 receptor activation have been described in venous and arterial beds.[180,218] A critical role for the EP_4 receptor in regulating the peri-natal closure of the pulmonary ductus arteriosus has also been suggested by the recent studies of mice with targeted disruption of the EP_4 receptor gene.[140,236] On a 129 strain background, $EP_4-/-$ mice had nearly 100% peri-natal mortality due to persistent patent ductus arteriosus.[236] Interestingly, when bred on a mixed genetic background, only 80% of $EP_4-/-$ mice died whereas ~21% underwent closure of the ductus and survived.[140] Preliminary studies in these survivors support an important role for the EP_4 receptor as a systemic vasodepressor[237]; however, their heterogeneous genetic background complicates the interpretation of these results because survival may select for modifier genes that not only allow ductus closure but also alter other hemodynamic responses.

Other roles for the EP_4 receptor in controlling blood pressure have been suggested, including the ability to stimulate aldosterone release from zona glomerulosa cells.[238] In the kidney, EP_4 receptor mRNA expression is primarily in the glomerulus, where its precise function is uncharacterized[235,239] but might contribute to regulation of the renal microcirculation as well as renin release.[240] Recent studies in mice with genetic deletion of selective prostanoid receptors indicated that $EP_4-/-$ mice, as well as IP$-/-$ mice to a lesser extent, failed to increase renin production in response to loop diuretic administration, indicating that macula densa-derived PGE2 increased renin primarily through EP4 activation.[241] This corresponds to recent studies suggesting EP_4 receptors are expressed in cultured podocytes and juxtaglomerular apparatus cells.[202,240] Finally, the EP4 receptor in the renal pelvis may participate in regulation of salt excretion by altering afferent renal nerve output.[242]

Regulation of Renal Function by EP Receptors

PGE_2 exerts myriad effects in the kidney, presumably mediated by EP receptors. PGE_2 not only dilates the glomerular microcirculation and vasa rectae, supplying the renal medulla,[243] but also modulates salt and water transport in the distal tubule (see Fig. 11-5).[244] The maintenance of normal renal function during physiologic stress is particularly dependent on endogenous prostaglandin synthesis. In this setting, the vasoconstrictor effects of angiotensin II, catecholamines, and vasopressin are more effectively buffered by prostaglandins in the kidney than in other vascular beds, preserving normal renal blood flow, glomerular filtration rate (GFR), and salt excretion. Administration of cyclooxygenase inhibiting NSAIDs in the setting of volume depletion interferes with these dilator effects and may result in a catastrophic decline in GFR, resulting in overt renal failure.[245]

Other evidence points to vasoconstrictor and prohypertensive effects of endogenous PGE_2. PGE_2 stimulates renin release from the juxtaglomerular apparatus[246] leading to a subsequent increase in the vasoconstrictor, angiotensin II. In conscious dogs, chronic intra-renal PGE2 infusion increases renal renin secretion resulting in hypertension.[247] Treatment of salt depleted rats with indomethacin not only decreases plasma renin activity, but also reduces blood pressure, suggesting prostaglandins support blood pressure during salt depletion, via their capacity to increase renin.[248] Direct vasoconstrictor effects of PGE_2 on vasculature have also been observed.[210] It is conceivable these latter effects might predominate in circumstances where the kidney is exposed to excessively high perfusion pressures. Thus depending on the setting, the primary effect of PGE_2 may be either to increase or decrease vascular tone, effects that appear to be mediated by distinct EP receptors.

Renal Cortical Hemodynamics

The expression of the EP_4 receptor in the glomerulus suggests it may play an important role regulating renal hemodynamics. Prostaglandins regulate the renal cortical microcirculation and as alluded to earlier, both glomerular constrictor and dilator effects of prostaglandins have been observed.[210,249] In the setting of volume depletion, endogenous PGE_2 helps maintain GFR by dilating the afferent arteriole.[249] Some data suggest roles for EP and IP receptors coupled to increased cAMP generation in mediating vasodilator effects in the preglomerular circulation.[42,240,250] PGE_2 exerts a dilator effect on the afferent arteriole but not the efferent arteriole, consistent with the presence of an EP_2 or EP_4 receptor in the preglomerular microcirculation.

Renin Release

Other data suggest the EP_4 receptor may also stimulate renin release. Soon after the introduction of NSAIDs it was recognized that endogenous prostaglandins play an important role in stimulating renin release.[42] Treatment of salt depleted rats with indomethacin not only decreases plasma renin activity, but also causes blood pressure to fall, suggesting prostaglandins support blood pressure during salt depletion, via their capacity to increase renin. Prostanoids also play a central role in the pathogenesis of renovascular hypertension, and administration of NSAIDs lowers blood pressure in both animals and humans with renal artery stenosis.[251] PGE_2 induces renin release in isolated pre-glomerular juxtaglomerular apparatus cells.[246] Like the effect of β-adrenergic agents, this effect appears to be through a cAMP coupled response, supporting a role for an EP_4 or EP_2 receptor.[246] EP_4 receptor mRNA has been detected in microdissected JGAs,[252] supporting the possibility that renal EP_4 receptor activation contributes to enhanced renin release. Finally regulation of plasma renin activity and intra-renal renin mRNA does not appear to be different in wild-type and EP_2 knockout mice,[253] arguing against a major role for the EP_2 receptor in regulating renin release. Conversely, one report suggests EP_3 receptor mRNA is localized to the macula densa, suggesting this cAMP inhibiting receptor may also contribute to the control of renin release.[239]

Renal Microcirculation

The EP_2 receptor also appears to play an important role in regulating afferent arteriolar tone.[249] In the setting of systemic hypertension, the normal response of the kidney is to increase salt excretion, thereby mitigating the increase in blood pressure. This so-called pressure natriuresis plays a key role in the ability of the kidney to protect against hypertension.[254] Increased blood pressure is accompanied by increased renal perfusion pressure and enhanced urinary PGE_2 excretion.[255] Inhibition of prostaglandin synthesis markedly blunts (although it does not eliminate) pressure natriuresis.[256] The mechanism by which PGE_2 contributes to pressure natriuresis may involve changes in resistance of the renal medullary microcirculation.[257] PGE_2 directly dilates descending vasa recta, and increased medullary blood flow may contribute to increased interstitial pressure observed as renal perfusion pressure increases, leading to enhanced salt excretion.[243] The identity of the dilator PGE_2 receptor controlling the contractile properties of the descending vasa recta remains uncertain, but EP_2 or EP_4 receptors seem likely candidates.[180] Recent studies demonstrating salt sensitive hypertension in mice with targeted disruption of the EP_2 receptor[217] suggests the EP_2 receptor facilitates the ability of the kidney to increase sodium excretion, thereby protecting systemic blood pressure from a high salt diet. Given its defined role in vascular smooth muscle,[217] these effects of the EP_2 receptor disruption seem more likely to relate to its effects on renal vascular tone. In particular, loss of a vasodilator effect in the renal medulla might modify pressure natriuresis and could contribute to hypertension in EP_2 knockout mice. Nonetheless a role for either the EP_2 or EP_4 receptor in regulating renal medullary blood flow remains to be established. In conclusion, direct vasomotor effects of EP_4 receptors as well as effects on renin release may play critical roles in regulating systemic blood pressure and renal hemodynamics.

Effects on Salt and Water Transport

COX-1 and COX-2 metabolites of arachidonate have important direct epithelial effects on salt and water transport in along the nephron.[258] Thus, functional effects can be observed that are thought to be independent of any hemodynamic changes produced by these compounds. Because biologically active arachidonic acid metabolites are rapidly metabolized, they act predominantly in an autocrine or paracrine fashion

and, thus, their locus of action will be quite close to their point of generation. Thus, one can expect that direct epithelial effects of these compounds will result when they are produced by the tubule cells themselves or the neighboring interstitial cells and the tubules possess an appropriate receptor for the ligand.

Proximal Tubule

Neither the proximal convoluted tubule nor the proximal straight tubule appears to produce amounts of biologically active cyclooxygenase metabolites of arachidonic acid. As will be discussed in a subsequent section, the dominant arachidonate metabolites produced by proximal convoluted and straight tubules are metabolites of the cytochrome P-450 pathway.[259]

Early whole animal studies suggested that PGE_2 might have an action in the proximal tubule because of its effects on urinary phosphate excretion. PGE_2 blocked the phosphaturic action of calcitonin infusion in thyroparathyroidectomized rats. Nevertheless, studies utilizing in vitro perfused proximal tubules failed to show an effect of PGE_2 on sodium chloride or phosphate transport in the proximal convoluted tubule. More recent studies suggest PGE_2 may play a key role in the phosphaturic action of FGF23,[260] because phosphaturia in hyp mice with X-linked hyperphosphaturia is associated with markedly increased urine PGE_2 excretion and phosphaturia was normalized by indomethacin.[261] Nevertheless, there are very little data on the actions of other cyclooxygenase metabolites in proximal tubules and scant molecular evidence for expression of classic G-protein coupled prostaglandin receptors in this segment of the nephron.

Loop of Henle

The nephron segments making up the loop of Henle also display limited metabolism of exogenous arachidonic acid through the cyclooxygenase pathway, although given the realization that COX-2 is expressed in this segment, it is of note that PGE_2 was uniformly greater in the cortical segment than the medullary thick ascending limb. The thick ascending limb has been shown to exhibit PGE_2 receptors in high density.[262] Studies have also demonstrated high expression levels of mRNA for the EP_3 receptor in medullary TAL of both rabbit and rat[201] (see earlier section on the EP_3 receptor). Subsequent to the demonstration that PGE_2 inhibits sodium chloride absorption in the medullary thick ascending limb of the rabbit TAL perfused in vitro, it was shown that PGE_2 blocks ADH but not cyclic AMP stimulated sodium chloride absorption in the medullary thick ascending limb of the mouse. It is likely that the mechanism involves activation of G_i and inhibition of adenyl cyclase by PGE_2, possibly via the EP_3 receptors expressed in this segment.

Collecting Duct System

In vitro perfusion studies of rabbit cortical collecting tubule demonstrated that PGE_2 directly inhibits sodium transport in the collecting duct when applied to the basolateral surface of this nephron segment. It is now apparent that PGE_2 utilizes multiple signal transduction pathways in the cortical collecting duct, including those that modulate intracellular cyclic AMP levels and Ca^{++}. PGE_2 can stimulate or suppress cyclic AMP accumulation. The latter may also involve stimulation of phosphodiesterase. Although modulation of cyclic AMP levels appears to play an important role in PGE_2 effects on water transport in the cortical collecting duct (see following section), it is less clear that PGE_2 affects sodium transport via modulation of cyclic AMP levels.[199] PGE_2 has been shown to increase cell calcium possibly coupled with PKC activation in in vitro perfused cortical collecting ducts.[263] This effect may be mediated by the EP_1 receptor subtype coupled to phosphatidylinositol hydrolysis.[206]

Water Transport

Vasopressin regulated water transport in the collecting duct is markedly influenced by cyclooxygenase products, especially prostaglandins. When cyclooxygenase inhibitors are administered to humans, rats, or dogs, the antidiuretic action of arginine vasopressin is markedly augmented. Because vasopressin also stimulates endogenous PGE_2 production by the collecting duct, these results suggest that PGE_2 participates in a negative feedback loop, whereby endogenous PGE_2 production dampens the action of AVP.[264] In agreement with this model, the early classical studies of Grantham and Orloff directly demonstrated that PGE_1 blunted the water permeability response of the cortical collecting duct to vasopressin. In these early studies, the action of PGE_1 appeared to be at a precyclic AMP step. Interestingly, when administered by itself PGE_1 modestly augmented basal water permeability. These earlier studies have been confirmed with respect to PGE_2. PGE_2 also stimulates basal hydraulic conductivity and suppresses the hydraulic conductivity response to AVP in rabbit cortical collecting duct.[265,266] Inhibition of both AVP stimulated cAMP generation and water permeability appears to be mediated by the EP_1 and EP_3 receptors, whereas the increase in basal water permeability may be mediated by the EP_4 receptor.[229] These data are consistent with functional redundancy between the EP_1 and EP_3 with respect to their effects on vasopressin stimulated water absorption in the collecting duct.

Metabolism of Prostaglandins

15-keto Dehydrogenase

The half life of prostaglandins is 3 to 5 minutes and that of TxA_2 is approximately 30 seconds. Elimination of PGE_2, $PGF_{2\alpha}$ and PGI_2 proceeds through enzymatic and non-enzymatic pathways, whereas that of TxA_2 is non-enzymatic. The end products of all of these degradative reactions generally possess minimal biologic activity, although this is not uniformly the case (see later discussion). The principal enzyme involved in the transformation of PGE_2, PGI_2, and $PGF_{2\alpha}$ is 15-hydroxyprostaglandin dehydrogenase (PGDH), which converts the 15 alcohol group to a ketone.[267]

15-PGDH is an $NAD^+/NADP^+$-dependent enzyme that is 30 to 49 times more active in the kidney of the young rat (3 weeks of age) than in the adult. It is mainly localized in cortical and juxtamedullary zones,[268] with little activity detected in papillary slices. Its K_m for PGE_2 is 8.4 μM and 22.6 μM for $PGF_{2\alpha}$.[267] Disruption of this gene in mice results in persistent patent ductus arteriosus PDA, thought to be a result of failure of circulating PGE_2 levels to fall in the immediate peripartum period.[269] Thus administration of cyclooxygenase inhibiting NSAIDs rescues the knockout mice by decreasing prostaglandins and allowing the animals to survive.

Subsequent catalysis of 15-hydroxy products by a delta-13 reductase leads to the formation of 13,14 dihydro compounds. PGI_2 and TxA_2 undergo rapid degradation to 6-keto-PGF_{1a} and TxB_2 respectively.[267] These stable metabolites are usually measured and their rates of formation taken as representative of those of the parent molecules.

ω/ω-1-Hydroxylation of Prostaglandins

Both PGA_2 and PGE_2 have been shown to undergo hydroxylation of the terminal or sub-termi nal carbons by a cytochrome P450 dependent mechanism.[270] This reaction may be mediated by a CYP4A family members or CYP4F enzyme. Both CYP4A[271] and CYP4F members have been mapped along the nephron.[272] Some of these derivatives have been shown to exhibit biological activity.

Cyclopentenone Prostaglandins

The cyclopentenone prostaglandins include PGA_2, a PGE_2 derivative, and PGJ_2, a derivative of PGD_2. Although it remains uncertain whether these compounds are actually produced in vivo, this possibility has received increasing attention because some cyclopentenone prostanoids been shown to be activating ligands for nuclear transcription factors, including PPARδ and PPARγ.[273–275] The realization that the antidiabetic thiazolidinedione drugs act through PPARγ to exert their antihyperglycemic and insulin sensitizing effects[276] has generated intense interest in the possibility that the cyclopentenone prostaglandins might serve as the endogenous ligands for these receptors. An alternative biologic activity of these compounds has been recognized in their capacity to covalently modify thiol groups, forming adducts with cysteine of several intracellular proteins including thioredoxin 1, vimentin, actin, and tubulin.[277] Studies regarding biological activity of cyclopentenone prostanoids abound and the reader is referred to several excellent sources in the literature.[278–280] Although evidence supporting the presence of these compounds in vivo exists,[281] it remains uncertain whether they can form enzymatically or are an unstable spontaneous dehydration product of the E and D ring prostaglandins.[282]

Non-enzymatic Metabolism of Arachidonic Acid

It has long been recognized that oxidant injury can result in peroxidation of lipids. In 1990, Morrow and Roberts reported that a series of prostaglandin-like compounds can be produced by free radical catalyzed peroxidation of arachidonic acid that is independent of cyclooxygenase activity.[283] These compounds, which are termed "isoprostanes", are increasingly utilized as a sensitive marker of oxidant injury in vitro and in vivo.[284] In addition, at least two of these compounds, 8-iso-$PGF_{2\alpha}$ (15-F_2-isoprostane) and 8-iso-PGE_2 (15-E_2-isoprostane) are potent vasoconstrictors when administered exogenously.[285] 8-iso-$PGF_{2\alpha}$ has been shown to constrict the renal microvasculature and decrease GFR, an effect that is prevented by thromboxane receptor antagonism.[286] However, the role of endogenous isoprostanes as mediators of biologic responses remains unclear.

Prostaglandin Transport and Urinary Excretion

It is notable that most of the prostaglandin synthetic enzymes have been localized to the intracellular compartment, yet extracellular prostaglandins are potent autocoids and paracrine factors. Thus, prostanoids must be transported extracellularly to achieve efficient metabolism and termination of their signaling. Similarly, enzymes that metabolize PGE_2 to inactive compounds are also intra-cellular, requiring uptake of the prostaglandin for its metabolic inactivation. The molecular basis of these extrusion and uptake processes are only now being defined.

As a fatty acid, prostaglandins may be classified as an organic anion at physiological pH. Early microperfusion studies documented that basolateral PGE_2 could be taken up into proximal tubules cells and actively secreted into the lumen. Furthermore this process could be inhibited by a variety of inhibitors of organic anion transport including PAH, probenecid, and indomethacin. Studies of basolateral renal membrane vesicles also supported the notion that this transport process was via an electroneutral anion exchanger. These studies are of note because renal prostaglandins enter the urine in Henle's loop, and late proximal tubule secretion could provide an important entry mechanism.

Recently a molecule that mediates PGE_2 uptake in exchange for lactate has been cloned and christened "PGT" for prostaglandin transporter.[287] PGT is a member of SLC21/SLCO:

organic anion transporting family (http://www.ncbi.nlm.nih.gov/entrez/viewer.fcgi?db=nucleotide&val=5032094) and its cDNA encodes a transmembrane protein of 100 amino acids that exhibits broad tissue distribution heart, placenta, brain, lung, liver, skeletal muscle, pancreas, kidney, spleen, prostate, ovary, small intestine, and colon.[288-290] Immunocytochemical studies of PGT expression in rat kidneys suggest expression primarily in glomerular endothelial and mesangial cells, arteriolar endothelial and muscularis cells, principal cells of the collecting duct, medullary interstitial cells, medullary vasa rectae endothelia, and papillary surface epithelium.[291] PGT appears to mediate PGE_2 uptake rather than release,[292] allowing target cells to metabolize this molecule and terminate signaling.[293]

Other members of the organic cation/anion/zwitterion transporter family SLC22 family have also been shown to transport prostaglandins[287] and have been suggested to mediate prostaglandin excretion into the urine. Specifically OAT1 (http://www.ncbi.nlm.nih.gov/entrez/viewer.fcgi?db=nucleotide&val=24497474) and OAT3 (http://www.ncbi.nlm.nih.gov/entrez/viewer.fcgi?db=nucleotide&val=24497498) are localized on the basolateral proximal tubule membrane, where they likely participate in urinary excretion of PGE_2.[294,295] Conversely members of the multidrug resistance protein (MRP) have been shown to transport prostaglandins in an ATP dependent fashion.[296,297] MRP2 (also designated ABBC2) is expressed in kidney proximal tubule brush borders and may contribute to the transport (and urinary excretion) of glutathione conjugated prostaglandins.[298,299] This transporter has more limited tissue expression, restricted to the kidney, liver, and small intestine and could contribute not only to renal PAH excretion but also to prostaglandin excretion as well.[300]

INVOLVEMENT OF CYCLOOXYGENASE METABOLITES IN RENAL PATHOPHYSIOLOGY

Experimental and Human Glomerular Injury

Glomerular Inflammatory Injury

Cyclooxygenase metabolites have been implicated in functional and structural alterations in glomerular and tubulointerstitial inflammatory diseases.[301] Essential fatty acid deficiency totally prevents the structural and functional consequences of administration of nephrotoxic serum (NTS) to rats, an experimental model of antiglomerular basement membrane glomerulonephritis.[302] Changes in arteriolar tone during the course of this inflammatory lesion are mediated principally by locally released COX and lipoxygenase (LO) metabolites of AA.[302]

TxA2 release appears to play an essential role in mediating the increased renovascular resistance observed during the early phase of this disease. Subsequently, increasing rates of PGE_2 generation may account for progressive dilation of renal arterioles and increases in renal blood flow at later stages of the disease. Consistent with this hypothesis, TxA_2 antagonism ameliorated the falls in RBF and GFR two hours post-NTS administration, but not at one day. During the later, heterologous, phase of NTS, COX metabolites mediate both the renal vasodilation as well as the reduction in K_f that characterize this phase.[302] The net functional result of COX inhibition during this phase of experimental glomerulonephritis, therefore, would depend on the relative importance of renal perfusion versus the preservation of K_f to the maintenance of GFR. Evidence also indicates that COX metabolites

are mediators of pathologic lesions and the accompanying proteinuria in this model. COX-2 expression in the kidney increases in experimental anti-GBM glomerulonephritis[303,304] and after systemic administration of lipopolysaccharide.[305]

A beneficial effect of fish oil diets (enriched in eicosapentaenoic acid), with an accompanying reduction in the generation of COX products, has been demonstrated on the course of genetic murine lupus (MRL-lpr mice). In subsequent studies, enhanced renal TxA_2 and PGE_2 generation was demonstrated in this model, as well as in NZB mice, another genetic model of lupus. In addition, studies in humans demonstrated an inverse relation between TxA_2 biosynthesis and glomerular filtration rate and improvement of renal function following short-term therapy with a thromboxane receptor antagonist in patients with lupus nephritis. More recently, studies have indicated that in humans, as well as NZB mice, COX-2 expression was up-regulated in patients with active lupus nephritis, with colocalization to infiltrating monocytes, suggesting that monocytes infiltrating the glomeruli contribute to the exaggerated local synthesis of TXA_2.[306,307] COX-2 inhibition selectively decreased thromboxane production, and chronic treatment of NZB mice with a COX-2 inhibitor and mycophenolate mofetil significantly prolonged survival.[307] Taken together, these data, as well as others from animal and human studies support a major role for the intrarenal generation of TxA_2 in mediating renal vasoconstriction during inflammatory and lupus-associated glomerular injury.

The demonstration of a functionally significant role for COX metabolites in experimental and human inflammatory glomerular injury has raised the question of the cellular sources of these eicosanoids in the glomerulus. In addition to infiltrating inflammatory cells, resident glomerular macrophages, glomerular mesangial cells, and glomerular epithelial cells represent likely sources for eicosanoid generation. In the anti-Thy1.1 model of mesangioproliferative glomerulonephritis, COX-1 staining was transiently increased in diseased glomeruli at day 6, and was localized mainly to proliferating mesangial cells. COX-2 expression in the macula densa region also transiently increased at day 6.[308,309] Glomerular COX-2 expression in this model has been controversial, with one group reporting increased podocyte COX-2 expression[304] and two other groups reporting minimal, if any glomerular COX-2 expression.[308,309] However, it is of interest that selective COX-2 inhibitors have been reported to inhibit glomerular repair in the anti-Thy1.1 model.[309] In both anti-Thy1.1 and anti-GBM models of glomerulonephritis, the non-selective COX inhibitor, indomethacin, increased monocyte chemoattractant protein-1 (MCP-1), suggesting that prostaglandins may repress recruitment of monocytes/macrophages in experimental glomerulonephritis.[310]

A variety of cytokines have been reported to stimulate PGE2 synthesis and COX-2 expression in cultured mesangial cells. Furthermore, complement components, in particular C5b-9, which are known to be involved in the inflammatory models described earlier, have been implicated in the stimulation of PGE_2 synthesis in glomerular epithelial cells. Cultured GEC express predominantly COX-1, but exposure to C5b-9 significantly increased COX-2 expression.

Glomerular Non-Inflammatory Injury

Studies have suggested that prostanoids may also mediate altered renal function and glomerular damage following subtotal renal ablation, and glomerular prostaglandin production may be altered in such conditions. Glomeruli from remnant kidneys, as well as animals fed a high protein diet, have increased prostanoid production. These studies suggested an increase in cyclooxygenase enzyme activity per se rather than, or in addition to, increased substrate availability because increases in prostanoid production were noted when excess exogenous arachidonic acid was added.

Following subtotal renal ablation, there are selective increases in renal cortical and glomerular COX-2 mRNA and immunoreactive protein expression, without significant alterations in COX-1 expression.[311] This increased COX-2 expression was most prominent in the macula densa and surrounding cTALH. In addition, COX-2 immunoreactivity was also present in podocytes of remnant glomeruli, and increased prostaglandin production in isolated glomeruli from remnant kidneys was inhibited by a COX-2 selective inhibitor but was not decreased by a COX-1 selective inhibitor.[311] Of interest, Weichert and colleagues have recently reported that in the fawn-hooded rat, which develops spontaneous glomerulosclerosis, there is increased cTALH/macula densa COX-2 and nNOS and juxtaglomerular cell renin expression preceding development of sclerotic lesions.[312]

When given 24 hours after subtotal renal ablation, a nonselective NSAID, indomethacin, normalized increases in renal blood flow and single nephron GFR; similar decreases in hyperfiltration were noted when indomethacin was given acutely to rats 14 days after subtotal nephrectomy, although in this latter study, the increased glomerular capillary pressure (P_{GC}) was not altered because both afferent and efferent arteriolar resistances increased. Previous studies have also suggested that non-selective cyclooxygenase inhibitors may acutely decrease hyperfiltration in diabetes and inhibit proteinuria and/or structural injury; more recent studies have indicated selective COX-2 inhibitors will decrease the hyperfiltration seen in experimental diabetes or increased dietary protein.[313,314] Of note, NSAIDs have also been reported to be effective in reducing proteinuria in patients with refractory nephrotic syndrome.

The prostanoids involved have not yet been completely characterized, although it is presumed that vasodilatory prostanoids are involved in mediation of the altered renal hemodynamics. Defective autoregulation of renal blood flow due to decreased myogenic tone of the afferent arteriole is seen after either subtotal ablation or excessive dietary protein and is corrected by inhibition of cyclooxygenase activity. In these hyperfiltering states, tubuloglomerular feedback (TGF) is reset at a higher distal tubular flow rate. Such a resetting dictates that afferent arteriolar vasodilatation will be maintained in the face of increased distal solute delivery. It has previously been shown that the alterations in TGF sensitivity after reduction in renal mass are prevented with the non-selective cyclooxygenase inhibitor, indomethacin. An important role has been suggested for neuronal nitric oxide synthase, which is localized to the macula densa, in the vasodilatory component of TGF.[315–317] Of interest, studies by Ishihara and co-workers have determined that this nNOS-mediated vasodilation is inhibited by the selective COX-2 inhibitor, NS398, suggesting that COX-2-mediated prostanoids may be essential for arteriolar vasodilation.[45,318]

Administration of COX-2 selective inhibitors decreased proteinuria and inhibited development of glomerular sclerosis in rats with reduced functioning renal mass.[319,320] In addition, COX-2 inhibition decreased mRNA expression of TGF-β1 and types III and IV collagen in the remnant kidney.[319] Similar protection was observed with administration of nitroflurbiprofen (NOF), a NO-releasing NSAID without gastrointestinal toxicity.[321] Prior studies have also demonstrated that thromboxane synthase inhibitors retarded progression of glomerulosclerosis, with decreased proteinuria and glomerulosclerosis in rats with remnant kidneys and in diabetic nephropathy, in association with increased renal prostacyclin production and lower systolic blood pressure.[322,323] Studies in models of type I and type II diabetes have indicated that COX-2 selective inhibitors retarded pro-

gression of diabetic nephropathy.[324,325] Schmitz and associates confirmed increases in thromboxane B_2 excretion in the remnant kidney and correlated decreased arachidonic and linoleic acid levels with increased thromboxane production because the thromboxane synthase inhibitor U63557A restored fatty acid levels and retarded progressive glomerular destruction.[322]

Enhanced glomerular synthesis and/or urinary excretion of both PGE_2 and TxA_2 have been demonstrated in passive Heymann nephritis (PHN), and Adriamycin-induced glomerulopathies in rats. Both COX-1 and COX-2 expression are increased in glomeruli with PHN.[326] Both thromboxane synthase inhibitors and selective COX-2 inhibitors also decreased proteinuria in PHN.

In contrast to the putative deleterious effects of thromboxane, the prostacyclin analog, cicaprost, retarded renal damage in uninephrectomized dogs fed a high sodium and high protein diet, an effect that was not mediated by amelioration of systemic hypertension.[327]

Prostanoids have also been shown to alter extracellular matrix production by mesangial cells in culture. Thromboxane A_2 stimulates matrix production by both TGF-β-dependent and -independent pathways.[328] PGE_2 has been reported to decrease steady state mRNA levels of alpha 1(I) and alpha 1(III) procollagens, but not alpha 1(IV) procollagen and fibronectin mRNA, and to reduce secretion of all studied collagen types into the cell culture supernatants. Of interest, this effect did not appear to be mediated by cAMP.[329] PGE_2 has also been reported to increase production of matrix metalloproteinase-2 and to mediate angiotensin II-induced increases in MMP-2.[330] Whether vasodilatory prostaglandins mediate decreased fibrillar collagen production and increased matrix degrading activity in glomeruli in vivo has not yet been studied; however, there is compelling evidence in nonrenal cells that prostanoids may either mediate or modulate matrix production.[331] Cultured lung fibroblasts isolated from patients with idiopathic pulmonary fibrosis exhibit decreased ability to express COX-2 and to synthesize PGE_2.[332]

Acute Renal Failure (ARF)

When cardiac output is compromised, as in extracellular fluid volume depletion or congestive heart failure, systemic blood pressure is preserved by the action of high circulating levels of systemic vasoconstrictors (norepinephrine, angiotensin II, AVP). Amelioration of their effects within the renal vasculature serves to blunt the development of otherwise concomitant marked depression of renal blood flow. Intrarenal generation of vasodilator products of AA, including PGE_2 and PGI_2, is a central part of this protective adaptation. Increased renal vascular resistance induced by exogenously administered angiotensin II or renal nerve stimulation (increased adrenergic tone) is exaggerated during concomitant inhibition of prostaglandin synthesis. Experiments in animals with volume depletion have demonstrated the existence of intrarenal AVP-prostaglandin interactions similar to those described earlier for angiotensin II. Studies in patients with congestive heart failure have confirmed that enhanced prostaglandin synthesis is crucial in protecting kidneys from various vasoconstrictor influences in this condition.

Acute renal failure accompanying the acute administration of endotoxin in rats is characterized by progressive reductions in RBF and GFR in the absence of hypotension. Renal histology in such animals is normal, but cortical generation of COX metabolites is markedly elevated. A number of reports have provided evidence for a role for TxA_2-induced renal vasoconstriction in this model of renal dysfunction.[333] In addition, roles for PGs and TxA_2 in modulating or mediating renal injury have been suggested in ischemia/reperfusion[334] and models of toxin-mediated acute tubular injury including those induced by uranyl nitrate,[335] amphotericin B,[336] aminoglycosides,[337] and glycerol.[338] In experimental acute renal failure, administration of vasodilator prostaglandins has been shown to ameliorate injury.[339]

Urinary Tract Obstruction

Following induction of chronic (more than 24 hours) ureteral obstruction, renal PG and TxA_2 synthesis is markedly enhanced, particularly in response to stimuli such as endotoxin or bradykinin. Enhanced prostanoid synthesis likely arises from infiltrating mononuclear cells, proliferating fibroblast-like cells, interstitial macrophages, and interstitial medullary cells. Considerable evidence, derived from studies utilizing specific enzyme inhibitors, suggests a causal relationship between increased renal generation of this eicosanoid and the intense vasoconstriction that characterizes the hydronephrotic or post-obstructed kidney (reviewed in Ref. 301). In this sense, therefore, hydronephrotic injury can be regarded as a form of sub-acute inflammatory insult in which intrarenal eicosanoid generation from infiltrating leukocytes contributes to the pathophysiologic process. Finally, TxA_2 has been implicated in the resetting of the tubuloglomerular feedback mechanism observed in hydronephrotic kidneys.[340] Recent studies have also suggested that selective COX-2 inhibitors may prevent renal damage in response to unilateral ureteral obstruction.[341,342]

Allograft Rejection and Cyclosporine Nephrotoxicity

Allograft Rejection

Coffman and colleagues demonstrated that acute administration of a TxA_2 synthesis inhibitor was associated with significant improvement in rat renal allograft function.[343] A number of other experimental and clinical studies have also demonstrated increased TxA_2 synthesis during allograft rejection,[344,345] leading some to suggest that increased urinary TxA2 excretion may be an early indicator in renal and cardiac allograft rejection.

Calcineurin Inhibitor Nephrotoxicity

Numerous investigators have demonstrated effects for cyclosporine A (CY-A) on renal prostaglandin/TxA_2 synthesis, and provided evidence for a major role for renal and leukocyte TxA_2 synthesis in mediating acute as well as chronic CY-A nephrotoxicity in rats.[346] Fish oil-rich diets, TxA_2 antagonists, or administration of CY-A in fish oil as vehicle have all been shown to reduce renal TxA_2 synthesis and afford protection against nephrotoxicity. Moreover, CY-A has been reported to decrease renal COX-2 expression.[347]

Hepatic Cirrhosis and Hepatorenal Syndrome

Patients with cirrhosis of the liver show an increased renal synthesis of vasodilating PGs, as indicated by the high urinary excretion of PGs and/or their metabolites. Urinary excretion of 2–3-dinor 6-keto-$PGF_{1\alpha}$, an index of systemic PGI_2 synthesis, is increased in patients with cirrhosis and hyperdynamic circulation, thus raising the possibility that systemic synthesis of PGI_2 may contribute to the arterial vasodilatation of these patients. Inhibition of cyclooxygenase activity in these patients may cause a profound reduction in renal blood flow and glomerular filtration rate, a reduction in sodium excretion, and an impairment of free water clearance.[348] The sodium-retaining properties of NSAIDs are particularly exaggerated in patients with cirrhosis of the liver, attesting to the dependence of renal salt excretion on vasodilatory PGs. In the kidneys of rats with cirrhosis, COX-2 expression increases while COX-1 expression is unchanged; however, in these animals, selective inhibition of COX-1 leads to impaired renal hemodynamics and natriuresis, whereas COX-2 inhibition has no effect.[349,350]

Diminished renal PG synthesis has been implicated in the pathogenesis of the severe sodium retention seen in hepatorenal syndrome, as well as in the resistance to diuretic therapy.[351,352] There is reduced renal synthesis of vasodilating PGE_2 in the face of activation of endogenous vasoconstrictors and a maintained or increased renal production of thromboxane A_2.[348,353] Therefore, an imbalance between vasoconstricting systems and the renal vasodilator PGE_2 has been proposed as a contributing factor to the renal failure observed in this condition. However, administration of exogenous prostanoids to patients with cirrhosis is not effective either in ameliorating renal function or in preventing the deleterious effect of NSAIDs.[348]

Diabetes Mellitus

In the streptozotocin-induced model of diabetes in rats, COX-2 expression is increased in the cTALH/macula densa region.[313,357] COX-2 immunoreactivity has also been detected in the macula densa region in human diabetic nephropathy.[354] Studies suggest that vasodilator prostanoids, PGI_2 and PGE_2, play an important role in the hyperfiltration seen early in diabetes mellitus.[355] In streptozotocin-induced diabetes in rats, previous studies indicated that non-selective cyclooxygenase inhibitors acutely decrease hyperfiltration in diabetes and inhibit proteinuria and/or structural injury,[356] and more recent studies have also indicated that acute administration of a selective COX-2 inhibitor decreased hyperfiltration.[313] Chronic administration of a selective COX-2 inhibitor significantly decreased proteinuria and reduced extracellular matrix deposition, as indicated by decreases in immunoreactive fibronectin expression and in mesangial matrix expansion. In addition, COX-2 inhibition reduced expression of TGF-β, PAI-1, and VEGF in the kidneys of the diabetic hypertensive animals.[357] The vasoconstrictor thromboxane A_2 may play a role in the development of albuminuria and basement membrane changes with diabetic nephropathy. In addition, administration of a selective PGE_2 EP1 receptor antagonist prevented development of experimental diabetic nephropathy.[358] In contrast to the proposed detrimental effects of these "vasoconstrictor" prostanoids, administration of a prostacyclin analog decreased hyperfiltration and reduced macrophage infiltration in early diabetic nephropathy by increasing eNOS expression in afferent arterioles and glomerular capillaries.[359]

Pregnancy

Most, but not all, investigators do not report increases in vasodilator PG synthesis or suggest an essential role for prostanoids in the mediation of the increased GFR and RPF of normal pregnancy[360]; however, diminished synthesis of PGI_2 has been demonstrated in humans and in animal models of pregnancy-induced hypertension.[361] In the latter, inhibition of TxA_2 synthetase has been associated with resolution of the hypertension, suggesting a possible pathophysiologic role.[362] A moderate beneficial effect of reducing TxA_2 generation, while preserving PGI_2 synthesis, by low dose (60–100 mg/day) aspirin therapy has been demonstrated in patients at high risk for pregnancy-induced hypertension and pre-eclampsia.[363,364]

THE LIPOXYGENASE PATHWAY

The lipoxygenase enzymes metabolize arachidonic acid to form leukotrienes (LTs), hydroxyeicosatetraenoic acids (HETEs), and lipoxins (LXs) (Fig. 11–13). These lipoxygenase metabolites are primarily produced by leukocytes, mast cells, and macrophages in response to inflammation and injury. There are three lipoxygenase enzymes, 5-, 12-, and 15-lipoxygenase, so named for the carbon of arachidonic acid where they insert an oxygen. The lipoxygenases are products of separate genes and have distinct distributions and patterns of regulation. Glomeruli, mesangial cells, cortical tubules, and vessels also produce the 12-lipoxygenase (12-LOX) product, 12(S)-HETE and the 15-LOX product, 15-HETE. Recent studies have localized 15-LO mRNA primarily to the distal nephron, and 12-LO mRNA to the glomerulus. 5-LO mRNA and 5-Lipoxygenase Activating Protein (FLAP) mRNA were expressed in the glomerulus and the vasa recta.[365] In polymorphonuclear leukocytes (PMNs) macrophages and mast cells, 5-lipoxygenase (5-LO) mediates the formation of leukotrienes.[366] 5-LO, which is regulated by FLAP, catalyzes the conversion of arachidonic acid to 5-HpETE and then to leukotriene A_4 (LTA$_4$).[367] LTA$_4$ is then further metabolized to either the peptidyl-leukotrienes (LTC$_4$ and LTD$_4$) by glutathione-S-transferase or to LTB$_4$ by LTA$_4$ hydrolase. Although glutathione-S-transferase expression is limited to inflammatory cells, LTA$_4$ hydrolase is also expressed in glomerular mesangial cells and endothelial cells[368]; PCR analysis has actually demonstrated ubiquitous LTA$_4$ hydrolase mRNA expression throughout the rat nephron.[365] Leukotriene C4 synthase mRNA could not be found in any nephron segment.[365]

Recently two cysteinyl leukotriene receptors (CysLTR) have been cloned and have been identified as members of the G protein coupled superfamily of receptors. They have been localized to vascular smooth muscle and endothelium of the pulmonary vasculature.[369–371] In the kidney the cysteinyl leukotriene receptor type 1 is expressed in the glomerulus, whereas cysteinyl receptor type 2 mRNA has not been detected in any nephron segment to date.[365]

The peptidyl-leukotrienes are potent mediators of inflammation and vasoconstrictors of vascular, pulmonary, and gastrointestinal smooth muscle. In addition, they increase vascular permeability and promote mucus secretion.[372] Because of the central role that peptidyl-leukotrienes play in the inflammatory trigger of asthma exacerbation, effective receptor antagonists have been developed and are now an important component of management of asthma.[373]

In the kidney, LTD$_4$ administration has been shown to decrease renal blood flow and GFR, and peptidyl leukotrienes are thought to be mediators of decreased RBF and GFR associated with acute glomerular inflammation. Micropuncture studies revealed that the decreases in GFR are the result of both afferent and arteriolar vasoconstriction, with more pronounced efferent vasoconstriction and a decrease in K$_f$.

In addition both LTC$_4$ and LTD$_4$ increase proliferation of cultured mesangial cells. The LTB$_4$ receptor is also a seven-transmembrane G protein coupled receptor. On PMNs, receptor activation promotes chemotaxis, aggregation and attachment to endothelium. In the kidney LTB$_4$ mRNA is localized to the glomerulus.[365] A second, low affinity LTB4 receptor is also expressed,[374] which may mediate calcium influx into PMNs, thereby leading to activation. LTB$_4$ receptor blockers lessen acute renal ischemic-reperfusion injury[375] and nephrotoxic nephritis in rats,[376] and PMN infiltration and structural and functional evidence of organ injury by ischemia/reperfusion are magnified in transgenic mice overexpressing the LTB$_4$ receptor.[377] In addition to activation of cell surface receptors, LTB$_4$ has also been shown to be a ligand for the nuclear receptor PPARα.[378]

15-lipoxygenase (15-LO) leads to the formation of 15-S-HETE. In addition, dual oxygenation in activated PMNs and macrophages by 5- and 15-LO leads to formation of the lipoxins. LX synthesis also can occur via transcellular metabolism of the leukocyte-generated intermediate, LTA$_4$, by 12-LO in platelets or adjoining cells including glomerular endothelial cells.[379,380]

15-S-HETE is a potent vasoconstrictor in the renal microcirculation[381]; however, 15-LO-derived metabolites

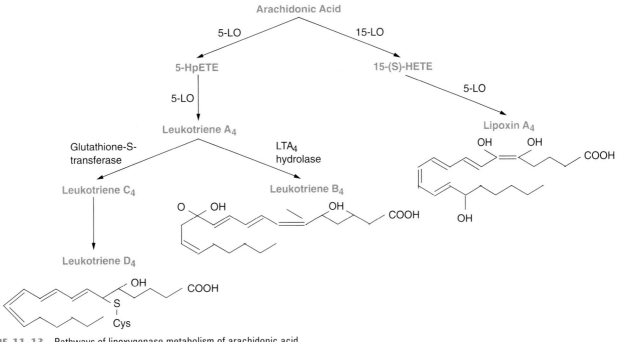

FIGURE 11–13 Pathways of lipoxygenase metabolism of arachidonic acid.

antagonize proinflammatory actions of leukotrienes, both by inhibiting PMN chemotaxis, aggregation, and adherence and by counteracting the vasoconstrictive effects of the peptidyl-leukotrienes.[382,383] Administration of 15-S-HETE reduced LTB_4 production by glomeruli isolated from rats with acute nephrotoxic serum-induced glomerulonephritis, and it has been proposed that 15-LO may regulate 5-LO activity in chronic glomerular inflammation because it is known that in experimental glomerulonephritis, lipoxin A_4 (LXA_4) administration increased renal blood flow and GFR in large part by inducing afferent arteriolar vasodilation, an effect mediated in part by release of vasodilator prostaglandins. LXA_4 also antagonized the effects of LTD_4 to decrease GFR, although not renal blood flow, even though administration of LXA_4 and LXB_4 directly into the renal artery induced vasoconstriction. Glomerular micropuncture studies revealed that LXA_4 led to moderate decreases in K_f.[382] Lipoxins signal through a specific G-protein coupled receptor G protein–coupled receptor denoted ALXR. This receptor is related at the nucleotide sequence level to both chemokine and chemotactic peptide receptors, such as N-formyl peptide receptor.[384] It is also noteworthy that in isolated perfused canine renal arteries and veins, LTC_4 and LTD_4 were found to be vasodilators, which were partially dependent upon an intact endothelium and was mediated by nitric oxide production.[385]

Recently, a potential interaction between cyclooxygenase- and lipoxygenase-mediated pathways has been reported. Whereas aspirin inhibits prostaglandin formation by both COX-1 and COX-2, aspirin-induced acetylation converts COX-2 to a selective generator of 15-R-HETE. This product can then be released, taken up in a transcellular route by PMNs and converted to 15-epi-lipoxins, which have similar biological actions as the lipoxins.[386]

Similar to 15-HETE, 12(S)-HETE also potently vasoconstricts glomerular and renal vasculature.[379] 12(S)-HETE increases protein kinase C and depolarizes cultured vascular smooth muscle cells. Afferent arteriolar vasoconstriction and increases in smooth muscle calcium in response to 12(S)-HETE, were partially inhibited by voltage-gated L-type calcium channel inhibitors.[387] 12(S)-HETE has also been proposed to be an angiogenic factor because in cultured endothelial cells, 12-LO inhibition reduces cell proliferation and 12-LO overexpression stimulates cell migration and endothelial tube formation.[388] 12/15 LO inhibitors and elective elimination of the leukocyte 12-LO enzyme also ameliorate the development of diabetic nephropathy in mice.[389] There is also interaction between 12/15-LO pathways and TGF-β-mediated pathways in the diabetic kidney.[390] 12(S)-HETE has also been proposed to be a mediator of renal vasoconstriction by angiotensin II, with inhibition of the 12-LO pathway attenuating angiotensin II-mediated afferent arteriolar vasoconstriction and decreased renal blood flow.[391] Lipoxygenase inhibition also blunted renal arcuate artery vasoconstriction by norepinephrine and KCl.[392] However, 12-LO products have also been implicated as inhibitors of renal renin release.[393,394]

Although the major significance of LO products in the kidney derives from their release from infiltrating leukocytes or resident cells of macrophage/monocyte origin, there is evidence to suggest that intrinsic renal cells are capable of generating LTs and LXs either directly or through transcellular metabolism of intermediates.[395] Human and rat glomeruli can generate 12- and 15-HETE, though the cells of origin are unclear. LTB_4 can be detected in supernatants of normal rat glomeruli, and its synthesis could be markedly diminished by maneuvers that depleted glomeruli of resident macrophages, such as irradiation or fatty acid deficiency. In addition, 5, 12, and 15-HETEs were detected from pig glomeruli, and their structural identity confirmed by mass spectrometry. 12-LO products are increased in mesangial cells exposed to

hyperglycemia and in diabetic nephropathy.[396] Glomeruli subjected to immune injury release LTB_4,[397] and LTB_4 generation was suppressed by resident macrophage depletion. Synthesis of peptido-LTs by inflamed glomeruli has also been demonstrated,[398] but leukocytes could not be excluded as its primary source LXA_4 is generated by immune-injured glomeruli.[399] Rat mesangial cells generate LXA_4 when provided with LTA_4 as substrate, thereby providing a potential intraglomerular source of LXs during inflammatory reactions. In non-glomerular tissue, 12-HETE production has been reported from rat cortical tubules and epithelial cells and 12- and 15-HETE from rabbit medulla.

Biological Activities of Lipoxygenase Products in the Kidney

In early experiments, systemic administration of LTC_4 in the rat and administration of LTC_4 and LTD_4 in the isolated perfused kidney revealed potent renal vasoconstrictor actions of these eicosanoids. Subsequently, micropuncture measurements revealed that LTD_4 exerts preferential constrictor effects on post-glomerular arteriolar resistance and depresses K_f and GFR. The latter is likely due to receptor-mediated contraction of glomerular mesangial cells, which has been demonstrated for LTC_4 and LTD_4 in vitro (see above). These actions of LTD_4 in the kidney are consistent with its known smooth-muscle contractile properties. LTB_4, a potent chemotactic and leukocyte-activating agent, is devoid of constrictor action in the normal rat kidney. Lipoxin A_4 dilates afferent arterioles when infused into the renal artery, without affecting efferent arteriolar tone. This results in elevations in intraglomerular pressure and plasma flow rate, thereby augmenting GFR.

Involvement of Lipoxygenase Products in Renal Pathophysiology

Increased generation rates of LTC_4 and LTD_4 have been documented in glomeruli from rats with immune complex nephritis and mice with spontaneously developing lupus nephritis.[366,399] Moreover, results from numerous physiologic studies utilizing specific LTD_4 receptor antagonists have provided strong evidence for the release of these eicosanoids during glomerular inflammation. In four animal models of glomerular immune injury (anti-GBM nephritis, anti-Thy1.1 antibody-mediated mesangiolysis, passive Heymann nephritis, and murine lupus nephritis) acute antagonism of LTD_4 by receptor binding competition or inhibition of LTD_4 synthesis led to highly significant increases in GFR in nephritic animals.[400] The principal mechanism underlying the improvement in GFR was reversal of the depressed values of the glomerular ultrafiltration coefficient (K_f), which is characteristically compromised in immune injured glomeruli. In other studies in PHN, Katoh and colleagues provided evidence that endogenous LTD_4 not only mediates reductions in K_f and GFR, but that LTD_4-evoked increases in intraglomerular pressure underlie, to a large extent, the accompanying proteinuria.[400] Cysteinyl-leukotrienes have been implicated in cyclosporine nephrotoxicity.[401] Of interest, 5-lipoxygenase deficiency accelerates renal allograft rejection.[402]

LTB_4 synthesis, measured in the supernates of isolated glomeruli, is markedly enhanced early in the course of several forms of glomerular immune injury.[403] Cellular sources of LTB_4 in injured glomeruli include PMNs and macrophages. All studies concur as to the *transient* nature of LTB_4 release. LTB_4 production decreases 24 hours after onset of the inflammation, which coincides with macrophage infiltration, a major source of 15-LO activity.[404] 15-HPETE incubation decreased lipopolysaccharide-induced tumor necrosis factor (TNF) expression in a human monocytic cell line,[405] and HVJ-liposome-mediated glomerular transfection of 15-LO in rats decreased markers of injury (BUN, proteinuria) and accelerated functional (GFR, renal blood flow) recovery in experimental glomerulonephritis.[406] In addition, MK501, a FLAP antagonist, restored size selectivity and decreased glomerular permeability in acute GN.[407]

The suppression of LTB$_4$ synthesis beyond the first 24 hours of injury is rather surprising, since both PMN and macrophages are capable of effecting the total synthesis of LTB$_4$ (they contain the two necessary enzymes that convert arachidonic acid to LTB$_4$, namely 5-LO and LTA$_4$-hydrolase). It has therefore been suggested, based on in vitro evidence that the major route for LTB$_4$ synthesis in inflamed glomeruli is through transcellular metabolism of leukocyte-generated LTA$_4$ to LTB$_4$ by LTA$_4$-hydrolase present in glomerular mesangial, endothelial, and epithelial cells. Since the transformation of LTA$_4$ to LTB$_4$ is rate-limiting, regulation of LTB$_4$ synthetic rate might relate to regulation of LTA$_4$-hydrolase gene expression or catalytic activity in these parenchymal cells, rather than to the number of infiltrating leukocytes. In any case, leukocytes represent an indispensable source for LTA$_4$, the initial 5-LO product and the precursor for LTB$_4$, since endogenous glomerular cells do not express the 5-LO gene.[408] Thus, it was demonstrated that the polymorphonuclear (PMN) cell-specific activator, N-Formyl-Met-Leu-Phe, stimulated LTB$_4$ production from isolated perfused kidneys harvested from NTS-treated rats to a significantly greater degree than from control animals treated with non-immune rabbit serum.[409] The renal production of LTB$_4$ correlated directly with renal myeloperoxidase activity, suggesting interdependence of LTB$_4$ generation and PMN infiltration.

The acute and long-term significance of LTB$_4$ generation in conditioning the extent of glomerular structural and functional deterioration has been highlighted in studies in which LTB$_4$ was exogenously administered or in which its endogenous synthesis was inhibited. Intrarenal administration of LTB$_4$ to rats with mild NTS-induced injury was associated with an increase in PMN infiltration, reduction in renal plasma flow rate, and marked exacerbation of the fall in glomerular filtration rate, the latter correlating strongly with the number of infiltrating PMNs/glomerulus, while inhibition of 5-lipoxygenase led to preservation of GFR and abrogation of proteinuria.[409] Similarly, both 5-LO knockout mice and wild type mice treated with the 5-LO inhibitor, zileuton, had reduced renal injury in response to ischemia/reperfusion.[410] Thus, while devoid of vasoconstrictor actions in the normal kidney, increased intrarenal generation of LTB$_4$ during early glomerular injury amplifies leukocyte-dependent reductions in glomerular perfusion and filtration rates and inflammatory injury, likely due to enhancement of PMN recruitment/activation.

THE CYTOCHROME P450 PATHWAY

Following their elucidation and characterization as endogenous metabolites of arachidonic acid, numerous studies have investigated the possibility that cytochrome P450 (CYP450) arachidonic acid metabolites subserve physiologic and/or pathophysiologic roles in the kidney (Fig. 11–14). In whole animal physiology, these compounds have been implicated in the mediation of release of peptide hormones, regulation of vascular tone, and regulation of volume homeostasis. On the cellular level, CYP arachidonic acid metabolites have been proposed to regulate ion channels and transporters and to act as mitogens.

CYP450 monooxygenases are mixed-function oxidases that utilize molecular oxygen and NADPH as cofactors[411,412] and will add an oxygen molecule to arachidonic acid in a regio- and stereo-specific geometry. CYP450 monooxygenase pathways metabolize arachidonic acid to generate HETEs and epoxyeicosatrienoic acids (EETs), the latter of which can be hydrolyzed to dihydroxyeicosatrienoic acids

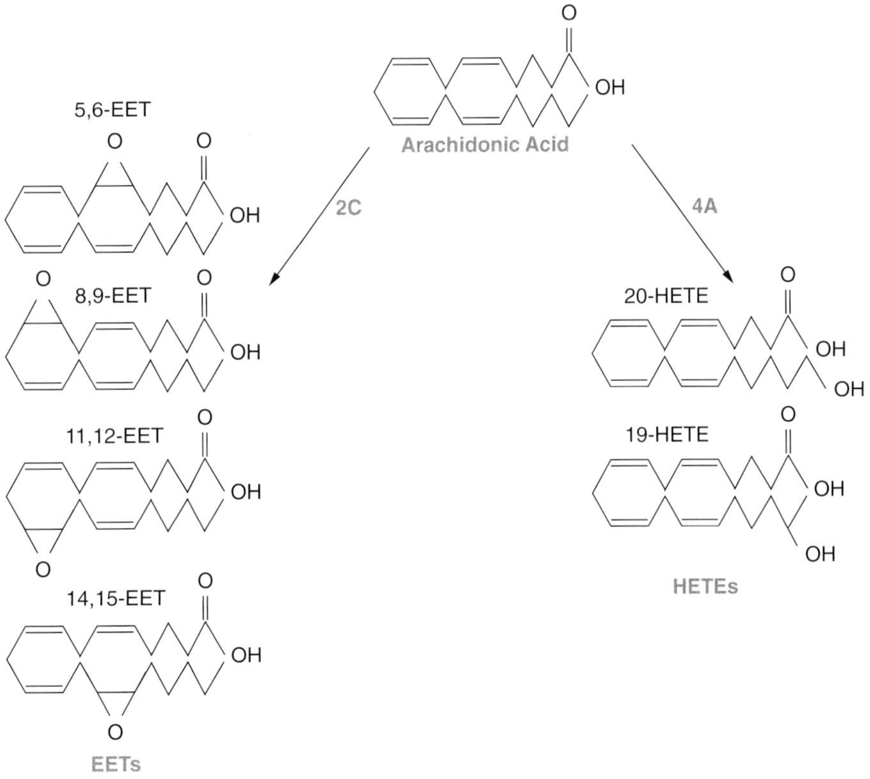

FIGURE 11–14 Pathways of CYP450 metabolism of arachidonic acid.

(DHETs).[411–413] The kidney displays one of the highest CYP450 activities of any organ and produces CYP450 arachidonic acid metabolites in significant amounts.[387,411,414] HETEs are formed primarily via CYP450 hydroxylase enzymes and EETs and DHETs are formed primarily via CYP450 epoxygenase enzymes.[414] The CYP450 4A gene family is the major pathway for synthesis of hydroxylase metabolites, especially 20-HETE and 19-HETE,[413,414] whereas the production of epoxygenase metabolites is primarily via the 2C gene family.[387,411] A member of the 2J family that is an active epoxygenase is also expressed in the kidney.[415] CYP450 enzymes have been localized to both vasculature and tubules.[413] The 4A family of hydroxylases is expressed in preglomerular renal arterioles, glomeruli, proximal tubules, the TALH, and macula densa.[416]

The 2C and 2J families of epoxygenases are expressed at highest levels in proximal tubule and collecting duct.[415,417] When isolated nephron segments expressing CYP450 protein have been incubated with arachidonic acid, production of CYP450 arachidonic acid metabolites can be detected. 20-HETE and EETs are both produced in the afferent arterioles,[418] glomerulus,[419] and proximal tubule.[420] 20-HETE is the predominant CYP450 AA metabolite produced by the TALH and in the pericytes surrounding vasa recta capillaries,[421,422] whereas EETs are the predominant CYP450 AA metabolites produced by the collecting duct.[423]

Renal production of both epoxygenase and hydroxylase metabolites has been shown to be regulated by hormones and growth factors, including angiotensin II, endothelin, bradykinin, parathyroid hormone, and epidermal growth factor.[387,412,413] Alterations in dietary salt intake also modulate CYP450 expression and activity.[424] Alterations in the production of CYP450 metabolites have also been reported with uninephrectomy, diabetes mellitus, and hypertension.[412,413]

Vasculature

20-HETE

In rat and dog renal arteries and afferent arterioles, 20-HETE is a potent vasoconstrictor,[418] whereas it is a vasodilator in rabbit renal arterioles. The vasoconstriction is associated with membrane depolarization and a sustained rise in intracellular calcium. 20-HETE is produced in the smooth muscle cells, and its afferent arteriolar vasoconstrictive effects are mediated by closure of K_{Ca} channels through a tyrosine kinase- and ERK-dependent mechanism (Fig. 11–15).

An interaction between CYP450 arachidonic acid metabolites and nitric oxide has also been demonstrated. NO can inhibit the formation of 20-HETE in renal VSM cells; a significant portion of NO's vasodilator effects in the preglomerular vasculature appear to be mediated by the inhibition of tonic 20-HETE vasoconstriction, and inhibition of 20-HETE formation attenuates the pressor response and fall in renal blood flow seen with NO synthase inhibition.[425,426]

Epoxides

Unlike CYP450 hydroxylase metabolites, epoxygenase metabolites of arachidonic acid increase renal blood flow and glomerular filtration rate.[387,412,413] 11,12-EET and 14,15-EET vasodilate the preglomerular arterioles independently of COX activity, whereas 5,6-EET and 8,9-EET cause COX-dependent vasodilation or vasoconstriction.[427] It is possible that these COX-dependent effects are mediated by COX conversion of 5,6-EET and 8,9-EET to prostaglandin-or thromboxane-like compounds.[428] EETs are produced primarily in the endothelial cells and exert their vasoactive effects on the adjacent smooth muscle cells. In this regard, it has been suggested that EETs, and specifically 11,12-EET, may serve as an endothelium-derived hyperpolarizing factor (EDHF) in the renal microcirculation.[387,429] EET-induced vasodilation is mediated by activation of K_{Ca} channels, through cAMP-dependent stimulation of protein kinase C.

CYP450 metabolites may serve as either second messengers or modulators of the actions of hormonal and paracrine agents. Vasopressin increases renal production of CYP450 metabolites, and increases in intracellular calcium and proliferation in cultured renal mesangial cells are augmented by EET administration.[430] CYP450 metabolites also may serve to modulate the renal hemodynamic responses of endothelin-1, with 20-HETE as a possible mediator of the vasoconstrictive effects and EETs counteracting the vasoconstriction.[431,432] Formation of 20-HETE does not affect the ability of ET-1 to increase free intracellular calcium transients in renal vascular smooth muscle intracellular but appears to enhance the sustained elevations that represent calcium influx through voltage-sensitive channels.

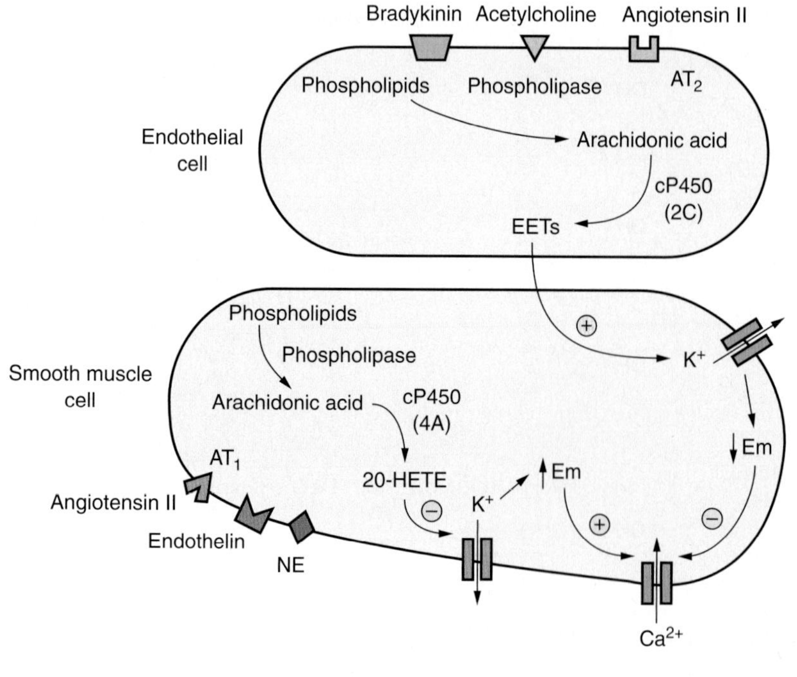

FIGURE 11–15 Proposed interactions of CYP450 arachidonic acid metabolites derived from vascular endothelial cells and smooth muscle cells to regulate vascular tone.

CYP450 metabolites have also been implicated in mediation of renal vascular responses to angiotensin II. In the presence of AT$_1$ receptor blockers, angiotensin II produces an endothelial-dependent vasodilation in rabbit afferent arterioles that is dependent on CYP450 epoxygenase metabolites production by AT$_2$ receptor activation.[433] With intact AT$_1$ receptors, angiotensin II increases 20-HETE release from isolated preglomerular microvessels through an endothelium-independent mechanism.[434] Angiotensin II's vasoconstrictive effects are in part the result of 20-HETE-mediated inhibition of K$_{Ca}$, which enhances sustained increases in intracellular calcium concentration by calcium influx through voltage-sensitive channels. Inhibition of 20-HETE production reduces the vasoconstrictor response to ANG II by >50% in rat renal interlobular arteries in which the endothelium has been removed.[434]

Autoregulation
CYP450 metabolites of AA have been shown to be mediators of renal blood flow autoregulatory mechanisms. When prostaglandin production was blocked in canine arcuate arteries, arachidonic acid administration enhanced myogenic responsiveness, and renal blood flow autoregulation was blocked by CYP450 inhibitors.[387,413] Similarly, in the rat juxtamedullary preparation, selective blockade of 20-HETE formation significantly decreased afferent arteriolar vasoconstrictor responses to elevations in perfusion pressure, and inhibition of epoxygenase activity enhanced vasoconstriction,[435] suggesting that 20-HETE is involved in afferent arteriolar autoregulatory adjustment, whereas release of vasodilatory epoxygenase metabolites in response to increases in renal perfusion pressure acts to attenuate the vasoconstriction. In vivo studies have also implicated 20-HETE as a mediator of the autoregulatory response to increased perfusion pressure.[436] Bradykinin-induced efferent arteriolar vasodilation has been shown to be mediated in part by direct release of EETs from this vascular segment. In addition, bradykinin-induced release of 20-HETE from the glomerulus can modulate the EET-mediated vasodilation.[437]

Tubuloglomerular Feedback
CYP450 metabolites may also be involved in the tubuloglomerular feedback response.[413] As noted, 20-HETE is produced by both the afferent arteriole and macula densa, and studies have suggested the possibility that 20-HETE may either serve as a vasoconstrictive mediator of tubuloglomerular feedback (TGF) released by the macula densa or a second messenger in the afferent arteriole in response to mediators released by the macula densa, such as adenosine or ATP.[438] 20-HETE may also be a mediator of regulation of intrarenal distribution of blood flow.[439,440]

Tubules

20-HETE and EETs both inhibit tubular sodium reabsorption.[412,413] Renal cortical interstitial infusion of the nonselective CYP450 inhibitor 17-ODYA increases papillary blood flow, renal interstitial hydrostatic pressure, and sodium excretion without affecting total renal blood flow or glomerular filtration rate. High dietary salt intake in rats increases expression of the renal epoxygenase 2C23 and production and urinary excretion of EETs, while decreasing 20-HETE production in renal cortex.[411,424] 14,15-EET has also been shown to inhibit renin secretion[441]; furthermore, clotrimazole, which is a relatively selective epoxygenase inhibitor, induced hypertension in rats fed a high salt diet, suggesting a role in regulation of blood pressure.[424]

Proximal Tubule
The proximal tubule contains the highest concentration of CYP450 within the mammalian kidney and expresses minimal cyclooxygenase and lipoxygenase activity. The 4A

CYP450 family of hydroxylases that produce 19- and 20-HETE is highly expressed in mammalian proximal tubule.[271] CYP450 enzymes of both the 2C and 2J family that catalyze the formation of EETs are also expressed in the proximal tubule.[411] Both EETs and 20-HETE have been shown to be produced in the proximal tubule and have been proposed to be modulators of sodium reabsorption in the proximal tubule.

Studies in isolated perfused proximal tubule indicate that 20-HETE inhibits sodium transport whereas 19-HETE stimulates sodium transport, suggesting that 19-HETE may serve as competitive antagonist of 20-HETE.[420,442] Administration of EETs inhibits amiloride-sensitive sodium transport in primary cultures of proximal tubule cells[443] and in LLC-PK1 cells, a non-transformed, immortalized cell line from pig kidney with proximal tubule characteristics.[444,445]

20-HETE has been proposed to be a mediator of hormonal inhibition of proximal tubule reabsorption by PTH, dopamine, angiotensin II, and EGF. Although the mechanisms of 20-HETE's inhibition have not yet been completely elucidated, there is evidence that it can inhibit Na$^+$/K$^+$-ATPase activity by phosphorylation of the Na$^+$/K$^+$-ATPase alpha subunit through a protein kinase C dependent pathway.[446,447]

Epoxyeicosatrienoic acids (EETs) may also serve as second messengers in the proximal tubule for EGF[448] and angiotensin II.[449] In the proximal tubule, angiotensin II has been noted to exert a biphasic response on net sodium uptake via AT1 receptors, with low (10^{-10}–10^{-11}) concentrations stimulating and high (10^{-7}) concentrations inhibiting net uptake.[449] Such high concentrations are not normally seen in plasma but may exist in the proximal tubule lumen as a result of the local production of angiotensin II by proximal tubule.[450] The mechanisms by which CYPP450 AA metabolites modulate proximal tubule reabsorption have not been completely elucidated, and may involve both luminal (NHE3) and basolateral (Na$^+$/K$^+$ATPase) transporters.[443,446] CYP450 arachidonic acid metabolites may modulate the proximal tubule component of the pressure-natriuresis response.[451]

TALH
20-HETE also serves as a second messenger to regulation transport in the thick ascending limb. It is produced in this nephron segment[416] and can inhibit net Na-K-Cl cotransport, by direct inhibition of the transporter and by blocking the 70-pS apical K$^+$ channel.[452,453] In addition, 20-HETE has been implicated as a mediator of the inhibitory effects of angiotensin II[454] and bradykinin[455] on TALH transport.

Collecting Duct
In the collecting duct, EETs and/or their diol metabolites serve as inhibitors of the hydroosmotic effects of vasopressin, as well as inhibitors of sodium transport in this segment.[423,456] The latter effects were specific for 5,6-EET and were blocked by cyclooxygenase inhibitors.[456] Patch clamp studies have indicated that the eNaC sodium channel activity in the cortical collecting duct is inhibited by 11,12-EET.[457]

Role in Mitogenesis

In rat mesangial cells, endogenous non-cyclooxygenase metabolites of arachidonic acid modulate the proliferative responses to phorbol esters, vasopressin, and EGF, and agonist-induced expression of the immediate early response genes c-fos and Egr-1 is inhibited by ketoconazole or nordihydroguaiaretic acid (NDGA), but not specific lipoxygenase inhibitors.[458] EET-mediated increases in rat mesangial cell proliferation was the first direct evidence that CYP450 arachidonic acid metabolites are cellular mitogens.[459] In cultured rabbit proximal tubule cells, CYP450 inhibitors blunted EGF-stimulated proliferation in proximal tubule cells.[448] In LLCPKcl$_4$, EETs were found to be potent mitogens, cytoprotective agents, and second messengers for EGF signaling. 14,15-EET-mediated signaling and mitogenesis are dependent upon EGF receptor transactivation, which is mediated by metalloproteinase-dependent release of HB-EGF.[460] In addition to the EETs, 20-HETE has been shown to increase thymidine incorporation in primary cultures of rat proximal tubule and LLC-PK1 cells[461] and vascular smooth muscle cells.[462]

Role in Hypertension

There is increasing evidence that the renal production of CYP450 AA metabolites is altered in a variety of models of hypertension and that blockade of the formation of compounds can alter blood pressure in several of these models. CYP450 AA metabolites may have both pro- and antihypertensive properties. At the level of the renal tubule, both 20-HETE and EETs inhibit sodium transport. However, in the vasculature, 20-HETE promotes vasoconstriction and hypertension, whereas EETs are endothelial-derived vasodilators that have antihypertensive properties. Rats fed a high salt diet increase expression of the CYP450 epoxygenase 2C23[463] and develop hypertension if treated with a relatively selective epoxygenase inhibitor. Because EETs have antihypertensive properties, efforts are underway to develop selective inhibitors of soluble epoxide hydrolase (sEH), which converts active EETs to their inactive metabolites, DHETs, and thereby increase EET levels. Studies in rats indicated that one such sEH inhibitor, 1-cyclohexyl-3-dodecylurea, lowered blood pressure and reduced glomerular and tubulointerstitial injury in an angiotensin II-mediated model of hypertension in rats.[464]

In DOCA/salt hypertension, administration of a CYP450 inhibitor prevented the development of hypertension.[465,466] Angiotensin II stimulates the formation of 20-HETE in the renal circulation,[467] and 20-HETE synthesis inhibition attenuates angiotensin II mediated renal vasoconstriction[434] and reduced angiotensin II-mediated hypertension.[466]

The CYP450 4A2 gene is regulated by salt and is overexpressed in spontaneously hypertensive rats (SHR),[468] and production of both 20HETE and diHETEs is increased and production of EETs is reduced.[271,469] CYP450 inhibitors or antisense oligonucleotides directed against CYP4A1 and 4A2 lowered blood pressure in SHR.[470,471] Conversely, recent studies in humans have indicated that a variant of the human CYP4A11 with reduced 20-HETE synthase activity is associated with hypertension.[472]

In Dahl salt sensitive rats (Dahl S), pressure-natriuresis in response to salt loading is shifted such that the kidney requires a higher perfusion pressure to excrete the same amount of sodium as normotensive salt resistant (Dahl R) rats,[411-413] which is due at least in part to increased TALH reabsorption. The production of 20-HETE and expression of CYP4A protein are reduced in the outer medulla and TALH of Dahl S rats relative to Dahl R, which is consistent with the observed effect of 20-HETE to inhibit TALH transport. In addition, Dahl S rats do not increase EET production in response to salt loading.

Studies have indicated that angiotensin II acts on AT_2 receptors on renal vascular endothelial cells to release EETs that may then counteract AT_1-induced renal vasoconstriction and may influence pressure natriuresis.[427,473,474] AT_2 receptor knockout mice develop hypertension,[475] which is associated with blunted pressure natriuresis, reduced renal blood flow, and glomerular filtration rate and defects in kidney 20-HETE production.[475]

ACKNOWLEDGMENTS

The writing of this chapter was supported by grants from the Veterans Administration and National Institute of Diabetes and Digestive and Kidney Diseases (NIDDK) to RCH (DK39261 and DK62794) and MDB (DK37097 and DK39261).

References

1. Harris RC, Breyer MD: Arachidonic acid metabolites and the kidney. *In* Brenner BM (ed): The Kidney. Philadelphia, W.B. Saunders, 2004, pp 727–776.
2. Murakami M, Kudo I: Phospholipase A2. J Biochem (Tokyo) 131:285–292, 2002.
3. Boulven I, Palmier B, Robin P, et al: Platelet-derived growth factor stimulates phospholipase C-gamma 1, extracellular signal-regulated kinase, and arachidonic acid release in rat myometrial cells: Contribution to cyclic 3′,5′-adenosine monophosphate production and effect on cell proliferation. Biol Reprod 65:496–506, 2001.
4. Fujishima H, Sanchez Mejia RO, Bingham CO, 3rd, et al: Cytosolic phospholipase A2 is essential for both the immediate and the delayed phases of eicosanoid generation in mouse bone marrow-derived mast cells. Proc Natl Acad Sci U S A 96:4803–4807, 1999.
5. Balsinde J, Winstead MV, Dennis EA: Phospholipase A(2) regulation of arachidonic acid mobilization. FEBS Lett 531:2–6, 2002.
6. Murakami M, Yoshihara K, Shimbara S, et al: Cellular arachidonate-releasing function and inflammation-associated expression of group IIF secretory phospholipase A2. J Biol Chem 277:19145–19155, 2002.
7. Smith WL, Langenbach R: Why there are two cyclooxygenase isozymes. J Clin Invest 107:1491–1495, 2001.
8. Fitzpatrick FA, Soberman R: Regulated formation of eicosanoids. J Clin Invest 107:1347–1351, 2001.
9. FitzGerald GA, Patrono C: The coxibs, selective inhibitors of cyclooxygenase-2. N Engl J Med 345:433–442, 2001.
10. Bonazzi A, Mastyugin V, Mieyal PA, et al: Regulation of cyclooxygenase-2 by hypoxia and peroxisome proliferators in the corneal epithelium. J Biol Chem 275:2837–2844, 2000.
11. Hayama M, Inoue R, Akiba S, et al: ERK and p38 MAP kinase are involved in arachidonic acid release induced by H(2)O(2) and PDGF in mesangial cells. Am J Physiol Renal Physiol 282:F485–491, 2002.
12. Basavappa S, Pedersen SF, Jorgensen NK, et al: Swelling-induced arachidonic acid release via the 85-kDa cPLA2 in human neuroblastoma cells. J Neurophysiol 79:1441–1449, 1998.
13. ω-3 fatty acids are those in which the double-bond is three carbons from the terminal (omega) carbon, i.e. that furthest from the carboxy-group atom. AA is thus an n-6 fatty acid)
14. Hansen RA, Ogilvie GK, Davenport DJ, et al: Duration of effects of dietary fish oil supplementation on serum eicosapentaenoic acid and docosahexaenoic acid concentrations in dogs. Am J Vet Res 59:864–868, 1998.
15. Grande JP, Donadio JV, Jr: Dietary fish oil supplementation in IgA nephropathy: a therapy in search of a mechanism? Nutrition 14:240–242, 1998.
16. Kujubu DA, Fletcher BS, Varnum BC, et al: TIS10, a phorbol ester tumor promoter-inducible mRNA from Swiss 3T3 cells, encodes a novel prostaglandin synthase/cyclooxygenase homologue. J Biol Chem 266:12866–12872, 1991.
17. O'Banion M, Winn V, Young D: cDNA cloning and functional activity of a glucocorticoid-regulated inflammatory cyclooxygenase. Proc Natl Acad Sci U S A 89:4888–4892, 1992.
18. Jang BC, Munoz-Najar U, Paik JH, et al: Leptomycin B, an inhibitor of the nuclear export receptor CRM1, inhibits COX-2 expression. J Biol Chem 31:2773–2776, 2003.
19. Dixon DA, Tolley ND, King PH, et al: Altered expression of the mRNA stability factor HuR promotes cyclooxygenase-2 expression in colon cancer cells. J Clin Invest 108:1657–1665, 2001.
20. Inoue H, Taba Y, Miwa Y, et al: Transcriptional and posttranscriptional regulation of cyclooxygenase-2 expression by fluid shear stress in vascular endothelial cells. Arterioscler Thromb Vasc Biol 22:1415–1420, 2002.
21. Hla T, Bishop-Bailey D, Liu CH, et al: Cyclooxygenase-1 and -2 isoenzymes. Int J Biochem Cell Biol 31:551–557, 1999.
22. Mestre JR, Mackrell PJ, Rivadeneira DE, et al: Redundancy in the signaling pathways and promoter elements regulating cyclooxygenase-2 gene expression in endotoxin-treated macrophage/monocytic cells. J Biol Chem 276:3977–3982, 2001.
23. Tanabe T, Tohnai N: Cyclooxygenase isozymes and their gene structures and expression. Prostaglandins Other Lipid Mediat 68–69:95–114, 2002.
24. Inoue H, Tanabe T: Transcriptional role of the nuclear factor kappa B site in the induction by lipopolysaccharide and suppression by dexamethasone of cyclooxygenase-2 in U937 cells. Biochem Biophys Res Commun 244:143–148, 1998.
25. Dixon DA, Kaplan CD, McIntyre TM, et al: Post-transcriptional control of cyclooxygenase-2 gene expression. The role of the 3′-untranslated region. J Biol Chem 275:11750–11757, 2000.
26. Vezza R, Mezzasoma AM, Venditti G, et al: Prostaglandin endoperoxides and thromboxane A2 activate the same receptor isoforms in human platelets. Thromb Haemost 87:114–121, 2002.
27. Garavito MR, Malkowski MG, DeWitt DL: The structures of prostaglandin endoperoxide H synthases-1 and -2. Prostaglandins Other Lipid Mediat 68–69:129–152, 2002.
28. Kalgutkar AS, Crews BC, Rowlinson SW, et al: Aspirin-like molecules that covalently inactivate cyclooxygenase-2. Science 280:1268–1270, 1998.
29. Yu Y, Fan J, Chen X-S, et al: Genetic model of selective COX2 inhibition reveals novel heterodimer signaling. Nat Med 12:699–704, 2006.
30. Crofford LJ: Specific cyclooxygenase-2 inhibitors: what have we learned since they came into widespread clinical use? Curr Opin Rheumatol 14:225–230, 2002.
31. Li S, Ballou LR, Morham SG, et al: Cyclooxygenase-2 mediates the febrile response of mice to interleukin-1beta. Brain Res 910:163–173., 2001.

32. Turini ME, DuBois RN: Cyclooxygenase-2: A therapeutic target. Annu Rev Med 53:35–57, 2002.

33. Pasinetti GM: From epidemiology to therapeutic trials with anti-inflammatory drugs in Alzheimer's disease: The role of NSAIDs and cyclooxygenase in beta-amyloidosis and clinical dementia. J Alzheimers Dis 4:435–445, 2002.

34. Harris RC, McKanna JA, Akai Y, et al: Cyclooxygenase-2 is associated with the macula densa of rat kidney and increases with salt restriction. J Clin Invest 94:2504–2510, 1994.

35. Zhang M-Z, Lopez-Sanchez P, McKanna JA, Harris RC: Regulation of cyclooxygenase expression by vasopressin in renal medulla. Endocrinology 145:1402–1409, 2004.

36. Guan Y, Chang M, Cho W, et al: Cloning, expression, and regulation of rabbit cyclooxygenase-2 in renal medullary interstitial cells. Am J Physiol 273:F18–26, 1997.

37. Yang T, Schnermann JB, Briggs JP: Regulation of cyclooxygenase-2 expression in renal medulla by tonicity in vivo and in vitro. Am J Physiol 277:F1–9, 1999.

38. Nantel F, Meadows E, Denis D, et al: Immunolocalization of cyclooxygenase-2 in the macula densa of human elderly. FEBS Lett 457:475–477, 1999.

39. Adegboyega PA, Ololade O: Immunohistochemical expression of cyclooxygenase-2 in normal kidneys. Appl Immunohistochem Mol Morphol 12:71–74, 2004.

40. Khan KN, Stanfield KM, Harris RK, et al: Expression of cyclooxygenase-2 in the macula densa of human kidney in hypertension, congestive heart failure, and diabetic nephropathy. Ren Fail 23:321–330, 2001.

41. Komhoff M, Jeck ND, Seyberth HW, et al: Cyclooxygenase-2 expression is associated with the renal macula densa of patients with Bartter-like syndrome. Kidney Int 58:2420–2424, 2000.

42. Schnermann J: Juxtaglomerular cell complex in the regulation of renal salt excretion. Am J Physiol 274:R263–279, 1998.

43. Schnermann J, Traynor T, Pohl H, et al: Vasoconstrictor responses in thromboxane receptor knockout mice: Tubuloglomerular feedback and ureteral obstruction. Acta Physiol Scand 168:201–207, 2000.

44. Qi Z, Hao CM, Langenbach RI, et al: Opposite effects of cyclooxygenase-1 and -2 activity on the pressor response to angiotensin II. J Clin Invest 110:61–69, 2002.

45. Ichihara A, Imig JD, Inscho EW, et al: Cyclooxygenase-2 participates in tubular flow-dependent afferent arteriolar tone: Interaction with neuronal NOS. Am J Physiol 275:F605–612, 1998.

46. Perazella MA, Tray K: Selective cyclooxygenase-2 inhibitors: A pattern of nephrotoxicity similar to traditional nonsteroidal anti-inflammatory drugs. Am J Med 111:64–67, 2001.

47. Peti-Peterdi J, Komlosi P, Fuson AL, et al: Luminal NaCl delivery regulates basolateral PGE2 release from macula densa cells. J Clin Invest 112:76–82, 2003.

48. Cheng HF, Wang JL, Zhang MZ, et al: Role of p38 in the regulation of renal cortical cyclooxygenase-2 expression by extracellular chloride [see comments]. J Clin Invest 106:681–688, 2000.

49. Yang T, Park JM, Arend L, et al: Low chloride stimulation of prostaglandin E2 release and cyclooxygenase- 2 expression in a mouse macula densa cell line. J Biol Chem 275:37922–37929, 2000.

50. Zhang MZ, Yao B, McKanna JA, et al: Cross talk between the intrarenal dopaminergic and cyclooxygenase-2 systems. Am J Physiol Renal Physiol 288:F840–845, 2005.

51. Schnermann J: Juxtaglomerular cell complex in the regulation of renal salt excretion. Am J Physiol 274:R263–279, 1998.

52. Cheng HF, Wang JL, Zhang MZ, et al: Angiotensin II attenuates renal cortical cyclooxygenase-2 expression. J Clin Invest 103:953–961, 1999.

53. Harding P, Sigmon DH, Alfie ME, et al: Cyclooxygenase-2 mediates increased renal renin content induced by low-sodium diet. Hypertension 29:297–302, 1997.

54. Stichtenoth DO, Marhauer V, Tsikas D, et al: Effects of specific COX-2-inhibition on renin release and renal and systemic prostanoid synthesis in healthy volunteers. Kidney Int 68:2197–2207, 2005.

55. Harris RC, Breyer MD: Physiological regulation of cyclooxygenase-2 in the kidney. Am J Physiol Renal Physiol 281:F1–11, 2001.

56. Traynor TR, Smart A, Briggs JP, et al: Inhibition of macula densa-stimulated renin secretion by pharmacological blockade of cyclooxygenase-2. Am J Physiol 277:F706–710, 1999.

57. Cheng HF, Wang JL, Zhang MZ, et al: Genetic deletion of COX-2 prevents increased renin expression in response to ACE inhibition. Am J Physiol Renal Physiol 280:F449–456, 2001.

58. Yang T, Endo Y, Huang YG, et al: Renin expression in COX-2-knockout mice on normal or low-salt diets. Am J Physiol Renal Physiol 279:F819–825, 2000.

59. Cheng HF, Wang SW, Zhang MZ, et al: Prostaglandins that increase renin production in response to ACE inhibition are not derived from cyclooxygenase-1. Am J Physiol Regul Integr Comp Physiol 283:R638–646, 2002.

60. Athirakul K, Kim HS, Audoly LP, et al: Deficiency of COX-1 causes natriuresis and enhanced sensitivity to ACE inhibition. Kidney Int 60:2324–2329, 2001.

61. Wang JL, Cheng HF, Harris RC: Cyclooxygenase-2 inhibition decreases renin content and lowers blood pressure in a model of renovascular hypertension. Hypertension 34:96–101, 1999.

62. Fujino T, Nakagawa N, Yuhki K, et al: Decreased susceptibility to renovascular hypertension in mice lacking the prostaglandin I2 receptor IP. J Clin Invest 114:805–812, 2004.

63. Hao CM, Yull F, Blackwell T, et al: Dehydration activates an NF-kappaB-driven, COX2-dependent survival mechanism in renal medullary interstitial cells. J Clin Invest 106:973–982, 2000.

64. Khan KN, Stanfield KM, Trajkovic D, et al: Expression of cyclooxygenase-2 in canine renal cell carcinoma. Vet Pathol 38:116–119, 2001.

65. Bishop-Bailey D, Calatayud S, Warner TD, et al: Prostaglandins and the regulation of tumor growth. J Environ Pathol Toxicol Oncol 21:93–101, 2002.

66. Toyota M, Shen L, Ohe-Toyota M, et al: Aberrant methylation of the Cyclooxygenase 2 CpG island in colorectal tumors. Cancer Res 60:4044–4048, 2000.

67. Ichitani Y, Holmberg K, Maunsbach AB, et al: Cyclooxygenase-1 and cyclooxygenase-2 expression in rat kidney and adrenal gland after stimulation with systemic lipopolysaccharide: In situ hybridization and immunocytochemical studies. Cell Tissue Res 303:235–252, 2001.

68. Yang T, Huang Y, Heasley LE, et al: MAPK mediation of hypertonicity-stimulated cyclooxygenase-2 expression in renal medullary collecting duct cells [In Process Citation]. J Biol Chem 275:23281–23286, 2000.

69. Rocca B, Secchiero P, Ciabattoni G, et al: Cyclooxygenase-2 expression is induced during human megakaryopoiesis and characterizes newly formed platelets. Proc Natl Acad Sci U S A 99:7634–7639, 2002.

70. Taniura S, Kamitani H, Watanabe T, et al: Transcriptional regulation of cyclooxygenase-1 by histone deacetylase inhibitors in normal human astrocyte cells. J Biol Chem 277:16823–16830, 2002.

71. Brater DC: Effects of nonsteroidal anti-inflammatory drugs on renal function: Focus on cyclooxygenase-2-selective inhibition. Am J Med 107:65S–70S; discussion 70S–71S, 1999.

72. Catella-Lawson F, McAdam B, Morrison BW, et al: Effects of specific inhibition of cyclooxygenase-2 on sodium balance, hemodynamics, and vasoactive eicosanoids. J Pharmacol Exp Ther 289:735–741, 1999.

73. Whelton A, Fort JG, Puma JA, et al: Cyclooxygenase-2–specific inhibitors and cardiorenal function: A randomized, controlled trial of celecoxib and rofecoxib in older hypertensive osteoarthritis patients. Am J Ther 8:85–95, 2001.

74. Swan SK, Rudy DW, Lasseter KC, et al: Effect of cyclooxygenase-2 inhibition on renal function in elderly persons receiving a low-salt diet. A randomized, controlled trial. Ann Intern Med 133:1–9, 2000.

75. Rossat J, Maillard M, Nussberger J, et al: Renal effects of selective cyclooxygenase-2 inhibition in normotensive salt-depleted subjects. Clin Pharmacol Ther 66:76–84, 1999.

76. Stokes JB: Effect of prostaglandin E2 on chloride transport across the rabbit thick ascending limb of Henle. J Clin Invest 64:495–502, 1979.

77. Whelton A, Schulman G, Wallemark C, et al: Effects of celecoxib and naproxen on renal function in the elderly. Arch Intern Med 160:1465–1470, 2000.

78. Muscara MN, Vergnolle N, Lovren F, et al: Selective cyclo-oxygenase-2 inhibition with celecoxib elevates blood pressure and promotes leukocyte adherence. Br J Pharmacol 129:1423–1430, 2000.

79. Atta MG, Whelton A: Acute renal papillary necrosis induced by ibuprofen. Am J Ther 4:55–60, 1997.

80. DeBroe M, Elseviers M: Analgesic nephropathy. N Engl J Med 338:446–452, 1998.

81. Segasothy M, Samad S, Zulfigar A, et al: Chronic renal disease and papillary necrosis associated with the long-term use of nonstroidal anti-inflammatory drugs as the sole or predominant analgesic. Am J Kidney Dis 24:17–24, 1994.

82. Black HE: Renal toxicity of non-steroidal anti-inflammatory drugs. Toxicol Pathol 14:83–90, 1986.

83. Hao CM, Redha R, Morrow J, et al: Peroxisome proliferator-activated receptor delta activation promotes cell survival following hypertonic stress. J Biol Chem 277:21341–21345, 2002.

84. Akhund L, Quinet RJ, Ishaq S: Celecoxib-related renal papillary necrosis. Arch Intern Med 163:114–115, 2003.

85. Ahmad SR, Kortepeter C, Brinker A, et al: Renal failure associated with the use of celecoxib and rofecoxib. Drug Saf 25:537–544, 2002.

86. Kleinknecht D: Interstitial nephritis, the nephrotic syndrome, and chronic renal failure secondary to nonsteroidal anti-inflammatory drugs. Semin Nephrol 15:228–235, 1995.

87. Henao J, Hisamuddin I, Nzerue CM, et al: Celecoxib-induced acute interstitial nephritis. Am J Kidney Dis 39:1313–1317, 2002.

88. Alper AB, Jr., Meleg-Smith S, Krane NK: Nephrotic syndrome and interstitial nephritis associated with celecoxib. Am J Kidney Dis 40:1086–1090, 2002.

89. Tietjen DP: Recurrence and specificity of nephrotic syndrome due to tolmetin. Am J Med 87:354–355, 1989.

90. Radford MG, Jr., Holley KE, Grande JP, et al: Reversible membranous nephropathy associated with the use of nonsteroidal anti-inflammatory drugs. JAMA 276:466–469, 1996.

91. Peruzzi L, Gianoglio B, Porcellini MG, et al: Neonatal end-stage renal failure associated with maternal ingestion of cyclo-oxygenase-type-2 selective inhibitor nimesulide as tocolytic [letter; comment]. Lancet 354:1615, 1999.

92. Komhoff M, Wang JL, Cheng HF, et al: Cyclooxygenase-2-selective inhibitors impair glomerulogenesis and renal cortical development. Kidney Int 57:414–422, 2000.

93. Dinchuk JE, Car BD, Focht RJ, et al: Renal abnormalities and an altered inflammatory response in mice lacking cyclooxygenase II. Nature 378:406–409, 1995.

94. Morham SG, Langenbach R, Loftin CD, et al: Prostaglandin synthase 2 gene disruption causes severe renal pathology in the mouse. Cell 83:473–482, 1995.

95. Langenbach R, Morham SG, Tiano HF, et al: Prostaglandin synthase 1 gene disruption in mice reduces arachidonic acid-induced inflammation and indomethacin-induced gastric ulceration. Cell 83:483–492, 1995.

96. Zhang MZ, Wang JL, Cheng HF, et al: Cyclooxygenase-2 in rat nephron development. Am J Physiol 273:F994–1002, 1997.

97. Avner ED, Sweeney WE, Jr, Piesco NP, et al: Growth factor requirements of organogenesis in serum-free metanephric organ culture. In Vitro Cell Dev Biol 21:297–304, 1985.

98. Sugimoto Y, Narumiya S, Ichikawa A: Distribution and function of prostanoid receptors: Studies from knockout mice. Prog Lipid Res 39:289–314, 2000.

99. Bagi Z, Erdei N, Toth A, et al: Type 2 diabetic mice have increased arteriolar tone and blood pressure: enhanced release of COX-2 derived constrictor prostaglandins. Arterioscler Thromb Vasc Biol 25:1610–1616, 2005.

100. McAdam BF, Catella-Lawson F, Mardini IA, et al: Systemic biosynthesis of prostacyclin by cyclooxygenase (COX)-2: The human pharmacology of a selective inhibitor of COX-2. Proc Natl Acad Sci U S A 96:272–277, 1999.

101. Fitzgerald GA: Coxibs and cardiovascular disease. N Engl J Med 351:1709–1711, 2004.

102. Bea F, Blessing E, Bennett BJ, et al: Chronic inhibition of cyclooxygenase-2 does not alter plaque composition in a mouse model of advanced unstable atherosclerosis. Cardiovasc Res 60:198–204, 2003.

103. Pratico D, Tillmann C, Zhang ZB, et al: Acceleration of atherogenesis by COX-1-dependent prostanoid formation in low density lipoprotein receptor knockout mice. Proc Natl Acad Sci U S A 98:3358–3363, 2001.

104. Burleigh ME, Babaev VR, Oates JA, et al: Cyclooxygenase-2 promotes early athero-sclerotic lesion formation in LDL receptor-deficient mice. Circulation 105:1816–1823, 2002.

105. Belton OA, Duffy A, Toomey S, et al: Cyclooxygenase isoforms and platelet vessel wall interactions in the apolipoprotein E knockout mouse model of atherosclerosis. Circulation 108:3017–3023, 2003.

106. Burleigh ME, Babaev VR, Yancey PG, et al: Cyclooxygenase-2 promotes early athero sclerotic lesion formation in ApoE-deficient and C57BL/6 mice. J Mol Cell Cardiol 39:443–452, 2005.

107. Egan KM, Wang M, Fries S, et al: Cyclooxygenases, thromboxane, and atherosclerosis: Plaque destabilization by cyclooxygenase-2 inhibition combined with thromboxane receptor antagonism. Circulation 111:334–342, 2005.

108. Hansson GK: Inflammation, atherosclerosis and coronary artery disease. N Engl J Med 352:1685–1695, 2005.

109. Okahara K, Sun B, Kambayashi J: Upregulation of prostacyclin synthesis-related gene expression by shear stress in vascular endothelial cells. Arterioscler Thromb Vasc Biol 18:1922–1926, 1998.

110. Guan Z, Buckman SY, Miller BW, et al: Interleukin-1beta-induced cyclooxygenase-2 expression requires activation of both c-Jun NH2-terminal kinase and p38 MAPK signal pathways in rat renal mesangial cells. J Biol Chem 273:28670–28676, 1998.

111. Soler M, Camacho M, Sola R, et al: Mesangial cells release untransformed prostaglan-din H2 as a major prostanoid. Kidney Int 59:1283–1289, 2001.

112. Guan Y, Zhang Y, Schneider A, et al: Urogenital distribution of a mouse membrane-associated prostaglandin E(2) synthase. Am J Physiol Renal Physiol 281:F1173–1177, 2001.

113. Hao CM, Komhoff M, Guan Y, et al: Selective targeting of cyclooxygenase-2 reveals its role in renal medullary interstitial cell survival. Am J Physiol 277:F352–359, 1999.

114. Chevalier D, Lo-Guidice JM, Sergent E, et al: Identification of genetic variants in the human thromboxane synthase gene (CYP5A1). Mutat Res 432:61–67, 2001.

115. Nusing R, Fehr PM, Gudat F, et al: The localization of thromboxane synthase in normal and pathological human kidney tissue using a monoclonal antibody Tu 300. Virchows Arch 424:69–74, 1994.

116. Wilcox CS, Welch WJ: Thromboxane synthase and TP receptor mRNA in rat kidney and brain: Effects of salt intake and ANG II. Am J Physiol Renal Physiol 284:F525–F531, 2003.

117. Quest DW, Wilson TW: Effects of ridogrel, a thromboxane synthase inhibitor and receptor antagonist, on blood pressure in the spontaneously hypertensive rat. Jpn J Pharmacol 78:479–486, 1998.

118. Yokoyama C, Yabuki T, Shimonishi M, et al: Prostacyclin-deficient mice develop ischemic renal disorders, including nephrosclerosis and renal infarction. Circulation 106:2397–2403, 2002.

119. Murata T, Ushikubi F, Matsuoka T, et al: Altered pain perception and inflammatory response in mice lacking prostacyclin receptor. Nature 388:678–682, 1997.

120. Urade Y, Eguchi N: Lipocalin-type and hematopoietic prostaglandin D synthases as a novel example of functional convergence. Prostaglandins Other Lipid Mediat 68–69:375–382, 2002.

121. Urade Y, Hayaishi O: Prostaglandin D synthase: Structure and function. Vitam Horm 58:89–120, 2000.

122. Eguchi N, Minami T, Shirafuji N, et al: Lack of tactile pain (allodynia) in lipocalin-type prostaglandin D synthase-deficient mice. Proc Natl Acad Sci U S A 96:726–730, 1999.

123. Vitzthum H, Abt I, Einhellig S, et al: Gene expression of prostanoid forming enzymes along the rat nephron. Kidney Int 62:1570–1581, 2002.

124. Ogawa M, Hirawa N, Tsuchida T, et al: Urinary excretions of lipocalin-type prosta-glandin D2 synthase predict the development of proteinuria and renal injury in OLETF rats. Nephrol Dial Transplant 21:924–934, 2006.

125. Ragolia L, Palaia T, Hall CE, et al: Accelerated glucose intolerance, nephropathy, and atherosclerosis in prostaglandin D2 synthase knock-out mice. J Biol Chem 280:29946–29955, 2005.

126. Watanabe K: Prostaglandin F synthase. Prostaglandins Other Lipid Mediat 68–69:401–407, 2002.

127. Roberts LJ, 2nd, Seibert K, Liston TE, et al: PGD2 is transformed by human coronary arteries to 9 alpha, 11 beta-PGF2, which contracts human coronary artery rings. Adv Prostaglandin Thromboxane Leukot Res 17A:427–429, 1987.

128. Sharif NA, Xu SX, Williams GW, et al: Pharmacology of [3H]prostaglandin E1/[3H]prostaglandin E2 and [3H]prostaglandin F2alpha binding to EP3 and FP prostaglandin receptor binding sites in bovine corpus luteum: characterization and correlation with functional data. J Pharmacol Exp Ther 286:1094–1102, 1998.

129. Wallner EI, Wada J, Tramonti G, et al: Relevance of aldo-keto reductase family members to the pathobiology of diabetic nephropathy and renal development. Ren Fail 23:311–320, 2001.

130. Siragy HM, Inagami T, Ichiki T, et al: Sustained hypersensitivity to angiotensin II and its mechanism in mice lacking the subtype-2 (AT2) angiotensin receptor. Proc Natl Acad Sci U S A 96:6506–6510, 1999.

131. Siragy HM, Senbonmatsu T, Ichiki T, et al: Increased renal vasodilator prostanoids prevent hypertension in mice lacking the angiotensin subtype-2 receptor. J Clin Invest 104:181–188, 1999.

132. Siragy HM, Carey RM: The subtype 2 angiotensin receptor regulates renal prostaglan-din F2 alpha formation in conscious rats. Am J Physiol 273:R1103–1107, 1997.

133. Tanikawa N, Ohmiya Y, Ohkubo H, et al: Identification and characterization of a novel type of membrane-associated prostaglandin E synthase. Biochem Biophys Res Commun 291:884–889, 2002.

134. Jakobsson PJ, Thoren S, Morgenstern R, et al: Identification of human prostaglandin E synthase: A microsomal, glutathione-dependent, inducible enzyme, constituting a potential novel drug target. Proc Natl Acad Sci U S A 96:7220–7225, 1999.

135. Trebino CE, Stock JL, Gibbons CP, et al: Impaired inflammatory and pain responses in mice lacking an inducible prostaglandin E synthase. Proc Natl Acad Sci U S A 100:9044–9049, 2003.

136. Engblom D, Saha S, Engstrom L, et al: Microsomal prostaglandin E synthase-1 is the central switch during immune-induced pyresis. Nat Neurosci 6:1137–1138, 2003.

137. Ouellet M, Falgueyret JP, Hien Ear P, et al: Purification and characterization of recom-binant microsomal prostaglandin E synthase-1. Protein Expr Purif 26:489–495, 2002.

138. Uematsu S, Matsumoto M, Takeda K, et al: Lipopolysaccharide-dependent prostaglan-din E(2) production is regulated by the glutathione-dependent prostaglandin E(2) synthase gene induced by the Toll-like receptor 4/MyD88/NF-IL6 pathway. J Immunol 168:5811–5816, 2002.

139. Dinchuk JE, Car BD, Focht RJ, et al: Renal abnormalities and an altered inflammatory response in mice lacking cyclooxygenase II. Nature 378:406–409, 1995.

140. Nguyen M, Camenisch T, Snouwaert JN, et al: The prostaglandin receptor EP4 triggers remodelling of the cardiovascular system at birth. Nature 390:78–81, 1997.

141. Tanioka T, Nakatani Y, Semmyo N, et al: Molecular identification of cytosolic prosta-glandin E2 synthase that is functionally coupled with cyclooxygenase-1 in immediate prostaglandin E2 biosynthesis. J Biol Chem 275:32775–32782, 2000.

142. Zhang Y, Schneider A, Rao R, et al: Genomic structure and genitourinary expression of mouse cytosolic prostaglandin E(2) synthase gene. Biochim Biophys Acta 1634:15–23, 2003.

143. Murakami M, Nakatani Y, Tanioka T, et al: Prostaglandin E synthase. Prostaglandins Other Lipid Mediat 68–69:383–399, 2002.

144. Hirata M, Hayashi Y, Ushikubi F, et al: Cloning and expression of cDNA for a human thromboxane A2 receptor. Nature 349:617–620, 1991.

145. Raychowdhury MK, Yukawa M, Collins LJ, et al: Alternative splicing produces a divergent cytoplasmic tail in the human endothelial thromboxane A2 receptor [pub-lished erratum appears in J Biol Chem 270:7011, 1995]. J Biol Chem 269:19256–19261, 1994.

146. Pierce KL, Regan JW: Prostanoid receptor heterogeneity through alternative mRNA splicing. Life Sci 62:1479–1483, 1998.

147. Wilson RJ, Rhodes SA, Wood RL, et al: Functional pharmacology of human prostanoid EP2 and EP4 receptors. Eur J Pharmacol 501:49–58, 2004.

148. Morinelli TA, Oatis JE, Jr, Okwu AK, et al: Characterization of an 125I-labeled throm-boxane A2/prostaglandin H2 receptor agonist. J Pharmacol Exp Ther 251:557–562, 1989.

149. Narumiya S, Sugimoto Y, Ushikubi F: Prostanoid receptors: Structures, properties, and functions. Physiol Rev 79:1193–1226, 1999.

150. Abramovitz M, Adam M, Boie Y, et al: The utilization of recombinant prostanoid receptors to determine the affinities and selectivities of prostaglandins and related analogs [In Process Citation]. Biochim Biophys Acta 1483:285–293, 2000.

151. Audoly LP, Rocca B, Fabre JE, et al: Cardiovascular responses to the isoprostanes iPF(2alpha)-III and iPE(2)-III are mediated via the thromboxane A(2) receptor in vivo. Circulation 101:2833–2840, 2000.

152. Welch WJ: Effects of isoprostane on tubuloglomerular feedback: Roles of TP receptors, NOS, and salt intake. Am J Physiol Renal Physiol 288:F757–762, 2005.

153. Morrow JD: Quantification of isoprostanes as indices of oxidant stress and the risk of atherosclerosis in humans. Arterioscler Thromb Vasc Biol 25:279–286, 2005.

154. Abe T, Takeuchi K, Takahashi N, et al: Rat kidney thromaboxane A2 receptor: Molecu-lar cloning signal transduction and intrarenal expression localization. J Clin Invest 96:657–664, 1995.

155. Namba T, Sugimoto Y, Hirata M, et al: Mouse thromboxane A2 receptor: cDNA cloning, expression and northern blot analysis. Biochem Biophys Res Commun 184:1197–1203, 1992.

156. Hirata T, Kakizuka A, Ushikubi F, et al: Arg60 to Leu mutation of the human throm-boxane A2 receptor in a dominantly inherited bleeding disorder. J Clin Invest 94:1662–1667, 1994.

157. Mannon RB, Coffman TM, Mannon PJ: Distribution of binding sites for thromboxane A2 in the mouse kidney. Am J Physiol 271:F1131–1138, 1996.

158. Thomas DW, Mannon RB, Mannon PJ, et al: Coagulation defects and altered hemo-dynamic responses in mice lacking receptors for thromboxane A2. J Clin Invest 102:1994–2001, 1998.

159. Spurney RF, Onorato JJ, Albers FJ, et al: Thromboxane binding and signal transduc-tion in rat glomerular mesangial cells. Am J Physiol 264:F292–299, 1993.

160. Nasjletti A, Arthur C: Corcoran Memorial Lecture. The role of eicosanoids in angiotensin-dependent hypertension. Hypertension 31:194–200, 1998.

161. Kawada N, Dennehy K, Solis G, et al: TP receptors regulate renal hemodynamics during angiotensin II slow pressor response. Am J Physiol Renal Physiol 287:F753–759, 2004.

162. Boffa J-J, Just A, Coffman TM, et al: Thromboxane receptor mediates renal vasocon-striction and contributes to acute renal failure in endotoxemic mice. J Am Soc Nephrol 15:2358–2365, 2004.

163. Welch WJ, Peng B, Takeuchi K, et al: Salt loading enhances rat renal TxA2/PGH2 receptor expression and TGF response to U-46,619. Am J Physiol 273:F976–983, 1997.

164. Welch WJ, Wilcox CS: Potentiation of tubuloglomerular feedback in the rat by throm-boxane mimetic. Role of macula densa. J Clin Invest 89:1857–1865, 1992.

165. Coffman TM, Spurney RF, Mannon RB, et al: Thromboxane A2 modulates the fibrinolytic system in glomerular mesangial cells. Am J Physiol 275:F262–269, 1998.

166. Kiriyama M, Ushikubi F, Kobayashi T, et al: Ligand binding specificities of the eight types and subtypes of the mouse prostanoid receptors expressed in Chinese hamster ovary cells. Br J Pharmacol 122:217–224, 1997.

167. Namba T, Oida H, Sugimoto Y, et al: cDNA cloning of a mouse prostacyclin receptor: Multiple signaling pathways and expression in thymic medulla. J Biol Chem 269:9986–9992, 1994.

168. Boie Y, Rushmore TH, Darmon-Goodwin A, et al: Cloning and expression of a cDNA for the human prostanoid IP receptor. J Biol Chem 269:12173–12178, 1994.

169. Oida H, Namba T, Sugimoto Y, et al: In situ hybridization studies on prostacyclin receptor mRNA expression in various mouse organs. Br J Pharmacol 116:2828–2837, 1995.

170. Nasrallah R, Hebert RL: Prostacyclin signaling in the kidney: Implications for health and disease. Am J Physiol Renal Physiol 289:F235–246, 2005.

171. Edwards A, Silldforff EP, Pallone TL: The renal medullary microcirculation. Front Biosci 5:E36–52, 2000.

172. Bugge JF, Stokke ES, Vikse A, et al: Stimulation of renin release by PGE2 and PGI2 infusion in the dog: Enhancing effect of ureteral occlusion or administration of ethacrynic acid. Acta Physiol Scand 138:193–201, 1990.

173. Ito S, Carretero OA, Abe K, et al: Effect of prostanoids on renin release from rabbit afferent arterioles with and without macula densa. Kidney Int 35:1138–1144, 1989.

174. Chaudhari A, Gupta S, Kirschenbaum M: Biochemical evidence for PGI2 and PGE2 receptors in the rabbit renal preglomerular microvasculature. Biochim Biophys Acta 1053:156–161, 1990.

175. Francois H, Athirakul K, Howell D, et al: Prostacyclin protects against elevated blood pressure and cardiac fibrosis. Cell Metab 2:201–207, 2005.

176. Hébert R, Regnier L, Peterson L: Rabbit cortical collecting ducts express a novel prostacyclin receptor. Am J Physiol 268:F145–154, 1995.

177. Komhoff M, Lesener B, Nakao K, et al: Localization of the prostacyclin receptor in human kidney. Kidney Int 54:1899–1908, 1998.

178. Tone Y, Inoue H, Hara S, et al: The regional distribution and cellular localization of mRNA encoding rat prostacyclin synthase. Eur J Cell Biol 72:268–277, 1997.

179. Hirata M, Kakizuka A, Aizawa M, et al: Molecular characterization of a mouse prostaglandin D receptor and functional expression of the cloned gene. Proc Natl Acad Sci U S A 91:11192–11196, 1994.

180. Coleman RA, Grix SP, Head SA, et al: A novel inhibitory prostanoid receptor in piglet saphenous vein. Prostaglandins 47:151–168, 1994.

181. Oida H, Hirata M, Sugimoto Y, et al: Expression of messenger RNA for the prostaglandin D receptor in the leptomeninges of the mouse brain. FEBS Lett 417:53–56, 1997.

182. Boie Y, Sawyer N, Slipetz DM, et al: Molecular cloning and characterization of the human prostanoid DP receptor. J Biol Chem 270:18910–18916, 1995.

183. Urade Y, Hayaishi O: Prostaglandin D2 and sleep regulation. Biochim Biophys Acta 1436:606–615, 1999.

184. Sri Kantha S, Matsumura H, Kubo E, et al: Effects of prostaglandin D2, lipoxins and leukotrienes on sleep and brain temperature of rats. Prostaglandins Leukot Essent Fatty Acids 51:87–93, 1994.

185. Matsuoka T, Hirata M, Tanaka H, et al: Prostaglandin D2 as a mediator of allergic asthma. Science 287:2013–2017, 2000.

186. Rao PS, Cavanagh D, Dietz JR, et al: Dose-dependent effects of prostaglandin D2 on hemodynamics, renal function, and blood gas analyses. Am J Obstet Gynecol 156:843–851, 1987.

187. Hirai H, Tanaka K, Takano S, et al: Cutting edge: Agonistic effect of indomethacin on a prostaglandin D2 Receptor, CRTH2. J Immunol 168:981–985, 2002.

188. Abramovitz M, Boie Y, Nguyen T, et al: Cloning and expression of a cDNA for the human prostanoid FP receptor. J Biol Chem 269:2632–2636, 1994.

189. Woodward DF, Fairbairn CE, Lawrence RA: Identification of the FP-receptor as a discrete entity by radioligand binding in biosystems that exhibit different functional rank orders of potency in response to prostanoids. Adv Exp Med Biol 400A:223–227, 1997.

190. Pierce KL, Bailey TJ, Hoyer PB, et al: Cloning of a carboxyl-terminal isoform of the prostanoid FP receptor. J Biol Chem 272:883–887, 1997.

191. Pierce KL, Fujino H, Srinivasan D, et al: Activation of FP prostanoid receptor isoforms leads to Rho-mediated changes in cell morphology and in the cell cytoskeleton. J Biol Chem 274:35944–35949, 1999.

192. Fujino H, Srinivasan D, Regan JW: Cellular conditioning and activation of beta-catenin signaling by the FPB prostanoid receptor. J Biol Chem 277:48786–48795, 2002.

193. Sugimoto Y, Yamasaki A, Segi E, et al: Failure of parturition in mice lacking the prostaglandin F receptor. Science 277:681–683, 1997.

194. Hasumoto K, Sugimoto Y, Gotoh M, et al: Characterization of the mouse prostaglandin F receptor gene: A transgenic mouse study of a regulatory region that controls its expression in the stomach and kidney but not in the ovary. Genes Cells 2:571–580, 1997.

195. Chen J, Champa-Rodriguez ML, Woodward DF: Identification of a prostanoid FP receptor population producing endothelium-dependent vasorelaxation in the rabbit jugular vein. Br J Pharmacol 116:3035–3041, 1995.

196. Muller K, Krieg P, Marks F, et al: Expression of PGF(2alpha) receptor mRNA in normal, hyperplastic and neoplastic skin. Carcinogenesis 21:1063–1066, 2000.

197. Linden C, Alm A: Prostaglandin analogues in the treatment of glaucoma. Drugs Aging 14:387–398, 1999.

198. Hebert RL, Carmosino M, Saito O, et al: Characterization of a rabbit PGF2alpha (FP) receptor exhibiting Gi-restricted signaling and that inhibits water absorption in renal collecting duct. J Biol Chem 280:35028–35037, 2005.

199. Hebert RL, Jacobson HR, Fredin D, et al: Evidence that separate PGE2 receptors modulate water and sodium transport in rabbit cortical collecting duct. Am J Physiol 265:F643–650, 1993.

200. Funk C, Furchi L, FitzGerald G, et al: Cloning and expression of a cDNA for the human prostaglandin E receptor EP₁ subtype. J Biol Chem 268:26767–26772, 1993.

201. Breyer MD, Jacobson HR, Davis LS, et al: In situ hybridization and localization of mRNA for the rabbit prostaglandin EP3 receptor. Kidney Int 44:1372–1378, 1993.

202. Bek M, Nusing R, Kowark P, et al: Characterization of prostanoid receptors in podocytes. J Am Soc Nephrol 10:2084–2093, 1999.

203. Breshnahan BA, Keleflotis D, Stratidakis I, et al: PGF2alpha-induced signaling events in glomerular mesangial cells. Proc Soc Exp Biol Med 212:165–173, 1996.

204. Breyer MD, Breyer RM: G protein-coupled prostanoid receptors and the kidney. Annu Rev Physiol 63:579–605, 2001.

205. Toh H, Ichikawa A, Narumiya S: Molecular evolution of receptors for eicosanoids. FEBS Lett 361:17–21, 1995.

206. Guan Y, Zhang Y, Breyer RM, et al: Prostaglandin E2 inhibits renal collecting duct Na+ absorption by activating the EP1 receptor. J Clin Invest 102:194–201, 1998.

207. Coleman RA, Kennedy I, Humphrey PPA, et al: Prostanoids and their receptors. In Emmet JC (ed): Comprehensive Medicinal Chemistry (vol 3). Oxford, Pergammon Press, 1990, pp 643–714.

208. Ishibashi R, Tanaka I, Kotani M, et al: Roles of prostaglandin E receptors in mesangial cells under high-glucose conditions. Kidney Int 56:589–600, 1999.

209. Inscho E, Carmines P, Navar L: Prostaglandin influences on afferent arteriolar responses to vasoconstrictor agonists. Am J Physiol 259:F157–163, 1990.

210. Zhang Y, Guan Y, Scheider A, et al: Characterization of murine vasopressor and vasodepressor prostaglandin E2 receptors. Hypertension 35:1129–1134, 2000.

211. Stock JL, Shinjo K, Burkhardt J, et al: The prostaglandin E2 EP1 receptor mediates pain perception and regulates blood pressure. J Clin Invest 107:325–331, 2001.

212. Tsuboi K, Sugimoto Y, Ichikawa A: Prostanoid receptor subtypes. Prostaglandins Other Lipid Mediat 68–69:535–556, 2002.

213. Regan JW, Bailey TJ, Pepperl DJ, et al: Cloning of a novel human prostaglandin receptor with characteristics of the pharmacologically defined EP2 subtype. Mol Pharmacol 46:213–220, 1994.

214. Nishigaki N, Negishi M, Honda A, et al: Identification of prostaglandin E receptor 'EP2 cloned from mastocytoma cells as EP4 subtype. FEBS Lett 364:339–341, 1995.

215. Guan Y, Stillman BA, Zhang Y, et al: Cloning and expression of the rabbit prostaglandin EP2 receptor. BMC Pharmacol 2:14, 2002.

216. Katsuyama M, Ikegami R, Karahashi H, et al: Characterization of the LPS-stimulated expression of EP2 and EP4 prostaglandin E receptors in mouse macrophage-like cell line, J774.1 [in process citation]. Biochem Biophys Res Commun 251:727–731, 1998.

217. Kennedy C, Schneider A, Young-Siegler A, et al: Regulation of renin and aldosterone levels in mice lacking the prostaglandin EP2 receptor. J Am Soc Nephrol 10:348A, 1999.

218. Coleman RA, Smith WL, Narumiya S: VIII. International union of pharmacology classification of prostanoid receptors: Properties, distribution, and structure of the receptors and their subtypes. Pharmacol Rev 46:205–229, 1994.

219. Boie Y, Stocco R, Sawyer N, et al: Molecular cloning and characterization of the four rat prostaglandin E2 prostanoid receptor subtypes. Eur J Pharmacol 340:227–241, 1997.

220. Breyer RM, Emeson RB, Tarng JL, et al: Alternative splicing generates multiple isoforms of a rabbit prostaglandin E2 receptor. J Biol Chem 269:6163–6169, 1994.

221. Kotani M, Tanaka I, Ogawa Y, et al: Molecular cloning and expression of multiple isoforms of human prostaglandin E receptor EP3 subtype generated by alternative messenger RNA splicing: multiple second messenger systems and tissue-specific distributions. Mol Pharmacol 48:869–879, 1995.

222. Irie A, Sugimoto Y, Namba T, et al: Third isoform of the prostaglandin-E-receptor EP3 subtype with different C-terminal tail coupling to both stimulation and inhibition of adenylate cyclase. Eur J Biochem 217:313–318, 1993.

223. Aoki J, Katoh H, Yasui H, et al: Signal transduction pathway regulating prostaglandin EP3 receptor-induced neurite retraction: requirement for two different tyrosine kinases. Biochem J 340:365–369, 1999.

224. Hasegawa H, Negishi M, Ichikawa A: Two isoforms of the prostaglandin E receptor EP3 subtype different in agonist-independent constitutive activity. J Biol Chem 271:1857–1860, 1996.

225. Breyer MD, Davis L, Jacobson HR, et al: Differential localization of prostaglandin E receptor subtypes in human kidney. Am J Physiol 270:F912–918, 1996.

226. Taniguchi S, Watanabe T, Nakao A, et al: Detection and quantitation of EP3 prostaglandin E2 receptor mRNA along mouse nephron segments by RT-PCR. Am J Physiol 266:C1453–1458, 1994.

227. Good DW, George T: Regulation of HCO3- absorption by prostaglandin E2 and G-proteins in rat medullary thick ascending limb. Am J Physiol 270:F711–717, 1996.

228. Good D: PGE2 reverses AVP inhibition of HCO3- absorption in rat MTAL by activation of protein kinase C. Am J Physiol 270:F978–985, 1996.

229. Sakairi Y, Jacobson HR, Noland TD, et al: Luminal prostaglandin E receptors regulate salt and water transport in rabbit cortical collecting duct. Am J Physiol 269:F257–265, 1995.

230. Athirakul K, Oliverio M, Fleming E, et al: Modulation of urinary concentrating mechanisms by the EP₃ receptor for prostaglandin (PG) E₂. J Am Soc Nephrol 8:(in press), 1997.

231. Ushikubi F, Segi E, Sugimoto Y, et al: Impaired febrile response in mice lacking the prostaglandin E receptor subtype EP3. Nature 395:281–284, 1998.

232. Audoly LP, Ruan X, Wagner VA, et al: Role of EP(2) and EP(3) PGE(2) receptors in control of murine renal hemodynamics. Am J Physiol Heart Circ Physiol 280:H327–333, 2001.

233. Castleberry TA, Lu B, Smock SL, et al: Molecular cloning and functional characterization of the canine prostaglandin E(2) receptor EP4 subtype. Prostaglandins 65:167–187, 2001.

234. Bastien L, Sawyer N, Grygorczyk R, et al: Cloning, functional expression, and characterization of the human prostaglandin E₂ receptor EP₂ subtype. J Biol Chem 269:11873–11877, 1994.

235. Breyer RM, Davis LS, Nian C, et al: Cloning and expression of the rabbit prostaglandin EP4 receptor. Am J Physiol 270:F485–493, 1996.

236. Segi E, Sugimoto Y, Yamasaki A, et al: Patent ductus arteriosus and neonatal death in prostaglandin receptor EP4-deficient mice. Biochem Biophys Res Commun 246:7–12, 1998.

237. Audoly LP, Tilley SL, Goulet J, et al: Identification of specific EP receptors responsible for the hemodynamic effects of PGE2. Am J Physiol 277:H924–930, 1999.

238. Csukas S, Hanke C, Rewolinski D, et al: Prostaglandin E2-induced aldosterone release is mediated by an EP2 receptor. Hypertension 31:575–581, 1998.

239. Sugimoto Y, Namba T, Shigemoto R, et al: Distinct cellular localization of mRNAs for three subtypes of prostaglandin E receptor in kidney. Am J Physiol 266:F823–828, 1994.

240. Jensen BL, Stubbe J, Hansen PB, et al: Localization of prostaglandin E(2) EP2 and EP4 receptors in the rat kidney. Am J Physiol Renal Physiol 280:F1001–1009, 2001.

241. Nusing RM, Treude A, Weissenberger C, et al: Dominant role of prostaglandin E2 EP4 receptor in furosemide-induced salt-losing tubulopathy: A model for hyperprostaglandin E syndrome/antenatal Bartter syndrome. J Am Soc Nephrol 16:2354–2362, 2005.

242. Kopp UC, Cicha MZ, Nakamura K, et al: Activation of EP4 receptors contributes to prostaglandin E2-mediated stimulation of renal sensory nerves. Am J Physiol Renal Physiol 287:F1269–1282, 2004.

243. Silldorf E, Yang S, Pallone T: Prostaglandin E2 abrogates endothelin-induced vasoconstriction in renal outer medullary descending vasa recta of the rat. J Clin Invest 95:2734–2740, 1995.

244. Breyer M, Breyer R, Fowler B, et al: EP1 receptor antagonists block PGE2 dependent inhibition of Na+ absorption in the cortical collecting duct. J Am Soc Nephrol 7:1645, 1996.

245. Schlondorff D: Renal complications of nonsteroidal anti-inflammatory drugs. Kidney Int 44:643–653, 1993.

246. Jensen B, Schmid C, Kurtz A: Prostaglandins stimulate renin secretion and renin mRNA in mouse renal juxtaglomerular cells. Am J Physiol 271:F659–669, 1996.

247. Hockel G, Cowley A: Prostaglandin E2-induced hypertension in conscious dogs. Am J Physiol 237:H449–454, 1979.

248. Francisco L, Osborn J, Dibona G: Prostaglandins in renin release during sodium deprivation. Am J Physiol 243:F537–F542, 1982.

249. Imig JD, Breyer MD, Breyer RM: Contribution of prostaglandin EP(2) receptors to renal microvascular reactivity in mice. Am J Physiol Renal Physiol 283:F415–422, 2002.

250. Schnermann J: Cyclooxygenase-2 and macula densa control of renin secretion. Nephrol Dial Transplant 16:1735–1738, 2001.

251. Imanishi M, Tsuji T, Nakamura S, et al: Prostaglandin i(2)/e(2) ratios in unilateral renovascular hypertension of different severities. Hypertension 38:23–29, 2001.

252. Jensen BL, Mann B, Skott O, et al: Differential regulation of renal prostaglandin receptor mRNAs by dietary salt intake in the rat. Kidney Int 56:528–537, 1999.

253. Tilley SL, Audoly LP, Hicks EH, et al: Reproductive failure and reduced blood pressure in mice lacking the EP2 prostaglandin E2 receptor. J Clin Invest 103:1539–1545, 1999.

254. Guyton A: Blood pressure control-special role of the kidneys and body fluids. Science 252:1813–1816, 1991.

255. Carmines P, Bell P, Roman R, et al: Prostaglandins in the sodium excretory response to altered renal arterial pressure in dogs. Am J Physiol 248:F8–F14, 1985.

256. Roman R, Lianos E: Influence of prostaglandins on papillary blood flow and pressure-natriuretic response. Hypertension 15:29–35, 1990.

257. Pallone TL, Silldorff EP: Pericyte regulation of renal medullary blood flow. Exp Nephrol 9:165–170, 2001.

258. Breyer MD, Breyer RM: Prostaglandin E receptors and the kidney. Am J Physiol Renal Physiol 279:F12–23, 2000.

259. Roman RJ: P-450 metabolites of arachidonic acid in the control of cardiovascular function. Physiol Rev 82:131–185, 2002.

260. Syal A, Schiavi S, Chakravarty S, et al: Fibroblast growth factor-23 increases mouse PGE2 production in vivo and in vitro. Am J Physiol Renal Physiol 290:F450–455, 2005.

261. Baum M, Loleh S, Saini N, et al: Correction of proximal tubule phosphate transport defect in Hyp mice in vivo and in vitro with indomethacin. Proc Natl Acad Sci U S A 100:11098–11103, 2003.

262. Eriksson LO, Larsson B, Andersson KE: Biochemical characterization and autoradiographic localization of [3H]PGE2 binding sites in rat kidney. Acta Physiol Scand 139:405–415, 1990.

263. Hebert RL, Jacobson HR, Breyer MD: Prostaglandin E2 inhibits sodium transport in rabbit cortical collecting duct by increasing intracellular calcium. J Clin Invest 87:1992–1998, 1991.

264. Breyer MD, Jacobson HR, Hebert RL: Cellular mechanisms of prostaglandin E2 and vasopressin interactions in the collecting duct. Kidney Int 38:618–624, 1990.

265. Nadler SP, Hebert SC, Brenner BM: PGE₂, forskolin, and cholera toxin interactions in rabbit cortical collecting tubule. Am J Physiol 250:F127–F135, 1986.

266. Hebert RL, Jacobson HR, Breyer MD: PGE2 inhibits AVP-induced water flow in cortical collecting ducts by protein kinase C activation. Am J Physiol 259:F318–F325, 1990.

267. Tai HH, Ensor CM, Tong M, et al: Prostaglandin catabolizing enzymes. Prostaglandins Other Lipid Mediat 68–69:483–493, 2002.

268. Sakuma S, Fujimoto Y, Hikita E, et al: Effects of metal ions on 15-hydroxy prostaglandin dehydrogenase activity in rabbit kidney cortex. Prostaglandins 40:507–514, 1990.

269. Coggins KG, Latour A, Nguyen MS, et al: Metabolism of PGE2 by prostaglandin dehydrogenase is essential for remodeling the ductus arteriosus. Nat Med 8:91–92, 2002.

270. Oliw E: Oxygenation of polyunsaturated fatty acids by cytochrome P450 monooxygenases. Prog Lipid Res 33:329–354, 1994.

271. Schwartzman ML, da Silva JL, Lin F, et al: Cytochrome P450 4A expression and arachidonic acid omega-hydroxylation in the kidney of the spontaneously hypertensive rat. Nephron 73:652–663, 1996.

272. Stec DE, Flasch A, Roman RJ, et al: Distribution of cytochrome P-450 4A and 4F isoforms along the nephron in mice. Am J Physiol Renal Physiol 284:F95–102, 2003.

273. Yu K, Bayona WK, CB, Harding H, et al: Differential activation of peroxisome proliferator activated receptors by eicosanoids. J Biol Chem 270:23975–23983, 1995.

274. Forman B, Tontonoz P, Chen J, et al: 15-deoxy-δ12,14-Prostaglandin J2 is a ligand for the adipocyte determination factor PPAR-gamma. Cell 83:803–812, 1995.

275. Kliewer S, Lenhard J, Wilson T, et al: A prostaglandin J₂ metabolite binds peroxisome proliferator-activated receptor gamma and promotes adipocyte differentiation. Cell 83:813–819, 1995.

276. Witzenbichler B, Asahara T, Murohara T, et al: Vascular endothelial growth factor-C (VEGF-C/VEGF-2) promotes angiogenesis in the setting of tissue ischemia. Am J Pathol 153:381–394, 1998.

277. Stamatakis K, Sanchez-Gomez FJ, Perez-Sala D: Identification of novel protein targets for modification by 15-Deoxy-{Delta}12,14-Prostaglandin J2 in mesangial cells reveals multiple interactions with the cytoskeleton. J Am Soc Nephrol 17:89–98, 2006.

278. Straus DS, Glass CK: Cyclopentenone prostaglandins: new insights on biological activities and cellular targets. Med Res Rev 21:185–210, 2001.

279. Negishi M, Katoh H: Cyclopentenone prostaglandin receptors. Prostaglandins Other Lipid Mediat 68–69:611–617, 2002.

280. Rossl A, Kapahl P, Natoli G, et al: Anti-inflammatory cyclopentenone prostaglandins are direct inhibitors of IκB kinase. Nature 403:103–108, 2000.

281. Shibata T, Kondo M, Osawa T, et al: 15-Deoxy-Delta 12,14-prostaglandin J2. A prostaglandin D2 metabolite generated during inflammatory processes. J Biol Chem 277:10459–10466, 2002.

282. Fam SS, Murphey LJ, Terry ES, et al: Formation of highly reactive A-ring and J-ring isoprostane-like compounds (A4/J4-neuroprostanes) in vivo from docosahexaenoic acid. J Biol Chem 277:36076–36084, 2002.

283. Morrow J, Harris TM, Roberts LJ 2nd: Noncyclooxygenase oxidative formation of a series of novel prostaglandins: Analytical ramifications for measurement of eicosanoids. Anal Biochem 184:1–10, 1990.

284. Roberts L, Morrow J: Products of the isoprostane pathway: unique bioactive compounds and markers of lipid peroxidation. Cell Mol Life Sci 59:808–820, 2002.

285. Morrow JD, Roberts LJ: The isoprostanes: unique bioactive products of lipid peroxidation. Prog Lipid Res 36:1–21, 1997.

286. Takahashi K, Nammour T, Fukunaga M, et al: Glomerular actions of a free radical-generated novel prostaglandin, 8-epi-prostaglandin F2 alpha, in the rat. Evidence for interaction with thromboxane A2 receptors. J Clin Invest 90:136–141, 1992.

287. Schuster VL: Prostaglandin transport. Prostaglandins Other Lipid Mediat 68–69:633–647, 2002.

288. Chan BS, Satriano JA, Pucci M, et al: Mechanism of prostaglandin E2 transport across the plasma membrane of HeLa cells and Xenopus oocytes expressing the prostaglandin transporter "PGT". J Biol Chem 273:6689–6697, 1998.

289. Lu R, Kanai N, Bao Y, et al: Cloning, in vitro expression, and tissue distribution of a human prostaglandin transporter cDNA(hPGT). J Clin Invest 98:1142–1149, 1996.

290. Kanai N, Lu R, Satriano JA, et al: Identification and characterization of a prostaglandin transporter. Science 268:866–869, 1995.

291. Bao Y, Pucci ML, Chan BS, et al: Prostaglandin transporter PGT is expressed in cell types that synthesize and release prostanoids. Am J Physiol Renal Physiol 282:F1103–1110, 2002.

292. Chi Y, Khersonsky SM, Chang Y-T, et al: Identification of a new class of prostaglandin transporter inhibitors and characterization of their biological effects on prostaglandin E2 transport. J Pharmacol Exp Ther 316:1346–1350, 2006.

293. Nomura T, Chang HY, Lu R, et al: Prostaglandin signaling in the renal collecting duct: Release, reuptake, and oxidation in the same cell. J Biol Chem 280:28424–28429, 2005.

294. Kimura H, Takeda M, Narikawa S, et al: Human organic anion transporters and human organic cation transporters mediate renal transport of prostaglandins. J Pharmacol Exp Ther 301:293–298, 2002.

295. Sauvant C, Holzinger H, Gekle M: Prostaglandin E2 inhibits its own renal transport by downregulation of organic anion transporters rOAT1 and rOAT3. J Am Soc Nephrol 17:46–53, 2006.

296. Touhey S, O'Connor R, Plunkett S, et al: Structure-activity relationship of indomethacin analogues for MRP-1, COX-1 and COX-2 inhibition. identification of novel chemotherapeutic drug resistance modulators. Eur J Cancer 38:1661–1670, 2002.

297. Homem de Bittencourt PI, Jr., Curi R: Antiproliferative prostaglandins and the MRP/GS-X pump role in cancer immunosuppression and insight into new strategies in cancer gene therapy. Biochem Pharmacol 62:811–819, 2001.

298. Jedlitschky G, Keppler D: Transport of leukotriene C4 and structurally related conjugates. Vitam Horm 64:153–184, 2002.

299. Nies AT, Konig J, Cui Y, et al: Structural requirements for the apical sorting of human multidrug resistance protein 2 (ABCC2). Eur J Biochem 269:1866–1876, 2002.

300. Van Aubel RA, Peters JG, Masereeuw R, et al: Multidrug resistance protein mrp2 mediates ATP-dependent transport of classic renal organic anion p-aminohippurate. Am J Physiol Renal Physiol 279:F713–717, 2000.

301. Klahr S, Morrissey JJ: The role of growth factors, cytokines, and vasoactive compounds in obstructive nephropathy. Semin Nephrol 18:622–632, 1998.

302. Takahashi K, Kato T, Schreiner GF, et al: Essential fatty acid deficiency normalizes function and histology in rat nephrotoxic nephritis. Kidney Int 41:1245–1253, 1992.

303. Chanmugam P, Feng L, Liou S, et al: Radicicol, a protein tyrosine kinase inhibitor, suppresses the expression of mitogen-inducible cyclooxygenase in macrophages stimulated with lipopolysaccharide and in experimental glomerulonephritis. J Biol Chem 270:5418–5426, 1995.

304. Hirose S, Yamamoto T, Feng L, et al: Expression and localization of cyclooxygenase isoforms and cytosolic phospholipase A2 in anti-Thy-1 glomerulonephritis. J Am Soc Nephrol 9:408–416., 1998.

305. Yang T, Sun D, Huang YG, et al: Differential regulation of COX-2 expression in the kidney by lipopolysaccharide: role of CD14. Am J Physiol 277:F10–16, 1999.

306. Tomasoni S, Noris M, Zappella S, et al: Upregulation of renal and systemic cyclooxygenase-2 in patients with active lupus nephritis. J Am Soc Nephrol 9:1202–1212, 1998.

307. Zoja C, Benigni A, Noris M, et al: Mycophenolate mofetil combined with a cyclooxygenase-2 inhibitor ameliorates murine lupus nephritis. Kidney Int 60:653–663, 2001.

308. Hartner A, Pahl A, Brune K, et al: Upregulation of cyclooxygenase-1 and the PGE2 receptor EP2 in rat and human mesangioproliferative glomerulonephritis. Inflamm Res 49:345–354, 2000.

309. Kitahara M, Eitner F, Ostendorf T, et al: Selective cyclooxygenase-2 inhibition impairs glomerular capillary healing in experimental glomerulonephritis. J Am Soc Nephrol 13:1261–1270, 2002.

310. Schneider A, Harendza S, Zahner G, et al: Cyclooxygenase metabolites mediate glomerular monocyte chemoattractant protein-1 formation and monocyte recruitment in experimental glomerulonephritis. Kidney Int 55:430–441, 1999.

311. Wang J-L, Cheng H-F, Zhang M-Z, et al: Selective increase of cyclooxygenase-2 expression in a model of renal ablation. Am J Physiol 275:F613–F622, 1998.

312. Weichert W, Paliege A, Provoost AP, et al: Upregulation of juxtaglomerular NOS1 and COX-2 precedes glomerulosclerosis in fawn-hooded hypertensive rats. Am J Physiol Renal Physiol 280:F706–714, 2001.

313. Komers R, Lindsley JN, Oyama TT, et al: Immunohistochemical and functional correlations of renal cyclooxygenase-2 in experimental diabetes. J Clin Invest 107:889–898, 2001.

314. Bing Y, Xu J, Qi Z, et al: The role of renal cortical cyclooxygenase-2 (COX-2) expression in hyperfiltration in rats with high protein intake. Am J Physiol Renal Physiol 291:F368–374, 2006.

315. Wilcox CS, Welch WJ, Murad F, et al: Nitric oxide synthase in macula densa regulates glomerular capillary pressure. Proceedings of the National Academy of Sciences of the United States of America 89:11993–11997, 1992.

316. Welch WJ, Wilcox CS, Thomson SC: Nitric oxide and tubuloglomerular feedback. Semin Nephrol 19:251–262, 1999.

317. Thorup C, Erik A, Persson G: Macula densa derived nitric oxide in regulation of glomerular capillary pressure. Kidney Int 49:430–436, 1996.

318. Ichihara A, Imig JD, Navar LG: Cyclooxygenase-2 modulates afferent arteriolar responses to increases in pressure. Hypertension 34:843–847, 1999.

319. Wang J-L, Cheng H-F, Sheppel S, et al: The cyclooxygenase-2 inhibitor, SC58326, decreases proteinuria and retards progression of glomerulosclerosis in the rat remnant kidney. Kidney Int 57:2334–2342, 2000.

320. Goncalves AR, Fujihara CK, Mattar AL, et al: Renal expression of COX-2, ANG II, and AT1 receptor in remnant kidney: Strong renoprotection by therapy with losartan and a nonsteroidal anti-inflammatory. Am J Physiol Renal Physiol 286:F945–954, 2004.

321. Fujihara CK, Malheiros DM, Donato JL, et al: Nitroflurbiprofen, a new nonsteroidal anti-inflammatory, ameliorates structural injury in the remnant kidney. Am J Physiol 274:F573–579, 1998.

322. Schmitz PG, Krupa SM, Lane PH, et al: Acquired essential fatty acid depletion in the remnant kidney: Amelioration with U-63557A. Kidney Int 46:1184–1191, 1994.

323. Stahl RA, Thaiss F, Wenzel U, et al: A rat model of progressive chronic glomerular sclerosis: The role of thromboxane inhibition. J Am Soc Nephrol 2:1568–1577, 1992.

324. Cheng HF, Wang CJ, Moeckel GW, et al: Cyclooxygenase-2 inhibitor blocks expression of mediators of renal injury in a model of diabetes and hypertension. Kidney Int 62:929–939, 2002.

325. Dey A, Maric C, Kaesemeyer WH, et al: Rofecoxib decreases renal injury in obese Zucker rats. Clin Sci (Lond) 107:561–570, 2004.

326. Takano T, Cybulsky AV: Complement C5b-9-mediated arachidonic acid metabolism in glomerular epithelial cells: Role of cyclooxygenase-1 and -2. Am J Pathol 156:2091–2101, 2000.

327. Villa E, Martinez J, Ruilope L, et al: Cicaprost, a prostacyclin analog, protects renal function in uninephrectomized dogs in the absence of changes in blood pressure. Am J Hypertension 6:253–257, 1992.

328. Studer R, Negrete H, Craven P, et al: Protein kinase C signals thromboxane induced increases in fibronectin synthesis and TGF-beta bioactivity in mesangial cells. Kidney Int 48:422–430, 1995.

329. Zahner G, Disser M, Thaiss F, et al: The effect of prostaglandin E2 on mRNA expression and secretion of collagens I, III, and IV and fibronectin in cultured rat mesangial cells. J Am Soc Nephrol 4:1778–1785, 1994.

330. Singhal P, Sagar S, Garg P, et al: Vasoactive agents modulate matrix metalloproteinase-2 activity by mesangial cells. Am J Med Sci 310:235–241, 1995.

331. Varga J, Diaz-Perez A, Rosenbloom J, Jimenez SA: PGE$_2$ causes a coordinate decrease in the steady state levels of fibronectin and types I and III procollagen mRNAs in normal human dermal fibroblasts. Biochem Biophys Res Comm 147:1282–1288, 1987.

332. Wilborn J, Crofford LJ, Burdick MD, et al: Cultured lung fibroblasts isolated from patients with idiopathic pulmonary fibrosis have a diminished capacity to synthesize prostaglandin E2 and to express cyclooxygenase-2. J Clin Invest 95:1861–1868, 1995.

333. Wise WC, Cook JA, Tempel GE, et al: The rat in sepsis and endotoxic shock. Prog Clin Biol Res 299:243–252, 1989.

334. Ruschitzka F, Shaw S, Noll G, et al: Endothelial vasoconstrictor prostanoids, vascular reactivity, and acute renal failure. Kidney Int Suppl 67:S199–201, 1998.

335. Chaudhari A, Kirschenbaum MA: Altered glomerular eicosanoid biosynthesis in uranyl nitrate-induced acute renal failure. Biochim Biophys Acta 792:135–140, 1984.

336. Hardie WD, Ebert J, Frazer M, et al: The effect of thromboxane A2 receptor antagonism on amphotericin B-induced renal vasoconstriction in the rat. Prostaglandins 45:47–56, 1993.

337. Higa EM, Schor N, Boim MA, et al: Role of the prostaglandin and kallikrein-kinin systems in aminoglycoside-induced acute renal failure. Braz J Med Biol Res 18:355–365, 1985.

338. Papanicolaou N, Hatziantoniou C, Bariety J: Selective inhibition of thromboxane synthesis partially protected while inhibition of angiotensin II formation did not protect rats against acute renal failure induced with glycerol. Prostaglandins Leukot Med 21:29–35, 1986.

339. Vargas AV, Krishnamurthi V, Masih R, et al: Prostaglandin E1 attenuation of ischemic renal reperfusion injury in the rat. J Am Coll Surg 180:713–717, 1995.

340. Morsing P, Stenberg A, Persson AE: Effect of thromboxane inhibition on tubuloglomerular feedback in hydronephrotic kidneys. Kidney Int 36:447–452, 1989.

341. Miyajima A, Ito K, Asano T, et al: Does cyclooxygenase-2 inhibitor prevent renal tissue damage in unilateral ureteral obstruction? J Urol 166:1124–1129, 2001.

342. Ozturk H, Ozdemir E, Otcu S, et al: Renal effects on a solitary kidney of specific inhibition of cyclooxygenase-2 after 24 h of complete ureteric obstruction in rats. Urol Res 30:223–226, 2002.

343. Coffman TM, Yarger WE, Klotman PE: Functional role of thromboxane production by acutely rejecting renal allografts in rats. J Clin Invest 75:1242–1248, 1985.

344. Tonshoff B, Busch C, Schweer H, et al: In vivo prostanoid formation during acute renal allograft rejection. Nephrol Dial Transplant 8:631–636, 1993.

345. Coffman TM, Yohay D, Carr DR, et al: Effect of dietary fish oil supplementation on eicosanoid production by rat renal allografts. Transplantation 45:470–474, 1988.

346. Coffman TM, Carr DR, Yarger WE, et al: Evidence that renal prostaglandin and thromboxane production is stimulated in chronic cyclosporine nephrotoxicity. Transplantation 43:282–285, 1987.

347. Hocherl K, Dreher F, Vitzthum H, et al: Cyclosporin A suppresses cyclooxygenase-2 expression in the rat kidney. J Am Soc Nephrol 13:2427–2436, 2002.

348. Laffi G, La Villa G, Pinzani M, et al: Arachidonic acid derivatives and renal function in liver cirrhosis. Semin Nephrol 17:530–548, 1997.

349. Lopez-Parra M, Claria J, Planaguma A, et al: Cyclooxygenase-1 derived prostaglandins are involved in the maintenance of renal function in rats with cirrhosis and ascites. Br J Pharmacol 135:891–900, 2002.

350. Bosch-Marce M, Claria J, Titos E, et al: Selective inhibition of cyclooxygenase 2 spares renal function and prostaglandin synthesis in cirrhotic rats with ascites. Gastroenterology 116:1167–1175, 1999.

351. Medina JF, Prieto J, Guarner F, et al: Effect of spironolactone on renal prostaglandin excretion in patients with liver cirrhosis and ascites. J Hepatol 3:206–211, 1986.

352. Epstein M, Lifschitz M: Renal eicosanoids as determinants of renal function in liver disease. Hepatology 7:1359–1367, 1987.

353. Moore K, Ward PS, Taylor GW, et al: Systemic and renal production of thromboxane A2 and prostacyclin in decompensated liver disease and hepatorenal syndrome. Gastroenterology 100:1069–1077, 1991.

354. Khan KN, Stanfield KM, Harris RK, et al: Expression of cyclooxygenase-2 in the macula densa of human kidney in hypertension, congestive heart failure, and diabetic nephropathy. Ren Fail 23:321–330, 2001.

355. DeRubertis FR, Craven PA: Eicosanoids in the pathogenesis of the functional and structural alterations of the kidney in diabetes. Am J Kidney Dis 22:727–735, 1993.

356. Hommel E, Mathiesen E, Arnold-Larsen S, et al: Effects of indomethacin on kidney function in type 1 (insulin-dependent) diabetic patients with nephropathy. Diabetologia 30:78–81, 1987.

357. Cheng HF, Wang CJ, Moeckel GW, et al: Cyclooxygenase-2 inhibitor blocks expression of mediators of renal injury in a model of diabetes and hypertension. Kidney Int 62:929–939, 2002.

358. Makino H, Tanaka I, Mukoyama M, et al: Prevention of diabetic nephropathy in rats by prostaglandin E receptor EP1-selective antagonist. J Am Soc Nephrol 13:1757–1765, 2002.

359. Yamashita T, Shikata K, Matsuda M, et al: Beraprost sodium, prostacyclin analogue, attenuates glomerular hyperfiltration and glomerular macrophage infiltration by modulating ecNOS expression in diabetic rats. Diabetes Res Clin Pract 57:149–161, 2002.

360. Baylis C: Cyclooxygenase products do not contribute to the gestational renal vasodilation in the nitric oxide synthase inhibited pregnant rat. Hypertens Pregnancy 21:109–114, 2002.

361. Khalil RA, Granger JP: Vascular mechanisms of increased arterial pressure in preeclampsia: lessons from animal models. Am J Physiol Regul Integr Comp Physiol 283: R29–45, 2002.

362. Keith JC, Jr., Thatcher CD, Schaub RG: Beneficial effects of U-63,557A, a thromboxane synthetase inhibitor, in an ovine model of pregnancy-induced hypertension. Am J Obstet Gynecol 157:199–203, 1987.

363. Klockenbusch W, Rath W: [Prevention of pre-eclampsia by low-dose acetylsalicylic acid—a critical appraisal]. Z Geburtshilfe Neonatol 206:125–130, 2002.

364. Heyborne KD: Preeclampsia prevention: lessons from the low-dose aspirin therapy trials. Am J Obstet Gynecol 183:523–528, 2000.

365. Reinhold SW, Vitzthum H, Filbeck T, et al: Gene expression of 5-, 12-, and 15-lipoxygenases and leukotriene receptors along the rat nephron. Am J Physiol Renal Physiol 290:F864–872, 2006.

366. Clarkson MR, McGinty A, Godson C, et al: Leukotrienes and lipoxins: Lipoxygenase-derived modulators of leukocyte recruitment and vascular tone in glomerulonephritis. Nephrol Dial Transplant 13:3043–3051, 1998.

367. Dixon RA, Diehl RE, Opas E, et al: Requirement of a 5-lipoxygenase-activating protein for leukotriene synthesis. Nature 343:282–284, 1990.

368. Albrightson CR, Short B, Dytko G, et al: Selective inhibition of 5-lipoxygenase attenuates glomerulonephritis in the rat. Kidney Int 45:1301–1310, 1994.

369. Lynch KR, O'Neill GP, Liu Q, et al: Characterization of the human cysteinyl leukotriene CysLT1 receptor. Nature 399:789–793, 1999.

370. Sarau HM, Ames RS, Chambers J, et al: Identification, molecular cloning, expression, and characterization of a cysteinyl leukotriene receptor. Mol Pharmacol 56:657–663, 1999.

371. Hui Y, Funk CD: Cysteinyl leukotriene receptors. Biochem Pharmacol 64:1549–1557, 2002.

372. Bigby TD: The yin and the yang of 5-lipoxygenase pathway activation. Mol Pharmacol 62:200–202, 2002.

373. Hallstrand TS, Henderson WR, Jr: Leukotriene modifiers. Med Clin North Am 86:1009–1033, vi, 2002.

374. Yokomizo T, Kato K, Terawaki K, et al: A second leukotriene B(4) receptor, BLT2. A new therapeutic target in inflammation and immunological disorders. J Exp Med 192:421–432, 2000.

375. Noiri E, Yokomizo T, Nakao A, et al: An in vivo approach showing the chemotactic activity of leukotriene B(4) in acute renal ischemic-reperfusion injury. Proc Natl Acad Sci U S A 97:823–828, 2000.

376. Suzuki S, Kuroda T, Kazama JI, et al: The leukotriene B4 receptor antagonist ONO-4057 inhibits nephrotoxic serum nephritis in WKY rats. J Am Soc Nephrol 10:264–270, 1999.

377. Chiang N, Gronert K, Clish CB, et al: Leukotriene B4 receptor transgenic mice reveal novel protective roles for lipoxins and aspirin-triggered lipoxins in reperfusion. J Clin Invest 104:309–316, 1999.

378. Devchand PR, Keller H, Peters JM, et al: The PPARalpha-leukotriene B4 pathway to inflammation control. Nature 384:39–43, 1996.

379. Badr KF: Glomerulonephritis: roles for lipoxygenase pathways in pathophysiology and therapy. Curr Opin Nephrol Hypertens 6:111–118, 1997.

380. Papayianni A, Serhan CN, Brady HR: Lipoxin A4 and B4 inhibit leukotriene-stimulated interactions of human neutrophils and endothelial cells. J Immunol 156:2264–2272, 1996.

381. Nassar GM, Badr KF: Role of leukotrienes and lipoxygenases in glomerular injury. Miner Electrolyte Metab 21:262–270, 1995.

382. Katoh T, Takahashi K, DeBoer DK, et al: Renal hemodynamic actions of lipoxins in rats: a comparative physiological study. Am J Physiol 263:F436–442, 1992.

383. Brady HR, Lamas S, Papayianni A, et al: Lipoxygenase product formation and cell adhesion during neutrophil-glomerular endothelial cell interaction. Am J Physiol 268:F1–12, 1995.

384. Chiang N, Fierro IM, Gronert K, et al: Activation of lipoxin A(4) receptors by aspirin-triggered lipoxins and select peptides evokes ligand-specific responses in inflammation. J Exp Med 191:1197–1208, 2000.

385. Pawloski JR, Chapnick BM: Leukotrienes C4 and D4 are potent endothelium-dependent relaxing agents in canine splanchnic venous capacitance vessels. Circ Res 73:395–404, 1993.

386. Claria J, Lee MH, Serhan CN: Aspirin-triggered lipoxins (15-epi-LX) are generated by the human lung adenocarcinoma cell line (A549)-neutrophil interactions and are potent inhibitors of cell proliferation. Mol Med 2:583–596, 1996.

387. Imig JD: Eicosanoid regulation of the renal vasculature. Am J Physiol Renal Physiol 279:F965–981, 2000.

388. Nie D, Tang K, Diglio C, et al: Eicosanoid regulation of angiogenesis: role of endothelial arachidonate 12-lipoxygenase. Blood 95:2304–2311, 2000.

389. Ma J, Natarajan R, LaPage J, et al: 12/15-lipoxygenase inhibitors in diabetic nephropathy in the rat. Prostaglandins Leukot Essent Fatty Acids 72:13–20, 2005.

390. Kim YS, Xu ZG, Reddy MA, et al: Novel interactions between TGF-[beta]1 actions and the 12/15-lipoxygenase pathway in mesangial cells. J Am Soc Nephrol 16:352–362, 2005.

391. Imig JD, Deichmann PC: Afferent arteriolar responses to ANG II involve activation of PLA2 and modulation by lipoxygenase and P-450 pathways. Am J Physiol 273:F274–282, 1997.

392. Wu XC, Richards NT, Michael J, et al: Relative roles of nitric oxide and cyclo-oxygenase and lipoxygenase products of arachidonic acid in the contractile responses of rat renal arcuate arteries. Br J Pharmacol 112:369–376, 1994.

393. Stern N, Nozawa K, Kisch E, et al: Tonic inhibition of renin secretion by the 12 lipoxygenase pathway: Augmentation by high salt intake. Endocrinology 137:1878–1884, 1996.

394. Antonipillai I, Nadler J, Vu EJ, et al: A 12-lipoxygenase product, 12-hydroxyeicosatetraenoic acid, is increased in diabetics with incipient and early renal disease. J Clin Endocrinol Metab 81:1940–1945, 1996.

395. Brady HR, Papayianni A, Serhan CN: Transcellular pathways and cell adhesion as potential contributors to leukotriene and lipoxin biosynthesis in acute glomerulonephritis. Adv Exp Med Biol 400B:631–640, 1997.

396. Kang SW, Adler SG, Nast CC, et al: 12-lipoxygenase is increased in glucose-stimulated mesangial cells and in experimental diabetic nephropathy. Kidney Int 59:1354–1362, 2001.

397. Rahman MA, Nakazawa M, Emancipator SN, et al: Increased leukotriene B4 synthesis in immune injured rat glomeruli. J Clin Invest 81:1945–1952, 1988.

398. Badr KF: Five-lipoxygenase products in glomerular immune injury. J Am Soc Nephrol 3:907–915, 1992.

399. Papayianni A, Serhan CN, Phillips ML, et al: Transcellular biosynthesis of lipoxin A4 during adhesion of platelets and neutrophils in experimental immune complex glomerulonephritis. Kidney Int 47:1295–1302, 1995.

400. Katoh T, Lianos EA, Fukunaga M, et al: Leukotriene D4 is a mediator of proteinuria and glomerular hemodynamic abnormalities in passive Heymann nephritis. J Clin Invest 91:1507–1515, 1993.

401. Butterly DW, Spurney RF, Ruiz P, et al: A role for leukotrienes in cyclosporine nephrotoxicity. Kidney Int 57:2586–2593, 2000.

402. Goulet JL, Griffiths RC, Ruiz P, et al: Deficiency of 5-lipoxygenase accelerates renal allograft rejection in mice. J Immunol 167:6631–6636, 2001.

403. Fauler J, Wiemeyer A, Marx KH, et al: LTB4 in nephrotoxic serum nephritis in rats. Kidney Int 36:46–50, 1989.

404. Lianos EA: Synthesis of hydroxyeicosatetraenoic acids and leukotrienes in rat nephrotoxic serum glomerulonephritis. Role of anti-glomerular basement membrane antibody dose, complement, and neutrophiles. J Clin Invest 82:427–435, 1988.

405. Ferrante JV, Huang ZH, Nandoskar M, et al: Altered responses of human macrophages to lipopolysaccharide by hydroperoxy eicosatetraenoic acid, hydroxy eicosatetraenoic acid, and arachidonic acid. Inhibition of tumor necrosis factor production. J Clin Invest 99:1445–1452, 1997.

406. Munger KA, Montero A, Fukunaga M, et al: Transfection of rat kidney with human 15-lipoxygenase suppresses inflammation and preserves function in experimental glomerulonephritis. Proc Natl Acad Sci U S A 96:13375–13380, 1999.

407. Guasch A, Zayas CF, Badr KF: MK-591 acutely restores glomerular size selectivity and reduces proteinuria in human glomerulonephritis. Kidney Int 56:261–267, 1999.

408. Makita N, Funk CD, Imai E, et al: Molecular cloning and functional expression of rat leukotriene A4 hydrolase using the polymerase chain reaction. FEBS Lett 299:273–277, 1992.

409. Yared A, Albrightson-Winslow C, Griswold D, et al: Functional significance of leukotriene B4 in normal and glomerulonephritic kidneys. J Am Soc Nephrol 2:45–56, 1991.

410. Patel NS, Cuzzocrea S, Chatterjee PK, et al: Reduction of renal ischemia-reperfusion injury in 5-lipoxygenase knockout mice and by the 5-lipoxygenase inhibitor zileuton. Mol Pharmacol 66:220–227, 2004.

411. Capdevila JH, Harris RC, Falck JR: Microsomal cytochrome P450 and eicosanoid metabolism. Cell Mol Life Sci 59:780–789, 2002.

412. Capdevila JH, Falck JR, Harris RC: Cytochrome P450 and arachidonic acid bioactivation. Molecular and functional properties of the arachidonate monooxygenase. J Lipid Res 41:163–181, 2000.

413. Roman RJ: P-450 metabolites of arachidonic acid in the control of cardiovascular function. Physiol Rev 82:131–185, 2002.

414. McGiff JC, Quilley J: 20-HETE and the kidney: resolution of old problems and new beginnings. Am J Physiol 277:R607–623, 1999.

415. Ma J, Qu W, Scarborough PE, et al: Molecular cloning, enzymatic characterization, developmental expression, and cellular localization of a mouse cytochrome P450 highly expressed in kidney. J Biol Chem 274:17777–17788, 1999.

416. Ito O, Alonso-Galicia M, Hopp KA, et al: Localization of cytochrome P-450 4A isoforms along the rat nephron. Am J Physiol 274:F395–404, 1998.

417. Yokose T, Doy M, Taniguchi T, et al: Immunohistochemical study of cytochrome P450 2C and 3A in human non-neoplastic and neoplastic tissues. Virchows Arch 434:401–411, 1999.

418. Imig JD, Zou AP, Stec DE, et al: Formation and actions of 20-hydroxyeicosatetraenoic acid in rat renal arterioles. Am J Physiol 270:R217–227, 1996.

419. Ito O, Roman RJ: Regulation of P-450 4A activity in the glomerulus of the rat. Am J Physiol 276:R1749–1757, 1999.

420. Quigley R, Baum M, Reddy KM, et al: Effects of 20-HETE and 19(S)-HETE on rabbit proximal straight tubule volume transport. Am J Physiol Renal Physiol 278:F949–953, 2000.

421. Escalante B, Erlij D, Falck JR, et al: Effect of cytochrome P450 arachidonate metabolites on ion transport in rabbit kidney loop of Henle. Science 251:799–802, 1991.

422. Ito O, Roman RJ: Role of 20-HETE in elevating chloride transport in the thick ascending limb of Dahl SS/Jr rats. Hypertension 33:419–423, 1999.

423. Hirt DL, Capdevila J, Falck JR, et al: Cytochrome P450 metabolites of arachidonic acid are potent inhibitors of vasopressin action on rabbit cortical collecting duct. J Clin Invest 84:1805–1812, 1989.

424. Makita K, Falck JR, Capdevila JH: Cytochrome P450, the arachidonic acid cascade, and hypertension: New vistas for an old enzyme system. FASEB J 10:1456–1463, 1996.

425. Alonso-Galicia M, Sun CW, Falck JR, et al: Contribution of 20-HETE to the vasodilator actions of nitric oxide in renal arteries. Am J Physiol 275:F370–378, 1998.

426. Sun CW, Alonso-Galicia M, Taheri MR, et al: Nitric oxide-20-hydroxyeicosatetraenoic acid interaction in the regulation of K+ channel activity and vascular tone in renal arterioles. Circ Res 83:1069–1079, 1998.

427. Imig JD, Navar LG, Roman RJ, et al: Actions of epoxygenase metabolites on the preglomerular vasculature. J Am Soc Nephrol 7:2364–2370, 1996.

428. Katoh T, Takahashi K, Capdevila J, et al: Glomerular stereospecific synthesis and hemodynamic actions of 8,9-epoxyeicosatrienoic acid in rat kidney. Am J Physiol 261:F578–586, 1991.

429. Campbell WB, Gauthier KM: What is new in endothelium-derived hyperpolarizing factors? Curr Opin Nephrol Hypertens 11:177–183, 2002.

430. Vazquez B, Rios A, Escalante B: Arachidonic acid metabolism modulates vasopressin-induced renal vasoconstriction. Life Sci 56:1455–1466, 1995.

431. Imig JD, Pham BT, LeBlanc EA, et al: Cytochrome P450 and cyclooxygenase metabolites contribute to the endothelin-1 afferent arteriolar vasoconstrictor and calcium responses. Hypertension 35:307–312, 2000.

432. Oyekan AO, Youseff T, Fulton D, et al: Renal cytochrome P450 omega-hydroxylase and epoxygenase activity are differentially modified by nitric oxide and sodium chloride. J Clin Invest 104:1131–1137, 1999.

433. Arima S, Endo Y, Yaoita H, et al: Possible role of P-450 metabolite of arachidonic acid in vasodilator mechanism of angiotensin II type 2 receptor in the isolated micro-perfused rabbit afferent arteriole. J Clin Invest 100:2816–2823, 1997.

434. Alonso-Galicia M, Maier KG, Greene AS, et al: Role of 20-hydroxyeicosatetraenoic acid in the renal and vasoconstrictor actions of angiotensin II. Am J Physiol Regul Integr Comp Physiol 283:R60–68, 2002.

435. Imig JD, Falck JR, Inscho EW: Contribution of cytochrome P450 epoxygenase and hydroxylase pathways to afferent arteriolar autoregulatory responsiveness. Br J Pharmacol 127:1399–1405, 1999.

436. Zou AP, Drummond HA, Roman RJ: Role of 20-HETE in elevating loop chloride reabsorption in Dahl SS/Jr rats. Hypertension 27:631–635, 1996.

437. Wang H, Garvin JL, Falck JR, et al: Glomerular cytochrome P-450 and cyclooxygenase metabolites regulate efferent arteriole resistance. Hypertension 46:1175–1179, 2005.

438. Schnermann J: Adenosine mediates tubuloglomerular feedback. Am J Physiol Regul Integr Comp Physiol 283:R276–277; discussion R278–279, 2002.

439. Zou AP, Imig JD, Kaldunski M, et al: Inhibition of renal vascular 20-HETE production impairs autoregulation of renal blood flow. Am J Physiol 266:F275–282, 1994.

440. Hercule HC, Oyekan AO: Cytochrome P450 omega/omega-1 hydroxylase-derived eicosanoids contribute to endothelin(A) and endothelin(B) receptor-mediated vaso-constriction to endothelin-1 in the rat preglomerular arteriole. J Pharmacol Exp Ther 292:1153–1160, 2000.

441. Henrich WL, Falck JR, Campbell WB: Inhibition of renin release by 14,15-epoxyeicosatrienoic acid in renal cortical slices. Am J Physiol 258:E269–274, 1990.

442. Alonso-Galicia M, Falck JR, Reddy KM, et al: 20-HETE agonists and antagonists in the renal circulation. Am J Physiol 277:F790–796, 1999.

443. Romero MF, Madhun ZT, Hopfer U, et al: An epoxygenase metabolite of arachidonic acid 5,6 epoxy-eicosatrienoic acid mediates angiotensin-induced natriuresis in proxi-mal tubular epithelium. Adv Prostaglandin Thromboxane Leukot Res 21A:205–208, 1991.

444. Escalante BA, Staudinger R, Schwartzman M, et al: Amiloride-sensitive ion transport inhibition by epoxyeicosatrienoic acids in renal epithelial cells. Adv Prostaglandin Thromboxane Leukot Res 23:207–209, 1995.

445. Staudinger R, Escalante B, Schwartzman ML, et al: Effects of epoxyeicosatrienoic acids on 86Rb uptake in renal epithelial cells. J Cell Physiol 160:69–74, 1994.

446. Nowicki S, Chen SL, Aizman O, et al: 20-Hydroxyeicosa-tetraenoic acid (20 HETE) activates protein kinase C. Role in regulation of rat renal Na+,K+-ATPase. J Clin Invest 99:1224–1230, 1997.

447. Carroll MA, Balazy M, Margiotta P, et al: Cytochrome P-450-dependent HETEs: profile of biological activity and stimulation by vasoactive peptides. Am J Physiol 271:R863–869, 1996.

448. Burns KD, Capdevila J, Wei S, et al: Role of cytochrome P-450 epoxygenase metabo-lites in EGF signaling in renal proximal tubule. Am J Physiol 269:C831–840, 1995.

449. Houillier P, Chambrey R, Achard JM, et al: Signaling pathways in the biphasic effect of angiotensin II on apical Na/H antiport activity in proximal tubule. Kidney Int 50:1496–1505, 1996.

450. Navar LG, Lewis L, Hymel A, et al: Tubular fluid concentrations and kidney contents of angiotensins I and II in anesthetized rats. J Am Soc Nephrol 5:1153–1158, 1994.

451. Zhang YB, Magyar CE, Holstein-Rathlou NH, et al: The cytochrome P-450 inhibitor cobalt chloride prevents inhibition of renal Na,K-ATPase and redistribution of apical NHE-3 during acute hypertension. J Am Soc Nephrol 9:531–537, 1998.

452. Escalante B, Erlij D, Falck JR, et al: Ion transport inhibition in the medullary thick ascending limb of Henle's loop by cytochrome P450-arachidonic acid metabolites. Adv Prostaglandin Thromboxane Leukot Res 21A:209–212, 1991.

453. Wang W, Lu M, Balazy M: Phospholipase A2 is involved in mediating the effect of extracellular Ca2+ on apical K+ channels in rat TAL. Am J Physiol 273:F421–429, 1997.

454. Good DW, George T, Wang DH: Angiotensin II inhibits HCO-3 absorption via a cyto-chrome P-450-dependent pathway in MTAL. Am J Physiol 276:F726–736, 1999.

455. Grider JS, Falcone JC, Kilpatrick EL, et al: P450 arachidonate metabolites mediate bradykinin-dependent inhibition of NaCl transport in the rat thick ascending limb. Can J Physiol Pharmacol 75:91–96, 1997.

456. Sakairi Y, Jacobson HR, Noland TD, et al: 5,6-EET inhibits ion transport in collecting duct by stimulating endogenous prostaglandin synthesis. Am J Physiol 268:F931–939, 1995.

457. Wei Y, Lin DH, Kemp R, et al: Arachidonic acid inhibits epithelial Na channel via cytochrome P450 (CYP) epoxygenase-dependent metabolic pathways. J Gen Physiol 124:719–727, 2004.

458. Sellmayer A, Uedelhoven WM, Weber PC, et al: Endogenous non-cyclooxygenase metabolites of arachidonic acid modulate growth and mRNA levels of immediate-early response genes in rat mesangial cells. J Biol Chem 266:3800–3807, 1991.

459. Harris RC, Homma TJ, Jacobson HR, Capdevila J: Epoxyeicosatrienoic acids are mito-gens for rat mesangial cells: Signal transduction pathways. J Cell Physiol 144:429–443, 1990.

460. Chen JK, Capdevila J, Harris RC: Heparin-binding EGF-like growth factor mediates the biological effects of P450 arachidonate epoxygenase metabolites in epithelial cells. Proc Natl Acad Sci U S A 99:6029–6034, 2002.

461. Lin F, Rios A, Falck JR, et al: 20-Hydroxyeicosatetraenoic acid is formed in response to EGF and is a mitogen in rat proximal tubule. Am J Physiol 269:F806–816, 1995.

462. Uddin MR, Muthalif MM, Karzoun NA, et al: Cytochrome P-450 metabolites mediate norepinephrine-induced mitogenic signaling. Hypertension 31:242–247, 1998.

463. Holla VR, Makita K, Zaphiropoulos PG, et al: The kidney cytochrome P-450 2C23 arachidonic acid epoxygenase is upregulated during dietary salt loading. J Clin Invest 104:751–760, 1999.

464. Imig JD: Epoxide hydrolase and epoxygenase metabolites as therapeutic targets for renal diseases. Am J Physiol Renal Physiol 289:F496–503, 2005.

465. Oyekan AO, McAward K, Conetta J, et al: Endothelin-1 and CYP450 arachidonate metabolites interact to promote tissue injury in DOCA-salt hypertension. Am J Physiol 276:R766–775, 1999.

466. Muthalif MM, Benter IF, Khandekar Z, et al: Contribution of Ras GTPase/MAP kinase and cytochrome P450 metabolites to deoxycorticosterone-salt-induced hypertension. Hypertension 35:457–463, 2000.

467. Croft KD, McGiff JC, Sanchez-Mendoza A, et al: Angiotensin II releases 20-HETE from rat renal microvessels. Am J Physiol Renal Physiol 279:F544–551, 2000.

468. Iwai N, Inagami T: Identification of a candidate gene responsible for the high blood pressure of spontaneously hypertensive rats. J. Hypertension 10:1155–1157, 1992.

469. Stec DE, Trolliet MR, Krieger JE, et al: Renal cytochrome P4504A activity and salt sensitivity in spontaneously hypertensive rats. Hypertension 27:1329–1336, 1996.

470. Wang MH, Zhang F, Marji J, et al: CYP4A1 antisense oligonucleotide reduces mesen-teric vascular reactivity and blood pressure in SHR. Am J Physiol Regul Integr Comp Physiol 280:R255–261, 2001.

471. Su P, Kaushal KM, Kroetz DL: Inhibition of renal arachidonic acid omega-hydroxylase activity with ABT reduces blood pressure in the SHR. Am J Physiol 275:R426–438, 1998.

472. Gainer JV, Bellamine A, Dawson EP, et al: Functional variant of CYP4A11 20-hydroxyeicosatetraenoic acid synthase is associated with essential hypertension. Circulation 111:63–69, 2005.

473. Imig JD, Zou AP, Ortiz de Montellano PR, et al: Cytochrome P-450 inhibitors alter afferent arteriolar responses to elevations in pressure. Am J Physiol 266:H1879–1885, 1994.

474. Muller C, Endlich K, Helwig JJ: AT2 antagonist-sensitive potentiation of angiotensin II-induced constriction by NO blockade and its dependence on endothelium and P450 eicosanoids in rat renal vasculature. Br J Pharmacol 124:946–952, 1998.

475. Gross V, Schunck WH, Honeck H, et al: Inhibition of pressure natriuresis in mice lacking the AT2 receptor. Kidney Int 57:191–202, 2000.

Extracellular Fluid and Edema Formation

Karl L. Skorecki • Joseph Winaver • Zaid A. Abassi

CONTROL OF EXTRACELLULAR FLUID VOLUME

The volume of extracellular fluid (ECF) is maintained within narrow limits in normal human subjects, despite day-to-day variations in dietary intake of salt and water over a wide range. Plasma volume, in turn determined by the total ECF volume and the partitioning of this volume between extravascular and intravascular compartments according to the dictates of the Starling relationship, also remains remarkably constant despite alterations in dietary salt intake (Fig. 12–1). The relationship of ECF volume and, in particular, the volume of the plasma compartment to overall vascular capacitance determines such fundamental indices of cardiovascular performance as mean arterial blood pressure and left ventricular filling volume. Given the rigorous defense of ECF sodium (Na^+) concentration, mediated mainly by osmoregulatory mechanisms concerned with external water balance (see Chapter 13), the quantity of Na^+ determines the volume of this compartment. Surfeits or deficits of total body water alter serum Na^+ concentration and osmolality but contribute little to determining the volume of the ECF. As vascular capacitance and Na^+ intake change in response to a given physiologic or pathologic stimulus, the renal excretion of Na^+ adjusts to restore ECF volume to a level appropriate to the renewed setting of vascular capacitance.

The overall relationship among Na^+ intake, ECF volume, and Na^+ excretion can be considered in pharmacokinetic terms. Such consideration has led to a shifting steady-state model for overall Na^+ homeostasis,[1] as opposed to the constant "set-point" model (see also Reinhardt and Seeliger[2] and references therein). According to the shifting steady-state model, in any given steady state, total daily Na^+ intake and excretion are equal. Acute deviations from a preexisting steady state, consequent to an alteration in Na^+ intake or extrarenal excretion, results in an adjustment in renal Na^+ excretion. This adjustment in renal Na^+ excretion occurs as a result of a new total body Na^+ content and ECF volume, and it aims to restore the preexisting steady state. This differs from the "set-point" model, in which the control system aims to reach a constant total body Na^+ ("set-point").[2] The establishment of a new steady-state level of Na^+ intake and excretion in the shifting steady-state model reflects a new total body Na^+ content and ECF volume. Alternatively, an alteration in the capacitance of the extracellular compartment can also result in an adjustment in renal Na^+ excretion, whose aim is to restore the preexisting relationship of volume to capacitance. It is clear that the operation of such a system for Na^+ homeostasis requires (1) sensors that detect changes in ECF volume relative to vascular and interstitial capacitance and (2) effector mechanisms that ultimately modify the rate of Na^+ excretion by the kidney to meet the demands of volume homeostasis. Adjustments in effector mechanisms occur in response to perceived alterations in sensor input, with the aim of optimizing circulatory performance. Derangements in either sensor or effector mechanisms can lead to disordered Na^+ balance and disruption of circulatory integrity. Thus, inability of the kidney to precisely adjust the rate of Na^+ excretion to a given Na^+ intake may result in the development of positive or negative total body Na^+ balance. These perturbations, when present over extended periods, may be clinically manifested as hypertension or edema formation in the case of positive Na^+ balance or hypotension and hypovolemia in the case of negative Na^+ balance.

The purpose of this chapter is to summarize current understanding of the various sensor and effector mechanisms thought to be involved in the normal regulation of ECF volume and the disturbances in the mechanisms that occur in edema-forming states, namely, congestive heart failure (CHF) and cirrhosis with ascites.

Afferent Limb: Sensors for Fluid Homeostasis

Fluid homeostasis is essential to the maintenance of circulatory stability, so it is hardly surprising that volume detectors reside at several sites within the vascular bed (Table 12–1). For this discussion, it is useful to consider the afferent sensing sites as comprising cardiopulmonary and arterial baroreceptors as well as renal, central nervous system (CNS), and hepatic sensors. Each compartment can be viewed as reflecting a unique characteristic of overall circulatory function, such as cardiac filling, cardiac output, renal perfusion, and fluid transudation into the interstitial space. Sensors within each compartment monitor a physical parameter (e.g., stretch, tension) that serves as an index of circulatory function within that compartment. The mechanisms by which these sensors operate are not fully elucidated, though our understanding has progressed significantly in recent years. In the past, it was assumed that mechanosensing is performed by afferent sensory nerve endings found primarily in blood vessel walls. However, it is now known that the endothelium may also participate in the process of mechanosensing.[3] The mechanisms involved include stretch-activated ion channels, protein kinases associated with the cytoskeleton, integrin-cytoskeletal interactions, cytoskeletal-nuclear interactions, and generation of reactive oxygen species.[3] It is also known that mechanical stretch and tension impinging on blood vessel cells can result in altered gene expression, mediated through specific recognition motifs within the upstream promoter elements of responsive genes.[4] In

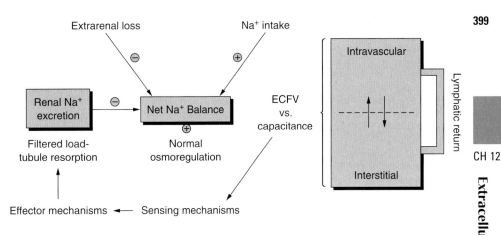

FIGURE 12–1 Overall scheme for body Na⁺ balance and partitioning of extracellular fluid volume (ECFV). In the setting of normal osmoregulation, extracellular Na⁺ content is the primary determinant of ECFV. Overall Na⁺ homeostasis depends on the balance between losses (extrarenal and renal) and intake. Renal Na⁺ excretion is determined by the balance between filtered load and tubule reabsorption. This latter balance is modulated under the influence of effector mechanisms, which, in turn, are responsive to sensing mechanisms that monitor the relation between ECFV and capacitance.

TABLE 12–1	**Mechanisms for Sensing Regional Changes in Body Fludi Volume**

Cardiopulmonary volume sensors
   Atria (neural/humoral pathways)
   Ventricular and pulmonary sensing sites

Arterial volume sensors
   Carotid and aortic arch baroreceptors
   Renal volume sensors

Central nervous system sensors

Hepatic volume sensors

turn, signals emanating from afferent sites engage efferent mechanisms that effect compensatory changes in renal Na⁺ excretion. Volume expansion results in an integrated sequence of neural reflexes and hormonal responses that enhances the renal excretion of salt and water. Conversely, the reflex response to volume contraction is renal conservation of salt and water.

Cardiopulmonary Volume Sensors

Atrial Sensors

The cardiac atria possess the distensibility and the compliance necessary to monitor changes in intrathoracic venous volume. Henry and colleagues[5] demonstrated that left atrial distention induces diuresis, as a part of a "volume reflex." Goetz and associates[6] provided a clear demonstration of the effectiveness of changes in atrial transmural pressure in controlling Na⁺ and water excretion in conscious dogs. Since that time, diuresis and natriuresis as a consequence of increasing atrial wall tension and the role of the atria in overall volume homeostasis have been clearly established. In humans, the role of the atria in volume homeostasis can best be illustrated by studies utilizing maneuvers that alter atrial volume and size, such as head-out water immersion (HWI) and exposure to head-down tilt, which causes a redistribution of blood and fluid from the peripheral to the central circulation and nonhypotensive lower body negative pressure (LBNP) that unloads the cardiopulmonary baroreceptors.[7–9] HWI results in increases in central blood volume, central venous pressure, and right atrial and pulmonary arterial transmural pressure gradients. After immersion, brisk natriuresis and diuresis ensue, with an increase in fractional excretion of Na⁺ comparable with that resulting from saline loading.[7] In contrast, the application of nonhypotensive LBNP results in a redistribution of blood to the lower limbs, thereby reducing central venous pressure and cardiac filling pressures without causing detectable changes in arterial pressure or heart rate. This maneuver has been shown by echocardiography to reduce

atrial diameter. In normal human subjects, LBNP has been shown to result in antidiuresis and antinatriuresis without a significant change in renal plasma flow (RPF).[8] These findings point clearly to an atrial sensing mechanism for central venous volume that influences renal Na⁺ and water excretion. Higher degrees of LBNP, at the hypotensive range, have been used as a model to study the cardiovascular adjustments during progression of acute hemorrhagic shock in humans.[10] Nevertheless, the use of these maneuvers to selectively load or unload the cardiopulmonary volume receptors must be faced with caution. In particular, HWI has been shown to cause, in addition to central hypervolemia, a significant degree of hemodilution.[11] The external hydrostatic pressure of the water reduces the hydrostatic pressure gradient across the capillary wall in the legs, resulting in a net transfer of fluids from the interstitial compartment to the intravascular compartment. The central blood volume expansion is therefore associated with hemodilution and a significant decrease in the colloid osmotic pressure (COP). The importance of hemodilution and the resultant decrease in COP in mediating the natriuresis of volume expansion was underscored by Cowley and Skelton.[12] They suggested that the decrease in COP, rather than stimulation of the cardiopulmonary volume receptors, was the predominant cause of natriuresis during saline infusions in dogs. Supporting this notion are the findings of Johansen and co-workers,[13] who demonstrated that preventing hemodilution by placing an inflated (80 mm Hg), tight cuff during HWI abolished the natriuresis. These findings suggest that, during HWI, the combined effects of hemodilution and central blood volume expansion, with their associated neuronal and endocrine changes, play a pivotal role in the initiation of natriuresis.

NEURAL PATHWAYS. Neural receptors responsive to mechanical stretch or transmural pressure have been described in the atria. These are thought to be branching ends of small medullated fibers running in the vagus nerve.[14] Two populations have been described. Type A receptors, concentrated at the entrance of the great veins into the atria, discharge once per cardiac cycle, beginning with atrial systole. The activity of these receptors is not affected by atrial volume. On the other hand, the activity of type B receptors, which discharge with atrial filling, correlates well with atrial size.[14] Stretch and tension signals detected at these sites are believed to travel along cranial nerves IX and X to the hypothalamic and medullary centers, in which a series of responses are initiated: inhibition of release of antidiuretic hormone (ADH), mostly left atrium[15]; a selective decrease in renal but not lumbar sympathetic nerve discharge[16,17]; and decreased tone in precapillary and postcapillary resistance vessels in the peripheral vascular bed, the latter influencing the magnitude of transudation of interstitial fluid. Reduction in central venous pressure and atrial size by LBNP exerts a stimulatory effect on renal nerve activity in humans, as assessed by renal norepinephrine (NE) spillover and plasma NE concentration.[9,18] Chronic atrial stretch results in adaptation and downward resetting of these neural responses. Thus, it was demonstrated in rhesus monkeys exposed to 10 degrees of head-down tilt that such an adaptation was responsible for a "shift to the left" in the relationship of urinary Na^+ excretion versus central venous pressure during saline infusion.[19] This suggests that the kidney responds with natriuresis at a significantly lower cardiac filling pressure under these conditions. Of note, cardiac denervation studies in canine models have shown that cardiac nerves are not essential for stimulating plasma renin activity and Na^+ retention after an acute deficit, but they are of importance in the restoration of steady-state Na^+ balance after repletion.[20] Similarly, disruption of long-term suppression of the renin-angiotensin-aldosterone system (RAAS) in response to chronic volume expansion occurs after cardiac transplantation in humans.[21]

HUMORAL PATHWAYS. Early experiments showed that interruption of neural pathways during atrial distention did not completely abolish the natriuresis and diuresis associated with this maneuver, indicating that additional factors were operative. These studies suggested a direct humoral mechanism that emanates from the heart and responds to fullness of the circulation. These findings, and the subsequent discovery by de Bold and colleagues[22] in 1981 of a factor in atrial extracts with strong natriuretic and vasodepressor activity, led to the eventual isolation and characterization of natriuretic peptides (NPs) of cardiac origin.[23] The first and best characterized of these is atrial natriuretic peptide (ANP). This 28–amino acid peptide belongs to the NP family, which comprises at least two additional structurally related peptides B- and C-type NPs (BNP and CNP, respectively) encoded by different genes.[24–26] The NPs are discussed in later sections of this chapter, as are effector mechanism for natriuresis induced by these peptides.

Numerous studies in animal models and in human subjects confirmed that a directly induced increment in atrial pressure or stretch results in a sharp release of ANP. It has been estimated that, for each rise of 1 mm Hg in atrial pressure, there is an associated rise of approximately 10 to 15 pmol/L in plasma ANP concentration.[27] This release occurs by a process of cleavage of mature circulating 28–amino acid COOH-terminus peptide, from prohormone located in preformed stores within atrial granules. Stretch-activated ANP release from atrial myocytes is thought to occur in two steps: a Ca^{2+}-sensitive and K^+ channel–dependent release of ANP from myocytes into the surrounding intercellular space, followed by a Ca^{2+}-independent translocation of the released ANP into the atrial lumen.[28] K^+-adenosine triphosphate (ATP) channel blockers such as glibenclamide can block stretch-activated ANP release.[29] Maneuvers that activate the afferent mechanism for release of ANP include intravascular volume expansion by supine posture, HWI, saline administration, exercise, angiotensin II (AII) administration, tachycardia, and ventricular dysfunction.[25,27] In contrast, a decline in plasma ANP concentration follows volume-depleting maneuvers such as Na^+ restriction, furosemide administration, and the reduction in central venous pressure associated with application of LBNP. Whereas the understanding of effects of acute alterations in atrial pressure/volume on ANP release is well established, the role of this peptide in the long-term regulation of volume homeostasis remains controversial.[30,31] In particular, a role for the NPs in the long-term of chronic response to changes in dietary salt intake could not be demonstrated. In a study in humans with incremental levels of dietary Na^+ intake, it was demonstrated that plasma ANP reflected the steady-state Na^+ balance, so that the higher the salt intake, the greater the initial plasma ANP level.[32] However, the main finding in this study was the contrasting ANP response to

acute oral compared with intravenous Na^+ loading: Plasma ANP increased significantly after intravenous saline infusion but not after the oral Na^+ loading.[32] In other studies in humans exposed to intravenous volume expansion and oral Na^+ loading, no direct correlation could be found between the change in plasma ANP level and the degree of natriuresis.[30,33,34] The application of gene-targeting technology in mice provided novel insights regarding the diverse biologic functions of the NP family and their receptors, guanylate cyclases A and B (GC-A and GC-B, respectively). John and co-workers[35] demonstrated that ANP-gene knockout mice displayed a reduced natriuretic response to acute ECF volume expansion compared with the wild-type mice. However, when the mice were maintained on a high-NaCl (8.0%) or low-NaCl (0.008%) diet for 1 week, their cumulative Na^+ and water excretions were comparable with those of wild-type mice. The main perturbation observed in mice with ANP-gene disruption was a significant increase in mean arterial pressure (MAP).[35] Additional studies demonstrated that disruption of the gene for ANP or its receptor, GC-A, demonstrated that this system is essential for maintenance of normal blood pressure but, in addition, exerts local antihypertrophic effects on the heart. Disruption of the genes encoding for the other members of the NP family, BNP and CNP or the GC-B, demonstrated that these peptides are probably not involved in the physiologic regulation of renal Na^+ excretion, but instead exert local paracrine/autocrine cyclic guanosine monophosphate (cGMP)–mediated effects on cellular proliferation and differentiation in various tissues (for recent reviews, see Kuhn[26,36]). It appears, therefore, that regulation of ECF volume and blood pressure is only one facet of the diverse biologic actions of the NP family.

Ventricular and Pulmonary Sensors

Ventricular receptors have usually been regarded solely in the context of reflex changes in heart rate and peripheral vascular resistance (PVR). However, several studies in the past suggested that nerve terminals in ventricles and in the pulmonary vasculature may be involved in sensing changes in blood volume. Increased left ventricular pressure in conscious dogs was found to cause a reflex inhibition of plasma renin activity,[37] and a coronary baroreceptor reflex, linking increased coronary artery pressure to decreased lumbar and renal sympathetic discharge, has also been detected.[38] In the lung, unmyelinated juxtapulmonary capillary (J) receptors have been found (adjacent to pulmonary capillaries) in the interstitium of the lungs.[14] The position of these receptors makes them ideally suited to detect interstitial edema before fluid enters the alveolar space. These afferent nerves join those from the atria in cranial nerves IX and X. Nevertheless, the role played by these ventricular and pulmonary receptors to overall regulation of ECF volume and Na^+ remains to be determined.

Arterial Sensors

The low-pressure receptors described previously assess the fullness of the capacitance system of the vascular tree and may be geared to defend against excessive ECF expansion with the attendant deleterious consequences of pulmonary and systemic venous congestion. However, a primary role of the cardiovascular system is to optimize tissue perfusion. Therefore, it seems logical that sensing mechanisms within the arterial circuit should also have input into overall volume homeostasis and serve to defend primarily against perceived depletion of ECF volume relative to capacitance. An increase in arterial pressure causes vascular distention and baroreceptor deformation. This depolarizes the nerve endings by opening mechanosensitive ion channels and triggers action potential discharge. Baroreceptor activity and sensitivity can be further modified during sustained increases in arterial pressure and in pathologic states associated with endothelial dysfunction, oxidative stress, and platelet activation.[39,40] Evidence favoring the presence of volume-sensitive receptors in the arterial circuit in humans originally derived from the classic observations by Epstein and co-workers[41] in subjects with arteriovenous (AV) fistulas. Closure of fistulas resulted in prompt natriuresis without changes in glomerular filtration rate (GFR) or RPF, whereas re-establishment of fistula patency reduced urinary Na+ excretion. These responses occurred in spite of a decline in hydraulic pressures in the atria and pulmonary vasculature with fistula closure, suggesting that underfilling of the arterial tree signals the kidney to retain Na+ and vice versa. Such sensors in the arterial (high-pressure) circulation exist in the carotid sinus and aortic arch as well as in the renal vasculature.

Carotid Baroreceptor

Histologic and molecular analysis of the carotid baroreceptor has indicated a large content of elastic tissue in the tunica media, which renders the vessel wall in the region highly distensible to changes in intraluminal pressure, thereby facilitating transmission of the stimulus intensity to sensory nerve terminals. Afferent signals from the baroreceptors are integrated in the nucleus tractus solitarius (NTS).[42] Mapping of the neural projections emanating from the carotid baroreceptor in the NTS of the medulla has been greatly facilitated by measurement of changes in the level of expression of the c-fos proto-oncogene after selective baroreceptor stimulation, which may vary according to different pressure thresholds.[43]

Occlusion of the common carotid artery was used in the past to alter renal sympathetic activity and Na+ excretion by the kidney in experimental animals. Common carotid arterial occlusion enhances the activity of the sympathetic nervous system (SNS) and augments renal sympathetic nerve activity. Interestingly, carotid occlusion is sometimes associated with a large natriuresis despite augmented renal sympathetic activation. This is most likely secondary to increases in arterial pressure that result in pressure natriuresis. Moreover, it has been demonstrated in humans that carotid baroreflexes may be modified by maneuvers that alter vascular volume. For example, in normal human subjects, high salt intake blunts the carotid baroreceptors.[44]

Renal Sensors

In addition to its role as a major effector target responding to signals indicating the need for adjustments in Na+ excretion, the kidney participates in the afferent limb of volume homeostasis. The sensor and effector limbs for volume homeostasis are juxtaposed in the kidney. Therefore, volume expansion and depletion may be sensed through alterations in glomerular hemodynamics and possibly renal interstitial pressure that result simultaneously in adjustments in physical forces governing tubule Na+ handling. These are described in greater detail later.

The kidney, along with other organs, has the ability to maintain constant blood flow and GFR at varying arterial pressures. This phenomenon, termed *autoregulation* (see also Chapter 3), operates over a wide range of alterations in renal perfusion pressure (RPP). Changes in RPP are "sensed" by smooth muscle elements that serve as baroreceptors in the afferent glomerular arteriole and respond by adjusting transmural pressure and tension across the arteriolar wall (myogenic response).[45] In addition to this myogenic reflex component, the juxtaglomerular apparatus–dependent tubuloglomerular feedback (TGF) contributes to the maintenance of volume homeostasis.[45-47] These mechanisms serve to minimize the changes in RPF and GFR when renal perfusion pressure is altered and thus maintain the filtered load of Na+. The juxtaglomerular apparatus is important not only because

of the TGF mechanism but also because of its involvement in the generation and release of renin from the kidney.[45,47] The physiologic control of renin release from the cells in the juxtaglomerular apparatus is exerted in three ways, all of which vary with ECF volume, thereby defining the juxtaglomerular apparatus as an important sensing site for volume homeostasis. First, renin secretion has been shown to be inversely related to perfusion pressure and directly related to intrarenal tissue pressure. The release of renin is further augmented when RPP falls below the autoregulatory range. A second mechanism influencing renin secretion is solute delivery to the macula densa. An increase in NaCl delivery passing the macula densa results in inhibition of renin release, whereas a decrease has the opposite effect. Sensing at the macula densa site is mediated by the entry of NaCl, through the Na,K,2Cl co-transport mechanism, which further leads to alterations in intracellular calcium concentration.[48] Prostaglandin E$_2$ (PGE$_2$) and adenosine are also involved in the release of renin.[48] A third mechanism involved in renin secretion concerns the influence of renal nerves.[49] Renal nerve stimulation increases the release of renin via direct activation of β-adrenoceptors on juxtaglomerular granular cells. This activation is followed promptly by release of renin, an effect that can be dissociated from major changes in renal hemodynamics. Sympathetic stimulation also affects intrarenal baroreceptor input, the composition of the fluid delivered to the macula densa, and the renal actions of AII, such that renal nerves may serve primarily to potentiate other controlling signals.[49]

Central Nervous System Sensors

Several studies in the past suggested that certain areas in the CNS may act as sensors to detect alterations in body salt balance. This hypothesis was based primarily on experiments showing that intracerebral administration of hypertonic saline solutions was associated with alterations in renal salt excretion (CNS-induced natriuresis) or in renal nerve activity.[50,51] The activity of various neuroendocrine systems in the CNS, in particular the RAAS and ANP, may be also influenced by alterations in Na+ balance. Thus, it was demonstrated that alterations in dietary Na+ intake may regulate the contribution of brain AII in the modulation of baroreflex regulation of renal sympathetic nerve activity.[52] Indeed, administration of AII into the cerebral ventricles impairs baroreflex regulation of renal sympathetic nerve activity.[52] Neurons that release ANP (ANPergic neurons) are located in the paraventricular nucleus and in a region extending to the anteroventral third ventricle (AV3V). These neurons act to inhibit water and salt intake by blocking the action of AII.[53,54] Stimulation of neurons in the AV3V region causes natriuresis and an increase in circulating ANP, whereas lesions in the AV3V region and caudally in the median eminence or neural lobe decrease resting ANP release and the response to blood volume expansion.[53,54]

However, despite the substantial evidence linking the CNS with the regulation of ECF volume homeostasis, the nature of the sensing mechanisms and their mode of operation remain largely unknown.

Role of the Gastrointestinal Tract in the Regulation of Extracellular Fluid Volume and Sodium Balance

Under normal physiologic conditions, intake of Na+ and water reaches the ECF by absorption from the gastrointestinal tract (GIT). It is, therefore, reasonable to assume that some sensing and controlling mechanisms may exist within the GIT itself that participate in the regulation of ECF volume and Na+ balance. Experimental evidence supporting the latter contention has accumulated in the past 4 decades. Early studies in humans suggested that urinary excretion of an oral Na+ load may be faster and more pronounced than the response to the same Na$^+$ load given by intravenous infusion.[55] Similarly, studies in experimental animals demonstrated that infusions of hypertonic NaCl directly into the portal vein caused a greater natriuresis than a similar infusion into the femoral vein. These findings were interpreted to suggest the presence of Na$^+$-sensing mechanisms in the splanchnic and/or portal circulations in the GIT. Several mechanisms of neural and hormonal origin have been proposed.

Hepatic Receptors

Two main neural reflexes have been described.[56,57] The "hepatorenal" and "hepatointestinal" reflexes originate from receptors in the hepatoportal region. They transduce portal plasma Na$^+$ concentration into hepatic afferent nerve activity and reflexively augment renal Na$^+$ excretion and attenuate intestinal Na$^+$ absorption before a measurable increase in systemic Na$^+$ concentration takes place. Studies in conscious rabbits subjected to intravenous infusion of 20% NaCl solution demonstrated that this procedure caused a marked decrease in renal nerve activity and increased urinary Na$^+$ excretion.[58] Similar findings were reported in other species, supporting a role of the "hepatorenal reflex" in the regulation of renal nerve activity and augmentation of urinary Na$^+$ excretion.[56,57] In addition, signals originating in hepatoportal sensors can also control the intestinal absorption of an Na$^+$ load. The intraportal infusion of 9% NaCl solution causes depression of Na$^+$ absorption across the jejunum.[59] The afferent limbs of this reflex, referred to as the *hepatointestinal reflex,* are the hepatic nerves, and the efferent limbs travel through the vagus nerve. The chemical inactivation of the NTS abolishes the depressing effect of intraportal NaCl infusion on jejunal absorption, suggesting that the NTS is involved in the hepatointestinal reflex. In conclusion, specialized receptors in the hepatoportal region transfer the signal of an increased portal plasma Na$^+$ concentration into an increase in hepatic afferent nerve activity. These afferent signals, in turn, activate the hepatorenal reflex (augmentation of renal Na$^+$ excretion) and the hepatointestinal reflex (suppression of salt absorption across the intestine). It has been suggested that the hepatoportal receptor senses the Na$^+$ concentration via the bumetanide-sensitive Na$^+$K$^+$2Cl$^-$ cotransporter, because the responses of hepatic afferent nerve activity to intraportal hypertonic NaCl injection were suppressed by intraportal infusion of furosemide or bumetanide.[60]

In addition to chemoreceptors (i.e., Na$^+$ sensors) in the hepatoportal area, the normal human liver also contains mechanoreceptors (baroreceptors). Increased intrahepatic hydrostatic pressure has been shown in the past to be associated with enhanced renal sympathetic activity and renal Na$^+$ retention in various experimental models.[61,62] Convincing evidence for a role of the intrahepatic baroreceptors in the modulation of renal salt retention was provided in 1987 by Levy and Wexler.[61] These investigators used the model of thoracic caval constriction in dogs to raise intrahepatic pressure without driving fluid from the vascular space as ascites. When venous pressure was increased by 6.6 cm H$_2$O, Na$^+$ balance studies showed a positive cumulative balance that could be prevented by liver denervation.[61] Although the nature of the volume- and Na$^+$-sensing mechanism has not been clarified, it is thought to play an important role in the pathogenesis of primary renal Na$^+$ retention associated with intrahepatic hypertension (see Renal Sodium Retention and Edema Formation in Cirrhosis with Ascites).

Guanylin Peptides: Intestinal Natriuretic Hormones

In addition to the Na$^+$-sensing mechanisms in the liver and GIT, an effector hormonal mechanism linking the gut with the kidney has been sought to account for the phenomenon of postprandial natriuresis. As pointed out previously, it has been suggested in the past that the natriuretic response of the kidney to an Na$^+$ load is more rapid when the load is delivered orally than when the same load is administered intravenously.[55] Although the latter finding remains controversial,[63] in the past decade, a novel family of cGMP-regulating peptides has been identified that may act as "intestinal natriuretic hormones."[36,64-67] Guanylin and uroguanylin, the main representatives of the family, are small, heat-stable peptides with intramolecular disulfide bridges that share similarity with the bacterial heat-stable enterotoxins that cause "traveler's diarrhea." Guanylin and uroguanylin were first isolated from rat jejunum and opossum urine, respectively.[68,69] In the intestine, guanylin and uroguanylin modulate epithelial ion and water transport by a local mechanism of action, which involves binding to and activation of the receptor guanylyl cyclase-C (GC-C), a transmembrane 1050- to 1053-amino acid protein that is present in the intestinal brush border. Guanylin apparently plays a regulatory role in intestinal fluid and electrolyte transport through the second messenger cGMP. GC-C is structurally similar to the membrane-bound GC-A and GC-B, which serve as receptors of the NP family.[64,67] In addition to these secretory effects, studies in mice with targeted inactivation of the guanylin gene suggest that this intestinal peptide has an important role in controlling intestinal epithelial cell proliferation and differentiation, via GC-C.[36]

It has been suggested that guanylin peptides, in particular uroguanylin, may also serve in intrarenal signaling pathways influencing cGMP production in renal cells, thus linking the digestive system and the kidney in the control of Na$^+$ homeostasis.[65-67,70] The following arguments favor the latter hypothesis.[34,36] First, intestinal guanylin and uroguanylin mRNA levels are modulated by oral salt intake. Second, both peptides may be detected in the circulation, and high concentrations of uroguanylin are excreted in the urine. Moreover, these hormones stimulate renal electrolyte excretion by inducing natriuresis, kaliuresis, and diuresis.[67] Finally, Lorenz and co-workers[71] recently showed that mice lacking the uroguanylin gene displayed an impaired natriuretic response to oral salt loading, but not to intravenous NaCl infusion. Interestingly, uroguanylin knockout mice exhibited an increase of 10 to 15 mm Hg in their MAP, regardless of the level of dietary salt intake. Taken together, these data highly suggest a role, at least for uroguanylin, as a natriuretic hormone, which adjusts urinary Na$^+$ excretion to balance the levels of NaCl absorbed via the GIT.[66] The importance of this system in the control of renal Na$^+$ excretion in humans awaits further clarification.

Efferent Limb: Effectors for Fluid Homeostasis

Major renal effector mechanisms include glomerular filtration, peritubular and luminal factors, and humoral and neural mechanisms (Table 12–2).

In humans, normal glomerular filtration leads to the delivery of approximately 4000 mmol of Na$^+$/day for downstream processing by the tubules. Of this quantity, the vast majority (>99%) is reabsorbed, leaving the small remainder to escape into the final urine. It is clear from this simple calculation that even minute changes in the relationship between filtered load and fraction of Na$^+$ reabsorbed can exert a profound cumulative influence on overall Na$^+$ balance. However, even marked perturbations in GFR are not necessarily associated with drastic alterations in urinary Na$^+$ excretion, and hence, overall Na$^+$ balance is most often preserved. This preservation of Na$^+$ homeostasis is the consequence of appropriate adjustments in two important protective mechanisms, namely, TGF control of GFR acting through macula densa[47] and

TABLE 12–2	Major Renal Effector Mechanisms for Body Fluid Volume Homeostasis

Glomerular filtration rate

Peritubular and luminal factors
  Peritubular capillary Starling forces
  Luminal composition
  Medullary interstitial composition
  Transtubular ion gradients

Humoral effector mechanisms
  Renin-angiotensin-aldosterone system
  Antidiuretic hormone
  Prostaglandins
  Natriuretic peptides
  Endothelium-derived factors
    Endothelins
    Nitric oxide (endothelium-derived relaxing factor)

Renal nerves

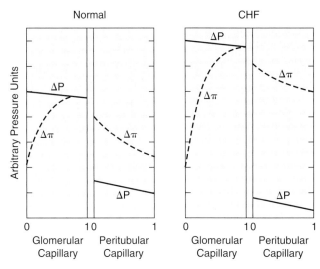

DIMENSIONLESS DISTANCES ALONG CAPILLARY SEGMENTS

FIGURE 12–2 The glomerular and peritubular microcirculations. *Left,* Approximate transcapillary pressure profiles for the glomerular and peritubular capillaries in normal humans. Vessel lengths are given in normalized, nondimensional terms, with 0 being the most proximal portion of the capillary bed and 1 the most distal portion. Thus, 0 for the glomerulus corresponds to the afferent arteriolar end of the capillary bed, and 1 to the efferent arteriolar end. The transcapillary hydraulic pressure difference (ΔP) is relatively constant with distance along the glomerular capillary, and the net driving force for ultrafiltration ($\Delta P - \Delta\pi$) diminishes primarily as a consequence of the increase in the opposing colloid osmotic pressure difference ($\Delta\pi$), the latter resulting in the formation of an essentially protein-free ultrafiltrate. As a result of the hydraulic pressure drop along the efferent arteriole, the net driving pressure in the peritubular capillaries ($\Delta P - \Delta\pi$) becomes negative, favoring reabsorption. *Right,* The hemodynamic alterations that are believed to occur in the renal microcirculation in congestive heart failure (CHF). The fall in renal plasma flow (RPF) in CHF is associated with a compensatory increase in ΔP for the glomerular capillary, favoring a greater-than-normal rise in the plasma protein concentration and, hence, $\Delta\pi$ along the glomerular capillary. This increase in the value of $\Delta\pi$ by the distal end of the glomerular capillary also translates to an increase in $\Delta\pi$ in the peritubular capillaries, resulting in the increase in the net driving pressure, responsible for enhanced proximal tubule fluid absorption, that is believed to take place in CHF. The increased peritubular capillary absorptive force in CHF also probably results from the decline in ΔP, a presumed consequence of the rise in renal vascular resistance. (From Humes HD, Gottlieb M, Brenner BM: The Kidney in Congestive Heart Failure: Contemporary Issues in Nephrology, Vol 1. New York, Churchill Livingstone, 1978, pp 51–72.)

glomerular-tubule balance (GTB). The latter term describes the ability of proximal tubular reabsorption to adapt proportionally to the changes in filtered load.

Indeed, numerous studies in the past revealed that the modest changes in GFR that accompany volume expansion and depletion maneuvers are not sufficient to explain the accompanying adjustments in urinary Na^+ excretion. Rather, these studies suggested that local intrarenal factors, acting at the level of the coupling of tubule reabsorption to glomerular filtration, are responsible for regulating urinary Na^+ excretion, responding to afferent limb signals that are responsive to volume perturbation. In the following sections, these intrarenal physical factors, acting at the level of the proximal tubule and beyond, are discussed. In addition, the neural and humoral factors that modulate tubule transport, through these physical factors or through direct epithelial transport effects, are considered.

Intrarenal Physical Factors
Peritubular Factors
Infusions of saline or albumin solutions to experimental animals and humans have been frequently used as a tool to study the mechanisms of the natriuretic response to ECF volume expansion. These experiments were performed usually on an acute basis and, therefore, may bear little relevance to the chronic regulation of ECF Na^+ balance. Nevertheless, the findings in many of these investigations led to the notion that alterations in hydraulic and oncotic pressures (Starling forces) in the peritubular capillary play an important role in the regulation of Na^+ and water transport, in particular at the proximal nephron.

The peritubular capillary network is anatomically connected in series with the glomerular capillary bed through the efferent arteriole, so that changes in the physical determinants of GFR critically influence Starling forces in the peritubular capillaries. In the proximal tubule, the relation of hydraulic and oncotic driving forces to the transcapillary fluid flux is given by the Starling relationship: $APR = K_r[(\pi_c - \pi_i) - (P_c - P_i)]$, in which APR is the absolute rate of reabsorption of proximal tubule absorbate by the peritubular capillary; K_r is the capillary reabsorption coefficient (the product of capillary hydraulic conductivity and absorptive surface area); π_c and P_c are the local capillary oncotic and hydraulic pressures, respectively; and π_i and P_i are the corresponding interstitial pressures. π_i and P_c are forces that oppose fluid absorption, whereas π_c and P_i tend to favor uptake of reabsorbate. The simultaneous determination of these driving forces

allows an analysis of the net pressure favoring fluid absorption or filtration.

As a consequence of the anatomic relationship of the postglomerular efferent arteriole to the peritubular capillary, the hydraulic pressure in the peritubular capillary is significantly lower than in the glomerular capillary. The function of the efferent arteriole as a resistance vessel contributes to a decrease in hydraulic pressure between the glomerulus and the peritubular capillary. Also, because the peritubular capillary receives blood from the glomerulus, the plasma oncotic pressure is high at the outset as a result of prior filtration of protein-free fluid. It follows that the greater the GFR relative to plasma flow rate (the filtration fraction), the greater the efferent arteriolar plasma protein concentration and the lower the proximal peritubule capillary hydraulic pressure, consequently favoring enhanced proximal fluid reabsorption (Fig. 12–2). Therefore, in contradistinction to the glomerular and peripheral capillary, the peritubular capillary is characterized by high values of $(\pi_c - \pi_i)$, which greatly exceed $(P_c - P_i)$, resulting in net reabsorption of fluid. The relation of proximal reabsorption to filtration fraction may contribute to Na^+-retaining and edema-forming states, such as CHF (see Fig. 12–2).

Compelling experimental evidence for the relationship between proximal peritubular Starling forces and proximal fluid reabsorption came from a series of a series of in vivo micropuncture and microperfusion studies by Brenner and colleagues.[72–75] In the earlier studies, rat efferent arterioles were perfused with various oncotic solutions, and it was shown that APR varied directly with the oncotic force of the perfusate and with constancy of GFR, thus providing evidence that changes in efferent arteriolar protein concentration directly modify proximal reabsorption independent of GFR.[72] To determine whether primary decreases in GFR regulate APR through effects on efferent arteriolar protein concentration, rats were studied after partial aortic constriction, a maneuver that reduced the single-nephron GFR (SNGFR) and the APR proportionately and decreased filtration fraction. APR was maintained at control levels with iso-oncotic albumin infusions that returned the efferent arteriolar plasma protein concentration to normal without changing GFR. In this way, the GTB could be modified by the prevailing peritubular oncotic pressure, with the link between GFR and APR again being related to changes in filtration fraction and peritubular capillary oncotic pressure. From these studies, the role of peritubular forces in the setting of increased ECF volume can be summarized as follows:

1. Acute saline expansion results in dilution of plasma proteins and reduction in efferent arteriolar oncotic pressure. SNGFR and peritubular capillary hydraulic pressures may be increased as well, but the decrease in peritubular oncotic pressure in itself results in a decreased net peritubular capillary reabsorptive force and decreased APR. GTB is disrupted because APR falls despite the tendency for SNGFR to rise.
2. Iso-oncotic plasma infusions tend to raise SNGFR and peritubular capillary hydraulic pressures but lead to relative constancy of efferent arteriolar oncotic pressure. APR may therefore decrease slightly, resulting in less disruption of GTB and natriuresis of lesser magnitude than that observed with saline expansion.
3. Hyperoncotic expansion usually increases SNGFR (because of volume expansion) as well as APR, the latter resulting from increased efferent arteriolar oncotic pressure. GTB therefore tends to be better preserved than with iso-oncotic plasma or saline expansion.

The possibility that changes in peritubular COP may alter proximal fluid reabsorption was also demonstrated in several studies using the in vitro isolated perfused tubule model.[76] Thus, an extensive literature from several laboratories supported the view that movements of fluid and electrolytes across the peritubular basement membrane into the surrounding capillary bed could be modulated by alterations in proximal peritubular capillary Starling forces. Moreover, these studies indicated that the effects might be mediated through corresponding alterations in physical parameters in the peritubular interstitial compartment. Ultrastructural data for the rat suggest that the peritubular capillary wall is in tight apposition to the tubule basement membrane for about 60% of the tubule basal surface. However, irregularly shaped wide portions of peritubular interstitium also exist over about 42% of the tubule basal surface, so a major part of reabsorbed fluid has to cross a true interstitial space before entering the peritubular capillaries. Alterations in the physical properties of the interstitial compartment could conceivably modulate either passive or active components of net proximal tubule fluid transport. The accepted formulation had been that Starling forces in the peritubular capillary regulate the rate of volume entry from the peritubular interstitium into the capillary. Any change in this rate of flux could lead to changes in

interstitial pressure that secondarily modify proximal tubule solute transport. This formulation could explain why experimental maneuvers that were known to raise renal interstitial hydrostatic pressure (e.g., infusion of renal vasodilators, renal venous constriction, renal lymph ligation), were associated with a natriuretic response, whereas the opposite effect was obtained with renal decapsulation (see also the section on the role of renal interstitial pressure the mechanism of pressure natriuresis).

In theory, interstitial forces could influence active reabsorption of Na^+, passive reabsorption, or the rate of back-flux through the paracellular shunt pathway. Because of the relatively highly permeability of the proximal, alterations in bidirectional paracellular flux have been thought to play a dominant role in transducing the effect of alterations in Starling forces on proximal tubular net reabsorption, though the magnitude of these effects and the mechanisms involved were not fully elucidated.[77] The discovery of the claudin family of adhesion molecules as an integral component of the tight junction has shed additional light on these processes.[78–80] Instead of a "passive" structure, the tight junction is now considered to be a dynamic, multifunctional complex that may be amenable to physiologic regulation by cellular second messengers or in pathologic states.[78,79] Among the 24 known mammalian claudin-family members, at least 3, claudin-2, -10, and -11 are located in the proximal nephron of the mouse and others at more distal nephron sites.[80,81] Claudin-2 is selectively expressed in the proximal nephron.[82] The claudin-family members are thus important candidates for the future study of the influence of Starling forces on fluid reasbsorption.

Although paracellular transport was believed to be mediated primarily through passive forces, some evidence also suggests the contribution of active transport processes. Thus, in the presence of active transport, the effects of proteins on fluid transport are enhanced. In addition, studies by Berry and colleagues[83] demonstrated no effect on the permeability properties of the proximal tubule and no effect on passive water and solute fluxes. The only active flux modulated by changes in peritubular protein was that of NaCl. On the basis of these observations, peritubular protein concentration would not likely be affecting Na^+,K^+-ATPase or the Na^+/H^+ antiporter because one would expect consequent effects on Na^+ bicarbonate absorption.[84]

Luminal Factors in Glomerular-Tubular Balance

Although a considerable amount of data supports the role of peritubular capillary and interstitial Starling forces in the regulation of proximal tubule transport, some studies either have not found such effects or have suggested the presence of additional mechanisms.

Since the early 1970s, studies utilizing tubular perfusion with plasma ultrafiltrate or native tubular fluid suggested that some constituents of this fluid or intraluminal flow rate per se may be important modulators of proximal fluid reabsorption, independent of peritubular Starling forces (see Romano and co-workers[85] and references therein). The flow-dependence of proximal reabsorption was likewise supported by studies in isolated perfused proximal tubules of the rabbit nephron.[86] A key observation indicated that the presence of a transtubular anion gradient, normally present in the late portion of the proximal nephron, was necessary for the flow-dependence to occur.[87] A potential mechanism for modulation of proximal Na^+ reabsorption in response to changes in filtered load depends on the close coupling of Na^+ transport with the cotransport of glucose, amino acids, and other organic solutes. The increased delivery of organic solutes that accompanies increases in GFR might help to augment the rates at which both the solutes and the Na^+ chloride are reabsorbed. The dependence of GTB on transtubular anion

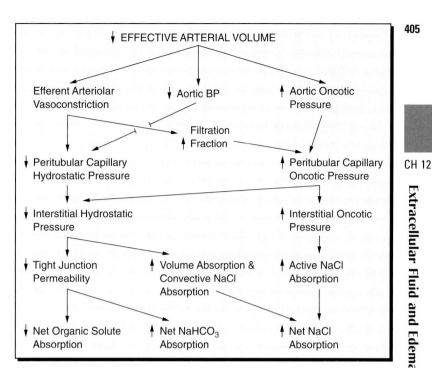

FIGURE 12–3 Effects of hemodynamic changes on proximal tubule solute transport: a summary. (From Seldin DW, Preisig PA, Alpern RJ: Regulation of proximal reabsorption by effective arterial blood volume. Semin Nephrol 11:212–219, 1991.)

gradient was explained by the ability of the $Cl^-HCO_3^-$ gradient, generated by the preferential reabsorption of Na^+ with bicarbonate in the early proximal tubule, to enhance the "passive" component of Na^+ and fluid reabsorption in the proximal nephron. Irrespective of the exact mechanism, an important notion emerged, namely, that states of ECF volume expansion impaired the integrity of the GTB, thus allowing increased delivery of salt and fluid to more distal parts of the nephron.

Figure 12–3 presents a schematic outline of the major factors acting on the proximal nephron during a decrease in ECF and effective circulating volume.

Physical Factors Acting beyond the Proximal Tubule

An extensive series of experimental studies showed that the final urinary excretion of Na^+, in response to volume expansion or depletion, can be dissociated from the amount delivered out of the superficial proximal nephron, suggesting that more distal and/or deeper segments of the nephron contribute to the modulation of Na^+ and water excretion. Several sites along the nephron, such as loop of Henle, distal nephron, and cortical and papillary collecting ducts, were found, by micropuncture and microcatheterization techniques, to increase or decrease the rate of Na^+ reabsorption in response to enhanced delivery from early segments of the nephron. However, direct evidence that these transport processes are mediated by changes in Starling forces per se is lacking. A detailed description of these experiments is not given in the present chapter, but may be found in previous editions of this book as well as in review articles.[88]

In summary, the following generalizations regarding the intrarenal control of Na^+ excretion apply. Provided that ECF volume is held relatively constant, an increase in GFR leads to little or no increase in salt excretion because of a close coupling between the GFR and the intrarenal physical forces acting at the peritubular capillary to control APR. In addition, changes in the filtered load of small organic solutes, and perhaps other as-yet-uncharacterized glomerulus-borne substances in tubule fluid, may influence APR. To the extent that changes, if any, in the load of Na^+ delivered to more distal segments also occur, these are matched by more or less parallel changes in distal reabsorptive rates, to ensure a high degree of GTB for the kidney as a whole. Conversely, ECF volume expansion leads to large increases in Na^+ excretion even in the presence of reduced GFR. Changes in Na^+ reabsorption in the proximal tubule alone cannot account for this natriuresis of volume expansion, and a variety of mechanisms for suppressing Na^+ reabsorption at more distal sites have been invoked.

Mechanism of Pressure Natriuresis: Role of Renal Medullary Hemodynamics and Interstitial Pressure in Control of Sodium Excretion

The idea that changes in renal medullary hemodynamics may be involved in the natriuresis evoked by volume expansion was initially proposed in the 1960s by Earley and Friedler.[89] According to their theory, ECF volume expansion results in an increase in medullary plasma flow (MPF) with a subsequent loss of medullary hypertonicity, thereby decreasing water reabsorption in the thin descending loop of Henle. The decrease in water reabsorption in the thin descending limb lowers the Na^+ concentration in the fluid entering the ascending loop of Henle, thus decreasing the transepithelial driving force for salt transport in this nephron segment. At the same time, a similar mechanism was proposed to explain the natriuresis involved in the pressure-natriuresis phenomenon. It was reasoned that increases in RPP produce a parallel increase in MPF that eliminates the medullary osmotic gradient.

The concept that alterations in the solute composition of the renal medulla and papilla play a key role in regulation of Na^+ transport gained significant support in the 1970s and 1980s, when several micropuncture studies suggested that volume expansion, renal vasodilatation, and increased RPP produced a greater inhibition of salt reabsorption in the loops of Henle of juxtamedullary nephrons than in superficial nephrons. Although measurements of MPF in experimental animals undergoing volume expansion and renal vasodilatation supported the possibility of redistribution of intrarenal blood flow toward the medulla, the validity of the methodologies for intrarenal blood flow measurements used at that time was questioned. The application of newer techniques that allowed a more reliable estimation of changes in medullary blood flow, such as laser-Doppler flowmetry and videomicroscopy, resulted in a renewal of interest in the role of medullary hemodynamics in the control of Na⁺ excretion, especially in the context of the pressure-natriuresis relationship.[90–93]

Elevation in blood pressure has been recorded, although not always, following expansion of the ECF and salt loading, though it is not a consistent observation in all studies.[30,93] This increase in blood pressure and RPP may lead to an increase in Na⁺ excretion by the kidney, a phenomenon termed *pressure-natriuresis.* The importance of pressure-natriuresis in the long-term control of arterial blood pressure and ECF volume regulation was first recognized by Guyton and associates.[93,94] According to this view, the kidneys play a dominant role in controlling arterial pressure by virtue of their ability to alter Na⁺ excretion in response to changes in arterial blood pressure. For instance, an increase in RPP results in a concomitant increase in Na⁺ excretion, thereby decreasing circulating blood volume and restoring arterial pressure. It was soon recognized that the coupling between arterial pressure and Na⁺ excretion occurred in the setting of preserved autoregulation (i.e., in the absence of changes in total RPF, GFR, or filtered load of Na⁺). Although the mechanism responsible for pressure-natriuresis in a setting of high-efficiency autoregulation is unclear, the possibility that the pressure-natriuresis mechanism is triggered by changes in medullary circulation received considerable attention.[89,91,95,96] Laser-Doppler flowmetry and servonull measurements of capillary pressure in volume-expanded rats revealed that papillary blood flow was directly related to RPP over a wide range of pressures studied. In contrast, cortical blood flow was well autoregulated, indicating that during alterations in RPP renal medullary blood flow may not be autoregulated to the same extent as cortical blood flow. As mentioned earlier, increase in medullary plasma flow might lead to medullary "washout" with a consequent reduction in the driving force for Na⁺ reabsorption in the ascending loop of Henle, particularly in the deep nephrons. In addition, the increase in medullary perfusion may be associated with a rise in renal medullary interstitial hydrostatic pressure. Indeed, various physiologic and pharmacologic maneuvers that increase P_i, such as ECF volume expansion, infusion of renal vasodilatory agents, long-term mineralocorticoid escape, and hilar lymph ligation, result in a significant increase in Na⁺ excretion. Numerous studies established that pressure-natriuresis is associated with elevated P_i that is most evident in the volume-expanded state (see reviews by Granger and colleagues[97,98] and references therein). Moreover, prevention of the increase in P_i by removal of the renal capsule significantly attenuated, but did not completely block, the natriuretic response to elevations in RPP. Thus, as depicted in Figure 12–4, elevation in renal perfusion pressure is associated with an increase in medullary blood flow and increased vasa recta capillary pressure, which result in an increase in medullary P_i. This increase of interstitial pressure is thought to be transmitted to the renal cortex in the encapsulated kidney and to provide a signal that inhibits Na⁺ reabsorption along the nephron. In that regard, the renal medulla may be viewed as a sensor that can detect changes in RPP and initiate the pressure-natriuresis mechanism.

It has been suggested that changes in systemic pressure are transmitted to the medullary circulation via shunt pathways connecting preglomerular vessels of juxtamedullary nephrons directly to the postglomerular vasa recta capillaries.[89] This might explain how changes in systemic pressures are transmitted to the medulla when RPF and GFR are well autoregulated. Alternatively, it has been suggested more recently that the process of autoregulation of renal blood flow (RBF) leads to increased shear stress in the preglomerular vasculature, so that release of nitric oxide (NO) (see later) and perhaps cytochrome P-450 products of arachidonic acid

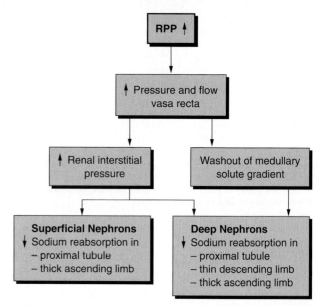

FIGURE 12–4 Role of the renal medulla in modulating tubular reabsorption of Na⁺ in response to changes in renal perfusion pressure (RPP). (Adapted from Cowley AW Jr: Role of the renal medulla in volume and arterial pressure regulation. Am J Physiol 273:R1–R15, 1997.)

metabolism, drive the cascade of events that inhibit Na⁺ reabsorption.[99,100]

Although a substantial amount of experimental data supports the association between changes in P_i and urinary Na⁺ excretion, the mechanisms by which these changes decrease tubular Na⁺ reabsorption, as well as the nephron sites responding to the alterations in P_i, have not been fully clarified.[98] As pointed out earlier, it was postulated that elevations in P_i may increase passive back-leak or the paracellular pathway hydraulic conductivity, with a resultant increase in back-flux of Na⁺ through the paracellular pathways.[97] However, the absolute changes in P_i, in the range of 3 to 8 mm Hg in response to increments of about 50 to 90 mm Hg in RPP, are probably not sufficient to account for the decrease in tubular Na⁺ reabsorption even in the proximal tubule, the nephron segment with the highest transepithelial hydraulic conductivity.[90] Nevertheless, considerable evidence from micropuncture studies indicate that pressure-natriuresis is associated with significant changes in proximal fluid reabsorption particularly in deep nephrons, with enhanced delivery to the loop of Henle, although alterations in the pars recta and thin descending limb must also be considered.[97] Pressure-induced changes in tubular reabsorption may also occur in more distal parts of the nephron, such as the ascending loop of Henle, distal nephron, and collecting duct.[101] Therefore, elevations in RPP can affect tubular Na⁺ reabsorption by both proximal and distal mechanisms.

The finding that small changes in P_i are associated with significant alterations in tubular Na⁺ reabsorption led to the hypothesis that the changes in P_i may be amplified by various hemodynamic, hormonal, and paracrine factors.[85,89,91,95,97] Specifically, the phenomenon of pressure-natriuresis is particularly demonstrable in states of volume expansion and renal vasodilatation and is significantly attenuated in states of volume depletion.[97] Among a variety of hormonal and paracrine systems that have been documented to play a role in modulating the pressure-natriuresis relationship, changes in the activity of the RAAS and local production of prostaglandins (PGs) within the kidney received considerable attention over the years.[97] Removal of the influence of AII, by either angiotensin-converting enzyme (ACE) inhibitors or angiotensin type 1 (AT$_1$) receptor antagonists, potentiates the pressure-natriuretic response, and inhibitors of cyclooxygenase attenuate it.[97,102] It is important to note, however, that pharmacologic blockade of these systems only attenuates but does not completely eliminate the pressure-natriuresis response, indicating that they act as modulators and not as mediators of the phenomenon.

In recent years, the importance of the endothelial-derived factors in the regulation of renal circulation and excretory function has been recognized. Evidence suggests a role of endothelium-derived NO and P-450 eicosanoids in the mechanism of pressure-natriuresis.[90,95,99] NO, generated in large amounts in the renal medulla, appears to play a critical role in the regulation of medullary blood flow and Na$^+$ excretion.[96,103] Several studies showed that inhibition of intrarenal NO production can reduce Na$^+$ excretion and markedly suppress the pressure-natriuretic response, whereas administration of the NO precursor improves transmission of perfusion pressure into the renal interstitium and normalizes the defect in pressure-natriuresis response in Dahl salt-sensitive rats.[90,101,104,105] Likewise, a positive correlation between urinary excretion of nitrites and nitrates (metabolites of NO) and changes in renal arterial pressure or urinary Na$^+$ excretion was observed in the dog.[106] The P-450 eicosanoids are additional endothelium-derived factor(s) that may participate in the mechanism of pressure-natriuresis.[99,100] The importance of these agents in the regulation of renal Na$^+$ transport and of renal and systemic hemodynamics, has been recently underscored.[107] Taken together, these observations support the hypothesis that alterations in the production of renal NO and eicosanoids may be involved in mediation of the pressure-induced natriuretic response. It is tempting to speculate that acute elevation in RPP in the autoregulatory range results in increased blood flow velocity and shear stress, leading to increased endothelial release of NO. Enhanced renal NO production may increase urinary Na$^+$ excretion either by acting directly on tubular Na$^+$ reabsorption or through its vasodilatory effect on renal vasculature.

Finally, McDonough and co-workers[108,109] reported that, in response to an increase in RPP, the apical Na$^+$/H$^+$ exchanger in the proximal tubules may be redistributed out of the brush border into intracellular compartments. Concomitantly, basolateral Na$^+$-K$^+$-ATPase activity significantly decreased. Although not fully elucidated, the mechanisms of these cellular events may be related directly to the change in P$_i$ or to changes in intrarenal paracrine agents described previously.

A major assumption of the pressure-natriuresis theory indicates that changes in systemic and renal perfusion pressure mediate the natriuretic response by the kidney. As pointed out in a recent comprehensive review by Bie,[30] acute regulatory changes in renal salt excretion may occur without a measurable elevation in arterial blood pressure.[2,30,110,111] Interestingly, in many of these studies, the natriuresis was accompanied by a decrease in the activity of the RAAS without changes in plasma ANP levels.[2,30,110–112] Thus, whereas increases in arterial blood pressure can drive renal Na$^+$ excretion, other "pressure-independent" control mechanisms must operate as well to mediate the "volume-natriuresis."[30]

Humoral Mechanisms
Renin-Angiotensin-Aldosterone System
The RAAS plays an integral role in the regulation of ECF volume, Na$^+$ homeostasis, and cardiac function.[113] This system is activated in situations that compromise hemodynamic stability, such as loss of blood volume, reduced ECF volume, low Na$^+$ intake, hypotension, and increase in sympathetic nerve activity. The RAAS comprises of a coordinated hormonal cascade whose synthesis is initiated by the release of renin from the juxtaglomerular apparatus in response to reduced renal perfusion or fall in arterial pressure.[114]

Messenger RNA (mRNA) for renin exists in juxtaglomerular cells and in renal tubule cells.[115] Renin acts on its circulating substrate, namely angiotensinogen, which is produced and secreted mainly by the liver but also by the kidney.[113] ACE, which cleaves angiotensin I (AI) to AII, exists in large amounts in the lung but also on endothelial cells of the vasculature and cell membrane of the brush border of the proximal nephron, heart, and brain.[113] AII is considered to be the principal effector of the RAAS, although it is recognized that few smaller metabolic products of AII may have biologic activities.[116] Nonrenin (cathepsin G, plasminogen-activating factor, tonin) and non-ACE pathways (chymase, cathepsin G) also exist in these tissues and may contribute to tissue AII synthesis.[113,114] In addition to its important function as a circulating hormone, AII produced locally acts as a paracrine agent in an organ-specific mode, which might be dissociated from its systemic vasoconstrictor action.[117,118] In that respect, the properties of AII as a growth-promoting agent in the cardiovascular system and the kidney have been increasingly appreciated.[113,119,120] For instance, local generation of AII in the kidney results in higher intrarenal levels of this peptide in proximal tubular fluid, interstitial fluid, and renal medulla compared with circulating levels. The epithelial cells of the proximal nephron may be an important source for the in situ generation of AII, because these cells show abundant expression of the mRNA for angiotensinogen.[121,122] Furthermore, AII is apparently secreted from tubular epithelial cells into the lumen of the proximal nephron.[123] This may account for the high proximal tubular fluid concentrations of AII—approximately 1000 times higher than the plasma levels of the peptide.[123,124] Moreover, recent data demonstrated that the mechanisms regulating intrarenal levels of AII may be dissociated from those controlling the systemic concentrations of the peptide.[125]

The biologic actions of AII are mediated through activation of at least two receptors subtypes, AT$_1$ and AT$_2$, encoded by different genes residing on different chromosomes.[126,127] Both receptors have been cloned and were found to be G-protein–coupled, seven-transmembrane polypeptides containing approximately 360 amino acids.[113,127–129] In the adult organism, the AT$_1$ receptor subtype mediates most of the biologic activities of AII, whereas the AT$_2$ receptor, expressed primarily in the fetal life, appears to play an important role in cell development and apoptosis.[130,131] AT$_1$ is expressed in the vascular poles of glomeruli, juxtaglomerular apparatus, and mesangial cells, whereas AT$_2$ is localized to renal arteries and tubular structure, at a small population.[132] Besides their functional distinction, the two receptor types employ different signal transduction pathways. Stimulation of the AT$_1$ receptor activates phospholipase A$_2$, C, and D, resulting in increased cytosolic Ca^{2+} and inositol triphosphate (IP$_3$) and inhibition of adenylate cyclase. In contrast, activation of the AT$_2$ receptor results in increased NO and bradykinin (BK) levels, leading to elevated cGMP concentrations and vasodilation.[133]

Besides being an important source of several components of the RAAS, the kidney acts a major target organ to the principal hormonal mediators of this cascade, AII and aldosterone. In the past, it was believed that the major contribution of AII to Na$^+$ homeostasis was the result of its actions as a circulating vasoconstrictor hormone and through stimulation of aldosterone release with subsequent tubular action of aldosterone. However, evidence indicates that AII, via AT$_1$ receptors, exerts multiple direct intrarenal influences, including renal vasoconstriction, stimulation of tubular epithelial Na$^+$ reabsorption, augmentation of TGF sensitivity, modulation of pressure-natriuresis, and stimulation of mitogenic pathways.[113] Moreover, exogenous infusion of AII that results in relatively low circulating levels of AII (picomolar range) is highly effective in modulating renal hemodynamic and tubular function compared with the 10- to 100-fold higher concentrations required for its extrarenal effects. Thus, the kidney appears to be uniquely sensitive to the actions of AII. Furthermore, the synergistic interactions that exist between the renal vascular and tubular actions of AII significantly amplify the influence of AII on Na^+ excretion.[134] Among the direct renal actions of AII, the effect of the peptide on renal hemodynamics appears to be of critical importance. AII elicits a dose-dependent decrease in RBF but slightly augments GFR, owing to its preferential vasoconstrictive effect on efferent arteriole, and therefore increases filtration fraction. As noted previously, the increase in filtration fraction in response to AII can be attributed to a predominant increase in efferent arteriolar resistance exerted by the peptide,[135] which may further modulate peritubular Starling forces, such as decreasing hyraulic pressure and increasing COP in the interstitium. These peritubular changes eventually lead to enhanced proximal Na^+ and fluid reabsorption. It is important to note, however, that changes in preglomerular resistance have also been described during AII infusion or blockade.[136,137] These may be secondary to changes in either systemic arterial pressure (myogenic reflex) or increased sensitivity of TGF, because AII does not alter preglomerular resistance when RPP is clamped or adjustments in TGF are prevented.[137] In addition, AII may affect GFR by reducing glomerular ultrafiltration coefficient, thereby altering the filtered load of Na^+.[138,139] This effect is believed to reflect the action of the hormone on mesangial cell contractility and increasing permeability to macromolecules.[136] Finally, AII may also influence Na^+ excretion through its action on medullary circulation. Because AII receptors are present in high abundance in the renal medulla, this peptide may contribute significantly to the regulation of medullary blood flow.[136,140] Indeed, use of fiberoptic probes revealed that AII usually reduces cortical blood flow and medullary blood flow and decreases Na^+ and water excretion.[113,132] As pointed out earlier, changes in medullary blood flow may affect medullary tonicity, which determines the magnitude of passive salt reabsorption in the loop of Henle, and also modulate pressure-natriuresis through renal interstitial pressure.[89,91]

The other well-characterized renal effect of AII is a direct action on tubule epithelial transport systems. Infusions of AII to achieve systemic concentrations of 10^{-12} to 10^{-11} M markedly stimulated Na^+ and water transport, independent of changes in renal or systemic hemodynamics.[113,141] AII exerts a dose-dependent biphasic effect on proximal Na^+ reabsorption. Peritubular capillary infusion with solutions containing low concentrations of AII (10^{-12}–10^{-10} M) stimulated Na^+ reabsorption, whereas perfusion with solutions containing higher concentrations of AII ($>10^{-7}$ M) inhibited proximal Na^+ reabsorption rate. Similar observations were reported in vitro in isolated perfused rabbit proximal tubule. Quan and Baum[142] demonstrated that addition of either the AT_1 receptor antagonist losartan or the ACE inhibitor enalaprilat directly into the luminal fluid of the proximal nephron resulted in a significant decrease in proximal fluid reabsorption, indicating tonic regulation of proximal tubule transport by endogenous AII. Several studies provided insight into the specific mechanisms by which AII influences proximal tubule transport. These studies showed that AII enhances proximal tubular Na^+ transport through actions at both luminal and basolateral membrane sites. AII increases Na^+ and HCO_3^- reabsorption by stimulation of the apical membrane Na^+/H^+ exchanger, basolateral membrane $Na^+/(3)HCO_3^-$ symporter, and Na^+,K^+-ATPase.[143,144] Thus, AII can affect Na^+ chloride absorption by two mechanisms. Activation of the Na^+/H^+ antiporter can directly increase Na^+ chloride absorption. In addition, conditions that increase the rate of Na^+ bicarbonate absorption can stimulate passive Na^+ chloride absorption by increasing the concentration gradient for passive Cl^- diffusion.[84] Sodium

reabsorption is further promoted by the action of AII on the Na^+,K^+-ATPase in the medullary thick ascending limb of henle's loop (TALH).[113] Although the issue of distal action of AII was controversial in the past, more recent studies indicated that AII also regulates Na^+ and bicarbonate reabsorption in distal segments of the nephron by modulating Na^+/H^+ exchange and the amiloride-sensitive Na^+ channel.[142,145–147] In this context, Wang and Giebisch[147] demonstrated that AII stimulates volume reabsorption in the late distal tubule not only via the acid-base transporter but also via Na^+ channels.[147] Most recently, using isolated perfused cortical collecting duct segments dissected from rabbit kidneys, Peti-Peterdi and colleagues[148] clearly showed that AII directly stimulates the Na^+ channel activity in this segment.

Two additional mechanisms may amplify the antinatriuretic effects of AII mediated by the direct actions of the peptide on renal hemodynamics and tubular transport. The first relates to the increased sensitivity of the TGF mechanism in the presence of AII, and the second to the effect of AII on the pressure-natriuresis relationship. The decrease in distal delivery produced by the action of AII on renal hemodynamics and proximal fluid reabsorption could elicit afferent arteriolar vasodilation via the TGF mechanism, which, in turn, could antagonize the AII-mediated increase in proximal reabsorption. This effect, however, is minimized because AII increases the responsiveness of the TGF mechanism, thus maintaining GFR at a lower delivery rate to the macula densa.[149] In addition, infusions of AII have been shown to blunt the pressure-natriuresis relationship and to shift the relationship between Na^+ excretion and arterial pressure toward higher pressures.[113,150] This "shift to the right" in the pressure natriuresis curve may be viewed as an important Na^+-conserving mechanism in situations of elevated arterial pressure.

The pharmacologic development of ACE inhibitors and highly specific AII receptor antagonists provided additional insight into the mechanisms of action of AII in the kidney and further suggested that most of the known intrarenal actions of AII, particularly regulation of renal hemodynamics and proximal tubule reabsorption of Na^+, HCO_3^-, are mediated by the AT_1 receptor.[142,151] However, recent functional studies showed that some part of the AII at the renal level is mediated by AT_2 receptors.[133] AT_2 receptor subtype plays a counterregulatory protective role against the AT_1 receptor–mediated antinatriuretic and pressor actions of AII. The accepted concept that AI is merely converted to AII was revised through the demonstration that AI is also a substrate for the formation of Ang-(1-7).[152] Moreover, a recently discovered homolog of ACE, ACE2, is responsible for the formation of Ang-(1-7) from AII and for the conversion of AI to Ang-(1-9), which may be converted to Ang-(1-7) by ACE.[152,153] Ang-(1-7) may play an important role as regulator of cardiovascular and renal function. Ang-(1-7) possesses opposite effects to those of AII, including vasodilatation, diuresis, and antihypertrophic action.[154] Thus, these relatively newly discovered components of the RAAS—ACE2 and Ang-(1-7)—may play a role as negative regulators of the classic ACE system.[153]

Finally, aldosterone, the second active component of the RAAS, plays an important physiologic role in the regulation of ECF and Na^+ homeostasis.[155] The primary sites of aldosterone action are the principal cells of the cortical collecting tubule and convoluted distal tubule, inwhich this hormone promotes the reabsorption of Na^+ and the secretion of K^+ and protons.[155,156] Mineralocorticoids may also enhance electrogenic Na^+ transport, but not K^+ secretion, in the inner medullary collecting duct (IMCD).[157] Aldosterone exerts its effects on ionic transport by increasing the number of open Na^+ and K^+ channels in the luminal membrane and the activity of Na^+-K^+-ATPase in the basolateral membrane.[158] The effect of aldosterone on Na^+ permeability appears to be the primary event because blockade of Na^+ channels with amiloride prevents the initial increase in Na^+ permeability and Na^+-K^+-ATPase activity.[159-161] This effect on Na^+ permeability is mediated by several potential mediators including changes in intracellular Ca^{2+} levels, changes in intracellular pH, and methylation of channel proteins, thus increasing mean open probability of the Na^+ channel.[159,160] However, the long-term effect of aldosterone on Na^+-K^+-ATPase activity involves de novo protein synthesis and is regulated at the transcriptional level by serum and glucocorticoid-induced kinase-1 (SGK-1).[162,163] The Na^+-retaining effect of aldosterone in the collecting tubule occurs in association with an increase in the transepithelial potential difference, which favors K^+ excretion. In terms of overall body fluid homeostasis, the actions of aldosterone in the defense of ECF result from the net loss of an osmotically active particle primarily confined to the intracellular compartment (K^+) and its replacement with a corresponding particle primarily confined to the ECF (Na^+). The effect of a given circulating level of aldosterone on overall Na^+ excretion depends on the volume of filtrate reaching the collecting duct and the composition of luminal and intracellular fluids. As noted earlier, this delivery of filtrate is in turn determined by other effector mechanisms (AII, sympathetic nerve activity, and peritubular physical forces) acting at more proximal nephron sites. It is not surprising that Na^+ balance can be regulated for a wide range of intake, even in subjects without adrenal glands, and despite fixed low or high supplemental doses of mineralocorticoids. Under these circumstances, other effector mechanisms predominate in controlling urinary Na^+ excretion, although often in a setting of altered ECF volume and/or K^+ concentration.

In terms of blood pressure maintenance, systemic vasoconstriction—another major extrarenal action of AII—may be considered the appropriate response to perceived ECF volume contraction. As mentioned previously, higher concentrations of AII are required to elicit this response than those that govern renal antinatriuretic actions of AII, a situation analogous to the discrepancy between antidiuretic and pressor actions of vasopressin. Transition from an antinatriuretic to a natriuretic action of AII at high infusion rates can be attributed almost entirely to a concomitant rise in blood pressure.[150] Over the past few years, increasing evidence suggests that, besides the adrenal glomerulosa, aldosterone may also be produced by the heart and vasculature. It exerts powerful effects on blood vessels,[164] independent of actions that can be attributed to the blood pressure rise via regulation of salt and water balance. As observed with AII, aldosterone also possesses significant mitogenic properties. It directly increases the expression and production of transforming growth factor-β and thus is involved in the development of glomerulosclerosis, hypertension, and cardiac injury/hypertrophy.[113,155,164]

In summary, AII, the principal effector of the RAAS, regulates extracellular volume and renal Na^+ excretion through intrarenal and extrarenal mechanisms. The intrarenal hemodynamic and tubular actions of the peptide and its main extrarenal actions (systemic vasoconstriction and aldosterone release) act in concert to adjust urinary Na^+ excretion under a variety of circumstances associated with alterations in ECF volume. Many of these mechanisms are synergistic and tend to amplify the overall influence of the RAAS.

Antidiuretic Hormone

ADH is a nonapeptide (9 a.a) hormone, synthesized in the brain and secreted from the posterior pituitary gland into the circulation in response to an increase in plasma osmolality (via osmoreceptor stimulation) or a decrease in effective circulating volume and blood pressure (via baroreceptor stimulation).[165] Thus, ADH plays a major role in the regulation of water balance and the support of blood pressure and circulating volume. ADH exerts its biologic actions through at least

three different G-protein–coupled receptors.[166] Two of these receptors, V_{1A} and V_2, are abundantly expressed in the cardiovascular system and the kidney and mediate the two main biologic actions of the hormone, namely, vasoconstriction and increased water reabsorption by the kidney. The V_{1A} receptor operates through the phosphoinositide signaling pathway, causing release of intracellular Ca^{2+} ions. Found in the vascular smooth muscle cells, hepatocytes, and platelets, it mediates vasoconstriction, glycogenolysis, and platelet aggregation, respectively. The V_2 receptor, found mainly in the renal collecting duct epithelial cells, is linked to the adenylate cyclase pathway, utilizing cyclic adenosine monophosphate (cAMP) as its second messenger. Activation of this receptor leads to increased synthesis and recruitment of aquaporin II (AQP II) water channels into the apical membrane of collecting duct cells, thus increasing the water permeability of the collecting duct.[167]

Under physiologic conditions, the ADH primarily functions to regulate water content in the body by adjusting water reabsorption in the collecting duct according to plasma tonicity. A change in plasma tonicity by as little as 1% causes a parallel change in ADH release. In turn, this alters the water permeability of the collecting duct. ADH's antidiuretic action results from complex effects of this hormone on principal cells of the collecting duct.[167] (1) ADH provokes the insertion of AQP II water channels into the luminal membrane (short-term response) and increases synthesis of AQP II mRNA and protein (long-term response)—both responses increase water permeability along the collecting duct.[167,168] This is considered in detail in Chapter 9. Briefly, activation of V_2 receptors localized to the basolateral membrane of the principal cells increases cytosolic cAMP, which stimulates the activity of protein kinase A. The latter triggers an unidentified phosphorylation cascade that promotes the translocation of AQP II from intracellular stores to the apical membrane, which allows the reabsorption of water from the lumen to the cells. Then, the water exits the cell to the hypertonic interstitium via AQP III and AQP IV, localized at the basolateral membrane.[169,170] (2) ADH increases the permeability of the IMCD to urea, via activation of the urea transporter (UT-A1), enabling the accumulation of the urea in the interstitium, where it contributes along with Na^+ to the hypertonicity of the medullary interstitium, which is a prerequisite for maximum urine concentration and water reabsortpion.[167] ADH exerts several effects on Na^+ handling at different segments of the nephron, where it increases the Na^+ reabsorption via activation of epithelial Na^+ channel (EnaC) mainly in the cortical and outer medullary collecting duct (OMCD).[167] In addition, ADH may influence renal hemodynamics and reduce RPF, especially to the inner medulla.[171] The latter is mediated by the V_{1A}-receptor and may be modulated by the local release of NO and PGs. At higher concentrations (pathophysiologic range), ADH may also decrease total RPF and GFR, as a part of the generalized vasoconstriction induced by the peptide.[167]

A third receptor for ADH, V_3 (V_{1B}), is found predominantly in the anterior pituitary and is involved in the regulation of adrenocorticotropic hormone (ACTH) release.

In addition to its renal effects, ADH also regulates extrarenal vascular tone through the V_{1A} receptor. Stimulation of this receptor by ADH results in a potent arteriolar vasoconstriction in various vascular beds with a significant increase in systemic vascular resistance (SVR). However, physiologic increases in ADH do not usually cause a significant increase in blood pressure, because ADH also potentiates the sinoaortic baroreflexes that subsequently reduce heart rate and cardiac output.[172] Nevertheless, at supraphysiologic concentrations of ADH, such as occur when effective circulating volume is severely compromised (e.g., shock, CHF), ADH plays an important role in supporting arterial pressure and maintaining adequate perfusion to vital organs such as the brain and myocardium. ADH also has a direct, V_1 receptor–mediated, inotropic effect in the isolated heart.[173] In vivo, however, ADH has been reported to decrease myocardial function,[174] the latter attributed due to either cardioinhibitory reflexes or coronary vasoconstriction induced by the peptide. More importantly, ADH has been shown to stimulate cardiomyocyte hypertrophy and protein synthesis in neonatal rat cardiomyocytes and in intact myocardium through a V_1-dependent mechanism.[175,176] These effects are very similar to those obtained with exposure of cardiomyocytes to AII or catecholamines, although not necessarily through the same cellular mechanisms. By this growth-promoting property, ADH may contribute to the induction of cardiac hypertrophy and remodeling.

Controversy exists regarding the effect of ADH on natriuresis, with some authors finding a natriuretic response with infusions and others finding Na^+ retention.[177,178] These variations may be due to species differences. Blandford and colleagues[179] infused rats with a specific antagonist of V_2 receptors, resulting in increased Na^+ and water excretion, and suggested that the endogenous activity of ADH is one of Na^+ retention. However, in terms of overall volume homeostasis, the predominant influence related to ADH arises indirectly from water accumulation or blood pressure changes. The systemic vasoconstrictor actions of ADH are the effects that would be expected to defend blood pressure in the presence of perceived ECF volume contraction. However, in this regard, potential hypertensive effects of ADH are buffered by a concomitant increase in baroreflex-mediated sympathoinhibition or by an increase in PGE_2, resulting in a blunting of vasoconstriction, and by a direct vasodepressor action of V_2 receptor activation.[178,180,181]

Prostaglandins (see also Chapter 11)

PGs in the kidney regulate renal function including hemodynamics, renin secretion, growth response, tubular transport processes, and immune response in both health and disease states (Table 12–3).[182] Currently, two known principal isoforms of cycloxygenase (COX-1 and COX-2) metabolize arachidonic acid released from membrane phospholipids to PGs (see also Chapter 11). Recently, an additional splice variant of the COX-1 gene, COX-3, isoforms was identified.[182] COX-1 and COX-2 catalyze the synthesis of PGH_2, which then converted into the various prostanoids.[183] COX-1 is constitutively expressed in many cell types, with abundant expresson in renal cells where high immunoreactive levels are found, especially in the collecting duct and medullary interstitial cells of most species.[184] In contrast, the expression of COX-2 is inducible and cell-type specific, with prominent renal expression levels varying among species.[185,186] Published studies in dog, rat, and rabbit revealed COX-2 expression in medullary interstitial cells, cells of the TALH, and cells of the macula densa, where expression has been shown to be regulated in response to varying salt intake.[187–189] Lower levels of COX-2 were detected in the tubular epithelial cells of the collecting duct.[186,190] In human and monkey, COX-2 is expressed in the glomerular podocytes and blood vessels.[186] However, a more recent study in humans older than 60 years detected COX-2 in the macula densa and medullary interstitial cells.[189] Furthermore, the profile of sensitivity to pharmacologic inhibitors differs between the two isoforms.[191,192] The principal eicosanoid metabolites of cyclooxygenase in the kidney are PGI_2 (human) and PGE_2 (rat), with smaller amounts of $PGF_{2\alpha}$, PGD_2, and thromboxane A_2 (TXA_2).[184] Metabolism of arachidonic acid by other pathways (lipoxygenase, epoxygenase) leads to other products of importance in the modulation of nephron function.[184] The major sites for PG production (and hence for local actions) are the renal arteries and arterioles and glomeruli in the cortex and the renal medullary interstitial cells in the medulla, with additional contributions from epithelial cells of the cortical and medullary collecting tubules.[184,186,193] Studies have revealed that PGI_2 and PGE_2 are the prominent products in the cortex of normal kidney, with PGE_2 predominating in the medulla.[184]

The two major roles for the contribution of PGs to volume homeostasis are related to their effect on RBF, on one hand, and on their effect on tubular handling of salt and water, on the other. Table 12–3 lists target structures, mode of action, and major biologic effects of the renal active PGs and TXA_2. Some of the information provided by this table is still subject to active research. In balance, it appears that PGI_2 and PGE_2 have a predominantly vasodilating and natriuretic activity; they also interfere with action of ADH and tend to stimulate renin secretion. TxA_2 has been shown to cause vasoconstriction; the importance of the physiologic effects of TxA_2 on the kidney is still controversial. The end result of the stimulation of PG secretion in the kidney eventually leads to vasodilation, increased renal perfusion, natriuresis, and facilitation of water excretion.

The role of PGs acting as vasodilators in the glomerular microcirculation has been extensively characterized and well established. The cellular targets for vasoactive hormones in the glomerular microcirculation are vascular smooth muscle of the afferent and efferent arteriole and mesangial cells within the glomerulus. Action at these sites governs renal vascular resistance (RVR), glomerular function, and downstream microcirculatory function in peritubular capillaries and vasa recta. In vivo studies showed that intrarenal

TABLE 12–3	Major Renal Biologic Effects of Prostaglandins and Thromboxane		
Agent	**Target Structure**	**Mode of Action**	**Direct Consequences**
PGE_2, PGI_2	Intrarenal arterioles	Vasodilation	Increased renal perfusion (more pronounced in inner cortical and medullary regions)
PGI_2	Glomeruli	Vasodilation	Increased filtration rate
PGE_2, PGI_2	Efferent arterioles	Vasodilation	Increased Na^+ excretion through increased postglomerular perfusion
PGE_2, PGI_2, $PGF_{2\alpha}$	Distal tubules	Decreased transport	Increased Na^+ excretion, decreased maximum medullary hypertonicity
PGE_2, PGI_2, $PGF_{2\alpha}$	Distal tubules	Inhibition of cAMP synthesis	Interference with ADH action
PGE_2, PGI_2	Juxtaglomerular apparatus	cAMP stimulation (?)	Increased rennin release
TxA_2	Intrarenal arterioles	Vasoconstriction	Decreased renal perfusion

ADH, antidiuretic hormone; cAMP, cyclic adenosine monophosphate; PGE, prostaglandin E; PGI, prostaglandin I; TxA₂, thromboxane A_2.

infusions of PGE₂ and PGI₂ cause vasodilation and increased RPF.[184] In agreement with these findings, in vitro experiments with isolated renal microvessels showed that both PGE₂ and PGE₁ attenuate AII-induced afferent arteriolar vasoconstriction and PGI₂ antagonizes AII-induced efferent arteriolar vasoconstriction.[194] Similarly, PGE₂ has been shown to counteract AII-induced contraction of isolated glomeruli and glomerular mesangial cells in culture, and conversely, cyclooxygenase inhibition augments these contractile responses. An inhibitory counterregulatory role of PGs with respect to renal nerve stimulation has been demonstrated in micropuncture studies.[195] Therefore, the elimination of the vasorelaxant action of PGE₂ and PGI₂ at these target sites by treatment with selective and nonselective cyclooxygenase inhibitors is believed to result in an augmented fall in glomerular blood flow. However, this occurs mainly in the setting of heightened vasoconstrictor input, such as occurs during states of real or perceived volume depletion.[184,186,192] These conditions, which include overt dehydration, CHF, liver cirrhosis, nephrotic syndrome, and adults older than 60 years, are invariably associated with activation of pressor mechanisms RAAS, CNS, and ADH.[196] The renal vasoconstrictive influences of NE and AII are mitigated by their simultaneous stimulation of vasodilatory renal prostaglandins.[196,197] RBF and GFR are thus maintained, averting prerenal azotemia or even ischemic damage to the renal parenchyma. When this PG-mediated counterregulatory mechanism is suppressed by drugs that inhibit cyclooxygenase (e.g., nonsteroidal anti-inflammatory drugs [NSAIDs]), an impairment of renal hemodynamics develops, thereby leading to rapid deterioration in renal function. Although the introduction of selective COX-2 inhibitors has been associated with clear-cut decrease in gastrointestinal bleeding, it is becoming increasingly apparent that COX-2 inhibitors can cause a spectrum of renal effects nearly identical to those observed with the classic, nonselective NSAIDs.[198,199] These adverse effects are not surprising in light of the recent laboratory observations indicating that COX-2 is constitutively expressed in the kidney and plays a critical role in regulating renal hemodynamics, excretory function, and renin secretion.[198,199] COX-2–derived prostanoids are required for preservation of RPF and GFR, especially in states of ECF volume deficit, and also promote natriuresis and stimulate renin secretion during low Na⁺ intake or the use of loop diuretics.[186,200] Selective COX-2 inhibitors decrease GFR, and renal perfusion and may cause acute renal injury. Moreover, COX-2 inhibitors such as celecoxib or rofecoxib caused Na⁺ and K⁺ retention, edema formation, CHF, and hypertension similar to the nonselective COX inhibitors diclofenac and naproxen.[186,192] Thus, acute Na⁺ retention by NSAIDs in volume-depleted healthy adults is extensively mediated by inhibition of COX-2.

Whereas the role of PGs in modulating glomerular vasoreactivity in states of varying salt balance is firmly established, the effects of PGs on salt excretion per se are less well established. Certainly, the aforementioned vascular effects of PGs can be expected to have secondary effects on tubule function through the various physical factors described previously in this chapter. One particular consequence of PG-induced renal vasodilatation may be medullary interstitial solute washout. Such a change in medullary interstitial composition could potentially account for the observed increase in urinary Na⁺ excretion with intrarenal infusion of PGE₂.[184,201] Studies by Haas and colleagues[202] showed that the natriuretic response to PGE₂ may be attenuated by preventing an increase in renal interstitial hydraulic pressure, even in the presence of a persistent increase in RBF. The same group demonstrated in rats that the natriuresis usually accompanying direct expansion of renal interstitial volume can be significantly attenuated by inhibition of PGs synthesis. These findings are consistent with the proposal that changes in PGs have a significant effect

on renal Na⁺ excretion. A number of micropuncture and microcatheterization studies in vivo suggested effects of PGs on urinary Na⁺ excretion independent of hemodynamic changes.[184] Motivated by such findings, investigators sought direct effects of PGs on epithelial transport in individual isolated perfused tubule preparations, taken from various nephron segments. These studies showed that the effects of PGE₂ on transport processes vary considerably in different nephron segments.[203] In the medullary TALH and the collecting tubule, PGE₂ has been reported to cause a decrease in the reabsorption of water, Na⁺, and chloride.[203] This inhibition of Na⁺ reabsorption in the medullary TALH and in the cortical collecting duct is correlated with reduced Na⁺,K⁺-ATPase activity. In contrast, in the distal convoluted tubule, PGE₂ caused increased Na⁺,K⁺-ATPase activity.[203] Most likely, the net effects of locally produced PGs on tubular Na⁺ handling is inhibitory because complete blockade of PGs synthesis by indomethacin in rats receiving a normal or salt-loaded diet increased fractional Na⁺ reabsorption and enhanced the activity of the renal medullary Na⁺,K⁺-ATPase.[204] In addition, PGs diminish the renal response to ADH.[194,205] Several studies revealed that PGE₂ inhibits ADH-stimulated Na⁺ chloride reabsorption in the medullary TALH and ADH-stimulated water reabsorption at the collecting duct.[194,206] Both of these effects would tend to antagonize the overall hydroosmotic response to ADH. However, because no such effect is seen in the cortical TALH, which is capable of augmenting Na⁺ chloride reabsorption in response to an increased delivered load, and the effects of PGs on solute transport in the collecting tubule remain controversial, no conclusions can be reached with respect to the contribution of direct epithelial effects of PGs to overall Na⁺ excretion.[194]

Similarly, it is not surprising that whole animal and clinical balance studies that have examined the effect of PG infusion or prostaglandin synthesis inhibition on urinary Na⁺ excretion, or that have attempted to correlate changes in urinary PG excretion with changes in salt balance, also yielded conflicting and inconclusive results. One complicating feature stems from the fact that PG excretion rates vary with urine flow rates. Nevertheless, one conclusion can be stated with confidence: PGs have an important influence on urinary Na⁺ excretion, precisely in the settings in which they are important in preserving GFR, namely, states of vasoconstrictor hormone activation (e.g., Na⁺-depletion states). A particularly striking illustration of this role emerged from studies using HWI by Epstein and co-workers.[207] In these studies, the natriuretic response to HWI was accompanied by an increase in urinary PG excretion. However, inhibition of cyclooxygenase did not blunt the natriuretic response to this central volume-expanding maneuver in salt-replete subjects but did blunt the natriuretic response in salt-depleted individuals.

The influence of changes in Na⁺ intake on renal COX-1 and COX-2 expressions has been studied intensively in the last few years. The expression of COX-2 in the macula densa and TALH is increased by low-salt diet. Similar alteration in COX-2 was reported by inhibition of renin angiotensin aldosterone and by renal hypoperfusion.[185,189] In contrast, a high-salt diet has been reported to decrease COX-2 expression in the renal cortex.[185,189] None of these changes on Na⁺ intake affected the expression of COX-1 in the cortex of the kidney. In the renal medulla, whereas low-salt diet down-regulated both COX-1 and COX-2, high-salt diet enhanced the expression of these cyclooxygenase isoforms.[189] In vitro studies showed that high osmolarity of the medium of cultured IMCD cells induces the expression of COX-2.[186] Infusion of nimesulide (a selective COX-2 inhibitor) into anesthetized dogs on normal Na⁺ diet reduced urinary Na⁺ excretion and urine flow rate, despite the lack of effect on renal hemodynamics or systemic blood pressure.[186] Collectively, these findings suggest that COX-2 is distinctly regulated in the renal cortex and medulla and that its expression is altered by Na^+ intake on the one hand and that COX-2 inhibition hampers the urinary Na^+ excretion, on the other hand.

Finally, it should be recalled that in addition to the hemodynamically mediated and potential direct epithelial effects of PGs already enumerated, PGs may mediate observed physiologic responses to other hormonal agents. The intermediacy of PGs in renin release responses has already been cited. As another example, some, but not all, of the known physiologic effects of BK and other products of the kallikrein-kinin system are mediated through BK-stimulated PG production (e.g., inhibition of ADH-stimulated osmotic water permeability in the cortical collecting tubule).[194] In addition, some of the renal and systemic actions of AII are mediated via various PG production by both COX-1 and COX-2. For instance, COX-2 inhibitors or COX-2 knockout dramatically augment the pressor effects of AII and reduced medullary blood flow of this hormone.[208] In contrast, in COX-1–deficient mice, AII did not reduce the medullary blood flow, suggesting synthesis of COX-2–dependent vasodilators. Moreover, the diuretic and natriuretic effects of AII were absent in COX-2 deficiency. The authors concluded that COX-1 and COX-2 exert opposite effects on systemic and renal function: COX-2 mediates the vasodilatory and natriuretic effects of AII, whereas COX-2 mediates the pressor effect of AII.[208]

The Natriuretic Peptide Family

Major advances have taken place in our understanding of the physiologic and pathophysiologic roles of the NP family in the regulation of Na^+ and water balance since the discovery of ANP by de Bold and colleagues.[209] ANP is an endogenous 28–amino acid peptide secreted mainly by the right atrium. Besides ANP, the NP family contains at least two other members, BNP and CNP.[27] Although encoded by different genes, these peptides share a high similarity in chemical structure, gene regulation, and degradation pathways, yielding a unique hormonal system that exerts various biologic actions on the renal, cardiac, and blood vessel tissues.[210,211] ANP plays an important role in blood pressure and volume homeostasis owing to its ability to induce natriuretic/diuretic and vasodilatory responses.[212–214] BNP has an amino acid sequence similar to that of ANP, with an extended NH_2-terminus. In humans, BNP is produced from proBNP, which contains 108 amino acids and, following a proteolytic process, releases a mature 32–amino acid molecule and N-terminal fragment into the circulation. Although BNP was originally cloned from the brain, it is now considered a circulating hormone produced mainly in the cardiac ventricles.[215] CNP, which is produced mostly by endothelial cells, shares the ring structure common to all NP members; however, it lacks the C-terminal tail (Fig. 12–5A).

The biologic effects of the NPs are mediated by binding the peptide to specific membrane receptors localized to numerous tissues, including vasculature, renal artery, glomerular mesangial and epithelial cells, collecting duct, adrenal zona glomerulosa, and CNS.[210] At least three different subtypes of NP receptors have been identified: NP-A, NP-B, and NP-C (see Fig. 12–5B).[216] NP-A and NP-B, single transmembrane proteins with a molecular weight (MW) of ~120 to 140 kDa, mediate most of the biologic effects of NPs. Both are coupled to GC, which contains the protein kinase and GC domains in their intracellular portions.[211,217,218] After binding to their receptors, all NPs isoforms (ANP, BNP, and CNP) markedly increase cGMP in target tissues and in plasma. Therefore, analogs of cGMP or inhibition of degradation of this second messenger mimic the vasorelaxant and renal effects of these peptides. The third class of NP-binding sites, NP-C (MW of 60–70 kDa), are believed to serve as clearance receptors because they are not coupled to any known second messenger system.[219] ANP-C receptors are the most abundant

type of NP receptors in many key target organs of these peptides.[219] Additional routes for the removal of NPs includes enzymatic degradation by neutral endopeptidase 24.11 (NEP), a metalloproteinase located mainly in the lung and the kidney.[220]

ATRIAL NATRIURETIC PEPTIDE. Both in vivo and in vitro studies, in humans as well as in experimental animals, established the role of ANP in the regulation of ECF volume and the control of blood pressure by acting on all organs/tissues involved in the homeostasis of Na^+ and blood pressure[212,221,222] (Table 12–4).

Therefore, it is not surprising that ANP and NH_2-terminal ANP levels are increased in (1) conditions associated with enhanced atrial pressure, (2) systolic or diastolic cardiac dysfunction, (3) cardiac hypertrophy/remodeling, and (4) severe myocardial infarction (MI).[222–225] In the kidney, ANP exerts hemodynamic/glomerular effects that increase Na^+ and water delivery to the tubule, in combination with inhibitory effects on tubular Na^+ and water reabsorption, leading to remarkable diuresis and natriuresis.[222,226] In addition to its powerful diuretic and natriuretic activities, ANP also relaxes vascular smooth muscle, thus acting as antagonist to vasoconstriction. The vasodilatory actions of ANP appear to be most evident in the context of antagonizing the concomitant action of such vasoconstrictive influences as AII, endothelin (ET), ADH, and α_1-adrenergic input.[27,221,226] In addition, ANP reduces cardiac output by shifting fluid from the intravascular to the extravascular compartment, an effect medicated by increased capillary hydraulic conductivity to water.[212] In this context, ANP provokes vasodilation, which leads to reduced preload and subsequently to a fall in cardiac output.[27,226,227] ANP inhibits the activity of vasoconstrictor systems, such as the RAAS, the SNS, ADH, and ET system, and acts on the CNS to modulate vasomotor tone, thirst, and ADH release.[27,226] ANP has also been shown to exert antiproliferative, growth-regulatory properties in cultured glomerular mesangial cells, vascular smooth muscle cells (VSMC), and endothelial cells.[27,226] Within the kidney, ANP causes afferent vasodilation and efferent vasoconstriction, thus leading to a rise in glomerular capillary pressure, GFR, and filtration fraction (FF).[228,229] In combination with increased medullary blood flow, these hemodynamic effects enhance diuresis and natriuresis. However, the overall natriuretic effect of ANP infusion does not require these changes in glomerular function (except for larger doses of the peptide). At the tubular level, ANP inhibits the stimulatory effect AII on Na^+,H^+ exchanger localized to the luminal side of the proximal tubule.[230,231] Likewise, ANP, acting via cGMP, inhibits thiazide-sensitive Na^+,Cl^- cotransporter in the distal tubule and Na^+ channels in the collecting duct, along with inhibition of ADH-induced AQP II incorporation in the apical membrane of these segments of the nephron[228,232–234] (see Table 12–4).

BRAIN NATRIURETIC PEPTIDE. Administration of BNP to human subjects induces natriuretic, endocrine, and hemodynamic responses similar to those induced by ANP.[235] It is well established that BNP is produced and secreted in small amounts by the atrium, compared with the ventricles, which are the major sites of its production.[215] Increased volume or pressure overload states such as CHF and hypertension enhance the secretion of BNP from the ventricles. Despite the comparable elevation in plasma levels of ANP and BNP in patients with CHF and other chronic volume-expanded conditions, acute intravenous saline loading or infusion of pressor doses of AII yields different patterns of ANP and BNP secretion.[224,236] Whereas plasma levels of ANP increase rapidly, the changes in plasma BNP of atrial origin are negligible, supporting the fact that the atrium contains tiny amounts of BNP, in contrast to the high abundance of ANP.[236] Moreover, plasma levels of BNP rise with age. Whereas circulating BNP levels are 26±2 pg/mL in subjects aged 55 to 64

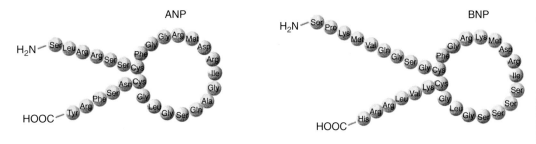

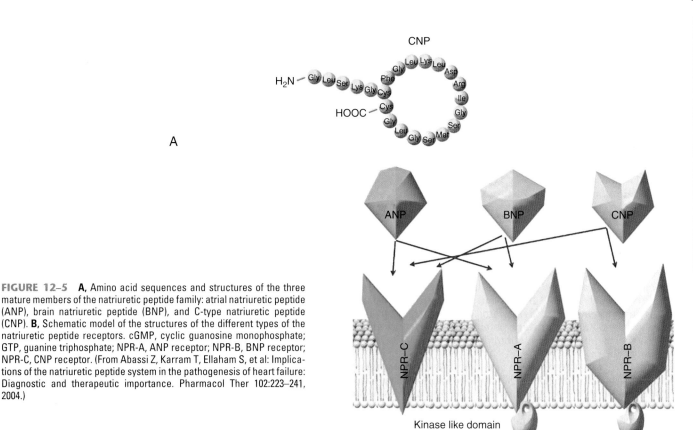

FIGURE 12–5 **A,** Amino acid sequences and structures of the three mature members of the natriuretic peptide family: atrial natriuretic peptide (ANP), brain natriuretic peptide (BNP), and C-type natriuretic peptide (CNP). **B,** Schematic model of the structures of the different types of the natriuretic peptide receptors. cGMP, cyclic guanosine monophosphate; GTP, guanine triphosphate; NPR-A, ANP receptor; NPR-B, BNP receptor; NPR-C, CNP receptor. (From Abassi Z, Karram T, Ellaham S, et al: Implications of the natriuretic peptide system in the pathogenesis of heart failure: Diagnostic and therapeutic importance. Pharmacol Ther 102:223–241, 2004.)

TABLE 12–4	Physiologic Actions of the Natriuretic Peptides
Target organ	**Biologic Effects**
Kidney	Increased glomerular filtration rate by inducing vasodilation of afferent arteriole and vasoconstriction of efferent arteriole Induction of natriuresis by inhibiting Na^+, H^+ exchanger in proximal tubule, Na^+, Cl^- cotransporter in distal tubule, and Na^+ channels in collecting duct Induction of diuresis owing to inhibition of ADH-induced aquaporin II incorporation into collecting duct apical membrane
Cardiac	Reduction in preload leading to reduced cardiac output Inhibition of cardiac remodeling
Hemodynamic	Vasorelaxation Elevating capillary hydraulic conductivity Decreased cardiac preload and afterload

Endocrine	Suppression of
	  Renin-angiotensin-aldosterone axis
	  Sympathetic outflow
	  ADH
	  Endothelin

Mitogenesis	Inhibition of mitogenesis in vascular smooth muscle cells Inhibition of growth factor–mediated hypertrophy in cardiac fibroblasts

years, they increase to 31 ± 2 and 64 ± 6 pg/mL in patients aged 65 to 74 years and 75 years or older, respectively.[237]

Animal and human studies demonstrated the natriuretic effects of pharmacologic doses of BNP. When administered to normal volunteers and hypertensive subjects at low doses, BNP induces a significant increase in urinary Na^+ excretion and to a lesser extent in urinary flow.[236] Significant natriuresis and diuresis were observed following the infusion of either ANP or BNP to normal subjects. The combination of ANP and BNP did not produce a synergistic renal effect, suggesting that these peptides share similar mechanisms of action.[236] Moreover, in similarity to ANP, BNP exerts a hypotensive effect in both animals and human subjects. For instance, transgenic mice that overexpress the BNP gene exhibit significant and lifelong hypotension to the same extent as transgenic mice that overexpress the ANP gene.[27] Therefore, it is clear that BNP induces its biologic actions through mechanisms similar to those of ANP.[27,236] This notion is supported by several findings: (1) Both ANP and BNP act via the same receptors, and both induce similar renal, cardiovascular, and endocrine actions in association with an increase in cGMP production[238] (see Table 12–4); (2) BNP suppresses the ACTH-induced aldosterone generation by cultured human adrenal cells.[236] Similar results were observed when BNP was infused in vivo.[239] The latter may be attributed to the inhibitory effects of BNP on renin secretion, as was shown in dogs.[238] In contrast, when BNP was given to humans, no significant change in plasma renin activity (PRA) was obtained. Similar to ANP, the hemodynamic effects of BNP vary according to the dose range and the species. When injected as a bolus at high doses, BNP caused a profound fall in systolic blood pressure; however, when infused at low doses, this peptide failed to change blood pressure or heart rate.[27] The effects of BNP have been utilized in the clinical setting in the treatment of the volume overload state of CHF, though recent studies showed a potentially deleterious effect of such therapy on renal function, as is outlined later in the section on CHF.

C-TYPE NATRIURETIC PEPTIDE. Although CNP is considered a neurotransmitter in the CNS, most recently it has been shown that endothelial cells produce considerable amounts of this NP, where it plays a role in the local regulation of vascular tone.[240] Smaller amounts of CNP are produced in kidney, heart ventricles, and intestine.[241,242] In addition, CNP has been found in human plasma, which could be of endothelial or cardiac origin. The physiologic stimuli for CNP production have not been identified, although enhanced CNP mRNA expression has been reported after volume overload.[27] Intravenous infusion of CNP decreases blood pressure, cardiac output, urinary volume, and Na^+ excretion. Furthermore, the hypotensive effects of CNP are less than those of ANP and BNP, but strongly stimulate cGMP production and inhibit VSMC proliferation.[27] Although all three NP forms inhibit the RAAS, CNP (unlike ANP and BNP) failed to induce significant hemodynamic changes in sheep, such as depression of cardiac output, reduction in blood pressure, and plasma volume contraction,[27,243] supporting the widely accepted concept that ANP and BNP are the major circulating NPs, whereas CNP is largely considered a local regulator of vascular structure/tone. Although all forms of NPs exist in the brain, their role and significance in the regulation of salt and water balance are not understood.

Taken together, the various biologic actions of NPs lead to reduction of effective volume, an expected response to perceived overfilling of the central intrathoracic circulation. Furthermore, all NPs counteract the adverse effects of RAAS, suggesting that the two systems are acting oppositely in the regulation of body fluid and cardiovascular homeostasis. Collectively, NPs are believed to participate in the regulation of Na^+ and water balance and blood pressure.

Endothelium-Derived Factors

The endothelium has been recognized as a major source of active substances that regulate the vascular tone in health and disease.[244–248] The most known representatives of these substances are: ET, NO (or as originally termed, endothelium-derived relaxing factor [EDRF]), and PGI_2. It is now well established that these vasoconstricting and vasodilating factors regulate the perfusion pressure of multiple organ systems that are strongly involved in water and Na^+ balance, such as the kidney, heart, and vasculature.

This section summarizes some of the concepts regarding actions of ET and EDRF/NO relevant to volume homeostasis.

ENDOTHELIN. The ET system consists of three vasoactive peptides, namely endothelin 1 (ET-1), endothelin 2 (ET-2), and endothelin 3 (ET-3). These peptides are synthesized and released mainly by endothelial cells and act in a paracrine/autocrine mode of action.[249–251] ET-1, the major representative of the ET family, is the most potent vasoconstrictor known at present.[252] All ETs are synthesized by proteolytic cleavage from specific preproETs that are further cleaved to form a 37–39–amino acid precursor, called big ET. Big ET is then converted into the biologically active, 21–amino acid peptide by a highly specific endothelin-converting-enzyme (ECE), a phosphoramidon-sensitive membrane-bound metalloprotease. To date, two isoforms of ECE have been identified: ECE-1 and ECE-2.[253] Four differentially spliced isoforms of ECE-1—ECE-1a, ECE-1b, ECE-1c, ECE-1d, are expressed in a variety of tissues including endothelial cells, and process big ET both intracellularly and on the cell surface. ECE-2 is localized mainly to VSMC, and is most likely an intracellular enzyme.[253] In ECE-1 knockout mice, tissue levels of ET-1 are reduced by about one third, suggesting that ECE independent pathways are involved in the synthesis of this peptide.[254] Recently, Wypij and co-workers[255] reported that chymase generates $ET-1_{1-21}$ as well as $ET-1_{1-31}$ peptide. The ETs bind to two distinct receptors, designated ETA and ETB.[251,253] The ETA receptor shows a higher affinity for ET-1 than ET-2 and ET-3. The ETB receptor shows equal affinity for each of the three ETs. Both receptors are expressed in a variety of tissues, including blood vessels, kidney, myocardium, lung, and brain.[250–253] The vasoconstrictor response to ET is induced by a ETA receptor–mediated increase in cytosolic Ca^{2+}. The endothelium-dependent relaxation is mediated by the ETB receptors via an NO-coupled mechanism. ET is detectable in the plasma of human subjects and many experimental animals and therefore may also act as a circulating vasoactive hormone.[249,252] The best known action of ET-1 is vasoconstriction, and its role in vascular homeostasis has been established.[251,253] In addition, accumulating evidence indicates that it has a variety of effects on the kidney.[250] The kidney is both a source of ET production (mainly the inner medulla) and an important target organ of the peptide. ET-1 is synthesized by the endothelial cells of the renal vessels, and ET-1 and ET-3 are produced by various cell types of the nephron.[256] Three major aspects of renal function are affected by ET: (1) renal vascular and mesangial cell tone, (2) renal tubular transport of salt and water, and (3) proliferation and mitogenesis of glomerular mesangial cells. Both ETA and ETB receptors are present in the glomerulus, renal vessels, and tubular epithelial cells, but the vast majority of the ETB subtype are found within the medulla.[250] The renal vasculature appears to be most sensitive to the vasoconstrictor action of ET-1 as compared with other vascular beds. Infusion of ET-1 into the renal artery of anesthetized rabbits decreases RPF, GFR, natriuresis, and urine volume.[257] Micropuncture studies demonstrated that ET-1 increases afferent and efferent arteriolar resistance (afferent more than efferent), resulting in a reduction in glomerular plasma flow rate. In addition, the ultrafiltration coefficient K_f is reduced owing to contraction of the mesangial cells, resulting in a diminished SNGFR. The profound reduction of RPF and concomitant lesser reduction in GFR should result in a rise in FF, but the effect of ET-1 on the FF appears to be variable, with some groups using low doses in a canine model reporting a rise[258] and others reporting no significant effect.[259] Infusion of ET-1 for 8 days into conscious dogs increased plasma levels of ET by two- to threefold and resulted in increased RVR and decreased GFR and RPF.[260] Interestingly, the effect of ET on regional intrarenal blood flow is not homogenous. By using laser-doppler flowmetry, Gurbanov and colleagues[261] reported that administration of ET-1 in control rats produced a sustained cortical vasoconstriction and a transient medullary vasodilatory response. These results are in line with previous studies reporting that the medulla predominantly expresses ETB receptors, whereas the cortical vasculature contains a high density of ETA-binding sites.[250]

The effect of ET on Na^+ and water excretion varies and depends on the dose and the source of ET. Systemic infusion of ET in high doses results in a profound antinatriuretic and antidiuretic effect, apparently secondary to the decrease in GFR and RBF.[262] However, in low doses or when produced locally in tubular epithelial cells, ET has been claimed to decrease the reabsorption of salt and water, suggesting the presence of ET-1 target sites on renal tubules.[263] Also, administration of the ET precursor, big ET, has been shown to cause natriuresis, supporting the notion of a direct inhibitory autocrine action of ET on tubular salt reabsorption. Hoffman and colleagues[264] observed that the natriuretic and diuretic actions of big ET-1 can be significantly reduced by ETB-specific blocker, A-192621. Similar results were reported by Pollock[265] when the same ETB antagonist was given chronically via osmotic minipump. Furthermore, Gariepy and co-workers[266] recently demonstrated that ETB knockout rats have salt-sensitive hypertension and that the luminal ENaC blocker amiloride restores normal arterial pressure in these rats, suggesting that in vivo ETB in the collecting duct tonically inhibits ENaC activity, the final regulator of Na^+ balance. Similarly, mice with collecting duct–specific knockout of the ET-1 gene have impaired Na^+ excretion in response to Na^+ load and develop hypertension with high salt intake.[250] The mice also have heightened sensitivity to ADH and reduced ability to excrete acute water load. These findings are in line with in vitro observations that ETB mediates the inhibitory effects of ET-1 on ion and water transport in various medullary tubular segments.[250,267] For instance ET-1 in vitro can inhibit Na^+ or water transport in the collecting duct and TALH.[250] Thus, if vascular and mesangial ET exerts a greater physiologic effect than tubule-derived ET, then RBF is diminished and net fluid retention occurs, whereas if the tubule-derived ET effect predominates, salt and water excretion is increased.

The ability of ET-1 to inhibit the hydro-osmotic effect of ADH is firmly established. Oishi and co-workers[268] examined the response of the isolated perfused IMCD to ET-1 and showed that ADH-stimulated water permeability was reversibly inhibited. The precise mechanism remains to be determined. However, ET-1 reduces ADH-stimulated cAMP accumulation and water permeability in the IMCD.[250] In addition, ET-1 mitigates the hydro-osmotic effect of ADH in the cortical collecting duct and the OMCD. Moreover, studies in rabbit cortical collecting duct indicate that ET-1 may inhibit luminal amiloride-sensitive Na^+ channels by a Ca^{2+}-dependent effect. Taking into account that the medulla contains ETB receptors and the highest ET concentrations in the body and that ETs also inhibit Na^+,K^+-ATPase in IMCD,[250] collectively, these effects may contribute to the diuretic and natriuretic actions of locally produced ET-1. This may also explain the natriuretic effect of ET-1 reported by some investigators, despite the reduction in RBF and GFR.[267]

Renal ET production is modulated differently than that in the vasculature. Whereas the vascular (and mesangial) ET generation is controlled by thrombin, AII, and transforming growth factor–β, the renal tubule ET production is under unique control. The nature of such regulation was initially derived from studies examining urinary ET excretion, which was entirely of renal origin.[269] Volume expansion in humans increased urinary ET excretion, suggesting an inhibitory action of renal ET on water reabsorption, particularly in collecting duct.[250] Today, it is believed that water balance regulates nephron ET production, but it is uncertain whether Na^+ balance has a direct impact. However, most recently, Sasser and colleagues[270] and Pollock and Pollock[271] provided evidence that ET-1 plays an important role in the response to high salt and that urinary ET-1 excretion is elevated in rats on a high-salt diet. Water balance may modulate collecting duct fluid reabsorption by altering the medullary tonicity. For instance, increasing the media tonicity with NaCl, raffinose, or mannitol decreased ET-1 synthesis by rat IMCD, Madin-Darby Canine Kidney cell line (MDCK), and M1 cortical collecting duct cells.[250] Moreover, inducing medullary hypotonicity, as occurred in water load, is most likely associated with augmented synthesis/release of medullary ET, thus provoking water loss. In contrast, medullary hypertonicity during dehydration probably reduces the generation of ET by the collecting duct and thus enhances fluid retention. Although not well established, the existence of such a system, in which collecting duct ET participates in the renal regulation of salt and water transport, is a tempting hypothesis.

NITRIC OXIDE. NO, originally described as the EDRF, is a diffusable gaseous molecule produced in endothelial cells of the renal vasculature as well as in tubular epithelial and mesangial cells from its precursor L-arginine by the enzyme NO synthase (NOS), which exists in three distinct isoforms: NOS 1 (bNOS), NOS 2 (iNOS), and NOS 3 (eNOS).[272] The use of selective NOS inhibitors and knockout mice has improved the ability to investigate the individual role of the NOS isoforms in the regulation of renal function.[273] However, it is difficult to identify the role of NO produced by a given isoform in a given cell type. Therefore, we refer to the renal effects of NO regardless of its enzymatic isoform source.

In the past decade, evidence has been provided regarding the importance of locally produced NO in the regulation of renal function, including RPF, salt excretion, and renin release as well as the long-term control of blood pressure.[273–275] NO has been shown to exert a tonic vasodilatory action on afferent arterioles and to mediate the renal vasorelaxant action of acetylcholine and BK.[273,275] The action of NO is mediated by activation of a soluble GC in adjacent VSMCs, thereby increasing intracellular levels of its second messenger, cGMP.[276,277] Evidence now indicates that all NOS isoforms are present in the human and other mammalian kidney.[273,276–278] Recent studies have shown that renal NOS activity is regulated by several humoral factors such as aldosterone and salt intake (see later).[273]

NO plays an important role in the regulation of renal hemodynamics and excretory function,[279] best evidenced by the fact that inhibiting of intrarenal NO production results in increased blood pressure and kindey function.[280,281] Infusion of NOS inhbitor, N_G monomethyl-L-arginine (L-NMMA), into one kidney of anesthetized dogs resulted in a dose-dependent decrease in urinary cGMP levels; decreases in RPF and GFR, antinatriuresis, and antidiuresis; and a decline in fractional Na^+ excretion in that kidney compared with the one on the contralateral side.[281] In addition, acute NO blockade amplifies the renal vasoconstriction action of AII in isolated micoperfused rabbit afferent arterioles[282] and conscious rats,[283] suggesting that NO and AII interact in the control of renal vasculature. This notion is supported by the findings that L-NMMA–induced vasoconstriction, decreased RBF, and reduced hydraulic coefficient, K_f, were prevented when the RAAS was blocked, suggesting that some of the major effects of NO are to counterbalance the vasoconstrictive action of AII. In addition, it is evident that NO plays a significant role in regulating TGF and in modulating renin secretion by the juxtaglomerular apparatus.[273,284] Inhibition of the NO system by nonselective blockers of NOS results in attenuation of the activity of TGF, augmentation of both its vasoconstriction and its vasodilator capacities, and stimulation of renin secretion.[273,284] Most likely, bNOS, which localizes to the macula densa, is the major NOS isoform responsible for TGF behavior.[279]

The involvement of the NO system in the regulation of Na^+ balance is well described. In a study by Salazar and colleagues,[285] conscious dogs were utilized to examine the role of NO in mediating the arterial pressure and renal excretory response to a prolonged increase in Na^+ intake. These investigators demonstrated that, with a normal Na^+ diet, NO inhibition induced a significant decrease in natriuresis and diuresis without a change in pressure. In dogs receiving a high-Na^+ diet and treated with an NO inhibitor, both arterial pressure and cumulative Na^+ balance were higher than in dogs receiving a comparable diet but untreated with NO inhibitors. Shultz and Tolins[286] demonstrated that exposure of rats to high-salt intake (1% NaCl drinking water) for 2 weeks induced increased serum concentration and urinary excretion of the NO metabolic products, $NO_2 + NO_3$. Urinary NO_2 and NO_3 and Na^+ excretion are significantly correlated. The increase in urinary NO metabolites is attributed to the enhanced expression of all three NOS isoforms in the renal medulla by high-salt intake.[273] These findings suggest that NO may have a role in promoting diuresis and natriuresis in both normal and increased salt intake/volume-expanded states.[286,287] In line with this notion, using micropuncture technique, Eitle and co-workers[288] showed that NO, like ANP, was able to inhibit proximal tubular fluid absorption via a cGMP-mediated mechanism. As mentioned earlier, L-nitroarginine methyl ester (L-NAME) infused directly into the renal medullary interstitium of anesthetized rats reduced the papillary blood flow, in association with decreased Na^+ and water excretion, indicating that NO exerts a tonic influence on renal medullary circulation and Na^+ excretion.[289] It should emphasized that high levels of eNOS in the renal medulla, on one hand, and with the inhibitory effect of NO on Na^+,K^+-ATPase in the collecting duct, on the other.[290] The renal NO system interacts with the local ET system at different levels.[267] The inhibition of NOS by L-NAME or of ETB receptor by A-192621 (highly selective ETB antagonist) abolished the diuretic and natriuretic effects of big ET-1 in the kidneys of anesthetized rats.[264,291] These findings indicate that NO mediates the diuretic and natriuretic action of locally produced ET-1 in the renal inner medulla. Likewise, substantial evidence indicates that NO inhibits the ADH-enhanced Na^+ reabsorption and hydro-osmotic water permeability of the cortical collecting duct.[292] Additional support for the involvement of the NO system in Na^+ homeostasis is derived from several studies that examined the mechanism of salt-sensitive hypertension. According to these studies, NOS activity, mainly of neural-type (bNOS), is significantly lower in salt-sensitive rats that were maintained on a high-salt diet than in salt-resistant animals.[293,294] In another study, the impaired activity of NOS in salt-sensitive rats was evidenced by a decreased urinary nitrate plus nitrite excretion.[293,295] Intravenous administration of L-arginine increased NO production and prevented the development of salt-induced hypertension in Dahl-sensitive rats.[295] These findings suggest that bNOS plays an important role in Na^+ handling and that decreases in bNOS activity may in part be involved in the mechanism of salt hypertension. The involvement of NO in the abnormality of Na^+ handling in this disease state could emerge from an inadequate direct effect on tubular pumps responsible for Na^+ reabsorption in proximal and distal segments. However, it may also be influenced by attenuated inhibitory actions of NO on renin secretion and TGF. In this context, recent studies concluded that NO of macula densa origin blunts the TGF vasoconstriction during high-salt intake in salt-resistant rats, whereas in salt-sensitive rats, this response is lost and thus may contribute to salt retention and subsequently to hypertension.[296]

Renal Nerves

Extensive autonomic innervation of the kidney makes an important contribution to the physiologic regulation of all aspects of renal function.[195] Sympathetic nerves, predominantly adrenergic, have been observed at all segments of the renal vasculature and tubule.[297] Adrenergic nerve endings reach VSMCs and mesangial cells, cells of the juxtaglomerular apparatus, and all segments of the tubule: proximal, loop of Henle, and distal. Only the basolateral membrane separates the nerve endings from the tubular cells.[298] Initial studies determined that the greatest innervation was found in the renal vasculature, mostly at the level of the afferent arterioles followed by the efferent arterioles and outer medullary descending vasa recta.[299] However, high-density tubular innervation was found in the ascending limb of the loop of Henle and the lowest density was observed in the collecting duct, inner medullary vascular elements, and papilla.[298,300] It is inferred that the magnitude of the tubular response to renal nerve activation may be proportional to the differential density of innervation.

Consistent with these anatomic observations, stimulation of the renal nerve results in vasoconstriction of afferent and efferent arterioles.[195,300] Pharmacologic evidence obtained in a variety of experimental animals indicates that the renal vasoconstriction generated by the renal nerves is mediated by the activation of postjunctional α_1-adrenoreceptors.[301] The presence of high-affinity adrenergic receptors in the nephron also supports a significant role of the renal nerves in tubule function. The α_1-adrenergic and most of the α_2-adrenergic receptors are found in the proximal tubule and have been localized in the basolateral membranes.[302] In the rat, β-adrenoreceptors have been found in the cortical TALH and have been subtyped as β_1-adrenoceptors.[303] The predominant neurotransmitters in renal sympathetic nerves are noradrenaline and, to a lesser extent. dopamine and acetylcholine.[300]

It is widely believed that changes in the activity of the renal sympathetic nerve play an important role in controlling body fluid homeostasis.[195,297,304] Renal sympathetic nerve activity can influence renal function and Na^+ excretion through several mechanisms: (1) changes in renal and glomerular hemodynamics, (2) effect on renin release from juxtaglomerular cells with increased formation of AII, and (3) direct effect on renal tubular fluid and electrolyte reabsorption.[195] Whether renal hemodynamics is influenced by changes in renal nerve activity within the physiologic range is a matter of debate.[197] Application of graded direct electrical renal nerve stimulation produces frequency-dependent changes in RBF and GFR, renal tubule Na^+ and water reabsorption, and renin secretion.[297,305] The lowest frequency (0.5–1.0 Hz) stimulates renin secretion, followed by increases in renal tubule Na^+ and water reabsorption at frequencies of 1.0 to 2.5 Hz. Increasing the frequency of stimulation to 2.5 Hz and higher results in decreases in RBF and GFR.[195,305] The decrease in SNGFR in response to enhanced renal nerve activity has been attributed to a combination of increases in both afferent and efferent glomerular resistance and decreases in glomerular capillary hydrostatic pressure (ΔP) and glomerular ultrfiltration coefficient.[195,197,297,306] Micropuncture experiments before and after renal nerve stimulation at different frequencies in Munich-Wistar rats revealed that the effector loci for vasomotor control by renal nerves localize to the afferent and efferent arteriole.

In addition, although urine flow and Na$^+$ excretion declined with renal nerve stimulation, there was no change in absolute proximal fluid reabsorption rate, suggesting that increased reabsorption occurs in the more distal segments of the nephron. However, earlier studies in the rat found alterations in proximal fluid reabsorption in response to renal nerve stimulation or acute denervation.

Studies of the response of the kidney to reflex activation of renal nerves are also supportive of a role for the SNS in regulating renal hemodynamic function and Na$^+$ excretion.[298] DiBona and colleagues[195] measured renal nerve activity in rats receiving different Na$^+$ diets in response to isotonic saline volume expansion and furosemide-induced volume contraction. A low-Na$^+$ diet resulted in a reduction in right atrial pressure and an increase in renal nerve activity. The high-Na$^+$ diet resulted in opposite changes, that is, an increase in right atrial pressure and a reduction in renal nerve activity. Thus, the relationship between atrial pressure and renal sympathetic nerve activity is both linear and bidirectional, with a gain of approximately –20%/mm Hg rise in atrial pressure.[195,307] Other studies in conscious animals, utilizing maneuvers such as HWI and left atrial balloon inflation,[308] support the importance of reflex regulation of renal nerve activity. Collectively, these studies demonstrate the reciprocal relationship between ECF volume and renal nerve activity, consistent with the role of central cardiopulmonary mechanoreceptors governing renal nerve activity. These authors also demonstrated that the contribution of efferent renal nerve activity is of greater significance during conditions of dietary Na$^+$ restriction when the need for renal Na$^+$ conservation is maximal. When this linkage between the renal SNS and the excretory kidney function is defected, abnormalities in the regulation of ECF volume and blood pressure may develop.[300,309]

Several studies that have examined the response of denervated kidneys to various physiologic maneuvers also indicated a role for renal nerves in regulating renal hemodynamic function and Na$^+$ excretion. Early studies showed that acute denervation of the kidney is associated with increased urine flow and Na$^+$ excretion.[195] Micropuncture techniques showed that, in euvolemic animals, elimination of renal innervation does not alter any of the determinants of SNGFR, indicating that renal nerves contribute little to the vasomotor tone of normal animals under baseline physiologic conditions. Yet, absolute proximal reabsorption was significantly reduced, in the absence of changes in peritubular capillary oncotic pressure, hydraulic pressure, and renal interstitial pressure.[195] Other studies showed that the decrease in tubular electrolyte and water reabsorption following renal denervation is not limited to the proximal nephron, but occurs also in the loop of Henle and the distal nephron segments.[195,310] In another micropuncture study, measurements obtained before and after denervation in control rats and rats with experimental CHF or acute volume depletion demonstrated that denervation resulted in diuresis and natriuresis in normal rats but failed to alter any of the parameters of renal cortical microcirculation.[311] In contrast, in rats with CHF, denervation caused an amelioration of renal vasoconstriction, by decreasing afferent and efferent arteriolar resistance, and again a natriuresis. This study indicates that in situations in which efferent neural tone is heightened above baseline level, renal nerve activity may profoundly influence renal circulatory dynamics. However, although the basal level of renal nerve activity in normal rats or conscious animal is apparently insufficient to influence renal hemodynamics, it is sufficient to exert a tonic stimulation on renal tubular epithelial Na$^+$ reabsorption and renin release.[195]

Clinical studies, in which guanethidine was given to achieve autonomic blockade or in patients with idiopathic autonomic insufficiency, revealed that intact adrenergic innervation is required for the normal renal adaptive response to dietary Na$^+$ restriction.[312] More direct examination of efferent renal sympathetic nerve activity in humans has been made possible by the measurement of renal NE spillover methodology to elucidate the kinetics of NE release. A study by Friberg and associates[313] determined that, in normal subjects, a low-Na$^+$ diet resulted in a fall in urinary Na$^+$ excretion and an increase in NE spillover, with no change in cardiac NE uptake, which supports the concept of a true increase of efferent renal nerve activity secondary to Na$^+$ restriction. Further evidence that the SNS plays a role in Na$^+$ balance in humans comes from a study by McMurray and co-workers,[314] who demonstrated that low-dose infusion of NE to normal salt-replete volunteers resulted in a physiologic plasma increment of this neurotransmitter in asscociation with antinatriuretic. This reduction in Na$^+$ excretion occurred without any change in GFR but was associated with a significant decline in Li$^+$ clearance, an indication of reduced proximal tubule reabsorption.

The cellular mechanisms mediating the tubular actions of NE are believed to include stimulation of Na$^+$,K$^+$-ATPase activity and Na$^+$/H$^+$ exchange in the proximal tubular epithelial cells.[195] It is assumed that α_1-adrenoreceptor stimulation, acting via phospholipase C, causes an increase in intracellular Ca^{2+} that activates Ca^{2+}/calmodulin–dependent calcineurin (phosphatase). Calcineurin dephosphorylates Na$^+$-K$^+$-ATPase from its inactive phosphorylated form to its active dephosphorylated form.[315] The stimulatory effect of renal nerve on Na$^+$/H$^+$ antiport is mediated through stimulation of α_2-adrenoreceptor.[195]

In addition to its direct action on epithelial cell transport and renal hemodynamics, interactions of renal nerve input with other effector mechanisms may contribute to the regulation of renal handling of Na$^+$. Efferent sympathetic nerve activity influences the rate of renin secretion from the kidney by a variety of mechanisms, directly or by interacting with the renal tubule macula densa and vascular baroreceptor mechanisms for renin secretion.[195] The increase in renin secretion is mediated primarily by direct stimulation of β_1-adrenergic receptors located on juxtaglomerular granular cells.[195] Sympathetic activation of renin release is augmented during RPP reduction.[195] Studies in the isolated perfused rat kidney suggest that intrarenal generation of AII has an important prejunctional action on renal sympathetic nerve terminal to facilitate NE release during renal nerve stimulation.[195] However, the physiologic significance of this facilitatory interaction on tubular Na$^+$ reabsorption remains controversial. Thus, administration of an ACE inhibitor or an AII receptor antagonist attenuated the antinatriuretic response to electrical renal nerve stimulation in anesthetized rats.[195] In contrast, when nonhypotensive hemorrhage was used to produce reflex increase in renal sympathetic activity in conscious dogs, the associated antinatriuresis was unaffected by ACE inhibition or AII receptor blockade.[316]

Sympathetic activity is also a stimulus for the production and release of renal PGs, coupled in series to the adrenergic-mediated renal vasoconstriction.[195] Evidence indicates that renal vasodilatory PGs attenuate the renal hemodynamic vasoconstrictive response to activation of the renal adrenergic system in vivo and on isolated renal arterioles.[195] Micropuncture experiments in Munich-Wistar rats provided evidence that the primary factor responsible for the reduction in the glomerular ultrafiltration coefficient during renal nerve stimulation may be AII rather than NE and that endogenously produced PGs neutralize the vasoconstrictive effects of renal nerve stimulation at an intraglomerular locus rather than at the arteriolar level.

Another interaction examined is that between the renal SNS and ADH. Studies in conscious animals showed that ADH exerted a dose-related effect on arterial baroreflex, such that low doses of ADH may sensitize the central baroreflex neurons to afferent input, whereas higher doses caused direct excitations of these neurons, resulting in a reduction in sympathetic outflow.[195] Nishida and colleagues[317] demonstrated that ADH suppresses renal sympathetic outflow and determined that this response depends on the number of afferent inputs from baroreceptors. Simon and associates[318] examined the plasma ADH response to renal nerve stimulation in conscious, baroreceptor-intact, Wistar rats. Renal nerve stimulation resulted in an elevated plasma concentration of ADH and a rise in arterial pressure.

Many studies demonstrated, in both normal and pathologic situations, that increased renal nerve sympathetic activity can antagonize the natriuretic/diuretic response to ANP and that removal of the influence of sympathetic activity enhances the natriuretic action of the peptide.[228,319,320] Awazu and co-workers[321] noted that, in Wistar rats, renal denervation increased ANP receptors and cGMP generation in glomeruli, resulting in an increase in ultrafiltration coefficient after ANP infusion.

In summary, evidence indicates that the renal sympathetic nerves can regulate urinary Na^+ and water excretion by changing RVR, by influencing renin release from the juxtaglomerular granular cells, and through a direct effect on tubular epithelial cells. These effects may be modulated via interactions with various other hormonal systems including ANP, PGs and ADH.

Other Factors

KININS. The kallikrein-kinin system (KKS) is a complex cascade responsible for the generation and release of vasoactive kinins, that is, BK and related peptides.[322] This endogenous metabolic system includes precursors of kinins, known as kininogen, and tissue and circulatory kallikreins. Kinins are produced by many cell types in the body and can be detected in secretory products such as urine, saliva, and sweat, interstitial fluid, and rarely, venous blood. That renal KKS can produce local concentrations of BK much higher than those present in blood is well known.[323] Kinins play an important role in hemodynamic and excretory processes through their receptors that include BK-B_1, and BK-B_2. The BK-B_2 receptors mediate most of the actions of kinins and are located mainly in kidney, although they are also detectable in heart, lung, brain, uterus, and testes. Activation of BK-B_2 receptors results in vasodilation most likely via an NO- or arachidonic acid metabolites–dependent mechanism.[322,324,325] BK is known for its multiple effects on the cardiovascular system, particularly vasodilation and plasma extravasation.[322]

Besides the vasculature, the kidney is an important target organ of kinins, where they induce diuresis and natriuresis via activation of BK-B_2 receptors. These effects are attributaed to an increase in RBF and to inhibition of Na^+ and water reabsorption in the distal nephron.[323,326] The latter effect is secondary to the observed action of kinins in reducing vascular resistance. Unlike many vasodilators, BK increases RBF without significantly affecting GFR or Na^+ reabsorption at the proximal tubule level, but with a marked decrease in the water and salt reabsorption in the distal portions of the nephron, thus contributing to increased urine volume and Na^+ excretion. Several studies that utilized transgenic animals enriched our understanding of the physiologic role of the kinins and the interaction between the KKS and the RAAS.[323] For instance, in the kidney, AII acting via AT_2 receptor stimulates a vasodilator cascade of BK, NO, and cGMP, which is tonically activated only during conditions of increased AII, such as Na^+ depletion.[327] In the absence of the AT_2 receptor, pressor and antinatriuretic hypersensitivity to AII is associated with BK and NO deficiency.[326] Furthermore, the involvement of the renal kinins in pressure natriuresis phenomenon

has been documented.[98] The heptapeptide angiotensin (Ang)-(1–7) is currently considered one of the biologically active end products of the RAAS.[323] BK mediates the biologic actions of Ang-(1–7), because rats transgenic to kallikrein gene display significant augmentation in the diuretic and natriuretic actions of Ang-(1–7).[323] Because ACE is involved in the degradation of kinins, ACE inhibitors not only attenuate the formation of AII but also may lead to the accumulation of kinins. Therefore, the latter are believed to be responsible in part for the beneficial effects of ACE inhibitors in patients with CHF.[328] Based on that, the KKS is believed to play a pivotal role in the regulation of fluid and electrolyte balance, mostly through its renal actions.

ADRENOMEDULLIN. Human adrenomedullin (AM) is a 52–amino acid peptide that was discovered over a decade ago by Kitamura and associates[329] in extracts of human pheochromocytoma. AM shares structural homology with calcitonin gene–related peptide and amylin.[329,330] Like the calcitonin gene, the AM gene is situated in a single locus of chromosome 11. Besides human AM, the amino acid sequence of AM has been determined in many species including rat, canine, mouse, porcine, and bovine. AM is produced from a 185 a.a. preprohormone that also contains a unique 20 a.a. sequence in the NH_2-terminus and termed *proadrenomedulin NH_2-terminal 20 peptide (PAMP)*. PAMP exists in vivo and has biologic activity similar to that of AM. AM-mRNA is expressed in several tissues including atrium, ventricles, vascular tissue, lung, kidney, pancreas, ventricle, smooth muscle cells, small intestine, and brain. The synthesis and secretion of AM are stimulated by chemical factors and physical stress. Among these stimulants are cytokines, corticosteroids, thyroid hormones, AII, NE, ET, BK, and shear stress.[331] AM immunoreactivity has been localized in most of the body tissues.[330,332] For instance, high concentrations of AM are present in pheochromocytoma, adrenal medulla, cardiac atria, pituitary gland, and at lower levels in cardiac ventricles, VSMC, endothelial cells, renal distal and collecting tubules, digestive, respiratory, reproductive, and endocrine systems.[331,332] Interestingly, endothelial cells produce and secrete AM in amounts comparable to that of ET.[330] In contrast to the other tissues, the AM synthesized in the adrenal medulla is stored in granules and secreted in a controlled pathway.[331] AM acts through a membrane receptor that consists of 395 a.a. that structurally resembles G-protein–linked receptor, containing seven transmembrane domains. AM receptors comprise the calcitonin receptor–like receptor and a family of receptor-activity–modifying protein (RAMPs 1–3).[333] Activation of these receptors increases intracellular cAMP, which most likely serves as a second messenger for the peptide.[330,334] Since its discovery, AM has undergone intensive investigation in regard to possible participation in the regulation of cardiovascular and volume homeostatsis.[335,336] Multiple biologic actions of AM have been reported. The most impressive biologic effect of AM is long-lasting and dose-dependent vasodilation of the vascular system including coronary arteries.[330,334,335] Injection of AM into anesthetized rats, cats, or conscious sheep, induced a potent and long-lasting hypotensive response associated with reduction in vascular resistance in the kidney, brain, lung, hind limbs, and mesentery.[331] The hypotensive action of AM is accompanied by increases in heart rate and cardiac output owing to positive inotropic effects.[331] The vasodilating effect of AM can be blocked by inhibiting NOS, suggesting that NO partly mediates the decrease in systemic vascular resistance.[330] Besides its hypotensive action, AM increases RBF via preglomerular and postglomerular arteriolar vasodilation.[334,337] The AM-induced hyperperfusion is associated with a dose-dependent diuresis and natriuresis.[331,334] These effects result from a decrease in tubular Na^+ reabsorption despite the AM-induced hyperfiltration.[337] Similar to natriuretic peptides, AM suppresses aldosterone secretion in response to AII and high potassium.[330] Furthermore, in cultured VSMC, AM inhibits ET production induced by various stimuli.[331] AM acts in the CNS to inhibit both water and salt intake.[338] In the hypothalamus, AM inhibits the secretion of ADH, an effect that may contribute to its diuretic and natriuretic actions.[338] Taken together, these findings show that AM is a vasoactive peptide of potential importance that may be involved in the physiologic control of renal, adrenal, vascular, and cardiac function. Furthermore, the existence of AM-like immunoreactivity in the glomerulus and in the distal tubule, in association with detectable amounts of AM mRNA in the kidney, suggests that AM plays a renal paracrine role.[339]

UROTENSIN. Urotensin-II (U-II) is a cyclic peptide originally isolated from the caudal neurosecretory organ of teleost fish.[340,341] The human isoform was cloned in 1999 and has been identified as the natural ligand for the orphan G-protein–coupled receptor GPR-14.[342-345] The U-II/GPR-14 system is expressed in the CNS, the cardiovascular system, and the kidney of various mammalian species, including humans.[345-349] In the human kidney, immunoreactive staining for U-II was detected in the epithelial cells of the tubules, mostly in the distal tubule, with moderate staining in the endothelial cells of the renal capillaries.[350] In addition, in fish, some evidence indicates that U-II modulates transepithelial ion (Na+/Cl−) transport.[351,352] Human U-II (hU-II) possesses potent vasoactive properties, although these effects are largely dependent on the species and the vascular bed examined.[342,353]

In the original study by Ames and colleagues,[342] hU-II induced a potent vasoconstrictor effect on isolated arteries from nonhuman primates that was an order of magnitude greater than that of ET-1. Since then, hU-II has been considered the most potent mammalian vasoconstrictor identified so far.[342,353,354] However, careful analysis of the literature reveals that this general notion may be unjustified and that U-II may exert both vasoconstrictor and vasodilatory effects. These actions depend largely on the animal species as well as on the vascular bed examined.[353,354] In the rat, the predominant cardiovascular actions of U-II are hyperemic vasodilatation in the mesenteric and hindquarter vascular beds, associated with hypotension and dose-dependent tachycardia.[355] Gibson[356] showed that U-II at low concentrations caused relaxation of noradrenaline-precontracted aortic stripes of rats in an endothelium-dependent manner. Evidence also indicates that hU-II may act as a potent vasodilator of human small pulmonary arteries and abdominal resistance arteries.[357] Likewise, in the isolated perfused rat heart, U-II elicited a sustained coronary vasodilatation through factors such as COX products and NO.[358] These findings may suggest that, although the direct effect of U-II on large vessels is contraction, U-II also relaxes blood vessels by the release of vasodilators from endothelium.[359]

The involvement of the U-II system in the regulation of renal function in mammals has not been thoroughly investigated. Recently, Zhang and associates[360] demonstrated that hU-II is an NO-dependent renal vasodilator and acts a natriuretic peptide in the rat kidney. Also, recent evidence by Clozel and co-workers[361] suggests that the UT-II system may be involved in the pathogenesis of the no-reflow phenomenon of renal ischemia induced by clamping of the renal artery.

DIGITALIS-LIKE FACTOR. Hamlyn and co-workers[362-364] identified an endogenous ouabain-like compound in human and other mammalian plasma that interacts with the cardenolide receptor on the Na+,K+-ATPase pump and whose mechanism of inhibition was strikingly similar to that of the digitalis glycosides used in the treatment of CHF and certain cardiac arrhythmias. This substance, which was later termed *endogenous digitalis-like factor (EDLF),* is secreted by the adrenal cortex. The physiologic role of the EDLF has not yet been fully elucidated. However, initial studies hypothesized that natriuretic hormone and the vascular Na+,K+-ATPase inhibitor are the same factor and, furthermore, that this factor played a causative role in the pathophysiology of certain types of hypertension. Indeed, prolonged elevation of circulating EDLF in the rat produces sustained hypertension.[365] Similarly, among white patients with essential hypertension, a large fraction has high circulating concentrations of EDLF.[365] Moreover, owing to its inhibitory action on the Na+ pump, EDLF increases cytosolic stores of Ca2+ in many types of cells, including VSMC, leading to an increase in vascular resistance.[366] In newborns, the inhibition of renal Na+,K+-ATPase may enhance elimination of surplus Na+.[367]

NEUROPEPTIDE Y. Neuropeptide Y (NPY), a 36-residue peptide, is a sympathetic co-transmitter stored and released together with noradrenaline by adrenergic nerve terminals of the SNS. Structurally, NPY shares high homology with two other members of the pancreatic polypeptide family, peptide YY (PYY) and pancreatic polypeptide (PP). These two closely related peptides are produced and released by the intestinal endocrine cells and pancreatic islet cells, respectively, and act as hormones.[368,369] Although NPY was originally isolated from the brain and is highly expressed in the CNS, it has been clearly demonstrated that NPY exhibits a wide spectrum of biologic activities in peripheral organs such as the cardiovascular system, the GIT, and the kidney.[370-372] Numerous studies utilizing both in vivo and in vitro techniques demonstrated the capacity of the NPY to reduce RBF and increase RVR in various species including rat, rabbit, pig, and humans.[372] Despite of the potent vasoconstrictor effect of this peptide on renal vasculature, this effect does not appear to be associated with a similar reduction in GFR. Indeed, most of the studies in which this parameter was evaluated show only minor or no alterations in GFR in response to NPY administration. Considering the potent renal vasoconstrictor action of NPY, a decrease in electrolyte and water excretion could be expected following the administration of the peptide.[372] However, the available data at present suggest that NPY may exert either a natriuretic[373] or an antinatriuretic[374] action, depending on the experimental conditions and the species utilized.

Collectively, numerous studies using physiologic and pharmacologic approaches indicated that this peptide has the capacity to alter renal function. In particular, these studies suggest that NPY may exert renal vasoconstrictor and tubular actions that are species dependent and may also influence renin secretion by the kidney. The question of whether NPY plays an important role in the physiologic regulation of renal hemodymaics and electrolyte excretion remains largely unanswered at present.

PATHOPHYSIOLOGY OF EDEMA FORMATION

Generalized edema formation, the clinical hallmark of ECF volume expansion, represents the accumulation of excessive volumes of fluid in the interstitial compartment and is invariably associated with renal Na+ retention. It occurs most commonly in response to CHF, cirrhosis with ascites, and the nephrotic syndrome. In CHF and cirrhosis with ascites, the primary disturbance leading to Na+ retention does not originate within the kidney. Instead, renal Na+ retention is the response to a disturbance of the circulation induced by disease of the heart or liver. In the nephrotic syndrome, glomerular injury accompanied by heavy proteinuria is associated with Na+ retention and leads to a profound disturbance in circulatory homeostasis. In each of these conditions, the renal effector mechanisms that normally operate to conserve Na+ and protect against an Na+ deficit are exaggerated and continue despite subtle or overt expansion of ECF volume.

Local Mechanisms in Interstitial Fluid Accumulation

Transcapillary fluid and solute transport can be viewed as consisting of two types of flow, convective and diffusive. Bulk water movement occurs via convective transport induced by hydraulic and osmotic pressure gradients.[375] Capillary hydraulic pressure is under the influence of a number of factors, including systemic arterial and venous blood pressures, local blood flow, and the resistances imposed by the pre- and postcapillary sphincters. Systemic arterial blood pressure, in turn, is determined by cardiac output, intravascular volume, and SVR; systemic venous pressure is determined by right atrial pressure, intravascular volume, and venous capacitance. Na$^+$ balance is a key determinant of these latter hemodynamic parameters. It should also be noted that, conversely, the massive accumulation of fluid in the peripheral interstitial compartment (anasarca) can itself diminish venous compliance and, hence, alter overall cardiovascular performance.[376]

The balance of Starling forces prevailing at the arteriolar end of the capillary ($\Delta P > \Delta\pi$) favors the net filtration of fluid into the interstitium. Net outward movement of fluid along the length of the capillary is associated with an axial decrease in the capillary hydraulic pressure and an increase in the plasma COP. Nevertheless, the local transcapillary hydraulic pressure gradient continues to exceed the opposing COP gradient throughout the length of the capillary bed in several tissues, such that filtration occurs along its entire length.[377] In such capillary beds, a substantial volume of filtered fluid must, therefore, return to the circulation via lymphatics. Given this importance of lymphatic drainage, the ability of lymphatics to expand and proliferate and the ability of lymphatic flow to increase in response to increased interstitial fluid formation provide protective mechanisms for minimizing edema formation.

Other mechanisms for minimizing edema formation have also been identified. Precapillary vasoconstriction tends to lower capillary hydraulic pressure and diminish the filtering surface area in a given capillary bed. Indeed, excessive precapillary vasodilatation in the absence of appropriate microcirculatory myogenic reflex regulation appears to account for lower extremity interstitial edema associated with Ca^{2+} entry blocker vasodilator therapy.[378] Increased net filtration itself is associated with dissipation of capillary hydraulic pressure, dilution of interstitial fluid protein concentration, and a corresponding rise in intracapillary plasma protein concentration. The resulting change in the profile of Starling forces associated with increased filtration, therefore, tends to mitigate against further interstitial fluid accumulation.[379,380] Interstitial fluid pressure is normally subatmospheric. Furthermore, even small increases in interstitial fluid volume tend to augment tissue hydraulic pressure, again opposing further transudation of fluid into the interstitial space.[381]

The appearance of generalized edema, therefore, implies one or more disturbances in microcirculatory hemodynamics associated with expansion of the ECF volume: increased venous pressure transmitted to the capillary, unfavorable adjustments in pre- and postcapillary resistances, or lymphatic flow inadequate to drain the interstitial compartment and replenish the intravascular compartment. Insofar as the continued net accumulation of interstitial fluid without renal Na$^+$ retention might result in prohibitive intravascular volume contraction and cessation of interstitial fluid formation, generalized edema, therefore, implies substantial renal Na$^+$ retention. Indeed, the volume of accumulated interstitial fluid required for clinical detection of generalized edema (>2–3 L) necessitates that all states of generalized edema are associated with expansion of ECF volume and, hence, body exchangable

Na$^+$ content. In conclusion,t all states of generalized edema reflect past or ongoing renal Na$^+$ retention.

Renal Sodium Retention and Edema Formation in Congestive Heart Failure

CHF is a clinical syndrome in which the heart is unable to satisfy the requirements of peripheral tissues for oxygen and other nutrients. This happens most commonly in the setting of a decrease in cardiac output (low-output CHF), but may occur as well when cardiac output is increased, for example, in patients with AV fistula, hyperthyroidism, and beriberi (high-output CHF). In both situations, the kidney responds in a similar manner, that is, by avidly retaining Na$^+$ and water despite expansion of the ECF volume.

The syndrome of CHF encompasses pathophysiologic alterations related to a reduction of the distending pressure within the arterial circuit and those that are related to increases in the volume of blood and the filling pressures in the atrium and great veins, behind the failing ventricle. In response to these changes, a series of adjustments occur that result from the operation of circulatory and neurohumoral compensatory mechanisms. These adjustments may be viewed teleologically as tending to support arterial pressure and maintain perfusion to critical organs such as the heart and brain. As long as these adaptations are able to maintain their compensatory role, they may prove to be beneficial (compensated CHF). However, with the development of CHF, excessive activation of these systems may become detrimental by further promoting peripheral vasoconstriction and increasing the abnormal loading conditions in the failing heart. At this turning point, a vicious circle is created (decompensated CHF) in which the "compensatory" mechanisms themselves contribute to further deterioration of the cardiovascular system.

From the standpoint of ECF volume homeostasis, two key abnormalities occur in CHF: (1) The perception of an inadequate circulating volume by various sensors within the circulation. (2) A disturbance in the effector arm of volume control, with excessive activation of antinatriuretic vasoconstrictor systems and failure of natriuretic vasodilatory mechanisms, shifting the balance between these systems toward Na$^+$ and water retention by the kidney.

Afferent Limb of Volume Homeostasis in Congestive Heart Failure: Abnormalities in Sensing Mechanisms

What constitutes the afferent signal for the continued retention of Na$^+$ and water by the kidney in CHF has been the focus of interest and debate for many years.[382-385] The observation that the kidney is intrinsically normal in CHF but continues to retain Na$^+$ and water avidly, despite expansion of the extracellular volume, indicated that it must be responding to "inadequate" signals from the volume regulatory system. This suggests either that a critical sensing area in the vascular tree is "underfilled" or that some sensing mechanisms of body fluid volume fail to detect appropriately the elevated circulating volume. Compelling evidence suggests that both mechanisms may contribute to development of salt and water retention and edema formation in CHF.

The recognition of the important role of arterial underfilling in mediating renal salt and water retention dates back to the concepts of "backward failure" and "forward failure" formulated by Starling,[386] Harrison,[387] and Stead and Ebert[388] as well as the concept of "effective circulating volume" suggested in 1948 by Peters.[389] According to the theory of "backward failure," accumulation of blood behind the failing myocardium results in venous congestion with increased capillary pressure, leading to transudation of fluid into the interstitium with edema formation and depletion of plasma volume. The decrease in plasma volume then initiates renal Na^+ and water retention. In contrast, the concept of "forward failure" emphasized the importance of the failure of the heart as a pump in supplying adequate blood flow to the tissues, similar to the mechanism of acute circulatory failure (shock), such that the kidneys are no longer able to excrete salt in a normal manner. Evidently, both mechanisms contain elements of "underfilling" of the arterial circulation.

Many early studies showed that cardiac output was reduced in CHF, in agreement with both the "backward" and "forward" concepts. Thus, the notion that a decrease in cardiac output might be the signal dictating renal Na^+ retention in CHF found increasing support over the years.[390,391] However, it was soon recognized that situations associated with high cardiac output, such as AV fistula, may be associated with renal salt and water retention and identical neurohormonal responses to those observed in low-output CHF.[41]

Schrier[383-385,392] refined the concept of arterial underfilling in a unifying hypothesis of body fluid volume regulation to explain the continued renal Na^+ and water retention in various edematous disorders. According to this view, the relative fullness of the arterial circulation, as determined by the relation between cardiac output and peripheral arterial resistance, constitutes the primary afferent signal for renal retention of salt and water. A decrease in cardiac output is the most obvious reason for arterial underfilling. However, a decrease in peripheral arterial resistance, as a result of diversion of blood flow from the arterial to venous circuit, may provide another afferent signal for arterial underfilling, which causes retention of salt and water by the kidney. Thus, arterial underfilling, caused by either an absolute decrease in cardiac output (low-output CHF) or diversion of blood flow through anatomic or physiologic AV shunt (high-output CHF), initiates the sequence of adaptive neurohormonal and renal hemodynamic responses that result in enhanced Na^+ and water reabsorption by the kidney. In that respect, activation of neurohormonal and hemodynamic compensatory mechanisms in CHF is not different from those occurring in true hypovolemia. It is important to note, however, that in contrast to true volume-depletion states, CHF is associated with a rise in intracardiac pressures, which, in theory, should promote natriuresis by activating cardiopulmonary reflexes and the release of ANP. In that respect, the increase in intracardiac pressures in CHF may be substantially higher than in other edema-forming states. Given the potency of these important volume-regulatory cardiopulmonary reflexes, it is conceivable that the blunted natriuresis associated with CHF reflects a disturbance in the afferent signaling mechanisms emanating from these volume-sensing sites.

As previously discussed, the sensory information that initiates the neurohumoral responses to changes in volume homeostasis originates from mechanosensitive nerve endings located in the cardiac atria, ventricles, and pulmonary circulation (cardiopulmonary receptors) and the arterial baroreceptors located in the aortic arch and carotid sinus. Information from these nerve endings is carried by the vagal and glossopharyngeal nerves to centers in the medulla and brainstem. In the normal situation, the prevailing discharge from these receptors exerts a tonic restraining effect on the heart and circulation by inhibiting the sympathetic outflow and augmenting parasympathetic activity. In addition, changes in transmural pressure across the atria and great vessels also influence the secretion of ADH and renin and the release of ANP.

In CHF, it is widely accepted that both the cardiopulmonary reflexes and the arterial baroreflexes are blunted, such that they can no longer exert an adequate tonic inhibitory effect on sympathetic outflow.[393,394] As a result of the diminished inhibitory input from these receptors sites, the SNS is activated, and the secretion of ADH and renin may be augmented, thus promoting Na^+ and water retention by the kidney despite a high circulating volume. Gabrielsen and co-workers[395] demonstrated that neuroendocrine link between volume sensing and renal Na^+ excretion is preserved in compensated CHF. However, the natriuretic response to volume expansion is modulated by the prevailing AII and aldosterone concentrations. Inhibition of AII formation by an ACE inhibitor increased Na^+ excretion to the same extent found in control subjects. In contrast, renal free water clearance is attenuated in response to volume expansion in compensated CHF despite normal plasma levels of ADH.

Greenberg and colleagues[396] were the first to report that the firing of atrial receptors in response to saline infusion was markedly attenuated over a wide range of central venous pressures in dogs with CHF induced by pulmonic valve stenosis and tricupid regurgitation. These findings were confirmed and extended in an aortocaval fistula canine model of CHF by Zucker and co-workers[397] who demonstrated a reduced firing of type B left atrial receptors in response to dextran volume expansion in the dogs with CHF. In addition, sonomicrometry of the left atrial appendage demonstrated reduced atrial compliance and microscopy indicated loss of nerve ending arborization.

Such an attenuated sensitivity of cardiopulmonary reflexes may explain the clinical observation indicating a sustained activation of the SNS in CHF patients with venous congestion,[398] a situation that would normally result in suppression of NE release. Likewise, studies using maneuvers that selectively altered central cardiac filling pressures (i.e., head-up tilt or LBNP) showed that patients with CHF, in contrast to normal subjects, usually do not demonstrate significant alterations in limb blood flow, circulating catecholamines, ADH, or renin activity in response to postural stimuli.[399,400] This diminished reflex responsiveness may be most impaired in patients with the greatest ventricular dysfunction.

In addition to the dysfunction of the cardiopulmonary reflexes, abnormalities in the arterial baroreflex control of the cardiovascular system also exist in CHF.[393,394,401] Ferguson and associates[402] demonstrated a high baseline muscle sympathetic activity in patients with CHF who failed to respond to activation and deactivation of arterial baroreceptors by infusion of phenylephrine and Na^+ nitroprusside, respectively. Depressed function of carotid and aortic baroreceptors were also reported in experimental models of cardiac failure.[403,404] These changes were associated with a resetting of receptor threshold to higher levels and a reduced range of pressures over which the receptors function.

Multiple abnormalities have been described in cardiopulmonary and arterial baroreceptor control of renal sympathetic activity in CHF. DiBona and co-workers[405] demonstrated in rats with coronary ligation an increased basal level of efferent renal sympathetic activity that failed to suppress normally during volume expansion. Similar observations were reported by Dibner-Dunlap and Thames[406] in sinoaortic denervated dogs with pacing-induced CHF. In this experimental model, cardiopulmonary receptors were stimulated by volume expansion, and left atrial baroreceptors were stimulated by inflating small balloons at the left atrial-pulmonary vein junctions. With both stimuli, a marked attenuation of the cardiopulmonary baroreflex control of the efferent renal sympathetic activity was found. In a more recent study, DiBona & Sawin[407] performed simultaneous recordings of efferent renal sympathetic activity with either single aortic or single vagal nerve units in a rat model of CHF. This study demonstrated that the abnormal regulation of efferent renal sympathetic activity was due to impaired function of both the aortic and the cardiopulmonary baroreflexes. These investigators reported later that the defect in cardiopulmonary baroreceptor was functionally more important than that in arterial baroreceptors in mediating the augmented efferent renal sympathetic activity.[408]

Several mechanisms have been implicated in the pathogenesis of the abnormalities in cardiopulmonary and arterial baroreflexes in CHF. Zucker and co-workers[397] suggested that loss of compliance in the dilated hearts as well as gross changes in the morphology of the receptors themselves were the mechanisms underlying the depressed atrial receptor discharge in dogs with aortocaval fistula. Additional studies in dogs with pacing-induced CHF raised the possibility that the decrease in carotid sinus baroreceptors sensitivity might be related to augmented Na^+,K^+-ATPase activity in the baroreceptor membranes.[403,409] Local perfusion of the carotid sinus with the cardiac glycoside ouabain led to a significant improvement of baroreceptor function.[403] Recent studies also demonstrated a role for AII in modulating baroreflex function, suggesting that increased activity of this peptide could be involved in the abnormal reflex regulation in CHF. Specifically, intracerebral or systemic administration of the AT_1 receptor antagonist losartan to rats with CHF significantly improved arterial baroreflex control of renal sympathetic activity.[394] Similarly, Murakami and colleagues[410] demonstrated that intravenous infusion of another AT_1 receptor antagonist, L-158,809, resulted in a significant enhancement of baroreflex control of heart rate in conscious rabbits with CHF. In addition, Dibner-Dunlap and co-workers[411] reported that treatment with the ACE inhibitor enalaprilat augmented arterial and cardiopulmonary baroreflex control of sympathetic nerve activity in patients with CHF. Taken together, these data support the possibility that high endogenous levels of AII in CHF may contribute to the depressed baroreflex sensitivity observed in CHF.

Although most of the studies indicated that the defects in the baroreflex function in CHF reside primarily in the afferent limb of the reflex arch, presumably at the receptor level, it has been suggested that alterations in more central sites may also be involved. As noted earlier, intracerebroventricular administration of an AT_1 antagonist improved baroreflex sensitivity in rats with CHF, suggesting that AII may also act on a central component of the reflex arch.[394] Indeed, in a study in which AII was injected into the vertebral artery of normal rabbits, a significant attenuation in arterial baroreflex function was observed.[412] Furthermore, this effect of AII could be blocked by prazosin, suggesting that the modulation of baroreflex function was mediated via a central α_1-adrenoreceptor.

As pointed out earlier, the blunted cardiopulmonary and arterial baroreceptor sensitivity in CHF may lead to an increase not only in total sympathetic outflow but also in ADH release and renin secretion. However, compared with the influence on sympathetic outflow, less information links the abnormalities in cardiopulmonary and arterial baroreflexes with enhanced ADH release and renin secretion in CHF.

The discovery that ANP is localized at some of the critical volume-sensing sites in the heart raised the possibility that alterations in secretory capacity of this hormone may exist in CHF. Thus, it was suggested that plasma ANP-atrial stretch relationship could be altered in CHF owing to limited reserve of the hormone in atrial storage as a result of a tonically increased stimulus for release of the hormone.[413] However, it is unlikely that such a defect could contribute significantly to salt and water retention in CHF for the following reasons. (1) Numerous studies in patients and animal models with CHF consistently demonstrated that circulating levels of the hormone are not depressed but rather elevated in CHF in proportion to the severity of cardiac dysfunction.[414–417] (2) It appears that cardiac ventricles become a major source of peptide secretion in CHF, as evidenced by increased tissue immunoreactive ANP and ANP mRNA in ventricles of patients and experimental models of CHF.[418–420] (3) Na^+ reten-

tion of CHF is not reversed when plasma ANP levels are further increased by exogenous administration of the peptide. The failure of ANP infusion to induce appropriate natriuretic and diuretic responses in patients[421] and experimental models of CHF[422,423] indicates that the main abnormality in CHF is the development of "resistance" to ANP rather than impaired secretion of the peptide.

The disturbances in the sensing mechanisms that initiate and maintain renal Na^+ retention in CHF are summarized in Figure 12–6. As indicated, a decrease in cardiac output or a diversion of systemic blood flow (anatomic or physiologic) diminishes the blood flow to the critical sites of the arterial circuit with pressure- and flow-sensing capabilities. The perception of diminished blood flow culminates in renal Na^+ retention, mediated by effector mechanisms to be described. An increase in systemic venous pressure promotes the transudation of fluid from the intravascular to the interstitial compartment by increasing the peripheral transcapillary hydraulic pressure gradient. These processes augment the perceived loss of volume and flow in the arterial circuit. In addition, distortion of the pressure-volume relationships as a result of chronic dilatation in the cardiac atria attenuates the normal natriuretic response to central venous congestion. This attenuation is manifested predominantly as diminished neural suppressive response to atrial stretch, which results in increased sympathetic nerve activity and augmented release of renin and ADH.

Efferent Limb of Volume Homeostasis in Congestive Heart Failure: Abnormalities in Effector Mechanisms

CHF is also characterized by a series of adaptive changes in the efferent limb of volume control. In many respects, these effector mechanisms for Na^+ retention are similar to those that govern renal function in states of true Na^+ depletion. These include adjustments in glomerular hemodynamics and tubule transport, which, in turn, are brought about by alterations in neural, humoral, and paracrine systems. However, in contrast to true volume depletion, CHF is also associated with activation of vasodilatory natriuretic agents, which tend to oppose the effects of the vasoconstrictor antinatriuretic systems. The final effect on urinary Na^+ excretion is determined by the balance between these antagonistic effector systems, which, in turn, may shift during the evolution of cardiac failure toward a dominance of Na^+-retaining systems. The abnormal regulation of the efferent limb of volume control reflects not only the exaggerated activity of the antinatriuretic systems but also the failure of natriuretic vasodilatory systems that are activated in the course of the deterioration in cardiac function.

Alterations in Glomerular Hemodynamics

CHF in patients and experimental models is characterized by significant alterations in renal hemodynamics that include an increase in RVR, reduced GFR, but an even more marked reduction of RPF, so that the FF is increased.[424–427] At the single-nephron level in rats with CHF induced by coronary ligation, Ichikawa and colleagues[428] demonstrated that SNGFR was lower than in control rats, but glomerular plasma flow was disproportionately reduced such that single-nephron filtration fraction (SNFF) was markedly elevated. Ultrafiltration coefficient was diminished, and both afferent and efferent arteriolar resistances were elevated, accounting for the diminished single-nephron glomerular plasma flow. The rise in SNFF was due to a disproportionate increase in efferent arteriolar resistance. Similar alterations in glomerular hemodynamics have been reported by Nishikimi and Frolich[429] in rats with aortocaval fistula, a high output failure model. In Figure 12–7, a comparison of the glomerular capillary hemodynamic profile in the normal (left) versus the CHF state (right) is

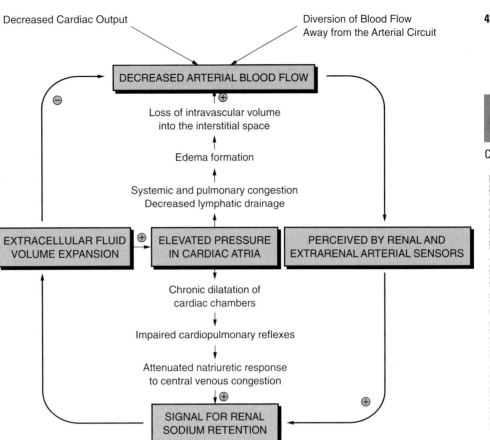

FIGURE 12–6 Sensing mechanisms that initiate and maintain renal Na⁺ retention in CHF. (Adapted from Skorecki KL, Brenner BM: Body fluid homeostasis in congestive heart failure and cirrhosis with ascites. Am J Med 72:323–338, 1982.)

FIGURE 12–7 Peritubular control of proximal tubule fluid reabsorption. Current concept of the role of peritubular capillary physical forces in the regulation of proximal tubule. Fluid reabsorption for the normal state *(left)* and in patients with CHF *(right)* is depicted. ΔP and $\Delta\pi$ are the transcapillary hydraulic and oncotic pressure differences across the peritubular capillary, respectively. The increase in filtration fraction causes $\Delta\pi$ to rise in CHF. The increase in renal vascular resistance in CHF is believed to reduce ΔP. Both the increase in $\Delta\pi$ and the fall in ΔP enhance peritubular capillary uptake of proximal reabsorbate and thus increase absolute Na⁺ reabsorption by the proximal tubule. (From Humes HD, Gottlieb M, Brenner BM: The Kidney in Congestive Heart Failure: Contemporary Issues in Nephrology, Vol 1. New York, Churchill Livingstone, 1978, pp 51–72.)

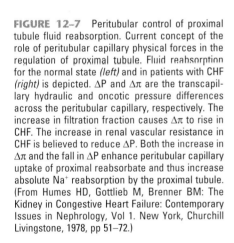
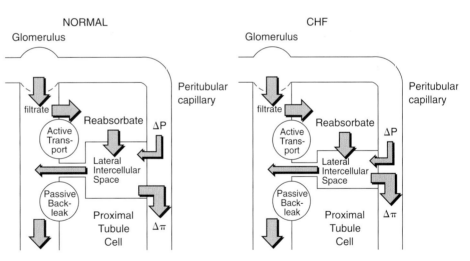

illustrated on the left graph of each panel. First, the transmural hydraulic pressure gradient ΔP declines along the distance of the glomerular capillary in both the normal and the CHF states, but compared with the normal state, ΔP in CHF is much higher because of the increased efferent arteriolar resistance. Second, the transmural plasma COP gradient $\Delta\pi$ increases over the length of the glomerular capillary in both states as fluid is filtered in the Bowman space, but it increases to a greater extent in CHF because of the increased filtration fraction. It is evident that a major component of the glomerular hemodynamic alterations in CHF emanates from the disproportionate increase in efferent compared with afferent arteriolar resistance. As outlined in a previous section of this chapter, this alteration is mediated principally by the action

of AII. The preferential efferent vasoconstriction induced by AII is considered to be an important adjustment in glomerular hemodynamics to preserve GFR in the presence of reduced RPF.[430–432] A study by Cody and associates[433] emphasized the importance of this mechanism in the regulation of glomerular filtration in patients with chronic CHF. In these patients, failure to maintain GFR was correlated with a diminished RPF as well as an impaired ability to maintain an adequately high FF. Thus, individuals with the greatest impairment of GFR had the greatest increase in overall RVR and the lowest FF. Moreover, because of the dependency of GFR on AII-induced efferent arteriolar vasoconstriction in CHF, removal of the influence of AII, for example, by ACE inhibitors, may result in a marked decline in renal function, particularly in patients with preexisting renal failure, massive diuretic treatment, and limited cardiac reserve.[431,434]

Alterations in Tubular Reabsorption

A direct consequence of the glomerular hemodynamic alterations that have been outlined is an increase in the fractional reabsorption of filtered Na^+ at the level of the proximal tubule. In Figure 12–2, a comparison of the peritubular capillary hemodynamic profile between the normal state *(left)* and the CHF state *(right)* is shown on the right graph of each panel. Compared with the normal state, in CHF, the average value of $\Delta\pi$ along the peritubular capillary is increased and that of ΔP is decreased. This favors fluid movement into the capillary and may also reduce back-leakage of fluid into the tubule via paracellular pathways, promoting overall net reabsorption. The peritubular control of proximal fluid reabsorption in normal and CHF states is illustrated schematically in Figure 12–7.

The contribution of enhanced fractional proximal Na^+ reabsorption in CHF and its dependence on abnormal glomerular hemodynamics have been demonstrated in a number of early experimental and clinical studies. Studies using mannitol infusion in conjunction with clearance techniques,[435] pharmacologic blockade of distal nephron transport,[436] and mineralocorticoid escape with deoxycorticosterone acetate (DOCA)[437] all provided indirect evidence for enhanced proximal Na^+ reabsorption and a consequent decrease in delivery of Na^+ to more distal sites. Evidence for the dependence of enhanced proximal fractional Na^+ reabsorption on altered glomerular hemodynamics in CHF was likewise obtained in the coronary ligation model of MI in rats by Ichikawa and co-workers.[428] When the increased SNFF was restored toward normal (with the use of an ACE inhibitor), there was a normalization of proximal peritubular capillary Starling forces and Na^+ reabsorption.

Notwithstanding the importance of physical factors in determining the increase in proximal reabsorption, the contribution of other factors, such as the direct actions of the renal nerve and of AII on proximal Na^+ transport, should not be underestimated. Thus, AII may act by modulating physical factors through its effect on efferent resistance, as well as by augmenting directly proximal epithelial transport, thereby amplifying the overall increase proximal Na^+ reabsorption.

Distal nephron sites also participate in the enhanced tubule Na^+ reabsorption in experimental models of CHF. Micropuncture studies in dogs and in rats with AV fistulas[438,439] and in dogs with pericardial constriction[440] or chronic partial thoracic vena caval obstruction[441] demonstrated enhanced distal nephron Na^+ reabsorption. Levy[442] showed that the inability of dogs with chronic vena cava obstruction to excrete an Na^+ load is a consequence of enhanced reabsorption of Na^+ at the loop of Henle. Furthermore, the mechanism leading to the augmented reabsorption of Na^+ by the loop of Henle in dogs with constriction of the vena cava seems to involve physical factors determined by renal hemodynamics, much as in the case of the proximal tubule.[443] Specifically, renal vasodilatation and elevation of RPP in dogs with vena cava constriction served to prevent the enhanced reabsorption of filtrate by the loop of Henle, thereby permitting a normal natriuretic response to saline loading.

Humoral Mechanisms

The homeostatic responses to myocardial failure include activation of vasoconstrictive/antinatriuretic systems, such as RAAS, SNS, ADH, and ETs, which increase vascular resistance and enhance renal water and salt reabsorption. In addition, several vasodilatory/natriuretic substances, such as NPS, NO, prostaglandins PGs, AM, and U-II, are also activated. It is recognized that salt and water homeostasis is largely determined by the fine balance between these vasoconstrictive/antinatriuretic and vasodilator/natriuretic systems, and that the development of positive Na^+ balance and edema formation in CHF represents a turning point at which the balance is in favor of the former (Fig. 12–8). This

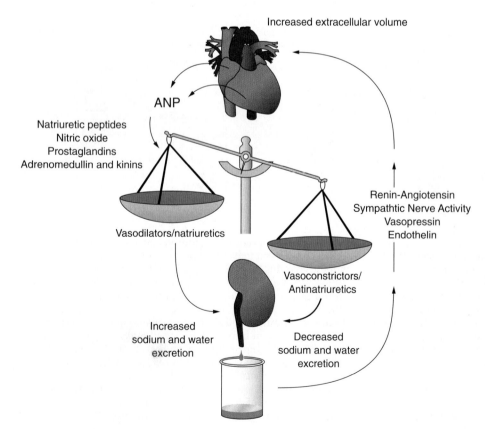

Increased extracellular volume

ANP

Natriuretic peptides
Nitric oxide
Prostaglandins
Adrenomedullin and kinins

Vasodilators/natriuretics

Renin-Angiotensin
Sympathtic Nerve Activity
Vasopressin
Endothelin

Vasoconstrictors/
Antinatriuretics

Increased
sodium and water
excretion

Decreased
sodium and water
excretion

FIGURE 12–8 Efferent limb of extracellular fluid (ECF) volume control in CHF. Volume homeostasis in CHF is determined by the balance between the natriuretic and the antinatriuretic forces. In decompensated CHF, enhanced activities of the Na^+-retaining systems overwhelm the effects of the vasodilatory/natriuretic systems, leading to a net reduction in Na^+ excretion and an increase in ECF volume. (Adapted from Winaver J, Hoffman A, Abassi Z, et al: Does the heart's hormone, ANP, help in congestive heart failure? News Physiol Sci 10:247–253, 1995.)

aspect of CHF became of special interest in the last few years, since a large-scale study on 1906 patients with CHF revealed that impaired renal function is a stronger predictor of mortality than impaired cardiac function.[444] These and other reports confirm that, in CHF, the activation of neurohormonal systems in association with renal dysfunction is strictly related to long-term mortality.[445]

Vasoconstrictive/Antinatriuretic Systems

RENIN-ANGIOTENSIN-ALDOSTERONE SYSTEM. The activity of the RAAS is enhanced in most patients with CHF in correlation with the severity of cardiac dysfunction.[446] Therefore, the activity of this system provides a prognostic index in the CHF patients. It has become increasingly apparent that, despite providing initial benefits in hemodynamic support, continued activation of RAAS contributes to the progression and worsening of CHF.[153,447] RAAS activation induces direct systemic vasoconstriction and activates other neurohormonal systems such as ADH, which contribute to maintaining adequate intravascular volume.[448] However, numerous studies in patients and in experimental models of CHF established the deleterious role of the RAAS in the progression of cardiovascular and renal dysfunction in CHF.[153,449] In particular, the kidney is highly sensitive to the action of the vasoconstrictor agents, especially AII, and a decrease in RPF is one of the most common pathophysiologic alterations in clinical and experimental CHF. Micropuncture techniques demonstrated that rats with chronic stable CHF display depressed glomerular plasma flow rates and SNGFR, as well as elevated efferent arteriolar resistance and FF. Direct renal administration of an ACE inhibitor did not affect renal function in sham-operated control rats but it did normalized it in the rats with experimental CHF. Utilizing a different model of CHF, induced by surgical creation of an aortocaval fistula, our group[450] showed that only a certain percentage of animals with AV fistula developed Na+ retention, whereas the rest maintained Na+ balance. The former subgroup is characterized by a marked increase in PRA and plasma aldosterone levels. In contrast, PRA and aldosterone levels in compensated animals were not different compared with those in sham-operated controls. Treatment with the ACE inhibitor enalapril resulted in a dramatic natriuretic response in rats with Na+ retention. The finding that animals with AV fistula either develop Na+ retention or maintain normal Na+ balance was previously demonstrated in dogs with CHF due to AV fistula.[451] A similar trend was also observed in patients with CHF. Whereas most CHF patients maintain normal Na+ balance when placed on a low-salt diet, about 50% of patients develop positive Na+ balance when fed a normal-salt diet. A common feature of both animals and patients with Na+ retention was the activation of the RAAS. In dogs with experimental high-output CHF, the initial period of Na+ retention was associated with a profound activation of the RAAS, and the return to normal Na+ balance was accompanied by a progressive fall in PRA. In sum, these findings clearly demonstrate that activation of the RAAS contributes to the pathogenesis of Na+ and water retention in CHF. The deleterious effects of the RAAS on renal function are not surprising in light of the previously mentioned actions of AII and aldosterone on kidney hemodynamics and excretory function. Activation of AII in response to the decreased pumping capacity of the failing myocardium promotes systemic vasoconstriction in association with the preferential renal vasoconstrictive action on the efferent and afferent arteries and glomerular mesangial cells.[113,153,452] In addition, AII exerts both a negative influence on renal cortical circulation in rats with CHF and increases tubular Na+ reabsorption directly and indirectly by augmenting aldosterone release.[452] In combination, these hemodynamic and tubular actions lead to avid Na+ and water retention, thus promoting circulatory congestion and edema formation.

Whereas most studies related renal Na+ retention in CHF to elevated levels of renin, AII, or aldosterone,[453] other studies found no consistent relationship between RAAS and positive Na+ balance.[454] For instance, in dogs with pulmonary artery or thoracic inferior vena cava constriction, the RAAS was activated to a striking degree during the early phase of constriction and was necessary for the support of systemic blood pressure.[455] Administration of the ACE inhibitor captopril resulted in systemic hypotension. Over subsequent days, Na+ retention and ECF volume expansion were pronounced and inhibition of converting-enzyme activity was no longer accompanied by significant hypotension.[455] However, animals with severe impairment of cardiac output remained sensitive to the hypotensive effects of ACE inhibition. Similarly, among patients with CHF, PRA and levels of vasoconstrictor hormones were most elevated in patients with acute, severe, and poorly compensated CHF.[455] Levels declined when CHF became stable in the chronic stage. The foregoing experimental and clinical data therefore indicate that the influence of the RAAS in maintaining circulatory homeostasis may depend on the stage of CHF, being most pronounced in acute and decompensated CHF, and least pronounced in chronic stable CHF. However, even though the circulating RAAS is not activated in chronic stable CHF, alterations in renal function can still be corrected by ACE inhibition.[456] Therefore, it has been hypothesized that activation of local RAAS in certain tissues including heart, vasculature, kidney and brain may occur in the absence of alterations in the circulating hormone. Schunkert and associates[457] studied the relative status of the circulating and intrarenal RAAS by examining the intrarenal expressions of renin and angiotensinogen mRNA in rats with stable compensated CHF 12 weeks after experimental MI induced by coronary artery ligation. Compared with sham-operated control rats, the chronic CHF rats demonstrated no significant difference in the components of the circulating RAAS. However, there was a significant increase in the renal angiotensinogen mRNA level in the CHF rats and a parallel increase in renal AII concentrations, directly correlated with infarct size, suggesting that the magnitude of activation of the tissue RAAS is influenced by the degree of CHF. Long-term ACE inhibition in CHF rats increased renal renin mRNA and enzyme levels but normalized renal angiotensinogen mRNA levels.[457] In this context, although originally the RAAS was viewed solely as an endocrine system, increasing evidence suggests that all its components reside within several individual organs, such as kidney, lung, heart, and VSMCs.[118,153] Moreover, several studies suggested that, in addition to the mechanical stress exerted on the myocardium due to AII-mediated increased afterload, activation of the local RAAS in these tissues may play a crucial role in the pathogenesis of CHF.[117,458] In turn, pressure overload activates the production of locally AII, perhaps more than circulating AII, owing to up-regulation of angiotensinogen and tissue ACE.[153] Local AII acts via AT-1 in a functionally independent paracrine/autocrine fashion, where it is believed to play a significant role in the development of cardiac hypertrophy (owing to its growth properties), remodeling and fibrosis, and in the reduced coronary flow, hallmarks of severe CHF.[459,460] In support of these observations are the well-established beneficial effects of ACE inhibitors and AT1 blockers (ARBs) in humans and animals with CHF, that is, improved cardiac function, prolonged survival, prevention of end-organ damage, and prevention or regression of cardiac hypertrophy.[114,153] In addition, ACE inhibitors and ARBs may offer benefits with respect to endothelial dysfunction, vascular remodeling, and potentiation of the vasodilatory effects of the KKS.[113,114,461,462] A significant component of these salutary effects emanate from the blockade of the local RAAS rather than the circulating system.[114,153] Similar to AII, the other component of the RAAS, namely, aldosterone seems also to

426

CH 12

act directly on the myocardium.[463] The role of aldosterone in cardiac remodeling has emerged in the last few years. It is widely accepted that structural remodeling of the interstitial collagen matrix is regulated by both AII and aldosterone. Moreover, cardiac aldosterone production is increased in patients with CHF, especially when caused by systolic dysfunction. Convincing evidence for the local production of aldosterone was provided by the finding that CYP11B2 mRNA (aldosterone synthase) is expressed in cultured neonatal rat cardiac myocytes. The adverse contribution of aldosterone to the functional and structural alterations of the failing heart was elegantly proved by the use of eplerenone, a specific aldosterone antagonist, in which it prevented progressive left ventricular systolic and diastolic dysfunction in association with reducing interstitial fibrosis, cardiomyocyte hypertrophy, and left ventricular chamber sphericity in dogs with CHF. Similarly, Delyani and co-workers[464] reported that eplerenone attenuated the development of ventricular remodeling and reactive but not reparative fibrosis after MI in rats. These findings are in agreement with the results observed in clinical trials. The Randomized Aldactone Evaluation Study (RALES) showed that therapy with spironolactone reduced overall mortality in patients with advanced CHF by 30% compared with placebo.[465] Recently, the EPHESUS study showed that addition of eplerenone to optimal medical therapy reduces morbidity and mortality among patients with acute MI complicated by left ventricular dysfunction and CHF.[466]

Based on the maladaptive actions of locally produced or circulatory AII, one may envision that blocking the formation of this peptide may improve cardiorenal functions in CHF. Indeed, many studies indicate that ACE inhibition improves renal function in patients with CHF and is responsible for the improved cardiac performance and increasing life expectancy of these patients,[467–469] whereas others report that renal functional deterioration is a frequent complication.[434] The latter may stem from the beneficial effect of AII in helping to maintain glomerular capillary pressure, and thus the GFR, by its preferential constricting action on the efferent arterioles.[434] Studies of experimental CHF in animals demonstrated similar variability.[470] Some of these discrepancies might be attributable to differences in study design, specific drug use, titration of dose, and hypotensive response. In an elegant study examining this issue,[471] detailed analysis of renal function (using inulin and p-aminohippurate clearance) was performed for patients with CHF in New York Heart Association (NYHA) functional classes II and III. After ACE inhibition, a small but insignificant decrease in GFR occurred and a concomitant but not statistically significant increase in RPF with no change in plasma creatinine. Because patients with CHF are unable to escape from the Na$^+$-retaining action of aldosterone and continue to retain Na$^+$ in response to aldosterone, blockade of the latter by spironolactone has substantial natriuresis in these patients.[446] In recent years and with the development of selective nonpeptide orally active ARBs, several studies indicated beneficial effects of these drugs on cardiac performance, comparable with those of ACE inhibition.[114,472] At the renal level, losartan was able to induce a significant natriuretic response in rats with decompensated CHF, induced by the placement of an aortocaval fistula.[473] In a model of ovine heart failure, acute administration of losartan was able to maintain GFR and urinary Na$^+$ excretion despite a fall in RPP.[474] Likewise, in dogs with CHF due to rapid atrial pacing, chronic administration of TVC-116, another AII antagonist, prevented the decrease in GFR, RPF, and Na$^+$ excretion.[475] Recent clinical studies found no differences between the efficacies of captopril and losartan on cardiac and renal functions in patients with CHF.[114,446,476] Overall, the effect of AII receptor blockade or ACE inhibition on renal function in CHF depends on a multiplicity of interacting factors. On the

TABLE 12–5 Converting-Enzyme Inhibition in Congestive Heart Failure

Factors favoring deterioration in renal function
  Evidence of Na$^+$ depletion or poor renal perfusion
    Large doses of diuretics
    Increased urea-to-creatinine ratio
    Mean arterial pressure < 80 mm Hg
  Evidence of maximal neurohumoral activation
    Presence of hyponatremia secondary to ADH activation
  Interruption of counterregulatory mechanisms
    Coadministration of prostaglandin inhibitors
    Presence of adrenergic dysfunction (e.g., diabetes mellitus)

Factors favoring improvement in renal function
  Maintenance of Na$^+$ balance
    Reduction in diuretic dosage
    Increase in Na$^+$ intake
    Mean arterial pressure > 80 mm Hg
  Minimal neurohumoral activation
  Intact counterregulatory mechanisms

one hand, RBF may improve as a result of lower efferent arteriolar resistance. Systemic vasodilatation may be associated with a rise in cardiac output. Under such circumstances, reversal of hemodynamically mediated effects of AII on Na$^+$ reabsorption would promote natriuresis. On the other hand, the aim of AII-induced elevation of the SNFF is to preserve GFR in the presence of diminished RPF. In patients with precarious renal hemodynamics, a fall in systemic arterial pressure below the autoregulatory range combined with removal of the AII effect on glomerular hemodynamics may cause severe deterioration of renal function. The net result depends on the integrated sum of these physiologic effects, which, in turn, depends on the severity and stage of heart disease (Table 12–5).

As noted previously, in addition to its renal and cardiovascular hemodynamic effects, the RAAS is involved directly in the exaggerated Na$^+$ reabsorption by the tubule in CHF. The most active component of this system, that is, AII, has a dose-dependent direct epithelial effect on the proximal tubule that favors active Na$^+$ reabsorption.[143,144,477] The predominant effect of the RAAS on distal nephron function is mediated by the action of the second active component, that is, aldosterone, which acts on cortical and medullary portions of the collecting duct to enhance Na$^+$ reabsorption, as outlined in a previous section. Numerous studies reported elevated plasma aldosterone concentration or urinary aldosterone secretion or natriuretic effects of pharmacologic aldosterone antagonists in animal models and human subjects with CHF, despite further activation of other antinatriuretic systems, supporting the pivotal role of this steroid hormone in the mediation of Na$^+$ retention in CHF.[478] Variabilities in the relative importance of mineralocorticoid action in the Na$^+$ retention of CHF emerging from these reports should be interpreted in light of the same considerations regarding stage and severity of disease that were noted with respect to the hemodynamic actions of AII.

Further evidence about the involvement of the RAAS in the development of positive Na$^+$ balance can be gleaned from studies showing that the renal and hemodynamic response to ANP is impaired in CHF.[450] And administration of either losartan or ACE inhibitor restored the blunted response to ANP (for further details, see section on The Natriuretic Peptides).[450] Recent studies have demonstrated that omapatrilat, a mixed inhibitor of ACE and NEP, has hemodynamic and clinical benefits in patients with CHF, compared with ACE inhibitors.[213,223] Interestingly, the rate of renal dysfunction was significantly less in those on omapatrilat.[223] This is of potential beneficial value because renal function frequently deteriorates during the progression of chronic CHF, and renal impairment is one of the most powerful predictors of prognosis in patients with CHF.[223,444] Although patients with CHF have low serum osmolarity, they display increased thirst, most likely owing to the high concentrations of AII, which stimulate thirst center cells in the hypothalamus.[446] This behavior may contribute to the positive water balance and hyponatremia in these patients.

SYMPATHETIC NERVOUS SYSTEM. Patients with CHF experience progressive activation of the SNS with progressive decline of cardiac function.[479] Elevated plasma NE levels are frequently observed in CHF and a strong consensus exists as to the adverse influence of sympathetic overactivity on the progression and outcome of patients with CHF.[480] Thus, sympathetic neural activity is significantly correlated to intracardiac pressures, cardiac hypertrophy, and left ventricular ejection fraction (LVEF).[479] Direct intraneural recordings in patients with CHF also showed increased neural traffic, which correlated with the increased plasma NE levels.[481] Activation of the SNS not only precedes the appearance of congestive symptoms but also is preferentially directed toward the heart and kidney. Clinical investigations revealed that patients with mild CHF have higher plasma NE in the coronary sinus than in the renal vein.[482] At the early stages, increased activity of SNS in CHF restores the hemodynamic abnormalities including hypoperfusion, diminished plasma volume, and impaired cardic function by producing vasoconstriction and avid Na^+ reabsorption.[459,479] However, chronic exposure to this system induces several long-term adverse myocardial effects including induction of apoptosis and hypertrophy, with an overall reduction in cardiac function, which reduces contractility. Some of these effects may be mediated, in turn, by activation of the RAAS.[446,459]

Measurements using catecholamine spillover techniques revealed that the basal sympathetic outflow to the kidney is significantly increased in patients with CHF.[479,480] The activation of the SNS and increased efferent renal sympathetic activity may be involved in the alterations in renal function in CHF. For example, exaggerated renal sympathetic nerve activity contributes to the increased renal vasoconstriction, avid Na^+ and water retention, renin secretion, and attenuation of the renal actions of ANP.[228] Experimental studies demonstrated that renal denervation of rats with experimental CHF due to coronary artery ligation resulted in an increase in RPF and SNGFR and a decrease in afferent and efferent arteriolar resistance.[311] Similarly, in dogs with low cardiac output induced by vena cava constriction, administration of a ganglionic blocker resulted in a marked increase in Na^+ excretion.[480] In rats with CHF induced by coronary ligation, the decrease in renal sympathetic nerve activity in response to an acute saline load was less than that of control rats.[307] Bilateral renal denervation restored the natriuretic response to volume expansion, implicating increased renal sympathetic nerve activity in the Na^+ avidity characteristic of CHF.[480] Studies in dogs with high-output CHF induced by aortocaval fistula demonstrated that total postprandial urinary Na^+ excretion was approximately twofold higher in renal-denervated dogs compared with control dogs with intact nerves.[483] In line with these observations, clinical investigation showed that administration of α-adrenoreceptor blocker dibenamine to patients with CHF caused an increase in fractional Na^+ excretion, without a change in RPF or GFR. Treatment with ibopamine, an oral dopamine analog, resulted in vasodilation and positive inotropic and diuretic effects in patients with CHF.[484] Marenzi and associates[445] found that, for a given degree of cardiac dysfunction, the concentration of NE is significantly higher in patients with concomitant abnormal renal function than in patients with preserved renal function. These findings are similar to those observed by Hillege and colleagues[444] and suggest that the association between renal function and

prognosis in patients with CHF is linked by neurohormonal activation, including CNS.

An additional mechanism by which renal sympathetic activity may affect renal hemodynamics and Na^+ excretion in CHF is through its antagonistic interaction with ANP. ANP has sympathoinhibitory effects.[228] In contrast, CNS that retains water and salt in CHF plays a role in reducing renal responsiveness to ANP. For example, it has been demonstrated that the blunted diuretic/natriuretic response to ANP in rats with CHF could be restored by prior renal denervation,[485] or administration of clonidine,[486] a centrally acting $α_2$-adrenoreceptor agonist, which decreases renal sympathetic nerve activity in CHF. These experimental and clinical data indicate that the SNS may play a role in the regulation of Na^+ excretion and glomerular hemodynamics in CHF, either by a direct renal action or by attenuating the action of ANP. However, other studies failed to show an ameliorative effect of renal denervation on renal hemodynamics and Na^+ excretion in CHF. Thus, in a study by Mizelle and colleagues,[487] no differences in renal hemodynamics or electrolyte excretion between innervated and denervated kidneys occurred following chronic unilateral denervation in conscious dogs with CHF induced by rapid ventricular pacing. Similarly, in dogs with reduced cardiac output due to pulmonary constriction, no significant differences in renal hemodynamics or Na^+ excretion occurred between the denervated and the intact kidney.[488] These discrepant results are probably due to species differences, the presence or absence of anesthesia, and the method of inducing CHF. It is also possible that high circulating catecholamines could interfere with the effects of renal denervation.

In summary, the perturbation in the efferent limb of volume homeostasis in CHF is a result of a complex interplay of the SNS and several other neurohormonal mechanisms on the glomeruli and the renal tubules.

ANTIDIURETIC HORMONE. Since the early 1980s, numerous studies demonstrated that plasma levels of ADH are elevated in patients with CHF, mostly in advanced CHF with hyponatremia, but also in asymptomatic patients with left ventricular dysfunction.[489–492] Potentially, these high circulating levels of ADH could adversely affect the kidney and the cardiovascular system in CHF. The mechanisms underlying the enhanced secretion of ADH in CHF are related to non-osmotic factors such as attenuated compliance of the left atrium, hypotension, and activation of the RAAS.[384,493] In a study by Pruszczynski and colleagues[494] in patients with CHF, baseline plasma ADH levels were higher and were not suppressed after administration of an oral water load, although marked hypo-osmolality occurred. Although impairment of the baroreflex control mechanism for ADH release could be involved in this phenomenon, a study in humans with CHF by Manthey and co-workers[495] found an intact reflex response of ADH to baroreceptor unloading. An early study suggested that AII may stimulate the release of ADH,[496] implicating an additional mechanism for increased ADH in CHF; however, a later study indicated that AII does not release ADH.[497] Bichet and colleagues[498] noted that treatment with captopril or with prazosin resulted in suppression of ADH and improved water excretion in response to water loading in patients with CHF. It is likely that improved cardiac function in response to afterload reduction was responsible for removal of the nonosmotic stimulus to ADH release. It is noteworthy that the observed decline in MAP was considered too small to have an effect on the hormone. This suggests that hemodynamic variables other than MAP alone (e.g., pulse pressure, stroke volume) that improve with afterload reduction therapy may have been sufficient to abrogate the nonosmotic stimulus for ADH release.

The most recognized renal effect of ADH in CHF is the development of hyponatremia, which usually occurs in advanced stages of the disease and may occur at concentrations much lower than those required for vasoconstriction.[499] This phenomenon has been attributed to water retention by the kidney owing to sustained release of ADH, irrespective of plasma osmolality. This notion has been demonstrated in both animal and human studies. In a study by Pruszczynski and colleagues,[494] free water clearance and minimal urine osmolality were markedly impaired in patients with CHF compared with control subjects, and only in control subjects was the plasma ADH level correlated with plasma osmolality. Because many patients with CHF have positive water balance that results in hyponatremia, it is reasonable to attribute the hyponatremia to the elevated plasma levels of this neuropeptide.[500] Mulinari and associates[501] demonstrated that administration of an ADH antagonist with dual V_1/V_2 antagonism to rats with ischemic CHF induced by left coronary ligation resulted in a rise in cardiac output, a decline in PVR, and an increase in urine output of 4- to 10-fold over baseline, confirming the role of ADH in the water retention and the increased vascular resistance of CHF. Recent reports provided further insights into the mechanisms of ADH-mediated water retention in experimental CHF. These studies in animal models of CHF also demonstrated an increased renal expression of AQP II in these animals, suggesting that this may also contribute to the enhanced water reabsorption in the collecting duct.[502] It is, therefore, not surprising that initial studies showed that administration of V_2 vasopressin receptor antagonists of peptidic and nonpeptidic nature to rats with inferior vena cava constriction,[503] dogs with CHF induced by rapid pacing,[504] and rats with CHF induced by coronary ligation[499] resulted in correction of the impaired urinary dilution in response to acute water load. The mechanism underlying these expected findings relies on the fact AQP II are expressed in the collecting duct and mediate the antidiuretic action of ADH.[505] Furthermore, the expression of AQP II and its immunoreactive levels has been reported to be elevated in the kidney of rats with experimental CHF induced by coronary artery ligation.[506,507] Oral treatment of these rats with V_2 antagonist (OPC31260) induced significant diuresis, a decrease in urinary osmolarity, and increased plasma osmolarity, which were associated with down-regulation of renal AQP II.[506] These findings indicate a major role for ADH in the up-regulation of AQP II water channels and subsequently enhanced water retention in experimental CHF. In agreement with the studies in experimental animals, several recent clinical studies demonstrated that chronic treatment with selective V_2 and dual V_{1a}/V_2 antagonists may be beneficial in the correction of hyponatremia in CHF.[500,508,509] For instance, administration of the oral selective V_2 receptor antagonist VPA-985 to patients with CHF for 7 days at incremental doses induced significant diuretic response accompanied by increase in plasma Na^+ concentration and decreased urine osmolarity.[214] Similarly, when YM087, an orally V_1/V_2 antagonist was given orally to patients with CHF, it increased plasma Na^+, reduced osmolarity of the urine, and increased urine output.[491,500] Interestingly, Eisenman and colleagues[510] demonstrated that low doses of ADH can restore urinary flow in patients with end-stage CHF. This effect may be due to activation of V_1 receptor subtype secondary to ANP release. It should be emphasized that, despite the promising therapeutic potential of the nonpeptidic ADH antagonist, care must be taken to avoid excessive or too rapid an aquaretic response, because this may predispose the patients to very serious CNS or even hemodynamic complications, as outlined in Chapter 13.

However, in addition to hyponatremia, CHF is characterized by other alterations in renal function. These include a decrease in RBF in particular to the renal cortex, a decrease in GFR, and Na^+ retention by the kidney. To what extent, if at all, enhanced levels of ADH are involved in these renal manifestations remains largely unknown.

In addition, ADH can impair cardiac function indirectly through its effect on SVR (increased cardiac afterload) as well as by V_2-receptor–mediated water retention leading to systemic and pulmonary congestion (increased preload). In addition, ADH, through a direct endocrine action on cardiomycytes, could contribute to cardiac remodeling, dilatation, and hypertrophy, that might be further exacerbated by the aforementioned abnormalities in preload and afterload.

The notion that ADH may potentially contribute to the alterations in renal and cardiac function in CHF through the mechanisms previously discussed is indeed supported by several in vitro and in vivo studies.[492] Yet, given that other vasoconstrictor systems may share similar actions in CHF, the key question about the relative role of the increased endogenous ADH, compared with other systems, remains largely unanswered. To answer this question, efficient tools to block the biologic activities of ADH are required.

In the past, a number of cyclic and linear derivatives of the natural hormone were designed in an attempt to create effective antagonists of the ADH receptors.[511] Although these compounds provided valuable tools for the classification and for mapping the distribution of the ADH receptors, they were largely inefficient as blockers because of their short half-life and the fact that they had agonistic effects as well, especially in humans. In the 1990s, significant progress was made in the development and synthesis of highly selective and potent antagonists for the V_{1A}, V_2, and most recently, for the V_{1B} receptor subtypes.[512] Likewise, mixed V_{1A}/V_2 receptor antagonists are now available. These compounds are small nonpeptide molecules, are orally active, lack agonist effects, and display high affinity and specificity to their corresponding receptors.[512,513] The term *Vaptan* has been coined to name the members of this new class of drugs. Several of these compounds have been utilized in experimental models of CHF and were found to produce hemodynamic improvement with transient decrease in SVR, increase cardiac output, and improve water diuresis.[504,514–516]

However, these studies examined primarily the acute effects of the drugs, and only limited and incomplete data are available at present on the long-term effects of the drugs in experimental CHF.[517,518] Similarly, in patients with CHF, there are only initial reports dealing mainly with the improvement in hyponatremia induced by the drugs.[508,509] One additional study reported a beneficial action of a dual V_{1A}/V_2 antagonist on right atrial pressure and pulmonary wedge pressure, but no change in cardiac output or SVR.[519]

In summary, from reviewing the current literature, it is clear that additional data are necessary to clarify the role of ADH in CHF as well as the efficacy of these drugs as a novel treatment in CHF. The question not only is of academic interest but also has important therapeutic implications, given that mortality in CHF remains high despite the effective use of ACE inhibitors.

Collectively, these data suggest that ADH is involved in the pathogenesis of water retention and hyponatremia that characterize CHF and that vasopressin receptor antagonist results in remarkable diuresis in both experimental and clinical CHF.

ENDOTHELIN. Recent evidence implicated ET-1 in the development and progression of CHF. Furthermore, this peptide is probably involved in the reduced renal function that characterizes the cardiorenal state, by inducing renal modeling, interstitial fibrosis, glomerulosclerosis, hypoperfusion/hypofiltration, and positive salt and water balance.[251,256] The pathophysiologic role of ET-1 in CHF is supported by two major lines of evidence: (1) Several studies demonstrated that the ET system is activated in CHF.[247,262,520] (2) Some clinical and experimental studies showed that ET-1 receptor antagonists modify this pathophysiologic process. The first line of evidence is based on the demonstration that plasma ET-1 and big ET-1 concentrations in both clinical CHF and experimental models of CHF are elevated and correlate with hemodynamic severity and symptoms.[521,522] Cavero and co-workers[523] reported that plasma immunoreactive ET-1 levels are elevated two- to three-fold above normal in dogs with CHF induced by rapid ventricular pacing. Elevated circulating ET-1 levels have also been reported in patients with CHF.[251,521] A negative correlation between plasma ET-1 concentration and LVEF has been reported.[524] In another study, the degree of pulmonary hypertension was the strongest predictor of plasma ET-1 level in patients with CHF.[525,526] Moreover, the 1-year mortality rate among patients who have had an MI strongly correlates with plasma levels of ET measured 3 days after the infarction.[527] These prognostic reports are in line with the observation that plasma ET-1 is elevated only in patients with moderate and severe CHF, but not in patients with asymptomatic CHF. The mechanisms underlying the increased plasma levels of ET-1 have not been clarified, although this may be due to either enhanced synthesis of the peptide in the lungs, heart, and circulation by several stimuli such as AII and thrombin or decreased clearance of the peptide by the pulmonary system.[251,522,528] Parallel to ET-1, ETA receptors are up-regulated, whereas ETB are down-regulated in the failing human heart.[528,529] Whether the activation of ET-1 system in CHF has any pathophysiologic significance is another area of debate. However, increasing plasma ET-1 levels in normal animals to concentrations found in CHF is associated with significant reduction in RBF and increased vascular resistance.[530] Bearing in mind that CHF is characterized by reduced RBF associated with increased vascular resistance along elevated levels of ET-1, it is appealing that a cause-and-effect relationship exists between these hemodynamic abnormalities and ET-1 in this disease state. This notion became evident with the development of numerous selective and highly specific ET receptor antagonists.[531-534] Experimental studies demonstrated that acute administration of bosentan, a mixed ET_A/ET_B receptor antagonist, significantly improved renal cortical perfusion in rats with severe decompensated CHF induced by aortocaval fistula formation.[535] Similarly, tezosentan, a dual parenteral ET receptor antagonist, reversed the profoundly increased RVR and improved RBF and Na^+ excretion in rats with CHF induced by MI.[536] This conclusion gained further support from several studies that showed that chronic blockade of ETA by selective antagonists[537,538] or by dual ETA/ETB receptor antagonists[539] attenuates the magnitude of Na^+ retention and prevents the decline in GFR in experimental CHF. These effects are in line with recent observations that infusion of ET-1 to normal rats produced a sustained cortical vasoconstrictor and a transient medullary vasodilatory response.[261,494] In contrast, rats with decompensated CHF displayed severely blunted cortical vasoconstriction, but significantly prolonged and preserved medullary vasodilation.[290] The significance of these attenuated renovascular effects of ET-1 and big ET in CHF experimental animals is uncertain, but the effect could probably result from activation of vasodilatory systems such as PGs and NO. Indeed, the medullary tissue of rats with decompensated CHF contains higher eNOS immunoreactive levels compared with that in sham controls.[290] These findings indicate that ET may be involved in the altered renal hemodynamics and the pathogenesis of cortical vasoconstriction in CHF.

Initial clinical studies showed that acute ET antagonism by bosentan decreased vascular resistance and increased cardiac index and cardiac output in patients with CHF, suggesting that ET-1 plays a role in the pathogenesis of CHF by increasing SVR.[540] However, in contrast to early studies, recent comprehensive clinical trials demonstrated no benefits from treating CHF patients with bosentan, which actually increased hepatic transaminases and mortality rate.[541] Unfortunately, none of these studies examined whether these antagonists

have any beneficial effects on renal function. However, given the marked vasoconstrictor and mitogenic properties of ET-1 and the increased local cardiac-pulmonary-renal production of this peptide in CHF, it is appealing to assume that ET-1 contributes directly and indirectly to the enhanced Na^+ retention and edema formation by aggravating kidney and heart functions, respectively.[529,539,542-544] However, establishing the importance of ET in the renal hemodynamic and excretory dysfunction in CHF requires further study.

Vasodilatory/Natriuretic Systems

THE NATRIURETIC PEPTIDE SYSTEM. Renal Na^+ and water retention in decompensated cardiac failure occurs despite expansion of the ECF volume and in the face of activiation of the NP system. Actually, CHF is the most prominent example of a clinical condition that involves abnormalities in the NP system. Several clinical and experimental studies implicated both ANP and BNP in the pathophysiology of the deranged cardiorenal axis in CHF.

ATRIAL NATRIURETIC PEPTIDE. Although initially considered to be a state of ANP deficiency, it soon became evident that plasma levels of ANP levels are frequently elevated in patients with CHF and positively correlate with the severity of cardiac failure as well as with the elevated atrial pressure and other parameters of left ventricular dysfunction.[414,417,545] Actually, the highest concentrations of ANP in the circulation occur in CHF. The high levels of plasma ANP are attributed to increased production rather than to decreased clearance. Although volume-induced atrial stretch is the main source for the elevated circulating ANP levels in CHF, enhanced synthesis and release of the hormone by the ventricular tissue in response to AII and ET also contribute to this phenomenon.[546,547]

Despite the high levels of this potent natriuretic and diuretic agent, patients and experimental animals with CHF retain salt and water owing to attenuated renal responsiveness to NPs. Infusion of pharmacologic doses of synthetic ANP to experimental animals[548] and to patients with CHF[421,549] also consistently demonstrated an attenuated renal response compared with normal control subjects. However, other beneficial effects accompany the infusion of ANP to patients with CHF, such as hemodynamic improvement and inhibition of activated neurohumoral systems. Hirsch and co-workers[550] showed in patients with CHF and Kanamori and associates[551] showed in dogs with CHF that ANP is a weak counterregulatory hormone, insufficient to overcome the substantial vasoconstriction mediated by the SNS, the RAAS, and ADH. However, despite the blunted renal response to ANP in CHF, elimination of the source of production of this peptide by surgical means aggravates the activation of these vasoconstrictive hormones in this disease state. For instance, Lohmeier and colleagues[552] demonstrated that atrial appendectomy to eliminate the source of ANP production in dogs with CHF due to rapid pacing resulted in substantial increments in PRA and plasma NE as well as marked Na^+ and water retention—suggesting that ANP plays a critical role as a suppressor of Na^+-retaining systems. Therefore, the increase in circulating NPs is still considered an important adaptive or compensatory mechanism aimed at reducing PVR and effective blood volume. Actually, the Na^+ balance in the initial compensated phase of CHF has been attributed in part to the elevated levels of ANP and BNP.[213] This notion is supported by the findings that inhibition of NP receptors in experimental CHF induces Na^+ retention.[515,553] Furthermore, NPs inhibit the systemic vasoconstrictive effect of AII,[554] AII-stimulated proximal tubule Na^+ reabsorption,[230] AII-enhanced secretion of aldosterone,[554] and the secretion of ET.[555] Therefore, NPs in CHF are an ideal counterregulatory hormone, influencing RPF and Na^+ excretion either through their direct renal actions or through inhibition of release or action of other vasoconstrictive agents. Moreover, besides these cardiovascular and endocrine effects,

TABLE 12–6	Possible Mechanisms Underlying the Renal Resistance to Natriuretic Peptides in Congestive Heart Failure
Release of less active forms of ANP, such as β-ANP and proANP	
Down-regulation of natriuretic peptide receptors coupled to guanylate cyclase	
Decreased renal perfusion pressure	
Increased degradation of natriuretic peptides by neutral endopeptidase and of its second messenger, cGMP, by specific phosphodiesterases	
Activation of antagonizing hormonal systems, such as renin-angiotensin-aldosterone system, sympathetic nervous system, ET, and ADH	

ANP, antinatriuretic peptide; cGMP, cyclic guanosine monophosphate; ET, endothelin.

NPs likely play an important role in promoting salt and water excretion by the kidney in the face of myocardial failure. Indeed, studies in an experimental model of CHF demonstrated that inhibition of the NPs by either specific antibodies to their receptors or the ANP receptor antagonist HS-142–1 causes further impairment in renal function, as expressed by increased RVR and decreased GFR, RBF, urine flow, Na+ excretion, and activation of the RAAS.[228,555]

A key question, then, related to why salt and water retention occurs in overt CHF, despite the remarkable activation of the NP system?

Several mechanisms have been suggested to explain this apparent discrepancy (Table 12–6):

1. Appearance of abnormal circulating peptides such as β-ANP and inadequate secretory reserves compared with the degree of CHF. However, the fact that circulating levels of native biologically active NPs are clearly elevated in CHF indicates that these putative factors cannot account for the exaggerated salt and water retention.

2. Decreased availability of NPs. Because NPs are removed from the circulation by two means, that is, NEP and clearance receptors, increased activity of these routes may theoretically contribute to the decreased effects of these peptides.[228] So far, no convincing evidence suggests that up-regulation of clearance receptors exist in the renal tissue of CHF animals or patients, although increased abundance of clearance receptors for NPs in platelets of patients with advanced CHF has been reported.[556] In contrast, several studies demonstrated that expression and activity of NEP are enhanced in experimental CHF.[557,558] This may contribute to increased elimination of NPs, thus leading to reduced availability of these peptides and consequently to renal resistance to these hormones. Further support for this notion comes from numerous reports wherein NEP inhibition by pharmacologic means has been shown to improve the vascular and renal response to NPs in CHF (see later).

   It is widely accepted today that the development of renal hyporesponsiveness represents a critical point in the development of positive salt balance and edema formation in advanced CHF. Some studies suggested that renal resistance to ANP actions may present even in the early presymptomatic stage of the disease.[559]

3. Activation of antinatriuretic systems. The ability of NPs to antagonize the renal effects of AII may be limited in the presence of markedly impaired RPF such as in CHF.[560] Abassi and co-workers[451] demonstrated that chronic blockade of the RAAS by enalapril partially but significantly improved the natriuretic response to endogenous and exogenous ANP in rats with CHF induced by aortocaval fistula. The improvement in renal response to ANP was more evident in rats with decompensated CHF than in rats with compensated CHF. It should be emphasized that decompensated CHF is characterized by profound activation of RAAS. These findings are in line with the fact that activation of RAAS in CHF largely contributes to Na+ and water retention by antagonizing the renal actions of ANP. Actually, AII, the main active component of the RAAS, counteracts the natriuretic effects of ANP even under normal conditions.[561] Potential mechanisms of this phenomenon may include AII-induced afferent and efferent vasoconstriction, mesangial cell contraction, activation of cGMP phosphodiesterases that attenuate the accumulation of the second messenger of NPs in target organs, and finally, stimulation of Na+,H+-exchanger and Na+ channels in the proximal tubule and collecting duct.[451] The mechanisms underlying the attenuated renal effects of ANP in CHF are not completely understood.

In addition, activation of the SNS antagonizes the renal effects of ANP. Although ANP has inhibitory effects on SNS, the latter is activated in CHF. Overactivity of the SNS leads to vasoconstriction of the peripheral circulation as well as the afferent and efferent arterioles, leading to reduction of RFF and eventually of GFR. These actions, besides direct stimulatory effects of SNS on Na+ reabsorption in the proximal tubule and loop of Henle, contribute to the attenuated renal responsiveness to ANP in CHF. Moreover, the SNS-induced renal hypoperfusion/hypofiltration stimulates renin secretion, thus aggravating the positive Na+ and water balance. A study by Feng and colleagues[486] in a rat model of CHF induced by coronary artery ligation demonstrated that the diuretic and natriuretic response to ANP was increased after pharmacologic sympathetic inhibition using low-dose clonidine. A similar response was produced by bilateral renal denervation procedure in rats with ischemic CHF.[485] The beneficial effects of renal denervation could be attributed to up-regulation of NP receptors and cGMP production, as has been demonstrated in normal rats.[321]

The fact that the NP system plays a beneficial role, counteracting the adverse effects of Na+-retaining and vasoconstrictive hormonal systems in CHF, provides a possible rationale for the use of these peptides in the therapy of CHF. Thus, either increasing the activity of the NPs or reducing the influence of the antinatriuretic systems by pharmacologic means may achieve a shift in the balance in favor of Na+ excretion in CHF. In the interplay between the RAAS and ANP in CHF, the approaches used in experimental studies and in clinical practice included reducing the activity of the RAAS by means of ACE inhibitors or AII receptor antagonists, increasing the activity of ANP or its second messenger, cGMP, or combinations of approaches:

A. Administration of NPs. As noted previously, circulating levels of NPs are elevated in CHF in proportion to the severity of the disease. However, the renal actions of these peptides are attenuated and even blunted in severe CHF. Nevertheless, several studies demonstrated that elimination of

NP action using blockers of NPR-A or surgical removal of the atrium aggravates renal function and cardiac performance in experimental CHF.[552,555] Therefore, increasing the circulating levels of NPs by the administration of exogenous synthetic peptides was tested in both clinical and experimental CHF and appears to be beneficial under certain circumstances. For example, intravenous administration of ANP to patients with acute CHF improved their clinical status.[562] Similarly, injection of BNP reduced pulmonary arterial pressure, pulmonary capillary wedge pressure (PCWP), right atrial pressure, and systemic blood pressure, in association with increased cardiac output and diuresis.[563,564] In light of its beneficial effects, BNP (nesiritide) was approved for the treatment of acute decompensated CHF in the United States in 2001. The observation that these effects occur despite the presence of elevated endogenous levels of NPs suggests that a relative deficiency of these peptides may exist in CHF. Owing to their peptidic nature, NPs are susceptible to degradation by NEP, thus limiting their clinical use to intravenous administration only.

B. Inhibitors of the RAAS system. With regard to ACE inhibitors, a large body of evidence attests to their beneficial effects on renal function in CHF. ACE inhibitors decrease mortality and cardiovascular morbidity in various disease states, including post–MI and CHF.[565] These beneficial effects are not surprising in light of the maladaptive actions of locally produced or circulating AII and aldosterone. Further evidence regarding the involvement of the RAAS in the development of positive Na^+ balance can be inferred from studies showing that the renal and hemodynamic response to ANP is impaired in the AV fistula model of CHF[451,473] and in the coronary ligation model[566] and that administration of either losartan or ACE inhibitor restores this blunted response to ANP.[451,473,567] Of note, both of these therapeutic agents were able to restore the urinary excretion of cGMP in rats with decompensated CHF, suggesting that RAAS contributes to the renal hyporesponsiveness to ANP in CHF by attenuating the generation of this second messenger.[451,473] This effect is consistent with the observation that AII induces down-regulation of natriuretic peptide receptor (NPR) in the glomerulus and blood vessels[568] or activation of cGMP phosphodiesterase at these tissues.[569]

In addition, the other active component of the RAAS, namely, the aldosterone, plays a pivotal role in the pathogenesis of CHF as well, but by distinct mechanisms. Besides promoting Na^+ retention, aldosterone contributes to vascular and cardiac remodeling by inducing perivascular and interstitial fibrosis.[570] Therefore, the addition of small doses of spironolactone to standard therapy substantially reduces the mortality rate and morbidity in CHF patients.[465]

C. NEP inhibitors. Correcting the imbalance between the RAAS and the NP systems may also be achieved by enhancing the activity of ANP or cGMP.[571,572] This approach utilizes pharmacologic agents that either inhibit the enzymatic degradation of ANP by NEP or block the ANP clearance receptors. Several specific and differently structured NEP inhibitors have been developed in recent years.[573] Most of the studies that examined the renal and cardiac effects of pharmacologic NEP inhibition in CHF have revealed an enhancement in plasma ANP and BNP levels in association with vasodilation, natriuresis, diuresis, and subsequently in reduction in cardiac preload and afterload. Seymour and colleagues[574] demonstrated that inhibition of NEP in dogs with pacing-induced CHF protected endogenous ANP from degradation and caused a sustained natriuretic response. Using rats with CHF induced by aorto-caval fistula, Wilkins and associates[575] reported that thiorphan, an NEP inhibitor, enhanced the natriuretic action of ANP in association with increased urinary cGMP excretion. Similar results were reported by Margulies and colleagues,[576] who found that acute inhibition of NEP in dogs with severe CHF produced a dose-related increase in urine flow and Na^+ excretion. Because NEP degrades other peptides (e.g., kinins), the latter may also be involved in the beneficial effects of NEP-Is. Candoxatril, the first NEP inhibitor to be released for clinical trials, produces favorable hemodynamic and neurohormonal effects in patients with CHF.[577,578] However, acute NEP inhibition in mild CHF results in marked increases in RPF and Na^+ excretion, which exceed the increase observed either in control animals or in severe CHF, suggesting a potential therapeutic role for NEP inhibition to enhance renal function in mild CHF.[579] In later studies of CHF, apparently the more marked activation of the RAAS serves to attenuates the beneficial renal and hemodynamic actions of NEP-Is, suggesting that mechanisms other than exaggerated NEP activity are involved in the renal resistance to NPs. Moreover, NEP inhibitors do not reduce afterload. Based on the foregoing, it is predicted that a combination of RAAS and NEP inhibitors should be more effective than each treatment alone.[580] Indeed, Margulies and co-workers[580] reported that AII inhibition potentiated the renal response to NEP inhibition by SQ 28,603 (an NEP inhibitor) in dogs with CHF. These findings led to the development of dual NEP and ACE inhibitors.[581] The beneficial effects of these compounds have been evaluated. NEP inhibition prevents the ACE blocker–induced decrease in GFR in dogs with pacing-induced CHF,[576,580] suggesting that concurrent inhibition of both NEP and ACE may effectively treat cardiovascular disorders without compromising renal function.

D. Vasopeptidase inhibitors (VPIs). The realization that ACE and NEP are involved in the biosynthesis/metabolism of peptides that play a major role in regulating cardiovascular and renal function led to the development of a novel class of drugs, the VPIs, that blocks the activity of both ACE and NEP. Thus, VPIs are novel, highly selective inhibitors of both ACE and neutral NEP. The most famous representative of this family of drugs, omapatrilat (BMS-186716, Vanlev), was synthesized by Robl and associates.[582] Since then, numerous VPIs have been synthesized by a number of pharmaceutical companies.[583,584] The dual inhibitory actions of these compounds are supposed to offer potential hemodynamic and neurohormonal advantages over the inhibition of either enzymatic system alone. Therefore, it is conceivable that VPIs may be highly beneficial in the treatment of clinical disorders characterized by the activation of ACE and NEP, such as CHF and hypertension. Indeed, recent results in both experimental and clinical CHF suggest beneficial hemodynamic and renal effects mediated by the synergistic ACE and NEP inhibition offered by this drug.[585–592] For example, short-term administration of omapatrilat to cardiomyopathic hamsters reduced left ventricular systolic and end-diastolic pressure in association with a 40% increase in cardiac output and a decrease in PVR.[593] These effects were more potent than those obtained with NEP-I or ACE-I. Long-term treatment of these hamsters with omaptrilat improved the cardiac geometry and survival rate compared with captopril treatment.[594] Using a different experimental model of CHF, Troughton and colleagues[587,588] showed that omapatrilat reduced cardiac mass and improved cardiac function in both mild and severe heart failure. These results are in agreement with previous studies[585,586] demonstrating that aladotril or alatriopril (mixed inhibitor of NEP and ACE) significantly increased cardiac output and attenuated cardiac hypertrophy in experimental CHF induced by pacing or coronary ligation.

At the renal level, administration of omapatrilat to dogs with CHF induced significant increases in Na$^+$ excretion and GFR that were greater than the increase produced by ACE-I alone.[595] When given in the presence of HS-142 (a blocker of NPR), the renal actions of omapatrilat were significantly attenuated, indicating that NPs partially mediate these effects.

Evaluation of cardiac and renal response to omapatrilat in patients with CHF revealed beneficial effects similar to those observed in experimental CHF. In a study that included 48 CHF patients (NYHA classes II–IV), McClean and co-workers[590] demonstrated that treatment with omapatrilat for 3 months increased ejection fraction from 24% to 28%, accompanied by a significant natriuresis. The same trend, that is, improvement in left ventricular function was obtained when omapatrilat was tested in a larger population of CHF patients ($n=369$).[591] Improvement in the clinical status of these patients was accompanied by a reduction of the elevated circulating levels of the prognostic marker BNP. However, decreases in systolic and MAP were observed in CHF patients after long-term treatment with high doses of omapatrilat.[591]

The IMPRESS study reported a greater improvement in NYHA class and reduction in combined mortality/hospitalization end points for patients with systolic CHF receiving omapatrilat (40 mg/day) compared with lisinopril, an ACE inhibitor (20 mg/day),[592] given for 24 weeks. Interestingly, the one parameter that best differentiated omapatrilat from lisinopril in this study was renal function. In particular, renal function was preserved to a greater extent with omapatrilat compared with that obtained by the ACE inhibitor therapy. Such renoprotection was also observed in experimental CHF, wherein acute VPI, but not ACE inhibition, increased the GFR.[583] However, in some studies NEP and ACE inhibition failed to improve CHF signs or symptoms.[596–598] To further establish the superiority of omapatrilat to conventional therapy in CHF, a comprehensive study (the OVERTURE) was carried out.[598] In this study,

5770 patients with CHF with NYHA classes II to IV were randomized to either omapatrilat (40 mg once daily) or enalapril (10 mg twice daily) therapy. After about 14.5 months, omapatrilat reduced the risk for death and hospitalization in chronic CHF subjects, but was not more effective than enalapril alone in reducing primary clinical events. Both drugs were well tolerated, but marked elevation of creatinine was less common with omapatrilat compared with ACE inhibitor therapy. In contrast, hypotension and dizziness were more frequent with omapatrilat therapy compared with the ACE inhibitor. An additional fatal reported complication of omapatrilat is the development of angioedema. Although this phenomenon has been well established in patients on ACE-I (0.1%–0.5%), it occurs at greater rates (three times) in patients treated with omapatrilat, especially when the starting dose was greater than 20 mg/day. The incidence of omapatrilat-induced angioedema was higher among African-Americans and African-Caribbeans.[599] The mechanisms underlying this life-threatening side effect of omapatrilat are not fully characterized. However, it is widely believed that BK and its metabolite Des-Arg^9-BK are implicated in VPI-induced angioedema.[599] Because VPIs inhibit both enzymes that inactivate BK (ACE and NEP), they may increase the plasma concentrations of BK dramatically.

VPIs are also expected to be of potential therapeutic benefit in hypertension. Several studies have shown greater blood pressure–reducing properties of VPIs in a number of populations when compared with other conventional antihypertensive agents, such as ACE inhibitors and calcium channel antagonists. Omapatrilat has demonstrated long-lasting (>24 hours) and dose-dependent hypotensive effects in all tested models of hypertension, independent of the status of the RAAS or the degree of salt retention.[583,584] Treatment of hypertensive patients with omapatrilat for 6 weeks had a greater lowering effect on systolic and diastolic blood pressure compared with lisinopril or amlodipine.[600] The preferential effect of omapatrilat on systolic blood pressure suggests that this compound improves the compliance and remodeling of large blood vessels. When administered in combination with hydrochlorothiazide (diuretic agent) to hypertensive patients, omapatrilat reduced systolic and diastolic blood pressure to a greater extent than hydrochlorothiazide alone.[601] Similarly, other members of the VPI family, sampatrilat and fasidotril, provoked significant hypotensive effects in hypertensive black and white patients.[223,602] The results of a comprehensive trial (Omapatrilat Cardiovascular Treatment Assessment Versus Enalapril [OCTAVE]) in which 25,302 hypertensive patients who were treated with either omaptrilat (initially 10 mg and titrated to a maximum of 80 mg) or enalapril (initially 5 mg and titrated to a maximum of 40 mg) for 24 weeks demonstrated that omapatrilat provided superior antihypertensive efficacy when used in a setting resembling clinical practice.[603] However, angioedema was more common than with enalapril, although life-threatening angioedema was rare. A higher incidence of angioedema was evident in black hypertensive patients as well as in smokers.

In summary, the obtained clinical and experimental results indicate that VPIs confer advantage in CHF and hypertensive patients over ACE inhibition alone. However, similar to ACE inhibitors, VPIs have adverse side effects, particulary angioedema. Nevertheless, in light of the encouraging beneficial cardiac and vascular effects of VPIs, the latter may serve as a therapeutic tool for the treatment of various cardiovascular diseases.

BRAIN NATRIURETIC PEPTIDE. As noted previously, BNP (32 amino acids in human) is structurally similar to ANP, but is produced mainly by the ventricles in response to ventricular stretch and pressure overload.[236,604–606] Similar to ANP, plasma levels of BNP are elevated in patients with CHF in proportion to the severity of myocardial systolic and diastolic dysfunction.[559,607–614] Wei and co-workers[615] reported that plasma levels of BNP are elevated only in patients with severe CHF, whereas the circulating concentrations of ANP are high in mild and severe cases. Similar results were obtained by Rademaker and colleagues,[616] who demonstrated that acute rapid atrial pacing in conscious sheep increased the secretion of ANP and BNP by 8.6- and 3.6-fold, respectively; whereas chronic rapid pacing elevated plasma levels of ANP and BNP by 7.8- and 9-fold, respectively. The extreme elevation of plasma BNP in severe CHF probably stems from the increased synthesis of BNP, predominantly by the hypertrophied ventricular tissue, although the contribution of the atria cannot be understated.[617] Asymptomatic experimental left ventricular dysfunction in dogs was not associated with enhanced expression of BNP in the ventricles, although the atrial tissue significantly increased the expression of this peptide in both mild and overt CHF.[617]

Plasma levels of ANP and NH_2-terminal ANP increase early in the course of CHF.[618] Lerman and co-workers[619] and Hall and associates[620] demonstrated that left ventricular dysfunction is associated with increased plasma levels of NT-proANP (1–98 NH_2-terminal). In this context, several studies showed that plasma ANP levels correlate with the severity of symptomatic CHF,[621] suggesting that the concentration of circulating ANP may serve as a diagnostic tool in the determination of cardiac dysfunction and as a prognostic marker in the prediction of survival of patients with CHF with a sensitivity and specificity of more than 90%.[611] Although echocardiography remains the gold standard for the evaluation of left ventricular dysfunction, numerous studies introduced plasma levels of BNP as a reliable marker for the diagnosis and management of CHF. Actually, in the past few years, the superiority of BNP to ANP as a diagnostic and prognostic factor in CHF has been supported by numerous clinical studies.[612,622–624] These and other studies showed that systemic BNP concentrations are significantly elevated in overt CHF, and these concentrations reflect left ventricular function with fidelity.[607,625] Patients diagnosed with CHF have a mean BNP value of 1076±138 pg/mL compared with 38±4 pg/mL in non-CHF subjects presenting to the urgent care unit.[237,624] Moreover, plasma levels of BNP correlate with NYHA class number, in which circulating levels of BNP range between ~200 pg/mL in class I and ~1000 pg/mL in class IV CHF patients.[237] Luchner and associates,[626] in their study on NT-proBNP after MI, observed an increase in NT-proBNP in subjects with MI. This increase was particularly pronounced in the presence of significant left ventricular dysfunction and renal dysfunction. Patients with an EF of less than 35% were detected by NT-proBNP with sensitivity, specificity, and negative predictive value of 75%, 62%, and 99%, respectively, at an optimal cutoff of 44 pmol/L. Patients with concomitant left ventricular hypertrophy were detected with sensitivity, specificity, and negative predictive value of 90%, 80%, and 99.9%, respectively, at a cutoff of 76 pmol/L. Similar results were obtained for patients with concomitant renal dysfunction at a cutoff of 162 pmol/L. These authors concluded that NT-proBNP is a marker of integrated cardiorenal function and a potential diagnostic tool for the detection and exclusion of impaired let ventricular function, particularly in the presence of concomitant left ventricular hypertrophy or renal dysfunction.[626] Similarly, de Lemos and associates[627] demonstrated the ability of circulating BNP, measured within a few days of acute coronary syndromes, to predict risk of mortality, clinical CHF, and new MI, suggesting that activation of this neurohormonal axis may be a common feature among patients at high risk for death after acute MI. Most recently, Richards and co-workers[628] showed that plasma BNP (or NH_2-terminal BNP) and LVEF are complementary independent predictors of major adverse events on follow-up after MI. For example, elevated BNP predicted new MI only in patients with LVEF<40%. LVEF<40% coupled to elevated NT-BNP over the group median conferred a substantially 3-year increased risk of death, CHF, and new MI of 37%, 18%, and 26%, respectively. These findings indicate that combined measurement of these two parameters provides risk stratification substantially better than that provided by either alone. The plasma level of BNP is a powerful marker for prognosis and risk stratification in the setting of CHF.[629,630] According to Harrison and colleagues,[631] BNP levels greater than 240 pg/ml are associated with high relative risk of 6 months' death in CHF dyspneic patients. Similarly, Berger and co-workers[632] found that BNP levels were the only independent predictor of sudden death in arrhythmic CHF patients with an ejection fraction of less than 35%. According to this study, the cut-off value was 130 mg/mL, which is comparable with those suggested by others ~80 to 100 pg/mL.[629,630,633]

As many as 40% to 50% of patients with a diagnosis of CHF have normal systolic function, which implicates diastolic dysfunction as the most likely potential abnormality responsible for this disorder. Diastolic heart failure cannot be distinguished from systolic heart failure on the basis of history, physical examination, chest x-ray, and electrocardiogram alone. As a result, indirect and noninvasive assessments of left ventricular filling dynamics have been used to characterize diastolic properties, especially echocardiographic Doppler transmitral velocity measurements. There are four distinct echocardiographic patterns: normal, delayed relaxation, pseudonormal, and restrictive. BNP release appears to be directly proportional to ventricular volume expansion and pressure overload, and elevated BNP levels in patients with normal systolic function correlate with diastolic abnormalities on Doppler studies. Thus, BNP represents a circulating plasma marker providing positive evidence of the presence of diastolic dysfunction, even in asymptomatic patients. Conversely, a reduction in BNP levels with treatment are associated with a reduction in left ventricular filling pressures, a lower readmission rate, and a better prognosis, such that monitoring of BNP levels may provide valuable information regarding treatment efficacy and expected patient outcomes.[237,634]

In addition, plasma levels of BNP are useful in distinguishing dyspnea caused by CHF or disorders other than CHF, such as pulmonary causes.[629,630,633,635] Dao and colleagues[633] reported that patients presenting to urgent care units owing to CHF have BNP plasma levels 28-fold those obtained in a non-CHF group. BNP at the cut-off point of 80 pg/mL was highly selective and sensitive for the diagnosis of CHF. According to this study, which included 250 patients, BNP values lower than 80 pg/mL have a negative predictive value of 98% for CHF diagnosis. Plasma levels of BNP in patients with dyspnea owing to CHF were sixfold those obtained in patients without CHF (675 compared with 110 pg/mL). Moderate values of BNP were observed in patients with mild left ventricular dysfunction (346 pg/mL). It is widely believed that a BNP level below 50 pg/mL has strong negative predictive value

(96%) in the assessment of patients with dyspnea caused by a disorder of noncardiac origin. In line with this conclusion, the diagnostic accuracy, sensitivity, specificity of BNP at a cut-off of 100 pg/mL were 83.4%, 90%, and 74%, respectively.[629,630] According to this and other studies,[610] the predictive accuracy of circulating BNP for the diagnosis of CHF equals and even exceeds the accuracy of classic examinations such as x-ray and physical examination. In a large-scale study, Maisel and colleagues[629,630] reported that a single determination of circulating BNP level was more accurate than both the National Health and Nutrition Examination score and Framingham clinical parameters (the most established criteria in use for the diagnosis of CHF) in differentiating dyspnea of cardiac versus noncardiac origin. This conclusion was supported by a recent prospective, randomized, and controlled study of 452 patients who presented to the emergency department with acute dyspnea. Half of the patients were randomly assigned to a diagnostic strategy involving the measurement of BNP levels with the use of a rapid bedside assay (BNP group), and half of the patients were assessed in a conventional manner (control group). In addition, the median time of discharge and cost of treatment were significantly higher in the former group compared with the latter. Again, measurement of BNP levels for the diagnosis of acute dyspnea of cardiac etiology should be assessed in conjunction with other conventional clinical parameters and not alone.

In addition to diagnostic and prognostic applications, circulating BNP and its NT-proBNP have been used as a guide in determining the therapeutic efficacy of typically prescribed drugs for CHF patients, including ACE inhibitors, diuretics, digitalis, and β-blockers.[587,588] Kawai and associates[636] reported that plasma BNP correlates with left ventricular end-diastolic dimension, LVEF, and left ventricular mass in patients with idiopathic dilated cardiomyopathy and that administration of carvedilol to these patients for 6 months improved these parameters in most patients in association with decreased BNP levels in responders. Similarly, Motwani and colleagues[637] found that BNP, but not ANP, accurately reflects the improvement in the ejection fraction of patients treated with ACE inhibitor following MI. In treated as well as untreated patients with CHF, high levels of BNP are an independent predictor of mortality. Maeda and co-workers[638] demonstrated that plasma levels of BNP and interleukin-6 are independent risk factors for morbidity and mortality in patients with CHF after 3 months of optimized treatment.

Taken together, these and other findings suggest that a simple and rapid determination of plasma levels of BNP in patients with CHF can be used to assess cardiac dysfunction and serve as a diagnostic and prognostic marker. In addition, measurements of plasma BNP may be useful in titrating relevant therapy. In this context, Troughton and associates[587,588] reported that the first cardiovascular event after 6 months of therapy was less frequent in CHF patients whose plasma BNP levels decreased in response to medical treatment.

However, it should be emphasized that measurement of plasma levels of either ANP and BNP outside of the broader clinical context is of limited diagnostic value, because the concentrations of these peptides in the circulation are affected by several factors, including age, salt intake, gender, and hemodynamic status. Therefore, a combination of conventional parameters such as clinical and echocardiographic measures taken together with plasma levels of BNP yield better clinical guidelines in patients with CHF than utilizing each tool alone.[639] This approach gained further support from a recently published study by Tang and co-workers,[640] who reported that in the ambulatory care setting, patients with asymptomatic and symptomatic chronic stable systolic heart failure present a wide range of plasma BNP levels. Nevertheless, still 21% of symptomatic patients display BNP plasma levels below 100 pg/mL.

In light of the reports that BNP is less susceptible to degradation by NEP 24.11 compared with ANP,[641,642] it is not surprising that, on a mole-to-mole basis, BNP is a more biologically potent natriuretic agent than the latter.[641] With this in mind, the efficacy of exogenous human BNP was examined in patients with decompensated CHF.[643] Bolus or sustained infusion of BNP (nesiritide) for short (minutes to hours) and long (hours to days) periods to patients with decompensated CHF (mostly NYHA classes III and IV) resulted in substantial beneficial hemodynamic changes. These changes included reductions in elevated right atrial pressure, pulmonary artery pressure (PAP), PCWP, MAP, and SVR, in association with increased cardiac index, urinary flow rate, and Na^+ excretion without activation of neurohumoral systems.[563,644-648] The hemodynamic and natriuretic effects of exogenous BNP administration were significantly greater than those obtained following the use of similar doses of ANP in patients with CHF.[644] These effects of BNP were associated with enhanced release of cGMP. Comparable results were reported by Abraham and colleagues,[649] who found that BNP infusion to patients with CHF improved cardiac performance and suppressed plasma levels of NE and aldosterone, but only one third of the patients showed increased Na^+ excretion. The attenuated natriuretic response to BNP in these patients is not surprising in light of the structural similarity between ANP and BNP and the fact that both peptides share the same mechanism of action. Similar attenuated renal responsiveness to BNP, despite elevated plasma levels of this peptide, was reported by Hoffman and co-workers[650] in rats with CHF induced by the placement of aortocaval fistula. When BNP was given at low and high subcutaneous doses for 10 days to dogs with experimental CHF, cardiac filling pressure was reduced in association with increased urinary Na^+ excretion, urine flow, and RPF.[651] After 10 days of treatment, cardiac output was increased and RVR and PCWP decreased, suggesting that chronic administration of BNP via a subcutaneous route may be used as a novel strategy for the treatment of CHF. It should be noted, however, that one of the most adverse effects of recombinant BNP (nesiritide) is dose-related hypotension.[564] The later adverse effect may impose serious problem when nesiritide is given with other vasodilators, such as ACE-I.[618] Nevertheless, when acutely infused into patients with decompensated CHF, nesiritide was less tachycardic or arrhythmogenic than dobutamine.[632]

When comparing intravenous nesiritide with nitroglycerin in treating patients with CHF, nesiritide displayed more prominent hemodynamic effects, such as reduction in PCWP, compared to standard care plus nitroglycerin or placebo, and these effects were sustained for at least 24 hours. Symptomatic effects, such as improvement in dyspnea, were observed with both drugs, although more pronounced following administration of nesiritide. The hemodynamic and symptomatic improvement with nesiritide, coupled with a safety profile similar to that of nitroglycerin, suggests that nesiritide, along with diuretics, is a useful addition to the initial therapy of patients hospitalized with acutely decompensated CHF.[652]

C-TYPE NATRIURETIC PEPTIDE. Although CNP is synthesized mainly by endothelial cells, small amounts are also produced by cardiac tissue.[653] In contrast to other NPs, CNP is predominantly a vasodilator and has little effect on urinary flow and Na^+ excretion, and in some cases, even reduces these parameters.[654-656] However, the production of CNP by the endothelium in proximity to its receptors in VSMC suggests that this peptide may play a role in the control of vascular tone and growth.[657] In contrast to ANP and BNP, plasma levels of CNP are not increased in CHF; however, local concentrations of CNP are elevated in the myocardium in this disease state.[615] In a recent large study ($n=305$), Wright and associates[658] demonstrated that plasma levels of CNP are elevated in patients with symptomatic CHF and that the use of BNP as a predictor for CHF shows a significant relation to concurrent plasma CNP. These findings suggest a possible peripheral vascular compensatory response to CHF by overexpression of this vasodilatory peptide. Most recently,[653] it has been demonstrated that CNP possesses an inhibitory effect on cultured cardiac myocyte hypertrophy, suggesting that overexpression of CNP in the myocardium during CHF may be involved in counteracting cardiac remodeling.

NITRIC OXIDE. Recent studies showed that endothelial dysfunction has a fundamental impact on the development of impaired cardiac performance with all the concomitant adverse systemic consequences. It is widely believed that endothelial dysfunction contributes to the increase in vascular resistance in CHF[245,247,659] and to the impaired endothelium-dependent vascular responses in correlation to the clinical severity of cardiac dysfunction.[247,659–661] Thus, the response to acetylcholine, an endothelium-dependent vasodilator that acts by releasing NO, was found to be markedly attenuated in patients and experimental animals with CHF. Similar observations were reported in isolated vessels from animals with CHF examined in vitro. The mechanisms mediating the impaired activity of the NO system in CHF are largely unknown. Several potential mechanisms have been offered as an explanation. These include a reduction in shear stress associated with the decreased cardiac output,[247] downregulation of NOS, decreased availability of the NO precursor L-arginine,[660,662] increased levels of dimethyl arginine and overriding activity of counterregulatory vasoconstrictor systems such as the RAAS.[660,663]

In view of the importance of NO in regulating RBF, it is possible that altered activity of the NO system may be involved in the pathogenesis of the renal hypoperfusion in CHF. The latter possibility is supported by our findings that rats with CHF induced by aortocaval fistula have attenuated NO-mediated renal vasodilation.[663] Moreover, this impairment could be reversed by pretreatment with an AT_1 receptor antagonist, suggesting that AII may be involved in mediating the impaired NO-dependent renal vasodilatation.[663] The resulting imbalance between NO and excessive activation of the RAAS and ET systems explains some of the beneficial effects of ACE-inhibitors, ARBs, and aldosterone antagonists.[664] A blunted response to endothelium-dependent vasodilators has been generally equated with a decrease in NOS activity and NO generation. However, several studies demonstrated that patients with CHF have higher plasma levels of $NO_2 + NO_3$ and exhibit augmented responsivness to inhibitors of NOS, suggesting that NO generation and release are enhanced in CHF.[660,665–668] According to these studies, the NO system in CHF represents another failing counterregulatory mechanisms in the face of the activated vsoconstrictors. In line with this concept, most recently, Abassi and co-workers[290] demonstrated that rats with experimental CHF induced by aortocaval fistula express higher abundance of eNOS-mRNA and protein immunoreactivity in the kidney, particularly in the renal medulla. It was speculated that the overexpression of eNOS in the renal medulla may play an important role in the preservation of intact medullary perfusion. In addition, the increased eNOS levels in the cortex, although to a lesser extent than in the medulla, may serve a compensatory mechanism in ameliorating the severe cortical vasoconstriction.

An additional issue worthy of consideration is the fact that the myocardium contains all the three isoforms of NOS, and the locally generated NO is believed to play a modulatory role on cardiac function.[278,446] Thus, it might be that alterations in the cardiac NO system in CHF contribute to the pathogenesis of cardiac dysfunction and, therefore, indirectly contribute to the impaired renal function.[669] Indeed, increasing evidence indicates that iNOS and eNOS overexpression occurs in failing myocardium. The deleterious actions of the

increased NO levels on ventricle contractility is well documented.[278] Based on the foregoing, achieving NO balance by either NO donors or selective NOS inhibitors has emerged as one of the most important therapeutic concepts in addressing and correcting the pathophysiology of CHF.[670] Although early clinical trials have yielded encouraging initial results, extensive efforts remain to be investigated in order to verify whether this treatment option is feasible/beneficial.

In summary, the endothelium-dependent vasodilatation is attenuated in various vascular beds in CHF. This attenuation may occur in the presence of increased NO production, suggesting that the vascular NO may be another example of failed vasodilator system in CHF.

PROSTAGLANDINS. Although the PGs have little contribution to kidney function in euvolemic and unstressed states, they play an important role in maintaining renal function during setting of pathophysiologic compromise, including CHF. As previously noted, when RBF is impaired, hypoperfusion of the kidney or activation of the RAAS stimulates the release of PGs that exert a vasodilator effect predominantly at the level of the afferent arteriole and promote Na^+ excretion by inhibiting Na^+ transport in TALH and medullary collecting duct.[671–673] Two previous observations suggested a compensatory role of PGs in experimental and clinical CHF: First, plasma levels of PGE_2, PGE_2 metabolites, and 6-keto-PGF_1 were elevated in CHF patients compared with normal subjects.[674] Moreover, studies in experimental and human CHF demonstrated a direct linear relationship between the PRA and AII concentrations and levels of circulating and urinary PGE_2 and PGI_2 metabolites.[675] This correlation probably reflects both stimulation of PG synthesis by AII and increased release of renin induced by PGs. A similar counterregulatory role of PGs with respect to the other vasoconstrictors (catecholamines and ADH) may also be inferred. An inverse correlation between serum Na^+ concentrations and plasma levels of PGE_2 metabolites has been demonstrated. The second approach that established the protective role of renal and vascular prostaglandins in CHF was derived from studies of nonsteroidal anti-inflammaatory drugs (NSAIDs), which inhibit the synthesis of PGs. In various experimental models of CHF, inhibition of PG synthesis was associated with adverse renal hemodynamic consequences.[470,495,674] In one of these studies,[470] using a rapid ventricular pacing canine model of CHF, the induction of CHF was associated with an elevation in urinary excretion of PGE_2. Administration of indomethacin was associated with a significant increase in body weight, serum creatinine, and urea and a significant decline in urine flow rate. In another study of experimental chronic moderate CHF,[676] increased urinary excretion of PGE_2 was obtained. Administration of indomethacin was associated with a profound increase in RVR and a resultant decrease in RBF, mainly related to afferent arteriolar constriction. On the basis of these observations, it is not surprising to find that patients with hyponatremia accompanied by the most striking activation of the SNS and the RAAS were most susceptible to adverse glomerular hemodynamic consequences after the administration of indomethacin.[674] In this regard, Townend and colleagues[677] demonstrated that administration of indomethacin to patients with chronic CHF resulted in a significant decrease in RBF and GFR in association with reduced urinary Na^+ excretion. These effects were prevented by intravenous infusion of PGE_2. In the same study, the authors showed that pretreatment of these patients with indomethacin prior to captopril administration attenuated the captopril-induced increase in RBF. These results suggest that PGs have a significant role in the regulation of renal function in patients with CHF. In addition, these results indicate that captopril-induced improvement in renal hemodynamics is mediated in part by an increase in PG synthesis. In this context, renal PGs also play an important role in mediating the natriuretic effects of ANP in dogs with experimental CHF induced by an AV fistula.[678] According to this study indomethacin reduced ANP-induced Na^+ excretion and creatinine clearance in these dogs by 75% and 35%, respectively, suggesting a substantial role of PGs in determining their nartiuretic responsiveness to this hormone. Collectively, both human and animal studies indicate that CHF is a "prostaglandin-dependent" state, in which elevated AII and enhanced renal sympathetic nerve activity stimulate renal synthesis of PGE_2 and PGI_2 that would counteract the vasoconstrictor effects of these stimuli to maintain GFR and RBF. Therefore, administration of NSAIDs to patients or animals with CHF would leave these vasoconstrictor systems unopposed, leading to hypoperfusion/hypofiltration and subsequently to Na^+ and water retention.[671]

In recent years, several studies reported a close relationship between the consumption of NSAIDs and a significant worsening of chronic CHF, especially in elderly patients taking diuretics.[679,680] The exacerbation of this condition was reported in patients taking either nonselective COX inhibitors or selective COX-2 inhibitors. The deleterious effects of the latter on cardiac and renal functions are in line with the relatively high abundance of COX-2 in renal tissue and to a lesser extent in the myocardium and with the observation that the renal immunoreactive levels of this isoform are enhanced in experimental CHF.[190] Moreover, the significant increase in the risk of MI with COX-2 inhibitors—rofecoxib and celecoxib—raised serious safety problems in the use of these drugs and led to their withdrawal from the market.[681,682]

In summary, patients with preexisting CHF or hypertension are at high risk to develop volume overload, edema formation, and deterioration of cardiac function following the use of COX-2 inhibitors to the same or even higher frequencies than observed with use of conventional NSAIDs.

ADRENOMEDULLIN. Evidence suggests that AM plays a role in the pathophysiology of CHF. Compared with healthy subjects, in CHF patients, plasma levels of the mature form of AM as well as the glycine extended AM (AM-gly) are elevated in proportion to the severity of cardiac and hemodynamic impairment.[331,338,683] For instance, plasma levels of AM in subjects with severe CHF are fivefold higher than in controls, and plasma levels of the peptide fell with effective anti-CHF treatment, such as with carvedilol.[336,684–686] The origin of the increased circulating AM appears to be the failing myocardium itself including both the ventricles and, to a lesser extent, the atria.[335] In addition, plasma AM levels correlate with plasma concentrations of NE, ANP, BNP, PAP, PCWP, and PRA in these patients, indicating that the more severe the disease the higher the plasma AM levels measured.[687,688] Moreover, Jougasaki and associates[686,689] reported that ventricular and renal tissue AM were significantly increased in dogs with CHF induced by rapid ventricular pacing, compared with normals.

The years following the discovery of AM witnessed intensive investigation in regard to its involvement in the pathophysiology of positive salt and water balance characterizing CHF. Both experimental and clinical studies showed that infusion of AM produced beneficial renal effects in states of volume overload of cardiac origin. For example, brief administration (90 min) of AM into sheep with CHF due to rapid pacing produced a threefold increase in sodium excretion with maintenance of urine output and a rise in creatinine clearance compared with baseline levels in normal sheep.[690] Chronic administration of AM for 4 days in sheep with CHF produced a significant and sustained increase in cardiac output in association with enhanced urine volume.[335] In light of the positive results in experimental CHF, the effects of acute infusion of AM into patients with CHF have been examined. However, the results obtained were less encouraging as compared with normal subjects. For example, acute administration of AM to patients with CHF resulted in increased forearm blood flow but to a lesser extent than in normal subjects, suggesting that the AM vascular effects are significantly attenuated in CHF.[691] In addition, Lainchbury and colleagues[692] demonstrated that AM has no significant effect on urine volume and Na^+ excretion in patients with CHF, but remarkably reduced plasma aldosterone levels. Nagaya and co-workers[693] extended this study and found that intravenous infusion of human AM into patients with CHF predominantly improved cardiac function as expressed by increased cardiac stroke index, dilatation of the resistant arteries, and urinary Na^+ excretion. The improvement in cardiac function following AM infusion is not surprising in light of its beneficial effects on pre- and afterload and cardiac contractility.[331] Collectively, the vasodilatory and natriuretic activities of AM, and its origin from the failing heart, suggest that AM acts as a compensatory agent to balance the elevation in SVR and volume expansion in this disease state. However, most recently, the complementary interactions between AM and other vasoactive substances such as ET, NPs and NO in myocardial dysfunction were assessed. Indeed, AM in combination with other therapies such as ACE and NEP inhibitors resulted in hemodynamic and renal benefits greater than those achieved by the agents administered separately.[335]

In summary, the alterations in the efferent limb of volume regulation in CHF include enhanced activities of vasoconstrictor/Na^+-retaining systems as well as activation of counterregulatory vasodilatory/natriuretic systems. The magnitude of Na^+ excretion by the kidney and, therefore, the disturbance in volume homeostasis in CHF are largely determined by the balance between these antagonistic systems. In the early stages of CHF, the balancing effect of the vasodilatory/natriuretic systems is of importance in the maintenance of circulatory and renal function. However, with the progression of CHF, there is a shift of this balance, with dysfunction of the vasodilatory/natriuretic systems and marked activation of the vasoconstrictor/antinatriuretic systems. These disturbances are translated at the renal circulatory and tubular level to alterations that result in avid retention of salt and water, thereby leading to edema formation.

UROTENSIN. A role of the U-II/GPR-14 in the pathogenesis of CHF has been suggested, based on the following findings: First, some but not all studies reported that plasma levels of U-II are elevated in patients with CHF, correlating with other markers, such as NH_2-terminal BNP and ET-1.[340,694,695] In addition, strong expression of U-II was demonstrated in the myocardium of patients with end-stage CHF, in correlation with the impairment of cardiac function.[696] This suggests that upregulation of the U-II/GPR-14 system could play a part in the cardiac dysfunction associated with CHF.

In view of the documented vasoactive and natriuretic properties of U-II and the finding that the U-II/GPR-14 system may be up-regulated in CHF, several studies examined a possible role of U-II in the regulation of renal function in CHF. A recent set of studies in rats with aortocaval fistula as an experimental model of CHF showed that hU-II acts primarily as a renal vasodilator.[697] Moreover, the renal vasodilatory properties of the peptide are augmented in rats with experimental CHF, apparently by an NO-dependent mechanism. Finally, hU-II increased GFR only in rats with CHF, but did not alter urinary Na^+ excretion, in either control or CHF rats. However, in contrast to the negligible renal vasodilatory effect in control rats, the peptide produced a prominent and prolonged decrease in RVR associated with a significant increase in RPF and in GFR in rats with experimental CHF. Thus, under these conditions of increased baseline renal vascular tone, hU-II has the capacity to act as a potent vasodilator in the kidney. Furthermore, our findings suggest that this increase in renal perfusion is dependent in part on NO production. This is consistent with the finding of Zhang and co-workers[360] regarding the importance of NO in the mediation of hU-II–induced renal vasodilatation.

In summary, several reports suggest that the U-II/GPR-14 system may participate in the control of renal hemodynamics in the rat. This regulation may be significantly altered in rats with experimental CHF, which could contribute to the adaptive changes in renal function and renal hemodynamic responses in CHF.

NEUROPEPTIDE Y AND HEART FAILURE. Because many neurohormonal mediators have been implicated in the pathogenesis of CHF, it is of no surprise that NPY has also been a subject of investigation in this condition, especially because NPY colocalization and release with the adrenergic neurotransmitters suggested excessive corelease with NE from the activated peripheral sympathetic system.[698] Indeed, numerous reports demonstrated elevated plasma levels of NPY of patients with CHF, regardless of the etiology of the disease.[699–701] This increase correlates with the severity the disease, suggesting that NPY might serve as an independent prognostic factor for CHF severity and outcome.[702]

Although circulating levels of NPY are elevated in patients with CHF, little information is available concerning the local concentrations of NPY in the myocardium. It appears, however, that NPY levels are not elevated and, in fact, might be rather lower than normal, as is also the case with NE, suggesting that NPY depletion might follow the state of the SNS in general.[703] The functional significance of elevated local or systemic levels of NPY in the circulation of patients with CHF is not entirely clear and can only be speculated upon at this time. In light of the complex physiologic actions of NPY, it may be involved in the regulation of cardiac actions. Recent studies by groups of Haramati and Zukowska brought new insights into the role of NPY receptors in chronic CHF. By utilizing an AV fistula to induce CHF in rats, the investigators found that cardiac Y1 receptor gene expression decreases in proportion to the severity of cardiac hypertrophy and decompensation.[704] Interestingly, at the same time, Y2 receptor expression was shown to increase markedly in failing hearts.[704] Similar patterns of receptor expression change were observed in the kidneys and were also proportional to the degree of renal failure.[704] Because Y1 receptor appears to mediate known NPY growth-promoting activities in blood vessels[705,706] and myocytes,[707] this receptor may play a pathogenic role in development of cardiac hypertrophy in the failing heart. Y2 receptor activation is also strongly implicated in the angiogenic activity of NPY,[708] suggesting that up-regulation of this receptor may play an important compensatory role aimed at improving angiogenesis in the ischemic heart.

Furthermore, NPY was shown in experimental models of CHF to exert diuretic and natriuretic properties,[709] most likely owing to increasing the release of ANP and inhibiting the RAAS,[710] thereby facilitating water and electrolyte clearance and reducing congestion. Because the RAAS and the SNS play an important role in the progression of CHF, the higher circulating levels of NPY could be considered as a counteracting mechanism to potentially reduce the progression of CHF. However, NPY acting via Y1 receptors is also a potent mediator of vascular constriction, which could contribute to increases in vascular resistance, including coronary vessel constriction with compromise of cardiac blood flow and blood flow to other essential organs.

In summary, a potential role of NPY in the pathogenesis of CHF progression, cardiac, and salt and water homeostasis via actions on vascular, cardiomyocyte, and kidney functions exerted via multiple receptors (Y1, Y2, and Y5) requires further investigation.

Renal Sodium Retention and Edema Formation in Cirrhosis with Ascites

Afferent Limb of Volume Homeostasis in Cirrhosis

Abnormalities in renal Na^+ and water excretion are commonly found in cirrhosis, in humans as well as in experimental animal models.[711,712] Avid Na^+ and water retention may lead eventually to ascites, a common complication of cirrhosis and a major cause of morbidity and mortality, with the occurrence of spontaneous bacterial peritonitis, variceal bleeding, and development of the hepatorenal syndrome.[713,714] In similarity to CHF, the pathogenesis of the renal water and Na^+ retention in cirrhosis is related not to an intrinsic abnormality of the kidney but to extrarenal mechanisms that regulate renal Na^+ and water handling. Indeed, when kidneys from cirrhotic patients are transplanted into recipients with normal liver function, renal Na^+ and water retention no longer occurs.

Several formulations have been proposed over the years to explain the mechanism(s) by which patients with cirrhosis develop positive Na^+ balance and ascites formation. Two major theories put forward to explain the mechanisms of Na^+ and water retention in cirrhosis are the "overflow" and the "underfilling" theories of ascites formation. Whereas the occurrence of primary renal Na^+ and water retention and plasma volume expansion prior to ascites formation was favored by the "overflow" hypothesis, the classic "underfilling" theory posits that ascites formation causes hypovolemia that further initiates secondary renal Na^+ and water retention. In 1988, Schrier and co-workers[715] proposed the "peripheral arterial vasodilatation hypothesis" as a mechanism that could explain the retention of Na^+ and water in cirrhosis. This concept was promoted in the 1990s as a unifying hypothesis of the disturbance in body fluid volume homeostatsis to explain the mechanism of renal Na^+ and water retention also in diverse states of edema formation, in addition to cirrhosis, including pregnancy.[383,716,717] At the same time, the importance of NO as a cardinal player in the hemodynamic abnormalities that mediate salt and water retention in cirrhosis became increasingly evident.[718,719] The contribution of this molecule, as well as other vasodilatory mechanisms, to generation of the "hyperdynamic" circulation in cirrhosis was further supported by numerous other investigators (see Iwakiri and Groszmann[720]).

In the next sections, these theories are briefly presented, followed by a description of the efferent limb of the volume control system in the regulation of renal handling of Na^+ in cirrhosis.

The "Overflow" and "Underfilling" Concepts: Role in Disturbed Volume Regulation and Ascites Formation in Cirrhosis

Based on studies in patients with cirrhosis, Lieberman and co-workers[721] postulated that non–volume-dependent renal Na^+ retention is the primary disturbance in Na^+ homeostasis in cirrhosis. In their view, this renal Na^+ retention leads to total plasma volume expansion, including its nonsplanchnic component. The predilection of the renal salt and water retention to cause ascites was explained by the local alteration of Starling forces in the portosplanchnic bed ("overflow" concept).

Strong support for the overflow theory came from the extensive and carefully designed experiments by Levy and co-workers in dogs with experimental cirrhosis (see review by Levy[722] and references therein). They studied sequentially the events that led to Na^+ retention and ascites after the institution of dimethylnitrosamine cirrhosis in the dog. They were also able to measure directly the changes in volume of the vascular compartments after salt retention. These studies indicated that renal Na+ retention and volume expansion may precede formation of ascites by 10 days. The Na+ retention was reported to occur independent of changes in cardiac output, MAP, splanchnic blood volume, hepatic arterial blood flow, GFR, RPF, aldosterone, and increased renal sympathetic nerve activity.[723] Also, elimination of ascites in these cirrhotic dogs with the LeVeen shunt did not prevent salt retention during liberal salt intake. Taken together, these studies supported the view that the initiating event in the renal Na+ retention of cirrhosis is not related to "underfilling." Rather, primary renal Na+ retention has been suggested as a cause.

In a series of additional studies in dogs with experimental cirrhosis, intrahepatic hypertension, secondary to hepatic venous outflow obstruction, was suggested to be of primary importance in the induction of salt retention by the kidney.[724] In dogs with cirrhosis due to common bile duct ligation and portocaval anastomosis, Levy's group[724] demonstrated that Na+ retention and ascites formation occurred only in dogs with partially or fully occluded portocaval fistulae, but not in dogs with patent portocaval anastomosis and normal intahepatic pressure.

For intrahepatic hypertension to act as a primary stimulus for renal Na+ retention, without the intermediary of underfilling, it is necessary to invoke the hepatic volume-sensing mechanisms mentioned earlier in this chapter. In particular, a sensing mechanism that specifically responds to elevated hepatic venous pressure with increased hepatic afferent nerve activity could be a candidate. The relays for these impulses consist of two hepatic autonomic nerve plexuses, one surrounding the hepatic artery and the other the portal vein. Kostreva and co-workers[725] delineated a neural reflex pathway composed of these elements that connects hepatic venous congestion to enhanced renal and cardiopulmonary sympathetic activity. Occlusion of the inferior vena cava at the diaphragm was associated with a rise in hepatic, portal, and renal venous pressures and resulted in markedly increased hepatic afferent nerve traffic and renal and cardiopulmonary sympathetic efferent nerve activity. Section of the anterior hepatic nerves eliminated the reflex increase in renal efferent nerve activity.[725] Similarly, Levy and Wexler[61] showed that denervation of the liver of dogs with vena cava constriction increases urinary Na+ excretion. Such neural networks, or alternatively other, as yet undefined humoral pathways, could provide an anatomic or physiologic basis for the primary effects of alterations in intrahepatic hemodynamics on renal function. This mechanism implies that renal Na+ retention could be a consequence of disturbed hepatic function, independent of input from extrahepatic volume sensors. As a result, renal Na+ retention would occur without reduction and possibly in the face of expansion of all vascular compartments.

In contrast, the classic "underfilling" theory suggested that, during the development of cirrhosis, true hypovolemia may occur as a result of transudation of fluid and its accumulation in the peritoneal cavity, mostly in the form of ascites. As a result, true intravascular hypovolemia develops, which, in turn, is sensed by the various components of the afferent volume control system described in previous sections of this chapter. The kidney then responds normally to the perceived hypovolemia by increasing Na+ and water reabsorption along the nephron, through activation of the efferent limb of the volume control system. This response includes activation of the RAAS and the SNS, as well as the nonosmotic release of ADH. This sequence of events results in enhanced renal water and Na+ retention, failure to escape from the Na+-retaining effect of aldosterone, and an impaired capacity to excrete solute-free water. However, such a mechanism would eventually result in further accumulation of Na+ and water and the development of positive Na+ balance.

Several mechanisms were offered to account for the development of the hypovolemia. One such mechanism arose as a consequence of the disruption in the normal Starling relationships that govern fluid movement in the hepatic sinusoids. These, unlike capillaries elsewhere in the body, are highly permeable to plasma proteins. As a result, partitioning of ECF between the intravascular (intrasinusoidal) and the interstitial (space of Disse and lymphatic) compartments of the liver is determined predominantly by the hydraulic pressure gradient along the length of the hepatic sinusoids. Obstruction to hepatic venous outflow promotes enhanced efflux of a protein-rich filtrate into the space of Disse and results in augmented hepatic lymph formation. Such augmented hepatic lymph flow, the main source of ascites formation, has been observed in human subjects with cirrhosis as well as in experimental models of liver disease. Vastly increased hepatic lymph formation is accompanied by increased flow through the thoracic duct. When the rate of enhanced hepatic lymph formation exceeds the capacity for return to the intravascular compartment via the thoracic duct, hepatic lymph accumulates in the form of ascites and the intravascular compartment is further compromised. As liver disease progresses, a fibrotic process surrounds the Kupffer cells lining the sinusoids, rendering the sinusoids less permeable to serum proteins. Under such circumstances, termed *capillarization of sinusoids,* a decrease in oncotic pressure also promotes transudation of ECF within the hepatic lymph space, much as it does in other vascular beds.

Additional consequences of intrahepatic hypertension have also been postulated to contribute to perceived volume contraction. Among these, transmission of elevated intrasinusoidal pressures to the portal vein leads to expansion of the splanchnic venous system, collateral vein formation, and portosystemic shunting. This results in increased vascular capacitance and diversion of blood flow from the arterial circuit.[726] Vasodilatation was believed to occur not only in the splanchnic circulation but in the systemic circulation as well and was attributed to refractoriness to the pressor effects of vasoconstrictor hormones such as AII and catecholamines, probably due to an as-yet-undefined uncoupling effect of bile salts.[727]

Along with diminished hepatic reticuloendothelial cell function, portosystemic shunting allows various products of intestinal metabolism and absorption to bypass the liver and escape hepatic elimination. Among these, endotoxins have been considered to contribute to perturbations in renal function in cirrhosis, possibly secondary to the hemodynamic consequences of endotoxemia or through direct renal effects.[728]

Elevated levels of conjugated bilirubin and bile acids may result from intrahepatic cholestasis or extrahepatic biliary obstruction. In experimental studies of bile duct ligation, it is difficult to distinguish the effects on renal function of jaundice itself from the effects of cirrhosis that ensue after the bile duct ligation. However, it has been shown that bile acids actually decrease proximal tubular reabsorption of Na+, a direct renal action that would tend to promote natriuresis.[729] Nevertheless, the diuretic-like effect of bile salts may also contribute to the underfilling state in cirrhotic patients.[729,730]

Hypoalbuminemia was proposed as another factor that could contribute to the development of hypovolemia, by diminishing the colloid osmotic forces in the systemic capillaries and hepatic sinusoids. Hypoalbuminemia was believed to occur as a result of decreased synthesis of albumin by the liver as well as dilution caused by ECF volume expansion. The development of hypoalbuminemia is a relatively late event in the course of chronic liver disease.

Likewise, a relative impairment of cardiac function could contribute to diminished arterial blood pressure in some cirrhotic patients.[730–732] Thus, in some patients, tense ascites

TABLE 12–7	Possible Etiologic Factors Causing "Underfilling" of the Circulation in Patients With Cirrhosis

Peripheral vasodilatation and blunted vasoconstrictor response to reflex, chemical, and hormonal influences

Opening arteriovenous shunts, particularly in the portal circulation

Increase in the vascular capacity of the portal as well as the nonportal circulation

Hypoalbuminemia

Impaired left ventricular performance, "cirrhotic cardiomyopathy"

Diminished venous return secondary to advanced tense ascites

Occult gastrointestinal bleeding from ulcers, gastritis, or varices

Volume losses due to vomiting and excessive use of diuretics

reduce venous return (preload) to the heart. Other factors in patients with chronic liver disease may adversely affect cardiac performance, and the concomitant cardiac dysfunction has been termed *cirrhotic cardiomyopathy,* although the mechanisms behind the cardiac abnormalities are only partly understood.[731,732]

Finally, volume depletion in cirrhotic patients may be aggravated by vomiting, occult variceal bleeding, and excessive use of diuretics. It is not surprising, therefore, that patients with cirrhosis tolerate hemorrhage or fluid loss very poorly, and they are prone to suffer cardiovascular collapse in the setting of hemodynamic disturbances.

Table 12–7 summarizes the various etiologic factors contributing to underfilling of the circulation in patients with advanced liver disease.

Two major arguments have been provided in support of the traditional underfilling theory. First, the progression of cirrhosis is characterized by increased neurohumoral activity with stimulation of the RAAS, increased sympathetic activity, and elevated plasma ADH levels. These classic markers of hypovolemia could not be explained by the overflow hypothesis. Second, a salutary improvement in volume homeostasis was observed after volume replenishment in these patients. For example, volume expansion could suppress the RAAS, increase the GFR, and cause a natriuresis and a negative salt balance in patients with cirrhosis. Indeed, several maneuvers of volume expansion, such as reinfusion of ascitic fluid, placement of peritoneojugular LeVeen shunt, HWI, were found to cause a brisk diuretic/natriuretic response in patients with cirrhosis, thus supporting the underfilling concept. Conversely, the main argument against the underfilling theory was that actual measurements of volume content in body fluid compartments failed to show true hypovolemia in most patients with compensated cirrhosis. In fact, when plasma volume was measured in patients with cirrhosis, it was found to be increased, and this increase in many circumstances antedated the formation of ascites.[716] In addition, although volume repletion by diverse measures, as described previously, could result in a dramatic improvement and natriuresis, such an improvement is at best temporary and occurs only in a subset of affected patients. Only 30% to 50% of cirrhotic patients exhibit natriuresis during volume expansion or HWI, although the latter procedure effectively suppresses the RAAS. Some of the variability could be due to the fact that the degree of volume replenishment achieved was inadequate in those who failed to respond. Nevertheless, it appears that underfilling cannot be the entire explanation

for the renal Na^+ and water retention that characterizes the cirrhotic patient. Moreover, it may occur only in a limited proportion of patients with cirrhosis, perhaps at a specific stage of their disease.

"Peripheral Arterial Vasodilatation Hypothesis" and the Hyperdynamic Circulation of Cirrhosis

In 1988, Schrier and associates[715] proposed that primary peripheral vasodilatation, initially in the splanchnic vascular bed and later in the systemic circulation, leads to a "relative underfilling" of the arterial circulation. As a result of the discrepancy between the blood volume and the capacitance of the arterial circulation, this perceived underfilling unloads the arterial high-pressure baroreceptors as well as other volume receptors, which, in turn, stimulate a compensatory neurohumoral response. The latter includes activation of the RAAS and the SNS, as well as the nonosmotic release of ADH.[383,715,717,733] The "relative" rather than the "absolute" underfilling leads to the apparent decrease in the effective arterial blood volume (EABV) and initiates the compensatory neurohumoral response. According to this theory, the main mechanism initiating the abnormal Na^+ and water retention and ascites formation is splanchnic vasodilatation.[715] Thus, increased hepatic resistance to portal flow causes a gradual development of portal hypertension, collateral vein formation, and shunting of blood to the systemic circulation. As portal hypertension develops, local production of vasodilators, mainly NO, increases, leading to splanchnic vasodilatation.[715,719] In the early stages of cirrhosis, arterial pressure is maintained through increases in plasma volume and cardiac output, in the form of a "hyperdynamic" circulation. However, as the disease progresses, vasodilatation in the splanchnic vascular bed, and presumably in other vascular beds, is so pronounced that EABV decreases markedly, leading to a sustained neurohumoral activation that further results in Na^+ and fluid retention.[715,734] This hypothesis could, therefore, potentially explain the increased cardiac output and the enhanced neurohumoral changes over the entire spectrum of cirrhosis.[716] Moreover, it is now believed that the vasodilatation in cirrhotic patients is not confined only to the splanchnic circulation but may occur in other vascular beds, such as the peripheral systemic and pulmonary circulations as well.[720] Thus, decreases in SVR associated with low arterial blood pressure and high cardiac output are clinical manifestations of the hyperdynamic circulation that are commonly seen in patients with cirrhosis. Indeed, the combination of "warm extremities, cutaneous vascular spiders, wide pulse pressure, and capillary pulsations in the nail bed" has been known in cirrhotic patients from the early 1950s.[718,720]

Pulmonary vasodilatation, associated with the hepatopulmonary syndrome, one of the most severe complications of chronic liver disease, may also be a considered an example of the hyperdynamic circulation caused by increased production of NO (and possibly also carbon monoxide [CO]) in the lung.[720,735] It has been also suggested that the hepatorenal syndrome may develop when the heart is not able to compensate any longer for the progressive decrease in peripheral resistance.[736] Thus, the hyperdynamic syndrome of chronic liver disease should be considered as a "progressive vasodilatory syndrome" that finally leads to multiorgan involvement, as suggested recently by Iwasaki and Groszmann.[720] As pointed out earlier, increased production of NO in the splanchnic vasculature plays a cardinal role in initiating this process.

Role of Nitric Oxide in the Hyperdynamic Circulation of Cirrhosis

Considerable evidence now indicates that aberrations in the endothelial vasodilator NO system are involved in the pathogenesis of the hyperdynamic circulation and Na^+ and water retention in cirrhosis.[716,719,720,737] NO is produced in excess by the vasculature of different animal models of portal hypertension, when measured by various methods,[738-740] as well as in cirrhotic patients.[741-743] In the carbon tetrachloride rat model of cirrhosis, this increased production of NO can be detected early in the course of the disease. Niederberger and colleagues[740] demonstrated that cGMP, the intracellular messenger of NO, was already increased in the aorta of cirrhotic rats without ascites when the cirrhotic rats begin to retain Na[+]. This increased vascular NO production is supported by in vitro or combined in vivo and in vitro studies that have demonstrated an increased production of NO by the vessels of cirrhotic animals and a role for NO in the impaired vascular responsiveness to vasoconstrictors.[744,745] Moreover, removal of the vascular endothelial layer has been demonstrated to abolish the difference in vascular reactivity between cirrhotic and control vessels.

Inhibition of NOS has beneficial effects in experimental models of cirrhosis. Niederberger and colleagues[746] reversed the high NO production in cirrhotic rats with ascites to normal control levels, by using 7 days of low-dose L-NAME treatment. This normalization of NO production corrected the hyperdynamic circulation. Further studies confirmed that normalization of NO production was accompanied by a marked increase in urinary Na[+] and water excretion and a concomitant decrease of ascites in cirrhotic rats.[747] These effects of NO inhibition and reversal of the hyperdynamic circulation were associated with a decrease in PRA and in the concentrations of aldosterone and vasopressin.

In patients with cirrhosis, the vascular hyporesponsiveness of the forearm circulation to noradrenaline has been shown to be reversed by the administration of the NOS inhibitor, L-NMMA, further supporting the increased vascular synthesis of NO in cirrhosis.[748] Inhibition of NO production also corrected the hypotension of cirrhosis. Similar observations, namely, correction of the hyperdynamic circulatory syndrome by inhibition of NOS activity, were reported in a more recent study in patients with compensated cirrhosis.[749] An improvement in renal function and Na[+] excretion was also observed in these patients, as well as a decrease in plasma NE levels.

The main source of the increased systemic vascular NO generation in cirrhosis has been demonstrated to be eNOS in the arterial and splanchnic circulations.[719,750] The up-regulation of eNOS appears to be, at least in part, caused by increased shear stress as a result of portal venous hypertension with increased flow in the splanchnic circulation.[719,720,737] However, in the rat with portal vein ligation, eNOS up-regulation and increased NO release in the superior mesenteric arteries were found to precede the development of the hyperdynamic splanchnic circulation.[751,752]

Interestingly, in contrast to the increased NO generation in the splanchnic and systemic circulation, there is also evidence for impaired NO production and "endothelial dysfunction" in the intrahepatic microcirculation in cirrhotic rats.[737,753,754] The mechanisms of this paradoxical behavior of the intrahepatic vascular bed is unknown. However, it has been speculated that this "intrahepatic endothelial dysfunction" and NO deficiency may play a significant role in the pathogenesis of the increased hepatic vascular resistance, as well as in the increased intrahepatic thrombosis and collagen synthesis in cirrhosis (for review, see Wiest and Groszman[737]). Indeed, it is currently believed that the increase in intrahepatic vascular resistance is not merely due to mechanical distortion of the vasculature by fibrosis. Rather, a dynamic process, due to contraction of myofibroblasts and stellate cells, is believed to determine the degree of intrahepatic vascular resistance.[712,737] The decrease in NO production due to endothelial dysfunction may shift the balance in favor of vasocostictors (ET, leukotrienes, thromboxane A_2, AII,

etc.), thus causing an increase in intrahepatic vascular resistance.[737] Indeed, studies utilizing in vivo gene transfer techniques, for delivery of either eNOS or neuronal NOS (nNOS), to livers of rats with experimental cirrhosis, showed that this maneuver is associated with a decrease in portal hyprtension.[755,756]

It has been clearly shown that eNOS protein is increased in animal models of portal hypertension and that this increase is already detectable in cirrhotic rats without ascites.[737,757] However, Iwakiri and co-workers[758] demonstrated that mice with targeted deletion of eNOS alone, or with combined deletion of eNOS and iNOS, may develop a hyperdynamic circulation associated with portal hypertension. The latter finding suggests that other vasodilatory agents may be activated in these mice. Indeed, some evidence indicates that PGI_2,[759] endothelium-derived hyperpolarizing factor (EDHF),[760] CO,[761] AM,[762] and other vasodilators may participate in the pathogenesis of the hyperdynamic circulation in experimental cirrhosis (see Iwakiri and Groszmann[720]).

Some evidence also suggests that another isoform of NOS, nNOS, may be involved in the generation of the hyperdynamic circulation and fluid retention in experimental cirrhosis.[763] Increased expression of nNOS has recently been suggested to partially compensate for the endothelial isoform deficiency in the eNOS knockout mice.[764] In contrast, the role of iNOS remains controversial. Vallance and Moncada[765] postulated that endotoxin-mediated induction of iNOS might play a role in the pathogenesis of the arterial vasodilation in cirrhosis. However, in more recent studies, the results were inconclusive, with some groups showing an increased iNOS in arteries of animals with experimental biliary cirrhosis[766] but not in other forms of experimental cirrhosis.[750,757] Although nonspecific inhibition of NOS may correct the hyperdynamic circulation, use of drugs that preferentially inhibit iNOS and cytokine production has shown varying results, ranging from an amelioration[767] to no effect.[744]

Several cellular mechanisms have been implicated in the up-regulation of eNOS activity in experimental cirrhosis. Elevated shear stress due to the hyperdynamic circulation and portal hypertension may be involved, because this is a well-documented mechanism that up-regulates transcription of the eNOS gene. However, it is believed that additional factors related to the hepatic dysfunction could further stimulate this up-regulation. For example, the activity of eNOS may be regulated at a post-transcripional level by tetrahydrobiopterin (BH_4).[768] It has been shown in rats with experimental cirrhosis that circulating endotoxins may increase the enzymatic production of BH_4, thereby enhancing the activity of eNOS in the mesenteric vascular bed.[769] Evidence also indicates that the activity of eNOS in experimental cirrhosis may be modulated by protein-protein interactions, for example, caveolin[754] and heat-shock protein 90 (HSP90),[770] as well as by direct phosphorylation of eNOS protein.[771] However, the relative contribution of the latter mechanisms to the activation of eNOS in cirrhosis remains to be determined.

Efferent Limb of Volume Homeostasis in Cirrhosis: Abnormalities in Effector Humoral Mechanisms

The efferent limb of the volume regulation in cirrhosis consists of factors similar to those described in CHF. Neurohumoral activation and alterations in circulating levels of vasoactive substances are believed to play a major role in promoting the enhanced Na[+] and water reabsorption by the kidney.[711,712,716-718,772,773] The RAAS and the SNS, together with ANP, are considered to be the main endogenous neurohumoral systems involved in Na[+] and volume homeostasis in this disease state. There is, however, evidence that other systems, such as renal PGs and ET, might contribute as well.

Vasoconstrictive and Antinatriuretic Systems

RENIN-ANGIOTENSIN-ALDOSTERONE SYSTEM. The renal and extrarenal sites and actions of AII and aldosterone that promote renal Na$^+$ retention were considered in previous sections of this chapter. Extrarenal vascular, glomerular microcirculatory, and direct tubular actions are all involved and are mutually interdependent. Both clinical and experimental evidence suggest that the RAAS contributes to Na$^+$ and fluid retention in cirrhosis. Indeed, elevated PRA and aldosterone levels were noted in parallel with the progressive severity of cirrhosis and the increase in Na$^+$ retention. In humans, activation of the RAAS is more commonly noted in patients with ascites than in preascitic patients. It was, therefore, assumed that activation of the RAAS occurs in a relatively advanced stage of the disease. Studies in animal models of cirrhosis tended, in general, to support this notion by showing the temporal relationship between Na$^+$ retention and activation of RAAS.[774] Whereas there is no doubt that the RAAS plays a dominant role in the mechanism of Na$^+$ retention in patients with cirrhosis and ascites, evidence suggests that increased activity of this system may also contribute earlier, in the preascitic phase of the disease.[775] At this early phase, patients with cirrhosis may develop positive Na$^+$ balance, but their PRA and aldosterone levels are maintained within normal range or even depressed. This finding was believed for years to support the role of the overflow theory in the mechanism of ascites formation. However, Bernardi and co-workers[776] found an elevated aldosterone level in preascitic cirrhotic patients that was inversely correlated with renal Na$^+$ excretion, particularly when the patients were standing. This suggested that aldosterone-dependent, Na$^+$ retention can develop in preascitic cirrhosis during standing and that posture-induced activation of the RAAS could already exist at this stage of the disease. Another study demonstrated that renal Na$^+$ retention induced by LBNP was associated with a prominent increase in renal renin and AII excretion.[777] Moreover, the same group reported that treatment with the AII receptor antagonist losartan at low dose that did not affect systemic and renal hemodynamics or glomerular filtration was associated with a significant natriuretic response.[778] The mechanism by which losartan induced natriuresis in the face of PRA within the normal range was attributed the action of losartan on the local intrarenal RAAS.[778,779] Indeed, it has been demonstrated in rats with chronic bile duct ligation that activation of the intrarenal RAAS may occur prior to the circulating system.[780] In addition, losartan has been shown to cause a decrease in portal pressure in cirrhotic patients with portal hypertension.[781]

The mechanisms of the postural-induced activation of RAAS at this early stage of the disease as well as the beneficial effects of low-dose losartan treatment in these patients require further investigation.

In contrast, in advanced cirrhosis with ascites, attempts to inhibit AII in Na$^+$-retaining cirrhotic patients yielded variable results. Administration of captopril to cirrhotic patients with ascites resulted in a decrease in both GFR and urinary Na$^+$ excretion, even when given in low doses.[782] At this stage of the disease, activation of the RAAS serves to support arterial pressure and maintain adequate circulation. Removal of these actions of the RAAS, either by blocking AII formation or by blocking of its receptor, may lead to deterioration with a profound decrease in RPP. This formulation might be important in the pathogenesis of the hepatorenal syndrome, which is regularly preceded by a state of Na$^+$ retention and may be precipitated by a hypovolemic insult. Abnormalities of the renal circulation characteristic of this syndrome include marked diminution of RPF with renal cortical ischemia and increased RVR, abnormalities consistent with the known actions of AII on the renal microcirculation. It is not surprising, then, that several groups correlated activation of the RAAS with worsening hepatic hemodynamics and decreased survival in patients with cirrhosis. For this reason, ACE inhibitors and ARBs are best avoided in patients with cirrhosis and ascites.

SYMPATHETIC NERVOUS SYSTEM. Activation of the SNS is a common feature in patients with chronic liver disease and cirrhosis with ascites.[783] Circulating NE levels, as well as urinary excretion of catecholamines and their metabolites, are elevated in patients with cirrhosis and usually correlate with the severity of the disease. Moreover, plasma NE in patients with decompensated cirrhosis may reach levels found in ischemic heart disease and is considered to be a grave prognostic sign associated with a high degree of mortality.[783] The source of the increased NE levels is enhanced SNS activity, rather than reduced disposal, with nerve terminal spillover from the liver, heart, kidney, muscle, and cutaneous innervation.[783–785] A causal relationship between the elevated SNS activity and the impaired Na$^+$ and water was suggested by Bichet and associates.[786] In this study, it was demonstrated that increased sympathetic activity, as assessed by plasma levels of NE, correlates closely with Na$^+$ and water retention in cirrhotic patients and thus may be of pathogenetic importance. Evidence also suggests the existence of an increase in efferent renal sympathetic tone in cirrhosis, based on direct recordings in experimental animals, as shown by DiBona and co-workers.[787] The same group also demonstrated a defect in the arterial and cardiopulmonary baroreflex control of renal sympathetic nerve activity, in rats with experimental cirrhosis.[788] This can explain why volume expansion fails to suppress the enhanced renal sympathetic activity in cirrhosis.

Concomitant with the increase in NE release, cardiovascular responsiveness to reflex autonomic stimulation may be impaired in patients with cirrhosis.[789] This includes impaired vasoconstrictor response to a variety of stimuli, such as mental arithmetic, LBNP, and the Valsalva maneuver. This interference in the peripheral and central autonomic nervous system in cirrhosis could be explained partially by increased occupancy of endogenous catecholamine receptors, by down-regulation of the adrenergic receptors, or by a defect at the level of postreceptor signaling.[773,783] It is also possible that the excessive NO-dependent vasodilatation found in cirrhosis could account for the vascular hyporesponsiveness. This assumption is supported by the finding that the hyporesponsiveness to pressor agents is not limited to NE but may be observed in response to AII in patients and experimental animals.[727,790]

It has been also suggested that metabolic derangements due to hepatic dysfunction may be an additional cause for sympathetic overactivity in cirrhosis.[783] In particular, alterations in glucose metabolism, hypoglycemia, and hyperinsulinemia are known to stimulate the activity of the SNS. However, overt hypoglycemia is seldom observed in patients with compensated cirrhosis. Hypoxia is an additional potential factor that may stimulate the SNS in patients with cirrhosis. A negative correlation was found between circulating NE levels and arterial oxygen tension in patients with cirrhosis.[791] Moreover, inhalation of oxygen significantly reduced the circulating levels of NE, suggesting a causal relationship between hypoxia and increased SNS activity in these patients.

The increase in renal sympathetic tone and plasma NE levels could contribute to the antinatriuresis of cirrhosis by decreasing total RBF, or its intrarenal distribution, or by acting directly at the tubular epithelial level to enhance Na$^+$ reabsorption. It is indeed known that patients with compensated cirrhosis may have a decreased RBF even in early stages, and during the progression of the disease, RBF tends to decline further concomitant with the increase in sympathetic activity.[783]

In parallel with the increase in sympathetic activity, patients with progressive cirrhosis show also an increase in the activities of two other important pressor systems, namely, the RAAS and ADH.[716,773] The marked neurohumoral activation that occurs at relatively advanced stages of cirrhosis probably represent a shift toward a decompensation, characterized by a severe decrease in effective blood volume and perhaps true volume depletion. In this setting, activation of the three pressor systems represents an attempt to support mean arterial blood pressure. A correlation also exists between plasma NE and ADH levels, suggesting that the increased activity of the SNS may stimulate the release of ADH.[716,786] A direct relationship also exists between plasma NE and the activity of the RAAS, which may imply that the three systems are activated by the same mechanisms and operate in concert to counteract the low arterial blood pressure and the decrease in effective blood volume.[383,715,716,783]

ANTIDIURETIC HORMONE. Patients with advanced hepatic cirrhosis frequently demonstrate a disturbed capacity to regulate water excretion by the kidney and, consequently, develop water retention with hyponatremia.[716,792] Nonosmotic release of ADH is believed to play a dominant role in the mechanism of water retention and the development of hyponatremia in these patients.[715,717,792]

Bichet and co-workers[793] subjected patients with cirrhosis to a standard oral water load and demonstrated that those who were unable to normally excrete the water load had high immunoreactive levels of ADH compared with those patients who exhibited a normal response. These patients also had higher plasma renin and aldosterone levels and lower urinary Na+ excretion, suggesting that the inability to suppress vasopressin was secondary to a decrease in effective arterial blood volume.[793]

Elevated plasma levels of ADH in association with overexpression of hypothalamic ADH mRNA were found in rats with experimental cirrhosis, together with a diminished pituitary ADH content.[794] This suggests an increased synthesis and release of ADH in this experimental model of cirrhosis. In addition, Fujita and colleagues[795] reported that the expression of AQP II, the ADH-regulated water channel in the collecting duct, was significantly increased in rats with CCl_4-induced cirrhosis. This finding seems to be a consequence of the increased ADH secretion, because blocking of ADH action by an ADH receptor antagonist, OPC-31260, significantly diminished AQP II expression. It is, therefore, possible that up-regulation of AQP II plays an important role in water retention associated with hepatic cirrhosis as well as in other pathologic states.[795]

As noted in a previous section of this chapter, the biologic actions of ADH are mediated through at least two G-protein–coupled receptors. It is believed that ADH supports arterial blood pressure through its action on the V_1 receptors found on the VSMCs, whereas the V_2 receptor is responsible for water transport in the collecting duct.[716,717] The development of selective blockers of these receptors provided clear evidence for the role of ADH in the induction of water abnormalities in cirrhosis.[796] Indeed, compelling evidence now indicates that the administration of a V_2 receptor antagonist to cirrhotic patients increased urine volume and decreased urine osmolality (for review, see Ferguson and colleagues[796]). Serum Na+ concentrations can also be corrected in hyponatremic cirrhotic patients by V_2 receptor antagonists.[214,796] Similarly, in rats with experimental cirrhosis, treatment with selective nonpeptide V_2 receptor antagonists proved to exert beneficial effects by increasing urine flow and decreasing urine osmolality.[797,798] It appears that this new class of aquaretic agents may have important clinical applications in the future in the treatment of patients with liver cirrhosis.

The role of the V_1 receptor was studied by Claria and co-workers[799] in rats with cirrhosis and ascites. They administered a selective antagonist of the vascular effect of vasopressin after blocking the actions of AII with saralasin and demon-strated a pronounced fall in arterial blood pressure. This suggests that ADH, acting via its V_1 receptor, is important for the maintenance of arterial pressure and circulatory integrity in cirrhosis.[799] Moreover, it argues against the use of nonselective ADH receptor antagonists that block both receptor subtypes in patients with cirrhosis.

ADH increases the synthesis of the vasodilatory PGs (PGE_2 and PGI_2) in several vascular beds, including the kidney. This, in turn, may inhibit the vasoconstrictor action as well as the hydro-osmotic effect of ADH. The modulation of ADH effects by PGE_2 is of particular importance in pathophysiologic situations, including cirrhosis. It is known that many patients with cirrhosis and ascites are able to generate positive free water clearance (C_{H_2O}) and dilute the urine after a water load, despite an impaired ability to suppress ADH.[792] Perez-Ayuso and associates[800] offered an explanation for the latter finding by showing that urinary PGE_2 was markedly increased in cirrhotic patients with positive free water clearance. Because PGE_2 inhibits the hydro-osmotic effect of ADH, it was suggested that, in cirrhotic patients with ascites and positive free water clearance, urinary diluting capacity is enhanced after a water load by increased synthesis of PGE_2 in the collecting duct.[792,800]

ENDOTHELINS. Plasma levels of immunoreactive ET (irET) are markedly elevated in patients with cirrhosis and ascites and in the hepatorenal syndrome[801–805] However, the role of ET in the pathogenesis of fluid and Na+ retention in cirrhosis is controversial. Specifically, the causal relationship between an increased level of serum ET and the hemodynamic disturbances in cirrhotic patients (characterized by systemic and splanchnic vasodilation, salt and water retention, and renal vasoconstriction) is still under debate.

Although ETs function as autocrine or paracrine agents by interacting with specific receptors located at or near the site of synthesis, a fraction may be released to the general circulation (spillover), where it can have systemic effects. Indeed, a number of studies have shown that there is a net hepatosplanchnic release of ETs in cirrhosis that correlates positively with portal pressure and cardiac output and inversely with central blood volume.[802,803,806] Increased local intrahepatic production of ET in the liver is also believed to contribute to the development of portal hypertension, probably through contraction of the stellate cells and a concomitant decrease in sinusoidal blood flow.[806]

In an attempt to provide further insight into the pathogenic significance of ET-1 in cirrhosis, Martinet and co-workers[807] measured ET-1 and its precursor, big ET-1, in the systemic circulation as well as in the splanchnic and renal venous beds of patients with cirrhosis and refractory ascites before and after transjugular intrahepatic portosystemic shunt (TIPS) to provide relief of portal hypertension. They found that the blood levels of both peptides were higher in the vena cava, hepatic vein, portal vein, and renal vein of cirrhotic patients compared with normal controls. One to 2 months after the TIPS procedure, creatinine clearance and urinary Na+ excretion increased, accompanied by a significant reduction of ET-1 and big ET-1 in portal and renal veins. The authors suggested that splanchnic and renal hemodynamic changes occurring in patients with cirrhosis and refractory ascites could be related to the production of ET-1 by the splanchnic and renal vascular beds. However, because the status of other hormones (e.g., renin, aldosterone) was altered as well, it is hard to attribute the change in hemodynamic variables after TIPS to an isolated change in the level of ETs. An opposite effect, namely, an increase in plasma ET-1, was recently reported in response to acute temporary occlusion of TIPS by angioplasty balloon, with a transient increase in portal pressure.[808] Interestingly, this was associated with a marked reduction of RPF and increased generation of ET-1 by the kidney.

Because the kidney is uniquely sensitive to the vasoconstrictor effect of ET-1, it was suggested that ET-1 may play an important role in the pathogenesis of the hepatorenal syndrome.[803,804] This is supported by the finding that the high plasma ET-1 levels in patients with the hepatorenal syndrome decreased within 1 week after successful orthotopic liver transplantation and that this decrease in circulating ET-1 was accompanied by an improvement in renal function.[809] Recently, the importance of the intrarenal ET system was demonstrated in a rat model of acute liver failure induced by galactosamine, in which renal failure also develops.[810] This experimental model shares some of the hallmarks of the hepatorenal syndrome in humans, in particular the marked reduction in renal function with normal renal histology. Plasma concentrations of ET-1 were increased twofold following the onset of liver and renal failure, and there was significant up-regulation of the ETA receptor in the renal cortex. Administration of bosentan, a nonselective ET receptor antagonist, prevented the development of renal failure when given before or 24 hours after the onset of liver injury.[810] It is possible that activation of the intrarenal ET system may play a role in the pathogenesis of the hepatorenal syndrome. From that point of view, ET antagonists may represent a potentially beneficial therapy for hepatorenal syndrome.[714] However, at present, not enough clinical evidence exists to support this view.

Vasodilators and Natriuretic Systems

PROSTAGLANDINS. The important contribution of PGs to the maintenance of renal function in cirrhosis was noted in previous sections of this chapter, with regard to their modulating effects on the renal hydro-osmotic effect of ADH. Patients with decompensated cirrhosis with ascites, but without renal failure, excrete greater amounts of vasodilatory PGs than do healthy subjects, suggesting that renal production of PGs is increased.[196,811] Likewise, in experimental animal models of cirrhosis, mostly rats with CCl_4-induced cirrhosis, there is evidence for increased synthesis and activity of renal and vascular PGs.[811,812]

One may conceive of renal PGs as constituting critical modulators of renal function during disease states involving volume contraction. In the setting of decompensated cirrhosis (presence of ascites and increased activity of endogenous vasoconstrictor systems), the ability to enhance PG synthesis constitutes a compensatory or adaptive response to incipient renal ischemia. The corollary of this formulation is that administration of agents that impair such an adaptation by inhibiting PG synthesis might result in a clinically important deterioration of renal function, primarily in patients with low effective blood volume who are retaining Na^+ avidly. Indeed, in several investigations, administration of nonselective inhibitors of COX, such as the NSAIDs indomethacin and ibuprofen, resulted in a significant decrement in GFR and RPF in patients with cirrhosis and ascites, in contrast to healthy subjects. The decrement in renal hemodynamics varies directly with the degree of Na^+ retention and the extent of neurohumoral activation, so that patients with high plasma renin and NE levels are particularly sensitive to these adverse effects.[811,813] However, the deleterious effects of NSAIDs on renal function were also observed in cirrhotic patients without ascites.[196,814]

In contrast to nonazotemic patients with cirrhosis and ascites, it has been suggested that patients with hepatorenal syndrome have reduced renal synthesis of vasodilatory PGs.[815] This renal PG "deficiency" may be an important factor in the pathogenesis of hepatorenal syndrome that exacerbates renal vasoconstriction and Na^+ and fluid retention.[811] Yet, an attempt to improve renal function in these patients by treatment with intravenous infusion of PGE_2 or its oral analog, misoprostol, was unsuccessful.[816]

It is now accepted that renal production of PGs is mediated by two isoforms of COX (i.e., COX-1 and COX-2). In contrast to other organs, both isoforms of COX are constitutively expressed in the kidney, but in different locations (see Chapter 11). It was recently demonstrated, by Western blotting analysis, that the COX-2 isoform is strongly up-regulated in kidneys from rats with CCl_4-induced cirrhosis with ascites.[811] The mechanism(s) responsible for this finding is not clear, although it should be mentioned that up-regulation of COX-2 in the kidney was observed in other situations associated with a decrease in effective arterial blood volume, such as low-salt diet and high-output CHF. Nevertheless, despite the increase in COX-2 expression, it is beleived that maintenance of renal function in cirrhosis is dependent primarily on COX-1-derived PGs.[811] This assumption is based on the finding that administration of SC-236, a selective COX-2 antagonist, spared renal function in cirrhotic rats with ascites, whereas nonselective inhibition of COX led to deterioration in renal function.[811,817] Further support for this notion was obtained recently in cirrhotic patients with ascites treated for a short duration with celecoxib, a selective COX-2 antagonist.[818] It was shown that short-term administration of celecoxib did not impair renal function in nonazotemic patients with cirrhosis and ascites, as opposed to the nonselective COX antagonist naproxen.[818] It should be emphasized that, in these studies, in both patients and experimental animals, administration of the selective COX-2 inhibitor was carried out on a short-term basis. Additional, long-term, studies are required in order to establish the safety of these drugs in patients with advanced cirrhosis.

NATRIURETIC PEPTIDES. Plasma levels of ANP are elevated in patients with cirrhosis, despite the reduction in effective circulating volume in the late stages of the disease.[819,820] In the preascitic stage of cirrhosis, the increase in plasma ANP may be important for the maintenance of Na^+ homeostasis, but with the progression of the disease, the patients develop resistance to the natriuretic action of the peptide.[819,820] Although it was suggested that reduced clearance may contribute to the increased levels of ANP in cirrhosis,[821] it appears that the high levels of ANP reflect mostly an increased cardiac release rather than impaired clearance of the peptide. In particular, intra-atrial processing of pro-ANP was found to be normal in cirrhotic dogs. Cardiac ANP mRNA levels were found to be increased by 2.8 to 4.1 times in cirrhotic rats compared with controls.[822]

The stimulus for increased cardiac ANP synthesis and release in cirrhosis has not been fully clarified. Overfilling of the circulation in early cirrhosis, secondary to intrahepatic hypertension–related renal Na^+ retention, could be responsible for the increased plasma ANP concentrations at these early stages. Indeed, some studies measured increased left atrial size, in association with increased intervascular volume and plasma ANP concentration, in both ascitic and nonascitic alcoholic cirrhosis patients.[823] Wong and co-workers[824] measured central blood volume (CBV), that is, the volume of the cardiac chambers, pulmonary circulation, and thoracic vessels, by radionuclide angiography in patients with cirrhosis. Interestingly, the preascitic patients had a significantly elevated CBV with higher left and right pulmonary volumes, despite having normal blood pressure, and normal renin, aldosterone, and NE levels.[824] Such an increase in CBV may trigger the release of ANP, as shown by numerous HWI studies in the past.[823] More recently, Wong and colleagues[825] examined the status of Na^+ homeostasis in preascitic cirrhosis by investigating renal Na^+ handling in patients with proven cirrhosis without ascites who submitted to a high-Na^+ diet for 5 weeks. The authors demonstrated that high Na^+ intake results in weight gain and positive Na^+ balance for 3 weeks, returning to a complete Na^+ balance thereafter. Thus, despite continued high Na^+ intake, preascitic patients reach a new steady state of Na⁺ balance, thereby preventing fluid retention and the development of ascites. Interestingly, the RAAS and the SNS were suppressed, whereas the ANP concentration was elevated, suggesting that ANP plays an important role in preventing the transition of these patients from the preascitic stage to ascites.[825]

The factors responsible for maintaining relatively high levels of ANP during the later stages of cirrhosis, associated with arterial underfilling, have not been determined. However, ANP levels do not increase further as patients proceed from early compensated to late decompensated stages of cirrhosis.

As pointed out earlier, with the progression of the disease, many patients with cirrhosis and ascites lose their ability to respond normally to exogenous administration of ANP or to the high endogenous levels of the peptide.[819,820] An extensive series of investigations have been done in many laboratories to document and determine the potential basis for this apparent resistance to ANP. Documentation of ANP resistance was obtained in a study by Skorecki and colleagues,[826] who used HWI in a series of patients with cirrhosis. All study subjects experienced with HWI an increase in ANP and in plasma and urinary cGMP, the second messenger for ANP action, but not all subjects responded with a natriuresis. Those who developed natriuresis were termed "responders" as opposed to "nonresponders," who failed to increase urinary Na⁺ excretion. No difference in the cGMP response was observed between the responders and the nonresponders. In subsequent human and animal studies that examined the renal response to volume expansion or to infusion of ANP, a similar heterogeneity of response was observed, with nonresponders experiencing equivalent increases in ANP and cGMP but also tending to have more severe and advanced disease.[827–829] The potential mechanisms responsible for the diminished natriuretic response in this subgroup of patients are discussed later. Nevertheless, the findings suggest that the interference with the natriuretic action of ANP occurs at a late stage of cellular signaling, beyond cGMP production, because both ANP release and cGMP generation in response to HWI remained intact in the nonresponders.

A number of experimental interventions were shown to ameliorate ANP resistance in cirrhosis. These included infusion of endopeptidase inhibitors, BK, kininase II inhibitors, mannitol; renal sympathetic denervation; peritoneovenous shunting; and orthotopic liver transplantation.[830–834] Analysis of these and other studies suggests that antinatriuretic factors counterbalance and overcome the natriuretic effect of ANP in later stages of cirrhosis.[828] In particular, the two best-studied antinatriuretic systems in cirrhosis are the SNS and RAAS. As discussed previously, the activation of the SNS in cirrhosis is characterized by an increase in circulating NE and increased efferent renal nerve sympathetic activity. When excessive, both may lead to a decrease in RPF and excessive proximal reabsorption of Na⁺. Indeed, Koepke and associates[835] demonstrated that renal denervation reversed the blunted diuretic and natriuretic responses to ANP in cirrhotic rats. With respect to the RAAS, excessive activation of the system and failure to suppress the RAAS with HWI or ANP infusion was clearly associated with resistance to the natriuretic effects of ANP.[826] Furthermore, infusion of AII mimicked the nonresponder state by causing patients in the early stages of cirrhosis who still responded to ANP to become unresponsive[836] (Fig. 12–9). This effect of AII infusion was reversible and occurred at both proximal (decreased distal delivery of Na⁺) and distal nephron sites to abrogate ANP-induced natriuresis. The importance of distal Na⁺ delivery was further confirmed in other studies, which showed that the administration of mannitol to increase distal delivery (as measured by lithium clearance) resulted in an improved natriuretic response to ANP.[832,837]

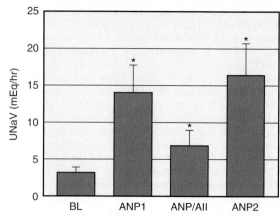

FIGURE 12–9 Effect of antiotensin II (AII) infusion in atrial natriuretic peptide (ANP)–induced natriuresis, showing Na⁺ excretion during the four experimental protocols. Response was defined by a natriuresis greater than 0.83 mmol/hr (20 mmol/day). Note that urinary sodium excretion dropped to almost baseline with combined ANP/AII infusion and returned to ANP levels when AII was discontinued. *P<.05 from previous phase of experiment. ANP/AII, infusion of ANP and AII combined; ANPI, ANP infusion alone; ANP2, ANP alone; BL, baseline. (Adapted from Tobe SW, Blendis LM, Morali GA, et al: Angiotensin II modulates ANP induced natriuresis in cirrhosis with ascites. Am J Kidney Dis 21:472–479, 1993.)

Altogether, five possible factors in ANP resistance were postulated by Warner and colleagues[828]: (1) impaired delivery of salt and water to distal nephron sites that are normally responsive to ANP; (2) the presence of antinatriuretic forces favoring Na⁺ retention that override the natriuretic effects of ANP and its distal site of action in the medullary collecting duct; (3) down-regulation of a population of ANP receptors at a distal nephron site, not reflected in plasma or urinary cGMP concentrations (which are elevated in concert with the elevated ANP); (4) biochemical abnormalities in the biologic responsiveness to ANP at a site parallel to or beyond the level of cGMP production (e.g., enhanced degradation); and (5) decreased delivery or effect of permissive cofactors that allow appropriate ANP action at its distal nephron site (e.g., PGs and kinins; salutary effect of endopeptidase and kininase inhibitors). Most of the current evidence does not favor an abnormality in ANP receptor number or action, but rather favors a combined effect of decreased delivery of Na⁺ to ANP-responsive distal nephron sites (glomerulotubular imbalance due to abnormal systemic hemodynamics and activation of the RAAS) together with an effective antinatriuretic factor overcoming the natriuretic action of ANP at its site of action in the medullary collecting tubule. Therefore, when mannitol was coadministered with ANP to responder patients with cirrhosis, a marked natriuresis was observed, suggesting that increased distal tubular Na⁺ delivery is essential for the expression of the renal actions of ANP.[837] Nonresponder cirrhotic patients did not show increased Na⁺ delivery to the distal tubule in response to a similar maneuver. There was no difference in the increase of urinary cGMP excretion between responders and nonresponders, indicating that the ANP receptors in the collecting duct are not defective.

An overall formulation for the role of ANP in cirrhosis is summarized in Figure 12–10. Na⁺ retention is initiated early in cirrhosis as a result of hepatic venous outflow block or peripheral vasodilatation. In early disease, this results in intravascular volume expansion and a subsequent rise in plasma ANP. This increase is sufficient to counterbalance the antinatriuretic influences, resulting in Na⁺ balance, albeit at the expense of an expanded intravascular volume. Secondary to peripheral vasodilatation, the circulation may become progressively more underfilled at later stages of the disease,

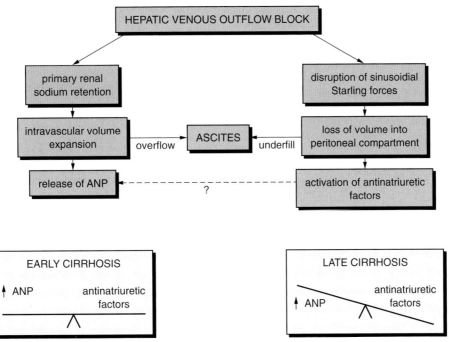

FIGURE 12–10 Working formulation for the role of atrial natriuretic peptide (ANP) in the renal Na⁺ retention of cirrhosis. The primary hepatic abnormality that is necessary and sufficient for renal Na⁺ retention is hepatic venous outflow blockade. In early disease, this signals renal Na⁺ retention with consequent intravascular volume expansion and a compensatory rise in plasma ANP levels. At this stage of disease, the rise in ANP is sufficient to counterbalance the primary antinatriuretic or renal Na⁺-retaining influences; however, it does so at the expense of an expanded intravascular volume with the potential for overflow ascites. With progression of disease, disruption of intrasinusoidal Starling forces and loss of volume from the vascular compartment into the peritoneal compartment occur. This underfilling of the circulation may attenuate further increases in ANP levels and promote the activation of antinatriuretic factors. Whether the antinatriuretic factors activated by underfilling are the same as or different from those that promote primary renal Na⁺ retention in early disease remains to be determined. At this later stage of disease, increased levels of ANP may not be sufficient to counterbalance antinatriuretic forces. (From Warner LC, Leung WM, Campbell P, et al: The role of resistance to atrial natriuretic peptide in the pathogenesis of sodium retention in hepatic cirrhosis. In American Society of Hypertension Series, Vol 3: Advances in Atrial Peptide Research. New York, Raven Press, 1989, pp 185–204.)

thereby activating antinatriuretic factors. With further progression of cirrhosis, a disruption of intrasinusoidal Starling forces occurs, increasing the potential for volume loss into the peritoneal compartment and causing ascites. The underfilling of the circulation may attenuate further increases in ANP levels and promote the activation of antinatriuretic factors. At this later stage of disease, increased levels of ANP may not be sufficient to counterbalance the antinatriuretic influences. ANP resistance ensues, leading to a state of persistently positive Na⁺ balance and clinical decompensation.

BNP levels have also been found to be elevated in patients with cirrhosis and ascites, and similar to ANP, its natriuretic effect is also blunted in cirrhotic patients with Na⁺ retention ascites.[838] Recent findings in patients with nonalcoholic cirrhosis suggest that plasma BNP levels may correlate with the severity of the disease and that BNP might be of prognostic value in the progression of cirrhosis.[839] However, additional studies are required in order to establish the prognostic value of BNP in cirrhosis, as already recognized for CHF.

In summary, two general explanations of Na⁺ retention complicating cirrhosis have been offered. The overflow mechanism of ascites formation in cirrhosis originally offered by Lieberman and Reynolds[721] envisions a volume-independent stimulus for renal Na⁺ retention. Possible mediators include adrenergic reflexes activated by hepatic sinusoidal hypertension and increased systemic concentrations of an unidentified antinatriuretic factor as a result of impaired liver metabolism. The underfilling theory, in contrast, postulates "effective" vascular volume depletion. According to the peripheral arterial vasodilation hypothesis, reduced SVR lowers blood pressure and activates arterial baroreceptors, initiating Na⁺ retention. The retained fluid extravasates from the hypertensive splanchnic circulation, preventing

arterial repletion, and Na⁺ retention and ascites formation continues.

It is quite obvious that neither the underfilling nor the overflow theory can account exclusively for all the observed derangements in volume regulation in cirrhosis. Rather, it is possible that elements of the two concepts may occur simultaneously or sequentially in cirrhosis patients (see Fig. 12–10). Thus, sufficient evidence suggests that, early in cirrhosis, intrahepatic hypertension due to hepatic venous outflow block signals primary renal Na⁺ retention with consequent intravascular volume expansion. Whether, at this stage, underfilling of the arterial circuit consequent to vasodilatation also applies remains to be determined. Owing to expansion of the intrathoracic venous compartment at this stage, plasma ANF levels rise. The rise in ANP levels is sufficient to counterbalance the renal Na⁺ retaining forces; however, it does so at the expense of an expanded intravascular volume, with the potential for overflow ascites. The propensity for the accumulation of volume in the peritoneal compartment and the splanchnic bed results from altered intrahepatic hemodynamics. With progression of disease, there are disruptions of intrasinusoidal Starling forces and loss of volume from the vascular compartment into the peritoneal compartment. These events coupled with other factors such as portosystemic shunting, hypoalbuminemia, and vascular refractoriness to pressor hormones, lead to underfilling of the arterial circuit, without the necessity for measurable underfilling of the venous compartment.

This underfilling of the circulation may attenuate further increases in ANP levels and promote the activation of antinatriuretic factors. Whether these antinatriuretic factors activated by underfilling are the same as or different from those that promote primary renal Na⁺ retention in early disease remains to be determined. At this later stage of disease, elevated levels of ANP may not be sufficient to counterbalance antinatriuretic influences.

It should be noted that, in early cirrhosis, salt retention is isotonic and accompanied by ECF expansion and normonatremia. However, with advancing cirrhosis, defective water excretion supervenes, resulting in hyponatremia, reflecting combined ECF and ICF space expansion. However, it is worth emphasizing that impaired water excretion and hyponatremia in cirrhotic patients with ascites is a marker of the severity of the same accompanying hemodynamic abnormalities that initiate Na^+ retention and eventuate in hepatorenal failure. The pathogenesis is primarily related to nonosmotic stimuli for release of vasopressin acting together with additional factors such as impaired distal Na^+ delivery. It was demonstrated that certain models of hepatic cirrhosis are associated with increased expression of both AQP II mRNA and AQP II immunoreactivity in the collecting duct. These changes in AQP II density may contribute to the positive water balance and hyponatremia in cirrhosis, although additional studies are needed to fully clarify this matter. The development of new aquaretic drugs that are very effective and the correction of the increased production of NO could provide new perspectives in the treatment of renal Na^+ and water retention in cirrhosis.

References

1. Bonventre JV, Leaf A: Sodium homeostasis: Steady states without a set point. Kidney Int 21:880–883, 1982.
2. Reinhardt HW, Seeliger E: Toward an integrative concept of control of total body sodium. News Physiol Sci 15:319–325, 2000.
3. Ali MH, Schumacker PT: Endothelial responses to mechanical stress: Where is the mechanosensor? Crit Care Med 30:S198–S206, 2002.
4. Sumpio BE, Du W, Galagher G, et al: Regulation of PDGF-B in endothelial cells exposed to cyclic strain. Arterioscler Thromb Vasc Biol 18:349–355, 1998.
5. Henry JP, Gauer OH, Reeves JL: Evidence of the atrial location of receptors influencing urine flow. Circ Res 4:85–90, 1956.
6. Goetz KL, Hermreck AS, Slick GL, Starke HS: Atrial receptors and renal function in conscious dogs. Am J Physiol 219:1417–1423, 1970.
7. Epstein M: Renal effects of head-out water immersion in humans: A 15-year update. Physiol Rev 72:563–621, 1992.
8. Miller JA, Floras JS, Skorecki KL, et al: Renal and humoral responses to sustained cardiopulmonary baroreceptor deactivation in humans. Am J Physiol 260:R642–R648, 1991.
9. Wurzner G, Chiolero A, Maillard M, et al: Renal and neurohormonal responses to increasing levels of lower body negative pressure in men. Kidney Int 60:1469–1476. 2001.
10. Cooke WH, Ryan KL, Convertino VA: Lower body negative pressure as a model to study progression to acute hemorrhagic shock in humans. J Appl Physiol 96:1249–1261, 2004.
11. Johansen LB: Hemodilution and natriuresis of intravascular volume expansion in humans. Dan Med Bull 47:283–295, 2000.
12. Cowley AW Jr, Skelton MM: Dominance of colloid osmotic pressure in renal excretion after isotonic volume expansion. Am J Physiol 261:H1214–H1225, 1991.
13. Johansen LB, Pump B, Warberg J, et al: Preventing hemodilution abolishes natriuresis of water immersion in humans. Am J Physiol 275:R879–R888, 1998.
14. Paintal AS: Vagal sensory receptors and their reflex effects. Physiol Rev 53:159–227, 1973.
15. Quail AW, Woods RL, Korner PI: Cardiac and arterial baroreceptor influences in release of vasopressin and renin during hemorrhage. Am J Physiol 252:H1120–H1126, 1987.
16. DiBona GF, Sawin LL: Renal nerve activity in conscious rats during volume expansion and depletion. Am J Physiol 248:F15–F23, 1985.
17. Myers BD, Peterson C, Molina C, et al: Role of cardiac atria in the human renal response to changing plasma volume. Am J Physiol 254:F562–F573, 1988.
18. Tidgren B, Hjemdahl P, Theodorsson E, Nussberger J: Renal responses to lower body negative pressure in humans. Am J Physiol 259:F573–F579, 1990.
19. Convertino VA, Ludwig DA, Elliott JJ, Wade CE: Evidence for central venous pressure resetting during initial exposure to microgravity. Am J Physiol Regul Integr Comp Physiol 281:R2021–R2028, 2001.
20. Kaczmarczyk G, Schmidt E: Sodium homeostasis in conscious dogs after chronic cardiac denervation. Am J Physiol 258:F805–F811, 1990.
21. Braith RW, Mills RM Jr, Wilcox CS, et al: Fluid homeostasis after heart transplantation: The role of cardiac denervation. J Heart Lung Transplant 15:872–880, 1996.
22. de Bold AJ, Borenstein HB, Veress AT, Sonnenberg H: A rapid and potent natriuretic response to intravenous injection of atrial myocardial extract in rats. Life Sci 28:89–94, 1981.
23. de Bold AJ, de Bold ML: Determinants of natriuretic peptide production by the heart: Basic and clinical implications. J Investig Med 53:371–377, 2005.
24. Beltowski J, Wojcicka G: Regulation of renal tubular sodium transport by cardiac natriuretic peptides: Two decades of research. Med Sci Monit 8:RA39–RA52, 2002.
25. Levin ER, Gardner DG, Samson WK: Natriuretic peptides. N Engl J Med 339:321–328, 1998.
26. Kuhn M: Molecular physiology of natriuretic peptide signalling. Basic Res Cardiol 99:76–82, 2004.
27. Espiner EA, Richards AM, Yandle TG, Nicholls MG: Natriuretic hormones. Review. Endocrinol Metab Clin North Am 24:1481–509, 1995.
28. Cho KW, Kim SH, Seul KH, et al: Effect of extracellular calcium depletion on the two-step ANP secretion in perfused rabbit atria. Regul Pept 52:129–137, 1994.
29. Kim SH, Cho KW, Chang SH, et al: Glibenclamide suppresses stretch-activated ANP secretion: Involvements of K+ATP channels and L-type Ca_2^+ channel modulation. Pflugers Arch 434:362–372, 1997.
30. Bie P, Wamberg S, Kjolby M: Volume natriuresis vs. pressure natriuresis. Acta Physiol Scand 181:495–503, 2004.
31. Lohmeier TE, Mizelle HL, Reinhart GA: Role of atrial natriuretic peptide in long-term volume homeostasis. Clin Exp Pharmacol Physiol 22:55–61, 1995.
32. Singer DR, Markandu ND, Buckley MG, et al: Contrasting endocrine responses to acute oral compared with intravenous sodium loading in normal humans. Am J Physiol 274:F111–F119, 1998.
33. Andersen LJ, Norsk P, Johansen LB, et al: Osmoregulatory control of renal sodium excretion after sodium loading in humans. Am J Physiol 275:R1833–R1842, 1998.
34. Andersen LJ, Andersen JL, Pump B, Bie P: Natriuresis induced by mild hypernatremia in humans. Am J Physiol Regul Integr Comp Physiol 282:R1754–R1761, 2002.
35. John SW, Veress AT, Honrath U, et al: Blood pressure and fluid-electrolyte balance in mice with reduced or absent ANP. Am J Physiol 271:R109–R114, 1996.
36. Kuhn M: Cardiac and intestinal natriuretic peptides: Insights from genetically modified mice. Peptides 26:1078–1085, 2005.
37. Gorman AJ, Chen JS: Reflex inhibition of plasma renin activity by increased left ventricular pressure in conscious dogs. Am J Physiol 256:R1299–R1307, 1989.
38. Drinkhill MJ, McMahon NC, Hainsworth R: Delayed sympathetic efferent responses to coronary baroreceptor unloading in anaesthetized dogs. J Physiol (Lond) 497:261–269, 1996.
39. Chapleau MW, Li Z, Meyrelles SS, et al: Mechanisms determining sensitivity of baroreceptor afferents in health and disease. Ann N Y Acad Sci 940:1–19, 2001.
40. Parati G, Di Rienzo M, Mancia G: Dynamic modulation of baroreflex sensitivity in health and disease. Ann N Y Acad Sci 940:469–487, 2001.
41. Epstein FH, Post RS, McDowell M: The effects of an arteriovenous fistula on renal hemodynamics and electrolyte excretion. J Clin Invest 32:233–241, 1953.
42. Andresen MC, Doyle MW, Jin YH, Bailey TW: Cellular mechanisms of baroreceptor integration at the nucleus tractus solitarius. Ann N Y Acad Sci 940:132–141, 2001.
43. Dean C, Seagard JL: Mapping of carotid baroreceptor subtype projections to the nucleus tractus solitarius using c-fos immunohistochemistry. Brain Res 758:201–208, 1997.
44. Creager MA, Roddy MA, Holland KM, et al: Sodium depresses arterial baroreceptor reflex function in normotensive humans. Hypertension 17:989–996, 1991.
45. Navar LG: Integrating multiple paracrine regulators of renal microvascular dynamics. Am J Physiol 274:F433–F444, 1998.
46. Schnermann J: Juxtaglomerular cell complex in the regulation of renal salt excretion. Am J Physiol 274:R263–R279, 1998.
47. Schnermann J: Homer W. Smith Award lecture. The juxtaglomerular apparatus: From anatomical peculiarity to physiological relevance. J Am Soc Nephrol 14:1681–1694, 2003.
48. Persson AE, Ollerstam A, Liu R, Brown R: Mechanisms for macula densa cell release of renin. Acta Physiol Scand 181:471–474, 2004.
49. DiBona GF: Nervous kidney. Interaction between renal sympathetic nerves and the renin-angiotensin system in the control of renal function. Hypertension 36:1083–1088, 2000.
50. Bolanos L, Colina I, Purroy A: Intracerebroventricular infusion of hypertonic NaCl increases urinary cGMP in healthy and cirrhotic rats. Arch Physiol Biochem 107:323–333, 1999.
51. Hansell P, Isaksson B, Sjoquist M: Renal dopamine and noradrenaline excretion during CNS-induced natriuresis in spontaneously hypertensive rats: Influence of dietary sodium. Acta Physiol Scand 168:257–266, 2000.
52. DiBona GF: Central angiotensin modulation of baroreflex control of renal sympathetic nerve activity in the rat: Influence of dietary sodium. Acta Physiol Scand 177:285–289, 2003.
53. McCann SM, Franci CR, Favaretto AL, et al: Neuroendocrine regulation of salt and water metabolism. Braz J Med Biol Res 30:427–441, 1997.
54. Antunes-Rodrigues J, de Castro M, Elias LL, et al: Neuroendocrine control of body fluid metabolism. Physiol Rev 84:169–208, 2004.
55. Carey RM: Evidence for a splanchnic sodium input monitor regulating renal sodium excretion in man. Lack of dependence upon aldosterone. Circ Res 43:19–23, 1978.
56. Hosomi H, Morita H: Hepatorenal and hepatointestinal reflexes in sodium homeostasis. News Physiol Sci 11:103–107, 1996.
57. Morita H, Matsuda T, Tanaka K, Hosomi H: Role of hepatic receptors in controlling body fluid homeostasis. Jpn J Physiol 45:355–368, 1995.
58. Morita H, Nishida Y, Hosomi H: Neural control of urinary sodium excretion during hypertonic NaCl load in conscious rabbits: Role of renal and hepatic nerves and baroreceptors. J Auton Nerv Syst 34:157–169, 1991.
59. Morita H, Ohyama H, Hagiike M, et al: Effects of portal infusion of hypertonic solution on jejunal electrolyte transport in anesthetized dogs. Am J Physiol 259:R1289–R1294, 1990.
60. Morita H, Fujiki N, Hagiike M, et al: Functional evidence for involvement of bumetanide-sensitive $Na^+K^+2Cl^-$ cotransport in the hepatoportal Na^+ receptor of the Sprague-Dawley rat. Neurosci Lett 264:65–68, 1999.

61. Levy M, Wexler MJ: Sodium excretion in dogs with low-grade caval constriction: Role of hepatic nerves. Am J Physiol 253:F672–F678, 1987.

62. Koyama S, Kanai K, Aibiki M, Fujita T: Reflex increase in renal nerve activity during acutely altered portal venous pressure. J Auton Nerv Syst 23:55–62, 1988.

63. Andersen LJ, Jensen TU, Bestle MH, Bie P: Gastrointestinal osmoreceptors and renal sodium excretion in humans. Am J Physiol Regul Integr Comp Physiol 278:R287–R294, 2000.

64. Forte LR, London RM, Krause WJ, Freeman RH: Mechanisms of guanylin action via cyclic GMP in the kidney. Annu Rev Physiol 62:673–695, 2000.

65. Forte LR, London RM, Freeman RH, Krause WJ: Guanylin peptides: Renal actions mediated by cyclic GMP. Am J Physiol Renal Physiol 278:F180–F191, 2000.

66. Forte LR Jr: Uroguanylin: Physiological role as a natriuretic hormone. J Am Soc Nephrol 16:291–292, 2005.

67. Sindic A, Schlatter E: Cellular effects of guanylin and uroguanylin. J Am Soc Nephrol 17:607–616, 2006.

68. Currie MG, Fok KF, Kato J, et al: Guanylin: An endogenous activator of intestinal guanylate cyclase. Proc Natl Acad Sci U S A 89:947–951, 1992.

69. Hamra FK, Forte LR, Eber SL, et al: Uroguanylin: Structure and activity of a second endogenous peptide that stimulates intestinal guanylate cyclase. Proc Natl Acad Sci U S A 90:10464–10468, 1993.

70. Sindic A, Schlatter E: Mechanisms of actions of guanylin peptides in the kidney. Pflugers Arch 450:283–291, 2005.

71. Lorenz JN, Nieman M, Sabo J, et al: Uroguanylin knockout mice have increased blood pressure and impaired natriuretic response to enteral NaCl load. J Clin Invest 112:1244–1254, 2003.

72. Brenner BM, Troy JL: Postglomerular vascular protein concentration: Evidence for a causal role in governing fluid reabsorption and glomerulotublar balance by the renal proximal tubule. J Clin Invest 50:336–349, 1971.

73. Ichikawa I, Brenner BM: Mechanism of inhibition of proximal tubule fluid reabsorption after exposure of the rat kidney to the physical effects of expansion of extracellular fluid volume. J Clin Invest 64:1466–1474, 1979.

74. Skorecki KL, Brenner BM: Body fluid homeostasis in man. A contemporary overview. Am J Med 70:77–88, 1981.

75. Ichikawa I, Brenner BM: Importance of efferent arteriolar vascular tone in regulation of proximal tubule fluid reabsorption and glomerulotubular balance in the rat. J Clin Invest 65:1192–1201, 1980.

76. Imai M, Kokko JP: Effect of peritubular protein concentration on reabsorption of sodium and water in isolated perfused proximal tubules. J Clin Invest 51:314–325, 1972.

77. Garcia NH, Ramsey CR, Knox FG: Understanding the role of paracellular transport in the proximal tubule. News Physiol Sci 13:38–43, 1998.

78. Schneeberger EE, Lynch RD: The tight junction: A multifunctional complex. Am J Physiol Cell Physiol 286:C1213–C1228, 2004.

79. Van Itallie CM, Anderson JM: The molecular physiology of tight junction pores. Physiol (Bethesda) 19:331–338, 2004.

80. Yu AS: Claudins and epithelial paracellular transport: The end of the beginning. Curr Opin Nephrol Hypertens 12:503–509, 2003.

81. Kiuchi-Saishin Y, Gotoh S, Furuse M, et al: Differential expression patterns of claudins, tight junction membrane proteins, in mouse nephron segments. J Am Soc Nephrol 13:875–886, 2002.

82. Enck AH, Berger UV, Yu AS: Claudin-2 is selectively expressed in proximal nephron in mouse kidney. Am J Physiol Renal Physiol 281:F966–F974, 2001.

83. Berry CA, Rector FC Jr: Mechanism of proximal NaCl reabsorption in the proximal tubule of the mammalian kidney. Semin Nephrol 11:86–97, 1991.

84. Seldin DW, Preisig PA, Alpern RJ: Regulation of proximal reabsorption by effective arterial blood volume. Semin Nephrol 11:212–219, 1991.

85. Romano G, Favret G, Damato R, Bartoli E: Proximal reabsorption with changing tubular fluid inflow in rat nephrons. Exp Physiol 83:35–48, 1998.

86. Schafer JA: Transepithelial osmolality differences, hydraulic conductivities, and volume absorption in the proximal tubule. Annu Rev Physiol 52:709–726, 1990.

87. Andreoli TE: An overview of salt absorption by the nephron. J Nephrol 12(suppl 2):S3–S15, 1999.

88. Jamison RL, Sonnenberg H, Stein JH: Questions and replies: Role of the collecting tubule in fluid, sodium, and potassium balance. Am J Physiol Renal Physiol 237:F247–F261, 1979.

89. Earley LE, Friedler RM: Changes in renal blood flow and possibly the intrarenal distribution of blood during the natriuresis accompanying saline loading in the dog. J Clin Invest 44:929–941, 1965.

90. Cowley AW Jr: Role of the renal medulla in volume and arterial pressure regulation. Am J Physiol 273:R1–R15, 1997.

91. Navar LG, Majid DS: Interactions between arterial pressure and sodium excretion. Curr Opin Nephrol Hypertens 5:64–71, 1996.

92. Roman RJ, Zou AP: Influence of the renal medullary circulation on the control of sodium excretion. Am J Physiol 265:R963–R973, 1993.

93. Hall JE: The kidney, hypertension, and obesity. Hypertension 41:625–633, 2003.

94. Guyton AC: Blood pressure control—Special role of the kidneys and body fluids. Science 252:1813–1816, 1991.

95. Cowley AW Jr, Mattson DL, Lu S, Roman RJ: The renal medulla and hypertension. Hypertension 25:663–673, 1995.

96. Mattson DL: Importance of the renal medullary circulation in the control of sodium excretion and blood pressure. Am J Physiol Regul Integr Comp Physiol 284:R13–R27, 2003.

97. Granger JP: Pressure natriuresis. Role of renal interstitial hydrostatic pressure. Hypertension 19:I9–I17, 1992;

98. Granger JP, Alexander BT, Llinas M: Mechanisms of pressure natriuresis. Curr Hypertens Rep 4:152–159, 2002.

99. Evans RG, Majid DS, Eppel GA: Mechanisms mediating pressure natriuresis: What we know and what we need to find out. Clin Exp Pharmacol Physiol 32:400–409, 2005.

100. Dos Santos EA, Dahly-Vernon AJ, Hoagland KM, Roman RJ: Inhibition of the formation of EETs and 20-HETE with 1-aminobenzotriazole attenuates pressure natriuresis. Am J Physiol Regul Integr Comp Physiol 287:R58–R68, 2004.

101. Majid DS, Navar LG: Blockade of distal nephron sodium transport attenuates pressure natriuresis in dogs. Hypertension 23:1040–1045, 1994.

102. Kline RL, Liu F: Modification of pressure natriuresis by long-term losartan in spontaneously hypertensive rats. Hypertension 24:467–473, 1994.

103. Cowley AW Jr, Mori T, Mattson D, Zou AP: Role of renal NO production in the regulation of medullary blood flow. Am J Physiol Regul Integr Comp Physiol 284:R1355–R1369, 2003.

104. Salom MG, Lahera V, Miranda-Guardiola F, Romero JC: Blockade of pressure natriuresis induced by inhibition of renal synthesis of nitric oxide in dogs. Am J Physiol 262:F718–F722, 1992.

105. Patel AR, Granger JP, Kirchner KA: L-Arginine improves transmission of perfusion pressure to the renal interstitium in Dahl salt-sensitive rats. Am J Physiol 266:R1730–R1735, 1994.

106. Majid DS, Godfrey M, Grisham MB, Navar LG: Relation between pressure natriuresis and urinary excretion of nitrate/nitrite in anesthetized dogs. Hypertension 25:860–865, 1995.

107. Sarkis A, Lopez B, Roman RJ: Role of 20-hydroxyeicosatetraenoic acid and epoxyeicosatrienoic acids in hypertension. Curr Opin Nephrol Hypertens 13:205–214, 2004.

108. Magyar CE, Zhang Y, Holstein-Rathlou NH, McDonough AA: Proximal tubule Na transporter responses are the same during acute and chronic hypertension. Am J Physiol Renal Physiol 279:F358–F369, 2000.

109. McDonough AA, Leong PK, Yang LE: Mechanisms of pressure natriuresis: How blood pressure regulates renal sodium transport. Ann N Y Acad Sci 986:669–677, 2003.

110. Rasmussen MS, Simonsen JA, Sandgaard NC, et al: Mechanisms of acute natriuresis in normal humans on low sodium diet. J Physiol 546:591–603, 2003.

111. Sandgaard NC, Andersen JL, Bie P: Hormonal regulation of renal sodium and water excretion during normotensive sodium loading in conscious dogs. Am J Physiol Regul Integr Comp Physiol 278:R11–R18, 2000.

112. Seeliger E, Wronski T, Ladwig M, et al: The "body fluid pressure control system" relies on the renin-angiotensin-aldosterone system: Balance studies in freely moving dogs. Clin Exp Pharmacol Physiol 32:394–399, 2005.

113. Brewster UC, Setaro JF, Perazella MA: The renin-angiotensin-aldosterone system: Cardiorenal effects and implications for renal and cardiovascular disease states. Am J Med Sci 326:15–24, 2003.

114. Schmieder RE: Mechanisms for the clinical benefits of angiotensin II receptor blockers. Am J Hypertens 18:720–730, 2005.

115. Inagami T, Mizuno K, Naruse K, et al: Intracellular formation and release of angiotensins from juxtaglomerular cells. Kidney Int 38(suppl 30):S33–S37, 1990.

116. Ardaillou R, Chansel D: Synthesis and effects of active fragments of angiotensin II. Review. Kidney Int 52:1458–1468, 1997.

117. Dzau VJ: Tissue renin-angiotensin system in myocardial hypertrophy and failure. Review. Arch Intern Med 153:937–942, 1993.

118. Dzau VJ: Circulating versus local renin-angiotensin system in cardiovascular homeostasis. Review. Circulation 77(suppl I):I-4–I-13, 1988.

119. Wolf G, Ziyadeh FN: Renal tubular hypertrophy induced by angiotensin II. Semin Nephrol 17:448–454, 1997.

120. Re RN: The clinical implication of tissue renin angiotensin systems. Curr Opin Cardiol 16:317–327, 2001.

121. Ingelfinger JR, Zuo WM, Fon EA, et al: In situ hybridization evidence for angiotensinogen messenger RNA in the rat proximal tubule. An hypothesis for the intrarenal renin angiotensin system. J Clin Invest 85:417–423, 1990.

122. Terada Y, Tomita K, Nonoguchi H, Marumo F: PCR localization of angiotensin II receptor and angiotensinogen mRNAs in rat kidney. Kidney Int 43:1251–1259, 1993.

123. Braam B, Mitchell KD, Fox J, Navar LG: Proximal tubular secretion of angiotensin II in rats. Am J Physiol 264:F891–F898, 1993.

124. Seikaly MG, Arant BSJ, Seney FDJ: Endogenous angiotensin concentrations in specific intrarenal fluid compartments of the rat. J Clin Invest 86:1352–1357, 1990.

125. Navar LG, Imig JD, Zou L, Wang CT: Intrarenal production of angiotensin II. Review. Semin Nephrol 17:412–422, 1997.

126. Goodfriend TL, Elliott ME, Catt KJ: Angiotensin receptors and their antagonists. Review. N Engl J Med 334:1649–1654, 1996.

127. Griendling KK, Lassegue B, Alexander RW: Angiotensin receptors and their therapeutic implications. Review. Annu Rev Pharmacol Toxicol 36:281–306, 1996.

128. Sasaki K, Yamano Y, Bardhan S, et al: Cloning and expression of a complementary DNA encoding a bovine adrenal angiotensin II type-1 receptor. Nature 351:230–233, 1991.

129. Mukoyama M, Nakajima M, Horiuchi M, et al: Expression cloning of type 2 angiotensin II receptor reveals a unique class of seven-transmembrane receptors. J Biol Chem 268:24539–24542, 1993.

130. Dzau VJ: Molecular biology of angiotensin II biosynthesis and receptors. Can J Cardiol 11(suppl F):21F–26F, 1995.

131. Horiuchi M, Hayashida W, Kambe T, et al: Angiotensin type 2 receptor dephosphorylates Bcl-2 by activating mitogen-activated protein kinase phosphatase-1 and induces apoptosis. J Biol Chem 272:19022–19026, 1997.

132. Arendshorst WJ, Brannstrom K, Ruan X: Actions of angiotensin II on the renal microvasculature. J Am Soc Nephrol 10(suppl 1):S149–S161,1999.

133. Arima S, Ito S: New insights into actions of the renin-angiotensin system in the kidney: Concentrating on the Ang II receptors and the newly described Ang-(1–7) and its receptor. Semin Nephrol 21:535–543, 2001.

134. Mitchell KD, Braam B, Navar LG: Hypertensinogenic mechanism mediated by renal actions of renin-angiotensin system. Hypertension 19(suppl I):I-18–I-27, 1992.

135. Edwards RM: Segmental effects of norepinephrine and angiotensin II on isolated renal microvessels. Am J Physiol 244:F526–F534, 1983.

136. Navar LG, Inscho EW, Majid SA, et al: Paracrine regulation of the renal microcirculation. Review. Physiol Rev 76:425–536, 1996.

137. Hall JE, Granger JP: Renal hemodynamic actions of angiotensin II: Interaction with tubuloglomerular feedback. Am J Physiol 245:R166–R173, 1983.

138. Ichikawa I, Yoshioka T, Fogo A, Kon V: Role of angiotensin II in altered glomerular hemodynamics in congestive heart failure. Kidney Int 30(suppl):S123–S126, 1990.

139. Blantz RC, Konnen KS, Tucker BJ: Angiotensin II effects upon the glomerular microcirculation and ultrafiltration coefficient of the rat. J Clin Invest 57:419–434, 1976.

140. Chou SY, Porush JG, Faubert PF: Renal medullary circulation: Hormonal control. Review. Kidney Int 37:1–13, 1990.

141. Cogan MG: Angiotensin II: A powerful controller of sodium transport in the early proximal tubule. Review. Hypertension 15:451–458, 1990.

142. Quan A, Baum M: Endogenous production of angiotensin II modulates rat proximal tubule transport. J Clin Invest 97:2878–2882, 1996.

143. Saccomani G, Mitchell KD, Navar LG: Angiotensin II stimulation of Na$^{(+)}$-H$^+$ exchange in proximal tubule cells. Am J Physiol 258:F1188–F1195, 1990.

144. Geibel J, Giebisch G, Boron WF: Angiotensin II stimulates both Na$^{(+)}$-H$^+$ exchange and Na$^+$/HCO$_3^-$ cotransport in the rabbit proximal tubule. Proc Natl Acad Sci U S A 87:7917–7920, 1990.

145. Barreto-Chaves ML, Mello-Aires M: Effect of luminal angiotensin II and ANP on early and late cortical distal tubule HCO$_3^-$ reabsorption. Am J Physiol 271:F977–F984, 1996.

146. Levine DZ, Iacovitti M, Buckman S, Burns KD: Role of angiotensin II in dietary modulation of rat late distal tubule bicarbonate flux in vivo. J Clin Invest 97:120–125, 1996.

147. Wang T, Giebisch G: Effects of angiotensin II on electrolyte transport in the early and late distal tubule in rat kidney. Am J Physiol 271:F143–F149, 1996.

148. Peti-Peterdi J, Warnock DG, Bell PD: Angiotensin II directly stimulates ENaC activity in the cortical collecting duct via AT(1) receptors. J Am Soc Nephrol 13:1131–1135, 2002.

149. Braam B, Mitchell KD, Koomans HA, Navar LG: Relevance of the tubuloglomerular feedback mechanism in pathophysiology. Editorial. Review. J Am Soc Nephrol 4:1257–1274, 1993.

150. Hall JE: Control of sodium excretion by angiotensin II: Intrarenal mechanisms and blood pressure regulation. Review. Am J Physiol 250:R960–R972, 1986.

151. Xie MH, Liu FY, Wong PC, et al: Proximal nephron and renal effects of DuP 753, a nonpeptide angiotensin II receptor antagonist. Kidney Int 38:473–479, 1990.

152. Ferrario CM: Angiotensin-converting enzyme 2 and angiotensin-(1–7)—An evolving story in cardiovascular regulation. Hypertension 47:515–521, 2006.

153. Pagliaro P, Penna C: Rethinking the renin-angiotensin system and its role in cardiovascular regulation. Cardiovasc Drugs Ther 19:77–87, 2005.

154. Donoghue M, Hsieh F, Baronas E, et al: A novel angiotensin-converting enzyme–related carboxypeptidase (ACE2) converts angiotensin I to angiotensin 1–9. Circ Res 87:E1–E9, 2000.

155. Goodfriend TL: Aldosterone—A hormone of cardiovascular adaptation and maladaptation. J Clin Hypertens 8(2):133–139, 2006.

156. Doucet A, Katz AI: Mineralocorticoid receptors along the nephron: [3H]aldosterone binding in rabbit tubules. Am J Physiol 241:F605–F611, 1981.

157. Husted RF, Laplace JR, Stokes JB: Enhancement of electrogenic Na$^+$ transport across rat inner medullary collecting duct by glucocorticoid and by mineralocorticoid hormones. J Clin Invest 86:498–506, 1990.

158. Olsen ME, Hall JE, Montani JP, et al: Mechanisms of angiotensin II natriuresis and antinatriuresis. Am J Physiol 249:F299–F307, 1985.

159. Garty H: Regulation of Na$^+$ permeability by aldosterone. Review. Semin Nephrol 12:24–29, 1992.

160. Duchatelle P, Ohara A, Ling BN, et al: Regulation of renal epithelial sodium channels. Review. Mol Cell Biochem 114:27–34, 1992.

161. Hayhurst RA, O'Neil RG: Time-dependent actions of aldosterone and amiloride on Na$^+$-K$^+$-ATPase of cortical collecting duct. Am J Physiol 254:F689–F696, 1988.

162. Bastl CP, Hayslett JP: The cellular action of aldosterone in target epithelia. Editorial. Kidney Int 42:250–264, 1992.

163. Horisberger JD, Rossier BC: Aldosterone regulation of gene transcription leading to control of ion transport. Review. Hypertension 19:221–227, 1992.

164. Schiffrin EL: Effects of aldosterone on the vasculature. Hypertension 47:312–318, 2006.

165. Robertson GL: Physiology of ADH secretion. Kidney Int 32:S20–S26, 1987.

166. Birnbaumer M: Vasopressin receptors. Trends Endocrinol Metab 11:406–410, 2000.

167. Bankir L: Antidiuretic action of vasopressin: Quantitative aspects and interaction between V1a and V2 receptor–mediated effects. Cardiovasc Res 51:372–390, 2001.

168. Friedrich EB, Muders F, Luchner A, et al: Contribution of the endothelin system to the renal hypoperfusion associated with experimental congestive heart failure. J Cardiovasc Pharmacol 34:612–617, 1999.

169. Birnbaumer M: The V2 vasopressin receptor mutations and fluid homeostasis. Cardiovasc Res 51:409–415, 2001.

170. Kwon TH, Hager H, Nejsum LN, et al: Physiology and pathophysiology of renal aquaporins. Semin Nephrol 21:231–238, 2001.

171. Cowley AW: Control of the renal medullary circulation by vasopressin V-1 and V-2 receptors in the rat. Exp Physiol 85:223S–231S, 2000.

172. Goldsmith SR: Vasopressin as vasopressor. Am J Med 82:1213–1219, 1987.

173. Walker BR, Childs ME, Adams EM: Direct cardiac effects of vasopressin—Role of V1-vasopressinergic and V2-vasopressinergic receptors. Am J Physiol 255:H261–H265, 1988.

174. Cheng CP, Igarashi Y, Klopfenstein HS, et al: Effect of vasopressin on left-ventricular performance. Am J Physiol 264:H53–H60, 1993.

175. Nakamura Y, Haneda T, Osaki J, et al: Hypertrophic growth of cultured neonatal rat heart cells mediated by vasopressin V-1A receptor. Eur J Pharmacol 391:39–48, 2000.

176. Fukuzawa J, Haneda T, Kikuchi K: Arginine vasopressin increases the rate of protein synthesis in isolated perfused adult rat heart via the V-1 receptor. Mol Cell Biochem 195:93–98, 1999.

177. Andersen SE, Engstrom T, Bie P: Effects on renal sodium and potassium excretion of vasopressin and oxytocin in conscious dogs. Acta Physiol Scand 145:267–274, 1992.

178. Inaba M, Katayama S, Itabashi A, et al: Effects of arginine vasopressin on blood pressure and renal prostaglandin E2 in rabbits. Endocrinol Jpn 38:505–509, 1991.

179. Blandford DE, Smyth DD: Role of vasopressin in response to intrarenal infusions of alpha-2 adrenoceptor agonists. J Pharmacol Exp Ther 255:264–270, 1990.

180. Abboud FM, Floras JS, Aylward PE, et al: Role of vasopressin in cardiovascular and blood pressure regulation. Review. Blood Vessels 27:106–115, 1990.

181. Bichet DG, Razi M, Lonergan M, et al: Hemodynamic and coagulation responses to 1-desamino[8-D-arginine] vasopressin in patients with congenital nephrogenic diabetes insipidus. N Engl J Med 318:881–887, 1988.

182. Nasrallah R, Hebert RL: Prostacyclin signaling in the kidney: Implications for health and disease. Am J Physiol Renal Physiol 289:F235–F246, 2005.

183. Kraemer SA, Meade EA, DeWitt DL: Prostaglandin endoperoxide synthase gene structure: Identification of the transcriptional start site and 5′-flanking regulatory sequences. Arch Biochem Biophys 293:391–400, 1992.

184. Simmons DL, Botting RM, Hla T: Cyclooxygenase isozymes: The biology of prostaglandin synthesis and inhibition. Pharmacol Rev 56:387–437, 2004.

185. Harris RC, Breyer MD: Physiological regulation of cyclooxygenase-2 in the kidney. Am J Physiol Renal Physiol 281:F1–F11, 2001.

186. Kramer BK, Kammerl MC, Komhoff M: Renal cyclooxygenase-2 (COX-2)—Physiological, pathophysiological, and clinical implications. Kidney Blood Press Res 27:43–62, 2004.

187. Harris RC, McKanna JA, Akai Y, et al: Cyclooxygenase-2 is associated with the macula densa of rat kidney and increases with salt restriction. J Clin Invest 94:2504–2510, 1994.

188. Yang T, Singh I, Pham H, et al: Regulation of cyclooxygenase expression in the kidney by dietary salt intake. Am J Physiol 274:F481–F489, 1998.

189. Harris RC: Cyclooxygenase-2 in the kidney. J Am Soc Nephrol 11:2387–2394, 2000.

190. Abassi Z, Brodsky S, Gealekman O, et al: Intrarenal expression and distribution of cyclooxygenase isoforms in rats with experimental heart failure. Am J Physiol Renal Physiol 280:F43–F53, 2001.

191. Patrignani P, Tacconelli S, Sciulli MG, Capone ML: New insights into COX-2 biology and inhibition. Brain Res Brain Res Rev 48:352–359, 2005.

192. Warner TD, Mitchell JA: Cyclooxygenases: New forms, new inhibitors, and lessons from the clinic. FASEB J 18:790–804, 2004.

193. Zusman RM, Keiser HR: Prostaglandin biosynthesis by rabbit renomedullary interstitial cells in tissue culture. Stimulation by angiotensin II, bradykinin, and arginine vasopressin. J Clin Invest 60:215–223, 1977.

194. Bonilla-Felix M: Development of water transport in the collecting duct. Am J Physiol Renal Physiol 287:F1093–F1101, 2004.

195. DiBona GF, Kopp UC: Neural control of renal function. Review. Physiol Rev 77:75–197, 1997.

196. Laffi G, La Villa G, Pinzani M, et al: Arachidonic acid derivatives and renal function in liver cirrhosis. Semin Nephrol 17:530–548, 1997.

197. Kon V: Neural control of renal circulation. Review. Miner Electrolyte Metab 15:33–43, 1989.

198. Perazella MA, Eras J: Are selective COX-2 inhibitors nephrotoxic? Am J Kidney Dis 35:937–940, 2000.

199. Breyer MD, Hao C, Qi Z: Cyclooxygenase-2 selective inhibitors and the kidney. Curr Opin Crit Care 7:393–400, 2001.

200. Venkatachalam MA, Kreisberg JI: Agonist-induced isotonic contraction of cultured mesangial cells after multiple passage. Am J Physiol 249:C48–C55, 1985.

201. Baer PG, Navar LG: Renal vasodilation and uncoupling of blood flow and filtration rate autoregulation. Kidney Int 4:12–21, 1973.

202. Haas JA, Hammond TG, Granger JP, et al: Mechanism of natriuresis during intrarenal infusion of prostaglandins. Am J Physiol 247:F475–F479, 1984.

203. Bonvalet JP, Pradelles P, Farman N: Segmental synthesis and actions of prostaglandins along the nephron. Am J Physiol 253(3 pt 2):F377–F387. 1987.

204. Rubinger D, Wald H, Scherzer P, Popovtzer MM: Renal sodium handling and stimulation of medullary Na-K-ATPase during blockade of prostaglandin synthesis. Prostaglandins 39:179–194, 1990.

205. Culpepper RM, Andreoli TE: Interactions among prostaglandin E$_2$, antidiuretic hormone, and cyclic adenosine monophosphate in modulating Cl$^-$ absorption in single mouse medullary thick ascending limbs of Henle. J Clin Invest 71:1588–1601, 1983.

206. Hebert RL, Jacobson HR, Breyer MD: PGE$_2$ inhibits AVP-induced water flow in cortical collecting ducts by protein kinase C activation. Am J Physiol 259:F318–F325, 1990.

207. Epstein M, Lifschitz MD, Hoffman DS, Stein JH: Relationship between renal prostaglandin E and renal sodium handling during water immersion in normal man. Circ Res 45:71–80, 1979.

208. Qi Z, Hao CM, Langenbach RI, et al: Opposite effects of cyclooxygenase-1 and -2 activity on the pressor response to angiotensin II. J Clin Invest 110:61–69, 2002.

209. Debold AJ, Borenstein HB, Veress AT, Sonnenberg H: A rapid and potent natriuretic response to intravenous-injection of atrial myocardial extract in rats. Life Sci 28:89–94, 1981.

210. Ballermann BJ, Brenner BM: Role of atrial peptides in body-fluid homeostasis. Circ Res 58:619–630, 1986.

211. Brenner BM, Ballermann BJ, Gunning ME, Zeidel ML: Diverse biological actions of atrial natriuretic peptide. Review. Physiol Rev 70:665–699, 1990.

212. Curry FR: Atrial natriuretic peptide: An essential physiological regulator of transvascular fluid, protein transport, and plasma volume. J Clin Invest 115(6):1458–1461, 2005.

213. Abassi Z, Karram T, Ellaham S, et al: Implications of the natriuretic peptide system in the pathogenesis of heart failure: Diagnostic and therapeutic importance. Pharmacol Ther 102:223–241, 2004.

214. Wong F, Blei AT, Blendis LM, Thuluvath PJ: A vasopressin receptor antagonist (VPA-985) improves serum sodium concentration in patients with hyponatremia: A multicenter, randomized, placebo-controlled trial. Hepatology 37:182–191, 2003.

215. Ogawa Y, Nakao K, Mukoyama M, et al: Natriuretic peptides as cardiac hormones in normotensive and spontaneously hypertensive rats. The ventricle is a major site of synthesis and secretion of brain natriuretic peptide. Circ Res 69:491–500,1991.

216. Pandey KN: Biology of natriuretic peptides and their receptors. Peptides 26:901–932, 2005.

217. Martin ER, Lewicki JA, Scarborough RM, Ballermann BJ: Expression and regulation of ANP receptor subtypes in rat renal glomeruli and papillae. Am J Physiol 257: F649–F657, 1989.

218. Inagami T, Naruse M, Hoover R: Endothelium as an endocrine organ. Review. Annu Rev Physiol 57:171–189, 1995.

219. Maack T: Receptors of atrial-natriuretic-factor. Annu Rev Physiol 54:11–27, 1992.

220. Roques BP, Noble F, Dauge V, et al: Neutral endopeptidase 24.11: Structure, inhibition, and experimental and clinical pharmacology. Review. Pharmacol Rev 45:87–146, 1993.

221. Inagami T: Atrial natriuretic factor as a volume regulator. Review. J Clin Pharmacol 34:424–426, 1994.

222. Silver MA: The natriuretic peptide system: Kidney and cardiovascular effects. Curr Opin Nephrol Hypertens 15:14–21, 2006.

223. Sagnella GA: Atrial natriuretic peptide mimetics and vasopeptidase inhibitors. Cardiovasc Res 51:416–428, 2001.

224. Sagnella GA: Measurement and significance of circulating natriuretic peptides in cardiovascular disease. Clin Sci 95:519–529, 1998.

225. Dietz JR: Mechanisms of atrial natriuretic peptide secretion from the atrium. Cardiovasc Res 68:8–17, 2005.

226. Espiner EA: Physiology of natriuretic peptides [see comments]. Review. J Intern Med 235:527–541, 1994.

227. Kleinert HD, Maack T, Atlas SA, et al: Atrial natriuretic factor inhibits angiotensin-, norepinephrine-, and potassium-induced vascular contractility. Hypertension 6: I143–I147, 1984.

228. Charloux A, Piquard F, Doutreleau S, et al: Mechanisms of renal hyporesponsiveness to ANP in heart failure. Eur J Clin Invest 33:769–778, 2003.

229. Cogan MG: Atrial natriuretic factor can increase renal solute excretion primarily by raising glomerular filtration. Am J Physiol 250:F710–F714, 1986.

230. Harris PJ, Thomas D, Morgan TO: Atrial natriuretic peptide inhibits angiotensin-stimulated proximal tubular sodium and water reabsorption. Nature 326:697–698, 1987.

231. Garvin JL: Inhibition of Jv by ANF in rat proximal straight tubules requires angiotensin. Am J Physiol 257:F907–F911, 1989.

232. Zeidel ML, Brady HR, Kone BC, et al: Endothelin, a peptide inhibitor of Na($^+$)-K($^+$)-ATPase in intact renaltubular epithelial cells. Am J Physiol 257:C1101–C1107, 1989.

233. Sonnenberg H: The physiology of atrial natriuretic factor. Review. Can J Physiol Pharmacol 65:2021–2023, 1987.

234. Sonnenberg H, Honrath U, Chong CK, Wilson DR: Atrial natriuretic factor inhibits sodium transport in medullary collecting duct. Am J Physiol 250:F963–F966, 1986.

235. Holmes SJ, Espiner EA, Richards AM, et al: Renal, endocrine, and hemodynamic effects of human brain natriuretic peptide in normal man. J Clin Endocrinol Metab 76:91–96, 1993.

236. Davidson NC, Struthers AD: Brain natriuretic peptide. Editorial. Review. J Hypertens 12:329–336, 1994.

237. Maisel AS, Koon J, Krishnaswamy P, et al: Utility of B-natriuretic peptide as a rapid, point-of-care test for screening patients undergoing echocardiography to determine left ventricular dysfunction. Am Heart J 141:367–374, 2001.

238. Akabane S, Matsushima Y, Matsuo H, et al: Effects of brain natriuretic peptide on renin secretion in normal and hypertonic saline-infused kidney. Eur J Pharmacol 198:143–148, 1991.

239. Hashiguchi T, Higuchi K, Ohashi M, et al: Effect of porcine brain natriuretic peptide (pBNP) on human adrenocortical steroidogenesis. Clin Endocrinol (Oxf) 31:623–630, 1989.

240. Scotland RS, Cohen M, Foster P, et al: C-type natriuretic peptide inhibits leukocyte recruitment and platelet-leukocyte interactions via suppression of P-selectin expression. Proc Natl Acad Sci U S A 102:14452–14457, 2005.

241. Komatsu Y, Nakao K, Suga S, et al: C-type natriuretic peptide (CNP) in rats and humans. Endocrinology 129:1104–1106, 1991.

242. Ueda S, Minamino N, Aburaya M, et al: Distribution and characterization of immunoreactive porcine C-type natriuretic peptide. Biochem Biophys Res Commun 175:759–767, 1991.

243. Needleman P, Blaine EH, Greenwald JE, et al: The biochemical pharmacology of atrial peptides. Review. Annu Rev Pharmacol Toxicol 29:23–54, 1989.

244. Vane JR, Anggard EE, Botting RM: Regulatory functions of the vascular endothelium. Review. N Engl J Med 323:27–36, 1990.

245. Luscher TF: The endothelium and cardiovascular disease—A complex relation. Editorial; comment. N Engl J Med 330:1081–1083, 1994.

246. Griendling KK, Alexander RW: Endothelial control of the cardiovascular system: Recent advances. Review. FASEB J 10:283–292, 1996.

247. Vanhoutte PM: Endothelium-dependent responses in congestive heart failure. J Mol Cell Cardiol 28:2233–2240, 1996.

248. Luscher TF: The endothelium in hypertension: Bystander, target or mediator? Review. J Hypertens Suppl 12:S105–S116, 1994.

249. Masaki T: Possible role of endothelin in endothelial regulation of vascular tone. Review. Annu Rev Pharmacol Toxicol 35:235–255, 1995.

250. Kohan DE: The renal medullary endothelin system in control of sodium and water excretion and systemic blood pressure. Curr Opin Nephrol Hypertens 15:34–40, 2006.

251. Brunner F, Bras-Silva C, Cerdeira AS, Leite-Moreira AF: Cardiovascular endothelins: Essential regulators of cardiovascular homeostasis. Pharmacol Ther 111:508–531, 2006.

252. Levin ER: Endothelins. Review. N Engl J Med 333:356–363, 1995.

253. Schiffrin EL: Vascular endothelin in hypertension. Vasc Pharmacol 43:19–29, 2005.

254. Yanagisawa H, Yanagisawa M, Kapur RP, et al: Dual genetic pathways of endothelin-mediated intercellular signaling revealed by targeted disruption of endothelin-converting enzyme-1 gene. Development 125:825–836, 1998.

255. Wypij DM, Nichols JS, Novak PJ, et al: Role of mast cell chymase in the extracellular processing of big-endothelin-1 to endothelin-1 in the perfused rat lung. Biochem Pharmacol 43:845–853, 1992.

256. Kedzierski RM, Yanagisawa M: Endothelin system: The double-edged sword in health and disease. Annu Rev Pharmacol Toxicol 41:851–876, 2001.

257. Katoh T, Chang N, Uchida S, et al: Direct effects of endothelin in the rat kidney. Am J Physiol 258:F397–F402, 1990.

258. Tsuchiya K, Naruse M, Sanaka T, et al: Effects of endothelin on renal hemodynamics and excretory functions in anesthetized dogs. Life Sci 46:59–65, 1990.

259. Stacy DL, Scott JW, Granger JP: Control of renal function during intrarenal infusion of endothelin. Am J Physiol 258:F1232–F1236, 1990.

260. Wilkins FCJ, Alberola A, Mizelle HL, et al: Systemic hemodynamics and renal function during long-term pathophysiological increases in circulating endothelin. Am J Physiol 268:R375–R381, 1995.

261. Gurbanov K, Rubinstein I, Hoffman A, et al: Differential regulation of renal regional blood flow by endothelin-1. Am J Physiol 271:F1166–F1172, 1996.

262. Clavell AL, Burnett JCJ: Physiologic and pathophysiologic roles of endothelin in the kidney. Review. Curr Opin Nephrol Hypertens 3:66–72, 1994.

263. Kon V, Yoshioka T, Fogo A, Ichikawa I: Glomerular actions of endothelin in vivo. J Clin Invest 83:1762–1767, 1989.

264. Hoffman A, Haramati A, Dalal I, et al: Diuretic-natriuretic actions and pressor effects of big-endothelin (1–39) in phosphoramidon-treated rats. Proc Soc Exp Biol Med 205:168–173, 1994.

265. Pollock DM: Contrasting pharmacological ETB receptor blockade with genetic ETB deficiency in renal responses to big ET-1. Physiol Genomics 6:39–43, 2001.

266. Gariepy CE, Ohuchi T, Williams SC, et al: Salt-sensitive hypertension in endothelin-B receptor–deficient rats. J Clin Invest 105:925–933, 2000.

267. Abassi ZA, Ellahham S, Winaver J, Hoffman A. The intrarenal endothelin system and hypertension. News Physiol Sci 16:152–156, 2001.

268. Oishi R, Nonoguchi H, Tomita K, Marumo F: Endothelin-1 inhibits AVP-stimulated osmotic water permeability in rat inner medullary collecting duct. Am J Physiol 261: F951–F956, 1991.

269. Abassi ZA, Tate JE, Golomb E, Keiser HR: Role of neutral endopeptidase in the metabolism of endothelin. Hypertension 20:89–95, 1992.

270. Sasser JM, Pollock JS, Pollock DM: Renal endothelin in chronic angiotensin II hypertension. Am J Physiol Regul Integr Comp Physiol 283:R243–R248, 2002.

271. Pollock DM, Pollock JS: Evidence for endothelin involvement in the response to high salt. Am J Physiol Renal Physiol 281:F144–F150, 2001.

272. Kone BC, Baylis C: Biosynthesis and homeostatic roles of nitric oxide in the normal kidney. Review. Am J Physiol 272:F561–F578, 1997.

273. Herrera M, Garvin JL: Recent advances in the regulation of nitric oxide in the kidney. Hypertension 45:1062–1067, 2005.

274. Baylis C, Qiu C: Importance of nitric oxide in the control of renal hemodynamics. Review. Kidney Int 49:1727–1731, 1996.

275. Imig JD, Roman RJ: Nitric oxide modulates vascular tone in preglomerular arterioles. Hypertension 19:770–774, 1992.

276. Kone BC: Nitric oxide in renal health and disease. Review. Am J Kidney Dis 30:311–333, 1997.

277. Bachmann S, Mundel P: Nitric oxide in the kidney: Synthesis, localization, and function. Review. Am J Kidney Dis 24:112–129, 1994.

278. Schulz R, Rassaf T, Massion PB, et al: Recent advances in the understanding of the role of nitric oxide in cardiovascular homeostasis. Pharmacol Ther 108:225–256, 2005.

279. Blantz RC, Deng A, Lortie M, et al: The complex role of nitric oxide in the regulation of glomerular ultrafiltration. Kidney Int 61:782–785, 2002.

280. McKee M, Scavone C, Nathanson JA: Nitric oxide, cGMP, and hormone regulation of active sodium transport. Proc Natl Acad Sci U S A 91:12056–12060, 1994.

281. Siragy HM, Johns RA, Peach MJ, Carey RM: Nitric oxide alters renal function and guanosine 3′,5′-cyclic monophosphate. Hypertension 19:775–779, 1992.

282. Ito S, Arima S, Ren YL, et al: Endothelium-derived relaxing factor/nitric oxide modulates angiotensin II action in the isolated microperfused rabbit afferent but not efferent arteriole. J Clin Invest 91:2012–2019, 1993.

283. Baylis C, Harvey J, Engels K: Acute nitric oxide blockade amplifies the renal vasoconstrictor actions of angiotension II. J Am Soc Nephrol 5:211–214, 1994.

284. Thorup C, Persson AE: Inhibition of locally produced nitric oxide resets tubuloglomerular feedback mechanism. Am J Physiol 267:F606–F611, 1994.

285. Salazar FJ, Alberola A, Pinilla JM, et al: Salt-induced increase in arterial pressure during nitric oxide synthesis inhibition. Hypertension 22:49–55, 1993.

286. Shultz PJ, Tolins JP: Adaptation to increased dietary salt intake in the rat. Role of endogenous nitric oxide. J Clin Invest 91:642–650, 1993.

287. Alberola A, Pinilla JM, Quesada T, et al: Role of nitric oxide in mediating renal response to volume expansion. Hypertension 19:780–784, 1992.

288. Eitle E, Hiranyachattada S, Wang H, Harris PJ: Inhibition of proximal tubular fluid absorption by nitric oxide and atrial natriuretic peptide in rat kidney. Am J Physiol 43:C1075–C1080, 1998.

289. Mattson DL, Roman RJ, Cowley AW Jr: Role of nitric oxide in renal papillary blood flow and sodium excretion. Hypertension 19:766–769, 1992.

290. Abassi Z, Gurbanov K, Rubinstein I, et al: Regulation of intrarenal blood flow in experimental heart failure: Role of endothelin and nitric oxide. Am J Physiol 274: F766–F774, 1998.

291. Hoffman A, Abassi ZA, Brodsky S, et al: Mechanisms of big endothelin-1–induced diuresis and natriuresis: Role of ET(B) receptors. Hypertension 35:732–739, 2000.

292. Garcia NH, Stoos BA, Carretero OA, Garvin JL: Mechanism of the nitric oxide–induced blockade of collecting duct water permeability. Hypertension 27:679–683, 1996.

293. Tolins JP, Shultz PJ: Endogenous nitric oxide synthesis determines sensitivity to the pressor effect of salt. Kidney Int 46:230–236, 1994.

294. Ikeda Y, Saito K, Kim JI, Yokoyama M: Nitric oxide synthase isoform activities in kidney of Dahl salt-sensitive rats. Hypertension 26:1030–1034, 1995.

295. Hu L, Manning RDJ: Role of nitric oxide in regulation of long-term pressure-natriuresis relationship in Dahl rats. Am J Physiol 268:H2375–H2383, 1995.

296. Wilcox CS, Welch WJ: TGF and nitric oxide: Effects of salt intake and salt-sensitive hypertension. Kidney Int Suppl 55:S9–S13, 1996.

297. Denton KM, Luff SE, Shweta A, Anderson WP: Differential neural control of glomerular ultrafiltration. Clin Exp Pharmacol Physiol 31(5–6):380–386, 2004.

298. DiBona GF: Neural control of the kidney: Functionally specific renal sympathetic nerve fibers. Am J Physiol Regul Integr Comp Physiol 279:R1517–R1524, 2000.

299. Barajas L, Powers K: Monoaminergic innervation of the rat kidney: A quantitative study. Am J Physiol 259:F503–F511, 1990.

300. Eppel GA, Malpas SC, Denton KM, Evans RG: Neural control of renal medullary perfusion. Clin Exp Pharmacol Physiol 31(5–6):387–396, 2004.

301. Jeffries WB, Pettinger WA: Adrenergic signal transduction in the kidney. Review. Miner Electrolyte Metab 15:5–15, 1989.

302. Matsushima Y, Akabane S, Ito K: Characterization of alpha 1- and alpha 2-adrenoceptors directly associated with basolateral membranes from rat kidney proximal tubules. Biochem Pharmacol 35:2593–2600, 1986.

303. Summers RJ, Stephenson JA, Kuhar MJ: Localization of beta adrenoceptor subtypes in rat kidney by light microscopic autoradiography. J Pharmacol Exp Ther 232:561–569, 1985.

304. DiBona GF, Sawin LL: Role of renal nerves in sodium retention of cirrhosis and congestive heart failure. Am J Physiol 260:R298–R305, 1991.

305. DiBona GF: Dynamic analysis of patterns of renal sympathetic nerve activity: Implications for renal function. Exp Physiol 90(2):159–161, 2005.

306. Kon V, Ichikawa I: Effector loci for renal nerve control of cortical microcirculation. Am J Physiol 245:F545–F553, 1983.

307. DiBona GF: Role of renal nerves in edema formation. NIPS 9:183–188, 1994.

308. Miki K, Hayashida Y, Shiraki K: Cardiac-renal-neural reflex plays a major role in natriuresis induced by left atrial distension. Am J Physiol 264:R369–R375, 1992.

309. DiBona GF: Sympathetic nervous system and the kidney in hypertension. Curr Opin Nephrol Hypertens 11:197–200, 2002.

310. Wang T, Chan YL: Neural control of distal tubular bicarbonate and fluid transport. Am J Physiol 257:F72–F76, 1989.

311. Kon V, Yared A, Ichikawa I: Role of renal sympathetic nerves in mediating hypoperfusion of renal cortical microcirculation in experimental congestive heart failure and acute extracellular fluid volume depletion. J Clin Invest 76:1913–1920, 1985.

312. Gill JR, Bartter FC: Adrenergic nervous system in sodium metabolism. II. Effects of guanethidine on the renal response to sodium deprivation in normal man. N Engl J Med 275:1466–1471, 1966.

313. Friberg P, Meredith I, Jennings G, et al: Evidence for increased renal norepinephrine overflow during sodium restriction in humans. Hypertension 16:121–130, 1990.

314. McMurray JJ, Seidelin PH, Balfour DJ, Struthers AD: Physiological increases in circulating noradrenaline are antinatriuretic in man. J Hypertens 6:757–761, 1988.

315. Aperia A, Ibarra F, Svensson LB, et al: Calcineurin mediates alpha-adrenergic stimulation of Na⁺,K⁺-ATPase activity in renal tubule cells. Proc Natl Acad Sci U S A 89:7394–7397, 1992.

316. Nelson LD, Osborn JL: Role of intrarenal ANG II in reflex neural stimulation of plasma renin activity and renal sodium reabsorption. Am J Physiol 265:R392–R398, 1993.

317. Nishida Y, Bishop VS: Vasopressin-induced suppression of renal sympathetic outflow depends on the number of baroafferent inputs in rabbits. Am J Physiol 263:R1187–R1194, 1992.

318. Simon JK, Kasting NW, Ciriello J: Afferent renal nerve effects on plasma vasopressin and oxytocin in conscious rats. Am J Physiol 256:R1240–R1244, 1989.

319. Koepke JP, DiBona GF: Blunted natriuresis to atrial natriuretic peptide in chronic sodium-retaining disorders. Am J Physiol 252:F865–F871, 1987.

320. Pollock DM, Arendshorst WJ: Effect of acute renal denervation and ANF on renal function in adult spontaneously hypertensive rats. Am J Physiol 261:R835–R841, 1991.

321. Awazu M, Kon V, Harris RC, et al: Renal sympathetic nerves modulate glomerular ANP receptors and filtration. Am J Physiol 261:F29–F35, 1991.

322. Moreau ME, Garbacki N, Molinaro G, et al: The kallikrein-kinin system: Current and future pharmacological targets. J Pharm Sci 99:6–38, 2005.

323. Souza Dos Santos RA, Passaglio KT, Pesquero JB, et al: Interactions between angiotensin-(1–7), kinins, and angiotensin II in kidney and blood vessels. Hypertension 38:660–664, 2001.

324. Cachofeiro V, Nasjletti A: Increased vascular responsiveness to bradykinin in kidneys of spontaneously hypertensive rats. Effect of N omega-nitro-L-arginine. Hypertension 18:683–688, 1991.

325. Marcondes S, Antunes E: The plasma and tissue kininogen-kallikrein-kinin system: Role in the cardiovascular system. Curr Med Chem Cardiovasc Hematol Agents 3(1):33–44, 2005.

326. Margolius HS: Theodore Cooper Memorial Lecture. Kallikreins and kinins. Some unanswered questions about system characteristics and roles in human disease. Review. Hypertension 26:221–229, 1995.

327. Carey RM, Jin X, Wang Z, Siragy HM: Nitric oxide: A physiological mediator of the type 2 (AT2) angiotensin receptor. Acta Physiol Scand 168:65–71, 2000.

328. Liu YH, Yang XP, Sharov VG, et al: Effects of angiotensin-converting enzyme inhibitors and angiotensin II type 1 receptor antagonists in rats with heart failure. Role of kinins and angiotensin II type 2 receptors. J Clin Invest 99:1926–1935, 1997.

329. Kitamura K, Sakata J, Kangawa K, et al: Cloning and characterization of cDNA encoding a precursor for human adrenomedullin [published erratum appears in Biochem Biophys Res Commun 202(1):643, 1994]. Biochem Biophys Res Commun 194:720–725, 1993.

330. Kitamura K, Eto T: Adrenomedullin—Physiological regulator of the cardiovascular system or biochemical curiosity? Review. Curr Opin Nephrol Hypertens 6:80–87, 1997.

331. Kitamura K, Kangawa K, Eto T: Adrenomedullin and PAMP: Discovery, structures, and cardiovascular functions. Microsc Res Tech 57:3–13, 2002.

332. Hanna FW, Buchanan KD: Adrenomedullin: A novel cardiovascular regulatory peptide. Review. Q J Med 89:881–884, 1996.

333. Mukoyama M, Sugawara A, Nagae T, et al: Role of adrenomedullin and its receptor system in renal pathophysiology. Peptides 22:1925–1931, 2001.

334. Schell DA, Vari RC, Samson WK: Adrenomedullin: A newly discovered hormone controlling fluid and electrolyte homeostasis. Trends Endocrinol Metab 7:7–13, 1996.

335. Rademaker MT, Cameron VA, Charles CJ, et al: Adrenomedullin and heart failure. Regul Pept 112:51–60, 2003.

336. Richards AM, Nicholls MG, Lewis L, Lainchbury JG: Adrenomedullin. Editorial. [published erratum appears in Clin Sci (Colch) 91(4):525, 1996]. Review. Clin Sci (Colch) 91:3–16, 1996.

337. Hirata Y, Hayakawa H, Suzuki Y, et al: Mechanisms of adrenomedullin-induced vasodilation in the rat kidney. Hypertension 25:790–795, 1995.

338. Taylor MM, Samson WK: Adrenomedullin and the integrative physiology of fluid and electrolyte balance. Microsc Res Tech 57:105–109, 2002.

339. Jougasaki M, Wei CM, Aarhus LL, et al: Renal localization and actions of adrenomedullin: A natriuretic peptide. Am J Physiol 268:F657–F663, 1995.

340. Ng LL, Loke I, O'Brien RJ, et al: Plasma urotensin in human systolic heart failure. Circulation 106(23):2877–2880, 2002.

341. Conlon JM, Yano K, Waugh D, Hazon N: Distribution and molecular forms of urotensin II and its role in cardiovascular regulation in vertebrates. J Exp Zool 275:226–238, 1996.

342. Ames RS, Sarau HM, Chambers JK, et al: Human urotensin-II is a potent vasoconstrictor and agonist for the orphan receptor GPR14. Nature 401:282–286, 1999.

343. Coulouarn Y, Lihrmann I, Jegou S, et al: Cloning of the cDNA encoding the urotensin II precursor in frog and human reveals intense expression of the urotensin II gene in motoneurons of the spinal cord. Proc Natl Acad Sci U S A 95(26):15803–15808, 1998.

344. Liu QY, Pong SS, Zeng ZZ, et al: Identification of urotensin II as the endogenous ligand for the orphan G-protein–coupled receptor GPR14. Biochem Biophys Res Commun 266:174–178, 1999.

345. Nothacker HP, Wang ZH, McNeil AM, et al: Identification of the natural ligand of an orphan G-protein–coupled receptor involved in the regulation of vasoconstriction. Nature Cell Biol 1:383–385, 1999.

346. Marchese A, Heiber M, Nguyen T, et al: Cloning and chromosomal mapping of 3 novel genes, Gpr9, Gpr10, and Gpr14 encoding receptors related to interleukin-8, neuropeptide-Y, and somatostatin receptors. Genomics 29:335–344, 1995.

347. Matsushita M, Shichiri M, Imai T, et al: Co-expression of urotensin II and its receptor (GPR14) in human cardiovascular and renal tissues. J Hypertens 19:2185–2190, 2001.

348. Tal M, Naim M: A novel 7-helix receptor cloned from circumvallate sensory taste papillae of the rat. Chem Senses 20:108, 1995.

349. Totsune K, Takahashi K, Arihara Z, et al: Role of urotensin II in patients on dialysis. Lancet 358:810–811, 2001.

350. Shenouda A, Douglas SA, Ohlstein EH, Giaid A: Localization of urotensin-II immunoreactivity in normal human kidneys and renal carcinoma. J Histochem Cytochem 50:885–889, 2002.

351. Bern HA, Pearson D, Larson BA, Nishioka RS: Neurohormones from fish tails: The caudal neurosecretory system. I. "Urophysiology" and the caudal neurosecretory system of fishes. Recent Prog Horm Res 41:533–552, 1985.

352. Loretz CA, Bern HA: Stimulation of sodium-transport across the teleost urinary-bladder by urotensin-II. Gen Comp Endocrinol 43:325–330, 1981.

353. Douglas S, Aiyar NV, Ohlstein EH, Willette RN: Human urotensin-II, the most potent mammalian vasoconstrictor identified, represents a novel therapeutic target in the treatment of cardiovascular disease. Eur Heart J 21:495, 2000.

354. Douglas SA: Human urotensin-II as a novel cardiovascular target: "Heart" of the matter or simply a fishy "tail"? Curr Opin Pharm 3:159–167, 2003.

355. Gardiner SM, March JE, Kemp PA, et al: Depressor and regionally-selective vasodilator effects of human and rat urotensin II in conscious rats. Br J Pharm 132:1625–1629, 2001.

356. Gibson A: Complex effects of gillichthys urotensin-II on rat aortic strips. Br J Pharmacol 91:205–212, 1987.

357. Stirrat A, Gallagher M, Douglas SA, et al: Potent vasodilator responses to human urotensin-II in human pulmonary and abdominal resistance arteries. Am J Physiol Heart Circ Physiol 280:H925–H928, 2001.

358. Katano Y, Ishihata A, Aita T, et al: Vasodilator effect of urotensin II, one of the most potent vasoconstricting factors, on rat coronary arteries. Eur J Pharmacol 402:R5–R7, 2000.

359. Hasegawa K, Kobayashi Y, Kobayashi H: Vasodepressor effects of urotensin-II in rats. Neuroendocrinol Lett 14:357–363, 1992.

360. Zhang AY, Chen YF, Zhang DX, et al: Urotensin II is a nitric oxide–dependent vasodilator and natriuretic peptide in the rat kidney. Am J Physiol Renal Physiol 285: F792–F798, 2003.

361. Clozel M, Binkert C, Birker-Robaczewska M, et al: Pharmacology of the urotensin-II receptor antagonist palosuran (ACT-058362; 1-[2-(4-benzyl-4-hydroxy-piperidin-1-yl)-ethyl]-3-(2-methyl-quinolin-4-yl)-urea sulfate salt): First demonstration of a pathophysiological role of the urotensin system. J Pharmacol Exp Ther 311:204–212, 2004;

362. Hamlyn JM, Blaustein MP, Bova S, et al: Identification and characterization of a ouabain-like compound from human plasma [published erratum appears in Proc Natl Acad Sci U S A 88(21):9907, 1991]. Proc Natl Acad Sci U S A 88:6259–6263, 1991.

363. Hamlyn JM, Harris DW, Clark MA, et al: Isolation and characterization of a sodium pump inhibitor from human plasma. Hypertension 13:681–689, 1989.

364. Hamlyn JM, Harris DW, Ludens JH: Digitalis-like activity in human plasma. Purification, affinity, and mechanism. J Biol Chem 264:7395–7404, 1989.

365. Hamlyn JM, Hamilton BP, Manunta P: Endogenous ouabain, sodium balance and blood pressure: A review and a hypothesis [see comments]. Review. J Hypertens 14:151–167, 1996.

366. Blaustein MP: Endogenous ouabain: Role in the pathogenesis of hypertension. Review. Kidney Int 49:1748–1753, 1996.

367. Kolbel F, Schreiber V: The endogenous digitalis-like factor. Review. Mol Cell Biochem 160–161:111–115, 1996.

368. Hazelwood RL: The pancreatic-polypeptide (pp-fold) family—Gastrointestinal, vascular, and feeding behavioral implications. Proc Soc Exp Biol Med 202:44–63, 1993.

369. Larhammar D: Evolution of neuropeptide Y, peptide YY and pancreatic polypeptide. Regul Pept 62:1–11, 1996.

370. Persson PB, Gimpl G, Lang RE: Importance of neuropeptide Y in the regulation of kidney function. Ann N Y Acad Sci 611:156–165, 1990.

371. Bischoff A, Michel MC: Renal effects of neuropeptide Y. Pflugers Arch 435:443–453, 1998.

372. Winaver J, Abassi Z: Role of neuropeptide Y in the regulation of kidney function. EXS 95:123–132, 2006.

373. Smyth DD, Blandford DE, Thom SL: Disparate effects of neuropeptide-Y and clonidine on the excretion of sodium and water in the rat. Eur J Pharmacol 152:157–162, 1988.

374. Echtenkamp SF, Dandridge PF: Renal actions of neuropeptide-Y in the primate. Am J Physiol 256:F524–F531, 1989.

375. Crone C, Christensen O: Transcapillary transport of small solutes and water. Int Rev Physiol 18:149–213, 1979.

376. Magrini F, Niarchos AP: Hemodynamic effects of massive peripheral edema. Am Heart J 105:90–97, 1983:

377. Intaglietta M, Zweifach BW: Microcirculatory basis of fluid exchange. Adv Biol Med Phys 15:111–159, 1974.

378. Gustafsson D: Microvascular mechanisms involved in calcium antagonist edema formation. J Cardiovasc Pharmacol 10(suppl 1):S121–S131, 1987.

379. Aukland K, Nicolaysen G: Interstitial fluid volume: Local regulatory mechanisms. Physiol Rev 61:556–643, 1981.

380. Fauchald P: Colloid osmotic pressures, plasma volume and interstitial fluid volume in patients with heart failure. Scand J Clin Lab Invest 45:701–706, 1985.

381. Brace RA, Guyton AC: Effect of hindlimb isolation procedure on isogravimetric capillary pressure and transcapillary fluid dynamics in dogs. Circ Res 38:192–196, 1976.

382. Andreoli TE: Edematous states: An overview. Review. Kidney Int Suppl 59:S2–S10, 1997.

383. Schrier RW: A unifying hypothesis of body fluid volume regulation. The Lilly Lecture. J R Coll Physicians Lond 26:295–306, 1992.

384. Schrier RW: Pathogenesis of sodium and water retention in high-output and low-output cardiac failure, nephrotic syndrome, cirrhosis, and pregnancy (1) [published erratum appears in N Engl J Med 320(10):676, 1989]. Review. N Engl J Med 319:1065–1072, 1988.

385. Schrier RW: A unifying hypothesis of body fluid volume regulation. J R Coll Physicians (Lond) 26:295–306, 1992.

386. Starling EH: Physiological factors involved in the causation of dropsy. Lancet 1:1407–1410, 1896.

387. Harrison TR: The pathogenesis of congestive heart failure. Medicine 14:255, 1935.

388. Stead EA, Ebert RV: Shock syndrome produced by failure of the heart. Arch Intern Med 69:75–89, 1942.

389. Peters JP: The role of sodium in the production of edema. N Engl J Med 239:353–362, 1948.

390. Borst JG, deVries LA: Three types of "natural" diuresis. Lancet 2:1–6, 1950.

391. Priebe HJ, Heimann JC, Hedley-Whyte J: Effects of renal and hepatic venous congestion on renal function in the presence of low and normal cardiac output in dogs. Circ Res 47:883–890, 1980.

392. Schrier RW: Body fluid volume regulation in health and disease: A unifying hypothesis. Review. Ann Intern Med 113:155–159, 1990.

393. Zucker IH, Wang W, Brandle M, et al: Neural regulation of sympathetic nerve activity in heart failure. Review. Prog Cardiovasc Dis 37:397–414, 1995.

394. Thames MD, Kinugawa T, Smith ML, Dibner-Dunlap ME: Abnormalities of baroreflex control in heart failure. Review. J Am Coll Cardiol 22(suppl A):56A–60A, 1993.

395. Gabrielsen A, Bie P, Holstein-Rathlou NH, et al: Neuroendocrine and renal effects of intravascular volume expansion in compensated heart failure. Am J Physiol Regul Integr Comp Physiol 281:R459–R467, 2001.

396. Greenberg TT, Richmond WH, Stocking RA, et al: Impaired atrial receptor responses in dogs with heart failure due to tricuspid insufficiency and pulmonary artery stenosis. Circ Res 32:424–433, 1973.

397. Zucker IH, Earle AM, Gilmore JP: The mechanism of adaptation of left atrial stretch receptors in dogs with chronic congestive heart failure. J Clin Invest 60:323–331, 1977.

398. Hasking GJ, Esler MD, Jennings GL, et al: Norepinephrine spillover to plasma in patients with congestive heart failure: Evidence of increased overall and cardiorenal sympathetic nervous activity. Circulation 73:615–621, 1986.

399. Goldsmith SR, Francis GS, Levine TB, Cohn JN: Regional blood flow response to orthostasis in patients with congestive heart failure. J Am Coll Cardiol 1:1391–1395, 1983.

400. Creager MA, Faxon DP, Rockwell SM, et al: The contribution of the renin-angiotensin system to limb vasoregulation in patients with heart failure: Observations during orthostasis and alpha-adrenergic blockade. Clin Sci 68:659–667, 1985.

401. Eckberg DL, Drabinsky M, Braunwald E: Defective cardiac parasympathetic control in patients with heart disease. N Engl J Med 285:877–883, 1971.

402. Ferguson DW, Berg WJ, Roach PJ, et al: Effects of heart failure on baroreflex control of sympathetic neural activity [see comments]. Am J Cardiol 69:523–531, 1992.

403. Wang W, Chen JS, Zucker IH: Carotid sinus baroreceptor sensitivity in experimental heart failure [see comments]. Circulation 81:1959–1966, 1990.

404. Dibner-Dunlap ME, Thames MD: Baroreflex control of renal sympathetic nerve activity is preserved in heart failure despite reduced arterial baroreceptor sensitivity. Circ Res 65:1526–1535, 1989.

405. DiBona GF, Herman PJ, Sawin LL: Neural control of renal function in edema-forming states. Am J Physiol 254:R1017–R1024, 1988.

406. Dibner-Dunlap ME, Thames MD: Control of sympathetic nerve activity by vagal mechanoreflexes is blunted in heart failure. Circulation 86:1929–1934, 1992.

407. DiBona GF, Sawin LL: Reflex regulation of renal nerve activity in cardiac failure. Am J Physiol 266:R27–R39, 1994.

408. DiBona GF, Sawin LL: Increased renal nerve activity in cardiac failure: Arterial vs. cardiac baroreflex impairment. Am J Physiol 268:R112–R116, 1995.

409. Zucker IH, Wang W, Brandle M: Baroreflex abnormalities in congestive heart failure. NIPS 8:87–90, 1993.

410. Murakami H, Liu JL, Zucker IH: Blockade of AT1 receptors enhances baroreflex control of heart rate in conscious rabbits with heart failure. Am J Physiol 271:R303–R309, 1996.

411. Dibner-Dunlap ME, Smith ML, Kinugawa T, Thames MD: Enalaprilat augments arterial and cardiopulmonary baroreflex control of sympathetic nerve activity in patients with heart failure. J Am Coll Cardiol 27:358–364, 1996.

412. Nishida Y, Ryan KL, Bishop VS: Angiotensin II modulates arterial baroreflex function via a central alpha 1-adrenoceptor mechanism in rabbits. Am J Physiol 269:R1009–R1016, 1995.

413. Volpe M, Tritto C, De Luca N, et al: Failure of atrial natriuretic factor to increase with saline load in patients with dilated cardiomyopathy and mild heart failure. J Clin Invest 88:1481–1489, 1991.

414. Raine AE, Erne P, Burgisser E, et al: Atrial natriuretic peptide and atrial pressure in patients with congestive heart failure. N Engl J Med 315:533–537, 1986.

415. Burnett JCJ, Kao PC, Hu DC, et al: Atrial natriuretic peptide elevation in congestive heart failure in the human. Science 231:1145–1147, 1986.

416. Tikkanen I, Fyhrquist F, Metsarinne K, Leidenius R: Plasma atrial natriuretic peptide in cardiac disease and during infusion in healthy volunteers. Lancet 2:66–69, 1985.

417. Shenker Y, Sider RS, Ostafin EA, Grekin RJ: Plasma levels of immunoreactive atrial natriuretic factor in healthy subjects and in patients with edema. J Clin Invest 76:1684–1687, 1985.

418. Thibault G, Nemer M, Drouin J, et al: Ventricles as a major site of atrial natriuretic factor synthesis and release in cardiomyopathic hamsters with heart failure. Circ Res 65:71–82, 1989.

419. Edwards BS, Ackermann DM, Lee ME, et al: Identification of atrial natriuretic factor within ventricular tissue in hamsters and humans with congestive heart failure. J Clin Invest 81:82–86, 1988.

420. Saito Y, Nakao K, Arai H, et al: Augmented expression of atrial natriuretic polypeptide gene in ventricle of human failing heart. J Clin Invest 83:298–305, 1989.

421. Cody RJ, Atlas SA, Laragh JH, et al: Atrial natriuretic factor in normal subjects and heart failure patients. Plasma levels and renal, hormonal, and hemodynamic responses to peptide infusion. J Clin Invest 78:1362–1374, 1986.

422. Scriven TA, Burnett JCJ: Effects of synthetic atrial natriuretic peptide on renal function and renin release in acute experimental heart failure. Circulation 72:892–897, 1985.

423. Winaver J, Hoffman A, Burnett JC, Haramati A: Hormonal determinants of sodium-excretion in rats with experimental high-output heart-failure. Am J Physiol 254:R776–R784, 1988.

424. Merrill AJ: Mechanisms of salt and water retention in heart failure. Am J Med 6:357, 1949.

425. Vander AJ, Malvin RL, Wilde WS, Sullivan LP: Reexamination of salt and water retention in CHF. Am J Med 25:497, 1958.

426. Barger AC: Renal hemodynamic factors in congestive heart failure. Ann N Y Acad Sci 139:276–284, 1966.

427. Hostetter TH, Pfeffer JM, Pfeffer MA, et al: Cardiorenal hemodynamics and sodium excretion in rats with myocardial infarction. Am J Physiol 245:H98–H103, 1983.

428. Ichikawa I, Pfeffer JM, Pfeffer MA, et al: Role of angiotensin II in the altered renal function of congestive heart failure. Circ Res 55:669–675, 1984.

429. Nishikimi T, Frohlich ED: Glomerular hemodynamics in aortocaval fistula rats: Role of renin-angiotensin system. Am J Physiol 264:R681–R686, 1993.

430. Packer M: Adaptive and maladaptive actions of angiotensin II in patients with severe congestive heart failure. Review. Am J Kidney Dis 10(suppl 1):66–73, 1987.

431. Suki WN: Renal hemodynamic consequences of angiotensin-converting enzyme inhibition in congestive heart failure. Review. Arch Intern Med 149:669–673, 1989.

432. Badr KF, Ichikawa I: Prerenal failure: A deleterious shift from renal compensation to decompensation. Review. N Engl J Med 319:623–629, 1988.

433. Cody RJ, Ljungman S, Covit AB, et al: Regulation of glomerular filtration rate in chronic congestive heart failure patients. Kidney Int 34:361–367, 1988.

434. Packer M, Lee WH, Medina N, et al: Functional renal insufficiency during long-term therapy with captopril and enalapril in severe chronic heart failure. Ann Intern Med 106:346–354, 1987.

435. Bell NH, Schedl HP: An explanation for abnormal water retention and hypoosmolality in CHF. Am J Med 36:351, 1964.

436. Bennett WM, Bagby GCJ, Antonovic JN, Porter GA: Influence of volume expansion on proximal tubular sodium reabsorption in congestive heart failure. Am Heart J 85:55–64, 1973.

437. Johnston CI, Davis JO, Robb CA, Mackenzie JW: Plasma renin in chronic experimental heart failure and during renal sodium "escape" from mineralocorticoids. Circ Res 22:113–125, 1968.

438. Schneider EG, Dresser TP, Lynch RE, Knox FG: Sodium reabsorption by proximal tubule of dogs with experimental heart failure. Am J Physiol 220:952–957, 1971.

439. Stumpe KO, Solle H, Klein H, Kruck F: Mechanism of sodium and water retention in rats with experimental heart failure. Kidney Int 4:309–317, 1973.

440. Mandin H, Davidman M: Renal function in dogs with acute cardiac tamponade. Am J Physiol 234:F117–F122, 1978.

441. Auld RB, Alexander EA, Levinsky NG: Proximal tubular function in dogs with thoracic caval obstruction. J Clin Invest 50:2150, 1964.

442. Levy M: Effects of acute volume expansion and altered hemodynamics on renal tubular function in chronic caval dogs. J Clin Invest 51:922–938, 1972.

443. Friedler RM, Belleau LJ, Martino JA, Earley LE: Hemodynamically induced natriuresis in the presence of sodium retention resulting from constriction of the thoracic inferior vena cava. J Lab Clin Med 69:565–583, 1967.

444. Hillege HL, Girbes AR, de Kam PJ, et al: Renal function, neurohormonal activation, and survival in patients with chronic heart failure. Circulation 102:203–210, 2000.

445. Marenzi G, Lauri G, Guazzi M, et al: Cardiac and renal dysfunction in chronic heart failure: Relation to neurohumoral activation and prognosis. Am J Med Sci 321:359–366, 2001.

446. Schrier RW, Abraham WT: Hormones and hemodynamics in heart failure. N Engl J Med 341:577–585, 1999.

447. Packer M: The neurohormonal hypothesis—A theory to explain the mechanism of disease progression in heart-failure. J Am Coll Cardiol 20:248–254, 1992.

448. Chatterjee K: Neurohormonal activation in congestive heart failure and the role of vasopressin. Am J Cardiol 95:8B–13B, 2005.

449. Cadnapaphornchai MA, Gurevich AK, Weinberger HD, Schrier RW: Pathophysiology of sodium and water retention in heart failure. Cardiology 96:122–131, 2001.

450. Winaver J, Hoffman A, Abassi Z, Haramati A: Does the heart's hormone, ANP, help in congestive heart failure? News Physiol Sci 10:247–253, 1995.

451. Abassi Z, Haramati A, Hoffman A, et al: Effect of converting-enzyme inhibition on renal response to ANF in rats with experimental heart failure. Am J Physiol 259:R84–R89, 1990.

452. Dzau VJ: Renin-angiotensin system and renal circulation in clinical congestive heart failure. Review. Kidney Int Suppl 20:S203–S209, 1987.

453. Cannon PJ, Martinez-Maldonado M: The pathogenesis of cardiac edema. Semin Nephrol 3:211–224, 1983.

454. Abassi Z, Winaver J, Skorecki K: Control of extracellular fluid volume and the pathophysiology of edema formation. In Brenner BM (ed): Brenner & Rector's The Kidney, Vol 1, 7th ed. Philadelphia, Saunders, 2004, pp 777–855.

455. Dzau VJ, Colucci WS, Hollenberg NK, Williams GH: Relation of the renin-angiotensin-aldosterone system to clinical state in congestive heart failure. Circulation 63:645–651, 1981.

456. Cleland JG, Dargie HJ: Heart failure, renal function, and angiotensin converting enzyme inhibitors. Review. Kidney Int Suppl 20:S220–S228, 1987.

457. Schunkert H, Ingelfinger JR, Hirsch AT, et al: Evidence for tissue-specific activation of renal angiotensinogen mRNA expression in chronic stable experimental heart failure. J Clin Invest 90:1523–1529, 1992.

458. Weber KT: Extracellular matrix remodeling in heart failure: A role for de novo angiotensin II generation. Review. Circulation 96:4065–4082, 1997.

459. Kjaer A, Hesse B: Heart failure and neuroendocrine activation: Diagnostic, prognostic and therapeutic perspectives. Clin Physiol 21:661–672, 2001.

460. Pieruzzi F, Abassi ZA, Keiser HR: Expression of renin-angiotensin system components in the heart, kidneys, and lungs of rats with experimental heart failure. Circulation 92:3105–3112, 1995.

461. Wells G, Little WC: Current treatment and future directions in heart failure. Curr Opin Pharmacol 2:148–153, 2002.

462. Krum H: New and emerging pharmacological strategies in the management of chronic heart failure. Curr Opin Pharmacol 1:126–133, 2001.

463. Brilla CG, Zhou G, Matsubara L, Weber KT: Collagen metabolism in cultured adult rat cardiac fibroblasts: Response to angiotensin II and aldosterone. J Mol Cell Cardiol 26:809–820, 1994.

464. Delyani JA, Robinson EL, Rudolph AE: Effect of a selective aldosterone receptor antagonist in myocardial infarction. Am J Physiol Heart Circ Physiol 281:H647–H654, 2001.

465. Pitt B, Zannad F, Remme WJ, et al: The effect of spironolactone on morbidity and mortality in patients with severe heart failure. Randomized Aldactone Evaluation Study Investigators. N Engl J Med 341:709–717, 1999.

466. Pitt B, White H, Nicolau J, et al: EPHESUS Investigators: Eplerenone reduces mortality 30 days after randomization following acute myocardial infarction in patients with left ventricular systolic dysfunction and heart failure. J Am Coll Cardiol 46:425–431, 2005.

467. Pfeffer MA, Braunwald E, Moye LA, et al: Effect of captopril on mortality and morbidity in patients with left ventricular dysfunction after myocardial infarction. Results of the Survival and Ventricular Enlargement Trial. The SAVE Investigators [see comments]. N Engl J Med 327:669–677, 1992.

468. The CONSENSUS Trial Study Group: Effects of enalapril on mortality in severe congestive heart failure. Results of the Cooperative North Scandinavian Enalapril Survival Study (CONSENSUS). N Engl J Med 316:1429–1435, 1987.

469. The SDI: Effect of enalapril on mortality and the development of heart failure in asymptomatic patients with reduced left ventricular ejection fractions. N Engl J Med 327:685–691, 1992.

470. Riegger GA, Elsner D, Hildenbrand J, et al: Prostaglandins, renin and atrial natriuretic peptide in the control of the circulation and renal function in heart failure in the dog. Prog Clin Biol Res 301:455–458, 1989.

471. Dietz R, Nagel F, Osterziel KJ: Angiotensin-converting enzyme inhibitors and renal function in heart failure. Am J Cardiol 70:119C–125C, 1992.

472. Awan NA, Mason DT: Direct selective blockade of the vascular angiotensin II receptors in therapy for hypertension and severe congestive heart failure. Review. Am Heart J 131:177–185, 1996.

473. Abassi ZA, Kelly G, Golomb E, et al: Losartan improves the natriuretic response to ANF in rats with high-output heart failure. J Pharmacol Exp Ther 268:224–230, 1994.

474. Fitzpatrick MA, Rademaker MT, Charles CJ, et al: Angiotensin II receptor antagonism in ovine heart failure: Acute hemodynamic, hormonal, and renal effects. Am J Physiol 263:H250–H256, 1992.

475. Maeda Y, Wada A, Tsutamoto T, et al: Chronic effects of ANG II antagonist in heart failure: Improvement of cGMP generation from ANP. Am J Physiol 272:H2139–H2145, 1997.

476. Pitt B, Segal R, Martinez FA, et al: Randomised trial of losartan versus captopril in patients over 65 with heart failure (Evaluation of Losartan in the Elderly Study, ELITE). Lancet 349:747–752, 1997.

477. Harris PJ, Navar LG: Tubular transport responses to angiotensin. Review. Am J Physiol 248:F621–F630, 1985.

478. Hensen J, Abraham WT, Durr JA, Schrier RW: Aldosterone in congestive heart failure: Analysis of determinants and role in sodium retention. Am J Nephrol 11:441–446, 1991.

479. Davila DF, Nunez TJ, Odreman R, de Davila CAM: Mechanisms of neurohormonal activation in chronic congestive heart failure: Pathophysiology and therapeutic implications. Int J Cardiol 101:343–346, 2005.

480. Kaye D, Esler M: Sympathetic neuronal regulation of the heart in aging and heart failure. Cardiovasc Res 66:256–264, 2005.

481. Leimbach WNJ, Wallin BG, Victor RG, et al: Direct evidence from intraneural recordings for increased central sympathetic outflow in patients with heart failure. Circulation 73:913–919, 1986.

482. Esler M, Lambert G, Brunner-La Rocca HP, et al: Sympathetic nerve activity and neurotransmitter release in humans: Translation from pathophysiology into clinical practice. Acta Physiol Scand 177:275–284, 2003.

483. Villarreal D, Freeman RH, Johnson RA, Simmons JC: Effects of renal denervation on postprandial sodium excretion in experimental heart failure. Am J Physiol 266:R1599–R1604, 1994.

484. Lieverse AG, van Veldhuisen DJ, Smit AJ, et al: Renal and systemic hemodynamic effects of ibopamine in patients with mild to moderate congestive heart failure. J Cardiovasc Pharmacol 25:361–367, 1995.

485. Pettersson A, Hedner J, Hedner T: Renal interaction between sympathetic activity and ANP in rats with chronic ischaemic heart failure. Acta Physiol Scand 135:487–492, 1989.

486. Feng QP, Hedner T, Hedner J, Pettersson A: Blunted renal response to atrial natriuretic peptide in congestive heart failure rats is reversed by the alpha 2-adrenergic agonist clonidine. J Cardiovasc Pharmacol 16:776–782, 1990.

487. Mizelle HL, Hall JE, Montani JP: Role of renal nerves in control of sodium excretion in chronic congestive heart failure. Am J Physiol 256:F1084–F1093, 1989.

488. Lohmeier TE, Reinhart GA, Mizelle HL, et al: Influence of the renal nerves on sodium excretion during progressive reductions in cardiac output. Am J Physiol 269:R679–R690, 1995.

489. Szatalowicz VL, Arnold PE, Chaimovitz C, et al: Radioimmunoassay of plasma arginine vasopressin in hyponatremic patients with congestive heart-failure. N Engl J Med 305:263–266, 1981.

490. Goldsmith SR, Francis GS, Cowley AW, et al: Increased plasma arginine vasopressin levels in patients with congestive heart-failure. J Am Coll Cardiol 1:1385–1390, 1983.

491. Lee CR, Watkins ML, Patterson JH, et al: Vasopressin: A new target for the treatment of heart failure. Am Heart J 146:9–18, 2003.

492. Goldsmith SR, Gheorghiade M: Vasopressin antagonism in heart failure. J Am Coll Cardiol 46(10):1785–1791, 2005.

493. Dietz R, Haass M, Osterziel KJ: Atrial natriuretic factor and arginine vasopressin. Prog Cardiol 4:113–133, 1994.

494. Pruszczynski W, Vahanian A, Ardaillou R, Acar J: Role of antidiuretic hormone in impaired water excretion of patients with congestive heart failure. J Clin Endocrinol Metab 58:599–605, 1984.

495. Manthey J, Dietz R, Opherk D, et al: Baroreceptor-mediated release of vasopressin in patients with chronic congestive heart failure and defective sympathetic responsiveness [see comments]. Am J Cardiol 70:224–228, 1992.

496. Bonjour JP, Malvin RL: Stimulation of ADH release by the renin-angiotensin system. Am J Physiol 218:1555–1559, 1970.

497. Henrich WL, Walker BR, Handelman WA, et al: Effects of angiotensin II on plasma antidiuretic hormone and renal water excretion. Kidney Int 30:503–508, 1986.

498. Bichet DG, Kortas C, Mettauer B, et al: Modulation of plasma and platelet vasopressin by cardiac function in patients with heart failure. Kidney Int 29:1188–1196, 1986.

499. Martin PY, Schrier RW: Sodium and water retention in heart failure: Pathogenesis and treatment. Review. Kidney Int 51(suppl 59):S57–S61, 1997.

500. Kalra PR, Anker SD, Coats AJ: Water and sodium regulation in chronic heart failure: The role of natriuretic peptides and vasopressin. Cardiovasc Res 51:495–509, 2001.

501. Mulinari RA, Gavras H, Wang YX, et al: Effects of a vasopressin antagonist with combined antipressor and antiantidiuretic activities in rats with left ventricular dysfunction. Circulation 81:308–311, 1990.

502. Ishikawa SE, Schrier RW: Pathophysiological roles of arginine vasopressin and aquaporin-2 in impaired water excretion. Clin Endocrinol (Oxf) 58(1):1–17, 2003.

503. Ishikawa S, Saito T, Okada K, et al: Effect of vasopressin antagonist on water excretion in inferior vena cava constriction. Kidney Int 30:49–55, 1986.

504. Naitoh M, Suzuki H, Murakami M, et al: Effects of oral AVP receptor antagonists OPC-21268 and OPC-31260 on congestive heart failure in conscious dogs. Am J Physiol 267:H2245–H2254, 1994.

505. Verbalis JG: Vasopressin V-2 receptor antagonists. J Mol Endocrinol 29:1–9, 2002.

506. Xu DL, Martin PY, Ohara M, et al: Upregulation of aquaporin-2 water channel expression in chronic heart failure rat. J Clin Invest 99:1500–1505, 1997.

507. Kim JK, Michel JB, Soubrier F, et al: Arginine vasopressin gene expression in chronic cardiac failure in rats. Kidney Int 38:818–822, 1990.

508. Gheorghiade M, Niazi I, Ouyang J, et al: Vasopressin V-2–receptor blockade with tolvaptan in patients with chronic heart failure—Results from a double-blind, randomized trial. Circulation 107:2690–2696, 2003.

509. Gheorghiade M, Gattis WA, O'Connor CM, et al: Effects of tolvaptan, a vasopressin antagonist, in patients hospitalized with worsening heart failure—A randomized controlled trial. JAMA 291:1963–1971, 2004.

510. Eisenman A, Armali Z, Enat R, et al: Low-dose vasopressin restores diuresis both in patients with hepatorenal syndrome and in anuric patients with end-stage heart failure. J Intern Med 246:183–190, 1999.

511. Manning M, Sawyer WH: Discovery, development, and some uses of vasopressin and oxytocin antagonists. J Lab Clin Med 114:617–632, 1989.

512. Serradeil-Le Gal C, Wagnon J, Valette G, et al: Nonpeptide vasopressin receptor antagonists: Development of selective and orally active V1a, V2 and V1b receptor ligands. Prog Brain Res 139:197–210, 2002.

513. Thibonnier M, Coles P, Thibonnier A, Shoham M: Molecular pharmacology and modeling of vasopressin receptors. Prog Brain Res 139:179–196, 2002.

514. Wada K, Tahara A, Arai Y, et al. Effect of the vasopressin receptor antagonist conivaptan in rats with heart failure following myocardial infarction. Eur J Pharmacol 450:169–177, 2002.

515. Yatsu T, Tomura Y, Tahara A, et al: Cardiovascular and renal effects of conivaptan hydrochloride (YM087), a vasopressin V-1A and V-2 receptor antagonist, in dogs with pacing-induced congestive heart failure. Eur J Pharmacol 376:239–246, 1999.

516. Yatsu T, Kusayama T, Tomura Y, et al: Effect of conivaptan, a combined vasopressin V-1a and V-2 receptor antagonist, on vasopressin-induced cardiac and haemodynamic changes in anaesthetised dogs. Pharmacol Res 46:375–381, 2002.

517. Burrell LM, Phillips PA, Risvanis J, et al: Long-term effects of nonpeptide vasopressin V-2 antagonist OPC-31260 in heart failure in the rat. Am J Physiol Heart Circ Physiol 44:H176–H182, 1998.

518. Van Kerckhoven R, Saxena PR, Schoemaker RG: Chronic vasopressin V-1a– but not V-2–receptor antagonism prevents heart failure in chronically infarcted rats. J Mol Cell Cardiol 34:A93, 2002.

519. Udelson JE, Smith WB, Hendrix GH, et al: Acute hemodynamic effects of conivaptan, a dual V-1A and V-2 vasopressin receptor antagonist, in patients with advanced heart failure. Circulation 104:2417–2423, 2001.

520. Love MP, McMurray JJ: Endothelin in chronic heart failure: Current position and future prospects. Review. Cardiovasc Res 31:665–674, 1996.

521. McMurray JJ, Ray SG, Abdullah I, et al: Plasma endothelin in chronic heart failure. Circulation 85:1374–1379, 1992.

522. von Lueder TG, Kjekshus H, Edvardsen T, et al: Mechanisms of elevated plasma endothelin-1 in CHF: Congestion increases pulmonary synthesis and secretion of endothelin-1. Cardiovasc Res 63:41–50, 2004.

523. Cavero PG, Miller WL, Heublein DM, et al: Endothelin in experimental congestive heart failure in the anesthetized dog. Am J Physiol 259:F312–F317, 1990.

524. Hiroe M, Hirata Y, Fujita N, et al: Plasma endothelin-1 levels in idiopathic dilated cardiomyopathy. Am J Cardiol 68:1114–1115, 1991.

525. Wei CM, Lerman A, Rodeheffer RJ, et al: Endothelin in human congestive heart failure. Circulation 89:1580–1586, 1994.

526. Cody RJ, Haas GJ, Binkley PF, et al: Plasma endothelin correlates with the extent of pulmonary hypertension in patients with chronic congestive heart failure [published erratum appears in Circulation 87(3):1064, 1993]. Circulation 85:504–509, 1992.

527. Omland T, Lie RT, Aakvaag A, et al: Plasma endothelin determination as a prognostic indicator of 1-year mortality after acute myocardial infarction [see comments]. Circulation 89:1573–1579, 1994.

528. Spieker LE, Noll G, Ruschitzka FT, Luscher TF: Endothelin receptor antagonists in congestive heart failure: A new therapeutic principle for the future? J Am Coll Cardiol 37:1493–1505, 2001.

529. Giannessi D, Del Ry S, Vitale RL: The role of endothelins and their receptors in heart failure. Pharmacol Res 43:111–126, 2001.

530. Lerman A, Kubo SH, Tschumperlin LK, Burnett JCJ: Plasma endothelin concentrations in humans with end-stage heart failure and after heart transplantation [see comments]. J Am Coll Cardiol 20:849–853, 1992.

531. Webb DJ, Monge JC, Rabelink TJ, Yanagisawa M: Endothelin: New discoveries and rapid progress in the clinic. Trends Pharmacol Sci 19:5–8, 1998.

532. Warner TD, Elliott JD, Ohlstein EH: California dreamin' 'bout endothelin: Emerging new therapeutics. Trends Pharmacol Sci 17:177–181, 1996.

533. Bax WA, Saxena PR: The current endothelin receptor classification: Time for reconsideration? Review. Trends Pharmacol Sci 15:379–386, 1994.

534. Douglas SA: Clinical development of endothelin receptor antagonists. Trends Pharmacol Sci 18:408–412, 1997.

535. Gurbanov K, Rubinstein I, Hoffman A, et al: Bosentan improves renal regional blood flow in rats with experimental congestive heart failure. Eur J Pharmacol 310:193–196, 1996.

536. Qiu C, Ding SS, Hess P, et al: Endothelin mediates the altered renal hemodynamics associated with experimental congestive heart failure. J Cardiovasc Pharmacol 38:317–324, 2001.

537. Borgeson DD, Grantham JA, Williamson EE, et al: Chronic oral endothelin type A receptor antagonism in experimental heart failure. Hypertension 31:766–770, 1998.

538. Bauersachs J, Braun C, Fraccarollo D, et al: Improvement of renal dysfunction in rats with chronic heart failure after myocardial infarction by treatment with the endothelin A receptor antagonist, LU 135252. J Hypertens 18:1507–1514, 2000.

539. Ding SS, Qiu C, Hess P, et al: Chronic endothelin receptor blockade prevents renal vasoconstriction and sodium retention in rats with chronic heart failure. Cardiovasc Res 53:963–970, 2002.

540. Kiowski W, Sutsch G, Hunziker P, et al: Evidence for endothelin-1–mediated vasoconstriction in severe chronic heart failure. Lancet 346:732–736, 1995.

541. Packer M, Mcmurray J, Massie BM, et al: Clinical effects of endothelin receptor antagonism with bosentan in patients with severe chronic heart failure: Results of a pilot study. J Card Fail 11:12–20, 2005.

542. Brown LA, Nunez DJ, Brookes CI, Wilkins MR: Selective increase in endothelin-1 and endothelin A receptor subtype in the hypertrophied myocardium of the aorto-venacaval fistula rat. Cardiovasc Res 29:768–774, 1995.

543. Colucci WS: Myocardial endothelin. Does it play a role in myocardial failure? Editorial; comment. Circulation 93:1069–1072, 1996.

544. Sakai S, Miyauchi T, Sakurai T, et al: Endogenous endothelin-1 participates in the maintenance of cardiac function in rats with congestive heart failure. Marked increase in endothelin-1 production in the failing heart [see comments]. Circulation 93:1214–1222, 1996.

545. Rodeheffer RJ, Tanaka I, Imada T, et al: Atrial pressure and secretion of atrial natriuretic factor into the human central circulation. J Am Coll Cardiol 8:18–26, 1986.

546. Hensen J, Abraham WT, Lesnefsky EJ, et al: Atrial natriuretic peptide kinetic studies in patients with cardiac dysfunction. Kidney Int 41:1333–1339, 1992.

547. Poulos JE, Gower WR, Sullebarger JT, et al: Congestive heart failure: Increased cardiac and extracardiac atrial natriuretic peptide gene expression. Cardiovasc Res 32:909–919, 1996.

548. Moe GW, Forster C, de Bold AJ, Armstrong PW: Pharmacokinetics, hemodynamic, renal, and neurohormonal effects of atrial natriuretic factor in experimental heart failure. Clin Invest Med 13:111–118, 1990.

549. Eiskjaer H, Bagger JP, Danielsen H, et al: Attenuated renal excretory response to atrial natriuretic peptide in congestive heart failure in man. Int J Cardiol 33:61–74, 1991.

550. Hirsch AT, Creager MA, Dzau VJ: Relation of atrial natriuretic factor to vasoconstrictor hormones and regional blood flow in congestive heart failure. Am J Cardiol 63:211–216, 1989.

551. Kanamori T, Wada A, Tsutamoto T, Kinoshita M: Possible regulation of renin release by ANP in dogs with heart failure. Am J Physiol 268:H2281–H2287, 1995.

552. Lohmeier TE, Mizelle HL, Reinhart GA, et al: Atrial natriuretic peptide and sodium homeostasis in compensated heart failure. Am J Physiol 271:R1353–R1363, 1996.

553. Stevens TL, Burnett JC, Kinoshita M, et al: A functional-role for endogenous atrial-natriuretic-peptide in a canine model of early left-ventricular dysfunction. J Clin Invest 95:1101–1108, 1995.

554. Laragh JH: Atrial natriuretic hormone, the renin-aldosterone axis, and blood pressure-electrolyte homeostasis. Review. N Engl J Med 313:1330–1340, 1985.

555. Wada A, Tsutamoto T, Matsuda Y, Kinoshita M: Cardiorenal and neurohumoral effects of endogenous atrial natriuretic peptide in dogs with severe congestive heart failure using a specific antagonist for guanylate cyclase–coupled receptors. Circulation 89:2232–2240, 1994.

556. Andreassi MG, Del Ry S, Palmieri C, et al: Up-regulation of "clearance" receptors in patients with chronic heart failure: A possible explanation for the resistance to biological effects of cardiac natriuretic hormones. Eur J Heart Fail 3:407–414, 2001.

557. Wegner M, Hirth-Dietrich C, Stasch JP: Role of neutral endopeptidase 24.11 in AV fistular rat model of heart failure. Cardiovasc Res 31:891–898, 1996.

558. Knecht M, Pagel I, Langenickel T, et al: Increased expression of renal neutral endopeptidase in severe heart failure. Life Sci 71:2701–2712, 2002.

559. Clerico A, Iervasi G, Del Chicca MG, et al: Circulating levels of cardiac natriuretic peptides (ANP and BNP) measured by highly sensitive and specific immunoradiometric assays in normal subjects and in patients with different degrees of heart failure. J Endocrinol Invest 21:170–179, 1998.

560. Sosa RE, Volpe M, Marion DN, et al: Relationship between renal hemodynamic and natriuretic effects of atrial natriuretic factor. Am J Physiol 250:F520–F524, 1986.

561. Showalter CJ, Zimmerman RS, Schwab TR, et al: Renal response to atrial natriuretic factor is modulated by intrarenal angiotensin-II. Am J Physiol 254:R453–R456, 1988.

562. Costello-Boerrigter LC, Boerrigter G, Burnett JC: Revisiting salt and water retention: New diuretics, aquaretics, and natriuretics. Med Clin North Am 87:475–491, 2003.

563. Colucci WS, Elkayam U, Horton DP, et al: Intravenous nesiritide, a natriuretic peptide, in the treatment of decompensated congestive heart failure. Nesiritide Study Group. N Engl J Med 343:246–253, 2000.

564. Colucci WS: Nesiritide for the treatment of decompensated heart failure. J Card Fail 7:92–100, 2001.

565. Laverman GD, Remuzzi G, Ruggenenti P: ACE inhibition versus angiotensin receptor blockade: Which is better for renal and cardiovascular protection? J Am Soc Nephrol 15:S64–S70, 2004.

566. Kohzuki M, Hodsman GP, Johnston CI: Attenuated response to atrial natriuretic peptide in rats with myocardial infarction. Am J Physiol 256:H533–H538, 1989.

567. Raya TE, Lee RW, Westhoff T, Goldman S: Captopril restores hemodynamic responsiveness to atrial natriuretic peptide in rats with heart failure. Circulation 80:1886–1892, 1989.

568. Gauquelin G, Schiffrin EL, Garcia R: Downregulation of glomerular and vascular atrial natriuretic factor receptor subtypes by angiotensin II. J Hypertens 9(12):1151–1160, 1991.

569. Haneda M, Kikkawa R, Maeda S, et al: Dual mechanism of angiotensin-II inhibits ANP-induced mesangial cGMP accumulation. Kidney Int 40:188–194, 1991.

570. Rocha R, Stier CT: Pathophysiological effects of aldosterone in cardiovascular tissues. Trends Endocrinol Metab 12:308–314, 2001.

571. Walter M, Unwin R, Nortier J, Deschodt-Lanckman M: Enhancing endogenous effects of natriuretic peptides: Inhibitors of neutral endopeptidase (EC.3.4.24.11) and phosphodiesterase. Review. Curr Opin Nephrol Hypertens 6:468–473, 1997.
572. Wilkins MR, Needleman P: Effect of pharmacological manipulation of endogenous atriopeptin activity on renal function. Review. Am J Physiol 262:F161–F167, 1992.
573. Sybertz EJJ, Chiu PJ, Watkins RW, Vemulapalli S: Neutral metalloendopeptidase inhibition: A novel means of circulatory modulation. J Hypertens Suppl 8:S161–S167, 1990.
574. Seymour AA, Asaad MM, Lanoce VM, et al: Inhibition of neutral endopeptidase 3.4.24.11 in conscious dogs with pacing induced heart failure. Cardiovasc Res 27:1015–1023, 1993.
575. Wilkins MR, Settle SL, Stockmann PT, Needleman P: Maximizing the natriuretic effect of endogenous atriopeptin in a rat model of heart failure. Proc Natl Acad Sci U S A 87:6465–6469, 1990.
576. Margulies KB, Burnett JCJ: Neutral endopeptidase 24.11: A modulator of natriuretic peptides. Review. Semin Nephrol 13:71–77, 1993.
577. Goetz KL: Evidence that atriopeptin is not a physiological regulator of sodium excretion. Review. Hypertension 15:9–19, 1990.
578. Anderson J, Struthers A, Christofides N, Bloom S: Atrial natriuretic peptide: An endogenous factor enhancing sodium excretion in man. Clin Sci (Colch) 70:327–331, 1986.
579. Chen HH, Schirger JA, Chau WL, et al: Renal response to acute neutral endopeptidase inhibition in mild and severe experimental heart failure. Circulation 100:2443–2448, 1999.
580. Margulies KB, Perrella MA, McKinley LJ, Burnett JCJ: Angiotensin inhibition potentiates the renal responses to neutral endopeptidase inhibition in dogs with congestive heart failure. J Clin Invest 88:1636–1642, 1991.
581. Blaine EH: Atrial natriuretic factor plays a significant role in body fluid homeostasis. Hypertension 15:2–8, 1990.
582. Robl JA, Sun CQ, Stevenson J, et al: Dual metalloprotease inhibitors: Mercaptoacetyl-based fused heterocyclic dipeptide mimetics as inhibitors of angiotensin-converting enzyme and neutral endopeptidase. J Med Chem 40:1570–1577, 1997.
583. Burnett JC: Vasopeptidase inhibition. Curr Opin Nephrol Hypertens 9:465–468, 2000.
584. Bralet J, Schwartz JC: Vasopeptidase inhibitors: An emerging class of cardiovascular drugs. Trends Pharmacol Sci 22:106–109, 2001.
585. Bralet J, Marie C, Mossiat C, et al: Effects of alatriopril, a mixed inhibitor of atriopeptidase and angiotensin I-converting enzyme, on cardiac-hypertrophy and hormonal responses in rats with myocardial-infarction—Comparison with captopril. J Pharmacol Exp Ther 270:8–14, 1994.
586. Marie C, Mossiat C, Lecomte JM, et al: Hemodynamic effects of acute and chronic treatment with aladotril, a mixed inhibitor of neutral endopeptidase and angiotensin I-converting enzyme, in conscious rats with myocardial infarction. J Pharmacol Exp Ther 275(3):1324–1331, 1995.
587. Troughton RW, Rademaker MT, Powell JD, et al: Beneficial renal and hemodynamic effects of omapatrilat in mild and severe heart failure. Hypertension 36(4):523–530. 2000.
588. Troughton RW, Frampton CM, Yandle TG, et al: Treatment of heart failure guided by plasma aminoterminal brain natriuretic peptide (N-BNP) concentrations. Lancet 355:1126–1130, 2000.
589. Klapholz M, Thomas I, Eng C, et al: Effects of omapatrilat on hemodynamics and safety in patients with heart failure. Am J Cardiol 88:657–661, 2001.
590. McClean DR, Ikram H, Garlick AH, et al: The clinical, cardiac, renal, arterial and neurohormonal effects of omapatrilat, a vasopeptidase inhibitor, in patients with chronic heart failure. J Am Coll Cardiol 36:479–486, 2000.
591. McClean DR, Ikram H, Mehta S, et al: Vasopeptidase inhibition with omapatrilat in chronic heart failure: Acute and long-term hemodynamic and neurohumoral effects. J Am Coll Cardiol 39:2034–2041, 2002.
592. Rouleau JL, Pfeffer MA, Stewart DJ, et al: Comparison of vasopeptidase inhibitor, omapatrilat, and lisinopril on exercise tolerance and morbidity in patients with heart failure: IMPRESS randomised trial. Lancet 356:615–620, 2000.
593. Trippodo NC, Robl JA, Asaad MM, et al: Cardiovascular effects of the novel dual inhibitor of neutral endopeptidase and angiotensin-converting enzyme Bms-182657 in experimental-hypertension and heart-failure. J Pharmacol Exp Ther 275:745–752, 1995.
594. Trippodo NC, Fox M, Monticello TM, et al: Vasopeptidase inhibition with omapatrilat improves cardiac geometry and survival in cardiomyopathic hamsters more than does ACE inhibition with captopril. J Cardiovasc Pharmacol 34:782–790, 1999.
595. Chen HH, Lainchbury JG, Matsuda Y, et al: Endogenous natriuretic peptides participate in renal and humoral actions of acute vasopeptidase inhibition in experimental mild heart failure. Hypertension 38:187–191, 2001.
596. Cleland, JG, Swedberg K: Lack of efficacy of neutral endopeptidase inhibitor ecadotril in heart failure. The International Ecadotril Multi-centre Dose-ranging Study Investigators. Lancet 351(9116):1657–1658, 1998.
597. O'Connor CM, Gattis WA, Gheorghiade M, et al: A randomized trial of ecadotril versus placebo in patients with mild to moderate heart failure: The US Ecadotril Pilot Safety Study. Am Heart J 138:1140–1148, 1999.
598. Packer M, Califf RM, Konstam MA, et al: Comparison of omapatrilat and enalapril in patients with chronic heart failure: The Omapatrilat Versus Enalapril Randomized Trial of Utility in Reducing Events (OVERTURE). Circulation 106:920–926, 2002.
599. Messerli FH, Nussberger J: Vasopeptidase inhibition and angio-oedema. Lancet 356:608–609, 2000.
600. Ruilope LM, Palatini P, Grossman E, et al: Randomized double-blind comparison of omapatrilat with amlodipine in mild-to-moderate hypertension. J Hypertens 18:S95–S96, 2000.
601. Ferdinand KC: Advances in antihypertensive combination therapy: Benefits of low-dose thiazide diuretics in conjunction with omapatrilat, a vasopeptidase inhibitor. J Clin Hypertens 3(5):307–312, 2001.
602. Corti R, Burnett JC, Rouleau JL, et al: Vasopeptidase inhibitors—A new therapeutic concept in cardiovascular disease? Circulation 104:1856–1862, 2001.
603. Kostis OB, Packer M, Black HR, et al: Omapatrilat and enalapril in patients with hypertension: The Omapatrilat Cardiovascular Treatment Vs. Enalapril (OCTAVE) Trial. Am J Hypertens 17:103–111, 2004.
604. Nakagawa O, Ogawa Y, Itoh H, et al: Rapid transcriptional activation and early messenger-RNA turnover of brain natriuretic peptide in cardiocyte hypertrophy—Evidence for brain natriuretic peptide as an emergency cardiac hormone against ventricular overload. J Clin Invest 96:1280–1287, 1995.
605. Yoshimura M, Yasue H, Okumura K, et al: Different secretion patterns of atrial-natriuretic-peptide and brain natriuretic peptide in patients with congestive-heart-failure. Circulation 87:464–469, 1993.
606. Maeda K, Tsutamoto T, Wada A, et al: Plasma brain natriuretic peptide as a biochemical marker of high left ventricular end-diastolic pressure in patients with symptomatic left ventricular dysfunction. Am Heart J 135:825–832, 1998.
607. Yasue H, Yoshimura M, Sumida H, et al: Localization and mechanism of secretion of B-type natriuretic peptide in comparison with those of A-type natriuretic peptide in normal subjects and patients with heart failure. Circulation 90:195–203, 1994.
608. Wallen T, Landahl S, Hedner T, et al: Brain natriuretic peptide predicts mortality in the elderly. Heart 77:264–267, 1997.
609. Cowie MR, Struthers AD, Wood DA, et al: Value of natriuretic peptides in assessment of patients with possible new heart failure in primary care. Lancet 350:1349–1353, 1997.
610. McDonagh TA, Robb SD, Murdoch DR, et al: Biochemical detection of left-ventricular systolic dysfunction. Lancet 351:9–13, 1998.
611. Davis M, Espiner E, Richards G, et al: Plasma brain natriuretic peptide in assessment of acute dyspnoea. Lancet 343:440–444, 1994.
612. Yamamoto K, Burnett JC Jr, Jougasaki M, et al: Superiority of brain natriuretic peptide as a hormonal marker of ventricular systolic and diastolic dysfunction and ventricular hypertrophy. Hypertension 28:988–994, 1996.
613. Yu CM, Sanderson JE, Shum IO, et al: Diastolic dysfunction and natriuretic peptides in systolic heart failure. Higher ANP and BNP levels are associated with the restrictive filling pattern. Eur Heart J 17:1694–1702, 1996.
614. Bettencourt P, Ferreira A, Dias P, et al: Evaluation of brain natriuretic peptide in the diagnosis of heart failure. Cardiology 93:19–25, 2000.
615. Wei CM, Heublein DM, Perrella MA, et al: Natriuretic peptide system in human heart failure. Circulation 88:1004–1009, 1993.
616. Rademaker MT, Charles CJ, Espiner EA, et al: Natriuretic peptide responses to acute and chronic ventricular pacing in sheep. Am J Physiol 270:H594–H602, 1996.
617. Luchner A, Stevens TL, Borgeson DD, et al: Differential atrial and ventricular expression of myocardial BNP during evolution of heart failure. Am J Physiol 274:H1684–H1689, 1998.
618. Bhatia V, Nayyar P, Dhindsa S: Brain natriuretic peptide in diagnosis and treatment of heart failure. J Postgrad Med 49(2):182–185, 2003.
619. Lerman A, Gibbons RJ, Rodeheffer RJ, et al: Circulating N-terminal atrial-natriuretic-peptide as a marker for symptomless left-ventricular dysfunction. Lancet 341:1105–1109, 1993.
620. Hall C, Rouleau JL, Moye L, et al: N-terminal proatrial natriuretic factor. An independent predictor of long-term prognosis after myocardial infarction. Circulation 89:1934–1942, 1994.
621. Gottlieb SS, Kukin ML, Ahern D, Packer M: Prognostic importance of atrial natriuretic peptide in patients with chronic heart failure. J Am Coll Cardiol 13:1534–1539, 1989.
622. Grantham JA, Burnett JCJ: BNP: Increasing importance in the pathophysiology and diagnosis of congestive heart failure. Editorial; comment. Circulation 96:388–390, 1997.
623. Tsutamoto T, Wada A, Maeda K, et al: Attenuation of compensation of endogenous cardiac natriuretic peptide system in chronic heart failure: Prognostic role of plasma brain natriuretic peptide concentration in patients with chronic symptomatic left ventricular dysfunction [see comments]. Circulation 96:509–516, 1997.
624. Chen HH, Burnett JC: The natriuretic peptides in heart failure: Diagnostic and therapeutic potentials. Proc Assoc Am Physicians 111:406–416, 1999.
625. Richards AM, Nicholls MG, Yandle TG, et al: Plasma N-terminal pro-brain natriuretic peptide and adrenomedullin: New neurohormonal predictors of left ventricular function and prognosis after myocardial infarction. Circulation 97:1921–1929, 1998.
626. Luchner A, Hengstenberg C, Lowel H, et al: N-terminal pro-brain natriuretic peptide after myocardial infarction: A marker of cardio-renal function. Hypertension 39:99–104, 2002.
627. de Lemos JA, Morrow DA, Bentley JH, et al: The prognostic value of B-type natriuretic peptide in patients with acute coronary syndromes. N Engl J Med 345:1014–1021, 2001.
628. Richards AM, Nicholls MG, Espiner EA, et al: B-type natriuretic peptides and ejection fraction for prognosis after myocardial infarction. Circulation 107:2786–2792, 2003.
629. Maisel A: B-type natriuretic peptide measurements in diagnosing congestive heart failure in the dyspneic emergency department patient. Rev Cardiovasc Med 3(4): S10–S17, 2002.
630. Maisel A: B-type natriuretic peptide levels: Diagnostic and prognostic in congestive heart failure—What's next? Circulation 105:2328–2331, 2002.
631. Harrison A, Morrison LK, Krishnaswamy P, et al: B-type natriuretic peptide predicts future cardiac events in patients presenting to the emergency department with dyspnea. Ann Emerg Med 39:131–138, 2002.
632. Berger R, Huelsman M, Strecker K, et al: B-type natriuretic peptide predicts sudden death in patients with chronic heart failure. Circulation 105:2392–2397, 2002.
633. Dao Q, Krishnaswamy P, Kazanegra R, et al: Utility of B-type natriuretic peptide in the diagnosis of congestive heart failure in an urgent-care setting. J Am Coll Cardiol 37:379–385, 2001.

634. Lubien E, DeMaria A, Krishnaswamy P, et al: Utility of B-natriuretic peptide in detecting diastolic dysfunction: Comparison with Doppler velocity recordings. Circulation 105:595–601, 2002.

635. McCullough PA: B-type natriuretic peptides. A diagnostic breakthrough in heart failure. Minerva Cardioangiol 51(2):121–129, 2003.

636. Kawai K, Hata K, Takaoka H, et al: Plasma brain natriuretic peptide as a novel therapeutic indicator in idiopathic dilated cardiomyopathy during beta-blocker therapy: A potential of hormone-guided treatment. Am Heart J 141:925–932, 2001.

637. Motwani JG, McAlpine H, Kennedy N, Struthers AD: Plasma brain natriuretic peptide as an indicator for angiotensin-converting-enzyme inhibition after myocardial infarction. Lancet 341:1109–1113, 1993.

638. Maeda K, Tsutamoto T, Wada A, et al: High levels of plasma brain natriuretic peptide and interleukin-6 after optimized treatment for heart failure are independent risk factors for morbidity and mortality in patients with congestive heart failure. J Am Coll Cardiol 36:1587–1593, 2000.

639. Packer M: Should B-type natriuretic peptide be measured routinely to guide the diagnosis and management of chronic heart failure? Circulation 108(24):2950–2953, 2003.

640. Tang WH, Girod JP, Lee MJ, et al: Plasma B-type natriuretic peptide levels in ambulatory patients with established chronic symptomatic systolic heart failure. Circulation 108(24):2964–2966, 2006.

641. Mattingly MT, Brandt RR, Heublein DM, et al: Presence of C-type natriuretic peptide in human kidney and urine. Kidney Int 46:744–747, 1994.

642. Kenny AJ, Bourne A, Ingram J: Hydrolysis of human and pig brain natriuretic peptides, urodilatin, C-type natriuretic peptide and some C-receptor ligands by endopeptidase 24.11. Biochem J 291(pt 1):83–88, 1993.

643. Vallon V, Peterson OW, Gabbai FB, et al: Interactive control of renal function by alpha 2-adrenergic system and nitric oxide: Role of angiotensin II. J Cardiovasc Pharmacol 26:916–922, 1995.

644. Saito Y, Nakao K, Nishimura K, et al: Clinical application of atrial natriuretic polypeptide in patients with congestive heart failure: Beneficial effects on left ventricular function. Circulation 76:115–124, 1987.

645. Marcus LS, Hart D, Packer M, et al: Hemodynamic and renal excretory effects of human brain natriuretic peptide infusion in patients with congestive heart failure. A double-blind, placebo-controlled, randomized crossover trial. Circulation 94:3184–3189, 1996.

646. Hobbs RE, Miller LW, Bott-Silverman C, et al: Hemodynamic effects of a single intravenous injection of synthetic human brain natriuretic peptide in patients with heart failure secondary to ischemic or idiopathic dilated cardiomyopathy. Am J Cardiol 78:896–901, 1996.

647. Abraham WT, Lowes BD, Ferguson DA, et al: Systemic hemodynamic, neurohormonal, and renal effects of a steady-state infusion of human brain natriuretic peptide in patients with hemodynamically decompensated heart failure. J Card Fail 4:37–44, 1998.

648. Mills RM, LeJemtel TH, Horton DP, et al: Sustained hemodynamic effects of an infusion of nesiritide (human b-type natriuretic peptide) in heart failure: A randomized, double-blind, placebo-controlled clinical trial. Natrecor Study Group. J Am Coll Cardiol 34:155–162, 1999.

649. Abraham WT, Hensen J, Schrier RW: Elevated plasma noradrenaline concentrations in patients with low-output cardiac failure: Dependence on increased noradrenaline secretion rates. Clin Sci (Colch) 79:429–435, 1990.

650. Hoffman A, Grossman E, Keiser HR: Increased plasma levels and blunted effects of brain natriuretic peptide in rats with congestive heart failure. Am J Hypertens 4:597–601, 1991.

651. Chen HH, Grantham JA, Schirger JA, et al: Subcutaneous administration of brain natriuretic peptide in experimental heart failure. J Am Coll Cardiol 36:1706–1712, 2000.

652. Young JB, Abraham WT, Stevenson LW, et al: Intravenous nesiritide vs nitroglycerin for treatment of decompensated congestive heart failure—A randomized controlled trial. JAMA 287:1531–1540, 2002.

653. Tokudome T, Horio T, Soeki T, et al: Inhibitory effect of C-type natriuretic peptide (CNP) on cultured cardiac myocyte hypertrophy: Interference between CNP and endothelin-1 signaling pathways. Endocrinology 145:2131–2140, 2004.

654. Sudoh T, Minamino N, Kangawa K, Matsuo H: C-type natriuretic peptide (CNP): A new member of natriuretic peptide family identified in porcine brain. Biochem Biophys Res Commun 168:863–870, 1990.

655. Stingo AJ, Clavell AL, Aarhus LL, Burnett JCJ: Cardiovascular and renal actions of C-type natriuretic peptide. Am J Physiol 262:H308–H312, 1992.

656. Clavell AL, Stingo AJ, Wei CM, et al: C-type natriuretic peptide: A selective cardiovascular peptide. Am J Physiol 264:R290–R295, 1993.

657. Barr CS, Rhodes P, Struthers AD: C-type natriuretic peptide. Review. Peptides 17:1243–1251, 1996.

658. Wright SP, Prickett TCR, Doughty RN, et al: Amino-terminal pro-C-type natriuretic peptide in heart failure. Hypertension 43:94–100, 2004.

659. Celermajer DS: Endothelial dysfunction: Does it matter? Is it reversible? J Am Coll Cardiol 30:325–333, 1997.

660. Mendes Ribeiro AC, Brunini TM, Ellory JC, Mann GE: Abnormalities in L-arginine transport and nitric oxide biosynthesis in chronic renal and heart failure. Cardiovasc Res 49:697–712, 2001.

661. Kubo SH, Rector TS, Bank AJ, et al: Endothelium-dependent vasodilation is attenuated in patients with heart failure. Circulation 84:1589–1596, 1991.

662. Hanssen H, Brunini TM, Conway M, et al: Increased L-arginine transport in human erythrocytes in chronic heart failure. Clin Sci 94:43–48, 1998.

663. Abassi ZA, Gurbanov K, Mulroney SE, et al: Impaired nitric oxide-mediated renal vasodilation in rats with experimental heart failure: Role of angiotensin II. Circulation 96:3655–3664, 1997.

664. Bauersachs J, Schafer A: Endothelial dysfunction in heart failure: Mechanisms and therapeutic approaches. Curr Vasc Pharmacol 2(2):115–124, 2004.

665. Drexler H, Hayoz D, Munzel T, et al: Endothelial function in chronic congestive heart failure. Am J Cardiol 69:1596–1601, 1992.

666. Drexler H, Holtz J: Endothelium dependent relaxation in chronic heart failure. Cardiovasc Res 28:720–721, 1994.

667. Habib F, Dutka D, Crossman D, et al: Enhanced basal nitric oxide production in heart failure: Another failed counter-regulatory vasodilator mechanism? [see comments]. Lancet 344:371–373, 1994.

668. Winlaw DS, Smythe GA, Keogh AM, et al: Increased nitric oxide production in heart failure. Lancet 344:373–374, 1994.

669. Cooke JP, Dzau VJ: Derangements of the nitric oxide synthase pathway, L-arginine, and cardiovascular diseases. Editorial; comment. Review. Circulation 96:379–382, 1997.

670. Tang WHW, Francis GS: The year in heart failure. J American Coll Cardiol 46:2125–2133, 2005.

671. Zambraski EJ: The effects of nonsteroidal anti-inflammatory drugs on renal function: Experimental studies in animals. Review. Semin Nephrol 15:205–213, 1995.

672. Anand IS, Chugh SS: Mechanisms and management of renal dysfunction in heart failure. Review. Curr Opin Cardiol 12:251–258, 1997.

673. Edwards RM: Effects of prostaglandins on vasoconstrictor action in isolated renal arterioles. Am J Physiol 248:F779–F784, 1985.

674. Dzau VJ, Packer M, Lilly LS, et al: Prostaglandins in severe congestive heart failure. Relation to activation of the renin-angiotensin system and hyponatremia. N Engl J Med 310:347–352, 1984.

675. Castellani S, Paladini B, Paniccia R, et al: Increased renal formation of thromboxane A2 and prostaglandin F2 alpha in heart failure. Am Heart J 133:94–100, 1997.

676. Riegger AJ: [Role of prostaglandins in regulation of kidney function in heart failure]. Review. German. Herz 16:116–123, 1991.

677. Townend JN, Doran J, Lote CJ, Davies MK: Peripheral haemodynamic effects of inhibition of prostaglandin synthesis in congestive heart failure and interactions with captopril. Br Heart J 73:434–441, 1995.

678. Villarreal D, Freeman RH, Habibullah AA, Simmons JC: Indomethacin attenuates the renal actions of atrial natriuretic factor in dogs with chronic heart failure. Am J Med Sci 314:67–72, 1997.

679. Page J, Henry D: Consumption of NSAIDs and the development of congestive heart failure in elderly patients: An underrecognized public health problem. Arch Intern Med 160:777–784, 2000.

680. Heerdink ER, Leufkens HG, Herings RM, et al: NSAIDs associated with increased risk of congestive heart failure in elderly patients taking diuretics. Arch Intern Med 158:1108–1112, 1998.

681. Solomon SD, Wittes J: Cardiovascular risk associated with celecoxib—The authors reply. N Engl J Med 352:2649, 2005.

682. Waxman HA: The lessons of Vioxx—Drug safety and sales. N Engl J Med 352(25):2576–2578, 2005.

683. Eto T, Kitamura K: Adrenomedullin and its role in renal diseases. Nephron 89:121–134, 2001.

684. Edwards RM, Trizna W, Aiyar N: Adrenomedullin: A new peptide involved in cardiorenal homeostasis? Review. Exp Nephrol 5:18–22, 1997.

685. Kobayashi K, Kitamura K, Etoh T, et al: Increased plasma adrenomedullin levels in chronic congestive heart failure. Am Heart J 131:994–998, 1996.

686. Jougasaki M, Rodeheffer RJ, Redfield MM, et al: Cardiac secretion of adrenomedullin in human heart failure. J Clin Invest 97:2370–2376, 1996.

687. Nishikimi T, Saito Y, Kitamura K, et al: Increased plasma levels of adrenomedullin in patients with heart failure. J Am Coll Cardiol 26:1424–1431, 1995.

688. Kato J, Kobayashi K, Etoh T, et al: Plasma adrenomedullin concentration in patients with heart failure. J Clin Endocrinol Metab 81:180–183, 1996.

689. Jougasaki M, Stevens TL, Borgeson DD, et al: Adrenomedullin in experimental congestive heart failure: Cardiorenal activation. Am J Physiol 273:R1392–R1399, 1997.

690. Rademaker MT, Charles CJ, Lewis LK, et al: Beneficial hemodynamic and renal effects of adrenomedullin in an ovine model of heart failure. Circulation 96:1983–1990, 1997.

691. Nakamura M, Yoshida H, Makita S, et al: Potent and long-lasting vasodilatory effects of adrenomedullin in humans. Comparisons between normal subjects and patients with chronic heart failure. Circulation 95:1214–1221, 1997.

692. Lainchbury JG, Cooper GJS, Coy DH: Adrenomedullin: A hypotensive hormone in man. Clin Sci 92:467–472, 1997.

693. Nagaya N, Satoh T, Nishikimi T, et al: Hemodynamic, renal, and hormonal effects of adrenomedullin infusion in patients with congestive heart failure. Circulation 101:498–503, 2000.

694. Richards AM, Nicholls MG, Lainchbury JG, et al: Plasma urotensin II in heart failure. Lancet 360:545–546, 2002.

695. Russell FD, Meyers D, Galbraith AJ, et al: Elevated plasma levels of human urotensin-II immunoreactivity in congestive heart failure. Am J Physiol Heart Circ Physiol 285:H1576–H1581, 2003.

696. Douglas SA, Tayara L, Ohlstein EH, et al: Congestive heart failure and expression of myocardial urotensin II. Lancet 359:1990–1997, 2002.

697. Ovcharenko E, Abassi Z, Rubinstein I, et al: Renal effects of human urotensin-II in rats with experimental congestive heart failure. Nephrol Dial Transplant 5:1205–1211, 2006.

698. Zukowska Z, Feuerstein GZ: NPY family of peptides, receptors and processing enzymes. In Zukowska Z, Feuerstein GZ (eds): NPY Family of Peptides in Neurobiology, Cardiovascular and Metabolic Disorders: From Genes to Therapeutics. Boston, EXS Birkhauser, 2005, pp 7–33.

699. Liu JJ, Shi SG, Han QD: Evaluation of plasma neuropeptide Y levels in patients with congestive heart failure. Zhonghua Nei Ke Za Zhi 33(10):687–689, 1994.

700. Madsen BK, Husum D, Videbaek R, et al: Plasma-immunoreactive neuropeptide-Y in congestive-heart-failure at rest and during exercise. Scand J Clin Lab Invest 53:569–576, 1993.

CH 12

701. Ullman B, Jensenurstad M, Hulting J, Lundberg JM: Neuropeptide-Y, noradrenaline and invasive hemodynamic data in mild-to-moderate chronic congestive-heart-failure. Clin Physiol 13:409–418, 1993.

702. Ullman B, Hulting J, Lundberg JM: Prognostic value of plasma neuropeptide-Y in coronary-care unit patients with and without acute myocardial-infarction. Eur Heart J 15:454–461, 1994.

703. Anderson FL, Port JD, Reid BB, et al: Myocardial catecholamine and neuropeptide-Y depletion in failing ventricles of patients with idiopathic dilated cardiomyopathy—Correlation with beta-adrenergic-receptor down-regulation. Circulation 85:46–53, 1992.

704. Feuerstein GZ, Lee WL: Neuropeptide Y and the heart: implication for myocardial infarction and heart failure. EXS 95:123–132, 2006.

705. Pons J, Kitlinska J, Ji H, et al:. Mitogenic actions of neuropeptide Y in vascular smooth muscle cells: Synergetic interactions with the beta-adrenergic system. Can J Physiol Pharmacol 81:177–185, 2003.

706. Li LJ, Lee EW, Ji H, Zukowska Z: Neuropeptide Y-induced acceleration of postangio-plasty occlusion of rat carotid artery. Arterioscler Thromb Vasc Biol 23:1204–1210, 2003.

707. Millar BC, Schluter KD, Zhou XJ, et al: Neuropeptide-Y stimulates hypertrophy of adult ventricular cardiomyocytes. Am J Physiol 266:C1271–C1277, 1994.

708. Lee EW, Michalkiewicz M, Kitlinska J, et al: Neuropeptide Y induces ischemic angio-genesis and restores function of ischemic skeletal muscles. J Clin Invest 111:1853–1862, 2003.

709. Allen JM, Raine AEG, Ledingham JGG, Bloom SR: Neuropeptide-Y—A novel renal peptide with vasoconstrictor and natriuretic activity. Clin Sci 68:373–377, 1985.

710. Waeber B, Burnier M, Nussberger J, Brunner HR: Role of atrial natriuretic peptides and neuropeptide Y in blood pressure regulation. Horm Res 34(3–4):161–165, 1990.

711. Cardenas A, Gines P: Pathogenesis and treatment of fluid and electrolyte imbalance in cirrhosis. Semin Nephrol 21:308–316, 2001.

712. Cardenas A, Arroyo V: Mechanisms of water and sodium retention in cirrhosis and the pathogenesis of ascites. Best Pract Res Clin Endocrinol Metab 17:607–622, 2003.

713. Gines P, Guevara M, Arroyo V, Rodes J: Hepatorenal syndrome. Lancet 362:1819–1827, 2003.

714. Moller S, Bendtsen F, Henriksen JH: Pathophysiological basis of pharmacotherapy in the hepatorenal syndrome. Scand J Gastroenterol 40:491–500, 2005.

715. Schrier RW, Arroyo V, Bernardi M, et al: Peripheral arterial vasodilation hypothesis: A proposal for the initiation of renal sodium and water retention in cirrhosis. Hepatology 8:1151–1157, 1988.

716. Schrier RW, Ecder T: Gibbs memorial lecture. Unifying hypothesis of body fluid volume regulation: Implications for cardiac failure and cirrhosis. Mt Sinai J Med 68:350–361, 2001.

717. Schrier RW, Gurevich AK, Cadnapaphornchai MA: Pathogenesis and management of sodium and water retention in cardiac failure and cirrhosis. Semin Nephrol 21:157–172, 2001.

718. Martin PY, Schrier RW: Pathogenesis of water and sodium retention in cirrhosis. Kidney Int Suppl 59:S43–S49, 1997.

719. Martin PY, Gines P, Schrier RW: Nitric oxide as a mediator of hemodynamic abnor-malities and sodium and water retention in cirrhosis. N Engl J Med 339:533–541, 1998.

720. Iwakiri Y, Groszmann RJ: The hyperdynamic circulation of chronic liver diseases: From the patient to the molecule. Hepatology 43:S121–S131, 2006.

721. Lieberman FL, Denison EK, Reynolds RB: The relationship of plasma volume, portal hypertension, ascites and renal sodium retention in cirrhosis: The overflow theory of ascites formation. Ann N Y Acad Sci 170:202–212, 1970.

722. Levy M: Pathogenesis of sodium retention in early cirrhosis of the liver: Evidence for vascular overfilling. Semin Liver Dis 14:4–13, 1994.

723. Levy M: Sodium retention in dogs with cirrhosis and ascites: Efferent mechanisms. Am J Physiol 233:F586–F592, 1977.

724. Unikowsky B, Wexler MJ, Levy M: Dogs with experimental cirrhosis of the liver but without intrahepatic hypertension do not retain sodium or form ascites. J Clin Invest 72:1594–1604, 1983.

725. Kostreva DR, Castaner A, Kampine JP: Reflex effects of hepatic baroreceptors on renal and cardiac sympathetic nerve activity. Am J Physiol 238:R390–R394, 1980.

726. Sikuler E, Kravetz D, Groszmann RJ: Evolution of portal hypertension and mecha-nisms involved in its maintenance in a rat model. Am J Physiol 248:G618–G625, 1985.

727. Bomzon A, Rosenberg M, Gali D, et al: Systemic hypotension and decreased pressor response in dogs with chronic bile duct ligation. Hepatology 6:595–600, 1986.

728. Levy M, Wexler MJ: Subacute endotoxemia in dogs with experimental cirrhosis and ascites: Effects on kidney function. Can J Physiol Pharmacol 62:673–677, 1984.

729. Better OS, Guckian V, Giebisch G, Green R: The effect of sodium taurocholate on proximal tubular reabsorption in the rat kidney. Clin Sci (Lond) 72:139–141, 1987.

730. Green J, Better OS: Systemic hypotension and renal failure in obstructive jaundice—Mechanistic and therapeutic aspects. J Am Soc Nephrol 5:1853–1871, 1995.

731. Ma Z, Lee SS: Cirrhotic cardiomyopathy: Getting to the heart of the matter. Hepatology 24:451–459, 1996.

732. Moller S, Henriksen JH: Cirrhotic cardiomyopathy: A pathophysiological review of circulatory dysfunction in liver disease. Heart 87:9–15, 2002.

733. Schrier RW, Niederberger M, Weigert A, Gines P: Peripheral arterial vasodilatation: Determinant of functional spectrum of cirrhosis. Semin Liver Dis 14:14–22, 1994.

734. Gines P, Cardenas A, Arroyo V, Rodes J: Management of cirrhosis and ascites. N Engl J Med 350:1646–1654, 2004.

735. Fallon MB: Mechanisms of pulmonary vascular complications of liver disease: Hepa-topulmonary syndrome. J Clin Gastroenterol 39:S138–S142, 2005.

736. Ruiz-del-Arbol L, Monescillo A, Arocena C, et al: Circulatory function and hepatore-nal syndrome in cirrhosis. Hepatology 42:439–447, 2005.

737. Wiest R, Groszmann RJ: The paradox of nitric oxide in cirrhosis and portal hyperten-sion: Too much, not enough. Hepatology 35:478–491, 2002.

738. Claria J, Jimenez W, Ros J, et al: Pathogenesis of arterial hypotension in cirrhotic rats with ascites: Role of endogenous nitric oxide. Hepatology 15:343–349, 1992.

739. Lee FY, Colombato LA, Albillos A, Groszmann RJ: N omega-nitro-L-arginine admin-istration corrects peripheral vasodilation and systemic capillary hypotension and ameliorates plasma volume expansion and sodium retention in portal hypertensive rats. Hepatology 17:84–90, 1993.

740. Niederberger M, Gines P, Tsai P, et al: Increased aortic cyclic guanosine monophos-phate concentration in experimental cirrhosis in rats: Evidence for a role of nitric oxide in the pathogenesis of arterial vasodilation in cirrhosis. Hepatology 21:1625–1631, 1995.

741. Laffi G, Foschi M, Masini E, et al: Increased production of nitric oxide by neutrophils and monocytes from cirrhotic patients with ascites and hyperdynamic circulation. Hepatology 22:1666–1673, 1995.

742. Sogni P, Garnier P, Gadano A, et al: Endogenous pulmonary nitric oxide production measured from exhaled air is increased in patients with severe cirrhosis. J Hepatol 23:471–473, 1995.

743. Guarner C, Soriano G, Tomas A, et al: Increased serum nitrite and nitrate levels in patients with cirrhosis: Relationship to endotoxemia. Hepatology 18:1139–1143, 1993.

744. Weigort AL, Martin PY, Niederberger M, et al: Endothelium-dependent vascular hypo-responsiveness without detection of nitric oxide synthase induction in aortas of cir-rhotic rats. Hepatology 21:1856–1862, 1995.

745. Ros J, Jimenez W, Lamas S, et al: Nitric oxide production in arterial vessels of cirrhotic rats. Hepatology 21:554–560, 1995.

746. Niederberger M, Martin PY, Gines P, et al: Normalization of nitric oxide production corrects arterial vasodilation and hyperdynamic circulation in cirrhotic rats. Gastro-enterology 109:1624–1630, 1995.

747. Martin PY, Ohara M, Gines P, et al: Nitric oxide synthase (NOS) inhibition for one week improves renal sodium and water excretion in cirrhotic rats with ascites. J Clin Invest 101:235–242, 1998.

748. Campillo B, Chabrier PE, Pelle G, et al: Inhibition of nitric oxide synthesis in the forearm arterial bed of patients with advanced cirrhosis. Hepatology 22:1423–1429, 1995.

749. La Villa G, Barletta G, Pantaleo P, et al: Hemodynamic, renal, and endocrine effects of acute inhibition of nitric oxide synthase in compensated cirrhosis. Hepatology 34:19–27, 2001.

750. Martin PY, Xu DL, Niederberger M, et al: Upregulation of endothelial constitutive NOS: A major role in the increased NO production in cirrhotic rats. Am J Physiol 270:F494–F499, 1996.

751. Wiest R, Shah V, Sessa WC, Groszmann RJ: NO overproduction by eNOS precedes hyperdynamic splanchnic circulation in portal hypertensive rats. Am J Physiol 276: G1043–G1051, 1999.

752. Wiest R, Groszmann RJ: Nitric oxide and portal hypertension: Its role in the regulation of intrahepatic and splanchnic vascular resistance. Semin Liver Dis 19:411–426, 1999.

753. Gupta TK, Toruner M, Chung MK, Groszmann RJ: Endothelial dysfunction and decreased production of nitric oxide in the intrahepatic microcirculation of cirrhotic rats. Hepatology 28:926–931, 1998.

754. Shah V, Toruner M, Haddad F, et al: Impaired endothelial nitric oxide synthase activ-ity associated with enhanced caveolin binding in experimental cirrhosis in the rat. Gastroenterology 117:1222–1228, 1999.

755. Yu Q, Shao R, Qian HS, et al: Gene transfer of the neuronal NO synthase isoform to cirrhotic rat liver ameliorates portal hypertension. J Clin Invest 105:741–748, 2000.

756. Van de CM, Omasta A, Janssens S, et al: In vivo gene transfer of endothelial nitric oxide synthase decreases portal pressure in anaesthetised carbon tetrachloride cir-rhotic rats. Gut 51:440–445, 2002.

757. Cahill PA, Redmond EM, Hodges R, et al: Increased endothelial nitric oxide synthase activity in the hyperemic vessels of portal hypertensive rats. J Hepatol 25:370–378, 1996.

758. Iwakiri Y, Cadelina G, Sessa WC, Groszmann RJ: Mice with targeted deletion of eNOS develop hyperdynamic circulation associated with portal hypertension. Am J Physiol Gastrointest Liver Physiol 283:G1074–G1081, 2002.

759. Sitzmann JV, Campbell K, Wu Y, St Clair C: Prostacyclin production in acute, chronic, and long-term experimental portal hypertension. Surgery 115:290–294, 1994.

760. Barriere E, Tazi KA, Rona JP, et al: Evidence for an endothelium-derived hyperpolar-izing factor in the superior mesenteric artery from rats with cirrhosis. Hepatology 32:935–941, 2000.

761. Chen YC, Gines P, Yang J, et al: Increased vascular heme oxygenase-1 expression contributes to arterial vasodilation in experimental cirrhosis in rats. Hepatology 39:1075–1087, 2004.

762. Kojima H, Sakurai S, Uemura M, et al: Adrenomedullin contributes to vascular hypo-reactivity in cirrhotic rats with ascites via a release of nitric oxide. Scand J Gastroen-terol 39:686–693, 2004.

763. Xu L, Carter EP, Ohara M, et al: Neuronal nitric oxide synthase and systemic vasodila-tion in rats with cirrhosis. Am J Physiol Renal Physiol 279:F1110–F1115, 2000.

764. Biecker E, Neef M, Sagesser H, et al: Nitric oxide synthase 1 is partly compensating for nitric oxide synthase 3 deficiency in nitric oxide synthase 3 knock-out mice and is elevated in murine and human cirrhosis. Liver Int 24:345–353, 2004.

765. Vallance P, Moncada S: Hyperdynamic circulation in cirrhosis: A role for nitric oxide? Lancet 337:776–778, 1991.

766. Moreau R, Barriere E, Tazi KA, et al: Terlipressin inhibits in vivo aortic iNOS expression induced by lipopolysaccharide in rats with biliary cirrhosis. Hepatology 36:1070–1078, 2002.
767. Lopez-Talavera JC, Cadelina G, Olchowski J, et al: Thalidomide inhibits tumor necrosis factor alpha, decreases nitric oxide synthesis, and ameliorates the hyperdynamic circulatory syndrome in portal-hypertensive rats. Hepatology 23:1616–1621, 1996.
768. Sessa WC: eNOS at a glance. J Cell Sci 117:2427–2429, 2004.
769. Wiest R, Cadelina G, Milstien S, et al: Bacterial translocation up-regulates GTP-cyclohydrolase I in mesenteric vasculature of cirrhotic rats. Hepatology 38:1508–1515, 2003.
770. Shah V, Wiest R, Garcia-Cardena G, et al: Hsp90 regulation of endothelial nitric oxide synthase contributes to vascular control in portal hypertension. Am J Physiol 277: G463–G468, 1999.
771. Iwakiri Y, Tsai MH, McCabe TJ, et al: Phosphorylation of eNOS initiates excessive NO production in early phases of portal hypertension. Am J Physiol Heart Circ Physiol 282:H2084–H2090, 2002.
772. Moller S, Henriksen JH: Neurohumoral fluid regulation in chronic liver disease. Scand J Clin Lab Invest 58:361–372, 1998.
773. Moller S, Bendtsen F, Henriksen JH: Vasoactive substances in the circulatory dysfunction of cirrhosis. Scand J Clin Lab Invest 61:421–429, 2001.
774. Lopez C, Jimenez W, Arroyo V, et al: Temporal relationship between the decrease in arterial pressure and sodium retention in conscious spontaneously hypertensive rats with carbon tetrachloride-induced cirrhosis. Hepatology 13:585–589, 1991.
775. Bernardi M, Trevisani F, Gasbarrini A, Gasbarrini G: Hepatorenal disorders: Role of the renin-angiotensin-aldosterone system. Semin Liver Dis 14:23–34, 1994.
776. Bernardi M, Di Marco C, Trevisani F, et al: Renal sodium retention during upright posture in preascitic cirrhosis. Gastroenterology 105:188–193, 1993.
777. Wong F, Sniderman K, Blendis L: The renal sympathetic and renin-angiotensin response to lower body negative pressure in well-compensated cirrhosis. Gastroenterology 115:397–405, 1998.
778. Wong F, Liu P, Blendis L: The mechanism of improved sodium homeostasis of low-dose losartan in preascitic cirrhosis. Hepatology 35:1449–1458, 2002.
779. Bernardi M: Renal sodium retention in preascitic cirrhosis: Expanding knowledge, enduring uncertainties. Hepatology 35:1544–1547, 2002.
780. Ubeda M, Matzilevich MM, Atucha NM, et al: Renin and angiotensinogen mRNA expression in the kidneys of rats subjected to long-term bile duct ligation. Hepatology 19:1431–1436, 1994.
781. Schneider AW, Kalk JF, Klein CP: Effect of losartan, an angiotensin II receptor antagonist, on portal pressure in cirrhosis. Hepatology 29:334–339, 1999.
782. Gentilini P, Romanelli RG, La Villa G, et al: Effects of low-dose captopril on renal hemodynamics and function in patients with cirrhosis of the liver. Gastroenterology 104:588–594, 1993.
783. Henriksen JH, Moller S, Ring-Larsen H, Christensen NJ: The sympathetic nervous system in liver disease. J Hepatol 29:328–341, 1998.
784. Floras JS, Legault L, Morali GA, et al: Increased sympathetic outflow in cirrhosis and ascites: Direct evidence from intraneural recordings. Ann Intern Med 114:373–380, 1991.
785. Moller S, Henriksen JH: Circulatory abnormalities in cirrhosis with focus on neurohumoral aspects. Semin Nephrol 17:505–519, 1997.
786. Bichet DG, Van Putten VJ, Schrier RW: Potential role of increased sympathetic activity in impaired sodium and water excretion in cirrhosis. N Engl J Med 307:1552–1557, 1982.
787. DiBona GF, Sawin LL, Jones SY: Characteristics of renal sympathetic nerve activity in sodium-retaining disorders. Am J Physiol 271:R295–R302, 1996.
788. Rodriguez-Martinez M, Sawin LL, DiBona GF: Arterial and cardiopulmonary baroreflex control of renal nerve activity in cirrhosis. Am J Physiol 268:R117–R129, 1995.
789. Laffi G, Lagi A, Cipriani M, et al: Impaired cardiovascular autonomic response to passive tilting in cirrhosis with ascites. Hepatology 24:1063–1067, 1996.
790. Ryan J, Sudhir K, Jennings G, et al: Impaired reactivity of the peripheral vasculature to pressor agents in alcoholic cirrhosis. Gastroenterology 105:1167–1172, 1993.
791. Moller S, Becker U, Schifter S, et al: Effect of oxygen inhalation on systemic, central, and splanchnic haemodynamics in cirrhosis. J Hepatol 25:316–328, 1996.
792. Arroyo V, Claria J, Salo J, Jimenez W: Antidiuretic hormone and the pathogenesis of water retention in cirrhosis with ascites. Semin Liver Dis 14:44–58, 1994.
793. Bichet D, Szatalowicz V, Chaimovitz C, Schrier RW: Role of vasopressin in abnormal water excretion in cirrhotic patients. Ann Intern Med 96:413–417, 1982.
794. Kim JK, Summer SN, Howard RL, Schrier RW: Vasopressin gene expression in rats with experimental cirrhosis. Hepatology 17:143–147, 1993.
795. Fujita N, Ishikawa SE, Sasaki S, et al: Role of water channel AQP-CD in water retention in SIADH and cirrhotic rats. Am J Physiol 269:F926–F931, 1995.
796. Ferguson JW, Therapondos G, Newby DE, Hayes PC: Therapeutic role of vasopressin receptor antagonism in patients with liver cirrhosis. Clin Sci (Lond) 105:1–8, 2003.
797. Tsuboi Y, Ishikawa S, Fujisawa G, et al: Therapeutic efficacy of the non-peptide AVP antagonist OPC-31260 in cirrhotic rats. Kidney Int 46:237–244, 1994.
798. Jimenez W, Gal CS, Ros J, et al: Long-term aquaretic efficacy of a selective nonpeptide V(2)-vasopressin receptor antagonist, SR121463, in cirrhotic rats. J Pharmacol Exp Ther 295:83–90, 2000.
799. Claria J, Jimenez W, Arroyo V, et al: Effect of V1-vasopressin receptor blockade on arterial pressure in conscious rats with cirrhosis and ascites. Gastroenterology 100:494–501, 1991.
800. Perez-Ayuso RM, Arroyo V, Camps J, et al: Evidence that renal prostaglandins are involved in renal water metabolism in cirrhosis. Kidney Int 26:72–80, 1984.
801. Salo J, Francitorra A, Follo A, et al: Increased plasma endothelin in cirrhosis. Relationship with systemic endotoxemia and response to changes in effective blood volume. J Hepatol 22:389–398, 1995.
802. Gerbes AL, Moller S, Gulberg V, Henriksen JH: Endothelin-1 and -3 plasma concentrations in patients with cirrhosis: Role of splanchnic and renal passage and liver function. Hepatology 21:735–739, 1995.
803. Moller S, Henriksen JH: Endothelins in chronic liver disease. Scand J Clin Lab Invest 56:481–490, 1996.
804. Moore K, Wendon J, Frazer M, et al: Plasma endothelin immunoreactivity in liver disease and the hepatorenal syndrome. N Engl J Med 327:1774–1778, 1992.
805. Bernardi M, Gulberg V, Colantoni A, et al: Plasma endothelin-1 and -3 in cirrhosis: Relationship with systemic hemodynamics, renal function and neurohumoral systems. J Hepatol 24:161–168, 1996.
806. Moore K: Endothelin and vascular function in liver disease. Gut 53:159–161, 2004.
807. Martinet JP, Legault L, Cernacek P, et al: Changes in plasma endothelin-1 and big endothelin-1 induced by transjugular intrahepatic portosystemic shunts in patients with cirrhosis and refractory ascites. J Hepatol 25:700–706, 1996.
808. Kapoor D, Redhead DN, Hayes PC, et al: Systemic and regional changes in plasma endothelin following transient increase in portal pressure. Liver Transpl 9:32–39, 2003.
809. Bachmann-Brandt S, Bittner I, Neuhaus P, et al: Plasma levels of endothelin-1 in patients with the hepatorenal syndrome after successful liver transplantation. Transpl Int 13:357–362, 2000.
810. Anand R, Harry D, Holt S, et al: Endothelin is an important determinant of renal function in a rat model of acute liver and renal failure. Gut 50:111–117, 2002.
811. Claria J, Arroyo V: Prostaglandins and other cyclooxygenase-dependent arachidonic acid metabolites and the kidney in liver disease. Prostaglandins Other Lipid Mediat 72:19–33, 2003.
812. Niederberger M, Gines P, Martin PY, et al: Increased renal and vascular cytosolic phospholipase A2 activity in rats with cirrhosis and ascites. Hepatology 27:42–47, 1998.
813. Epstein M: Renal prostaglandins and the control of renal function in liver disease. Am J Med 80:46–55, 1986.
814. Wong F, Massie D, Hsu P, Dudley F: Indomethacin-induced renal dysfunction in patients with well-compensated cirrhosis. Gastroenterology 104:869–876, 1993.
815. Govindarajan S, Nast CC, Smith WL, et al: Immunohistochemical distribution of renal prostaglandin endoperoxide synthase and prostacyclin synthase: Diminished endoperoxide synthase in the hepatorenal syndrome. Hepatology 7:654–659, 1987.
816. Gines A, Salmeron JM, Gines P, et al: Oral misoprostol or intravenous prostaglandin E2 do not improve renal function in patients with cirrhosis and ascites with hyponatremia or renal failure. J Hepatol 17:220–226, 1993.
817. Bosch-Marce M, Claria J, Titos E, et al: Selective inhibition of cyclooxygenase 2 spares renal function and prostaglandin synthesis in cirrhotic rats with ascites. Gastroenterology 116:1167–1175, 1999.
818. Claria J, Kent JD, Lopez-Parra M, et al: Effects of celecoxib and naproxen on renal function in nonazotemic patients with cirrhosis and ascites. Hepatology 41:579–587, 2005.
819. Wong F, Blendis L: Pathophysiology of sodium retention and ascites formation in cirrhosis: Role of atrial natriuretic factor. Semin Liver Dis 14:59–70, 1994.
820. Levy M: Atrial natriuretic peptide: Renal effects in cirrhosis of the liver. Semin Nephrol 17:520–529, 1997.
821. Moreau R, Pussard E, Brenard R, et al: Clearance of atrial natriuretic peptide in patients with cirrhosis. Role of liver failure. J Hepatol 13:351–357, 1991.
822. Poulos JE, Gower WR, Fontanet HL, et al: Cirrhosis with ascites: Increased atrial natriuretic peptide messenger RNA expression in rat ventricle. Gastroenterology 108:1496–1503, 1995.
823. Rector WG Jr, Adair O, Hossack KF, Rainguet S: Atrial volume in cirrhosis: Relationship to blood volume and plasma concentration of atrial natriuretic factor. Gastroenterology 99:766–770, 1990.
824. Wong F, Liu P, Tobe S, et al: Central blood volume in cirrhosis: Measurement with radionuclide angiography. Hepatology 19:312–321, 1994.
825. Wong F, Liu P, Blendis L: Sodium homeostasis with chronic sodium loading in preascitic cirrhosis. Gut 49:847–851, 2001.
826. Skorecki KL, Leung WM, Campbell P, et al: Role of atrial natriuretic peptide in the natriuretic response to central volume expansion induced by head-out water immersion in sodium-retaining cirrhotic subjects. Am J Med 85:375–382, 1988.
827. Epstein M, Loutzenhiser R, Norsk P, Atlas S: Relationship between plasma ANF responsiveness and renal sodium handling in cirrhotic humans. Am J Nephrol 9:133–143, 1989.
828. Warner L, Skorecki K, Blendis LM, Epstein M: Atrial natriuretic factor and liver disease. Hepatology 17:500–513, 1993.
829. Legault L, Warner LC, Leung WM, et al: Assessment of atrial natriuretic peptide resistance in cirrhosis with head-out water immersion and atrial natriuretic peptide infusion. Can J Physiol Pharmacol 71:157–164, 1993.
830. MacGilchrist A, Craig KJ, Hayes PC, Cumming AD: Effect of the serine protease inhibitor, aprotinin, on systemic haemodynamics and renal function in patients with hepatic cirrhosis and ascites. Clin Sci (Lond) 87:329–335, 1994.
831. Legault L, Cernacek P, Levy M: Attempts to alter the heterogeneous response to ANP in sodium-retaining caval dogs. Can J Physiol Pharmacol 70:897–904, 1992.
832. Morali GA, Tobe SW, Skorecki KL, Blendis LM: Refractory ascites: Modulation of atrial natriuretic factor unresponsiveness by mannitol. Hepatology 16:42–48, 1992.
833. Piccinni P, Rossaro L, Graziotto A, et al: Human natriuretic factor in cirrhotic patients undergoing orthotopic liver transplantation. Transpl Int 8:51–54, 1995.
834. Tobe SW, Morali GA, Greig PD, et al: Peritoneovenous shunting restores atrial natriuretic factor responsiveness in refractory hepatic ascites. Gastroenterology 105:202–207, 1993.
835. Koepke JP, Jones S, DiBona GF: Renal nerves mediate blunted natriuresis to atrial natriuretic peptide in cirrhotic rats. Am J Physiol 252:R1019–R1023, 1987.

836. Tobe SW, Blendis LM, Morali GA, et al: Angiotensin II modulates atrial natriuretic factor–induced natriuresis in cirrhosis with ascites. Am J Kidney Dis 21:472–479, 1993.

837. Abraham WT, Lauwaars ME, Kim JK, et al: Reversal of atrial natriuretic peptide resistance by increasing distal tubular sodium delivery in patients with decompensated cirrhosis. Hepatology 22:737–743, 1995.

838. La Villa G, Riccardi D, Lazzeri C, et al: Blunted natriuretic response to low-dose brain natriuretic peptide infusion in nonazotemic cirrhotic patients with ascites and avid sodium retention. Hepatology 22:1745–1750, 1995.

839. Yildiz R, Yildirim B, Karincaoglu M, et al: Brain natriuretic peptide and severity of disease in non-alcoholic cirrhotic patients. J Gastroenterol Hepatol 20:1115–1120, 2005.

CHAPTER 13

Disorders of Water Balance

Joseph G. Verbalis • Tomas Berl

Disorders of body fluids are among the most commonly encountered problems in clinical medicine, largely because many different disease states can potentially disrupt the finely balanced mechanisms that control the intake and output of water and solute. Because body water is the primary determinant of the osmolality of the extracellular fluid (ECF), disorders of water metabolism can be broadly divided into hyperosmolar disorders, in which there is a deficiency of body water relative to body solute, and hypoosmolar disorders, in which there is an excess of body water relative to body solute. Because sodium is the main constituent of plasma osmolality, these disorders are typically characterized by hypernatremia and hyponatremia, respectively. Before discussing specific aspects of these disorders, this chapter first briefly reviews the regulatory mechanisms underlying water metabolism, which, in concert with sodium metabolism, maintains body fluid homeostasis.

BODY FLUIDS: COMPARTMENTALIZATION, COMPOSITION, AND TURNOVER

Water constitutes approximately 55% to 65% of body weight (BW), varying with age, sex, and amount of body fat, and therefore constitutes the largest single constituent of the body. Total body water (TBW) is distributed between the intracellular fluid (ICF) and the ECF compartments. Estimates of the relative sizes of these two pools differ significantly depending on the tracer used to measure the ECF volume, but most studies in animals and humans have indicated that 55% to 65% of TBW resides in the ICF and 35% to 45% in the ECF. Approximately 75% of the ECF compartment is interstitial fluid and only 25% is intravascular fluid (i.e., blood volume).[1,2] Figure 13–1 summarizes the estimated body fluid spaces of an average weight adult.

The solute composition of the ICF and ECF differs considerably because most cell membranes possess multiple transport systems that actively accumulate or expel specific solutes. Thus, membrane-bound Na^+/K^+-ATPase maintains Na^+ in a primarily extracellular location and K^+ in a primarily intracellular location.[3] Similar transporters effectively result in confining Cl^- largely to the ECF and Mg^{2+}, organic acids, and phosphates to the ICF. Glucose, which requires an insulin-activated transport system to enter most cells, is present in significant amounts only in the ECF because it is rapidly converted intracellularly to glycogen or metabolites.[4] HCO_3^- is present in both compartments, but is approximately three times more concentrated in the ECF. Urea is unique among the major naturally occurring solutes in that it diffuses freely across most cell membranes[5]; therefore, it is present in similar concentrations in virtu-

ally all body fluids, except in the renal medulla where it is concentrated by urea transporters (see Chapter 9).

Despite very different solute compositions, both the ICF and the ECF have an equivalent osmotic pressure,[6] which is a function of the total concentration of all solutes in a fluid compartment because most biologic membranes are semipermeable (i.e., freely permeable to water but not to aqueous solutes). Thus, water will flow across membranes into a compartment with a higher solute concentration until a steady state is reached at which the osmotic pressures have equalized on both sides of the cell membrane.[7] An important consequence of this thermodynamic law is that the volume of distribution of body Na^+ and K^+ is actually the TBW rather than just the ECF or ICF volume, respectively.[8] For example, any increase in ECF sodium concentration (Na^+) will cause water to shift from the ICF to the ECF until the ICF and ECF osmotic pressures are equal, thereby effectively distributing the Na^+ across both extracellular and intracellular water.

Osmolality is defined as the concentration of all of the solutes in a given weight of water. The total solute concentration of a fluid can be determined and expressed in several different ways. The most common method is to measure its freezing point or vapor pressure, because these are colligative properties of the number of free solute particles in a volume of fluid,[9,10] and to express the result relative to a standard solution of known concentration using units of either osmolality (milliosmoles of solute per kilogram of water, mOsm/kg H_2O), or osmolarity (milliosmoles of solute per liter of water, mOsm/L H_2O). Plasma osmolality can be measured directly as described previously or calculated by summing the concentrations of the major solutes present in the plasma:

$$P_{osm} \text{ (mOsm/kg } H_2O) = 2 \times \text{plasma } Na^+ \text{ (mEq/L)} + \text{glucose (mg/dL)}/18 + \text{BUN (mg/dL)}/2.8$$

where BUN is the blood urea nitrogen. Both methods produce comparable results under most conditions (the value obtained using this formula is generally within 1% to 2% of that obtained by direct osmometry), as will simply doubling the plasma Na^+ because

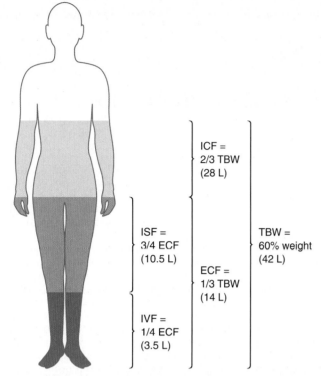

FIGURE 13–1 Schematic representation of body fluid compartments in humans. The *shaded areas* depict the approximate size of each compartment as a function of body weight. The *numbers* indicate the relative sizes of the various fluid compartments and the approximate absolute volumes of the compartments (in liters) in a 70-kg adult. ECF, extracellular fluid; ICF, intracellular fluid; ISF, interstitial fluid; IVF, intravascular fluid; TBW, total body water. (From Verbalis JG: Body water and osmolality. *In* Wilkinson B, Jamison R [eds]: Textbook of Nephrology. London, Chapman & Hall, 1997, pp 89–94.)

valent increase in plasma anions, but in this case, the effective osmolality will also be elevated by 20 mOsm/kg H_2O because the Na^+ and accompanying anions will largely remain restricted to the ECF owing to the relative impermeability of cell membranes to Na^+ and other ions. Thus, elevations of solutes such as urea, unlike elevations of sodium, do not cause cellular dehydration and, consequently, do not activate mechanisms that defend body fluid homeostasis by increasing body water stores.

Both body water and solutes are in a state of continuous exchange with the environment. The magnitude of the turnover varies considerably depending on physical, social, and environmental factors, but in healthy adults, it averages 5% to 10% of the total body content each day. For the most part, daily intake of water and electrolytes is not determined by physiologic requirements but is more a function of dietary preferences and cultural influences. Healthy adults have an average daily fluid ingestion of approximately 2 to 3 L, but with considerable individual variation; approximately one third of this is derived from food or the metabolism of fat and the rest from discretionary ingestion of fluids. Similarly, of the 1000 mOsm of solute ingested or generated by the metabolism of nutrients each day, nearly 40% is intrinsic to food, another 35% is added to food as a preservative or flavoring, and the rest is mostly urea. In contrast to the largely unregulated nature of basal intakes, the urinary excretion of both water and solute is highly regulated to preserve body fluid homeostasis. Thus, under normal circumstances, almost all ingested Na^+, Cl^- and K^+, as well as both ingested and metabolically generated urea, are excreted in the urine under the control of specific regulatory mechanisms. Other ingested solutes, for example, divalent minerals, are excreted primarily by the gastrointestinal tract. Urinary excretion of water is also tightly regulated by the secretion and renal effects of arginine vasopressin (AVP), which is discussed in greater detail in Chapters 8 and 9 and the following section.

sodium and its accompanying anions are the predominant solutes present in plasma. However, the total osmolality of plasma is not always equivalent to the *effective* osmolality, often referred to as the *tonicity* of the plasma, because the latter is a function of the relative solute permeability properties of the membranes separating the two compartments. Solutes that are impermeable to cell membranes (e.g., Na^+, mannitol) are restricted to the ECF compartment and are effective solutes because they create osmotic pressure gradients across cell membranes, leading to osmotic movement of water from the ICF to the ECF compartments. Solutes that are permeable to cell membranes (e.g., urea, ethanol, methanol) are ineffective solutes because they do not create osmotic pressure gradients across cell membranes and therefore are not associated with such water shifts.[11] Glucose is a unique solute because at normal physiologic plasma concentrations, it is taken up by cells via active transport mechanisms and therefore acts as an ineffective solute, but under conditions of impaired cellular uptake (e.g., insulin deficiency), it becomes an effective extracellular solute.[12]

The importance of this distinction between total and effective osmolality is that only the effective solutes in plasma are determinants of whether clinically significant hyperosmolality or hypoosmolality is present. An example of this is uremia: A patient with a urea concentration that has increased by 56 mg/dL will have a corresponding 20 mOsm/kg H_2O elevation in plasma osmolality, but the effective osmolality will remain normal because the increased urea is proportionally distributed across both the ECF and the ICF. In contrast, a patient whose plasma Na^+ has increased by 10 mEq/L will also have a 20 mOsm/kg H_2O elevation of plasma osmolality, because the increased cation must be balanced by an equi-

WATER METABOLISM

Water metabolism is responsible for the balance between the intake and the excretion of water. Each side of this balance equation can be considered to consist of a *regulated* and an *unregulated* component, the magnitudes of which can vary quite markedly under different physiologic and pathophysiologic conditions. The unregulated component of water intake consists of the intrinsic water content of ingested foods, the consumption of beverages primarily for reasons of palatability or desired secondary effects (e.g., caffeine), or for social or habitual reasons (e.g., alcoholic beverages), whereas the regulated component of water intake consists of fluids consumed in response to a perceived sensation of thirst. Studies of middle-aged subjects have shown mean fluid intakes of 2.1 L/24 hr, and analysis of the fluids consumed indicated that the vast majority of the fluid ingested is determined by influences such as meal-associated fluid intake, taste, or psychosocial factors rather than true thirst.[13]

The unregulated component of water excretion occurs via insensible water losses from a variety of sources (cutaneous losses from sweating, evaporative losses in exhaled air, gastrointestinal losses) as well as the obligate amount of water that the kidneys must excrete to eliminate solutes generated by body metabolism, whereas the regulated component of water excretion comprises the renal excretion of free water in excess of the obligate amount necessary to excrete metabolic solutes. Unlike solutes, a relatively large proportion of body water is excreted by evaporation from skin and lungs. This amount varies markedly depending on several factors, including dress, humidity, temperature, and exercise.[14] Under the sedentary and temperature-controlled indoor conditions typical of modern urban life, daily insensible water loss in healthy adults is minimal at approximately 10 ml/kg BW (0.7 L in a 70-kg man or woman). However, insensible losses can increase to twice this level (i.e., 20 ml/kg BW) simply under conditions of increased activity and temperature; and if environmental temperature or activity is even greater, such as in arid environments, the rate of insensible water loss can even approximate the maximal rate of free water excretion by the kidney.[14] Thus, in quantitative terms, insensible loss and the factors that influence it can be just as important to body fluid homeostasis as regulated urine output. Another major determinant of unregulated water loss is the rate of urine solute excretion, which cannot be reduced below a minimal obligatory level required to excrete the solute load. The volume of urine required depends not only on the solute load but also on the degree of antidiuresis. At a typical basal level of urinary concentration (urine osmolality = 600 mOsm/kg H_2O) and a typical solute load of 900 to 1200 mOsm/day, a 70-kg adult would require a total urine volume of 1.5 to 2.0 L (21–28 ml/kg BW) to excrete the solute load. However, under conditions of maximal antidiuresis (urine osmolality = 1200 mOsm/kg H_2O), the same solute load would require a minimal obligatory urine output of only 0.75 to 1.0 L/day, and conversely, a decrease in urine concentration to minimal levels (urine osmolality=60 mOsm/kg H_2O) would obligate a proportionally larger urine volume of 15 to 20 L/day to excrete the same solute load.

The previous discussion serves to emphasize that both water intake and water excretion have very substantial unregulated components, and these can vary tremendously as a result of factors that are unrelated to maintenance of body fluid homeostasis. In effect, the regulated components of water metabolism are those that act to maintain body fluid homeostasis by compensating for whatever perturbations result from unregulated water losses or gains. Within this framework, it is clear that the two major mechanisms responsible for regulating water metabolism are pituitary secretion and renal effects of AVP and thirst, each of which is discussed in greater detail.

Arginine Vasopressin Synthesis and Secretion

The primary determinant of free water excretion in animals and humans is the regulation of urinary water excretion by circulating levels of AVP in plasma. The renal effects of AVP are covered extensively in Chapters 8 and 9. This chapter focuses on the regulation of AVP synthesis and secretion from the neurohypophysis.

Structure and Synthesis
Before AVP was biochemically characterized, early studies used the general term "antidiuretic hormone" (ADH) to describe this substance. Now that AVP is known to be the only naturally occurring antidiuretic substance, it is more appropriate to refer to it by its correct hormonal designation. AVP is a 9–amino acid peptide synthesized in the hypothalamus. It is a composed of a 6–amino acid ringlike structure formed by a disulfide bridge, with a 3–amino acid tail at the end of which the COOH-terminal group is amidated. Substitution of lysine for arginine in position 8 yields lysine vasopressin, the ADH found in pigs and other members of the suborder Suina. Substitution of isoleucine for phenylalanine at position 3 and of leucine for arginine at position 8 yields oxytocin, a hormone found in all mammals as well as many submammalian species.[15] Oxytocin has weak antidiuretic activity[16] but is a potent constrictor of smooth muscle in mammary glands and uterus. As implied by their names, AVP and lysine vasopressin also cause constriction of blood vessels, which was the property that led to their original

discovery in the late 19th century,[17] but this pressor effect occurs only at concentrations many times those required to produce antidiuresis and is probably of little physiologic or pathologic importance in humans except under conditions of severe hypotension and hypovolemia, in which it acts to supplement the vasoconstrictive actions of angiotensin II (Ang II) and the sympathetic nervous system.[18] The multiple actions of AVP are mediated by different G-protein–coupled receptors, designated V_{1a}, V_{1b}, and V_2.

AVP and oxytocin are produced by the *neurohypophysis,* often referred to as the *posterior pituitary gland* because the neural lobe is located centrally and posterior to the adenohypophysis, or anterior pituitary gland, in the sella turcica. However, it is important to understand that the posterior pituitary gland consists only of the distal axons of the magnocellular neurons that compose the neurohypophysis. The cell bodies of these axons are located in specialized (magnocellular) neural cells located in two discrete areas of the hypothalamus, the paired supraoptic (SON) and paraventricular (PVN) nuclei (Fig. 13–2). In adults, the posterior pituitary is connected to the brain by a short stalk through the diaphragm sellae. The neurohypophysis is supplied with blood by branches of the superior and inferior hypophysial arteries, which arise from the posterior communicating and intracavernous portion of the internal carotid artery. In the posterior pituitary, the arterioles break up into localized capillary networks that drain directly into the jugular vein via the sellar, cavernous, and lateral venous sinuses. Many of the neurosecretory neurons that terminate higher in the infundibulum and median eminence originate in parvicellular neurons in the PVN and are functionally distinct from the magnocellular neurons that terminate in the posterior pituitary because they primarily enhance secretion of adrenocorticotropin hormone (ACTH) from the anterior pituitary. AVP-containing neurons also project from parvicellular neurons of the PVN to other areas of the brain, including the limbic system, the nucleus tractus solitarius, and the lateral gray matter of the spinal cord. The functions of these extrahypophysial projections are still under study.

The genes encoding the AVP and oxytocin precursors are located in close proximity on chromosome 20 but are expressed in mutually exclusive populations of neurohypophyseal neurons.[19] The AVP gene consists of approximately 2000 base pairs and contains three exons separated by two intervening sequences (Fig. 13–3). Each exon encodes one of the three functional domains of the pre-prohormone, although small parts of the nonconserved sequences of neurophysin are located in the first and third exons that code for AVP and the C-terminal glycoprotein, respectively. The untranslated 5′-flanking region, which regulates expression of the gene, shows extensive sequence homology across several species but is markedly different from the otherwise closely related gene for oxytocin. This promoter region of the AVP gene in the rat contains several putative regulatory elements, including a glucocorticoid response element, a cyclic adenosine monophosphate (cAMP) response element, and four activating protein (AP)-2–binding sites.[20] Recent experimental data indicated that the DNA sequences between the AVP and the oxytocin genes, the intergenic region, contain critical sites for cell-specific expression of these two hormones.[21]

The gene for AVP is also expressed in a number of other neurons, including but not limited to the parvicellular neurons of the paraventricular and suprachiasmatic nuclei. Oxytocin and AVP genes are also expressed in several peripheral tissues, including the adrenal medulla, ovary, testis, thymus, and certain sensory ganglia.[22] However, the AVP mRNA in these tissues appears to be shorter (620 bases) than its hypothalamic counterpart (720 bases), apparently because of tissue-specific differences in the length of the polyA tails. More importantly, the levels of AVP in peripheral tissues are

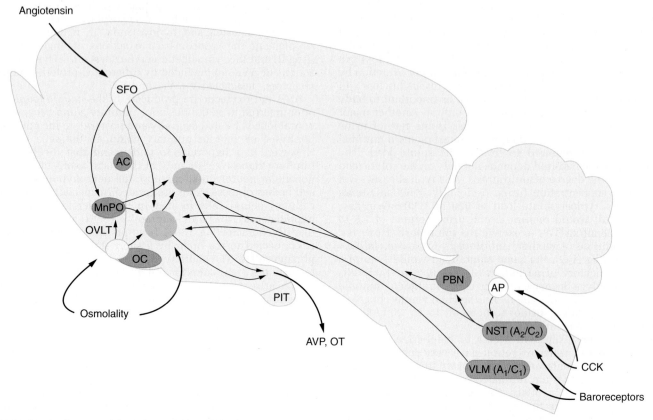

FIGURE 13–2 Summary of the main anterior hypothalamic pathways that mediate secretion of arginine vasopressin (AVP) and oxytocin (OT). The vascular organ of the lamina terminalis (OVLT) is especially sensitive to hyperosmolality. Hyperosmolality also activates other neurons in the anterior hypothalamus, such as those in the subfornical organ (SFO) and median preoptic nucleus (MnPO), and magnocellular neurons, which are intrinsically osmosensitive. Circulating angiotensin II (Ang II) activates neurons of the SFO, an essential site of Ang II action, as well as cells throughout the lamina terminalis and MnPO. In response to hyperosmolality or Ang II, projections from the SFO and OVLT to the MnPO activate excitatory and inhibitory interneurons that project to the supraoptic nucleus (SON) and paraventricular nucleus (PVN) to modulate direct inputs to these areas from the circumventricular organs. Cholecystokinin (CCK) acts primarily on gastric vagal afferents that terminate in the nucleus of the solitary tract (NST), but at higher doses, it can also act at the area postrema (AP). Although neurons are apparently activated in the ventrolateral medulla (VLM) and NST, most neurohypophyseal secretion appears to be stimulated by monosynaptic projections from A_2/C_2 cells, and possibly also noncatecholaminergic somatostatin/inhibin B cells, of the NST. Baroreceptor-mediated stimuli, such as hypovolemia and hypotension, are more complex. The major projection to magnocellular AVP neurons appears to arise from A_1 cells of the VLM that are activated by excitatory interneurons from the NST. Other areas, such as the parabrachial nucleus (PBN), may contribute multisynaptic projections. Cranial nerves IX and X, which terminate in the NST, also contribute input to magnocellular AVP neurons. It is unclear whether baroreceptor-mediated secretion of oxytocin results from projections from VLM neurons or from NST neurons. AC, anterior commissure; OC, optic chiasm; PIT, anterior pituitary. (From Stricker EM, Verbalis JG: Water intake and body fluids. *In* Squire LR, Bloom FE, McConnell SK, et al [eds]: Fundamental Neuroscience. San Diego, Academic Press, 2003, pp 1011–1029.)

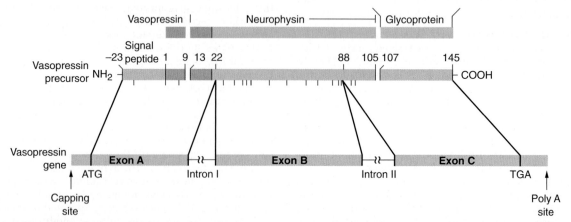

FIGURE 13–3 The arginine vasopressin (AVP) gene and its protein products. The three exons encode a 145–amino acid prohormone with an NH_2-terminal signal peptide. The prohormone is packaged into neurosecretory granules of magnocellular neurons. During axonal transport of the granules from the hypothalamus to the posterior pituitary, enzymatic cleavage of the prohormone generates the final products: AVP, neurophysin, and a COOH-terminal glycoprotein. When afferent stimulation depolarizes the AVP-containing neurons, the three products are released into capillaries of the posterior pituitary. (Adapted from Richter D, Schmale H: The structure of the precursor to arginine vasopressin, a model preprohormone. Prog Brain Res 60:227–233, 1983.)

generally two to three orders of magnitude lower than in the neurohypophysis, suggesting that AVP in these tissues likely has paracrine rather than endocrine functions. This is consistent with the observation that destruction of the neurohypophysis essentially eliminates AVP from the plasma despite the presence of these multiple peripheral sites of AVP synthesis.

Secretion of AVP and its associated neurophysin occurs by a calcium-dependent exocytotic process similar to that described for other neurosecretory systems. Secretion is triggered by propagation of an electrical impulse along the axon that causes depolarization of the cell membrane, an influx of Ca^{2+}, fusion of secretory granules with the cell membrane, and extrusion of their contents. This view is supported by the observation that AVP, neurophysin, and the copeptin glycoprotein are released simultaneously by many stimuli.[23] However, at the physiologic pH of plasma, there is no binding of either AVP or oxytocin to their respective neurophysins, so after secretion each peptide circulates independently in the bloodstream.[24]

Stimuli for secretion of AVP or oxytocin also stimulate transcription and increase the mRNA content of both prohormones in the magnocellular neurons. This has been well documented in rats, in which dehydration, which stimulates secretion of AVP, accelerates transcription and increases the levels of AVP (and oxytocin) mRNA,[25,26] and hypoosmolality, which inhibits secretion of AVP, produces a decrease in the content of AVP mRNA.[27] These and other data indicate that the major control of AVP synthesis resides at the level of transcription.[28]

Antidiuresis occurs via interaction of the circulating hormone with AVP V_2 receptors in the kidney, which results in increased water permeability of the collecting duct through the insertion of the aquaporin-2 (AQP2) water channel into the apical membranes of collecting tubule principal cells (see Chapters 8 and 9). The importance of AVP for maintaining water balance is underscored by the fact that the normal pituitary stores of this hormone are very large, allowing more than a week's supply of hormone for maximal antidiuresis under conditions of sustained dehydration.[28] Knowledge of the different conditions that stimulate pituitary AVP release in humans is therefore essential for understanding water metabolism.

Osmotic Regulation

AVP secretion is influenced by many different stimuli, but since the pioneering studies of antidiuretic hormone secretion by Verney, it has been clear that the most important under physiologic conditions is the osmotic pressure of plasma. With further refinement of radioimmunoassays for AVP, the unique sensitivity of this hormone to small changes in osmolality, as well as the corresponding sensitivity of the kidney to small changes in plasma AVP levels, has become apparent. Although the magnocellular neurons themselves have been found to have intrinsic osmoreceptive properties,[29] research over the last several decades has clearly shown that the most sensitive osmoreceptive cells that are able to sense small changes in plasma osmolality and transduce these changes into AVP secretion are located in the anterior hypothalamus, likely in or near the circumventricular organ called the *organum vasculosum of the lamina terminalis* (OVLT) (see Fig. 13–2). Perhaps the strongest evidence for location of the primary osmoreceptors in this area of the brain are the multiple studies that have demonstrated that destruction of this area disrupts osmotically stimulated AVP secretion and thirst without affecting the neurohypophysis or its response to nonosmotic stimuli.[30,31]

Although some debate still exists with regard to the exact pattern of osmotically stimulated AVP secretion, most studies to date have supported the concept of a discrete

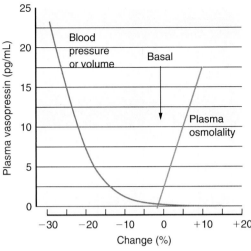

FIGURE 13–4 Comparative sensitivity of AVP secretion in response to increases in plasma osmolality versus decreases in blood volume or blood pressure in human subjects. The *arrow* indicates the low plasma AVP concentrations found at basal plasma osmolality Note that AVP secretion is much more sensitive to small changes in blood osmolality than to changes in volume or pressure. (Adapted from Robertson GL: Posterior pituitary. *In* Felig P, Baxter J, Frohman LA [eds]: Endocrinology and Metabolism. New York, McGraw Hill, 1986, pp 338–386.)

osmotic threshold for AVP secretion above which a linear relationship between plasma osmolality and AVP levels occurs (Fig. 13–4).[32] At plasma osmolalities below a threshold level, AVP secretion is suppressed to low or undetectable levels; above this point, AVP secretion increases linearly in direct proportion to plasma osmolality. The slope of the regression line relating AVP secretion to plasma osmolality can vary significantly across individual human subjects, in part because of genetic factors[33] but also in relation to other factors. In general, each 1 mOsm/kg H_2O increase in plasma osmolality causes an increase in plasma AVP level ranging from 0.4 to 1.0 pg/mL. The renal response to circulating AVP is similarly linear, with urinary concentration that is directly proportional to AVP levels from 0.5 to 4 to 5 pg/mL, after which urinary osmolality is maximal and cannot increase further despite additional increases in AVP levels (Fig. 13–5). Thus, changes of as little as 1% in plasma osmolality are sufficient to cause significant increases in plasma AVP levels with proportional increases in urine concentration, and maximal antidiuresis is achieved after increases in plasma osmolality of only 5 to 10 mOsm/kg H_2O (i.e., 2%–4%) above the threshold for AVP secretion.

However, even this analysis underestimates the sensitivity of this system to regulate free water excretion. Urinary osmolality is directly proportional to plasma AVP levels as a consequence of the fall in urine flow induced by the AVP, but urine volume is inversely related to urine osmolality (see Fig. 13–5). An increase in plasma AVP concentration from 0.5 to 2 pg/mL has a much greater relative effect to decrease urine flow than does a subsequent increase in AVP concentration from 2 to 5 pg/mL, thereby magnifying the physiologic effects of small initial changes in plasma AVP levels. Furthermore, the rapid response of AVP secretion to changes in plasma osmolality coupled with the short half-life of AVP in human plasma (10–20 min) allows the kidneys to respond to changes in plasma osmolality on a minute-to-minute basis. The net result is a finely tuned osmoregulatory system that adjusts the rate of free water excretion accurately to the ambient plasma osmolality primarily via changes in pituitary AVP secretion.

The set-point of the osmoregulatory system also varies from person to person. In healthy adults, the osmotic threshold for

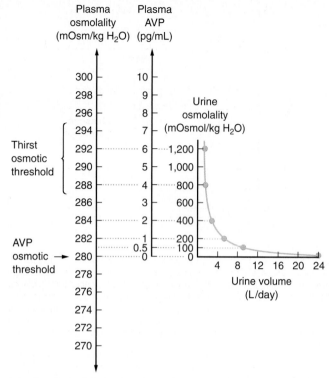

FIGURE 13–5 Relationship of plasma osmolality, plasma AVP concentrations, urine osmolality, and urine volume in humans. Note that the osmotic threshold for AVP secretion defines the point at which urine concentration begins to increase, but the osmotic threshold for thirst is significantly higher and approximates the point at which maximal urine concentration has already been achieved. Note also that, because of the inverse relation between urine osmolality and urine volume, changes in plasma AVP concentrations have much larger effects on urine volume at low plasma AVP concentrations than at high plasma AVP concentrations. (Adapted from Robinson AG: Disorders of antidiuretic hormone secretion. J Clin Endocrinol Metab 14:55–88, 1985.)

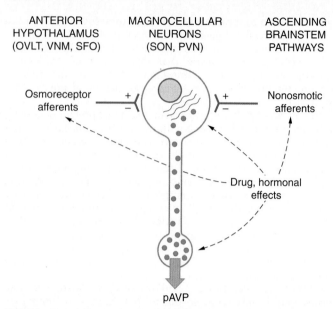

FIGURE 13–6 Schematic model of the regulatory control of the neurohypophysis. The secretory activity of individual magnocellular neurons is determined by an integration of the activities of both excitatory and inhibitory osmotic and nonosmotic afferent inputs. Superimposed on this are the effects of hormones and drugs, which can act at multiple levels to modulate the output of the system. (Adapted from Verbalis JG: Osmotic inhibition of neurohypophyseal secretion. Ann N Y Acad Sci 689:227–233, 1983.)

AVP secretion ranges from 275 to 290 mOsm/kg H_2O (averaging approximately 280–285 mOsm/kg H_2O). Similar to sensitivity, individual differences in the set-point of the osmoregulatory system are relatively constant over time and appear to be genetically determined.[33] However, multiple factors, in addition to genetic influences, can alter either the sensitivity and/or the set-point of the osmoregulatory system for AVP secretion.[33] Foremost among these are acute changes in blood pressure, effective blood volume or both, which are discussed in the following section. Aging has been found to increase the sensitivity of the osmoregulatory system in multiple studies.[34,35] Metabolic factors such as serum Ca^{2+} and various drugs can alter the slope of the plasma AVP-osmolality relationship as well.[36] Lesser degrees of shifting of the osmsensitivity and set-point for AVP secretion have been noted with alterations in gonadal hormones. Some studies have found increased osmosensitivity in women, particularly during the luteal phase of the menstrual cycle,[37] and in estrogen-treated men,[38] but these effects were relatively minor; others have found no significant sex differences.[33] The set-point of the osmoregulatory system is reduced more dramatically and reproducibly during pregnancy.[39] Recent evidence has suggested the possible involvement of the placental hormone relaxin[40] rather than gonadal steroids or human chorionic gonadotropin hormone in pregnancy-associated resetting of the osmostat for AVP secretion. That multiple factors can influence the set-point and sensitivity of osmotically regulated AVP secretion is not surprising in view of the fact that AVP secretion reflects a balance of bimodal inputs, that is, both inhibitory as well as stimulatory,[41] from multiple different afferent inputs to the neurohypophysis (Fig. 13–6).[42]

Understanding the osmoregulatory mechanism also requires addressing the observation that AVP secretion is not equally sensitive to all plasma solutes. Sodium and its anions, which normally contribute more than 95% of the osmotic pressure of plasma, are the most potent solutes in terms of their capacity to stimulate AVP secretion and thirst, although certain sugars such as mannitol and sucrose are also equally effective when infused intravenously.[11] In contrast, increases in plasma osmolality caused by noneffective solutes such as urea or glucose cause little or no increase in plasma AVP levels in humans or animals.[11,43] These differences in response to various plasma solutes are independent of any recognized nonosmotic influence, indicating that they are a property of the osmoregulatory mechanism itself. According to current concepts, the osmoreceptor neuron is stimulated by osmotically induced changes in its water content. In this case, the stimulatory potency of any given solute would be an inverse function of the rate at which it moves from the plasma to the inside of the osmoreceptor neuron. Solutes that penetrate slowly, or not at all, create an osmotic gradient that causes an efflux of water from the osmoreceptor, and the resultant shrinkage of the osmoreceptor neuron activates a stretch-inactivated noncationic channel that initiates depolarization and firing of the neuron.[44] Conversely, solutes that penetrate the cell readily create no gradient and, thus, have no effect on the water content and cell volume of the osmoreceptors. This mechanism agrees well with the observed relationship between the effect of certain solutes like Na^+, mannitol, and glucose on AVP secretion and the rate at which they penetrate the blood-brain barrier.

Many neurotransmitters have been implicated in mediating the actions of the osmoreceptors on the neurohypophysis. The SON is richly innervated by multiple pathways, including acetylcholine, catecholamines, glutamate, gamma-aminobutyric acid (GABA), histamine, opioids, Ang II, and dopamine (see review[45]). Studies have supported a potential role for all of these, and yet others, in the regulation of AVP secretion, as has local secretion of AVP into the hypothalamus from dendrites of the AVP-secreting neurons.[46] Although it remains unclear which of these are involved in the normal physiologic control of AVP secretion, in view of the likelihood that the osmoregulatory system is bimodal and integrated with multiple different afferent pathways (see Fig. 13–6), it seems likely that magnocellular AVP neurons are influenced by a complex mixture of neurotransmitter systems rather than only a few.

Nonosmotic Regulation

HEMODYNAMIC CHANGES. Not surprisingly, hypovolemia is also a potent stimulus for AVP secretion in humans,[32,47] because an appropriate response to volume depletion should include renal water conservation. In humans as well as multiple animal species, lowering blood pressure suddenly by any of several methods increases plasma AVP levels by an amount that is proportional to the degree of hypotension achieved.[32,48] This stimulus-response relationship follows a distinctly exponential pattern, such that small reductions in blood pressure, of the order of 5% to 10%, usually have little effect on plasma AVP, whereas blood pressure decreases of 20% to 30% result in hormone levels many times those required to produce maximal antidiuresis (see Fig. 13–4). The AVP response to acute reductions in blood volume appears to be quantitatively and qualitatively similar to the response to blood pressure. In rats, plasma AVP increases as an exponential function of the degree of hypovolemia. Thus, little increase in plasma AVP can be detected until blood volume falls by 5% to 8%; beyond that point, plasma AVP increases at an exponential rate relation to the degree of hypovolemia and usually reaches levels 20 to 30 times normal when blood volume is reduced by 20% to 40%.[49,50] The volume-AVP relation has not been as thoroughly characterized in other species, but it appears to follow a similar pattern humans.[51] Conversely, acute increases in blood volume or pressure suppress AVP secretion. This response has been characterized less well than that of hypotension or hypovolemia, but it seems to have a similar quantitative relationship (i.e., relatively large changes, of the order of 10%–15%, are required to alter hormone secretion appreciably).[52]

The minimal to absent effect of small changes in blood volume and pressure on AVP secretion contrasts sharply with the extraordinary sensitivity of the osmoregulatory system (see Fig. 13–4). Recognition of this difference is essential for understanding the relative contribution of each system to control AVP secretion under physiologic and pathologic conditions. Because day-to-day variations of TBW rarely exceed 2% to 3%, their effect on AVP secretion must be mediated largely, if not exclusively, by the osmoregulatory system. Nonetheless, modest changes in blood volume and pressure do, in fact, influence AVP secretion indirectly, even though they are weak stimuli by themselves. This occurs via shifting the sensitivity of AVP secretion to osmotic stimuli so that a given increase in osmolality will cause a greater secretion of AVP during hypovolemic conditions than during euvolemic states (Fig. 13–7).[53,54] In the presence of a negative hemodynamic stimulus, plasma AVP continues to respond appropriately to small changes in plasma osmolality and can still be fully suppressed if the osmolality falls below the new (lower) set-point. The retention of the threshold function is a vital aspect of the interaction because it ensures that the capacity to regulate the osmolality of body fluids is not lost even in the presence of significant hypovolemia or hypotension. Consequently, it is reasonable to conclude that the major effect of moderate degrees of hypovolemia on both AVP secretion and thirst is to modulate the gain of the osmoregulatory responses, with direct effects on thirst and AVP secretion occurring only during more severe degrees of hypo-

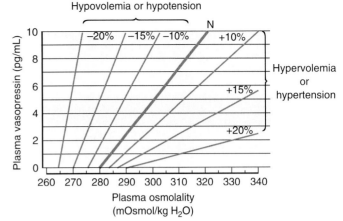

FIGURE 13–7   The relation between the osmolality of plasma and the concentration of AVP in plasma is modulated by blood volume and pressure. The *line labeled N* shows plasma AVP concentration across a range of plasma osmolality in an adult with normal intravascular volume (euvolemic) and normal blood pressure (normotensive). The *lines to the left of N* show the relationship between plasma AVP concentration and plasma osmolality in adults whose low intravascular volume (hypovolemia) or blood pressure (hypotension) is 10%, 15%, and 20% below normal. *Lines to the right of N* indicate volumes and blood pressures 10%, 15%, and 20% above normal. Note that hemodynamic influences do not disrupt the osmoregulation of AVP but rather raise or lower the set-point, and possibly the sensitivity as well, of AVP secretion in proportion to the magnitude of the change in blood volume or pressure. (Adapted from Robertson GL, Athar S, Shelton RL: Osmotic control of vasopressin function. *In* Andreoli TE, Grantham JJ, Rector FC Jr [eds]: Disturbances in Body Fluid Osmolality. Bethesda, MD, American Physiological Society, 1977, p 125.)

volemia (e.g., >10%–20% reductions in blood pressure or volume).

These hemodynamic influences on AVP secretion are mediated at least in part by neural pathways that originate in stretch-sensitive receptors, generally called *baroreceptors,* in the cardiac atria, aorta, and carotid sinus (see Fig. 13–2). Afferent nerve fibers from these receptors ascend in the vagus and glossopharyngeal nerves to the nuclei of the tractus solitarius (NTS) in the brainstem.[55] A variety of postsynaptic pathways from the NTS then project, both directly and indirectly via the ventrolateral medulla and the lateral parabrachial nucleus, to the PVN and SON in the hypothalamus.[56] Early studies suggested that the input from these pathways was predominantly inhibitory under basal conditions, because interrupting them acutely resulted in large increases in plasma AVP levels as well as in arterial blood pressure.[57] However, as for most neural systems including the neurohypophysis, innervation is complex and consists of both excitatory and inhibitory inputs. Consequently, different effects have been observed under different experimental conditions.

The baroreceptor mechanism also appears to mediate a large number of pharmacologic and pathologic effects on AVP secretion (Table 13–1). Among them are diuretics, isoproterenol, nicotine, prostaglandins, nitroprusside, trimethaphan, histamine, morphine, and bradykinin, all of which stimulate AVP at least in part by lowering blood volume or pressure,[47] and norepinephrine, which suppresses AVP by raising blood pressure.[58] In addition, upright posture, sodium depletion, congestive heart failure, cirrhosis, and nephrosis likely stimulate AVP secretion by reducing effective circulating blood volume.[59,60] Symptomatic orthostatic hypotension, vasovagal reactions, and other forms of syncope more markedly stimulate AVP secretion via greater and more acute decreases in blood pressure, with the exception of orthostatic hypotension associated with loss of afferent baroregulatory function.[61] Almost every hormone, drug, or condition that affects blood volume or pressure will also affect AVP secretion, but in most cases, the degree of change of blood pressure or volume is modest and will result in a shift of the set-point and/or sensitivity of the osmoregulatory response rather than marked stimulation of AVP secretion (see Fig. 13–7).

TABLE 13–1	Drugs and Hormones That Affect Vasopressin Secretion
Stimulatory	**Inhibitory**
Acetylcholine	Norepinephrine
Nicotine	Fluphenazine
Apomorphine	Haloperidol
Morphine (high doses)	Promethazine
Epinephrine	Oxilorphan
Isoproterenol	Butorphanol
Histamine	Opioid agonists
Bradykinin	Morphine (low doses)
Prostaglandin	Ethanol
β-Endorphin	Carbamazepine
Cyclophosphamide IV	Glucocorticoids
Vincristine	Clonidine
Insulin	Muscimol
2-Deoxyglucose	Phencyclidine
Angiotensin II	Phenytoin
Lithium	
Corticotropin-releasing factor	
Naloxone	
Cholecystokinin	

DRINKING. Peripheral neural sensors other than baroreceptors can also affect AVP secretion. In humans as well as dogs, drinking lowers plasma AVP before there is any appreciable decrease in plasma osmolality or serum Na+. This is clearly a response to the act of drinking itself because it occurs independently of the composition of the fluid ingested,[62,63] although it may be influenced by the temperature of the fluid because the degree of suppression appears to be greater in response to colder fluids.[64] The pathways responsible for this effect have not been delineated, but likely include sensory afferent originating in the oropharynx and transmitted centrally via the glossopharyngeal nerve.

NAUSEA. Among other nonosmotic stimuli to AVP secretion in humans, nausea is the most prominent. The sensation of nausea, with or without vomiting, is by far the most potent stimulus to AVP secretion known in humans. Whereas 20% increases in osmolality will typically elevate plasma AVP levels to the range of 5 to 20 pg/mL, and 20% decreases in blood pressure to 10 to 100 pg/mL, nausea has been described to cause AVP elevations in excess of 200 to 400 pg/mL.[65] The pathway mediating this effect has been mapped to the chemoreceptor zone in the area postrema of the brainstem in animal studies (see Fig. 13–2). It can be activated by a variety of drugs and conditions, including apomorphine, morphine, nicotine, alcohol, and motion sickness. Its effect on AVP is instantaneous and extremely potent (Fig. 13–8), even when the nausea is transient and not accompanied by vomiting or changes in blood pressure. Pretreatment with fluphenazine, haloperidol, or promethazine in doses sufficient to prevent nausea completely abolishes the AVP response. The inhibitory effect of these dopamine antagonists is specific for emetic stimuli, because they do not alter the AVP response to osmotic and hemodynamic stimuli. Water loading blunts, but does not abolish, the effect of nausea on AVP release, suggesting that osmotic and emetic influences interact in a manner similar to that for osmotic and hemodynamic pathways. Species differences also affect emetic stimuli. Whereas dogs and cats appear to be even more sensitive than humans to emetic stimulation of AVP release, rodents have little or no AVP response but release large amounts of oxytocin instead.[66]

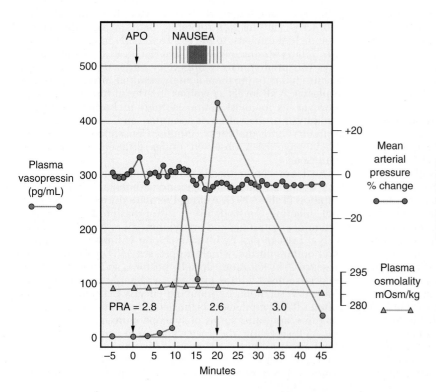

FIGURE 13–8 Effect of nausea on AVP secretion. Apomorphine was injected at the point indicated by the *vertical arrow*. Note that the rise in plasma AVP coincided with the occurrence of nausea and was not associated with detectable changes in plasma osmolality or blood pressure. (Adapted from Robertson GL: The regulation of vasopressin function in health and disease. Recent Prog Horm Res 33:333, 1977.)

The emetic response probably mediates many pharmacologic and pathologic effects on AVP secretion. In addition to the drugs and conditions already noted, it may be responsible at least in part for the increase in AVP secretion that has been observed with vasovagal reactions, diabetic ketoacidosis, acute hypoxia, and motion sickness. Because nausea and vomiting are frequent side effects of many other drugs and diseases, many additional situations likely occur as well. The reason for this profound stimulation is not known (although it has been speculated that the AVP response assists evacuation of stomach contents via contraction of gastric smooth muscle, AVP is not necessary for vomiting to occur), but it is probably responsible for the intense vasoconstriction that produces the pallor often associated with this state.

HYPOGLYCEMIA. Acute hypoglycemia is a less potent but reasonably consistent stimulus for AVP secretion.[67,68] The receptor and pathway that mediate this effect are unknown; however, they appear separate from those of other recognized stimuli, because hypoglycemia stimulates AVP secretion even in patients who have selectively lost the capacity to respond to hypernatremia, hypotension, or nausea.[68] The factor that actually triggers the release of AVP is likely intracellular deficiency of glucose or ATP, because 2-deoxyglucose is also an effective stimulus.[69] Generally, more than 20% decreases in glucose are required to significantly increase plasma AVP levels; the rate of fall in glucose is probably the critical stimulus, however, because the rise in plasma AVP is not sustained with persistent hypoglycemia.[67] However, glucopenic stimuli are of unlikely importance in the physiology or pathology of AVP secretion, because there are probably few drugs or conditions that lower plasma glucose rapidly enough to stimulate release of the hormone, and furthermore, because this effect is transient.

RENIN-ANGIOTENSIN SYSTEM. The renin-angiotensin system has also been intimately implicated in the control of AVP secretion.[70] Animal studies have indicated dual sites of action. Blood-borne Ang II stimulates AVP secretion by acting in the brain at the circumventricular subfornical organ (SFO),[71] a small structure located in the dorsal portion of the third cerebral ventricle (see Fig. 13–2). Because circumventricular organs lack a blood-brain barrier, the densely expressed Ang II AT_1 receptors of the SFO can detect very small increases in blood levels of Ang II.[72] Neural pathways from the SFO to the hypothalamic SON and PVN mediate AVP secretion and also appear to use Ang II as a neurotransmitter.[73] This accounts for the observation that the most sensitive site for angiotensin-mediated AVP secretion and thirst is intracerebroventricular injection into the cerebrospinal fluid. Further evidence in support of Ang II as a neurotransmitter is that intraventricular administration of angiotensin receptor antagonists inhibits the AVP response to osmotic and hemodynamic stimuli.[74] The level of plasma Ang II required to stimulate AVP release is quite high, leading some to argue that this stimulus is active only under pharmacologic conditions. This is consistent with observations that even pressor doses of Ang II increase plasma AVP only about two- to fourfold[70] and may account for the failure of some investigators to demonstrate stimulation of thirst by exogenous angiotensin. However, this procedure may underestimate the physiologic effects of angiotensin, because the increased blood pressure caused by exogenously administered Ang II appears to blunt the induced thirst via activation of inhibitory baroreceptive pathways.[75]

STRESS. Nonspecific stress caused by factors such as pain, emotion, or physical exercise has long been thought to cause AVP secretion, but it has never been determined whether this effect is mediated by a specific pathway or is secondary to the hypotension or nausea that often accompanies stress-induced vasovagal reactions. In rats[76] and humans,[77] a variety of noxious stimuli capable of activating the pituitary-adrenal axis and sympathetic nervous system do not stimulate AVP

secretion unless they also lower blood pressure or alter blood volume. The marked rise in plasma AVP elicited by manipulation of the abdominal viscera in anesthetized dogs has been attributed to nociceptive influences,[78] but mediation by emetic pathways cannot be excluded in this setting. Endotoxin-induced fever stimulates AVP secretion in rats, and recent data support possible mediation of this effect by circulating cytokines such as interleukin-1 (IL-1) and IL-6.[79] Clarification of the possible role of nociceptive and thermal influences on AVP secretion is particularly important in view of the frequency with which painful or febrile illnesses are associated with osmotically inappropriate secretion of the hormone.

HYPOXIA AND HYPERCAPNIA. Acute hypoxia and hypercapnia also stimulate AVP secretion.[80,81] In conscious humans, however, the stimulatory effect of moderate hypoxia (arterial partial pressure of oxygen [PaO_2] > 35 mm Hg) is inconsistent, and seems to occur mainly in subjects who develop nausea or hypotension. In conscious dogs, more severe hypoxia (PaO_2 < 35 mm Hg) consistently increases AVP secretion without reducing arterial pressure.[82] Studies of anesthetized dogs suggest that the AVP response to acute hypoxia depends on the level of hypoxemia achieved. At a PaO_2 of 35 mm Hg or lower, plasma AVP increases markedly even though there is no change or even an increase in arterial pressure, but less severe hypoxia (PaO_2 > 40 mm Hg) has no effect on AVP levels.[83] These results indicate that there is likely a hypoxemic threshold for AVP secretion and suggest that severe hypoxemia alone may also stimulate AVP secretion in humans. If so, it may be responsible, at least in part, for the osmotically inappropriate AVP elevations noted in some patients with acute respiratory failure.[84] In conscious or anesthetized dogs, acute hypercapnia, independent of hypoxia or hypotension, also increases AVP secretion.[82,83] It has not been determined whether this response also exhibits threshold characteristics or otherwise depends on the degree of hypercapnia, nor is it known whether hypercapnia has similar effects on AVP secretion in humans or other animals. The mechanisms by which hypoxia and hypercapnia release AVP remain undefined, but they likely involve peripheral chemoreceptors and/or baroreceptors, because cervical vagotomy abolishes the response to hypoxemia in dogs.[85]

DRUGS. As is discussed more extensively in the clinical disorders, a variety of drugs, including nicotine, also stimulate AVP secretion (see Table 13–1). Drugs and hormones can potentially affect AVP secretion at many different sites, as depicted in Figure 13–6. As already discussed, many excitatory stimulants such as isoproterenol, nicotine, high doses of morphine and cholecystokinin act, at least in part, by lowering blood pressure and/or producing nausea. Others, like substance P, prostaglandin, endorphin, and other opioids, have not been studied sufficiently to define their mechanism of action, but they may also work by one or both of the same mechanisms. Inhibitory stimuli similarly have multiple modes of action. Vasopressor drugs like norepinephrine inhibit AVP secretion indirectly by raising arterial pressure. In low doses, a variety of opioids of all subtypes including morphine, met-enkephalin and kappa-agonists inhibit AVP secretion in rats and humans.[86] Endogenous opioid peptides interact with the magnocellular neurosecretory system at several levels to inhibit basal as well as stimulated secretion of AVP and oxytocin. Opioid inhibition of AVP secretion has been found to occur in isolated posterior pituitary tissue, and the action of morphine as well as several opioid agonists such as butorphanol and oxilorphan likely occurs via activation of kappa-opioid receptors located on nerve terminals of the posterior pituitary.[87] The well-known inhibitory effect of alcohol on AVP secretion may be mediated, at least in part, by endogenous opiates, because it is due to an elevation in the osmotic threshold for AVP release[88] and can be blocked in part by treatment with naloxone.[89] Carbamazepine inhibits AVP secretion by diminishing the sensitivity of the osmoregulatory system; this effect occurs independently of changes in blood volume, blood pressure, or blood glucose.[90] Other drugs that inhibit AVP secretion include clonidine, which appears to act via both central and peripheral adrenoreceptors,[91] muscimol,[92] which acts as a GABA antagonist, and phencyclidine,[93] which probably acts by raising blood pressure. However, despite the importance of these stimuli during pathologic conditions, none of them is a significant determinant of physiologic regulation of AVP secretion in humans.

Distribution and Clearance

Plasma AVP concentration is determined by the difference between the rates of secretion from the posterior pituitary gland and removal of the hormone from the vascular compartment via metabolism and urinary clearance. In healthy adults, intravenously injected AVP distributes rapidly into a space equivalent in size to the ECF compartment. This initial, or mixing, phase has a half-life between 4 and 8 minutes and is virtually complete in 10 to 15 minutes. The rapid mixing phase is followed by a second, slower decline that corresponds to the metabolic clearance of AVP. Most studies of this phase have yielded mean values of 10 to 20 minutes by both steady-state and non–steady-state techniques,[32] consistent with the observed rates of change in urine osmolality after water loading and injection of AVP, which also support a short half-life.[94] In pregnant women, the metabolic clearance rate of increases nearly fourfold,[95] which becomes significant in the pathophysiology of gestational diabetes insipidus (GDI) (see later discussion). Smaller animals such as rats clear AVP much more rapidly than humans because their cardiac output is higher relative to their BW and surface area.[94]

Although many tissues have the capacity to inactivate AVP, metabolism in vivo appears to occur largely in liver and kidney.[94] The enzymatic processes by which the liver and kidney inactivate AVP involve an initial reduction of the disulfide bridge followed by aminopeptidase cleavage of the bond between amino acid residues 1 and 2. The extent of further degradation and the peptide products that escape into plasma and urine are currently unknown. Some AVP is excreted intact in the urine, but there is disagreement about the amounts and the factors that affect it. For example, in healthy, normally hydrated adults, the urinary clearance of AVP ranges from 0.1 to 0.6 mL/kg/min under basal conditions and has never been found to exceed 2 mL/kg/min, even in the presence of solute diuresis.[32] The mechanisms involved in the excretion of AVP have not been defined with certainty, but the hormone is probably filtered at the glomerulus and variably reabsorbed at sites along the nephron. The latter process may be linked to the reabsorption of Na^+ or other solutes in the proximal nephron, because the urinary clearance of AVP has been found to vary by as much as 20-fold in direct relation to the solute clearance.[32] Consequently, measurements of urinary AVP excretion in humans do not provide a consistently reliable index of changes in plasma AVP, and should be interpreted cautiously when glomerular filtration or solute clearance is inconstant or abnormal.

Thirst

Thirst is the body's defense mechanism to increase water consumption in response to perceived deficits of body fluids. It can be most easily defined as a consciously perceived desire for water. True thirst must be distinguished from other determinants of fluid intake such as taste, dietary preferences, and social customs, as discussed previously. Thirst can be stimulated in animals and humans either by intracellular dehydration caused by increases in the effective osmolality of the ECF or by intravascular hypovolemia caused by losses

of ECF.[96,97] As would be expected, many of these same variables provoke AVP secretion. Of these, hypertonicity is clearly the most potent. Similar to AVP secretion, substantial evidence to date has supported mediation of osmotic thirst by osmoreceptors located in the anterior hypothalamus of the brain,[30,31] whereas hypovolemic thirst appears to be stimulated both via activation of low- and/or high-pressure baroreceptors[98] and circulating Ang II.[99]

OSMOTIC THIRST. In healthy adults, an increase in effective plasma osmolality of only 2% to 3% above basal levels produces a strong desire to drink.[100] This response is not dependent on changes in ECF or plasma volume, because it occurs similarly whether plasma osmolality is raised by infusion of hypertonic solutions or by water deprivation. The absolute level of plasma osmolality at which a person develops a conscious urge to seek and drink water is called the *osmotic thirst threshold.* It varies appreciably among individuals, likely as a result of by genetic factors,[33] but in healthy adults, it averages approximately 295 mOsm/kg H_2O. Of physiologic significance is the fact that this level is above the osmotic threshold for AVP release and approximates the plasma osmolality at which maximal concentration of the urine is normally achieved (see Fig. 13–5).

The brain pathways that mediate osmotic thirst have not been well defined, but it is clear that initiation of drinking requires osmoreceptors located in the anteroventral hypothalamus in the same area as the osmoreceptors that control osmotic AVP secretion are located.[30,31] Whether the osmoreceptors for AVP and thirst are the same cells or simply located in the same general area remains unknown. However, the properties of the osmoreceptors are very similar. Ineffective plasma solutes such as urea and glucose, which have little or no effect on AVP secretion, are equally ineffective at stimulating thirst, whereas effective solutes such as NaCl and mannitol are.[11,101] The sensitivities of the thirst and AVP osmoreceptors cannot be compared precisely, but they are probably similar. Thus, in healthy adults, the intensity of thirst increases rapidly in direct proportion to serum Na^+ or plasma osmolality and generally becomes intolerable at levels only 3% to 5% above the threshold level.[102] Water consumption also appears to be proportional to the intensity of thirst, in both humans and animals and, under conditions of maximal osmotic stimulation, can reach rates as high as 20 to 25 L/day. The dilution of body fluids by ingested water complements the retention of water that occurs during AVP-induced antidiuresis, and both responses occur concurrently when drinking water is available.

As with AVP secretion, the osmoregulation of thirst appears to be bimodal, because a modest decline in plasma osmolality induces a sense of satiation and reduces the basal rate of spontaneous fluid intake.[102,103] This effect is sufficient to prevent hypotonic overhydration even when antidiuresis is fixed at maximal levels for prolonged periods, suggesting that osmotically inappropriate secretion of ADH (SIADH) should not result in the development of hyponatremia unless the satiety mechanism is impaired or fluid intake is inappropriately high for some other reason, such as the unregulated components of fluid intake discussed earlier.[103] Also similar to AVP secretion, thirst can be influenced by oropharyngeal or upper gastrointestinal receptors that respond to the act of drinking itself.[63] In humans, however, the rapid relief provided by this mechanism lasts only a matter of minutes and thirst quickly recurs until enough of the water is absorbed to lower plasma osmolality to normal. Therefore, although local oropharyngeal sensations may have a significant short-term influence on thirst, the hypothalamic osmoreceptors ultimately determine the volume of water intake in response to dehydration.

HYPOVOLEMIC THIRST. In contrast, the threshold for producing hypovolemic, or extracellular, thirst is significantly higher in both animals and humans. Studies in several species have shown that sustained decreases in plasma volume or blood pressure of at least 4% to 8%, and in some species 10% to 15%, are necessary to consistently stimulate drinking.[104,105] In humans, the degree of hypovolemia or hypotension required to produce thirst has not been precisely defined, but it has been difficult to demonstrate any effects of mild to moderate hypovolemia to stimulate thirst independently of osmotic changes occurring with dehydration. This blunted sensitivity to changes in ECF volume or blood pressure in humans probably represents an adaptation that occurred as a result of the erect posture of primates, which predisposes them to wider fluctuations in blood and atrial filling pressures as a result of orthostatic pooling of blood in the lower body; stimulation of thirst (and AVP secretion) by such transient postural changes in blood pressure might lead to overdrinking and inappropriate antidiuresis in situations in which the ECF volume was actually normal but only transiently maldistributed. Consistent with a blunted response to baroreceptor activation, recent studies have also shown that systemic infusion of Ang II to pharmacologic levels is a much less potent stimulus to thirst in humans[106] than in animals, in which it is one of the most potent dipsogens known. Nonetheless, this response is not completely absent in humans, as demonstrated by rare cases of polydipsia in patients with pathologic causes of hyperreninemia.[107] The pathways by which hypovolemia or hypotension produces thirst have not been well-defined, but probably involve the same brainstem baroreceptive pathways that mediate hemodynamic effects on AVP secretion,[98] as well as a likely contribution from circulating levels of Ang II in some species.[108]

Integration of Arginine Vasopressin Secretion and Thirst

A synthesis of what is presently known about the regulation of AVP secretion and thirst in humans leads to a relatively simple but elegant system to maintain water balance. Under normal physiologic conditions, the sensitivity of the osmoregulatory system for AVP secretion accounts for maintenance of plasma osmolality within narrow limits by adjusting renal water excretion to small changes in osmolality. Stimulated thirst does not represent a major regulatory mechanism under these conditions, and unregulated fluid ingestion supplies adequate water in excess of true "need," which is then excreted in relation to osmoregulated pituitary AVP secretion. However, when unregulated water intake cannot adequately supply body needs in the presence of plasma AVP levels sufficient to produce maximal antidiuresis, then plasma osmolality rises to levels that stimulate thirst (see Fig. 13–5), and water intake increases proportional to the elevation of osmolality above this thirst threshold.

In such a system, thirst essentially represents a back-up mechanism called into play when pituitary and renal mechanisms prove insufficient to maintain plasma osmolality within a few percent of basal levels. This arrangement has the advantage of freeing humans from frequent episodes of thirst that would require a diversion of activities toward behavior oriented to seeking water when water deficiency is sufficiently mild to be compensated for by renal water conservation but would stimulate water ingestion once water deficiency reaches potentially harmful levels. Stimulation of AVP secretion at plasma osmolalities below the threshold for subjective thirst acts to maintain an excess of body water sufficient to eliminate the need to drink whenever slight elevations in plasma osmolality occur. This system of differential effective thresholds for thirst and AVP secretion nicely complements many studies that have demonstrated excess unregulated, or "need-free," drinking in both humans and

animals. Only when this mechanism becomes inadequate to maintain body fluid homeostasis does thirst-induced regulated fluid intake become the predominant defense mechanism for the prevention of severe dehydration.

DISORDERS OF INSUFFICIENT ARGININE VASOPRESSIN OR ARGININE VASOPRESSIN EFFECT

Disorders of insufficient AVP or AVP effect are associated with inadequate urine concentration and increased urine output (polyuria). If thirst mechanisms are intact, this is accompanied by compensatory increases in fluid intake (polydipsia) as a result of stimulated thirst in order to preserve body fluid homeostasis. The net result is polyuria and polydipsia with preservation of normal plasma osmolality and serum electrolyte concentrations. However, if thirst is impaired or if fluid intake is insufficient for any reason to compensate for the increased urine excretion, then hyperosmolality and hypernatremia can result, with the consequent complications associated with these disorders. The quintessential disorder of insufficient AVP is diabetes insipidus (DI), which is a clinical syndrome characterized by excretion of abnormally large volumes of urine (i.e., diabetes) that is dilute (i.e., hypotonic) and devoid of taste from dissolved solutes (e.g., insipid), in contrast to the hypertonic sweet-tasting urine characteristic of diabetes mellitus (i.e., honey, in Greek).

Several different pathophysiologic mechanisms can cause hypotonic polyuria (Table 13–2). Central (also called hypothalamic, neurogenic, or neurohypophyseal) DI (CDI) is due to inadequate secretion, and usually deficient synthesis of, AVP in the hypothalamic neurohypophyseal system. Lack of AVP-stimulated activation of the V_2 subtype of AVP receptors in the kidney collecting tubules (see Chapters 8 and 9) causes excretion of large volumes of dilute urine. In most cases, thirst mechanisms are intact, leading to compensatory polydipsia. However, in a variant of CDI called osmoreceptor dysfunction, thirst is also impaired, leading to hypodipsia. DI of pregnancy is a transient disorder due to an accelerated metabolism of AVP as a result of increased activity of the enzyme oxytocinase/vasopressinase in the serum of pregnant females, again leading to polyuria and polydipsia; accelerated metabolism of AVP during pregnancy may also cause a patient with subclinical DI from other causes to shift from a relatively asymptomatic state to a symptomatic state as a result of the more rapid AVP degradation. Nephrogenic DI (NDI) is due to inappropriate renal responses to AVP. This produces excretion of dilute urine despite normal pituitary AVP secretion and secondary polydipsia, similar to CDI. The final cause of hypotonic polyuria, primary polydipsia, differs significantly from the other causes because it is not due to deficient AVP secretion or impaired renal responses to AVP, but rather to excessive ingestion of fluids. This can result from either an abnormality in the thirst mechanism, in which case it is sometimes called dipsogenic DI, or to psychiatric disorders, in which case it is generally referred to as psychogenic polydipsia.

Central Diabetes Insipidus

Etiology

CDI is caused by inadequate secretion of AVP from the posterior pituitary in response to osmotic stimulation. In most cases, this is due to destruction of the neurohypophysis by a variety of acquired or congenital anatomic lesions that destroy or damage the neurohypophysis by pressure or infiltration (see Table 13–2). The severity of the resulting hypotonic

TABLE 13–2 Etiologies of Hypotonic Polyuria

Central (neurogenic) diabetes insipidus
Congenital (congenital malformations, autosomal dominant,
    arginine vasopressin (AVP)–neurophysin gene mutations)
Drug-/toxin-induced (ethanol, diphenylhydantoin, snake venom)
Granulomatous (histiocytosis, sarcoidosis)
Neoplastic (craniopharyngioma, germinoma, lymphoma,
    leukemia, meningioma, pituitary tumor; metastases)
Infectious (meningitis, tuberculosis, encephalitis)
Inflammatory/autoimmune (lymphocytic
    infundiculoneurohypophysitis)
Trauma (neurosurgery, deceleration injury)
Vascular (cerebral hemorrhage or infarction, brain death)
Idiopathic

Osmoreceptor dysfunction
Granulomatous (histiocytosis, sarcoidosis)
Neoplastic (craniopharyngioma, pinealoma, meningioma,
    metastases)
Vascular (anterior communicating artery aneurysm/ligation,
    intrahypothalamic hemorrhage)
Other (hydrocephalus, ventricular/suprasellar cyst, trauma,
    degenerative diseases)
Idiopathic

Increased AVP metabolism
Pregnancy

Nephrogenic diabetes insipidus
Congenital (X-linked recessive, AVP V_2 receptor gene mutations,
    autosomal recessive or dominant, aquaporin-2 water channel
    gene mutations)
Drug-induced (demeclocycline, lithium, cisplatin,
    methoxyflurane)
Hypercalcemia
Hypokalemia
Infiltrating lesions (sarcoidosis, amyloidosis)
Vascular (sickle cell anemia)
Mechanical (polycystic kidney disease, bilateral ureteral
    obstruction)
Solute diuresis (glucose, mannitol, sodium, radiocontrast dyes)
Idiopathic

Primary polydipsia
Psychogenic (schizophrenia, obsessive-compulsive behaviors)
Dipsogenic (downward resetting of thirst threshold, idiopathic or
    similar lesions as with central DI)

diuresis depends on the degree of destruction of the neurohypophysis, leading to either complete or partial deficiency of AVP secretion.

Despite the wide variety of lesions that can potentially cause CDI, it is much more common to *not* have CDI in the presence of such lesions than to actually produce the syndrome. This apparent inconsistency can be understood by considering several common principles of neurohypophyseal physiology and pathophysiology that are relevant to all of these etiologies. The first is that the synthesis of AVP occurs in the hypothalamus (see Fig. 13–2); the posterior pituitary simply represents the site of storage and secretion of the neurosecretory granules that contain AVP. Consequently, lesions contained within the sella turcica that destroy only the posterior pituitary generally do not cause CDI because the cell bodies of the magnocellular neurons that synthesize AVP remain intact and the site of release of AVP shifts more superiorly, typically into the blood vessels of the median eminence at the base of the brain. Perhaps the best examples of this phenomenon are large pituitary macroadenomas that completely destroy the anterior and posterior pituitary. DI is a distinctly unusual presentation for such pituitary adenomas, because destruction of the posterior pituitary by such slowly enlarging intrasellar lesions merely destroys the nerve terminals, but not the cell bodies, of the AVP neurons. As this

occurs, the site of release of AVP shifts more superiorly to the pituitary stalk and median eminence. Sometimes this can be detected on noncontrast magnetic resonance imaging (MRI) as a shift of the pituitary "bright spot" more superiorly to the level of the infundibulum or median eminence,[109] but often, this process is too diffuse to be detected in this manner. The occurrence of DI from a pituitary adenoma is so uncommon, even with macroadenomas that completely obliterate sellar contents sufficiently to cause panhypopituitarism, that its presence should lead to consideration of alternative diagnoses, such as craniopharyngioma, which often causes damage to the median eminence by virtue of adherence of the capsule to the base of the hypothalamus, more rapidly enlarging sellar/suprasellar masses that do not allow sufficient time for shifting the site of AVP release more superiorly (e.g., metastatic lesions), or granulomatous disease with more diffuse hypothalamic involvement (e.g., sarcoidosis, histiocytosis). With very large pituitary adenomas that produce ACTH deficiency, it is actually more likely that patients will present with hypoosmolality from an SIADH-like picture as a result of the impaired free water excretion that accompanies hypocortisolism, as is discussed later.

A second general principle is that the capacity of the neurohypophysis to synthesize AVP is greatly in excess of the body's daily needs for maintenance of water homeostasis. Carefully controlled studies of surgical section of the pituitary stalk in dogs have clearly demonstrated that destruction of 80% to 90% of the magnocellular neurons in the hypothalamus is required to produce polyuria and polydipsia in this species.[110] Thus, even lesions that do cause destruction of the AVP magnocellular neuron cell bodies must cause a large degree of destruction to produce DI. The most illustrative example of this is surgical section of the pituitary stalk in humans. Necropsy studies of these patients have revealed atrophy of the posterior pituitary and loss of the magnocellular neurons in the hypothalamus.[111] This loss of magnocellular cells presumably results from retrograde degeneration of neurons whose axons were cut during surgery. As is generally true for all neurons, the likelihood of retrograde neuronal degeneration depends on the proximity of the axotomy, in this case, section of the pituitary stalk, to the cell body of the neuron. This was shown clearly in studies of human subjects in whom section of the pituitary stalk at the level of the diaphragm sella (i.e., a low stalk section) produced transient but not permanent DI, whereas section at the level of the infundibulum (i.e., a "high" stalk section) was required to cause permanent DI in most cases.[112]

In recent years, several genetic causes of AVP deficiency have also been characterized. Prior to the application of techniques for amplification of genomic DNA, the only experimental model to study the mechanism of hereditary hypothalamic DI was the Brattleboro rat, a strain that was found serendipitously to have CDI.[113] In this animal, the disease demonstrates a classic pattern of autosomal recessive inheritance in which DI is expressed only in the homozygotes. The hereditary basis of the disease has been found to be a single base deletion producing a translational frame shift beginning in the third portion of the neurophysin coding sequence. Because the gene lacks a stop codon, there is a modified neurophysin, no glycopeptide, and a long polylysine tail.[114] Although the mutant prohormone accumulates in the endoplasmic reticulum, sufficient AVP is produced by the normal allele that the heterozygotes are asymptomatic. In contrast, most all families with genetic CDI in humans that have been described to date demonstrate an autosomal dominant mode of inheritance.[115–117] In this case, DI is expressed despite the expression of one normal allele, which is sufficient to prevent the disease in the heterozygous Brattleboro rats. Numerous studies have been directed at understanding this apparent anomaly. Two potentially important clues as to the etiology of the DI in familial genetic CDI are that (1) severe to partial deficiencies of AVP and overt signs of DI do not develop in these patients until several months to several years after birth and then gradually progress over the ensuing decades,[115,118] suggesting adequate initial function of the normal allele with later decompensation and (2) a limited number of autopsy studies suggested that some of these cases are associated with gliosis and a marked loss of magnocellular AVP neurons in the hypothalamus,[119] although other studies have shown normal neurons with decreased expression of AVP, or no hypothalamic abnormality. In most of these cases, the hyperintense signal normally emitted by the neurohypophysis in T1-weighted MRI (see later discussion) is also absent, although some exceptions have been reported.[120] Another interesting, but as yet unexplained, observation is that some adults in these families have been described in whom DI was clinically apparent during childhood but who went into remission as adults, without evidence that their remissions could be attributed to renal or adrenal insufficiency or to increased AVP synthesis.[121]

The autosomal dominant form of familial CDI is caused by diverse mutations in the gene that codes for the AVP-neurophysin precursor (Fig. 13–9). All of the mutations identified to date have been in the coding region of the gene and affect only one allele. They are located in all three exons and are predicted to alter or delete amino acid residues in the signal peptide, AVP, and neurophysin moieties of the precursor. Only the C-terminus glycopeptide, or copeptin moiety, has not been found to be affected. Most are missense mutations, but nonsense mutations (premature stop codons) and deletions also occur. One characteristic shared by all the mutations is that they are predicted to alter or delete one or more amino acids known, or reasonably presumed, to be crucial for processing, folding, and oligomerization of the precursor protein in the endoplasmic reticulum.[115,117] Because of the related functional effects of the mutations, the common clinical characteristics of the disease, the dominant-negative mode of transmission, and the autopsy and hormonal evidence of postnatal neurohypophysial degeneration, it has been postulated that all of the mutations act by causing production of an abnormal precursor protein that accumulates and eventually kills the neurons because it cannot be correctly processed, folded, and transported out of the endoplasmic reticulum. Expression studies of mutant DNA from several human mutations in cultured neuroblastoma cells

support this misfolding/neurotoxicity hypothesis by demonstrating abnormal trafficking and accumulation of mutant prohormone in the endoplasmic reticulum with low or absent expression in the Golgi apparatus, suggesting difficulty with packaging into neurosecretory granules.[122] However, cell death may not be necessary to decrease available AVP. Normally, proteins retained in the endoplasmic reticulum are selectively degraded, but if excess mutant is produced and the selective normal degradative process is overwhelmed, an alternate nonselective degradative system (autophagy) is activated. As more and more mutant precursor builds up in the endoplasmic reticulum, normal wild type is trapped with the mutant protein and degraded by the activated nonspecific degradative system. In this case, the amount of AVP that matures and is packaged would be markedly reduced.[123,124] This explanation is consistent with those cases in which little pathology is found in the magnocellular neurons and also with cases of DI in which some small amount of AVP can still be detected.

Idiopathic forms of AVP deficiency represent a large pathogenic category in both adults and children. A recent study in children revealed that over half (54%) of all cases of CDI were classified as idiopathic.[125] These patients do not have historical or clinical evidence of any injury or disease that can be linked to their DI, and MRI of the pituitary-hypothalamic area generally reveals no abnormality other than absence of the posterior pituitary bright spot and sometimes varying degrees of thickening of the pituitary stalk. Several lines of evidence have suggested that many of these patients may have had an autoimmune destruction of the neurohypophysis to account for their DI. First, the entity of lymphocytic infundibuloneurohypophysitis has been documented to be present in a subset of patients with idiopathic DI.[126] Lymphocytic infiltration of the anterior pituitary, lymphocytic hypophysitis, has been recognized as a cause of anterior pituitary deficiency for many years, but it was not until an autopsy called attention to a similar finding in the posterior pituitary of a patient with DI that this pathology was recognized to occur in the neurohypophysis as well.[127] Since that initial report, a number of similar cases have been described, including cases in the postpartum period, which is characteristic of lymphocytic hypophysitis.[128] With the advent of MRI, *lymphocytic infundibuloneurohypophysitis* has been diagnosed based on the appearance of a thickened stalk and/or enlargement of the posterior pituitary mimicking a pituitary tumor. In these

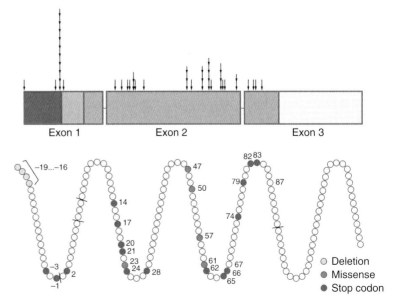

FIGURE 13–9 Location and type of mutations in the gene that codes for the AVP-neurophysin precursor in kindreds with the autosomal, dominant form of familial central diabetes insipidus (CDI). *Each arrow* indicates the location of the mutation in a different kindred. The various portions of the precursor protein are designated by the abbreviations AVP, vasopressin; CP, copeptin; NP, neurophysin; SP, signal peptide. Deletion and missense mutations are those expected to remove or replace one or more amino acid residues in the precursor. Those designated stop codons are expected to cause premature termination of the precursor. Note that none of the mutations causes a frame shift or affects the part of the gene that encodes the copeptin moiety, that all of the stop codons are in the distal part of the neurophysin moiety, and that only one of the mutations affects the AVP moiety. All these findings are consistent with the concept that the mutant precursor is produced but cannot be folded properly because of interference with either (1) the binding of AVP to neurophysin, (2) the formation of intrachain disulfide bonds, or (3) the extreme flexibility or rigidity normally required at crucial places in the protein. (Adapted from Rittig S, Robertson GL, Siggaard C, et al: Identification of 13 new mutations in the vasopressin-neurophysin gene in 17 kindreds with familial autosomal dominant neurohypophyseal DI. Am J Hum Genet 58:107, 1996; and Hansen LK, Rittig S, Robertson GL: Genetic basis of familial neurohypophyseal diabetes insipidus. Trends Endocrinol Metab 8:363, 1997.)

cases, the characteristic bright spot on MRI T1-weighted images is lost. The enlargement of the stalk can so mimic a neoplastic process that some of these patients were operated based on a suspicion of a pituitary tumor, but with the finding of lymphocytic infiltration of the pituitary stalk. Since then, a number of patients with a suspicion of infundibuloneuro-hypophysitis and no other obvious cause of DI have been followed and have shown regression of the thickened pituitary stalk over time.[125,126] Several cases have been reported with the coexistence of CDI and adenohypophysitis, and these presumably represent cases of combined lymphocytic infundibuloneurohypophysitis and hypophysisis.[129,130] A second line of evidence supporting an autoimmune etiology in many cases of idiopathic DI stems is the finding of AVP antibodies in the serum of an many as one third of patients with idiopathic DI and two thirds of those with Langerhans cell histiocytosis X, but not in patients with DI caused by tumors.[131] More recently, 878 patients with autoimmune endocrine diseases, but without hypothalamic DI, were screened, and 9 patients were found to have AVP antibodies; upon further testing, 4 of these patients were found to have partial DI and 5 were normal. After a 4-year follow-up, 3 of the normal subjects also had developed partial DI and 1 had progressed to complete DI, but interestingly 2 of the patients who had partial DI at entry were treated with desmopressin (desamino-8-d-arginine vasopressin [DDAVP]) and after 1 year became negative for AVP antibodies and had recovered normal posterior pituitary function.[132]

Pathophysiology

The normal inverse relationship between urine volume and urine osmolality (see Fig. 13–5) means that initial decreases in maximal AVP secretion will not cause an increase in urine volume sufficient to be detected clinically by polyuria. In general, basal AVP secretion must fall to less than 10% to 20% of normal before basal urine osmolality decreases to less than 300 mOsm/kg H_2O and urine flow increases to symptomatic levels (i.e., >50 ml/kg BW/day). This resulting loss of body water produces a slight rise in plasma osmolality that stimulates thirst and induces a compensatory polydipsia. The resultant increase in water intake restores balance with urine output and stabilizes the osmolality of body fluids at a new, slightly higher but still normal level. As the AVP deficit increases, this new steady-state level of plasma osmolality approximates the osmotic threshold for thirst (see Fig. 13–5). It is important to recognize that the deficiency of AVP need not be complete for polyuria and polydipsia to occur; it is only necessary that the maximal plasma AVP concentration achievable at or below the osmotic threshold for thirst is inadequate to concentrate the urine.[133] The degree of neuro-hypophysial destruction at which such failure occurs varies considerably from person to person, largely because of individual differences in the set-point and sensitivity of the osmoregulatory system.[33] In general, functional tests of AVP levels in patients with DI of variable severity, duration, and cause indicate that AVP secretory capacity must be reduced by at least 75% to 80% for significant polyuria to occur, which also agrees with neuroanatomic studies of cell loss in the SON of dogs with experimental pituitary stalk section[110] and of patients who had undergone pituitary surgery.[111]

Because renal mechanisms for sodium conservation are unimpaired with impaired or absent AVP secretion, there is no accompanying sodium deficiency. Although untreated DI can lead to both hyperosmolality and volume depletion, until the water losses become severe, volume depletion is minimized by osmotic shifts of water from the ICF compartment to the more osmotically concentrated ECF compartment. This phenomenon is not as evident following increases in ECF Na^+ concentration, because such osmotic shifts result in a slower increase in the serum Na^+ than would otherwise occur.

However, when nonsodium solutes such as mannitol are infused, this effect is more obvious owing to the progressive dilutional decrease in serum Na^+ caused by translocation of intracellular water to the ECF compartment. Because patients with DI do not have impaired urine Na^+ conservation, the ECF volume is generally not markedly decreased and regulatory mechanisms for maintenance of osmotic homeostasis are primarily activated: stimulation of thirst and AVP secretion (to whatever degree the neurohypophysis is still able to secrete AVP). In cases where AVP secretion is totally absent (complete DI), patients are dependent entirely on water intake for maintenance of water balance. However, in cases in which some residual capacity to secrete AVP remains (partial DI), plasma osmolality can eventually reach levels that allow moderate degrees of urinary concentration (see Fig. 13–10).

The development of DI following surgical or traumatic injury to the neurohypophysis represents a unique situation and can follow any of several different well-defined patterns. In some patients, polyuria develops 1 to 4 days after injury and resolves spontaneously. Less often, the DI is permanent and continues indefinitely (see previous discussion on the relation between the level of pituitary stalk section and the development of permanent DI). Most interestingly, a *"triphasic" response* can occur as a result of pituitary stalk transection.[112] The initial DI (first phase) is due to axon shock and lack of function of the damaged neurons. This phase lasts from several hours to several days, and then is followed by an antidiuretic phase (second phase) that is due to the uncontrolled release of AVP from the disconnected and degenerating posterior pituitary or from the remaining severed neurons.[134] Overly aggressive administration of fluids during this second phase does not suppress the AVP secretion and can lead to hyponatremia. The antidiuresis can last from 2 to 14 days, after which DI recurs following depletion of the AVP from the degenerating posterior pituitary gland (third phase).[135] Recently, transient hyponatremia without preceding or subsequent DI has been reported following transphenoidal surgery for pituitary microadenomas,[136] which generally occurs 5 to 10 days postoperatively. The incidence may be as high as 30% when such patients are carefully followed, although majority of cases are mild and self-limited.[137,138] This is due to inappropriate AVP secretion via the same mechanism as in the triphasic response, except that in these cases only the second phase occurs (*"isolated second phase"*) because the initial neural lobe/pituitary stalk damage is not sufficient to impair AVP secretion sufficiently to produce clinical manifestations of DI.[139]

Once a deficiency of AVP secretion has been present for more than a few days or weeks, it rarely improves even if the underlying cause of the neurohypophysial destruction is eliminated. The major exception to this is in patients with postoperative DI, in which spontaneous resolution is the rule. Although recovery from DI that persists more than several weeks postoperatively is less common, nonetheless well-documented cases of long-term recovery have been reported.[135] The reason for amelioration and resolution is apparent from pathologic and histologic examination of neurohypophyseal tissue following pituitary stalk section.[140,141] Neurohypophyseal neurons that have intact perikarya are able to regenerate axons and form new nerve terminal endings capable of releasing AVP into nearby capillaries. In animals, this may be accompanied by a bulbous growth at the end of the severed stalk, which represents a new, albeit small, neural lobe. In humans, the regeneration process appears to proceed more slowly, and formation of a new neural lobe has not been noted. Nonetheless, histologic examination of a severed human stalk from a patient 18 months after hypophysectomy has demonstrated reorganization of neurohypophyseal fibers with neurosecretory granules in close proximity to nearby

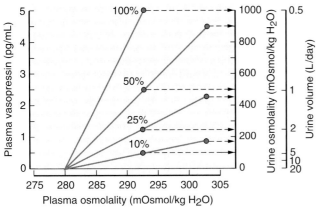

FIGURE 13–10 Relation between plasma AVP levels, urine osmolality, and plasma osmolality in subjects with normal posterior pituitary function (100%) compared with patients with graded reductions in AVP-secreting neurons (to 50%, 25%, and 10% of normal). Note that the patient with a 50% secretory capacity can achieve only half the plasma AVP level and half the urine osmolality of normal subjects at a plasma osmolality of 293 mOsm/kg H_2O, but with increasing plasma osmolality, this patient can nonetheless eventually stimulate sufficient AVP secretion to reach a near maximal urine osmolality. In contrast, patients with more severe degrees of AVP-secreting neuron deficits are unable to reach maximal urine osmolalities at any level of plasma osmolality. (Adapted from Robertson GL: Posterior pituitary. In Felig P, Baxter J, Frohman LA [eds]: Endocrinology and Metabolism. New York, McGraw Hill, 1986, pp 338–386.)

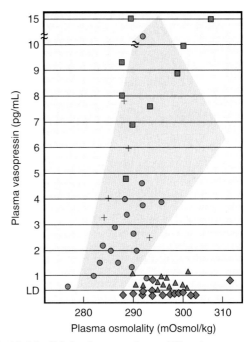

FIGURE 13–11 Relation between plasma AVP and concurrent plasma osmolality in patients with polyuria of diverse causes. All measurements were made at the end of a standard dehydration test. The *shaded area* represents the range of normal. In patients with severe (◆) or partial (▲) central DI, plasma AVP was almost always subnormal relative to plasma osmolality. In contrast, the values from patients with dipsogenic (○) or nephrogenic (■) DI were consistently within or above the normal range. (From Robertson GL: Diagnosis of diabetes insipidus. In Czernichow AP, Robinson A [eds]: Diabetes Insipidus in Man: Frontiers of Hormone Research. Basel, S Karger, 1985, p 176.)

blood vessels, closely resembling the histology of a normal posterior pituitary.[141]

Recognition of the fact that almost all patients with CDI retain a limited capacity to secrete some AVP allows an understanding some otherwise perplexing features of the disorder. For example, in many patients, restricting water intake long enough to raise plasma osmolality by only 1% to 2% induces sufficient AVP secretion to concentrate the urine (Figs. 13–10 and 13–11). As the plasma osmolality increases further, some patients with partial DI can even secrete enough AVP to achieve near maximal urine osmolalities (Fig. 13–12). However, this should not cause confusion about the diagnosis of DI, because in such patients, the urine osmolality will still be inappropriately low at plasma osmolalities within normal ranges, and they will respond to exogenous AVP administration with further increases in urine osmolality. These responses to dehydration illustrate the relative nature of the AVP deficiency in most cases and underscore the importance of the thirst mechanism to restrict the use of residual secretory capacity under basal conditions of ad libitum water intake.

CDI is also associated with changes in the renal response to AVP. The most obvious change is a reduction in maximal concentrating capacity, which has been attributed to washout of the medullary concentration gradient caused by the chronic polyuria. The severity of this defect is proportional to the magnitude of the polyuria and is independent of its cause.[133] Because of this, the level of urinary concentration achieved at maximally effective levels of plasma AVP is reduced in all types of DI. In patients with CDI, this concentrating abnormality is offset to some extent by an apparent increase in renal sensitivity to low levels of plasma AVP (see Fig. 13–12). The cause of this supersensitivity is unknown, but it may reflect upward regulation of AVP V_2 receptor expression or function secondary to a chronic deficiency of the hormone.[142]

Osmoreceptor Dysfunction

Etiology

Extensive literature in animals indicates that the primary osmoreceptors that control AVP secretion and thirst are

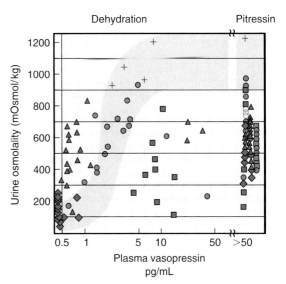

FIGURE 13–12 Relation between urine osmolality and concurrent plasma AVP in patients with polyuria of diverse causes. All measurements were made at the end of a standard dehydration test. The *shaded area* represents the range of normal. In patients with severe (◆) or partial (▲) central DI, urine osmolality is normal or supranormal relative to plasma AVP when the latter is submaximal. In patients with nephrogenic DI (■), urine osmolality is always subnormal for plasma AVP. In patients with dipsogenic DI (○), the relation is normal at submaximal levels of plasma AVP but is usually subnormal when plasma AVP is high. (From Robertson GL: Diagnosis of diabetes insipidus. In Czernichow AP, Robinson A [eds]: Diabetes Insipidus in Man: Frontiers of Hormone Research. Basel, S Karger, 1985, p 176.)

CH 13

located in the anterior hypothalamus; lesions of this region in animals, the so-called *AV3V area,* cause hyperosmolality through a combination of impaired thirst and osmotically stimulated AVP secretion.[30,31] Initial reports in humans described this syndrome as "essential hypernatremia,"[143] and subsequent studies used the term "adipsic hypernatremia" in recognition of the profound thirst deficits found in most of the patients.[144] Based on the known pathophysiology, all of these syndromes can be grouped together as disorders of *osmoreceptor dysfunction.*[145] Although the pathologies responsible for this condition can be quite varied, all of the cases reported to date have been due to various degrees of osmoreceptor destruction associated with a variety of different brain lesions, as summarized in Table 13–2. Many of these are the same types of lesions that can cause CDI, but in contrast to CDI, these lesions usually occur more rostrally in the hypothalamus, consistent with the anterior hypothalamic location of the primary osmoreceptor cells (see Fig. 13–2). One lesion unique to this disorder is an anterior communicating cerebral artery aneurysm. Because the small arterioles that feed the anterior wall of the third ventricle originate from the anterior communicating cerebral artery, an aneurysm in this region,[146] but more often following surgical repair of such an aneurysm that typically involves ligation of the anterior communicating artery,[147] produces infarction of the part of the hypothalamus containing the osmoreceptor cells.

Pathophysiology

The cardinal defect of patients with this disorder is lack of the osmoreceptors that regulate thirst. With rare exceptions, the osmoregulation of AVP is also impaired, although the hormonal response to nonosmotic stimuli remains intact (Fig. 13–13).[148,149] Four major patterns of osmoreceptor dysfunction have been described as characterized by defects in thirst and/or AVP secretory responses: (1) upward resetting of the osmostat for both thirst and AVP secretion (normal AVP and thirst responses but at an abnormally high plasma osmo-

lality), (2) partial osmoreceptor destruction (blunted AVP and thirst responses at all plasma osmolalities), (3) total osmoreceptor destruction (absent AVP secretion and thirst regardless of plasma osmolality), and (4) selective dysfunction of thirst osmoregulation with intact AVP secretion.[145] Regardless of the actual pattern, the hallmark of this disorder is an abnormal thirst response in addition to variable defects in AVP secretion. Because of this, such patients fail to drink sufficiently as their plasma osmolality rises, and as a result, the new set-point for plasma osmolality rises far above the normal thirst threshold. Unlike patients with CDI whose polydipsia maintains their plasma osmolality within normal ranges, patients with osmoreceptor dysfunction typically have osmolalities in the range of 300 to 340 mOsm/kg H_2O. This again underscores the critical role played by normal thirst mechanisms in maintaining body fluid homeostasis; intact renal function alone is insufficient to maintain plasma osmolality within normal limits in such cases.

The rate of development and the severity of hyperosmolality and hypertonic dehydration in patients with osmoreceptor dysfunction are influenced by a number of factors. First is the ability to maintain some degree of osmotically stimulated thirst and AVP secretion, which will determine the new set-point for plasma osmolality. Second are environmental influences that affect the rate of water output. When physical activity is minimal and ambient temperature is not elevated, the overall rates of renal and insensible water loss are low and the patient's diet may be sufficient to maintain a relatively normal balance for long periods of time. Anything that increases perspiration, respiration, or urine output greatly accelerates the rate of water loss and thereby uncovers the patient's inability to mount an appropriate compensatory increase in water intake.[14] Under these conditions, severe and even fatal hypernatremia can develop relatively quickly. When the dehydration is only moderate (plasma osmolality 300–330 mOsm/kg H_2O), the patient is usually asymptomatic and signs of volume depletion are minimal, but if the dehydration becomes severe, the patient can exhibit symptoms and signs of hypovolemia, including weakness, postural dizziness, paralysis, confusion, coma, azotemia, hypokalemia, hyperglycemia, and secondary hyperaldosteronism (see subsequent section on Clinical Manifestations). In severe cases, there may also be rhabdomyolysis with marked serum elevations in muscle enzymes and occasionally acute renal failure.

However, a third factor also influences the degree of hyperosmolality and dehydration present in these patients. For all cases of osmoreceptor dysfunction, it is important to remember that afferent pathways from the brainstem to the hypothalamus remain intact; therefore, these patients will usually have normal AVP and renal concentrating responses to baroreceptor-mediated stimuli such as hypovolemia and hypotension (see Fig. 13–13)[149] or to other nonosmotic stimuli such as nausea (see Fig. 13–8).[144,148] This has the effect of preventing severe dehydration, because, as hypovolemia develops, this will stimulate AVP secretion via baroreceptive pathways through the brainstem (see Fig. 13–2). Although protective, this effect often causes confusion, because at some times, these patients appear to have DI, yet at other times, they can concentrate their urine quite normally. Nonetheless, the presence of refractory hyperosmolality with absent or inappropriate thirst should alert clinicians to the presence of osmoreceptor dysfunction regardless of apparent normal urine concentration at some times.

In a few patients with osmoreceptor dysfunction, forced hydration has been found to lead to hyponatremia in association with inappropriate urine concentration.[143,144] This paradoxical defect resembles that seen in the SIADH and has been postulated to be due to two different pathogenic mechanisms. One is continuous or fixed secretion of AVP because of loss

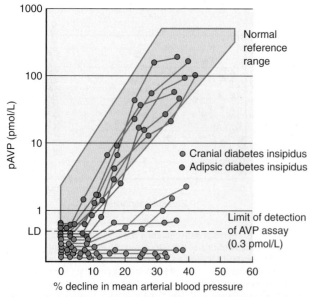

FIGURE 13–13 Plasma AVP responses to arterial hypotension produced by infusion of trimethephan in patients with central DI ("cranial diabetes insipidus") and osmoreceptor dysfunction ("adipsic diabetes insipidus). Normal responses in healthy volunteers are shown by the *shaded area.* Note that despite absent or markedly blunted AVP responses to hyperosmolality, patients with osmoreceptor dysfunction respond normally to baroreceptor stimulation induced by hypotension. (From Baylis PH, Thompson CJ: Diabetes insipidus and hyperosmolar syndromes. *In* Becker KL [ed]: Principles and Practice of Endocrinology and Metabolism. Philadelphia, JB Lippincott, 1995, p 257.)

of the capacity for osmotic inhibition and stimulation of hormone secretion. These observations, as well as electrophysiologic data,[41] strongly suggest that the osmoregulatory system is bimodal (i.e., it is composed of inhibitory as well as stimulatory input to the neurohypophysis [see Fig. 13–6]). The other cause of the diluting defect appears to be hypersensitivity to the antidiuretic effects of AVP, because in some patients, urine osmolality may remain high even when the hormone is undetectable.[144]

Hypodipsia is also a common occurrence in elderly persons in the absence of any overt hypothalamic lesion.[150] In such cases, it is not clear whether the defect is in the hypothalamic osmoreceptors, in their projections to the cortex, or in some other regulatory mechanism. However, in most cases, the osmoreceptor is likely not involved, because both basal and stimulated plasma AVP levels have been found to be normal, or even hyperresponsive, in relation to plasma osmolality in aged humans, with the exception of only a few studies that showed decreased plasma levels of AVP relative to plasma osmolality.[151]

Gestational Diabetes Insipidus

Etiology
A relative deficiency of plasma AVP can also result from an increase in the rate of AVP metabolism.[95,152] This condition has been observed only in pregnancy, and therefore, it is generally referred to as *gestational DI*. It is due to the action of a circulating enzyme called cysteine aminopeptidase ("oxytocinase" or "vasopressinase") that is normally produced by the placenta in order to degrade circulating oxytocin and prevent premature uterine contractions.[153] Because of the close structural similarity between AVP and oxytocin, this enzyme degrades both peptides. In some patients, plasma levels of oxytocinase/vasopressinase are markedly elevated above those found normally in pregnancy.[152,154] In others, however, oxytocinase/vasopressinase levels are relatively normal, but the effect of the increase in AVP metabolism may be exacerbated by an underlying subclinical deficiency of AVP secretion.[155] Some of these patients have been noted to have accompanying preeclampsia, acute fatty liver, and coagulopathies, but causal relations between the DI and these abnormalities have not been identified. The relationship of this disorder to the transient NDI of pregnancy[156] is not clear.

Pathophysiology
The pathophysiology of GDI is similar to that of CDI. The only exception is that the polyuria is usually not corrected by administration of AVP, because this is rapidly degraded just as is endogenous AVP, but it can be controlled by treatment with DDAVP, the AVP V_2 receptor agonist that is more resistant to degradation by oxytocinase/vasopressinase.[153] It should be remembered that patients with partial CDI in whom only low levels of AVP can be maintained, or patients with compensated NDI in whom the lack of response of the kidney to AVP may be not be absolute, can be relatively asymptomatic with regard polyuria, but with accelerated destruction of AVP during pregnancy, the underlying DI may become manifest. Consequently, patients presenting with GDI should not be assumed so simply have excess oxytocinase/vasopressinase; rather, these patients should be evaluated for other possible underlying pathologic diagnoses (see Table 13–2).[155]

Nephrogenic Diabetes Insipidus

Etiology
Resistance to the antidiuretic action of AVP is usually due to some defect within the kidney, and is commonly referred to

as NDI. It was first recognized in 1945 in several patients with the familial, sex-linked form of the disorder. Subsequently, additional kindreds with the X-linked form of familial NDI were identified. Clinical studies of NDI indicate that symptomatic polyuria is present from birth, plasma AVP levels are normal or elevated, resistance to the antidiuretic effect of AVP can be partial or virtually complete, and the disease affects mostly males and is usually, although not always,[157] mild or absent in carrier females. More than 90% of cases of congenital NDI are caused by mutations of the AVP V_2 receptor (see review[158] and Chapter 40). Most mutations occur in the part of the receptor that is highly conserved among species and/or is conserved among similar receptors, for example, homologies with AVP V_{1a} or oxytocin receptors. The effect of some of these mutations on receptor synthesis, processing, trafficking, and function has been studied by in vitro expression.[159,160] These types of studies show that the various mutations cause several different defects in cellular processing and function of the receptor but can be classified into four general categories based on differences in transport to the cell surface and AVP binding and/or stimulation of adenylyl cyclase: (1) the mutant receptor is not inserted in the membrane; (2) the mutant receptor is inserted in the membrane but does not bind or respond to AVP; (3) the mutant receptor is inserted in the membrane and binds AVP but does not activate adenylyl cyclase; or (4) the mutant protein is inserted into the membrane and binds AVP but responds subnormally in terms of adenylyl cyclase activation. Several recent studies have shown a relation between the clinical phenotype and the genotype and/or cellular phenotype.[159,161] Approximately 10% of the V_2 receptor defects causing congenital NDI are believed to be de novo. This high incidence of de novo cases coupled with the large number of mutations that have been identified hinders the clinical use of genetic identification, because it is necessary to sequence the entire open reading frame of the receptor gene rather than short sequences of DNA; nonetheless, use of automated gene sequencing techniques in selected families has been shown to successfully identify mutations in both patients with clinical disease and asymptomatic carriers.[162] Although most female carriers of the X-linked V_2 receptors defect have no clinical disease, some females have been reported with symptomatic NDI.[157] Carriers can have a decreased maximum urine osmolality in response to plasma AVP levels, but are generally asymptomatic because of absence of overt polyuria. Occasionally, a girl manifests severe NDI due to a V_2 receptor mutation, which is likely due to inactivation of the normal X chromosome.[163]

Congenital NDI can also result from mutations of the autosomal gene that codes for AQP2, the protein that forms the water channels in renal medullary collecting tubules. When the proband is a girl, it is likely the defect is a mutation of the AQP2 gene on chromosome 12, Q12–13[164] More than 20 different mutations of the AQP2 gene have been described (see review[165] and Chapter 40). The patients may be heterozygous for two different recessive mutations[166] or homozygous for the same abnormality from both parents.[167] Because most of these mutations are recessive, the patients usually do not present with a family history of DI unless consanguinity is present. Functional expression studies of these mutations show that all of them result in varying degrees of reduced water transport, because the mutant aquaporins either are not expressed in normal amounts, are retained in various cellular organelles, or simply do not function effectively as water channels. Regardless of the type of mutation, the phenotype of NDI from AQP2 mutations is identical to that produced by V_2 receptor mutations. Some of the defects in cellular routing and water transport can be reversed by treatment with chemicals that act like "chaperones,"[168] suggesting that misfolding of the mutant AQP2 may be responsible for misrouting.

CH 13

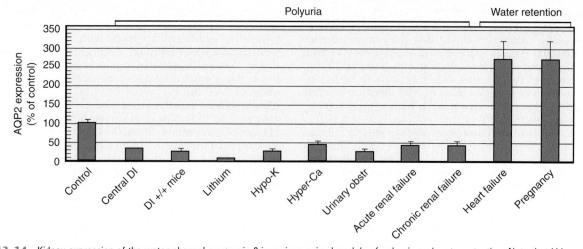

FIGURE 13–14 Kidney expression of the water channel aquaporin-2 in various animal models of polyuria and water retention. Note that kidney aquaporin-2 expression is uniformly down-regulated relative to levels in controls in all animal models of polyuria, but up-regulated in animal models of inappropriate antidiuresis. DI +/+, genetic diabetes insipidus; Hyper-Ca, hypercalcemia; Hypo-K, hypokalemia; Urinary obstr, ureteral obstruction. (From Nielsen S, Kwon TH, Christensen BM, et al: Physiology and pathophysiology of renal aquaporins. J Am Soc Nephrol 10:647–663, 1999.)

Similar salutary effects of chaperones have been found to reverse defects in cell surface expression and function of selected mutations of the AVP V_2 receptor.[169]

NDI can also be caused by a variety of drugs, diseases, and metabolic disturbances, among them lithium, hypokalemia, and hypercalcemia (see Table 13–2). Some of these disorders (e.g., polycystic kidney disease) act to distort the normal architecture of the kidney and interfere with the normal urine concentration process. However, experimental studies in animal models have suggested that many have in common a down-regulation of AQP2 expression in the renal collecting tubules (Fig. 13–14, see also Chapters 8 and 9).[170,171] The polyuria associated with potassium deficiency develops in parallel with decreased expression of kidney AQP2, and repletion of potassium reestablishes the normal urinary concentrating mechanism and normalizes renal expression of AQP2.[172] Similarly, hypercalcemia has also been found to be associated with down-regulation of AQP2.[173] A low-protein diet diminishes the ability to concentrate the urine primarily by a decreased delivery of urea to the inner medulla, thus decreasing medullary concentration gradient, but rats on a low-protein diet also appear to down-regulate AQP2, which could be an additional component of the decreased ability to concentrate the urine.[174] Bilateral urinary tract obstruction causes inability to produce a maximum concentration of the urine, and rat models have demonstrated a down-regulation of AQP2, which persists for several days after release of the obstruction.[175] However, it is not yet clear which of these effects on AQP2 expression are primary or secondary and what cellular mechanism(s) are responsible for the down-regulation of AQP2 expression.

Administration of lithium to treat psychiatric disorders is the most common cause of drug-induced NDI and illustrates the multiple mechanisms likely involved in producing this disorder. As many as 10% to 20% of patients on chronic lithium therapy develop some degree of NDI.[176] Lithium is known to interfere with the production of cAMP[177] and produces a dramatic (95%) reduction in kidney AQP2 levels in animals.[178] The defect of aquaporins is slow to correct both in experimental animals and in humans, and in some cases, it can be permanent[179] in association with glomerular or tubulointerstitial nephropathy.[180] Several other drugs that are known to induce renal concentrating defects have also been associated with abnormalities of AQP2 synthesis.[181]

Pathophysiology

Similar to CDI, renal insensitivity to the antidiuretic effect of AVP also results in the excretion of an increased volume of dilute urine, a decrease in body water, and a rise in plasma osmolality, which by stimulating thirst induces a compensatory increase in water intake. As a consequence, the osmolality of body fluid stabilizes at a slightly higher level that approximates the osmotic threshold for thirst. As in patients with CDI, the magnitude of polyuria and polydipsia varies greatly depending on a number of factors, including the degree of renal insensitivity to AVP, individual differences in the set-points and sensitivity of thirst and AVP secretion, as well as total solute load. It is important to note that the renal insensitivity to AVP need not be complete for polyuria to occur; it is only necessary that the defect be great enough to prevent concentration of the urine at plasma AVP levels achievable under ordinary conditions of ad libitum water intake (i.e., at plasma osmolalities near the osmotic threshold for thirst). Calculations similar to those used for states of AVP deficiency indicate that this requirement is not met until the renal sensitivity to AVP is reduced by more than 10-fold. Because renal insensitivity to the hormone is often incomplete, especially in cases of acquired rather than congenital NDI, many patients with NDI are able to concentrate their urine to varying degrees when they are deprived of water or given large doses of DDAVP.

New knowledge about the renal concentration mechanism from studies of AQP2 expression in experimental animals (see Chapters 8 and 9) has suggested that a form of NDI is likely associated with all types of DI, as well as with primary polydipsia. Brattleboro rats have been found to have low levels of kidney AQP2 expression compared to Long-Evans control rats; AQP2 levels are corrected by treatment with AVP or DDAVP, but this process takes 3 to 5 days, during which time urine concentration remains subnormal despite pharmacologic concentrations of AVP.[182] Similarly, physiologic suppression of AVP by chronic overadministration of water produces a down-regulation of AQP2 in the renal collecting duct.[182] Clinically, it is well known that patients with both CDI and primary polydipsia often fail to achieve maximally concentrated urine when they are given DDAVP during a water deprivation test to differentiate among the various causes of DI. This effect has long been attributed to a "washout" of the medullary concentration gradient as a result of the high urine flow rates in polyuric patients, but based on the results of animal studies, it seems certain that at least part of the decreased response to AVP is due to a down-regulation of kidney AQP2 expression. This also explains why it takes time, typically several days, to restore normal urinary concentration after patients with primary polydipsia and CDI are treated with water restriction or antidiuretic therapy.[183]

Primary Polydipsia

Etiology

Excessive fluid intake also causes hypotonic polyuria and, by definition, polydipsia. Consequently, this disorder must be differentiated from the various causes of DI. Furthermore, it is apparent that despite normal pituitary and kidney function, patients with this disorder share many characteristics of both CDI (i.e., AVP secretion is suppressed as a result of the decreased plasma osmolality) and NDI (kidney AQP2 expression is decreased as a result of the suppressed plasma AVP levels). Many different names have been used to describe patients with excessive fluid intake, but *primary polydipsia* remains the best descriptor, because it does not presume any particular etiology for the increased fluid intake. Primary polydipsia is often due to a severe mental illness such as schizophrenia, mania, or an obsessive-compulsive disorder,[184] in which case, it is called *psychogenic polydipsia*. These patients usually deny true thirst and attribute their polydipsia to bizarre motives such as a need to cleanse their body of poisons. Series of polydipsic patients in psychiatric hospital have shown an incidence as high as 42% of patients with some form of polydipsia, and in most reported cases, there is no obvious explanation for the polydipsia.[185] However, primary polydipsia can also be caused by an abnormality in the osmoregulatory control of thirst, in which case it has been termed *dipsogenic DI*.[186] These patients have no overt psychiatric illness and invariably attribute their polydipsia to a nearly constant thirst. Dipsogenic DI is usually idiopathic, but it can also be secondary to organic structural lesions in the hypothalamus identical to any of the disorders described as causes of CDI, such as neurosarcoidosis of the hypothalamus, tuberculous meningitis, multiple sclerosis, or trauma. Consequently, all polydipsic patients should be evaluated with an MRI scan of the brain before concluding that excessive water intake is due to an idiopathic or psychiatric cause. Primary polydipsia can also be produced by drugs that cause a dry mouth or by any peripheral disorder causing pathologic elevations of renin and/or angiotensin.[107] Finally, primary polydipsia is sometimes caused by physicians, nurses, lay practitioners, or health writers who recommend a high fluid intake for valid (e.g., recurrent nephrolithiasis) or unsubstantiated reasons of health.[187] These patients lack overt signs of mental illness but also deny thirst and usually attribute their polydipsia to habits acquired from years of adherence to their drinking regimen.

Pathophysiology

The pathophysiology of primary polydipsia is essentially the reverse of that in CDI: The excessive intake of water expands and slightly dilutes body fluids, suppresses AVP secretion, and dilutes the urine. The resultant increase in the rate of water excretion balances the increase in intake, and the osmolality of body water stabilizes at a new, slightly lower level that approximates the osmotic threshold for AVP secretion. The magnitude of the polyuria and polydipsia varies considerably, depending on the nature or intensity of the stimulus to drink. In patients with abnormal thirst, the polydipsia and polyuria are relatively constant from day to day. However, in patients with psychogenic polydipsia, water intake and urine output tend to fluctuate widely, and at times can be quite large.

Occasionally, fluid intake rises to such extraordinary levels that the excretory capacity of the kidneys is exceeded and dilutional hyponatremia develops.[188] There is little question that excessive water intake alone can sometimes be sufficient to override renal excretory capacity and produce severe hyponatremia. Although the water excretion rate of normal adult kidneys can generally exceed 20 L/day, maximum hourly rates rarely exceed 1000 mL/hr. Because many psychiatric patients drink predominantly during the day or during intense drinking binges,[189] they can transiently achieve symptomatic levels of hyponatremia with total daily volumes of water intake under 20 L if it is ingested sufficiently rapidly. This likely accounts for many of the cases in which such patients present with maximally dilute urine, accounting for as many as 50% of patients in some studies, and correct quickly via a free water diuresis.[190] The prevalence of this disorder based on hospital admissions for acute symptomatic hyponatremia may have been underestimated, because studies of polydipsic psychiatric patients have shown a marked diurnal variation in serum Na^+ (from 141 mEq/L at 7 AM to 130 mEq/L at 4 PM), suggesting that many such patients drink excessively during the daytime but then correct themselves via a water diuresis at night.[191] This and other considerations have led to defining this disorder as the *psychosis, intermittent hyponatremia, polydipsia* (PIP) syndrome.[189]

However, many other cases of hyponatremia with psychogenic polydipsia have been found to meet the criteria for a diagnosis of SIADH, suggesting the presence of nonosmotically stimulated AVP secretion. As might be expected, in the face of much higher than normal water intakes, virtually any impairment of urinary dilution and water excretion can exacerbate the development of a positive water balance and thereby produce hypoosmolality. Acute psychosis itself can also cause AVP secretion,[192] which often appears to take the form of a reset osmostat.[184] It is therefore apparent that no single mechanism can completely explain the occurrence of hyponatremia in polydipsic psychiatric patients, but the combination of higher than normal water intakes plus modest elevations of plasma AVP levels from a variety of potential sources appears to account for a significant portion of such cases.

Clinical Manifestations

The characteristic clinical symptoms of DI are the polyuria and polydipsia that result from the underlying impairment of urinary concentrating mechanisms, which have already been covered in the previous section discussing pathophysiology of specific types of DI. Interestingly, patients with DI typically describe a craving for cold water, which appears to quench their thirst better.[64] Patients with CDI also typically describe a precipitous onset of their polyuria and polydipsia, which simply reflects the fact that urinary concentration can be maintained fairly well until the number of AVP-producing neurons in the hypothalamus decreases to 10% to 15% of normal, after which plasma AVP levels decrease to the range at which urine output increases dramatically.

However, patients with DI, and particularly those with osmoreceptor dysfunction syndromes, can also present with varying degrees of hyperosmolality and dehydration, depending on their overall hydration status. It is therefore important to be aware of the clinical manifestations of hyperosmolality as well. These can be divided into the signs and symptoms produced by dehydration, which are largely cardiovascular, and those caused by the hyperosmolality itself, which are predominantly neurologic and reflect brain dehydration as a result of osmotic water shifts out of the central nervous system (CNS). Cardiovascular manifestations of hypertonic dehydration include hypotension, azotemia, acute tubular necrosis secondary to renal hypoperfusion or rhabdomyolysis, and shock.[193,194] Neurologic manifestations range from nonspecific symptoms such as irritability and cognitive dysfunction to more severe manifestations of *hypertonic encephalopathy* such as disorientation, decreased level of consciousness, obtundation, chorea, seizures, coma, focal neurologic deficits, subarachnoid hemorrhage, and cerebral infarction.[193,195] The severity of symptoms can be roughly correlated with the degree of hyperosmolality, but individual variability is marked, and for any single patient, the level of serum Na^+ at which symptoms will appear cannot be accurately predicted. Similar to hypoosmolar syndromes, the length of time over which hyperosmolality develops can markedly affect the clinical symptomatology. Rapid development of severe hyperosmolality is frequently associated with marked neurologic symptoms, whereas gradual development over several days or weeks generally causes milder symptoms.[193-196] In this case, the brain counteracts osmotic shrinkage by increasing intracellular content of solutes. These include electrolytes such as potassium and a variety of *organic osmolytes,* which previously had been called "idiogenic osmoles"; for the most part, these are the same organic osmolytes that are lost from the brain during adaptation to hypoosmolality.[197] The net effect of this process is to protect the brain against excessive shrinkage during sustained hyperosmolality. However, once the brain has adapted by increasing its solute content, rapid correction of the hyperosmolality can produce brain edema, because it takes a finite time (24–48 hr in animal studies) to dissipate the accumulated solutes, and until this process has been completed, the brain will accumulate excess water as plasma osmolality is normalized.[198] This effect is most often seen in dehydrated pediatric patients who can develop seizures with rapid rehydration,[199] but it has been described only rarely in adults, including the most severely hyperosmolar patients with nonketotic hyperglycemic hyperosmolar coma.

Differential Diagnosis

Before beginning involved diagnostic testing to differentiate among the various forms of DI and primary polydipsia, the presence of true hypotonic polyuria should be established by measurement of a 24-hour urine for volume and osmolality. Generally accepted standards are that 24-hour urine volume should exceed 50 mL/kg BW with an osmolality less than 300 mOsm/kg H_2O.[200] Simultaneously, there should be a determination of whether the polyuria is due to an osmotic agent such as glucose, or intrinsic renal disease. Routine laboratory studies and the clinical setting will generally distinguish these disorders; diabetes mellitus and other forms of solute diuresis usually can be excluded by the history, a routine urinalysis for glucose, or measurement of the solute excretion rate (urine osmolality x urine volume in liters <15 mOsm/kg BW/day). There is universal agreement that the diagnosis of DI requires stimulating AVP secretion osmotically and then measuring the adequacy of the secretion by either direct measurement of plasma AVP levels or indirect assessment by urine osmolality.

In a patient who is already hyperosmolar with submaximally concentrated urine (i.e., urine osmolality <800 mOsm/kg H_2O), the diagnosis is straightforward and simple: Primary polydipsia is ruled out by the presence of hyperosmolality,[200] confirming a diagnosis of DI. CDI can then be distinguished from NDI by evaluating the response to administered AVP (5 units SC) or, preferably, the AVP V_2 receptor agonist DDAVP (1–2 μg subcutaneously or intravenously). A significant increase in urine osmolality within 1 to 2 hours after injection indicates insufficient endogenous AVP secretion and, therefore, CDI, whereas an absent response indicates renal resistance to AVP effects and, therefore, NDI. Although conceptually simple, interpretational difficulties can arise because the water diuresis produced by AVP deficiency in DDI produces a washout of the renal medullary concentrating gradient as well as down-regulation of kidney AQP2 water channels, as discussed previously, so that initial increases in urine osmolality in response to administered AVP or DDAVP are not as great as would be expected. Generally, increases of urine osmolality greater than 50% reliably indicate CDI and responses of less than 10% indicate NDI, but responses between 10% and 50% are indeterminate.[133] For this reason, plasma AVP levels should be measured to aid in this distinction: Hyperosmolar patients with NDI will have clearly elevated AVP levels, whereas those with CDI will have absent (complete) or blunted (partial) AVP responses relative to their plasma osmolality (Fig. 13–15). Because it will not be known beforehand which patients will have diagnostic versus indeterminate responses to AVP or DDAVP, a plasma AVP level should be drawn prior to AVP or DDAVP administration in patients presenting with hyperosmolality and inadequately concentrated urine without a solute diuresis.

Because patients with DI have intact thirst mechanisms, most often they do not present with hyperosmolality, but rather with a normal plasma osmolality and serum Na^+ and

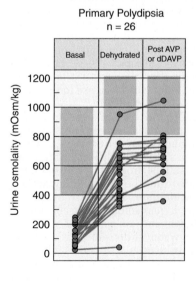

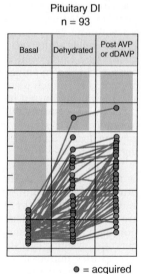

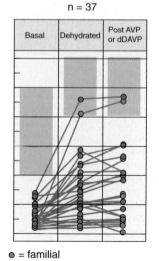

● = acquired   ○ = familial

FIGURE 13–15 Effects of fluid deprivation and subsequent AVP (Pitressin) administration on urine osmolality in 156 patients with polyuria of diverse causes. The *shaded areas* indicate the range of values in healthy adults. Note that, although AVP responses tended to be greater in patients with central (neurogenic) DI, the overlap between the three groups was significant.

symptoms of polyuria and polydipsia. In these cases, it is most appropriate to perform a *fluid deprivation test.* The relative merits of the indirect fluid deprivation test (the Miller-Moses test[201]) versus direct measurement of plasma AVP levels after a period of fluid deprivation[133] has been debated in the literature for the last 2 decades, with substantial pros and cons in support of each of these tests. The standard indirect test has a long track record of successfully making an appropriate diagnosis in the large majority of cases, generally yields interpretable results by the end of the test, and does not require sensitive assays for the notoriously difficult measurement of plasma AVP levels.[202,203] However, maximum urine concentrating capacity is well known to be variably reduced in all forms of DI as well as primary polydipsia,[133] and as a result, the absolute levels of urine osmolality achieved during fluid deprivation and after AVP administration are reduced to overlapping degrees in patients with partial CDI, partial NDI, and primary polydipsia (see Fig. 13–15). Measurements of basal plasma osmolality or serum Na^+ are of little use, because they also overlap considerably among these disorders.[200] And although association with certain diseases, surgical procedures, or family history often helps to differentiate among these disorders, sometimes the clinical setting may not be helpful because certain diseases such as sarcoidosis, tuberculous meningitis, and other hypothalamic pathologies can cause more than one type of DI (see Table 13–2). Consequently, a simpler approach that has been proposed is to measure plasma or urine AVP before and during a suitable osmotic stimulus such as fluid restriction or hypertonic NaCl infusion and plot the results as a function of the concurrent plasma osmolality or plasma sodium concentration (see Figs. 13–11 and 13–12).[204,205] Using a highly sensitive and validated research assay for plasma AVP determinations, this approach has been shown to provide a definite diagnosis of most cases if the final level of plasma osmolality or sodium achieved is above the normal range (>295 mOsm/kg H_2O or 145 mmol/L, respectively). The diagnostic effectiveness of this approach derives from the fact that the magnitude of the AVP response to osmotic stimulation is not appreciably diminished by chronic overhydration[184] or dehydration. Hence, the relationship of plasma AVP to plasma osmolality is usually within or above normal limits in NDI and primary polydipsia. In most cases, these two disorders can then be distinguished by measuring urine osmolality before and after the dehydration test and relating these values to the concurrent plasma AVP concentrations (see Fig. 13–12). However, because maximal concentrating capacity can be severely blunted in patients with primary polydipsia, it is often better to analyze the relationship under basal, nondehydrated conditions when plasma AVP is not elevated. Because of the solute diuresis that often ensues following infusion of hypertonic NaCl, measurements of urine osmolality or AVP excretion are unreliable indicators of changes in hormone secretion and are of little or no diagnostic value when this procedure is used to increase osmolality to greater than 295 mOsm/kg H_2O. Given the proven usefulness of both the indirect and the direct approaches, a combined fluid deprivation test that synthesizes the crucial aspects of both tests can easily be performed (Table 13–3) and, in many cases, will allow interpretation of both the plasma AVP levels and the response to an AVP challenge.

With use of the fluid deprivation test with plasma AVP determinations, greater than 95% of all cases of polyuria and polydipsia can be diagnosed accurately. A useful approach in the remaining indeterminate cases is to conduct a closely monitored trial with standard therapeutic doses of DDAVP. If this treatment abolishes thirst and polydipsia as well as polyuria for 48 to 72 hours without producing water intoxication, the patient most likely has uncomplicated CDI. Conversely, if the treatment abolishes the polyuria but has no or a lesser

TABLE 13–3 Fluid Deprivation Test for the Diagnosis of Diabetes Insipidus

Procedure

1. Initiation of the deprivation period depends on the severity of the DI; in routine cases, the patient should be made NPO after dinner, whereas in cases with more severe polyuria and polydipsia, this may be too long a period without fluids and the water deprivation should be begun early on the morning (e.g., 6 AM) of the test.
2. Obtain plasma and urine osmolality, serum electrolytes and a plasma AVP level at the start of the test.
3. Measure urine volume and osmolality hourly or with each voided urine.
4. Stop the test when body weight decreases by ≥3%, the patient develops orthostatic blood pressure changes, the urine osmolality reaches a plateau (i.e., <10% change over two or three consecutive measurements), or the serum Na^+ >145 mmol/L.
5. Obtain plasma and urine osmolality, serum electrolytes, and a plasma AVP level at the end of the test, when the plasma osmolality is elevated, preferably >300 mOsm/kg H_2O.
6. If the serum Na^+ <146 mmol/L or the plasma osmolality <300 mOsm/kg H_2O when the test is stopped, then consider a short infusion of hypertonic saline (3% NaCl at a rate of 0.1 ml/kg/min for 1–2 hr) to reach these endpoints.
7. If hypertonic saline infusion is not required to achieve hyperosmolality, administer AVP (5 U) or DDAVP (1 μg) SC and continue following urine osmolality and volume for an additional 2 hr.

Interpretation

1. An unequivocal urine concentration after AVP/DDAVP (>50% increase) indicates CDI and an unequivocal absence of urine concentration (<10%) strongly suggests nephrogenic DI (NDI) or primary polydipsia (PP).
2. Differentiating between NDI and PP, as well as for cases in which the increase in urine osmolality after AVP/DDAVP administration is more equivocal (e.g., 10%–50%), is best done using the relation between plasma AVP levels and plasma osmolality obtained at the end of the dehydration period and/or hypertonic saline infusion and the relation between plasma AVP levels and urine osmolality under basal conditions (see Figs. 13–11 and 13–12).

effect on thirst or polydipsia and results in the development of hyponatremia, it is more likely that the patient has some form of primary polydipsia. If DDAVP has no effect over this time interval, even when given by injection, it is virtually certain that the patient has some form of NDI.

As might be expected, most patients with DI will also exhibit a subnormal increase in AVP secretion in response to nonosmotic stimuli, such as hypotension, nausea, and hypoglycemia.[204] For diagnostic purposes, however, these nonosmotic tests of neurohypophyseal function do not provide any advantage over dehydration or hypertonic NaCl infusion, because orthostatic, emetic, and glucopenic stimuli are difficult to control or quantitate and generally cause a markedly variable AVP response. A more fundamental disadvantage with all nonosmotic stimuli is the possibility of a false-positive or false-negative results, because there are patients who exhibit little or no rise in AVP after hypotension or emesis yet lack polyuria and have a normal response to osmotic stimuli. Conversely, patients with osmoreceptor dysfunction exhibit little or no AVP response to hypertonic NaCl but have a normal increase in response to induced hypotension (see Fig. 13–13).[149]

MRI has also proved to be useful in diagnosing DI. In normal subjects, the posterior pituitary produces a characteristic bright signal in the posterior part of the sella turcica similar on T1-weighted images, usually best seen in sagittal views.[206] This was originally believed to represent fatty tissue, but more recent evidence indicates that the bright spot is actually due to the stored hormone in neurosecretory granules.[207] An experimental study done in rabbits subjected to dehydration for varying periods of time showed a linear correlation between pituitary AVP content and the signal intensity of the posterior pituitary by MRI.[208] As might be expected from the fact that destruction of more than 85% to 90% of the neurohypophysis is necessary to produce clinical symptomatology of DI, this signal has been found to be most always absent in patients with CDI in multiple studies.[209] However, as with any diagnostic test, clinical usefulness is dependent on the sensitivity and specificity of the test. Although earlier studies using small numbers of subjects demonstrated the presence of the bright spot in all normal subjects, subsequent larger studies reported an age-related absence of a pituitary bright spot in up to 20% of normal subjects.[210] Conversely, some studies have reported the presence of a bright spot in patients with clinical evidence of DI.[211] This may be because some patients with partial CDI have not yet progressed to the point of depletion of all neurohypophyseal reserves of AVP or because a persistent bright spot in patients with DI might be due to pituitary content of oxytocin rather than AVP. In support of this, it is known that oxytocinergic neurons are more resistant to destruction by trauma than are vasopressinergic neurons in both rats[212] and humans.[23] The presence of a positive posterior pituitary bright spot has been variably reported in other polyuric disorders. In primary polydipsia, the bright spot is usually seen,[209] consistent with studies in animals in which even prolonged lack of secretion of AVP caused by hyponatremia did not cause a decreased content of AVP in the posterior pituitary.[27] In NDI, the bright spot has been reported to be absent in some patients but present in others.[120] Consequently, specificity is lacking to use the MRI routinely as a diagnostic screening test for DI. Nonetheless, the sensitivity is sufficient to allow an approximately 95% probability that a patient with a bright spot on MRI does not have CDI. Thus, MRI is more useful for ruling out than for ruling in a diagnosis of CDI.

Additional useful information can be gained through the MRI via assessment of the pituitary stalk. Enlargement of the stalk beyond 2 to 3 mm is generally considered to be pathologic[213] and can be due to multiple disease processes.[214] Consequently, when the MRI reveals thickening of the stalk, especially with absence of the posterior pituitary bright spot, systemic diseases should be searched for diligently, including cerebrospinal fluid and plasma beta-human chorionic gonadotropin and alpha-fetoprotein measurement for evaluation of suprasellar germinoma, chest imaging and cerebrospinal fluid and plasma angiotensin-converting enzyme (ACE) levels for evaluation of sarcoidosis, and bone and skin surveys for evaluation of histiocytosis. When a diagnosis is still in doubt, the MRI should be repeated every 3 to 6 months. Continued enlargement, especially in children over the first 3 years of follow-up, suggest a germinoma and mandates a biopsy, whereas a decrease in the size of the stalk over time is more indicative of an inflammatory process such as lymphocytic infundibuloneurohypophysitis.[215]

Therapy

The general goals of treatment of all forms of DI are (1) a correction of any preexisting water deficits and (2) a reduction in the ongoing excessive urinary water losses. The specific therapy required (Table 13–4) will vary according to both the type of DI present and the clinical situation. Awake, ambulatory patients with normal thirst have relatively little body water deficit, but benefit greatly by alleviation of the polyuria and polydipsia that disrupt their normal activities. In contrast, comatose patients with acute DI after head trauma are unable to drink in response to thirst,

TABLE 13–4	Therapies for the Treatment of Diabetes Insipidus

Water

Antidiuretic agents
Arginine vasopressin (Pitressin)
1-Deamino-8-D-arginine vasopressin (Desmopressin; DDAVP)

Antidiuresis-enhancing agents
Chlorpropamide
Prostaglandin synthetase inhibitors (indomethacin, ibuprofen, tolmetin)

Natriuretic agents
Thiazide diuretics
Amiloride

and in these patients, progressive hyperosmolality can be life-threatening.

The TBW deficit in a hyperosmolar patient can be estimated using the formula:

$$\text{TBW deficit} = 0.6 \times \text{premorbid weight} \times (1 - 140/\text{Na}^+)$$

where Na^+ is the serum sodium concentration in mmol/L and weight is in kg. This formula depends on three assumptions: (1) TBW is approximately 60% of the premorbid BW, (2) no body solute was lost as the hyperosmolality developed, and (3) the premorbid serum Na^+ was 140 mEq/L.

To reduce the risk of CNS damage from protracted exposure to severe hyperosmolality, in most cases, the plasma osmolality should be rapidly lowered in the first 24 hours to the range of 320 to 330 mOsm/kg H_2O, or by approximately 50%. Plasma osmolality may be estimated most easily as twice the serum Na^+ if there is no hyperglycemia, and measured osmolality may be substituted if azotemia is not present. As discussed earlier, the brain increases intracellular osmolality by increasing content of a variety organic osmolytes as a protection against excessive shrinkage during hyperosmolality.[197] Because these osmolytes cannot be immediately dissipated, further correction to a normal plasma osmolality should be spread over the next 24 to 72 hours to avoid producing cerebral edema during treatment.[198] This is especially important in children,[216] in whom several studies have indicated that limiting correction of hypernatremia to a maximal rate of no greater than 0.5 mmol/L/hr prevents the occurrence of symptomatic cerebral edema with seizures.[199,217] In addition, the possibility of associated thyroid or adrenal insufficiency should also be kept in mind, because patients with CDI caused by hypothalamic masses can have associated deficiencies of anterior pituitary function.

The previous formula does not take into account ongoing water losses and is, at best, a rough estimate. Frequent serum and urine electrolyte determinations should be made, and the administration rate of oral water, or intravenous 5% dextrose in water, should be adjusted accordingly. Note, for example, that the estimated deficit of a 70-kg patient whose serum Na^+ is 160 mEq/L is 5.25 L of water. In such an individual, administration of water at a rate greater than 200 mL/hr would be required simply to correct the established deficit over 24 hours. Additional fluid would be needed to keep up with ongoing losses until a definitive response to treatment has occurred. The therapeutic agents available for the treatment of DI are shown in Table 13–4. Water should be considered a therapeutic agent because, when ingested or infused in sufficient quantity, there is no abnormality of body fluid volume or composition.

As noted previously, in most patients with DI, thirst remains intact, and the patients will drink sufficient fluid to maintain a relatively normal fluid balance. Patients with known DI should therefore be treated in order to decrease the patient's polyuria and polydipsia to acceptable levels that allow the patient to maintain a normal lifestyle. Because the major goal of therapy is improvement in symptomatology, the therapeutic regimen prescribed should be individually tailored to each patient in order to accommodate her or his needs. The safety of the prescribed agent and use of a regimen that avoids potential detrimental effects of overtreatment are primary considerations because of the relatively benign course of DI in most cases, and the potential adverse consequences of hyponatremia. Available treatments are summarized later, and their use is discussed separately for different types of DI.

ARGININE VASOPRESSIN (PITRESSIN). Pitressin is a synthetic form of naturally occurring human AVP. The aqueous solution contains 20 units/mL. Because of the drug's relatively short half-life (2–4-hour duration of antidiuretic effect) and propensity to cause acute increases in blood pressure when given as a bolus intravenously, this route of administration should generally be avoided. This agent is mainly used for acute situations such as postoperative DI. However, repeated dosing is required, unless a continuous infusion is used, and the frequency of dosing or infusion rate must be titrated to achieve the desired reduction in urine output (see subsequent discussion of postoperative DI).

DESMOPRESSIN. DDAVP is an agonist of the AVP V_2 receptor that was developed for therapeutic use because it has a significantly longer half-life than AVP (8–20-hr duration of antidiuretic effect) and is devoid of the latter's pressor activity by virtue of absence of activation of AVP V_{1a} receptors on vascular smooth muscle.[218] As a result of these advantages, it is the drug of choice for both acute and chronic administration in patients with CDI.[219] Several different preparations are available. The intranasal form is provided as an aqueous solution containing 100 µg/mL in a bottle with either a calibrated rhinal tube, which requires specific training to use appropriately, or a nasal spray delivering a metered dose of 10 µg in 0.1 mL. An oral preparation is also available in doses of 0.1 or 0.2 mg. Neither the intranasal or the oral preparations should be utilized in an acute emergency setting, where it is essential that the patient achieve a therapeutic dose of the drug; in this case, the parenteral form should always be used. This is supplied as a solution containing 4 µg/mL and may be given by intravenous, intramuscular, or subcutaneous route. The parenteral form is approximately 5 to 10 times more potent than the intranasal preparation, and the recommended dosage is 1 to 2 µg every 8 to 12 hours. For both the intranasal and the parenteral preparations, increasing the dose generally has the effect of prolonging the duration of antidiuresis for several hours rather than increasing its magnitude; consequently, altering the dose can be useful to reduce the required frequency of administration. However, given the cost of the drug, it is often more cost-effective, and sometimes more efficacious, to use a smaller dose more frequently than a larger dose less frequently.

CHLORPROPAMIDE (DIABINESE). Primarily used as an oral hypoglycemic agent, this sulfonylurea also potentiates the hydro-osmotic effect of AVP in the kidney. Chlorpropamide has been reported to reduce polyuria by 25% to 75% in patients with CDI. This effect appears to be independent of the severity of the disease and is associated with a proportional rise in urine osmolality, correction of dehydration, and elimination of the polydipsia similar to that caused by small doses of AVP or DDAVP.[200] The major site of action of chlorpropamide appears to be at the renal tubule to potentiate the hydro-osmotic action of circulating AVP, but there is also evidence of a pituitary effect to increase release of AVP as well; the latter effect may account for the observation that chlorpropamide can produce significant antidiuresis even in patients with severe CDI and presumed near-total AVP defi-

ciency.[200] The usual dose is 250 to 500 mg/day with a response noted in 1 to 2 days and a maximum antidiuresis in 4 days. It should be remembered that this is an off-label use of chlorpropamide; it should not be used in pregnancy or in children, it should never be used in an acute emergency setting in which achievement of rapid antidiuresis is necessary, and it should be avoided in patients with concurrent hypopituitarism because of the increased risk of hypoglycemia. Other sulfonylureas share chlorpropamide's effect but are generally less potent. In particular, the newer generation oral hypoglycemic agents such as glipizide and glyburide are virtually devoid of any AVP-potentiating effects.

PROSTAGLANDIN SYNTHASE INHIBITORS. Prostaglandins have complex effects both in the CNS and in the kidney, most of which are incompletely understood at this time owing to the variety of different prostaglandins and their multiplicity of cellular effects. In the brain, intracerebroventricular infusion of E prostaglandins stimulate AVP secretion[220] and administration of prostaglandin synthase inhibitors attenuate osmotically stimulated AVP secretion.[221] However, in the kidney, prostaglandin E_2 (PGE_2) has been reported to inhibit AVP-stimulated generation of cAMP in the cortical collecting tubule by interacting with Gi.[222] Thus, the effect of prostaglandin synthetase inhibitors to sensitize AVP effects in the kidney likely result from enhanced cAMP generation upon AVP binding to the V_2 receptor. The predominant renal effects of these agents is demonstrated by the fact that clinically they successfully reduce urine volume and free water clearance even in patients with NDI of different etiologies.[223,224]

NATRIURETIC AGENTS. Thiazide diuretics have a paradoxical antidiuretic effect in patients with CDI.[225] However, given the better antidiuretic agents available for treatment of CDI, its main therapeutic use is in NDI. Hydrochlorothiazide at doses of 50 to 100 mg/day usually reduces urine output by approximately 50%, and efficacy can be further enhanced by restricting sodium intake. Unlike DDAVP or the other antidiuresis-enhancing drugs, these agents are equally effective in most forms of NDI (see later).

Central Diabetes Insipidus

Patients with CDI should generally be treated with intranasal or oral DDAVP. Unless the hypothalamic thirst center is also affected by the primary lesion causing superimposed osmoreceptor dysfunction, these patients will develop thirst when the plasma osmolality increases by only 2% to 3%.[200] Severe hyperosmolality is therefore not a risk in the patient who is alert, ambulatory, and able to drink in response to perceived thirst. Polyuria and polydipsia are thus inconvenient and disruptive, but not life-threatening. However, hypoosmolality is largely asymptomatic and may be progressive if water intake continues during a period of continuous antidiuresis. Therefore, treatment must be designed to minimize polyuria and polydipsia but without an undue risk of hyponatremia from overtreatment.

Treatment should be individualized to determine optimal dosage and dosing interval. Although tablets offer greater convenience and are generally preferred by patients, it is useful to start with the nasal spray initially because of greater consistency of absorption and physiologic effect, and then switch to the oral tablets only after the patient is comfortable with use of the intranasal preparation to produce antidiuresis; having tried both preparations, the patient can then chose which he or she prefers for long-term usage. Because of variability in response among patients, it is desirable to determine the duration of action of individual doses in each patient.[226] A satisfactory schedule can generally be determined using modest doses, and the maximum dose needed is rarely above 0.2 mg orally or 10 µg (one nasal spray) given two, or occasionally three, times daily.[227] Even in these cases, multiple small doses may be preferred because of the relatively high cost of DDAVP. In selected cases, chlorprop-amide may lower the required DDAVP dose and produce an additional, though limited, economy. These doses generally produce plasma DDAVP levels many times those required to produce maximum antidiuresis but obviate the need for more frequent treatment. Rarely, once-daily dosing suffices. In a few patients, the effect of intranasal or oral DDAVP is erratic, probably as a result of variable interference with absorption from the gastrointestinal tract or nasal mucosa. This variability can be reduced and the duration of action prolonged by administering the drug on an empty stomach[228] or after thorough cleansing of the nostrils. Resistance caused by antibody production has not been reported to date.

Hyponatremia is a rare complication of DDAVP therapy and occurs only if the patient is continually antidiuretic while maintaining a fluid intake sufficient to become volume expanded and natriuretic. Absence of thirst in this circumstance is protective; but also, most patients with DI on standard therapy are not continuously maximally antidiuretic. There are reports of hyponatremia in patients with normal AVP function, and presumably normal thirst, when they are given DDAVP to treat hemophilia and von Willebrand's disease,[229] and in children treated with DDAVP for primary enuresis.[230] In these cases, the hyponatremia can develop rapidly and is often first noted by the onset of convulsions and coma.[231] Severe hyponatremia in patients with DI being treated with DDAVP can be avoided by monitoring serum electrolytes frequently during initiation of therapy. Patients who show a tendency to develop low serum sodium concentrations that do not respond to recommended decreases in fluid intake should then be instructed to delay a scheduled dose of DDAVP once or twice a week so that polyuria recurs, thereby allowing any excess retained fluid to be excreted.[203]

Acute postsurgical DI occurs relatively frequently following surgery that involves the suprasellar hypothalamic area, but several confounding factors must be considered. These patients often receive stress doses of glucocorticoids, and the resulting hyperglycemia with glucosuria may confuse a diagnosis of DI. Thus, the blood glucose must first be brought under control to eliminate an osmotic diuresis as the cause of the polyuria. In addition, excess fluids administered intravenously may be retained perioperatively, but then excreted normally postoperatively. If this large output is matched with continued intravenous input, an incorrect diagnosis of DI may be made based on the resulting polyuria. Therefore, if the serum Na+ is not elevated concomitantly with the polyuria, the rate of parenterally administered fluid should be slowed with careful monitoring of serum Na+ and urine output to establish the diagnosis. Once a diagnosis of DI is confirmed, the only acceptable pharmacologic therapy is an antidiuretic agent. However, because many neurosurgeons fear water overload and brain edema after this type of surgery, the patient is sometimes treated with only intravenous fluid replacement for a considerable time before the institution of ADH therapy (see the potential benefits of this approach later in this chapter). If the patient is awake and able to respond to thirst, one can treat with an ADH and allow the patient's thirst to be the guide for water replacement. However, if the patient is unable to respond to thirst, either because of a decreased level of consciousness or from hypothalamic damage to the thirst center, fluid balance must be maintained by intravenously administered fluid. The urine osmolality and serum Na+ must be checked every several hours during the initial therapy, and then at least daily until stabilization or resolution of the DI. Caution must also be exercised regarding the volume of water replacement, because excess water administered during continued administration of AVP or DDAVP can create a syndrome of inappropriate antidiuresis and potentially severe hyponatremia. Recent studies in

experimental animals have indicated that DDAVP-induced hyponatremia markedly impairs survival of vasopressin neurons after pituitary stalk compression,[212] suggesting that overhydration with subsequent decreased stimulation of the neurohypophysis may also increase the likelihood of permanent DI postoperatively.

Postoperatively, DDAVP may be given parenterally in a dose of 1 to 2 μg subcutaneously, intramuscularly, or intravenously. The intravenous route is preferable, because it obviates any concern about absorption, is not associated with significant pressor activity, and has the same total duration of action as the other parenteral routes. A prompt reduction in urine output should occur, and the duration of antidiuretic effect is generally 6 to 12 hours. Usually, the patient is hypernatremic with relatively dilute urine when therapy is started. One should follow the urine osmolality and urine volume to be certain the dose was effective, and check the serum Na+ at frequent intervals to ensure some improvement of hypernatremia. It is generally advisable to allow some return of the polyuria before administration of subsequent doses of DDAVP, because postoperative DI is often transient and return of endogenous AVP secretion will become apparent by a lack of return of the polyuria. Also, in some cases, transient postoperative DI is part of a "triphasic" pattern that has been well described following pituitary stalk transection (see previous discussion). Because of this possibility, allowing a return of polyuria before redosing with DDAVP will allow earlier detection of a potential second phase of inappropriate antidiuresis and decrease the likelihood of producing symptomatic hyponatremia by continuing antidiuretic therapy and intravenous fluid administration when it is not required. Some clinicians have recommended using a continuous intravenous infusion of a dilute solution of AVP to control DI postoperatively. Algorithms for continuous AVP infusion in postoperative and posttraumatic DI in pediatric patients have begun at infusion rates of 0.25 to 1.0 mU/kg/hr and titrated the rate using urine specific gravity (goal of 1.010–1.020) and urine volume (goal 2–3 mL/kg/hr) as a guide to adequacy of the antidiuresis.[232,233] Although pressor effects have not been reported at these infusion rates and the antidiuretic effects are quickly reversible in 2 to 3 hours, it should be remembered that use of continuous infusions versus intermittent dosing will not allow an assessment of when the patent has recovered from transient DI or entered the second phase of a triphasic response. If DI persists, the patient should eventually be switched to maintenance therapy with intranasal or oral preparations of DDAVP for treatment chronic DI.

Acute traumatic DI can occur after injuries to the head, usually a motor vehicle accident. DI is more common with deceleration injuries that result in a shearing action on the pituitary stalk and/or cause hemorrhagic ischemia of the hypothalamus and/or posterior pituitary.[135] Similar to the onset of postsurgical DI, posttraumatic DI is usually recognized by hypotonic polyuria in the face of an increased plasma osmolality. The clinical management is similar to that of postsurgical DI as outlined previously, except that the possibility of anterior pituitary insufficiency must also be considered in such cases, and the patient should be given stress doses of glucocorticoids (e.g., hydrocortisone, 100 mg intravenously every 8 hr) until anterior pituitary function can be definitively evaluated.

Osmoreceptor Dysfunction

Acutely, patients with hypernatremia due to osmoreceptor dysfunction should be treated the same as any hyperosmolar patient by replacing the underlying free water deficit as described at the beginning of this section. The long-term management of osmoreceptor dysfunction syndromes requires a thorough search for a potentially treatable causes (see Table

13–2) in conjunction with the use of measures to prevent recurrence of dehydration. Because the hypodipsia cannot be cured, and rarely if ever improves spontaneously, the mainstay of management is education of the patient and her or his family about the importance of continuously regulating her or his fluid intake in accordance with the hydration status. This is never accomplished easily in such patients, but can be done most efficaciously by establishing a daily schedule of water intake based on changes in BW and regardless of the patient's thirst. In effect, a "prescription" for daily fluid intake must be written for these patients, because they will not drink spontaneously. In addition, if the patient has polyuria, DDAVP should also be given as for any patient with DI. The success of this regimen should be monitored periodically (weekly at first, later every month depending on the stability of the patient) by measuring serum Na^+. In addition, the target weight (at which hydration status and serum Na^+ concentration are normal) may need to be recalculated periodically to allow for growth in children or changes in body fat in adults.

Gestational Diabetes Insipidus

The polyuria of GDI is usually not corrected by administration of AVP itself because this is rapidly degraded by high circulating levels of oxytocinase/vasopressinase just as is endogenous AVP. The treatment of choice is DDAVP, because this synthetic AVP V_2 receptor agonist is not destroyed by the cysteine aminopeptidase (oxytocinase/vasopressinase) in the plasma of pregnant women[234] and to date appears to be safe for both the mother and the child.[235,236] DDAVP has only 2% to 25% the oxytocic activity of AVP[219] and can be used with minimal stimulation of the oxytocin receptors in the uterus. Doses should be titrated to individual patients, because higher doses and more frequent dosing intervals are sometimes required because of the increased degradation of the peptide. However, physicians should remember that the naturally occurring volume expansion and reset osmostat that occurs in pregnancy maintains the serum Na^+ at a lower level during pregnancy.[39] During delivery, these patients can maintain adequate oral intake and continued administration of DDAVP, but physicians should be cautious about overadministration of fluid parenterally during delivery because these patients will not be able to excrete the fluid and will be susceptible to the development of water intoxication and hyponatremia. After delivery, oxytocinase/vasopressinase decreases in plasma within several days and, depending on the etiology of the DI, the patients may have disappearance of the disorder or become asymptomatic with regard to fluid intake and urine volume.[237]

Nephrogenic Diabetes Insipidus

By definition, patients with NDI are resistant to the effects of AVP. Some patients with NDI can be treated by eliminating the drug (e.g., lithium) or disease (e.g., hypercalcemia) responsible for the disorder. For many others, however, including those with the genetic forms, the only practical form of treatment at present is to restrict sodium intake and administer a thiazide diuretic either alone[225] or in combination with prostaglandin synthetase inhibitors[238] or amiloride.[239,240] The natriuretic effect of the thiazide class of diuretics is conferred by their ability to block sodium absorption in the renal cortical diluting site. When combined with dietary sodium restriction, the drugs cause modest hypovolemia. This stimulates isotonic proximal tubular solute reabsorption and diminishes solute delivery to the more distal diluting site, where experimental studies have indicated that thiazides also act to enhance water reabsorption in the inner medullary collecting duct independently of AVP.[241] Together, these effects markedly diminish renal diluting ability and free water clearance independently of any action of AVP. Thus, agents of this class are the mainstay of therapy for NDI. Monitoring for hypokalemia is recommended, and potassium supplementation is occasionally required. Any drug of the thiazide class may be used with equal potential for benefit, and the clinicians should use the one with which they are most familiar from use in other conditions. Care must be exercised when treating patients taking lithium with diuretics, because the induced contraction of plasma volume may increase lithium concentrations and worsen potential toxic effects of the therapy. In the acute setting, diuretics are of no use in NDI and only free water administration can reverse hyperosmolality.

Indomethacin, tolmetin, and ibuprofen have been used in this setting,[238,242,243] although the last may be less effective than the others. The combination of thiazides and a nonsteroidal anti-inflammatory agent will not increase urinary osmolality above that of plasma, but the lessening of polyuria is nonetheless beneficial to patients. In many cases, the combination of thiazides with the potassium-sparing diuretic amiloride is preferred in order to lessen the potential side effects associated with long-term use of nonsteroidal anti-inflammatory agents.[239,240] Amiloride also has the advantage of decreasing lithium entrance into cells in the distal tubule, and because of this, may have a preferable action for the treatment of lithium-induced NDI.[244,245]

Although DDAVP is generally not effective in NDI, a few patients may have receptor mutations that allow partial responses to AVP or DDAVP,[246] with increases in urine osmolality following much higher doses of these agents than typically used to treat central DI (e.g., 6–10 μg), and it is generally worth a trial of DDAVP at these doses to ascertain whether this is a potential useful therapy in selected patients in whom the responsivity of other affected family members is not already known. Potential therapies involving administration of chaperones to bypass defects in cellular routing of misfolded aquaporin[168] and AVP V_2 receptor[169] proteins is an exciting, but uncertain, future possibility.[158]

Primary Polydipsia

At present, no completely satisfactory treatment for primary polydipsia exists. Fluid restriction would seem to be the obvious treatment of choice. However, patients with a reset thirst threshold will be resistant to fluid restriction because of the resulting thirst from stimulation of brain thirst centers at higher plasma osmolalities.[247] In some cases, the use of alternative methods to ameliorate the sensation of thirst (e.g., wetting the mouth with ice chips or using sour candies to increase salivary flow) can help to reduce fluid intake. Fluid intake in patients with psychogenic causes of polydipsia is driven by psychiatric factors that have responded variably to behavioral modification and pharmacologic therapy. Several recent reports have suggested potential efficacy of the antipsychotic drug clozapine as an agent to reduce polydipsia and prevent recurrent hyponatremia in at least a subset of these patients.[248] Administration of any ADH or thiazides to decrease polyuria is hazardous because they invariably produce water intoxication.[200,249] Therefore, if the diagnosis of DI is uncertain, any trial of antidiuretic therapy should be conducted with close monitoring, preferably in the hospital with frequent evaluation of fluid balance and serum electrolytes. If a patient with primary polydipsia is troubled by nocturia, this may be reduced or eliminated by administering a small dose of DDAVP at bedtime; because thirst and fluid intake are reduced during sleep, this treatment is less likely to cause water intoxication provided the dose is titrated to allow resumption of a water diuresis as soon as the patient awakens the next morning. However, this approach cannot be recommended for patients with psychogenic polydipsia because of the unpredictability of their fluid intake.

DISORDERS OF EXCESS ARGININE VASOPRESSIN OR ARGININE VASOPRESSIN EFFECT

The disorders of the renal concentrating mechanism that have been described may be associated with water depletion and hypernatremia. In contrast, disorders in the renal diluting mechanism frequently present as hyponatremia and hypo-osmolality. Hyponatremia is among the most common electrolyte disorders encountered in clinical medicine, with an incidence of 0.97% and a prevalence of 2.48% in hospitalized adult patients when plasma Na^+ concentration below 130 mEq/L is the diagnostic criterion,[250] and as high as 15% to 30% if a sodium of less than 135 mEq/L is used.[251] The prevalence may be somewhat lower in the hospitalized pediatric population (between 0.34% and 1.38%),[252] but the incidence is higher than originally recognized in the geriatric population.[251,253]

As serum osmolality is most often measured to assist in the evaluation of hyponatremic disorders, it is useful to bear in mind the basic relationship of plasma osmolality to Na^+ concentration. As reviewed in the introduction to this chapter, Na^+ and its associated anions account for nearly all of the osmotic activity of plasma. Therefore, changes in plasma Na^+ are usually associated with comparable changes in plasma osmolality. The osmolality calculated from the concentrations of Na^+, urea, and glucose is usually in close agreement with that obtained from a measurement of osmolality.[254] When the measured osmolality exceeds the calculated osmolality by more than 10 mOsm/kg H_2O, an osmolar gap is said to be present.[254] This occurs in two circumstances: (1) with a decrease in the water content of serum and (2) on addition of a solute other than urea or glucose to the serum. A decrease in the water content of serum is usually due to its displacement by excessive amounts of protein or lipids, as may occur in severe hyperglobulinemia or hyperlipidemia. Normally, 92% to 94% plasma volume is water, the remaining 6% to 8% being lipids and protein. Because of its ionic nature, Na^+ dissolves only in the water phase of plasma. Thus, when a greater than normal proportion of plasma is accounted for by solids, the concentration of Na^+ in plasma water remains normal, but the concentration in the total volume, as measured by flame photometry, is artifactually low. Such a discrepancy can be avoided if the Na^+ concentration is measured with an ion-selective electrode that is now widely available.[255] The sample needs to remain undiluted (direct potentiometry) for accurate measurement of the serum Na^+ concentration. Whereas the flame photometer measures the concentration of Na^+ in the total volume, the ion-selective electrode measures it in plasma water. Normally, the difference is only 3 mEq/L, but in the setting under discussion, the difference may be much greater. Likewise, because the large lipid and protein molecules contribute only minimally to the total osmolality, the measurement of osmolality by freezing point depression remains normal in these patients. The hyponatremia associated with normal osmolality has been termed *factitious* or *pseudohyponatremia*. The most common causes of pseudohyponatremia are primary or secondary hyperlipidemic disorders. The serum need not appear lipemic as increments in cholesterol alone can cause the same discrepancy.[255] Plasma protein elevations above 10 g/dL, as seen in multiple myeloma or macroglobulinemia, can also cause pseudohyponatremia. More recently the administration of intravenous immune globulin has been reported to be associated with hyponatremia without hypo-osmolality in several patients.[256]

The second setting in which an osmolar gap occurs is the presence in plasma of an exogenous low-molecular-weight substance such as ethanol, methanol, ethylene glycol, or mannitol.[257] Undialyzed patients with chronic renal failure, as well as critically ill patients,[258] also have an increment in the osmolar gap of unknown cause. Whereas all of these exogenous substances, as well as glucose and urea, elevate measured osmolality, the effect they have on the plasma concentration of Na^+ and intracellular hydration depends on the solute in question. As previously discussed, substances such as glucose, in the presence of relative insulin deficiency, do not penetrate cells readily and remain in the ECF. As a consequence, they draw water from the cellular compartment, causing cell shrinkage, and this translocation of water commensurately decreases the extracellular concentration of Na^+. In this setting, therefore, the plasma Na^+ concentration may be low while plasma osmolality is high. It is said that for every 100 mg/dL rise in plasma glucose, the osmotic shift of water causes plasma Na^+ to drop by 1.6 mEq/L. However, a more recent assessment suggests that this may represent an underestimate of the decrease caused by hyperglycemia, and suggests a 2.4-mEq/L correction factor.[259] Similar "translocational" hyponatremia occurs with mannitol or maltose or with the absorption of glycine during transurethral prostate resection, as well as in gynecologic and orthopedic procedures. A potential toxicity for glycine in this setting also requires consideration.[260] The introduction of new bipolar retroscopes that allow for the use of NaCl as irrigants should translate into the disappearance of this clinical entity. When the plasma solute is readily permeable (e.g., urea, ethylene glycol, methanol, ethanol), it enters the cell and so does not establish an osmotic gradient for water movement. There is no cellular dehydration despite the hypertonic state, and the plasma Na^+ concentration remains unchanged. The relationship between plasma osmolality and the plasma Na^+ concentration in the presence of various substances is summarized in Table 13–5.

Variables That Influence Water Excretion

In considering clinical disorders that result from excessive or inappropriate secretion of AVP, it is also helpful to remember the other variables that influence water excretion (Fig. 13–16). These factors fall into three categories.

FLUID DELIVERY FROM THE PROXIMAL TUBULE. In spite of the fact that proximal fluid reabsorption is iso-osmotic and therefore does not contribute directly to urine dilution, the volume of tubule fluid that is delivered to the distal nephron determines in large measure the volume of dilute urine that can be excreted. Thus, if glomerular filtration is decreased or proximal tubule reabsorption is greatly enhanced, the resulting diminution in the amount of fluid delivered to the distal tubule itself limits the rate of renal water excretion even if other components of the diluting mechanism are intact.

TABLE 13–5	Relationship Between Serum Tonicity and Sodium Concentration in the Presence of Other Substances	
Condition or Substance	**Serum Tonicity**	**Serum Sodium**
Hyperglycemia	↑	↓
Mannitol, maltose, glycine	↑	↓
Azotemia (high blood urea)	↑	↔
Ingestion of ethanol, methanol, ethylene glycol	↑	↔
Elevated serum lipid/protein	↔	↓

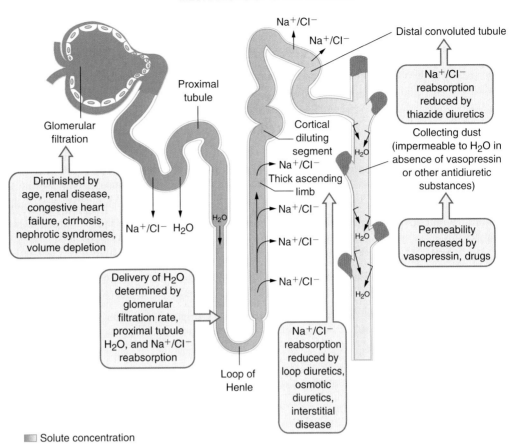

FIGURE 13-16 Urinary dilution mechanisms. Normal determinants of urinary dilution and disorders causing hyponatremia. (From Cogan M: Normal water homeostasis. *In* Cogan M [ed]: Fluid and Electrolytes. Norwalk, CT, Appleton & Lange, 1991, pp 98-106.)

Solute concentration

DILUTION OF TUBULAR FLUID. The excretion of urine that is hypotonic to plasma requires that some segment of the nephron reabsorb solute in excess of water. The water impermeability of the entire ascending limb of Henle, as well as the capacity of its thick segment to reabsorb NaCl, actively endows this segment of the nephron with the characteristics required for the diluting process. Thus, the transport of NaCl by the $Na^+/K^+/2Cl^-$ cotransporter converts the hypertonic tubule fluid that is delivered from the descending limb of the loop of Henle to a distinctly hypotonic fluid (100 mOsm/kg H_2O). Interference with the reabsorption of Na^+ and Cl^- in the ascending limb therefore impairs urine dilution.

WATER IMPERMEABILITY OF THE COLLECTING DUCT. The excretion of urine, which is more dilute than the fluid that is delivered to the distal convoluted tubule, requires continued solute reabsorption and minimal water reabsorption in the terminal segments of the nephron. Because the water permeability of the collecting duct epithelium is primarily dependent on the presence or absence of AVP, the hormone plays a pivotal role in determining the fate of the fluid delivered to the collecting duct and, thus, the concentration or dilution of the final urine. In the absence of AVP, the collecting duct remains essentially impermeable to water, even though some water is still reabsorbed. The continued reabsorption of solute then results in the excretion of a maximally dilute urine (~50 mOsm/kg H_2O). As the medullary interstitium is always hypertonic, the absence of circulating AVP, which renders the collecting duct impermeable to water, is critical to the normal diluting process.

This diluting mechanism allows the intake and subsequent excretion of large volumes of water without major alterations in the tonicity of body water.[261] Rarely, this limit can be exceeded, causing water intoxication. Much more commonly,

however, hyponatremia occurs at lower rates of water intake, owing either to an intrarenal defect in urine dilution or to the persistent secretion of AVP in the circulation. In the latter case, because hypo-osmolality normally suppresses AVP secretion,[262] the hypo-osmolar state frequently reflects the persistent secretion of AVP in response to hemodynamic or other nonosmolar stimuli.[262]

ETIOLOGY OF HYPONATREMIA

The serum Na^+ concentration is determined by the body's content of sodium, potassium, and TBW. Thus:

$$\text{Serum } Na^+ = \frac{\text{Total body } Na^+ + \text{total body } K^+}{\text{TBW}}$$

This formula has been simplified from the observations made by Edelman in the 1950s. This simplification introduces some errors in the prediction of changes in serum sodium based on the previous formula and has been subject of some reinterpretation by Nguyen and Kurtz.[263] Whereas their revision of the formula is more accurate, as pointed out by Sterns, there are so many inaccuracies in the measurements of sodium, potassium, and water losses as well as intake that there is no substitute for frequent measurements of serum sodium concentration in rapidly changing clinical settings.[264]

As the previous relationship depicts, hyponatremia can therefore occur by an increase in TBW, a decrease in body solutes (either Na^+ or K^+), or any combination of these. In most cases, more than one of these mechanisms is operant. Therefore, an alternative approach is presented here. In approaching the hyponatremic patient, the physician's first task is to ensure that hyponatremia in fact reflects a hypo-osmotic state

486

and is not a consequence of the causes of pseudohyponatremia or translocational hyponatremia, discussed earlier. Thereafter, an assessment of ECF volume provides a useful working classification of hyponatremia as it can be associated with decreased, normal, or high total body sodium[265,266]: (1) hyponatremia with ECF volume depletion, (2) hyponatremia with excess ECF volume, and (3) hyponatremia with normal ECF volume.

Hyponatremia with Extracellular Fluid Volume Depletion

Patients with hyponatremia who have ECF volume depletion have sustained a deficit in total body Na⁺ that exceeds the deficit in water. The decrease in ECF volume is manifested by physical findings such as flat neck veins, decreased skin turgor, dry mucous membranes, orthostatic hypotension, and tachycardia.

If sufficiently severe, volume depletion is a potent stimulus to AVP release. When the osmoreceptor and volume receptor receive opposing stimuli, the former remains fully active but the set-point of the system is lowered. Thus, in the presence of hypovolemia, AVP is secreted and water is retained despite hypo-osmolality. Whereas the hyponatremia in this setting clearly involves a depletion of body solutes, a concomitant failure to excrete water is critical to the process.

As shown in Figure 13–17, an examination of the urinary Na⁺ concentration is helpful in assessing whether the fluid losses are renal or extrarenal in origin. A urinary Na⁺ concentration of less than 20 mEq/L reflects a normal renal response to volume depletion and points to an extrarenal source of fluid loss. This is most commonly seen in patients with gastrointestinal disease with vomiting or diarrhea. Other causes include loss of fluid into the third space, such as the abdominal cavity in pancreatitis or the bowel lumen with ileus. Burns and muscle trauma can also be associated with large fluid and electrolyte losses. Because many of these pathologic states are associated with thirst, an increase in either orally or parenterally taken free water leads to hyponatremia. Hypovolemic hyponatremia in patients whose urinary Na⁺ concentration is greater than 20 mEq/L points to the kidney as the source of the fluid losses.

Diuretic-induced hyponatremia, a commonly observed clinical entity, accounts for a significant proportion of symptomatic hyponatremia in hospitalized patients. It occurs almost exclusively with thiazide rather than loop diuretics, most likely because the former have no effect on urine concentrating ability but the latter do. The hyponatremia is usually evident within 14 days but can occur up to 2 years later in most patients.[267] Underweight women appear to be particularly prone to this complication,[268] and advanced age has been found to be a risk factor in some,[267,269] but not all,[268] studies. A careful study on diluting ability in the elderly revealed that thiazide diuretics exaggerate the already slower recovery from hyponatremia induced by water ingestion in this population.[270] Diuretics can cause hyponatremia by a variety of mechanisms[271]: (1) volume depletion, which results in impaired water excretion by both enhanced AVP release and decreased fluid delivery to the diluting segment; (2) a direct effect of diuretics on the diluting segment; and (3) K⁺ depletion causing a decrease in the water permeability of the collecting duct as well as an increase in water intake. K⁺ depletion leads to hyponatremia independent of the Na⁺ depletion that frequently accompanies diuretic use.[272] The concomitant administration of K⁺-sparing diuretics does not prevent the development of hyponatremia. Although the diagnosis of diuretic-induced hyponatremia is frequently obvious, surreptitious diuretic abuse is being increasingly recognized and should be considered in patients in whom other electrolyte abnormalities and high urinary Cl⁻ excretion suggest this possibility.

Salt-losing nephropathy occurs in some patients with advanced renal insufficiency. In the majority of these patients,

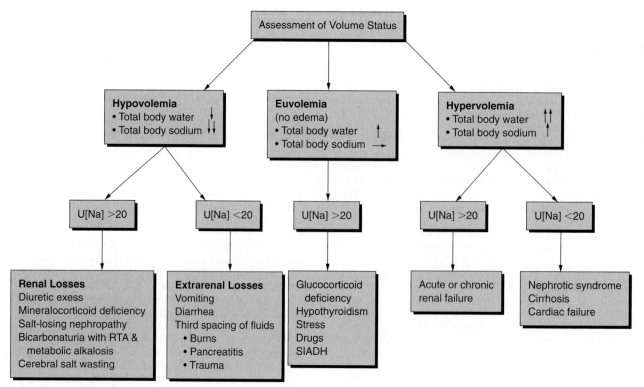

FIGURE 13–17 Diagnostic approach to the hyponatremic patient. (Modified from Halterman R, Berl T: Therapy of dysnatremic disorders. *In* Brady H, Wilcox C [eds]: Therapy in Nephrology and Hypertension. Philadelphia, WB Saunders, 1999, p 256.)

the Na$^+$-wasting tendency is not one that manifests itself at normal rates of sodium intake; however, some patients with interstitial nephropathy, medullary cystic disease, polycystic kidney disease, or partial urinary obstruction with sufficient Na$^+$ wasting exhibit hypovolemic hyponatremia.[273] Patients with proximal renal tubular acidosis exhibit renal sodium and potassium wasting despite modest renal insufficiency because bicarbonaturia obligates these cation losses.

It has long been recognized that adrenal insufficiency is associated with impaired renal water excretion and hyponatremia. This diagnosis should be considered in the volume-contracted hyponatremic patient whose urinary Na$^+$ concentration is not low, particularly when the serum K$^+$, BUN, and creatinine levels are elevated. Separate mechanisms for mineralocorticoid and glucocorticoid deficiency have been defined.[274]

Observations in glucocorticoid-replete adrenalectomized experimental animals provide evidence to support a role of mineralocorticoid deficiency in the abnormal water excretion, as both AVP release and intrarenal factors appear to be causal mechanisms. Thus, conscious adrenalectomized dogs given physiologic doses of glucocorticoids develop hyponatremia. Either saline or physiologic doses of mineralocorticoids corrected the defect in association with both ECF volume repletion and improvement in renal hemodynamics. Immunoassayable AVP levels were elevated in a similarly treated group of mineralocorticoid-deficient dogs despite hypo-osmolality.[275] The decreased ECF volume thus provides the nonosmotic stimulus of AVP release. More direct evidence for the role of AVP was provided in studies employing an AVP antagonist. When glucocorticoid-replete, adrenally insufficient rats were given an AVP antagonist, the minimal urine osmolality was significantly lowered.[276] Urine dilution was not corrected, in contrast to mineralocorticoid-replete rats, supporting a role for an AVP-independent mechanism. This is in concert with studies of adrenalectomized homozygous Brattleboro rats, which also have a defect in water excretion that can be partially corrected by mineralocorticoids or by normalization of volume. In summary, therefore, the mechanism of the defect in water excretion associated with mineralocorticoid deficiency is mediated by AVP and by AVP-independent intrarenal factors, both of which are activated by decrements of ECF volume, rather than by deficiency of the hormone per se.

The presence in the urine of an osmotically active nonreabsorbable or poorly reabsorbable solute causes renal excretion of Na$^+$ and culminates in volume depletion. Glycosuria secondary to uncontrolled diabetes mellitus, mannitol infusion, or urea diuresis after relief of obstruction is a common setting for this disorder. In patients with diabetes, the Na$^+$ wasting caused by the glycosuria can be aggravated by ketonuria because hydroxybutyrate and acetoacetate also cause urinary electrolyte losses. In fact, ketonuria can contribute to the renal Na$^+$ wasting and hyponatremia seen in starvation and alcoholic ketoacidosis. Na$^+$ and water excretion are also increased when a nonreabsorbable anion appears in the urine. This is observed principally with the metabolic alkalosis and bicarbonaturia that accompany severe vomiting or nasogastric suction. In these patients, the excretion of HCO$_3^-$ requires, for the maintenance of electroneutrality, the excretion of cations, including Na$^+$ and K$^+$. Whereas the renal losses in these clinical settings may be hypotonic, the volume contraction–stimulated thirst and water intake can result in the development of hyponatremia.

Cerebral salt wasting is a rare syndrome described primarily in patients with subarachnoid hemorrhage; it leads to renal salt wasting and volume contraction.[277] Although hyponatremia is increasingly reported in these patients, true cerebral wasting is probably less common than reported.[278] In fact, one critical review found no conclusive evidence for

volume contraction or renal salt wasting in any of the patients.[279] The mechanism of this natriuresis is unknown but the increased release of natriuretic peptides has been suggested.[280]

Hyponatremia with Excess Extracellular Fluid Volume

In the advanced stages, the edematous states listed in Figure 13–17 are associated with a decrease in plasma Na$^+$ concentration. Patients have an increase in total body Na$^+$ content, but the rise in TBW exceeds that of Na$^+$. With the exception of renal failure, these states are characterized by avid Na$^+$ retention (urinary Na$^+$ concentration <10 mEq/L). This avid retention may be obscured by the concomitant use of diuretics, which are frequently used in treating these patients. In fact, these agents can further contribute to the abnormal water excretion seen in these states.

Congestive Heart Failure

The common association between congestive heart failure and Na$^+$ and water retention is well established. A mechanism mediated by decreased delivery of tubule fluid to the distal nephron or increased release of AVP has been proposed. In an experimental model of low cardiac output, both AVP and diminished delivery to the diluting segment were found to be important in mediating the abnormality in water excretion. It thus appears that the decrement in "effective" blood volume and the decrease in arterial filling are sensed by aortic and carotid sinus baroreceptors and most likely stimulate AVP release.[281]

This stimulation must supersede the inhibition of AVP release that accompanies at least acute distention of the left atrium. In fact, there is evidence that chronic distention of the atria blunts the sensitivity for the receptor, so high-pressure baroreceptors can act in an uninhibited manner to stimulate AVP release. The importance of AVP in the abnormal dilution in experimental models of heart failure is underscored by the total correction of the water excretory defect by an AVP antagonist in rats with inferior vena cava constriction.[282]

High plasma AVP levels have been demonstrated in patients with congestive heart failure, in both the presence and the absence of diuretics.[283] Likewise, the hypothalamic mRNA message for the AVP pre-prohormone is elevated in rats with chronic cardiac failure.[284] Although these human studies do not exclude a role for intrarenal factors in the pathogenesis of the abnormal water retention, they complement the experimental observations that demonstrate an important role for AVP in the process. It is most likely that nonosmotic pathways, whose activation is suggested by the increase in sympathetic activity seen in congestive heart failure,[285] are the mediators of AVP release. These hormonal factors, by decreasing the glomerular filtration rate (GFR) and enhancing tubular Na$^+$ reabsorption, decrease distal fluid delivery, further contributing to the hyponatremia. The degree of neurohumoral activation correlates with the clinical severity of left ventricular dysfunction.[286] The degree of hyponatremia is a powerful prognostic factor in these patients.[287] The role of the vasopressin-regulated water channel (AQP2) has been examined in heart failure as well. Two groups have described an up-regulation of this water channel in rats with heart failure.[288,289] In the latter study,[289] the V$_2$ receptor antagonist OPC31260 reversed the up-regulation, suggesting that a receptor-mediated function, most likely enhanced cAMP generation, is responsible for the process. In fact, a selective V$_2$ antagonist decreases AQP2 excretion[290] and increases urine flow in patients with heart failure.

Hepatic Failure

Patients with advanced cirrhosis and ascites frequently present with hyponatremia as a consequence of their inability to excrete a water load.[291] The classic view suggests that a decrement in effective arterial volume leads to avid Na^+ and water retention in an attempt to restore volume toward normal.[292] In this regard, a number of the pathologic derangements in cirrhosis—including splanchnic venous pooling, diminished plasma oncotic pressure secondary to hypoalbuminemia, and the decrease in peripheral resistance—could all contribute to a decrease in effective blood volume.[293] This classic theory was challenged by observations that suggest primary renal Na^+ retention—the overflow hypothesis.[294] A proposal that unifies these views has been put forth: Na^+ retention occurs early but is a consequence of the severe vasodilation-mediated arterial underfilling.[295]

As with cardiac failure, the relative role of intrarenal and extrarenal factors in impaired water excretion has been a matter of controversy. The observation that expansion of intravascular volume with saline, mannitol, ascites fluid, water immersion, or peritoneovenous shunting improves water excretion in cirrhosis could be interpreted as implicating an intrarenal mechanism in the impaired water excretion, as these maneuvers increase GFR and improve distal delivery. Such maneuvers could also suppress baroreceptor-mediated AVP release and cause an osmotic diuresis, which would also improve water excretion.[292] Experimental models of deranged liver function, including acute portal hypertension by vein constriction, bile duct ligation, and chronic cirrhosis produced by administration of carbon tetrachloride, have demonstrated a predominant role for AVP secretion in the pathogenesis of the disorder. In this latter model, an increment in hypothalamic AVP mRNA has been demonstrated.[296] A study employing an AVP antagonist also points to a central role for AVP in the process.[297] As was the case in heart failure, increased expression of AQP2 has also been reported in the cirrhotic rat,[298] but dysregulation of AQP1 and AQP3 is also present in carbon tetrachloride (CCl_4^-)–induced cirrhosis.[299] In contrast, in the common bile duct model of cirrhosis, no increase in AQP2 is observed.[300]

Although patients with cirrhosis who have no edema or ascites excrete a water load normally, those with ascites usually do not. Several studies have demonstrated elevated AVP levels in such patients.[291] Patients who had a defect in water excretion had higher levels of AVP, plasma renin activity, plasma aldosterone, and norepinephrine,[301] as well as lower rates of PGE_2 production. Likewise, their serum albumin was lower, as was their urinary excretion of Na^+, all suggesting a decrease in effective blood volume. As is the case in heart failure, sympathetic tone is high in cirrhosis.[302] In fact, the plasma concentration of norepinephrine, a good index of baroreceptor activity in humans, appears to correlate well with the levels of AVP and the excretion of water. These studies, therefore, offer strong support for the view that effective arterial blood volume is contracted, rather than expanded, in decompensated cirrhosis.[295] This view is further strengthened by observations of subjects during head-out water immersion. This maneuver, which translocates fluid to the central blood volume, caused a decrease in AVP levels and improved water excretion,[303] but in this study, peripheral resistance decreased further. By combining head-out water immersion with norepinephrine administration in an effort to increase systemic pressure and peripheral resistance, water excretion was completely normalized.[304] Such observations underline the critical role of peripheral vasodilation in the process. The observation that inhibition of nitric oxide corrects the arterial hyporesponsiveness to vasodilators[305] and the abnormal water excretion in cirrhotic rats provides evidence for a role of nitric oxide in the vasodilation.[306,307]

Nephrotic Syndrome

The incidence of hyponatremia in the nephrotic syndrome is lower than in either congestive heart failure or cirrhosis, most likely as a consequence of the higher blood pressure, higher GFR, and more modest impairment in Na^+ and water excretion than in the other groups of patients.[308] As lipids are frequently elevated, a direct measurement of plasma osmolality should be done. Diminished excretion of free water was first noted in children with the nephrotic syndrome, and since then, other investigators[309] have noted elevated levels of AVP in these patients. In view of the alterations in Starling forces that accompany hypoalbuminemia and allow transudation of salt and water across capillary membranes to the interstitial space, patients with the nephrotic syndrome have been believed to have intravascular volume contraction. Increased levels of humoral markers of decreased effective blood volume also support this underfilling theory.[310] The possibility that this nonosmotic pathway stimulates AVP release was suggested by studies in which head-out water immersion and blood volume expansion[309] increased water excretion in nephrotic subjects. However, these pathogenic events may not be applicable to all patients with the disorder. Some patients with the nephrotic syndrome in fact have increased plasma volumes with suppressed plasma renin activity and aldosterone levels.[311] The cause of these discrepancies is not immediately evident, but this overfill view has been subject to some criticism.[312] It is most likely that the underfilling mechanism is operant in patients with normal GFR and with the histologic lesion of minimal-change disease and that hypervolemia may be more prevalent in patients with underlying glomerular pathology and decreased renal function. In such patients, an intrarenal mechanism probably causes Na^+ retention, as has been described in an experimental model of nephrotic syndrome.[313] Also, in contrast to the increase in AQP2 found in the previously described Na^{2+}- and water-retaining states, in two models of nephrotic syndrome induced with either puromycin aminonucleoside[314] or doxorubicin (Adriamycin),[315] the expression of the water channel was decreased. The animals were not hyponatremic and most likely had expanded ECF volumes to explain the discrepancy.

Renal Failure

Hyponatremia with edema can occur with either acute or chronic renal failure. It is clear that in the setting of either experimental or human renal disease, the ability to excrete free water is maintained better than the ability to reabsorb water. Nonetheless, the patient's GFR rate still determines the maximal rate of free water formation; thus, whenever minimal urine osmolality is reduced to 150 to 250 mOsm/kg H_2O and fractional water excretion approaches 20% to 30% of the filtered load, the uremic patient with a GFR of 2 mL/min can excrete only 300 mL/day. Intake of more fluid culminates in hyponatremia. Thus, a decrement in GFR rate with an increase in thirst underlies the hyponatremia of patients with renal insufficiency.[316]

Hyponatremia with Normal Extracellular Fluid Volume

Figure 13–17 lists the clinical entities that have to be considered in patients with hyponatremia whose volume is neither contracted nor expanded and who are, at least by clinical assessment, euvolemic. These entities are considered individually.

Glucocorticoid Deficiency

Considerable evidence exists for an important role for glucocorticoids in the abnormal water excretion of adrenal insufficiency.[317] The water excretory defect of anterior pituitary insufficiency, and particularly corticotropin deficiency, is associated with elevated AVP levels[318,319] and corrected by physiologic doses of glucocorticoids. Likewise, adrenalectomized dogs receiving replacement of mineralocorticoids have abnormal water excretion. The relative importance of intrarenal factors and AVP in defective water excretion has been a matter of considerable controversy. Studies employing a sensitive radioimmunoassay for plasma AVP and the Brattleboro rat with hypothalamic DI have provided evidence that both factors are involved. Support for a role for AVP has been obtained in studies of conscious adrenalectomized, mineralocorticoid-replaced dogs[320] and rats[321] and with the use of an inhibitor of the hydro-osmotic effect of AVP.[276] As plasma AVP was elevated despite a fall in plasma osmolality, the hormone's release may have been nonosmotically mediated. Although in both of these studies ECF volume was normal, a decrease in systemic pressure and cardiac function[320,321] could well have provided the hemodynamic stimulus for AVP release. In addition, there may be a direct effect of glucocorticoids that inhibits vasopressin secretion. In this regard, vasopressin gene expression is increased in glucocorticoid-deficient rats.[322] The presence of a glucocorticoid-responsive element on the AVP gene promoter may be responsible for the inhibition of vasopressin gene transcription by glucocorticoids.[323] Also, glucocorticoid receptors are present in magnocellular neurons and they are increased during hypo-osmolality.[324]

A role for AVP-independent intrarenal factors was defined in the antidiuretic-deficient, adrenalectomized Brattleboro rat[321] and with the AVP inhibitor.[276] It appears that prolonged glucocorticoid deficiency (14–17 days) is accompanied by decreases in renal hemodynamics that impair water excretion. A direct effect of glucocorticoid deficiency that enhances water permeability of the collecting duct has been proposed, but such a view is not supported by studies of anuran membranes that suggest that glucocorticoids enhance rather than inhibit water movement. Also, in vitro perfusion studies of the collecting duct of adrenalectomized rabbits show an impaired rather than enhanced AVP response,[325] a defect that may be related to enhanced cAMP metabolism.[326] In fact, AQP2 and AQP3 abundance appears not to be sensitive to glucocorticoid.[327] In summary, the defect in glucocorticoid deficiency is primarily AVP-dependent, and an AVP-independent pathway becomes evident with more prolonged hormone deficiency. It appears likely that alterations in systemic hemodynamics account for the nonosmotic release of AVP, but a direct effect of glucocorticoid hormone in AVP release has not been entirely excluded. The AVP-independent renal mechanism is probably caused by alterations in renal hemodynamics and not by a direct increase in collecting duct permeability. It must be noted that secondary hypoadrenalism, as occurs in hypopituitarism, can also be associated with hyponatremia.[328,329]

Hypothyroidism

Patients and experimental animals with hypothyroidism often have impaired water excretion and sometimes develop hyponatremia.[317,330] The dilution defect is reversed by treatment with thyroid hormones. Both decreased delivery of filtrate to the diluting segment and persistent secretion of AVP, alone or combination, have been proposed as mechanisms responsible for the defect.

Hypothyroidism has been shown to be associated with decreases in GFR and renal plasma flow.[330] In the AVP-free Brattleboro rat, the decrement in maximal free water excretion can be entirely accounted for by the decrease in GFR. The osmotic threshold for AVP release appears not to be altered in hypothyroidism.[331] The normal suppression of AVP release with water loading and the normal response to hypertonic saline,[332] coupled with the failure to observe upregulation of hypothalamic AVP gene expression in

hypothyroid rats,[333] supports an AVP-independent mechanism. There is, however, also evidence for a role of AVP in impairing water excretion in hypothyroidism. Thus, in both experimental animals[334] and humans with advanced hypothyroidism,[330] elevated AVP levels were measured in the basal state and after a water load. Although increased sensitivity to AVP in hypothyroidism has been proposed, experimental evidence suggests the contrary, as urine osmolality is relatively low for the circulating levels of the hormone,[334] and AVP-stimulated cyclase is impaired in the renal medulla of hypothyroid rats,[335] possibly leading to decreased AQP2 expression.[336] However, the predominant defect is one of water of excretion with increased AQP2 expression and reversal with a V_2 antagonist.[337] It appears, therefore, that diminished distal fluid delivery and persistent AVP release mediate the impaired water excretion in this disorder, but the relative contributions of these two factors remain undefined and may depend on the severity of the endocrine disorder.

Psychosis—Primary Polydipsia

It has long been recognized that patients with psychiatric disease demonstrate generous water intake. Although such polydipsia is normally not associated with hyponatremia, it has been observed that these patients are at increased risk of developing hyponatremia when they are acutely psychotic.[338] Most patients have schizophrenia, but some have psychotic depression. The frequency of hyponatremia in this population of patients is unknown, but in a survey conducted in one large psychiatric hospital, 20 polydipsic patients with a plasma Na+ concentration below 124 mEq/L were reported,[339] and another survey found hyponatremia in 8 of 239 patients.[340] Elucidation of the mechanism of the impaired water excretion has been confounded by antipsychotic drug treatment (see later). The relative contributions of the pharmacologic agent and the psychosis are therefore difficult to define, as thiazides and carbamazepine are frequently implicated.[341] Nonetheless, there are several reports of psychotic patients who suffered water intoxication when free of medication.[342]

The mechanism responsible for the hyponatremia in psychosis appears to be multifactorial.[184] In a comprehensive study of water metabolism in eight psychotic hyponatremic patients and seven psychotic normonatremic control subjects, no unifying defect emerged. The investigators found a small defect in osmoregulation that caused AVP to be secreted at plasma osmolalities somewhat lower than those of the control group, but they did not observe a true resetting of the osmostat. Also, the hyponatremic patients had a mild urine dilution defect even in the absence of AVP. When AVP was present, the renal response was somewhat enhanced, suggesting increased renal sensitivity to the hormone. Psychotic exacerbations appear to be associated with increased vasopressin levels in schizophrenic patients with hyponatremia.[343] Finally, thirst perception is also increased, as excessive water intake that exceeds excretory capacity is responsible for most episodes of hyponatremia in these patients. However, concurrent nausea caused increased vasopressin levels in some of the subjects.[344] Although each of these derangements by itself would remain clinically unimportant, it is possible that, during exacerbation of the psychosis, the defects are more pronounced and that, in combination, they can culminate in hyponatremia.[345]

Hyponatremia also supervenes in beer drinkers (so-called beer potomania). Although this has been ascribed to an increase in fluid intake in the setting of very low solute intake,[346] a recent report suggests that such patients may also have sustained significant solute losses.[347]

Postoperative Hyponatremia

The incidence of hospital-acquired hyponatremia is high, both in adults[205] and in children,[348] and it is particularly

CH 13

prevalent in the postoperative stage[349,350] (incidence ~4%). The majority of affected patients appear clinically euvolemic and have measurable levels of AVP in their circulation.[349,351] Although this occurs primarily as a consequence of administration of hypotonic fluids,[352] a decrease in serum Na^+ can occur in this high AVP state, even when isotonic fluids are given.[353] Hyponatremia has also been reported following cardiac catherization in patients receiving hypotonic fluids.[354] Although the presence of hyponatremia is a marker for poor outcome, this is a consequence not of the hyponatremia per se but of the severe underlying diseases associated with it. As discussed in more detail later, there is, however, a subgroup of postoperative patients—almost always premenstrual women—who develop catastrophic neurologic events, frequently accompanied by seizures and hypoxia.[355,356]

Strenuous Exercise

There is increasing recognition that strenuous exercise, such as military training[357] and marathons and triathlons,[358] can cause hyponatremia that is frequently symptomatic. A review of 57 such patients found a mean serum Na^+ of 121 mEq/L.[359] A recent prospective study of 488 runners in the Boston Marathon revealed that 13% of the runners had a sodium level less than 130 mEq/L. The multivariate analysis revealed that weight gain related to excessive fluid intake was the strongest single predictor of the hyponatremia. Longer racing times and very low body mass indexes (BMIs) were also predictors.[360] Composition of the consumed fluids and use of nonsteroidal anti-inflammatory agents was not predictive. Symptomatic hyponatremia is even more frequent in ultraendurance events.[361]

Pharmacologic Agents

Table 13–6 lists drugs associated with water retention. Some of the more clinically important ones are discussed here. An increasing number of patients who are receive vasopressin for indications such as von Willebrand disease[362] and nocturnal enuresis[363,364] are developing severe hyponatremia.

CHLORPROPAMIDE. The incidence of at least mild hyponatremia in patients taking chlorpropamide may be as high as

TABLE 13–6 Drugs Associated with Hyponatremia

Antidiuretic hormone analogs
Desmopressin acetate
Oxytocin

Drugs that enhance arginine vasopressin (AVP)
Chlorpropamide
Clofibrate
Carbamazepine, oxycarbazepine
Vincristine
Nicotine
Narcotics (μ-opioid receptors)
Antipsychotics, antidepressants
Ifosfamide

Drugs that potentiate renal action of AVP
Chlorpropamide
Cyclophosphamide
Nonsteroidal anti-inflammatory drugs
Acetaminophen

Drugs that cause hyponatremia by unknown mechanisms
Haloperidol
Fluphenazine
Amitriptyline
Thioridazine
Selective serotonin reuptake inhibitors
Ecstasy (amphetamine-related)

Data from Berl T, Schrier RW: Disorders of water metabolism. In Schrier RW (ed): Renal and Electrolyte Disorders, 6th ed. Philadelphia, Lippincott Williams & Wilkins, 2003.

7%, but severe hyponatremia (<130 mEq/L) occurs in 2% of patients so treated.[365] As noted earlier, the drug exerts its action primarily by potentiating the renal action of AVP.[366] Studies of toad urinary bladder have demonstrated that, although chlorpropamide alone has no effect, it enhances both AVP- and theophylline-stimulated water flow but decreases cAMP-mediated flow. The enhanced response may be due to up-regulation of the hormone's receptor.[367] Alternatively, studies of chlorpropamide-treated animals suggest that the drug enhances solute reabsorption in the medullary ascending limb (thereby increasing interstitial tonicity and the osmotic drive for water reabsorption) rather than a cAMP-mediated alteration in collecting duct water permeability.[368]

CARBAMAZEPINE AND OXYCARBAZEPINE. The anticonvulsant drug carbamazepine is known to possess antidiuretic properties. The incidence of hyponatremia in carbamazepine-treated patients was believed to be as high as 21%, but a survey of patients with mental retardation reported an incidence of 5%.[369] Cases continue to be reported.[370] The antiepileptic oxcarbazepine, of the same class as carbamazepine, has also been reported to cause hyponatremia.[371] Evidence exists for both a mechanism mediated by AVP release[90] and for renal enhancement of the hormone's action[372] to explain carbamazepine's antidiuretic effect. The drug also decreases the sensitivity of the vasopressin response to osmotic stimulation.[373]

PSYCHOTROPIC DRUGS. An increasing number of psychotropic drugs have been associated with hyponatremia, and in fact, they are frequently implicated to explain the water intoxication in psychotic patients. Among the agents implicated are the phenothiazines,[374] the butyrophenone haloperidol,[375] and the tricyclic antidepressants.[376] Recently, an increasing number of cases of amphetamine (Ecstasy)-related hyponatremia have been described.[377,378] Likewise, the widely used antidepressants fluoxetine,[379] sertraline,[380] and paroxetine[381] have been associated with hyponatremia. In this latter study involving 75 patients, 12% developed hyponatremia (Na<135 mmol/L). The elderly appear to be particularly susceptible,[382,383] with an incidence as high as 22% to 28%.[384,385] The tendency for these drugs to cause hyponatremia is further compounded by their anticholinergic effect. By drying the mucous membranes, they stimulate water intake. The role of the drugs in impaired water excretion has not, in most cases, been dissociated from the role of the underlying disorder for which the drug is given. Furthermore, evaluation of the effect of the drugs on AVP release has frequently revealed a failure to increase the levels of the hormone, particularly if mean arterial pressure remained unaltered. Therefore, although a clinical association between antipsychotic drugs and hyponatremia is frequently encountered, the pharmacologic agents themselves may not be the principal factors responsible for the water retention.[184]

ANTINEOPLASTIC DRUGS. Several drugs used in cancer therapy cause antidiuresis. The effect of vincristine may be mediated by the drug's neurotoxic effect on the hypothalamic microtubule system, which then alters normal osmoreceptor control of AVP release.[386] A recent retrospective survey suggests that this may be more common in Asians given the drug.[387] The mechanism of the diluting defect that results from cyclophosphamide administration is not fully understood. It may act, at least in part, to enhance action, because the drug does not increase hormone levels.[388] It is known that the antidiuresis has its onset 4 to 12 hours after injection of the drug, lasts as long as 12 hours, and seems to be temporally related to excretion of a metabolite. The importance of anticipating potentially severe hyponatremia in cyclophosphamide-treated patients who are vigorously hydrated to avert urologic complications cannot be overstated. The synthetic analog of cyclophosphamide, ifosfamide, has also been associated with hyponatremia and AVP release.[389]

NARCOTICS. Since the 1940s, it has been known that the administration of opioid agonists, such as morphine, reduces urine flow by causing the release of an antidiuretic substance. The possibility that endogenous opioids could serve as potential neurotransmitters has been suggested by the finding of enkephalins in nerve fibers projecting from the hypothalamus to the pars nervosa. However, the reported effects vary and range from stimulation to no change and even to inhibition of AVP release. The reasons for these diverse observations may be that the opiates and their receptors are widely distributed in the brain, implying that the site of action of the opiate can differ markedly depending on the route of administration. Likewise, there are multiple opiate peptides and receptor types. It has now been defined that agonists of μ-receptors have antidiuretic properties whereas Δ receptors have the opposite effect.

MISCELLANEOUS. Several case reports suggest an association between the use of ACE inhibitors and hyponatremia.[390-392] Of interest is that all three reported patients were women in their 60s. The use of ACE inhibition was also a concomitant risk factor for the development of hyponatremia in a survey of veterans who received chlorpropamide.[365] However, given the widespread use of these agents, the incidence of hyponatremia must be vanishingly low. Likewise, an association with angiotensin receptor blockers has to date not been reported.

Recently four patients have been reported to develop hyponatremia during amiodorone loading.[393]

Syndrome of Inappropriate Antidiuretic Hormone Secretion

Clinical Characteristics

SIADH is the most common cause of hyponatremia in hospitalized patients.[250] As first described by Schwartz and associates[394] in two patients with bronchogenic carcinoma and later further characterized by Bartter and Schwartz,[395] patients with this syndrome have serum hypo-osmolality when excreting urine that is less than maximally dilute (>50 mOsm/kg H_2O). Thus, a diagnostic criterion for this syndrome is the presence of inappropriate urinary concentration. The development of hyponatremia with a dilute urine (<100 mOsm/kg H_2O) should raise suspicion of a primary polydipsic disorder. Although large volumes of fluid need to be ingested to overwhelm normal water excretory ability, if there are concomitant decreases in solute intake, this volume need not be excessively high.[396] In SIADH, the urinary Na^+ is dependent on intake, because Na^+ balance is well maintained. As such, urinary Na^+ concentration is usually high, but it may be low in patients with the syndrome who are receiving a low-sodium diet. The presence of Na^+ in the urine is helpful in excluding extrarenal causes of hypovolemic hyponatremia, but low urinary Na^+ concentration does not exclude SIADH. Before the diagnosis of SIADH is made, other causes for a decreased diluting capacity, such as renal, pituitary, adrenal, thyroid, cardiac, or hepatic disease, must be excluded. In addition, nonosmotic stimuli for AVP release, particularly hemodynamic derangements (e.g., due to hypotension, nausea, or drugs), need to be ruled out. Another clue to the presence of the syndrome is the finding of hypouricemia. In one study, 16 of 17 patients had levels below 4 mg/dL, whereas in 13 patients with hyponatremia of other causes the level was greater than 5 mg/dL. This hypouricemia appears to occur as a consequence of increased urate clearance.[397] The measurement of an elevated level of AVP confirms the clinical diagnosis. It must be noted, however, that the majority of patients with SIADH have AVP levels in the "normal" range (≤10 pg/mL); the presence of any AVP is, however, abnormal in the hypo-osmolar state. As the presence of hyponatre-

mia is itself evidence for abnormal dilution, a formal urine-diluting test need not be performed. The water test is helpful in determining whether an abnormality remains in a patient whose serum Na^+ has been corrected by water restriction. Because Brattleboro rats receiving vasopressin,[398] as well as an animal model of SIADH, display up-regulation of AQP2 expression, the excretion of AQP2 has been investigated as a marker for the persistent secretion of ADH. The excretion of the water channel remains elevated in patients with SIADH; however, this is not specific to this entity, as a similar pattern was observed in patients with hyponatremia due to hypopituitarism.[399]

Pathophysiology

In 1953, Leaf and associates[400] described the effects of chronic AVP administration on Na^+ and water balance. They noted that high-volume water intake was required for the development of hyponatremia. Concomitant with the water retention, an increment in urinary Na^+ excretion was noted. The relative contributions of the water retention and Na^+ loss to the development of hyponatremia were subsequently investigated. Acute water loading causes transient natriuresis but, when water intake is increased more slowly, no significant negative Na^+ loss can be documented. Such studies clearly demonstrate that the hyponatremia is in large measure a consequence of water retention; however, it must be noted that the net increase in water balance fails to account entirely for the decrement in serum Na^+.[400] In a carefully studied model of SIADH secretion in rats, the retained water was found to be distributed in the intracellular space and to be in equilibrium with the tonicity of ECF.[401] The natriuresis and kaliuresis that occur early in the development of this model contribute to a decrement of body solutes and in part account for the observed hyponatremia.[402] Studies involving analysis of whole-body water and electrolyte content demonstrate that the relative contributions of water retention and solute losses vary with the duration of induced hyponatremia; the former is central to the process, but with more prolonged hyponatremia, Na^+ depletion becomes predominant.[403] In this regard, it has even been suggested that the natriuresis and volume contraction are an important component of the syndrome that maintains the secretion of AVP[404] with atrial natriuretic peptide as a mediator of the Na^+ loss.[405] Therefore, although natriuresis frequently accompanies the syndrome, the secretion of ADH is essential. Finally, patients with the syndrome must also have a defect in thirst regulation whereby the osmotic inhibition of water intake is not operant. The mechanism of this failure to suppress thirst is not fully understood.

After the initial retention of water, loss of Na^+, and development of hyponatremia, continued administration of AVP is accompanied by the reestablishment of Na^+ balance and a decline in the hydro-osmotic effect of the hormone. The integrity of renal regulation of Na^+ balance is manifested by the ability to conserve Na^+ during Na^+ restriction and by the normal excretion of an Na^+ load. Thus, the mechanisms that regulate Na^+ excretion are intact. Loss of the hydro-osmotic effect of AVP, albeit to varying degrees, is evident in many studies,[400,402] because urine flow increased and urine osmolality decreased despite continued administration of the hormone (Fig. 13–18). This effect has been termed *vasopressin escape*.[406] Several studies have demonstrated that hypotonic expansion rather than chronic administration of AVP per se is needed for escape to occur, as the escape phenomenon is seen only when positive water balance is achieved.[406]

The cellular mechanisms responsible for vasopressin escape have been the subject of some investigation. Studies of broken epithelial cell preparations of the toad urinary bladder revealed down-regulation of AVP receptors[407] as well

A

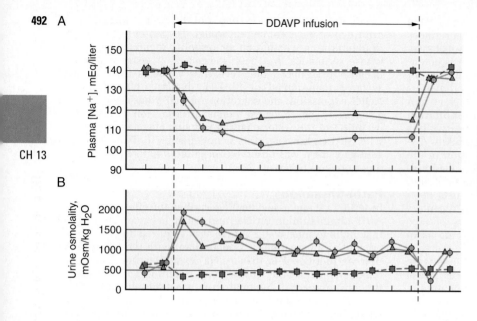

B

FIGURE 13–18 Effects of desmopressin (DDAVP) and water administration to two normal rats (*circles* and *triangles*). Note that urine osmolality decreases and serum Na⁺ stabilizes. Sham-treated control subjects are depicted by *squares*. (From Verbalis JG, Drutarosky M: Adaptation to chronic hypo-osmolality in rats. Kidney Int 34:351, 1988.)

as vasopressin binding in the inner medulla.[408] Post-cAMP mechanisms are probably also operant. In this regard, a decrease in expression of AQP2 has been reported in the process of escape from DDAVP-induced antidiuresis, without a concomitant change in basolateral AQP3 and AQP4.[409,410] The decrement in AQP2 was associated with decreased V_2 responsiveness.[409] The distal tubule also has an increase in sodium transporters, including the α- and γ-subunits of the epithelial sodium channel and the thiazide sensitive Na⁺/Cl⁻ cotransporter.[411] In addition to a renal mechanism, it appears that chronic hyponatremia causes a decrement in hypothalamic mRNA production, a process that could ameliorate the syndrome in the clinical setting.[27]

Clinical Settings

It is now apparent that the previously described pathophysiologic sequence occurs in a variety of clinical settings characterized by persistent AVP secretion. Since the original report of Schwartz and co-workers,[394] the syndrome has been described in an increasing number of clinical settings (Table 13–7). These fall into three general categories[412]: (1) malignancies, (2) pulmonary disease, and (3) CNS disorders. In addition, an increasing number of patients with acquired immunodeficiency syndrome have been reported to have hyponatremia. The frequency may be as high as 35% of hospitalized patients with the disease, and in as many as two thirds, SIADH may be the underlying cause.[413] As was noted previously, hyponatremia caused by excessive water repletion can occur after moderate and severe exercise.[358,359,414,415] Finally, it is increasingly recognized that an idiopathic form is common in the elderly.[416–419] As many as 25% of elderly patients admitted to a rehabilitation center had serum Na⁺ values less than 135 mEq/L.[417] In a significant proportion of these patients, no underlying cause is unveiled. This may be related to an increase in AQP2 production and excretion in this age group.[420]

A material with antidiuretic properties has been extracted from some of the tumors or metastases of patients with malignancy-associated SIADH. Not all patients with the syndrome have AVP in their tumors. A number of the tumors have also been found to produce the carrier hormone of AVP, neurophysin, suggesting that repression of normal genetic information has occurred. Of the tumors that cause SIADH secretion, bronchogenic carcinoma, and particularly small cell lung cancer, is the most common, with a reported inci-

dence of 11%.[421] It appears that patients with bronchogenic carcinoma have higher plasma AVP levels in relation to plasma osmolality, even if they do not manifest the full-blown SIADH, although in patients with the syndrome, the levels of the hormone are higher. The possibility that the hormone could serve as a marker of bronchogenic carcinoma has been suggested, and in fact, SIADH has been reported occasionally to precede the diagnosis of the tumor by several months.[422] In view of the potential to treat patients with this tumor, it is important that patients with unexplained SIADH be fully investigated and evaluated for the presence of this malignancy. Head and neck malignancies are the second most common tumors associated with the syndrome, as it occurs in approximately 3% of such patients.

The mechanism whereby AVP is produced in other pulmonary disorders is not known, but the associated abnormalities in blood gases could act as mediators of the effect. Antidiuretic activity has also been assayed in tuberculous lung tissue. The syndrome can also occur in the setting of miliary rather than only lung-limited tuberculosis.[423] In CNS disorders, AVP is most likely released from the neurohypophysis. Studies of monkeys have shown that elevations of intracranial pressure cause AVP secretion, and this may be the mechanism that mediates the syndrome in at least some CNS disorders. The magnocellular vasopressin secreting cells in the hypothalamus are subject to numerous excitatory inputs, and therefore, it is conceivable that a large variety of neurologic disorders can cause the secretion of the hormone.

Finally, hyponatremia was described recently in two infants with undetectable AVP levels who were found to have a gain of function mutation at the X-linked vasopressin receptor wherein in codon 137 a missense mutation resulted in the change from arginine to cysteine or leucine. The authors termed this nephrogenic syndrome of inappropriate antidiuresis (NSIAD).[424]

Robertson and colleagues have studied osmoregulation of AVP secretion in a large group of patients with SIADH.[425] In the great majority, the plasma AVP concentration was inadequately suppressed relative to the hypotonicity present. In most patients, the plasma AVP concentration ranged between 1 and 10 pg/mL, the same range as in normally hydrated healthy adults. Inappropriate secretion, therefore, can often be demonstrated only by measuring AVP under hypotonic conditions. Even with this approach, however, abnormalities

TABLE 13–7	**Disorders Associated with the Syndrome of Inappropriate Antidiuretic Hormone Secretion**		
Carcinomas	**Pulmonary Disorders**	**Central Nervous System Disorders**	**Other**
Bronchogenic carcinoma	Viral pneumonia	Encephalitis (viral or bacterial)	AIDS
Carcinoma of the duodenum	Bacterial	Meningitis (viral, bacterial, tuberculous, fungal)	Prolonged exercise
Carcinoma of the pancreas	Pneumonia	Carcinoma of the ureter	Idiopathic (in elderly)
Thymoma	Pulmonary abscess	Head trauma	Nephrogenic
Carcinoma of the stomach	Tuberculosis	Brain abscess	
Lymphoma	Aspergillosis	Guillain-Barré syndrome	
Ewing sarcoma	Positive pressure breathing	Acute intermittent porphyria	
Carcinoma of the bladder	Asthma	Subarachnoid hemorrhage or subdural hematoma	
Prostatic carcinoma	Pneumothorax	Cerebellar and cerebral atrophy	
Oropharyngeal tumor	Mesothelioma Cystic fibrosis	Cavernous sinus thrombosis Neonatal hypoxia Shy-Drager syndrome Rocky Mountain spotted fever Delirium tremens Cerebrovascular accident (cerebral thrombosis or hemorrhage) Acute psychosis Peripheral neuropathy Multiple sclerosis	

Data from Berl T, Schrier RW: Disorders of water metabolism. *In* Schrier RW (ed): Renal and Electrolyte Disorders, 6th ed. Philadelphia, Lippincott Williams & Wilkins, 2003.

in plasma AVP were not apparent in almost 10% of the patients with clinical evidence of SIADH. To better define the nature of the osmoregulatory defect in these patients, plasma AVP was measured during infusion of hypertonic saline. When this method of analysis was applied to 25 patients with SIADH, four different types of osmoregulatory defects were identified.

As shown in Figure 13–19, in the type A osmoregulatory defect, infusion of hypertonic saline was associated with large and erratic fluctuations in plasma AVP, which bore no relationship to the rise in plasma osmolality. This pattern was found in 6 of 25 patients studied, who had acute respiratory failure, bronchogenic carcinoma, pulmonary tuberculosis, schizophrenia, or rheumatoid arthritis. This pattern indicates that the secretion of AVP either had been totally divorced from osmoreceptor control or was responding to some periodic nonosmotic stimulus.

A completely different type of osmoregulatory defect is exemplified by the type B response, as depicted in Figure 13–19. The infusion of hypertonic saline resulted in prompt and progressive rises in plasma osmolality. Regression analysis showed that the precision and sensitivity of this response were essentially the same as those in healthy subjects, except that the intercept or threshold value at 253 mOsm/kg was well below the normal range. This pattern, which reflects the resetting of the osmoreceptor, was found in 9 of the 25 patients who had a diagnosis of bronchogenic carcinoma, cerebrovascular disease, tuberculous meningitis, acute respiratory

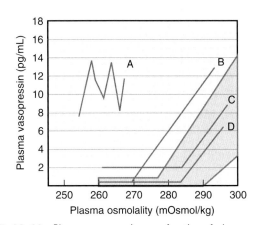

FIGURE 13–19 Plasma vasopressin as a function of plasma osmolality during the infusion of hypertonic saline in four groups of patients with clinical syndrome of inappropriate antidiuretic hormone (SIADH). The *shaded area* indicates the range of normal values. See text for description of each group. (From Zerbe R, Stropes L, Robertson G: Vasopressin function in the syndrome of inappropriate antidiuresis. Annu Rev Med 31:315, 1980.)

disease, or carcinoma of the pharynx. Another patient has been reported with hyponatremia and acute idiopathic polyneuritis who reacted in an identical manner to the hypertonic saline infusion and was determined to have resetting of the osmoreceptor. Because their threshold function is retained when they receive a water load, this patient and others with reset osmostats have been able to dilute their urine maximally and sustain a urine flow sufficient to prevent a further increase in body water. Thus, an abnormality in AVP regulation can exist in spite of the ability to maximally dilute the urine and excrete a water load.

In the type C response (see Fig. 13–19), plasma AVP was elevated initially but did not change during the infusion of hypertonic saline until plasma osmolality reached the normal range. At that point, plasma AVP began to rise appropriately, indicating a normally functioning osmoreceptor mechanism. This response was found in 8 of the 25 patients with the diagnosis of CNS disease, bronchogenic carcinoma, carcinoma of the pharynx, pulmonary tuberculosis, or schizophrenia. Its pathogenesis is unknown, but the authors speculate that it may be due to a constant, nonsuppressible leak of AVP despite otherwise normal osmoregulatory function. Unlike type B, the resetting type of defect, the type C response results in impaired urine dilution and water excretion at all levels of plasma osmolality.

In the type D response (see Fig. 13–19), the osmoregulation of AVP appears to be completely normal despite a marked inability to excrete a water load. The plasma AVP is appropriately suppressed under hypotonic conditions and does not rise until plasma osmolality reaches the normal threshold level. When this procedure is reversed by water loading, plasma osmolality and plasma AVP again fall normally, but urine dilution does not occur, and the water load is not excreted. This defect was present in 2 of 25 patients with the diagnosis of bronchogenic carcinoma, indicating that, in these patients, the antidiuretic defect is caused by some abnormality other than SIADH. It could be due either to increased renal tubule sensitivity to AVP or to the existence of an antidiuretic substance other than AVP. Alternatively, it is possible that the presently available assays are not sufficiently sensitive to detect significant levels of AVP. Perhaps some of these subjects have the nephrogenic syndrome of antidiuresis described previously.[424]

It is of interest that patients with bronchogenic carcinoma, which has generally been believed to be associated with ectopic production of AVP, manifested every category of osmoregulatory defect, including the reset osmostat. It has been suggested that many of these tumors probably cause SIADH secretion not by producing the hormone ectopically but rather by interfering with the normal osmoregulation of AVP secretion from the neurohypophysis through direct invasion of the vagus nerve, metastatic implants in the hypothalamus, or some other more generalized neuropathic changes.

Symptoms, Morbidity, and Mortality

The majority of patients with hyponatremia appear to be asymptomatic. However, a recent case-control study of 122 elderly patients with a mean serum sodium of 126 mmol/L suggests that such patients are not truly asymptomatic. Thus, when compared with 244 age-matched controls, they had a 67-fold greater risk for sustaining falls, and neuropsychiatric testing revealed subtle abnormalities.[426] Other clinical manifestations of hyponatremia usually occur only at a serum Na+ concentration below 125 mmol/L. Although gastrointestinal complaints occur early, the majority of the manifestations are neuropsychiatric, including lethargy, psychosis, and seizures, designated as *hyponatremic encephalopathy*.[427,428] In its severe form, hyponatremic encephalopathy can cause brainstem compression leading to pulmonary edema and hypoxemia,[94,429] which may be, at least in part, mediated by AQP4.[430] In fact, in a retrospective study of 168 hyponatremic patients, most of them acute, a strong association existed between the development of hypoxemia and the risk of mortality (13-fold).[431] Finally, a number of hyponatremic patients have been reported to also develop rhabdomyolysis.[414]

The development of symptoms also depends on the age, gender, and magnitude and acuteness of the process. Elderly persons and young children with hyponatremia are most likely to develop symptoms. It has also become apparent that neurologic complications occur more frequently in menstruating women. In a case-control study, Ayus and colleagues[356] noted that, despite an approximately equal incidence of postoperative hyponatremia in males and females, 97% of those with permanent brain damage were women and 75% of them were menstruant. However, this view is not universally held, as others have not found increased postoperative hyponatremia in this population,[432] and the aforementioned retrospective study did not reveal a gender or age association with mortality.[431]

The degree of clinical impairment is related not to the absolute measured level of lowered serum Na+ concentration but to both the rate and the extent of the drop in ECF osmolality. In a survey of hospitalized hyponatremic patients (serum Na+ level <128 mEq/L), 46% had CNS symptoms and 54% were asymptomatic.[433] It is of note, however, that the authors believed that the hyponatremia was the cause of the symptoms in only 31% of the symptomatic patients. In this subgroup of symptomatic patients, the mortality was no different from that of asymptomatic patients (9%–10%). In contrast, the mortality of patients whose CNS symptoms were not caused by hyponatremia was high (64%), suggesting that the mortality of these patients is more often due to the associated disease than to the electrolyte disorder itself. This is in agreement with the report of Anderson,[250] who noted a 60-fold increase in mortality in hyponatremic patients over that of normonatremic control subjects. In the hyponatremic patients, death frequently occurred after the plasma Na+ concentration was returned toward normal and was due to progression of severe underlying disease; this suggests that the hyponatremia is an indicator of severe disease and poor prognosis. In fact, a number of recent studies further point out that even mild hyponatremia is an independent predictor of higher mortality in a number of disorders. These include patients with acute ST elevation myocardial infarctions,[434] heart failure,[435] and liver disease.[436,437] In fact, these authors have concluded that the addition of the hyponatremia to the model end stage liver disease (MELD) score (employed as a system to assign priority for liver transplantation) predicts outcome more precisely than the now-used MELD score.

The mortality of acute symptomatic hyponatremia has been noted to be as high as 55% and as low as 5%.[438,439] The former reflects the observation of few symptomatic hyponatremic patients in a consultative setting, the latter the estimate from a broad-based literature survey. Equally controversial is the mortality rate associated with hyponatremia in children. One series found no in-hospital deaths attributable to hyponatremia, but others described an 8.4% mortality in such postoperative children and estimated that more than 600 children die as a result of hyponatremia in the United States yearly.[252] Hospital-acquired hyponatremia may have contributed to the morbidity and mortality associated with La Crosse encephalitis in children.[440] The mortality associated with chronic hyponatremia has been reported to be between 14% and 27%.[441,442]

The observed CNS symptoms are most likely related to the cellular swelling and cerebral edema that result from acute lowering of ECF osmolality, which leads to movement of water into cells. In fact, such cerebral edema occasionally causes herniation, as has been noted in postmortem examination of both humans and experimental animals. The increase in brain water is, however, much less marked than would be predicted from the decrease in tonicity were the brain to operate as a passive osmometer. The volume regulatory responses that protect against cerebral edema, and which probably occur throughout the body, have been extensively studied and reviewed.[443] Studies of rats demonstrate a prompt loss of both electrolyte and organic osmolytes after the onset

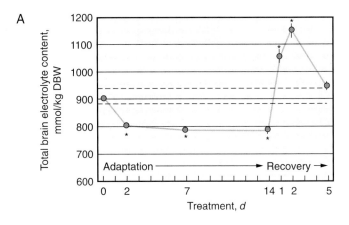

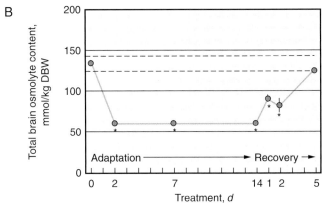

FIGURE 13–20 Comparison of changes in brain electrolyte (**A**) and organic osmolyte (**B**) contents during adaptation to hyponatremia and after rapid correction of hyponatremia in rats. Both electrolytes and organic osmolytes are lost quickly after the induction of hyponatremia beginning on day 0. Brain content of both solutes remains depressed during maintenance of hyponatremia from days 2 through 14. After rapid correction of the hyponatremia on day 14, electrolytes reaccumulate rapidly and overshoot normal brain contents on the first 2 days after correction, before returning to normal levels by the 5th day after correction. In contrast, brain organic osmolytes recover much more slowly and do not return to normal brain contents until the 5th day after correction. The *dashed lines* indicate ±SEM from the mean values of normonatremic rats on day 0. *P<.01 compared with brain contents of normonatremic rats. DBW, dry brain weight. (Data from Verbalis JG, Gullans SR: Hyponatremia causes large sustained reductions in brain content of multiple organic osmolytes in rats. Brain Res 567:274, 1991; and Verbalis JG, Gullans SR: Rapid correction of hyponatremia produces differential effects on brain osmolyte and electrolyte reaccumulation in rats. Brain Res 606:19, 1993.)

of hyponatremia.[443,444] Some of the osmolyte losses occur within 24 hours,[445] but the loss of water becomes more marked in subsequent days (Fig. 13–20). The rate at which the brain restores the lost electrolytes and osmolytes when hyponatremia is corrected is of great pathophysiologic importance. Na⁺ and Cl⁻ recover quickly and even overshoot.[444–446] However, the reaccumulation of osmolytes is considerably delayed (see Fig. 13–20). This process is likely to account for the more remarked cerebral dehydration that accompanies the correction in previously adapted animals.[447] It has been observed that urea may prevent the myelinosis associated with this pathology. This may well be due to the more rapid reaccumulation of organic osmolytes, and particularly myoinositol, in the azotemic state.[448]

Treatment

Treatment of hyponatremia is a subject of considerable interest and has been discussed in a companion to this chapter[449] and in other reviews.[450] The therapeutic strategy is dictated by the underlying cause of the disorder, as well as (1) the presence or absence of symptoms, (2) the duration of

the disorder, and (3) the risk for neurologic complications. Although the ultimate goal, whenever possible, is to identify and treat the underlying pathologic condition, this is not always entirely possible (especially in SIADH), so a general approach to the management of categories of hyponatremia has been developed.[449]

SYMPTOMATIC HYPONATREMIA. The therapeutic approach to symptomatic hyponatremia has been a subject of great controversy[438,439,447–454] emanating from the observation that neurologic disorders supervene both in untreated acutely hyponatremic patients and occasionally in the course of treatment of the hyponatremia. The neurologic symptoms that occur in acutely hyponatremic patients[355,356] and in elderly persons taking thiazide diuretics[455] usually include apathy, confusion, nausea, vomiting, and frequently seizures. The mortality rate in this group is high and the majority of survivors have significant neurologic residua. The possibility that this permanent neurologic damage is a consequence of post-anoxic encephalopathy has been suggested. In fact, there is evidence from experimental animals to support the view that, when hypoxia is combined with hyponatremia, the adaptive mechanisms are abrogated, leading to an increase in brain edema and mortality,[456] perhaps explaining the previously mentioned association of hypoxemia with high mortaltity.[431] The cause of the female preponderance among those who suffer permanent neurologic damage is unknown, but it has been suggested that the adaptive mechanisms whereby the brain decreases its volume in acute hyponatremia are less efficient and could be inhibited by sex hormones. In this regard, it is of interest that estrogens appear to alter the function of the Na⁺,K⁺-ATPase in rat brain synaptosomes,[457] a process that could delay cell volume regulation in response to hypotonicity. Nonetheless, a combination of factors, including AVP via a V₁ receptor[458] atrial natriuretic peptide,[459] hypoxia, and sex hormones, all contribute to alterations in cellular adaptation and vascular reactivity culminating in severe, often fatal, cerebral edema.

In view of the devastating neurologic consequences that can be associated with acute symptomatic hyponatremia, it has been suggested that such patients' metabolic disorder should be corrected rapidly[431,460] (Fig. 13–21). In fact, the observation of Ayus and associates[461] demonstrated the safety of this approach. Nonetheless, the increasing number of patients who have been reported to develop a neurologic syndrome suggestive of central pontine myelinolysis in the course of treatment of hyponatremia cannot be ignored.[451] This syndrome has been recently reviewed.[462] The clinical picture is not that of the classic syndrome described in malnourished alcoholics, and the demyelinating lesions are frequently extrapontine in both humans,[451] including children,[463] and experimental animals.[448] It appears that the demyelinating syndrome is most likely to occur in patients whose hyponatremia is more chronic and is corrected once the adaptive process has set in.[447] A disruption of the blood-brain barrier and alterations in cortical and subcortical blood flow may be involved in the pathogenesis of this disorder.

Although small lesions produce minimal symptoms, patients with more extensive disease have flaccid quadriplegia, dysphagia, and dysarthria. Patients with extrapontine demyelination can present with an atypical picture that includes disorders of movements, mutism, and catatonia. The disorder was considered uniformly fatal, but it is now recognized that most patients survive, including some with complete recovery.[464] The diagnosis is now best made with MRI, with diffusion-weighted MRI showing lesions within 24 hours of symptoms.[465] The factors that predispose to these neurologic complications have not been fully delineated. In the view of some, the rate of correction is critical,[438] a view supported by data from experimental animals.[461] Other data suggest that the process is independent of the rate of correc-

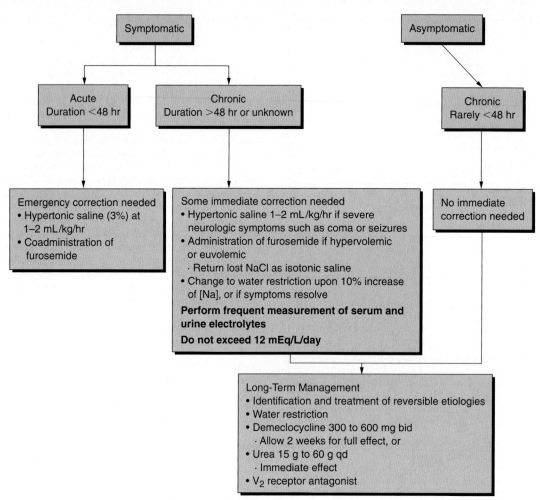

FIGURE 13–21   Treatment of severe euvolemic hyponatremia. (From Thurman J, Halterman R, Berl T: Therapy of dysnatremic disorders. *In* Brady H, Wilcox C [eds]: Therapy in Nephrology and Hypertension, 2nd ed. Philadelphia, Saunders, 2003.)

tion and is due to the absolute change in serum Na⁺ over a given time period.[451] This concept is also supported by experimental data.[466] These two variables are not entirely independent, and therefore, attention to both correction rate and magnitude is indicated. In this regard, in experimental animals,[467] correction at an excessive rate (>2 mEq/L/hr) and magnitude (>20 mEq/L/24 hr) was associated with the development of cerebral lesions (Fig. 13–22). Others would propose more conservative correction rates of approximately 0.4 mEq/L/hr and 12 mEq/L in any 24-hour period.[468]

In summary, rapid correction is indicated for patients with acute (<48 hr) and symptomatic hyponatremia (see Fig. 13–21). This should probably aim to raise serum Na⁺ concentrations by approximately 1 to 2 mEq/L/hr until seizures subside. This correction can be achieved by administration of hypertonic saline with the concomitant administration of furosemide, which impairs free water reabsorption and lowers urine osmolality, induces excretion of Na⁺ in a much larger volume of urine, and leads to a much greater negative water balance. This allows more rapid correction of the plasma Na⁺ concentration. Although full correction in this setting is safe, it is not necessary. Several formulas have been suggested to predict the increased serum Na⁺ that accompanies administration of intravenous fluids.[266] These formulas operate well in static conditions but fail to account for ongoing water and solute losses. A comprehensive formula that incorporates these variables has been proposed.[469] Although probably accurate, its complexity makes it difficult to employ in practice. A tonicity, solutes, and water balance approach that monitors the Na⁺, K⁺, and water infused and excreted best predicts changes in serum sodium.[470]

Example: A 70-kg man has a serum Na⁺ concentration of 110 mEq/L. Assuming that 60% of BW is water,

$$TBW = 70 \times 0.6 = 42 \text{ L}$$

Serum Na⁺ concentration =

$$\frac{\text{Total body cation (Na}^+ + \text{K}^+\text{) content}}{TBW}$$

In this patient,

$$\text{Total body cation content} = 42 \text{ L} \times 110 \text{ mEq/L}$$
$$= 4620 \text{ mEq}$$

Over the next 2 hours, the patient receives 200 mL of 3% NaCl and excretes 1000 mL of urine. The urinary Na⁺ is 70 mEq/L and the urinary K⁺ is 39 mEq/L. In this case, there is no net cation gain or loss, as 100 mEq of Na⁺ was given (the Na⁺ content of 200 mL of 3% NaCl) and 100 mEq of cation was excreted. However, TBW has decreased by 800 mL (1000 mL excreted −200 mL given with the hypertonic saline). Thus, the 4620 mEq of body cations is now in 41.2 L, which would increase serum Na⁺ to 112 mEq/L (4620/41.2). The rate at which serum Na⁺ will rise therefore depends not only on the volume of hypertonic saline administered but also on the volume and cation content of urine excreted. Because Na⁺ and K⁺ balance is maintained, cation excretion is dependent on the amount infused, but the urine volume is in large measure determined by the kidney's ability to generate free water. Concomitant administration of loop diuretics would increase free water excretion and therefore the rate of correction, if needed.

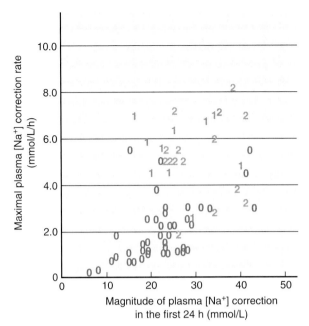

FIGURE 13–22 Incidence of demyelinative lesions in individual rats as a function of both the maximal rate of correction of hyponatremia and the magnitude of the increase in plasma Na⁺ concentration over the first 24 hours of the correction. Each rat in one of the three correction groups (water restriction, water diuresis, and hypertonic saline) is plotted as a function of the maximal rate of increase in plasma Na⁺ achieved in any 4-hour period during the correction *(abscissa)* and the total magnitude of the increase in plasma Na⁺ achieved during the first 24 hours of the correction *(ordinate)*. Rats are represented by their neuropathology score (0, no demyelinative lesions; 1, focal demyelinative lesions; 2, diffuse demyelinative lesions). (Data from Verbalis JG, Martinez AJ: Neurological and neuropathological sequelae of correction of chronic hyponatremia. Kidney Int 39:1274, 1991.)

The excess water that must be excreted to achieve an increment in Na⁺ can likewise be calculated. Assuming that a patient weighs 70 kg when the serum Na⁺ is 115 mEq/L, the excess water that needs to be excreted to correct the hyponatremia to 130 mEq/L can be estimated as follows:

$$TBW = \text{body weight (kg)} \times 60\%$$

or in this case,

$$TBW = 70 \times 0.6 = 42 \text{ L}$$

$$\text{Excess water} = \underset{(TBW)}{TBW} - (\text{actual plasma Na}^+/\text{desired Na}^+)$$

$$\text{Excess water} = 42 - [(115/130)(42)] = 42 - 37.2 = 4.8 \text{ L}$$

During therapy, serum and urine electrolytes should be monitored frequently to avoid overcorrection. Once symptoms have decreased and a small degree of correction has been achieved, further therapy can proceed more slowly with either decreased rates of saline or fluid restriction alone.

Because of the increased risk of osmotic demyelination syndrome, the treatment of symptomatic patients with chronic hyponatremia calls for careful monitoring and restraint. In general, treatment with hypertonic saline to raise serum Na⁺ concentrations by approximately 10 mEq/L (i.e., 10%), at a rate not to exceed 1 mEq/L/hr is probably safe and usually sufficient for amelioration of symptoms. This is rarely necessary, and should be employed only when the patient has seizures. Even more so than in the acutely symptomatic group, care should be taken to avoid an absolute increase in Na⁺ concentration greater than 12 mEq/L/day. After this degree of correction, therapy should continue with water restriction. Such an approach should be accompanied by a vanishingly low incidence of myelinolysis. The issue of spon-

taneous correction at an undesirably rapid rate by the onset of a water diuresis is deserving of consideration because brain damage can ensue in this setting. There are some clinical settings in which correction of hyponatremia can occur at a very rapid rate with institution of therapy. If the previous parameters have been exceeded and correction has been proceeded more rapidly than discussed (usually because of excretion of hypotonic urine), the events leading to demyelination may be reversed by readministration of hypotonic fluids and DDAVP. This is suggested from animal studies[471] and case reports in humans,[472] even when overtly symptomatic.[473]

"ASYMPTOMATIC HYPONATREMIA." The cornerstone of the treatment of "asymptomatic" hyponatremia is water restriction (see Fig. 13–21). The extent of this restriction depends on the particular patient's degree of diluting impairment. Thus, for some patients, restriction to 1000 mL/day is adequate and achieves negative water balance and an increase in serum Na⁺ concentration. If, in another patient, such a volume exceeds the total renal and extrarenal water losses, no improvement will be noted and even greater restriction of water intake is necessary. A guide to the degree of water restriction required to improve the hyponatremia can be assessed from the concentration of Na⁺ and K⁺ in the urine.[474]

In practical terms, severe water restriction is difficult to enforce for prolonged periods, especially in the outpatient setting. Pharmacologic agents that antagonize AVP action and maneuvers that increase solute excretion have allowed patients with SIADH to drink more water. The two most commonly employed agents are lithium and dimethylchlortetracycline.

Despite the well-established effect of lithium to antagonize AVP action, its use in SIADH has been superseded by the less toxic and perhaps more effective use of demeclocycline.[475] This agent, in doses between 600 and 1200 mg/day, is effective in inhibiting AVP action and restores serum Na⁺ to normal levels within 5 to 14 days, permitting unrestricted water intake. The mechanism whereby demeclocycline exerts this effect is not known. Toxicity in patients with cirrhosis has been well recognized. A nonpharmacologic alternative to the treatment of these patients involves an increase in solute intake and excretion. Because the level of urine concentration is more or less fixed in many patients with SIADH, urine flow is extremely dependent on solute excretion and increasing the solute load therefore increases fluid loss. Thus, administration of urea (30–60 g dissolved in 100 mL of water) once a day was successful in patients with the syndrome.[476] With the exception of one patient who had headaches but who responded to an alteration in dosing schedule, no reactions were noted, although gastrointestinal disturbances would not be unexpected.

The use of furosemide (40 mg/day) and high salt intake (200 mEq/day), an extension of the treatment of acute symptomatic hyponatremia to the chronic management of euvolemic hyponatremia, has also been reported to be successful.[477] In general, all these treatments are in one manner or another unsatisfactory, and therefore, the emergence of vasopressin antagonists to treat these disorders represents an important improvement in the armamentarium.

VASOPRESSIN ANTAGONISTS. The development of antagonists to the vasopressor and antidiuretic properties of AVP has potential therapeutic implications for the management of patients with excess AVP. Initial attempts to develop such agents were met with problems related to agonist effects and species specificity. More recently nonpeptide AVP selective V_2 and combined V_{1a}/V_2 have been developed. These agents antagonize both endogenous and exogenous AVP, causing water diuresis in the absence of alterations in filtration rate or solute excretion.[478] The antagonists block the action of AVP to stimulate adenylate cyclase in cortical, medullary, and papillary collecting ducts; to interfere with binding of radioactive AVP in papillary membranes; and to block AVP-mediated water flow in isolated rabbit collecting ducts.[479] The antagonist appears to bind to the transmembrane region of the receptor blocking the binding of AVP to the receptor.[480] The development of a number of oral antagonists of the V_2 receptors[478,481] is extremely promising, particularly as they have been found effective in a rat model of SIADH,[482] as well as in patients with SIADH.[483-485] In one study, the V_1 and V_2 antagonist conivaptan has been administered for 3 months.[486] The agent was well tolerated and maintained a normal serum Na^+. An intravenous preparation of this drug has now been approved by the U.S. food and Drug Administration (FDA) for use in hospitalized patients with euvolemic and hypervolemic hyponatremia. Vasopressin antagonists appear to also cause an aquaresis in other disorders characterized by high AVP levels such as cirrhosis[487,488] as well as in heart failure.[489,490] A potential role for these compounds in the treatment of heart failure has been considered.[491] A large scale trial (EVEREST) demonstrated short-term improvement in dyspnea,[492] but no long-term survival benefit.[493] The potential therapeutic role of the antagosits in the treatment of water-retaining disorders will await further experience and the delineations of potential toxicities. Nonetheless, they clearly usher in a new era in the treatment of these disorders.

References

1. Edelman IS, Leibman J: Anatomy of body water and electrolytes. Am J Med 27:256, 1959.
2. Fanestil DD: Compartmentation of body water. In Narins RG (ed): Clinical Disorders of Fluid and Electrolyte Metabolism. New York, McGraw-Hill, 1994, pp 3–20.
3. Thomas RC: Electrogenic sodium pump in nerve and muscle cells. Physiol Rev 52:563, 1972.
4. Czech MP: The molecular basis of insulin action. Annu Rev Biochem 46:359, 1977.
5. Wolf AV, McDowell ME: Apparent and osmotic volumes of distribution of sodium, chloride, sulfate and urea. Am J Physiol 176:207, 1954.
6. Maffly RH, Leaf A: The potential of water in mammalian tissues. J Gen Physiol 42:1257, 1959.
7. Leaf A, Chatillon JY, Tuttle EPJ: The mechanism of the osmotic adjustment of body cells as determined in vivo by the volume of distribution of a large water load. J Clin Invest 33:1261, 1954.
8. Rose BD: New approach to disturbances in the plasma sodium concentration. Am J Med 81:1033–1040, 1986.
9. Foster KG: Relation between the colligative properties and chemical composition of sweat. J Physiol (Lond) 155:490, 1961.
10. Hendry EB: Osmolarity of human serum and of chemical solutions of biologic importance. Clin Chem 7:156, 1961.
11. Zerbe RL, Robertson GL: Osmoregulation of thirst and vasopressin secretion in human subjects: Effect of various solutes. Am J Physiol 244:E607–E614, 1983.
12. Vokes TP, Aycinena PR, Robertson GL: Effect of insulin on osmoregulation of vasopressin. Am J Physiol 252:E538–E548, 1987.
13. de Castro J: A microregulatory analysis of spontaneous fluid intake in humans: Evidence that the amount of liquid ingested and its timing is mainly governed by feeding. Physiol Behav 3:705–714, 1988.
14. Adolph EF: Physiology of Man in the Desert. New York, Hafner Publishing, 1969.
15. Du Vigneaud V: Hormones of the posterior pituitary gland: Oxytocin and vasopressin. In DuVigneaud V, Bing RJ, Oncley JL (eds): The Harvey Lectures, 1954–55. New York, Academic Press, 1956, pp 1–28.
16. Edwards BR, LaRochelle FT Jr: Antidiuretic effect of endogenous oxytocin in dehydrated Brattleboro homozygous rats. Am J Physiol 247:F453–F465, 1984.
17. Oliver G, Schaefer EA: On the physiological actions of extracts of the pituitary body and certain other glandular organs. J Physiol (Lond) 18:277–279, 1895.
18. Cowley AW Jr: Vasopressin and blood pressure regulation. Clin Physiol Biochem 6:150–162, 1988.
19. Mohr E, Bahnsen U, Kiessling C, et al: Expression of the vasopressin and oxytocin genes in rats occurs in mutually exclusive sets of hypothalamic neurons. FEBS Lett 242:144–148, 1988.
20. Mohr E, Richter D: Sequence analysis of the promoter region of the rat vasopressin gene. FEBS Lett 260:305–308, 1990.
21. Gainer H, Yamashita M, Fields RL, et al: The magnocellular neuronal phenotype: Cell-specific gene expression in the hypothalamo-neurohypophysial system. Prog Brain Res 139:1–14, 2002.
22. Richter D: Molecular events in expression of vasopressin and oxytocin and their cognate receptors. Am J Physiol 255:F207–F219, 1988.
23. Robinson AG, Haluszczak C, Wilkins JA, et al: Physiologic control of two neurophysins in humans. J Clin Endocrinol Metab 44:330–339, 1977.
24. Nowycky MC, Seward EP, Chernevskaya NI: Excitation-secretion coupling in mammalian neurohypophysial nerve terminals. Cell Mol Neurobiol 18:65–80, 1998.
25. Herman JP, Schafer MK, Watson SJ, et al: In situ hybridization analysis of arginine vasopressin gene transcription using intron-specific probes. Mol Endocrinol 5:1447–1456, 1991.
26. Majzoub JA, Rich A, van Boom J, et al: Vasopressin and oxytocin mRNA regulation in the rat assessed by hybridization with synthetic oligonucleotides. J Biol Chem 258:14061–14064, 1983.
27. Robinson AG, Roberts MM, Evron WA, et al: Hyponatremia in rats induces downregulation of vasopressin synthesis. J Clin Invest 86:1023–1029, 1990.
28. Fitzsimmons MD, Roberts MM, Robinson AG: Control of posterior pituitary vasopressin content: Implications for the regulation of the vasopressin gene. Endocrinology 134:1874–1878, 1994.
29. Leng G, Mason WT, Dyer RG: The supraoptic nucleus as an osmoreceptor. Neuroendocrinology 34:75–82, 1982.
30. Buggy J, Jonhson AK: Preoptic-hypothalamic periventricular lesions: Thirst deficits and hypernatremia. Am J Physiol 233:R44–R52, 1977.
31. Thrasher TN, Keil LC, Ramsay DJ: Lesions of the organum vasculosum of the lamina terminalis (OVLT) attenuate osmotically-induced drinking and vasopressin secretion in the dog. Endocrinology 110:1837–1839, 1982.
32. Robertson GL: The regulation of vasopressin function in health and disease. Rec Prog Horm Res 33:333–385, 1976.
33. Zerbe RL, Miller JZ, Robertson GL: The reproducibility and heritability of individual differences in osmoregulatory function in normal human subjects. J Lab Clin Med 117:51–59, 1991.
34. Helderman JH, Vestal RE, Rowe JW, et al: The response of arginine vasopressin to intravenous ethanol and hypertonic saline in man: The impact of aging. J Gerontol 33:39–47, 1978.
35. Ledingham JGG, Crowe MJ, Forsling ML: Effects of aging on vasopressin secretion, water excretion, and thirst in man. Kidney Int Suppl 32:S90, 1987.
36. Baylis PH: Osmoregulation and control of vasopressin secretion in healthy humans. Am J Physiol 253:R671–R678, 1987.
37. Vokes TJ, Weiss NM, Schreiber J, et al: Osmoregulation of thirst and vasopressin during normal menstrual cycle. Am J Physiol 254:R641–R647, 1988.
38. Vallotton MB, Merkelbach U, Gaillard RC: Studies of the factors modulating antidiuretic hormone excretion in man in response to the osmolar stimulus: Effects of oestrogen and angiotensin II. Acta Endocrinol (Copenh) 104:295–302, 1983.
39. Davison JM, Gilmore EA, Durr J, et al: Altered osmotic thresholds for vasopressin secretion and thirst in human pregnancy. Am J Physiol 246:F105–F109, 1984.
40. Weisinger RS, Burns P, Eddie LW, et al: Relaxin alters the plasma osmolality-arginine vasopressin relationship in the rat. J Endocrinol 137:505–510, 1993.
41. Leng G, Brown CH, Bull PM, et al: Responses of magnocellular neurons to osmotic stimulation involves coactivation of excitatory and inhibitory input: An experimental and theoretical analysis. J Neurosci 21:6967–6977, 2001.
42. Verbalis JG: Osmotic inhibition of neurohypophysial secretion. Ann N Y Acad Sci 689:146–160, 1993.
43. Thrasher TN: Osmoreceptor mediation of thirst and vasopressin secretion in the dog. Fed Proc 41:2528–2532, 1982.
44. Bourque CW, Voisin DL, Chakfe Y: Stretch-inactivated cation channels: Cellular targets for modulation of osmosensitivity in supraoptic neurons. Prog Brain Res 139:85–94, 2002.
45. Sladek CD, Kapoor JR: Neurotransmitter/neuropeptide interactions in the regulation of neurohypophyseal hormone release. Exp Neurol 171:200–209, 2001.
46. Ludwig M, Sabatier N, Dayanithi G, et al: The active role of dendrites in the regulation of magnocellular neurosecretory cell behavior. Prog Brain Res 139:247–256, 2002.
47. Schrier RW, Berl T, Anderson RJ: Osmotic and nonosmotic control of vasopressin release. Am J Physiol 236:F321–F332, 1979.
48. Raff H, Merrill D, Skelton M, et al: Control of ACTH and vasopressin in neurohypophysectomized conscious dogs. Am J Physiol 249:R281–R284, 1985.
49. Dunn FL, Brennan TJ, Nelson AE, et al: The role of blood osmolality and volume in regulating vasopressin secretion in the rat. J Clin Invest 52:3212–3219, 1973.
50. Stricker EM, Verbalis JG: Interaction of osmotic and volume stimuli in regulation of neurohypophyseal secretion in rats. Am J Physiol 250:R267–R275, 1986.
51. Goldsmith SR, Francis GS, Cowley AW, et al: Response of vasopressin and norepinephrine to lower body negative pressure in humans. Am J Physiol 243:H970–H973, 1982.
52. Goldsmith SR, Cowley AW Jr, Francis GS, et al: Effect of increased intracardiac and arterial pressure on plasma vasopressin in humans. Am J Physiol 246:H647–H651, 1984.
53. Robertson GL, Athar S: The interaction of blood osmolality and blood volume in regulating plasma vasopressin in man. J Clin Endocrinol Metab 42:613–620, 1976.
54. Quillen EW Jr, Cowley AW Jr: Influence of volume changes on osmolality-vasopressin relationships in conscious dogs. Am J Physiol 244:H73–H79, 1983.
55. Andresen MC, Doyle MW, Jin YH, et al: Cellular mechanisms of baroreceptor integration at the nucleus tractus solitarius. Ann N Y Acad Sci 940:132–141, 2001.
56. Renaud LP: CNS pathways mediating cardiovascular regulation of vasopressin. Clin Exp Pharmacol Physiol 23:157–160, 1996.
57. Blessing WW, Sved AF, Reis DJ: Destruction of noradrenergic neurons in rabbit brainstem elevates plasma vasopressin, causing hypertension. Science 217:661–663, 1982.
58. Berl T, Cadnapaphornchai P, Harbottle JA, et al: Mechanism of suppression of vasopressin during alpha-adrenergic stimulation with norepinephrine. J Clin Invest 53:219–227, 1974.
59. Schrier RW: Pathogenesis of sodium and water retention in high-output and low-output cardiac failure, nephrotic syndrome, cirrhosis, and pregnancy (1). N Engl J Med 319:1065–1072, 1988.
60. Schrier RW: Pathogenesis of sodium and water retention in high-output and low-output cardiac failure, nephrotic syndrome, cirrhosis, and pregnancy (2). N Engl J Med 319:1127–1134, 1988.

61. Zerbe RL, Henry DP, Robertson GL: Vasopressin response to orthostatic hypotension. Etiologic and clinical implications. Am J Med 74:265–271, 1983.
62. Seckl JR, Williams TD, Lightman SL: Oral hypertonic saline causes transient fall of vasopressin in humans. Am J Physiol 251:R214–R217, 1986.
63. Thompson CJ, Burd JM, Baylis PH: Acute suppression of plasma vasopressin and thirst after drinking in hypernatremic humans. Am J Physiol 252:R1138–R1142, 1987.
64. Salata RA, Verbalis JG, Robinson AG: Cold water stimulation of oropharyngeal receptors in man inhibits release of vasopressin. J Clin Endocrinol Metab 65:561–567, 1987.
65. Rowe JW, Shelton RL, Helderman JH, et al: Influence of the emetic reflex on vasopressin release in man. Kidney Int 16:729–735, 1979.
66. Verbalis JG, McHale CM, Gardiner TW, et al: Oxytocin and vasopressin secretion in response to stimuli producing learned taste aversions in rats. Behav Neurosci 100:466–475, 1986.
67. Baylis PH, Robertson GL: Rat vasopressin response to insulin-induced hypoglycemia. Endocrinology 107:1975–1979, 1980.
68. Baylis PH, Zerbe RL, Robertson GL: Arginine vasopressin response to insulin-induced hypoglycemia in man. J Clin Endocrinol Metab 53:935–940, 1981.
69. Thompson DA, Campbell RG, Lilavivat U, et al: Increased thirst and plasma arginine vasopressin levels during 2-deoxy-D-glucose–induced glucoprivation in humans. J Clin Invest 67:1083–1093, 1981.
70. Keil LC, Summy-Long J, Severs WB: Release of vasopressin by angiotensin II. Endocrinology 96:1063–1065, 1975.
71. Ferguson AV, Renaud LP: Systemic angiotensin acts at subfornical organ to facilitate activity of neurohypophysial neurons. Am J Physiol 251:R712–R717, 1986.
72. McKinley MJ, McAllen RM, Pennington GL, et al: Physiological actions of angiotensin II mediated by AT1 and AT2 receptors in the brain. Clin Exp Pharmacol Physiol Suppl 3:S99–104, 1996.
73. McKinley MJ, Allen AM, Mathai ML, et al: Brain angiotensin and body fluid homeostasis. Jpn J Physiol 51:281–289, 2001.
74. Yamaguchi K, Sakaguchi T, Kamoi K: Central role of angiotensin in the hyperosmolality- and hypovolaemia-induced vasopressin release in conscious rats. Acta Endocrinol (Copenh) 101:524–530, 1982.
75. Stocker SD, Stricker EM, Sved AF: Acute hypertension inhibits thirst stimulated by ANG II, hyperosmolality, or hypovolemia in rats. Am J Physiol Regul Integr Comp Physiol 280:R214–R224, 2001.
76. Keil LC, Severs WB: Reduction in plasma vasopressin levels of dehydrated rats following acute stress. Endocrinology 100:30–38, 1977.
77. Edelson JT, Robertson GL: The effect of the cold pressor test on vasopressin secretion in man. Psychoneuroendocrinology 11:307–316, 1986.
78. Ukai M, Moran WH Jr, Zimmermann B: The role of visceral afferent pathways on vasopressin secretion and urinary exeretory patterns during surgical stress. Ann Surg 168:16–28, 1968.
79. Chikanza IC, Petrou P, Chrousos G: Perturbations of arginine vasopressin secretion during inflammatory stress. Pathophysiologic implications. Ann N Y Acad Sci 917:825–834, 2000.
80. Baylis PH, Stockley RA, Heath DA: Effect of acute hypoxaemia on plasma arginine vasopressin in conscious man. Clin Sci Mol Med 53:401–404, 1977.
81. Claybaugh JR, Hansen JE, Wozniak DB: Response of antidiuretic hormone to acute exposure to mild and severe hypoxia in man. J Endocrinol 77:157–160, 1978.
82. Rose CE Jr, Anderson RJ, Carey RM: Antidiuresis and vasopressin release with hypoxemia and hypercapnia in conscious dogs. Am J Physiol 247:R127–R134, 1984.
83. Raff H, Shinsako J, Keil LC, et al: Vasopressin, ACTH, and corticosteroids during hypercapnia and graded hypoxia in dogs. Am J Physiol 244:E453–E458, 1983.
84. Farber MO, Weinberger MH, Robertson GL, et al: Hormonal abnormalities affecting sodium and water balance in acute respiratory failure due to chronic obstructive lung disease. Chest 85:49–54, 1984.
85. Anderson RJ, Pluss RG, Berns AS, et al: Mechanism of effect of hypoxia on renal water excretion. J Clin Invest 62:769–777, 1978.
86. Miller M: Role of endogenous opioids in neurohypophysial function of man. J Clin Endocrinol Metab 50:1016–1020, 1980.
87. Oiso Y, Iwasaki Y, Kondo K, et al: Effect of the opioid kappa-receptor agonist U50488H on the secretion of arginine vasopressin. Study on the mechanism of U50488H-induced diuresis. Neuroendocrinology 48:658–662, 1988.
88. Eisenhofer G, Johnson RH: Effect of ethanol ingestion on plasma vasopressin and water balance in humans. Am J Physiol 242:R522–R527, 1982.
89. Oiso Y, Robertson GL: Effect of ethanol on vasopressin secretion and the role of endogenous opioids. *In* Schrier R (ed): Water Balance and Antidiuretic Hormone. New York, Raven Press, 1985, pp 265–269.
90. Stephens WP, Coe JY, Baylis PH: Plasma arginine vasopressin concentrations and antidiuretic action of carbamazepine. BMJ 1:1445–1447, 1978.
91. Reid IA, Ahn JN, Trinh T, et al: Mechanism of suppression of vasopressin and adrenocorticotropic hormone secretion by clonidine in anesthetized dogs. J Pharmacol Exp Ther 229:1–8, 1984.
92. Iovino M, De Caro G, Massi M, et al: Muscimol inhibits ADH release induced by hypertonic sodium chloride in rats. Pharmacol Biochem Behav 19:335–338, 1983.
93. Zerbe RL, Bayorh MA, Quirion R, et al: The role of vasopressin suppression in phencyclidine-induced diuresis. Pharmacology 26:73–78, 1983.
94. Lausen HD: Metabolism of the neurohypophyseal hormones. *In* Greep RO, Astwood EB, Knobil E, et al (eds): Handbook of Physiology. Washington, DC, American Physiological Society, 1974, pp 287–393.
95. Davison JM, Sheills EA, Barron WM, et al: Changes in the metabolic clearance of vasopressin and in plasma vasopressinase throughout human pregnancy. J Clin Invest 83:1313–1318, 1989.
96. Andersson B: Thirst—and brain control of water balance. Am Sci 59:408–415, 1971.
97. Fitzsimons JT: Thirst. Physiol Rev 52:468–561, 1972.
98. Quillen EW, Reid IA, Keil LC: Carotid and arterial baroreceptor influences on plasma vasopressin and drinking. *In* Cowley AWJ, Liard JF, Ausiello DA (eds): Vasopressin: Cellular and Integrative Functions. New York, Raven Press, 1988, pp 405–411.
99. Stricker EM, Verbalis JG: Water intake and body fluids. *In* Zigmond MJ, Bloom FE, Landis SC, et al (eds): Fundamental Neuroscience. San Diego, Academic Press, 1999, pp 1111–1126.
100. Phillips PA, Rolls BJ, Ledingham JG, et al: Osmotic thirst and vasopressin release in humans: A double-blind crossover study. Am J Physiol 248:R645–R650, 1985.
101. Szczepanska-Sadowska E, Kozlowski S: Equipotency of hypertonic solutions of mannitol and sodium chloride in eliciting thirst in the dog. Pflugers Arch 358:259–264, 1975.
102. Robertson GL: Disorders of thirst in man. *In* Ramsay DJ, Booth DA (eds): Thirst: Physiological and Psychological Aspects. London, Springer-Verlag, 1991, pp 453–477.
103. Verbalis JG: Inhibitory controls of drinking. *In* Ramsay DJ, Booth DA (eds): Thirst: Physiological and Psychological Aspects. London, Springer-Verlag, 1991, pp 313–334.
104. Fitzsimons JT: Drinking by rats depleted of body fluid without increases in osmotic pressure. J Physiol (Lond) 159:297–309, 1961.
105. Thrasher TN, Keil LC, Ramsay DJ: Hemodynamic, hormonal, and drinking responses to reduced venous return in the dog. Am J Physiol 243:R354–R362, 1982.
106. Phillips PA, Rolls BJ, Ledingham JG, et al: Angiotensin II–induced thirst and vasopressin release in man. Clin Sci (Lond) 68:669–674, 1985.
107. Rogers PW, Kurtzman NA: Renal failure, uncontrollable thirst, and hyperreninemia. Cessation of thirst with bilateral nephrectomy. JAMA 225:1236–1238, 1973.
108. Stricker EM, Sved AF: Thirst. Nutrition 16:821–826, 2000.
109. Root AW, Martinez CR, Muroff LR: Subhypothalamic high-intensity signals identified by magnetic resonance imaging in children with idiopathic anterior hypopituitarism. Evidence suggestive of an "ectopic" posterior pituitary gland. Am J Dis Child 143:366–367, 1989.
110. Heinbecker P, White HL: Hypothalamico-hypophyseal system and its relation to water balance in the dog. Am J Physiol 133:582–593, 1941.
111. Maccubbin DA, Van Buren JM: A quantitative evaluation of hypothalamic degeneration and its relation to diabetes insipidus following interruption of the human hypophyseal stalk. Brain 86:443, 1963.
112. Lippsett MB, MacLean IP, West CD, et al: An analysis of the polyuria induced by hypophysectomy in man. J Clin Endocrinol Metab 16:183–195, 1956.
113. Valtin H, North WG, Edwards BR, Gellai M: Animal models of diabetes insipidus. *In* Czernichow P, Robinson AG (eds): Diabetes insipidus in man. Basel, Karger, 1985, pp 105–126.
114. Schmale H, Richter D: Single base deletion in the vasopressin gene is the cause of diabetes insipidus in Brattleboro rats. Nature 308:705–709, 1984.
115. Hansen LK, Rittig S, Robertson GL: Genetic basis of familial neurohypophyseal diabetes insipidus. Trends Endocrinol Metab 8:363, 1997.
116. Repaske DR, Phillips JA, III, Kirby LT, et al: Molecular analysis of autosomal dominant neurohypophyseal diabetes insipidus. J Clin Endocrinol Metab 70:752–757, 1990.
117. Rittig S, Robertson GL, Siggaard C, et al: Identification of 13 new mutations in the vasopressin-neurophysin ii gene in 17 kindreds with familial autosomal dominant neurohypophyseal diabetes insipidus. Am J Hum Genet 58:107–117, 1996.
118. Repaske DR, Medlej R, Gultekin EK, et al: Heterogeneity in clinical manifestation of autosomal dominant neurohypophyseal diabetes insipidus caused by a mutation encoding ala-1-val in the signal peptide of the arginine vasopressin/neurophysin ii/copeptin precursor. J Clin Endocrinol Metab 82:51–56, 1997.
119. Bergeron C, Kovacs K, Ezrin C, et al: Hereditary diabetes insipidus: An immunohistochemical study of the hypothalamus and pituitary gland. Acta Neuropathol (Berl) 81:345–348, 1991.
120. Maghnie M, Villa A, Arico M, et al: Correlation between magnetic resonance imaging of posterior pituitary and neurohypophyseal function in children with diabetes insipidus. J Clin Endocrinol Metab 74:795–800, 1992.
121. Kaplowitz PB, D'Ercole AJ, Robertson GL: Radioimmunoassay of vasopressin in familial central diabetes insipidus. J Pediatr 100:76–81, 1982.
122. Siggaard C, Rittig S, Corydon TJ, et al: Clinical and molecular evidence of abnormal processing and trafficking of the vasopressin preprohormone in a large kindred with familial neurohypophyseal diabetes insipidus due to a signal peptide mutation. J Clin Endocrinol Metab 84:2933–2941, 1999.
123. Si-Hoe SL, de Bree FM, Nijenhuis M, et al: Endoplasmic reticulum derangement in hypothalamic neurons of rats expressing a familial neurohypophyseal diabetes insipidus mutant vasopressin transgene. FASEB J 14:1680–1684, 2000.
124. Davies J, Murphy D: Autophagy in hypothalamic neurones of rats expressing a familial neurohypophysial diabetes insipidus transgene. J Neuroendocrinol 14:629–637, 2002.
125. Maghnie M, Cosi G, Genovese E, et al: Central diabetes insipidus in children and young adults. N Engl J Med 343:998–1007, 2000.
126. Imura H, Nakao K, Shimatsu A, et al: Lymphocytic infundibuloneurohypophysitis as a cause of central diabetes insipidus. N Engl J Med 329:683–689, 1993.
127. Kojima H, Nojima T, Nagashima K, et al: Diabetes insipidus caused by lymphocytic infundibuloneurohypophysitis. Arch Pathol Lab Med 113:1399–1401, 1989.
128. Van Havenbergh T, Robberecht W, Wilms G, et al: Lymphocytic infundibulohypophysitis presenting in the postpartum period: Case report. Surg Neurol 46:280–284, 1996.
129. Nishioka H, Ito H, Sano T, et al: Two cases of lymphocytic hypophysitis presenting with diabetes insipidus: A variant of lymphocytic infundibulo-neurohypophysitis. Surg Neurol 46:285–290, 1996.
130. Thodou E, Asa SL, Kontogeorgos G, et al: Clinical case seminar: lymphocytic hypophysitis: Clinicopathological findings. J Clin Endocrinol Metab 80:2302–2311, 1995.
131. Scherbaum WA, Bottazzo GF, Czernichow P: Role of autoimmunity in central diabetes insipidus. *In* Czernichow P, Robinson AG (eds): Diabetes insipidus in man. Basel, Karger, 1985, pp 232–239.

132. De Bellis A, Colao A, Di Salle F, et al: A longitudinal study of vasopressin cell anti-bodies, posterior pituitary function, and magnetic resonance imaging evaluations in subclinical autoimmune central diabetes insipidus. J Clin Endocrinol Metab 84:3047–3051, 1999.

133. Zerbe RL, Robertson GL: A comparison of plasma vasopressin measurements with a standard indirect test in the differential diagnosis of polyuria. N Engl J Med 305:1539–1546, 1981.

134. Hollinshead WH: The interphase of diabetes insipidus. Mayo Clin Proc 39:92–100, 1964.

135. Verbalis JG, Robinson AG, Moses AM: Postoperative and post-traumatic diabetes insipidus. In Czernichow P, Robinson AG (eds): Diabetes Insipidus in Man. Basel, Karger, 1984, pp 247–265.

136. Cusick JF, Hagen TC, Findling JW: Inappropriate secretion of antidiuretic hormone after transsphenoidal surgery for pituitary tumors. N Engl J Med 311:36–38, 1984.

137. Olson BR, Rubino D, Gumowski J, et al: Isolated hyponatremia after transsphenoidal pituitary surgery. J Clin Endocrinol Metab 80:85–91, 1995.

138. Olson BR, Gumowski J, Rubino D, et al: Pathophysiology of hyponatremia after trans-sphenoidal pituitary surgery. J Neurosurg 87:499–507, 1997.

139. Ultmann MC, Hoffman GE, Nelson PB, et al: Transient hyponatremia after damage to the neurohypophyseal tracts. Neuroendocrinology 56:803–811, 1992.

140. Daniel PM, Prichard MM: Regeneration of hypothalamic nerve fibres after hypophy-sectomy in the goat. Acta Endocrinol (Copenh) 64:696–704, 1970.

141. Daniel PM, Prichard MM: The human hypothalamus and pituitary stalk after hypoph-ysectomy or pituitary stalk section. Brain 95:813–824, 1972.

142. Block LH, Furrer J, Locher RA, et al: Changes in tissue sensitivity to vasopressin in hereditary hypothalamic diabetes insipidus. Klin Wochenschr 59:831–836, 1981.

143. DeRubertis FR, Michelis MF, Davis BB: "Essential" hypernatremia. Report of three cases and review of the literature. Arch Intern Med 134:889–895, 1974.

144. Halter JB, Goldberg AP, Robertson GL, et al: Selective osmoreceptor dysfunction in the syndrome of chronic hypernatremia. J Clin Endocrinol Metab 44:609–616, 1977.

145. Baylis PH, Thompson CJ: Osmoregulation of vasopressin secretion and thirst in health and disease. Clin Endocrinol (Oxf) 29:549–576, 1988.

146. Takaku A, Shindo K, Tanaka S, et al: Fluid and electrolyte disturbances in patients with intracranial aneurysms. Surg Neurol 11:349–356, 1979.

147. McIver B, Connacher A, Whittle I, et al: Adipsic hypothalamic diabetes insipidus after clipping of anterior communicating artery aneurysm. BMJ 303:1465–1467, 1991.

148. DeRubertis FR, Michelis MF, Beck N, et al: "Essential" hypernatremia due to ineffec-tive osmotic and intact volume regulation of vasopressin secretion. J Clin Invest 50:97–111, 1971.

149. Smith D, McKenna K, Moore K, et al: Baroregulation of vasopressin release in adipsic diabetes insipidus. J Clin Endocrinol Metab 87:4564–4568, 2002.

150. Phillips PA, Bretherton M, Johnston CI, et al: Reduced osmotic thirst in healthy elderly men. Am J Physiol 261:R166–R171, 1991.

151. Hodak SP, Verbalis JG: Abnormalities of water homeostasis in aging. Endocrinol Metab Clin North Am 34:1031–1046, 2005.

152. Durr JA, Hoggard JG, Hunt JM, et al: Diabetes insipidus in pregnancy associated with abnormally high circulating vasopressinase activity. N Engl J Med 316:1070–1074, 1987.

153. Durr JA: Diabetes insipidus in pregnancy. Am J Kidney Dis 9:276–283, 1987.

154. Gordge MP, Williams DJ, Huggett NJ, et al: Loss of biological activity of arginine vasopressin during its degradation by vasopressinase from pregnancy serum. Clin Endocrinol (Oxf) 42:51–58, 1995.

155. Baylis PH, Thompson C, Burd J, et al: Recurrent pregnancy-induced polyuria and thirst due to hypothalamic diabetes insipidus: An investigation into possible mecha-nisms responsible for polyuria. Clin Endocrinol (Oxf) 24:459–466, 1986.

156. Barron WM, Cohen LH, Ulland LA, et al: Transient vasopressin-resistant diabetes insipidus of pregnancy. N Engl J Med 310:442–444, 1984.

157. van Lieburg AF, Verdijk MA, Schoute F, et al: Clinical phenotype of nephrogenic diabetes insipidus in females heterozygous for a vasopressin type 2 receptor mutation. Hum Genet 96:70–78, 1995.

158. Morello JP, Bichet DG: Nephrogenic diabetes insipidus. Annu Rev Physiol 63:607–630, 2001.

159. Sadeghi H, Robertson GL, Bichet DG, et al: Biochemical basis of partial nephrogenic diabetes insipidus phenotypes. Mol Endocrinol 11:1806–1813, 1997.

160. Wildin RS, Cogdell DE, Valadez V: AVPR2 variants and V2 vasopressin receptor func-tion in nephrogenic diabetes insipidus. Kidney Int 54:1909–1922, 1998.

161. Pasel K, Schulz A, Timmermann K, et al: Functional characterization of the molecular defects causing nephrogenic diabetes insipidus in eight families. J Clin Endocrinol Metab 85:1703–1710, 2000.

162. Wildin RS, Cogdell DE: Clinical utility of direct mutation testing for congenital nephrogenic diabetes insipidus in families. Pediatrics 103:632–639, 1999.

163. Chan Seem CP, Dossetor JF, Penney MD: Nephrogenic diabetes insipidus due to a new mutation of the arginine vasopressin V2 receptor gene in a girl presenting with non-accidental injury. Ann Clin Biochem 36(pt 6):779–782, 1999.

164. Deen PM, Knoers NV: Vasopressin type-2 receptor and aquaporin-2 water channel mutants in nephrogenic diabetes insipidus. Am J Med Sci 316:300–309, 1998.

165. Knoers NV, Deen PM: Molecular and cellular defects in nephrogenic diabetes insipi-dus. Pediatr Nephrol 16:1146–1152, 2001.

166. Canfield MC, Tamarappoo BK, Moses AM, et al: Identification and characterization of aquaporin-2 water channel mutations causing nephrogenic diabetes insipidus with partial vasopressin response. Hum Mol Genet 6:1865–1871, 1997.

167. van Os CH, Deen PM: Aquaporin-2 water channel mutations causing nephrogenic diabetes insipidus. Proc Assoc Am Physicians 110:395–400, 1998.

168. Tamarappoo BK, Verkman AS: Defective aquaporin-2 trafficking in nephrogenic dia-betes insipidus and correction by chemical chaperones. J Clin Invest 101:2257–2267, 1998.

169. Morello JP, Salahpour A, Laperriere A, et al: Pharmacological chaperones rescue cell-surface expression and function of misfolded V2 vasopressin receptor mutants. J Clin Invest 105:887–895, 2000.

170. Knepper MA, Verbalis JG, Nielsen S: Role of aquaporins in water balance disorders. Curr Opin Nephrol Hypertens 6:367–371, 1997.

171. Nielsen S, Kwon TH, Christensen BM, et al: Physiology and pathophysiology of renal aquaporins. J Am Soc Nephrol 10:647–663, 1999.

172. Marples D, Frokiaer J, Dorup J, et al: Hypokalemia-induced downregulation of aqua-porin-2 water channel expression in rat kidney medulla and cortex. J Clin Invest 97:1960–1968, 1996.

173. Earm JH, Christensen BM, Frokiaer J, et al: Decreased aquaporin-2 expression and apical plasma membrane delivery in kidney collecting ducts of polyuric hypercalce-mic rats. J Am Soc Nephrol 9:2181–2193, 1998.

174. Sands JM, Naruse M, Jacobs JD, et al: Changes in aquaporin-2 protein contribute to the urine concentrating defect in rats fed a low-protein diet. J Clin Invest 97:2807–2814, 1996.

175. Frokiaer J, Christensen BM, Marples D, et al: Downregulation of aquaporin-2 parallels changes in renal water excretion in unilateral ureteral obstruction. Am J Physiol 273:F213–F223, 1997.

176. Bendz H, Aurell M: Drug-induced diabetes insipidus: Incidence, prevention and management. Drug Saf 21:449–456, 1999.

177. Christensen S, Kusano E, Yusufi AN, et al: Pathogenesis of nephrogenic diabetes insipidus due to chronic administration of lithium in rats. J Clin Invest 75:1869–1879, 1985.

178. Marples D, Christensen S, Christensen EI, et al: Lithium-induced downregulation of aquaporin-2 water channel expression in rat kidney medulla. J Clin Invest 95:1838–1845, 1995.

179. Bendz H, Sjodin I, Aurell M: Renal function on and off lithium in patients treated with lithium for 15 years or more. A controlled, prospective lithium-withdrawal study. Nephrol Dial Transplant 11:457–460, 1996.

180. Markowitz GS, Radhakrishnan J, Kambham N, et al: Lithium nephrotoxicity: A pro-gressive combined glomerular and tubulointerstitial nephropathy. J Am Soc Nephrol 11:1439–1448, 2000.

181. Fernandez-Llama P, Andrews P, Ecelbarger CA, et al: Concentrating defect in experi-mental nephrotic syndrome: Altered expression of aquaporins and thick ascending limb Na⁺ transporters. Kidney Int 54:170–179, 1998.

182. Terris J, Ecelbarger CA, Nielsen S, et al: Long-term regulation of four renal aquaporins in rats. Am J Physiol 271:F414–F422, 1996.

183. Harrington AR, Valtin H: Impaired urinary concentration after vasopressin and its gradual correction in hypothalamic diabetes insipidus. J Clin Invest 47:502, 1968.

184. Goldman MB, Luchins DJ, Robertson GL: Mechanisms of altered water metabolism in psychotic patients with polydipsia and hyponatremia. N Engl J Med 318:397–403, 1988.

185. de Leon J, Verghese C, Tracy JI, et al: Polydipsia and water intoxication in psychiatric patients: A review of the epidemiological literature. Biol Psychol 35:408–419, 1994.

186. Robertson GL: Differential diagnosis of polyuria. Annu Rev Med 39:425–442, 1988.

187. Valtin H: "Drink at least eight glasses of water a day." Really? Is there scientific evi-dence for "8 x 8"? Am J Physiol Regul Integr Comp Physiol 283:R993–R1004, 2002.

188. Goldman MB, Robertson GL, Luchins DJ, et al: The influence of polydipsia on water excretion in hyponatremic, polydipsic, schizophrenic patients. J Clin Endocrinol Metab 81:1465–1470, 1996.

189. Vieweg WV, Carey RM, Godleski LS, et al: The syndrome of psychosis, intermittent hyponatremia, and polydipsia: Evidence for diurnal volume expansion. Psychol Med 8:135–144, 1990.

190. Cheng JC, Zikos D, Skopicki HA, et al: Long-term neurologic outcome in psychogenic water drinkers with severe symptomatic hyponatremia: the effect of rapid correction. Am J Med 88:561–566, 1990.

191. Vieweg WV, Robertson GL, Godleski LS, et al: Diurnal variation in water homeostasis among schizophrenic patients subject to water intoxication. Schizophr Res 1:351–357, 1988.

192. Goldman MB, Robertson GL, Luchins DJ, et al: Psychotic exacerbations and enhanced vasopressin secretion in schizophrenic patients with hyponatremia and polydipsia. Arch Gen Psychiatry 54:443–449, 1997.

193. Adrogue HJ, Madias NE: Hypernatremia. N Engl J Med 342:1493–1499, 2000.

194. Palevsky PM, Bhagrath R, Greenberg A: Hypernatremia in hospitalized patients. Ann Intern Med 124:197–203, 1996.

195. Riggs JE: Neurologic manifestations of fluid and electrolyte disturbances. Neurol Clin 7:509–523, 1989.

196. Palevsky PM: Hypernatremia. Semin Nephrol 18:20–30, 1998.

197. Gullans SR, Verbalis JG: Control of brain volume during hyperosmolar and hypoos-molar conditions. Annu Rev Med 44:289–301, 1993.

198. Ayus JC, Armstrong DL, Arieff AI: Effects of hypernatraemia in the central nervous system and its therapy in rats and rabbits. J Physiol 492(pt 1):243–255, 1996.

199. Kahn A, Brachet E, Blum D: Controlled fall in natremia and risk of seizures in hyper-tonic dehydration. Intensive Care Med 5:27–31, 1979.

200. Robertson GL: Diabetes insipidus. Endocrinol Metab Clin North Am 24:549–572, 1995.

201. Miller M, Dalakos T, Moses AM, et al: Recognition of partial defects in antidiuretic hormone secretion. Ann Intern Med 73:721–729, 1970.

202. Moses AM: Clinical and laboratory observations in the adult with diabetes insipidus and related syndromes. In Czernichow P, Robinson AG (eds): Diabetes Insipidus in Man. Karger, Basel, 1985, pp 156–175.

203. Robinson AG: Disorders of antidiuretic hormone secretion. Clin Endocrinol Metab 14:55–88, 1985.

204. Baylis PH, Gaskill MB, Robertson GL: Vasopressin secretion in primary polydipsia and cranial diabetes insipidus. Q J Med 50:345–358, 1981.

205. Milles JJ, Spruce B, Baylis PH: A comparison of diagnostic methods to differentiate diabetes insipidus from primary polyuria: A review of 21 patients. Acta Endocrinol (Copenh) 104:410–416, 1983.

206. Fujisawa I, Asato R, Nishimura K, et al: Anterior and posterior lobes of the pituitary gland: Assessment by 1.5 T MR imaging. J Comput Assist Tomogr 11:214–220, 1987.

207. Arslan A, Karaarslan E, Dincer A: High intensity signal of the posterior pituitary. A study with horizontal direction of frequency-encoding and fat suppression MR techniques. Acta Radiol 40:142–145, 1999.

208. Kurokawa H, Fujisawa I, Nakano Y, et al: Posterior lobe of the pituitary gland: Correlation between signal intensity on T1-weighted MR images and vasopressin concentration. Radiology 207:79–83, 1998.

209. Moses AM, Clayton B, Hochhauser L: Use of T1-weighted MR imaging to differentiate between primary polydipsia and central diabetes insipidus. Comment. [see comments]. AJNR Am J Neuroradiol 13:1273–1277, 1992.

210. Brooks BS, el Gammal T, Allison JD, et al: Frequency and variation of the posterior pituitary bright signal on MR images. AJNR Am J Neuroradiol 10:943–948, 1989.

211. Maghnie M, Genovese E, Bernasconi S, et al: Persistent high MR signal of the posterior pituitary gland in central diabetes insipidus. AJNR Am J Neuroradiol 18:1749–1752, 1997.

212. Dohanics J, Hoffman GE, Verbalis JG: Chronic hyponatremia reduces survival of magnocellular vasopressin and oxytocin neurons following axonal injury. J Neurosci 16:2372–2380, 1996.

213. Bonneville JF, Cattin F, Dietemann JL: The pituitary stalk. In Bonneville JF (ed): Computed Tomography of the Pituitary Gland. New York, Springer-Verlag, 1986, pp 106–114.

214. Leger J, Velasquez A, Garel C, et al: Thickened pituitary stalk on magnetic resonance imaging in children with central diabetes insipidus. J Clin Endocrinol Metab 84:1954–1960, 1999.

215. Czernichow P, Garel C, Leger J: Thickened pituitary stalk on magnetic resonance imaging in children with central diabetes insipidus. Horm Res 53(suppl 3):61–64, 2000.

216. Bruck E, Abal G, Aceto T,Jr: Pathogenesis and pathophysiology of hypertonic dehydration with diarrhea. A clinical study of 59 infants with observations of respiratory and renal water metabolism. Am J Dis Child 115:122–144, 1968.

217. Blum D, Brasseur D, Kahn A, et al: Safe oral rehydration of hypertonic dehydration. J Pediatr Gastroenterol Nutr 5:232–235, 1986.

218. Fjellestad-Paulsen A, Hoglund P, Lundin S, et al: Pharmacokinetics of 1-deamino-8-D-arginine vasopressin after various routes of administration in healthy volunteers. Clin Endocrinol (Oxf) 38:177–182, 1993.

219. Robinson AG: DDAVP in the treatment of central diabetes insipidus. N Engl J Med 294:507–511, 1976.

220. Sklar AH, Schrier RW: Central nervous system mediators of vasopressin release. Physiol Rev 63:1243–1280, 1983.

221. Hoffman PK, Share L, Crofton JT, et al: The effect of intracerebroventricular indomethacin on osmotically stimulated vasopressin release. Neuroendocrinology 34:132–139, 1982.

222. Nadler SP, Hebert SC, Brenner BM: PGE$_2$, forskolin, and cholera toxin interactions in rabbit cortical collecting tubule. Am J Physiol 250:F127–F135, 1986.

223. Allen HM, Jackson RL, Winchester MD, et al: Indomethacin in the treatment of lithium-induced nephrogenic diabetes insipidus. Arch Intern Med 149:1123–1126, 1989.

224. Delaney V, de Pertuz Y, Nixon D, et al: Indomethacin in streptozocin-induced nephrogenic diabetes insipidus. Am J Kidney Dis 9:79–83, 1987.

225. Magaldi AJ: New insights into the paradoxical effect of thiazides in diabetes insipidus therapy. Nephrol Dial Transplant 15:1903–1905, 2000.

226. Richardson DW, Robinson AG: Desmopressin. Ann Intern Med 103:228–239, 1985.

227. Lam KS, Wat MS, Choi KL, et al: Pharmacokinetics, pharmacodynamics, long-term efficacy and safety of oral 1-deamino-8-D-arginine vasopressin in adult patients with central diabetes insipidus. Br J Clin Pharmacol 42:379–385, 1996.

228. Rittig S, Jensen AR, Jensen KT, et al: Effect of food intake on the pharmacokinetics and antidiuretic activity of oral desmopressin (DDAVP) in hydrated normal subjects. Clin Endocrinol (Oxf) 48:235–241, 1998.

229. Dunn AL, Powers JR, Ribeiro MJ, et al: Adverse events during use of intranasal desmopressin acetate for haemophilia A and von Willebrand disease: A case report and review of 40 patients. Haemophilia 6:11–14, 2000.

230. Robson WL, Norgaard JP, Leung AK: Hyponatremia in patients with nocturnal enuresis treated with DDAVP. Eur J Pediatr 155:959–962, 1996.

231. Schwab M, Wenzel D, Ruder H: Hyponatraemia and cerebral convulsion due to short term DDAVP therapy for control of enuresis nocturna. Eur J Pediatr 155:46–48, 1996.

232. Lugo N, Silver P, Nimkoff L, et al: Diagnosis and management algorithm of acute onset of central diabetes insipidus in critically ill children. J Pediatr Endocrinol Metab 10:633–639, 1997.

233. Ralston C, Butt W: Continuous vasopressin replacement in diabetes insipidus. Arch Dis Child 65:896–897, 1990.

234. Davison JM, Sheills EA, Philips PR, et al: Metabolic clearance of vasopressin and an analogue resistant to vasopressinase in human pregnancy. Am J Physiol 264:F348–F353, 1993.

235. Kallen BA, Carlsson SS, Bengtsson BK: Diabetes insipidus and use of desmopressin (minirin) during pregnancy. Eur J Endocrinol 132:144–146, 1995.

236. Ray JG: DDAVP use during pregnancy: An analysis of its safety for mother and child. Obstet Gynecol Surv 53:450–455, 1998.

237. Iwasaki Y, Oiso Y, Kondo K, et al: Aggravation of subclinical diabetes insipidus during pregnancy. N Engl J Med 324:522–526, 1991.

238. Libber S, Harrison H, Spector D: Treatment of nephrogenic diabetes insipidus with prostaglandin synthesis inhibitors. J Pediatr 108:305–311, 1986.

239. Kirchlechner V, Koller DY, Seidl R, et al: Treatment of nephrogenic diabetes insipidus with hydrochlorothiazide and amiloride. Arch Dis Child 80:548–552, 1999.

240. Uyeki TM, Barry FL, Rosenthal SM, et al: Successful treatment with hydrochlorothiazide and amiloride in an infant with congenital nephrogenic diabetes insipidus. Pediatr Nephrol 7:554–556, 1993.

241. Cesar KR, Magaldi AJ: Thiazide induces water absorption in the inner medullary collecting duct of normal and Brattleboro rats. Am J Physiol 277:F756–F760, 1999.

242. Usberti M, Dechaux M, Guillot M, et al: Renal prostaglandin E2 in nephrogenic diabetes insipidus: Effects of inhibition of prostaglandin synthesis by indomethacin. J Pediatr 97:476–478, 1980.

243. Chevalier RL, Rogol AD: Tolmetin sodium in the management of nephrogenic diabetes insipidus. J Pediatr 101:787–789, 1982.

244. Batlle DC, von Riotte AB, Gaviria M, et al: Amelioration of polyuria by amiloride in patients receiving long-term lithium therapy. N Engl J Med 312:408–414, 1985.

245. Singer I, Oster JR, Fishman LM: The management of diabetes insipidus in adults. Arch Intern Med 157:1293–1301, 1997.

246. Postina R, Ufer E, Pfeiffer R, et al: Misfolded vasopressin V2 receptors caused by extracellular point mutations entail congenital nephrogenic diabetes insipidus. Mol Cell Endocrinol 164:31–39, 2000.

247. Robertson GL: Abnormalities of thirst regulation. Kidney Int 25:460–469, 1984.

248. Canuso CM, Goldman MB: Clozapine restores water balance in schizophrenic patients with polydipsia-hyponatremia syndrome. J Neuropsychiatry Clin Neurosci 11:86–90, 1999.

249. Robertson GL: Dipsogenic diabetes insipidus: A newly recognized syndrome caused by a selective defect in the osmoregulation of thirst. Trans Assoc Am Phys 100:241–249, 1987.

250. Anderson RJ: Hospital-associated hyponatremia. Kidney Int 29:1237, 1986.

251. Hawkins RC: Age and gender as risk factors for hyponatremia and hypernatremia. Clin Chim Acta 337:169–172, 2003.

252. Wattad A, Chiang ML, Hill LL: Hyponatremia in hospitalized children. Clin Pediatr (Phila) 31:153, 1992.

253. Saito T: Hyponatremia in elderly patients. Intern Med 40:851, 2001.

254. Kumar S, Berl T: Sodium. Lancet 352:220–228, 1998.

255. Turchin A, Seifter JL, Seely EW: Clinical problem-solving. Mind the gap. N Engl J Med 349:1465–1469, 2003.

256. Steinberger BA, Ford SM, Coleman TA: Intravenous immunoglobulin therapy results in post-infusional hyperproteinemia, increased serum viscosity, and pseudohyponatremia. Am J Hematol 73:97–100, 2003.

257. Perez-Perez AJ, Pazos B, Sobrado J, et al: Acute renal failure following massive mannitol infusion. Am J Nephrol 22:573–575, 2002.

258. Guglielminotti J, Pernet P, Maury E, et al: Osmolar gap hyponatremia in critically ill patients: Evidence for the sick cell syndrome? Crit Care Med 30:1051–1055, 2002.

259. Hillier TA, Abbott RD, Barrett EJ: Hyponatremia: Evaluating the correction factor for hyperglycemia. Am J Med 106:399–403, 1999.

260. Ayus JC, Arieff AI: Glycine-induced hypo-osmolar hyponatremia. Arch Intern Med 557:223, 1997.

261. Berl T, Schrier RW: Disorders of water metabolism. In Schrier RW (ed): Renal and Electrolyte Disorders, 6th ed. Philadelphia, Lippincott Williams & Wilkins, 2003.

262. Robertson GL: Physiopathology of ADH secretion. In Tolis G, Labrie F, Martin JB, et al (eds): Clinical Neuroendocrinology: A Pathophysiological Approach. New York, Raven Press, 1070, p 247.

263. Nguyen MK, Kurtz I: New insights into the pathophysiology of the dysnatremias: A quantitative analysis. Am J Physiol Renal Physiol 287:F172–F180, 2004.

264. Sterns R: Sodium and water balance disorders. Neph SAP 5:35–50, 2006.

265. Parikh C, Kumar S, Berl T: Disorders of water metabolism. In Johnson RR, Feehaly J (eds): Comprehensive Clinical Nephrology, 3rd ed. St Louis, CV Mosby, 2007 (in press).

266. Androgue HJ, Madias NE. Hyponatremia. N Engl J Med 342:1581–1589, 2000.

267. Chow KM, Kwan BC, Szeto CC: Clinical studies of thiazide-induced hyponatremia. J Natl Med Assoc 96:1305–1308, 2004.

268. Sonnenblick M, Friedlander Y, Rosin AJ: Diuretic induced severe hyponatremia. Review and analysis of 129 reported patients. Chest 103:601, 1993.

269. Sharabi Y, Illan R, Kamari Y, et al: Diuretic induced hyponatraemia in elderly hypertensive women. J Hum Hypertens 16:631–635, 2002.

270. Clark B, Shannon R, Rosa R, Epstein F: Increased susceptibility to thiazide induced hyponatremia in the elderly. J Am Soc Nephrol 5:1106, 1994.

271. Berl T: Water metabolism in potassium depletion. Miner Electrolyte Metab 4:209, 1980.

272. Fichman MP, Vorherr H, Kleeman CR, Tefler N: Diuretic induced hyponatremia. Ann Intern Med 75:853, 1971.

273. Danovitch GM, Bourgoignie J, Bricker NS: Reversibility of the salt losing tendency of chronic renal failure. N Engl J Med 296:14, 1977.

274. Schrier RW, Linas SL: Mechanisms of the defect in water excretion in adrenal insufficiency. Miner Electrolyte Metab 4:1, 1980.

275. Boykin J, McCool A, Robertson G, et al: Mechanisms of impaired water excretion in mineralocorticoid deficient dogs. Miner Electrolyte Metab 2:310, 1979.

276. Schrier RW: Body water homeostasis: Clinical disorders of urinary dilution and concentration. J Am Soc Nephrol 17:1820–1832, 2006.

277. Palmer BF: Hyponatremia in patients with central nervous system disease: SIADH versus CSW. Trends Endocrinol Metab 14.182–187, 2003.

278. Bohn S, Carlotti P, Cusimono M, et al: Cerebral salt wasting: Truth, fallacies, theories and challenges. Crit Care Med 30:2575, 2002.

279. Oh MS, Carroll HJ: Cerebral salt-wasting syndromes. Crit Care Clin 17:125–138, 2001.

280. McGirt MJ, Blessing R, Nimjee SM, et al: Correlation of serum brain natriuretic peptide with hyponatremia and delayed ischemic neurological deficits after subarachnoid hemorrhage. Neurosurgery 54:1369–1373; discussion 1373–1364, 2004.

281. Schrier RW, Gurevich AK, Cadnapaphornchai MA: Pathogenesis and management of sodium and water retention in cardiac failure and cirrhosis. Semin Nephrol 2:157–172, 2002.

282. Ishikawa S, Saito S, Okada K, et al: Effect of vasopressin antagonist on water excretion in vena cava constriction. Kidney Int 30:49, 1986.

283. Szatalowicz VL, Arnold PE, Chaimovitz C, et al: Radioimmunoassay of plasma arginine vasopressin in hyponatremic patients with congestive heart failure. N Engl J Med 305:263, 1981.

284. Kim JK, Michel JB, Soubrier F, Schrier RW: Arginine vasopressin gene expression in chronic cardiac failure in rats. Kidney Int 38:818, 1990.

285. Ferguson DW, Berg WJ, Sanders JS: Clinical and hemodynamic correlates of sympathetic nerve activity in normal humans and patients with heart failure. Evidence from direct microneurographic recordings. J Am Coll Cardiol 16:1125, 1990.

286. Benedict C, Johnston D, Weiner D, et al: Relation of neurohumoral activation to clinical variables and degrees of ventricular dysfunction. J Am Coll Cardiol 23:1410, 1994.

287. Lee W, Packer M: Prognostic importance of serum sodium concentration and its modification by converting enzyme inhibitors. Circulation 73:257, 1986.

288. Nielsen S, Torris D, Andersen C: Congestive heart failure in rats is associated with increased expression and targeting of aquaporin 2 water channel in collecting duct. Proc Natl Acad Sci U S A 94:5450, 1997.

289. Xu DL, Martin P-Y, Ohara M, et al: Upregulation of aquaporin 2 water channel expression in chronic heart failure rat. J Clin Invest 99:1500, 1997.

290. Martin PY, Abraham WT, Lieming X, et al: Selective V_2-receptor vasopressin antagonism decreases urinary aquaporin-2 excretion in patients with chronic heart failure. J Am Soc Nephrol 10:2165–2170, 1999.

291. Gines P, Berl T, Bernardi M, et al: Hyponatremia in cirrhosis: From pathogenesis to treatment. Hepatology 28:851–864, 1998.

292. Schrier RW: Mechanisms of disturbed renal water excretion in cirrhosis. Gastroenterology 84:870, 1983.

293. Arroyo V, Jimenez W: Complications of cirrhosis: Renal and circulatory dysfunction, light shadows in an important clinical problem. J Hepatol 32(suppl 1):157, 2000.

294. Unikowsky B, Wexler JJ, Levy M: Dogs with experimental cirrhosis of the liver but without intrahepatic hypertension do not retain sodium or form ascites. J Clin Invest 72:1594, 1983.

295. Rahman SN, Abraham W, Schrier RW: Peripheral arterial vasodilation in cirrhosis. Gastroenterol Int 5:192, 1992.

296. Kim J, Summer S, Howard R, Schrier RW: Vasopressin gene expression in rats with experimental cirrhosis. Hepatology 17:143, 1993.

297. Claria J, Jimenez W, Arroyo V, et al: Blockade of the hydroosmotic effect of vasopressin normalizes water excretion in cirrhotic rats. Gastroenterology 97:1294, 1989.

298. Fujita N, Ishikawa S, Sasaki S: Role of water channel AQP-CD in water retention in SIADH and cirrhotic rats. Am J Physiol 269:F926, 1994.

299. Fernandez-Llama P, Jimenez W, Bosch-Marce M, et al: Dysregulation of renal aquaporins and Na-Cl cotransporter in CCl4-induced cirrhosis. Kidney Int 58:216–228, 2000.

300. Fernandez-Llama, P, Turner R, Dibona G, Knepper MA: Renal expression of aquaporins in liver cirrhosis induced by chronic common bile duct ligation in rats. J Am Soc Nephrol 10:1950–1957, 1999.

301. Bichet D, Van Putten VJ, Schrier RW: Potential role of increased sympathetic activity in impaired sodium and water excretion in cirrhosis. N Engl J Med 307:1552, 1982.

302. Floras J, Legaut L, Morali GA: Increased sympathetic outflow in cirrhosis and ascites. Direct evidence from intraneural recordings. Ann Intern Med 114:373, 1991.

303. Bichet DG, Groves BM, Schrier RW: Mechanism of improvement of water and sodium excretion by enhancement of central hemodynamics in decompensated cirrhosis. Kidney Int 24:788, 1983.

304. Shapiro M, Nichols K, Groves B, Schrier RW: Interrelationship between cardiac output and vascular resistance as determinants of effective arterial blood volume in cirrhotic patients. Kidney Int 28:201, 1985.

305. Weigert A, Martin P, Niederberger M: Edothelium-dependent vascular hyporesponsiveness without detection of nitric oxide synthase induction in aorta of cirrhotic rats. Hepatology 22:1856, 1997.

306. Martin P-Y, Ohara M, Gines P: Nitric oxide synthase (NOS) inhibition for one week improves sodium and water retention in cirrhotic rats with ascites. J Clin Invest 201:235, 1998.

307. Martin P-Y, Gines P, Schrier RW: Nitric oxide as a mediator of hemodynamic abnormalities and sodium and water retention in cirrhosis. N Engl J Med 339:533, 1998.

308. Abraham W, Cadnapopornchai M, Schrier RW: Cardiac failure, liver disease and nephrotic syndrome. In Schrier RW, Gottschalk CW (eds): Disease of the Kidney, 7th ed. Philadelphia, Lippincott Williams & Wilkins, 2001, pp 2465.

309. Usberti M, Federico S, Mecariello S, et al: Role of plasma vasopressin in the impairment of water excretion in nephrotic syndrome. Kidney Int 25:422, 1984.

310. Kimagi H, Onayma K, Isehi K: Role of renin-angiotensin-aldosterone in minimal change nephrotic syndrome. Clin Nephrol 25:229, 1985.

311. Meltzer JI, Keim HJ, Laragh JH, et al: Nephrotic syndrome: Vasoconstriction and hypervolemic types indicated by renin-sodium profiling. Ann Intern Med 91:688, 1979.

312. Schrier RW, Fasset RG: A critique of the overfill hypothesis of sodium and water retention in the nephrotic syndrome. Kidney Int 53:1111, 1998.

313. Ichikawa I, Rennke HG, Hoyer JR, et al: Role of intrarenal mechanisms in the impaired salt excretion in experimental nephrotic syndrome. J Clin Invest 71:91, 1983.

314. Apostol E, Ecelbarger CA, Terris J, et al: Reduced renal medullary water channel expression in puromycin aminonucleoside–induced nephrotic syndrome. J Am Soc Nephrol 8:15–24, 1997.

315. Fernandez-Llama P, Andrews P, Ecelbarger CA, et al: Concentrating defect in experimental nephrotic syndrone: Altered expression of aquaporins and thick ascending limb Na^+ transporters. Kidney Int 54:170–179, 1998.

316. Gross P, Raascher W: Vasopressin and hyponatremia in renal insufficiency. Contrib Nephrol 50:54, 1986.

317. Weiss NM, Robertson GL: Water metabolism in endocrine disorders. Semin Nephrol 4:303, 1987.

318. Ishikawa S, Fujisawa G, Tsuboi Y, et al: Role of antidiuretic hormone in hyponatremia in patients with isolated adrenocorticotropic hormone deficiency. Endocrinol Jpn 38:325, 1991.

319. Oelkers W: Hyponatremia and inappropriate secretion of vasopressin in patients with hypopituitarism. N Engl J Med 321:492, 1989.

320. Boykin J, de Torrente A, Erickson A, et al: Role of plasma vasopressin in impaired water excretion of glucocorticoid deficiency. J Clin Invest 62:738, 1978.

321. Linas SL, Berl T, Robertson GL, et al: Role of vasopressin in the impaired water excretion of glucocorticoid deficiency. Kidney Int 18:58, 1980.

322. Pyo HI, Summer SN, Kim JK: Vasopressin gene expression in glucocorticoid hormone deficient rats. Ann N Y Acad Sci 689:659, 1993.

323. Kim JK, Summer SN, Wood WM, et al: Role of glucocorticoid hormones in arginine vasopressin gene regulation. Biochem Biophys Res Commun 289:1252–1256, 2001.

324. Berghorn KA, Knapp LT, Hoffman GE, Sherman TG: Induction of glucocorticoid receptor expression in hypothalamus neurons during chronic hypoosmolality. Endocrinology 136:804, 1995.

325. Schwartz MJ, Kokko JP: Urinary concentrating defect of adrenal insufficiency. Permissive role of adrenal steroids on the hydroosmotic response across the rabbit collecting tubule. J Clin Invest 66:234, 1980.

326. Jackson BA, Braun-Werness J, Kusano E, Dousa T: Concentrating defect in adrenalectomized rat. J Clin Invest 72:997, 1983.

327. Kwon TH, Nielson J, Masilamani S, et al: Regulation of collection duct AQP3 expression response to mineralocorticoid. Am J Physiol Renal Physiol 283:F1403–F1421, 2002.

328. Olchovsky D, Ezra D, Vered I, et al: Symptomatic hyponatremia as a presenting sign of hypothalamic-pituitary disease: A syndrome of inappropriate secretion of antidiuretic hormone (SIADH)—like glucocorticosteroid responsive condition. J Endocrinol Invest 28:151–156, 2005.

329. Diederich S, Franzen NF, Bahr V, et al: Severe hyponatremia due to hypopituitarism with adrenal insufficiency: Report on 28 cases. Eur J Endocrinol 148:609–617, 2003.

330. Hanna F, Scanlon M: Hyponatremia, hypothyroidism and role of arginine vasopressin. Lancet 350:755, 1997.

331. Hochberg Z, Benderly A: Normal osmotic threshold for vasopressin release in the hyponatremia of hypothyroidism. Horm Res 18:128, 1983.

332. Iwasaki Y, Oiso Y, Yamauchi K: Osmoregulation of plasma vasopressin in myxedema. J Clin Endocrinol Metab 70:534, 1990.

333. Howard R, Summer S, Rossi N: Short term hypothyroidism and vasopressin gene expression in the rat. Am J Kidney Dis 19:573, 1992.

334. Seif SM, Robinson AG, Zenser TV, et al: Neurohypophyseal peptides in hypothyroid rats: Plasma levels and kidney response. Metabolism 28:137, 1979.

335. Harckom TM, Kim JK, Palumbo PJ, et al: Medullary effect of thyroid function on enzymes of the vasopressin-sensitive adenosine 3′,5′-monophosphate system in renal medulla. Endocrinology 102:1475, 1978.

336. Cadnapaphornchai MA, Kim YW, Gurevich AK, et al: Urinary concentrating defect in hypothyroid rats: Role of sodium, potassium, 2-chloride co-transporter, and aquaporins. J Am Soc Nephrol 14:566–574, 2003.

337. Chen YC, Cadnapaphornchai MA, Yang J, et al: Nonosmotic release of vasopressin and renal aquaporins in impaired urinary dilution in hypothyroidism. Am J Physiol Renal Physiol 289:F672–F678, 2005.

338. Riggs AT, Dysken MW, Kim SW, Opsahl JA: A review of disorders of water homeostasis in psychiatric patients. Psychosomatics 32:133, 1991.

339. Hariprasad MK, Eisinger RP, Nadler IM, et al: Hyponatremia in psychogenic polydipsia. Arch Intern Med 140:1639–1642, 1980.

340. Jose CJ, Perez Crult J: Incidence and morbidity of self-induced water intoxication in state mental hospital patients. Am J Psychiatry 136:221, 1979.

341. Shah PJ, Greenberg WM: Water intoxication precipitated by thiazide diuretics in polydipsic psychiatric patients. Am J Psychiatry 148:1424–1425, 1991.

342. Brows RP, Koesis JM, Cohen SK: Delusional depression and inappropriate antidiuretic hormone secretion. Biol Psychiatry 18:1059, 1983.

343. Goldman MB, Robertson GL, Luchins DJ, et al: Psychotic exacerbations and enhanced vasopressin secretion in schizophrenic patients with hyponatremia and polydipsia. Arch Gen Psychiatry 54:443–449, 1997.

344. Kawai N, Atsuomi B, Toshihito S, Hiroyasu S: Roles of arginine vasopressin and atrial natriuretic peptide in polydipsia-hyponatremia of schizophrenic patients. Psychiatry Res 101:37–45, 2001.

345. Berl T: Psychosis and water balance. N Engl J Med 318:441, 1988.

346. Fenves AZ, Thomas S, Knochel JP: Beer potomania: Two cases and review of the literature. Clin Nephrol 45:61–64, 1996.

347. Musch W, Xhaet O, Decaux G: Solute loss plays a major role in polydipsia-related hyponatraemia of both water drinkers and beer drinkers. QJM 96:421–426, 2003.

348. Hoorn EJ, Geary D, Robb M, et al: Acute hyponatremia related to intravenous fluid administration in hospitalized children: An observational study. Pediatrics 113:1279–1284, 2004.

349. Chung H-M, Kluge R, Schrier RW, Anderson RJ: Post-operative hyponatremia. Arch Intern Med 146:333, 1986.

350. Tambe AA, Hill R, Livesley PJ: Post-operative hyponatraemia in orthopaedic injury. Injury 34:253–255, 2003.

351. Anderson RJ, Chung H-M, Kluge R, Schrier RW: Hyponatremia: A prospective analysis of its epidemiology and the pathogenetic role of vasopressin. Ann Intern Med 102:164, 1985.

352. Shafiee MA, Charest AF, Cheema-Dhadli S, et al: Defining conditions that lead to the retention of water: The importance of the arterial sodium concentration. Kidney Int 67:613–621, 2005.

353. Steele A. Growishankar A, Abramson S, et al: Postoperative hyponatremia despite near isotonic saline infusion. A phenomenon of desalination. Ann Intern Med 126:20, 1997.

354. Aronson D, Dragu RE, Nakhoul F, et al: Hyponatremia as a complication of cardiac catheterization: a prospective study. Am J Kidney Dis 40:940–946, 2002.

355. Arieff AI: Permanent neurological disability from hyponatremia in healthy women undergoing elective surgery. N Engl J Med 314:1529, 1986.

356. Ayus JC, Wheeler J, Arieff AI: Postoperative hyponatremic encephalopathy in menstruant women. Ann Intern Med 117:891, 1992.

357. O'Brien KK, Montain SJ, Corr WP, et al: Hypernatremia associated with hyponatremia in US Army trainees. Mil Med 166:405–410, 2001.

358. Davis DP, Videen JS, Marino A, et al: Exercise associated hyponatremia in marathon runners: A two year experience. J Emerg Med 21:47–57, 2001.

359. Montain SJ, Sawka MN, Wenger CB: Hyponatremia associated with exercise: Risk factors and pathogenesis. Exerc Sports Sci Rev 29:113–117, 2001.

360. Almond CS, Shin AY, Fortescue EB, et al: Hyponatremia among runners in the Boston Marathon. N Engl J Med 352:1550–1556, 2005.

361. Noakes TD, Sharwood K, Collins M, et al.: The dipsomania of great distance: Water intoxication in an Ironman triathlete. Br J Sports Med 38:E16, 2004.

362. Bertholini DM, Butler CS: Severe hyponatraemia secondary to desmopressin therapy in von Willebrand's disease. Anaesth Intensive Care 28:199–201, 2000.

363. Schwab M, Wenzel D, Ruder H: Hyponatraemia and cerebral convulsion due to short term DDAVP therapy for control of enuresis nocturna. Eur J Pediatr 155:46–48, 1996.

364. Shindel A, Tobin G, Klutke C: Hyponatremia associated with desmopressin for the treatment of nocturnal polyuria. Urology 60:344, 2002.

365. Hirokawa CA, Gray DR: Chlorpropamide-induced hyponatremia in the veteran population. Ann Pharmacother 26:1243, 1992.

366. Mendoza SA, Brown CF Jr: Effect of chlorpropamide on osmotic water flow across toad bladder and the response to vasopressin, theophylline and cyclic AMP. J Clin Endocrinol Metab 38:883–889, 1974.

367. Durr JA, Hensen J, Ehnis T, et al: Chlorpropamide upregulates antidiuretic hormone receptors and unmasks constitutive receptor signaling. Am J Physiol Renal Physiol 278:F799–F808, 2000.

368. Kusano B, Brain-Werness JL, Vich DJ, et al: Chlorpropamide action on renal concentrating mechanism in rats with hypothalamic diabetes insipidus. J Clin Invest 72:1298, 1983.

369. Kastner T, Friedman DL, Pond WS: Carbamazepine-induced hyponatremia in patients with mental retardation. Am J Ment Retard 96:536, 1992.

370. Cooney JA: Carbamazepine and SIADH. Am J Psychiatry 147:1101, 1990.

371. Steinhoff BJ, Stoll KD, Stodieck SR, Paulus W: Hyponatremic coma under oxcarbazepine therapy. Epilepsy Res 11:67, 1995.

372. Meinders HE, Cejka V, Robertson GL: Antidiuretic action of carbamazepine. Clin Sci Mol Med 47:289, 1974.

373. Gold PW, Robertson GL, Ballenger J, et al: Carbamazepine diminishes the sensitivity of the plasma arginine vasopressin response to osmotic stimulation. J Clin Endocrinol Metab 57:952, 1983.

374. Kosten TR, Camp W: Inappropriate secretion of antidiuretic hormone in a patient receiving piperazine phenothiazines. Psychosomatics 21:351, 1980.

375. Peck V, Shenkman L: Haloperidol-induced syndrome of inappropriate secretion of antidiuretic hormone. Clin Pharmacol Ther 26:442, 1979.

376. Beckstrom D, Reding R, Cerletti J: Syndrome of inappropriate antidiuretic hormone secretion associated with amitriptyline administration. JAMA 241:133, 1979.

377. Cherney DZ, Davids MR, Halperin ML: Acute hyponatremia and "ecstasy": Insights from a quantative and integrated analysis. Q J Med 95:475–483, 2002.

378. Budisavljevic MN, Stewart L, Sahn SA, et al: Hyponatremia associated with 3,4-methylenedioxymethylamphetamine ("Ecstasy") abuse. Am J Med Sci 326:89–93, 2003.

379. Vishwanath BM, Vavalgund A, Cusando W, et al: Fluoxetine as a cause of SIADH. Am J Psychiatry 148:542, 1991.

380. Kessler J, Samuels S: Sertraline and hyponatremia. Letter. N Engl J Med 335:524, 1996.

381. Fabian TJ, Amico JA, Kroboth PD, et al: Paroxetine-induced hyponatremia in the elderly due to the syndrome of inappropriate secretion of antidiuretic hormone (SIADH). J Geriatr Psychiatry Neurol 16:160–164, 2003.

382. Spigset O, Hedermalm K: Hyponatremia in relation to treatment with antidepressants. Pharmacotherapy 17:348, 1997.

383. Kirby D, Harrigan S, Ames D: Hyponatremia in elderly psychiatric patients treated with selective serotonin reuptake inhibitors and venlafaxine: A retrospective controlled study in an inpatient unit. Int J Geriatr Psychiatry 17:231–237, 2002.

384. Strachan J, Shepherd J: Hyponatraemia associated with the use of selective serotonin reuptake inhibitors. Aust N Z J Psychiatry 32:295–298, 1998.

385. Bouman WP, Pinner G, Johnson H: Incidence of selective serotonin reuptake inhibitor (SSRI) induced hyponatraemia due to the syndrome of inappropriate antidiuretic hormone (SIADH) secretion in the elderly. Int J Geriatr Psychiatry 13:12–15, 1998.

386. Robertson GL, Bhoopalam N, Zelkowitz LJ: Vincristine neurotoxicity and abnormal secretion of antidiuretic hormone. Arch Intern Med 132:717, 1973.

387. Hammond IW, Ferguson JA, Kwong K, et al: Hyponatremia and syndrome of inappropriate anti-diuretic hormone reported with the use of vincristine: An over-representation of Asians? Pharmacoepidemiol Drug Saf 11:229–234, 2002.

388. Bode U, Seif SM, Levine AS: Studies on the antidiuretic effect of cyclophosphamide vasopressin release and sodium excretion. Med Pediatr Oncol 8:295, 1980.

389. Culine S, Ghosn M, Droz J: Inappropriate antidiuretic hormone secretion induced by ifosfamide. Eur J Cancer 26:922, 1990.

390. Subramanian D, Ayus JC: Case report: Severe symptomatic hyponatremia associated with lisinopril therapy. Am J Med Sci 303:177, 1992.

391. Castrillon JL, Mediavilla A, Mendez MA, et al: Syndrome of inappropriate antidiuretic hormone secretion (SIADH) and enalapril. J Intern Med 233:89, 1993.

392. Gonzalex-Martinez H, Gaspard JJ, Espino DV: Hyponatremia due to enalapril in an elderly patient. A case report. Arch Fam Med 2:791, 1993.

393. Aslam MK, Gnaim C, Kutnick J, et al: Syndrome of inappropriate antidiuretic hormone secretion induced by amiodarone therapy. Pacing Clin Electrophysiol 27:831–832, 2004.

394. Schwartz WB, Bennett W, Curelop S, Bartter FC: A syndrome of renal sodium loss and hyponatremia probably resulting from inappropriate secretion of antidiuretic hormone. Am J Med 23:529, 1957.

395. Bartter FE, Schwartz WB: The syndrome of inappropriate secretion of antidiuretic hormone. Am J Med 42:790, 1967.

396. Thaler S, Teitelbaum I, Berl T: "Beer potamania" in beer drinkers. Effect of low dietary solute intake. Am J Kidney Dis 31:1028, 1998.

397. Passamonte PM: Hypouricemia, inappropriate secretion of antidiuretic hormone, and small cell carcinoma of the lung. Arch Intern Med 144:1569, 1984.

398. DiGiovanni SR, Nielsen S, Christensen E, et al: Regulation of collection duct water channel expression by vasopressin in Brattleboro rat. Proc Natl Acad Sci U S A 91:8984, 1994.

399. Saito T, Ishikawa S, Ando F, et al: Exaggerated urinary excretion of aquaporin 2 in the pathological state of impaired water excretion dependent upon arginine vasopressin. J Clin Endocrinol Metab 83:4043, 1998.

400. Leaf A, Bartter FC, Santos RF, Woony O: Evidence in man that urine electrolyte loss induced by Pitressin is a function of water retention. J Clin Invest 32:868, 1953.

401. Verbalis J: An experimental model of syndrome of inappropriate antidiuretic hormone secretion in the rat. Am J Physiol 247:E540, 1984.

402. Verbalis JG, Drutarosky M: Adaptation to chronic hypoosmolality in rats. Kidney Int 34:351, 1988.

403. Verbalis JG: Pathogenesis of hyponatremia in an experimental model of inappropriate antidiuresis. Am J Physiol 267:R1617, 1994.

404. Nelson PB, Seif SM, Maroon JC, Robinson AG: Hyponatremia in intracranial disease: Perhaps not the syndrome of inappropriate secretion of antidiuretic hormone. J Neurosurg 55:938, 1991.

405. Diringer MN, Lim JS, Kirsch JR, Hanley DF: Suprasellar and intraventricular blood predicts elevated plasma atrial natriuretic factor in subarachnoid hemorrhage. Stroke 22:577, 1991.

406. Anderson RJ: Arginine vasopressin escape. In vivo and in vitro studies. In Cowley AW, Liard JK, Ausiello DA (eds): Vasopressin: Cellular and Integrative Function. New York, Raven Press, 1988, p 215.

407. Eggena P, Ma CL: Downregulation of vasopressin receptors in toad bladder. Am J Physiol 250:C453, 1986.

408. Tian Y, Sandberg K, Murase T, et al: VasopressinR_x receptor binding is downregulated during renal escape from vasopressin antidiuresis. Endocrinology 141:307, 2000.

409. Ecelbarger C, Chou C, Lee A, et al: Escape from vasopressin-induced antidiuresis: Role of vasopressin resistance of the collecting duct. Am J Physiol 274:F1161, 1998.

410. Ecelbarger C, Nielsen S, Olson BR, et al: Role of renal aquaporins in escape from vasopressin antidiuresis in rat. J Clin Invest 99:1852, 1997.

411. Ecelbarger C, Verbalis J, Knepper M: Increased abundance of distal sodium transporters in rat kidney during vasopressin escape. J Am Soc Nephrol 12:207, 2001.

412. Berl T, Schrier RW. Disorders of water metabolism. In Schrier RW (ed): Renal and Electrolyte Disorders, 6th ed. Philadelphia, Lippincott, Williams & Wilkins, 2003, p 1.

413. Tang WW, Kaptein EM, Feinstein EI, Massry SG: Hyponatremia in hospitalized patients with the acquired immunodeficiency syndrome and the AIDS related complex. Am J Med 94:169, 1993.

414. Putterman C, Levy L, Rubinger D: Transient exercise induced water intoxication and rhabdomyolysis. Am J Kidney Dis 21:206, 1993.

415. Irving RA, Noakes TD, Buck R, et al: Evaluation of renal function and fluid homeostasis during recovery from exercise induced hyponatremia. J Appl Physiol 70:342, 1991.

416. Miller M, Hecker MS, Friedlander DA, et al: Apparent idiopathic hyponatremia in an ambulatory geriatric population. J Am Geriatr Soc 44:404–408, 1996.

417. Anpalahan M: Chronic idiopathic hyponatremia in older people due to the syndrome of inappropriate antidiuretic hormone secretion (SIADH) possibly related to aging. J Am Geriatr Soc 49:788–792, 2001.

418. Hirshberg B, Ben-Yehuda A: The syndrome of inappropriate antidiuretic hormone secretion in the elderly. Am J Med 103:270–273, 1997.

419. Arinzon Z, Feldman J, Jarchowsky J, et al: A comparative study of the syndrome of inappropriate antidiuretic hormone secretion in community-dwelling patients and nursing home residents. Aging Clin Exp Res 15:6–11, 2003.

420. Ishikawa SE, Saito T, Fukagawa A, et al: Close association of urinary excretion of aquaporin-2 with appropriate and inappropriate arginine vasopressin-dependent antidiuresis in hyponatremia in elderly subjects. J Clin Endocrinol Metab 86:1665–1671, 2001.

421. List AF, Hainsworth JD, Davis BW, et al: The syndrome of inappropriate secretion of antidiuretic hormone (SIADH) in small cell lung cancer. J Clin Oncol 4:1191, 1986.

422. Coyle S, Penney MD, Masters PW, Walker BE: Early diagnosis of ectopic arginine vasopressin secretion. Clin Chem 39:152, 1993.

423. Hussain SF, Irfan M, Abbasi M, et al: Clinical characteristics of 110 miliary tuberculosis patients from a low HIV prevalence country. Int J Tuberc Lung Dis 8:493–499, 2004.

424. Feldman BJ, Rosenthal SM, Vargas GA, et al: Nephrogenic syndrome of inappropriate antidiuresis. N Engl J Med 352:1884–1890, 2005.

425. Zerbe R, Stropes L, Robertson G: Vasopressin function in the syndrome of inappropriate antidiuresis. Annu Rev Med 31:315, 1980.

426. Renneboog B, Musch W, Vandemergel X, et al: Mild chronic hyponatremia is associated with falls, unsteadiness, and attention deficits. Am J Med 119:e71–78, 2006.

427. Fraser CL, Arieff AI: Epidemiology, pathophysiology, and management of hyponatremic encephalopathy. Am J Med 102:67, 1997.

428. Verbalis JG: SIADH and other hypoosmolar disorders. *In* Schrier RW (ed): Diseases of the Kidney and Urinary Tract. Philadelphia, Lippincott Williams & Wilkins, 2007, pp 2219–2248.

429. Ayus JC, Varon J, Arieff AI: Hyponatremia, cerebral edema, and noncardiogenic pulmonary edema in marathon runners. Ann Intern Med 132:711–714, 2000.

430. Manley GT, Fujimura M, Ma T, et al: Aquaporin-4 deletion in mice reduces brain edema after acute water intoxication and ischemic stroke. Nat Med 6:159–163, 2000.

431. Nzerue CM, Baffoe-Bonnie H, You W, et al: Predictors of outcome in hospitalized patients with severe hyponatremia. J Natl Med Assoc 95:335–343, 2003.

432. Wijdicks EF, Larson TS: Absence of postoperative hyponatremia syndrome in young, healthy females. Ann Neurol 35:626, 1994.

433. Baran D, Hutchinson TA: The outcome of hyponatremia in a general hospital population. Clin Nephrol 22:72, 1984.

434. Goldberg A, Hammerman H, Petcherski S, et al: Prognostic importance of hyponatremia in acute ST-elevation myocardial infarction. Am J Med 117:242–248, 2004.

435. Lee DS, Austin PC, Rouleau JL, et al: Predicting mortality among patients hospitalized for heart failure: Derivation and validation of a clinical model. JAMA 290:2581–2587, 2003.

436. Ruf AE, Dremers WK, Chavez LL, et al: Addition of serum sodium into the MELD score predicts waiting list mortality better than MELD alone. Liver Transpl 11:336–343, 2005.

437. Heuman DM, Abou-Assi SG, Habib A, et al: Persistent ascites and low serum sodium identify patients with cirrhosis and low MELD scores who are at high risk for early death. Hepatology 40:802–810, 2004.

438. Sterns RH: Severe symptomatic hyponatremia: Treatment and outcome. Ann Intern Med 107:656, 1987.

439. Berl T: Treating hyponatremia. What is all the controversy about? Ann Intern Med 113:417, 1990.

440. McJunkin JE, de los Reyes EC, Irazuzta JE, et al: La Crosse encephalitis in children. N Engl J Med. 34:801–807, 2001.

441. Tierney WM, Martin DK, Greenlee MC, et al: The prognosis of hyponatremia in hospital admission. J Gen Intern Med 1:380, 1986.

442. Sterns RH: The treatment of hyponatremia. Am J Med 88:557, 1990.

443. Pasantes-Morales H, Franco R, Ordaz B, et al: Mechanisms counteracting swelling in brain cells during hyponatremia. Arch Med Res 33:237–244, 2002.

444. Lien YH, Shapiro UI, Chan L: Study of brain electrolytes and organic osmolytes during correction of chronic hyponatremia. Implication for the pathogenesis of central pontine myelinolysis. J Clin Invest 88:303, 1991.

445. Verbalis JG, Gullans SR: Hyponatremia causes large sustained reductions in brain content of multiple organic osmolytes in rats. Brain Res 567:274, 1991.

446. Verbalis JG, Gullans SR: Rapid correction of hyponatremia produces differential effects on brain osmolyte and electrolyte reaccumulation in rats. Brain Res 606:19, 1993.

447. Berl T: Treating hyponatremia. Are we damned if we do and damned if we don't? Kidney Int 37:1008, 1990.

448. Soupart A, Silver S, Schroeder B, et al: Rapid (24 hour) reaccumulation of brain organic osmolytes (particularly *myo*-inositol) in azotemic rats after correction of chronic hyponatremia. J Am Soc Nephrol 13:1433–1441, 2002.

449. Thurman J, Halterman R, Berl T: Treatment of dysnatremic disorders in therapy in nephrology and hypertension. *In* Brady H, Wilcox C (eds): Therapy in Nephrology and Hypertension. Philadelphia, WB Saunders, 2003.

450. Gross P: Treatment of severe hyponatremia. Kidney Int 60:2417–2427, 2001.

451. Sterns RH, Riggs JE, Schochet SS: Osmotic demyelination syndrome following correction of hyponatremia. N Engl J Med 314:1535, 1986.

452. Oh MS, Kim HJ, Carroll HJ: Recommendation for treatment of symptomatic hyponatremia. Nephrology 70:143, 1995.

453. Ayus JC, Krothapalli RK, Arieff AI: Treatment of symptomatic hyponatremia and its relation to brain damage. N Engl J Med 317:1190, 1987.

454. Ayus JC, Arieff AI: Chronic hyponatremic encephalopathy in postmenopausal women: Association of therapies with morbidity and mortality. JAMA 281:2299–2304, 1999.

455. Ashouri OS: Severe diuretic induced hyponatremia in the elderly: A series of eight patients. Arch Intern Med 146:1355, 1986.

456. Vexler Z, Ayus C, Roberts T, et al: Hypoxic and ischemic hypoxia exacerbates injury associated with metabolic encephalopathy in laboratory animals. J Clin Invest 93:256, 1994.

457. Fraser CL, Sarnacki P: Na$^+$-K$^+$-ATPase pump function in male rat brain synaptosomes is different from that of females. Am J Physiol 257:E284, 1989.

458. Dickinson LD, Betz AL: Attenuated development of ischemic brain edema in vasopressin deficient rats. J Cereb Blood Flow Metab 12:681, 1992.

459. Rosenberg GA, Scremin O, Estrada E, Kyner WT: Arginine vasopressin V_1 antagonist and atrial natriuretic peptide reduce hemorrhagic brain edema in rats. Stroke 23:1767, 1992.

460. Ayus JC, Arieff AI: Pathogenesis and prevention of hyponatremic encephalopathy. Endocrinol Metab Clin North Am 22:425, 1993.

461. Ayus JC, Krothapalli RK, Armstrong DL: Rapid correction of severe hyponatremia in the rat: Histopathological changes in the brain. Am J Physiol 248:F711, 1985.

462. Martin RJ: Central pontine and extrapontine myelinolysis: The osmotic demyelination syndromes. J Neurol Neurosurg Psychiatry 75(suppl 3):iii22–iii28, 2004.

463. Tan H, Onbas O: Central pontine myelinolysis central pontine myelinolysis manifesting with massive myoclonus. Pediatr Neurol 31:64–66, 2004.

464. Menger H, Jorg J: Outcome of central pontine and extrapontine myelinolysis. J Neurol 246:700–705, 1999.

465. Ruzek KA, Campeau NG, Miller GM: Early diagnosis of central pontine myelinolysis with diffusion-weighted imaging. AJNR Am J Neuroradiol 25:210–213, 2004.

466. Soupart A, Penninck R, Stenuit R, et al: Treatment of chronic hyponatremia in rats by intravenous saline: Comparison of rate versus magnitude of correction. Kidney Int 41:1662, 1992.

467. Verbalis JG, Martinez AJ: Neurological and neuropathological sequelae of correction of chronic hyponatremia. Kidney Int 39:1274, 1991.

468. Sterns RH: Severe hyponatremia. The case for conservative management. Crit Care Med 20:534, 1992.

469. Barsoum NR, Levine BS: Current prescriptions for the corrections of hyponatremia and hypernatremia: Are they too simple? Nephrol Dial Transplant 17:1176–1180, 2002.

470. Carlotti AP, Bohn D, Mallie JP, Halperin ML: Tonicity balance, and not electrolyte-free water calculations, more accurately guides therapy for acute changes in natremia. Intensive Care Med 27:921–924, 2001.

471. Soupart A, Pennirek U, Creniar L, et al: Prevention of brain demyelination in rats after excessive correction of chronic hyponatremia by serum sodium lowering. Kidney Int 45:193, 1994.

472. Coldszmidt MA, Iliescu EA: DDAVP to prevent rapid correction in hyponatremia. Clin Nephrol 53:226–229, 2000.

473. Oya S, Tsutsumi K, Ueki K, Kirino T: Reinduction of hyponatremia to treat central pontine myelinolysis. Neurology 57:1931–1932, 2001.

474. Furst H, Hallows KR, Post J, et al: The urine/plasma electrolyte ratio: A predictive guide to water restriction. Am J Med Sci 319:240–244, 2000.

475. Forrest JN, Cox M, Hong C, et al: Superiority of demeclocycline over lithium in the treatment of chronic syndrome of inappropriate secretion of antidiuretic hormone. N Engl J Med 298:173, 1978.

476. Decaux G, Genette F: Urea for long term treatment of syndrome of inappropriate secretion of antidiuretic hormone. BMJ 283:1081, 1981.

477. Decaux G, Waterlot Y, Genette F, Mockel J: Treatment of the syndrome of inappropriate secretion of antidiuretic hormone with furosemide. N Engl J Med 304:329, 1981.

478. Greenberg A, Verbalis JG: Vasopressin receptor antagonists. Kidney Int 69:2124–2130, 2006.

479. Kim JK, Dillingham MD, Summer SN, et al: Effects of vasopressin antagonist on the cellular action of vasopressin binding, adenylate cyclase activation and water flux. J Clin Invest 76:1530, 1985.

480. Macion-Dazard R, Callahan N, Xu Z, et al: Mapping the binding site of six nonpeptide antagonists to the human V2-renal vasopressin receptor. J Pharmacol Exp Ther 316:564–571, 2006.

481. Ohnishi A, Orita Y, Okahara R: Potent aquaretic agent: A novel nonpeptide selective vasopressin antagonist OPC 31260 in man. J Clin Invest 92:2653, 1993.

482. Fujisawa G, Ishikawa S, Okada K, Saito T: Therapeutic efficacy of non-peptide ADH antagonist OPC-31260 in SIADH rats. Kidney Int 44:19, 1993.

483. Saito T, Ishikawa S, Abe K: Acute aquaresis by the nonpeptide arginine vasopressin antagonist OPC 31260 improves hyponatremia in patients with the syndrome of inappropriate secretion of antidiuretic hormone. J Clin Endocrinol Metab 82:1054, 1997.

484. Schrier RW, Gross P, Gheorghiade M, et al: Tolvaptan, a selective oral vasopressin V2-receptor antagonist, for hyponatremia. N Engl J Med 355:2099–2112, 2006.

485. Decaux G: Difference in solute excretion during correction of hyponatremic patients with cirrhosis or syndrome of inappropriate secretion of antidiuretic hormone by oral vasopressin V_2 receptor antagonist VPA-985. J Lab Clin Med 138:18–21, 2001.

486. Decaux G: Long-term treatment of patients with inappropriate secretion of antidiuretic hormone by the vasopressin receptor antagonist conivaptan, urea, or furosemide. Am J Med 110:582–584, 2001.

487. Guyader D, Patat A, Ellis-Grosse EJ, Orczyk GP: Pharmacodynamic effects of a nonpeptide antidiuretic hormone V_2 antagonist in cirrhotic patients with ascites. Hepatology 36(5):1197–1205, 2002.

488. Gerbes AL, Gulberg V, Gines P, et al: Therapy of hyponatremia in cirrhosis with a vasopressin receptor antagonist: A randomized double blind multicenter trial. Gastroenterology 124:933–939, 2003.

489. Abraham WT, Shamshirsaz AA, McFann K, et al: Aquaretic effect of lixivaptan, an oral, non-peptide, selective V2 receptor vasopressin antagonist, in New York Heart Association functional class II and III chronic heart failure patients. J Am Coll Cardiol 47:1615–1621, 2006.

490. Gheorghiade M, Niazi I, Ouyang J, et al: Vasopressin V2-receptor blockade with tolvaptan in patients with chronic heart failure: Results from a double-blind, randomized trial. Circulation 107:2690–2696, 2003.

491. Gheorghiade M, Gattis WA, O'Connor CM, et al: Effects of tolvaptan, a vasopressin antagonist, in patients hospitalized with worsening heart failure: A randomized controlled trial. JAMA 291:1963–1971, 2004.

492. Gheorghiade M, Konstam MA, Burnett JC, Jr., et al: Short-term clinical effects of tolvaptan, an oral vasopressin antagonist, in patients hospitalized for heart failure: the EVEREST Clinical Status Trials. JAMA 297:1332–1343, 2007.

493. Konstam MA, Gheorghiade M, Burnett JC, Jr., et al: Effects of oral tolvaptan in patients hospitalized for worsening heart failure: the EVEREST Outcome Trial. JAMA 297:1319–1331, 2007.

CHAPTER 14

Disorders of Acid-Base Balance

Thomas D. DuBose, Jr.

The appropriate diagnosis and management of acid-base disorders in acutely ill patients requires accurate and timely interpretation of the specific acid-base disorder. Appropriate interpretation requires simultaneous measurement of plasma electrolytes and arterial blood gases (ABGs), as well as an appreciation by the clinician of the physiologic adaptations and compensatory responses that occur with specific acid-base disturbances. In most circumstances, these compensatory responses can be predicted through an analysis of the prevailing disorder in a stepwise sequence.

The maintenance of systemic pH requires the integration of a number of physiologic mechanisms, including cellular and extracellular buffering and the compensatory actions of the kidneys and lungs.

This chapter reviews acid-base homeostasis as a consequence of acid-base chemistry and physiology but places major emphasis on the pathophysiologic basis, diagnosis, and management of clinical acid-base disorders. The diagnosis of acid-base disorders is reviewed in detail, with emphasis on a simple stepwise approach, founded on appreciation of the predictable compensatory responses to primary acid-base disturbances.

▐ ACID-BASE HOMEOSTASIS

Acid-base homeostasis operates to maintain systemic arterial pH within a narrow range. Although the normal range for clinical laboratories is between 7.35 and 7.45 pH units, pH in vivo in an individual subject is maintained in a much more narrow range. This degree of tight regulation is accomplished through (1) chemical buffering in the extracellular fluid (ECF) and the intracellular fluid (ICF) and (2) regulatory responses that are under the control of the respiratory and renal systems. Those chemical buffers, respiration, and renal processes efficiently dispose of the physiologic daily load of carbonic acid (as volatile CO_2) and nonvolatile acids and defend against the occasional addition of pathologic quantities of acid and alkali. Therefore, chemical buffers within the extracellular and intracellular compartments serve to blunt changes in pH that would occur with retention of either acids or bases. In addition, the control of CO_2 tension (P_{CO_2}) by the central nervous system and respiratory system and the control of the plasma HCO_3^- by the kidneys constitute the regulatory processes that act in concert to stabilize the arterial pH.

The major buffer system in the body comprises a base (H^+ acceptor), which is predominantly HCO_3^-, and an acid (H^+ donor), which is predominantly carbonic acid (H_2CO_3):

$$H^+ + HCO_3^- \Leftrightarrow H_2CO_3 \quad (1)$$

Extracellular H^+ concentration ($[H^+]_e$) throughout the body is constant in the steady state. The HCO_3^-/H_2CO_3 ratio is proportional to the ratio of all the other extracellular buffers (B^-/HB) such as PO_4^{3-} and plasma proteins:

$$[H^+]_e \propto \frac{HCO_3^-}{H_2CO_3} \propto \frac{B^-}{HB} \quad (2)$$

The intracellular H^+ concentration ($[H^+]_i$), or pH_i, is also relatively stable, maintaining, under most circumstances, a fairly constant relationship to the extracellular H^+ concentration. Both cellular ion exchange mechanisms and intracellular buffers (hemoglobin, tissue proteins, organophosphate complexes, and bone apatite) participate in the blunting of changes in both $[H^+]_i$ and $[H^+]_e$. Extracellular and intracellular buffers provide the *first line of defense* against addition of acid or base to the body (see Mechanisms of pH Buffering, later).

The second line of defense is the respiratory system. Pulmonary participation in acid-base homeostasis relies on the excretion of CO_2 by the lungs. The reaction is catalyzed by the enzyme carbonic anhydrase:

$$H^+ + HCO_3^- \leftrightarrow H_2CO_3 \xleftarrow[\text{anhydrase}]{\text{Carbonic}} H_2O + CO_2 \quad (3)$$

Large amounts of CO_2 (10–12 mol/day) accumulate as metabolic end products of tissue metabolism. This CO_2 load is transported in the blood to the lungs as hemoglobin-generated HCO_3^- and hemoglobin-bound carbamino groups.[1]

$$\text{Metabolism} \to CO_2 \xleftrightarrow[\text{transport}]{\text{Blood}} \text{Lungs} \quad (4)$$

Conventionally, H^+ concentration is expressed in two different ways, either directly as $[H^+]$ or indirectly as pH. The relationship between these two factors can be written in mathematically equivalent forms:

$$pH = -\log_{10}[H^+] \tag{5}$$

$$[H^+] \, (Eq/L) = 10^{-pH} \tag{6}$$

When $[H^+]$ is expressed (for numeric convenience) in nanomoles per liter (nmol/L) or nanometers (nM), then

$$[H^+] = 10^{9-pH} \tag{7}$$

Buffer Systems

Acid-base chemistry deals with molecular interactions that involve the transfer of H^+. A large variety of molecules, both inorganic and organic, contain hydrogen atoms that can dissociate to yield H^+. As defined classically, an acid is a molecular species that can function as an H^+ donor; a base is a molecular species that can serve as an H^+ acceptor. The relationship between an undissociated acid (HA) and its conjugate, disassociated base (A^-) may be represented as

$$HA \Leftrightarrow H^+ + A^- \tag{8}$$

Besides the many inorganic and organic acid-base substances encountered in biologic systems, many protein molecules (e.g., hemoglobin) contain acidic groups that may dissociate, yielding a corresponding conjugate base.

Mechanisms of pH Buffering

Buffer systems are critical to the physiology and pathophysiology of acid-base homeostasis and, in their broadest definition, are systems that attenuate the pH change in a solution or tissue by reversibly combining with or releasing H^+. Thus, the pH change of a solution during addition of acid or base equivalents, in the presence of a buffer system, is smaller than would have occurred if no buffer systems were present. The acid or base load can be **extrinsic,** such as during systemic acid or base infusion, or **intrinsic,** resulting from net generation of new acid or base equivalents that are added to the extracellular or intracellular space.

Chemical Equilibria of Physicochemical Buffer Systems

As an example of a physicochemical buffer pair, consider a neutral weak acid (HA) and its conjugate weak base (A^-). Examples of such buffer pairs include acetic acid and acetate and the carboxyl groups on proteins. Another example of a physicochemical buffer pair is a neutral weak base (B) and its conjugate weak acid (BH^+):

$$BH^+ \Leftrightarrow B + H^+ \tag{9}$$

Examples of such buffer pairs are NH_3 and NH_4^+ and the imidazole group in proteins. A rigorous analysis of the kinetics of reversible reactions in solution yields the law of mass action, which states that, at equilibrium (i.e., when the velocities of the forward and backward reactions are equal), the ratio of the concentration products of opposing reactions is a constant.

$$K_a' = \frac{[H^+][A^-]}{HA} \tag{10}$$

$$K_b' = \frac{[H^+][B^-]}{BH} \tag{11}$$

K_a' and K_b' are the equilibrium or dissociation constants for Equations 10 and 11, respectively.

Taking logarithms of both sides of Equations 10 and 11 and defining $pK_a' = -\log_{10}(K_a')$ and $pK_b' = -\log_{10}(K_b')$ yields

$$pH = pK_a' + \log_{10}\frac{[A^-]}{[HA]} \tag{12}$$

$$pH = pK_b' + \log_{10}\frac{[B^-]}{[BH]} \tag{13}$$

The dissociation constants K_a' and K_b' provide an estimate of the strength of the acid and base, respectively. From Equations 12 and 13, it can be seen that the buffer pairs are half dissociated at $pH = pK'$. In other words, pK' of a buffer pair is defined as the pH at which 50% of the buffer pair exists as the weak acid (HA) and 50% as the anion (A^-).

Chemical Equilibria for the Carbon Dioxide–Bicarbonate System

When CO_2 is dissolved in water, H_2CO_3 is formed according to the reaction

$$CO_2 + H_2O \Leftrightarrow H_2CO_3 \tag{14}$$

The rate of this reaction, in the absence of the enzyme carbonic anhydrase, is slow, with a half-time of about 8 seconds at 37°C. The major portion of CO_2 remains as dissolved CO_2; only about 1 part in 1000 forms H_2CO_3, a nonvolatile acid. Because H_2CO_3 is a weak acid, it dissociates to yield H^+ and HCO_3^-.

$$H_2CO_3 \Leftrightarrow H^+ + HCO_3^- \tag{15}$$

The concentration of dissolved CO_2 is given by Henry's law:

$$[CO_2]_{dis} = \alpha_{CO_2} PCO_2 \tag{16}$$

where α_{CO_2} is the physical solubility coefficient for CO_2, which has a value of 0.0301 mmol/L in most body fluids, including plasma. Because the concentration of H_2CO_3 is low and proportional to the concentration of dissolved CO_2, Equations 14 and 15 can be combined and treated as a single reaction:

$$CO_2 + H_2O \Leftrightarrow H^+ + HCO_3^- \tag{17}$$

The equilibrium constant for this reaction is given by

$$K = \frac{[H^+][HCO_3^-]}{[CO_2][H_2O]} \tag{18}$$

Defining $K' = K[H_2O]$ as the apparent equilibrium constant and using Equation 17,

$$K' = \frac{[H^+][HCO_3^-]}{\alpha_{CO_2} PCO_2} \tag{19}$$

Taking logarithms of both sides of Equation 19 and recognizing that $pK' = -\log_{10}(K')$, the familiar Henderson-Hasselbalch equation is derived:

$$pH = pK' + \log_{10}\frac{[HCO_3^-]}{(\alpha_{CO_2} PCO_2)} \tag{20}$$

Using $pK' = 6.1$ in Equation 20, the Henderson equation is derived, which may be utilized in clinical interpretation of acid-base data:

$$[H^+](nmol/L) = 24\frac{PCO_2(mmHg)}{[HCO_3^-](mM)} \tag{21}$$

The Physiologic Advantage of an Open Buffer System

The quantitative behavior of an open system buffer pair differs considerably from that in which the buffer pair is confined to a closed system. In an open system, the buffer pair may be envisioned as occurring in two separate but communicating compartments (internal and external). The external compartment provides an effective infinite reservoir of the uncharged buffer pair component, to which the barrier between the internal and the external compartments (e.g., plasma cell membrane, vascular capillary endothelium) is freely permeable.

Physiologically, the most important open system buffer is the CO_2-HCO_3^- system. Adjustments in alveolar ventilation serve to maintain a constant $PaCO_2$:

$$\text{acid } (H^+)\downarrow \qquad\qquad \uparrow\uparrow \text{ (expired gas)}$$
$$H^+ + HCO_3^- \rightarrow H_2CO_3 \rightarrow H_2O + CO_2 \qquad (22)$$

The CO_2-HCO_3^- buffer system has a pK' of 6.1 and a base-to-acid ($[HCO_3^-]/[H_2CO_3]$) ratio of 20:1 at pH 7.4. Because buffer efficiency is greatest in the pH range near pK_a', it appears at first glance that the CO_2-HCO_3^- system would not function as an effective buffer in the physiologic pH range. The potency and efficacy of the CO_2-HCO_3^- buffer system are due largely to the augmentation of buffer capacity that accompanies operation in an open system. Because CO_2 is freely diffusible across biologic barriers and cell membranes, its concentration in biologic fluids can be modulated rapidly through participation of the respiratory system. When acid (H^+) is added to an HCO_3^--containing fluid, H^+ combines with HCO_3^- to generate H_2CO_3, which, in the presence of the enzyme carbonic anhydrase, is rapidly dehydrated to CO_2 (Equation 22). The CO_2 produced can escape rapidly from the fluid and be excreted in the lung, preventing accumulation of CO_2 concentrations in biologic fluids.

Regulation of Buffers

The plasma HCO_3^- concentration is protected by both metabolic and renal regulatory mechanisms. In addition, the pH of blood can be affected by respiratory adjustments in $PaCO_2$. Primary changes in $PaCO_2$ may result in acidosis or alkalosis, depending on whether CO_2 is elevated above or depressed below the normal value: 40 mm Hg. Such disorders are termed *respiratory acidosis* and *respiratory alkalosis,* respectively. A primary change in the plasma HCO_3^- concentration owing to metabolic or renal factors results in commensurate changes in ventilation. The respiratory response to acidemia or alkalemia blunts the change in blood pH that would occur otherwise. Such respiratory alterations that adjust blood pH toward normal are referred to as *secondary* or *compensatory* alterations, because they occur in response to primary metabolic changes.

Human subjects are confronted, under most physiologic circumstances, with an acid challenge. "Acid production" in biologic systems is represented by the milliequivalents (mEq) of protons (H^+) added to body fluids. Conversely, proton removal is equivalent to equimolar addition of base, OH^- (generation of HCO_3^- from dissolved CO_2). Metabolism generates a daily load of relatively strong acids (lactate, citrate, acetate, and pyruvate), which must be removed by other metabolic reactions. The oxidation of these organic acids in the Krebs cycle, for example, generates CO_2, which must be excreted by the lungs. The oxidation of carbon-containing fuels produces as much as 16,000 to 20,000 mmol of CO_2 gas daily. Nevertheless, the complete combustion of carbon involves the intermediate generation and metabolism of 2000 to 3000 mmol of relatively strong organic acids, such as lactic acids, tricarbox-

ylic acids, keto acids, or other acids, depending on the type of fuel consumed. These organic acids do not accumulate in the body under most circumstances, with concentrations remaining in the low millimolar range. However, if production and consumption rates become mismatched, these organic acids can accumulate (e.g., lactic acid accumulation with strenuous exertion). Correspondingly, the HCO_3^- in the ECF will decline as the organic acid concentration increases. During recovery, the organic acids reenter metabolic pathways to CO_2 production, removal of H^+, and generation of HCO_3^-. Nevertheless, if the organic anions are excreted (e.g., ketonuria), these entities are no longer available for regeneration of HCO_3^-. The metabolism of some body constituents such as proteins, nucleic acids, and small fractions of lipids and certain carbohydrates generates specific organic acids that cannot be burned to CO_2 (e.g., uric, oxalic, glucoronic, hippuric acids). In addition, the inorganic acids H_2SO_4 and H_3PO_4, derived respectively from sulfur-containing amino acids and organophosphates, must be excreted by the kidneys or the gastrointestinal tract.

In summary, in the steady state, as a result of the buffering power of the HCO_3^-/H_2CO_3 buffer system and its preeminence over other body buffer systems, addition or removal of H^+ results in equimolar changes in the HCO_3^- concentration according to the relationship outlined in Equation 3. Moreover, because this buffer system is open to air, the concentration of CO_2 remains essentially fixed. Therefore, the evidence for H^+ addition or removal can be found in reciprocal changes in the numerator of the Henderson-Hasselbach equation (Equation 20), or the $[HCO_3^-]$.

Integration of Regulatory Processes

Three physiologic processes militate against changes in the HCO_3^-/CO_2 ratio: (1) metabolic regulation, (2) respiratory regulation, and (3) renal regulation. Metabolic regulation is of minor importance in terms of overall physiologic regulation of acid-base balance. Nevertheless, regulatory enzymes, whose activity may be pH sensitive, may catalyze metabolic reactions that either generate or consume organic acids. Such a process constitutes a negative feedback regulatory system. The best example is phosphofructokinase, the pivotal enzyme in the glycolytic pathway, the activity of which is inhibited by low pH and enhanced by high pH. Therefore, an increase in pH_i accelerates glycolysis and generates pyruvate and lactate. It follows, therefore, that the generation of lactate in patients with lactic acidosis and the generation of keto acids in patients with ketoacidosis are impeded by acidemia.

Because, under most circumstances, CO_2 excretion and CO_2 production are matched, the usual steady-state $PaCO_2$ is maintained at 40 mm Hg. Underexcretion of CO_2 produces hypercapnia, and overexcretion produces hypocapnia. Production and excretion are again matched but at a new steady-state PCO_2. Therefore, the arterial PCO_2 ($PaCO_2$) is regulated primarily by neurorespiratory factors and is not subject to regulation by the rate of metabolic CO_2 production. Hypercapnia is primarily the result of hypoventilation, not increased CO_2 production. Increases or decreases in PCO_2 represent derangements of control of neurorespiratory regulation or can result from compensatory changes in response to a primary alteration in the plasma HCO_3^- concentration.

RENAL REGULATION

Although temporary relief from changes in the pH of body fluids may be derived from chemical buffering or respiratory compensation, the ultimate defense against addition of nonvolatile acid or of alkali resides in the kidneys. The addition of a strong acid (HA) to the ECF titrates plasma HCO_3^-:

$$HA + NaHCO_3 \Leftrightarrow NaA + H_2O + CO_2 \qquad (23)$$

The CO_2 is expired by the lungs, and body HCO_3^- buffer stores are diminished. This process occurs constantly as endogenous metabolic acids are generated. To maintain a normal plasma HCO_3^- in the face of constant accession of metabolic acids, the kidneys must (1) conserve the HCO_3^- present in glomerular filtrate and (2) regenerate the HCO_3^- decomposed by reaction with metabolic acids (Equation 23). For more detail, see Chapter 7.

The first process (HCO_3^- reclamation) is accomplished predominantly in the proximal tubule, with an additional contribution by the loop of Henle and a minor contribution by more distal nephron segments. Under most circumstances, the filtered load of HCO_3^- is absorbed almost completely, especially during an acid load. Nevertheless, when less acid is generated or if the plasma HCO_3^- concentration increases above the normal value of 25 mEq/L, HCO_3^- will be excreted efficiently into the urine. The second process, HCO_3^- regeneration, is represented by the renal output of acid or net acid excretion (Fig. 14–1).

$$\text{Net acid excretion} = NH_4^+ + \text{titratable acid} - HCO_3^- \qquad (24)$$

On balance, each milliequivalent of net acid excreted corresponds to 1 mEq of HCO_3^- returned to the ECF. This process of HCO_3^- regeneration is necessary to replace the HCO_3^- lost by the entry of fixed acids into the ECF or, less commonly, that HCO_3^- excreted in stool or urine. Because a typical North American diet generates fixed acids at 50 to 70 mEq/day, net acid excretion must be affected to maintain acid-base balance. Therefore, net acid excretion approximates 50 to 70 mEq/day. If acid production remained stable and unabated by net acid excretion, metabolic acidosis would ensue. Conversely, an increase in net acid excretion above the level of net acid production results in metabolic alkalosis.

Daily acid-base balance can be estimated, therefore, by subtracting net acid excretion plus any base absorbed from the gut from the amount of acid produced daily. The daily production of acid is represented by the amount of H_2SO_4 and noncombustible organic acids generated. In other words, net acid production is represented by the milliequivalents of SO_4^{2-} and organic acid anions (A^-) excreted in the urine. It has been confirmed in patients ingesting an artificial diet that urinary $[NH_4^+ + TA - HCO_3]$ is equal to urinary $[SO_4^{2-} + \text{organic } A^- + \text{dietary phosphoester-derived } H^+]$.[1]

SYSTEMIC RESPONSE TO CHANGES IN CARBON DIOXIDE TENSION

Generation of Respiratory Acidosis or Alkalosis: Acute Response

Intrinsic disturbances in the respiratory system can alter the relationship of CO_2 production and excretion and give rise to abnormal values of $PaCO_2$. Some stimuli evoke a primary increase in ventilation, which lowers systemic $PaCO_2$. These stimuli include hypoxemia, fever, anxiety, central nervous system disease, acute cardiopulmonary processes, septicemia, liver failure, pregnancy, and drugs (e.g., salicylates).[2] Conversely, $PaCO_2$ increases if the respiratory system is depressed by suppression of the respiratory control center or of the respiratory apparatus itself (neuromuscular, parenchymal, and airway components).[3] In both kinds of acute respiratory disorders, CO_2 is added to or subtracted from the body until the $PaCO_2$ assumes a new steady state so that pulmonary CO_2 excretion equals CO_2 production.

The accumulation or loss of CO_2 causes changes in blood pH within minutes. The plasma HCO_3^- decreases slightly as the $PaCO_2$ is reduced in acute respiratory alkalosis and increases slightly in acute respiratory acidosis.[1–4] The small changes in HCO_3^- concentration are due to buffering by nonbicarbonate buffers.[1–4] The estimated change in blood HCO_3^- concentration is approximately equal to 0.1 mEq/L of $[HCO_3^-]$ for each millimeter of mercury increase in PCO_2 and 0.25 mEq/L for each millimeter of mercury decrease in PCO_2.[3] Acute alterations in PCO_2 in either direction within the physiologic range do not change the blood HCO_3^- concentration by more than a total of about 4 to 5 mEq/L from normal. Organic acid

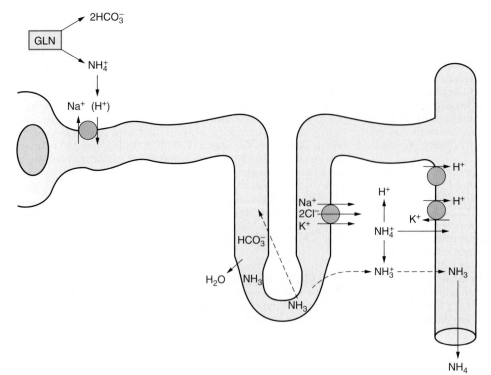

FIGURE 14–1 Synchrony of regulation of ammonium production (from glutamine [GLN] precursors, and excretion). Process allows generation of "new" HCO_3^- by the kidney. NH_4^+ excretion is regulated in response to changes in systemic acid-base and K^+ balance. Segmental contributions include: proximal convoluted tubule, proximal straight tubule, thin descending limb, thick ascending limb, and medullary collecting duct. Up-regulated by acidosis and hypokalemia. Inhibited by hyperkalemia.

production, especially of lactic and citric acids, increases modestly during acute hypocapnia, decreasing the blood HCO_3^- concentration and blunting the respiratory response to metabolic alkalosis.[1-4]

Chronic Response

Although the blood pH is relatively poorly defended during acute changes in $PaCO_2$, during chronic changes, the kidneys are recruited to excrete or retain HCO_3^- and return blood pH toward normal. The persistence of hypocapnia reduces renal bicarbonate absorption to achieve a further decrease in the plasma HCO_3^- concentration. Hypocapnia decreases renal HCO_3^- reabsorption[2] by inhibiting acidification in both the proximal[4] and the distal nephrons. The resulting decrease in plasma HCO_3^- concentration is equal to about 0.4 to 0.5 mEq/ L for each millimeter of mercury decrease in PCO_2^3. Thus, the arterial pH falls toward but not completely back to normal.

Several hours to days are required for full expression of the renal response to chronic hypocapnia,[3,4] which includes a reduction in the rate of H^+ secretion, an increase in urine pH, a decrease in NH_4^+ and titratable acid excretion, and a modest bicarbonaturia (see Chapter 7). An increase in blood Cl^- concentration occurs simultaneously by means of several mechanisms: a shift of Cl^- out of red blood cells, ECF volume contraction, and enhanced Cl^- reabsorption.

An overshoot in HCO_3^- generation and sustained reabsorption may occur on occasion so that blood pH may become alkaline with severe chronic hypercapnia (values $\leq$ 70 mm Hg).[3,4] One example of this phenomenon is the increment in renal HCO_3^- generation caused by nocturnal CO_2 retention in patients with obstructive sleep apnea. Both blood PCO_2 and HCO_3^- concentration increase during the night. Later in the morning, alkalotic blood gas values are often obtained, because $PaCO_2$ has declined more rapidly than HCO_3^- concentration to values characteristic of wakefulness. In chronic hypercapnia, the blood HCO_3^- concentration increases about 0.25 to 0.50 mEq/L for each millimeter of mercury elevation in $PaCO_2$.[3,4]

The increase in generation of HCO_3^- by the kidney during chronic hypercapnia takes several days for completion. The mechanism of HCO_3^- retention involves increased H^+ secretion by both proximal and distal nephron segments, regardless of sodium bicarbonate or sodium chloride intake, mineralocorticoid levels, or K^+ depletion.[1,3-5]

Chronic hypercapnia results in sustained increases in renal cortical PCO_2, and the increase in renal cortical PCO_2 that occurs with chronic hypercapnia stimulates acidification.[4,5] The increased PCO_2 enhances distal H^+ secretion so that increased NH_4^+ excretion occurs even with a low-salt diet or with hypoxemia. However, if hyperkalemia ensues or is present initially, the renal adaptation to chronic hypercapnia is blunted significantly. Hyperkalemia decreases NH_4^+ production and excretion even in the face of acidemia.[5,6] The effect of an elevated PCO_2 to augment tubule HCO_3^- reabsorption may also be mediated by hemodynamic changes, especially by systemic vasodilatation, so that a decreased effective ECF status is sensed by the kidney. Hypercapnia also decreases proximal sodium chloride reabsorption and causes a chloriuresis, which can further compromise ECF.[4,5] If the hemodynamic alterations induced by hypercapnia are corrected, the direct influence of acute hypercapnia, to increase net renal HCO_3^- transport, is abated. Over time, an adaptation occurs in the proximal nephron: HCO_3^- reabsorption is stimulated after several days of hypercapnia.[7] The cellular mechanism by which chronic hypercapnia enhances H^+ secretion by the distal nephron appears to involve an increase in the number of H^+ pumps (H^+-ATPase and H^+,K^+-ATPase) inserted into the apical membrane of proximal tubules and collecting ducts.[8]

In summary, although primary alterations in systemic $PaCO_2$ cause relatively marked changes in blood pH, renal homeostatic mechanisms allow the blood pH to return toward normal over a sufficient period. The renal response to chronic hypercapnia is manifest primarily by an increase in net acid excretion and HCO_3^- absorption, which is accomplished by augmented H^+ secretion in both the proximal and the distal nephrons.

SYSTEMIC RESPONSE TO ADDITION OF NONVOLATILE ACIDS

In addition to large quantities of CO_2, the metabolic processes of the body produce a smaller quantity of nonvolatile acids. The lungs readily excrete CO_2, and this process can respond rapidly to changes in production. In contrast, the kidneys must excrete nonvolatile acids through a much slower adaptive response. The time course of compensation for addition of acid or alkali to the body is displayed schematically in Figure 14–2. The hypothetical completion of each process is plotted as a function of time and proceeds in the following sequence: (1) distribution and buffering in the ECF, (2) cellular buffering, (3) respiratory compensation, and (4) renal acid or base excretion.

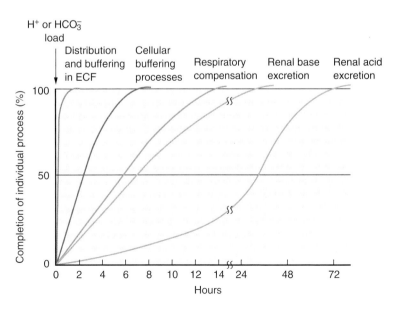

FIGURE 14–2 Time course of acid-base compensatory mechanisms. In response to a metabolic acid or alkaline load, component approaches to completion of the distribution and extracellular buffering mechanisms, of cellular buffering events, and of respiratory and renal regulatory processes are presented as a function of time. ECF, extracellular fluid.

Pathologically, acid loads may be derived from endogenous acid production (e.g., generation of keto acids and lactic acids) or loss of base (e.g., diarrhea) or from exogenous sources (e.g., ammonium chloride or toxin ingestion). Under normal physiologic circumstances, a daily input of acid derived from the diet and metabolism confronts the body. The net result of these processes amounts to about 1.0 mEq of new H^+ per kilogram per day.[1,4]

Sulfuric acid is formed when organic sulfur from methionine and cysteine residues of proteins are oxidized to SO_4^{2-}. The metabolism of sulfur-containing amino acids is the primary source of acid in the usual Western diet, accounting for approximately 50%. The quantity of sulfuric acid generated is equal to the SO_4^{2-} excreted in the urine.

Organic acids are derived from intermediary metabolites formed by partial combustion of dietary carbohydrates, fats, and proteins as well as from nucleic acids (uric acid). Organic acid generation contributes to net endogenous acid production when the conjugate bases are excreted in the urine as organic anions. If full oxidation of these acids can occur, however, H^+ is reclaimed and eliminated as CO_2 and water. The net amount of H^+ added to the body from this source can be estimated by the amount of organic anions excreted in the urine.

Phosphoric acid can be derived from hydrolysis of PO_4^{3-} esters in proteins and nucleic acids if it is not neutralized by mineral cations (e.g., Na^+, K^+, and Mg^{2+}). The contribution of dietary phosphates to acid production is dependent on the kind of protein ingested. Some proteins generate phosphoric acid, whereas others generate only neutral phosphate salts.[1,4] Hydrochloric acid is generated by metabolism of cationic amino acids (lysine, arginine, and some histidine residues) into neutral products. Other potential acid or base sources in the diet can be estimated from the amount of unidentified cations and anions ingested.

Potential sources of bases are also found in the diet (e.g., acetate, lactate, citrate) and can be absorbed to neutralize partially the H^+ loads from the three sources just mentioned. These potential base equivalents may be estimated by subtracting the unmeasured anions in the stool ($Na^+ + K^+ + Ca^{2+} + Mg^{2+} - Cl^- - 1.8P$) from those measured in the diet. The net base absorbed by the gastrointestinal tract is derived from the anion gap (AG) of the diet minus that of the stool. Acid production is partially offset by HCO_3^- produced when organic anions combine with H^+ and are oxidized to CO_2 and H_2O or when dibasic phosphoesters combine with H^+ during hydrolysis. The gastrointestinal tract may modify the amount of these potential bases reabsorbed under particular circumstances of acidosis or growth. It has been confirmed in patients ingesting an artificial diet that urinary $[NH_4^+ + TA - HCO_3]$ is equal to urinary $[SO_4^{2-} + \text{organic } A^- + \text{dietary phosphoester-derived } H^+]$.[1,4,9]

In summary, dietary foodstuffs contain many sources of acids and bases. These can be estimated by the urinary excretion of SO_4^{2-} and organic anions minus the unmeasured anions. The usual North American diet represents a daily source of acid generation for which the body must compensate constantly.

Hepatic and Renal Roles in Acid-Base Homeostasis

The generation of acid by protein catabolism is balanced by the generation of new HCO_3^- through renal NH_4^+ and titratable acid excretion. Hepatic protein catabolism, with the exception of sulfur- and PO_4^{3-}-containing amino acids, can be considered a neutral process. The products of these neutral reactions are HCO_3^- and NH_4^+ (Fig. 14–3). Most of the NH_4^+ produced by metabolism of amino acids reacts with HCO_3^- or

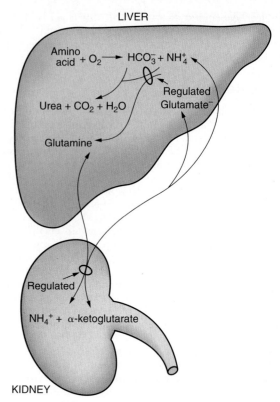

Figure 14–3 Hepatic and renal roles in NH_4^+ and acid balance. Virtually all NH_4^+ produced by metabolism of amino acids reacts with HCO_3^- to form urea, a process that has no impact on acid-base balance. A small fraction of this NH_4^+ is diverted to glutamine synthesis. This diversion is influenced by the local pH and acidemia-promoting and alkalemia-inhibiting glutamine synthesis. Glutamine circulates to the kidney, where it can be deaminated to form glutamate, initiating a process that eventually generates HCO_3^- through metabolism of α-ketoglutarate. If glutamine is not deaminated, it returns to the liver and is deaminated there to contribute to NH_4^+ to the urea synthetic pool. (Adapted from Gennari FJ, Maddox DA: Renal regulation of acid-base homeostasis: Integrated response. *In* Seldin DW, Giebisch GH [eds]: The Kidney: Physiology and Pathophysiology, 3rd ed. New York, Lippincott Williams and Wilkins, 2000.)

forms urea and, thus, has no impact on acid-base balance. A portion of this NH_4^+ is diverted to glutamine synthesis, the amount of which is regulated by pH. Acidemia promotes and alkalemia inhibits glutamine synthesis. Glutamine enters the circulation and reaches the kidney, where it is deaminated to form glutamate. Renal glutamine deamination results in NH_4^+ production and initiates a metabolic process that generates new HCO_3^- through α-ketoglutarate. Glutamine deamination in the kidney is also highly regulated by systemic pH, so that acidemia augments and alkalemia inhibits NH_4^+ and HCO_3^- production. The ultimate control, however, resides in the renal excretion of NH_4^+, because the NH_4^+ must be excreted to escape entry into the hepatic urea synthetic pool. Hepatic urea synthesis would negate the new HCO_3^- realized from α-ketoglutarate in the kidney. Hepatic regulation of NH_4^+ metabolic pathways appears to facilitate glutamine production when NH_4^+ excretion is stimulated by acidemia or, conversely, blunts glutamine production when excretion is inhibited by alkalemia.[9]

Neurorespiratory Response to Acidemia

A critically important response to an acid load is the neurorespiratory control of ventilation. Although the precise mechanism for this response is debated,[1,3,4,9] the prevailing view is that a fall in systemic arterial pH is sensed by the

Primary Acid-Base Disorders	Primary Defect	Effect on pH	Compensatory Response	Expected Range of Compensation	Limits of Compensation
Respiratory acidosis	Alveolar hypoventilation ($\uparrow$ P_{CO_2})	$\downarrow$	$\uparrow$ Renal HCO_3^- reabsorption (HCO_3^- $\uparrow$)	Acute $\Delta[HCO_3^-] = +1$ mEq/L for each $\uparrow$ ΔP_{CO_2} of 10 mm Hg Chronic $\Delta[HCO_3^-] = +4$ mEq/L for each $\uparrow$ ΔP_{CO_2} of 10 mm Hg	$[HCO_3^-] = 38$ mEq/L $[HCO_3^-] = 45$ mEq/L
Respiratory alkalosis	Alveolar hyperventilation ($\downarrow$ P_{CO_2})	$\uparrow$	$\downarrow$ Renal HCO_3^- reabsorption (HCO_3^- $\downarrow$)	Acute $\Delta[HCO_3^-] = -2$ mEq/L for each $\downarrow$ ΔP_{CO_2} of 10 mm Hg Chronic $\Delta[HCO_3^-] = -5$ mEq/L for each $\downarrow$ ΔP_{CO_2} of 10 mm Hg	$[HCO_3^-] = 18$ mEq/L $[HCO_3^-] = 15$ mEq/L
Metabolic acidosis	Loss of HCO_3^- or gain of H^+ ($\downarrow$ HCO_3^-)	$\downarrow$	Alveolar hyperventilation to $\uparrow$ pulmonary CO_2 excretion ($\downarrow$ P_{CO_2})	$P_{CO_2} = 1.5[HCO_3^-] + 8 \pm 2$ $P_{CO_2} = $ last 2 digits of pH $\times$ 100 $P_{CO_2} = 15 + [HCO_3^-]$	$P_{CO_2} = 15$ mm Hg
Metabolic alkalosis	Gain of HCO_3^- or loss of H^+ ($\uparrow$ HCO_3^-)	$\uparrow$	Alveolar hypoventilation to $\downarrow$ pulmonary CO_2 excretion ($\uparrow$ P_{CO_2})	$P_{CO_2} = + 0.6$ mm Hg for $\Delta[HCO_3^-]$ of 1 mEq/L $P_{CO_2} = 15 + [HCO_3^-]$	$P_{CO_2} = 55$ mm Hg

TABLE 14-1 Acid-Base Abnormalities and Appropriate Compensatory Responses for Simple Disorders

Adapted from Bidani A, Tauzon DM, Heming TA: Regulation of whole body acid-base balance. In DuBose TD, Hamm LL (eds): Acid-Base and Electrolyte Disorders: A Companion to Brenner and Rector's The Kidney. Philadelphia, WB Saunders, 2002, pp 1–21.

chemoreceptors that stimulate ventilation and, therefore, reduce $PaCO_2$. The fall in blood pH that would otherwise occur in uncompensated metabolic acidosis is, therefore, blunted. The pH is not restored to normal; however, $PaCO_2$ declines by an average of 1.25 mm Hg for each 1.0 mEq/L drop in HCO_3^- concentration. The appropriate $PaCO_2$ in steady-state metabolic acidosis can be estimated from the prevailing HCO_3^- concentration according to the expression[10]:

$$PaCO_2 = 1.5 [HCO_3^-] + 8 \ (\pm 2 \text{ mm Hg}) \qquad (25)$$

It is convenient to remember that the predicted (or compensatory) $PaCO_2$ is also roughly equal to addition to the serum $[HCO_3^-]$ of the number 15 (valid in pH range of 7.2–7.5). Because the $PaCO_2$ cannot fall below about 10 to 12 mm Hg, the blood pH is less well defended by respiration after very large reductions in the plasma HCO_3^- concentration (Table 14–1). Approximately 12 to 24 hours is required to achieve full respiratory compensation for metabolic acidosis (see Fig. 14–2).

Renal Excretion

As already discussed, the kidneys eliminate the acid that is produced daily by metabolism and diet and have the capacity to increase urinary net acid excretion (and, hence, HCO_3^- generation) in response to endogenous or exogenous acid loads. Renal excretion of acid is usually matched to the net production of metabolic and dietary acids, about 55 to 70 mEq/day, so little disturbance in systemic pH or HCO_3^- concentration occurs.

As an acid load is incurred, the kidneys respond to restore homeostasis by increasing NH_4^+ excretion (titratable acid excretion has limited capacity for regulation). With continued acid loading, renal net acid excretion increases over the course of 3 to 5 days (see Fig. 14–2) but does not quite achieve the level of acid production. Progressive positive acid balance ensues, buffered presumably by bone carbonate.

Thus, the renal response to an acid load requires (1) reclamation of the filtered HCO_3^- by the proximal tubule and (2)

augmentation of NH_4^+ production and excretion by the distal nephron. In this way, the kidneys efficiently retain all filtered base and attempt to generate enough new base to restore the arterial pH toward normal.

In summary, acidosis enhances proximal HCO_3^- absorption, decreasing delivery of HCO_3^- out of the proximal tubule, and enhances distal acidification. Net acid excretion is increased by stimulation of NH_4^+ production and excretion. Hyperaldosteronism and the effect of nonreabsorbable anions can act synergistically to strengthen the renal defense to an acid challenge.

SYSTEMIC RESPONSE TO GAIN OF ALKALI

Whereas the major goal of the body in defense of an acid challenge is to conserve body buffer stores and to generate new base, the response to an alkali load is to eliminate base as rapidly as possible. The response is dependent on the same three responses outlined for defense of an acid challenge, namely, cellular buffering and distribution within the ECF, respiratory, and renal excretion.

Distribution and Cellular Buffering

Ninety-five percent of a base load in the form of HCO_3^- is distributed in the ECF within about 25 minutes[1,4,9,11] (see Fig. 14–2). Simultaneously, the various processes of cellular buffering serve to dissipate this HCO_3^- load. Cellular buffering of the HCO_3^- load has a half-time of 3.3 hours. The apparent distribution volume for the administered HCO_3^- is inversely proportional to the preexisting plasma HCO_3^- concentration. A lesser fraction of base is buffered via cellular processes than occurs when a comparable amount of acid is administered (see Fig. 14–2). Two thirds of the administered HCO_3^- is retained in the ECF; a third is buffered in cells, principally by Na^+/H^+ exchange, and a small amount is buffered by increased lactate production and Cl^-/HCO_3^- exchange.[1] Modest hypokalemia as a result of K^+ shifts into cells and is approximately equal to 0.4 to 0.5 mEq/L of K^+ per 0.1 unit pH increase above 7.40.

In summary, the cellular defense against an alkaline load is somewhat less effective than the defense against an acid load. There is also poorer stabilization of intracellular pH in the alkaline than in the acid range.[1,11]

Respiratory Compensation

The pulmonary response to an acute increase in HCO_3^- concentration is biphasic. Neutralization of sodium bicarbonate by buffers (H^+ buffer$^-$) results in CO_2 liberation and an increase in PCO_2:

$$Na^+HCO_3^- + H^+ \text{ buffer}^- \Leftrightarrow Na^+ \text{ buffer}^- + H_2CO_3 \Leftrightarrow H_2O + CO_2 \quad (26)$$

The increased PCO_2 stimulates ventilation acutely to return PCO_2 toward normal. If the pulmonary system is compromised or the ventilation rate controlled artifically, increased CO_2 production from infused sodium bicarbonate can lead to hazardous hypercapnia.[1,4,11]

About an hour after an abrupt increment in the HCO_3^- concentration, when the increased generation of CO_2 subsides, stimulation of respiration is transformed into suppression of respiration, and PCO_2 increases. This secondary hypercapnic response takes several hours and partially compensates for the elevated HCO_3^- concentration so that arterial pH is returned toward (although not completely to) normal (see Fig. 14–2).

The hypercapnic response to metabolic alkalosis is difficult to predict reliably. Attempts to substantiate a role for K^+ deficiency in preventing hypoventilation have not been illuminating.[9,11,12] Moreover, studies of alkalotic patients taking diuretics demonstrate a predictable hypoventilatory response and cast doubt on a significant role of K^+ deficiency to blunt alkalosis-induced hypoventilation.[11] Most studies have found that an increase in PCO_2 regularly occurs in response to alkalosis. The hypoventilatory response can lead to borderline or even frank hypoxemia in patients with chronic lung disease.[11,12] In general, the increase in $PaCO_2$ can be predicted to equal 0.75 mm Hg per 1.0 mEq/L increase in plasma HCO_3^-; or more simply, add the value of 15 to the measured plasma $[HCO_3^-]$[12] to predict the expected $PaCO_2$ (see Table 14–1).

Renal Excretion

With Extracellular Volume Expansion

Addition of sodium bicarbonate to the body results in prompt cellular buffering and respiratory compensation. However, as with an acid load, the kidneys have the ultimate responsibility for the disposal of base and restoration of base stores to normal. The renal response is more rapid with HCO_3^- addition than with acid ingestion (see Fig. 14–2). The speed and efficiency with which HCO_3^- can be excreted by the kidneys are such that it is difficult to render a patient with normal renal function more than mildly alkalotic on a chronic basis, even when as much as 24 mEq/kg/day of sodium bicarbonate is ingested for several weeks.[11,12] A pulse base load is excreted almost entirely within 24 hours.

The proximal tubule is responsible principally for HCO_3^- excretion when the blood HCO_3^- concentration increases. Absolute proximal HCO_3^- reabsorption does not increase in proportion to HCO_3^- load in the rat kidney because of suppression of proximal acidification by alkalemia[5] so that HCO_3^- delivery to the distal nephron increases. The limited capacity of the distal nephron to secrete H^+ can be overwhelmed easily, and bicarbonaturia increases progressively. NH_4^+ and titratable acid excretion are mitigated in response to the increasing urine pH.[5,12]

Acute graded HCO_3^- loads that concomitantly increase ECF also function in human subjects to increase urinary HCO_3^- excretion progressively as plasma HCO_3^- concentration increases.[5] In summary, an acute base load is excreted entirely, and the blood HCO_3^- concentration is returned to normal within 12 to 24 hours because of depression of fractional proximal HCO_3^- reabsorption. In addition to suppression of reabsorption of the filtered HCO_3^- load, direct HCO_3^- secretion in the CCT has been proposed as another mechanism for mediating HCO_3^- disposal during metabolic alkalosis.[12]

The increased delivery of HCO_3^- out of the proximal tubule in response to an increased blood HCO_3^- concentration (and, hence, filtered HCO_3^- load) in the setting of ECF expansion facilitates HCO_3^- excretion and the return of blood pH toward normal. However, other factors may independently enhance distal H^+ secretion sufficiently to prevent HCO_3^- excretion and thus counterbalance the suppressed fractional proximal HCO_3^- reabsorptive capacity. Under these circumstances, the alkalosis is maintained. For example, in the setting of primary hyperaldosteronism, despite the expanded ECF, a stable mild alkalotic condition persists in most experimental models owing to augmented collecting duct H^+ secretion.[12] In such cases, concurrent hypokalemia facilitates the generation and maintenance of metabolic alkalosis by enhancing NH_4^+ production and excretion.[5,12] Moreover, chronic hypokalemia dramatically enhances the abundance and functionality of the colonic H^+,K^+-ATPase isoform in the medullary collecting tubule, thus increasing rather than decreasing bicarbonate absorption.[12–15] Enhanced nonreabsorbable anion delivery, as with drug anions, also increases net collecting tubule H^+ secretion by increasing the effective luminal negative potential difference or by suppressing HCO_3^- secretion in the cortical collecting duct (CCD).

With Extracellular Volume Contraction and Potassium Ion Deficiency

The renal response to an increase in plasma HCO_3^- concentration can be modified significantly in the presence of ECF contraction and K^+ depletion.[15,16] Because the volume of distribution of Cl^- is approximately equal to ECF, the depletion of the ECF is roughly equivalent to the depletion of Cl^-. The critical role of effective ECF and K^+ stores in modifying net HCO_3^- reabsorption has been demonstrated in numerous experimental models.

Deficiency of both Cl^- and K^+ is common in metabolic alkalosis because of renal and/or gastrointestinal losses that occur concurrently with the generation of the alkalosis.[14,16] With Cl^- depletion alone, the normal bicarbonaturic response to an increase in plasma HCO_3^- is prevented and metabolic alkalosis can develop. K^+ depletion, even without mineralocorticoid administration, can cause metabolic alkalosis in rats and humans. When Cl^- and K^+ depletion coexist, severe metabolic alkalosis may develop in all species studied.

Two general mechanisms exist by which the bicarbonaturic response to hyperbicarbonatemia can be prevented by Cl^- and/or K^+ depletion: (1) As the plasma HCO_3^- concentration increases, there is a reciprocal fall in GFR. If the fall in glomerular filtration rate (GFR) were inversely proportional to the rise in the plasma HCO_3^- concentration, the filtered HCO_3^- load would not exceed the normal level. In this case, normal rates of proximal and distal HCO_3^- reabsorption would suffice to prevent bicarbonaturia. (2) Cl^- deficiency or K^+ deficiency increases overall renal HCO_3^- reabsorption in the setting of a normal GFR and high filtered HCO_3^- load. In this case, overall renal HCO_3^- reabsorption and, therefore, acidification would be increased. An increase in renal acidification might occur as a result of an increase in H^+ secretion by the proximal or the distal nephron or by both nephron segments.[12–14]

The possibility that Cl^- or K^+ depletion might decrease GFR or increase proximal HCO_3^- reabsorption has been evaluated in experimental animals. That extracellular and plasma volume depletion decreases GFR is well described. GFR can also be decreased by K^+ depletion in rats and dogs. The reduction in GFR by K^+ depletion is assumed to be the result of increased production of the vasoconstrictors angiotensin II and thromboxane B_2.[13,15] These results, taken together, provide support for the first mechanism: that metabolic alkalosis can be maintained by a depression in GFR.[12–16]

The combination of an elevated and stable plasma HCO_3^- concentration, negligible urinary HCO_3^- excretion, and normal or only slightly depressed GFR suggests that renal HCO_3^- reabsorption is enhanced. An increase in renal acidification appears to be a major mechanism by which metabolic alkalosis is maintained in chronic models of this disorder. Animals with experimental forms of chronic metabolic alkalosis display increased HCO_3^- reabsorption in both the proximal and the distal tubules. The increase in HCO_3^- absorption in the proximal tubule is due, at least in part, to an increase in the delivered load of HCO_3^-. The augmented HCO_3^- absorption in distal nephron segments appears to be due to a primary increase in H^+ secretion that is independent of the HCO_3^- load delivered. Recent studies have demonstrated clearly that chronic hypokalemia up-regulates "colonic" H^+,K^+-ATPase mRNA and protein expression in the renal medulla, concomitant with an increase in H^+ secretion in the outer medullary collecting duct (OMCD) and IMCD. Chronic hypokalemia dramatically enhances the abundance and function of the colonic isoform of the H^+,K^+-ATPase in the medullary collecting tubule. Therefore, up-regulation of the H^+,K^+-ATPase by hypokalemia may be a significant factor in the maintenance of chronic metabolic alkalosis.[13,17,18]

The maintenance of a high plasma HCO_3^- concentration by the kidney can be repaired by repletion of Cl^-.[19] The mechanism by which Cl^- repairs metabolic alkalosis could include normalization of the low GFR that was induced by ECF repletion. In addition, Cl^- repletion might result in a decrease in proximal HCO_3^- reabsorption, an increase in HCO_3^- secretion by the distal nephron, or other less well-defined mechanisms that favor enhanced Cl^- reabsorption in preference to HCO_3^- reabsorption.

Repletion of K^+ alone (without Cl^- repletion) only partially corrects metabolic alkalosis. Indeed, several experimental studies have shown that Cl^- repletion can repair the alkalosis despite persisting K^+ deficiency. Full correction of metabolic alkalosis by Cl^- but not K^+ supplementation does not necessarily prove that K^+ deficiency has no role in maintaining the alkalosis. In fact, in most studies of repair of hyperbicarbonatemia by Cl^- repletion alone (without K^+ repletion), normalization of blood pH occurred only after significant volume expansion occurred. There is complete agreement that, with simultaneous repair of K^+ and Cl^- deficiencies in metabolic alkalosis, correction of the alteration in renal HCO_3^- reabsorption ensues as a result of normalization of GFR, which allows increased HCO_3^--delivery from the proximal tubule and, thus, excretion of the excess HCO_3^-.

In summary, the physiologic response by the kidney to a base load associated with volume expansion is to excrete the base. Base is retained, however, if there is enhanced distal HCO_3^- reabsorption as a result of K^+ and/or Cl^- deficiency.

The four cardinal acid-base disorders reviewed thus far, and the predicted compensatory responses and their limits, are summarized in Table 14–1.

STEPWISE APPROACH TO THE DIAGNOSIS OF ACID-BASE DISORDERS (Table 14–2)

Suspicion that an acid-base disorder exists is usually based on clinical judgment or on the finding of an abnormal blood pH, $PaCO_2$, or HCO_3^- concentration. Obviously, acid-base dis-

TABLE 14–2	Systematic Method for Diagnosis of Simple and Mixed Acid-Base Disorders

1. Obtain arterial blood gas and electrolyte panel simultaneously.

2. Compare the $[HCO_3^-]$ measured on the electrolyte panel with the calculated value from the arterial blood gas. Because the latter is obtained by the Henderson-Hasselbach equation, agreement of two values rules out laboratory error or error due to time discrepancy between the drawing of blood gas and electrolytes.

3. Calculate the anion gap (correct for low albumin if necessary).

4. Appreciate the four major categories of high anion gap acidoses:
   Ketoacidosis
   Lactic acid acidosis
   Renal failure acidosis
   Toxins and poisons

5. Appreciate the two major causes of non–anion gap acidoses:
   Gastrointestinal loss of HCO_3^-
   Renal loss of HCO_3^-

6. Estimate the compensatory response for either PCO_2 or HCO_3^- (see Table 14–1).

7. Compare the ΔAG and the ΔHCO_3^- (see text).

8. Compare the $\Delta[Cl^-]$ and the ΔNa^+ (see text).

orders require careful analysis of laboratory parameters along with the clinical processes occurring in the patient as revealed in the history and physical examination.

Step 1: Obtain Arterial Blood Gas and Electrolyte Values Simultaneously

To avoid errors in diagnosis, ABGs should be measured simultaneously with the plasma electrolyte panel in all patients with component acid-base abnormalities. This is necessary because changes in plasma HCO_3^-, Na^+, K^+, and Cl^- do not allow precise diagnosis of specific acid-base disturbances. When obtaining ABGs, care should be taken to obtain the arterial blood sample without excessive heparin.

Step 2: Verify Acid-Base Laboratory Values

A careful analysis of the blood gas indices (pH, $PaCO_2$) should begin with a check to determine whether the concomitantly measured plasma HCO_3^- (total CO_2 concentration from the electrolyte panel) is consistent. In the determination of ABGs by the clinical laboratory, both pH and $PaCO_2$ are measured, but the reported HCO_3^- concentration is calculated from the Henderson-Hasselbalch equation (Equation 20) by the blood gas analyzer. The calculated value for HCO_3^- or (total CO_2) reported with the blood gas panel should be compared with the measured HCO_3^- concentration (total CO_2) obtained on the electrolyte panel. The two values should agree within ± 2 to 3 mEq/L. If these values do not agree, the clinician should suspect that the samples were not obtained simultaneously or that a laboratory error is present. The stepwise analysis of all available laboratory values to determine whether the patient has a **mixed** or **simple** acid-base disturbance is emphasized in the following sections.

On occasion, it may be necessary to compute the third value (pH, PCO_2, or HCO_3^-) when only two are available. From the Henderson equation, derived previously in this chapter

(Equation 21), several caveats of clinical significance are apparent. First, the normal H^+ concentration in blood is 40 nM (conveniently remembered as the last two digits of the normal blood pH, 7.40), and the corresponding H^+ concentration at a pH of 7.00 is 100 nM. Second, the H^+ concentration increases by about 10 nM for each decrease in the blood pH of 0.10 unit (in the range 7.20–7.50). An acidotic patient with a pH of 7.30 (a reduction of 0.10 pH unit, or an increase of 10 nM H^+ concentration to 50 nM) and a P_{CO_2} of 25 mm Hg would have a HCO_3^- concentration of 12 mEq/L:

$$[HCO_3^-] = \frac{24 \times P_aCO_2}{[H^+]} = \frac{24 \times 25}{50} = 12 \text{ mEq/L} \qquad (27)$$

Although the Henderson equation and H^+ concentration have been suggested as the most physiologic way to portray acid-base equilibrium, the logarithmic transformation of the Henderson equation to the familiar Henderson-Hasselbalch equation is used more commonly (see Equation 20). This equation is useful because acidity is measured in the clinical laboratory as pH rather than H^+ concentration.

Implicit in Equations 20 and 21 is the concept that the final pH, or H^+ concentration, is determined by the ratio of HCO_3^- and P_aCO_2, not by the absolute amount of either. Thus, a normal concentration of HCO_3^- does not necessarily mean that the pH is normal, neither does a normal P_aCO_2 denote a normal pH. Conversely, a normal pH does not imply that either HCO_3^- or P_aCO_2 is normal.

Step 3: Define the Limits of Compensation to Distinguish Simple from Mixed Acid-Base Disorders

After verifying the blood acid-base values by either the Henderson equation (Equation 21) or the Henderson-Hasselbalch equation (Equation 20), one can define the precise acid-base disorder. If the HCO_3^- concentration is low and the Cl^- concentration is high, either chronic respiratory alkalosis or hyperchloremic metabolic acidosis is present. ABG determi-

nation serves to differentiate the two conditions. Although both have a decreased P_aCO_2, the pH is high with a primary respiratory disorder and low in a metabolic disorder. Chronic respiratory acidosis and metabolic alkalosis are both associated with high HCO_3^- and low Cl^- concentration in plasma. Again, a pH measurement distinguishes the two conditions. In many clinical situations, however, a mixture of acid-base disorders may exist. Diagnosis of these disturbances requires additional information and a more complex analysis of data.

A convenient, but not always reliable, approach is an acid-base map, such as the one displayed in Figure 14–4, which defines the 95% confidence limits of simple acid-base disorders.[1,4,20] If the arterial acid-base values fall within one of the shaded bands in Figure 14–4, one may assume that a simple acid-base disturbance is present, and a tentative diagnostic category can be assigned. Values that fall outside the shaded areas imply, but do not prove, that a mixed disorder exists.

The two broad types of acid-base disorders are metabolic and respiratory. Metabolic acidosis and alkalosis are disorders characterized by primary disturbances in the concentration of HCO_3^- in plasma (numerator of Equation 20), whereas respiratory disorders involve primarily alteration of P_aCO_2 (denominator of Equation 20). The most commonly encountered clinical disturbances are simple acid-base disorders, that is, one of the four cardinal acid-base disturbances— metabolic acidosis, metabolic alkalosis, respiratory acidosis, or respiratory alkalosis—occurring in a pure or simple form. More complicated clinical situations, especially in severely ill patients, may give rise to **mixed acid-base disturbances.**[20] The possible combinations of mixed acid-base disturbances are outlined in Table 14–2. To appreciate and recognize a mixed acid-base disturbance, it is important to understand the physiologic compensatory responses that occur in the simple acid-base disorders. Primary respiratory disturbances (denominator of Equation 20) invoke secondary metabolic responses (numerator of Equation 20), and primary metabolic disturbances evoke a predictable respiratory response (see Table 14–1). To illustrate, metabolic acidosis as a result of

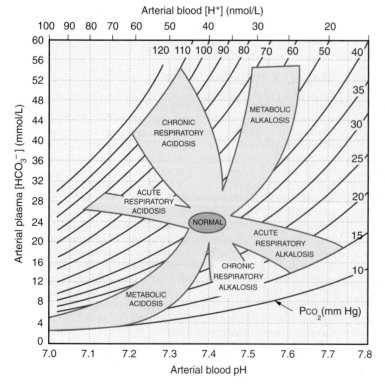

Figure 14–4 Acid-base nomogram (map). *Shaded areas* represent the 95% confidence limits of the normal respiratory and metabolic compensations for primary acid-base disturbances. Data falling *outside the shaded areas* denote a mixed disorder if a laboratory error is not present (see text).

gain of endogenous acids (e.g., lactic acid or ketoacidosis) lowers the concentration of HCO_3^- in ECF and, thus, extracellular pH. As a result of **acidemia,** the medullary chemoreceptors are stimulated and invoke an increase in ventilation. As a result of the hypocapnic response, the ratio of HCO_3^- to $PaCO_2$ and the subsequent pH are returned toward, but not completely to, normal. The degree of compensation expected in a simple form of metabolic acidosis can be predicted from the relationship depicted in Equation 26. Thus, a patient with metabolic acidosis and a plasma HCO_3^- concentration of 12 mEq/L would be expected to have a $PaCO_2$ between 24 and 28 mm Hg. Values of $PaCO_2$ below 24 or greater than 28 mm Hg define a **mixed metabolic-respiratory disturbance** (metabolic acidosis and respiratory alkalosis or metabolic acidosis and respiratory acidosis, respectively). Therefore, by definition, mixed acid-base disturbances exceed the physiologic limits of compensation. Similar considerations are examined for each type of acid-base disturbance as these disorders are discussed in detail separately. It should be emphasized that compensation is a predictable physiologic consequence of the primary disturbance and does not represent a secondary acidosis or alkalosis (see Fig. 14–4 and Table 14–1). As emphasized in the following sections, the recognition of mixed disturbances demands of the alert physician consideration of additional clinical disorders that may require immediate attention or additional therapy.

Clinical and Laboratory Parameters in Acid-Base Disorders

For correct diagnosis of a simple or mixed acid-base disorder, it is imperative that a careful history is obtained. Patients with pneumonia, sepsis, or cardiac failure frequently have respiratory alkalosis, and patients with chronic obstructive pulmonary disease or a sedative drug overdose often display a respiratory acidosis. The patient's drug history assumes importance because patients taking loop or thiazide diuretics may have a metabolic alkalosis and patients receiving acetazolamide frequently have a metabolic acidosis. Physical findings are often helpful as well. Tetany may occur with alkalemia, cyanosis with respiratory acidosis, and volume contraction with metabolic alkalosis. The initial suspicion can then be supported or ruled out by laboratory data. Knowledge of the limits of compensation may be helpful in this regard. For example, the plasma HCO_3^- concentration rarely falls below 12 to 15 mEq/L as a result of compensation for a respiratory alkalosis and rarely exceeds 45 mEq/L as a result of compensation for respiratory acidosis.[20]

The plasma K^+ value is often useful but should be considered only in conjunction with the knowledge of the HCO_3^- concentration and blood pH. It is generally appreciated that the serum K^+ value can be altered by primary acid-base disturbances as a result of shifts of K^+ either into the extracellular compartment or into the intracellular compartment. Metabolic acidosis leads to hyperkalemia as a result of cellular shifts whereby H^+ is exchanged for K^+ or Na^+. It has been reported that for each decrease in blood pH of 0.10 pH unit, the K^+ concentration should increase by 0.6 mEq/L. Thus, a patient with a pH of 7.20 would be expected to have a plasma K^+ value of 5.2 mEq/L. However, considerable variation in this relationship has been reported in several conditions, especially diabetic ketoacidosis (DKA) and lactic acidosis, which are often associated with K^+ depletion. The lack of correlation between the degree of acidemia and the plasma K^+ level is a result of several factors, including the nature and cellular permeability of the accompanying anion, the magnitude of the osmotic diuresis, the level of renal function, and the degree of catabolism. It is important to appreciate that the relationship between arterial blood pH and plasma K^+ is complex and, therefore, often variable. Nevertheless, the failure of a patient with severe metabolic acidosis to exhibit hyperkalemia or, conversely, the failure of a patient with severe metabolic alkalosis to exhibit hypokalemia suggests a significant derangement of body K^+ homeostasis. Furthermore, the combination of a low plasma K^+ and elevated HCO_3^- suggests metabolic alkalosis, whereas the combination of an elevated plasma K^+ and low HCO_3^- suggests metabolic acidosis.

It is helpful to compare the serum Cl^- concentration with the Na^+ concentration. The serum Na^+ concentration changes only as a result of changes in hydration. The Cl^- concentration changes for two reasons: (1) changes in hydration and (2) changes in acid-base balance. Thus, changes in Cl^- not reflected by proportional changes in Na^+ suggest the presence of an acid-base disorder. For example, consider a patient with a history of vomiting, volume depletion, a Cl^- concentration of 85 mEq/L, and a Na^+ concentration of 130 mEq/L. In this case, both Na^+ and Cl^- are reduced, but the reduction in Cl^- is proportionally greater (15% versus 7%). A disproportionate decrease in Cl^- suggests metabolic alkalosis or respiratory acidosis, and a disproportionate increase in Cl^- suggests metabolic acidosis or respiratory alkalosis.

Step 4: Calculate the Anion Gap

All evaluations of acid-base disorders should include a simple calculation of the AG. The AG is calculated from the serum electrolytes and is defined as:

$$AG = Na^+ - (Cl^- + HCO_3^-) = 10 \pm 2 \text{ mEq/L} \quad (28)$$

The AG represents the unmeasured anions normally present in plasma and unaccounted for by the serum electrolytes that are measured on the electrolyte panel. The unmeasured anions normally present in serum include anionic proteins (principally albumin and, to lesser extent, α and β globulins), PO_4^{3-}, SO_4^{2-}, and organic anions. When acid anions, such as acetoacetate and lactate, are produced endogenously in excess and accumulate in ECF, the AG increases above the normal value. This is referred to as a **high anion gap** acidosis.[20,21] If it is assumed that the serum albumin is within the normal range, for each milliequivalent per liter increase in the AG, there should be an equal decrease in the plasma HCO_3^- concentration. Serum protein at 1 g/dL has a negative charge equivalence of approximately 1.7 to 2.4 mEq/L.[22] The contribution of other unmeasured anions includes PO_4^{3-} (2 mEq/L), SO_4^{2-} (1 mEq/L), and lactate and other organic anions (5 mEq/L).

An increase in the AG may be due to a decrease in unmeasured cations or an increase in unmeasured anions. Combined severe hypocalcemia and hypomagnesemia represent a decrease in the contribution of unmeasured cation (Table 14–3). In addition, the AG may increase secondary to an increase in anionic albumin, as a consequence of either an increased albumin concentration or alkalemia.[20,21] The increased AG in severe alkalemia can be explained in part by the effect of alkaline pH on the electrical charge of albumin.

A decrease in the AG can be generated by an increase in unmeasured cations or a decrease in the unmeasured anions (see Table 14–3). A decrease in the AG can result from (1) an increase in unmeasured cations (Ca^{2+}, Mg^{2+}, K^+) or (2) the addition to the blood of abnormal cations, such as Li^+ (Li^+ intoxication) or cationic immunoglobulins (immunoglobulin G as in plasma cell dyscrasias). Because albumin is the major unmeasured anion, the AG will also decrease if the quantity of albumin is low (e.g., nephrotic syndrome, protein malnutrition).[22] In general, each decline in the serum albumin by 1 g/dL from the normal value of 4.5 g/dL decreases the AG by 2.5 mEq/L. Therefore, when hypoalbuminemia exists, it is possible to underestimate the AG and even miss an increased AG unless correction for the low albumin and its effect on the AG is taken into account. For example, in a patient with

TABLE 14–3 The Anion Gap

$$\text{Anion gap} = Na^+ - (Cl^- + HCO_3^-) = 9 \pm 3 \text{ mEq/L}$$

Decreased anion gap	Increased anion gap
Increased cations (not Na⁺)	**Increased anions (not Cl⁻ or HCO₃⁻)**
↑ Ca^{2+}, Mg^{2+}	↑ Albumin concentration
↑ Li^+	Alkalosis
↑ IgG	↑ Inorganic anions
Decreased anions (not Cl⁻ or HCO₃⁻)	Phosphate
↓ Albumin concentration hypoalbuminemia)*	Sulfate
Acidosis	↑ Organic anions
Laboratory error	L-Lactate
Hyperviscosity	D-Lactate
Bromism	Ketones
	Uremic
	↑ Exogenously supplied anions
	Toxins
	Salicylate
	Paraldehyde
	Ethylene glycol
	Propylene glycol
	Methanol
	Toluene
	Pyroglutamic acidosis
	↑ Unidentified anions
	Toxins
	Uremic
	Hyperosmolar, nonketotic states
	Myoglobinuric acute renal failure
	Decreased cations (not Na⁺)
	↓ Ca^{2+}, Mg^{2+}

*For each decline in albumin by 1 g/dL from normal (4.5 g/dL), anion gap decreases by 2.5 mEq/L.

an albumin of 1.5 and an uncorrected AG of 10 mEq/L, the corrected AG would be 17.5 mEq/L.

Laboratory errors can create a falsely low AG. Hyperviscosity and hyperlipidemia lead to an underestimation of the true Na^+ concentration, and bromide (Br^-) intoxication causes an overestimation of the true Cl^- concentration.[20]

In the presence of a normal serum albumin, elevation of unmeasured anions is usually due to addition to the blood of non–Cl^--containing acids. Thus, in most clinical circumstances, a high AG indicates that a metabolic acidosis is present. The anions accompanying such acids include inorganic (PO_4^{3-}, SO_4^{2-}), organic (keto acids, lactate, uremic organic anions), exogenous (salicylate or ingested toxins with organic acid production), or unidentified anions.[20] When these non–Cl^--containing acids are added to blood in excess of the rate of removal, HCO_3^- is titrated (consumed), and the accompanying anion is retained to balance the preexisting cationic (Na^+) charge:

$$H^+anion^- + NaHCO_3 \Leftrightarrow H_2O + CO_2 + Na^+ anion^- \quad (29)$$

The preexisting Cl^- concentration is unchanged when the new acid anion is added to the blood. Therefore, the high AG acidoses exhibit normochloremia as well as a high gap. If the kidney does not excrete the anion, the magnitude of the decrement in HCO_3^- concentration will match the increment in the AG. If the retained anion can be metabolized to HCO_3^- directly or indirectly (e.g., ketones or lactate, after successful treatment), normal acid-base balance is restored as the AG returns toward the normal value. Alternatively, if the anion can be excreted, ECF contraction occurs, leading to renal sodium chloride retention. Cl^- replaces the excreted anion, and hyperchloremic acidosis emerges as the anion is excreted and the AG disappears.

In summary, after the titration of HCO_3^-, the ability of the kidney to excrete the anion of an administered acid determines the type of acidosis that develops. If the anion is fil-

tered and is nonreabsorbable (e.g., SO_4^{2-}) ECF contraction, Cl^- retention, and hyperchloremic acidosis with a normal AG develop (non-AG acidosis). Conversely, if the anion is poorly filtered (e.g., uremic anions) or is produced endogenously, filtered, and reabsorbed (e.g., lactate and other organic anions), no change in Cl^- concentration occurs. The retained anion replaces the HCO_3^- lost when titrated by acid, creating a high-AG acidosis.

Superimposition of a High Anion Gap Acidosis on a Preexisting Acid-Base Disorder

By definition, a high AG acidosis has two identifying features: a low HCO_3^- concentration and an elevated AG. This means, therefore, that the elevated AG will remain evident even if another disorder coincides to modify the HCO_3^- concentration independently. Simultaneous metabolic acidosis of the high AG variety plus either metabolic alkalosis or chronic respiratory acidosis illustrates such a situation. The HCO_3^- concentration may be normal or even high in such a setting. However, the AG is normal, and the Cl^- concentration is relatively depressed. Consider a patient with chronic obstructive pulmonary disease with a compensated respiratory acidosis ($PaCO_2$ of 65 mm Hg and HCO_3^- concentration of 40 mEq/L) in whom acute bronchopneumonia and respiratory decompensation develop. If this patient presents with an HCO_3^- concentration of 24 mEq/L, Na^+ of 145 mEq/L, K^+ of 4.8 mEq/L, and Cl^- of 96 mEq/L, it would be incorrect to assume that this "normal" HCO_3^- concentration represents improvement in acid-base status toward normal. Indeed, the arterial pH would probably be low (~7.1), as a result of a more serious degree of hypercapnia than observed previously (e.g., if the PCO_2 increased from 65 to 80 mm Hg as a result of pneumonia). Even without blood gas measurements, prompt recognition that the AG was elevated to 25 mEq/L should suggest that a life-threatening lactic acidosis was superimposed on a pre-existing chronic respiratory acidosis, necessitating immediate therapy.

Similarly, a normal arterial HCO_3^- concentration, $PaCO_2$, and pH do not ensure the absence of an acid-base disturbance. For example, an alcoholic who has been vomiting may develop a metabolic alkalosis with a pH of 7.55; HCO_3^- concentration of 40 mEq/L; PCO_2 of 48 mm Hg; and Na^+ of 135 mEq/L, Cl^- of 80 mEq/L, and K^+ of 2.8 mEq/L. If such a patient were then to develop a superimposed alcoholic ketoacidosis with a β-hydroxybutyrate concentration of 15 mM; the arterial pH would fall to 7.40, HCO_3^- concentration to 25 mEq/L, and PCO_2 to 40 mm Hg. Although the blood gas values are normal, the AG (assuming no change in Na^+, or Cl^-) is elevated (25 mEq/L), indicating the existence of a mixed metabolic acid-base disorder (mixed metabolic alkalosis and metabolic acidosis). The combination of metabolic acidosis and metabolic alkalosis is not uncommon and is most easily recognized when the AG is elevated but the HCO_3^- concentration and pH are near normal ($\Delta AG > \Delta HCO_3^-$).

Mixed Acid-Base Disorders

Mixed acid-base disorders—defined as independently co-existing disorders, not merely compensatory responses—are often seen in patients in critical care units and can lead to dangerous extremes of pH. A patient with DKA (metabolic acidosis) may develop an independent respiratory problem, leading to respiratory acidosis or alkalosis. Patients with underlying pulmonary disease may not respond to metabolic acidosis with an appropriate ventilatory response because of insufficient respiratory reserve. Such imposition of respiratory acidosis on metabolic acidosis can lead to severe acidemia and a poor outcome. When metabolic acidosis and metabolic alkalosis coexist in the same patient, the pH may be normal or near normal. When the pH is normal, an elevated AG denotes the presence of a metabolic acidosis. A discrepancy in the ΔAG (prevailing minus normal AG) and the ΔHCO_3^- (normal minus prevailing HCO_3^-) indicates the presence of a mixed high gap acidosis—metabolic alkalosis (see example later). A diabetic patient with ketoacidosis may have renal dysfunction resulting in simultaneous metabolic acidosis. Patients who have ingested an overdose of drug combinations such as sedatives and salicylates may have mixed disturbances as a result of the acid-base response to the individual drugs (metabolic acidosis mixed with respiratory acidosis or respiratory alkalosis, respectively). Even more complex are triple acid-base disturbances. For example, patients with metabolic acidosis due to alcoholic ketoacidosis may develop metabolic alkalosis owing to vomiting and superimposed respiratory alkalosis owing to the hyperventilation of hepatic dysfunction or alcohol withdrawal. Conversely, when hyperchloremic acidosis and metabolic alkalosis occur concomitantly, the increase in Cl^- is out of proportion to the change in HCO_3^- concentration ($\Delta Cl^- > \Delta HCO_3^-$).[20]

In summary, an AG exceeding that expected for a patient's albumin concentration and blood pH denotes the existence of either a simple high AG metabolic acidosis or a complex acid-base disorder in which an organic acidosis is superimposed on another acid-base disorder.

Step 5: Recognize Conditions Causing Acid-Base Abnormalities with High or Normal Anion Gap

Appreciation that the AG is elevated requires knowledge of the four causes of a high AG acidosis: (1) ketoacidosis, (2)

TABLE 14–4	Clinical Causes of High Anion Gap and Normal Anion Gap Acidosis

High anion gap acidosis
  Ketoacidosis
    Diabetic ketoacidosis (acetoacetate)
    Alcoholic ketoacidosis (β-hydroxybutyrate)
    Starvation ketoacidosis
  Lactic acid acidosis
    L-Lactic acid acidosis (types A and B)
    D-Lactic acid acidosis
  Toxins
    Ethylene glycol
    Methyl alcohol
    Salicylate
    Propylene glycol
    Pyroglutamic acidosis

Normal anion gap acidosis
  Gastrointestinal loss of HCO_3^- (negative urine anion gap)
    Diarrhea
    Fistulae external
  Renal loss of HCO_3^- or failure to excrete NH_4^+ (positive urine anion gap = low net acid excretion)
    Proximal renal tubular acidosis (RTA)
    Acetazolamide (or other carbonic anlydrase inhibitor)
    Classic distal renal tubular acidosis (low serum K^+)
    Generalized distal renal tubular defect (high serum K^+)
  Miscellaneous
    NH_4Cl ingestion
    Sulfur ingestion
    Dilutional acidosis

lactic acid acidosis, (3) renal failure acidosis, and (4) toxin-induced metabolic acidosis (Table 14–4). Accordingly, if the AG is normal in the face of metabolic acidosis, a hyperchloremic or non-AG acidosis exists. The specific causes of hyperchloremic acidosis that must be appreciated are outlined in a following section. Table 14–4 displays the directional changes in pH, PCO_2, and HCO_3^- for the four simple acid-base disorders. With this stepwise approach, in the next sections, the specific causes of the major types of acid-base disorders are reviewed in detail.

RESPIRATORY DISORDERS

Respiratory Acidosis

Respiratory acidosis occurs as the result of severe pulmonary disease, respiratory muscle fatigue, or depression in ventilatory control. The increase in $PaCO_2$ owing to reduced alveolar ventilation is the primary abnormality leading to acidemia. In acute respiratory acidosis, there is an immediate compensatory elevation (due to cellular buffering mechanisms) in HCO_3^-, which increases 1 mEq/L for every 10 mm Hg increase in $PaCO_2$. In chronic respiratory acidosis (>24 hr), renal adaption is achieved and the HCO_3^- increases by 4 mEq/L for every 10 mm Hg increase in $PaCO_2$. The serum bicarbonate will usually not increase above 38 mEq/L, however.

The clinical features of respiratory acidosis vary according to severity, duration, the underlying disease, and whether there is accompanying hypoxemia. A rapid increase in $PaCO_2$ may result in anxiety, dyspnea, confusion, psychosis, and hallucinations and may progress to coma. Lesser degrees of dysfunction in chronic hypercapnia include sleep disturbances, loss of memory, daytime somnolence, and personality changes. Coordination may be impaired, and motor disturbances such as tremor, myoclonic jerks, and asterixis may develop. The sensitivity of the cerebral vasculature to the

TABLE 14–5 Respiratory Acid-Base Disorders

Alkalosis	**Acidosis**
Central nervous system stimulation	Central
Pain	Drugs (anesthetics, morphine, sedatives)
Anxiety, psychosis	Stroke
Fever	Infection
Cerebrovascular accident	Airway
Meningitis, encephalitis	Obstruction
Tumor	Asthma
Trauma	Parenchyma
Hypoxemia or tissue hypoxia	Emphysema/chronic obstructive
High altitude, ↓ $PaCO_2$	pulmonary disease
Pneumonia, pulmonary edema	Pneumoconiosis
Aspiration	Bronchitis
Severe anemia	Adult respiratory distress syndrome
Drugs or hormones	Barotrauma
Pregnancy, progesterone	Mechanical ventilation
Salicylates	Hypoventilation
Nikethamide	Permissive hypercapnia
Stimulation of chest receptors	Neuromuscular
Hemothorax	Poliomyelitis
Flail chest	Kyphoscoliosis
Cardiac failure	Myasthenia
Pulmonary embolism	Muscular dystrophies
Miscellaneous	Multiple sclerosis
Septicemia	Miscellaneous
Hepatic failure	Obesity
Mechanical hyperventilation	Hypoventilation
Heat exposure	
Recovery from metabolic acidosis	

vasodilating effects of CO_2 can cause headaches and other signs that mimic increased intracranial pressure, such as papilledema, abnormal reflexes, and focal muscle weakness.

The causes of respiratory acidosis are displayed in Table 14–5 *(right column)*. A reduction in ventilatory drive from depression of the respiratory center by a variety of drugs, injury, or disease can produce respiratory acidosis. Acutely, this may occur with general anesthetics, sedatives, β-adrenergic blockers, and head trauma. Chronic causes of respiratory center depression include sedatives, alcohol, intracranial tumors, and the syndromes of sleep-disordered breathing, including the primary alveolar and obesity-hypoventilation syndromes. Neuromuscular disorders involving abnormalities or disease in the motor neurons, neuromuscular junction, and skeletal muscle can cause hypoventilation. Although a number of diseases should be considered in the differential diagnosis, drugs and electrolyte disorders should always be ruled out. Mechanical ventilation when not properly adjusted and supervised may result in respiratory acidosis. This occurs if carbon dioxide production suddenly rises (because of fever, agitation, sepsis, or overfeeding) or if alveolar ventilation falls because of worsening pulmonary function. High levels of positive end-expiratory pressure in the presence of reduced cardiac output may cause hypercapnia as a result of large increases in alveolar dead space. Permissive hypercapnia has been utilized in the critical care setting with increasing frequency with the rationale of mitigating the barotrauma and volutrauma associated with high airways pressure and peak airways pressure in mechanically ventilated patients with respiratory distress syndrome.[23,24] Acute hypercapnia of any cause can lead to severe acidemia, neurologic dysfunction, and death. However, when carbon dioxide levels are allowed to increase gradually, the resulting acidosis is less severe, and the elevation in arterial PCO_2 is tolerated more readily. Although hypercapnia is not the goal of this approach, but secondary to the attempt to limit airway pressures, the arterial pH will decline, and the degree of acidemia may be called to the attention of the nephrologist

intensivist. Furthermore, the magnitude of the acidemia associated with permissive hypercapnia may be augmented if superimposed on metabolic acidosis, such as lactic acid acidosis. This combination is not uncommon in the setting of the critical care unit. Bicarbonate therapy may be indicated with mixed metabolic acidosis–respiratory acidosis, but the goal of therapy with alkali is to not raise the bicarbonate and pH to normal. With low tidal volume ventilation, a reasonable therapeutic target for arterial pH is approximately 7.30.[23] Moreover, with hypercapnia in the range of 60 mm Hg, a larger amount of bicarbonate will be necessary to achieve this goal. Bicarbonate administration will further increase the PCO_2, especially in patients on fixed rates of ventilation, and add to the magnitude of the hypercapnia. Use of a continuous bicarbonate infusion in this setting should be avoided if possible.

Disease and obstruction of the airways, when severe or long-standing, causes respiratory acidosis. Acute hypercapnia follows sudden occlusion of the upper airway or the more generalized bronchospasm that occurs with severe asthma, anaphylaxis, and inhalational burn or toxin injury. Chronic hypercapnia and respiratory acidosis occur in end-stage obstructive lung disease.[3]

Restrictive disorders involving both the chest wall and the lungs can cause acute and chronic hypercapnia. Rapidly progressing restrictive processes in the lung can lead to respiratory acidosis because the high cost of breathing causes ventilatory muscle fatigue. Intrapulmonary and extrapulmonary restrictive defects present as chronic respiratory acidosis in their most advanced stages.

The diagnosis of respiratory acidosis requires, by definition, the measurement of arterial $PaCO_2$ and pH. Detailed history and physical examination often provide important diagnostic clues to the nature and duration of the acidosis. When a diagnosis of respiratory acidosis is made, its cause should be investigated. Pulmonary function studies, including spirometry, diffusing capacity for carbon monoxide, lung volumes, and arterial $PaCO_2$ and oxygen saturation usually provide adequate assessment of whether respiratory acidosis is secondary to lung disease. Workup for nonpulmonary causes should include a detailed drug history, measurement of hematocrit, and assessment of upper airway, chest wall, pleura, and neuromuscular function.[3]

The treatment of respiratory acidosis depends on its severity and rate of onset. Acute respiratory acidosis can be life-threatening, and measures to reverse the underlying cause should be simultaneous with restoration of adequate alveolar ventilation to relieve severe hypoxemia and acidemia. Temporarily, this may necessitate tracheal intubation and assisted mechanical ventilation. Oxygen should be carefully titrated in patients with severe chronic obstructive pulmonary disease and chronic CO_2 retention who are breathing spontaneously. When oxygen is used injudiciously, these patients may experience progression of the respiratory acidosis. Aggressive and rapid correction of hypercapnia should be avoided because the falling $PaCO_2$ may provoke the same complications noted with acute respiratory alkalosis (i.e., cardiac arrhythmias, reduced cerebral perfusion, and seizures). It is advisable to lower the $PaCO_2$ gradually in chronic respiratory acidosis, aiming to restore the $PaCO_2$ to baseline levels while at the same time providing sufficient chloride and potassium to enhance the renal excretion of bicarbonate.[3]

Chronic respiratory acidosis is frequently difficult to correct, but general measures aimed at maximizing lung function with cessation of smoking, use of oxygen, bronchodilators, corticosteroids, diuretics, and physiotherapy can help some patients and can forestall further deterioration. The use of respiratory stimulants may prove useful in selected cases, particularly if the patient appears to have hypercapnia out of proportion to his or her level of lung function.

Respiratory Alkalosis

Alveolar hyperventilation decreases $PaCO_2$ and increases the $HCO_3^-/PaCO_2$ ratio, thus increasing pH (alkalemia). Nonbicarbonate cellular buffers respond by consuming HCO_3^-. Hypocapnia develops whenever a sufficiently strong ventilatory stimulus causes CO_2 output in the lungs to exceed its metabolic production by tissues. Plasma pH and HCO_3^- concentration appear to vary proportionately with $PaCO_2$ over a range from 40 to 15 mmHg. The relationship between arterial hydrogen ion concentration and $PaCO_2$ is about 0.7 nmol/L/mm Hg (or 0.01 pH unit/mm Hg) and that for plasma $[HCO_3^-]$ is 0.2 mEq/L/mm Hg, or the $[HCO_3^-]$ will decrease ~2 mEq/L for each 10 mm Hg.[2]

Beyond 2 to 6 hours, sustained hypocapnia is further compensated by a decrease in renal ammonium and titratable acid excretion and a reduction in filtered HCO_3^- reabsorption. The full expression of renal adaptation may take several days and depends on a normal volume status and renal function. The kidneys appear to respond directly to the lowered $PaCO_2$ rather than the alkalemia per se. A 1 mm Hg fall in $PaCO_2$ causes a 0.4 to 0.5 mEq/L drop in HCO_3^- and a 0.3 nmol/L fall (or 0.003 unit rise in pH) in hydrogen ion concentration, or the $[HCO_3^-]$ will decrease 4 mEq/L for each 10 mm Hg decrease in $PaCO_2$.[2]

The effects of respiratory alkalosis vary according to duration and severity but, in general, are primarily those of the underlying disease. A rapid decline in $PaCO_2$ may cause dizziness, mental confusion, and seizures, even in the absence of hypoxemia, as a consequence of reduced cerebral blood flow. The cardiovascular effects of acute hypocapnia in the awake human are generally minimal, but in the anesthetized or mechanically ventilated patient, cardiac output and blood pressure may fall because of the depressant effects of anesthesia and positive-pressure ventilation on heart rate, systemic resistance, and venous return. Cardiac rhythm disturbances may occur in patients with coronary artery disease as a result of changes in oxygen unloading by blood

from a left shift in the hemoglobin-oxygen dissociation curve (Bohr effect). Acute respiratory alkalosis causes minor intracellular shifts of sodium, potassium, and phosphate and reduces serum-free calcium by increasing the protein-bound fraction. Hypocapnia-induced hypokalemia is usually minor.[2]

Respiratory alkalosis is the most common acid-base disturbance encountered in critically ill patients and, when severe, portends a poor prognosis. Many cardiopulmonary disorders manifest respiratory alkalosis in their early to intermediate stages. Hyperventilation usually results in hypocapnia. The finding of normocapnia and hypoxemia may herald the onset of rapid respiratory failure and should prompt an assessment to determine whether the patient is becoming fatigued. Respiratory alkalosis is a common occurrence during mechanical ventilation.

The causes of respiratory alkalosis are summarized in Table 14–5 (*left column*). The hyperventilation syndrome may mimic a number of serious conditions and be disabling. Paresthesias, circumoral numbness, chest wall tightness or pain, dizziness, inability to take an adequate breath, and rarely, tetany may be themselves sufficiently stressful to perpetuate a vicious circle. ABG analysis demonstrates an acute or chronic respiratory alkalosis, often with hypocapnia in the range of 15 to 30 mm Hg and no hypoxemia. Central nervous system diseases or injury can produce several patterns of hyperventilation with sustained arterial $PaCO_2$ levels of 20 to 30 mm Hg. Conditions such as hyperthyroidism, high caloric loads, and exercise raise the basal metabolic rate, but usually, ventilation rises in proportion so that ABGs are unchanged and respiratory alkalosis does not develop. Salicylates, the most common cause of drug-induced respiratory alkalosis, stimulate the medullary chemoreceptor directly. The methylxanthine drugs, theophylline and aminophylline, stimulate ventilation and increase the ventilatory response to carbon dioxide. High progesterone levels increase ventilation and decrease the arterial $PaCO_2$ by as much as 5 to 10 mm Hg. Thus, chronic respiratory alkalosis is an expected feature of pregnancy. Respiratory alkalosis is a prominent feature in liver failure, and its severity correlates well with the degree of hepatic insufficiency and mortality. Respiratory alkalosis is common in patients with gram-negative septicemia, and it is often an early finding, before fever, hypoxemia, and hypotension develop. It is presumed that some bacterial product or toxin acts as a respiratory center stimulant, but the precise mechanism remains unknown.

The diagnosis of respiratory alkalosis requires measurement of arterial pH and $PaCO_2$ (higher and lower than normal, respectively). The plasma potassium concentration is often reduced, and the serum chloride concentration increased. In the acute phase, respiratory alkalosis is not associated with increased renal bicarbonate excretion, but within hours, net acid excretion is reduced. In general, the bicarbonate concentration falls by 2.0 mEq/L for each 10 mm Hg decrease in $PaCO_2$. Chronic hypocapnia reduces the serum bicarbonate concentration by 5.0 mEq/L for each 10 mm Hg decrease in $PaCO_2$. It is unusual to observe a plasma bicarbonate concentration below 12 mEq/L as a result of a pure respiratory alkalosis.

When a diagnosis of hyperventilation or respiratory alkalosis is made, its cause should be investigated. The diagnosis of hyperventilation syndrome is made by exclusion. In difficult cases, it may be important to rule out other conditions such as pulmonary embolism, coronary artery disease, and hyperthyroidism.

The treatment of respiratory alkalosis is primarily directed toward alleviation of the underlying disorder. Because respiratory alkalosis is rarely life-threatening, direct measures to correct it will be unsuccessful if the stimulus remains unchecked. If respiratory alkalosis complicates ventilator management, changes in dead space, tidal volume, and frequency can minimize the hypocapnia. Patients with the hyperventilation syndrome may benefit from reassurance, rebreathing from a paper bag during symptomatic attacks, and attention to underlying psychologic stress. Antidepressants and sedatives are not recommended, although in a few patients, β-adrenergic blockers may help to ameliorate distressing peripheral manifestations of the hyperadrenergic state.

METABOLIC DISORDERS

Metabolic Acidosis

Metabolic acidosis occurs as a result of a marked increase in endogenous production of acid (such as L-lactic acid and keto acids), loss of HCO_3^- or potential HCO_3^- salts (diarrhea or renal tubular acidosis [RTA]), or progressive accumulation of endogenous acids, when excretion is impaired because of renal insufficiency.[19]

The AG, when corrected for the prevailing albumin concentration (Equation 28),[20,21] serves a useful role in the initial differentiation of the metabolic acidoses and should always be calculated. A metabolic acidosis with a normal AG (hyperchloremic, or non-AG acidosis) suggests that HCO_3^- has been effectively replaced by Cl^-. Thus, the AG will not change.

In contrast, metabolic acidosis with a high AG (see Table 14–3) indicates addition of an acid other than hydrochloric acid or its equivalent to the ECF. If the attendant non-Cl^- acid anion cannot be readily excreted and is retained after HCO_3^- titration, the anion replaces titrated HCO_3^- without disturbing the Cl^- concentration (Equation 29). Hence, the acidosis is normochloremic and the AG increases. The relationship between the rate of addition to the blood of a non–Cl^--containing acid, and the rate of excretion of the accompanying anion with secondary Cl^- retention determines whether the resultant metabolic acidosis is expressed as a high AG or hyperchloremic variety.[19,20]

Hyperchloremic (Normal Anion Gap) Metabolic Acidoses

The diverse clinical disorders that may result in a hyperchloremic metabolic acidosis are outlined in Table 14–6. Because a reduced plasma HCO_3^- and elevated Cl^- concentration may also occur in chronic respiratory alkalosis, it is important to confirm the acidemia by measuring arterial pH. Hyperchloremic metabolic acidosis occurs most often as a result of loss of HCO_3^- from the gastrointestinal tract or as a result of a renal acidification defect. The majority of disorders in this category can be reduced to two major causes: (1) loss of bicarbonate from the gastrointestinal tract (diarrhea) or from the kidney (proximal RTA) or (2) inappropriately low renal acid excretion (classic distal RTA [cDRTA], or renal failure). Hypokalemia may accompany both gastrointestinal loss of HCO_3^- and proximal and cDRTA. Therefore, the major challenge in distinguishing these causes is to be able to define whether the response of renal tubular function to the prevailing acidosis is appropriate (gastrointestinal origin) or inappropriate (renal origin).

Diarrhea results in the loss of large quantities of HCO_3^- and HCO_3^- decomposed by reaction with organic acids. Because diarrheal stools contain a higher concentration of HCO_3^- and decomposed HCO_3^- than plasma, volume depletion and metabolic acidosis develop. Hypokalemia exists because large quantities of K^+ are lost from stool and because volume depletion causes elaboration of renin and aldosterone, enhancing renal K^+ secretion. Instead of an acid urine pH as might be logically anticipated with chronic diarrhea, a pH of 6.0 or more may be found. This occurs because chronic metabolic acidosis and hypokalemia increase renal NH_4^+

TABLE 14–6	Differential Diagnosis of Hyperchloremic Metabolic Acidosis

Gastrointestinal bicarbonate loss
Diarrhea
External pancreatic or small bowel drainage
Uterosigmoidostomy, jejunal loop
Drugs
    Calcium chloride (acidifying agent)
    Magnesium sulfate (diarrhea)
    Cholestyramine (bile acid diarrhea)

Renal acidosis
Hypokalemia
    Proximal RTA (type II)
    Distal (classic) RTA (type I)
Hyperkalemia
    Generalized distal nephron dysfunction (type IV RTA)
        Mineralocorticoid deficiency
        Mineralocorticoid resistance (PHA I—autosomal dominant)
        Voltage defects (PHA I—autosomal recessive)
        PHA II
        ↓ Na^+ delivery to distal nephron
        Tubulointerstitial disease
    Drug-induced hyperkalemia
        Potassium-sparing diuretics (amiloride, triamterene, spironolactone)
        Trimethoprim
        Pentamidine
        ACE inhibitors and ARBs
        NSAIDs
        Cyclosporine, tacrolimus
Normokalemia
    Early renal insufficiency

Other
Acid loads (ammonium chloride, hyperalimentation)
Loss of potential bicarbonate: ketosis with ketone excretion
Dilution acidosis (rapid saline administration)
Hippurate
Cation exchange resins

ACE, angiotensin-converting enzyme; ARBs, angiotensin II receptor blockers; NSAIDs, nonsteroidal anti-inflammatory drugs; PHA, pseudohypoaldosteronism.

synthesis and excretion, thus providing more urinary buffer, accommodating an increase in urine pH. Therefore, the urine pH may not be less than 5.5. Nevertheless, metabolic acidosis caused by gastrointestinal losses with a high urine pH can be differentiated from RTA. Because urinary NH_4^+ excretion is typically low in RTA and high in patients with diarrhea,[5,6,25] the level of urinary NH_4^+ excretion (not usually measured by clinical laboratories) in metabolic acidosis can be assessed indirectly[6] by calculating the urine anion gap (UAG):

$$UAG = [Na^+ + K^+]_u - [Cl^-]_u \qquad (30)$$

where u denotes the urine concentration of these electrolytes. The rationale for using the UAG as a surrogate for ammonium excretion is that, in chronic metabolic acidosis, ammonium excretion should be elevated if renal tubular function is intact. Because ammonium is a cation, it should balance part of the negative charge of chloride in the previous expression. Therefore, the UAG should become progressively negative as the rate of ammonium excretion increases in response to acidosis or to acid loading.[6,19] Because NH_4^+ can be assumed to be present if the sum of the major cations ($Na^+ + K^+$) is less than the sum of major anions in urine, a negative UAG (usually in the range of −20 to −50 mEq/L) provides evidence that sufficient NH_4^+ is present in the urine, as might obtain with an extrarenal origin of the hyperchloremic acidosis. Conversely, urine estimated to contain little or no NH_4^+ has more $Na^+ + K^+$ than Cl^- (UAG is positive)[6,19,25] and would suggest a renal mechanism for the hyperchloremic acidosis, such as in cDRTA (with hypokalemia) or hypoaldosteronism with hyperkalemia. Note that this qualitative test is useful only in the differential diagnosis of a hyperchloremic metabolic acidosis. If the patient has ketonuria or drug anions in large quantity (penicillins or aspirin) in the urine, the test is not reliable.

In this situation, the urinary ammonium ($U_{NH_4^+}$) may be estimated additionally from the measured urine osmolality (U_{osm}), urine [$Na^+ + K^+$], which will take into account the salts of ß-hydroxybutyrate and other keto acids, and urine urea and glucose (all expressed in mmol/L):

$$U_{NH_4^+} = 0.5 \ (U_{osm} - [2 \ (Na^+ + K^+)_u + urea_u + glucose_u] \quad (31)$$

Urinary ammonium concentrations of 75 mEq/L or more would be anticipated if renal tubular function is intact and the kidney is responding to the prevailing metabolic acidosis by increasing ammonium production and excretion. Conversely, values below 25 mEq/L denote inappropriately low urinary ammonium concentrations.

In addition to the UAG, the fractional excretion of Na^+ may be helpful and would be expected to be low (<1%–2%) in patients with HCO_3^- loss from the gastrointestinal tract but usually exceeds 2% to 3% in RTA.[6,25]

Gastrointestinal HCO_3^- loss, as well as proximal RTA (type 2) and cDRTA (type 1), results in ECF contraction and stimulation of the renin-aldosterone system, leading typically to hypokalemia. The serum K^+ concentration, therefore, serves to distinguish these disorders with a low K^+ from either generalized distal nephron dysfunction (e.g., type 4 RTA), in which the renin–aldosterone–distal nephron axis is abnormal and hyperkalemia exists, and the acidosis of glomerular insufficiency, in which normokalemia is the rule.

In addition to gastrointestinal tract HCO_3^- loss, external loss of pancreatic and biliary secretions can cause a hyperchloremic acidosis. Cholestyramine, calcium chloride, and magnesium sulfate ingestion can also result in a hyperchloremic metabolic acidosis (see Table 14–6), especially in patients with renal insufficiency. Coexistent L-lactic acidosis is common in severe diarrheal illnesses but will raise the AG.

Severe hyperchloremic metabolic acidosis with hypokalemia may occur on occasion in patients with ureteral diversion procedures. Because the ileum and the colon are both endowed with Cl^-/HCO_3^- exchangers, when the Cl^- from the urine enters the gut, the HCO_3^- concentration increases as a result of the exchange process.[19] Moreover, K^+ secretion is stimulated, which, together with HCO_3^- loss, can result in a hyperchloremic hypokalemic metabolic acidosis. This defect is particularly common in patients with ureterosigmoidostomies and is more common with this type of diversion because of the prolonged transit time of urine caused by stasis in the colonic segment.

Dilutional acidosis, acidosis caused by exogenous acid loads and the posthypocapnic state, can usually be excluded by history. When isotonic saline is infused rapidly, particularly in patients with temporary or permanent renal functional impairment, the serum HCO_3^- declines reciprocally in relation to Cl^-.[19] Addition of acid or acid equivalents to blood results in metabolic acidosis. Examples include infusion of arginine or lysine hydrochloride during parenteral hyperalimentation or ingestion of ammonium chloride. A similar situation may arise from endogenous addition of keto acids during recovery from ketoacidosis when the sodium salts of ketones may be excreted by the kidneys and lost as potential HCO_3^-.[26]

This sequence may also occur in mild, chronic ketoacidosis in which renal ketone excretion is high and may be accentuated by a defect in tubule ketone reabsorption.[27] The plasma ketone concentration is maintained at low levels. Continued titration of HCO_3^- with Cl^- retention and excretion of potential base (ketones) may result in hyperchloremic acidosis. Metabolism of sulfur to sulfuric acid and excretion of SO_4^{2-} with Cl^- retention represents another example of a hyperchloremic acidosis resulting from increased acid loading and anion excretion.[26]

Loss of functioning renal parenchyma in progressive renal disease is known to be associated with metabolic acidosis. Typically, the acidosis is hyperchloremic when the GFR is between 20 and 50 mL/min but may convert to the typical high AG acidosis of uremia with more advanced renal failure, that is, when the GFR is less than 20.[28] It is generally assumed that such progression is observed more commonly in patients with tubulointerstitial forms of renal disease, but hyperchloremic metabolic acidosis can occur with advanced glomerular disease. The principal defect in acidification of advanced renal failure is that ammoniagenesis is reduced in proportion to the loss of functional renal mass. In addition, medullary NH_4^+ accumulation and trapping in the outer medullary collecting tubule may be impaired.[28] Because of adaptive increases in K^+ secretion by the collecting duct and colon, the acidosis of chronic renal insufficiency is typically normokalemic.[28] Hyperchloremic metabolic acidosis associated with hyperkalemia is almost always associated with a generalized dysfunction of the distal nephron.[6,25] However, K^+-sparing diuretics, triamterene, pentamidine, cyclosporine, tacrolimus, nonsteroidal anti-inflammatory drugs, angiotensin-converting enzyme (ACE) inhibitors, angiotensin II receptor blockers (ARBs), β-blockers, and heparin may mimic or cause this disorder, resulting in hyperkalemia and a hyperchloremic acidosis.[6,25] Such drugs should be discontinued before the diagnosis of a nonreversible, generalized defect of the distal nephron is considered. Drug-induced hyperkalemic metabolic acidosis almost always occurs in the face of renal functional impairment of some degree and is most common in patients prone to develop hyporeninemic hypoaldosteronism (e.g., diabetic nephropathy).

Disorders of Impaired Renal Bicarbonate Reclamation: Proximal Renal Tubular Acidosis
Physiology

Because the first phase of acidification by the nephron involves reabsorption of the filtered HCO_3^-, 80% of the filtered HCO_3^- is normally returned to the blood by the proximal convoluted tubule.[5]

If the capacity of the proximal tubule is reduced, less of the filtered HCO_3^- is reabsorbed in this segment and more is delivered to the more distal segments. This increased HCO_3^- delivery overwhelms the limited capacity for bicarbonate reabsorption by the distal nephron, and bicarbonaturia ensues, net acid excretion ceases, and metabolic acidosis follows. Enhanced Cl^- reabsorption, stimulated by ECF volume contraction, results in a hyperchloremic form of chronic metabolic acidosis. With progressive metabolic acidosis, the filtered HCO_3^- load declines progressively. As the plasma HCO_3^- concentration decreases, the absolute amount of HCO_3^- entering the distal nephron eventually reaches the low level approximating the distal HCO_3^- delivery in normal individuals (at the normal threshold). At this point, the quantity of HCO_3^- entering the distal nephron can be reabsorbed completely (Fig. 14–5), and the urine pH declines. A new steady state in which acid excretion equals acid production then prevails. The serum HCO_3^- concentration usually reaches a nadir of 15 to 18 mEq/L, so that systemic acidosis is not progressive. Therefore, in proximal RTA, in the steady state, the serum HCO_3^- is low and the urine pH is acid (<5.5). With bicarbonate administration, the amount of bicarbonate in the urine increases $FE_{HCO_3^-}$ 10% to 15% and the urine pH becomes alkaline.[25]

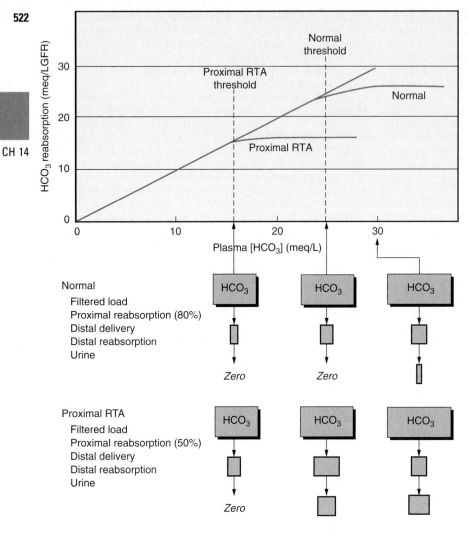

Figure 14–5 Schematic representation of the single-nephron correlates of whole-kidney HCO_3^- titration curves *(top)* in normal subjects and in patients with proximal renal tubular acidosis (proximal RTA). The impact of these relationships on bicarbonaturia is displayed below the graph. Bicarbonate will not appear in the urine when reabsorption is complete at the plasma HCO_3^- concentration threshold, and distal H+ secretory processes are capable of reabsorbing the HCO_3^- delivered out of the proximal nephron. The relationship shows that the fractional proximal HCO_3^- reabsorptive capacity is reduced in patients with proximal RTA (50% versus the normal 80%), so the new steady state is achieved at the expense of systemic metabolic acidosis.

Pathogenesis of Proximal Renal Tubular Acidosis

Proximal RTA can present in two ways: one in which acidification is the only defective function and one in which there is a more generalized proximal tubule dysfunction. A proximal tubule defect involving only acidification is rare. Such a disorder would be assumed to involve a selective defect in the Na^+/H^+ antiporter, the H^+-ATPase, or the $Na^+/HCO_3^-/CO_3^{2-}$ symporter. Abnormalities of cell depolarization or abnormalities of the enzymes carbonic anhydrase II or IV could also cause a selective defect.[25]

In contradistinction to a selective defect, the majority of cases of proximal RTA fit into the category of generalized proximal tubule dysfunction with glycosuria, aminoaciduria, hypercitraturia, and phosphaturia, often referred to as the *Fanconi syndrome.* Numerous experimental studies in animal models demonstrate that the nephropathies associated with maleic acid and cystine involve disruption of active transcellular absorption of HCO_3^-, amino acids, and other solutes. Such a defect could be due to a generalized disorder of the Na^+-coupled apical membrane transporters, a selective disorder of the basolateral Na^+,K^+-ATPase, or a specific metabolic disorder that lowers intracellular adenosine triphosphate (ATP) concentrations.

Development of the Fanconi syndrome by intracellular PO_4^{3-} depletion has also been proposed in hereditary fructose intolerance, in which ingestion of fructose leads to accumulation of fructose 1-phosphate in the proximal tubule. Because these patients lack the enzyme fructose 1-phosphate aldolase, fructose 1-phosphate cannot be further metabolized and intracellular PO_4^{3-} is sequestered in this form. The renal lesion is confined to the proximal tubule because this is the only segment in the kidney that possesses the enzyme fructokinase. Administration of large parenteral loads of fructose to rats leads to high intracellular concentrations of fructose 1-phosphate and low concentrations of ATP and guanosine triphosphate (GTP), as well as of total adenine nucleotides. Prior PO_4^{3-} loading prevents reductions in intracellular ATP, total adenine nucleotides, and PO_4^{3-}.[25,29] Numerous investigators have noted an association between vitamin D deficiency and a proximal RTA with aminoaciduria and hyperphosphaturia. In these studies, correction of the vitamin D deficiency has allowed correction of the proximal tubule dysfunction.[25] Similar results have been obtained in patients with vitamin D–dependent and vitamin D–resistant rickets treated with dihydrotachysterol.[25] The mechanisms involved in the proximal tubule dysfunction are not yet clear.

Another model for isolated proximal tubule acidosis is inherited carbonic anhydrase deficiency. Sly and associates[30] have reported an inherited syndrome with osteopetrosis, cerebral calcification, and RTA caused by an inherited deficiency of carbonic anhydrase II. These patients may have combined proximal and distal RTA but have no other evidence for proximal tubule dysfunction and carbonic anhydrase IV is intact.[30] As already discussed, carbonic anhydrase II is present in the cytoplasm of renal cells, and thus, an acidification defect occurring in association with its deficiency is not unexpected. A defect of carbonic anhydrase IV (the membrane-bound form) has not been reported.

Clinical Spectrum

In general, proximal RTA is more common in children. The two most common causes of acquired proximal RTA in adults are multiple myeloma, in which increased excretion of immunoglobulin light chains injures the proximal tubule epithelium. The light chains that cause injury may have a biochemical characteristic in the variable domain that is resistant to degradation by proteases in lysosomes in proximal tubule cells. Accumulation of the variable domain fragments may be responsible for the impairment in tubular function. In contrast, idiopathic RTA, ifosfamide, lead intoxication, and cystinosis are more common causes in children. Certain chemotherapeutic agents (ifosfamide) also cause proximal RTA. Carbonic anhydrase inhibitors cause pure bicarbonate wasting but not the Fanconi syndrome, by contrast. A comprehensive list of the disorders associated with proximal RTA is displayed in Table 14–7.[25] Some of the entries on this list are no longer seen and are of only historic interest. For example, application of sulfanilamide to the skin of patients with large surface area burns is no longer practiced in most centers. Sulfanilamide, a carbonic anhydrase inhibitor, is absorbed from burned skin. Pharmaceutical manufacturing techniques have improved, and outdated tetracycline is no longer associated with proximal RTA. Some of the agents or associated disorders on this list—such as ifosfamide, Sjögren's syndrome, renal transplantation, and amyloidosis—also appear as causes of distal RTA (see Table 14–7).

Diagnosis

The diagnosis of proximal RTA relies initially on the documentation of a chronic hyperchloremic metabolic acidosis. These patients generally present in the steady state with a chronic metabolic acidosis, an acid urine pH, and a low fractional excretion of HCO_3^-. With alkali therapy or slow infusion of sodium bicarbonate intravenously, when the plasma HCO_3^- increases above the threshold in these patients, bicarbonaturia ensues, and the urine becomes alkaline (Fig. 14–6). By increasing the plasma bicarbonate concentration toward normal (18–20 mEq/L) with an intravenous infusion of sodium bicarbonate at a rate of 0.5 to 1.0 mEq/kg/hr, the urine pH, even if initially acid, will increase once the reabsorptive threshold for bicarbonate has been exceeded. Thus, the urine pH will exceed 7.5 and the fractional excretion of bicarbonate (FE_{HCO3^-}) will increase to 15 to 20 percent.

The hyperchloremic metabolic acidosis is usually seen in association with hypokalemia. If bicarbonate administration has been high in an attempt to repair the acidosis, the bicarbonaturia will drive kaliuresis and the hypokalemia may be severe.[25] Patients with proximal tubule dysfunction exhibit intact distal nephron function (generate steep urine pH gradients and titrate luminal buffers) when the serum HCO_3^- concentration and, hence, distal HCO_3^- delivery are sufficiently reduced. A low HCO_3^- threshold exists. Below this plasma HCO_3^- concentration, distal acidification can compensate for defective proximal acidification, although at the expense of systemic metabolic acidosis. When the plasma HCO_3^- concentration is raised to normal values, a large fraction of the filtered HCO_3^- is inappropriately excreted because the limited reabsorptive capacity of the distal nephron cannot compensate for the reduced proximal nephron reabsorption.

Associated Characteristics

K^+ excretion is typically high in patients with proximal RTA, especially during $NaHCO_3$ administration.[25] Kaliuresis is promoted by the increased delivery of a relatively impermeant anion, HCO_3^-, to the distal nephron in the setting of secondary hyperaldosteronism, which is due to mild volume

TABLE 14–7	Disorders with Dysfunction of Renal Acidification—Defective HCO₃⁻ Reclamation: Proximal Renal Tubular Acidosis

Selective (unassociated with Fanconi syndrome)
  Primary
    Transient (infants)
    Idiopathic or genetic
  Carbonic anhydrase deficiency, inhibition, or alteration
    Drugs
      Acetazolamide
      Sulfanilamide
      Mafenide acetate
    Carbonic anhydrase II deficiency with osteopetrosis
    (Sly syndrome)

Generalized (associated with Fanconi syndrome)
  Primary (without associated systemic disease)
    Genetic
    Sporadic
  Genetically transmitted systemic diseases
    Cystinosis
    Lowe syndrome
    Wilson syndrome
    Tyrosinemia
    Galactosemia
    Hereditary fructose intolerance (during fructose ingestion)
    Metachromatic leukodystrophy
    Pyruvate carboxylase deficiency
    Methylmalonic academia
  Dysproteinemic states
    Multiple myeloma
    Monoclonal gammopathy
  Secondary hyperparathyroidism with chronic hypocalcemia
    Vitamin D deficiency or resistance
    Vitamin D dependency
  Drugs or toxins
    Ifosfamide
    Outdated tetracycline
    3-Methylchromone
    Streptozotocin
    Lead
    Mercury
  Tubulointerstitial diseases
    Sjögren syndrome
    Medullary cystic disease
    Renal transplantation
  Other renal and miscellaneous diseases
    Nephrotic syndrome
    Amyloidosis
    Paroxysmal nocturnal hemoglobinuria

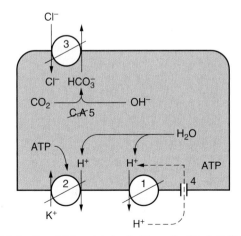

Figure 14–6 Type A intercalated cell of the collecting duct displaying five pathophysiologic defects that could result in classic distal RTA: (1) Defective H^+-ATPase, (2) defective H^+,K^+-ATPase, (3) defective HCO_3^--Cl^- exchanger, (4) H^+ leak pathway, and (5) defective intracellular carbonic anhydrase (type 2).

depletion. Therefore, correction of acidosis in such patients leads to an exaggeration of the kaliuresis and K^+ deficiency.

If the acidification defect is part of a generalized proximal tubule dysfunction (Fanconi syndrome), such patients will have hypophosphatemia, hyperphosphaturia, hypouricemia, hyperuricosuria, glycosuria, aminoaciduria, hypercitraturia, hypercalciuria, and proteinuria.

Although Ca^{2+} excretion may be high in patients with proximal RTA, nephrocalcinosis and renal calculi are rare. This may be related to the high rate of citrate excretion in patients with proximal RTA compared with most patients with acidosis from other causes. Osteomalacia, rickets, abnormal gut Ca^{2+} and phosphorus absorption, and abnormal vitamin D metabolism in children are common, although not invariantly present. Adults tend to have osteopenia without pseudofractures.[25]

The proximal reabsorption of filtered low-molecular-weight proteins may also be abnormal in proximal RTA. Lysozymuria and increased urinary excretion of immunoglobulin light chains can occur.[25]

Treatment

The magnitude of the bicarbonaturia (>10% of the filtered load) at a normal HCO_3^- concentration requires that large amounts of HCO_3^- be administered. At least 10 to 30 mEq/kg/day of HCO_3^- or its metabolic equivalent (citrate) is required to maintain plasma HCO_3^- concentration at normal levels. Correcting the HCO_3^- to near normal values (22–24 mEq/L) is desirable in children to preserve normal growth. Correction to this level is less desirable in adults. Large supplements of K^+ are often necessary because of the kaliuresis induced by high distal HCO_3^- delivery when the plasma HCO_3^- concentration is normalized. Thiazides have proved useful in diminishing therapeutic requirements for HCO_3^- supplementation by causing ECF contraction to stimulate proximal absorption. However, K^+ wasting continues to be a problem, often requiring the addition of a K^+-sparing diuretic.[25] Vitamin D and PO_4^{3-} may be supplemented and in some patients even improve the acidification defect. Fructose should be restricted in patients with fructose intolerance.[29]

Disorders of Impaired Net Acid Excretion with Hypokalemia: Classic Distal Renal Tubule Acidosis
Pathophysiology

The mechanisms involved in the pathogenesis of hypokalemic cDRTA have been more clearly elucidated by appreciation of the genetic and molecular bases of the inherited forms of this disease in the recent years. The observation that these patients tend to be hypokalemic (rather than hyperkalemic) demonstrates that generalized CCT dysfunction or aldosterone deficiency is not causative. Most studies suggest that the acquired or inherited forms of cDRTA are due to defects in the basolateral HCO_3^-/Cl^- exchanger, or subunits of the H^+-ATPase. Other examples include an abnormal leak pathway (e.g., amphoteriein B)[6,19,25] or abnormalities of the H^+,K^+-ATPase. Defects in either of these transport pathways or an increase in apical membrane permeability are displayed in Figure 14–6, which depicts acid-base transporters of a type A intercalated cell in the medullary collecting duct and the possible abnormalities causing cDRTA. The classic feature of this entity is an inability to acidify the urine maximally (to <pH 5.5) in the face of systemic acidosis.[6,25]

The pathogenesis of the acidification defect in most patients is evident by the response of the urine P_{CO_2} to sodium bicarbonate infusion. When normal subjects are given large infusions of sodium bicarbonate to produce a high HCO_3^- excretion, distal nephron H^+ secretion leads to the generation of a high P_{CO_2} in the renal medulla and final urine.[31] The magnitude of the urinary P_{CO_2} (often referred to as the urine minus blood P_{CO_2} or U – B P_{CO_2}) can be used as an index of distal nephron H^+ secretory capacity.[32,33] The U – B P_{CO_2} is generally subnormal in classic hypokalemic distal RTA, with the notable exception of amphotericin B–induced distal RTA, which remains as the most common example of the "gradient" defect.[31,33,34]

INHERITED DEFECTS IN THE BICARBONATE/CHLORINE ION EXCHANGER. Recently, three groups have independently demonstrated an association between mutations in the *AE-1* gene, which encodes the basolateral HCO_3^-/Cl^- exchanger in the collecting duct, and the occurrence of autosomal dominant cDRTA (Example 3 in Fig. 14–6).[35–38] Surprisingly, however, when these point mutations were expressed in vitro, abnormalities in HCO_3^-/Cl^- exchange have not been observed. It was hypothesized that misdirection of the HCO_3^-/Cl^- exchanger to the apical, rather than the basolateral, membrane might obtain in this disorder, resulting in impaired net H^+ secretion.[36,37,39] For a more detailed discussion, the reader is referred to a recent review by Alper.[40]

HYDROGEN ION–SECRETORY DEFECTS (INHERITED AND ACQUIRED). Alternatively, the rate of proton secretion could be affected by an abnormality in a specific transporter or mechanism involved in apical membrane proton extrusion. These include the apical H^+-ATPase or the H^+- K^+-ATPase (see Fig. 14–6). Impairment of the H^+-ATPase in cDRTA has been documented in both acquired and inherited disorders. Acquired defects of H^+-ATPase have been demonstrated in renal biopsy specimens of patients with Sjögrens syndrome with evidence of classic hypokalemic distal RTA.[25] These biopsy specimens revealed an absence of H^+-ATPase protein in the apical membrane of type A intercalated cells. Karet and colleagues[41] have described two different mutations in the *ATP6B1* gene encoding the B1-subunit of the H^+-ATPase. One defect is associated with sensorineural deafness (rd RTA 1), and the other with normal hearing (rd RTA 2).[42] The former recessive disorder is manifest in the first year of life as a failure to thrive, bilateral sensorineural hearing deficits, hyperchloremic, hypokalemic metabolic acidosis, severe nephrolithiasis, nehrocalcinosis, and osteodystrophy. Interestingly, the H^+-ATPase is critical for maintaining pH in the cochlea and endolymph, and its loss in this disorder explains the loss of hearing as well as the renal tubule acidification defect. The latter defect is rare but is associated with normal hearing and has been localized to chromosome 7q 33–34. This group also identified the gene, *ATP6N1B,* which encodes an 840–amino acid novel kidney-specific isoform of ATP6N1A, the 116-kD noncatalytic accessory subunit of the proton pump. Through this work, they described a new kidney-specific proton pump accessory subunit that was highly expressed in proton-secreting cells in the distal nephron.[43,44]

The genetic and molecular basis of distal RTA is outlined in Table 14–8.

Alternatively, abnormalities in the H^+,K^+-ATPase could result in both hypokalemia and metabolic acidosis. A role for H^+,K^+-ATPase involvement in cDRTA was suggested by the observation that chronic administration of vanadate in rats decreased H^+,K^+-ATPase activity and was associated with metabolic acidosis, hypokalemia, and an inappropriately alkaline urine.[45] In addition, an unusually high incidence of hypokalemic distal RTA (endemic RTA) has been observed in northeastern Thailand. To date, no genetic linkages between H^+,K^+-ATPase genes and inherited forms of cDRTA have been documented. Nevertheless, Schwartz and colleagues have presumed such an abnormality in an infant with severe metabolic acidosis and hypokalemia.[25]

Patients with impaired collecting duct H^+ secretion and cDRTA also exhibit uniformly low excretory rates of NH_4^+ when the degree of systemic acidosis is taken into account.[5,6,25] Low NH_4^+ excretion equates with inappropriately low renal regeneration of HCO_3^-, indicating that the kidney is respon-

TABLE 14–8	Genetic and Molecular Bases of Distal Renal Tubular Acidoses
Classic distal RTA	
Inherited	
Autosomal dominant	Defect in AE-1 gene encodes for a single missense mutation (R589H) in the HCO_3^-/Cl^- exchanger (band 3 protein)
	Transporter may be misstargeted to apical membrane
	Other missense mutations reported in some families (R589C and S613F)
Autosomal recessive	
With deafness	Mutations in ATP6B1, encoding B-subunit of the collecting duct apical H^+-ATPase, maps to chromosome 7q33-34. Progressive sensorineural hearing loss (rd RTA1)
With normal hearing	Linkage to segment of 7q33-34 distinct from ATP6N1B (rd RTA2)
Carbonic anhydrase II deficiency	Defect in carbonic anhydrase II in RBC, bone, kidney
Endemic (Northeastern Thailand)	Possible abnormality in H^+,K^+-ATPase?
Acquired	Reduced expression of H^+-ATPase (Sjögren)
Generalized distal nephron Dysfunction	
Pseudohypoaldosteronism type I	
Autosomal recessive	Missense mutation with loss of function of ENaC maps to chromosome 16p12.2-13.11 in six families and to 12p13.1-pter in five additional families
Autosomal dominant	Heterozygous mutations of MLR; two frameshift mutations, two premature termination codons, and one splice donor mutation of the mineralocorticoid receptor gene (MLR)
Pseudohypoaldosteronism type II	WNK1 and WNK4 defect increases function of NCCT to increase NaCl absorption

sible for causing or perpetuating the chronic metabolic acidosis. Low NH_4^+ excretion in classic hypokalemic distal RTA occurs because of the failure to trap NH_4^+ in the medullary collecting duct as a result of higher than normal tubule fluid pH in this segment and loss of the disequilibrium pH (pH > 6.0).[46] The high urine pH indicates impaired H^+ secretion.

In summary, hypokalemic distal RTA is characterized by inability to acidify the urine below pH 5.5. In some patients, this is attributable to an enhanced leakage pathway (amphotericin B lesion) or, in rare patients, without exposure to the antibiotic.[47] However, in most patients, the defect cannot be attributed to such a leak. In these patients, a decreased rate of distal H^+ secretion is the likely mechanism. When the defect is a result of an abnormal H^+-ATPase, hypokalemia occurs secondarily as a result of volume depletion–induced hyperreninemic hyperaldosteronism and acidosis that accompanies this disorder.

Clinical Spectrum and Associated Features
The hallmark of classic hypokalemic distal RTA has been the inability to acidify the urine appropriately during spontaneous or chemically induced metabolic acidosis. The defect in acidification by the collecting duct impairs NH_4^+ and titratable acid excretion and results in positive acid balance, hyperchloremic metabolic acidosis, and volume depletion.[25,48–50] Moreover, medullary interstitial disease, which commonly occurs in conjunction with distal RTA, may impair NH_4^+ excretion by interrupting the medullary countercurrent system for NH_4^+.[6,25,48,49] Hypokalemia and hypercalciuria are typically present,[6] but proximal tubule reabsorptive function is preserved. The dissolution of bone, which may on occasion accompany distal RTA, appears to be the result of chronic positive acid balance that causes Ca^{2+}, Mg^{2+}, and PO_4^{3-}

wasting.[25] Because chronic metabolic acidosis also decreases renal production of citrate,[5,6,25] the resulting hypocitraturia in combination with hypercalciuria creates an environment favorable for urinary stone formation and nephrocalcinosis. Nephrocalcinosis appears to be a reliable marker for cDRTA, because nephrocalcinosis does not occur in proximal RTA or with generalized dysfunction of the nephron associated with hyperkalemia.[6,25] Nephrocalcinosis probably aggravates further the reduction in net acid excretion by impairing the transfer of ammonia from the loop of Henle into the collecting duct. Pyelonephritis is a common complication of distal RTA, especially in the presence of nephrocalcinosis, and eradication of the causative organism may be difficult.[25] Distal RTA occurs frequently in patients with Sjögren's syndrome.[51]

The clinical spectrum of cDRTA is outlined in detail in Table 14–9.[6,25,50]

Treatment
Correction of chronic metabolic acidosis can usually be achieved in patients with cDRTA by administration of alkali in an amount sufficient to neutralize the production of metabolic acids derived from the diet.[25] In adult patients with distal RTA, this is may be equal to no more than 1 to 3 mEq/kg/day.[52] In growing children, endogenous acid production is usually between 2 and 3 mEq/kg/day but may, on occasion, exceed 5 mEq/kg/day. Larger amounts of bicarbonate must be administered to correct the acidosis and maintain normal growth.[6,25] The various forms of alkali replacement are outlined in Table 14–10.

In adult patients with distal RTA, correction of acidosis with alkali therapy reduces urinary K^+ excretion, and prevents hypokalemia and Na^+ depletion.[25] Therefore, in most adult patients with distal RTA, K^+ supplementation is not

TABLE 14–9	Disorders with Dysfunction of Renal Acidification— Selective Defect in Net Acid Excretion: Classic Distal Renal Tubular Acidosis

Primary
Familial
  1. Autosomal dominant
    a. *AE 1* gene
  2. Autosomal recessive
    a. With deafness (rd RTA1 or *ATP6B1* gene)
    b. Without deafness (rd RTA2 or *ATP6N1B*)
Sporadic

Endemic
Northeastern Thailand

Secondary to systemic disorders
Autoimmune diseases

Hyperglobulinemic purpura	Fibrosing alveolitis
Cryoglobulinemia	Chronic active hepatitis
Sjögren syndrome	Primary biliary cirrhosis
Thyroiditis	Polyarthritis nodosa
HIV nephropathy	

Hypercalciuria and nephrocalcinosis

Primary hyperparathyroidism	Vitamin D intoxication
Hyperthyroidism	Idiopathic hypercalciuria
Medullary sponge kidney	Wilson disease
Fabry disease	Hereditary fructose intolerance
X-linked hypophosphatemia	

Drug- and toxin-induced disease

Amphotericin B	Toluene
Cyclamate	Mercury
Hepatic cirrhosis	Vanadate lithium
Ifosfamide	Classic analgesic nephropathy
Foscarnet	

Tubulointerstitial diseases

Balkan nephropathy	Kidney transplantation
Chronic pyelonephritis	Leprosy
Obstructive uropathy	Jejunoileal bypass with hyperoxaluria
Vesicoureteral reflux	

Associated with genetically transmitted diseases

Ehlers-Danlos syndrome	Hereditary elliptocytosis
Sickle cell anemia	Marfan syndrome
Medullary cystic disease	Jejunal bypass with hyperoxaluria
Hereditary sensorineural deafness	Carnitine palmitoyltransferase
Osteopetrosis with carbonic anhydrase II deficiency	

TABLE 14–10	Forms of Alkali Replacement

Shohl solution

Na$^+$ citrate 500 mg	Each 1 mL contains 1 mEq sodium and is equivalent of
Citric acid 334 mg/5 mL	1 mEq of bicarbonate

NaHCO$_3$ tablets

	3.9 mEq/tablet (325 mg)
	7.8 mEq/tablet (650 mg)

Baking soda   60 mEq/tsp
K-Lyte   25–50 mEq/tablet

Polycitra (K-Shohl solution)

Na$^+$ citrate 500 mg	Each 1 mL contains 1 mEq potassium and 1 mEq sodium
K$^+$ citrate 550 mg	and is equivalent to 2 mEq bicarbonate
Citric acid 334 mg/5 mL	

Polycitra K crystals

K$^+$ citrate 3300 mg	Each packet contains 30 mEq potassium and is equivalent
Citric acid 1002 mg/packet	to 30 mEq bicarbonate

Urocit K tablets

Potassium citrate	5 or 10 mEq/tablet

necessary. Frank wasting of K$^+$ may occur in a minority of adult patients and in some children in association with secondary hyperaldosteronism despite correction of the acidosis by alkali therapy requiring K$^+$ supplementation. If required, potassium can be administered as potassium bicarbonate (K-Lyte 25 or 50 mEq), potassium citrate (Urocit K), or polycitra (K-Shohls).[6,25]

Maintenance of a normal serum bicarbonate with alkali therapy also raises urinary citrate, reduces urinary calcium, lowers the frequency of nephrolithiasis, and tends to correct bone disease and restore normal growth in children.[52,53] Therefore, every attempt should be made to correct and maintain a near-normal serum [HCO_3^-] in all patients with cDRTA.

Severe hypokalemia with flaccid paralysis, metabolic acidosis, and hypocalcemia may occur in some patients under extreme circumstances and require immediate therapy. Because the hypokalemia may result in respiratory depression, increasing systemic pH with alkali therapy may worsen the hypokalemia. Therefore, immediate intravenous potassium replacement should be achieved prior to alkali administration.

Disorders of Impaired Net Acid Excretion with Hyperkalemia: Generalized Distal Nephron Dysfunction (Type 4 Renal Tubular Acidosis)

The coexistence of hyperkalemia and hyperchloremic acidosis suggests a generalized dysfunction in the cortical and medullary collecting tubules. In the differential diagnosis, it is important to evaluate the functional status of the renin-aldosterone system and of ECF volume. The specific disorders causing hyperkalemic hyperchloremic metabolic acidosis are outlined in detail in Table 14–11.[6,25]

The regulation of potassium excretion is primarily the result of regulation of potassium secretion, which responds to hyperkalemia, aldosterone, sodium delivery, and nonreabsorbable anions in the CCD. Therefore, a clinical estimate of K^+ transfer into that segment could be helpful to recognize hyperkalemia of renal origin. An abnormally low fractional excretion of potassium or transtubular potassium gradient (TTKG) in the face of hyperkalemia defines hyperkalemia of renal origin. When the TTKG is low in a hyperkalemic patient (<8), it reveals that the collecting tubule is not responding appropriately to the prevailing hyperkalemia and that potassium secretion is impaired. In contrast, in hyperkalemia of nonrenal origin, the kidney should respond by increasing K^+ secretion, as evidenced by a sharp increase in the TTKG. The TTKG assumes no significant net addition or absorption of K^+ between the CCD and the final urine, that CCD tubular fluid osmolality is approximately the same as plasma osmolality, that "osmoles" are not extracted between CCD and final urine, and that plasma [K^+] approximates peritubular fluid [K^+]. Under certain clinical conditions, it is important to note that some or none of these assumptions may be entirely correct. With high urine flow rates, for example, the TTKG underestimates K^+ secretory capacity in the hyperkalemic patient.

Hyperkalemia should also be regarded as an important mediator of the renal response to acid-base balance. Potassium status can affect distal nephron acidification by both direct and indirect mechanisms. First, the level of potassium in systemic blood is an important determinant of aldosterone elaboration, which is also an important determinant of distal H^+ secretion. Chronic potassium deficiency was demonstrated in studies in our laboratory to stimulate ammonium production while chronic hyperkalemia suppressed ammoniagenesis.[54,55] These changes in ammonium production may also affect medullary interstitial ammonium concentration and buffer availability.[55] Hyperkalemia has no effect on ammonium transport in the superficial proximal tubule but markedly impairs ammonium absorption in the thick ascending limb of henle's loop (TALH), reducing inner medullary concentrations of total ammonia and decreasing secretion of NH_3 into the IMCD. The mechanism for impaired absorption of NH_4^+ in the TALH is competition between K^+ and NH_4^+ for the K^+ secretory site on the Na^+-Cl^--$2K^+$ transporter.[56,57] Hyperkalemia may also decrease entry of NH_4^+ into the medullary collecting duct through competition of NH_4^+ and K^+ for the K^+-secretory site on the basolateral membrane sodium pump (Fig. 14–7).[57]

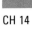

TABLE 14–11	Disorders with Dysfunction of Renal Acidification: Generalized Abnormality of Distal Nephron with Hyperkalemia

Mineralocorticoid deficiency
Primary mineralocorticoid deficiency
  Combined deficiency of aldosterone, desoxycorticosterone, and cortisol
    Addison disease
    Bilateral adrenalectomy
    Bilateral adrenal destruction
    Hemorrhage or carcinoma
  Congenital enzymatic defects
    21-Hydroxylase deficiency
    3β-Hydroxydehydrogenase deficiency
    Desmolase deficiency
  Isolated (selective) aldosterone deficiency
    Chronic idiopathic hypoaldosteronism
    Heparin (low molecular weight or unfractionated) in critically ill patient
    Familial hypoaldosteronism
    Coricosterone methyloxidase deficiency, types 1 and 2
    Primary zona glomerulosa defect
    Transient hypoaldosteronism of infancy
    Persistent hypotension and/or hypoxemia in critically ill patient
  Angiotensin II–converting enzyme inhibition
    Endogenous
    Angiotensin-converting enzyme inhibitors (ACE-I) and AT_1 receptor antagonists (ARB)
Secondary mineralocorticoid deficiency
  Hyporeninemic hypoaldosteronism
    Diabetic nephropathy
    Tubulointerstitial nephropathies
    Nephrosclerosis
    Nonsteroidal anti-inflammatory agents
    Acquired immunodeficiency syndrome
    IgM monoclonal gammopathy

Mineralocorticoid resistance
  PHA I—autosomal dominant (hMR defect)

Renal tubular dysfunction (voltage defect)
  PHA I—autosomal recessive
  PHA II—autosomal dominant
  Drugs that interfere with Na^+ channel function in CCT
    Amiloride
    Triamterene
    Trimethoprim
    Pentamidine
  Drugs that interfere with Na^+, K^+-ATPase in CCT
    Cyclosporine, tacrolimus
  Drugs that inhibit aldosterone effect on CCT
    Spironolactone
  Disorders associated with tubulointerstitial nephritis and renal insufficiency
    Lupus nephritis
    Methicillin nephrotoxicity
    Obstructive nephropathy
    Kidney transplant rejection
    Sickle cell disease
    William syndrome with uric acid nephrolithiasis

In summary, hyperkalemia may have a dramatic impact on ammonium production and excretion (Table 14–12). Chronic hyperkalemia decreases ammonium production in the proximal tubule and whole kidney, inhibits absorption of NH_4^+ in the medullary TALH (mTALH), reduces medullary interstitial concentrations of NH_4^+ and NH_3, and decreases entry of NH_4^+ and NH_3 into the medullary collecting duct. This same series of events leads, in the final analysis, to a marked reduction in urinary ammonium excretion ($U_{Am}V$). The potential for development of a hyperchloremic metabolic acidosis is greatly augmented when a reduction in functional renal mass

528

CH 14

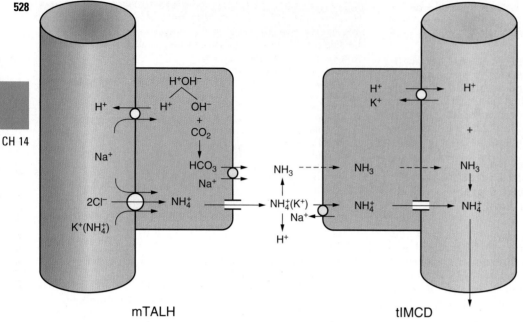

mTALH

tIMCD

Figure 14–7 Relationship between NH_4^+ transport in the medullary thick ascending limb of Henle's loop (mTALH) and the terminal inner medullary collecting duct (tIMCD). This integrated process allows for both countercurrent multiplication of $NH_3 \leftrightarrow NH_4^+$, achieving higher levels in the inner medulla, and facilitated entry of NH_3/NH_4^+ into the tIMCD, bypassing the distal tubule and cortical collecting tubule (CCT), thus trapping NH_4^+ for excretion. The sites at which K^+ competes with NH_4^+ transport are displayed to emphasize that hyperkalemia impairs NH_4^+ production and transport.

TABLE 14–12	Effects of Hyperkalemia on Ammonium Excretion
Decrease in ammonium production	
Decrease in NH_4^- absorption thick ascending limb of henle	
Decrease in interstitial NH_4^+ concentration	
Impaired countercurrent multiplication	
Decrease in NH_3/NH_4^+ secretion into outer and inner medullary collecting ducts	

coexists (GFR < 60 mL/min) with hyperkalemia, or in the presence of aldosterone deficiency or resistance.

Clinical Disorders
Generalized distal nephron dysfunction is manifest as a hyperchloremic, hyperkalemic metabolic acidosis in which urinary ammonium excretion is invariably depressed (positive UAG) and renal function often compromised. Although hyperchloremic metabolic acidosis and hyperkalemia occur with regularity in advanced renal insufficiency, patients selected because of severe hyperkalemia (>5.5 mEq/L) with, for example, diabetic nephropathy and tubulointerstitial disease have hyperkalemia that is disproportionate to the reduction in glomerular filtration rate. The TTKG and/or the FE_K^+ is usually low in patients with this disorder. In such patients, a unique dysfunction of potassium and acid secretion by the collecting tubule coexists and can be attributed to either mineralocorticoid deficiency, resistance to mineralocorticoid, or a specific type of renal tubular dysfunction (voltage defects). The clinical spectrum of generalized abnormalities in the distal nephron is summarized in Table 14–11.

Primary Mineralocorticoid Deficiency
A number of factors modulate aldosterone secretion: angiotensin II, adrenocorticotropic hormone (ACTH), endothelin, dopamine, acetylcholine, epinephrine, plasma K^+, and Mg^{2+}. However, angiotensin II and plasma K^+ remain the principal modulators of aldosterone production and secretion. Destruction of the adrenal cortex by hemorrhage, infection, invasion

by tumors, or autoimmune processes results in Addison's disease. This causes combined glucocorticoid and mineralocorticoid deficiency and is recognized clinically by hypoglycemia, anorexia, weakness, hyperpigmentation, and a failure to respond to stress. These defects can occur in association with renal salt wasting and hyponatremia, hyperkalemia, and metabolic acidosis. The most common congenital adrenal defect in steroid biosynthesis is 21-hydroxylase deficiency, which is associated with salt wasting, hyperkalemia, and metabolic acidosis in a fraction of the patients. Causes of Addison's disease include tuberculosis, autoimmune adrenal failure, fungal infections, adrenal hemorrhage, metastasis, lymphoma, AIDS, amyloidosis, and drug toxicity (ketoconazole, fluconozole, phenytoin, rifampin, and barbiturates). These disorders are associated with low plasma aldosterone levels and high levels of plasma renin activity.[25] The metabolic acidosis of mineralocorticoid deficiency results from a decrease in hydrogen ion secretion in the collecting duct secondary to decreased H^+-ATPase pump number and function. The hyperkalemia of mineralocorticoid deficiency decreases ammonium production and excretion.

Hyporeninemic Hypoaldosteronism
In contrast to patients with the primary adrenal disorder, patients in this group will exhibit low plasma renin activity, are usually older (mean age 65 yr), and frequently have mild to moderate renal insufficiency (70%) and acidosis (50%) in association with chronic hyperkalemia in the range of 5.5 to 6.5 mEq/L (Table 14–13).[25] Although the hyperkalemia may be asymptomatic, it is important to recognize that both the metabolic acidosis and the hyperkalemia are out of proportion to the level of reduction in GFR. The most frequently associated renal diseases are diabetic nephropathy and tubulointerstitial disease. Additional disorders associated with hyporeninemic hypoaldosteronism include tubulointerstitial nephritis, systemic lupus erythematosis, and HIV. For 80% to 85% of such patients, there is a reduction in plasma renin activity that cannot be stimulated by the usual physiologic maneuvers. Because approximately 30% of patients with hyporeninemic hypoaldosteronism are hypertensive, the finding of a low plasma renin in such patients suggests a volume-dependent form of hypertension with physiologic suppression of renin elaboration.

TABLE 14–13	Hyporeninemic Hypoaldosteronism: Typical Clinical Features

Mean age 65 yr

Asymptomatic hyperkalemia (75%)
   Weakness (25%)
   Arrhythymia (25%)

Hyperchloremic metabolic acidosis (>50%)

Renal insufficiency (70%)

Diabetes mellitus (50%)

Cardiac disorders
   Arrhythmia (25%)
   Hypertension (75%)
   Congestive heart failure (50%)

TABLE 14–14	Isolated Hypoaldosteronism in the Critically Ill Patient

Elevated adrenocorticotropic hormone (ACTH) and cortisol levels in association with a decrease in aldosterone elaboration

Inhibition of aldosterone synthase
   Heparin
   Hypoxia
   Cytokines
   Atrial natriuretic peptide

Manifestations of hypoaldosteronism
   Hyperkalemia
   Metabolic acidosis

Potentiated by K^+-sparing diuretics, K^+ loads in parenteral nutrition, or heparin

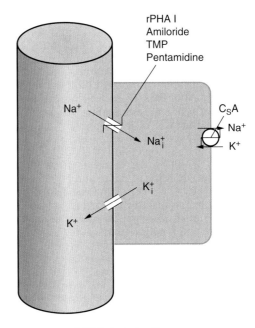

CCT (principal cell)

Figure 14–8 Examples of "voltage" defects in the CCT causing abnormal Na^+ transport (and K^+ secretion) across the apical membrane of a principal cell: (1) the Na^+ channel (ENaC) is blocked or occupied by amiloride, trimethoprim, or pentamidine or is inoperative (autosomal recessive PHA-I), and (2) inhibition of basolateral Na^+,K^+-ATPase activity by calcineurin-cyclosporine (C_sA). As a consequence of impaired Na^+ uptake, transepithelial K^+ secretion is compromised, leading to hyperkalemia. The pathogenesis of metabolic acidosis, when present, is the result of the unfavorable voltage (which impairs H^+ secretion by the type A intercalated cell, not shown) or the inhibition of NH_4^+ production and transport and the H^+,K^+-ATPase as a consequence of hyperkalemia.

Impaired ammonium excretion is the combined result of hyperkalemia, impaired ammoniagenesis, a reduction in nephron mass, reduced proton secretion, and impaired transport of ammonium by nephron segments in the inner medulla.[6,25,58] Hyperchloremic metabolic acidosis occurs in approximately 50% of patients with hyporeninemic hypoaldosteronism. Drugs, which may result in similar manifestations, are reviewed later.

Isolated Hypoaldosteronism in Critically Ill Patients

Isolated hypoaldosteronism, which may occur in critically ill patients, particularly in the setting of severe sepsis or cardiogenic shock, is manifest by markedly elevated ACTH and cortisol levels in concert with a decrease in aldosterone elaboration in response to angiotensin II. This may be secondary to selective inhibition of aldosterone synthase as a result of hypoxia or in response to cytokines such as tumor necrosis factor (TNF)-α or interleukin (IL)-1 or, alternatively, as a result of high circulating levels of atrial natriuretic peptide (ANP).[6,25,59] ANP, a powerful suppressor of aldosterone secretion, may be elevated in congestive heart failure (CHF), with atrial arrhythmias, in subclinical cardiac disease, and in volume expansion. The tendency to manifest the features of hypoaldosteronism, including hyperkalemia and metabolic acidosis, is often potentiated by the administration of potassium-sparing diuretics or potassium loads in parenteral nutrition solutions or as a result of heparin administration. The latter suppresses aldosterone synthesis in the critically ill patient (Table 14–14).

Resistance to Mineralocorticoid and Voltage Defects

Autosomal dominant pseudohypoaldosteronism type I (PHA) is the prototypical example of renal resistance to aldosterone

action. This disorder, which is clinically less severe than the autosomal recessive form discussed later, is associated with hyperkalemia (which can be attributed to impaired potassium secretion), renal salt wasting, elevated levels of renin and aldosterone, and hypotension. Physiologic mineralocorticoid replacement therapy does not correct the hyperkalemia. The autosomal dominant disorder has been shown to be the result of a mutation in the intracellular mineralocorticoid receptor (hMR) in the collecting tubule.[60] Unlike the autosomal recessive disorder, this defect is not expressed in organs other than the kidney and becomes less severe with advancing age. Because the decrease in mineralocortoid reduces apical Na^+ absorption and activity of the epithelial sodium channel (EnaC), transepithelial potential difference declines and K^+ secretion is impaired.

The prototype for a "voltage" defect is autosomal recessive PHA I (Fig. 14–8). This disorder is the result of a loss of function mutation of the gene that encodes one of the subunits of the α, β, or γ subunit of the ENaC.[61–65] Children with this disorder have severe hyperkalemia and renal salt wasting because of impaired sodium absorption in principal cells of the CCT. In addition, the hyperchloremic metabolic acidosis may be severe and is associated with hypotension and marked elevations of plasma renin and aldosterone. These children also manifest vomiting, hyponatremia, failure to thrive, and respiratory distress. The latter is due to involvement of ENaC in the alveolus, preventing Na^+ and water absorption in the lungs.[64,66] Patients with this disease respond to a high salt intake and correction of the hyperkalemia. Unlike the autosomal dominant form, autosomal recessive PHA I persists throughout life.

A number of additional adult patients have been reported with a rare form of autosomal dominant low-renin hypertension, which is invariably associated with hyperkalemia, hyperchloremic metabolic acidosis, mild volume expansion, normal renal function, and low aldosterone levels. This syndrome has been designated *familial hyperkalemic hypertension,* but is also known as *pseudohypoaldosteronism type II* (PHA II),[67] or *Gordon's syndrome.* Lifton's group[68,69] identified two genes causing PHA II. Both genes encode members of the WNK family of serine-threonine kinases. WNK1 and WNK4 localize to the CCT. WNK4 negatively regulates surface expression of the Na^+-Cl^- co-transporter in the connecting tubule (NCCT).[69] Loss of regulation of NCCT by WNK4 mutation appears to result in an increase in NCCT function, volume expansion, shunting of voltage, and therefore, reduced K^+ secretion in the CCT.[69-71] PHA II may be distinguished from selective hypoaldosteronism by the presence of normal renal function and hypertension, the absence of diabetes mellitus and salt wasting, and a kaliuretic response to mineralocorticoids. The acidosis in these patients is mild and can be accounted for by the magnitude of hyperkalemia; the acidosis and renal potassium excretion are resistant to mineralocorticoid administration. Thiazide diuretics consistently correct the hyperkalemia and metabolic acidosis, as well as the hypertension, plasma aldosterone, and plasma renin levels.

Secondary Renal Diseases Associated with Acquired Voltage Defects

In addition to the previous discussion on inherited voltage defects, Table 14–15 outlines a number of acquired renal disorders due to drugs or tubulointerstitial diseases, which are often associated with hyperkalemia.[25] Examples of the former include amiloride and the structurally related compounds, trimethoprim (TMP), and pentamidine. As discussed earlier, this explains the occurrence of hyperkalemic hyperchloremic acidosis in patients receiving higher doses of these agents. TMP and pentamidine occupy the Na^+ channel, as does amiloride, causing hyperkalemia, which contributes to the acidosis. Additional drugs not related to amiloride include cyclooxygenase (COX)-2 inhibitors, cyclosporine, tacrolimus, and nonsteroidal anti-inflammatory durgs (NSAIDs).[72,73] In these disorders, the frequency with which hyperkalemia is associated with metabolic acidosis and decreased net acid excretion as a result of impaired ammonium production or excretion cannot be presumed to be a result of the severity of

impairment in renal function. Hyperkalemia which is out of proportion to the degree of renal insufficiency is typically observed with the nephropathies associated with sickle cell, HIV disease, systemic lupus erythematosis, obstructive uropathy; acute and chronic renal allograft rejection, hypoaldosteronism, multiple myeloma, and amyloidosis.[25,74] Tubulointerstitial disease with hyperkalemia and hyperchloremic metabolic acidosis with or without salt wasting may be associated with analgesic abuse, sickle cell disease, obstructive uropathy, nephrolithiasis, nephrocalcinosis, and hyperuricemia.[25]

Hyperkalemic Distal Renal Tubular Acidosis

A generalized defect in CCD secretory function that results in hyperkalemic hyperchloremic metabolic acidosis has been delineated as *hyperkalemic distal RTA* because of the coexistence of an inability to acidify the urine ($U_{pH} > 5.5$) during spontaneous acidosis or following an acid load and hyperkalemia. The hyperkalemia is the result of impaired renal K^+ secretion and the TTKG or FE_{K^+} is invariably lower than expected for hyperkalemia. Urine ammonium excretion is reduced, but aldosterone levels may be low, normal, or even increased. Hyperkalemic distal RTA may be observed in a wide variety of renal diseases including systemic lupus erythematosis, sickle cell disease, obstructive uropathy, transplantation, and amyloidosis. Drugs may be associated with a number of tubular defects that can be manifest as hyperkalemic distal RTA (see later). Hyperkalemic distal RTA can be distinguished from selective hypoaldosteronism because plasma renin and aldosterone levels are usually high or normal. Typically in selective hypoaldosteronism, the U_{pH} is low and the defect in urinary acidification can be attributed to the decrease in ammonium excretion. In contrast with hypokalemic or cDRTA, patients with hyperkalemic distal RTA do not increase H^+ or K^+ excretion in response to nonreabsorbable anions (SO_4^{2-}) or furosemide.

Drug-induced Renal Tubular Secretory Defects

IMPAIRED RENIN-ALDOSTERONE ELABORATION. Drugs may impair renin or aldosterone elaboration or produce mineralocorticoid resistance and mimic the clinical manifestations of the acidification defect seen in the generalized form of distal RTA with hyperkalemia (see Table 14–15). COX inhibitors (NSAIDs or COX-2-I) can generate hyperkalemia and metabolic acidosis as a result of inhibition of renin release.[73] β-Adrenergic antagonists cause hyperkalemia as a result of altered potassium distribution and by interference with the renin-aldosterone system. Heparin impairs aldosterone synthesis as a result of direct toxicity to the zona glomerulosa and inhibition of aldosterone synthase. ACE inhibitors and ARBs interrupt the rennin-aldosterone system and result in hypoaldosteronism with hyperkalemia and acidosis, particularly in the patient with advanced renal insufficiency or in patients with a tendency to develop hyporeninemic hypoaldosteronism (diabetic nephropathy). The combination of potassium-sparing diuretics and ACE inhibitors should be avoided judiciously in diabetics.

INHIBITORS OF POTASSIUM SECRETION IN THE COLLECTING DUCT. Spironolactone acts as a competitive inhibitor of aldosterone and inhibits aldosterone biosynthesis. This drug may be a frequent cause of hyperkalemia and metabolic acidosis when administered to patients with significant renal insufficiency, in patients with advanced liver disease, or in patients unrecognized renal hemodynamic compromise. Similarly, amiloride and triamterine may be associated with hyperkalemia but through an entirely different mechanism. Both potassium-sparing diuretics occupy and thus block the apical Na^+-selective channel (ENaC) in the collecting duct principal cell (see Fig. 14–8). Occupation of ENaC inhibits Na^+ absorp-

---

TABLE 14–15 Causes of Drug-induced Hyperkalemia

Impaired renin-aldosterone elaboration/function
Cyclooxygenase inhibitors (NSAIDs)
β-Adrenergic antagonists
Spironolactone
Converting-enzyme inhibitors and ARBs
Heparin

Inhibitors of renal potassium secretion
Potassium-sparing diuretics (amiloride, triamterine)
Trimethoprim
Pentamidine
Cyclosporine
Digitalis overdose
Lithium

Altered potassium distribution
Insulin antagonists (somatostatin, diazoxide)
β-Adrenergic antagonists
α-Adrenergic agonists
Hypertonic solutions
Digitalis
Succinylcholine
Arginine hydrochloride, lysine hydrochloride

TABLE 14–16	Hyperkalemic Hyperchloremic Metabolic Acidosis with Trimethoprim
Occurs in 20% of HIV patients on trimethoprin-sulfamethoxazole (TMP-SMX)	
More prevalent with higher doses (>20 mg/kg/day)	
Hyperkalemia most frequent complication	
Seen in children and older HIV-negative patients on "conventional" doses	
Reversible	
Etiology of metabolic acidosis	
Voltage defect	
Hyperkale	
Decreased ammonium production/excretion	

TABLE 14–17	Treatment of Generalized Dysfunction of the Nephron with Hyperkalemia
Alkali therapy (Shohl solution or $NaHCO_3$)	
Loop diuretic (furosemide, bumetanide)	
Sodium polystyrene sulfonate (Kayexalate)	
Low-potassium diet	
Fludrocortisone (0.1–0.3 mg/day) Avoid in hypertension, volume expansion, heart failure Combine with loop diuretic	
Avoid drugs associated with hyperkalemia	
In PHA I, add NaCl supplement	

tion and reduces the negative transepithelial voltage, which alters the driving force for K^+ secretion. Amiloride is the prototype for a growing number of agents, including TMP and pentamidine, that act similarly to cause hyperkalemia, particularly in patients with AIDS. TMP and pentamidine are related structurally to amiloride and triamterene. The protonated forms of both TMP and pentamidine have been demonstrated by Kleyman and Ling[75] to inhibit ENaC in A6 distal nephron cells. This effect in A6 cells has been verified in rat late distal tubules perfused in vivo.[77] Hyperkalemia has been observed in 20% to 50% of HIV-infected patients receiving high-dose TMP–sulfamethoxazole (SMX) or TMP-dapsone for the treatment of opportunistic infections and as many as 100% of patients with AIDS-associated infections (Pneumocystis carinii) receiving pentamidine for more than 6 days.[77] The pathophysiologic basis of the hyperkalemia and metabolic acidosis from TMP is displayed in Table 14–16. Because both TMP and pentamidine decrease the electrochemical driving force for both K^+ and H^+ secretion in the CCT, metabolic acidosis may accompany the hyperkalemia even in the absence of severe renal failure, adrenal insufficiency, tubulointerstitial disease, or hypoaldosteronism. Whereas it has been assumed that such a "voltage" defect could explain the decrease in H^+ secretion, it is likely that, in addition, hyperkalemia plays a significant role in the development of metabolic acidosis by direct inhibition of ammonium production and excretion (see Fig. 14–7 and Table 14–12). Cyclosporine (CsA) or tacrolimus (FK 506) may be associated with hyperkalemia in the transplant recipient as a result of inhibition of the basolateral Na^+,K^+-ATPase, thereby decreasing intracellular $[K^+]$ and the transepithelial potential, which together decrease the driving force for K^+ secretion (see Fig. 14–8).[73] It has been suggested that the specific mechanism of inhibition of the Na^+ pump is through inhibition by these agents of calcineurin activity.[78] Either drug could also decrease the filtered load of K^+ through hemodynamic mechanisms such as vasoconstriction, which decrease GFR and alter the filtration fraction.

Treatment
In hyperkalemic hyperchloremic metabolic acidosis, documentation of the underlying disorder is necessary and therapy should be based on a precise diagnosis if possible. Of particular importance is a careful drug and dietary history. Contributing or precipitating factors should be considered, including low urine flow or decreased distal Na^+ delivery, a rapid decline in GFR (especially in acute superimposed on chronic renal failure), hyperglycemia or hyperosmolality, and unsus-

pected sources of exogenous K^+ intake.[25] The workup should include evaluation of the TTKG or the fractional excretion of potassium, an estimate of renal ammonium excretion (UAG, osmolar gap, and urine pH), and evaluation of plasma renin activity and aldosterone secretion. The latter may be obtained under stimulated conditions with dietary salt restriction and furosemide-induced volume depletion and the response of potassium excretion to furosemide and fludrocortisone.

The decision to treat is often based on the severity of the hyperkalemia. Reduction in serum potassium will often improve the metabolic acidosis by increasing ammonium excretion as potassium levels return to the normal range. Correction of hyperkalemia with sodium polystyrene can correct the metabolic acidosis as the serum potassium declines.[6,25] Patients with combined glucocorticoid and mineralocorticoid deficiency should receive both adrenal steroids in replacement dosages. Additional measures may include laxatives, alkali therapy, or treatment with a loop diuretic to induce renal potassium and salt excretion (Table 14–17). Volume depletion should be avoided unless the patient is volume overexpanded or hypertensive. Supraphysiologic doses of mineralocorticoids are rarely necessary and, if administered, should be done cautiously in combination with a loop diuretic to avoid volume overexpansion or aggravation of hypertension and to increase potassium excretion.[25] Infants with autosomal recessive or dominant PHA I should receive salt supplements in amounts sufficient to correct the volume depletion, hypotension, and other features of the syndrome and to allow normal growth. In contrast, patients with PHA II should receive thiazide diuretics along with dietary salt restriction. Although it may be prudent to discontinue drugs that are identified as the most likely cause of the hyperkalemia, this may not always be feasible in the patient with a life-threatening disorder, for example, during TMP-SMX or pentamidine therapy in the AIDS patient with Pneumocystis carinii pneumonia. Based on the previous analysis of the mechanism by which TMP and pentamidine cause hyperkalemia (voltage defect), it might also be reasoned that the delivery to the CCD of a poorly reabsorbed anion might improve the electrochemical driving force favoring K^+ and H^+ secretion. The combined use of acetazolamide along with sufficient sodium bicarbonate to deliver HCO_3^- to the CCT and thereby increase the negative transepithelial voltage could theoretically increase K^+ and H^+ secretion. Obviously with such an approach, aggravation of metabolic acidosis by excessive acetazolamide or insufficient $NaHCO_3$ administration must be avoided.

Distinguishing the Types of Renal Tubular Acidosis
The contrasting findings and diagnostic features of the three types of RTA discussed in this chapter are summarized in Table 14–18:

TABLE 14–18	Contrasting Features and Diagnostic Studies in Renal Tubular Acidosis		
Finding	Type of RTA		
	Proximal	*Classic Distal*	*Generalized Distal Dysfunction*
Plasma [K$^+$]	Low	Low	High
Urine pH with acidosis	<5.5	>5.5	<5.5 or >5.5
Urine net charge	Positive	Positive	Positive
Fanconi lesion	Present	Absent	Absent
Fractional bicarbonate excretion	10%–15%	2%–5%	5%–10%
U–B PCO_2 H$^+$-ATPase defect HCO$_3^-$-Cl$^-$ defect Amphotericin B	Normal	Low* Low High Normal	Low
Response to therapy	Least readily	Readily	Less readily
Associated features	Fanconi syndrome	Nephrocalcinosis/ hyperglobulinemia	Renal insufficiency

U-B PCO_2, urine-blood CO_2 tension.
*See specific defects below.

Disorders of Impaired Net Acid Excretion and Impaired Bicarbonate Reclamation with normokalemia: Acidosis of Progressive Renal Failure

A reduction in functional renal mass by disease has long been known to be associated with acidosis.[28] The metabolic acidosis is initially hyperchloremic in nature (GFR in the range of 20–30 mL/min) but may convert to the normochloremic, high AG variety as renal insufficiency progresses and GFR falls below 15 mL/min.[28,79]

The major defect in acidification is due to impaired net acid excretion. When the plasma HCO$_3^-$ concentration is in the normal range, urine pH is relatively high (≥6.0), and net acid excretion is low. Unlike patients with distal RTA, patients with primary renal disease have a normal ability to lower the urine pH during acidosis.[28] The distal H$^+$ secretory capacity is qualitatively normal and can be increased by buffer availability in the form of PO$_4^{3-}$ or by nonreabsorbable anions. Also in contrast to distal RTA, the U − B PCO_2 gradient is normal in patients with reduced GFR, reflecting intact distal H$^+$ secretory capacity.

The principal defect in net acid excretion in patients with reduced GFR is thus not an inability to secrete H$^+$ in the distal nephron, but rather an inability to produce or to excrete NH$_4^+$. Consequently, the kidneys cannot quantitatively excrete all the metabolic acids produced daily, and metabolic acidosis supervenes.[28]

Although the acidosis of chronic progressive kidney disease is rarely severe, the argument can be made that the progressive dissolution of bone[28] and the impaired hydroxylation of 25-hydroxycholecalciferol by acidosis[28,79] warrant treatment.

Moreover, chronic metabolic acidosis due to chronic progressive kidney disease prior to dialysis has other deleterious effects including: insulin resistance, suppression of the growth hormone/insulin-like growth factor (IGF)-1 cascade, increased levels of glucocorticoids, protein degradation, and muscle wasting. The latter is a result of activation of the ubiquitin-proteosome pathway. In general, it is accepted that alkali therapy helps to reverse these deleterious effects. An amount of alkali slightly in excess (1–2 mEq/kg/day) of dietary metabolic acid production usually restores acid-base equilibrium and prevents acid retention.[28] Fear of Na$^+$ retention in chronic

renal failure as a result of sodium bicarbonate administration appears ill founded. Unlike the case in sodium chloride therapy, patients with chronic renal disease retain administered sodium bicarbonate only as long as acidosis is present. Further sodium bicarbonate then exceeds the reabsorptive threshold and is excreted without causing an increase in weight or in blood pressure unless very large amounts are administered.

The clinical guidelines endorsed by the National Kidney Foundation (K/DOQI [Kidney disease outcomes quality initiative]) recommend monitoring of total CO_2 in patients with chronic kidney disease (CKD) with a goal of maintaining the [HCO$_3^-$] above 22 mEq/L. Such therapy is based on the view that chronic metabolic acidosis has an adverse impact on muscle and bone metabolism.

Also of concern in chronic progressive kidney disease is the use of sevelamer hydrochloride, which has been shown in patients on chronic hemodialysis to result in significantly lower [HCO$_3^-$] compared with Ca^{2+}-containing phosphate binders.[80] Although related to a lower intake of potential alkali, sevelamer may also provide an acid load.[81] Therefore, the clinician should be alert for changes in the [HCO$_3^-$] in the face of sevelamer treatment. A number of potential mechanisms exist for the acidosis associated with sevelamer. This agent binds monovalent phosphate in exchange for chloride in the gastrointestinal tract. For each molecule of monovalent phosphate bound, one molecule of HCl is liberated. Upon entry into the small intestine, exposure to pancreatic secretion of bicarbonate would result in the binding of bicarbonate by the polymer in exchange for chloride—much like the mechanism in chloride diarrhea. There may be other drug effects on bicarbonate in the colon as well.[82] As kidney disease progresses below a GFR of 15 mL/min, the non-AG acidosis typically evolves into the usual high AG acidosis of end-stage renal disease (see later).[80]

High Anion Gap Acidoses

The addition to the body of an acid load in which the attendant non-Cl$^-$ anion is not excreted rapidly results in the development of a high AG acidosis. The normochloremic acidosis is maintained as long as the anion that was part of the original acid load remains in the blood. AG acidosis is caused by the accumulation of organic acids. This may occur if the anion does not undergo glomerular filtration (e.g., uremic acid anions), if the anion is filtered but is readily reabsorbed, or if, because of alteration in metabolic pathways (ketoacidosis, L-lactic acidosis), the anion cannot be utilized. Theoretically, with a pure AG acidosis, the increment in the AG (ΔAG) above the normal value of 10 mEq/L should equal the decrease in bicarbonate concentration (ΔHCO$_3^-$) below the normal value of 25 mEq/L. When this relationship is considered, circumstances in which the increment in the AG exceeds the decrement in bicarbonate (ΔAG > ΔHCO$_3^-$) suggest the coexistence of a metabolic alkalosis. Such findings are not unusual when uremia leads to vomiting, for example.

Identification of the underlying cause of a high AG acidosis is facilitated by consideration of the clinical setting and associated laboratory values. The common causes are outlined in Table 14–19 and include: (1) lactic acid acidosis (e.g., L-lactic acidosis and D-lactic acidosis), (2) ketoacidosis (e.g., diabetic, alcoholic, and starvation ketoacidoses), (3) toxin- or poison-induced acidosis (e.g., ethylene glycol, methyl alcohol, or toluene poisoning), and (4) uremic acidosis. Initial screening to differentiate the high AG acidoses should include: (1) a history or other evidence of drug and toxin ingestion and ABG measurement to detect coexistent respiratory alkalosis (salicylates), (2) historical evidence of diabetes mellitus (DKA), (3) evidence of alcoholism or increased levels of β-hydroxybutyrate (alcoholic ketoacidosis), (4) observation for clinical signs of uremia and determination of the blood urea nitrogen and creatinine (uremic acidosis), (5) inspection of the urine for oxalate crystals (ethylene glycol), and finally, (6) recognition of the numerous settings in which lactic acid levels may be increased (hypotension, cardiac failure, ischemic bowel, intestinal obstruction and bacterial overgrowth, leukemia, cancer, and with certain drugs).

Lactic Acidosis
Physiology
Lactic acid can exist in two forms: L-lactate and D-lactate. In mammals, only the levorotary form is a product of metabolism. D-Lactate can accumulate in humans as a byproduct of metabolism by bacteria, which accumulate and overgrow in the gastrointestinal tract with jejunal bypass or short bowel syndrome. Thus, D-lactic acid acidosis is a rare cause of a high AG acidosis. Hospital chemical laboratories measure routinely L-lactic acid levels, not D-lactic acid levels. Thus, most of the remarks that follow apply to L-lactic acid metabolism and acidosis except as noted. L-lactic acidosis is one of the most common forms of a high AG acidosis.

Although lactate metabolism bears a close relationship to that of pyruvate,[83] lactic acid is in a metabolic cul-de-sac with pyruvate as its only outlet. In most cells, the major metabolic pathway for pyruvate is oxidation in the mitochondria to acetyl coenzyme A by the enzyme pyruvate dehydrogenase within the mitochordria. The overall reaction is usually expressed as:

$$\text{Pyruvate}^- + \text{NADH} \leftrightarrow \text{lactate}^- + \text{NAD} + \text{H}^+ \quad (32)$$

Normally, this cytosolic reaction catalyzed by the enzyme lactate dehydrogenase (LDH) is close to equilibrium, so that the law of mass action applies and the equation is rearranged as:

$$[\text{Lactate}^-] = K_{eq}[\text{pyruvate}^-][\text{H}^+]\frac{[\text{NADH}]}{[\text{NAD}^+]} \quad (33)$$

The lactate concentration is a function of the equilibrium constant (K_{eq}), the pyruvate concentration, the cytosolic pH, and the intracellular redox state represented by the pyridine nucleotide concentration ratio [NADH]/[NAD$^+$].[83]

After rearranging the mass action equation, the ratio of lactate concentration to pyruvate concentration may be expressed as

TABLE 14–19	Metabolic Acidosis with High Anion Gap

Conditions associated with type A lactic acidosis
  Hypovolemic shock
  Cholera
  Septic shock
  Cardiogenic shock
    Low-output heart failure
    High-output heart failure
  Regional hypoperfusion
  Severe hypoxia
    Severe asthma
    Carbon monoxide poisoning
    Severe anemia

Conditions associated with type B lactic acidosis
  Liver disease
  Diabetes mellitus
  Catecholamine excess
    Endogenous
    Exogenous
  Thiamine deficiency
  Intracellular inorganic phosphate depletion
    Intravenous fructose
    Intravenous xylose
    Intravenous sorbitol
  Alcohols and other ingested compounds metabolized
    by alcohol
    Dehydrogenase
    Ethanol
    Methanol
    Ethylene glycol
    Propylene glycol
  Mitochondrial toxins
    Salicylate intoxication
    Cyanide poisoning
    2,4-Dinitrophenol ingestion
    Non-nucleoside antireverse transcriptase drugs
  Other drugs
  Malignancy
  Seizure
  Inborn errors of metabolism

D-Lactic acidosis
  Short-bowel syndrome
  Ischemic bowel
  Small bowel obstruction

Ketoacidosis
  Diabetic
  Alcoholic
  Starvation

Other toxins
  Salicylates
  Paraldehyde
  Pyroglutamic acid

Uremia (late renal failure)

$$\frac{[\text{Lactate}^-]}{[\text{Pyruvate}^-]} = K_{eq}[\text{H}^+]\frac{[\text{NADH}]}{[\text{NAD}^+]} \quad (34)$$

Because K_{eq} and intracellular H$^+$ concentration are relatively constant, the normal lactate-to-pyruvate concentration ratio (1.0/0.1 mEq/L) is proportional to the NADH/NAD$^+$ concentration ratio. The lactate-to-pyruvate ratio is regulated by the oxidation-reduction potential of the cell, therefore.

NADH/NAD$^+$ is also involved in many other metabolic redox reactions.[83] Moreover, the steady-state concentrations of all these redox reactants are related to one another. Important in considerations in acid-base pathophysiology are the redox pairs β-hydroxybutyrate–acetoacetate and ethanol-acetaldehyde. The ratio of the reduced to the oxidized forms of these molecules is thus a function of the cellular redox potential:

$$\frac{[NADH]}{[NAD^+]} \approx \frac{[Lactate^-]}{[Pyruvate^-]} \approx$$

$$\frac{[\beta - hydroxybutyrate^-]}{[acetoacetate^-]} \propto \frac{[ethanol]}{[acetaldehyde]} \quad (35)$$

If the lactate concentration is high compared with that of pyruvate, NAD^+ would be depleted, and the $NADH/NAD^+$ ratio would increase. Likewise, all the other related redox ratios previously listed would be similarly affected; that is, both the β-hydroxybutyrate/acetoacetate and the ethanol-to-acetaldehyde ratios would increase. In clinical practice, these considerations are of practical importance. If lactate levels are increased as a result of lactic acidosis concurrently with ketone overproduction as a result of diabetic acidosis, the ketones exist primarily in the form of β-hydroxybutyrate. Tests for ketones that measure only acetoacetate (such as the nitroprusside reaction, e.g., Acetest tablets and reagent sticks), therefore, may be misleadingly low or even negative despite high total ketone concentrations. Similarly, high levels of alcohol plus ketones shift the redox ratio, so that the $NADH/NAD^+$ ratio is increased. Again, ketones would then be principally in the form of β-hydroxybutyrate. This situation is commonly found in alcoholic ketoacidosis (AKA), in which qualitative ketone tests that are more sensitive to acetoacetate are frequently only trace positive or negative, despite markedly increased β-hydroxybutyrate levels.

The L-lactate concentration can be increased in two ways relative to the pyruvate concentration. First, when pyruvate production is increased at a constant intracellular pH and redox stage, the lactate concentration increases at a constant lactate-to-pyruvate ratio of 10. In contrast, states in which the production of lactate exceeds the ability to convert to pyruvate, so that the $NADH/NAD^+$ redox ratio is increased, an increased L-lactate concentrations is observed, but with a lactate-to-pyruvate ratio greater than 10. This defines an *excess lactate* state.

Therefore, the concentration of lactate must be viewed in terms of cellular determinants (e.g., the intracellular pH and redox state) as well as the total body production and removal rates. Normally, the rates of lactate entry and exit from the blood are in balance, so that net lactate accumulation is zero. This dynamic aspect of lactate metabolism is termed the *Cori cycle*:

$$2Lactate^- + 2H^+ \xleftarrow[\text{Muscle, brain, skin, red blood cells, gut}]{\text{Liver, kidney, heart}} Glucose \quad (36)$$

As can be envisioned by this relationship, either net overproduction of lactic acid from glucose by some tissues or underutilization by others results in net addition of L-lactic acid to the blood and lactic acid acidosis. However, ischemia accelerates both lactate production and decreases, simultaneously, lactate utilization.

The production of lactic acid has been estimated to be about 15 to 30 mEq/kg/day in normal humans.[28] This enormous quantity contrasts with total ECF buffer base stores of about 10 to 15 mEq/kg and with enhanced production can accumulate. The rate of lactic acid production can be increased with ischemia, seizures, extreme exercise, leukemia, and alkalosis.[83] The increase in production occurs principally through enhanced phosphofructokinase activity.

Decreased lactate consumption more commonly leads to L-lactic acidosis. The principal organs for lactate removal during rest are the liver and kidneys. Both the liver and the kidneys and perhaps muscle have the capacity for increased lactate removal under the stress of increased lactate loads.[83] Hepatic utilization of lactate can be impeded by several factors: poor perfusion of the liver; defective active transport of lactate into cells, or inadequate metabolic conversion of lactate into pyruvate because of altered intracellular pH, redox state, or enzyme activity. Examples of impaired hepatic lactate removal include primary diseases of the liver, enzymatic defects, tissue anoxia or ischemia, severe acidosis, altered redox states, as occurs with alcohol intoxication, fructose, or administration of nucleoside analog reverse transcriptase inhibitors (NRTIs) such as zidovudine and stavudine in patients with HIV infection[83–85] and biguanides such as phenformin or metformin.[83,86,87] Deaths have been reported due to refractory lactic acidosis secondary to thiamine deficiency in patients receiving parenteral nutrition formulations without thiamine.[88] Thiamine is a cofactor for pyruvate dehydrogenase that catalyzes the oxidative decarboxylation of pyruvate to acetyl coenzyme A under aerobic conditions. Pyruvate cannot be metabolized in this manner with thiamine deficiency, converting excess pyruvate to hydrogen ions and lactate.

The quantitative aspects of normal lactate production and consumption in the Cori cycle demonstrate how the development of lactic acidosis can be the most rapid and devastating form of metabolic acidosis.[83,89]

Diagnosis

Because lactic acid has a pK_a of 3.8, lactic acid addition to the blood leads to a reduction in blood HCO_3^- concentration and an equivalent elevation in lactate concentration; which is associated with an increase in the AG. Lactate concentrations are mildly increased in various nonpathologic states (e.g., exercise), but the magnitude of the elevation is generally small. In practical terms, a lactate concentration greater than 4 mEq/L (normal is 1 mEq/L) is generally accepted as evidence that the metabolic acidosis is ascribable to net lactic acid accumulation.

Clinical Spectrum

In the classical classification of the L-lactic acidoses (see Table 14–19), type A L-lactic acidosis is due to tissue hypoperfusion or acute hypoxia, whereas type B L-lactic acidosis is associated with common diseases, drugs and toxins, and hereditary and miscellaneous disorders.[83]

Tissue underperfusion and acute underoxygenation at the tissue level (tissue hypoxia) are the most common causes of type A lactic acidosis. Severe arterial hypoxemia even in the absence of decreased perfusion can generate L-lactic acidosis. Inadequate cardiac output, of either the low-output or the high-output variety, is the usual pathogenetic factor. The prognosis is related directly to the increment in plasma L-lactate and the severity of the acidemia.[83,87,89]

Numerous medical conditions (without tissue hypoxia) predispose to type B L-lactic acidosis (see Table 14–19). Hepatic failure reduces hepatic lactate metabolism, and leukemia increases lactate production. Severe anemia, especially as a result of iron deficiency or methemoglobulinemia, may cause lactic acidosis. Among the most common causes of L-lactic acid acidosis is bowel ischemia and infarction in patients in the medical intensive care unit. Malignant cells produce more lactate than normal cells even under aerobic conditions. This phenomenon is magnified if the tumor expands rapidly and outstrips the blood supply. Therefore, exceptionally large tumors may be associated with severe L-lactic acid acidosis. Seizures, extreme exertion, heat stroke, and tumor lysis syndrome may all cause L-lactic acidosis.

Several drugs and toxins predispose to L-lactic acidosis (see Table 14–19). Of these, metformin and other biguanides (such as phenformin) are the most widely reported.[83,86,87] The occurrence of phenformin-induced lactic acidosis prompted the withdrawal of the drug from U.S. markets in 1977. Although much less frequent with metformin than with phenformin, metformin-induced lactic acidosis has been reported in association with volume depletion and with contrast dye administration. Fructose causes intracellular ATP depletion and lactate accumulation.[83] Inborn errors of metabolism may also cause lactic acidosis, primarily by blocking gluconeogenesis or by inhibiting the oxidation of pyruvate.[83] Carbon monoxide poisoning produces lactic acidosis frequently by reduction of the oxygen-carrying capacity of hemoglobin. Cyanide binds cytochrome a and a_3 and blocks the flow of electrons to oxygen. Nucleoside analogs in patients with HIV infections can induce toxic effects on mitochondria by inhibiting DNA polymerase gamma. Hyperlactatemia is common with NRTI therapy, especially stavudine and zidovudine, but the serum L-lactate is usually only mildly elevated and compensated.[83–85,90] Nevertheless, with severe concurrent illness, pronounced lactic acidosis may occur in association with hepatic steatosis.[83,85] This combination carries a high mortality. Propylene glycol is used as a vehicle for intravenous medications and some cosmetics and is metabolized to lactic acid in the liver by alcohol dehydrogenase. The lactate is metabolized to pyruvic acid and shunted to the glycolytic pathway. Scattered case reports have described hyperosmolality with or without L-lactic acidosis when propylene glycol was used as a vehicle to deliver topical silver sulfadiazine cream, intravenous diazepam or lorazepam (in alcohol withdrawal), intravenous nitroglycerin, and etomidate.[91,92] A prospective study of nine patients receiving high-dose lorezepam infusions[91] showed elevated plasma propylene levels and an elevated osmolar gap. Six of nine patients had moderate degrees of metabolic acidosis.[91]

Associated Clinical Features

Hyperventilation, abdominal pain, and disturbances in consciousness are frequently present, as are signs of inadequate cardiopulmonary function in type A L-lactic acidosis. Leukocytosis, hyperphosphatemia, hyperuricemia, and hyperaminoacidemia (especially alanine) are common, and hypoglycemia may occur.[83] Hyperkalemia may or may not accompany acute lactic acidosis.

Treatment of L-Lactic Acidosis

GENERAL SUPPORTIVE CARE. The overall mortality in L-lactic acidosis is 60% to 70% but approaches 100% with coexisting hypotension.[83] Therapy for this condition has not advanced substantively for the last 2 decades. The basic principle and only effective form of therapy for L-lactic acidosis is that the underlying condition initiating the disruption in normal lactate metabolism must first be corrected. In type A L-lactic acidosis, cessation of acid production by improving tissue oxygenation, restoration of the circulating fluid volume, improvement or augmentation of cardiac function, resection of ischemic tissue, and amelioration of sepsis are necessary in many cases. Septic shock requires control of the underlying infection and volume resuscitation in hypovolomic shock. Hypothetically, interruption of the cytokine cascade may be advantageous but not yet applicable. High L-lactate levels portend a poor prognosis almost uniformly, and sodium bicarbonate is of little value. Vasoconstricting agents are problematic because they may potentiate the hypoperfused state. Dopamine is preferred to epinephrine if pressure support is required, but the vasodilator nitroprusside has been suggested because it may enhance cardiac output and hepatic and renal blood flow to augment lactate removal.[83] Nevertheless, nitroprusside therapy may result in cyanide toxicity and has no proven efficacy in the treatment of this disorder.

ALKALI THERAPY. Alkali therapy is generally advocated for acute, severe acidemia (pH < 7.1) to improve inotropy and lactate utilization. However, in experimental models and clinical examples of lactic acidosis, it has been shown that

$NaHCO_3$ therapy in large amounts can depress cardiac performance and exacerbate the acidemia. Parodoxically, bicarbonate therapy activates phosphofructokinase, thereby increasing lactate production. The use of alkali in states of moderate L-lactic acidemia is controversial, therefore, and it is generally agreed that attempts to normalize the pH or HCO_3^- concentration by intravenous $NaHCO_3$ therapy is both potentially deleterious and practically impossible. Thus, raising the plasma HCO_3^- to approximately 15 to 17 mEq/L and the pH to 7.2 to 7.25 is a reasonable goal to improve tissue pH. Constant infusion of hypertonic bicarbonate has many disadvantages and is discouraged.

Fluid overload occurs rapidly with $NaHCO_3$ administration because of the massive amounts required in some cases. In addition, central venoconstriction and decreased cardiac output are common. The accumulation of lactic acid may be relentless and may necessitate diuretics, ultrafiltration, or dialysis. Hemodialysis can simultaneously deliver HCO_3^-, remove lactate, remove excess ECF volume, and correct electrolyte abnormalities. The use of continuous renal replacement therapy as a means of lactate removal and simultaneous alkali addition is a promising adjunctive treatment in critically ill patients with L-lactic acidosis.

If the underlying cause of the L-lactic acidosis can be remedied, blood lactate will be reconverted to HCO_3^-. HCO_3^- derived from lactate conversion and any new HCO_3^- generated by renal mechanisms during acidosis and from exogenous alkali therapy are additive and may result in an overshoot alkalosis.

OTHER AGENTS. Dichloroacetate, an activator of pyruvate dehydrogenase, was suggested in an uncontrolled study as a potentially useful therapeutic agent. In experimental L-lactic acidosis, dichloroacetate stimulated lactate consumption in muscle and, hence, decreased lactate production and improved survival. In nonacidotic diabetic patients, it successfully lowered lactate as well as glucose, lipid, and amino acid levels. Despite encouraging results of short-term clinical use in acute lactic acidosis, a prospective multicenter trial failed to substantiate any beneficial effect of dichloroacetate therapy.[93] The drug cannot be used chronically. Methylene blue was once advocated as a means of reversing the altered redox state to enhance lactate metabolism. There is no evidence from controlled studies supporting its use. THAM (0.3 M tromethamine) or other preparations of this type are not effective.[83] Tribonat, a mixture of THAM, acetate, $NaHCO_3$, and phosphate, although apparently an effective clinical buffer, has shown no survival advantage in limited clinical trials.[94] Ringer's lactate and lactate-containing peritoneal dialysis solutions should be avoided.

D-LACTIC ACIDOSIS. The manifestations of D-lactate acid acidosis are typically episodic encephalopathy and high AG acidosis in association with short bowel syndrome. Features include slurred speech, confusion, cognitive impairment, clumsiness, ataxia, hallucinations, and behavioral disturbances. D-Lactic acidosis has been described in patients with bowel obstruction, jejunal bypass, short bowel, or ischemic bowel disease. These disorders have in common ileus or stasis associated with overgrowth of flora in the gastrointestinal tract and is exacerbated by a high-carbohydrate diet.[83] D-Lactate, therefore, occurs when fermentation by colonic bacteria in the intestine accumulates and can be absorbed into the circulation. D-Lactate is not measured by the typical clinical laboratory that reports the L-isomer. The disorder should be suspected in patients with an unexplained AG acidosis and some of the typical features noted previously. While waiting for results of specific testing, the patient should be made NPO. Serum D-lactate levels of greater than 3 mmol/L confirm the diagnosis. Treatment with a low-carbohydrate diet and antibiotics (neomycin, vancomycin, or metronidazole) is often effective.[95–98]

Ketoacidosis

Diabetic Ketoacidosis

DKA is due to increased fatty acid metabolism and the accumulation of keto acids (acetoacetate and β-hydroxybutyrate) as a result of insulin deficiency or resistance in association with elevated glucagon levels. DKA is usually seen in insulin-dependent diabetes mellitus in association with cessation of insulin or an intercurrent illness, such as an infection, gastroenteritis, pancreatitis, or myocardial infarction, which increases insulin requirements temporarily and acutely. The accumulation of keto acids accounts for the increment in the AG, which is accompanied, most often, by evidence of hyperglycemia (glucose > 300 mg/dL). In comparison to patients with AKA, described later, DKA is associated with metabolic profiles characterized by a higher plasma glucose, lower β-hydroxybutyrate-to-acetoacetate and lactate-to-pyruvate ratios.[27,98,99]

TREATMENT OF DIABETIC KETOACIDOSIS. Most, if not all, patients with DKA require correction of the volume depletion that almost invariably accompanies the osmotic diuresis and ketoacidosis. In general, it seems prudent to initiate therapy with intravenous isotonic saline at a rate of 1000 mL/hr, especially in the severely volume-depleted patient. When the pulse and blood pressure have stabilized and the corrected serum Na^+ concentration is in the range 130 to 135 mEq/L, switch to 0.45% sodium chloride. Ringer lactate should be avoided. If the blood glucose level falls below 300 mg/dL, 0.45% sodium chloride with 5% dextrose should be administered.[27,98]

Low-dose intravenous insulin therapy (0.1 U/kg/hr) smoothly corrects the biochemical abnormalities and minimizes hypoglycemia and hypokalemia.[27,98] Usually, in the first hour, a loading dose of the same amount is given initially as a bolus intravenously. Intramuscular insulin is not effective in patients with volume depletion, which often occurs in ketoacidosis.

Total body K^+ depletion is usually present, although the K^+ level on admission may be elevated or normal. A normal or reduced K^+ value on admission indicates severe K^+ depletion and should be approached with caution. Administration of fluid, insulin, and alkali may cause the K^+ level to plummet. When the urine output has been established, 20 mEq of potassium chloride should be administered in each liter of fluid as long as the K^+ value is less than 4.0 mEq/L. Equal caution should be exercised in the presence of hyperkalemia, especially if the patient has renal insufficiency, because the usual therapy does not always correct hyperkalemia. Never administer potassium chloride empirically.

The young patient with a pure AG acidosis ($\Delta AG = \Delta HCO_3^-$) usually does not require exogenous alkali because the metabolic acidosis should be entirely reversible. Elderly patients, patients with severe high AG acidosis (pH < 7.15), or patients with a superimposed hyperchloremic component may receive small amounts of sodium bicarbonate by slow intravenous infusion (no more than 44–88 mEq in 60 min). Thirty minutes after this infusion is completed, ABGs should be repeated. Alkali administration can be repeated if the pH is 7.20 or less or if the patient exhibits a significant hyperchloremic component but is rarely necessary. The AG should be followed closely during therapy because it is expected to decline as ketones are cleared from plasma and herald an increase in plasma HCO_3^- as the acidosis is repaired. Therefore, it is not necessary to monitor blood ketone levels continuously. Hypokalemia and other complications of alkali therapy dramatically increase when amounts of sodium bicarbonate exceeding 400 mEq are administered. However, the effect of alkali therapy on arterial blood pH needs to be reassessed regularly, and the total administered kept at a minimum, if necessary.[27,98,99]

Routine administration of PO_4^{3-} (usually as potassium phosphate) is not advised because of the potential for hyperphosphatemia and hypocalcemia.[27,98] A significant proportion of patients with DKA have significant hyperphosphatemia before initiation of therapy. In the volume-depleted, malnourished patient, however, a normal or elevated PO_4^{3-} concentration on admission may be followed by a rapid fall in plasma PO_4^{3-} levels within 2 to 6 hours after initiation of therapy.

Alcoholic Ketoacidosis

Some chronic alcoholics, especially binge drinkers, who discontinue solid food intake while continuing alcohol consumption develop this form of ketoacidosis when alcohol ingestion is curtailed abruptly.[27,98,99] Usually the onset of vomiting and abdominal pain with dehydration leads to cessation of alcohol consumption before presentation to the hospital.[27,99] The metabolic acidosis may be severe but is accompanied by only modestly deranged glucose levels, which are usually low but may be slightly elevated.[27,99] Typically, insulin levels are low and levels of triglyceride, cortisol, glucagon, and growth hormone are increased. The net result of this deranged metabolic state leads to ketosis. The acidosis is primarily due to elevated ketone levels, which exist predominantly in the form of β-hydroxybutyrate because of the altered redox state induced by the metabolism of alcohol. Compared with patients with DKA, patients with AKA have lower plasma glucose concentrations and higher β-hydroxybutyrate-to-acetoacetate and lactate-to-pyruvate levels.[27,99] This disorder is not rare and is underdiagnosed. The clinical presentation in AKA may be complex because a mixed disorder is often present and due to metabolic alkalosis (vomiting), respiratory alkalosis (alcoholic liver disease), lactic acid acidosis (hypoperfusion), and hyperchloremic acidosis (renal excretion of ketoacids). Finally, the osmolar gap is elevated if the blood alcohol level is elevated, but the differential should always include ethylene glycol and/or methanol intoxication.

TREATMENT. Therapy includes intravenous glucose and saline administration, but insulin should be avoided. K^+, PO_4^{3-}, Mg^{2+}, and vitamin supplementation (especially thiamine) are frequently necessary. Glucose in isotonic saline, not saline alone, is the mainstay of therapy. Because of superimposed starvation, patients with AKA often develop hypophosphatemia within 12 to 18 hours of admission. Treatment with glucose-containing intravenous fluids increases the risk for severe hypophosphatemia. Levels should be checked on admission and at 4, 6, 12, and 18 hours. Profound hypophosphatemia may provoke aspiration, platelet dysfunction, and rhabdomyolysis. Therefore, phosphate replacement should be provided promptly when indicated. Hypokalemia and hypomagnesemia are also common and should not be overlooked.[27,99]

Starvation Ketoacidosis

Ketoacidosis occurs within the first 24 to 48 hours of fasting, is accentuated by exercise and pregnancy, and is rapidly reversible by glucose or insulin. Starvation-induced hypoinsulinemia and accentuated hepatic ketone production have been implicated pathogenetically.[27,99] Fasting alone can increase ketoacid levels, although not usually above 10 mEq/L. High-protein, weight-loss diets typically cause mild ketosis but not ketoacidosis. Patients typically respond to glucose and saline infusion.

Drug- and Toxin-induced Acidosis

Salicylate

Intoxication by salicylates, although more common in children than in adults, may result in the development of a high AG metabolic acidosis, but the acid-base abnormality most commonly associated with salicylate intoxication in adults is respiratory alkalosis due to direct stimulation of the respiratory center by salicylates.[98] Adult patients with salicylate intoxication usually have pure respiratory alkalosis or mixed respiratory alkalosis–metabolic acidosis.[98] Metabolic acidosis occurs due to uncoupling of oxidative phosphorylation and enhances the transit of salicylates into the central nervous system. Only part of the increase in the AG is due to the increase in plasma salicylate concentration, because a toxic salicylate level of 100 mg/dL would account for an increase in the AG of only 7 mEq/L. High ketone concentrations have been reported to be present in as many as 40% of adult salicylate-intoxicated patients, sometimes as a result of salicylate-induced hypoglycemia.[100] L-Lactic acid production is also often increased, partly as a direct drug effect[98] and partly as a result of the decrease in PCO_2 induced by salicylate. Proteinuria and pulmonary edema may occur.

TREATMENT. General treatment should always consist of initial vigorous gastric lavage with isotonic saline followed by administration of activated charcoal per nasogastric tube. Treatment of the metabolic acidosis may be necessary because acidosis can enhance the entry of salicylate into the central nervous system. Alkali should be given cautiously and frank alkalemia should be avoided. Coexisting respiratory alkalosis can make this form of therapy hazardous. The renal excretion of salicylate is enhanced by an alkaline diuresis accomplished with intravenous $NaHCO_3$. Caution is urged if the patient exhibits concomitant respiratory alkalosis with frank alkalemia because $NaHCO_3$ may cause severe alkalosis and hypokalemia may result from alkalinization of the urine. To minimize the administration of $NaHCO_3$, acetazolamide may be administered to the alkalemic patient, but this can cause acidosis and impair salicylate elimination. Hemodialysis may be necessary for severe poisoning, especially if renal failure coexists, is preferred with severe intoxication (>700 mg/L), and is superior to hemofiltration, which does not correct the acid-base abnormality.[98,100]

Toxin-Induced Metabolic Acidoses

THE OSMOLAR GAP IN TOXIN-INDUCED ACIDOSIS. Under most physiologic conditions, Na^+, urea, and glucose generate the osmotic pressure of blood. Serum osmolality is calculated according to the expression:

$$\text{Osmolality} = 2[Na^+] + \frac{\text{BUN}}{2.8} + \frac{\text{glucose (mg/dL)}}{18} \quad (37)$$

The calculated and determined osmolalities should agree within 10 to 15 mOsm/kg. When the measured osmolality exceeds the calculated osmolality by more than 15 to 20 mOsm/kg, one of two circumstances prevails. First, the serum Na^+ may be spuriously low, as occurs with hyperlipidemia or hyperproteinemia (pseudohyponatremia); or second, osmolytes other than sodium salts, glucose, or urea have accumulated in plasma. Examples include infused mannitol, radiocontrast media, or other solutes, including the alcohols, ethylene glycol, and acetone, that can increase the osmolality in plasma. In these examples, the difference between the osmolality calculated from Equation 37 and the measured osmolality is proportional to the concentration of the unmeasured solute. Such differences in these clinical circumstances have been referred to as the **osmolar gap.** With an appropriate clinical history and index of suspicion, the **osmolar gap** becomes a very reliable and helpful screening tool in toxin-associated high AG acidosis.

ETHANOL. Ethanol, after absorption from the gastrointestinal tract, is oxidized to acetaldehyde, acetyl coenzyme A, and CO_2. A blood ethanol level over 500 mg/dL is associated with high mortality. Acetaldehyde levels do not increase appreciably unless the load is exceptionally high or the acetaldehyde dehydrogenase step is inhibited by compounds such as disulfiram, insecticides, and sulfonylurea hypoglycemia agents. Such agents in the presence of ethanol result in severe toxic-

ity. The association of ethanol with the development of AKA and lactic acidosis has been discussed in the previous section, but in general, ethanol intoxication does not cause a high AG acidosis.

ETHYLENE GLYCOL. Ingestion of ethylene glycol, used in antifreeze, leads to a high AG metabolic acidosis in addition to severe central nervous system, cardiopulmonary, and renal damage.[98,101,102] The high AG is attributable to ethylene glycol metabolites, especially oxalic acid, glycolic acid, and other incompletely identified organic acids.[102] L-Lactic acid production also increases as a result of a toxic depression in the reaction rates of the citric acid cycle and altered intracellular redox state.[102] Recognizing oxalate crystals in the urine facilitates diagnosis, as does fluoresence of urine by a Wood's light if the ingested ethylene glycol contains a fluorescent vehicle.[101,102] A disparity between the measured blood osmolality and that calculated (high **osmolar gap**) is often present. Treatment includes prompt institution of osmotic diuresis, thiamine and pyridoxine supplements, 4-methylpyrazole (fomepizole),[103] or ethyl alcohol and dialysis.[98,101,103] Ethanol or fomepizole should be given intravenously. Competitive inhibition of alcohol dehydrogenase with one of these agents is absolutely necessary in all patients to lessen toxicity because ethanol and fomepizole compete for metabolic conversion of ethylene glycol and alters the cellular redox state. Fomepizole (initiated as a loading dose of 7 mg/kg) offers the advantages of a predictable decline in ethylene glycol levels without the adverse effect of excessive obtundation, as seen with ethyl alcohol infusion. When these measures have been accomplished, hemodialysis should be initiated to remove the ethylene glycol metabolites. At this juncture the intravenous ethanol infusion should be increased to allow maintenance of the blood alcohol level in the range of 100 to 150 mg/dL or greater than 22 mmol/L.

METHANOL. Methanol (wood alcohol) ingestion causes metabolic acidosis in addition to severe optic nerve and central nervous system manifestations resulting from its metabolism to formic acid from formaldehyde.[98,101] Lactic acids and keto acids as well as other unidentified organic acids may contribute to the acidosis. Because of the low molecular mass of methanol (32 Da), an osmolar gap is usually present. Therapy is generally similar to that for ethylene glycol intoxication, including general supportive measures, ethanol or fomepizole administration, and sometimes, hemodialysis.[103]

ISOPROPYL ALCOHOL. Rubbing alcohol poisoning is usually the result of accidental oral ingestion or absorption through the skin. Although isopropyl alcohol is metabolized by the enzyme alcohol dehydrogenase, as are methanol and ethanol, isopropyl alcohol is *not metabolized to a strong acid* and *does not elevate the AG.* Isopropyl alcohol is metabolized to acetone, and the osmolar gap increases as the result of accumulation of both acetone and isopropyl alcohol. Despite a positive nitroprusside reaction from acetone, the AG, as well as the blood glucose, is typically normal, not elevated, and the plasma HCO_3^- is not depressed. Thus, isopropyl alcohol intoxication does not typically cause metabolic acidosis. Treatment is supportive, with attention to removal of unabsorbed alcohol from the gastrointestinal tract and administration of intravenous fluids. Hemodialysis is effective but not usually necessary. Although patients with significant isopropyl alcohol intoxication (blood levels > 100 mg/dL) may develop cardiovascular collapse and lactic acidosis, watchful waiting with a conservative approach (intravenous. fluids, electrolyte replacement, and tracheal intubation) is often sufficient. Very severe intoxication (>400 mg/dL) is an indication for hemodialysis.[98]

PARALDEHYDE. Intoxication with paraldehyde is now very rare, but is a result of acetic acid accumulation, the metabolic product of the drug from acetaldehyde and other organic acids.

PYROGLUTAMIC ACIDOSIS. Pyroglutamic acid, or 5-oxoproline, is an intermediate in the γ-glutamyl cycle for the synthesis of glutathione. Acetaminophen ingestion can rarely deplete glutathione, resulting in increased formation of γ-glutamyl cysteine, which is metabolized to pyroglutamic acid.[104] Accumulation of this intermediate, first appreciated in the rare patient with congenital glutathione synthetase deficiency, has been observed recently in an acquired variety. Those patients observed thus far have severe high AG acidosis and alterations in mental status.[104] Many were septic and receiving full therapeutic doses of acetaminophen. All had elevated blood levels of pyroglutamic acid, which increased in proportion to the increase in the AG. It is conceivable that the heterozygote state for glutathione synthetase deficiency could predispose to proglutamic acidosis, because only a minority of critically ill patients on acetaminophen develop this newly appreciated form of metabolic acidosis.[104]

Uremia

Advanced renal insufficiency eventually converts the hyperchloremic acidosis discussed earlier to a typical high AG acidosis.[28] Poor filtration plus continued reabsorption of poorly identified uremic organic anions contributes to the pathogenesis of this metabolic disturbance.

Classic uremic acidosis is characterized by a reduced rate of NH_4^+ production and excretion because of cumulative and significant loss of renal mass.[4,5,19,28] Usually, acidosis does not occur until a major portion of the total functional nephron population (>75%) has been destroyed, because of the ability of surviving nephrons to increase ammoniagenesis. Eventually, however, there is a decrease in total renal ammonia excretion as renal mass is reduced to a level at which the GFR is 20 mL/min or less. PO_4^{3-} balance is maintained as a result of both hyperparathyroidism, which decreases proximal PO_4^{3-} absorption, and an increase in plasma PO_4^{3-} as GFR declines. Protein restriction and the administration of phosphate biners reduce the availability of PO_4^{3-}.

TREATMENT OF ACIDOSIS OF CHRONIC RENAL FAILURE. The uremic acidosis of renal failure requires oral alkali replacement to maintain the HCO_3^- concentration above 20 mEq/L. This can be accomplished with relatively modest amounts of alkali (1.0–1.5 mEq/kg/day). Shohl solution or sodium bicarbonate tablets (325- or 650-mg tablets) are equally effective. It is assumed that alkali replacement serves to prevent the harmful effects of prolonged positive H^+ balance, especially progressive catabolism of muscle and loss of bone. Because sodium citrate (Shohl solution) has been shown to enhance the absorption of aluminum from the gastrointestinal tract, it should never be administered to patients receiving aluminum-containing antacids because of the risk of aluminum intoxication. When hyperkalemia is present, furosemide (60–80 mg/day) should be added. An occasional patient may require chronic sodium polystyrene sulfonate (Kayexalate) therapy orally (15–30 g/day). The pure powder preparation is better tolerated long term than the commercially available syrup preparation and avoids sorbitol (which may cause bowel necrosis). The powder may be obtained from www.drugstore.com (454 g for $246).

Metabolic Alkalosis

Diagnosis of Simple and Mixed Forms of Metabolic Alkalosis

Metabolic alkalosis is a primary acid-base disturbance that is manifest in the most pure or simple form as alkalemia (elevated arterial pH) and an increase in $PaCO_2$ as a result of compensatory alveolar hypoventilation. Metabolic alkalosis is one of the more common acid-base disturbances in hospitalized patients, and occurs as both a simple and a mixed disorder.[11,104]

A patient with a high plasma HCO_3^- concentration and a low plasma Cl^- concentration has either metabolic alkalosis or chronic respiratory acidosis. The arterial pH establishes the diagnosis, because it is increased in metabolic alkalosis and is typically decreased in respiratory acidosis. Modest increases in the $PaCO_2$ are expected in metabolic alkalosis. A combination of the two disorders is not unusual, because many patients with chronic obstructive lung disease are treated with diuretics, which promote ECF contraction, hypokalemia, and metabolic alkalosis. Metabolic alkalosis is also frequently observed not as a pure or simple acid-base disturbance, but in association with other disorders such as respiratory acidosis, respiratory alkalosis, and metabolic acidosis **(mixed disorders). Mixed metabolic alkalosis–metabolic acidosis can be appreciated only if the accompanying metabolic acidosis is a high AG acidosis.** The mixed disorder can be appreciated by comparison of the increment in the AG above the normal value of 10 mEq/L (ΔAG = Patient's AG − 10), with the decrement in the $[HCO_3^-]$ below the normal value of 25 mEq/L (ΔHCO_3^- = 25 − Patient's HCO_3^-). A mixed metabolic alkalosis–high AG metabolic acidosis is recognized because the delta values are not similar. Often, there is no bicarbonate deficit, yet the AG is significantly elevated. Thus, in a patient with an AG of 20 but a near-normal bicarbonate, mixed metabolic alkalosis–metabolic acidosis should be considered. Common examples include renal failure acidosis (uremic) with vomiting or DKA with vomiting.

Respiratory compensation for metabolic alkalosis is less predictable than for metabolic acidosis. In general the anticipated PCO_2 can be estimated by adding 15 to the patient's serum $[HCO_3^-]$ in the range of HCO_3^- from 25 to 40 mEq/L. Further elevation in PCO_2 is limited by hypoxemia and, to some extent, hypokalemia, which accompanies metabolic alkalosis with regularity. Nevertheless, if a patient has a PCO_2 of only 40 mm Hg while the $[HCO_3^-]$ is frankly elevated (e.g., 35 mEq/L) and the pH is in the alkalemic range, then respiratory compensation is inadequate and a mixed metabolic alkalosis–respiratory alkalosis exists.

In assessing a patient with metabolic alkalosis, two questions must be considered: (1) What is the source of alkali gain (or acid loss) that **generated** the alkalosis? (2) What renal mechanisms are operating to prevent excretion of excess HCO_3^-, thereby **maintaining**, rather than correcting, the alkalosis? In the following discussion, the entities responsible for generating alkalosis are discussed individually and reference is made to the mechanisms necessary to sustain the increase in blood HCO_3^- concentration in each case. The general mechanisms responsible for the **maintenance of alkalosis** have been discussed in detail earlier in this chapter, but are a result of the combined effects of chloride, ECF volume, and potassium depletion (Fig. 14–9).

Hypokalemia is an important participant in the maintenance phase of metabolic alkalosis and has selective effects on (1) H^+ secretion and (2) ammonium excretion. The former is a result predominantly of stimulation of the H^+,K^+-ATPase in type A intercalated cells of the collecting duct. The latter is a direct result of enhanced ammoniagenesis and ammonium transport (proximal convoluted tubule, TALH, medullary collecting duct) in response to hypokalemia. Finally, hyperaldosteronism (primary or secondary) participates in sustaining the alkalosis by increasing activity of the H^+,K^+-ATPase in type A-IC cells as well as the ENaC and the Na^+,K^+-ATPase in principal cells in the collecting duct. The net result of the latter process is to stimulate K^+ secretion through K^+ selective channels in this same cell, thus maintaining the alkalosis.[105]

Under normal circumstances, the kidneys display an impressive capacity to excrete HCO_3^-. For HCO_3^- to be added to the ECF, HCO_3^- must be administered exogenously or retained in some manner. Thus, **the development of meta-**

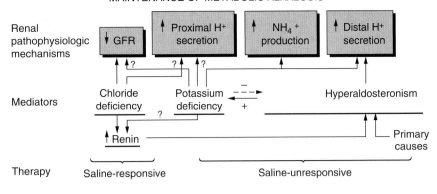

Figure 14–9 Pathophysiologic basis and approach to treatment of maintenance phase of chronic metabolic alkalosis. Paradoxical stimulation of bicarbonate absorption (H⁺ secretion) and NH₄⁺ production and excretion is the combined result of Cl⁻ deficiency, K⁺ deficiency, and secondary hyperaldosteronism. GFR, glomerular filtration rate.

bolic alkalosis represents a failure of the kidneys to eliminate HCO_3^- at the normal capacity. The kidneys retain, rather than excrete, the excess alkali and maintain the alkalosis if one of several mechanisms is operative (see Fig. 14–9):

1. Cl⁻ deficiency (ECF contraction) exists concurrently with K⁺ deficiency to decrease GFR and/or enhance proximal and distal HCO_3^- absorption. This combination of disorders evokes secondary hyperreninemic hyperaldosteronism and stimulates H⁺ secretion in the collecting duct and ammoniagenesis. Repair of the alkalosis may be accomplished by saline and K⁺ administration.

2. Hypermineralocorticoidism and hypokalemia are induced by autonomous factors unresponsive to increased ECF. The stimulation of distal H⁺ secretion is then sufficient to reabsorb the increased filtered HCO_3^- load and to overcome the decreased proximal HCO_3^- reabsorption caused by ECF expansion. Repair of the alkalosis in this case rests with removal of the excess autonomous mineralocorticoid; saline is ineffective.

The various causes of metabolic alkalosis are summarized in Table 14–20. In attempting to establish the cause of metabolic alkalosis, it is necessary to assess the status of the ECF, blood pressure, serum K⁺, and renin-aldosterone system. For example, the presence of hypertension and hypokalemia in an alkalotic patient would suggest either some form of primary mineralocorticoid excess (see Table 14–20) or a hypertensive patient on diuretics. Low plasma renin activity and normal urinary Na⁺ and Cl⁻ values in a patient not taking diuretics would also indicate a primary mineralocorticoid excess syndrome. The combination of hypokalemia and alkalosis in a normotensive, nonedematous patient can pose a difficult diagnostic problem. The possible causes to be considered include Bartter or Gitelman syndrome, Mg²⁺ deficiency, surreptitious vomiting, exogenous alkali, and diuretic ingestion. Urine electrolyte determinations and urine screening for diuretics are helpful diagnostic tools (Table 14–21). If the urine is alkaline, with high values for Na⁺ and K⁺ concentrations but low values for Cl⁻ concentration, the diagnosis is usually either active (continuous) vomiting (overt or surreptitious) or alkali ingestion. On the one hand, if the urine is relatively acid, with low concentrations of Na⁺, K⁺, and Cl⁻, the most likely possibilities are prior (discontinuous) vomiting, the posthypercapnic state, or prior diuretic ingestion. If, on the other hand, the urinary Na⁺, K⁺, and Cl⁻ concentrations are not depressed, one must consider Mg²⁺ deficiency, Bartter or Gitelman syndrome, or current diuretic ingestion. In addition to a low serum Mg²⁺, in most patients, Gitelman syndrome is characterized by a low urine Ca²⁺. In contrast, the urine calcium is elevated in Bartter syndrome. The diagnostic approach to metabolic alkalosis is summarized in the flow diagram in Figure 14–10.

TABLE 14–20	Causes of Metabolic Alkalosis

Exogenous HCO_3^- loads
Acute alkali administration
Milk-alkali syndrome

Effective ECV contraction, normotension, K⁺ deficiency, and secondary hyperreninemic hyperaldosteronism
Gastrointestinal origin
  Vomiting
  Gastric aspiration
  Congenital chloridorrhea
  Villous adenoma
    Combined administration of sodium polystyrene sulfonate (Kayexalate and aluminum hydroxide)
Renal origin
  Diuretics (especially thiazides and loop diuretics)
  Edematous states
  Posthypercapnic state
  Hypercalcemia-hypoparathyroidism
  Recovery from lactic acidosis or ketoacidosis
  Nonreabsorbable anions such as penicillin, carbenicillin
  Mg²⁺ deficiency
  K⁺ depletion
  Bartter syndrome (loss of function mutations in TALH)
  Gitelman syndrome (loss of function mutation in Na⁺-Cl⁻ cotransporter)
  Carbohydrate refeeding after starvation

ECV expansion, hypertension, K⁺ deficiency, and hypermineralocorticoidism
Associated with high renin
  Renal artery stenosis
  Accelerated hypertension
  Renin-secreting tumor
  Estrogen therapy
Associated with low renin
  Primary aldosteronism
    Adenoma
    Hyperplasia
    Carcinoma
    Glucocorticoid suppressible
  Adrenal enzymatic defects
    11β-Hydroxylase deficiency
    17α-Hydroxylase deficiency
  Cushing syndrome or disease
    Ectopic corticotropin
    Adrenal carcinoma
    Adrenal adenoma
    Primary pituitary
  Other
    Licorice
    Carbenoxolone
    Chewer's tobacco
    Lydia Pincham tablets

Gain of function mutation of ENaC with ECF volume expansion, hypertension, K⁺ deficiency, and hyporeninemic hypoaldosteronism
Liddle's syndrome

Exogenous Bicarbonate Loads

Chronic administration of alkali to individuals with normal renal function results in minimal, if any, alkalosis. In patients with chronic renal insufficiency, however, overt alkalosis can develop after alkali administration, presumably because the capacity to excrete HCO_3^- is exceeded or because coexistent hemodynamic disturbances have caused enhanced fractional HCO_3^- reabsorption.

TABLE 14–21	Diagnosis of Metabolic Alkalosis
Saline-Responsive Alkalosis	**Saline-Unresponsive Alkalosis**
Low Urinary [Cl⁻] (<10 mEq/L)	*High or Normal Urinary [Cl⁻] (>15–20 mEq/L)*
Normotensive	Hypertensive
Vomiting	Primary aldosteronism
Nasogastric aspiration	Cushing syndrome
Diuretics (distant)	Renal artery stenosis
Posthypercapnia	Renal failure plus alkali therapy
Villous adenoma	Normotensive
Bicarbonate therapy of	Mg^{2+} deficiency
organic acidosis	Severe K^+ deficiency
K^+ deficiency	Bartter syndrome
Hypertensive	Gitelman syndrome
Liddle's syndrome	Diuretics (recent)

Bicarbonate and Bicarbonate-Precursor Administration

The propensity of patients with ECF contraction or renal disease plus alkali loads to develop alkalosis is exemplified by patients who receive oral or intravenous HCO_3^-, acetate loads in parenteral hyperalimentation solutions, sodium citrate loads (regional anticoagulation, transfusions, or infant formula), or antacids plus cation exchange resins. The use of trisodium citrate solution for anticoagulation regionally has been reported as a cause of metabolic alkalosis in patients on continuous renal replacement therapy.[106,107] Citrate metabolism consumes a hydrogen ion and, thereby, generates HCO_3^- in liver and skeletal muscle. Dilute (0.1 N) HCl is often required for correction in this setting.[107] The risk for alkalosis, in my experience, is reduced when anticoagulant citrate dextrose formula A (ACD-A) is used because less bicarbonate is generated in comparison to hypertonic trisodium citrate administration.

Milk-Alkali Syndrome

Another cause is a long-standing history of excessive ingestion of milk and antacids. Milk-alkali syndrome is making a comeback because of the use of calcium supplementation (e.g., calcium carbonate) in women for osteoporosis treatment or prevention. Older women with poor dietary intake ("tea and toasters") are especially prone. In Asia, betel nut chewing is a cause because the erosive nut is often wrapped in calcium hydroxide. Both hypercalcemia and vitamin D excess have been suggested to increase renal HCO_3^- reabsorption. Patients

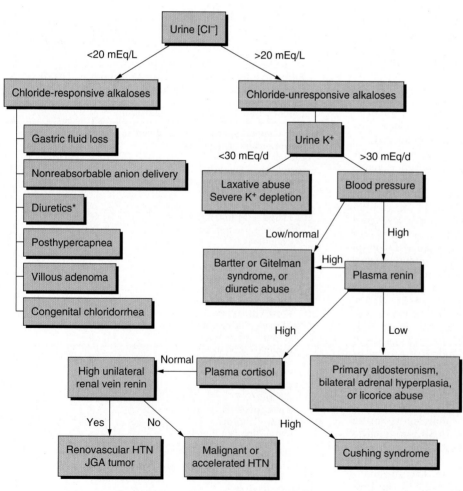

Figure 14–10 Diagnostic algorithm for metabolic alkalosis, based on the spot urine Cl⁻ and K⁺ concentration. JGA, juxtaglomerular apparatus; HTN, hypertension.

* After diuretic therapy

with these disorders are prone to develop nephrocalcinosis, renal insufficiency, and metabolic alkalosis.[105] Discontinuation of alkali ingestion or administration is usually sufficient to repair the alkalosis.

Normal Blood Pressure, Extracellular Volume Contraction, Potassium Depletion, and Hyperreninemic Hyperaldosteronism

Gastrointestinal Origin

VOMITING AND GASTRIC ASPIRATION. Gastrointestinal loss of H^+ results in retention of HCO_3^- in the body fluids. Increased H^+ loss through gastric secretions can be caused by vomiting for physical or psychiatric reasons, through nasogastric tube aspiration, or by a gastric fistula (see Table 14–20).[105]

The fluid and sodium chloride loss in vomitus or in nasogastric suction results in ECF contraction with an increase in plasma renin activity and aldosterone.[105] These factors decrease GFR and enhance the capacity of the renal tubule to reabsorb HCO_3^-.[11] During the active phase of vomiting, there is continued addition of HCO_3^- to plasma in exchange for Cl^-. The plasma HCO_3^- concentration increases to a level that exceeds the reabsorptive capacity of the proximal tubule. The excess sodium bicarbonate enters the distal tubule, where, under the influence of the increased level of aldosterone, K^+ and H^+ secretion is stimulated. Because of ECF contraction and hypochloremia, the kidney avidly conserves Cl^-. Consequently, in this disequilibrium state generated by active vomiting, the urine contains large quantities of Na^+, K^+, and HCO_3^- but has a low concentration of Cl^-. On cessation of vomiting, the plasma HCO_3^- concentration falls to the HCO_3^- threshold, which is markedly elevated by the continued effects of ECF contraction, hypokalemia, and hyperaldosteronism. The alkalosis is maintained at a slightly lower level than during the phase of active vomiting, and the urine is now relatively acidic with low concentrations of Na^+, HCO_3^-, and Cl^-.

Correction of the ECF contraction with sodium chloride may be sufficient to reverse these events, with restoration of normal blood pH even without repair of K^+ deficits.[11] Good clinical practice, however, dictates K^+ repletion as well.

Congenital Chloridorrhea

This rare autosomal recessive disorder is associated with severe diarrhea, fecal acid loss, and HCO_3^- retention. The pathogenesis is due to loss of the normal ileal HCO_3^-/Cl^- anion exchange mechanism so that Cl^- cannot be reabsorbed. The parallel Na^+/H^+ ion exchanger remains functional, allowing Na^+ to be reabsorbed and H^+ to be secreted. Subsequently, net H^+ and Cl^- exit in the stool, causing Na^+ and HCO_3^- retention in the ECF.[11,105] Alkalosis results and is sustained by concomitant ECF contraction with hyperaldosteronism and K^+ deficiency. Therapy consists of oral supplements of sodium and potassium chloride. The use of proton-pump inhibitors has been advanced as a means of reducing chloride secretion by the parietal cells and, thus, reducing the diarrhea.[108]

Villous Adenoma

Metabolic alkalosis has been described in cases of villous adenoma and is ascribed to high adenoma-derived K^+ secretory rates. K^+ and volume depletion likely cause the alkalosis, because colonic secretion is alkaline.

Renal Origin

Diuretics

Drugs that induce chloriuresis without bicarbonaturia, such as thiazides and loop diuretics (furosemide, bumetanide, and torsemide), acutely diminish the ECF space without altering the total body HCO_3^- content. The HCO_3^- concentration in the blood and ECF increases. The PCO_2 does not increase commensurately, and a "contraction" alkalosis results.[105] The

degree of alkalosis is usually small, however, because of cellular and non-HCO_3^- ECF buffering processes.[11,105]

Administration of diuretics chronically tends to generate an alkalosis by increased distal salt delivery, so that both K^+ and H^+ secretion is stimulated. Diuretics, by blocking Cl^- reabsorption in the distal tubule or by increasing H^+ pump activity, may also stimulate distal H^+ secretion and increase net acid excretion. Maintenance of alkalosis is ensured by the persistence of ECF contraction, secondary hyperaldosteronism, K^+ deficiency, enhanced ammonium production, stimulation of the H^+,K^+-ATPase, and the direct effect of the diuretic as long as diuretic administration continues. Repair of the alkalosis is achieved by providing Cl^- to normalize the ECF deficit.

Edematous States

In diseases associated with edema formation (congestive heart failure, nephrotic syndrome, cirrhosis), effective ECF is diminished, although total ECF is increased. Common to these diseases is diminished renal plasma flow and GFR with limited distal Na^+ delivery. Net acid excretion is usually normal, and alkalosis does not develop, even with an enhanced proximal HCO_3^- reabsorptive capacity. However, the distal H^+ secretory mechanism is primed by hyperaldosteronism to excrete excessive net acid if GFR can be increased to enhance distal Na^+ delivery or if K^+ deficiency or diuretic administration supervenes.

Posthypercapnia

Prolonged CO_2 retention with chronic respiratory acidosis enhances renal HCO_3^- absorption and the generation of new HCO_3^- (increased net acid excretion). If the PCO_2 is returned to normal, metabolic alkalosis, caused by the persistently elevated HCO_3^- concentration, emerges. Alkalosis develops immediately if the elevated PCO_2 is abruptly returned toward normal by a change in mechanically controlled ventilation. There is a brisk bicarbonaturic response proportional to the change in PCO_2. The accompanying cation is predominantly K^+, especially if dietary potassium is not limited. Secondary hyperaldosteronism in states of chronic hypercapnia may be responsible for this pattern of response. Associated ECF contraction does not allow complete repair of the alkalosis by normalization of the PCO_2 alone. Alkalosis persists until Cl^- supplementation is provided. Enhanced proximal acidification as a result of conditioning induced by the previous hypercapnic state may also contribute to the maintenance of the posthypercapnic alkalosis.[5]

Bartter Syndrome

Both classic Bartter syndrome and the antenatal Bartter are inherited as autosomal recessive disorders and involve impaired TALH salt absorption, which results in salt wasting, volume depletion, and activation of the renin-angiotensin system.[109] These manifestations are the result of loss of function mutations of one of the genes that encode three transporters involved in vectorial NaCl absorption in the TALH. The most prevalent disorder is a mutation of the gene NKCC2 that encodes the bumetanide-sensitive Na^+-$2Cl^-$-K^+ cotransporter on the apical membrane. A second mutation has been discovered in the gene KCNJ1 which encodes the ATP-sensitive apical K^+ conductance channel (ROMK) that operates in parallel with the Na^+-$2Cl^-$-K^+ transporter to recycle K^+. Both defects can be associated with classic Bartter syndrome. A third mutation of the CLCNKb gene encoding the voltage-gated basolateral chloride channel (ClC-Kb) is associated only with classic Bartter syndrome and is milder and rarely associated with nephrocalcinosis. All three defects have the same net effect, loss of Cl^- transport in the TALH.[110]

Antenatal Bartter syndrome has been observed in consanguineous families in association with sensorineural deafness; a syndrome linked to chromosome 1p31. The responsible gene, *BSND,* encodes a subunit, barttin, that colocalizes with the CLC-Kb channel in the TALH and K-secreting epithelial cells in the inner ear. Barttin appears to be necessary for function of the voltage-gated chloride channel. Expression of ClC-Kb is lost when coexpressed with mutant barttins. Thus, mutations in *BSND* represent a fourth category of patients with Bartter syndrome.[109]

Such defects would predictably lead to ECF contraction, hyperreninemic hyperaldosteronism, and increased delivery of Na^+ to the distal nephron and, thus, alkalosis and renal K^+ wasting and hypokalemia. Secondary overproduction of prostaglandins, juxtaglomerular apparatus hypertrophy, and vascular pressor unresponsiveness would then ensue. Most patients have hypercalciuria and normal serum magnesium levels, which distinguishes this disorder from Gitelman syndrome.

Bartter syndrome is inherited as an autosomal recessive defect, and most patients studied with mutations in these genes have been homozygotes or compound heterozygotes for different mutations in one of these genes. A few patients with the clinical syndrome have no discernible mutation in any of these four genes. Plausible explanations include unrecognized mutations in other genes, a dominant-negative effect of a heterozygous mutation, or other mechanisms. Recently, two groups of investigators have reported features of Bartter syndrome in patients with autosomal dominant hypocalcemia and activating mutations in the calcium-sensing receptor (CaSR). Activation of the CaSR on the basolateral cell surface of the TALH inhibits function of ROMK. Thus, mutations in CaSR may represent a fifth gene associated with the Bartter syndrome.[90]

The pathophysiologic basis of the myriad manifestations of Bartter syndrome is displayed in Figure 14–11. Historically, many of these features (e.g., elevated PGE_2 and kallikreins), once considered potentially causative, are now realized to be secondary to the genetic defects in TALH solute transport.

Distinction from surreptitious vomiting, diuretic administration, and laxative abuse is necessary to make the diagnosis of Bartter syndrome. The finding of a low urinary Cl^- concentration is helpful in identifying the vomiting patient. The urinary Cl^- concentration in Bartter syndrome would be expected to be normal or increased, rather than depressed.

The therapy of Bartter syndrome is generally focused on repair of the hypokalemia by inhibition of the renin-angio-

tensin-aldosterone or the prostaglandin-kinin system. K^+ supplementation, Mg^{2+} repletion, propranolol, spironolactone, prostaglandin inhibitors, and ACE inhibitors have been used with limited success.

Gitelman Syndrome

Patients with Gitelman syndrome resemble the Bartter syndrome phenotype in that an autosomal recessive chloride-resistant metabolic alkalosis is associated with hypokalemia, a normal to low blood pressure, volume depletion with secondary hyperreninemic hyperaldosteronism, and juxtaglomerular hyperplasia.[110,111] However, hypocalciuria and symptomatic hypomagnesemia are consistently useful in distinguishing Gitelman syndrome from Bartter syndrome on clinical grounds.[11] These unique features mimic the effect of chronic thiazide diuretic administration. A number of missense mutations in the gene *SLC12A3,* which encodes the thiazide-sensitive sodium-chloride cotransporter in the distal convoluted tubule, have been described and account for the clinical features including the classic finding of hypocalciuria.[112] However, it is not clear why these patients have pronounced hypomagnesemia. A recent study has demonstrated that peripheral blood mononuclear cells from patients with Gitelman syndrome express mutated *NCCT* mRNA. In a large consanguineous Bedouin family, missense mutations were noted in *CLCNKb* but the clinical features overlapped between Gitelman and Bartter syndrome.

Gitelman syndrome becomes symptomatic later in life and is associated with milder salt wasting than that occurring with the Bartter syndrome. A large study of adults with proven Gitelman syndrome and *NCCT* mutations showed that salt craving, nocturia, cramps, and fatigue were more common than in sex- and age-matched controls.[112] Women experienced exacerbation of symptoms during menses, and many had complicated pregnancies.

Treatment of Gitelman syndrome, as with Bartter syndrome, consists of liberal dietary sodium and potassium salts, but with the addition of magnesium supplementation in most patients. ACE inhibitors have been suggested as helpful in selected patients but may cause frank hypotension.

After Treatment of Lactic Acidosis or Ketoacidosis

When an underlying stimulus for the generation of lactic acid or keto acid is removed rapidly, as occurs with repair of circulatory insufficiency or with insulin, the lactate or ketones can be metabolized to yield an equivalent amount of HCO_3^-. Thus, the initial process of HCO_3^- titration that induced the metabolic acidosis is effectively reversed. In the oxidative metabolism of ketones or lactate, HCO_3^- is not directly produced; rather, H^+ is consumed by metabolism of the organic anions, with the liberation of an equivalent amount of HCO_3^-. This process regenerates HCO_3^- if the organic acids can be metabolized to HCO_3^- before their renal excretion. Other sources of new HCO_3^- are additive with the original amount of HCO_3^- regenerated by organic anion metabolism to create a surfeit of HCO_3^-. Such sources include (1) new HCO_3^- added to the blood by the kidneys as a result of enhanced net acid excretion during the preexisting acidotic period and (2) alkali therapy during the treatment phase of the acidosis. The coexistence of acidosis-induced ECF contraction and K^+ deficiency acts to sustain the alkalosis.[11,105]

Nonreabsorbable Anions and Magnesium Ion Deficiency

Administration of large amounts of nonreabsorbable anions, such as penicillin or carbenicillin, can enhance distal acidification and K^+ excretion by increasing the luminal potential difference attained[105] or possibly by allowing Na^+ delivery to the CCT without Cl^-, thus favoring H^+ secretion without Cl^--dependent HCO_3^- secretion.[105] Mg^{2+} deficiency also results in

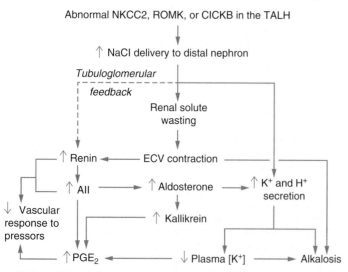

Figure 14–11 Schematic representation of the pathogenesis of Bartter syndrome. The primary defect is impairment of solute reabsorption in the thick ascending limb of Henle's loop (TALH) as a result of an inherited loss of function mutation of NKCC2 (or BSC-1), ROMK, or ClCKB channel. These mutations impair the function of the Na^+-$2Cl^-$-K^+ transporter.

hypokalemic alkalosis by enhancing distal acidification through stimulation of renin and hence aldosterone secretion.

Potassium Ion Depletion

Pure K^+ depletion causes metabolic alkalosis, although generally of only modest severity. One reason that the alkalosis is usually mild is that K^+ depletion also causes positive sodium chloride balance with or without mineralocorticoid administration. The salt retention, in turn, antagonizes the degree of alkalemia. When access to salt as well as to K^+ is restricted, more severe alkalosis develops. Activation of the renal H^+,K^+-ATPase in the collecting duct by chronic hypokalemia likely plays a role in maintenance of the alkalosis. Specifically, chronic hypokalemia has been shown to markedly increase the abundance of the colonic H^+,K^+-ATPase mRNA and protein in the OMCD. In animals, the alkalosis is maintained in part by reduction in GFR without a change in tubule HCO_3^- transport. In humans, the pathophysiologic basis of the alkalosis has not been well defined. Alkalosis associated with severe K^+ depletion, however, is resistant to salt administration. Only repair of the K^+ deficiency corrects the alkalosis.

Extracellular Volume Expansion, Hypertension, and Hypermineralocorticoidism (see Table 14–18)

As previously discussed, mineralocorticoid administration increases net acid excretion and tends to create metabolic alkalosis. The degree of alkalosis is augmented by the simultaneous increase in K^+ excretion leading to K^+ deficiency and hypokalemia. Salt intake for sufficient distal Na^+ delivery is also a prerequisite for the development of both the hypokalemia and the alkalosis. Hypertension develops partly as a result of ECF expansion from salt retention. The alkalosis is not progressive and is generally mild. Volume expansion tends to antagonize the decrease in GFR and/or increase in tubule acidification induced by hypermineralocorticoidism and K^+ deficiency.

Increased mineralocorticoid hormone levels may be the result of autonomous primary adrenal overproduction of mineralocorticoid or of secondary aldosterone release by primary renal overproduction of renin. In both examples, the normal feedback by ECF on net mineralocorticoid production is disrupted and volume retention results in hypertension. These disorders are considered in detail in Chapters 15, 42, and 43.

High Renin

States associated with inappropriately high renin levels may be associated with hyperaldosteronism and alkalosis. Renin levels are elevated because of primary elaboration of renin or, secondarily, by diminished effective circulating blood volume. Total ECF may not be diminished. Examples of high-renin hypertension include renovascular, accelerated, and malignant hypertension. Estrogens increase renin substrate and, hence, angiotensin II formation. Primary tumor overproduction of renin is another rare cause of hyperreninemic hyperaldosterone-induced metabolic alkalosis.[105]

Low Renin

In these disorders, primary adrenal overproduction of mineralocorticoid suppresses renin elaboration. Hypertension occurs as the result of mineralocorticoid excess with volume overexpansion.

PRIMARY ALDOSTERONISM. Tumor involvement (adenoma or, rarely, carcinoma) or hyperplasia of the adrenal gland is associated with aldosterone overproduction. Mineralocorticoid administration or excess production (primary aldosteronism of Cushing's syndrome and adrenal cortical enzyme defects) increases net acid excretion and may result in metabolic alkalosis, which may be worsened by associated K^+

deficiency. ECF volume expansion from salt retention causes hypertension and antagonizes the reduction in GFR and/or increases tubule acidification induced by aldosterone and by K^+ deficiency. The kaliuresis persists and causes continued K^+ depletion with polydipsia, inability to concentrate the urine, and polyuria. Increased aldosterone levels may be the result of autonomous primary adrenal overproduction or of secondary aldosterone release due to renal overproduction of renin. In both situations, the normal feedback of ECF volume on net aldosterone production is disrupted, and hypertension from volume retention can result. The glucocorticoid-remediable form is an autosomal dominant form.

GLUCOCORTICOID-REMEDIABLE HYPERALDOSTERONISM. This is an autosomal dominant form of hypertension, the features of which resemble those of primary aldosteronism (hypokalemic metabolic alkalosis and volume-dependent hypertension). In this disorder, however, glucocorticoid administration corrects the hypertension as well as the excessive excretion of 18-hydroxysteroid in the urine. Lifton has demonstrated that this disorder results from unequal crossing over between the two genes located in close proximity on chromosome 8.[113] This region contains the glucocorticoid-responsive promoter region of the gene encoding 11-β-hydroxylase (CYP11B1) where it is joined to the structural portion of the CYP11B2 gene encoding aldosterone synthase.[113] The chimeric gene produces excess amounts of aldosterone synthase, unresponsive to serum potassium or renin levels, but it is suppressed by glucocorticoid administration. Although a rare cause of primary aldosteronism, the syndrome is important to distinguish because treatment differs and it can be associated with severe hypertension, stroke, and accelerated hypertension during pregnancy.

CUSHING DISEASE OR SYNDROME. Abnormally high glucocorticoid production caused by adrenal adenoma or carcinoma or to ectopic corticotropin production causes metabolic alkalosis. The alkalosis may be ascribed to coexisting mineralocorticoid (deoxycorticosterone and corticosterone) hypersecretion. Alternatively, glucocorticoids may have the capability of enhancing net acid secretion and NH_4^+ production, which may be due to occupancy of cellular mineralocorticoid receptors.

MISCELLANEOUS CONDITIONS. Ingestion of licorice, carbenoxolone, chewer's tobacco, or nasal spray can cause a typical pattern of hypermineralocorticoidism. These substances inhibit 11 β-hydroxysteroid dehydrogenase (which normally metabolizes cortisol to an inactive metabolite), so that cortisol is allowed to occupy type I renal mineralocorticoid receptors, mimicking aldosterone. Genetic apparent mineralocorticoid excess resembles excessive ingestion of licorice: volume expansion, low renin, low aldosterone levels, and a salt-sensitive form of hypertension, which may include metabolic alkalosis and hypokalemia. The hypertension responds to thiazides and spironolactone but without abnormal steroid products in the urine. Licorice and carbenoxolone contain glycyrrhetinnic acid, which inhibits 11 β-hydroxysteroid dehydrogenase. This enzyme is responsible for converting cortisol to cortisone, an essential step in protecting the mineralocorticoid receptor from cortisol, and protects normal subjects from exhibiting apparent mineralcorticoid excess. Without the renal-specific form of this enzyme, monogenic hypertension develops.

LIDDLE'S SYNDROME. Liddle's syndrome is associated with severe hypertension presenting in childhood, accompanied by hypokalemic metabolic alkalosis. These features resemble primary hyperaldosteronism, but the renin and aldosterone levels are suppressed (pseudohyperaldosteronism).[113] The defect is constitutive activation of the ENaC at the apical membrane of principal cells in the CCD. Liddle originally described patients with low renin and low aldosterone levels that did not respond to spironolactone. The defect in **Liddle's**

syndrome is inherited as an autosomal dominant form of monogenic hypertension and has been localized to chromosome 16q. Subsequently, this disorder has been attributed to an inherited abnormality in the gene that encodes the β- or the γ-subunit the renal ENaC. Either mutation results in deletion of the cytoplasmic tails of the β- or γ-subunits, respectively. The C-termini contain PY amino acid motifs that are highly conserved, and essentially all mutations in Liddle syndrome patients involve disruption or deletion of this motif. These PY motifs are important in regulating the number of sodium channels in the luminal membrane by binding to the WW domains of the Nedd4-like family of ubiquitin-protein ligases.[114] Disruption of the PY motif dramatically increases the surface localization of ENaC complex, because these channels are not internalized or degraded (Nedd4 pathway), but remain activated on the cell surface.[114] Persistent Na^+ absorption eventuates in volume expansion, hypertension, hypokalemia, and metabolic alkalosis.[113]

Symptoms and Treatment
Symptoms
Symptoms of metabolic alkalosis include changes in central and peripheral nervous system function similar to those in hypocalcemia: mental confusion, obtundation, and a predisposition to seizures, paresthesias, muscular cramping, and even tetany. Aggravation of arrhythmias and hypoxemia in chronic obstructive pulmonary disease is also a problem. Related electrolyte abnormalities including hypokalemia and hypophosphatemia are common, and patients may present with symptoms of these deficiencies.

Treatment
The maintenance of metabolic alkalosis represents a failure of the kidney to excrete bicarbonate efficiently because of chloride or potassium deficiency or continuous mineralocorticoid elaboration or both. Treatment is primarily directed at correcting the underlying stimulus for HCO_3^- generation and to restore the ability of the kidney to excrete the excess bicarbonate. Assistance is gained in the diagnosis and treatment of metabolic alkalosis by paying attention to the urinary chloride, the arterial blood pressure, and the volume status of the patient (particularly the presence or absence of orthostasis) (see Fig. 14–10). Particularly helpful in the history is the presence or absence of vomiting, diuretic use, or alkali therapy. A high urine chloride and hypertension suggests that mineralocorticoid excess is present. If primary aldosteronism is present, correction of the underlying cause will reverse the alkalosis (adenoma, bilateral hyperplasia, Cushing's syndrome). Patients with bilateral adrenal hyperplasia may respond to spironolactone. Normotensive patients with a high urine chloride may have Bartter or Gitelman syndrome if diuretic use or vomiting can be excluded. A low urine chloride and relative hypotension suggests a chloride responsive metabolic alkalosis such as vomiting or nasogastric suction. [H^+] loss by the stomach or kidneys can be mitigated by the use of proton-pump inhibitors or the discontinuation of diuretics. The second aspect of treatment is to remove the factors that sustain HCO_3^- reabsorption, such as ECF volume contraction or K^+ deficiency. Although K^+ deficits should be repaired, NaCl therapy is usually sufficient to reverse the alkalosis if ECF volume contraction is present, as indicated by a low urine [Cl^-].

Patients with CHF or unexplained volume overexpansion represent special challenges in the critical care setting. Patients with a low urine chloride concentration, usually indicative of a "chloride-responsive" form of metabolic alkalosis, may not tolerate normal saline infusion. Renal HCO_3^- loss can be accelerated by administration of acetazolamide (250–500 mg intravenously), a carbonic anhydrase inhibitor, if associated conditions preclude infusion of saline (elevated

pulmonary capillary wedge pressure, or evidence of CHF).[105] Acetazolamide is usually very effective in patients with adequate renal function, but can exacerbate urinary K^+ losses. Dilute hydrochloric acid (0.1 N HCl) is also effective and must be infused centrally. It can cause hemolysis and may be difficult to titrate. If used, the goal should not be to restore the pH to normal, but to a pH of approximately 7.50. Hemodialysis against a dialysate low in [HCO_3^-] and high in [Cl^-] can be effective when renal function is impaired. Patients receiving continuous renal replacement therapy in the intensive care unit typically develop metabolic alkalosis with high bicarbonate dialysate or when citrate regional anticoagulation is employed. Therapy should include reduction of alkali loads via dialysis by reducing the bicarbonate concentration in the dialysate, or if citrate is being used, by infusion of 0.1 N HCl postfiltration.

References

1. Bidani A, Tauzon DM, Heming TA: Regulation of whole body acid-base balance. *In* DuBose TD, Hamm LL (eds): Acid-Base and Electrolyte Disorders: A Companion to Brenner and Rector's The Kidney. Philadelphia, WB Saunders, 2002, pp 1–21.
2. Madias NE, Adrogue HJ: Respiratory alkalosis. *In* DuBose TD, Hamm LL (eds): Acid-Base and Electrolyte Disorders: A Companion to Brenner and Rector's The Kidney. Philadelphia, WB Saunders, 2002, pp 147–164.
3. Toews GB: Respiratory acidosis. *In* DuBose TD, Hamm LL (eds): Acid-Base and Electrolyte Disorders: A Companion to Brenner and Rector's The Kidney. Philadelphia, WB Saunders, 2002, pp 129–146.
4. Bidani A, DuBose TD Jr: Acid-base regulation: Cellular and whole body. *In* Arieff AI, DeFronzo RA (eds): Fluid, Electrolyte, and Acid Base Disorders, 2nd ed. New York, Churchill Livingstone, 1995, p 69.
5. Alpern RJ, Hamm LL: Urinary acidification. *In* DuBose TD, Hamm LL (eds): Acid-Base and Electrolyte Disorders: A Companion to Brenner and Rector's The Kidney. Philadelphia, WB Saunders, 2002, pp 23–40.
6. DuBose TD, McDonald GA: Renal tubular acidosis. *In* DuBose TD, Hamm LL (eds): Acid-Base and Electrolyte Disorders: A Companion to Brenner and Rector's The Kidney. Philadelphia, WB Saunders, 2002, pp 189–206.
7. Krapf R: Mechanisms of adaptation to chronic respiratory acidosis in the proximal tubule. J Clin Invest 83:890–896, 1989.
8. Schwartz GJ, Al-Awqati Q: Carbon dioxide causes exocytosis of vesicles containing H^+ pumps in isolated perfused proximal and collecting tubules. J Clin Invest 75:1638–1644, 1985.
9. Gennari FJ, Maddox DA: Renal regulation of acid-base homeostasis: Integrated response. *In* Seldin DW, Giebisch G (eds): The Kidney: Physiology and Pathophysiology, 3rd ed. Philadelphia, Lippincott Williams and Wilkins, 2000, pp 2015–2054.
10. Albert MS, Dell RB, Winters RW: Quantitative displacement of acid-base equilibrium in metabolic acidosis. Ann Intern Med 66:312, 1967.
11. Galla JH: Metabolic alkalosis. *In* DuBose TD, Hamm LL (eds): Acid-Base and Electrolyte Disorders: A Companion to Brenner and Rector's The Kidney. Philadelphia, WB Saunders, 2002, pp 109–128.
12. DuBose TD: Metabolic alkalosis. *In* Greenberg A (ed): Primer on Kidney Diseases. Philadelphia, Elsevier Saunders, 2005, pp 90–96.
13. DuBose TD Jr, Codina J, Burges A, Pressley TA: Regulation of H^+,K^+-ATPase expression in kidney. Am J Physiol 269:F500, 1995.
14. Wesson DE: Na/H exchange and H-K-ATPase increase distal tubule acidification in chronic alkalosis. Kidney Int 53:945–951, 1998.
15. Wesson DE, Dolson GM: Endothelin-1 increases rat distal tubule acidification in vivo. Am J Physiol 273:F586–F594, 1997.
16. Wesson DE: Combined K^+ and Cl^- repletion corrects augmented H^+ secretion by distal tubules in chronic alkalosis. Am J Physiol 266:F592–F603, 1994.
17. Guntupalli J, Onuigbo M, Wall SM, et al: Adaptation to low K^+ media increases H^+,K^+-ATPase but not Na^+,K^+-ATPase-mediated pH_i recovery in $OMCD_1$ cells. Am J Physiol 273:C558–C571, 1997.
18. Wall SM, Mehta P, DuBose TD Jr: Dietary K^+ restriction upregulates total and Sch-28080-sensitive bicarbonate absorption in rat tIMCD. Am J Physiol 275:F543–F549, 1998.
19. Krapf R, Alpern RJ, Seldin DW: Clinical syndromes of metabolic acidosis. *In* Seldin DW, Giebisch G (eds): The Kidney, 3rd ed. Philadelphia, Lippincott Williams and Wilkins, 2000, pp 2055–2072.
20. Emmett M: Diagnosis of simple and mixed disorders. *In* DuBose TD, Hamm LL (eds): Acid-Base and Electrolyte Disorders: A Companion to Brenner and Rector's The Kidney. Philadelphia, WB Saunders, 2002, pp 41–54.
21. Oh MS, Carroll HJ: The anion gap. N Engl J Med 297:814, 1977.
22. Feldman M, Soni N, Dickson B: Influence of hypoalbuminemia or hyperalbuminemia on the serum anion gap. J Lab Clin Med 146:317–320, 2005.
23. Acute Respiratory Distress Syndrome Network: Ventilation with lower tidal volumes as compared with traditional tidal volumes for acute lung injury and the acute respiratory distress syndrome. N Engl J Med 342:1301, 2000.
24. Slutsky AS, Tremblay LN: Multiple system organ failure. Is mechanical ventilation a contributing factor? Am J Respir Crit Care Med 157:1721–1725, 1998.

25. DuBose TD, Alpern RJ: Renal tubular acidosis. *In* Scriver CR, Beaudet AL, Sly WS, Valle D (eds): The Metabolic and Molecular Bases of Inherited Disease, 8th ed. New York, McGraw-Hill, 2001, pp 4983–5021.

26. Wong KM, Chak WL, Cheung CY, et al: Hypokalemic metabolic acidosis attributed to cough mixture abuse. Am J Kidney Dis 38:390, 2001.

27. Halperin M, Kamel KS, Cherny DZI: Ketoacidosis. *In* DuBose TD, Hamm LL (eds): Acid-Base and Electrolyte Disorders: A Companion to Brenner and Rector's The Kidney. Philadelphia, WB Saunders, 2002, pp 67–82.

28. Gautheir P, Simon EE, Lemann J: Acidosis of chronic renal failure. *In* DuBose TD, Hamm LL (eds): Acid-Base and Electrolyte Disorders: A Companion to Brenner and Rector's The Kidney. Philadelphia, WB Saunders, 2002, pp 207–216.

29. Morris RC Jr, Nigon K, Reed EB: Evidence that the severity of depletion of inorganic phosphate determines the severity of the disturbance of adenine nucleotide metabolism in the liver and renal cortex of the fructose-loaded rat. J Clin Invest 61:209, 1978.

30. Sly WS, Whyte MP, Sundaram V, et al: Carbonic anhydrase II deficiency in 12 families with the autosomal recessive syndrome of osteopetrosis with renal tubular acidosis and cerebral calcification. N Engl J Med 313:139, 1985.

31. Morris RC Jr: Renal tubular acidosis. Mechanisms, classification and implications. N Engl J Med 281:1405, 1969.

32. DuBose TD Jr: Hydrogen ion secretion by the collecting duct as a determinant of the urine to blood PCO_2 gradient in alkaline urine. J Clin Invest 69:145, 1982.

33. DuBose TD Jr, Caflisch CR: Validation of the difference in urine and blood CO_2 tension during bicarbonate loading as an index of distal nephron acidification in experimental models of distal renal tubular acidosis. J Clin Invest 75:1116, 1985.

34. Batlle DC: Segmental characterization of defects in collecting tubule acidification. Kidney Int 30:546–554, 1986.

35. Bruce LJ, Cope DL, Jones GK, et al: Familial distal renal tubular acidosis is associated with mutations in red cell anion exchanger (Band 3, *AE1*) gene. J Clin Invest 100:1693, 1997.

36. Alper SL: Genetic diseases of acid-base transporters. Annu Rev Physiol 64:899, 2002.

37. Karet FE, Gainza FJ, Gyory AZ, et al: Mutations in the chloride-bicarbonate exchanger gene AE1 cause autosomal dominant but not autosomal recessive distal renal tubular acidosis. Proc Natl Acad Sci U S A 95:6337, 1998.

38. Jarolim P, Shayakul C, Prabakaran D, et al: Autosomal dominant distal renal tubular acidosis is associated in three families with heterozygosity for the R589H mutation in the AE1 (band 3) Cl⁻/HCO₃⁻ exchanger. J Biol Chem 273:6380, 1998.

39. DuBose TD: Autosomal dominant distal renal tubular acidosis and the *AE1* gene. Am J Kidney Dis 33:1191–1197, 1999.

40. Alper SL: Molecular physiology of SLC4 anion exchangers. Exp Physiol 91:153–161, 2006.

41. Karet FE, Finberg KE, Nelson RD, et al: Mutations in the gene encoding B1 subunit of H⁺-ATPase cause renal tubular acidosis with sensorineural deafness. Nat Genet 21:84, 1999.

42. Karet FE, Finberg KE, Nayir A, et al: Localization of a gene for autosomal recessive distal renal tubular acidosis with normal hearing (rdRTA2) to 7q33–34. Am J Hum Genet 65:1656, 1999.

43. Smith AN, Finberg KE, Wagner CA, et al: Molecular cloning and characterization of Atp6n1b. J Biol Chem 276:42382, 2001.

44. Smith AN, Skaug J, Choate KA, et al: Mutations in *Atp6n1b*, encoding a new kidney vacuolar proton pump 116-kD subunit, cause recessive distal renal tubular acidosis with preserved hearing. Nat Genet 26:71, 2000.

45. Kaitwatcharachai C, Vasuvattakul S, Yenchitsomanuas P, et al: Distal renal tubular acidosis and high urine carbon dioxide tension in a patient with Southeast Asian ovalocytosis. Am J Kidney Dis 33:1147–1152, 1999.

46. DuBose TD Jr, Lucci MS, Hogg RJ, et al: Comparison of acidification parameters in superficial and deep nephrons of the rat. Am J Physiol 244:F497, 1983.

47. Bonilla-Felix M: Primary distal renal tubular acidosis as a result of a gradient defect. Am J Kidney Dis 27:428, 1996.

48. DuBose TD Jr, Good DW: Role of the thick ascending limb and inner medullary collecting duct in the regulation of urinary acidification. Semin Nephrol 11:120, 1991.

49. DuBose TD Jr, Good DW, Hamm LL, Wall SM: Ammonium transport in the kidney: New physiologic concepts and their clinical implications. J Am Soc Nephrol 1:1193, 1991.

50. Laing CM, Toye AM, Capasso G, Unwin RJ: Renal tubular acidosis: Developments in our understanding of the molecular basis. Int J Biochem Cell Biol 37:1151–1161, 2005.

51. Pessler F, Emery H, Dai L, et al: The spectrum of renal tubular acidosis in paediatric Sjogren syndrome. Rheumatology 45:85–91, 2006.

52. Morris RC Jr, Sebastian A: Alkali therapy in renal tubular acidosis: Who needs it? J Am Soc Nephrol 13:2186–2188, 2002.

53. Wrong O, Henderson JE, Kaye M: Distal renal tubular acidosis: Alkali heals osteomalacia and increases net production of 1,25-dihydroxyvitamin D. Nephron Physiol 101:72–76, 2005.

54. DuBose TD Jr, Good DW: Effects of chronic chloride depletion metabolic alkalosis on proximal tubule transport and renal production of ammonium. Am J Physiol Renal Fluid Electrol Physiol 269:F508, 1995.

55. DuBose TD Jr, Good DW: Chronic hyperkalemia impairs ammonium transport and accumulation in the inner medulla of the rat. J Clin Invest 90:1443, 1992.

56. Good DW: Ammonium transport by the thick ascending limb of Henle's loop. Annu Rev Physiol 56:623, 1994.

57. Watts BA, Good DW: Effects of ammonium on intracellular pH in rat medullary thick ascending limb: Mechanisms of apical membrane NH₄⁺ transport. J Gen Physiol 103:917, 1994.

58. DuBose TD Jr, Caflisch CR: Effect of selective aldosterone deficiency on acidification in nephron segments of the rat inner medulla. J Clin Invest 82:1624, 1988.

59. Antonipillai I, Wang Y, Horton R: Tumor necrosis factor and interleukin-1 may regulate renin secretion. Endocrinology 126:273, 1990.

60. Geller DS, Rodriguez-Soriano J, Valla Boado A, et al: Mutations in the mineralocorticoid receptor gene cause autosomal dominant pseudohypoaldosteronism type 1. Nat Genet 19:279, 1998.

61. Chang SS, Grunder S, Hanukoglu A, et al: Mutations in subunits of the epithelial sodium channel cause salt wasting with hyperkalemic acidosis, pseudohypoaldosteronism type 1. Nat Genet 12:248, 1996.

62. Grunder S, Firsou D, Chang SS, et al: A mutation causing pseudohypoaldosteronism type 1 identifies a conserved gyycine that is involved in the gating of the epithelial sodium channel. EMBO J 16:899, 1997.

63. Viemann M, Peter M, Lopez-Siguero JP, et al: Evidence for genetic heterogeneity of pseudohypoaldosteronism type 1: Identification of a novel mutation in the human mineralocorticoid receptor in one sporadic case and no mutations in two autosomal dominant kindreds. J Clin Endocrinol Metab 86:2056, 2001.

64. Adachi M, Tachibana K, Asakura Y, et al: Compound heterozygous mutations in the gamma subunit gene of ENaC (1627delG and 1570–1G–>A) in one sporadic Japanese patient with a systemic form of pseudohypoaldosteronism type 1. J Clin Endocrinol Metab 86:9, 2001.

65. Thomas CP, Zhou J, Liu KZ, et al: Systemic pseudohypoaldosteronism from deletion of the promoter region of the human beta epithelial Na⁺ channel subunit. Am J Respir Cell Mol Biol 27:314–319, 2002.

66. Barker PM, Nguyen MS, Gatzy JT, et al: Role of gamma ENaC subunit in lung liquid clearance and electrolyte balance in newborn mice: Insights into perinatal adapation and pseudohypoaldosteronism. J Clin Invest 102:1634, 1998.

67. Achard JM, Disse-Nicodem S, Fiquet-Kempf B, Jeunemaitre X: Phenotypic and genetic heterogeneity of familial hyperkalaemic hypertension (Gordon sydrome). Clin Exp Pharmacol Physiol 28:1048, 2001.

68. Wilson FH, Disse-Nicodeme S, Choate KA, et al: Human hypertension caused by mutations in WNK kinases. Science 293:1107–1112, 2001.

69. Wilson FH, Kahle KT, Sabath E, et al: Molecular pathogenesis of inherited hypertension with hyperkalemia: The Na-Cl cotransporter is inhibited by wild-type but not mutant WNK4. Proc Natl Acad Sci U S A 100:680–684, 2003.

70. Kahle KT, Macgregor GG, Wilson FH, et al: Paracellular Cl⁻ permeability is regulated by WNK4 kinase: Insight into normal physiology and hypertension. Proc Natl Acad Sci U S A 101:14877–14882, 2004.

71. Kahle KT, Wilson FH, Leng Q, et al: WNK4 regulates the balance between renal NaCl reabsorption and K⁺ secretion. Nat Genet 35:372–376, 2003.

72. Braden GL, O'Shea MH, Mulhern JG, Germain MJ: Acute renal failure and hyperkalaemia associated with cyclooxygenase-2 inhibitors. Nephrol Dial Transplant 19:1149–1153, 2004.

73. Caliskan Y, Kalayoglu-Besisik S, Sargin D, Ecder T: Cyclosporine-associated hyperkalemia: Report of four allogeneic blood stem-cell transplant cases. Transplantation 75:1069–1072, 2003.

74. Caramelo C, Bello E, Ruiz E, et al: Hyperkalemia in patients infected with the human immunodeficiency virus: Iinvolvement of a systemic mechanism. Kidney Int 56:198–205, 1999.

75. Schlanger LE, Kleyman TR, Ling BN: K⁺-Sparing diuretic actions of trimethoprim: Inhibition of Na⁺ channels in A6 distal nephron cells. Kidney Int 45:1070–1076, 1994.

76. Kleyman TR, Roberts C, Ling BN: A mechanism for pentamidine-induced hyperkalemia: Inhibition of distal nephron sodium transport. Ann Intern Med 122:103–106, 1995.

77. Valazquez H, Perazella MN, Wright FS, Ellison DH: Renal mechanisms of trimethoprim-induced hyerkalemia. Ann Intern Med 19193:296–301, 1993.

78. Sands JM, McMahon SJ, Tumlin JA: Evidence that the inhibition of Na⁺/K⁺-ATPase activity by FK506 involves calcineurin. Kidney Int 46:647–652, 1994.

79. Kraut JA, Kurtz I: Metabolic acidosis of CKD: Diagnosis, clinical characteristics, and treatment. Am J Kidney Dis 45:978–993, 2005.

80. Qunibi WY, Hootkins RE, McDowell LL, et al: Treatment of hyperphosphatemia in hemodialysis patients: The Calcium Acetate Renagel Evaluation (CARE Study). Kidney Int 65:1914–1926, 2004.

81. Sonikan MA, Pani IT, Iliopoulos AN, et al: Metabolic acidosis aggravation and hyperkalemia in hemodialysis patients treated by sevelamer hydrochloride. Ren Fail 27:143–147, 2005.

82. Wrong O, Harland C: Sevelamer-induced acidosis. Kidney Int 67:776–777, 2005.

83. Laski ME, Wesson DE: Lactic acidosis. *In* DuBose TD, Hamm LL (eds): Acid-Base and Electrolyte Disorders: A Companion to Brenner and Rector's The Kidney. Philadelphia, WB Saunders, 2002, pp 68–83.

84. John M, Mallal S: Hyperlactatemia syndromes in people with HIV infection. Curr Opin Infect Dis 15:23, 2002.

85. Cote HC, Brumme ZL, Craig KJ, et al: Changes in mitochondrial DNA as a marker of nucleoside toxicity in HIV-infected patients. N Engl J Med 346:811, 2002.

86. Lalau JD, Race JM: Lactic acidosis in metformin therapy. Drug 1:55, 1999.

87. Calabrese AT, Coley KC, DaPos SV, et al: Evaluation of prescribing practices: Risk of lactic acidosis with metformin therapy. Arch Intern Med 62:434–437, 2002.

88. Romanski SA, McMahon MM: Metabolic acidosis and thiamine deficiency. Mayo Clin Proc 74:259–263, 1999.

89. Luft FC: Lactic acidosis update for critical care clinicians. J Am Soc Nephrol 12:S15, 2001.

90. Gerard Y, Maulin L, Yazdanpanah T, et al: Symptomatic hyperlactataemia: An emerging complication of antiretroviral therapy. AIDS 14:2723–2730, 2000.

91. Wilson KC, Reardon C, Farber HW: Propylene glycol toxicity in a patient receiving intravenous diazepam. N Engl J Med 343:815, 2000.

92. Arroliga AC, Shehab N, McCarthy K, Gonzales JP: Relationship of continuous infusion lorazepam to serum propylene glycol concentration in critically ill adults. Crit Care Med 32:1709–1714, 2004.

93. Stacpoole PW, Wright EC, Baumgartner TG, et al: A controlled clinical trial of dichloroacetate for treatment of lactic acidosis in adults. The Dichloroacetate–Lactic Acidosis Study Group. N Engl J Med 327:1564, 1992.

94. Bjerneroth G: Alkaline buffers for correction of metabolic acidosis during cardiopulmonary resuscitation with focus on Tribonat—A review. Resuscitation 37:161–171, 1998.

95. Uchida H, Yamamoto H, Kisaki Y, et al: D-Lactic acidosis in short-bowel syndrome managed with antibiotics and probiotics. J Pediatr Surg 39:634–636, 2004.

96. Jorens PG, Demey HE, Schepens PJ, et al: Unusual D-lactic acid acidosis from propylene glycol metabolism in overdose. J Toxicol Clin Toxicol 42:163–169, 2004.

97. Lalive PH, Hadengue A, Mensi N, et al: Recurrent encephalopathy after small bowel resection. Implication of D-lactate. Rev Neurol (Paris) 157:679, 2001.

98. Whitney GM, Szerlip HM. Acid-base disorders in the critical care setting. In DuBose TD, Hamm LL (eds): Acid-Base and Electrolyte Disorders: A Companion to Brenner and Rector's The Kidney. Philadelphia, WB Saunders, 2002, pp 165–187.

99. Umpierrez GE, DiGirolamo M, Tuvlin JA, et al: Differences in metabolic and hormonal milieu in diabetic- and alcohol-induced ketoacidosis. J Crit Care 15:52, 2000.

100. Proudfoot AT, Krenzelok EP, Brent J, Vale JA: Does urine alkalinization increase salicylate elimination? If so, why? Toxicol Rev 22:129–136, 2003.

101. Sterns RH: Fluid, electrolyte, and acid-base disturbances. Neph SAP 2:4–5, 2003.

102. Fraser AD: Clinical toxicologic implications of ethylene glycol and glycolic acid poisoning. Ther Drug Monit 24:232–238, 2002.

103. Brent J, McMartin K, Phillips S, et al: Fomepizole for the treatment of methanol poisoning. N Engl J Med 344:424–429, 2001.

104. Mizock BA, Belyaev S, Mecher C: Unexplained metabolic acidosis in critically ill patients: The role of pyroglutamic acid. Intensive Care Med 30:502–505, 2004.

105. DuBose TD: Metabolic alkalosis. In Greenberg A (ed): Primer on Kidney Diseases. Philadelphia, Elsevier Saunders, 2005, pp 90–96.

106. Gupta M, Wadhwa NK, Bukovsky R: Regional citrate anticoagulation for continuous venovenous hemodiafiltration using calcium-containing dialysate. Am J Kidney Dis 43:67–73, 2004.

107. Meier-Kriesche H, Gitomer J, Finkel K, DuBose T: Increased total to ionized calcium ratio during continuous venovenous hemodialysis with regional citrate anticoagulation. Crit Care Med 29:748–752, 2001.

108. Aichbichler BW, Zerr CH, Santa Ana CA, et al: Proton-pump inhibition of gastric chloride secretion in congenital chloridorrhea. N Engl J Med 336:106, 1997.

109. Simon DB, Karet FE, Rodriguez-Soriano J, et al: Genetic heterogeneity of Bartter's syndrome revealed by mutations in the K+ channel, ROMK. Nat Genet 14:152–156, 1996.

110. Herbert SC, Gullans SR: The molecular basis of inherited hypokalemic alkalosis: Bartter's and Gitelman's syndromes. Am J Physiol Renal Physiol 271:F957–F959, 1996.

111. Shaer AJ: Inherited primary renal tubular hypokalemic alkalosis: A review of Gitelman and Bartter syndromes. Am J Med Sci 322:316–332, 2001.

112. Monkawa T, Kurihara I, Kobayashi K, et al: Novel mutations in thiazide-sensitive Na-Cl cotransporter gene of patients with Gitelman's syndrome. J Am Soc Nephrol 11:65, 2000.

113. Toka HR, Luft FC: Monogenic forms of human hypertension. Semin Nephrol 22:81, 2002.

114. Kamynina E, Staub O: Concerted action of ENaC, Nedd4-2, and Sgkl in transepithelial Na+ transport. Am J Physiol Renal Physiol 283:F377, 2002.

CHAPTER 15

Disorders of Potassium Balance

David B. Mount • Kambiz Zandi-Nejad

The diagnosis and management of potassium disorders are central skills in clinical nephrology, relevant not only to consultative nephrology but also to dialysis and renal transplantation. An understanding of the underlying physiology is an obligatory component of the approach to hyperkalemic and hypokalemic patients. This chapter reviews those aspects of the physiology of potassium homeostasis judged to be relevant to the understanding of potassium disorders; a more detailed review is provided in Chapter 5.

The physiology and pathophysiology of potassium disorders continue to evolve at a rapid rate. The ever-expanding armamentarium of drugs with a potential to affect serum potassium (K^+) has both complicated clinical analysis and provided new insight. The evolving molecular understanding of rare disorders affecting serum K^+ has also uncovered novel pathways of regulation; whereas none of these disorders constitute a "public health menace",[1] they are experiments of nature that have provided new windows on critical aspects of potassium homeostasis. Finally, the increasing availability of knockout and transgenic mice with precisely defined genetic modifications has provided the unprecedented opportunity to extend the relevant molecular physiology to whole-animal studies. These advances can be incorporated into an increasingly mechanistic, molecular understanding of potassium disorders.[1a]

NORMAL POTASSIUM BALANCE

The dietary intake of potassium ranges from <35 to >110 mmoles/day in U.S. men and women. Despite this widespread variation in intake, homeostatic mechanisms precisely maintain serum K^+ between 3.5 and 5.0 mmol/L. In a healthy individual at steady state, the entire daily intake of potassium is excreted, approximately 90% in the urine and 10% in the stool. More than 98% of total body potassium is intracellular, chiefly in muscle (Fig. 15–1). Buffering of extracellular K^+ by this large intracellular pool plays a crucial role in the regulation of serum K^+.[2] Thus within 60 minutes of an intravenous load of 0.5 mmol/kg of K^+-Cl^- only 41% appears in the urine, yet serum

K^+ rises by no more than 0.6 mmol/L[3]; adding the equivalent 35 millimoles exclusively to the extracellular space of a 70 kg man would be expected to raise serum K^+ by ~2.5 mmol/L.[4] Changes in cellular distribution also defend serum K^+ during K^+ depletion. For example, military recruits have been shown to maintain a normal serum K^+ after 11 days of basic training, despite a profound K^+ deficit generated by renal and extra-renal loss.[5] The rapid exchange of intracellular K^+ with extracellular K^+ plays a crucial role in maintaining serum K^+ within such a narrow range; this is accomplished by overlapping and synergistic[6] regulation of a number of renal and extra-renal transport pathways.

Potassium Transport Mechanisms (see Chapter 5)

The intracellular accumulation of K^+ against its electrochemical gradient is an energy-consuming process, mediated by the ubiquitous Na^+/K^+-ATPase enzyme. The Na^+/K^+-ATPase functions as an electrogenic pump, given that the stoichiometry of transport is three intracellular Na^+ ions to two extracellular K^+ ions. The enzyme complex is made up of a tissue-specific combination of multiple α-, β-, and γ-subunits, which are further subject to tissue-specific patterns of regulation.[7] The Na^+/K^+-ATPase proteins share significant homology with the corresponding subunits of the H^+/K^+-ATPase enzymes (see later discussion on potassium reabsorption in the distal nephron). Cardiac glycosides (i.e., digoxin and ouabain) bind to the α subunits of Na^+/K^+-ATPase at an exposed extracellular hairpin loop that also contains the major binding sites for extracellular K^+.[8] The binding of digoxin and K^+ to the Na^+/K^+-ATPase complex is thus mutually antagonistic, explaining in part the potentiation of digoxin toxicity by hypokalemia.[9] Although the four α subunits have equivalent affinity for ouabain, they differ significantly in intrinsic K^+/ouabain antagonism.[10] Ouabain binding to isozymes containing the ubiquitous α-1 subunit is relatively insensitive to K^+ concentrations within the physiological range, such that this isozyme is protected from digoxin under conditions wherein cardiac α-2 and α-3 subunits, the probable therapeutic

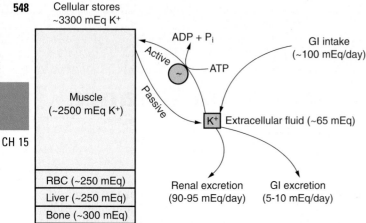

FIGURE 15–1 Body K⁺ distribution and cellular K⁺ flux.

targets,[11] are inhibited.[10] Genetic reduction in cardiac α-1 content has a negative ionotropic effect,[11] such that the relative resistance of this subunit to digoxin at physiological serum K⁺ likely has an additional cardioprotective effect. Notably, the digoxin/ouabain binding site of α subunits is highly conserved, suggesting a potential role in the physiological response to endogenous ouabain/digoxin-like compounds. Recently, "knockin" mice have been generated that express α-2 subunits with engineered resistance to ouabain. These mice are strikingly resistant to ouabain-induced hypertension[12] and to adrenocorticotropic hormone (ACTH)-dependent hypertension,[13] the latter known to involve an increase in circulating ouabain-like glycosides. This provocative data lends new credence to the highly controversial role of such ouabain-like molecules in hypertension and cardiovascular disease. Furthermore, modulation of the K⁺-dependent binding of circulating ouabain-like compounds to Na⁺/K⁺-ATPase may underlie at least some of cardiovascular complications of hypokalemia.[14]

Skeletal muscle contains as much as 75% of body potassium (see Fig. 15–1), and exerts considerable influence on extracellular K⁺. Exercise is thus a well-described cause of transient hyperkalemia; interstitial K⁺ in human muscle can reach levels as high as 10 mM after fatiguing exercise.[15] Not surprisingly, therefore, changes in skeletal muscle Na⁺/K⁺-ATPase activity and abundance are major determinants of the capacity for extra-renal K⁺ homeostasis. Hypokalemia induces a marked decrease in muscle K⁺ content and Na⁺/K⁺-ATPase activity,[16] an "altruistic"[2] mechanism to regulate serum K⁺. This is primarily due to dramatic decreases in the protein abundance of the α-2 subunit of Na⁺/K⁺-ATPase.[17] In contrast, hyperkalemia due to potassium loading is associated with adaptive *increases* in muscle K⁺ content and Na⁺/K⁺-ATPase activity.[18] These interactions are reflected in the relationship between physical activity and the ability to regulate extracellular K⁺ during exercise.[19] For example, exercise training is associated with increases in muscle Na⁺/K⁺-ATPase concentration and activity, with reduced interstitial K⁺ in trained muscles[20] and an enhanced recovery of serum K⁺ after defined amounts of exercise.[19]

Potassium can also accumulate in cells by coupling to the gradient for Na⁺ entry, entering via the electroneutral Na⁺-K⁺-2Cl⁻ cotransporters NKCC1 and NKCC2. The NKCC2 protein is found only at the apical membrane of thick ascending limb (TAL) and macula densa cells (see Figs. 15–2 and 15–9), where it functions in transepithelial salt transport and tubular regulation of renin release.[20] In contrast, NKCC1 is widely expressed in multiple tissues,[21] including muscle. The cotransport of K⁺-Cl⁻ by the four K⁺-Cl⁻ cotransporters (KCC1-

4) can also function in the transfer of K⁺ across membranes; although the KCCs typically function as efflux pathways driven by the electrochemical gradient,[22] they can mediate influx when extracellular K⁺ increases.[21] Whereas the collective role of NKCC1 and the four KCCs in regulating intracellular Cl⁻ activity is increasingly accepted,[21] their function in potassium homeostasis is as yet unclear.

The efflux of K⁺ out of cells is largely accomplished by K⁺ channels, which comprise the largest family of ion channels in the human genome. There are three major subclasses of mammalian K⁺ channels; the six-transmembrane domain (TMD) family,[23] which encompasses both the voltage-sensitive and Ca²⁺-activated K⁺ channels, the two-pore, four TMD family,[24] and the two TMD family of inward rectifying K⁺ (Kir) channels.[25] There is tremendous genomic variety in human K⁺ channels, with 26 separate genes encoding principal subunits of the voltage-gated Kv channels and 16 genes encoding the principal Kir subunits. Further complexity is generated by the presence of multiple accessory subunits and alternative patterns of mRNA splicing. Not surprisingly, an increasing number and variety of K⁺ channels have been implicated in the control of K⁺ homeostasis and the membrane potential of excitable cells such as muscle and heart.

Factors Affecting Internal Distribution of Potassium

A number of hormones and physiological conditions have acute effects on the distribution of K⁺ between the intracellular and extracellular space (Table 15–1). Some of these factors are of particular clinical relevance, and are therefore reviewed in detail.

Insulin

The effect of insulin to decrease serum K⁺ has been known since the early twentieth century.[26] The impact of insulin on plasma K⁺ and plasma glucose is separable at multiple levels, suggesting independent mechanisms.[16,27] Notably, the hypokalemic effect of insulin is not renal-dependent.[28] Insulin and K⁺ appear to form a feedback loop of sorts, in that increases in serum K⁺ have a marked stimulatory effect on insulin levels.[16,29] Inhibition of basal insulin secretion in normal subjects by somatostatin infusion increases serum K⁺ by up to 0.5 mmol/L, in the absence of a change in urinary excretion, emphasizing the crucial role of circulating insulin in the regulation of serum K⁺.[30]

Insulin stimulates the uptake of K⁺ by several tissues, most prominently liver, skeletal muscle, cardiac muscle, and fat.[16,31] It does so by activating several K⁺ transport pathways, with particularly well-documented effects on the Na⁺/K⁺-ATPase.[32] Insulin activates Na⁺-H⁺ exchange and/or Na⁺-K⁺-2Cl⁻ cotransport in several tissues; although the ensuing increase in intracellular Na⁺ was postulated to have a secondary activating effect on Na⁺/K⁺-ATPase,[33] it is clear that this is not the primary mechanism in most cell types.[34] Insulin induces translocation of the Na⁺/K⁺-ATPase α-2 subunit to the plasma membrane of skeletal muscle cells, with a lesser effect on the α-1 subunit.[35] This translocation is dependent on the activity of phosphoinositide-3 kinase (PI-3) kinase,[35] which itself also binds to a proline-rich motif in the N-terminus of the α subunit.[36] The activation of PI3-kinase by insulin thus induces phosphatase enzymes to dephosphorylate a specific serine residue adjacent to the PI3-kinase binding domain. Trafficking of Na⁺/K⁺-ATPase to the cell surface also appears to require the phosphorylation of an adjacent tyrosine residue, perhaps catalyzed by the tyrosine kinase activity of the insulin receptor itself.[37] Insulin-stimulated K⁺ uptake, measured in rats using a "K⁺ clamp" technique, is rapidly reduced by 2 days of K⁺ depletion, before a modest drop in plasma K⁺,[38] and in the *absence* of a change in plasma K⁺ in rats

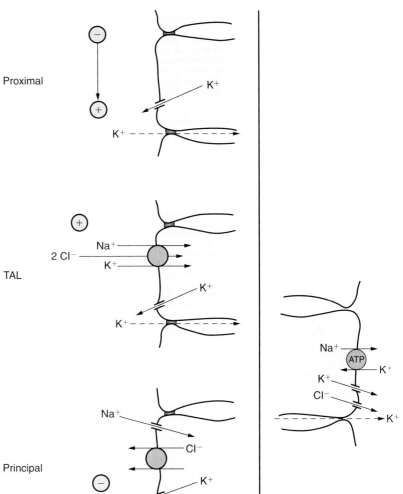

Proximal

TAL

Principal

Intercalated

FIGURE 15-2 Schematic cell models of potassium transport along the nephron. Cell types are as specified; TAL refers to thick ascending limb. Note the differences in luminal potential difference along the nephron. (From Giebisch G: Renal potassium transport: Mechanisms and regulation. Am J Physiol 274: F817–833, 1998.)

subject to a lesser K+ restriction for 14 days.[6] Insulin-mediated K+ uptake is thus modulated by the factors that preserve plasma K+ in the setting of K+ deprivation.

In addition to mediating the direct cellular entry of K+, Na+/K+-ATPase and other pathways activated by insulin induce a hyperpolarization of the plasma membrane,[39] resulting in increased *passive* entry of K+. Electroneutral transport pathways are also activated by insulin in peripheral tissue, including Na+-K+-2Cl− cotransport in adipocytes[40] and K+-Cl− cotransport in skeletal muscle.[41]

Sympathetic Nervous System

The sympathetic nervous system plays a prominent role in regulating the balance between extracellular and intracellular K+. Again, as is the case for insulin, the effect of catecholamines on plasma K+ has been known for some time[42]; however, a complicating issue is the differential effect of stimulating α- and β-adrenergic receptors (Table 15–2). Uptake of K+ by liver and muscle, with resultant hypokalemia, is stimulated via β2 receptors.[43,44] The hypokalemic effect of catecholamines appears to be largely independent of changes in circulating insulin,[45] and has been reported in nephrectomized animals.[46] The cellular mechanisms whereby catecholamines induce K^+ uptake in muscle include an activation of the Na^+/K^+-ATPase,[47] likely via increases in cyclic-AMP.[48] However, β-adrenergic receptors in skeletal muscle also activate the inwardly directed Na^+-K^+-$2Cl^-$ cotransporter NKCC1, which may account for as much as one third of the uptake response to catecholamines.[16,49]

In contrast to β-adrenergic stimulation, α-adrenergic agonists impair the ability to buffer increases in K^+ induced via intravenous loading or by exercise[50]; the cellular mechanisms whereby this occurs are not known. It is thought that β-adrenergic stimulation increases K^+ uptake during exercise to avoid hyperkalemia, whereas α-adrenergic mechanisms help blunt the ensuing post-exercise nadir.[50] The clinical consequences of the sympathetic control of extra-renal K^+ homeostasis are reviewed elsewhere in this chapter.

Acid-Base Status

The association between changes in pH and serum K^+ was observed some time ago.[51] It has long been held that acute disturbances in acid-base equilibrium results in changes in plasma K^+, such that alkalemia shifts K^+ into cells whereas acidemia is associated with K^+ release from the cells.[52,53] It is thought that this effective K^+-H^+ exchange helps maintain extracellular pH. Rather limited data exists for the durable concept that a change of 0.1 unit in plasma pH will result in 0.6 mmol/L change in plasma K^+ in the opposite direction.[54] However, despite the complexities of changes in K^+ homeostasis associated with various acid-base disorders, a few general observations can be made. The induction of metabolic acidosis by the infusion of mineral acids (NH_4^+-Cl^- or H^+-Cl^-) consistently increases serum K^+,[52-56] whereas organic acidosis generally fails to increase serum K^+.[53,55,57,58] Notably, a more recent report failed to detect an increase in plasma K^+ in normal human subjects with acute acidosis secondary to duodenal NH_4^+-Cl^- infusion, in which a modest acidosis was accompanied by an increase in circulating insulin.[59] However, as noted by Adrogué and Madias,[60] the concomitant infusion of 350 ml of D5W in these fasting subjects may have served to increase circulating insulin, thus blunting the potential hyperkalemic response to NH_4^+-Cl^-. Clinically, use of the oral phosphate binder sevelamer in patients with end-stage renal disease (ESRD) is associated with acidosis, due to effective gastrointestinal absorption of H^+-Cl^-; in hemodialysis patients this acidosis has been associated with an increase in serum K^+,[61] which is ameliorated by an increase in dialysis bicarbonate concentration.[62] Metabolic alkalosis induced by sodium-bicarbonate infusion usually results in a modest reduction in plasma K^+.[52-54,56,63] Respiratory alkalosis reduces serum K^+, by a magnitude comparable to that of metabolic alkalosis.[52-54,64] Finally, acute respiratory acidosis increases serum K^+; the absolute increase is smaller than that induced by metabolic acidosis secondary to inorganic acids.[52-54] Again, however, some studies have failed to show a change in serum K^+ following acute respiratory acidosis.[53,65]

TABLE 15–1	Factors Affecting K^+ Distribution between Intracellular and Extracellular Compartments
Acute	
Factor	**Effect on Potassium**
Insulin	Enhanced cell uptake
β-Catecholamines	Enhanced cell uptake
α-Catecholamines	Impaired cell uptake
Acidosis	Impaired cell uptake
Alkalosis	Enhanced cell uptake
External potassium balance	Loose correlation
Cell damage	Impaired cell uptake
Hyperosmolality	Enhanced cell efflux
Chronic	
Factor	**Effect on ATP Pump Density**
Thyroid	Enhanced
Adrenal steroids	Enhanced
Exercise (training)	Enhanced
Growth	Enhanced
Diabetes	Impaired
Potassium deficiency	Impaired
Chronic renal failure	Impaired

From Giebisch G: Renal potassium transport: Mechanisms and regulation. Am J Physiol 274:F817–833, 1998.

TABLE 15–2	Sustained Effects of β– and α–Adrenergic Agonists and Antagonists on Serum K^+
Catecholamine Specificity	**Sustained Effect on Serum K^+**
$β_1$+$β_2$ agonist (epinephrine, isoproterenol)	Decrease*
Pure $β_1$ agonist (ITP)	None
Pure $β_2$ agonist (salbutamol, soterenol, terbutaline)	Decrease
$β_1$+$β_2$ Antagonist (propranolol, sotalol)	Increase; blocks effect of β agonists
$β_1$ Antagonist (practolol, metoprolol, atenolol)	None; does not block effect of β agonists
$β_2$ Antagonist (butoxamine, H 35/25)	Blocks hypokalemic effect of β agonists
α Agonist (phenylephrine)	Increase
α Antagonist (phenoxybenzamine)	None; blocks effect of α agonist

ITP, isopropylamino-3-(2thiazoloxy)-2-propanol.
*Results refer to the late (after 5 min), sustained effect.

Potassium Secretion in the Distal Nephron

The proximal tubule and loop of Henle mediate the bulk of potassium reabsorption, such that a considerable fraction of filtered potassium is reabsorbed prior to entry into the superficial distal tubules.[66] Renal potassium excretion is primarily determined by regulated secretion in the distal nephron, specifically within the connecting segment (CNT) and cortical collecting duct (CCD). The principal cells of the CCD and CNT play a dominant role in K+ excretion; the relevant transport pathways are shown in Figures 15–2 and 15–3. Apical Na+ entry via the amiloride-sensitive epithelial Na+ channel (ENaC)[67] results in the generation of a lumen-negative potential difference in the CNT and CCD, which drives passive K+ exit through an expanding list of apical K+ channels. A criti-

cal consequence of this relationship is that K+ secretion is dependent on delivery of adequate luminal Na+ to the CNT and CCD[68,69]; K+ secretion by the CCD essentially ceases as luminal Na+ drops below 8 mmol/L.[70] Dietary Na+ intake also influences K+ excretion, such that excretion is enhanced by excess Na+ intake and reduced by Na+ restriction (Fig. 15–4).[68,69] Basolateral exchange of Na+ and K+ is mediated by the Na+/K+-ATPase, providing the driving force for both Na+ entry and K+ exit at the apical membrane (see Figs. 15–2 and 15–3).

Electrophysiological characterization has documented the presence of several subpopulations of apical K+ channels in the CCD and CNT, most prominently a small-conductance (SK) 30 pS channel[71,72] and a large-conductance, Ca2+-activated 150 pS ("maxi-K") channel.[72,73] The higher density and higher open probability of the SK channel suggests that it likely mediates K+ secretion under baseline conditions, hence its frequent designation as the "secretory" K+ channel. The characteristics of the SK channel are particularly close

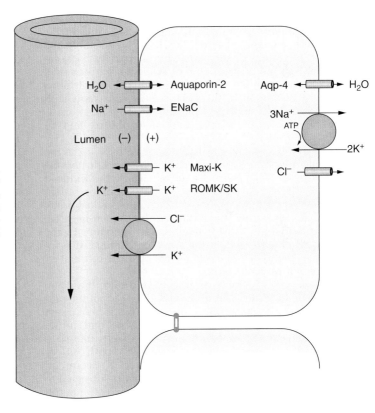

FIGURE 15–3 K+ secretory pathways in principal cells of the connecting segment (CNT) and cortical collecting duct (CCD). The absorption of Na+ via the amiloride-sensitive epithelial sodium channel (ENaC) generates a lumen-negative potential difference, which drives K+ excretion through the apical secretory K+ channel ROMK. Flow-dependent K+ secretion is mediated by an apical voltage-gated, calcium-sensitive maxi-K channel.

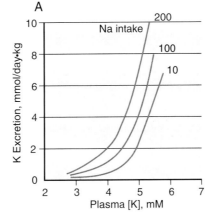
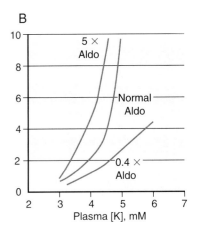

FIGURE 15–4 **A,** Relationship between steady-state serum K+ and urinary K+ excretion in the dog, as a function of dietary Na+ intake (mmol/day). Animals were adrenalectomized and replaced with aldosterone, dietary K+ and Na+ content were varied as specified. (From Young DB, Jackson TE, Tipayamontri U, Scott RC: Effects of sodium intake on steady-state potassium excretion. Am J Physiol 246:F772–778, 1984.) **B,** Relationship between steady-state serum K+ and urinary K+ excretion as a function of circulating aldosterone. Animals were adrenalectomized and variably replaced with aldosterone, dietary K+ content was varied. (From Young DB: Quantitative analysis of aldosterone's role in potassium regulation. Am J Physiol 255:F811–822, 1988.)

to those of the K⁺ channel ROMK, encoded by the *Kcnj1* gene,[74] and ROMK protein has been localized at the apical membrane of principal cells.[75] Definitive evidence that ROMK is the SK channel was obtained from mice with a targeted deletion of both alleles of the *Kcnj1* gene; no 30 pS K⁺ channels were found in apical membranes from the CCD of these mice, with an intermediate channel density in heterozygous mice.[73] The observation that ROMK knockout mice are normokalemic with an *increased* excretion of K⁺ serves to emphasize that there is considerable redundancy in distal K⁺ secretory pathways[73]; recent data suggest that distal K⁺ excretion in these mice is primarily mediated by maxi-K/BK channel activity (see later discussion).[76]

Alternative apical K⁺ secretory pathways in the CNT and/or CCD include the Ca²⁺-activated maxi-K channel,[71] voltage-sensitive channels such as Kv1.3,[77,78] KCNQ1, and double-pore K⁺ channels such as TWIK-1.[24] Maxi-K channels, also known as "BK" channels, have a heteromeric structure, encompassing functional α-subunits that form the ion channel pore and modulatory β-subunits that affect the biophysical and pharmacological characteristics of the channel complex.[71] Maxi-K α-subunit transcripts are expressed in multiple nephron segments, and channel protein is detectable at the apical membrane of principal and intercalated cells in the CCD and CNT.[71] Increased distal flow has a well-established stimulatory effect on K⁺ secretion, due in part to both enhanced delivery and absorption of Na⁺ and to increased removal of secreted K⁺.[16,68,69] The pharmacology of flow-dependent K⁺ secretion in the CCD is most consistent with maxi-K channels,[79] and flow-dependent K⁺ secretion is reduced in mice with targeted deletion of the α1 and β1 subunits.[71]

The role of the Kv1.3 and KCNQ1 channels in K⁺ secretion is less clear. However, Kv1.3 is activated by the aldosterone-induced kinase SGK (serum and glucocorticoid-induced kinase, see discussion on control of potassium secretion: aldosterone),[80] and may serve as a "brake" on aldosterone-stimulated K⁺ excretion by reducing the lumen-negative potential difference.[77] KCNQ1 mediates K⁺ secretion in the inner ear and is expressed at the apical membrane of principal cells in the CCD[81]; the role of this channel in renal K⁺ excretion is not as yet known.

In addition to K⁺ channels, a series of studies in the distal nephron have suggested a role for apical K⁺-Cl⁻ cotransport in K⁺ secretion.[22,68,82] In rat distal tubules, a mixture of distal convoluted tubule (DCT), connecting segment, and initial collecting duct, a reduction in luminal Cl⁻ markedly increases K⁺ secretion.[16,83] The replacement of luminal Cl⁻ with SO₄⁻ or gluconate has the same stimulatory effect on K⁺ secretion; analogous results have been reported in humans subjected to dietary modulation of excreted anions.[84] This electroneutral component of K⁺ secretion is not influenced by luminal Ba²⁺,[16,83] which inhibits K⁺ secretion through apical K⁺ channels. These findings have been extended to the rabbit CCD, where a decrease in luminal Cl⁻ from 112 mmol/L to 5 mmol/L increases K⁺ secretion by 48%.[85] A reduction in basolateral Cl⁻ also decreases K⁺ secretion without an effect on transepithelial voltage or Na⁺ transport, and the direction of K⁺ flux can be reversed by a lumen-to-bath Cl⁻ gradient, resulting in K⁺ absorption.[85] In perfused CCDs from rats treated with mineralocorticoid, vasopressin increases K⁺ secretion[86]; because this increase in K⁺ secretion is resistant to luminal Ba²⁺ (2 mmol/L), vasopressin may stimulate Cl⁻-dependent K⁺ secretion.[85] Recent pharmacological studies are consistent with K⁺-Cl⁻ cotransport mediated by the KCCs[22,82]; of the three renal KCCs only KCC1 is apically expressed along the nephron (D.B.M., unpublished observations). Other functional possibilities for Cl⁻-dependent K⁺ secretion include the parallel operation of apical H⁺-K⁺-exchange and Cl⁻-HCO₃⁻ exchange in type B intercalated cells.[87]

Potassium Reabsorption in the Distal Nephron

In addition to secretion, the distal nephron is capable of considerable reabsorption, particularly during restriction of dietary K⁺.[16,66,88,89] This reabsorption is accomplished primarily by intercalated cells in the outer medullary collecting duct (OMCD), via the activity of apical H⁺/K⁺-ATPase pumps (see Fig. 15–2). H⁺/K⁺-ATPase constitutes the third major class of apical K⁺ transport in the distal nephron, with evolving roles in distal bicarbonate and K⁺ reabsorption.[90] The H⁺/K⁺-ATPase enzymes are of course central to gastric acid secretion, and the availability of pharmacological inhibitors such as omeprazole was critical to the initial identification of their role in K⁺ homeostasis.[88,89]

Like the Na⁺/K⁺-ATPases, H⁺/K⁺-ATPase enzymes are members of the P-type family of ion transport ATPases. Although the HKα-1 ("gastric") and HKα-2 ("colonic") subunits are the best known, humans also have an HKα-4 subunit.[91] Within the kidney, the HKα-1 subunit is expressed at the apical membrane of at least a subset of type A intercalated cells in the distal nephron.[16,91] HKα-2 distribution in the distal nephron is more diffuse, with robust expression at the apical membrane of type A and B intercalated cells and connecting segment cells, with lesser expression in principal cells.[92,93] Finally, the human HKα-4 subunit is detectable in intercalated cells of human kidneys.[91] The various H⁺/K⁺-ATPase holoenzymes differ in pharmacological behavior, such that those assembled with the gastric HKα-1 are classically sensitive to the H⁺/K⁺-ATPase inhibitors SCH-28080 and omeprazole and resistant to ouabain, whereas the colonic HKα-2 subunit is usually *sensitive* to ouabain and *resistant* to SCH-28080.[16,94] This pharmacology has helped clarify the role of individual subunits in H⁺/K⁺-ATPase activity of the distal nephron, in both normal and K⁺-restricted animals.

K⁺ deprivation induces a significant absorptive flux of K⁺ in the inner stripe of the outer medulla, which is largely inhibited by omeprazole and SCH-28080.[16,88] Although both HKα-1 and HKα-2 are constitutively expressed in the distal nephron, tubule perfusion of normal animals suggests a functional dominance of omeprazole/SCH-28080-sensitive, ouabain-resistant H⁺/K⁺-ATPase activity, consistent with holoenzymes containing HKα-1. K⁺ depletion significantly increases the overall activity of H⁺/K⁺-ATPase in the collecting duct, with the emergence of a ouabain-sensitive H⁺/K⁺-ATPase activity.[16] The limitations of the available pharmacology notwithstanding, these data suggest a dominance of HKα-2 during K⁺ depletion. This conclusion is supported by the dramatic up-regulation of HKα-2 transcript and protein in the outer and inner medulla during K⁺ depletion, as reported by multiple laboratories.[16,95,96] In contrast, HKα-1 abundance is minimally affected by K⁺ depletion.[95,96]

The preceding discussion suggests that the HKα-2 H⁺/K⁺-ATPase plays a major role in K⁺ reabsorption by the distal nephron, serving to limit kaliuresis during K⁺ depletion. Indeed, mice with a homozygous targeted deletion of HKα-2 exhibit lower plasma and muscle K⁺ than wild-type litter mates when maintained on a K⁺-deficient diet. However, this appears to be due to marked loss of K⁺ in the colon rather than kidney because renal K⁺ excretion is appropriately reduced in the K⁺-depleted mutant mice.[97] Presumably the lack of an obvious renal phenotype in either HKα-1[98] or HKα-2[97] knockout mice reflects the marked redundancy in the expression of HKα subunits in the distal nephron. Indeed, collecting ducts from the HKα-1 knockout mice have significant residual ouabain-resistant and SCH-28080-sensitive H⁺/K⁺-ATPase activities, consistent with the expression of other HKα subunits that confer characteristics similar to the "gastric" H⁺/K⁺-ATPase.[99] However, more recent data from HKα-1 and HKα-2 knockout mice suggest that compensatory mechanisms in these mice are not accounted for by ATPase-type mechanisms.[100]

In an alternative approach, transgenic mice have been generated with generalized over-expression of a "gain-of-function" mutation in H⁺/K⁺-ATPase. These mice globally over-express a mutant form of the HKβ subunit, in which a tyrosine-to-alanine mutation within the C-terminal tail abrogates regulated endocytosis from the plasma membrane. The gastric glands of these mice constitutively express H⁺/K⁺-ATPase at the plasma membrane, with significant gastric hyperacidity.[101] They also have higher plasma K⁺'s than their wild-type litter mates, with approximately half the fractional excretion of urinary K⁺,[102] consistent with increased distal K⁺ reabsorption. These transgenic mice thus provide indirect evidence for the role of H⁺/K⁺-ATPase in K⁺ homeostasis.

Control of Potassium Secretion: Aldosterone

Aldosterone is well established as an important regulatory factor in K⁺ excretion. However, an increasingly dominant theme is that it plays a permissive and synergistic role (see next section).[77,103,104] This is reflected clinically in the frequent absence of hyperkalemia or hypokalemia in disorders associated with a deficiency or an overabundance of circulating aldosterone, respectively (see Hyperaldosteronism and Hypoaldosteronism). Regardless, it is clear that aldosterone and downstream effectors of this hormone have clinically relevant effects on K⁺ secretion, and that the ability to excrete K⁺ is modulated by systemic aldosterone levels (see Fig. 15–4).

Aldosterone has no effect on the density of apical SK channels,[105] despite the fact that it increases transcript levels of the ROMK (*KCNJ1*) gene that encodes this channel.[106,107] Aldosterone does however induce a marked increase in the density of apical Na⁺ channels in the CNT and CCD,[105] thus increasing the driving force for apical K⁺ excretion. The apical amiloride-sensitive epithelial Na⁺ channel is composed of three subunits, α-, β-, and γ-, that assemble together to synergistically traffic to the cell membrane and mediate Na⁺ transport.[67] Aldosterone activates this channel complex by multiple mechanisms. First, it uniquely induces transcription of the α-ENaC subunit, via a glucocorticoid-response element in the channel's promoter.[108] This is reflected in an increased abundance of α-ENaC protein in response to either exogenous aldosterone or dietary Na⁺-Cl⁻ restriction[109]; the response of α-ENaC to Na⁺-Cl⁻ restriction is blunted by spironolactone, indicating that the effect is dependent on the mineralocorticoid receptor.[110] Second, aldosterone and dietary Na⁺-Cl⁻ restriction stimulate a significant redistribution of ENaC subunits in the CNT and early CCD, from a largely cytoplasmic location during dietary Na⁺-Cl⁻ excess to a purely apical

distribution after aldosterone or Na⁺-Cl⁻ restriction.[110–112] The leading mechanism whereby aldosterone promotes the intracellular redistribution of ENaC subunits has emerged over the past 6 to 7 years, in a spectacular convergence of human genetics and physiology. An aldosterone-induced kinase has thus been shown to regulate the interaction between ENaC channels and proteins discovered through the identification of disease-associated mutations in Liddle syndrome.

In cell culture systems, aldosterone strongly and rapidly induces a serine-threonine kinase called SGK-1 (serum and glucocorticoid-induced kinase-1)[113]; co-expression of SGK with ENaC subunits results in a dramatic activation of the channel due to increased expression at the plasma membrane.[111] Rapid induction of SGK-1 by aldosterone has also been shown in vivo,[114] where it appears to correlate with the redistribution of channel protein to the plasma membrane.[111] Unlike the effect on α-ENaC induction, spironolactone does not interfere with intracellular redistribution of ENaC subunits during dietary Na⁺-Cl⁻ restriction[110]; this is consistent with the observation that SGK-1 also functions in the activation of ENaC by other hormones, including vasopressin and insulin.[16,115]

The mechanism underlying the effect of SGK-1 on surface expression of ENaC was recently uncovered via the pathobiology of Liddle syndrome (see also discussion on Liddle syndrome). With one exception,[116] autosomal dominant mutations in the β- and γ-ENaC subunits associated with Liddle syndrome affect a so-called PPxY motif in the cytoplasmic C-terminus of the channel proteins, resulting in a gain of function. This PPxY motif was shown to bind to WW domains of the ubiquitin-ligase Nedd4[117] and the related protein Nedd4-2; the latter turns out to be the likely physiological regulator of ENaC.[118] Co-expression of Nedd4-2 or Nedd4 with wild-type ENaC channel results in a marked inhibition of channel activity due to retrieval from the cell membrane, whereas channels bearing Liddle syndrome mutations are resistant.[119] Nedd4-2 is thought to ubiquitinate ENaC subunits, resulting in the removal of channel subunits from the cell membrane and degradation in the proteosome[119,120]; direct inhibition of channel activity by WW domains may also play a role.[121] The circle between ENaC, aldosterone, and SGK-1 was ultimately closed with the observation that Nedd4-2 is a phosphorylation substrate for the latter, such that phosphorylation of Nedd4-2 by SGK abrogates its inhibitory effect on ENaC (Fig. 15–5).[122] Aldosterone thus rapidly induces a kinase that inhibits Nedd4-2–dependent retrieval of ENaC from the apical membrane. Aldosterone evidently stimulates Nedd4-2 phosphorylation in vivo[123] and reduces Nedd4-2 protein expression in cultured CCD cells.[124]

The importance of SGK-1 in K⁺ and Na⁺ homeostasis is illustrated by the phenotype of SGK-1 knockout mice.[125,126] On a normal diet, homozygous SGK-1 –/– mice exhibit normal blood pressure and a normal serum K⁺, with only a mild

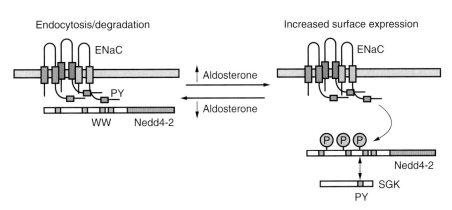

FIGURE 15–5 Coordinated regulation of ENaC by the aldosterone-induced SGK kinase and the ubiquitin ligase Nedd4-2. Nedd4-2 binds via its WW domains to ENaC subunits via their "PPXY" domains (denoted PY here), ubiquitinating the channel subunits and targeting them for removal from the cell membrane and destruction in the proteosome. Aldosterone induces the SGK kinase, which phosphorylates and inactivates Nedd4-2, thus increasing surface expression of ENaC channels. Mutations that cause Liddle syndrome affect the interaction between ENaC and Nedd4-2. (From Snyder PM, Olson DR, Thomas BC: Serum and glucocorticoid-regulated kinase modulates Nedd4-2-mediated inhibition of the epithelial Na⁺ channel. J Biol Chem 277:5–8, 2002.)

Endocytosis/degradation

Increased surface expression

ENaC

ENaC

Aldosterone

Aldosterone

PY

WW   Nedd4-2

Nedd4-2

SGK

PY

elevation of circulating aldosterone. However, dietary Na$^+$-Cl$^-$ restriction of these mice results in relative Na$^+$-wasting and hypotension, marked weight loss, and a drop in glomerular filtration rate (GFR), despite considerable increases in circulating aldosterone.[126] In addition, dietary K$^+$ loading over 6 days leads to a 1.5 mM increase in plasma K$^+$, also accompanied by a considerable increase in circulating aldosterone (~fivefold greater than that of wild-type litter mate controls).[125] This hyperkalemia occurs despite evident increases in apical ROMK expression, compared with the normokalemic litter mate controls. The amiloride-sensitive, lumen-negative potential difference generated by ENaC is reduced in SGK-1 knockout mice,[125] resulting in a decreased driving force for distal K$^+$ secretion and the observed susceptibility to hyperkalemia.

Another novel mechanism whereby aldosterone activates ENaC involves proteolytic cleavage of the channel by serine proteases. A "channel activating protease" that increases channel activity of ENaC was identified some time ago in *Xenopus laevis* A6 cells.[127] The mammalian ortholog, denoted CAP1[128] or prostasin,[129] is an aldosterone-induced protein in principal cells.[129] Urinary excretion of CAP1 is increased in hyperaldosteronism, with a reduction after adrenalectomy. CAP1 is membrane-associated, via a glycosylphosphatidylinositol (GPI) linkage[127]; mammalian principal cells also express two transmembrane proteases, denoted CAP2 and CAP3, with homology to CAP1.[130] All three of these proteases activate ENaC by increasing the open probability of the channel, rather than by increasing expression at the cell surface.[130] Because SGK increases channel expression at the cell surface,[111] one would expect synergistic activation by co-expressed CAP1-3 and SGK; this is indeed the case.[130] Therefore, aldosterone activates ENaC by at least three separate synergistic mechanisms; induction of α-ENaC, induction of SGK/repression of Nedd4-2, and induction of the channel-activating proteases (CAP1-3).

Aldosterone also has significant effects on the basolateral membrane of principal cells, with dramatic changes in cellular morphology and length of basolateral membranes in response to the hormone.[131,132] This is accompanied by an increase in basolateral Na$^+$/K$^+$-ATPase activity, although it has been difficult to determine how much of these cellular and functional changes are due to enhanced Na$^+$ entry via apical ENaC.[133,134] It is however known that aldosterone increases the expression of the Na$^+$/K$^+$-ATPase α-1 and β-1 subunits in the CCD[135]; these effects are evidently independent of ENaC activity.[134]

Control of Potassium Secretion: The Effect of K$^+$ Intake

Despite the evident importance of aldosterone in regulating K$^+$ excretion, it is clear that other factors play important, synergistic roles. Chief among these is peritubular K$^+$, induced experimentally by increases in K$^+$ intake or by variation in tubule perfusion conditions.[103,104,136] A high K$^+$ diet in adrenalectomized animals increases apical Na$^+$ reabsorption and K$^+$ secretion in the CCD, a qualitatively similar response to that induced by aldosterone.[137] When peritubular K$^+$ is increased, there is a significant activation of basolateral Na$^+$/K$^+$-ATPase, accompanied by a secondary activation of apical Na$^+$ and K$^+$ channels.[138] Increased dietary K$^+$ also significantly increases the density of SK channels in the CCD of normal, along with a modest increase in Na$^+$ channel (ENaC) density.[105] Notably, this increase in ENaC and SK density in the CCD occurs within hours of assuming a high K$^+$ diet, with a minimal associated increase in circulating aldosterone.[139] In contrast, a week of low Na$^+$-Cl$^-$ intake, with almost a 1000-fold increase in aldosterone, has no effect on SK channel

density; nor for that matter does 2 days of aldosterone infusion, despite the development of hypokalemia.[139] Therefore, despite the important role of aldosterone in "setting the stage" for K$^+$ secretion, other factors affect the density and activity of apical K$^+$ secretory channels in response to increases in dietary K$^+$.

Considerable progress has recently been made in defining the signaling pathways that regulate the activity of ROMK, the SK channel, in response to changes in dietary K$^+$. It appears that dietary K$^+$ intake impacts on trafficking of the ROMK channel protein to the plasma membrane of principal cells, with a marked increase in the relative proportion of intracellular channel protein in K$^+$-depleted animals[140,141] and clearly defined expression at the plasma membrane of CCD cells from animals on a high-K$^+$ diet.[141] The membrane insertion and activity of ROMK is affected considerably by the tyrosine phosphorylation status of the channel protein, such that phosphorylation of tyrosine residue 337 stimulates endocytosis and dephosphorylation induces exocytosis[142,143]; this tyrosine phosphorylation appears to play a dominant role in the regulation of ROMK by dietary K$^+$.[144] Whereas the levels of protein tyrosine phosphatase-1D do not vary with K$^+$ intake, intra-renal activity of the cytoplasmic tyrosine kinases c-src and c-yes are inversely related to dietary K$^+$ intake, with a decrease under high K$^+$ conditions and a marked increase after several days of K$^+$ restriction.[145,146] Localization studies indicate co-expression of c-src with ROMK in TAL and principal cells of the CCD.[141] Moreover, inhibition of protein tyrosine phosphatase activity, leading to a dominance of tyrosine phosphorylation, dramatically increases the proportion of intracellular ROMK in the CCD of animals on a high-K$^+$ diet.[141]

As reviewed earlier, maxi-K channels in the CNT and CCD play an important role in the flow-activated component of distal K$^+$ excretion. Flow-stimulated K$^+$ secretion by the CCD of both mice 76 and rats[147] is enhanced on a high-K$^+$ diet, with an absence of flow-dependent K$^+$ secretion in rats on a low-K$^+$ diet.[147] This is accompanied by commensurate changes in transcript levels for α- and β$_{2-4}$-subunits of the maxi-K channel proteins in micro-dissected CCDs (β$_1$ subunits are restricted to the CNT[71]), with a marked induction by dietary K$^+$ loading and reduction by K$^+$ deprivation. Trafficking of maxi-K subunits is also affected by dietary K$^+$, with largely intracellular distribution of α-subunits in K$^+$-restricted rats and prominent apical expression in K$^+$-loaded rats.[147]

The upstream K$^+$-dependent stimuli that affect the trafficking and expression of ROMK and maxi-K channels in the distal nephron are not as yet known. However, a landmark study recently implicated the intra-renal generation of superoxide anions in the activation of cytoplasmic tyrosine kinases and downstream phosphorylation of the ROMK channel protein by K$^+$ depletion.[148] What might the circulating factor(s) be that respond to reduced dietary K$^+$, leading to increases in intra-renal superoxides and a reduced kaliuresis? Potential candidates include angiotensin II (ATII) and growth factors such as IGF-1.[148] Regardless, reports of a marked post-prandial kaliuresis in sheep, independent of changes in plasma K$^+$ or aldosterone, have led to the suggestion that an enteric or hepatoportal K$^+$ "sensor" controls kaliuresis via a sympathetic reflex.[149] These investigators have reported similar data for humans ingesting oral K$^+$-citrate.[150] More recently, Morita and colleagues[151] suggested that a bumetanide-sensitive hepatoportal K$^+$ sensor induces a significant kaliuresis in response to infusion of K$^+$-Cl$^-$ into rat portal vein, but not the inferior vena cava. Changes in dietary K$^+$ absorption may thus have a direct "anticipatory" effect on K$^+$ homeostasis, in the absence of changes in plasma K$^+$. Such a "feedforward" control has the theoretical advantage of greater stability because it operates prior to changes in plasma K$^+$, which induce the "feedback" element of control.[152] Notably, changes in ROMK phosphorylation status and insulin-sensitive muscle uptake can be seen in K⁺-deficient animals in the absence of a change in plasma K⁺,[6] suggesting that upstream activation of the major mechanisms that serve to reduce K⁺ excretion (reduced K⁺ secretion in the CNT/CCD, decreased peripheral uptake, and increased K⁺ reabsorption in the OMCD) does not require changes in plasma K⁺.

Finally, we should note in this context that new evidence has stimulated a reappraisal of the role of the CNT in regulated K⁺ and Na⁺ handling by the kidney (see also Chapter 5). It has recently been appreciated that the density of both Na⁺ and K⁺ channels is considerably greater in the CNT than in the CCD[72,153]; the capacity of the CNT for Na⁺ reabsorption may be as much as 10 times greater than that of the CCD.[153] Indeed, it is likely that, under basal conditions of high Na⁺-Cl⁻ and low K⁺ intake, the bulk of aldosterone-stimulated Na⁺ and K⁺ transport has occurred prior to the entry of tubular fluid into the CCD.[154] The recruitment of ENaC subunits in response to dietary Na⁺ restriction begins in the CNT, with progressive recruitment of subunits in the CCD at lower levels of dietary Na⁺.[112] With respect to K⁺ secretion, unlike the marked increase seen in the CCD,[105,139] the density of SK channels in the CNT is not increased by high dietary K⁺ loading; again, this is consistent with progressive, axial recruitment of transport capacity for Na⁺ and K⁺ along the distal nephron.

Urinary Indices of Potassium Excretion

A bedside test to directly measure distal tubular K⁺ excretion in humans would be ideal, however for obvious reasons this not technically feasible. A widely used surrogate is the "transtubular K⁺ gradient" (TTKG), which is defined as follows:

$$TTKG = \frac{[K^+]_{urine} \times Osm_{blood}}{[K^+]_{blood} \times Osm_{urine}}$$

The expected values of the TTKG are largely based on historical data, and are <3 in the presence of hypokalemia and >7 to 8 in the presence of hyperkalemia.[155] Clearly water absorption in the CCD and medullary collecting duct is an important determinant of the absolute K⁺ concentration in the final urine, hence the use of a ratio of urine:plasma osmolality. Indeed, water absorption may in large part determine the TTKG, such that it far exceeds the limiting K⁺ gradient.[156] The TTKG may be less useful in patients ingesting diets of changing K⁺ and mineralocorticoid intake.[157] There is however a linear relationship between serum aldosterone and the TTKG, suggesting that it provides a rough approximation of the ability to respond to aldosterone with a kaliuresis.[158] Moreover, the determination of urinary electrolytes provides measurement of urinary Na⁺, which will determine whether significant pre-renal stimuli are limiting distal Na⁺ delivery and thus K⁺ excretion (see also Fig. 15–4). Urinary electrolytes also afford the opportunity to calculate the urinary anion gap, an indirect index of urinary NH₄⁺ content and thus the ability to respond to an acidemia.[159] Restraint is always advised, however, to avoid excessive flights of fancy in the physiological interpretation of urinary electrolytes.

Regulation of Renal Renin and Adrenal Aldosterone

Modulation of the renin-angiotensin-aldosterone (RAS) axis has profound clinical effects on K⁺ homeostasis. Although multiple tissues are capable of renin secretion, renin of renal origin has a dominant physiological impact. Renin secretion by juxtaglomerular cells within the afferent arteriole is initiated in response to a signal from the macula densa,[160] specifically a decrease in luminal chloride[161] transported through the Na⁺-K⁺-2Cl⁻ cotransporter (NKCC2) at the apical membrane of macula densa cells.[21] In addition to this macula densa signal, decreased renal perfusion pressure and renal sympathetic tone stimulate renal renin secretion.[16] The various inhibitors of renin release include angiotensin II, endothelin,[162] adenosine,[163] ANP,[164,165] TNF-α,[166] and vitamin D.[167] The cGMP-dependent protein kinase type II (cGKII) tonically inhibits renin secretion, in that renin secretion in response to several stimuli is exaggerated in homozygous cGKII knockout mice.[168] Activation of cGKII by atrial natriuretic peptide (ANP) or nitric oxide (or both) has a marked inhibitory effect on the release of renin from juxtaglomerular cells.[164,165] Local factors that stimulate renin release from juxtaglomerular cells include prostaglandins,[169] adrenomedullin,[170] and catecholamines (β-1 receptors).[171]

The relationship between renal renin release, the RAS, and cycloogenase-2 (COX-2) is particularly complex.[172] COX-2 is heavily expressed in the macula densa,[173] with a significant recruitment of COX-2⁽⁺⁾ cells seen with salt restriction or furosemide treatment.[16,173] Reduced intracellular chloride in macula densa cells appears to stimulate COX-2 expression via p38 MAP kinase,[174] whereas both aldosterone and angiotensin II (ATII) reduce its expression.[172] Prostaglandins derived from COX-2 in the macula densa play a dominant role in the stimulation of renal renin release by salt restriction, furosemide, renal artery occlusion, or angiotensin converting enzyme (ACE) inhibition.[16,175]

Renin released from the kidney ultimately stimulates aldosterone release from the adrenal via angiotensin II. Hyperkalemia per se is also an independent and synergistic stimulus (Fig. 15–6) for aldosterone release from the adrenal gland,[16,176] although dietary K⁺ loading is less potent than dietary Na⁺-Cl⁻ restriction in increasing circulating aldosterone.[103] ATII and K⁺ both activate Ca²⁺ entry in adrenal glomerulosa cells, via voltage-sensitive T-type Ca²⁺ channels.[16,177] Elevations in extracellular K⁺ thus depolarize glomerulosa cells and activate these Ca²⁺ channels, which are independently and synergistically activated by ATII.[177] The physiological importance of the K⁺-dependent stimulation of adrenal aldosterone release is vividly illustrated by the phenotype of mice with a targeted deletion of the KCNE1 K⁺ channel subunit. These mice have an exaggerated adrenal release of aldosterone when placed on a high K⁺ diet.[178] The KCNE1 gene is expressed in adrenal glomerulosa cells, where it

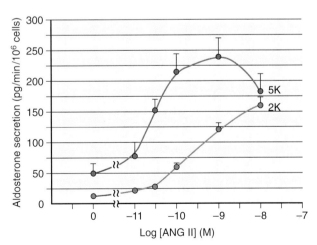

FIGURE 15–6 Synergistic effect of increased extracellular K⁺ and angiotensin II (ANGII) in inducing aldosterone release from bovine adrenal glomerulosa cells. Dose response curves for ANGII were performed at extracellular K⁺ of 2 mmol/l (○) and 5 mmol/l (●). (From Chen XL, Bayliss DA, Fern RJ, Barrett PQ: A role for T-type Ca²⁺ channels in the synergistic control of aldosterone production by ANG II and K⁺. Am J Physiol 276:F674–683, 1999.)

presumably affects the electrophysiological response to increased extracellular K^+.[178]

The adrenal release of aldosterone due to increased K^+ is dependent on an intact *adrenal* renin-angiotensin system,[179] particularly during Na^+ restriction. ACE inhibitors and angiotensin-receptor blockers (ARBs) thus completely abrogate the effect of high K^+ on salt-restricted adrenals.[180] Other clinically relevant activators of adrenal aldosterone release include prostaglandins[181] and catecholamines,[182] via increases in cyclic-AMP.[183,184] Finally, ANP exerts a potent negative effect on aldosterone release induced by K^+ and other stimuli,[185] at least in part by inhibiting early events in aldosterone synthesis.[186] ANP is therefore capable of inhibiting both renal renin release and adrenal aldosterone release, functions that may be central to the pathophysiology of hyporeninemic hypoaldosteronism.

CONSEQUENCES OF HYPOKALEMIA AND HYPERKALEMIA

Consequences of Hypokalemia

Excitable Tissues: Muscle and Heart

Hypokalemia is a well-described risk factor for both ventricular and atrial arrhythmias.[187–189] For example, in patients undergoing cardiac surgery, a serum K^+ of <3.5 mmol/L is a predictor of serious intra-operative arrhythmia, perioperative arrhythmia, and post-operative atrial fibrillation.[190] Moderate hypokalemia does not, however, appear to increase the risk of serious arrhythmia during exercise stress testing.[191] Electrocardiographic changes in hypokalemia include broad flat T waves, ST depression, and QT prolongation; these are most marked when serum K^+ is <2.7 mmol/L.[192,193] Hypokalemia, often accompanied by hypomagnesemia, is an important cause of the long QT syndrome (LQTS), either alone or in combination with drug toxicity[194] or with LQTS-associated mutations in cardiac K^+ and Na^+ channels.[195,196]

In muscle, hypokalemia causes hyperpolarization, thus impairing the capacity to depolarize and contract. Weakness and paralysis is therefore a not-infrequent consequence of hypokalemia of diverse etiologies.[197,198] On an historical note, the realization in 1946 that K^+ replacement reversed the hypokalemic diaphragmatic paralysis induced by management of diabetic ketoacidosis was a milestone in diabetes care.[199] Pathologically, muscle biopsies in hypokalemic myopathy demonstrate phagocytosis of degenerating muscle fibers, fiber regeneration, and atrophy of type 2 fibers.[200] Most patients with significant myopathy will have elevations in creatine kinase, and hypokalemia of diverse etiologies predisposes to rhabdomyolysis with acute renal failure.

Renal Consequences

Hypokalemia causes a host of structural and functional changes in the kidney, which are reviewed in detail elsewhere.[201] In humans, the renal pathology includes a relatively specific proximal tubular vacuolization,[201,202] interstitial nephritis,[203] and renal cysts.[204] Hypokalemic nephropathy can cause end-stage renal disease, mostly in patients with long-standing hypokalemia due to eating disorders and/or laxative abuse[205]; acute renal failure with proximal tubular vasculopathy has also been described.[206] In animal models, hypokalemia increases susceptibility to acute renal failure induced by ischemia, gentamicin, and amphotericin.[16] Potassium restriction in rats induces cortical ATII and medullary endothelin-1 expression, with an ischemic pattern of renal injury.[207] Morphological changes in this model are prevented by blockade of endothelin[208] and ATII type 1 (AT_1)[209] receptors.

The prominent functional changes in renal physiology that are induced by hypokalemia include Na^+-Cl^- retention, polyuria,[202] phosphaturia,[210] hypocitraturia,[211] and increased ammoniagenesis.[201] K^+ depletion in rats causes proximal tubular hyper-absorption of Na^+-Cl^-, in association with an up-regulation of ATII,[207] AT_1 receptor,[212] and the α_2-adrenergic receptor[213] in this nephron segment. NHE3, the dominant apical Na^+ entry site in the proximal tubule, is massively (>700%) up-regulated in K^+-deficient rats,[214] which is consistent with the observed hyper-absorption of both Na^+-Cl^- and bicarbonate.[201] Polyuria in hypokalemia is due to polydipsia[215] and to a vasopressin-resistant defect in urinary concentrating ability.[201] This renal concentrating defect is multifactorial, with evidence for both a reduced hydro-osmotic response to vasopressin in the collecting duct[201] and decreased Na^+-Cl^- absorption by the TAL.[216] K^+ restriction has been shown to result in a rapid, reversible decrease in the expression of aquaporin-2 in the collecting duct,[217] beginning in the CCD and extending to the medullary collecting duct within the first 24 hours.[218] In the TAL, the marked reductions seen during K^+ restriction in both the apical K^+ channel ROMK and the apical Na^+-K^+-$2Cl^-$ cotransporter NKCC2[140,214] reduce Na^+-Cl^- absorption, and thus inhibit countercurrent multiplication and the driving force for water absorption by the collecting duct.

Cardiovascular Consequences

A large body of experimental and epidemiological evidence implicates hypokalemia or reduced dietary K^+ (or both) in the genesis or worsening of hypertension, heart failure, and stroke.[219] K^+ depletion in young rats induces hypertension,[220] with a salt sensitivity that persists after K^+ levels are normalized; presumably this salt sensitivity is due to the significant tubulointerstitial injury induced by K^+ restriction.[207] Short-term K^+ restriction in healthy humans and patients with essential hypertension also induces Na^+-Cl^- retention and hypertension,[221–223] and abundant epidemiological data links dietary K^+ deficiency or hypokalemia with hypertension or both.[189,219] Correction of hypokalemia is particularly important in hypertensive patients treated with diuretics; blood pressure in this setting is improved with the establishment of normokalemia,[224] and the cardiovascular benefits of diuretic agents are blunted by hypokalemia.[225,226] Finally, K^+ depletion may play important roles in the pathophysiology and progression of heart failure.[219]

Consequences of Hyperkalemia

Excitable Tissues: Muscle and Heart

Hyperkalemia constitutes a medical emergency, primarily due to its effect on the heart. Mild increases in extracellular K^+ affect the repolarization phase of the cardiac action potential, resulting in changes in T wave morphology or direction.[227] Mild to moderate hyperkalemia depresses intracardiac conduction, with progressive prolongation of the PR and QRS intervals.[228] Severe hyperkalemia results in loss of the P wave and a progressive widening of the QRS complex; fusion with T waves causes a "sine-wave" sinoventricular rhythm. Cardiac arrhythmias associated with hyperkalemia include sinus bradycardia, sinus arrest, slow idioventricular rhythms, ventricular tachycardia, ventricular fibrillation, and asystole.[227,229] The differential diagnosis and treatment of a wide-complex tachycardia in hyperkalemia can be particularly problematic; moreover, hyperkalemia potentiates the blocking effect of lidocaine on the cardiac Na^+ channel, such that use of this agent may precipitate asystole or ventricular fibrillation in this setting.[230] Classically, the electrocardiographic manifestations in hyperkalemia progress as shown in Table 15–3. However, these changes are notoriously insensitive, such that only 55% of patients with serum $K^+ > 6.8$ mmol/L in one case series manifested peaked T waves.[231] Hemodialysis patients[232] and patients with chronic renal failure[233] in par-

TABLE 15–3 The Approximate Relationship between Hyperkalemic Electrocardiographic Changes and Serum K⁺

Serum K⁺	ECG Abnormality
Mild hyperkalemia 5.5–6.5 mmol/L	Tall peaked T waves with narrow base, best seen in precordial leads
Moderate hyperkalemia 6.5–8.0 mmol/L	Peaked T waves; Prolonged PR interval; Decreased amplitude of P waves; Widening of QRS complex
Moderate hyperkalemia >8.0 mmol/L	Absence of P wave; Intraventricular blocks, fascicular blocks, bundle branch blocks, QRS axis shift; Progressive widening of the QRS complex; "Sine-wave" pattern (sinoventricular rhythm), ventricular fibrillation, asystole

From Mattu A, Brady WJ, Robinson DA: Electrocardiographic changes and hyperkalemia. Am J Emerg Med 18:721–729, 2000.

ticular may not demonstrate electrocardiographic changes, perhaps due to concomitant abnormalities in serum Ca²⁺. Care should also be taken to adequately distinguish the symmetrically peaked, "church steeple", T waves induced by hyperkalemia from T wave changes due to other causes.[234]

Hyperkalemia can also rarely present with ascending paralysis,[16] denoted "secondary hyperkalemic paralysis" to differentiate it from familial hyperkalemic periodic paralysis (HYPP). This presentation of hyperkalemia can mimic Guillain-Barré syndrome, and may include diaphragmatic paralysis and respiratory failure.[235] Hyperkalemia from a diversity of causes can cause paralysis, as reviewed by Evers and colleagues.[236] The mechanism is not entirely clear; however, nerve conduction studies in one case suggest a neurogenic mechanism, rather than a direct effect on muscle excitability.[236]

In contrast to secondary hyperkalemic paralysis, HYPP is a primary myopathy. Patients with HYPP develop myopathic weakness during hyperkalemia induced by increased K⁺ intake or rest after heavy exercise.[237] The hyperkalemic trigger in HYPP serves to differentiate this syndrome from hypokalemic periodic paralysis (HOKP); a further distinguishing feature is the presence of myotonia in HYPP.[237] Depolarization of skeletal muscle by hyperkalemia unmasks an inactivation defect in a tetrodotoxin-sensitive Na⁺ channel in patients with HYPP, and autosomal dominant mutations in the SCN4A gene encoding this channel cause most forms of the disease.[238] Mild muscle depolarization (5–10 mV) in HYPP results in a persistent inward Na⁺ current through the mutant channel; the normal, allelic SCN4 channels quickly recover from inactivation and can then be re-activated, resulting in myotonia. When muscle depolarization is more marked (i.e., 20–30 mV) all of the Na⁺ channels are inactivated, rendering the muscle inexcitable and causing weakness (Fig. 15–7). Related disorders due to mutations within the large SCN4A channel protein include HOKP type II,[239] paramyotonia congenita,[238] and K⁺-aggravated myopathy.[238] American thoroughbred quarter horses have a high incidence (4.4%) of HYPP, due to a mutation in equine SCN4A traced to the sire "Impressive" (see Fig. 15–7).[238] Finally, loss-of-function mutations in the muscle-specific K⁺ channel subunit "MinK-related peptide 2" (MiRP2) have also been shown to cause HYPP; MiRP2 and the associated Kv3.4 K⁺ channel play a role in setting the resting membrane potential of skeletal muscle.[240]

Renal Consequences

Hyperkalemia has a significant effect on the ability to excrete an acid urine, due to interference with the urinary excretion

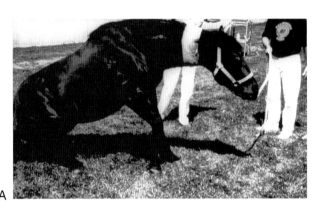

A

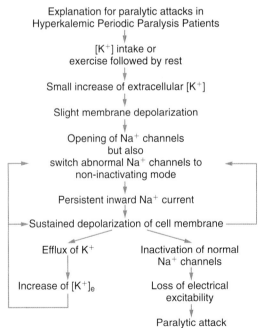

Explanation for paralytic attacks in Hyperkalemic Periodic Paralysis Patients

[K⁺] intake or exercise followed by rest → Small increase of extracellular [K⁺] → Slight membrane depolarization → Opening of Na⁺ channels but also switch abnormal Na⁺ channels to non-inactivating mode → Persistent inward Na⁺ current → Sustained depolarization of cell membrane → Efflux of K⁺ → Increase of [K⁺]ₑ; Inactivation of normal Na⁺ channels → Loss of electrical excitability → Paralytic attack

B

FIGURE 15–7 Hyperkalemic periodic paralysis (HYPP) due to mutations in the voltage-gated Na⁺ channel of skeletal muscle. **A,** This disorder is particularly common in thoroughbred quarter horses; an affected horse is shown during a paralytic attack, triggered by rest after heavy exercise (picture courtesy of Dr. Eric Hoffman). **B,** Mechanistic explanation for muscle paralysis in HYPP. (From Lehmann-Horn F, Jurkat-Rott K: Voltage-gated ion channels and hereditary disease. Physiol Rev 79:1317–1372, 1999.)

of ammonium (NH_4^+). Whereas *hypokalemia* increases NH3 production by the proximal tubule, hyperkalemia does not affect proximal tubular ammoniagenesis; urinary excretion of NH_4^+ is however reduced.[241] The TAL absorbs NH_4^+ from the tubular lumen, followed by countercurrent multiplication and ultimately excretion from the medullary interstitium.[242] The NH_4^+ ion has the same ionic radius as K^+, and can be transported in lieu of K^+ by NKCC2,[243] the apical Na^+-K^+/NH_4^+-$2Cl^-$ cotransporter of the TAL, in addition to a number of other pathways. As is the case for other cations, countercurrent multiplication of NH_4^+ by the TAL greatly increases the concentration of NH_4^+/NH_3 available for secretion in the collecting duct. The NH_4^+ produced by the proximal tubule in response to acidosis is thus reabsorbed across the TAL, concentrated by countercurrent multiplication in the medullary interstitium, and secreted in the collecting duct. The capacity of the TAL to reabsorb NH_4^+ is increased during acidosis, due to induction of NKCC2 expression.[243] Hyperkalemia in turn appears to inhibit renal acid excretion by competing with NH_4^+ for reabsorption by the TAL[244]; this may be a major factor in the acidosis associated with various defects in K^+ excretion.[245]

CAUSES OF HYPOKALEMIA

Epidemiology

Hypokalemia is a relatively common finding in both outpatients and inpatients, perhaps the most common electrolyte abnormality encountered in clinical practice.[246] When defined as a serum K^+ of less than 3.6 mmol/L, it is found in up to 20% of hospitalized patients.[247] Hypokalemia is usually mild, with K^+ levels in the 3.0 to 3.5 mmol/L range, but in up to 25% it can be moderate to severe (<3.0 mmol/L).[247,248] It is a particularly prominent problem in patients receiving thiazide diuretics for hypertension, with an incidence of up to 48% (average 15%–30%).[224,249,250] The thiazide-type diuretic metolazone is frequently utilized in the management of heart failure refractory to loop diuretics alone, causing moderate ($K^+ \leq 3.0$ mmol/L) or severe ($K^+ \leq 2.5$ mmol/L) hypokalemia in approximately 40% and 10% of patients, respectively.[251] Hypokalemia is also a common finding in patients receiving peritoneal dialysis, with 10% to 20% requiring potassium supplementation.[252] Hypokalemia *per se* can increase in-hospital mortality rate up to 10-fold,[248] likely due to the profound effects on arrhythmogenesis, blood pressure, and cardiovascular morbidity.[219,253]

Spurious Hypokalemia

Delayed sample analysis is a well-recognized cause of spurious hypokalemia, due to increased cellular uptake; this may become clinically relevant if ambient temperature is increased.[254–256] Very rarely, patients with profound leukocytosis due to acute leukemia present with artifactual hypokalemia caused by time-dependent uptake of K^+ by the large white cell mass.[254] Such patients do not develop clinical or electrocardiographic complications of hypokalemia, and serum K^+ is normal if measured immediately after venipuncture.

Redistribution and Hypokalemia

Manipulation of the factors affecting internal distribution of K^+ (see discussion of factors affecting internal distribution of potassium) can cause hypokalemia, due to redistribution of K^+ between the extracellular and intracellular compartments. Endogenous insulin is rarely a cause of hypokalemia;

however, administered insulin is a frequent cause of iatrogenic hypokalemia,[247] and may be a factor in the "dead in bed syndrome" associated with aggressive glycemic control.[257] Alterations in the activity of the endogenous sympathetic nervous system can cause hypokalemia in several settings, including alcohol withdrawal,[258] acute myocardial infarction,[219,259] and head injury.[260,261] Redistributive hypokalemia after severe head injury can be truly profound, with reported serum K^+ of 1.2[260] and 1.9,[261] and marked rebound hyperkalemia after repletion. Due to their ability to activate both Na^+/K^+-ATPase[47] and the Na^+-K^+-$2Cl^-$ cotransporter NKCC1,[16,49] β_2 agonists are powerful activators of cellular K^+ uptake. These agents are chiefly encountered in the therapy of asthma; however, tocolytics such as ritodrine can induce hypokalemia and arrhythmias during maternal labor.[262] Occult sources of sympathomimetics, such as pseudoephedrine and ephedrine in cough syrup[198] or dieting agents, are an overlooked cause of hypokalemia. Finally, downstream activation of cyclic-AMP by xanthines such as theophylline[16,263] and dietary caffeine[264] may induce hypokalemia, and may synergize in this respect with β_2 agonists.[265]

Whereas β_2 agonists activate K^+ uptake via the Na^+/K^+-ATPase, one would expect that inhibition of passive K^+ efflux would also lead to hypokalemia; this is accomplished by barium, a potent inhibitor of K^+ channels. This rare cause of hypokalemia is usually due to ingestion of the rodenticide barium carbonate, either unintentionally or during a suicide attempt.[266] Suicidal ingestion of barium-containing shaving powder[267] and hair remover[268] has also been described. Treatment of barium poisoning with K^+ likely serves to both increase serum K^+ and to displace barium from affected K^+ channels[266]; hemodialysis is also an effective treatment.[269] Barium salts are widely used in industry, and poisoning has been described by various mechanisms in industrial accidents.[16,270] Hypokalemia is also common with chloroquine toxicity or overdose,[271] although the mechanism is not entirely clear.

Hypokalemic Periodic Paralysis

The periodic paralyses have both genetic and acquired causes, and are further subdivided into hyperkalemic and hypokalemic forms.[16,237,238,266] The genetic and secondary forms of hyperkalemic paralysis are discussed earlier (see discussion on consequences of hyperkalemia). Autosomal dominant mutations in the *CACNA1S* gene encoding the α1 subunit of L-type calcium channels are the most common genetic cause of hypokalemic periodic paralysis (HOKP type I), whereas type II HOKP is due to mutations in the *SCN4A* gene encoding the skeletal Na^+ channel.[239] In Andersen syndrome, autosomal dominant mutations in the *KCNJ2* gene encoding the inwardly rectifying K^+ channel Kir2.1 cause periodic paralysis, cardiac arrhythmias, and dysmorphic features.[272] Paralysis in Andersen syndrome can be normokalemic, hypokalemic, or hyperkalemic; however, the symptomatic trigger is consistent within individual kindreds.[272]

The pathophysiology of HOKP is not entirely clear. Reversible attacks of paralysis with hypokalemia are typically precipitated by rest after exercise and meals rich in carbohydrate.[266] Although the induction of endogenous insulin by carbohydrate meals is thought to reduce serum K^+, insulin can precipitate paralysis in HOKP in the absence of significant hypokalemia.[273] The generation of action potentials and muscle contraction are reduced in type I and II HOKP muscle fibers exposed to insulin in vitro[239,274]; this effect is seen at an extracellular K^+ of 4.0 mmol/L and is potentiated as K^+ decreases.[274] Mutations in type I HOKP have relatively modest effects on L-type calcium channel activity, and type I HOKP may in fact be an "indirect channelopathy" wherein subtle changes in intracellular Ca^{2+} signaling exert downstream effects on the expression or function of other ion channels. Consistent with this hypothesis, type I HOKP muscles have a reduced activity of ATP-sensitive, inward rectifying K^+ channels (K_{ATP}),[275] which likely contributes to hypokalemia due to the resultant unopposed activity of muscle Na^+/K^+-ATPase.[276] Insulin inhibits the remaining K_{ATP} activity in muscle fibers of both type I HOKP patients 274 and hypokalemic rats,[277] resulting in a depolarizing shift towards the equilibrium potential for the Cl^- ion (approximately 50 mV); at this potential, voltage-dependent Na^+ channels are largely inactivated, resulting in paralysis.

Paralysis is associated with multiple other causes of hypokalemia, both acquired and genetic.[197,198,266,278] Renal causes of hypokalemia with paralysis include Fanconi syndrome,[279] Gitelman syndrome,[197,278] and the various causes of hypokalemic distal renal tubular acidosis.[266,280,281] The activity and regulation of skeletal muscle K_{ATP} channels is aberrant in animal models of hypokalemia, suggesting a parallel muscle physiology to that of genetic HOKP (see earlier discussion). However, the pathophysiology of thyrotoxic periodic paralysis (TPP), a particularly important cause of hypokalemic paralysis, is distinctly different from that of HOKP; for example, despite the clinical similarities between the two syndromes, thyroxine has no effect on HOKP.

Thyrotoxic periodic paralysis is classically seen in patients of Asian origin, but also occurs at higher frequencies in Hispanic patients.[282] Patients typically present with weakness of the extremities and limb girdles, with attacks occurring most frequently between 1 AM and 6 AM. As in HOKP, attacks may be precipitated by rest, and almost never occur during vigorous activity. Again, carbohydrate-rich meals may also provoke an episode of TPP. Clinical signs and symptoms of hyperthyroidism are not invariably present.[282,283] Hypokalemia is profound, ranging between 1.1 and 3.4 mol/L, and is frequently accompanied by hypophosphatemia and hypomagnesemia[282]; all three abnormalities presumably contribute to the associated weakness. The hypokalemia in TPP is most likely due to both direct and indirect activation of the Na^+/K^+-ATPase, given the evidence for increased activity in erythrocytes and platelets in TPP patients.[284,285] Thyroid hormone clearly induces expression of multiple subunits of the Na^+/K^+-ATPase in skeletal muscle.[286] Increases in β-adrenergic response due to hyperthyroidism also play an important role because high-dose propranolol (3 mg/kg) rapidly reverses the hypokalemia, hypophosphatemia, and paralysis seen in acute attacks.[287,288] Of particular importance, no rebound hyperkalemia is associated with this treatment, whereas aggressive K^+ replacement in TPP is associated with an incidence of ~25%.[289]

Non-renal Potassium Loss

The loss of K^+ from skin is typically low, with the exception of extremes in physical exertion.[5] Direct gastric loss of K^+ due to vomiting or nasogastric suctioning is also typically minimal, however the ensuing hypochloremic alkalosis results in persistent kaliuresis due to secondary hyperaldosteronism and bicarbonaturia.[290,291] Intestinal loss of K^+ due to diarrhea is a quantitatively important cause of hypokalemia, given the worldwide prevalence of diarrheal disease, and may be associated with acute complications such as myopathy and flaccid paralysis.[292] The presence of a non-anion gap metabolic acidosis with a negative urinary anion gap[159] (consistent with an intact ability to increase NH_4^+ excretion) should strongly suggest diarrhea as a cause of hypokalemia. Non-infectious gastrointestinal processes such as celiac disease,[293] ileostomy,[294] and chronic laxative abuse can present with acute hypokalemic syndromes or with chronic complications such as end-stage renal disease.[16]

Renal Potassium Loss

Drugs

Diuretics are an especially important cause of hypokalemia, due to their ability to increase distal flow rate and distal delivery of Na^+ (see discussion on potassium secretion in the distal nephron). Thiazides generally cause more hypokalemia[16,295] than do loop diuretics, despite their lower natriuretic efficacy. One potential explanation is the differential effect of loop diuretics and thiazides on calcium excretion. Whereas thiazides and loss-of-function mutations in the Na^+-Cl^- cotransporter decrease Ca^{2+} excretion,[296] loop diuretics cause a significant calciuresis.[297] Increases in luminal Ca^{2+} in the distal nephron serve to reduce the lumen-negative driving force for K^+ excretion,[298] perhaps by direct inhibition of ENaC in principal cells. A mechanistic explanation is provided by the presence of apical calcium-sensing receptor (CaSR) in the collecting duct[299]; analogous to the evident decrease in the apical trafficking of aquaporin-2 induced by luminal Ca^{2+}, tubular Ca^{2+} may stimulate endocytosis of ENaC via the CaSR and thus limit generation of the lumen-negative potential difference that is so critical for distal K^+ excretion. Regardless of the underlying mechanism, the increase in distal delivery of Ca^{2+} induced by loop diuretics may serve to blunt kaliuresis; such a mechanism would not occur with thiazides, which reduce distal delivery of Ca^{2+}, with unopposed activity of ENaC and increased kaliuresis.

Other drugs associated with hypokalemia due to kaliuresis include high doses of penicillin-related antibiotics, thought to increase obligatory K^+ excretion by acting as non-reabsorbable anions in the distal nephron; in addition to penicillin, implicated antibiotics include nafcillin, dicloxacillin, ticarcillin, oxacillin, and carbenicillin.[300] Increased distal delivery of other anions such as SO_4^{2-} and HCO_3^- also induces a kaliuresis. The usual explanation is that K^+ excretion increases so as to balance the negative charge of these non-reabsorbable anions. However, increased delivery of such anions will also increase the electrochemical gradient for K^+-Cl^- exit via apical K^+-Cl^- cotransport or parallel K^+-H^+ and Cl^--HCO_3^- exchange[22,68,82] (see also discussion on potassium secretion in the distal nephron).

Several tubular toxins result in both K^+ and magnesium wasting. These include gentamicin, which can cause tubular toxicity with hypokalemia that can masquerade as Bartter syndrome (BS).[301] Other drugs that can caused mixed magnesium and K^+ wasting include amphotericin, foscarnet,[302] cisplatin,[16,303] and ifosfamide.[304] Aggressive replacement of magnesium is obligatory in the management of combined hypokalemia and hypomagnesemia; successful K^+ replacement depends on management of the hypomagnesemia.

Hyperaldosteronism

Increases in circulating aldosterone (hyperaldosteronism) may be primary or secondary. Increased levels of circulating renin in secondary forms of hyperaldosteronism leads to increased ATII and thus aldosterone, and can be associated with hypokalemia; causes include renal artery stenosis,[305] Page kidney (renal compression by a subcapsular mass or hematoma, with hyperreninemia),[306] a paraneoplastic process,[307] or renin-secreting renal tumors.[308] The incidence of hypokalemia in renal artery stenosis is thought to be <20%.[305] An unusual but under-appreciated presentation of renal artery stenosis and renal ischemia is the "hyponatremic hypertensive syndrome", in which concurrent hypokalemia may be profound.[309]

Primary hyperaldosteronism may be genetic or acquired. Hypertension and hypokalemia, generally attributed to increases in circulating 11-deoxycorticosterone,[310] are seen in patients with congenital adrenal hyperplasia due to defects in either steroid 11β-hydroxylase[310] or steroid 17α-hydroxylase[311]; deficient 11β-hydroxylase results in virilization and other signs of androgen excess,[310] whereas reduced sex steroids in 17α-hydroxylase deficiency result in hypogonadism.[311] The two major forms of isolated primary hyperaldosteronism are denoted familial hyperaldosteronism type I (FHI, also known as glucocorticoid-remediable hyperaldosteronism or GRA)[312] and familial hyperaldosteronism type II (FHII), in which aldosterone production is not repressible by exogenous glucocorticoids. Patients with FHII are clinically indistinguishable from sporadic forms of primary hyperaldosteronism due to bilateral adrenal hyperplasia; a gene has been localized to chromosome 7p22 by linkage analysis, but has yet to be characterized.[313]

Patients with FHI/GRA are generally hypertensive, typically presenting at an early age; the severity of hypertension is however variable, such that some affected individuals are normotensive.[312] Aldosterone levels are modestly elevated and regulated solely by ACTH. The diagnosis is confirmed by dexamethasone suppression test, with suppression of aldosterone to <4 ng/dL consistent with the diagnosis.[314] Patients also have high levels of abnormal "hybrid" 18-hydroxylated steroids, generated by transformation of steroids typically formed in the zona fasciculata by aldosterone synthase, an enzyme that is normally expressed in the zona glomerulosa.[315,316] FHI has been shown to be caused by a chimeric gene duplication between the homologous 11β-hydroxylase (CYP11B1) and aldosterone synthase (CYP11B2) genes, fusing the ACTH-responsive 11β-hydroxylase promoter to the coding region of aldosterone synthase; this chimeric gene is thus under the control of ACTH and expressed in a glucocorticoid-repressible fashion.[315] Ectopic expression of the hybrid CYP11B1- CYP11B1 gene in the zona fasciculata has been reported in a single case where adrenal tissue became available for molecular analysis.[317]

Although the initial patients reported with FHI were hypokalemic, the majority are in fact normokalemic,[316,318] albeit perhaps with a propensity to develop hypokalemia while on thiazide diuretics.[316] Patients with FHI are able to appropriately increase K+ excretion in response to K+ loading or fludrocortisone, but fail to increase serum aldosterone in response to hyperkalemia.[319] This may reflect the ectopic expression of the chimeric aldosterone synthase in the adrenal fasciculata, which likely lack the appropriate constellation of ion channels to respond to increases in extracellular K+ with an increase in aldosterone secretion.

Acquired causes of primary hyperaldosteronism include aldosterone-producing adenomas (APA), primary or unilateral adrenal hyperplasia (PAH), idiopathic hyperaldosteronism (IHA) due to bilateral adrenal hyperplasia, and adrenal carcinoma; APA and IHA account for close to 60% and 40%, respectively, of diagnosed hyperaldosteronism.[320,321] A rare case involving paraneoplastic over-expression of aldosterone synthase in lymphoma has also been described.[322] Because surgery can be curative in APA, adequate differentiation of APA from IHA is critical; this may require both adrenal imaging and adrenal venous sampling (Fig. 15–8). Contemporary reports have emphasized the continued importance of adrenal vein sampling in subtype differentiation.[323,324]

Increasing utilization of the plasma aldosterone (PAC)/plasma renin activity (PRA) ratio in hypertension clinics has led to reports of a much higher incidence of primary hyperaldosteronism than previously appreciated, with incidence rates in hypertension ranging from zero to 72%[325]; however, the prevalence was 3.2% in a large, multicenter study of

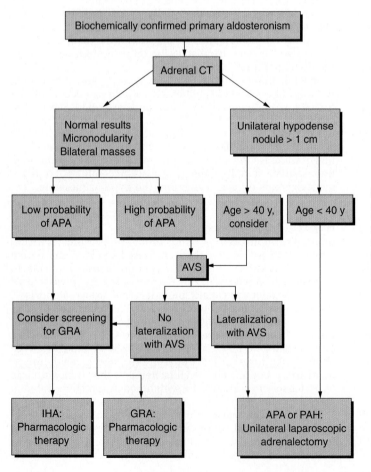

FIGURE 15–8 Diagnostic algorithm in patients with primary hyperaldosteronism. Adrenal adenoma (APA) must be distinguished from glucocorticoid remediable hyperaldosteronism (FHI or GRA), primary or unilateral adrenal hyperplasia (PAH), and idiopathic hyperaldosteronism (IHA). This requires computed axial tomography (CT), adrenal venous sampling (AVS), and the relevant diagnostic biochemical and hormonal assays (see text). (From Young WF, Jr: Adrenalectomy for primary aldosteronism. Ann Intern Med 138(2):157–159, 2003.)

patients with mild to moderate hypertension without hypokalemia.[326] The true incidence of hypokalemia in patients with acquired forms of primary hyperaldosteronism remains difficult to evaluate, due to a variety of factors. First, historically, patients have only been screened for hyperaldosteronism when hypokalemia is present, hence even recent case series from clinics with such a referral pattern may suffer from a selection bias; other recent series have concentrated on hypertensive patients, also a selection bias. Second, the incidence of hypokalemia is higher in adrenal adenomas than in IHA, likely due to higher average levels of aldosterone.[321] Third, because increased kaliuresis in hyperaldosteronism can be induced by dietary Na^+-Cl^- loading or diuretics, dietary factors or medications (or both) may play a role in the incidence of hypokalemia at presentation. Regardless, it is clear that hypokalemia is not a universal feature of primary hyperaldosteronism; this is perhaps not unexpected because aldosterone does not appear to affect the hypokalemic response of H^+/K^+-ATPase,[327] the major reabsorptive pathway for K^+ in the distal nephron (see discussion on K^+ reabsorption in the distal nephron). A related issue is whether primary hyperaldosteronism is under-diagnosed when hypokalemia is used as a criterion for further investigation; the utility of the PAC/PRA ratio in screening for hyperaldosteronism is an active and controversial issue in hypertension research.[325,326]

Finally, hypokalemia may also occur with systemic increases in glucocorticoids.[328,329] In *bona fide* Cushing syndrome caused by increases in pituitary ACTH the incidence of hypokalemia is only 10%,[328] whereas it is 57%[329] to 100%[328] in patients with ectopic ACTH, despite a similar incidence of hypertension. Indirect evidence suggests that the activity of renal 11β-hydroxysteroid dehydrogenase-2 (11βHSD-2) is reduced in patients with ectopic ACTH compared with Cushing syndrome,[330] resulting in a syndrome of apparent mineralocorticoid excess (see later discussion). Whether this reflects a greater degree of saturation of the enzyme by circulating cortisol or direct inhibition of 11βHSD-2 by ACTH is not entirely clear, and there is evidence for both mechanisms[329]; however, indirect indices of 11βHSD-2 activity in patients with ectopic ACTH expression correlate with hypokalemia and other measures of mineralocorticoid activity.[331] Similar mechanisms likely underlie the severe hypokalemia reported in patients with familial glucocorticoid resistance, in which loss-of-function mutations in the glucocorticoid receptor result in marked hypercortisolism without Cushingoid features, accompanied by very high ACTH levels.[332]

Syndromes of Apparent Mineralocorticoid Excess

The syndromes of "apparent mineralocorticoid excess" (AME) have a self-explanatory label. In the classic form of AME, recessive loss-of-function mutations in the 11β-hydroxysteroid dehydrogenase-2 (*11βHSD-2*) gene cause a defect in the peripheral conversion of cortisol to the inactive glucocorticoid cortisone; the resulting increase in the half-life of cortisol is associated with a marked decrease in synthesis, such that plasma levels of cortisol are normal and patients are not Cushingoid.[333] The 11βHSD-2 protein is expressed in epithelial cells that are targets for aldosterone; in the kidney, these include cells of the distal convoluted tubule (DCT), connecting segment (CNT), and CCD.[334] Because the mineralocorticoid receptor (MR) has equivalent affinity for aldosterone and cortisol, generation of cortisone by 11βHSD-2 serves to protect mineralocorticoid-responsive cells from illicit activation by cortisol.[335] In patients with AME, the unregulated mineralocorticoid effect of glucocorticoids results in hypertension, hypokalemia, and metabolic alkalosis, with suppressed PRA and aldosterone.[333] Biochemical studies of mutant enzymes usually indicate a complete loss of function; lesser enzymatic defects in patients with AME are associated with altered

ratios of urinary cortisone/cortisol metabolites,[336] lesser impairment in the peripheral conversion of cortisol to cortisone,[337] and/or older age at presentation.[338]

Mice with a homozygous targeted deletion of *11βHSD-2* exhibit hypertension, hypokalemia, and polyuria; the polyuria is likely secondary to the hypokalemia (see discussion on renal consequences of hypokalemia), which reaches 2.4 mmol/ml in *11βHSD-2*–null mice.[339] As expected, both PRA and plasma aldosterone in the *11βHSD-2*-null mice are profoundly suppressed, with a decreased urinary Na^+/K^+ ratio that is increased by dexamethasone (given to suppress endogenous cortisol). These knockout mice have significant nephromegaly, due to a massive hypertrophy and hyperplasia of distal convoluted tubules. The relative effect of genotype on the morphology of cells in the DCT, CNT, and CCD was not determined by the appropriate phenotypic studies[340]; however, it is known that both the DCT and the CCD are target cells for aldosterone[109,341] and both cell types express 11βHSD-2. The induction of ENaC activity by unregulated glucocorticoid likely causes the Na^+ retention and the marked increase in K^+ excretion in *11βHSD-2*-null mice; distal tubular micropuncture studies in rats treated with a systemic inhibitor of 11βHSD-2 are consistent with such a mechanism.[342] In addition, the cellular "gain of function" in the DCT would be expected to be associated with hypercalciuria, given the phenotype of pseudohypoaldosteronism type II and Gitelman syndrome (see later discussion on hereditary tubular causes of hyperkalemia and Gitelman syndrome); indeed, patients with AME are reported to exhibit nephrocalcinosis.[333]

Pharmacological inhibition of 11βHSD-2 is also associated with hypokalemia and AME. The most infamous offender is licorice, in its multiple guises (licorice root, tea, candies, herbal remedies, etc.). The early observations that licorice required small amounts of cortisol to exert its kaliuretic effect, in the Addisonian absence of endogenous glucocorticoid,[343] presaged the observations that its active ingredients (glycyrrhetinic/glycyrrhizinic acid and carbenoxolone) inhibit 11βHSD-2 and related enzymes.[333] Licorice intake remains considerable in European countries, particularly Iceland, Netherlands, and Scandinavia[344]; Pontefract cakes, eaten both as sweets and as a laxative, are a continued source of licorice in the United Kingdom,[344] whereas it is an ingredient in several popular sweeteners and preservatives in Malaysia.[345] Glycyrrhizinic acid is used in Japan to manage hepatitis, and has been under evaluation elsewhere for the management of hepatitis C; AME has been reported with its use for this indication.[346] Glycyrrhizinic acid is also a component of Chinese herbal remedies, prescribed for disorders such as for allergic rhinitis.[347] Carbenoxolone is in turn utilized in some countries in the management of peptic ulcer disease.[333]

Finally, a rare, mechanistically distinct form of AME has been reported, due to a gain-of-function mutation in the mineralocorticoid receptor (MR).[348] A single kindred was thus described with autosomal dominant inheritance of severe hypertension and hypokalemia; the causative mutation involves a serine residue that is conserved in the MR from multiple species, yet differs in other nuclear steroid receptors. This mutation results in constitutive activation of the MR in the absence of ligand, and induces significant affinity for progesterone.[348] The MR is thus constitutively "on" in these patients, with a marked stimulation by progesterone; of interest, pregnancies in the affected female members of the family have all been complicated by severe hypertension, due to marked increases in serum progesterone induced by the gravid state.[348]

Liddle Syndrome

Liddle syndrome constitutes an autosomal dominant gain-in-function of ENaC, the amiloride-sensitive Na^+ channel of the CNT and CCD.[349] Patients manifest severe hypertension with hypokalemia, unresponsive to spironolactone yet sensitive to triamterene and amiloride. Liddle syndrome could therefore also be classified as a syndrome of apparent mineralocorticoid excess. Both hypertension and hypokalemia are variable aspects of the Liddle phenotype; consistent features include a blunted aldosterone response to ACTH and reduced urinary aldosterone excretion.[350,351] The vast majority of mutations target the C-terminus of either the β- or γ-ENaC subunit. ENaC channels containing Liddle syndrome mutations are constitutively over-expressed at the cell membrane[352,353]; unlike wild-type ENaC channels, they are not sensitive to inhibition by intracellular Na^+,[354] an important regulator of endogenous channel activity in the CCD.[355] The mechanism whereby mutations in the C-terminus of ENaC subunits lead to this channel phenotype are discussed earlier in this chapter (see Fig. 15–5 and discussion of control of potassium secretion: aldosterone). In addition to effects on interaction with Nedd4-2–dependent retrieval from the plasma membrane, Liddle-associated mutations increase proteolytic cleavage of ENaC at the cell membrane[356]; as discussed earlier, aldosterone-induced "channel-activating proteases" activate ENaC channels at the plasma membrane. This important result provides a mechanistic explanation for the longstanding observation that Liddle-associated mutations in ENaC appear to have a dual activating effect, on both the open probability of the channel (i.e., on channel activity) and on expression at the cell membrane.[352]

Given the overlapping and synergistic mechanisms that regulate ENaC activity, it stands to reason that mutations in ENaC that give rise to Liddle syndrome might do so by a variety of means. Indeed, mutation of a residue within the extracellular domain of ENaC increases open probability of the channel without changing surface expression; the patient with this mutation has a typical Liddle syndrome phenotype.[116] Extensive searches for more common mutations and polymorphisms in ENaC subunits that correlate with blood pressure in the general population have essentially been negative. However, there are a handful of genetic studies that correlate specific variants in ENaC subunits with biochemical evidence of greater in vivo activity of the channel (i.e., a suppressed PRA and aldosterone or increased ratios of urinary K^+: aldosterone/PRA, or both).[357,358]

Familial Hypokalemic Alkalosis: Bartter Syndrome

Bartter and Gitelman syndromes are the two major variants of familial hypokalemic alkalosis; Gitelman syndrome is a much more common cause of hypokalemia than is Bartter syndrome (BS).[359] Whereas a clinical subdivision of these syndromes has been used in the past, a genetic classification is increasingly in use, due in part to phenotypic overlap. Patients with "classic" BS typically suffer from polyuria and polydipsia, and manifest a hypokalemic, hypochloremic alkalosis. They may have an increase in urinary calcium (Ca^{2+}) excretion, and 20% are hypomagnesemic.[360] Other features include marked elevation of serum ATII, serum aldosterone, and plasma renin. Patients with "antenatal" BS present earlier in life with a severe systemic disorder characterized by marked electrolyte wasting, polyhydramnios, and significant hypercalciuria with nephrocalcinosis. Prostaglandin synthesis and excretion is significantly increased, and may account for much of the systemic symptoms. Decreasing prostaglandin synthesis by cyclooxygenase inhibition can improve polyuria in patients with BS, by reducing the amplifying inhibition of urinary concentrating mechanisms by prostaglandins. Indomethacin also increases serum K^+ and decreases plasma renin activity, but does not correct the basic tubular defect. Of interest, COX-2 immunoreactivity is increased in the TAL and macula densa of patients with BS,[361] and recent reports indicate a clinical benefit of COX-2 inhibitors.[362]

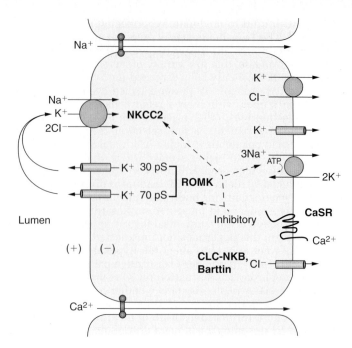

FIGURE 15–9 Bartter syndrome and the thick ascending limb. Bartter syndrome can result from loss-of-function mutations in the Na^+-K^+-$2Cl^-$ cotransporter NKCC2, the K^+ channel subunit ROMK, or the Cl^- channel subunits CLC-NKB and Barttin (Bartter syndrome types I to IV, respectively). Gain-of-function mutations in the calcium-sensing receptor CaSR can also cause a Bartter syndrome phenotype (type V); the CaSR has an inhibitory effect on salt transport by the thick ascending limb, targeting several transport pathways. ROMK encodes the low conductance 30 pS K^+ channel in the apical membrane, and also appears to function as a critical subunit of the higher conductance 70 pS channel. The loss of K^+ channel activity Bartter syndrome type II leads to reduced apical K^+ recycling and reduced Na^+-K^+-$2Cl^-$ cotransport. Decreased apical K^+ channels also lead to a decrease in the lumen-positive potential difference, which drives paracellular Na^+, Ca^{2+}, and Mg^{2+} transport.

Early studies in Bartter syndrome suggested that these patients had a defect in the function of the TAL.[363] Many of the clinical features are mimicked by the administration of loop diuretics, to which at least a subset of patients with antenatal BS do not respond.[364] The apical Na^+-K^+-$2Cl^-$ cotransporter (NKCC2, SLC12A1) of the mammalian TAL[21] (Fig. 15–9) was thus an early candidate gene. In 1996, disease-associated mutations were found in the human NKCC2 gene in four kindreds with antenatal BS[365]; in the genetic classification of BS, these patients are considered to have BS type I. Although the functional consequences of disease-associated NKCC2 mutations have not been comprehensively studied, the first[365] and subsequent reports[366,367] include patients with frameshift mutations and premature stop codons that predict the absence of a functional NKCC2 protein.

Bartter syndrome is a genetically heterogeneous disease. Given the role of apical K^+ permeability in the TAL, encoded at least in part by ROMK,[73,75] this K^+ channel was another early candidate gene. K^+ recycling via the Na^+-K^+-$2Cl^-$ cotransporter and apical K^+ channels generates a lumen-positive potential difference in the TAL, which drives the paracellular transport of Na^+ and other cations[368] (see Fig. 15–9). Multiple disease-associated mutations in ROMK have been reported in patients with BS type II, most of whom exhibit the antenatal phenotype.[369] Finally, mutations in BS type III have been reported in the chloride channel CLC-NKB,[370] which is expressed at the basolateral membrane of at least the thick ascending limb and distal convoluted tubule.[371] Patients with mutations in CLC-NKB typically have the classic Bartter phenotype, with a relative absence of nephrocalcinosis. In a significant fraction of patients with BS the NKCC2, ROMK, and CLC-NKB genes are not involved.[370] For example, a subset of patients with associated sensorineural deafness exhibit linkage to chromosome 1p31[372]; the gene for this syndrome, denoted Barttin, is an obligatory subunit for the CLC-NKB chloride channel.[373] The occurrence of deafness in these patients suggests that Barttin functions in the regulation or function of Cl^- channels in the inner ear. Notably, the CLC-NKB gene is immediately adjacent that for another epithelial Cl^- channel, denoted CLC-NKA; digenic inactivation was recently described in two siblings with deafness and BS,[374] suggesting that CLC-NKA plays an important role in Barttin-dependent Cl^- transport in the inner ear.

Patients with activating mutations in the calcium-sensing receptor (CaSR) were recently described with autosomal dominant hypocalcemia and hypokalemic alkalosis.[375,376] The CaSR is heavily expressed at the basolateral membrane of the TAL,[377] where it is thought to play an important inhibitory role in regulating the transcellular transport of both Na^+-Cl^- and Ca^{2+}. For example, activation of the basolateral CaSR in the TAL is known to reduce apical K^+ channel activity,[378] which would induce a Bartter-like syndrome (see Fig. 15–9). Genetic activation of the CaSR by these mutations was also expected to increase urinary Ca^{2+} excretion, by inhibiting generation of the lumen-positive potential difference that drives paracellular Ca^{2+} transport in the TAL. In addition, the "set-point" of the CaSR response to Ca^{2+} in the parathyroid is shifted to the left, inhibiting PTH secretion by this gland. No doubt the positional cloning of other BS genes will have a considerable impact on mechanistic understanding of the TAL.

Despite the reasonable correlation between the disease gene involved and the associated subtype of familial alkalosis, there is significant phenotypic overlap and phenotypic variability in hereditary hypokalemic alkalosis. For example, patients with mutations in CLC-NKB most frequently exhibit classic BS, but can present with a more severe antenatal phenotype, or even with a phenotype similar to Gitelman syndrome.[379,380] With respect to BS due to mutations in NKCC2, a number of patients have been described with variant presentations, including an absence of hypokalemia.[367] Two brothers were recently described with a late onset of mild BS; these patients were found to be compound heterozygotes for a mutant form of NKCC2 that exhibits partial function, with a loss-of-function mutation on the other NKCC2 allele.[381]

Bartter syndrome type II is particularly relevant to K^+ homeostasis, given that ROMK is the SK secretory channel of the CNT and CCD (see discussion on potassium secretion in the distal nephron). Patients with BS type II typically have slightly higher serum K^+ than the other genetic forms of BS[369,380]; patients with severe (9.0 mmol/l), transient, neonatal hyperkalemia have also been described.[382] It is likely that this reflects a transient, developmental deficit in the other K^+ channels involved in distal K^+ secretion, including the apical maxi-K channel responsible for flow-dependent K^+ secretion in the distal nephron.[71,79] Distal K^+ secretion in ROMK knockout mice is primarily mediated by maxi-K/BK channel activity,[76] such that developmental deficits in this channel would indeed lead to hyperkalemia in BS type II. The mammalian TAL has two major apical K^+ conductances, the 30 pS channel corresponding to ROMK, and a 70 pS channel[383]; both are thought to play a role in transepithelial salt transport by the TAL. ROMK is evidently a subunit of the 70 pS channel, given the absence of this conductance in TAL segments of ROMK knockout mice.[384] The identity of the other putative subunit of this 70 pS channel is not as yet known; one would assume that deficiencies in this gene would also be a cause of BS.

Finally, BS must be clinically differentiated from the various causes of "pseudo-Bartter" syndrome; these commonly include laxative abuse, furosemide abuse, and bulimia (see discussion on the clinical approach to hypokalemia). Other reported causes include gentamicin nephrotoxicity,[301] Sjögren syndrome,[385] and cystic fibrosis (CF).[386,387] Fixed loss of Na^+-Cl^- in sweat is likely the dominant predisposing factor for hypokalemic alkalosis in patients with CF; patients with this presentation generally respond promptly to intravenous fluids and electrolyte replacement. However, the CFTR protein co-associates with ROMK in the TAL, and confers sensitivity to both ATP and glibenclamide to apical K^+ channels in this nephron segment.[388] Lu and colleagues[388] have proposed that this interaction serves to modulate the response of ROMK to cAMP and vasopressin, such that K^+ excretion in CFTR deficiency would not be appropriately reduced during water diuresis, thus predisposing such patients to the development of hypokalemic alkalosis.

Familial Hypokalemic Alkalosis: Gitelman Syndrome

A major advance in the understanding of hereditary alkaloses was the realization that a subset of patients exhibit marked hypocalciuria, rather than the hypercalciuria typically seen in BS; patients in this hypocalciuric subset are universally hypomagnesemic.[296] Such patients are now clinically classified as suffering from Gitelman syndrome. Although plasma renin activity may be increased, renal prostaglandin excretion is not elevated in these hypocalciuric patients,[389] another distinguishing feature between Bartter and Gitelman syndromes. Gitelman syndrome (GS) is a milder disorder than BS; however, patients do report significant morbidity, mostly related to muscular symptoms and fatigue.[390] The QT interval is frequently prolonged in GS, suggesting an increased risk of cardiac arrhythmia.[391] A more exhaustive cardiac evaluation of a large group of patients failed to detect significant abnormalities of cardiac structure or rhythm.[392] However, presyncope or ventricular tachycardia (or both) has been observed in at least two patients with GS[196,393] one with concomitant long QT syndrome due to a mutation in the cardiac KCNQ1 K^+ channel.[196]

The hypocalciuria detected in GS was an expected consequence of inactivating the thiazide-sensitive Na^+-Cl^- cotransporter NCC (SLC12A2), and loss-of-function mutations in the human gene have been reported[394]; many of these mutations lead to a defect in cellular trafficking when introduced into the human NCC protein.[395] GS is genetically homogeneous, except for the occasional patient with mutations in CLC-NKB and an overlapping phenotype.[196,379,380] The NCC protein has been localized to the apical membrane of epithelial cells in the distal convoluted tubule (DCT) and connecting segment. A mouse strain with targeted deletion of the *Slc12a2* gene encoding NCC exhibits hypocalciuria and hypomagnesemia, with a mild alkalosis and marked increase in circulating aldosterone.[396] These knockout mice exhibit marked morphological defects in the early DCT,[396] with both a reduction in absolute number of DCT cells and changes in ultrastructural appearance. That GS is a disorder of cellular development or cellular apoptosis (or both) should perhaps not be a surprise, given the observation that thiazide treatment promotes marked apoptosis of this nephron segment.[397] This cellular deficit leads to downregulation of the DCT magnesium channel TRPM6,[398] resulting in the magnesium wasting and hypomagnesemia seen in GS. The downstream CNT tubules are hypertrophied in NCC-deficient mice,[396] reminiscent of the hypertrophic DCT and CNT segments seen in furosemide-treated animals.[399] These CNT cells also exhibit an increased expression of ENaC at their apical membranes, versus litter mate controls[396]; this is likely due to activation of SGK1-

dependent trafficking of ENaC by the increase in circulating aldosterone (see discussion on control of potassium secretion: aldosterone).

Hypokalemia does not occur in NCC −/− mice on standard rodent diet, but emerges on a K^+ restricted diet; plasma K^+ of these mice is ~1 mM lower than K^+-restricted litter mate controls.[400] Several mechanisms account for the hypokalemia seen in GS and NCC −/− mice. The distal delivery of both Na^+ and fluid is decreased in NCC −/− mice, at least on a normal diet; however, the increased circulating aldosterone and CNT hypertrophy likely compensate, leading to increased kaliuresis. As discussed earlier for thiazides, decreased luminal Ca^{2+} in NCC-deficiency may augment baseline ENaC activity,[298] further exacerbating the kaliuresis. Of particular interest, NCC-deficient mice develop considerable polydipsia and polyuria on a K^+-restricted diet[400]; this is reminiscent perhaps of the polydipsia that has been implicated in thiazide-associated hyponatremia.[401]

Hypocalciuria in GS is not accompanied by changes in serum calcium, phosphate, vitamin D, or PTH,[402] suggesting a direct effect on renal calcium transport. The late DCT is morphologically intact in NCC-deficient mice, with preserved expression of the epithelial calcium channel (ECAC1 or TRPV5) and the basolateral Na^+-Ca^{2+} exchanger.[396] Furthermore, the hypocalciuric effect of thiazides persists in mice deficient in TRPV5,[398] arguing against the putative effects of this drug on distal Ca^{2+} absorption. Rather, several lines of evidence argue that the hypocalciuria of GS and thiazide treatment is due to increased absorption of Na^+ by the proximal tubule,[396,398] with secondary increases in proximal Ca^{2+} absorption. Regardless, reminiscent of the clinical effect of thiazides on bone,[403] there are clear differences in bone density between affected and unaffected members of specific Gitelman kindreds. Thus homozygous patients have much higher bone densities than unaffected wild-type family members, whereas heterozygotes have intermediate values for both bone density and calcium excretion.[402] An interesting association has repeatedly been described between chondrocalcinosis, the abnormal deposition of calcium pyrophosphate dihydrate (CPPD) in joint cartilage, and Gitelman syndrome.[404] Patients have also been reported with ocular choroidal calcification.[405]

Finally, as in Bartter syndrome, there are reports of acquired tubular defects that mimic GS. These include patients with hypokalemic alkalosis, hypomagnesemia, and hypocalciuria after chemotherapy with cisplatin.[406] Patients have also been described with acquired GS due to Sjögren syndrome and tubulointerstitial nephritis[407,408] with a documented absence of coding sequence mutations in NCC.[408]

Magnesium Deficiency

Magnesium deficiency results in refractory hypokalemia, particularly if the serum Mg^{2+} is less than 0.5 mg/dl[247]; hypomagnesemic patients are thus refractory to K^+ replacement in the absence of Mg^{2+} repletion.[409,410] Magnesium deficiency is also a common concomitant of hypokalemia, in part because associated tubular disorders (e.g., aminoglycoside nephrotoxicity) may cause both a kaliuresis and magnesium wasting. Serum Mg^{2+} must thus be checked on a routine basis, along with other electrolytes.[246,411] Magnesium depletion has inhibitory effects on muscle Na^+/K^+-ATPase activity,[412] resulting in significant efflux from muscle and a secondary kaliuresis. Furthermore, it has been suggested that the repletion of intracellular K^+ is impaired in hypomagnesemia, even in normokalemic patients.[411] Decreased intracellular Mg^{2+} enhances K^+ efflux from the cytoplasm of cardiac and perhaps skeletal myocytes, likely due to both intracellular blockade of K^+ channels and inhibition of the Na^+/K^+-ATPase; serum K^+ levels thus remain normal at the expense of intracellular K^+.[16,411] This phenomenon is particularly important in patients

with cardiac disease taking both diuretics and digoxin. In such patients hypokalemia and arrhythmias will respond to correction of magnesium deficiency and potassium supplementation.[16,411]

The Clinical Approach to Hypokalemia

The initial priority in the evaluation of hypokalemia is an assessment for signs and/or symptoms (muscle weakness, ECG changes, etc.) suggestive of an impending emergency that requires immediate treatment. The cause of hypokalemia is usually obvious from history, physical examination, basic laboratory tests, or all three. However, persistent hypokalemia despite appropriate initial intervention requires a more rigorous workup; in most cases, a systematic approach reveals the underlying cause (Fig. 15–10).

The history should focus on medications (e.g., diuretics, laxatives, antibiotics, herbal medications), diet and dietary supplements (e.g., licorice), and associated symptoms (e.g., diarrhea). During the physical examination, particular attention should be paid to blood pressure, volume status, and signs suggestive of specific disorders associated with hypokalemia (hyperthyroidism, Cushing syndrome, etc.). Initial laboratory tests should include electrolytes, BUN, creatinine, serum osmolality, Mg^{2+}, and Ca^{2+}, a complete blood count, and urinary pH, osmolality, creatinine, and electrolytes. Serum and urine osmolality are required for calculation of the transtubular K^+ gradient[155] (see discussion of urinary indices of potassium excretion). Further tests such as urinary Mg^{2+} and Ca^{2+} and plasma renin and aldosterone levels may be necessary in specific cases (see Fig. 15–10). The timing and evolution of hypokalemia is also helpful in differentiating the cause, particularly in hospitalized patients; for example, hypokalemia due to transcellular shift usually occurs in a matter of hours.[413]

The most common causes of chronic, diagnosis-resistant hypokalemia are Gitelman syndrome (GS), surreptitious vomiting, and diuretic abuse.[414] Alternatively, an associated acidosis would suggest the diagnosis of hypokalemic distal or proximal renal tubular acidosis. Hypokalemia occurred in 5.5% of patients with eating disorders in an American study from the mid 1990s,[415] mostly in those with surreptitious vomiting (bulimia) or laxative abuse (the purging[291] subtype of anorexia nervosa). These patients may have a constellation of associated symptoms and signs, including dental erosion and depression.[416] Hypokalemic patients with bulimia will have an associated metabolic alkalosis, with an obligatory natriuresis accompanying the loss of bicarbonate; urinary Cl^- is typically <10 mmol/L, and this clue can often yield the diagnosis.[414,417] Urinary electrolytes are however generally unremarkable in unselected, mostly normokalemic patients with bulimia.[416] Urinary excretion of Na^+, K^+, and Cl^- is high in patients who abuse diuretics, albeit not to the levels seen in GS. Marked variability in urinary electrolytes is an important clue for diuretic abuse, which can be verified with urinary drug screens. Clinically, nephrocalcinosis is very common in furosemide abuse, due to the increase in urinary calcium excretion.[418] Differentiation of GS from Bartter syndrome (BS) requires a 24-hour urine to assess calcium excretion, since hypocalciuria is a distinguishing feature for the former[296]; patients with GS are also invariably hypomagnesemic. Bartter syndrome must be differentiated from "pseudo-Bartter" syndrome due to gentamicin toxicity,[301,419] mutations in CFTR, the cystic fibrosis gene,[386,387] or Sjögren syndrome with tubulointerstitial nephritis.[385] Acquired forms of GS have in turn been reported after cisplatin therapy[406] and in patients with Sjögren syndrome.[407,408] Finally, although laxative abuse is perhaps a less common cause of chronic hypokalemia, an accompanying metabolic acidosis with a negative urinary anion gap should raise the diagnostic suspicion of this cause.[159]

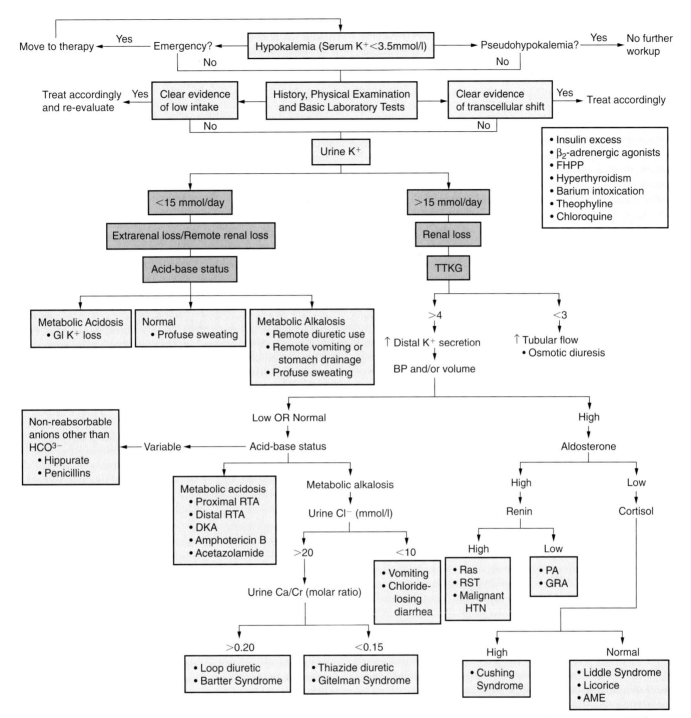

FIGURE 15–10 The diagnostic approach to hypokalemia. See text for details. FHPP: familial hypokalemic periodic paralysis; GI: gastrointestinal; TTKG: transtubular potassium gradient; CCD: cortical collecting duct; BP: blood pressure; RTA: renal tubular acidosis; DKA: diabetic ketoacidosis; RAS: renal artery stenosis; RST: renin secreting tumor; HTN: hypertension; PA: primary aldosteronism; GRA: glucocorticoid remediable aldosteronism; AME: apparent mineralocorticoid excess.

TREATMENT OF HYPOKALEMIA*

The goals of therapy in hypokalemia are to prevent life-threatening conditions (diaphragmatic weakness, rhabdomyolysis, and cardiac arrhythmias), to replace any K^+ deficit, and to diagnose and correct the underlying cause. The urgency of therapy depends on the severity of hypokalemia, associated conditions and settings (e.g., a patient with heart failure on digoxin, or a patient with hepatic encephalopathy), and the

rate of decline in serum K^+. A rapid drop to less than 2.5 mmol/L poses a high risk of cardiac arrhythmias and calls for urgent replacement.[420] Although replacement is usually limited to patients with a true deficit, it should be considered in patients with hypokalemia due to redistribution (e.g., hypokalemic periodic paralysis) when serious complications such as muscle weakness, rhabdomyolysis, and cardiac arrhythmias are present or imminent.[421] The risk of arrhythmia from hypokalemia is highest in older patients, patients with evidence of organic heart disease, and patients on digoxin or antiarrhythmic drugs.[246] In these high-risk patients, an increased incidence of arrhythmias may occur at even mild to modest degrees of hypokalemia.

---

* All the recommended doses are for adults.

It is also crucial to diagnose and eliminate the underlying cause, so as to tailor therapy to the pathophysiology involved. For example, the risk of overcorrection or rebound hyperkalemia in hypokalemia caused by redistribution is particularly high, with the potential for fatal hyperkalemic arrhythmias.[247,260,421,422] When increased sympathetic tone or increased sympathetic response is thought to play a dominant role, the use of non-specific β-adrenergic blockade with propranolol generally avoids this complication and should be considered; the relevant causes of hypokalemia include thyrotoxic periodic paralysis,[287] theophylline overdose,[423] and acute head injury.[260]

K[+] replacement is the mainstay of therapy in hypokalemia. However, hypomagnesemic patients can be refractory to K[+] replacement alone,[410] such that concomitant Mg[2+] deficiency should always be addressed with oral or parenteral repletion. To prevent hyperkalemia due to excessive supplementation, the deficit and the rate of correction should be estimated as accurately as possible. Renal function, medications, and co-morbid conditions such as diabetes (with a risk of both insulinopenia and autonomic neuropathy) should also be considered, so as to gauge the risk of overcorrection. The goal is to raise the serum K[+] to a safe range rapidly and then replace the remaining deficit at a slower rate over days to weeks.[246,247,421] In the absence of abnormal K[+] redistribution, the total deficit correlates with serum K[+][247,421,424] such that serum K[+] drops by approximately 0.27 mmol/L for every 100-mmol reduction in total-body stores. Loss of 400 to 800 mmol of body K[+] results in a reduction in serum K[+] by approximately 2.0 mmol/L[424]; these parameters can be used to estimate replacement goals.

Although the treatment of asymptomatic patients with borderline or low normal serum K[+] remains controversial, supplementation is recommended in patients with serum K[+] lower than 3 mmol/L. In high-risk patients (i.e., those with heart failure, cardiac arrhythmias, myocardial infarction, ischemic heart disease, or taking digoxin), serum K[+] should be maintained at ≥4.0 mmol/L[246] or even ≥4.5 mmol/L.[253] Patients with severe hepatic disease may not be able to tolerate mild-to-moderate hypokalemia due to the associated augmentation in ammoniagenesis, and thus serum K[+] should be maintained at approximately 4.0 mmol/L.[425,426] In asymptomatic patients with mild-to-moderate hypertension, an attempt should be made to maintain serum K[+] above 4.0 mmol/L[246] and potassium supplementation should be considered when serum K[+] falls below 3.5 mmol/L.[246] Notably, prospective studies have shown an inverse relationship between dietary potassium intake and both fatal and nonfatal stroke, independent of the associated anti-hypertensive effect.[246,427,428]

Potassium is available in the form of potassium chloride, potassium phosphate, potassium bicarbonate or its precursors (potassium citrate, potassium acetate), and potassium gluconate.[246,247,421] Potassium phosphate is indicated when phosphate deficit accompanies K[+] depletion (e.g., in diabetic ketoacidosis).[421] Potassium bicarbonate (or its precursors) should be considered in patients with hypokalemia and metabolic acidosis.[246,421] Potassium chloride should otherwise be the default salt of choice in most patients, for several reasons. First, metabolic alkalosis typically accompanies chloride loss from renal (e.g., diuretics) or upper gastrointestinal routes (e.g., vomiting), and contributes significantly to renal K[+] wasting.[247] In this setting, replacing chloride along with K[+] is essential in treating the alkalosis and preventing further kaliuresis; because dietary K[+] is mainly in the form of potassium phosphate or potassium citrate, it usually does not suffice. Second, potassium bicarbonate may offset the benefits of K[+] administration by aggravating concomitant alkalosis. Third, potassium chloride raises serum K[+] at a faster rate than does potassium bicarbonate, a factor that is crucial in patients with marked hypokalemia and related symptoms. In all likelihood, this faster rise in serum K[+] occurs because Cl[−] is mainly an extracellular fluid anion that does not enter cells to the same extent as bicarbonate, keeping the administered K[+] in the extracellular fluid compartment.[429]

Parenteral (intravenous) K[+] administration should be limited to patients unable to utilize the enteral route or when the patient is experiencing associated signs and symptoms. However, rapid correction of hypokalemia through oral supplementation is possible and may be faster than intravenous K[+] supplementation, due to limitations in the rapidity of intravenous K[+] infusion. For example, serum K[+] can be increased by 1 mmol/L to 1.4 mmol/L in 60 to 90 minutes, following the oral intake of 75 mmol of K[+][430]; the ingestion of approximately 125 to 165 mmol of K[+] as a single oral dose can increase serum K[+] by approximately 2.5 to 3.5 mmol/L in 60 to 120 minutes.[431] The oral route is thus both effective and appropriate in patients with asymptomatic severe hypokalemia. If the patient is experiencing life-threatening signs and symptoms of hypokalemia, however, the maximum possible IV infusion of K[+] should be administered acutely for symptom control, followed by rapid oral supplementation.

The usual intravenous dose is 20 to 40 mmol of K[+]-Cl[−] in a liter of vehicle solution.[421] The vehicle solution should be dextrose-free to prevent a transient reduction in serum K[+] level of 0.2 to 1.4 mmol/L, due to an enhanced endogenous insulin secretion induced by the dextrose.[432] Higher concentrations of K[+]-Cl[−] (up to 400 mmol/L, as 40 mmol in 100 ml of normal saline) have been used in life-threatening conditions.[433,434] In these cases, the amount of K[+] per intravenous bag should be limited (e.g., 20 mmol in 100 ml of saline solution) to prevent inadvertent infusion of a large dose.[434,435] These solutions are best given through a large central vein. Femoral veins are preferable because infusion through upper body central lines can acutely increase the local concentration of K[+] with deleterious effects on cardiac conduction.[434,435] As a general rule and to avoid venous pain, irritation, and sclerosis, concentrations of more than 60 mmol/L should not be given through a peripheral vein.[421] Although the recommended rate of administration is 10 to 20 mmol/hour, rates of 40 to 100 mmol/hour or even higher (for a short period) have been used in patients with life-threatening conditions.[433,435-437] However, a rapid increase in serum K[+] associated with electrocardiographic (ECG) changes may occur with higher rates of infusion (e.g., ≥80 mmol/hour).[438] Intravenous administration of K[+] at a rate of more than 10 mmol/hour requires continuous ECG monitoring.[421] In patients receiving such high infusion rates, close monitoring of the appropriate physiologic consequences of hypokalemia is essential; after these effects have abated, the rate of infusion should be decreased to the standard dose of 10 to 20 mmol/hour.[435] It is important to remember that volume expansion in patients with moderate-to-severe hypokalemia and Cl[−]-responsive metabolic alkalosis should be performed cautiously and with close follow-up of serum K[+] because bicarbonaturia associated with volume expansion may aggravate renal K[+] wasting and hypokalemia.[420] In patients with combined severe hypokalemia and hypophosphatemia (e.g., diabetic ketoacidosis), intravenous K[+] phosphate can be used. However, this solution should be infused at a rate of less than 50 mmol over 8 hours to prevent the risk of hypocalcemia and metastatic calcification.[420] A combination of potassium phosphate and potassium chloride may be necessary to correct hypokalemia effectively in these patients.

The easiest and most straightforward method of oral K[+] supplementation is to increase dietary intake of potassium-rich foods[247] (Table 15–4). A recent study compared the effectiveness of diet vs medication supplementation in cardiac surgery patients receiving diuretics in hospital and found no difference between the two groups in respect to maintenance of serum K[+]. However, limitations of this study include a small number of subjects, relatively short duration, and lack of information on acid-base status, making it less than conclusive and not generalizable.[439] Regardless, dietary K^+ is mainly in the form of potassium phosphate or potassium citrate and is inadequate in the majority of patients who have concomitant K^+ and Cl^- deficiency. Most patients will therefore need to combine a high-K^+ diet with a prescribed dose of K^+-Cl^-.[247] Salt substitutes are an inexpensive and potent source of K^+-Cl^-; each gram contains 10 to 13 mmol of K^+.[440] However, patients, particularly those with an impaired ability to excrete potassium, must be counseled regarding the appropriate amount and the potential for hyperkalemia.[441] Potassium chloride is also available in either liquid or tablet form

TABLE 15–4 Foods with High Potassium Content

Highest content (>1000 mg [25 mmol]/100 g)
  Dried figs
  Molasses
  Seaweed

Very high content (>500 mg [12.5 mmol]/100 g)
  Dried fruits (dates, prunes)
  Nuts
  Avocados
  Bran cereals
  Wheat germ
  Lima beans

High content (>250 mg [6.2 mmol]/100 g)
  Vegetables
    Spinach
    Tomatoes
    Broccoli
    Winter squash
    Beets
    Carrots
    Cauliflower
    Potatoes
  Fruits
    Bananas
    Cantaloupe
    Kiwis
    Oranges
    Mangos
  Meats
    Ground beef
    Steak
    Pork
    Veal
    Lamb

From Gennari FJ: Hypokalemia. N Engl J Med 339:451–458, 1998.

(Table 15–5).[246] In general, the available preparations are well absorbed.[247] Liquid forms are less expensive but are less well tolerated. Slow-release forms are more palatable and better tolerated; however, they have been associated with gastrointestinal ulceration and bleeding, ascribed to local accumulation of high concentrations of K^+.[247,435] Notably, this risk is rather low, and lower still with the microencapsulated forms.[247] The chance of overdose and hyperkalemia is higher with slow-release formulations; unlike the immediate release forms these tablets are less irritating to the stomach and less likely to induce vomiting.[442] The usual dose is 40 to 100 mmol of K^+ (as K^+-Cl^-) per day, divided in 2 to 3 doses, in patients taking diuretics[247] (K^+-Cl^- can be toxic in doses of more than 2 mmol/Kg[442]). This dose is effective in maintaining serum K^+ in up to 90%; however, in the 10% of patients who remain hypokalemic, increasing the oral dose or adding a K^+-sparing diuretic is an appropriate choice.[247]

In addition to potassium supplementation, strategies to minimize K^+ losses should be considered. These measures may include minimizing the dose of non-K^+-sparing diuretics, restricting Na^+ intake, and using a combination of non-K^+-sparing and K^+-sparing medications (e.g., angiotensin-converting enzyme inhibitors, angiotensin receptor blockers, K^+-sparing diuretics, β-blockers).[224,246] The use of a K^+-sparing diuretic is of particular importance in hypokalemia resulting from primary hyperaldosteronism and related disorders, such as Liddle syndrome and AME; K^+ supplementation alone may be ineffective in these settings.[443–445] In patients with hypokalemia due to loss through upper gastrointestinal secretion (continuous nasogastric tube suction, continuous or self-induced vomiting), proton-pump inhibitors are reportedly useful in helping to correct the metabolic alkalosis and reduce hypokalemia.[446]

CAUSES OF HYPERKALEMIA

Epidemiology

Hyperkalemia is usually defined as a potassium level of 5.5 mmol/L or higher,[447,448] although in some studies 5.0 to 5.4 mmol/L qualifies for the diagnosis.[449] Hyperkalemia has been reported in 1.1% to 10% of all hospitalized patients,[231,447–451] with approximately 1.0% of patients (8% to 10% of hyperkalemic patients) having significant hyperkalemia ($\geq$6.0 mmol/L).[447] Hyperkalemia has been associated with a higher mortality rate (14.3% to 41%),[447,448,450] accounting for approximately 1 death per 1000 patients in one case series

TABLE 15–5 Oral Preparations of Potassium Chloride

Supplement	Attributes
Controlled-release microencapsulated tablets	Disintegrate better in stomach than encapsulated microparticles; less adherent and less cohesive
Encapsulated controlled-release microencapsulated particles	Fewer erosions than wax-matrix tablets
Potassium chloride elixir	Inexpensive, tastes bad, poor compliance; few erosions; immediate effect
Potassium chloride (effervescent tablets) for solution	Convenient, but more expensive than elixir; immediate effect
Wax-matrix extended-release tablets	Easier to swallow; more gastrointestinal tract erosions compared with microencapsulated formulations

From Cohn JN, Kowey PR, Whelton PK, Prisant LM: New guidelines for potassium replacement in clinical practice: A contemporary review by the National Council on Potassium in Clinical Practice. Arch Intern Med 160:2429–2436, 2000.

from the mid 1980s.[452] In most hospitalized patients, the pathophysiology of hyperkalemia is multifactorial, with reduced renal function, medications, older age (≥60 years), and hyperglycemia being the most common contributing factors.[231,447,448] However, in one study of patients younger than 60 years, ESRD was the most common cause.[453]

In patients with ESRD, the prevalence of hyperkalemia is 5% to 10%.[454–456] Hyperkalemia accounts for or contributes to 1.9% to 5% of deaths among patients with ESRD.[231,456] Hyperkalemia is the reason for emergency hemodialysis in 24% of patients with ESRD on hemodialysis[456] and renal failure is the most common cause of hyperkalemia diagnosed in the emergency room.[454] A recent study reported the prevalence of marked hyperkalemia ($K^+ \geq 5.8$ mmol/L) to be approximately 1% in a general medicine outpatient setting. Alarmingly, the management was often suboptimal, with approximately 25% of the patients lacking any follow-up, ECGs performed in only 36% of cases, and frequent delays in repeating serum K^+.[457]

Pseudohyperkalemia

Factitious or pseudohyperkalemia is an artifactual increase in serum K^+ due to the release of K^+ during or after venipuncture. There are several potential causes for pseudohyperkalemia.[458] First, forearm contraction,[459] fist clenching,[16] or tourniquet use[458] may increase K^+ efflux from local muscle and thus raise the measured serum K^+. Second, thrombocytosis,[460] leukocytosis,[461] and/or erythrocytosis[462] may cause pseudohyperkalemia due to release from these cellular elements. Third, acute anxiety during venipuncture may provoke a respiratory alkalosis and hyperkalemia due to redistribution.[52–54,64] Fourth, mechanical and physical factors may induce pseudohyperkalemia after blood has been drawn. For example, pneumatic tube transport has been shown to induce pseudohyperkalemia in one patient with leukemia and massive leukocytosis.[463] Cooling of blood prior to the separation of cells from plasma or serum is also a well-recognized cause of artefactual hyperkalemia.[464] The converse is the risk of increased uptake of K^+ by cells at high ambient temperatures, leading to normal values for hyperkalemic patients or spurious hypokalemia (or both) in patients who are normokalemic.[255,256] This issue is particularly important for outpatient primary practice samples that are transported off-site and analyzed at a central facility[255,256,465]; this phenomenon leads to "seasonal pseudohyperkalemia",[255] with fluctuations of outpatient samples as a function of season and ambient temperature.

Finally, patients have been described with hereditary forms of pseudohyperkalemia, caused by increase in passive K^+ permeability of erythrocytes. Abnormal red cell morphology, varying degrees of hemolysis, and/or perinatal edema can accompany hereditary pseudohyperkalemia, whereas in many kindreds there are no overt hematological consequences. Plasma K^+ increases in pseudohyperkalemia patient samples that have been left at room temperature, due to abnormal K^+ permeability of erythrocytes. Several subtypes have been defined, based on differences in the temperature-dependence curve of this red cell leak pathway.[466,467] The disorder is genetically heterogeneous, with a recently characterized gene on chromosome 17q21 and uncharacterized loci on chromosomes 16q23-ter[468] and 2q35-36.[466] Of particular interest, 11 pedigrees of patients with autosomal dominant hemolysis, pseudohyperkalemia, and temperature-dependent loss of red cell K^+ were recently found to have heterozygous mutations in the *SLC4A1* gene on chromosome 17q21, which encodes the band 3 anion exchanger, AE1.[467] The mutations that were detected all cluster within exon 17 of the gene,[467] between transmembrane domains 8 and 10 of the AE1 protein. These mutations reduce anion transport in both red cells and

Xenopus oocytes injected with AE1, with the novel acquisition of a non-selective transport pathway for both Na^+ and K^+. Pseudohyperkalemia in these patients thus results from a genetic event that endows AE1 with the ability to transport K^+; that single point mutations can convert an anion exchanger to a non-selective cation channel serves to underline the narrow boundaries that separate exchangers and transporters from ion channels.[467]

Excess Intake of Potassium and Tissue Necrosis

Increased intake of even small amounts of K^+ may provoke severe hyperkalemia in patients with predisposing factors. For example, the oral administration of 32 millimoles to a diabetic patient with hyporeninemic hypoaldosteronism resulted in an increase in serum K^+ from 4.9 mmol/l to a peak of 7.3 mmol/l, within 3 hours.[469] Increased intake or changes in intake of dietary sources rich in K^+ (see Table 15–4) may also provoke hyperkalemia in susceptible patients. Very rarely, marked intake of K^+, for example in sports beverages,[470] may provoke severe hyperkalemia in individuals free of predisposing factors. Other occult sources of K^+ must also be considered, including salt substitutes,[440] alternative medicines,[471] and alternative diets.[472] Geophagia with ingestion of K^+-rich clay,[473] and cautopyreiophagia[474] (ingestion of burnt matchsticks), are two forms of pica that have been reported to cause hyperkalemia in dialysis patients. Sustained-release K^+-Cl^- tablets can cause hyperkalemia in suicidal overdoses.[442] Such pills are radio-opaque, and may thus be seen on radiographs; whole bowel irrigation should be used for gastrointestinal decontamination.[442] Iatrogenic causes include simple over-replacement with K^+-Cl^- or administration of a potassium-containing medication, such as K^+-penicillin, to a susceptible patient.

Red cell transfusion is a well-described cause of hyperkalemia, typically seen in children or in massive transfusions. Risk factors for transfusion-related hyperkalemia include the rate and volume of the transfusion, the use of a central venous infusion and/or pressure pumping, the use of irradiated blood, and the age of the blood infused[16]; whereas 7-day-old blood has a free K^+ concentration of ~23 mmol/L, this rises to the 50 mmol/L range in 42-day-old blood.[475]

Tissue necrosis is an important cause of hyperkalemia. Hyperkalemia due to rhabdomyolysis is particularly common, due the enormous store of K^+ in muscle (see Fig. 15–1). In many cases, volume depletion, medications (statins in particular), and metabolic predisposition contribute to the genesis of rhabdomyolysis. Hypokalemia is an important metabolic predisposing factor in rhabdomyolysis (see discussion on consequences of hypokalemia); others include hypophosphatemia, hypernatremia and hyponatremia, and hyperglycemia. Those patients with hypokalemia-associated rhabdomyolysis in whom redistribution is the cause of hypokalemia are at particular risk of subsequent hyperkalemia, as rhabdomyolysis evolves and renal function worsens.[16,268] Finally, massive release of K^+ and other intracellular contents may occur as a result of acute tumor lysis.[469]

Redistribution and Hyperkalemia

Several different mechanisms can induce an efflux of intracellular K^+, resulting in hyperkalemia. Increases in serum K^+ due to hypertonic mannitol or hypertonic saline[476] are generally attributed to a "solvent drag" effect, as water moves out of cells in response to the osmotic gradient. Severe hyperkalemia and ventricular tachycardia is a well-described complication of mannitol for the management or prevention of cerebral edema.[477] Diabetics are prone to severe hyperkalemia in response to intravenous hypertonic glucose in the absence of adequate co-administered insulin, due to a similar osmotic effect.[478,479] Finally, a retrospective report recently documented considerable increases in serum K+ after IV contrast dye in five patients with chronic kidney disease, four on dialysis, and one with stage IV CKD[480]; again, the acute osmolar load was the likely cause of the acute hyperkalemia in these patients. The implications of this provocative, preliminary study are not entirely clear. However, one would expect the development or worsening of hyperkalemia in dialysis patients exposed to large volumes of hyperosmolar contrast dye.

Two reports have appeared regarding the risk of hyperkalemia with epsilon-aminocaproic acid,[481,482] a cationic amino acid that is structurally similar to lysine and arginine. Cationic but not anionic amino acids induce efflux of K+ from cells, although the transport pathways involved are unknown.[16]

Muscle plays a dominant role in extra-renal K+ homeostasis, primarily via regulated uptake by the Na+/K+-ATPase. Although exercise is a well-described cause of acute hyperkalemia, this effect is usually transient and clinical relevance is difficult to judge. ESRD patients on dialysis do not have an exaggerated increase in serum K+ with maximal exercise, perhaps due to greater insulin, catecholamine, and aldosterone responses to exercise and/or to their pre-existing hyperkalemia.[483] The results and design of this and other studies of exercise-associated hyperkalemia in ESRD have been criticized by a more recent report, which linked abnormal extra-renal K+ homeostasis to increased fatigue in ESRD.[484] Regardless, however, exercise-associated hyperkalemia is not a major clinical cause of hyperkalemia. Dialysis patients are however susceptible to modest increases in serum K+ after prolonged fasting, due to the relative insulinopenia in this setting.[485] This may be clinically relevant in pre-operative ESRD patients, for whom intravenous glucose infusions +/– insulin are appropriate preventive measures for the development of hyperkalemia.[485]

Digoxin inhibits Na+/K+-ATPase and thus impairs the uptake of K+ by skeletal muscle (see discussion on factors affecting internal distribution of potassium), such that digoxin overdose can result in hyperkalemia. The skin and venom gland of the cane toad *Bufo marinus* contains high concentrations of bufadienolide, a structurally similar glycoside. The direct ingestion of such toads[486] or of toad extracts can result in fatal hyperkalemia. In particular, certain herbal aphrodisiac pills contain appreciable amounts of toad venom, and have lead to several case reports in the United States.[16,487] Patients may have detectable serum levels using standard digoxin assays, since bufadienolide is immunologically similar to digoxin. Moreover, treatment with digoxin-specific Fab fragment, indicated for management of digoxin overdoses, may be effective and life-saving in bufadienolide toxicity.[16,487] Finally, fluoride ions also inhibit Na+/K+-ATPase, such that fluoride poisoning is typically associated with hyperkalemia.[488]

Succinylcholine depolarizes muscle cells, resulting in the efflux of K+ through acetylcholine receptors (AChRs) and a rapid, but usually transient hyperkalemia. The use of this agent is contraindicated in patients who have sustained thermal trauma, neuromuscular injury (upper or lower motor neuron), disuse atrophy, mucositis, or prolonged immobilization in an ICU setting; the efflux of K+ induced by succinylcholine is enhanced in these patients and can result in significant hyperkalemia.[489] These disorders share a 2- to 100-fold upregulation of AChRs at the plasma membrane of muscle cells, with loss of the normal clustering at the neuromuscular junction.[489] Depolarization of these up-regulated AChRs by succinylcholine results in an exaggerated efflux of K+ through the receptor-associated cation channels that are

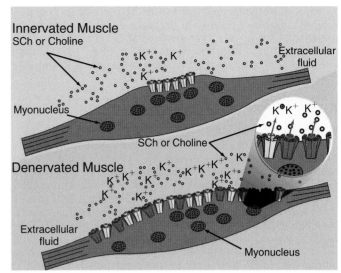

FIGURE 15–11 Succinylcholine-induced efflux of potassium is increased in denervated muscle. In innervated muscle, succinylcholine interacts with the entire plasma membrane, but depolarizes only the junctional ($\alpha1$, $\beta1$, δ, and ϵ-multicolored) acetylcholine receptors (AChRs); this leads to a modest, transient hyperkalemia. With denervation, there is a considerable up-regulation of muscle AChRs, with increased extra-junctional AChRs ($\alpha1$, $\beta1$, δ, and γ-multicolored) and acquisition of homomeric, neuronal-type $\alpha7$-AChRs. Depolarization of denervated muscle leads to an exaggerated K+ efflux, due to the up-regulation and redistribution of these AChRs. In addition, choline generated from metabolism of succinylcholine maintains the depolarization mediated via $\alpha7$-AChRs, thus enhancing and prolonging the K+ efflux after paralysis has subsided. (From Martyn JA, Richtsfeld M: Succinylcholine-induced hyperkalemia in acquired pathologic states: Etiologic factors and molecular mechanisms. Anesthesiology 104:158–169, 2006.)

spread throughout the muscle cell membrane (Fig. 15–11). Concomitant upregulation of the neuronal $\alpha7$ AChR subunit has also been observed in denervated muscle; the $\alpha7$-containing AChR is a homomeric, pentameric channel that depolarizes in response to both succinylcholine and choline, its metabolite.[489] Depolarization $\alpha7$-AChRs in response to choline is furthermore not subject to desensitization, and may explain in part the hyperkalemic effect that persists in some patients well after the paralytic effect of succinylcholine has subsided.[489] Consistent perhaps with this neuromuscular pathophysiology, patients with renal failure do not appear to have an increased risk of succinylcholine-associated hyperkalemia.[490]

A recent report of three patients suggested the possibility that drugs that share the ability to open K_{ATP} channels may have an under appreciated propensity to cause hyperkalemia in critically ill patients. The implicated drugs included cyclosporin, isoflurane, and nicorandil.[491] These patients exhibited hyperkalemia that resisted usual therapies (insulin/dextrose +/– hemofiltration), with a temporal hypokalemic response to the K_{ATP} inhibitor glibenclamide (glyburide). The daring, off-label use of glibenclamide was presumably instigated by the senior author's observation that cyclosporin activates K_{ATP} channels in vascular smooth muscle.[492] K_{ATP} channels are widely distributed, including in skeletal muscle,[493] such that activation of such channels is indeed a plausible cause of acute hyperkalemia. However, it remains to be seen whether this is a common or important mechanism for acute hyperkalemia.

Finally, β-blockers cause hyperkalemia in part by inhibiting cellular uptake, but also through hyporeninemic hypoaldosteronism induced by effect of these drugs on both renal renin release and adrenal aldosterone release (see discussion of regulation of renal renin and adrenal aldosterone release).

Labetalol, a broadly reactive sympathetic blocker, is a particularly common cause of hyperkalemia in susceptible patients.[16,494] However, both non-specific and cardio-specific β-blockers have been shown to reduce PRA, ANG-II, and aldosterone,[495] such that β-blockade in general will increase susceptibility to hyperkalemia.

Reduced Renal Potassium Excretion

Hypoaldosteronism

Aldosterone promotes kaliuresis by activating apical amiloride-sensitive Na^+ currents in the CNT and CCD and thus increasing the lumen-negative driving force for K^+ excretion (see discussion of control of potassium excretion: aldosterone). Aldosterone release from the adrenal may be reduced by hyporeninemic hypoaldosteronism and its multiple causes, by medications, or due to isolated deficiency of ACTH. The isolated loss in pituitary secretion of ACTH leads to a deficit in circulating cortisol; variable defects in other pituitary hormones are likely secondary to this reduction in cortisol.[496] Concomitant hyporeninemic hypoaldosteronism is frequent,[497] however hyperkalemia is perhaps less common in secondary hypoaldosteronism than in Addison disease.[496]

Primary hypoaldosteronism may be genetic or acquired.[498] The X-linked disorder adrenal hypoplasia congenita (AHC) is caused by loss-of-function mutations in the transcriptional repressor Dax-1. Patients with AHC present with primary adrenal failure and hyperkalemia either shortly after birth or much later in childhood.[499] This bimodal presentation pattern does not appear to be influenced by *Dax-1* genotype; rather, if patients survive the early neonatal period they will then miss being diagnosed until much later in life, presenting either with delayed puberty (see later discussion) or with an adrenal crisis. The steroidogenic factor-1 (SF-1), a functional partner for Dax-1, is also required for adrenal development in both mouse and humans. Both genes are involved in gonadal development, with *Dax-1* deficiency leading to hypogonadotropic hypogonadism[499] and *SF-1* deficiency causing male-to-female sex reversal, in addition to adrenal insufficiency.

Reduced steroidogenesis causes two other important forms of primary hypoaldosteronism.[498] Congenital lipoid adrenal hyperplasia (lipoid CAH) is a severe autosomal recessive syndrome characterized by impaired synthesis of mineralocorticoids, glucocorticoids, and gonadal steroids.[16] Patients present in early infancy with adrenal crisis, including severe hyperkalemia.[500] Genotypically male 46,XY patients with lipoid CAH have female external genitalia, due to the developmental absence of testosterone. Lipoid CAH is caused by loss-of-function mutations in steroidogenic acute regulatory protein, a small mitochondrial protein that helps shuttle cholesterol from the outer to the inner mitochondrial membrane, thus initiating steroidogenesis[501]; some patients may alternatively have mutations in the side-chain cleavage P450 enzyme.[502] The classic, salt-wasting form of congenital adrenal hyperplasia due to 21-hydroxlase deficiency is associated with marked reductions in both cortisol and aldosterone, leading to adrenal insufficiency.[503] Concomitant over-production of androgenic steroids results in virilization in female patients with this form of CAH.

Isolated deficits in aldosterone synthesis with hyperreninemia are caused by loss-of-function mutations in aldosterone synthase, although genetic heterogeneity has recently been reported.[504] Patients typically present in childhood with volume depletion and hyperkalemia.[505] Much like pseudohypoaldosteronism due to loss-of-function mutations in the MR (see later discussion), patients tend to become asymptomatic in adulthood. Acquired hyperreninemic hypoaldosteronism has been described in critical illness,[16] type II diabetes,[506] amyloidosis due to familial Mediterranean fever,[507] and after metastasis of carcinoma to the adrenal gland.[16] Finally, aldosterone synthesis is selectively reduced by heparin, with a 7% incidence of hyperkalemia associated with heparin therapy.[508] Both unfractionated[508] and low-molecular weight[16,509] heparin can cause hyperkalemia. Heparin reduces the adrenal aldosterone response to both ANGII and hyperkalemia, resulting in hyperreninemic hyperaldosteronism. Histological findings in experimental animals include a marked diminution in size of the zona glomerulosa and an attenuated hyperplastic response to salt depletion.[508]

Most primary adrenal insufficiency is due to autoimmunity, either in Addison disease or in the context of a polyglandular endocrinopathy.[498,510] The antiphospholipid syndrome may also cause bilateral adrenal hemorrhage and adrenal insufficiency.[511] Another renal syndrome in which there should be a high index of suspicion for adrenal insufficiency is renal amyloidosis.[512] Finally, HIV has surpassed tuberculosis as the most important infectious cause of adrenal insufficiency. The most common cause of adrenalitis in HIV disease is CMV, however a long list of infectious, degenerative, and infiltrative processes may involve the adrenal glands in these patients.[513] Although the adrenal involvement in HIV is usually subclinical, adrenal insufficiency may be precipitated by stress, drugs such as ketoconazole that inhibit steroidogenesis, or the acute withdrawal of steroid agents such as megestrol.

Contemporary estimates of the risk of hyperkalemia with Addison disease are lacking, however the incidence is likely 50% to 60%.[16] The absence of hyperkalemia in such a high percentage of hypoadrenal patients underscores the importance of aldosterone-independent modulation of K^+ excretion by the distal nephron. A high K^+ diet and high peritubular K^+ serves to increase apical Na^+ reabsorption and K^+ secretion in the CNT and CCD (see discussion on Control of potassium excretion); in most patients with reductions in circulating aldosterone this homeostatic mechanism would appear to be sufficient to regulate serum K^+ to within normal limits.

Hyporeninemic Hypoaldosteronism

Hyporeninemic hypoaldosteronism[514] is a very common predisposing factor in several large, overlapping subsets of hyperkalemic patients; diabetics,[515] the elderly,[16,185,516] and patients with renal insufficiency.[16] Hyporeninemic hypoaldosteronism has also been described in systemic lupus erythematosus (SLE),[517] multiple myeloma,[518] and acute glomerulonephritis.[519] Classically, patients should have suppressed plasma renin activity (PRA) and aldosterone, which cannot be activated by typical maneuvers such as furosemide or sodium restriction.[514] Approximately 50% have an associated acidosis, with a reduced renal excretion of NH_4^+, a positive urinary anion gap, and urine pH <5.5.[159,520] Although the generation of this acidosis is clearly multi-factorial,[521] strong clinical[520,522,523] and experimental[244] evidence suggests that hyperkalemia *per se* is the dominant factor, due to competitive inhibition of NH_4^+ transport in the thick ascending limb and reduced distal excretion of NH_4^+[245] (see also discussion on consequences of hyperkalemia).

Several factors account for the reduced PRA in diabetic patients with hyporeninemic hypoaldosteronism.[515] First, many patients have an associated autonomic neuropathy, with impaired release of renin during orthostatic challenges.[16] Failure to respond to isoproterenol with an increase in PRA, despite an adequate cardiovascular response, suggests a post-receptor defect in the ability of the juxtaglomerular apparatus to respond to β-adrenergic stimuli[16] (see also discussion on regulation of renal renin). Second, the conversion of pro-renin to active renin is impaired in some diabetics,[515] despite adequate release of pro-renin in response to furosemide[16]; this suggests a defect in the normal processing of pro-renin. Third, as is the case with perhaps all patients with hyporeninemic hypoaldosteronism (see later), many diabetic patients appear to be volume expanded, with subsequent suppression of PRA.

The most attractive current hypothesis for the suppression of PRA in hyporeninemic hypoaldosteronism is that primary volume expansion increases circulating atrial natriuretic peptide (ANP), which then exerts a negative effect on both renal renin release and adrenal aldosterone release (see also discussion on regulation of renal renin and adrenal aldosterone). There is evidence that these patients are volume-expanded, and many will respond to either Na^+-Cl^- restriction or to furosemide with an increased PRA (i.e., renin is physiologically rather than pathologically suppressed).[524-526] Patients with hyporeninemic hypoaldosteronism due to a diversity of underlying causes have elevated ANP levels,[16,185,519,525,527] which is also an indicator of their underlying volume expansion. Patients who respond to furosemide with an increase in PRA exhibit a concomitant decrease in ANP.[525] Furthermore, the infusion of exogenous ANP can suppress the adrenal aldosterone response to both hyperkalemia[185] and dietary Na^+-Cl^- depletion.[528]

Acquired Tubular Defects and Potassium Excretion

Unlike hyporeninemic hypoaldosteronism, hyperkalemic distal renal tubular acidosis is associated with a normal or increased aldosterone and/or PRA. Urine pH in these patients is greater than 5.5, and they are unable to increase acid or K^+ excretion in response to furosemide, Na^+-SO_4^{2-}, or fludrocortisone.[529-531] Classic causes include SLE,[529] sickle cell anemia,[16,531] and amylodosis.[16]

Hereditary Tubular Defects and Potassium Excretion

Hereditary tubular causes of hyperkalemia have overlapping clinical features with hypoaldosteronism; hence the shared label "pseudohypoaldosteronism" (PHA). PHA-I has both an autosomal recessive and an autosomal dominant form. The autosomal dominant form is due to loss-of-function mutations in the mineralocorticoid receptor.[532] These patients require aggressive salt supplementation during early childhood; however, similar to the hypoaldosteronism due to mutations in aldosterone synthase, they typically become asymptomatic in adulthood.[349] Of interest, the lifelong increases in circulating aldosterone, ANGII, and renin seen in this syndrome do not appear to have untoward cardiovascular consequences.[532]

The recessive form of PHA-I is caused by various combinations of mutations in all three subunits of ENaC, resulting in impairment in its channel activity.[349] Patients with this syndrome present with severe neonatal salt wasting, hypotension, and hyperkalemia; in contrast to the autosomal dominant form of PHA-I, the syndrome does not improve in adulthood.[349] One unexpected result in the physiological characterization of ENaC was that mice with a targeted deletion of the α-ENaC subunit were found to die within 40 hours of birth due to pulmonary edema.[533] Patients with recessive PHA-I may have pulmonary symptoms, which can occasionally be very severe[534]; however, it appears that, unlike in ENaC-deficient mice, the modest residual activity associated with heteromeric PHA-I channels is generally sufficient to mediate pulmonary Na^+ and fluid clearance in humans with loss-of-function mutations in ENaC.[535] PHA-I has also had a significant impact on the understanding of the biophysical properties of the ENaC channels, since the functional characterization of one specific PHA-I mutation lead to the characterization of a domain in ENaC subunits that determines channel gating.[536]

Pseudohypoaldosteronism type II (PHA-II) (also known as Gordon syndrome and "hereditary hypertension with hyper-

kalemia") is in every respect the "mirror image" of Gitelman syndrome; the clinical phenotype includes hypertension, hyperkalemia, hyperchloremic metabolic acidosis, suppressed PRA and aldosterone, hypercalciuria, and reduced bone density.[537] PHA-II behaves like a gain-of-function in the thiazide-sensitive Na^+-Cl^- cotransporter NCC, and treatment with thiazides typically results in resolution of the entire clinical picture.[537] PHA-II is an extreme form of hyporeninemic hypoaldosteronism due to volume expansion; aggressive salt restriction decreases ANP levels and increases PRA, with resolution of the hypertension, hyperkalemia, and metabolic acidosis.[527] Characterization of the diseases genes for this disorder has also revealed a direct effect of PHA-II on Na^+, Cl^-, and K^+ handling by the distal nephron.

PHA-II is an autosomal dominant syndrome, with as many as three genetic loci.[16] In a landmark paper, mutations in two related serine-threonine kinases were detected in various kindreds with PHA-II.[538] The catalytic sites of these kinases lack specific catalytic lysines conserved in other kinases, hence the designation "WNK" (with no lysine). Whereas PHA-II mutations in WNK4 affect the C-terminus of the coding sequence, large intronic deletions in the WNK1 gene result in increased expression. Both kinases are expressed within the distal nephron, in both DCT and CCD cells; whereas WNK1 localizes to the cytoplasm and basolateral membrane, WNK4 protein is found at the apical tight junctions.[538] WNK1 is also expressed at the basolateral membrane of other epithelial tissues, suggesting a more generalized role in epithelial salt transport.[539] Consistent with the physiological gain-of-function in NCC, WNK4 co-expression inhibits this transporter, and both kinase-dead and disease-associated mutations abolish the effect.[540,541] WNK1 in turn has no effect on NCC, but abrogates the inhibitory effect of WNK4.[542] These observations are consistent with the molecular genetics of PHA-II,[538] suggesting that heterozygous loss-of-function and gain-of-function mutations in WNK4 and WNK1, respectively, cause the disorder. WNK4 reportedly interacts directly with the NCC protein.[540] However, the WNK kinases appear to exert their effect on NCC and other cation-chloride cotransporters via the phosphorylation and activation of the SPAK and OSRI serine/threonine kinases, which in turn phosphorylate the transporter proteins.[543-545]

A unified picture has yet to emerge of the roles of WNK1/4 and associated signaling pathways in the regulation of distal Na^+, Cl^-, and K^+ handling. Analysis is further complicated by the transcriptional complexity of the WNK1 gene, which has at least three separate promoters and a number of alternative splice forms. In particular, the predominant intra-renal WNK1 isoform is generated by a distal nephron transcriptional site that bypasses the N-terminal exons that encode the kinase domain, yielding a kinase-deficient "short" form of the protein.[546] It is however reported that both WNK1[547] and WNK4[548] inhibit ROMK, the secretory K^+ channel; disease-associated mutations in WNK4 increase its inhibitory effect,[548] suggesting a direct inhibition of distal K^+ secretion in PHA-II. WNK4 also increases paracellular Cl^- permeability in transfected epithelial cells, with loss of this effect in cells expressing kinase-dead WNK4 and an augmentation of the effect in cells expressing PHA-II-associated mutations.[549] An increase in paracellular Cl^- permeability in the CNT and CCD is expected to reduce the lumen-negative potential difference; again, this effect of disease-associated mutations in WNK4 is expected to inhibit distal K^+ secretion.

Medication-related Hyperkalemia

Non-Steroidal Anti-Inflammatories

Hyperkalemia is a well-recognized complication of nonsteroidal anti-inflammatories (NSAIDs). NSAIDs cause hyperkalemia by a variety of mechanisms, as would be predicted from the relevant physiology. By decreasing glomerular filtration rate and increasing sodium retention they decrease distal delivery of Na^+ and reduce distal flow rate. Moreover, the flow-activated apical maxi-K channel in the CNT and CCD is activated by prostaglandins,[550] hence NSAIDs will reduce its activity and the flow-dependent component of K^+ excretion.[71,79] NSAIDs are also a classic cause of hyporeninemic hypoaldosteronism.[551,552] The administration of indomethacin to normal volunteers thus attenuates furosemide-induced increases in plasma renin activity (PRA).[175,553] Finally, NSAIDs would not cause hyperkalemia with such regularity if they did not also blunt the adrenal response to hyperkalemia, which is at least partially dependent on prostaglandins acting though prostaglandin EP2 receptors and cyclic-AMP.[184]

The physiology reviewed earlier in this chapter (discussion of regulation of renal renin and adrenal aldosterone) would suggest that COX-2 inhibitors are equally likely to cause hyperkalemia. Indeed, COX-2 inhibitors can clearly cause sodium retention and a decrease in glomerular filtration rate,[554,555] suggesting NSAID-like effects on renal pathophysiology. COX-2-derived prostaglandins stimulate renal renin release[16] and COX-2 inhibitors reduce PRA in both dogs[556] and humans.[175] Salt restriction potentiates the hyperkalemia seen in dogs treated with COX-2 inhibitors,[556] such that hypovolemic patients may be particularly prone to hyperkalemia in this setting. Not surprisingly, clinical reports have begun to emerge of hyperkalemia and acute renal failure associated with COX-2 inhibitors.[16,557,558] Where the data have been reported, circulating PRA or aldosterone (or both) have been reduced in hyperkalemia associated with COX-2 inhibitors.[557,558]

Cyclosporin and Tacrolimus
Both cyclosporin (CsA)[559] and tacrolimus[560] cause hyperkalemia; the risk of sustained hyperkalemia may be higher in renal transplant patients treated with tacrolimus than in those treated with CsA.[561] CsA is perhaps the most versatile of all drugs in the variety of mechanisms whereby it causes hyperkalemia. It causes hyporeninemic hypoaldosteronism[562] due in part to its inhibitory effect on COX-2 expression in the macula densa.[563] CsA inhibits apical SK secretory K^+ channels in the distal nephron,[564] in addition to basolateral Na^+-K^+-APTase.[16] Finally, CsA causes redistribution of K^+ and hyperkalemia, particularly when used in combination with β-blockers.[565] A provocative but preliminary report has linked acute hyperkalemia secondary to CsA to indirect activation of K_{ATP} channels (see also earlier discussion)[491]; this is particularly intriguing given the reported response to K_{ATP} inhibition with glibenclamide infusion.

ENaC Inhibition
Inhibition of apical ENaC activity in the distal nephron by amiloride and other K^+-sparing diuretics predictably results in hyperkalemia. Amiloride is structurally similar to the antibiotics trimethoprim (TMP) and pentamidine, which can also inhibit ENaC.[566-568] Trimethoprim thus inhibits Na^+ reabsorption and K^+ secretion in perfused CCDs.[569] Both TMP/SMX (Bactrim) and pentamidine were reported to cause hyperkalemia during high-dose treatment of *Pneumocystis* pneumonia in HIV patients,[16,568] who are otherwise predisposed to hyperkalemia. However, this side effect is not restricted to high-dose intravenous therapy; in a study of hospitalized patients treated with standard doses of trimethoprim, significant hyperkalemia occurred in greater than 50%, with severe hyperkalemia (>5.5 mmol/l) in 21%.[570] Risk factors for hyperkalemia due to normal-dose TMP include renal insufficiency[570] and hyporeninemic hypoaldosteronism.[571]

Whereas TMP and pentamidine directly inhibit ENaC, a novel, indirect mechanism causing hyperkalemia has recently emerged.[16,572] Aldosterone induces expression of the membrane associated proteases CAP1-3 (see discussion on control of potassium excretion: aldosterone). Nafamostat, a protease inhibitor this widely used in Japan for pancreatitis and other indications, is known to cause hyperkalemia[572]; indirect evidence suggests that the mechanism involves inhibition of amiloride-sensitive Na^+ channels in the CCD.[16] Treatment of rats with nafamostat was also shown to reduce the urinary excretion of CAP1/prostasin, in contrast to the reported effect of aldosterone.[129] Thus inhibition of the protease activity of CAP1, and/or other proteases, by nafamostat appears to abrogate its activating effect on ENaC (Fig. 15–12), and may reduce expression of the protein in the CCD.[573]

ACE Inhibitors, Mineralocorticoid, and Angiotensin Antagonists
Hyperkalemia is a predictable and common effect of both ACE inhibition and antagonism of the mineralocorticoid receptor[16] (Fig. 15–13). ARBs appear to have a

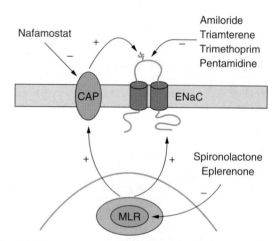

FIGURE 15–12 Pharmacological inhibition of the epithelial Na^+ channel ENaC. Whereas amiloride and related compounds directly inhibit the channel, the protease inhibitor nafamostat inhibits membrane-associated proteases such as CAP1, thus indirectly inhibiting the channel. Spironolactone and related drugs inhibit the mineralocorticoid receptor, thus reducing transcription of the α-subunit of ENaC, the ENaC-activating kinase SGK, and several other target genes (see text for details).

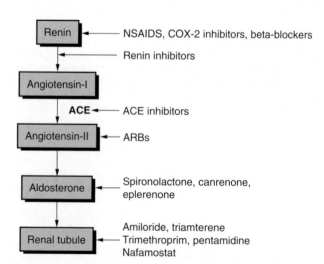

FIGURE 15–13 Medications that target the renin-angiotensin-aldosterone axis are common causes of hyperkalemia, as are drugs that inhibit epithelial Na^+ channels (ENaC) in the renal tubule (CNT or CCD).

lesser effect on plasma K^+ in patients with renal insufficiency.[574] Of note, renin-inhibitors constitute a forthcoming class of agents that also target the renin-angiotensin-aldosterone axis[575]; these drugs are also likely to affect serum K^+. As with many other causes of hyperkalemia, that induced by pharmacological targeting of the rennin-angiotensin-aldosterone axis depends on concomitant inhibition of the adrenal aldosterone release by hyperkalemia; the adrenal release of aldosterone due to increased K^+ is clearly dependent on an intact adrenal renal-angiotensin system, such that this response is abrogated by systemic ACE inhibitors and ARBs[179] (see discussion on regulation of renal renin and adrenal aldosterone release).

The increasing rationale to combine spironolactone with ACE-inhibitors or ARBs,[576,577] along with the emergence of mineralocorticoid receptor antagonists with perhaps a greater potential for hyperkalemia,[578] may magnify the potential for serious hyperkalemia. This is particularly true when higher than recommended doses are utilized.[16] The prevalence of hyperkalemia associated with the combined use of mineralocorticoid receptor antagonists and ACE-inhibitors/ARBs appears to be much higher in clinical practice (~10%)[579] than what has been reported in large clinical trials ($\leq2\%$).[574,577,580] Notably, Juurlink and colleagues studied the correlation between the rate of spironolactone prescription for patients with heart failure on ACE-inhibitors, following the publication of The Randomized Aldactone Evaluation Study (RALES),[577] with hyperkalemia and associated morbidity.[581] This provocative study found an abrupt increase in the rate of prescription for spironolactone after release of RALES, with a temporal correlation to increases in the rate of admissions with hyperkalemia[581]; the association remained statistically significant for admissions where hyperkalemia was the primary diagnosis.[582]

Given the mounting evidence supporting the combined use of ACE-inhibitors, ARBs, and/or mineralocorticoid receptor antagonists, it is prudent to systematically adhere to measures that will minimize the chance of associated hyperkalemia, therefore allowing patients to benefit from the cardiovascular effects of these agents. The patients at risk for the development of hyperkalemia in response to drugs that target the renin-angiotensin-aldosterone axis, singly or in combination therapy, are those in whom the ability of kidneys to excrete the potassium load is markedly diminished due to one or a combination of the following: (1) decreased delivery of sodium to the cortical collecting duct (as in congestive heart failure, volume depletion, etc.), (2) decreased circulating aldosterone (hyporeninemic hypoaldosteronism, drugs such as heparin or ketoconazole, etc.), (3) inhibition of amiloride-sensitive Na^+ channels in the CNT and CCD, by co-administration of TMP/SMX, pentamidine, or amiloride, (4) chronic tubulointerstitial disease, with associated dysfunction of the distal nephron, and (5) increased potassium intake (salt substitutes, diet, etc.). In these susceptible patients, the following approach is recommended to prevent or minimize the occurrence of hyperkalemia in response to medications that interfere with the renin-angiotensin-aldosterone system[583,584]:

A. Estimate glomerular filtration rate using MDRD equation, Cockroft-Gault equation, and/or 24-hour creatinine clearance.

B. Inquire about diet and dietary supplements (e.g., salt substitutes, licorice) and prescribe a low potassium diet.

C. Inquire about medications, particularly those that can interfere with renal K^+ excretion (e.g., NSAIDS, COX-2 inhibitors, K^+-sparing diuretics) and, if appropriate, discontinue these agents.

D. Continue or initiate loop or thiazide-like diuretics.

E. Correct acidosis with sodium bicarbonate.

F. Initiate treatment with a low dose of only one of the agents (i.e., of ACE-inhibitors, ARB, or mineralocorticoid receptor antagonists).

G. Check serum K^+ 3 to 5 days after initiation of the therapy and each dose increment, followed by another measurement one week later.

H. If the serum K^+ is >5.6, ACE-inhibitors, ARBs, and/or mineralocorticoid receptor blockers should be stopped and patient be treated for hyperkalemia.

I. If serum K^+ is increased but <5.6 mmol/L, reduce the dose and reassess the possible contributing factors. If the patient is on a combination of ACE-inhibitors, ARBs, and/or mineralocorticoid receptor blockers, all but one should be stopped and potassium rechecked.

J. A combination of a mineralocorticoid receptor blocker and either an ACE-inhibitor or an ARB should not be prescribed to patients with stage IV or V of chronic kidney disease.

K. The dose of spironolactone in combination with ACE-inhibitors or ARBs should be no more than 25 mg/day.

The Clinical Approach to Hyperkalemia

The first priority in the management of hyperkalemia is to assess the need for emergency treatment (ECG changes, $K^+\geq6.0$ mmol/L). This should be followed by a comprehensive workup to determine the cause (Fig. 15–14). History and physical examination should focus on medications (e.g., angiotensin converting enzyme inhibitors, NSAIDs, trimethoprim/sulfamethoxazole), diet and dietary supplements (e.g., salt substitute), risk factors for kidney failure, reduction in urine output, blood pressure, and volume status. Initial laboratory tests should include electrolytes, BUN, creatinine, serum osmolality, Mg^{2+}, and Ca^{2+}, a complete blood count, and urinary pH, osmolality, creatinine, and electrolytes. Serum and urine osmolality are required for calculation of the transtubular K^+ gradient (see discussion on urinary indices of potassium excretion).

MANAGEMENT OF HYPERKALEMIA*

Indications for the hospitalization of patients with hyperkalemia are poorly defined, in part because there is no universally accepted definition for mild, moderate, or severe hyperkalemia. The clinical sequelae of hyperkalemia, which are primarily cardiac and neuromuscular, depend on many other variables (e.g., plasma calcium level, acid-base status, chronicity), in addition to the absolute value of serum K^+[451,585]; these issues are likely to influence management decisions. Severe hyperkalemia (serum $K^+\geq8.0$ mmol/L), ECG changes other than peaked T waves, acute deterioration of renal function, and the existence of additional medical problems have been suggested as appropriate criteria for hospitalization.[451] However, hyperkalemia in patients with any ECG manifestation should be considered a true medical emergency and treated urgently.[229,449,586] Given the limitations of ECG changes as a predictor of cardiac toxicity (see discussion on consequences of hyperkalemia), patients with severe hyperkalemia ($K^+\geq6$ to 6.5 mmol/L) in the absence of ECG changes should also be aggressively treated.[228,229,449,587,588]

Urgent management of hyperkalemia constitutes a 12-lead electrocardiogram, admission to the hospital, continuous ECG monitoring, and immediate treatment. The management of hyperkalemia is generally divided into three categories: (1) antagonism of the cardiac effects of hyperkalemia, (2) rapid reduction in K^+ by redistribution into cells, and (3) removal of K^+ from the body. The necessary measures to treat the underlying conditions causing hyperkalemia should be

---

*All the recommended doses are for adults.

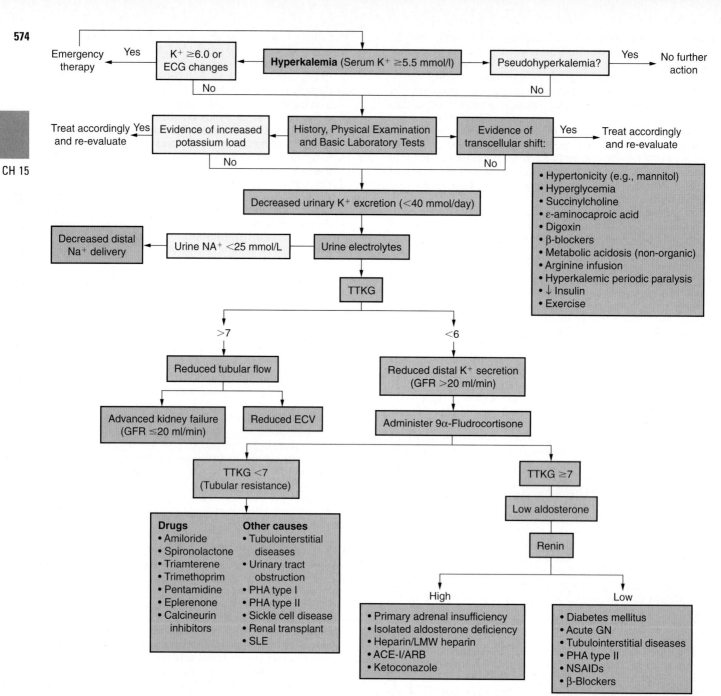

FIGURE 15–14 The diagnostic approach to hyperkalemia. See text for details. ECG: electrocardiogram; TTKG: transtubular potassium gradient; CCD: cortical collecting duct; GFR: glomerular filtration rate; ECV: effective circulatory volume; acute GN: acute glomerulonephritis; HIV: human immunodeficiency virus; NSAIDs: non-steroidal anti-inflammatory drugs; LMW heparin: low molecular weight heparin; ACE-I: angiotensin converting enzyme inhibitor; ARB: angiotensin II receptor blocker; PHA: pseudohypoaldosteronism; SLE: systemic lupus erythematosus.

undertaken to minimize the factors that are contributing to hyperkalemia and to prevent future episodes.[229] Dietary restriction (usually 60 meq/day) with emphasis on K+ content of total parenteral nutrition (TPN) solutions and enteral feeding products (typically 25 to 50 mmol/L) and adjustment of medications and intravenous fluids are necessary; hidden sources of K+, such as intravenous antibiotics, should not be overlooked.[229,589]

Antagonism of Cardiac Effects: Calcium

Intravenous calcium is the first-line drug in the emergency management of hyperkalemia, even for patients with normal calcium levels. The mutually antagonistic effects of calcium and K+ on the myocardium and the protective role of Ca²⁺ in hyperkalemia have long been known.[590] Calcium raises the action potential threshold and reduces excitability, without changing the resting membrane potential.[591] By restoring the difference between resting and threshold potentials, Ca²⁺ reverses the depolarization blockade due to hyperkalemia.[591]

Calcium is available as calcium chloride or calcium gluconate (10 ml ampules of 10% solutions) for intravenous infusion. Each milliliter of 10% calcium gluconate or calcium chloride has 8.9 mg (0.22 mmol) and 27.2 mg (0.68 mmol) of elemental calcium, respectively.[592] Calcium gluconate[593] is less irritating to the veins and can be used through a peripheral intravenous (IV) line; calcium chloride can cause tissue necrosis if it extravasates, and requires a central line. A study of patients undergoing cardiac surgery with extracorporeal perfusion (with concomitant high gluconate infusion) suggested that the increase in the ionized calcium level is significantly lower with calcium gluconate.[594] This finding was attributed to a requirement for hepatic metabolism in the release of ionized calcium from calcium gluconate, such that less ionized calcium would be bioavailable in cases of liver failure or diminished hepatic perfusion.[594] However, further studies in vitro,[595] in animals,[596] in humans with normal hepatic function,[596] and during the anhepatic stage of liver transplantation[597] have shown equal and rapid dissociation of ionized calcium from equal doses of calcium chloride and calcium gluconate, indicating that release of ionized calcium from calcium gluconate is independent of hepatic metabolism.

The recommended dose is 10 mL of 10% calcium gluconate (3 mL to 4 mL of calcium chloride), infused intravenously over 2 to 3 minutes and under continuous ECG monitoring. The effect of the infusion starts in 1 to 3 minutes and lasts 30 to 60 minutes.[456,588] The dose should be repeated if there is no change in ECG findings or if they recur after initial improvement.[456,588] However, calcium should be used with extreme caution in patients taking digoxin, because hypercalcemia potentiates the toxic effects of this drug on the myocardium.[593] In this case, 10 mL of 10% calcium gluconate should be added to 100 mL of 5% dextrose in water and infused over 20 to 30 minutes to avoid hypercalcemia and to allow for an even distribution of calcium in the extracellular compartment.[454,587,591] To prevent the precipitation of calcium carbonate, calcium should not be administered in solutions containing bicarbonate.

Redistribution of K+ into Cells

Sodium bicarbonate, β_2 agonists, and insulin with glucose are all used in the management of hyperkalemia to induce redistribution of K+. Of these treatments, insulin with glucose is the most constant and reliable, whereas bicarbonate is the most controversial. However, these are all temporary measures and should not be substituted for the definitive therapy of hyperkalemia, which is removal of K+ from the body.

Insulin and Glucose
Insulin has the ability to lower serum K+ by shifting K+ into cells, particularly into skeletal myocytes and hepatocytes (see discussion on factors affecting internal distribution). This effect is reliable, reproducible, dose dependent,[456] and effective, even for patients with chronic kidney disease and ESRD[598–600] and in the anhepatic stage of liver transplantation.[601] The effect of insulin on serum K+ is independent of age, of adrenergic activity,[602] and of its hypoglycemic effect, which in fact may be impaired in patients with chronic kidney disease or ESRD.[27,598,603]

Insulin can be administered with glucose as a constant infusion or as a bolus injection.[599,600] The recommended dose for insulin with glucose infusion is 10 units of regular insulin in 500 mL of 10% dextrose, given over 60 minutes (there is no further drop in serum K+ after 90 minutes of insulin infusion[591,602]). However, a bolus injection is easier to administer, particularly under emergency conditions.[229] The recommended dose is 10 units of regular insulin administered intravenously followed immediately by 50 ml of 50% dextrose (25 g of glucose).[586,599,604,605] The effect of insulin on serum K+ begins in 10 to 20 minutes, peaks at 30 to 60 minutes, and lasts for 4 to 6 hours.[456,587,599,606] In almost all patients, the serum K+ drops by 0.5 to 1.2 mmol/L after this treatment.[600,601,605,606] The dose can be repeated as necessary.

Despite glucose administration, hypoglycemia may occur in up to 75% of patients treated with the bolus regimen described above, typically 1 hour after the infusion.[599] The likelihood of hypoglycemia is greater when the dose of glucose given is less than 30 g.[454] To prevent this, infusion of 10% dextrose at 50 ml/hr to 75 ml/hr and close monitoring of the blood glucose is recommended.[586,604] Administration of glucose without insulin is not recommended because the endogenous insulin release may be variable.[485] Glucose in the absence of insulin may in fact increase serum K+ by increasing plasma osmolality.[478,479,604] In hyperglycemic patients with glucose levels of ≥200 to 250 mg/dl, insulin should be administered without glucose and with close monitoring of serum glucose.[591] Combined treatment with β_2-agonists, in addition to their synergism with insulin in lowering serum K+, may reduce the level of hypoglycemia.[599] Of note, the combined regimen may increase the heart rate by 15.1 ± 6.0 beats per minute.[599]

β_2 Adrenergic Agonists
β_2-agonists are an important but under-utilized group of agents for the acute management of hyperkalemia. They exert their effect by activating Na+/K+-ATPase and the NKCC1 Na^+-K^+-$2Cl^-$ cotransporter, shifting K+ into hepatocytes and skeletal myocytes (see also discussion on factors affecting internal distribution). Albuterol (Salbutamol), a selective β_2-agonist, is the most widely studied and used. It is available in oral, inhaled, and intravenous forms; both the intravenous and inhaled or nebulized forms are effective.[607]

The recommended dose for intravenous administration, which is not available in the United States, is 0.5 mg of albuterol in 100 ml of 5% dextrose, given over 10 to 15 minutes.[591,607,608] Its K+-lowering effect starts in few minutes and is maximal at about 30 to 40 minutes,[607,608] lasting for 2 to 6 hours.[454] It reduces serum K+ levels by approximately 0.9 to 1.4 mmol/L.[454]

The recommended dose for inhaled albuterol is 10 to 20 mg of nebulized albuterol in 4 ml of normal saline, inhaled over 10 minutes.[599] (Nebulized levalbuterol is as effective as albuterol.[609]) Its kaliopenic effect starts at about 30 minutes, reaches its peak at about 90 minutes,[599,607] and lasts for 2 to 6 hours.[454,607] Inhaled albuterol reduces serum K+ levels by approximately 0.5 mmol/L to 1.0 mmol/L[454]; albuterol administered by metered-dose inhaler with spacer reduced serum K+ level by approximately 0.4 mmol/L.[610] Albuterol (in inhaled or parenteral form) and insulin with glucose have an additive effect on reducing serum K+ levels, by approximately 1.2 mmol/L to 1.5 mmol/L in total.[454,599,606] However, a subset of patients with ESRD (~20% to 40%) are not responsive to the K+-lowering effect of albuterol ($\Delta K \leq 0.4$ mmol/L); albuterol (or other β_2-agonists) should not be used as a single agent in the management of hyperkalemia.[456,485] In an attempt to reduce pharmacokinetic variability, a recent study tested the effects of "weight-based dosing" on serum K+ levels, using 7 μg/kg of subcutaneous terbutaline (a β_2-agonist) in a group of ESRD patients.[611] The results showed a significant decline in serum K+ levels in almost all patients (mean 1.31 mmol/L $\pm$ 0.5 mmol/L, range 0.5 mmol/L to 2.3 mmol/L) in 30 to 90 minutes; of note, heart rate increased by an average of 25.8 ± 10.5 beats per minute (range 6.5 to 48).[611]

Treatment with albuterol may result in an increase in serum glucose (~2 mmol/L to 3 mmol/L) and heart rate. The increase in heart rate is more pronounced with the intravenous form (~20 beats per minute) than with the inhaled form (~6 to 10 beats per minute).[485,607] There is no significant increase in systolic or diastolic blood pressure with nebulized or intravenous administration of albuterol.[607] However, it is prudent to use these agents with extreme caution in patients with ischemic heart disease.[454]

Sodium Bicarbonate

Bicarbonate prevailed as a preferred treatment modality of hyperkalemia for decades. For example, in a survey of nephrology-training program directors in 1989, it was ranked as the second-line treatment, after Ca^{2+}.[612] Its use to manage acute hyperkalemia was mainly based on small older uncontrolled clinical studies with a very limited number of patients,[54,63,613] in which bicarbonate was typically administered as a long infusion over many hours (contrary to IV push, which later became the routine).[614] One of these studies, which is frequently quoted, concluded that the K^+-lowering effect of bicarbonate is independent of changes in pH.[63] However, confounding variables included the duration of infusion, the use of glucose-containing solutions, and infrequent monitoring of serum K^+.[63,615]

The role of bicarbonate in the acute management of hyperkalemia has been challenged.[600,614,616] Blumberg and colleagues compared different K^+-lowering modalities (Fig. 15–15) and showed that bicarbonate infusion (isotonic or hypertonic) for up to 60 minutes had no effect on serum K^+ in their cohort of ESRD patients on hemodialysis.[600] These observations were later confirmed by others, who failed to show any acute (60 to 120 minutes) K^+-lowering effects for bicarbonate.[614–616]

A few studies have shown that metabolic acidosis may attenuate the physiologic responses to insulin and β_2 agonists.[456,616] The combined effect of bicarbonate and insulin with glucose has been studied, with conflicting results.[616] In addition, bicarbonate and albuterol co-administration failed to show any additional benefit over albuterol alone.[616]

In summary, it appears that bicarbonate administration, especially as a single agent, has no role in the acute management of hyperkalemia. It also may reduce serum ionized calcium levels and cause volume overload, issues of relevance in patients with renal failure.[456,587] The acute effect of bicarbonate infusion on serum K^+ levels in severely acidemic patients is not clear; however, it may be of some benefit in this setting, particularly if acidemia is judged to require bicarbonate.[229,586]

Removal of Potassium

Diuretics

Diuretics have a relatively modest effect on urinary K^+ excretion in patients with chronic kidney disease,[617] particularly in an acute setting.[588] However, these medications are useful in correcting hyperkalemia in patients with the syndrome of hyporeninemic hypoaldosteronism,[618] and selective renal K^+ secretory problems (e.g., after transplantation or administration of trimethoprim).[619,620] In patients with impaired renal function, use of the following agents is recommended: (1) oral diuretics with the highest bioavailability (e.g., torsemide) and the least renal metabolism (e.g., torsemide, bumetanide) in order to minimize the chance of accumulation and toxicity, (2) intravenous agents (short-term treatment) with the least hepatic metabolism (e.g., furosemide rather than bumetanide), (3) combinations of loop and thiazide-like diuretics for better efficacy, although this may decrease glomerular filtration rate due to activation of tubuloglomerular feedback,[621] (4) the maximal effective "ceiling" dose.[617,621]

Mineralocorticoids

Limited data are available on the role of mineralocortoids in the management of acute hyperkalemia.[519,622] However, these agents may be useful in managing chronic hyperkalemia in patients with hypoaldosteronism with or without hyporeninism, those with systemic lupus erythematosus,[623] kidney transplant patients on cyclosporine,[624] and ESRD patients on hemodialysis with interdialytic hyperkalemia.[625,626] A recent study, powered to detect a 0.7 mmol/L reduction in serum K^+, examined the effect of 0.1 mg/day of fludrocortisone in patients on chronic hemodialysis; this showed a non-significant reduction in serum K^+ in the treated group (4.8±0.5 mmol/L) vs the control group (5.2±0.7 mmol/L).[627] The recommended dose is 0.1 mg/day to 0.3 mg/day of fludrocortisone, a synthetic glucocorticoid with potent mineralocorticoid activity and moderate glucocorticoid activity (0.3 mg of fludrocortisone is equal to 1 mg of prednisone with regard to glucocorticoid activity).[519,624–626] In patients with ESRD on hemodialysis, this regimen reduces serum K^+ by 0.5 mmol/L to 0.7 mmol/L and has not been associated with significant changes in blood pressure or weight (i.e., surrogate for fluid retention).[625] Overall, the available data are limited for the use of fludrocortisone in hyperkalemia, and close monitoring of blood pressure and weight after initiation of these medications is prudent, especially in non-ESRD patients.

Cation-Exchange Resins

Ion-exchange resins are cross-linked polymers containing acidic or basic structural units that can exchange either anions or cations on contact with a solution. They are capable of binding to a variety of mono- and divalent cations. Cation-exchange resins are classified based on the cation (i.e., hydrogen, ammonium, sodium, potassium, or calcium) that is cycled during the synthesis of the resin to saturate sulfonic or carboxylic groups. Elkinton and colleagues in 1950 successfully used a carboxylic resin in ammonium cycle in three patients with hyperkalemia.[628] However, hydrogen- or ammonium-cycled resins were associated with metabolic acidosis[629] and mouth ulcers,[630] making the sodium-cycled resins preferable. Sodium-cycled resins were associated with volume overload in some cases.[629] Calcium-cycled resins may have other potential benefits, including a phosphate-lowering effect; however, this requires large, potentially toxic, doses of resin.[631] Moreover, these resins have been associated with hypercalcemia.[632]

Sodium polystyrene sulfonate (SPS, Kayexalate) exchanges Na^+ for K^+ in the gastrointestinal tract, mainly in the

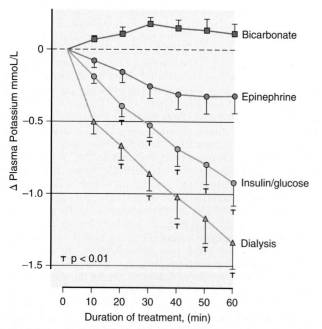

FIGURE 15–15 Changes in serum K^+ during intravenous infusion of bicarbonate, epinephrine, or insulin in glucose, and during hemodialysis. (From Blumberg A, Weidmann P, Shaw S, Gnadinger M: Effect of various therapeutic approaches on plasma potassium and major regulating factors in terminal renal failure. Am J Med 85:507–512, 1988.)

colon[586,630,633] and has been shown to increase the fecal excretion of K+.[630] To prevent constipation and to facilitate the passage of the resin through the gastrointestinal tract, Flinn and co-workers added sorbitol to the resin.[634]

The current recommended dose is 15 to 30 grams of powder in water or preferably 70% sorbitol one to four times a day. A ready-made suspension is also available as 15 g of SPS per 60 ml of suspension. Its effect on K+ is slow, and the full effect may take up to 4 to 24 hours.[587,588] Thus it should be used only in conjunction with other measures in the management of acute hyperkalemia. Each gram of resin binds 0.5 to 1.2 mEq of K+ in exchange for 2 to 3 mEq of Na+.[588,630,635,636] The discrepancy is caused in part by the binding of small amounts of other cations.[630]

The role of resins and their effect on potassium has recently been re-examined. One study of healthy subjects compared the rate of fecal excretion of K+ by different laxatives with or without resin (SPS) and found that the combination of phenolphthalein/docusate with resin produced greater fecal excretion of K+ (49 mmol in 12 hours) than did phenolphthalein/docusate alone (37 mmol in 12 hours) or other laxative-resin combinations.[635] Earlier studies, mostly before the era of chronic hemodialysis, used multiple doses of the exchange resin orally or rectally as an enema and were associated with declines in serum K+ of 1 mEq per liter and 0.8 mEq per liter in 24 hours, respectively.[630] However, with the advent of chronic hemodialysis, it has become common to order only a single dose of resin-cathartic in the management of acute hyperkalemia. A recent study has questioned the efficacy of this practice, evaluating the effect of four single-dose resin-cathartic regimens on serum K+ levels of six patients with chronic kidney disease on maintenance hemodialysis; none of the regimens used reduced the serum K+ below the initial baseline.[636] Notably, the subjects in this study were normokalemic. However, when dialysis is not immediately feasible or appropriate, repeated doses of Kayexalate may be required for an adequate effect.

Kayexalate can be administered rectally as a retention enema in patients unable to take or tolerate the oral form. The recommended dose is 30 to 50 grams of resin as an emulsion in 100 mL of an aqueous vehicle every 6 hours. It should be administered warm (body temperature), after a cleansing enema with body-temperature tap water, through a rubber tube placed at about 20 cm from the rectum with the tip well into the sigmoid colon. The emulsion should be introduced by gravity, flushed with an additional 50 ml to 100 ml of non-sodium-containing fluid, retained for at least 30 to 60 minutes, and followed by a cleansing enema (250 ml to 1000 ml of body-temperature tap water).[637] We do not recommend using emulsion in sorbitol because multiple cases of colonic necrosis secondary to SPS-sorbitol have been attributed to the sorbitol.[588,638]

Ischemic colitis and colonic necrosis are the most serious complications of SPS[638,639]; they are more common with the enema form, and have been attributed to the sorbitol content.[638] However, in at least some of these cases, the enemas, including the pre-administration and post administration cleansing enemas, were not administered as recommended by the manufacturer, which might have been protective.[637] The actual incidence of colonic necrosis following Kayexalate enemas is unknown. In a retrospective study by Gerstman and colleagues, the overall incidence was 0.27%, whereas postoperative incidence was higher (1.8%).[640] The incidence in transplant patients has been estimated at about 1%.[641] Postoperative ileus and the direct toxic effect of sorbitol have been suggested as potential cofactors for necrosis. This complication can also occur with oral administration of SPS in sorbitol, although the incidence tends to be much lower, and can affect both the upper and the lower gastrointestinal tract.[640–642] A case of colonic necrosis following oral SPS

(without sorbitol) was reported.[643] Other potential complications, although rare, include reduction of serum calcium,[644] volume overload,[629] interference with lithium absorption,[645] and iatrogenic hypokalemia.[637]

Dialysis

All modes of acute renal replacement therapies are effective in removing K+. Continuous hemodiafiltration is increasingly used in the management of critically ill and hemodynamically unstable patients.[646] Peritoneal dialysis, although not very effective in an acute setting, has been utilized effectively in cardiac arrest complicating acute hyperkalemia.[647] Peritoneal dialysis is capable of removing significant amounts of K+ (5 mmol/hour or 240 mmol in 48 hours) using 2-liter exchanges, with each exchange taking almost an hour.[591] However, hemodialysis is the preferred mode when rapid correction of a hyperkalemic episode is desired.[648]

An average 3- to 5-hour hemodialysis session removes approximately 40 mmol to 120 mmol of K+.[648–656] Approximately 15% of the total K+ removal results from ultrafiltration, with the remaining clearance from dialysis.[652,657] Of the total K+ removed, about 40% is from extracellular space, and the remainder is from intracellular compartments.[650,652,653] In most patients, the greatest decline in serum K+ (1.2 mmol/l to 1.5 mmol/l) and the largest amount of K+ removed occur during the first hour; the serum K+ usually reaches its nadir at about 3 hours. Despite a relatively constant serum K+, K+ removal continues until the end of the hemodialysis session, although at significantly lower rate.[651,652,656]

The amount of K+ removed depends primarily on the type and surface area of the dialyzer used, blood flow rate, dialysate flow rate, dialysis duration, and serum to dialysate K+ gradient. However, about 40% of the difference in removal cannot be explained by the previously mentioned factors, and may instead be related to the relative distribution of K+ between intracellular and extracellular spaces.[650] Glucose-free dialysates are more efficient in removing K+.[650,653] This effect may be caused by alterations in endogenous insulin levels, with concomitant intracellular shift of K+; the insulin level is 50% lower when glucose-free dialysates are utilized.[650] Furthermore, these findings imply that K+ removal may be greater if hemodialysis is performed in a fasting state.[657] Treatment with β2-agonists also reduces the total K+ removal, by approximately 40%.[648] The change in pH during dialysis has been thought to have no significant effect on K+ removal.[648,657] A recent study evaluated this issue in detail, examining the effect of dialysate bicarbonate concentration on both serum K+ and K+ removal. Dialysates with bicarbonate concentration of 39 mmol/L (high), 35 mmol/L (standard), and 27 mmol/L (low) were utilized. The use of high concentration of bicarbonate was associated with a more rapid decline in serum K+; this was statistically significant for high vs both standard and low bicarbonate dialysates, at 60 and 240 minutes. However, the total amount of K+ removed was higher with the low bicarbonate dialysate (116.4±21.6 mmol/dialysis) in comparison to standard (73.2±12.8 mmol/dialysis) and high (80.9±15.4 mmol/dialysis) bicarbonate dialysates; all statistically not significant.[658] Therefore, whereas high-bicarbonate dialysis may *acutely* have a more rapid effect on serum K+, this advantage is potentially mitigated by a lesser total removal of the ion over the course of a typical treatment session.

One of the major determinants of total K+ removal is the K+ gradient between the serum and dialysate. Dialysates with a lower K+ concentration are more effective at reducing serum K+.[651,655] However, a rapid decline in the level of serum K+ can be of concern. An acute decrease in serum K+ can be associated with rebound hypertension (i.e., a significant increase in blood pressure 1 hour after dialysis),[649] which is attributed in part to the peripheral vasoconstriction that is a direct result of the change in serum K[+].[649] On the other hand, a low serum K[+] can alter the rate of tissue metabolism—the so-called Solandt effect[659]—and decrease tissue oxygen consumption, promoting arteriolar constriction.[649] This vasoconstriction, in turn, may reduce the efficiency of dialysis[660]; a randomized, prospective study did not, however, confirm this finding.[651] The difference may have been due to the glucose content of the dialysate (i.e., 200 mg/dL in the former and zero in the latter study); the glucose can increase the insulin level and thereby muscle blood flow.[661] This effect can later be attenuated by a rapid decline in serum K[+].[651]

Several studies have found an increased incidence of significant arrhythmia with hemodialysis, occurring during or immediately after treatment[662-664]; an incidence of up to 76% has been reported.[665] However, many investigators do not consider the hemodialysis procedure to be significantly arrhythmogenic.[666-668] Some have suggested that a relationship exists between decreases in K[+], dialysate K[+], and the incidence of significant arrhythmias.[662] Despite the controversy, it seems prudent to recommend that dialysates with a very low K[+] (0 mmol/L or 1 mmol/L) be used cautiously, particularly in high-risk patients. This definition includes those patients receiving digoxin; those with a history of arrhythmia, coronary artery disease, left ventricular hypertrophy, or high systolic blood pressure; and those of an advanced age. Continuous cardiac monitoring for all patients dialyzed against a 0 mmol/L or 1 mmol/L K[+] bath is recommended.[456] To minimize the risk of the previously mentioned complications without significantly affecting dialytic efficacy, we recommend the use of a graded reduction in the dialysate K[+] concentration, particularly in high-risk patients.[456,669] For example in a patient with a serum K[+] of 8.5 mmol/L we initiate dialysis with a 4 mmol/L K[+] dialysate and reduce the K[+] concentration of the dialysate over the course of the dialysis treatment, by 1 mmol/L every hour to a final K[+] concentration of 1 mmol/L. However, for those hyperkalemic patients with life-threatening arrhythmias (sinus bradycardia, sinus arrest, slow idioventricular rhythms, ventricular tachycardia, ventricular fibrillation, and asystole[227,229]), initiation with a low-K[+] dialysate may be appropriate, followed by a graded approach once the acute arrhythmia has resolved.

A rebound increase in serum K[+] can occur after hemodialysis. This phenomenon can be especially marked in cases of massive release from devitalized tissues (e.g., tumor lysis, rhabdomyolysis), requiring frequent monitoring of serum K[+] and further hemodialysis. However, a rebound increase may also occur in ESRD patients during regular maintenance hemodialysis, despite technically adequate treatment,[652] particularly in those patients with a high pre-dialysis K[+]. Factors attenuating K[+] removal and thus increasing the risk and magnitude of postdialysis rebound include; pretreatment with β2-agonists[648]; pretreatment with insulin and glucose, eating early during the dialysis treatment[657]; a high pre-dialysis serum K[+] [652]; and higher dialysate Na[+] concentrations.[654]

References

1. Warnock DG, Bubien JK: Liddle's syndrome: A public health menace? Am J Kidney Dis 25:924–927, 1995.
1a. Giebisch G, Krapf R, Wagner C: Renal and extrarenal regulation of potassium. Kidney Int 72:397–410, 2007
2. McDonough AA, Thompson CB, Youn JH: Skeletal muscle regulates extracellular potassium. Am J Physiol Renal Physiol 282:F967–974, 2002.
3. Williams ME, Rosa RM, Silva P, et al: Impairment of extrarenal potassium disposal by alpha-adrenergic stimulation. N Engl J Med 311:145–149, 1984.
4. Rosa RM, Epstein FH: Extrarenal potassium metabolism. In Seldin DW, Giebisch G (eds): The Kidney: Physiology and Pathophysiology, Vol 2. Philadelphia, Lippincott Williams & Wilkins, 2000, pp 1552–1573.
5. Knochel JP, Dotin LN, Hamburger RJ: Pathophysiology of intense physical conditioning in a hot climate. I. Mechanisms of potassium depletion. J Clin Invest 51:242–255, 1972.
6. Chen P, Guzman JP, Leong PK, et al: Modest dietary K[+] restriction provokes insulin resistance of cellular K[+] uptake and phosphorylation of renal outer medulla K[+] channel without fall in plasma K[+] concentration. Am J Physiol Cell Physiol 290:C1355–1363, 2006.
7. Therien AG, Blostein R: Mechanisms of sodium pump regulation. Am J Physiol Cell Physiol 279:C541–566, 2000.
8. Lingrel JB, Croyle ML, Woo AL, Arguello JM: Ligand binding sites of Na,K-ATPase. Acta Physiol Scand Suppl 643:69–77, 1998.
9. McDonough AA: Significance of sodium pump isoforms in digitalis therapy. J Mol Cell Cardiol 27:1001–1009, 1995.
10. Crambert G, Hasler U, Beggah AT, et al: Transport and pharmacological properties of nine different human Na, K-ATPase isozymes. J Biol Chem 275:1976–1986, 2000.
11. James PF, Grupp IL, Grupp G, et al: Identification of a specific role for the Na,K-ATPase alpha 2 isoform as a regulator of calcium in the heart. Mol Cell 3:555–563, 1999.
12. Dostanic I, Paul RJ, Lorenz JN, et al: The alpha2-isoform of Na-K-ATPase mediates ouabain-induced hypertension in mice and increased vascular contractility in vitro. Am J Physiol Heart Circ Physiol 288:H477–485, 2005.
13. Dostanic-Larson I, Van Huysse JW, Lorenz JN, Lingrel JB: The highly conserved cardiac glycoside binding site of Na,K-ATPase plays a role in blood pressure regulation. Proc Natl Acad Sci U S A 102:15845–15850, 2005.
14. Akimova O, Tremblay J, Hamet P, Orlov SN: The Na(+)/K(+)-ATPase as [K(+)](o) sensor: Role in cardiovascular disease pathogenesis and augmented production of endogenous cardiotonic steroids. Pathophysiology 13:209–216, 2006.
15. Juel C, Pilegaard H, Nielsen JJ, Bangsbo J: Interstitial K(+) in human skeletal muscle during and after dynamic graded exercise determined by microdialysis. Am J Physiol Regul Integr Comp Physiol 278:R400–406, 2000.
16. Mount DB, Zandi-Nejad K: Disorders of potassium balance. In Brenner BM (ed): Brenner and Rector's The Kidney. Philadelphia, WB Saunders, 2004, pp 997–1040.
17. Clausen T: Clinical and therapeutic significance of the Na[+],K[+] pump*. Clin Sci (Lond) 95:3–17, 1998.
18. Bundgaard H, Schmidt TA, Larsen JS, Kjeldsen K: K[+] supplementation increases muscle [Na[+]-K[+]-ATPase] and improves extrarenal K[+] homeostasis in rats. J Appl Physiol 82:1136–1144, 1997.
19. McKenna MJ: Effects of training on potassium homeostasis during exercise. J Mol Cell Cardiol 27:941–949, 1995.
20. Nielsen JJ, Mohr M, Klarskov C, et al: Effects of high-intensity intermittent training on potassium kinetics and performance in human skeletal muscle. J Physiol 554:857–870, 2004.
21. Hebert SC, Mount DB, Gamba G: Molecular physiology of cation-coupled Cl- cotransport: The SLC12 family. Pflugers Arch 447 580–593, 2004.
22. Mount DB, Gamba G: Renal K-Cl cotransporters. Curr Opin Nephrol Hypertens 10:685–692, 2001.
23. Yellen G: The voltage-gated potassium channels and their relatives. Nature 419:35–42, 2002.
24. Lesage F, Lazdunski M: Molecular and functional properties of two-pore-domain potassium channels. Am J Physiol Renal Physiol 279:F793–801, 2000.
25. Reimann F, Ashcroft FM: Inwardly rectifying potassium channels. Curr Opin Cell Biol 11:503–508, 1999.
26. Briggs AP, Koechig I, Doisy EA, Weber CJ: Some changes in the composition of blood due to the injection of insulin. J Biol Chem 58:721–730, 1924.
27. Ferrannini E, Taddei S, Santoro D, et al: Independent stimulation of glucose metabolism and Na[+]-K[+] exchange by insulin in the human forearm. Am J Physiol 255:E953–958, 1988.
28. Rossetti L, Klein-Robbenhaar G, Giebisch G, et al: Effect of insulin on renal potassium metabolism. Am J Physiol 252:F60–64, 1987.
29. Dluhy RG, Axelrod L, Williams GH: Serum immunoreactive insulin and growth hormone response to potassium infusion in normal man. J Appl Physiol 33:22–26, 1972.
30. DeFronzo RA, Sherwin RS, Dillingham M, et al: Influence of basal insulin and glucagon secretion on potassium and sodium metabolism. Studies with somatostatin in normal dogs and in normal and diabetic human beings. J Clin Invest 61:472–479, 1978.
31. DeFronzo RA, Felig P, Ferrannini E, Wahren J: Effect of graded doses of insulin on splanchnic and peripheral potassium metabolism in man. Am J Physiol 238:E421–427, 1980.
32. Clausen T, Everts ME: Regulation of the Na,K-pump in skeletal muscle. Kidney Int 35:1–13, 1989.
33. Rosic NK, Standaert ML, Pollet RJ: The mechanism of insulin stimulation of (Na[+],K[+])-ATPase transport activity in muscle. J Biol Chem 260:6206–6212, 1985.
34. Li D, Sweeney G, Wang Q, Klip A: Participation of PI3K and atypical PKC in Na[+]-K[+]-pump stimulation by IGF-I in VSMC. Am J Physiol 276:H2109–2116, 1999.
35. Al-Khalili L, Yu M, Chibalin AV: Na(+),K(+)-ATPase trafficking in skeletal muscle: Insulin stimulates translocation of both alpha(1)- and alpha(2)-subunit isoforms. FEBS Lett 536 198–202, 2003.
36. Yudowski GA, Efendiev R, Pedemonte CH, et al: Phosphoinositide-3 kinase binds to a proline-rich motif in the Na[+], K[+]-ATPase alpha subunit and regulates its trafficking. Proc Natl Acad Sci U S A 97:6556–6561, 2000.
37. Feraille E, Carranza ML, Gonin S, et al: Insulin-induced stimulation of Na[+],K[+]-ATPase activity in kidney proximal tubule cells depends on phosphorylation of the alpha-subunit at Tyr-10. Mol Biol Cell 10:2847–2859, 1999.
38. Choi CS, Thompson CB, Leong PK, et al: Short-term K(+) deprivation provokes insulin resistance of cellular K(+) uptake revealed with the K(+) clamp. Am J Physiol Renal Physiol 280:F95–F102, 2001.
39. Clausen T, Flatman JA: Effects of insulin and epinephrine on Na[+]-K[+] and glucose transport in soleus muscle. Am J Physiol 252:E492–499, 1987.
40. Sargeant RJ, Liu Z, Klip A: Action of insulin on Na(+)-K(+)-ATPase and the Na(+)-K(+)-2Cl- cotransporter in 3T3-L1 adipocytes. Am J Physiol 269:C217–225, 1995.

41. Weil-Maslansky E, Gutman Y, Sasson S: Insulin activates furosemide-sensitive K⁺ and Cl- uptake system in BC3H1 cells. Am J Physiol 267:C932–939, 1994.

42. D'Silva JL: The action of adrenaline on serum potassium. J Physiol 82:393–398, 1934.

43. Reid JL, Whyte KF, Struthers AD: Epinephrine-induced hypokalemia: The role of beta adrenoceptors. Am J Cardiol 57:23F-27F, 1986.

44. Brown MJ, Brown DC, Murphy MB: Hypokalemia from beta2-receptor stimulation by circulating epinephrine. N Engl J Med 309:1414–1419, 1983.

45. Pettit GW, Vick RL: An analysis of the contribution of the endocrine pancreas to the kalemotropic actions of catecholamines. J Pharmacol Exp Ther 190:234–242, 1974.

46. Olsson AM, Persson S, Schoder R: Effects of terbutaline and isoproterenol on hyperkalemia in nephrectomized rabbits. Scand J Urol Nephrol 12:35–38, 1978.

47. Ballanyi K, Grafe P: Changes in intracellular ion activities induced by adrenaline in human and rat skeletal muscle. Pflugers Arch 411:283–288, 1988.

48. Scheid CR, Fay FS: Beta-adrenergic stimulation of 42K influx in isolated smooth muscle cells. Am J Physiol 246:C415–421, 1984.

49. Gosmanov AR, Wong JA, Thomason DB: Duality of G protein-coupled mechanisms for beta-adrenergic activation of NKCC activity in skeletal muscle. Am J Physiol Cell Physiol 283:C1025–1032, 2002.

50. Williams ME, Gervino EV, Rosa RM, et al: Catecholamine modulation of rapid potassium shifts during exercise. N Engl J Med 312:823–827, 1985.

51. Fenn WO, Cobb DM: The potassium equilibrium in muscle. J Gen Physiol 17:629–656, 1934.

52. Simmons DH, Avedon M: Acid-base alterations and plasma potassium concentration. Am J Physiol 197:319–326, 1959.

53. Adrogue HJ, Madias NE: Changes in plasma potassium concentration during acute acid-base disturbances. Am J Med 71:456–467, 1981.

54. Burnell JM, Villamill MF, Uyeno BT, Scribner BH: The effect in humans of extracellular PH change on the relationship between serum potassium concentration and intracellular potassium. J Clin Invest 35:935–939, 1956.

55. Oster JR, Perez G, Castro A, Vaamonde CA: Plasma potassium response to acute metabolic acidosis induced by mineral and nonmineral acids. Miner Electrolyte Metab 4:28–36, 1980.

56. Abrams WB, Lewis DW, Bellet S: The effect of acidosis and alkalosis on the plasma potassium concentration and the electrocardiogram of normal and potssium depleted dogs. Am J Med Sci 222:506–515, 1951.

57. Fulop M: Serum potassium in lactic acidosis and ketoacidosis. N Engl J Med 300:1087–1089, 1979.

58. Orringer CE, Eustace JC, Wunsch CD, Gardner LB: Natural history of lactic acidosis after grand-mal seizures A model for the study of an anion-gap acidosis not associated with hyperkalemia. N Engl J Med 297:796–799, 1977.

59. Wiederseiner JM, Muser J, Lutz T, et al: Acute metabolic acidosis: Characterization and diagnosis of the disorder and the plasma potassium response. J Am Soc Nephrol 15:1589–1596, 2004.

60. Adrogue HJ, Madias NE: PCO₂ and [K⁺]p in metabolic acidosis: Certainty for the first and uncertainty for the other. J Am Soc Nephrol 15:1667–1668, 2004.

61. Sonikian MA, Pani IT, Iliopolous AN, et al: Metabolic acidosis aggravation and hyperkaliemia in hemodialysis patients treated by sevelamer hydrochloride. Ren Fail 27:143–147, 2005.

62. Sonikian M, Metaxaki P, Vlassopoulos D, et al: Long-term management of sevelamer hydrochloride-induced metabolic acidosis aggravation and hyperkalemia in hemodialysis patients. Ren Fail 28:411–418, 2006.

63. Fraley DS, Adler S: Correction of hyperkalemia by bicarbonate despite constant blood pH. Kidney Int 12:354–360, 1977.

64. Krapf R, Caduff P, Wagdi P, et al: Plasma potassium response to acute respiratory alkalosis. Kidney Int 47:217–224, 1995.

65. Natalini G, Serramondi V, Fassini P, et al: Acute respiratory acidosis does not increase plasma potassium in normokalaemic anaesthetized patients. A controlled randomized trial. Eur J Anaesthesiol 18:394–400, 2001.

66. Malnic G, Klose RM, Giebisch G: Micropuncture study of renal potassium excretion in the rat. Am J Physiol 206:674–686, 1964.

67. Canessa CM, Schild L, Buell G, et al: Amiloride-sensitive epithelial Na⁺ channel is made of three homologous subunits. Nature 367:463–467, 1994.

68. Giebisch G: Renal potassium transport: Mechanisms and regulation. Am J Physiol 274:F817–833, 1998.

69. Muto S: Potassium transport in the mammalian collecting duct. Physiol Rev 81:85–116, 2001.

70. Stokes JB: Potassium secretion by cortical collecting tubule: Relation to sodium absorption, luminal sodium concentration, and transepithelial voltage. Am J Physiol 241:F395–402, 1981.

71. Pluznick JL, Sansom SC: BK channels in the kidney: Role in K⁺ secretion and localization of molecular components. Am J Physiol Renal Physiol 291:F517–529, 2006.

72. Frindt G, Palmer LG: Apical potassium channels in the rat connecting tubule. Am J Physiol Renal Physiol 287:F1030–1037, 2004.

73. Lu M, Wang T, Yan Q, et al: Absence of small conductance K⁺ channel (SK) activity in apical membranes of thick ascending limb and cortical collecting duct in ROMK (Bartter's) knockout mice. J Biol Chem 277:37881–37887, 2002.

74. Palmer LG, Choe H, Frindt GL: Is the secretory K channel in the rat CCT ROMK? Am J Physiol 273:F404–410, 1997.

75. Xu JZ, Hall AE, Peterson LN, et al: Localization of the ROMK protein on apical membranes of rat kidney nephron segments. Am J Physiol 273:F739–F748, 1997.

76. Bailey MA, Cantone A, Yan Q, et al: Maxi-K channels contribute to urinary potassium excretion in the ROMK-deficient mouse model of Type II Bartter's syndrome and in adaptation to a high-K diet. Kidney Int 70:51–59, 2006.

77. Giebisch GH: A trail of research on potassium. Kidney Int 62:1498–1512, 2002.

78. Giebisch G: Renal potassium channels: Function, regulation, and structure. Kidney Int 60:436–445, 2001.

79. Woda CB, Bragin A, Kleyman TR, Satlin LM: Flow-dependent K⁺ secretion in the cortical collecting duct is mediated by a maxi-K channel. Am J Physiol Renal Physiol 280:F786–793, 2001.

80. Gamper N, Fillon S, Feng Y, et al: K(⁺) channel activation by all three isoforms of serum- and glucocorticoid-dependent protein kinase SGK. Pflugers Arch 445:60–66, 2002.

81. Zheng W, Verlander VW, Lynch IJ, et al: Cellular distribution of the potassium channel, KCNQ1, in normal mouse kidney. Am J Physiol Renal Physiol 292:F456–F466, 2006.

82. Amorim JB, Bailey MA, Musa-Aziz R, et al: Role of luminal anion and pH in distal tubule potassium secretion. Am J Physiol Renal Physiol 284:F381–388, 2003.

83. Ellison DH, Velazquez H, Wright FS: Unidirectional potassium fluxes in renal distal tubule: Effects of chloride and barium. Am J Physiol 250:F885–894, 1986.

84. Carlisle EJ, Donnelly SM, Ethier JH, et al: Modulation of the secretion of potassium by accompanying anions in humans. Kidney Int 39:1206–1212, 1991.

85. Wingo CS: Reversible chloride-dependent potassium flux across the rabbit cortical collecting tubule. Am J Physiol 256:F697–704, 1989.

86. Schafer JA, Troutman SL: Potassium transport in cortical collecting tubules from mineralocorticoid-treated rat. Am J Physiol 253:F76–88, 1987.

87. Zhou X, Xia SL, Wingo CS: Chloride transport by the rabbit cortical collecting duct: Dependence on H,K-ATPase. J Am Soc Nephrol 9:2194–21202, 1998.

88. Wingo CS, Armitage FE: Rubidium absorption and proton secretion by rabbit outer medullary collecting duct via H-K-ATPase. Am J Physiol 263:F849–857, 1992.

89. Okusa MD, Unwin RJ, Velazquez H, et al: Active potassium absorption by the renal distal tubule. Am J Physiol 262:F488–493, 1992.

90. DuBose TD, Jr, Gitomer J, Codina J: H⁺,K⁺-ATPase. Curr Opin Nephrol Hypertens 8:597–602, 1999.

91. Kraut JA, Helander KG, Helander HF, et al: Detection and localization of H⁺-K⁺-ATPase isoforms in human kidney. Am J Physiol Renal Physiol 281:F763–768, 2001.

92. Verlander JW, Moudy RM, Campbell WG, et al: Immunohistochemical localization of H-K-ATPase alpha(2c)-subunit in rabbit kidney. Am J Physiol Renal Physiol 281:F357–365, 2001.

93. Fejes-Toth G, Naray-Fejes-Toth A: Immunohistochemical localization of colonic H-K-ATPase to the apical membrane of connecting tubule cells. Am J Physiol Renal Physiol 281:F318–325, 2001.

94. Sangan P, Thevananther S, Sangan S, et al: Colonic H-K-ATPase alpha- and beta-subunits express ouabain-insensitive H-K-ATPase. Am J Physiol Cell Physiol 278:C182–189, 2000.

95. Kraut JA, Hiura J, Besancon M, et al: Effect of hypokalemia on the abundance of HK alpha 1 and HK alpha 2 protein in the rat kidney. Am J Physiol 272:F744–750, 1997.

96. Codina J, Delmas-Mata JT, DuBose, TD Jr: Expression of HKalpha2 protein is increased selectively in renal medulla by chronic hypokalemia. Am J Physiol 275:F433–440, 1998.

97. Meneton P, Schultheis PJ, Greeb J, et al: Increased sensitivity to K⁺ deprivation in colonic H,K-ATPase-deficient mice. J Clin Invest 101:536–542, 1998.

98. Spicer Z, Miller ML, Andringa A, et al: Stomachs of mice lacking the gastric H,K-ATPase alpha -subunit have achlorhydria, abnormal parietal cells, and ciliated metaplasia. J Biol Chem 275:21565–21565, 2000.

99. Petrovic S, Spicer Z, Greeley T, et al: Novel Schering and ouabain-insensitive potassium-dependent proton secretion in the mouse cortical collecting duct. Am J Physiol Renal Physiol 282:F133–143, 2002.

100. Dherbecourt O, Cheval L, Bloch-Faure M, et al: Molecular identification of Sch28080-sensitive K-ATPase activities in the mouse kidney. Pflugers Arch 451:769–775, 2006.

101. Courtois-Coutry N, Roush D, Rajendran V, et al: A tyrosine-based signal targets H/K-ATPase to a regulated compartment and is required for the cessation of gastric acid secretion. Cell 90:501–510, 1997.

102. Wang T, Courtois-Coutry N, Giebisch G, Caplan MJ: A tyrosine-based signal regulates H-K-ATPase-mediated potassium reabsorption in the kidney. Am J Physiol 275:F818–826, 1998.

103. Palmer LG, Frindt G: Aldosterone and potassium secretion by the cortical collecting duct. Kidney Int 57:1324–1328, 2000.

104. Gennari FJ, Segal AS: Hyperkalemia: An adaptive response in chronic renal insufficiency. Kidney Int 62:1–9, 2002.

105. Palmer LG, Antonian L, Frindt G: Regulation of apical K and Na channels and Na/K pumps in rat cortical collecting tubule by dietary K. J Gen Physiol 104:693–710, 1994.

106. Beesley AH, Hornby D, White SJ: Regulation of distal nephron K⁺ channels (ROMK) mRNA expression by aldosterone in rat kidney. J Physiol 509 (Pt 3):629–634, 1998.

107. Wald H, Garty H, Palmer LG, Popovtzer MM: Differential regulation of ROMK expression in kidney cortex and medulla by aldosterone and potassium. Am J Physiol 275:F239–245, 1998.

108. Mick VE, Itani RA, Loftus RW, et al: The alpha-subunit of the epithelial sodium channel is an aldosterone-induced transcript in mammalian collecting ducts, and this transcriptional response is mediated via distinct cis-elements in the 5′-flanking region of the gene. Mol Endocrinol 14:575–588, 2001.

109. Masilamani S, Kim GH, Mitchell C, et al: Aldosterone-mediated regulation of ENaC alpha, beta, and gamma subunit proteins in rat kidney. J Clin Invest 104:R19–23, 1999.

110. Nielsen J, Kwon TH, Masilimani S, et al: Sodium transporter abundance profiling in kidney: Effect of spironolactone. Am J Physiol Renal Physiol 283:F923–933, 2002.

111. Loffing J, Zecevic M, Feraille E, et al: Aldosterone induces rapid apical translocation of ENaC in early portion of renal collecting system: Possible role of SGK. Am J Physiol Renal Physiol 280:F675–682, 2001.

112. Loffing J, Pietri L, Aregger F, et al: Differential subcellular localization of ENaC subunits in mouse kidney in response to high- and low-Na diets. Am J Physiol Renal Physiol 279:F252–258, 2000.

580

113. Naray-Fejes-Toth A, Canessa C, Cleaveland ES, et al: sgk is an aldosterone-induced kinase in the renal collecting duct. Effects on epithelial na⁺ channels. J Biol Chem 274:16973–16978, 1999.

114. Bhargava A, Fullerton MJ, Myles K, et al: The serum- and glucocorticoid-induced kinase is a physiological mediator of aldosterone action. Endocrinology 142:1587–1594, 2001.

115. Alvarez de la Rosa D, Canessa CM: Role of SGK in hormonal regulation of epithelial sodium channel in A6 cells. Am J Physiol Cell Physiol 284:C404–414, 2003.

116. Hiltunen TP, Hannila-Handelberg T, Petajaniemi N, et al: Liddle's syndrome associated with a point mutation in the extracellular domain of the epithelial sodium channel gamma subunit. J Hypertens 20:2383–2390, 2002.

117. Staub O, Dho S, Henry P, et al: WW domains of Nedd4 bind to the proline-rich PY motifs in the epithelial Na⁺ channel deleted in Liddle's syndrome. EMBO J 15:2371–2380, 1996.

118. Kamynina E, Tauxe C, Staub O: Distinct characteristics of two human Nedd4 proteins with respect to epithelial Na(⁺) channel regulation. Am J Physiol Renal Physiol 281:F469–477, 2001.

119. Goulet CC, Volk KA, Adams CM, et al: Inhibition of the epithelial Na⁺ channel by interaction of Nedd4 with a PY motif deleted in Liddle's syndrome. J Biol Chem 273:30012–30017, 1998.

120. Staub O, Gautschi I, Ishikawa T, et al: Regulation of stability and function of the epithelial Na⁺ channel (ENaC) by ubiquitination. EMBO J 16:6325–6336, 1997.

121. Henry PC, Kanelis V, O'Brien MC, et al: Affinity and specificity of interactions between Nedd4 isoforms and ENaC. J Biol Chem 278:20019–20028, 2003.

122. Snyder PM, Olson DR, Thomas BC: Serum and glucocorticoid-regulated kinase modulates Nedd4-2-mediated inhibition of the epithelial Na⁺ channel. J Biol Chem 277:5–8, 2002.

123. Flores SY, Loffing-Cueni D, Kamynina E, et al: Aldosterone-induced serum and glucocorticoid-induced kinase 1 expression is accompanied by Nedd4-2 phosphorylation and increased Na⁺ transport in cortical collecting duct cells. J Am Soc Nephrol 16:2279–2287, 2005.

124. Loffing-Cueni D, Flores SY, Sauter D, et al: Dietary sodium intake regulates the ubiquitin-protein ligase nedd4-2 in the renal collecting system. J Am Soc Nephrol 17:1264–1274, 2006.

125. Huang DY, Wulff P, Volkl H, et al: Impaired regulation of renal K⁺ elimination in the sgk1-knockout mouse. J Am Soc Nephrol 15:885–891, 2004.

126. Wulff P, Vallon V, Huang DY, et al: Impaired renal Na(⁺) retention in the sgk1-knockout mouse. J Clin Invest 110:1263–1268, 2002.

127. Vallet V, Chraibi A, Gaeggeler HP, et al: An epithelial serine protease activates the amiloride-sensitive sodium channel. Nature 389:607–610, 1997.

128. Vuagniaux G, Vallet V, Jaeger NF, et al: Activation of the amiloride-sensitive epithelial sodium channel by the serine protease mCAP1 expressed in a mouse cortical collecting duct cell line. J Am Soc Nephrol 11:828–834, 2000.

129. Narikiyo T, Kitamuara K, Adachi M, et al: Regulation of prostasin by aldosterone in the kidney. J Clin Invest 109:401–408, 2002.

130. Vuagniaux G, Vallet V, Jaeger NF, et al: Synergistic activation of ENaC by three membrane-bound channel-activating serine proteases (mCAP1, mCAP2, and mCAP3) and serum- and glucocorticoid-regulated kinase (Sgk1) in Xenopus Oocytes. J Gen Physiol 120:191–201, 2002.

131. Wade JB, Stanton BA, Field MJ, et al: Morphological and physiological responses to aldosterone: Time course and sodium dependence. Am J Physiol 259:F88–94, 1990.

132. Stanton B, janzen A, Klein-Robbenhaar G, et al: Ultrastructure of rat initial collecting tubule: Effect of adrenal corticosteroid treatment. J Clin Invest 75:1327–1334, 1985.

133. Palmer LG, Antonian L, Frindt, G: Regulation of the Na-K pump of the rat cortical collecting tubule by aldosterone. J Gen Physiol 102:43–57, 1993.

134. Summa V, Mordasini D, Roger F, et al: Short term effect of aldosterone on Na,K-ATPase cell surface expression in kidney collecting duct cells. J Biol Chem 276:47087–47093, 2001.

135. Welling PA, Caplan M, Sutters M, Giebisch G: Aldosterone-mediated Na/K-ATPase expression is alpha 1 isoform specific in the renal cortical collecting duct. J Biol Chem 268:23469–23476, 1993.

136. Muto S, Giebisch G, Sansom S: An acute increase of peritubular K stimulates K transport through cell pathways of CCT. Am J Physiol 255:F108–114, 1988.

137. Muto S, Sansom S, Giebisch G: Effects of a high potassium diet on electrical properties of cortical collecting ducts from adrenalectomized rabbits. J Clin Invest 81:376–380, 1988.

138. Muto S, Asano Y, Seldin D, Giebisch G: Basolateral Na⁺ pump modulates apical Na⁺ and K⁺ conductances in rabbit cortical collecting ducts. Am J Physiol 276:F143–158, 1999.

139. Palmer LG, Frindt G: Regulation of apical K channels in rat cortical collecting tubule during changes in dietary K intake. Am J Physiol 277:F805–812, 1999.

140. Mennitt PA, Frindt G, Silver RB, Palmer LG: Potassium restriction downregulates ROMK expression in rat kidney. Am J Physiol Renal Physiol 278:F916–924, 2000.

141. Lin DH, Sterling H, Yang B, et al: Protein tyrosine kinase is expressed and regulates ROMK1 location in the cortical collecting duct. Am J Physiol Renal Physiol 286:F881–892, 2004.

142. Lin DH, Serling H, Lorea KM, et al: K depletion increases protein tyrosine kinase-mediated phosphorylation of ROMK. Am J Physiol Renal Physiol 283:F671–677, 2002.

143. Sterling H, Lin DH, Gu RM, et al: Inhibition of protein-tyrosine phosphatase stimulates the dynamin-dependent endocytosis of ROMK1. J Biol Chem 277:4317–4323, 2002.

144. Lin DH, Sterling H, Wang WH: The protein tyrosine kinase-dependent pathway mediates the effect of K intake on renal K secretion. Physiology (Bethesda) 20:140–146, 2005.

145. Wang W, Lerea KM, Chan M, Giebisch G: Protein tyrosine kinase regulates the number of renal secretory K channels. Am J Physiol Renal Physiol 278:F165–171, 2000.

146. Wei Y, Bloom P, Lin D, et al: Effect of dietary K intake on apical small-conductance K channel in CCD: Role of protein tyrosine kinase. Am J Physiol Renal Physiol 281:F206–212, 2001.

147. Najjar F, Zhou H, Morimoto T, et al: Dietary K⁺ regulates apical membrane expression of maxi-K channels in rabbit cortical collecting duct. Am J Physiol Renal Physiol 289:F922–932, 2005.

148. Babilonia E, Wei Y, Sterling H, et al: Superoxide anions are involved in mediating the effect of low K intake on c-Src expression and renal K secretion in the cortical collecting duct. J Biol Chem 280:10790–10796, 2005.

149. Rabinowitz L: Aldosterone and potassium homeostasis. Kidney Int 49:1738–1742, 1996.

150. Calo L, Borsatti A, Favaro S, Rabinowitz L: Kaliuresis in normal subjects following oral potassium citrate intake without increased plasma potassium concentration. Nephron 69:253–258, 1995.

151. Morita H, Fujiki N, Miyahara T, et al: Hepatoportal bumetanide-sensitive K(⁺)-sensor mechanism controls urinary K(⁺) excretion. Am J Physiol Regul Integr Comp Physiol 278:R1134–1139, 2000.

152. McDonough AA, Youn JH: Role of muscle in regulating extracellular [K⁺]. Semin Nephrol 25: 335–342, 2005.

153. Frindt G, Palmer LG: Na channels in the rat connecting tubule. Am J Physiol Renal Physiol 286:F669–6674, 2004.

154. Meneton P, Loffing J, Warnock DG: Sodium and potassium handling by the aldosterone-sensitive distal nephron: The pivotal role of the distal and connecting tubule. Am J Physiol Renal Physiol 287:F593–601, 2004.

155. Ethier JH, Kamel KS, Magner PO, et al: The transtubular potassium concentration in patients with hypokalemia and hyperkalemia. Am J Kidney Dis 15:309–315, 1990.

156. Weinstein AM: A mathematical model of rat cortical collecting duct: Determinants of the transtubular potassium gradient. Am J Physiol Renal Physiol 280:F1072–1092, 2001.

157. Chacko M, Fordtran JS, Emmett M: Effect of mineralocorticoid activity on transtubular potassium gradient, urinary [K]/[Na] ratio, and fractional excretion of potassium. Am J Kidney Dis 32:47–51, 1998.

158. Joo KW, Chang SH, Lee JG, et al: Transtubular potassium concentration gradient (TTKG) and urine ammonium in differential diagnosis of hypokalemia. J Nephrol 13:120–125, 2000.

159. Batlle DC, Hizon M, Cohen E, et al: The use of the urinary anion gap in the diagnosis of hyperchloremic metabolic acidosis. N Engl J Med 318:594–599, 1988.

160. Skott O, Briggs JP: Direct demonstration of macula densa-mediated renin secretion. Science 237:1618–1620, 1987.

161. Lorenz JN, Weihprecht H, Schnermann J, et al: Renin release from isolated juxtaglomerular apparatus depends on macula densa chloride transport. Am J Physiol 260:F486–493, 1991.

162. Wagner C, Jensen BL, Kramer BK, Kurtz A: Control of the renal renin system by local factors. Kidney Int Suppl 67:S78–83, 1998.

163. Schweda F, Wagner C, Kramer BK, et al: Preserved macula densa-dependent renin secretion in A1 adenosine receptor knockout mice. Am J Physiol Renal Physiol 284:F770–777, 2003.

164. Kurtz A, Della Bruna R, Pfeilschifter J, et al: Atrial natriuretic peptide inhibits renin release from juxtaglomerular cells by a cGMP-mediated process. Proc Natl Acad Sci U S A 83:4769–4773, 1986.

165. Henrich WL, McAlister EA, Smith PB, et al: Direct inhibitory effect of atriopeptin III on renin release in primate kidney. Life Sci 41:259–264, 1987.

166. Todorov V, Muller M, Schweda F, Kurtz A: Tumor necrosis factor-alpha inhibits renin gene expression. Am J Physiol Regul Integr Comp Physiol 283:R1046–1051, 2002.

167. Li YC, Kong J, Wei M, et al: 1,25-Dihydroxyvitamin D(3) is a negative endocrine regulator of the renin-angiotensin system. J Clin Invest 110:229–238, 2002.

168. Wagner C, Pfeifer A, Ruth P, et al: Role of cGMP-kinase II in the control of renin secretion and renin expression. J Clin Invest 102:1576–1582, 1998.

169. Jensen BL, Schmid C, Kurtz A: Prostaglandins stimulate renin secretion and renin mRNA in mouse renal juxtaglomerular cells. Am J Physiol 271:F659–669, 1996.

170. Jensen BL, Kramer BK, Kurtz A: Adrenomedullin stimulates renin release and renin mRNA in mouse juxtaglomerular granular cells. Hypertension 29:1148–1155, 1997.

171. Boivin V, Jahns R, Gambaryan S, et al: Immunofluorescent imaging of beta 1- and beta 2-adrenergic receptors in rat kidney. Kidney Int 59:515–531, 2001.

172. Harris RC: Interactions between COX-2 and the renin-angiotensin system in the kidney. Acta Physiol Scand 177:423–427, 2003.

173. Harris RC, McKanna JA, Akai Y, et al: Cyclooxygenase-2 is associated with the macula densa of rat kidney and increases with salt restriction. J Clin Invest 94:2504–2510, 1994.

174. Cheng HF, Wang JL, Zhang MZ, et al: Role of p38 in the regulation of renal cortical cyclooxygenase-2 expression by extracellular chloride. J Clin Invest 106:681–688, 2000.

175. Stichtenoth DO, Marhauer V, Tsikas D, et al: Effects of specific COX-2-inhibition on renin release and renal and systemic prostanoid synthesis in healthy volunteers. Kidney Int 68:2197–2207, 2005.

176. Dluhy RG, Axelrod L, Underwood RH, Williams GH: Studies of the control of plasma aldosterone concentration in normal man II. Effect of dietary potassium and acute potassium infusion. J Clin Invest 51:1950–1957, 1972.

177. Chen XL, Bayliss DA, Fern RJ, Barrett PQ: A role for T-type Ca²⁺ channels in the synergistic control of aldosterone production by ANG II and K⁺. Am J Physiol 276:F674–683, 1999.

178. Arrighi I, Bloch-Faure M, Grahammer F, et al: Altered potassium balance and aldosterone secretion in a mouse model of human congenital long QT syndrome. Proc Natl Acad Sci U S A 98:8792–8797, 2001.

179. Hilbers U, Peters J, Bornstein SR, et al: Local renin-angiotensin system is involved in K⁺-induced aldosterone secretion from human adrenocortical NCI-H295 cells. Hypertension 33:1025–1030, 1999.

180. Mazzocchi G, Malendowicz LK, Markowska A, et al: Role of adrenal renin-angiotensin system in the control of aldosterone secretion in sodium-restricted rats. Am J Physiol Endocrinol Metab 278:E1027–1030, 2000.

181. Saruta T, Kaplan NM: Adrenocortical steroidogenesis: the effects of prostaglandins. J Clin Invest 51:2246–2251, 1972.

182. Gordon RD, Kuchel O, Liddle GW, Island DP: Role of the sympathetic nervous system in regulating renin and aldosterone production in man. J Clin Invest 46:599–605, 1967.

183. Gupta P, Franco-Saenz R, Mulrow PJ: Regulation of the adrenal renin angiotensin system in cultured bovine zona glomerulosa cells: Effect of catecholamines. Endocrinology 130:2129–2134, 1992.

184. Csukas S, Hanke CJ, Rewolinski D, Campbell WB: Prostaglandin E2-induced aldosterone release is mediated by an EP2 receptor. Hypertension 31:575–581, 1998.

185. Clark BA, Brown RS, Epstein FH: Effect of atrial natriuretic peptide on potassium-stimulated aldosterone secretion: Potential relevance to hypoaldosteronism in man. J Clin Endocrinol Metab 75:399–403, 1992.

186. Cherradi N, Brandenburger Y, Rossier MF, et al: Atrial natriuretic peptide inhibits calcium-induced steroidogenic acute regulatory protein gene transcription in adrenal glomerulosa cells. Mol Endocrinol 12:962–972, 1998.

187. Cohen JD, Neaton JD, Prineas RJ, Daniels KA: Diuretics, serum potassium and ventricular arrhythmias in the Multiple Risk Factor Intervention Trial. Am J Cardiol 60:548–554, 1987.

188. Strickberger SA, Miller CB, Levine JH: Multifocal atrial tachycardia from electrolyte imbalance. Am Heart J 115:680–682, 1988.

189. He FJ, MacGregor GA: Fortnightly review: Beneficial effects of potassium. BMJ 323:497–501, 2001.

190. Wahr JA, Parks R, Boisvert D, et al: Preoperative serum potassium levels and perioperative outcomes in cardiac surgery patients Multicenter Study of Perioperative Ischemia Research Group. JAMA 281:2203–2210, 1999.

191. Modesto KM, Mollert JE, Freeman WK, et al: Safety of exercise stress testing in patients with abnormal concentrations of serum potassium. Am J Cardiol 97:1247–1249, 2006.

192. Slovis C, Jenkins R: ABC of clinical electrocardiography: Conditions not primarily affecting the heart. BMJ 324:1320–1323, 2002.

193. Schwartz AB: Potassium-related cardiac arrhythmias and their treatment. Angiology 29:194–205, 1978.

194. Roden DM: A practical approach to torsade de pointes. Clin Cardiol 20:285–290, 1997.

195. Berthet M, Denjoy I, Donger C, et al: C-terminal HERG mutations: The role of hypokalemia and a KCNQ1-associated mutation in cardiac event occurrence. Circulation 99:1464–1470, 1999.

196. Darbar D, Sile S, Fish FA, George AL, Jr: Congenital long QT syndrome aggravated by salt-wasting nephropathy. Heart Rhythm 2:304–306, 2005.

197. Tang NL, Hui J, To KF, et al: Severe hypokalemic myopathy in Gitelman's syndrome. Muscle Nerve 22:545–547, 1999.

198. Wong KM, Chak WL, Cheung CY, et al: Hypokalemic metabolic acidosis attributed to cough mixture abuse. Am J Kidney Dis 38:390–394, 2001.

199. Tattersall RB: A paper which changed clinical practice (slowly) Jacob Holler on potassium deficiency in diabetic acidosis (1946). Diabet Med 16:978–984, 1999.

200. Comi G, Testa D, Cornelio F, et al: Potassium depletion myopathy: A clinical and morphological study of six cases. Muscle Nerve 8:17–21, 1985.

201. Mujais SK, Katz AI: Potassium deficiency. In Seldin DW, Giebisch G (eds): The Kidney: Physiology and Pathophysiology, Vol 2. Philadelphia, Lippincott Williams & Wilkins, 2000, pp 1615–1646.

202. Schwartz WB, Relman AS: Effects of electrolyte disorders on renal structure and function. N Engl J Med 276:383–389 1967.

203. Cremer W, Bock KD: Symptoms and course of chronic hypokalemic nephropathy in man. Clin Nephrol 7:112–119, 1977.

204. Torres VE, Young WF, Jr, Offord KP, Hattery RR: Association of hypokalemia, aldosteronism, and renal cysts. N Engl J Med 322:345–351, 1990.

205. Yasuhara D, Naruo T, Taguchi S, et al: "End-stage kidney" in longstanding bulimia nervosa. Int J Eat Disord 38:383–385, 2005.

206. Menahem SA, Perry GJ, Dowling J, Thomson NM: Hypokalaemia-induced acute renal failure Nephrol Dial Transplant 14:2216–2218, 1999.

207. Suga SI, Phillips MI, Ray PE, et al: Hypokalemia induces renal injury and alterations in vasoactive mediators that favor salt sensitivity. Am J Physiol Renal Physiol 281, F620–629, 2001.

208. Suga S, Yasui N, Yashihara F, et al: Endothelin a receptor blockade and endothelin B receptor blockade improve hypokalemic nephropathy by different mechanisms. J Am Soc Nephrol 14:397–406, 2003.

209. Suga S, Mazzali M, Ray PE, et al: Angiotensin II type 1 receptor blockade ameliorates tubulointerstitial injury induced by chronic potassium deficiency. Kidney Int 61:951–958, 2002.

210. Zajicek HK, Wang H, Puttaparthi K, et al: Glycosphingolipids modulate renal phosphate transport in potassium deficiency. Kidney Int 60:694–704, 2001.

211. Levi M, McDonald LA, Preisig PA, Alpern RJ: Chronic K depletion stimulates rat renal brush-border membrane Na-citrate cotransporter. Am J Physiol 261:F767–773, 1991.

212. Fryer JN, Burns KD, Ghorbani M, Levine DZ: Effect of potassium depletion on proximal tubule AT1 receptor localization in normal and remnant rat kidney. Kidney Int 60:1792–1799, 2001.

213. Huang L, Wei YY, Momose-Hotokezaka A, et al: Alpha 2B-adrenergic receptors: Immunolocalization and regulation by potassium depletion in rat kidney. Am J Physiol 270:F1015–1026, 1996.

214. Elkjaer ML, Kwon TH, Wang W, et al: Altered expression of renal NHE3, TSC, BSC-1, and ENaC subunits in potassium depleted rats. Am J Physiol Renal Physiol 283: F1376–1388, 2002.

215. Berl T, Linas SL, Aisenbrey GA, Anderson RJ: On the mechanism of polyuria in potassium depletion: The role of polydipsia. J Clin Invest 60:620–625, 1977.

216. Gutsche HU, Peterson LN, Levine DZ: In vivo evidence of impaired solute transport by the thick ascending limb in potassium-depleted rats. J Clin Invest 73:908–916, 1984.

217. Marples D, Frokiaer J, Dorup J, et al: Hypokalemia-induced downregulation of aquaporin-2 water channel expression in rat kidney medulla and cortex. J Clin Invest 97:1960–1968, 1996.

218. Amlal H, Krane CM, Chen Q, Soleimani M: Early polyuria and urinary concentrating defect in potassium deprivation. Am J Physiol Renal Physiol 279:F655–663, 2000.

219. Coca SG, Perazella MA, Buller GK: The cardiovascular implications of hypokalemia. Am J Kidney Dis 45:233–247, 2005.

220. Ray PE, Suga S, Liu XH, et al: Chronic potassium depletion induces renal injury, salt sensitivity, and hypertension in young rats. Kidney Int 59:1850–1858, 2001.

221. Krishna GG, Chusid P, Hoeldtke RD: Mild potassium depletion provokes renal sodium retention. J Lab Clin Med 109:724–730, 1987.

222. Krishna GG, Miller E, Kapoor S: Increased blood pressure during potassium depletion in normotensive men. N Engl J Med 320:1177–1182, 1989.

223. Coruzzi P, Brambilla L, Brambilla V, et al: Potassium depletion and salt sensitivity in essential hypertension. J Clin Endocrinol Metab 86:2857–2862, 2001.

224. Kaplan NM, Carnegie A, Raskin P, et al: Potassium supplementation in hypertensive patients with diuretic-induced hypokalemia. N Engl J Med 312:746–749, 1985.

225. Franse LV, Pahor M, Di Bari M, et al: Hypokalemia associated with diuretic use and cardiovascular events in the Systolic Hypertension in the Elderly Program. Hypertension 35:1025–1030, 2000.

226. Cohen HW, Madhavan S, Alderman MH: High and low serum potassium associated with cardiovascular events in diuretic-treated patients. J Hypertens 19:1315–1323, 2001.

227. Mattu A, Brady WJ, Robinson DA: Electrocardiographic manifestations of hyperkalemia. Am J Emerg Med 18:721–729, 2000.

228. Parham WA, Mehdirad AA, Biermann KM, Fredman CS: Hyperkalemia revisited. Tex Heart Inst J 33:40–47, 2006.

229. Greenberg A: Hyperkalemia: Treatment options. Semin Nephrol 18:46–57, 1998.

230. McLean SA, Paul ID, Spector PS: Lidocaine-induced conduction disturbance in patients with systemic hyperkalemia. Ann Emerg Med 36:615–618, 2000.

231. Acker CG, Johnson JP, Palevsky PM, Greenberg A: Hyperkalemia in hospitalized patients: Causes, adequacy of treatment, and results of an attempt to improve physician compliance with published therapy guidelines. Arch Intern Med 158:917–924, 1998.

232. Aslam S, Friedman EA, Ifudu O: Electrocardiography is unreliable in detecting potentially lethal hyperkalaemia in haemodialysis patients. Nephrol Dial Transplant 17:1639–1642, 2002.

233. Szerlip HM, Weiss J, Singer I: Profound hyperkalemia without electrocardiographic manifestations. Am J Kidney Dis 7:461–465, 1986.

234. Somers MP, Brady, WJ, Perron AD, Mattu A: The prominant T wave: Electrocardiographic differential diagnosis. Am J Emerg Med 20:243–251, 2002.

235. Freeman SJ, Fale AD: Muscular paralysis and ventilatory failure caused by hyperkalaemia. Br J Anaesth 70:226–227, 1993.

236. Evers S, Engelien A, Karsch V, Hund M: Secondary hyperkalaemic paralysis. J Neurol Neurosurg Psychiatry 64:249–252, 1998.

237. Miller TM, Dias da Silva MR, Miller HA, et al: Correlating phenotype and genotype in the periodic paralyses. Neurology 63:1647–1655, 2004.

238. Lehmann-Horn F, Jurkat-Rott K: Voltage-gated ion channels and hereditary disease. Physiol Rev 79:1317–1372, 1999.

239. Jurkat-Rott K, Mitrovic N, Hang C, et al: Voltage-sensor sodium channel mutations cause hypokalemic periodic paralysis type 2 by enhanced inactivation and reduced current. Proc Natl Acad Sci U S A 97:9549–9554, 2000.

240. Abbott GW, Butler MH, Bendahhou S, et al: MiRP2 forms potassium channels in skeletal muscle with Kv34 and is associated with periodic paralysis. Cell 104:217–231, 2001.

241. DuBose TD, Jr, Good DW: Effects of chronic hyperkalemia on renal production and proximal tubule transport of ammonium in rats. Am J Physiol 260:F680–687, 1991.

242. Good DW: Ammonium transport by the thick ascending limb of Henle's loop. Ann Rev Physiol 56:623–647, 1994.

243. Attmane-Elakeb A, Mount DB, Sibella V, et al: Stimulation by in vivo and in vitro metabolic acidosis of expression of rBSC1, the Na-K(NH4)-2Cl cotransporter of the rat medullary thick ascending limb. J Biol Chem 273:33681–33691, 1998.

244. DuBose TD, Jr, Good DW: Chronic hyperkalemia impairs ammonium transport and accumulation in the inner medulla of the rat. J Clin Invest 90:1443–1449, 1992.

245. DuBose TD: Hyperkalemic hyperchloremic metabolic acidosis: Pathophysiologic insights. Kidney Int 51:591–602, 1997.

246. Cohn JN, Kowey PR, Whelton PK, Prisant LM: New guidelines for potassium replacement in clinical practice: A contemporary review by the National Council on Potassium in Clinical Practice. Arch Intern Med 160:2429–2436, 2000.

247. Gennari FJ: Hypokalemia. N Engl J Med 339:451–458, 1998.

248. Paltiel O, Salakhov, E, Ronen I, et al: Management of severe hypokalemia in hospitalized patients: A study of quality of care based on computerized databases. Arch Intern Med 161:1089–1095, 2001.

249. Morgan DB, Davidson C: Hypokalaemia and diuretics: An analysis of publications. Br Med J 280: 905–908, 1980.

250. Schnaper HW, Freis ED, Friedman RG, et al: Potassium restoration in hypertensive patients made hypokalemic by hydrochlorothiazide. Arch Intern Med 149:2677–2681, 1989.

251. Rosenberg J, Gustafsson F, Galatius S, Hildebrandt PR: Combination therapy with metolazone and loop diuretics in outpatients with refractory heart failure: An observational study and review of the literature. Cardiovasc Drugs Ther 19:301–306, 2005.

252. Tziviskou E, Musso C, Bellizzi V, et al: Prevalence and pathogenesis of hypokalemia in patients on chronic peritoneal dialysis: One center's experience and review of the literature. Int Urol Nephrol 35:429–434, 2003.

253. Macdonald JE, Struthers AD: What is the optimal serum potassium level in cardio-vascular patients? J Am Coll Cardiol 43:155–161, 2004.

254. Masters PW, Lawson N, Marenah CB, Maile LJ: High ambient temperature: A spurious cause of hypokalaemia. BMJ 312:1652–1653, 1996.

255. Sinclair D, Briston P, Young R, Pepin N: Seasonal pseudohyperkalaemia. J Clin Pathol 56:385–388, 2003.

256. Ulahannan TJ, McVittie J, Keenan J: Ambient temperatures and potassium concentrations. Lancet 352:1680–1681, 1998.

257. Heller SR, Robinson RT: Hypoglycaemia and associated hypokalaemia in diabetes: Mechanisms, clinical implications and prevention. Diabetes Obes Metab 2:75–82, 2000.

258. Laso FJ, Gonzalez-Buitrago JM, Martin-Ruiz C, et al: Inter-relationship between serum potassium and plasma catecholamines and 3':5' cyclic monophosphate in alcohol withdrawal. Drug Alcohol Depend 26:183–188, 1990.

259. Madias JE, Shah B, Chintalapally G, et al: Admission serum potassium in patients with acute myocardial infarction: Its correlates and value as a determinant of in-hospital outcome. Chest 118: 904–913, 2000.

260. Schaefer M, Link J, Hannemann L, Rudolph KH: Excessive hypokalemia and hyperkalemia following head injury. Intensive Care Med 21:235–237, 1995.

261. Tse HF, Yeung CK: From profound hypokalemia to fatal rhabdomyolysis after severe head injury. Am J Med 109:599–600, 2000.

262. Braden GL, von Oeyen PT, Germain MJ, et al: Ritodrine- and terbutaline-induced hypokalemia in preterm labor: Mechanisms and consequences. Kidney Int 51:1867–1875, 1997.

263. Amitai Y, Lovejoy FH, Jr: Hypokalemia in acute theophylline poisoning. Am J Emerg Med 6: 214–218, 1988.

264. Rice JE, Faunt JD: Excessive cola consumption as a cause of hypokalaemic myopathy. Intern Med J 31:317–318, 2001.

265. Whyte KF, Reid C, Addis GJ, et al: Salbutamol induced hypokalaemia: The effect of theophylline alone and in combination with adrenaline. Br J Clin Pharmacol 25:571–578, 1988.

266. Ahlawat SK, Sachdev A: Hypokalaemic paralysis. Postgrad Med J 75:193–197, 1999.

267. Downs JC, Milling D, Nichols CA: Suicidal ingestion of barium-sulfide-containing shaving powder. Am J Forensic Med Pathol 16:56–61, 1995.

268. Sigue G, Gamble L, Pelitere M, et al: From profound hypokalemia to life-threatening hyperkalemia: A case of barium sulfide poisoning. Arch Intern Med 160:548–551, 2000.

269. Wells JA, Wood KE: Acute barium poisoning treated with hemodialysis. Am J Emerg Med 19: 175–177, 2001.

270. Jacobs IA, Taddeo J, Kelly K, Valenziano C: Poisoning as a result of barium styphnate explosion. Am J Ind Med 41:285–288, 2002.

271. Bradberry SM, Vale JA: Disturbances of potassium homeostasis in poisoning. J Toxicol Clin Toxicol 33:295–310, 1995.

272. Plaster NM, Tawil R, Tristani-Firouzi M, et al: Mutations in Kir21 cause the developmental and episodic electrical phenotypes of Andersen's syndrome. Cell 105:511–519, 2001.

273. Ruff RL: Skeletal muscle sodium current is reduced in hypokalemic periodic paralysis. Proc Natl Acad Sci U S A 97:9832–9833, 2000.

274. Ruff RL: Insulin acts in hypokalemic periodic paralysis by reducing inward rectifier K⁺ current. Neurology 53:1556–1563, 1999.

275. Tricarico D, Servidei S, Tonali P, et al: Impairment of skeletal muscle adenosine triphosphate-sensitive K⁺ channels in patients with hypokalemic periodic paralysis. J Clin Invest 103:675–682, 1999.

276. Renaud JM: Modulation of force development by Na⁺, K⁺, Na⁺ K⁺ pump and KATP channel during muscular activity. Can J Appl Physiol 27:296–315, 2002.

277. Tricarico D, Capriulo R, Conte Camerino D: Insulin modulation of ATP-sensitive K⁺ channel of rat skeletal muscle is impaired in the hypokalaemic state. Pflugers Arch 437:235–240, 1999.

278. Cheng NL, Kao MC, Hsu YD, Lin SH: Novel thiazide-sensitive Na-Cl cotransporter mutation in a Chinese patient with Gitelman's syndrome presenting as hypokalaemic paralysis. Nephrol Dial Transplant 18:1005–1008, 2003.

279. Yang SS, Chu P, Lin YF, et al: Aristolochic acid-induced Fanconi's syndrome and nephropathy presenting as hypokalemic paralysis. Am J Kidney Dis 39:E14, 2002.

280. Feldman M, Prikis M, Athanauiou Y, et al: Molecular investigation and long-term clinical progress in Greek Cypriot families with recessive distal renal tubular acidosis and sensorineural deafness due to mutations in the ATP6V1B1 gene. Clin Genet 69:135–144, 2006.

281. Kim CJ, Woo YJ, Ma JS, et al: Hypokalemic paralysis and rhabdomyolysis in distal renal tubular acidosis. Pediatr Int 47:211–213, 2005.

282. Manoukian MA, Foote JA, Crapo LM: Clinical and metabolic features of thyrotoxic periodic paralysis in 24 episodes. Arch Intern Med 159:601–606, 1999.

283. Goh SH: Thyrotoxic periodic paralysis: Reports of seven patients presenting with weakness in an Asian emergency department. Emerg Med J 19:78–79, 2002.

284. Chan A, Shinde R, Chow CC, et al: In vivo and in vitro sodium pump activity in subjects with thyrotoxic periodic paralysis. BMJ 303:1096–1099, 1991.

285. Lam KS, Yeung RT, Benson EA, Wang C: Erythrocyte sodium-potassium pump in thyrotoxic periodic paralysis. Aust N Z J Med 19:6–10, 1989.

286. Azuma KK, Hensley CB, Tang MJ, McDonough AA: Thyroid hormone specifically regulates skeletal muscle Na(⁺)-K(⁺)-ATPase alpha 2- and beta 2-isoforms. Am J Physiol 265:C680–687, 1993.

287. Lin SH, Lin YF: Propranolol rapidly reverses paralysis, hypokalemia, and hypophosphatemia in thyrotoxic periodic paralysis. Am J Kidney Dis 37:620–623, 2001.

288. Birkhahn RH, Gaeta TJ, Melniker L: Thyrotoxic periodic paralysis and intravenous propranolol in the emergency setting. J Emerg Med 18:199–202, 2000.

289. Ko GT, Chow CC, Yeung VT, et al: Thyrotoxic periodic paralysis in a Chinese population. QJM 89:463–468, 1996.

290. Kassirer JP, Schwartz WB: The response of normal man to selective depletion of hydrochloric acid Factors in the genesis of persistent gastric alkalosis. Am J Med 40:10–18, 1966.

291. Coghill NF, McAllen PM, Edwards F: Electrolyte losses associated with the taking of purges investigated with aid of sodium and potassium radioisotopes. BMJ 1:14–19, 1959.

292. Orman RA, Lewis JB, Jr: Flaccid quadriparesis associated with Yersinia enterocolitis-induced hypokalemia. Arch Intern Med 149:1193–1194, 1989.

293. Wolf I, Mouallem M, Farfel Z: Adult celiac disease presented with celiac crisis: Severe diarrhea, hypokalemia, and acidosis. J Clin Gastroenterol 30:324–326, 2000.

294. Diekmann F, Rudolph B, Plauth M, et al: Hypokalemic nephropathy after pelvic pouch procedure and protective loop ileostomy. Z Gastroenterol 39:579–582, 2001.

295. Halpern MT, Irwin DE, Brown RE, et al: Patient adherence to prescribed potassium supplement therapy. Clin Ther 15:1133–1145; discussion 1120, 1993.

296. Bettinelli A, Bianchetti MG, Girardin E, et al: Use of calcium excretion values to distinguish two forms of primary renal tubular hypokalemic alkalosis: Bartter and Gitelman syndromes [see comments]. J Pediatr 120:38–43, 1992.

297. Suki WN, Yium JJ, Von Minden M, et al: Acute treatment of hypercalcemia with furosemide. N Engl J Med 283:836–840, 1970.

298. Okusa MD, Velazquez H, Ellison DH, Wright FS: Luminal calcium regulates potassium transport by the renal distal tubule. Am J Physiol 258:F423–428, 1990.

299. Sands JM, Naruse M, Baum M, et al: Apical extracellular calcium/polyvalent cation-sensing receptor regulates vasopressin-elicited water permeability in rat kidney inner medullary collecting duct. J Clin Invest 99:1399–1405, 1997.

300. Johnson DW, Kay TD, Hawley CM: Severe hypokalaemia secondary to dicloxacillin. Intern Med J 32:357–358, 2002.

301. Landau D, Kher KK: Gentamicin-induced Bartter-like syndrome. Pediatr Nephrol 11:737–740, 1997.

302. Malin A, Miller RF: Foscarnet-induced hypokalaemia. J Infect 25:329–330, 1992.

303. Milionis HJ, Bourantas CL, Siamopoulos KC, Elisaf MS: Acid-base and electrolyte abnormalities in patients with acute leukemia Am J Hematol 62:201–207, 1999.

304. Husband DJ, Watkin SW: Fatal hypokalaemia associated with ifosfamide/mesna chemotherapy Lancet 1:1116, 1988.

305. Bunchman TE, Sinaiko AR: Renovascular hypertension presenting with hypokalemic metabolic alkalosis Pediatr Nephrol 4:169–170, 1990.

306. Pintar TJ, Zimmerman S: Hyperreninemic hypertension secondary to a subcapsular perinephric hematoma in a patient with polyarteritis nodosa. Am J Kidney Dis 32:503–507, 1998.

307. Ringrose TR, Phillips PA, Lindop GB: Renin-secreting adenocarcinoma of the colon. Ann Intern Med 131:794–795, 1999.

308. Corvol P, Pinet F, Plouin PF, et al: Renin-secreting tumors Endocrinol Metab Clin North Am 23: 255–270, 1994.

309. Nicholls MG: Unilateral renal ischemia causing the hyponatremic hypertensive syndrome in children—more common than we think? Pediatr Nephrol 21:887–890, 2006.

310. White PC: Steroid 11 beta-hydroxylase deficiency and related disorders. Endocrinol Metab Clin North Am 30:61–79, vi, 2001.

311. Goldsmith O, Solomon DH, Horton R: Hypogonadism and mineralocorticoid excess The 17-hydroxylase deficiency syndrome. N Engl J Med 277:673–677, 1967.

312. Dluhy RG, Lifton RP: Glucocorticoid-remediable aldosteronism J Clin Endocrinol Metab 84:4341–4344, 1999.

313. So A, Duffy DL, Gordon RD, et al: Familial hyperaldosteronism type II is linked to the chromosome 7p22 region but also shows predicted heterogeneity. J Hypertens 23:1477–1484, 2005.

314. Litchfield WR, New MI, Coolidge C, et al: Evaluation of the dexamethasone suppression test for the diagnosis of glucocorticoid-remediable aldosteronism. J Clin Endocrinol Metab 82:3570–3573, 1997.

315. Lifton RP, Dluhy RG, Powers M, et al: A chimaeric 11 beta-hydroxylase/aldosterone synthase gene causes glucocorticoid-remediable aldosteronism and human hypertension. Nature 355:262–265, 1992.

316. Rich GM, Ulick S, Cooke S, et al: Glucocorticoid-remediable aldosteronism in a large kindred: Clinical spectrum and diagnosis using a characteristic biochemical phenotype. Ann Intern Med 116:813–820, 1992.

317. Pascoe L, Jeunemaitre X, Lebrethon MC, et al: Glucocorticoid-suppressible hyperaldosteronism and adrenal tumors occurring in a single French pedigree. J Clin Invest 96:2236–2246, 1995.

318. Jamieson A, Slutsker L, Inglis G, et al: Clinical, biochemical and genetic features of five extended kindred's with glucocorticoid-suppressible hyperaldosteronism. Endocr Res 21:463–469, 1995.

319. Litchfield WR, Coolidge C, Silva P, et al: Impaired potassium-stimulated aldosterone production: A possible explanation for normokalemic glucocorticoid-remediable aldosteronism. J Clin Endocrinol Metab 82:1507–1510, 1997.

320. Ghose RP, Hall PM, Bravo EL: Medical management of aldosterone-producing adenomas. Ann Intern Med 131:105–108, 1999.

321. Blumenfeld JD, Sealey JE, Schlussel Y, et al: Diagnosis and treatment of primary hyperaldosteronism. Ann Intern Med 121:877–885, 1994.

322. Mulatero P, Rabbia F, Veglio F: Paraneoplastic hyperaldosteronism associated with non-Hodgkin's lymphoma. N Engl J Med 344:1558–1559, 2001.

323. Nwariaku FE, Miller BS, Auchus R, et al: Primary hyperaldosteronism: Effect of adrenal vein sampling on surgical outcome. Arch Surg 141:497–502; discussion 502–503, 2006.

324. Young WF, Stanson AW, Thompson GB, et al: Role for adrenal venous sampling in primary aldosteronism. Surgery 136:1227–1235, 2004.

325. Montori VM, Young WF, Jr: Use of plasma aldosterone concentration-to-plasma renin activity ratio as a screening test for primary aldosteronism. A systematic review of the literature. Endocrinol Metab Clin North Am 31:619–632, xi, 2002.

326. Williams JS, Williams GH, Raji A, et al: Prevalence of primary hyperaldosteronism in mild to moderate hypertension without hypokalaemia. J Hum Hypertens 20:129–136, 2006.
327. Eiam-Ong S, Kurtzman NA, Sabatini S: Regulation of collecting tubule adenosine triphosphatases by aldosterone and potassium. J Clin Invest 91:2385–23892, 1993.
328. Howlett TA, Drury PL, Perry L, et al: Diagnosis and management of ACTH-dependent Cushing's syndrome: Comparison of the features in ectopic and pituitary ACTH production. Clin Endocrinol (Oxf) 24:699–713, 1986.
329. Torpy, DJ, Mullen N, Ilias I, Nieman LK: Association of hypertension and hypokalemia with Cushing's syndrome caused by ectopic ACTH secretion: A series of 58 cases. Ann N Y Acad Sci 970:134–144, 2002.
330. Stewart PM, Walker BR, Holder G, et al: 11 beta-Hydroxysteroid dehydrogenase activity in Cushing's syndrome: Explaining the mineralocorticoid excess state of the ectopic adrenocorticotropin syndrome. J Clin Endocrinol Metab 80:3617–3620, 1995.
331. Koren W, Grienspuhn A, Kuzneetsov SR, et al: Enhanced Na^+/H^+ exchange in Cushing's syndrome reflects functional hypermineralocorticoidism. J Hypertens 16:1187–1191, 1998.
332. Mendonca BB, Leite MV, de Castro M, et al: Female pseudohermaphroditism caused by a novel homozygous missense mutation of the GR gene. J Clin Endocrinol Metab 87:1805–1809, 2002.
333. White PC, Mune T, Agarwal AK: 11 beta-Hydroxysteroid dehydrogenase and the syndrome of apparent mineralocorticoid excess. Endocr Rev 18:135–156, 1997.
334. Bostanjoglo M, Reeves WB, Reilly RF, et al: 11Beta-hydroxysteroid dehydrogenase, mineralocorticoid receptor, and thiazide-sensitive Na-Cl cotransporter expression by distal tubules [published erratum appears in J Am Soc Nephrol 9(11):2179, 1998]. J Am Soc Nephrol 9:1347–1358, 1998.
335. Funder JW, Pearce PT, Smith R, Smith AI: Mineralocorticoid action: Target tissue specificity is enzyme, not receptor, mediated. Science 242:583–585, 1988.
336. Li A, Tedde R, Krozowski ZS, et al: Molecular basis for hypertension in the "type II variant" of apparent mineralocorticoid excess. Am J Hum Genet 63:370–379, 1998.
337. Wilson RC, Dave-Sharma S, Wei JQ, et al: A genetic defect resulting in mild low-renin hypertension. Proc Natl Acad Sci U S A 95:10200–10205, 1998.
338. Nunez BS, Rogerson FM, Mune T, et al: Mutants of 11beta-hydroxysteroid dehydrogenase (11-HSD2) with partial activity: Improved correlations between genotype and biochemical phenotype in apparent mineralocorticoid excess. Hypertension 34:638–642, 1999.
339. Kotelevtsev Y, Brown RW, Fleming S, et al: Hypertension in mice lacking 11beta-hydroxysteroid dehydrogenase type 2. J Clin Invest 103:683–689, 1999.
340. Loffing J, Loffing-Cueni D, Valderrabano V, et al: Distribution of transcellular calcium and sodium transport pathways along mouse distal nephron. Am J Physiol Renal Physiol 281:F1021–1027, 2001.
341. Kim GH, Masilamani S, Turner R, et al: The thiazide-sensitive Na-Cl cotransporter is an aldosterone-induced protein. Proc Natl Acad Sci U S A 95:14552–14557, 1998.
342. Biller KJ, Unwin RJ, Shirley DG: Distal tubular electrolyte transport during inhibition of renal 11beta-hydroxysteroid dehydrogenase. Am J Physiol Renal Physiol 280: F172–179, 2001.
343. Borst JGG, Ten Holt SP, de Vries LA, Molhysen JA: Syngergistic action of liquorice and cortisone in Addison's and Simmond's disease. Lancet 1:657–663, 1953.
344. Woywodt A, Herrmann A, Haller H, Haubitz M: Severe hypokalaemia: is one reason enough? Nephrol Dial Transplant 19:2914–2917, 2004.
345. Hamidon BB, Jeyabalan V: Exogenously-induced apparent hypermineralocorticoidism associated with ingestion of "asam boi". Singapore Med J 47:156–158, 2006.
346. van Rossum TG, de Jong FH, Hop WC, et al: "Pseudo-aldosteronism" induced by intravenous glycyrrhizin treatment of chronic hepatitis C patients. J Gastroenterol Hepatol 16:789–795, 2001.
347. Iida R, Otsuka Y, Matsumoto K, et al: Pseudoaldosteronism due to the concurrent use of two herbal medicines containing glycyrrhizin: Interaction of glycyrrhizin with angiotensin-converting enzyme inhibitor. Clin Exp Nephrol 10:131–135, 2006.
348. Geller DS, Farhi A, Pinkerton N, et al: Activating mineralocorticoid receptor mutation in hypertension exacerbated by pregnancy. Science 289:119–123, 2000.
349. Lifton RP, Gharavi AG, Geller DS: Molecular mechanisms of human hypertension. Cell 104:545–556, 2001.
350. Findling JW, Raff H, Hansson JH, Lifton RP: Liddle's syndrome: Prospective genetic screening and suppressed aldosterone secretion in an extended kindred. J Clin Endocrinol Metab 82:1071–1074, 1997.
351. Botero-Velez M, Curtis JJ, Warnock DG: Brief report: Liddle's syndrome revisited—a disorder of sodium reabsorption in the distal tubule. N Engl J Med 330:178–181, 1994.
352. Firsov D, Schild L, Gautschi I, et al: Cell surface expression of the epithelial Na channel and a mutant causing Liddle syndrome: A quantitative approach. Proc Natl Acad Sci U S A 93:15370–15375, 1996.
353. Pradervand S, Vandewalle A, Bens M, et al: Dysfunction of the epithelial sodium channel expressed in the kidney of a mouse model for Liddle syndrome. J Am Soc Nephrol 14:2219–2228, 2003.
354. Kellenberger S, Gautschi I, Rossier BC, Schild L: Mutations causing Liddle syndrome reduce sodium-dependent downregulation of the epithelial sodium channel in the Xenopus oocyte expression system. J Clin Invest 101:2741–2750, 1998.
355. Frindt G, Silver RB, Windhager EE, Palmer LG: Feedback regulation of Na channels in rat CCT II Effects of inhibition of Na entry. Am J Physiol 264:F565–574, 1993.
356. Knight KK, Olson DR, Zhou R, Snyder PM: Liddle's syndrome mutations increase Na^+ transport through dual effects on epithelial Na^+ channel surface expression and proteolytic cleavage. Proc Natl Acad Sci U S A 103:2805–2808, 2006.
357. Hannila-Handelberg T, Kontula K, Tikkanen I, et al: Common variants of the beta and gamma subunits of the epithelial sodium channel and their relation to plasma renin and aldosterone levels in essential hypertension. BMC Med Genet 6:4, 2005.
358. Ambrosius WT, Bloem LJ, Zhou L, et al: Genetic variants in the epithelial sodium channel in relation to aldosterone and potassium excretion and risk for hypertension. Hypertension 34:631–637, 1999.
359. Gladziwa U, Schwarz R, Gitter AH, et al: Chronic hypokalaemia of adults: Gitelman's syndrome is frequent but classical Bartter's syndrome is rare. Nephrol Dial Transplant 10:1607–1613, 1995.
360. Guay-Woodford LM: Bartter syndrome: Unraveling the pathophysiologic enigma. Am J Med 105:151–161, 1998.
361. Komhoff M, Jeck ND, Seyberth HW, et al: Cyclooxygenase-2 expression is associated with the renal macula densa of patients with Bartter-like syndrome. Kidney Int 58:2420–2424, 2000.
362. Reinalter SC, Jeck N, Brochhauser C, et al: Role of cyclooxygenase-2 in hyperprostaglandin E syndrome/antenatal Bartter syndrome. Kidney Int 62:253–260, 2002.
363. Gill JR, Jr, Bartter FC: Evidence for a prostaglandin-independent defect in chloride reabsorption in the loop of Henle as a proximal cause of Bartter's syndrome. Am J Med 65:766–772, 1978.
364. Kockerling A, Reinalter SC, Seyberth HW: Impaired response to furosemide in hyperprostaglandin E syndrome: Evidence for a tubular defect in the loop of Henle. J Pediatr 129:519–528, 1996.
365. Simon DB, Karet FE, Hamdan JM, et al: Bartter's syndrome, hypokalaemic alkalosis with hypercalciuria, is caused by mutations in the Na-K-2Cl cotransporter NKCC2. Nat Genet 13:183–188, 1996.
366. Vargas-Poussou R, Feldmann D, Vollmer M, et al: Novel molecular variants of the Na-K-2Cl cotransporter gene are responsible for antenatal Bartter syndrome. Am J Hum Genet 62:1332–1340, 1998.
367. Bettinelli A, Ciarmatori S, Cesario L, et al: Phenotypic variability in Bartter syndrome type I. Pediatr Nephrol 14:940–945, 2000.
368. Sun A, Grossman EB, Lombardi M, Hebert SC: Vasopressin alters the mechanism of apical Cl- entry from Na^+:Cl- to Na^+:K^+:2Cl- cotransport in mouse medullary thick ascending limb. J Membr Biol 120:83–94, 1991.
369. Simon DB, Karet FE, Rodriguez-Soriano J, et al: Genetic heterogeneity of Bartter's syndrome revealed by mutations in the K^+ channel, ROMK. Nat Genet 14:152–156, 1996.
370. Simon DB, Bindra RS, Mansfield TA, et al: Mutations in the chloride channel gene, CLCNKB, cause Bartter's syndrome type III. Nat Genet 17:171–178, 1997.
371. Vandewalle A, Cluzeaud F, Bens M, et al: Localization and induction by dehydration of ClC-K chloride channels in the rat kidney. Am J Physiol 272:F678–688, 1997.
372. Vollmer M, Jeck N, Lemmink HH, et al: Antenatal Bartter syndrome with sensorineural deafness: Refinement of the locus on chromosome 1p31. Nephrol Dial Transplant 15:970–974, 2000.
373. Estevez R, Boettger T, Stein V, et al: Barttin is a Cl- channel beta-subunit crucial for renal Cl- reabsorption and inner ear K^+ secretion. Nature 414:558–561, 2001.
374. Schlingmann KP, Konrad M, Jeck N, et al: Salt wasting and deafness resulting from mutations in two chloride channels. N Engl J Med 350:1314–1319, 2004.
375. Watanabe S, Fukumoto S, Chang H, et al: Association between activating mutations of calcium-sensing receptor and Bartter's syndrome. Lancet 360:692–694, 2002.
376. Vargas-Poussou R, Huang C, Hulin P, et al: Functional characterization of a calcium-sensing receptor mutation in severe autosomal dominant hypocalcemia with a Bartter-like syndrome. J Am Soc Nephrol 13:2259–2266, 2002.
377. Riccardi D, Hall AE, Chattopadhyay N, et al: Localization of the extracellular $Ca2^+$/polyvalent cation-sensing protein in rat kidney. Am J Physiol 274:F611–622, 1998.
378. Wang WH, Lu M, Hebert SC: Cytochrome P-450 metabolites mediate extracellular $Ca(2^+)$-induced inhibition of apical K^+ channels in the TAL. Am J Physiol 271:C103–111, 1996.
379. Konrad M, Vollmer M, Lemmick HH, et al: Mutations in the chloride channel gene CLCNKB as a cause of classic Bartter syndrome. J Am Soc Nephrol 11:1449–1459, 2000.
380. Peters M, Jeck N, Reinalter S, et al: Clinical presentation of genetically defined patients with hypokalemic salt-losing tubulopathies. Am J Med 112:183–190, 2002.
381. Pressler CA, Heinzinger J, Jeck N, et al: Late-onset manifestation of antenatal Bartter syndrome as a result of residual function of the mutated renal Na^+-K^+-2Cl- Co-transporter. J Am Soc Nephrol 17:2136–2142, 2006.
382. Finer G, Shalev H, Birk OS, et al: Transient neonatal hyperkalemia in the antenatal (ROMK defective) Bartter syndrome. J Pediatr 142:318–323, 2003.
383. Lu M, Wang W: Two types of $K(^+)$ channels are present in the apical membrane of the thick ascending limb of the mouse kidney. Kidney Blood Press Res 23:75–82, 2000.
384. Lu M, Wang T, Yan Q, et al: ROMK is required for expression of the 70-pS K channel in the thick ascending limb. Am J Physiol Renal Physiol 286:F490–495, 2004.
385. Casatta L, Ferraccioli GF, Bartoli E: Hypokalaemic alkalosis, acquired Gitelman's and Bartter's syndrome in chronic sialoadenitis. Br J Rheumatol 36:1125–1128, 1997.
386. Bates CM, Baum M, Quigley R: Cystic fibrosis presenting with hypokalemia and metabolic alkalosis in a previously healthy adolescent. J Am Soc Nephrol 8:352–355, 1997.
387. Dave S, Honney, S, Raymond J, Flume PA: An unusual presentation of cystic fibrosis in an adult. Am J Kidney Dis 45:e41–44, 2005.
388. Lu M, Leng Q, Egan ME, et al: CFTR is required for PKA-regulated ATP sensitivity of Kir11 potassium channels in mouse kidney. J Clin Invest 116:797–807, 2006.
389. Luthy C, Bettinelli A, Iselin S, et al: Normal prostaglandinuria E2 in Gitelman's syndrome, the hypocalciuric variant of Bartter's syndrome. Am J Kidney Dis 25:824–828, 1995.
390. Cruz, DN, Shaer AJ, Bia MJ, et al: Gitelman's syndrome revisited: An evaluation of symptoms and health-related quality of life. Kidney Int 59:710–717, 2001.
391. Bettinelli A, Tosetto C, Colussi G, et al: Electrocardiogram with prolonged QT interval in Gitelman disease. Kidney Int 62:580–584, 2002.

392. Foglia PE, Bettinelli A, Tosetto C, et al: Cardiac work up in primary renal hypokalae-mia-hypomagnesaemia (Gitelman syndrome). Nephrol Dial Transplant 19:1398–1402, 2004.

393. Pachulski RT, Lopez, F, Sharaf R: Gitelman's not-so-benign syndrome. N Engl J Med 353:850–851, 2005.

394. Simon DB, Nelson-Williams C, Bia MJ, et al: Gitelman's variant of Bartter's syndrome, inherited hypokalaemic alkalosis, is caused by mutations in the thiazide-sensitive Na-Cl cotransporter. Nat Genet 12:24–30, 1996.

395. De Jong JC, Van Der Vliet WA, Van Den Heuvel LP, et al: Functional expression of mutations in the human NaCl cotransporter: Evidence for impaired routing mechanisms in Gitelman's Syndrome. J Am Soc Nephrol 13:1442–1448, 2002.

396. Loffing J, Vallon V, Loffing-Cueni D, et al: Altered renal distal tubule structure and renal Na($^+$) and Ca(2^+) handling in a mouse model for Gitelman's syndrome. J Am Soc Nephrol 15:2276–2288, 2004.

397. Loffing J, Loffing-Cueni D, Hegyi I, et al: Thiazide treatment of rats provokes apoptosis in distal tubule cells. Kidney Int 50:1180–1190, 1996.

398. Nijenhuis T, Vallon V, van der kemp AW, et al: Enhanced passive Ca2^+ reabsorption and reduced Mg2^+ channel abundance explains thiazide-induced hypocalciuria and hypomagnesemia. J Clin Invest 115:1651–1658, 2005.

399. Kaissling B, Stanton BA: Adaptation of distal tubule and collecting duct to increased sodium delivery I. Ultrastructure Am J Physiol 255:F1256–1268, 1988.

400. Morris RG, Hoorn EJ, Knepper MA: Hypokalemia in a mouse model of Gitelman's syndrome. Am J Physiol Renal Physiol 290:F1416–1420, 2006.

401. Friedman E, Shadel M, Halkin H, Farfel Z: Thiazide-induced hyponatremia. Reproducibility by single dose rechallenge and an analysis of pathogenesis. Ann Intern Med 110:24–30, 1989.

402. Cruz, D, Simon D, Lifton RP: Inactivating mutations in the Na-Cl cotransporter is associated with high bone density. J Am Soc Nephrol 10:597A, 1999.

403. Cauley JA, Cummings SR, Seeley DG, et al: Effects of thiazide diuretic therapy on bone mass, fractures, and falls. The Study of Osteoporotic Fractures Research Group. Ann Intern Med 118:666–673, 1993.

404. Cobeta-Garcia JC, Gascon A, Iglesias E, Estopinan V: Chondrocalcinosis and Gitelman's syndrome A new association? Ann Rheum Dis 57:748–749, 1998.

405. Vezzoli G, Soldati L, Jansen A, Pierro L: Choroidal calcifications in patients with Gitelman's syndrome. Am J Kidney Dis 36:855–858, 2000.

406. Panichpisal K, Angulo-Pernett F, Selhi S, Nugent KM: Gitelman-like syndrome after cisplatin therapy: A case report and literature review. BMC Nephrol 7:10, 2006.

407. Schwarz, C, Barisani T, Bauer E, Druml W: A woman with red eyes and hypokalemia: A case of acquired Gitelman syndrome. Wien Klin Wochenschr 118:239–242, 2006.

408. Chen YC, Chang WC, Yang AH, et al: Primary Sjogren's syndrome associated with Gitelman's syndrome presenting with muscular paralysis. Am J Kidney Dis 42:586–590, 2003.

409. Rodriguez, M, Solanki DL, Whang R: Refractory potassium repletion due to cisplatin-induced magnesium depletion. Arch Intern Med 149:2592–2594, 1989.

410. Whang R, Flink EB, Dyckner T, et al: Magnesium depletion as a cause of refractory potassium repletion. Arch Intern Med 145:1686–1689, 1985.

411. Whang R, Whang DD, Ryan MP: Refractory potassium repletion. A consequence of magnesium deficiency. Arch Intern Med 152:40–45, 1992.

412. Dorup I, Clausen T: Correlation between magnesium and potassium contents in muscle: Role of Na($^+$)-K$^+$ pump. Am J Physiol 264:C457–463, 1993.

413. Groeneveld JH, Sijpkens YW, Lin SH, et al: An approach to the patient with severe hypokalaemia: The potassium quiz. QJM 98:305–316, 2005.

414. Reimann D, Gross P: Chronic, diagnosis-resistant hypokalaemia. Nephrol Dial Transplant 14: 2957–2961, 1999.

415. Greenfeld D, Mickley, D, Quinlan DM, Roloff P: Hypokalemia in outpatients with eating disorders. Am J Psychiatry 152:60–63, 1995.

416. Crow, SJ, Rosenberg ME, Mitchell JE, Thuras P: Urine electrolytes as markers of bulimia nervosa. Int J Eat Disord 30:279–287, 2001.

417. Woywodt A, Herrmann A, Eisenberger U, et al: The tell-tale urinary chloride. Nephrol Dial Transplant 16:1066–1068, 2001.

418. Kim YG, Kim B, Kim MK, et al: Medullary nephrocalcinosis associated with long-term furosemide abuse in adults. Nephrol Dial Transplant 16:2303–2309, 2001.

419. Holmes AM, Hesling CM, Wilson TM: Drug-induced secondary hyperaldosteronism in patients with pulmonary tuberculosis. Q J Med 39:299–315, 1970.

420. Kone BC: Hypokalemia in Acid-base and Electrolyte Disorders: A companion to Brenner, Rector's The Kidney. DuBose TD Jr, Hamm LL (eds). Philadelphia, WB Saunders, 2002, pp 381–394.

421. Kim GH, Han JS: Therapeutic approach to hypokalemia. Nephron 92 Suppl 1:28–32, 2002.

422. Zydlewski AW, Hasbargen JA: Hypothermia-induced hypokalemia. Mil Med 163:719–721, 1998.

423. Kearney, TE, Manoguerra AS, Curtis GP, Ziegler MG: Theophylline toxicity and the beta-adrenergic system. Ann Intern Med 102:766–769, 1985.

424. Sterns RH, Cox, M, Feig PU, Singer I: Internal potassium balance and the control of the plasma potassium concentration. Medicine (Baltimore) 60:339–354, 1981.

425. Gabduzda GJ, Hall PW, 3rd: Relation of potassium depletion to renal ammonium metabolism and hepatic coma. Medicine (Baltimore) 45:481–490, 1966.

426. Jaeger P, Karlmark B, Giebisch G: Ammonium transport in rat cortical tubule: relationship to potassium metabolism. Am J Physiol 245:F593–600, 1983.

427. Khaw, KT, Barrett-Connor E: Dietary potassium and stroke-associated mortality. A 12-year prospective population study. N Engl J Med 316:235–240, 1987.

428. Ascherio A, Rimm EB, Hernan MA, et al: Intake of potassium, magnesium, calcium, and fiber and risk of stroke among US men. Circulation 98:1198–1204, 1998.

429. Villamil MF, Deland EC, Henney, RP, Maloney, JV, Jr: Anion effects on cation movements during correction of potassium depletion. Am J Physiol 229:161–166, 1975.

430. Nicolis GL, Kahn T, Sanchez, A, Gabrilove JL: Glucose-induced hyperkalemia in diabetic subjects. Arch Intern Med 141:49–53, 1981.

431. Keith NM, Osterberg AE, Burchell HB: Some effects of potassium salts in man. Ann Intern Med 16:879, 1942.

432. Kunin AS, Surawicz, B, Sims EAH: Decrease in serum potassium concentrations and appearance of cardiac arrhythmias during infusion of potassium with glucose in potassium-depleted patients. N Engl J Med 266:228–233, 1962.

433. Hamill RJ, Robinson LM, Wexler HR, Moote C: Efficacy and safety of potassium infusion therapy in hypokalemic critically ill patients. Crit Care Med 19:694–699, 1991.

434. Kruse JA, Carlson RW: Rapid correction of hypokalemia using concentrated intravenous potassium chloride infusions. Arch Intern Med 150:613–617, 1990.

435. Rose BD, Post TW: Hypokalemia. In Rose BD, Post TW (eds): Clinical Physiology of Acid-base and Electrolyte Disorders, Vol 1. New York, McGraw-Hill, pp 836–887.

436. Pullen H, Doig A, Lambie AT: Intensive intravenous potassium replacement therapy. Lancet 2: 809–811, 1967.

437. Abramson E, Arky R: Diabetic acidosis with initial hypokalemia. Therapeutic implications. JAMA 196:401–403, 1966.

438. Seftel HC, Kew MC: Early and intensive potassium replacement in diabetic acidosis. Diabetes 15: 694–696, 1966.

439. Norris W, Kunzelman KS, Bussell S, et al: Potassium supplementation, diet vs pills: A randomized trial in postoperative cardiac surgery patients. Chest 125:404–409, 2004.

440. Sopko JA, Freeman RM: Salt substitutes as a source of potassium. JAMA 238:608–610, 1977.

441. Doorenbos CJ, Vermeij CG: Danger of salt substitutes that contain potassium in patients with renal failure. BMJ 326:35–36, 2003.

442. Su M, Stork C, Ravuri S, et al: Sustained-release potassium chloride overdose. J Toxicol Clin Toxicol 39:641–648, 2001.

443. Ganguly A, Weinberger MH: Triamterene-thiazide combination: Alternative therapy for primary aldosteronism. Clin Pharmacol Ther 30:246–250, 1981.

444. Brown JJ, Davies DL, Ferriss JB, et al: Comparison of surgery and prolonged spironolactone therapy in patients with hypertension, aldosterone excess, and low plasma renin. Br Med J 2:729–734, 1972.

445. Griffing GT, Cole AG, Aurecchia AJ, et al: Amiloride in primary hyperaldosteronism. Clin Pharmacol Ther 31:56–61, 1982.

446. Eiro M, Katoh T, Watanabe T: Use of a proton-pump inhibitor for metabolic disturbances associated with anorexia nervosa. N Engl J Med 346:140, 2002.

447. Stevens MS, Dunlay, RW: Hyperkalemia in hospitalized patients. Int Urol Nephrol 32:177–180, 2000.

448. Moore ML, Bailey RR: Hyperkalaemia in patients in hospital. N Z Med J 102:557–558, 1989.

449. Rastegar A, Soleimani M, Rastergar A: Hypokalaemia and hyperkalaemia. Postgrad Med J 77, 759–764, 2001.

450. Paice B, Gray JM, McBride D, et al: Hyperkalaemia in patients in hospital. Br Med J (Clin Res Ed) 286:1189–1192, 1983.

451. Charytan D, Goldfarb DS: Indications for hospitalization of patients with hyperkalemia. Arch Intern Med 160:1605–1611, 2000.

452. Ponce SP, Jennings AE, Madias NE, Harrington JT: Drug-induced hyperkalemia. Medicine (Baltimore) 64:357–370, 1985.

453. Borra S, Shaker R, Kleinfeld M: Hyperkalemia in an adult hospitalized population. Mt Sinai J Med 55:226–229, 1988.

454. Ahee P, Crowe AV: The management of hyperkalaemia in the emergency department. J Accid Emerg Med 17:188–191, 2000.

455. Allon M, Dunlay R, Copkney C: Nebulized albuterol for acute hyperkalemia in patients on hemodialysis. Ann Intern Med 110:426–429, 1989.

456. Ahmed J, Weisberg LS: Hyperkalemia in dialysis patients. Semin Dial 14:348–356, 2001.

457. Moore CR, Lin JJ, O'Connor N, Halm EA: Follow-up of markedly elevated serum potassium results in the ambulatory setting: Implications for patient safety. Am J Med Qual 21:115–124, 2006.

458. Wiederkehr MR, Moe OW: Factitious hyperkalemia. Am J Kidney Dis 36, 1049–1053, 2000.

459. Skiner S: A cause of erroneous potassium levels. Lancet 277:478–480, 1961.

460. Graber M, Subramani K, Corish D, Schwab A: Thrombocytosis elevates serum potassium. Am J Kidney Dis 12:116–120, 1988.

461. Bellevue R, Dosik H, Spergel G, Gussoff BD: Pseudohyperkalemia and extreme leukocytosis. J Lab Clin Med 85:660–664, 1975.

462. Sevastos N, Theodossiades G, Savvas SP, et al: Pseudohyperkalemia in patients with increased cellular components of blood. Am J Med Sci 331:17–21, 2006.

463. Kellerman PS, Thornbery JM: Pseudohyperkalemia due to pneumatic tube transport in a leukemic patient. Am J Kidney Dis 46:746–748, 2005.

464. Oliver TK, Jr, Young GA, Bates GD, Adamo JS: Factitial hyperkalemia due to icing before analysis. Pediatrics 38:900–902, 1966.

465. Seamark D, Backhouse S, Barber P, et al: Transport and temperature effects on measurement of serum and plasma potassium. J R Soc Med 92:339–341, 1999.

466. Carella M, d'Adamo AP, Grootenboer-Mignot S, et al: A second locus mapping to 2q35–36 for familial pseudohyperkalaemia. Eur J Hum Genet 12:1073–1076, 2004.

467. Bruce LJ, Robinson HC, Guizouarn H, et al: Monovalent cation leaks in human red cells caused by single amino-acid substitutions in the transport domain of the band 3 chloride-bicarbonate exchanger, AE1. Nat Genet 37:1258–1263, 2005.

468. Iolascon A, Stewart GW, Ajetunmobi JF, et al: Familial pseudohyperkalemia maps to the same locus as dehydrated hereditary stomatocytosis (hereditary xerocytosis). Blood 93:3120–3123, 1999.

469. Arrambide K, Toto RD: Tumor lysis syndrome. Semin Nephrol 13:273–280, 1993.

470. Parisi A, Alabiso A, Sacchetti M, et al: Complex ventricular arrhythmia induced by overuse of potassium supplementation in a young male football player. Case report. J Sports Med Phys Fitness 42:214–216, 2002.

471. Mueller BA, Scott MK, Sowinski KM, Prag KA: Noni juice (Morinda citrifolia): Hidden potential for hyperkalemia? Am J Kidney Dis 35:310–312, 2000.

472. Nagasaki A, Takamine W, Takasu N: Severe hyperkalemia associated with "alternative" nutritional cancer therapy. Clin Nutr 24:864–865, 2005.

473. Gelfand MC, Zarate A, Knepshield JH: Geophagia A cause of life-threatening hyperkalemia in patients with chronic renal failure. JAMA 234:738–740, 1975.

474. Abu-Hamdan DK, Sondheimer JH, Mahajan SK: Cautopyreiophagia. Cause of life-threatening hyperkalemia in a patient undergoing hemodialysis. Am J Med 79:517–519, 1985.

475. Baz, EM, Kanazi GE, Mahfouz, RA, Obeid MY: An unusual case of hyperkalaemia-induced cardiac arrest in a paediatric patient during transfusion of a "fresh" 6-day-old blood unit. Transfus Med 12:383–386, 2002.

476. Moreno M, Murphy C, Goldsmith C: Increase in serum potassium resulting from the administration of hypertonic mannitol and other solutions. J Lab Clin Med 73:291–298, 1969.

477. Hirota K, Hara T, Hosoi S, et al: Two cases of hyperkalemia after administration of hypertonic mannitol during craniotomy. J Anesth 19:75–77, 2005.

478. Goldfarb S, Strunk B, Singer I, Goldberg M: Paradoxical glucose-induced hyperkalemia Combined aldosterone-insulin deficiency. Am J Med 59:744–750, 1975.

479. Magnus Nzerue C, Jackson E: Intractable life-threatening hyperkalaemia in a diabetic patient. Nephrol Dial Transplant 15:113–114, 2000.

480. Sirken G, Raja R, Garces J, et al: Contrast-induced translocational hyponatremia and hyperkalemia in advanced kidney disease. Am J Kidney Dis 43:e31–35, 2004.

481. Perazella MA, Biswas P: Acute hyperkalemia associated with intravenous epsilon-aminocaproic acid therapy. Am J Kidney Dis 33:782–785, 1999.

482. Nzerue CM, Falana B: Refractory hyperkalaemia associated with use of epsilon-aminocaproic acid during coronary bypass in a dialysis patient. Nephrol Dial Transplant 17:1150–1151, 2002.

483. Clark BA, Shannon C, Brown RS, Gervino EV: Extrarenal potassium homeostasis with maximal exercise in end-stage renal disease. J Am Soc Nephrol 7:1223–1227, 1996.

484. Sangkabutra T, Crankshaw GP, Schneider P, et al: Impaired K$^+$ regulation contributes to exercise limitation in end-stage renal failure. Kidney Int 63:283–290, 2003.

485. Allon M: Hyperkalemia in end-stage renal disease: Mechanisms and management. J Am Soc Nephrol 6:1134–1142, 1995.

486. Chi HT, Hung DZ, Hu WH, Yang DY: Prognostic implications of hyperkalemia in toad toxin intoxication. Hum Exp Toxicol 17:343–346, 1998.

487. Gowda RM, Cohen RA, Khan IA: Toad venom poisoning: resemblance to digoxin toxicity and therapeutic implications. Heart 89:e14, 2003.

488. Baltazar RF, Mower MM, Reider R, et al: Acute fluoride poisoning leading to fatal hyperkalemia. Chest 78:660–663, 1980.

489. Martyn JA, Richtsfeld M: Succinylcholine-induced hyperkalemia in acquired pathologic states: Etiologic factors and molecular mechanisms. Anesthesiology 104:158–169, 2006.

490. Thapa S, Brull SJ: Succinylcholine-induced hyperkalemia in patients with renal failure: An old question revisited. Anesth Analg 91:237–241, 2000.

491. Singer M, Coluzzi F, O'Brien A, Clapp LH: Reversal of life-threatening drug-related potassium-channel syndrome by glibenclamide. Lancet 365:1873–1875, 2005.

492. Wilson AJ, Jabr RI, Clapp LH: Calcium modulation of vascular smooth muscle ATP-sensitive K($^+$) channels: Role of protein phosphatase-2B. Circ Res 87:1019–1025, 2000.

493. Nielsen JJ, Kristensen M, Hellsten Y, et al: Localization and function of ATP-sensitive potassium channels in human skeletal muscle. Am J Physiol Regul Integr Comp Physiol 284:R558–563, 2003.

494. McCauley J, Murray J, Jordan M, et al: Labetalol-induced hyperkalemia in renal transplant recipients. Am J Nephrol 22:347–351, 2002.

495. Blumenfeld JD, Sealey JE, Mann SJ, et al: Beta-adrenergic receptor blockade as a therapeutic approach for suppressing the renin-angiotensin-aldosterone system in normotensive and hypertensive subjects. Am J Hypertens 12:451–459, 1999.

496. Yamamoto T, Fukuyama J, Hasegawa K, Sugiura M: Isolated corticotropin deficiency in adults. Report of 10 cases and review of literature. Arch Intern Med 152:1705–1712, 1992.

497. Mansiere TJ, Estep H: Pseudo-Addison's disease Isolated corticotropin deficiency associated with hyporeninemic hypoaldosteronism. Arch Intern Med 146:996–997, 1986.

498. Fujieda K, Tajima T: Molecular basis of adrenal insufficiency. Pediatr Res 57:62R-69R, 2005.

499. Achermann JC, Meeks JJ, Jameson JL: Phenotypic spectrum of mutations in DAX-1 and SF-1 Mol Cell Endocrinol 185:17–25, 2001.

500. Fujieda K, Tajima T, Nakae J, et al: Spontaneous puberty in 46,XX subjects with congenital lipoid adrenal hyperplasia. Ovarian steroidogenesis is spared to some extent despite inactivating mutations in the steroidogenic acute regulatory protein (StAR) gene. J Clin Invest 99:1265–1271, 1997.

501. Bose HS, Sugawara T, Strauss JF, 3rd, Miller WL: The pathophysiology and genetics of congenital lipoid adrenal hyperplasia. International Congenital Lipoid Adrenal Hyperplasia Consortium. N Engl J Med 335:1870–1878, 1996.

502. Hiort O, Holterhus PM, Werner R, et al: Homozygous disruption of P450 side-chain cleavage (CYP11A1) is associated with prematurity, complete 46,XY sex reversal, and severe adrenal failure. J Clin Endocrinol Metab 90:538–541, 2005.

503. Speiser PW: Congenital adrenal hyperplasia owing to 21-hydroxylase deficiency. Endocrinol Metab Clin North Am 30:31–59, vi, 2001.

504. Kayes-Wandover KM, Tannin GM, Shulman D, et al: Congenital hyperreninemic hypoaldosteronism unlinked to the aldosterone synthase (CYP11B2) gene. J Clin Endocrinol Metab 86:5379–5382, 2001.

505. Kayes-Wandover KM, Schindler RE, Taylor HC, White PC: Type 1 aldosterone synthase deficiency presenting in a middle-aged man. J Clin Endocrinol Metab 86:1008–1012, 2001.

506. Morimoto S, Kim KS, Yamamoto I, et al: Selective hypoaldosteronism with hyperreninemia in a diabetic patient. J Clin Endocrinol Metab 49:742–747, 1979.

507. Agmon D, Green J, Platau E, Better OS: Isolated adrenal mineralocorticoid deficiency due to amyloidosis associated with familial Mediterranean fever. Am J Med Sci 288:40–43, 1984.

508. Oster JR, Singer I, Fishman LM: Heparin-induced aldosterone suppression and hyperkalemia. Am J Med 98:575–586, 1995.

509. Koren-Michowitz M, Avni B, Michowitz Y, et al: Early onset of hyperkalemia in patients treated with low molecular weight heparin: A prospective study. Pharmaco-epidemiol Drug Saf 13:299–302, 2004.

510. Oelkers W: Adrenal insufficiency. N Engl J Med 335:1206–1212, 1996.

511. Espinosa G, Santos E, Cervera R, et al: Adrenal involvement in the antiphospholipid syndrome: Clinical and immunologic characteristics of 86 patients. Medicine (Baltimore) 82:106–118, 2003.

512. Danby P, Harris KP, Williams B, et al: Adrenal dysfunction in patients with renal amyloid. Q J Med 76:915–922, 1990.

513. Mayo J, Collazos J, Martinez E, Ibarra S: Adrenal function in the human immunodeficiency virus-infected patient. Arch Intern Med 162:1095–1098, 2002.

514. Schambelan M, Stockigt JR, Biglieri EG: Isolated hypoaldosteronism in adults A renin-deficiency syndrome. N Engl J Med 287:573–578, 1972.

515. Lush DJ, King JA, Fray JC: Pathophysiology of low renin syndromes: Sites of renal renin secretory impairment and prorenin overexpression. Kidney Int 43:983–999, 1993.

516. Michelis MF: Hyperkalemia in the elderly. Am J Kidney Dis 16:296–299, 1990.

517. Lee FO, Quismorio FP, Jr, Troum OM, et al: Mechanisms of hyperkalemia in systemic lupus erythematosus. Arch Intern Med 148:397–401, 1988.

518. Shaked Y, Blau A, Shpilberg O, Samra Y: Hyporeninemic hypoaldosteronism associated with multiple myeloma: 11 years of follow-up. Clin Nephrol 40:79–82, 1993.

519. Don BR, Schambelan M: Hyperkalemia in acute glomerulonephritis due to transient hyporeninemic hypoaldosteronism. Kidney Int 38:1159–1163, 1990.

520. Szylman P, Better OS, Chaimowitz C, Rosler A: Role of hyperkalemia in the metabolic acidosis of isolated hypoaldosteronism. N Engl J Med 294:361–365, 1976.

521. DuBose TD, Jr, Caflisch CR: Effect of selective aldosterone deficiency on acidification in nephron segments of the rat inner medulla. J Clin Invest 82:1624–1632, 1988.

522. Matsuda O, Nonoguchi H, Tomita K, et al: Primary role of hyperkalemia in the acidosis of hyporeninemic hypoaldosteronism. Nephron 49:203–209, 1988.

523. Sebastian A, Schambelan M, Lindenfeld S, Morris RC, Jr: Amelioration of metabolic acidosis with fludrocortisone therapy in hyporeninemic hypoaldosteronism. N Engl J Med 297:576–583, 1977.

524. Sebastian A, Schambelan M: Amelioration of type 4 renal tubular acidosis in chronic renal failure with furosemide. Kidney Int 12:534, 1977.

525. Chan R, Sealey JE, Michelis MF, et al: Renin-aldosterone system can respond to furosemide in patients with hyperkalemic hyporeninism. J Lab Clin Med 132:229–235, 1998.

526. Oh MS, Carroll HJ, Clemmons JE, et al: A mechanism for hyporeninemic hypoaldosteronism in chronic renal disease. Metabolism 23:1157–1166, 1974.

527. Klemm SA, Gordon RD, Tunny, TJ, Finn WL: Biochemical correction in the syndrome of hypertension and hyperkalaemia by severe dietary salt restriction suggests renin-aldosterone suppression critical in pathophysiology. Clin Exp Pharmacol Physiol 17:191–195, 1990.

528. Tuchelt H, Eschenhagen G, Bahr V, et al: Role of atrial natriuretic factor in changes in the responsiveness of aldosterone to angiotensin II secondary to sodium loading and depletion in man. Clin Sci (Lond) 79:57–65, 1990.

529. DeFronzo RA, Cooke CR, Goldberg M, et al: Impaired renal tubular potassium secretion in systemic lupus erythematosus. Ann Intern Med 86:268–271, 1977.

530. DeFronzo RA, Taufield PA, Black H, et al: Impaired renal tubular potassium secretion in sickle cell disease. Ann Intern Med 90:310–316, 1979.

531. Batlle D, Itsarayoungyuen K, Arruda JA, Kurtzman NA: Hyperkalemic hyperchloremic metabolic acidosis in sickle cell hemoglobinopathies. Am J Med 72:188–192, 1982.

532. Geller DS, Zhang J, Zennaro MC, et al: Autosomal dominant pseudohypoaldosteronism type 1: Mechanisms, evidence for neonatal lethality, and phenotypic expression in adults. J Am Soc Nephrol 17:1429–1436, 2006.

533. Hummler E, Barker P, Gatzy J, et al: Early death due to defective neonatal lung liquid clearance in alpha- ENaC-deficient mice. Nat Genet 12:325–328, 1996.

534. Akcay A, Yavuz T, Semiz S, et al: Pseudohypoaldosteronism type 1 and respiratory distress syndrome. J Pediatr Endocrinol Metab 15:1557–1561, 2002.

535. Bonny O, Chraibi A, Loffing J, et al: Functional expression of a pseudohypoaldosteronism type I mutated epithelial Na$^+$ channel lacking the pore-forming region of its alpha subunit. J Clin Invest 104:967–974, 1999.

536. Grunder S, Jaeger NF, Gautschi I, et al: Identification of a highly conserved sequence at the N-terminus of the epithelial Na$^+$ channel alpha subunit involved in gating. Pflugers Arch 438:709–715, 1999.

537. Mayan H, Vered I, Mouallem M, et al: Pseudohypoaldosteronism type II: Marked sensitivity to thiazides, hypercalciuria, normomagnesemia, and low bone mineral density. J Clin Endocrinol Metab 87:3248–3254, 2002.

538. Wilson FH, Disse-Nicodeme S, Choate KA, et al: Human hypertension caused by mutations in WNK kinases. Science 293:1107–1112, 2001.

539. Choate KA, Kahle KT, Wilson FH, et al: WNK1, a kinase mutated in inherited hypertension with hyperkalemia, localizes to diverse Cl- -transporting epithelia. Proc Natl Acad Sci U S A 100:663–668, 2003.

540. Wilson FH, Kahle KT, Sabath E, et al: Molecular pathogenesis of inherited hypertension with hyperkalemia: The Na-Cl cotransporter is inhibited by wild-type but not mutant WNK4. Proc Natl Acad Sci U S A 100:680–684, 2003.

541. Golbang AP, Cope G, Hamad A, et al: Regulation of the expression of the Na/Cl cotransporter (NCCT) by WNK4 and WNK1: Evidence that accelerated

dynamin-dependent endocytosis is not involved. Am J Physiol Renal Physiol 291: F1369–F1376, 2006.

542. Yang CL, Angell J, Mitchell R, Ellison DH: WNK kinases regulate thiazide-sensitive Na-Cl cotransport. J Clin Invest 111:1039–1145, 2003.

543. Vitari AC, Deak M, Morrice NA, Alessi DR: The WNK1 and WNK4 protein kinases that are mutated in Gordon's hypertension syndrome phosphorylate and activate SPAK and OSR1 protein kinases. Biochem J 391:17–24, 2005.

544. Gagnon KB, England R, Delpire E: Characterization of SPAK and OSR1, regulatory kinases of the Na-K-2Cl cotransporter. Mol Cell Biol 26:689–698, 2006.

545. Moriguchi T, Urushiyama S, Hisamoto N, et al: WNK1 regulates phosphorylation of cation-chloride-coupled cotransporters via the STE20-related kinases, SPAK and OSR1. J Biol Chem 280:42685–42693, 2005.

546. Delaloy C, Lu J, Houot AM, et al: Multiple promoters in the WNK1 gene: One controls expression of a kidney-specific kinase-defective isoform. Mol Cell Biol 23:9208–9221, 2003.

547. Lazrak A, Liu Z, Huang CL: Antagonistic regulation of ROMK by long and kidney-specific WNK1 isoforms. Proc Natl Acad Sci U S A 103:1615–1620, 2006.

548. Kahle KT, Wilson FH, Leng Q, et al: WNK4 regulates the balance between renal NaCl reabsorption and K+ secretion. Nat Genet 35:372–376, 2003.

549. Kahle KT, Macgregor GG, Wilson FH, et al: Paracellular Cl- permeability is regulated by WNK4 kinase: Insight into normal physiology and hypertension. Proc Natl Acad Sci U S A 101:14877–14882, 2004.

550. Ling BN, Webster CL, Eaton DC: Eicosanoids modulate apical Ca(2+)-dependent K+ channels in cultured rabbit principal cells. Am J Physiol 263:F116–126, 1992.

551. Mactier RA, Khanna R: Hyperkalemia induced by indomethacin and naproxen and reversed by fludrocortisone. South Med J 81:799–801, 1988.

552. Tan SY, Shapiro R, Franco R, et al: Indomethacin-induced prostaglandin inhibition with hyperkalemia A reversible cause of hyporeninemic hypoaldosteronism. Ann Intern Med 90:783–785, 1979.

553. Tan SY, Mulrow PJ: Inhibition of the renin-aldosterone response to furosemide by indomethacin. J Clin Endocrinol Metab 45:174–176, 1977.

554. Harris RC, Jr: Cyclooxygenase-2 inhibition and renal physiology. Am J Cardiol 89:10D–17D, 2002.

555. Swan SK, Rudy DW, Lasseter KC, et al: Effect of cyclooxygenase-2 inhibition on renal function in elderly persons receiving a low-salt diet: A randomized, controlled trial. Ann Intern Med 133:1–9, 2000.

556. Roig F, Llinas MT, Lopez R, Salazar FJ: Role of cyclooxygenase-2 in the prolonged regulation of renal function. Hypertension 40:721–728, 2002.

557. Braden GL, O'Shea MH, Mulhern JG, Germain MJ: Acute renal failure and hyperkalaemia associated with cyclooxygenase-2 inhibitors. Nephrol Dial Transplant 19:1149–1153, 2004.

558. Lam Q, Schneider HG: Hyperkalaemia with cyclooxygenase-2 inhibition and hypoaldosteronism Intern Med J 35:572–573, 2005.

559. Perazella MA: Drug-induced hyperkalemia: Old culprits and new offenders. Am J Med 109:307–14, 2000.

560. Oishi M, Yagi T, Urishihara N, et al: A case of hyperkalemic distal renal tubular acidosis secondary to tacrolimus in living donor liver transplantation. Transplant Proc 32:2225–2226, 2000.

561. Higgins R, Ramaiyan K, Dasgupta T, et al: Hyponatraemia and hyperkalaemia are more frequent in renal transplant recipients treated with tacrolimus than with cyclosporin: Further evidence for differences between cyclosporin and tacrolimus nephrotoxicities. Nephrol Dial Transplant 19:444–450, 2004.

562. Bantle JP, Nath KA, Sutherland DE, et al: Effects of cyclosporine on the renin-angiotensin-aldosterone system and potassium excretion in renal transplant recipients. Arch Intern Med 145:505–508, 1985.

563. Hocherl K, Dreher F, Vitzthum H, et al: Cyclosporine A suppresses cyclooxygenase-2 expression in the rat kidney. J Am Soc Nephrol 13:2427–2436, 2002.

564. Ling BN, Eaton DC: Cyclosporin A inhibits apical secretory K+ channels in rabbit cortical collecting tubule principal cells. Kidney Int 48:974–984, 1993.

565. Pei Y, Richardson R, Greenwood C, et al: Extrarenal effect of cyclosporine A on potassium homeostasis in renal transplant recipients. Am J Kidney Dis 22:314–319, 1993.

566. Choi MJ, Fernandez PC, Patnaik A, et al: Brief report: Trimethoprim-induced hyperkalemia in a patient with AIDS. N Engl J Med 328:703–736, 1993.

567. Kleyman TR, Roberts C, Ling BN: A mechanism for pentamidine-induced hyperkalemia: Inhibition of distal nephron sodium transport. Ann Intern Med 122:103–106, 1995.

568. Velazquez, H, Perazella MA, Wright FS, Ellison DH: Renal mechanism of trimethoprim-induced hyperkalemia. Ann Intern Med 119:296–301, 1993.

569. Muto S, Tsuruoka S, Miyata Y, et al: Effect of trimethoprim-sulfamethoxazole on Na and K+ transport properties in the rabbit cortical collecting duct perfused in vitro. Nephron Physiol 102:51–60, 2006.

570. Alappan R, Perazella MA, Buller GK: Hyperkalemia in hospitalized patients treated with trimethoprim-sulfamethoxazole. Ann Intern Med 124:316–320, 1996.

571. Elisaf M, Terrovitou C, Tomos P, Siamopoulos KC: Severe hyperkalaemia after cotrimoxazole administration in a patient with hyporeninaemic hypoaldosteronism. Nephrol Dial Transplant 12:1254–1255, 1997.

572. Kitagawa H, Chang H, Fujita T: Hyperkalemia due to nafamostat mesylate. N Engl J Med 332: 687, 1995.

573. Iwashita K, Kitamura K, Narikiyo T, et al: Inhibition of prostasin secretion by serine protease inhibitors in the kidney. J Am Soc Nephrol 14:11–16, 2003.

574. Bakris GL, Siomos M, Richardson D, et al: ACE inhibition or angiotensin receptor blockade: Impact on potassium in renal failure VAL-K Study Group. Kidney Int 58:2084–2092, 2000.

575. Azizi M: Renin inhibition. Curr Opin Nephrol Hypertens 15:505–510, 2006.

576. Rossing K, Schjoedt KJ, Smidt UM, et al: Beneficial effects of adding spironolactone to recommended antihypertensive treatment in diabetic nephropathy: A randomized, double-masked, cross-over study. Diabetes Care 28:2106–2112, 2005.

577. Pitt B, Zannad F, Remme WJ, et al: The effect of spironolactone on morbidity and mortality in patients with severe heart failure Randomized Aldactone Evaluation Study Investigators. N Engl J Med 341:709–717, 1999.

578. Pitt B, Remme W, Zannad F, et al: Eplerenone a selective aldosterone blocker, in patients with left ventricular dysfunction after myocardial infarction. N Engl J Med 348:1309–1321, 2003.

579. Gross P, Pistrosch F: Hyperkalaemia: Again. Nephrol Dial Transplant 19:2163–2166, 2004.

580. Bakris GL, Weir MR: Angiotensin-converting enzyme inhibitor-associated elevations in serum creatinine: Is this a cause for concern? Arch Intern Med 160:685–693, 2000.

581. Juurlink DN, Mamdani MM, Lee DS, et al: Rates of hyperkalemia after publication of the Randomized Aldactone Evaluation Study. N Engl J Med 351:543–551, 2004.

582. Goldfarb DS: Hyperkalemia after the publication of RALES. N Engl J Med 351: 2448–2450; author reply 2448–2450, 2004.

583. Zandi-Nejad K, Brenner BM: Strategies to retard the progression of chronic kidney disease. Med Clin North Am 89:489–509, 2005.

584. Palmer BF: Managing hyperkalemia caused by inhibitors of the renin-angiotensin-aldosterone system. N Engl J Med 351:585–592, 2004.

585. Levinsky NG: Management of emergencies. VI Hyperkalemia. N Engl J Med 274:1076–1077, 1966.

586. Allon M: Treatment and prevention of hyperkalemia in end-stage renal disease. Kidney Int 43:1197–1209, 1993.

587. Kim HJ, Han SW: Therapeutic approach to hyperkalemia. Nephron 92 Suppl 1:33–40, 2002.

588. Evans KJ, Greenberg A: Hyperkalemia: A review. J Intensive Care Med 20:272–290, 2005.

589. Rose BD, Post TW: Hyperkalemia. In Rose BD, Post TW (eds): Clinical Physiology of Acid-base and Electrolyte Disorders, Vol 1. New York, McGraw-Hill, 2001, pp 888–930.

590. Winkler AW, Hoff HE, Smith PK: Factors affecting the toxicity of potassium. Am J Physiol 127:430–436, 1939.

591. Pergola PE, DeFronzo R: Clinical disorders of hyperkalemia. In Seldin GW, Giebisch G (eds): The Kidney: Physiology and Pathophysiology, Vol 2. Philadelphia, Lippincott, Williams & Wilkins, 2000, pp 1647–1700.

592. Davey M, Caldicott D: Calcium salts in management of hyperkalaemia. Emerg Med J 19:92–93, 2002.

593. Bower JO, Mengle HAK: The additive effects of calcium and digitalis. JAMA 106: 1151–1153, 1936.

594. White RD, Goldsmith RS, Rodriguez R, et al: Plasma ionic calcium levels following injection of chloride, gluconate, and gluceptate salts of calcium. J Thorac Cardiovasc Surg 71:609–613, 1976.

595. Bull J, Band DM: Calcium and cardiac arrest. Anaesthesia 35:1066–1067, 1980.

596. Cote CJ, Drop LJ, Daniels AL, Hoaglin DC: Calcium chloride versus calcium gluconate: Comparison of ionization and cardiovascular effects in children and dogs. Anesthesiology 66:465–470, 1987.

597. Martin TJ, Kang Y, Robertson KM, et al: Ionization and hemodynamic effects of calcium chloride and calcium gluconate in the absence of hepatic function. Anesthesiology 73:62–65, 1990.

598. Alvestrand A, Wahren J, Smith D, DeFronzo RA: Insulin-mediated potassium uptake is normal in uremic and healthy subjects. Am J Physiol 246:E174–180, 1984.

599. Allon M, Copkney C: Albuterol and insulin for treatment of hyperkalemia in hemodialysis patients. Kidney Int 38:869–872, 1990.

600. Blumberg A, Weidmann P, Shaw S, Gnadinger M: Effect of various therapeutic approaches on plasma potassium and major regulating factors in terminal renal failure. Am J Med 85:507–512, 1988.

601. De Wolf A, Frenette L, Kang Y, Tang C: Insulin decreases the serum potassium concentration during the anhepatic stage of liver transplantation. Anesthesiology 78:677–682, 1993.

602. Minaker KL, Rowe JW: Potassium homeostasis during hyperinsulinemia: Effect of insulin level, beta-blockade, and age. Am J Physiol 242:E373–377, 1982.

603. Smith D, DeFronzo RA: Insulin resistance in uremia mediated by postbinding defects. Kidney Int 22:54–62, 1982.

604. Perazella MA: Approach to hyperkalemic end-stage renal disease patients in the emergency department. Conn Med 63:131–136, 1999.

605. Emmett M: Non-dialytic treatment of acute hyperkalemia in the dialysis patient. Semin Dial 13:279–280, 2000.

606. Lens XM, Montoliu J, Cases A, et al: Treatment of hyperkalaemia in renal failure: Salbutamol v insulin. Nephrol Dial Transplant 4:228–232, 1989.

607. Liou HH, Chaing SS, Wu SC, et al: Hypokalemic effects of intravenous infusion or nebulization of salbutamol in patients with chronic renal failure: Comparative study. Am J Kidney Dis 23:266–271, 1994.

608. Montoliu J, Lens XM, Revert L: Potassium-lowering effect of albuterol for hyperkalemia in renal failure. Arch Intern Med 147:713–717, 1987.

609. Ostovar H, Jones J, Brown M: Best evidence topic report Nebulised levalbuterol or albuterol for lowering serum potassium. Emerg Med J 22:366–367, 2005.

610. Mandelberg A, Krupnik Z, Houri S, et al: Salbutamol metered-dose inhaler with spacer for hyperkalemia: How fast? How safe? Chest 115:617–622, 1999.

611. Sowinski KM, Cronin D, Mueller BA, Kraus MA: Subcutaneous terbutaline use in CKD to reduce potassium concentrations. Am J Kidney Dis 45:1040–1045, 2005.

612. Iqbal Z, Friedman EA: Preferred therapy of hyperkalemia in renal insufficiency: Survey of nephrology training-program directors. N Engl J Med 320:60–61, 1989.

613. Schwarz KC, Cohen BD, Lubash GD, Rubin AL: Severe acidosis and hyperpotassemia treated with sodium bicarbonate infusion. Circulation 19:215–220, 1959.

614. Blumberg A, Weidmann P, Ferrari P: Effect of prolonged bicarbonate administration on plasma potassium in terminal renal failure. Kidney Int 41:369–374, 1992.

615. Gutierrez R, Schlessinger F, Oster JR, et al: Effect of hypertonic versus isotonic sodium bicarbonate on plasma potassium concentration in patients with end-stage renal disease. Miner Electrolyte Metab 17:297–302, 1991.

616. Allon M, Shanklin N: Effect of bicarbonate administration on plasma potassium in dialysis patients: Interactions with insulin and albuterol. Am J Kidney Dis 28:508–514, 1996.

617. Suki WN: Use of diuretics in chronic renal failure. Kidney Int Suppl 59:S33–35, 1997.

618. Sebastian A, Schambelan M, Sutton JM: Amelioration of hyperchloremic acidosis with furosemide therapy in patients with chronic renal insufficiency and type 4 renal tubular acidosis. Am J Nephrol 4:287–300, 1984.

619. DeFronzo RA, Goldberg M, Cooke CR, et al: Investigations into the mechanisms of hyperkalemia following renal transplantation. Kidney Int 11:357–365, 1977.

620. Reiser IW, Chou SY, Brown MI, Porush JG: Reversal of trimethoprim-induced antikaliuresis. Kidney Int 50:2063–2069, 1996.

621. Wilcox CS: New insights into diuretic use in patients with chronic renal disease. J Am Soc Nephrol 13:798–805, 2002.

622. Sherman DS, Kass CL, Fish DN: Fludrocortisone for the treatment of heparin-induced hyperkalemia. Ann Pharmacother 34:606–610, 2000.

623. Dreyling KW, Wanner C, Schollmeyer P: Control of hyperkalemia with fludrocortisone in a patient with systemic lupus erythematosus. Clin Nephrol 33:179–183, 1990.

624. Petersen KC, Silberman H, Berne TV: Hyperkalaemia after cyclosporin therapy. Lancet 1:1470, 1984.

625. Furuya R, Kumagai H, Sakao T, et al: Potassium-lowering effect of mineralocorticoid therapy in patients undergoing hemodialysis. Nephron 92:576–581, 2002.

626. Imbriano LJ, Durham JH, Maesaka JK: Treating interdialytic hyperkalemia with fludrocortisone. Semin Dial 16:5–7, 2003.

627. Kaisar MO, Wiggins KJ, Sturtevant JM, et al: A randomized controlled trial of fludrocortisone for the treatment of hyperkalemia in hemodialysis patients. Am J Kidney Dis 47:809–814, 2006.

628. Elkinton JR, Clark JK, Squires RD: Treatment of potassium retention in uremia with cation exchange resin: Preliminary report. Am J Med Sci 220:547–552, 1950.

629. Berlyne GM, Janabi K, Shaw AB: Dangers of resonium A in the treatment of hyperkalemia in renal failure. Lancet 1:167–169, 1966.

630. Scherr L, Ogden DA, Mead AW: Management of hyperkalemia with cation-exchange resin. N Engl J Med 264:115–119, 1961.

631. Monzu B, Caramelo C, Traba ML, Garvia R: Effect of potassium-chelating resins on phosphorus absorption. Nephron 68:148, 1994.

632. Papadimitriou M, Gingell JC, Chisholm GD: Hypercalcaemia from calcium ion-exchange resin in patients on regular haemodialysis. Lancet 2:948–950, 1968.

633. Agarwal R, Afzalpurkar R, Fordtran JS: Pathophysiology of potassium absorption and secretion by the human intestine. Gastroenterology 107:548–571, 1994.

634. Flinn RB, Merrill JP, Welzant WR: Treatment of the oliguric patient with a new sodium-exchange resin and sorbitol. N Engl J Med 264:111–115, 1961.

635. Emmett M, Hootkins RE, Fine KD, et al: Effect of three laxatives and a cation exchange resin on fecal sodium and potassium excretion. Gastroenterology 108:752–760, 1995.

636. Gruy-Kapral C, Emmett M, Santa Ana CA, et al: Effect of single dose resin-cathartic therapy on serum potassium concentration in patients with end-stage renal disease. J Am Soc Nephrol 9:1924–1930, 1998.

637. Gales MA, Gales BJ, Dyer ME, Orr SR: Rectally administered sodium polystyrene sulfonate. Am J Health Syst Pharm 52:2813–2815, 1995.

638. Lillemoe KD, Romolo JL, Hamilton SR, et al: Intestinal necrosis due to sodium polystyrene (Kayexalate) in sorbitol enemas: Clinical and experimental support for the hypothesis. Surgery 101:267–272, 1987.

639. Dardik A, Moosinger RC, Efron G, et al: Acute abdomen with colonic necrosis induced by Kayexalate-sorbitol. South Med J 93:511–513, 2000.

640. Gerstman BB, Kirkman R, Platt R: Intestinal necrosis associated with postoperative orally administered sodium polystyrene sulfonate in sorbitol. Am J Kidney Dis 20:159–161, 1992.

641. Rashid A, Hamilton SR: Necrosis of the gastrointestinal tract in uremic patients as a result of sodium polystyrene sulfonate (Kayexalate) in sorbitol: An underrecognized condition. Am J Surg Pathol 21:60–69, 1997.

642. Roy-Chaudhury P, Meisels IS, Freedman S, et al: Combined gastric and ileocecal toxicity (serpiginous ulcers) after oral kayexalate in sorbital therapy. Am J Kidney Dis 30:120–122, 1997.

643. Cheng ES, Stringer KM, Pegg SP: Colonic necrosis and perforation following oral sodium polystyrene sulfonate (Resonium A/Kayexalate) in a burn patient. Burns 28:189–190, 2002.

644. Ng YY, Wu SC, Cheng CT, et al: Reduction of serum calcium by sodium sulfonated polystyrene resin. J Formos Med Assoc 89:399–402, 1990.

645. Linakis JG, Hull AM, Lacoutoure PG, et al: Sodium polystyrene sulfonate treatment for lithium toxicity: Effects on serum potassium concentrations. Acad Emerg Med 3:333–337, 1996.

646. Amaya F, Fukui M, Tsuruta H, et al: Simulation of potassium extraction by continuous haemodiafiltration. Anaesth Intensive Care 30:198–201, 2002.

647. Jackson MA, Lodwick R, Hutchinson SG: Hyperkalaemic cardiac arrest successfully treated with peritoneal dialysis. BMJ 312:1289–1290, 1996.

648. Allon M, Shanklin N: Effect of albuterol treatment on subsequent dialytic potassium removal. Am J Kidney Dis 26:607–613, 1995.

649. Dolson GM, Ellis KJ, Bernardo MV, et al: Acute decreases in serum potassium augment blood pressure. Am J Kidney Dis 26:321–326, 1995.

650. Sherman RA, Hwang ER, Bernholc AS, Eisinger RP: Variability in potassium removal by hemodialysis. Am J Nephrol 6:284–288, 1986.

651. Zehnder C, Gutzwiller JP, Huber A, et al: Low-potassium and glucose-free dialysis maintains urea but enhances potassium removal. Nephrol Dial Transplant 16:78–84, 2001.

652. Blumberg A, Roser HW, Zehnder C, Muller-Brand J: Plasma potassium in patients with terminal renal failure during and after haemodialysis; relationship with dialytic potassium removal and total body potassium. Nephrol Dial Transplant 12:1629–1634, 1997.

653. Ward RA, Wathen RL, Williams TE, Harding GB: Hemodialysate composition and intradialytic metabolic, acid-base and potassium changes. Kidney Int 32:129–135, 1987.

654. De Nicola L, Bellizzi V, Minutolo R, et al: Effect of dialysate sodium concentration on interdialytic increase of potassium. J Am Soc Nephrol 11:2337–2343, 2000.

655. Hou S, McElroy PA, Nootens J, Beach M: Safety and efficacy of low-potassium dialysate. Am J Kidney Dis 13:137–143, 1989.

656. Williams AJ, Barnes JN, Cunningham J, et al: Effect of dialysate buffer on potassium removal during haemodialysis. Proc Eur Dial Transplant Assoc Eur Ren Assoc 21:209–214, 1985.

657. Allon M: Medical and dialytic management of hyperkalemia in hemodialysis patients. Int J Artif Organs 19:697–699, 1996.

658. Heguilen RM, Sciurano C, Bellusci AD, et al: The faster potassium-lowering effect of high dialysate bicarbonate concentrations in chronic haemodialysis patients. Nephrol Dial Transplant 20:591–597, 2005.

659. Solandt DY: The effect of potassium on the excitability and resting metabolism of frog's muscle. J Physiol (Lond) 86:162–170, 1936.

660. Dolson GM, Adrogue HJ: Low dialysate [K⁺] decreases efficiency of hemodialysis and increases urea rebound. J Am Soc Nephrol 9:2124–2128, 1998.

661. Baron AD: Hemodynamic actions of insulin. Am J Physiol 267:E187–202, 1994.

662. Morrison G, Michelson EL, Brown S, Morganroth J: Mechanism and prevention of cardiac arrhythmias in chronic hemodialysis patients. Kidney Int 17:811–819, 1980.

663. Kimura K, Tabei K, Asano Y, Hosoda S: Cardiac arrhythmias in hemodialysis patients. A study of incidence and contributory factors. Nephron 53:201–207, 1989.

664. Ramirez G, Brueggemeyer CD, Newton JL: Cardiac arrhythmias on hemodialysis in chronic renal failure patients. Nephron 36:212–218, 1984.

665. Rombola G, Colussi G, De Ferrari ME, et al: Cardiac arrhythmias and electrolyte changes during haemodialysis. Nephrol Dial Transplant 7:318–322, 1992.

666. Weber H, Schwarzer C, Stummvoll HK, et al: Chronic hemodialysis: High risk patients for arrhythmias? Nephron 37:180–185, 1984.

667. Wizemann V, Kramer W, Funke T, Schutterle G: Dialysis-induced cardiac arrhythmias: fact or fiction? Importance of preexisting cardiac disease in the induction of arrhythmias during renal replacement therapy. Nephron 39:356–360, 1985.

668. Kyriakidis M, Voudiclaris S, Kremastinos D, et al: Cardiac arrhythmias in chronic renal failure? Holter monitoring during dialysis and everyday activity at home. Nephron 38:26–29, 1984.

669. Redaelli B, Locatelli F, Limido D, et al: Effect of a new model of hemodialysis potassium removal on the control of ventricular arrhythmias. Kidney Int 50:609–617, 1996.

CHAPTER 16

Disorders of Calcium, Magnesium, and Phosphate Balance

Martin R. Pollak • Alan S. L. Yu • Eric N. Taylor

DISORDERS OF CALCIUM HOMEOSTASIS

The extracellular calcium concentration is tightly maintained and reflects the actions of multiple hormones (including parathyroid hormone [PTH], calcitonin, and vitamin D) on multiple tissues (including bone, intestine, kidney, and parathyroid). This homeostatic system is modulated by dietary and environmental factors (including vitamins, hormones, medications, and mobility). Disorders of extracellular calcium homeostasis may be regarded as perturbations of this homeostatic system, either at the level of the genes controlling this system (as in, for example, familial hypocalciuric hypercalcemia, pseudohypoparathyroidism, or vitamin D–dependent rickets) or perturbations of this system induced by nongenetic means (as in lithium toxicity or postsurgical hypoparathyroidism).

The normal total extracellular calcium concentration is 9 mg/dL to 10.5 mg/dL. Approximately 50% of serum calcium is bound to serum proteins, a small amount is complexed to anions, and the remainder exists as free ionized calcium. It is the ionized calcium concentration that is pathophysiologically relevant. Alterations in blood pH can alter ionized calcium: acidosis decreases Ca^{2+}/albumin binding; alkalosis increases it. Although in most instances an alteration in ionized calcium is reflected by altered total calcium, such may not be the case when an abnormality in serum protein concentrations is present.[1] A useful rule is to add 0.8 mg/dL for every 1 mg depression in serum albumin below 4 mg/dL to "correct" for hypoalbuminemia.

Hypercalcemia

Hypercalcemia results from an alteration in the net fluxes of extracellular calcium at the organs responsible for calcium homeostasis: bone, gut, and kidney. Most commonly, increased osteoclastic bone resorption is responsible, as in hyperparathyroidism (HPT) or excess parathyroid hormone–related protein (PTHrP) production in malignancy. Excess circulating 1,25-dihydroxyvitamin D (1,25[OH]$_2$D) from various causes also may contribute to excess bone resorption. Increased intestinal calcium absorption may lead to the development of hypercalcemia, as in vitamin D overdose or milk-alkali syndrome. In general, the kidney does not contribute to hypercalcemia; rather, it defends against the development of hypercalcemia. Typically, hypercalciuria precedes hypercalcemia. Extracellular calcium itself in fact appears to have a calciuric effect on the renal tubule by its direct action on the calcium-sensing receptor (CaR) of the thick ascending limb (TAL). Thus, in most hypercalcemic states, renal calcium handling is subject to competing influences: excess PTH or PTHrP acts on the PTH/PTHrP receptor to promote renal calcium reabsorption; excess calcium acts on the calcium receptor to promote calcium excretion.[2]

In rare cases, the kidney can actively contribute to the development of hypercalcemia. As opposed to primary HPT and humoral hypercalcemia of malignancy, where increases in renal calcium excretion are observed, renal calcium excretion is not elevated in familial hypocalciuric hypercalcemia because of a defective renal response to calcium itself. The hypercalcemia associated with thiazide use is also mediated by the kidney: in both thiazide use and its genetic counterpart Gitelman syndrome,[3] renal calcium excretion is decreased. Hyper-

calcemia is common, with an annual incidence in the population estimated to be on the order of 0.1% to 0.2% and a prevalence of about 1%.[4–6]

Signs and Symptoms
The clinical manifestations of hypercalcemia relate more to the degree of hypercalcemia and rate of increase than the underlying cause. Neuromuscular sequelae are common, as are altered mental status, depression, fatigue, and muscle weakness. Frequently observed gastrointestinal complications include constipation, nausea, and vomiting. Peptic ulcer disease is a rare complication; pancreatitis is exceedingly rare. Even very mild hypercalcemia may be of clinical significance inasmuch as some studies have suggested an increased cardiovascular risk from quite mild, but prolonged calcium elevations.[7]

Hypercalcemia causes polyuria and polydipsia, and significant hypercalcemia can lead to severe dehydration. Nephrolithiasis and nephrocalcinosis are common complications of hypercalcemia seen in 15% to 20% of cases of primary HPT. Hypercalcemia causes a shortened QT interval on electrocardiograms as a result of an increased rate of cardiac repolarization. Heart block and other arrhythmias also may be observed.

Diagnosis
Primary HPT and malignancy-associated hypercalcemia are responsible for the vast majority of cases of hypercalcemia, each contributing roughly an equal number. It is generally easy to differentiate these two entities. Hypercalcemia is only rarely an early finding in occult malignancy. PTH levels are essential in the diagnosis of hypercalcemia. In primary HPT, serum PTH is usually frankly elevated; in malignancy-associated hypercalcemia and in most other causes, PTH levels are low. In addition, PTHrP can now be assayed by commercial clinical laboratories; an elevated PTHrP level indicates humoral hypercalcemia of malignancy (although some forms of malignancy-associated hypercalcemia are not mediated by this circulating hormone).

Approximately 10% of cases of hypercalcemia are due to other causes. Of particular importance in the evaluation of a hypercalcemic patient are the family history (because of familial syndromes, including multiple endocrine neoplasia type I [MEN-I], MEN-II, and familial hypocalciuric hypercalcemia), medication history (because of the several medication-induced forms of hypercalcemia), and the presence of other disease (such as granulomatous or malignant disease).

Causes

Primary Hyperparathyroidism

Primary HPT is caused by excess PTH secretion and consequent hypercalcemia and hypophosphatemia (Table 16-1). It is the underlying cause of approximately 50% of hypercalcemic cases. Its manifestation has shifted markedly over the past half century as measurement of serum calcium has become routine. Thus, the diagnosis is now usually suggested by the incidental finding of hypercalcemia rather than any of the sequelae of PTH excess or marked hypercalcemia. Hypercalcemia may be quite mild and intermittent. The estimated prevalence of HPT is on the order of 1%, but may be as high as 2% in postmenopausal women.[6,8] The annual incidence is approximately 0.03% to 0.04%.[8-10] Most individuals (95%) have four parathyroid glands located adjacent to the thyroid. A single enlarged parathyroid gland is the cause of primary HPT in 80% to 90% of cases.

Most cases of primary HPT are due to a single benign adenoma, whereas in about 15% of cases, four-gland hyperplasia is responsible. The disease is about three times more common in women than men. The genetic alterations underlying parathyroid adenomas are being elucidated. Rearrangements and overexpression of the PRAD-1/cyclin D1 oncogene have been observed in about one fifth of parathyroid adenomas.[11,12] The MEN-I gene menin is inactivated in about 15% of adenomas.[13,14] Other chromosomal regions may also harbor parathyroid tumor suppressor genes.[15]

Substantial controversy surrounds the potential relation between primary HPT and increased mortality. Some data suggest that primary HPT may be associated with hypertension,[16,17] dyslipidemia,[18] diabetes,[19] increased thickness of the carotid artery,[20] and increased mortality,[21-24] primarily from cardiovascular disease.[25,26] The morbidity from primary HPT can be substantial. Although the usual manifestation is the incidental finding of hypercalcemia, primary HPT may be associated with altered mental status, depression, joint pain, or constipation.

The classic bone lesion in primary HPT, osteitis fibrosa cystica, is now rarely seen. Diffuse osteopenia is more common.[27] Even in asymptomatic patients, increased rates of bone turnover are always present.[28]

Standard therapy for primary HPT remains surgery.[29] It is generally agreed that parathyroidectomy is indicated in patients with severe hypercalcemia, bone disease, or symptoms. In 2002, a National Institutes of Health consensus conference updated guidelines for the management of asymptomatic HPT.[29] Surgery was suggested for individuals with serum calcium levels greater than 1 mg/dL above normal, a history of life-threatening hypercalcemia, renal insufficiency, kidney stones, reduced bone mass, or hypercalciuria (~400 mg calcium per 24 hours). Medical surveillance was considered a reasonable alternative for individuals older than 50 years with no obvious symptoms. Such patients should receive close follow-up, including periodic measurements of bone density, renal function, and serum calcium. Although surgery remains the definitive treatment, calcimimetic agents hold promise as a potential treatment.[30-32] Modern surgical techniques make parathyroidectomy safe even in elderly individuals.[32a]

Preoperative localization of the parathyroid glands has generally been considered unnecessary in uncomplicated patients undergoing surgery for the first time. However, there is increasing enthusiasm for the use of technetium 99m scintigraphy for preoperative localization of parathyroid adenomas.[29] If a single adenoma is visualized, minimally invasive parathyroidectomy may be an option: this procedure requires the surgeon to visualize only one gland as long as resection results in a substantial intra-operative decline in PTH. Otherwise, all four parathyroid glands should be surgically identified. Although excision of a single enlarged gland is curative, the finding of more than one enlarged gland raises the possibility of diffuse parathyroid hyperplasia and MEN. When all glands are enlarged, removal of $3\frac{1}{2}$ glands or all 4 glands with forearm autotransplantation of a portion of the gland is advocated.[33] Recurrence of HPT is rare after identification and removal of one enlarged gland.[34]

If the initial exploration failed and hypercalcemia persists or recurs, preoperative parathyroid localization should be performed.[29] Techniques used include ultrasound, arteriography, magnetic resonance imaging, venous sampling, intraoperative PTH monitoring, and technetium sestamibi scanning. Complications are greater with re-exploration of the neck than after the initial operation.

Carcinoma

Although estimates vary, parathyroid carcinoma probably accounts for less than 1% of primary HPT.[35] The diagnosis of parathyroid carcinoma may be difficult to make in the absence of metastases because the histologic appearance may be similar to that of atypical adenomas.[36] In general, parathyroid carcinoma is not aggressive, and survival is common if the entire gland can be removed.[37] Mutations of the HRPT2 tumor suppressor gene likely play an important role in the pathogenesis of parathyroid carcinoma.[38]

Malignancy

Humoral hypercalcemia of malignancy (HHM) generally refers to the syndrome of malignancy-associated hypercalcemia caused by secretion of PTHrP. HHM accounts for approximately 80% of cases of hypercalcemia-associated malignancy. Numerous types of malignancies are associated with HHM and secretion of PTHrP, including squamous, renal cell, breast, and ovarian carcinomas. Lymphomas associated with

---

TABLE 16–1 Causes of Hypercalcemia

Common
  Primary hyperparathyroidism
    Adenoma
    Carcinoma
    Hyperplasia
  Malignancy
    Humoral hypercalcemia
    Lytic bone disease
    Ectopic 1,25(OH)$_2$vitamin D production

Less common
  Inherited disease
    Multiple endocrine neoplasia type I, II
    Familial hypocalciuric hypercalcemia
    Other
  Granulomatous disease
  Drug induced
    Lithium
    Vitamin D
    Thiazides
    Aminophylline
    Estrogens
    Vitamin A
  Milk-alkali syndrome
  Non-parathyroid endocrinopathies
  Immobilization
  Renal failure
  Neonatal hypercalcemia

human T-lymphotropic virus type I (HTLV-I) infection may cause PTHrP-mediated HHM, and other non-Hodgkin lymphomas may be associated with PTHrP-mediated hypercalcemia as well.[39] Patients are hypercalcemic and hypophosphatemic and demonstrate increased osteoclastic bone resorption, increased urinary cyclic adenosine monophosphate (cAMP), and hypercalciuria. Malignancy is generally advanced at the time of diagnosis of HHM. HHM is not typically a manifestation of occult malignancy.

PTHrP is a large protein encoded by a gene on chromosome 12; it is similar to PTH only at the NH_2 terminus, where the initial eight amino acids are identical.[40] PTHrP is widely expressed in a variety of tissues, including keratinocytes, mammary gland, placenta, cartilage, nervous system, vascular smooth muscle, and various endocrine sites.[41] PTH and PTHrP interact with the PTH receptor with equal affinity. Injection of PTHrP produces hypercalcemia in rats[42] and essentially reproduces the entire clinical syndrome of HHM, but other circulating factors such as cytokines may also be important. Normal circulating levels of PTHrP are negligible; it is probably unimportant in normal calcium homeostasis. However, mice with a targeted disruption in the PTHrP gene show a lethal defect in bone development,[43] thus demonstrating its importance in normal physiology.

Other forms of malignancy-associated hypercalcemia may be humoral in nature. Malignant lymphomas have been reported to produce $1,25(OH)_2D$[44–46] in sufficient quantity to lead to elevated levels and hypercalcemia secondary to bone resorption and increased intestinal calcium absorption. Ectopic production of PTH itself by a nonparathyroid tumor may occur, but it is rare.[47]

Bone is a frequent site of metastatic disease. Osteolytic metastases may produce severe pain, pathologic fractures, and hypercalcemia. Advanced breast and prostate cancer almost invariably spreads to bone. Hypercalcemia in breast cancer is associated with the presence of both extensive osteolytic metastases and HHM. Bisphosphonate administration is effective therapy for this form of hypercalcemia. In many cancers, bisphosphonates delay the appearance of skeletal complications of metastatic disease,[48] but research on the possible antitumor activity of this class of medication has produced conflicting results.[49]

Extensive bone destruction is seen in multiple myeloma.[50] Although bone lesions develop in all patients with myeloma, hypercalcemia does not develop in every patient, and the degree of hypercalcemia and bone destruction do not correlate well.[51] Some degree of renal impairment is common in multiple myeloma, and hypercalcemia rarely develops in the absence of any renal insufficiency. Conversely, hypercalcemia is a common cause of renal insufficiency in myeloma patients. Treatment with bisphosphonates appears to protect against the development of skeletal complications (including hypercalcemia) in patients with myeloma and lytic bone lesions.[52]

Inherited Disease
Familial Hyperparathyroid Syndromes
Familial isolated hyperparathyroidism (FIHP) and familial hypocalciuric hypercalcemia (FHH) (see later) are the major nonsyndromic familial hypercalcemic disorders. Both can cause mild hypercalcemia, and both follow autosomal dominant transmission. Because their treatment is different, correct diagnosis is important. FIHP is characterized by hypercalcemia, elevated levels of PTH, and parathyroid tumors in one or more glands. More than 70 families with FIHP have been reported.[53]

The genes involved in syndromic forms of hyperparathyroid disease (see later) also appear to be responsible for some cases of parathyroid-limited familial disease.[54] Some patients with FIHP have a defect on chromosome 1 similar to

that in the familial hyperparathyroidism-jaw tumor syndrome (HRPT2 gene),[55] but the majority do not.[56] In addition, mutations in the MEN1 gene may explain some cases of FIHP.[57,58]

Jansen-type metaphyseal chondrodysplasia is a rare disorder characterized by bone deformity (chondrodysplasia), dwarfism, and severe hypercalcemia. PTH and PTHrP levels are undetectable. The cause of this disease has been shown to be constitutive activation of the PTH/PTHrP receptor.[59,60]

Multiple Endocrine Neoplasias
MEN-I is the most common form of familial HPT.[61] It is an autosomal dominant disorder characterized by tumors of the parathyroid gland, pituitary, and pancreas. Primary HPT is almost always present, whereas pancreatic and pituitary tumors are more likely to be absent. Primary HPT is caused by diffuse hyperplasia of all four glands in most cases. Treatment of the HPT is surgical: subtotal parathyroidectomy or total parathyroidectomy with autotransplantation of a portion of the excised parathyroid gland in the forearm.

The gene defect in MEN-I was mapped by linkage analysis to chromosome 11q13.[62] The responsible gene has been identified[63] and is termed menin; it encodes a 610 amino acid nuclear protein peptide without obvious similarity to known proteins.[64] Genetic evidence suggests that menin is a tumor suppressor gene.[65] A large number of distinct mutations have been described.[66]

MEN-IIA is also characterized by parathyroid hyperplasia and autosomal dominant inheritance. Associated findings are medullary thyroid carcinoma in all cases and pheochromocytoma in many, either of which may be lethal. Linkage analysis localized the gene defect to chromosome 10, and the RET proto-oncogene, which encodes a tyrosine kinase, has been identified as the MEN-IIA gene.[67] Within affected kindreds, genetic testing is supplanting calcitonin assays to aid in presymptomatic diagnosis and early treatment.[68] Diagnosis and management of MEN-I and MEN-II differ; these differences are summarized in an international consensus report.[69]

Hyperparathyroidism–jaw tumor syndrome is a rare autosomal dominant disorder characterized by severe hypercalcemia, parathyroid adenoma, and fibro-osseous jaw tumors.[70] The responsible gene, HRPT2, is a tumor suppressor gene located on chromosome 1q25-32.[71]

Familial Hypocalciuric Hypercalcemia and Neonatal Severe Hyperparathyroidism
Familial benign hypercalcemia (FHH) is a rare inherited condition with autosomal dominant inheritance.[72] The hypercalcemia is typically mild to moderate (10.5 mg/dL to 12 mg/dL), and affected patients do not exhibit the typical complications associated with elevated serum calcium concentrations. Both total and ionized calcium concentrations are elevated, but the PTH level is generally "inappropriately normal," although mild elevations have also been reported. Urinary calcium excretion is not elevated, as would be expected in hypercalcemia of other causes. The renal calcium–to–creatinine clearance ratio is usually less than 0.01. Bone mineral density is normal, as are vitamin D levels.

In most families with FHH, the disease is due to inactivating defects in the extracellular calcium receptor (CaR) located on chromosome 3q. CaR is widely expressed in mammalian tissues. In the kidney, CaR is expressed throughout the nephron, but particularly strongly in the TAL. The fact that relative hypocalciuria persists even after parathyroidectomy in FHH patients confirms the role of CaR in regulating renal calcium handling.[73] Inactivating mutations, most of which are missense, have been found throughout the large predicted structure of the CaR protein.[74,75] Expression studies of mutant CaRs have shown great variability in their effect on calcium responsiveness. In some cases, CaR mutations only slightly shift the set-point of half-maximal response to calcium; other mutations appear to render the receptor largely inactive.[76-78] In about 15% of cases, CaR mutations have not been found in patients with typical features of FHH. In some of these cases, CaR mutations may be in noncoding sequence; in others, different gene defects may be responsible. Thus, mutational analysis is not yet a tool for clinical diagnosis of FHH. Differentiating primary HPT from FHH is critically important because the hypercalcemia in FHH is benign and does not respond to subtotal parathyroidectomy.

Two copies of CaR alleles bearing inactivating mutations cause neonatal severe hyperparathyroidism (NSHPT). This rare disorder, most often reported in the offspring of consanguineous FHH parents, is characterized by severe hyperparathyroid hyperplasia, PTH elevation, and elevated extracellular calcium.[79-81] In a few affected infants, only one defective allele has been found, but it is unclear whether the finding of only one defective allele is due to the presence of an undetected defect in the other CaR allele. Treatment is total parathyroidectomy followed by vitamin D and calcium supplementation. This disease is usually lethal without surgical intervention.

Medications

Hypercalcemia is a long-recognized and well-described consequence of lithium therapy.[82] Series of lithium-treated patients report about 5% to 10% with hypercalcemia, often with elevated PTH levels. Lithium probably acts through an interaction with the extracellular CaR to alter the set-point for PTH secretion in relation to extracellular calcium.[83,84] The effect of lithium on PTH function occurs immediately. Hypercalcemia is reversible in most patients after discontinuing lithium, although lithium-independent hyperparathyroidism may develop after prolonged treatment.[85]

Vitamin A intoxication, on the order of 100,000 U/day, may cause hypercalcemia, presumably from increased osteoclast-mediated bone resorption.[86,87] Vitamin A analogs, used in the management of dermatologic and hematologic malignant disease, have also been reported to cause hypercalcemia.[88,89] Estrogens (and antiestrogens) used in the management of breast cancer may rarely cause hypercalcemia.[90]

Hypercalcemia is a well-recognized complication of thiazide diuretics.[91,92] Although these agents clearly have a hypocalciuric effect, it is not clear whether the renal action alone is responsible for the hypercalcemia observed.[93,94] Because thiazides may exacerbate borderline hypercalcemia of other causes, severe hypercalcemia in a thiazide-treated patient should prompt further investigation. Theophylline has been reported to cause mild hypercalcemia,[95] but the cause is not known.

Milk-Alkali Syndrome

The syndrome of hypercalcemia, alkalosis, and renal insufficiency caused by the ingestion of large amounts of calcium and antacids is known as the milk-alkali syndrome.[96] As calcium supplementation in the form of calcium carbonate has become popular, the incidence of milk-alkali syndrome has increased: in some reports it is now the third leading cause of hypercalcemia after primary hyperparathyroidism and malignancy, accounting for up to 12% of cases.[97,98] The pathogenesis of the milk-alkali syndrome is unclear, and requires the ingestion of much more calcium than contained in a normal calcium-supplemented diet, on the order of 5 g/day. In susceptible individuals, increased alkali intake, hypercalcemia, and a concomitant reduction in GFR engender a metabolic alkalosis that inhibits renal calcium excretion[99] and further perpetuates the syndrome. The diagnosis is made largely by the history and may not be obvious because of atypical dietary sources of calcium and alkali.

Vitamin D Intoxication

Hypercalcemia may develop in individuals ingesting vitamin D or vitamin D analogs, including $1,25(OH)_2D$.[100] Hypercalcemia has been caused by accidental overdose of vitamin D from fortified cow's milk,[101] and an outbreak of hypercalcemia and hypervitaminosis D from fortified milk has been reported.[102] Serum $25(OH)D$ is elevated and immunoreactive parathyroid hormone (iPTH) is depressed in this setting. However, vitamin D well in excess of the normal recommended daily allowance is required for this form of hypercalcemia to develop. The diagnosis is made by the history and detection of elevated $25(OH)D$ levels. Treatment consists of calciuresis, volume expansion, and if necessary, glucocorticoids.

Immobilization

Although the mechanism is not well understood, immobilization can produce increased rates of bone resorption, decreased rates of bone formation, and hypercalcemia.[103] Typically, this entity is seen days to weeks after start of complete bed rest. The hypercalcemia is reversible with resumption of activity. Biochemically, this form of hypercalcemia is characterized by low PTH and $1,25(OH)_2D$ levels. Bisphosphonates may help decrease the hypercalcemia and osteopenia in this setting.[104]

Granulomatous Disease

Hypercalcemia is a frequent complication of sarcoidosis and occurs in 10% of patients; hypercalciuria is more common and is seen in up to 50% of patients during the course of their disease.[105] Patients with sarcoidosis often have increased sensitivity to vitamin D, and hypercalcemia may develop in normocalcemic patients after minimally increased intake of vitamin D or sunlight exposure. The cause of hypercalcemia is increased production of $1,25(OH)_2D$ from nonrenal sites.[106] Macrophages from sarcoid granulomas may 1-hydroxylate $25(OH)D$ to produce calcitriol.[107] Bone mineral content tends to be reduced in these patients. Serum calcium should be measured, but hypercalciuria may precede hypercalcemia and may be an earlier indicator of this complication. Standard treatment consists of administration of glucocorticoids, which decreases the abnormal $1,25(OH)_2D$ production.[108] Chloroquine and ketoconazole, which also decrease $1,25(OH)_2D$ production, have likewise been shown to be efficacious.[109,110]

Other granulomatous disorders are also associated with altered vitamin D metabolism and hypercalcemia.[111] Leprosy, silicone-induced granulomas, disseminated candidiasis, disseminated coccidioidomycosis, acquired immune deficiency syndrome (AIDS) with pulmonary Pneumocystis carinii infection, and Wegener granulomatosis have all been reported to cause this syndrome. The development of hypercalcemia in patients with pulmonary tuberculosis is frequently mentioned, but most studies of infected patients in fact suggest it to be a rare problem.[112]

Nonparathyroid Enodcrinopathies

Mild hypercalcemia is common in thyrotoxicosis.[113] Bone turnover is increased and PTH and $1,25(OH)_2D$ levels are decreased.[114] Pheochromocytoma may be associated with hypercalcemia[115]; most commonly, it is due to coincident PTH and MEN-IIA. Adrenal insufficiency,[116] pancreatic islet cell tumors,[117] growth hormone administration,[118] and acromegaly[119] have all been associated with hypercalcemia.

Childhood Hypercalcemia

Williams syndrome is an inherited disorder with a frequency of 1 in 10,000 that is manifested in infancy as supravalvular aortic stenosis, elfin facial features, and hypercalcemia.[120] The hypercalcemia is generally self-limited. Deletions at the elastin locus on chromosome 7 seem to be responsible for this disease,[121] but the cause of the hypercalcemia is unknown. Childhood HPT is rare; a severe recessive form of HPT results from mutations in CaR (see earlier). Infantile subcutaneous fat necrosis, caused by perinatal problems, may be associated with hypercalcemia mediated by abnormal vitamin D metabolism.[122]

Management of Hypercalcemia

Whereas treatment of chronic hypercalcemia ultimately depends on therapy specific to the underlying cause, immediate therapy is required for patients with acute severe hypercalcemia (or an acute worsening of chronic hypercalcemia). Immediate measures are generally not called for with asymptomatic mild or moderate calcium elevations.[123] Other considerations may be relevant to the decision to initiate aggressive therapy (is the cause of the hypercalcemia reversible, or is it a result of a terminal condition such as widely metastatic cancer?).

Some degree of volume depletion is almost always present with severe hypercalcemia (~14 mg/dL). Volume repletion and induction of saline diuresis are central to successful therapy (Table 16–2). Generally, large volumes of 0.9% sodium chloride are administered intravenously to increase urine calcium excretion. Loop diuretics given concurrently can increase the calciuresis by inhibiting calcium reabsorption in the TAL. Thiazide diuretics, which have a hypocalciuric effect, are not appropriate. Care must be taken to monitor the patient's volume status closely during the administration of large amounts of saline and diuretic, particularly in hospitalized patients with cardiac or pulmonary disease.

Bisphosphonates are pyrophosphate analogs with a high affinity for hydroxyapatite. These compounds inhibit osteoclast function in areas of high bone turnover.[124] Newer-generation bisphosphonates such as pamidronate and clodronate are more potent than etidronate at blocking osteoclastic bone resorption and do not cause significant demineralization as etidronate does at high doses.[104] A single intravenous dose of 30 mg to 90 mg may be effective in normalizing the serum calcium level for many weeks. These drugs appear to be particularly efficacious in patients with breast cancer. Fever is observed in about one fifth of patients. Zoledronic acid may be more effective than pamidronate as treatment of hypercalcemia.[125]

The thyroid C cell–derived polypeptide calcitonin is an effective inhibitor of osteoclast bone resorption. It has a rapid onset, but its effect is transient. Given as 4 to 8 U salmon calcitonin per kilogram subcutaneously, this drug has minimal toxicity but is of limited use as sole therapy for hypercalcemia.[126]

TABLE 16–2 Management of Hypercalcemia
Hydration
Saline diuresis
Bisphosphonates
Calcitonin
Gallium nitrate
Glucocorticoids
Phosphate
Dialysis

Correction of underlying cause(s)
    Mobilization
    Parathyroidectomy
    Discontinue contributing medications
    Chemotherapy

Gallium nitrate inhibits bone resorption by increasing the solubility of hydroxyapatite crystals. It is given as a 5-day infusion, and the hypocalcemic effect is not generally observed until the end of this period. Gallium nitrate is effective, but can be nephrotoxic.[127,128] Other therapies for hypercalcemia, such as Plicamycin, chelation with EDTA, and intravenous phosphate, have adverse side effect profiles and are no longer recommended.

Glucocorticoids are useful therapy for hypercalcemia of a specific subset of causes. It is most effective in hematologic malignancies (multiple myeloma, Hodgkin disease) and disorders of vitamin D metabolism (granulomatous disease, vitamin D toxicity).[108,129]

In severely hypercalcemic patients, hemodialysis or peritoneal dialysis with a low- or no-calcium dialysate is an effective treatment and should be regarded as a first-line therapy for chronic dialysis patients.[130,131] Therapies for the management of hypercalcemia continue to evolve. Noncalcemic analogs of calcitriol, such as 22-oxacalcitriol, may reduce the release of PTHrP in patients with HHM.[132] Manipulation of the Ca^{2+}/PTH response with calcimimetic agents such as cinacalcet holds promise as a treatment for primary and secondary HPT.[30–32,132a,132b]

Hypocalcemia

At any given subnormal extracellular calcium level, the clinical manifestations may vary greatly (Table 16–3). The marked chronic hypocalcemia commonly seen in chronic dialysis patients, for example, is frequently asymptomatic. When present, symptoms of chronic hypocalcemia are predominantly neurologic and neuromuscular. The most common clinical manifestations are muscle cramps and numbness in the digits. Severe hypocalcemia can cause laryngeal spasm, carpopedal spasm, bronchospasm, seizures, and even respiratory arrest. Mental changes include irritability, depression, and decreased cognitive capacity. The electrocardiogram may show shortening of the QT interval and arrhythmias. Overt heart failure is seen rarely.[133] Bedside signs of hypocalcemia include ipsilateral facial muscle twitching in response to tapping the facial nerve (Chvostek sign) and carpal spasm induced by brachial artery occlusion (Trousseau sign). The Chvostek sign is often present in the absence of hypocalcemia; both these well-known signs are often negative in hypocalcemic patients. Long-standing hypocalcemia may result in dry skin, coarse hair, alopecia, and brittle nails. Teeth can be absent or hypoplastic. Calcifications of the basal ganglia and cerebral cortex may be detected by computed tomography in chronic hypocalcemia.[134] Bone disease may be observed, but its findings differ in the various causes of hypocalcemia (see later).

Ionized calcium is the pathophysiologically relevant biochemical measurement. Although total calcium generally reflects the ionized level, this measurement may be altered in chronic illness, where hypoalbuminemia may lead to decreased total calcium but normal ionized calcium measurements. Clinicians also should be aware of pseudohypocalcemia: some gadolinium-based contrast agents used in magnetic resonance angiography interfere with colorimetric assays for calcium, resulting in a marked reduction in the measured calcium concentration.[135]

The most common causes of hypocalcemia in the nonacute setting are hypoparathyroidism, hypomagnesemia, renal failure, and vitamin D deficiencies (Table 16–4). These entities should be considered early in the diagnosis of hypocalcemic individuals. It is conceptually and clinically useful to subclassify hypocalcemic individuals into those with elevated PTH levels and those with either subnormal or "inappropriately normal" PTH concentrations, as in primary

TABLE 16-3	Major Inherited or Genetic Disorders Affecting Parathyroid Hormone Secretion or Responsiveness
Isolated hypercalcemia	
FHH (HHC1)	MIM 145980, 601199
NSHPT	MIM 239200
FIHP (HPRT1)	MIM 145000
Syndromic hypercalcemia	
MENI	MIM 13100
MENII	MIM 171400
HPT-JT (HPRT2)	MIM 145001
Jansen	MIM 168468
Isolated hypocalcemia	
ADH	MIM 146200, 601199
PTH gene	MIM 168450
PsHP Ib	MIM 603233
X-linked (HYPX)	MIM 307700
Syndromic hypocalcemia	
PsHP Ia (AHO)	MIM 103580
Autoimmune polyglandular syndrome I	MIM 240300
DiGeorge (DGS)	MIM 188400
Barakat syndrome	MIM 146255
Kenny-Caffey syndrome	MIM 127000
Kearns-Sayre syndrome	MIM 530000
Hypoparathyroidism with short stature, mental retardation	MIM 241410

ADH, antidiuretic hormone; AHO, Albright hereditary osteodystrophy; FHH, familial hypocalciuric hypercalcemia; FIHP, familial isolated hyperparathyroidism; HPT-JT, hyperparathyroidism–jaw tumor syndrome; MEN, multiple endocrine neoplasia; MIM, mendelian inheritance in man number; NSHPT, neonatal severe hyperparathyroidism; PsHP, pseudohypoparathyroidism; PTH, parathyroid hormone.

TABLE 16-4	Major Clinical Features of Hypocalcemia
Neuromuscular irritability
Tetany
Seizures
Anxiety/depression
Paresthesias
Bronchospasm
Laryngospasm
Prolonged QT interval on ECG

TABLE 16-5	Causes of Chronic Hypocalcemia

I. Hypoparathyroidism
Altered Ca2+/PTH set-point (CaR mutations)
PTH gene defects
Post-surgical
Neck irradiation
Infiltrative disease
Hypomagnesemia/hypermagnesemia
Autoimmune disease

II. Parathyroid hormone resistance
Pseudohypoparathyroidism
Pseudopseudohypoparathyroidism
Hypomagnesemia

III. Other
Vitamin D deficiency
Altered vitamin D metabolism
Drug induced

hypoparathyroidism. A thorough medical history and physical examination are diagnostically important because hypocalcemia can be caused by postsurgical, pharmacologic, inherited, developmental, and nutritional problems, in addition to being part of complex syndromes.

Genetic Disorders of Parathyroid Hormone Dysfunction or Altered Responsiveness
Calcium Receptor Mutations
The most proximal component of the PTH axis is extracellular calcium itself, which regulates PTH activity by interaction with the extracellular CaR on the surface of parathyroid cells (Table 16–5). Just as defects in this receptor at the gene level can make the parathyroid gland hyporesponsive to calcium (as in FHH and NSHPT, discussed earlier), mutations in CaR can also activate CaR or cause CaR to be hyperresponsive to extracellular calcium.[136] The phenotype seen is essentially the opposite of FHH and has been termed both autosomal dominant hypoparathyroidism and autosomal hypocalcemia. CaR mutations associated with this phenotype continue to be reported both in familial cases and in isolated individuals presumed to have de novo mutations.[75]

Individuals with this condition typically have mildly or moderately depressed serum calcium concentrations, low or "inappropriately normal" PTH levels, and occasionally, hypomagnesemia. Urine calcium concentrations are greater than in hypoparathyroidism of other causes, almost certainly because of the effect of an activated renal CaR. Management of the hypocalcemia with vitamin D and calcium supplementation in these patients can result in frank hypercalciuria and nephrocalcinosis.[137] Thus, medical intervention is warranted only for patients with severe symptomatic hypocalcemia. CaR mutations probably represent the most common cause of genetic hypoparathyroidism.[138]

Parathyroid Hormone Gene Abnormalities
Although most patients with familial hypoparathyroidism do not appear to have defects in the pre-pro-PTH gene,[139] both autosomal dominant and recessive inheritance of hypoparathyroidism has been reported in families with PTH gene mutations.[140,141]

X-Linked Hypoparathyroidism

An X-linked form of hypoparathyroidism has been described. The apparent absence of parathyroid tissue in affected patients suggests a role for the responsible gene in parathyroid development: the SOX3 gene recently has been implicated.[142]

Syndromic Hypoparathyroidism

Patients with DiGeorge syndrome exhibit heart defects, thymic aplasia, facial anomalies, and neonatal hypoparathyroidism[143] resulting from defective third and fourth branchial pouch development. Most cases are sporadic, but autosomal dominant families have been observed.[144] Chromosome 22q11 mutations are the most common cause, but several other chromosomal abnormalities have also been associated with DiGeorge syndrome. The phrase CATCH22 has been introduced to describe the syndrome of cardiac anomalies, abnormal facies, thymic aplasia, cleft palate, and hypocalcemia associated with chromosome 22 deletions. These deletions generally contain several genes, and although the precise genetic etiology of the DiGeorge syndrome and CATCH22 remains the subject of active investigation, the Tbx1 gene appears to play a major role.[145] Symptomatic hypocalcemia may be the major clinical feature of chromosome 22 deletions.[146] Hypoparathyroidism also occurs in several disorders of mitochondrial dysfunction[147] and in the autoimmune polyendocrinopathy known as APECED[148] (see later). Kenny-Caffey syndrome, a recessive disorder in which hypoparathyroidism is associated with osteosclerosis, mental retardation, and growth failure, has been shown to result from mutations in the TBCE gene encoding a chaperone protein important in tubulin folding.[149]

Inherited Disorders of Parathyroid Hormone Resistance

Individuals with pseudohypoparathyroidism (PsHP) are hypocalcemic because of resistance to the effects of PTH. Typically, PsHP patients have elevated PTH levels. PsHP is now recognized as a heterogeneous group of related disorders.[150] The patients first described by Albright exhibited a pattern of features that included short stature, round face, mental retardation, brachydactyly, and the lack of a phosphaturic response to parathyroid extract.

PsHP type I refers to complete resistance to the effects of PTH, as demonstrated by the failure of patients to increase serum calcium, urinary cAMP, and phosphate in response to PTH infusion.[151] The somatic features originally described (termed Albright hereditary osteodystrophy [AHO]) together with the biochemical features are referred to as PsHP type Ia. The presence of the biochemical features of PTH resistance without the somatic features (AHO) is referred to as PsHP type Ib. Patients with pseudo-pseudohypoparathyroidism (PPsHP) are not hypocalcemic, nor do they demonstrate the other biochemical feature seen in PsHP, but they do have the somatic features of AHO.

PsHP-Ia results from a loss-of-function mutation of the GNAS1 gene, which encodes the stimulatory G protein α-subunit $G_s\alpha$ (the PTH receptor utilizes the adenylyl cyclase pathway).[152] Promoter specific genomic imprinting of GNAS1 has been established and provides the probable explanation for the complex phenotypic expression of the dominantly inherited genetic defect. Maternal transmission of the mutation causes PsHP-Ia; paternal transmission leads to PPsHP.[153]

Like PsHP-Ia, PsHP-Ib follows autosomal dominant inheritance. The biochemical features of hypocalcemia and a defective urine cAMP and phosphaturic response to PTH are present, but the somatic features (AHO) are absent. Disease expression appears to be due to mutations that affect the regulatory elements of GNAS1.[154,155] PsHP-Ib is maternally transmitted.

Of particular note, these three disorders are not the only clinical manifestations of GNAS gene defects. In McCune-Albright syndrome, which is characterized by endocrine hyperfunction and fibrous dysplasia, somatic mutations in GNAS lead to constitutive $G_s\alpha$ activity.[156] Temperature-sensitive mutations in GNAS were found in two hypocalcemic patients exhibiting resistance to some hormones (PTH, thyroid-stimulating hormone) and independence from the effects of others (luteinizing hormone) that lead to precocious puberty.[157]

Patients with PsHP type Ic exhibit the features of PsHP type I, but without defective $G_s\alpha$ activity or GNAS mutations. Presumably, some other component of the PTH/PTHrP receptor signaling pathway is defective.[158] PsHP type II is a heterogeneous group of disorders characterized by a reduced phosphaturic response to PTH but a normal increase in urinary cAMP.[159] The cause is unclear but may be a defect in the intracellular response to cAMP or some other component of the PTH signaling pathway. PsHP type II does not appear to follow a clear familial pattern.

Acquired Hypoparathyroidism

Surgical hypoparathyroidism is the most common cause of acquired hypoparathyroidism. It is observed after total thyroidectomy for cancer or thyrotoxicosis, radical neck dissection, and repeated operations for parathyroid adenoma removal. Hypoparathyroidism may result from inadvertent removal of the parathyroids, damage from bleeding, or devascularization. Transient hypoparathyroidism and hypocalcemia are quite common after total thyroidectomy.[160–162] They may result from a rapid reduction in thyroid hormone–mediated bone resorption or from temporary damage to the parathyroids. Removal of a single hyperfunctioning parathyroid adenoma can result in transient hypocalcemia because of hypercalcemia-induced suppression of PTH secretion from the normal glands.

Acquired hypoparathyroidism from nonsurgical causes is rare, with the exception of magnesium deficiency (see the next section). Although metal overload diseases (hemochromatosis, Wilson disease) and granulomatous or neoplastic invasion of the parathyroid are often mentioned as causes of hypoparathyroidism, these entities are quite rare. Miliary tuberculosis and amyloidosis are exceedingly rare causes of infiltrative hypoparathyroidism. Alcohol consumption has been reported to cause transient hypocalcemia.[163]

Magnesium-Related Disorders

Interestingly, both hypomagnesemia and hypermagnesemia are associated with hypocalcemia. Mg^{2+} is an extracellular CaR agonist, though less potent than calcium. Acute infusion of Mg or hypermagnesemia inhibits PTH secretion.[164] Chronic severe hypomagnesemia results in hypocalcemia, not from an effect on CaR but from intracellular Mg^{2+} depletion and its effect on PTH gland function.[165] In addition, hypomagnesemia also alters end-organ responsiveness to PTH.[166] Typically, these patients have low or inappropriately normal PTH levels for the degree of hypocalcemia observed.[167] Severe hypocalcemia is seen as a consequence of hypomagnesemia only when the Mg^{2+} deficiency is severe. The appropriate therapy is Mg repletion; in the absence of adequate Mg repletion, the hypocalcemia is resistant to PTH or to vitamin D therapy.

Mg^{2+} excess can also cause hypoparathyroidism. Clinically, this condition occurs in the acute setting. High doses of intravenous magnesium sulfate are used in obstetrics. The effect of acute hypermagnesemia may be a result of CaR-mediated inhibition of PTH secretion.[168]

Autoimmune Disease

Autoimmune disease may cause hypoparathyroidism as an isolated finding or as a component of a syndrome of multiple endocrinopathies. Type I polyglandular autoimmune syndrome, also referred to as APECED (autoimmune polyendocrinopathy, candidiasis, ectodermal dystrophy syndrome), is a recessive disorder.[169] Its cardinal features are childhood onset of hypoparathyroidism in association with adrenal insufficiency and mucocutaneous candidiasis (thus the older acronym HAM), although a great deal of clinical variability is seen. The gene for APECED, mapped to chromosome 21q in multiple families, has been identified. This gene, termed AIRE for autoimmune regulator, appears to be a transcription factor.[170]

Autoantibodies against parathyroid tissue have been reported in a significant percentage of cases of hypoparathyroidism, but the causative role of these antibodies is unclear. CaR has been identified as a possible autoantigen in some cases of autoimmune hypoparathyroidism (either isolated or polyglandular).[171]

Vitamin D-Related Disorders

Several inherited and acquired disorders of vitamin D metabolism or deficiency can lead to hypocalcemia, though usually not as an isolated finding. Because vitamin D_3 is normally produced by the skin from 7-dehydrocholesterol in the presence of sunlight, vitamin D deficiency requires both dietary deficiency and lack of exposure to the sun. Prolonged vitamin D deficiency causes rickets (a disorder of mineralization of growing bone) and osteomalacia (a disorder of mineralization of formed bone). Elevation of PTH levels is generally observed.[172] The diagnosis is confirmed by measurement of serum 25(OH)D levels.

Despite routine dietary supplementation in milk and other foods, vitamin D deficiency appears to be relatively common in certain populations. A study of hospitalized patients found a high prevalence of vitamin D deficiency, even in younger patients without risk factors who were consuming the recommended daily allowance of vitamin D_3.[173] Similarly, in nursing home residents with vitamin D–supplemented diets, hypovitaminosis D is common. Breast-feeding infants of mothers with diets low in vitamin D are also susceptible. In urban populations with low exposure to sunlight, vitamin D deficiency is common.

Vitamin D deficiency is a frequent complication of gastrointestinal disease.[174] Hypovitaminosis D and osteomalacia are commonly seen after gastrectomy, often occurring many years after surgery.[175] The cause of osteomalacia and hypocalcemia involves impaired absorption of vitamin D, impaired calcium absorption, increased vitamin D catabolism, and patient avoidance of milk products.

Vitamin D deficiency is seen in diseases of the intestine, including Crohn disease, celiac sprue, and intestinal resection,[176,177] and is not uncommon. Causes may include altered enterohepatic circulation of 25(OH)D and 1,25(OH)$_2$D. Treatment of celiac disease with appropriate dietary changes reverses the osteopenia and biochemical abnormalities.

Hepatobiliary disease is a relatively rare cause of vitamin D deficiency and osteopenia. More commonly, the hypocalcemia in this group of patients results from hypoalbuminemia. Causes of vitamin D deficiency include impaired hepatic 25-hydroxylation of vitamin D, malabsorption of vitamin D (possibly resulting from impaired bile salt synthesis), and poor nutritional status. Therapy with vitamin D and calcium is not fully effective.[178]

Vitamin D deficiency with hypocalcemia is commonly seen in patients with renal insufficiency (see Chapter 52) and is due in part to impaired 1α-hydroxylation of vitamin D. Patients with nephrotic syndrome may have decreased 25(OH)D levels as a result of urinary loss, hypocalcemia, and secondary HPT.[179]

Disorders of altered vitamin D metabolism represent a second group of vitamin D–related hypocalcemias. They may be acquired or inherited. Medications, most notably anticonvulsants, may interfere with the metabolism of vitamin D.[180] Phenytoin and phenobarbital appear to stimulate the conversion of 25(OH)D to inactive metabolites.[181]

The vitamin D–dependent rickets (VDDR type I and II) are hypocalcemic disorders of vitamin D metabolism. In VDDR-I, which is characterized by autosomal recessive, childhood-onset rickets, secondary HPT, and aminoaciduria, the biochemical abnormality is defective 1α-hydroxylation of 25(OH)D. The gene for 25(OH)D–1α-hydroxylase has been cloned and found to be defective in VDDR-I patients.[182]

VDDR-II (also called hereditary vitamin D-resistant rickets), like type I, is an autosomal recessive disorder. Affected patients have extreme elevations in 1,25(OH)$_2$D levels, in addition to alopecia and the abnormalities seen in VDDR-I.[183] Biochemically, the disorder results from end-organ resistance to 1,25(OH)$_2$D. A number of different mutations have been found in the vitamin D receptor gene of affected individuals.[184]

Medications

Medication-induced hypocalcemia is a relatively rare cause of hypocalcemia. Bisphosphonates, calcimimetics, mithramycin, and calcitonin, all of which may be used in the management of hypercalcemia or to inhibit bone resorption, may depress serum calcium to subnormal levels.

Citrate administration during transfusion of citrated blood or plasmapheresis may cause hypocalcemia. Transfusions of citrated blood rarely cause significant hypocalcemia, but it may occur in the course of massive transfusion.[185] Similarly, significant hypocalcemia occurs but is rare after plasmapheresis.[186]

Foscarnet (trisodium phosphoformate), which is used in the management of viral opportunistic infections, can cause hypocalcemia through the chelation of extracellular calcium ions, and normal total calcium measurements may not reflect ionized hypocalcemia.[187] As stated previously, anticonvulsants, particularly phenytoin and phenobarbital, appear to interfere with vitamin D metabolism.[181] Fluoride overdose is an exceedingly rare cause of hypocalcemia.

Other drugs associated with hypocalcemia include anti-infectious agents (pentamidine, ketoconazole) and chemotherapeutic agents (asparaginase, cisplatin, WR-2721, doxorubicin).

Miscellaneous Causes

Hypocalcemia is common in acute pancreatitis and is a poor prognostic indicator.[188] It is probably due to calcium chelation by free fatty acids generated by the action of pancreatic lipase. Severe hyperphosphatemia may cause hypocalcemia, particularly in patients with renal failure. This association is observed in several clinical settings. Soft tissue calcification and hypocalcemia have been reported in the management of hypophosphatemia.[189] Enemas containing phosphate and infant formulas supplemented with phosphate have been reported to cause hypocalcemia. Massive tumor lysis, particularly from rapidly growing hematologic malignancies, may cause hyperphosphatemia, hyperuricemia, and hypocalcemia.[190] The early phase of rhabdomyolysis may include severe hyperphosphatemia and associated hypocalcemia, in contrast to the recovery phase, when hypercalcemia is common. In hemodialysis patients, hypocalcemia is common and may result at least in part from reduced renal phosphate clearance and consequent hyperphosphatemia and reduced 1,25(OH)$_2$D production (see Chapter 52).

Critical Illness

In complicated, critically ill patients, total calcium measurements may be poor indicators of the ionized calcium concentration because a large number of factors that may interfere with or alter calcium/protein binding may be present (albumin infusion, citrate, intravenous fluids, acid/base disturbances, dialysis therapy). Thus, it is particularly important to measure ionized calcium in this setting. In fact, hypocalcemia has been reported to be present in over 70% of intensive care unit patients.[191] Hypocalcemia is frequently noted in both gram-negative sepsis and toxic shock syndrome.[192] The cause in unknown, but a direct effect of interleukin-1 on parathyroid function may be partly responsible.[193]

Neonatal Hypocalcemia

In the first few days of life, infants normally have serum calcium levels significantly lower than normal adult levels. More severe hypocalcemia is referred to as neonatal hypocalcemia and is generally divided into early neonatal and late neonatal hypocalcemia by pediatricians.[194] Early-onset hypocalcemia, which appears in the first 3 to 4 days of life, is often associated with maternal gestational diabetes, prematurity, or other perinatal problems. The hypocalcemia may be severe enough to cause neuromuscular dysfunction, including seizures, but it is self-limited.

Late neonatal hypocalcemia, which occurs within the first 5 to 10 days of life, is rarer. It is observed in infants receiving cow's milk or infant formula with a high phosphate concentration[195]; hypomagnesemia may be responsible in some cases. Other forms of late-onset hypocalcemia may be observed in infants of hypercalcemic mothers, presumably as a result of secondary hypoparathyroidism in the fetus.[196]

Management of Hypocalcemia

Treatment of acute hypocalcemia depends on the severity of the depression in serum calcium and the presence of clinical manifestations. Oral calcium supplementation may be sufficient treatment for mild hypocalcemia; severe hypocalcemia with evidence of neuromuscular effects or tetany is treated with intravenous calcium. Typically, 1 g to 3 g of intravenous calcium gluconate is given over a period of 10 to 20 minutes, followed by slow intravenous infusion. Dialysis may be appropriate if hyperphosphatemia is also present. Correction of hypomagnesemia and hyperphosphatemia should also be undertaken when present.

Treatment of chronic hypocalcemia depends on the underlying cause, for instance, correction of hypomagnesemia or vitamin D deficiency. The principal therapy for primary disorders of parathyroid dysfunction or PTH resistance is dietary calcium supplementation and vitamin D therapy. Correction of serum calcium to the low-normal range is generally advised; correction to normal levels may lead to frank hypercalciuria.

DISORDERS OF MAGNESIUM HOMEOSTASIS

Hypomagnesemia and Magnesium Deficiency

The terms "hypomagnesemia" and "Mg^{2+} deficiency" tend to be used interchangeably. However, there is a complex relationship between total body Mg^{2+} stores, serum Mg^{2+} concentrations, and the Mg^{2+} level in different intracellular compartments. Because extracellular fluid Mg^{2+} accounts for only 1% of total body Mg^{2+}, it is hardly surprising that serum Mg^{2+} concentrations have been found to correlate poorly with overall Mg^{2+} status. Indeed, in patients with Mg^{2+} deficiency, serum Mg^{2+} concentrations may be normal or may seriously underestimate the severity of the Mg^{2+} deficit.[197] However, no satisfactory clinical test to assay body Mg^{2+} stores is available.

The Mg^{2+} tolerance test is generally thought to be the best test of overall Mg^{2+} status. It is based on the observation that Mg^{2+}-deficient patients tend to retain a greater proportion of a parenterally administered Mg^{2+} load and excrete less in the

urine than normal individuals do.[198] Studies in Mg^{2+}-deficient rats indicate that the administered Mg^{2+} is rapidly diverted to non–extracellular fluid stores, so the low urinary excretion is due to a small filtered load of Mg^{2+} delivered to the nephron.[199] By contrast, in normal rats given intravenous Mg^{2+}, the serum concentration and therefore the filtered load rise dramatically, and Mg^{2+} spills into the urine because of the "threshold" effect. Clinical studies indicate that the results of an Mg^{2+} tolerance test correlate well with Mg^{2+} status as assessed by skeletal muscle Mg^{2+} content and exchangeable Mg^{2+} pools. However, the test is invalid in patients who have impaired renal function or a renal Mg^{2+}-wasting syndrome or in patients who are taking diuretics or other medications that induce renal Mg^{2+} wasting. For this reason and also because of the time and effort required to perform the Mg^{2+} tolerance test, it is used infrequently in clinical practice.

The serum Mg^{2+} concentration, though an insensitive measure of Mg^{2+} deficit, remains the only practical test of Mg^{2+} status in widespread use. Surveys of serum Mg^{2+} levels in hospitalized patients indicate a high incidence of hypomagnesemia (presumably an underestimate of the true incidence of Mg^{2+} deficiency), ranging from 11% in general inpatients[200] to 60% in patients admitted to intensive care units.[201] Furthermore, among intensive care unit patients, hypomagnesemia was associated with increased mortality when compared with patients who have normomagnesemia.[201]

Etiology and Diagnosis

Mg^{2+} deficiency may be caused by decreased intake or intestinal absorption; increased losses via the gastrointestinal tract, kidneys, or skin; or rarely, sequestration in the bone compartment. The first step in determining the etiology is to distinguish between renal Mg^{2+} wasting and extrarenal causes of Mg^{2+} loss by performing a quantitative assessment of urinary Mg^{2+} excretion. The fractional excretion of magnesium ($FeMg^{2+}$) from a random urine specimen can be calculated in the standard fashion after multiplying the plasma magnesium concentration by 0.7 (because about 30% of circulating magnesium is bound to plasma protein and remains unfiltered). In general, a $FeMg^{2+}$ of more than 3% in an individual with normal GFR is indicative of inappropriate urinary magnesium loss.[202] The $FeMg^{2+}$ is likely superior to the urinary magnesium to creatinine molar ratio for this purpose. Alternatively, a 24-hour urine collection can be obtained: the kidneys can normally reduce the 24-hour urinary magnesium excretion to less than 24 mg in states of magnesium deficiency.[203] If renal Mg^{2+} wasting has been excluded, the losses must be extrarenal in origin and the underlying cause can usually be identified from the case history.

Extrarenal Causes
Nutritional Deficiency

Human Mg^{2+} deprivation studies have demonstrated that induction of Mg^{2+} deficiency by dietary means in normal individuals is surprisingly difficult because nearly all foods contain significant amounts of Mg^{2+} and renal adaptation to conserve Mg^{2+} is very efficient. Nevertheless, Mg^{2+} deficiency of nutritional origin can be observed, particularly in two clinical settings: alcoholism and parenteral feeding.

In chronic alcoholics, the intake of ethanol substitutes for the intake of important nutrients. Approximately 20% to 25% of alcoholics are frankly hypomagnesemic, and most can be shown to be Mg^{2+} deficient with the Mg^{2+} tolerance test.[198] Of note, some evidence suggests that alcohol also may impair renal magnesium conservation.[204]

Patients receiving parenteral nutrition have a particularly high incidence of hypomagnesemia.[205] In general, these patients are sicker than the average inpatient and are more likely to have other conditions associated with an Mg^{2+} deficit and ongoing Mg^{2+} losses. However, even for nutritionally replete subjects, the daily Mg^{2+} requirement to maintain Mg^{2+} balance is increased during parenteral feeding, for unclear reasons. Furthermore, hypomagnesemia may also be a consequence of the refeeding syndrome.[206] In this condition, overzealous parenteral feeding of severely malnourished patients causes hyperinsulinemia, as well as rapid cellular uptake of glucose and water, together with phosphorus, potassium, and Mg^{2+}.

Intestinal Malabsorption
Generalized malabsorption syndromes caused by conditions such as celiac disease, Whipple disease, and inflammatory bowel disease are frequently associated with intestinal Mg^{2+} wasting and Mg^{2+} deficiency.[207] In fat malabsorption with concomitant steatorrhea, free fatty acids in the intestinal lumen may combine with Mg^{2+} to form nonabsorbable soaps, a process known as saponification, thus contributing to impaired Mg^{2+} absorption. Indeed, the severity of hypomagnesemia in patients with malabsorption syndrome correlates with the fecal fat excretion rate, and in rare patients, reduction of dietary fat intake alone, which reduces steatorrhea, can correct the hypomagnesemia. Previous intestinal resection, particularly of the distal part of the small intestine, is also an important cause of Mg^{2+} malabsorption[208] and a confounding factor in many studies of patients with Crohn disease. Similarly, Mg^{2+} deficiency can be a late complication of jejunoileal bypass surgery performed for the management of obesity.

Diarrhea and Gastrointestinal Fistula
The Mg^{2+} concentration of diarrheal fluid is high and ranges from 1 mg/dL to 16 mg/dL,[208] so Mg^{2+} deficiency may occur in patients with chronic diarrhea of any cause, even in the absence of concomitant malabsorption,[197] and in patients who abuse laxatives. By contrast, secretions from the upper gastrointestinal tract are low in Mg^{2+} content, and significant Mg^{2+} deficiency is therefore rarely observed in patients with an intestinal, biliary, or pancreatic fistula, ileostomy, or prolonged gastric drainage (except as a consequence of malnutrition).[208]

Cutaneous Losses
Hypomagnesemia may be observed after prolonged intense exertion. For example, serum Mg^{2+} concentrations fall 20% on average after a marathon run.[209] About a quarter of the decrement in serum Mg^{2+} can be accounted for by losses in sweat, which can contain up to 0.5 mg/dL of Mg^{2+}, with the remainder most likely being due to transient redistribution into the intracellular space. Hypomagnesemia occurs in 40% of patients with severe burn injuries during the early period of recovery. The major cause is loss of Mg^{2+} in the cutaneous exudate, which can exceed 1 g/day.[210]

Redistribution to Bone Compartment
Hypomagnesemia may occasionally accompany the profound hypocalcemia of hungry bone syndrome observed in some patients with HPT and severe bone disease immediately after parathyroidectomy.[211] In such cases, a high bone turnover state exists, and sudden removal of excess PTH is believed to result in virtual cessation of bone resorption, with a continued high rate of bone formation and consequent sequestration of both Ca^{2+} and Mg^{2+} into bone mineral.

Renal Magnesium Wasting
The diagnosis of renal Mg^{2+} wasting is made by demonstrating an inappropriately high rate of renal Mg^{2+} excretion in the face of hypomagnesemia, as detailed previously.

Polyuria
Renal Mg^{2+} wasting occurs with osmotic diuresis, as in the severe hyperglycemic state of diabetic ketoacidosis.[212,213] Indeed, the estimated average Mg^{2+} deficit at initial evaluation varies from 200 mg to 500 mg.[212,213] Hypermagnesuria also occurs during the polyuric phase of recovery from acute renal failure in a native kidney, during recovery from ischemic injury in a transplanted kidney, and in postobstructive diuresis. In such cases, it is likely that residual tubule reabsorptive defects persisting from the primary renal injury play as important a role as polyuria itself in inducing renal Mg^{2+} wasting.

Extracellular Fluid Volume Expansion
Chronic therapy with Mg^{2+}-free parenteral fluids, either crystalloid or hyperalimentation,[205] can cause renal Mg^{2+} wasting, in part because of expansion of extracellular fluid volume. Renal Mg^{2+} wasting is also characteristic of hyperaldosteronism.[214]

Defective Na Reabsorption in Distal Nephron
Loop diuretics inhibit the apical membrane $Na^+/K^+/2Cl^-$ cotransporter of the TAL and abolish the transepithelial potential difference, thereby inhibiting paracellular Mg^{2+} reabsorption. Hypomagnesemia is therefore a frequent finding in patients receiving chronic loop diuretic therapy.[215] Thiazides inhibit renal Mg^{2+} reabsorption by an incompletely understood mechanism. Thiazide-induced hypomagnesemia has been suggested to increase the risk of arrhythmias in hypertensive patients. However, in a cohort of participants from the Multiple Risk Factor Intervention Trial treated chronically with chlorthalidone, the degree of hypomagnesemia was clinically and statistically insignificant.[216]

Hypercalcemia
Elevated serum ionized Ca^{2+} levels directly induce renal Mg^{2+} wasting and hypomagnesemia,[217] a phenomenon that is most clearly observable in the setting of hypercalcemia caused by malignant bone metastases. In HPT, the situation is more complicated because the hypercalcemia-induced tendency to Mg^{2+} wasting is counteracted by the action of PTH, which stimulates Mg^{2+} reabsorption, so renal Mg^{2+} handling is usually normal and Mg^{2+} deficiency is rare.[218]

Tubule Nephrotoxins
Cisplatin, a widely used chemotherapeutic agent for solid tumors, frequently causes renal Mg^{2+} wasting. All patients receiving monthly cycles of cisplatin at a dose of 50 mg/m² become hypomagnesemic during treatment.[219] The occurrence of Mg^{2+} wasting does not appear to correlate with the incidence of cisplatin-induced acute renal failure.[220] Renal magnesuria continues after cessation of the drug for a mean of 4 to 5 months, but it can persist for years.[220] Although the nephrotoxic effects of cisplatin are manifested histologically as acute tubular necrosis confined to the S3 segment of proximal tubule, the magnesuria does not correlate temporally with the clinical development of acute renal failure secondary to acute tubular necrosis. Furthermore, patients who become hypomagnesemic are also subject to the development of hypocalciuria, thus suggesting that the reabsorption defect may actually be in the distal convoluted tubule (DCT), as with Gitelman syndrome. Carboplatin, an analog of cisplatin, appears to be considerably less nephrotoxic and rarely causes either acute renal failure or hypomagnesemia.[221] Of interest, recent data suggest that cisplatin also may impair intestinal absorption of magnesium.[222]

Amphotericin B is a well-recognized tubule nephrotoxin that can cause renal K^+ wasting, distal renal tubular acidosis, and acute renal failure, with tubule necrosis and Ca^{2+} deposition noted in the DCT and TAL on renal biopsy. Amphotericin B causes renal Mg^{2+} wasting and hypomagnesemia that is related to the cumulative dose administered, but these effects may be observed after as little as a 200 mg total dose.[223] Interestingly, the amphotericin-induced magnesuria is accompanied by the reciprocal development of hypocalciuria, so as

CH 16

with cisplatin, the serum Ca^{2+} concentration is usually preserved, again suggesting that the functional tubule defect resides in the DCT.

Aminoglycosides cause a syndrome of renal Mg^{2+} and K^+ wasting with hypomagnesemia, hypokalemia, hypocalcemia, and tetany. Hypomagnesemia may occur despite levels in the appropriate therapeutic range.[224] Most patients reported had delayed onset of hypomagnesemia occurring after at least 2 weeks of therapy, and they received total doses in excess of 8 g, thus suggesting that it is the cumulative dose of aminoglycoside that is the key predictor of toxicity. In addition, no correlation has been found between the occurrence of aminoglycoside-induced acute tubular necrosis and hypomagnesemia. Mg^{2+} wasting persists after cessation of the aminoglycoside, often for several months. All aminoglycosides in clinical use have been implicated, including gentamicin, tobramycin, and amikacin, as well as neomycin when administered topically for extensive burn injuries. This form of symptomatic aminoglycoside-induced renal Mg^{2+} wasting is now relatively uncommon because of heightened general awareness of its toxicity. However, asymptomatic hypomagnesemia can be observed in one third of individuals treated with a single course of an aminoglycoside at standard doses (3 to 5 mg/kg/day for a mean of 10 days). In these cases, the hypomagnesemia occurs on average 3 to 4 days after the start of therapy and readily reverses after cessation of therapy.[225]

Intravenous pentamidine causes hypomagnesemia as a result of renal Mg^{2+} wasting in most patients, typically in association with hypocalcemia.[226] The average onset of symptomatic hypomagnesemia occurs after 9 days of therapy, and the defect persists for at least 1 to 2 months after discontinuation of pentamidine. Hypomagnesemia is also observed in two thirds of AIDS patients with cytomegalovirus retinitis treated intravenously with the pyrophosphate analog foscarnet.[227] As with aminoglycosides and pentamidine, foscarnet-induced hypomagnesemia is often associated with significant hypocalcemia.

Cyclosporine causes renal Mg^{2+} wasting and hypomagnesemia in patients after renal and bone marrow transplantation.[228,229] Mg^{2+} loss does not correlate either with serum trough cyclosporine levels or with the development of cyclosporin-induced renal failure. Interestingly, the development of hypomagnesemia correlates temporally with the onset and severity of neurologic symptoms such as ataxia, tremor, depression, and transient dysphasia. These symptoms had previously been attributed to direct cyclosporine neurotoxic-

ity, but they may well be a secondary consequence of cyclosporine-induced Mg^{2+} deficiency. Interestingly, some studies have shown that Mg^{2+} supplementation may help prevent cyclosporine nephrotoxicity.[230]

Tubulointestinal Nephropathies

Renal Mg^{2+} wasting has occasionally been reported in patients with acute or chronic tubulointerstitial nephritis not caused by nephrotoxic drugs, for example, in chronic pyelonephritis and acute renal allograft rejection. Other manifestations of tubule dysfunction, such as salt wasting, hypokalemia, renal tubular acidosis, and Fanconi syndrome, also may be present and provide clues to the diagnosis.

Inherited Renal Magnesium Wasting Disorders

Primary magnesium-wasting disorders are rare.[231] Though fairly heterogeneous, these patients can be broadly classified into distinct clinical syndromes by their genetic and phenotypic patterns (Table 16–6). Genetic studies are helping to clarify the genetic and molecular etiologies and, in turn, elucidate the mechanism of renal and intestinal magnesium handling (see Chapter 5).

Isolated Familial Hypomagnesemia

Isolated familial hypomagnesemia is most commonly manifested in childhood as tetany or seizures.[232,233] Laboratory investigation reveals hypomagnesemia with inappropriate magnesuria, but usually no other electrolyte or renal disturbances, and renal biopsy findings are normal by light and electron microscopy, as well as by standard immunofluorescence studies. Both autosomal dominant and recessive forms exist.[232,233]

A locus for autosomal dominant hypomagnesemia was mapped to chromosome 11q23 by a genome-wide linkage scan in two large families with this condition. Subsequently, the gene responsible was identified as FXYD2, which encodes the sodium-potassium-adenosinetriphosphatase (Na^+,K^+-ATPase) α-subunit.[234] The absence of hypomagnesemia in individuals with large deletions at this locus suggested a gain-of-function rather than loss-of-function disease mechanism. Expression studies indicated that the identified Gly41Arg mutation may lead to defective posttranslational processing of the protein, which is expressed in the distal convoluted tubule.[234,235] The dominant form of isolated hypomagnesemia is genetically heterogeneous: FXYD2 has been excluded as the responsible locus in a large family with dominant hypomagnesemia, low bone mass, relatively low

TABLE 16–6	Classification and Clinical Features of Inherited Renal Mg^{2+} Wasting Disorders			
	Isolated Familial Hypomagnesemia (Recessive)	Isolated Familial Hypomagnesemia (Dominant)	Hypomagnesemia with Hypocalcemia	Familial Hypomagnesemia with Hypercalciuria
MIM number	248250	154020	602014	603959
Fluid and electrolyte abnormalities	—	Hypocalciuria	Hypocalcemia, hypercalciuria	Hypocalcemia Distal renal tubular acidosis Nephrogenic diabetes insipidus
Gene	?	FXYD2, other(s)	TRPM6	CLDN16
Locus		11q23	9q22	3q27
Structural renal abnormalities	—	—	—	Nephrocalcinosis
Chronic renal failure	No	No	No	Yes
Extrarenal manifestations	—	—	—	Ocular abnormalities
Pattern of inheritance	AR	AD	AR	AR

AD, autosomal dominant; AR, autosomal recessive. Urinary magnesium wasting can be observed in Gitelman and Bartter syndromes. These entities are discussed in Chapter 21.

PTH levels, and hypermagnesuria.[236] The gene responsible for the autosomal recessive form is unknown.[231]

Hypomagnesemia with Hypercalciuria and Nephrocalcinosis

Familial hypomagnesemia with hypercalciuria is characterized by renal Mg^{2+} wasting in association with significant hypercalciuria.[231] The major cause of morbidity in this disorder is probably the hypercalciuria, which leads to hypocalcemia and renal calculi in some cases and to nephrocalcinosis in all. In turn, nephrocalcinosis and renal stone disease are thought to be the cause of recurrent urinary tract infections, distal renal tubular acidosis (usually incomplete), nephrogenic diabetes insipidus, and progressive renal impairment, which may lead to end-stage renal failure. The tendency to tissue calcium deposition may also be manifested as calcification of the basal ganglia and chondrocalcinosis with crystal arthropathy. In addition, the condition is associated with several ocular abnormalities, including corneal calcification, chorioretinitis, keratoconus, macular colobomas, nystagmus, and myopia.

By means of a genome-wide scan in 12 families with recessive hypomagnesemia and hypercalciuria, Simon and co-workers[237] identified a locus on chromosome 3q and determined that the gene responsible was a member of the claudin family of cell junction proteins, claudin-16 (CLDNN16), also known as paracellin (PCLN1). PCLN1 is a tight-junction protein expressed only in the TAL and DCT and facilitates the passive, paracellular reabsorption of both magnesium and calcium.[238]

Affected patients show marked hypomagnesemia and hypercalciuria with associated nephrocalcinosis and progressive renal insufficiency. In studies of phenotype and genotype, affected patients were often initially evaluated in childhood for hematuria and urinary tract infections. Treatment with thiazides and magnesium supplementation did not prevent the progression of renal failure, which occurred in 11 of 33 patients at a median age of 14.5 years.[239] In these patients, a large fraction of mutant alleles shared a Leu151Phe mutation, thus suggesting a founder effect. Studies have suggested an increase in urine calcium and magnesium excretion in heterozygotes for CLDN16 mutations.

Hypomagnesemia with Hypocalcemia

Primary hypomagnesemia with hypocalcemia is inherited as an autosomal recessive trait. A locus was identified on chromosome 9q22 by genetic mapping in inbred Bedouin kindreds.[240] Subsequently, the gene responsible was identified as TRPM6, a member of the TRP family of ion channels.[241] TRPM6 is expressed in renal tubules and throughout the intestine, although the major problem appears to stem from altered intestinal magnesium absorption. TRPM6 is regulated by dietary magnesium and by estrogens.[241a]

The hypomagnesemia in this condition is severe, with seizures being a frequent finding in infants. High doses of enteral magnesium can help keep the serum calcium level near the normal range (presumably via paracellular absorption) and decrease complications.

Bartter/Gitelman Syndromes

Classic Bartter syndrome (see Chapter 15) is an autosomal recessive disorder characterized by Na^+ wasting, hypokalemic metabolic alkalosis, and hypercalciuria, and it usually occurs in infancy or early childhood. Most Bartter syndrome kindreds result from inactivating mutations in one of the three transport proteins that mediate the TAL NaCl reabsorption/apical K^+ recycling pathway, namely, the apical $Na^+/K^+/2Cl^-$ cotransporter (BSC1), the apical inwardly rectifying K^+ channel (ROMK1), or the basolateral Cl^- channel (CLC-Kb). All Bartter syndrome patients are by definition hypercalciuric, and in addition, one third has hypomagnesemia with

inappropriate magnesuria, consistent with loss of the TAL transepithelial potential difference that drives paracellular divalent cation reabsorption. Thus, the physiology of Bartter syndrome is essentially identical to that of chronic loop diuretic therapy.

Gitelman syndrome (see Chapter 15) is a variant of Bartter syndrome that is distinguished primarily by hypocalciuria (urinary calcium-to-creatinine ratio, 0.07 mg/mg). Patients with Gitelman syndrome are identified later in life, usually after the age of 6 years, have milder symptoms, and generally have preserved urinary concentrating ability. The genetic defect in these families is caused by inactivating mutations in the DCT electroneutral thiazide-sensitive NaCl cotransporter TSC. The difference in the nephron segment site of the NaCl reabsorption defect can explain the difference between classic Bartter and Gitelman syndromes in urinary concentrating ability (NaCl reabsorption in the medullary TAL, but not the DCT, contributes to the medullary interstitium concentrating gradient) and Ca^{2+} excretion (NaCl reabsorption is required for generation of the driving force for Ca^{2+} reabsorption in the TAL, but not the DCT), and these in turn mirror the differences observed with chronic loop and thiazide diuretic therapy. Interestingly however, renal Mg^{2+} wasting and hypomagnesemia are universally found in patients with Gitelman syndrome.

Ca^{2+}-Sensing Disorders

In FHH, the hypercalcemia is due to inactivating mutations in CaR (discussed earlier). As a consequence of the inactivated CaR, the normal magnesuric response to hypercalcemia is impaired,[242] and thus these patients are paradoxically mildly hypermagnesemic. Activating mutations in CaR cause the opposite syndrome, autosomal dominant hypoparathyroidism. As might be expected, most such patients are mildly hypomagnesemic, presumably because of TAL Mg^{2+} wasting.[137]

Clinical Manifestations

Hypomagnesemia may cause symptoms and signs of disordered cardiac, neuromuscular, and central nervous system function (Table 16–7). It is also associated with an imbalance of other electrolytes such as K^+ and Ca^{2+}. However, many patients with hypomagnesemia are completely asymptomatic.[243]

TABLE 16–7 Clinical Manifestations of Mg^{2+} Deficiency

Cardiac
  Electrocardiographic abnormalities
    Non-specific T wave changes
    U waves
    Prolonged QT and QU interval
    Repolarization alternans
  Arrhythmias
    Ventricular ectopy
    Monomorphic ventricular tachycardia
    Torsades de pointes
    Ventricular fibrillation
    Enhanced digitalis toxicity

Neuromuscular
  Muscle weakness
  Muscle tremor and twitching
  Positive Trousseau and Chvostek signs
  Tetany
  Vertical and horizontal nystagmus
  Paresthesias
  Generalized seizures
  Multifocal motor seizures

Metabolic
  Hypokalemia
  Hypocalcemia

Thus, the clinical importance of hypomagnesemia remains controversial. Furthermore, many of the cardiac and neurologic manifestations attributed to Mg^{2+} deficiency may also be explained by the frequent coexistence of hypokalemia and hypocalcemia in the same patient.

Cardiovascular System

Mg^{2+} has protean and complex effects on myocardial ion fluxes, among which its effect on the sodium pump (Na^+,K^+-ATPase) is probably the most important. Because Mg^{2+} is an obligate cofactor in all reactions that require adenosine triphosphate (ATP), it is essential for the activity of Na^+,K^+-ATPase.[244] During Mg^{2+} deficiency, Na^+,K^+-ATPase function is impaired. The intracellular K^+ concentration falls, which may potentially result in a relatively depolarized resting membrane potential, so the excitation threshold for activation of an action potential is more easily attainable and thus predisposes to ectopic excitation and tachyarrhythmias.[245] Furthermore, the magnitude of the outward K^+ gradient is decreased, thereby reducing the driving force for the K^+ efflux needed to terminate the cardiac action potential, and as a result, repolarization is delayed.

Electrocardiographic changes may be observed with isolated hypomagnesemia and usually reflect abnormal cardiac repolarization, including bifid T waves and other nonspecific abnormalities in T wave morphology, U waves, prolongation of the QT or QU interval, and rarely, electrical alternation of the T or U wave.[246]

Numerous anecdotal reports indicate that hypomagnesemia alone can predispose to cardiac tachyarrhythmias, particularly of ventricular origin, including torsades de pointes, monomorphic ventricular tachycardia, and ventricular fibrillation, which may be resistant to standard therapy and respond only to Mg^{2+} repletion.[246] Many of the reported patients also had a prolonged QT interval, an abnormality that is known to predispose to torsades de pointes and may also increase the period of vulnerability to R-on-T phenomena. In the setting of exaggerated cardiac excitability, hypomagnesemia may be the trigger for other types of ventricular tachyarrhythmias.[246] In addition, hypomagnesemia facilitates the development of digoxin cardiotoxicity.[247] Because both cardiac glycosides and Mg^{2+} depletion inhibit Na^+,K^+-ATPase, their additive effects on intracellular K^+ depletion may account for their enhanced toxicity in combination.

The existence of occasional patients with clear hypomagnesemia-induced arrhythmias is undisputed. However, the magnitude of the risk for arrhythmias in patients with hypomagnesemia in general, the issue of whether mild hypomagnesemia carries the same risk as severe hypomagnesemia does, and the relative importance of Mg^{2+} deficiency versus coexistent hypokalemia or intrinsic cardiac disease in the pathogenesis of the arrhythmia remain highly controversial. In a frequently cited study by Dyckner[248] of 342 patients with acute myocardial infarction admitted to a coronary care unit, complex ventricular ectopy, ventricular tachycardia, and ventricular fibrillation were three times more frequent during the first 24 hours in hypomagnesemic than in patients with normomagnesemia. In a control group of patients without myocardial infarction, ventricular ectopy and arrhythmias were not associated with hypomagnesemia. The major difficulty in interpreting this study stems from the failure to control for hypokalemia, a well-established risk factor for ventricular arrhythmias. Indeed, the prevalence of hypokalemia was high (30%) in the hypomagnesemic patients with ventricular arrhythmias and exceeded its prevalence in those without arrhythmias (10%), so the serum K^+ concentration was almost certainly an important confounder. The value of magnesium administration after cardiac surgery is also controversial.[249,250]

Data on magnesium deficiency and arrhythmia in individuals without overt heart disease is provocative. In one small prospective study, low dietary magnesium appeared to increase the risk for supraventricular and ventricular ectopy despite the absence of frank hypomagnesemia, hypokalemia, and hypocalcemia.[251] In the Framingham Offspring Study, lower levels of serum magnesium were associated with higher prevalence of ventricular premature complexes.[252]

Neuromuscular System

Symptoms and signs of neuromuscular irritability, including tremor, muscle twitching, the Trousseau and Chvostek signs, and frank tetany, may develop in patients with isolated hypomagnesemia.[253] Hypomagnesemia is also frequently manifested as seizures, which may be generalized and tonic-clonic in nature or multifocal motor seizures, and they are sometimes triggered by loud noises.[253] Interestingly, noise-induced seizures and sudden death are also characteristic of mice made hypomagnesemic by dietary Mg^{2+} deprivation. The effects of Mg^{2+} deficiency on brain neuronal excitability are thought to be mediated by N-methyl-D-aspartate (NMDA)-type glutamate receptors. Glutamate is the principal excitatory neurotransmitter in the brain; it acts as an agonist at NMDA receptors and opens a cation conductance channel that depolarizes the postsynaptic membrane. Extracellular Mg^{2+} normally blocks NMDA receptors, so hypomagnesemia may release the inhibition of glutamate-activated depolarization of the postsynaptic membrane and thereby trigger epileptiform electrical activity.[254] Vertical nystagmus is a rare, but diagnostically useful neurologic sign of severe hypomagnesemia.[255] In the absence of a structural lesion of the cerebellar or vestibular pathways, the only recognized metabolic causes are Wernicke encephalopathy and severe Mg^{2+} deficiency.[255]

Electrolyte Homeostasis

Patients with hypomagnesemia are frequently also hypokalemic. Many of the conditions associated with hypomagnesemia that have been outlined earlier can cause simultaneous Mg^{2+} and K^+ loss. However, hypomagnesemia by itself can induce hypokalemia in both humans and experimental animals, and such patients are often refractory to K^+ repletion until their Mg^{2+} deficit is corrected.[256] The cause of the hypokalemia appears to be depletion of intracellular K^+ as a result of impaired Na^+,K^+-ATPase function, together with renal K^+ wasting; the K^+ leaked from cells is lost in the urine.[245] The physiologic mechanism for renal K^+ wasting in hypomagnesemia is unknown.

Hypocalcemia is present in approximately half of patients with hypomagnesemia.[243] The major cause is impairment of PTH secretion by Mg^{2+} deficiency, which is reversed within 24 hours by Mg^{2+} repletion.[166] In addition, hypomagnesemic patients also have low circulating $1,25(OH)_2D$ levels and end-organ resistance to both PTH and vitamin D.[166]

Treatment

Mg^{2+} deficiency may sometimes be prevented. Individuals whose dietary intake has been reduced or who are being maintained by parenteral nutrition should receive Mg^{2+} supplementation. The recommended daily allowance of Mg^{2+} in adults is 420 mg (35 mEq) for men and 320 mg (27 mEq) for women.[257] Thus, in the absence of dietary Mg^{2+} intake, an appropriate supplement would therefore be one 140 mg tablet of Mg oxide four to five times daily or the equivalent dose of an alternative oral Mg^{2+}-containing salt. Because the oral bioavailability of Mg^{2+} is approximately 33% in patients with normal intestinal function, the equivalent parenteral maintenance requirement of Mg^{2+} would be 10 mEq daily.

Once symptomatic Mg^{2+} deficiency develops, patients should clearly be repleted with Mg^{2+}. However, the importance of treating asymptomatic Mg^{2+} deficiency remains controversial. Given the clinical manifestations outlined earlier, it seems prudent to replete all Mg^{2+}-deficient patients with a significant underlying cardiac or seizure disorder, patients with concurrent severe hypocalcemia or hypokalemia, and patients with isolated asymptomatic hypomagnesemia if it is severe (~1.4 mg/dL).

Intravenous Replacement
In the inpatient setting, the intravenous route of administration of Mg^{2+} is favored because it is highly effective, inexpensive, and usually well tolerated. The standard preparation is $MgSO_4 \cdot 7H_2O$. The initial rate of repletion depends on the urgency of the clinical situation. In a patient who is actively seizing or who has a cardiac arrhythmia, 8 mEq to 16 mEq (1 g to 2 g) may be administered intravenously over a 2- to 4-minute period; otherwise, a slower rate of repletion is safer. Because the added extracellular Mg^{2+} equilibrates slowly with the intracellular compartment and because renal excretion of extracellular Mg^{2+} exhibits a threshold effect, approximately 50% of parenterally administered Mg^{2+} is excreted into urine.[258] A slower rate and prolonged course of repletion would be expected to decrease these urinary losses and therefore be much more efficient and effective at repleting body Mg^{2+} stores. The magnitude of the Mg^{2+} deficit is difficult to gauge clinically and cannot be readily deduced from the serum Mg^{2+} concentration. In general, though, the average deficit can be assumed to be 1 to 2 mEq/kg body weight.[258] A simple regimen for nonemergency Mg^{2+} repletion is to administer 64 mEq (8 g) of $MgSO_4$ over the first 24 hours and then 32 mEq (4 g) daily for the next 2 to 6 days. It is important to remember that serum Mg^{2+} levels rise early whereas intracellular stores take longer to replete, so Mg^{2+} repletion should continue for at least 1 to 2 days after the serum Mg^{2+} level normalizes. In patients with renal Mg^{2+} wasting, additional Mg^{2+} may be needed to replace ongoing losses. In patients with a reduced glomerular filtration rate (GFR), the rate of repletion should be reduced by 25% to 50%,[258] the patient should be carefully monitored for signs of hypermagnesemia, and the serum Mg^{2+} level should be checked frequently.

The main adverse effects of Mg^{2+} repletion are due to hypermagnesemia as a consequence of an excessive rate or amount of Mg^{2+} administered. These effects include facial flushing, loss of deep tendon reflexes, hypotension, and atrioventricular block. Monitoring of tendon reflexes is a useful bedside test to detect Mg^{2+} overdose. In addition, intravenous administration of large amounts of $MgSO_4$ results in an acute decrease in the serum ionized Ca^{2+} level[259] related to increased urinary Ca^{2+} excretion and complexing of Ca^{2+} by sulfate. Thus, in an asymptomatic patient who is already hypocalcemic, administration of $MgSO_4$ may further lower the ionized Ca^{2+} level and thereby precipitate tetany.[260] Administration of Mg^{2+} with sulfate as the anion may have an additional theoretical disadvantage. Because sulfate cannot be reabsorbed in the distal tubule, it favors the development of a negative luminal electrical potential, thereby increasing K^+ secretion. In Mg^{2+}-depleted rats with hypokalemia, repletion with Mg^{2+} in the form of a nonsulfate salt was associated with correction of the hypokalemia, whereas repletion with $MgSO_4$ resulted in persistent hypokalemia and kaliuresis.[261]

Oral Replacement
Oral Mg^{2+} administration is used either initially for repletion of mild cases of hypomagnesemia or for continued replacement of ongoing losses in the outpatient setting after an initial course of intravenous repletion. A number of oral Mg^{2+} salts are available, but little is known about their relative oral bioavailability or efficacy, and all of them cause diarrhea in high doses. Mg hydroxide and Mg oxide are alkalinizing salts

with the potential to cause systemic alkalosis, whereas the sulfate and gluconate salts may potentially exacerbate K^+ wasting, as discussed earlier. The appropriate dose of each salt can be estimated, if ongoing losses are known, by determining its content of elemental Mg^{2+} and assuming a bioavailability of approximately 33% for normal intestinal function. In patients with intestinal Mg^{2+} malabsorption, this dose may need to be increased twofold to fourfold.

Potassium-Sparing Diuretics
In patients with inappropriate renal Mg^{2+} wasting, potassium-sparing diuretics that block the distal tubule epithelial Na^+ channel, such as amiloride and triamterene, may reduce renal Mg^{2+} losses.[262] These drugs may be particularly useful in patients who are refractory to oral repletion or require such high doses of oral Mg^{2+} that diarrhea develops. In rats, amiloride and triamterene can be demonstrated to reduce renal Mg^{2+} clearance at baseline and after induction of Mg^{2+} diuresis by furosemide, but the mechanism is unknown. One possibility is that these drugs, by reducing luminal Na^+ uptake and inhibiting the development of a negative luminal transepithelial potential difference, may favor passive reabsorption of Mg^{2+} in the late distal tubule or collecting duct.

Hypermagnesemia
Etiology
In states of body Mg^{2+} excess, the kidney has a very large capacity for Mg^{2+} excretion. Once the apparent renal threshold is exceeded, most of the excess filtered Mg^{2+} is excreted unchanged into the final urine; the serum Mg^{2+} concentration is then determined by the GFR. Thus, hypermagnesemia generally occurs in two clinical settings: compromised renal function and excessive Mg^{2+} intake.

Renal Insufficiency
In chronic renal failure, the remaining nephrons adapt to the decreased filtered load of Mg^{2+} by markedly increasing their fractional excretion of Mg^{2+}.[263] As a consequence, serum Mg^{2+} levels are usually well maintained until the creatinine clearance falls below about 20 mL/min.[263] Even in advanced renal insufficiency, significant hypermagnesemia is rare unless the patient has received exogenous Mg^{2+} in the form of antacids, cathartics, or enemas. Increasing age is an important risk factor for hypermagnesemia in individuals with apparently normal renal function; it presumably reflects the decline in GFR that normally accompanies old age.[264]

Excessive Mg^{2+} Intake
Hypermagnesemia can occur in individuals with a normal GFR when the rate of Mg^{2+} intake exceeds the renal excretory capacity. It has been reported with excessive oral ingestion of Mg^{2+}-containing antacids and cathartics and with the use of rectal Mg sulfate enemas and is common with large parenteral doses of Mg^{2+}, such as those given for preeclampsia. Toxicity from enterally administered Mg^{2+} salts is particularly common in patients with inflammatory disease, obstruction, or perforation of the gastrointestinal tract, presumably because Mg^{2+} absorption is enhanced.

Miscellaneous
Modest elevations in serum Mg^{2+} (less than 4 mEq/L) have occasionally been described in patients receiving lithium therapy, as well as in postoperative and in those with bone metastases, milk-alkali syndrome, FHH,[242] hypothyroidism, pituitary dwarfism, and Addison disease. In most patients cases, the mechanism is unknown.

Clinical Manifestations
Mg^{2+} toxicity is a serious and potentially fatal condition. Progressive hypermagnesemia is usually associated with a

predictable sequence of symptoms and signs.[265] Initial manifestations, observed once the serum Mg^{2+} level exceeds 4 mg/dL to 6 mg/dL, are hypotension, nausea, vomiting, facial flushing, urinary retention, and ileus. If untreated, it may progress to flaccid skeletal muscular paralysis and hyporeflexia, bradycardia and bradyarrhythmias, respiratory depression, coma, and cardiac arrest. An abnormally low (or even negative) serum anion gap may be a clue to hypermagnesemia,[264] but it is not consistently observed and probably depends on the nature of the anion that accompanies the excess body Mg^{2+}.

Cardiovascular System
Hypotension is one of the earliest manifestations of hypermagnesemia,[266] is often accompanied by cutaneous flushing, and is thought to be due to vasodilatation of vascular smooth muscle and inhibition of norepinephrine release by sympathetic postganglionic nerves. Electrocardiographic changes are common but nonspecific.[266] Sinus or junctional bradycardia may develop, as well as varying degrees of sinoatrial, atrioventricular, and His bundle conduction block. Cardiac arrest as a result of asystole is often the terminal event.

Nervous System
High levels of extracellular Mg^{2+} inhibit acetylcholine release from the neuromuscular end-plate,[267] leading to the development of flaccid skeletal muscle paralysis and hyporeflexia when serum Mg^{2+} exceeds 8 mg/dL to 12 mg/dL. Respiratory depression is a serious complication of advanced Mg^{2+} toxicity.[266] Smooth muscle paralysis also occurs and is manifested as urinary retention, intestinal ileus, and pupillary dilatation. Signs of central nervous system depression, including lethargy, drowsiness, and eventually coma, are well described in severe hypermagnesemia, but they may also be entirely absent.

Treatment
Mild cases of Mg^{2+} toxicity in individuals with good renal function may require no treatment other than cessation of Mg^{2+} supplements because renal Mg^{2+} clearance is usually quite rapid. The normal half-life of serum Mg^{2+} is approximately 28 hours. In the event of serious toxicity, particularly cardiac toxicity, temporary antagonism of the effect of Mg^{2+} may be achieved by the administration of intravenous Ca^{2+} (1 g of calcium chloride infused into a central vein over a period of 2 to 5 minutes or calcium gluconate infused through a peripheral vein, repeated after 5 minutes if necessary).[265] Renal excretion of Mg^{2+} can be enhanced by saline diuresis and by the administration of furosemide, which inhibits tubule reabsorption of Mg^{2+} in the medullary TAL.

In patients with renal failure, the only way to clear the excess Mg^{2+} may be by dialysis. The typical dialysate for hemodialysis contains 0.6 mg/dL to 1.2 mg/dL of Mg^{2+}, but Mg^{2+}-free dialysate can also be used and is generally well tolerated except for muscle cramps.[268] Hemodialysis is extremely effective at removing excess Mg^{2+} and can achieve clearances of up to 100 mL/min.[268] As a rough rule of thumb, the expected change in serum Mg^{2+} after a 3- to 4-hour dialysis session with a high-efficiency membrane is approximately one third to one half the difference between the dialysate Mg^{2+} concentration and predialysis serum ultra-filterable Mg^{2+} (estimated at 70% of total serum Mg^{2+}).[268] Note that when hemodialysis is performed against a bath with the same total concentration of Mg^{2+} as in serum, net transfer of Mg^{2+} into the patient occurs because the ultra-filterable (and therefore free) Mg^{2+} concentration in serum is less than the total concentration and thus the gradient of free Mg^{2+} is directed from dialysate to blood. Peritoneal dialysis is also effective at Mg^{2+} removal.[269]

DISORDERS OF PHOSPHATE HOMEOSTASIS

Hyperphosphatemia

Hyperphosphatemia is generally defined as serum phosphate levels elevated above 5 mg/dL. The threshold for labeling a child as hyperphosphatemic is higher because children tend to have higher phosphate levels than adults do. Whereas the normal range of blood phosphorus for adult men and women is 4.5 mg/dL to 5.2 mg/dL, for children, the upper range of normal is 6 mg/dL. In infants, phosphorus levels as high as 7.4 mg/dL are considered normal.[270] The serum phosphorus level usually exhibits diurnal variation. Typically, phosphorus levels are lowest in the late morning and peak in the first morning hours.[271] Hemolysis in the blood specimen can lead to spuriously elevated measurements of phosphorus.

Causes
The clinical causes of hyperphosphatemia can be broadly classified into one of three groups: reduced phosphate excretion, excess intake of phosphorus, and redistribution of cellular phosphorus (Table 16–8).

Decreased Renal Phosphate Excretion
Renal Insufficiency
Decreased renal function is by far the most common cause of hyperphosphatemia. Increased fractional excretion of PO_4 is able to compensate until GFR falls and normal PO_4 excretion can no longer be maintained. Increases in serum phosphorus levels are observed even among individuals with mild to moderate chronic kidney disease.[272] Hyperphosphatemia is observed in acute kidney injury as well as chronic disease. Hyperphosphatemia caused by decreased renal function is not discussed in detail here because it is reviewed extensively in Chapter 52 in the context of renal osteodystrophies.

Hypoparathyroidism and Pseudohypoparathyroidism
Decreased renal excretion of phosphate may also occur in the setting of reduced PTH (hypoparathyroidism) or an altered renal response to PTH (PsHP). These entities are discussed earlier in this chapter. In primary hypoparathyroidism, circulating phosphorus generally reaches a higher than normal steady-state level (6 mg/dL to 7 mg/dL), with a low serum calcium level. Patients with PsHP typically have increased PTH levels, but serum chemistries are similar to those seen in hypoparathyroidism.

Acromegaly
Some patients with acromegaly demonstrate hyperphosphatemia. Parathyroid function is usually normal or slightly increased in acromegaly.[119] The hyperphosphatemia observed appears to result from increased proximal tubule phosphate

---

TABLE 16–8 Causes of Hyperphosphatemia

Decreased renal excretion of phosphorus
  Renal insufficiency
  Hypoparathyroidism, pseudohypoparathyroidism
  Acromegaly
  Tumoral calcinosis

Redistribution of phosphorus
  Tumor lysis syndrome
  Respiratory acidosis

Exogenous phosphorus administration
  Ingestion of phosphate containing enemas
  IV phosphate

reabsorption. Growth hormone directly stimulates proximal tubule phosphorus reabsorption and increases the T_m for phosphorus.[273]

Familial Tumoral Calcinosis

Familial tumoral calcinosis is a rare autosomal recessive disorder. The hyperphosphatemia that characterizes the disease is a result of increased proximal tubular reabsorption of phosphorus. Often, increased serum 1,25-$(OH)_2D$ levels are observed.[274] The disease is genetically heterogeneous: defects have been described in the GALNT3 gene,[275] which encodes a glycosyltransferase, and in the FGF-23 gene.[276,277] Mutations in the GALNT3 or FGF23 genes may lead to deficiency of FGF-23, an important promoter of urinary phosphate excretion. If so, familial tumoral calcinosis may be the phenotypic opposite of X-linked and autosomal dominant hypophosphatemic rickets (see later discussion).

Together, a normal serum calcium concentration and elevated serum phosphorus lead to an elevated calcium phosphate product and soft tissue calcium phosphate deposition. Though usually periarticular, the calcifications can occur as paraspinal or extradural masses. Decreasing phosphorus intake by ingestion of a low-phosphate diet or the addition of phosphate binders, as well as the use of acetazolamide, has been reported to be effective treatment.[278]

Bisphosphonates

Bisphosphonates can cause hyperphosphatemia. In a study by Walton and colleagues,[279] altered renal phosphate handling with bisphosphonate treatment was suggested by the absence of altered urine phosphate excretion despite increased plasma phosphate. Studies in humans have shown that various members of this class of medication cause a similar increase in tubule reabsorption of phosphate.[280]

Increased Phosphorus Intake

Exogenous intake of phosphorus sufficient to cause clincally significant hyperphosphatemia is rare in the absence of underlying kidney disease. However, oral sodium phosphate administration for bowel preparation has been recognized as a cause of hyperphosphatemia for some time. Even individuals with normal baseline kidney function develop transient hyperphosphatemia.[280a] Caution is required in the administration of phosphate-containing enemas to children and individuals with chronic kidney disease.

Phosphate Nephropathy

Administration of oral sodium phosphate solutions has been increasingly recognized as a cause of acute renal failure (so-called "phosphate nephropathy").[280b] In a review of over 7000 kidney biopsies processed at their center, Markowitz and colleagues found 16 cases where patients had developed renal failure and intrarenal calcium-phosphate deposits after oral sodium phosphate administration for colonoscopy.[280c] This syndrome may occur in individuals with good baseline kidney function. Kidney injury in this setting does not typically recover.

Redistribution of Phosphorus
Respiratory Acidosis

Chronic respiratory acidosis can lead to hyperphosphatemia, renal PTH resistance, and hypocalcemia.[281] The effect is more pronounced in acute respiratory acidosis. Respiratory acidosis does not appear to significantly alter the renal handling of phosphorus. Rather, efflux of phosphate from cells into the extracellular space is probably responsible for the hyperphosphatemia of respiratory acidosis.[282]

Tumor Lysis

Tumor lysis syndrome is a well-described complication of the treatment of hematologic malignancies.[190] It is seen after the treatment of various forms of lymphoma and lymphoblastic leukemia, and when a particularly heavy tumor burden is present, it may occur spontaneously before treatment. Patients with tumor lysis syndrome have elevated lactate dehydrogenase, uric acid, and phosphate levels shortly after chemotherapy. Lymphoblasts are particularly high in phosphorus. The lactate dehydrogenase level before the initiation of therapy correlates with the development of hyperphosphatemia and azotemia.[283] Hyperphosphatemia is seen in essentially all patients with Burkitt lymphoma after treatment if they had any preexisting kidney disease and in approximately 30% of patients with normal renal function.

In general, common practice is to induce high urine output and phosphate excretion before chemotherapy with a large volume of intravenous fluid. Bicarbonate infusion is often given but requires caution because in the presence of a high calcium phosphate product, the risk of nephrocalcinosis is increased. Hemodialysis is often used in the setting of acute kidney injury with hyperphosphatemia. Continuous dialysis modalities (continuous arteriovenous hemodialysis [CAVHD], continuous venovenous hemodialysis [CVVHD]) that can provide high and continued clearance may be the preferred treatment for patients with tumor lysis and acute kidney injury.

Pseudohyperphosphatemia

Incorrect hyperphosphatemic laboratory readings from patient samples may occur in certain settings as a result of interference with the analysis. This problem is most common in the case of paraproteinemia (as in multiple myeloma or Waldenström macroglobulinemia).[284] Hyperlipidemia, hyperbilirubinemia, and sample dilution problems are rare causes.

Clinical Manifestations and Treatment

Most of the major clinical manifestations of hyperphosphatemia stem from hypocalcemia, discussed earlier in this chapter. Hyperphosphatemia is also important in the development of secondary HPT, as discussed in Chapter 52. Hyperphosphatemia leads to secondary hypocalcemia by causing calcium precipitation, by decreasing the production of 1,25$(OH)_2D$, and by decreasing intestinal calcium absorption. Ectopic calcification is the other important clinical manifestation of hyperphosphatemia. When the product of serum calcium and serum phosphorus (expressed in milligrams per deciliter) exceeds 70, the risk for ectopic calcium precipitation is significant. The skin, vasculature, cornea, and joints are often affected in this setting.

Treatment of chronic hyperphosphatemia is generally accomplished through dietary phosphate restriction and oral phosphate binders. Chronic hyperphosphatemia is most commonly observed in association with renal insufficiency and end-stage kidney disease and is discussed in Chapter 52. Chronic hyperphosphatemia also may be seen in association with tumoral calcinosis and is treated similarly, with a reduction in dietary phosphate and administration of oral phosphate binders.

Acute hyperphosphatemia in association with hypocalcemia requires rapid attention. Severe hyperphosphatemia in patients with reduced renal function or acute kidney injury, particularly in those with tumor lysis syndrome, may require hemodialysis or a continuous form of renal replacement therapy. Volume expansion may increase urinary phosphate excretion, as can administration of acetazolamide.

Hypophosphatemia

Only a small percentage (about 1%) of total body phosphorus is extracellular. Thus, although hypophosphatemia may reflect total body phosphorus depletion, such need not be the case. Hypophosphatemia is relatively common in hospitalized patients and is present in a significant fraction of chronic alcoholics.[285] Later, we discuss hypophosphatemia in terms of its underlying cause: increased renal excretion (acquired or inherited), decreased intestinal absorption, and shifts of phosphorus from the extracellular compartment.

Clinical Manifestations

Mild hypophosphatemia does not typically cause symptoms. Patients with symptoms usually have serum phosphate levels below 1 mg/dL. Severe hypophosphatemia can have significant clinical consequences, including disturbances in multiple cellular functions and organ systems.

The clinical manifestations of hypophosphatemia and phosphorus depletion generally result from a decrease in intracellular ATP levels. In addition, erythrocytes experience a decrease in 2,3-diphosphoglycerate levels, which increases hemoglobin-oxygen affinity and alters oxygen transport efficiency.[286]

Hematologic consequences include a predisposition to hemolysis, thought to result from increased red cell rigidity.[287] Hemolysis is not typically seen in the absence of other exacerbating features. White cell phagocytosis can be diminished. Presumably, impaired ATP production diminishes the phagocytic capability.[288]

Severe hypophosphatemia impairs muscle function. Again, this sequela is a result of ATP depletion. Overt heart failure and respiratory failure as a result of decreased muscle performance may be observed.[289,290] Hypophosphatemia may also affect skeletal and smooth muscle performance. Proximal myopathies and intestinal effects of hypophosphatemia have been described.

Rhabdomyolysis is a well-recognized complication of severe hypophosphatemia.[291] Because cell breakdown may lead to the release of intracellular phosphate, normophosphatemia or hyperphosphatemia in this setting may mask the existence of true phosphate depletion.

Chronic phosphate depletion alters bone and kidney function, and hypophosphatemia leads to increased bone resorption. If phosphate depletion is prolonged, rickets and osteomalacia may result. Hypophosphatemia leads to decreased proximal tubule reabsorptive function.[292] A decrease in renal conservation of calcium is also observed, and at times frank hypercalciuria develops. This hypercalciuria is not solely the result of renal calcium handling but also reflects increased calcium release from bone and increased intestinal calcium absorption.[293]

Diagnosis

The probable cause of hypophosphatemia may be immediately apparent from the clinical findings (e.g., in a malnourished patient with alcoholism or anorexia). Shifts of phosphorus from the extracellular to the intracellular space generally occur in the acute setting (respiratory alkalosis, treatment of diabetic ketoacidosis). In hospitalized patients, hypophosphatemia caused by shifts of phosphorus into the intracellular compartment are much more common than hypophosphatemia caused by renal losses.[294] In situations where the underlying diagnosis is not immediately apparent, it can be clinically useful to determine the rate of urine phosphorus excretion. High urine phosphorus in the face of hypophosphatemia suggests HPT, a renal tubule defect, or a form of rickets.

Causes of Hypophosphatemia
Increased Renal Excretion

As discussed in Chapter 5 in detail, renal phosphate excretion plays a major role in regulating phosphate metabolism (Table 16–9). Most renal reabsorption of phosphate occurs in the proximal tubule by means of sodium-dependent phosphate transporters (type I cotransporters). Serum phosphate depletion leads to stimulation of phosphate reabsorption. PTH also regulates renal phosphate reabsorption. Phosphate depletion itself decreases proximal tubule and distal nephron phosphate reabsorption. Hypophosphatemia caused by increased urinary phosphate excretion is generally the result

TABLE 16–9	Causes of Hypophosphatemia

I. Increased urinary phosphate excretion
  Hyperparathyroidism
  Inherited defects
  Volume expansion
  Vitamin D deficiency (or resistance)
  Fanconi syndrome
  Acetazolamide
  Post-renal transplant	

II. Decreased GI absorption of phosphate
  Inadequate phosphate intake
  Chronic diarrhea
  Phosphate-binding antacids
  Chronic alcoholism	

III. Altered phosphorus distribution
  Acute respiratory alkalosis
  "Hungry bone syndrome" (post-parathyroidectomy)
  Management of diabetic ketoacidosis
  Refeeding of malnourished patients, alcoholics
  Leukemia	

of either excess PTH or an inherited disorder of renal phosphate handling in the proximal tubule.

Hyperparathyroidism

Both primary and secondary HPT may lead to hyperphosphaturia and hypophosphatemia. Primary HPT is discussed earlier in this chapter. Excess PTH directly decreases renal phosphate reabsorption, thereby leading to increased renal phosphate excretion and hypophosphatemia. The degree of hypophosphatemia observed is highly variable. The secondary HPT observed in patients with chronic kidney disease is typically associated with hyperphosphatemia because of a decreased ability of the kidney to excrete phosphorus. However, other forms of secondary HPT (typically from decreased intestinal calcium absorption and vitamin D deficiency) may be manifested as hypophosphatemia.

Acute Renal Failure and Recovery from Acute Tubular Necrosis

Hyperphosphatemia is the typical derangement of phosphate metabolism observed in patients with acute kidney injury. However, confounding factors in the setting of critical illness may contribute to the development of hypophosphatemia in some instances: administration of phosphate-binding antacids, refeeding syndrome, and mechanically induced respiratory alkalosis. In addition, during the diuretic phase of recovery from acute tubular necrosis, significant urinary losses of phosphate may lead to hypophosphatemia. Similarly, significant urinary phosphate losses leading to frank hypophosphatemia may be seen after recovery from obstructive uropathy.

Renal Transplantation

Hypophosphatemia is well described in patients after renal transplantation, and a typically mild to moderate form develops in a high fraction of recipients.[295] Severe hypophosphatemia and phosphate depletion is uncommon. Persistent secondary HPT does not appear to be the sole mechanism of hypophosphatemia. Renal tubule dysfunction in the allograft leading to hyperphosphaturia is a contributory factor,[295] and excess FGF-23 may play a role in the etiology.[296] Therapy with diuretics and immunosuppressive medications also contributes to post-transplant hypophosphatemia.

Fanconi Syndrome

Increased urine phosphorus excretion is a typical feature of the defect in proximal tubule transport known as Fanconi syndrome.[297] Hypophosphatemia is usually observed in association with glucosuria, uricosuria, aminoaciduria, and proximal renal tubular acidosis.

Decreased Intestinal Absorption
Malnutrition
Malnutrition from poor phosphate intake is not a common cause of hypophosphatemia. Increased renal reabsorption of phosphorus can compensate for all but the most severe decreases in oral phosphate intake. Most dietary phosphate comes from protein. Children from parts of the world where protein malnutrition is common are most susceptible to this problem.

Malabsorption
More common is hypophosphatemia resulting from malabsorption. Most phosphorus absorption occurs in the duodenum and jejunum, and intestinal disorders affecting the small intestine may lead to hypophosphatemia.[298] Heavy use of phosphate-binding antacids may also result in hypophosphatemia. Hypophosphatemia can develop quickly, even in patients given a relatively moderate, but sustained dosage. Prolonged use of phosphate-binding antacids can lead to clinically significant osteomalacia.[299]

Vitamin D-Mediated Disorders
Vitamin D is critical for normal control of phosphorus. Deficiency of vitamin D leads to decreased intestinal absorption of phosphorus. In addition, vitamin D deficiency leads to hypocalcemia, HPT, and a consequent PTH-mediated increase in renal phosphorus excretion. The vitamin D deficiency and resistance syndromes known as rickets are characterized by hypophosphatemia, hypocalcemia, and bone disease.

Redistribution
Respiratory Alkalosis
Respiratory alkalosis decreases serum phosphorus levels. When the alkalosis is prolonged and severe, phosphorus levels can drop below 1 mg/dL.[300] In mechanically ventilated patients, hypophosphatemia is common, and urinary phosphate excretion drops to undetectable levels. This drop in phosphaturia contrasts with the high urine phosphate excretion and hypophosphatemia that may be observed with metabolic alkalosis from sodium bicarbonate administration. It has been suggested that in the hypophosphatemia seen in respiratory alkalosis, carbon dioxide diffusion from the intracellular space increases intracellular pH, stimulates glycolysis, and increases the formation of phosphorylated carbohydrates, thereby leading to a fall in extracellular phosphorus levels.[301]

Refeeding
In chronically malnourished individuals, rapid refeeding can result in significant hypophosphatemia. The mechanism is related to increased cellular phosphate uptake and utilization. The incidence of refeeding-related hypophosphatemia is quite high in hospitalized patients receiving parenteral nutrition, as high as one in three in one series.[302] Refeeding after even very short periods of starvation can lead to hypophosphatemia.[303] Adequate phosphate in the parenteral nutrition formulation generally prevents this complication. In most patients, 13.6 mEq phosphorus per liter appears to be adequate. Even higher amounts may be required in patients with diabetes or chronic alcoholism. Hypophosphatemia and phosphate depletion are common in individuals with anorexia nervosa, and phosphorus supplementation is required in over 25% of such patients during hospitalization and refeeding.[304]

Special Situations: Alcoholism and Diabetes
Hypophosphatemia is a particularly common and often severe problem in alcoholic patients with poor intake, vitamin D deficiency, and heavy use of phosphate-binding antacids.[305] Alcohol-induced proximal tubule dysfunction also contributes to phosphate depletion.[204] Phosphorus deficiency is often not manifested as hypophosphatemia immediately at initial evaluation for medical care. Typically, refeeding or administration of intravenous glucose (or both) in this patient population stimulates shifts of phosphorus into cells and thereby leads to the development of severe hypophosphate-

mia. Hypophosphatemic alcoholics are at particular risk for rhabdomyolysis.

In uncontrolled diabetes, increased urine phosphate excretion can be observed, and in diabetic ketoacidosis, phosphate is released from cells and excreted in urine.[306] Although serum phosphate levels may be normal, total phosphate stores are usually low. During treatment of diabetic ketoacidosis, the development of hypophosphatemia is extremely common.[307] Administration of insulin stimulates the cellular uptake of phosphorus, and thus the serum phosphate level can fall dramatically with treatment.[308] However, routine administration of phosphate in this setting before the development of frank hypophosphatemia is discouraged because it may lead to significant hypocalcemia.[309]

Drug-induced Hypophosphatemia
In addition to the phosphate-binding antacids mentioned earlier, other medications may cause hypophosphatemia. Diuretics, particularly those acting on the proximal nephron, may result in hypophosphatemia. Corticosteroids both decrease intestinal phosphorus absorption and increase renal phosphorus excretion and thus may cause mild to moderate hypophosphatemia.[310] Agents that damage the proximal tubule (such as certain antineoplastic agents) may lead to phosphate wasting. Hypophosphatemia has also been reported in acetaminophen toxicity, but the mechanism is not clear. Theophylline administered in the setting of acute bronchospasm is associated with hypophosphatemia, apparently by causing phosphorus flux into the intracellular compartment.

Miscellaneous
Moderate and at times severe hypophosphatemia may be observed in acute leukemia and in the leukemic phases of lymphomas.[311] It is thought that rapid cell growth with consequent phosphorus utilization is responsible for the drop in extracellular phosphorus. Toxic shock may be associated with hypophosphatemia. In one study of 22 women with toxic shock syndrome, hypophosphatemia and hypocalcemia were common features.[312] The underlying mechanism is not clear. Rapid volume expansion diminishes proximal tubule sodium phosphate reabsorption and may lead to transient hypophosphatemia.[313] Hepatic disease may cause hypophosphatemia; hypophosphatemia is an almost universal observation after hepatic lobectomy for liver transplantation. Hypophosphatemia is frequently observed in the setting of sepsis, but the complicated clinical picture in septic patients makes it difficult to attribute the hypophosphatemia to a unique mechanism. Hypophosphatemia is seen in patients with heat stroke, as well as hyperthermia. In this setting, renal phosphorus excretion is increased.

Inherited Disorders
X-Linked Hypophosphatemia
X-linked hypophosphatemia (XLH) is a rare X-linked dominant disorder characterized by hypophosphatemia, rickets and osteomalacia, growth retardation, decreased intestinal calcium and phosphate absorption, and decreased renal phosphate reabsorption (Table 16–10). Penetrance is high, and both females and males are affected. Serum calcium levels are normal. Genotype does not predict phenotype severity.[314]

The gene responsible, PHEX, is named for its putative function: phosphate regulating gene with homology to endopeptidases on the X chromosome. PHEX was identified by positional cloning.[315] Well over 100 independent PHEX mutations have been described.[316]

The term phosphatonin refers to a circulating factor or factors with phosphaturic activity. PHEX mutations are thought to inactivate this activity and thereby lead to increased serum phosphatonin activity and increased urine phosphate excretion. The hyp mouse, like humans with XLH, has a defect in the PHEX gene. Transplantation studies of normal and hyp mouse kidneys supported the idea that an

TABLE 16–10	Inherited Hypophosphatemia		
Name	Gene	Mendelian Inheritance in Man Number
Hypophosphatemic rickets with hypercalciuria	SLC34A3	241530
X-linked hypophosphatemia	PHEX	307800
Autosomal dominant hypophosphatemic rickets	FGF-23	193100
Nephrolithiasis, osteoporosis, and hypophosphatemia	NPT2	182309
Autosomal recessive hypophosphatemic rickets	DMP1	241520
Renal hypophosphatemia with intracerebral calcifications	?	241519

altered circulating activity rather than a kidney defect was responsible for the phenotype.[317] PHEX is not expressed in the kidney; its predominant expression is in bone.[318]

FGF-23 has received considerable attention as a candidate phosphatonin. FGF-23 is a PHEX substrate,[319] and FGF-23 mutations have been shown to cause autosomal dominant hypophosphatemic rickets. Of interest, normal or slightly reduced plasma 1,25(OH)$_2$D levels, despite the presence of hypophosphatemia, suggest that 1,25(OH)$_2$D synthesis is abnormal in XLH. FGF-23 may down-regulate 1-alpha hydroxylase.[320]

Treatment of XLH patients with oral phosphate and calcitriol improves their growth rate. Treatment does not reduce renal phosphate excretion. The goal of therapy is to allow normal growth and reduce bone pain.[321]

Autosomal Dominant Hypophosphatemic Rickets

Autosomal dominant hypophosphatemic rickets (ADHR) is an extremely rare disorder of phosphate wasting with variable penetrance. The phenotype is similar to that of XLH. Some individuals are initially seen in childhood with lower extremity deformities, as well as rickets and phosphate wasting. Others have bone pain, weakness, and phosphate wasting as adolescents or adults. In some individuals with early-onset disease, the phosphate wasting returns to normal after puberty.

The ADHR locus was mapped to chromosome 12p13.3 and subsequently identified as FGF-23.[322] Mutations on FGF-23 appear to interfere with proteolytic cleavage by PHEX.[323]

FGF-23 is a substrate for the XLH gene product PHEX, and it directly inhibits renal phosphate reabsorption. In addition, FGF-23 is responsible for tumor-induced osteomalacia (TIO) (also called oncogenic hypophosphatemic osteomalacia).[324] TIO is an acquired hypophosphatemic disorder seen in association with mesenchymal tumors. Whereas mutations in FGF-23 cause ADHR, overexpression of FGF-23 by tumor causes TIO. FGF-23 is probably not the only phosphatonin, and other factors with appropriate biologic characteristics have been identified.[325] The anti-aging protein Klotho regulates FGF23 action.[325a,325b] Tumors causing this syndrome are usually benign. The diagnosis may be made by detection of osteomalacia and phosphate wasting, which suggest the presence of a responsible tumor.

Other candidate phosphatonins are under study. The bone-expressed gene MEPE, or matrix extracellular phosphoglycoprotein, is a strong candidate as another phosphaturic factor in TIO.[326]

Hereditary Hypophosphatemic Rickets with Hypercalciuria

Hereditary hypophosphatemic rickets with hypercalciuria (HHRH) is a rare autosomal recessive syndrome characterized by rickets, short stature, renal phosphate wasting, and hypercalciuria. HHRH is caused by mutations in SLC34A3, the gene encoding the renal sodium-phosphate cotransporter NaP(i)-IIc.[327] Unlike X-linked hypophosphatemia and autosomal dominant hypophosphatemic rickets, patients have an appropriate elevation in 1,25(OH)$_2$D, which results in hypercalciuria. Patients are treated with phosphorus supplementation.

Although defects in the NPT2 gene, which encodes the type IIa sodium-phosphate cotransporter, are not the cause of HHRH, mutations have been found in two patients with nephrolithiasis, osteoporosis, and hypophosphatemia. Sodium-dependent phosphate uptake was impaired in oocytes expressing the mutant NPT2.[328]

Other Mendelian Forms of Hypophosphatemia

An unusual form of mendelian hypophosphatemia was reported by Stamp and Baker.[329] Children of a consanguineous mating demonstrated hypophosphatemia as well as childhood rickets, deafness, and high bone density. Recessive inheritance was suggested by the absence of disease in both parents. Mutations in the DMP1 gene are responsible for disease in at least some families with this disorder.[329a]

Chitayat and co-workers[330] described a family with apparent recessive inheritance of renal hypophosphatemia, facial anomalies, intracerebral calcifications, and recurrent dental abscesses. Affected children had normal calcium, vitamin D, and PTH levels but significant hypophosphatemia. The inheritance pattern was consistent with autosomal recessive transmission.

Treatment

As noted, serum levels of phosphorus may not be a good reflection of total body stores. Therefore, it is essentially impossible to predict the amount of phosphorus necessary to correct phosphorus deficiency and hypophosphatemia. The clinical circumstances will suggest whether severe underlying phosphate deficiency is present. In chronically malnourished patients (e.g., anorectics, alcoholics), significant phosphorus repletion will be necessary, whereas in patients who are hypophosphatemic from other causes (antacid ingestion, acetazolamide use), correction of the underlying problem may be sufficient.

In mild or moderate hypophosphatemia (~2 mg/dL), oral repletion with low-fat milk (containing 0.9 mg phosphorus per milliliter) is effective. In individuals intolerant of milk, potassium phosphate or sodium phosphate preparations can be used. Intravenous phosphorus repletion is generally reserved for individuals with severe (~1 mg/dL) hypophosphatemia. One standard regimen is to administer 2.5 mg/kg body mass of elemental phosphorus over a 6-hour period for severe asymptomatic hypophosphatemia and

5 mg/kg body mass of elemental phosphorus over a 6-hour period for severe symptomatic hypophosphatemia.[331] Intravenous phosphorus repletion is generally safe and effective.[332] Malnourished patients receiving hyperalimentation should have adequate phosphorus supplementation to avoid the frequently observed refeeding hypophosphatemia.

References

1. Ladenson JH, Lewis JW, Boyd JC: Failure of total calcium corrected for protein, albumin, and pH to correctly assess free calcium status. J Clin Endocrinol Metab 46:986–993, 1978.
2. Motoyama HI, Friedman PA: Calcium-sensing receptor regulation of PTH-dependent calcium absorption by mouse cortical ascending limbs. Am J Physiol Renal Physiol 283:F399–406, 2002.
3. Simon DB, Nelson-Williams C, Bia MJ, et al: Gitelman's variant of Bartter's syndrome, inherited hypokalaemic alkalosis, is caused by mutations in the thiazide-sensitive Na-Cl cotransporter. Nat Genet 12:24–30, 1996.
4. Palmer M, Jakobsson S, Akerstrom G, Ljunghall S: Prevalence of hypercalcaemia in a health survey: A 14-year follow-up study of serum calcium values. Eur J Clin Invest 18:39–46, 1988.
5. Christensson T, Hellstrom K, Wengle B, et al: Prevalence of hypercalcaemia in a health screening in Stockholm. Acta Med Scand 200:131–137, 1976.
6. Lundgren E, Rastad J, Thrufjell E, et al: Population-based screening for primary hyperparathyroidism with serum calcium and parathyroid hormone values in menopausal women. Surgery 121:287–294, 1997.
7. Lind L, Skarfors E, Berglund L, et al: Serum calcium: A new, independent, prospective risk factor for myocardial infarction in middle-aged men followed for 18 years. J Clin Epidemiol 50:967–973, 1997.
8. Melton LR: The epidemiology of primary hyperparathyroidism in North America. J Bone Miner Res 17 Suppl 2:N12–17, 2002.
9. Wermers RA, Khosla S, Atkinson EJ, et al: The rise and fall of primary hyperparathyroidism: A population-based study in Rochester, Minnesota, 1965–1992. Ann Intern Med 126:433–440, 1997.
10. Wermers RA, Khosla S, Atkinson EJ, et al: Incidence of primary hyperparathyroidism in Rochester, Minnesota, 1993–2001: An update on the changing epidemiology of the disease. J Bone Miner Res 21:171–177, 2006.
11. Hsi ED, Zukerberg LR, Yang WI, Arnold A: Cyclin D1/PRAD1 expression in parathyroid adenomas: An immunohistochemical study. J Clin Endocrinol Metab 81:1736–1739, 1996.
12. Hemmer S, Wasenius VM, Haglund C, et al: Deletion of 11q23 and cyclin D1 overexpression are frequent aberrations in parathyroid adenomas. Am J Pathol 158:1355–1362, 2001.
13. Heppner C, Kester MB, Agarwal SK, et al: Somatic mutation of the MEN1 gene in parathyroid tumours. Nat Genet 16:375–378, 1997.
14. Farnebo F, Teh BT, Kytola S, et al: Alterations of the MEN1 gene in sporadic parathyroid tumors [see comments]. J Clin Endocrinol Metab 83:2627–2630, 1998.
15. Arnold A, Shattuck TM, Mallya SM, et al: Molecular pathogenesis of primary hyperparathyroidism. J Bone Miner Res 17 Suppl 2:N30–36, 2002.
16. Lind L, Hvarfner A, Palmer M, et al: Hypertension in primary hyperparathyroidism in relation to histopathology. Eur J Surg 157:457–459, 1991.
17. Lind L, Jacobsson S, Palmer M, et al: Cardiovascular risk factors in primary hyperparathyroidism: A 15-year follow-up of operated and unoperated cases. J Intern Med 230:29–35, 1991.
18. Hagstrom E, Lundgren E, Lithell H, et al: Normalized dyslipidaemia after parathyroidectomy in mild primary hyperparathyroidism: Population-based study over five years. Clin Endocrinol (Oxf) 56:253–260, 2002.
19. Procopio M, Magro G, Cesario F, et al: The oral glucose tolerance test reveals a high frequency of both impaired glucose tolerance and undiagnosed Type 2 diabetes mellitus in primary hyperparathyroidism. Diabet Med 19:958–961, 2002.
20. Nuzzo V, Tauchmanova L, Fonderico F, et al: Increased intima-media thickness of the carotid artery wall, normal blood pressure profile and normal left ventricular mass in subjects with primary hyperparathyroidism. Eur J Endocrinol 147:453–459, 2002.
21. Palmer M, Adami HO, Bergstrom R, et al: Survival and renal function in untreated hypercalcaemia. Population-based cohort study with 14 years of follow-up. Lancet 1:59–62, 1987.
22. Leifsson BG, Ahren B: Serum calcium and survival in a large health screening program. J Clin Endocrinol Metab 81:2149–2153, 1996.
23. Hedback G, Oden A: Increased risk of death from primary hyperparathyroidism—an update. Eur J Clin Invest 28:271–276, 1998.
24. Palmer M, Adami HO, Bergstrom R, et al: Mortality after surgery for primary hyperparathyroidism: A follow-up of 441 patients operated on from 1956 to 1979. Surgery 102:1–7, 1987.
25. Stefenelli T, Abela C, Frank H, et al: Cardiac abnormalities in patients with primary hyperparathyroidism: Implications for follow-up. J Clin Endocrinol Metab 82:106–112, 1997.
26. Nilsson IL, Yin L, Lundgren E, et al: Clinical presentation of primary hyperparathyroidism in Europe—nationwide cohort analysis on mortality from nonmalignant causes. J Bone Miner Res 17 Suppl 2:N68–74, 2002.
27. Silverberg SJ, Shane E, de la Cruz L, et al: Skeletal disease in primary hyperparathyroidism [see comments]. J Bone Miner Res 4:283–291, 1989.
28. Bilezikian JP, Silverberg SJ, Shane E, et al: Characterization and evaluation of asymptomatic primary hyperparathyroidism. J Bone Miner Res 6 Suppl 2:S85–89; discussion S121–124, 1991.
29. Bilezikian JP, Potts JT, Jr., Fuleihan Gel H, et al: Summary statement from a workshop on asymptomatic primary hyperparathyroidism: A perspective for the 21st century. J Clin Endocrinol Metab 87:5353–5361, 2002.
30. Shoback DM, Bilezikian JP, Turner SA, et al: The calcimimetic cinacalcet normalizes serum calcium in subjects with primary hyperparathyroidism. J Clin Endocrinol Metab 88:5644–5649, 2003.
31. Silverberg SJ, Bone HG, 3rd, Marriott TB, et al: Short-term inhibition of parathyroid hormone secretion by a calcium-receptor agonist in patients with primary hyperparathyroidism. N Engl J Med 337:1506–1510, 1997.
32. Peacock M, Bilezikian JP, Klassen PS, et al: Cinacalcet hydrochloride maintains long-term normocalcemia in patients with primary hyperparathyroidism. J Clin Endocrinol Metab 90:135–141, 2005.
32a. Politz D, Norman J: Hyperparathyroidism in patients over 80: clinical characteristics and their ability to undergo outpatient parathyroidectomy. Thyroid 17:333–339, 2007.
33. Saxe AW, Brennan MF: Reoperative parathyroid surgery for primary hyperparathyroidism caused by multiple-gland disease: Total parathyroidectomy and autotransplantation with cryopreserved tissue. Surgery 91:616–621, 1982.
34. Rudberg C, Akerstrom G, Palmer M, et al: Late results of operation for primary hyperparathyroidism in 441 patients. Surgery 99:643–651, 1986.
35. Ruda JM, Hollenbeak CS, Stack BC, Jr: A systematic review of the diagnosis and treatment of primary hyperparathyroidism from 1995 to 2003. Otolaryngol Head Neck Surg 132:359–372, 2005.
36. Anderson BJ, Samaan NA, Vassilopoulou-Sellin R, et al: Parathyroid carcinoma: Features and difficulties in diagnosis and management. Surgery 94:906–915, 1983.
37. Hoelting T, Weber T, Herfarth C: Surgical treatment of parathyroid carcinoma (review). Oncol Rep 8:931–934, 2001.
38. Shattuck TM, Valimaki S, Obara T, et al: Somatic and germ-line mutations of the HRPT2 gene in sporadic parathyroid carcinoma. N Engl J Med 349:1722–1729, 2003.
39. Kremer R, Shustik C, Tabak T, et al: Parathyroid-hormone-related peptide in hematologic malignancies. Am J Med 100:406–411, 1996.
40. Grill V, Ho P, Body JJ, et al: Parathyroid hormone-related protein: elevated levels in both humoral hypercalcemia of malignancy and hypercalcemia complicating metastatic breast cancer. J Clin Endocrinol Metab 73:1309–1315, 1991.
41. Strewler GJ, Nissenson RA: Parathyroid-hormone-related protein. In Favus MJ (ed): Primer on the Metabolic Bone Diseases and Disorders of Mineral Metabolism. Philadelphia, Lippincott-Raven, 1996.
42. Stewart AF, Mangin M, Wu T, et al: Synthetic human parathyroid hormone-like protein stimulates bone resorption and causes hypercalcemia in rats. J Clin Invest 81:596–600, 1988.
43. Karaplis AC, Luz A, Glowacki J, et al: Lethal skeletal dysplasia from targeted disruption of the parathyroid hormone-related peptide gene. Genes Dev 8:277–289, 1994.
44. Breslau NA, McGuire JL, Zerwekh JE, et al: Hypercalcemia associated with increased serum calcitriol levels in three patients with lymphoma. Ann Intern Med 100:1–6, 1984.
45. Rosenthal N, Insogna KL, Godsall JW, et al: Elevations in circulating 1,25-dihydroxyvitamin D in three patients with lymphoma-associated hypercalcemia. J Clin Endocrinol Metab 60:29–33, 1985.
46. Fetchick DA, Bertolini DR, Sarin PS, et al: Production of 1,25-dihydroxyvitamin D3 by human T cell lymphotrophic virus-I-transformed lymphocytes. J Clin Invest 78:592–596, 1986.
47. Nussbaum SR, Gaz RD, Arnold A: Hypercalcemia and ectopic secretion of parathyroid hormone by an ovarian carcinoma with rearrangement of the gene for parathyroid hormone. N Engl J Med 323:1324–1328, 1990.
48. Ross JR, Saunders Y, Edmonds PM, et al: Systematic review of role of bisphosphonates on skeletal morbidity in metastatic cancer. BMJ 327:469, 2003.
49. Neville-Webbe H, Holen I, Coleman R: The anti-tumour activity of bisphosphonates. Cancer Treat Rev 28:305–319, 2002.
50. Mundy GR: Myeloma bone disease. Eur J Cancer 34:246–251, 1998.
51. Durie BG, Salmon SE, Mundy GR: Relation of osteoclast activating factor production to extent of bone disease in multiple myeloma. Br J Haematol 47:21–30, 1981.
52. Berenson J, Hillner B, Kyle R, et al: American Society of Clinical Oncology clinical practice guidelines: The role of bisphosphonates in multiple myeloma. J Clin Oncol 20:3719–3736, 2002.
53. Huang S-M, Duh QY, Shaver J, et al: Familial hyperparathyroidism without multiple endocrine neoplasia. World J Surg 21:22–29, 1997.
54. Simonds W, James-Newton L, Agarwal S, et al: Familial isolated hyperparathyroidism: Clinical and genetic characteristics of 36 kindreds. Medicine (Baltimore) 81:1–26, 2002.
55. Teh BT, Farnebo F, Twigg S, et al: Familial isolated hyperparathyroidism maps to the hyperparathyroidism- jaw tumor locus in 1q21–q32 in a subset of families. J Clin Endocrinol Metab 83:2114–2120, 1998.
56. Simonds WF, Robbins CM, Agarwal SK, et al: Familial isolated hyperparathyroidism is rarely caused by germline mutation in HRPT2, the gene for the hyperparathyroidism-jaw tumor syndrome. J Clin Endocrinol Metab 89:96–102, 2004.
57. Teh BT, Esapa CT, Houlston R, et al: A family with isolated hyperparathyroidism segregating a missense MEN1 mutation and showing loss of the wild-type alleles in the parathyroid tumors. Am J Hum Genet 63:1554–1549, 1998.
58. Villablanca A, Wassif W, Smith T, et al: Involvement of the MEN1 gene locus in familial isolated hyperparathyroidism. Eur J Endocrinol 147:313–322, 2002.
59. Schipani E, Langman CB, Parfitt AM, et al: Constitutively activated receptors for parathyroid hormone and parathyroid hormone-related peptide in Jansen's metaphyseal chondrodysplasia [see comments]. N Engl J Med 335:708–714, 1996.
60. Schipani E, Kruse K, Juppner H: A constitutively active mutant PTH-PTHrP receptor in Jansen-type metaphyseal chondrodysplasia. Science 268:98–100, 1995.

61. Guo S, Sawicki M: Molecular and genetic mechanisms of tumorigenesis in multiple endocrine neoplasia type-1. Mol Endocrinol 15:1653–1664, 2001.

62. Bystrom C, Larsson C, Blomberg C, et al: Localization of the MEN1 gene to a small region within chromosome 11q13 by deletion mapping in tumors. Proc Natl Acad Sci U S A 87:1968–1972, 1990.

63. Lemmens I, Van de Ven WJ, Kas K, et al: Identification of the multiple endocrine neoplasia type 1 (MEN1) gene. The European Consortium on MEN1. Hum Mol Genet 6:1177–1183, 1997.

64. Guru SC, Goldsmith PK, Burns AL, et al: Menin, the product of the MEN1 gene, is a nuclear protein. Proc Natl Acad Sci U S A 95:1630–1634, 1998.

65. Marx SJ, Agarwal SK, Kester MB, et al: Germline and somatic mutation of the gene for multiple endocrine neoplasia type 1 (MEN1). J Intern Med 243:447–453, 1998.

66. Bassett JH, Forbes SA, Pannett AA, et al: Characterization of mutations in patients with multiple endocrine neoplasia type 1. Am J Hum Genet 62:232–244, 1998.

67. Donis-Keller H, Dou S, Chi D, et al: Mutations in the RET proto-oncogene are associated with MEN 2A and FMTC: Hum Mol Genet 2:851–856, 1993.

68. Marx SJ, Simonds WF, Agarwal SK, et al: Hyperparathyroidism in hereditary syndromes: special expressions and special managements. J Bone Miner Res 17 Suppl 2: N37–43, 2002.

69. Brandi M, Gagel R, Angeli A, et al: Guidelines for diagnosis and therapy of MEN type 1 and type 2. J Clin Endocrinol Metab 86:5658–5671, 2001.

70. Jackson CE, Norum RA, Boyd SB, et al: Hereditary hyperparathyroidism and multiple ossifying jaw fibromas: A clinically and genetically distinct syndrome. Surgery 108:1006–12; discussion 1012–1013, 1990.

71. Carpten J, Robbins C, Villablanca A, et al: HRPT2, encoding parafibromin, is mutated in hyperparathyroidism-jaw tumor syndrome. Nat Genet 32:676–680, 2002.

72. Marx SJ, Attie MF, Levine MA, et al: The hypocalciuric or benign variant of familial hypercalcemia: Clinical and biochemical features in fifteen kindreds. Medicine (Baltimore) 60:397–412, 1981.

73. Attie M, Gill J, Stock J, et al: Urinary calcium excretion in familial hypocalciuric hypercalcemia. Persistence of relative hypocalciuria after induction of hypoparathyroidism. J Clin Invest 72:667–676, 1983.

74. Pollak MR, Seidman CE, Brown EM: Three inherited disorders of calcium sensing. Medicine (Baltimore) 75:115–123, 1996.

75. Hendy GN, D'Souza-Li L, Yang B, et al: Mutations of the calcium-sensing receptor (CASR) in familial hypocalciuric hypercalcemia, neonatal severe hyperparathyroidism, and autosomal dominant hypocalcemia. Hum Mutat 16:281–296, 2000.

76. Bai M, Quinn S, Trivedi S, et al: Expression and characterization of inactivating and activating mutations in the human Ca2+o-sensing receptor. J Biol Chem 271:19537–19545, 1996.

77. Bai M, Pearce SH, Kifor O, et al: In vivo and in vitro characterization of neonatal hyperparathyroidism resulting from a de novo, heterozygous mutation in the Ca2+-sensing receptor gene: Normal maternal calcium homeostasis as a cause of secondary hyperparathyroidism in familial benign hypocalciuric hypercalcemia. J Clin Invest 99:88–96, 1997.

78. Bai M, Janicic N, Trivedi S, et al: Markedly reduced activity of mutant calcium-sensing receptor with an inserted Alu element from a kindred with familial hypocalciuric hypercalcemia and neonatal severe hyperparathyroidism. J Clin Invest 99:1917–1925, 1997.

79. Pollak MR, Brown EM, Chou YH, et al: Mutations in the human Ca(2+)-sensing receptor gene cause familial hypocalciuric hypercalcemia and neonatal severe hyperparathyroidism. Cell 75:1297–1303, 1993.

80. Marx S, Fraser D, Rapoport A: Familial hypocalciuric hypercalcemia. Mild expression of the gene in heterozygotes and severe expression in homozygotes. Am J Med 78:15–22, 1985.

81. Pollak M, Chou Y-H, Marx S, et al: Familial hypocalciuric hypercalcemia and neonatal severe hyperparathyroidism. Effects of mutant gene dosage on phenotype. J Clin Invest 93:1108–1112, 1994.

82. Herman SP: Lithium, hypercalcemia, and hyperparathyroidism. Biol Psychiatry 16:593–595, 1981.

83. Spiegel AM, Rudorfer MV, Marx SJ, Linnoila M: The effect of short term lithium administration on suppressibility of parathyroid hormone secretion by calcium in vivo. J Clin Endocrinol Metab 59:354–357, 1984.

84. McHenry CR, Racke F, Meister M, et al: Lithium effects on dispersed bovine parathyroid cells grown in tissue culture. Surgery 110:1061–1066, 1991.

85. Mallette LE, Eichhorn E: Effects of lithium carbonate on human calcium metabolism. Arch Intern Med 146:770–776, 1986.

86. Fishbane S, Frei GL, Finger M, et al: Hypervitaminosis A in two hemodialysis patients. Am J Kidney Dis 25:346–349, 1995.

87. Ragavan VV, Smith JE, Bilezikian JP: Vitamin A toxicity and hypercalcemia. Am J Med Sci 283:161–164, 1982.

88. Suzumiya J, Asahara F, Katakami H, et al: Hypercalcaemia caused by all-trans retinoic acid treatment of acute promyelocytic leukaemia: Case report [letter] [see comments]. Eur J Haematol 53:126–127, 1994.

89. Valentic JP, Elias AN, Weinstein GD: Hypercalcemia associated with oral isotretinoin in the treatment of severe acne. JAMA 250:1899–1900, 1983.

90. Larsen W, Fellowes G, Rickman LS: Life-threatening hypercalcemia and tamoxifen. Am J Med 88:440–442, 1990.

91. Duarte CG, Winnacker JL, Becker KL, Pace A: Thiazide-induced hypercalcemia. N Engl J Med 284:828–830, 1971.

92. Christensson T, Hellstrom K, Wengle B: Hypercalcemia and primary hyperparathyroidism. Prevalence in patients receiving thiazides as detected in a health screen. Arch Intern Med 137:1138–1142, 1977.

93. Parfitt AM: The interactions of thiazide diuretics with parathyroid hormone and vitamin D: Studies in patients with hypoparathyroidism. J Clin Invest 51:1879–1888, 1972.

94. Popovtzer MM, Subryan VL, Alfrey AC, et al: The acute effect of chlorothiazide on serum-ionized calcium. Evidence for a parathyroid hormone-dependent mechanism. J Clin Invest 55:1295–1302, 1975.

95. McPherson ML, Prince SR, Atamer ER, et al: Theophylline-induced hypercalcemia. Ann Intern Med 105:52–54, 1986.

96. Burnett CH, Commons RR, Albright F, et al: Hypercalcemia without hypercalciuria or hypophosphatemia, calcinosis and renal insufficiency: A syndrome following prolonged intake of milk and alkali. N Engl J Med 240:787, 1949.

97. Picolos MK, Lavis VR, Orlander PR: Milk-alkali syndrome is a major cause of hypercalcaemia among non-end-stage renal disease (non-ESRD) inpatients. Clin Endocrinol (Oxf) 63:566–576, 2005.

98. Beall DP, Scofield RH: Milk-alkali syndrome associated with calcium carbonate consumption. Report of 7 patients with parathyroid hormone levels and an estimate of prevalence among patients hospitalized with hypercalcemia. Medicine (Baltimore) 74:89–96, 1995.

99. Sutton RA, Wong NL, Dirks JH: Effects of metabolic acidosis and alkalosis on sodium and calcium transport in the dog kidney. Kidney Int 15:520–533, 1979.

100. Bell NH, Stern PH: Hypercalcemia and increases in serum hormone value during prolonged administration of 1alpha,25-dihydroxyvitamin D. N Engl J Med 298:1241–1243, 1978.

101. Jacobus CH, Holick MF, Shao Q, et al: Hypervitaminosis D associated with drinking milk [see comments]. N Engl J Med 326:1173–1177, 1992.

102. Blank S, Scanlon KS, Sinks TH, et al: An outbreak of hypervitaminosis D associated with the overfortification of milk from a home-delivery dairy. Am J Public Health 85:656–659, 1995.

103. Stewart AF, Adler M, Byers CM, et al: Calcium homeostasis in immobilization: An example of resorptive hypercalciuria. N Engl J Med 306:1136–1140, 1982.

104. Singer FR, Minoofar PN: Bisphosphonates in the treatment of disorders of mineral metabolism. Adv Endocrinol Metab 6:259–288, 1995.

105. Studdy PR, Bird R, Neville E, James DG: Biochemical findings in sarcoidosis. J Clin Pathol 33:528–533, 1980.

106. Barbour GL, Coburn JW, Slatopolsky E, et al: Hypercalcemia in an anephric patient with sarcoidosis: Evidence for extrarenal generation of 1,25-dihydroxyvitamin D. N Engl J Med 305:440–443, 1981.

107. Mason RS, Frankel T, Chan YL, et al: Vitamin D conversion by sarcoid lymph node homogenate. Ann Intern Med 100:59–61, 1984.

108. Sandler LM, Winearls CG, Fraher LJ, et al: Studies of the hypercalcaemia of sarcoidosis: Effect of steroids and exogenous vitamin D3 on the circulating concentrations of 1,25- dihydroxy vitamin D3. Q J Med 53:165–180, 1984.

109. Adams JS, Sharma OP, Diz MM, Endres DB: Ketoconazole decreases the serum 1,25-dihydroxyvitamin D and calcium concentration in sarcoidosis-associated hypercalcemia. J Clin Endocrinol Metab 70:1090–1095, 1990.

110. O'Leary TJ, Jones G, Yip A, et al: The effects of chloroquine on serum 1,25-dihydroxyvitamin D and calcium metabolism in sarcoidosis. N Engl J Med 315:727–730, 1986.

111. Fuss M, Pepersack T, Gillet C, et al: Calcium and vitamin D metabolism in granulomatous diseases. Clin Rheumatol 11:28–36, 1992.

112. Kelestimur F, Guven M, Ozesmi M, Pasaoglu H: Does tuberculosis really cause hypercalcemia? J Endocrinol Invest 19:678–681, 1996.

113. Burman KD, Monchik JM, Earll JM, Wartofsky L: Ionized and total serum calcium and parathyroid hormone in hyperthyroidism. Ann Intern Med 84:668–671, 1976.

114. Mundy GR, Shapiro JL, Bandelin JG, et al: Direct stimulation of bone resorption by thyroid hormones. J Clin Invest 58:529–534, 1976.

115. Stewart AF, Hoecker JL, Mallette LE, et al: Hypercalcemia in pheochromocytoma. Evidence for a novel mechanism. Ann Intern Med 102:776–779, 1985.

116. Diamond T, Thornley S: Addisonian crisis and hypercalcaemia. Aust N Z J Med 24:316, 1994.

117. Mao C, Carter P, Schaefer P, et al: Malignant islet cell tumor associated with hypercalcemia. Surgery 117:37–40, 1995.

118. Knox JB, Demling RH, Wilmore DW, et al: Hypercalcemia associated with the use of human growth hormone in an adult surgical intensive care unit. Arch Surg 130:442–445, 1995.

119. Aloia J, Powell D, Mendizibal E, Roginsky M: Parathyroid function in acromegaly. Horm Res 6:145–149, 1975.

120. Grimm T, Wesselhoeft H: The genetic aspects of Williams-Beuren syndrome and the isolated form of the supravalvular aortic stenosis. Investigation of 128 families (author's transl)]. Z Kardiol 69:168–172, 1980.

121. Perez Jurado LA, Peoples R, Kaplan P, et al: Molecular definition of the chromosome 7 deletion in Williams syndrome and parent-of-origin effects on growth. Am J Hum Genet 59:781–792, 1996.

122. Cook JS, Stone MS, Hansen JR: Hypercalcemia in association with subcutaneous fat necrosis of the newborn: Studies of calcium-regulating hormones. Pediatrics 90:93–96, 1992.

123. Bilezikian JP: Management of acute hypercalcemia [see comments]. N Engl J Med 326:1196–1203, 1992.

124. Sato M, Grasser W, Endo N, et al: Bisphosphonate action. Alendronate localization in rat bone and effects on osteoclast ultrastructure. J Clin Invest 88:2095–2105, 1991.

125. Major P, Lortholary A, Hon J, et al: Zoledronic acid is superior to pamidronate in the treatment of hypercalcemia of malignancy: A pooled analysis of two randomized, controlled clinical trials. J Clin Oncol 19:558–567, 2001.

126. Deftos LJ, First BP: Calcitonin as a drug. Ann Intern Med 95:192–197, 1981.

127. Chitambar CR: Gallium nitrate revisited. Semin Oncol 30:1–4, 2003.

128. Cvitkovic F, Armand JP, Tubiana-Hulin M, et al: Randomized, double-blind, phase II trial of gallium nitrate compared with pamidronate for acute control of cancer-related hypercalcemia. Cancer J 12:47–53, 2006.

129. Seymour JF, Gagel RF: Calcitriol: The major humoral mediator of hypercalcemia in Hodgkin's disease and non-Hodgkin's lymphomas. Blood 82:1383–1394, 1993.

130. Cardella CJ, Birkin BL, Rapoport A: Role of dialysis in the treatment of severe hypercalcemia: Report of two cases successfully treated with hemodialysis and review of the literature. Clin Nephrol 12:285–290, 1979.

131. Kaiser W, Biesenbach G, Kramar R, Zazgornik J: Calcium free hemodialysis: an effective therapy in hypercalcemic crisis—report of 4 cases. Intensive Care Med 15:471–474, 1989.

132. Falzon M, Zong J: The noncalcemic vitamin D analogs EB1089 and 22-oxacalcitriol suppress serum-induced parathyroid hormone-related peptide gene expression in a lung cancer cell line. Endocrinology 139:1046–1053, 1998.

132a. Lomonte C, Antonelli M, Losurdo N, et al: Cinacalcet is effective in relapses of secondary hyperparathyroidism after parathyroidectomy. Nephrol Dial Transplant 2007 Apr 20; [Epub ahead of print].

132b. Sloand JA, Shelly MA: Normalization of lithium-induced hypercalcemia and hyperparathyroidism with cinacalcet hydrochloride. Am J Kidney Dis 48:832–837, 2006.

133. Connor TB, Rosen BL, Blaustein MP, et al: Hypocalcemia precipitating congestive heart failure. N Engl J Med 307:869–872, 1982.

133a. Kazmi AS, Wall BM: Reversible congestive heart failure related to profound hypocalcemia secondary to hypoparathyroidism. Am J Med Sci 333:226–229, 2007.

134. Illum F, Dupont E: Prevalences of CT-detected calcification in the basal ganglia in idiopathic hypoparathyroidism and pseudohypoparathyroidism. Neuroradiology 27:32–37, 1985.

135. Prince MR, Erel HE, Lent RW, et al: Gadodiamide administration causes spurious hypocalcemia. Radiology 227:639–646, 2003.

136. Pollak MR, Brown EM, Estep HL, et al: Autosomal dominant hypocalcaemia caused by a Ca(2+)-sensing receptor gene mutation. Nat Genet 8:303–307, 1994.

137. Pearce SH, Williamson C, Kifor O, et al: A familial syndrome of hypocalcemia with hypercalciuria due to mutations in the calcium-sensing receptor. N Engl J Med 335:1115–1122, 1996.

138. Watanabe S, Fukumoto S, Chang H, et al: Association between activating mutations of calcium-sensing receptor and Bartter's syndrome. Lancet 360:692–694, 2002.

139. Ahn TG, Antonarakis SE, Kronenberg HM, et al: Familial isolated hypoparathyroidism: A molecular genetic analysis of 8 families with 23 affected persons. Medicine (Baltimore) 65:73–81, 1986.

140. Arnold A, Horst SA, Gardella TJ, et al: Mutation of the signal peptide-encoding region of the preproparathyroid hormone gene in familial isolated hypoparathyroidism. J Clin Invest 86:1084–1087, 1990.

141. Parkinson DB, Thakker RV: A donor splice site mutation in the parathyroid hormone gene is associated with autosomal recessive hypoparathyroidism. Nat Genet 1:149–152, 1992.

142. Bowl MR, Nesbit MA, Harding B, et al: An interstitial deletion-insertion involving chromosomes 2p25.3 and Xq27.1, near SOX3, causes X-linked recessive hypoparathyroidism. J Clin Invest 115:2822–2831, 2005.

143. Raatikka M, Rapola J, Tuuteri L, et al: Familial third and fourth pharyngeal pouch syndrome with truncus arteriosus: DiGeorge syndrome. Pediatrics 67:173–175, 1981.

144. Scambler PJ, Carey AH, Wyse RK, et al: Microdeletions within 22q11 associated with sporadic and familial DiGeorge syndrome. Genomics 10:201–206, 1991.

145. Yagi H, Furutani Y, Hamada H, et al: Role of TBX1 in human del22q11.2 syndrome. Lancet 362:1366–1373, 2003.

146. Scire G, Dallapiccola B, Iannetti P, et al: Hypoparathyroidism as the major manifestation in two patients with 22q11 deletions. Am J Med Genet 52:478–482, 1994.

147. Zupanc ML, Moraes CT, Shanske S, et al: Deletion of mitochondrial DNA in patients with combined features of Kearns-Sayre and MELAS syndromes. Ann Neurol 29:680–683, 1991.

148. Neufeld M, Maclaren N, Blizzard R: Two types of autoimmune Addison's disease associated with different polyglandular autoimmune (PCA) syndromes. Medicine (Baltimore) 60:355–362, 1981.

149. Parvari R, Hershkovitz E, Grossman N, et al: Mutation of TBCE causes hypoparathyroidism-retardation-dysmorphism and autosomal recessive Kenny-Caffey syndrome. Nat Genet 32:448–452, 2002.

150. Ringel MD, Schwindinger WF, Levine MA: Clinical implications of genetic defects in G proteins. The molecular basis of McCune-Albright syndrome and Albright hereditary osteodystrophy. Medicine (Baltimore) 75:171–184, 1996.

151. Chase LR, Melson GL, Aurbach GD: Pseudohypoparathyroidism: Defective excretion of 3',5'-AMP in response to parathyroid hormone. J Clin Invest 48:1832–1844, 1969.

152. Farfel Z, Brickman AS, Kaslow HR, et al: Defect of receptor-cyclase coupling protein in pseudohypoparathyroidism. N Engl J Med 303:237–242, 1980.

153. Nakamoto JM, Sandstrom AT, Brickman AS, et al: Pseudohypoparathyroidism type Ia from maternal but not paternal transmission of a Gsalpha gene mutation. Am J Med Genet 77:261–267, 1998.

154. Bastepe M, Frohlich LF, Hendy GN, et al: Autosomal dominant pseudohypoparathyroidism type Ib is associated with a heterozygous microdeletion that likely disrupts a putative imprinting control element of GNAS. J Clin Invest 112:1255–1263, 2003.

155. Bastepe M, Frohlich LF, Linglart A, et al: Deletion of the NESP55 differentially methylated region causes loss of maternal GNAS imprints and pseudohypoparathyroidism type Ib. Nat Genet 37:25–27, 2005.

156. Weinstein LS, Shenker A, Gejman PV, et al: Activating mutations of the stimulatory G protein in the McCune-Albright syndrome [see comments]. N Engl J Med 325:1688–1695, 1991.

157. Iiri T, Herzmark P, Nakamoto JM, et al: Rapid GDP release from Gs alpha in patients with gain and loss of endocrine function [see comments]. Nature 371:164–168, 1994.

158. Farfel Z, Brothers VM, Brickman AS, et al: Pseudohypoparathyroidism: Inheritance of deficient receptor-cyclase coupling activity. Proc Natl Acad Sci U S A 78:3098–3102, 1981.

159. Drezner M, Neelon FA, Lebovitz HE: Pseudohypoparathyroidism type II: A possible defect in the reception of the cyclic AMP signal. N Engl J Med 289:1056–1060, 1973.

160. See AC, Soo KC: Hypocalcaemia following thyroidectomy for thyrotoxicosis. Br J Surg 84:95–97, 1997.

161. Demeester-Mirkine N, Hooghe L, Van Geertruyden J, De Maertelaer V: Hypocalcemia after thyroidectomy. Arch Surg 127:854–858, 1992.

162. Yamashita H, Noguchi S, Tahara K, et al: Postoperative tetany in patients with Graves' disease: a risk factor analysis. Clin Endocrinol (Oxf) 47:71–77, 1997.

163. Laitinen K, Lamberg-Allardt C, Tunninen R, et al: Transient hypoparathyroidism during acute alcohol intoxication. N Engl J Med 324:721–727, 1991.

164. Cholst IN, Steinberg SF, Tropper PJ, et al: The influence of hypermagnesemia on serum calcium and parathyroid hormone levels in human subjects. N Engl J Med 310:1221–1225, 1984.

165. Quitterer U, Hoffmann M, Freichel M, Lohse MJ: Paradoxical block of parathormone secretion is mediated by increased activity of G alpha subunits. J Biol Chem 276:6763–6769, 2001.

166. Rude RK, Oldham SB, Singer FR: Functional hypoparathyroidism and parathyroid hormone end-organ resistance in human magnesium deficiency. Clin Endocrinol (Oxf) 5:209–224, 1976.

167. Elisaf M, Milionis H, Siamopoulos KC: Hypomagnesemic hypokalemia and hypocalcemia: Clinical and laboratory characteristics. Miner Electrolyte Metab 23:105–112, 1997.

168. Brown E, Vassilev P, Hebert S: Calcium ions as extracellular messengers. Cell 83:679–682, 1995.

169. Betterle C, Greggio NA, Volpato M: Clinical review 93: Autoimmune polyglandular syndrome type 1. J Clin Endocrinol Metab 83:1049–1055, 1998.

170. Heino M, Peterson P, Kudoh J, et al: APECED mutations in the autoimmune regulator (AIRE) gene. Hum Mutat 18:205–211, 2001.

171. Li Y, Song YH, Rais N, et al: Autoantibodies to the extracellular domain of the calcium sensing receptor in patients with acquired hypoparathyroidism [see comments]. J Clin Invest 97:910–914, 1996.

172. Preece MA, Tomlinson S, Ribot CA, et al: Studies of vitamin D deficiency in man. Q J Med 44:575–589, 1975.

173. Thomas MK, Lloyd-Jones DM, Thadhani RI, et al: Hypovitaminosis D in medical inpatients [see comments]. N Engl J Med 338:777–783, 1998.

174. Honasoge M, Rao DS: Metabolic bone disease in gastrointestinal, hepatobiliary, and pancreatic disorders and total parenteral nutrition. Curr Opin Rheumatol 7:249–254, 1995.

175. Morgan DB, Paterson CR, Woods CG, et al: Search for osteomalacia in 1228 patients after gastrectomy and other operations on the stomach. Lancet 2:1085–1088, 1965.

176. Hajjar ET, Vincenti F, Salti IS: Gluten-induced enteropathy. Osteomalacia as its principal manifestation. Arch Intern Med 134:565–566, 1974.

177. Parfitt AM, Miller MJ, Frame B, et al: Metabolic bone disease after intestinal bypass for treatment of obesity. Ann Intern Med 89:193–199, 1978.

178. Crippin JS, Jorgensen RA, Dickson ER, Lindor KD: Hepatic osteodystrophy in primary biliary cirrhosis: Effects of medical treatment. Am J Gastroenterol 89:47–50, 1994.

179. Barragry JM, France MW, Carter ND, et al: Vitamin-D metabolism in nephrotic syndrome. Lancet 2:629–632, 1977.

180. Hahn TJ: Drug-induced disorders of vitamin D and mineral metabolism. Clin Endocrinol Metab 9:107–127, 1980.

181. Hahn TJ, Birge SJ, Scharp CR, Avioli LV: Phenobarbital-induced alterations in vitamin D metabolism. J Clin Invest 51:741–748, 1972.

182. Kitanaka S, Takeyama K, Murayama A, et al: Inactivating mutations in the 25-hydroxyvitamin D3 1alpha-hydroxylase gene in patients with pseudovitamin D-deficiency rickets [see comments]. N Engl J Med 338:653–661, 1998.

183. Brooks MH, Bell NH, Love L, et al: Vitamin-D-dependent rickets type II: Resistance of target organs to 1,25-dihydroxyvitamin D. N Engl J Med 298:996–999, 1978.

184. Haussler MR, Haussler CA, Jurutka PW, et al: The vitamin D hormone and its nuclear receptor: Molecular actions and disease states. J Endocrinol 154 Suppl:S57–73, 1997.

185. Rudolph R, Boyd CR: Massive transfusion: Complications and their management. South Med J 83:1065–1070, 1990.

186. Silberstein LE, Naryshkin S, Haddad JJ, Strauss JF: Calcium homeostasis during therapeutic plasma exchange. Transfusion 26:151–155, 1986.

187. Jacobson MA, Gambertoglio JG, Aweeka FT, et al: Foscarnet-induced hypocalcemia and effects of foscarnet on calcium metabolism. J Clin Endocrinol Metab 72:1130–1135, 1991.

188. Ranson JH, Rifkind KM, Roses DF, et al: Prognostic signs and the role of operative management in acute pancreatitis. Surg Gynecol Obstet 139:69–81, 1974.

189. Chernow B, Rainey TG, Georges LP, O'Brian JT: Iatrogenic hyperphosphatemia: A metabolic consideration in critical care medicine. Crit Care Med 9:772–774, 1981.

190. Zusman J, Brown DM, Nesbit ME: Hyperphosphatemia, hyperphosphaturia and hypocalcemia in acute lymphoblastic leukemia. N Engl J Med 289:1335–1340, 1973.

191. Zivin JR, Gooley T, Zager RA, Ryan MJ: Hypocalcemia: A pervasive metabolic abnormality in the critically ill. Am J Kidney Dis 37:689–698, 2001.

192. Sperber SJ, Blevins DD, Francis JB: Hypercalcitoninemia, hypocalcemia, and toxic shock syndrome. Rev Infect Dis 12:736–739, 1990.

193. Boyce BF, Yates AJ, Mundy GR: Bolus injections of recombinant human interleukin-1 cause transient hypocalcemia in normal mice. Endocrinology 125:2780–2783, 1989.

194. Mimouni F, Tsang RC: Neonatal hypocalcemia: To treat or not to treat? (A review). J Am Coll Nutr 13:408–415, 1994.

195. Specker BL, Tsang RC, Ho ML, et al: Low serum calcium and high parathyroid hormone levels in neonates fed 'humanized' cow's milk-based formula. Am J Dis Child 145:941–945, 1991.

196. Thomas BR, Bennett JD: Symptomatic hypocalcemia and hypoparathyroidism in two infants of mothers with hyperparathyroidism and familial benign hypercalcemia [see comments]. J Perinatol 15:23–26, 1995.

197. Lim P, Jacob E: Tissue magnesium level in chronic diarrhea. J Lab Clin Med 80:313–321, 1972.

610

CH 16

198. Ryzen E, Elbaum N, Singer FR, Rude RK: Parenteral magnesium tolerance testing in the evaluation of magnesium deficiency. Magnesium 4:137–147, 1985.

199. Carney SL, Wong NL, Quamme GA, Dirks JH: Effect of magnesium deficiency on renal magnesium and calcium transport in the rat. J Clin Invest 65:180–188, 1980.

200. Wong ET, Rude RK, Singer FR, Shaw ST, Jr: A high prevalence of hypomagnesemia and hypermagnesemia in hospitalized patients. Am J Clin Pathol 79:348–352, 1983.

201. Tong GM, Rude RK: Magnesium deficiency in critical illness. J Intensive Care Med 20:3–17, 2005.

202. Elisaf M, Panteli K, Theodorou J, Siamopoulos KC: Fractional excretion of magnesium in normal subjects and in patients with hypomagnesemia. Magnes Res 10:315–20, 1997.

203. Sutton RA, Domrongkitchaiporn S: Abnormal renal magnesium handling. Miner Electrolyte Metab 19:232–40, 1993.

204. De Marchi S, Cecchin E, Basile A, et al: Renal tubular dysfunction in chronic alcohol abuse—effects of abstinence. N Engl J Med 329:1927–1934, 1993.

205. Dickerson RN, Brown RO: Hypomagnesemia in hospitalized patients receiving nutritional support. Heart Lung 14:561–569, 1985.

206. Bowling TE, Silk DB: Refeeding remembered. Nutrition 11:32–34, 1995.

207. Booth CC, Babouris N, Hanna S, MacIntyre I: Incidence of hypomagnesaemia in intestinal malabsorption. Br Med J 2:141–144, 1963.

208. Thorén L: Magnesium deficiency in gastrointestinal fluid loss. Acta Chir Scand Suppl 306:1–65, 1963.

209. Cohen L, Zimmerman AL: Changes in serum electrolyte levels during marathon running. S Afr Med J 53:449–453, 1978.

210. Berger MM, Rothen C, Cavadini C, Chiolero RL: Exudative mineral losses after serious burns: A clue to the alterations of magnesium and phosphate metabolism. Am J Clin Nutr 65:1473–1481, 1997.

211. Davies DR, Friedman M: Complications after parathyroidectomy: Fractures from low calcium and magnesium convulsions. J Bone Joint Surg Br 48B:117–126, 1966.

212. Nabarro JDN, Spencer AG, Stowers JM: Metabolic studies in severe diabetic ketosis. Q J Med 82:225–243, 1952.

213. Martin HE, Smith K, Wilson ML: The fluid and electrolyte therapy of severe diabetic acidosis and ketosis: A study of twenty-nine episodes (twenty-six patients). Am J Med 24:376–389, 1958.

214. Mader IJ, Iseri LT: Spontaneous hypopotassemia, hypomagnesemia, alkalosis and tetany due to hypersecretion of corticosterone-like mineralocorticoid. Am J Med 19:976–988, 1955.

215. Dyckner T, Wester PO: Renal excretion of electrolytes in patients on long-term diuretic therapy for arterial hypertension and/or congestive heart failure. Acta Med Scand 218:443–448, 1985.

216. Kuller L, Farrier N, Caggiula A, et al: Relationship of diuretic therapy and serum magnesium levels among participants in the Multiple Risk Factor Intervention Trial. Am J Epidemiol 122:1045–1059, 1985.

217. Quamme GA: Effect of hypercalcemia on renal tubular handling of calcium and magnesium. Can J Physiol Pharmacol 60:1275–1280, 1982.

218. Johansson G, Danielson BG, Ljunghall S: Magnesium homeostasis in mild-to-moderate primary hyperparathyroidism. Acta Chir Scand 146:85–91, 1980.

219. Buckley JE, Clark VL, Meyer TJ, Pearlman NW: Hypomagnesemia after cisplatin combination chemotherapy. Arch Intern Med 144:2347–2348, 1984.

220. Brock PR, Koliouskas DE, Barratt TM, et al: Partial reversibility of cisplatin nephrotoxicity in children. J Pediatr 118:531–534, 1991.

221. Ettinger L, Gaynon P, Krailo M, et al: A phase II study of carboplatin in children with recurrent or progressive solid tumors. A report from the Childrens Cancer Group. Cancer 73:1297–1301, 1994.

222. Lajer H, Kristensen M, Hansen HH, et al: Magnesium and potassium homeostasis during cisplatin treatment. Cancer Chemother Pharmacol 55:231–236, 2005.

223. Barton CH, Pahl M, Vaziri ND, Cesario T: Renal magnesium wasting associated with amphotericin B therapy. Am J Med 77:471–474, 1984.

224. Wilkinson R, Lucas GL, Heath DA, et al: Hypomagnesaemic tetany associated with prolonged treatment with aminoglycosides. Br Med J 292:818–819, 1986.

225. Zaloga GP, Chernow B, Pock A, et al: Hypomagnesemia is a common complication of aminoglycoside therapy. Surg Gynecol Obstet 158:561–565, 1984.

226. Mani S: Pentamidine-induced renal magnesium wasting [letter]. AIDS 6:594–595, 1992.

227. Palestine AG, Polis MA, De Smet MD, et al: A randomized, controlled trial of foscarnet in the treatment of cytomegalovirus retinitis in patients with AIDS. Ann Intern Med 115:665–673, 1991.

228. Barton CH, Vaziri ND, Martin DC, et al: Hypomagnesemia and renal magnesium wasting in renal transplant recipients receiving cyclosporine. Am J Med 83:693–699, 1987.

229. June CH, Thompson CB, Kennedy MS, et al: Profound hypomagnesemia and renal magnesium wasting associated with the use of cyclosporine for marrow transplantation. Transplantation 39:620–624, 1985.

230. Yuan J, Zhou J, Chen BC, et al: Magnesium supplementation prevents chronic cyclosporine nephrotoxicity via adjusting nitric oxide synthase activity. Transplant Proc 37:1892–1895, 2005.

231. Konrad M, Weber S: Recent advances in molecular genetics of hereditary magnesium-losing disorders. J Am Soc Nephrol 14:249–260, 2003.

232. Geven WB, Monnens LA, Willems HL, et al: Renal magnesium wasting in two families with autosomal dominant inheritance. Kidney Int 31:1140–1144, 1987.

233. Geven WB, Monnens LA, Willems JL, et al: Isolated autosomal recessive renal magnesium loss in two sisters. Clin Genet 32:398–402, 1987.

234. Meij IC, Koenderink JB, van Bokhoven H, et al: Dominant isolated renal magnesium loss is caused by misrouting of the Na(+),K(+)-ATPase gamma-subunit. Nat Genet 26:265–266, 2000.

235. Meij IC, Koenderink JB, De Jong JC, et al: Dominant isolated renal magnesium loss is caused by misrouting of the Na+,K+-ATPase gamma-subunit. Ann N Y Acad Sci 986:437–443, 2003.

236. Kantorovich V, Adams J, Gaines J, et al: Genetic heterogeneity in familial renal magnesium wasting. J Clin Endocrinol Metab 87:612–617, 2002.

237. Simon DB, Lu Y, Choate KA, et al: Paracellin-1, a renal tight junction protein required for paracellular Mg^{2+} resorption. Science 285:103–106, 1999.

238. Kausalya PJ, Amasheh S, Gunzel D, et al: Disease-associated mutations affect intracellular traffic and paracellular Mg^{2+} transport function of Claudin-16. J Clin Invest 116:878–891, 2006.

239. Weber S, Schneider L, Peters M, et al: Novel paracellin-1 mutations in 25 families with familial hypomagnesemia with hypercalciuria and nephrocalcinosis. J Am Soc Nephrol 12:1872–1881, 2001.

240. Walder R, Shalev H, Brennan T, et al: Familial hypomagnesemia maps to chromosome 9q, not to the X chromosome: Genetic linkage mapping and analysis of a balanced translocation breakpoint. Hum Mol Genet 6:1491–1497, 1997.

241. Walder R, Landau D, Meyer P, et al: Mutation of TRPM6 causes familial hypomagnesemia with secondary hypocalcemia. Nat Genet 31:171–174, 2002.

241a. Groenestege WM, Hoenderop JG, van den Heuvel L, et al: The epithelial Mg^{2+} channel transient receptor potential melastatin 6 is regulated by dietary Mg^{2+} content and estrogens. J Am Soc Nephrol 17:1035–1043, 2006.

242. Kristiansen JH, Brochner Mortensen J, Pedersen KO: Familial hypocalciuric hypercalcaemia I: Renal handling of calcium, magnesium and phosphate. Clin Endocrinol (Oxf) 22:103–116, 1985.

243. Kingston ME, Al-Siba'i MB, Skooge WC: Clinical manifestations of hypomagnesemia. Crit Care Med 14:950–954, 1986.

244. Skou JC: The influence of some cations on an adenosine triphosphatase from peripheral nerves. Biochim Biophys Acta 23:394–401, 1957.

245. Whang R, Morosi HJ, Rodgers D, Reyes R: The influence of sustained magnesium deficiency on muscle potassium repletion. J Lab Clin Med 70:895–902, 1967.

246. Agus ZS: Hypomagnesemia. J Am Soc Nephrol 10:1616–1622, 1999.

247. Seller RH, Cangiano J, Kim KE, et al: Digitalis toxicity and hypomagnesemia. Am Heart J 79:57–68, 1970.

248. Dyckner T: Serum magnesium in acute myocardial infarction. Relation to arrhythmias. Acta Med Scand 207:59–66, 1980.

249. England MR, Gordon G, Salem M, Chernow B: Magnesium administration and dysrhythmias after cardiac surgery. A placebo-controlled, double-blind, randomized trial. JAMA 268:2395–402, 1992.

250. Hazelrigg SR, Boley TM, Cetindag IB, et al: The efficacy of supplemental magnesium in reducing atrial fibrillation after coronary artery bypass grafting. Ann Thorac Surg 77:824–830, 2004.

251. Klevay L, Milne D: Low dietary magnesium increases supraventricular ectopy. Am J Clin Nutr 75:550–554, 2002.

252. Tsuji H, Venditti FJ, Jr, Evans JC, et al: The associations of levels of serum potassium and magnesium with ventricular premature complexes (the Framingham Heart Study). Am J Cardiol 74:232–235, 1994.

253. Vallee BL, Wacker WEC, Ulmer DD: The magnesium-deficiency tetany syndrome in man. N Engl J Med 262:155–161, 1960.

254. Mody I, Lambert JD, Heinemann U: Low extracellular magnesium induces epileptiform activity and spreading depression in rat hippocampal slices. J Neurophysiol 57:869–888, 1987.

255. Saul RF, Selhorst JB: Downbeat nystagmus with magnesium depletion. Arch Neurol 38:650–652, 1981.

256. Whang R, Whang DD, Ryan MP: Refractory potassium repletion. A consequence of magnesium deficiency. Arch Intern Med 152:40–45, 1992.

257. Dietary Reference Intakes: Calcium, Phosphorus, Magnesium, Vitamin D and Fluoride. In Board IoMFaN (ed). Washington, DC: National Academy Press, 1999.

258. Oster JR, Epstein M: Management of magnesium depletion. Am J Nephrol 8:349–354, 1988.

259. Eisenbud E, LoBue CC: Hypocalcemia after therapeutic use of magnesium sulfate. Arch Intern Med 136:688–691, 1976.

260. Navarro J, Oster JR, Gkonos PJ, et al: Tetany induced on separate occasions by administration of potassium and magnesium in a patient with hungry-bone syndrome. Miner Electrolyte Metab 17:340–344, 1991.

261. Farkas RA, McAllister CT, Blachley JD: Effect of magnesium salt anions on potassium balance in normal and magnesium-depleted rats. J Lab Clin Med 110:412–417, 1987.

262. Bundy JT, Connito D, Mahoney MD, Pontier PJ: Treatment of idiopathic renal magnesium wasting with amiloride. Am J Nephrol 15:75–77, 1995.

263. Coburn JW, Popovtzer MM, Massry SG, Kleeman CR: The physicochemical state and renal handling of divalent ions in chronic renal failure. Arch Intern Med 124:302–311, 1969.

264. Clark BA, Brown RS: Unsuspected morbid hypermagnesemia in elderly patients. Am J Nephrol 12:336–343, 1992.

265. Mordes JP, Wacker WE: Excess magnesium. Pharmacol Rev 29:273–300, 1977.

266. Touyz RM: Magnesium in clinical medicine. Front Biosci 9:1278–1293, 2004.

267. del Castillo J, Engbaek L: The nature of the neuromuscular block produced by magnesium. J Physiol 124:370–384, 1954.

268. Kelber J, Slatopolsky E, Delmez JA: Acute effects of different concentrations of dialysate magnesium during high-efficiency dialysis. Am J Kidney Dis 24:453–460, 1994.

269. Boen ST: Kinetics of peritoneal dialysis. 40:243–287, 1961.

270. Burritt M, Slockbower J, Forsman R, et al: Pediatric reference intervals for 19 biologic variables in healthy children. Mayo Clin Proc 65:329–336, 1990.

271. Markowitz M, Rotkin L, Rosen J: Circadian rhythms of blood minerals in humans. Science 213:672–674, 1981.

272. Hsu CY, Chertow GM: Elevations of serum phosphorus and potassium in mild to moderate chronic renal insufficiency. Nephrol Dial Transplant 17:1419–1425, 2002.

273. Quigley R, Baum M: Effects of growth hormone and insulin-like growth factor I on rabbit proximal convoluted tubule transport. J Clin Invest 88:368–374, 1991.

274. Mitnick P, Goldfarb S, Slatopolsky E, et al: Calcium and phosphate metabolism in tumoral calcinosis. Ann Intern Med 92:482–487, 1980.

275. Topaz O, Shurman DL, Bergman R, et al: Mutations in GALNT3, encoding a protein involved in O-linked glycosylation, cause familial tumoral calcinosis. Nat Genet 36:579–581, 2004.

276. Araya K, Fukumoto S, Backenroth R, et al: A novel mutation in fibroblast growth factor 23 gene as a cause of tumoral calcinosis. J Clin Endocrinol Metab 90:5523–5527, 2005.

277. Chefetz I, Heller R, Galli-Tsinopoulou A, et al: A novel homozygous missense mutation in FGF23 causes Familial Tumoral Calcinosis associated with disseminated visceral calcification. Hum Genet 118:261–266, 2005.

278. Yamaguchi T, Sugimoto T, Imai Y, et al: Successful treatment of hyperphosphatemic tumoral calcinosis with long-term acetazolamide. Bone 16:247S-250S, 1995.

279. Walton R, Russell R, Smith R: Changes in the renal and extrarenal handling of phosphate induced by disodium etidronate (EHDP) in man. Clin Sci Mol Med 49:45–56, 1975.

280. McCloskey E, Yates A, Gray R, et al: Diphosphonates and phosphate homoeostasis in man. Clin Sci (Lond) 74:607–612, 1988.

280a. Gumurdulu Y, Serin E, Ozer B, et al: Age as a predictor of hyperphosphatemia after oral phosphosoda administration for colon preparation. J Gastroenterol Hepatol 19:68–72, 2004.

280b. Desmeules S, Bergeron MJ, Isenring P: Acute phosphate nephropathy and renal failure. N Engl J Med 349:1006–1007, 2003.

280c. Markowitz GS, Stokes MB, Radhakrishnan J, D'Agati VD: Acute phosphate nephropathy following oral sodium phosphate bowel purgative: an underrecognized cause of chronic renal failure. J Am Soc Nephrol 16:3389–3396, 2005.

281. Krapf R, Jaeger P, Hulter H: Chronic respiratory alkalosis induces renal PTH-resistance, hyperphosphatemia and hypocalcemia in humans. Kidney Int 42:727–734, 1992.

282. Thompson C, Kemp G, Radda G: Changes in high-energy phosphates in rat skeletal muscle during acute respiratory acidosis. Acta Physiol Scand 146:15–19, 1992.

283. Tsokos G, Balow J, Spiegel R, Magrath I: Renal and metabolic complications of undifferentiated and lymphoblastic lymphomas. Medicine (Baltimore) 60:218–229, 1981.

284. Larner A: Pseudohyperphosphatemia. Clin Biochem 28:391–393, 1995.

285. Knochel J: The pathophysiology and clinical characteristics of severe hypophosphatemia. Arch Intern Med 137:203–220, 1977.

286. Lichtman M, Miller D, Cohen J, Waterhouse C: Reduced red cell glycolysis, 2, 3-diphosphoglycerate and adenosine triphosphate concentration, and increased hemoglobin-oxygen affinity caused by hypophosphatemia. Ann Intern Med 74:562–568, 1971.

287. Jacob H, Amsden T: Acute hemolytic anemia with rigid red cells in hypophosphatemia. N Engl J Med 285:1446–1450, 1971.

288. Craddock P, Yawata Y, VanSanten L, et al: Acquired phagocyte dysfunction. A complication of the hypophosphatemia of parenteral hyperalimentation. N Engl J Med 290:1403–1407, 1974.

289. Newman J, Neff T, Ziporin P: Acute respiratory failure associated with hypophosphatemia. N Engl J Med 296:1101–1103, 1977.

290. Fuller T, Nichols W, Brenner B, Peterson J: Reversible depression in myocardial performance in dogs with experimental phosphorus deficiency. J Clin Invest 62:1194–1200, 1978.

291. Knochel J: Hypophosphatemia and rhabdomyolysis. Am J Med 92:455–457, 1992.

292. Goldfarb S, Westby G, Goldberg M, Agus Z: Renal tubular effects of chronic phosphate depletion. J Clin Invest 59:770–779, 1977.

293. Coburn J, Massry S: Changes in serum and urinary calcium during phosphate depletion: studies on mechanisms. J Clin Invest 49:1073–1087, 1970.

294. Juan D, Elrazak M: Hypophosphatemia in hospitalized patients. JAMA 242:163–164, 1979.

295. Torres A, Lorenzo V, Salido E: Calcium metabolism and skeletal problems after transplantation. J Am Soc Nephrol 13:551–558, 2002.

296. Bhan I, Shah A, Holmes J, et al: Post-transplant hypophosphatemia: Tertiary 'hyperphosphatoninism'? Kidney Int 70:1486–1494, 2006.

297. Roth K, Foreman J, Segal S: The Fanconi syndrome and mechanisms of tubular transport dysfunction. Kidney Int 20:705–716, 1981.

298. Gannage M, Abikaram G, Nasr F, Awada H: Osteomalacia secondary to celiac disease, primary hyperparathyroidism, and Graves' disease. Am J Med Sci 315:136–139, 1998.

299. Chines A, Pacifici R: Antacid and sucralfate-induced hypophosphatemic osteomalacia: A case report and review of the literature. Calcif Tissue Int 47:291–295, 1990.

300. Mostellar ME, Tuttle EP: Effects of alkalosis on plasma concentration and urinary excretion of urinary phosphate in man. J Clin Invest 43:138–149, 1964.

301. Brautbar N, Leibovici H, Massry S: On the mechanism of hypophosphatemia during acute hyperventilation: Evidence for increased muscle glycolysis. Miner Electrolyte Metab 9:45–50, 1983.

302. ChrisAnderson D, Heimburger D, Morgan S, et al: Metabolic complications of total parenteral nutrition: Effects of a nutrition support service. JPEN J Parenter Enter Nutr 20:206–210, 1996.

303. Marik P, Bedigian M: Refeeding hypophosphatemia in critically ill patients in an intensive care unit. A prospective study. Arch Surg 131:1043–1047, 1996.

304. Ornstein R, Golden N, Jacobson M, Shenker I: Hypophosphatemia during nutritional rehabilitation in anorexia nervosa: Implications for refeeding and monitoring. J Adolesc Health 32:83–88, 2003.

305. Knochel J: Hypophosphatemia in the alcoholic. Arch Intern Med 140:613–615, 1980.

306. Seldin DW, Tarail R: The metabolism of glucose and electrolytes in diabetic acidosis. J Clin Invest 552–560, 1950.

307. Atchley DW, Loeb RF, Richards DW: On diabetic acidosis. A detailed study of electrolyte balances following the withdrawal and reestablishment of insulin therapy. J Clin Invest 12:297, 1933.

308. Kebler R, McDonald F, Cadnapaphornchai P: Dynamic changes in serum phosphorus levels in diabetic ketoacidosis. Am J Med 79:571–576, 1985.

309. Fisher J, Kitabchi A: A randomized study of phosphate therapy in the treatment of diabetic ketoacidosis. J Clin Endocrinol Metab 57:177–180, 1983.

310. Turner S, Kiebzak G, Dousa T: Mechanism of glucocorticoid effect on renal transport of phosphate. Am J Physiol 243:C227–236, 1982.

311. Zamkoff K, Kirshner J: Marked hypophosphatemia associated with acute myelomonocytic leukemia. Indirect evidence of phosphorus uptake by leukemic cells. Arch Intern Med 140:1523–1524, 1980.

312. Chesney P, Davis J, Purdy W, et al: Clinical manifestations of toxic shock syndrome. JAMA 246:741–748, 1981.

313. Suki W, Martinez-Maldonado M, Rouse D, Terry A: Effect of expansion of extracellular fluid volume on renal phosphate handling. J Clin Invest 48:1888–1894, 1969.

314. Dixon P, Christie P, Wooding C, et al: Mutational analysis of PHEX gene in X-linked hypophosphatemia. J Clin Endocrinol Metab 83:3615–3623, 1998.

315. The HYP Consortium: A gene (PEX) with homologies to endopeptidases is mutated in patients with X-linked hypophosphatemic rickets. The HYP Consortium. Nat Genet 11:130–136, 1995.

316. Sabbagh Y, Jones A, Tenenhouse H: PHEXdb, a locus-specific database for mutations causing X-linked hypophosphatemia. Hum Mutat 16:1–6, 2000.

317. Nesbitt T, Coffman T, Griffiths R, Drezner M: Crosstransplantation of kidneys in normal and Hyp mice. Evidence that the Hyp mouse phenotype is unrelated to an intrinsic renal defect. J Clin Invest 89:1453–1459, 1992.

318. Meyer M, Meyer RJ: MRNA expression of Phex in mice and rats: The effect of low phosphate diet. Endocrine 13:81–87, 2000.

319. Bowe A, Finnegan R, Jan dBS, et al: FGF-23 inhibits renal tubular phosphate transport and is a PHEX substrate. Biochem Biophys Res Commun 284:977–981, 2001.

320. Shimada T, Hasegawa H, Yamazaki Y, et al: FGF-23 is a potent regulator of vitamin D metabolism and phosphate homeostasis. J Bone Miner Res 19:429–435, 2004.

321. Sullivan W, Carpenter T, Glorieux F, et al: A prospective trial of phosphate and 1,25-dihydroxyvitamin D3 therapy in symptomatic adults with X-linked hypophosphatemic rickets. J Clin Endocrinol Metab 75:879–885, 1992.

322. Autosomal dominant hypophosphataemic rickets is associated with mutations in FGF23. The ADHR Consortium. Nat Genet 26:345–348, 2000.

323. White K, Carn G, Lorenz-Depiereux B, Benet-Pages A, et al: Autosomal-dominant hypophosphatemic rickets (ADHR) mutations stabilize FGF-23. Kidney Int 60:2079–2086, 2001.

324. Shimada T, Mizutani S, Muto T, et al: Cloning and characterization of FGF23 as a causative factor of tumor-induced osteomalacia. Proc natl. Acad Sci U S A 98:6500–6505, 2001.

325. Schiavi S, Moe O: Phosphatonins: A new class of phosphate-regulating proteins. Curr Opin Nephrol Hypertens 11:423–430, 2002.

325a. Urakawa I, Yamazaki Y, Shimada T, et al: Klotho converts canonical FGF receptor into a specific receptor for FGF23. Nature 444:770–774, 2006.

325b. Torres PU, Prie D, Molina-Bletry V, et al: Klotho: an antiaging protein involved in mineral and vitamin D metabolism. Kidney Int 71:730–737, 2007.

326. Rowe P, de ZP, Dong R, et al: MEPE, a new gene expressed in bone marrow and tumors causing osteomalacia. Genomics 67:54–68, 2000.

327. Bergwitz C, Roslin NM, Tieder M, et al: SLC34A3 mutations in patients with hereditary hypophosphatemic rickets with hypercalciuria predict a key role for the sodium-phosphate cotransporter NaPi-IIc in maintaining phosphate homeostasis. Am J Hum Genet 78:179–192, 2006.

328. Prie D, Huart V, Bakouh N, et al: Nephrolithiasis and osteoporosis associated with hypophosphatemia caused by mutations in the type 2a sodium-phosphate cotransporter. N Engl J Med 347:983–991, 2002.

329. Stamp T, Baker L: Recessive hypophosphataemic rickets, and possible aetiology of the 'vitamin D-resistant' syndrome. Arch Dis Child 51:360–365, 1976.

329a. Feng JQ, Ward LM, Liu S, et al: Loss of DMP1 causes rickets and osteomalacia and identifies a role for osteocytes in mineral metabolism. Nat Genet 38:1310–1315, 2006.

330. Chitayat D, McGillivray B, Rothstein R, et al: Familial renal hypophosphatemia, minor facial anomalies, intracerebral calcifications, and non-rachitic bone changes: Apparently new syndrome? Am J Med Genet 35:406–414, 1990.

331. Lentz R, Brown D, Kjellstrand C: Treatment of severe hypophosphatemia. Ann Intern Med 89:941–944, 1978.

332. Perreault M, Ostrop N, Tierney M: Efficacy and safety of intravenous phosphate replacement in critically ill patients. Ann Pharmacother 31:683–688, 1997.

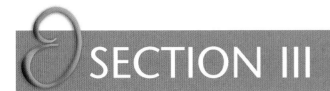

SECTION III

Epidemiology and Risk Factors in Kidney Disease

CHAPTER 17

Epidemiology of Kidney Disease

Josef Coresh • Joseph A. Eustace

Insight into the occurrence and consequences of kidney disease has rapidly progressed over the last decade. Pivotal to this improved understanding has been recently developed and widely disseminated guidelines providing a standardized definition and staging scheme for chronic kidney disease (CKD), a term used to encompass the entire spectrum of renal dysfunction. The prevalence of CKD has historically been underappreciated on both the population and the clinical levels. When used in isolation, serum creatinine is an inadequate screening tool, especially in the elderly and other groups with reduced muscle mass. The development and ongoing refinement of equations to estimate glomerular filtration rates (GFRs) and the growing appreciation of the need to uniformly calibrate serum creatinine assays is improving the diagnosis and staging of CKD. Moreover, it presents us with multiple, and as yet unmet, challenges as to how we develop the resources and care structures necessary to manage this now-visible substantial population with CKD in the face of clear evidence of complications but limited clinical trial data on efficacious interventions. A major concern in this regard is the inequalities that abound in CKD. Both within the United States and abroad, kidney disease afflicts the socially and economically disadvantaged, affecting those persons who have less access to preventive services and who are less equipped to achieve the many lifestyle modifications that are essential to the successful prevention and management of CKD.

The most evident, and for a long time, sole manifestation of the epidemic of kidney disease was those subjects treated with renal replacement therapy, the prevalence of which is predicted to continue to increase. In a global context, several countries have incidence and prevalence rates that are equal to that of the United States, whereas many more have rates that are rapidly increasing. The previous exponential increase in incidence of treated end-stage renal disease (ESRD) in the United States has decreased to the point at which age- and race-adjusted rates have been constant since 2000. Ominously, the ongoing increase of type 2 diabetes and obesity within the general population, if left uncontrolled, may serve to reignite this epidemic, as will the aging of the population and growth of high-risk minority groups. Renal transplantation continues to be the optimal management strategy for kidney failure; however, its broader application is hindered by the limited number of available grafts. Innovative strategies to overcome this shortage have been developed but suffer from a lack of uniform implementation. Survival rates for patients treated with either dialysis or transplantation have steadily improved over time but, despite much progress, still remain markedly reduced compared with rates in the general population. Renal replacement therapy prolongs life but does not restore a normal life expectancy.

The consequences of CKD are many and complex and include hypertension, anemia, acidosis, the interrelated phenomena of renal malnutrition and inflammation, and varied consequences of aberrant bone mineral metabolism. Increased awareness of CKD has led to greater recognition of the burden of illness that accompanies its progression, that contributes to its outcome, and that develops long before the point of actual kidney failure. Hypertension, despite its impact on both renal and patient survival, remains underdiagnosed and, even when noted in conjunction with kidney disease, is still often undertreated. A better understanding of the epidemiology of these complications, in addition to the traditional study of their pathophysiology, is essential if we are to develop successful, rational, and cost-effective strategies to improve the outcome of CKD.

Numerous studies over the last several years have unequivocally proved that kidney disease is a major risk factor for cardiovascular events. Thus, the most common conclusion for a patient with advanced CKD is progression not to dialysis but to death from cardiovascular disease. Much of the attention has focused on ischemic heart disease and, to a lesser extent, on heart failure. The relationship of CKD with stroke, peripheral vascular disease, and sudden cardiac death remains less fully understood. Similarly, whereas much attention has focused on novel cardiovascular risk factors in CKD, we still know far too little about the role and optimal management of traditional well-established risk factors, although they are likely to explain much of the increased association between diseases of the heart and those of the kidney.

DEFINITION AND STAGING OF CHRONIC KIDNEY DISEASE

In 2002, The National Kidney Foundation's (NKF) "Kidney Disease Outcomes Quality Initiative (KDOQI)" proposed a definition and classification scheme of CKD[1] that has since been widely adopted both within and outside of the United States.[2–6] This has provided standardization to a terminology that previously was both ambiguous and confusing.[7] The NKF guidelines define CKD on the basis of kidney damage and/or reduced kidney function. Kidney damage may be confirmed through a variety of methods including histologic evidence of kidney disease, abnormalities in the composition of blood or urine, or abnormal findings on renal imaging. Proteinuria is the most frequent early indicator of kidney damage. Given the complex relationship between hypertension and kidney disease, and the uncertainty as to which of the two conditions developed first, from the definition viewpoint, hypertension alone is not taken as a sufficient indicator of kidney damage.

A major obstacle to the wider recognition of CKD has been the clinical reliance on isolated unstandardized serum creatinine levels as a marker of kidney function and the frequent tendency to dismiss mild elevation in serum creatinine as clinically insignificant and so to systematically underestimate the severity of CKD even when the condition is recognized. The use of isolated serum creatinine levels as a measure of renal function is fraught with limitations.[8] The degree of elevation in serum creatinine is dependent not only on the decrement in GFR but also on creatinine generation rates, which vary substantially with age, race, gender, and diet.[1] As a result, a considerable proportion of patients, especially elderly women and individuals with low muscle mass, have a clinically significant reduction in renal function but have serum creatinine values that fall within the population reference range.[9]

Not surprisingly, the use of unadjusted serum creatinine measurements as a screening tool for early CKD is insensitive and results in the widespread misclassification.[10–12] To avoid this, renal function should instead be quantified by the actual measurement or estimation of the GFR.[1,13] Given that the absolute GFR is expected to vary with body size, the GFR is usually indexed to some measure of body size, traditionally to 1.73 m^2 of body surface area, which in an earlier time was the average adult body surface area. In clinical practice, the assessment of GFR is most readily and reliably achieved using estimation equations, such as the Cockcroft-Gault equation or the Modification of Diet in Renal Disease (MDRD) Study equation. The Cockcroft-Gault equation calculates unadjusted creatinine clearance, using serum creatinine, age, gender, and body weight.[14] The formula was developed in 1976 from a sample of 249 men, and uses an empirical adjustment factor for women, based on a theoretical 15% lower muscle mass in women relative to men; the equation tends to overestimate renal function in subjects who are edematous or obese and underestimates renal function in the elderly.[15–18] The modified MDRD equation was developed from 1628 subjects enrolled in the baseline period of the MDRD study.[1] It estimates GFR adjusted to body surface area and is calculated from the subject's serum creatinine, age, race, and gender. Although mathematically somewhat complicated, it can be readily calculated with the aid of a simple computer or at several web sites [www.nephron.com; www.renal.org/eGFRcalc/GFR.pl; and www.kidney.org/professionals/KDOQI]. Ideally, estimated GFR (eGFR) should be reported automatically as part of the standardized biochemistry report, in conjunction with appropriate caveats as to its interpretation.[19–22] A new version of the formula has been developed

suitable for use with creatinine assay methods standardized to reference methods.[23,24] This demonstrates nearly unbiased estimates across all age groups, although, as with the original abbreviated MDRD equation, its accuracy remains limited in subjects with near-normal renal function.[15,25,26]

The MDRD equation has been independently validated in several different populations, including transplant recipients.[15,16,18,25,27–29] The equation underestimates GFR when it is normal or mildly reduced.[18,25,26,30] In addition, the source population will have an impact on the relationship between measured and eGFR.[24,26] Whether it is better to develop separate equations for different populations while correcting for limited GFR spread in healthy populations or to use a single equation and interpret the resulting estimated GFR with the source population and individual patient characteristics in mind is uncertain. A National Institutes of Health (NIH)–sponsored initiative, "The Chronic Kidney Disease Epidemiology Collaboration," is attempting to further refine the accuracy and precision of GFR estimation equations.[18] Regardless of the equation used, an additional major limitation to current clinical practice is the lack of standardization in serum creatinine assays,[13,31–33] levels of which can vary in clinically meaningful amounts between different laboratories and over time. Attempts to produce a uniform standard for serum creatinine is a major ongoing challenge in the early and reliable recognition of CKD.[33,34] An additional approach especially for the identification of early stages of kidney damage and in the elderly has been the measurement of cystatin C, which is superior to serum creatinine in being less dependent on muscle mass, age, sex, and race. This is a major advantage in predicting risk of events among elderly individuals with higher GFR.[35] For estimating GFR, cystatin C is superior to unadjusted serum creatinine measurements. Its advantage relative to creatinine-based estimation equations is less dramatic, and its utility in routine clinical practice requires further evaluation.[36] Cystatin C–based estimates of GFR will require knowledge of the source population in their interpretation, and there is evidence that organ receipients have higher cystatin C levels at the same GFR.[37]

For operational purposes, CKD is defined as the presence, for at least 3 months, of evidence of kidney damage with an abnormal GFR or, alternatively, by a GFR below 60 mL/min/1.73 m^2 body surface area.[1] A cutoff of 60 mL/min/1.73 m^2 is selected because it represents a decrement to approximately half of normal renal function and because its use avoids the classification of many older individuals who may have mild reductions in their GFR.[38] Whether such reductions truly represent a physiologic alteration or are the consequence of occult pathology is unknown. The accurate assessment of CKD is similarly difficult during and immediately after pregnancy, as GFR increases substantially during the first and second trimesters of pregnancy and may not return to its previous or new baseline level until several weeks postpartum.[39–42]

The NKF guidelines use a five-stage schema based on the reduction in GFR to help classify the severity of CKD. An international position statement added modifiers for noting whether a patient is treated with dialysis or transplantation (Table 17–1). The presence of hypertension should be noted independently of the CKD stage (Table 17–2). This staging system represents a measure of the "azotemic burden" resulting from the degree of kidney dysfunction, which is largely independent of the underlying etiology or renal pathology. Its use is validated by the established relationships between the number and the severity of complications that develop in parallel with increasing stage of CKD.[1] In essence, this staging system recognizes that the progressive decrement in renal function gives rise to common complications (e.g., hypertension, anemia, hyperparathyroidism) and management issues (e.g., hepatitis B vaccination, dietary modification, patient education) that are independent of the underlying condition that caused the kidney damage. This staging system complements and in no way replaces traditional classification schema, such as those based on clinical features (e.g., the presence and severity of proteinuria) or on pathophysiologic mechanisms (e.g., immune complex deposition on renal biopsy). These earlier classification systems provide important information regarding the rate of progression, long-term prognosis, and management of a given condition, whereas the CKD stage is informative regarding the likely complications and non–disease-specific management steps that relate to the current level of renal function.

Stage 5 CKD representing kidney failure is defined either by GFR below 15 mL/min/1.73 m² or by the need for dialysis. Following renal transplantation, patients are defined by the stage according to the posttransplant GFR.[43] It is unclear, however, whether the relationship between complications and CKD stage posttransplantation is identical to that reported with decrements in native kidney function. In a study of 459 renal transplant recipients, the definition of CKD was met in 90% of patients, with 60% of subjects having stage 3 CKD.[44] A higher stage was associated with significantly higher rates of hypertension, number of antihypertensive medications, and presence of anemia.

Incidence of Chronic Kidney Disease

Estimating the incidence of CKD requires a large cohort followed for many years with several estimates of kidney function. Among 2585 Framingham participants with baseline eGFR greater than 60, and a mean age of 43 years, 9.4% developed CKD, defined by eGFR less than 60, over a mean follow-up period of 18 years.[45] Risk was related to baseline GFR, diabetes, hypertension, low high-density lipoprotein (HDL) and smoking. Among 10,661 white and 3859 African American participants in the Atherosclerosis Risk in Communities (ARIC) study, age 45 to 64 years, the incidence of a 0.4 mg/dL rise in creatinine or hospitalization or death with CKD was 4.4/1000 person-years in whites and 8.8/1000 person-years in African Americans.[46] Risk was related to age, male gender, African American race, diabetes, hypertension, coronary heart disease at baseline, dyslipidemia, low GFR, elevated body mass index, and apo E genotype. Studies of CKD incidence are limited and complicated because creatinine assay calibration often changes over time by amounts of comparable magnitude to creatinine changes associated with the progression of CKD. Conversely, prevalence data are becoming more widely available.

Prevalence of Stages 1 to 4 Chronic Kidney Disease

The occurrence of kidney damage and CKD in the general population is important because only a minority of patients progress to kidney failure and are thereby identified on national ESRD registries. Instead, the majority of patients with CKD die from competing mortality[47,48] or else maintain relatively stable, although reduced, renal function[47,49] and suffer the consequences of CKD without ever progressing to the need for dialysis. Thus, ESRD registries provide only limited insight into the true burden of morbidity and mortality associated with CKD. Several challenges limit the better description of CKD in the absence of renal replacement therapy. The early stages of kidney dysfunction are often clinically silent, especially when the condition is only slowly progressive and complications have a gradual onset. The symptoms that do ultimately arise are usually nonspecific,

TABLE 17–1	**Stages of Chronic Kidney Disease**	
Stage	**Description**	**GFR (mL/min/1.73 m²)**
1	Kidney damage with normal or ↑ GFR	≥90
2	Kidney damage with mild ↓ GFR	60–89
3	Moderate ↓ GFR	30–59
4	Severe ↓ GFR	15–29
5	Kidney failure	<15 (or dialysis)

Chronic kidney disease is defined as either kidney damage or GFR <60 mL/min/1.73 m² for ≥3 months. Kidney damage is defined as pathologic abnormalities or markers of damage, including abnormalities in blood or urine tests or imaging studies.
From National Kidney Foundation: K/DOQI clinical practice guidelines for chronic kidney disease: Evaluation, classification and stratification. Am J Kidney Dis 39(suppl 1):S1–S266, 2002.

TABLE 17–2	**Definition and Stages of Chronic Kidney Disease**			
GFR (mL/min/1.73 m²)	**With Kidney Damage***		**Without Kidney Damage***	
	With HBP†	*Without HBP†*	*With HBP†*	*Without HBP†*
≥90	1	1	"High blood pressure"	"Normal"
60–89	2	2	"High blood pressure with ↓ GFR"	"↓ GFR"‡
30–59	3	3	3	3
15–29	4	4	4	4
<15 (or dialysis)	5	5	5	5

Shaded area represents chronic kidney disease; *numbers* designate state of chronic kidney disease.
*Kidney damage is defined as pathologic abnormalities or markers of damage, including abnormalities in blood or urine tests or imaging studies.
†High blood pressure (HBP) is defined as ≥140/90 in adults and >90th percentile for height and gender in children.
‡May be normal in infants and in the elderly.
From National Kidney Foundation: K/DOQI clinical practice guidelines for chronic kidney disease: Evaluation, classification and stratification. Am J Kidney Dis 39(suppl 1):S1–S266, 2002.

are often recognized late, and even then, are typically nonspecific and commonly attributed to comorbidities or age-related frailty.[50] As a consequence, hospital-based case series tend to be unrepresentative of the broader spectrum of CKD.

Table 17–3 summarizes the literature on the prevalence of decreased kidney function in large studies conducted recently.[4,11,51–64] Interpretation of the studies should take into account the source population, sampling methods, thresholds for defining different aspects of CKD, creatinine calibration, and the strong age dependence of measures of CKD. The latter is particularly strong because prevalence of disease can vary by an order of magnitude from young adults to older subgroups of the population. Large cross-sectional health surveys using probability sampling allow for estimates that represent the entire population (National Health and Nutrition Examination Survey [NHANES],[51] The Inter Asia study,[59] and AusDiab[4]). These estimates are least likely to be biased for common conditions but require a dedicated research setting. Alternatively, large amounts of data have been collected in screening programs of unselected groups (e.g., The Okinawa Screening Project[62]), high-risk subgroups (e.g., Kidney Early Evaluation Program [KEEP][54]), and the databases of large clinical practices or laboratories.[50,53,65,66] A major advantage of surveys of a random sample of the population is that, with the use of appropriately adjusted weights to control for nonresponse bias and missing data, they allow inferences to be drawn regarding the national prevalence of CKD. In addition, they provide relatively unbiased estimates of the concurrent complication rates. Such surveys have the limitation that, as they are cross-sectional, they measure prevalence, which represents both the rate of occurrence of new cases and the duration of established disease. Milder cases of longer duration due to either better survival or slow progression will influence prevalence more than incidence. To the extent that sicker individuals in stages 4 and 5 CKD are less likely to participate in surveys, prevalence estimates will be too low. The results of health screenings, especially if focused to a particular disease, may be strongly influenced by differential participation rates, with health-conscious subjects being more likely and those with less insight or interest in their long-term health being less likely to participate. Estimates based on clinical or laboratory databases are less informative because they require that the subject first come to medical attention, a major limitation in an often asymptomatic condition such as CKD.

All prevalence estimates show a strong age dependence consistent with the most common forms of CKD being progressive and increasing with age. Several of the initial studies examining the prevalence of CKD were based on elevated serum creatinine levels.[65,67–69] With the increased recognition of the many limitations of this approach, more recent surveys have instead used estimation equations with attention to creatinine assay calibration. The diagnosis of stages 1 and 2 CKD requires the presence of kidney damage in addition to a reduced GFR. From an epidemiologic perspective, the most commonly used surrogate for kidney damage in this setting has been albuminuria. Other potential markers of kidney

TABLE 17–3	Prevalence Studies of Chronic Kidney Disease							
Study	Source Population	Country or Region (age, yr)	N	Proteinuria/ Albuminuria (Cutoff) (%)	Hematuria (%)	GFR ≤ 60 mL/min/1.73 m²		
						Overall (%)	Age Dependence (%)	
NHANES III[51]	GP (PS)	US 1988–1994 (20+)	15,488	4.4 (>30 mg/g)	NA	4.4[c]	0.2–25.8	
NHANES 99–00[51]	GP (PS)	US 1999–2000 (20+)	4,101	5.6 (>30 mg/g)	NA	3.8[c]	0.5–23.1	
REGARDS[52]	GP (PS)	Southeastern US (45+)	20,667	NA	NA	43.3[c]	19.3–71.0	
Kaiser[53]	Clinical	US Northern California (20+)	1,120,295	NA	NA	17.5[c]	Strong	
KEEP[54]	High risk	US	11,246	32.5	3	14.9	Strong	
NEOERICA[55]	Clinical	UK region (0–90+)	28,862	NA	NA	4.9	0.2–33.4	
Salford[11]	Diabetes	UK Salford region (adult)	7,596	9	NA	27.5	Strong	
SAPALDIA[56]	GP (PS)	Swiss 1991 (adult)	6,317	NA	NA	NA	0–35	
HUNT II[57]	GP (Cohort)	Norway, Nord-Trondelag 1995–97 (20+)	65,181	5.9 (>30 mg/g)	NA	4.4[c]	0.2–18.6	
Ausdiab[4]	GP (PS)	Australia (25+)	11,247	2.4 (>200 mg/g)	4.6	11.2	0–54.8	
Aboriginies[58]	High risk (V)	Australia, Tiwi (18+)	237	44	—	12	Strong	
InterAsia[59]	GP (PS)	China (35–74)	15,540	NA	NA	2.5[c]	0.7–8.1	
Beijing[60]	GP (V)	China, Beijing (40+)	2,310	8.4 (S)	0.7	4.9[c]	0.3–11.5	
Okinawa[61]	GP (V)	Japan, Okinawa (30–79)	6,980	NA	NA	NA	NA	
Okinawa Screening[62]	GP (V)	Japan, Okinawa GHMA (20+)	95,255	47.4 (≥1+)	NA	42.6	Strong	
Karachi[63]	GP (V)	Pakistan, Karachi (40+)	1,166	NA	NA	10	6–21.2	
Thailand EGA[64]	Workplace	Thailand, Nonthaburi 1985 (35–55)	3,499	2.64 (1+)	NA	1.7	Strong	

Source population: GP, general population; PS, probability sampling survey design; V, volunteer sample; Cohort, an existing cohort; Clinical and Workplace populations without specific criteria are noted.
S, Albuminuria sex-specific definition: >17 mg/g in men and >25 mg/g in women.
[c], some calibration of the serum creatinine assay to the MDRD equation laboratory.
Age dependence shows the prevalence from youngest to the oldest age group studied.

damage include renal imaging[70] or hematuria, although the latter is less specific for CKD because the bleeding may often originate from the lower genitourinary tract rather than the kidney.

Over the last several years, the NHANES have provided a wealth of information regarding the prevalence of CKD and its complications within the United States. The third NHANES was conducted between 1998 and 1994 and included over 15,488 subjects who were older than 20 years and who had available laboratory data. The serum creatinine value that was used to estimate GFR was recalibrated to the original assay used to develop the MDRD equation. Kidney damage was identified using spot urine protein-to-creatinine ratios and adjusted for the estimated degree of persistence over time, based on results from a subsample of 1241 subjects who underwent repeat proteinuria testing approximately 2 weeks after the original test. Recent NHANES are carried out in 2-year intervals starting in 1999 to 2000 using similar methods as NHANES III. The smaller sample size ($n = 4101$) in 1999 to 2000 resulted in less precision in prevalence estimates. Updated results for NHANES 1999–2004 with calibration to standard creatinine should be available by 2008 and preliminary analysis suggest the prevalence of CKD has risen.

In NHANES III, the mean (standard error [se]) prevalence estimate for KDOQI-defined mild, moderate, and severe levels of decreased kidney function was 31.2% (0.78), 4.2% (0.25), and 0.19% (0.03).[51,71] In NHANES 1999 to 2000, the mean (se) prevalence of mildly reduced GFR had significantly increased to 36.3% (1.26), but estimates were otherwise similar for moderate and severe reductions in GFR at 3.7% (0.37) and 0.13% (0.06), respectively.[51] Both surveys showed similar declines in eGFR with age. In NHANES III, the median (95% confidence interval [CI]) eGFR for subjects aged 20 to 29 years was 113 mL/min/1.73 m^2 (112–114) and for those aged 70 years and above it was 75 ml/min/1.73 m^2 (73–77). Approximately one quarter of all subjects aged over 70 had an eGFR of below 60 mL/min/1.73 m^2. Decreased kidney function was more common in women than in men, but this difference disappeared with adjustment for age differences. Early stages of kidney damage were more common among non-Hispanic whites than among non-Hispanic blacks. Odds ratio of CKD in blacks as compared with whites, adjusted for age, gender, history of hypertension, use of hypertensive medications, and history of diabetes in normal, mild, moderate, and severe reductions in GFR were 1.0 (reference), 0.37 (0.32–0.43), 0.56 (0.44–0.71) and 1.1 (0.51–2.37), respectively.[71] Prevalence was lowest for Mexican Americans. The extent to which these differences from the pattern of ESRD incidence reflect limitations of equations to estimate GFR or a shorter duration due

to more rapid progression or poorer survival in different subgroups is uncertain.

In NHANES III, approximately 11.7% of subjects had abnormal urine albumin-to-creatinine ratios and the prevalence was higher at lower levels of kidney function. In the subsample of NHANES III that underwent repeat urine testing, macroalbuminuria always persisted on repeat testing, whereas microalbuminuria persisted in only 54% of patients with an eGFR of greater than 90 mL/min/1.73 m^2 and 73% of those with a GFR of 60 to 89. These findings may reflect an initial false-positive result, a subsequent false-negative result, or the presence of intermittent proteinuria—the significance of which is unknown. It is notable that, given the differences in muscle mass between the sexes, the urine protein-to-creatinine threshold level used to define microalbuminuria should ideally be gender specific, at approximately 17 to 250 mg/g creatinine in men and 25 to 355 mg/g creatinine in women.[72] Such gender specific cutoffs have not entered standard clinical practice. The most widely used non–gender-specific cutoff is an albumin-to-creatinine ratio greater than or equal to 30 mg/g for microalbuminuria. Using this cutoff, the overall prevalence of albuminuria rose significantly from 8.2% in 1988 to 1994 to 10.1% in 1999 to 2000, $P = .01$, and the estimated proportion of the U.S. population with CKD stages 1 to 4 was 8.8% in 1988 to 1994 and 9.4% in 1999 to 2000 (Table 17–4).

Internationally, it is clear that both proteinuria and decreased eGFR are quite common in many settings (see Table 17–3). However, it is hard to relate the prevalence of these markers of CKD to rates of ESRD due to methodologic differences between studies and different reports. A focused comparison of Norway to the United States revealed very similar prevalence rates of albuminuria and CKD stage 3, despite markedly higher treated ESRD incidence in the United States than in Norway. This suggests that factors determining progression from CKD to ESRD, not the least of which are treatment availability and patient management, will be important to understand.[57] It is also clear that CKD prevalence rates are substantial in countries with low income in which ESRD treatment is very limited or not available, such as Pakistan.[63]

Incidence of End-Stage Renal Disease in the United States

Much more precise data are available on the occurrence of treated ESRD compared with earlier stages of CKD. In the United States, ESRD is tracked by the U.S. Renal Disease

TABLE 17–4	**Trends in the Prevalence of Chronic Kidney Disease in the U.S.**				
CKD		**Prevalence (%)**		**Prevalence Ratio (95% CI)[†]**	**No. in U.S. in 2000,[‡] Thousands (95% CI)**
Stage	**Description**	**1988–1994***	**1999–2000***		
1	GFR ≥90 and persistent albuminuria[†]	2.2	2.8	1.26 (1.00–1.59)	5,600 (4,000–7,200)
2	GFR 60–89 and persistent albuminuria[†]	2.2	2.8	1.27 (1.00–1.61)	5,700 (4,200–7,200)
3	GFR 30–59	4.2	3.7	0.88 (0.67–1.10)	7,400 (6,000–8,900)
4	GFR 15–29	0.19	0.13[§]	0.68 (0.07–1.44)	300 (24–500)
Total	Stages 1–4	8.8	9.4	1.07 (0.93–1.22)	19,000 (16,300–21.600)

ACR, albumin-to-creatinine ratio; CKD, chronic kidney disease; CI, confidence interval; GFR in ml/min per 1.73 m^2; MEC, mobile examination center; NHANES, National Health and Nutrition Examination Survey.

*MEC examined respondents with nonmissing serum creatinine measures and estimated GFR >15 and for albuminuria nonmissing ACR data, nonpregnant and not in menses.

[†]Bootstrap CI estimates include variability in the persistence estimates of albuminuria but assume persistence to be the same in the two surveys.

[‡]Based on NHANES 1999–2000 prevalence and 200,948,641 adults age 20 yr and older in 2000 census.

[§]From Coresh J, Byrd-Holt D, Astor BC, et al: Chronic kidney disease awareness, prevalence, and trends among U.S. adults, 1999 to 2000. J Am Soc Nephrol 16(1):180–188, 2005.

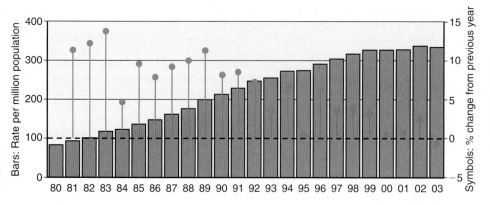

FIGURE 17-1 Adjusted U.S. incidence rates of ESRD and annual percent change. (From U.S. Renal Data System: USRDS 2005 Annual Data Report: Atlas of End-Stage Renal Disease in the United States. Bethesda, MD, National Institutes of Health, National Institute of Diabetes and Digestive and Kidney Diseases, 2005, p 68.)

Registry (USRDS) and detailed reports are published annually. The 2005 report includes data up until 2003 and is the year referred to in the following text, unless otherwise stated. In that year, 102,567 new patients commenced treatment with renal replacement therapy in the United States, equivalent to an age-, gender-, and race-adjusted rate of 338 per million population (pmp). Throughout most of the 1980s and early 1990s, the incidence of ESRD increased by 5% to 10% over consecutive years, resulting in an adjusted incidence rate for 1981, 1991, and 2001 of 91, 223, and 334 pmp, respectively (Fig. 17–1). However, in the last several years, this rate of increase has leveled off, and in 2003, for the first time, the adjusted incidence rate actually decreased, albeit marginally, by 2 pmp. The rate for 2004 has decreased by 0.9%. Despite this recent stabilization in the ESRD incidence rate, the absolute number of patients commencing renal replacement therapy continues to rise, increasing by 2% in 2003, in keeping with the overall population aging and growth, particularly among minorities within the United States. Furthermore, even with the stabilization of the incidence rate, on the basis of the anticipated demographic changes in general population and of the sustained increase in diabetes, it is estimated that, by 2015, the incidence (95% CI) rate for ESRD will have increased to 136,166 (110,989–164,550) cases per year.[73]

Trends and Determinants of End-Stage Renal Disease Incidence Rates

The reasons underlying the epidemic growth in incident ESRD and the more recent stabilization of this trend are not completely understood. The incidence of renal replacement therapy will vary with the prevalence of CKD in the general population, the rate of progression of CKD to ESRD, the rate of acceptance of patients onto renal replacement programs, and effects of competing causes of mortality, which result in the death of patients prior to the initiation of dialysis. Furthermore, the relative impact of these different factors with regard to increasing incidence may differ substantially by race.[74]

PREVALENCE OF CHRONIC KIDNEY DISEASE. As described earlier, the prevalence of CKD in the general U.S. population as estimated from the NHANES has not demonstrated the dramatic increase seen in ESRD prevalence. Whereas recent analysis of 12,866 enrollees of the Multiple Risk Factor Intervention Trial (MRFIT) study confirmed that the presence of proteinuria and a low GFR (<60) were strongly and independently associated with the 25-year risk of developing ESRD,[75] it is clear that only a minority of such patients progress to ESRD, with the remainder presumably demonstrating relatively stable or only slowly deteriorating renal function[47,49] or else succumbing to competing mortality.[47,48] The last 2 decades have witnessed an epidemic growth in the number of subjects with type 2 diabetes, typically in association with

obesity and increasingly sedentary lifestyles within the population.[76] Given the relatively slow natural history of diabetic glomerulosclerosis, it is possible that we are only beginning to see the impact of this increase in diabetes on the occurrence of kidney failure and that this may in part be responsible for the increased prevalence of proteinuria and early stages of CKD seen in NHANES 1999 to 2000 relative to the 1988 to 1994 survey.[51] Thus, although changes in the prevalence of CKD do not appear to explain the dramatic growth in ESRD seen over the last 2 decades, there is the ominous possibility that an increased prevalence of diabetes will considerably escalate future rates. Ethnic differences in CKD prevalence rates reflect differences in CKD and ESRD incidence rates, as discussed previously.[51,71,77] U.S. NHANES data through 2004 should be published in 2008.

RATE OF PROGRESSION OF CHRONIC KIDNEY DISEASE. The rate of progression of CKD is influenced by a wide range of potentially modifiable risk factors, including blood pressure control[78-81]; proteinuria[80,82]; hyperglycemia[83-85]; dietary intake[82,86,87]; obesity[88]; the activity of the renin-angiotensin-aldosterone system[89-91]; smoking[15,92-95]; illicit drug use[96]; socioeconomic factors, including issues such as access to care[97-101]; and possibly hyperlipidemia[102,103] and anemia[104]; as well as exposure to potential environmental or industrial toxins.[105,106] Multiple opportunities thereby exist to intervene and change the natural history of the renal decline, especially through the focus of tight blood pressure control and inhibition of the renin-angiotensin-aldosterone system. It is suggested that the recent improvement in the incidence rate of ESRD seen in the USRDS reflects better secondary prevention of kidney damage, such as through the increased use of angiotensin-converting enzyme (ACE) inhibition, as well as better glycemic and overall blood pressure management.[66] In keeping with this, the incidence rates of ESRD for type 1 diabetes have steadily declined over the last decades in U.S. whites, though not in blacks.[66] In a Finnish cohort of all patients with type 1 diabetes, diagnosed between 1965 and 1999 (n = 20,005), and followed for a total of 346,851 patient-years, the incidence of ESRD decreased steadily over time; the relative risk for ESRD in 1965 to 1969, 1970 to 1974, 1975 to 1979, and 1980 to 1999 was 1.0 (reference), 0.78, 0.72, and 0.47, respectively, (P trend <.001).[107] The control of type 2 diabetes, which is by far the more common form of diabetes, is much more problematic, in part due to the fact that it represents a combined glycemic, ischemic, and hypertensive renal injury as well as presenting a far greater challenge in early recognition and appropriate management.

The race- and age-adjusted incidence of ESRD is higher in men (413 pmp) than in women (280 pmp), a differential that has increased over time (Fig. 17–2). Whereas several studies have suggested that women progress less quickly to ESRD than do men,[108,109] an observation that is supported by several animal models,[110] this has not been a uniform finding in all human studies.[111] Indeed, in a patient level meta-analysis of trials of nondiabetic subjects examining the effect of ACE inhibition on progression of CKD, the mean systolic blood pressure and proteinuria were greater in women than in men. There was no significant difference in the rate of progression by gender in an unadjusted analysis, the relative risk being 0.98. However, after adjustment for baseline variables, changes in ACE inhibitor use, and changes in blood pressure over follow up, the relative risk (95% CI) for progression in females compared with males was 1.36 (1.06–1.75).[112] As the mean (standard deviation [sd]) age of women in this study was 53 (13), the majority of the women were likely to have been post-menopausal, and these observations may not extend to younger women. In light of these results, whether the lower incidence of ESRD in women relative to men represents a true biologic effect of gender or is the result of underdiagnosis or undertreatment of ESRD in women requires further evaluation.

ACCEPTANCE FOR DIALYSIS. The occurrence of renal failure increases dramatically with increasing age. The race- and gender-adjusted treated ESRD incidence rate is currently almost 30-fold higher for those in their 8th decade of life (1703 pmp) compared with those in their 20s (58 pmp) (Fig. 17–3). Traditionally, older subjects, especially those with significant comorbidities, may not have been offered or may not have been willing to accept dialysis. More recently, whether because of better management of comorbidities, higher patient expectations, or greater availability of renal replacement therapy, this has substantially changed. Whereas the adjusted, age-specific incidence rate for those younger than 65 has decreased since 2000 (currently 606 pmp), the rate for those aged 65 to 74 and those older than 74 years has continued to steadily increase and is currently 1435 pmp and 1687 pmp, respectively. The hypothesis that part of this sustained increase has been due to the acceptance of older and sicker patients onto renal replacement programs is supported by the increased burden of comorbidities, indicated by administrative billing codes in a random 5% of Medicare enrollees.[66] Increased acceptance of patients onto dialysis is less likely to contribute to the increase seen in younger subjects, the majority of whom have traditionally been offered dialysis, if deemed medically appropriate.

COMPETING MORTALITY. The mortality rates for patients with advanced CKD prior to initiation of renal replacement therapy are very high.[47,48] This has a dramatic potential influence on the numbers of patients with progressive kidney disease who survive long enough to require dialysis. Analysis linking NHANES and USRDS data estimated that improved survival from myocardial infarction and stroke explained only 4.8% of the increase in incident ESRD from 1978 to 1991 compared with 28% due to the higher prevalence of diabetes and 8% from U.S. population growth.[113] However, the time period examined may have predated the period of increased recognition and better management of patients with CKD, and similarly, this analysis does not quantify the effects of the primary prevention of cardiovascular disease or competing mortality from other causes such as infection or cancer.

Variation in End-Stage Renal Disease Incidence Rates

Adjusted ESRD incidence rate differs substantially by race, with African Americans having a 3.5-fold higher age- and gender-adjusted incidence rate (996 pmp) than do whites (259 pmp); rates for Native Americans (504 pmp) are midway between those of whites and blacks; and the rate in Asians (346 pmp) is closer to that of whites (see Fig. 17–3). One examination of the excess risk of ESRD in blacks compared with whites suggests differences in socioeconomic factors explained 12%, lifestyle differences 24%, and clinical differences 32%, whereas all three groups of factors combined explained 44% of this excess risk. Thus, some but not all of the excess risk in blacks compared with whites is understood.[101] Some of this unexplained excess may relate to residual confounding, owing to imprecision in the measurement of known risk factors; however, it is possible that some of the

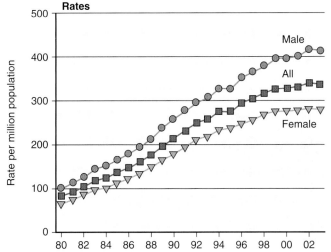

FIGURE 17–2 Adjusted U.S. incidence rates of ESRD by gender. (From U.S. Renal Data System: USRDS 2005 Annual Data Report: Atlas of End-Stage Renal Disease in the United States. Bethesda, MD, National Institutes of Health, National Institute of Diabetes and Digestive and Kidney Diseases, 2005, p 68.)

FIGURE 17–3 Adjusted U.S. ESRD incidence rates by age and race/ethnicity. (From U.S. Renal Data System: USRDS 2005 Annual Data Report: Atlas of End-Stage Renal Disease in the United States. Bethesda, MD, National Institutes of Health, National Institute of Diabetes and Digestive and Kidney Diseases, 2005, p 36.)

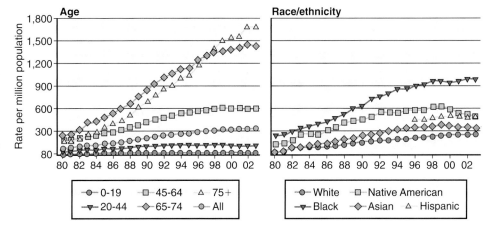

unexplained excess relates to genetic factors and/or to genetic-environmental interactions. The observation of higher rates of kidney failure, in many cases from different etiologies, in some families; especially within African Americans, further supports a genetic component to this increased risk.[114,115] The age- and gender-adjusted incidence rate is similarly higher in Hispanics (496 pmp) than in those of non-Hispanic ethnicity (323 pmp).

Substantial geographical variability exists in the adjusted ESRD incidence rate, with over 2.5-fold difference in incidence rates despite adjusting for demographic differences; the rate is highest in South Dakota (411 pmp) and lowest in Wyoming (166 pmp). Incidence rates are also significantly higher in urban than in rural settings. This may be due to a movement of patients on treatment from rural to urban environments or to limited access to care in rural settings, with reduced opportunities for disease recognition and management. Similar findings were observed in a nested case-control study of patients developing ESRD based on an NHANES II study in which living in a more heavily populated than a less heavily populated area was associated with a relative risk of kidney failure (95% CI) of 4.33 (2.09–8.97).[116]

Prevalence of End-Stage Renal Disease in the United States

In 2003, a total of 324,826 patients were treated with renal replacement therapy in the United States, equivalent to a rate per million population of 1496. The prevalence of ESRD has grown consistently over the last several decades, as a result of both the increased incidence rate and better survival rates. The current prevalence is five times higher than in 1980. However, more recently, as seen with the incidence rate, the rate of increase has stabilized, with recent annual increases of less than 4% per year (Fig. 17–4). Prevalence rates are higher in urban than in rural areas and vary substantially across states, with the highest rates seen in the Southwest and Midwest.[66]

The median age of the prevalent ESRD population is 58.2 years, and it has remained relatively constant over the last decade; it is 6.6 years younger than the average age of persons starting dialysis, owing to the higher mortality in older patients. Whereas the prevalence rate for those younger than 65 has remained stable over the last decade, the rate for those aged 65 to 74 (5300 pmp) has increased by two thirds, and for those aged 75 years and older (4609 pmp) has nearly doubled (Fig. 17–5). However, owing to the age structure of the underlying general U.S. population, in terms of actual number of patients, the highest count is for those aged 45 to 64, whose prevalence rate has been consistently between 37 and 42 pmp over the last 2 decades.

There is a slightly larger differential between blacks and whites with regard to the age and gender-adjusted prevalence—4700 pmp versus 1096 pmp, a 4-fold difference—as compared with the incidence rate, for which there is a 3.5-fold differential. The difference is due to better survival rates among blacks on dialysis. The adjusted prevalence rate for Hispanics is 46% higher than for non-Hispanics and mirrors the difference in their respective incidence rate, whereas the prevalence in men (1806 pmp) is 1.5-fold higher than in women (1242 pmp).

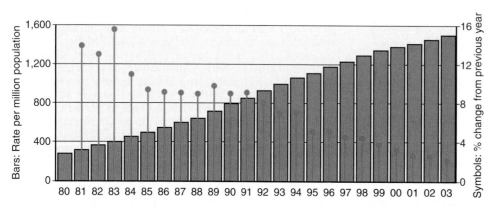

FIGURE 17–4 Adjusted U.S. prevalence rates of ESRD and annual percent change. (From U.S. Renal Data System: USRDS 2005 Annual Data Report: Atlas of End-Stage Renal Disease in the United States. Bethesda, MD, National Institutes of Health, National Institute of Diabetes and Digestive and Kidney Diseases, 2005, p 72.)

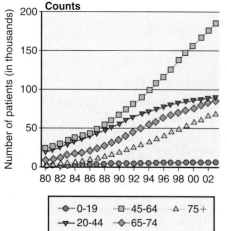

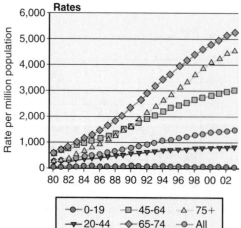

FIGURE 17–5 Prevalent U.S. ESRD counts and adjusted rates by age. (From U.S. Renal Data System: USRDS 2005 Annual Data Report: Atlas of End-Stage Renal Disease in the United States. Bethesda, MD, National Institutes of Health, National Institute of Diabetes and Digestive and Kidney Diseases, 2005, p 72.)

Incidence and Prevalence of End-Stage Renal Disease: Global Comparisons

The occurrence of ESRD varies widely between different countries and, on many occasions, within different regions of the same country (Fig. 17–6). In addition to variability in the general factors that determine the incidence of ESRD, which are discussed previously, international comparison of incidence and prevalence rates may be complicated by different

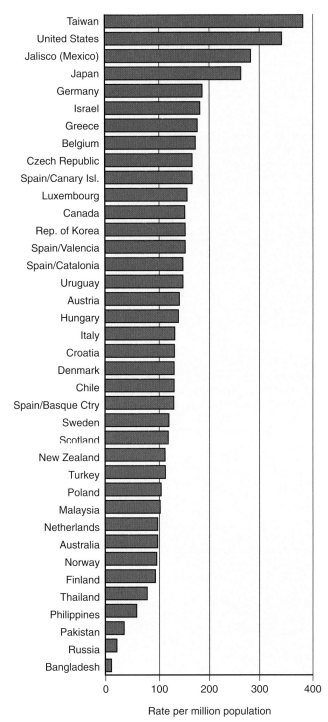

FIGURE 17–6 International comparison of ESRD incidence rates in 2003. (From U.S. Renal Data System: USRDS 2005 Annual Data Report: Atlas of End-Stage Renal Disease in the United States. Bethesda, MD, National Institutes of Health, National Institute of Diabetes and Digestive and Kidney Diseases, 2005, p 218.)

administrative definitions of ESRD and in the classification of the underlying cause of kidney failure, as well as by variability in the completeness and accuracy of the reported data. As a result, direct comparison of the data from different national registries must be undertaken with caution. However, within these limitations, the increase in ESRD in Europe has mirrored the U.S. experience, although absolute rates are lower. It is as yet unclear whether the rising incidence of ESRD in Europe is starting to slow, as has occurred in the United States in the last several years.[117]

The age- and gender-adjusted incidence rates for Western Europe between 1990 and 1999 increased 47% from 79.4 pmp in 1990 up to 117 pmp in 1998. Thus, the age- and gender-adjusted incidence rates in Europe are about one third those of the United States. The incidence rates in Western Europe increased linearly by approximately 4.8% per year. As occurred in the United States, rates increased faster in men than in women and were more marked in older age groups. Incidence in those aged over 75 increased 3-fold from 141 to 540 pmp; as in the United States, there is widespread variability between countries in Europe, especially for older subjects. During the 1990s, the incidence rate for patients older than 75 increased 2-fold in the Netherlands, 6.5-fold in Scotland, 9-fold in Denmark, and 30-fold in Finland.[117]

The annual incidence rate of ESRD in Japan increased roughly threefold between 1982 (81 pmp) and 2001 (252 pmp). The unadjusted rate in Taiwan is similar to that of the United States (331 pmp) and has continued to increase at almost double the U.S. rate over the last several years.[66] The unadjusted incidence rate in Australia and New Zealand is considerably less than the aforementioned rates at 92 and 107 pmp, respectively.[118] In Australia, the annual incidence rates increased by twofold. This is largely reflected in the increase of those aged over 65, with rates of those younger than 65 being relatively stable. As in the United States, racial minorities in people of native descent such as the Australian Aboriginals or the New Zealand Maori islanders bear a disproportionate degree of the overall burden of ESRD.[119]

DIALYSIS MODALITY

In 2003, 91% of the incident U.S. ESRD population were treated with hemodialysis, 7% by peritoneal dialysis, and 2% by preemptive transplantation. Of the prevalent population, 65.5% are treated by in-center hemodialysis, 0.3% by home hemodialysis, 5.7% by peritoneal dialysis (2.5% with cycler-based therapy, 3.2% with manual, noncycler therapy), and 28.5% with transplantation. There has been a renewed interest in the potential benefits of more frequent dialysis, using short daily dialysis or quotidian nocturnal dialysis, spurred by promising initial results from what have, in general, been small and poorly controlled studies.[120–126] This has led to the establishment of an NIH trial to quantify the potential benefits of more frequent dialysis.[127]

Substantial racial differences exist in renal replacement therapy; white patients make up 55% of prevalent hemodialysis patients but 75% of the prevalent transplant population; African Americans account for 38% of prevalent hemodialysis population but only 18% of the transplant population. Over the last decade, substantial changes in dialysis provider characteristics have occurred in the United States with a sustained growth in large dialysis corporations. Currently, approximately 63% of prevalent hemodialysis and 60% of prevalent peritoneal dialysis patients are dialysed in a chain-owned facility, percentages that have increased from 52% and 47%, respectively, 5 years ago (Fig. 17–7). These large chains, the majority of which are for-profit corporations, clearly have an enormous influence on practice patterns and outcomes in ESRD patients, for better or for worse. Concerns

CH 17

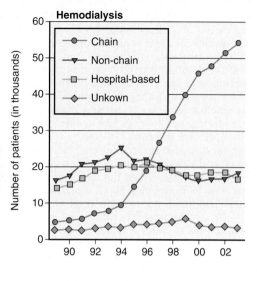

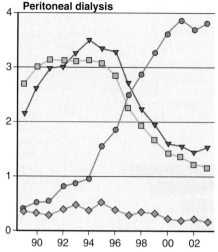

FIGURE 17–7 Incident dialysis patient counts in the United States by first modality and unit type. (From U.S. Renal Data System: USRDS 2005 Annual Data Report: Atlas of End-Stage Renal Disease in the United States. Bethesda, MD, National Institutes of Health, National Institute of Diabetes and Digestive and Kidney Diseases, 2005, p 104.)

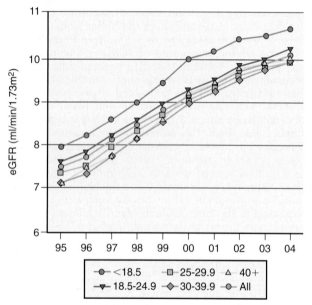

FIGURE 17–8 Estimated GFR (eGFR) at initiation of ESRD treatment in the United States by body mass index (kg/m²). (From U.S. Renal Data System: USRDS 2005 Annual Data Report: Atlas of End-Stage Renal Disease in the United States. Bethesda, MD, National Institutes of Health, National Institute of Diabetes and Digestive and Kidney Diseases, 2005, p 92.)

have been raised that the latter effect is more likely and that a for-profit chain affiliation may be associated with decreased indicators of quality of care, such as the probability of entering the transplant wait list[128] and higher adjusted mortality rates compared with those of not-for-profit institutions, relative hazard (95% CI): 1.08 (1.04–1.13), P < .001.[129]

DIALYSIS SURVIVAL

Improved survival rates have contributed to the increased number of prevalent patients on dialysis. In 2003, the number of new patients exceeded by 17,911 the number of established patients who died. The adjusted mortality rate (adjusted for age, race, ethnicity, gender, primary renal diagnosis, and years on dialysis) decreased from 224.3/1000 patient-years at risk in 1993 to 210.7/1000 patient-years in 2003, a 6.1% reduction. Some of this difference may reflect a recent secular trend toward earlier initiation of dialysis with better preserved GFR (Fig. 17–8) with the resulting potential for "lead

time bias" in the comparisons of survival rates from earlier time periods. Against this, early initiation of dialysis has not to date been shown to improve survival[130] and is typically associated with greater degrees of comorbidity, with sicker patients needing to commence dialysis earlier. However, the determination of incident comorbidity is based on the Center for Medicaid and Medicare Services "Medical Evidence Form" (Form 2728), which at least initially was relatively inaccurate and insensitive.[131] More recently, the policy to publish the outcomes of individual dialysis units, which are adjusted for comorbidity using the information provided in Form 2728, has provided a powerful incentive for units to more accurately and fully report comorbidity. Thus, although it is likely that the current incident population has more comorbidities than was historically the case, reliably quantifying this effect is difficult.

The overwhelming primary cause of death in patients treated with dialysis is due to premature and often accelerated cardiovardiovascular disease. In recognition of this, a recent position statement from the American Heart Association recommended that patients with ESRD be considered to be at "highest risk" with regard to future cardiovascular events.[132] Moreover, overwhelming evidence now indicates that the entire spectrum of CKD is associated with increased rates of cardiovascular disease.[133–135] Some of the absolute increase in cardiovascular risk seen with reduced renal function is the result of the very high prevalence of traditional Framingham risk factors in patients with CKD.[136,137] In early CKD, these traditional risk factors appear to have the same relationship with cardiovascular disease as has been described in the general population,[137] but in ESRD, the relationship for some risk factors, most notably hypertension and cholesterol, alters and becomes more U shaped, with lower in addition to higher levels being associated with higher risk. It has been postulated that this increased risk of cardiovascular disease seen with low levels of total cholesterol[138,139] and low blood pressure levels[140–142] may be due to reverse causation and the presence of uncontrolled confounding. Although some authors have referred to this observation as "reverse epidemiology," the term is somewhat misleading because, by definition, observational studies can only demonstrate the presence of an association and thus are unable to directly determine causality, be it in a forward or a reverse direction.

In addition to traditional risk factors, a wide array of novel cardiovascular risk factors cluster in CKD and are implicated in increased cardiovascular risk. A wealth of observational data has associated the presence of anemia with poor cardiovascular outcomes. However, the currently available clinical trial evidence suggests that much of this association is not directly causal in nature.[143–146] Thus, whereas the correction of anemia remains a cornerstone of the management of CKD with regard to symptom control and quality of life issues, there remains to date no convincing evidence that extending erythropoietin therapy to beyond its current targets exerts a cardioprotective effect. A major potential confounder of the association of anemia with cardiovascular disease is the presence of inflammation and associated malnutrition, both of which are powerful predictors of poor long-term survival on dialysis.[147–149] With the initiation of dialysis, nutritional status typically improves but then often slowly deteriorates over time with increasing dialysis vintage.[150,151] Strategies to counteract this progressive nutritional deterioration are currently lacking. It is of note, however, that despite the negative effects of obesity on long-term health in the general population and the transplant population,[152,153] obese dialysis patients have better outcomes relative to nonoverweight subjects.[154,155] This may relate to obese subjects effectively having a better nutritional reserve at the start of dialysis or obesity marking patients with fewer comorbidities that result in weight loss. Thus, the mechanisms and ramifications of this paradoxical association require further exploration.

The mortality rate seen with CKD reflects both an increased prevalence of cardiovascular disease and an increased case fatality rate. The latter may result from the severity of the cardiovascular disease, the presence of extensive comorbidities, or a greater degree of therapeutic nihilism in the management of patients with CKD. Several studies have supported this last contention.[156–159]

Mortality rates in ESRD steadily increase with increasing age, from 102/1000 patient-years in 20- to 44-year-olds to 427/1000 patient-years for those older than 75. The 2003 crude mortality rate for males and females was 229.4 and 239.3, with adjusted rates of 210.9 and 211.1; both the crude and the adjusted rates are higher for whites than for blacks. The adjusted mortality rate is significantly worse for those whose primary renal diagnosis is diabetes (253/1000 patient-years) compared with those whose cause of ESRD is attributed to hypertension (194/1000 patient-years) or glomerulonephritis (157/1000 patient-years).

Modality-specific mortality rates for 2001 to 2003 were 194.7/1000 patient-years in peritoneal dialysis compared with 235.4/1000 patient-years for hemodialysis. Considerable caution is needed in interpreting these data. Despite being adjusted for demographic characteristics, the data nevertheless suffer from a major degree of persistent confounding owing to the substantial differences in clinical characteristics between the two modalities at initiation of dialysis, both in terms of comorbidity and in level of residual renal function.[160,161] In addition, these analyses do not control for switches in dialysis modality over time, with substantially more switching occurring for sick subjects from peritoneal dialysis to hemodialysis than vice versa. A moderately sized prospective observational cohort study compared survival in peritoneal dialysis and hemodialysis among subjects in the mid and late 1990s and reported worse apparent survival for the peritoneal dialysis group when controlling for many of the parameters previously discussed.[162] However, these reports predate the more recent developments in clinical practice and the introduction of newer, more biocompatible dialysate solutions.[163] Observational studies cannot prove causation, particularly in the face of strong confounding. However, a randomized interventional trial to definitively compare modalities is unlikely to be conducted.

More recent USRDS data suggest that the age-, race-, and gender-adjusted 5-year mortality difference between hemodialysis and peritoneal dialysis has decreased over time (Fig. 17–9). This improvement has been more marked in peritoneal dialysis, in which crude mortality has reduced by 12% since 1985 compared with an 8% reduction over the same time period for hemodialysis. The mortality rate for diabetics initiating peritoneal dialysis in 1994 to 1998 (22.8%) was lower than for those initiating hemodialysis (26.7%). For nondiabetics, 5-year survival rates were better in peritoneal dialysis (41.1%) than for hemodialysis (39%). Whether these improvements reflect a secular change in selection criteria, as the numbers of patients treated with peritoneal dialysis has decreased over time, or whether it is indeed a result of improved medical management or technical advance remains speculative.

The general trend toward overall improvements in survival rates in both dialysis modalities over the last 2 decades obscures significant technique-specific interactions between mortality rates and duration on dialysis (vintage) (Fig. 17–10). In hemodialysis, prior to 1993, mortality rates were substan-

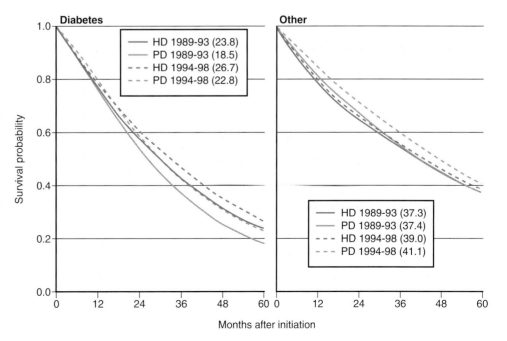

FIGURE 17–9 Adjusted 5-year survival of U.S. incident dialysis patients by modality and primary diagnosis. HD, hemodialysis; PD, peritoneal dialysis. (From U.S. Renal Data System: USRDS 2005 Annual Data Report: Atlas of End-Stage Renal Disease in the United States. Bethesda, MD, National Institutes of Health, National Institute of Diabetes and Digestive and Kidney Diseases, 2005, p 131.)

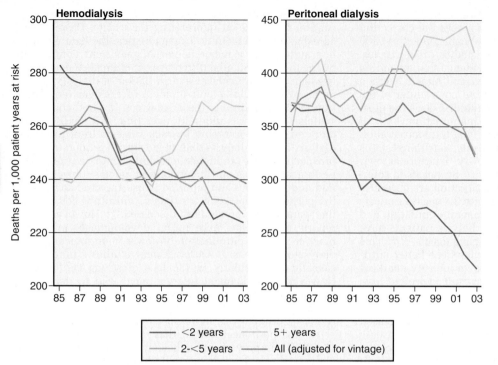

FIGURE 17–10 Adjusted all-cause mortality in U.S. prevalent dialysis patients by number of years on dialysis (vintage) and calendar year. (From U.S. Renal Data System: USRDS 2005 Annual Data Report: Atlas of End-Stage Renal Disease in the United States. Bethesda, MD, National Institutes of Health, National Institute of Diabetes and Digestive and Kidney Diseases, 2005, p 131.)

tially higher for those who had been dialyzed for less than 2 years compared with those who had been on therapy for more than 5 years. In 1993, the rates for the two vintages were approximately similar. Since that time, mortality rates for those treated for less than 2 years have progressively declined, and for those of older vintage have steadily risen. In peritoneal dialysys, the 1985 mortality rate was similar for those dialyzed less than 2 years and for those dialyzed for more than 5 years, and since that date, mortality in the less than 2-year vintage patients has decreased while that of those dialyzed for longer than 5 years has increased. The improvement has been attributed to efforts such as improvements in pre-ESRD care and widespread provision of higher dialysis doses, although whether these associations are causal or coincidental is unproved. The trend toward poorer longer-term survival is concerning. It was unclear whether this reflected a carry-over effect from earlier periods of possibly less optimal clinical practice or if it suggests that recent improvements were merely postponing mortality to a slightly later time period. However, the most recent USRDS report found that rates for older vintages have actually stabilized in hemodialysis patients and are decreasing in peritoneal dialysis subjects. Further data are required to see if this trend continues.

The USRDS tracks survival of incident patients, starting from 90 days following initiation of dialysis. A general trend is evident in the all-cause as well as for both cardiovascular-specific and infectious-specific mortality rates for event rates to peak at approximately 6 months of follow-up by USRDS (i.e., approximately 9 months after the initiation of dialysis). Rates sharply decline over the following 3 to 6 months, with a subsequent more gradual increase in mortality. These trends have persisted over time, although at lower absolute rates. Patients on peritoneal dialysis tend to have lower initial event rates than in those treated with hemodialysis, but have no initial fall, instead demonstrating a monotonic trend toward increasing event rates over time. Understanding the degree to which these differences represent differences in clinical practices as opposed to being the result of different selection biases is important.

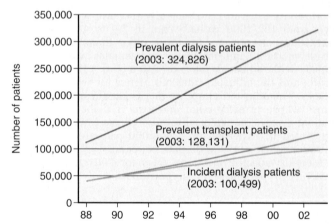

FIGURE 17–11 Incident and prevalent U.S. dialysis patient counts and prevalent transplant patient counts. (From U.S. Renal Data System: USRDS 2005 Annual Data Report: Atlas of End-Stage Renal Disease in the United States. Bethesda, MD, National Institutes of Health, National Institute of Diabetes and Digestive and Kidney Diseases, 2005, p 67.)

The overall impact that having ESRD has on long-term patient outcomes is perhaps most clearly seen in the examination of estimated remaining years of life. When adjusted for gender, the expected remaining life span for a 60- to 64-year-old white dialysis patient is 3.9 years, less than one fifth that of a similarly aged member of the general population (20.5 yr), and the estimated remaining years of life for a similarly aged black subject (4.9 yr) is less than one quarter that of a similarly aged black subject without ESRD (18.5 yr).

TRANSPLANTATION

In 2003, 14,853 renal transplants were performed in the United States. The number of transplants has slowly increased over time. However, this increase has been overshadowed by the far greater increase in the number of patients starting dialysis (Fig. 17–11). Thus, in 2003, the number of patients

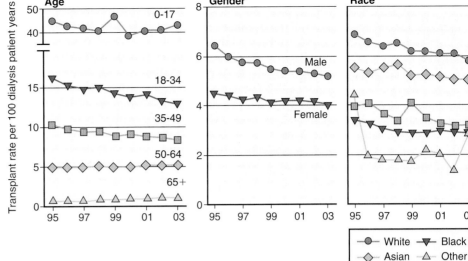

FIGURE 17–12 Transplantation rates in the United States by age, gender, and race. N Am, North American. (From U.S. Renal Data System: USRDS 2005 Annual Data Report: Atlas of End-Stage Renal Disease in the United States. Bethesda, MD, National Institutes of Health, National Institute of Diabetes and Digestive and Kidney Diseases, 2005, p 148.)

transplanted (16,043) was one seventh the number of patients who commenced renal replacement therapy and two thirds the number of patients (23,488) who were added to the transplant waiting list. The transplantation rate, expressed as transplants per 100 wait-listed patient-years has decreased to 5.7 in 2003, resulting in longer median wait-list times. Median wait-list time has progressively increased over the last decade, with little variation by gender and substantially shorter wait-list times in whites than in other racial groups (Fig. 17–12).

Transplant rates are highest in patients aged less than 18 years and decrease with advancing age. Rates have remained relatively constant in subjects aged less than 50 years but have doubled over the last decade in those aged 50 to 64 and tripled in those aged 65 and older. Striking gender and racial inequalities remain in current transplant rates, with male patients being wait listed and transplanted relatively more frequently than females and white patients being severalfold more likely to receive a transplant than African Americans. These racial disparities in transplantation rates appear to stem from both clinical characteristics that appropriately influence the subjects candidacy for transplantation and apparent overutilization in whites and underutilization in blacks.[164] These inequalities have narrowed somewhat over time as transplant rates in whites and males have decreased, while those in blacks and in women have remained steady. Similar racial inequalities are evident on a global basis. Indigenous Australians represent less than 2% of the Australian population, account for 8% to 10% of incident dialysis patients, but receive transplants at only one third the rate of nonindigenous patients.[119] There is also widespread geographic variability in rates of transplant wait listing, median wait-list times, and transplantation rates, with an over twofold difference in transplantation rates between states. Transplantation rates are highest in the upper Midwest states such as Iowa and Minnesota. These differentials have led some patients to be listed in multiple organ procurement areas.

Much of the increase in the absolute number of transplants performed in the United States over the last decade is a result of an increase in living donation rates, now representing over 50% of transplant donations (Fig. 17–13). Living donation has the advantages of planned elective surgery, reduced cold ischemia time, decreased wait-list time, and closer human leukocyte antigen (HLA) matching.[165] Living kidney donation has excellent outcomes when there is less optimal HLA matching, as may occur with unrelated donors.[166] Live dona-

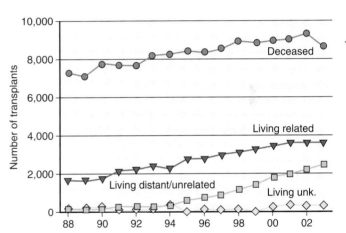

FIGURE 17–13 Number of transplants in the United States by donor type. Living unk, living unknown. (From U.S. Renal Data System: USRDS 2005 Annual Data Report: Atlas of End-Stage Renal Disease in the United States. Bethesda, MD, National Institutes of Health, National Institute of Diabetes and Digestive and Kidney Diseases, 2005, p 147.)

tion is not without risk to the donor.[167] As a result, careful physical and psychological evaluation of potential donors is necessary. Some of this risk may be counterbalanced by emotional benefits experienced by the donor.[168] The risks to the live donor are likely to be greater and less appropriately balanced in paid organ donors. Despite serious ethical objections, paid organ donation is common in several areas.[169–171]

Cadaveric donation rates increased by less than 10% from 1994 (n = 7700) to 2003 (n = 8389) and have more recently decreased. In contrast, living donor transplantation numbers doubled from 3007 to 6464 over the same decade. Some of this increase may be the result of technical advances in harvesting the donor kidney, especially with the use of laparoscopic organ harvesting that has led to a reduction in patient discomfort and recovery time.[172,173] Donor characteristics differ in deceased versus living donors. Deceased donation rates are highest in donors aged 45 to 59 years old, and in men compared with women; rates are higher for whites than for blacks, and lowest in Asians. In contrast, living donation rates are highest in older donors (those aged 60–69), higher in women than in men, and similar in whites and blacks, who in turn, have higher rates than Asians or Native Americans. Attempts to increase the number of deceased donor transplants have led to several novel strategies including the use of less optimal allografts. In 2000, the United Network of Organ Sharing (UNOS) established an Extended Criteria Donors (ECD) based on the presence of several characteristics that are associated with an approximately 70% higher failure rate than that found with non-ECD kidneys. Additional strategies have included increased use of marginal kidneys by transplanting both kidneys that are judged to be individually inadequate for use separately and the use of non–heart-beating donors—as distinct from the more usual situation of donation from a patient who is brain dead but whose cardiorespiratory circulation is maintained through artificial life support. Whereas non–heart-beating donation is associated with poorer initial graft function, the long-term outcomes may nonetheless be acceptable.[174] The increased complexity of non–heart-beating donation, especially regarding diagnosis of death, obtaining informed consent, and the timely initiation of organ preservation measures, poses major challenges to its wider utilization.[175] Wider utilization of living donation is limited by unaltered requirements for appropriate tissue cross matching. Based on blood type frequencies in the United States, it is estimated that there is a 35% chance that any two individuals will be ABO incompatible and a 30% chance that persons awaiting transplantation will be highly sensitized owing to allo-HLA antibodies—measured as high levels of panel reactive antibodies (PRA). High PRA levels may result from previous pregnancies, blood transfusions, or prior transplants. Desensitization protocols, based on the use of plasmapheresis and adjunct immunotherapy, have helped overcome these barriers and so facilitate successful transplantation in subjects with high PRA levels,[176–180] with ABO-incompatible donors,[181–183] or both.[184] An alternative approach is that of paired organ exchanges between two or more pairs of donors and recipients, in which a donor is willing to donate a kidney but is an unsuitable match for the desired recipient and therefore provides his or her kidney to an alternative recipient who has a donor who gifts his or her kidney to the original potential recipient.[185,186] Such paired donation procedures increase the complexity of the transplant procedure, not least because the several surgeries need to be conducted simultaneously.[187] The impact of such paired exchanges on the ever-increasing waiting list for transplantation has to date been limited and is likely to remain so in the absence of national strategies to help optimize their implementation and execution.[186] Ominously, it has been suggested that, even in the event of a substantial increase in the allograft availability, the greater availability of organs, especially in the setting of improved outcomes post-transplantation, is likely to encourage an even higher proportion of dialysis patients to opt for transplantation.[188]

TRANSPLANT OUTCOMES

The reduction in acute rejection rates and improvement in short-term graft survival have been a dramatic success story in the field of transplantation. The 1-year graft and patient survival for a deceased donor transplant is 88% and 95%, the comparable figures for a living donor are 94% and 98%.[66] Transplantation offers a significant survival advantage over continued dialysis (Fig. 17–14). This advantage persists even when accounting for selection biases by use of the transplant wait-listed population as a comparison population.[189–191] This advantage also extends to elderly patients who are considered medically fit for transplantation.[192] Preemptive kidney transplant—transplantation without preceding dialysis—also enjoys superior outcomes over transplant following initial

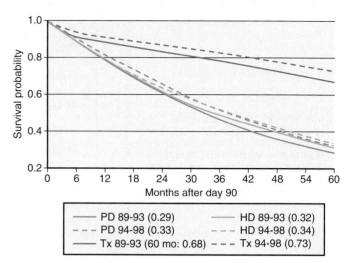

FIGURE 17–14 Adjusted 5-year survival in U.S. incident ESRD by first modality. HD, hemodialysis; PD, peritoneal dialysis; Tx, transplant. (From U.S. Renal Data System: USRDS 2005 Annual Data Report: Atlas of End-Stage Renal Disease in the United States. Bethesda, MD, National Institutes of Health, National Institute of Diabetes and Digestive and Kidney Diseases, 2005, p 27.)

dialysis.[193] The cumulative rejection rates in the first 6 months are now less than 20%. These steady improvements in patient and graft survival have derived from better tissue cross matching,[176] the improved ability to quickly and accurately diagnose complications such as acute humoral rejection,[194,195] standardization of diagnostic criteria of complications,[196] better antirejection therapy[165,197,198] and improved antimicrobial prophylaxis.[199] Unfortunately, the long-term graft outcome has failed to improve to a comparable degree.[200,201] One-year conditional graft half-life (the expected length for which half of all grafts that survive 1 year will remain functional) has remained essentially unchanged over the last decade, although this coincides with the increased use of less optimal grafts. The rate of graft failure due to death with a functioning graft has remained constant at 3.4/100 patient-years, whereas the rate of graft failure in surviving patients has steadily declined and is now only slightly greater than the rate of graft failure due to death with function. The rate of death with a functioning graft was similar for men and women, although approximately twofold higher for blacks that for whites or Asians. The proportion of patients who received preemptive retransplant—without any interim return to dialysis—has increased slightly and now represents approximately 10% of all graft failures. Of the patients who return to dialysis, approximately half go on to a subsequent transplant while the remainder stay and ultimately die on dialysis.

The most common cause of death in transplant recipients is cardiovascular disease, which accounts for 43.5% of those with a known cause of death (Fig. 17–15). The risk of cardiovascular mortality in transplant subjects is substantially less than that in dialysis patients but is still higher than race-, age-, and gender-matched rates in the general public. Some improvement in survival of successful transplants is expected on the grounds of the extensive cardiovascular evaluation performed prior to transplant wait listing. However, this survival benefit persists in comparison with transplant wait-listed subjects, who continue on dialysis having undergone a similar initial evaluation as part of their transplant evaluation. Such subjects thereby form a fairer, though still imperfect, control group. The wait-listed population remains a somewhat biased comparator, as it is, by definition, enriched with subjects who have been on the waiting list longer, for example, due to higher PRA status, and who thus may have a higher cardiovascular risk profile. In comparison to the

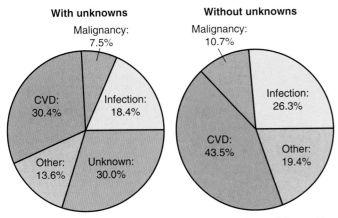

With unknowns

Malignancy:
7.5%

CVD:
30.4%

Infection:
18.4%

Other:
13.6%

Unknown:
30.0%

Without unknowns

Malignancy:
10.7%

Infection:
26.3%

CVD:
43.5%

Other:
19.4%

FIGURE 17–15 Causes of death among U.S. transplant recipients with a functioning graft. CVD, cardiovascular disease. (From U.S. Renal Data System: USRDS 2005 Annual Data Report: Atlas of End-Stage Renal Disease in the United States. Bethesda, MD, National Institutes of Health, National Institute of Diabetes and Digestive and Kidney Diseases, 2005, p 152.)

sive increase in all countries. The rate of increase has slowed in the United States with age-specific rates stabilizing, but the total number of cases requiring dialysis is projected to continue increasing substantially. Outcomes on dialysis have improved but are still inferior to outcomes with transplantation. Finally, the complications of CKD include but are clearly not limited to progression to kidney failure requiring renal replacement. These complications, which include hypertension, anemia, acidosis, poor nutrition, mineralization abnormalities, cardiovascular disease, and increased risk of mortality, suggest the need for a wider approach to kidney disease that is not limited to subspecialty care. Strategies for decreasing the progression of kidney disease as well as strategies for controlling metabolic complications at all stages of kidney disease need to be developed, evaluated, and implemented to improve outcomes in CKD.

629

CH 17

Epidemiology of Kidney Disease

References

1. National Kidney Foundation: K/DOQI clinical practice guidelines for chronic kidney disease: Evaluation, classification and stratification. Am J Kidney Dis 39(suppl 1): S1–S266, 2002.
2. Levey AS, Coresh J, Balk E, et al: National Kidney Foundation practice guidelines for chronic kidney disease: Evaluation, classification, and stratification. Ann Intern Med 139:137–147, 2003.
3. Levey AS, Eckardt KU, Tsukamoto Y, et al: Definition and classification of chronic kidney disease: A position statement from Kidney Disease: Improving Global Outcomes (KDIGO). Kidney Int 67:2089–2100, 2005.
4. Chadban SJ, Ierino FL: Welcome to the era of CKD and the eGFR. Estimating glomerular filtration rate using a simplified formula will lead to a vast increase in detection of chronic kidney disease in Australia. Med J Aust 183:117–118, 2005.
5. Snyder S, Pendergraph B: Detection and evaluation of chronic kidney disease. Am Fam Physician 72:1723–1732, 2005.
6. MacGregor MS, Boag DE, Innes A: Chronic kidney disease: Evolving strategies for detection and management of impaired renal function. QJM 99:365–375, 2006.
7. Hsu CY, Chertow GM: Chronic renal confusion: Insufficiency, failure, dysfunction, or disease. Am J Kidney Dis 36:415–418, 2000.
8. Hsu CY, Chertow GM, Curhan GC: Methodological issues in studying the epidemiology of mild to moderate chronic renal insufficiency. Kidney Int 61:1567–1576, 2002.
9. Swedko PJ, Clark HD, Paramsothy K, et al: Serum creatinine is an inadequate screening test for renal failure in elderly patients. Arch Intern Med 163:356–360, 2003.
10. Akbari A, Swedko PJ, Clark HD, et al: Detection of chronic kidney disease with laboratory reporting of estimated glomerular filtration rate and an educational program. Arch Intern Med 164:1788–1792, 2004.
11. Middleton RJ, Foley RN, Hegarty J, et al: The unrecognized prevalence of chronic kidney disease in diabetes. Nephrol Dial Transplant 21:88–92, 2006.
12. Duncan L, Heathcote J, Djurdjev O, et al: Screening for renal disease using serum creatinine: Who are we missing? Nephrol Dial Transplant 16:1042–1046, 2001.
13. Van BW, Vanholder R, Veys N, et al: The importance of standardization of creatinine in the implementation of guidelines and recommendations for CKD: Implications for CKD management programmes. Nephrol Dial Transplant 21:77–83, 2006.
14. Cockcroft DW, Gault MH: Prediction of creatinine clearance from serum creatinine. Nephron 16:31–41, 1976.
15. Hallan S, Astor B, Lydersen S: Estimating glomerular filtration rate in the general population: The second Health Survey of Nord-Trondelag (HUNT II). Nephrol Dial Transplant 21:1525–1533, 2006.
16. Froissart M, Rossert J, Jacquot C, et al: Predictive performance of the Modification of Diet in Renal Disease and Cockcroft-Gault equations for estimating renal function. J Am Soc Nephrol 16:763–773, 2005.
17. Cirillo M, Anastasio P, De Santo NG: Relationship of gender, age, and body mass index to errors in predicted kidney function. Nephrol Dial Transplant 20:1791–1798, 2005.
18. Coresh J, Stevens L: Kidney function estimating equations: Where do we stand? Curr Opin Nephrol Hypertens 15:276–284, 2006.
19. Eknoyan G, Hostetter T, Bakris GL, et al: Proteinuria and other markers of chronic kidney disease: a position statement of the National Kidney Foundation (NKF) and the National Institute of Diabetes and Digestive and Kidney Diseases (NIDDK). Am J Kidney Dis 42:617–622, 2003.
20. Anavekar N, Bais R, Carney S, et al: Chronic kidney disease and automatic reporting of estimated glomerular filtration rate: A position statement. Clin Biochem Rev 26:81–86, 2005.
21. Mathew TH: Chronic kidney disease and automatic reporting of estimated glomerular filtration rate: A position statement. Med J Aust 183:138–141, 2005.
22. Thorp ML, Eastman L: Potential application of the National Kidney Foundation's chronic kidney disease guidelines in a managed care setting. Am J Manag Care 10:417–422, 2004.
23. Levey AS, Coresh J, Greene T, et al: Using standardized serum creatinine valves in the modification of diet in renal disease study equation for estimating glomerular filtration rate. Ann Intern Med 145:247–254, 2006.
24. Stevens LA, Coresh J, Greene T, et al: Assessing kidney function: Measured and estimated glomerular filtration rate. N Engl J Med 354:2473–2483, 2006.

transplant wait-listed population, rates of cardiovascular death, censored for graft loss, among transplant recipients peak during the first 3 months postengraftment and thereafter gradually decline while the rates progressively increase for wait-listed subjects who continue on dialysis.[202]

The etiology of cardiovascular disease in the transplant population is multifactorial. Although much of the increased risk may relate to carryover effects from earlier periods on dialysis or with lesser degrees of CKD, an element of the increased risk remains attributable to the transplantation period. Hypertension often persists following renal transplantation, despite improvements in volume control. It is associated with both donor and recipient characteristics and may be exacerbated by the use of corticosteroids and calcineurin inhibitors. Post-transplant hypertension is associated with both poor cardiovascular outcomes[203] and chronic allograft nephropathy and, despite the close monitoring of transplant patients, is still often poorly controlled.[44,204,205]

Infection accounts for 26.3% of the remaining patients and malignancy for 10.7%. Unfortunately, in approximately 30% of transplant patients, the cause of death is unknown. This figure increases with increasing durations of follow up.

The outcome of extended criteria grafts has been examined in a retrospective cohort study based on USRDS data. This examined the 3-year survival among 7790 ECDs versus 41,052 patients receiving standard therapy. It demonstrated initial early excess perioperative mortality, with cumulative survival not equalizing until 3.5 years post-transplantation. Long-term survival was 17% lower for ECD recipients. Subgroups with significant benefit from ECD were those over 40, unsensitized subjects, and those with diabetes. In organ procurement areas with long median wait times (>1350 days), the relative risk reduction (95% CI) in mortality with ECDs was 27% (17%–36%), P < .001. In areas with shorter wait list times, only diabetics demonstrated a benefit with extended criteria donation.[206]

CONCLUSION

The epidemiology of CKD has advanced into recognition of the high prevalence of earlier stages of CKD marked by kidney damage and moderate reductions in GFR. Estimates of the prevalences of CKD are becoming increasingly available internationally but still suffer from limited standardization. The epidemiology of treated kidney failure is more mature, with widely available data internationally showing a progres-

25. Poggio ED, Nef PC, Wang XL, et al: Performance of the Cockcroft-Gault and modification of diet in renal disease equations in estimating GFR in ill hospitalized patients. Am J Kidney Dis 46:242–252, 2005.

26. Rule AD, Larson TS, Bergstralh EJ, et al: Using serum creatinine to estimate glomerular filtration rate: Accuracy in good health and in chronic kidney disease. Ann Intern Med 141:929–937, 2004.

27. Mariat C, Alamartine E, Afiani A, et al: Predicting glomerular filtration rate in kidney transplantation: Are the K/DOQI guidelines applicable? Am J Transplant 5:2698–2703, 2005.

28. Poge U, Gerhardt T, Palmedo H, et al: MDRD equations for estimation of GFR in renal transplant recipients. Am J Transplant 5:1306–1311, 2005.

29. Lewis J, Agodoa L, Cheek D, et al: Comparison of cross-sectional renal function measurements in African Americans with hypertensive nephrosclerosis and of primary formulas to estimate glomerular filtration rate. Am J Kidney Dis 38:744–753, 2001.

30. Verhave JC, Fesler P, Ribstein J, et al: Estimation of renal function in subjects with normal serum creatinine levels: Influence of age and body mass index. Am J Kidney Dis 46:233–241, 2005.

31. Miller WG, Myers GL, Ashwood ER, et al: Creatinine measurement: State of the art in accuracy and interlaboratory harmonization. Arch Pathol Lab Med 129:297–304, 2005.

32. Murthy K, Stevens LA, Stark PC, et al: Variation in the serum creatinine assay calibration: A practical application to glomerular filtration rate estimation. Kidney Int 68:1884–1887, 2005.

33. Myers GL, Miller WG, Coresh J, et al: Recommendations for improving serum creatinine measurement: A report from the laboratory working group of the National Kidney Disease Education Program. Clin Chem 52:5–18, 2006.

34. Lamb EJ, Tomson CR, Roderick PJ: Estimating kidney function in adults using formulae. Ann Clin Biochem 42:321–345, 2005.

35. Shlipak M, Katz R, Sarnak M, et al: Cystatin C and prognosis for cardiovascular and kidney outcomes in elderly persons without chronic kidney disease. Ann Int Med 145:237–246, 2006.

36. Shlipak MG, Praught ML, Sarnak MJ: Update on cystatin C: New insights into the importance of mild kidney dysfunction. Curr Opin Nephrol Hypertens 15:270–275, 2006.

37. Rule AD, Bergstralh EJ, Slezak JM, et al: Glomerular filtration rate estimated by cystatin C among different clinical presentations. Kidney Int 69:399–405, 2006.

38. Hoang K, Tan JC, Derby G, et al: Determinants of glomerular hypofiltration in aging humans. Kidney Int 64:1417–1424, 2003.

39. Baylis C: Glomerular filtration rate in normal and abnormal pregnancies. Semin Nephrol 19:133–139, 1999.

40. Moran P, Baylis PH, Lindheimer MD, et al: Glomerular ultrafiltration in normal and preeclamptic pregnancy. J Am Soc Nephrol 14:648–652, 2003.

41. Babay Z, Al-Wakeel J, Addar M, et al: Serum cystatin C in pregnant women: Reference values, reliable and superior diagnostic accuracy. Clin Exp Obstet Gynecol 32:175–179, 2005.

42. Conrad KP: Mechanisms of renal vasodilation and hyperfiltration during pregnancy. J Soc Gynecol Investig 11:438–448, 2004.

43. Marcen R, Pascual J, Tenorio M, et al: Chronic kidney disease in renal transplant recipients. Transplant Proc 37:3718–3720, 2005.

44. Karthikeyan V, Karpinski J, Nair RC, et al: The burden of chronic kidney disease in renal transplant recipients. Am J Transplant 4:262–269, 2004.

45. Fox CS, Larson MG, Leip EP, et al: Predictors of new-onset kidney disease in a community-based population. JAMA 291:844–850, 2004.

46. Hsu CC, Kao WH, Coresh J, et al: Apolipoprotein E and progression of chronic kidney disease. JAMA 293:2892–2899, 2005.

47. Eriksen BO, Ingebretsen OC: The progression of chronic kidney disease: A 10-year population-based study of the effects of gender and age. Kidney Int 69:375–382, 2006.

48. Foley RN, Murray AM, Li S, et al: Chronic kidney disease and the risk for cardiovascular disease, renal replacement, and death in the United States Medicare population, 1998 to 1999. J Am Soc Nephrol 16:489–495, 2005.

49. Rottey S, Vanholder R, De Schoenmakere G, et al: Progression of renal failure in patients with compromised renal function is not always present: Evaluation of underlying disease. Clin Nephrol 54:1–10, 2000.

50. Stevens LA, Fares G, Fleming J, et al: Low rates of testing and diagnostic codes usage in a commercial clinical laboratory: Evidence for lack of physician awareness of chronic kidney disease. J Am Soc Nephrol 16:2439–2448, 2005.

51. Coresh J, Byrd-Holt D, Astor BC, et al: Chronic kidney disease awareness, prevalence, and trends among U.S. adults, 1999 to 2000. J Am Soc Nephrol 16(1):180–188, 2005.

52. McClellan W, Warnock DG, McClure L, et al: Racial differences in the prevalence of chronic kidney disease among participants in the Reasons for Geographic and Racial Differences in Stroke (REGARDS) cohort study. J Am Soc Nephrol 17:1710–1715, 2006.

53. Go AS, Chertow GM, Fan DJ, et al: Chronic kidney disease and the risks of death, cardiovascular events, and hospitalization. N Engl J Med 351:1296–1305, 2004.

54. McGill JB, Brown WW, Chen SC, et al: Kidney Early Evaluation Program (KEEP). Findings from a community screening program. Diabetes Educ 30:196–206, 2004.

55. de Lusignan S, Chan T, Stevens P, et al: Identifying patients with chronic kidney disease from general practice computer records. Fam Pract 22:234–241, 2005.

56. Nitsch D, Dietrich DF, Von EA, et al: Prevalence of renal impairment and its association with cardiovascular risk factors in a general population: Results of the Swiss SAPALDIA study. Nephrol Dial Transplant 21:935–944, 2006.

57. Hallan SI, Coresh J, Astor BC, et al: International comparison of the relationship of chronic kidney disease prevalence and end-stage renal disease risk. J Am Soc Nephrol 17:2275–2284, 2006.

58. McDonald SP, Maguire GP, Hoy WE: Renal function and cardiovascular risk markers in a remote Australian Aboriginal community. Nephrol Dial Transplant 18:1555–1561, 2003.

59. Chen J, Wildman RP, Gu D, et al: Prevalence of decreased kidney function in Chinese adults aged 35 to 74 years. Kidney Int 68:2837–2845, 2005.

60. Li ZY, Xu GB, Xia TA, et al: Prevalence of chronic kidney disease in a middle and old-aged population of Beijing. Clin Chim Acta 366:209–215, 2006.

61. Tanaka H, Shiohira Y, Uezu Y, et al: Metabolic syndrome and chronic kidney disease in Okinawa, Japan. Kidney Int 69:369–374, 2006.

62. Iseki K, Kinjo K, Iseki C, et al: Relationship between predicted creatinine clearance and proteinuria, and the risk of developing ESRD in Okinawa, Japan. Am J Kidney Dis 44:806–814, 2004.

63. Jafar TH: Hypertension and kidney disease in Asia. Curr Opin Nephrol Hypertens 15:291–295, 2006.

64. Domrongkitchaiporn S, Sritara P, Kitiyakara C, et al: Risk factors for development of decreased kidney function in a southeast Asian population: A 12-year cohort study. J Am Soc Nephrol 16:791–799, 2005.

65. Nissenson AR, Pereira BJ, Collins AJ, et al: Prevalence and characteristics of individuals with chronic kidney disease in a large health maintenance organization. Am J Kidney Dis 37:1177–1183, 2001.

66. U.S. Renal Data Systems: USRDS 2005 Annual Data Report: Atlas of End-Stage Renal Disease in the United States. Bethesda, MD, National Institutes of Health, National Institute of Diabetes and Digestive and Kidney Diseases, 2005.

67. Culleton BF, Larson MG, Evans JC, et al: Prevalence and correlates of elevated serum creatinine levels: The Framingham Heart Study. Arch Intern Med 159:1785–1790, 1999.

68. Iseki K: The okinawa screening program. J Am Soc Nephrol 14:S127–S130, 2003.

69. Jones CA, McQuillan GM, Kusek JW, et al: Serum creatinine levels in the US population: Third National Health and Nutrition Examination Survey. Am J Kidney Dis 32:992–999, 1998.

70. Manley JA, O'Neill WC: How echogenic is echogenic? Quantitative acoustics of the renal cortex. Am J Kidney Dis 37:706–711, 2001.

71. Coresh J, Astor BC, Greene T, et al: Prevalence of chronic kidney disease and decreased kidney function in the adult US population: Third National Health and Nutrition Examination Survey. Am J Kidney Dis 41:1–12, 2003.

72. Knight EL, Curhan GC: Albuminuria: Moving beyond traditional microalbuminuria cut-points. Curr Opin Nephrol Hypertens 12:283–284, 2003.

73. Gilbertson DT, Liu J, Xue JL, et al: Projecting the number of patients with end-stage renal disease in the United States to the year 2015. J Am Soc Nephrol 16:3736–3741, 2005.

74. Hall YN, Hsu CY, Iribarren C et al: The conundrum of increased burden of end-stage renal disease in Asians. Kidney Int 68:2310–2316, 2005.

75. Ishani A, Grandits GA, Grimm RH, et al: Association of single measurements of dipstick proteinuria, estimated glomerular filtration rate, and hematocrit with 25-year incidence of end-stage renal disease in the Multiple Risk Factor Intervention Trial. J Am Soc Nephrol 17:1444–1452, 2006.

76. Hu FB, Manson JE, Stampfer MJ, et al: Diet, lifestyle, and the risk of type 2 diabetes mellitus in women. N Engl J Med 345:790–797, 2001.

77. Hsu CY, Lin F, Vittinghoff E, et al: Racial differences in the progression from chronic renal insufficiency to end-stage renal disease in the United States. J Am Soc Nephrol 14:2902–2907, 2003.

78. Sarnak MJ, Greene T, Wang X, et al: The effect of a lower target blood pressure on the progression of kidney disease: Long-term follow-up of the modification of diet in renal disease study. Ann Intern Med 142:342–351, 2005.

79. Young JH, Klag MJ, Muntner P, et al: Blood pressure and decline in kidney function: Findings from the Systolic Hypertension in the Elderly Program (SHEP). J Am Soc Nephrol 13:2776–2782, 2002.

80. Agodoa LY, Appel L, Bakris GL, et al: Effect of ramipril vs amlodipine on renal outcomes in hypertensive nephrosclerosis: A randomized controlled trial. JAMA 285:2719–2728, 2001.

81. Bakris GL, Weir MR, Shanifar S, et al: Effects of blood pressure level on progression of diabetic nephropathy: Results from the RENAAL study. Arch Intern Med 163:1555–1565, 2003.

82. Klahr S, Levey AS, Beck GJ, et al: The effects of dietary protein restriction and blood-pressure control on the progression of chronic renal disease. Modification of Diet in Renal Disease Study Group. N Engl J Med 330:877–884, 1994.

83. UK Prospective Diabetes Study (UKPDS) Group: Intensive blood-glucose control with sulphonylureas or insulin compared with conventional treatment and risk of complications in patients with type 2 diabetes (UKPDS 33). Lancet 352:837–853, 1998.

84. Brancati FL, Whelton PK, Randall BL, et al: Risk of end-stage renal disease in diabetes mellitus: A prospective cohort study of men screened for MRFIT. Multiple Risk Factor Intervention Trial. JAMA 278:2069–2074, 1997.

85. The Diabetes Control and Complications Trial Research Group: The effect of intensive treatment of diabetes on the development and progression of long-term complications in insulin-dependent diabetes mellitus. N Engl J Med 329:977–986, 1993.

86. Weir MR, Fink JC: Salt intake and progression of chronic kidney disease: an overlooked modifiable exposure? A commentary. Am J Kidney Dis 45:176–188, 2005.

87. Mandayam S, Mitch WE: Dietary protein restriction benefits patients with chronic kidney disease. Nephrology (Carlton) 11:53–57, 2006.

88. Kramer H, Luke A, Bidani A, et al: Obesity and prevalent and incident CKD: The Hypertension Detection and Follow-Up Program. Am J Kidney Dis 46:587–594, 2005.

89. Zandi-Nejad K, Brenner BM: Strategies to retard the progression of chronic kidney disease. Med Clin North Am 89:489–509, 2005.

90. De Zeeuw D, Lewis EJ, Remuzzi G, et al: Renoprotective effects of renin-angiotensin-system inhibitors. Lancet 367:899–900, 2006.

CH 17

91. Forman JP, Brenner BM: "Hypertension" and "microalbuminuria": The bell tolls for thee. Kidney Int 69:22–28, 2006.

92. Ejerblad E, Fored CM, Lindblad P, et al: Association between smoking and chronic renal failure in a nationwide population-based case-control study. J Am Soc Nephrol 15:2178–2185, 2004.

93. Haroun MK, Jaar BG, Hoffman SC, et al: Risk factors for chronic kidney disease: A prospective study of 23,534 men and women in Washington County, Maryland. J Am Soc Nephrol 14:2934–2941, 2003.

94. Stengel B, Tarver-Carr ME, Powe NR, et al: Lifestyle factors, obesity and the risk of chronic kidney disease. Epidemiology 14:479–487, 2003.

95. Warmoth L, Regalado MM, Simoni J, et al: Cigarette smoking enhances increased urine albumin excretion as a risk factor for glomerular filtration rate decline in primary hypertension. Am J Med Sci 330:111–119, 2005.

96. Vupputuri S, Batuman V, Muntner P, et al: The risk for mild kidney function decline associated with illicit drug use among hypertensive men. Am J Kidney Dis 43:629–635, 2004.

97. Powe NR: To have and have not: Health and health care disparities in chronic kidney disease. Kidney Int 64:763–772, 2003.

98. Klag MJ, Whelton PK, Randall BL, et al: End-stage renal disease in African-American and white men. 16-year MRFIT findings. JAMA 277:1293–1298, 1997.

99. Garg PP, Diener-West M, Powe NR: Income-based disparities in outcomes for patients with chronic kidney disease. Semin Nephrol 21:377–385, 2001.

100. Bommer J: Prevalence and socio-economic aspects of chronic kidney disease. Nephrol Dial Transplant 17(suppl 11):8–12, 2002.

101. Tarver-Carr ME, Powe NR, Eberhardt MS, et al: Excess risk of chronic kidney disease among African-American versus white subjects in the United States: A population-based study of potential explanatory factors. J Am Soc Nephrol 13:2363–2370, 2002.

102. Hunsicker LG, Adler S, Caggiula A, et al: Predictors of the progression of renal disease in the Modification of Diet in Renal Disease Study. Kidney Int 51:1908–1919, 1997.

103. Sahadevan M, Kasiske BL: Hyperlipidemia in kidney disease: Causes and consequences. Curr Opin Nephrol Hypertens 11:323–329, 2002.

104. Rossert J, Levin A, Roger SD, et al: Effect of early correction of anemia on the progression of CKD. Am J Kidney Dis 47:738–750, 2006.

105. Muntner P, He J, Vupputuri S, et al: Blood lead and chronic kidney disease in the general United States population: Results from NHANES III. Kidney Int 63:1044–1050, 2003.

106. Weaver VM, Jaar BG, Schwartz BS, et al: Associations among lead dose biomarkers, uric acid, and renal function in Korean lead workers. Environ Health Perspect 113:36–42, 2005.

107. Finne P, Reunanen A, Stenman S, et al: Incidence of end-stage renal disease in patients with type 1 diabetes. JAMA 294:1782–1787, 2005.

108. Neugarten J, Acharya A, Silbiger SR: Effect of gender on the progression of nondiabetic renal disease: A meta-analysis. J Am Soc Nephrol 11:319–329, 2000.

109. Seliger SL, Davis C, Stehman-Breen C: Gender and the progression of renal disease. Curr Opin Nephrol Hypertens 10:219–225, 2001.

110. Sandberg K, Ji H: Sex and the renin angiotensin system: Implications for gender differences in the progression of kidney disease. Adv Ren Replace Ther 10:15–23, 2003.

111. Li PK, Ho KK, Szeto CC, et al: Prognostic indicators of IgA nephropathy in the Chinese—Clinical and pathological perspectives. Nephrol Dial Transplant 17:64–69, 2002.

112. Jafar TH, Schmid CH, Stark PC, et al: The rate of progression of renal disease may not be slower in women compared with men: a patient-level meta analysis Nephrol Dial Transplant 18:2047–2053, 2003.

113. Muntner P, Coresh J, Powe NR, et al: The contribution of increased diabetes prevalence and improved myocardial infarction and stroke survival to the increase in treated end-stage renal disease. J Am Soc Nephrol 14:1568–1577, 2003.

114. Jurkovitz C, Franch H, Shoham D, et al: Family members of patients treated for ESRD have high rates of undetected kidney disease. Am J Kidney Dis 40:1173–1178, 2002.

115. Lei HH, Perneger TV, Klag MJ, et al: Familial aggregation of renal disease in a population-based case-control study. J Am Soc Nephrol 9:1270–1276, 1998.

116. Powe NR, Tarver-Carr ME, Eberhardt MS, et al: Receipt of renal replacement therapy in the United States: A population-based study of sociodemographic disparities from the Second National Health and Nutrition Examination Survey (NHANES II). Am J Kidney Dis 42:249–255, 2003.

117. Stengel B, Billon S, Van Dijk PC, et al: Trends in the incidence of renal replacement therapy for end-stage renal disease in Europe, 1990–1999. Nephrol Dial Transplant 18:1824–1833, 2003.

118. McDonald SP, Russ GR, Kerr PG, et al: ESRD in Australia and New Zealand at the end of the millennium: a report from the ANZDATA registry. Am J Kidney Dis 40:1122–1131, 2002.

119. Cass A, Devitt J, Preece C, et al: Barriers to access by Indigenous Australians to kidney transplantation: The IMPAKT study. Nephrology (Carlton) 9(suppl 4):S144–S146, 2004.

120. McFarlane PA, Bayoumi AM, Pierratos A, et al: The quality of life and cost utility of home nocturnal and conventional in-center hemodialysis. Kidney Int 64:1004–1011, 2003.

121. Pierratos A: Daily hemodialysis: an update. Curr Opin Nephrol Hypertens 11:165–171, 2002.

122. Ting GO, Kjellstrand C, Freitas T, et al: Long-term study of high-comorbidity ESRD patients converted from conventional to short daily hemodialysis. Am J Kidney Dis 42:1020–1035, 2003.

123. Chan CT, Floras JS, Miller JA, et al: Regression of left ventricular hypertrophy after conversion to nocturnal hemodialysis. Kidney Int 61:2235–2239, 2002.

124. Fagugli RM, Reboldi G, Quintaliani G, et al: Short daily hemodialysis: Blood pressure control and left ventricular mass reduction in hypertensive hemodialysis patients. Am J Kidney Dis 38:371–376, 2001.

125. Spanner E, Suri R, Heidenheim AP, et al: The impact of quotidian hemodialysis on nutrition. Am J Kidney Dis 42:30–35, 2003.

126. Pierratos A: Daily nocturnal home hemodialysis. Kidney Int 65:1975–1986, 2004.

127. Briggs JP: Evidence-based medicine in the dialysis unit: A few lessons from the USRDS and the NCDS and HEMO trials. Semin Dial 17:136–141, 2004.

128. Garg PP, Frick KD, Diener-West M, et al: Effect of the ownership of dialysis facilities on patients' survival and referral for transplantation. N Engl J Med 341:1653–1660, 1999.

129. Devereaux PJ, Schunemann HJ, Ravindran N, et al: Comparison of mortality between private for-profit and private not-for-profit hemodialysis centers: A systematic review and meta-analysis. JAMA 288:2449–2457, 2002.

130. Kazmi WH, Gilbertson DT, Obrador GT, et al: Effect of comorbidity on the increased mortality associated with early initiation of dialysis. Am J Kidney Dis 46:887–896, 2005.

131. Longenecker JC, Coresh J, Klag MJ, et al: Validation of comorbid conditions on the end-stage renal disease medical evidence report: The CHOICE study. Choices for Healthy Outcomes in Caring for ESRD. J Am Soc Nephrol 11:520–529, 2000.

132. Sarnak MJ, Levey AS, Schoolwerth AC, et al: Kidney disease as a risk factor for development of cardiovascular disease: A statement from the American Heart Association Councils on Kidney in Cardiovascular Disease, High Blood Pressure Research, Clinical Cardiology, and Epidemiology and Prevention. Circulation 108:2154–2169, 2003.

133. Collins AJ, Li S, Gilbertson DT, et al: Chronic kidney disease and cardiovascular disease in the Medicare population. Kidney Int Suppl S24–S31, 2003.

134. Henry RM, Kostense PJ, Bos G, et al: Mild renal insufficiency is associated with increased cardiovascular mortality: The Hoorn Study. Kidney Int 62:1402–1407, 2002.

135. Muntner P, He J, Hamm L, et al: Renal insufficiency and subsequent death resulting from cardiovascular disease in the United States. J Am Soc Nephrol 13:745–753, 2002.

136. Longenecker JC, Coresh J, Powe NR, et al: Traditional cardiovascular disease risk factors in dialysis patients compared with the general population: The CHOICE Study. J Am Soc Nephrol 13:1918–1927, 2002.

137. Muntner P, He J, Astor BC, et al: Traditional and nontraditional risk factors predict coronary heart disease in chronic kidney disease: Results from the Atherosclerosis Risk in Sommunities study. J Am Soc Nephrol 16:529–538, 2005.

138. Iseki K, Yamazato M, Tozawa M, et al: Hypocholesterolemia is a significant predictor of death in a cohort of chronic hemodialysis patients. Kidney Int 61:1887–1893, 2002.

139. Liu Y, Coresh J, Eustace JA, et al: Association between cholesterol level and mortality in dialysis patients: Role of inflammation and malnutrition. JAMA 291:451–459, 2004.

140. Foley RN, Herzog CA, Collins AJ: Blood pressure and long-term mortality in United States hemodialysis patients: USRDS Waves 3 and 4 Study. Kidney Int 62:1784–1790, 2002.

141. Port FK, Hulbert-Shearon TE, Wolfe RA, et al: Predialysis blood pressure and mortality risk in a national sample of maintenance hemodialysis patients. Am J Kidney Dis 33:507–517, 1999.

142. Zager PG, Nikolic J, Brown RH, et al: "U" curve association of blood pressure and mortality in hemodialysis patients. Medical Directors of Dialysis Clinic, Inc. Kidney Int 54:561–569, 1998.

143. Roger SD, McMahon LP, Clarkson A, et al: Effects of early and late intervention with epoetin alpha on left ventricular mass among patients with chronic kidney disease (stage 3 or 4): Results of a randomized clinical trial. J Am Soc Nephrol 15:148–156, 2004.

144. Foley RN, Parfrey PS, Morgan J, et al: Effect of hemoglobin levels in hemodialysis patients with asymptomatic cardiomyopathy. Kidney Int 58:1325–1335, 2000.

145. Levin A, Djurdjev O, Thompson C, et al: Canadian randomized trial of hemoglobin maintenance to prevent or delay left ventricular mass growth in patients with CKD. Am J Kidney Dis 46:799–811, 2005.

146. Phrommintikul A, Haas SJ, Elsik M, Krum H: Mortality and target haemoglobin concentrations in anaemic patients with chronic kidney disease treated with erythropoietin: a meta-analysis. Lancet 369:381–388, 2007.

147. Port FK, Ashby VB, Dhingra RK, et al: Dialysis dose and body mass index are strongly associated with survival in hemodialysis patients. J Am Soc Nephrol 13:1061–1066, 2002.

148. Kopple JD, Zhu X, Lew NL, et al: Body weight-for-height relationships predict mortality in maintenance hemodialysis patients. Kidney Int 56:1136–1148, 1999.

149. Mittman N, Avram MM, Oo KK, et al: Serum prealbumin predicts survival in hemodialysis and peritoneal dialysis: 10 years of prospective observation. Am J Kidney Dis 38:1358–1364, 2001.

150. Chertow GM, Johansen KL, Lew N, et al: Vintage, nutritional status, and survival in hemodialysis patients. Kidney Int 57:1176–1181, 2000.

151. Rocco MV, Dwyer JT, Larive B, et al: The effect of dialysis dose and membrane flux on nutritional parameters in hemodialysis patients: Results of the HEMO Study. Kidney Int 65:2321–2334, 2004.

152. Baum CL, Thielke K, Westin E, et al: Predictors of weight gain and cardiovascular risk in a cohort of racially diverse kidney transplant recipients. Nutrition 18:139–146, 2002.

153. Meier-Kriesche HU, Arndorfer JA, Kaplan B: The impact of body mass index on renal transplant outcomes: A significant independent risk factor for graft failure and patient death. Transplantation 73:70–74, 2002.

154. Kalantar-Zadeh K, Abbott KC, Salahudeen AK, et al: Survival advantages of obesity in dialysis patients. Am J Clin Nutr 81:543–554, 2005.

632

155. Snyder JJ, Foley RN, Gilbertson DT, et al: Body size and outcomes on peritoneal dialysis in the United States. Kidney Int 64:1838–1844, 2003.

156. Shlipak MG, Heidenreich PA, Noguchi H, et al: Association of renal insufficiency with treatment and outcomes after myocardial infarction in elderly patients. Ann Intern Med 137:555–562, 2002.

157. Wright RS, Reeder GS, Herzog CA, et al: Acute myocardial infarction and renal dysfunction: A high-risk combination. Ann Intern Med 137:563–570, 2002.

158. Reddan DN, Szczech L, Bhapkar MV, et al: Renal function, concomitant medication use and outcomes following acute coronary syndromes. Nephrol Dial Transplant 20:2105–2112, 2005.

159. Trespalacios FC, Taylor AJ, Agodoa LY, et al: Incident acute coronary syndromes in chronic dialysis patients in the United States. Kidney Int 62:1799–1805, 2002.

160. Foley RN: Comparing the incomparable: Hemodialysis versus peritoneal dialysis in observational studies. Perit Dial Int 24:217–221, 2004.

161. Vonesh EF, Snyder JJ, Foley RN, et al: The differential impact of risk factors on mortality in hemodialysis and peritoneal dialysis. Kidney Int 66:2389–2401, 2004.

162. Jaar BG, Coresh J, Plantinga LC, et al: Comparing the risk for death with peritoneal dialysis and hemodialysis in a national cohort of patients with chronic kidney disease. Ann Intern Med 143:174–183, 2005.

163. Schulman G: Mortality and treatment modality of end-stage renal disease. Ann Intern Med 143:229–231, 2005.

164. Epstein AM, Ayanian JZ, Keogh JH, et al: Racial disparities in access to renal transplantation—Clinically appropriate or due to underuse or overuse? N Engl J Med 343:1537–1544, 2000.

165. Magee CC, Pascual M: Update in renal transplantation. Arch Intern Med 164:1373–1388, 2004.

166. Gjertson DW, Cecka JM: Living unrelated donor kidney transplantation. Kidney Int 58:491–499, 2000.

167. Matas AJ, Bartlett ST, Leichtman AB, et al: Morbidity and mortality after living kidney donation, 1999–2001: Survey of United States transplant centers. Am J Transplant 3:830–834, 2003.

168. Fehrman-Ekholm I, Brink B, Ericsson C, et al: Kidney donors don't regret: Follow-up of 370 donors in Stockholm since 1964. Transplantation 69:2067–2071, 2000.

169. Goyal M, Mehta RL, Schneiderman LJ, et al: Economic and health consequences of selling a kidney in India. JAMA 288:1589–1593, 2002.

170. Jha V: Paid transplants in India: The grim reality. Nephrol Dial Transplant 19:541–543, 2004.

171. Kreis H: The question of organ procurement: beyond charity. Nephrol Dial Transplant 20:1303–1306, 2005.

172. Schweitzer EJ, Wilson J, Jacobs S, et al: Increased rates of donation with laparoscopic donor nephrectomy. Ann Surg 232:392–400, 2000.

173. Wolf JS Jr, Merion RM, Leichtman AB, et al: Randomized controlled trial of hand-assisted laparoscopic versus open surgical live donor nephrectomy. Transplantation 72:284–290, 2001.

174. Rudich SM, Kaplan B, Magee JC, et al: Renal transplantations performed using non–heart-beating organ donors: Going back to the future? Transplantation 74:1715–1720, 2002.

175. Vanrenterghem Y: Cautious approach to use of non-heart-beating donors. Lancet 356:528, 2000

176. Fuggle SV, Martin S: Toward performing transplantation in highly sensitized patients. Transplantation 78:186–189, 2004.

177. Montgomery RA, Zachary AA: Transplanting patients with a positive donor-specific crossmatch: A single center's perspective. Pediatr Transplant 8:535–542, 2004.

178. Jordan SC, Tyan D, Stablein D, et al: Evaluation of intravenous immunoglobulin as an agent to lower allosensitization and improve transplantation in highly sensitized adult patients with end-stage renal disease: report of the NIH IG02 trial. J Am Soc Nephrol 15:3256–3262, 2004.

179. Glotz D, Antoine C, Julia P, et al: Desensitization and subsequent kidney transplantation of patients using intravenous immunoglobulins (IVIg). Am J Transplant 2:758–760, 2002.

180. Lorenz M, Regele H, Schillinger M, et al: Peritransplant immunoadsorption: A strategy enabling transplantation in highly sensitized crossmatch-positive cadaveric kidney allograft recipients. Transplantation 79:696–701, 2005.

181. Stegall MD, Dean PG, Gloor JM: ABO-incompatible kidney transplantation. Transplantation 78:635–640, 2004.

182. Gloor JM, Lager DJ, Moore SB, et al: ABO-incompatible kidney transplantation using both A2 and non-A2 living donors. Transplantation 75:971–977, 2003.

183. Sonnenday CJ, Warren DS, Cooper M, et al: Plasmapheresis, CMV hyperimmune globulin, and anti-CD20 allow ABO-incompatible renal transplantation without splenectomy. Am J Transplant 4:1315–1322, 2004.

184. Warren DS, Zachary AA, Sonnenday CJ, et al: Successful renal transplantation across simultaneous ABO incompatible and positive crossmatch barriers. Am J Transplant 4:561–568, 2004.

185. Delmonico FL, Morrissey PE, Lipkowitz GS, et al: Donor kidney exchanges. Am J Transplant 4:1628–1634, 2004.

186. Segev DL, Gentry SE, Warren DS, et al: Kidney paired donation and optimizing the use of live donor organs. JAMA 293:1883–1890, 2005.

187. Ross LF, Zenios S: Practical and ethical challenges to paired exchange programs. Am J Transplant 4:1553–1554, 2004.

188. Wolfe R: The state of kidney transplantation in the United States. Semin Dial 18:453–455, 2005.

189. McDonald SP, Russ GR: Survival of recipients of cadaveric kidney transplants compared with those receiving dialysis treatment in Australia and New Zealand, 1991–2001. Nephrol Dial Transplant 17:2212–2219, 2002.

190. Wolfe RA, Ashby VB, Milford EL, et al: Comparison of mortality in all patients on dialysis, patients on dialysis awaiting transplantation, and recipients of a first cadaveric transplant. N Engl J Med 341:1725–1730, 1999.

191. Meier-Kriesche HU, Ojo AO, Port FK, et al: Survival improvement among patients with end-stage renal disease: Trends over time for transplant recipients and waitlisted patients. J Am Soc Nephrol 12:1293–1296, 2001.

192. Oniscu GC, Brown H, Forsythe JL: How great is the survival advantage of transplantation over dialysis in elderly patients? Nephrol Dial Transplant 19:945–951, 2004.

193. Mange KC, Joffe MM, Feldman HI: Effect of the use or nonuse of long-term dialysis on the subsequent survival of renal transplants from living donors. N Engl J Med 344:726–731, 2001.

194. Collins AB, Schneeberger EE, Pascual MA, et al: Complement activation in acute humoral renal allograft rejection: Diagnostic significance of C4d deposits in peritubular capillaries. J Am Soc Nephrol 10:2208–2214, 1999.

195. Watschinger B, Pascual M: Capillary C4d deposition as a marker of humoral immunity in renal allograft rejection. J Am Soc Nephrol 13:2420–2423, 2002.

196. Racusen LC, Halloran PF, Solez K: Banff 2003 meeting report: New diagnostic insights and standards. Am J Transplant 4:1562–1566, 2004.

197. Denton MD, Magee CC, Sayegh MH: Immunosuppressive strategies in transplantation. Lancet 353:1083–1091, 1999.

198. Hariharan S, Johnson CP, Bresnahan BA, et al: Improved graft survival after renal transplantation in the United States, 1988 to 1996. N Engl J Med 342:605–612, 2000.

199. Brennan DC: Cytomegalovirus in renal transplantation. J Am Soc Nephrol 12:848–855, 2001.

200. Meier-Kriesche HU, Schold JD, Srinivas TR, et al: Lack of improvement in renal allograft survival despite a marked decrease in acute rejection rates over the most recent era. Am J Transplant 4:378–383, 2004.

201. Meier-Kriesche HU, Schold JD, Kaplan B: Long-term renal allograft survival: Have we made significant progress or is it time to rethink our analytic and therapeutic strategies? Am J Transplant 4:1289–1295, 2004.

202. Meier-Kriesche HU, Schold JD, Srinivas TR, et al: Kidney transplantation halts cardiovascular disease progression in patients with end-stage renal disease. Am J Transplant 4:1662–1668, 2004.

203. Kasiske BL, Chakkera HA, Roel J: Explained and unexplained ischemic heart disease risk after renal transplantation. J Am Soc Nephrol 11:1735–1743, 2000.

204. Castillo-Lugo JA, Vergne-Marini P: Hypertension in kidney transplantation. Semin Nephrol 25:252–260, 2005.

205. Tutone VK, Mark PB, Stewart GA, et al: Hypertension, antihypertensive agents and outcomes following renal transplantation. Clin Transplant 19:181–192, 2005.

206. Merion RM, Ashby VB, Wolfe RA, et al: Deceased-donor characteristics and the survival benefit of kidney transplantation. JAMA 294:2726–2733, 2005.

CH 17

CHAPTER 18

Risk Factors and Kidney Disease

Vandana Menon • Mark J. Sarnak • Andrew S. Levey

Chronic kidney disease (CKD) is a public health problem with increasing prevalence, poor outcomes, and high costs.[1,2] The major adverse outcomes of CKD include loss of kidney function sometimes leading to kidney failure, complications of decreased kidney function, and also development of cardiovascular disease and premature death.[3] Improving outcomes in CKD requires an integrated approach to prevention, detection, evaluation, and management, as exists for other chronic diseases, such as hypertension, diabetes, hypercholesterolemia, and obesity. A comprehensive analysis of risk factors for the development and progression of CKD is imperative to inform clinical practice and health policy.

FRAMEWORK FOR NATURAL HISTORY, DEFINITION, AND CLASSIFICATION OF CHRONIC KIDNEY DISEASE

Figure 18–1 shows the natural history of CKD and provides a framework for a public health approach to improving outcomes in kidney disease.[4-6] Shaded ellipses denote stages of kidney disease, kidney damage, decreased glomerular filtration rate (GFR), and kidney failure; unshaded ellipses represent antecedents or outcomes of CKD. Thick arrows between ellipses represent transitions between stages, and can be considered as risk factors for adverse outcomes: susceptibility factors (black), initiation factors (dark gray), progression factors (light gray), and end-stage factors (white). Complications refer to all complications of CKD and its treatment, including complications of decreased GFR (hypertension, anemia, malnutrition, bone disease, neuropathy, and decreased quality of life), and cardiovascular disease. Increasing thickness of arrows connecting later stages of kidney disease to complications represents the increased risk as kidney disease progresses. Below each ellipse are actions to improve outcomes specific for each stage.

Chronic kidney disease is defined as functional or structural abnormalities of the kidneys for three or more months, irrespective of cause (Table 18–1). Proteinuria is the most common marker of kidney damage.[4,7] Glomerular filtration rate is estimated from serum creatinine and equations using age,

sex, race, and body size.[8] Patients with CKD can be classified according to severity based on the level of GFR (Table 18–2). Qualitatively, stages 1 and 2 represent kidney damage, stages 3 and 4 represent decreased kidney function, and stage 5 is kidney failure, usually with signs and symptoms of uremia requiring kidney replacement therapies such as dialysis or transplantation.

This definition and classification enable identification and staging of the severity of kidney disease based on objective criteria, without the need for specialized laboratory studies or specialist evaluation of the cause of disease. In addition, the definition and classification facilitate study of risk factors in large clinical databases and populations based on commonly available clinical data. Indeed, there has been a large increase in the number of studies on risk factors for kidney disease in the past few years. In this chapter, we will use the term "risk factors" to include conditions that increase risk for the development of kidney disease, as well as those that increase risk of adverse outcomes associated with CKD. Accordingly, these can be defined as susceptibility and initiation factors that help to define persons at increased risk for developing CKD and progression, and end-stage factors that define persons at risk for increasing kidney damage, decline in GFR and development of associated complications (Table 18–3). This chapter will briefly review basic concepts of epidemiologic investigation and provide an overview of the current evidence regarding the epidemiology of risk factors in CKD.

EPIDEMIOLOGIC METHODS FOR RISK FACTOR IDENTIFICATION

In this section, we review epidemiologic methods that are used to identify and confirm relationships between putative risk factors and development of disease.

Definition of a Risk Factor

The purpose of epidemiologic investigation is to identify a profile of variables that characterize the disease under study. The associations identified between the characteristics and disease may be due to chance, may represent a non-causal relationship, or

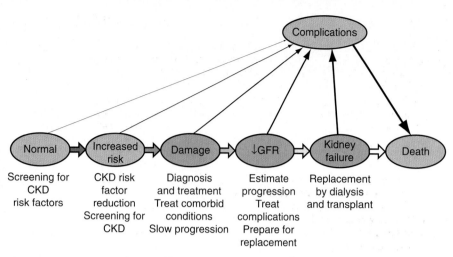

FIGURE 18–1 Stages in progression of CKD and therapeutic strategies. (From Kidney Disease Outcome Quality Initiative: K/DOQI clinical practice guidelines for chronic kidney disease: Evaluation, classification, and stratification. Am J Kidney Dis 39:S1–246, 242 [Figure 1]; Levey AS, Eckardt KU, Tsukamoto Y, et al: Definition and classification of chronic kidney disease: A position statement from Kidney Disease: Improving Global Outcomes (KDIGO). Kidney Int 67:2089–2100, 2005; Coresh J, Astor BC, Greene T, et al: Prevalence of chronic kidney disease and decreased kidney function in the adult U.S. population: Third National Health and Nutrition Examination Survey. Am J Kidney Dis 41:1–12, 2003.)

TABLE 18–1	Definition of Chronic Kidney Disease
Criteria	

Kidney damage for ≥3 months, with or without decreased GFR
- Pathological abnormalities
- Markers of kidney damage
  - Urinary abnormalities (proteinuria)
  - Blood abnormalities (renal tubular syndromes)
  - Imaging abnormalities
- Kidney transplantation

GFR <60 ml/min/1.73 m² for ≥3 months, with or without kidney damage

GFR, glomerular filtration rate.
Kidney Disease Outcome Quality Initiative: K/DOQI clinical practice guidelines for chronic kidney disease: Evaluation, classification, and stratification. Am J Kidney Dis 39(2 Suppl 2):S1–246, 2002 [Table 2].

TABLE 18–2	National Kidney Foundation Kidney Disease Outcomes Quality Initiative Classification, Prevalence, and Action Plan for Stages of Chronic Kidney Disease			
Stage*	Description	GFR ml/min/1.73 m²	Prevalence, n (%)†	Actions‡
—	At increased risk	≥60 (with chronic kidney disease risk factors)	—	Screening; chronic kidney disease risk reduction
1	Kidney damage with normal or increased GFR	≥90	5,900,000 (3.3)	Diagnosis and treatment; treatment of comorbid conditions; slowing progression; cardiovascular disease risk reduction
2	Kidney damage with mild decreased GFR	60–89	5,300,000 (3.0)	Estimating progression
3	Moderately decreased GFR	30–59	7,600,000 (4.3)	Evaluating and treating complications
4	Severely decreased GFR	15–29	400,000 (0.2)	Preparation for kidney replacement therapy
5	Kidney failure	<15 or dialysis	300,000 (0.1)	Kidney replacement therapy (if uremia present)

GFR, glomerular filtration rate.
Modified from National Kidney Foundation: K/DOQI clinical practice guidelines on hypertension and antihypertensive agents in chronic kidney disease. Am J Kidney Dis 43(5 Suppl 1):S1–290, 2004 [Table 2, Table 51].
*Stages 1 to 5 indicate patients with chronic kidney disease; the row without a stage number indicates persons at increased risk for developing chronic kidney disease. Chronic kidney disease is defined as either kidney damage or GFR less than 60 mL/min per 1.73 m² for 3 or more months. Kidney damage is defined as pathologic abnormalities or markers of damage, including abnormalities in blood or urine tests or imaging studies.
†Prevalence for stage 5 is from the U.S. Renal Data System (1998); it includes approximately 230,000 patients treated with dialysis and assumes 70,000 additional patients not receiving dialysis. Prevalence for stages 1 to 4 is from the Third National Health and Nutrition Examination Survey (1988 to 1994). Population of 177 million adults age 20 or more years. Glomerular filtration rate is estimated from serum creatinine measurements by using the Modification of Diet in Renal Disease study equation based on age, sex, race, and calibration for serum creatinine. For stages 1 and 2, kidney damage is estimated by using untimed urine samples to determine the albumin-creatinine ratios; greater than 17 mg/g in men or greater than 25 mg/g in women on two measurements indicates kidney damage. The proportion of persons at risk for chronic kidney disease has not been estimated accurately.
‡Includes actions from preceding stages.

TABLE 18–3 Risk Factors for Chronic Kidney Disease and its Outcomes

Risk Factor	Definition	Examples
Susceptibility factors	Increase susceptibility to kidney damage	Older age, family history of chronic kidney disease, reduction in kidney mass, low birthweight, U.S. racial or ethnic minority status, low income or education
Initiation factors	Directly initiate kidney damage	Diabetes, high blood pressure, autoimmune diseases, systemic infections, urinary tract infections, urinary stones, lower urinary tract obstruction, drug toxicity
Progression factors	Cause worsening kidney damage and faster decline in kidney function after initiation of kidney damage	Higher level of proteinuria, systolic blood pressure, poor glycemic control in diabetes, smoking
End-stage factors	Increase morbidity and mortality in kidney failure	Lower dialysis dose (Kt/V), temporary vascular access, anemia, low serum albumin level, late referral

Kt/V, dialyzer urea clearance multiplied by time divided by volume of distribution of urea.
Modified and reprinted with permission from Levey AS, Coresh J, Balk E, et al: National Kidney Foundation practice guidelines for chronic kidney disease: evaluation, classification, and stratification. Ann Intern Med 139:137–147, 2003; Kidney Disease Outcome Quality Initiative: K/DOQI clinical practice guidelines for chronic kidney disease: Evaluation, classification, and stratification. Am J Kidney Dis 39:S1–246, 2002.

TABLE 18–4 Bradford-Hill Criteria of Causality

Criteria	Explanation
Strength of association	Stronger the association the more likely the relationship is causal
Consistency	A causal association is consistent when replicated in different populations and studies
Specificity	A single putative cause produces a single effect
Temporality	Exposure precedes outcome (i.e., risk factor predates disease)
Biological gradient	Increasing exposure to risk factor increases risk of disease and reduction in exposure reduces risk
Plausibility	The observed association is consistent with biological mechanisms of disease processes
Coherence	The observed association is compatible with existing theory and knowledge within a given field
Experimental evidence	The factor under investigation is amenable to modification by an appropriate experimental approach
Analogy	An established cause and effect relationship exists for a similar exposure or disease

Modified from Hill AB: The environment and disease: Association or causation? Proc R Soc Med 58:295–300, 1965.

may signify a true risk factor. The latter implies the presence of a cause and effect relationship between the variable and disease of interest. Identification of risk factors is a key step in understanding pathways leading to development of disease and therefore for the formulation of effective strategies to prevent development and retard progression.

Bradford-Hill criteria provide guidelines for inferring causation when an association is observed and specify the minimal conditions that must be met to establish a causal relationship between the putative risk factor (exposure) and disease (outcome) (Table 18–4).[9] In a complex disease such as CKD with its multifactorial etiology, most risk factors studied may not meet all these criteria. However, they form a good framework to evaluate the adequacy of existing evidence for or against a causal association between risk factors under investigation and CKD.

Sources of Evidence for Identification of Risk Factors

Analytical epidemiology studies examine associations between putative risk factor exposures and health outcomes and can be broadly classified as observational and experimental. The three basic observational study designs include cross-sectional studies, case control studies, and prospective or cohort studies, and the main experimental study design is a randomized controlled trial (Table 18–5).[10,11]

Cross-Sectional Studies
In this type of study the relationship between exposure and outcome of interest in a given study population is assessed at a single point in time. Cross-sectional studies are the simplest study design and offer a quick first look at associations. However, a major shortcoming of cross-sectional studies is that the relationships detected using this study design by definition cannot fulfill Hill's criteria of temporality. Because this study design involves a snap shot of the association being studied, with both disease and exposure being assessed simultaneously, it cannot establish the temporal sequence required to establish causality. In other words, cross-sectional studies do not determine whether the exposure preceded outcome. Nevertheless, this study design is useful for the preliminary examination of plausible relationships and hypothesis generation.

Case-Control Studies
In this study design associations between exposure and disease are assessed by comparing rates of exposure in groups with and without disease. The measure of association between the risk factor and disease obtained from a case-control study is the odds ratio. In the simplest design, individuals with

TABLE 18–5 Comparison of Observational Study Designs

	Cross-Sectional	Case-Control	Cohort
Study population	Cases (individuals with disease) and controls (individuals without disease) ascertained by single examination of population	Cases (individuals with disease) selected based on selection criteria formulated by investigator and controls (individuals without disease) selected to resemble cases	Defined population followed-up for pre defined time period, cases and controls ascertained during follow-up.
Exposure	Exposure ascertained by single examination of population	Past exposure predating development of disease, measured, or reconstructed	Exposure measured before development of disease
Statistical analysis	Odds Ratio provides estimate of relative risk of exposure	Odds Ratio provides estimate of relative risk of disease	Direct measures of incidence and relative risk

From Fletcher RH, Fletcher SW, Wagner EH: Clinical Epidemiology, The Essentials. Philadelphia: Lippincott Williams & Wilkins, 1996.

TABLE 18–6 Examples of Epidemiologic Studies Involving Patients with Kidney Disease*

Study Design	Examples
Prospective cohorts	Population Based Cohorts
	Atherosclerosis Risk in Communities Study (ARIC)
	Framingham Heart Study
	Cardiovascular Health Study (CHS)
	Multi-Ethnic Study of Atherosclerosis (MESA)
	Health, Aging and Body Composition (Health ABC)
	Coronary Artery Risk Development in Young Adults (CARDIA)
	Cohorts of Patients with Kidney Disease
	Chronic Renal Insufficiency Cohort (CRIC)
	Cardiovascular Risk in Birmingham (CRIB)
	United States Renal Data System (USRDS)
	Choices for Healthy Outcomes in Caring for End Stage Renal Disease (CHOICE)
Intervention trials	Trials in Patients with Kidney Disease
	Modification of Diet in Renal Disease Study (MDRD)
	African American Study of Kidney Disease (AASK)
	Study of Heart and Renal Protection (SHARP)
	Prevention of Renal and Vascular Endstage Disease Intervention Trial (PREVEND IT)
	The Microalbuminuria Captopril Study
	Gruppo Italiano di Studi Epidemiologici in Nefrologia (GISEN)
	Deutsche Diabetes Dialyse Studie (4D)
	Reduction of Endpoints in NIDDM with the Angiotensin II Antagonist Losartan (RENAAL)
	Irbesartan in Diabetic Nephropathy Trial (IDNT)
	Hemodialysis Study (HEMO)
	The Ramipril Efficacy In Nephropathy (REIN)
	Post Hoc Analysis of Trials in Populations with CVD or CVD Risk Factors
	Heart Outcomes Prevention Evaluation Trial (HOPE)
	Cholesterol and Recurrent Events Trial (CARE)
	Antihypertensive and Lipid-Lowering Treatment to Prevent Heart Attack Trial (ALLHAT)

*This is not an exhaustive list.

(cases) and without (controls) the disease are identified at a given time point from a study population. Rates of past exposure to the risk factor of interest are measured and compared between these groups. A major issue with case-control studies includes exposure identification bias or recall bias whereby because the exposure occurred in the past there may be imperfect ascertainment of the level of exposure.

Cohort Studies

In a cohort study, also termed prospective study, a study population consisting of individuals with and without exposure to the risk factor of interest is followed into the future and rates of disease occurrence are compared between the two groups. A major advantage of a cohort study is the ability

to obtain direct measures of disease occurrence or incidence and of the risk of developing disease. The measure of association obtained from a cohort study is a relative risk. A cohort study is of benefit to confirm associations observed in cross-sectional or case-control studies. Table 18–6, although by no means exhaustive, lists examples of important cohort studies that have provided key information regarding risk factor relationships in CKD. One potential problem with cohort studies is the issue of confounding. A confounder is a variable that is associated with both the exposure and the outcome under study (Fig. 18–2). The presence of confounding can alter (i.e., strengthen, weaken, or mask) the association between the exposure of interest and outcome. One analytical approach for dealing with confounding is to adjust or control for poten-

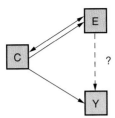

FIGURE 18-2 The confounder (C) is causally associated with the outcome of interest (Y) and either causally or noncausally associated with exposure (E); these associations may distort the association of interest: whether E causes Y. (From Szklo M, Nieto JF: Epidemiology Beyond the Basics. Gaithersburg: Aspen Publishers, Inc. [Figure 5–1, page 181], 2000.)

tially confounding variables in multivariable regression analyses. However, it must be emphasized that statistical adjustment may not completely mitigate the effects of confounding and imperfect adjustment may result in residual confounding.

Randomized Controlled Trials

In this experimental study design a defined study population is randomly assigned to different interventions. After a fixed follow-up period, rates of pre-defined outcomes are compared between the study arms. In variations of this theme, comparisons can be made between existing treatments and new ones, treated versus untreated, etc. In addition, certain study questions may require blinding or masking; in a single blind study, participants are unaware of their assignment to treatment or control arms, whereas in a double blind study neither participants nor data collectors are aware of study assignment. Blinding in drug therapy trials is often achieved by using a placebo. Table 18–6 lists some examples of important randomized controlled trials that have investigated interventions for patients with CKD. The randomized trial is considered the gold standard for evaluating interventions and associations as it minimizes many of the biases associated with observational study designs and is the only study design that fulfills the Bradford Hill criteria of experimental evidence. In particular, these studies have an advantage over observational study designs of minimizing the effects of confounding because successful randomization should ensure the uniform distribution of known and unknown confounders between the different study arms. However, it must be noted that although randomized trials provide a high level of evidence for evaluating therapeutic agents they are less definitive in terms of assessing risk factor associations. This is attributable to the fact that several interventions affect multiple risk factors, for example angiotensin converting enzyme (ACE) inhibitors reduce blood pressure and proteinuria and statins improve lipid profiles and reduce levels of C-reactive protein, and thus it is difficult to isolate the association between one particular risk factor and outcome.

Data from clinical trials are also used for subgroup and post hoc analyses. In subgroup analyses, a subset of the original participants is selected for study. Post hoc analyses refer to an unplanned exploration of data to try and find associations between variables of interest. Subgroup analyses may be determined a priori or may be post hoc. For example, the Heart Outcomes and Prevention Evaluation (HOPE) study was a randomized trial that investigated the effects of ramipril and vitamin E on major cardiovascular outcomes in 9297 high-risk patients.[12] The study had an upper limit for serum creatinine concentrations of 2.3 mg/dL and found a benefit of ramipril on CVD mortality with a hazard ratio of 0.74. In a post hoc subgroup analysis, the investigators examined the impact of ramipril on prevention of CVD outcomes in 980 patients with mild kidney dysfunction defined as serum

creatinine >1.4 mg/dL[13] and found a benefit for ramipril with a hazard ratio of 0.59 for CVD mortality. Although this was an important analysis demonstrating benefit of a specific intervention in a high-risk group of patients, subgroups and post hoc analyses are problematic in many ways. They may lack statistical power and thus be vulnerable to type 2 errors where one incorrectly fails to reject a null hypothesis or conversely when multiple hypotheses are tested, especially in a large dataset, there is an increased chance of a type 1 error (where one incorrectly rejects a true null hypothesis) unless the conventional cut off of $P < 0.05$ is lowered. Predetermined analyses can be planned to minimize the risk of type 1 and type 2 errors. For example, if the subgroup analysis had been planned in advance, the investigators may have stratified by kidney function or performed power analyses for this particular subgroup of interest. However, despite these caveats, subgroup and post hoc analyses of large clinical trials are valuable in hypothesis generation and for exploratory analyses. Finally, participants from the different arms of randomized clinical trials are often combined and analyzed as a cohort. Examples of randomized clinical trials that have yielded prospective cohort data include the Modification of Diet in Renal Disease (MDRD) Study and the Multiple Risk Factor Intervention Trial (MRFIT).

Types of Risk Factors in Chronic Kidney Disease

In this section, we define the different types of risk factor relationships involved in the development and progression of CKD. By definition, studies of risk factors for susceptibility and initiation of kidney disease require study in populations without kidney disease, whereas studies of risk factors for progression and end-stage factors are conducted in populations with CKD. In later sections of the chapter, we will discuss individual risk factors for CKD. The distinction as to the type of risk factor is inherently complicated by limitations of study designs; in particular, without appropriate ascertainment for the earlier stages of CKD, it is difficult to determine whether risk factors for later stages of CKD affect susceptibility, initiation, or progression.

Susceptibility Factors

As defined in Table 18–3 and depicted in Figure 18–1, a susceptibility factor is one that increases susceptibility to kidney damage following exposure to an initiation factor. For example, susceptibility to urinary tract infections is in part determined by host factors that influence pathogen recognition and pathogen-induced signaling. Recently, Toll-like receptors have been identified in the uroepithilia that are important for pathogen recognition and activation of the immune response. Thus, genetic polymorphisms that downregulate the activity of these receptors may make an individual more susceptible to urinary tract infections.[14] An ideal study design to detect susceptibility factors would involve identifying a large cohort of individuals who are free of kidney disease and are exposed to an initiation factor and following them for an extended period of time to determine risk factors associated with development of kidney damage (Table 18–7). The large sample size and extended follow-up time entailed by this approach has the disadvantage of costs and logistic difficulties. Much of our current understanding regarding susceptibility factors is derived from case-control studies; unfortunately, this design usually cannot distinguish susceptibility from initiation factors.

Initiation Factors

An initiation factor is one that directly initiates kidney damage, such as diabetes, hypertension, urinary tract infection, or a toxic drug, in an individual who is susceptible to

TABLE 18–7 Ideal Study Design for Risk Factor Identification

Risk Factors	Study Design	Populations	Outcome	Indicator
Susceptibility	Prospective Randomized controlled trial	Free of kidney disease and exposure to initiation factor	Kidney damage	Microalbuminuria Proteinuria
Initiation	Prospective Randomized controlled trial	Free of kidney disease and susceptible to kidney disease	Kidney damage	Microalbuminuria Proteinuria
Progression	Prospective Randomized controlled trial	Earlier stages of kidney disease	Worsening kidney disease	Microalbuminuria → proteinuria Microalbuminuria → reduced GFR Worsening GFR Kidney failure
End-stage including development of cardiovascular disease	Prospective Randomized controlled trial	Earlier stages of kidney disease Kidney failure	Morbidity Complications Mortality Cardiovascular disease	Biomarkers/surrogate markers Comorbid illness Hospitalization Death

GFR, glomerular filtration rate.

kidney damage. Given the lack of a "cure" or means to reverse kidney damage, the identification and amelioration of initiation factors is crucial to prevent the development of CKD and its associated adverse outcomes. While case-control studies are hypothesis generating, the ideal study design for identification of initiation factors is a prospective cohort study (see Table 18–7). This would entail identifying and following a cohort of individuals free of kidney disease at baseline, with known susceptibility factors, and with and without exposure to the putative initiation factor, for the development of incident kidney disease defined as development of microalbuminuria, proteinuria, or reduced GFR.

Progression Factors

Progression factors worsen the kidney damage caused by initiation factors and lead to further decline in kidney function. Progression factors may also be termed perpetuation factors and this term better reflects the self-perpetuating nature of progressive kidney disease. Prospective cohort studies as well as clinical trials help to establish risk factor relationships between putative progression factors and kidney disease (see Table 18–7). The identification of progression factors using a cohort study design involves identification and follow-up of a cohort of patients with early-stage CKD to estimate rates of progression of disease. Alternatively, a clinical trial can be used to provide experimental evidence of a risk factor relationship (i.e., that the modification of the putative progression factor in a randomized controlled trial results in prevention of progression of disease). This would entail identification of a group of individuals in the earlier stages of CKD. Participants are randomly assigned to an intervention arm that receives the therapy designed to modify the risk factor under investigation, and a control arm that does not receive the study intervention, and rates of progression are compared between the two arms. Indicators of progression may include progression of microalbuminuria to overt proteinuria or reduced GFR, rate of decrease of GFR, or development of kidney failure necessitating dialysis or transplantation.

End-Stage Factors

End-stage factors are those that exacerbate the morbidity and mortality associated with kidney failure. As with progression factors, ideal study designs for studying end-stage factors include prospective cohort studies and randomized controlled trials (see Table 18–7). In a prospective study, a cohort of patients with kidney failure is followed to determine factors associated with adverse outcomes including morbidity and mortality. Alternatively, patients with kidney failure are randomized to receive interventions targeted at modifying putative end-stage factors and improving mortality and morbidity. Examples of indicators of morbidity include hospitalizations, poor quality of life measures, and cardiovascular disease complications.

CARDIOVASCULAR DISEASE AND CHRONIC KIDNEY DISEASE (see Chapter 48)

It is well established that patients with kidney failure are at high risk of cardiovascular mortality (Fig. 18–3).[15–17] Patients with CKD experience a high rate of fatal and nonfatal cardiovascular disease events prior to reaching kidney failure.[18–20] Patients in all stages of CKD are therefore considered in the "highest risk group" for development of cardiovascular disease and CKD is recognized as a cardiovascular risk equivalent.[21–23]

An investigation of the natural history of disease in a large cohort of patients with CKD stages 2 to 4 demonstrated that death was a more likely outcome than progression to kidney failure in every stage of CKD (Table 18–8).[24] There was a higher baseline prevalence of cardiovascular disease in patients who died, compared with those who survived, suggesting that cardiovascular disease accounted for a large proportion of the deaths. Thus, most patients in the earlier stages of CKD do not progress to kidney failure because of mortality due to cardiovascular disease; consequently, in studies of patients with earlier stages of CKD, cardiovascular disease is a major "competing outcome or risk" with kidney failure.

The relationship between CKD and cardiovascular disease is complex; CKD is a risk factor for cardiovascular disease and cardiovascular disease may be a risk factor for CKD (Fig. 18–4). Several cardiovascular risk factors promote the development and progression of both CKD and cardiovascular disease; declining kidney function, in turn, is associated with elevated levels of cardiovascular risk factors[25] (Table 18–9). As noted in Table 18–10, several potential mechanisms underlie this complex relationship.[26]

An abundance of evidence exists in support of an association between reduced kidney function and cardiovascular disease morbidity and mortality.[23] Data from several population-based epidemiologic studies, such as the Atherosclerosis Risk In Communities Study,[20] Cardiovascular Health Study,[18,27,28] and the Hoorn Study,[29] show an association

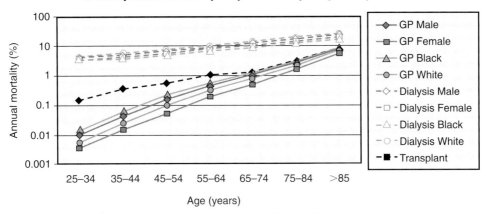

FIGURE 18–3 Cardiovascular mortality defined by death due to arrhythmias, cardiomyopathy, cardiac arrest, myocardial infarction, atherosclerotic heart disease, and pulmonary edema in the general population (GP) (NCHS multiple cause of mortality data files ICD 9 codes 402, 404, 410–414, and 425–429, 1993) compared with kidney failure treated by dialysis or kidney transplant (USRDS special data request HCFA form 2746 #s 23, 26–29, and 31, 1994–1996). Data are stratified by age, race, and gender. CVD mortality is underestimated in kidney transplant recipients due to incomplete ascertainment of cause of death. (From Foley RN, Parfrey PS, Sarnak MJ: Clinical epidemiology of cardiovascular disease in chronic renal disease. Am J Kidney Dis 32(5 Suppl 3):S112–119, 1998; Sarnak MJ, Levey AS, Schoolwerth AC, et al: Kidney disease as a risk factor for development of cardiovascular disease: A statement from the American Heart Association Councils on Kidney in Cardiovascular Disease, High Blood Pressure Research, Clinical Cardiology, and Epidemiology and Prevention. Circulation 108:2154–2169 [Figure 1, page 2155], 2003.)

TABLE 18–8	Competing Risks of Death and Kidney Failure in Chronic Kidney Disease			
End Points	GFR 60–89 No Proteinuria (n = 14,202)	Stage 2 GFR 60–89, Proteinuria (n = 1741)	Stage 3 GFR 30–59 (n = 11,278)	Stage 4 GFR 15–29 (n = 777)
Dis-enrolled from plan	14.9	16.2	10.3	6.6
Died (prior to transplant/dialysis)	10.2	19.5	24.3	45.7
Received a transplant	0.01	0.2	0.2	2.3
Initiated dialysis	0.06	0.9	1.1	17.6
None of the above through June 30, 2001	74.8	63.3	64.2	27.8

From Keith DS, Nichols GA, Gullion CM, et al: Longitudinal follow-up and outcomes among a population with chronic kidney disease in a large managed care organization. Arch Intern Med 164:659–663 [Table 2], 2004.

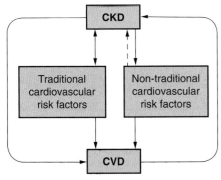

FIGURE 18–4 Chronic kidney disease (CKD) is a risk factor for cardiovascular disease (CVD) and cardiovascular disease may be a risk factor for progression of chronic kidney disease. Traditional cardiovascular disease risk factors promote the development and progression of both chronic kidney disease and cardiovascular disease. Declining kidney function is associated with elevated levels of traditional and nontraditional cardiovascular disease risk factors. It remains unknown whether nontraditional cardiovascular disease risk factors (dotted arrow) are important risk factors for progression of kidney disease. (From Menon V, Gul A, Sarnak MJ: Cardiovascular risk factors in chronic kidney disease. Kidney Int 68:1413–1418 [Figure 1], 2005.)

between reduced kidney function and risk of all-cause and cardiovascular disease mortality that persists after adjustment for traditional cardiovascular disease risk factors. In the Second National Health And Nutrition Examination Survey Mortality Study, patients with GFR <70 ml/min had a 68% higher risk of cardiovascular disease mortality compared with subjects with normal GFR.[30] In a pooled analysis of community-based studies including Atherosclerosis Risk in Communities Study, Cooperative Health Study, Framingham Heart Study, and the Framingham Offspring Study, CKD, defined as GFR of 15 to 60 ml/min/1.73m², was an independent predictor of a composite outcome of all-cause mortality as well as fatal and nonfatal cardiovascular disease events.[31] Finally, a study of over 1 million members of a large healthcare system demonstrated an independent graded association between reduced GFR and fatal and nonfatal cardiovascular events[32] (Fig. 18–5). Possible explanations for the observed independent association between reduced GFR and cardiovascular disease are presented in Table 18–11.

Evidence from several studies has established urinary albumin excretion as an independent predictor of cardiovascular outcomes.[23,33–42] The association between albumin excretion and cardiovascular disease appears to extend well below current definitions and cut offs for microalbuminuria and is independent of traditional cardiovascular risk factors

TABLE 18–9 Manifestations of Cardiovascular Disease in Chronic Kidney Disease and Associated Putative Risk Factors

Pathology	Traditional Risk Factors	Non-traditional Risk Factors
Cardiomyopathy	Older age Hypertension Valvular disease Dyslipidemia Smoking Diabetes	Albuminuria Reduced glomerular filtration rate Anemia Inflammation Arteriosclerosis Extracellular fluid volume overload Abnormal calcium/phosphate metabolism
Atherosclerosis	Older age Male gender Hypertension Diabetes Dyslipidemia Smoking Physical inactivity LVH	Albuminuria Reduced glomerular filtration rate Anemia Inflammation Oxidative stress Endothelial dysfunction Homocysteine Lipoprotein (a) Malnutrition Thrombogenic factors Sympathetic activity Insulin resistance/metabolic syndrome
Arteriosclerosis	Older age Male gender Smoking Hypertension Diabetes Dyslipidemia	Albuminuria Reduced glomerular filtration rate Endothelial dysfunction Abnormal calcium/phosphate metabolism Metabolic syndrome

From Menon V, Gul A, Sarnak MJ: Cardiovascular risk factors in chronic kidney disease. Kidney Int 68:1413–1418, 2005.

TABLE 18–10 Potential Mechanisms for Increased Cardiovascular Disease Risk in Chronic Kidney Disease

1. Chronic kidney disease is associated with an increase in prevalence of cardiovascular disease risk factors and these cardiovascular disease risk factors promote development and progression of CKD.
2. Cardiovascular disease is a risk factor for CKD.
3. Chronic kidney disease is an independent risk factor for cardiovascular disease.

CKD, chronic kidney disease.
From Menon V, Sarnak MJ: The epidemiology of chronic kidney disease stages 1 to 4 and cardiovascular disease: A high-risk combination. Am J Kidney Dis 45:223–232 [p 225], 2005.

TABLE 18–11 Possible Explanations for the Observed Independent Association between Kidney Dysfunction and Cardiovascular Disease

Reduced Glomerular Filtration Rate	Albuminuria
Reduced GFR is associated with an increased level of nontraditional risk factors that are frequently not adjusted for in analyses.[153]	Microalbuminuria may be a marker of generalized endothelial dysfunction and vascular permeability.[188,189]
Reduced GFR may be a marker of the severity of diagnosed vascular disease or of undiagnosed vascular disease.	Microalbuminuria may be associated with other traditional and nontraditional cardiovascular disease risk factors.[188,190]
Reduced GFR may be a measure of residual confounding from traditional risk factors.[25]	Microalbuminuria may be a precursor for the development of early or incipient kidney disease.[39]
Patients with reduced GFR may not receive the benefits of optimal therapies such as aspirin, beta blockers, angiotensin converting enzyme inhibitors.[191]	

GFR, glomerular filtration rate.

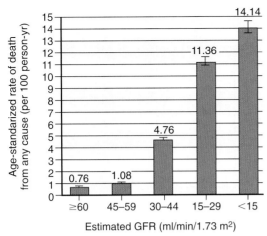

A   No. of Events   25,803   11,569   7802   4408   1842

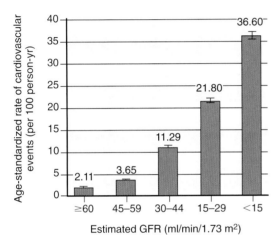

B   No. of Events   73,108   34,690   18,580   8809   3824

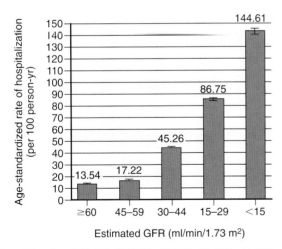

C   No. of Events   366,757   106,543   49,177   20,581   11,593

FIGURE 18–5 Age-standardized rates of death from any cause (Panel A), cardiovascular events (Panel B), and hospitalization (Panel C), according to the estimated GFR among 1,120,295 ambulatory adults. A cardiovascular event was defined as hospitalization for coronary heart disease, heart failure, ischemic stroke, and peripheral arterial disease. Error bars represent 95% confidence intervals (CI). The rate of events is listed above each bar. (From Age-Standardized Rates of Death from Any Cause (Panel A), Cardiovascular Events (Panel B), and Hospitalization (Panel C), According to the Estimated GFR. From Go AS, Chertow GM, Fan D, et al: Chronic kidney disease and the risks of death, cardiovascular events, and hospitalization. N Engl J Med 351:1296–1305 [Figure 1], 2004.)

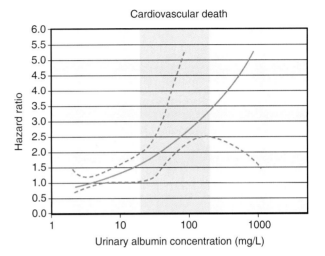

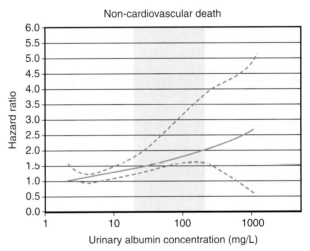

FIGURE 18–6 Adjusted effect of UAC on hazard function. Solid line shows estimated relation when logarithmic hazard is modeled as linear function of log(UAC). Dotted lines are 95% confidence limits for more general functional relation, as estimated by P-splines. Hatched area represents upper and lower limit of current definition of microalbuminuria (20 mg/L to 200 mg/L). (From Hillege HL, Fidler V, Diercks GFH, et al for the Prevention of Renal and Vascular End Stage Disease (PREVEND) Study Group: Urinary albumin excretion predicts cardiovascular and noncardiovascular mortality in general population. Circulation 106:1777–1782 [Figure 1], 2002.)

(Fig. 18–6). Potential reasons for the observed relationship between microalbuminuria and cardiovascular disease are presented in Table 18–11.

Given the close correlation between cardiovascular disease and CKD, we have organized the following discussion to reflect the association between these chronic diseases. Consequently, we have categorized risk factors for CKD as cardiovascular disease risk factors, kidney-related risk factors, and non-kidney–related risk factors.

CARDIOVASCULAR DISEASE RISK FACTORS AS RISK FACTORS FOR CHRONIC KIDNEY DISEASE

In this section we review the evidence relating cardiovascular disease risk factors to CKD. Although many of the risk factors discussed in this section may also promote the development of cardiovascular disease in individuals with CKD this is discussed in detail in Chapter 48. Therefore, we limit our focus to the role of cardiovascular disease risk factors in promoting the development and progression of CKD.

Hypertension

Hypertension is well recognized as a risk factor for the development and progression of kidney disease. Several large prospective studies, including the MRFIT and the Systolic Hypertension in the Elderly Program, have established a strong relationship between hypertension and rate of decline in kidney function and development of kidney failure.[43-48] Degree of blood pressure control appears to be an important determinant of rate of progression of kidney disease among treated patients with hypertension.[49] Systolic and diastolic blood pressure were demonstrated to be significant predictors for the development of microalbuminuria in several prospective studies of diabetic and non-diabetic populations.[50-52]

Data from randomized controlled trials examining the effect of blood pressure control on progression of kidney disease is less consistent. In the Modification of Diet in Renal Disease (MDRD) Study, a randomized, controlled trial of 840 persons with predominantly nondiabetic kidney disease and a GFR of 13 to 55 mL/min per 1.73 m[2], strict blood pressure control did not slow progression of kidney disease over the 2.2-year follow-up period of the trial; however, in long-term follow-up the low target blood pressure slowed the progression of kidney disease in patients irrespective of cause of kidney disease, baseline GFR, or degree of proteinuria.[53,54] In contrast, in the African American Study of Kidney Disease (AASK), 1094 African Americans with hypertensive renal disease were randomly assigned to usual or lower mean arterial pressure goals and to initial treatment with a beta-blocker, an ACE inhibitor, or a dihydropyridine calcium channel blocker, and followed up for 3 to 6.4 years. The lower blood pressure goal did not appear to confer any additional benefit of slowing progression of hypertensive nephrosclerosis, although ACE inhibitors appeared to be more effective than beta-blockers or dihydropyridine calcium channel blockers in slowing GFR decline.[55] One hypothesis to explain these discrepant results is that higher blood pressure is a stronger risk factor in patients with higher levels of proteinuria[56] (Fig. 18-7), as was seen in the MDRD Study compared with AASK.[57] Similarly, a randomized controlled trial studied the effect of adding calcium channel blocker to achieve a lower blood pressure goal in patients with non-diabetic proteinuric nephropathies receiving background ACE-inhibitor therapy. This study was unable to demonstrate any additional benefit from further blood pressure reduction on progression of kidney disease,[58] possibly because of a lower than anticipated difference in achieved blood pressure between the two groups.[57] Thus, although there is consensus that high blood pressure is deleterious and promotes kidney injury and progression of kidney disease, further research is required to establish the ideal goal for target blood pressure.[57]

Diabetes

Diabetic kidney disease accounts for almost half of all incident cases of kidney failure in the United States.[59,60] Several studies have established the role of diabetes as a predominant

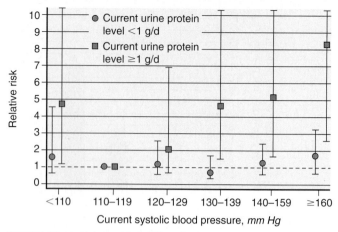

FIGURE 18-7 Relative risk for kidney disease progression based on current level of systolic blood pressure and current urine protein excretion. The relative risk for patients with a current urine protein excretion of 1.0 g/d or greater represents 9336 patients (223 events), and the relative risk for patients with a current urine protein excretion less than 1.0 g/d represents 13,274 visits (88 events). The reference group for each is defined at a systolic blood pressure of 110 mm Hg to 119 mm Hg. Confidence intervals are truncated, as shown. Results are from a single multivariable model including two levels for urine protein excretion, six levels for systolic blood pressure, and the interaction of current systolic blood pressure and current urine protein excretion. Covariates include assignment to angiotensin-converting enzyme inhibitor versus control group, sex, age, baseline systolic blood pressure, baseline diastolic blood pressure, baseline urine protein excretion, baseline serum creatinine concentration (<2.0 or ≥2.0 mg/dL [<177 or ≥177 μmol/L]), interaction of baseline serum creatinine and baseline urine protein excretion, interaction of baseline serum creatinine and current urine protein excretion, and study terms. (From Jafar TH, Stark PC, Schmid CH, et al: Progression of chronic kidney disease: The role of blood pressure control, proteinuria, and angiotensin-converting enzyme inhibition: A patient-level meta-analysis. Ann Intern Med 139:244–252 [Figure 1], 2003.)

contributory factor for the development of CKD. In a population-based case-control study of White and African American individuals with type 1 and type 2 diabetes, the overall population-attributable risk for kidney failure was 42%.[61] In the United Kingdom Prospective Diabetes Study (UKPDS), 10 years after diagnosis of diabetes, the prevalence of microalbuminuria was 25%, of macroalbuminuria was 5.3%, and of elevated plasma creatinine or kidney failure was 0.8%.[62] In the Framingham Heart Study offspring cohort, baseline dysglycemia was associated with future risk of developing CKD.[63]

Among patients with diabetes, there appears to be a strong relationship between poor metabolic control and the risk for development of diabetic kidney disease. A Danish prospective study examined the incidence of diabetic kidney disease in patients with onset of type 1 diabetes between 1965 and 1979 followed up until death or until 1991. The cumulative incidence of diabetic kidney disease was 17%, and 19% to 28% of the patients had persistent microalbuminuria.[64] The primary risk factor for the development of kidney complications was long-term glycemic control. A Swedish population-based cohort study demonstrated dramatic decreases in the cumulative incidence of diabetic kidney disease with improved metabolic control.[65] In a prospective study of type 1 diabetes, glycemic control was the major determinant for the development of microalbuminuria.[66]

Evidence from intervention trials supports the data from observational studies regarding the importance of glycemic control. In the Diabetes Control and Complications Trial (DCCT), 1441 patients with type 1 diabetes and with and without retinopathy at baseline were randomized to receive intensive or conventional therapy. After a mean follow-up

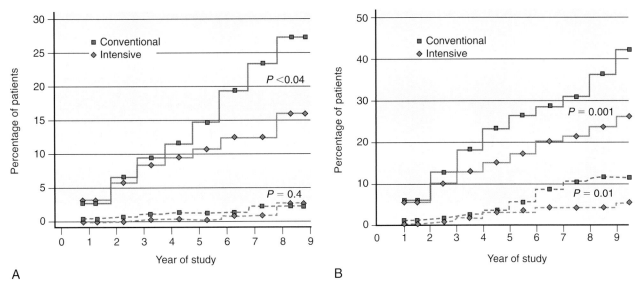

FIGURE 18–8 Cumulative incidence of urinary albumin excretion in patients with IDDM receiving intensive or conventional therapy. In the primary-prevention cohort (Panel A), intensive therapy reduced the adjusted mean risk of microalbuminuria by 34% (*P* < 0.04). In the secondary-intervention cohort (Panel B), patients with urinary albumin excretion of ≥40 mg per 24 hours at baseline were excluded from the analysis of the development of microalbuminuria. Intensive therapy reduced the adjusted mean risk of albuminuria by 56% (*P* = 0.01) and the risk of microalbuminuria by 43% (*P* = 0.001), as compared with conventional therapy. (From The Diabetes Control and Complications Trial Research Group: The effect of intensive treatment of diabetes on the development and progression of long-term complications in insulin-dependent diabetes mellitus. N Engl J Med 329:977–986 [Figure 3], 1993.)

of 6.5 years, intensive therapy reduced the occurrence of microalbuminuria by 39%, and albuminuria by 54%[67] (Fig. 18–8). Thus reducing the incidence of diabetes and improving metabolic control among patients with diabetes are key components of any strategy aimed at reducing the burden of CKD.

However, only one third of patients with newly diagnosed diabetes develop diabetic kidney disease, strongly suggesting the possibility of a major contribution of susceptibility factors to the pathogenesis of this disease. In the Inception Cohort Study, a prospective observational study of an inception cohort of 286 patients newly diagnosed with type 1 diabetes, baseline factors independently associated with development of persistent microalbuminuria included baseline urinary albumin excretion rate, male gender, mean arterial blood pressure, and haemoglobin A_{1c} concentration.[51] Furthermore, progression of diabetic kidney disease also appears to be influenced by factors other than the level of glycemic control. For example, in the Reduction of End Points in NIDDM with the Angiotensin II Receptor Antagonist Losartan (RENAAL) study, which included 1513 patients with type 2 diabetes and nephropathy proteinuria, serum creatinine, serum albumin, and hemoglobin level were associated with increased risk of doubling of serum creatinine, dialysis, or transplantation for patients in whom blood pressure was controlled.[68] Diabetic nephropathy is discussed in detail in Chapter 36.

Smoking

Several observational studies have suggested a link between smoking and CKD. In cross-sectional analysis of a population sample of 28,409 individuals, former and current smoking was associated with an approximately threefold increased risk of proteinuria.[69] Similar results were seen in an Australian population-based sample where the investigators found a graded relationship between smoking and proteinuria.[70] A European, multi-center, case-control study of men on dialysis demonstrated an increased risk of kidney failure among smokers.[71] Smoking was also a risk factor for kidney function decline in diabetic kidney disease[72] and essential hyperten-

sion.[73] Prospective studies have reproduced these findings. The population-based Prevention of Renal and Vascular End Stage Disease Study (PREVEND) noted that smoking was an independent predictor for the development of microalbuminuria and reduced GFR among healthy individuals.[74] Similar results were obtained from the Framingham Offspring Study.[75] In a prospective study of patients with CKD, smoking cessation was associated with decreased rate of progression and postponement of kidney failure over a 2-year follow-up period.[76] These data collectively suggest that smoking not only induces direct kidney injury but also potentiates kidney damage in the presence of other susceptibility and initiation factors.

Dyslipidemia

Several, but admittedly not all, studies suggest that dyslipidemia may promote development and progression of kidney disease.[77] In the Physician's Health Study, over a 14-year follow-up period, dyslipidemia was associated with increased risk of developing decreased kidney function (defined as creatinine >1.5 mg/dl) in men with normal kidney function at baseline[78] (Fig. 18–9). In the Atherosclerosis Risk In Communities (ARIC) Study, high triglycerides and low high-density lipoprotein cholesterol were associated with an increased risk of developing decreased kidney function.[79] A study evaluating risk factors for incident CKD (defined as GFR <60 ml/min/1.73 m^2) in patients with essential hypertension and normal glomerular filtration at baseline, noted that higher mean total cholesterol during follow up was a significant risk factor for the development of CKD.[80] In a hospital-based cohort, hypercholesterolemia was associated with a twofold increase in the risk of developing CKD.[81] Finally, low high-density lipoprotein cholesterol was an independent risk factor for the development of incident CKD (GFR <60 ml/min/1.73 m^2) in the Framingham Offspring Study.[75]

Few randomized controlled trials have evaluated the effect of cholesterol lowering on the progression of CKD. The Cholesterol and Recurrent Events (CARE) Study was a randomized double-blind placebo controlled trial of pravastatin

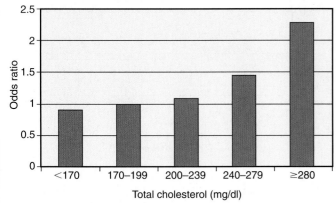

FIGURE 18–9 Association between total cholesterol categories and increased serum creatinine (≥1.5 mg/dl), adjusted for age (P for trend = 0.01). (From Schaeffner ES, Kurth T, Curhan GC, et al: Cholesterol and the risk of renal dysfunction in apparently healthy men. J Am Soc Nephrol 14:2084–2091 [Figure 1], 2003.)

versus placebo in participants with previous myocardial infarction and total plasma cholesterol <240 mg/dl. In a post hoc subgroup analysis of this trial, pravastatin appeared to slow the rate of loss of kidney function in a subset of 690 individuals with estimated GFR <60 ml/min/1.73m^2.[82] In contrast, post hoc subgroup analysis of the Veterans Affairs High-Density Lipoprotein Intervention (VA-HIT) Trial, a randomized double-blind trial of gemfibrozil versus placebo in men with coronary disease, failed to demonstrate any benefit of gemfibrozil on progression of kidney disease in 399 participants with GFR of 30 to 60 ml/min/1.73 m^2.[83] A meta-analysis of 13 prospective controlled trials concluded that treatment for hyperlipidemia may be associated with lower rate of decline in GFR and may decrease proteinuria compared with controls.[84] There is a need for a large randomized controlled trial in patients with CKD to provide definitive answers regarding whether treatment of hyperlipidemia retards the development and progression of CKD, and to identify optimal agents and target lipid levels.

Obesity

The emergence of obesity as a growing public health problem has led to its investigation as a risk factor for kidney disease. In a retrospective cohort study from Japan, a higher baseline body mass index was associated with increased risk for development of kidney failure.[85] In a small prospective study of patients who underwent unilateral nephrectomy, baseline obesity defined as body mass index >30 kg/m^2 was associated with higher risk for the development of proteinuria and reduced kidney function.[86] Similarly, in a cohort of incident patients with biopsy-proven immunoglobulin A nephropathy, body mass index ≥25 kg/m^2 at baseline was associated with the development of hypertension and kidney dysfunction.[87] Obesity also appears to predispose to the development of focal segmental glomerulosclerosis.[88] In a large retrospective cohort study of over 300,000 adults, there was a strong and graded independent relationship between body mass index and risk for kidney failure.[89] This relationship was present in subgroups based on race, gender, age, and comorbid conditions such as diabetes and hypertension. Several studies have also suggested a benefit of weight loss on preserving kidney function in obese patients.[90,91] Further studies are required to confirm a pathophysiologic role for obesity in CKD and to demonstrate the benefits of weight loss in preventing progression of CKD.

Metabolic Syndrome

The metabolic syndrome is a clustering of risk factors that include abdominal obesity, dyslipidemia, hypertension, insulin resistance, hyperfiltration, and prothrombotic and proinflammatory states. Abundant data exist from observational studies in support of metabolic syndrome as a risk factor for the development of CKD. The association between the metabolic syndrome and CKD (defined as either GFR <60 ml/min/1.73 m^2 or microalbuminuria) was assessed in cross-sectional analyses of the Third National Health and Nutrition Examination Survey (NHANES III).[92] The prevalence of CKD or microalbuminuria was higher among participants with two or more components of the metabolic syndrome compared with those with zero or one component. There was a linear relationship between presence of CKD and number of components of metabolic syndrome. In prospective analysis of 10,096 nondiabetic participants from the ARIC Study with normal baseline kidney function, after 9 years of follow-up, participants with metabolic syndrome had a 43% increased risk of developing CKD after adjusting for potential confounders.[93] This increased risk persisted after adjustment for the subsequent development of diabetes and hypertension during follow-up suggesting that metabolic syndrome is an independent risk factor for the development of kidney disease. Although observational evidence points to an association, there are no intervention trials aimed at studying the effect of treating metabolic syndrome on the risk of developing incident CKD. Such a trial would entail a complicated study design with multiple risk factor interventions. Glomerular hyperfiltration has also been identified as a new market of metabolic risk.[93a]

Cardiovascular Disease as a Risk Factor for Chronic Kidney Disease

Few studies have evaluated whether the presence of cardiovascular disease is an independent risk factor for progression of CKD and development of kidney failure. Patients with heart failure have decreased kidney perfusion that at times may lead to kidney failure and patients with coronary disease have a higher prevalence of renovascular disease, which in turn may promote progression of kidney disease.[94] In a Canadian cohort of patients in different stages of CKD, the presence of cardiovascular disease at baseline increased the probability of progression to kidney failure by 50%[95] (Fig. 18–10). The magnitude of this effect persisted after multivariable adjustment for other established risk factors. In Medicare beneficiaries hospitalized for heart failure or myocardial infarction, there was a high prevalence of CKD stage 3 to 4 with more than half the cohort having reduced GFR.[96] The presence of CKD was associated with increased readmission and mortality rates, and a high risk for developing kidney failure. In a large cohort of hypertensive men, new-onset myocardial infarction doubled the future risk of kidney failure and heart failure increased the risk fivefold.[97] Thus, as described earlier, there is a complex interrelationship between cardiovascular disease and CKD resulting in a high-risk combination.

■ KIDNEY DISEASE-RELATED RISK FACTORS

In this section, we review risk factors for progression that are related to the characteristics of kidney disease and its treatment.

Proteinuria/Microalbuminuria

The National Kidney Foundation Kidney Disease Outcomes Quality Initiative guidelines define microalbuminuria as albumin excretion in 24-hour urine excretion of 30 to 300 mg/

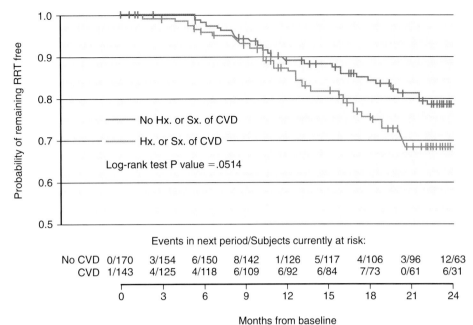

FIGURE 18–10 Kaplan-Meier curves of time to RRT by cardiovascular disease status at baseline. (From Levin A, Djurdjev O, Barrett B, et al: Cardiovascular disease in patients with chronic kidney disease: Getting to the heart of the matter. Am J Kidney Dis 38:1398–1407, 2001.)

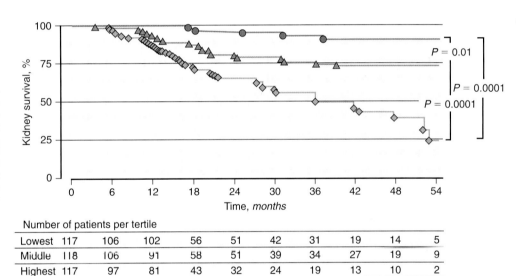

FIGURE 18–11 Progression to end-stage renal failure per tertile of baseline urinary protein excretion rate. Symbols are: (●) lowest; (▲) middle; (○) highest tertile. (From Ruggenenti P, Perna A, Mosconi L, et al., Gruppo Italiano di Studi Epidemiologici in N: Urinary protein excretion rate is the best independent predictor of ESRF in non-diabetic proteinuric chronic nephropathies. Kidney Int 53:1209–1216, 1998.)

day, or a spot urine albumin-to-creatinine ratio of 30 to 300 mg/g (some consider sex-specific cut-off values of 17 to 250 mg/g in men and 25 to 355 mg/g in women), or albumin concentration of >3 mg/dl in a spot urine specimen using an albumin-specific dipstick.[4] Albuminuria, macroalbuminuria, or clinical proteinuria is defined as urinary albumin excretion in excess of 300 mg/day, spot urine albumin-to-creatinine ratio above the microalbuminuria range, or ≥1+ tested in a spot urine sample using a conventional dipstick.

As described in an earlier section, there is abundant evidence in support of a strong and independent association between microalbuminuria and cardiovascular disease. In addition, a growing body of work that suggests that microalbuminuria or elevated urinary albumin excretion may be the earliest pathological marker of early kidney damage and may be a risk factor for the progression of diabetic and non-diabetic CKD. Microalbuminuria was inversely correlated to level of GFR in a cross-sectional analysis of 7728 individuals without diabetes.[98] In a prospective study of 537 patients with type 1 diabetes, 25% progressed to persistent

microalbuminuria or macroalbuminuria during a 10-year follow-up period.[52] Similarly, in 286 newly diagnosed patients with type 1 diabetes, baseline urinary albumin excretion rate was a strong predictor for the development of persistent microalbuminuria.[51] In post hoc subgroup analysis of 7674 participants of the HOPE trial with albuminuria data available at baseline and at follow-up, baseline microalbuminuria was associated with a 17.5-fold increased risk for clinical proteinuria in individuals without and with diabetes.[39,99] A higher baseline level of proteinuria and an increase in proteinuria during follow-up appear to be risk factors for faster kidney disease progression. For example, the rate of GFR decline was related to reduction in proteinuria in both the MDRD Study and the AASK Study.[100,101] Similarly in the Ramipril Efficacy In Nephropathy (REIN) study of 352 patients with proteinuric non-diabetic chronic nephropathies, proteinuria was a strong predictor for the development of kidney failure[102] (Fig. 18–11). As described in Chapter 54, the effectiveness of agents that reduce the activity of the renin-angiotensin-aldosterone system (RAAS) on the progression of kidney disease appears to be mediated in part by lowering urine protein excretion.[102a]

Renin-Angiotensin-Aldosterone System Activity

The RAAS is a key regulator of blood pressure and has been implicated in hypertensive end-organ damage via its role in fluid and electrolyte balance, vasoconstrictor properties, and hypertrophic effects on the cardiovascular system. These hemodynamic effects suggest a role for RAAS in mediating kidney damage and the progression of kidney disease.[103] Several guidelines recommend ACE inhibitors and angiotensin receptor blockers (ARB) as first-line anti-hypertensive agents for patients with diabetic and non-diabetic kidney disease.[21,104,105] In addition, nonhemodynamic properties of the RAAS including oxidative stress, inflammation, and endothelial dysfunction,[106] may contribute to kidney damage. These pleiotropic effects indicate a potential benefit of RAAS blockade beyond its antihypertensive and antiproteinuric actions.

Several clinical trials demonstrate a beneficial effect of ACE inhibitors on kidney outcomes that was independent of blood pressure reduction and partly accounted for by their antiproteinuric effects.[107–109] In data from the Collaborative Study Group, a randomized, controlled trial comparing captopril with placebo in patients with type 1 diabetes and overt kidney disease, captopril treatment was associated with a 50% reduction in the risk of the composite outcome of death, dialysis, and transplantation. This effect appeared to be independent of blood pressure.[110] In the Irbesartan Diabetic Nephropathy Trial (IDNT), 1715 hypertensive patients with kidney disease due to type 2 diabetes were assigned to irbesartan, amlodipine, or placebo with a target blood pressure of 135/85 mm Hg or less in all groups. The irbesartan arm had a lower risk of doubling of serum creatinine and kidney failure endpoints. These differences appeared to be independent of the blood pressures that were achieved in each arm.[111] In the RENAAL Study, a clinical trial in patients with type 2 diabetic kidney disease, losartan, an angiotensin II receptor antagonist, reduced the incidence of doubling of the serum creatinine concentration, kidney failure, and decreased level of proteinuria by 35%. The benefit of losartan on kidney outcomes exceeded that attributable to changes in blood pressure.[112] Similarly, in the REIN study where 352 patients were stratified by baseline proteinuria and assigned to ramipril or placebo plus conventional antihypertensive therapy with target diastolic blood pressure of under 90 mm Hg, ramipril reduced proteinuria and GFR decline beyond that expected with blood pressure reductions.[108] In contrast, in post hoc analyses of the Antihypertensive and Lipid-Lowering Treatment to Prevent Heart Attack Trial (ALLHAT), where hypertensive participants with one other coronary heart disease risk factor were randomized to chlorthalidone, amlodipine, or lisinopril, there was no difference in kidney outcomes of halving of GFR or kidney failure between the groups.[113]

Two meta-analyses demonstrated a benefit with ACE-inhibitor use on progression of kidney disease. ACE-inhibitor use was associated with decreased progression to macroalbuminuria in a meta-analysis of individual patient level data from 698 normotensive patients with type 1 diabetes mellitus and microalbuminuria, independent of blood pressure lowering.[114] These results were reproduced and extended by the ACE Inhibition in Progressive Renal Disease (AIPRD) Study Group with a patient-level meta-analysis of 1860 subjects with non-diabetic kidney disease, which demonstrated a benefit of ACE inhibitors in slowing the progression of non-diabetic kidney disease, defined as doubling of creatinine or kidney failure, which appeared to be independent of their effects on blood pressure and proteinuria.[115]

It appears clear that ACE inhibitors are the anti-hypertensive agents of choice in CKD due to the additional benefits derived from their ability to decrease urinary albumin excretion and other potential pleiotropic effects resulting from RAAS blockade. Clinical trials with appropriate comparators, which are specifically designed to study the effects of this class of drugs on kidney outcomes are needed to better define the mechanisms underlying the protective effects of these agents.

Dietary Protein

Several studies support the premise that dietary protein restriction delays the progression of CKD. In a cross-sectional analysis of data from the NHANES III, there was a correlation between dietary protein intake assessed from 24-hour dietary recall and albuminuria.[116] In the Nurse's Health Study, lower protein intake was associated with preservation of kidney function in women with reduced kidney function at baseline.[117] However, the MDRD Study was unable to demonstrate definitively that dietary protein restriction retards the progression of kidney disease in patients with CKD stage 3 to 4.[53] The lack of an effect appeared to be due to a short-term effect of dietary protein restriction to lower GFR and inadequate follow-up after the short-term effect.[118] In two meta-analyses, Foque and coworkers demonstrated a benefit of low-protein diets on progression of kidney disease for patients with diabetic and non-diabetic kidney disease.[119,120] In a meta-analysis of 13 randomized trials, low-protein diets were associated with reduced rate of GFR decline.[121] Low-protein diets also appeared to reduce risk of kidney failure and death in a meta-analysis of 1413 patients with non-diabetic kidney disease and 108 patients with diabetic kidney disease.[122] Furthermore this effect appeared to be independent of blood pressure in both groups and glycemic control in patients with diabetes. Although these studies appear to support a role for dietary protein restriction in delaying progression of kidney disease, as stated in the National Kidney Foundation guidelines, these data are by no means conclusive.[4]

Low Serum Albumin

Several observational studies suggest an association between low serum albumin and faster progression of kidney disease. In the Modification of Diet in Renal Disease Study, low serum albumin at baseline was associated with a higher rate of decline of GFR in multivariate analyses.[47] In post hoc analysis from the Collaborative Study Group, low serum albumin was a predictor of loss of kidney function for patients with established diabetic kidney disease.[123] Similar results were found in a Japanese cohort of patients with type 2 diabetes.[124] However, there are no clinical trials evaluating whether a high serum albumin is protective against loss of kidney function.

Reduction in Kidney Mass

Acquired or congenital oligonephropathy with a concomitant reduction in total glomerular surface area available for filtration may induce systemic and glomerular hypertension, which leads to glomerular sclerosis and kidney injury, and the development of CKD.[125] The pathophysiologic process hypothesized to increase susceptibility, to initiate kidney damage, or to promote progression in this condition is glomerular hyperfiltration caused by a disparity between the need for excretion of wastes and the number of nephrons. The predominant cause of congenital oligonephropathy is low birthweight and this is discussed in more detail in the next section. Acquired causes of oligonephropathy include accidents, surgery, malignancies, and other pathology. Evidence regarding associations between reduced kidney mass and the development of CKD comes from autopsy studies, animal studies, and a few case control and cohort studies.

In whole kidney autopsy studies, female gender, older age, certain racial groups, and lower birthweight were associated with lower glomerular number.[126] In a uninephrectomized rat model, neonatal reduction of nephron mass was associated with the development of salt-sensitive hypertension and reduced kidney function in adulthood.[127] In a case-control study comparing kidneys of adults with primary hypertension or left ventricular hypertrophy, and age, gender, height, and weight matched normotensive controls, hypertension was associated with significantly fewer glomeruli per kidney and higher glomerular volume.[128] Whereas many studies of kidney donors have noted higher blood pressure and urinary albumin following nephrectomy, one study found a higher risk of proteinuria and hypertension.[129] These data, although not conclusive, collectively support the hypothesis that reduced nephron number may lead to hypertension and kidney damage. A more detailed discussion of low nephron endowment as a risk factor for CKD is presented in Chapter 19.

Primary Hyperfiltration States

In this category we include those conditions in which glomerular hyperfiltration results from alterations in metabolism rather than reduction in nephron number. Examples of physiologic states leading to hyperfiltration include pregnancy,[130] and high protein intake[131]; examples of pathologic states include type and type 2 diabetes,[132] obesity,[133] sickle cell disease,[134] and glycogen storage diseases.[135] As with congenital or acquired oligonephropathy, it is unclear whether the hyperfiltration associated with these conditions is a susceptibility factor, is directly involved in the initiation of kidney injury, or promotes faster progression.

Anemia

Several observational studies have established that anemia is prevalent in the earlier stages of CKD and pervasive in kidney failure.[24,136-138] Other studies have demonstrated that anemia is associated with a faster progression of kidney failure; for example, the randomized cohort of the RENAAL study, each 1 g/dL decrease in hemoglobin concentration from baseline was associated with an 11% increase in the risk of developing kidney failure over a mean follow-up time of 3.4 years.[139] The severity of anemia is closely related to both the duration and stage of CKD. Given this close correlation, it is inherently difficult to establish causality and resolve whether anemia is a risk factor for progression or a marker for more severe kidney disease. A few clinical trials examining the effect of treatment of anemia on progression of kidney disease have demonstrated a benefit of anemia correction with erythropoietin[140,141] or iron.[142] However in other trials designed to study safety of erythropoietin, where kidney endpoints were not the primary outcomes, there was no effect on rate of decline in kidney function.[143-149] Three ongoing trials of cardiovascular disease, the Trial to Reduce Cardiovascular Events with Aranesp Therapy (TREAT),[150] Correction of Hemoglobin and Outcomes in Renal Insufficiency (CHOIR),[151] and Cardiovascular Risk Reduction by Early Anemia Treatment with Epoetin Beta (CREATE),[152] may provide more data regarding the utility of anemia correction in slowing progression of kidney disease as a secondary outcome.

Kidney Disease-Related Nontraditional Cardiovascular Disease Risk Factors

Nontraditional or novel risk factors for CVD are those that were not described in the Framingham study. Several of these

TABLE 18–12 Traditional and Nontraditional Cardiovascular Risk Factors in Chronic Kidney Disease

Traditional Risk Factors	Nontraditional Risk Factors
Older age	Albuminuria/Proteinuria
Male sex	Homocysteine
Hypertension	Lipoprotein (a) and apolipoprotein (a) isoforms
Higher LDL cholesterol	Lipoprotein remnants
Low HDL cholesterol	Anemia
Diabetes	Abnormal calcium/phosphate metabolism
Smoking	Extracellular fluid overload
Physical inactivity	Oxidative stress
Menopause	Inflammation (C-reactive protein)
Family history of cardiovascular disease	Malnutrition Thrombogenic factors
LVH	Sleep disturbances Altered nitric oxide/endothelin balance

HDL, high-density lipoprotein; LDL, low-density lipoprotein; LVH, left ventricular hypertrophy.
From Sarnak MJ, Levey AS: Cardiovascular disease and chronic renal disease: A new paradigm. Am J Kidney Dis 35:S117–131 [Table 4], 2000.

TABLE 18–13 Criteria for Nontraditional Risk Factors

1. A biologically plausible role for the factor in promoting cardiovascular risk

2. A dose response relationship between level of the risk factor and severity of kidney disease

3. An association between the factor and cardiovascular disease in CKD

4. Evidence from clinical trials that treatment of the risk factor decreases cardiovascular risk

CKD, chronic kidney disease.
From Sarnak MJ, Levey AS, Schoolwerth AC, et al: Kidney disease as a risk factor for development of cardiovascular disease: A statement from the American Heart Association Councils on Kidney in Cardiovascular Disease, High Blood Pressure Research, Clinical Cardiology, and Epidemiology and Prevention. Circulation 108:2154–2169 [Page 2158], 2003.

novel risk factors increase in prevalence as kidney function declines and thus may potentially contribute to the excess risk of cardiovascular disease seen in CKD 15[153] (Table 18–12). A scientific statement from the American Heart Association defines four criteria for a nontraditional risk factor (Table 18–13).[23] There are limited trial data evaluating these nontraditional factors as risk factors for the development and progression of CKD.

Several cross-sectional studies have suggested that many of these factors such as markers of inflammation, oxidative stress, and endothelial dysfunction, homocysteine, and lipoprotein (a)[153-159] are elevated in CKD; however, few prospective studies and no intervention trials have investigated their role in the progression of kidney disease. In cross-sectional analyses of NHANES III data, there was a direct correlation between prevalence of CKD and markers of insulin resistance such as levels of serum insulin, C-peptide, glycosylated hemoglobin, and Homeostasis Model Assessment-insulin resistance.[160] In long-term prospective follow-up of the randomized cohort of the MDRD Study, leptin, C-reactive protein, homocysteine, cysteine, and B vitamins were not associated with progression of kidney disease.[161,162] In contrast, data from the Cardiovascular Health Study demonstrated an association between rate of GFR decline and level of inflammatory and prothrombotic markers including C-reactive protein, white blood cell count, factor VII, and fibrinogen.[163] In a cohort of 131 patients with incident kidney disease, asymmetric dimethyl arginine, a marker of endothelial function, was an independent predictor for the development of kidney failure.[164] At this point, there is insufficient evidence in support of or against a role for nontraditional risk factors in CKD. Further laboratory, observational, and experimental studies are necessary to investigate nontraditional risk factors both from a pathophysiologic and therapeutic perspective.

Other Kidney Disease-Related Risk Factors

Other kidney disease-related risk factors for CKD include autoimmune disorders, chronic infections, drug toxicity, especially anti-inflammatory drugs, endogenous nephrotoxins (e.g., paraproteins), exogenous nephrotoxins, nephrolithiasis, inherited disorders, and cystic diseases (Table 18–14). These topics are covered in detail in other chapters.

OTHER RISK FACTORS FOR CHRONIC KIDNEY DISEASE

In this section, we review other significant risk factors for development or progression of CKD.

Family History

There are several hereditary kidney diseases that follow specific inheritance patterns and are due to single gene mutations. Examples of these include autosomal dominant polycystic kidney disease types 1 and 2 involving polycystin the protein product of the PKD 1 and 2 genes[165,166] and x-linked Fabry disease involving the human α-galactosidase A gene.[167] These genetic factors would appear to be initiation factors as all affected individuals acquire the disease. Although the majority of kidney diseases are not associated with identifiable genetic defects, the presence of familial aggregation of kidney disease suggests a multifactorial etiology involving a genetic component with regard to susceptibility.[75,168–170]

Data in support of family history as a risk factor for the development of CKD come from case-control and prospective studies. In a population-based case-control study, prevalence of kidney disease among first-degree relatives was compared between 689 incident kidney failure patients with nonhereditary kidney disease, and 361 population-based controls.[171] After adjustment for other covariates including sociodemographic variables, and family history of diabetes and hypertension, having two or more affected first-degree relatives was associated with a 10-fold increase in the odds of kidney failure. Thus in this study, family history could potentially be a susceptibility factor (siblings of affected individuals are more susceptible to disease), an initiation factor (family history increases vulnerability to other insults or injury), or a progression factor (family history promotes progression to end-stage disease). Faronato and colleagues compared albumin excretion rate among siblings of probands with type 2 diabetes, with and without albuminuria.[172] Siblings of probands with albuminuria had an almost four times increased odds of abnormal albumin excretion rates compared with siblings of probands without albuminuria after adjustment for several confounding variables including age, history and duration of hypertension, glycated haemoglobin A_{1c}, duration of diabetes, body mass index, smoking, and alcohol. In addition, non-diabetic siblings of probands with albuminuria had high normal albumin excretion rates compared with non-diabetic siblings of probands without albuminuria. In this example, family history of albuminuria appears to be a susceptibility factor that increases susceptibility to kidney injury secondary to diabetes and an initiation factor in non-diabetic siblings. Freedman and colleagues[173] demonstrated that in a cohort of 4365 incident dialysis patients, 20% of these individuals reported a family history of kidney failure among first or second-degree relatives. These data collectively suggest that inherent genetic factors may play a role in the initiation, susceptibility, and progression of kidney disease irrespective of the underlying cause of kidney disease.

Low Birthweight (see Chapter 19)

Intrauterine growth retardation or low birthweight (or both) appears to be associated with reduced nephron number. In

TABLE 18–14	Percentage of Incident End-Stage Kidney Disease from 1990–2000 Due to Non-diabetic Kidney Disease by Race/Ethnicity				
Non-diabetic Kidney Disease	**Whites**	**Blacks**	**Asians**	**Native Americans**	**Hispanics**
Hypertension	24.0%	32.9%	23.5%	11.0%	16.5%
Glomerulonephritis/vasculitis	12.0%	10.4%	17.3%	10.4%	11.2%
Interstitial nephritis	4.8%	2.0%	2.9%	1.8%	2.4%
Cystic disease/hereditary	3.8%	1.5%	2.2%	1.2%	2.5%
Cancers/tumors	2.4%	1.3%	0.8%	0.8%	1.0%
Miscellaneous	3.7%	4.7%	1.6%	1.7%	2.1%
Unknown	5.7%	5.1%	5.5%	3.9%	4.1%
Total	56.5%	57.95%	53.8%	30.8%	39.8%

Adapted from the U.S. Renal Data System, USRDS: 2002 Annual Data Report: Atlas of End-Stage Renal Disease in the United States. Bethesda, MD, National Institutes of Health, National Institute of Diabetes and Digestive and Kidney Diseases, 2002.

an autopsy study of 35 neonates who died within 2 weeks of birth and who were free of congenital abnormalities of the genito-urinary tract, low birthweight was associated with reduced glomerular number and increased glomerular volume.[174] In a study using serial ultrasounds to estimate kidney size at 0, 3, and 18 months, in infants who were small or appropriate for gestational age, low birthweight was associated with smaller kidneys at birth and impaired kidney growth.[175] As discussed in greater detail in Chapter 19, these findings have led to the hypothesis that congenital retardation of kidney development may contribute to the pathogenesis of CKD.

The relationship between birthweight and kidney function has been assessed in several prospective studies. In a cohort of 422 young adults whose gestational age was <32 weeks at birth, there was a positive correlation between birthweight and GFR, and a negative correlation of birthweight with serum creatinine concentration and albumin creatinine ratio.[176] In a cohort of African Americans and whites, higher birthweight was associated with an increase in the number of glomeruli.[177] Epidemiologic studies in Pima Indians and Australian Aboriginals, racial groups at high risk for kidney disease, demonstrated that low birthweight was associated with albuminuria and kidney damage.[178,179] Thus the weight of existing evidence appears to support a relationship between low birthweight and reduced kidney size and therefore increased susceptibility to kidney disease. Putative mechanisms for impaired nephrogenesis in the setting of intra uterine growth retardation include malnutrition, protein and vitamin deficiencies, maternal hyperglycemia, smoking, alcohol ingestion, and iron deficiency.

Racial Factors

Rates of kidney failure are higher among African Americans compared with whites.[180] The basis of this racial difference is unclear and possibly reflects both genetic etiology, as well as lifestyle and environmental differences. Although this is an inherently difficult question to resolve, a few prospective studies have attempted to investigate race as an independent risk factor for kidney disease.

In prospective analysis of 9802 African American and White adults who participated in NHANES II, during 10 years of follow-up African Americans had an almost threefold increased risk for a composite outcome of kidney failure or dying from kidney disease (Fig. 18–12).[181] Only half of this excess risk was explained by identifiable sociodemographic, lifestyle, and clinical factors. The results of this study indicated that race or factors associated with it could potentially be involved in susceptibility to kidney disease, and in the initiation and progression of kidney disease. The effect of race on the development of earlier stages of kidney disease, defined as serum creatinine ≥1.5 mg/dl in men and ≥1.2 mg/dl in women, was studied in a cohort of individuals aged 18 to 30 years.[182] In univariate analyses black race was associated with increased risk of developing kidney disease; however, in multivariable analysis this relationship was attenuated in women but remained significant in men. Similarly, data from the Atherosclerosis Risk in Communities Study, a population-based cohort, showed that while African American race was associated with increased odds of developing reduced kidney function (defined as increase in serum creatinine of 0.4 mg/dl), 80% of the excess risk was attributable to sociodemographic, environmental, and behavioral factors, and comorbid conditions.[183] In these examples, race and race-related factors may be susceptibility or initiation factors for the development of kidney disease.

There is a racial difference in the rate of progression of kidney disease and potentially also with regard to develop-

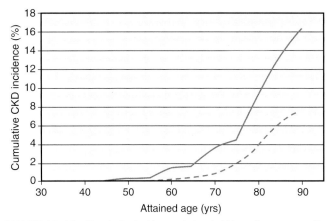

FIGURE 18–12 Cumulative incidence of chronic kidney disease, according to race and attained age, in NHANES II, 1976 to 1992. Results are weighted to the general United States population. Solid line, African Americans; dashed line, whites. The cumulative incidence of CKD among African Americans was significantly higher than that among whites (log-rank test, $P < 0.001$). (From Tarver-Carr ME, Powe NR, Eberhardt MS, et al: Excess risk of chronic kidney disease among African-American *versus* white subjects in the United States: A population-based study of potential explanatory factors. J Am Soc Nephrol 13:2363–2370 [Figure 1, p 2366], 2002.)

ment of cardiovascular disease. In a birth cohort analysis using data from the NHANES III, Hsu and colleagues[184] noted that although the prevalence of CKD was similar among black and white adults, the incidence rate of kidney failure was much higher among the blacks. Thus, for 100 blacks with CKD in 1991, there were five incident cases of kidney failure in 1996, compared with 1 incident case per 100 whites. Kiberd and co-workers[185] modeled the cumulative lifetime risk of kidney failure and found the risk was higher for African American men and women compared with whites. These data suggest a role for race and race-related factors in the progression of kidney disease. In summary, although it appears that racial disparities beyond differences in other known potential risk factors exist in the development and progression of kidney disease, the exact mechanisms for this excess risk remain unresolved.

Other Non-Kidney Related Factors

Other non-kidney related risk factors for CKD that we have not discussed include male gender and older age. These topics are covered in detail in Chapters 20 and 21.

CONCLUSION

Given our current state of knowledge regarding risk factors for CKD, it is estimated that a significant portion of the U.S. population is vulnerable to the development and progression of kidney disease (Table 18–15). Despite progress in the management of kidney failure, gains in reducing the incidence, prevalence, morbidity, and mortality attributable to CKD have been inadequate. As summarized in this chapter, several modifiable risk factors appear to be involved in the development and progression of kidney disease. These data imply that early interventions targeting these risk factors can prevent the development of CKD and delay its progression, as well as reduce associated adverse outcomes. Therefore, a better understanding of these risk factor associations and the identification of as-yet unrecognized mechanisms of development and progression are crucial to reduce the risk of developing

TABLE 18–15 Prevalence of Individuals at Risk for Chronic Kidney Disease

Risk Factor	Prevalence	
	Estimated %	Estimated N
Diabetes mellitus	Diagnosed: 5.1% of adults age ≥ 20 Undiagnosed: 2.7% of adults age ≥ 20	10.2 million 5.4 million
Hypertension	24.0% of adults age ≥18	43.1 million
Systemic lupus erythematosus	~0.05% definite or suspected	~239,000
Functioning kidney graft	~0.03%	88,311 as of 12/31/98
African American	12.3%	34.7 million
Hispanic or Latino (of any race)	12.5%	35.3 million
American Indian and Alaska Native	0.9%	2.5 million
Age 60–70	7.3%	20.3 million
Age ≥ 70	9.2%	25.5 million
Acute kidney failure	~0.14%	~363,000 non-federal hospital stays in 1997
Daily NSAID use	~5.2% with rheumatoid arthritis or osteoarthritis (assumed daily use) ~30% yearly use	~13 million assumed daily use ~75 million yearly use

From Kidney Disease Outcome Quality Initiative: 2002 K/DOQI clinical practice guidelines for chronic kidney disease: Evaluation, classification, and stratification. Am J Kidney Dis 39:S1–246 [Table 42, p S74], 2002.

kidney disease and to improve outcomes in patients with kidney disease.

References

1. United States Renal Data System: Excerpts from the 2000 U.S. Renal Data System Annual Report: Atlas of End Stage Renal Disease in the United States. Am J Kidney Dis 36:S1-S279, 2000.
2. Hunsicker LG: The consequences and costs of chronic kidney disease before ESRD. J Am Soc Nephrol 15(5):1363–1364, 2004.
3. Special report from the National Kidney Foundation Task Force on Cardiovascular Disease: Controlling the epidemic of cardiovascular disease in chronic renal disease: What do we know? What do we need to learn? Where do we go from here? Am J Kidney Dis 32(5):S1-S199, 1998.
4. Kidney Disease Outcome Quality Initiative: K/DOQI clinical practice guidelines for chronic kidney disease: Evaluation, classification, and stratification. Am J Kidney Dis 39(2 Suppl 2):S1–246, 2002.
5. Coresh J, Astor BC, Greene T, et al: Prevalence of chronic kidney disease and decreased kidney function in the adult U.S. population: Third National Health and Nutrition Examination Survey. Am J Kidney Dis 41(1):1–12, 2003.
6. Levey AS, Eckardt KU, Tsukamoto Y, et al: Definition and classification of chronic kidney disease: A position statement from Kidney Disease: Improving Global Outcomes (KDIGO). Kidney Int 67(6):2089–2100, 2005.
7. Keane WF, Eknoyan G: Proteinuria, albuminuria, risk, assessment, detection, elimination (PARADE): A position paper of the National Kidney Foundation. Am J Kidney Dis 35(5):1004–1010, 1999.
8. Levey AS, Bosch JP, Lewis JB, et al: A more accurate method to estimate glomerular filtration rate from serum creatinine: A new prediction equation. Modification of Diet in Renal Disease Study Group. Ann Intern Med 130(6):461–470, 1999.
9. Hill AB: The environment and disease: Association or causation? Proc R Soc Med 58:295–300, 1965.
10. Gordis L: Epidemiology, 2nd ed. Philadelphia, WB Saunders, 2000.
11. Szklo M, Nieto JF: Epidemiology Beyond the Basics. Gaithersburg, Aspen Publishers, Inc., 2000.
12. The Heart Outcomes Prevention Evaluation Study, Investigators: Effects of an angiotensin-converting-enzyme inhibitor, ramipril, on cardiovascular events in high-risk patients. N Engl J Med 342(3):145–153, 2000.
13. Mann JF, Gerstein HC, Pogue J, et al: Renal insufficiency as a predictor of cardiovascular outcomes and the impact of ramipril: The HOPE randomized trial. Ann Intern Med 134(8):629–636, 2001.
14. Anders H-J, Patole PS: Toll-like receptors recognize uropathogenic Escherichia coli and trigger inflammation in the urinary tract. Nephrol Dial Transplant 20(8):1529–1532, 2005.
15. Coresh J, Astor B, Sarnak MJ: Evidence for increased cardiovascular disease risk in patients with chronic kidney disease. Curr Opin Nephrol Hypertens 13(1):73–81, 2004.
16. Cheung AK, Sarnak MJ, Yan G, et al: Atherosclerotic cardiovascular disease risks in chronic hemodialysis patients. Kidney Int 58(1):353–362, 2000.
17. Foley RN, Parfrey PS, Sarnak MJ: Clinical epidemiology of cardiovascular disease in chronic renal disease. Am J Kidney Dis 32(5 Suppl 3):S112–119, 1998.
18. Fried LF, Shlipak MG, Crump C, et al: Renal insufficiency as a predictor of cardiovascular outcomes and mortality in elderly individuals. J Am Coll Cardiol 41(8):1364–1372, 2003.
19. Jungers P, Massy ZA, Khoa TN, et al: Incidence and risk factors of atherosclerotic cardiovascular accidents in predialysis chronic renal failure patients: A prospective study. Nephrol Dial Transplant 12(12):2597–2602, 1997.
20. Manjunath G, Tighiouart H, Ibrahim H, et al: Level of kidney function as a risk factor for atherosclerotic cardiovascular outcomes in the community. J Am Coll Cardiol 41(1):47–55, 2003.
21. Chobanian AV, Bakris GL, Black HR, et al: The Seventh Report of the Joint National Committee on Prevention, Detection, Evaluation, and Treatment of High Blood Pressure: The JNC 7 report. JAMA 289(19):2560–2572, 2003.
22. Mosca L, Appel LJ, Benjamin EJ, et al: Evidence-based guidelines for cardiovascular disease prevention in women. Circulation 109(5):672–693, 2004.
23. Sarnak MJ, Levey AS, Schoolwerth AC, et al: Kidney disease as a risk factor for development of cardiovascular disease: A statement from the American Heart Association Councils on Kidney in Cardiovascular Disease, High Blood Pressure Research, Clinical Cardiology, and Epidemiology and Prevention. Circulation 108(17):2154–2169, 2003.
24. Keith DS, Nichols GA, Gullion CM, et al: Longitudinal follow-up and outcomes among a population with chronic kidney disease in a large managed care organization. Arch Intern Med 164(6):659–663, 2004.
25. Foley RN, Wang C, Collins AJ: Cardiovascular risk factor profiles and kidney function stage in the US general population: The NHANES III study. Mayo Clin Proc 80(10):1270–1277, 2005.
26. Menon V, Gul A, Sarnak MJ: Cardiovascular risk factors in chronic kidney disease. Kidney Int 68(4):1413–1418, 2005.
27. Manjunath G, Tighiouart H, Coresh J, et al: Level of kidney function as a risk factor for cardiovascular outcomes in the elderly. Kidney Int 63(3):1121–1129, 2003.
28. Shlipak MG, Fried LF, Stehman-Breen C, et al: Chronic renal insufficiency and cardiovascular events in the elderly: Findings from the Cardiovascular Health Study. Am J Geriatr Cardiol 13(2):81–90, 2004.
29. Henry RM, Kostense PJ, Bos G, et al: Mild renal insufficiency is associated with increased cardiovascular mortality: The Hoorn Study. Kidney Int 62(4):1402–1407, 2002.
30. Muntner P, He J, Hamm L, et al: Renal insufficiency and subsequent death resulting from cardiovascular disease in the United States. J Am Soc Nephrol 13(3):745–753, 2002.
31. Weiner DE, Tighiouart H, Amin MG, et al: Chronic kidney disease as a risk factor for cardiovascular disease and all-cause mortality: A pooled analysis of community-based studies. J Am Soc Nephrol 15(5):1307–1315, 2004.
32. Go AS, Chertow GM, Fan D, et al: Chronic kidney disease and the risks of death, cardiovascular events, and hospitalization. N Engl J Med 351(13):1296–1305, 2004.
33. Arnlov J, Evans JC, Meigs JB, et al: Low-grade albuminuria and incidence of cardiovascular disease events in nonhypertensive and nondiabetic individuals: The Framingham Heart Study. Circulation 112(7):969–975, 2005.
34. Borch-Johnsen K, Feldt-Rasmussen B, Strandgaard S, et al: Urinary albumin excretion. An independent predictor of ischemic heart disease. Arterioscler Thromb Vasc Biol 19(8):1992–1997, 1999.
35. Dinneen SF, Gerstein HC: The association of microalbuminuria and mortality in non-insulin-dependent diabetes mellitus. A systematic overview of the literature. Arch Intern Med 157(13):1413–1418, 1997.

36. Freedman BI, Langefeld CD, Lohman KK, et al: Relationship between albuminuria and cardiovascular disease in type 2 diabetes. J Am Soc Nephrol 16:2156–2161, 2005.

37. Hillege HL, Fidler V, Diercks GFH, et al: Urinary albumin excretion predicts cardiovascular and noncardiovascular mortality in general population. Circulation 106(14):1777–1782, 2002.

38. Klausen K, Borch-Johnsen K, Feldt-Rasmussen B, et al: Very low levels of microalbuminuria are associated with increased risk of coronary heart disease and death independently of renal function, hypertension, and diabetes. Circulation 110(1):32–35, 2004.

39. Mann JF, Yi QL, Gerstein HC: Albuminuria as a predictor of cardiovascular and renal outcomes in people with known atherosclerotic cardiovascular disease. Kidney Int 66(s92):S59-S62, 2004.

40. Nakamura S, Kawano Y, Inenaga T, et al: Microalbuminuria and cardiovascular events in elderly hypertensive patients without previous cardiovascular complications. Hypertens Res 26(8):603–608, 2003.

41. Wachtell K, Ibsen H, Olsen MH, et al: Albuminuria and cardiovascular risk in hypertensive patients with left ventricular hypertrophy: The LIFE study. Ann Intern Med 139(11):901–906, 2003.

42. Gerstein HC, Mann JF, Yi Q, et al: Albuminuria and risk of cardiovascular events, death, and heart failure in diabetic and nondiabetic individuals. JAMA 286(4):421–426, 2001.

43. Pascual JM, Rodilla E, Gonzalez C, et al: Long-term impact of systolic blood pressure and glycemia on the development of microalbuminuria in essential hypertension. Hypertension 45:1125–1130, 2005.

44. Klag MJ, Whelton PK, Randall BL, et al: Blood pressure and end-stage renal disease in men. N Engl J Med 334(1):13–18, 1996.

45. Haroun MK, Jaar BG, Hoffman SC, et al: Risk factors for chronic kidney disease: A prospective study of 23,534 men and women in Washington County, Maryland. J Am Soc Nephrol 14(11):2934–2941, 2003.

46. Hsu c-y, McCulloch CE, Darbinian J, et al: Elevated blood pressure and risk of end-stage renal disease in subjects without baseline kidney disease. Arch Intern Med 165(8):923–928, 2005.

47. Hunsicker LG, Adler S, Caggiula A, et al: Predictors of the progression of renal disease in the Modification of Diet in Renal Disease Study. Kidney Int 51(6):1908–1919, 1997.

48. Young JH, Klag MJ, Muntner P, et al: Blood pressure and decline in kidney function: Findings from the Systolic Hypertension in the Elderly Program (SHEP). J Am Soc Nephrol 13(11):2776–2782, 2002.

49. Vupputuri S, Batuman V, Muntner P, et al: Effect of blood pressure on early decline in kidney function among hypertensive men. Hypertension 42(6):1144–1149, 2003.

50. Ramirez SP, McClellan W, Port FK, Hsu SI: Risk factors for proteinuria in a large, multiracial, southeast Asian population. J Am Soc Nephrol 13(7):1907–1917, 2002.

51. Hovind P, Tarnow L, Rossing P, et al: Predictors for the development of microalbuminuria and macroalbuminuria in patients with type 1 diabetes: Inception Cohort Study. BMJ 328(7448):1105–1100, 2004.

52. Rossing P, Hougaard P, Parving H-H: Risk factors for development of incipient and overt diabetic nephropathy in type 1 diabetic patients: A 10-year prospective observational study. Diabetes Care 25(5):859–864, 2002.

53. Klahr S, Levey AS, Beck GJ, et al: The effects of dietary protein restriction and blood-pressure control on the progression of chronic renal disease. Modification of Diet in Renal Disease Study Group. N Engl J Med 330(13):877–884, 1994.

54. Sarnak MJ, Greene T, Wang X, et al: The effect of a lower target blood pressure on the progression of kidney disease: Long-term follow-up of the modification of diet in renal disease study. Ann Intern Med 142(5):342–351, 2005.

55. Wright JT, Jr, Bakris G, Greene T, et al: Effect of blood pressure lowering and antihypertensive drug class on progression of hypertensive kidney disease. Results from the AASK trial. JAMA 288(19):2421–2431, 2002.

56. Jafar TH, Stark PC, Schmid CH, et al: Progression of chronic kidney disease: The role of blood pressure control, proteinuria, and angiotensin-converting enzyme inhibition: A patient-level meta-analysis. Ann Intern Med 139(4):244–252, 2003.

57. Levey AS, Mulrow CD: An editorial update: What level of blood pressure control in chronic kidney disease? Ann Intern Med 143(1):79–81, 2005.

58. Ruggenenti P, Perna A, Loriga G, et al: Blood-pressure control for renoprotection in patients with non-diabetic chronic renal disease (REIN-2): multicentre, randomised controlled trial. Lancet 365:939–946, 2005.

59. American Diabetes Association. Diabetic Nephropathy, 2002.

60. US Renal Data Systems: USRDS 2003 Annual Data Report: Atlas of End Stage Renal Diseases in the United States. Bethesda, MD: National Institutes of Health. The National Institute of Diabetes and Digestive and Kidney Disease. Division of Kidney, Urologic, and Hematologic Diseases, 2003.

61. Perneger TV, Brancati FL, Whelton PK, Klag MJ: End-stage renal disease attributable to diabetes mellitus. Ann Intern Med 121(12):912–918, 1994.

62. Adler AI, Stevens RJ, Manley SE, et al: Development and progression of nephropathy in type 2 diabetes: The United Kingdom Prospective Diabetes Study (UKPDS 64). Kidney Int 63(1):225–232, 2003.

63. Fox CS, Larson MG, Leip EP, et al: Glycemic status and development of kidney disease: The Framingham Heart Study. Diabetes Care 28(10):2436–2440, 2005.

64. Rossing P, Rossing K, Jacobsen P, Parving HH: Unchanged incidence of diabetic nephropathy in IDDM patients. Diabetes 44(7):739–743, 1995.

65. Bojestig M, Arnqvist HJ, Hermansson G, et al: Declining incidence of nephropathy in insulin-dependent diabetes mellitus. N Engl J Med 330(1):15–18, 1994.

66. Powrie JK, Watts GF, Ingham JN, et al: Role of glycaemic control in development of microalbuminuria in patients with insulin dependent diabetes. BMJ 309(6969):1608–1612, 1994.

67. The Diabetes Control and Complications Trial Research Group: The effect of intensive treatment of diabetes on the development and progression of long-term complications in insulin-dependent diabetes mellitus. N Engl J Med 329(14):977–986, 1993.

68. Keane WF, Brenner BM, de Zeeuw D, et al: The risk of developing end-stage renal disease in patients with type 2 diabetes and nephropathy: The RENAAL study. Kidney Int 63(4):1499–1507, 2003.

69. Halimi JM, Giraudeau B, Vol S, et al: Effects of current smoking and smoking discontinuation on renal function and proteinuria in the general population. Kidney Int 58(3):1285–1292, 2000.

70. Briganti EM, Branley P, Chadban SJ, et al: Smoking is associated with renal impairment and proteinuria in the normal population: The AusDiab kidney study. Australian Diabetes, Obesity and Lifestyle Study. Am J Kidney Dis 40(4):704–712, 2002.

71. Orth SR, Stockmann A, Conradt C, et al: Smoking as a risk factor for end-stage renal failure in men with primary renal disease. Kidney Int 54(3):926–931, 1998.

72. Chuahirun T, Wesson DE: Cigarette smoking predicts faster progression of type 2 established diabetic nephropathy despite ACE inhibition. Am J Kidney Dis 39(2):376–382, 2002.

73. Regalado M, Yang S, Wesson DE: Cigarette smoking is associated with augmented progression of renal insufficiency in severe essential hypertension. Am J Kidney Dis 35(4):687–694, 2000.

74. Pinto-Sietsma SJ, Mulder J, Janssen WM, et al: Smoking is related to albuminuria and abnormal renal function in nondiabetic persons. Ann Intern Med 133(8):585–591, 2000.

75. Fox CS, Larson MG, Leip EP, et al: Predictors of new-onset kidney disease in a community-based population. JAMA 291(7):844–850, 2004.

76. Schiffl H, Lang SM, Fischer R: Stopping smoking slows accelerated progression of renal failure in primary renal disease. J Nephrol 15(3):270–274, 2002.

77. Cases A, Coll E: Dyslipidemia and the progression of renal disease in chronic renal failure patients. Kidney Int Suppl 99:S87–93, 2005.

78. Schaeffner ES, Kurth T, Curhan GC, et al: Cholesterol and the risk of renal dysfunction in apparently healthy men. J Am Soc Nephrol 14(8):2084–2091, 2003.

79. Muntner P, Coresh J, Smith JC, et al: Plasma lipids and risk of developing renal dysfunction: The atherosclerosis risk in communities study. Kidney Int 58(1):293–301, 2000.

80. Segura J, Campo C, Gil P, et al: Development of chronic kidney disease and cardiovascular prognosis in essential hypertensive patients. J Am Soc Nephrol 15(6):1616–1622, 2004.

81. Hsu CY, Bates DW, Kuperman GJ, Curhan GC: Diabetes, hemoglobin A(1c), cholesterol, and the risk of moderate chronic renal insufficiency in an ambulatory population. Am J Kidney Dis 36(2):272–281, 2000.

82. Tonelli M, Moye L, Sacks FM, et al: Effect of pravastatin on loss of renal function in people with moderate chronic renal insufficiency and cardiovascular disease. J Am Soc Nephrol 14(6):1605–1613, 2003.

83. Tonelli M, Collins D, Robins S, et al: Effect of gemfibrozil on change in renal function in men with moderate chronic renal insufficiency and coronary disease. Am J Kidney Dis 44(5):832–839, 2004.

84. Fried LF, Orchard TJ, Kasiske BL: Effect of lipid reduction on the progression of renal disease: A meta-analysis. Kidney Int 59(1):260–269, 2001.

85. Iseki K, Ikemiya Y, Kinjo K, et al: Body mass index and the risk of development of end-stage renal disease in a screened cohort. Kidney Int 65(5):1870–1876, 2004.

86. Praga M, Hernandez E, Herrero JC, et al: Influence of obesity on the appearance of proteinuria and renal insufficiency after unilateral nephrectomy. Kidney Int 58(5):2111–2118, 2000.

87. Bonnet F, Deprele C, Sassolas A, et al: Excessive body weight as a new independent risk factor for clinical and pathological progression in primary IgA nephritis. Am J Kidney Dis 37(4):720–727, 2001.

88. Kambham N, Markowitz GS, Valeri AM, et al: Obesity-related glomerulopathy: an emerging epidemic. Kidney Int 59(4):1498–1509, 2001.

89. Hsu C-y, McCulloch CE, Iribarren C, et al: Body mass index and risk for end-stage renal disease. Ann Intern Med 144(1):21–28, 2006.

90. Chagnac A, Weinstein T, Herman M, et al: The effects of weight loss on renal function in patients with severe obesity. J Am Soc Nephrol 14(6):1480–1486, 2003.

91. Morales E, Valero MA, Leon M, et al: Beneficial effects of weight loss in overweight patients with chronic proteinuric nephropathies. Am J Kidney Dis 41(2):319–327, 2003.

92. Chen J, Muntner P, Hamm LL, et al: The metabolic syndrome and chronic kidney disease in U.S. adults. Ann Intern Med 140(3):167–174, 2004.

93. Kurella M, Lo JC, Chertow GM: Metabolic syndrome and the risk for chronic kidney disease among nondiabetic adults. J Am Soc Nephrol 16(7):2134–2140, 2005.

93a. Tomaszewski M, Charchor FJ, Maric C, et al: Glomerular hyperfiltration: a new marker of metabolic risk. Kidney Int 71:816–821, 2007.

94. Buller CE, Nogareda JG, Ramanathan K, et al: The profile of cardiac patients with renal artery stenosis. J Am Coll Cardiol 43(9):1606–1613, 2004.

95. Levin A, Djurdjev O, Barrett B, et al: Cardiovascular disease in patients with chronic kidney disease: Getting to the heart of the matter. Am J Kidney Dis 38(6):1398–1407, 2001.

96. McClellan WM, Langston RD, Presley R: Medicare patients with cardiovascular disease have a high prevalence of chronic kidney disease and a high rate of progression to end-stage renal disease. J Am Soc Nephrol 15(7):1912–1919, 2004.

97. Perry HM, Jr, Miller JP, Fornoff JR, et al: Early predictors of 15-year end-stage renal disease in hypertensive patients. Hypertension 25(4 Pt 1):587–594, 1995.

98. Pinto-Sietsma SJ, Janssen WM, Hillege HL, et al: Urinary albumin excretion is associated with renal functional abnormalities in a nondiabetic population. J Am Soc Nephrol 11(10):1882–1888, 2000.

99. Mann JFE, Gerstein HC, Yi Q-L, et al: Development of renal disease in people at high cardiovascular risk: Results of the HOPE Randomized Study. J Am Soc Nephrol 14(3):641–647, 2003.

100. Peterson JC, Adler S, Burkart JM, et al: Blood pressure control, proteinuria, and the progression of renal disease. The Modification of Diet in Renal Disease Study. Ann Intern Med 123(10):754–762, 1995.
101. Lea J, Greene T, Hebert L, et al: The relationship between magnitude of proteinuria reduction and risk of end-stage renal disease: Results of the African American Study of Kidney Disease and Hypertension. Arch Intern Med 165(8):947–953, 2005.
102. Ruggenenti P, Perna A, Mosconi L, Gruppo Italiano di Studi Epidemiologici in N: Urinary protein excretion rate is the best independent predictor of ESRF in non-diabetic proteinuric chronic nephropathies. Kidney Int 53(5):1209–1216, 1998.
102a. Eijkelkamp WB, Zhang Z, Remuzzi G, et al: Albuminuria is a target for renoprotective therapy independent from blood pressure in patients with type 2 diabetic nephropathy. J Am Soc Nephrol 18:1540–1546, 2007.
103. Remuzzi G, Bertani T: Pathophysiology of progressive nephropathies. N Engl J Med 339(20):1448–1456, 1998.
104. Standards of medical care in diabetes. Diabetes Care 28 Suppl 1:S4-S36, 2005.
105. National Kidney Foundation: K/DOQI clinical practice guidelines on hypertension and antihypertensive agents in chronic kidney disease. Am J Kidney Dis 43(5 Suppl 1):S1–290, 2004.
106. Schmidt-Ott KM, Kagiyama S, Phillips MI: The multiple actions of angiotensin II in atherosclerosis. Regul Pept 93(1–3):65–77, 2000.
107. Agodoa LY, Appel L, Bakris GL, et al: Effect of ramipril vs amlodipine on renal outcomes in hypertensive nephrosclerosis: A randomized controlled trial. JAMA 285(21):2719–2728, 2001.
108. The GISEN Group (Gruppo Italiano di Studi Epidemiologici in Nefrologia): Randomised placebo-controlled trial of effect of ramipril on decline in glomerular filtration rate and risk of terminal renal failure in proteinuric, non-diabetic nephropathy. Lancet 349(9069):1857–1863, 1997.
109. Ruggenenti P, Perna A, Gherardi G, et al: Renal function and requirement for dialysis in chronic nephropathy patients on long-term ramipril: REIN follow-up trial. Gruppo Italiano di Studi Epidemiologici in Nefrologia (GISEN). Ramipril Efficacy in Nephropathy. Lancet 352(9136):1252–1256, 1998.
110. Lewis EJ, Hunsicker LG, Bain RP, Rohde RD: The effect of angiotensin-converting-enzyme inhibition on diabetic nephropathy. The Collaborative Study Group. N Engl J Med 329(20):1456–1462, 1993.
111. Lewis EJ, Hunsicker LG, Clarke WR, et al: Renoprotective effect of the angiotensin-receptor antagonist irbesartan in patients with nephropathy due to type 2 diabetes. N Engl J Med 345(12):851–860, 2001.
112. Brenner BM, Cooper ME, de Zeeuw D, et al: Effects of losartan on renal and cardiovascular outcomes in patients with type 2 diabetes and nephropathy. N Engl J Med 345(12):861–869, 2001.
113. Rahman M, Pressel S, Davis BR, et al: Renal outcomes in high-risk hypertensive patients treated with an angiotensin-converting enzyme inhibitor or a calcium channel blocker vs a diuretic: A report from the Antihypertensive and Lipid-Lowering Treatment to Prevent Heart Attack Trial (ALLHAT). Arch Intern Med 165(8):936–946, 2005.
114. ACE Inhibitors in Diabetic Nephropathy Trialist Group: Should all patients with type 1 diabetes mellitus and microalbuminuria receive angiotensin-converting enzyme inhibitors? A meta-analysis of individual patient data. Ann Intern Med 134(5):370–379, 2001.
115. Jafar TH, Schmid CH, Landa M, et al: Angiotensin-converting enzyme inhibitors and progression of nondiabetic renal disease. A meta-analysis of patient-level data. Ann Intern Med 135(2):73–87, 2001.
116. Wrone EM, Carnethon MR, Palaniappan L, Fortmann SP: Association of dietary protein intake and microalbuminuria in healthy adults: Third National Health and Nutrition Examination Survey. Am J Kidney Dis 41(3):580–587, 2003.
117. Knight EL, Stampfer MJ, Hankinson SE, et al: The impact of protein intake on renal function decline in women with normal renal function or mild renal insufficiency. Ann Intern Med 138(6):460–467, 2003.
118. Levey AS, Greene T, Beck GJ, et al: Dietary protein restriction and the progression of chronic renal disease: What have all of the results of the MDRD study shown? Modification of Diet in Renal Disease Study group. J Am Soc Nephrol 10(11):2426–2439, 1999.
119. Fouque D, Laville M, Boissel JP, et al: Controlled low protein diets in chronic renal insufficiency: Meta-analysis. BMJ 304(6821):216–220, 1992.
120. Fouque D, Wang P, Laville M, Boissel JP: Low protein diets delay end-stage renal disease in non-diabetic adults with chronic renal failure. Nephrol Dial Transplant 15(12):1986–1992, 2000.
121. Kasiske BL, Lakatua JD, Ma JZ, Louis TA: A meta-analysis of the effects of dietary protein restriction on the rate of decline in renal function. Am J Kidney Dis 31(6):954–961, 1998.
122. Pedrini MT, Levey AS, Lau J, et al: The effect of dietary protein restriction on the progression of diabetic and nondiabetic renal diseases: A meta-analysis. Ann Intern Med 124(7):627–632, 1996.
123. Breyer JA, Bain RP, Evans JK, et al: Predictors of the progression of renal insufficiency in patients with insulin-dependent diabetes and overt diabetic nephropathy. The Collaborative Study Group. Kidney Int 50(5):1651–1658, 1996.
124. Yokoyama H, Tomonaga O, Hirayama M, et al: Predictors of the progression of diabetic nephropathy and the beneficial effect of angiotensin-converting enzyme inhibitors in NIDDM patients. Diabetologia 40(4):405–411, 1997.
125. Brenner BM, Chertow GM: Congenital oligonephropathy and the etiology of adult hypertension and progressive renal injury. Am J Kidney Dis 23(2):171–175, 1994.
126. Hoy WE, Hughson MD, Bertram JF, et al: Nephron number, hypertension, renal disease, and renal failure. J Am Soc Nephrol 16:2557–2564, 2005.
127. Woods LL, Weeks DA, Rasch R: Hypertension after neonatal uninephrectomy in rats precedes glomerular damage. Hypertension 38(3):337–342, 2001.
128. Keller G, Zimmer G, Mall G, et al: Nephron number in patients with primary hypertension. N Engl J Med 348(2):101–108, 2003.
129. Hakim RM, Goldszer RC, Brenner BM: Hypertension and proteinuria: Long-term sequelae of uninephrectomy in humans. Kidney Int 25(6):930–936, 1984.
130. Conrad KP, Novak J, Danielson LA, et al: Mechanisms of renal vasodilation and hyperfiltration during pregnancy: Current perspectives and potential implications for preeclampsia. Endothelium 12(1–2):57–62, 2005.
131. Skov AR, Toubro S, Bulow J, et al: Changes in renal function during weight loss induced by high vs low-protein low-fat diets in overweight subjects. Int J Obes Relat Metab Disord 23(11):1170–1177, 1999.
132. Parving H-H, Mauer M, Ritz E: Diabetic nephropathy. *In* Brenner BM (ed), Brenner and Rector's The Kidney, 7th ed. Philadelphia, Elsevier, 2004, pp 1177–1818.
133. Chagnac A, Weinstein T, Herman M, et al: The effects of weight loss on renal function in patients with severe obesity. J Am Soc Nephrol 14(6):1480–1486, 2003.
134. Kenneth I, Ataga EPO: Renal abnormalities in sickle cell disease. Am J Hematol 63(4):205–211, 2000.
135. Lee PJ, Dalton RN, Shah V, et al: Glomerular and tubular function in glycogen storage disease. Pediatr Nephrol 9(6):705–710, 1995.
136. Wheeler DC, Townend JN, Landray MJ: Cardiovascular risk factors in predialysis patients: Baseline data from the Chronic Renal Impairment in Birmingham (CRIB) study. Kidney Int Suppl (84):S201–203, 2003.
137. Muntner P, He J, Astor BC, et al: Traditional and Nontraditional Risk Factors Predict Coronary Heart Disease in Chronic Kidney Disease: Results from the Atherosclerosis Risk in Communities Study. J Am Soc Nephrol 16(2):529–538, 2005.
138. Levin A, Thompson CR, Ethier J, et al: Left ventricular mass index increase in early renal disease: Impact of decline in hemoglobin. Am J Kidney Dis 34(1):125–134, 1999.
139. Mohanram A, Zhang Z, Shahinfar S, et al: Anemia and end-stage renal disease in patients with type 2 diabetes and nephropathy. Kidney Int 66(3):1131–1138, 2004.
140. Kuriyama S, Tomonari H, Yoshida H, et al: Reversal of anemia by erythropoietin therapy retards the progression of chronic renal failure, especially in nondiabetic patients. Nephron 77(2):176–185, 1997.
141. Jungers P, Choukroun G, Oualim Z, et al: Beneficial influence of recombinant human erythropoietin therapy on the rate of progression of chronic renal failure in predialysis patients. Nephrol Dial Transplant 16(2):307–312, 2001.
142. Silverberg DS, Iaina A, Peer G, et al: Intravenous iron supplementation for the treatment of the anemia of moderate to severe chronic renal failure patients not receiving dialysis. Am J Kidney Dis 27(2):234–238, 1996.
143. Albertazzi A, Di Liberato L, Daniele F, et al: Efficacy and tolerability of recombinant human erythropoietin treatment in pre-dialysis patients: Results of a multicenter study. Int J Artif Organs 21(1):12–18, 1998.
144. Hayashi T, Suzuki A, Shoji T, et al: Cardiovascular effect of normalizing the hematocrit level during erythropoietin therapy in predialysis patients with chronic renal failure. Am J Kidney Dis 35(2):250–256, 2000.
145. Roth D, Smith RD, Schulman G, et al: Effects of recombinant human erythropoietin on renal function in chronic renal failure predialysis patients. Am J Kidney Dis 24(5):777–784, 1994.
146. Portoles J, Torralbo A, Martin P, et al: Cardiovascular effects of recombinant human erythropoietin in predialysis patients. Am J Kidney Dis 29(4):541–548, 1997.
147. The US Recombinant Human Erythropoietin Predialysis Study Group: Double-blind, placebo-controlled study of the therapeutic use of recombinant human erythropoietin for anemia associated with chronic renal failure in predialysis patients. Am J Kidney Dis 18(1):50–59, 1991.
148. Austrian Multicenter Study Group of r-HuEPO in Predialysis Patients: Effectiveness and safety of recombinant human erythropoietin in predialysis patients. Nephron 61(4):399–403, 1992.
149. Abraham PA, Opsahl JA, Rachael KM, et al: Renal function during erythropoietin therapy for anemia in predialysis chronic renal failure patients. Am J Nephrol 10(2):128–136, 1990.
150. Rao M, Pereira BJ: Prospective trials on anemia of chronic disease: The Trial to Reduce Cardiovascular Events with Aranesp Therapy (TREAT). Kidney Int Suppl (87):S12–19, 2003.
151. Reddan DN, Singh AK, Group tCS: Can risk factor modification provide meaningful benefit? The Correction of Hemoglobin and Outcomes in Renal Insufficiency (CHOIR) Study. Paper presented at: The American Society of Nephrology Renal Week; 2003; San Diego, CA.
152. Macdougall IC: CREATE: New strategies for early anaemia management in renal insufficiency. Nephrol Dial Transplant 18 Suppl 2:ii13–16, 2003.
153. Muntner P, Hamm LL, Kusek JW, et al: The prevalence of nontraditional risk factors for coronary heart disease in patients with chronic kidney disease. Ann Intern Med 140(1):9–17, 2004.
154. Knight EL, Rimm EB, Pai JK, et al: Kidney dysfunction, inflammation, and coronary events: A prospective study. J Am Soc Nephrol 15(7):1897–1903, 2004.
155. Annuk M, Zilmer M, Lind L, et al: Oxidative stress and endothelial function in chronic renal failure. J Am Soc Nephrol 12(12):2747–2752, 2001.
156. Oberg BP, McMenamin E, Lucas FL, et al: Increased prevalence of oxidant stress and inflammation in patients with moderate to severe chronic kidney disease. Kidney Int 65(3):1009–1016, 2004.
157. Stuveling EM, Bakker SJL, Hillege HL, et al: Biochemical risk markers: A novel area for better prediction of renal risk? Nephrol Dial Transplant 20(3):497–508, 2005.
158. Menon V, Wang X, Greene T, et al: Homocysteine in chronic kidney disease: Effect of low protein diet and repletion with B vitamins. Kidney Int 67(4):1539–1546, 2005.
159. Kronenberg F, Kuen E, Ritz E, et al: Lipoprotein(a) serum concentrations and apolipoprotein(a) phenotypes in mild and moderate renal failure. J Am Soc Nephrol 11(1):105–115, 2000.
160. Chen J, Muntner P, Hamm LL, et al: Insulin resistance and risk of chronic kidney disease in nondiabetic U.S. adults. J Am Soc Nephrol 14(2):469–477, 2003.
161. Sarnak MJ, Poindexter A, Wang SR, et al: Serum C-reactive protein and leptin as predictors of kidney disease progression in the Modification of Diet in Renal Disease Study. Kidney Int 62(6):2208–2215, 2002.

162. Sarnak MJ, Wang SR, Beck GJ, et al: Homocysteine, cysteine, and B vitamins as predictors of kidney disease progression. Am J Kidney Dis 40(5):932–939, 2002.

163. Fried L, Solomon C, Shlipak M, et al: Inflammatory and prothrombotic markers and the progression of renal disease in elderly individuals. J Am Soc Nephrol 15(12):3184–3191, 2004.

164. Ravani P, Tripepi G, Malberti F, et al: Asymmetrical dimethylarginine predicts progression to dialysis and death in patients with chronic kidney disease: A competing risks modeling approach. J Am Soc Nephrol 16(8):2449–2455, 2005.

165. The European Polycystic Kidney Disease Consortium: The polycystic kidney disease 1 gene encodes a 14 kb transcript and lies within a duplicated region on chromosome 16. Cell 77(6):881–894, 1994.

166. Peters DJ, Spruit L, Saris JJ, et al: Chromosome 4 localization of a second gene for autosomal dominant polycystic kidney disease. Nat Genet 5(4):359–362, 1993.

167. Eng CM, Desnick RJ: Molecular basis of Fabry disease: Mutations and polymorphisms in the human alpha-galactosidase A gene. Hum Mutat 3(2):103–111, 1994.

168. Jurkovitz C, Franch H, Shoham D, et al: Family members of patients treated for ESRD have high rates of undetected kidney disease. Am J Kidney Dis 40(6):1173–1178, 2002.

169. Paterson AD, Magistroni R, He N, et al: Progressive loss of renal function is an age-dependent heritable trait in type 1 autosomal dominant polycystic kidney disease. J Am Soc Nephrol 16(3):755–762, 2005.

170. Spray BJ, Atassi NG, Tuttle AB, Freedman BI: Familial risk, age at onset, and cause of end-stage renal disease in white Americans. J Am Soc Nephrol 5(10):1806–1810, 1995.

171. Lei HH, Perneger TV, Klag MJ, et al: Familial aggregation of renal disease in a population-based case-control study. J Am Soc Nephrol 9(7):1270–1276, 1998.

172. Faronato PP, Maioli M, Tonolo G, et al: Clustering of albumin excretion rate abnormalities in Caucasian patients with NIDDM. The Italian NIDDM Nephropathy Study Group. Diabetologia 40(7):816–823, 1997.

173. Freedman BI, Soucie JM, McClellan WM: Family history of end-stage renal disease among incident dialysis patients. J Am Soc Nephrol 8(12):1942–1945, 1997.

174. Manalich R, Reyes L, Herrera M, et al: Relationship between weight at birth and the number and size of renal glomeruli in humans: A histomorphometric study. Kidney Int 58(2):770–773, 2000.

175. Schmidt IM, Chellakooty M, Boisen KA, et al: Impaired kidney growth in low-birth-weight children: Distinct effects of maturity and weight for gestational age. Kidney Int 68(2):731–740, 2005.

176. Keijzer-Veen MG, Schrevel M, Finken MJJ, et al: Microalbuminuria and lower glomerular filtration rate at young adult age in subjects born very premature and after intrauterine growth retardation. J Am Soc Nephrol 16(9):2762–2768, 2005.

177. Hughson M, Farris AB, 3rd, Douglas-Denton R, et al: Glomerular number and size in autopsy kidneys: The relationship to birthweight. Kidney Int 63(6):2113–2122, 2003.

178. Hoy WE, Rees M, Kile E, et al: Low birthweight and renal disease in Australian aborigines. Lancet 352(9143):1826–1827, 1998.

179. Nelson RG, Morgenstern H, Bennett PH: Birthweight and renal disease in Pima Indians with type 2 diabetes mellitus. Am J Epidemiol 148(7):650–656, 1998.

180. Klag MJ, Whelton PK, Randall BL, et al: End-stage renal disease in African-American and white men. 16-year MRFIT findings. JAMA 277(16):1293–1298, 1997.

181. Tarver-Carr ME, Powe NR, Eberhardt MS, et al: Excess risk of chronic kidney disease among African-American versus white subjects in the United States: A population-based study of potential explanatory factors. J Am Soc Nephrol 13(9):2363–2370, 2002.

182. Stehman-Breen CO, Gillen D, Steffes M, et al: Racial differences in early-onset renal disease among young adults: The coronary artery risk development in young adults (CARDIA) study. J Am Soc Nephrol 14(9):2352–2357, 2003.

183. Krop JS, Coresh J, Chambless LE, et al: A community-based study of explanatory factors for the excess risk for early renal function decline in blacks vs whites with diabetes: The Atherosclerosis Risk in Communities study. Arch Intern Med 159(15):1777–1783, 1999.

184. Hsu CY, Lin F, Vittinghoff E, Shlipak MG: Racial differences in the progression from chronic renal insufficiency to end-stage renal disease in the United States. J Am Soc Nephrol 14(11):2902–2907, 2003.

185. Kiberd BA, Clase CM: Cumulative risk for developing end-stage renal disease in the US population. J Am Soc Nephrol 13(6):1635–1644, 2002.

186. Fletcher RH, Fletcher SW, Wagner EH: Clinical Epidemiology, The Essentials. Philadelphia, Lippincott Williams & Wilkins, 1996.

187. Menon V, Sarnak MJ: The epidemiology of chronic kidney disease stages 1 to 4 and cardiovascular disease: A high-risk combination. Am J Kidney Dis 45(1):223–232, 2005.

188. Stehouwer CD, Gall MA, Twisk JW, et al: Increased urinary albumin excretion, endothelial dysfunction, and chronic low-grade inflammation in type 2 diabetes: Progressive, interrelated, and independently associated with risk of death. Diabetes 51(4):1157–1165, 2002.

189. Paisley KE, Beaman M, Tooke JE, et al: Endothelial dysfunction and inflammation in asymptomatic proteinuria. Kidney Int 63(2):624–633, 2003.

190. Jensen JS, Borch-Johnsen K, Jensen G, Feldt-Rasmussen B: Atherosclerotic risk factors are increased in clinically healthy subjects with microalbuminuria. Atherosclerosis 112(2):245–252, 1995.

191. McCullough PA, Sandberg KR, Borzak S, et al: Benefits of aspirin and beta-blockade after myocardial infarction in patients with chronic kidney disease. Am Heart J 144(2):226–232, 2002.

192. Sarnak MJ, Levey AS: Cardiovascular disease and chronic renal disease: A new paradigm. Am J Kidney Dis 35(4 Suppl 1):S117–131, 2000.

193. U.S. Renal Data Systems: USRDS 2002 Annual Data Report: Atlas of End Stage Renal Diseases in the United States. Bethesda, MD: National Institutes of Health. The National Institute of Diabetes and Digestive and Kidney Disease. Division of Kidney, Urologic, and Hematologic Diseases, 2002.

CHAPTER 19

Nephron Endowment

Valerie A. Luyckx • Barry M. Brenner

Genetic factors are important determinants of development and function of major organ systems as well as of susceptibility to disease. Rare genetic and congenital abnormalities leading to abnormal kidney development are associated with the occurrence of subsequent renal dysfunction, often manifest in very early in life.[1,2] Most renal disease in the general population, however, is not ascribable to genetic mutations, with the most common causes of end-stage renal disease (ESRD) worldwide being the polygenic disorders of diabetes and hypertension. Hypertension and renal disease prevalence vary among populations from different ethnic backgrounds, with very high rates being observed among Aboriginal Australians, Native Americans, and people of African descent.[3–6] Similarly, renal disease in hypertension and diabetes appear to "run" in families. It is well established that lifestyle factors pose significant risk for the development and persistence of hypertension and diabetes in the general population, with increasing obesity being the most concerning, especially in the developing world.[7] Searches for specific genetic polymorphisms or mutations, however, have not yielded smoking "genes" except in rare kindreds, but instead point to a likely complex interplay between polygenic predisposition and environmental factors in the development of diabetes, hypertension, and renal disease.[7–10] Furthermore, evidence highlighting the far-reaching effects of the intrauterine environment on organ development, organ function, and subsequent susceptibility to adult disease is becoming more and more compelling. These data suggest that fetal development may be the first in a succession of "hits" that ultimately manifests in overt disease expression. This chapter outlines the effects of fetal programming on renal development (nephrogenesis), nephron endowment, and the risks of hypertension and kidney disease in later life. Low birth weight also predicts later-life diabetes, and therefore, renal function may be affected indirectly as well, through fetal programming effects on other organ systems that are beyond the scope of this discussion.[11,12]

FETAL PROGRAMMING OF ADULT DISEASE

The process through which an environmental insult experienced early in life, particularly in utero, can predispose to adult disease is known as *fetal programming* or *developmental plasticity*. Fetal programming refers to the observation that an environmental stimulus experienced during a critical period of development in utero can induce long-term structural and functional effects in the developing organism.[13] Developmental plasticity is the process whereby different phenotypes may result on a background of a single genotype in response to different environmental stimuli experienced during intrauterine life.[14] These phenomena are intimately linked and have far-reaching implica-tions in that their effects can be transferred and perpetuated across generations.[15]

The association between adverse intrauterine events, for which low birth weight may be a surrogate marker, and subsequent cardiovascular disease has long been recognized.[13,14,16,17] Adults of low birth weight have higher cardiovascular morbidity and mortality than those of normal birth weight.[18] Subsequently, a large body of evidence from different populations has not only confirmed these initial findings but also expanded them to include other conditions such as hypertension, impaired glucose tolerance, type 2 diabetes, obesity, and chronic kidney disease.[13,19–23] Of these, the relation between low birth weight and subsequent hypertension has been the most studied, as demonstrated in Figure 19–1.[22–26] It is important to note that reported blood pressures tend to be higher in infants, children, and young adults of low birth weight compared with normal birth weight, but do not reach overt hypertensive ranges until well into adulthood in most studies.[26–28] Blood pressures are also highest in those of low birth weight who "caught up" fastest in postnatal weight.[26] The differences in blood pressure between people of low birth weight and those of normal birth weight also become amplified with age, with the result that adults who had been of low birth weight often develop overt hypertension, which increases with age.[29]

NEPHRON NUMBER

The kidney is the organ central to the development of hypertension. The relationship between renal sodium handling, intravascular fluid volume homeostasis, and hypertension is well accepted.[30,31] In addition, all known monogenetic mutations associated with hypertension involve proteins expressed in the kidney.[32,33] That factors intrinsic to the kidney itself affect blood pressure has been demonstrated clinically in renal transplantation, in which the blood pressure in the recipient after transplantation has been shown to be related to the blood pressure or hypertension risk factors of the donor: that is, hypertension "follows" the kidney.[34]

In 1988 Garcia and colleagues[35,36] proposed that a congenital (programmed) varia-

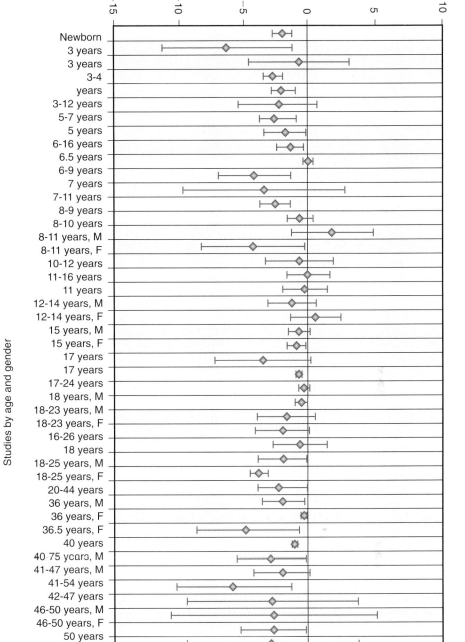

CH 19

Nephron Endowment

FIGURE 19–1 Studies reporting multiple regression analysis of change in systolic blood pressure (mm Hg) per kg increase in birth weight in children, adolescents, and adults. (For complete citations for individual studies, please refer to original reference, Figure 1, p 819.) (Adapted from Huxley RR, Shiell AW, Law CM: The role of size at birth and postnatal catch-up growth in determining systolic blood pressure: A systematic review of the literature. J Hypertens 18:815–831, 2000.)

tion in nephron number may be a factor explaining why some individuals are susceptible to hypertension and renal injury whereas others may seem relatively resistant under similar circumstances (e.g., sodium excess or diabetes mellitus). A reduction in nephron number and whole kidney glomerular surface area would result in reduced sodium excretory capacity enhancing susceptibility to hypertension and reduced renal reserve limiting compensation for renal injury. This hypothesis is attractive in that an association between a reduced nephron number and low birth weight, a surrogate marker of an adverse intrauterine environment, for example, may explain some of the differences in hypertension and renal disease prevalence observed among populations of different ethnicity, among whom those who tend to have lower birth weights often have higher prevalences and more rapid progression of renal disease.[37-40] Recent evidence is also pointing not only to an association with low birth weight and subsequent renal disease but also to high birth weight being a risk factor, especially for diabetic nephropathy.[5,38]

An obstacle to investigation of the nephron number hypothesis has been the difficulty of accurately counting nephron numbers.[41] Review of early studies shows that humans were believed to have an average of approximately one million nephrons per kidney.[42] Such studies, however, were performed using techniques such as acid-maceration or traditional stereologic analysis, which are prone to bias because of required assumptions, extrapolations, and operator sensitivity.[41-43] More recently, an unbiased fractionator-sampling/dissector-counting method has been developed that is believed to be more objective and reproducible.[41-43] It is important to recognize that all reported glomerular counting techniques have been performed on autopsy samples and that, to date, no validated technique permits determination of nephron number in vivo. Basgen and associates[44] attempted to develop an in vivo glomerular counting method and compared the fractionator technique with a combined renal biopsy/magnetic resonance imaging (MRI) method on excised canine kidneys. These authors found a good agreement of glomerular number on average between the two methods, but within kidneys, there was a 36% difference, potentially making the renal biopsy/MRI technique less useful in individuals. It is possible that with some refinement this technique may become more accurate and provide a useful technique to determine glomerular numbers in vivo.

Using the fractionator technique, among 37 normal Danish adults, the average glomerular (nephron) number was reported to be 617,000 per kidney (range 331,000–1,424,000).[42] These authors also reported a positive correlation between glomerular number and kidney weight, which has subsequently been used as a surrogate marker for nephron number in vivo. Another study including 78 kidneys from subjects of multiple ethnic origins from the United States and Australia showed somewhat similar results, with a mean of 784,909 glomeruli per kidney, but with a very wide range, from 210,332 to 1,825,380.[45] In both studies, numbers of viable glomeruli were reduced in kidneys from older subjects, owing to age-related glomerulosclerosis and obsolescence.[42,45] Glomerular number, therefore, appears to vary by up to eightfold within the normal population. The variability of mean nephron number reported in presumed normal subjects in different studies, from 617,000 to 1,429,200, should raise a note of caution about the fractionator technique.[42,46] Whether these differences reflect true differences in the populations studied or are reflections of small samples sizes will become clearer with time as more studies accumulate or as better techniques evolve.

It is known that persons born with severe nephron deficits, for example, unilateral renal agenesis, bilateral renal hypoplasia, and oligomeganephronia, develop progressive pro-teinuria, glomerulosclerosis, and renal dysfunction with time.[47-51] Similarly, people born with nephron numbers at or below the median level may be more susceptible to superimposed postnatal factors that act as subsequent "hits"; thus, a significant proportion of the population may be at risk for the development of hypertension and renal disease.[43] This may be a plausible hypothesis given that some 30% of the world's adult population is hypertensive.[7] Drawing on experimental data in animals, surgical removal of more than one kidney under different circumstances and in different species does not always lead to the development of hypertension and renal disease.[43] In humans, uninephrectomy is accompanied by compensatory hypertrophy and function of the remaining contralateral kidney, often with little adverse clinical consequence, although progressive hypertension and proteinuria have been reported.[52,53] Of interest, however, uninephrectomy on postnatal day 1 in rats or fetal uninephrectomy in sheep, that is, loss of nephrons at a time when nephrogenesis is not yet completed, does lead to adult hypertension prior to any evidence of renal injury.[54-56] These data support the hypothesis that intrauterine or congenital reduction in nephron number, that is, before nephrogenesis is completed, may be associated with different compensatory mechanisms or a reduced compensatory capacity than occurs in response to later nephron loss, resulting in subsequent development or risk of hypertension. In support of this hypothesis, kidneys from rats that underwent uninephrectomy at 3 days of age showed a similar total glomerular number, but a significantly reduced number of mature glomeruli compared with those who underwent nephrectomy at 120 days of age.[57] Furthermore, the mean glomerular volume in neonatally nephrectomized rats increased by 59% versus 20% in the adult nephrectomized rats, indicating a likely greater burden of compensatory hypertrophy and hyperfunction in response to neonatal nephrectomy.

Nephron Number and Glomerular Volume

Despite the large variation in nephron number seen in the normal population, it has been noted consistently that glomerular volume varies inversely with glomerular number as shown in Figure 19–2.[46,58,59] This observation suggests that larger glomeruli may reflect compensatory hyperfiltration and hypertrophy in subjects with fewer nephrons.[45,59] In fact, Hoy and co-workers[58] found that, although mean glomerular volume was increased in subjects with reduced nephron numbers, total glomerular tuft volume (a surrogate for total filtration surface area) was not different among groups with different nephron numbers (Table 19–1). This observation suggests that total filtration surface area may initially be maintained in the setting of a reduced nephron number but at the expense of glomerular hypertension and hypertrophy, which are maladaptive and predictors of poor outcomes.[60-62] Consistent with this possibility, glomerulomegaly is common in renal biopsies from Australian Aborigines, a population with high rates of low birth weight and renal disease, and has also been associated with faster rate of decline of glomerular filtration rate (GFR) in Pima Indians.[63-65] Furthermore, in a study of donor kidneys, maximal planar area of glomeruli was found to be higher in kidneys from African Americans compared with whites and a predictor of poorer transplant function.[62] In populations at high risk of kidney failure, therefore, large glomeruli are a common finding at early stages of renal disease and may reflect programmed reductions in nephron number in these populations in which access to prenatal and subsequent health care is often suboptimal.[66-68]

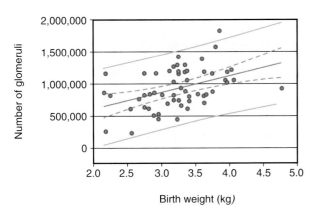 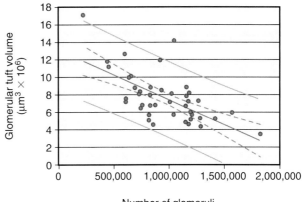

FIGURE 19-2   Birth weight, glomerular number, and glomerular volume in adults. (From Hughson M, Farris AB, Douglas-Denton R, et al: Glomerular number and size in autopsy kidneys: The relationship to birth weight. Kidney Int 63:2113–2122, 2003.)

TABLE 19-1	Glomerular Characteristics by Birth Weight in Humans			
Birth Weight	N	No Glomeruli*	Mean Glomerular Tuft Volume ($\mu m^2 \times 10^6$)	Total Glomerular Tuft Volume (cm²)
2.65 Kg (1.81–3.12)	29	770,860 (658,757–882,963)	9.2	6.7
3.27 Kg (3.18–3.38)	28	965,729 (885,714–1,075,744)	7.2	6.8
3.93 Kg (3.41–4.94)	30	1,005,356 (900,094–1,110,599)	6.9	6.6

*Adjusted for age, gender, race, and body surface area.
From Hoy WE, Hughson MD, Bertram JF, et al: Nephron number, hypertension, renal disease, and renal failure. J Am Soc Nephrol 16:2557–2564, 2005.

EVIDENCE FOR FETAL PROGRAMMING AND THE KIDNEY

Low birth weight is defined by the World Health Organization as a birth weight less than 2500 grams. Low birth weight can be the result of intrauterine growth restriction (IUGR; birth weight <10th percentile for gestational age) or premature birth. Low birth weight associated with IUGR generally reflects intrauterine stress during late gestation as opposed to low birth weight of prematurity, which may be an appropriate weight for the duration of gestation. Full-term birth low birth weight (i.e., IUGR) has the strongest association with adult disease.[69] Low birth weight is more common among African Americans, Native Americans, and Aboriginal Australians than among whites, the former being populations with disproportionately high rates of hypertension, chronic kidney disease, type 2 diabetes, and cardiovascular disease.[4,38,70,71]

Multiple animal models have demonstrated the association of low birth weight (induced by gestational exposure to low-protein diet, uterine ischemia, dexamethasone, vitamin A deprivation) with subsequent hypertension.[72–78] The link between adult hypertension and low birth weight in these animal models appears to be mediated, at least in part, by an associated congenital nephron deficit occurring with IUGR.[72,75,77] Vehaskari and colleagues[75] demonstrated an almost 30% reduction in glomerular number in offspring of pregnant rats fed a low-protein diet compared with a normal-protein diet during pregnancy. As shown in Figure 19–3, the maternal low-protein–fed offspring had systolic blood pressures that were 20 to 25 mm Hg higher by 8 weeks of age.[75] Similarly, Celsi and associates[72] found that prenatal adminis-

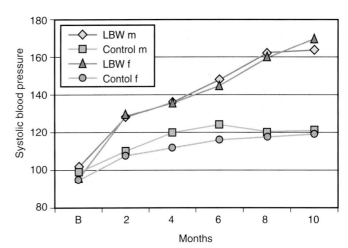

FIGURE 19-3   Fetal programming of hypertension in low-birth-weight rats. (Adapted from Vehaskari VM, Aviles DH, Manning J: Prenatal programming of adult hypertension in the rat. Kidney Int 59:238–245, 2001.)

tration of dexamethasone in rats was also associated with low birth weight and fewer glomeruli compared with controls. In these nephron-deficient rats, GFR was reduced, albuminuria was increased, and urinary sodium excretion was lower than those with a greater nephron complement.[72] These findings in animals lend credence to the hypothesis that a congenital deficit in nephron number, resulting in a decreased filtration surface area and thus a limitation in renal sodium excretion, is an independent factor determining susceptibility to essential hypertension. Low nephron number alone, however, does not account for all observed programmed hypertension. Langely-Evans and co-workers[24] reported that supplementation of a low-protein diet during gestation with glycine, urea, or alanine resulted in a normalization of nephron number in the offspring but only a normalization of blood pressure in those supplemented with glycine. This finding suggests that there may be factors leading to intrauterine programming of hypertension in addition to, or independent of, nephron number.

Programming of Nephron Number in Humans

As mentioned previously, nephron numbers vary widely in the normal human population (Fig. 19–2; see also Table 19–1). More and more data are emerging supporting a direct relationship between nephron number and birth weight and an inverse relationship between nephron number and glomerular volume.[59,79,80] After analysis of 56 kidneys, Hughson and colleagues[80] reported a linear relationship between glomerular number and birth weight and calculated a regression coefficient predicting an increase of 257,426 glomeruli per kilogram increase in birth weight. The applicability of the regression coefficient in populations in which the distribution of nephron number appears bimodal, however, may not be valid. It has also been calculated that in the normal population without renal disease, approximately 4500 glomeruli are lost per kidney per year after the age of 18.[58] Glomerular numbers tend to be lower in females than in males. A kidney starting with a lower nephron number, therefore, would conceivably reach a critical reduction of nephron mass, either with age or in response to an renal insult, earlier than a kidney with a greater nephron complement, contributing to hypertension and/or renal dysfunction.

Kidney development in the human begins during the 9th week of gestation and continues until the 34th to 36th week.[58] Nephron number at birth is, therefore, largely dependent on the intrauterine environment and gestational age. It is generally believed that no new nephrons are formed in humans after birth. In an attempt to investigate whether glomerulogenesis does indeed continue postnatally in premature infants, Rodriguez and colleagues[81] studied kidneys at autopsy from 56 extremely premature infants compared with 10 full-term infants as controls. The radial glomerular counts were lower in premature versus full-term infants and correlated with gestational age. Furthermore, evidence of active glomerulogenesis, indicated by the presence of basophilic S-shaped bodies immediately under the renal capsule, was found in premature infants who died before 40 days but absent in those who died after 40 days of life. The authors concluded that nephrogenesis may continue for up to 40 days after birth in premature infants. Interestingly, these authors also stratified their cases by presence or absence of renal failure in the infants. Among infants surviving longer than 40 days, those with renal failure (serum creatinine ≥2.0 mg/dL) had significantly fewer glomeruli than those without renal failure. This cross-sectional observation may suggest that renal failure inhibited glomerulogenesis or, conversely, that fewer glomeruli lowered the threshold to develop renal failure in these extremely ill infants. Those premature infants surviving longer than 40 days without renal failure exhibited glomerulomegaly, which may reflect, at least in the short term, a compensatory renoprotective response. In contrast to these findings, Hinchliffe and associates[82,83] studied nephron number in premature or full-term stillbirths or infants who died at 1 year of age and who were born with either appropriate weight for gestational age or small for gestational age. At

both time points, growth-restricted infants had fewer nephrons than controls. In addition, the number of nephrons in growth-restricted infants dying at 1 year of age had not increased compared with the growth-restricted stillbirths, demonstrating a lack of postnatal compensation in nephron number (Fig. 19–4A). Manalich and co-workers[59] examined the kidneys of neonates dying within 2 weeks of birth in relation to their birth weights (Fig. 19–4B). A significant direct correlation was found between glomerular number and birth weight. In addition, there was also a strong inverse correlation between glomerular volume and glomerular number independent of sex and race. These studies, therefore, support the hypothesis that an adverse intrauterine environment, manifest as low birth weight, in infants, is associated with a congenital reduction in nephron number and an early, compensatory increase in glomerular volume.

Renal mass is known to be proportional to nephron number, and renal volume is proportional to renal mass; therefore, renal volume has been analyzed as a surrogate for nephron endowment in infants in vivo.[42] Renal volume was found to be reduced by anthropomorphic and Doppler flow measurements performed in utero in fetuses subjected to growth restriction.[84] A subsequent analysis of kidney size and growth postnatally, as assessed by ultrasound, in 178 children born premature or small for gestational age as compared with 717 mature children with appropriate weight for gestational age at 0, 3, and 18 months, found that weight for gestational age was positively associated with kidney volume at all three time points.[85] Slight catch-up kidney growth was observed in growth-retarded infants but not in premature infants. In Australian Aboriginal children, low birth weight was also found to be associated with lower renal volumes on ultrasound.[86] A smaller kidney size, therefore, may be a surrogate marker of a reduced nephron endowment, but it must be borne in mind that the growth in kidney size on ultrasound cannot distinguish between the components of normal growth with age and renal hypertrophy.

In a population of 140 adults aged 18 to 65 years old, who died of various causes, a significant correlation was also observed between birth weight and glomerular number.[79] Glomerular volume was again found to be inversely correlated with glomerular number. Mean glomerular numbers did not differ statistically among African American and white subjects, although the distribution among African Americans appeared bimodal, with a few outliers having very high nephron numbers, and several subjects having nephron numbers below 500,000. No white subject had fewer than 500,000 nephrons. Significantly, however, none of the subjects in this study had been of low birth weight; therefore, no conclusion can be drawn as to whether an association with low birth weight and nephron number exists in either population group.[87] In a European study among 26 subjects with non-insulin–dependent diabetes compared with 19 age-matched nondiabetic controls, no difference in glomerular number was found, but again, all subjects had birth weights above 3000 g, and therefore, the impact of low birth weight on nephron number could not be assessed.[88]

In support of the potential association of nephron number and hypertension, a German study of whites aged 35 to 59 years who died in accidents found that, in 10 subjects with a history of essential hypertension, the number of glomeruli per kidney was significantly lower, and glomerular volume significantly higher, than in 10 normotensive-matched controls (Fig. 19–5).[46] Birth weights were not reported in this study, but the authors concluded that a reduced nephron number is associated with susceptibility to essential hypertension. Similarly, among a subset of 63 subjects in whom mean arterial pressures and birth weights were available, Hughson and co-workers[79] reported a significant correlation between birth weight and glomerular number, mean arterial

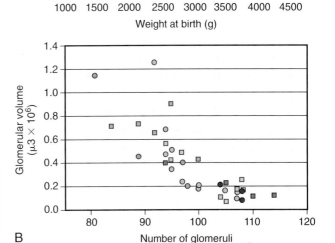

FIGURE 19–4 **A,** Effect of IUGR on nephron number in humans. (a) Nephron number in relation to gestational age; (b) lack of postnatal catch-up in nephron number. **B,** Birth weight, glomerular volume, and glomerular number in neonates. (A, From Hinchliffe SA, Lynch MR, Sargent PH, et al: The effect of intrauterine growth retardation on the development of renal nephrons. Br J Obstet Gynaecol 99:296–301, 1992; B, From Manalich R, Reyes L, Herrera M, et al: Relationship between weight at birth and the number and size of renal glomeruli in humans: A histomorphometric study. Kidney Int 58:770–773, 2000.)

pressure and glomerular number, and mean arterial pressure and birth weight among the white but not the African American subjects. Among African Americans having nephron numbers below the mean, however, twice as many were hypertensive as normotensive, suggesting a possible contribution of lower nephron number in this group as well.[79] In addition, glomerular volumes were found to be higher among the hypertensive African American subjects compared with hypertensive whites.[79] A similar finding was reported among donor kidney biopsies, in which maximal planar area of glomeruli was found to be higher in African Americans than in whites.[62] In this study, glomerulomegaly emerged as an independent predictor of poor allograft function.

Programming of Renal Function and Disease

Experimental Evidence

As opposed to infants of low birth weight, in whom nephron numbers have been shown to be reduced, in adults, there are no data on nephron number specifically in those who had been of low birth weight. The association between nephron number and birth weight, however, does appear to be a consistent finding in infants, so the extrapolation seems reasonable that nephron numbers would also remain reduced in

adults of low birth weight.[80] The determination of nephron number in vivo, as mentioned previously, is difficult and not yet reliable enough; therefore, the most utilized in vivo surrogate marker available at present is birth weight. In some animal models, low nephron numbers have been observed also in the setting of normal birth weight; therefore, among humans, if birth weight is the only surrogate marker used, the impact of nephron number on any outcome is likely to be underestimated.[89] Glomerulomegaly is also consistently observed in the setting of a low nephron number. Although this may be a compensatory mechanism to restore filtration surface area, it is conceivable that renal reserve in these kidneys in reduced.[58] If this is the case, these kidneys may be expected to be less able to compensate further in the setting of additional renal insults and to begin to manifest signs of renal dysfunction (i.e., proteinuria, elevations in serum creatinine, and hypertension).

In a provocative study, diabetes was induced by streptozotocin injection in subgroups of low-birth-weight (induced by maternal protein restriction) and normal-birth-weight rats.[90] Low-birth-weight rats, as expected, were found to have reduced nephron numbers and higher blood pressures compared with those of normal birth weight. Among those rendered diabetic, there was a greater proportional increase in renal size and glomerular hypertrophy in the low-birth-weight rats than in normal-birth-weight controls after 1 week

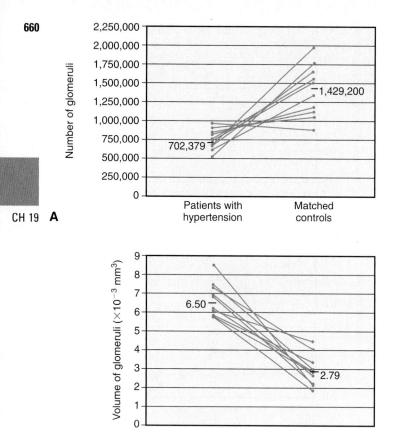

A

B

FIGURE 19–5 Nephron number (**A**) and glomerular volume (**B**) in Caucasian subjects with primary hypertension compared with controls. (From Keller G, Zimmer G, Mall G, et al: Nephron number in patients with primary hypertension. N Engl J Med 348:101–108, 2003.)

(Fig. 19–6).[90] This study demonstrates that the renal response to injury in the setting of a reduced nephron number may be exaggerated and could lead to accelerated loss of renal function. Subsequently, the same authors[91] published outcomes in low-birth-weight versus normal-birth-weight diabetic rats at 40 weeks. Histologically, the podocyte density was reduced and the average area covered by each podocyte was greater in the low-birth-weight diabetic rats than in the normal-birth-weight controls. These findings correlated with urine albumin excretion rate, which was higher in low-birth-weight diabetic rats, although this did not reach statistical significance. In support of the role of altered podocyte physiology in renal disease progression, similar findings were observed in the Munich Wistar-Fromter rat, a strain that has congenitally reduced nephron numbers and develops spontaneous renal disease (see later).[92] Whether these podocyte changes are secondary to an increase in glomerular pressure in the setting of reduced nephron numbers or a primary programmed structural change leading to glomerular injury is not yet known.

As mentioned previously, hypertension has frequently been reported in low-birth-weight rats and sheep, but is not universally observed.[13,24,25,72,93] Some authors have reported the presence of salt-sensitive hypertension in rats in which low birth weight was induced by maternal uterine artery ligation, whereas others report no salt-sensitivity in rats in which low birth weight was induced by maternal protein restriction.[94,95] GFR measured in rats in which low birth weight was induced by maternal protein restriction was found to be reduced, concomitant with a reduction in nephron number.[76,96] Of interest, GFR was reduced by 10%, although nephron number was reduced by 25%, implying some degree of compensatory hyperfunction per nephron (Fig. 19–7).[25] In contrast, in low-birth-weight rats exposed to prenatal dexamethasone and subsequently fed a high-protein diet, GFR was similar to that in normal-birth-weight controls.[97] Nephron numbers were reduced by 13% in only male low-birth-weight rats. This study may suggest that there is a threshold reduction in nephron number above which compensation is adequate or that the high-protein diet induced supranormal GFRs in both groups, masking subtle differences in baseline GFR. Another study that measured GFR in low-birth-weight rats, this time induced by maternal uterine artery ligation

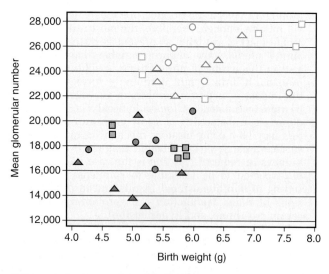

Solid symbols—Low protein diet offspring
Open symbols—Normal protein diet offspring

A

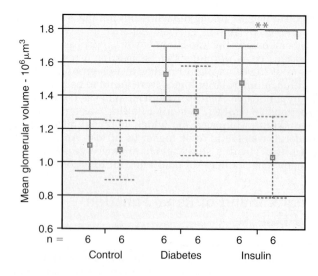

— Low protein diet offspring; - - Normal protein diet offspring

B

FIGURE 19–6 **A and B,** Influence of glomerular number on adaptation to diabetes in rats. (From Jones SE, Bilous RW, Flyvbjerg A, Marshall SM: Intra-uterine environment influences glomerular number and the acute renal adaptation to experimental diabetes. Diabetologia 44:721–728, 2001.)

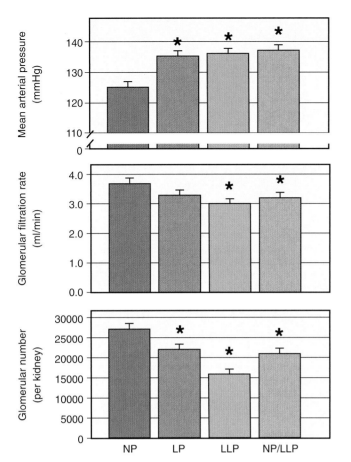

NP = 19% protein diet; LP = 8.5% protein diet; LLP = 5% protein diet; NP/LLP = 5% in last 1/2 of pregnancy.
*P < 0.05

FIGURE 19–7 Increased blood pressure, decreased glomerular filtration rate, and glomerular number in low-birth-weight adult male rats. (From Vehaskari VM, Woods LL: Prenatal programming of hypertension: Lessons from experimental models. J Am Soc Nephrol 16:2545–2556, 2005.)

fore, does appear to predispose to progressive renal functional decline.

Evidence in Humans

One consequence of glomerular hyperfiltration is microalbuminuria. Studies from several countries have demonstrated an increased prevalence of microalbuminuria and proteinuria among adults who had been of low birth weight.[4,5,64,100–102] In long-term follow-up studies of children who had been extremely low-birth-weight premature infants, weighing less than 1000 g a birth, serum creatinine was found to be higher and GFR reduced compared with those in age-matched normal-birth-weight children at ages 6 to12 years.[103] Another study compared blood pressures and renal function in females in their mid-20s who had been preterm, small-for-gestational-age, or normal full-term infants.[104] Blood pressures were significantly higher among those who had been preterm compared with the normal-birth-weight controls. There was no statistically significant difference in GFR or urinary albumin excretion between the groups, but GFR tended to be lower in the small-for-gestational-age group and albuminuria higher in the preterm and small-for-gestational-age groups. This study included fewer than 20 subjects in each group, which might suggest that, with larger numbers, statistical significance may have been reached. In a similar study, 422 19-year-old subjects who had been very premature were stratified according to whether they had been appropriate weight or small for gestational age at birth.[105] Birth weight was found to be negatively associated with serum creatinine and albuminuria and positively associated with GFR. The authors concluded that IUGR is associated with poorer renal function in young adults. Prematurity itself may therefore be associated with poor long-term renal function in some studies, a risk that is increased when there is associated IUGR.

Analysis of 724 subjects aged 48 to 53, who had been subjected to malnutrition in midgestation during the Dutch famine, revealed an increased prevalence of microalbuminuria (12%) when compared with those subjected to malnutrition during early gestation (9%), late gestation (7%), or not exposed to famine (4–8%).[106] Interestingly, size at birth was not associated with the observed increase in microalbuminuria, suggesting that renal development may have been irreversibly affected in midgestation, although subsequent intrauterine whole-body growth was able to catch up with restoration of more normal nutrition. These data further emphasize the need for other surrogate markers of the intrauterine environment in addition to birth weight. Furthermore, among all subjects who had microalbuminuria in this cohort, systolic and diastolic blood pressures were increased, glucose intolerance was more prevalent, and GFRs were increased, indicating a degree of compensatory hyperfiltration.

The association between low birth weight and subsequent metabolic syndrome has been well described in many populations around the world.[14,18] Whether very early renal dysfunction, manifest as microalbuminuria, is a trigger or a consequence of the metabolic syndrome is a topic of significant interest. Recent evidence points to improved cardiovascular outcomes associated with reduction in microalbuminuria, which may support the former possibility, although experimental evidence also supports simultaneous programming of the endocrine pancreas and cardiovascular system during fetal development.[107]

It is not easy to dissect the relative contributions of genetics and the fetal environment to the ultimate manifestation of disease. To address this question, Gielen and colleagues[108] studied 653 twins, comprising 265 twin pairs and 123 individuals whose twin did not participate in the study. Creatinine clearance was significantly lower in low-birth-weight than in normal-birth-weight twins. Furthermore, intrapair

during gestation, also failed to demonstrate a difference in GFR in low-birth-weight rats, but they were significantly hypertensive compared with normal-birth-weight controls.[98] Conceivably, in this study, the higher intraglomerular pressure due to elevated blood pressure and reduced nephron mass in low-birth-weight rats may have led to a compensatory increase in single-nephron GFR (SNGFR) and, thus, normalization of whole-kidney GFR. In another study, low-birth-weight rats, which had been subjected to gestational protein restriction, had significantly higher blood pressures and urinary protein excretion at 20 weeks of age than controls, although again GFR was not different.[99] Definitive understanding of the pathophysiologic impact of a reduction in nephron number is difficult to elucidate from the existing literature comprising very varied experimental conditions. Ooverall, however, it is possible that, although whole-kidney GFR may not change, SNGFR is likely to be increased in the setting of a reduced nephron number. In support of this possibility, the Munich-Wistar-Fromter rat is known to develop spontaneously progressive glomerular injury. Interestingly, compared with the control Wistar rat strain, nephron numbers have been found to be significantly reduced, urine protein excretion and systolic blood pressure to be significantly higher, and by micropuncture study, the SN GFR was found to be significantly elevated. A "naturally" occurring (i.e., not experimentally induced) congenital nephron deficit, there-

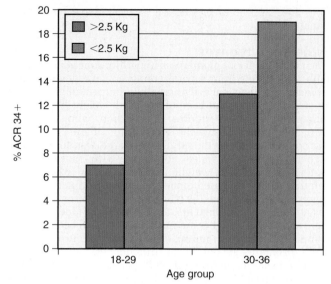

FIGURE 19–8 Birth weight and albumin-to-creatinine ratio in Tiwi adults. (From Hoy WE, Mathews JD, McCredie DA, et al: The multidimensional nature of renal disease: Rates and associations of albuminuria in an Australian Aboriginal community. Kidney Int 54:1296–1304, 1998.)

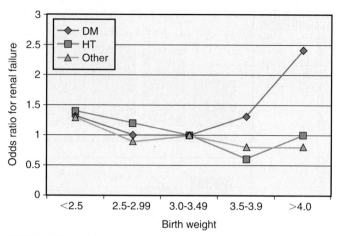

FIGURE 19–9 Birth weight and risk of end-stage renal disease. (From Lackland DT, Bendall HE, Osmond C, et al: Low birth weights contribute to high rates of early-onset chronic renal failure in the Southeastern United States. Arch Intern Med 160:1472–1476, 2000.)

birth weight differences were positively correlated with GFR in both monozygotic and dizygotic twin pairs, tha tis, the twin with a higher birth weight had a higher creatinine clearance. These authors concluded that fetoplacental factors have a greater impact than genetic factors on adult renal function.

Early compelling evidence of the relationship between birth weight and renal function was published by Hoy and associates[4,64,101,102] in the Australian Aboriginal population. These authors found that the odds ratio for overt albuminuria was 2.8 in those who had been of low birth weight with a reference value of 1.0 for those of normal birth weight (Fig. 19–8).[101] Furthermore, in addition to the association of albuminuria with low birth weight, the degree of albuminuria predicted loss of renal function and was strongly correlated with both renal and nonrenal deaths.[64,65] Similarly, among Pima Indians with type 2 diabetes, the prevalence of albuminuria was 63% in those who had a birth weight less than 2500 g, 41% in those of normal birth weight, and 64% among those of high birth weight (≥4500 g).[5] After controlling for maternal diabetes, the odds of albuminuria among those of high birth weight was not increased, indicating a major role for gestational exposure to diabetes in programming of renal disease risk. This finding has been confirmed in other studies.[109] Gestational hyperglycemia often results in high birth weight, and as is discussed later, is also associated with a reduced nephron number in the offspring.

A handful of studies have examined the relationship between birth weight and diabetic nephropathy and found an increased susceptibility among subjects who had been of low birth weight.[5,110–113] Among women with type 1 diabetes mellitus, nephropathy was present in 75% of those with a birth weight below the 10th percentile (≤2700 g), compared with 35% of those with birth weights above the 90th percentile (≥4000 g).[112] This relationship was not present in men, however, but men with diabetic nephropathy were significantly shorter than those without nephropathy, possibly indicating some degree of growth restriction.[111,112]

A variety of generally small studies have reported a greater severity of renal disease and more rapid progression of diverse renal diseases, including immunoglobulin A (IgA) nephropathy, membranous nephropathy, minimal change disease, nephrotic syndrome, and chronic pyelonephritis, among children and adults who had been of low birth weight.[110,113–117] Lackland and co-workers[40] examined the relationship of birth weight and ESRD in 1230 dialysis patients and 2460 age- and sex-matched normal controls in South Carolina. This population has a high prevalence of ESRD among young patients, in whom 70% is attributable to hypertension or diabetes. In this cohort, the odds ratio for ESRD was 1.4 (1.1–1.8) among those with birth weights under 2500 g compared with those of normal birth weight. This association was consistent for all causes of ESRD and was not affected by family history of ESRD.[40,118] Interestingly, the odds ratio for diabetic renal disease was 2.4 for those having birth weights greater than 4000 g (Fig. 19–9). Although maternal diabetic status is not given, such high birth weights suggest intrauterine exposure to hyperglycemia and its role in programming of renal disease. Epidemiologic data are, therefore, accumulating in support of the impact of fetal programming on subsequent renal disease.

PROPOSED MECHANISMS OF FETAL PROGRAMMING OF NEPHRON NUMBER

Kidney development is a complex process involving tightly controlled expression of many genes and constant remodeling.[119] Many experimental models, as outlined in Table 19–2, have been shown to result in a reduced nephron number. In many of the experimental models of programming, as mentioned previously, a reduced nephron number is often associated with low birth weight and, in some cases, with subsequent hypertension and evidence of renal injury. Interestingly, in normal rat litters, those pups with naturally occurring low birth weight (i.e., birth weights < –2 SD from the mean) were found to have a 13% reduction in nephron number, which was also associated with glomerulomegaly and proteinuria.[120] Low birth weight in rodents, therefore, may be associated with a low nephron number even under nonexperimental conditions. Low birth weight in humans is often associated with poor maternal nutrition, smoking, alcohol ingestion, infections, and low socioeconomic status, all factors that, in turn, may affect nephrogenesis.[58] In humans, kidney development begins around 8 weeks of gestation and continues until 36 weeks. Approximately two thirds of the nephrons develop during the last trimester of gestation, making this the window most susceptible to adverse effects, but earlier insults can also

TABLE 19-2	Nephron Endowment				
Model	Subject	Nephron Number (%)	BW	BP	Renal Function
Maternal calorie restriction[129,130,156]	Rat	↓ 20–40	↓	↑	↓ GFR proteinuria
Uterine artery ligation[120,137,187,188]	Rat	↓ 20–30	↓	↑	Impaired proteinuria
Low-protein diet[24,25,99,128]	Rat	↓ 25 ↓ 17 ↓ 16	↓/↔	↑	↓ GFR proteinuria ↓ Longevity
Iron deficiency[124]	Rat	↓ 22	↓	↑	NA
Vitamin A deficiency[125]	Rat	↓ 20	↔	NA	NA
Glucocorticoids[72,77,140,189]	Rat	↓ 20	↔	↑	Glomerulosclerosis ↑ Collagen deposition
	Sheep	↓ 38	↔	↑	
Maternal diabetes[145]	Rat	↓ 10–35	↔	NA	NA
Gentamicin[149]	Rat	↓ 10–20	↓	NA	NA
β-Lactams[150]	Rat	↓ 5–10	↔	NA	Tubular dilatation Interstitial inflammation
Cyclosporine[152,153]	Rabbits	↓ 25–33	↓/↔	↑	↓ GFR ↑ RVR proteinuria
Dahl salt-sensitive[35]	Rat	↓ 15	↔	↑ With Na intake	Accelerated FSGS
Munich-Wistar-Fromter rat[35,190]	Rat	↓ 40		↑ With age	↑ SNGFR FSGS
Milan hypertensive rat[35]	Rat	↓ 17		↑	NA
PVG/c [35]	Rat	↑ 122		Resistant	Resistant to FSGS
Os/+ mouse[191]	Mouse	↓ 50		NA	Glomerular hypertrophy
PAX2 mutations[134,135]	Mouse	↓ 22		NA	Renal coloboma syndrome in humans
GDNF heterozygote[138,139]	Mouse	↓ 30	↔	↑	Normal GFR Enlarged glomeruli
c-ret null mutant[119]	Mouse	↓	NA	NA	Severe renal dysplasia
hIGFBP-1 overexpression[146]	Mouse	↓ 18–25	↓	NA	Glomerulosclerosis
Bcl-2 deficiency[133]	Mouse	↓	NA	NA	↑ Urea and creatinine
BF-2 null mutant[119]	Mouse	↓ 75	NA	NA	NA
BMP 7 null mutant[119]	Mouse	↓	NA	NA	Small kidneys
p53 transgenic[136]	Mouse	↓ 50	NA	NA	Glomerular hypertrophy Renal failure
Intrauterine growth retardation[59,82]	Human 0–1 yr	↓ 13–35	↓	NA	NA
Hypertensive vs. normotensive Caucasian[46,79]	Human 35–59 yr	↓ 19–50	NA	↑	No ↑ glomerulosclerosis
Hypertensive vs. normotensive African American[79]	Human 35–59 yr	NS ↓	NA	↑	No ↑ glomerulosclerosis
Aboriginal Australians[43]	Human 0–85 yr	↓ 23	↓	NA	Glomerular hypertrophy

BP, blood pressure; BW, birth weight; FSGS, focal segmental glomerulosclerosis; GFR, glomerular filtration rate; NA, not assessed; NS, nonsignificant; RVR, renal vascular resistance; SNGFR, single-nephron GFR.
Adapted from Brenner BM, Garcia DL, Anderson S: Glomeruli and blood pressure. Less of one, more the other? Am J Hypertens 1:335–347, 1988; and Kett MM, Bertram JF: Nephron endowment and blood pressure: What do we really know? Curr Hypertens Rep 6:133–139, 2004.

have a major impact on subsequent nephrogenesis.[82,121] In rodents, nephrogenesis continues for up to 10 days after birth, but from most animal studies, the major impact is noted when environmental stimuli are manipulated when nephrogenesis is most active, that is, mid to late gestation.[121]

Three processes determine ultimate nephron number: branching of the ureteric bud, condensation of mesenchymal cells, and conversion of mesenchymal condensates into epithelium.[119] It has been estimated that a 2% decrease in ureteric bud branching efficiency would result in a 50% reduction in final nephron complement after 20 generations of branching.[122] The specific molecular mechanisms whereby nephron numbers may be affected and/or function altered, however, are not yet completely understood. Several potential

TABLE 19–3	Experimental Models and Proposed Mechanisms of Intrauterine Programming of Renal Development
Experimental Model	**Possible Mechanism of Nephron Number Reduction**
Maternal low-protein diet	↑ Apoptosis in metanephrons and postnatal kidney Altered gene expression in developing kidney Altered gene methylation ↓ Placental 11-βHSD2 expression
Maternal vitamin A restriction	↓ Branching of ureteric bud ? Maintenance of spatial orientation of vascular development ↓ c-ret expression
Maternal iron restriction	? Reduced oxygen delivery ? Altered glucocorticoid responsiveness ? Altered micronutrient availability
Gestational glucocorticoid exposure	↑ Fetal glucocorticoid exposure ? Enhanced tissue maturation ↑ Glucocorticoid receptor expression ↑ 1α- and 1β ATPase expression ↓ Renal and adrenal 11-βHSD2 expression
Uterine artery ligation/ embolization	↑ Pro-apoptotic gene expression in developing kidney: casepase-3, Bax, p53 ↓ Antiapoptotic gene expression: PAX2, bcl-2 Altered gene methylation
Maternal diabetes/ hyperglycemia	↓ IGF-II/mannose-6-phosphate receptor expression Altered IGF-II activity/bioavailability
Gestational drug exposure • Gentamicin • β-Lactams • Cyclosporine	↓ Branching morphogenesis ↑ Mesenchymal apoptosis Arrest of nephron formation

mechanisms have been proposed and investigated thus far, as summarized in Table 19–3 and discussed later.

Maternal Nutrient Restriction

Experimental alterations in maternal dietary composition at different stages of gestation have been shown to program embryonic kidney gene expression early in the course of gestation, which later affects nephron number.[123] Fetal nutrient supply is also affected by alterations in placental blood flow. Maternal *protein restriction* during pregnancy has been the most widely studied model, but manipulations at different times of gestation and for different periods during gestation make results not always easy to compare and interpret. Furthermore, not all low-protein diets have the same programming effects. It has been proposed that relative deficiencies of specific amino acids—methionine or glycine, for example—may have a greater impact on organ development than total protein restriction per se.[24] Such effects have been proposed to be mediated largely by changes in DNA methylation, depending on amino acid availability, resulting in epigenetic changes in gene expression.[13]

Maternal *iron restriction* during pregnancy in rats also leads to a reduction in birth weight and nephron number and the development of subsequent hypertension in the offspring.[124] The authors suggest that fetal anemia may result in reduced tissue oxygen delivery, altered fetal kidney glucocorticoid sensitivity, or altered availability of other micronutrients that may affect nephrogenesis. These hypotheses remain to be proved.

Maternal *vitamin A restriction* has also been associated with a reduction in nephron number in the offspring.[78,125] Severe vitamin A deficiency during pregnancy is associated with congenital malformations and renal defects in the offspring. Vitamin A and all-*trans* retinoic acid have been shown to stimulate nephrogenesis through modulation of ureteric

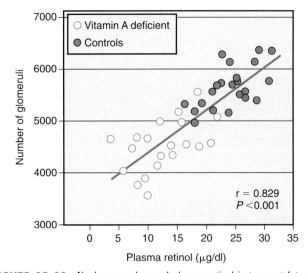

FIGURE 19–10 Nephron number and plasma retinol in term rat fetuses. (From Merlet-Benichou C: Influence of fetal environment on kidney development. Int J Dev Biol 43:453–456, 1999.)

bud branching capacity in ureteric epithelial cell culture and in maintenance of spatial organization of blood vessel development in cultured renal cortical explants.[125] In vivo, a vitamin A–deficient diet sufficient to reduce circulating vitamin A levels by 50% in pregnant rats resulted in a 25% reduction in nephron number in the offspring.[125] Intriguingly, supplementation of vitamin A increased nephron numbers. Analysis of 21-day-old fetal rats (just before birth) revealed a direct correlation between plasma retinol concentration and nephron number, as shown in Figure 19–10.[125] The reduction in nephron number in the setting of vitamin A deficiency is likely mediated at least in part by modulation of genes regulating branching morphogenesis.[125] These genes are discussed in detail later. It is interesting to note that smoking and alcohol intake are associated with reduced levels of circulating vitamin A, and both, in pregnancy, are associated with infant low birth weight. There has been a single abstract suggesting an impact of maternal alcohol ingestion on kidney development, but it is not known whether the effects are mediated by associated vitamin A deficiency or other mechanisms.[58] Subtle differences in vitamin A level during pregnancy, therefore, may be a significant factor contributing to the wide distribution of nephron number in the general population.[58]

Increased Apoptosis in the Kidney

Total calorie restriction and maternal dietary protein restriction in animals result in low birth weight of offspring and frequently associated hypertension and reduced nephron numbers.[13,75,126–130] Vehaskari and colleagues[75] reported a 29% reduction in nephron number in low-birth-weight rat offspring of mothers subjected to a 6% low-protein diet compared with a 20% normal-protein diet during pregnancy. Associated with this reduction, systolic blood pressures were 20 to 25 mm Hg higher at 8 weeks in pups from the low-protein-diet group than in the normal-protein-diet group (see Fig. 19–3). These authors also found that, despite the kidneys' looking histologically normal at 8 weeks' postnatally, there was evidence of increased apoptosis without an increase in proliferation in the low-protein-diet group. Welham and co-workers[126] examined embryonic metanephroi to evaluate at which stage of development a low-protein diet affects nephrogenesis. At embryonic day 13, the metanephros has just formed, the ureteric bud has branched once, branch tips are surrounded by condensed mesenchyme that later transforms into tubule epithelium, and the ureteric stalk is surrounded by loose stromal mesenchyme.[123] By day 15, multiple branching cycles have occurred and primitive nephrons begin to be formed.[123] The authors, therefore, examined metanephroi at these two time points. At embryonic day 13, there was no difference in the number of cells in metanephroi from embryos whose mothers had received a normal-protein diet compared with those eating a reduced-protein diet. At day 15, however, there were significantly fewer cells per metanephros in the low-protein group compared with the normal-protein group. Furthermore, when they examined apoptosis at these two time points, they observed a significant increase in the numbers of apoptotic cells in the low-protein group at day 13 but not at day 15. The authors concluded that the increase in early (day 13) apoptosis was most likely responsible for the reduced cell numbers later (day 15). As mentioned previously, Vehaskari and colleagues[75] noted an increase in apoptosis at 8 weeks postnatally in offspring of low-protein-diet–fed rats; therefore, there may be successive waves of apoptosis at different stages of nephrogenesis that may affect final nephron endowment.

Welham and co-workers[126] described an increase in apoptosis in both the condensing and the loose mesenchyme of the metanephros but did not measure the relative amount of cell death in each compartment. They therefore suggest two possible mechanisms whereby an increase in apoptosis observed in the offspring of low-protein-diet–fed dams at embryonic day 13 could lead to a reduction in nephron number: (1) directly through loss of actual nephron precursors (i.e., in the condensing mesenchyme) or (2) indirectly through loss of cells in the loose mesenchyme (i.e., the stromal compartment, which supports nephrogenesis but does not contribute actual cells to the final epithelial lineage).[126] These hypotheses are as yet unproved, but evidence for impact of changes in the supporting metanephric

stroma on nephron development and number is emerging. Mice deficient in the BF-2 transcription factor, expressed in metanephric stroma, have abnormal kidney development and reduced nephron numbers, associated with slower differentiation of condensed mesenchyme into tubule epithelium and decreased ureteric branching.[131] Nephron development therefore depends upon a close relationship between tubule epithelial precursors and surrounding tissue matrix. Both compartments are therefore likely to be susceptible to programming effects.

Other studies have suggested that altered regulation of apoptosis in the developing kidney may be due to down-regulation of anti-apoptotic factors (e.g., Pax-2 or Bcl-2) and/or up-regulation of pro-apoptotic factors in response to environmental or other stimuli (e.g., Bax, p53).[126,132–134] Humans with haploinsufficiency of PAX2 have renal coloboma syndrome, which includes renal hypoplasia and early renal failure as well as optic nerve colobomas.[134,135] PAX2 is an anti-apoptotic transcriptional regulator that is highly expressed in the branching ureteric bud as well as in foci of induced nephrogenic mesenchyme during kidney development.[134] Heterozygous mice with Pax2 mutations were found to be very small at birth and to have significant reductions in nephron number. In addition, there was a significant increase in apoptotic cell death in the developing kidneys. Subsequently, the same group[135] demonstrated that loss of Pax2 anti-apoptotic activity reduced ureteric bud branching and increased ureteric bud apoptosis. Similarly, loss of the anti-apoptotic factor Bcl-2 or gain of function of the pro-apoptotic factor p53 are also associated with a significant reduction in nephron number, associated with increased apoptosis in metanephric blastemas, in Bcl-2 knockout mice and p53 transgenic mice.[133,136]

Mutant mouse models, however, although providing evidence that an increase in apoptosis results in reduced nephron numbers, do not address the impact of environmental factors in renal programming. Pham and associates[137] examined gene expression in the kidneys of growth-retarded offspring of rats subjected to uterine artery ligation during gestation. These authors found a 25% reduction in glomerular number, associated with increased evidence of apoptosis and increased pro-apoptotic caspase-3 activity in the kidney at birth. Furthermore, they found evidence of increased mRNA expression of the pro-apoptotic genes Bax and p53 and a decreased expression of the anti-apoptotic gene Bcl-2. These authors also found evidence of hypomethylation of the p53 gene, which in addition to a decrease in Bcl-2 expression, would lead to an increase in p53 activity. Alteration in gene methylation has also been proposed as a mechanism of protein-diet–induced programming effects, as mentioned previously. The increase in apoptotic activity in the developing kidney subjected to varied gestational insults therefore appears to be a consistent finding and mediated via modulation of gene expression in a number of different pathways.

Glial-Cell Line–derived Neurotrophic Factor and c-ret Receptor Function

Glial-cell line–derived neurotrophic factor (GDNF), signaling through its receptor-tyrosine kinase Ret, is known to be a key ligand-receptor interaction driving initiation of ureteric bud branching. C-ret is expressed on the tips of the ureteric bud branches, and knockout of this receptor in mice leads to severe renal dysplasia and reduction in nephron number.[119] Homozygous GDNF null mutant mice have complete renal agenesis and die shortly after birth.[138] Heterozygous GDNF mice exhibit reduced branching morphogenesis and have approximately 30% fewer nephrons than wild-type mice.[138,139] These mice also develop spontaneous

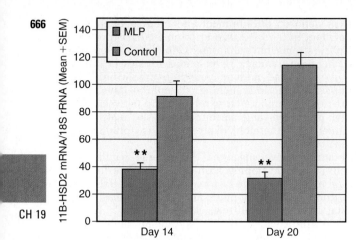

MLP—maternal low protein-fed rats; Control—maternal control fed rats

FIGURE 19–11 Decreased expression of placental 11bHSD2 in placentas of mothers fed low-protein diets during gestation. (From Bertram C, Trowern AR, Copin N, et al: The maternal diet during pregnancy programs altered expression of the glucocorticoid receptor and type 2 11beta-hydroxysteroid dehydrogenase: Potential molecular mechanisms underlying the programming of hypertension in utero. Endocrinology 142:2841–2853, 2001.)

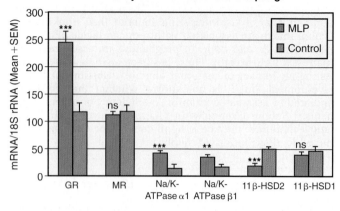

MLP—maternal low protein-fed rats; Control—maternal control fed rats. GR—glucocorticoid receptor; MR—mineralocorticoid receptor
**P <0.01; ***P <0.001

FIGURE 19–12 Programming of glucocorticoid sensitivity. (From Bertram C, Trowern AR, Copin N, et al: The maternal diet during pregnancy programs altered expression of the glucocorticoid receptor and type 2 11beta-hydroxysteroid dehydrogenase: Potential molecular mechanisms underlying the programming of hypertension in utero. Endocrinology 142:2841–2853, 2001.)

hypertension and glomerulomegaly with time. As described previously, maternal dietary vitamin A has a significant impact on nephrogenesis (see Fig. 19–10). In cultured metanephroi, the expression of c-ret was found to be regulated by retinoic acid supplementation in a dose-dependent manner.[78] GDNF expression was not affected by vitamin A fluctuations. Modulation of c-ret expression is therefore likely to be a significant pathway through which vitamin A availability regulates nephrogenesis.

Fetal Exposure to Glucocorticoids

Under normal circumstances, the fetus is protected from exposure to excess maternal corticosteroids by the placental enzyme 11β-hydroxysteroid dehydrogenase type 2 (11β-HSD2), which metabolizes corticosterone to the inert 11-dehydrocorticosterone.[13] Prenatal administration of dexamethasone, a steroid not metabolized by 11β-HSD2, was found to lead to fetal growth restriction, a 20% to 60% reduction in nephron number, glomerulomegaly, and subsequent hypertension in rats and sheep.[72,77,97,140] Similar effects have been seen with lower levels of placental 11β-HSD2 in rats and humans with mutations in the 11β-HSD2 gene, in whom birth weights are low and hypertension develops prematurely.[141,142] Interestingly, maternal low-protein diet during gestation has been shown to result in decreased placental expression of 11β-HSD2, therefore likely increasing the exposure of the fetus to maternal corticosteroids (Fig. 19–11).[24,143] Treatment of pregnant rats fed a low-protein diet with an inhibitor of steroid synthesis abrogates the programming of hypertension in the offspring, suggesting a prominent role for fetal steroid exposure in the low-protein-diet model.[13,24] Excessive fetal steroid exposure may then drive inappropriate gene expression and affect growth and nephrogenesis, potentially through more rapid maturation of tissue structures.[24]

In an attempt to examine the molecular mechanisms through which glucocorticoid exposure may program hypertension, Bertram and associates[143] examined expression of steroid-responsive receptors in offspring of rats fed a low-protein diet during gestation. These authors found a greater than twofold increase in fetal and neonatal glucocorticoid receptor mRNA expression in offspring of mothers fed a low-

protein diet compared with those fed a normal-protein diet. This difference increased to threefold as the offspring aged. In addition, the expression of the corticosteroid responsive renal Na/K-ATPase α1- and β1-subunits were also increased in these offspring (Fig. 19–12). Expression of the mineralocorticoid receptors was not different among the two groups. Interestingly, levels of 11β-HSD2 in offspring kidney and adrenal were significantly reduced during fetal and postnatal life in those exposed to a low-protein diet in utero. These authors conclude that the observed changes would result in marked increases in glucocorticoid action in these tissues and is likely a significant mediator of programmed hypertension.[143] The mechanism of glucocorticoid-mediated reduction in nephron number has not yet been elucidated.

Fetal Exposure to Hyperglycemia and the Role of Insulin-like Growth Factors and Their Receptors

As discussed previously, in the South Carolina dialysis population and the Pima Indian population in Arizona, high birth weight is associated with an increased susceptibility to proteinuria and renal disease (see Fig. 19–9).[5,38,109] High birth weight is a complication of gestational hyperglycemia and diabetes and may therefore also be a surrogate marker of abnormal intrauterine programming. To address the question of whether gestational diabetes affects nephrogenesis in the offspring, Amri and co-workers[144] studied offspring of rats rendered hyperglycemic during pregnancy either by inducing diabetes mellitus with streptozotocin or by infusing glucose from gestational days 12 to 16. Nephron numbers in offspring exposed to maternal hyperglycemia were reduced by 10% to 35%, and the degree of nephron number reduction correlated with the degree of maternal hyperglycemia (Fig. 19–13). Furthermore, in vitro culture of metanephroi subjected to varying glucose concentrations demonstrated that tight glucose control is necessary for optimal metanephric growth and differentiation.

Offspring of diabetic pregnancies have a higher incidence of congenital malformations, resulting for defects in early organogenesis.[145] Furthermore, it is known that expression

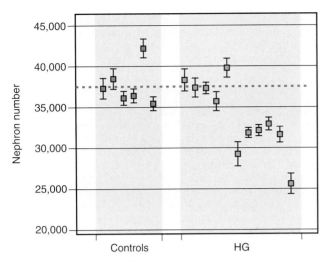

HG-hyperglycemia. Dotted line represents mean value in control group

FIGURE 19–13 Effects of maternal hyperglycemia on nephron number in rat offspring. (From Amri K, Freund N, Vilar J, et al: Adverse effects of hyperglycemia on kidney development in rats: In vivo and in vitro studies. Diabetes 48:2240–2245, 1999.)

and bioavailability of the insulin-like growth factors (IGFs) are altered in diabetic pregnancies, and that IGFs and their binding proteins are important regulators of fetal development.[145] The impact of maternal diabetes on metanephros expression of IGFs and their receptors was studied in rats in which diabetes was induced by streptozotocin compared with gestational-age–matched normal controls.[145] In metanephroi from offspring subjected to maternal diabetes, there was no significant change in IGF-1 or -II or insulin receptor expression at any stage. Throughout nephrogenesis, however, there was a significantly increased expression of the IGF-II/mannose-6-phosphate receptor. The authors postulate that as this receptor tightly regulates the action of IGF-II, a reduction in its expression may lead to enhanced activity of IGF-II, a critical player in renal development. The same group of investigators have examined the impact of IGF binding protein-1 on nephrogenesis in genetically modified mice.[146] Overexpression of human IGF binding protein-1 in adult mice results in glomerulosclerosis. Offspring of females overexpressing human IGF binding protein-1 were found to be growth restricted and to have an 18% to 25% reduction in nephron number depending on whether human IGF binding protein-1 was overexpressed in the mother only, fetus only, or both. When metanephroi from these mice were cultured in the presence of IGF-I or IGF-II, the authors found that IGF-II increased nephron numbers by 25% to 40% in a concentration dependent manner, whereas IGF-1 had no effect.[146] This study did not involve maternal diabetes or hyperglycemia, but the findings are consistent for a role of increased IGF-II activity in nephrogenesis.

Fetal Drug Exposure

Several medications commonly used during pregnancy have been studied for their effects on nephrogenesis. The aminoglycoside antibiotic *gentamicin,* administered to pregnant rats, results in a permanent nephron deficit in the offspring.[147] In subsequent experiments, the same authors demonstrated a significant reduction in nephron number in metanephric explants cultured in the presence of gentamicin.[148] In cultured metanephroi, within 8 hours of administration, gentamicin was localized to the growing tips of ureteric buds and the surrounding blastema, and within 24 hours, the presence

of gentamicin was associated with a significant reduction in the number of branching points.[149] These data suggest that the reduction in nephron number observed after administration of gentamicin during pregnancy is a result of a decrease in branching morphogenesis.

Another group of antibiotics that has been shown to result in impaired nephrogenesis is the *β-lactams.*[150] Administration of ampicillin to pregnant rats leads to an 11% average reduction in nephron number in the offspring, as well as evidence of focal cystic tubule dilatation and interstitial inflammation. The administration of ceftriaxone in vivo did not result in a nephron deficit, but histologically, there was evidence of renal interstitial inflammation. The penicillins were also found to inhibit nephrogenesis in cultured metanephroi in vitro in a dose-dependent fashion, an effect that was less evident with ceftriaxone. Importantly, nephrogenesis was affected even at therapeutic doses of penicillins in the rats, which warrants further research on such frequently used antibiotics in human pregnancy. The mechanism whereby these antibiotics reduce nephron number is likely through an increase in apoptosis observed in the induced mesenchyme in exposed developing kidneys.[78]

The immunosuppressive medication *cyclosporine* is a known nephrotoxin in humans; it crosses the placenta.[151] Women treated with this medication may have successful pregnancies, but its effect on the fetal kidney is not well described, although infants tend to have birth weights in the low range.[151] The effects of administration of this medication in varying doses and at different stages of gestation were evaluated in pregnant rabbits compared with rabbits receiving either vehicle or no drug.[152] Cyclosporine administration in the later period, but not the earlier period, of gestation resulted in smaller litters and growth-restricted pups. All pups exposed to cyclosporine in utero had a 25% to 33% reduction in nephron number compared with controls. The reduction in nephron number was accompanied by glomerulomegaly and was independent of birth weight. At 1 month of age, these kidneys also demonstrated foci of glomerulosclerosis. Subsequent functional evaluation of the kidneys of rabbits exposed to cyclosporine in utero demonstrated a reduction in GFR at 18 and 35 weeks of age and an increase in proteinuria at 11, 18, and 35 weeks of age.[153] Rabbits exposed to cyclosporine in utero developed spontaneous hypertension by 11 weeks of age, which worsened progressively with time.[153] It is important to recognize that, despite reduction in nephron number from birth, renal function did not deteriorate until later, an important factor to bear in mind when evaluating children exposed to cyclosporine in utero. Nephron formation was found to be arrested, potentially due to inhibition of conversion of metanephric mesenchyme to epithelium in the presence of cyclosporine.[78]

PROGRAMMED CHANGES WITHIN THE KIDNEY

The kidney is one of the major organs influencing blood pressure, and programming of hypertension does appear to be at least in part mediated by nephron endowment. That congenitally acquired nephron number is not the sole programmable factor responsible for subsequent hypertension has been shown in offspring of low-protein-diet–fed rats in whom diets were supplemented with glycine, alanine, or urea.[24] As mentioned previously, nephron number was restored in all offspring, but hypertension was prevented only in the glycine supplementation group. In humans, in the two studies that have examined nephron number in relation to presence or absence of essential hypertension, a relationship was found among whites but was weaker for African Americans.[46,79] These studies suggest that programming of hypertension may occur in the absence of an alteration in nephron number. The pressure-natriuresis curve is shifted to the right in most forms of hypertension, and prenatally programmed hypertension has been demonstrated by some investigators to be salt sensitive.[25,94,96,154] A reduction in filtration surface area associated with a reduction in nephron number is one plausible hypothesis to explain this observation, but other programmed effects have also been described that are likely to influence blood pressure and sodium homeostasis.

Renal Vascular Reactivity

An increase in baseline renal vascular resistance has been described by several authors using different models of fetal programming.[153,155,156] In addition, renal arterial responses to β-adrenergic stimulation and sensitivity to adenylyl cyclase were found to be increased in 21-day-old growth-restricted offspring of mothers subjected to uterine artery ligation during gestation.[157] The renal expression of β₂-adrenoreceptor mRNA was increased in the pups of rats subjected to reduced uteroplacental blood flow, but there was also evidence of adaptations to the signal transduction pathway contributing to the β-adrenergic hyper-responsiveness observed. Intriguingly, these findings were much more marked in the right compared with the left kidney, an observation that remains unexplained but that is not without precedent: asymmetry of renal blood flow was found in 51% of a cohort of hypertensives without renovascular disease.[157,158] Functionally, in this study, the growth-restricted rats had reduced glomerular numbers, exhibited hyperfiltration and hyperperfusion, and had significantly increased proteinuria compared with the controls.

Renin-Angiotensin System

All of the components of the renin-angiotensin system are expressed in the developing kidney.[159] The importance of angiotensin II in nephrogenesis was demonstrated by the administration of the angiotensin II subtype 1 receptor (AT1R) blocker losartan to normal rats during the first 12 days of life (while nephrogeneisis is proceeding), which resulted in a reduction in final nephron number and subsequent development of hypertension.[160] Interestingly, administration of an angiotensin-converting enzyme inhibitor (ACEI), captopril, or losartan to low-birth-weight rats from 2 to 4 weeks of age, abrogated the development of adult hypertension in these animals.[13,161] These data suggest upregulation of the AT1R postnatally, which could be a result of increased glucocorticoid exposure.[13] In support of this hypothesis, administration of angiotensin II or ACEI to adult rats subjected to a low-protein diet in utero resulted in a more exaggerated hypertensive or hypotensive response than in control rats.[13,162-164]

In neonates and young offspring of rats subjected to gestational protein restriction, renal renin, AT1R, and angiotensin II mRNA and protein levels have all been found to be reduced compared with control rats, but the AT1R expression increases above control levels as the rats reach the prehypertensive stage.[25,76,160,163-165] The renal expression of the angiotensin II subtype 2 receptor (AT2R) has been found to be downregulated in young rats and up-regulated in neonatal sheep, an effect that may reflect different stages of renal maturation at birth among these species.[89,162] Angiotensin II can stimulate the expression of Pax-2 (an anti-apoptotic factor) through AT2R.[166] AT2R expression, therefore, is likely to affect nephrogenesis and kidney development, but its role in programming is still unclear. Overall, programmed suppression of the intrarenal renin-angiotensin system during nephrogenesis is likely to contribute to the reduction in nephron number under adverse circumstances, and postnatal up-regulation of the AT1R, possibly mediated by an increase in glucocorticoid activity or sensitivity, may contribute to the subsequent development of hypertension.

Altered Sodium Handling by the Kidney

Another contributor to a shift of the pressure-natriuresis curve to the right is an alteration of sodium transporter expression or activity in the kidney. Administration of dexamethasone to pregnant rats was associated with growth retardation in the offspring, lower nephron number, reduction in GFR, higher blood pressure, lower urinary sodium excretion rate, reduced fractional excretion of sodium, and higher tissue sodium content in liver and skeletal muscle.[72] Similar findings were seen in growth-retarded piglets in which low nephron number was associated with a reduced GFR but a normal fractional excretion of sodium.[167] A lower fractional excretion of sodium in the presence of reduced GFR is strong evidence of sodium retention by the kidney. Consistent with these whole-kidney observations, Vehaskari and colleagues[168] found significant increases in expression of sodium co-transporters Na-K-2Cl (bumetanide-sensitive co-transporter, BSC1, 302%) and Na-Cl (thiazide-sensitive co-transporter, TSC, 157%) in the offspring of rats fed a protein-restricted diet during gestation compared with normals (Fig. 19–14). Other authors reported an increase in glucocorticoid receptor expression and expression of the glucocorticoid responsive α₁- and β₁-subunits of Na-K-ATPase in offspring of pregnant rats fed a low-protein diet (see Fig. 19–12).[143] Taken together, these data suggest that an increased sodium avidity of the fetally programmed kidney, possibly in the setting of an increase in background glucocorticoid activity, is a likely contributor to the development of adult hypertension. This hypothesis requires further validation.

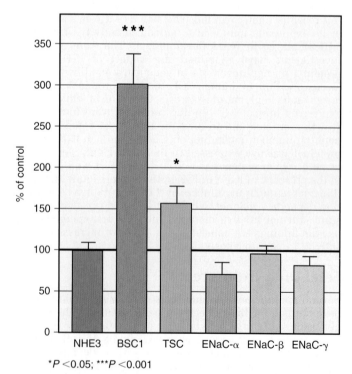

*P <0.05; ***P <0.001

FIGURE 19–14 Apical Na transporter expression in 4-week-old offspring from maternal low-protein diet. (From Vehaskari VM, Woods LL: Prenatal programming of hypertension: Lessons from experimental models. J Am Soc Nephrol 16:2545–2556, 2005.)

IMPACT OF NEPHRON ENDOWMENT ON TRANSPLANTATION OUTCOMES

Prescription of donor kidneys is largely decided based on immunologic matching. In animal experiments of renal transplantation, however, the impact of transplanted nephron mass, independent of immunologic factors, on the subsequent development of chronic allograft nephropathy has been demonstrated.[169–173] Despite such evidence, prescription of kidneys on the basis of the physiologic capacity of the donor organ to meet the metabolic needs of the recipient has not generally been considered.[174] More and more data are accumulating, however, suggesting a significant impact of transplanted renal mass on long-term post-transplantation outcomes.

Demographic and anthropomorphic factors associated with late renal allograft loss include donor age, sex, and race, as well as recipient body surface area (BSA).[175–177] In general, kidneys from older, female, and African American donors fare worse and tend to have lower nephron numbers than younger, white, and male donors.[42,62,178,179] Indirectly, these observations suggest that the intrinsic nephron endowment of the transplanted kidney is likely to play a role in the development of chronic allograft nephropathy. To investigate this question, several investigators have compared recipient and donor BSA as surrogates for metabolic demand and kidney size; others have used kidney weights or renal volumetric measurements by ultrasound as surrogates for nephron mass.

Mismatches between donor kidney size and recipient BSA have an impact on long-term allograft outcomes. A retrospective analysis of 32,083 patients who received a first cadaver kidney found that large recipients of kidneys from small donors had a 43% increased risk of late allograft failure compared with medium-sized recipients receiving kidneys from medium-sized donors.[180] The best outcomes tended to be in small recipients receiving kidneys from large donors. Other smaller, and often single-center studies have not consistently found similar results.[180] One such study analyzed 378 paired recipients of cadaver kidneys from 189 donors, in which one recipient had a high and the other a low BSA.[181] These authors did not find a significant association between allograft loss and the ratio between donor and recipient BSA.[181] Importantly, however, the BSA ranges in the "larger" and "smaller" groups overlapped in this study, limiting the power to detect a true effect. Another interesting study evaluated outcomes in patients receiving cadaveric kidneys from donors either below or above 60 years of age.[182] Kidneys from older donors have fewer viable nephrons and may be less able to recover from transplant-related injury.[42,183] The recipients were also subdivided into two groups according to mean body mass index (BMI) and mean BSA.[182] The authors found that, in patients receiving kidneys from donors over age 60, there was a positive correlation between BMI and BSA and nadir creatinine. At 5 years, graft survival was significantly better in those with smaller BMI and BSA. This study demonstrates that an older kidney with fewer nephrons transplanted into a smaller recipient functions better than an older kidney given to a larger recipient.

Kidney size, however, may not always be directly proportional to BSA; therefore, ratios of donor to recipient BSA may not be an ideal method of estimating nephron mass to recipient mismatch. Kidney weight, however, is an acceptable surrogate for nephron mass.[42,184] Using this parameter, Kim and associates[185] analyzed the ratio of donor kidney weight to recipient body weight (DKW/RBW) in 259 live-donor transplants. These authors found that a higher DKW/RBW of greater than 4.5 g/kg was significantly associated with improved allograft function at 3 years compared with a ratio

of less than 3.0 g/kg. A similar study including 964 recipients of cadaveric kidneys, in whom proteinuria and Cockroft-Gault creatinine clearances were also calculated, found that 10% of the subjects were "strongly" mismatched, having a DKW/RBW ratio of less than 2 g/kg.[179] The DKW/RBW ratio was lowest when male recipients received kidneys from female donors. The risk of having proteinuria higher than 0.5 g/kg was significantly greater, and developed earlier, in those with DKW/RBW below 2 g/kg as compared with those with higher ratios. In fact, proteinuria was present in 50% of those with DKW/RBW less than 2 g/kg, 33% of those with DKW/RBW of 2 to 4 g/kg, and 23% in those with DKW/RBW of 4 g/kg or lower. Furthermore, calculated creatinine clearance, although fraught with imprecision, increased progressively in the subgroup with DKW/RBW less than 2 g/kg, suggesting glomerular hyperfiltration in response to the increased metabolic demand placed on the small kidney by the larger recipient. GFRs remained stable post-transplantation in those with DKW/RBW of 4 g/kg or lower. At 5 years follow-up, however, there was no difference in graft survival among the three DKW/RBW groups, but the authors concede that it is likely that longer follow-up is needed to determine the true impact of donor to recipient mismatch.[179] Other investigators have used renal ultrasonography to measure cadaveric transplant kidney (Tx) cross-sectional area in relation to recipient body weight (W) to calculate a "nephron dose index," Tx/W.[186] These authors found that, during the first 5 years after transplantation, serum creatinine was significantly lower in patients with a high Tx/W compared with those with lower values, with a trend toward better graft survival. Therefore, the ratio between renal mass and the recipient's metabolic needs does appear to be a determinant of long-term allograft function. A small kidney transplanted into a large recipient may not have an adequate capacity to meet the metabolic needs of the recipient without imposing glomerular hyperfiltration, which ultimately leads to further nephron loss and eventual allograft failure.[23,183]

Transplanted nephron mass not only may be a function of congenital endowment and attrition of nephrons with age but also is affected by peritransplant renal injury (i.e., donor hypotension, prolonged cold and warm ischemia, nephrotoxic immunosuppressive drugs). All of these factors need to be closely considered, in addition to immunologic matching, in selection of appropriate recipients in whom the allograft is likely to function for the longest time and therefore provide best possible improvement in quality of life.

CONCLUSION

The association between an adverse fetal environment and subsequent hypertension and kidney disease in later life is now quite compelling and appears to be mediated, at least in part, by impaired nephrogenesis. Concomitant glomerular hypertrophy and altered expression of sodium transporters in the programmed kidney also contribute to the vicious circle of glomerular hypertension, glomerular injury, and sclerosis, leading to worsening hypertension and ongoing renal injury (Fig. 19–15). The number of nephrons in humans varies widely, suggesting that a significant proportion of the general population, especially in areas where high or low birth weights are prevalent, may be at increased risk of developing later-life hypertension and renal dysfunction. Measurement of nephron number in vivo remains an obstacle, with the best surrogate markers thus far being a low birth weight, a high birth weight, and in the absence of other known renal diseases, a reduced kidney volume on ultrasound, especially in children, and glomerular enlargement on kidney biopsy. A kidney with a reduced complement of nephrons would have less renal reserve to adapt to dietary excesses or to compensate for renal

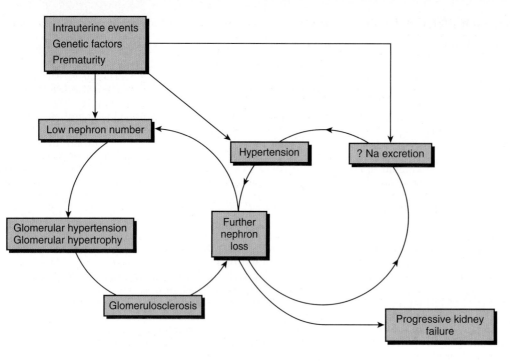

FIGURE 19-15 Proposed mechanism of fetal programming of hypertension and renal disease. (Adapted from Zandi-Nejad K, Luyckx VA, Brenner BM: Adult hypertension and kidney disease: The role of fetal programming. Hypertension 47:502–508, 2006.)

injury. The molecular mechanisms through which fetal programming exerts its effects on nephrogenesis are varied and likely complementary and intertwined. The fact that even seemingly minor influences, such as composition of maternal diet during fetal life, can have major consequences on renal development in the offspring underscores the critical importance of optimization of perinatal care.

References

1. Kemper MJ, Muller-Wiefel DE: Renal function in congenital anomalies of the kidney and urinary tract. Curr Opin Urol 11:571–575, 2001.
2. Rodriguez MM: Developmental renal pathology: Its past, present, and future. Fetal Pediatr Pathol 23:211–229, 2004.
3. Lackland DT: Mechanisms and fetal origins of kidney disease. J Am Soc Nephrol 16:2531–2532, 2005.
4. Hoy WE, Rees M, Kile E, et al: Low birthweight and renal disease in Australian aborigines. Lancet 352:1826–1827, 1998.
5. Nelson RG, Morgenstern H, Bennett PH: Birth weight and renal disease in Pima Indians with type 2 diabetes mellitus. Am J Epidemiol 148:650–656, 1998.
6. Hall YN, Hsu CY, Iribarren C, et al: The conundrum of increased burden of end-stage renal disease in Asians. Kidney Int 68:2310–2316, 2005.
7. Kaplan NM, Opie LH: Controversies in hypertension. Lancet 367:168–176, 2006.
8. Lifton RP, Gharavi AG, Geller DS: Molecular mechanisms of human hypertension. Cell 104:545–556, 2001.
9. Hubner N, Yagil C, Yagil Y: Novel integrative approaches to the identification of candidate genes in hypertension. Hypertension 47:1–5, 2006.
10. Bianchi G: Genetic variations of tubular sodium reabsorption leading to "primary" hypertension: from gene polymorphism to clinical symptoms. Am J Physiol Regul Integr Comp Physiol 289:R1536–R1549, 2005.
11. Hales CN, Barker DJ: Type 2 (non-insulin-dependent) diabetes mellitus: The thrifty phenotype hypothesis. Diabetologia 35:595–601, 1992.
12. Hales CN, Barker DJ, Clark PM, et al: Fetal and infant growth and impaired glucose tolerance at age 64. BMJ 303:1019–1022, 1991.
13. McMillen IC, Robinson JS: Developmental origins of the metabolic syndrome: Prediction, plasticity, and programming. Physiol Rev 85:571–633, 2005.
14. Barker DJ: Developmental origins of adult health and disease. J Epidemiol Community Health 58:114–115, 2004.
15. Drake AJ, Walker BR: The intergenerational effects of fetal programming: Non-genomic mechanisms for the inheritance of low birth weight and cardiovascular risk. J Endocrinol 180:1–16, 2004.
16. Kermack WO, McKendrick AG, McKinlay PL: Death-rates in Great Britain and Sweden. Some general regularities and their significance. Lancet i:698–703, 1934.
17. Forsdahl A: Are poor living conditions in childhood and adolescence an important risk factor for arteriosclerotic heart disease? Br J Prev Soc Med 31:91–95, 1977.
18. Barker DJ, Hales CN, Fall CH, et al: Type 2 (non-insulin-dependent) diabetes mellitus, hypertension and hyperlipidaemia (syndrome X): Relation to reduced fetal growth. Diabetologia 36:62–67, 1993.
19. Bellinger L, Langley-Evans SC: Fetal programming of appetite by exposure to a maternal low protein diet in the rat. Clin Sci (Lond) 109:413–420, 2005.
20. Gardner DS, Tingey K, Van Bon BW, et al: Programming of glucose-insulin metabolism in adult sheep after maternal undernutrition. Am J Physiol Regul Integr Comp Physiol 289:R947–R954, 2005.
21. Wust S, Entringer S, Federenko IS, et al: Birth weight is associated with salivary cortisol responses to psychosocial stress in adult life. Psychoneuroendocrinology 30:591–598, 2005.
22. Zandi-Nejad K, Luyckx VA, Brenner BM: Adult hypertension and kidney disease: The role of fetal programming. Hypertension 47:502–508, 2006.
23. Luyckx VA, Brenner BM: Low birth weight, nephron number, and kidney disease. Kidney Int Suppl S68–S77, 2005.
24. Langley-Evans S, Langley-Evans A, Marchand M: Nutritional programming of blood pressure and renal morphology. Arch Physiol Biochem 111:8–16, 2003.
25. Vehaskari VM, Woods LL: Prenatal programming of hypertension: Lessons from experimental models. J Am Soc Nephrol 16:2545–2556, 2005.
26. Huxley RR, Shiell AW, Law CM: The role of size at birth and postnatal catch-up growth in determining systolic blood pressure: A systematic review of the literature. J Hypertens 18:815–831, 2000.
27. Barker DJ, Osmond C, Golding J, et al:. Growth in utero, blood pressure in childhood and adult life, and mortality from cardiovascular disease. BMJ 298:564–567, 1989.
28. Launer LJ, Hofman A, Grobbee DE: Relation between birth weight and blood pressure: Longitudinal study of infants and children. BMJ 307:1451–1454, 1993.
29. Law CM, de Swiet M, Osmond C, et al: Initiation of hypertension in utero and its amplification throughout life. BMJ 306:24–27, 1993.
30. Guyton AC, Young DB, DeClue JW, et al: Fluid balance, renal function, and blood pressure. Clin Nephrol 4:122–126, 1975.
31. Guyton AC, Coleman TG, Young DB, et al: Salt balance and long-term blood pressure control. Annu Rev Med 31:15–27, 1980.
32. Lifton RP, Wilson FH, Choate KA, Geller DS: Salt and blood pressure: New insight from human genetic studies. Cold Spring Harb Symp Quant Biol 67:445–450, 2002.
33. Xu J, Li G, Wang P, et al: Renalase is a novel, soluble monoamine oxidase that regulates cardiac function and blood pressure. J Clin Invest 115:1275–1280, 2005.
34. Guidi E, Bianchi G, Rivolta E, et al: Hypertension in man with a kidney transplant: Role of familial versus other factors. Nephron 41:14–21, 1985.
35. Brenner BM, Garcia DL, Anderson S: Glomeruli and blood pressure. Less of one, more the other? Am J Hypertens 1:335–347, 1988.
36. Brenner BM, Chertow GM: Congenital oligonephropathy and the etiology of adult hypertension and progressive renal injury. Am J Kidney Dis 23:171–175, 1994.
37. Hsu CY, Lin F, Vittinghoff E, Shlipak MG: Racial differences in the progression from chronic renal insufficiency to end-stage renal disease in the United States. J Am Soc Nephrol 14:2902–2907, 2003.
38. Lackland DT, Bendall HE, Osmond C, et al: Low birth weights contribute to high rates of early-onset chronic renal failure in the Southeastern United States. Arch Intern Med 160:1472–1476, 2000.
39. Lackland DT, Egan BM, Ferguson PL: Low birth weight as a risk factor for hypertension. J Clin Hypertens (Greenwich) 5:133–136, 2003.
40. Lackland DT, Egan BM, Syddall HE, Barker DJ: Associations between birth weight and antihypertensive medication in black and white Medicaid recipients. Hypertension 39:179–183, 2002.
41. Bertram JF: Counting in the kidney. Kidney Int 59:792–796, 2001.
42. Nyengaard JR, Bendtsen TF: Glomerular number and size in relation to age, kidney weight, and body surface in normal man. Anat Rec 232:194–201, 1992.
43. Kett MM, Bertram JF: Nephron endowment and blood pressure: What do we really know? Curr Hypertens Rep 6:133–139, 2004.

44. Basgen JM, Steffes MW, Stillman AE, Mauer SM: Estimating glomerular number in situ using magnetic resonance imaging and biopsy. Kidney Int 45:1668–1672, 1994.
45. Hoy WE, Douglas-Denton RN, Hughson MD, et al: A stereological study of glomerular number and volume: Preliminary findings in a multiracial study of kidneys at autopsy. Kidney Int Suppl S31–S37, 2003.
46. Keller G, Zimmer G, Mall G, et al: Nephron number in patients with primary hypertension. N Engl J Med 348:101–108, 2003.
47. Rugiu C, Oldrizzi L, Lupo A, et al. Clinical features of patients with solitary kidneys. Nephron 43:10–15, 1986.
48. Morita T, Wenzl J, McCoy J, et al: Bilateral renal hypoplasia with oligomeganephronia: Quantitative and electron microsopic study. Am J Clin Pathol 59:104–112, 1973.
49. Kiprov DD, Colvin RB, McCluskey RT: Focal and segmental glomerulosclerosis and proteinuria associated with unilateral renal agenesis. Lab Invest 46:275–281, 1982.
50. Elfenbein IB, Baluarte HJ, Gruskin AB: Renal hypoplasia with oligomeganephronia: Light, electron, fluorescent microscopic and quantitative studies. Arch Pathol 97:143–149, 1974.
51. Bhathena DB, Julian BA, McMorrow RG, Baehler RW: Focal sclerosis of hypertrophied glomeruli in solitary functioning kidneys of humans. Am J Kidney Dis 5:226–232, 1985.
52. Kasiske BL, Ma JZ, Louis TA, Swan SK: Long-term effects of reduced renal mass in humans. Kidney Int 48:814–819, 1995.
53. Flanigan WJ, Burns RO, Takacs FJ, Merril JP: Serial studies of glomerular filtration rate and renal plasma flow in kidney transplant donors, identical twins, and allograft recipients. Am J Surg 116:788–794, 1968.
54. Woods LL: Neonatal uninephrectomy causes hypertension in adult rats. Am J Physiol 276:R974–R978, 1999.
55. Woods LL, Weeks DA, Rasch R: Hypertension after neonatal uninephrectomy in rats precedes glomerular damage. Hypertension 38:337–342, 2001.
56. Moritz KM, Wintour EM, Dodic M: Fetal uninephrectomy leads to postnatal hypertension and compromised renal function. Hypertension 39:1071–1076, 2002.
57. Nyengaard JR: Number and dimensions of rat glomerular capillaries in normal development and after nephrectomy. Kidney Int 43:1049–1057, 1993.
58. Hoy WE, Hughson MD, Bertram JF, et al: Nephron number, hypertension, renal disease, and renal failure. J Am Soc Nephrol 16:2557–2564, 2005.
59. Manalich R, Reyes L, Herrera M, et al: Relationship between weight at birth and the number and size of renal glomeruli in humans: A histomorphometric study. Kidney Int 58:770–773, 2000.
60. Abdi R, Dong VM, Rubel JR, et al: Correlation between glomerular size and long-term renal function in patients with substantial loss of renal mass. J Urol 170:42–44, 2003.
61. Abdi R, Slakey D, Kittur D, et al: Baseline glomerular size as a predictor of function in human renal transplantation. Transplantation 66:329–333, 1998.
62. Abdi R, Slakey D, Kittur D, et al: Heterogeneity of glomerular size in normal donor kidneys: Impact of race. Am J Kidney Dis 32:43–46, 1998.
63. Lemley KV: A basis for accelerated progression of diabetic nephropathy in Pima Indians. Kidney Int Suppl S38–S42, 2003.
64. Hoy WE, Wang Z, VanBuynder P, et al: The natural history of renal disease in Australian Aborigines. Part 1. Changes in albuminuria and glomerular filtration rate over time. Kidney Int 60:243–248, 2001.
65. Hoy WE, Wang Z, VanBuynder P, et al: The natural history of renal disease in Australian Aborigines. Part 2. Albuminuria predicts natural death and renal failure. Kidney Int 60:249–256, 2001.
66. Schmidt K, Pesce C, Liu Q, et al: Large glomerular size in Pima Indians: Lack of change with diabetic nephropathy. J Am Soc Nephrol 3:229–235, 1992.
67. Young RJ, Hoy WE, Kincaid-Smith P, et al: Glomerular size and glomerulosclerosis in Australian Aborigines. Am J Kidney Dis 36:481–489, 2000.
68. Lu MC, Halfon N: Racial and ethnic disparities in birth outcomes: A life-course perspective. Matern Child Health J 7:13–30, 2003.
69. Yiu V, Buka S, Zurakowski D, et al: Relationship between birthweight and blood pressure in childhood. Am J Kidney Dis 33:253–260, 1999.
70. Fang J, Madhavan S, Alderman MH: The influence of maternal hypertension on low birth weight: Differences among ethnic populations. Ethn Dis 9:369–376, 1999.
71. Fuller KE: Low birth-weight infants: The continuing ethnic disparity and the interaction of biology and environment. Ethn Dis 10:432–445, 2000.
72. Celsi G, Kistner A, Aizman R, et al: Prenatal dexamethasone causes oligonephronia, sodium retention, and higher blood pressure in the offspring. Pediatr Res 44:317–322, 1998.
73. Gilbert T, Lelievre-Pegorier M, Merlet-Benichou C: Long-term effects of mild oligonephronia induced in utero by gentamicin in the rat. Pediatr Res 30:450–456, 1991.
74. Langley-Evans SC: Intrauterine programming of hypertension in the rat: Nutrient interactions. Comp Biochem Physiol A Physiol 114:327–333, 1996.
75. Vehaskari VM, Aviles DH, Manning J: Prenatal programming of adult hypertension in the rat. Kidney Int 59:238–245, 2001.
76. Woods LL, Ingelfinger JR, Nyengaard JR, Rasch R: Maternal protein restriction suppresses the newborn renin-angiotensin system and programs adult hypertension in rats. Pediatr Res 49:460–467, 2001.
77. Ortiz LA, Quan A, Weinberg A, Baum M: Effect of prenatal dexamethasone on rat renal development. Kidney Int 59:1663–1669, 2001.
78. Merlet-Benichou C: Influence of fetal environment on kidney development. Int J Dev Biol 43:453–456, 1999.
79. Hughson MD, Douglas-Denton R, Bertram JF, Hoy WE: Hypertension, glomerular number, and birth weight in African Americans and white subjects in the southeastern United States. Kidney Int 69:671–678, 2006.
80. Hughson M, Farris AB, Douglas-Denton R, et al: Glomerular number and size in autopsy kidneys: The relationship to birth weight. Kidney Int 63:2113–2122, 2003.
81. Rodriguez MM, Gomez AH, Abitbol CL, et al: Histomorphometric analysis of postnatal glomerulogenesis in extremely preterm infants. Pediatr Dev Pathol 7:17–25, 2004.
82. Hinchliffe SA, Lynch MR, Sargent PH, et al: The effect of intrauterine growth retardation on the development of renal nephrons. Br J Obstet Gynaecol 99:296–301, 1992.
83. Hinchliffe SA, Howard CV, Lynch MR, et al: Renal developmental arrest in sudden infant death syndrome. Pediatr Pathol 13:333–343, 1993.
84. Silver LE, Decamps PJ, Korst LM, et al: Intrauterine growth restriction is accompanied by decreased renal volume in the human fetus. Am J Obstet Gynecol 188:1320–1325, 2003.
85. Schmidt IM, Damgaard IN, Boisen KA, et al: Increased kidney growth in formula-fed versus breast-fed healthy infants. Pediatr Nephrol 19:1137–1144, 2004.
86. Spencer J, Wang Z, Hoy W: Low birth weight and reduced renal volume in Aboriginal children. Am J Kidney Dis 37:915–920, 2001.
87. Pesce C, Schmidt K, Fogo A, et al: Glomerular size and the incidence of renal disease in African Americans and Caucasians. J Nephrol 7:355–358, 1994.
88. Nyengaard JR, Bendtsen TF, Mogensen CE: Low birth weight—Is it associated with few and small glomeruli in normal subjects and NIDDM patients? Diabetologia 39:1634–1637, 1996.
89. Gilbert JS, Lang AL, Grant AR, Nijland MJ: Maternal nutrient restriction in sheep: Hypertension and decreased nephron number in offspring at 9 months of age. J Physiol 565:137–147, 2005.
90. Jones SE, Bilous RW, Flyvbjerg A, Marshall SM: Intra-uterine environment influences glomerular number and the acute renal adaptation to experimental diabetes. Diabetologia 44:721–728, 2001.
91. Jones SE, White KE, Flyvbjerg A, Marshall SM: The effect of intrauterine environment and low glomerular number on the histological changes in diabetic glomerulosclerosis. Diabetologia 49:191–199, 2006.
92. Macconi D, Bonomelli M, Benigni A, et al: Pathophysiologic implications of reduced podocyte number in a rat model of progressive glomerular injury. Am J Pathol 168:42–54, 2006.
93. Holemans K, Gerber R, Meurrens K, et al: Maternal food restriction in the second half of pregnancy affects vascular function but not blood pressure of rat female offspring. Br J Nutr 81:73–79, 1999.
94. Sanders MW, Fazzi GE, Janssen GM, et al: High sodium intake increases blood pressure and alters renal function in intrauterine growth-retarded rats. Hypertension 46:71–75, 2005.
95. Zimanyi MA, Bertram JF, Black MJ: Does a nephron deficit in rats predispose to salt-sensitive hypertension? Kidney Blood Press Res 27:239–247, 2004.
96. Woods LL, Weeks DA, Rasch R: Programming of adult blood pressure by maternal protein restriction: Role of nephrogenesis. Kidney Int 65:1339–1348, 2004.
97. Martins JP, Monteiro JC, Paixao AD: Renal function in adult rats subjected to prenatal dexamethasone. Clin Exp Pharmacol Physiol 30:32–37, 2003.
98. Alexander BT: Placental insufficiency leads to development of hypertension in growth-restricted offspring. Hypertension 41:457–462, 2003.
99. Nwagwu MO, Cook A, Langley-Evans SC: Evidence of progressive deterioration of renal function in rats exposed to a maternal low-protein diet in utero. Br J Nutr 83:79–85, 2000.
100. Yudkin JS, Martyn CN, Phillips DI, Gale CR: Associations of micro-albuminuria with intra-uterine growth retardation. Nephron 89:309–314, 2001.
101. Hoy WE, Rees M, Kile E, et al: A new dimension to the Barker hypothesis: Low birthweight and susceptibility to renal disease. Kidney Int 56:1072–1077, 1999.
102. Hoy WE, Mathews JD, McCredie DA, et al: The multidimensional nature of renal disease: Rates and associations of albuminuria in an Australian Aboriginal community. Kidney Int 54:1296–1304, 1998.
103. Rodriguez-Soriano J, Aguirre M, Oliveros R, Vallo A: Long-term renal follow-up of extremely low birth weight infants. Pediatr Nephrol 20:579–584, 2005.
104. Kistner A, Celsi G, Vanpee M, Jacobson SH: Increased blood pressure but normal renal function in adult women born preterm. Pediatr Nephrol 15:215–220, 2000.
105. Keijzer-Veen MG, Schrevel M, Finken MJ, et al: Microalbuminuria and lower glomerular filtration rate at young adult age in subjects born very premature and after intrauterine growth retardation. J Am Soc Nephrol 16:2762–2768, 2005.
106. Painter RC, Roseboom TJ, van Montfrans GA, et al: Microalbuminuria in adults after prenatal exposure to the Dutch famine. J Am Soc Nephrol 16:189–194, 2005.
107. Ibsen H, Olsen MH, Wachtell K, et al: Reduction in albuminuria translates to reduction in cardiovascular events in hypertensive patients: Losartan Intervention for Endpoint Reduction in Hypertension Study. Hypertension 45:198–202, 2005.
108. Gielen M, Pinto-Sietsma SJ, Zeegers MP, et al. Birth weight and creatinine clearance in young adult twins: Influence of genetic, prenatal, and maternal factors. J Am Soc Nephrol 16:2471–2476, 2005.
109. Nelson RG, Morgenstern H, Bennett PH: Intrauterine diabetes exposure and the risk of renal disease in diabetic Pima Indians. Diabetes 47:1489–1493, 1998.
110. Sandeman D, Reza M, Phillips DI, et al: Why do some Type 1 diabetic patients develop nephropathy? A possible role of birth weight. Diabet Med 9:36A, 1992.
111. Rossing P, Tarnow L, Nielsen FS, et al: Short stature and diabetic nephropathy. BMJ 310:296–297, 1995.
112. Rossing P, Tarnow L, Nielsen FS, et al: Low birth weight. A risk factor for development of diabetic nephropathy? Diabetes 44:1405–1407, 1995.
113. Garrett P, Sandeman D, Reza M, et al. Weight at birth and renal disease in adulthood. Nephrol Dial Transplant 8:920, 1993.
114. Zidar N, Avgustin Cavic M, Kenda RB, Ferluga D: Unfavorable course of minimal change nephrotic syndrome in children with intrauterine growth retardation. Kidney Int 54:1320–1323, 1998.
115. Zidar N, Cavic MA, Kenda RB, et al: Effect of intrauterine growth retardation on the clinical course and prognosis of IgA glomerulonephritis in children. Nephron 79:28–32, 1998.
116. Duncan RC, Bass PS, Garrett PJ, Dathan JR: Weight at birth and other factors influencing progression of idiopathic membranous nephropathy. Nephrol Dial Transplant 9:875, 1994.

117. Na YW, Yang HJ, Choi JH, et al: Effect of intrauterine growth retardation on the progression of nephrotic syndrome. Am J Nephrol 22:463–467, 2002.

118. Fan ZJ, Lackland DT, Kenderes B, et al: Impact of birth weight on familial aggregation of end-stage renal disease. Am J Nephrol 23:117–120, 2003.

119. Clark AT, Bertram JF: Molecular regulation of nephron endowment. Am J Physiol 276: F485–F497, 1999.

120. Schreuder MF, Nyengaard JR, Fodor M, et al: Glomerular number and function are influenced by spontaneous and induced low birth weight in rats. J Am Soc Nephrol 16:2913–2919, 2005.

121. Simeoni U, Zetterstrom R: Long-term circulatory and renal consequences of intrauterine growth restriction. Acta Paediatr 94:819–824, 2005.

122. Sakurai H, Nigam SK: In vitro branching tubulogenesis: Implications for developmental and cystic disorders, nephron number, renal repair, and nephron engineering. Kidney Int 54:14–26, 1998.

123. Welham SJ, Riley PR, Wade A, et al: Maternal diet programs embryonic kidney gene expression. Physiol Genomics 22:48–56, 2005.

124. Lisle SJ, Lewis RM, Petry CJ, et al: Effect of maternal iron restriction during pregnancy on renal morphology in the adult rat offspring. Br J Nutr 90:33–39, 2003.

125. Merlet-Benichou C, Vilar J, Lelievre-Pegorier M, Gilbert T: Role of retinoids in renal development: Pathophysiological implication. Curr Opin Nephrol Hypertens 8:39–43, 1999.

126. Welham SJ, Wade A, Woolf AS: Protein restriction in pregnancy is associated with increased apoptosis of mesenchymal cells at the start of rat metanephrogenesis. Kidney Int 61:1231–1242, 2002.

127. Langley-Evans SC, Jackson AA: Rats with hypertension induced by in utero exposure to maternal low-protein diets fail to increase blood pressure in response to a high salt intake. Ann Nutr Metab 40:1–9, 1996.

128. Langley SC, Jackson AA: Increased systolic blood pressure in adult rats induced by fetal exposure to maternal low protein diets. Clin Sci (Lond) 86:217–222; discussion 121, 1994.

129. Lucas SR, Costa Silva VL, Miraglia SM, et al: Functional and morphometric evaluation of offspring kidney after intrauterine undernutrition. Pediatr Nephrol 11:719–723, 1997.

130. Almeida JR, Mandarim-de-Lacerda CA: Maternal gestational protein-calorie restriction decreases the number of glomeruli and causes glomerular hypertrophy in adult hypertensive rats. Am J Obstet Gynecol 192:945–951, 2005.

131. Hatini V, Huh SO, Herzlinger D, et al: Essential role of stromal mesenchyme in kidney morphogenesis revealed by targeted disruption of Winged Helix transcription factor BF-2. Genes Dev 10:1467–1478, 1996.

132. Torban E, Eccles MR, Favor J, Goodyer PR: PAX2 suppresses apoptosis in renal collecting duct cells. Am J Pathol 157:833–842, 2000.

133. Sorenson CM, Rogers SA, Korsmeyer SJ, Hammerman MR: Fulminant metanephric apoptosis and abnormal kidney development in bcl-2-deficient mice. Am J Physiol 268:F73–F81, 1995.

134. Porteous S, Torban E, Cho NP, et al: Primary renal hypoplasia in humans and mice with PAX2 mutations: Evidence of increased apoptosis in fetal kidneys of Pax2(1Neu) +/- mutant mice. Hum Mol Genet 9:1–11, 2000.

135. Dziarmaga A, Clark P, Stayner C, et al: Ureteric bud apoptosis and renal hypoplasia in transgenic PAX2-Bax fetal mice mimics the renal-coloboma syndrome. J Am Soc Nephrol 14:2767–2774, 2003.

136. Godley LA, Kopp JB, Eckhaus M, et al: Wild-type p53 transgenic mice exhibit altered differentiation of the ureteric bud and possess small kidneys. Genes Dev 10:836–850, 1996.

137. Pham TD, MacLennan NK, Chiu CT, et al: Uteroplacental insufficiency increases apoptosis and alters p53 gene methylation in the full-term IUGR rat kidney. Am J Physiol Regul Integr Comp Physiol 285:R962–R970, 2003.

138. Cullen-McEwen LA, Drago J, Bertram JF: Nephron endowment in glial cell line-derived neurotrophic factor (GDNF) heterozygous mice. Kidney Int 60:31–36, 2001.

139. Cullen-McEwen LA, Kett MM, Dowling J, et al: Nephron number, renal function, and arterial pressure in aged GDNF heterozygous mice. Hypertension 41:335–340, 2003.

140. Wintour EM, Moritz KM, Johnson K, et al: Reduced nephron number in adult sheep, hypertensive as a result of prenatal glucocorticoid treatment. J Physiol 549:929–935, 2003.

141. Seckl JR, Meaney MJ: Glucocorticoid programming. Ann N Y Acad Sci 1032:63–84, 2004.

142. Dave-Sharma S, Wilson RC, Harbison MD, et al: Examination of genotype and phenotype relationships in 14 patients with apparent mineralocorticoid excess. J Clin Endocrinol Metab 83:2244–2254, 1998.

143. Bertram C, Trowern AR, Copin N, et al: The maternal diet during pregnancy programs altered expression of the glucocorticoid receptor and type 2 11beta-hydroxysteroid dehydrogenase: Potential molecular mechanisms underlying the programming of hypertension in utero. Endocrinology 142:2841–2853, 2001.

144. Amri K, Freund N, Vilar J, et al: Adverse effects of hyperglycemia on kidney development in rats: In vivo and in vitro studies. Diabetes 48:2240–2245, 1999.

145. Amri K, Freund N, Van Huyen JP, et al: Altered nephrogenesis due to maternal diabetes is associated with increased expression of IGF-II/mannose-6-phosphate receptor in the fetal kidney. Diabetes 50:1069–1075, 2001.

146. Doublier S, Amri K, Seurin D, et al: Overexpression of human insulin-like growth factor binding protein-1 in the mouse leads to nephron deficit. Pediatr Res 49:660–666, 2001.

147. Gilbert T, Lelievre-Pegorier M, Merlet-Benichou C: Immediate and long-term renal effects of fetal exposure to gentamicin. Pediatr Nephrol 4:445–450, 1990.

148. Gilbert T, Gaonach S, Moreau E, Merlet-Benichou C: Defect of nephrogenesis induced by gentamicin in rat metanephric organ culture. Lab Invest 70:656–666, 1994.

149. Gilbert T, Cibert C, Moreau E, et al: Early defect in branching morphogenesis of the ureteric bud in induced nephron deficit. Kidney Int 50:783–795, 1996.

150. Nathanson S, Moreau E, Merlet-Benichou C, Gilbert T: In utero and in vitro exposure to beta-lactams impair kidney development in the rat. J Am Soc Nephrol 11:874–884, 2000.

151. McKay DB, Josephson MA: Pregnancy in recipients of solid organs—Effects on mother and child. N Engl J Med 354:1281–1293, 2006.

152. Tendron A, Decramer S, Justrabo E, et al: Cyclosporin A administration during pregnancy induces a permanent nephron deficit in young rabbits. J Am Soc Nephrol 14:3188–3196, 2003.

153. Tendron-Franzin A, Gouyon JB, Guignard JP, et al: Long-term effects of in utero exposure to cyclosporin A on renal function in the rabbit. J Am Soc Nephrol 15:2687–2693, 2004.

154. Manning J, Vehaskari VM: Postnatal modulation of prenatally programmed hypertension by dietary Na and ACE inhibition. Am J Physiol Regul Integr Comp Physiol 288: R80–R84, 2005.

155. Paixao AD, Maciel CR, Teles MB, Figueiredo-Silva J: Regional Brazilian diet-induced low birth weight is correlated with changes in renal hemodynamics and glomerular morphometry in adult age. Biol Neonate 80:239–246, 2001.

156. Franco Mdo C, Arruda RM, Fortes ZB, et al: Severe nutritional restriction in pregnant rats aggravates hypertension, altered vascular reactivity, and renal development in spontaneously hypertensive rats offspring. J Cardiovasc Pharmacol 39:369–377, 2002.

157. Sanders MW, Fazzi GE, Janssen GM, et al: Reduced uteroplacental blood flow alters renal arterial reactivity and glomerular properties in the rat offspring. Hypertension 43:1283–1289, 2004.

158. van Onna M, Houben AJ, Kroon AA, et al: Asymmetry of renal blood flow in patients with moderate to severe hypertension. Hypertension 41:108–113, 2003.

159. Guron G, Friberg P: An intact renin-angiotensin system is a prerequisite for normal renal development. J Hypertens 18:123–137, 2000.

160. Woods LL, Rasch R: Perinatal ANG II programs adult blood pressure, glomerular number, and renal function in rats. Am J Physiol 275:R1593–R1599, 1998.

161. Langley-Evans SC, Jackson AA: Captopril normalises systolic blood pressure in rats with hypertension induced by fetal exposure to maternal low protein diets. Comp Biochem Physiol A Physiol 110:223–228, 1995.

162. McMullen S, Gardner DS, Langley-Evans SC: Prenatal programming of angiotensin II type 2 receptor expression in the rat. Br J Nutr 91:133–140, 2004.

163. Sahajpal V, Ashton N: Renal function and angiotensin AT1 receptor expression in young rats following intrauterine exposure to a maternal low-protein diet. Clin Sci (Lond) 104:607–614, 2003.

164. Sahajpal V, Ashton N: Increased glomerular angiotensin II binding in rats exposed to a maternal low protein diet in utero. J Physiol 563:193–201, 2005.

165. Vehaskari VM, Stewart T, Lafont D, et al: Kidney angiotensin and angiotensin receptor expression in prenatally programmed hypertension. Am J Physiol Renal Physiol 287: F262–267, 2004.

166. Zhang SL, Moini B, Ingelfinger JR: Angiotensin II increases Pax-2 expression in fetal kidney cells via the AT2 receptor. J Am Soc Nephrol 15:1452–1465, 2004.

167. Bauer R, Walter B, Bauer K, et al: Intrauterine growth restriction reduces nephron number and renal excretory function in newborn piglets. Acta Physiol Scand 176:83–90, 2002.

168. Manning J, Beutler K, Knepper MA, Vehaskari VM: Upregulation of renal BSC1 and TSC in prenatally programmed hypertension. Am J Physiol Renal Physiol 283:F202–206, 2002.

169. Azuma H, Nadeau K, Mackenzie HS, et al: Nephron mass modulates the hemodynamic, cellular and molecular response of the rat renal allograft. Transplantation 63:519–528, 1997.

170. Mackenzie HS, Azuma H, Rennke HG, et al: Renal mass as a determinant of late allograft outcome: Insights from experimental studies in rats. Kidney Int 48:S-38—S-42, 1995.

171. Heeman UW, Azuma H, Tullius SG, et al: The contribution of reduced functioning mass to chronic kidney allograft dysfunction in rats. Transplantation 58:1317–1321, 1994.

172. Mackenzie HS, Azuma H, Troy JL, et al: Augmenting kidney mass at transplantation abrogates chronic renal allograft injury in rats. Proc Assoc Am Phys 108:127–133, 1996.

173. Mackenzie HS, Tullius SG, Heeman UW, et al: Nephron supply is a major determinant of long-term renal allograft outcome in rats. J Clin Invest 94:2148–2152, 1994.

174. Brenner BM, Milford EL: Nephron underdosing: A programmed cause of chronic renal allograft failure. Am J Kidney Dis 21:66–72, 1993.

175. Chertow GM, Milford EL, Mackenzie HS, Brenner BM: Antigen-independent determinants of cadaveric kidney transplant failure. JAMA 276:1732–1736, 1996.

176. Chertow GM, Brenner BM, Mori M, et al: Antigen-independent determinants of graft survival in living-related kidney transplantation. Kidney Int 52:S-84–S-86, 1997.

177. Chertow GM, Brenner BM, Mackenzie HS, Milford EL: Non-immunologic predictors of chronic renal allograft failure: Data from the United Network of Organ Sharing. Kidney Int 48:S-48–S-51, 1995.

178. Fulladosa X, Moreso F, Narvaez JA, et al: Estimation of total glomerular number in stable renal transplants. J Am Soc Nephrol 14:2662–2668, 2003.

179. Giral M, Nguyen JM, Karam G, et al: Impact of graft mass on the clinical outcome of kidney transplants. J Am Soc Nephrol 16:261–268, 2005.

180. Kasiske BL, Snyder JJ, Gilbertson D: Inadequate donor size in cadaver kidney transplantation. J Am Soc Nephrol 13:2152–2159, 2002.

181. Gaston RS, Hudson SL, Julian BA, et al: Impact of donor/recipient size matching on outcomes in renal transplantation. Transplantation 61:383–388, 1996.

182. Nakatani T, Sugimura K, Kawashima H, et al: The influence of recipient body mass on the outcome of cadaver kidney transplants. Clin Exp Nephrol 6:158–162, 2002.

183. Vazquez MA, Jeyarajah DR, Kielar ML, Lu CY: Long-term outcomes of renal transplantation: A result of the original endowment of the donor kidney and the inflammatory

response to both alloantigens and injury. Curr Opin Nephrol Hypertens 9:643–648, 2000.

184. Taal MW, Tilney NL, Brenner BM, Mackenzie HS: Renal mass: An important determinant of late allograft outcome. Transpl Rev 12:74–84, 1998.

185. Kim YS, Kim MS, Han DS, et al: Evidence that the ratio of donor kidney weight to recipient body weight, donor age, and episodes of acute rejection correlate independently with live-donor graft function. Transplantation 72:280–283, 2002.

186. Nicholson ML, Windmill DC, Horsburgh T, Harris KPG: Influence of allograft size to recipient body-weight ratio on the long-term outcome of renal transplantation. Br J Surg 87:314–319, 2000.

187. Mitchell EK, Louey S, Cock ML, et al: Nephron endowment and filtration surface area in the kidney after growth restriction of fetal sheep. Pediatr Res 55:769–773, 2004.

188. Merlet-Benichou C, Gilbert T, Muffat-Joly M, et al: Intrauterine growth retardation leads to a permanent nephron deficit in the rat. Pediatr Nephrol 8:175–180, 1994.

189. Ortiz LA, Quan A, Zarzar F, et al: Prenatal dexamethasone programs hypertension and renal injury in the rat. Hypertension 41:328–334, 2003.

190. Fassi A, Sangalli F, Maffi R, et al: Progressive glomerular injury in the MWF rat is predicted by inborn nephron deficit. J Am Soc Nephrol 9:1399–1406, 1998.

191. Zalups RK: The Os/+ mouse: A genetic animal model of reduced renal mass. Am J Physiol 264:F53–F60, 1993.

CHAPTER 20

Gender and Kidney Disease

Joel Neugarten • Sharon R. Silbiger • Ladan Golestaneh

GENDER AND RENAL DISEASE PROGRESSION

Many renal diseases show clear gender dimorphism.[1] Gender influences not only the incidence of renal disease but also its rate of progression. In animal models, such as aging, renal ablation, and polycystic kidney disease, male animals have a worse renal prognosis than females.[2,3] Female C57BL6 mice, normally resistant to sclerosis, develop progressive scarring after menopause.[4] Most of these studies evaluate the rate of progression of renal disease in the presence of sex hormone manipulation, such as oophorectomy, orchiectomy, or supplementation of testosterone or estrogen.[5–7] In most models, testosterone promotes renal disease progression, and estrogen slows progression[3,8–11] (Table 20–1). A notable exception is the deleterious effect that estrogen has in certain animals models of renal disease characterized by severe hyperlipidemia in which estrogen markedly exaggerates the lipid disturbance; a circumstance without human counterpart.

In humans, most literature supports the belief that women with certain renal diseases progress at a slower rate to end-stage renal disease (ESRD) than men, independent of the severity of hypertension or cholesterol levels.[12] This has been evidenced most clearly in membranous glomerulopathy, autosomal dominant polycystic kidney disease, and immunoglobulin A (IgA) nephropathy and has been confirmed by a recent meta-analysis.[12] Included in this meta-analysis is the Modification of Diet in Renal Disease study,[13] which evaluated renal disease progression in 840 participants, nearly 40% of whom were women, assigned to various dietary protein and blood pressure groups. Over the course of the study, the rate of deterioration of glomerular filtration rate (GFR) was slower in the women, but this difference was mitigated when corrected for differences in blood pressure, urinary protein excretion, and high-density lipoprotein (HDL) levels. More recently, two population-based studies from Scandinavia followed patients with chronic renal disease of various etiologies and concluded that male gender confers a poor renal prognosis.[14,15] Despite certain methodologic limitations, these studies are consistent with earlier observations showing a faster rate of progression of renal disease in men. Conversely, a few studies have concluded that there is no difference in the rate of renal disease progression between men and women or that women progress to renal failure at a faster rate than do men. A recent meta-analysis analyzed 11 randomized studies evaluating the effect of angiotensin-converting enzyme (ACE) inhibitors on the progression of nondiabetic renal disease.[16] After adjusting for differences in systolic blood pressure and urinary protein excretion, the authors concluded that women have a worse renal prognosis than men. However, most of the female participants in these studies were postmenopausal. Therefore, these data are entirely consistent with a renoprotective effect of female gender in premenopausal women, mediated by estrogen.

Because ESRD due to diabetes makes up a substantial fraction of all incident ESRD, the effect of gender on the progression of diabetic nephropathy merits separate consideration. In the Cohen diabetic rat, females have more rapidly progressive renal disease than do males.[17] In contrast, ovariectomy accelerates loss of renal function in female rats made diabetic with streptozotocin.[18] This effect is mitigated by estrogen supplementation, suggesting a beneficial effect of female sex hormones on the rate of renal disease progression in this model. Similarly, in the db/db rat, a model of type 2 diabetes, ovariectomy worsens diabetic renal pathology, whereas estrogen supplementation mitigates this effect.[19]

In humans, the influence of gender on the course of diabetic nephropathy is also unclear and is further complicated by interactions among gender, race, and age. According to recent data provided by the U.S. Centers for Disease Control and Prevention, the incidence of diagnosed diabetes in individuals 18 to 79 years of age is equivalent in men and women.[20] Among diabetics undergoing renal replacement therapy, the percentage of men and women is also nearly equal.[21] The age-adjusted incidence of diabetes-associated ESRD is highest among black men and lowest among white women.[20] The incidence of diabetes-associated ESRD is increasing at a much faster rate in white men than in white women, whereas in African Americans, the incremental rate in women exceeds that in men.[22]

Several studies suggest that males with type 1 diabetic nephropathy have a poorer renal prognosis than do females. Hovind and associates[23] studied proteinuric type 1 diabetics and concluded that males have a worse renal prognosis. In a study of the rate of progression of diabetic nephropathy in normotensive type 1 diabetics, the authors concluded that male sex is a "progression promoter."[24] Investigators analyzing the patient cohort of The Diabetes Control and Complications/Epidemiology of Diabetes Interventions and Complications (DCCT/EDIC) Trial concluded that, in type 1 diabetics, male sex was associated with higher urinary albumin excretion.[25] In another study using the DCCT database, Zhang and colleagues[26] found that, among those participants who exhibited good metabolic control, women had a higher risk of developing diabetic nephropathy, whereas among those manifesting extremely poor metabolic control, men had a higher risk of developing nephropathy. In contrast, analysis of a large trial in type 1 diabetics with nephropathy randomized to receive either captopril or placebo found no gender-related differences in the rate of renal disease progression.[27]

Data on the contribution of gender to the rate of progression of nephropathy in type 2 diabetics are limited. Although Torffvit and Agardh[28] concluded that gender had no effect on the rate of progression of nephropathy in type 2 diabetics, Ravid and colleagues[29] found that male sex was associated with the development of microalbuminuria and worsening serum creatinine. In con-

TABLE 20-1	Animal Models of Renal Disease: Effect of Gender	
Model	**Rate of Progression**	**Sex Hormone Effects**
Aging	↑ In males	T detrimental, E_2 beneficial
Renal ablation	↑ In males	T detrimental
PKD	↑ In males	E_2 beneficial
Hyperlipidemia	↑ In females in several models	E_2 detrimental in several models
Diabetes mellitus	Conflicting	Conflicting
Lupus nephritis	↑ In females	T beneficial, E_2 detrimental

↑, Faster rate of progression; E_2, estradiol; PKD, polycystic kidney disease; T, testosterone.

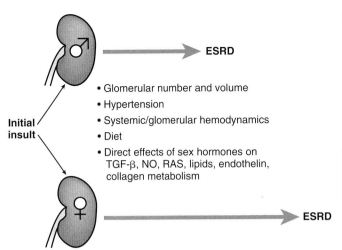

FIGURE 20-1 Factors contributing to gender-related differences in renal disease progression. NO, nitric oxide; RAS, renin-angiotensin system; TGF-β, transforming growth factor-beta.

trast, Nakano and co-workers[30] found that female, not male, gender was a strong predictor of ESRD in type 2 diabetics. Thus, the effect of gender on the progression of diabetic nephropathy remains to be determined.

A role for sex hormones in the pathogenesis of systemic lupus erythematosus (SLE) is suggested by the striking predominance of young women with this disorder.[31] Although gender disparity in the prevalence of SLE also exists before puberty and after menopause, it is markedly less pronounced.[31] These observations may be explained in part by the immunomodulating activity of sex hormones.[32] Estrogens enhance immune responsiveness, whereas androgens are immunosuppressive.[32] In this regard, female lupus patients have abnormal metabolism of estrogenic hormones and male lupus patients have reduced androgen levels.[32] In experimental models of lupus nephritis, androgenic hormones have a protective effect and estrogenic hormones exacerbate disease activity.[32] Most studies have shown that men with SLE, as compared with women with SLE, have a higher prevalence of renal disease, more aggressive nephritis, a higher risk of progressing to renal failure, and a higher renal mortality.[31] However, it should be noted that numerous other studies have failed to demonstrate any gender differences in the prevalence or course of renal disease in lupus patients.[33]

Factors Contributing to Gender-related Differences in Renal Disease Progression

Numerous mechanisms have been suggested to explain the protective effect of female gender on the progression of most nondiabetic renal diseases. These include differences between the sexes in renal structure, systemic and renal hemodynamics, diet, and blood pressure as well as direct effects of sex hormones on cellular processes (Fig. 20–1).

Kidney size and weight are greater in male than in female animals even when corrected for differences in body weight.[2] In addition, androgens increase kidney weight in a variety of animal models, predominantly by increasing proximal tubular bulk.[2] Several studies have examined kidney size, nephron number, and glomerular volume in men and women.[34-37] Hughson and colleagues[34] studied 104 African American and white adults at autopsy and found that women had 15% fewer glomeruli than did men but found no significant difference in mean glomerular volume. Nycngaard and Bendtsen[36] studied 36 autopsy specimens and found 10% fewer glomeruli in women compared with men, but the difference did not achieve statistical significance. Further analysis of these data

showed that body surface area, but not gender, was an independent determinant of kidney weight, glomerular size, and total glomerular volume.[37] However, because men are generally larger than women, these parameters also tend to be larger in men.

Although male animals may exhibit a higher total GFR than females, when corrected for kidney weight or body surface area, no significant difference exists between the sexes.[38] In humans, GFR in men and women is similar when corrected for body surface area.[39] In addition, neither testosterone nor estrogen has direct effects on GFR or renal blood flow.[40,41] Despite these data, evidence suggests that glomerular hemodynamic responses to angiotensin II (AII) may differ in men versus women. Healthy young adult men respond to an infusion of AII by increasing their filtration fraction, suggesting increased glomerular capillary pressure.[42] In contrast, women show no change in filtration fraction. This gender dimorphism may contribute to renoprotection in females by blunting elevations in glomerular capillary pressure and reducing glomerular hemodynamic stress. In a study of normotensive, nonproteinuric type 1 diabetic adolescents, the same investigators[43] found gender-related differences in the renal hemodynamic response to clamped euglycemia and clamped hyperglycemia. It was suggested that these differences may explain the lack of a consistent protective effect of female gender on the course of nephropathy in type 1 diabetics.

Excessive caloric intake or high dietary intake of protein, phosphorus, or sodium promotes the development and progression of renal disease in numerous experimental models. Protein loading increases GFR and glomerular transcapillary hydraulic pressure difference, which, if sustained, may ultimately be detrimental to the kidney. Men consume more calories and protein than do women, which may contribute to the adverse effect of male gender on renal disease progression.

Sex hormones have direct effects on the synthesis and activity of numerous cytokines and vasoactive agents, the serum level and oxidative state of lipids, and the generation and degradation of matrix components. Because these factors influence renal disease severity, interactions between these factors and estrogen may contribute to the renal protection afforded by female gender.

Nitric oxide (NO) contributes to the development and progression of renal injury in numerous experimental models.[2,44] In addition to its effects on the systemic and renal vasculature and on glomerular ultrafiltration,[45,46] NO induces apoptosis of mesangial and endothelial cells.[47] In cultured glomerular and vascular endothelial cells, physiologic concentrations of estrogen cause a rapid release of NO via estrogen receptor α.[48,49] The promoter region of the endothelial NO synthase (eNOS) gene contains an estrogen-responsive element, which may mediate estrogen-induced up-regulation of eNOS mRNA and protein levels.[50] Female rats express higher levels of eNOS than males, an effect that is reversed by ovariectomy.[49,51,52] Estradiol also increases local prostaglandin E_2 (PGE$_2$) and prostacyclin levels, which in turn activate NO synthase (NOS).[49] Although chronic NO inhibition in rats induces systolic hypertension in both sexes, only male rats develop proteinuria, which is prevented by orchiectomy.[53]

Sex hormones have profound effects on the renin-angiotensin system (RAS). Estrogen up-regulates the expression of angiotensinogen and angiotensin type 2 (AT-2) receptors, but down-regulates the expression of renin, ACE, and AII.[49,54–57] AT-1 receptors are also down-regulated in many but not all cell types.[49,54,56,58] In contrast, testosterone activates the RAS.[59–61] Renal angiotensinogen mRNA levels are higher in adult male rats than in females, an effect that is reversed by orchiectomy and restored by testosterone administration.[60] Prorenin and renin levels and plasma renin activity are higher in men than in women.[60] In cultured mesangial cells, dihydrotestosterone up-regulates the expression of AT-1 receptors.[60] As noted earlier, the effect of infused AII on renal hemodynamics also differs between men and women.[42] Clearly, interactions between sex hormones and the RAS may contribute to gender dimorphism in renal disease progression.

Although lipids promote renal injury in experimental models, their role in the progression of renal disease in humans is less clear. Premenopausal women have lower levels of total cholesterol and low density lipoproteins (LDLs) and higher levels of HDLs than age-matched men.[62] After menopause, this difference narrows, but estrogen replacement therapy returns lipids to premenopausal levels.[63] At high concentrations, estrogen has a direct inhibitory effect on lipid oxidation.[64] At physiologic concentrations, however, estrogen may promote oxidation.[65] Further studies are needed to determine whether estrogen reduces oxidative stress associated with renal injury in vivo. In contrast, testosterone has no effect on lipid oxidation.[64]

Estrogens exert numerous effects on mesangial cells that may slow renal disease progression (Table 20–2). Estrogens and selective estrogen receptor modulators suppress the synthesis of type I and type IV collagen by cultured mesangial cells.[66] Estrogen also up-regulates the activity of two collagen degrading enzymes, metalloproteinase-2 and metalloproteinase-9.[67,68] Another mechanism by which estrogen may ameliorate renal injury is via antagonism of the actions of transforming growth factor-β (TGF-β). In cultured mesangial cells, physiologic concentrations of estradiol inhibit the pro-fibrotic effects of TGF-β and reverse TGF-β–mediated mesangial cell apoptosis by interfering with the activity of protein kinase CK2.[69,70] In the TGF-β transgenic mouse, estradiol supplementation mitigates the extensive sclerosis that develops in untreated

males.[71,72] Because TGF-β and mesangial matrix accumulation contribute to progressive renal injury, the interaction of sex hormones with these factors may help explain gender-related differences in renal disease progression.

GENDER AND RENAL TRANSPLANTATION

An effect of gender on the outcome of renal transplantation was first noted in the 1980s. Despite extensive research and commentary, the precise nature of this effect and its underlying mechanisms have not been clearly elucidated.

Donor Gender

Donor gender has a significant impact on allograft survival. Analysis of death-censored data from nearly 125,000 first renal allograft recipients collected by the Collaborative Transplant Study confirmed earlier reports of lower graft survival in recipients of female compared with male donor kidneys.[73] Poorest graft and patient survival was observed among male recipients of female donor kidneys. Renal function was also superior in recipients of male donor kidneys irrespective of recipient gender. In this study, graft survival in recipients of female donor kidneys was inferior to recipients of male donor kidneys only when the female donor was below 45 years of age. This observation is in striking contrast to earlier reports from smaller registries indicating that the survival of female donor kidneys was inferior only in kidneys from older female donors. In these studies, kidneys from young female donors were found to have a survival rate equivalent to that of kidneys from young male donors. These markedly disparate observations cannot be easily reconciled.

A survival advantage for male donor kidneys has also been observed among recipients of a living donor kidney.[74,75] However, in another analysis of over 32,000 cadaver allograft recipients, the effect of donor gender on late graft survival was no longer significant after donor and recipient body surface area was taken into account.[76] The survival advantage associated with male donor kidneys was attributed in large part to favorable donor/recipient size-matching.

Mechanisms to Explain the Donor Gender Effect

Nephron Supply/Functional Demand Mismatch

It has been suggested that the diminished long-term survival of kidneys from female versus male donors may be explained by a mismatch between the donor's nephron supply and the recipient's functional demand.[77–79] A small kidney with fewer nephrons transplanted into a large recipient would be expected to undergo greater hypertrophy and enhanced hyperfiltration. Resultant hemodynamic-mediated glomerular injury might then give rise to progressive nephron loss leading to graft failure. Because females generally have smaller kidneys and fewer nephrons, transplantation of a female kidney into a male recipient may be functionally inadequate to meet the needs of the recipient.[34] The lower graft survival among recipients of kidneys from older female donors, demonstrated in some studies, may reflect age-related nephron loss, which exaggerates the mismatch between donor nephron number and recipient functional demand.[75]

The effect of donor gender on graft survival is already evident within 3 to 6 months post-transplantation.[75] It seems unlikely that hyperfiltration-induced glomerular injury due to size mismatch could entirely account for shortened graft survival in the very early post-transplant period because longer periods of hyperfiltration would presumably be required to damage the transplanted kidney. However, a reduced nephron reserve in female donor kidneys may enhance susceptibility to ischemic injury, acute rejection, or

TABLE 20–2	Direct Effects of Estradiol on Mesangial Cells
Reverses TGF-β–induced type I and type IV collagen synthesis	
Reverses TGF-β–induced apoptosis	
Increases collagenase activity	
Inhibits oxidation of LDL	
Affects cellular proliferation	

LDL, low-density lipoprotein; TGF-β, transforming growth factor-β.

cyclosporine nephrotoxlcity and accelerate allograft failure. In this context, grafts from female donors are less likely to survive after a rejection episode than are male donor kidneys.[75] This observation may be explained if compromise of the female donor kidney by rejection further reduces nephron number and exaggerates supply/demand mismatch.

The mismatch hypothesis also predicts that differences in graft loss between the sexes would increase steadily with increasing duration of exposure to hyperfiltration. Although some investigators have found that the survival advantage of male donor kidneys is exaggerated by the passage of time after transplantation,[80,81] others have found that the difference in survival is maximum soon after transplantation and then plateaus.[82]

Cyclosporine Nephrotoxicity

Donor gender was first recognized as a factor influencing graft survival in the early to mid 1980s, corresponding in time to the introduction and widespread use of cyclosporine.[75,82] Consistent with observations made by earlier investigators, we[82] found no effect of donor gender on allograft survival in recipients who were transplanted in the pre-cyclosporine era, whereas a clear effect was demonstrated in cyclosporine-treated recipients. Recipients treated with tacrolimus rather than cyclosporine also failed to show a donor gender effect.[83] The equivalence of graft survival between male and female donor kidneys in non–cyclosporine-treated recipients suggests that a mismatch between nephron supply and donor functional demand is alone insufficient to explain the adverse effect of female donor gender observed in cyclosporine-treated recipients.

Gender-related differences in susceptibility to cyclosporine nephrotoxicity or in the therapeutic response to cyclosporine may contribute to the shortened graft survival of female donor kidneys under cyclosporine immunosuppression. Whereas cyclosporine increases the survival of young female donor kidneys to the same extent as that of male donor kidneys, cyclosporine does not increase the survival of older female kidneys.[75] Enhanced susceptibility of older female kidneys to the nephrotoxic effects of cyclosporine may help explain this observation.[69]

Higher doses of cyclosporine are administered to male recipients, who generally weigh more than females.[75] Transplantation of a small female donor kidney into a male recipient results in the largest relative dosing of cyclosporine, which may enhance nephrotoxicity and explain the poor graft survival in this group.

Recipient Gender

Females show enhanced immune responsiveness.[75] In animal models, estrogen administration antagonizes the immuno-suppressive activity of cyclosporine and leads to shortened allograft survival.[75] Notwithstanding these observations, most studies have failed to show a significant effect of recipient gender on the outcome of renal transplantation.[75] Meier-Kriesche and co-workers[84,85] analyzed data from over 73,000 recipients of primary renal allografts and found that graft survival censored for death was no different in male versus female recipients. However, patient survival and uncensored graft survival were better in female recipients. Female recipients showed a 10% increased risk of acute rejection. However, this effect was offset by a 10% decreased risk of graft loss secondary to chronic allograft failure. Reduced risk of chronic allograft failure was observed only in female recipients above the age of 45. In contrast, the sex of the kidney donor was not a significant factor in determining chronic allograft failure.

The effect of gender and sex hormones on the development of chronic allograft nephropathy has been examined in numerous animal models.[75] These studies have consistently demonstrated that the progression of chronic allograft nephropathy is ameliorated by estrogen and accelerated by testosterone. However, these experimental data do not explain the observation made by Meier-Kriesche and associates[84,85] that only female recipients above the age of 45 demonstrate a reduced risk of chronic allograft failure.

GENDER AND HYPERTENSION

Epidemiology

Both the overall prevalence of hypertension and the incidence of uncontrolled hypertension are higher among men than women.[86–92] There is no difference in systemic blood pressure between prepubescent boys and girls, and it is only after puberty that boys exhibit higher blood pressure than girls.[88] Blood pressure increases in age in both men and women, but the rate of rise in blood pressure is steeper in women beginning in their 60s such that, after the 7th decade, women have higher systolic blood pressures and pulse pressures than men.[87]

Blood pressure tends to parallel estrogen levels, being lower during ovulation and in the luteal phase of the menstrual cycle than in the follicular phase.[93] Pregnancy is characterized by a marked elevation in the serum concentration of estrogen, associated with a decline in blood pressure. After menopause, the serum concentration of estradiol falls to levels similar to or lower than those found in men, associated with an elevation in blood pressure.[50] The increase in blood pressure observed after the onset menopause develops over 5 to 20 years. Other factors that may contribute to the development of postmenopausal hypertension include higher testosterone levels, higher body mass index, decreased renal function, endothelial dysfunction, and oxidative stress associated with aging as well as a higher incidence of co-morbid conditions including diabetes and atherosclerotic disease.[87,94]

Exogenous hormone intake and its effects on blood pressure are more complicated and do not parallel the seemingly clear-cut dose-response effect seen with endogenous estrogen levels.[93,95] A recent meta-analysis suggested a mild increase in blood pressure in women using oral contraceptives and a mild decrease in those using estrogen replacement therapy.[96] Women taking oral contraceptives are two to three times more likely to have high blood pressure than nonusers.[97] At the high levels of estrogen seen in oral contraceptives, estrogen may exert a vasoconstrictor effect via greater activation of the RAS and enhanced sympathetic tone.[17] At lower levels, comparable with those used in hormone replacement therapy, estrogen tends to reduce blood pressure via enhanced production of vasodilators. However, the clinical data on the effect of hormone replacement therapy on blood pressure are conflicting.[91,95,98]

The evidence supporting a benefit from treatment of hypertension is based on combined results for men and women. A recent meta-analysis of blood pressure–lowering treatments showed a lower absolute risk reduction in women than in men.[90,92] The benefits of adequate blood pressure control in women was reflected in a lower incidence of strokes but not in reduced mortality, whereas in men there was a significant reduction in mortality. Despite established benefit from treatment of hypertension, only about a quarter of treated hypertensive women achieve blood pressure control with prescribed antihypertensives.[86]

Factors Contributing to Gender-related Differences in Hypertension

Estrogen receptors α and β are found in vascular endothelial and smooth muscle cells, and both have been implicated in

TABLE 20–3 Role of Sex Hormones in the Pathogenesis of Hypertension

	RAS	Vascular Smooth Muscle	Endothelium	Oxidative Injury
Estrogen	↓ Renin, ACE, and AII levels ↓ AT-1 receptors in many cell types ↑ Angiotensinogen levels ↑ AT-2 receptors	↑ Opening of calcium-activated potassium channels	↑ eNOS levels and NOS activity ↑ NO and cGMP levels ↑ Prostacyclin and PGE$_2$ levels ↑ Kininogen, kallikrein, and bradykinin levels ↓ Endothelin levels ↓ Kininase (ACE) levels	↓ Oxygen free radicals (supraphysiologic concentrations of E$_2$) ↓ Experimental endothelial oxidative injury
Testosterone	↑ Proximal tubular sodium reabsorption ↑ Prorenin, renin, angiotensinogen, and AII levels ↑ Renin activity ↑ ACE activity ↑ AT-1 receptors	↑ Vasoconstriction induced by sympathetic hormones	↑ Endothelin levels and actions ↓ Adenosine-induced vasodilation ↓ NO levels and local actions	↑ Oxygen free radicals (direct and indirect actions)

AII, angiotensin II; ACE, angiotensin-converting enzyme; AT-1, angiotensin type 1 receptors; AT-2, angiotensin type 2 receptors; cGMP, cyclic guanosine monophosphate; E$_2$, estradiol; eNOS, endothelial nitric oxide synthase; NO, nitric oxide; PGE$_2$, prostaglandin E$_2$; RAS, renin-angiotensin system.

small vessel dilatation, as well as protection against endothelial injury.[50] Although the mechanisms that mediate the vascular effects of estrogen have not yet been fully elucidated, it appears that both genomic and nongenomic pathways are involved (Table 20–3). Estrogen induces vasodilatation and increases blood flow within 5 to 20 minutes of administration through both endothelium-dependent and endothelium-independent mechanisms.[49] Estrogen activates endothelium-dependent vascular relaxation factors including NO, cyclic guanosine monophosphate, and prostacyclin. As discussed earlier, estrogen up-regulates the NO pathway at multiple levels.

At physiologic concentrations, estrogen stimulates the opening of calcium-activated potassium channels, leading to smooth muscle relaxation and vasodilatation.[49] Vascular smooth muscle contraction in response to vasopressors is greater in the aorta of male rats compared with female rats and is enhanced in females by ovariectomy.[49,87] The ability of estrogen to directly inhibit vascular smooth muscle contraction is demonstrated by its vasodilatory effect on de-endothelialized coronary arteries.[49,87]

As discussed earlier, estrogen has profound effects on the RAS at multiple levels. In experimental models, estrogen replacement reduces AII levels associated with a reduction in blood pressure. Estrogen increases AT-2 receptor density in the renal medulla and down-regulates AT-1 receptor density in the kidney and in vascular smooth muscle.[49,54] Enhanced AT-2 receptor expression stimulates bradykinin synthesis, which in turn stimulates NO release and up-regulates PGE$_2$ expression.[50,87] Down-regulation of AT-1 receptor density antagonizes sodium retention and vasoconstriction.

Endothelin is a potent vasoconstrictor that enhances renal sodium reabsorption, promotes oxidative stress, and contributes to increased blood pressure.[49] Estradiol inhibits not only the synthesis of endothelin but also its vasoconstrictor effects.[49,87] Endothelin levels increase after menopause. Because AII stimulates endothelin synthesis, the ability of estrogen to decrease AII levels may contribute to a reduction in endothelin levels. Estrogen stimulates the synthesis of bradykinin, a vasorelaxant agent, and enhances its vasodepressor effects.[49,87,99] Estrogen also stimulates kallikrein and kininogen expression and reduces kininase (ACE) levels.[100]

Recent data indicate that oxidant injury to blood vessels may contribute to the development of hypertension. Estradiol is a potent antioxidant in supraphysiologic concentration and protects against endothelial damage mediated by oxidative stress in experimental models.[50] If estrogens were to exert antioxidative effects in vivo, these actions might contribute to the protective effect of female gender on the development of hypertension.[50,87]

The action of androgens to up-regulate vasoconstrictors, promote oxidative stress, and enhance sodium retention may contribute to the development and aggravation of hypertension[87] (see Table 20–3). Androgen receptors are found in proximal tubules and may directly increase proximal tubular sodium reabsorption. In animal models, castration of males shifts pressure-natriuresis curves toward those of intact females. Testosterone also stimulates tyrosine hydroxylase, which is the rate-limiting step for catecholamine synthesis, blocks adenosine-mediated vasodilatation, and enhances the contractile effects of endothelin.[52,59]

In genetic models of hypertension, castration of males attenuates the development of hypertension, and blockade of androgen receptors with flutamide reduces blood pressure to levels found in females.[87] Serum testosterone levels rise after the onset of menopause and may contribute to the development of hypertension in postmenopausal women. In this regard, women with virilizing tumors develop hypertension.

As discussed earlier, testosterone activates the RAS and increases efferent arteriolar resistance.[59] Stimulation of the RAS promotes oxidative stress and increases superoxide production, which in turn quenches NO; all of which decrease vascular response to vasodilators.[87] These effects may explain why androgen withdrawal enhances endothelium-dependent vasodilatation.[59]

The nonmodulator phenotype is an intermediate marker for hypertension and is characterized by a blunted natriuretic response to elevated pressure in the renal vasculature and higher than expected aldosterone levels in response to a salt load.[99,101] The nonmodulator phenotype is much more common in men than in women. As our awareness of genetic influences on the pathophysiology of hypertension increases, it is important to note that genetic polymorphisms in the ACE, AII, and AT-1 receptor genes have a more profound influence on the development of hypertension in men than in women.[99,101,102]

References

1. Silbiger S, Neugarten J: The impact of gender on the progression of chronic renal disease. Am J Kidney Dis 25:515–533, 1995.

2. Silbiger SR, Neugarten J: The role of gender in the progression of renal disease. Adv Renal Repl Ther 10:3–14, 2003.

3. Denton K, Baylis C: Physiological and molecular mechanisms governing sexual dimorphism of kidney, cardiac and vascular function. Am J Physiol Regul Integr Comp Physiol 292:R697–R699, 2007.

4. Zheng F, Plati AR, Potier M, et al: Resistance to glomerulosclerosis in B6 mice disappears after menopause. Am J Pathol 162:1339–1348, 2003.

5. Gilboa N, Magro AM, Han Y, Rudofsky VH: Contrasting effects of early and late orchiectomy on hypertension and renal disease in Fawn-hooded rats. Life Sci 41:1629–1634, 1987.

6. Baylis C, Corman G: The aging kidney: Insights from experimental studies. J Am Soc Nephrol 9:699–709, 1988.

7. Elliot SJ, Karl M, Berho M, et al: Estrogen deficiency accelerates progression of glomerulosclerosis in susceptible mice. Am J Pathol 162:1441–1448, 2003.

8. Baylis C: Age-dependent glomerular damage in the rat. Dissociation between glomerular injury and both glomerular hypertension and hypertrophy. Male gender as a primary risk factor. J Clin Invest 94:1823–1829, 1994.

9. Sakemi T, Ohtsuka N, Shouno Y, Morito F: Effect of ovariectomy on glomerular injury in hypercholesterolemic, female Imai rats. Nephron 72:72–78, 1996.

10. Gross M-L, Adamczak M, Rabe T, et al: Beneficial effects of estrogens on indices of renal damage in uninephrectomized SHRsp rats. J Am Soc Nephrol 15:348–358, 2004.

11. Tofovic SP, Dubey R, Salah EM, Jackson EK: 2-Hydroxyestradiol attenuates renal disease in chronic puromycin aminonucleoside nephropathy. J Am Soc Nephrol 13:2737–2747, 2002.

12. Neugarten J, Acharya A, Silbiger SR: Effect of gender on the progression of nondiabetic renal disease: A meta-analysis. J Am Soc Neprhol 11:319–329, 2000.

13. Coggins CH, Lewis JB, Caggiula AW, et al: Differences between women and men with chronic renal disease. Nephrol Dial Transplant 13:1430–1437, 1998.

14. Evans M, Fryzek JP, Elinder CG, et al: The natural history of chronic renal failure: Results from an unselected population-based inception cohort in Sweden. Am J Kidney Dis 46:863–870, 2005.

15. Eriksen BO, Ingebretsen OC: The progression of chronic kidney disease: A 10-year population-based study of the effects of gender and age. Kidney Int 69:375–382, 2006.

16. Jafar TH, Schmid CH, Stark PC, et al for the ACE Inhibition in Progressive Renal Disease (AIPRD) Study Group: The rate of progression of renal disease may not be slower in women compared with men: A patient-level meta-analysis. Nephrol Dial Transplant 18:2047–2053, 2003.

17. Rosenmann E, Yanko L, Cohen AM: Female sex hormone and nephropathy in Cohen diabetic rat (genetically selected sucrose-fed). Horm Metab Res 16:11–16, 1984.

18. Mankhey RW, Bhatti F, Maric C: 17β-Estradiol replacement improves renal function and pathology associated with diabetic nephropathy. Am J Physiol Renal Physiol 288:F399–F405, 2005.

19. Chin M, Isono M, Isshiki K, et al: Estrogen and raloxifene, a selective estrogen receptor modulator, ameliorate renal damage in db/db mice. Am J Pathol 166:1629–1636, 2005.

20. www.cdc.gov/diabetes/statistics/index.htm

21. U.S. Renal Data System: USRDS 2005 Annual Data Report: Atlas of End-Stage Renal Disease in the United States. Bethesda, MD, National Institutes of Health, National Institute of Diabetes and Digestive and Kidney Diseases, 2005, Table 2.a, p 74.

22. Jones CA, Krolewski AS, Rogus J, et al: Epidemic of end-stage renal disease in people with diabetes in the United States population: Do we know the cause? Kidney Int 67:1684–1691, 2005.

23. Hovind P, Tarnow L, Oestergaard PB, et al: Elevated vascular endothelial growth factor in type 1 diabetic patients with diabetic nephropathy. Kidney Int Suppl 75:S56–S61, 2000.

24. Jacobsen P, Rossing K, Tarnow K, et al: Progression of diabetic nephropathy in normotensive type 1 diabetic patients. Kidney Int Suppl 71:D101–D105, 1999.

25. Sibley SD, Thomas W, de Boer I, et al: Gender and elevated albumin excretion in the Diabetes Control and Complications Trial/Epidemiology of Diabetes Interventions and Complications (DCCT/EDIC) cohort: Role of obesity. Am J Kidney Dis 47:223–232, 2006.

26. Zhang L, Krzentowski G, Albert A, Lefebvre PJ: Factors predictive of nephropathy in DCCT type 1 diabetic patients with good or poor metabolic control. Diabet Med 20:580–585, 2003.

27. Breyer JA, Bain RP, Evans JK, et al, and The Collaborative Study Group: Predictors of the progression of renal insufficiency in patients with insulin-dependent diabetes and overt diabetic nephropathy. Kidney Int 50:1651–1658, 1996.

28. Torffvit O, Agardh CD: The impact of metabolic and blood pressure control on incidence and progression of nephropathy. A 10-year study of 385 type 2 diabetic patients. J Diabetes Complications 15:307–313, 2001.

29. Ravid M, Brosh D, Ravid-Safran D, et al: Main risk factors for nephropathy in type 2 diabetes mellitus are plasma cholesterol levels, mean blood pressure and hyperglycemia. Arch Intern Med 158:998–1004, 1998.

30. Nakano O, Ogihara M, Tamura C, et al: Reversed circadian blood pressure rhythm independently predicts end-stage renal failure in noninsulin-dependent diabetes mellitus subjects. J Diabetes Complications 13:224–231, 1999.

31. Molina JF, Drenkard C, Molina J, et al: Systemic lupus erythematosus in males: A study of 107 Latin American patients. Medicine 75:124–130, 1996.

32. Lahita RG: Sex hormones and the immune response-human studies. Baillieres Clin Rheumat 4.1:1–12, 1990.

33. Koh WH, Fong KY, Boey ML, Feng PH: Systemic lupus erythematosus in 61 Oriental males. A study of clinical and laboratory manifestations. Br J Rhematol 33:339–342, 1994.

34. Hughson MD, Douglas-Denton R, Bertram JF, Hoy WE: Hypertension, glomerular number, and birth weight in African Americans and white subjects in the southeastern United States. Kidney Int 69:671–678, 2006.

35. Hughson M, Farris AB, Douglas-Denton R, et al: Glomerular number and size in autopsy kidneys: The relationship to birth weight. Kidney Int 63:2113–2122, 2003.

36. Nyengaard JR, Bendtsen TF: Glomerular number and size in relation to age, kidney weight, and body surface in normal man. Anat Rec 232:194–201, 1992.

37. Neugarten J, Kasiske B, Silbiger SR. Nyengaard JR: Effects of sex on renal structure. Nephron 90:139–144, 2002.

38. Munger K, Baylis C: Sex differences in renal hemodynamics in rats. Am J Physiol 254:F223–F231, 1988.

39. Slack TK, Wilson DM: Normal renal function. C_{in} and C_{PAH} in healthy donors before and after nephrectomy. Mayo Clin Proc 51:296–300, 1976.

40. Klopp C, Young NF, Taylor HC: The effects of testosterone and of testosterone propionate on renal functions in man. J Clin Invest 24:189–191, 1945.

41. Dignam WS, Voskian J, Assali NS: Effects of estrogens on renal hemodynamics and excretion of electrolytes in human subjects. J Clin Endocrinol 16:1032–1041, 1956.

42. Miller JA, Abacta LA, Cattran DC: Impact of gender on renal response to angiotensin II. Kidney Int 55:278–285, 1999.

43. Cherney DZI, Sochett EB, Miller JA: Gender differences in renal response to hyperglycemia and angiotensin-converting enzyme inhibition in diabetes. Kidney Int 68:1722–1728, 2005.

44. Baylis C: Changes in renal hemodynamics and structure in the aging kidney: Sexual dimorphism and the nitric oxide system. Exp Gerontol 40:271–278, 2005.

45. Chambliss KL, Shaul PW: Estrogen modulation of endothelial nitric oxide synthase. Endocr Rev 23: 665–686, 2002.

46. Blantz RC, Deng A, Lortie M, et al: The complex role of nitric oxide in the regulation of glomerular ultrfiltration. Kidney Int 61:782–785, 2002.

47. Pautz A, Franzen R, Dorsch S, et al: Cross-talk between nitric oxide and superoxide determines ceramide formation and apoptosis in glomerular cells. Kidney Int 61:790–796, 2002.

48. Xiao S, Gillespie DG, Baylis C, et al: Effects of estradiol and its metabolites on glomerular endothelial nitric oxide synthesis and mesangial cell growth. Hypertension 37:645–650, 2001.

49. Thompson J, Khalil RA: Gender differences in the regulation of vascular tone. Clin Exp Pharmacol Physiol 30:1–15, 2003.

50. Mendelsohn M, Karas RH: Mechanisms of disease: The protective effects of estrogen on the cardiovascular system. N Engl J Med 340:1801–1811, 1999.

51. Neugarten J, Ding Q, Friedman A, et al: Sex hormone and renal nitric oxide synthases. J Am Soc Nephrol 8:1240–1246, 1997.

52. Lieberman EH, Gerhard MD, Uehata A, et al: Estrogen improves endothelium-dependent, flow-mediated vasodilation in postmenopausal women. Ann Intern Med 121:936–941, 1994.

53. Verhagen AM, Attia DM, Koomans HA, Joles JA: Male gender increases sensitivity to proteinuria induced by mild NOS inhibition in rats: Role of sex hormones. Am J Physiol 279:F664–F670, 2000.

54. Veille JC, Li P, Eisenach JC, et al: Effects of estrogen in nitric oxide biosynthesis and vasorelaxant activity in sheep uterine and renal arteries in vivo. Am J Obstet Gynecol 174:1043–1049, 1996.

55. Oelkers WK: Effects of estrogens and progestogens on the renin angiotensinogen system and blood pressure. Steroids 61.166–171, 1996.

56. Baiardi G, Macova M, Armando I, et al: Estrogen upregulates renal angiotensin II, AT_1 and AT_2 receptors in the rats. Regul Pept 124:7–17, 2005.

57. Gallagher PE, Li R, Lenhart JR, et al: Estrogen regulation of angiotensin-converting enzyme mRNA. Hypertension 33:323–328, 1999.

58. Nickenig G, Baumer AT, Grohe C, et al: Estrogen modulates AT1 receptors gene expression in vitro and in vivo. Circulation 97:2197–2201, 1998.

59. Reckelhoff JF, Yanes LL, Iliescu R, et al: Testosterone supplementation in aging men and women: Possible impact on cardiovascular-renal disease. Am J Physiol 289:F941–F948, 2005.

60. Ellison KE, Ingelfinger JR, Pivor M, Dzau VJ: Androgen regulation of rat renal angiotensinogen messenger RNA expression. J Clin Invest 83:1941–1945, 1989.

61. Chen YF, Naftilan AJ, Oparil S: Androgen-dependent angiotensinogen and renin messenger RNA expression in hypertensive rats. Hypertension 19:456–463, 1992.

62. Bittner V: Lipoprotein abnormalities related to women's health. Am J Cardiol 90(suppl):77i–84i, 2002.

63. Pickar JH, Wild RA, Walsh B, et al: Effects of different hormone replacement regimens on postmenopausal women with abnormal lipid levels. Menopause Study Group. Climacteric 1:26–32, 1998.

64. Silbiger S, Ghossein C, Neugarten J: Estradiol inhibits mesangial cell mediated oxidation of low density lipoprotein. J Lab Clin Med 126:385–391, 1995.

65. Chiang K, Parthasarathy S, Santanam N: Estrogen, neutrophils and oxidation. Life Sci 75:2425–2438, 2004.

66. Neugarten J, Acharya A, Lei J, Silbiger S: Selective estrogen receptor modulators suppress mesangial cell collagen synthesis. Am J Physiol Renal Physiol 279:F309–318, 2000.

67. Guccione M, Silbiger S, Lei J, Neugarten J: Estradiol upregulates mesangial cell MMP-2 activity via transcription factor AP-2. Am J Physiol Renal Physiol 282:F164–169, 2002.

68. Potier M, Elliot SJ, Tack I, et al: Expression and regulation of estrogen receptors in mesangial cells: Influence on matrix metalloproteinase-9. J Am Soc Nephrol 12:241–251, 2001.

680

69. Zdunek M, Silbiger S, Lei J, Neugarten J: Protein kinase CK2 mediates TGF-β1-stimulated type IV collagen gene transcription and its reversal by estradiol. Kidney Int 60:2097–2108, 2001.

70. Negulescu O, Bognar I, Lei J, et al: Estradiol reverses TGF-β1-induced mesangial cell apoptosis by a casein kinase 2-dependent mechanism. Kidney Int 62:1989–1998, 2002.

71. Blush J, Lei J, Ju W, et al: Estradiol reverses renal injury in Alb/TGF-β1 transgenic mice. Kidney Int 66:2148–2154, 2004.

72. Nielsen CB, Krag S, Ostergy R, et al: Transforming growth factor beta1-induced glomerulopathy is prevented by 17beta-estradiol supplementation Virchows Arch 444:561–566, 2004.

73. Zeier M, Dohler B, Opelz G, Ritz E: The effect of donor gender on graft survival. J Am Soc Nephrol 13:2570–2576, 2002.

74. Kayler LK, Ramussen CS, Dystra DM, et al: Gender imbalance and outcomes in living donor renal transplantation in the United States. Am J Transplant 3:452–458, 2003.

75. Neugarten J, Silbiger SR: The impact of gender on renal transplantation. Transplantation 58:1145–1152, 1994.

76. Kasiske BL, Snyder JJ, Gilbertson D: Inadequate donor size in cadaveric kidney transplantation. J Am Soc Nephrol 13:2152–2159, 2002.

77. Brenner BM, Milford EL: Nephron underdosing: A programmed cause of chronic renal allograft failure. Am J Kidney Dis 21(suppl 2):66–72, 1993.

78. Brenner BM, Cohen RA, Milford EL: In renal transplantation, one size may not fit all. J Am Soc Nephrol 3:162–169, 1992.

79. Terasaki PI, Cecka JM, Takemoto S, et al: Overview. In Terasaki PI (ed): Clinical Transplants 1988. Los Angeles: UCLA Tissue Typing Laboratory, 1990, p 409.

80. Chertow GM, Milford EL, Mackenzie HS, Brenner BM: Antigen-independent determinants of cadaveric kidney transplant failure. JAMA 276:1732–1736, 1996.

81. Chertow GM, Brenner BM, Mackenzie HS, Milford EL: Non-immunologic predictors of chronic renal allograft failure; Data from the United Network of Organ Sharing. Kidney Int 48(suppl. 52):S48–S51, 1995.

82. Neugarten J, Srinivas T, Tellis V, et al: The effect of donor gender on renal allograft survival. J Am Soc Nephrol 7:318–324, 1996.

83. Shapiro R, Vivas C, Scantlebury VP, et al: "Suboptimal" kidney donors: The experience with tacrolimus-based immunosuppression. Transplantation 62:1242–1246, 1996.

84. Meier-Kriesche HU, Ojo AO, Leavey SF, et al: Differences in etiology for graft loss in female renal transplant recipients. Transplant Proc 33:1288–1290, 2001.

85. Meier-Kriesche HU, Ojo AO, Leavey SF, et al: Gender differences in the risk for chronic renal allograft failure. Transplantation 71:429–432, 2001.

86. Burt VL, Whelton P, Roccella EJ, et al: Prevalence of hypertension in the US adult population: Results from the Third National Health and Nutrition Examination Survey, 1988–1991. Hypertension 25:305–313, 1995.

87. Reckelhoff J: Gender differences in the regulation of blood pressure. Hypertension 37:1199–1208, 2001.

88. Ahimastos AA, Formosa M, Dart AM, Kingwell BA: Gender differences in large artery stiffness pre- and post puberty. J Clin Endocrinol Metab 88:5375–5380, 2003.

89. Anastos K, Charney P, Charon RA, et al: Hypertension in women: What is really known? The Women's Caucus, Working Group on Women's Health of the Society of General Internal Medicine. Ann Intern Med 115:287–293, 1991.

90. Quan A, Kerlikowske K, Gueyffier F, Boissel JP, INDIANA Investigators: Pharmacotherapy for hypertension in women of different races. Cochrane Database Syst Rev Issue 2, 2000.

91. Wassertheil-Smoller S, Anderson G, Psaty BM, et al: Hypertension and its treatment in postmenopausal women: Baseline data from the Women's Health Initiative. Hypertension 36:780–789, 2000.

92. Gueyffier F, Boutitie F, Boissel JP, et al: Effect of antihypertensive drug treatment on cardiovascular outcomes in women and men. A meta-analysis of individual patient data from randomized controlled trials. The INDIANA investigators. Ann Intern Med 126:761–767, 1997.

93. Dubey RK, Oparil S, Imthurn B, Jackson EK: Sex hormones and hypertension. Cardiovasc Res 53:688–708, 2002.

94. Reckelhoff J, Fortepiani LA: Novel mechanisms responsible for postmenopausal hypertension. Hypertension 43:918–923, 2004.

95. Harvey PJ, Wing LM, Savage J, Molloy D: The effects of different types and doses of estrogen replacement therapy on clinic and ambulatory blood pressure and the renin-angiotensin system in normotensive postmenopausal women. J Hypertens 17:405–411, 1999.

96. Pechere-Bertschi A, Burnier M: Female sex hormones, salt, and blood pressure regulation. Am J Hypertens 17:994–1001, 2004.

97. Friedman GD: Oral contraceptives and hypertension. Contrib Nephrol 8:213–220, 1977.

98. The Writing Group for the PEPI Trial: Effects of estrogen or estrogen/progestin regimens on heart disease risk factors in postmenopausal women. The Postmenopausal Estrogen/Progestin Interventions (PEPI) Trial. JAMA 273:199–208, 1995.

99. Fischer M, Baessler A, Schunkert H: Renin angiotensin system and gender differences in the cardiovascular system. Cardiovasc Res. 53:672–677, 2002.

100. Madeddu P, Emanueli C, Song Q, et al: Regulation of bradykinin B2-receptor expression by oestrogen. Br J Pharmacol 121:1763–1769, 1997.

101. O'Donnell CJ, Lindpaintner K, Larson MG, et al: Evidence for association and genetic linkage of the angiotensin-converting enzyme locus with hypertension and blood pressure in men but not women in the Framingham heart study. Circulation 97:1766–1772, 1998.

102. Pechere-Bertschi A, Burnier M: Gonadal steroids, salt-sensitivity and renal function. Curr Opin Nephrol Hypertens 16:16–21, 2007.

Aging and Kidney Disease

Devasmita Choudhury • Moshe Levi

Structural and functional changes associated with biologic aging in the kidney are most evident in the presence of significant physiological and pathophysiological perturbations. Despite aging, the kidney functions to maintain appropriate internal milieu until renal reserve is challenged. Older kidneys seem to adapt less well and recover more slowly in the presence of intervening infections, immunologic processes, exposure to drugs and toxins, or other organ failure. This can be seen with healthy donor kidneys from those older than 55 years of age, which are more likely to fail from chronic allograft nephropathy than younger donor kidneys.[1-5] With a growing older adult population (>65 years), expected to be 54 million by year 2010,[6] and five times greater prevalence of end stage renal disease (ESRD)[7] added to the independent risk of renal failure[6] contributing to mortality, basic knowledge of anatomic, physiologic, and pathologic physiologic changes associated with renal aging may be helpful to avoid disastrous outcomes in the elderly. Renal senescence can now be probed with molecular technology to better understand basic mechanisms such that newer interventions can be entertained to prevent loss of renal function in the elderly. The goal of this chapter then is to provide current understanding of the effect of aging on renal function and disease.

STRUCTURAL CHANGES

Gross and Microscopic

With advancing age, there is a decrease in renal mass as well as weight, size, and volume as noted by radiographic[8] and postmortem studies. Kidney weights of 250 gm to 270 gm in young adulthood decrease over years to 200 gm by the ninth decade. When adjusted for concurrent decrease in body surface area with aging, this decrease may be age appropriate.

Variable sclerotic changes in the walls of the larger renal vessels can be made worse by hypertension.[9] Changes in the aging intrarenal vasculature however can occur, independent of hypertension and other renal diseases. Increased arteriosclerosis of interlobular and arcuate arteries can be seen in older healthy donor kidney biopsies in comparison to younger donors. Sections of human cortical arteries from age 6 to 70 years reveal progressive arterionephrosclerosis with increased fibrointima and medial sclerosis.[10]

Underlying glomerulosclerosis and tubulointerstitial fibrosis may lead to the decrease in renal size and weight noted. Histology reveals a 30% to 50% decrease in cortical glomerular number by age 70 from ischemic changes. There is loss of glomerular tuft lobulation, increased mesangial volume, and capillary collapse with obliteration in the obsolescent glomeruli. There are hyaline deposits in residual glomeruli and Bowman space with little cellular response. Fibrous intimal thickening, medial sclerosis, as well as hyalinosis of both arteries and arterioles is seen (Fig. 21–1).[10-12] Both glomerular and peritubular capillary density is decreased.[13] This may be explained by decreased concentration in proangiogenic vascular endothelial growth factor as well as increased expres-

sion of antiangiogenic factor, thrombospondin-1 as demonstrated in aging rats.[13] These changes in addition to basement membrane wrinkling and thickening of both glomeruli and tubules lead to progressive reduction and simplification of vascular channels.[14,15] Blood flow is then shunted from afferent to efferent arterioles of the juxtamedullary glomeruli, favoring the renal medulla. The arteriolar Vera rectae remain intact to provide adequate blood flow to the medulla.

Renal tubules, lessening in size and number, atrophy to form distal diverticula. These outpouchings may signify formation of early renal cysts as seen in aging kidneys.[16] Collection of debris and bacteria in these structures may then lead to infection and possible pyelonephritis.

Tubulointerstitial fibrosis characterizes the aging renal extracellular matrix and may precede development of focal glomerulosclerosis and tubular atrophy.[17,18] Studies from aging rodents suggest that tubulointerstitial fibrosis may be the result of an active process with associated interstitial inflammation, fibroblast activation, and accelerated apoptosis.[19] The presence of focal tubular proliferation, myofibroblast activation, macrophage infiltration, and increased immunostaining for adhesive proteins osteopontin and intracellular adhesion molecule-1 (ICAM-1) as well as collagen IV deposition are found in aging rat kidneys. Peritubular capillary ischemia and injury with altered endothelial nitric oxide expression (eNOS) is believed to trigger this inflammatory process with subsequent development of focal glomerulosclerosis or tubular atrophy.[20] Collagen-1 protein accumulation increased with age and correlated with the extent of interstitial fibrosis when renal tissue from autopsies was examined.[20,21] Therefore collagen-1 may be an important component of age-associated interstitial fibrosis.

Histological changes may reflect changes at the molecular level. Cell cycle inhibitor, p16INK4a, inversely correlates with cell cycle replication, and is increased with both age and glomerulosclerosis and tubulointerstitial fibrosis.[22] Interestingly telomere length also appears to shorten in an age-dependent fashion in the renal cortex faster than the renal medulla. Telomere DNA repeats is thought to act as mitotic clocks for reflecting replicative senescence

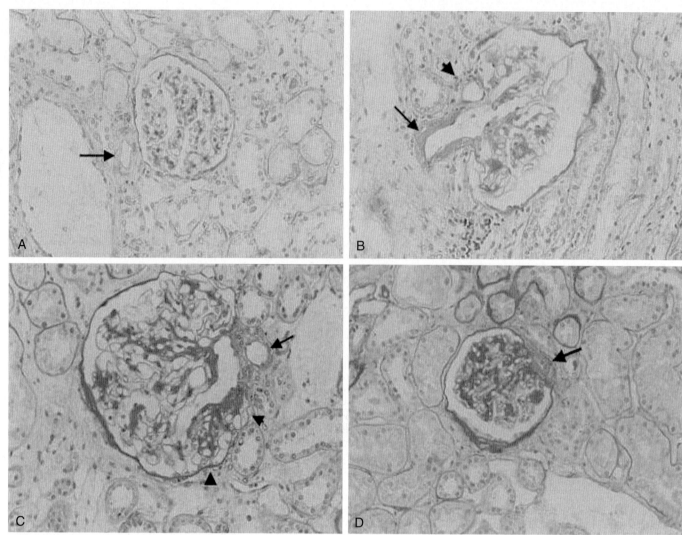

FIGURE 21–1 Glomerular and arteriolar types. **A,** A normal glomerulus and its associated afferent arteriole (arrow) without hyaline deposits. **B,** A hypertrophic glomerulus, which although not particularly large in this plane of section, demonstrates the massive dilatation of hilar capillary and its first branches. Peripheral capillaries are dilated and a channel (arrowhead) leading to the efferent arteriole is also dilated. The dilated afferent arteriole (arrow) shows a massive nonobstructive hyaline deposit. **C,** A focal segmental glomerulosclerosis (FSGS)-type glomerulus shows mesangial increase and sclerosis with capsular adhesions, particularly at hilus (arrowheads). Its associated afferent arteriole (arrow) shows nonobstructive deposits. **D,** An ischemic glomerulus shows collapsing capillary loops with resulting small capillary lumens. Its afferent arteriole (arrow) is without deposits. All were stained with periodic acid-Schiff.[250] (Reprinted with permission from Hill GS, Heudes D, Bariety J: Morphometric study of arterioles and glomeruli in the aging kidney suggests focal loss of autoregulation. Kidney Int 63:1027–1036, 2003.)

of the cell. Critical telomere shortening is seen in the renal cortex in aging. However rodent studies indicate that environmental stresses may contribute more to renal senescence than telomere shortening.[23]

MEDIATORS AND POTENTIAL MODULATORS OF AGE-ASSOCIATED RENAL FIBROSIS

Mediators associated with renal fibrosis (Fig. 21–2) such as angiotensin II, transforming growth factor-β (TGF-β), nitric oxide (NO), advanced glycosylation end products (AGE), oxidative stress, and lipids are also evident in kidneys of aging animals and may be targets for modulating progression of sclerosis. Longitudinal studies in healthy elderly indicate that up to one third of individuals have little functional change in creatinine clearance whereas two thirds show decline in function.[24] Thus it is possible that various factors

hasten sclerosis in some more than others. The ability to modify these factors may result then in preventing progressive age-related decline in renal function.

Angiotensin II

Diverse biologic effects of angiotensin II on the kidney including proximal tubular transport of sodium and water,[25] glomerular and tubular growth,[26–28] decreased nitric oxide (NO) synthesis,[29] immunomodulation, growth factor induction, and accumulation of extracellular matrix proteins can affect glomerulosclerosis and tubulointerstitial fibrosis. Hemodynamic effects of angiotensin II in aging nephrons maintain filtration pressure with preferential efferent arteriolar vasoconstriction. This effect however is also implicated with inducing intraglomerular hypertension and subsequent glomerular damage.[30] With use of angiotensin converting enzyme inhibitors (ACEIs) in aged rats, there is decrease intra renal vascular resistance (RVR) and intracapillary pressure, which decreases protein leak in aging rodents.[31] Chronic ACEI use

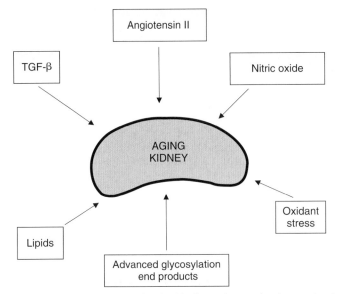

FIGURE 21–2 Factor associated with the pathogenesis of age-related glomerulosclerosis and tubulointerstitial fibrosis. TGF-β, transforming growth factor-β.

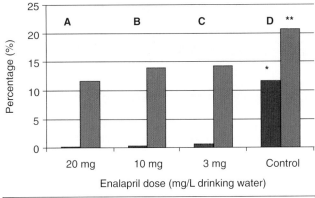

Enalapril dose	Glomerulosclerosis (%)	Mesangial area per glomerulus (%)
20 mg/L	0.1 ± 0.1	11.6 ± 4.8
10 mg/L	0.3 ± 0.1	13.9 ± 2.9
3 mg/L	0.6 ± 0.2	14.2 ± 3.1
Control	11.6 ± 1.9	20.6 ± 1.9

FIGURE 21–3 Effects of angiotensin converting enzyme on renal aging. Enalapril administered to drinking water in aging mice. Group A (n = 16), B (n = 17), C (n = 16), D (n = 10). **P < 0.01, Group A, B, C compared with D. *P < 0.001, Group A, B, C compared with D. (Figure drawn from data from Ferder L, Inserra F, Romano L, et al: Decreased glomerulosclerosis in aging by angiotensin-converting enzyme inhibitors. J Am Soc Nephrol 5:1147–1152, 1994.)

decreases postprandial hyperfiltration, thus decreasing filtered load.[32] Glomerular capillary size selectivity or change in the distribution of negative charge within the glomerular barrier may also be affected with ACEI.[31,33] ACEI-treated aged mice are noted to have a decrease in glomerular area, mesangial area, and overall total decrease in glomerulosclerosis in comparison to age-matched and sex-matched untreated mice (Fig. 21–3).[33–37] It is interesting to note that although systemic

changes in renin and angiotensin converting enzymes may not be evident with aging, there is intrarenal downregulation of renin mRNA and angiotensin converting enzyme level with aging.[38]

Nonhemodynamic growth effects of angiotensin II stimulate profibrotic cytokines. Angiotensin II induces synthesis and autocrine action of TGF-β to stimulate collagen IV transcription in the medullary collecting tubule.[39,40] Angiotensin II also promotes monocyte-macrophage influx, stimulates mRNA and protein expression of the chemokine RANTES in endothelial cells, and inhibits NO.[41] NO inhibition leads to transcription of the proinflammatory chemokine, monocyte chemoattractant protein-1 (MCP-1). Tubulointerstitial fibrosis and α smooth muscle cell actin was significantly reduced when ACEI enalapril-treated aged rats were compared with either calcium channel blocker nifedipine-treated aged rats or untreated aged rats despite similar blood pressure control.[42]

Another nonhemodynamic effect of angiotensin II in the aged kidney may be matrix accumulation by stimulating plasminogen activator inhibitor-1 (PAI-1) from the endothelium.[43] Increased PAI-1 levels inhibit tissue plasminogen activator and urokinase-plasminogen activator and leads to decreased proteolysis and fibrinolysis with increased matrix accumulation.[44] Angiotensin antagonist treated rats had regression of age-related glomerular and vascular sclerosis with decrease in collagen content.[45] Use of angiotensin II antagonists also prevented age-associated decrease in mitochondrial energy production by lessening the age-related increases in mitochondrial oxidants.[46]

The *klotho* gene that is primarily expressed in the kidney and its protein product are associated with suppression of premature aging and arteriosclerosis. Angiotensin II appears to downregulate this gene expression. Mouse *klotho* gene transfer, via adenovirus vector into male Sprague-Dawley rats, ameliorated angiotensin II-mediated renal morphologic damage. Also klotho mRNA downregulation was reversed with the angiotensin II receptor blocker losartan but not by use of other antipressor agents such as hydralazine.[47] Taken together, these animal data suggest benefits of angiotensin II antagonism in elderly with age-related renal functional decline although conclusive data in humans is lacking.

TGF-β

Renal fibrosis seen with aging may be the result of normal or pathologic tissue repair or both. Response to injury is wound healing and tissue repair. Persistent injury or insult may lead to tissue fibrosis. TGF-β, an active modulator of tissue repair, is associated with the structural changes of renal scarring as seen in the aging kidney. A number of factors can stimulate TGF-β including increased angiotensin II activity, abnormal glucose metabolism, platelet-derived growth factors, hypoxic or oxidative stress, mesangial stretch, and increased levels of advanced glycosylation end products (AGE). TGF-β induces gene transcription and production of matrix proteins collagen III, IV, I, fibronectin, tenascin, osteonectin, osteopontin, thrombospondin, and matrix glycosaminoglycans.[48] In addition, TGF-β inhibits collagenase and metalloproteinase (MMP) inhibitors.[49] The net result is accumulation of extracellular matrix proteins with subsequent glomerulosclerosis and tubulointerstitial nephritis.[49–52] TGF-β mRNA is increased in the renal interstitium of aged rats.[18,53] Down-regulation of TGF-β via angiotensin II antagonism results in decreased interstitial fibrosis.[53] Although increased expression of TGF-β may in part mediate age-related sclerosis, direct evidence is not available. Identification and use of antisense oligonucleotides inhibiting TGF-β expression, or function such as decorin may provide better understanding of the role TGF-β plays in aging sclerosis and prevention. Recently identified functions of relaxin, a peptide hormone produced by the pregnant ovary and prostate, include antifibrotic properties. Via direct actions on TGF-β–stimulated fibroblasts to decrease collagen 1 and 3, treatment with relaxin of relaxin-deficient 12-month-old male knockout mice improved established interstitial fibrosis, glomerulosclerosis, and cortical thickening with a decrease in collagen content.[54] Future studies may further clarify the clinical use of this peptide in aging renal sclerosis.

Nitric Oxide

The role of nitric oxide goes beyond affecting vascular reactivity. NO acts to decrease fibrosis by inhibiting the family of transcription factors NF-κB, which in the presence of reactive oxygen intermediates stimulates MCP-1 and promotes influx of monocyte-macrophages leading to inflammation and injury.[55,56] However, in the aging vasculature, levels of nitric oxide are decreased as seen in urinary excretion of stable NO oxidation products (nitrites and nitrates) in aged rats.[57,58] Oxidant stress may also induce NADPH oxidase-mediated NO scavenging and NO depletion in aged kidneys.[59] In addition there is decreased expression of eNOS in peritubular capillaries of aged rats.[19] This can lead to chronic tubulointerstitial ischemia and fibrosis. L-arginine dietary supplementation in aging rats improves renal plasma flow (RPF) and glomerular filtration rate (GFR) and decreases proteinuria and glomerulosclerosis.[60] Supplementation with L-arginine also significantly decreases kidney collagen and N-ε-(carboxymethyl) lysine accumulation.[61] Suspected factors imposing on the age-related decrease in eNOS are increased angiotensin II activity, increased AGE levels, hypoxia, oxidative stress, and dietary protein intake.[58,62–65] Angiotensin II antagonists and or dietary protein restriction is associated with significant increases and normalization of urinary NO excretion.[58]

Advanced Glycosylation End Products

Cross links of glycosylated proteins, lipids, and nucleic acids (AGE) slowly accumulate and produce damage to the vascular and renal tissue with aging.[66,67] In the presence of hyperglycemia, these end products accumulate more rapidly and accelerate tissue damage.[68] These glycated proteins decrease vascular elasticity, induce endothelial cell permeability, and increase monocyte chemotactic activity via AGE-receptor ligand binding, which stimulates macrophage activation and secretion of cytokines and growth factors. AGE accumulation in the vascular endothelium and basement membrane results in defective NO vasodilation, possibly due to chemical inactivation of endothelium-derived relaxing factor.[69–72] Similar perturbations of the vascular endothelium are evident in diabetic patients and those with age-related vasculopathy. Both biochemical assays and histochemical studies have demonstrated increased levels of AGE and AGE-receptor (RAGE) in aged kidneys of animals.[66] AGE deposition in the kidney is associated with increased mesangial matrix, increased basement thickening, increased vascular permeability, and induction of platelet-derived growth factor and TGF-β, resulting in glomerulosclerosis and tubulointerstitial fibrosis.[69] Several factors contribute to AGE and RAGE accumulation including age-related decline in GFR and increased oxidative stress causing oxidative modifications of glycated proteins and accumulation of N-ε-(carboxymethyl) lysine. With age-related insulin resistance there is abnormal glucose metabolism and glycation of proteins. Recent studies also suggest that lifelong AGE-enriched food consumption and smoking can lead to increased AGE loads and increased AGE accumulation in tissues.[73,74]

Although mesangial cell response to AGE/RAGE interaction are increased in the kidney in the presence of hyperglycemia and oxidative stress, a newly identified mesangial cell receptor, AGE-R1, may act to counterregulate the proinflammatory mesangial cell response to increased AGE. Supersaturation and possible receptor downregulation, under increased AGE burden, may prevent appropriate opposing regulatory control of this receptor.[75] In addition, whether aging itself affects mesangial cell receptor expression or activity must be understood. Intuitively then, mechanisms that can increase AGE-R1 antioxidant mesangial receptor activity may be future targets in decreasing AGE-associated tissue changes seen with aging kidneys.

Studies using long-term aminoguanidine treatment in aged rats and rabbits, show marked decreased in glomerulosclerosis and proteinuria,[76] as well as a decrease in age-related arterial stiffening and cardiac hypertrophy.[77] Furthermore, AGE-associated changes in vascular permeability, and abnormal vasodilation to acetylcholine and nitroglycerin were reversed in aminoguanidine-treated animals.[78] In addition, mononuclear cell migration activity was prevented in these animals.

Calorie restriction also seems to decrease the burden of AGE and other glycated proteins including N-ε-(carboxymethyl) lysine and pentosidine in rats restricted to 60% of the ad libitum dietary intake of control rats with improved life span.[79,80] AGE content in renal glomeruli and abdominal aorta of lean 30-month-old rats restricted to even 30% caloric intake was decreased compared to ad libitum control similar aged rats[81] (Fig. 21–4). Future studies may delineate the role of decreasing the burden of AGE in aging individuals.

Oxidative Stress

Tissue injury in aging can occur from free radical production and or antioxidant enzyme deficiency with subsequent lipid peroxidation and oxidative stress.[82–85] Increased urinary oxidized amino acid levels in aged rats indicate the presence of increased oxidized skeletal muscle proteins.[86] Aged kidneys indicate the presence of increased levels of reactive oxygen species and thiobarbiturate acid reactive substances (TBARS), substances associated with lipid oxidative damage.[87] In addition, other markers of oxidative stress and lipid peroxidation such as isoprostanes, AGE, RAGE, increased heme oxygenase, are also noted in aged rats.[88] Experimental studies evaluating oxidant stress on *klotho* gene expression in mouse medullary IMCD3 cells show reduced klotho expression[89] suggesting another possible mechanism toward renal aging. When an antioxidant vitamin E-enriched diet is fed to aged rats, markers of oxidative stress are lessened, with improvements noted in renal plasma flow (RPF), glomerular filtration rate (GFR), as well as decreased glomerulosclerosis.[88] Studies indicate that ACEI can increase antioxidant enzyme activity and block TGF-β induction by reactive oxygen species.[90,91] In addition the anti-oxidant taurine also blocks reactive oxygen species in cultured mesangial cells.[92] A superoxide scavenger, tempol, restored the NO-mediated response of angiotensin II receptor blocker to suppress oxygen consumption in renal cortical tissue.[59] These findings suggest the possibility of both angiotensin II antagonists and anti-oxidants as potential therapeutic options in the future. Furthermore, calorie restriction is also noted to decrease age-related oxidant stress via suppressing activation of mitogen activated protein kinase (MAPK) cellular signaling pathways, as well as mitochondrial lipid peroxidation, and membrane damage with decrease in apoptosis[93,94] suggesting perhaps the need for dietary discrimination in the prevention of age-associated renal sclerosis.

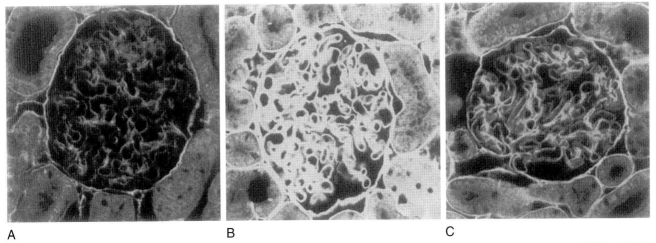

FIGURE 21–4   Immunolocalization of advanced glycosylation end products (AGE) in the renal cortex of 10-month-old (**A**) and 30-month-old (**B**) female WAG/Rij rats fed ad libitum and 30-month-old animals food restricted by 30% (**C**) age localized predominantly in extracellular matrix. Increased AGE accumulation was evident in tubular basement membranes, mesangial matrix, glomerular basement membranes, and Bowman capsule between 10-month-old and 30-month-old rats fed ad libitum. Such accumulation was mostly prevented in food-restricted animals. Magnification ×350. (Reprinted with permission from Teillet L, Verbeke P, Gouraud S, et al: Food restriction prevents advanced glycation end product accumulation and retards kidney aging in lean rats. J Am Soc Nephrol 11:1488–1497, 2000.)

Lipids

Cholesterol accumulation in the kidney occurs with aging and may contribute to the progression of glomerulosclerosis and proteinuria.[95,96] Sterol regulatory element binding proteins 1 and 2 (SREBP-1 and SREBP-2), key regulators of fatty acid and cholesterol synthesis, are associated with increased synthesis and renal accumulation of triglyceride and cholesterol in aged rats.[96] In addition, serum leptin levels are also increased in aging.[96] The presence of oxidative stress and increases in AGE level in aging may further contribute to increased levels of modified low density lipoproteins (LDL), lipoprotein (a).[97–99] Associated with increased free oxygen radical formation, increased expression of growth factors such as platelet-derived growth factor and TGF-β, inhibition of NO synthesis, migration and adherence of monocytes, and growth of mesangial and vascular cells, these lipids can add to the pathogenic role of aging-related renal disease progression. Calorie restriction in aging rats have shown not only decreases in extracellular matrix accumulation and expression of growth factors, but also significant decreases in renal nuclear SREBP-1 and SREBP-2 abundance and renal triglyceride and cholesterol accumulation.[96]

Similar changes of glomerulosclerosis and tubulointerstitial fibrosis occur from lipo-oxidative stress with high cholesterol feeding in type 2 diabetic rats.[100] When treated with 3–hydroxy-3-methylglutaryl-coenzyme A (HMG-CoA) reductase inhibitor for 12 months, streptozotocin-induced diabetic rats decrease urine albumin excretion and glomerular volume compared with untreated rats.[101] Both diabetic and nondiabetic patients treated long term with HMG-CoA reductase inhibitors and or peroxisome proliferator activated receptor-α (PPAR-α) agonists seem to decrease proteinuria and partially preserve GFR.[102–104] Further studies defining their role in the prevention of age-related renal changes in humans must be done.

FUNCTIONAL CHANGES

Renal Plasma Flow

Changes in renal plasma flow as measured by paraaminohippurate clearance note a 10% decrease per decade increase from the third to ninth decade.[105] Xenon washout scans demonstrate a preferential decrease in cortical blood flow with medullary flow preserved, paralleling the histological changes observed with aging. Although changes in cardiac output may possibly be contributing the decrease in RPF, there seems to be a small but definite decrease in the renal fraction of the cardiac output.[106,107] Changes in anatomic and vascular responsiveness seen with aging may explain this decrease.

When vasodilation is assessed in elderly healthy subjects with infusion intra-arterial acetylcholine, or intravenous infusion of pyrogen or atria natriuretic peptide (ANP), vascular response is altered.[108] Older subject have a blunted response in comparison to younger counterparts. This is also noted with infusion of amino acids, where RPF is unchanged whereas filtration fraction (FF) increases with increases in GFR.[109] With the addition of dopamine and amino acid, older subjects increase RPF and GFR although the response is less in older subjects than younger subjects (Fig. 21–5).[9]

Abnormal intrarenal signaling in the older subjects may lead to impaired vasorelaxation.[110] Stimulation of the renal sympathetic system results in exaggerated vasoconstriction.[111,112] Mediators of vasorelaxation, such as vasodilatory prostacyclin (PGI2) are decreased in aged human vascular cells and aged rat kidneys compared with vasoconstrictive thromboxanes.[113,114] Older subjects also excrete less vasodilatory natriuretic prostaglandins. With inhibition of angiotensin II, vasodilation appears to be exaggerated or preserved.[115,116] RPF increases significantly in aged rats.[117] This allows for speculation for possibly a greater role for angiotensin II-mediated vasoconstriction in the aging renal vessels; however, intra-arterial angiotensin infusion leads to similar vasoconstrictive responses in both young and older human subjects. With preserved vasoconstriction and blunted vasodilation, it is possible that the aged kidney remains in a state of renal vasodilation to compensate for underlying sclerotic damage.

Similar changes with intravenous glycine infusion are observed in aged rats that histologically correlate with progressive glomerulosclerosis.[118] With competitive inhibition of endothelium-derived relaxing factor, NO, there is a significant increase in vasoconstriction, increased RVR, and decreased RPF in aged rats versus younger rats.[119] Micropuncture demonstrates no age-associated changes in magnitude of pressor or vasoconstriction with angiotensin II infusion in

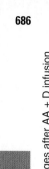

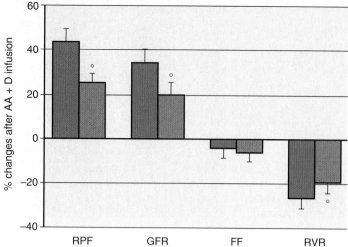

FIGURE 21–5 Percent changes in renal plasma flow (RPF), glomerular filtration rate (GFR), filtration fraction (FF), and renal vascular resistance (RVR) in younger (blue bars) and older (red bars) subjects ($P<0.05$ for the difference in changes between the two groups). (Reprinted from Fuiano G, Sund S, Mazza G, et al: Renal hemodynamic response to maximal vasodilating stimulus in healthy older subjects. Kidney Int 59:1052–1058, 2001.)

rats. Both pre-glomerular and efferent arteriolar resistances increase whereas RPF and glomerular plasma flow decrease accompanied by a rise in glomerular hydraulic pressure gradient and increased filtration fraction in both young and older rats. Single nephron GFR (SNGFR) and GFR are lower in older rats with noted decrease in glomerular capillary ultrafiltration coefficient (Kf), with no change in these parameters in the younger rats. Angiotensin II-mediated glomerular mesangial cell contraction and decrease in Kf likely translates to decreased filtration surface.[120] Studies in healthy transplant donors suggest that a drop in Kf with age may be the function of both underlying structural changes lowering single nephron Kf and a decrease in the number of functioning glomeruli.[105]

Despite a linear decrease in RPF, filtration fraction increases with age.[105] Preserved medullary flow in relation to decreased cortical flow may allow for a higher juxtamedullary FF than cortical nephrons.

Glomerular Filtration Rate

Changes in GFR can be expected with gradual renal senescence. Factors including race, gender, genetic variation, and underlying risk factors for renal disease all contribute to the rate of GFR decline in the elderly. Increased arterial stiffness, as reflected by elevated pulse pressure in older individuals, also appears to inversely correlate with age-related loss in GFR.[121] Retinal microvascular abnormalities indicative of systemic microvascular disease in elderly participants of the Cardiovascular Health Study are associated with greater decline in GFR.[122]

Methodological variations differ in gauging the rate of change. A decrease in urea clearance was noted in the late 1930s and confirmed with noted decreases in inulin, creatinine, and iothalamate clearances with increasing age.[105] Iohexol clearances indicate a drop of 1.0 ml/min/1.73 m² per year.[123] Despite normal protein intake, the decrease in inulin clearance in older subjects without renal disease is less than younger controls. Creatinine clearance drops from 0.8 ml/min/1.73 m² per year from age 40 to age 80 years in healthy elderly subjects.[124] However, a parallel rise in serum creatinine is not seen because muscle mass concomitantly decreases with age. Clinically this translates to an overestimation of GFR in older patients when using serum creatinine alone to assess medication dosing or renal risk to the aged kidney for ischemic, toxic, or metabolic events. Commonly used formulas (Table 21–1) to estimate GFR frequently overestimate or underestimate GFR in the older subjects (Fig. 21–6).[6,125,126]

TABLE 21–1	Commonly Used Formulas to Estimate Glomerular Flow Rate (GFR)

1. Creatinine clearance (mL/min/1.73 m²) = $(1.33 - 0.64) \times$ age*

2. Creatinine clearance (ml/min) = $\dfrac{(140 - \text{age}) \times \text{weight (kg)}}{72 \times \text{serum creatinine (mg/dl)}}$*

3. GFR = $170 \times [P_{cr}]^{-0.999} \times [\text{age}]^{-0.0176} \times [0.762 \text{ if patient is female}] \times [1.180 \text{ if patient is black}] \times [\text{SUN}]^{-0.0170} \times [\text{alb}]^{+0.318}$

*15% less in females.

Formula 1 from Rowe JW, Andrew R, Tobin JD, et al: Age-adjusted standards for creatinine clearance. Ann Intern Med 84:567–569, 1976. Formula 2 from Cockcroft DW, Gault MH: Prediction of creatinine clearance from serum creatinine. Nephron 16:31–41, 1976. Formula 3 from Levey AS, Bosch J, Lewis JB, et al: A more accurate method to estimate glomerular filtration rate from serum creatinine: A new prediction equation. Ann Intern Med 130:461–470, 1999.

The GFR formula derived from the Modification of Diet in Renal Disease (MDRD) study appears to more closely proximate GFR changes in aged subjects.[126] Newer markers such as serum 2-(alpha-mannopyranosyl)-L-tryptophan (MTP)[127] and cystatin C are being considered for estimating GFR. Cystatin C, an endogenous cysteine proteinase with a constant rate of production by nucleated cells, freely filtered, reabsorbed, and catabolized, but not secreted by the renal tubules is being evaluated more closely for accuracy in predicting GFR in the elderly.[128] Future widespread availability of this marker may increase its applicability in estimating GFR in the elderly.

Routine 24-hour creatinine clearance to estimate GRF may be cumbersome with measurement precision dependent on the volume collected, diet, and other factors. Radionuclide clearances with technetium 99m-labelled diethylenetriamine-pentacetic acid (99mTc-DTPA)125-iothalamte or radiocontrast clearance with single injection iohexol x-ray fluorescence analysis can also be done.[129] However expense, radioactivity exposure, and test availability may be limiting factors.

Although some studies suggest a bias toward slower decline with being female, the role of gender with declining GFR in the elderly population is not yet clear. Genetic variance and race seem however to suggest a greater loss of GFR in aging African Americans and those of Japanese origin than whites.[130,131] The presence of hypertension,[132,133] and other risk factors including glucose intolerance,[134] frank diabetes, systemic or renal atherosclerosis, and abnormal lipid metabolism add to a greater rate of GFR decline in the elderly.

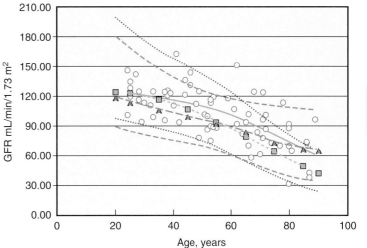

○   Inulin clearance in healthy men (Davies & Shock 1950)
— ▲ — NHANES III GFR calculation (median, 5th, 95th %iles)
- - ■ - - NHANES III Cockroft-Gault (median, 5th, 95th %iles)

FIGURE 21–6 Percentiles of glomerular filtration rate (GFR) and Cockcroft-Gault creatinine clearance (CCr) by age, plotted on the same graph as data from 1950 on inulin clearance in healthy men by Davies and Shock (J Clin Invest 29:496, 1950). Percentiles are calculated using a fourth-order polynomial weighted quantile regression. The solid line shows a polynomial regression to the inulin data. Dashed lines without symbols show the fifth and ninety-fifth percentiles for GFT estimates. (Reprinted from Coresh J, Astor BC, Greene T, et al: Prevalence of chronic kidney disease and decreased kidney function in the US population: Third National Health and Nutrition Examination Survey. Am J Kidney Dis 41:1–12, 2003.)

Sodium Conservation

Tubular efficiency in conserving filtered sodium declines with aging. This is seen with sodium restriction in older healthy subjects who take twice as long to decrease urinary sodium excretion in comparison to younger subjects under similar conditions. Subjects ≥60 years take almost 31 hours to decrease urinary sodium compared with 17.6 hours in those ≤30 years old.[135] Distal sodium conservation may be diminished (Fig. 21–7).[136] Age-related changes in interstitial scarring, decreased nephron number, and increased medullary flow likely increase solute load per nephron as observed in patients with chronic renal failure.

In addition, both levels and responses to hormones that regulate tubular sodium reabsorption change with aging. Concentration of plasma renin and aldosterone are decreased in aging healthy elderly subjects. A 30% to 50% lower basal renin activity is noted despite normal levels of renin substrate. Maneuvers such as upright position, 10 meq/day sodium intake, furosemide administration, and air jet stress that stimulate renin secretion further amplifies age-related differences in plasma renin activity.[137,138] Decreased juxtamedullary single nephron renin content,[139] down-regulation of renin mRNA abundance, and decreased renal angiotensin converting enzyme levels and decreased type-1 angiotensin receptor mRNA are found in aged rats.[38,140] Both pre and post hemorrhage plasma renin content are decreased in 15-month-old rats in comparison to 3-month-old rats.[38] Sodium deprivation with a resultant fall in mean arterial pressure revealed a blunted response to plasma renin activity with delayed fall in urinary sodium excretion.[141] Normal aging adults have decreased conversion of inactive to active renin when plasma renin substrate is measured.[142]

Plasma aldosterone also decreases in parallel with aging with a fall of 30% to 50% seen in older adults versus younger counterparts. Because infusion of adrenocorticotropic hormone produces an appropriate aldosterone and cortisol response, aldosterone deficiency with aging is more likely related to a renin-angiotensin deficiency and not an intrinsic adrenal defect.[143] Interestingly the sluggish response to dietary sodium restriction can be reproduced by ACE inhibition and blocking of the renin-angiotensin-aldosterone system (RAAS).[144] Tubular sensitivity to aldosterone infusion appears appropriate with increased sodium reabsorption noted, lending further support to an abnormal RAAS response

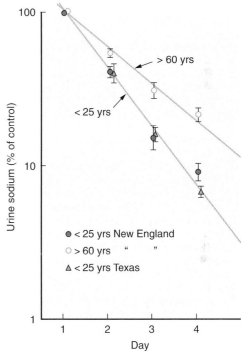

FIGURE 21–7 Response of urinary sodium excretion to restriction of sodium intake in normal humans. The mean half-time (t1/2) for eight subjects older than 60 years was 30.9±2.8 hours, exceeding the mean t1/2 of 17.6±0.7 hours for subjects younger than 25 years of age (P<0.01). When younger subjects were separated by geographic area, the mean t1/2 for the Texas group (>17.9±0.7 hours) was similar to that of the New England group (>15.6±1.4 hours; P<0.3). (Reprinted from Macias Nunez JF, Garcia Iglesias C, Bondia Roman A, et al: Renal handling of sodium in old people: A functional study. Age Ageing 7:178–181, 1978.)

as an important factor leading to delayed sodium conservation with aging.

Sodium Excretion

Tubular natriuretic capacity is also blunted with aging. This is seen with sodium loading or volume expansion in healthy elderly.[145,146] A 2 liter saline load is excreted much slower with a greater amount excreted overnight in adults over 40 years of age than gender-, size-, and race-matched younger adults.[130,147] This circadian variation in sodium excretion with older adults may add to the higher frequency of nocturia seen in this population.

Studies implicate a diminished response to atrial natriuretic peptide (ANP), an important factor in the control of sodium excretion. ANP via specific cell surface receptors on the renal microvasculature and tubular epithelium induces hyperfiltration, inhibits luminal membrane sodium channels and reabsorption, and suppresses renin release. Released from atrial myocytes in response to atrial stretch, ANP is rapidly degraded but serum half-life can be prolonged with selective blockade of degradative enzymes or clearance receptors.[148] Healthy older adults have elevated basal levels three to five times those of healthy young adults.[149,150] Stimulation of ANP with increased salt load, head-out body water immersion leads to higher levels in older versus younger individuals.[151] Decreased salt intake results in similar ANP levels in old and young adults. This suggests intact ANP release with aging. However, higher basal levels may be a result of decreased metabolic clearance with aging.[152,153] A decrease in GFR with aging may not be the etiology, given that patients with chronic kidney disease and low GFR do not have high ANP levels.[154] However, endopeptidases, degradative enzymes in the renal proximal brush border, which degrade ANP, may be decreased with aging. Rats with reduced renal mass when infused with endopeptidase inhibitors, phosphoramidon, have increased urinary cGMP (ANP second messenger) and urinary salt excretion.[155] Similarly renal endopeptidase inhibition by candoxatril in class II New York Heart Association congestive heart failure patients significantly increased ANP and cGMP levels as well as urinary sodium excretion without changes in renal hemodynamics.[156] Metabolic clearance of low level ANP infusate is decreased in older compared with younger subjects.[152]

Some investigators propose that higher ANP levels may be homeostatic to reduced renal sensitivity with aging.[145,146] A blunted response to incremental increases in ANP infusion is seen with older adults who do not continue to increase urinary sodium beyond 2 ng/kg/min, whereas younger subjects have progressive increase in their urinary sodium excretion with increased ANP infusion (Fig. 21–8).[145] Baseline cGMP and ANP second messenger levels may not change with age. Although cGMP[157] increases with low-dose ile-ANP administration, increased urinary sodium is not seen in older subjects.[152] This suggests a possible post-cGMP problem.

Simultaneous measurements in plasma renin and aldosterone during ANP infusion notes that natriuretic properties of ANP is different from that of inhibiting sodium reabsorption via suppression of RAAS. Each property of ANP appears to be influenced differently by age.[145,152]

Urinary Concentration

The ability to maximize urinary concentration is diminished with aging (Fig. 21–9).[124,158] Appropriate urinary concentration under hyperosmolar and water-deprived conditions depends on intact osmoreceptor and volume receptor sensitivity of arginine vasopressin (AVP) release in addition to an intact collecting tubule response to AVP under maximum medullary tonicity. With aging, a combination of processes appears to impair water conservation.

Both volume pressure and osmotic stimulation of AVP release is intact in the elderly with osmoreceptor AVP sensitivity enhanced.[159,160] Basal circulating AVP levels are also increased after 24 hours of water deprivation in older adults.[161,162] Intrarenal resistance to AVP infusion in healthy older adults is suspected given that decreased concentrating capacity is not corrected with AVP infusion.[163] A medullary "washout" is suggested with increased medullary blood flow in the aged kidney, increased solute excretion and osmolar clearance as well as decreased urine osmolality in elderly healthy subjects deprived of water for 12 hours overnight.[124] Water diuresis in older adults demonstrates decreased sodium chloride transport in the ascending loop of Henle.[164] Studies in aged rats however suggest AVP resistance in the collecting tubules. Solute free water formation after 40 hours dehydration and exogenous AVP is normal; however, solute free water reabsorption is impaired. Solute content in the inner medulla is identical in young and older rats. This suggests intact ascending limb solute transport but diminished collecting tubule water transport.[165]

Investigation of collecting tubule response to AVP suggests no change in receptor number or affinity for AVP.[166] However, greater amounts of AVP are required to increase cAMP, which is decreased in older animals.[167,168] Post receptor guanine nucleotide-binding protein (Gs) is also decreased in aging kidneys.[169] Stimulation of the G proteins with cholera toxin and using forskolin to stimulate adenylate cyclase at the level of the catalytic unit and G protein interaction resulted in significantly lower adenylate cyclase stimulation from older rabbit cortical collecting tubule (CCT).[170] Thus an inadequate AVP response in the CCT in aging may be located to the level of interaction of Gs catalytic subunit of adenylate cyclase.

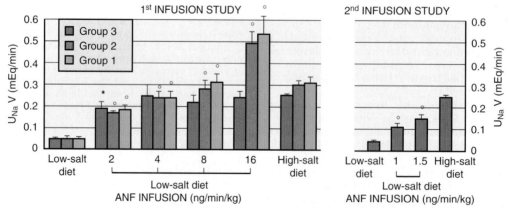

FIGURE 21–8 Urinary sodium excretion (UnaV) with a low-salt diet (in basal condition and during infusion of atrial natriuretic factor (ANF)) and with a high-salt diet in young (group 1), middle age (group 2), and elderly (group 3) subjects. The columns represent means and the bars SE. °$P<0.05$ versus other steps and low-salt diet, *$P<0.01$ versus low-salt diet. (Reprinted from Leosco D, Ferrara N, Landino P, et al: Effects of age on the role of atrial natriuretic factor in renal adaptation to physiologic variations of dietary salt intake. J Am Soc Nephrol 7:1045–1051, 1996.)

A

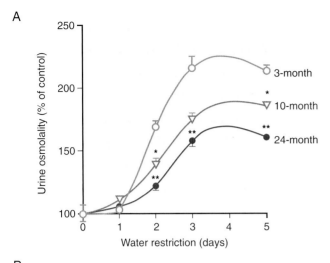

B

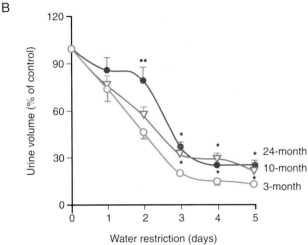

FIGURE 21-9 Age-related changes in urine osmolality (**A**) and urine volume (**B**) after mild water restriction. Urine osmolality and volume in the water restricted rats were expressed s a percentage of the non dehydrated rats of each age group. Values are expressed as means±SE (n=12; *$P<0.05$ compared with 3-month-old rats, **$P<0.05$ compared with 3-month-old and 10-month-old rats). (Reprinted from Tian Y, Serino R, Verbalis JG: Downregulation of renal vasopressin V2 receptor and aquaporin-2 expression parallels age-associated defects in urine concentration. Am J Physiol Renal Physiol 287. F797–805, 2004.)

Evaluation of collecting duct water channel activity in older rats is notable for decreased expression of aquaporin-2 (AQP-2)[158] (Fig. 21–10) and aquaporin-3 (AQP-3) in medullary collecting duct of older rats compared to younger rats whereas papillary cAMP content was not different.[171] V2 mRNA abundance is also decreased in aged rats under baseline conditions despite equivalent plasma AVP concentration as in young rats.[158] Furthermore, V2 receptors on basolateral membranes in dehydrated older and younger rats have similar levels of downregulation.[172] This in part may explain the low water permeability in the inner medullary collecting duct and decreased urinary concentration seen with aging.

Decreased urea transporters, UT-A1 and UT-B-1, expression is also seen in the renal medulla of older rats with decrease papillary osmolality whether food restricted on ad libitum diet.[173] Deamino-8-D arginine vasopressin (DDAVP) infusion improved papillary urea accumulation and improved urine osmolality and flow rates with up-regulation of urea transporters.[174] These data suggest another mechanism by which urinary concentration may be affected in aging kidneys.

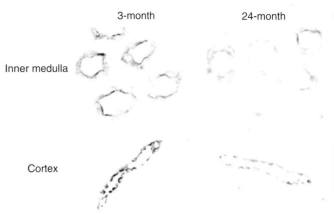

FIGURE 21-10 Immunohistolocalization of AQP2 under baseline conditions. AQP2 staining in both the inner medulla (top) and cortex (bottom) is less intense in 24-month-old rats compared with 3-month-old F344BN rats. Staining of the apical membrane is specifically reduced by visual inspection, particularly in the inner medulla (original magnification ×400). (Reprinted with permission from Tian Y, Serino R, Verbalis JG: Downregulation of renal vasopressin V2 receptor and aquaporin-2 expression parallels age-associated defects in urine concentration. Am J Physiol Renal Physiol 287:F797–805, 2004.)

Urinary Dilution

An impairment in urinary diluting capacity is seen with aging when older individuals undergo water diuresis.[175] The minimum osmolality reached in subjects older than 70 years is 92 mOsm/kgH$_2$O compared with 52 mOsm/kgH$_2$O in subjects younger than 40 years. Oral water loading of 20 ml/kg plus overnight fast from fluids in older versus younger adults results in free water clearance of 6.0±0.6 ml/min in the elderly compared to 10.1±0.8 ml/min in the young. Various factors including appropriate solute extraction, adequate AVP suppression must occur with the distally delivered filtered load. Although a decline in GFR may be contributing, solute free water clearance is decreased despite correction for GFR.[175] Other factors including appropriate AVP suppression or solute extraction (or both) in the ascending loop need further clarification.

Acid-Base Balance

Although homeostatic acid base balance is maintained in the elderly, acid loading reveals an impaired ability to excrete the acid load. Age-associated loss of renal mass and decrease in GFR may be contributing. Constant endogenous acid production from a steady-state acid diet leads to worsening of a low-grade metabolic acidosis with age. Changes in both blood pH and plasma HCO$_3$ correlate with changes in GFR with age (Fig. 21–11). A reciprocal increase in plasma chloride concentration as noted with early renal disease or renal tubular acidosis is seen.[176] Ammonia excretion appears to account for less of the total acid excretion in older adults than younger adults. With glutamine intake, ammonium excretion increased in equal amounts and with the same rapidity in both older and younger subjects.[177] However, ammonium loading in older patients resulted in reduced ammonium excretion with inability to reach minimal urinary pH despite correction for GFR[178] suggesting a possible intrinsic tubular defect. This is confirmed by animal studies of ammonium loading. Sodium-hydrogen exchanger activity, a major regulator of proximal tubular transport was similarly enhanced in young and aged rages.[179] Phosphate transport was reduced to the same extent in both groups.[179] Thus impaired ammonium excretion may mediate the age-related renal impairment to metabolic acidosis.

690

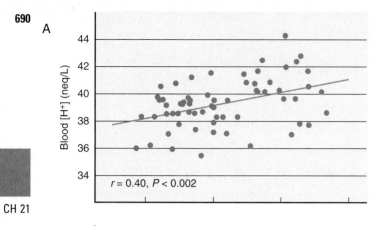

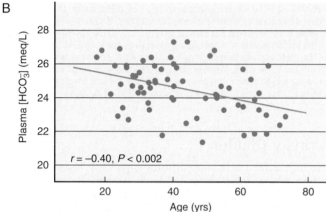

FIGURE 21–11 Relation between blood pH ((H+)b) and age (**A**), and between plasma bicarbonate concentration ((HCO3–)p) and age (**B**), in normal adult humans (n=64). Each data point represents the mean steady-state value in a subject eating a constant diet. Regression equations: (H+)b=0.045×age+37.2 (HCO3–)p=−0.038×age+26.0. (Reprinted from Frassetto LA, Morris RC, Jr, Sebastian A: Effect of age on blood acid-base composition in adult humans: Role of age-related renal functional decline. Am J Physiol 271:F1114–1122, 1996.)

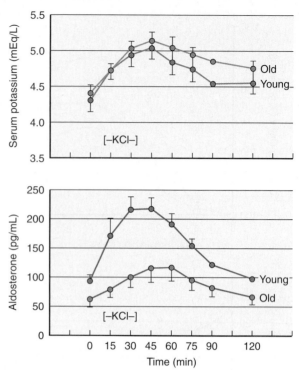

FIGURE 21–12 Serum potassium and aldosterone levels before, during, and after infusion of potassium chloride (0.05 mEq/kg body weight over 45 minutes) in six healthy young and six healthy elderly men. Changes in serum potassium levels were similar, but elderly subjects have lower aldosterone responses (P<0.005) by analysis of variance. (Reprinted from Mulkerrin E, Epstein FH, Clark BA: Aldosterone responses to hyperkalemia in healthy elderly humans. J Am Soc Nephrol 6:1459–1462, 1995.)

The subtle degree of metabolic acidosis that exists in the elderly is not associated with laboratory abnormalities in serum bicarbonate or pH. However, bone demineralization and muscle wasting, complications of chronic metabolic acidosis, are common in the elderly. Increased protein intake increases endogenous acid production. Underlying metabolic acidosis regulated calcium and alkali mobilization from bone and inhibits renal calcium reabsorption. Acidosis-induced enhanced muscle breakdown is medicated by activation of an ATP-dependent ubiquitin and proteasome pathway.[180] In industrialized nations, increased protein intake in the elderly in conjunction with aging and impaired acid excretion, may be associated with negative calcium balance, osteoporosis, and increased incidence of fractures and muscle wasting despite eubicarbonatemia.[181] Studies in postmenopausal women have noted improved nitrogen and calcium balance with potassium bicarbonate supplementation.[182] Whether bicarbonate supplementation should be recommended as an intervention in the elderly to prevent complications of subtle acidosis remains to be determined.

Potassium Balance

Total body potassium decreases with advancing age and loss of muscle mass and is more pronounced in women than men. Plasma renin and aldosterone levels parallel this decrease.[183] As a result, a relative hypoaldosteronism predisposes the

elderly to hyperkalemia. Potassium infusion results in a blunted aldosterone response in the elderly (Fig. 21–12).[184] Potassium excretion on high potassium diet was less efficient in older rats. The rise in plasma potassium was also higher when KCL infusion was given. Bilateral nephrectomy and high k feeding along with KCL infusion, revealed inability of the older rats to decrease serum potassium. Sodium-potassium exchange pump (Na+-K+ ATPase) activity was decreased by 38% in the medulla of the older rats.[185] No effect of aging was noted with insulin-mediated potassium uptake in humans.[186] Exercise-mediated potassium increase in the elderly suggest an impaired β-adrenergic-induced increase in the adenylate cyclase system yielding a decreased activity of the Na+K+ ATPase pump in skeletal muscle.[187]

Defect in renal acidification and also of the RAAS in the elderly may contribute to the increased incidence of type 4 renal tubular acidosis (RTA) or syndrome of hyporeninemic hypoaldosteronism in this population. Given problems with chronic potassium adaptation with aging, medications inhibiting the RAAS including ACEIs, heparin, cyclosporine, tacrolimus, β-blockers, spirolactone, and NSAIDs can increase the risk of hyperkalemia in older adults. In addition, sodium channel blockers such as trimethoprim, pentamidine, amiloride, and triamterene can add to the underlying defects in potassium excretion in the elderly.

Calcium Balance

Calcium reabsorption in the renal tubules is unaffected with aging though calcium metabolism is impaired. Both reabsorption and excretion of calcium is appropriate in aged rats under conditions of either decreased or increased dietary calcium.[188] The absolute filtered load and proximal reabsorption of calcium per nephron is unaffected between young and aged rats.[189]

Intestinal calcium reabsorption is decreased with aging and correlates with decrease 1-α-hydroxlase activity, decreased 1.25-dihydroxy-cholecalciferol (1,25(OH)2D3), and increased basal parathyroid hormone (PTH) levels. The 1,25(OH)2D3—dependent calcium binding protein declines with age in parallel with the age-related drop in calcium absorption.[188,190] PTH infusion stimulated less renal 1,25(OH)2D3 production in healthy elderly although final concentrations were not different between the older and younger groups. Urinary cAMP and fractional phosphorus excretion also increased similarly in both groups, suggesting that the renal response to PTH infusion is intact with aging.[191] However, calcium regulation of PTH release may be altered with aging shown by calcium gluconate infusion and sodium ethylenediamene tetraacetic acid (NaEDTA) infusion in relation to PTH response. Serum concentration of PTH reflects an increase in both the set point for calcium and the number of parathyroid cells. It is not clear if the G protein-coupled calcium-sensing receptor (CaSR), which alters the set point for PTH seen in primary and secondary uremic hyperparathyroidism, plays a role in the increase in the set point for PTH release seen with aging.[192]

Phosphate Balance

Metabolic balance and clearance studies in humans and rats reveal an age-related decrease in intrinsic capacity of renal tubules to reabsorb phosphate.[192,193] Renal adaptation to a low phosphate diet is impaired with age.[95,194] In addition, there is an age-related decrement in intestinal phosphate absorption. Maximum inorganic phosphate (Pi) transport capacity (TmPi) assessed in parathyroidectomized aged rats infused with graded levels of Pi shows a significant drop in TmPi with age. Parathyroid hormone infusion in these rats reveals an appropriate further drop in TmPi; however, the magnitude of the response decreased with age.[193]

A similar age-related impairment in phosphate transport has also been demonstrated in primary cultures of renal tubule cells from young and adult rats.[195] In agreement with the in vivo studies,[194] there is a decrease in maximum velocity of sodium-dependent phosphate transport (Na/Pi cotransport) and decreased ability to adapt to low-phosphate culture media in renal tubular cells cultured from old rats compared with young adult rats. This is accompanied by a decrease in type IIa Na/Pi cotransporter cortical mRNA level and apical brush border membrane protein abundance in aged rats.[196]

An additional factor that may play a role in the decrease in Na/Pi cotransport is the age-related increase in membrane cholesterol content.[197] In vitro cholesterol enrichment of isolated brush border membranes of young adult rats reproduces the age-related impairment in V_{max} of Na/Pi cotransport activity.[197] Direct changes in opossum kidney cell cholesterol content appears to affect Na/Pi cotransport activity by changing expression of the apical membrane type II Na/Pi cotransport protein.[198] Thus changes in membrane cholesterol content with aging may play a role in phosphate transport.

The role of vitamin D (1,25(OH)2D3) metabolism with aging and its effect on intestinal phosphate transport must be considered given that vitamin D-deficient animals improve both renal and intestinal phosphate transport when given vitamin D replacement.[199–201] The changes in phosphate transport associated with vitamin D parallel significant changes in brush border membrane lipid composition and fluidity.[202] This suggests that 1,25(OH)2D3 may possibly act via lipid modulating effects on the aged to improve renal and intestinal transport of phosphate (and calcium).

Osmolar Disorders

Hyponatremia
Hyponatremia is a common finding in geriatric patients with the greatest prevalence in chronic care facilities. Enhanced osmotic AVP release and impaired diluting capacity predisposes the elderly to a higher incidence of hyponatremia.[203] The idiopathic form of syndrome of anti-diuretic hormone secretion can be easily found among many older ambulatory clinic patients.[204] Thiazide diuretic use in older adults further impairs an already present dilution defect and is implicated in 20% to 30% of the cases of hyponatremia.[205] Deficient prostaglandin synthesis with aging may increase thiazide susceptibility to hyponatremia as water diuresis is impaired with inhibition of prostaglandin synthesis.[205] Other common medications including sulfonylureas, chlorpropramide, tolbutamide, or NSAIDs potentiate peripheral AVP action and can be synergistic in decreasing water excretion. Medications that lead to a nonosmotic release of AVP or potentiation of AVP action on the renal tubules by medications can also worsen or exacerbate hyponatremia in the elderly and should be used carefully (Table 21–2).

Significant or acute hyponatremia frequently leads to a myriad of signs and symptoms including apathy, disorientation, lethargy, muscle cramps, anorexia, nausea, agitation, depressed tendon reflexes, pseudobulbar palsy, and seizures. This results from an osmotic shift of water from the

CH 21

Aging and Kidney Disease

TABLE 21–2	Mechanisms by which Drugs Can Lead to Impaired Water Metabolism		
Inhibit AVP Release	**Inhibit Peripheral Action of AVP**	**Potentiate AVP Release**	**Potentiate Peripheral Action of AVP**
Fluphenazine	Lithium	Nicotine	Tolbutamide
Haloperidol	Colchicine	Vincristine	Chlorpropramide
Promethazine	Vinblastine	Histamine	Nonsteroidal anti-inflammatory drugs
Morphine (low doses)	Demeclocycline	Morphine (high doses)	
Alcohol	Glyburide	Epinephrine	
Carbamazepine	Methoxyflurane	Cyclophosphamide	
Norepinephrine	Acetohexamide	Angiotensin	
Cisplatinum	Propoxyphene	Bradykinin	
Clonidine	Loop diuretics		
Glucocorticoids			

AVP, arginine vasopressin.

691

extracellular to the intracellular space. Prompt recognition and appropriate initiation of therapy is necessary to avoid severe neurological sequelae including central pontine myelinolysis.

Hypernatremia

Susceptibility to hypernatremia is common for the elderly with impaired renal concentrating and sodium conserving ability. Thirst followed by fluid intake usually defends against hypernatremia and free water loss. However, the thirst mechanism is frequently decreased in the elderly. In addition, altered levels of consciousness or immobility often prevent geriatric patient's access to free water replacement. Significant hypernatremia can be lethal in some cases with mortality as high as 46% to 70%.[206] Acute increases in serum sodium concentrations more than 160 mEq/l is associated with a 75% mortality rate.

Medications that can cloud the sensorium (e.g., sedatives, tranquilizers) and inhibit thirst or further inhibit AVP action in the renal tubules such as lithium or demeclocycline should be given with caution. Use of osmotic diuretics, parenteral high protein or glucose feedings, and bowel cathartics must be monitored carefully. Geriatric patients with systemic illnesses, infections, dementia, fevers, or neurological disorders that impair AVP release are at high risk for dehydration and hypernatremia. Cellular dehydration can lead to severe obtundation, stupor, coma, seizures, and death. Therefore cautious review and monitoring of electrolytes and medications in older particularly debilitated patients is necessary.

AGING AND RENAL DISEASE

Acute Renal Failure

With aging, susceptibility to acute renal failure (ARF) is greater. Prospective studies note ARF to be 3.5 times more common over age 70 years.[207] Underlying prevalence of systemic diseases in older patients of atherosclerosis, hypertension, diabetes, heart failure, and malignancy precludes increased medical and surgical interventions further exacerbating common causes of ARF. Cholesterol embolization to the kidney, both spontaneous and post procedure, occurs more commonly in those with generalized atherosclerosis. Acute vasculitis and rapidly progressive glomerulonephritis can lead to significant morbidity and cannot be overlooked as the number of older adults increase.

Vomiting, diarrhea, overzealous use of diuretics, bleeding, medication, and/or sepsis- induced renal hypoperfusion or low cardiac output lead to 50% prevalence of pre-renal azotemia in the elderly.[207,208] Impaired urinary concentration, thirst, and sodium conservation likely contribute to greater susceptibility. In addition, impaired autoregulation, decreased RPF, and renal reserve make the aging kidney more vulnerable to acute changes in volume. Medications such as prostaglandin inhibitors (NSAIDs), angiotensin antagonists (ACEIs and ARBs), and α-adrenergic blockers frequently necessary for rheumatologic, cardiovascular, or genitourinary disorders in the elderly can further compromise renal vaso-regulatory mechanisms. Careful volume management, drug discontinuation, and improvement in cardiac output often lead to renal recovery.

Although prerenal azotemia is frequently reversible, some instances can lead to acute tubular necrosis (ATN). Evolution to ATN is more common in older than younger patients (23% versus 15%, respectively).[209] Moreover traditional indices to distinguish prerenal process from other intrinsic renal etiologies such as fractional sodium excretion (FeNa) should be carefully interpreted in the elderly. Despite volume depletion, older patients may not have the capacity to conserve adequate tubular sodium to achieve a FeNa less than 1. Thus an elevated FeNa from preexisting tubular defects may be present despite underlying hypoperfusion.[210]

Surgical complications account for 30% of ARF in the elderly. Hypotension pre or post surgery, postoperative fluid losses from gastrointestinal drainage, dysarrhythmias, and myocardial infarction are common postsurgical complications leading to ARF in older patients.

Septic complications during hospitalization also account for one third of ARF prevalence in the elderly. Endotoxin-mediated renal vasoconstriction from gram negative sepsis increases susceptibility for ATN. Associated multi-organ failure or peri-operative sepsis increases catabolic demands, which carry a poor prognosis in the elderly.[211–213] Hemodynamic instability, along with the need for complicated nephrotoxic antibiotic regimens such as use of aminoglycosides or amphoteracin, can prolong renal dysfunction. Biochemical and tubular alterations with aging may enhance toxic effects of antibiotics. Age is a well-known risk factor for aminoglycoside-induced nephrotoxicity.[214] Thus, careful dosing and monitoring of antibiotics is necessary in the elderly. Bedside estimates of GFR using creatinine-based formulas may be helpful (see Table 21–1). Use of serum creatinine alone may be highly unreliable.

Various common infections such as staphylococci, streptococci, legionella, cytomegalovirus, human immunodeficiency virus, as well as common antibiotics, β-lactams, sulfonamides, and numerous other medications lead to interstitial inflammation and nephritis.[215] Activated macrophages during tubulointerstitial inflammation release degradative enzymes resulting in injury to intact basement membranes, which can hamper regeneration of tubular segments. Loss of functioning nephrons, with failure of the remaining nephrons to compensate, results in a fall in GFR.[215] An atypical presentation of acute interstitial nephritis can be seen with NSAIDs and angiotensin II antagonists presenting as nephrotic proteinuria only with or without pyuria. Renal biopsy lesions are of minimal change or membranous pathology with NSAIDs,[216] particularly propionic acid derivatives, and membranous lesions with the ACEI captopril.

Acute and prolonged vasoconstriction from radiocontrast infusion can significantly impair renal function in the elderly.[217] An acute reversible rise in serum creatinine within 1 to 4 days after contrast injection can be attributed to the contrast dye. The osmotic load delivered to the macula densa may trigger tubuloglomerular feedback with renin release and drop in GFR.[218]

Experimental studies in aging rodents indicated a greater propensity for ischemic and toxic ARF.[219,220] Renal artery occlusion leads to a more severe decline and slower recovery of renal function in older versus younger rats.[221,222] Changes in renal hemodynamics with aging rats may be more at play than underlying glomerulosclerosis. Older rats increase renal vascular resistance (RVR) with renal artery clamping to a greater extent than younger rats. Euvolemic men on a constant sodium diet also have increased RVR with blunted response to orthostatic change.[223] A predisposition to hypoxic renal injury in older adults is demonstrated by inability to improve medullary oxygenation with water diuresis as in younger adults.[224] Older cardiopulmonary bypass patients without acute renal failure also have greater excretion of kidney specific proteins (N-acetyl-β-glucosaminadase, alpha-1-microglobulin, glutathione transferase-pi (GST-pi), glutathione-alpha (GST-alpha)) as well as higher fractional sodium excretion post surgery to pre surgery in comparison to similar younger patients.[225] Oxygen free radicals can be generated during hemodynamically mediated ischemic ARF.[226] Infusion of a free radical scavenger, superoxide dismutase, markedly improves renal hemodynamics in ischemic aged rats (Fig. 21–13).[221]

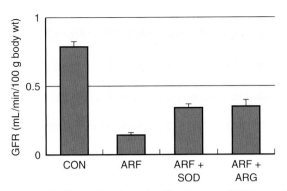

FIGURE 21-13 Change in glomerular filtration rate (GFR) in aged (18-month-old) rats measured under basal conditions (CON) 1 day after acute renal failure (ARF); with super oxide dismutase infusion 1 day after ARF (ARF+SOD); and with pretreatment with L-arginine and ARF (ARF+ARG). (Redrawn from Sabbatini M, Sansone G, Uccello F, et al: Functional versus structural changes in the pathophysiology of acute ischemic renal failure in aging rats. Kidney Int 45:1355–1361, 1994.)

Biochemical and metabolic alterations of aging tubular cells may also make aged kidneys more prone to ischemic injury. Renal cortical slices of older rats exposed to anoxia have impaired uptake of paraaminohippurate and tetraethylammonium in comparison to younger rats.[220]

Atheroembolic renal disease can be a complication after intra-arterial cannulation in elderly with generalized atherosclerosis. Spontaneous cholesterol embolization may also occur[233]; however, cholesterol embolization is more common after manipulation of the arterial vasculature for radiographic or surgical intervention such as carotid, coronary, renal or abdominal angiography; aortic surgery; percutaneous transluminal angioplasty of coronary or renal arteries. Embolization of cholesterol plaques can also be triggered by the use of anticoagulants and or fibrinolytic agents.[238] Renal failure is frequently progressive and irreversible and not necessarily associated with other systemic symptoms findings of purpura, livido reticularis of the abdominal and lumbar wall and or lower extremities, Hollenhorst plaques with retinal ischemia, gastrointestinal bleeding, pancreatitis, myocardial infarction, cerebral infarction, and distal ischemic necrosis of the toes. Laboratory clues of low complement, eosinophilia, and eosinophiluria may not necessarily be present. Therapy remains primarily supportive with necessary avoidance or clear procedural and or anticoagulation benefits and risks outlined.

Acute renal failure from urethral or ureteral obstruction can present with either complaints of dysuria, hesitancy, dribbling, incontinence, or as only a rise in blood urea nitrogen and serum creatinine. Prostatic hypertrophy, either benign or malignant, strictures, uroepithelial malignancies, pelvic tumors of the uterus or cervix can present commonly in the form of acute renal failure in the elderly.[239] Retroperitoneal fibrosis, metastatic tumors, and lymphomas may also result in ureteral obstruction and loss of renal function in the elderly. Medications such as anticholinergic agents, central nervous system inhibition leading to bladder detrusor muscle overactivity in elderly patients with cerebrovascular accident, Parkinson disease, and Alzheimer disease can lead to bladder outlet obstruction with subsequent renal failure. Similarly, detrusor underactivity from injury to nerves supplying the bladder or autonomic neuropathy as seen in diabetes or chronic alcoholism also leads to outlet bladder obstruction. Prolapse of pelvic structures in post menopausal women with atrophy of supporting tissues under low estrogen levels can also lead to obstructive nephropathy. Prolonged obstruction can result frequently in irreversible renal loss. Therefore prompt medication review and evaluation including post void residual, noncontrast renal imaging with ultrasonography, CT, or MRI scan with urologic evaluation for decompression may be necessary in older individuals presenting with acute renal failure.

Although older individuals face both greater risk[207] and require longer time to recover from acute renal failure,[240] age alone does not determine the survival of patients with acute renal failure and should not be used as a discriminating factor in therapeutic decisions concerning ARF.[211,241,242] Most of the older patients respond well to treatment of ARF with dialysis if necessary to alleviate uremic symptoms and complications of ARF such as volume overload, bleeding, disorientation, catabolic state, and electrolyte disturbances.

The role of nitric oxide (NO) in aging vasculature may have a pronounced role in maintaining renal perfusion. Intrarenal levels of NO and acetylcholine-induced vasodilation are reduced in aging rodent kidneys.[227] NO production from isolated conduit arteries also decreases with aging.[228–230] L-arginine, NO synthase substrate, levels are low in both aged rats and aging humans.[230,231] However, gene expression regulating substrate synthesis does not appear to be affected with aging.[232] Urinary nitrate, nitrite and cGMP, a marker for NO production was lower in healthy aged subjects despite a fall in blood pressure while on a low sodium diet, suggesting age-dependent decrease in clearance.[233] It is possible that renal endothelial NO production is maximized in normal aging to maintain stable renal function. This may explain the blunted vasodilator response observed in the elderly. NO measurements in face of renal ischemia have yet to be done in humans.

L-arginine feeding prior to renal occlusion results in significant improvements in GFR and RPF with decreased RVR in older rats. When NOS inhibitor, L-NAME was given to these rats, these hemodynamic changes were abolished.[221] Whether higher protein intake affected these results is unclear as protein restricted aged rats maintain urinary excretion of nitrate and nitrite similar to controls.[58] L-arginine supplementation in drinking water of aged animals appears to limit structural changes in the aging glomerular basement membrane.[60,61] Whether beneficial effects of low-protein diet on age-related glomerulosclerosis is in some way related to NO is not yet clear. Recent studies of ischemic acute renal failure in aged and young rats with suggest improved NO availability with increase in eNOS mRNA and protein in older animals via partial inhibition of RhoA protein activation, decreasing renal vasoconstriction and significantly attenuating ischemic lesions.[234]

NOS inhibitor, N (G), N (G')-asymmetric dimethylarginine (ADMA) is significantly elevated in aged rats compared to younger control rats despite similar levels of L-arginine.[235] ADMA levels are also increased with age in humans.[236] Increased ADMA levels can then decrease NO synthesis in endothelial cells thus impairing endothelium-dependent vasodilation[235] predisposing the aged kidney to ischemia. High ADMA levels with increased RVR and decreased effective renal plasma flow are noted in healthy older adults in comparison to younger adults. Even greater ADMA levels are noted in hypertensive elderly suggesting that endogenous NOS inhibition may be important in decreased renal perfusion and increased blood pressure seen with aging.[237]

Renovascular Disease

Renovascular atherosclerotic disease leads to hypertension and progressive ischemic renal failure with ESRD in up to 15% of patients. Prevalence of renovascular disease over age 65 years is estimated at 6.8%.[243] Lesions in the renal arteries leading to stenosis, as well as complex intrarenal vascular lesions and atheromatous embolization represent the spectrum of this disease in the elderly.[244] New onset or sudden worsening of underlying hypertension or renal failure in those with generalized atherosclerosis should bring attention to this disease. An underlying angiographic stenosis in the renal arteries of 75% or greater usually leads to eventual occlusion with loss of GFR.[245] Azotemic patients with high-grade stenosis in a solitary kidney or unilateral renal artery occlusion and contralateral stenosis are at greatest risk for renal failure.[246] Bilateral renal artery stenosis is associated with a crude mortality of 45% at 5 years.[247]

Smoking is noted to be an independent risk factor and predictor in the progression of both macrovascular and microvascular renal disease and renal artery stenosis in the elderly.[248] In the Cardiovascular Health Study cohort, a multivariate "best fit" model adjusted for gender, race, weight, age, and baseline serum creatinine of nondiabetic patients >65 years suggests that the number of cigarettes smoked daily is independently associated with an increase in serum creatinine.[249] Smoking increases epinephrine and norepinephrine release in addition to interfering with both endothelial metabolism of prostacyclin, thromboxane A2 as well as vascular response to acetylcholine, NO, and endothelin-1 (ET-1). ET-1, a potent vasoconstrictor with mitogenic and atherogenic activity on vascular smooth muscle, may be important in mediating renal arteriolar thickening. ET-1 levels are increased in active smokers and the protein is up-regulated in healthy aging rodents.[250,251]

Diagnosis of clinically significant renovascular disease involves a combination of both functional and radiological evaluations. An increase in serum creatinine with use of angiotensin II antagonists (ACEI or ARB) may provide a clinical clue to the presence of functional stenoses in bilateral renovascular disease or unilateral atherosclerotic stenosis in a solitary functional kidney.[252] Angiotensin II antagonism interferes with necessary efferent autoregulatory vasoconstriction, which maintains GFR despite decreased renal perfusion from renal artery stenosis. Renal scintigraphy with technetium 99m-labelled diethylenetriamine-pentacetic acid (99mTc-DTPA) or technetium-mercaptoacetythiglycine (99-Tc-Mag3) before and after ACEI administration can be useful to increase clinical suspicion for a significant functional unilateral renal artery stenosis.[253,254] Duplex ultrasound scanning of renal arteries is used in some centers with reliability to provide both noninvasive imaging of stenoses and data on blood flow velocity to determine stenosis significance.[255] Recently imaging with magnetic resonance angiography is being used to visualize stenosis anatomy. CO_2 angiography is also useful to evaluate anatomy in the presence of decreased GFR. Contrast angiography remains the gold standard with visualization of the renal and intrarenal vasculature because lesions in distal renal branches and microvasculature can also lead to hypertension and ischemic renal failure.[256]

Arterial manipulation of diffuse atherosclerotic vessels can lead to irreversible and often progressive renal failure that occurs 1 to 4 weeks after arterial manipulation and is often secondary to cholesterol embolization with or without systemic manifestations. Cholesterol crystals lodge in arteries with diameters of 100 μm to 200 μm or smaller, including glomerular tufts.[257] Biconvex clefts with surrounding inflammation are seen on renal biopsy as the lipid material dissolves during tissue fixation. Management is supportive with blood pressure control, avoidance of other nephrotoxic insults, and anticoagulation.

Percutaneous transluminal angioplasty (PTA) or surgical revascularization can be considered when technically feasible to preserve renal function and improve blood pressure control in patients with significant atherosclerotic renovascular disease. The presence of collateral circulation in some may protect renal parenchymal ischemia despite progressive occlusive disease.[258] Although reversibility of renal failure is noted with angioplasty or surgical revascularization (or both) of renal artery stenosis by some, a creatinine ≥2.5 mg/dL may predict poorer outcome including no improvement in blood pressure, need for dialysis, and death seen within months after a technically successful PTA.[259,260] Lesions amenable to angioplasty are more commonly unilateral, nonostial, and technically feasible to approach. Repeat angioplasty may be necessary in at least 20% of patients. Surgical revascularization is recommended for ostial, bilateral lesions or those completely occluded. Predictors of poor outcome are initial serum creatinine ≥3.2 mg/dl, need for surgical repair, and high-grade unilateral stenosis. Bilateral renal artery repair and unchanged or improved post operative response are favorable outcomes after surgical repair.[261]

Acute Glomerulonephritis

Rapidly progressive glomerulonephritis (RPGN) generally characterizes acute glomerulonephritis in the elderly. A rapid decline in renal function associated with active nephritic urine sediment (hematuria, pyuria, red blood cell casts, and moderate to severe proteinuria) with histological findings of more than 50% glomerular crescents is seen. An immune pathogenesis is most likely though direct evidence may not be always be evident. RPGN immune histology can broadly be categorized into 3 types: type 1—presence of anti-glomerular antibodies; type 2—with granular immune deposits; type 3—with no immune deposits seen; however, circulating anti-neutrophilic cytoplasmic antibodies may be present. The latter two immune processes are more prevalent in the elderly.[262,263] In a case series biopsy of 115 older patients, 19 patients were noted to have RPGN. Of these 19 patients, 9 patients had granular IgG deposits, 6 had no immune deposits found on histology, and 3 patients were noted to have antiglomerular basement membrane antibodies.[264] Other case series have suggested pauci-immune crescentic glomerulonephritis as the most common form of acute glomerulonephritis in adults over age 60 years presenting with acute renal failure.[265,266] Renal prognosis of RPGN in the elderly is poor. Risks and benefits of treatment with pulse steroids, cyclophosphamide, and/or plasmapheresis must be individualized in the elderly given medication side effects.

Poststreptococcal diffuse proliferative glomerulonephritis usually occurs in association with streptococcal infections of the throat and skin. Incidence in patients older than 55 years is as high as 22.6%.[267] Supportive renal management is usually recommended with an expected generally favorable renal outcome.

Chronic Glomerulonephritis

Nephrotic proteinuria and nephrotic syndrome often lead to renal biopsy in the elderly. Both registry and collected case series data from different countries reveal idiopathic membranous nephropathy as the most common histological finding followed by minimal change pathology (Table 21–3).[264,268–277] Nephrotic syndrome may coexist or precede a malignancy in the elderly in up to 20% of patients. The association between membranous lesions and malignancy is presumed to be mediated in part via immune response to tumor associated antigens.[278] Solid tumors of lung, colon, rectum, kidney, breast, and stomach have most commonly been associated with membranous lesions on biopsy. Minimal change pathology has also been associated with both Hodgkin and non-Hodgkin lymphoma in the elderly. A higher risk of renal failure, more severe proteinuria, and lower albumin level is also found in the elderly with minimal change than in younger patients.[279] Given a greater predisposition to underlying malignancy in the elderly, a thorough history, physical examination, and basic screening for underlying malignancy should be done in elderly presenting with nephrotic syndrome.

TABLE 21–3 Histologic Lesions in 545 Elderly Patients with Primary Nephrotic Syndrome

Authors	Minimal Change	Membranous Glomerulonephritis	Mesangial Proliferative Glomerulonephritis	Membranoproliferative Glomerulonephritis	Glomerulosclerosis	Chronic Glomerulonephritis
Fawcett et al., 1971	6	5	—	4	16	5
Huriet et al., 1975	4	2	—	6	—	—
Moorthy and Zimmerman, 1980	9	15	7	2	1	—
Ishimuto et al., 1981	1	6	—	2	7	—
Lustig et al., 1982	2	16	—	2	3	—
Zech et al., 1982	19	31	2	4	—	3
Kingswood et al., 1984	2	16	11	3	—	—
Murphy et al., 1987	2	2	—	2	—	—
Sato et al., 1987	7	30	12	7	1	—
Johnston et al., 1992	35	116	18	—	5	—
Ozono et al., 1994	6	26	—	8	—	—
Shin et al., 2001	14	27	—	8	6	1
Total	107 (19%)	292 (54%)	50 (9%)	48 (9%)	39 (7%)	9 (2%)

Prednisone therapy alone for membranous lesions did not affect the rate of renal function loss when compared younger patients; however, the incidence of chronic renal failure was greater in the elderly, possibly from a decreased functional reserve. Treatment with prednisone and cytotoxic agents may induce partial or complete remission; however, use of these agents in the elderly must be carefully and individually considered given risks of infection. Steroid use alone may have a more favorable response in elderly with minimal change disease.[280,281]

Other common causes of nephrosis in the elderly include systemic amyloidosis both primary and secondary to paraproteinemic processes. Approximately 40% to 68% patients with primary amyloidosis present with paraproteinemia. Serum and urine electrophoresis should be checked in elderly presenting with unexplained nephrotic syndrome. Abnormal test findings should prompt a bone marrow biopsy to rule out multiple myeloma. Although abdominal fat pad aspiration examined with Congo red stain may be useful in some hands to diagnose primary amyloidosis, renal biopsy is often done to confirm in this diagnosis. Kidney biopsy specimens in older adults presenting with unexplained nephrotic syndrome should routinely be stained with Congo red and examined under electron microscopy for amyloid fibrils. Treatment with Melphalan and prednisone may delay the progression to ESRD.

A small percentage of elderly patients presenting with nephrotic syndrome have a generalized glomerulosclerosis on biopsy. Because filtration fraction is greater in the juxtamedullary glomeruli of the elderly, these may be more affected. Immunofluorescence staining is notable for IgM and third complement component, C3. This pathology is frequently seen as the end result of other glomerulopathies and secondary to advanced systemic diseases including hypertension, as hyperfiltration hastens the sclerotic process. Glomerular enlargement and segmental sclerosis may be adaptive. Interestingly, renal histology in healthy aging rats is similar to human glomerulosclerosis.

Chronic Renal Failure

Progression of underlying medical diseases common with increasing age frequently leads to chronic renal failure with aging. Approximately 6.6 million elderly people have GFR <60 ml/min/1.73 m^2 per NHANES III data.[282] The presence of longstanding diabetes, hypertension, chronic glomerulonephritis, atherosclerotic ischemic renovascular disease, and obstructive uropathy are prevalent diagnoses associated with chronic renal failure in the elderly. Furthermore, the level of GFR is an independent risk for de novo cardiovascular disease and all-cause mortality in individuals over 65 years of age.[283] Decompensating medical illness can sometimes herald renal failure progression rather than frank uremia. Volume overload with symptoms of heart failure, gastrointestinal bleeding, hypertension, and gradual confusion can be presenting signs in older individuals approaching renal loss. Actual renal reserve may be underestimated by laboratory serum creatinine measurements given gradual loss of muscle mass in the elderly.

Renal Replacement Therapy

Age alone does not preclude renal replacement therapy. Elderly patients without other major organ dysfunction seem to adjust and tolerate dialysis fairly well. Approximately 55% of the current ESRD population is older than 60 years of age.[284–286] Although longevity is less than younger ESRD patients, life expectancy on dialysis for the older population is not significantly reduced. Octogenarians on hemodialysis are found to have 24-month median survival.[287] Older patients on shorter treatment schedules are more likely to die from increased risk for silent ischemia during hypotensive episodes, more common with shorter treatments.[288,289] Chronic ambulatory peritoneal dialysis (CAPD) can be an alternative to hemodialysis particularly for those with hemodynamic instability on hemodialysis.[285,290] Differences in the number of episodes of peritonitis, or type of organism, or likelihood of technique failure are not significant between younger and older patients. Catheter replacement is in fact less likely in the older than younger patients.[290,291]

Neither dialysis mode, peritoneal nor hemodialysis, is clearly demonstrated to be superior to the other in the elderly.[292–294] Evaluation of CMS data suggest that older patients, particularly patients with diabetes may have lower relative risk of death on hemodialysis than peritoneal dialysis.[295] Dialysis modality should be individualized in the elderly taking into consideration underlying medical and psychosocial factors. Patients with widespread vascular disease or inability to maintain vascular access or those with hemodynamic instability during hemodialysis may benefit from peritoneal dialysis. Hemodialysis may be more appropriate for deconditioned patients or those with a precarious home situation that prevents adequate self care dialysis. Socialization during in-center hemodialysis may be important for lonely or depressed elderly patients. Co-morbidity of malnutrition, malignancy, infection, vascular disease, and withdrawal from dialysis contribute to ESRD mortality in the elderly.

Renal Transplantation

Medically eligible elderly patients can undergo successful renal transplantation. Age alone generally is not exclusion for renal transplantation in the elderly.[296,297] Donor age is more significant in determining delayed graft function than recipient age (Fig. 21–14).[4] Analytic decision models for quality-adjusted life expectancy for selected elderly patients younger than 70 years and with few co-morbidities project 1.1 years of life expectancy gain with transplantation.[298] Patients over 60 years of age matched for demographics and co-morbidities with anticipated 80% or more 5-year survival who have undergone rigorous pre-transplant screening have increased survival advantage over ESRD patients on dialysis. Preoperative 1-, 3-, and 5-year survival was 98%, 95%, and 90% respectively for elderly transplant patients compared to 92%, 62%, and 27% respectively for elderly dialysis patients.[299] Post-transplant 1-year patient survival and allograft survival rates are similar between young and elderly patients. Cardiovascular and infection related patient mortality is major

reasons for allograft loss after transplantation in older individuals.[297,300] Age seems to be an independent risk for infection-associated death in the elderly transplant patient.[301] Acute rejection episodes are also noted to be fewer in older individuals.[302] Thus mortality risk given biologic age and co-morbidities must be carefully considered when considering renal transplantation in the elderly.

Urinary Tract Infection

Urinary tract infection is quite common in the older population. Numerous factors contribute to increased prevalence. Altered bladder function, immune senescence and decreased defenses, changes in pelvic musculature, prostate size and concomitant illnesses such as cerebrovascular accident or dementia can lead to poor hygiene, impaired mobility, and neurogenic as well as obstructive bladder dysfunction. Lower prostatic secretions in elderly men predispose to lower urinary tract infections. Prostatic microcalculi can harbor bacteria and provide nidus for prostatic infections. Decreased estrogen levels in postmenopausal women change pH of vaginal secretions leading to vaginal colonization of bacteria and cystitis. Intravaginal estrogen may prevent recurrent urinary tract infection in these women.

Prevalence of asymptomatic bacteriuria can range from 20% in older men to 25% in both men and women living in extended care facilities. Thirty percent to 50% of older hospitalized patients also have bacteriuria. Creatinine clearance is decreased in older patients with bacteriuria compared with nonbacteriuric older individuals. Although the mechanism is not clear, chronic pyelonephritis and glomerulosclerosis may contribute. Underlying predisposing illness leading to chronic bacteriuria frequently leads to decreased survival as treatment for asymptomatic bacteriuria does not result in improved survival.[303] As treatment failure and relapse is high,[304] treatment for asymptomatic bacteriuria in the elderly is not necessary in the absence of renal or urologic abnormalities. Given the possibility of resistant bacterial strains, use of long-term suppressive antibiotic therapy must be determined.

Acquired Renal Cysts

Number of simple renal cysts increase with age. Incidental cysts are being detected with increased frequency as abdominal imaging procedures for other diagnostic purposes are done. Microdissection of the distal renal tubule in adults and those older than 50 years reveals greater ectasia, diverticula, and microscopic cysts in comparison to 20-year-olds. These findings morphologically lead to larger cysts with age. Postmortem studies reveal at lease one cyst in at least 50% of older patients. Sonographic evidence suggest a 22% prevalence for acquired cysts in subjects ≥70 years of age, with 0% prevalence in the 15- to 29-year age group.[305] Acquired cysts are usually painless, simple, and asymptomatic. With bleeding into the cyst, or cyst infection, there may be associated lumbar pain, hematuria. Associated renin-dependent

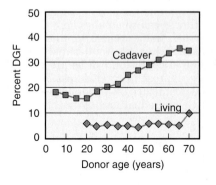
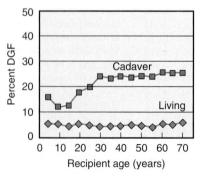

FIGURE 21–14 Effect of donor age on delayed graft function (DGF) of first transplants (1996–2000). (Reprinted from Cecka JM: The UNOS renal transplant registry. Clin Transpl:1–18, 2001.)

hypertension can also be present. Cysts with smooth clear walls, fluid-filled without internal echoes, usually require no further follow-up. Cysts filled with debris and or internal echoes, thick walls, or occurring in association with a possible renal mass are considered to be complicated acquired cysts. Complicated cysts must be followed carefully with further investigation with cyst puncture, angiography, or surgical exploration as indicated.

Acknowledgments

The authors thank Masuma Hussain and the Library and Medical Media staff at the Dallas VA Medical Center with expert help with obtaining the references, creating the endnote library, and preparing the figures.

References

1. Prommool S, Jhangri GS, Cockfield SM, Halloran PF: Time dependency of factors affecting renal allograft survival. J Am Soc Nephrol 11:565–573, 2000.
2. Terasaki PI, Gjertson DW, Cecka JM, et al: Significance of the donor age effect on kidney transplants. Clin Transplant 11:366–372, 1997.
3. Kasiske BL, Snyder J: Matching older kidneys with older patients does not improve allograft survival. J Am Soc Nephrol 13:1067–1072, 2002.
4. Cecka JM: The UNOS renal transplant registry. Clin Transpl:1–18, 2001.
5. Asderakis A, Dyer P, Augustine T, et al: Effect of cold ischemic time and HLA matching in kidneys coming from "young" and "old" donors: Do not leave for tomorrow what you can do tonight. Transplantation 72:674–678, 2001.
6. Coresh J, Astor BC, Greene T, et al: Prevalence of chronic kidney disease and decreased kidney function in the adult US population: Third National Health and Nutrition Examination Survey. Am J Kidney Dis 41:1–12, 2003.
7. Executive summary. United States Renal Data System 1999 Annual Data Report. Am J Kidney Dis 34:S9–S19, 1999.
8. Gourtsoyiannis N, Prassopoulos P, Cavouras D, Pantelidis N: The thickness of the renal parenchyma decreases with age: A CT study of 360 patients. AJR Am J Roentgenol 155:541–544, 1990.
9. Fuiano G, Sund S, Mazza G, et al: Renal hemodynamic response to maximal vasodilating stimulus in healthy older subjects. Kidney Int 59:1052–1058, 2001.
10. Tracy RE, Berenson G, Wattigney W, Barrett TJ: The evolution of benign arterionephrosclerosis from age 6 to 70 years. Am J Pathol 136:429–439, 1990.
11. Melk A, Halloran PF: Cell senescence and its implications for nephrology. J Am Soc Nephrol 12:385–393, 2001.
12. Hill GS, Heudes D, Bariety J: Morphometric study of arterioles and glomeruli in the aging kidney suggests focal loss of autoregulation. Kidney Int 63:1027–1036, 2003.
13. Kang DH, Anderson S, Kim YG, et al: Impaired angiogenesis in the aging kidney: vascular endothelial growth factor and thrombospondin-1 in renal disease. Am J Kidney Dis 37:601–611, 2001.
14. Lindeman RD, Goldman R: Anatomic and physiologic age changes in the kidney. Exp Gerontol 21:379–406, 1986.
15. Takazakura E, Sawabu N, Handa A, et al: Intrarenal vascular changes with age and disease. Kidney Int 2:224–230, 1972.
16. Baert L, Steg A: Is the diverticulum of the distal and collecting tubules a preliminary stage of the simple cyst in the adult? J Urol 118:707–710, 1977.
17. Abrass CK, Adcox MJ, Raugi GJ: Aging-associated changes in renal extracellular matrix. Am J Pathol 146:742–752, 1995.
18. Ding G, Franki N, Kapasi AA, et al: Tubular cell senescence and expression of TGF-beta1 and p21(WAF1/CIP1) in tubulointerstitial fibrosis of aging rats. Exp Mol Pathol 70:43–53, 2001.
19. Thomas SE, Anderson S, Gordon KL, et al: Tubulointerstitial disease in aging: evidence for underlying peritubular capillary damage, a potential role for renal ischemia. J Am Soc Nephrol 9:231–242, 1998.
20. Gagliano N, Arosio B, Santambrogio D, et al: Age-dependent expression of fibrosis-related genes and collagen deposition in rat kidney cortex. J Gerontol A Biol Sci Med Sci 55:B365–B372, 2000.
21. Eikmans M, Baelde HJ, de Heer E, Bruijn JA: Effect of age and biopsy site on extracellular matrix mRNA and protein levels in human kidney biopsies. Kidney Int 60:974–981, 2001.
22. Melk A, Schmidt BM, Takeuchi O, et al: Expression of p16INK4a and other cell cycle regulator and senescence associated genes in aging human kidney. Kidney Int 65:510–520, 2004.
23. Melk A, Kittikowit W, Sandhu I, et al: Cell senescence in rat kidneys in vivo increases with growth and age despite lack of telomere shortening. Kidney Int 63:2134–2143, 2003.
24. Lindeman RD, Tobin J, Shock NW: Longitudinal studies on the rate of decline in renal function with age. J Am Geriatr Soc 33:278–285, 1985.
25. Cogan MG: Angiotensin II: A powerful controller of sodium transport in the early proximal tubule. Hypertension 15:451–458, 1990.
26. Norman JT: The role of angiotensin II in renal growth. Ren Physiol Biochem 14:175–185, 1991.
27. Maric C, Aldred GP, Antoine AM, et al: Effects of angiotensin II on cultured renomedullary interstitial cells are mediated by AT1A receptors. Am J Physiol 271:F1020–F1028, 1996.
28. Wolf G, Ziyadeh FN, Zahner G, Stahl RA: Angiotensin II is mitogenic for cultured rat glomerular endothelial cells. Hypertension 27:897–905, 1996.
29. Wolf G, Ziyadeh FN, Schroeder R, Stahl RA: Angiotensin II inhibits inducible nitric oxide synthase in tubular MCT cells by a posttranscriptional mechanism. J Am Soc Nephrol 8:551–557, 1997.
30. Anderson S, Brenner BM: Effects of aging on the renal glomerulus. Am J Med 80:435–442, 1986.
31. Heudes D, Michel O, Chevalier J, et al: Effect of chronic ANG I-converting enzyme inhibition on aging processes. I. Kidney structure and function. Am J Physiol 266:R1038–R1051, 1994.
32. Corman B, Chami-Khazraji S, Schaeverbeke J, Michel JB: Effect of feeding on glomerular filtration rate and proteinuria in conscious aging rats. Am J Physiol 255:F250–F256, 1988.
33. Remuzzi A, Puntorieri S, Battaglia C, et al: Angiotensin converting enzyme inhibition ameliorates glomerular filtration of macromolecules and water and lessens glomerular injury in the rat. J Clin Invest 85:541–549, 1990.
34. Zoja C, Remuzzi A, Corna D, et al: Renal protective effect of angiotensin-converting enzyme inhibition in aging rats. Am J Med 92:60S–63S, 1992.
35. Anderson S, Rennke HG, Zatz R: Glomerular adaptations with normal aging and with long-term converting enzyme inhibition in rats. Am J Physiol 267:F35–F43, 1994.
36. Michel JB, Heudes D, Michel O, et al: Effect of chronic ANG I-converting enzyme inhibition on aging processes. II. Large arteries. Am J Physiol 267:R124–R135, 1994.
37. Ferder L, Inserra F, Romano L, et al: Decreased glomerulosclerosis in aging by angiotensin-converting enzyme inhibitors. J Am Soc Nephrol 5:1147–1152, 1994.
38. Jung FF, Kennefick TM, Ingelfinger JR, et al: Down-regulation of the intrarenal renin-angiotensin system in the aging rat. J Am Soc Nephrol 5:1573–1580, 1995.
39. Wolf G, Killen PD, Neilson EG: Intracellular signaling of transcription and secretion of type IV collagen after angiotensin II-induced cellular hypertrophy in cultured proximal tubular cells. Cell Regul 2:219–227, 1991.
40. Wolf G, Zahner G, Schroeder R, Stahl RA: Transforming growth factor beta mediates the angiotensin-II-induced stimulation of collagen type IV synthesis in cultured murine proximal tubular cells. Nephrol Dial Transplant 11:263–269, 1996.
41. Wolf G, Ziyadeh FN, Thaiss F, et al: Angiotensin II stimulates expression of the chemokine RANTES in rat glomerular endothelial cells. Role of the angiotensin type 2 receptor. J Clin Invest 100:1047–1058, 1997.
42. Inserra F, Romano LA, de Cavanagh EM, et al: Renal interstitial sclerosis in aging: Effects of enalapril and nifedipine. J Am Soc Nephrol 7:676–680, 1996.
43. Vaughan DE, Lazos SA, Tong K: Angiotensin II regulates the expression of plasminogen activator inhibitor-1 in cultured endothelial cells. A potential link between the renin-angiotensin system and thrombosis. J Clin Invest 95:995–1001, 1995.
44. Fogo AB: The role of angiotensin II and plasminogen activator inhibitor-1 in progressive glomerulosclerosis. Am J Kidney Dis 35:179–188, 2000.
45. Ma LJ, Nakamura S, Aldigier JC, et al: Regression of glomerulosclerosis with high-dose angiotensin inhibition is linked to decreased plasminogen activator inhibitor-1. J Am Soc Nephrol 16:966–976, 2005.
46. de Cavanagh EM, Piotrkowski B, Basso N, et al: Enalapril and losartan attenuate mitochondrial dysfunction in aged rats. FASEB J 17:1096–1098, 2003.
47. Mitani H, Ishizaka N, Aizawa T, et al: In vivo klotho gene transfer ameliorates angiotensin II-induced renal damage. Hypertension 39:838–843, 2002.
48. Roberts AB, McCune BK, Sporn MB: TGF-beta: Regulation of extracellular matrix. Kidney Int 41:557–559, 1992.
49. Wolf G: Link between angiotensin II and TGF-beta in the kidney. Miner Electrolyte Metab 24:174–180, 1998.
50. Noble NA, Border WA: Angiotensin II in renal fibrosis: should TGF-beta rather than blood pressure be the therapeutic target? Semin Nephrol 17:455–466, 1997.
51. Peters H, Noble NA, Border WA: Transforming growth factor-beta in human glomerular injury. Curr Opin Nephrol Hypertens 6:389–393, 1997.
52. Frishberg Y, Kelly CJ: TGF-beta and regulation of interstitial nephritis. Miner Electrolyte Metab 24:181–189, 1998.
53. Ruiz-Torres MP, Bosch RJ, O'Valle F, et al: Age-related increase in expression of TGF-beta1 in the rat kidney: Relationship to morphologic changes. J Am Soc Nephrol 9:782–791, 1998.
54. Samuel CS, Zhao C, Bond CP, et al: Relaxin-1-deficient mice develop an age-related progression of renal fibrosis. Kidney Int 65:2054–2064, 2004.
55. Wolf G: Molecular mechanisms of angiotensin II in the kidney: Emerging role in the progression of renal disease: Beyond haemodynamics. Nephrol Dial Transplant 13:1131–1142, 1998.
56. Satriano JA, Shuldiner M, Hora K, et al: Oxygen radicals as second messengers for expression of the monocyte chemoattractant protein, JE/MCP-1, and the monocyte colony-stimulating factor, CSF-1, in response to tumor necrosis factor-alpha and immunoglobulin G. Evidence for involvement of reduced nicotinamide adenine dinucleotide phosphate (NADPH)-dependent oxidase. J Clin Invest 92:1564–1571, 1993.
57. Hill C, Lateef AM, Engels K, et al: Basal and stimulated nitric oxide in control of kidney function in the aging rat. Am J Physiol 272:R1747–R1753, 1997.
58. Sonaka I, Futami Y, Maki T: L-arginine-nitric oxide pathway and chronic nephropathy in aged rats. J Gerontol 49:B157–B161, 1994.
59. Adler S, Huang H, Wolin MS, Kaminski PM: Oxidant stress leads to impaired regulation of renal cortical oxygen consumption by nitric oxide in the aging kidney. J Am Soc Nephrol 15:52–60, 2004.
60. Reckelhoff JF, Kellum JA, Jr, Racusen LC, Hildebrandt DA: Long-term dietary supplementation with L-arginine prevents age-related reduction in renal function. Am J Physiol 272:R1768–R1774, 1997.
61. Radner W, Hoger H, Lubec B, et al: L-arginine reduces kidney collagen accumulation and N-epsilon-(carboxymethyl)lysine in the aging NMRI-mouse. J Gerontol 49:M44–M46, 1994.

62. Nakayama I, Kawahara Y, Tsuda T, et al: Angiotensin II inhibits cytokine-stimulated inducible nitric oxide synthase expression in vascular smooth muscle cells. J Biol Chem 269:11628–11633, 1994.

63. Arima S, Ito S, Omata K, et al, Abe K: High glucose augments angiotensin II action by inhibiting NO synthesis in in vitro microperfused rabbit afferent arterioles. Kidney Int 48:683–689, 1995.

64. Hogan M, Cerami A, Bucala R: Advanced glycosylation endproducts block the antiproliferative effect of nitric oxide. Role in the vascular and renal complications of diabetes mellitus. J Clin Invest 90:1110–1115, 1992.

65. McQuillan LP, Leung GK, Marsden PA, et al: Hypoxia inhibits expression of eNOS via transcriptional and posttranscriptional mechanisms. Am J Physiol 267:H1921–H1927, 1994.

66. Verbeke P, Perichon M, Borot-Laloi C, et al: Accumulation of advanced glycation endproducts in the rat nephron: Link with circulating AGEs during aging. J Histochem Cytochem 45:1059–1068, 1997.

67. Schleicher ED, Wagner E, Nerlich AG: Increased accumulation of the glycoxidation product N(epsilon)-(carboxymethyl)lysine in human tissues in diabetes and aging. J Clin Invest 99:457–468, 1997.

68. Raj DS, Choudhury D, Welbourne TC, Levi M: Advanced glycation end products: A nephrologist's perspective. Am J Kidney Dis 35:365–380, 2000.

69. Vlassara H: Advanced glycosylation in nephropathy of diabetes and aging. Adv Nephrol Necker Hosp 25:303–315, 1996.

70. Bucala R, Tracey KJ, Cerami A: Advanced glycosylation products quench nitric oxide and mediate defective endothelium-dependent vasodilatation in experimental diabetes. J Clin Invest 87:432–438, 1991.

71. McVeigh GE, Brennan GM, Johnston GD, et al: Impaired endothelium-dependent and independent vasodilation in patients with type 2 (non-insulin-dependent) diabetes mellitus. Diabetologia 35:771–776, 1992.

72. Gascho JA, Fanelli C, Zelis R: Aging reduces venous distensibility and the venodilatory response to nitroglycerin in normal subjects. Am J Cardiol 63:1267–1270, 1989.

73. He C, Sabol J, Mitsuhashi T, Vlassara H: Dietary glycotoxins: Inhibition of reactive products by aminoguanidine facilitates renal clearance and reduces tissue sequestration. Diabetes 48:1308–1315, 1999.

74. Cerami C, Founds H, Nicholl I, et al: Tobacco smoke is a source of toxic reactive glycation products. Proc Natl Acad Sci U S A 94:13915–13920, 1997.

75. Lu C, He JC, Cai W, et al: Advanced glycation endproduct (AGE) receptor 1 is a negative regulator of the inflammatory response to AGE in mesangial cells. Proc Natl Acad Sci U S A 101:11767–11772, 2004.

76. Li YM, Steffes M, Donnelly T, et al: Prevention of cardiovascular and renal pathology of aging by the advanced glycation inhibitor aminoguanidine. Proc Natl Acad Sci U S A 93:3902–3907, 1996.

77. Corman B, Duriez M, Poitevin P, et al: Aminoguanidine prevents age-related arterial stiffening and cardiac hypertrophy. Proc Natl Acad Sci U S A 95:1301–1306, 1998.

78. Vlassara H, Fuh H, Makita Z, et al: Exogenous advanced glycosylation end products induce complex vascular dysfunction in normal animals: a model for diabetic and aging complications. Proc Natl Acad Sci U S A 89:12043–12047, 1992.

79. Cefalu WT, Bell-Farrow AD, Wang ZQ, et al: Caloric restriction decreases age-dependent accumulation of the glycoxidation products, N epsilon-(carboxymethyl) lysine and pentosidine, in rat skin collagen. J Gerontol A Biol Sci Med Sci 50:B337–B341, 1995.

80. Novelli M, Masiello P, Bombara M, Bergamini E: Protein glycation in the aging male Sprague-Dawley rat: effects of antiaging diet restrictions. J Gerontol A Biol Sci Med Sci 53:B94–B101, 1998.

81. Teillet L, Verbeke P, Gouraud S, et al: Food restriction prevents advanced glycation end product accumulation and retards kidney aging in lean rats. J Am Soc Nephrol 11:1488–1497, 2000.

82. Xia E, Rao G, Van Remmen H, et al: Activities of antioxidant enzymes in various tissues of male Fischer 344 rats are altered by food restriction. J Nutr 125:195–201, 1995.

83. Oppenheim RW: Related mechanisms of action of growth factors and antioxidants in apoptosis: An overview. Adv Neurol 72:69–78, 1997.

84. Papa S, Skulachev VP: Reactive oxygen species, mitochondria, apoptosis and aging. Mol Cell Biochem 174:305–319, 1997.

85. Beckman KB, Ames BN: The free radical theory of aging matures. Physiol Rev 78:547–581, 1998.

86. Leeuwenburgh C, Hansen PA, Holloszy JO, Heinecke JW: Oxidized amino acids in the urine of aging rats: Potential markers for assessing oxidative stress in vivo. Am J Physiol 276:R128–R135, 1999.

87. Ruiz-Torres P, Lucio J, Gonzalez-Rubio M, et al: Oxidant/antioxidant balance in isolated glomeruli and cultured mesangial cells. Free Radic Biol Med 22:49–56, 1997.

88. Reckelhoff JF, Kanji V, Racusen LC, et al: Vitamin E ameliorates enhanced renal lipid peroxidation and accumulation of F2-isoprostanes in aging kidneys. Am J Physiol 274:R767–R774, 1998.

89. Mitobe M, Yoshida T, Sugiura H, et al: Oxidative stress decreases klotho expression in a mouse kidney cell line. Nephron Exp Nephrol 101:e67–e74, 2005.

90. Ushio-Fukai M, Zafari AM, Fukui T, et al: p22phox is a critical component of the superoxide-generating NADH/NADPH oxidase system and regulates angiotensin II-induced hypertrophy in vascular smooth muscle cells. J Biol Chem 271:23317–23321, 1996.

91. de Cavanagh EM, Inserra F, Ferder L, et al: Superoxide dismutase and glutathione peroxidase activities are increased by enalapril and captopril in mouse liver. FEBS Lett 361:22–24, 1995.

92. Cruz CI, Ruiz-Torres P, del Moral RG, et al: Age-related progressive renal fibrosis in rats and its prevention with ACE inhibitors and taurine. Am J Physiol Renal Physiol 278:F122–F129, 2000.

93. Kim HJ, Jung KJ, Yu BP, et al: Influence of aging and calorie restriction on MAPKs activity in rat kidney. Exp Gerontol 37:1041–1053, 2002.

94. Lee JH, Jung KJ, Kim JW, et al: Suppression of apoptosis by calorie restriction in aged kidney. Exp Gerontol 39:1361–1368, 2004.

95. Levi M, Jameson DM, van der Meer BW: Role of BBM lipid composition and fluidity in impaired renal Pi transport in aged rat. Am J Physiol 256:F85–F94, 1989.

96. Jiang T, Liebman SE, Lucia MS, et al: Calorie restriction modulates renal expression of sterol regulatory element binding proteins, lipid accumulation, and age-related renal disease. J Am Soc Nephrol 16:2385–2394, 2005.

97. Wanner C, Greiber S, Kramer-Guth A, et al: Lipids and progression of renal disease: role of modified low density lipoprotein and lipoprotein(a). Kidney Int Suppl 63: S102–S106, 1997.

98. Kamanna VS, Roh DD, Kirschenbaum MA: Hyperlipidemia and kidney disease: Concepts derived from histopathology and cell biology of the glomerulus. Histol Histopathol 13:169–179, 1998.

99. Wu ZL, Liang MY, Qiu LQ: Oxidized low-density lipoprotein decreases the induced nitric oxide synthesis in rat mesangial cells. Cell Biochem Funct 16:153–158, 1998.

100. Dominguez JH, Tang N, Xu W, et al: Studies of renal injury III: Lipid-induced nephropathy in type II diabetes. Kidney Int 57:92–104, 2000.

101. Kim SI, Han DC, Lee HB: Lovastatin inhibits transforming growth factor-beta1 expression in diabetic rat glomeruli and cultured rat mesangial cells. J Am Soc Nephrol 11:80–87, 2000.

102. Lam KS, Cheng IK, Janus ED, Pang RW: Cholesterol-lowering therapy may retard the progression of diabetic nephropathy. Diabetologia 38:604–609, 1995.

103. Tonolo G, Ciccarese M, Brizzi P, et al: Reduction of albumin excretion rate in normotensive microalbuminuric type 2 diabetic patients during long-term simvastatin treatment. Diabetes Care 20:1891–1895, 1997.

104. Fried LF, Orchard TJ, Kasiske BL: Effect of lipid reduction on the progression of renal disease: a meta-analysis. Kidney Int 59:260–269, 2001.

105. Hoang K, Tan JC, Derby G, et al: Determinants of glomerular hypofiltration in aging humans. Kidney Int 64:1417–1424, 2003.

106. Kenney WL, Ho CW: Age alters regional distribution of blood flow during moderate-intensity exercise. J Appl Physiol 79:1112–1119, 1995.

107. Minson CT, Wladkowski SL, Cardell AF, et al: Age alters the cardiovascular response to direct passive heating. J Appl Physiol 84:1323–1332, 1998.

108. Mulkerrin EC, Brain A, Hampton D, et al: Reduced renal hemodynamic response to atrial natriuretic peptide in elderly volunteers. Am J Kidney Dis 22:538–544, 1993.

109. Clark B: Biology of renal aging in humans. Adv Ren Replace Ther 7:11–21, 2000.

110. Fliser D, Zeier M, Nowack R, Ritz E: Renal functional reserve in healthy elderly subjects. J Am Soc Nephrol 3:1371–1377, 1993.

111. Lakatta EG: Cardiovascular regulatory mechanisms in advanced age. Physiol Rev 73:413–467, 1993.

112. Moritoki H, Yoshikawa T, Hisayama T, Takeuchi S: Possible mechanisms of age-associated reduction of vascular relaxation caused by atrial natriuretic peptide. Eur J Pharmacol 210:61–68, 1992.

113. Sato I, Kaji K, Morita I, et al: Augmentation of endothelin-1, prostacyclin and thromboxane A2 secretion associated with in vitro ageing in cultured human umbilical vein endothelial cells. Mech Ageing Dev 71:73–84, 1993.

114. Rathaus M, Greenfeld Z, Podjarny E, et al: Altered prostaglandin synthesis and impaired sodium conservation in the kidneys of old rats. Clin Sci (Lond) 83:301–306, 1992.

115. Naeije R, Fiasse A, Carlier E, et al: Systemic and renal haemodynamic effects of angiotensin converting enzyme inhibition by zabicipril in young and in old normal men. Eur J Clin Pharmacol 44:35–39, 1993.

116. Hollenberg NK, Moore TJ: Age and the renal blood supply: renal vascular responses to angiotensin converting enzyme inhibition in healthy humans. J Am Geriatr Soc 42:805–808, 1994.

117. Baylis C: Renal responses to acute angiotensin II inhibition and administered angiotensin II in the aging, conscious, chronically catheterized rat. Am J Kidney Dis 22:842–850, 1993.

118. Baylis C, Fredericks M, Wilson C, et al: Renal vasodilatory response to intravenous glycine in the aging rat kidney. Am J Kidney Dis 15:244–251, 1990.

119. Tank JE, Vora JP, Houghton DC, Anderson S: Altered renal vascular responses in the aging rat kidney. Am J Physiol 266:F942–F948, 1994.

120. Zhang XZ, Qiu C, Baylis C: Sensitivity of the segmental renal arterioles to angiotensin II in the aging rat. Mech Ageing Dev 97:183–192, 1997.

121. Verhave JC, Fesler P, du Cailar G, et al: Elevated pulse pressure is associated with low renal function in elderly patients with isolated systolic hypertension. Hypertension 45:586–591, 2005.

122. Edwards MS, Wilson DB, Craven TE, et al: Associations between retinal microvascular abnormalities and declining renal function in the elderly population: The Cardiovascular Health Study. Am J Kidney Dis 46:214–224, 2005.

123. Back SE, Ljungberg B, Nilsson-Ehle I, et al: Age dependence of renal function: Clearance of iohexol and p-amino hippurate in healthy males. Scand J Clin Lab Invest 49:641–646, 1989.

124. Rowe JW, Shock NW, DeFronzo RA: The influence of age on the renal response to water deprivation in man. Nephron 17:270–278, 1976.

125. Lew SW, Bosch JP: Effect of diet on creatinine clearance and excretion in young and elderly healthy subjects and in patients with renal disease. J Am Soc Nephrol 2:856–865, 1991.

126. Levey AS, Bosch JP, Lewis JB, et al: A more accurate method to estimate glomerular filtration rate from serum creatinine: a new prediction equation. Modification of Diet in Renal Disease Study Group. Ann Intern Med 130:461–470, 1999.

127. Yonemura K, Takahira R, Yonekawa O, et al: The diagnostic value of serum concentrations of 2-(alpha-mannopyranosyl)-L-tryptophan for normal renal function. Kidney Int 65:1395–1399, 2004.

128. Dharnidharka VR, Kwon C, Stevens G: Serum cystatin C is superior to serum creatinine as a marker of kidney function: a meta-analysis. Am J Kidney Dis 40:221–226, 2002.

129. Baracskay D, Jarjoura D, Cugino A, et al: Geriatric renal function: Estimating glomerular filtration in an ambulatory elderly population. Clin Nephrol 47:222–228, 1997.
130. Luft FC, Fineberg NS, Miller JZ, et al: The effects of age, race and heredity on glomerular filtration rate following volume expansion and contraction in normal man. Am J Med Sci 279:15–24, 1980.
131. Tauchi H, Tsuboi K, Okutomi J: Age changes in the human kidney of the different races. Gerontologia 17:87–97, 1971.
132. Fliser D, Franek E, Joest M, et al: Renal function in the elderly: impact of hypertension and cardiac function. Kidney Int 51:1196–1204, 1997.
133. Tolbert EM, Weisstuch J, Feiner HD, Dworkin LD: Onset of glomerular hypertension with aging precedes injury in the spontaneously hypertensive rat. Am J Physiol Renal Physiol 278:F839–F846, 2000.
134. Ribstein J, Du Cailar G, Mimran A: Glucose tolerance and age-associated decline in renal function of hypertensive patients. J Hypertens 19:2257–2264, 2001.
135. Epstein M, Hollenberg NK: Age as a determinant of renal sodium conservation in normal man. J Lab Clin Med 87:411–417, 1976.
136. Macias Nunez JF, Garcia Iglesias C, Bondia Roman A, et al: Renal handling of sodium in old people: a functional study. Age Ageing 7:178–181, 1978.
137. Bauer JH: Age-related changes in the renin-aldosterone system. Physiological effects and clinical implications. Drugs Aging 3:238–245, 1993.
138. Baylis C, Engels K, Beierwaltes WH: Beta-adrenoceptor-stimulated renin release is blunted in old rats. J Am Soc Nephrol 9:1318–1320, 1998.
139. Hayashi M, Saruta T, Nakamura R, et al: Effect of aging on single nephron renin content in rats. Ren Physiol 4:17–21, 1981.
140. Lu X, Li X, Li L, et al: Variation of intrarenal angiotensin II and angiotensin II receptors by acute renal ischemia in the aged rat. Ren Fail 18:19–29, 1996.
141. Jover B, Dupont M, Geelen G, et al: Renal and systemic adaptation to sodium restriction in aging rats. Am J Physiol 264:R833–R838, 1993.
142. Tsunoda K, Abe K, Goto T, et al: Effect of age on the renin-angiotensin-aldosterone system in normal subjects: Simultaneous measurement of active and inactive renin, renin substrate, and aldosterone in plasma. J Clin Endocrinol Metab 62:384–389, 1986.
143. Weidmann P, de Chatel R, Schiffmann A, et al: Interrelations between age and plasma renin, aldosterone and cortisol, urinary catecholamines, and the body sodium/volume state in normal man. Klin Wochenschr 55:725–733, 1977.
144. Mimran A, Ribstein J, Jover B: Aging and sodium homeostasis. Kidney Int Suppl 37: S107–S113, 1992.
145. Leosco D, Ferrara N, Landino P, et al: Effects of age on the role of atrial natriuretic factor in renal adaptation to physiologic variations of dietary salt intake. J Am Soc Nephrol 7:1045–1051, 1996.
146. Pollack JA, Skvorak JP, Nazian SJ, et al: Alterations in atrial natriuretic peptide (ANP) secretion and renal effects in aging. J Gerontol A Biol Sci Med Sci 52:B196–B202, 1997.
147. Luft FC, Grim CE, Fineberg N, Weinberger MC: Effects of volume expansion and contraction in normotensive whites, blacks, and subjects of different ages. Circulation 59:643–650, 1979.
148. Brenner BM, Ballermann BJ, Gunning ME, Zeidel ML: Diverse biological actions of atrial natriuretic peptide. Physiol Rev 70:665–699, 1990.
149. Ohashi M, Fujio N, Nawata H, et al: High plasma concentrations of human atrial natriuretic polypeptide in aged men. J Clin Endocrinol Metab 64:81–85, 1987.
150. Haller BG, Zust H, Shaw S, et al: Effects of posture and ageing on circulating atrial natriuretic peptide levels in man. J Hypertens 5:551–556, 1987.
151. Tajima F, Sagawa S, Iwamoto J, et al: Renal and endocrine responses in the elderly during head-out water immersion. Am J Physiol 254:R977–R983, 1988.
152. Or K, Richards AM, Espiner EA, et al: Effect of low dose infusions of ile-atrial natriuretic peptide in healthy elderly males. Evidence for a postreceptor defect. J Clin Endocrinol Metab 76:1271–1274, 1993.
153. Gillies AH, Crozier IG, Nicholls MG, et al: Effect of posture on clearance of atrial natriuretic peptide from plasma. J Clin Endocrinol Metab 65:1095–1097, 1987.
154. Rascher W, Tulassay T, Lang RE: Atrial natriuretic peptide in plasma of volume-overloaded children with chronic renal failure. Lancet 2:303–305, 1985.
155. Lafferty HM, Gunning M, Silva P, et al: Enkephalinase inhibition increases plasma atrial natriuretic peptide levels, glomerular filtration rate, and urinary sodium excretion in rats with reduced renal mass. Circ Res 65:640–646, 1989.
156. Kimmelstiel CD, Perrone R, Kilcoyne L, et al: Effects of renal neutral endopeptidase inhibition on sodium excretion, renal hemodynamics and neurohormonal activation in patients with congestive heart failure. Cardiology 87:46–53, 1996.
157. Tan AC, Hoefnagels WH, Swinkels LM, et al: The effect of volume expansion on atrial natriuretic peptide and cyclic guanosine monophosphate levels in young and aged subjects. J Am Geriatr Soc 38:1215–1219, 1990.
158. Tian Y, Serino R, Verbalis JG: Downregulation of renal vasopressin V2 receptor and aquaporin-2 expression parallels age-associated defects in urine concentration. Am J Physiol Renal Physiol 287:F797–F805, 2004.
159. Helderman JH, Vestal RE, Rowe JW, et al: The response of arginine vasopressin to intravenous ethanol and hypertonic saline in man: The impact of aging. J Gerontol 33:39–47, 1978.
160. Ishikawa S, Fujita N, Fujisawa G, et al: Involvement of arginine vasopressin and renal sodium handling in pathogenesis of hyponatremia in elderly patients. Endocr J 43:101–108, 1996.
161. Phillips PA, Bretherton M, Risvanis J, et al: Effects of drinking on thirst and vasopressin in dehydrated elderly men. Am J Physiol 264:R877–R881, 1993.
162. Faull CM, Holmes C, Baylis PH: Water balance in elderly people: Is there a deficiency of vasopressin? Age Ageing 22:114–120, 1993.
163. Miller JH, Shock NW: Age differences in the renal tubular response to antidiuretic hormone. J Gerontol 8:446–450, 1953.
164. Macias Nunez JF, Garcia Iglesias C, Tabernero Romo JM, et al: Renal management of sodium under indomethacin and aldosterone in the elderly. Age Ageing 9:165–172, 1980.
165. Bengele HH, Mathias RS, Perkins JH, Alexander EA: Urinary concentrating defect in the aged rat. Am J Physiol 240:F147–F150, 1981.
166. Davidson YS, Davies I, Goddard C: Renal vasopressin receptors in ageing C57BL/Icrfat mice. J Endocrinol 115:379–385, 1987.
167. Beck N, Yu BP: Effect of aging on urinary concentrating mechanism and vasopressin-dependent cAMP in rats. Am J Physiol 243:F121–F125, 1982.
168. Goddard C, Davidson YS, Moser BB, et al: Effect of ageing on cyclic AMP output by renal medullary cells in response to arginine vasopressin in vitro in C57BL/Icrfat mice. J Endocrinol 103:133–139, 1984.
169. Liang CT, Barnes J, Hanai H, Levine MA: Decrease in Gs protein expression may impair adenylate cyclase activation in old kidneys. Am J Physiol 264:F770–F773, 1993.
170. Wilson PD, Dillingham MA: Age-associated decrease in vasopressin-induced renal water transport: A role for adenylate cyclase and G protein malfunction. Gerontology 38:315–321, 1992.
171. Preisser L, Teillet L, Aliotti S, et al: Downregulation of aquaporin-2 and -3 in aging kidney is inde-pendent of V(2) vasopressin receptor. Am J Physiol Renal Physiol 279: F144–F152, 2000.
172. Terashima Y, Kondo K, Inagaki A, et al: Age-associated decrease in response of rat aquaporin-2 gene expression to dehydration. Life Sci 62:873–882, 1998.
173. Combet S, Teillet L, Geelen G, et al: Food restriction prevents age-related polyuria by vasopressin-dependent recruitment of aquaporin-2. Am J Physiol Renal Physiol 281: F1123–F1131, 2001.
174. Combet S, Geffroy N, Berthonaud V, et al: Correction of age-related polyuria by dDAVP: molecular analysis of aquaporins and urea transporters. Am J Physiol Renal Physiol 284:F199–F208, 2003.
175. Crowe MJ, Forsling ML, Rolls BJ, et al: Altered water excretion in healthy elderly men. Age Ageing 16:285–293, 1987.
176. Frassetto LA, Morris RC, Jr, Sebastian A: Effect of age on blood acid-base composition in adult humans: Role of age-related renal functional decline. Am J Physiol 271: F1114–F1122, 1996.
177. Adler S, Lindeman RD, Yiengst MJ, et al: Effect of acute acid loading on urinary acid excretion by the aging human kidney. J Lab Clin Med 72:278–289, 1968.
178. Agarwal BN, Cabebe FG: Renal acidification in elderly subjects. Nephron 26:291–295, 1980.
179. Prasad R, Kinsella JL, Sacktor B: Renal adaptation to metabolic acidosis in senescent rats. Am J Physiol 255:F1183–F1190, 1988.
180. Mitch WE, Medina R, Grieber S, et al: Metabolic acidosis stimulates muscle protein degradation by activating the adenosine triphosphate-dependent pathway involving ubiquitin and proteasomes. J Clin Invest 93:2127–2133, 1994.
181. Alpern RJ, Sakhaee K: The clinical spectrum of chronic metabolic acidosis: Homeostatic mechanisms produce significant morbidity. Am J Kidney Dis 29:291–302, 1997.
182. Sebastian A, Morris RC, Jr: Improved mineral balance and skeletal metabolism in postmenopausal women treated with potassium bicarbonate. N Engl J Med 331:279, 1994.
183. Weidmann P, De Myttenaere-Bursztein S, Maxwell MH, de Lima J: Effect on aging on plasma renin and aldosterone in normal man. Kidney Int 8:325–333, 1975.
184. Mulkerrin E, Epstein FH, Clark BA: Aldosterone responses to hyperkalemia in healthy elderly humans. J Am Soc Nephrol 6:1459–1462, 1995.
185. Bengele HH, Mathias R, Perkins JH, et al: Impaired renal and extrarenal potassium adaptation in old rats. Kidney Int 23:684–690, 1983.
186. Minaker KL, Rowe JW: Potassium homeostasis during hyperinsulinemia: Effect of insulin level, beta-blockade, and age. Am J Physiol 242:E373–E377, 1982.
187. Ford GA, Blaschke TF, Wiswell R, Hoffman BB: Effect of aging on changes in plasma potassium during exercise. J Gerontol 48:M140–M145, 1993.
188. Armbrecht HJ, Zenser TV, Gross CJ, Davis BB: Adaptation to dietary calcium and phosphorus restriction changes with age in the rat. Am J Physiol 239:E322–E327, 1980.
189. Corman B, Roinel N: Single-nephron filtration rate and proximal reabsorption in aging rats. Am J Physiol 260:F75–F80, 1991.
190. Armbrecht HJ, Zenser TV, Bruns ME, Davis BB: Effect of age on intestinal calcium absorption and adaptation to dietary calcium. Am J Physiol 236:E769–E774, 1979.
191. Halloran BP, Lonergan ET, Portale AA: Aging and renal responsiveness to parathyroid hormone in healthy men. J Clin Endocrinol Metab 81:2192–2197, 1996.
192. Portale AA, Lonergan ET, Tanney DM, Halloran BP: Aging alters calcium regulation of serum concentration of parathyroid hormone in healthy men. Am J Physiol 272: E139–E146, 1997.
193. Mulroney SE, Woda C, Haramati A: Changes in renal phosphate reabsorption in the aged rat. Proc Soc Exp Biol Med 218:62–67, 1998.
194. Kiebzak GM, Sacktor B: Effect of age on renal conservation of phosphate in the rat. Am J Physiol 251:F399–F407, 1986.
195. Chen ML, King RS, Armbrecht HJ: Sodium-dependent phosphate transport in primary cultures of renal tubule cells from young and adult rats. J Cell Physiol 143:488–493, 1990.
196. Sorribas V, Lotscher M, Loffing J, et al: Cellular mechanisms of the age-related decrease in renal phosphate reabsorption. Kidney Int 50:855–863, 1996.
197. Levi M, Baird BM, Wilson PV: Cholesterol modulates rat renal brush border membrane phosphate transport. J Clin Invest 85:231–237, 1990.
198. Breusegem SY, Halaihel N, Inoue M, et al: Acute and chronic changes in cholesterol modulate Na-Pi cotransport activity in OK cells. Am J Physiol Renal Physiol 289: F154–F165, 2005.
199. Brandis M, Harmeyer J, Kaune R, et al: Phosphate transport in brush-border membranes from control and rachitic pig kidney and small intestine. J Physiol 384:479–490, 1987.
200. Kurnik BR, Hruska KA: Effects of 1,25-dihydroxycholecalciferol on phosphate transport in vitamin D-deprived rats. Am J Physiol 247:F177–F184, 1984.

201. Liang CT, Barnes J, Cheng L, et al: Effects of 1,25-(OH)2D3 administered in vivo on phosphate uptake by isolated chick renal cells. Am J Physiol 242:C312–C318, 1982.

202. Brasitus TA, Dudeja PK, Eby B, Lau K: Correction by 1–25-dihydroxycholecalciferol of the abnormal fluidity and lipid composition of enterocyte brush border membranes in vitamin D-deprived rats. J Biol Chem 261:16404–16409, 1986.

203. Beck LH, Lavizzo-Mourey R: Geriatric hypernatremia [corrected]. Ann Intern Med 107:768–769, 1987.

204. Miller M, Hecker MS, Friedlander DA, Carter JM: Apparent idiopathic hyponatremia in an ambulatory geriatric population. J Am Geriatr Soc 44:404–408, 1996.

205. Clark BA, Shannon RP, Rosa RM, Epstein FH: Increased susceptibility to thiazide-induced hyponatremia in the elderly. J Am Soc Nephrol 5:1106–1111, 1994.

206. Snyder NA, Feigal DW, Arieff AI: Hypernatremia in elderly patients. A heterogeneous, morbid, and iatrogenic entity. Ann Intern Med 107:309–319, 1987.

207. Pascual J, Orofino L, Liano F, et al: Incidence and prognosis of acute renal failure in older patients. J Am Geriatr Soc 38:25–30, 1990.

208. McInnes EG, Levy DW, Chaudhuri MD, Bhan GL: Renal failure in the elderly. Q J Med 64:583–588, 1987.

209. Macias-Nunez JF, Lopez-Novoa JM, Martinez-Maldonado M: Acute renal failure in the aged. Semin Nephrol 16:330–338, 1996.

210. Zarich S, Fang LS, Diamond JR: Fractional excretion of sodium. Exceptions to its diagnostic value. Arch Intern Med 145:108–112, 1985.

211. Gentric A, Cledes J: Immediate and long-term prognosis in acute renal failure in the elderly. Nephrol Dial Transplant 6:86–90, 1991.

212. Klouche K, Cristol JP, Kaaki M, et al: Prognosis of acute renal failure in the elderly. Nephrol Dial Transplant 10:2240–2243, 1995.

213. Santacruz F, Barreto S, Mayor MM, et al: Mortality in elderly patients with acute renal failure. Ren Fail 18:601–605, 1996.

214. Moore RD, Smith CR, Lipsky JJ, et al: Risk factors for nephrotoxicity in patients treated with aminoglycosides. Ann Intern Med 100:352–357, 1984.

215. Michel DM, Kelly CJ: Acute interstitial nephritis. J Am Soc Nephrol 9:506–515, 1998.

216. Kleinknecht D: Interstitial nephritis, the nephrotic syndrome, and chronic renal failure secondary to nonsteroidal anti-inflammatory drugs. Semin Nephrol 15:228–235, 1995.

217. Rich MW, Crecelius CA: Incidence, risk factors, and clinical course of acute renal insufficiency after cardiac catheterization in patients 70 years of age or older. A prospective study. Arch Intern Med 150:1237–1242, 1990.

218. Porter GA: Radiocontrast-induced nephropathy. Nephrol Dial Transplant 9 Suppl 4:146–156, 1994.

219. Beierschmitt WP, Keenan KP, Weiner M: Age-related increased susceptibility of male Fischer 344 rats to acetaminophen nephrotoxicity. Life Sci 39:2335–2342, 1986.

220. Miura K, Goldstein RS, Morgan DG, et al: Age-related differences in susceptibility to renal ischemia in rats. Toxicol Appl Pharmacol 87:284–296, 1987.

221. Sabbatini M, Sansone G, Uccello F, et al: Functional versus structural changes in the pathophysiology of acute ischemic renal failure in aging rats. Kidney Int 45:1355–1361, 1994.

222. Zager RA, Alpers CE: Effects of aging on expression of ischemic acute renal failure in rats. Lab Invest 61:290–294, 1989.

223. Adachi T, Kawamura M, Owada M, Hiramori K: Effect of age on renal functional and orthostatic vascular response in healthy men. Clin Exp Pharmacol Physiol 28:877–880, 2001.

224. Prasad PV, Epstein FH: Changes in renal medullary pO2 during water diuresis as evaluated by blood oxygenation level-dependent magnetic resonance imaging: Effects of aging and cyclooxygenase inhibition. Kidney Int 55:294–298, 1999.

225. Boldt J, Brenner T, Lang J, et al: Kidney-specific proteins in elderly patients undergoing cardiac surgery with cardiopulmonary bypass. Anesth Analg 97:1582–1589, 2003.

226. Paller MS, Hoidal JR, Ferris TF: Oxygen free radicals in ischemic acute renal failure in the rat. J Clin Invest 74:1156–1164, 1984.

227. Long DA, Mu W, Price KL, Johnson RJ: Blood vessels and the aging kidney. Nephron Exp Nephrol 101:e95–e99, 2005.

228. Kung CF, Luscher TF: Different mechanisms of endothelial dysfunction with aging and hypertension in rat aorta. Hypertension 25:194–200, 1995.

229. Luscher TF, Bock HA: The endothelial L-arginine/nitric oxide pathway and the renal circulation. Klin Wochenschr 69:603–609, 1991.

230. Reckelhoff JF, Kellum JA, Blanchard EJ, et al: Changes in nitric oxide precursor, L-arginine, and metabolites, nitrate and nitrite, with aging. Life Sci 55:1895–1902, 1994.

231. Sarwar G, Botting HG, Collins M: A comparison of fasting serum amino acid profiles of young and elderly subjects. J Am Coll Nutr 10:668–674, 1991.

232. Mistry SK, Greenfeld Z, Morris SM, Jr., Baylis C: The 'intestinal-renal' arginine biosynthetic axis in the aging rat. Mech Ageing Dev 123:1159–1165, 2002.

233. Cronin RE: Renal failure following radiologic procedures. Am J Med Sci 298:342–356, 1989.

234. Sabbatini M, Pisani A, Uccello F, et al: Atorvastatin improves the course of ischemic acute renal failure in aging rats. J Am Soc Nephrol 15:901–909, 2004.

235. Xiong Y, Yuan LW, Deng HW, et al: Elevated serum endogenous inhibitor of nitric oxide synthase and endothelial dysfunction in aged rats. Clin Exp Pharmacol Physiol 28:842–847, 2001.

236. Miyazaki H, Matsuoka H, Cooke JP, et al: Endogenous nitric oxide synthase inhibitor: A novel marker of atherosclerosis. Circulation 99:1141–1146, 1999.

237. Kielstein JT, Bode-Boger SM, Frolich JC, et al: Asymmetric dimethylarginine, blood pressure, and renal perfusion in elderly subjects. Circulation 107:1891–1895, 2003.

238. Gupta BK, Spinowitz BS, Charytan C, Wahl SJ: Cholesterol crystal embolization-associated renal failure after therapy with recombinant tissue-type plasminogen activator. Am J Kidney Dis 21:659–662, 1993.

239. Feest TG, Round A, Hamad S: Incidence of severe acute renal failure in adults: results of a community based study. BMJ 306:481–483, 1993.

240. Arora P, Kher V, Kohli HS, et al: Acute renal failure in the elderly: Experience from a single centre in India. Nephrol Dial Transplant 8:827–830, 1993.

241. Druml W, Lax F, Grimm G, et al: Acute renal failure in the elderly 1975–1990. Clin Nephrol 41:342–349, 1994.

242. Pascual J, Liano F, Ortuno J: The elderly patient with acute renal failure. J Am Soc Nephrol 6:144–153, 1995.

243. Hansen KJ, Edwards MS, Craven TE, et al: Prevalence of renovascular disease in the elderly: A population-based study. J Vasc Surg 36:443–451, 2002.

244. Edwards MS, Hansen KJ, Craven TE, et al: Relationships between renovascular disease, blood pressure, and renal function in the elderly: a population-based study. Am J Kidney Dis 41:990–996, 2003.

245. Jacobson HR: Ischemic renal disease: An overlooked clinical entity? Kidney Int 34:729–743, 1988.

246. Connolly JO, Higgins RM, Walters HL, et al: Presentation, clinical features and outcome in different patterns of atherosclerotic renovascular disease. QJM 87:413–421, 1994.

247. Baboolal K, Evans C, Moore RH: Incidence of end-stage renal disease in medically treated patients with severe bilateral atherosclerotic renovascular disease. Am J Kidney Dis 31:971–977, 1998.

248. Appel RG, Bleyer AJ, Reavis S, Hansen KJ: Renovascular disease in older patients beginning renal replacement therapy. Kidney Int 48:171–176, 1995.

249. Bleyer AJ, Shemanski LR, Burke GL, et al: Tobacco, hypertension, and vascular disease: risk factors for renal functional decline in an older population. Kidney Int 57:2072–2079, 2000.

250. Haak T, Jungmann E, Raab C, Usadel KH: Elevated endothelin-1 levels after cigarette smoking. Metabolism 43:267–269, 1994.

251. Barton M, Lattmann T, d'Uscio LV, et al: Inverse regulation of endothelin-1 and nitric oxide metabolites in tissue with aging: Implications for the age-dependent increase of cardiorenal disease. J Cardiovasc Pharmacol 36:S153–S156, 2000.

252. van de Ven PJ, Beutler JJ, Kaatee R, et al: Angiotensin converting enzyme inhibitor-induced renal dysfunction in atherosclerotic renovascular disease. Kidney Int 53:986–993, 1998.

253. Erbsloh-Moller B, Dumas A, Roth D, et al: Furosemide-131I-hippuran renography after angiotensin-converting enzyme inhibition for the diagnosis of renovascular hypertension. Am J Med 90:23–29, 1991.

254. Prigent A: The diagnosis of renovascular hypertension: the role of captopril renal scintigraphy and related issues. Eur J Nucl Med 20:625–644, 1993.

255. Olin JW, Piedmonte MR, Young JR, et al: The utility of duplex ultrasound scanning of the renal arteries for diagnosing significant renal artery stenosis. Ann Intern Med 122:833–838, 1995.

256. Bleyer AJ, Chen R, D'Agostino RB, Jr, Appel RG: Clinical correlates of hypertensive end-stage renal disease. Am J Kidney Dis 31:28–34, 1998.

257. Meyrier A: Renal vascular lesions in the elderly: Nephrosclerosis or atheromatous renal disease? Nephrol Dial Transplant 11 Suppl 9:45–52, 1996.

258. Schlanger LE, Haire HM, Zuckerman AM, et al: Reversible renal failure in an elderly woman with renal artery stenosis. Am J Kidney Dis 23:123–126, 1994.

259. Zeller T: Renal artery stenosis: Epidemiology, clinical manifestation, and percutaneous endovascular therapy. J Interv Cardiol 18:497–506, 2005.

260. Dorros G, Jaff M, Mathiak L, et al: Four-year follow-up of Palmaz-Schatz stent revascularization as treatment for atherosclerotic renal artery stenosis. Circulation 98:642–647, 1998.

261. Marone LK, Clouse WD, Dorer DJ, et al: Preservation of renal function with surgical revascularization in patients with atherosclerotic renovascular disease. J Vasc Surg 39:322–329, 2004.

262. Furci L, Medici G, Baraldi A, et al: Rapidly progressive glomerulonephritis in the elderly. Long-term results. Contrib Nephrol 105:98–101, 1993.

263. Jeffrey RF, Gardiner DS, More IA, et al: Crescentic glomerulonephritis: Experience of a single unit over a five year period. Scott Med J 37:175–178, 1992.

264. Moorthy AV, Zimmerman SW: Renal disease in the elderly: Clinicopathologic analysis of renal disease in 115 elderly patients. Clin Nephrol 14:223–229, 1980.

265. Bergesio F, Bertoni E, Bandini S, et al: Changing pattern of glomerulonephritis in the elderly: A change of prevalence or a different approach? Contrib Nephrol 105:75–80, 1993.

266. Haas M, Spargo BH, Wit EJ, Meehan SM: Etiologies and outcome of acute renal insufficiency in older adults: A renal biopsy study of 259 cases. Am J Kidney Dis 35:433–447, 2000.

267. Washio M, Oh Y, Okuda S, et al: Clinicopathological study of poststreptococcal glomerulonephritis in the elderly. Clin Nephrol 41:265–270, 1994.

268. Davison AM, Johnston PA: Glomerulonephritis in the elderly. Nephrol Dial Transplant 11 Suppl 9:34–37, 1996.

269. Prakash J, Singh AK, Saxena RK, Usha: Glomerular diseases in the elderly in India. Int Urol Nephrol 35:283–288, 2003.

270. Fawcett IW, Hilton PJ, Jones NF, Wing AJ: Nephrotic syndrome in the elderly. Br Med J 2:387–388, 1971.

271. Lustig S, Rosenfeld JB, Ben-Bassat M, Boner G: Nephrotic syndrome in the elderly. Isr J Med Sci 18:1010–1013, 1982.

272. Kingswood JC, Banks RA, Tribe CR, et al: Renal biopsy in the elderly: Clinicopathological correlations in 143 patients. Clin Nephrol 22:183–187, 1984.

273. Murphy PJ, Wright G, Rai GS: Nephrotic syndrome in the elderly. J Am Geriatr Soc 35:170–173, 1987.

274. Zech P, Colon S, Pointet P, et al: The nephrotic syndrome in adults aged over 60: Etiology, evolution and treatment of 76 cases. Clin Nephrol 17:232–236, 1982.

275. Shin JH, Pyo HJ, Kwon YJ, et al: Renal biopsy in elderly patients: Clinicopathological correlation in 117 Korean patients. Clin Nephrol 56:19–26, 2001.

276. Ozono Y, Harada T, Yamaguchi K, et al: Nephrotic syndrome in the elderly—clinicopathological study. Nippon Jinzo Gakkai Shi 36:44–50, 1994.

277. Johnston P: The nephrotic syndrome in the elderly: Clinicopathologic correlations in 317 patients. Geriatr Nephrol Urol 2:85, 1992.

278. Donadio JV, Jr: Treatment of glomerulonephritis in the elderly. Am J Kidney Dis 16:307–311, 1990.

279. Nolasco F, Cameron JS, Heywood EF, et al: Adult-onset minimal change nephrotic syndrome: A long-term follow-up. Kidney Int 29:1215–1223, 1986.

280. Zent R, Nagai R, Cattran DC: Idiopathic membranous nephropathy in the elderly: A comparative study. Am J Kidney Dis 29:200–206, 1997.

281. Ponticelli C, Altieri P, Scolari F, et al: A randomized study comparing methylprednisolone plus chlorambucil versus methylprednisolone plus cyclophosphamide in idiopathic membranous nephropathy. J Am Soc Nephrol 9:444–450, 1998.

282. K/DOQI clinical practice guidelines for chronic kidney disease: Evaluation, classification, and stratification. Am J Kidney Dis 39:S1–S266, 2002.

283. Manjunath G, Tighiouart H, Coresh J, et al: Level of kidney function as a risk factor for cardiovascular outcomes in the elderly. Kidney Int 63:1121–1129, 2003.

284. Agodoa LY, Eggers PW: Renal replacement therapy in the United States: Data from the United States Renal Data System. Am J Kidney Dis 25:119–133, 1995.

285. Nissenson AR: Dialysis therapy in the elderly patient. Kidney Int Suppl 40:S51–S57, 1993.

286. Port FK: Morbidity and mortality in dialysis patients. Kidney Int 46:1728–1737, 1994.

287. Peri UN, Fenves AZ, Middleton JP: Improving survival of octogenarian patients selected for haemodialysis. Nephrol Dial Transplant 16:2201–2206, 2001.

288. Lowrie EG, Lew NL: Death risk in hemodialysis patients: The predictive value of commonly measured variables and an evaluation of death rate differences between facilities. Am J Kidney Dis 15:458–482, 1990.

289. Capuano A, Sepe V, Cianfrone P, et al: Cardiovascular impairment, dialysis strategy and tolerance in elderly and young patients on maintenance haemodialysis. Nephrol Dial Transplant 5:1023–1030, 1990.

290. Ismail N, Hakim RM, Oreopoulos DG, Patrikarea A: Renal replacement therapies in the elderly: Part 1. Hemodialysis and chronic peritoneal dialysis. Am J Kidney Dis 22:759–782, 1993.

291. Wolcott DL, Nissenson AR: Quality of life in chronic dialysis patients: A critical comparison of continuous ambulatory peritoneal dialysis (CAPD) and hemodialysis. Am J Kidney Dis 11:402–412, 1988.

292. Balaskas EV, Yuan ZY, Gupta A, et al: Long-term continuous ambulatory peritoneal dialysis in diabetics. Clin Nephrol 42:54–62, 1994.

293. Lunde NM, Port FK, Wolfe RA, Guire KE: Comparison of mortality risk by choice of CAPD versus hemodialysis among elderly patients. Adv Perit Dial 7:68–72, 1991.

294. Maiorca R, Vonesh EF, Cavalli P, et al: A multicenter, selection-adjusted comparison of patient and technique survivals on CAPD and hemodialysis. Perit Dial Int 11:118–127, 1991.

295. Vonesh EF, Snyder JJ, Foley RN, Collins AJ: The differential impact of risk factors on mortality in hemodialysis and peritoneal dialysis. Kidney Int 66:2389–2401, 2004.

296. Cantarovich D, Baranger T, Tirouvanziam A, et al: One-hundred and five cadaveric kidney transplants with cyclosporine in recipients more than 60 years of age. Transplant Proc 25:1323, 1993.

297. Ismail N, Hakim RM, Helderman JH: Renal replacement therapies in the elderly: Part II. Renal transplantation. Am J Kidney Dis 23:1–15, 1994.

298. Jassal SV, Krahn MD, Naglie G, et al: Kidney transplantation in the elderly: A decision analysis. J Am Soc Nephrol 14:187–196, 2003.

299. Johnson DW, Herzig K, Purdie D, et al: A comparison of the effects of dialysis and renal transplantation on the survival of older uremic patients. Transplantation 69:794–799, 2000.

300. Nyberg G, Nilsson B, Hallste G, et al: Renal transplantation in elderly patients: Survival and complications. Transplant Proc 25:1062–1063, 1993.

301. Meier-Kriesche HU, Ojo A, Hanson J, et al: Increased immunosuppressive vulnerability in elderly renal transplant recipients. Transplantation 69:885–889, 2000.

302. Becker BN, Ismail N, Becker YT: Renal transplantation in the older end stage renal disease patient. Semin Nephrol 16:353–362, 1996.

303. Abrutyn E, Mossey J, Berlin JA, et al: Does asymptomatic bacteriuria predict mortality and does antimicrobial treatment reduce mortality in elderly ambulatory women? Ann Intern Med 120:827–833, 1994.

304. Stamm WE, Hooton TM: Management of urinary tract infections in adults. N Engl J Med 329:1328–1334, 1993.

305. Kissane JM: The morphology of renal cystic disease. Perspect Nephrol Hypertens 4:31–63, 1976.

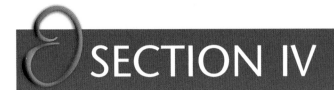

SECTION IV

Pathogenesis of Renal Disease

CHAPTER 22

Approach to the Patient with Kidney Disease

Ramesh Saxena • Robert D. Toto

Kidney disease manifests in many ways. A patient may be completely asymptomatic or may be desperately ill with a life-threatening emergency. Nephrologists must know how to recognize and deal with various presentations and be familiar with and adept at evaluating and managing them. In general, a careful and thorough history and physical examination coupled with routine laboratory testing and renal ultrasonography are sufficient to direct further evaluation in order to make an accurate diagnosis. At present, these techniques constitute the mainstay for diagnosis of most genetic renal diseases as well. In the future, however, genetic testing will provide more direct and accurate diagnosis of many renal diseases.

A greater appreciation for the prevalence of chronic kidney disease (CKD) in the population has led to improvements in identification and diagnosis of CKDs and slowing down their progression to end-stage renal disease (ESRD). This chapter is divided into two sections, presentations of patients with kidney disease and methods of evaluation of acute kidney injury (AKI) and CKD.

PRESENTATIONS IN KIDNEY DISEASE

Differentiating AKI and CKD is an important distinction (Table 22–1). Kidney disease progresses toward the end stage in most patients with CKD (see Chapters 17 and 18). In contrast, most patients with AKI recover renal function, which returns to normal with no long-term sequelae. However, outcome in AKI depends on three factors: (1) early recognition, (2) establishment of cause, and (3) appropriate clinical management.[1–5] Evaluation is similar for AKI and CKD but must be performed much more rapidly in patients with AKI. Moreover, diagnostic tools may differ to some extent. For these reasons, the evaluation procedures for AKD and CKD overlap to some extent but are described separately in order of urgency.

ACUTE KIDNEY INJURY

AKI is defined as a sudden decrease in kidney function. Early manifestations of AKI vary and depend in part on context and underlying cause.[6] For example, some patients with toxic nephropathies (e.g., induced by nonsteroidal anti-inflammatory drugs [NSAIDs]) may be completely asymptomatic, so that kidney failure is discovered through laboratory evaluation (Table 22–2). In contrast, AKI due to acute hemolytic uremic syndrome (HUS) may manifest as oliguria, symptoms and signs of volume overload, life-threatening electrolyte abnormalities, and severe neurologic dysfunction.[1]

History

The nephrologist must perform a careful history to determine the cause of AKI. The history should initially focus on causes of kidney hypoperfusion and nephrotoxin exposure. Detailed history of recent events causing alterations in cardiovascular and volume status and use of drugs or toxins should be sought. Presenting complaints of patients suffering from volume depletion leading to kidney hypoperfusion include orthostatic dizziness, presyncope, and syncope. Common causes of volume depletion, such as vomiting, diarrhea, excessive sweating, burns, and renal salt wasting (e.g., diabetic ketoacidosis), must be investigated. In contrast, presenting complaints in patients with renal hypoperfusion due to primary (e.g., glomerulonephritis, HUS, atheroembolic renal disease) or secondary (e.g., congestive heart failure) renal sodium–retaining states include headaches (caused by hypertension), dyspnea, and peripheral edema due to extracellular fluid volume expansion. A history of recent trauma with or without blood loss or muscle trauma should raise the possibility of ischemia, myoglobin-induced tubular necrosis, or both. Fever, rash, and joint pains are associated with lupus nephritis, systemic necrotizing vasculitides, endocarditis, drug allergy, and infectious diseases (e.g., Hantavirus), all of which are causes of intrinsic kidney failure.[7–10] A history of dyspnea or hemoptysis may be a sign of Goodpasture syndrome, Wegener granulomatosis, Churg-Strauss vasculitis, lupus nephritis, or pulmonary edema due to volume overload associated with an acute glomerulonephritis.[10,11]

TABLE 22–1 Differentiation of Acute from Chronic Kidney Disease

History	Long-standing history suggests chronic kidney disease
Renal osteodystrophy	Radiographic evidence of osteitis fibrosa cystica, osteomalacia
Renal size (length)	
Small kidneys (e.g., <9 cm)	Chronic kidney disease of any cause
Normal or enlarged kidney disease (9–12 cm)	Acute kidney injury of any cause
	Chronic kidney disease
	Human immunodeficiency virus (HIV) nephropathy
	Diabetic nephrophathy
	Amyloidosis
Enlarged kidneys (>12 cm)	Autosomal dominant polycystic kidney disease
	Tuberous sclerosis
	Obstructive nephropathy
Renal biopsy	Histologic diagnosis

TABLE 22–2 Presentations of Renal Failure

Symptomatic presentation
General
  Fatigue
  Weakness
Cardiovascular
  Hypertension
  Pulmonary congestion
  Cough
  Dyspnea
  Hemoptysis
Neurologic
  Encephalopathy
  Seizure
  Peripheral neuropathy
Gastrointestinal
  Anorexia
  Nausea
  Vomiting
  Abdominal pain
  Bleeding
Muscoloskeletal
  Muscle weakness
  Periarticular or articular pain
  Bone pain
Genitourinary
  Hematuria
  Dysuria
Cutaneous
  Pruritus
  Necrosis
  Vasculitis
  Bruising

Asymptomatic presentation
Hypertension
Proteinuria
Hematuria
Abnormal renal imaging findings

In the hospital setting, meticulous review of medical records in patients with AKI should include a careful search for ischemic and nephrotoxic insults.[12] Postoperative AKI often develops as a consequence of an ischemic or nephrotoxic event.[13,14] Abdominal pain and flank pain are signs of AKI. Obstructive uropathies, acute inflammation of the kidney causing renal enlargement that stretches the renal capsule, can cause pain. Flank pain may also be observed in renal vein thrombosis. Upper quadrant pain may also a sign of acute renal infarction (e.g., renal artery emboli). Prominent neurologic signs are often observed in thrombotic thrombocytopenic purpura (TTP), HUS, toxic nephropathies, and some poisonings such as with aspirin.[15,16] Constitutional and nonspecific symptoms, such as malaise, weakness, fatigue, anorexia, nausea, and vomiting, are common in patients with AKI but do not alone establish an etiologic diagnosis.

A history of nephrotoxin exposure is an extremely important component of the evaluation of a patient with AKI.[12] Both endogenous and exogenous toxins can give rise to renal failure (Table 22–3). Myoglobin, hemoglobin, and light chains are nephrotoxic. Therefore, muscle damage, hemolysis, and myeloma should be considered in the patient with AKI.[17-21] The search should include a careful examination not only for known nephrotoxins such as NSAIDs,[22,23] acetaminophen,[12] angiotensin-converting enzyme (ACE) inhibitors,[24,25] antibiotics,[12,20,26] calcineurin inhibitors,[27-29] mannitol and intravenous immunoglobulin,[30,31] high-dose vitamin K in transplant recipients,[32] interferon-α,[33] chemotherapeutic agents including cisplatin and others,[12,34] radiocontrast agents,[35-37] diuretics[12] but also any agent that may be new to the patient's regimen. This search is important because drugs that uncommonly cause AKI may otherwise be overlooked (e.g., anticonvulsants, antidepressants).

In addition, over-the-counter drugs, including acetaminophen, herbal and health care products,[38,39] antibiotics, antihypertensives, and poisons, should be considered in all patients in whom the cause of AKI is not readily apparent. For example, occult ingestion of ethylene glycol can lead to AKI from nephrocalcinosis.[40] In this situation, patients survive the initial metabolic acidosis and present 1 to 2 weeks after the ingestion. Cancers, including solid tumors and lymphoma, may cause intrinsic renal failure as a result of hypercalcemia or tumor infiltration.[41]

Endogenous nephrotoxins include abnormal proteins, myoglobin, hemoglobin, uric acid, and calcium-phosphorus complexes. Tumor lysis, usually occurring in patients with bulky abdominal lymphomas, can be caused by acute uric acid nephropathy or deposition of calcium and phosphorus, leading to severe, even anuric AKI.[42] AKI may be the presenting finding in patients with nontraumatic rhabdomyolysis, from cocaine use, infections or tonic-clonic seizures. Hemoglobinuric renal failure may be the initial presentation in a severe episode of acute intravascular hemolysis.[18,19] Occupational exposure to heavy metals can cause acute tubular necrosis (ATN). This disorder can be observed in welders and miners after exposure to mercury, lead, cadmium, or other metals.[12,43] In addition, infections can cause renal failure either by direct renal damage or by immune-mediated mechanisms.[10,44,45] A history of acquired immunodeficiency syndrome (AIDS) may be a clue to the cause of AKI due to underlying disease or to nephrotoxic drugs such as reverse transcriptase inhibitors, antibiotics, or chemotherapeutic agents.[46]

A history of the color and volume of the patient's urine as well as the pattern of urination can be useful in some settings. For example, abrupt anuria suggests urinary obstruction, severe acute glomerulonephritis, or vascular obstruction due to renal artery emboli or atherosclerotic occlusion of the aortorenal bifurcation.[16,47,48] Also, patients with anti–glomerular basement membrane (anti-GBM)–mediated crescentic glomerulonephritis may present with anuria and require dialysis.[48] History of gradually diminishing urine output may indicate urethral stricture or, in an older man, bladder outlet obstruction due to prostate enlargement. Gross hematuria in the setting of ARF suggests acute glomerulonephritis or ureteral obstruction by tumor, blood clots, or renal papillae.[49,50]

TABLE 22–3	Some Substances Reported to Cause Acute Kidney Injury

Endogenous substances
Myoglobin
Uric acid
Calcium phosphorus
Light chains
Atheroemboli

Exogenous substances
Antibiotics
  Aminoglycosides
  Penicillins
  Cephalosporins
  Fluoroquinolones
  Sulfa drugs
  Pentamidine
  Foscarnet
  Cidofivir
  Acyclovir
Angiotensin-converting enzyme inhibitors
Angiotensin II receptor 1 antagonists
Analgesics and nonsteroidal anti-inflammatory drugs
  Acetaminophen
  Aspirin
  Nonselective cyclooxygenase inhibitors
  Cyclooxygenase-2 inhibitors
Calcineurin inhibitors
Cyclosporine
Tacrolimus
Chemotherapeutic agents
  Cisplatin
  Mitomycin C
  Methotrexate
  Cystosine arabinoside
  Interleukin-2
Reverse transcriptase inhibitors
  Indinavir
  Stavudine
  Mannitol
Immunomodulatory agents
  Interferon-α
Therapeutic immunoglobulins
Radiocontrast agents
Heavy metals and poisons
  Mercury
  Arsenic
  Cadmium
  Lead
  Ethylene glycol
Antidepressants and anticonvulsants
  Celexa
  Phenytoin
  Carbamazepine

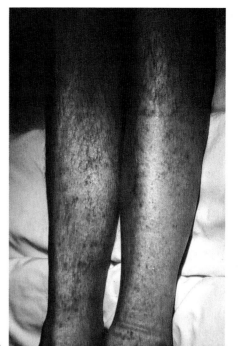
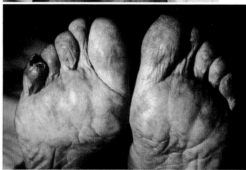

FIGURE 22–1 **A,** Pretibial purpura in a patient with glomerulonephritis due to systemic necrotizing vasculitis. **B,** Digital infarction of the fifth digit, typical of systemic atheroembolism syndrome.

Physical Examination

The physical examination can provide many clues to the underlying cause of and potential therapy for AKI. Careful examination of organ systems as described in this section may help direct the nephrologist to the correct diagnosis.

Skin

Petechiae, purpura, and ecchymoses are clues to inflammatory and vascular causes of kidney failure, including infectious diseases, TTP, and disseminated intravascular coagulation (DIC). Cutaneous infarcts may result from embolic phenomena, and cutaneous vasculitis manifesting as palpable purpura occurs in patients with septic shock, atheroembolic disease, systemic vasculitis, and infective endocarditis and should be looked for (Fig. 22–1).[51] Diffuse erythematous maculopapular rash may be observed in cases of drug-induced (e.g., sulfa drug) allergic interstitial nephritis or in systemic collagen vascular disease such as systemic lupus erythematosus. Reduced skin turgor is a common finding in prerenal ARF caused by volume depletion, although this sign is less reliable in the elderly.

Eye

Search for uveitis (interstitial nephritis and necrotizing vasculitis), ocular muscle paralysis (ethylene glycol poisoning and necrotizing vasculitis), signs of severe hypertension, atheroembolic lesions (Hollenhorst crystals), Roth spots (endocarditis), and cytoid bodies (cotton-wool exudates are seen in acute lupus nephritis). Ophthalmoplegia may be present in patients with systemic necrotizing vasculitis. Conjunctivitis can be a result of vasculitis or drug toxicity or a manifestation of ESRD ("red eyes of renal failure"), the latter due to conjunctival calcium deposition.

Cardiovascular and Volume Status

Meticulous and accurate assessment of the cardiovascular and volume status is the most important aspect in the diagnosis and initial management of AKI. Pulse rate and blood pressure (BP) should be measured in the supine and standing (or seated with legs dangling) positions whenever possible in patients with suspected volume depletion. Close inspection of jugular venous pulse level as well as heart and lungs and detection of peripheral edema are essential. Evidence for volume depletion, including orthostatic hypotension, dry mucous membranes, and decreased skin turgor, as well as signs of sepsis, congestive heart failure, and cardiac tamponade should be sought in patients with low BP or overt hypotension. However, it is often difficult to assess the volume status from physical findings alone in older patients as well as in patients with heart failure, severe liver disease, obesity, and severe edematous states. In some cases, it may be necessary to place a central venous catheter (e.g., pulmonary artery catheter) to measure right heart pressures, cardiac output, and systemic vascular resistance.

In a hypotensive, oliguric patient, volume status can vary greatly. Despite similar decreases in effective arterial blood volume, hypotension and oliguria may be present in patients with severe congestive heart failure (extracellular volume expansion) and those with severe volume depletion. Measurement of BP, urine output, and urine sodium concentration does not distinguish these two conditions, yet the management of congestive heart failure is quite different from that of volume depletion. Patients with heart failure may need vasodilators, inotropic agents, and diuretics, whereas those with volume depletion need infusions of large volumes of fluid such as saline, blood products, or both (Tables 22–4 and 22–5).

In severe hypertension, AKI may be due to malignant nephrosclerosis (e.g., essential hypertension, scleroderma), glomerulonephritis, or atheroembolic disease.[48,49,51-53] Cardiac murmurs are associated with endocarditis or atrial myxoma, which can cause AKI owing to fulminant glomerulonephritis. A pericardial friction rub in a patient with new renal failure may be a sign of impending cardiac tamponade and is an indication for emergency dialysis. In this situation, progressive hypotension is dramatic but can be temporarily stabilized by a rapid intravenous bolus infusion of fluids.

Abdomen

Abdominal examination may reveal a palpable bladder (urinary obstruction). Also, tenderness in the upper quadrants can be associated with ureteral obstruction or renal infarction. Ascites may be observed in fulminant hepatic failure, severe nephrotic syndrome, and Budd-Chiari syndrome, all of which are associated with AKI. Abdominal bruit evokes the diagnosis of severe atherosclerotic disease, which can engender renal failure from renal artery stenosis, thrombosis of the aortorenal bifurcation, or atheroembolic renal disease. Flank mass can be a sign of renal obstruction

from tumor or retroperitoneal fibrosis.[54] In addition, a tense, distended abdomen in a patient who has just undergone surgery raises the possibility of abdominal compartment syndrome.[55,56]

Extremities

Examination of the extremities for signs of edema, evidence of tissue ischemia, muscle tenderness (e.g., rhabdomyolysis causing myoglobinuric renal failure), and arthritis (e.g., systemic lupus erythematosus, rheumatoid arthritis, relapsing polychondritis, infections) may provide clues to the diagnosis of renal failure. Nail signs of hypoalbuminemia (paired bands of pallor in the nailbed [Muerhcke lines]) may be a clue to underlying nephrotic syndrome, which may predispose the patient to ATN.

Neuropsychiatric Features

Neuropsychiatric abnormalities are common in AKI. They range from signs of uremic encephalopathy (confusion, somnolence, stupor, coma, seizures) to focal neurologic abnormalities in specific diseases such as the vasculitides, systemic lupus erythematosus, and infection. As previously mentioned, cranial nerve palsies can be seen in patients with ethylene glycol poisoning and vasculitides, including Wegener granulomatosis and polyarteritis nodosa. Altered and changing mental status is common in thrombotic microangiopathies and systemic atheroembolism.

TABLE 22–4	Evaluation of Cardiovascular and Volume Status	
Volume Depletion		**Volume Overload**
Hypotension (± orthostatic)		Hypertension
Decreased skin turgor		Edema, ascites, pleural effusions
Dry mucous membranes		S_3 gallop
Normal or decreased jugular venous pulse		Elevated jugular venous pulse
Absence of sweat		
Clear lungs, no volume overload on chest radiograph		Rales, volume overload on chest radiograph

TABLE 22–5	Impact of Physical Examination on the Management of Two Prerenal Patients with Different Volume Status	
Parameter	**Patient 1 (Volume Depletion)**	**Patient 2 (Cardiogenic Shock)**
Blood pressure (mm Hg)	90/60	90/60
Urine output (mL/hr)	20	20
Urine sodium (mEg/L)	<20	<20
Physical findings	Decreased turgor, no sweat	S_3 gallop, rales, peripheral edema
Pulmonary capillary wedge pressure (cm H_2O)	2	30
Right atrial pressure (cm H_2O)	2	15
Cardiac index (L/min/1.73 m²)	2.1	1.5
Systemic vascular resistance (dynes/cm⁻⁵)	2590	2933
Management	Intravenous saline, ± inotrope	Inotrope, vasodilator, diuretic

Urinalysis (see also Chapters 23 and 24)

The urinalysis is essential in the evaluation of AKI and should be performed by the nephrologist.[57] Abnormal urinary sediment strongly suggests an intrarenal cause for kidney failure. Gross color changes in the urine may be seen with various intrinsic renal diseases. For example, the urine of a patient with ATN frequently appears "dirty" brown and opaque on gross examination owing to the presence of tubular casts.[1] Reddish-brown urine or "Coca-Cola" urine is a characteristic of some patients with acute glomerulonephritis and of those with pigment-associated tubular necroses, including myoglobinuria and hemoglobinuria. Bilious urine in patients with combined liver and renal disease appears yellow-brown owing to bile pigments.

Qualitative assessments for proteinuria and heme pigment are helpful in identifying glomerulonephritis, interstitial nephritis, and toxic and infectious causes of tubular necrosis. Microscopic examination of urine sediment after centrifugation is extremely helpful for differentiating prerenal from intrarenal causes of kidney failure (Fig. 22–2). As shown in Table 22–6, the urine sediment in ATN typically has granular "muddy brown" casts and renal tubular cells. Interstitial nephritis is often accompanied by pyuria, microhematuria, eosinophiluria, and fine granular and white blood cell casts. Glomerulonephritis is heralded by hematuria with dysmorphic red blood cells (RBCs) and RBC casts. In addition, granular casts, fat globules, and oval fat bodies may be seen in glomerulopathies associated with heavy proteinuria. Uric acid crystals suggest ATN associated with acute uric acid nephropathy from tumor lysis syndrome. Calcium oxalate crystals may be present in ethylene glycol poisoning with AKI due to nephrocalcinosis, and acetaminophen crystals may be observed in acute acetaminophen poisoning.

Blood Tests (see also Chapter 24)

Increases in blood urea nitrogen (BUN) and serum creatinine (Cr) levels are hallmarks of kidney failure. The rate of rise in BUN and Cr levels varies considerably from patient to patient. The normal BUN/Cr ratio of 10:1 is usually maintained in cases of intrinsic AKI (see Table 22–6). The ratio is usually elevated (>20:1) in prerenal conditions and in some patients with obstructive uropathy. Also, in patients with significant upper gastrointestinal bleeding, the BUN/Cr ratio may increase further as digested blood proteins are absorbed and metabolized by the liver. In contrast, the BUN/Cr ratio may be reduced in liver failure, malnutrition, and rhabdomyolysis. In these conditions, low BUN/Cr ratio occurs as a result of a relative decrease in urea production, an increase in Cr production, or both.

Hypofiltration and abnormal tubular function lead to hyperkalemia, hypocalcemia, and hyperphosphatemia. Serum potassium concentration is frequently elevated in patients with AKI as a result of hypofiltration, decreased tubular secretion, and in some cases, excessive cellular release (e.g., rhabdomyolysis). Hypokalemia may be observed with severe volume depletion (e.g., from vomiting, diarrhea, diuretics). Hypocalcemia and hyperphosphatemia result from hypofiltration and complexation as well as hypovitaminosis D. Hypercalcemia is observed in patients with myeloma and other cancers, milk-alkali syndrome, hypervitaminosis D, and other hypercalcemic states that cause volume depletion.[58]

Anemia is almost invariably seen in AKI. Clues to the cause of ARF can be obtained from examination of the peripheral blood smear. For example, the presence of schistocytes suggests TTP, HUS, malignant hypertension, and DIC. Spherocytes are common in the immunohemolytic anemia of lupus nephritis. Ghost cells or cells containing malarial parasites substantiate the diagnosis of hemoglobin-induced AKI.

Hyperuricemia is also common in AKI and is not diagnostic of tumor lysis syndrome.[42] When the diagnosis of tumor lysis

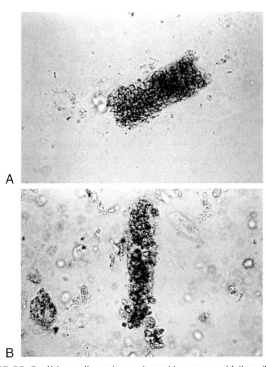

FIGURE 22–2 Urine sediment in a patient with acute renal failure, illustrating fine **(A)** and coarse **(B)** granular casts typical of acute tubular necrosis.

TABLE 22–6	Urine Tests in the Differential Diagnosis of Acute Kidney Injury			
Diagnosis	**Urinalysis**	**Urine-to-Plasma Osmolality**	**Una (mEq/L)**	**Fractional Excretion of Na**
Prerenal	Normal	>1.0	<20	<1.0
Acute tubular necrosis	Granular casts, epithelial cells	≤1.0	>20	>1.0
Interstitial nephritis	RBCs, WBCs, ± eosinophils, granular casts	≤1.0	>20	>1.0
Glomerulonephritis	RBCs, RBC casts, marked proteinuria	>1.0	<20	<1.0
Vascular disorders	Normal or RBCs, proteinuria	>1.0	<20	<1.0
Postrenal	Normal or RBCs, casts, pyuria	<1.0	>20	>1.0

RBC, red blood cell; Una, urine sodium concentration; WBC, white blood cell.

syndrome is entertained, urinalysis and urine chemistry evaluation are essential.

Urine Chemistry Evaluation (see also Chapters 23 and 24)

Urine electrolyte measurement in a patient with ARF is performed to test functional integrity of the renal tubules. The single most informative test is the fractional excretion of sodium (FENa), defined as

$$FENa = \frac{Urine\ Na \times Plasma\ Cr}{Urine\ Cr \times Plasma\ Na} \times 100$$

In prerenal azotemia, the FENa is usually less than 1.0%, and in ATN, it is usually greater than 1.0%. Exceptions to this general rule occur in some patients with ATN due to severe burns, radiocontrast nephropathy, or underlying liver disease. FENa may be less than 1.0% in these conditions owing to the combination of severe renal vasoconstriction, low tubular flow rate, and focal or patchy tubular injury. FENa is typically less than 1.0% in patients with acute glomerulonephritis, because tubular function remains intact with increased, rather than decreased, proximal tubular sodium reabsorption. Also, FENa is most accurate for differentiating prerenal from intrarenal ARF when determined in a patient with hypotension and oliguria. Because of these limitations, FENa alone should not be used in assessing the cause of AKI.

Urine-to–plasma osmolality ratio (U/P Osm) is another useful test of tubular function in the setting of AKI. With intact tubular function, the urinary osmolality exceeds plasma osmolality three- to fourfold, whereas when tubules are damaged and concentrating capacity is impaired, urine is isosthenuric to plasma. Therefore, a U/P Osm value of 1 or less is consistent with ATN, and a value greater than 1 is consistent with a prerenal cause. If the urine is scant in amount and sample volume is low, routine urinalysis is the best diagnostic test. Diagnosis of acute uric acid nephropathy can be substantiated by the urine uric acid–to–urine creatinine ratio. A value greater than 1 suggests this diagnosis.[1] Urine uric acid–to–urine creatinine ratio can be used to help differentiate acute uric acid nephropathy from other causes in patients with malignancy. A ratio of urine uric acid–to–creatinine greater than 1 suggests acute uric acid nephropathy, and a ratio less than 1, other causes.

Assessing Urine Output

Whereas knowledge of the urine output is not particularly helpful in diagnosing the cause of AKI, it is very important for directing management and for predicting outcome. Anuria is defined as urine output less than 100 mL/day. Oliguric renal failure is defined as a 24-hour urine output between 100 and 400 mL/day. Nonoliguric renal failure is defined as urine output greater than 400 mL/day. In patients with suprapubic discomfort and an obviously distended bladder or in patients with a history of declining urine output or documented oliguria, a bladder catheter should be temporarily placed to relieve or rule out bladder outlet obstruction. Patients with oliguric renal failure are easier to manage and have a lower overall mortality rate than those with oliguria or anuria (see discussions on management and survival in accompanying sections). Also, measurement of subsequent daily urine output is important for management of patients.

Fluid Challenge

In patients with suspected prerenal cause of renal failure from significant intravascular volume depletion, an intravenous infusion of normal saline (or colloid such as albumin, dextran, or blood products) may be helpful. In this circumstance, a fluid challenge should improve renal blood flow with correction of renal failure and increased urine output. This maneuver usually consists of an infusion of 1 to 2 L of normal saline administered over 1 to 4 hours. The actual rate prescribed depends on repeated bedside evaluation and clinical judgment. Failure of this maneuver to improve the vital signs and urine output can help point to intrarenal or postrenal causes of renal failure. Caution must be exercised during fluid challenge because of the potential for producing pulmonary edema in patients with congestive heart failure or intrarenal failure, which are unlikely to improve with volume expansion. Therefore, the rate of fluid challenge should be adjusted and the patient should be carefully and repeatedly examined to reduce the risk of precipitating pulmonary edema.

Imaging (see also Chapter 27)

Renal Ultrasonography and Doppler Flow Scanning

Ultrasonography should be performed whenever urinary tract obstruction is considered in the differential diagnosis of AKI. The test is readily available, noninvasive, accurate, reliable, and very reproducible.[59] In some cases, such as ureteral encasement by tumor or fibrosis, ureteral and renal pelvis dilatation may not be detected by ultrasonography. Increased echogenicity of renal parenchyma is a common and nonspecific indicator of intrinsic renal disease. In some cases of ATN, renal parenchymal echogenicity may be normal.

Renal blood flow is reduced in most cases of AKI regardless of the etiology. Doppler flow scanning can detect low renal blood flow and abnormal flow associated with renal artery stenosis. Absence of renal blood flow on Doppler scanning suggests complete thrombosis of the renal circulation.[59]

Nuclear Scan

Radionuclide imaging with ^{99m}Tc-labeled diethylene-triaminepenta-acetic acid (^{99m}Tc-DTPA) or I^{131}-labeled iodo-hippurate (I^{131}-Hippuran) or Mag3 scans can be used to assess renal blood flow and tubular function in AKI. However, the utility of this evaluation is similar to that of Doppler flow scanning. Unfortunately, marked delay in tubular excretion of nuclide occurs in both prerenal and intrarenal diseases; thus, this technique is of little value in the evaluation of most patients with AKI. However, it is helpful if it reveals a complete absence of blood flow.

Computed Tomography and Magnetic Resonance Imaging

Computed tomography (CT) or magnetic resonance imaging (MRI) may be useful in detecting parenchymal renal disease and obstructive uropathy. These modalities are of limited value and in most cases do not provide more information with regard to renal blood flow than does Doppler flow scanning. However, an increase in T2-weighted signal on an MRI may be seen in some cases of acute tubulointerstitial nephritis (Fig. 22–3). Magnetic resonance venography is helpful in the evaluation of renal vein thrombosis.

Lately, an increasing number of reports have suggested an association between exposure to gadolinium-containing contrast agents during MRI studies and nephrogenic fibrosing dermopathy/nephrogenic systemic fibrosis (NFD/NSF), a progressive debilitating in patients with CKD and ESRD.[60] In light of these reports, the Food and Drug Administration has issued a public health advisory regarding the use of agents in CKD patients and has recommended the physicians to carefully weigh risks and benefits of using gadolinium in patients with moderate CKD (GFR < 60 ml/min/1.73 m²) to ESRD. It also recommends considering prompt dialysis to eliminate the contrast agent although there are no published data to suggest utility of dialysis to prevent NSF.

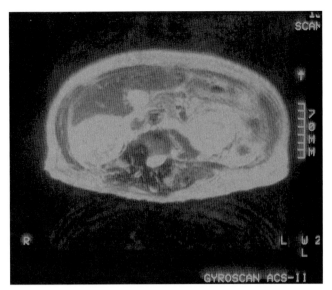

FIGURE 22–3 T2-weighted magnetic resonance image of a patient with biopsy-proven acute tubulointerstitial nephritis. Note increased signal diffusely throughout the cortex of both kidneys.

TABLE 22–7 Risk Factors for Chronic Kidney Disease

Established risk factors*
Age
Gender (male predilection)
Race (African American, Hispanic, Native American)
High blood pressure
Diabetes mellitus
Obesity
Metabolic syndrome
Proteinuria
Family history of kidney disease
Smoking
Atherosclerosis
Exposure to nephrotoxins such as analgesics, aristolochic acid, heavy metals
Dyslipidemia
Reduced nephron number at birth
Recurrent urinary tract infection

Emerging risk factors*
Oxidative stress
Elevated plasma homocysteine level
Anemia
Prothrombotic factors (e.g., plasminogen inhibitor activator-1)

*See also Chapter 18.

CH 22

Approach to the Patient with Kidney Disease

Renal Angiography

A renal angiogram is helpful in patients with AKI due to vascular disorders, including renal artery stenosis with AKI from ACE inhibition, renal artery emboli, and aortic atherosclerosis with acute aortorenal occlusion, as well as in cases of systemic necrotizing vasculitides such as polyarteritis nodosa and Takayasu arteritis. Takayasu arteritis can affect the distal aorta and manifest as advanced renal failure.

Renal Biopsy

When clinical, biochemical, and noninvasive imaging studies are insufficient for diagnosis and management of AKI, a renal biopsy should be considered. Some studies show that biopsy in the setting of AKI often has unexpected findings.[52,61-63] Renal biopsy is considered the "gold standard" for diagnostic accuracy in AKI, but in clinical practice, it is not often performed. An exception is biopsy of a renal transplant, which is performed relatively commonly in patients with AKI because of the need to exclude transplant rejection as the cause.

Patients presenting with the clinical syndrome of rapidly progressive glomerulonephritis should undergo percutaneous renal biopsy as soon as possible unless there is an overt contraindication. This condition is considered a medical emergency because effective kidney-preserving therapy may be indicated and, if so, should be instituted as soon as possible.[63] For example, in a febrile patient with endocarditis who is receiving broad-spectrum antibiotics, a biopsy may be necessary to distinguish between glomerulonephritis and acute tubulointerstitial nephritis. These conditions require different therapeutic interventions.

CHRONIC KIDNEY DISEASE

Patients with CKD most often present with nonspecific complaints or are asymptomatic and are referred to a nephrologist because of abnormal blood or urine findings.[64] As with AKD, it is important to establish the cause of CKD. Once this has been accomplished, further evaluation may be important in order to maximize the potential to preserve or restore glomerular filtration rate (GFR). Evaluation methods for CKD are similar to those for AKI; however, specific evaluations based on cause and chronicity are essential in patients with CKD. In particular, evaluation of cardiovascular risk factors is criti-

cal because of the high rate of cardiovascular complications in CKD.[65-68] This section focuses on CKD in the pre-ESRD period.

Establishing Chronicity of Disease

History and measurement of renal size are helpful in establishing chronicity of kidney disease.[59] It is important to note that no specific blood or urine test unequivocally differentiates AKD from CKD. For example, a common misconception is that very high blood levels of urea nitrogen or very low levels of blood hemoglobin signify CKD. Similarly, other biochemical markers such as parathyroid hormone level or phosphate concentration should not be used to establish chronicity of kidney disease. Cr concentration in the fingernail can establish Chronicity, but the determination is not widely available in practice.[69]

History

In symptomatic patients with CKD, symptoms have often been present for months or years.[70] Urinary symptoms suggesting CKD include difficulty with urination, history of urinary tract infections, passage of kidney stones, dribbling, dysuria, and especially, nocturia. The last, a common symptom in CKD, is usually found when sought during history taking. Other long-standing symptoms associated with kidney disease are often present in patients with nocturia. However, the history does not always distinguish AKD from CKD. Reasons for the lack of specificity include poor patient recall and patient adaptation to slow development of uremia and lack of recognition of subtle symptoms or changes in behavior. Thus, patients with CKD may appear to present with very recent onset of symptoms that belies chronicity. Furthermore, compensatory mechanisms in the kidney and extrarenal adaptation to the uremic milieu account for the fact that many patients with CKD are asymptomatic, even in later stages of the disease (Table 22–7).[70] This is unfortunate because late nephrology referral and evaluation of patients with CKD are associated with greater morbidity and mortality.[71] For this reason, referral of patients in early stages of CKD (1 to 3; see later) has been suggested.[72]

A common early sign of uremic encephalopathy is sleep disturbance. Typically, patients have difficulty falling asleep, awaken during the night, and again have difficulty falling asleep, with subsequent early morning awakening accompanied by daytime sleeping. Subsequent loss of short-term memory, difficulty concentrating, and episodes of confusion occur. Because patients are often unaware of these abnormalities, the history should be supplemented by interviewing a family member whenever possible.

A history of recent infection, chronic rash, or long-standing arthritis may indicate a primary renal or systemic disease that is chronic in nature. A history of human immunodeficiency virus (HIV) infection should be sought in patients with proteinuria and CKD of unknown cause. Routine inquiry into the following risk factors should be conducted: hypertension, diabetes mellitus, congestive heart failure, chronic liver disease, known or suspected hepatitis B or C infection, and rheumatologic diseases. A previous history of urologic disorders or procedures may provide clues to the detection and diagnosis of obstructive and reflux nephropathies and congenital anomalies of the urinary tract. For example, long-standing history of dysuria, nocturia, stranguria, recurrent bladder or kidney infection, trauma, and urinary frequency may indicate vesicoureteral reflux.[73] A history of abnormal findings on a urinalysis conducted as part of an entrance examination for education, military service, or other purposes may provide clues to diagnosis of CKD. A history of back pain or bone pain, particularly in an older patient with CKD, should raise the possibility of malignancy, especially multiple myeloma.

A history of nephrotoxin exposure is essential. Nephrotoxins take many forms, including prescription medication, over-the-counter drugs, and environmental substances. Recent or long-standing history of ingestion of combination analgesic agents (phenacetin, acetaminophen, aspirin) is important in establishing the diagnosis of analgesic nephropathy.[74] Environmental exposure to lead, arsenic, mercury, or silicon or ingestion of certain herbal remedies (e.g., slimming regimens containing aristolochic acid) can lead to the diagnosis of CKD.[43,75–79] Exposure to cancer chemotherapeutic agents, herbal remedies, over-the-counter drugs (such as pamidronate for chronic hypercalcemia or osteoporosis), lithium in patients with bipolar disorders, and cyclosporine in recipients of solid organ transplants can cause CKD.[12,80,81] A history of recurrent urinary tract infection with flank pain, fever, polyuria, and nocturia suggests chronic pyelonephritis.

A family pedigree should be constructed during the ascertainment of a family history in search for inherited diseases. Family history of common diseases, including diabetes and hypertension, should be explored as common causes (diabetes, hypertensive nephrosclerosis) of CKD aggregate in families.[82–85] African Americans have a higher incidence of CKD than whites, but the reasons for this discrepancy are incompletely understood.[86,87] Although genetic predisposition seems possible, it has yet to be proved. Family history of anemia and sickle cell disease is important, particularly in African American patients.[88] For approximately 50% of patients with CKD attributed to hypertension or diabetes, at least one family member has the disorder.[83,89] A pedigree comprising parents, grandparents, great-grandparents, siblings, and offspring is important for identifying autosomal dominant (e.g., autosomal dominant polycystic kidney disease), sex-linked (e.g., Fabry disease), Alport's syndrome, and autosomal recessive (e.g., medullary cystic disease) diseases. These diseases require radiologic evaluation and, often, renal biopsy to establish the diagnosis.[90] Detailed family history improves the diagnosis of genetic diseases and aids in future diagnostic and therapeutic interventions in CKD that will be based on genetic tests.

Physical Examination
BP should be measured in all patients undergoing evaluation for kidney disease. Standard technique for accurate measurement should be used (see later).

The skin should be examined for excoriations due to uremic pruritus, which are often seen on the back, torso, and lower extremities. Vitiligo and periungual fibromas may be seen in tuberous sclerosis. Neurofibromas may be a clue to renal disease caused by underlying renal artery stenosis in patients with neurofibromatosis. Hyperpigmented macules in the pretibial skin are often observed in patients with cryoglobulinemic disease, and livedo reticularis may be observed in those with atherosclerotic ischemic nephropathy. A general sallow appearance of the skin is also a common finding in patients with stage 5 CKD.

Funduscopic examination may demonstrate vascular findings, such as microaneurysms and proliferative retinopathy characteristic of diabetic retinopathy. Arteriolar narrowing, arteriovenous nicking, hemorrhage, and exudates consistent with hypertension are also common. Less common findings that are more difficult to demonstrate on routine examination are anterior lenticonus and retinal flecks characteristic of Alport syndrome. Angioid streaks may be present in those with Fabry disease. Ocular palsy may be present in patients with vasculitides (e.g., Wegener granulomatosis), and diffuse conjunctivitis is a sign of calcium-phosphorus deposition in CKD with secondary hyperparathyroidism.

High-tone sensorineural hearing loss is overt in about 50% of patients with Alport syndrome. Nasal and oropharyngeal ulcers may be present in those with active lupus nephritis. The presence of perforated nasal septum should raise the suspicion for Wegener granulomatosis in patients with hypertensive proteinuric renal disease. Examination for carotid bruit as a manifestation of underlying atherosclerosis may also provide a clue to the presence of renovascular hypertension and ischemic nephropathy as a cause of CKD.

Assessment of the cardiovascular and volume status is essential, because abnormal findings require early and rapid intervention before completion of the evaluation for CKD. For example, volume depletion in a patient with advanced CKD may be a "reversible" cause of ESRD. Cardiopulmonary examination for signs of volume overload is essential not only for diagnosis but also for subsequent evaluation and management of CKD. For example, many patients have underlying heart diseases such as left ventricular hypertrophy and heart failure. Cardiac murmurs may be present in patients with endocarditis or atrial myxoma associated with glomerulonephritis.

Abdominal examination should include a search for palpable kidneys, as observed in polycystic kidney disease and tuberous sclerosis. A flank mass can be found in patients with retroperitoneal fibrosis, lymphoma, or other tumors that can obstruct the ureters. A palpable bladder or enlarged prostate gland suggests chronic urinary outlet obstruction.

Musculoskeletal examination, including examination for edema, should be performed. Synovial thickening in small joints of the hands may be seen in systemic lupus erythematosus and rheumatoid arthritis, both of which may be associated with CKD. Clubbing may be a clue to bacterial endocarditis or chronic suppurative conditions (e.g., lung abscess) that may lead to development of secondary amyloidosis involving the kidney. Neurologic signs in patients with CKD include peripheral sensorimotor neuropathy and central nervous system manifestations. Generalized muscle weakness and diminished deep tendon reflexes are common.

Urinalysis
Urinalysis is not particularly useful for differentiating AKD from CKD. Similar findings, such as pyuria, hematuria, and proteinuria, indicating interstitial nephritis can be seen in AKI or CKD. Presence of oval fat bodies in the urine, signifying high-grade proteinuria, implies a glomerular disease, as does the presence of dysmorphic RBCs.[91,92] Calcium oxalate crystals may be seen in the urine of patients with hereditary

or secondary forms of oxalosis causing kidney disease. The presence of calcium phosphate and sodium urate crystals may signify previous stone disease as a cause of CKD. Triple phosphate crystals may suggest recurrent urinary tract infection and staghorn calculi causing CKD. As described later, proteinuria is an important finding in any patient with CKD.

Renal Osteodystrophy
Radiographic evidence for renal osteodystrophy is present in CKD but not in ARF. Elevated plasma parathyroid hormone concentration can be present in both AKI and CKD but is not sufficient evidence for the diagnosis of osteodystrophy. Radiographs of the shoulders, ribs, hands, and pelvis illustrating signs of osteitis fibrosa cystica strongly suggest CKD; this finding is rarely if ever observed in ARF. A possible exception may be a patient with parathyroid cancer in whom severe primary hyperparathyroidism may induce hypercalcemic AKI.

Renal Mensuration
The most sensitive and specific test for establishing the chronicity of kidney disease is measurement of renal size. Renal ultrasonography remains the technique of choice to screen for renal size abnormalities.[59] The details of this procedure are discussed in Chapter 27. The finding of small kidneys (i.e., small relative to body size) on renal ultrasonography (or other method, such as a plain film of the abdomen, CT and MRI scans) is a reliable indicator of CKD. However, it is important to note that kidney size varies from individual to individual and between evaluation methods (e.g., CT versus ultrasonography). In contrast to the finding of small kidneys as a sign of CKD, the finding of normal size or large kidneys is a sensitive but not specific sign of AKD. That is, patients with AKI have normal or enlarged kidneys; however, normal or enlarged kidneys are observed in many forms of CKD including HIV nephropathy, diabetic nephropathy, and autosomal dominant polycystic kidney disease (see Table 22–1). Enlarged multicystic kidneys are a highly characteristic feature of polycystic kidney disease, and ultrasonography is the screening procedure of choice for this disease (see Chapter 27).[59]

Renal Biopsy
Renal biopsy is the most definitive method of differentiating AKI from CKD.[62] A biopsy is used to establish diagnosis, determine treatment regimen, collect prognostic information, and track the clinical course of CKD, especially in glomerulonephritis. Histologic findings of chronicity include glomerulosclerosis, tubular atrophy, and interstitial fibrosis. The latter finding is the best indicator of chronicity and prognosticator of long-term outcome. Renal biopsy is a low-risk procedure in stable patients with CKD, including the elderly.[59]

Risk Factors for Chronic Kidney Disease
(see also Chapter 18)

It is now recognized that a number of factors increase the risk for development of CKD (see Table 22–7).[93–105] Among the strongest factors associated with increased risk for CKD are diabetes mellitus and hypertension.[106] Currently, nearly 50% of new cases of ESRD occur in diabetic patients, and 27% in hypertensive patients. Additional clinical factors associated with increased risk for CKD are autoimmune disease, chronic systemic infection, urinary tract infection, obstruction of the urinary tract, cancer, family history, reduced renal mass, low birth weight, drug exposure, and recovery after AKI (see later). Older age and ethnicity are also important.[106] It is well known that certain ethnic minorities have a markedly higher risk for CKD, including African Americans, Mexican Americans, Native Americans, Asians, and Pacific Islanders.[83,106–109]

Cigarette smoking, metabolic syndrome, and obesity as well as dyslipidemia have been linked with development of CKD.[110–112]

Prevalence of Chronic Kidney Disease
(see also Chapter 17)

It is estimated that approximately 20 million Americans have CKD.[106,113] Both the prevalence and the incidence of CKD are increasing.[106] The most common causes of CKD leading to ESRD are diabetes mellitus, hypertension, glomerulonephritis, and cystic kidney disease, which together account for 90% of all new cases of CKD. In the United States, estimates of prevalence of CKD vary from 10 to 20 million, depending on the definition. Confusion in terminology as well as methods for defining CKD and its severity have hampered our ability to identify patients and, therefore, how to approach the problem of CKD. The Kidney Disease Outcomes Quality Initiative (K/DOQI) clinical practice guidelines for CKD evaluation, classification, and stratification published by the National Kidney Foundation provide a framework designed to address the growing burden of CKD in the United States.[70] The guidelines emphasize the need for prevention, early diagnosis, and treatment of CKD.

Definition and Staging of Chronic Kidney Disease (see also Chapter 17)

CKD is defined as kidney damage with or without decreased GFR, manifested as either pathologic abnormalities or markers of kidney damage, including abnormalities in composition of blood or urine, abnormality renal imaging findings, and a GFR less than 60 mL/min 1.73 m². This broad definition includes patients with or without symptoms of kidney disease (Fig. 22–4).[70]

Staging of CKD is based on estimate of GFR (Table 22–8).[70] Observational studies, administrative databases, and clinical trials indicate that patients with CKD are at increased risk for both progression to ESRD and cardiovascular morbidity and mortality.[114,115] This situation is accounted for in part by the fact that many risk factors are common to both progression of kidney disease and cardiovascular complications, such as diabetes, hypertension, and dyslipidemia. However, even after adjustment for common risk factors, the incidence of myocardial infarction and cerebrovascular events is higher in patients with CKD, suggesting that CKD is a risk factor for cardiovascular disease.[116] Therefore, management of risk factors is paramount in this patient population.

Evaluation of Chronic Kidney Disease

Estimation of Glomerular Filtration Rate
(see also Chapter 23)
GFR is generally considered the best overall estimate of renal function and therefore should be used to evaluate onset and progression of kidney disease. In addition, estimating GFR is useful for determining dosage regimens for therapeutic agents whose excretion is primarily renal. This later consideration is very important not only in general medicine but also in geriatrics and oncology, specialties in which serum Cr concentration alone gives a poor estimate of renal function. Moreover, it is known that, as GFR declines, the number of complications and comorbidities associated with CKD increases.

Estimation of GFR can be accomplished by formal measurement of inulin or iothalamate or other clearance markers. These methods are most accurate but are also cumbersome, inconvenient, and expensive. Estimating GFR on the basis of a patient's age, gender, ethnicity, and serum Cr concentration

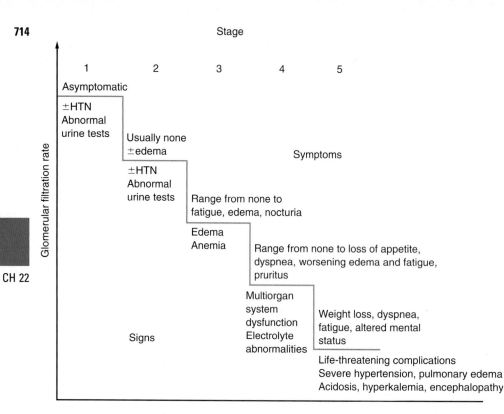

Stage

FIGURE 22–4 Clinical signs and symptoms in chronic kidney disease according to stage. With advancing stage, both symptoms and signs tend to worsen. HTN, hypertension.

TABLE 22–8	Staging of Chronic Kidney Disease		
Stage	Description	Estimated GFR*	Evaluation Plan
	At increased risk	>90 (with CKD risk factors)	Screening CKD risk reduction
1	Kidney damage with normal or increased GFR	≥90	Diagnose and treat cause, slow progression, evaluate risk of cardiovascular disease
2	Kidney damage with mild decrease in GFR	60–89	Estimate progression
3	Moderate decrease in GFR	30–59	Evaluate and treat complications
4	Severe decrease in GFR	15–29	Prepare for renal replacement therapy
5	Kidney failure	<15	Initiate renal replacement therapy

*GFR = $186 \cdot Scr^{-1.154} \cdot Age^{-0.203}$ [$\cdot$ 0.742 for female and/or $\cdot$ 1.210 for African American]
CKD, chronic kidney disease; GFR; glomerular filtration rate; Scr, serum creatinine level.

is a practical method that is gaining widespread acceptance.[116,117] This estimate is derived from regression models based on demographic, anthropometric, and biochemical data in participants in clinical trials who underwent repeated direct measurement of GFR by iothalamate clearance. Similar methods using Cr clearance as an estimate of GFR are based on regression models developed from 24-hour urine samples (detailed analysis of these methods is presented in Chapter 23). The most widely used estimate of GFR is based on data obtained in the Modification of Diet in Renal Disease (MDRD) Study, a large-scale clinical trial, sponsored by the National Institutes of Health, of diet and BP control in patients with established CKD.[118] The equation for estimating GFR based on these variables and the staging of CKD on basis of GFR, as recommended by the National Kidney Foundation, are outlined in Table 22–8.

An important aspect of this method of estimating GFR is the determination of serum Cr concentration for a single estimate of GFR as well as repeated measures over time. First, it should be remembered that measurement error could result in spurious overestimation or underestimation of GFR. In addition, laboratory methods for measuring serum Cr concentration vary, and the variations can result in substantial differences in estimated GFR (see equation in Table 22–8). For this reason, it is appropriate to measure serum Cr value in new patients in the nephrologist's own laboratory and to repeat the measurements in the same laboratory with the same method over time.

Second, dietary intake can have an important effect on serum Cr concentration. It is known that meals containing cooked meat can transiently but significantly raise serum Cr concentration. Calculation of GFR from a serum Cr value obtained after a patient has eaten a meal containing a large amount of Cr, which would yield a falsely high Cr value for that patient, would lead to a spurious underestimation of the patient's GFR. Therefore, it is important to measure serum

Cr concentration in a fasting blood specimen to increase the likelihood of an accurate estimate. Also, steady-state serum Cr concentration may change as a result of a long-term change in dietary protein intake.[117,119] Thus, high animal protein intake increases, and low animal protein intake decreases, the steady-state serum Cr. Estimating GFR at two time points in a patient who markedly alters his or her dietary animal protein intake in the interim may confound the interpretation of GFR estimation and lead to an erroneous conclusion regarding changes in the patient's renal function. Finally, it should be remembered that estimating GFR from serum Cr values is subject to inaccuracy and imprecision beyond changes in serum Cr concentration, errors in Cr measurement, and nonstandardization of methods for Cr measurement.[120]

Recently, cystatin C has been proposed as novel marker for kidney function. Cystatin C is an endogenous small-molecular-weight protein present in normal human plasma. Its production rate is relatively constant and independent of muscle mass, and it is excreted from the body by the kidney through filtration, not secretion. In these respects, it is a superior marker of filtration function than serum Cr. Moreover, in elderly individuals enrolled in the Cardiovascular Health Study, cystatin C appeared to be a better predictor of clinical outcomes than serum Cr.[121]

Hypertension (see also Chapter 42)

Ninety percent of patients with CKD experience hypertension (BP >130/80 mm Hg) during the course of the disease. Uncontrolled hypertension accelerates the rate of progression regardless of the cause of renal failure. Clinical trials and epidemiologic studies indicate that hypertension is a major risk factor for progressive kidney disease. Evaluation of subjects screened in a multiple risk factor intervention trial who were monitored over a 16-year period showed that (1) higher BP was a strong and independent risk factor for the development of ESRD and (2) the relative risk for ESRD increased with rising systolic BP independent of diastolic BP. In patients with type 2 diabetes mellitus, there is almost a linear relationship between increase in mean arterial BP and yearly decrease in GFR. Analysis of National Health and Nutrition Evaluation Survey (NHANES) III data suggests that adequate BP control is achieved in only 11% of patients with hypercreatininemia (serum Cr > 1.5 mg/dL).[122] More recent analysis of NHANES IV indicates that only 37% of hypertensive patients with CKD have BP controlled to a level of less than 130/80 mm Hg.[123] Risk factors for uncontrolled hypertension included age older than 65, black race, and presence of albuminuria. In general, older people with hypertension are unaware of their BP elevation, and the majority of those who are aware have poor control rates. CKD prevalence is higher in older age groups, in which systolic hypertension is very common. Currently, the median age of patients with CKD entering treatment programs in the United States is 64.8 years.[106]

Documentation of BP is essential in the assessment of CKD because this parameter is strongly associated with kidney disease progression and cardiovascular mortality. BP should be measured often with standardized techniques promulgated by the American Heart Association and National Heart Lung and Blood Institute. The goal BP for patients with CKD is 120 to 139 mm Hg systolic and 70 to 85 mm Hg diastolic, depending on the disease type. For example, goal BP for diabetic patients with hypertension is less than 130 mm Hg systolic and less than 80 mm Hg diastolic[124]; for patients with hypertensive nephrosclerosis, the goal BP is 130 to 140 mm Hg systolic and 80 to 89 mm Hg diastolic.[125]

Figure 22–5A illustrates the mean rate of decline in GFR plotted as a function of mean controlled systolic BP in nine clinical trials of both diabetic and nondiabetic patients with CKD. The dotted line labeled "Normal" indicates the normal rate of decline in GFR of about 0.75 mL/min/yr observed with aging alone in normal men older than 45 years. As can be seen in the graph, lower systolic BP values are associated with slower rate of decline in GFR. Figure 22–5B illustrates the hypothetical effect of lowering systolic BP from a range of 150 to 160 mm Hg to a range of 120 to 130 mm Hg on the decline in GFR in an individual patient. Although this figure is only an estimate, it serves as a reminder to the treating nephrologist and as an educational tool for patients about the importance and potential benefit of BP control in renal outcome.

Detection and Estimation of Proteinuria
(see also Chapter 23)

Evaluation of all patients with CKD should include testing for proteinuria. Strategies aimed at reducing proteinuria have been shown to slow the rate of decline in GFR in CKD due to hypertension, diabetes, and the glomerulonephritides.[125] Detection and quantification of microalbuminuria in patients with CKD and a negative urine protein dipstick test result should be performed on an initial visit. For the patient in whom a urine protein dipstick test result is positive, quantification of proteinuria should be performed as described later. For individuals referred for proteinuria with a negative urine protein dipstick test result but positive sulfosalicylic acid test result or a 24-hour urine sample demonstrating protein, a test for urine light chains should be performed. As discussed in Chapter 18, unrelenting proteinuria has been shown to greatly increase risk for progression of CKD in diabetic and nondiabetic nephropathies including the glomerulonephritides, hypertensive nephrosclerosis, and autosomal dominant polycystic kidney disease.

Proteinuria has been extensively studied as a marker for progression of renal disease. Clinical trials have shown that patients with impaired renal function and high-grade proteinuria (>1 g/day) progress at a faster rate than those with low-grade proteinuria (≤1 g/day).[99,104] For example, in both diabetic and nondiabetic patients with proteinuric renal disease, acceleration of renal disease progression correlates with the level of baseline proteinuria. Even in patients with controlled essential hypertension and no evidence of renal disease, the onset of proteinuria may be a marker of future decline of renal function. Also, the MDRD Study demonstrated that baseline proteinuria was an independent risk factor for progression of renal disease in nondiabetic patients and that the extent of proteinuria reduction might be a measure of the effectiveness of BP control.[126] Normal individuals excrete less than 150 mg/day of protein. Loss of protein (albumin) in the urine becomes apparent on reagent test strip tests when the urine contains 300 mg/L or more, or 300 mg or more albumin/g Cr (Table 22–9).

The recommended method of screening for abnormal albuminuria is to first measure albumin by urine dipstick test. If the result is negative, it is preferable to obtain a freshly voided morning urine sample ("spot" or "random") and send it to the laboratory for measurement of albumin and Cr and calculation of the albumin-to-Cr ratio. Collection of a 24-hour urine sample to screen for albuminuria is not recommended; instead, a random specimen should be collected for determination of urine albumin– or protein–to–urine creatinine ratio.[101] Under normal circumstances, urinary albumin, measured as the ratio of albumin to Cr, in a random urine sample is less than 30 mg/g Cr.

Microalbuminuria, defined as an albumin excretion in the range between 30 and 300 mg/g Cr, is not detected by the routine dipstick method (which, by the way, detects only albumin, not other proteins such as light chains). Macroalbuminuria is defined as an albumin excretion rate of more than 300 mg/g Cr. Both are markers for risk for progression of

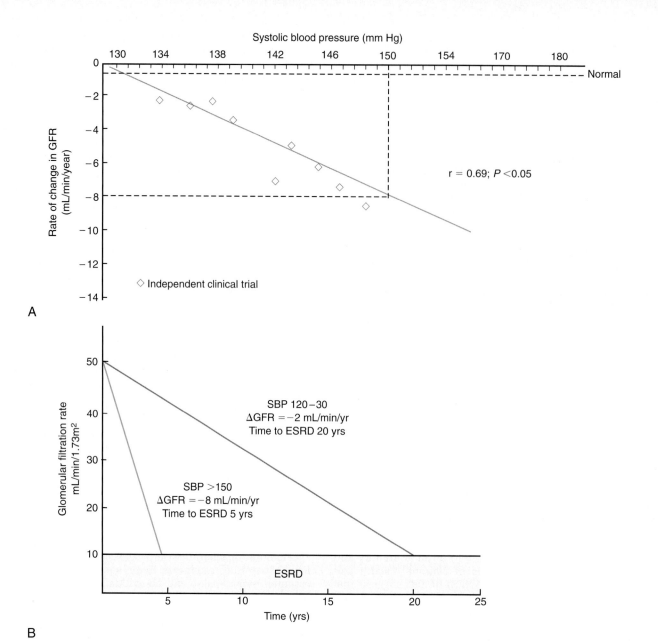

FIGURE 22–5 **A,** Relationship between blood pressure and decline in glomerular filtration rate (GFR) in chronic kidney disease, based on data from clinical trials (see text for details). Results from nine clinical trials, five in patients with diabetic nephropathy and four in patients with nondiabetic nephropathy, indicate that mean rate of decline in GFR is directly associated with level of mean systolic blood pressure (SBP) during the trial. Note that even at normal systolic blood pressure, the rate of decline in GFR in patients with nephropathy is more than twice that associated with aging in normal individuals (*dotted horizontal line*). **B,** Effect of an intervention that lowers blood pressure on the rate of decline in GFR and the time of onset of end-stage renal disease (ESRD) in a theoretical patient with chronic kidney disease and hypertension.

TABLE 22–9	Microalbuminuria and Macroalbuminuria	
	Microalbuminuria	**Macroalbuminuria**
Definition (mg albumin/mg creatinine)	>30–299	≥300
Routine dipstick test result	Negative	Positive
Renal significance	At risk for nephropathy	Marker of rapid progression
Effect on cardiovascular risk	Increased	Increased

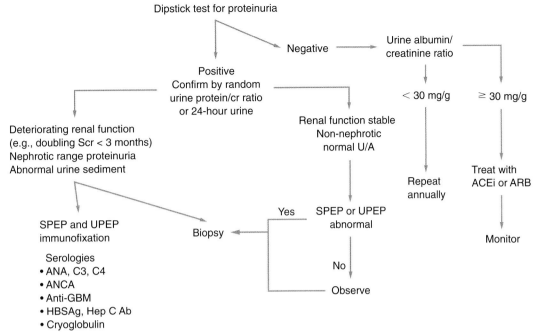

FIGURE 22–6 Algorithm for evaluation of proteinuria in chronic kidney disease. ACEi, angiotensin-converting enzyme inhibitors; ANA, antinuclear antibody; ANCA, antineutrophil cytoplasmic antibody; ARB, angiotensin type 1 receptor blocker; GBM, glomerular basement membrane; HBSAg, hepatitis surface B antigen; Hep C Ab, hepatitis C antibody; Scr, serum creatinine level; SPEP, serum protein electrophoresis; U/A, urinalysis; UPEP, urine protein electrophoresis.

nephropathy in patients with type 1 and type 2 diabetes and for increased risk of cardiovascular death.[94,127] Moreover, more than 300 mg/g of protein is associated with higher risk of progression of kidney disease in hypertensive nephrosclerosis.

A simple algorithm for screening and evaluation of proteinuria is illustrated in Figure 22–6. Monitoring proteinuria or albuminuria in CKD can be accomplished without 24-hour urine collection, but instead by repeated determinations of the urine albumin-to-Cr or urine protein–to-Cr. As with screening samples, these determinations should be performed on freshly voided morning urine samples.

Obesity
Two recent observational studies indicate that obesity may be an independent risk factor for development of CKD.[128,129] These studies raise the possibility that factors other than hypertension and diabetes obesity may play a role in development of kidney disease.

Cardiovascular Disease in Chronic Kidney Disease (see also Chapter 48)
CKD is an independent risk factor for cardiovascular disease and all-cause mortality.[115] Observational studies indicate that rates of both stroke and myocardial infarction are higher in patients with CKD before development of ESRD. For example, Go and co-workers[130] reported on the risk of all-cause mortality and cardiovascular hospitalizations among 1.2 million participants in the Northern California Kaiser-Permanente health care system. They found a graded increase in mortality and cardiovascular hospitalizations as estimated GFR declined. This association was independent of traditional cardiovascular risk factors. In prospective clinical trials, an increased serum Cr value at baseline raised risk for stroke, myocardial infarction, and all-cause cardiovascular mortality.[131] These data suggest that CKD, independent of common risk factors such as age, BP, diabetes, and proteinuria, may be an independent coronary heart disease risk factor.

CKD markedly increases the risk of cardiovascular death from cardiac events and stroke.[106,116] The mortality risk in patients with CVD is 10- to 30-fold higher than that in normal, age-matched populations. Median survival after an acute myocardial infarction in patients undergoing dialysis is less than 18 months, even in the thrombolytic era. Hypertensive patients with hypercreatininemia are at higher risk of myocardial infarction and stroke,[2] and diabetic patients with proteinuria are at greater risk for fatal myocardial infarction and stroke.[12] Prevalence of left ventricular hypertrophy and congestive heart failure is strikingly elevated in patients with CKD stages 2 through 5,[132] including those undergoing dialysis. Morbidity and mortality for congestive heart failure and coronary heart disease are also excessive in CKD.

Figure 22–7 illustrates that CVD and CKD may be manifestations of a similar disease process. Cardiovascular and renal disease have the following types of markers in common: clinical,[133,134] pathophysiologic (e.g., increased angiotensin II activity, up-regulation of inflammatory and fibrosis producing cytokines),[135] histopathologic, biochemical,[135] acute and chronic inflammation,[135] and subclinical signs of atherosclerosis (e.g., increased common carotid artery intima-media thickness).[136,137] Furthermore, the constellation of cardiovascular disease risk factors found in the obesity metabolic syndrome have been linked to higher risk for development of both cardiovascular disease and CKD.[138]

Assessing Comorbidity
Most patients with CKD have comorbidities, the number rising with increasing stage of CKD.[70] Extrarenal diseases play a key role in the progression of CKD as well as associated morbidity and mortality.[139]

Diabetes Mellitus
Diabetes accounts for nearly 50% of all new cases of ESRD in the United States and an increasing percentage of cases of ESRD around the world. Recognition of diabetes as a comorbidity is essential in evaluation of CKD.

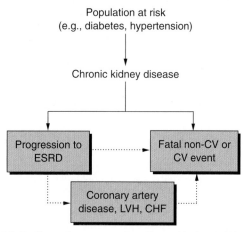

FIGURE 22-7 Competing outcomes in patients with chronic kidney disease (CKD). Cardiovascular disease and CKD may be manifestations of a similar disease process. Patients with CKD are at high risk for both fatal cardiovascular (CV) and noncardiovascular (non-CV) events as well as progression to end-stage renal disease (ESRD). Risk factors for these competing outcomes may be identical. CHF, congestive heart failure; LVH, left ventricular hypertrophy.

Assessment of blood glucose control by measurement of hemoglobin A_{1c} should be conducted in patients with diabetes mellitus, because hyperglycemia is associated with progression to nephropathy. Elevated plasma glucose raises the risk of progression to diabetic kidney disease in both type 1 and type 2 diabetes.[126,140] Undiagnosed and untreated, diabetic kidney disease progresses rapidly. It is critical to evaluate glycemic control and BP in diabetic patients, because optimal management of these risk factors can slow progression of kidney disease.

Cardiovascular morbidity is common in patients with CKD and the major cause of death.[124,141] Evaluation of cardiac status and function should include a careful history for coronary artery disease and congestive heart failure. This is particularly important in older patients with CKD, who are more than 100-fold more likely to die before development of ESRD than are age-matched normal persons.[141] In addition, diabetes is associated with many comorbidities that complicate the course of CKD, including high rates of heart failure and peripheral vascular disease complications.

Homocysteine
Studies in CKD and non-CKD populations indicate that hyperhomocysteinemia is a risk factor for cardiovascular death.[142] Plasma homocysteine concentration rises with decreasing renal function in CKD.[143] The mechanism of hyperhomocysteinemia in CKD is incompletely understood; however, abnormal enzyme activity, substrate limitation, and abnormal renal excretion have all been cited as possible causes.[144] Hyperhomocysteinemia is associated with progression of CKD in diabetic and nondiabetic patients but is not an independent risk factor.[145]

Current guidelines do not recommend measurement of homocysteine level, because whether long-term lowering of homocysteine reduces the risk of either cardiovascular disease or progression of CKD is not known.[145] Administration of folic acid, 5 mg/day, in patients with CKD can lower plasma homocysteine levels.[146] It remains to be determined whether this therapy decreases cardiovascular complications or affects progression of kidney disease in patients with CKD. Recently, intervention studies using homocysteine in the general population have not demonstrated a reduction in cardiovascular events.[147-149] However, the health risk of folic acid in doses of up to 5 mg/day is rather low, and the agent is inexpensive. Until clinical trials determine whether folic acid or other treatment of hyperhomocysteinemia is beneficial in patients

with CKD, clinical judgment should be used in determining whether to prescribe folic acid for this purpose.

Dyslipidemia
Fasting serum total cholesterol, low-density lipoprotein (LDL) cholesterol, and triglyceride levels should be measured in patients with CKD. Clinical evidence indicates that dyslipidemia may contribute to the onset and progression of CKD as well as of cardiovascular disease in patients with CKD.[150] Both hypertriglyceridemia and hypercholesterolemia have been associated with declining kidney function.[93,151] Dyslipidemia is believed to play a role in both the development of cardiovascular disease and the progression of renal disease in patients with pre-ESRD or kidney transplants regardless of the underlying cause (e.g., diabetes, hypertension).[93] The most common dyslipidemia observed in patients with CKD is atherogenic dyslipidemia—a combination of hypertriglyceridemia, low levels of high-density lipoprotein (HDL) cholesterol, and high levels of small, dense LDL particles.[152] In addition, isolated hypercholesterolemia and combined hypercholesterolemia and hypertriglyceridemia are common in patients with CKD and nephrotic syndrome.[153,154] Increased levels of lipoprotein (a) are also common in CKD.[155] Cardiovascular morbidity and mortality are increased in patients with hypercreatininemia (serum Cr level > 1.4 mg/dL), and most patients with CKD have multiple risk factors, including hypertension, proteinuria, metabolic syndrome, increased lipoprotein (a), hyperhomocysteinemia, anemia, and elevated calcium phosphorous product. Consequently, it is reasonable to expect that treatment of dyslipidemia in this population is at least as important as in populations without renal disorders.[156] Two recently completed double-blind randomized placebo-controlled clinical trials in hemodialysis patients and post-transplant patients failed to demonstrate a benefit of statin intervention for major cardiovascular morbidity and mortality.[157,158] There are no long-term cardiovascular outcome trials in predialysis populations that have demonstrated a benefit of any lipid-lowering treatment with statins or other lipid-lowering drugs.

Current evidence supports use of the Adult Treatment Program (ATP) III guidelines for coronary heart disease in the management of dyslipidemia in patients with CKD.[152] The ATP III guidelines focus on LDL cholesterol as the primary target but also recognize the importance of atherogenic dyslipidemia as a risk factor. As noted previously, this pattern of lipid levels is the most common dyslipidemia observed in patients with CKD, including those with type 2 diabetes.

Coronary risk equivalent is defined by the National Cholesterol Education Program (NCEP) as the level of risk equivalent to that of a patient with clinical coronary heart disease. CKD is emerging as a coronary heart disease risk equivalent,[115] although it has not yet been recognized as such by the NCEP. Several lines of evidence point to CKD as a coronary risk equivalent, including clinical trials showing high prevalence of diabetes mellitus (recognized as a coronary risk equivalent) in CKD epidemiologic studies[106,115,141,151,159] and a high prevalence of traditional and nontraditional risk factors for coronary artery disease (see Table 22-2). Finally, the prevalence and magnitude of major risk factors for coronary disease increase as renal failure progresses (e.g., hypertension, insulin resistance, hyperhomocysteinemia).[133]

Secondary Hyperparathyroidism and Vascular Calcification
Derangements in calcium and phosphorus metabolism that develop during the course of CKD are caused by multiple mechanisms, including alterations in dietary intake, development of secondary hyperparathyroidism and hypovitaminosis D, and alterations in calcium-sensing receptor and bone-associated proteins.[160] Serum calcium, phosphorus, parathyroid hormone, and 1,25-dihydroxyvitamin D_3 levels

should be measured in patients with CKD. Although the serum calcium level drops, the serum phosphorus level rises, leading to an abnormal increase in the calcium-phosphorus product, $[Ca] \times [Pi]$.[161,162] The normal product is about 40 mg^2/dL^2. Experimentally, even small increases in $[Ca] \times [Pi]$ may increase calcification of soft tissue, including vascular tissues. Furthermore, mobilization of calcium and phosphorus from bone as a consequence of elevated parathyroid hormone may worsen the increase in $[Ca] \times [Pi]$.[162] Also, patients with stages 3 through 5 CKD not on dialysis have an eightfold higher risk for increased coronary artery calcification as detected by electron-beam CT than those without CKD. This increase was largely due to the high calcium burden in coronary arteries of diabetics with CKD.[163–169] Hyperphosphatemia activates bone-associated proteins that increase smooth muscle cell proliferation and vascular calcification, including osteocalcin, bone morphogenetic protein 2a (BMP 2a), alkaline phosphatase, and osteonectin, but down-regulates p21, a cyclin-dependent kinase complex that inhibits proliferation.[162] The net effect is the development of renal osteodystrophy and vascular calcification. The latter consequence is ominous: It contributes to an acceleration in the rate of atherosclerosis and cardiovascular events in CKD. Increased $[C] \times [Pi]$ is associated with greater mortality in patients undergoing hemodialysis as well as with a higher increased coronary artery calcification score in such patients.[137,164–169] For this reason, levels of calcium, phosphorus, and calcium-phosphorus product should be evaluated and monitored in all patients with CKD, and early treatment to reduce an elevated $[Ca] \times [Pi]$ should be considered.[170] In addition, the majority of patients with CKD stage 3 (or higher) have vitamin D deficiency (low plasma 25(OH) vitamin D_3 level) in association with secondary hyperparathyroidism. Therefore, measurement of plasma 25(OH) vitamin is recommended by the National Kidney Foundation.[170] In this situation, repletion of 25(OH) vitamin D_3, the precursor of 1.25 $(OH)_2$ vitamin D_3 is recommended to correct vitamin D deficiency and secondary hyperparathyroidism. Outcomes trials in hemodialysis patient populations examining the role of hyperparathyroidism are limited. The Dialysis Cardiovascular Outcomes Revisited (DCOR) trial enrolled more than 2000 patients randomized either to the non–calcium-containing phosphate binder sevelamer HCl or to calcium-containing phosphate binders and followed them for 3 years.[171] The results indicate no overall benefit of sevelamer versus calcium-containing binder. However, in subgroup analysis, older (>65 yr) study participants randomized to sevelamer had fewer cardiovascular events.

Malnutrition

Malnutrition is common in patients with stages 4 and 5 CKD and is associated with reduced survival.[70,172,173] Patients with stages 4 and 5 CKD have reduced energy intake, abnormal levels and metabolism of plasma amino acids, and dysregulation in carbohydrate and lipid metabolism (see later). Clinical evidence indicates that estimation of dietary protein intake is an important component of evaluation of CKD. Malnutrition is identified clinically from a dietary history of decreased energy and nutrient intake along with weight loss, physical signs of muscle wasting, and declining serum albumin, transthyretin, and transferrin levels. Anthropometric analysis indicates that patients with stages 4 and 5 disease have abnormal decreases in midarm muscle circumference and increased scapular, brachial, and thigh skin fold thicknesses. Abnormal amino acid, carbohydrate, and lipid metabolism is also present in patients with stages 4 and 5 CKD.

Markers of Inflammation and Oxidative Stress

Currently, routine clinical determinations of markers of inflammation and oxidative stress are not recommended.

Intensive research is ongoing in an effort to elucidate the role of these factors in onset, progression, and complications of CKD.[174–176] There is little doubt that inflammation plays an important role in the development and progression of most CKDs. The kidney itself at end stage is characterized histologically in virtually all cases by hallmarks of chronic inflammation, including infiltration by white blood cells and fibrosis. Markers of inflammation, including C-reactive protein, interleukins 1 and 6, and tumor necrosis factor, are elevated in plasma of patients with CKD. These markers correlate with signs and symptoms of malnutrition and may play a pathogenetic role in development and persistence of malnutrition. Currently, these markers are used for experimental purposes but may become useful clinically in the future for monitoring nutrition as CKD progresses.

Metabolic Acidosis

Measurement of serum bicarbonate concentration as part of routine electrolyte analysis is essential in patients with CKD. When doubt exists as to the cause of low plasma bicarbonate value in a patient with CKD, arterial blood pH and PCO_2 should be measured to confirm the presence of metabolic acidosis, concomitant primary respiratory alkalosis, or both.

Treatment of metabolic acidosis to raise bicarbonate concentration above 22 mEq/L can reduce the risk of organ dysfunction caused by the effects of metabolic acidosis on brain, heart, bone, muscles, and liver. Metabolic acidosis develops in CKD as a result of failure of the kidney's normal acid excretion ability. The consequences of chronic metabolic acidosis due to renal failure include loss of calcium from bone, hypercalciuria, fatigue, dyspnea, weakness, and protein catabolism.[177] Metabolic acidosis activates ubiquitin-sensitive proteasome pathways and branched-chain amino acid dehydrogenate in skeletal muscle cells, leading to greater protein breakdown and decreasing hepatic albumin synthesis.[178,179] The precise pH level at which these events occur in humans is not known; however, general practice is to keep serum bicarbonate from declining below 22 mEq/L, and a normal value is desirable.

Anemia

Hemoglobin, serum iron, total iron-binding capacity, ferritin, and RBC indices and reticulocyte count must be measured as screening tests for anemia in all patients with CKD. Additional tests for other causes of anemia, such as vitamin B_{12}, folic acid, hemoglobin electrophoresis, and tests for hemolysis should be performed on the basis of the history, physical findings, and results of the initial screen for anemia. Anemia is a major risk factor for morbidity and mortality in CKD, and practice guidelines for its management have been published. Current guidelines define anemia as a blood hemoglobin concentration less than 11 g/dL in premenopausal women and less than 12 g/dL in men and postmenopausal women.[180] This definition has led to a higher prevalence of anemia diagnosis in women, because in normal premenopausal women, blood hemoglobin level is lower than that in men.[181]

Anemia develops in more than 90% of patients with CKD as kidney disease progresses, and is multifactorial.[70,182] The major factor in development of anemia is decreased blood level of erythropoietin due to reductions in renal synthesis and secretion of erythropoietin.[183] However, uremia contributes to this process in several ways, including direct inhibition of erythropoietin's effects on erythroprogenitor cells, anorexia leading to reduced intake of hemoglobin substrates (protein, vitamins, iron), decreased RBC life span, and reduced iron absorption. Low blood hemoglobin level due to reduced renal production of erythropoietin may begin in CKD as early as stage 2.[184,185] Reduced oxygen-carrying capacity consequent to anemia in CKD results in organ hypoxia, which in turn aggravates uremic symptoms such as fatigue,

720

deteriorating cognitive ability, dyspnea on exertion, and reduced physical ability.

Anemia also plays an important role in the development of congestive heart failure and left ventricular hypertrophy, the latter being observed in up to 40% of patients with stage 4 CKD and 80% of patients with stage 5 disease.[186–197] Left ventricular hypertrophy is associated with subsequent development of ischemic heart disease and congestive heart failure as well as sudden cardiac death.[198,199] Both hypertension and anemia are independent risk factors for left ventricular growth in CKD, and the increased risks attributed to hypertension and anemia are similar.

Anemia may also be a risk factor for progression of CKD. Several small studies indicate that treatment of anemia may slow the progression of CKD, and mild anemia (hemoglobin < 13.8 g/dL) is associated with a higher risk of ESRD in patients with type 2 diabetes and nephropathy.[200] In a recent study involving 88 patients, early treatment of anemia with erythropoietin decreased the incidence of ESRD after 3 years follow up. A higher hemoglobin was achieved and maintained during the study. Clinical trials to test whether treatment or prevention of anemia slows progression of CKD are in progress. Finally, anemia is an independent risk factor for all-cause mortality in patients with stage 5 CKD. Thus, for each 1 g/dL decrease in blood hemoglobin level below normal, mortality rate rises 18%.

Currently, practice guidelines recommend treatment of anemia attributed to erythropoietin deficiency with erythropoietin and iron (when indicated) to achieve a hemoglobin level of 12 g/dL for both men and women regardless of stage of CKD.[180] Therefore, patients with hemoglobin levels less than 11 g/dL are candidates for treatment. This issue is discussed in detail in Chapter 55.

CH 22

References

1. Esson ML, Schrier RW: Diagnosis and treatment of acute tubular necrosis. Ann Intern Med 137:744–752, 2002.
2. Paganini EP, Kanagasundaram NS, Larive B, Greene T: Prescription of adequate renal replacement in critically ill patients. Blood Purif 19:238–244, 2001.
3. Chertow GM, Levy EM, Hammermeister KE, et al: Independent association between acute renal failure and mortality following cardiac surgery. Am J Med 104:343–348, 1998.
4. Mehta RL, Pascual MT, Gruta CG, et al: Refining predictive models in critically ill patients with acute renal failure. J Am Soc Nephrol 13:1350–1357, 2002.
5. Brivet FG, Kleinknecht DJ, Loirat P, Landais PJ: Acute renal failure in intensive care units: Causes, outcome, and prognostic factors of hospital mortality. A prospective, multicenter study. French Study Group on Acute Renal Failure. Crit Care Med 24:192–198, 1996.
6. Thadhani R, Pascual M, Bonventre JV: Medical progress: Acute renal failure. N Engl J Med 334:1448–1460, 1996.
7. O'Hare A, Olson JL, Connolly MK, et al: Renal insufficiency with monoclonal gammopathy and urticarial vasculitis. Am J Kidney Dis 39:203–207, 2002.
8. Fechner FP, Faquin WC, Pilch BZ: Wegener's granulomatosis of the orbit: A clinicopathological study of 15 patients. Laryngoscope 112:1945–1950, 2002.
9. Austin HA: Clinical evaluation and monitoring of lupus kidney disease. Lupus 7:618–621, 1998.
10. Toto RD: Acute tubulointerstitial nephritis. Am J Med Sci 299:392–410, 1990.
11. Saxena R, Arvattsson B, Bygren P, Wieslander J: Circulating autoantibodies as serological markers in the differential dagnosis of pulmonary-renal syndrome. J Int Med 238:143–152, 1995.
12. Bennett WM: Drug nephrotoxicity: An overview. Ren Fail 19:221–224, 1997.
13. Hladunewich M, Rosenthal MH: Pathophysiology and management of renal insufficiency in the perioperative and critically ill patient. Anesthesiol Clin North Am 18:773–789, 2000.
14. Ouriel K, Geary K, Green RM, et al: Factors determining survival after ruptured aortic aneurysm: The hospital, the surgeon, and the patient. J Vasc Surg 11:493–496, 1990.
15. Hasegawa Y, Nagasawa T: [Thrombotic thrombocytopenic purpura]. Ryoikibetsu Shokogun Shirizu (31):152–154, 2000.
16. Remuzzi G, Ruggenenti P: The hemolytic uremic syndrome. Kidney Int 48:2–19, 1995.
17. Segasothy M, Swaminathan M, Kong NC: Acute renal failure in falciparum malaria. Med J Malaysia 49:412–415, 1994.
18. Valbonesi M, De Luigi MC, Lercari G, et al: Acute intravascular hemolysis in two patients transfused with dry-platelet units obtained from the same ABO incompatible donor. Int J Artif Organs 23:642–646, 2000.
19. Moore KP, Holt SG, Patel RP, et al: A causative role for redox cycling of myoglobin and its inhibition by alkalinization in the pathogenesis and treatment of rhabdomyolysis-induced renal failure. J Biol Chem 273:31731–31737, 1998.
20. De Vriese AS, Robbrecht DL, Vanholder RC, et al: Rifampicin-associated acute renal failure: Pathophysiologic, immunologic, and clinical features. Am J Kidney Dis 31:108–115, 1998.
21. Bruneel F, Gachot B, Wolff M, et al: Resurgence of blackwater fever in long-term European expatriates in Africa: Report of 21 cases and review. Clin Infect Dis 32:1133–1140, 2001.
22. Toto RD, Anderson SA, Brown-Cartwright D, et al: Effects of acute and chronic dosing of NSAIDs in patients with renal insufficiency. Kidney Int 30:760–768, 1986.
23. Sturmer T, Elseviers MM, De Broe ME: Nonsteroidal anti-inflammatory drugs and the kidney. Curr Opin Nephrol Hypertens 10:161–163, 2001.
24. Toto RD, Mitchell H, Milam C, Pettinger WA: Reversible renal insufficiency due to converting enzyme inhibitors in hypertensive nephrosclerosis. Ann Intern Med 115:513–519, 1991.
25. Bridoux F, Hazzan M, Pallot JL, et al: Acute renal failure after the use of angiotensin-converting-enzyme inhibitors in patients without renal artery stenosis. Nephrol Dial Transplant 7:100–104, 1992.
26. Schwarz A, Krause PH, Kunzendorf U, et al: The outcome of acute interstitial nephritis: Risk factors for the transition from acute to chronic interstitial nephritis. Clin Nephrol 54:179–190, 2000.
27. Mazzali M, Dias EP, Ribeiro-Alves MA, et al: Nonrecurrent hemolytic uremic syndrome (HUS de novo) as cause of acute renal failure after renal transplant. Ren Fail 19:271–277, 1997.
28. Suehiro A: [Thrombotic thrombocytopenic purpura: pathophysiology and treatment]. Rinsho Ketsueki 41:463–467, 2000.
29. Parving HH, Tarnow L, Nielsen FS, et al: Cyclosporine nephrotoxicity in type 1 diabetic patients: A 7-year follow-up study. Diabetes Care 22:478–483, 1999.
30. Ahsan N: Intravenous immunoglobulin induced-nephropathy: A complication of IVIG therapy. J Nephrol 11:157–161, 1998.
31. Cayco AV, Perazella MA, Hayslett JP: Renal insufficiency after intravenous immune globulin therapy: A report of two cases and an analysis of the literature. J Am Soc Nephrol 8:1788–1794, 1997.
32. Chung YC, Huang MT, Chang CN, et al: Prolonged nonoliguric acute renal failure associated with high-dose vitamin K administration in a renal transplant recipient. Transplant Proc 26:2129–2131, 1994.
33. Dimitrov Y, Heibel F, Marcellin L, et al: Acute renal failure and nephrotic syndrome with alpha interferon therapy. Nephrol Dial Transplant 12:200–203, 1997.
34. Daugaard G: Cisplatin nephrotoxicity: Experimental and clinical studies. Danish Med Bull 37:1–12, 1990.
35. Asif A, Garces G, Preston RA, Roth D: Current trials of interventions to prevent radiocontrast-induced nephropathy. Am J Therapeutics 12:127–132, 2005.
36. Morcos SJ: Prevention of contrast media-induced nephrotoxicity after angiographic procedures. J Vasc Interv Radiol 16:13–23, 2005.
37. Barrett BJ, Parfey PS: Preventing nephropathy induced by contrast medium. N Engl J Med 354:379–386, 2006.
38. Combest W, Newton M, Combest A, Kosier JH: Effects of herbal supplements on the kidney. Urol Nurs 26:381–386, 2005
39. Steenkamp V, Stewart MJ: Nephrotoxicity associated with exposure to plant toxins, with particular reference to Africa. Ther Drug Monit 27:270–277, 2005.
40. Aakervik O, Svendsen J, Jacobsen D: [Severe ethylene glycol poisoning treated with fomepizole (4-methylpyrazole)]. Tidsskr Nor Laegeforen 122:2444–2446, 2002.
41. van Gelder T, Michiels JJ, Mulder AH, et al: Renal insufficiency due to bilateral primary renal lymphoma. Nephron 60:108–110, 1992.
42. Arrambide K, Toto RD: Tumor lysis syndrome. Semin Nephrol 13:273–280, 1993.
43. Bhowmik D, Mathur R, Bhargava Y, et al: Chronic interstitial nephritis following parenteral copper sulfate poisoning. Ren Fail 23:731–735, 2001.
44. Stokes MB, Chawla H, Brody RI, et al: Immune complex glomerulonephritis in patients coinfected with human immunodeficiency virus and hepatitis C virus. Am J Kidney Dis 29:514–525, 1997.
45. Zikos D, Grewal KS, Craig K, et al: Nephrotic syndrome and acute renal failure associated with hepatitis A virus infection. Am J Gastroenterol 90:295–298, 1995.
46. Rao TK: Acute renal failure syndromes in human immunodeficiency virus infection. Semin Nephrol 18:378–395, 1998.
47. Ismail-Allouch M, Burke G, Nery J, et al: Rapidly progressive focal segmental glomerulosclerosis occurring in a living related kidney transplant donor: Case report and review of 21 cases of kidney transplants for primary FSGS. Transplant Proc 25:2176–2177, 1993.
48. Bolton WK: Rapidly progressive glomerulonephritis. Semin Nephrol 16:517–526, 1996.
49. Packham DK, Hewitson TD, Yan HD, et al: Acute renal failure in IgA nephropathy. Clin Nephrol 42:349–353, 1994.
50. Piqueras AI, White RH, Raafat F, et al: Renal biopsy diagnosis in children presenting with haematuria. Pediatr Nephrol 12:386–391, 1998.
51. Frock J, Bierman M, Hammeke M, Reyes A: Atheroembolic renal disease: Experience with 22 patients. Nebr Med J 79:317–321, 1994.
52. Preston RA, Stemmer CL, Materson BJ, et al: Renal biopsy in patients 65 years of age or older: An analysis of the results of 334 biopsies. J Am Geriatr Soc 38:669–674, 1990.
53. Lefebvre C, Lambert M, Pirson Y: [Pulmonary-renal syndrome: Diagnostic and therapeutic strategy.] Acta Clin Belg 50:94–102, 1995.
54. Monev S: Idiopathic retroperitoneal fibrosis: Prompt diagnosis preserves organ function. Cleve Clin J Med 69:160–166, 2002.
55. Surge M. Abdominal compartment syndrome. Curr Opin Crit Care 11:333–338, 2005.

56. Malbrain MLNG, Chiumello D, Pelosi P, et al: Incidence and prognosis of intraabdominal hypertension in a mixed population of critically ill patients: A multiple-center epidemiological study. Crit Care Med 33:315–322, 2005.
57. Hall PM: The clinical usefulness of urinalysis. Cleve Clin J Med 61:177–178, 1994.
58. Duthie JS, Solanki HP, Krishnamurthy M, Chertow BS: Milk-alkali syndrome with metastatic calcification. Am J Med 99:102–103, 1995.
59. O'Neill WC: Sonographic evaluation of renal failure. Review. Am J Kidney Dis 35:1021–1038, 2000.
60. Cheung S, Abramova L, Saath G, et al: Nephrogenic fibrosing dermopathy associated with exposure to gadolinium-containing contrast agents—St. Louis, Missouri, 2002–2006. MMWR 56:137–141, 2007.
61. Haas M, Spargo BH, Wit EJ, Meehan SM: Etiologies and outcome of acute renal insufficiency in older adults: A renal biopsy study of 259 cases. Am J Kidney Dis 35:433–447, 2000.
62. Korbet SM: Percutaneous renal biopsy. Semin Nephrol 22:254–267, 2002.
63. Solez K, Racusen LC: Role of the renal biopsy in acute renal failure. Contrib Nephrol (132):68–75, 2001.
64. Rahman M, Smith MC: Chronic renal insufficiency: A diagnostic and therapeutic approach. Arch Intern Med 158:1743–1752, 1998.
65. Go AS, Chertow GM, Fan D, et al: Chronic kidney disease and risks of death, cardiovascular events and hospitalization. N Engl J Med 351:1296–1305, 2004.
66. Anavekar NS, McMurray JJV, Velasquez EJ, et al: Relationship between renal dysfunction and cardiovascular outcomes after myocardial infarction. N Engl J Med 351:1285–1295, 2004.
67. Vanholder R, Massy Z, Argiles A, et al: Chronic kidney disease as cause of cardiovascular morbidity and mortality. Nephrol Dial Transplant 20:1048–1056, 2005.
68. Tomakova MP, Skali H, Kenchaiah S, et al: Chronic kidney disease, cardiovascular risk, and response to angiotensin-convertng enzyme inhibitionafter myocardial infarction: The Survival And Ventricular Enlargement (SAVE) study. Circulation 110:3667–3673, 2004.
69. Shand BI, Bailey MA, Bailey RR: Fingernail creatinine as a determinant of the duration of renal failure. Clin Nephrol 47:135–136, 1997.
70. K/DOQI Clinical Practice Guidelines for Chronic Kidney Disease: Evaluation, classification, and stratification. Kidney Disease Outcome Quality Initiative. Am J Kidney Dis 2002 39:S1–S246, 2002.
71. Sack AG: Impact of timing of nephrology referral and pre-ESRD care on mortality risk among new ESRD patients in the United States. Am J Kidney Dis 41:310–318, 2003.
72. Kinchen KS, Sadler J, Fink N, et al: The timing of specialist evaluation in chronic kidney disease and mortality. Ann Intern Med 137:479–486, 2002.
73. Kamil ES: Recent advances in the understanding and management of primary vesicoureteral reflux and reflux nephropathy. Curr Opin Nephrol Hypertens 9:139–142, 2000.
74. Fored CM, Ejerblad E, Lindblad P, et al: Acetaminophen, aspirin, and chronic renal failure. N Engl J Med 345:1801–1808, 2001.
75. Lin JL, Tan DT, Hsu KH, Yu CC: Environmental lead exposure and progressive renal insufficiency. Arch Intern Med 161:264–271, 2001.
76. Calvert GM, Steenland K, Palu S: End-stage renal disease among silica-exposed gold miners: A new method for assessing incidence among epidemiologic cohorts. JAMA 277:1219–1223, 1997.
77. Hogan SL, Satterly KK, Dooley MA, et al: Silica exposure in anti-neutrophil cytoplasmic autoantibody-associated glomerulonephritis and lupus nephritis. J Am Soc Nephrol 12:134–142, 2001.
78. Steenland K, Sanderson W, Calvert GM: Kidney disease and arthritis in a cohort study of workers exposed to silica. Epidemiology 12:405–412, 2001.
79. Cronin AJ, Maidment G, Cook T, et al: Aristolochic acid as a causative factor in a case of Chinese herbal nephropathy. Nephrol Dial Transplant 17:524–525, 2002.
80. Markowitz GS, Appel GB, Fine PL, et al: Collapsing focal segmental glomerulosclerosis following treatment with high-dose pamidronate. J Am Soc Nephrol 12:1164–1172, 2001.
81. Bennett WM, Burdmann EA, Andoh TF, et al: Nephrotoxicity of immunosuppressive drugs. Nephrol Dial Transplant 9(suppl 4):141–145, 1994.
82. Freedman BB, Wilson CH, Spray BJ, et al: Familial clustering of end-stage renal disease in blacks with lupus nephritis. Am J Kidney Dis 29:729–732, 1997.
83. Freedman BI, Soucie JM, McClellan WM: Family history of end-stage renal disease among incident dialysis patients. J Am Soc Nephrol 8:1942–1945, 1997.
84. Freedman BI, Bowden DW, Rich SS, Appel RG: Genetic initiation of hypertensive and diabetic nephropathy. Am J Hypertens 11:251–257, 1998.
85. Byrne C, Nedelman J, Luke RG: Race, socioeconomic status, and the development of end-stage renal disease. Am J Kidney Dis 23:16–22, 1994.
86. Longenecker JC, Coresh J, Klag MJ, et al: Validation of comorbid conditions on the end-stage renal disease medical evidence report: The CHOICE study. Choices for Healthy Outcomes in Caring for ESRD. J Am Soc Nephrol 11:520–529, 2000.
87. Tarver-Carr ME, Powe NR, Eberhardt MS, et al: Excess risk of chronic kidney disease among African-American versus white subjects in the United States: A population-based study of potential explanatory factors. J Am Soc Nephrol 13:2363–2370, 2002.
88. Falk RJ, Jennette JC: Sickle cell nephropathy. Adv Nephrol Necker Hosp 23:133–147, 1994.
89. Hsu SI, McClellan W, Ramirez SPB: Family history of renal disease is a predictor of proteinuria in a large multi-racial Southeast Asian population. Abstract. J Am Soc Nephrol 12:210A, 2001.
90. Torres VE, Harris PC: Mechanism of disease: Autosomal dominant and recessive polycystic kidney diseases. Nature Clin Prac Nephrol 2:40–55, 2006.
91. Hyodo T, Kumano K, Sakai T: Differential diagnosis between glomerular and nonglomerular hematuria by automated urinary flow cytometer: Kitasato University Kidney Center criteria. Nephron 82:312–323, 1999.
92. Singhal R, Mittal BV: Haematuria: Glomerular or non-glomerular? Indian J Pathol Microbiol 39:281–286, 1996.
93. Attman PO, Alaupovic P, Samuelsson O: Lipoprotein abnormalities as a risk factor for progressive nondiabetic renal disease. Kidney Int 56:S14–S17, 1999.
94. Bigazzi R, Bianchi S, Baldari D, Campese VM: Microalbuminuria predicts cardiovascular events and renal insufficiency in patients with essential hypertension. J Hypertens 16:1325–1333, 1998.
95. Cappelli P, Di Liberato L, Albertazzi A: Role of dyslipidemia in the progression of chronic renal disease. Ren Fail 20:391–397, 1998.
96. Foley RN, Parfrey PS, Sarnak MJ: Epidemiology of cardiovascular disease in chronic renal disease. J Am Soc Nephrol 9:S16–S23, 1998.
97. Goldfarb-Rumyantzev AS, Pappas L: Prediction of renal insufficiency in Pima Indians with nephropathy of type 2 diabetes mellitus. Am J Kidney Dis 40:252–264, 2002.
98. Hovind P, Tarnow L, Rossing P, et al: Progression of diabetic nephropathy: Role of plasma homocysteine and plasminogen activator inhibitor-1. Am J Kidney Dis 38:1376–1380, 2001.
99. Isreb MA, Daoud TM, Chatha MP, Leehey DJ: Risk factors for progression of renal disease in patients with type 2 diabetes. J Am Soc Nephrol 13:685A–686A, 2002.
100. Keane WF, Eknoyan G: Proteinuria, albuminuria, risk, assessment, detection, elimination (PARADE): A position paper of the National Kidney Foundation. Am J Kidney Dis 33:1004–1010, 1999.
101. Klag MJ, Whelton PK, Randall BL, et al: End-stage renal disease in African-American and white men: 16-year MRFIT findings. JAMA 277:1293–1298, 1997.
102. Krop JS, Coresh J, Chambless LE, et al: A community-based study of explanatory factors for the excess risk for early renal function decline in blacks vs whites with diabetes: The Atherosclerosis Risk in Communities study. Arch Intern Med 159:1777–1783, 1999.
103. Locatelli F, Alberti D, Graziani G, et al: Factors affecting chronic renal failure progression: Results from a multicentre trial. The Northern Italian Cooperative Study Group. Miner Electrolyte Metab 18:295–302, 1992.
104. Peterson JC, Adler S, Burkart JM, et al: Blood-pressure control, proteinuria, and the progression of renal-disease—The Modification of Diet in Renal Disease study. Ann Intern Med 123:754–762, 1995.
105. Stehouwer CD, Gall MA, Twisk JW, et al: Increased urinary albumin excretion, endothelial dysfunction, and chronic low-grade inflammation in type 2 diabetes: Progressive, interrelated, and independently associated with risk of death. Diabetes 51:1157–1165, 2002.
106. U.S. Renal Data System: USRDS 2005 Annual Data Report: Atlas of End-Stage Renal Disease in the United States. Bethesda, MD, National Institutes of Health, National Institute of Diabetes and Digestive and Kidney Diseases, 2005.
107. Coresh J, Jaar B: Further trends in the etiology of end-stage renal disease in African-Americans. Curr Opin Nephrol Hypertens 6:243–249, 1997.
108. Haywood LJ: Hypertension in minority populations: Access to care. Am J Med 88:17S–20S, 1990.
109. Pugh JA, Medina RA, Cornell JC, Basu S: NIDDM is the major cause of diabetic end-stage renal disease: More evidence from a tri-ethnic community. Diabetes 44:1375–1380, 1995.
110. Chuahirun T, Wesson DE: Cigarette smoking and increased urine albumin excretion are interrelated predictors of nephropathy progression in type 2 diabetes. Am J Kidney Dis 41:13–21, 2003.
111. Chen J, Muntner P, Hamm L, et al: The metabolic syndrome and chronic kidney disease in US adults. Ann Intern Med 140:167–174, 2004.
112. Hsu C-Y, McCulloch CE, Iribarren C, et al: Body mass index and risk for end-stage renal disease. Ann Intern Med 144:21–28, 2006.
113. Coresh J, Astor BC, Greene T, et al: Prevalence of chronic kidney disease and decreased kidney function in the adult US population. Third National Health and Nutrition Examination Survey. Am J Kidney Dis 41:1–12, 2003.
114. Jones CA, Francis ME, Eberhardt MS, et al: Microalbuminuria in the US population: Third National Health and Nutrition Examination Survey. Am J Kidney Dis 39:445–459, 2002.
115. Mann JFE, Gerstein HC, Pogue J, et al: Renal insufficiency as a predictor of cardiovascular outcomes and the impact of ramipril: The HOPE Randomized Trial. Ann Intern Med 134:629–636, 2001.
116. Muntner P, Coresh J, Klag MJ, et al: History of myocardial infarction and stroke among incident end-stage renal disease cases and population-based controls: An analysis of shared risk factors. Am J Kidney Dis 40:323–330, 2002.
117. Levey AS: Measurement of renal function in chronic renal disease. Kidney Int 38:167–184, 1990.
118. Levey AS, Bosch JP, Lewis JB, et al: A more accurate method to estimate glomerular filtration rate from serum creatinine: A new prediction equation. Modification of Diet in Renal Disease Study Group. Ann Intern Med 130:461–470, 1999.
119. Cockcroft DW, Gault MH: Prediction of creatinine clearance from serum creatinine. Nephron 16:31–41, 1979.
120. Toto RD, Kirk KA, Coresh J, et al: Evaluation of serum creatinine for estimating glomerular filtration rate in African Americans with hypertensive nephrosclerosis: Results from the African-American Study of Kidney Disease and Hypertension (AASK) Pilot Study. J Am Soc Nephrol 8:279–287, 1997.
121. Shlipak MG, Sarnak MJ, Katz R, et al: Cystatin C and the risk of death and cardiovascular events among elderly persons. N Engl J Med 351:2049–2060, 2005.
122. Coresh J, Wei GL, McQuillan G, et al: Prevalence of high blood pressure and elevated serum creatinine level in the United States: Findings from the Third National Health and Nutrition Examination Survey (1988–1994). Arch Intern Med 161:1207–1216, 2001.
123. Perlata CA, Hicks LS, Chertaw GM, et al: Control of hypertension in adults with chronic kidney disease in the United States. Hypertension 45:1119–1124, 2005.
124. Bakris GL, Williams M, Dworkin L, et al: Preserving renal function in adults with hypertension and diabetes: A consensus approach. National Kidney Foundation Hypertension and Diabetes Executive Committees Working Group. Am J Kidney Dis 36:646–661, 2000.

125. Wright JT Jr, Bakris G, Greene T, et al: Effect of blood pressure lowering and antihypertensive drug class on progression of hypertensive kidney disease: Results from the AASK trial. JAMA 288:2421–2431, 2002.

126. Intensive blood-glucose control with sulphonylureas or insulin compared with conventional treatment and risk of complications in patients with type 2 diabetes (UKPDS 33). UK Prospective Diabetes Study (UKPDS) Group. Lancet 352:837–853, 1998.

127. Adler AI, Stevens RJ, Manley SE, et al: Development and progression of nephropathy in type 2 diabetes. The United Kingdom Prospective Diabetes Study (UKPDS 64). Kidney Int 63:225–232, 2003.

128. Chen J, Munter P, Hamm L, et al: The metabolic syndrome and chronic kidney disease in US adults. Ann Intern Med 140:167–174, 2004.

129. Hsu C-Y, McCulloch CE, Iribarren C, et al: Body mass index and risk for end-stage renal disease. Ann Intern Med 144:21–28, 2006.

130. Go AS, Chertow GM, Fan D, et al: Chronic kidney disease and risks of death, cardiovascular events and hospitalization. N Engl J Med 351:1296–1305, 2004.

131. Shulman NB, Ford CE, Hall WD, et al: Prognostic value of serum creatinine and effect of treatment of hypertension on renal function. Results from the Hypertension Detection and Follow-up program. The Hypertension Detection and Follow-up Group. Hypertension 13(suppl 5):I80–I93, 1989.

132. Middleton RJ, Parfrey PS, Foley RN: Left ventricular hypertrophy in the renal patient. J Am Soc Nephrol 12:1079–1084, 2001.

133. Shlipak MG, Fried LF, Crump C, et al: Elevations of inflammatory and procoagulant biomarkers in elderly persons with renal insufficiency. Circulation 107:87–92, 2003.

134. Stenvinkel P, Heimburger O, Paultre F, et al: Strong association between malnutrition, inflammation, and atherosclerosis in chronic renal failure. Kidney Int 55:1899–1911, 1999.

135. Festa A, D'Agostino R, Howard G, et al: Chronic subclinical inflammation as part of the insulin resistance syndrome. The Insulin Resistance Atherosclerosis Study (IRAS). Circulation 102:42–47, 2000.

136. Panichi V, Migliori M, De Pietro S, et al: C-reactive protein as a marker of chronic inflammation in uremic patients. Blood Purif 18:183–190, 2000.

137. Goodman WG, Goldin J, Kuizon BD, et al: Coronary-artery calcification in young adults with end-stage renal disease who are undergoing dialysis. N Engl J Med 342:1478–1483, 2000.

138. Hayden JM, Reaven PD: Cardiovascular disease in diabetes mellitus type 2: A potential role for novel cardiovascular risk factors. Curr Opin Lipidol 11:519–528, 2000.

139. Miskulin DC, Meyer KB, Martin AA, et al: Comorbidity and its change predict survival in incident dialysis patients. Am J Kidney Dis 41:149–161, 2003.

140. The effect of intensive treatment of diabetes on the development and progression of long-term complications in insulin-dependent diabetes mellitus. The Diabetes Control and Complications Trial Research Group. N Engl J Med 329:977–986, 1993.

141. Sarnak MJ, Levey AS: Epidemiology, diagnosis, and management of cardiac disease in chronic renal disease. J Thromb Thrombolysis 10:169–180, 2000.

142. Brattstrom L, Wilcken DE: Homocysteine and cardiovascular disease: Cause or effect? Am J Clin Nutr 72:315–323, 2000.

143. Parsons DS, Reaveley DA, Pavitt DV, Brown EA: Relationship of renal function to homocysteine and lipoprotein(a) levels: The frequency of the combination of both risk factors in chronic renal impairment. Am J Kidney Dis 40:916–923, 2002.

144. Friedman AN, Bostom AG, Levey AS, et al: Plasma total homocysteine levels among patients undergoing nocturnal versus standard hemodialysis. J Am Soc Nephrol 13:265–268, 2002.

145. Beto JA, Bansal VK: Interventions for other risk factors: Tobacco use, physical inactivity, menopause, and homocysteine. Am J Kidney Dis 32:S172–S183, 1998.

146. Bostom AG, Shemin D, Gohh RY, et al: Treatment of mild hyper homocysteinemia in renal transplant recipients versus hemodialysis patients. Transplantation 69:2128–2131, 2000.

147. The Heart Outcomes Prevention Evaluation (HOPE) 2 Investigators: Homocysteine lowering with folic acid and B vitamins in vascular disease. N Engl J Med 354:1567–1577, 2006.

148. Bonaa KH, Njolstad I, Ueland PM, et al: Homocysteine lowering and cardiovascular events after acute nyocardial infarction. N Engl J Med 354:1578–1588, 2006.

149. Wrone EM, Hornberger JM, Zehnder JL, et al: Randomized trial of folic acid for prevention of cardiovascular events in end-stage renal disease. J Am Soc Nephrol 15:420–426, 2004.

150. Longenecker JC, Klag MJ, Marcovina SM, et al: Small apolipoprotein(a) size predicts mortality in end-stage renal disease: The CHOICE study. Circulation 106:2812–2818, 2002.

151. Muntner P, Coresh J, Smith JC, et al: Plasma lipids and risk of developing renal dysfunction: The Atherosclerosis Risk in Communities Study. Kidney Int 58:293–301, 2000.

152. Toto RD, Vega G, Grundy SM: Cholesterol management in patients with chronic kidney disease. In Brayd H, Wilcox C (eds): Therapy in Nephrology and Hypertension. Philadelphia and New York, Lippincott Williams & Wilkins, 2003, pp 631–639.

153. Toto RD, Grundy SM, Vega GL: Pravastatin treatment of very low density, intermediate density, and low density lipoproteins in hypercholesterolemia and combined hyperlipidemia secondary to the nephrotic syndrome. Am J Nephrol 70:12–17, 2000.

154. Vega GL, Toto RD, Grundy S: Metabolism of low-density lipoproteins in nephrotic dyslipidemia: Comparison of hypercholesterolemia alone and combined hyperlipidemia. Kidney Int 47:579–586, 1995.

155. Kronenberg F, Kuen E, Ritz E, et al: Lipoprotein(a) serum concentrations and apolipoprotein(a) phenotypes in mild and moderate renal failure. J Am Soc Nephrol 11:105–115, 2000.

156. Gundy SM: United States Cholesterol Guidelines 2001: Expanded scope of intensive low-density lipoprotein-lowering therapy. Am J Cardiol 88:23J–27J, 2001.

157. Wanner C, Krane V, Marz W, et al: Atorvastatin in patients with type 2 diabetes mellitus undergoing hemodialysis. N Engl J Med 353:238–248, 2005.

158. Holdaas H, Fellstrom B, Jardine AG, et al: Effect of fluvastatin on cardiac outcomes in renal transplant recipients: A multicenter, randomized, placebo-controlled trial. Lancet 361:2024–2031, 2003.

159. Lewis EJ, Hunsicker LG, Clarke WR, et al: Renoprotective effect of the angiotensin-receptor antagonist irbesartan in patients with nephropathy due to type 2 diabetes. N Engl J Med 345:851–860, 2001.

160. Ho LT, Sprague SM: Renal osteodystrophy in chronic renal failure. Semin Nephrol 22:488–493, 2002.

161. Chertow GM, Burke SK, Dillon MA, Slatopolsky E: Long-term effects of sevelamer hydrochloride on the calcium x phosphate product and lipid profile of haemodialysis patients. Nephrol Dial Transplant 14:2907–2914, 1999.

162. Cozzolino M, Dusso A, Slatopolsky E: Role of calcium-phosphorus product and bone-associated proteins in vascular calcification in renal failure. J Am Soc Nephrol 12:2511–2516, 2001.

163. Kramer H, Toto R, Peshock R, et al: Association between chronic kidney disease and coronary artery calcification. The Dallas Heart study. J Am Soc Nephrol 16:507–513, 2005.

164. Sigrist M, Bungay P, Taal MW, McIntyre CW: Vascular calcification and cardiovascular function in chronic kidney disease. Nephrol Dial Transplant 21:707–714, 2006.

165. Block GA, Port FK: Re-evaluation of risks associated with hyperphosphatemia and hyperparathyroidism in dialysis patients: Recommendations for a change in management. Am J Kidney Dis 35:1226–1237, 2000.

166. Goodman WG, Goldin J, Kuizon BD, et al: Coronary-artery calcification in young adults with end-stage renal disease who are undergoing dialysis. N Engl J Med 342:1478–1483, 2000.

167. Chertow GM, Burke SK, Raggi P: Sevelamer attenuates the progression of coronary and aortic calcification in hemodialysis patients. Kidney Int 62:245–252, 2002.

168. Raggi P, Boulay A, Chasan-Taber S, et al: Cardiac calcification in adult hemodialysis patients: A link between end-stage renal disease and cardiovascular disease? J Am Coll Cardiol 39:695–701, 2002.

169. Hsu CY, Cummings SR, McCulloch CE, Chertow GM: Bone mineral density is not diminished by mild to moderate chronic renal insufficiency. Kidney Int 61:1814–1820, 2002.

170. National Kidney Foundation Kidney Disease Outcomes Quality Initiative: Clinical practice guidelines for bone metabolism and disease in chronic kidney disease. Am J Kidney Dis 42(suppl 3):S1–S201, 2003.

171. Suki WN, Zabaneh R, Congiano J, et al: The DCOR trial—A prospective randomized trial assessing the impact on outcomes of sevelamer in dialysis patients. J Am Soc Nephrol 16:281A, 2005.

172. Lawson JA, Lazarus R, Kelly JJ: Prevalence and prognostic significance of malnutrition in chronic renal insufficiency. J Renal Nutr 11:16–22, 2001.

173. Chertow GM, Johansen KL, Lew N, et al: Vintage, nutritional status, and survival in hemodialysis patients. Kidney Int 57:1176–1181, 2000.

174. Festa A, D'Agostino R, Howard G, et al: Inflammation and microalbuminuria in non-diabetic and type 2 diabetic subjects: The Insulin Resistance Atherosclerosis Study. Kidney Int 58:1703–1710, 2000.

175. Fernandez-Real JM, Ricart W: Insulin resistance and inflammation in an evolutionary perspective: The contribution of cytokine genotype/phenotype to thriftiness. Diabetologia 42:1367–1374, 1999.

176. Panichi V, Migliori M, De Pietro S, et al: C-reactive protein as a marker of chronic inflammation in uremic patients. Blood Purif 18:183–190, 2000.

177. DuBose TDJ: Hyperkalemic hyperchloremic metabolic acidosis: Pathophysiologic insights. Kidney Int 51:591–602, 1997.

178. Mitch WE, Price SR: Mechanisms activated by kidney disease and the loss of muscle mass. Am J Kidney Dis 38:1337–1342, 2001.

179. Mitch WE: Insights into the abnormalities of chronic renal disease attributed to malnutrition. J Am Soc Nephrol 13(suppl 1):S22–S27, 2002.

180. IV: NKF-K/DOQI Clinical Practice Guidelines for Anemia of Chronic Kidney Disease: Update 2000. [Erratum appears in Am J Kidney Dis 38:442, 2001.] Am J Kidney Dis 37:S182–S238, 2001.

181. Hsu CY, McCulloch CE, Curhan GC: Epidemiology of anemia associated with chronic renal insufficiency among adults in the United States: Results from the Third National Health and Nutrition Examination Survey. J Am Soc Nephrol 13:504–510, 2002.

182. Astor BC, Muntner P, Levin A, et al: Association of kidney function with anemia: The Third National Health and Nutrition Examination Survey (1988–1994). Arch Intern Med 162:1401–1408, 2002.

183. Richardson D: Clinical factors influencing sensitivity and response to epoetin. Nephrol Dial Transplant 17(suppl 1):53–59, 2002.

184. Kazmi WH, Kausz AT, Khan S, et al: Anemia: An early complication of chronic renal insufficiency. Am J Kidney Dis 38:803–812, 2001.

185. Obrador G, Ruthazer R, Arora P, et al: Prevalence of and factors associated with suboptimal care before initiation of dialysis in the United States. J Am Soc Nephrol 10:1793–1800, 1999.

186. Besarab A, Levin A: Defining a renal anemia management period. Am J Kidney Dis 36:S13–S23, 2000.

187. Foley RN, Parfrey PS, Morgan J, et al: Effect of hemoglobin levels in hemodialysis patients with asymptomatic cardiomyopathy. Kidney Int 58:1325–1335, 2000.

188. Gotch FA, Levin NW, Port FK, et al: Clinical outcome relative to the dose of dialysis is not what you think: The fallacy of the mean. Editorial. Am J Kidney Dis 30:1–15, 1997.

189. Levin A: Anemia and left ventricular hypertrophy in chronic kidney disease populations: A review of the current state of knowledge. Kidney Int Suppl (80):35–38, 2002.

190. Levin A: The role of anaemia in the genesis of cardiac abnormalities in patients with chronic kidney disease. Nephrol Dial Transplant 17:207–210, 2002.

191. Levin A, Thompson CR, Ethier J, et al: Left ventricular mass index increase in early renal disease: Impact of decline in hemoglobin. Am J Kidney Dis 34:125–134, 1999.

192. Levin A: Anaemia in the patient with renal insufficiency: Documenting the impact and reviewing treatment strategies. Nephrol Dial Transplant 14:292–295, 1999.

193. Levin A, Djurdjev O, Barrett B, et al: Cardiovascular disease in patients with chronic kidney disease: Getting to the heart of the matter. Am J Kidney Dis 38:1398–1407, 2001.

194. Foley RN: Should hemoglobin be normalized in uremic patients? Clin Nephrol 58(suppl 1):S58–S61, 2002.

195. Foley RN, Parfrey PS, Harnett JD, et al: The impact of anemia on cardiomyopathy, morbidity and mortality in end-stage renal disease. Am J Kidney Dis 28:53–61, 1996.

196. Foley RN, Parfrey PS, Morgan J, et al: Effect of hemoglobin levels in hemodialysis patients with asymptomatic cardiomyopathy. Kidney Int 58:1325–1335, 2000.

197. Hegarty J, Foley RN: Anaemia, renal insufficiency and cardiovascular outcome. Nephrol Dial Transplant 16(suppl 1):102–104, 2001.

198. Levin A, Singer J, Thompson CR, et al: Prevalent left ventricular hypertrophy in the predialysis population: Identifying opportunities for intervention. Am J Kidney Dis 27:347–354, 1996.

199. Eknoyan G: The importance of early treatment of the anaemia of chronic kidney disease. Nephrol Dial Transplant 16(suppl 5):45–49, 2001.

200. Mohanram A, Zhang J, Shahinfar S, et al: Anemia and end-stage renal disease in patients with type 2 diabetes and nephropathy. Kidney Int 66:1131–1138, 2004.

CH 22

Approach to the Patient with Kidney Disease

CHAPTER 23

Laboratory Assessment of Kidney Disease: Clearance, Urinalysis, and Kidney Biopsy

Ajay K. Israni • Bertram L. Kasiske

DETECTION AND DIAGNOSIS OF KIDNEY DISEASE

Because patients in early stages of chronic kidney disease (CKD) often exhibit few signs and symptoms, tests for screening and diagnosis are critical in nephrology. Directly or indirectly, these tests measure kidney structure and function. Ideally, they should detect abnormalities early enough to alert patients and physicians to the potential need for therapy that may prevent morbidity and mortality associated with kidney disease. In addition, tests can help establish a specific diagnosis that will suggest the correct therapy and the likelihood of response to treatment.

Even in the absence of effective therapy, accurate diagnosis of kidney disease helps determine prognosis, which often serves a useful purpose in its own right. Tests to determine kidney structure and function can also be important for measuring disease progression. Once disease has been detected and therapy begun, it is desirable to determine whether the therapy has been effective, so that ineffective therapy can be discontinued or altered. In any case, it is important to predict the clinical course of disease to better inform patients and to help determine when renal replacement therapy may be appropriate.

Finally, data have now suggested that CKD is an important independent risk factor for cardiovascular disease. Individuals with mild to moderate reductions in kidney function are at increased risk for cardiovascular disease, **and this reduction in kidney function has an adverse effect on the prognosis of cardiovascular disease.**[1] Microalbuminuria, even in the absence of diabetes, has also been linked to cardiovascular disease.[2] Therefore, detecting kidney damage may help identify patients for cardiovascular disease risk factor management.

The tests that best detect abnormalities in kidney function are those that measure glomerular filtration rate (GFR). However, measurements of GFR may not be useful for screening purposes in many clinical settings. Patients with early kidney disease may have normal or even increased GFR. Because there is a large amount of physiologic variability among normal individuals, it is virtually impossible to define limits for normal GFR. Indeed, substantial differences in the amount of structural kidney damage can be demonstrated in patients with identical GFRs. Furthermore, measuring GFR is of little value in establishing a diagnosis once other abnormalities have been detected. Nevertheless, an accurate determination of GFR can provide useful prognostic information and can be particularly helpful in following the clinical course. Guidelines developed by the National Kidney Foundation's Kidney Disease and Outcomes Quality Initiative (K/DOQI) have defined stages of CKD largely on the basis of levels of GFR.[3]

Urinalysis is often the most useful test available for detecting early kidney abnormalities. Measuring urine protein level or examining the urine sediment can also help establish a diagnosis or aid the decision whether to subject a patient to biopsy. Examining the microscopic structure of kidney tissue is invaluable in detecting and diagnosing kidney disease. However, major limitations of kidney biopsy include the risk and inconvenience of the procedure as well as the potential for sampling errors. The careful selection of patients who undergo biopsy can be aided by measurements in urine that help screen for kidney injury.

The GFR measurement, urinalysis, and kidney biopsy serve complementary roles in the detection and diagnosis of kidney disease. However, the relative usefulness of these tests is, in large part, determined by their sensitivity and specificity. Sensitivity and specificity, in turn, depend on accuracy and precision. Moreover, the prevalence of abnormalities in the population of individuals being tested affects the clinical utility of each of these tests.

The *sensitivity*, or true-positive rate, of a test is the proportion of positive results in patients known to have disease (Table 23–1). The *specificity* is the proportion of negative results in disease-free individuals. The *false-positive rate* is the proportion of positive results in disease-free individuals; and the *false-negative rate* is the proportion of negative results in individuals with

Conflicts: Dr. Kasiske currently receives research support from the Merck/Schering Plough Joint Venture and Bristol-Myers Squibb. In the past 2 years, he received honoraria from Astra-Zenica, Bristol-Myers Squibb, Fujisawa, Merck, Pfizer, and Wyeth.

Dr. Israni currently receives research support from Roche and Bristol-Myers Squibb.

Support: Supported in part by NIH grant K23-DK062829 to Dr. Israni.

TABLE 23-1	Definitions of Parameters Commonly Used to Assess the Diagnostic Discrimination of a Clinical Test	
	Disease (Total = a + c)	**No Disease (Total = b + d)**
Test positive (Total = a + b)	a	b
Test negative (Total = c + d)	c	d

Sensitivity = a/(a + c)
Specificity = d/(b + d)
False-positive rate = 1 − specificity = b/(b + d)
False-negative rate = 1 − sensitivity = c/(a + c)
Positive predictive value = a/(a + b)
Negative predictive value = d/(c + d)

disease. *Positive predictive value* of a test refers to the proportion of individuals with a positive result who have the disease (i.e., the likelihood of disease if the result is positive). *Negative predictive value* refers to the proportion of individuals with a negative result who are disease-free.

The sensitivity and specificity of any test are ultimately dictated by its accuracy (determined by comparison with a "gold standard") and precision (determined by comparing repeated measurements using the same test). The accuracy and precision of a test that yields values on a continuum also depend on the cutoff value or values used to define what is abnormal. Often, the utility of a test can be determined by examining receiver-operating characteristic (ROC) curves generated for each test. ROC curves are plots of the true-positive rate (sensitivity) on the y axis and the false-positive rate (1 − specificity) on the x axis. A perfect test is one in which the ROC is described by a line in which all values for y are between 0 and 100 when x is 0, and all values for y are 100 when x is greater than 0. A worthless test is one in which the ROC curve is described by a line in which y is equal to x for all values of x and y. The utility of a given test depends on the extent to which the ROC curve resembles that of a perfect test.

Finally, the number of true-positive and false-positive results and the number of true-negative and false-negative results ultimately depend on the prevalence of dysfunction in the population being screened. Some simple algebraic calculations can easily demonstrate how the prevalence of a disease influences the diagnostic discrimination of a test. Take the case of a hypothetical test evaluating 100 individuals known to have a high prevalence (30%) of disease. The test would appear to be quite reasonable with a sensitivity of 0.90 and a specificity of 0.90. Among the 100 patients tested, a positive result would indicate a 79% likelihood that disease was present, whereas a negative result would indicate a 95% likelihood that disease was absent. If the same test were then applied to a general population of 10,000 individuals in whom the prevalence of disease was 0.3%, the sensitivity and specificity of the test would be unchanged. However, in this population, a positive result would indicate only a 2.6% likelihood of disease, and the number of false-positive results would greatly exceed the number of true-positive results.

This chapter reviews the usefulness and limitations of currently available techniques for measuring GFR, examining urine constituents, and assessing kidney structure. In reality, precise data on the sensitivity and specificity of tests of kidney structure and function are often not available, and even when they are, the prevalence (prior probability) of the outcome being measured can be only crudely estimated. Nevertheless, data on sensitivity and specificity are discussed when available. When possible, we make an empirical estimation of the effect of differences in the underlying

RENAL CLEARANCE—GLOMERULAR FILTRATION RATE

Historical Perspective

The modern era of kidney function assessment began with the measurement of urea. Urea was first isolated from human urine by Rouelle in 1773. In the early 1800s, Fourcroy coined the term "urée," carefully choosing a name that would avoid confusion with "urique," or uric acid. In 1827, Richard Bright observed that urea accumulated in the blood of patients with dropsy, and he linked this phenomenon to decreased urine urea concentration, proteinuria, and diseased kidneys. One year later, Wöhler synthesized urea from ammonium cyanate; in so doing, he helped discredit the doctrine of vitalism, which was then prevalent. In 1842, Dumas and Cahours demonstrated that urea was a product of dietary protein catabolism, and in 1903, Strauss introduced blood urea level as a diagnostic test for kidney disease.[4]

Homer Smith credited Ambard and Weill with one of the first attempts to measure kidney function with a "dynamic" test in 1912.[4] These researchers characterized kidney function (K) as blood urea concentration (B) divided by the product of the square root of the rate of urea excretion (D) times the square root of urine urea concentration (U), as follows:

$$K = B(\sqrt{D} \cdot \sqrt{U})$$

In 1926, Rehberg used exogenous creatinine to measure renal clearance (urine concentration of creatinine times urine flow rate divided by plasma concentration of creatinine) as an estimate of glomerular filtration. In 1928, Addis described kidney function as a urea excretion ratio, or the quantity of urea excreted divided by the concentration in blood. Around the same time, the concept of urea clearance as a measure of kidney function was described in detail by Möller, McIntosh, and Van Slyke.[4]

Overview

GFR is traditionally measured as the renal clearance of a particular substance, or marker, from plasma. The clearance of an indicator substance is the amount removed from plasma, divided by the average plasma concentration over the time of measurement. Clearance is expressed in moles or weight of the indicator per volume per time. It can be thought of as the volume of plasma that can be completely cleared of the indicator in a unit of time.

Under the right conditions, measuring the amount of an indicator in both plasma and urine can allow the accurate calculation of GFR (Fig. 23–1). Indeed, if we assume that there is no extrarenal elimination, tubular reabsorption, or tubular secretion of the marker, then GFR can be calculated as follows:

$$\text{Glomerular filtration rate} = (U \cdot V)/(P \cdot T)$$

where U is the urine concentration, V is the urine volume, and P is the average plasma concentration of the marker over the time (T) of the urine collection. Unfortunately, tubular secretion, tubular reabsorption, or both, of the indicator can cause renal clearance measurements to give estimates of the GFR that are falsely high or falsely low.

Under the right conditions, plasma concentrations of an indicator substance can be completely dependent on renal clearance and can accurately reflect GFR. When the amount of an indicator added to the plasma from an exogenous or endogenous source is constant, and when there is no extra-renal elimination, tubular secretion, or tubular reabsorption, then the GFR is equal to the inverse plasma concentration of the indicator multiplied by a constant. That constant is the amount excreted by glomerular filtration, which, under steady-state conditions, must equal the amount added to the plasma (see Fig. 23–1). In other words, under these conditions, $U \cdot V/T$ is equal to a constant (C) so that GFR = C/P, and changes in GFR must be inversely proportional to changes in P.

This information can be used to define the characteristics of an ideal indicator for measuring GFR (Tables 23–2 and 23–3). Although such an indicator does not exist, its definition can serve as a useful benchmark for comparing the advantages and disadvantages of tests designed to measure GFR. The ideal endogenous indicator would be produced at the same constant rate under all conditions, so that changes in the plasma levels are inversely proportional to changes in GFR multiplied by a constant. This constant would be uniquely determined for an individual patient by measuring the urine excretion rate of the marker (GFR equals the urine excretion rate divided by the plasma concentration). Thereafter, only a single plasma determination would be needed to accurately assess GFR in that patient, unless the renal function was changing so rapidly that a steady state was not achieved. An ideal exogenous indicator would have all of these same characteristics, but should also be safe, easy to administer, and inexpensive.

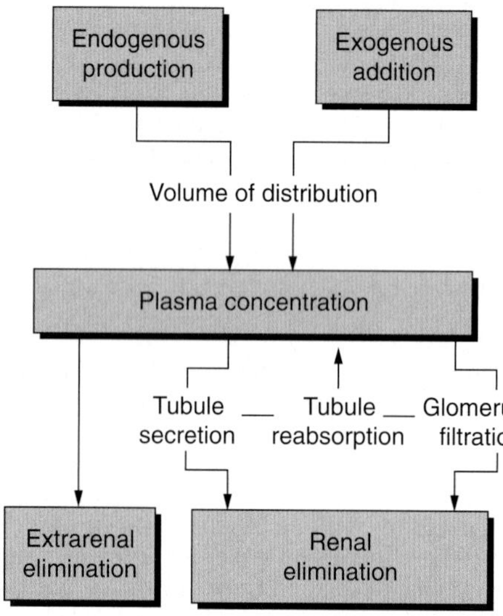

Whether endogenous or exogenous, an ideal indicator would distribute freely and instantaneously throughout the extracellular space. It would not bind to plasma proteins and would be freely filtered at the glomerulus. It would be subject to neither excretion nor reabsorption in the tubules or urinary collecting system. It would be completely resistant to degradation, and its elimination would be entirely dependent on glomerular filtration. It would be easy to measure in plasma and in urine, and nothing would interfere with the assay. Ideally, the inter- and intrapatient coefficient of variation would be low.

Obviously, the ideal marker for measuring GFR has yet to be discovered. Nevertheless, a mythical gold standard obeys principles that should be considered in any discussion of methods used to measure GFR. Actual methods will violate these principles in different ways and with different tradeoffs of accuracy and practicality. In the end, these tradeoffs can be tailored to the clinical situation, taking into account estimated prior probabilities, to achieve a maximum amount of information for a minimum cost. The question is not which test is best, but which test is best suited for the clinical situation at hand.

Plasma Urea

Urea was one of the first indicators used to measure GFR. Unfortunately, it shares few of the attributes of an ideal marker, and plasma urea has been shown to be a poor measure of GFR. Urea production is variable and is largely dependent on protein intake. Although one quarter of the urea produced is metabolized in the intestine, the ammonia produced is reconverted to urea. Thus, most of the urea is ultimately excreted by the kidneys. With a molecular weight of 60 Da, urea is freely filtered at the glomerulus. However, it can be readily reabsorbed, and the amount of tubular reabsorption is variable. Indeed, medullary collecting duct urea reabsorption is functionally linked to water reabsorption. In states of diuresis and low levels of antidiuretic hormone, the

FIGURE 23–1 Factors influencing the relationship between an indicator used to measure renal function and true glomerular filtration rate (GFR). When tubular secretion and reabsorption of the indicator are nil and plasma concentration is constant, then GFR is equal to renal elimination divided by plasma concentration. Also, if the sum of endogenous production and exogenous addition minus extrarenal elimination is constant, then renal elimination is constant and the GFR is inversely proportional to plasma concentration.

TABLE 23–2	Formulae for Estimating Glomerular Filtration Rate Using Serum Creatinine and Other Clinical Parameters		
Formula		**Units**	**Reference**
$(100/Cr) - 12$ *if male* $(80/Cr) - 7$ *if female*		ml/min/1.73 m²	Jelliffe[38]
$(Wt \cdot (29.3 - 0.203 \cdot Age)/(Cr \cdot 14.4)$, *if male* $(Wt \cdot (25.3 - 0.175 \cdot Age)/(Cr \cdot 14.4)$, *if female*		ml/min	Mawer[39,41]
$(98 - 16 \cdot (Age - 20)/20)/Cr$, *multiply by* 0.90 *if female*		ml/min/1.73 m²	Jelliffe[40]
$((140 - Age) \cdot (Wt))/(72 \cdot Cr)$, *multiply by* 0.85 *if female*		ml/min	Cockcroft and Gault[42]
$((145 - Age)/Cr) - 3$, *multiply by* 0.85 *if female*		ml/min/70 kg	Hull[43]
$(27 - (0.173 \cdot Age))/Cr$, *if male* $(27 - (0.175 \cdot Age))/Cr$, *if female*		ml/min	Bjornsson[46]
$7.58/(Cr \cdot 0.0884) - 0.103 \cdot Age + 0.096 \cdot Wt - 6.66$, *if male* $6.05/(Cr \cdot 0.0884) - 0.080 \cdot Age + 0.080 \cdot Wt - 4.81$, *if female*		ml/min/1.73 m² (height²)	Walser[52]
$170 \cdot Cr^{-.999} \cdot Age^{-.176} \cdot (0.762$ *if female*$) \cdot (1.180$ *if black*$) \cdot SUN^{-.170} \cdot Alb^{.318}$		ml/min/1.73 m²	Levey[53]

Alb, serum albumin (g/dL); Cr, serum creatinine (mg/dL); SUN, serum urea nitrogen (mg/dL); Wt, body weight (kg).

TABLE 23-3	Characteristics of an Ideal Endogenous or Exogenous Marker for Measuring Glomerular Filtration Rate
Constant production	
Safe	
Convenient	
Readily diffusible in extracellular space	
No protein binding and freely filterable	
No tubular reabsorption	
No tubular secretion	
No extrarenal elimination or degradation	
Accurate and reproducible assay	
No compounds interfere	
Inexpensive	
No influence on the GFR	

medullary collecting duct is relatively impermeable to urea. However, in states of decreased effective intravascular volume, low urine tubular flow, and increased antidiuretic hormone, urea reabsorption can be substantial.[4]

Plasma urea, or blood urea nitrogen (BUN), concentration is affected by a number of factors other than alterations in GFR. As indicated previously, increased plasma urea levels accompany decreased urine flow in patients with intravascular volume depletion, as occurs following the administration of diuretics. Congestive heart failure also raises plasma urea, probably by similar mechanisms. Increased plasma levels that are probably caused by increased production are seen with elevated dietary protein intake, gastrointestinal bleeding, and tetracycline use. On the other hand, reduced levels of plasma urea can be seen in patients with alcohol abuse and chronic liver disease.[4]

Some substances can interfere with the laboratory determination of urea. Substances that can give falsely high urea levels include acetohexamide, allantoin, aminosalicylic acid, bilirubin (very high levels), chloral hydrate, dextran, free hemoglobin, hydantoin derivatives, lipids (lipemia), sulfonamides, tetracycline, thiourea, and uric acid.[5] Substances that can give falsely low analytical values of urea include ascorbic acid, levodopa, lipids (lipemia), and streptomycin.[6]

Urea Clearance

Because of tubular urea reabsorption, renal urea clearance usually underestimates GFR. Urea clearance can be as little as one half or less of the GFR as measured by other techniques. As with plasma urea, the state of hydration can markedly influence urea clearance. However, the degree of underestimation of glomerular filtration and the tendency for urea clearance to vary with the state of hydration are both less in patients with markedly reduced renal function. Moreover, because creatinine clearance overestimates GFR, some investigators have suggested that the mean of creatinine and urea clearance would be a reasonable estimate of GFR, at least in patients with low levels of renal function.[4] In a large enough sample of patients, errors from tubular reabsorption of urea may negate errors from tubular secretion of creatinine, so that mean urea and creatinine clearances may better approximate the true GFR. However, the factors that affect tubular creatinine secretion and urea reabsorption are different, and any tendency for "two wrongs to make a right" would likely be coincidental and infrequent in a given patient.

Urea clearance determinations are made by measuring renal urea excretion. The accuracy of any clearance technique that relies on urine excretion measurements is compromised by problems associated with obtaining accurate urine collections. Twenty-four–hour collections are inconvenient and difficult for most patients to perform. Patients should be instructed to empty the bladder, note the time, and save all subsequent urine, including urine voided at exactly the same time 24 hours from the time of initiation. They should be warned to empty the bladder before defecation to avoid inadvertent loss of urine. The completeness of 24-hour urine collections can be examined by measuring creatinine excretion (see later). Shorter collection times enhance patient compliance but provide samples for only a portion of the day, during which GFR varies in a diurnal pattern. Incomplete bladder emptying can also reduce the accuracy of timed urine collections. Incomplete bladder emptying can be obviated by catheterization, but the discomfort, risk, and inconvenience often make it unacceptable.

Serum Creatinine

Creatinine is a metabolic product of creatine and phosphocreatine, both of which are found almost exclusively in muscle. Thus, creatinine production is proportional to muscle mass and varies little from day to day. However, production can change over longer periods of time if there is a change in muscle mass. Age- and gender-associated differences in creatinine production are also largely attributable to differences in muscle mass.[4] Although diet ordinarily accounts for a relatively small proportion of overall creatinine excretion, it is another source of variability in serum creatinine levels. Creatine from ingested meat is converted to creatinine and can be the source for up to 30% of total creatinine excretion. Thus, variability in meat intake can also contribute to variability in serum creatinine levels. The conversion of creatine to creatinine can occur with cooking. Because creatinine is readily absorbed from the gastrointestinal tract, ingesting cooked meat can lead to a rapid increase in serum creatinine levels.[4]

Creatinine is small (molecular weight 113 Da), does not bind to plasma proteins, and is freely filtered by the renal glomerulus. However, it has long been appreciated that creatinine is also secreted by the renal tubule. Secretion is a saturable process that probably occurs via the organic cation pathway and is blocked by some commonly used medications including cimetidine, trimethoprim, pyrimethamine, and dapsone.[4] If tubular secretion of creatinine were constant, differences in serum creatinine and renal clearance could still reflect differences in GFR. However, evidence suggests that the secretion of creatinine varies substantially in the same individuals over time, between individuals, and between laboratories.[7,8] Particularly troublesome is the fact that the proportion of total renal creatinine excretion due to tubular secretion increases with decreasing renal function[7,9]; this feature could have a dampening effect on serial measurements in individuals, because GFR could fall more rapidly than indicated by either serum creatinine or creatinine clearance.

Although proportional tubular secretion of creatinine increases with decreasing GFR, total urine creatinine excretion actually declines[7] owing to the fact that extrarenal creatinine degradation increases with declining renal function.[10,11] Indeed, it has been shown that increased extrarenal creatinine degradation may be sufficient to entirely account for the decrease in urine creatinine excretion associated with declining GFR.[10] The extrarenal degradation of creatinine has been attributed to its conversion to carbon dioxide and methylamine by bacteria in the intestine.[12] Because of the increase in extrarenal creatinine degradation with declining kidney function, plasma creatinine can be expected to underestimate declines in GFR.

A number of methods are used to measure creatinine.[13-17] The original Folin-Wu method used the Jaffé reaction, which has been used with various modifications since.[4] The method of Hare involved the isolation of creatinine by absorption on Lloyd's reagent.[14] The direct alkaline picrate method of Bonsnes and Taussky[13] has been used. This method involves the complexing of creatinine with alkaline picrate and measurement using a colorimetric technique. The Jaffé reaction has also been adapted for use on autoanalyzers. Other methods currently in use employ O-nitrobenzaldehyde (Sakaguchi reaction) and imidohydrolase.[17]

There is probably more variation in what laboratories report as the upper limit of normal for serum creatinine than for any other standard chemistry value.[18] In the absence of procedures to remove noncreatinine chromogens, the upper limit of the normal measured by the Jaffé reaction may be as high as 1.6 to 1.9 mg/dL for adults (to covert mg/dL to mmol/L, multiply by 88.4). The upper limit of normal for serum creatinine measured by autoanalyzer or the imidohydrolase method is usually 1.2 to 1.4 mg/dL. Some laboratories will report separate normal ranges for men and women and for adults and children. Besides differences in methods, differences in equipment may also affect plasma creatinine concentrations. Miller and co-workers[19] evaluated over 5000 laboratories using 20 different instruments to measure creatinine by up to three different alkaline picrate methods and found that the mean serum creatinine concentration on a standardized sample ranged from 0.84 to 1.21 mg/dL. The bias, which describes the systematic deviation from the gold standard measure related to the instrument manufacturer, was greater than that due to the alkaline picrate method.

A number of normal plasma constituents can interfere with creatinine measurement. Glucose, fructose, pyruvate, acetoacetate, uric acid, ascorbic acid, and plasma proteins can all cause the Jaffé colorimetric assay to yield falsely high creatinine values.[4] The low levels of these substances generally do not interfere with the Jaffé assay of creatinine in urine. Normally, interfering chromogens increase the creatinine result by about 20%, but in some disease states, the interference can be much greater. In diabetic ketoacidosis, for example, spurious elevations in serum creatinine can be significant. Cephalosporin antibiotics can also interfere with the Jaffé reaction.[20-23] One study showed that, in marked renal insufficiency, serum creatinine rises and noncreatinine chromogens contribute proportionally less to the total reaction.[24] In individuals with normal kidney function, noncreatinine chromogens made up 14% (range 4.5%-22.3%) of the total, whereas in individuals with serum creatinine levels ranging from 5.6 to 29.4 mg/dL, noncreatinine chromogens contributed only 5% (range 0%-14.6%) to the total measured level.[24] This same study found no effect of the noncreatinine chromogens on the variability of plasma values.

Several modifications in the classic Jaffé assay have been designed to remove interfering chromogens before analysis,[16] including deproteinization with specific adsorption of creatinine using Fuller earth and ion-exchange resins, the measurement of Jaffé-positive chromogens before and after the destruction of creatinine with bacteria, and dialysis separation. These methods have largely been replaced by less costly and more convenient autoanalyzer techniques. Autoanalyzer methods utilize the Jaffé reaction, but separate creatinine from noncreatinine chromogens by the rate of color development,[16] thus avoiding most of the interference seen with the standard Jaffé method.[25] However, very high serum bilirubin levels can cause falsely low creatinine levels.[26] Newer techniques measuring true serum creatinine give plasma levels that are slightly lower than those from the Jaffé assay method.[16] The imidohydrolase method can be perturbed by extremely high glucose levels,[17] and by the antifungal agent 5-flucytosine.[4] K/DOQI guidelines recommend that autoanalyzer manufacturers and clinical laboratories calibrate serum creatinine assays using an international standard.[3]

Serum creatinine is probably the most widely used indirect measure of GFR, its popularity attributable to convenience and low cost. Unfortunately, serum creatinine is very insensitive to even substantial declines in GFR. The GFR measured by more accurate techniques (described later) may be reduced by up to 50% before serum creatinine becomes elevated.[4] In addition, the correct interpretation of serum creatinine in the clinical setting is problematic. Failure to consider variation in creatinine production due to differences in muscle mass frequently leads to misinterpretation of serum creatinine levels. This confusion may be compounded by the use of standard normal ranges for serum creatinine levels that appear on routine laboratory reports. For example, a serum creatinine that falls in the "normal" range may indicate a normal GFR in a young, healthy individual. However, the same serum creatinine in an elderly individual could indicate a twofold reduction in GFR owing to a comparable reduction in muscle mass.[4] Therefore, K/DOQI guidelines recommend that clinical laboratories report serum creatinine with an estimated GFR using a serum creatinine–based formula[3] (see Table 23–2).

Muscle mass may also decline over a relatively short period of time. For example, significant declines in creatinine excretion were seen in patients undergoing kidney transplantation, especially those who had chronic declines in allograft function.[27] The decline in creatinine excretion was probably due to decreases in muscle mass from multiple causes, including the effects of corticosteroids. As a result of the reduction in muscle mass, changes in serum creatinine underestimated the amount of decline in kidney function.[4]

Failure to remember the potential effects of tubular secretion on serum creatinine, especially in patients with reduced kidney function, may lead the clinician to believe that renal function is better than it actually is. One study has suggested that tubular secretion of creatinine is significant in patients with nephritic syndrome and decreased serum albumin levels.[8] Moreover, the potential for interference from plasma constituents and medications requires the clinician to know what assay is being used to measure serum creatinine. One the basis of whether the reported upper limit of normal for adults is high (1.4–1.9 mg/dL) or low (1.2–1.4 mg/dL), it may sometimes be possible to correctly surmise whether an unmodified alkaline picrate–Jaffé reaction (higher normal limits) or a newer method that removes interference with chromogens (lower normal limits) is being used. The clinician should also be aware of the precision of the assay. Precision is commonly measured by the coefficient of variation, which is the mean of replicate samples divided by the standard deviation.

Creatinine Clearance

Measuring creatinine clearance obviates some of the problems of using serum creatinine as a marker of GFR but creates others. Differences in steady-state creatinine production due to differences in muscle mass that affect serum creatinine should not affect creatinine clearance. Extrarenal elimination of creatinine should have little influence on the ability of the creatinine clearance to estimate GFR. However, the reliability of creatinine clearance is greatly diminished by variability in tubular secretion of creatinine and by the inability of most patients to accurately collect timed urine samples. Indeed, some investigators[28,29] have argued that the creatinine clearance rate is a less reliable measure of GFR than serum creatinine and should be abandoned.

Tubular secretion of creatinine gives a creatinine clearance rate that overestimates the true GFR. The overestimation is reduced somewhat if serum and urine creatinine are both measured by the Jaffé method. As discussed, plasma constituents tend to falsely raise the serum creatinine level as measured by the Jaffé assay, while urine creatinine levels are largely unaffected. Thus, creatinine clearance determinations calculated from serum and urine creatinine levels measured with the Jaffé assay tend to be falsely low. In a given population of patients, this error will tend to cancel the error introduced by tubular creatinine secretion, and the creatinine clearance rate GFR. However, the two errors are independent, and the occurrence of opposing errors of the same magnitude in the same patient is largely a result of chance.[4]

Thus, variability in the precision of creatinine clearance rate as an estimate of true GFR is not reduced and may be increased by this fortuitous combination of errors. Indeed, the creatinine clearance rate determined in 30 patients with a total chromogen method was only 9% higher than inulin clearance, although the true creatinine clearance was 31% higher.[4] However, the correlation coefficient with inulin clearance compared with the true creatinine clearance was much better ($r = 0.96$) than the correlation coefficient for inulin clearance compared with the total chromogen creatinine clearance ($r = 0.86$), suggesting that the latter technique was more accurate but less precise.

Prolonged storage of the urine can introduce error in the creatinine clearance determination by perturbing urine creatinine levels. High temperature and low urine pH enhance the conversion of creatine to creatinine in urine.[30] Indeed, storing urine under adverse conditions for 24 hours was shown to cause a 20% increase in the amount of measured urine creatinine.[30] This problem can be obviated by refrigerating urine samples and by measuring the urine creatinine level without undue delay.

Tubular secretion of creatinine would cause little difficulty if it was constant, and a constant correction factor could be subtracted from creatinine clearance determinations to yield a more accurate estimate of GFR. Unfortunately, interpatient and intrapatient variability in tubular creatinine secretion makes such an approach impossible. The tendency for tubular secretion to rise proportionally with declining levels of kidney function, for example, decreases the usefulness of creatinine clearance determinations as accurate reflections of GFR in patients with kidney disease.[9]

As mentioned earlier for urea clearance, all renal clearance techniques that rely on measuring a marker of GFR in the urine are subject to the vagaries of urine collection. Variability in the adequacy of timed urine samples can introduce substantial error in the clearance determination. Having patients perform urine collections under direct supervision of trained personnel can enhance the accuracy of timed collections. However, decreasing the duration of urine collection may increase the contribution of errors due to incomplete bladder emptying, especially if urine volumes are not increased with water loading. In addition, short-interval urine collections negate the advantages of time-averaged GFR estimates made from 24-hour urine collection. The cost of the procedure can also be substantially higher if trained personnel are used to directly supervise urine collections in a clinic setting.

In principle, the renal clearance of creatinine is the urine creatinine excretion divided by the area under the plasma creatinine concentration time curve over the period of time in which the urine was sampled. In practice, creatinine clearance is usually measured by determining the urine creatinine excretion and sampling a single plasma creatinine value. It is then assumed that the plasma creatinine was constant over the time of the urine collection. Plasma creatinine remains relatively constant over 24 hours if food intake and activity are also constant.[31] However, in a 24-hour period, there may be substantial variability in plasma creatinine levels, largely due to effects of diet.[4] Thus, under usual clinical conditions, the assumption that plasma creatinine levels are constant during the period of urine collection may not valid and may, in fact, be a source of error.

The day-to-day coefficient of variation for serum creatinine is approximately 8%.[32,33] Because two creatinine determinations must be made to calculate a creatinine clearance, the coefficient of variation of the creatinine clearance should be higher than that of serum creatinine level. Indeed, the coefficient of variation of creatinine clearance could be expected to be at least 11.3% (the square root of 2 times the square of 8%). This is, in fact, similar to the coefficient of variation for creatinine clearance reported in at least one investigation.[33] Other researchers[34] have reported a day-to-day coefficient of variation for creatinine clearance, when carried out in the routine clinical setting, as high as 27%.

Cimetidine-Enhanced Creatinine Clearance

Because tubular secretion of creatinine is a major limitation of the creatinine clearance, several investigators[35,36] have tried to enhance the accuracy of creatinine clearance by blocking tubular creatinine secretion with the histamine-2 receptor antagonist cimetidine. In these studies, cimetidine substantially improved the creatinine clearance estimate of GFR in patients with mild to moderate renal impairment. However, in many patients, tubular secretion of creatinine was not completely blocked, and the cimetidine-enhanced creatinine clearance value still overestimated GFR in these individuals.

A cimetidine-enhanced creatinine clearance measurement requires little additional cooperation from the patient than a standard creatinine clearance. Cimetidine is very safe; indeed, one study reported that the incidence of adverse reactions during prolonged treatment of 622 patients with cimetidine (10.9%) was similar to that seen during treatment of 516 patients with placebo (10.1%).[37] Because the cimetidine-enhanced creatinine clearance rate can be measured in most clinical laboratories, it may especially useful for patients who live in areas in which more expensive GFR measurement techniques are not readily available. Although it will not replace other, more accurate methods for measuring GFR, the cimetidine-enhanced creatinine clearance could prove to be a cost-effective alternative in many clinical situations.

Serum Creatinine Formulas to Estimate Kidney Function

The need to collect a urine sample remains a major limitation of the creatinine clearance technique, with or without cimetidine enhancement. Therefore, many attempts have been made to mathematically transform or correct serum creatinine so that it may more accurately reflect GFR (see Table 23–2).[29,38–53] Under ideal conditions, GFR, as measured by a marker such as creatinine, should be equal to the inverse of the creatinine value multiplied by a constant rate of creatinine GFR. However, changes in creatinine production, extrarenal elimination, and tubular secretion of creatinine can all create errors in the use of inverse creatinine value to measure changes in GFR. Indeed, none of the shortcomings of using serum creatinine as a marker of GFR is avoided by using inverse creatinine value.[4]

One of the problems with using creatinine or its inverse as a measure of GFR is that interpatient and intrapatient differences in creatinine production often occur. Variations in creatinine production owing to age- and sex-related differences in muscle mass have been measured and have been incorporated in formulas to improve the ability of serum creatinine to estimate GFR. The most widely used formula is that of Cockcroft and Gault,[42] which reduces the variability of serum creatinine estimates of glomerular filtration measured in a population of men and women of different ages. However, the formula does not take into account differences in creatinine production between individuals of the same age and sex or even in the same individual over time.[45,47] The formula systematically overestimates GFR in individuals who are obese or edematous.[47] Moreover, it does not take into account extrarenal elimination, tubular handling, or inaccuracies in the laboratory measurement of creatinine that can contribute to error in the serum creatinine estimate of GFR. With readily available parameters and relative simplicity, the Cockcroft-Gault formula has maintained widespread support. In subjects screened for the African-American Study of Kidney Disease and Hypertension pilot study, outpatient 24-hour urine collections and timed creatinine clearances offered no more precision than the Cockcroft-Gault formula, despite requiring substantially more time and effort.[8]

The GFR has probably never been measured with more accuracy in a large population of patients than it was in the Modification of Diet in Renal Disease (MDRD) Study. The investigators[54] used the isotopically measured GFR determinations from the MDRD study to derive a formula for estimating GFR using only readily measurable clinical variables. Significantly, they derived the formula on a randomly selected subset of patients from the whole population, and then tested the formula in the remainder of the population. A formula, sometimes referred to as the MDRD study equation or the Levey formula, uses only serum chemistry values (creatinine, urea, and albumin) and patient characteristics (age, gender, and race). It was able to predict 90.3% of the variability in isotopically measured GFR in the validation sample (see Table 23–2).[53] A simplified version requiring only serum creatinine value, age, race, and gender was found to similarly correlate with measured GFR.[55]

Levey and colleagues[53] cautioned against the immediate application of theses formulas in patient subgroups not represented in the initial study, including individuals with normal kidney function, patients with type 1 diabetes, elderly persons, and kidney transplant recipients. It cannot be assumed that formulas to predict kidney function derived from data for one patient population will be valid when applied to another population. For example, few diabetic individuals were included in some of the original studies that examined formulas for predicting GFR. When these formulas were subsequently tested in diabetic patients, they were found by some investigators[56] to be inaccurate. Several small studies have indicated some degree of inaccuracy in the use of the MDRD equation for subjects with normal kidney function.[57] However, the National Kidney Foundation's K/DOQI guidelines consider the MDRD equation a reliable measure for GFR in adults,[3] and the European Best Practice Guidelines Expert Group on Hemodialysis prefers it over the Cockcroft-Gault equation for individuals with advanced kidney failure.[58]

Serum creatinine formulas to estimate the GFR may not be reliable in certain individuals. Individuals on a vegetarian diet, consuming creatinine supplements, with unusual muscle mass, with unusual weight (morbid obesity, amputation), or pregnant woman were not included in the study populations that were used to generate these formulas. Likewise, the formulas are not accurate for individuals with normal or near-normal kidney function[57,59] and ethnic groups.[60] Therefore, such individuals may have better measurement of clearance utilizing a 24-hour urine sample for creatinine clearance. For example, among healthy individuals such as kidney donors, the MDRD formula underestimated GFR.[59] In kidney transplant recipients, the MDRD provided variable results.[61]

Serum Cystatin C

Several low-molecular-weight (LMW) proteins have been evaluated as endogenous markers of GFR, with cystatin C commanding the most attention. The use of serum cystatin C as a marker of GFR was first suggested in 1985, when Simonsen and co-workers[62] demonstrated a correlation between reciprocal cystatin C values and ^{51}Cr-labeled ethylenediaminetetraacetic acid (^{51}Cr-EDTA) clearance. Since then, numerous investigators[63–66] have shown that cystatin C may be a particularly good marker of GFR. Cystatin C is a 13-kD basic protein of the cystatin superfamily of cysteine proteinase inhibitors. It is synthesized by all nucleated cells at a constant rate, fulfilling an important criterion for any endogenous marker of GFR.[67,68] In most studies, production of cystatin C is not altered by inflammatory processes,[62,63] by muscle mass,[69] or by gender.[70] One study did find higher levels of cystatin C in males, older patients, and those with greater height and weights. However, the study utilized 24-hour urine collections to determine creatinine clearance as the gold standard for kidney function.[71] Another study found that inflammation or immunosuppression therapy may affect cystatin C levels.[72] Concentrations of cystatin C are highest in the first days of life and rapidly decrease during the first 4 months, likely due to maturation of the glomerular filtration capacity.[73,74] In children older than 1 year, cystatin C levels stabilize and approximate those of adults.[73,74] An increase in levels after the 5th decade reflects the age-related decline in GFR and contrasts with stable serum creatinine values, presumably due to a decline in muscle mass with age.[75] Because of its LMW and positive charge at physiologic pH, cystatin C freely passes the glomerular filter. It is not secreted, but proximal tubular cells reabsorb and catabolize the filtered cystatin C, resulting in very low urinary concentrations.[63,76] Although calculation of GFR using urinary cystatin C is not possible, some investigators[77] have speculated that urinary cystatin C could serve as a marker for renal tubular dysfunction.

Cystatin C can be measured using any of a number of radioimmunoassays, fluorescent, or enzymatic immunoassays.[68] Because these methods are slow and relatively imprecise, widespread clinical use is not feasible. Latex immunoassays employing latex particles conjugated with cystatin C–specific antibody demonstrate greater precision, produce more consistent reference intervals, and are far quicker.[68] Particle-enhanced turbidimetric immunoassay (PETIA)[64,65,70] and particle-enhanced nephelometric immunoassay (PENIA)[75,78,79] are the two available versions of latex immunoassay. On the basis of a 2002 meta-analysis, immunonephelometric methods appear to be superior to other assays when measuring cystatin C.[80]

Studies in a number of patients have shown that serum cystatin C may be more sensitive and specific than serum creatinine value for signifying early changes in isotopically determined GFR.[65,66,72] ROC analysis of one of these studies demonstrated superiority of accuracy of cystatin C over creatinine in patients with reduced GFR.[64] In addition, small reductions in GFR appear to be detected more easily using cystatin C measurement than with creatinine determination.[65,66] Other studies have indicated that cystatin C determination has a greater ability to detect subclinical kidney dysfunction than using creatinine measurement.[81] Coll and colleagues[81] demonstrated that cystatin C levels rose when GFR fell to 88 mL/min/1.73 m^2 and that creatinine levels did not rise until GFR dropped to 75 mL/min/1.73 m^2. However, ROC analysis showed no difference in the diagnostic accuracy of the two tests.[81] Likewise, several other studies have not shown a significant difference between cystatin C and creatinine determinations, despite a trend toward greater accuracy with cystatin C.[82–84] A meta-analysis[80] incorporating studies published in 46 articles and 8 abstracts and using standard measures of GFR suggested superiority of reciprocal cystatin C value over reciprocal serum creatinine level as a marker of GFR.[80] Superior correlation coefficients and greater ROC-plot area under the curve (AUC) values were calculated for cystatin C. The authors of this meta-analysis speculated that prior studies indicating a lack of superiority of cystatin C could reflect a type II error or differences caused by assay methods.

Cystatin C has also been examined in a diverse number of groups. In children, cystatin C measurement appears to be at least as useful as serum creatinine determination in assessing GFR, although the number of children studied who were younger than 4 years is small. This age subgroup, for which serum creatinine levels have been unreliable, might arguably be most benefited by the measurement of cystatin C to evaluate GFR. Cystatin C has been favorably evaluated in other similar subgroups, including patients with cirrhosis,[83] spinal cord injury,[85] and rheumatoid arthritis,[86] as well as elderly patients.[87,88] In diabetic patients, results have been mixed.[89,90]

In kidney transplant recipients, cystatin C value has been found to be more sensitive than serum creatinine level in detecting decreases in GFR.[91,92] However, some investigators have shown that cystatin C values underestimate GFR in this population.[93] In one study, levels of cystatin C were significantly higher in 54 pediatric kidney transplant recipients than in 56 control subjects with similar GFR values.[93] The reason for this result is not clear. However, corticosteroids have been implicated, given the finding of elevation of cystatin C in asthmatic patients treated with corticosteroids[94] and in in vitro experiments demonstrating a dose-dependent rise in cystatin C production in HeLa cells treated with dezamethasone.[95] A case-control study of kidney transplant recipients showed a dose-dependent increase in cystatin C in individuals who were receiving corticosteroids compared with those who were not.[96] In contrast, corticosteroids did not raise levels of cystatin C in a group of children treated for nephritic syndrome.[97] Mixed conclusions of other studies evaluating cystatin C as a marker of GFR in transplant recipients[98] and the discrepancy in the effects of corticosteriods illustrate a need for further studies in this population. Furthermore, the cost of the cystatin C assay, the difficulty in making the assay universally available, and the potentially high intraindividual variability in the determination of cystatin C levels are all issues that require attention if this particular marker is to be used in clinical practice.[99,100] Currently, there is no standard for serum cystatin C measurement.[101]

Inulin

Inulin was once considered the gold standard of exogenously administered markers of GFR. However, the scarcity and high cost all but eliminated its routine use. Inulin (molecular weight 5200 Da) is a polymer of fructose found in tubers such as the dahlia, the Jerusalem artichoke, and chicory. Inulin is inert and does not bind to plasma proteins. It distributes in extracellular fluid, is freely filtered at the glomerulus, and is neither reabsorbed nor secreted by renal tubules.[102] Inulin is readily measured in plasma and urine by one of several colorimetric assays. These assays are time consuming but can be adapted for use on an autoanalyzer. Glucose is also detected in most inulin assays and must, therefore, be either removed beforehand or measured independently in the sample and subtracted. In any case, appropriate care must be taken in patients with high plasma or urine glucose levels, especially if the levels fluctuate during the GFR determination.

The renal clearance method for using inulin to measure GFR was originally developed and championed by Homer Smith. Over the years, this technique has been used by many clinical investigators and has been modified only slightly.

Generally, measurements are made under standardized conditions. Patients are typically studied in the morning, after an overnight fast. An oral water load of 10 to 15 mL/kg body weight is given before inulin is infused, and additional water is administered throughout the test to ensure a constant urine flow rate of at least 4 mL/min. When a good urine flow has been established, a loading dose of inulin is given, followed by a constant infusion to maintain plasma levels. Once a steady state has been achieved, several timed (generally 30-min) urine collections are carried out. Ideally, a bladder catheter is used to ensure the accuracy of the timed urine collections. Serial plasma levels of inulin are also measured.

Inulin clearance is calculated from the plasma level (time averaged), urine concentration, and urine flow rate. Usually, an average of three to five separate determinations is made. Each of these measurements is subject to inaccuracies; indeed, the coefficient of variation between clearance periods is 10%,[54] and the coefficient of variation of inulin clearance measured on different days in the same individual is approximately 7.5%.[54] No doubt, some of the variability in inulin clearance determinations made in the same individual are due to error in measurement, and some are due to true fluctuation in GFR (see later). It has been estimated that a difference of 20 mL/1.73 m^2/min in the values of inulin clearances measured in the same individual on 2 separate days predicts a real difference in GFR at $P < .05$.[4] A difference of 27 mL/1.73 m^2/min between measurements predicts a real difference at $P < .01$.[4]

The renal inulin clearance method has a number of drawbacks. Bladder catheterization is associated with some risk and is not readily accepted by many patients. Although inulin clearance measurements can be carried out using spontaneous voiding, incomplete bladder emptying can introduce additional variability. Unfortunately, no studies have compared inulin clearance results obtained using bladder catheterization with those obtained using spontaneous voiding. Problems with residual urine are most likely to occur in individuals with prostatism and in patients with neurogenic bladder dysfunction. High urine volumes probably help reduce the effect of incomplete bladder emptying, but water loading is itself uncomfortable for many patients. It has been noted that inulin clearance tends to decline during serial urine collections, in part as a result of the difficulty patients have in maintaining a high water intake throughout the procedure. Use of an intravenous cannula and a constant infusion is another source of discomfort and inconvenience. Thus, despite its accuracy, the renal inulin clearance technique is cumbersome and inconvenient.

To avoid problems related to urine collection, many investigators have turned to plasma clearance techniques. Plasma clearance can be measured with the use of either a constant infusion or a bolus injection.[103] If, during a constant infusion, both the distribution space and the plasma level of inulin are constant, the rate of infusion will be equal to the rate of elimination. The inulin clearance then becomes the rate of infusion divided by the plasma concentration. There is a high degree of correlation between results from this technique and those from the renal clearance method.[103] However, maintaining constant plasma concentrations is very difficult,[104,105] and the constant infusion technique is rarely used. The bolus injection technique has been used with inulin,[106] and this technique is discussed in greater detail in the section on radionuclide and radiocontrast markers of GFR.

As previously noted, a number of problems limit the usefulness of inulin as a marker of GFR. Although most data suggest that inulin is freely filtered and is not handled by the renal tubules, this indication may not be true in all clinical situations. For example, it has been suggested that impaired filtration, back-diffusion of inulin, or both can limit its usefulness in kidney transplant recipients.[107] However, the decline in the use of inulin as a marker of GFR has largely been due to its scarcity and cost.

Radionuclide and Radiocontrast Markers of Glomerular Filtration Rate

Any of several radionuclide-labeled and unlabeled radiocontrast markers of GFR can be used in either renal or plasma clearance studies. Estimating GFR by plasma clearance of an intravenous bolus injection of an indicator is convenient and has been used more often than constant infusion or renal clearance techniques. The assumptions underlying the measurement of renal clearance using a single injection technique are critical. Basically, renal clearance is measured as the plasma clearance, or the amount of indicator injected divided by the integrated area of the plasma concentration curve over time.[108] Because it is not possible to measure enough samples to accurately determine the area under the plasma concentration time curve, estimation of this area is based on mathematical formulations that describe the decline in plasma levels over time.

Models used to estimate plasma clearance assume that the volume of distribution and renal excretion are constant over time and that there is no extrarenal excretion. A constant renal excretion has been demonstrated for at least two indicators, ^{125}I-iothalamate and ^{51}Cr-EDTA.[109] However, underestimation of GFR with the use of technetium-radiolabeled diethylenetriaminepenta-acetic acid (^{125m}Tc-DTPA) may be due to plasma protein binding and decreasing renal clearance over time.[110,111] Other researchers[112] have shown that there is a small, constant overestimation of plasma compared with renal clearance of ^{51}Cr-EDTA.

Although the indicator is eliminated directly from the arterial circulation, it is injected intravenously, and blood samples to measure the plasma clearance are drawn from the venous compartment. The assumption that there is instantaneous equilibration between the arterial and the venous circulation is incorrect.[4] Thus, any method used to calculate renal clearance must correct for inaccuracies due to delayed equilibration between the venous and the arterial compartments.

Because it is not possible to measure the entire plasma concentration time curve, a limited number of samples must be measured, and an appropriate curve fitted to these points must be used to measure the plasma clearance. Both one- and two-compartment models have been used to measure plasma clearance (Fig. 23–2). In the two-compartment model, the first compartment can be thought of as corresponding to plasma and the second to extracellular fluid.[4] Two slopes and two intercepts are derived from plotting plasma values over time after injection.[113] One slope and intercept are derived from the initial data that fit a straight line when plotted on a logarithmic scale, and the other slope and intercept are derived from a line that fits the data of the terminal elimination phase.

Unfortunately, the two-compartment method, although more accurate than the one-compartment model, requires more frequent plasma sampling. Therefore, most investigators now use a one-compartment model, whereby only values measured during the terminal elimination phase (generally commencing 90–120 min after injection) are sampled. In this model, the slope and intercept of a line plotted on a logarithmic scale are used to calculate clearance by the formula:

$$\text{Clearance} = V_o \, (\ln(2))/t_{1/2}$$

where V_o is the volume of distribution, and $t_{1/2}$ is the half-time for decay in plasma levels. The value derived from this relationship is multiplied by a constant to correct for systematic errors attributable to overestimation of V_o and a higher con-

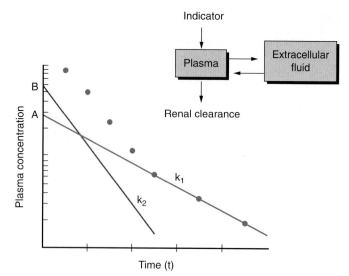

FIGURE 23–2 Plasma disappearance curve for the indicator of GFR after bolus intravenous administration. *Dots* represent measured concentrations. The line with slope k_1 and intercept A is the least-squares best fit of the terminal elimination phase. The line with slope k_2 and intercept B represents best fit of the difference between actual values and values calculated from the line fitted to the terminal elimination phase. GFR (one-compartment method) is calculated as Qk_1/A, where Q is the quantity of indicator administered. GFR (two-compartment method) is calculated as $Qk_1k_2/(Ak_2 + Bk_1)$.

centration of marker in venous compared with arterial blood. The clearance calculated using this simple monoexponential model is surprisingly accurate.[4] Also surprising is the fact that as few as two samples yield results that seem to be as accurate as multiple samples.[114]

Single-sample techniques have also been used to estimate plasma clearance.[115] One such method was based on the use of different sampling times dictated by the predicted GFR.[115] Tepe and co-workers[116] compared different sampling times using monoexponential models for GFR determinations in 139 subjects. They found that a single-sample method was accurate, and that sampling between 60 and 240 minutes after injection was optimal. Other researchers have confirmed that single-sample techniques can give reasonably accurate estimates of GFR that are generally suitable for clinical practice.[117,118] Nevertheless, multiple sampling yields a GFR determination that is more accurate than that obtained by single-sample techniques and may, therefore, be more suitable for clinical investigations that must detect small differences in changes in GFR between patients.[119] There is some controversy over the applicability of standard adult formulas for calculating GFR in children using single-sample techniques,[120,121] and further study is required.

Whether single or multiple samples are used with a monoexponential model, it is probably important that the sampling time be adjusted to the level of kidney function.[108,119] To sample after only 2 hours may be too soon for patients with normal to moderately decreased kidney function[109]; a sampling time of 4 to 5 hours after injection is probably more appropriate.[108] However, this interval may be too short in individuals with more marked declines in kidney function or in patients with ascites. In such patients, sampling times up to 24 hours may be appropriate.[108]

The use of radiolabeling and very sensitive high-performance liquid chromatography (HPLC) detection methods have reduced the amount of marker that needs to be administered, and this, in turn, has permitted subcutaneous administration.[122] It has been shown that reasonably predictable plasma concentrations can be achieved after subcutaneous injection of a radiolabeled marker such as ^{125}I-iothalamate. Thus, the renal clearance of such a marker can be measured after subcutaneous injection.

The measurement of plasma clearance need not require plasma sampling. A gamma camera positioned over the kidneys can be used to measure renal elimination of a radioactive indicator.[123,124] Quantitative renal imaging most commonly uses ^{99m}Tc-DTPA, radioiodinated iodohippuran (Hippuran), ^{123}I-ortho-iodohippurate, or ^{99m}Tc-mercaptoacetyltriglycine (MAG$_3$).[123,125] Estimation of GFR has now been combined with computed tomography (CT) using radiocontrast agents.[126] Magnetic resonance imaging (MRI) has also been proposed as a method for estimating GFR and renal blood flow.[127]

In general, GFR determination through quantitative renal imaging is not as precise as that arrived at through plasma sampling.[125,128] The advantage of quantitative renal imaging is that additional information pertaining to the anatomy of renal function can be obtained. Indeed, the "split function" or relative contribution to total GFR from each kidney can be calculated. This information can be important in the evaluation of some patients with renal vascular disease and can be crucial in certain circumstances (e.g., in deciding whether or not to carry out a unilateral nephrectomy). Although currently experimental, MRI techniques may someday provide quantitative information on regional cortical and medullary perfusion. Another potential application of techniques that measure isotopes externally may exploit the rapidity with which measurements can be obtained to monitor acute changes in kidney function. Indeed, miniaturized external monitoring devices have been applied to real-time monitoring of kidney function using ^{99m}Tc-DTPA.[129]

It is assumed that, whatever indicator is used to measure plasma clearance, it is not extensively protein bound, is freely filtered, is neither secreted nor reabsorbed by the tubules, and is eliminated only by the kidneys. A number of radionuclide and radiocontrast markers have been developed to measure GFR. In general, they share most of the characteristics of inulin that make it a good indicator of GFR. The popularity of these radionuclide-labeled agents is attributable to their ready availability, ease of administration, relatively low cost, and accuracy of laboratory assay.

Probably the most extensively investigated radionuclide-bound indicator of GFR has been ^{51}Cr-EDTA.[4] It is small (molecular weight 292 Da), appears to have little binding to plasma proteins, and is freely filtered by the glomerulus. Studies in humans have shown that the renal clearance of ^{51}Cr-EDTA is about 10% lower than that of inulin when both are measured simultaneously. Although the reason for these lower values is not known, it could be due to plasma protein binding, tubular reabsorption, or in vivo dissociation of the nuclide from EDTA.

Iothalamate sodium, a derivative of triiodobenzoic acid, is a high-osmolar, ionic radiocontrast agent. It is small (molecular weight 614 Da) and appears to be only slightly bound to plasma proteins. Several studies in humans have found that simultaneously measured renal clearances of ^{125}I-iothalamate and inulin are similar,[4] but whether this finding resulted from similar renal handling of inulin and iothalamate or whether there was a fortuitous cancellation of errors due, for example, to plasma protein binding countering the effects of tubular secretion is unclear. The use of ^{125}I-iothalamate to measure kidney function is generally considered safe, although there are virtually no long-term follow-up data. The potential problem of thyroid uptake and concentration of the radionuclide can be avoided by administering a large dose of oral iodine (Lugol's solution) prior to the procedure. The half-life of ^{125}I is approximately 60 days.[4]

DTPA (molecular weight 393 Da) has frequently been chelated to radionuclides for use in renal imaging.[123] The one most commonly used to measure GFR is ^{99m}Tc-DTPA.[130,131] The radiolabeling of DTPA with ^{99m}Tc must be carried out immediately before use owing to the chelate's instability. The half-life of ^{99m}Tc is only 6 hours, so samples must be counted soon after the procedure.[123] Protein binding of ^{99m}Tc-DTPA may be a significant source of error in some patients.[110,111] A comparison of clearance measurements based on whole plasma and protein-free, ultrafiltered plasma found significant differences, especially in patients taking multiple medications.[128]

All radionuclide markers are radioactive. This fact has begun to erode their acceptance by patients and has been subjected to close monitoring by regulatory agencies. In the United States, the storage and disposal of all radioactive waste has come under growing scrutiny and regulation, and the use of isotopes now requires that a number of conditions be met. The actual amount of radiation delivered to patients is generally considered to be less than the amount received while undergoing most standard radiologic procedures.[4] However, the isotope is concentrated in the urine, so that exposure of the urinary collecting system may be greater.[123] To alleviate this potential problem, patients are advised to maintain a high fluid intake and urine volume after the procedure. There are no long-term follow-up studies to assess the risk of this exposure of the collecting system to radiation. In theory, the use of radioisotopes in children and pregnant women may carry an increased risk of potential problems.

In an effort to avoid using radiolabeled compounds, techniques have been developed to measure low levels of iodine in urine and plasma. These techniques permit the use of unlabeled radiocontrast agents, which are inherently rich in iodine, to measure GFR. Radiocontrast agents are of LMW (600–1600 Da), are not protein bound, and are eliminated from plasma mainly by glomerular filtration. The HPLC assay has been used to measure renal clearance of iothalamate sodium (Conray), diatrizoate meglumine (Hypaque), and iohexol (Omnipaque). The sensitivity of the assay allows the use of as little as 1 mL of radiocontrast agent, which can be injected subcutaneously. However, the main disadvantage of HPLC is the expense, time, and labor needed to carry out the assay. A rapid and convenient method has been developed to measure relatively low concentrations of iodine with the use of x-ray fluorescence, and the method has been applied to the measurement of the plasma clearance of iohexol.[132,133]

The use of iohexol (molecular weight 821 Da) to measure GFR has grown in popularity, probably because of the low incidence of adverse effects, which is attributable to iohexol's low osmolality and nonionic properties. Plasma clearance determinations using iohexol appear to be comparable with those obtained with the use of other radionuclide-labeled markers and with inulin.[134,135] Up to 30 mL of iohexol may be required if samples are measured by x-ray fluorescence, but the amount administered is reduced in patients with decreased kidney function. As little as 5 mL may be needed if more sensitive techniques are used (e.g., HPLC). The technique appears to be safe, an observation that is not surprising because, even in very high-risk diabetic patients with markedly reduced kidney function, nephrotoxicity from radiocontrast agents occurred only at doses above those generally used to measure kidney function.[136]

The incidence of extrarenal adverse reactions from higher doses of nonionic radiocontrast agents used in radiographic procedures is low. All of the methods that use labeled or unlabeled radiocontrast agents share the risk of allergic reactions. Although this risk is small, none of these agents should be administered to patients who are allergic to iodine. Higher doses of iohexol can also be used when GFR is measured in conjunction with standard urography.[137] Extremely low levels of GFR can be measured, and the technique has been adapted to determining residual renal function in patients on maintenance hemodialysis.[138]

Normalizing Glomerular Filtration Rate

The measurement of GFR is usually better suited for monitoring disease progression than for detection or diagnosis, for two reasons. The first is the cost and inconvenience of the procedure. Second, the enormous physiologic variability of GFR in healthy individuals makes it difficult to define what a normal GFR should be for an individual patient.[4] An understanding of the factors that contribute to this normal variability is essential in interpreting any test of GFR.

A number of investigators have attempted to normalize GFR in populations of humans who have no known kidney disease. For years, body surface area (BSA) has been used to normalize GFR.[4] Usually, GFR is indexed to BSA; that is, GFR is expressed per unit of BSA. However, at least one report suggested that a regression relationship is more accurate than indexing for normalizing GFR to BSA.[139] The rationale has been that the weight of the kidney and the basal metabolic rate are proportional to BSA in normal individuals of different age and body size.[4] Generally, the DuBois formula for calculating BSA using power functions of height and weight has been used to estimate BSA.[4] This formula is less accurate at extremes of age. Obesity may also perturb the otherwise physiologic relationship between BSA and renal hemodynamic function.[140]

The argument has been made that extracellular fluid volume be used to normalize GFR,[141,142] because the purpose of the kidney is to maintain the composition of the extracellular fluid. A comparison of extracellular volume and calculated BSA in normalizing GFR found that the two methods yielded very similar results.[143] Like extracellular fluid volume, blood volume is also closely correlated to calculated BSA in adult men and women.[4] In addition, both kidney and glomerular size correlate to BSA.[144] Thus, to the extent that GFR may be expected to correlate to kidney and glomerular size, the use of BSA to normalize GFR seems to be sound.

Blood volume, extracellular fluid volume, and basal metabolic rate can be more accurately predicted with the use of indices of lean body mass than calculated BSA alone. Thus, measures of lean body mass could theoretically be better predictors of normal GFR, at least in adults. However, until this is clearly demonstrated to be the case, the more convenient calculated BSA will, no doubt, continue to be the standard for normalizing GFR.[4]

Although the variability of GFR measurements in normal individuals can be reduced by taking BSA differences into account, the residual variability is substantial. A number of factors may contribute to this variability. GFR normally declines with age, but does so to a variable extent.[4] It is well known that dietary protein intake can affect GFR.[145]

Similarly, salt intake, water consumption, posture, and normal diurnal variation can all affect GFR determinations in normal individuals.[4] In women, the menstrual cycle can affect GFR and may be an additional source of physiologic variability.[146]

The concept of "renal functional reserve" was introduced in studies that demonstrated higher GFR after an oral protein load.[147] This development led to an unfortunate confusion between increased function due to structural changes after a reduction in kidney mass and acute increases in GFR of a functional nature (e.g., after an oral protein load).[147] In theory, the normal intraindividual physiologic variability in GFR could be reduced if the measurement were made after an acute maneuver that maximized kidney function. However, there are inadequate data to determine whether this is the case. Moreover, such maneuvers substantially increase the complexity and expense of the measurement.

Applications

A number of factors should be considered in selecting a clinical test to measure GFR. Unfortunately, the necessary information on accuracy, precision, and expected prevalence of abnormal results is usually not available for each test in each specific clinical situation. However, recognition of how these factors affect the utility of a test, along with crude estimations of these critical parameters, can provide guidance in test selection. Finally, the usefulness of a test to measure GFR is dictated not only by issues of accuracy and precision but also by cost, safety, and convenience. In general, the tests that are most accurate and precise are also those that are most costly and inconvenient (Fig. 23–3).

No single test of GFR is ideally suited for every clinical and research application. Rather, the goal should be to select the most accurate and precise test to answer the question being addressed in the safest, most cost-effective, and convenient manner possible in the population being studied. In clinical practice, tests of GFR are most commonly used for (1) screening for the presence of kidney disease, (2) measuring disease progression to determine prognosis and effects of therapy, (3) confirming the need for treatment of end-stage renal disease with dialysis or transplantation, (4) estimating renal clearance of drugs to guide dosing, and (5) assessing GFR as a risk factor for cardiovascular disease. For research purposes, tests of GFR are most commonly asked to distinguish differences in the rate of change between two or more experimental groups.

Although precise data do not exist, it is probable that none of the currently available tests of renal function is very well suited for detecting early or mild kidney disease in the general population. Nevertheless, there is a legitimate need for tests to identify patients with moderate or marked declines in kidney function in high-risk situations. The cost and inconvenience of creatinine clearance and radionuclide measure-

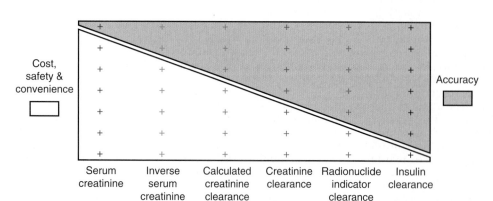

FIGURE 23–3 Conflict between practicality (cost, safety, and convenience) and accuracy of methods to estimate GFR. On one end of the spectrum, serum creatinine is most practical but least accurate. On the other end of the spectrum, inulin clearance is most accurate but least practical.

ments of GFR ordinarily preclude their use for these screening purposes. Therefore, serum creatinine has most often been used to screen for the presence of significant renal impairment. For example, serum creatinine is commonly used to screen for impaired renal function in order to identify patients who are at increased risk to develop radiocontrast-induced acute renal failure. Serum creatinine has been shown to be useful in this situation.[148,149] Clearly, the number of patients who receive radiocontrast agents would preclude the use of other, more expensive and inconvenient tests for this purpose. Similarly, the high prevalence of essential hypertension in the Western world renders radionuclide determinations of GFR impractical as a first-line screening procedure for a renal cause of hypertension in low-risk individuals.

In contrast to the situation for individuals who are unlikely to have kidney disease, the use of more expensive, but more accurate measures of GFR may be warranted in patients at high risk for kidney functional impairment. For example, the prevalence of kidney dysfunction in patients with systemic lupus erythematosus (SLE) and low serum complements may be high enough to justify the use of a radionuclide determination of GFR to screen for kidney dysfunction that could suggest a need for therapy or additional diagnostic tests. Similarly, the high incidence of both acute and chronic kidney allograft rejection could make the use of relatively complex tests of kidney function cost effective.

Much effort has been devoted to defining methods for measuring progression of CKD. It has been noted that plots of inverse serum creatinine over time can often be closely fitted (by least-squares method) to a straight line. The use of inverse creatinine value has generally been found to provide fits as good as or better than plots of logarithmically transformed serum creatinine values.[4] Serial inverse creatinine values can be corrected for changes in creatinine excretion (measured less frequently than serum creatinine) to reduce error attributable to changes in muscle mass over time.[150,151] Because changes in the rate of decline in inverse creatinine may indicate an effect of therapeutic intervention, a method developed to determine whether there is a "breakpoint" of two hinged regression lines has been applied to plots of inverse serum creatinine values.[152,153]

Changes in kidney function estimated by plots of serial inverse serum creatinine can vary substantially from changes estimated by radionuclide-determined GFR.[154,155] Correlation between radionuclide measurements of GFR and changes in creatinine clearance are no better and may be even worse than those for inverse creatinine.[155,156] Because spontaneous changes in the slope of inverse creatinine are frequent,[151,157] inverse serum creatinine plots are not reliable predictors of the time remaining to dialysis or transplantation or of changes in the rate of functional decline attributable to therapy.

Estimating renal clearance of drugs that are predominantly eliminated by glomerular filtration, in the absence of tubular secretion and reabsorption, is yet another potential application for tests of kidney function.[158,159] In principle, the rate of drug elimination is often proportional to the GFR. However, because most drugs are either weak acids or weak bases, changes in urine pH can alter tubular handling and affect the relationship between GFR and renal elimination. Competition of drugs for the same secretory pathway can also perturb renal elimination. Nevertheless, impaired renal function is the most common way in which the kidney affects drug levels, and GFR can approximate renal excretion of many drugs. Cost, convenience, and timeliness make creatinine clearance and radionuclide determinations of GFR impractical for guiding drug dosing. Most investigators have used formulas to calculate GFR calculated from age, sex, and serum creatinine values to dose drugs that are excreted primarily by the kidney.[160] Although the accuracy of these calculated clearances has been studied with the use of other measures of

kidney function as a gold standard, the ability of these formulas to predict pharmacokinetic profiles has not been determined for most therapeutic agents.

Many studies have attempted to examine changes in the rate of decline in GFR, determined by inverse creatinine plots or other techniques, to assess the effectiveness of therapeutic interventions. However, measuring changes in the rate of decline is problematic, as previously discussed. Moreover, it has also been shown that a substantial proportion of apparent amelioration in functional declines measured by inverse creatinine or radionuclide determinations of GFR can be attributed to regression to the mean.[156] Therefore, comparing the rate of change in GFR between two or more experimental groups has become the most reliable method for studying interventions designed to delay or prevent progression of CKD.[102,161] Generally, cost and inconvenience are subordinated to the increased accuracy and precision of radionuclide measurements of GFR in a clinical trial, and these tests are routinely used in that setting. A study of 2250 patients participating in two large, randomized, controlled trials confirmed the reliability of serial determinations of the renal clearance of subcutaneously injected (^{125}I)iothalamate.[162]

A doubling of serum creatinine has also been used as an end point in a number of clinical trials measuring progression of CKD. Using time to doubling of serum creatinine as an end point avoids the difficult-to-prove assumption that the rate of decline in kidney function is uniformly linear in all patients. It also avoids problems with premature patient dropout. Although the low cost and convenience of using time to doubling of serum creatinine makes this end point particularly attractive, it nevertheless has a number of important limitations.[163] First and foremost is the insensitivity of serum creatinine value to changes in GFR. False-positive results may also be problematic. It has been pointed out that changes in serum creatinine value would have given a positive result in the MDRD study, whereas no such benefit could be demonstrated when more accurate methods were used to measure changes in GFR.[163] Furthermore, variation in serum creatinine assays and calibration method can have an important impact on the ability to accurately predict levels of kidney function. Coresh and colleagues[55] analyzed frozen serum from both the MDRD study and the Third National Health and Nutrition Examination Survey (NHANES III) and showed substantial variation in calibration of serum creatinine among laboratories and through time. These errors in calibration became more important with progressively higher GFR values. Therefore, both research and clinical laboratories should consider calibrating serum creatinine to the MDRD study clinical laboratory,[55] although this may not be feasible.[164] Clearly, better techniques are still needed to measure the progression of CKD in clinical trials, techniques that can reduce the number of patients and duration of follow-up required to assess the effectiveness of therapies.

URINALYSIS

Historical Background

In common English usage, "urinalysis" is the chemical analysis of urine. However, analysis per se is "the identification or separation of ingredients of a substance," and as such, urinalysis can take on a much broader meaning. Historically, inspection of the urine for diagnosis is virtually as old as medicine itself. The connection between sweet-tasting urine and diabetes was made as early as 600 BC. Hippocrates used the appearance, color, and consistency of urine to diagnose disease and predict outcomes. In the Middle Ages, prognostication from the examination of urine was raised to an art by the "Pisse Prophets."[4]

The use of test strips dates back at least as far as the invention of litmus paper by Robert Boyle in about 1670. In 1848, Fehling described a chemical test for glucose in the urine, and in 1850, the French chemist Maumenté described a test strip for glucose. At about the same time, chemical tests for protein and blood were described. The early 1900s saw the development of primitive, multitest strips. It was not until 1956 that commercial urine tests strips resembling those used today were marketed.[4]

Overview

There are three ways to obtain a urine specimen: spontaneous voiding, ureteral catheterization, and percutaneous bladder puncture. Although the safety and utility of suprapubic needle aspiration of the bladder has been demonstrated, its use is generally reserved to situations in which urine cannot easily be obtained by other means. It may be particularly useful in infants, for example. Once a specimen is obtained, there are countless techniques for examining the urine and its contents.

This section reviews only those analytic techniques that are readily available and in common use and focuses on three broad areas: (1) chemical content, (2) protein composition, and (3) formed elements. The discussion of chemical content is limited to tests readily available through the use of reagent strips, such as specific gravity, pH, bilirubin, urobilinogen, nitrite, leukocyte esterase, glucose, and ketoacetate. More specific chemical tests (e.g., tests to diagnose metabolic disorders) are not discussed. Similarly, the measurement and interpretation of urine electrolyte composition are excluded from this section. The discussion on protein composition focuses on proteins from both tubular and glomerular sources. Formed elements include commonly encountered blood cells and casts.[4]

As with all laboratory procedures and clinical tests, the usefulness of urinalysis techniques depends not only on accuracy and precision but also on prior probabilities of the occurrence of positive results. Studies have found that routine hospital admission or preoperative urinalysis that includes both reagent strip testing and microscopic examination rarely lead to better patient outcomes and are generally not cost effective.[165–167] As a result, most investigators have concluded that routine urinalysis should be abandoned in this setting. Whether a more limited approach to routine screening that relies on reagent strip testing without microscopy is more effective remains to be determined.[168,169]

The probability of a positive result on urinalysis is no doubt greater for patients who are already known to have proteinuria than for otherwise normal patients routinely admitted to a medical ward. Therefore, the utility of examining the urine sediment may be quite different in patients with proteinuria and routinely admitted patients. In one study, in patients who were believed to have kidney disease and, therefore, underwent biopsy, urine microscopy was highly predictive of abnormal kidney histology.[170] Data such as these have led to the suggestion that examining the urine sediment is critical in assessing the implications of proteinuria.[171] Although accurate data on the sensitivity and specificity of urinalysis techniques are not available for most clinical conditions, an awareness of how individual tests are influenced by the underlying likelihood of disease can be helpful in determining the appropriate use of urinalysis and in assessing the implications of the results.

CHEMICAL CONTENT

Color

The color of urine is determined by chemical content, concentration, and pH. Urine may be almost colorless if the output is high and the concentration is low. Cloudy urine is generally the result of phosphates (usually normal) or leukocytes and bacteria (usually abnormal). Black urine is seen in alkaptonuria.[4] Acute intermittent porphyria frequently causes dark urine. A number of exogenous chemicals and drugs can make urine green, but green urine may also be associated with *Pseudomonas* bacteruria and urine bile pigments. The most common cause of red urine is hemoglobin. Red urine in the absence of red blood cells in the sediment usually indicates either free hemoglobin or myoglobin. Red urine and red sediment indicates hemoglobin. In contrast, red urine and clear sediment are most often the result of myoglobin but may also be seen in some porphyrias, or the use of bladder analgesic phenazopyridine, or a variety of other medications, food dyes, or ingestions of beets in some individuals. Finally, red-orange urine due to rafampin is one of the better-known drug effects. Among endogenous sources, bile pigments are the most common cause of orange urine.[4]

Specific Gravity

The measurement of the specific gravity is usually included as part of the standard urinalysis. Specific gravity is a convenient and rapidly obtained indicator of urine osmolality. It can be measured accurately with a refractometer or a hygrometer or more crudely estimated with a dipstick. The accuracy and usefulness of the reagent strip method has been debated.[172,173] Measurement of specific gravity by dipstick depends on the ionic strength of the urine and the fact that there is generally a linear relationship between ionic strength and osmolality in urine. The strip contains a polyionic polymer with binding sites saturated with hydrogen ions. The release of hydrogen ions when they are competitively replaced with urinary cations causes a change in the pH-sensitive indicator dye.[174] Specific gravity values measured by dipstick tend to be falsely high at urine pH less than 6 and falsely low if the pH is greater than 7.[175] The effects of albumin, glucose, and urea on osmolality are not reflected by changes in the dipstick specific gravity.[172] In newborns, specific gravity measurement with either a refractometer or a reagent strip is inaccurate.[176,177] The specific gravity of urine reflects the relative proportion of dissolved solutes to total volume and, as such, is a measure of urine concentration. The normal range for specific gravity is 1.003 to 1.030,[174,178] but values decrease with age as the kidney's ability to concentrate urine decreases. Specific gravity can be used to crudely estimate how the concentration of other urine constituents may reflect total excretion of those constituents[179] because specific gravity correlates inversely with 24-hour urine volume.[180] Indeed, self-monitoring of urine specific gravity may be useful for stone-forming patients, who benefit from maintaining a dilute urine.[173] Specific gravity can be affected by protein, glucose, mannitol, dextrans, diuretics, radiographic contrast media, and some antibiotics. Most clinical decisions should be based only on more accurate determinations of urine osmolality.

Urine pH

Urine pH is usually measured with a reagent test strip. Most commonly, the double indicators methyl red and bromthymol blue are used in the reagent strips to give a broad range of colors at different pH values. In conjunction with other specific urine and plasma measurements, urine pH is often invaluable in diagnosing systemic acid-base disorders. By itself, however, urine pH provides little useful diagnostic information. The normal range for urine pH is 4.5 to 7.8. A very alkaline urine (pH > 7.0) is suggestive of infection with a urea-splitting organism, such as *Proteus mirabilis*. Prolonged storage can lead to overgrowth of urea-splitting bacteria and a high urine pH. However, diet (vegetarian), diuretic therapy, vomiting, gastric suction, and alkali therapy can also cause a high urine pH. Low urine pH (pH < 5.0) is seen most commonly in metabolic acidosis. A higher value may indicate the presence of one of the forms of renal tubular acidosis. Acidic urine is also associated with the ingestion of large amounts of meat.[4]

Bilirubin and Urobilinogen

Only conjugated bilirubin is passed into the urine. Thus, the result of a reagent test for bilirubin is typically positive in patients with obstructive jaundice or in jaundice due to hepatocellular injury, whereas it is usually negative in patients with jaundice due to hemolysis. In patients with hemolysis, however, the urine urobilinogen result is often positive. Reagent test strips are very sensitive to bilirubin, detecting as little as 0.05 mg/dL. However, the detection of bilirubin in the urine is not very sensitive for detecting liver disease.[4] False-positive test results for urine bilirubin can occur if the urine is contaminated with stool. Prolonged storage and exposure to light can lead to false-negative results.[4]

Leukocyte Esterase and Nitrites

Dipstick screening for urinary tract infection has been recommended for high-risk individuals, but the issue is controversial. The U.S. Preventative Services Task Force has recommended screening for asymptomatic bacteriuria in pregnant women at 12 to 16 weeks' gestation. The Task Force stated that there was insufficient evidence to recommend for or against the routine screening of elderly women, women with diabetes, or children who are asymptomatic (http://www.ahrq.gov/clinic/3rduspstf/asymbac/asymbacrs.htm).[181] However, the American College of Physicians and the Canadian Task Force on the Periodic Health Examination have recommended that urinalysis not be used to screen for bacteriuria in asymptomatic persons. (http://www.ahrq.gov/clinic/3rduspstf/asymbac/asymbacrs.htm).[181] In children, routine screening for bacteriuria has also been controversial. The American Academy of Pediatrics recommends screening in infancy, early childhood, late childhood, and adolescence.[182] However, on the basis of a cost-effectiveness analysis, Kaplan and co-workers[183] suggested that a single screening test at school entry would be more effective. Whether dipstick screening for bacteriuria is sufficient (without microscopic examination) has also been debated.[184] Craver and co-workers[185] found that dipstick testing (with microscopic confirmation of positive results) was sufficient and cost-effective for children in an emergency department setting. In a study of 5486 urine samples, Bonnardeaux and co-workers[186] found that a negative dipstick result was probably sufficient to exclude microscopic abnormalities in the urine. Thus, it seems reasonable that a microscopic examination can be reserved for patients with an abnormal dipstick test result.

The esterase method relies on the fact that esterases are released from lysed urine granulocytes. These esterases liberate 3-hydroxy-5-phenyl pyrrole after substrate hydrolysis. The pyrrole reacts with a diazonium salt, yielding a pink to purple color.[187] The result is usually interpreted as negative, trace, small, moderate, or large. Urine that is allowed to stand indefinitely results in a greater lysis of leukocytes and a more intense reaction. False-positive results can occur with vaginal contamination. High levels of glucose, albumin, ascorbic acid, tetracycline, cephalexin, cephalothin, or large amounts of oxalic acid may inhibit the reaction.[188]

Urinary bacteria convert nitrates to nitrites. In the reagent strip test, nitrite reacts with an *p*-arsanilic acid to form a diazonium compound; further reaction with 1,2,3,4-tetrahydrobenzo(h)quinolin-3-ol, results in a pink color end point.[187,189] Results are usually interpreted as positive or negative. High specific gravity and ascorbic acid may interfere with the test. False-positive results are common and may be due to low urine nitrates resulting from low diet intake. It may take up to 4 hours to convert nitrate to nitrite, so inadequate bladder retention time can also give false-negative results.[189] Prolonged storage of the sample can lead to degradation of nitrites, another source of false-negative results. Finally, several potential urinary pathogens such as *Streptococcus faecalis*, other gram-positive organisms, *Neisseria gonorrhea*, and *Mycobacterium tuberculosis* do not convert nitrate to nitrite.[189]

Studies have examined the sensitivity and specificity of reagent strip tests for urinary tract infection in different clinical settings and patient populations, including patients attending general medicine clinic,[190] patients visiting an emergency department because of abdominal pain,[191] in children with neurogenic bladders,[192] in children attending a general medical outpatient clinic,[193] in men being screened for sexually transmitted disease,[194] and in women.[195] A meta-analysis of the results of 51 relevant studies compared the use of nitrite alone, leukocyte esterase alone, disjunctive pairing (either test result positive), and conjunctive pairing (both test result positive).[196] The ROC curves were fitted to the data using logistic transformations and weighted linear regression. This analysis indicated that the disjunctive pairing of both tests is the most accurate approach to screening for infection. However, when the likelihood of infection is high (e.g., when signs and symptoms are present), negative results of both tests are still inadequate to exclude infection. These tests, in combination with other clinical information, may be more useful in situations in which the likelihood of infection is low.

Glucose

Reagent strip measurement of urine glucose level, once used to monitor diabetic therapy, has been almost completely replaced by more reliable methods that measure finger-stick blood glucose level. Urine glucose is less accurately quantitated than blood glucose and is dependent on urine volume. In addition, the appearance of glucose in the urine always occurs later than blood glucose elevations. Thus, the value of the reagent strip glucose is limited almost entirely to screening.

Most reagent strips use a glucose oxidase/peroxidase method, which generally detects levels of glucose as low as 50 mg/dL.[197] Because the renal threshold for glucose is generally 160 to 180 mg/dL, the presence of detectable urine glucose indicates blood glucose in excess of 210 mg/dL. Large quantities of ketones, ascorbate, and pyridium metabolites may interfere with the color reaction,[197,198] and urine peroxide contamination may cause false-positive results. Nevertheless, the appearance of glucose in the urine is a specific indicator of high serum glucose levels. Glucosuria due to a low renal threshold for glucose reabsorption is rare. As a screening test for diabetes, fasting urine glucose testing has a specificity of 98% but a sensitivity of only 17%.[199]

Ketones

Ketones (acetoacetate and acetone) are generally detected with the nitroprusside reaction.[200] Ascorbic acid and phenazopyridine can give false-positive reactions. Beta-hydroxybutyrate (often 80% of total serum ketones in ketosis) is not normally detected by the nitroprusside reaction. Ketones may appear in the urine, but not in serum, with prolonged fasting or starvation. Ketones may also be measured in the urine in alcoholic or diabetic ketoacidosis.

Hemoglobin and Myoglobin

Reagent strips utilize the peroxidase-like activity of hemoglobin to catalyze the reaction of cumene hydroperoxide and 3,3',5,5'-tetramethylbenzidine. Hematuria, or contamination of the urine with menstrual blood, produces a positive reaction. Oxidizing contaminants and povidone iodine will cause false-positive reactions.[197] Myoglobin will also react positively.

Free hemoglobin is filtered at the renal glomerulus and, thus, will appear in the urine when the capacity for plasma protein binding with haptoglobin is exceeded. Some of the hemoglobin is catabolized by the proximal tubules. The principle cause of increased serum and urine free hemoglobin is hemolysis. Conversely, rhabdomyolysis gives rise to myoglobin. A positive dipstick test for hemoglobin in the absence of red blood cells in the urine sediment may suggest either hemolysis or rhabdomyolysis. Often, the clinical history provides important differential diagnostic information. Hemolysis can usually be diagnosed by examining the peripheral blood smear and measuring levels of lactate dehydrogenase, haptoglobin, and serum free hemoglobin. Rhabdomyolysis is accompanied by increased levels of serum creatine phosphokinase. In the end, specific assays for hemoglobin and myoglobin can be used to measure urine levels.

Protein

Normal Physiology

Normally, large quantities of large high-molecular-weight (HMW) plasma proteins traverse the glomerular capillaries, mesangium, or both without entering the urinary space. Both charge- and size-selective properties of the capillary wall prevent all but a tiny fraction of albumin, globulin, and other large plasma proteins from crossing. Smaller proteins (<20,000 Da) pass readily across the capillary wall. However, because the plasma concentration of these proteins is much lower than that of albumin and globulins, the filtered load is small. Moreover, LMW proteins are normally reabsorbed by the proximal tubule. Thus, proteins such as α_2-microglobulin, apoproteins, enzymes, and peptide hormones are normally excreted in only very small amounts in the urine.[4] Most healthy individuals excrete between 30 and 130 mg/day of protein, and the upper limit of normal total urine protein excretion is generally given as 150 to 200 mg/day for adults.[201] The upper limit of normal albumin excretion is usually given as 30 mg/day.[201]

A very small amount of protein that normally appears in the urine is the result of normal tubular secretion. Tamm-Horsfall protein is an HMW glycoprotein (23×10^6 Da) that is formed on the epithelial surface of the thick ascending limb of the loop of Henle and early distal convoluted tubule.[4] Tamm-Horsfall protein, also known as uromodulin, binds and inactivates the cytokines interleukin-1 and tumor necrosis factor.[202,203] Immunoglobulin A (IgA) and urokinase are also secreted by the renal tubule and appear in the urine in small amounts.[4]

From a consideration of normal physiology, it is apparent that abnormal amounts of protein may appear in the urine as the result of three mechanisms. First, a disruption of the capillary wall barrier may lead to a large amount of HMW plasma proteins that overwhelm the limited capacity of tubular reabsorption and cause protein to appear in the urine. The resulting proteinuria can be classified as glomerular in origin. Second, tubular damage or dysfunction can inhibit the normal resorptive capacity of the proximal tubule, resulting in increased amounts of mostly LMW proteins to appear in the urine. Such proteinuria can be classified as tubular proteinuria. Third, increased production of normal or abnormal plasma proteins can be filtered at the glomerulus and overwhelms the resorptive capacity of the proximal tubule. These filtered proteins can be especially numerous if their size is small or positively charged. Although increased urine protein excretion can also result from increased tubular production of protein, this is rarely the case.

Techniques to Measure Urine Protein

Protein can be measured in random samples, in timed or untimed overnight samples, or in 24-hour collections. Inaccurate urine collection is probably the greatest source of error in quantifying protein excretion in timed collections, particularly 24-hour collections. However, urine creatinine can be measured to judge the adequacy of the 24-hour collection. If creatinine excretion is similar to that in previous 24-hour samples, then the collection is likely to be reasonably accurate. If no other collections are available for comparison, then the adequacy of collection can be judged from the expected normal range of creatinine excretion. For hospitalized men ages 20 to 50 years, this range was found to be 18.5 to 25.0 mg/kg body weight/day, and for women of the same age, 16.5 to 22.4 mg/kg/day (Fig. 23–4). These values declined with age, so that for men ages 50 to 70 years, creatinine excretion was 15.7 to 20.2 mg/kg/day, and for women, 11.8 to 16.1 mg/kg/day (see Fig. 23–4). Patients who are malnourished or who may have reduced muscle mass for other reasons can be expected to have lower than normal creatinine excretion rates.[4]

Tests to accurately quantitate total protein concentration in urine rely on precipitation. In the commonly used sulfosalicylic acid method, sulfosalicylic acid is added to a sample of urine, and the turbidity is measured with a photometer or a nephelometer. Protein is quantified through comparison of the turbidity of the sample with that of a standard. This method lacks precision, and the coefficient of variation is as high as 20%. A number of proteins are detected with this method, including γ-globulin light chains and albumin. The

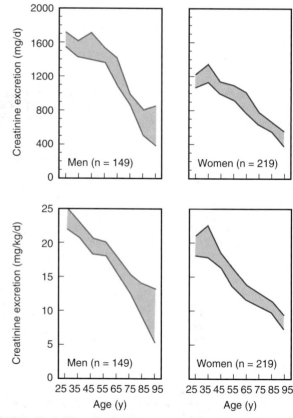

FIGURE 23–4 Age-related differences in urine creatinine excretion in normal men (left panels) and normal women (right panels). Shaded areas represent 95% confidence intervals calculated from the data of Kampmann J, Siersbæk-Nielson K, Kristensen M, Mølholm-Hansen J: Rapid evaluation of creatinine clearance. Acta Med Scand 196:517–520, 1974. Values in the upper panels are in mg/day and values in the lower panels are in mg/kg of body weight/day.

method is more sensitive to albumin than to globulins. Trichloroacetic acid can be used in place of sulfosalicylic acid to increase the sensitivity to γ-globulin. False-positive reactions may occur from high levels of tolmetin sodium (Tolectin), tolbutamide, antibiotics, and radiocontrast agents. Total protein can more accurately be quantified with the use of several monospecific antibodies to different types of urine protein, but this method is somewhat cumbersome and is seldom used in clinical laboratories.[4]

Total protein concentration in urine can be estimated with chemically impregnated plastic strips. Most dipstick reagents contain a pH-sensitive colorimetric indicator that changes color when negatively charged proteins bind to it. However, positively charged proteins are less readily detected. Positively charged immunoglobulin light chains, for example, may escape urine dipstick detection even when present in large amounts in the urine. A very high urine pH (>7.0) can also give false-positive results, as can contamination of the urine with blood. The dipstick technique is sensitive to very small urine protein concentrations (the lower limit of detection is 10–20 mg/dL). However, at these low levels, the major constituent of urine protein may be Tamm-Horsfall protein, and thus, a positive test result may not reflect kidney injury. This is especially likely to occur when the urine volume is low and the concentration is high. When urine volume is high and the urine is maximally dilute, however, a relatively large amount of protein can go undetected. Indeed, total protein excretion approaching 1 g/day may not be detected if urine output is high. If, for example, urine volume is 10 L/day, then the concentration of 1 g of protein would be 10 mg/dL, or below the limit of detection for most reagent strip tests of total protein.[4]

The consistency of results with the same sample assessed repeatedly or the precision of reagent strip tests of urine total protein concentration is generally poor.[204] Variability in interpretation both by the same technologist and among technologists has been examined and has been found to be relatively high. For example, at low levels of urine protein concentration (e.g., 6–39 mg/dL), inconsistent results between different technologists were seen in 19% to 56% of the determinations. At higher concentrations (e.g., 196–328 mg/dL), inconsistencies were seen in 19% to 44%.[4] Similar findings were reported in a later study that also found that inconsistencies depended somewhat on the experience of the operator and the type of reagent strip. Inconsistencies were found among experienced technologists in up to 33% of cases and among inexperienced technologists in up to 93% of cases.[204]

The sensitivity and specificity of reagent strip protein tests have also been assessed using more accurate quantitative determinations as gold standards. Interestingly, the sensitivity of these tests appears to be higher when assessed through the use of samples prepared by adding albumin and globulin to normal, protein-free urine than when assessed using actual patient specimens.[204] This difference likely reflects the inability of reagent strips to react to many of the heterogeneous proteins found in human urine. When 20 to 25 mg/dL is used as the limit of detection in clinical specimens, the sensitivity of reagent strips has been found to be only 32% to 46%, and the specificity was 97% to 100%.[204] The effect of the sensitivity and specificity on the utility of these reagent strip tests also, of course, depends on the prevalence of proteinuria in the population being screened. In a population with a low prevalence of disease, the low sensitivity of the reagent strip tests suggests that the majority of individuals with proteinuria would be missed.[4,204]

Urine albumin concentrations can be quantified by a number of assays including

1. Radioimmunoassay can be carried out using a double-antibody technique. Albumin in a urine sample competes with a known amount of radiola-

beled albumin for fixed binding sites of antibodies. Free albumin can be separated from bound albumin by immunoabsorption of the (albumin-bound) antibody. Albumin concentration in the sample is inversely proportional to the radioactivity.[205]

2. The immunoturbimetric technique depends on the turbidity of a solution when albumin in a sample of urine reacts with a specific antibody. The turbidity is measured with a spectrophotometer, and the absorbency is proportional to the albumin concentration.[206]

3. When albumin in the urine sample reacts with a specific antibody, it forms light-scattering antigen-antibody complexes that can be measured with a laser nephelometer. The amount of albumin is proportional to scatter in the signal.[207]

4. The competitive enzyme-linked immunosorbent assay (ELISA) has also been used to measure urine albumin.[208]

5. HPLC has also been used to measure urine albumin. This assay also measures the immuno-unreactive intact albumin that is not recognized by immunologic methods. However, the clinical significance of this immuno-unreactive intact albumin is not fully understood.[209]

Although the correlation between most of these quantitative assays is very good, a good correlation only indicates a strong linear relationship. For example, the correlation coefficients (r-values) between radioimmunoassay and immunoturbidimetry and that between radioimmunoassay and nephelometry were both 0.98.[210] Intra-assay coefficients of variation for immunoturbidimetry and nephelometry, respectively, were found to be 6.6% and 11.5% at low concentrations (10–60 mg/L) and 11.1% and 4.1% at high concentrations (90–120 mg/L), respectively.[210] Interassay coefficients of variation were 11.4% and 11.5% at low concentrations (10–60 mg/L) and 5.4% and 1.4% at high concentrations (90–120 mg/L), respectively, for these two techniques.[210] However, this study had few samples in the midrange of albumin concentration (16–90 mg/L), and here there were considerable different results between the radioimmunoassay and the nephelometry assay.[210] In another study, each assay varied from one another up to threefold between radioimmunoassay, immunoturbidimetry, nephelometry, and HPLC.[211] Other studies have also found similar variations between different immunoassays.[212] In contrast, the within-run coefficient of variation for an immunoturbidometric methods was found to be 3.5% at low albumin concentrations and 2.4% at high albumin concentrations.[213] The day-to-day coefficient of variation for the same assay was 5.1% at low or high albumin concentrations.[213] Therefore, ideally the same assay should be used when comparing the albuminuria results over time for a patient. The choice of assay used to measure albuminuria is largely determined by issues of accuracy, cost, and convenience.

Reagent strip methods have recently been developed to qualitatively screen for urine albumin excretion. The Albustix (Bayer Diagnostik, Munich, Germany) reagent strip uses a protein error of indicators method that causes color changes in the presence of albumin.[214] Trace reactions indicate urine albumin concentrations between 50 and 200 mg/L. Thus, more positive reactions can be used to indicate albumin concentrations higher than those generally found in patients with microalbuminuria. In one study, the sensitivity and specificity of the Albustix was found to be only 0.81 and 0.55, respectively.[214] Thus, there was almost a 50% chance of a false-negative result with the Albustix method.

Screening methods have been developed to measure albumin concentrations low enough to detect albumin excretion rates that are abnormal, but below the level of detection with standard reagent strips (i.e., in the microalbuminuria range).[210,215–220] One of the most extensively investigated methods to screen for microalbuminuria is the immunometric dipstick Micral-Test (Boehringer Mannheim, Mannheim, Germany).[210,217] The strip is made up of a series of reagent pads through which the urine sample passes sequentially. Urine is first drawn into a wick fleece and then passes into a buffer fleece that adjusts the sample pH. Next, it passes into a third pad, in which albumin in the sample is bound by a soluble conjugate of antibodies linked to the enzyme β-galactosidase. Excess antibody is then adsorbed on immobilized albumin in the next pad, so that only albumin bound to antibody and enzyme reaches the color pad. There the β-galactosidase reacts with a chemical substrate to produce a red dye, the intensity of which is proportional to the bound albumin concentration. The test strip must be read at precisely 5 minutes.[210,217]

Another qualitative test that has been examined in several investigations is the Micro-Bumintest (Ames, Miles, Elkhart, IN). This test uses a reagent tablet containing the indicator dye bromphenol blue. The intensity of the bluish-green color produced after a drop of urine is placed on the surface of the tablet is proportional to the concentration of albumin.[210] A latex agglutination method, Albusure (Cambridge Life Sciences, Cambridge, UK), binds albumin in the urine sample to latex.[214] Agglutination occurs when mixed with sheep antihuman antibody. When urine albumin concentrations are greater than 20 mg/L, agglutination is inhibited (antigen excess). Thus, agglutination indicates urine albumin concentration of less than 20 mg/L.

A number of studies have examined the sensitivity and specificity of screening methods designed to detect very low levels of albumin in urine.[210,215–220] Because these tests are only semiquantitative (i.e., nonparametric), a true coefficient of variation cannot be determined. Nevertheless, in one evaluation of the Micral-Test method, an estimated coefficient of variation of the same sample interpreted by different technicians was 12.4%.[219] Experience in reading the Micral-Test was shown to be important.[218] Observer concordance for the Micro-Bumintest was found to be 95% in one study.[215] A new version of the Micral-Test, Micral-Test II, has been described[221]; it is designed to react faster, to be less dependent on timing, and to allow a better color comparison to reduce observer variance. Indeed, in one study, the interobserver concordance was 93% with the Micral-Test II.[221]

Several studies have examined the sensitivity and specificity of the newer reagent strips that measure very low concentrations of urine albumin. Most of these investigations studied patients with diabetes, and most examined the Micral-Test,[210,216–218,222] the Micro-Bumintest,[210,215] or both. In general, these albumin reagent strip tests are more sensitive than standard dipsticks, but they also have a relatively high rate of false-positive results. Moreover, it should be remembered that, for the most part, these reagent strips were tested in populations of diabetic patients with a high prior probability of a positive result. The number of false-positive results would be expected to be much higher in populations in which the prevalence of albuminuria was lower. Because these strips may be in error owing to variation in urinary concentration, these should only be used to approximate urinary protein if the ability to directly measure protein is not available.[223,224]

All of the qualitative or semiquantitative urine protein and albumin screening tests discussed so far measure only total protein, or albumin concentration. The sensitivity and specificity of these tests can be markedly influenced by fluid intake, the state of diuresis, and the resulting urine concentration. Indeed, in one study, albumin concentration had a low discriminant value for detecting increased albumin excretion in a 12-hour timed urine sample (Fig. 23–5). In an effort to

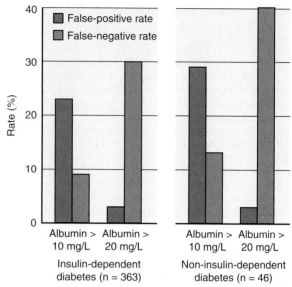

FIGURE 23–5 Comparison of false-positive and false-negative rates when urine albumin concentration was used to predict 12-hour (overnight) excretion greater than 15 μg/min in diabetics. At a concentration cutoff greater than 10 mg/L, the false-positive rate is high. At a concentration cutoff greater than 20 mg/L, the false-positive rate is reduced, but the false-negative rate is high. (Data from Kouri TT, Viikari JSA, Mattila KS, Irjala KMA: Invalidity of simple concentration-based screening tests for early nephropathy due to urinary volumes of diabetic patients. Diabetes Care 14:591–593, 1991.)

correct for problems arising out of variability in urine volume and concentration, many investigators have used the protein-to-creatinine or albumin-to-creatinine ratio in random, or timed urine collections. There is a high degree of correlation between 24-hour urine protein excretion and protein-to-creatinine ratios in random, single-voided urine samples in patients with a variety of kidney diseases.[225] It has been suggested that a protein-to-creatinine ratio of greater than 3.0 or 3.5 mg/mg or less than 0.2 mg/mg indicates protein excretion rates of greater than 3.0 or 3.5 g/24 hr or less than 0.2 g/24 hr, respectively.[225] However, few studies have systematically examined the sensitivity and specificity or defined optimal levels of detection for protein-to-creatinine ratios in large numbers of patients in different clinical settings.

Much of the data on the usefulness of albumin-to-creatinine ratios has been derived from studies of patients with type 1 or type 2 diabetes.[226–229] In most of these investigations, the sensitivity and specificity of albumin-to-creatinine ratios were determined using albumin excretion rates from timed urine collections as a standard. Data from several studies were combined to examine the true- and false-positive rates for albumin-to-creatinine ratios to detect albuminuria in overnight urine.[4] Independent of the albumin-to-creatinine ratio cutoff used, the sensitivities and specificities appeared to be reasonable.[4] Altogether, these data suggest that albumin-to-creatinine ratios may be useful as a screening test for kidney disease in populations in which the expected prevalence of disease is high (e.g., diabetic persons). Less clear is their potential usefulness in other patient populations in which the prior likelihood of disease may be lower than in patients with diabetes.[230] A cross-sectional study by Ruggenenti and co-workers[231] found that morning protein-to-creatinine ratios among 177 nondiabetic outpatients with CKD were predictive of declining kidney function. In kidney transplant recipients, protein-to-creatinine ratios have been shown to significantly correlate with measurements of 24-hour urine protein and appear useful as both screening devices and longitudinal tests for following the level of proteinuria.[232] Use of the protein-to-creatinine ratio has also proved reliable in detecting significant proteinuria in pregnant women,[233,234] but the threshold for identifying pregnant women with significant proteinuria is controversial.[235–237]

Although protein-to-creatinine or albumin-to-creatinine ratios may be more quantitative than a simple dipstick screening procedure, their use has a number of limitations. For example, obtaining protein-to-creatinine or albumin-to-creatinine ratios on morning, first-void samples may underestimate 24-hour protein excretion because of the reduction in proteinuria that normally occurs at night.[238] Storage time and temperature may also affect albumin levels in urine,[239] and specimens should be analyzed as soon as possible after collection. The fact that urine creatinine must be measured in addition to albumin introduces another source of error. Indeed, the combination of the errors of two measurements is greater than the error of either one alone (the coefficient of variation is the square root of the sum of the two coefficients of variations, each squared). Urine creatinine concentration is extremely variable, so that very different ratios can be obtained in individuals with similar protein excretion rates. Moreover, a number of variables that may interfere with creatinine determinations may affect the ratios.[240] Despite these limitations, the urine protein-to-creatinine or albumin-to-creatinine ratio may be useful, especially in individuals in whom urine collection is difficult or impossible. Given the day-to-day variability in albumin excretion and the potential limitations of albumin to creatinine ratio, the American Diabetic Association recommends that at least two or three samples in a 3- to 6-month period should show elevated levels before a patient is deemed to have microalbuminuria.[223]

A number of analytic tools have been developed to separate and identify individual urinary proteins.[241] These techniques include agarose gel electrophoresis, column gel chromatography, polyacrylamide gel electrophoresis, immunoelectrophoresis, and isoelectric focusing. Proteomic techniques employing mass spectrometry and peptide mass fingerprinting have expanded the number of identified urinary proteins.[242,243] However, these latter techniques are generally designed to identify, but not accurately quantitate, urine proteins. Some have been used in clinical laboratories to determine the selectivity of urine protein or to identify monoclonal immunoglobulin heavy and light chains. Otherwise, they have been largely confined to research applications.

Applications of Urine Protein Measurement
Screening for Kidney Disease

Although urine protein measurement can be used to assist in the diagnosis of kidney disease and to assess progression and response to therapy (discussed later), it is most commonly used as a screening test. Because screening tests are generally applied to relatively large numbers of patients, convenience and cost are major considerations. To make screening more convenient, a number of methods have been developed to measure urine protein in a single-voided, or "spot," urine sample, so that timed urine collections can be avoided.

In 1982, Viberti and co-workers[244] reported that clinical (Albustix-positive) proteinuria subsequently developed in patients with insulin-dependent diabetes in whom albumin excretion rates of 30 to 140 µg/min were measured by radioimmunoassay in timed overnight urine collections. In contrast, patients with less than 30 µg/min did not develop overt proteinuria.[244] Viberti and co-workers[244] coined the term "microalbuminuria" to indicate increased urine albumin excretion rates in patients with normal urine total protein. A more recent follow-up of the original cohort confirmed that the patients with microalbuminuria not only had a higher risk of developing overt proteinuria but also had a greater risk of dying from cardiovascular disease.[245] Similar findings have been reported by others in patients with insulin-dependent

and non–insulin-dependent diabetes.[246–249] Some investigators have used 15 to 150 µg/min to define microalbuminuria,[248] whereas others have used 20 to 200 µg/min.[249,250] Microalbuminuria has also been defined as urine albumin excretion of 30 to 300 mg/day.[201] Microalbuminuria has also been defined as a urine albumin-to-creatinine ratio of above 30 mg/g (or 0.03 mg/g) in an untimed urine sample but may vary by race and gender. Thus, others have defined microalbuminuria as 20 to 200 mg/g and 30 to 400 mg/g for males and females, respectively.[251] Whatever definition is used, microalbuminuria appears to be an important risk factor for end-organ damage in patients with diabetes. Similarly, in patients with essential hypertension, increased urine albumin excretion ratio (>30 mg/24 hr) is associated with increased cardiovascular mortality.

Most studies showing a relationship between microalbuminuria and end-organ damage have used quantitative techniques to measure urine albumin excretion. Although few studies have examined whether other screening techniques predict outcome, there is no reason to believe that the results cannot be extrapolated to other screening tests, taking differences in sensitivity and specificity into account. Indeed, albumin-to-creatinine ratios have been shown to predict the subsequent development of overt kidney disease. In a population of diabetic southwestern Native Americans, albumin-creatinine ratios of 0.03 to 0.30 mg/mg (microalbuminuria range) were a strong predictor of diabetic nephropathy.[252]

The recognition that microalbuminuria identifies diabetic patients at risk for subsequent renal and cardiovascular disease complications has given great impetus to developing effective screening tools. Borch-Johnsen and associates,[250] using published data, carried out a critical appraisal of screening for microalbuminuria in patients with diabetes. Making a number of assumptions, they performed a cost-benefit analysis of the impact of screening and antihypertensive treatment and concluded that screening and intervention programs are likely to lead to considerable reductions in cost and mortality.[250] Even though microalbuminuria has been recommended as a routine test to screen for early diabetic nephropathy, it is important to realize that there are some patients with either type 1 or type 2 diabetes who have decreased GFR due to diabetic nephropathy in the absence of microalbuminuria.[253,254]

The use of dipstick tests for total protein excretion and microalbuminuria to screen for renal disease has not been rigorously examined in nondiabetic patient populations. Epidemiologic data suggest that even in nondiabetics, proteinuria is a risk factor for cardiovascular disease,[2] perhaps because proteinuria is a sensitive indicator of kidney damage. However strong these correlations are statistically (low P-value), the amount of unexplained variability (low r-value) is great, suggesting that the sensitivity and specificity for proteinuria detection of kidney injury in the general population could be too low to make this a useful screening tool in an individual patient. Nevertheless, data to assess this are generally not available for individuals who are not diabetic. A cost-effectiveness analysis compared a strategy of annual screening with no screening for proteinuria at age 50 years followed by treatment with an angiotensin-converting enzyme inhibitor or an angiotensin II receptor blocker and found that annual screening was not cost-effective unless selectively directed toward high-risk groups of patients older than 60 years and patients with hypertension.[255] Regardless of whether or not measuring urine protein excretion in the general population is a cost-effective approach to the early detection of kidney disease, such screening may be useful when combined with other clinical parameters in estimating vascular disease risk. However, the prospective data needed to assess the utility of this application of urine protein excretion are also incomplete.

The appropriate manner in which to use various tests to screen for renal disease has not been extensively investigated. Because the number of false-positive results on dipstick tests for protein excretion is high, a positive test should probably be followed by tests designed to more accurately quantitate urine protein excretion. However, in some clinical circumstances, the likelihood that a positive dipstick test for urine protein excretion indicates CKD is so low that the screening test should be repeated at a later date before more costly quantitation procedures are undertaken. A positive dipstick test result for protein in a patient with a urinary tract infection, for example, could be dismissed if subsequent posttreatment tests are negative. Fever can cause tubular and glomerular proteinuria that most often disappears when the fever resolves. Congestive heart failure and seizures can also cause transient proteinuria. Light or strenuous exercise is often associated with urine protein excretion that resolves spontaneously.[4]

It seems clear that, even in the absence of identifiable causes of transient proteinuria, some individuals have increases in urine protein excretion that are not associated with kidney disease.[256] This proteinuria can be classified in two categories, intermittent or persistent and postural. Several dipstick measurements of urine protein over time can be made to determine whether an individual patient fits in either of these two distinct patterns. Intermittent proteinuria is less well characterized than postural proteinuria, but it appears to be relatively benign in otherwise normal individuals. It has been shown, for example, that mortality after more than 40 years of follow-up of college students with intermittently positive urine protein screens was no different than that of normal individuals. However, few histologic studies including sufficiently large numbers of patients have been carried out to precisely characterize intermittent proteinuria.[4]

Posture can cause an increase in urine protein excretion in otherwise normal individuals.[256] This postural proteinuria should be distinguished from the increase in proteinuria seen in patients with kidney disease who assume an upright posture. Postural proteinuria usually does not exceed 1 g/24 hr. It is usually diagnosed by detecting protein excretion during the day that is absent at night while the patient is recumbent. Kidney histology in patients with postural proteinuria is generally normal or nonspecific.[257,258] Patients with postural proteinuria have been shown to have an excellent long-term prognosis.[259] Indeed, six patients diagnosed by Thomas Addis had no evidence of kidney disease after 42 to 50 years of follow-up.[260] Even in individuals without postural proteinuria or renal disease, levels of urine protein excretion are lower at night than during the day.[261] Thus, the timing of urine collection is likely to influence the sensitivity and specificity of screening tests for urine protein excretion.

Diagnosis and Prognosis

Once proteinuria has been detected by screening, the clinician must not only confirm the results of screening but also precisely quantitate the amount of protein excretion in a timed urine collection. Quantifying urine protein excretion may help to distinguish glomerular from tubular proteinuria. If, for example, a patient's protein excretion is in the nephrotic range (e.g., >3 g/24 hr), a glomerular source is almost certain. Quantitation of urine protein excretion can also provide useful prognostic information and assist in monitoring the response to therapy.

After detection and quantification, determining the composition of urine protein may provide diagnostic information. Higher amounts of albumin and HMW proteins suggest glomerular proteinuria, whereas isolated increases in LMW protein fractions are more suggestive of tubular proteinuria. It is unusual for tubular proteinuria to exceed 1 to 2 g/day, and only a small fraction of protein excretion due to

tubular damage should be albumin. Tubular proteins are heterogeneous; however, α_2-microglobulin is often a major constituent.

β_2-Microglobulin is an LMW (11.8-kDa) protein that has been identified as the light chain of class I major histocompatibility antigens (e.g., human leukocyte antigens [HLAs] A, B, and C).[262] β_2-Microglobulin is most commonly measured in urine using radioimmunoassay or ELISA. It is freely filtered at the glomerulus and is avidly taken up and catabolized by the proximal tubule. Not surprisingly, therefore, detectable urinary levels of β_2-microglobulin have been associated with many pathologic conditions involving the proximal tubule, including aminoglycoside, Balkan endemic nephropathy, heavy metal nephropathies, radiocontrast nephropathy, and kidney transplant rejection.[263-268] β_2-Microglobulin has also been found to be useful in distinguishing upper from lower urinary tract infection.[269] Because urine β_2-microglobulin is a nonspecific marker of kidney tubular injury, it is not useful in differentiating among different causes of kidney disease. However, when the likely cause is already known, measurement of β_2-microglobulin may be useful in detecting and monitoring injury. Nevertheless, the sensitivity and specificity for this test of tubular injury have generally not been established in different clinical situations in which prior probabilities of various kidney disorders may strongly influence its usefulness. Thus, the test may be useful in monitoring factory workers exposed to heavy metals in whom other causes of tubular injury could be expected to be uncommon. Conversely, measuring β_2-microglobulin may be of limited value in diagnosing kidney transplant rejection, because other causes of tubular injury are common in transplant recipients.

Glomerular proteinuria can be further characterized as selective or nonselective. Patients with a clearance ratio of immunoglublin G (IgG; an HMW protein)–to-albumin that is less than 0.10 are said to have a selective glomerular proteinuria, whereas those with IgG-to-albumin clearance ratios of greater than 0.50 have a nonselective pattern. In general, selective proteinuria is more often seen in patients with minimal change disease and predicts a good response to treatment with corticosteroids.[4] The sensitivity and specificity of determining the selectivity of glomerular proteinuria have not been systematically examined in large numbers of patients with different kidney diseases. Moreover, the cost of the protein separation procedures has limited their widespread clinical use.

Plasma cell dyscrasias may produce monoclonal proteins, immunoglobulin, free light chains, and a combination of these. Light chains are filtered at the glomerulus and may appear in the urine as Bence Jones protein. The detection of urine immunoglobulin light chains can be the first clue to a number of important clinical syndromes associated with plasma cell dyscrasias that involve the kidney.[4] Unfortunately, urine immunoglobulin light chains may not be detected by reagent strip tests for protein. However, plasma cell dyscrasias may also manifest as proteinuria or albuminuria when the glomerular deposition of light chains causes disruption of the normally impermeable capillary wall.[270] The diagnosis of a plasma cell dyscrasia can be suspected when a tall, narrow band on electrophoresis suggests the presence of a monoclonal γ-globulin or immunoglobulin light chain. However, monoclonal proteins are best detected using serum and urine immunoelectrophoresis.[4]

Once patients have been screened and a diagnosis of kidney disease has been established, measuring the amount of urine protein can provide additional prognostic information and can be used to monitor the response to therapy. The amount of urine protein excretion has consistently been shown to predict subsequent disease progression in different clinical settings: for example, protein excretion correlated with progression in patients presenting with the nephrotic syndrome[271] and in patients with mild renal insufficiency of various causes.[272] Similar findings have been reported in patients with IgA nephropathy,[273–275] membranous nephropathy,[275–277] and type I membranoproliferative glomerulonephritis (GN).[275] The clinical course and effect of immunosuppressive therapy can also be monitored with sequential quantitation of urine protein excretion.[278]

Formed Elements

Urine Microscopy Methods

The examination of the urine by microscopy remains a useful qualitative and semiquantitative procedure. Efforts to more accurately quantitate formed elements in the urine have been made over the years. For example, Addis measured excretion rates of erythrocytes using timed urine collections. However, formed elements can quickly deteriorate in the urine, and timed collections are difficult for most patients to carry out with accuracy. Moreover, the excretion rate of many formed elements correlates with urine concentration, so that, often, little additional information is gained from the effort made to collect timed specimens.[4] For all of these reasons, the use of timed collections to obtain excretion rates of formed elements has not gained widespread acceptance. Quantifying the number of formed elements can still be carried out using untimed specimens and a counting chamber.

A number of conditions affect formed elements in the urine, and when possible, these conditions should be optimized. Contamination with bacteria can be minimized through careful attention to collection technique. A midstream, "clean-catch" specimen should be collected when possible; the patient should be instructed to retract foreskin and labia. A high urine concentration and a low urine pH help to preserve formed elements.[4] Thus, a first-void morning specimen, which is most likely to be acidic and concentrated, should be used whenever possible. Strenuous exercise and bladder catheterization can cause hematuria, and urine specimens collected to detect hematuria should not be obtained under these conditions. Urine should be examined as soon as possible after collection to avoid lysis of the formed elements and bacterial overgrowth. The specimen should not be refrigerated, because lowering the temperature causes the precipitation of phosphates and urates.

It is helpful to first measure the urine specific gravity and pH, so as to judge the density of formed elements according to the concentration and acidity of the specimen. Specimens from concentrated and acidic urine may be expected to have a greater density of formed elements than dilute and alkaline specimens from the same patients. Urine should be centrifuged at approximately 2000 revolutions per minute (rpm) for 5 to 10 minutes or 2500 to 3000 rpm for 3 to 5 minutes. The supernate should be carefully poured off, the pellet resuspended by gentle agitation, and a drop placed on a slide under a coverslip.

Most commonly, urine is examined under an ordinary bright-field microscope. However, polarized light can be used to identify anisotropic crystals, and phase-contrast microscopy can enhance the contrast of cell membranes. The urine should first be examined under low power (100x) to best judge the number of formed elements. These elements can then be examined in detail under high power (400x). Generally, the urine is examined unstained, but occasionally, stains can be helpful in distinguishing cell types.

Hematuria

Gross hematuria may first be detected by a change in urine color. Microscopic hematuria can be detected by dipstick methodology, microscopic examination, or both. These latter methods may be applied as diagnostic tests in patients with known kidney disease or as screening tools in normal or high-risk individuals. The sensitivity and specificity of screening tests for hematuria have not been thoroughly examined in many pertinent patient populations. Moreover, the cost-to-benefit ratio of screening is often unclear.

Who and when to screen for microscopic hematuria are controversial. The most cogent reason to screen for occult hematuria may be to facilitate the early, and potentially life-saving detection of urologic malignancies. A dipstick test in more than 10,000 adult men undergoing health screening was found to be positive in about 2.5%.[279] About one fourth of those who were investigated had cystoscopic abnormalities, including bladder neoplasms in 2 men. However, more than one third of those found to have occult hematuria in this retrospective study did not undergo further investigation. In study of over 2000 men, 4% were found to have occult hematuria, and 1 of these patients was found to have bladder carcinoma.[280] Higher detection rates have been reported by other investigators.[281] The U.S. Preventive Services Task Force no longer recommends screening for occult hematuria (www.preventiveservices.ahrq.gov).[181] The value of screening for occult hematuria in other populations is questionable,[282] and the role for occult hematuria screening to detect parenchymal kidney disease is unclear.

Even when the urine is red, or when a dipstick-screening test is positive, the sediment should be examined to determine whether red cells are present. Other pigments such as free hemoglobin and myoglobin can masquerade as hematuria. In addition, red blood cells can be detected in the urine sediment when screening tests are negative. An occasional red blood cell can be seen in normal individuals, but generally only one or two cells per high power field.

The differential diagnosis of hematuria is broad but for practical purposes can be categorized as originating in the upper or lower urinary tract. Hematuria that is accompanied by red blood cell casts, marked proteinuria, or both is most likely to be glomerular in origin. In the absence of these important findings, distinguishing glomerular from postglomerular bleeding can be difficult. Red blood cells originating in glomeruli have been reported to have a distinctive dysmorphic appearance that is most readily appreciated using phase-contrast microscopy.[283–285] Automated blood cell analysis has also been used to determine the number of dysmorphic red cells in urine.[206,207] In vitro studies suggest that pH and osmolality changes found in the distal tubule could explain the higher number of dysmorphic red blood cells in patients with glomerular disease.[288]

The clinical utility of tests to distinguish dysmorphic red cells in the urine has been examined in numerous studies.[287,289–293] Most investigators concluded that detecting dysmorphic red cells reliably identified patients with glomerular disease; however, one investigator-blinded, controlled trial found unacceptable interobserver variability.[290] A number of investigators have attempted to develop automated methods to detect glomerular hematuria.[294–296] These techniques employ cell counters or more sophisticated flow cytometry methods. However, the use of automated cell size determinations in individuals with low-grade hematuria may be particularly unreliable owing to interference from cell debris.[295] A meta-analysis of 21 published studies using predetermined criteria for evaluation of dysmorphic urine red cells was carried out.[297] All studies originated in referral centers. The weighted average sensitivity and specificity for dysmorphic red cell test detection of glomerular disease were (with 95% confidence intervals): 0.88 (0.86–0.91) and 0.95 (0.93–0.97), respectively. The sensitivity and specificity for the use of abnormal (automated) red blood cell volumes to detect glomerular disease were 1.00 (0.98–1.00) and 0.87 (0.80–0.91). The investigators in this meta-analysis concluded that the negative predictive value of these tests was probably not sufficient to rule out important urologic lesions, especially in a referral setting in which the prevalence of urologic disease may be relatively high.

The differential diagnosis of hematuria is broad (Table 23–4). Kidney vascular causes include arterial and venous thrombosis, ateriovenous malformations, arteriovenous fistula, and the nutcracker syndrome (compression of the left renal vein between the aorta and the superior mesenteric artery).[298] Most patients undergoing anticoagulant therapy who have hematuria can be found to have an underlying cause, especially if the hematuria is macroscopic. However, excessive anticoagu-

TABLE 23–4	Common Sources of Hematuria

Vascular
Coagulation abnormalities
Over anticoagulation
Arterial emboli or thrombosis
Ateriovenous malformations
Arteriovenous fistula
Nutcracker syndrome
Renal vein thrombosis
Loin-pain hematuria syndrome (vascular?)

Glomerular
IgA nephropathy
Thin basement membrane diseases (including Alport's syndrome)
Other causes of primary and secondary glomerulonephritis

Interstitial
Allergic interstitial nephritis
Analgesic nephropathy
Renal cystic diseases
Acute pyelonephritis
Tuberculosis
Renal allograft rejection

Uroepithelium
Malignancy
Vigorous exercise
Trauma
Papillary necrosis
Cystitis/urethritis/protatitis (usually caused by infection)
Parasitic diseases (e.g., schistosomiasis)
Nephrolithiasis or bladder calculi

Multiple sites or source unknown
Hypercalciuria
Hyperuricosuria
Sickle cell disease

lation or other coagulopathies can themselves be associated with hematuria. The source of hematuria in patients with sickle cell disease is often unclear, although occasionally, sickle cells may actually be seen in the urine.[299]

Worldwide, the most common cause of glomerular hematuria is probably IgA nephropathy.[300] However, thin basement membrane diseases and other causes of glomerular nephritis are common as well. The differential diagnosis of glomerular hematuria is influenced by the geographic locale and the clinical setting. Thus, in Asia, IgA nephropathy is a very common cause of microscopic hematuria.[300] However, in another report, 25 to 30 of otherwise normal candidates for kidney donation who had asymptomatic microscopic hematuria were found to have hereditary nephritis.[301] Interstitial nephritis, whether allergic or infectious, is frequently associated with microscopic hematuria. Uroepithelial causes of hematuria include nephrolithiasis, acute and chronic infections, and malignancies. Malignancies are more common in patients who are male, are older, have macroscopic versus microscopic hematuria, are white rather than black, or have a history of analgesic abuse or other toxic exposure.

A reasonable approach to the patient with asymptomatic hematuria is to first perform a thorough history and physical examination (Fig. 23–6). If the findings are unenlightening, important clues can sometimes be obtained by examining the urine. Red blood cell casts, significant proteinuria, or both may suggest a glomerular source for the hematuria. For the patients in whom glomerular proteinuria is likely, a kidney biopsy may give the diagnosis. If the source of proteinuria is not evident from the history, physical examination, or urinalysis, a renal ultrasound is probably a reasonable next step. In the young patient (e.g., <40 years) in whom renal ultrasonography findings are normal and who is otherwise at low risk for a uroepithelial malignancy, the next step can be 24-hour urine collection to exclude hypercalciuria and hyperuricosuria. If urinalysis tests are normal, it is reasonable to observe the patient without further evaluation. However, some patients may wish to undergo kidney biopsy to better understand the prognosis. Patients who are older than 40 years, have risk factors for uroepithelial malignancies, or both should undergo an intravenous pyelogram and, possibly, cystoscopy in addition to the renal ultrasonography.

Leukocyturia

The number of white blood cells that can normally be found in the urine is controversial. A conservative approach is to consider more than one per high-power field to be abnormal.

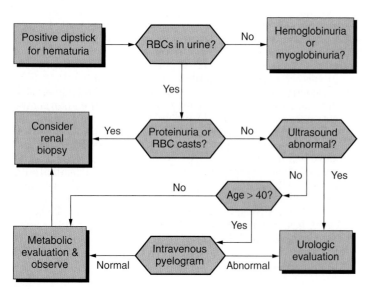

FIGURE 23–6 An approach to the patient with hematuria. RBCs, red blood cells.

The differential diagnosis of leukocyturia is broad. White blood cells can enter the urine from anywhere along the excretory system. The presence of other formed elements (e.g., proteinuria and casts) suggests a glomerular source. In the absence of other formed elements, the clinician must look beyond the urine sediment for additional clues to find the origin of urine leukocytes. Unlike red blood cells, there are no effective methods to identify the origin of white blood cells found in the urine. Contamination is a common cause of leukocyturia that should always be considered in the absence of other suggestive clinical findings.

Most often, leukocytes in the urine are polymorphonuclear. However, it should not be assumed that all urinary leukocytes are neutrophils. The presence of non-neutrophil white blood cells in the urine—for example, eosinophils—can sometimes be an important diagnostic clue. The association between eosinophiluria and drug-induced hypersensitivity reactions was first reported by Eisenstaedt, in 1951. Since then, a number of investigators have reported on the association between eosinophiluria and kidney disease.[4] Wright stain can be used to detect urine eosinophils, but a urine pH less than 7 inhibits Wright stain.[302] The use of Hansel stain improves the sensitivity of urinary eosinophil detection over the standard Wright stain.[303] In one retrospective investigation, the use of Hansel stain rather than Wright stain improved the sensitivity of using the presence of any urinary eosinophils for detecting acute interstitial nephritis from 25% to 63%[303]; the positive predictive value was improved from 25% to 50%.[303] However, not all patients in this study underwent renal biopsy to establish the diagnosis of interstitial nephritis, and the retrospective inclusion of only patients in whom urinary eosinophils were sought by clinicians makes interpretation of these data difficult. The true sensitivity and specificity of urinary eosinophils for detecting different clinical kidney diseases are unclear. Indeed, the list of diseases that may be associated with eosinophiluria is long and continues to grow (Table 23–5). Moreover, the sensitivity and specificity of eosinophiluria in detecting kidney disease can be expected to vary with the threshold value used.[304]

Other Cells

It is difficult to identify the origin of cells that are neither leukocytes nor red blood cells without special stains. Most common are probably squamous epithelial cells. These are shed from the bladder or urethra and are rarely pathologic. Renal tubular cells may appear whenever there has been tubular damage. Transitional epithelial cells are rare but may be seen with collecting system infection or neoplasias.

TABLE 23–5 Diseases Associated with Eosinophiluria[4]

Common
Acute allergic interstitial nephritis
Urinary tract infection (upper and lower tract)

Unusual
Acute tubular necrosis
Diabetic nephropathy
Focal segmental glomerulosclerosis
Polycystic kidney disease
Obstruction
Rapidly progressive glomerulonephritis
Postinfectious glomerulonephritis
IgA nephropathy
Acute cystitis
Acute prostatitis
Atheroembolic renal disease
Renal transplant rejection

From Silkensen JR, Kasiske BL: Laboratory assessment of renal disease: Clearance, urinalysis, and renal biopsy. In Brenner BM (ed): Brenner and Rector's The Kidney, 7th ed. Philadelphia, Saunders, 2004, p 1131.

Podocytes are normally absent or seen in small numbers in urine of normal individuals or those with inactive kidney disease. Although not visible utilizing a microscope, it is possible to visualize these podocytes in urine with immunofluoresence staining and after incubation with antihuman podocalyxin monoclonal antibody PHM-5 (Australian Monoclonal Development, Artarmon, New South Wales, Australia). The number of podocytes in urine or podocyturia increases with active kidney disease even before proteinuria appears and seems to improve with treatment.[305] The clinical utility of podocyturia is still being investigated and is not available in the clinical setting.

Urine Fat

In the absence of contamination, urinary lipids are almost always pathologic. Lipids are not usually seen as an isolated finding; however, their presence is rarely diagnostic. Lipids usually appear as free fat droplets or oval fat bodies. They have a distinctive appearance but are most readily seen under polarized light as doubly refractile "Maltese crosses." The Maltese cross is indicative of cholesterol and cholesterol esters. Maltese crosses can also be seen with some crystals and with starch granules. Neutral fat can be identified with special lipid stains. Urinary lipids are most commonly associated with proteinuria and are particularly common in patients with the nephrotic syndrome; they can also occur in the absence of heavy proteinuria.[4] Urine fat can also be seen in bone marrow or fat embolization syndromes.

Casts

Casts are cylindrical bodies severalfold larger than leukocytes and red blood cells. They form in distal tubules and collecting ducts where Tamm-Horsfall glycoprotein precipitates and entraps cells present in the urinary space.[4] Dehydration and the resulting increased tubular fluid concentration favor the formation of casts. An acid urine is also conducive to cast formation. Observing casts in the urine sediment often provides helpful diagnostic information. The differential diagnosis of cast formation is aided by first considering the type of cast found. A number of different types can be readily distinguished (Fig. 23–7; see also Color Plate IV).

Hyaline or finely granular casts can be seen in normal individuals and provide little useful diagnostic information. Cellular casts are generally more helpful. Red blood cell casts, for example, are distinctive and most often indicate glomerular disease. White blood cell casts are most commonly associated with interstitial nephritis but can also be seen in GN. Casts made up of renal tubular epithelial cells are always indicative of tubular damage. Coarsely granular casts often result from the degeneration of different cellular casts. They also contain protein aggregates. Thus, the presence of granular casts is usually pathologic, but nonspecific. Waxy casts are also nonspecific. They are believed to result from the degeneration of cellular casts and, thus, can be seen in a variety of kidney diseases. Pigmented casts usually derive their distinctive color from bilirubin or hemoglobin, and they are found in hyperbilirubinemia and hemoglobinuria, respectively. Fatty casts contain lipid and oval fat bodies (see preceding section).

Crystals and Other Elements

A large variety of crystals can be seen in the urine sediment. Most result from urine concentration, acidification, and ex vivo cooling of the sample and have little pathologic significance. However, an experienced observer can gain useful information in patients with microhematuria, nephrolithiasis, or toxin ingestion by examining a freshly voided, warm specimen.[306] For example, a large number of calcium oxalate crystals may suggest ethylene glycol toxicity when seen in the right clinical setting. Another example, a large number of uric acid crystals in the setting of acute renal failure suggest tumor lysis syndrome. Calcium oxalate crystals are uniform, small, double pyramids that often appear as crosses in a

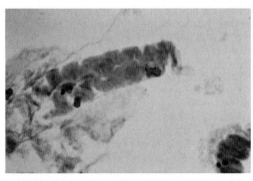

A

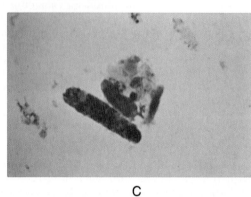

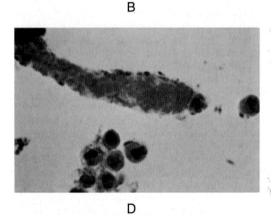

B

C

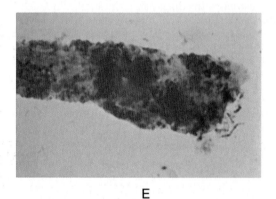

D

E

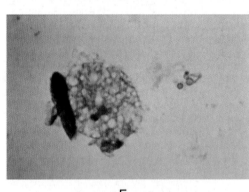

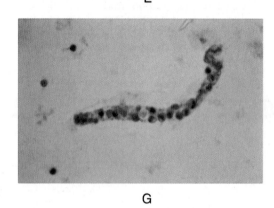

F

G

FIGURE 23-7 Abnormalities in urine sediment stained to enhance detail. **A,** Red blood cell cast (×900). **B,** Hyaline cast (×900). **C,** Hyaline and granular casts (×400). **D,** Coarse granular cast with adjacent white blood cells (×750). **E,** Fine and coarse granular cast (×900). **F,** Oval fat body with adjacent hyalin cast (×400). **G,** White blood cell cast (×400).

square. Calcium phosphate crystals, conversely, are usually narrow rectangular needles, often clumped in a flower-like configuration. Uric acid crystals form only in an acidic urine, which favors the conversion of relatively insoluble urate salts into insoluble uric acid. Calcium magnesium ammonium

pyrophosphate (so-called triple phosphate) crystals form domed rectangles that take on the appearance of coffin lids. These magnesium ammonium phosphate (struvite) and calcium carbonate-apatite stones occur when ammonia production is increased and the urine pH is elevated to decrease the solubility of phosphate. This combination of events occurs with urease-producing organisms in the urine, such as *Proteus* or *Klebsiella*.

Microorganisms

The most common cause of bacteria in the urine is contamination, particularly in specimens that have been improperly collected. The concomitant presence of leukocytes, however, suggests infection. Fungal elements can also be seen, especially in women. Like bacteria, fungi can be contaminants or pathogens. The most common protozoan seen in the urine is *Trichomonas vaginalis*. Urinary parasites are generally not seen in the urine sediment. In Africa and the Middle East, however, *Schistosoma haematobium* is common.

KIDNEY BIOPSY

Historical Perspective

The first biopsies of the kidney were likely surgical biopsies performed by the New York gynecologist and surgeon Michael Edelbohls. In 1904, he summarized his experience with therapeutic, surgical stripping of kidneys and mentions that "in a number of cases the diagnosis was confirmed by histological examination of kidney tissue." Percutaneous kidney biopsy was performed by Ball in 1934, using an aspiration technique to diagnose kidney tumors.[4] In the 1940s, kidney tissue was occasionally obtained accidentally during attempts to biopsy the liver. This development inspired Nils Awall, who began to biopsy the kidney in patients with kidney disease on a regular basis in 1944 (using x-ray guidance), although his results were not reported until 1952.[4]

Antonio Perez-Ara, a pathologist in Cuba, described the use of the cutting Vim-Silverman needle to obtain diagnostic kidney tissue in 1950. His work went largely unnoticed outside of Cuba and was unknown to Poul Iversen and Claus Brun when they began to conduct kidney biopsies in Copenhagen in 1949 using an aspiration needle. Their publication in 1951 brought kidney biopsy to the attention of clinicians everywhere. Biopsies were initially performed in the sitting position, but in the technique described by Robert Kark and Robert Muehrcke in 1954, patients were biopsied in the prone position, with the use of a Vim-Silverman needle and methods similar to those commonly used today. Their introduction of the Franklin-modified Vim-Silverman needle and the initial localization of the kidney with a small atraumatic needle resulted in a better core of tissue and an improved success rate.[4] Since these initial reports, the major advances that have been made center on improved localization of the kidney using ultrasound technology[307] and the introduction of more automated and smaller biopsy needles. Improved methods of tissue processing, staining, and the correlation of the light-microscopic findings with those of electron microscopy and immunofluorescence techniques[4] have led to dramatic increases in our knowledge of kidney disease.

Clinical Utility

A kidney biopsy may be obtained to help establish the diagnosis, suggest prognosis, or direct therapy. The information obtained from a biopsy is still largely qualitative. Although morphometric techniques have been developed to quantify histopathologic alterations, these techniques have been used almost exclusively in research.[308] Even in this setting, few data compare the reproducibility of different techniques to quantify kidney biopsy results.

Overall, relatively few studies have documented the reproducibility of the qualitative, clinical interpretation of kidney biopsy findings. Marcussen and co-workers[309] examined interobserver variation in the interpretation of biopsy specimens (light microscopy only) using the World Health Organization (WHO) classification of GN. One hundred biopsy specimens of a variety of glomerular diseases were circulated among members of a panel, who made their diagnosis without knowledge of the interpretation of other panel members. There was very good overall diagnostic agreement, with a κ statistic of 0.61. The highest κ values (best agreement) were reported for crescentic GN (0.81), endocapillary GN (0.79), and membranous GN (0.74), whereas the lowest values were for membranoproliferative GN (0.40) and diffuse mesangial proliferative GN (0.44).[309]

The reliability of the National Institutes of Heath histologic scoring system for lupus nephritis was shown to be only moderately reproducible in a nonreferral setting.[310] Probably as important, there is a virtual absence of data clearly indicating which specific renal histopathologic finding predicts progression of structural injury. In general, the relationship between the extent of tubulointerstitial and vascular damage is better correlated with the level of kidney function than is the extent of glomerular injury. A number of studies have inversely correlated the extent of tubulointerstitial damage and fibrosis with kidney function in a variety of kidney diseases.[4] Because biopsy results are largely qualitative, the sensitivity and specificity of biopsy findings are often unclear.

Indications

Since the 1960s, the kidney biopsy has been most instrumental in the development of our understanding of the various types of kidney histopathologic abnormalities that contribute to abnormalities of the urinary sediment. The use of this technique has not only improved our diagnostic acumen but also given new insights into the pathogenesis of human kidney disease. However, as our sophistication and knowledge of the various forms of kidney disease has expanded, questions regarding the routine use of kidney biopsy in all patients with clinical evidence of kidney disease have been articulated.

Paone and Meyer[311] conducted a retrospective evaluation to determine whether kidney biopsy findings influenced therapeutic judgments. Although a definite or probable diagnosis was ascertained in 77% of patients, therapy was modified in only 19%. In large part, changes in therapy based on biopsy findings were confined to patients with proteinuria, with little change seen in those with hematuria. Although therapy was also unaltered in those with acute or chronic kidney disease, it should be underscored that therapy for these indications is relatively nonspecific. Similarly, Cohen and associates,[312] Turner and colleagues,[313] and Shah and co-workers[314] reported the influence of the kidney histopathology results on physicians' judgments regarding diagnosis, prognosis, and treatment in patients with diverse types of kidney disease. They reported changes in judgments in more than one half of patients as a result of information gained directly from the biopsy results. Likewise, Richards and co-workers[315] conducted a prospective study of 276 biopsies and found that biopsy results altered management in 42% of cases. On the other hand, Whiting-O'Keefe and co-workers[316] retrospectively analyzed the case histories of 30 patients who underwent kidney biopsy for severe lupus nephritis. Knowledge of the kidney biopsy failed to improve predictive accuracy scores of estimates of future serum creatinine levels, urine protein levels, renal death, and long-term immunosuppressive therapy.

Questions about the role of kidney biopsy in patients with idiopathic nephrotic syndrome have also emerged.[317,318] Levey and colleagues[319] reported results of a decision analysis suggesting that initial therapy based on clinical data alone could avoid the use of kidney biopsy in all patients. However,

748

decision analysis cannot replace prospective trials, and additional studies detailing patient outcomes, quality of life, and complications of therapeutic misadventures are needed before biopsy is abandoned as a diagnostic technique in these patients. It is also important to recognize that kidney biopsy is relatively safe and provides a specific diagnosis that may quickly and efficiently define a therapeutic strategy.

At present, there are no specific clinical indications that mandate the use of kidney biopsy, and its utility must be taken in the context of the patients' needs in terms of diagnosis, prognosis, and therapy. Nonetheless, there are clinical settings in which kidney biopsy is likely to be most useful. In the following section, we provide some guidelines that may be used in defining the relative clinical value of a kidney biopsy.

Nephrotic Syndrome

The causes of the nephrotic syndrome are numerous, and the laboratory parameters consistent with this diagnosis are discussed elsewhere. The nephrotic syndrome is either primary or secondary, the latter reflecting either a systemic disease or drug toxicity. Once the secondary forms of the nephrotic syndrome are excluded by appropriate clinical or laboratory data, there remains a group of patients with idiopathic nephrotic syndrome who can be precisely differentiated only by kidney biopsy. This latter category includes minimal change glomerulopathy, focal glomerulosclerosis, and membranous nephropathy. The distribution of these entities is quite different in adults and children, and as a result, different approaches have emerged. In children with the idiopathic nephrotic syndrome, a kidney biopsy is generally not performed initially, and empirical steroid therapy is initiated. This is in large part due to the fact that minimal change glomerulopathy, which is sensitive to steroid therapy, accounts for nearly 80% of cases of the syndrome in children.[4] However, in children who have no response to an appropriate course of steroids or have frequent relapses over a year, a kidney biopsy may become indicated. This would allow specific diagnosis and the potential for tailoring therapy with more potent immunosuppressive therapy.

In the adult patient, minimal change disease is responsible for 20% to 25% of cases of idiopathic nephrotic syndrome; thus, a propensity for performance of a kidney biopsy has traditionally been followed.[311,320] Therefore, empirical treatment of adults, in the absence of a biopsy diagnosis in idiopathic nephrotic syndrome, would expose a high proportion of patients to the adverse effects of corticosteroids unnecessarily. The goals for therapy as well as disease-specific protocols have evolved over the past few years, making the rationale for an initial biopsy more compelling. Richards and colleagues[315] reported that a biopsy for nephrotic range proteinuria influenced management in 24 out of 28 cases (86%) that were biopsied.

In patients with evidence of elevated levels of serum or urinary light chains in association with proteinuria in the range seen in nephrotic syndrome, a kidney biopsy frequently helps to distinguish amyloidosis from light chain glomerulopathy. In the presence or absence of multiple myeloma, the detection of light chain deposits in the kidney biopsy specimen appears to have prognostic and therapeutic implications.[321]

Systemic Lupus Erythematosus

The diagnosis of SLE is generally established using a variety of clinical and laboratory criteria. Rarely, the diagnosis is first suggested by kidney biopsy findings, particularly when the laboratory test results are negative. However, the yield of kidney biopsy in this clinical situation is low and the information obtained that would affect therapy is relatively low. Kidney involvement in SLE correlates with overall prognosis;

the more severe the kidney involvement, the worse the prognosis.[4]

In SLE, the principal glomerular lesion is cellular proliferation, which is variably present in amount and distribution. These changes have most frequently formed the basis for a number of histologic classification schema,[4] the WHO classification being the most commonly used today. The WHO class is correlated with clinical features such as hypertension, urinary sediment, extent of proteinuria, and reduction in GFR as well as with prognosis. In this system, patients with minimal proliferative glomerular changes (class I) have the best prognosis, whereas those with diffuse proliferative changes (class IV) have the worst prognosis.[322] Hence, the treatment is different depending on the biopsy changes. When the types of SLE changes are not clinically evident, a renal biopsy is helpful.

In patients with diffuse proliferative glomerular changes, immunosuppressive therapy with high-dose prednisone has consistently demonstrated improved survival of kidney and patient, although no prospective trial has been performed.[4] It has been proposed that the biopsy results in this form of SLE may help in the selection of the dose and route of administration of steroids as well as the selection of other immunosuppressive drugs. However, this proposition has not been proved in controlled trials. Some,[323,324] but not all,[310,325,326] have found the morphologic findings of activity, chronicity of glomerular and interstitial lesions, or both are related to the risk of subsequent progression of kidney disease in a manner independent of their correlation with clinical indicators of severity of kidney disease. In addition, the intraobserver variability when these approaches are used in routine clinical settings makes their utility marginal at best.[310]

Currently, it appears that the use of more sophisticated quantitative analysis adds little to selection of therapy or prognosticating outcomes. Chagnac and co-workers[327] have performed morphometric studies of glomerular capillary surface area on serial biopsy specimens obtained from SLE patients. These investigators reported evidence of progressive loss of glomerular capillary surface area with no or minimal changes in proteinuria, GFR, or serum creatinine value. These studies would suggest that the kidney biopsy findings may be a more sensitive index of progression than clinical features alone. However, the lack of standardization of morphometric analysis and the time to perform these studies does not allow for their routine histopathologic use.

Rapidly Progressive Glomerulonephritis

In patients with abnormalities of the urinary sediment consistent with a nephritic syndrome and rapidly progressive loss of kidney function, a kidney biopsy may provide invaluable information. Commonly, patients with this syndrome demonstrate the histologic presence of crescents. Ellis is credited with first noting the relationship between the loss of kidney function and the presence of glomerular crescents.[4] Although the number of glomeruli with crescents is variable, most clinical studies that have evaluated outcomes report a poor prognosis when the proportion of glomeruli with circumferential crescents exceed 50%.[328] The pathogenesis of rapidly progressive-cresenteric GN is diverse and is most commonly seen with three types of immunologic injury: antiglomerular basement membrane antibody with or without pulmonary hemorrhage (Goodpasture's syndrome), immune complex disease, and the so-called pauci-immune GN. This last entity is the most frequently diagnosed disease, particularly when systemic illnesses are excluded. Recognition of the association between antineutrophilic cytoplasmic antibodies, systemic vasculitic syndromes, and pauci-immune cresenteric GN has provided new and important insights in the understanding of the pathogenesis of this disease as well as therapeutic strategies that are clinically useful.[329] Nonethe-

CH 23

less, the kidney biopsy still may provide important information about the severity of disease and, thus, has clinical management implications.

Post-Transplantation Biopsy

Biopsy of the transplanted kidney has been established as an important diagnostic and therapeutic technique in the management of patients in whom rejection of the kidney allograft is suspected. It has become particularly important in an era when the differential diagnosis of decreased allograft function includes nephrotoxicity from the immunosuppressive drugs that are most commonly used.[330] Although a variety of histologic techniques, including fine-needle aspiration cytology, have been used, the standard needle-core biopsy processed for conventional, light microscopic histology remains the most reliable technique for diagnosis in the setting of kidney allograft dysfunction.[331] Several classification systems have been proposed to standardize the interpretation of kidney allograft biopsy specimens, but the Banff classification scheme has been most widely adopted.[332] Studies have documented that the interpretation of allograft biopsy findings using the Banff classification system is relatively reproducible and correlates with clinical outcomes.[333] Studies have also examined the amount of tissue necessary to reach concordance in the interpretation of kidney allograft biopsy findings. For example, Sorof and associates[334] found that two cores (obtained with a 15-gauge needle) were needed to avoid missing moderate or severe acute rejection in almost 10% of cases.

Kidney allograft biopsy is generally safe. Most clinicians now carry out the procedure using spring-loaded, automated biopsy needles under direct ultrasound visualization. The principle complication is bleeding. In one study, risk factors for bleeding included biopsy within 30 days of transplantation and the use of a 14-gauge Vim-Silverman rather than an 18-gauge automated needle.[335] Other investigators have confirmed the safety and efficacy of allograft biopsy using 18-gauge, automated needles under direct ultrasound visualization.[336] Although the most common diagnosis resulting from kidney allograft biopsy is acute rejection, biopsies also play a role in differentiating between acute cellular and acute humoral rejection and also in determining the cause of proteinuria and chronic allograft dysfunction. Recurrence of the original glomerulopathy in the transplanted kidney has been observed with a variety of kidney diseases. Other than focal glomerulosclerosis, most of the other recurrent glomerulopathies appear to have little functional impact outcome after transplantation.[4] Biopsy findings, particularly the amount of interstitial fibrosis,[337] are useful in predicting the long-term function of the transplanted kidney independent of the underlying cause of kidney damage.

Asymptomatic Urinary Abnormalities

The finding of small quantities of isolated proteinuria is a common clinical problem. In a survey of 68,000 army recruits without a history of hypertension or kidney disease, only 1% were found to have isolated proteinuria.[338] Of the 45 patients who underwent biopsy, 33 (73%) had mild mesangial proliferation with or without glomerulosclerosis. If the proteinuria was intermittent or postural, significant glomerular lesions were infrequent. No lesion was serious enough to warrant therapy. Although no changes in kidney function were noted over a 3-year interval in these patients, longer-term follow-up has not been reported. At present, there is no evidence that a kidney biopsy provides more prognostic information than evaluation of the pattern of proteinuria and routine clinical follow-up.

Isolated hematuria occurs as commonly as isolated proteinuria.[339] Frequently, routine evaluation of the urinary tract will indicate the nonrenal source of the hematuria and kidney biopsy is not necessary. However, kidney biopsy has been proposed as an accurate and direct way to identify the cause of isolated hematuria. Kidney biopsy is abnormal in over 75% of patients with hematuria in whom proteinuria or reduced kidney function is present.[340] In this setting, IgA nephropathy is the most common diagnosis, although hereditary nephritis or thinning of the glomerular basement membrane is also seen.[340] Proven, effective, and specific therapies for such entities as IgA nephropathy have not as yet been developed, and thus, the utility of the biopsy to guide therapy has not been shown. Although a number of histopathologic changes predict renal outcomes, several clinical features such as reduced kidney function, proteinuria, and hypertension accurately predict a poor prognosis.[341] At present, additional therapeutic or prognostic information is not gained from a kidney biopsy. Richards and colleagues[315] reported in a study of 276 native kidney biopsies that the renal biopsies changed management in only 1 out of 36 cases of isolated hematuria. However, for some patients, the specific diagnosis may be useful for genetic counseling purposes such as in Alport's syndrome.

Other Indications

A kidney biopsy does not seem indicated in patients with chronic, end-stage renal failure, and biopsy in this setting is probably associated with an increased risk of complications. In patients with acute kidney injury, in whom no obvious cause for rapid deterioration in kidney function can be found, kidney biopsy may be indicated.[4] Biopsy in this setting appears valuable mostly for those few patients with acute allergic interstitial nephritis in whom a course of corticosteroids may be of benefit.

Cholesterol embolic acute renal failure without the typical clinical presentation has been more commonly observed in older patients with atherosclerotic disease, presenting a diagnostic challenge. Because some of these patients may regain kidney function after prolonged intervals, closer attention to kidney function while on dialysis is appropriate. However, a clear-cut case for the utility of a kidney biopsy for diagnosis, prognosis, or therapy has not been made in patients with acute kidney injury.[4]

Occasionally, patients with diabetes mellitus may be considered for kidney biopsy, particularly when they present with severe proteinuria in the absence of other manifestations of diabetic microvascular disease or when the duration of the disease is short. In this setting, other kidney diseases, such as idiopathic nephrotic syndrome, can be seen.[4]

Patient Preparation

Before biopsy, the patient should be evaluated for conditions that may increase the risk or worsen consequences of complications. Postbiopsy bleeding can necessitate nephrectomy, and the consequences of this complication are obviously greater in patients with only one functioning kidney. It was once believed that the presence of a solitary (native) kidney was an absolute contraindication to kidney biopsy.[342] However, the use of 18-gauge automated needles and direct ultrasound visualization have reduced the risk, and biopsy of a solitary kidney is no longer considered to be contraindicated.[343] Most clinicians consider the biopsy of a very small, shrunken kidney to be ill advised. In any case, a practical approach is to first visualize both kidneys with ultrasonography. If the kidneys are reasonable in size, the operator can proceed directly to biopsy under direct ultrasonographic guidance. This approach obviates the need for a second radiologic procedure to assess the size and number of kidneys.

Because bleeding is the major complication of biopsy, most clinicians obtain a coagulation profile. A platelet count, prothrombin time, and partial thromboplastin time (and, possibly, a bleeding time if the patient is uremic) can be used to screen for bleeding tendencies. Although the exact correlation between abnormalities in these coagulation screening tests and postbiopsy bleeding is not known, prudence would dictate that biopsies should be carried out with great reluctance in patients with coagulation abnormalities. Probably the most commonly encountered abnormality is a prolonged bleeding time caused by platelet dysfunction in patients who are uremic. A number of steps can be taken to correct the prolonged bleeding time associated with uremia. They include the use of fresh frozen plasma, arginine vasopressin, and estrogens.[344] If the patient is acutely uremic, hemodialysis is usually of value in improving the coagulopathy. Salicylates or nonsteriodal anti-inflammatory drugs should be discontinued, if possible, at least 1 to 2 weeks after the procedure.[345] For patients with bleeding diathesis or those undergoing anticoagulation for a thromboembolic disorder, the accepted approach is not clear. Guidelines devised for the management of anticoagulated patients before and after elective surgery are of uncertain relevance to a kidney biopsy, a closed procedure in which the level of hemostasis cannot be determined.[346] Suspending anticoagulation or treating the diathesis is feasible, although many investigators recommend open biopsy with direct visualization of the kidney.[347] Alternatively, transjugular kidney biopsy has been successfully performed in some institutions,[348] although some centers have reported significant rates of bleeding owing to capsular perforation.[348] Significant anemia that would substantially increase risk of bleeding should be corrected before a kidney biopsy is performed.

Uncontrolled hypertension can raise the risk of bleeding after biopsy.[349] Therefore, it is advisable to control blood pressure before the procedure is undertaken. Having the patient void immediately before the biopsy may help reduce the risk of inadvertently puncturing the bladder. Because a major complication of biopsy can require surgical intervention, it may be advisable to carry out the procedure with the patient fasting in order to reduce the potential risks of vomiting and aspiration during anesthesia induction. However, these risks must be weighed against the risk of hypoglycemia in diabetic patients and the rarity of complications requiring surgical intervention.

With the use of direct ultrasound visualization and 18-gauge, automated needles, the complication rate from biopsy has been reduced.[350,351] Indeed, it is now possible to perform biopsies safely in an outpatient setting,[351,352] making the procedure more convenient for both patients and clinicians and greatly reducing cost.

Localization

There are few controlled studies comparing the use of different radiographic localization techniques for percutaneous kidney biopsy. Fluoroscopy was used in the past, but adequate imaging of the kidneys often requires intravenous administration of contrast media, which can be nephrotoxic. CT can be used, but the inability to guide the biopsy needle in "real time" makes the procedure somewhat cumbersome.[353] The greatest value of CT is likely in morbidly obese patients,[354] a group in whom the use of ultrasonography is sometimes limited. Ultrasound with continuous visualization of the biopsy needle, however, usually provides adequate imaging[355] and is less costly than CT. It appears that newer techniques using direct ultrasonographic guidance are safer than older techniques; however, ultrasonographic guidance and automated needle devises were introduced simultaneously, making it difficult to determine which of these advances resulted in the apparent reduction in the rate of complications.[356]

Needle Selection

In the past, the Tru-Cut (Travenol) and the Franklin-modified Vim-Silverman needles were most commonly used to perform percutaneous kidney biopsies. Automated, spring-loaded biopsy devices have been developed.[356] Some studies, although largely uncontrolled, have suggested that the new automated devices may reduce the incidence of postbiopsy bleeding without reducing the chances of obtaining adequate tissue.[357] Automated devices have led to significantly larger sample sizes than with manual devices using comparable-gauged needles.[345] A prospective, randomized trial involving 100 consecutive allograft biopsy procedures showed a correlation between needle gauge and sample size, with 14-gauge needles providing the largest number of glomeruli per core and the greatest diagnostic success compared with 16-gauge and 18-gauge needles. The complication rates of the three groups were not significantly different, although the 14-gauge needle was associated with more pain.[358]

Processing of the Specimen

Proper interpretation of a kidney biopsy specimen optimally requires examination by light, immunofluorescence, and electron microscopy. Immediate placement of tissue in appropriate fixatives is important to obtain the best histologic-stained material. The availability of a pathologist experienced in processing kidney specimens is particularly helpful in preparing adequate kidney tissue. In general, obtaining two cores of cortical tissue usually provides sufficient material for all examinations. Each core is divided longitudinally with a razor blade in order to obtain glomeruli in each section. The majority of the tissue is processed for light microscopy, and the remainder for immunofluorescence and electron microscopy. If difficulty is encountered in obtaining sufficient tissue cores, the small fragments can be processed for electron microscopy, and the remainder processed for immunofluorescence microscopy.

Numerous fixatives are available for histologic preparation, and tissue for light microscopy is usually fixed in paraffin or plastic and cut in 2-μm-thick sections, which are routinely stained with hematoxylin and eosin, a silver methenamine stain, and a periodic acid–Schiff or trichrome stain. If amyloidosis is suspected, Congo red and thioflavin T stains are performed. Tissue for immunofluorescence microscopy is placed in pre-cooled isopentane and snap frozen in liquid nitrogen. Frozen sections are cut 4 μm thick and typically stained with fluoresceinated antisera against IgG, immunoglobulin M (IgM), IgA, complement components C3 and C4, fibrin/fibrinogen, and albumin. When indicated, antibodies for specific immunoglobulin light chains or specific cell surface markers can be used. The complement-split product C4d has been found to be an independent predictor of kidney allograft injury and a specific marker for antibody-dependent allograft injury.[359]

For electron microscopic studies, small (1-μm) pieces of the biopsy specimen are fixed in buffered glutaraldehyde or other suitable fixatives, dehydrated in graded alcohols, embedded in plastic, and sectioned. Ultrathin sections are stained with uranyl acetate and lead citrate and examined with a transmission electron microscope. Electron microscopy provides useful diagnostic information in nearly one half of all native kidney biopsy specimens.[360] However, to reduce cost, it is reasonable to set aside tissue for electron microscopy until the light-microscopic evaluation of tissue has been completed.

Complications

The most common complication of a kidney biopsy is hematuria. Microscopic hematuria occurs virtually in all patients, whereas gross hematuria occurs in less than 10% of patients. Gross hematuria has also been associated with intrarenal arteriovenous fistulas.[361] The presence of uncontrolled hypertension, anticoagulation, or azotemia increases the risk for hematuria.[362] Hematuria usually resolves spontaneously in 48 to 72 hours, although in approximately 0.5 % of patients, hematuria persists for 2 to 3 weeks.[342,361] Occasionally, gross hematuria occurs days after the biopsy, but it usually resolves within a few days with rest.[342] Transfusions are necessary in 0.1% to 3% of patients.[342] Surgery for persistent bleeding is required in less than 0.3% of patients.[342,361]

Perinephric hematomas occur commonly. In patients who are evaluated by CT immediately after kidney biopsy, hematomas were detected in 57% to 85% of patients.[363,364] Most of these are clinically occult, perhaps associated with only a fall in hemoglobin.[342] In 1% to 2% of patients, perinephric hematoma is manifested as flank pain and swelling associated with signs of volume contraction and a decrease in hematocrit. Rarely, these hematomas can become infected, requiring antibiotic therapy and surgical drainage,[361] and rarely, they lead to chronic hypertension owing to pressure-induced ischemia from a large subcapsular hematoma producing a persistent activation of the renin-angiotensin system.[365]

Less common complications of renal biopsy include arteriovenous fistulas, aneurysms, and infections. Arteriovenous fistulas can be demonstrated by arteriography in 15% to 18% of patients. They are usually clinically silent, and the majority spontaneously resolve in 2 years.[4] Postbiopsy aneurysms have been reported in less than 1% of patients.[342] Infections are unusual except in the presence of pyelonephritis. The development of sepsis and bacteremia after kidney biopsy has been reported.[4]

A number of unusual complications of kidney biopsy have been reported including ileus, lacerations of other abdominal organs, pneumothorax, ureteral obstruction, and dissemination of carcinoma. The mortality associated with 14,492 reported kidney biopsies is 0.12%,[361] although only 1 death have been reported since 1980.[345]

References

1. Sarnak MJ, Levey AS, Schoolwerth AC, et al: Kidney disease as a risk factor for development of cardiovascular disease: A statement from the American Heart Association Councils on Kidney in Cardiovascular Disease, High Blood Pressure Research, Clinical Cardiology, and Epidemiology and Prevention. Hypertension 42:1050–1065, 2003.
2. Gerstein HC, Mann JF, Yi Q, et al: Albuminuria and risk of cardiovascular events, death, and heart failure in diabetic and nondiabetic individuals. JAMA 286:421–426, 2001.
3. National Kidney Foundation Kidney: K/DOQI Clinical Practice Guidelines for Chronic Kidney Disease: Evaluation, classification and stratification. Am J Kidney Dis 39(suppl 1):S1–S266, 2002.
4. Silkensen, JR, Kasiske BL: Laboratory assessment of renal disease: Clearance, urinalysis, and renal biopsy. In Brenner BM (ed): Brenner and Rector's The Kidney, 7th ed. Philadelphia, Saunders, 2004, pp 1107–1150.
5. Young DS: Effects of Drugs on Clinical Laboratory Tests, 3rd ed. Washington, DC, American Association for Clinical Chemistry Press, 1990, p 3-356-3-357.
6. Young DS: Effects of Drugs on Clinical Laboratory Tests, 3rd ed. Washington, DC, American Association for Clinical Chemistry Press, 1990, p 3–359.
7. Levey AS, Berg RL, Gassman JJ, et al: Creatinine filtration, secretion and excretion during progressive renal disease. Kidney Int 36(suppl 27):S-73–S-80, 1989.
8. Coresh J, Toto RD, Kirk KA, et al: Creatinine clearance as a measure of GFR in screenees for the African-American Study of Kidney Disease and Hypertension pilot study. Am J Kidney Dis 32:32–42, 1998.
9. Shemesh O, Golbetz H, Kriss JP, Myers BD: Limitations of creatinine as a filtration marker in glomerulopathic patients. Kidney Int 28:830–838, 1985.
10. Mitch WE, Collier VU, Walser M: Creatinine metabolism in chronic renal failure. Clin Sci 58:327–335, 1980.
11. Hankins DA, Babb AL, Uvelli DA, Scribner BH: Creatinine degradation: I: The kinetics of creatinine removal in patients with chronic kidney disease. Int J Artif Organs 4:35–39, 1981.
12. Dunn SR, Gabuzda GM, Superdock KR, et al: Induction of creatininase activity in chronic renal failure: Timing of creatinine degradation and effect of antibiotics. Am J Kidney Dis 29:72–77, 1997.
13. Bonsnes RW, Taussky HH: On the colorimetric determination of creatinine by Jaffé reaction. J Biol Chem 158:581–591, 1945.
14. Hare RS: Endogenous creatinine in serum and urine. Proc Soc Exp Biol Med 74:148, 1950.
15. Mandel EE, Jones FL: Studies in nonprotein nitrogen: III. Evaluation of methods measuring creatinine. J Lab Clin Med 41:323–334, 1953.
16. Fabiny DL, Ertingshausen G: Automated reaction-rate method for determination of serum creatinine with the Centrichem. Clin Chem 17:696–700, 1971.
17. Toffaletti J, Blosser N, Hall T, et al: An automated dry-slid enzymatic method evaluated for measurement of creatinine in serum. Clin Chem 29:684–687, 1983.
18. Jacobs DS, De Mott WR, Strobel SL, Fody EP: Chemistry. In Jacobs DS, Kasten BL, De Mott WR, Wolfson WL (eds): Laboratory Test Handbook. Baltimore, Williams & Wilkins, 1990, pp 171–172.
19. Miller WG, Myers GL, Ashwood ER, et al: Creatinine measurement: State of the art in accuracy and interlaboratory harmonization. Arch Pathol Lab Med 129:297–304, 2005.
20. Swain RR, Briggs SL: Positive interference with the Jaffé reaction by cephalosporin antibiotics. Clin Chem 23:1340–1342, 1977.
21. Durham SR, Bignell AHC, Wise R: Interference of cefoxitin in the creatinine estimation and its clinical relevance. J Clin Pathol 32:1148–1151, 1979.
22. Saah AJ, Koch TR, Drusano GL: Cefoxitin falsely elevates creatinine levels. JAMA 247:205–206, 1982.
23. Young DS: Effects of Drugs on Clinical Laboratory Tests, 3rd ed. Washington, DC, American Association of Clinical Chemistry Press, 1990, pp 3–128.
24. Doolan PD, Alpen EL, Theil GB: A clinical appraisal of the plasma concentration and endogenous clearance of creatinine. Am J Med 32:65–79, 1962.
25. Gerard SK, Khayam-Bashi H: Characterization of creatinine error in ketotic patients: A prospective comparison of alkaline picrate methods with an enzymatic method. Am J Clin Pathol 84:659–664, 1985.
26. Osberg IM, Hammond KB: A solution to the problem of bilirubin interference with the kinetic Jaffé method for serum creatinine. Clin Chem 24:1196–1197, 1978.
27. Kasiske BL: Creatinine excretion after renal transplantation. Transplantation 48:424–428, 1989.
28. Payne RB: Creatinine clearance: A redundant clinical investigation. Ann Clin Biochem 23:243–250, 1986.
29. DeSanto NG, Coppola S, Anastasio P, et al: Predicted creatinine clearance to assess glomerular filtration rate in chronic renal disease in humans. Am J Nephrol 11:181–185, 1991.
30. Fuller NJ, Elia M: Factors influencing the production of creatinine: Implications for the determination and interpretation of urinary creatinine and creatine in man. Clin Chim Acta 175:199–210, 1988.
31. van Acker BAC, Koomen GCM, Koopman MG, et al: Discrepancy between circadian rhythms of inulin and creatinine clearance. J Lab Clin Med 120:400–410, 1992.
32. Morgan DB, Dillon S, Payne RB: The assessment of glomerular function: Creatinine clearance or plasma creatinine? Postgrad Med J 54:302–310, 1978.
33. Rosano TG, Brown HH: Analytical and biological variability of serum creatinine and creatinine clearance: Implications for clinical interpretation. Clin Chem 28:2330–2331, 1982.
34. Bröchner-Mortensen J, Rödbro P: Selection of routine method for determination of glomerular filtration rate in adult patients. Scand J Clin Lab Invest 36:35–43, 1976.
35. Roubenoff R, Drew H, Moyer M, et al: Oral cimetidine improves the accuracy and precision of creatinine clearance in lupus nephritis. Ann Intern Med 113:501–506, 1990.
36. van Acker BAC, Koomen GCM, Koopman MG, et al: Creatinine clearance during cimetidine administration for measurement of glomerular filtration rate. Lancet 340:1326–1329, 1992
37. Richter JM, Colditz GA, Huse DM, et al: Cimetidine and adverse reactions: A meta-analysis of randomized clinical trials of short-term therapy. Am J Med 87:278–284, 1989.
38. Jelliffe RW, Jelliffe SM: Estimation of creatinine clearance from changing serum-creatinine levels. Lancet 2:710, 1971.
39. Mawer GE, Knowles BR, Lucas SB, Stirland RM: Computer-assisted dosing of kanamycin for patients with renal insufficiency. Lancet 1:12–14, 1972.
40. Jelliffe RW: Creatinine clearance: Bedside estimate. Ann Intern Med 79:604, 1973.
41. Kampmann J, Siersbæk-Nielson K, Kristensen M, Mølholm-Hansen J: Rapid evaluation of creatinine clearance. Acta Med Scand 196:517–520, 1974.
42. Cockcroft DW, Gault MH: Prediction of creatinine clearance from serum creatinine. Nephron 16:31–41, 1976.
43. Hull JH, Hak LJ, Koch GG, et al: Influence of range of renal function and liver disease on predictability of creatinine clearance. Clin Pharmacol Ther 29:516–521, 1981.
44. Sawyer WT, Canaday BR, Poe TE, et al: A multicenter evaluation of variables affecting the predictability of creatinine clearance. Am J Clin Pathol 78:832–838, 1982.
45. Taylor GO, Bamgboye EA, Oyediran ABOO, Longe O: Serum creatinine and prediction formulae for creatinine clearance. Afr J Med Sci 11:175–181, 1982.
46. Bjornsson TD, Cocchetto DM, McGowan FX, et al: Nomogram for estimating creatinine clearance. Clin Pharmacokinet 8:365–369, 1983.
47. Rolin HA, III, Hall PM, Wei R: Inaccuracy of estimated creatinine clearance for prediction of iothalamate glomerular filtration rate. Am J Kidney Dis 4:48–54, 1984.
48. Gates GF: Creatinine clearance estimation from serum creatinine values: An analysis of three mathematical models of glomerular function. Am J Kidney Dis 5:199–205, 1985.
49. Sinton TJ, De Leacy EA, Cowley DM: Comparison of 51Cr EDTA clearance with formulae in the measurement of glomerular filtration rate. Pathology 18:445–447, 1986.
50. Trollfors B, Alestig K, Jagenburg R: Prediction of glomerular filtration rate from serum creatinine, age, sex and body weight. Acta Med Scand 221:495–498, 1987.
51. Gault MH, Longerich LL, Harnett JD, Wesolowski C: Predicting glomerular function from adjusted serum creatinine. Nephron 62:249–256, 1992.

52. Walser M, Drew HH, Guldan JL: Prediction of glomerular filtration rate from serum creatinine concentration in advanced chronic renal failure. Kidney Int 44:1145–1148, 1993.
53. Levey AS, Bosch JP, Lewis JB, et al: A more accurate method to estimate glomerular filtration rate from serum creatinine: A new prediction equation. Modification of Diet in Renal Disease Study Group. Ann Intern Med 130:461–470, 1999.
54. Levey AS: Use of glomerular filtration rate measurements to assess the progression of renal disease. Semin Nephrol 9:370–379, 1989.
55. Coresh J, Astor BC, McQuillan G, et al: Calibration and random variation of the serum creatinine assay as critical elements of using equations to estimate glomerular filtration rate. Am J Kidney Dis 39:920–929, 2002.
56. Waz WR, Feld LG, Quattrin T: Serum creatinine, height, and weight do not predict glomerular filtration rate in children with IDDM. Diabetes Care 16:1067–1070, 1993.
57. Vervoort G, Willems HL, Wetzels JF: Assessment of glomerular filtration rate in healthy subjects and normoalbuminuric diabetic patients: Validity of a new (MDRD) prediction equation. Nephrol Dial Transplant 17:1909–1913, 2002.
58. European Best Practice Guidelines for Haemodialysis (Part 1). Section I: Measurement of renal function, when refer and when to start dialysis. Nephrol Dial Transplant 17(suppl 7):7–15. 2002.
59. Lin J, Knight EL, Hogan ML, Singh AK: A comparison of prediction equations for estimating glomerular filtration rate in adults without kidney disease. J Am Soc Nephrol 14:2573–2580, 2003.
60. Li Z, Lew NL, Lazarus JM, Lowrie EG: Comparing the urea reduction ratio and the urea product as outcome-based measures of hemodialysis dose. Am J Kidney Dis 35:598–605, 2000.
61. Gaspari F, Ferrari S, Stucchi N, et al: Performance of different prediction equations for estimating renal function in kidney transplantation. Am J Transplant 4:1826–1835, 2004.
62. Simonsen O, Grubb A, Thysell H: The blood serum concentration of cystatin C (gamma-trace) as a measure of the glomerular filtration rate. Scand J Clin Lab Invest 45:97–101, 1985.
63. Grubb A: Diagnostic value of analysis of cystatin C and protein HC in biological fluids. Clin Nephrol 38(suppl 1):S20–S27, 1992.
64. Kyhse-Andersen J, Schmidt C, Nordin G, et al: Serum cystatin C, determined by a rapid, automated particle-enhanced turbidimetric method, is a better marker than serum creatinine for glomerular filtration rate. Clin Chem 40:1921–1926, 1994.
65. Newman DJ, Thakkar H, Edwsards RG, et al: Serum cystatin C measured by automated immunoassay: A more sensitive marker of changes in GFR than serum creatinine. Kidney Int 47:312–318, 1995.
66. Tian S, Kusano E, Ohara T, et al: Cystatin C measurement and its practical use in patients with various renal diseases. Clin Nephrol 48:104–108, 1997.
67. Randers E, Erlandsen EJ: Serum cystatin C as an endogenous marker of the renal function—A review. Clin Chem Lab Med 37:389–395, 1999.
68. Laterza OF, Price CP, Scott MG: Cystatin C: An improved estimator of glomerular filtration rate? Clin Chem 48:699–707, 2002.
69. Vinge E, Lindergard B, Nilsson-Ehle P, Grubb A: Relationships among serum cystatin C, serum creatinine, lean tissue mass and glomerular filtration rate in healthy adults. Scand J Clin Lab Invest 59:587–592, 1999.
70. Norlund L, Fex G, Lanke J, et al: Reference intervals for the glomerular filtration rate and cell-proliferation markers: Serum cystatin C and serum beta 2-microglobulin/cystatin C-ratio. Scand J Clin Lab Invest 57:463–470, 1997.
71. Knight EL, Verhave JC, Spiegelman D, et al: Factors influencing serum cystatin C levels other than renal function and the impact on renal function measurement. Kidney Int 65:1416–1421, 2004.
72. Rule AD, Bergstralh EJ, Slezak JM, et al: Glomerular filtration rate estimated by cystatin C among different clinical presentations. Kidney Int 69:399–405, 2006.
73. Bokenkamp A, Domanetzki M, Zinck R, et al: Reference values for cystatin C serum concentrations in children. Pediatr Nephrol 12:125–129, 1998.
74. Bokenkamp A, Domanetzki M, Zinck R, et al: Cystatin C—A new marker of glomerular filtration rate in children independent of age and height. Pediatrics 101:875–881, 1998.
75. Finney H, Newman DJ, Price CP: Adult reference ranges for serum cystatin C, creatinine and predicted creatinine clearance. Ann Clin Biochem 37(pt 1):49–59, 2000.
76. Tenstad O, Roald AB, Grubb A, Aukland K: Renal handling of radiolabelled human cystatin C in the rat. Scand J Clin Lab Invest 56:409–414, 1996.
77. Uchida K, Gotoh A: Measurement of cystatin-C and creatinine in urine. Clin Chim Acta 323:121–128, 2002.
78. Hayashi T, Nitta K, Hatano M, et al: The serum cystatin C concentration measured by particle-enhanced immunonephelometry is well correlated with inulin clearance in patients with various types of glomerulonephritis. Nephron 82:90–92, 1999.
79. Herget-Rosenthal S, Feldkamp T, Volbracht L, Kribben A: Measurement of urinary cystatin C by particle-enhanced nephelometric immunoassay: Precision, interferences, stability and reference range. Ann Clin Biochem 41:111–118, 2004.
80. Dharnidharka VR, Kwon C, Stevens G: Serum cystatin C is superior to serum creatinine as a marker of kidney function: A meta-analysis. Am J Kidney Dis 40:221–226, 2002.
81. Coll E, Botey A, Alvarez L, et al: Serum cystatin C as a new marker for noninvasive estimation of glomerular filtration rate and as a marker for early renal impairment. Am J Kidney Dis 36:29–34, 2000.
82. Stickle D, Cole B, Hock K, et al: Correlation of plasma concentrations of cystatin C and creatinine to inulin clearance in a pediatric population. Clin Chem 44:1334–1338, 1998.
83. Woitas RP, Stoffel-Wagner B, et al: Correlation of serum concentrations of cystatin C and creatinine to inulin clearance in liver cirrhosis. Clin Chem 46:712–715, 2000.
84. Donadio C, Lucchesi A, Ardini M, Giordani R: Cystatin C, beta 2-microglobulin, and retinol-binding protein as indicators of glomerular filtration rate: Comparison with plasma creatinine. J Pharm Biomed Anal 24:835–842, 2001.
85. Thomassen SA, Johannesen IL, Erlandsen EJ, et al: Serum cystatin C as a marker of the renal function in patients with spinal cord injury. Spinal Cord 40:524–528, 2002.
86. Mangge H, Liebmann P, Tanil H, et al: Cystatin C, an early indicator for incipient renal disease in rheumatoid arthritis. Clin Chim Acta 300:195–202, 2000.
87. Fliser D, Ritz E: Serum cystatin C concentration as a marker of renal dysfunction in the elderly. Am J Kidney Dis 37:79–83, 2001.
88. Shlipak MG, Sarnak MJ, Katz R, et al: Cystatin C and the risk of death and cardiovascular events among elderly persons. N Engl J Med 352:2049–2060, 2005.
89. Oddoze C, Morange S, Portugal H, et al: Cystatin C is not more sensitive than creatinine for detecting early renal impairment in patients with diabetes. Am J Kidney Dis 38:310–316, 2001.
90. Mussap M, Dalla VM, Fioretto P, et al: Cystatin C is a more sensitive marker than creatinine for the estimation of GFR in type 2 diabetic patients. Kidney Int 61:1453–1461, 2002.
91. Le Bricon T, Thervet E, Froissart M, et al: Plasma cystatin C is superior to 24-h creatinine clearance and plasma creatinine for estimation of glomerular filtration rate 3 months after kidney transplantation. Clin Chem 46:1206–1207, 2000.
92. Risch L, Herklotz R, Blumberg A, Huber AR: Effects of glucocorticoid immunosuppression on serum cystatin C concentrations in renal transplant patients. Clin Chem 47:2055–2059, 2001.
93. Bokenkamp A, Domanetzki M, Zinck R, et al: Cystatin C serum concentrations underestimate glomerular filtration rate in renal transplant recipients. Clin Chem 45:1866–1868, 1999.
94. Cimerman N, Brguljan PM, Krasovec M, et al: Serum cystatin C, a potent inhibitor of cysteine proteinases, is elevated in asthmatic patients. Clin Chim Acta 300:83–95, 2000.
95. Bjarnadottir M, Grubb A, Olafsson I: Promoter-mediated, dexamethasone-induced increase in cystatin C production by HeLa cells. Scand J Clin Lab Invest 55:617–623, 1995.
96. Risch L, Blumberg A, Huber A: Rapid and accurate assessment of glomerular filtration rate in patients with renal transplants using serum cystatin C. Nephrol Dial Transplant 14:1991–1996, 1999.
97. Bokenkamp A, van Wijk JA, Lentze MJ, Stoffel-Wagner B: Effect of corticosteroid therapy on serum cystatin C and beta2-microglobulin concentrations. Clin Chem 48:1123–1126, 2002.
98. Bokenkamp A, Ozden N, Dieterich C, et al: Cystatin C and creatinine after successful kidney transplantation in children. Clin Nephrol 52:371–376, 1999.
99. Keevil BG, Kilpatrick ES, Nichols SP, Maylor PW: Biological variation of cystatin C: Implications for the assessment of glomerular filtration rate. Clin Chem 44:1535–1539, 1998.
100. Deinum J, Derkx FH: Cystatin for estimation of glomerular filtration rate? Lancet 356:1624–1625, 2000.
101. Mussap M, Plebani M: Biochemistry and clinical role of human cystatin C. Crit Rev Clin Lab Sci 41:467–550, 2004.
102. Levey AS: Measurement of renal function in chronic renal disease. Kidney Int 38:167–184, 1990.
103. Schnurr E, Lahme W, Küppers H: Measurement of renal clearance of inulin and PAH in the steady state without urine collection. Clin Nephrol 13:26–29, 1980.
104. van Guldener C, Gans ROB, ter Wee PM: Constant infusion clearance is an inappropriate method for accurate assessment of an impaired glomerular filtration rate. Nephrol Dial Transplant 10:47–51, 1995.
105. van Acker BAC, Koomen GCM, Arisz L: Drawbacks of the constant-infusion technique for measurement of renal function. Am J Physiol 268(Renal Fluid Electrolyte Physiol 37):F543–F552, 1995.
106. Florijn KW, Barendregt JNM, Lentjex EGWM, et al: Glomerular filtration rate measurement by "single-shot" injection of inulin. Kidney Int 46:252–259, 1994.
107. Rosenbaum RW, Hruska KA, Anderson C, et al: Inulin: An inadequate marker of glomerular filtration rate in kidney donors and transplant recipients? Kidney Int 16:179–186, 1979.
108. Brochner-Mortensen J: Current status on assessment and measurement of glomerular filtration rate. Clin Physiol 5:1–17, 1984.
109. Pihl B: The single injection technique for determination of renal clearance. V. A comparison with the continuous infusion technique in the dog and in man. Scand J Urol Nephrol 8:147–154, 1974.
110. Carlsen JE, Moller ML, Lund JO, Trap-Jensen J: Comparison of four commercial Tc-99m(Sn)DTPA preparations used for the measurement of glomerular filtration rate: Concise communications. J Nucl Med 21:126–129, 1980.
111. Russell CD, Bischoff PG, Rowell KL, et al: Quality control of Tc-99m DTPA for measurement of glomerular filtration: Concise communication. J Nucl Med 24:722–727, 1983.
112. Sambataro M, Thomaseth K, Pacini G, et al: Plasma clearance rate of ^{51}Cr-EDTA provides a precise and convenient technique for measurement of glomerular filtration rate in diabetic humans. J Am Soc Nephrol 7:118–127, 1996.
113. Bianchi C, Donadio C, Tramonti G: Noninvasive methods for the measurement of total renal function. Nephron 28:53–57, 1981.
114. Gaspari F, Mosconi L, Viganò G, et al: Measurement of GFR with a single intravenous injection of nonradioactive iothalamate. Kidney Int 41:1081–1084, 1992.
115. Tauxe WN: Determination of glomerular filtration rate by single sample technique following injection of radioiodinated diatrizoate. J Nucl Med 27:45–50, 1986.
116. Tepe PG, Tauxe WN, Bagchi A, et al: Comparison of measurement of glomerular filtration rate by single sample, plasma disappearance slope/intercept and other methods. Eur J Nucl Med 13:28–31, 1987.
117. Rydström M, Tengström B, Cederquist I, Ahlmén J: Measurement of glomerular filtration rate by single-injection, single-sample techniques, using ^{51}Cr-EDTA or iohexol. Scand J Urol Nephrol 29:135–139, 1995.
118. Lundqvist S, Hietala SO, Groth S, Sjodin JG: Evaluation of single sample clearance calculations of 902 patients. A comparison of multiple and single sample techniques. Acta Radiol 38:68–72, 1997.

119. Gaspari F, Guerini E, Perico N, et al: Glomerular filtration rate determined from a single plasma sample after intravenous iohexol injection: Is it reliable? J Am Soc Nephrol 7:2689–2693, 1996.
120. Ham HR, Piepsz A: Feasibility of estimating glomerular filtration rate in children using single-sample adult technique. J Nucl Med 37:1808, 1996
121. Fleming JS, Waller DG: Feasibility of estimating glomerular filtration rate on children using single-sample adult technique. Letter. J Nucl Med 38:1665–1667, 1997.
122. Al-Uzri A, Holliday MA, Gambertoglio JG, et al: An accurate practical method for estimating GFR in clinical studies using a constant subcutaneous infusion. Kidney Int 41:1701–1706, 1992.
123. Sanger JJ, Kramer EL: Radionuclide quantitation of renal function. Urol Radiol 14:69–78, 1992.
124. Blaufox MD, Aurell M, Bubeck B, et al: Report of the Radionuclides in Nephrourology Committee on Renal Clearance. J Nucl Med 37:1883–1890, 1996.
125. Oriuchi N, Inoue T, Hayashi I, et al: Evaluation of gamma camera-based measurement of individual kidney function using iodine-123 orthoiodohippurate. Eur J Nucl Med 23:371–375, 1996.
126. Blomley MJK, Dawson P: Review article: The quantification of renal function with enhanced computed tomography. Br J Radiol 69:989–995, 1996.
127. Niendorf ER, Grist TM, Lee FT Jr, et al: Rapid in vivo measurement of single-kidney extraction fraction and glomerular filtration rate with MR imaging. Radiology 206:791–798, 1998.
128. Goates JJ, Morton KA, Whooten WW, et al: Comparison of methods for calculating glomerular filtration rate: Technetium-99m-DTPA scintigraphic analysis, protein-free and whole-plasma clearance of technetium-99m-DTPA and iodine-125-iothalamate clearance. J Nucl Med 31:424–429, 1990.
129. Rabito CA, Panico F, Rubin R, et al: Noninvasive, real-time monitoring of renal function during critical care. J Am Soc Nephrol 4:1421–1428, 1994.
130. Bianchi C, Bonadio M, Donadio C, et al: Measurement of glomerular filtration rate in man using DTPA-^{99m}Tc. Nephron 24:174–178, 1979.
131. Dubovsky EV, Russell CD: Quantitation of renal function with glomerular and tubular agents. Semin Nucl Med 12:308–329, 1982.
132. O'Reilly PH, Brooman PJC, Martin PJ, et al: Accuracy and reproducibility of a new contrast clearance method for the determination of glomerular filtration rate. BMJ 293:234–236, 1986.
133. O'Reilly PH, Jones DA, Farah NB: Measurement of the plasma clearance of urographic contrast media for the determination of glomerular filtration rate. J Urol 139:9–11, 1988.
134. Lewis R, Kerr N, Van Buren C, et al: Comparative evaluation of urographic contrast media, inulin, and ^{99m}Tc-DTPA clearance methods for determination of glomerular filtration rate in clinical transplantation. Transplantation 48:790–796, 1989.
135. Gaspari F, Perico N, Matalone M, et al: Precision of plasma clearance of iohexol for estimation of GFR in patients with renal disease. J Am Soc Nephrol 9:310–313, 1998.
136. Manske CL, Sprafka JM, Strony JT, Wang Y: Contrast nephropathy in azotemic diabetic patients undergoing coronary angiography. Am J Med 89:615–620, 1990.
137. Lundqvist S, Hietala S-O, Berglund C, Karp K: Simultaneous urography and determination of glomerular filtration rate. A comparison of total plasma clearances of iohexol and ^{51}Cr-EDTA in plegic patients. Acta Radiol 35:391–395, 1994.
138. Swan SK, Halstenson CE, Kasiske BL, Collins AJ: Determination of residual renal function with iohexol clearance in hemodialysis patients. Kidney Int 49:232–235, 1996.
139. Turner ST, Reilly SL: Fallacy of indexing renal and systemic hemodynamic measurements for body surface area. Am J Physiol 268(Regul Integr Comp Physiol 37):R978–R988, 1995.
140. Schmieder RE, Beil AH, Weihprecht H, Messerli FH: How should renal hemodynamic data be indexed in obesity? J Am Soc Nephrol 5:1709–1713, 1995.
141. Newman EV, Bordley J, Winternitz J: The interrelationships of glomerular filtration rate (mannitol clearance), extracellular fluid volume, surface area of the body, and plasma concentration of mannitol. Johns Hopkins Med J 75:253–268, 1944.
142. Peters AM, Allison H, Ussov WY: Simultaneous measurement of extracellular fluid distribution and renal function with a single injection of ^{99m}Tc DTPA. Nephrol Dial Transplant 10:1829–1833, 1995.
143. White AJ, Strydom WJ: Normalisation of glomerular filtration rate measurements. Eur J Nucl Med 18:385–390, 1991.
144. Kasiske BL, Umen AJ: The influence of age, sex, race, and body habitus on kidney weight in humans. Arch Pathol Lab Med 110:55–60, 1986.
145. King AJ, Levey AS: Dietary protein and renal function. J Am Soc Nephrol 3:1723–1737, 1993.
146. van Beek E, Houben AJHM, van Es PN, et al: Peripheral haemodynamics of renal function in relation to the menstrual cycle. Clin Sci 91:163–168, 1996.
147. Zuccalá A, Zucchelli P: Use and misuse of the renal functional reserve concept in clinical nephrology. Nephrol Dial Transplant 5:410–417, 1990.
148. Lautin EM, Freeman NJ, Schoenfeld AH, et al: Radiocontrast-associated renal dysfunction: Incidence and risk factors. AJR Am J Roentgenol 157:49, 1991.
149. D'Elia JA, Gleason RE, Alday M, et al.: Nephrotoxicity from angiographic contrast material. Am J Med 72:719, 1982.
150. Walser M, Drew HH, LaFrance ND: Creatinine measurements often yield false estimates of progression in chronic renal failure. Kidney Int 34:412–418, 1988.
151. Kasiske BL, Heim-Duthoy KL, Tortorice KL, Rao KV: The variable nature of chronic declines in renal allograft function. Transplantation 51:330–334, 1991.
152. Jones RH, Molitoris BA: A statistical method for determining the breakpoint of two lines. Anal Biochem 141:287–290, 1984.
153. Wright JP, Salzano S, Brown CB, El Nahas AM: Natural history of chronic renal failure: A reappraisal. Nephrol Dial Transplant 7:379–383, 1992.
154. Viberti GC, Bilous RW, Mackintosh D, Keen H: Monitoring glomerular function in diabetic nephropathy. Am J Med 74:256–264, 1983.
155. Walser M, Drew HH, LaFrance ND: Creatinine measurements often yielded false estimates of progression in chronic renal failure. Kidney Int 34:412–418, 1988.
156. Levey AS, Gassman JJ, Hall PM, Walker WG: Assessing the progression of renal disease in clinical studies: Effects of duration of follow-up and regression to the mean. J Am Soc Nephrol 1:1087–1094, 1991.
157. Shah BV, Levey AS: Spontaneous changes in the rate of decline in reciprocal serum creatinine: Errors in predicting the progression of renal disease from extrapolation of the slope. J Am Soc Nephrol 2:1186–1191, 1992.
158. Dettli L: Drug dosage in renal disease. Clin Pharmacokinet 1:126–134, 1983.
159. Reidenberg MM: Kidney function and drug action. N Engl J Med 313:816–817, 1985.
160. Maderazo EG, Sun H, Jay GT: Simplification of antibiotic dose adjustments in renal insufficiency: the DREM system. Lancet 340:767–770, 1992.
161. Walser M: Progression of chronic renal failure in man. Kidney Int 37:1195–1210, 1990.
162. Levey AS, Greene T, Schluchter MD, et al: Glomerular filtration rate measurements in clinical trials. J Am Soc Nephrol 4:1159–1171, 1993.
163. Rossing P: Doubling of serum creatinine: Is it sensitive and relevant? Nephrol Dial Transplant 13:244–246, 1998.
164. Murthy K, Stevens LA, Stark PC, Levey AS: Variation in the serum creatinine assay calibration: A practical application to glomerular filtration rate estimation. Kidney Int 68:1884–1887, 2005.
165. Kroenke K, Hanley JF, Copley JB, et al: The admission urinalysis: Impact on patient care. J Gen Intern Med 1:238–242, 1986.
166. Akin BV, Hubbell FA, Frye EB, et al: Efficacy of the routine admission urinalysis. Am J Med 82:719–722, 1987.
167. Mitchell N, Stapleton FB: Routine admission urinalysis examination in pediatric patients: A poor value. Pediatrics 86:345–349, 1990.
168. Schumann GB, Greenberg NF: Usefulness of macroscopic urinalysis as a screening procedure. Am J Clin Pathol 71:452–456, 1979.
169. Is routine urinalysis worthwhile? Lancet 1:747, 1988.
170. Györy AZ, Hadfield C, Lauer CS: Value of urine microscopy in predicting histological changes in the kidney: Double blind comparison. BMJ 288:819–822, 1984.
171. Morrin PAF: Urinary sediment in the interpretation of proteinuria. Ann Intern Med 98:254–255, 1983.
172. Assadi FK, Fornell L: Estimation of urine specific gravity in neonates with a reagent strip. J Pediatr 108:995–996, 1986.
173. Siegrist D, Hess B, Montandon M, et al: Spezifisches Gewicht des Urins—vergleichende Messungen mit Teststreifen und Refraktometer bei 340 Morgenurinproben. Schweiz Rundsch Med Prax 82:112–116, 1993.
174. Jacobs DS, De Mott WR, Willie GR: Urinalysis and clinical microscopy. *In* Jacobs DS, Kasten BL, De Mott WR, Wolfson WL (eds): Laboratory Test Handbook. Baltimore, Williams & Wilkins, 1990, pp 933–934.
175. Adams LJ: Evaluation of Ames Multistix^{R} SG for urine specific gravity versus refractometer specific gravity. Am J Pathol 80:871–873, 1983.
176. Benitez OA, Benitez M, Stijnen T, et al: Inaccuracy of neonatal measurement of urine concentration with a refractometer. J Pediatr 108:613–616, 1986.
177. Gouyon JB, Houchan N: Assessment of urine specific gravity by reagent strip test in newborn infants. Pediatr Nephrol 7:77–78, 1993.
178. Sheets C, Lyman JL: Urinalysis. Emerg Med Clin North Am 4:263–280, 1986.
179. Jung K: Enzyme activities in urine: How should we express their excretion? A critical literature review. Eur J Clin Chem Clin Biochem 29:725–729, 1991.
180. McCormack M, Dessureault J, Guitard M: The urine specific gravity dipstick: A useful tool to increase fluid intake in stone forming patients. J Urol 146:1475–1477, 1991.
181. The U.S. Preventive Services Task Force: Screening for asymptomatic bacteriuria, hematuria and proteinuria. Am Fam Physician 42:389–395, 1990.
182. American Academy of Pediatrics: American Academy of Pediatrics. Recommendations for preventive pediatric health care. *In* Policy Reference Guide: A Comprehensive Guide to AAP Policy statement, Elk Grove Village, IL, AAP, 1993.
183. Kaplan RE, Springate JE, Feld LG: Screening dipstick urinalysis: A time to change. Pediatrics 100:919–921, 1997.
184. Arant BS Jr: Screening for urinary abnormalities: Worth doing and worth doing well. Lancet 351:307–308, 1998.
185. Craver RD, Abermanis JG: Dipstick only urinalysis screen for the pediatric emergency room. Pediatr Nephrol 11:331–333, 1997.
186. Bonnardeaux A, Somerville P, Kaye M: A study on the reliability of dipstick urinalysis. Clin Nephrol 41:167–172, 1994.
187. Goldsmith BM, Campos JM: Comparison of urine dipstick, microscopy, and culture for the detection of bacteriuria in children. Clin Pediatr (Phila) 29:214–218, 1990.
188. Jacobs DS, De Mott WR, Willie GR: Urinalysis and clinical microscopy. *In* Jacobs DS, Kasten BL, De Mott WR, Wolfson WL (eds): Laboratory Test Handbook. Baltimore, Williams & Wilkins, 1990, pp 914–915.
189. Jacobs DS, De Mott WR, Willie GR: Urinalysis and clinical microscopy. *In* Jacobs DS, Kasten BL, De Mott WR, Wolfson WL (eds): Laboratory Test Handbook. Baltimore, Williams & Wilkins, 1990, p 919.
190. Ditchburn RK, Ditchburn JS: A study of microscopical and chemical tests for the rapid diagnosis of urinary tract infections in general practice [see comments]. Br J Gen Pract 40:406–408, 1990.
191. McGlone R, Lambert M, Clancy M, Hawkey PM: Use of Ames SG10 Urine Dipstick for diagnosis of abdominal pain in the accident and emergency department. Arch Emerg Med 7:42–47, 1990.
192. Liptak GS, Campbell J, Stewart R, Hulbert WC Jr: Screening for urinary tract infection in children with neurogenic bladders. Am J Phys Med Rehabil 72:122–126, 1993.
193. Lohr JA, Portilla MG, Geuder TG, et al: Making a presumptive diagnosis of urinary tract infection by using a urinalysis performed in an on-site laboratory. J Pediatr 122:22–25, 1993.

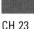

194. McNagny SE, Parker RM, Zenilman JM, Lewis JS: Urinary leukocyte esterase test: A screening method for the detection of asymptomatic chlamydial and gonococcal infections in men. J Infect Dis 165:573–576, 1992.

195. Blum RN, Wright RA: Detection of pyuria and bacteriuria in symptomatic ambulatory women. J Gen Intern Med 7:140–144, 1992.

196. Hurlbut TA, III, Littenberg B: The diagnostic accuracy of rapid dipstick tests to predict urinary tract infection. Am J Clin Pathol 96:582–588, 1991.

197. Jacobs DS, De Mott WR, Willie GR: Urinalysis and clinical microscopy. In Jacobs DS, Kasten BL, De Mott WR, Wolfson WL (eds): Laboratory Test Handbook. Baltimore, Williams & Wilkins, 1990, pp 906–909.

198. Brigden ML, Edgell D, McPherson M, et al: High incidence of significant urinary ascorbic acid concentrations in a west coast population—Implications for routine urinalysis. Clin Chem 38:426–431, 1992.

199. Singer DE, Coley CM, Samet JH, Nathan DM: Tests of glycemia in diabetes mellitus: Their use in establishing a diagnosis and in treatment. Ann Intern Med 110:125–137, 1989.

200. Jacobs DS, De Mott WR, Willie GR: Urinalysis and clinical microscopy. In Jacobs DS, Kasten BL, De Mott WR, Wolfson WL (eds): Laboratory Test Handbook. Baltimore, Williams & Wilkins, 1990, p 912.

201. Shihabi ZK, Konen JC, O'Connor ML: Albuminuria vs urinary total protein for detecting chronic renal disorders. Clin Chem 37:621–624, 1991.

202. Hession C, Decker JM, Sherblom AP, et al: Uromodulin (Tamm-Horsfall glycoprotein): A renal ligand for lymphokines. Science 237:1479–1484, 1987.

203. Pennica D, Kohr WJ, Kuang W-J, et al: Identification of human uromodulin as the Tamm-Horsfall urinary glycoprotein. Science 236:83–88, 1987.

204. Allen JK, Krauss EA, Deeter RG: Dipstick analysis of urinary protein. A comparison of Chemstrip-9 and Multistix-10SG. Arch Pathol Lab Med 115:34–37, 1991.

205. Rowe DJF, Dawnay A, Watts GF: Microalbuminuria in diabetes mellitus: Review and recommendations for the measurement of albumin in urine. Ann Clin Biochem 27:297–312, 1990.

206. Harmoinen A, Vuorinen P, Jokela H: Turbidimetric measurement of microalbuminuria. Clin Chim Acta 166:85–89, 1987.

207. Stamp RJ: Measurement of albumin in urine by end-point immunonephelometry. Ann Clin Biochem 25:442–443, 1988.

208. Neuman RG, Cohen MP: Improved competitive enzyme-linked immunoassay (ELISA) for albuminuria. Clin Chim Acta 179:229–238, 1989.

209. Comper WD, Osicka TM, Jerums G: High prevalence of immuno-unreactive intact albumin in urine of diabetic patients. Am J Kidney Dis 41:336–342, 2003.

210. Tiu SC, Lee SS, Cheng MW: Comparison of six commerical techniques in the measurement of microalbuminuria in diabetic patients. Diabetes Care 16:616–620, 1993.

211. Comper WD, Jerums G, Osicka TM: Differences in urinary albumin detected by four immunoassays and high-performance liquid chromatography. Clin Biochem 37:105–111, 2004.

212. Giampietro O, Penno G, Clerico A, et al: Which method for quantifying "micro-albuminuria" in diabetics? Comparison of several immunological methods (immuno-turbidimetric assay, immunonephelometric assay, radioimmunoassay and two semiquantitative tests) for measurement of albumin in urine. Acta Diabetol 28:239–245, 1992.

213. Ballantyne FC, Gibbons J, O'Reilly DS: Urine albumin should replace total protein for the assessment of glomerular proteinuria. Ann Clin Biochem 30(pt 1):101–103, 1993.

214. Sawicki PT, Heinemann L, Berger M: Comparison of methods for determination of microalbuminuria in diabetic patients. Diabet Med 6:412–415, 1989.

215. Tai J, Tze WJ: Evaluation of Micro-Bumintest reagent tablets for screening of microalbuminuria. Diabetes Res Clin Pract 9:137–142, 1990.

216. Bangstad HJ, Try K, Dahl-Jørgensen K, Hanssen KF: New semiquantitative dipstick test for microalbuminuria. Diabetes Care 14:1094–1097, 1991.

217. Marshall SM, Schearing PA, Alberti KG: Micral-test strips evaluated for screening for albuminuria. Clin Chem 38:588–591, 1992.

218. Poulsen PL, Hansen B, Amby T, et al: Evaluation of a dipstick test for microalbuminuria in three different clinical settings, including the correlation with urinary albumin excretion rate. Diabetes Metab 18:395–400, 1992.

219. Schaufelberger H, Caduff F, Engler H, Spinas GA: Evaluation eines Streifentests (Micral-Test^R) zur semiquantitativen Erfassung der mikroalbinurie in der praxis. Schweiz Med Wochenschr 122:576–581, 1992.

220. Schwab SJ, Dunn FL, Feinglos MN: Screening for microalbuminuria. Diabetes Care 15:1581–1584, 1992.

221. Mogensen CE, Viberti GC, Peheim E, et al: Multicenter evaluation of the Micral-Test II test strip, an immunologic rapid test for the detection of microalbuminuria. Diabetes Care 20:1642–1646, 1997.

222. Minetti EE, Cozzi MG, Granata S, Guidi E: Accuracy of the urinary albumin titrator stick "Micral-Test" in kidney-disease patients. Nephrol Dial Transplant 12:78–80, 1997.

223. Molitch ME, Defronzo RA, Franz MJ, et al: Nephropathy in diabetes. Diabetes Care 27(suppl 1):S79–S83, 2004.

224. Gross JL, de Azevedo MJ, Silveiro SP, et al: Diabetic nephropathy: Diagnosis, prevention, and treatment. Diabetes Care 28:164–176, 2005.

225. Schwab SJ, Christensen L, Dougherty K, Klahr S: Quantitation of proteinuria by the use of protein-to-creatinine ratios in single urine samples. Arch Intern Med 147:943–944, 1987.

226. Gatling W, Knight C, Hill RD: Screening for early diabetic nephropathy: Which sample to detect microalbuminuria? Diabet Med 2:451–455, 1985.

227. Marshall SM, Alberti KGMM: Screening for early diabetic nephropathy. Ann Clin Biochem 23:195–197, 1986.

228. Cohen DL, Close CF, Viberti GC: The variability of overnight urinary albumin excretion in insulin-dependent diabetic and normal subjects. Diabet Med 4:437–440, 1987.

229. Hutchison AS, O'Reilly DStJ, MacCuish AC: Albumin excretion rate, albumin concentration, and albumin creatinine ratio compared for screening diabetics for slight albuminuria. Clin Chem 34:2019–2021, 1988.

230. Sessoms S, Mehta K, Kovarsky J: Quantitation of proteinuria in systemic lupus erythematosus by use of a random, spot urine collection. Arthritis Rheum 26:918–920, 1983.

231. Ruggenenti P, Gaspari F, Perna A, Remuzzi G: Cross-sectional longitudinal study of spot morning urine protein:creatinine ratio, 24-hour urine protein excretion rate, glomerular filtration rate, and end-stage renal failure in chronic renal disease in patients without diabetes. BMJ 316:504–509, 1998.

232. Torng S, Rigatto C, Rush DN, et al: The urine protein to creatinine ratio (P/C) as a predictor of 24-hour urine protein excretion in renal transplant patients. Transplantation 72:1453–1456, 2001.

233. Ramos JG, Martins-Costa SH, Mathias MM, et al: Urinary protein/creatinine ratio in hypertensive pregnant women. Hypertens Pregnancy 18:209–218, 1999.

234. Rodriguez-Thompson D, Lieberman ES: Use of a random urinary protein-to-creatinine ratio for the diagnosis of significant proteinuria during pregnancy. Am J Obstet Gynecol 185:808–811, 2001.

235. Neithardt AB, Dooley SL, Borensztajn J: Prediction of 24-hour protein excretion in pregnancy with a single voided urine protein-to-creatinine ratio. Am J Obstet Gynecol 186:883–886, 2002.

236. Durnwald C, Mercer B: A prospective comparison of total protein/creatinine ratio versus 24-hour urine protein in women with suspected preeclampsia. Am J Obstet Gynecol 189:848–852, 2003.

237. Al RA, Baykal C, Karacay O, et al: Random urine protein-creatinine ratio to predict proteinuria in new-onset mild hypertension in late pregnancy. Obstet Gynecol 104:367–371, 2004.

238. Zuppi C, Baroni S, Scribano D, et al: Choice of time for urine collection for detecting early kidney abnormalities in hypertensives. Ann Clin Biochem 32:373–378, 1995.

239. Hara F, Nakazato K, Shiba K, et al: Studies of diabetic nephropathy. I. Effects of storage time and temperature on microalbuminuria. Biol Pharm Bull 17:1241–1245, 1994.

240. Watts GF, Pillay D: Effect of ketones and glucose on the estimation of urinary creatinine: Implications for microalbuminuria screening. Diabet Med 7:263–265, 1990.

241. Weber MH: Urinary protein analysis. J Chromatogr 429:315–344, 1988.

242. Vidal BC, Bonventre JV, Hong HS: Towards the application of proteomics in renal disease diagnosis. Clin Sci (Lond) 109:421–430, 2005.

243. Thongboonkerd V, Malasit P: Renal and urinary proteomics: Current applications and challenges. Proteomics 5:1033–1042, 2005.

244. Viberti GC, Jarrett RJ, Mahmud U, et al: Microalbuminuria as a predictor of clinical nephropathy in insulin-dependent diabetes mellitus. Lancet 1:1430–1431, 1982.

245. Messent JWC, Elliott TG, Hill RD, et al: Prognostic significance of microalbuminuria in insulin-dependent diabetes mellitus: A twenty-three year follow-up study. Kidney Int 41:836–839, 1992.

246. Mogensen CE: Microalbuminuria predicts clinical proteinuria and early mortality in maturity-onset diabetes. N Engl J Med 310:356–360, 1984.

247. Jarrett RJ, Viberti CG, Argyropoulos A, et al: Microalbuminuria predicts mortality in non-insulin-dependent diabetes. Diabet Med 1:17–19, 1984.

248. Mogensen CE, Christensen CK: Predicting diabetic nephropathy in insulin-dependent patients. N Engl J Med 311:89–93, 1984.

249. Mattock MB, Morrish NJ, Viberti G, et al: Prospective study of microalbuminuria as predictor of mortality in NIDDM. Diabetes 41:736–741, 1992.

250. Borch-Johnsen K, Wenzel H, Viberti GC, Mogensen CE: Is screening and intervention for microalbuminuria worthwhile in patients with insulin dependent diabetes? Br Med J 306:1722–1725, 1993.

251. Mattix HJ, Hsu CY, Shaykevich S, Curhan G: Use of the albumin/creatinine ratio to detect microalbuminuria: Implications of sex and race. J Am Soc Nephrol 13:1034–1039, 2002.

252. Nelson RG, Knowler WC, Pettitt DJ, et al: Assessment of risk of overt nephropathy in diabetic patients from albumin excretion in untimed urine specimens. Arch Intern Med 151:1761–1765, 1991.

253. Caramori ML, Fioretto P, Mauer M: Low glomerular filtration rate in normoalbuminuric type 1 diabetic patients: An indicator of more advanced glomerular lesions. Diabetes 52:1036–1040, 2003.

254. MacIsaac RJ, Tsalamandris C, Panagiotopoulos S, et al: Nonalbuminuric renal insufficiency in type 2 diabetes. Diabetes Care 27:195–200, 2004.

255. Boulware LE, Jaar BG, Tarver-Carr ME, et al: Screening for proteinuria in US adults: A cost-effectiveness analysis. JAMA 290:3101–3114, 2003.

256. Robinson RR: Nephrology Forum: Isolated proteinuria in asymptomatic patients. Kidney Int 18:395–406, 1980.

257. Robinson RR: Isolated proteinuria. Contrib Nephrol 24:53–62, 1981.

258. von Bonsdorff M, Koskenvuo K, Salmi HA, Pasternack A: Prevalence and causes of proteinuria in 20-year-old Finnish men. Scand J Urol Nephrol 15:285–290, 1981.

259. Springberg PD, Garrett LE Jr, Thompson AL Jr, et al: Fixed and reproducible orthostatic proteinuria: Results of a 20-year follow-up. Ann Intern Med 97:516–519, 1982.

260. Rytand DA, Spreiter S: Prognosis in postural (orthostatic) proteinuria. N Engl J Med 305:618–621, 1981.

261. Houser MT: Characterization of recumbent, ambulatory, and postexercise proteinuria in the adolescent. Pediatr Res 21:442–446, 1987.

262. Schardijn GHC, Statius van Eps LW: β2-Microglobulin: Its significance in the evaluation of renal function. Kidney Int 32:635–641, 1987.

263. Schentag JJ, Sutfin TA, Plaut ME, Jusko WJ: Early detection of aminoglycoside nephrotoxicity with urinary B-2 microglobulin. J Med 9:201–210, 1978.

264. Hall PW III, Dammin GJ: Balkan nephropathy. Nephron 22:281–300, 1978.

265. Taniguchi N, Tanaka M, Kishihara C, et al: Determination of carbonic anhydrase C and β2-microglobulin by radioimmunoassay in urine of heavy-metal-exposed subjects and patients with renal tubular acidosis. Environ Res 20:154–161, 1979.

266. Roxe DM, Siddiqui F, Santhanam S, et al: Rationale and application of beta-$_2$-microglobulin measurements to detect acute transplant rejection. Nephron 27:260–264, 1981.
267. Statius van Eps LW, Schardijn GHC: Value of determination of B2-microglobulin in toxic nephropathy and interstitial nephritis. Klin Wochenschr 18:673–678, 1984.
268. Bäckman L, Ringdén O, Björkhem I, Lindbäck B: Increased serum β_2-microglobulin during rejection, cyclosporine-induced nephrotoxicity and cytomegalovirus infection in renal transplant recipients. Transplantation 42:368–371, 1986.
269. Schardijn GHC, Statius van Eps LW, Pauw W, et al: Comparison of reliability of tests to distinguish upper from lower urinary tract infections. BMJ 289:284–287, 1984.
270. Buxbaum JN, Chuba JV, Hellman GC, et al: Monoclonal immunoglobulin deposition disease: Light chain and light and heavy chain deposition diseases and their relation to light chain amyloidosis. Ann Intern Med 112:455–464, 1990.
271. Hunt LP, Short CD, Mallick NP: Prognostic indicators in patients presenting with the nephrotic syndrome. Kidney Int 34:382–388, 1988.
272. Williams PS, Fass G, Bone JM: Renal pathology and proteinuria determine progression in untreated mild/moderate chronic renal failure. Q J Med 67:343–354, 1988.
273. Neelakantappa K, Gallo GAR, Baldwin DS: proteinuria in IgA nephropathy. Kidney Int 33:716–721, 1988.
274. Alamartine E, Sabatier J-C, Guerin C, et al: Prognostic factors in mesangial IgA glomerulonephritis: An extensive study with univariate and multivariate analyses. Am J Kidney Dis 18:12–19, 1991.
275. D'Amico G: Influence of clinical and histological features on actuarial renal survival in adult patients with idiopathic IgA nephropathy, membranous nephropathy, and membranoproliferative glomerulonephritis: Survey of the recent literature. Am J Kidney Dis 20:315–323, 1992.
276. Donadio JV Jr, Torres VE, Velosa JA, et al: Idiopathic membranous nephropathy: The natural history of untreated patients. Kidney Int 33:708–715, 1988.
277. Cattran DC, Pei Y, Greenwood C: Predicting progression in membranous glomerulonephritis. Nephrol Dial Transplant Suppl 1:48–52, 1992.
278. Brahm M, Brammer M, Balsløv JT, et al: Prognosis in glomerulonephritis. III. A longitudinal analysis of changes in serum creatinine and proteinuria during the course of disease: Effect of immunosuppressive treatment. Report from Copenhagen Study Group of Renal Diseases. J Intern Med 231:339–347, 1992.
279. Ritchie CD, Bevan EA, Collier SJ: Importance of occult haematuria found at screening. BMJ 292:681–683, 1986.
280. Thompson IM: The evaluation of microscopic hematuria: A population-based study. J Urol 138:1189–1190, 1987.
281. Messing EM, Vaillancourt A: Hematuria screening for bladder cancer. J Occup Med 32:838–845, 1990.
282. Lieu TA, Grasmeder HM III, Kaplan BS: An approach to the evaluation and treatment of microscopic hematuria. Pediatr Clin North Am 38:579–592, 1991.
283. Fairley KF, Birch DF: Hematuria: A simple method for identifying glomerular bleeding. Kidney Int 21:105–108, 1982.
284. Fassett RG, Horgan BA, Mathew TH: Detection of glomerular bleeding by phase-contrast microscopy. Lancet 1:1432–1434, 1982.
285. Van Iseghem PH, Hauglastaine D, Bollens W, Michielsen P: Urinary erythrocyte morphology in acute glomerulonephritis. BMJ 287:1183, 1983.
286. Shichiri M, Nishio Y, Suenaga M, et al: Red-cell volume distribution curves in diagnosis of glomerular and non-glomerular haematuria. Lancet 1:908–911, 1988.
287. Goldwasser P, Antignani A, Mittman N, et al: Urinary red cell size: Diagnostic value and determinants. Am J Nephrol 10:148–156, 1990.
288. Schramek P, Moritsch A, Haschkowitz H, et al: In vitro generation of dysmorphic erythrocytes. Kidney Int 36:72–77, 1989.
289. Thal SM, DeBellis CC, Iverson SA, Schumann GB: Comparison of dysmorphic erythrocytes with other urinary sediment parameters of renal bleeding. Am J Clin Pathol 86:784–787, 1986.
290. Raman GV, Pead L, Lee HA, Maskell R: A blind controlled trial of phase-contrast microscopy by two observers for evaluating the source of hematuria. Nephron 44:304–308, 1986.
291. Sayer J, McCarthy MP, Schmidt JD: Identification and significance of dysmorphic versus isomorphic hematuria. J Urol 143:545–548, 1990.
292. Marcussen N, Schumann JL, Schumann GB, et al: Analysis of cytodiagnostic urinalysis findings in 77 patients with concurrent renal biopsies. Am J Kidney Dis 20:618–628, 1992.
293. Dinda AK, Saxena S, Guleria S, et al: Diagnosis of glomerular haematuria: Role of dysmorphic red cell, G1 cell and bright-field microscopy. Scand J Clin Lab Invest 57:203–208, 1997.
294. Lettgen B, Hestermann C, Rascher W: Differentiation of glomerular and non-glomerular hematuria in children by measurement of mean corpuscular volume of urinary red cells using a semi-automated cell counter. Acta Paediatr 83:946–949, 1994.
295. Apeland T: Flow cytometry of urinary erythrocytes for evaluating the source of haematuria. Scand J Urol Nephrol 29:33–37, 1995.
296. Hyodo T, Kumano K, Haga M, et al: Analysis of urinary red blood cells of healthy individuals by an automated urinary flow cytometer. Nephron 75:451–457, 1997.
297. Offringa M, Benbassat J: The value of urinary red cell shape in the diagnosis of glomerular and post-glomerular haematuria. A meta-analysis. Postgrad Med J 68:648–654, 1992.
298. Shaper KR, Jackson JE, Williams G: The nutcracker syndrome: An uncommon cause of haematuria. Br J Urol 74:144–146, 1994.
299. Fogazzi GB, Leong SO, Cameron JS: Don't forget sickled cells in the urine when investigating a patient for haematuria. Nephrol Dial Transplant 11:723–725, 1996.
300. Tanaka H, Kim S-T, Takasugi M, Kuroiwa A: Isolated hematuria in adults: IgA nephropathy is a predominant cause of hematuria compared with thin glomerular basement membrane nephropathy. Am J Nephrol 16:412–416, 1996.
301. Sobh MA, Moustafa FE, el-Din Saleh MA, et al: Study of asymptomatic microscopic hematuria in potential living related kidney donors. Nephron 65:190–195, 1993.
302. Jacobs DS, De Mott WR, Willie GR: Urinalysis and clinical microscopy. *In* Jacobs DS, Kasten BL, De Mott WR, Wolfson WL (eds): Laboratory Test Handbook. Baltimore, Williams & Wilkins, 1990, pp 903–904.
303. Corwin HL, Bray RA, Haber MH: The detection and interpretation of urinary eosinophils. Arch Pathol Lab Med 113:1256–1258, 1989.
304. Corwin HL, Korbet SM, Schwartz MM: Clinical correlates of eosinophiluria. Arch Intern Med 145:1097–1099, 1985.
305. Yu D, Petermann A, Kunter U, et al: Urinary podocyte loss is a more specific marker of ongoing glomerular damage than proteinuria. J Am Soc Nephrol 16:1733–1741, 2005.
306. Jacobs DS, De Mott WR, Willie GR: Urinalysis and clinical microscopy. *In* Jacobs DS, Kasten BL, De Mott WR, Wolfson WL (eds): Laboratory Test Handbook. Baltimore, Williams & Wilkins, 1990, p 938.
307. Arenson AM: Ultrasound guided percutaneous renal biopsy. Australas Radiol 35:38–39, 1991.
308. Grimm PC, Nickerson P, Gough J, et al: Computerized image analysis of Sirius Red-stained renal allograft biopsies as a surrogate marker to predict long-term allograft function. J Am Soc Nephrol 14:1662–1668, 2003.
309. Marcussen N, Olsen S, Larsen S, et al: Reproducibility of the WHO classification of glomerulonephritis. Clin Nephrol 44:220–224, 1995.
310. Wernick RM, Smith DL, Houghton DC, et al: Reliability of histologic scoring for lupus nephritis: A community-based evaluation. Ann Intern Med 119:805–811, 1993.
311. Paone DB, Meyer LE: The effect of biopsy on therapy in renal disease. Arch Intern Med 141:1039–1041, 1981.
312. Cohen AH, Nast CC, Adler SG, Kopple JD: The clinical usefulness of kidney biopsies in the diagnosis and management of renal disease. Kidney Int 27:135, 1985.
313. Turner MW, Hutchinson TA, Barré PE, et al: A prospective study on the impact of the renal biopsy in clinical management. Clin Nephrol 26:217–221, 1986.
314. Shah RP, Vathsala A, Chiang GS, et al: The impact of percutaneous renal biopsies on clinical management. Ann Acad Med Singapore 22:908–911, 1993.
315. Richards NT, Darby S, Howie AJ, et al: Knowledge of renal histology alters patient management in over 40% of cases. Nephrol Dial Transplant 9:1255–1259, 1994.
316. Whiting-O'Keefe Q, Riccardi PJ, Henke JE, et al: Recognition of information in renal biopsies of patients with lupus nephritis. Ann Intern Med 96(pt 1):723–727, 1982.
317. Primack WA, Schulman SL, Kaplan BS: An analysis of the approach to management of childhood nephrotic syndrome by pediatric nephrologists. Am J Kidney Dis 23:524, 1994.
318. Adu D: The nephrotic syndrome: Does renal biopsy affect management? Nephrol Dial Transplant 11:12–14, 1996.
319. Levey AS, Lau J, Pauker SG, Kassirer JP: Idiopathic nephrotic syndrome: Puncturing the biopsy myth. Ann Intern Med 107:697–713, 1987.
320. Tomura S, Tsutani K, Sakuma A, Takeuchi J: Discriminant analysis in renal histological diagnosis of primary glomerular diseases. Clin Nephrol 23:55–62, 1985.
321. Ganeval D, Noel L-H, Preud'homme J-L, et al: Light-chain deposition disease: Its relation with AL-type amyloidosis. Kidney Int 26:1, 1984.
322. Schwartz MM, Lan SP, Bonsib SM, et al: Clinical outcome of 3 discrete glomerular lesions in severe lupus glomerulonephritis. The Lupus Nephritis Collaborative Study Group. Am J Kidney Dis 13:273–283, 1989.
323. Fries JF, Porta J, Liang MH: Marginal benefit of renal biopsy in systemic lupus erythematosus. Arch Intern Med 138:1386, 1978.
324. Whiting-O'Keefe Q, Henke JE, Shearn MA, et al: The information content from renal biopsy in systemic lupus erhythematosus. Ann Intern Med 96(pt 1):718–723, 1982.
325. Schwartz MM, Bernstein J, Hill GS, et al and Lupus Nephritis Collaborative Study Group: Predictive value of renal pathology in diffuse proliferative lupus glomerulonephritis. Kidney Int 36:891–896, 1989.
326. Schwartz MM, Lan SP, Bernstein J, et al: Role of pathology indices in the management of severe lupus glomerulonephritis. Lupus Nephritis Collaborative Study Group. Kidney Int 42:743–748, 1992.
327. Chagnac A, Kiberd BA, Farinas MC, et al: Outcome of acute glomerular injury in proliferative lupus nephritis. J Clin Invest 84:922–930, 1989.
328. Schwartz MM, Korbet SM: Crescentic glomerulonephritis. Prog Reprod Urinary Tract Pathol 1:163, 1989.
329. Falk RJ: ANCA-associated renal disease. Kidney Int 38:998, 1990.
330. Nankivell BJ, Borrows RJ, Fung CL, et al: The natural history of chronic allograft nephropathy. N Engl J Med 349:2326–2333, 2003.
331. Gray DWR, Richardson A, Hughes D, et al: A prospective, randomized, blind comparison of three biopsy techniques in the management of patients after renal transplantation. Transplantation 53:1226–1232, 1992.
332. Racusen LC, Colvin RB, Solez K, et al: Antibody-mediated rejection criteria—An addition to the Banff 97 classification of renal allograft rejection. Am J Transplant 3:708–714, 2003.
333. Solez K, Hansen HE, Kornerup HJ, et al: Clinical validation and reproducibility of the Banff schema for renal allograft pathology. Transplant Proc 27:1009–1011, 1995.
334. Wang HJ, Kjellstrand CM, Cockfield SM, Solez K: On the influence of sample size on the prognostic accuracy and reproducibility of renal transplant biopsy. Nephrol Dial Transplant 13:165–172, 1998.
335. Kolb LG, Velosa JA, Bergstralh EJ, Offord KP: Percutaneous renal allograft biopsy. A comparison of two needle types and analysis of risk factors. Transplantation 57:1742–1746, 1994.
336. Riehl J, Maigatter S, Kierdorf H, et al: Percutaneous renal biopsy: Comparison of manual and automated puncture techniques with native and transplanted kidneys. Nephrol Dial Transplant 9:1568–1574, 1994.
337. Diaz Encarnacion MM, Griffin MD, Slezak JM, et al: Correlation of quantitative digital image analysis with the glomerular filtration rate in chronic allograft nephropathy. Am J Transplant 4:248–256, 2004.

338. Sinniah R, Law CH, Pwee HS: Glomerular lesions in patients with asymptomatic persistent and orthostatic proteinuria discovered on routine medical examination. Clin Nephrol 7:1–14, 1977.

339. Sinniah R, Pwee HS, Lim CM: Glomerular lesions in asymptomatic microscopic hematuria discovered on routine medical examination. Clin Nephrol 5:216–228, 1976.

340. Copley JB, Hasbargen JA: Idiopathic hematuria: A prospective evaluation. Arch Intern Med 147:434–437, 1987.

341. Nomoto Y, Endoh M, Suga T, et al: Minimum requirements for renal biopsy size for patients with IgA nephropathy. Nephron 60:171–175, 1992.

342. Wickre CG, Golper TA: Complications of percutaneous needle biopsy of the kidney. Am J Nephrol 2:173–178, 1982.

343. Mendelssohn DC, Cole EH: Outcomes of percutaneous kidney biopsy, including those of solitary native kidneys. Am J Kidney Dis 26:580–585, 1995.

344. Shemin D, Elnour M, Amarantes B, et al: Oral estrogens decrease bleeding time and improve clinical bleeding in patients with renal failure. Am J Med 89:436–440, 1990.

345. Korbet SM: Percutaneous renal biopsy. Semin Nephrol 22:254–267, 2002.

346. Kearon C, Hirsh J: Management of anticoagulation before and after elective surgery. N Engl J Med 336:1506–1511, 1997.

347. Stiles KP, Yuan CM, Chung EM, et al: Renal biopsy in high-risk patients with medical diseases of the kidney. Am J Kidney Dis 36:419–433, 2000.

348. Abbott KC, Musio FM, Chung EM, et al: Transjugular renal biopsy in high-risk patients: An American case series. BMC Nephrol 3:5, 2002.

349. Christensen J, Lindequist S, Knudsen DU, Pedersen RS: Ultrasound-guided renal biopsy with biopsy gun technique—Efficacy and complications. Acta Radiol 36:276–279, 1995.

350. Doyle AJ, Gregory MC, Terreros DA: Percutaneous native renal biopsy: Comparison of a 1.2-mm spring-driven system with a traditional 2-mm hand-driven system. Am J Kidney Dis 23:498–503, 1994.

351. Voss DM, Lynn KL: Percutaneous renal biopsy: An audit of a 2-year experience with the Biopty gun. N Z Med J 108:8–10, 1995.

352. Fraser IR, Fairley CK: Renal biopsy as an outpatient procedure. Am J Kidney Dis 25:876–878, 1995.

353. Kudryk BT, Martinez CR, Gunasekeran S, Ramirez G: CT-guided renal biopsy using a coaxial technique and an automated biopsy gun. South Med J 88:543–546, 1995.

354. Lee SM, King J, Spargo BH: Efficacy of percutaneous renal biopsy in obese patients under computerized tomographic guidance. Clin Nephrol 35:123–129, 1991.

355. Burstein DM, Schwartz MM, Korbet SM: Percutaneous renal biopsy with the use of real-time ultrasound. Am J Nephrol 11:195–200, 1991.

356. Burstein DM, Korbet SM, Schwartz MM: The use of the automatic core biopsy system in percutaneous renal biopsies: A comparative study. Am J Kidney Dis 22:545–552, 1993.

357. Kim D, Kim H, Shin G, et al: A randomized, prospective, comparative study of manual and automated renal biopsies. Am J Kidney Dis 32:426–431, 1998.

358. Nicholson ML, Wheatley TJ, Doughman TM, et al: A prospective randomized trial of three different sizes of core-cutting needle for renal transplant biopsy. Kidney Int 58:390–395, 2000.

359. Mauiyyedi S, Crespo M, Collins AB, et al: Acute humoral rejection in kidney transplantation: II. Morphology, immunopathology, and pathologic classification. J Am Soc Nephrol 13:779–787, 2002.

360. Haas M: A reevaluation of routine electron microscopy in the examination of native renal biopsies. J Am Soc Nephrol 8:70–76, 1997.

361. Parrish AE: Complications of percutaneous renal biopsy: A review of 37 years' experience. Clin Nephrol 38:135–141, 1992.

362. Manno C, Strippoli GF, Arnesano L, et al: Predictors of bleeding complications in percutaneous ultrasound-guided renal biopsy. Kidney Int 66:1570–1577, 2004.

363. Ginsburg JC, Fransman SL, Singer MA, et.al: Use of computerized tomography (CT) to evaluate bleeding after renal biopsy. Nephron 26:240, 1980.

364. Alter AJ, Zimmerman S, Kirachaiwanich C: Computerized tomographic assessment of retroperitoneal hemorrhage after percutaneous renal biopsy. Arch Intern Med 140:1323, 1980.

365. McCune TR, Stone WJ, Breyer JA: Page kidney: Case report and review of the literature. Am J Kidney Dis 18:593–599, 1991.

366. Kouri TT, Viikari JSA, Mattila KS, Irjala KMA: Invalidity of simple concentration-based screening tests for early nephropathy due to urinary volumes of diabetic patients. Diabetes Care 14:591–593, 1991.

CHAPTER 24

Interpretation of Electrolyte and Acid-Base Parameters in Blood and Urine

K.S. Kamel • M.R. Davids • S.H. Lin • M.L. Halperin

An analysis of laboratory data in blood and urine is essential to make accurate diagnoses and to design optimal therapy for patients with disturbances of water, sodium (Na^+), potassium (K^+), and acid-base homeostasis.[1,2] Our clinical approach and interpretation of these tests rely heavily on an understanding of basic concepts in renal physiology. Hence we begin each section with concepts that help to identify the most important factor(s) that indicate how the kidneys regulate the excretion of these substances and then discuss the tools that utilize the laboratory data to help make a correct diagnosis; consults are presented to illustrate the utility of these tools. At the end of each section, all of the information is integrated to design a clinical approach.

Two principles will hold true throughout this chapter. First, there are *no normal values* for the urinary excretion of water and electrolytes because normal subjects in steady state excrete all ions that are consumed and not lost by non-renal routes. The urine also contains the major nitrogenous metabolic waste, urea—its rate of excretion depends largely on protein intake. Second, data should be interpreted with respect to the prevailing stimulus and the "expected" renal response. In this regard, urine collections done over short periods of time are more valuable than 24-hour urine collections because they more closely reflect the renal response to the prevailing stimulus at that time.

WATER AND SODIUM

In this section, we illustrate how to use information about the composition and volume of the urine in the differential diagnosis and management of disorders causing polyuria, an abnormal intracellular fluid (ICF) volume, and/or an abnormal extracellular fluid (ECF) volume.

Polyuria

There are three reasons why polyuria may be present; a water diuresis, an osmotic diuresis, and/or a renal medullary concentrating defect.

Water Diuresis
Concept SW-1
To move water across a membrane, there must be a channel that allows water to cross that lipid membrane and a driving force (a difference in concentration of "effective" osmoles).

Water Channels
Vasopressin is released when the concentration of Na^+ in plasma (P_{Na}) is >136 mmol/L. This hormone causes the insertion of aquaporin-2 water channels (AQP2) into the luminal membrane of the late distal nephron; AQP2 permit water to be reabsorbed when there is an osmotic driving force.[3] Even in the absence of vasopressin, there is a small degree of water permeability in the inner medullary collecting duct (MCD) (basal water permeability).[4]

Driving Force
Water will be drawn from a compartment with a lower to one with a higher "effective" osmolality; the magnitude of the force is enormous (~19 mm Hg per

mOsm/kg H_2O per osmol/L difference). In the renal cortex, fluid with an osmolality of ~100 mOsm/L enters the late distal convoluted tubule. When AQP2 are present in their luminal membranes, water is reabsorbed because the osmotic pressure difference is ~200 mOsm/L (interstitial osmolality equals the plasma osmolality (P_{osm}), which is ~300 mOsm/L for easy math). Hence the osmotic driving force is ~3800 mm Hg (19 mm Hg × 200 mOsm/L). In the renal inner medulla, the "effective" interstitial osmolality rises ~twofold (from 300 mOsm/L to 600 mOsm/L). Because this driving force is even larger, water will be absorbed rapidly until osmotic equilibrium is achieved.

Tools: Water Diuresis
Urine Flow Rate
When AQP2 are *not* present in the luminal membrane (absence of vasopressin actions), the urine volume will be equal to the volume of filtrate delivered to the late distal nephron (Fig. 24–1). In subjects consuming a typical western diet, the distal flow rate is high and the peak urine flow rate is 10 ml/min to 15 ml/min (~14 L/day to 21 L/day). If the urine volume is considerably <14 L/day, seek a reason for a low distal delivery of filtrate.

Urine Osmolality (U_{osm})
The U_{osm} is equal to the number of excreted osmoles divided by the urine volume. When the osmole excretion rate is 800 mosmol/day and vasopressin is absent, the U_{osm} will be 50 mOsm/L when the 24-hour urine volume is 16 L/day. A change in the U_{osm} in this setting reflects a change in the osmole excretion rate and/or the volume of filtrate delivered to the late distal nephron (which determines the urine volume), rather than a change in the concentrating ability of the kidney. In the above example, the U_{osm} will be 100 mOsm/L when the 24-hour urine volume is 8 L and the rate of excretion of osmoles has not changed. In both of these settings, there is still an enormous difference in osmolality between the luminal and interstitial fluid compartments due the absence of AQP2.

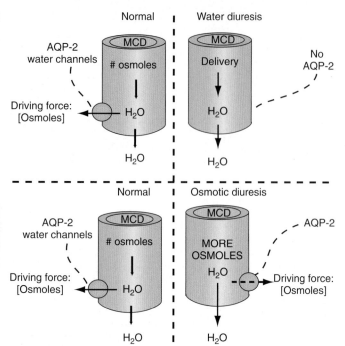

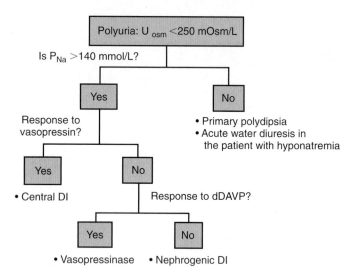

FIGURE 24–2 Approach to the patient with polyuria due to a water diuresis. To enter this flow chart, the patient must have a large urine volume with an osmolality that is distinctly lower than the P_{osm}. A bullet symbol denotes the final diagnostic categories.

CH 24

FIGURE 24–1 Major concept in the control of the excretion of water. The barrel-shaped structure represents the late distal nephron. The major concept is shown to the left of the vertical dashed line. When vasopressin acts, water channels (AQP2, shown by the circle) are inserted in the luminal membrane of collecting duct cells, making these nephron segments permeable to water. The driving force to reabsorb water is a high "effective" osmolality in the medullary interstitial compartment. In a water diuresis (top right portion), AQP2 are absent; hence the urine flow rate is regulated by the distal volume delivery. In contrast, during an osmotic diuresis (lower right portion), AQP2 are present so the urine flow rate is dependent on the number of "effective" osmoles delivered to this nephron segment and the osmolality in the medullary interstitial compartment.

Osmole Excretion Rate
This is simply the product of the U_{osm} and the urine flow rate. In subjects eating a typical western diet, this excretion rate is 600 mosmol/day to 900 mosmol/day. Electrolytes and urea each account for half of these osmoles. In absence of AQP2, a change in the rate of excretion of osmoles does *not* cause a change in urine volume; rather, there is a change in the U_{osm}. Nevertheless, the osmole excretion rate should be calculated in a patient with a water diuresis because it will influence the urine flow rate if vasopressin is given and acts.

Consult SW-1: Does This Patient Have Polyuria?
A 22-year-old female lives in a southern climate. She is concerned about her body image and runs several miles per day. To avoid "dehydration", she drinks large volumes of water, despite the absence of thirst. She consumes a low-salt diet because this helps her maintain her desired weight. She sought medical advice because she voided frequently, passing large volumes of urine each time. On the past two visits, her laboratory results were very similar; her P_{Na} was 130 mmol/L, the 24-hour urine volume was 5 L, and the U_{osm} was 80 mOsm/kg H_2O.

Questions
Does this patient have polyuria?
What risks might you anticipate with respect to her P_{Na}?

Discussion
Does This Patient Have Polyuria?
There are two definitions of polyuria:
Conventional definition: Polyuria is present when the urine volume is >2.5 or 3 L/day.

Physiology-based definition: Polyuria is present when the urine volume is "higher than expected" in a specific setting.

Using the conventional definition, polyuria is present in this patient. The polyuria is due to a water diuresis because the U_{osm} is low (Fig. 24–2). Because hyponatremia is present, polyuria is due to primary polydipsia.

Using the physiology-based definition, the "expected" urine flow rate in a normal adult that lacks vasopressin actions (P_{Na} is 130 mmol/L) should be at least 10 ml/min or ~14 L/day.[5] Hence a urine volume of 5 L/day in this setting is a *low* urine volume; in fact, she has a diminished ability to excrete water. Because of a low "effective" ECF volume due to ongoing losses of Na^+ and Cl^- in sweat, there would be an increased reabsorption of Na^+ upstream in the nephron, lowering the distal delivery of filtrate. The combination of this low distal delivery and the presence of basal water permeability in the medullary collecting duct, even in the absence of detectable levels of vasopressin in plasma,[4] leads to a diminished ability to excrete water, what we call "trickle-down" hyponatremia.[6] In support of presence of a low distal delivery of filtrate, her osmole excretion rate is low (80 mOsm/L × 5 L/day = 400 mosmol/day Vs the usual 600–900 mosmol/day) which suggests that there is a low rate of excretion of NaCl.

What Risks Might You Anticipate with Respect to Her P_{Na}?
Because this is a chronic condition, she is in balance and water intake must equal water loss. One route for water loss is her urine (5 L/day); she also has a large loss of water in sweat (volume is not known, perhaps 2 L/day to 3 L/day). Hence she has a daily intake and loss of 7 L to 8 L of water.

With such a large throughput of water, she could easily develop a large *positive* balance of water. This will cause acute hyponatremia, which leads to acute brain cell swelling. There are three possible causes for this large positive balance of water: first, she may drink >8 L of water on a given day (her water intake is not driven by thirst); second, she may lose less water in sweat (e.g., she did not run that day); third, water excretion may decrease suddenly due to a non-osmotic stimulus for the release of vasopressin (e.g., pain, nausea, anxiety, drugs such as "Ecstasy"[7]).

A different risk is osmotic demyelination, which may develop if she had a large *negative* balance of water and thereby, too rapid a rise in her P_{Na}, especially if she had a much lower P_{Na} for several days. Moreover, patients with a poor dietary intake are at greater risk of developing osmotic demyelination.[8] Because her urine flow rate is determined by the rate of delivery of filtrate to the distal nephron, this delivery may increase if she had a high salt intake (e.g., she ate pizza with anchovies) or was given an infusion of isotonic saline (see Fig. 24–1).

Consult SW-2: What Is "Partial" About Partial Central Diabetes Insipidus?

A 32-year-old healthy male had a recent basal skull fracture. His urine output is ~4-L/day—this is a consistent finding. The first morning P_{Na} is 143-mmol/L, his U_{osm} is 200 mOsm/kg H_2O in the 24-hour urine collection, and vasopressin levels in plasma were undetectable. When he was given dDAVP, his urine flow rate decreased to 0.5 ml/min and the U_{osm} rose to 900 mOsm/kg H_2O. Two other facts, however, deserve further analysis. First, he was thirsty in the morning when he woke up. Second, his sleep was not interrupted by a need to urinate. In fact his U_{osm} was ~425 mOsm/kg H_2O in several overnight urines. In random urine daytime collections, his U_{osm} was 900 mOsm/kg H_2O; his P_{Na} at those times was 137 mmol/L. Moreover, his urine flow rate fell to 0.5 ml/min and his U_{osm} rose to 900 mOsm/kg H_2O after an infusion of hypertonic saline.

Questions

Is this a water diuresis?
What are the best options for therapy?

Discussion
Is This A Water Diuresis?
U_{osm} and urine flow rate: Because his U_{osm} was 200 mOsm/kg H_2O and the urine volume was 4 L/day, this was a water diuresis with a normal osmole excretion rate (800 mosmol/day) (see Fig. 24–2).
Response to dDAVP: He had an adequate renal response to dDAVP because his U_{osm} rose to 900 mOsm/kg H_2O when this hormone was given—this ruled out nephrogenic diabetes insipidus (DI). Hence he has central DI. Because his urine volume was 4 L/day and not 10 L/day to 15 L/day, the diagnosis was "partial central DI".

Interpretation
Although the diagnosis of central DI was straightforward, there were two facts that have not yet been interpreted. First, because he was thirsty, his "osmostat" and thirst center as well as the fibers connecting them appear to be functionally intact (Fig. 24–3). Similarly, because he could excrete concentrated urine (his overnight U_{osm} was 425 mOsm/kg H_2O) when his P_{Na} was 143 mmol/L, his vasopressin release center was also functioning, but only when there was this "stronger stimulus" for the release of this hormone. Therefore a possible site for his lesion was destruction of some but not all of the fibers linking his "osmostat" to his vasopressin release center (Fig. 24–4).[9] This could also explain why polyuria was *not* present overnight. (He stopped his oral water intake several hours prior to going to sleep.) This challenged the diagnosis of partial central DI, or at least our concept of what that diagnosis really implies.

Primary Polydipsia
On first evaluation, because his P_{Na} was high enough to stimulate the release of vasopressin (143 mmol/L), primary polydipsia was not present at this time. In contrast, his U_{osm} was consistently ~90 mOsm/kg H_2O and his P_{Na} was 137 mmol/L during the daytime; this suggests that primary polydipsia was present while he was awake. Its basis probably reflects a "learned behavior" to avoid the very uncomfortable feeling of thirst. This interpretation provides a rationale to under-

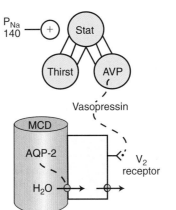

Disorders

1. Central diabetes insipidus
   - hypodipsia if involves the stat or thirst centers

2. Circulating vasopressinase

3. Nephrogenic diabetes insipidus

4. Decreased medullary osmolality

FIGURE 24–3 Lesion causing a water diuresis. The three circles represent areas in the hypothalamus; the top one labeled "stat" is the sensor ("osmostat"), which detects changes in cell volume in response to a change in the P_{Na}. These cells are linked to the thirst center (lower left) and to the vasopressin (AVP) release center (lower right). Non-osmotic stimuli also influence the release of vasopressin. Vasopressin causes the insertion of water channels in the late distal nephron (lower barrel-shaped structure). The diseases that can lead to an abnormally high urine output are shown to the right.

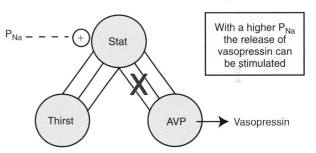

FIGURE 24–4 Lesion in the CNS causing partial central DI. The three circles represent areas in the hypothalamus, the top one labeled "stat" is the sensor ("osmostat"), the circle on the lower left is the thirst center, and the circle on the lower right is the vasopressin (AVP) release center. The X symbol represents the hypothetical lesion that leads to severing of some but not all of the fibers connecting the "osmostat" to the vasopressin release center.

stand the natural history of, and importantly the options for management for his partial central DI.

What Are The Best Options for Therapy?
The major point here is that a higher P_{Na} could stimulate the release of vasopressin. There are two ways to raise the P_{Na}: an input of NaCl or a water deficit. The patient selected oral NaCl tablets to raise his P_{Na} to control his daytime polyuria because of its rapid and reproducible onset. Moreover, this therapy avoids the risk of acute hyponatremia, which may occur if he was given dDAVP and drank an excessive quantity of water. In contrast, he selected water deprivation to raise his P_{Na} overnight to permit him to have undisturbed sleep; he was able to tolerate the thirst that developed.

Osmotic Diuresis with The "Expected" Medullary Osmolality
Concept SW-2
When AQP2 water channels are inserted into the luminal membrane of the late distal nephron, the U_{osm} is equal to the medullary interstitial osmolality.

The volume of an osmotic diuresis is directly proportional to the rate of excretion of osmoles and inversely proportional to the medullary interstitial osmolality. Because AQP2 are not present in late distal nephron in the absence of vasopressin, the rate of excretion of osmoles does *not* influence the urine volume in this setting. Therefore there cannot be an osmotic diuresis and a water diuresis in the *same patient* at the *same time* (see Fig. 24–1).

The medullary interstitial osmolality falls during an osmotic diuresis because there is less reabsorption of Na^+ and Cl^- in the medullary thick limb of the loop of Henle (mTAL), largely due to the fact that fluid entering the mTAL has a lower Na^+ concentration.[10]

The "expected" medullary interstitial osmolality is ~600 mOsm/kg H_2O at somewhat high osmole excretion rates and values are closer to the P_{osm} at much higher osmole excretion rates.[11]

Tools: Osmotic Diuresis

When evaluating the basis for a large urine volume in a patient with an osmotic diuresis, measure the concentrations of all major solutes in the urine (Fig. 24–5).

Osmole excretion rate: This rate should be much >1000 mosmol/day or 0.5 mosmol/min in an adult during an osmotic diuresis.

U_{osm}: The "expected" U_{osm} should be more than the P_{osm}; the absolute value depends on the osmole excretion rate and the medullary interstitial osmolality.

Nature of the urine osmoles: This should be determined by measuring the rate of excretion of the individual osmoles in the urine. As a quick test, however, deduce which solute may be responsible for the osmotic diuresis by measuring the concentrations of likely compounds in plasma (e.g., glucose and urea) and determine if mannitol or a lavage fluid solute was infused. Nevertheless, patients rarely are given a sufficiently large amount of mannitol to be the sole cause of a sustained osmotic diuresis. A saline- induced osmotic diuresis may occur if there was a large infusion of saline or in a patient with cerebral or nephrogenic salt wasting. To diagnose a state of salt wasting, there must be an appreciable excretion of Na^+ at a time when the "effective" arterial blood volume is *definitely* contracted.

Source of the urine osmoles: In a patient with a glucose or urea-induced osmotic diuresis, it is important to decide

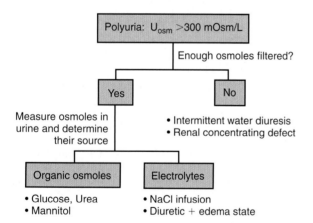

FIGURE 24–5 Approach to the patient with polyuria due to an osmotic diuresis. To enter this flow chart, the patient must have a large urine volume with an osmolality that is distinctly higher than the P_{osm}. A bullet symbol denotes the final diagnostic categories.

whether these osmoles were derived from catabolism of endogenous proteins.

Consult SW-3: An Unusually Large Osmotic Diuresis in A Diabetic Patient

A 50-kg, 14-year-old female has a long history of poorly controlled type 1 diabetes mellitus because she does not take insulin regularly. In the past 48 hours, she was thirsty, drank large volumes of fruit juice, and her urine volume was very high. On physical examination, there was no evidence to imply that her ECF volume was appreciably contracted. The urine flow rate was 10 ml/min over this 100-minute period. Other lab data include: pH 7.33, P_{HCO_3} 24 mmol/L, $P_{Anion\ gap}$ 16-mEq/L, P_K 4.8 mmol/L, $P_{Creatinine}$ 1.0 mg/dL (88 μmol/L) (close to her usual values), BUN 22 mg/dL (P_{Urea} 8 mmol/L), and hematocrit 0.45. Of note, there was no decrease in her glucose concentration in plasma ($P_{Glucose}$) despite the excretion of a large amount of glucose (Table 24–1).

Questions

What is the basis of the polyuria?
What dangers do you anticipate for this patient?

Discussion

What Is the Basis of the Polyuria?

Osmole excretion rate: The product of her U_{osm} (450 mOsm/L) and urine flow rate (10 ml/min) yields an osmole excretion rate of 4.5 mosmol/min, a value that is ninefold higher than the usual value in an adult (0.5 mosmol/min) (see Fig. 24–5).

U_{osm}: The U_{osm} of 450 mOsm/kg H_2O indicates that this polyuria is due to an osmotic diuresis. In addition, this U_{osm} is lower than "expected", probably reflecting the very high osmole excretion rate, which caused a larger fall in her medullary interstitial osmolality.

Urine flow rate: The urine flow rate was extremely high for two reasons: the very high osmole excretion rate and the lower than "expected" osmolality in her medullary interstitial compartment.

Nature of the urine osmoles: Because her GFR is modestly low and her $P_{Glucose}$ was extremely high (1260 mg/dL, 70 mmol/L), her filtered load of glucose will be markedly higher than the maximum tubular capacity for its reabsorption; hence, this is likely to be a glucose-induced osmotic diuresis (confirmed by a $U_{Glucose}$ that was 350 mmol/L).

Source of the urine osmoles: Of special emphasis, her $P_{Glucose}$ did not decline despite such a high rate of excretion of glucose. To put it into quantitative terms, the total content of glucose in her ECF compartment is 12.6 g (1260 mg/dL × 10 × 10 L ECFV/1000) while she excreted 54 g of glucose (5400 mg/dL × 10 × 1 L/1000). Therefore, she excreted an amount of glucose that is fourfold more than all the glucose she had in her ECF compartment. Accordingly, to maintain this degree of hyperglycemia, she needed an enormous input of glucose over a short period of time. The only likely source of such a large input of glucose was the glucose that was retained in her stomach. As a reference, 1 L of apple juice contains ~135 g of glucose. For ingested glucose to fuel an osmotic diuresis, this patient would need a rapid rate of gastric emptying. Although the usual effect of hyperglycemia

TABLE 24–1	Data for Consult SW-3					
		Admission		**100 min**	
		Plasma	**Urine**	**Plasma**	**Urine**
Glucose	mg/dL (mmol/L)	1260 (70)	5400 (300)	1260 (70)	5400 (300)
Na^+	mmol/L	125	50	123	50
Osmolality	mOsm/L	320	450	316	450

is to slow gastric emptying, for some reason this did *not* occur in this patient.[12]

What Dangers Do You Anticipate for This Patient?

Low ECF volume: Because glucose is an "effective" osmole in the ECF compartment, it helped to maintain her ECF volume. If she had discontinued her ingestion of glucose-containing beverages long before arriving in hospital, her ECF volume would now be obviously contracted because she would have excreted a large proportion of the glucose in her ECF compartment (e.g., at a rate faster than glucose entry from the GI tract).

Cerebral edema: Brain cell swelling may occur if there is a significant fall in her "effective" P_{osm} ($2 P_{Na} + P_{Glucose}$ in mmol/L terms).[13] This could occur if she excretes urine with a higher "effective" osmolality than the P_{osm}. This risk would be even greater if she had changed her intake to water rather than sugar-containing beverages.

Concept SW-4

Not all osmoles are equal in their ability to increase the urine volume.

The osmoles that cannot achieve equal concentrations in the lumen of the MCD and in the medullary interstitial compartment are called "effective" osmoles; they dictate what the urine flow rate will be when the MCD is permeable to water. Urea, on the other hand, may be an "*ineffective*" urine osmole in some circumstances and an "*effective*" urine osmole in other circumstances. Because cells in the papillary collecting duct have urea transporters in their membrane when vasopressin acts, urea is usually an "ineffective" osmole (same concentration on both sides of that membrane) and it does *not* cause water to be excreted. The net result of excreting a small *extra* amount of urea is a higher U_{osm}, but not a higher "effective" U_{osm} or a higher urine flow rate.[14] Therefore, it is more correct to say that the urine flow rate is directly proportional to the number of non-urea or "effective" urine osmoles and inversely proportional to their concentration in the medullary interstitial compartment (see following equation).

Urine flow rate = # "Effective" urine osmoles/
["effective" urine osmoles]

In contrast, when the rate of excretion of urea rises by a large amount, urea might not be absorbed fast enough to achieve equal concentrations on both sides of a membrane. Hence, urea may become an "effective" osmole in the inner MCD and obligate the excretion of water. The analysis is not always that simple because urea is a partially "effective" urine osmole if the rate of excretion of electrolytes is low.[14,15]

Tools

Urea Appearance Rate

The rate of appearance of urea can be determined from the amount of urea that is retained in the body plus the amount excreted in the urine over a given period of time. The former can be calculated from the rise in the concentration of urea in plasma (P_{Urea}) and assuming a volume of distribution of urea equal to total body water (~60% body weight).

Source of Urea

Close to 16% of the weight of protein is nitrogen. Therefore if 100 g of protein were oxidized, 16 g of nitrogen would be formed. Because the molecular weight of nitrogen is 14, there would be 1143 mmol of nitrogen produced. Since urea contains two atoms of nitrogen, 572 mmol urea are produced from the oxidation of 100 g of protein. In terms of lean body mass, because water is its main constituent (80% of weight), each kg has 800 g of water and 180 g of protein.[16] Therefore, breakdown of 1 kg of lean mass will produce ~1000 mmol of urea. One can use this calculation to determine if the source of urea was exogenous or from endogenous breakdown of protein.

Consult SW-4: Osmotic Diuresis with An Emphasis on The Rate of Excretion of Urea

A 70-kg male had a recent bone marrow transplant. He was given large doses of corticosteroids. His 24-hour urine volume was 6 L/day and his U_{osm} was 500 mOsm/kg H_2O. He did not receive mannitol, his $P_{Glucose}$ was 180 mg/dl (10 mmol/L), and his BUN was 210 mg/dL (P_{Urea} was 75 mmol/L).

Questions

What is the cause of polyuria?
What is the major aim of therapy with respect to urea excretion?

Discussion

What is the cause of the polyuria?
Osmole excretion rate: There is an osmotic diuresis because his osmole excretion rate was 3000 mosmol/day (6 L urine/day and U_{osm} of 500 mOsm/kg H_2O).

Nature of the Osmoles

His $P_{Glucose}$ was too low for high rates of glucosuria. On the other hand, his P_{Urea} was high enough (75 mmol/L) to produce a sufficient quantity of filtered urea to cause the osmotic diuresis—this was confirmed later when his U_{Urea} was measured (400 mmol/L). Because his urine volume was 6 L, he excreted ~2400 mmol of urea that day.

Source of the Urine Urea

These 2400 mmol of urea would be produced from the oxidation of 420 g of protein. On that day, he was given 60 g of protein by nasogastric tube so he oxidized approximately 360 g of endogenous protein. This excretion of urea represents the catabolism of 2 kg of lean body mass (360 g/180 g/kg). If this were to continue, he would ultimately undergo marked muscle wasting. This can cause a problem because of compromised respiratory muscle function leading to bronchopneumonia. Furthermore, this catabolic state could affect his immunological defense mechanisms.[17]

What Is the Major Aim of Therapy?

Once this metabolic problem is recognized, therapy must be more vigorous at the nutritional level. First, more exogenous calories and protein must be given. Second, therapy could include anabolic hormones such as high-dose insulin (with glucose to avoid hypoglycemia) or anabolic steroids and/or the provision of nutritional supplements such as glutamine to minimize endogenous protein catabolism.[17] Third, one should be cautious about continued use of high doses of the catabolic hormone, glucocorticoids.

Concept SW-5

If there is no change in the number of osmoles in the ICF compartment, the volume of the ICF compartment is inversely proportional to the P_{Na}.

When the P_{Na} rises, the cell volume shrinks and when the P_{Na} falls, the cell volume swells (Fig. 24–6). The volume of brain cells is most important in this regard because the brain is constrained by the rigid skull.

Tools

Tonicity Balance

To decide what the basis is for a change in the P_{Na} and to define the proper therapy to return the P_{Na}, ECF and ICF volumes to their normal value, separate balances for water and Na^+ *must* be calculated.[18] To perform this calculation, one must examine the volume and electrolyte composition of all the fluids ingested and infused and that of all outputs over the period when the P_{Na} changed (Fig. 24–7). In practical terms, a tonicity balance can be performed only in a hospital setting where inputs and outputs are accurately recorded. With regard to the output, this can be restricted to the urine in an acute setting. In a febrile patient or one who has been

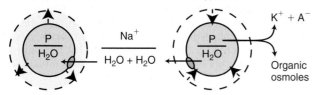

FIGURE 24–6 The P_{Na} reflects the ICF volume. The solid circle represents a cell. The ICF compartment contains macromolecular anions (P^-) that are restricted to this compartment along with its major effective osmole, K^+. The osmoles restricted to the ECF compartment are Na^+ and its attendant anions (Cl^- and HCO_3^-). Urea is not an effective osmole because there is a urea transporter that permits urea to achieve near-equal concentrations in the ECF and ICF compartments. There is osmotic equilibrium because water can cross the cell membrane rapidly through water channels (AQP1) in the cell membrane. The P_{Na} is inversely proportional to the ICF volume (e.g., in acute hyponatremia shown on the left). Exceptions to this rule are when there are other "effective" osmoles in the ECF compartment (e.g., glucose, mannitol) or when the number of "effective" osmoles changes in the ICF compartment (e.g., brain cell volume regulation in chronic hyponatremia [shown on the right], or during a seizure [not shown]).

in the ICU for a prolonged period, balance calculations will not be as accurate because sweat losses are not measured. For example, if the balance for water is recorded in the hospital chart, the clinician can determine why the P_{Na} changed.[18]

When calculating a Na^+ balance, be careful not to multiply the concentration of Na^+ in the terminal potion of a long urine collection period by the total urine volume because the urine composition may have changed during this time.

Calculation of An Electrolyte-Free Water Balance

To perform this calculation, one must also know the volume and the concentrations of $Na^+ + K^+$ in the input and in the urine. The first step is decide how much water is needed to convert all of the $Na^+ + K^+$ into an isotonic saline solution (e.g., 150 mmol in 1 L of water in molal terms if the P_{osm} is in the normal range). For example, if the concentration of $Na^+ + K^+$ in a urine sample were lower than in plasma, the remainder of the volume is called electrolyte-free water. Alternatively, had there been residual $Na^+ + K^+$, the excretion of the remaining electrolytes is given the very confusing name of "negative" electrolyte-free water. As shown in Table 24–2, an electrolyte-free water balance cannot distinguish between negative balances of water and positive balances for Na^+ as the cause of the rise in the P_{Na}. Accordingly, we do not use electrolyte-free water balances as they do *not* reveal the basis

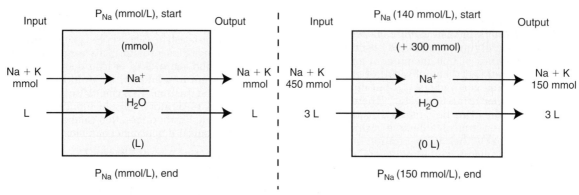

FIGURE 24–7 Calculation of a tonicity balance. The rectangle represents the body with its concentration of Na^+ in the ECF compartment at the beginning (written above this rectangle) and at the end (written below this rectangle) of this period where the tonicity balance is calculated. The input of $Na^+ + K^+$ and of water are shown on the left and their outputs are shown on the right of this rectangle. The essential data to calculate a tonicity balance are shown to the left of the vertical dashed line and actual values from Consult SW-5 are shown to the right of that line.

TABLE 24–2	Comparison of an Electrolyte-free Water Balance and a Tonicity Balance				
	Na + K (mmol)	Water (L)	EFW (L)	Therapy from Balances	
				EFW	Tonicity
Consult SW-5					
Input	450	3	0	+2 L	+0 L water
Output	150	3	2	? Na$^+$	−300 mmol Na$^+$
Balance	**+300**	**0**	**−2**		
Case if 4 L of isotonic saline were infused and the urine output was unchanged					
Input	600	4	0	+2 L	−1 L
Output	150	3	2	? Na$^+$	−450 mmol Na$^+$
Balance	**+450**	**+1**	**−2**		
Case if no intravenous fluid was administered and the urine output was unchanged					
Input	0	0	0	+2 L	+3 L
Output	150	3	2	? Na$^+$	+150 mmol Na$^+$
Balance	**−150**	**−3**	**−2**		

Three situations are described where the P_{Na} rose from 140 mmol/L to 150 mmol/L. The only difference is the volume of isotonic saline infused over the time period of observation. In all three settings, there is a negative balance of 2 L of electrolyte-free water. Nevertheless, the goals of therapy to correct the hypernatremia are clear only after a tonicity balance is calculated.
EFW, electrolyte-free water.

of the change in the P_{Na} and hence do *not* help with the design of therapy to return the volume and composition of the ECF and ICF compartments to their normal values.

Consult SW-5: A Water Diuresis and An Osmotic Diuresis in the Same Patient?

A craniopharyngioma was resected today from a 16-year-old male (weight 50 kg, total body water 30 L). During neurosurgery, his urine flow rate rose to 10 ml/min (3 L in 300 min) and his P_{Na} rose from 140 mmol/L to 150 mmol/L. Over this period, he received 3 L of isotonic saline. His U_{osm} was 120 mOsm/kg H_2O, and his urine $Na^+ + K^+$ concentration was 50 mmol/L. To confirm the diagnosis of central DI, he was given dDAVP; his urine flow rate fell to 6 ml/min, the U_{Na+K} rose to 175 mmol/L, and his U_{osm} was 375 mOsm/kg H_2O.

Questions

What is the "expected" renal response to dDAVP in this patient?
Why did his P_{Na} rise from 140 mmol/L to 150 mmol/L during his large water diuresis?

Discussion

What is the "Expected" Renal Response to dDAVP?

The initial information that will be available to assess the response to dDAVP is his urine flow rate; it is directly proportional to the osmole excretion rate and inversely proportional to the medullary interstitial osmolality.

Osmole excretion rate: The osmole excretion rate before dDAVP is given—it is equal to the product of the U_{osm} (120 mOsm/kg H_2O) and urine flow rate (10 ml/min), or 1.2 mosmol/min; this excretion rate is more than double the expected rate of 0.5 mosmol/min.

U_{osm}: There will be a delay before the actual value is known, but we can predict what it might be; the "expected" value is ~600 mOsm/kg H_2O in an osmotic diuresis, but because the preceding large water diuresis would have "washed out" or lowered the osmolality in the medullary interstitial compartment, a reasonable prediction would be ~400 mOsm/kg H_2O.

Nature of the osmoles: Prior to the administration of dDAVP, 5 of 6 of the osmoles in the urine were $Na^+ + K^+$ salts ($U_{Na} + U_K = 50$ mmol/L, U_{osm} 120 mOsm/kg H_2O). Because electrolytes are "effective" osmoles whereas urea is not usually an "effective" osmole when vasopressin acts, his "effective" osmole excretion rate is even higher than expected from the osmole excretion rate calculated earlier.

Summary: Based on all of the previous discussion, we would not be surprised to find a urine flow rate of ~5 ml/min after dDAVP acts. In fact, once the effect of the anesthetic agent that diminished the tone of venous capacitance vessels abates, there will be an even higher "effective" osmole excretion rate (i.e., a larger natriuresis driven by the higher central venous pressure).

Why Did His P_{Na} Rise from 140 mmol/L to 150 mmol/L during His Large Water Diuresis?

Tonicity balance: The patient received 3 L of water (as isotonic saline, but it is still 3 L of water in volume terms) and he excreted 3 L of urine (with a $U_{Na} + U_K$ of 50 mmol/L, but it too is still water in volume terms). Accordingly, there is a nil balance of water.

Balance data for $Na^+ + K^+$ reveal that he received 450 mmol (3 L × 150 mmol/L) and he excreted only 150 mmol (3 L × 50 mmol/L). Hence he has a positive balance of 300 mmol of $Na^+ + K^+$. Dividing this surplus by the total body water (30 L) suggests that the rise in P_{Na} should be 10 mmol/L, a value equal to the actual rise in the P_{Na}. Therefore the basis for the rise in P_{Na} was a gain of Na^+ and not a loss of water. The proper treatment to restore body tonicity and the volume and composition of the ECF and ICF compartments is to induce a loss of 300 mmol of Na^+.

Parenthetically, even if there were no measurements of Na^+ or K^+ in the urine, these values can be calculated for the period where one has the following measured values; the P_{Na} at the beginning and end of the balance period, water balance for that period, and the quantity of $Na^+ + K^+$ infused; details of the calculation and its verification can be found in Ref. 19.

Integration: Clinical Approach to the Patient with Polyuria

In a patient with polyuria, a water diuresis is present when the U_{osm} is appreciably <250 mOsm/L (see Fig. 24–2). To determine if it is due to a lack of vasopressin (central DI) or an inability of vasopressin to act (nephrogenic DI), this hormone should be administered. Patients with circulating vasopressinase (e.g., tissue necrosis) respond to the administration of dDAVP, but fail to respond to the administration of vasopressin. As shown in Consult SW-5, the "expected" response should be adjusted for the calculated osmole excretion rate and the lower medullary interstitial osmolality due to prior medullary wash out. Another caveat in interpreting the urine data after the administration of dDAVP is that in absence of vasopressin action, the urine flow rate is determined by of the distal delivery of filtrate. Therefore, a lower urine flow rate and a higher U_{osm} may be observed if there is diminished distal delivery of filtrate because of a fall in the GFR. The clinical clues for this scenario are a fall in blood pressure and a fall in the osmole excretion rate.

To diagnose an osmotic diuresis, vasopressin must act, the U_{osm} must exceed the P_{osm}, and the osmole excretion rate must be >1000 mosmol/day (see Fig. 24–5). Another factor that influences the urine flow rate in an osmotic diuresis is the medullary interstitial osmolality. To deduce which osmole is responsible for the osmotic diuresis, assess whether there is a high $P_{Glucose}$ or P_{Urea}, whether sufficient amount of mannitol was infused, whether the patient has received a large amount of saline; and/or whether the patient has renal or cerebral salt wasting. The diagnosis of an osmotic diuresis has several important implications for the patient. First, it can induce a loss of Na^+ in the urine, and thereby lead to contraction of the ECF volume (e.g., the patient with diabetic ketoacidosis [DKA]). Second, because the concentration of Na^+ in the urine is usually much less than the P_{Na}, the urinary loss can lead to the development of hypernatremia. Third, the source of the urine osmoles may be a high rate of excretion of glucose or urea that was derived from lean body mass (see "Consult SW-4").

To know whether a water or an osmotic diuresis will lead to a rise (or fall) in the P_{Na} and to design appropriate therapy, one should calculate separate balances for water and Na^+ (a tonicity balance).

Concentrating Defect in the Renal Medulla

There are two factors that influence the urine flow rate when vasopressin acts, the number of "effective" osmoles in the luminal fluid of the inner medullary collecting duct and the osmolality of the fluid in the medullary interstitial compartment. To illustrate the importance of each of these factors, consider a patient who has sickle cell anemia. In this disorder, there is obstruction of the blood vessels by sickled cells deep in the inner medulla. As a result, there is necrosis of the renal papilla. Since the inner medullary collecting duct is the nephron site where vasopressin causes the insertion of urea transporters, patients with papillary necrosis cannot reabsorb urea at appreciable rates when vasopressin acts. Therefore, urea becomes an "effective" urine osmole in this setting and it obligates the excretion of water. In addition, if urea cannot be reabsorbed as an isosmotic solution in the inner medullary collecting duct, this will prevent the

763

CH 24

Interpretation of Electrolyte and Acid-Base Parameters in Blood and Urine reabsorption of Na^+ and Cl^- from the thin ascending limb of the loop of Henle. Accordingly, the maximum medullary interstitial osmolality will be ~600 mOsm/kg H_2O. If this patient excretes 900 mosmol/day and *all* of the urine osmoles are "effective", the minimum urine volume will be 1.5 L/day. Contrast these numbers with a subject who has a similar osmole excretion rate (1/2 urea, 1/2 electrolytes) who has a normal papilla, but a maximum U_{osm} that is also 600 mosmol/kg H_2O. After vasopressin acts, there will be an insertion of urea transporters in the inner medullary collecting duct and the concentration of urea will be equal in the lumen of the inner medullary collecting duct and in the papillary interstitial compartment. Therefore, his rate of excretion of effective osmoles would be 1/2 of 900 mosmol/day or 450 mosmol/day. Accordingly, his daily urine volume would be 0.75 L (450 mosmol/600 mOsm/L), much less than in the patient with sickle cell anemia.

This example illustrates the complexities of a concentrating defect with a given maximum U_{osm} because if the lesion converts urinary urea into an "effective" urine osmole, the daily urine volume will increase ~ twofold.

Defense of the Extracellular Fluid Volume

Concept SW-6
The volume of the ECF compartment is largely determined by its quantity of Na^+.

The most reliable way to know how much Na^+ is present in the ECF compartment is to measure the P_{Na} and to multiply this value by the ECF volume. This requires a *quantitative* assessment of the ECF volume.

Concept SW-7
Na^+ wasting can only be diagnosed when there is excretion of too much Na^+; the term "wasting" implies that the ECF volume must be low.

To make a diagnosis of renal or cerebral salt wasting, one needs a *quantitative* estimate of the ECF volume.

Tools
Estimate the Extracellular Fluid Volume
The physical examination, the concentrations of K^+, HCO_3^-, creatinine, urea, and urate in plasma as well as the fractional excretions of the latter two are useful at times to imply that the "effective" ECF volume may be contracted. Nevertheless, none of the above provides a quantitative estimate of the ECF volume. For the latter, we rely on the hematocrit (or a change in the hematocrit with therapy in the patient who has anemia or erythrocytosis) (Table 24–3).

Sample calculation: In a normal adult, the usual hematocrit is 0.40; this represents a blood volume of 5 L (2 L of red blood cells (RBC) and 3 L of plasma; see following equation). Therefore, with a hematocrit of 0.50, there are still 2 L of RBC. Solving for "X"—the present blood volume—it is 4 L and the plasma volume is 2 L (+2 L RBC)—hence the plasma volume

is reduced by 1 L from its normal 3 L value. Ignoring changes in Starling forces for simplicity, the ECF volume should have declined to approximately two thirds of its normal volume.

$$\text{Hematocrit} (0.40) = 2 \text{ L RBC/Blood volume}$$
$$(2 \text{ L RBC} + 3 \text{ L plasma})$$

$$\text{Hematocrit} (0.50) = 2 \text{ L RBC/"X" L blood volume}$$

Basis for the Low Extracellular Fluid Volume
Measuring the urine electrolytes can be very helpful to gain insights into the basis for a contracted ECF volume (Table 24–4). As background, the expected response to a low "effective" arterial blood volume is to excrete as little Na^+ and Cl^- as possible. Because timed urine collections to calculate absolute rates of excretion of Na^+ and Cl^- are seldom obtained, clinicians should interpret the U_{Na} and U_{Cl} in a spot urine sample. A low U_{Na} or a low U_{Cl} (or both) does not necessarily indicate a low rate of excretion of Na^+ and/or Cl^- if the urine flow rate is high. To avoid this type of error, the U_{Na} and U_{Cl} should be related to the urine creatinine concentration ($U_{Creatinine}$).

A Low Rate of Excretion of Na^+ and Cl^-
This pattern may suggest a low intake of NaCl or that the effective arterial blood volume is contracted due to a loss of NaCl by a non-renal route (e.g., by sweating), or that there was a prior renal loss of Na^+ and Cl^- (e.g., remote use of diuretics).

A High Rate of Excretion of Na^+ but Little Excretion of Cl^-
In a patient with a low effective arterial blood volume, there is an anion other than Cl^- being excreted with Na^+. If the anion is HCO_3^- (the urine pH is alkaline), suspect recent vomiting. The anion could also be one that was ingested or administered (e.g., penicillin) in which case, the urine pH is usually less than 6.

A High Rate of Excretion of Cl^- but Little Excretion of Na^+
In this patient with a low "effective" arterial blood volume, there is a cation being excreted with Cl^- other than Na^+. Most often the cation is NH_4^+ and the setting is diarrhea or laxative abuse. Rarely the cation could be K^+ if KCl was ingested.

The Excretions of Na^+ and Cl^- Are Not Low
In a patient who has a low effective arterial blood volume, a high rate of excretion of both Na^+ and Cl^- suggests that the patient has a deficit of a stimulator of the reabsorption of Na^+

TABLE 24–3	Use of the Hematocrit to Estimate the Extracellular Fluid Volume	
Hematocrit	Hemoglobin (g/L)	% Change in ECF Volume
0.40	140	0
0.50	171	−33
0.60	210	−60

The assumptions made when using this calculation are that the patient did not have anemia or erythrocytosis, that the RBC volume is 2 L, and the plasma volume is 3 L (blood volume 5 L). The formula is: hematocrit = RBC volume/(RBC volume + plasma volume).
ECF, extracellular fluid.

TABLE 24–4	Urine Electrolytes in the Differential Diagnosis of Extracellular Fluid Volume Contraction	
Condition	**Urine Electrolyte**	
	Na⁺	**Cl⁻**
Vomiting		
Recent	High*	Low†
Remote	Low	Low
Diuretics		
Recent	High	High
Remote	Low	Low
Diarrhea or laxative abuse	Low	High
Bartter or Gitelman syndrome	High	High

*High = Urine concentration > 15 mmol/L.
†Low = Urine concentration < 15 mmol/L.
Adjust values for the urine electrolyte concentration when polyuria is present.

and Cl^- (e.g., aldosterone), the presence of an inhibitor of the reabsorption of NaCl (e.g., a diuretic), or an intrinsic renal lesion that is similar to having the actions of a diuretic (discussed later in "Potassium and Metabolic Alkalosis"). The pattern of excretion of electrolytes throughout the day can also be very important. For example, if there are times when the U_{Na} and U_{Cl} are both low, this suggests that the patient is taking a diuretic.

Fractional Excretion of Na^+ or Cl^-
On a typical western diet, the daily excretions of Na^+ and Cl^- are ~150 mmol. Because a normal GFR is ~180 L/day, the kidney filters ~27,000 mmol of Na^+ and 20,000 mmol of Cl^- per day (adjusting the P_{Na} and P_{Cl} per plasma water). Rather then expressing this function in fractional reabsorption terms (>99%), it is common to express them as fractional excretion terms (FE_{Na} ~ 0.5%, FE_{Cl} ~ 0.75%). To make this calculation of the fractional excretion as simple as possible, the urine to plasma ratio for creatinine is used (see following equation).

$$FE_{Na} = 100 \times (U_{Na}/P_{Na})/(U_{Creatinine}/P_{Creatinine})$$

There are three practical points to bear in mind when using the FE_{Na} or FE_{Cl}. First, the excretions of Na^+ and Cl^- are directly related to the dietary intake of NaCl. Hence a low FE_{Na} or FE_{Cl} may represent either a low effective arterial blood volume or a low intake of NaCl (or both). Second, the FE_{Na} *or* FE_{Cl} may be high in a patient with a low "effective" arterial blood volume when there is an unusually large excretion of another anion (e.g., HCO_3^-) in the case of Na^+ or another cation (e.g., NH_4^+) in the case of Cl^-. Third, the numeric values for the FE_{Na} and the FE_{Cl} will be twice as high in a euvolemic patient who consumes 150 mmol of NaCl daily if that patient has a GFR that is half of normal. Hence the clinical significance of these FE_{Na} and FE_{Cl} numeric values must be adjusted for the GFR at the time when the measurements are made. In addition, there are problems with respect to accuracy when creatinine is used to measure the GFR. Nevertheless, the use of these parameters may be of value in the differential diagnosis of pre-renal azotemia versus acute tubular necrosis (ATN).[20] The advantage of using these tests in this setting over the use of the U_{Na} and U_{Cl} is that the use of $U_{Creatinine}/P_{Creatinine}$ adjusts these concentration terms for water reabsorption in the nephron.

Determine the Nephron Site with an Abnormal Reabsorption of Na^+

Look for Failure to Reabsorb Other Substances
If a compound or ion that should have been reabsorbed in a given nephron segment is being excreted, one has presumptive evidence for a reabsorptive defect in that nephron segment. For example, if the defect is in the PCT, one might find glucosuria in the absence of hyperglycemia.

Compensatory Effects in Downstream Nephron Segments
When there is inhibition of the reabsorption of NaCl in upstream nephron segments, more NaCl is delivered to the CCD, where the reabsorption of Na^+ may occur in conjunction with K^+ secretion.

Consult SW-6: Assessment of the "Effective" Arterial Blood Volume
A 25-year-old female was assessed by her family physician because of progressive weakness. Although she admitted to being concerned about her body image, she denied vomiting or the intake of diuretics. Her blood pressure was 90/60 mm Hg, her pulse rate was 110 beats/min, and her jugular venous pressure was low. Acid-base measurements in arterial blood revealed a pH 7.39 and a PCO_2 of 39 mm Hg. In results from venous blood, her P_{HCO3} was 24 mmol/L, $P_{Anion\ gap}$ was

17 mEq/L, P_K was 1.9 mmol/L, hematocrit was 0.50, and her $P_{Albumin}$ was 5.0 g/dL (50 g/L). The urine electrolytes prior to therapy were U_{Na} 0 mmol/L, U_{Cl} 42 mmol/L, and U_K 23 mmol/L.

Questions
How severe is her degree of ECF volume contraction? What is the cause of her low ECF volume?

Discussion

How Severe Is Her Degree of extracellular Fluid Volume Contraction?
The elevated value for the hematocrit (0.50) provides quantitative information about her ECF volume (see Table 24–3)[21]; her ECF volume is reduced by 33% if she did not have anemia prior to therapy. If anemia were present, her ECF volume would be even more reduced.

What Is the Cause of Her Low Extracellular Fluid Volume?
The low U_{Na} implies that the "effective" arterial blood volume is low if the patient is not consuming a low salt diet. Nevertheless, the high U_{Cl} (42 mmol/L) does not necessarily indicate an intrinsic renal abnormality. Rather, the fact that her U_{Cl} exceeded the sum of her $U_{Na} + U_K$ suggested that there was another cation in that urine, most likely NH_4^+.

Interpretation
Calculating the content of HCO_3^- in her ECF reveals that she had a deficit of $NaHCO_3$ (see "Metabolic Acidosis" for more discussion). Loss of NaCl plus $NaHCO_3$ via the GI tract was suspected as the cause of contracted ECF volume. The patient later admitted to the frequent use of a laxative. Hence the hypokalemia and contracted effective ECF volume are easily accounted for. Hypokalemia stimulated ammoniagenesis, raising the rate of excretion of the cation NH_4^+; this obligated the excretion of Cl^- despite the presence of a low effective circulating volume.

POTASSIUM AND METABOLIC ALKALOSIS

We combine disorders of K^+ homeostasis and metabolic alkalosis in this section because a deficiency of KCl plays an important role in the pathophysiology of metabolic alkalosis.

Dyskalemias

Hypokalemia and hyperkalemia are common electrolyte disorders in clinical practice that may precipitate life-threatening cardiac arrhythmias. Data from urine measurements provide essential evidence to establish their underlying pathophysiology and to suggest options for therapy.

Concept K-1
There are two factors that influence the movement of K^+ across cell membranes: first, a driving force, which is the concentration difference for K^+ and the electrical voltage across cell membranes and second, the presence of open K^+ channels in cell membranes.

K^+ are kept inside the cells by a net negative interior voltage because the Na-K-ATPase is an electrogenic pump—exporting 3 Na^+ while importing 2 K^+.[22] The Na-K-ATPase can cause more K^+ ions to enter cells if there is a higher concentration of intracellular Na^+ or if this ion pump is activated by β_2-adrenergics, thyroid hormone, or insulin.[23] For the former to result in an increase in cell negative voltage, Na^+ entry into cells must be electroneutral (e.g., via the Na^+/H^+ exchanger (NHE) (Fig. 24–8). NHE is almost always *inactive* in cell membranes, but it becomes active if there is a high concentration of insulin and/or a high H^+ concentration in the ICF compartment.[24]

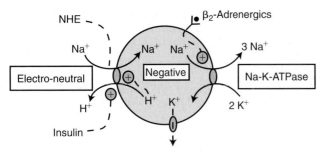

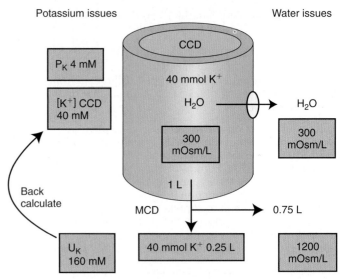

FIGURE 24–8 Factors influencing the movement of K^+ across cell membranes. The passive movement of K^+ across cell membranes requires a driving force (voltage and/or a concentration difference) and an open K^+ channel. The active transport of Na^+ from cells is by the electrogenic Na-K-ATPase increases the intracellular negative voltage. The source of the intracellular Na^+ is the electro-neutral entry of Na^+ via NHE (activated by insulin or a high ICF [H^+]) or the existing ICF Na^+ content. β_2 adrenergic agonists activate the Na-K-ATPase.

FIGURE 24–9 Non-invasive estimate of the flow rate and the [K^+] in the terminal CCD. The barrel-shaped structures represent the CCD and the arrow below it represents the medullary collecting duct (MCD). As shown in the right side of the CCD, when vasopressin acts, the P_{osm} and the osmolality in the luminal fluid in the terminal CCD are equal (e.g., 300 mOsm/kg H_2O); hence the flow rate in the terminal CCD is determined by the rate of delivery of osmoles. In the example shown on the left side, the luminal K^+ concentration is 40 mmol/L or 10-fold larger than the peritubular K^+ concentration of 4 mmol/L. When 1 L of fluid traverses the MCD, 75% of this water is reabsorbed (and no K^+ was reabsorbed or secreted in the MCD in this example). Hence the U_K is fourfold higher (40 mmol/L to 160 mmol/L) as is the U_{osm} (300 to 1200 mOsm/kg H_2O). To back-calculate the [K^+]$_{CCD}$, the U_K is divided by the (U/P)$_{osm}$.

Concept K-2

There is no normal rate of K^+ excretion in the urine because normal subjects in steady state excrete all the K^+ they eat and absorb from the GI tract.

In a patient with hypokalemia or hyperkalemia, the "expected" rate of K^+ excretion is the one observed when normal subjects were deprived of K^+ or given a large load of KCl.

Concept K-3

Chronic disorders of K^+ homeostasis are due to abnormal rates of renal excretion of K^+.

This regulation occurs primarily in the late cortical distal nephron including the cortical collecting duct (CCD). This process has two components—the secretion of K^+ by principal cells and the rate of flow traversing the CCD.

Tools

Rate of Excretion of K^+

The appropriate renal response is to excrete as little K^+ as possible when there is a deficit of K^+ (i.e., <15 mmol/day)[25] and to excrete as much K^+ as possible when there is a surplus of K^+ (i.e., >200 mmol/day).[26] A 24-hour urine collection is not necessary to assess the rate of excretion of K^+. Taking advantage of the fact that creatinine is excreted at a near-constant rate throughout the day (200 μmol/min/kg body weight or 20 mg/min/kg body weight),[27] the same information about the rate of excretion of K^+ from a 24-hour urine collection can be obtained by examining the $U_K/U_{Creatinine}$ ratio in a spot-urine. Furthermore, The $U_K/U_{Creatinine}$ has an advantage because the data are available very quickly and more relevant information is gathered because one knows the stimulus (P_K) influencing K^+ excretion at that time. On the other hand, it has a disadvantage because there is a diurnal variation in K^+ excretion,[28] but this does not negate the advantages. The expected $U_K/U_{Creatinine}$ ratio in a patient with hypokalemia is <15 mmol K^+/g creatinine (or 1.5 mmol K^+/mmol creatinine) whereas this ratio should be >200 mmol K^+/g creatinine (>20 in mmol K^+/mmol creatinine) in a patient with hyperkalemia.

Calculate the Components of the Rate of Excretion of K^+ in the terminal Cortical Collecting Duct

If the rate of K^+ excretion is inappropriate for the presence of hypokalemia or hyperkalemia, both components of the K^+ excretion formula (flow rate and [K^+]) should be examined in terms of events in the terminal CCD (see following equation).[29]

$$K^+ \text{ in the lumen of the CCD} = [K^+]_{CCD} \times \text{Flow rate}_{CCD}$$

<u>Flow rate in the terminal CCD:</u> When vasopressin acts, the luminal osmolality is equal to the P_{osm} and the flow rate in the terminal CCD is determined by the rate of delivery of osmoles because the luminal osmolality is relatively constant (equal to the P_{osm}) and all the luminal osmoles are "effective" ones in this nephron site. Therefore one can obtain a minimum estimate of the rate of flow in terminal CCD by dividing the rate of excretion of osmoles by the P_{osm} (see following equation) (Fig. 24–9). This provides a minimum estimate of flow rate in terminal CCD because of reabsorption of some osmoles in the medullary collecting duct.

$$\text{Flow rate}_{CCD} = (\text{Urine flow rate} \times U_{osm})/P_{osm}$$

The "usual" rate of osmole excretion is ~0.5 mosmol/min or 600 mosmol/day to 900 mosmol/day so a minimum estimate of flow rate in the terminal CCD is 2 L/day to 3 L/day. The major osmoles in the terminal CCD are urea and Na^+ plus Cl^-. Hence a low flow rate in the terminal CCD could be due to a low delivery of urea (low intake of proteins) and/or of Na^+ and Cl^- (low effective circulating volume, low intake of salt). On the other hand, a high flow rate in the CCD could be due to inhibition of the reabsorption of NaCl in an upstream nephron segment (a high salt intake, use of a diuretic [osmotic or pharmacologic]), or diseases that lead to an inhibition of reabsorption of NaCl in an upstream nephron segment (e.g., Bartter syndrome or Gitelman syndrome). During a water diuresis, while the rate of flow in the CCD is high, the rate of excretion of K^+ is not because vasopressin is required for K^+ secretion in the CCD.[30]

[K^+] in the lumen of the terminal CCD ([K^+]$_{CCD}$): A reasonable approximation of the [K^+]$_{CCD}$ can be obtained by adjusting the U_K for the amount of water reabsorbed in the MCD (see Fig. 24–9). The assumption here is that there is little K^+ secretion or reabsorption occurs in the MCD (reasonable in most circumstances; see the following equation).

$$[K^+]_{CCD} = [K^+]_{urine}/(U/P)_{Osm}$$

Transtubular [K^+] Gradient (TTKG)

To calculate the TTKG, divide the [K^+]$_{CCD}$ by the P_K (see following equation). The TTKG offers an advantage over the

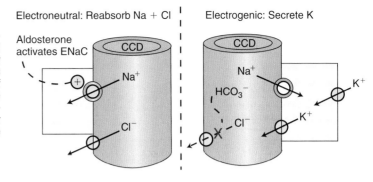

FIGURE 24–10 K$^+$ secretion in the cortical collecting duct. The barrel-shaped structures represent the CCD and the rectangles represent principal cells. Na$^+$ ions are reabsorbed via ENaC; their reabsorption is increased by aldosterone (the shaded enlarged circle). Net secretion of K$^+$ occurs through their specific ion channel (ROM-K). Electroneutral reabsorption of Na$^+$ and Cl$^-$ (shown to the left of the vertical dashed line) does not generate a lumen-negative voltage, which diminishes the secretion of K$^+$. Electrogenic reabsorption of Na$^+$ enhances the secretion of K$^+$ (e.g., HCO$_3^-$ and/or an alkaline luminal pH decreases the apparent permeability for Cl$^-$ in the CCD; this is shown to the right of the dashed vertical line).

TABLE 24–5	Plasma Renin and Aldosterone to Assess the Basis of Hypokalemia due to a Fast Na Type Lesion		
Adrenal gland lesion		Renin	Aldosterone
Primary hyperaldosteronism or adrenal tumor		Low	High
ACTH causes aldosterone synthesis (GRA)		Low	High
Kidney lesions			
Renal artery stenosis		High	High
Malignant hypertension		High	High
Renin-secreting tumor		High	High
Liddle syndrome		Low	Low
11β-HSDH fails to remove all cortisol			
Hereditary defect (AME)		Low	Low
Inhibition (e.g., licorice ingestion)		Low	Low
Saturated because of ectopic ACTH		Low	Usually low

For details, see text.
AME, apparent mineralocorticoid excess syndrome; 11β-HSDH, 11 β-hydroxysteroid dehydrogenase; GRA, glucocorticoid-remedial aldosteronism.

[K$^+$]$_{CCD}$ because it permits one to relate the [K$^+$]$_{CCD}$ to the P$_K$.[31] The expected value for the TTKG in a patient with hypokalemia due to a non-renal cause is <2, whereas the appropriate renal response to hyperkalemia is a TTKG > 7.

$$TTKG = [K^+]_{CCD}/P_K$$

Establish the Basis for the Abnormal [K$^+$]$_{CCD}$

The driving force for the net secretion of K$^+$ in the cortical distal nephron is a lumen-negative transepithelial voltage generated by the "electrogenic" reabsorption of Na$^+$ (i.e., Na$^+$ is reabsorbed faster than Cl$^-$) (Fig. 24–10). For secretion of K$^+$, open channels for K$^+$ must be in the luminal membrane.[32] In a patient with hypokalemia, a higher than expected [K$^+$]$_{CCD}$ implies that the lumen-negative voltage is abnormally more negative and that open luminal ROMK channels are present in the CCD.[32] The former could be due to reabsorbing Na$^+$ "faster" than Cl$^-$ in the CCD. The converse is true in a patient with hyperkalemia and a lower than expected [K$^+$]$_{CCD}$.

The clinical indices that help in this differential diagnosis of the pathophysiology of the abnormal rate of electrogenic reabsorption of Na$^+$ in CCD are an assessment of the ECF volume and the ability to conserve Na$^+$ and Cl$^-$ in response to a contracted effective arterial blood volume. The measurement of the activity of renin (P$_{renin}$) and the level of aldosterone in plasma (P$_{Aldosterone}$) are helpful in patients with hypokalemia (Table 24–5).[29]

Consult K-1: Hypokalemia and A Low Rate of Excretion of K$^+$

A 35-year-old obese, Asian male developed extreme weakness progressing to paralysis over a period of 12 hours. It was

TABLE 24–6	Data for Consult K-1					
		Blood	Urine			Blood
K$^+$	mmol/L	1.8	10	pH		7.40
Creatinine	mg/dL	0.6	1 g/L	PCO$_2$	mm Hg	40
Na$^+$	mmol/L	140	—	HCO$_3^-$	mmol/L	25
Cl$^-$	mmol/L	103	—	Glucose	mg/dL	84

preceded by his routine exercise after eating a carbohydrate-rich meal. He has had three similar attacks of paralysis in the past 6 months, but there was no family history of hypokalemia, paralysis, or hyperthyroidism. He denied the intake of laxatives and diuretic use, but he did take amphetamines to induce weight loss. On physical examination, he was alert and oriented; blood pressure was 150/70 mm Hg, heart rate was 124 beats/min, and respiratory rate was 18 per minute. Symmetrical flaccid paralysis with areflexia was present in all four limbs. There were no other abnormal findings on examination. The pH and PCO$_2$ in Table 24–6 were from arterial blood whereas all other data were from venous blood. The EKG showed prominent U waves. On subsequent evaluation, tests indicated thyroid function was normal.

Questions

Is there a medical emergency?
What is the basis of the hypokalemia?
What are the major options for therapy?

Discussion

Is There A Medical Emergency?
Because the EKG did not show significant changes due to hypokalemia and because respiratory muscle weakness was not evident from the arterial PCO$_2$, there were no emergencies that required urgent therapy (Fig. 24–11).

What Is the Basis of the Hypokalemia?
Rate of excretion of K$^+$: Because the time course was short, the major basis for his acute hypokalemia is a shift of K$^+$ into cells. In support of this diagnosis, his U$_K$/U$_{Creatinine}$ was <15 mmol/g creatinine (<1.5 in mmol/mmol terms).[33] There is a possible caveat—the low rate of excretion of K$^+$ may represent the normal renal response to a prior K$^+$ loss or an extrarenal loss of K$^+$. The absence of an acid-base disorder suggested also that the major basis for his hypokalemia is an acute shift of K$^+$ into cells (Table 24–7).[33]

Reasons for K$^+$ to shift into cells: There were reasons to believe that K$^+$ may have shifted into cells (e.g., a large carbohydrate intake [high insulin levels activate NHE]) and vigorous exercise (β$_2$ adrenergic agonists stimulate Na-K-ATPase). Notwithstanding, the stimulus for K$^+$ shift must be prolonged considering that his symptoms persisted for a long period of time. The absence of hypoglycemia made it unlikely that there was a prolonged excessive release of insulin. Long-term

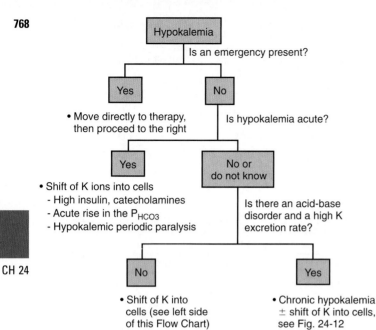

FIGURE 24–11 Initial approach to the patient with hypokalemia. In the initial approach, the major objectives are to rule out an emergency for which therapy must take precedence. The next step is to decide whether there is an important degree of shift of K^+ into cells. One must follow this up with an examination of the renal response to hypokalemia (see Figure 24–12).

TABLE 24–7	Plasma Acid-Base Status and Hypokalemia

Patients with metabolic alkalosis
  Vomiting, nasogastric suction, cationic resins, rare types of diarrhea
  Diuretic use or abuse
  Other disorders based on plasma renin activity
    Settings with a low renin activity in plasma
      (e.g., primary aldosteronism, glucocorticoid remediable hypertension, Liddle syndrome, apparent mineralocorticoid excess syndrome, Cushing syndrome, licorice)
    Settings with a high renin activity in plasma
      (e.g., renal artery stenosis, malignant hypertension, renin producing tumor, Bartter or Gitelman syndrome)

Patients with hyperchloremic metabolic acidosis
  Overproduction of hippuric acid (e.g., toluene abuse)
  GI loss of $NaHCO_3$ (e.g., diarrhea, laxative abuse, fistula, ileus, ureteral diversion)
  Reduced reabsorption of in the PCT (e.g., proximal RTA treated with large amounts of $NaHCO_3$, use of acetazolamide)
  Distal renal tubular acidosis
    Low excretion of NH_4^+ (e.g., usually low net distal H^+ secretion subtype, Sjögren syndrome, Southeast Asian Ovalocytosis with second mutation of Cl^-/HCO_3^- anion exchanger)

β-adrenergic stimulation can be caused by amphetamine that was used by this patient, or a large intake of caffeine, especially if the relevant cytochrome P_{450} for its metabolism is inhibited[34]; this was denied on careful questioning of the patient. There was no personal or family history of hypokalemic periodic paralysis (HPP) or hyperthyroidism.

Evidence for an adrenergic surge: On physical examination, there were findings supporting a high β-adrenergic state (e.g., tachycardia, systolic hypertension, and a wide pulse pressure). Other laboratory tests that suggest this diagnosis include the presence of hypophosphatemia with a low $U_{phosphate}/U_{calcium}$ ratio.[35]

Interpretation

The cause of the hypokalemia seemed to be an acute shift of K^+ into cells due to a large adrenergic surge due to the use of amphetamines.[34] (More detailed information about causes for an acute shift of K^+ into cells can be found in Ref. 33.)

What Are the Major Options for therapy?

Because the diagnosis was an acute shift of K^+ into cells due to a large adrenergic surge due to the amphetamines, he was treated with a non-selective ß-blocker and a moderate dose of K^+ supplementation[36]; the P_K returned to the normal range in 2 hours. Of great importance, large doses of K^+ should not be given because of the risk of life- threatening rebound hyperkalemia when the reason for this shift of K^+ abates.

Consult K-2: Hypokalemia and A High Rate of Excretion of K^+

A 76-year-old Asian male developed progressive muscle weakness over the past 6 hours that became so severe that he became unable to move. He had no other neurological symptoms. He denied nausea, vomiting, diarrhea, or the use of diuretics or laxatives. Hypokalemia (P_K 3.3 mmol/L) and hypertension were noted 1 year ago, but were not investigated further. His family history was negative for hypertension or hypokalemia. His blood pressure was 160/96 mm Hg and his heart rate was 70 per minute. Neurological examination revealed symmetric flaccid paralysis with areflexia, but no other findings. The laboratory data prior to therapy are shown in Table 24–8. Subsequent measurements indicated that his P_{renin} and $P_{Aldosterone}$ were low and his $P_{Cortisol}$ was in the normal range.

The patient was treated initially with intravenous KCl; the weakness improved when his P_K reached 2.5 mmol/L. He was continued on oral KCl supplementation. Two weeks later, his P_K and blood pressure had returned to normal levels, while his body weight decreased from 78 kg to 74 kg.

Question

What is the cause of hypokalemia in this patient?

Discussion

Excretion of K^+

The patient presented with an acute symptom—extreme weakness of both upper and lower limbs. There was little to support the diagnosis of HPP because he did not have previous attacks of paralysis and there was no evidence of thyrotoxicosis. Most importantly, his $U_K/U_{Creatinine}$ was 5, a value that is fivefold higher than what is expected if the major basis

		Blood	**Urine**			**Blood**	**Urine**
K$^+$	mmol/L	1.8	26	pH		7.55	—
Na$^+$	mmol/L	147	132	PCO$_2$	mm Hg	40	—
Cl$^-$	mmol/L	90	138	HCO$_3^-$	mmol/L	45	0
Creatinine	mg/dL	0.8	0.6 g/L	Osmolality	mOsm/L	302	482

TABLE 24–8 Data for Consult K-2

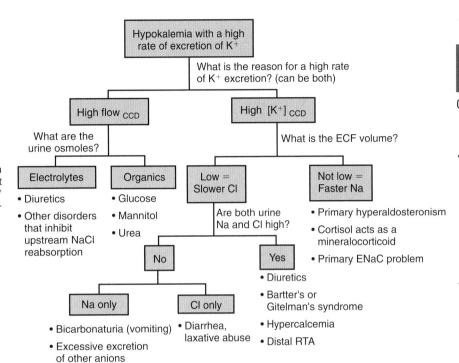

FIGURE 24–12 Renal causes of hypokalemia. In a patient with a high rate of excretion of K$^+$, one must examine both the flow rate and the concentration of K$^+$ in the luminal fluid exiting from the terminal CCD as discussed in the text.

for his hypokalemia was an acute shift of K$^+$ into cells (see Fig. 24–11). Moreover, he had metabolic alkalosis. Hence his hypokalemia was largely due to a disorder that caused excessive loss of K$^+$ into the urine.

Notwithstanding, his acute presentation with extreme weakness might be due to an acute shift of K$^+$ into cells in conjunction with a chronic disorder that caused excessive excretion of K$^+$. This component of an acute shift of K$^+$ into cells could have been induced by vigorous exercise and a large carbohydrate intake during breakfast prior to the onset of symptoms. Our approach to determine the pathophysiology of his hypokalemia will utilize the clinical tools discussed earlier and the step-by-step approach is illustrated in Figure 24–12.

Assess the [K$^+$]$_{CCD}$

The [K$^+$]$_{CCD}$ was very high in the presence of hypokalemia. This reflects a high lumen-negative voltage in the CCD, due to either a faster rate of reabsorption of Na$^+$ or a slower rate of reabsorption of Cl$^-$ (see Fig. 24–9).

Establish the Basis for the Abnormal [K$^+$]$_{CCD}$

On clinical assessment, his ECF volume was not contracted and he had hypertension. Therefore the increased lumen-negative voltage in his CCD was likely due to a faster rate of reabsorption of Na$^+$ (see Fig. 24–10). The differential diagnosis of disorders with a faster rate of reabsorption of Na$^+$ in the CCD is guided by measurements of the P$_{renin}$ and P$_{Aldosterone}$ (see Table 24–5).

Interpretation

Because both P$_{Aldosterone}$ and P$_{renin}$ were suppressed, the differential diagnosis was between disorders in which cortisol acts as mineralocorticoid and those with an open ENaC despite the undetectable levels of aldosterone. A chest radiograph did not reveal a lung mass and cortisol levels were not elevated. Inherited disorders where ENaC is constitutively active (Liddle syndrome) seemed unlikely considering the patient's age. Although the patient denied consuming licorice or chewing tobacco, it turned out that an herbal sweetener he used to sweeten his tea contained large amounts of glycyrrhizic acid (the active principle in licorice).[37] Discontinuing this intake led to a normal P$_K$ and a fall in his blood pressure.

Consult K-3: Hyperkalemia in A Patient Taking Trimethoprim

A 35-year-old cachectic male with HIV developed Pneumocystis carinii jerovici (PJP). On admission, he was febrile; his ECF volume and all plasma electrolyte values were in the normal range. He was treated with clotrimazole (sulfamethoxazole and trimethoprim). Three days later, he was noted to have low blood pressure, his "effective" arterial blood volume was low, and his P$_K$ rose to 6.8 mmol/L. His urine volume was 0.8 L/day and his U$_{osm}$ was 350 mOsm/L (Table 24–9).

Question

Why is hyperkalemia present?

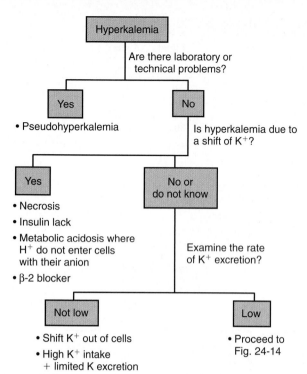

FIGURE 24–13 Initial steps in the patient with hyperkalemia. In the initial approach, the major objectives are to rule out an emergency for which therapy must take precedence. The next step is to decide whether there is an important degree of shift of K$^+$ out of cells. One must follow this up with an examination of the renal response to hyperkalemia (see Figure 24–14).

Discussion

The steps to follow are provided in Figures 24–13 and 24–14. Although an element of pseudohyperkalemia could be present in this cachectic patient, the presence of EKG changes indicated that he has true hyperkalemia.

Rate of Excretion of K$^+$

Because the rise in P$_K$ occurred over many days, one would be tempted to conclude that the major basis for the hyperkalemia was the low rate of excretion of K$^+$.

Shift of K$^+$ Out of Cells

Because the patient consumed little K$^+$, a shift of K$^+$ from cells rather than a large positive external balance for K$^+$ should be the major cause of hyperkalemia.[29] The likely cause of this exit of K$^+$ from cells could be cell necrosis, insulin deficiency, and/or hyperchloremic metabolic acidosis.[38] Insulin deficiency could be due to the α-adrenergic effect of adrenaline released in response to the low ECF volume.[39] Because the major basis of hyperkalemia is a shift of K$^+$ from cells, it would be an error to induce a large loss of K$^+$ when the total body K$^+$ surplus is small. It is important to realize that he could also have a defect in K$^+$ excretion.

Rate of Excretion of K$^+$

His U$_K$ was 14 mmol/L and his rate of excretion of K$^+$ was extremely low in the face of hyperkalemia (U$_K$/U$_{Creatinine}$ was 17.5 mmol/g).

Flow Rate in His Terminal Cortical Collecting Ducts

This flow rate was low because his rate of excretion of osmoles was only 0.2 mosmol/min (U$_{osm}$ 350 mOsm/kg H$_2$O and the urine flow rate was 0.6 ml/min)—this is less than half the usual rate of excretion of osmoles (0.5 mosmol/min).[28] It was likely that he had a low rate of production of urea (low

TABLE 24–9		Data for Consult K-3					
		Blood	**Urine**			**Blood**	**Urine**
K$^+$	mmol/L	6.8	14	pH		7.30	—
Na$^+$	mmol/L	130	80	PCO$_2$	mm Hg	30	—
Cl$^-$	mmol/L	105	63	HCO$_3^-$	mmol/L	15	0
Creatinine	mg/dL	0.9	0.8 g/L	BUN	mg/dL	14	420

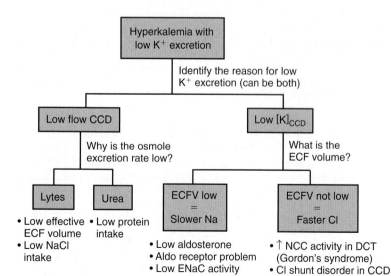

FIGURE 24–14 Renal causes for hyperkalemia and a low rate of K$^+$ excretion. In a patient with a hyperkalemia and a low rate of excretion of K$^+$, one must examine both the flow rate and the concentration of K$^+$ in the luminal fluid exiting from the terminal CCD as discussed in the text. NCC, Na, Cl, cotransporter.

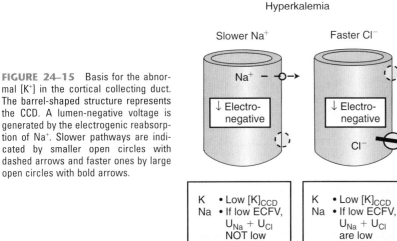

Hyperkalemia | Hypokalemia

Slower Na⁺ — Faster Cl⁻ | Faster Na⁺ — Slower Cl⁻

FIGURE 24–15 Basis for the abnormal [K⁺] in the cortical collecting duct. The barrel-shaped structure represents the CCD. A lumen-negative voltage is generated by the electrogenic reabsorption of Na⁺. Slower pathways are indicated by smaller open circles with dashed arrows and faster ones by large open circles with bold arrows.

K Na	• Low [K]$_{CCD}$ • If low ECFV, $U_{Na} + U_{Cl}$ NOT low
K Na	• Low [K]$_{CCD}$ • If low ECFV, $U_{Na} + U_{Cl}$ are low
K Na	• High [K]$_{CCD}$ • If low ECFV, $U_{Na} + U_{Cl}$ are low
K Na	• High [K]$_{CCD}$ • If low ECFV, $U_{Na} + U_{Cl}$ NOT low

TABLE 24–10 Renal Causes of a Dyskalemia

1. Hyperkalemia
(i) Slower reabsorption of Na⁺ in the CCD
   Low levels of aldosterone (e.g., Addison disease)
   Blockade of the aldosterone receptor (e.g., spironolactone)
   Low activity of ENaC (e.g., amiloride, trimethoprim)
(ii) Faster reabsorption of Cl⁻ in the CCD
   Gordon syndrome (e.g., WNK kinase mutations), drugs (e.g., cyclosporin)

2. Hypokalemia
(i) Faster reabsorption of Na⁺ in the CCD
   High aldosterone levels
   Cortisol acts as a mineralocorticoid
     Low 11-β hydroxysteroid dehydrogenase (11-βHSDH) activity (AME)
     Inhibitors of 11-βHSDH (e.g., licorice)
     Very high cortisol levels (e.g., ACTH-producing tumor)
   Constitutively active ENaC (e.g., Liddle syndrome)
   Artificial ENaC (e.g., amphotericin B)
(ii) Slower reabsorption of Cl⁻ in the CCD
   Delivery of Na⁺ to the CCD with little Cl⁻
   Higher delivery of Na⁺ and Cl⁻ to the CCD when ENaC is active (e.g., Bartter or Gitelman syndrome, loop or thiazide diuretic plus a contracted ECF volume)
   Inhibition of Cl⁻ reabsorption in the CCD (e.g., bicarbonaturia)

AME, Apparent mineralocorticoid excess syndrome; CCD, cortical collecting duct.
Chronic kidney disease is not included in this table as the mechanism is not well-defined.

protein intake) and a low excretion of NaCl (low effective arterial blood volume and low intake of NaCl).

The [K⁺]$_{CCD}$
His [K⁺]$_{CCD}$ was <2—this indicates a low rate of K⁺ secretion in his CCD, which implies a low lumen-negative voltage in the CCD due to less electrogenic reabsorption of Na⁺.

Establish the Basis for the Low [K⁺]$_{CCD}$
Because he had a low effective arterial blood volume and a U_{Na} and U_{Cl} that were inappropriately high in the presence of a contracted ECF volume, his low [K⁺]$_{CCD}$ was due to slower reabsorption of Na⁺ in the CCD (Fig. 24–15).

The major groups of disorders that can cause a slower reabsorption of Na⁺ in the CCD are listed in Table 24–10. Because he did not have a response to exogenous mineralocorticoids, the presumptive diagnosis was that his slower Na⁺ reabsorption was due to inhibition of ENaC by the trimethoprim that was used to manage his PJP.[40] Both his P_{renin} and

$P_{Aldosterone}$ (which became available later) were high as expected in this setting.

Interpretation
Renal salt wasting due to blockade of ENaC by trimethoprim led to the development of a contracted ECF volume. As a result, there was a shift of K⁺ out of cells probably because of inhibition of insulin release by α-adrenergics.[39] Because of the low ECF volume (and the low intake of proteins), there was a low rate of flow in the CCD. This low flow rate in the CCD, in addition to its effect to diminish the rate of K⁺ excretion, caused the trimethoprim concentration to be higher in the lumen of the CCD (same amount of trimethoprim in a smaller volume); hence trimethoprim became a more effective blocker of ENaC.

From a therapeutic point of view, the question arose as to whether trimethoprim should be discontinued. Because the drug was needed to manage his PJP, a means to remove its renal ENaC-blocking effect was sought. Increasing flow in the CCD using a loop diuretic plus the infusion of enough NaCl to re-expand his ECF volume should lower the concentration of trimethoprim in the lumen of the CCD (same amount of trimethoprim in a much larger volume). Inducing bicarbonaturia could also be considered to lower the concentration of H⁺ in the luminal fluid in the CCD and thereby the cationic form of the drug that blocks ENaC.[41]

Integration: Clinical Approach, Hypokalemia
The first step in the clinical approach to the patient with hypokalemia is to identify whether there is an emergency prior to therapy (cardiac arrhythmia and/or respiratory muscle weakness) and to anticipate and avoid dangers associated with therapy (e.g., administration of glucose leading to the release of insulin and a shift of K⁺ into cells).

The second step is to decide if a major basis for hypokalemia is an acute shift of K⁺ into cells (see Fig. 24–11). The time course, a family or past personal history of hypokalemia, and/or episodes of muscle weakness or paralysis, male gender, Asian ethnicity, as well as other issues from the history that suggest the presence of a cause for a K⁺ shift into cells are very helpful to make this decision. In addition, physical findings that suggest an adrenergic surge, the absence of an acid-base disorder (see Table 24–7), and a low $U_K/U_{Creatinine}$ are excellent indicators to suggest that the diagnosis might be a condition that caused an acute shift of K⁺ into cells.

The third step is to examine the rate of K excretion using the $U_K/U_{Creatinine}$ to identify renal causes for hypokalemia (see Fig. 24–12). A ratio >1.5 indicates a high rate of excretion of K⁺. At this point, a reason for this higher [K⁺]$_{CCD}$ should be sought—i.e., the reason why the voltage is more negative in the lumen of the CCD. This could be due to a faster rate of reabsorption of Na^+ or a slower rate of reabsorption of Cl^- in the CCD (see Fig. 24–15).

Patients with disorders that cause a faster reabsorption of Na^+ often have hypertension because they have an expanded ECF volume. The U_{Cl} reflects their intake of salt. Measurements of P_{renin} and $P_{Aldosterone}$ provide means to identify the cause in this group of patients (see Table 24–5).

Patients with disorders that cause a slower reabsorption of Cl^- (than Na^+) can be divided into three groups. First, there is a delivery of very little Cl^- to the CCD (e.g., delivery of Na^+ with HCO_3^- [recent vomiting] or a drug anion like penicillin); second, there is a decreased rate of reabsorption of Cl^- in the CCD (e.g., possibly due to the effect of HCO_3^- or an alkaline luminal pH[42]); third, there is a combination of a high delivery of Na^+ and Cl^- to the CCD due to inhibition of their absorption in an upstream nephron segment together with a higher capacity for the reabsorption of Na^+ than Cl^- in the CCD (e.g., release of aldosterone in response to a low ECF volume). Patients with a slow Cl^- type of lesion should have a high P_{renin}.

Integration: Clinical Approach, Hyperkalemia

It is imperative to recognize when hyperkalemia represents a medical emergency because therapy must then take precedence over diagnosis (see Fig. 24–13); this emergency is usually secondary to a cardiac arrhythmia. If there is no emergency present, the second step is to assess whether there is a component of pseudohyperkalemia (including hemolysis, megakaryocytosis, fragile leukemic cells, a K^+ channel disorder in red blood cells,[43] and excessive fist clenching during blood sampling[44]). Even without fist clenching, pseudohyperkalemia can be present in cachectic patients because the normal T-tubule architecture in skeletal muscle can be disturbed thus permitting more K^+ to be released into venous blood. (Normally K^+ is released during muscle depolarization into a region that does not mix appreciably with the circulating volume.) The third step is to determine if hyperkalemia is acute and/or occurred in absence of a large intake of K^+—if so, there is an important contribution of a shift of K^+ out of cells (see "Consult K-3"). If a shift of K^+ is likely, proceed to an analysis of factors that could either destroy cells or decrease the magnitude of the intracellular negative voltage.[38]

The fourth step is to examine the rate of excretion of K^+. If this rate is considerably <200 mmol/g creatinine (or <20 mmol K^+/mmol creatinine), it is inappropriately low for the presence of hyperkalemia. If so, the basis for the low rate of K^+ excretion should be examined by analyzing the two components of the K^+ excretion formula in terms of events in the terminal CCD. The flow rate in the terminal CCD should be assessed when vasopressin is acting ($U_{osm} > P_{osm}$) by calculating the osmole excretion rate (see Fig. 24–9). If the $[K^+]_{CCD}$ is low, seek the basis for a slower rate of electrogenic reabsorption of Na^+ in the CCD. In patients with few remaining nephrons, the flow rate is so rapid per nephron that this may limit K^+ secretion.

Slower Na^+ Type of Lesion

These patients will have a low effective ECF volume, their U_{Na} and U_{Cl} will not be very low, and their P_{renin} will be high. The basis could be a low $P_{Aldosterone}$ if there is a rise in the $[K^+]_{CCD}$ 2 hours after the administration of 100 µg of fludrocortisone in an adult; in addition, the U_{Na} and U_{Cl} should fall to very low values. This diagnosis can be confirmed by finding a low $P_{Aldosterone}$. On the other hand, if the patient did not respond to exogenous mineralocorticoids, the presumptive diagnosis would be that his slower Na^+ lesion would be due to blockade of the aldosterone receptor in principal cells (e.g., by drugs such as spironolactone), an aldosterone receptor

problem (e.g., inherited disorders), or a reduced activity of the epithelial Na^+ channel (ENaC) in principal cells (e.g., inherited disorder or blockade by cationic drugs such as amiloride, triamterene, or trimethoprim). If the P_{renin} is low in the presence of a low ECF volume, suspect that there is a defect in renin release from the juxtaglomerular apparatus.

Faster Cl^--Type of Lesion

The ECF volume in these patients tends to be expanded. Hypertension may be present if their blood pressure is more sensitive to blood volume than usual. The P_{renin} is suppressed and the $P_{Aldosterone}$ is low considering that hyperkalemia is present. This type of lesion could be due to an increased activity of the thiazide sensitive NaCl cotransporter in the distal convoluted tubule (e.g., Gordon syndrome or type II pseudohypoaldosteronism due to a mutation involving WNK-1 or WNK-4 kinases[45]). The decreased delivery of Na^+ and Cl^- to the CCD, together with a diminished activity of ENaC (because of low aldosterone level in response to expansion of the ECF volume), lead to a rate of reabsorption of Cl^- that cannot be less than that of Na^+ in the CCD. These patients are expected to have a have a rise in $[K^+]_{CCD}$ with the administration of a thiazide diuretic. A faster Cl^- type of lesion may result from increased permeability for Cl^- in CCD (e.g., the putative cause of hyperkalemia due to cyclosporin). A rise in the $[K^+]_{CCD}$ when there is bicarbonaturia suggests the diagnosis of a Cl^- shunt disorder.[46]

Metabolic Alkalosis

Metabolic alkalosis is a process that leads to a rise in the P_{HCO3} and the plasma pH. It is important to recognize that metabolic alkalosis is a diagnostic category with many different causes. Notwithstanding, metabolic alkalosis is included in this section on K^+ disorders because a deficiency of KCl plays an important role in its pathophysiology.[47] The following fundamental concepts are central to our understanding of why metabolic alkalosis develops. They also provide the basis for our clinical approach to this diagnostic category, and in the design of optimal therapy.

Concept M Alk-1

Because concentration terms have numerators and denominators, there are two ways to raise the P_{HCO3}: add more HCO_3^- or reduce the ECF volume (Fig. 24–16).

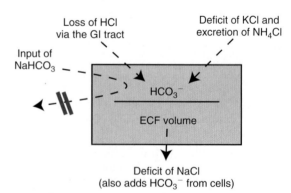

FIGURE 24–16 Basis for a high concentration of HCO_3^- in the ECF compartment. The rectangle represents the ECF compartment. The concentration of HCO_3^- is the ratio of the content of HCO_3^- in the ECF compartment (numerator) and the ECF volume (denominator). The major causes for a rise in the content of HCO_3^- in the ECF compartment are a deficit of HCl or a deficit of KCl (upper portion of the figure). The major cause for a fall in the ECF volume is a deficit of NaCl. An intake of $NaHCO_3$ (or Na^+ with potential alkali/bicarbonate) is not sufficient on its own to cause a sustained increase in the content of HCO_3^- in the ECF compartment, except if there also is a mechanism to diminish the renal excretion of $NaHCO_3$ (double bold lines on the left portion of the figure indicate the reduced renal output of $NaHCO_3$). As shown in Figure 24–17, a contracted ECF volume leads to the net addition of HCO_3^- to the ECF compartment.

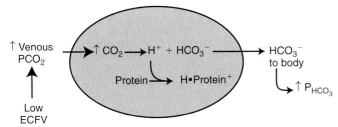

FIGURE 24–17 Addition of HCO_3^- to the ECF compartment when the venous PCO_2 is high. The oval represents a cell with its HCO_3^- and protein buffer systems. When the ECF volume is very contracted, rate of blood flow is reduced and more O_2 is extracted *from each liter* of blood flowing through the capillaries; this raises both the capillary blood and ICF PCO_2 (left portion of the figure). The higher PCO_2 in these cells drives the synthesis of H^+ and HCO_3^- ions; the H^+ bind to intracellular proteins while the HCO_3^- ions are exported to the ECF (right portion of the figure). This process reverses when a large volume of saline is infused and the venous PCO_2 declines.

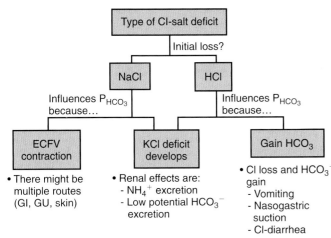

FIGURE 24–18 Pathophysiology of metabolic alkalosis due to a deficit of CL-salts. This Flow Chart is useful to understand how a deficit of each type of Cl^--containing compound contributes to the development of metabolic alkalosis.

When metabolic alkalosis is caused by a deficit of NaCl, the content of HCO_3^- in the ECF compartment is not elevated until the venous PCO_2 rises (Fig. 24–17).[21]

Concept M Alk-2
Electroneutrality must be present in every body compartment and in the urine. Therefore balances for Cl^--salts must be defined in electroneutral terms (i.e., HCl, KCl, and/or NaCl Fig. 24–18). It follows that "Cl-depletion" is *not* an adequate term to describe the pathophysiology of metabolic alkalosis because it ignores the need for electroneutrality.

Concept M Alk-3
Knowing balances for Na^+, K^+, and Cl^- permits one to deduce why the P_{HCO3} rose and what changes occurred in the composition of ECF and ICF compartments (see Fig. 24–16).

Concept M Alk-4
The kidney plays an important role in the pathophysiology of metabolic alkalosis largely because this organ determines the balance for K^+.

NaCl or HCl deficits, which can lead to a higher P_{HCO3}, can also lead to a secondary deficit of KCl and hypokalemia. A deficit of K^+ is associated with an acidified PCT cell pH and this can both initiate and sustain a high P_{HCO3} as a result of renal new HCO_3^- generation (higher excretion of NH_4^+), reduced excretion of dietary HCO_3^- in the form of organic anions,[48] and enhanced reabsorption of HCO_3^- in the PCT.

TABLE 24–11		Data for Consult Met Alk-1			
P_{Na}	mmol/L	140	pH		7.47
P_K	mmol/L	2.7	P_{HCO3}	mmol/L	37
P_{Cl}	mmol/L	90	Arterial PCO_2	mm Hg	47
Hematocrit		0.50			

Contrary to the widely held impression, there is no renal tubular maximum for the reabsorption of HCO_3^-.[49] Rather HCO_3^- ions are retained unless their reabsorption is inhibited (low angiotensin II because of ECF volume expansion and/or an alkaline PCT cell pH[50]). Said a different way, ingesting $NaHCO_3$ will not cause metabolic alkalosis because it expands the "effective" ECF volume, lowers angiotensin II, and raises the ICF pH in PCT cells. Nevertheless, $NaHCO_3$ can be retained when there is a significant decrease in its filtered load due to a large fall in the GFR.[49]

Tools
Quantitative Estimate of the Extracellular Fluid Volume
It is critical to know the ECF volume to determine the content of HCO_3^- in the ECF compartment and thereby why there was a rise in the P_{HCO3}. We rely on the hematocrit for this purpose (see Table 24–3) (or a change in the hematocrit with therapy in the patient who has anemia or erythrocytosis).

Balance Data for Na^+, K^+, and Cl^-
These data are essential to describe deficits in electroneutral terms, but they are rarely available in clinical medicine. Nevertheless, they can be inferred if one knows the new ECF volume and the P_{Na}, P_{Cl}, and P_{HCO3}. One cannot know the balances for K^+ from these calculations, but one can deduce their rough magnitude by comparing the differences in the content of Na^+ versus that of Cl^- and HCO_3^- in the ECF compartment.[51]

Consult Met Alk-1: Metabolic Alkalosis without Diuretics or Vomiting
After a forced 6-hour run in the desert in the heat of the day, this elite corps soldier was the only one in his squad who collapsed. Although he perspired profusely during the run, he had free access to water and glucose containing fluids. He did not vomit and denied the intake of medications. Physical examination revealed a markedly contracted ECF volume. Initial laboratory data are provided in Table 24–11.

Questions
What is the basis for the metabolic alkalosis?
What is the therapy for metabolic alkalosis in this patient?

Discussion
What is the basis for metabolic alkalosis?

Quantitative Estimate of the Extracellular Fluid Volume
Although this patient had an obvious degree of contraction of his ECF volume, the physical examination cannot provide a quantitative dimension for this deficit. To distinguish between HCl, KCl, and NaCl deficits, a quantitative analysis of the degree of contraction of the ECF volume is needed—his hematocrit of 0.50 provides this information (see Table 24–3). With a hematocrit of 0.50, his ECF volume decreased by one third, from its normal value of 15 L (as he weighed 80 kg) to ~10 L; accordingly, he lost 5 L of ECF in that period.

Balance Data for Na^+, K^+, and Cl^-
Deficit of HCl: There was no history of vomiting so this is very unlikely basis for the metabolic alkalosis.

Deficit of KCl: The basis of hypokalemia could be a shift of K^+ into cells or a loss of KCl in the urine. To lower the P_K to

2.7 mmol/L due to a deficit of KCl, especially in this muscular elite solider, the loss of KCl must be very large. Moreover, it is extremely unlikely that this happened over such a short period of time. Furthermore, even if there was a KCl deficit, it is difficult to attribute the rise in the P_{HCO3} to the formation of new HCO_3^- due to the renal effects of hypokalemia (high excretion of NH_4^+) because the time course is too short.

Deficit of NaCl: The decrease in his ECF volume was ~5 L. One can now calculate how much this degree of ECF volume contraction would raise his P_{HCO3} (divide the normal content of HCO_3^- in his ECF compartment [15 L × 25 mmol/L or 375 mmol] by his new ECF volume of 10 L = 37.5 mmol/L). This value is remarkably close to the observed 37 mmol/L. Therefore the major reason for his metabolic alkalosis is the NaCl deficit (a "contraction" form of metabolic alkalosis).

Balance for Na^+: Multiplying his P_{Na} (140 mmol/L) before the race times his normal ECF volume (15 L) yields a Na^+ content of ~2100 mmol in this compartment. After the race, his P_{Na} was 140 mmol/L and his ECF volume was 10 L; hence his ECF Na^+ content was now 1400 mmol. Accordingly, his deficit of Na^+ was ~700 mmol.

Balance for Cl^-: Multiplying his P_{Cl} before the race (103 mmol/L) times his normal ECF volume (15 L) yields a Cl^- content of ~1545 mmol in this compartment. After the race, his P_{Cl} was 90 mmol/L and his ECF volume was 10 L; hence his ECF Cl^- content was now 900 mmol. Accordingly, his deficit of Cl^- is ~645 mmol, a value that is similar to his deficit of Na^+.

Balance for K^+: It is possible to have a loss of KCl in sweat in patients with cystic fibrosis with concentrations of K^+ as high as 20 mmol/L to 30 mmol/L. Nevertheless, because there was little difference between the deficits of Na^+ and Cl^-, there is only a minor total body deficit of K^+. Accordingly, the major mechanism for hypokalemia is likely to be a shift of K^+ into cells (due to adrenergic surge and the alkalemia).

Interpretation

The deficits of Na^+ and Cl^- are similar in his ECF compartment. The next issue is to examine possible routes for a large loss of NaCl in such a short time period. Because both diarrhea and polyuria were not present, the only route for a large NaCl loss is via sweat. To have a high electrolyte concentration in sweat (e.g., ~70 mmol/L for Na^+ and Cl^-), the likely underlying lesion would be cystic fibrosis. Moreover, he would need to lose >1 L of sweat per hour. The diagnosis of cystic fibrosis was confirmed later by molecular studies.

What Is the Therapy for Metabolic Alkalosis in this Patient?

Knowing that the basis for the metabolic alkalosis is largely a deficit of NaCl, he will need to receive NaCl as his major treatment; the goal will be to replace the deficit that was calculated earlier, or ~700 mmol. If he had a reverse degree of hyponatremia (drank a large volume of water), he should be given hypertonic saline, especially because he may still have a large volume of water in his stomach. Thus acute hyponatremia should be added to the list of emergencies in this setting.

Integration: Clinical Approach; Metabolic Alkalosis

The initial first step is to establish whether the "effective" ECF volume is contracted (Fig. 24–19). Quantitative information can be obtained from the hematocrit or total protein concentration (or both). This permits one to know the relative importance of deficits of NaCl, HCl, and KCl, in the patient.

In the patient with a low ECF volume, the aim is to rule out first the two common causes of metabolic alkalosis: vomiting and diuretics. Although this may be evident from the clinical history, some patients may deny them; hence, measuring the urine electrolytes is particularly helpful (see Table 24–5). A very low U_{Cl} is expected when there is a deficit of HCl and/or NaCl. Nevertheless, the recent intake of diuretics

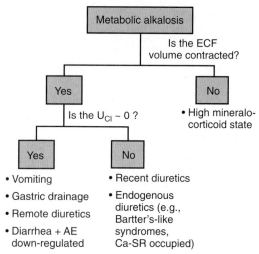

FIGURE 24–19 Clinical approach to the patient with metabolic alkalosis. Abbreviations: Ca-SR, calcium sensing receptor in thick ascending limb of the loop of Henle; AE, Cl^-/HCO_3^- anion exchanger.

will cause a higher excretion of Na^+ and Cl^-. Another group of causes for Na^+ and Cl^- wasting are patients with disorders of Bartter or Gitelman syndromes that lead to inhibition of reabsorption of Na^+ and Cl^-. The clue here is that these electrolytes will be present in every urine sample and urine tests for diuretics will be negative. A clinical picture that mimics Bartter syndrome may result from binding of cations to the calcium-sensing receptor in the thick ascending limb of the loop of Henle (high P_{Ca}, drugs like gentamicin or cisplatinum, and perhaps cationic proteins).

In the patient with a normal or high ECF volume, the basis of the metabolic alkalosis and a deficit of K^+ is a group of disorders of high primary mineralocorticoid activity. Many, but not all of these patients, will have hypertension.

If the cause of the metabolic alkalosis were an exogenous input of alkali in a patient with a marked reduction in GFR, the ECF volume may be expanded and the P_K will not be low; it is easy to recognize this subgroup.

METABOLIC ACIDOSIS

Metabolic acidosis is a process that leads to a fall in the P_{HCO3} and the plasma pH. Similar to metabolic alkalosis, metabolic acidosis represents a diagnostic category with many different causes. The risks for the patient and the treatment to be prescribed depend on the underlying disorder that caused the metabolic acidosis, the ill effects due to the H^+ load, and possible dangers associated with the anions accompanying these H^+.

Our goal is to provide a bedside approach when the patient first seeks medical attention.[52] The initial decisions are to determine if an emergency is present and to *anticipate and prevent* threats that may develop during therapy (Fig. 24–20). As in previous sections, we shall highlight the concepts that provide the underpinning for our approach. After each is defined, the laboratory tests that are needed to better define the problem will be outlined. Illustrative consults are used to emphasize the concepts and the utility of these tools.

Concept M Ac-1

The P_{HCO3} is the ratio of the *content* of HCO_3^- in the ECF compartment to the ECF volume.

There are two ways to lower the P_{HCO3}: decrease the content of HCO_3^- in, or raise the volume of the ECF compartment (see following equation).

$$[HCO_3^-]_{ECF} = \text{Content of } HCO_3^-$$
$$\text{in the ECF compartment/ECF volume}$$

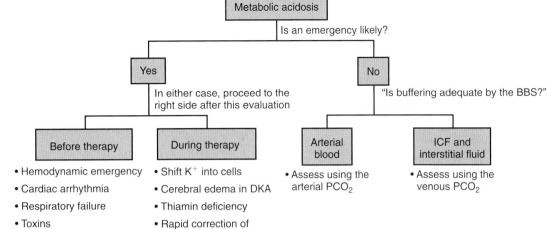

FIGURE 24–20 Initial steps in the patient with metabolic acidosis. The first step is to determine threats that are present prior to therapy and anticipate those that may develop during therapy (left side of the Flow Chart). The second step is to assess buffering by the BBS in both the ECF and ICF compartments (right side of the Flow Chart).

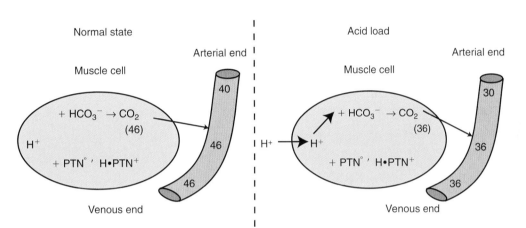

FIGURE 24–21 The BBS in cells; an emphasis on integrative physiology. The large oval represents a skeletal muscle cell and its capillary blood supply is represented by the curved cylindrical structure to its right. Because we are highlighting the BBS, the intracellular proteins are de-emphasized in this figure. The normal state is shown on the left and buffering of a H^+ load is shown on the right. Notice that a lower arterial PCO_2 resulting from hyperventilation favors the diffusion of CO_2 from cells into the capillary blood and the venous PCO_2 is virtually equal to the PCO_2 in cells. Hence new H^+ will be forced to react with HCO_3^- in cells because the PCO_2 in cells declines. Of even greater importance, the concentration of H^+ in cells did not rise appreciably and hence very few H^+ bind to proteins in cells.

It is important to distinguish between acidemia (lower plasma pH) and acidosis. Metabolic acidosis is a *process* that leads to a lower P_{HCO3} and pH in the ECF compartment; however, acidemia (i.e., a low P_{HCO3} and pH) might not be present if there is a loss of *both* NaCl and NaHCO$_3$ (i.e., a decrease in the in the ECF volume, a fall in its content of HCO_3^-, but not in its concentration) (e.g., the patient with cholera and immense losses of diarrhea fluid[21] and certain patients with DKA[53]). To make a diagnosis of metabolic acidosis in this setting, a quantitative estimate of the ECF volume is needed to assess the *content* of HCO_3^- in this compartment.

Tools
Quantitative Assessment of the Extracellular Fluid Volume
To provide quantitative information about the ECF volume, use the hematocrit or the concentration of total proteins in plasma. The assumption that must be made is that the patient did not have a preexisting anemia or a low plasma protein concentration.

Concept M Ac-2
H^+ must by removed by HCO_3^- to avoid its binding to intracellular proteins (Fig. 24–21). Because the vast majority of the bicarbonate buffer system (BBS) is located in the interstitial fluid and in the ICF compartment in skeletal muscle, it is

essential that the majority of H^+ removal take place by the BBS in this location (Fig. 24–22).

If buffering by the BBS were compromised in skeletal muscle, many more H^+ would be forced to bind to proteins in cells in vital organs (e.g., brain cells). If this occurred, these proteins would have a more positive charge ($H•PTN^+$), a change in their shape, and ultimately a diminution in their essential functions[54] (Fig. 24–23).

Tools to Assess the Removal of H^+ by the Bicarbonate Buffer System
Arterial PCO_2
To remove H^+ by the BBS in the ECF compartment, the arterial PCO_2 must be low as "expected" for the degree of acidemia. Nevertheless, although the arterial PCO_2 sets a *lower limit* on the possible value for the PCO_2 in cells, it is *not* a reliable indicator of the actual value of the intracellular PCO_2.

$$H^+ + HCO_3^- \rightarrow CO_2 + H_2O \text{ ("pulled" by a low } [CO_2])$$

Venous PCO_2
To remove H^+ by the BBS in the ICF compartment, the PCO_2 must be low in cells (see Fig. 24–21). The PCO_2 in cells is almost equal to the PCO_2 in capillaries draining individual organs. Because CO_2 is not added after the capillary, the *venous* PCO_2 will reflect the capillary PCO_2. There is, however, one caveat when using the venous PCO_2 to reflect PCO_2 in cells. If an appreciable quantity of blood shunts from the

CH 24

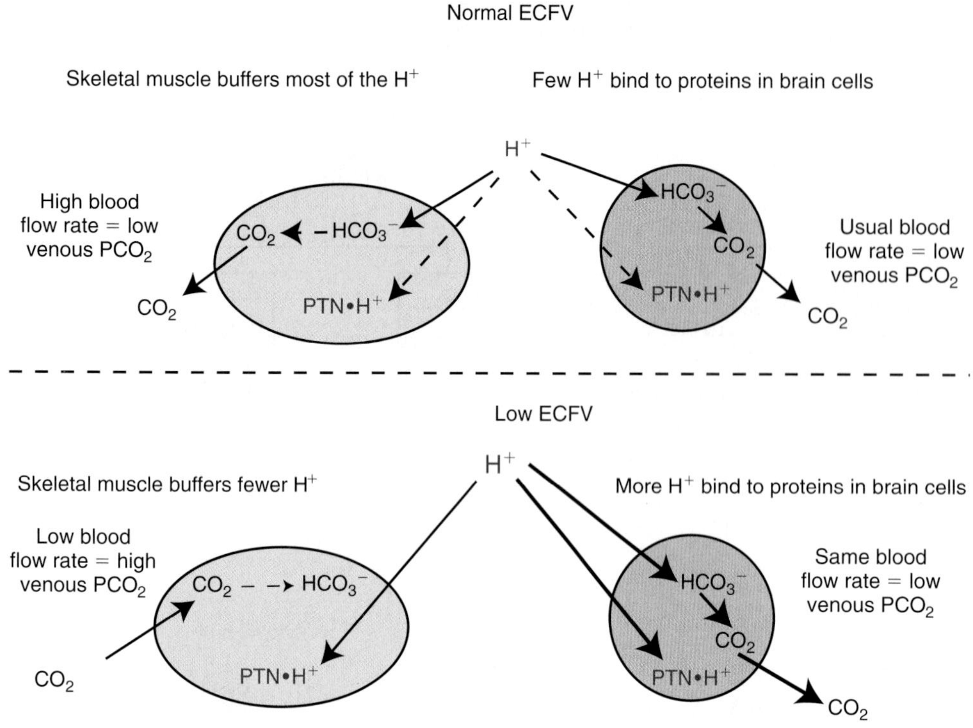

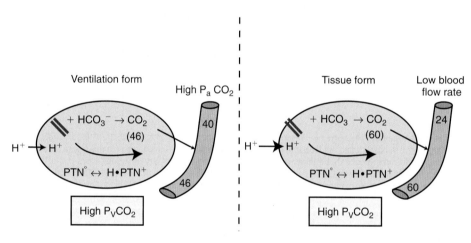

FIGURE 24-22 Buffering of H$^+$ by the BBS in vital organs in a patient with a contracted ECF volume. Skeletal muscle cells are shown to the left and brain cells to the right. When the ECF volume is low (below the horizontal dashed line), the PCO$_2$ in the venous blood draining muscle is high. This causes a high PCO$_2$ in muscle cells, which prevents H$^+$ from being buffered by its intracellular HCO$_3^-$. As a result, the concentration of H$^+$ in plasma rises and more H$^+$ will be buffered in brain cells. The latter have their usual BBS because the PCO$_2$ in venous blood draining the brain will change minimally with all but a very severe degree of ECF volume contraction as the *cerebral* blood flow rate is autoregulated. Because brain is 1/20 the size of muscle, it has far less HCO$_3^-$ and hence H$^+$ will bind to proteins in brain cells. In contrast, when intravenous saline is administered, blood flow to skeletal muscle rises, its venous PCO$_2$ falls, and more H$^+$ are removed by its BBS. As a result, the concentration of H$^+$ in the ECF compartment falls and H$^+$ are released from proteins in brain cells.

FIGURE 24-23 Failure of the BBS in a patient with metabolic acidosis. When faced with a H$^+$ load, failure of buffering in cells occurs when H$^+$ *cannot* be removed by reacting with HCO$_3^-$. Failure of the BBS to remove a H$^+$ load occurs when the tissue PCO$_2$ cannot fall because the *arterial* PCO$_2$ is not low enough (40 versus 24 mm Hg in this patient with metabolic acidosis, left of the dashed line) and/or the blood flow rate is low relative to the rate of CO$_2$ production (right of the dashed line). This rise in tissue PCO$_2$ increases the concentration of H$^+$ in cells, *pushing* H$^+$ to bind to intracellular proteins (H•PTN$^+$).

arterial to the venous circulation without passing through capillaries, the venous PCO$_2$ will not reflect the PCO$_2$ in cells.

The venous PCO$_2$ may be considerably higher than the arterial PCO$_2$ when a larger quantity of CO$_2$ is produced and/or there is a reduced blood flow to individual organs.[54] Venous PCO$_2$ measured in the brachial vein reflects the PCO$_2$ in skeletal muscle, the site where most of the buffering of H$^+$ should occur by the BBS. If this PCO$_2$ is high, there is failure of the BBS in muscle, which indicates that more of the H$^+$ load was buffered in vital organs (e.g., the brain). At the usual blood flow rate, the brachial venous PCO$_2$ is ~46 mm Hg when the arterial PCO$_2$ is 40 mm Hg, but much higher venous PCO$_2$ values were seen in patients with DKA and a very contracted ECF volume.[53] This tool can also be used during therapy; the high venous PCO$_2$ will fall appreciably when sufficient saline has been infused.

Consult M Ac-1: Hyperglycemia without Obvious Ketoacidosis

A 16-year-old, 50 kg, female had several past admissions for DKA because she failed to take her insulin on a regular basis. Her present illness began gradually. In response to thirst, she

drank predominantly large volumes of fruit juice and she voided frequently. On physical examination, her ECF volume was obviously contracted, but there was no odor of acetone on her breath and she was not breathing deeply or rapidly. She was easily roused and answered questions appropriately, but she seemed to be somewhat less alert than usual. The remainder of the physical examination was unremarkable. The pH and PCO$_2$ are from an *arterial* blood sample whereas the remainder of the data prior to therapy is from blood drawn from an antecubital vein; the *venous* PCO$_2$ was 69 mm Hg (Table 24-12).

Questions

Does this patient have metabolic acidosis?
Is her ability to buffer H$^+$ via BBS in skeletal muscle cells compromised?

Discussion

Does This Patient Have Metabolic Acidosis?

Her arterial pH, P$_{HCO3}$, and PCO$_2$ were in the normal range. However, the modestly elevated value for her anion gap in plasma (P$_{Anion\ gap}$) suggests that added acids were present and that she indeed had metabolic acidosis (see Fig. 24–20). Because her ECF volume is contracted, the quantity of HCO_3^- in her ECF compartment must be calculated. Using the hematocrit of 0.50 for this purpose, her plasma volume was 2 L instead of the normal value of 3 L—hence her ECF volume was reduced by ~33% (6.7 L instead of 10 L). This marked reduction of ECF volume was due to the urinary loss of NaCl during the osmotic diuresis. This low ECF volume and normal P_{HCO3} indicate that she had a significant deficit of HCO_3^- in her ECF compartment (6.7 L × 24 mmol/L = 160 mmol HCO_3^-) (Table 24–13).

Upon reflection, the modestly elevated value for her $P_{Anion\ gap}$ was due in large part to a high concentration of albumin in plasma ($P_{Albumin}$), which represents the contracted ECF volume, and not the addition of new acids (confirmed later because the concentrations of ketoacid anions, L-lactate, and D-lactate anions in plasma were not appreciably elevated). Thus she does have metabolic acidosis due to a deficit of $NaHCO_3$. This deficit represents an indirect loss of $NaHCO_3$ caused by the excretion of ketoacid anions along with Na^+ in the urine because the rate of excretion of NH_4^+ is not high early in the course of DKA (Fig. 24–24).

TABLE 24–12 Data for Consult M AC-1

Glucose	mg/dL	900	Glucose	mmol/L	50
Na^+	mmol/L	120	K^+	mmol/L	5.5
Cl^-	mmol/L	80	HCO_3^-	mmol/L	24
pH		7.40	PCO_2	mm Hg	40
Albumin	g/dL	5.1	Anion gap	mEq/L	16
Creatinine	mg/dL	2.0	Hematocrit		0.50
Creatinine	μmol/L	230			

TABLE 24–13 Balance of HCO_3^- in Her Extracellular Fluid Compartment

	ECF volume (L)	HCO_3^-		Ketoacid anions	
		(mmol/L)	mmol	(mmol/L)	mmol
	10	24	240	0	0
	6.7	24	160	1	7
Balance	−3.3		−80		+7

For details, see text.
ECF, extracellular fluid.

Is Her Ability to Buffer H^+ Via Bicarbonate Buffer System in Skeletal Muscle Cells Compromised?

Because her brachial venous PCO_2 was 69 mm Hg, buffering of H^+ by her BBS in the interstitial fluid and in muscle cells was compromised. Hence there would be more H^+ binding to intracellular protein in vital organs (e.g., brain and heart); we call this a "tissue form" of respiratory acidosis.[21] One of the results of this process is that there is a net addition of HCO_3^- to the ECF compartment (see Fig. 24–17).

The venous PCO_2 should fall once tissue perfusion improves. As a clinical guide, enough saline should be given to lower venous PCO_2 to a value less than 10 mm Hg higher than the arterial PCO_2.

Concept M Ac-3

When added acids are the cause of metabolic acidosis, one can detect the addition of H^+ by finding a fall in the P_{HCO3} along with the appearance of new anions. These new anions may remain in the body or be excreted (e.g., in the urine or diarrhea fluid).

Tools
Detect New Anions in Plasma

The accumulation of new anions in plasma can be detected from the calculation of the $P_{Anion\ gap}$ (Fig. 24–25). When using this calculation, one must adjust the $P_{Anion\ gap}$ for the concentration of the major unmeasured anion in plasma, albumin ($P_{Albumin}$). As a rough estimate, the baseline value for the $P_{Anion\ gap}$ rises (or falls) by 3 mEq/L to 4 mEq/L for every 10 g/L or 1 g/dL rise (or fall) in the $P_{Albumin}$.

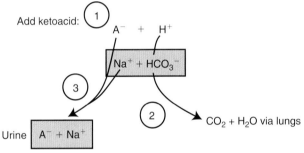

FIGURE 24–24 Ketoacidosis without high $P_{KETOACIDS}$ early in DKA. In the early stage of DKA, metabolic acidosis develops because ketoacids are produced (step 1), their H^+ titrate some of the HCO_3^- in the ECF compartment (larger rectangle), and the resultant CO_2 is exhaled (step 2). Because some of the filtered ketoacid anions (A^-) are not reabsorbed, they will be excreted, but they are not excreted with an equal quantity of NH_4^+ because the renal production of NH_4^+ has not yet increased. Hence these ketoacid anions are excreted largely with Na^+ derived from the ECF compartment (step 3). Overall, there is a net loss of $NaHCO_3$ from the ECF compartment.

FIGURE 24–25 Assessment of the anion gap in plasma. The normal values are shown in the left portion of the figure; the $P_{Anion\ gap}$ is the shaded area between the cation (left) and anion (right) columns. When L-lactic acid is added (middle portion of figure), the P_{HCO3} will fall, and the HCO_3^- will be replaced with L-lactate anions such that the rise in the $P_{Anion\ gap}$ equals the fall in the P_{HCO3}. A loss of $NaHCO_3$ is depicted in the right portion of the figure. Note that the P_{HCO3} fell and the P_{Cl} was elevated, but no new anions were added.

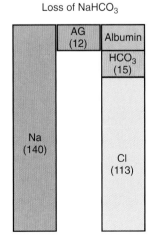

Another approach to detect new anions in plasma was recommended by Stewart[55]; it is called the strong ion difference (SID). This approach is rather complex and offers only a minor advantage over $P_{Anion\ gap}$ in that it includes a correction for the net negative charge on $P_{Albumin}$. It suffers from the same limitations as the $P_{Anion\ gap}$ in that it relies *only* on concentrations in plasma and it does not include information from the venous PCO_2 or the hematocrit. There are, however, additional weaknesses when using the SID approach in that it leads to misunderstandings concerning interpretations of acid-base physiology.[56]

Detect New Anions in the Urine

These anions can be detected with the urine net charge using a value for the concentration of NH_4^+ in the urine (U_{NH4}) that is estimated from the urine osmolal gap ($U_{osm\ gap}$) as discussed in the next section (see following equation). The nature of these new anions may sometimes be deduced by comparing their filtered load to their excretion rate. For example, when a very large proportion of new anions are excreted, suspect that this anion was secreted in the proximal convoluted tubule (PCT)[57] (see "Consult M Ac-2") or freely filtered and poorly reabsorbed by the PCT (e.g., reabsorption of ketoacid anions is inhibited by acetosalycilate anions). On the other hand, a very low excretion of new anions suggests that they were avidly reabsorbed in the PCT (e.g., L-lactate).

$$New\ urine\ anions = (U_{Na} + U_K + U_{NH4}) - U_{Cl}$$

Concept M Ac-4

The identification of new anions helps to predict important dangers for your patient. Examples include anions such as citrate that chelate ionized calcium in plasma,[58] anions that are excreted at a high rate and cause a very high rate of excretion of Na^+ and K^+ (see "Consult M Ac-2"), and those that suggest that toxins were produced during the metabolism of unusual alcohols (e.g., methanol, ethylene glycol metabolism).

Tools

Detect Toxic Alcohols

The presence of alcohols in plasma can be detected by finding a large increase in plasma osmolal gap ($P_{osm\ gap}$) (see following equation). This occurs because the compound is uncharged, has a low molecular weight, and because large quantities have been ingested.

$$P_{osm\ gap} = Measured\ P_{osm} - (2\ P_{Na} + P_{Glucose} + P_{Urea}),$$

all in mmol/L terms

Concept M Ac-5

The expected renal response to chronic metabolic acidosis is a high rate of excretion of NH_4^+.

In a patient with *chronic* metabolic acidosis, the expected rate of excretion of NH_4^+ should be >200 mmol/day.[59] We stress the term "chronic" because there is a lag period of a few days before high rates of excretion of NH_4^+ can be achieved.

Tools: Detect Urinary Ammonium
Urine Osmolal Gap

Because the $U_{osm\ gap}$ detects all NH_4^+ salts in the urine, it provides the best indirect estimate of the U_{NH4}, and hence, we no longer use the urine net charge (or urine anion gap) for this purpose (see following equation).[60] The premise of the test is that NH_4^+ is detected by its contribution to the U_{osm} (Fig. 24–26).

$$U_{osm\ gap} = Measured\ U_{osm} - calculated\ U_{osm}$$

$$Calculated\ U_{osm} = 2\ (U_{Na} + U_K) + U_{Urea} + U_{Glucose},$$

all in mmol/L terms

$$Urine\ NH_4^+ = U_{osm\ gap}/2$$

We use the $U_{NH4}/U_{Creatinine}$ ratio in a spot urine sample to assess the rate of excretion of NH_4^+. The rationale is that the rate of excretion of creatinine is relatively constant over the 24-hour period in complete, timed urine collections.[27] In a patient with chronic metabolic acidosis the expected renal response is $U_{NH4}/U_{Creatinine}$ ratio >150 mmol/g creatinine (>15 in mmol/mmol terms).

Consult M Ac-2: Metabolic Acidosis Due to Glue Sniffing

A 28-year-old male sniffs glue on a regular basis. He developed profound weakness over the course of 3 days. On physical examination, his ECF volume was obviously contracted. His pH and PCO_2 were from arterial blood and the other data were from venous blood; his venous PCO_2 was 70 mm Hg, $P_{Glucose}$ was 3.5 mmol/L (63 mg/dL), and his $P_{Albumin}$ was 4.5 g/dL (45 g/L) (Table 24–14).

Questions

What is the basis for the metabolic acidosis?
What dangers are implied from the high rate of excretion of anions in the urine?

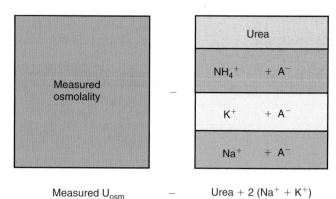

FIGURE 24–26 Use of the urine osmolal gap to reflect the concentration of NH_4^+ in the urine. Because most urine anions are monovalent, the U_{NH4} is equal to one half the $U_{osmolal\ gap}$.

TABLE 24–14	Data for Consult MAc-2						
		Blood	**Urine**			**Blood**	**Urine**
pH		7.30	6.0	PCO_2	mm Hg	30	—
HCO_3^-	mmol/L	15	<5	K^+	mmol/L	2.3	20
Na^+	mmol/L	120	50	Cl^-	mmol/L	90	0
Creatinine	mg/dL	1.7	3.0	Urea	mmol/L	2.5	50
Osmolality	mOsm/L	245	500	Hematocrit		0.50	—

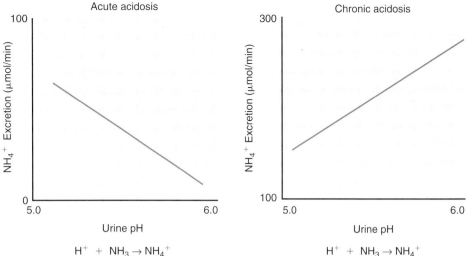

FIGURE 24-27 Failure of the urine pH to detect U_{NH4}. As shown on the left, the urine pH is low during acute metabolic acidosis due to enhanced distal H^+ secretion. The rate of excretion of NH_4^+ is only modestly high at this time due to the lag period before the rate of renal production of NH_4^+ is augmented. In contrast, during chronic metabolic acidosis shown on the right, the rate of renal production of NH_4^+ is very high and the availability of NH_3 in the medullary interstitial compartment provides more NH_3 in the lumen of the MCD than H^+ secretion in this nephron segment. Therefore note the much higher NH_4^+ excretion rate at a urine pH of 6.

Discussion

What Is the Basis for the Metabolic Acidosis?

Metabolic acidosis is present because of the low pH and P_{HCO3}. He also has a very low content of HCO_3^- in his ECF compartment because his P_{HCO3} is low and his ECF volume is contracted (hematocrit 0.50).

Detect new anions in plasma: Because there was no increase in the $P_{Anion\ gap}$ corrected for the $P_{Albumin}$, this suggested that the metabolic acidosis was not due to a gain of acids.

Detect new anions in the urine: For this, the U_{NH4} must be estimated using the $U_{osm\ gap}$. The measured U_{osm} was 500 mOsm/L and the calculated U_{osm} was 190 mOsm/L (2 × (U_{Na} 50 + U_K 20) + U_{urea} 50 mmol/L). Hence the $U_{osm\ gap}$ was 310 mOsm/L and the U_{NH4} was half of this value or 155 mmol/L (confirmed later by direct measurement). Therefore the patient had a high U_{NH4} and many unmeasured anions in the urine. Hence we deduced that there was overproduction of acids while the kidney excreted their accompanying anions. The high rate of excretion of the anions suggested that they were not only filtered but also secreted by PCT—this is the fate of hippurate anions.[61] Hippuric acid is the end product of the metabolism of toluene, a constituent of glue—hence the basis of the metabolic acidosis is overproduction of hippuric acid together with excretion of hippurate anions in the urine at a rate that exceeded the rate of excretion of NH_4^+.[57]

What Dangers Are Implied from the High Rate of Excretion of Anions in the Urine?

Hippurate is secreted by the PCT and it is excreted very rapidly. When the excretion of hippurate exceeds that of NH_4^+, this obligates the excretion of Na^+ and K^+, which may cause ECF volume contraction and hypokalemia (see Fig. 24-23). The presence of ECF volume contraction lowers the rate of excretion of NH_4^+ if it also leads to a low GFR.[62]

The higher rate of excretion of K^+ can lead to a cardiac arrhythmia and hypoventilation if it causes respiratory muscle weakness. Hypoventilation caused by muscle weakness, along with the low ECF volume, can lead to hypokalemia and, as a result, a high venous PCO_2 with diminished buffering of H^+ by the BBS in skeletal muscles and hence buffering of more H^+ in vital organs (e.g., the brain and the heart) (see Fig. 24-22).

Concept M Ac-6

A low rate of excretion of NH_4^+ could be due to a decreased medullary NH_3 or a decreased net H^+ secretion in distal nephron.

A low rate of ammoniagenesis could be due to due to an alkaline PCT cell (e.g., hyperkalemia, genetic, or acquired disorders compromising proximal H^+ secretion) or decreased

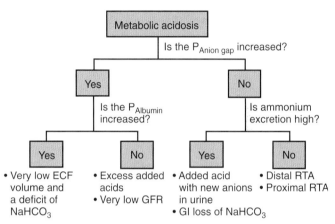

FIGURE 24-28 Basis of metabolic acidosis. One must use a definition of metabolic acidosis based not only the P_{HCO3} but also on the content of HCO_3^- in the ECF compartment.

availability of ADP reflecting less work performed in PCT cells because of a low filtered load of Na^+ due to a reduced GFR.[62] Another cause for a low rate of excretion of NH_4^+ is a low net secretion of H^+ in the distal nephron. This could be due to a H^+-ATPase defect (e.g., autoimmune and hypergammaglobulinemic disorders including Sjögren syndrome), back-leak of H^+ (e.g., drugs like amphotericin B), or disorders associated with the distal secretion of HCO_3^- (e.g., in certain patients with Southeast Asian Ovalocytosis (SAO)[63]).

Tools: Detect Why the Rate of Excretion of NH_4^+ is Low

Urine pH

The urine pH is *not* helpful to imply that the rate of excretion of NH_4^+ is low.[64] For example, at a urine pH of 6.0, the U_{NH4} can be 20 mmol/L or 200 mmol/L (Fig. 24-27). However, the basis for the low rate of excretion NH_4^+ may be deduced from the urine pH. A urine pH that is ~5 suggests that the basis for a low rate of excretion of NH_4^+ is due primarily to a decreased availability of NH_3 in the medullary interstitial compartment. On the other hand, a urine pH that is >7 suggests that NH_4^+ excretion is low because there is a defect in H^+ secretion and/or that there was a high rate of excretion of HCO_3^- in the distal nephron (Fig. 24-28).

Assess Distal H^+ Secretion

H^+ secretion in the distal nephron can be evaluated using the PCO_2 in alkaline urine (U_{PCO2}) (Fig. 24-29). A U_{PCO2} that is ~70 mm Hg in a second-voided alkaline urine implies that H^+

secretion in the distal nephron is likely to be normal whereas much lower U_{PCO_2} values suggest that distal H^+ secretion is impaired.[65] In patients with low net distal H^+ secretion, the U_{PCO_2} can be high if there is a lesion causing a back-leak of H^+ from the lumen of the collecting ducts (e.g., use of amphotericin B[66]) or distal secretion of HCO_3^- as in some patients with SAO who also have a second mutation in their HCO_3^-/Cl^- anion exchanger that leads to mis-targeting of the exchanger to the luminal membrane of the α-intercalated cells.[54,63] A caveat with this test is that the U_{PCO_2} is also influenced by the renal concentrating ability.[67]

Tools to Assess Proximal Cell pH

Fractional excretion of HCO_3^-: In patients with metabolic acidosis associated with a low capacity to reabsorb filtered HCO_3^- (e.g., disorders with defects in H^+ secretion in the PCT called proximal RTA), some would measure the fractional excretion of HCO_3^- after infusing $NaHCO_3$ to confirm this diagnosis. This is rarely needed in our opinion—often the results are far from clear (e.g., in a patient with an abnormal ECF volume or P_K) and, in addition, the test can impose a danger (e.g., in a patient with a low P_K). These patients will be detected clinically by failure to correct their metabolic acidosis despite being given large amounts of $NaHCO_3$.

Rate of citrate excretion: The rate of excretion of citrate is a marker of pH in cells of the PCT.[68] The daily rate of excretion of citrate in children and adults consuming their usual diet

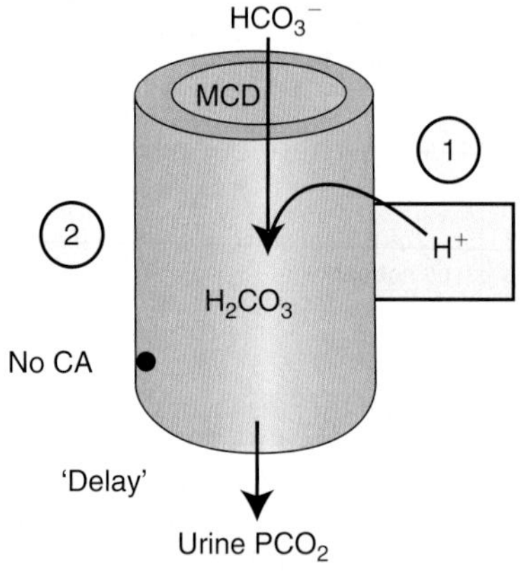

FIGURE 24–29 The basis for an increased PCO_2 in alkaline urine. When $NaHCO_3$ is given, there is a large delivery of HCO_3 to the distal nephron, which makes HCO_3^- virtually the only H^+ acceptor in its lumen. Because there is no luminal carbonic anhydrase (CA), the H_2CO_3 formed will be delivered downstream and form CO_2 plus water. Thus a urine PCO_2 that is appreciably higher than the plasma PCO_2 provides evidence for distal H^+ secretion. The PCO_2 in alkaline urine will be low if there is a lesion involving the H^+-ATPase or causes an alkaline cell pH in intercalated cells in the distal nephron. If the lesion is one that causes back-leak of H^+ or distal secretion of HCO_3^-, the urine PCO_2 will be high.

is ~400 mg (~2 mmol/g or 10 mmol of creatinine). Although the rate of excretion of citrate is very low during most forms of metabolic acidosis,[69] a notable exception is in patients with disorders causing an alkaline PCT cell pH.[70]

Consult M Ac-3: Determine the Cause of Hyperchloremic Metabolic Acidosis

A 23-year-old female suffers from Southeast Asian Ovalocytosis and was referred for assessment of hypokalemia. Her physical examination was unremarkable. Her laboratory results in plasma and a spot urine sample are summarized in Table 24–15. Her urine urea was 220 mmol/L and the urine was glucose-free.

Questions

What is the basis of the hyperchloremic metabolic acidosis? What is the basis for the low rate of excretion of NH_4^+?

Discussion

What Is the Basis of the Hyperchloremic Metabolic Acidosis?

Urine osmolar gap: The patient had a low U_{NH4} because her measured U_{osm} (450 mOsm/kg H_2O) was very similar to her calculated U_{osm} [420 mOsm/kg H_2O, i.e., 2 (U_{Na} 75 + U_K 35 mmol/L) + U_{Urea} (220 mOsm/kg H_2O) + $U_{Glucose}$ (0)]. In addition, her rate of excretion of NH_4^+ was low because the ratio of $U_{NH4}/U_{Creatinine}$ was very low. Because her GFR was not very low, the diagnosis is renal tubular acidosis (RTA).

What Is the Cause for the Low Rate of Excretion of NH_4^+?

Urine pH: Because the urine pH is 6.8, the basis for the low rate of NH_4^+ excretion is a low net secretion of H^+ in the distal nephron (Fig. 24–30).

Assess distal H^+ secretion: After hypokalemia was corrected, the PCO_2 in alkaline urine was 70 mm Hg.

Assess proximal cell pH: The rate of excretion of citrate was low. In addition, her P_{HCO3} remained in the normal range after the infusion of $NaHCO_3$.

Interpretation

The high urine pH and the low rate of excretion of NH_4^+ suggested that she had a defect in distal H^+ secretion. H^+ secretion by her PCT seemed to be intact (her P_{HCO3} remained in the normal range after initial therapy, $U_{citrate}$ was low, and her FE_{HCO3} was <3%). Because her U_{PCO2} was unexpectedly high and a back leak of H^+ type of defect is unlikely, perhaps her mutant Cl^-/HCO_3^- anion exchanger was targeted abnormally to the luminal membrane of α-intercalated cells. The U_{PCO2} would be high due to distal secretion of HCO_3^- by alkaline intercalated cells.

Integration: Clinical Approach to the Patient with Metabolic Acidosis

The first step in our clinical approach to the patient with metabolic acidosis is to establish that metabolic acidosis is present by finding either a low pH and P_{HCO3} or a low content of HCO_3^- in the ECF compartment. Our next step is to identify

TABLE 24–15		Data for Consult Mac-3					
		Plasma	Urine			Plasma	Urine
pH		7.35	6.8	PCO_2	mm Hg	30	—
HCO_3^-	mmol/L	15	10	K^+	mmol/L	3.1	35
Na^+	mmol/L	140	75	Cl^-	mmol/L	113	95
Anion gap	mEq/L	12	5	Creatinine	mg/dL	0.7	60
Osmolality	mOsm/L	290	450	Citrate	mg/dL	—	Low

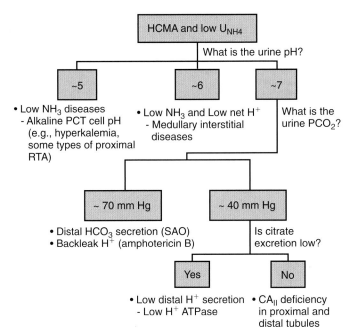

FIGURE 24-30 Approach to the patient with HCMA and a low excretion of NH_4^+. The initial approach to determine the pathophysiology in patients with HCMA and a low rate of excretion of NH_4^+ is based on the urine pH.

threats present before therapy begins *and* to anticipate and prevent dangers that may develop during the course of the illness or with its therapy (see Fig. 24-20). After the emergencies are considered, the arterial and venous PCO_2 should be assessed to examine the effectiveness of the BBS. If the venous PCO_2 is too high, the BBS cannot prevent H^+ from binding to ICF proteins (see Fig. 24-22).

The third step in our approach is to determine the basis of metabolic acidosis (see Fig. 24-28). The most important step is to hunt for new unmeasured anions in the plasma and the urine. This is followed by an assessment of the renal response to metabolic acidosis. If the rate of excretion of NH_4^+ is low (low $U_{osm\ gap}$) while the GFR is not very low, a diagnosis of RTA is suspected. To uncover the cause for the low rate of excretion of NH_4^+, the urine pH is the most important of the laboratory tests in the urine (see Fig. 24-30). The U_{PCO2} is helpful in the subgroup with a high urine pH and measuring the rate of excretion of citrate is useful to assess the pH in PCT cells.

CONCLUSION

Given the tremendous advances in our understanding of the integrative physiology of the topics covered in this chapter and the many new insights gained from molecular and genetic advances, clinicians should now pursue diagnoses right down to the enzyme or transporter that is defective. A physiology-based clinical approach is a crucial component to make more exact diagnoses and design more appropriate therapy for patients with disorders of water, Na^+, K^+, and/or acid-base homeostasis.

References

1. Kamel KS, Ethier JH, Richardson RMA, et al: Urine electrolytes and osmolality: When and how to use them. Am J Nephrol 10:89–102, 1990.
2. Halperin ML, Kamel KS: Use of the composition of the urine at the bedside: Emphasis on physiological principles to provide insights into diagnostic and therapeutic issues. *In* Seldin DW, Giebisch G (eds): Physiology and Pathology of Electrolyte Metabolism. The Kidney: Physiology and Pathophysiology. 3rd ed. New York, Raven Press, 2001.
3. Nielsen S, Frokiaer J, Marples D, et al: Aquaporins in the kidney: From molecules to medicine. Physiol Rev 82:205–244, 2002.
4. Halperin ML, Bichet DG, Oh MS: Integrative physiology of basal water permeability in the distal nephron: Implications for the syndrome of inappropriate secretion of antidiuretic hormone. Clin Nephrol 56:339–345, 2001.
5. Shafiee MA, Charest AF, Cheema-Dhadli S, et al: Defining conditions that lead to the retention of water: The importance of the arterial sodium concentration. Kidney Int 67:613–621, 2005.
6. Oh MS, Carroll HJ, Roy A, et al: Chronic hyponatremia in the absence of ADH: Possible role of decreased delivery of filtrate. J Am Soc Nephrol 8:108A, 1997.
7. Cherney DZI, Davids MR, Halperin ML: Acute hyponatraemia and MDMA ("Ecstasy"): Insights from a quantitative and integrative analysis. Quart J Med 95:475–483, 2002.
8. Laureno R, Karp BI: Pontine and extrapontine myelinolysis following rapid correction of hyponatremia. Lancet 1:1439–1441, 1988.
9. Kamel KS, Bichet DG, Halperin ML: Studies to clarify the pathophysiology of partial central diabetes insipidus. Am J Nephrol 37:1290–1293, 2001.
10. Spira A, Gowrishankar M, Halperin ML: Factors contributing to the degree of polyuria in a patient with diabetes mellitus in poor control. Am J Kidney Dis 30:829–835, 1997.
11. Deetjen P, Baeyer HV, Drexel H: Renal glucose transport. *In* Seldin D, Giebisch G (eds). The Kidney: Physiology and Pathophysiology. 2nd ed. New York, Raven Press, 1992, pp 2873–2888.
12. Davids MR, Edoute Y, Stock S, Halperin ML: Severe degree of hyperglycemia: Novel insights revealed by the use of simple principles of integrative physiology. Quart J Med 95:113–124, 2002.
13. Carlotti APCP, Bohn D, Halperin ML: Importance of timing of risk factors for cerebral oedema during therapy for diabetic ketoacidosis. Arch Dis Child 88:170–173, 2003.
14. Gowrishankar M, Lenga I, Cheung RY, et al: Minimum urine flow rate during water deprivation: Importance of the permeability of urea in the inner medulla. Kidney Int 53:159–166, 1998.
15. Gamble JL, McKhann CF, Butler AM, Tuthill E: An economy of water in renal function referable to urea. Am J Physiol 109:139–154, 1934.
16. Halperin ML, Rolleston FS: Clinical Detective Stories: A Problem-Based Approach to Clinical Cases in Energy and Acid-Base Metabolism. 1st ed. London, England, Portland Press, 1993.
17. Labow BI, Souba WW: Glutamine. World J Surg 24:1503–1513, 2000.
18. Carlotti APCP, Bohn D, Mallie J-P, Halperin ML: Tonicity balance and not electrolyte-free water calculations more accurately guide therapy for acute changes in natremia. Intensive Care Med 27:921–924, 2001.
19. Carlotti APCP, Bohn D, Rutka JT, et al: A method to estimate urinary electrolyte excretion in patients at risk for developing cerebral salt wasting. J Neurosurg 95:420–424, 2001.
20. Mitch WE, Collier VU, Walser M: Creatinine metabolism in chronic renal failure. Clin Sci 58:327–335, 1980.
21. Zalunardo N, Lemaire M, Davids MR, Halperin ML: Acidosis in a patient with cholera: A need to redefine concepts. Quart J Med 97:681–696, 2004.
22. Russell JM: Sodium-potassium-chloride cotransport. Physiol Rev 80:211–276, 2000.
23. Clausen T: Regulation of active Na^+-K^+ transport in skeletal muscle. Physiol Rev 66:542–580, 1986.
24. Solemani M, Burham C: Physiology and molecular aspects of the $Na^+:HCO_3^-$ contransporter in health and disease processes. Kidney Int 57:371–384, 2000.
25. Huth EJ, Squires RD, Elkinton JR: Experimental potassium depletion in normal human subjects. II. Renal and hormonal factors in the development of extracellular alkalosis during depletion. J Clin Invest 38:1149–1165, 1959.
26. Talbott JH, Schwab RS: Recent advances in the biochemistry and therapeutics of potassium salts. N Engl J Med 222:585–590, 1940.
27. Cockcroft DW, Gault MH: Prediction of creatinine clearance from serum creatinine. Nephron 16:31–41, 1976.
28. Steele A, deVeber H, Quaggin SE, et al: What is responsible for the diurnal variation in potassium excretion? Am J Physiol 36:R554–R560, 1994.
29. Halperin ML, Kamel KS: Potassium. Lancet 352:135–142, 1998.
30. Field MJ, Giebisch GJ: Hormonal control of renal potassium excretion. Kidney Int 27:379–387, 1985.
31. Ethier JH, Kamel KS, Magner PO, et al: The transtubular potassium concentration in patients with hypokalemia and hyperkalemia. Am J Kidney Dis 15(4):309–315, 1990.
32. Cheema-Dhadli S, Lin S-H, Chong CK, et al: Requirements for a high rate of potassium excretion in rats consuming a low electrolyte diet. J Physiol London 572.2:493–501, 2006.
33. Lin S-H, Lin Y-F, Halperin ML: Hypokalemia and paralysis: Clues on admission to help in the differential diagnosis. Quart J Med 94:133–139, 2001.
34. Alazami M, Lin S-H, Chu C-J, et al: Unusual causes of hypokalaemia and paralysis. Quart J Med 99:181–192, 2006.
35. Lin S-H, Chu P, Cheng C-J, et al: Early diagnosis of thyrotoxic periodic paralysis: Spot urine calcium to phosphate ratio. Crit Care Med 34:2984–2989, 2006.
36. Lin SH, Lin YF: Propranolol rapidly reverses paralysis, hypokalemia and hypophosphatemia in thyrotoxic periodic paralysis. Am J Kidney Dis 37:620–624, 2001.
37. Edwards CRW: Lessons from licorice. N Engl J Med 24:1242–1243, 1991.
38. Rosa RM, Williams ME, Epstein FH: Extrarenal potassium metabolism. *In* Seldin DW, Giebisch G (eds): The Kidney: Physiology and Pathophysiology. 2nd ed. New York, Raven Press, 1992, pp 2165–2190.
39. Porte DJ: Sympathetic regulation of insulin secretion. Arch Intern Med 123:252–260, 1969.
40. Choi MJ, Fernandez PC, Patnaik A, et al: Trimethoprim induced hyperkalemia in a patient with AIDS. N Engl J Med 328:703–706, 1993.
41. Schreiber MS, Chen C-B, Lessan-Pezeshki M, et al: Antikaliuretic action of trimethoprim is minimized by raising urine pH. Kidney Int 49:82–87, 1996.

42. Carlisle EJF, Donnelly SM, Ethier J, et al: Modulation of the secretion of potassium by accompanying anions in humans. Kidney Int 39:1206–1212, 1991.

43. Iolascon A, Stewart GW, Ajetunmobi JF, et al: Familial pseudohyperkalemia maps to the same locus as dehydrated hereditary stomatocytosis (hereditary xerocytosis). Blood 93:3120–3123, 1999.

44. Don BR, Sebastian A, Cheitlin M, et al: Pseudohyperkalemia caused by fist clenching during phlebotomy. N Engl J Med 322(18):1290–1292, 1990.

45. Kahle KT, Wilson FH, Lalioti M, et al: WNK kinases: Molecular regulators of integrated epithelial ion transport. Curr Opin Nephrol Hypertens (13):557–562, 2004.

46. Kamel K, Ethier JH, Quaggin S, et al: Studies to determine the basis for hyperkalemia in recipients of a renal transplant who are treated with cyclosporin. J Am Soc Nephrol 2:1279–1284, 1992.

47. Scheich A, Donnelly S, Cheema-Dhadli S, et al: Does saline "correct" the abnormal mass balance in metabolic alkalosis associated with chloride-depletion in the rat. Clin Invest Med 17:448–460, 1994.

48. Cheema-Dhadli S, Lin S-H, Halperin ML: Mechanisms used to dispose of a progressively increasing alkali load in the rat. Am J Physiol 282:F1049–F1055, 2002.

49. Rubin SI, Sonnenberg B, Zettle R, Halperin ML: Metabolic alkalosis mimicking the acute sequestration of HCl in rats: Bucking the alkaline tide. Clin Invest Med 17:515–521, 1994.

50. Cogan M: Angiotensin II: A powerful controller of sodium transport in the early proximal tubule. Hypertension 15:451–458, 1990.

51. Shafiee MA, Napolova O, Charest AF, Halperin ML: When is sodium chloride the physiologically appropriate treatment for patients with metabolic alkalosis. Indian J Nephrol 13:45–54, 2003.

52. Kamel KS, Halperin ML: An improved approach to the patient with metabolic acidosis: A need for four amendments. J Nephrol 19:S76–S85, 2006.

53. Napolova O, Urbach S, Davids MR, Halperin ML: How to assess the degree of extracellular fluid volume contraction in a patient with a severe degree of hyperglycemia. Nephrol Dial Trans 18:2674–2677, 2003.

54. Vasuvattakul S, Warner LC, Halperin ML: Quantitative role of the intracellular bicarbonate buffer system in response to an acute acid load. Am J Physiol 262:R305–R309, 1992.

55. Stewart PA: Modern quantitative acid-base chemistry. Can J Physiol Pharmacol 61:1444–1461, 1983.

56. Halperin ML, Goldstein MB, Kamel KS: Fluid, Electrolyte and Acid-Base Physiology; A Problem-Based Approach. Philadelphia, WB Saunders, 2006.

57. Carlisle EJF, Donnelly SM, Vasuvattakul S, et al: Glue-sniffing and distal renal tubular acidosis: Sticking to the facts. J Am Soc Nephrol 1:1019–1027, 1991.

58. DeMars C, Hollister K, Tomassoni A, et al: Citric acidosis: A life-threatening cause of metabolic acidosis. Ann Emerg Med 38:588–591, 2001.

59. Halperin ML: How much "new" bicarbonate is formed in the distal nephron in the process of net acid excretion? Kidney Int 35:1277–1281, 1989.

60. Dyck RF, Asthana S, Kalra J, et al: A modification of the urine osmolal gap: An improved method for estimating urine ammonium. Am J Nephrol 10:359–362, 1990.

61. Smith HW, Finfelstein N, Aliminosa L, et al: The renal clearances of substituted hippuric acid derivatives and other aromatic acids in dogs and man. J Clin Invest 24:388–404, 1945.

62. Halperin ML, Jungas RL, Pichette C, Goldstein MB: A quantitative analysis of renal ammoniagenesis and energy balance: A theoretical approach. Can J Physiol Pharmacol 60:1431–1435, 1982.

63. Kaitwatcharachai C, Vasuvattakul S, Yenchitsomanus P, et al: Distal renal tubular acidosis in a patient with southeast Asian ovalocytosis: Possible interpretations of a high urine PCO_2. Am J Kidney Dis 33:1147–1152, 1999.

64. Richardson RMA, Halperin ML: The urine pH: A potentially misleading diagnostic test in patients with hyperchloremic metabolic acidosis. Am J Kidney Dis 10:140–143, 1987.

65. Halperin ML, Goldstein MB, Haig A, et al: Studies on the pathogenesis of type I (distal) renal tubular acidosis as revealed by the urinary PCO_2 tensions. J Clin Invest 53:669–677, 1974.

66. Roscoe J, Goldstein M, Halperin M, et al: Effect of amphotericin B on urine acidification in rats: Implications for the pathogenesis of distal renal tubular acidosis. J Lab Clin Med 89:463, 1977.

67. Berliner RW, DuBose TDJ: Carbon dioxide tension of alkaline urine. In Seldin DW, Giebisch G (eds): The Kidney: Physiology and Pathophysiology. 2nd ed. New York, Raven Press, 1992, pp 2681–2694.

68. Simpson D: Citrate excretion: A window on renal metabolism. Am J Physiol 244:F223-F234, 1983.

69. Dedmond RE, Wrong O: The excretion of organic anion in renal tubular acidosis with particular reference to citrate. Clin Sci 22:19–32, 1962.

70. Halperin ML, Kamel KS, Ethier JH, Magner PO: What is the underlying defect in patients with isolated, proximal renal tubular acidosis? Am J Nephrol 9:265–268, 1989.

CHAPTER 25

Adaptation to Nephron Loss

Maarten W. Taal • Barry M. Brenner

The introduction of a classification system for chronic kidney disease (CKD) by the Kidney Disease Outcomes Quality Initiative (K/DOQI) and its adoption worldwide have made a valuable contribution to raising awareness of the problem of CKD.[1] Importantly the division of the spectrum of CKD into stages has emphasized the progressive nature of CKD and facilitated the development of stage-specific strategies for slowing the progression of CKD as well as managing the complications of chronic renal failure. These developments highlight the importance of understanding the mechanisms that contribute to CKD progression in order to inform strategies for slowing such progression. Central to these mechanisms are the adaptations observed in the kidney when nephrons are lost.

The kidney's primary function of maintaining constancy of the extracellular fluid volume and composition is remarkably well preserved until late in the course of CKD. When nephrons are lost through disease or surgical ablation, those remaining or least affected undergo remarkable physiological responses resulting in hypertrophy and hyperfunction that combine to compensate for the acquired loss of renal function. Effective kidney function requires close integration of glomerular and tubular functions. Indeed, the preservation of *glomerulotubular balance* seen until the terminal stages of CKD is fundamental to the *intact nephron hypothesis* of Bricker, which essentially states that as CKD advances, kidney function is supported by a diminishing pool of functioning (or hyperfunctioning) nephrons, rather than relatively constant numbers of nephrons, each with diminishing function. This concept has important implications for the mechanisms of disease progression in CKD.

Several decades ago, clinical studies of patients with CKD established that once glomerular filtration rate (GFR) fell below a critical level, a relentless progression to end-stage renal failure inevitably ensued, even when the initial disease activity had abated. The rate of decline of GFR in a given individual followed a near constant linear relationship with time, enabling remarkably accurate predictions of the date at which end-stage renal failure would be reached and renal replacement therapy required. Among patients with diverse renal diseases, the slope of the GFR/

time relationship was found to be a characteristic of individual patients rather than typical of their specific renal diseases. This observation suggested that the progressive nature of renal disease could be attributed to a final "common pathway" of mechanisms, independent of the primary cause of nephropathy.[2] Within this framework, Brenner and colleagues formulated a unifying hypothesis for renal disease progression based on the physiological adaptations observed in experimental models of CKD.[3] The central tenets of the common pathway theory state that CKD progression occurs, in general, through focal nephron loss and that the adaptive responses of surviving nephrons, although initially serving to increase single-nephron GFR and offset the overall loss in clearance, ultimately prove detrimental to the kidney. Over time, glomerulosclerosis and tubular atrophy further reduce nephron number, fueling a self-perpetuating cycle of nephron destruction culminating in uremia.

In this chapter we describe in detail the functional and structural adaptations observed in remaining nephrons following substantial reductions in functioning renal mass and the mechanisms thought to be responsible for them. We then consider how these changes may in time prove maladaptive and contribute to the progressive renal injury described above. Given the growing worldwide burden of CKD that causes substantial morbidity and mortality in individuals and threatens to overburden health care systems, it could be argued that the further elucidation of the mechanisms of CKD progression resulting in more effective interventions to slow its advance should remain among the highest priorities for nephrologists today.

STRUCTURAL AND FUNCTIONAL ADAPTATION OF THE KIDNEY TO NEPHRON LOSS

Alterations in Glomerular Physiology

Glomerular hemodynamic responses to nephron loss have been studied largely in animals subjected to surgical ablation of renal mass. It was recognized several decades ago that unilateral nephrectomy in rats resulted in a rapid increase in function of the remaining kidney, detectable 3 days after nephrectomy, such that the GFR achieved a maximum of 70% to 85% of the previous 2-kidney value after 2 to 3 weeks. As no new nephrons are formed in mature rodents, the observed rise in GFR represents an increase in the filtration rate of remaining nephrons.

Detailed study of glomerular hemodynamics was facilitated by the identification of a rat strain, Munich-Wistar, which is unique in bearing glomeruli on the kidney surface. This allowed micropuncture of the glomerulus and direct measurement of intraglomerular pressures as well as sampling of blood from afferent and efferent arterioles. These techniques made possible the study of mechanisms underlying the compensatory rise in GFR after renal mass ablation. Increases in whole kidney GFR at 2 to 4 weeks after unilateral nephrectomy were attributable to an increase in single nephron GFR (SNGFR) averaging 83%, achieved in large part by a rise in glomerular plasma flow rate (Q_A), which in turn, resulted from dilation of both afferent and efferent arterioles. Although systemic blood pressure was not elevated, glomerular capillary hydraulic pressure (P_{GC}) and the glomerular transcapillary pressure difference (ΔP) were increased significantly post uninephrectomy, accounting for an estimated 25% of the rise in SNGFR.[4] The glomerular ultrafiltration coefficient, K_f (the product of glomerular hydraulic permeability and surface area available for filtration), was unaltered at this stage but may become elevated later.[5]

With more extensive nephron loss, even greater compensatory increases in SNGFR were observed. In Munich-Wistar rats studied 7 days after unilateral nephrectomy and infarction of 5/6 of the contralateral kidney, SNGFR in the remnant was more than double that of 2-kidney controls. This increment was again attributable to large increases in Q_A, and a substantial rise in P_{GC}. Efferent and afferent arteriolar resistances were reduced to half or less of control values but the decrease in afferent arteriolar resistance was proportionately greater, accounting for the observed rise in P_{GC}.[6] Comparison of renal infarction versus surgical excision models of 5/6 nephrectomy subsequently found that changes in arteriolar resistance were similar but that P_{GC} was significantly more elevated in the infarction model, indicating that glomerular transmission of elevated systemic blood pressure (absent in the surgical excision model) also contributes to the increase in P_{GC}.[7] Changes in K_f after extensive renal mass ablation appear to be time-dependent, with a decrease reported at 2 weeks after surgery,[8] and an increase at 4 weeks.[9] Further studies indicated that glomerular hemodynamic responses to nephron loss seem to be similar between the superficial cortical and juxtamedullary nephrons.[10] The rise in SNGFR associated with renal mass ablation is often referred to as *glomerular hyperfiltration* and the elevated P_{GC} is termed *glomerular hypertension*. Together these terms encompass the central concepts underlying the hemodynamic adaptations in the remnant kidney.

Glomerular hemodynamic adaptations to nephron loss may show interspecies variation. In dogs, increases in SNGFR observed 4 weeks after 3/4 or 7/8 nephrectomy were attributable largely to increases in Q_A and K_f. In contrast to the findings in rodents, ΔP was only modestly elevated. After ablation of 7/8 of their renal mass, dogs developed a significant rise in P_{GC} independent of arterial pressure, again as a result of relatively greater relaxation of afferent versus efferent arterioles.[11]

In humans, the effects of nephron loss on the physiology of the remnant kidney have been studied mainly in healthy individuals undergoing donor nephrectomy for kidney transplantation. Inulin clearance studies of the earliest kidney donors revealed that total GFR in the donor's remaining kidney had increased to 65% to 70% of the previous 2-kidney value by 1 week post nephrectomy. A meta-analysis of data from 48 studies that included 2988 living kidney donors, estimated that GFR decreased, on average, by only 17 ml/min after uninephrectomy.[12] These observations imply that single kidney GFR (and therefore also the average SNGFR) increases by 30% to 40% after uninephrectomy in humans. There is currently no method for estimating SNGFR or P_{GC} in vivo and more detailed assessments of glomerular hemodynamics in humans have thus not yet been possible.

Mediators of the Glomerular Hemodynamic Responses to Nephron Loss

The factors that are sensed after renal mass ablation and serve as signals to initiate the adjustments in glomerular hemodynamics responsible for the increase in remnant kidney GFR remain to be identified. However, the effector mechanisms have been studied extensively and the hemodynamic changes can be attributed to the net effects of complex interactions of several factors, each having specific, and sometimes opposing actions on the various determinants of glomerular ultrafiltration. Several vasoactive substances, including angiotensin II (AII), aldosterone, natriuretic peptides (NP), endothelins (ET) eicosanoids and bradykinin, have been implicated. Moreover, sustained increases in SNGFR also require resetting of the autoregulatory mechanisms that normally govern GFR and renal plasma flow (RPF).

Renin-Angiotensin-Aldosterone System

Angiotensin II appears to play a critical role in the development of glomerular capillary hypertension following renal ablation and may also contribute to changes in K_f. Acute infusion of AII in normal rats results in a rise in P_{GC}, due to a greater increase in efferent than afferent resistance, and reductions in Q_A and K_f.[13,14] Chronic administration of AII for 8 weeks resulted in systemic hypertension, lowered single kidney GFR and, with the exception of K_f, elicited similar glomerular hemodynamic changes to those observed after acute infusion in both normal and uninephrectomized rats.[5] The importance of the influence of endogenous AII on glomerular hemodynamics in remnant kidneys was revealed by studies with pharmacological inhibitors of the renin-angiotensin system (RAS). Chronic treatment of 5/6 nephrectomized rats with either an angiotensin-converting enzyme inhibitor (ACEI)[15,16] or angiotensin II (subtype 1) receptor antagonist (AT₁RA)[17,18] results in normalization of P_{GC} through reduction in systemic blood pressure and dilatation of both afferent and efferent arterioles. SNGFR, however, remains elevated due to an increase in K_f. Furthermore, acute infusion of an ACEI or saralasin, a peptide analogue receptor antagonist of AII, was found to normalize P_{GC} in 5/6 nephrectomized rats through efferent arteriolar dilatation, without affecting mean arterial pressure (MAP).[8,19] It is unclear why these findings could not be confirmed with the AT₁RA, losartan.[20]

These effects of RAS inhibition imply that there is increased local activity of endogenous AII, yet plasma renin levels show only a transient increase following 5/6 nephrectomy.[7,21] This suggests differential regulation of the systemic versus intrarenal RAS and that AII is formed locally. Renin mRNA and protein levels are both increased in glomeruli adjacent to the infarction scar in 5/6 nephrectomized rats.[22–24] Furthermore renal renin mRNA levels are increased at day 3 and 7 after renal mass ablation by infarction but not when renal mass is excised surgically, suggesting that renal infarction activates the RAS by creating a margin of ischemic tissue around the organizing infarct and explaining the greater severity of hypertension as well as glomerulosclerosis associated with the infarction model.[7] Detailed studies of intrarenal AII levels following 5/6 nephrectomy achieved by infarction have confirmed these findings by showing higher AII levels in the peri-infarct portion of the kidney than the intact portion at all time points.[21] On the other hand, the studies also showed that the rise in intrarenal AII following 5/6 nephrectomy was transient. Whereas AII levels in the peri-infarct portion were elevated compared to sham-operated controls at 2 weeks after surgery, they were not statistically different at 5 or 7 weeks. In the intact portion of the remnant kidney, AII levels were similar to controls at 2 and 5 weeks and were lower at 7 weeks.[21] Sustained increases in intrarenal AII levels are therefore not required to maintain the hypertension and progressive renal injury characteristic of this model. Nevertheless, subsequent studies have shown that the renoprotective effects of ACEI and AT$_1$RA treatment are associated with a reduction in intrarenal AII levels in both the peri-infarct and intact portions of the remnant kidney.[25] In contrast, treatment with the dihydropyridine calcium antagonist, nifedipine, did not reduce proteinuria despite lowering blood pressure to the same levels as the RAS antagonists, and was associated with an increase in intrarenal AII.[25] Thus intrarenal AII appears to play a central role in the pathogenesis of hypertension and renal injury in this model even in the absence of sustained increases in AII levels. Further research is required to fully explain these findings. It could be argued that apparently normal intrarenal AII levels are inappropriately high in the context of the hypertension and extracellular fluid (ECF) volume expansion in these animals or that the average intrarenal AII-levels measured may have failed to detect important local elevations of AII.

Recently attention has focused on the potential role of aldosterone in progressive renal injury. In addition to evidence that aldosterone may exert profibrotic effects in the kidney (see later), recent observations suggest that it may also have important glomerular hemodynamic effects. Previous observations that the deoxycorticosterone–salt model of hypertension is associated with glomerular capillary hypertension prompted detailed studies of microperfused rabbit afferent and efferent arterioles that found dose-dependent constriction of both arterioles in response to nanomolar concentrations of aldosterone, with greater sensitivity observed in efferent arterioles.[26] These effects were not inhibited by spironolactone and were still present with albumin-bound aldosterone, indicating that they may be mediated by specific membrane receptors rather than the intracellular receptors responsible for most of the actions of aldosterone. Interestingly aldosterone may also counteract rabbit afferent arteriolar vasoconstriction via an NO-dependent pathway, an action that would also increase P$_{GC}$.[27,28]

Endothelins

Endothelins are potent vasoconstrictor peptides that act via at least two receptor subtypes, ET$_A$ and ET$_B$. ET receptors have been identified throughout the body and are most abundant in the lungs and kidneys. ET$_A$ receptors are primarily located on vascular smooth muscle cells and mediate vasoconstriction as well as cellular proliferation. ET$_B$ receptors are expressed on vascular endothelial and renal epithelial cells and appear to play a role as clearance receptors as well as mediating endothelium–dependent vasodilation via NO.[29–31] Renal production of endothelins is increased after 5/6 nephrectomy, raising the possibility that they may also contribute to the observed glomerular hemodynamic adaptations.[32,33] Acute and chronic infusion of endothelin elicits dose-dependent reductions in RPF and GFR in normal rats.[34–37] Despite some differences that were likely due to differences in experimental conditions and endothelin dose, most studies have reported greater increases in efferent than afferent arteriolar resistance resulting in an increase in P$_{GC}$.

The ultrafiltration coefficient (K$_f$) was significantly reduced and thus SNGFR was unchanged or was decreased.[38–41] On the other hand, blockade of endogenous endothelin actions in normal rats results in a large fall in P$_{GC}$ due mainly to a rise in afferent arteriolar resistance indicating that endogenous endothelin causes tonic dilation of the afferent arteriole via ET$_B$ receptors in normal rats.[42] The potential interaction between endothelins and other vasoactive molecules is illustrated by observations that chronic infusion of AII results in increased production of endothelin[43] and that endothelin-1 transgenic mice are not hypertensive but evidence induction of inducible nitric oxide synthase (iNOS) resulting in increased NO production as a probable counter-regulatory mechanism to maintain normal blood pressure.[44] Furthermore some of the glomerular hemodynamic effects of endothelin appear to be modulated by prostaglandins.[41] Detailed micropuncture studies to elucidate the role of endothelins in remnant kidney hemodynamics have not yet been published. These studies should be facilitated by the ongoing development of specific ET$_A$ and ET$_B$ receptor antagonists.

Natriuretic Peptides

Atrial natriuretic peptide (ANP) and other structurally related natriuretic peptides (NP), mediate, in large part, the functional adaptations in tubular sodium reabsorption that maintain sodium excretion in 5/6 nephrectomized rats[45] but also exert important hemodynamic effects. Circulating ANP levels are elevated in 5/6 nephrectomized rats and acute administration of a NP antagonist elicited profound decreases in GFR and RPF in 5/6 nephrectomized rats on high salt (but not low salt diet), indicating that NP play an important role in the observed hemodynamic responses to 5/6 nephrectomy.[46] Further insights into the renal hemodynamic effects of NP were gained from observations in normal rats infused with a synthetic ANP. Whole kidney and single nephron GFR increased by approximately 20% due entirely to a rise P$_{GC}$, resulting from significant afferent arteriolar dilatation and efferent arteriolar constriction.[47] In the experiments discussed earlier, some residual elevation in remnant kidney GFR appeared to persist even after the NP system was suppressed by sodium restriction or a NP receptor antagonist, suggesting that factors other than NP make contributions to glomerular hyperfiltration following renal mass ablation. The potential interaction between NP and other vasoactive molecules is illustrated by the observation that ANP infusion in normal rats induced an increase in renal nitric oxide synthase activity.[48]

Eicosanoids

Eicosanoids, another family of potent vasoactive molecules present in abundance in the kidney, may also play a role in mediating glomerular hyperfiltration. Urinary excretion per nephron of both vasodilator and vasoconstrictor prostaglandins is increased in rats and rabbits after renal mass ablation.[49–51] Infusion of PGE$_2$, PGI$_2$, or 6-keto PGE$_1$ into the renal artery elicits significant renal vasodilatation.[52] Whereas acute inhibition of prostaglandin synthesis by infusion of the cyclooxygenase (COX) inhibitor, indomethacin, had no effect on GFR or glomerular hemodynamics in normal rats, indomethacin lowered both SNGFR and Q$_A$ after 3/4 or 5/6 nephrectomy.[49,50] On the other hand, chronic treatment with a selective COX-2 inhibitor attenuated the systemic and glomerular hypertension observed in 5/6 nephrectomized rats but had no effect on GFR.[53] The relative effects of prostaglandin synthesis inhibitors on afferent and efferent arterioles may vary with time post nephrectomy. Afferent arteriolar constriction was the predominant finding reported at 24 hours post surgery, whereas constriction of both afferent and efferent arterioles was observed at 3 to 4 weeks.[49,50] Some contribution of thromboxanes to glomerular hemodynamic adjustments after 5/6 nephrectomized rats is suggested by the increase in GFR seen after acute infusion of a selective thromboxane synthesis inhibitor.[51] Thus different eicosanoids appear to exert opposite effects but the general impression is that the combined effects of vasodilator prostaglandins outweigh those of the vasoconstrictors. This interaction is illustrated by the observation that perfusion of isolated glomeruli with bradykinin resulted in vasodilation of the efferent arteriole that was completely blocked by a indomethacin but that this blockade was reversed by a specific antagonist of 20-hydroxyeicosatetraenoic acid (20-HETE), a vasocontrictor eicosanoid, indicating that the glomerulus produced both vasodilator and vasoconstrictor eicosanoids.[54]

Nitric Oxide

The extremely short half-life of nitric oxide (NO) precludes direct measurement of NO levels or administration of exogenous NO in experimental models. The actions of NO have thus been inferred from experiments with inhibitors of nitric oxide synthase (NOS). Intravenous infusion of NOS inhibitors results in systemic and renal vasoconstriction as well as a reduction in GFR in normal rats.[55,56] Thus, NO appears to exert a tonic effect on the physiological maintenance of systemic blood pressure and renal perfusion under resting conditions. It is unclear, however, whether NO plays a specific role in the adaptive hemodynamic changes that follow renal mass ablation. Indeed, renal expression of nitric oxide synthase and renal NO generation are reduced in 5/6 nephrectomized rats, whereas systemic production of NO is increased.[57,58] Mean arterial pressure and renal vascular resistance increased whereas RBF and GFR decreased to a similar extent after acute infusion of an endothelial NOS inhibitor, NG-monomethyl-L-arginine (L-NMMA), irrespective of whether given to normal rats or 3 to 4 weeks after unilateral or 5/6 nephrectomy.[56] Chronic NOS inhibition with L-NAME produced elevations in systemic blood pressure and P_{GC} in 5/6 nephrectomized rats without affecting GFR[59] whereas chronic treatment with aminoguanidine, an inhibitor of inducible NOS, had no effect on GFR, RPF, or P_{GC}.[58] On the other hand, renal NOS expression and activity are increased early after unilateral nephrectomy and pretreatment of rats with a subpressor dose of nitro-L-arginine methyl ester (L-NAME) prevents the early increase in RBF and decrease in renal vascular resistance usually observed after unilateral nephrectomy.[60,61] It therefore appears that NO plays a role in early hemodynamic adaptations to nephron loss resulting in an increase in RBF but in the longer term NO retains a tonic influence on systemic and renal hemodynamics without being a specific determinant of the adaptive changes in glomerular hemodynamics.

Bradykinin

Bradykinin is a potent vasodilatory peptide that is elevated in the remnant kidney[21] and may therefore contribute to hemodynamic adaptations after nephron loss. Acute and chronic infusion of bradykinin results in increased RPF but has no effect on GFR.[62,63] Micropuncture studies in intact animals are lacking but studies of isolated perfused afferent arterioles have shown that bradykinin induces a biphasic response with vasodilation at low concentrations and vasconstriction at higher concentrations. Both effects appear to be mediated by products of COX.[64] Similar experiments with efferent arterioles found dose-dependent vasodilation (no biphasic response) that was dependent on cytochrome P450 metabolites but independent of COX products or NO.[65] When glomeruli were perfused with bradykinin, vasodilation of efferent arterioles was again observed but was inhibited by a COX inhibitor indicating that bradykinin induces glomerular production of COX metabolites (prostaglandins) that also contribute to efferent arteriolar dilation.[54] Further

studies are required to elucidate the role of bradykinin after nephron loss.

Adjustments in Renal Autoregulatory Mechanisms

After extensive renal mass ablation, there is a marked readjustment of the autoregulatory mechanisms that control RPF and GFR.[66,67] The role of myogenic mechanisms is uncertain but detailed studies of afferent arteriolar myogenic responses suggest that the primary role of the myogenic response is to protect the glomerulus from elevations in systolic blood pressure.[68] The tubuloglomerular feedback system is reset after renal mass ablation to permit and sustain the elevations in SNGFR and P_{GC} described earlier.[69,70] Resetting appears to occur as early as 20 minutes after unilateral nephrectomy,[71] in proportion to the extent of renal ablation. The adjustments observed after uninephrectomy are of lesser magnitudes than those seen after 5/6 nephrectomy.[69]

Interaction of Multiple Factors

As is readily appreciated from the earlier discussion, the adjustments in glomerular hemodynamics seen after renal mass ablation represent the net effect of several endogenous vasoactive factors. Natriuretic peptides and vasodilator prostaglandins dilate the preglomerular vessels whereas bradykinin dilates both afferent and efferent arterioles. On the other hand AII, vasoconstrictor prostaglandins, and possibly endothelins constrict both afferent and efferent arterioles with a greater effect on the latter. A net fall in preglomerular vascular resistance is observed and efferent arteriolar resistance decreases to a lesser extent. Together with transmission of a greater proportion of the raised systemic blood pressure to the glomerular capillary network, these alterations in microvascular resistances result in the observed elevations in Q_A, P_{GC}, ΔP, and SNGFR (Table 25–1). The importance of multiple vasoactive factors is illustrated by the observation that treatment of 5/6 nephrectomized rats with omapatrilat, an inhibitor of both angiotensin-converting enzyme and neutral endopeptidase that results in reduced AII production as well as increased NP and bradykinin levels, lowered P_{GC} more than angiotensin-converting enzyme inhibition alone.[72] The complexity of factors involved is further illustrated by observations that other molecules involved in the modulation of progressive renal injury may exert hemodynamic effects by influencing the mediators discussed earlier. Acute infusion of hepatocyte growth factor (HGF) has been shown to induce a decline in blood pressure and GFR, an effect that is mediated by a short-term increase in endothelin-1 production.[73] In isolated perfused preparations, platelet-activating factor (PAF) at picomolar concentrations has been shown to induce glomerular production of NO, resulting in dilation of preconstricted efferent arterioles whereas at nanomolar concentrations, PAF constricts efferent arterioles through local release of COX metabolites.[74] The potential role of other recently identified vasoactive molecules such as urotensin II remains to be elucidated.[75]

Renal Hypertrophic Responses to Nephron Loss

The notion that a single kidney enlarges to compensate for the loss of its partner has been entertained since antiquity. Aristotle (384–322 BC) noted that a single kidney was able to sustain life in animals, and that such kidneys were enlarged. In preparation for the first human nephrectomy in 1869 a German surgeon, Gustav Simon, uninephrectomized dogs and noted a 1.5-fold increase in the size of the remaining kidney at 20 days.[76] Compensatory renal hypertrophy has been studied in a variety of species including toads, mice, rats, guinea-pigs, rabbits, cats, dogs, pigs, and baboons. The

CH 25

TABLE 25–1	Hemodynamic Effects of Vasoactive Molecules Mediating Glomerular Hemodynamic Adaptations after Partial Renal Mass Ablation							
	R_A	R_E	P_{GC}	Q_A	K_f	SNGFR	RPF	GFR
Angiotensin II[5,13–19]	↑	↑↑	↑	↓	↓↔	↓↔	↓	↔
Aldosterone[26–28]	↑	↑↑	↑	?	?	?	?	?
Endothelins[34–42]	↑↔	↑	↑↔	↓	↓↔	↓↔	↓	↓↔
Natriuretic peptides[46,47]	↓	↑ (?)	↑	↔	↔	↑	↑↔	↑
Prostaglandins[49–54]	↓	↓	↔	↑	↑	↑	↑	↑
Bradykinin[62–65]	↓↑	↓	?	?	?	?	↑	↔
Observed changes after partial renal ablation[6,7]	↓↓	↓	↑	↑	↑↓	↑	—	↓

P_{GC}, glomerular capillary hydraulic pressure; Q_A, glomerular plasma flow rate; K_f, glomerular ultrafiltration coefficient; SNGFR, single nephron GFR; RPF, renal plasma flow; GFR, glomerular filtration rate.

majority of experimental work has been conducted on rodents subjected to uninephrectomy, but hypertrophic responses have also been studied in response to unilateral ureteric obstruction or after nephrotoxin administration.[77]

Whole-Kidney Hypertrophic Responses

Among the earliest responses to unilateral nephrectomy are biochemical changes that precede cell growth. Increased incorporation of choline, a precursor of cell membrane phospholipid, has been detected as early as 5 minutes and increased choline kinase activity, at 2 hours after nephrectomy. Activity of ornithine decarboxylase, the enzyme catalyzing the first step of polyamine synthesis, is elevated at 45 to 120 minutes and polyamine levels peak at 1 to 2 days post nephrectomy. Early alterations in mRNA metabolism have also been observed. Although there is no change in the half-life or cytoplasmic distribution of mRNA, a near 25% increase in the fraction of newly synthesized poly(A)-deficient mRNA occurs within 1 hour of uninephrectomy and total RNA synthesis in the kidney increases by 25% to 100% relative to that in the liver. Ribosomal RNA synthesis is increased by 40% to 50% at 6 hours. The rate of protein synthesis is increased at 2 hours and is nearly doubled at 3 hours. Data on cyclic nucleotide levels, which are thought to affect cell growth and proliferation, are conflicting. Some studies report elevated levels of cGMP in the remaining kidney as early as 10 minutes after surgery, whereas others have found no consistent changes in cAMP or cGMP levels.[77] Genome-wide analysis of gene expression using cDNA microarrays in remaining rat kidneys up to 72 hours after uninephrectomy has revealed the dominant response to be suppression of genes responsible for inhibition of growth and apoptosis.[78]

Early biochemical changes are followed by a period of rapid growth. DNA synthesis is increased at 24 hours and increased numbers of mitotic figures are evident at 28 to 36 hours. Both reach a maximum increase of 5-fold to 10-fold at 40 to 72 hours. In rats, kidney weight is increased at 48 to 72 hours after uninephrectomy and achieves a 30% to 40% gain at 2 to 3 weeks (Fig. 25–1).[61,77] As nephron number is fixed shortly before birth in most species, this gain in kidney weight is attributable to increased nephron size. Growth is thought to occur largely through cell hypertrophy, accounting for 80% of the increase in renal mass seen in adult rats and, to a lesser extent, through hyperplasia. Hypertrophy is achieved largely through regulation of the G1 cell cycle kinase (cell cycle-dependent mechanism).[79] Renal mass continues to rise for 1 to 2 months until a 40% to 50% increase is achieved. The degree of compensatory growth is a function of the extent of renal ablation. Uninephrectomy has been shown to provoke an 81% increase of residual renal mass at 4 weeks compared

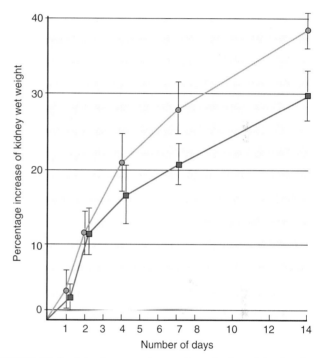

FIGURE 25–1 Rate of compensatory renal growth after unilateral nephrectomy (circles) and ureter ligation (squares). (Reproduced with permission from Dicker SE, Shirley DG: Compensatory hypertrophy of the contralateral kidney after unilateral ureteral ligation. J Physiol (Lond) 220:199–210, 1972.)

to an increase of 168% after 70% renal ablation. Normal controls gained 31% in kidney weight over the same period. Age diminishes renal hypertrophic responses: after uninephrectomy, greater increases in kidney weight and more extensive hyperplasia was observed in 5-day-old versus 55-day-old rats and aging rats exhibited gains in kidney weight of only one third to three quarters of those seen in younger controls.[77]

In humans, assessment of renal hypertrophy after nephrectomy is dependent on radiological studies. Ultrasound studies have reported increases of 19% to 100% in kidney volume[80] and in computed tomography studies, an increase of 30% to 53% in renal cross-sectional area.[81,82] The relatively small number of subjects included, wide variation in the time intervals between nephrectomy and assessment of renal size, and differing indications for nephrectomy make interpretation of these results difficult.

The principal morphometric change observed in glomeruli after uninephrectomy is an increase in volume. Glomerular enlargement appears to parallel whole-kidney growth and has been detected as early as 4 days after surgery.[83] The degree of enlargement of superficial and juxtamedullary glomeruli is similar. Proportionally similar increases in number and size of all cell types occur, with preservation of the relative volumes of different glomerular cells.[77] There is consensus that glomerular capillaries increase in length and number (i. e., more branching) but most studies show that diameter or cross-sectional surface area of the glomerular capillaries remains constant or increases only minimally.[84,85] Transplantation of hypertrophied kidneys into uninephrectomized recipients has demonstrated regression of glomerular hypertrophy within 3 weeks, yet the increase in capillary length was maintained.[85]

Glomerular hypertrophy, as evidenced by elevated RNA/DNA and protein/DNA ratios as well as by increased glomerular volume (V_G) on electron microscopy, has been detected at 2 days after 5/6 nephrectomy.[86] The initial increase in V_G was due, almost entirely, to increases in visceral epithelial cell volume, whereas at 14 days the increase in V_G was largely accounted for by mesangial matrix expansion. Although several studies report glomerular capillary lengthening after 5/6 nephrectomy, few have detected any increase in cross-sectional area or diameter of the glomerular capillaries.[87-90] These observations should, however, be considered in the light of important technical considerations. *In vitro* perfusion of isolated glomeruli demonstrates that V_G increases as perfusion pressure is raised through physiological and pathophysiological ranges. Moreover, glomerular capillary "compliance" in these studies was a function of the baseline V_G and glomeruli obtained from remnant kidneys post 5/6 nephrectomy had a higher compliance than those from control animals.[91] These findings have two important implications. First, although glomerular pressures are only minimally elevated after uninephrectomy, the glomerular capillary hypertension associated with more extensive renal ablation is likely to contribute significantly to the increase in V_G. Second, estimates of V_G in tissues that have not been perfusion-fixed at the appropriate blood pressure should be interpreted with caution. Direct comparison of V_G in perfusion-fixed versus immersion-fixed kidney from the same rats yielded estimates of V_G in immersion-fixed samples that were 61% lower than those from perfusion-fixed kidneys.[92]

Mechanisms of Renal Hypertrophy

Despite more than a century of research that has identified a large number of mediators or modulators of renal hypertrophy, the identities of the specific factors that regulate hypertrophy and the stimuli to which these factors respond remain elusive. Renal innervation does not appear to play a role as kidneys transplanted into bilaterally nephrectomized rats exhibit the same degree of hypertrophy after 3 weeks as kidneys remaining after uninephrectomy.[93] The absence of any reduction in renal hypertrophy when rats are treated with an ACEI after uninephrectomy indicates that the renin-angiotensin system also does not play a major role.[94] Several hypotheses have been advanced to account for the observed changes that are associated with renal hypertrophy and have been discussed in detail in other publications[76,77] but are summarized below. Currently, however, none is able to explain satisfactorily all of the reported observations.

Solute Load

The notion that hypertrophy after uninephrectomy is stimulated by the need for the remaining kidney to excrete larger amounts of metabolic waste products, necessitating more

excretory "work", was proposed by Sacerdotti in 1896. Subsequently, it became apparent that urea excretion is largely a function of glomerular filtration, whereas the main energy-requiring function of the renal tubules is reabsorption of filtered electrolytes (principally sodium) and water. The hypothesis was therefore modified to view hypertrophy as a response to the increased demand for water and solute reclamation imposed by increased SNGFR (solute load hypothesis). Several lines of evidence support the concepts underlying the "solute load hypothesis". After uninephrectomy RBF increased by 8% in the remaining kidney and preceded hypertrophy but treatment with a subpressor dose of the NOS inhibitor L-NAME prevented the rise in RBF and substantially attenuated increases in renal weight as well as glomerular and proximal tubule area at 7 days post nephrectomy.[61] In the remnant kidney, proximal tubule sodium absorption increases in parallel with GFR (glomerulotubular balance) and tubules continue to display enhanced fluid reabsorption *in vitro*, implying that the adaptive changes are intrinsic to the tubular epithelial cells. In chronic glomerulonephritis, a lesion characterized by marked heterogeneity in SNGFR, there is preservation of the SNGFR to proximal fluid reabsorption ratio and a close correlation between glomerular and proximal tubule hypertrophy. Moreover, sustained increases in GFR in the absence of renal mass ablation result in renal hypertrophy in some conditions, including pregnancy (in some but not all studies) and diabetes mellitus.[76]

On the other hand, experimental maneuvers dissociating renal solute load from hypertrophy appear to contradict the solute load hypothesis. Total diversion of urine from one kidney into the peritoneum by ureteroperitoneostomy is associated with an increase in GFR in the contralateral kidney of similar magnitude to that seen after uninephrectomy, but no increase in renal mass or mitotic activity. In another example, potassium depletion results in renal hypertrophy without any increase in GFR. Moreover, the findings that some of the early biochemical changes associated with hypertrophy precede increases in glomerular filtration or sodium reabsorption, argue against a causal association of hypertrophy and increased solute load. It is, however, possible to offer alternative explanations for each of the observations discussed earlier. Despite these conflicting data, there is nevertheless considerable evidence of an association between glomerular filtration rate and proximal tubule hypertrophy that may play a role in stimulating renal growth in the remnant kidney.[76]

Renotropic Factors

Failure of the "solute load hypothesis" to explain all of the experimental data has led others to propose instead that the primary stimulus for renal hypertrophy is a change in renal mass and that renal growth is under the control of specific growth and/or inhibitory factors. Evidence in support of this theory is derived from three types of experiment. In the first, a stable connection is established between the extracellular space and microcirculation of two animals (parabiosis) and the effects of renal mass ablation in one animal are assessed in the intact kidneys of its partner. Despite some inconsistencies due to variations in methodology these experiments generally found that uninephrectomy in one animal resulted in hypertrophy of the contralateral kidney and, to a lesser extent, of both kidneys of the parabiotic partner. Bilateral nephrectomy in one partner or triple nephrectomy produced incremental degrees of hypertrophy in the remaining kidney(s). Furthermore, the hypertrophy was rapidly reversed following cessation of cross circulation.[76]

A second strategy has been to inject serum or plasma from uninephrectomized animals into intact subjects and then assess renal hypertrophy by radiolabeled thymidine uptake or mitotic count. Although studies using single small intraperitoneal or subcutaneous doses were negative, the administration of repeated, large doses by intraperitoneal or intravenous routes elicited renal hypertrophy in most.[76]

The data that most consistently support the existence of a renotropic factor are derived from *in vitro* experiments in which renal tissues are incubated in the presence or absence of plasma or serum from rats subjected to renal mass ablation. Evidence for hypertrophy has generally been assessed by incorporation of radiolabelled thymidine or uridine into DNA or RNA, respectively. In general these experiments have shown increased uptake of radiolabeled nucleotides after incubation with serum from uninephrectomized animals. This effect appears to organ specific, but not species specific. That a tissue factor produced by kidneys and up-regulated after nephrectomy may be required for the activity of a circulating "renotropin", is suggested by experiments in which kidney extract from rats taken 20 hours after uninephrectomy, in the presence of normal rat serum, was found to stimulate ^{3}H thymidine incorporation in normal renal cortex but addition of the same extract in the absence of the serum tended to depress ^{3}H thymidine uptake. Serum taken from bilaterally nephrectomized animals lacks renotropic effects but these can be restored after dialysis of the serum, suggesting the presence of renotropin inhibitory factors that accumulate in the absence of renal function. Although the specific identity of renotropin remains elusive, several lines of evidence suggest that it is a small protein. Retention of activity after ultrafiltration, dialysis and removal of albumin from serum implies that renotropin is a molecule of 12 kDa to 25 kDa with no significant binding to albumin.[76,77]

Several hypotheses have been advanced to reconcile the earlier observed effects and operation of a putative renotropic system. It has variously been proposed that (1) renotropin is a circulating substance normally catabolized or excreted by the kidneys, (2) renal growth is regulated by a specific renotropin-producing tissue that is inhibited by a factor produced by normal kidneys, (3) renal growth is tonically inhibited by a substance produced by normal kidneys, a decrease in the levels of which induces an enzyme in the renal cortex that cleaves a circulating precursor of renotropin to produce the active molecule.[76,77]

Endocrine Effects

Several of the major endocrine systems influence renal growth but each lacks selective effects on the kidney. There is little evidence that any of these systems represent the specific mediators of compensatory renal hypertrophy. Whereas early experiments suggested that hypophysectomy inhibits compensatory hypertrophy after uninephrectomy, later studies that controlled for the reduction in renal mass that usually accompanies hypopituitarism, found a degree of hypertrophy comparable to that seen in normal rats. Nevertheless, specific renotropic activity has been identified in a sub-fraction of ovine pituitary extract associated with a lutropin-like substance.[76,77] Uninephrectomy is accompanied by a transient increase in the pulsatile release of growth hormone (GH) in male but not female rats suggesting a role for this hormone in the early phase of hypertrophy in males.[95] When the increase in GH was prevented by administration of an antagonist to GH-releasing factor or the effects of GH are blocked by a GH-receptor blocker, renal hypertrophy is significantly attenuated.[96,97] Adrenal hormones appear to play little role in renal hypertrophy. Adrenalectomy does not inhibit compensatory growth after uninephrectomy. Whereas renal weight relative to body weight is reduced in hypothyroidism and increased by excess thyroid hormone, compensatory hypertrophy still occurs in thyroidectomized rats. Progesterone and estradiol in excess or ovariectomy have little effect on renal weight, but testosterone appears to play a role, as evidenced by a fall in kidney/body weight after orchidectomy and an increase in kidney weight with excess testosterone. Whereas orchidectomy does not inhibit hypertrophy after uninephrectomy, exogenous testosterone did increase the degree of hypertrophy observed, in some, but not all studies.[76,77]

Growth Factors

Of the numerous growth factors and their receptors that have been localized in the kidney, at least four are associated with renal hypertrophy.[98,99] Several lines of evidence suggest a role for insulin-like growth factor-I (IGF-1). Renal IGF-1 levels were elevated at 1 to 5 days after uninephrectomy and started to decline within days in some[100,101] but not all studies.[102] In one study the level of renal IGF-1 expression was significantly correlated with the extent of renal mass ablation.[103] On the other hand, Shohat and colleagues found an increase in serum IGF-1 levels only at 10 days post nephrectomy, which was still present on day 60.[100] That IGF-1 may be induced independent of GH in the setting of renal hypertrophy is illustrated by preservation of the increase in renal IGF-1 in hypophysectomized[104] and GH-deficient rats.[105] Other molecules related to IGF function are also up-regulated: renal IGF-1 receptor gene expression was increased twofold to fourfold in female rats after uninephrectomy[95]; IGF-1 binding protein mRNA was up-regulated in the remnant kidney at 2 weeks after 5/6 nephrectomy[106]; analysis of the genome-wide transcriptional response to unilateral nephrectomy identified IGF-2 binding protein was one of the few activated genes.[78] Further evidence suggests that IGF-1 may in turn promote production of vascular endothelial growth factor (VEGF), suggesting that VEGF may be a down-stream mediator of IGF-1 effects, at least in the pathogenesis of diabetic retinopathy.[107] That VEGF is important for compensatory renal hypertrophy is confirmed by the observation that treatment of mice with VEGF antibodies after uninephrectomy completely prevented glomerular hypertrophy and inhibited renal growth at 7 days.[101] Epidermal growth factor (EGF) in the remaining kidney is increased on day 1 in mice[108] and by day 5 in rats.[109] In addition, EGF has been shown to induce IGF-I mRNA production in collecting duct cells in vitro, suggesting the existence of a local paracrine system.[110] Increased mRNA levels for both hepatocyte growth factor (HGF) and its receptor, c-met, have been demonstrated in the remaining kidney as early as 6 hours after uninephrectomy.[111,112] In another study the rise in HGF message was found to be non-specific, occurring in both liver and kidney, and also in sham-operated rats, whereas the increase in mRNA for c-met was specific for the outer renal medulla.[113] Despite these associations, the timing of the changes in growth factor levels remains unclear. Whereas some investigators report early increases,[108,114] several others report changes only at time points when significant hypertrophy is already present, thus failing to provide convincing evidence that they represent the proximal effectors in a renotropic system.[100,109]

Failure to identify a specific "renotropin" to date has led some to suggest instead that renal hypertrophy occurs as a result of increased sensitivity of renal cells to prevailing levels of growth promoting factors. This enhanced sensitivity, it is argued, may result from changes in the intracellular environment brought about by responses to increased glomerular filtration such as the increase in Na^+/H^+ exchange seen in proximal tubule cells after renal mass reduction.[76] As can readily be appreciated from the earlier discussion, many factors have been associated with compensatory renal hypertrophy but a unifying hypothesis that adequately accounts for them all remains elusive. It is likely that multiple pathways are involved. Some factors appear to control normal renal growth and may have a permissive or modulating role in compensatory hypertrophy, whereas others act as specific mediators of the dynamic processes that follow a reduction in renal mass.

ADAPTATION OF SPECIFIC TUBULE FUNCTIONS IN RESPONSE TO NEPHRON LOSS

As noted earlier, the bulk of the increase in renal mass following uninephrectomy is due to hypertrophy of the proximal nephron. The more distal nephron segments also enlarge, but to a lesser extent. In uninephrectomized rats, the proximal convoluted tubule is increased on average by 17% in luminal diameter and 35% in length, yielding a 96% increase in total volume; the distal convoluted tubule is enlarged by 12% in luminal diameter and 17% in length, yielding a 25% increase in total volume.[115] Maintenance of homeostasis for various solutes in the face of a declining GFR requires highly integrated responses from each tubule segment. Whereas some solutes including creatinine and urea are chiefly cleared by glomerular filtration and therefore rise gradually in plasma with declining GFR, for others, the tubule solute handling adapts so that plasma levels remain constant, virtually until end–stage renal failure is reached (Fig. 25–2).

Adaptation in Proximal Tubule Solute Handling

In renal ablation models, as with the increase in remnant kidney SNGFR, the extent to which proximal tubule enlarges is inversely proportional to the remnant kidney mass. Proximal tubule enlargement is associated with an increase in proximal fluid reabsorption. In studies of both animals and humans with reduced renal mass, the increase in proximal fluid reabsorption observed was found to be proportional

both to the increase in remnant kidney GFR and the increase in tubular volume.[116] Similarly, in proximal tubules isolated from remnant kidneys, the observed increase in transtubular fluid flux was proportional to the increases in size and protein content of the tubule epithelial cells.[117,118] Folding of the basolateral membrane of the proximal tubule epithelium was also found to increase, resulting in augmentation of the basolateral surface area, in proportion to the increase in cell volume.[119] This increase in surface area was accompanied by an increase in activity of Na-K-ATPase, the membrane pump that generates the main driving force for proximal tubule solute transport.[119]

Increases in proximal tubule size and surface area are not, however, the only determinants of increased transport activity in this nephron segment. Fluid reabsorption in isolated proximal tubule segments increases within 24 hours of nephrectomy (i.e., when GFR is already increasing, but well before significant hypertrophy occurs), implying an intrinsic tubular epithelial cell adaptation to nephron loss.[120] This observation also raises the possibility that the increases in proximal fluid reabsorption occurring in response to nephron loss are driven by the increase in SNGFR and further implies that the increased reabsorptive load could stimulate hypertrophy.[76,77] As solute reclamation is an energy-requiring process, it is not surprising that in uninephrectomized rabbits, the increase in proximal tubule volume was accompanied by a proportional increase in mitochondrial volume.[121] The observation that the increase in renal mass is outstripped by the rise in GFR in models of progressive nephron loss implies that renal energy consumption per unit of remnant renal mass increases as renal function declines.[115]

The rise in SNGFR that occurs in the remnant kidney presents increased loads of glucose, amino acids, and other solutes that would normally be reabsorbed entirely in the proximal tubule, provided the maximal transport capacity was not exceeded. Maximal proximal tubular reabsorptive capacities for glucose and amino acids have been shown to increase in proportion to tubule mass after partial renal ablation.[122] Some metabolic functions of proximal tubules are also augmented in the remnant kidney, so as to maintain adequate plasma levels of important metabolites including citrulline, arginine, and serine.[123] Other proximal tubule functions, however, are not adjusted in proportion to proximal tubule mass: fractional phosphate reabsorption is decreased whereas ammoniagenesis increases.[122,124,125] These adaptations are appropriate homeostatic responses that permit continued excretion of daily phosphate and acid loads, respectively, as the number of functioning nephrons declines.

Loop of Henle and Distal Nephron

Although there is little change in cross-sectional area in the thick ascending limb of the loop of Henle, fluid reabsorption in this segment also increases in proportion to SNGFR.[115] In contrast, both the distal tubule and the cortical collecting duct enlarge in response to nephron loss.[115] Unlike the proximal tubule, however, where the increased reabsorptive capacity is chiefly due to increased tubule dimensions, the increased reabsorptive capacity observed in the distal segments is far greater than would be expected for the corresponding increase in tubule volume, implying a major adaptive increase in active solute transport.[115] Levels of mRNA for the Na+/myo-inositol cotransporter (SMIT) and Na+/Cl-/betaine-gamma-amino-n-butyric acid transporter (BGT-1) are increased in the cortex and outer medulla of remnant kidneys from 5/6 nephrectomized rats.[126] Likewise, potassium secretion by the distal nephron increases in compensation for nephron loss, facilitated by an increased basolateral surface area of cortical collecting duct principal cells and an increase in Na-K-ATPase activity.[127,128]

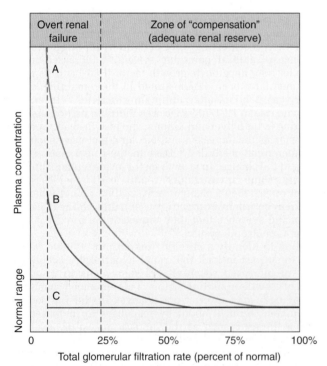

FIGURE 25-2 Representative patterns of adaptation for different types of solutes in body fluids in chronic renal failure. Pattern A: rise in serum concentration with each permanent reduction in GFR (e.g., creatinine); Pattern B: rise in serum concentration only after GFR falls below a critical value due to adaptive increases in tubular secretion (e.g., phosphate); Pattern C: serum concentration remains normal through almost entire period of progression of renal failure (e.g., sodium). (Modified from Bricker NS, Fine L: In Brenner BM, Rector FC (eds): The Kidney, 2nd ed. Philadelphia, WB Saunders, 1981.)

Glomerulotubular Balance

Micropuncture studies have confirmed that proximal fluid reabsorption remains proportional to glomerular filtration over a wide range of SNGFR in both glomerular and tubulointerstitial diseases.[129,130] This glomerulotubular balance is critical to the physiological integrity of remnant nephron function and hence extracellular fluid homeostasis. Compensatory increases in SNGFR in surviving nephrons must be accompanied by similar increases in proximal tubular solute and water reabsorption, so as to avoid overwhelming the distal nephron transport capacity and disrupting its regulation of the volume and composition of the final urine. Conversely, reductions in SNGFR in damaged nephrons must be matched by similar reductions in proximal fluid reabsorption so as to maintain adequate solute and water delivery to the distal tubule, again permitting excretion of urine of appropriate volume and composition.

Glomerulotubular balance is maintained as follows: the degree of single nephron hyperfiltration occurring as a consequence of nephron loss determines the passive Starling forces operating in the post-glomerular microcirculation, which in turn, govern net trans-tubular solute reabsorption.[131] Increases in SNGFR associated with an increased filtration fraction result in elevated post-glomerular capillary protein concentrations, which determine nonlinear increases in oncotic pressure, Π_E, the major determinant of peritubular capillary reabsorptive force (P_r). Reductions in SNGFR, in contrast, result in a lowered peritubular oncotic pressure, thereby reducing P_r. Thus, SNGFR and proximal fluid reabsorption remain in direct proportion to one another. Prevention of hyperfiltration by dietary protein restriction has been shown to abrogate the increase in proximal fluid reabsorption in the remnant kidney, underscoring the dependence of proximal tubular function on the level of glomerular filtration.[131] In the remnant kidney of rats subjected to extensive renal mass ablation, absolute fluid reabsorption was found to be markedly increased in proximal portions of both superficial and juxtamedullary nephrons, yet fluid delivery to the more distal segments of the nephron was also somewhat increased.[132] In the setting of nephron loss, sodium reabsorption by the loop of Henle has been shown to remain proportional to sodium delivery to that segment, indicating preservation of tubulo-tubular balance, a mechanism that maintains appropriate distal solute and water delivery in the face of progressive nephron loss. Until the adaptive capacities of these mechanisms are finally exhausted, the operation of glomerulotubular balance and tubulotubular balance ensures that the distal tubule mechanisms that determine final urine composition are not overwhelmed by unregulated distal delivery of water and solute.[133] In keeping with these physiological observations, morphologic studies have shown that within the same kidney, nephrons associated with damaged glomeruli are usually atrophic and presumably hypofunctioning, whereas those associated with healthier glomeruli are usually hypertrophic and hyperfunctioning.[134]

In order to maintain homeostasis in the face of continued food and water intake, specific mechanisms that enhance single nephron water and solute excretion must come into play, in addition to the adjustments in SNGFR and tubular reabsorption that occur in response to nephron loss. These mechanisms are not unique to the setting of renal insufficiency, however, and are also engaged when the normal kidney is challenged to excrete extraordinary loads of solute and water. In general, the adaptive physiology of the chronically injured kidney is adequate to preserve homeostasis for many solutes under baseline conditions, but the adaptive capacity may easily become overwhelmed by fluctuations in fluid intake and especially by increases in electrolyte and acid loads. Patients with chronic renal failure are therefore susceptible to develop volume overload, volume loss, hyperkalemia, and acidosis when the excretory capacity of the kidney is challenged by relatively modest increases in excretory demands.

Sodium Excretion and Extracellular Fluid Volume Regulation

In chronic renal failure, ECF volume is often maintained very close to normal until end-stage is reached.[135] This remarkable feat is accomplished by an increase in fractional sodium excretion (FE_Na) in inverse proportion to the decline in GFR.[136] Many studies have been carried out in an attempt to identify which nephron segments are responsible for the decrease in sodium reabsorption: micropuncture studies in uninephrectomized rats have shown that tubule fluid transit times, as well as the half-time for reabsorption of a stationary saline droplet in the proximal tubule lumen, were not different from controls[115]; in remnant kidneys of rats receiving high, normal, or low sodium diets, *absolute* sodium reabsorption was found to increase, but *fractional* sodium and fluid reabsorption were found to decrease in all groups[137]; micropuncture studies in dogs and rats have failed to detect significant reductions in fractional proximal tubule fluid and sodium reabsorption[138]; distal sodium delivery was found to be markedly increased in the rat remnant kidney[137]; increased solute transport activity has been demonstrated in distal tubule of uninephrectomized rats[115]; under conditions of hydropenia and salt loading, sodium reabsorption by the medullary collecting duct of the rat remnant kidney was markedly reduced.[139] Taken together, these data suggest that proximal fractional reabsorption remains largely unchanged, and that in the setting of renal insufficiency, adjustments in sodium excretion occur predominantly in the loop and distal nephron segments.[140]

In addition to load-dependent tubular adaptations in sodium handling, sodium excretion is also modulated by hormonal influences. Levels of natriuretic peptides (NP) are elevated in chronic renal failure as a result of reduced clearance and in response to alterations in sodium and volume status.[46,141] In rats with extensive renal mass ablation, plasma atrial natriuretic peptide (ANP) levels may be restored toward normal levels by dietary sodium restriction, but, in response to increases in sodium intake, they rise progressively along with sodium excretion.[142] The notion that ANP plays an important role in mediating adaptive changes in sodium excretion in the setting of renal ablation is confirmed by observations that administration of a NP receptor antagonist reduced both FE_Na and GFR in 5/6 nephrectomized rats receiving either normal or high salt diets, but did not alter these variables in rats fed low salt diets.[143] Significantly, NP not only modulate sodium excretion but may also contribute to the attendant glomerular hyperfiltration, and thereby further exacerbate renal injury (see earlier).

Systemic hypertension has also been proposed by Guyton and associates as a contributor to the increase in FE_Na observed with renal insufficiency.[144] Their hypothesis states that a constant sodium intake in the face of a reduced number of functioning nephrons leads to positive sodium balance as a result of reduced excretory capacity. Positive sodium balance leads to an increase in ECF volume and a rise in systemic blood pressure that, in turn, leads to an increase in FE_Na and re-establishes the steady state. In support of this hypothesis, salt intake has been shown to be critical to the development of hypertension in subtotally nephrectomized dogs[145] and uremic patients have been found to exhibit marked sodium retention when treated with vasodilating antihypertensive agents.[146] On the other hand, a lowered salt intake in 5/6 nephrectomized rats does not prevent the development of systemic hypertension,[89] suggesting that sodium excretion and hypertension are not always interdependent in the setting of extensive renal mass ablation. Sodium conservation, on the other hand, is also impaired with renal insufficiency and, in response to an acute reduction in sodium intake most patients were unable to reduce sodium excretion below 20 to 30 mEq/day.[147] The "salt-losing" tendency associated with CKD appears to be dependent on the salt load per nephron and may therefore be reversible with adequate dietary sodium restriction. Other factors modulating FE_{Na} in the setting of renal insufficiency include changes in sympathetic nervous system activity, aldosterone, prostaglandins, and parathyroid hormone levels.[140,148] Sodium homeostasis and volume regulation are discussed in further detail in Chapters 5 and 12.

Urinary Concentration and Dilution

Extracellular fluid homeostasis is usually well maintained until renal insufficiency is far advanced, when the ability of the kidney to excrete a volume load becomes significantly reduced.[140] Normal generation of solute-free water is about 12 mL per 100 mL of GFR, and is dependent on dilution of tubule fluid in the thick ascending limb, maintenance of low water permeability in the distal nephron segments in the absence of antidiuretic hormone (ADH), and decreased hypertonicity of the medullary interstitium during water diuresis. Although the single nephron capacity to excrete free water per milliliter of GFR is not reduced in patients with advanced renal disease,[149] the absolute reduction in GFR reduces the overall capacity of the kidney to excrete a water load. Patients with chronic renal failure therefore cannot adequately dilute their urine, and are prone to water intoxication and hyponatremia. Hypothetically, in addition to excretion of the equivalent of 2 L of "isotonic urine" per day (obligatory excretion of 600 mOsm/d), normal kidneys, with a GFR of 150 L/d, can excrete up to 18 L of free water, whereas failing kidneys, with a GFR of 15 L/d, can only excrete about 1.8 L of free water per day. The minimum urinary osmolality achievable by normal kidneys would therefore approach 30 mOsm/L (600 mOsm/20 L) whereas that of diseased kidneys would be 160 mOsm/L (600 mOsm/3.8 L).

Urinary concentration is also impaired in renal insufficiency. Normal urinary concentration requires preservation of the countercurrent mechanism in order to maintain hypertonicity of the medullary interstitium and normal water transport across the distal nephron segments in response to ADH. Maximal urinary osmolality in normal subjects is about 1200 mOsm/L. As GFR decreases, however, maximal urinary osmolality falls, and with a GFR of 15 mL/min is reduced to about 400 mOsm/L.[150] A normal individual can therefore excrete the obligatory daily 600 mOsm in as little as 0.5 L of urine, whereas the patient with a GFR of 15 mL/min can excrete the same load in a minimum of 1.5 L. Part of the defect in urinary concentration observed in renal injury may be attributed to the high solute load imposed per surviving nephron. In patients with chronic renal insufficiency, however, the osmotic effect of urea was shown to be inadequate to account fully for the reduction in maximal urine concentration, indicating that factors other than osmotic diuresis contribute to reduction in urinary concentrating ability in these patients.[150] Furthermore, in patients with chronic primary glomerulonephritis, reduction in urine concentrating capacity was found to correlate significantly with the degree of medullary fibrosis on renal biopsy,[151] suggesting that disruption of the medullary architecture, with the consequent loss of medullary hypertonicity, may result in disproportionate impairment of urinary concentrating ability at any given level of GFR. Consistent with this observation, patients with primary tubulointerstitial injury (e.g., analgesic

nephropathy and sickle cell disease) have markedly impaired urinary concentrating abilities, even early in the course of their illness.[150,152,153] Similarly, in animal experiments, surgical exposure of the renal papilla in intact hydropenic rats was found to lead to reduction in urinary osmolality because of the accompanying alterations in vasa recta flow and ensuing washout of medullary solutes.[154] Interestingly, similar exposure of papillae in rats with remnant kidneys did not affect urinary osmolality, presumably because medullary solute washout had already occurred due to the adaptive responses to nephron loss. Urinary concentration also depends on water reabsorption in the distal nephron segments of the remnant nephron. Reduction in water reabsorption may be the result of several mechanisms in the failing kidney. Defective cyclic AMP-mediated response to ADH may render the cortical collecting duct resistant to the effects of ADH, resulting in increased water delivery to the papillary collecting duct.[155] Urinary osmolality is inversely proportional to fractional water delivery to the papillary collecting duct in 5/6 nephrectomized rats, despite an increase in absolute water reabsorption per functioning collecting tubule when compared with controls.[154] Patients with renal insufficiency are therefore prone to volume depletion in the presence of water deprivation or impaired thirst mechanisms. More commonly, the inability to concentrate urine becomes manifest as nocturia, which develops as renal function deteriorates. Urinary concentrating and diluting mechanisms are discussed in further detail in Chapters 9 and 13.

Potassium Excretion

In order to maintain potassium homeostasis in the face of continued dietary intake and a reduced number of functioning nephrons, potassium excretion per nephron must increase. In both normal and diseased kidneys, almost all of the filtered potassium is reabsorbed in the proximal tubule and loop of Henle. Potassium excretion is therefore determined predominantly by distal secretion,[140] although a reduction in potassium reabsorption by the loop of Henle has been shown to contribute to increased potassium excretion in rats with reduced renal mass.[156] In both normal and partially nephrectomized dogs, urinary potassium excretion was found to correlate directly with serum potassium concentration.[157] Similarly, in intact and uninephrectomized rats, net potassium secretion in the distal convoluted tubule occurred only during potassium infusion, whereas potassium secretion by cortical collecting tubules (CCT) occurred under all conditions, and was greater after uninephrectomy.[158] Other studies have confirmed that the CCT is an important site of potassium secretion in the remnant kidney.[127,139] Secretion of potassium by CCT isolated from remnant kidneys of rabbits fed normal or high potassium diets, was shown to persist in vitro, and to be directly related to the dietary potassium content,[127] indicating an intrinsic tubular adaptation to potassium load. This adaptation was absent in CCT from rabbits in which dietary potassium had been reduced in proportion to the amount of renal mass lost. In addition to variation with dietary potassium load, the increase in potassium secretion by remnant CCT was also found to correlate with plasma aldosterone levels, but not with intracellular potassium concentration or Na-K-ATPase activity.[127] In contrast, however, others have reported an increase in cortical and outer medullary Na-K-ATPase activity in homogenates from rat remnant kidneys that was abrogated when potassium intake was reduced in proportion to the reduction in GFR.[159] Finally, the frequent occurrence of hyperkalemia in patients with chronic renal insufficiency after treatment with an aldosterone antagonist or an ACEI, suggests that "normal" aldosterone levels are required to maintain adequate potassium excretion in this population.[160] In general therefore, the increase in potassium secretion by surviving nephrons appears to be predominantly determined by the rise plasma potassium after potassium ingestion, and by intrinsic tubular adaptation to the increased filtered potassium load.[157,158] In both dogs and patients with chronic renal insufficiency, however, the kaliuretic response to an oral potassium load is attenuated compared to normals despite higher serum potassium levels.[157,161] The eventual, complete excretion of a potassium load, therefore, occurs at the expense of a sustained increase in serum potassium. Control of potassium excretion is discussed further in Chapters 5 and 15.

Acid-Base Regulation

Reduction of GFR in patients with chronic kidney disease is associated with the development of systemic metabolic acidosis, due to a reduction in serum bicarbonate concentration. Normal acid-base balance requires reabsorption of filtered bicarbonate, excretion of titratable acid, ammonia generation, and acidification of tubular luminal fluid by the distal nephron.[140] In chronic kidney disease, acidosis develops as a result of varying degrees of impairment in each of these processes.[162]

Reduction in renal ammonia synthesis is the greatest limitation to acid excretion in CKD. Low serum bicarbonate levels result in maintenance of acid urine, which stimulates proximal tubule ammoniagenesis and also protonates ammonia resulting in its entrapment as ammonium in the tubule lumen. Net ammonia production per hypertrophied proximal tubule has been shown to increase in response to nephron loss.[155] With decreasing GFR, however, this increase becomes inadequate to compensate for further nephron loss, and absolute ammonia excretion falls.[125] In addition, disruption of the tubulo-medullary ammonium concentration gradient as a result of structural injury may impair ammonia trapping and therefore reduce ammonium excretion.[125] Bicarbonate reabsorption by the nephron occurs predominantly in association with sodium reclamation in the proximal tubule and is dependent on generation of a proton gradient in the distal nephron. Conflicting data with respect to bicarbonate reabsorption in remnant kidneys may reflect species differences. In dogs with remnant kidneys, bicarbonate reabsorption was increased at both proximal and distal micropuncture sampling sites compared to intact controls.[163] In contrast, bicarbonate reabsorption per unit GFR is reduced in both humans and rats with CKD[140] and some patients with renal insufficiency demonstrate bicarbonate wasting until serum bicarbonate drops below 20 mEq/L.[164] Bicarbonate reabsorption is also reduced in the setting of hyperkalemia, increased extracellular fluid volume, and hyperparathyroidism, all of which may be present in patients with chronic renal insufficiency.[165–167] Distal urinary acidification tends to be relatively well preserved in patients with CKD and urinary pH, although higher than in normal individuals with experimental acidosis, is usually about 5.[168] Urinary excretion of titratable acid is also generally well preserved in the setting of nephron loss, as a consequence of increased fractional phosphate excretion.[122,125] As renal failure progresses, acid excretion becomes more dependent on excretion of titratable acid. Renal acidification mechanisms are discussed more comprehensively in Chapters 7 and 14.

Calcium and Phosphate

Derangements of calcium and phosphate metabolism occurring with renal insufficiency are not only the result of impaired urinary excretion of these solutes, but also of associated abnormalities in vitamin D metabolism and parathyroid hormone (PTH) secretion. With progressive renal dysfunction, 1-hydroxylation of vitamin D by the kidney decreases;

calcium absorption from the gut decreases; serum calcium tends to decrease; serum phosphate tends to increase; PTH secretion increases. In response to increased PTH, calcium is mobilized from bone, renal phosphate excretion is enhanced, and the steady state becomes re-established, with secondary hyperparathyroidism as the "trade-off".[169] In CKD, serum phosphate does not increase until GFR falls below 20 ml/min, and phosphate balance is maintained predominantly by an increase in fractional phosphate excretion.[170] With moderate renal insufficiency, therefore, filtered phosphate is not greatly increased and the increase in phosphate excretion must be achieved by a reduction in phosphate reabsorption per nephron.[171] With more severe reductions in GFR, however, phosphate excretion is maintained by an increase in serum phosphate as well as reduced reabsorption per nephron. Sodium-dependent phosphate transport measured in proximal tubular brush border membrane vesicles prepared from the remnant kidneys of dogs was shown to be decreased when compared to that in vesicles derived from normal dogs.[122] Interestingly, however, this decrease was abolished if the partially nephrectomized dog had also undergone parathyroidectomy, indicating that PTH plays an important role in proximal tubular adaptation to phosphate excretion. Studies of isolated proximal tubules from eu-parathyroid uremic rabbits showed a reduction in net phosphate flux per unit of reabsorptive surface area, and an increase in sensitivity to PTH.[124] The authors postulated that the number of PTH receptors per tubule must increase in the remnant kidney, concomitant with tubular hypertrophy. The levels of mRNA encoding the sodium coupled phosphate transporter, NaPi-2 are reduced by approximately 50% in remnant kidneys from 5/6 nephrectomized rats.[172] In contrast, tubules from hyperparathyroid uremic rabbits demonstrated reduced PTH sensitivity, consistent with down-regulation or persistent occupancy of the PTH receptors. On the other hand, studies in animals with reduced renal mass subjected to parathyroidectomy have shown that fractional excretion of phosphate remains inversely proportional to the reduction in GFR,[173] indicating that phosphate excretion is not entirely dependent on the presence of PTH. Whereas most of the reduction in phosphate reabsorption is achieved in the proximal tubule, there is also some evidence of increased fractional phosphate excretion by the distal tubule in uremic dogs and rats.[174] As kidney failure advances, renal 1-hydroxylation of vitamin D decreases, and as a result, calcium absorption from the gut is reduced.[175] In renal failure, fractional intestinal calcium absorption is inversely proportional to blood urea nitrogen.[175] Calcium excretion, on the other hand, varies widely in patients with renal disease, probably due to differences in diet, heterogeneity of vitamin D production, and predominance of glomerular versus tubulointerstitial injury.[176] In normal individuals, calcium excretion is mediated by suppression of PTH-induced reabsorption in the distal nephron, and by suppression of PTH-independent mechanisms in the thick ascending limb. In patients with CKD, fractional calcium excretion remains unchanged until GFR falls below 25 mL/min, when fractional excretion increases due to the obligatory solute diuresis.[140] Absolute calcium excretion, however, remains low. Hypocalciuria in patients with chronic renal insufficiency has been shown to be due, in part, to the attendant hyperparathyroidism.[177] Similar findings were obtained in rats with reduced renal mass, in which parathyroidectomy resulted in increased calcium excretion compared to non-parathyroidectomized controls.[178] Renal calcium clearance is increased in patients with tubulointerstitial disease and in rats with surgical papillectomy, suggesting that regulation of calcium reabsorption depends on intact medullary structures, and that regulation of calcium excretion may be largely modulated by the distal nephron segments.[140] The potential contribution of calcium and phosphate to renal disease progression are discussed later. Calcium and phosphate metabolism are also discussed in greater detail in Chapters 5 and 16.

LONG-TERM ADVERSE CONSEQUENCES OF ADAPTATIONS TO NEPHRON LOSS

The functional and structural adaptations to nephron loss described earlier may be regarded as a beneficial response that minimizes the resultant loss of total GFR. It has been appreciated for several decades, however, that rats subjected to partial nephrectomy subsequently develop hypertension, albuminuria, and progressive renal failure. Detailed histopathological studies in rat remnant kidneys after 5/6 nephrectomy revealed mesangial accumulation of hyaline material that progressively encroached on capillary lumina, obliterating Bowman's space and finally resulting in global sclerosis of the glomerulus. These findings, together with the observation that sclerosed glomeruli are a common finding in human CKD of diverse etiologies, led to the hypothesis that glomerular hyperfiltration ultimately results in damage to remaining glomeruli and contributes to a vicious cycle of progressive nephron loss. The 5/6 nephrectomy model has been extensively studied and considerable progress has been made in elucidating how the physiological adaptations of remaining nephrons that initially permit greatly augmented function per nephron, ultimately produce a complex series of adverse effects that eventuate in progressive renal injury and an inexorable decline in function.[6]

Hemodynamic Factors

As early as 1 week after extensive renal mass ablation, glomerular hyperfiltration and glomerular capillary hypertension were associated with morphological changes, including visceral epithelial cell cytoplasmic attenuation, protein reabsorption droplets and foot process fusion, mesangial expansion and focal lifting of endothelial cells from the basement membrane.[6] Evidence that these morphological changes were a consequence of the glomerular hemodynamic alterations was provided by studies in rats fed a low protein diet after 5/6 nephrectomy. This intervention prevented the hemodynamic changes, effectively normalizing Q_A, P_{GC}, and SNGFR, and abrogated the structural lesions observed in rats on standard diet.[6] Similar findings were subsequently described in a variety of animal models of CKD, including diabetic nephropathy[179,180] and deoxycorticosterone (DOCA)-salt hypertension.[181] Together, these observations led Brenner and colleagues to propose that the hemodynamic adaptations following renal mass ablation ultimately prove injurious to glomeruli and initiate processes that eventuate in glomerulosclerosis. The resulting obliteration of further glomeruli would induce hyperfiltration in remaining, less affected glomeruli, thereby establishing a vicious cycle of progressive nephron loss. These mechanisms constituted a "common pathway" for renal damage that could account for the inexorable progression of CKD, regardless of the cause of the initial renal injury.[3] The hypothesis also explained the finding of both atrophic and hypertrophic nephrons typically encountered in chronically diseased kidneys. Further evidence supportive of the "hyperfiltration hypothesis" was gleaned from the study of experimental diabetic nephropathy in which glomerular hyperfiltration was also found to be a forerunner of glomerular pathology.[6,180] Maneuvers such as unilateral nephrectomy, which exacerbates hyperfiltration in the remaining kidney, were also found to exacerbate diabetic renal injury.[182] Furthermore, when the kidney was shielded from elevated perfusion pressure and from glomerular capillary hypertension by creating unilateral renal artery stenosis, the ipsilateral kidney was protected against the development

of diabetic injury, which progressed unabated in the contralateral kidney.[183] In addition, when glomerular hyperfiltration was reversed in 5/6 nephrectomized rats by transplantation of an isogeneic kidney, hypertension and proteinuria were ameliorated, and glomerular injury was limited.[184] Similarly, augmenting renal mass in the Fisher→Lewis rat transplant model normalized P_{GC} and greatly reduced the development of chronic renal allograft injury.[185,186] Direct evidence that similar mechanisms may operate in human kidneys is derived from a study of 14 patients with solitary kidneys who had undergone varying degrees of partial nephrectomy of the remaining kidney for malignancy.[187] Before renal sparing surgery, proteinuria was absent in all patients. Although serum creatinine remained stable after an initial rise of 50% in 12 patients, the two patients subjected to the most extensive nephrectomy (75% and 67%, respectively) developed progressive renal failure and required long-term dialysis. Moreover, among the remaining patients, seven developed proteinuria, the levels of which were inversely related to the amount of renal tissue preserved. Renal biopsy specimens in four patients with moderate to severe proteinuria showed FSGS,[187] which later morphometric analysis revealed to involve virtually all glomeruli examined.[188]

The importance of glomerular hemodynamic factors in the development of progressive renal injury was further illustrated by studies that reported dramatic protective effects against the development of glomerulosclerosis after chronic inhibition of the RAS with either ACEI or AT_1RA treatment in 5/6 nephrectomized rats.[15–18] Micropuncture studies showed that like the low protein diet, the renoprotective effects of RAS inhibition were associated with near normalization of the P_{GC}, yet, in contrast to the effects of dietary protein restriction, SNGFR remained elevated.[189] This suggested that glomerular capillary hypertension, rather than hyperfiltration per se, was the key factor in the initiation and progression of glomerular injury. Confirmation of this view came from an experiment in which rats were treated with a combination of reserpine, hydralazine, and hydrochlorothiazide ("triple therapy") to lower arterial pressure to levels similar to those obtained with an ACEI. In contrast to the glomerular hemodynamic effects of the ACEI, however, triple therapy did not alleviate glomerular hypertension or proteinuria and glomerular injury progressed unabated[16,17] (Fig. 25–3). Interestingly, within the context of pharmacological inhibition of the RAS, the level to which systemic blood pressure is reduced remains a critical determinant of the extent of the renal protection conferred.[190] The effectiveness of both ACEI and AT_1RA in lowering glomerular pressure and ameliorating glomerular injury has since been observed in several other animal models of chronic kidney disease, including diabetic nephropathy,[179,191,192] hypertensive renal disease,[193,194] experimental chronic renal allograft failure (a model that lacks systemic hypertension but exhibits glomerular capillary hypertension),[195–197] age-related glomerulosclerosis,[198,199] and obesity-related glomerulosclerosis.[200] It is noteworthy that the phase of transition from an acute, nonhypertensive experimental injury induced by PAN administration, to a chronic nephropathy characterized by proteinuria and glomerulosclerosis, is also associated with the development of glomerular capillary hypertension.[201] That similar mechanisms are relevant in human CKD progression has been strongly suggested by the results of clinical trials showing substantial renoprotective effects with ACEI and AT_1RA treatment.[202–206] The importance of glomerular capillary hypertension has been further illustrated by studies of the effects of Omapatrilat, a vasopeptidase inhibitor. Micropuncture studies after 5/6 nephrectomy showed even greater lowering of P_{GC} with Omapatrilat than with ACEI treatment, despite equivalent effects on systemic blood pressure. In subsequent chronic studies, Omapatrilat produced more effective renoprotection

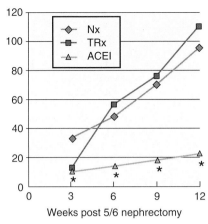

FIGURE 25-3 Proteinuria levels following 5/6 nephrectomy in untreated rats (NX) versus treatment with triple therapy (reserpine, hydralazine, and hydrochlorothiazide—TRx), (NX + TRx), or enalapril (NX + ACEI). Despite equivalent levels of blood pressure control, enalapril therapy almost completely prevented proteinuria and glomerulosclerosis whereas triple therapy afforded no renoprotection. (Reproduced with permission from Anderson S, Rennke HG, Brenner BM: Therapeutic advantage of converting enzyme inhibitors in arresting progressive renal disease associated with systemic hypertension in the rat. J Clin Invest 77:1993–2000, 1986.) *P < 0.05 versus untreated controls.

than the ACEI.[72] Thus, among the determinants of glomerular hyperfiltration, glomerular capillary hypertension has been identified as a critical factor in the initiation and progression of glomerular injury.

Mechanisms of Hemodynamically Induced Injury

Mechanical Stress
Several mechanisms have been proposed whereby elevated P_{GC} may result in glomerular cell injury. Experiments in isolated perfused rat glomeruli have reported significant increases in glomerular volume with increases in perfusion pressure over the normal and relevant abnormal range.[91] These increases in wall tension and glomerular volume can be predicted to result in stretching of glomerular cells. Experimental evidence suggests that such stretching may have adverse consequences for all three major cell types in the glomerulus. Furthermore, recent advances in the study of cellular responses to mechanical stress raise the possibility that glomerular hyperperfusion may also promote the development of glomerulosclerosis through more subtle and complex pathways that induce profibrotic phenotypic alterations in glomerular cells.[207]

Endothelial Cells
The vascular endothelium serves multiple complex functions including acting as a dynamic barrier to leukocytes and plasma proteins, secretion of vasoactive factors (prostacyclin, NO, and endothelin), conversion of AI to AII, and expression of cell adhesion molecules. It is also the first cellular structure in the kidney that encounters the mechanical forces imparted by glomerular hyperperfusion. After 5/6 nephrectomy, endothelial cells are activated or injured, resulting in detachment and exposure of the basement membrane. This in turn may induce platelet aggregation, deposition of fibrin, and intracapillary microthrombus formation.[6,208] It has been recognized for some time that segmental glomerulosclerosis is associated with focal obliteration of capillary loops[209] and that interstitial fibrosis is associated with loss of peritubular capillaries.[210] Recently it has been shown that this loss of capillaries in the remnant kidney is associated with a decrease

in endothelial cell proliferation and reduced constitutive expression of vascular endothelial growth factor (VEGF) by podocytes and renal tubule cells as well as increased expression of the anti-angiogenic factor, thrombospondin-1, by the renal interstitium.[211] Because VEGF is an important endothelial cell angiogenic, survival, and trophic factor, these findings suggest that capillary loss may be in part due to failure of recovery from hemodynamically mediated endothelial cell injury. Furthermore, short-term treatment of rats with VEGF ameliorated both glomerular and peritubular capillary loss after 5/6 nephrectomy.[212] This preservation of capillaries was associated with a trend toward less glomerulosclerosis and significantly less interstitial deposition of type III collagen, as well as better preservation of renal function. Long-term studies are required to evaluate further the potential benefit of improving renal angiogenesis in the setting of progressive renal injury.

Endothelial cells bear numerous receptors that allow them to detect and respond to changes in mechanical forces. Thus exposure of endothelial cells to changes in shear stress, cyclic stretch, or pulsatile barostress that result from glomerular hyperperfusion may induce changes in expression of genes involved in inflammation, cell cycle control, apoptosis, thrombosis, and oxidative stress.[213] The in vitro responses of endothelial cells to mechanical forces have largely been studied in the context of vascular remodeling and atherosclerosis but it can readily be appreciated that similar responses may impact on the development of inflammation and fibrosis within the remnant kidney. Of particular interest are observations that shear stress can stimulate endothelial expression of adhesion molecules[214] and proinflammatory cytokines.[215] It is clear from the earlier discussion why biomechanical activation has been described as an "emerging paradigm" in endothelial cell biology[216] but further studies focusing on glomerular endothelial responses to mechanical stress are required to elucidate the role of such mechanisms in progressive renal injury.

Mesangial Cells
Mesangial cells are closely associated with the capillaries in the glomerulus and are therefore also exposed to mechanical forces. Evidence from in vitro studies indicates that mesangial cells respond to changes in these mechanical forces in ways that may promote inflammation and fibrosis. Subjecting mesangial cells to cyclical stretch or strain has been shown to induce proliferation[217] and synthesis of extracellular matrix constituents.[218,219] Cyclical stretch also stimulates synthesis of intercellular cell adhesion molecule (ICAM)-1,[220] monocyte chemoattractant protein (MCP)-1,[220] transforming growth factor (TGF)-β,[221] and its receptor[222] as well as connective tissue growth factor (CTGF).[223] Cyclical stretch also activates the RAS in cultured mesangial cells[224] and AII in turn may induce TGF-β synthesis.[225] Mesangial cells cultured at ambient pressures of 50 mm Hg to 60 mm Hg (i.e., levels corresponding to glomerular capillary hypertension) also show enhanced synthesis and secretion of extracellular matrix when compared with cells grown at "normal" pressures of 40 mm Hg to 50 mm Hg.[226] Exposure of mesangial cells to barostress, achieved by culture under increased barometric pressure, stimulates expression of cytokines including platelet derived growth factor (PDGF)-B[227] and MCP-1.[228] Transduction of mechanical forces by mesangial cells has been associated with tyrosine phosphorylation[229] and protein kinase C–induced increases in S-6 kinase activity.[230]

Podocytes
A growing body of evidence attests to the importance of podocyte injury in a variety of renal diseases and in CKD progression.[231] Podocytes display morphological evidence of injury as early as 1 week after 5/6 nephrectomy[6] and 6 months

after uninephrectomy.[232] Increased numbers of podocytes have been observed in the urine from rats after 5/6 nephrectomy and in human CKD.[231] In 5/6 nephrectomized rats the number of podocytes correlated with the severity of proteinuria as well as mean arterial blood pressure, suggesting that podocyte loss may contribute to CKD progression.[233] The importance of podocyte injury in CKD progression is further supported by the observation that amelioration of glomerular damage in 5/6 nephrectomized rats treated with 1,25-dihydroxyvitamin D3 is associated with preservation of podocyte number as well as prevention of podocyte hypertrophy and injury.[234] It has been proposed that progressive loss of podocytes results in adhesions between exposed areas of glomerular basement membrane and parietal epithelial cells. Formation of adhesions between the glomerular tuft and Bowman's capsule in turn allows misdirection of protein-rich glomerular filtrate into the interstitium where it provokes inflammation that further contributes to nephron loss.[235] As podocytes are attached to the outer aspect of the glomerular basement membrane it is reasonable to expect that they would be exposed to increased mechanical forces resulting from glomerular hypertension. Confirmation that podocytes respond to such physical forces is derived from several in vitro experiments that examined podocyte responses to stretching. Activation of a voltage-sensitive potassium channels was observed in response to stretching of the podocyte cell membrane[236] and culture of podocytes under constant stretch inhibited podocyte proliferation.[237] Exposure to cyclical stretching that mimics pulsatile strain within the glomerulus has been shown to cause reorganization of the actin cytoskeleton,[238] up-regulation of COX-2 and E-prostanoid 4 receptor expression[239] as well as podocyte hypertrophy.[240] In another experiment cyclical stretching of podocytes was associated with increased production of AII and TGF-β as well as up-regulation of angiotensin subtype 1 receptors resulting in increased AII–dependent apoptosis.[241] Taken together these data suggest that stretch-induced podocyte injury is a further mechanism whereby glomerular hypertension contributes to glomerular injury.

Cellular Infiltration in Remnant Kidneys

Despite the lack of an obvious immune stimulus, an inflammatory cell infiltrate composed predominantly of macrophages and smaller numbers of lymphocytes is observed in remnant kidneys after 5/6 nephrectomy.[242] As discussed earlier it is possible that the glomerular hemodynamic adaptations to nephron loss may provoke an inflammatory cell response through the effects of mechanical forces on endothelial and mesangial cells. Thus up-regulation of renal endothelial adhesion molecules may facilitate egress of leukocytes from the circulation into the mesangium, where they may participate in further renal injury. The recruited cellular infiltrate may constitute an abundant source of potent pleiotropic cytokine products that in turn influence other infiltrating leukocytes, dendritic cells, and kidney cells, stimulating cell proliferation, elaboration of extracellular matrix components, and increased endothelial adhesiveness.[243] Evidence is now emerging that these proposed mechanisms, based largely on in vitro observations, are indeed relevant in vivo. In the 2-kidney, 1-clip model of renovascular hypertension, up-regulated expression of adhesion molecules and TGF-β as well as cell infiltration is observed only in the non-clipped kidney that is exposed to the hypertensive perfusion pressure.[244,245] In the 5/6 nephrectomy model, coordinated up-regulation of a variety of cell adhesion molecules, cytokines, and growth factors in association with macrophage infiltration has been observed at time points that precede the development of severe glomerulosclerosis.[246,247] Furthermore, the renoprotection afforded by ACEI or AT₁RA treatment in this model was associated with inhibition of cytokine up-regulation and prevention of renal infiltration by macrophages.[247,248]

Several lines of evidence suggest that this cellular infiltrate contributes to renal injury and is not merely a consequence of it. In one study, multiple linear regression analysis identified glomerular macrophage infiltration in the remnant kidney as a major determinant of mesangial matrix expansion and adhesion formation between Bowman's capsule and glomerular tufts.[242] Furthermore, depletion of leukocytes in rats by irradiation delayed the onset of glomerular injury after renal ablative surgery.[249] Several studies have reported amelioration of the cellular infiltrate and renal injury in the 5/6 nephrectomy model following treatment with the immunosuppressive agent, mycophenolate mofetil.[250-253] One study found that mycophenolate also lowers P_{GC}, which may account for some of its renoprotective effects.[254] Interestingly, the anti-inflammatory agent, nitroflurbiprofen, which is also a NO donor, has a modest effect to ameliorate remnant kidney injury following 5/6 nephrectomy.[255]

Infiltrating macrophages, although present in the glomeruli of remnant kidney, are chiefly distributed in the tubulointerstitial regions,[242,247] suggesting that they play a role in the development of the tubulointerstitial fibrosis that accompanies glomerulosclerosis. Further analysis of the cellular infiltrate has also identified mast cells in close proximity to areas of tubulointerstitial fibrosis.[256] It is possible that interstitial infiltrates are recruited as the result of tubulointerstitial cell activation by the downstream effects of cytokines released in the glomeruli. Alternatively it has been proposed that excessive uptake of filtered proteins by tubule epithelial cells stimulates expression of cell adhesion and chemoattractant molecules that recruit macrophages and other monocytic cells to tubulointerstitial areas.[257] The chemokine receptor CCR-1 has been shown to be important in interstitial but not glomerular recruitment of leukocytes. Treatment with a non-peptide CCR-1 antagonist has been shown to reduce interstitial macrophage infiltration and ameliorate interstitial fibrosis in the unilateral ureteric obstruction (UUO) model but data are still lacking in the 5/6 nephrectomy model.[258] Furthermore, antagonism of MCP-1 signaling through gene therapy-induced production of a mutant form of MCP-1 by skeletal muscle resulted in reduced interstitial macrophage infiltration and amelioration of interstitial fibrosis in mice after UUO.[259] Finally, overexpression of the anti-inflammatory cytokine interleukin-10 in rats using an adeno-associated virus serotype 1 vector system was associated with reduced interstitial infiltration and lower levels of MCP-1, RANTES, IFN-γ, and IL-2 expression after 5/6 nephrectomy as well as attenuation of proteinuria, glomerulosclerosis, and tubulointerstitial fibrosis.[260] The identification of renal tubule cells expressing α-smooth muscle actin after 5/6 nephrectomy has raised the possibility that tubule cells may undergo trans-diffrentiation to a myofibrobast phenotype that contributes to interstitial fibrosis.[261] Furthermore, the renoprotection observed with mycophenolate treatment in 5/6 nephrectomized rats is associated with reductions in interstitial myofibroblast infiltration and collagen type III deposition.[262]

The importance of inflammatory factors acting "downstream" from the hemodynamic changes in the common pathway mechanisms of CKD progression has further been demonstrated by studies using a peroxisome proliferator-activated receptor γ (PPARγ) receptor agonist.[263] These compounds are primarily used as antidiabetic agents that reduce insulin resistance in type 2 diabetes mellitus. The PPARγ receptor is a member of the nuclear receptor superfamily of transcriptional factors and in vitro studies suggest that PPARγ receptor agonists may have a wide range of effects including modulation of adipocyte differentiation, macrophage function, and activation of other transcription factors.[263] Rats treated with a PPARγ receptor agonist after 5/6 nephrectomy evidenced significant attenuation of the proteinuria and glomerulosclerosis observed in untreated rats, despite the failure of treatment to lower blood pressure. This renoprotection was observed in association with marked reductions in glomerular cell proliferation, glomerular macrophage infiltration, and renal expression of PAI-1 as well as TGF-β.[263] The authors speculate that some of these effects may have resulted from the known actions of PPARγ receptor activation to antagonize the activities of the transcription factors AP-1 and NF-κB.

Taken together these findings strongly support the hypothesis that in addition to direct glomerular cell injury, glomerular hemodynamic adaptations to nephron loss provoke a complex series of proiflammatory and profibrotic responses that further contribute to renal damage. Treatments that antagonize the mediators of these responses may therefore be of benefit in slowing the rate of progression of CKD.

Non-hemodynamic Factors in the Development of Nephron Injury Following Extensive Renal Mass Ablation

The weight of evidence in support of the hypothesis that glomerular hemodynamic adaptations are central to progressive renal injury does not exclude the possibility that the kidney may also be affected by a variety of factors not directly attributable to hemodynamic changes. These non-hemodynamic factors have been extensively studied in recent years and may offer new therapeutic targets for future renoprotective interventions.

Transforming Growth Factor-β
TGF-β is associated with chronic fibrotic states throughout the body, including CKD.[264] In vitro TGF-β elicits overproduction of extracellular matrix constituents by mesangial cells and its expression is increased in several experimental models of renal disease including diabetic nephropathy,[265] anti-Thy-1 glomerulonephritis,[266] Adriamycin-induced nephropathy,[267] and chronic allograft nephropathy[268] as well as in human glomerulonephritis,[269,270] HIV nephropathy,[271] diabetic nephropathy,[272] and chronic allograft nephropathy.[273] The role of TGF-β in renal fibrosis is further illustrated by experiments in which transfection of the gene for TGF-β into one renal artery produced ipsilateral renal fibrosis.[274] In 5/6 nephrectomized rats a twofold to threefold increase in remnant kidney mRNA levels for TGF-β was observed and in situ hybridization revealed elevations in TGF-β mRNA throughout glomeruli, tubules, and interstitium. Treatment with an ACEI or an AT₁RA resulted in substantial renal protection and prevented up-regulation of TGF-β.[247,248] Furthermore, in rats treated with an ACEI or an AT₁RA the extent of glomerulosclerosis correlated closely with remnant kidney TGF-β mRNA levels.[190] Several interventions that inhibit the effects of TGF-β have been shown to afford renoprotection in animal models of renal disease: transfection of the gene for decorin, a naturally occurring inhibitor of TGFβ, into skeletal muscle limited the progression of renal injury in anti Thy-1 glomerulonephritis[275]; administration of anti-TGF-β antibodies to salt-loaded Dahl-salt sensitive rats ameliorated the hypertension, proteinuria, glomerulosclerosis, and interstitial fibrosis typical of this model[276]; treatment with Tranilast [n-(3,4-dimethoxycin-namoyl) anthranilic acid; Pharm Chemical, Shanghai Lansheng Corporation, Shanghai, China], an inhibitor of TGF-β–induced extracellular matrix production, significantly reduced albuminuria, macrophage infiltration, glomerulosclerosis, and interstitial fibrosis in 5/6 nephrectomized rats[277]; transfer of an inducible gene for Smad 7, which blocks TGF-β signaling by inhibiting Smad 2/3 activation, inhibited proteinuria, fibrosis, and myofibroblast accumula-

tion after 5/6 nephrectomy[278]; two weeks of treatment with a polyamide compound designed to suppress transcription of the TGF-β gene, significantly reduced proteinuria and prevented up-regulation of TGF-β, connective tissue growth factor (CTGF), collagen type 1 α1, and fibronectin mRNA in the renal cortex as well as suppressing urinary TGF-β excretion and staining for TGF-β by immunofluorescence in salt-loaded Dahl-salt sensitive rats.[279] Another fibrogenic molecule, CTGF, has also been observed to be overexpressed in kidney biopsies from patients with a variety of renal diseases.[280] The specific induction of CTGF expression by exogenous TGF-β in mesangial cells[223,281] and fibroblasts,[282] together with the finding that blocking antibodies to TGF-β inhibited increased CTGF expression in mesangial cells exposed to high glucose concentrations,[281] suggests that CTGF may serve as a downstream mediator of the profibrotic effects of TGF-β.[283]

Angiotensin II
As discussed earlier, AII plays a central role in the glomerular hemodynamic adaptations observed after renal mass ablation. Angiotensin subtype 1 receptors are, however, distributed on many cell types within the kidney including mesangial, glomerular epithelial, endothelial, tubule epithelial and vascular smooth muscle cells suggesting multiple potential actions of AII within the kidney.[284] Experimental studies have revealed several non-hemodynamic effects of AII that may be important in CKD progression (Fig. 25–4): in isolated, perfused kidneys, infusion of AII results in loss of glomerular size permselectivity and proteinuria, an effect that has been attributed to both hemodynamic effects of AII resulting in elevations in P_{GC}, and a direct effect of AII on glomerular permselectivity.[285] Furthermore, overexpression of angiotensin subtype 1 receptors on podocytes resulted in albuminuria and focal segmental glomerulosclerosis in the absence of hypertension in transgenic rats.[286] In vitro AII has been shown to stimulate mesangial cell proliferation and induce expression of TGF-β, resulting in increased synthesis of extracellular matrix (ECM).[225] In vivo, transfection of rat kidneys with human genes for renin and angiotensinogen, resulted in glomerular ECM expansion within 7 days.[287] AII also stimulates production of plasminogen activator inhibitor-1 (PAI-1) by endothelial cells and vascular smooth muscle cells[288-290] and may therefore further increase accumulation of ECM through inhibition of ECM breakdown by matrix metalloproteinases that require conversion to an active form by plasmin. Other reports indicate that AII may directly induce the transcription of a variety of cell adhesion molecules and cytokines as well as activating the transcription factor, NF-κB[291-293] and directly stimulating monocyte activation.[294] AII infusion provoked up-regulation of COX-2 expression in rats that was not dependent on blood pressure elevation[295] and 5/6 nephrectomized rats evidenced AII–dependent up-regulation of interstitial COX-2 expression.[296] Finally, AII may have fibrogenic effects via mineralocorticoids (see later). Interestingly AII may also have antifibrotic effects via the angiotensin subtype 2 receptor (AT₂). AII appears to up-regulate AT₂ receptor expression via an AT₂ receptor-dependent mechanism after 5/6 nephrectomy and treatment with an AT₂ receptor antagonist exacerbates renal damage.[297] Furthermore overexpression AT₂ receptors in transgenic mice was associated with reduced albuminuria as well as decreased glomerular expression of platelet derived growth factor-BB chain and TGF-β after 5/6 nephrectomy.[298]

Aldosterone
Observations that aldosterone stimulates collagen synthesis in the myocardium and that spironolactone treatment affords survival benefit in addition to that achieved with ACEI alone in heart failure patients[299] gave impetus to studies investigating the potential role of aldosterone in renal fibrosis. In the

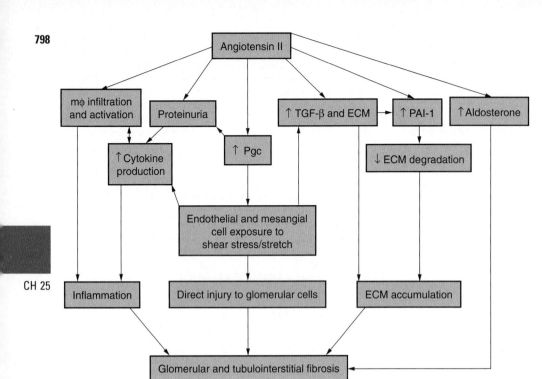

FIGURE 25–4 Scheme depicting the central role of angiotensin II, through hemodynamic and non-hemodynamic effects, in the pathogenesis of progressive renal injury and fibrosis following nephron loss. ECM, extracellular matrix; mφ, macrophage; PAI-1, plasminogen activator inhibitor-1; P_{GC}, glomerular capillary hydraulic pressure; TGF-β, transforming growth factor-β. (Reproduced and revised with permission from Taal MW, Brenner BM: Renoprotective benefits of RAS inhibition: From ACEI to angiotensin II antagonists. Kidney Int 57:1803–1817, 2000.)

remnant kidney model, adrenal hypertrophy and markedly elevated plasma aldosterone levels have been reported. Furthermore, administration of exogenous aldosterone during inhibition of the RAS with combination ACEI and AT_1RA therapy in the 5/6 nephrectomy model negates the renal protective effects of the latter.[300] Further evidence of the role of aldosterone was provided by experiments in which rats subjected to adrenelectomy after 5/6 nephrectomy received replacement glucocorticoid but not mineralocorticoid therapy, resulting in less severe renal injury than rats with intact adrenal glands.[301] Mechanisms whereby aldosterone may contribute to renal damage include hemodynamic effects (see earlier), mesangial cell proliferation,[302] and reactive oxygen species production[303] as well as increased production of PAI-1,[304,305] TGF-β,[306] and CTGF.[307,308] Early experimental use of aldosterone receptor blockers in 5/6 nephrectomized rats yielded only modest renoprotective effects[300,309] but one study has found significant amelioration of glomerulosclerosis in 5/6 nephrectomized rats treated with spironolactone, alone or in combination with triple antihypertensive therapy or an AT_1RA.[304] In some rats spironolactone was associated with apparent regression of glomerulosclerosis. Furthermore the observed renoprotection was associated with inhibition of renal cortex mRNA levels for PAI-1.[304] Spironolactone has also been shown to ameliorate renal damage in other experimental models including diabetic nephropathy,[307] radiation nephritis,[310] and stroke-prone hypertension.[311] Several small clinical trials have reported renoprotective benefits associated with spironolactone or other aldosterone receptor blockers, generally in combination with ACEI treatment.[312] In the largest study to date (reported only in abstract form) treatment of patients with type 2 diabetes and microalbuminuria with the aldosterone receptor blocker, eplerenone, was associated with greater reduction in albuminuria than ACEI treatment (62% versus 45%) and combination ACEI and eplerenone treatment resulted in an even greater reduction (74%).[313]

Hepatocyte Growth Factor

Investigations have shed light on the role of HGF as a potential anti-fibrotic factor in CKD. Initial studies focused on the property of HGF to ameliorate tubule cell injury in models of

renal ischemia[314,315] but studies in models of CKD suggest that HGF may also ameliorate chronic renal injury through its mitogenic, motogenic, morphogenic, and anti-apoptotic actions.[316] As discussed earlier, HGF is up-regulated in the remaining kidney after uninephrectomy and may play a role in compensatory renal hypertrophy.[111] Further studies have confirmed that HGF and its receptor, c-met, are also up-regulated in the remnant kidney after 5/6 nephrectomy.[317] Furthermore, blockade of HGF action with anti-HGF antibodies resulted in a more rapid decline in GFR and more severe renal fibrosis that was associated with increased ECM accumulation and a greater number of myofibroblasts in the interstitium and tubules. Moreover, in vitro studies revealed that HGF decreased ECM accumulation in proximal tubule cell cultures by increasing expression of collagenases such as matrix metalloproteinase-9 (MMP-9) and decreasing the expression of the endogenous inhibitors of MMPs, tissue inhibitors of matrix metalloproteinase-1 (TIMP-1), and TIMP-2.[317] Multiple experiments have confirmed the renoprotective effects of HGF: the renoprotective effects of ACEI and AT_1RA treatment are associated with increased renal expression on HGF mRNA[318]; treatment with anti-HGF antibodies resulted in increased TGF-β levels in a mouse model of chronic glomerulonephritis[319]; HGF treatment ameliorated the progression of chronic allograft nephropathy in a renal transplant model[320]; HGF blocked the TGF-β induced transdifferentiation of tubule epithelial cells to myofibroblasts[321]; exogenous HGF administration[321] or HGF over-expression[322] blocked myofibroblast activation and prevented interstitial fibrosis in the unilateral ureteric obstruction model; HGF gene transfer into skeletal muscle ameliorated glomerulosclerosis and interstitial fibrosis after 5/6 nephrectomy[323]; HGF treatment suppressed CTGF expression and attenuated renal fibrosis after 5/6 nephrectomy.[324] In contrast, other studies have reported adverse renal effects associated with excess HGF exposure: transgenic mice that over-expressed HGF developed progressive renal disease characterized by tubular hypertrophy, glomerulosclerosis, and cyst formation[325] and HGF administration resulted in more rapid deterioration of creatinine clearance as well as increased albuminuria in obese db diabetic mice.[326] Available evidence thus suggests that HGF may play a role in ameliorating chronic renal injury but inappropriate or excessive exposure to HGF may have adverse renal effects.

Bone Morphogenetic Protein-7

Bone morphogenetic protein (BMP)-7, also termed osteogenic protein-1, is a bone morphogen involved in embryonic development and tissue repair. Preliminary evidence suggests that BMP-7 may also play a role in renal repair. BMP-7 is down-regulated after acute renal ischaemia,[327] early in the course of experimental diabetes[328] and after 5/6 nephrectomy.[329] Furthermore administration of exogenous BMP-7 increased tubular regeneration after 5/6 nephrectomy,[329] attenuated interstitial inflammation and fibrosis after UUO,[330] and ameliorated glomerulosclerosis in rats with diabetic nephropathy.[331] In vitro experiments have identified several potential renoprotective effects attributable to BMP-7 including inhibition of proinflammatory cytokine as well as endothelin expression in tubule cells exposed to TNF-α,[332] reversal of renal tubule epithelial to mesenchymal cell transdifferentiation,[333] and antagonism of the fibrogenic effects of TGF-β in mesangial cells.[334] The renoprotective effect is further illustrated by the observation that expression of a transgene for BMP-7 in podocytes and proximal renal tubule cells was associated with prevention of podocyte drop-out as well as amelioration of albuminuria, glomerulosclerosis, and interstitial fibrosis after induction of diabetes.[335] Further experiments are required to evaluate the potential renoprotective effects of chronic BMP-7 administration after 5/6 nephrectomy.

Hypertrophy

The consistent observation of renal and in particular glomerular hypertrophy after renal mass reduction has prompted investigators to propose that processes involved in, or resulting from hypertrophy may contribute to progressive renal injury in CKD.[336] The well-documented observation that renal and glomerular hypertrophy precede the development of diabetic nephropathy and the finding of a positive association between glomerular size and early sclerosis in rats subjected to renal mass ablation[337] further suggests that hypertrophy may play a direct role in pathogenesis of glomerulosclerosis. Several clinical observations also support an association between glomerular hypertrophy and renal injury. Oligomeganephronia, a rare congenital condition in which nephron number 25% of normal or less, is characterized by marked hypertrophy of the remaining glomeruli and development of proteinuria and renal failure in adolescence, with FSGS as the typical renal biopsy finding.[338] In children with minimal change disease, a glomerulopathy generally associated with spontaneous remission and lack of progression to renal failure, investigators noted an association between glomerular size and the risk of developing FSGS and renal failure.[339]

Two forms of intervention have been employed in an attempt to interrupt the development of glomerular hypertrophy after renal mass reduction and thereby assess its role in renal disease progression. Rats subjected to 5/6 nephrectomy were compared to rats in which 2/3 of the left kidney was infarcted and the right ureter drained into the peritoneal cavity (an intervention that apparently results in decreased renal clearance without compensatory renal hypertrophy). Micropuncture studies confirmed similar degrees of elevation of P_{GC} and SNGFR in both models. At 4 weeks, however, the maximal planar area of the glomerulus was significantly less and glomerular injury, as assessed by sclerosis index, significantly reduced in ureteroperitoneostomized rats versus 5/6 nephrectomized controls. Accordingly, the authors concluded that glomerular hypertrophy was more important than glomerular capillary hypertension in the progression of glomerular injury in this model.[336] Dietary sodium restriction

has also been utilized to inhibit renal hypertrophy after 5/6 nephrectomy. Although sodium restriction had no effect on glomerular hemodynamics, glomerular volume was significantly reduced in 5/6 nephrectomized rats fed low versus normal sodium diets. Moreover, urinary protein excretion was lower and glomerulosclerosis was less severe in rats on restricted sodium intake.[89] These findings were extended by another study in which the effect of sodium restriction in preventing glomerular hypertrophy and ameliorating glomerular injury was confirmed, but that also found that these benefits were overcome by administration of an androgen that stimulated glomerular hypertrophy despite sodium restriction. Glomerular hemodynamics were similar among the groups.[340]

Glomerular hypertrophy may contribute to glomerulosclerosis through a number of different mechanisms. According to the Law of Laplace, the increase in glomerular volume could result in an increase in capillary wall tension only if the capillary wall diameter was also increased. Cyclic stretch would then exert stress capable of damaging epithelial, mesangial, and endothelial cells as described earlier. Alternatively, glomerulosclerosis may be viewed as a maladaptive growth response following loss of renal mass and resulting in excessive mesangial proliferation and extracellular matrix production.[336] In the past there has tended to be a dichotomy of viewpoints regarding the relative importance of hemodynamic factors or hypertrophy in the pathogenesis of glomerulosclerosis.[336,341] Proponents of the "hypertrophy hypothesis" pointed out that in some experiments a disassociation between glomerular hemodynamic changes and glomerulosclerosis has been observed and that in one study, antihypertensive therapy was renoprotective without lowering P_{GC}.[336] On the other hand, those favoring the "hemodynamic hypothesis" noted that treatment with an ACEI[16] or AT_1RA[18] in 5/6 nephrectomized rats resulted in renoprotection without preventing renal or glomerular hypertrophy and that many of the studies purporting to show a positive association between glomerular hypertrophy and sclerosis failed to report glomerular hemodynamic data. Furthermore, rats subjected to ureteroperitoneostomy developed significantly more glomerulosclerosis than sham-operated controls despite a lack of increase in glomerular size.[341] Several other observations suggests that hemodynamic factors override the potential role of hypertrophy in progressive renal damage: the renoprotection achieved after 5/6 nephrectomy by low protein diet (associated with prevention of glomerular hypertrophy) can be reversed by treatment with calcium channel blockers that inhibit renal autoregulation but have no effect on glomerular size[342]; comparison of rats subjected to 5/6 nephrectomy by excision versus infarction of 2/3 of the remaining kidney shows similar increases in glomerular volume but the infarction model is associated with more severe glomerular hypertension and glomerulosclerosis.[7] A growing appreciation of the complexity of the multiple adaptations that follow nephron loss has facilitated the development of a consensus view that continues to regard raised glomerular capillary pressure as a central factor in initiating glomerulosclerosis but also acknowledges that glomerular hypertrophy and other pathogenetic mechanisms may act in concert with hemodynamic factors in a complex interplay that eventuates in a vicious cycle of progressive renal damage (Fig. 25-5).[207,343]

Altered Glomerular Permselectivity to Proteins

Abnormal excretion of protein in the urine is the hallmark of experimental and clinical glomerular disease. Whereas immune complex deposition and resulting inflammation account for abnormal permeability of the glomerular filtration barrier to proteins in glomerulonephritis, studies in rats

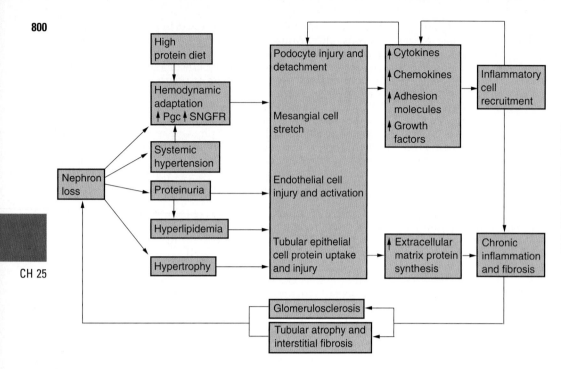

FIGURE 25–5 Scheme hypothesizing the interaction of hemodynamic and non-hemodynamic factors in the "common pathway" of mechanisms contributing to progressive nephron loss in chronic renal disease. P_{GC}, glomerular capillary hydraulic pressure; SNGFR, single nephron glomerular filtration rate. (Reproduced from Mackenzie HS, Taal MW, Luyckx VA: *In* Brenner BM (ed): The Kidney, 6th ed. Philadelphia, WB Saunders, 2000.)

subjected to extensive renal ablation have shown loss of glomerular barrier function to proteins of similar molecular size, yet in the apparent absence of primary immune-mediated renal injury or inflammatory response. Sieving studies using dextrans and other macromolecules in rats 7 or 14 days after 5/6 nephrectomy revealed loss of both size and charge-selectivity of the glomerular filtration barrier. Ultrastructural examination of the remnant kidneys revealed detachment of glomerular endothelial cells and visceral epithelial cells from the glomerular basement membrane. In addition, protein reabsorption droplets and attenuation of cytoplasm resulting in bleb formation was observed in podocytes. The authors concluded that the altered permselectivity may be due, in part, to separation of endothelial cells from the glomerular basement membrane allowing access of macromolecules and, in part, to loss of anionic sites in the lamina rara externa resulting in both loss of charge-selectivity and detachment of podocytes.[344] A direct role for AII in modulating glomerular capillary permselectivity is suggested by the observation of marked increases in urinary protein excretion during infusion of AII in normal rats. Although some investigators have attributed this to a direct effect of AII on the cellular components of the glomerular filtration barrier, resulting in opening of interendothelial junctions and epithelial cell disruption, others have shown that the increase in proteinuria may be accounted for almost completely by the associated hemodynamic changes, principally a reduction in Q_A and an increase in filtration fraction.[345] On the other hand, the notion that AII may mediate changes in glomerular permselectivity independent of its effects on glomerular hemodynamics is supported by studies in an isolated perfused rat kidney preparation in which infusion of AII augmented urinary protein excretion and enhanced the clearance of tracer macromolecules independent of any change in filtration fraction.[285]

Proteinuria, long considered simply a marker of glomerular injury, has also been implicated as an effector of injury processes involved in renal disease progression, especially those resulting in tubulointerstitial fibrosis.[346] In rats with aminonucleoside-induced nephrotic syndrome the proteinuric phase of the disease was associated with an acute interstitial nephritis, the intensity of which correlated closely with the severity of the proteinuria.[257] Furthermore, in an overload

proteinuria model induced by daily intraperitoneal administration of bovine serum albumin to uninephrectomized rats, proximal tubule cell injury and interstitial infiltration of macrophages and lymphocytes were evident after 1 week.[347] The severity of the proteinuria showed a positive correlation with the intensity of the infiltrate. At 4 weeks, focal areas of chronic interstitial inflammation were noted.[347] A causative association between excessive proteinuria and interstitial inflammation has been suggested by *in vitro* studies of proximal tubule epithelial cells cultured in media supplemented with high concentrations of albumin, immunoglobulin (Ig) G, or transferrin. Cellular uptake of these proteins was observed to increase secretion of endothelin-1,[348] MCP-1,[349] RANTES,[350] interleukin-8,[351] and fractaline.[352] Electrophoretic mobility shift assay of cell nucleus extracts revealed intense activation of the transcription factor NF-κB that was dependent on the concentration of protein in the medium.[350] Furthermore, the liberation of these molecules was noted to be predominantly from the basolateral aspect of the cells. This would be in keeping with secretion into the renal interstitium *in vivo*, thereby contributing to the development of tubulo-interstitial inflammation and fibrosis. Exposure of tubule cells to albumin has also been shown to result in increased levels of intracellular reactive oxygen species and activation of the signal transducer and activator of transcription (STAT) signaling pathway.[353] The STAT pathway in turn mediates a variety of cellular responses including proliferation and induction of cytokines as well as growth factors. Preliminary evidence suggests that exposure of tubule cells to albumin may also induce apoptosis.[354] Other experiments have found apoptosis in tubule cells exposed to high molecular weight plasma proteins but not smaller proteins.[355] Despite this evidence, other investigators have raised important concerns regarding the interpretation of these observations.[356] They point out that the concentrations of plasma proteins used *in vitro* were non-physiological and far exceeded those observed in proximal tubule fluid from experimental models of nephrotic syndrome. Furthermore many of the experiments were performed in cells that were routinely cultured in the presence of high concentrations of protein (serum) that may significantly alter their phenotype. Finally, not all investigators have been able to confirm the observations. In particular some have found proliferative or profibrotic responses when proximal tubule cells are exposed to serum or serum fractions, but no response after exposure to purified forms of albumin or transferrin, suggesting that factors other than albumin or transferrin may be involved.[357,358] Thus uncertainty remains regarding the potential tubulotoxic effect of filtered plasma proteins in proteinuric CKD and the specific identity of filtered molecules that may contribute to kidney damage.[356]

Several lines of evidence suggest that proteins other than albumin or immunoglobulin may indeed play a role in the progression of chronic nephropathies. It has been proposed that free fatty acids (FFA) bound to albumin may play an important role provoking a proinflammatory response in tubule cells. In one experiment albumin-bound fatty acids stimulated macrophage chemotactic activity whereas delipidated albumin did not.[359] Albumin-bound FFA has also been shown to activate peroxisome proliferator activated-receptors (PPAR)-γ and induce apoptosis in proximal tubule cells.[360] HDL and LDL have been identified in the urine, renal interstitium and tubule cells in renal biopsies of patients with nephrotic syndrome. In vitro, cultured human proximal tubule epithelial cells take up LDL and HDL.[361] Oxidized LDL may cause tubular cell injury and exposure of tubular epithelial cells to HDL is associated with increased synthesis of endothelin-1.[361,362] A role has also been proposed for other compounds bound to filtered proteins such as IGF-1, which has been detected in increased amounts in the proximal tubular fluid of rats with adriamycin nephrosis. Proximal tubule cells cultured in the presence of proximal tubular fluid from nephrotic rats exhibit enhanced cell proliferation and increased secretion of type I and type IV collagen. Both effects were inhibited by neutralizing IGF-1 receptor antibodies.[363] Other growth factors in plasma including HGF and TFG-β may also appear in glomerular ultrafiltrate with proteinuria and exert effects on tubule cells.[364] Furthermore cytokines produced in injured glomeruli may have downstream proinflammatory effects. Whereas complement components are normally absent from tubular fluid, C3 and C5b-9 neoantigen were observed along the luminal border of tubule epithelial cells in the protein overload proteinuria model. To examine the role of filtered complement in renal injury, rats with puromycin aminonucleoside nephrosis were subjected to complement depletion with cobra venom factor or inhibition of complement activation by administration of soluble recombinant human complement receptor type 1, before the onset of proteinuria. In control rats, proximal tubular degeneration, interstitial leukocyte infiltrate, and renal impairment (as assessed by inulin and para-aminohippurate (PAH) clearances) occurred at 7 days, together with positive staining for C3 and C5b-9 along the proximal tubule brush border. Both interventions were associated with significantly less tubulointerstitial pathology and greater clearance of PAH but not inulin, whereas the severity of the proteinuria was unaffected, suggesting that filtered complement plays a significant role in the tubulointerstitial injury associated with proteinuria.[365] A more selective approach, using recombinant complement inhibitory molecules targeted to proximal tubule cells with carrier antibodies to brush border antigen resulted in significant reduction of interstitial fibrosis in the same model.[366]

In experimental models of proteinuric renal disease, filtered proteins have also been found to accumulate in the glomerular mesangium[344] and may therefore contribute to glomerular as well as tubulointerstitial injury. Further support for this notion is derived from a meta-analysis of 57 studies of experimental CKD that found a consistent positive correlation between the severity of proteinuria and the extent of glomerulosclerosis.[367] Lipoproteins, in particular, accumulate in the glomeruli of patients with glomerulonephritis.[368,369] Furthermore, low density lipoprotein (LDL) stimulates

mesangial cells to proliferate in vitro[370,371] and enhances mesangial cell synthesis of the extracellular matrix protein, fibronectin.[372] LDL exposure is also associated with increased mesangial cell mRNA levels for MCP-1,[372] and PDGF.[371] Oxidation of LDL by mesangial cells or macrophages may enhance its toxicity.[370] Thus, accumulation of proteins in the mesangium may stimulate a number of different mechanisms that contribute to glomerulosclerosis.

The relevance of these findings to the processes occurring in vivo has been borne out by studies in rats. In the protein-overload model, the development of proteinuria at 1 week was associated with significant increases in TGF-β at both protein and mRNA levels, in interstitial as well as proximal tubule cells.[347] Similarly, renal cortical mRNA levels encoding the macrophage chemoattractant, osteopontin, were increased on day 4 and immunofluorescence localized increased osteopontin staining to cortical tubules at day 7. MCP-1 and osteopontin mRNA and protein levels were elevated at 2 and 3 weeks. Furthermore, a significant effect of proteinuria on molecules involved in ECM protein turnover was observed. Although mRNA levels for various renal matrix proteins were variable, staining for the proteins in the cortical interstitium increased progressively. Levels of mRNA for the protease inhibitors plasminogen activator inhibitor-1 (PAI-1) and tissue inhibitor of metalloproteinases-1 (TIMP-1) were elevated at 2 weeks, at which time significant renal fibrosis was present.[347] Gene expression profiling has identified over 100 genes that are up-regulated in the proximal tubule cells of mice exposed to overload proteinuria.[373] Consistent with the hypothesis that protein-bound FFA are important, rats receiving FFA-replete bovine serum albumin (BSA) developed more severe tubulointerstitial injury and more extensive macrophage infiltration than those receiving FFA-depleted BSA.[374,375] In other models of proteinuric renal disease including 5/6 nephrectomy and passive Heymann nephritis, accumulation of albumin and IgG by proximal tubule cells occurred before infiltration of the interstitium by macrophages and MHC-II positive mononuclear cells. The infiltrates localized to areas where proximal tubule cells stained positive for intracellular IgG, or where luminal casts were present. Furthermore, proximal tubule cells that stained positive for IgG also showed evidence of increased osteopontin production.[376] The IgG staining in proximal tubule cells was subsequently associated with peritubular accumulation of macrophages and α-smooth muscle actin positive cells as well as up-regulation of TFG-β mRNA in the tubular and infiltrating cells.[377] The importance of inflammatory factors in the development of interstitial fibrosis is illustrated by the observation that treatment of rats with experimental membranous nephropathy with rapamycin was associated with reduced expression of profibrotic and proinflammatory genes as well as amelioration of interstitial inflammation and fibrosis.[378] Further studies in the 5/6 nephrectomy model have suggested that tubulo-interstitial injury may play an important role in the decline of GFR, especially in the late stages of progressive renal injury.[379] By examining serial sections of remnant kidneys, the investigators were able to show that in association with a doubling in serum creatinine, there was a substantial increase in the proportion of glomeruli no longer connected to glomeruli (atubular glomeruli) or connected to atrophic tubules. The majority of these glomeruli were not globally sclerosed, implying that the tubular injury was responsible for the final loss of function in these glomeruli. The authors speculate that the absorption of excess filtered protein may play an important role in this tubular injury.[379] Finally evidence is accumulating of the role of proteinuria in the development of interstitial damage in human CKD. Among 215 patients with CKD, urine albumin to creatinine ratio (ACR) correlated with urinary MCP-1 levels and interstitial macrophage numbers. Furthermore urine ACR and interstitial macrophage number independently predicted renal survival.[380]

Establishing a cause-effect relationship between proteinuria and renal damage in humans is difficult but several clinical studies provide evidence in support of this notion. A meta-analysis of 17 clinical studies of CKD revealed a positive correlation between the severity of proteinuria and the extent of biopsy-proven glomerulosclerosis.[367] Observations from the Modification of Diet in Renal Disease (MDRD) trial also suggest that proteinuria is an independent determinant of CKD progression: greater levels of baseline proteinuria were strongly associated with more rapid declines in GFR; reduction of proteinuria, independent of reduction in blood pressure, was associated with lesser rates of decline in GFR. Furthermore, the degree of benefit achieved by lowering blood pressure below usual target levels, was highly dependent on the level of baseline proteinuria.[381] The severity of proteinuria at baseline has been shown to be the most important independent predictor of renal outcomes in randomized trials of ACEI or AT$_1$RA treatment in diabetic nephropathy[382] and non-diabetic CKD.[203] Furthermore the percentage reduction in proteinuria over the first 3 to 6 months as well as the absolute level of proteinuria at 3 or 6 months are strong independent predictors of the subsequent rate of decline in GFR among patients with diabetic nephropathy[382] and non-diabetic CKD.[383] A meta-analysis that included data from 1860 patients with non-diabetic CKD confirmed these findings and showed that during antihypertensive treatment, the current level of proteinuria was a powerful predictor of the combined end point of doubling of baseline serum creatinine or onset of ESRD (relative risk 5.56 for each 1.0 g/day of proteinuria).[384] Taken together, the evidence from experimental and clinical studies provides support for the hypothesis that impaired glomerular permselectivity results in excessive filtration of proteins and/or protein-bound molecules that contribute to kidney damage but many questions regarding the tubulotoxic potential of filtered plasma proteins and the identity of the specific molecules involved remain unanswered. Despite these uncertainties, the close association between the severity of proteinuria and renal prognosis implies that reduction of proteinuria should be regarded as an important independent therapeutic goal in clinical strategies seeking to slow the rate of progression of CKD.

INSIGHTS FROM MODIFIERS OF CHRONIC KIDNEY DISEASE PROGRESSION

Pharmacological Inhibition of the Renin-Angiotensin System

Experimental evidence showing a central role for AII in mechanisms of CKD progression through hemodynamic and non-hemodynamic effects has been borne out in randomized clinical trails of ACEI and AT$_1$RA treatment in patients with all forms of CKD. ACEI treatment has been shown to be renoprotective in patients with microalbuminuria and type 2 diabetes mellitus,[385] type 1 diabetes and overt nephropathy,[202] as well as non-diabetic CKD.[203,206,386,387] Treatment with an AT$_1$RA affords renoprotection in patients with type 2 diabetes and microalbuminuria[388] or overt nephropathy.[204,205] Furthermore at least one large randomized study has reported additional renoprotective benefit among patients with non-diabetic CKD who received combination ACEI and AT$_1$RA treatment versus monotherapy.[389] Evidence is also accumulating that AT$_1$RA treatment at doses higher than previously recommended affords additional renoprotection.[390] One meta-analysis has called into question the importance of RAS inhibition[391] but

it should be noted that this study was dominated by data from the Antihypertensive and Lipid Lowering Treatment to Prevent Heart Attack (ALLHAT) study, which found no difference in fatal coronary heart disease or non-fatal myocardial infarction among hypertensive patients with at least one cardiovascular risk factor randomized to treatment with a thiazide diuretic, a calcium channel blocker or an ACEI.[392] In a *post hoc* analysis there was also no difference in the secondary outcome of ESRD or >50% decrement in GFR but patients with serum creatinine >2 mg/dl were specifically excluded resulting in only a minority of patients (5662 of 33,357) having renal disease (estimated GFR < 60 ml/min/1.73m^2). Furthermore, there was no assessment of proteinuria.[393] Thus inclusion of the ALLHAT data was inappropriate and significantly affected the results of the meta-analysis.[394] Other meta-analyses that did not include ALLHAT data have shown significant renoprotective benefit in patients receiving ACEI treatment.[395,396] In summary there is now evidence from multiple randomized trials showing significant renoprotection associated with pharmacological inhibition of the RAS in a wide variety of forms of CKD, confirming that AII is a critical mediator of mechanisms of CKD progression in humans and providing support for the consensus that RAS inhibition should be central to treatment strategies for slowing CKD progression.[397] The role of RAS inhibitor treatment in achieving optimal renoprotection is discussed further in Chapter 54.

Arterial Hypertension

Malignant hypertension frequently leads to renal injury, but whether or not less severe forms of hypertension cause "hypertensive nephrosclerosis" remains a subject of debate.[398,399] An increased risk of developing progressive renal failure with higher levels of blood pressure has been observed in several population-based studies[400–403] and is exemplified by findings from the Multiple Risk Factors Intervention Trial (MRFIT).[404] In a population of 332,544 men there was a strong, graded relationship between blood pressure and the risk of developing or dying with ESRD over a 15- to 17-year follow-up period. Renal function was not assessed at screening or during follow-up, however, so it is not possible to establish with any certainty whether higher blood pressure initiated renal disease or accelerated a nephropathy that was already present. In one study the importance of hypertension as a risk factor for ESRD was further illustrated by the observation that lowering systolic blood pressure by 20 mm Hg reduced the risk of ESRD by two thirds.[401] Even small increases in blood pressure, below the threshold usually used to define hypertension, are associated with an increased risk of ESRD.[400,402,405] Hypertension has also been identified as a risk factor for developing albuminuria or renal impairment among patients with type 2 diabetes mellitus.[406]

Whereas the role of hypertension in initiating renal disease requires further clarification, there is clear evidence that hypertension accelerates the rate of progression of preexisting renal disease, most likely through transmission of raised hydraulic blood pressure to the glomerulus resulting in exacerbation of glomerular capillary hypertension associated with nephron loss.[2] Among patients with diabetic nephropathy and non-diabetic CKD, the initiation of antihypertensive therapy results in significant reductions in rates of GFR decline implying that hypertension, an almost universal consequence of impaired renal function, also contributes to the progression of CKD.[407] The potential impact of hypertension on the kidney is exemplified by case reports of patients with unilateral renal artery stenosis who manifested diabetic nephropathy or focal segmental glomerulosclerosis only in the non-stenotic kidney, and not in the stenotic side that was shielded from the hypertension.[408,409] Uncertainty remains, however, as to what level of blood pressure lowering is required to achieve optimal renoprotection. Several randomized trials have sought to resolve this issue. In the Modification of Diet in Renal Disease (MDRD) study patients with predominantly non-diabetic CKD were randomized to a target MAP of <92 mm Hg (equivalent to <125/75 mm Hg) versus <107 mm Hg (equivalent to 140/90 mm Hg). Whereas there was no difference between the overall rate of change in GFR during a mean of 2.2 years follow-up, patients randomized to the low blood pressure target evidenced an early rapid decrease in GFR, likely due to associated renal hemodynamic effects, which obscured a later significantly slower rate of GFR decline. Furthermore the effect of blood pressure control was strongly modulated by the severity of proteinuria. Among patients with >3 g/day of proteinuria at baseline, randomization to the low blood pressure target was associated with a significantly slower rate of GFR decline.[410] Secondary analysis also revealed significant correlations between the rate of GFR decline and *achieved* blood pressure, an effect that was more marked among those with greater baseline proteinuria.[411] In study 1 (patients with GFR of 25–55 ml/min/1.73m^2), rates of GFR decline increased above a MAP of 98 mm Hg among patients with baseline proteinuria of 0.25–3.0 g/day, and above 92 mm Hg in those with baseline proteinuria >3.0 g/day. In study 2 (patients with GFR of 13–24 ml/min/m^2), higher achieved blood pressure was associated with greater rates of GFR decline at all levels among patients with baseline proteinuria >1 g/day (Fig. 25–6). That the benefits of lower blood pressure may become evident only over a longer period is illustrated by the observation that further follow-up (mean 6.6 years) of patients from the MDRD study revealed a significant reduction in the risk of ESRD (adjusted HR 0.68; 95%CI 0.57–0.82) or a combined end point of ESRD or death (adjusted HR 0.77; 95%CI 0.65–0.91) among patients randomized to the low blood pressure target even though treatment and blood pressure data were not available beyond the 2.2 years of the original trial.[412] In the African American Study of Kidney Disease and Hypertension (AASK) no significant difference in the rate of GFR decline was observed between patients randomized to a MAP goals of ≤92 mm Hg versus 102 mm Hg to 107 mm Hg. It should be noted, however, that patients in AASK generally had low levels of baseline proteinuria (mean urine protein 0.38–0.63 g/day).[387] Thus the MDRD and AASK study results support the notion that lower blood pressure targets afford additional renoprotection in patients with more severe proteinuria. Because not all the patients in the MDRD study received ACEI treatment, it remained unclear to what extent the level of blood pressure attained is important in CKD patients receiving ACEI or AT$_1$RA treatment. Experimental studies have found systolic blood pressure to be a major determinant of glomerular injury in rats receiving either ACEI or AT$_1$RA treatment.[190,413] Moreover among patients with type 1 diabetes and established nephropathy receiving ACEI treatment, randomization to a low (MAP < 92 mm Hg) versus "usual" (MAP = 100–107 mm Hg) blood pressure target was associated with significantly lower levels of proteinuria after 2 years, although there was no significant difference in GFR decline.[414] On the other hand intensive blood pressure control was not associated with significantly improved renal function among patients with autosomal dominant polycystic kidney disease but, by the authors' own admission, the study may not have had adequate statistical power to detect such a difference.[415] Furthermore, additional blood pressure reduction with a calcium channel blocker in patients with non-diabetic CKD on ACEI treatment failed to produce additional renoprotection but the degree of additional blood pressure reduction was modest (4.1/2.8 mm Hg) and may have been insufficient to improve outcomes in patients already receiving optimal ACEI therapy.[416] On the other hand, secondary analysis of data from the Irbesartan Diabetic Nephropathy Trial (IDNT) did show greater renoprotection among patients who achieved lower blood pressure targets such that achieved systolic blood pressure (SBP) >149 mm Hg was associated with a 2.2-fold increased risk of developing ESRD or a doubling of serum creatinine versus achieved SBP < 134 mm Hg.[417] Importantly, the relationship between improved outcomes and lower achieved SBP persisted among those patients treated with irbesartan. A note of caution from this study was the observation that achieved SBP < 120 mm Hg was associated with increased all-cause mortality and no further improvement in renal outcomes.[417] Whereas the results of randomized trials comparing "low" and "usual" blood pressure targets among CKD patients have not yielded unequivocal results, the overall picture is one of lower blood pressure targets being associated with more effective renoprotection among those with more severe proteinuria. These observations have led to a consensus that blood pressure should be lowered to <130/80 mm Hg in all patients with CKD.[397] Available evidence also supports a somewhat lower target blood pressure of <125/75 mm Hg for patients with significant proteinuria (>1 g/day).[411,417]

Dietary Protein Intake

Increased dietary protein intake and intravenous protein loading in animals or humans with intact kidneys are

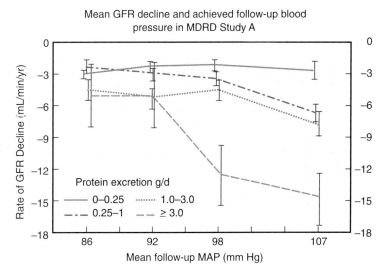

FIGURE 25–6 The interaction of blood pressure reduction and proteinuria at baseline on the rate of decline in glomerular filtration rate. (Reproduced with permission from Peterson JC, Adler S, Burkart JM, et al: Blood pressure control, proteinuria, and the progression of renal disease. The Modification of Diet in Renal Disease Study. Ann Intern Med 123:754–762, 1995.)

associated with increases in renal mass, renal blood flow, and GFR, as well as a decrease in renal vascular resistance. The magnitude of the increases in GFR and renal blood flow in response to a protein load is a function of renal reserve. In patients with renal insufficiency some studies have shown that the percentage increase in GFR in response to a protein meal is reduced in those with a lower baseline GFR.[418,419] In contrast, a study comparing the renal response to an oral protein load in patients with moderate and advanced renal failure found a similar percent increase in GFR over baseline in both groups, demonstrating that even with advanced renal disease, some renal reserve is still present and that elevated intake of dietary protein may have undesirable effects on glomerular hemodynamics at all levels of renal function.[420]

To understand the mechanisms whereby protein loading acutely augments renal function, various components of protein diets have been examined individually: administration of equivalent quantities of urea, sulfate, acid, and vegetable protein to dogs or humans all failed to reproduce a meat protein-induced rise in GFR.[421–423] In contrast, feeding or infusion of mixed or individual amino acids (e.g., glycine, L-arginine) was shown to effect increases in GFR of similar magnitude to those seen with meat ingestion.[424,425] Micropuncture experiments demonstrated that amino acid infusion resulted in increases in glomerular plasma flow and transcapillary hydraulic pressure difference, thereby raising SNGFR without affecting the ultrafiltration coefficient.[424] Interestingly, however, perfusion of the isolated kidney with an amino acid mixture resulted in only a modest increase in GFR.[426] Taken together, these observations suggest that amino acids themselves do not have a major direct effect on renal hemodynamics, but their effects appear to be mediated by an intermediate compound generated only in the intact organism. Glucagon, the secretion of which is stimulated by protein feeding, has been proposed as such a mediator. GFR and renal blood flow increase in response to glucagon infusion in dogs.[425] Furthermore, administration of the glucagon antagonist, somatostatin, consistently blocks amino acid-induced augmentation in renal function both in humans and rats.[424,427] Large protein meals are also rich in minerals, potassium, phosphate, and acids. Indeed, after feeding a protein meal to dogs, the excretions of sodium, potassium, phosphorus, and urea were found to increase in parallel to the increase in GFR.[421] On the other hand, sodium chloride reabsorption in the proximal tubule and loop of Henle was found to be increased in rats maintained on a high protein diet.[428] As result, less sodium and chloride would be delivered to the macula densa, thereby inhibiting tubulo-glomerular feedback and adding a further stimulus to renal hyperemia. Because dietary protein does not affect systemic blood pressure,[424] other factors have been suggested to contribute to the renal hemodynamic changes following a protein load. Administration of the nitric oxide inhibitor L-NMMA or non-steroidal anti-inflammatory agents have been shown to blunt the renal hyperemic response to an oral protein load in both rats and humans, invoking a role for nitric oxide and prostaglandins.[428,429] In addition, AII and endothelin have been proposed as mediators of protein-induced renal injury as low protein diets have been shown to reduce renal endothelin-1, endothelin receptors A and B, and AT$_1$ receptor mRNA expression in PAN-injected and normal rats.[430,431]

It has been proposed that the augmented renal function induced by dietary protein may be an evolutionary adaptation of the kidney to the intermittent heavy protein intake of the hunter-gatherer.[3] Renal hyperfunction following a protein load would serve to facilitate excretion of the waste products of protein catabolism and other dietary components thereby achieving homeostasis in the face of an abrupt increase in consumption in times of nutritional plenty; the subsequent decline of GFR to baseline during the intervals between meals would then favor mechanisms suited to conservation of fluid and electrolytes in times of scarcity. Persistent renal hyperfunction due to continuous excessive protein intake, however, leads to renal injury in experimental models. Laboratory animals with intact kidneys and ingesting food *ad libitum* become proteinuric and develop glomerulosclerosis with age.[3,131,432] This progression was significantly attenuated by feeding animals on alternate days only.[131] Furthermore, aging rats fed a high protein diet *ad libitum* showed marked acceleration and increased severity of renal injury compared to rats receiving a normal protein diet, whereas rats fed a low protein diet were protected from renal injury.[432] Similarly, in diabetic rats, progression of nephropathy was markedly accelerated in the setting of a high protein diet and substantially attenuated by a low protein diet.[180] In this study, kidney weight in high-protein-fed diabetic rats was significantly greater than in diabetic rats receiving normal protein diets, suggesting that protein-induced renal hypertrophy may itself contribute to acceleration of renal functional deterioration. As discussed earlier, the renoprotective effects of dietary protein restriction in experimental animals are associated with virtual normalization of P$_{GC}$ and SNGFR.[6]

Despite unambiguous evidence from experimental studies, confirmation of a beneficial effect of protein restriction in clinical trials has proved elusive. Following the publication of several smaller studies that generally suggested a beneficial effect from protein restriction but that suffered from deficiencies in design or patient compliance, a large, multicenter, randomized study, the MDRD study, was conducted to resolve the issue.[410] Five hundred eighty-five patients with moderate chronic renal failure (GFR = 25–55 ml/min/1.73m^2) were randomized to "usual" (1.3 g/kg/day) or "low" (0.58 g/kg/day) protein diet (study 1) and 255 patients with severe chronic renal failure (GFR = 13–24 ml/min/1.73m^2) to "low" (0.58 g/kg/day) or "very low" (0.28 g/kg/day) protein diet. All causes of CKD were included but patients with diabetes mellitus requiring insulin therapy were excluded. Patients were also assigned to different levels of blood pressure control. After a mean of 2.2 years follow-up, the primary analysis revealed no difference in the mean rate of GFR decline in study 1, and only a trend toward a slower rate of decline in the "very low" protein group in study 2. Secondary analyses of the MDRD data, however, revealed that dietary protein restriction probably did achieve beneficial effects. In study 1 "low" protein diet was associated with an initial reduction in GFR that likely resulted from the functional effects of decreased protein intake and not from loss of nephrons. This initial reduction in GFR obscured a later reduction in the rate of GFR decline that was evident after 4 months in the "low" protein group and that may have resulted in more robust evidence of renoprotection had follow-up been continued for a longer period.[433] Despite inconclusive findings in several of the individual studies, three meta-analyses have each concluded that dietary protein restriction is associated with a reduced risk of ESRD (odds ratio of 0.62 and 0.67, respectively)[434,435] as well as a modest reduction in the rate of estimated GFR decline (0.53 ml/min/year).[436] Whereas the renoprotective benefit of dietary protein restriction in humans appears modest, such dietary restriction is associated with other benefits including improvement in acidosis as well as reduction in phosphorus and potassium load. Thus comprehensive dietary intervention with a moderate restriction in dietary protein intake should remain an important part of the treatment of patients with CKD.[437] The interaction of diet and kidney disease is discussed further in Chapter 53.

Gender

Laboratory studies indicate that male animals appear to be at greater risk of developing renal disease and of disease progression than females. Age-associated glomerulosclerosis is much more pronounced in male than in female rats and it is notable that the male propensity for age-related glomerulosclerosis can be prevented by castration.[438] This gender difference was found to be independent of P_{GC} or glomerular hypertrophy, suggesting a role for the sex hormones as modulators of renal injury. Ovariectomy, on the other hand, had no effect on the development of glomerular injury seen in nonovariectomized female rats, implying that the presence of androgens, and not the lack of estrogens promotes renal injury.[438,439] By contrast, in the hypercholesterolemic Imai rat the development of spontaneous glomerulosclerosis in males can be significantly reduced by castration, or by administration of exogenous estrogens.[440,441] These data again suggest an important role for androgens in the development of renal injury, and raise the possibility that estrogens may to some extent counteract the adverse effects of androgens. In an apparently conflicting observation, female Nagase analbuminemic rats develop renal injury of greater severity than males, a characteristic that is ameliorated by ovariectomy.[442] These rats may be unique, however, in that triglyceride levels, which are higher in females, may have an independent and overriding effect on renal disease propensity. Glomerulosclerosis also develops to a significantly greater extent in male versus female rats subjected to extensive renal ablation.[443] This difference was independent of blood pressure and glomerular hypertrophy, but the degree of glomerulosclerosis and the extent of mesangial expansion each were found to correlate significantly with an increased expression of glomerular procollagen $\alpha1(IV)$ mRNA in males. Similarly, in aging Munich-Wistar rats, glomerular metalloproteinase activity was found to decrease with age in males but not in females or castrated rats, suggesting that suppression of metalloproteinase activity by androgens could account for the gender difference in disease susceptibility.[444] Finally, estrogens, but not androgens possess anti-oxidant activity and have been shown to inhibit mesangial cell LDL oxidation,[445] a property that may contribute to renoprotection.

Clinical studies suggest that humans also evidence a gender difference with respect to CKD progression. Data from the United States Renal Data System show a substantially higher incidence of ESRD among males (413/million population in 2003) versus females (280/million population)[446] and several studies have reported worse renal outcomes in males. In a Japanese community-based mass screening program the risk of developing ESRD (if baseline serum creatinine was greater than 1.2 mg/dl for males or 1 mg/dl for females) was almost 50% higher in men than in women.[447] In a large population-based study in the United States, male gender was associated with a significantly increased risk of ESRD or death associated with CKD.[402] Similarly, in France, studies of factors influencing development of ESRD in patients with moderate and severe renal disease found that disease progression was accelerated in males versus females, especially in those with chronic glomerulonephritis or ADPKD. Furthermore, the effect of hypertension as a risk factor for CKD progression appeared to be greater in males.[448,449] Other studies of patients with established CKD have reported a lower risk of ESRD among female patients with CKD stage 3[450] and a shorter time to renal replacement therapy among male patients with CKD stage 4 and 5.[451] One meta-analysis of 68 studies that included 11,345 patients with CKD reported a higher rate of decline in renal function in men[452] but another meta-analysis of individual patient data from 11 randomized trials evaluating the efficacy of ACEI treatment in CKD did not show an increased risk of doubling of serum creatinine or ESRD, or ESRD alone among men.[453] On the contrary, after adjustment for baseline variables including blood pressure and urinary protein excretion women evidenced a significantly higher risk of these end points than men.[453] One limitation of these studies is that the

menopausal status of the women was often not documented. In general, the prevalence of hypertension and uncontrolled hypertension is higher among men; men tend to consume more protein than women; the prevalence of dyslipidemias is greater in men than premenopausal women. All of these factors may contribute to the increased severity of renal disease observed in men but they do not explain all of the differences.[454,455] The role of gender in kidney disease is extensively reviewed in Chapter 20.

Nephron Endowment

Experimental and clinical studies have shown that the number of nephrons per kidney is variable and may be influenced by several factors during development *in utero*. Furthermore low nephron endowment predisposes individuals to CKD. It has been proposed that reduced nephron endowment results in an increase in single nephron GFR and therefore a reduction in renal reserve.[456] Whereas the glomerular hemodynamic changes associated with mild-moderate congenital nephron deficiencies may not in themselves be sufficient to provoke renal injury, they could be predicted to compound the effects of an acquired nephron loss and predispose the individual to progressive renal damage. Thus CKD should be viewed as a "multi-hit" process in which the first "hit" may be reduced nephron endowment.[457] Nephron endowment is discussed in detail in Chapter 19.

Ethnicity

African Americans comprise only 12.4% of the total U.S. population but account for 30.8% of the U.S. ESRD population.[458] In the age group from 20 to 44 years, there are 18 African Americans for every white patient with ESRD.[459] The reasons for this obvious discrepancy are complex and include both social and biological factors.[460,461] Interestingly, data from the Reasons for Geographic and Racial Differences in Stroke (REGARDS) Cohort Study show a lower prevalence of estimated GFR 50–59 ml/min/1.73m² among Africa American versus white subjects but a higher prevalence of estimated GFR 10–19 ml/min/1.73m² suggesting that African Americans have a lower risk of developing CKD but a higher risk of progression of CKD to ESRD.[462]

African Americans appear to be more susceptible to focal and segmental glomerulosclerosis (FSGS). One retrospective analysis of 340 routine kidney biopsies detected a significantly higher prevalence of FSGS and a significantly lower prevalence of membranous glomerulonephritis, IgA, and immunotactoid nephropathies among black versus white patients.[463] Similarly, among pediatric transplant recipients a higher proportion of African American and Hispanic children had FSGS as a primary diagnosis versus whites.[464] The same investigators found that despite similar treatment modalities and similar durations of nephrotic syndrome, black children with FSGS reached ESRD almost twice as frequently as white children.[464]

More significant in terms of patient numbers and morbidity, however, are the racial discrepancies in the incidence of ESRD due to hypertensive and diabetic nephropathies. Among hypertensive patients undergoing treatment, the risk of decline in renal function in black patients was found to be almost twice that of whites.[465] This finding of increased risk persisted after controlling for the effects of diabetes, blood pressure levels, heart failure, and male gender. Similarly, in the MRFIT trial, despite similar levels of blood pressure control in black versus white men, renal function deteriorated more rapidly in the black men.[466] MDRD study data showed the prevalence of hypertension to be higher in blacks versus whites among patients with CKD, despite a higher mean GFR in the black patients.[455] Hypertensive patients were found to have had more rapid progression of renal disease prior to entry into the study, suggesting that the higher prevalence of hypertension in black patients is likely to be a significant contributor to accelerated progression of CKD. On the other hand both higher mean arterial pressure and black race were independent predictors of a faster decline in GFR in the MDRD study.[467] In a large community-based epidemiological study, black patients were found to have a 5.6 times higher unadjusted incidence of hypertensive ESRD with respect to the entire study population.[468] This increased incidence was directly related to the prevalence of hypertension, severe hypertension, and diabetes in the study population, and inversely related to age at diagnosis of hypertension and socioeconomic status. After adjustment for these factors the risk of hypertensive ESRD remained 4.5 times greater among blacks compared to whites, providing further evidence that black patients have an increased susceptibility to renal disease beyond that attributable to their increased prevalence of hypertension and diabetes. Salt-sensitive hypertension, in particular, is more prevalent in the black population than in the white population.[469] Comparing renal responses to a high sodium intake in salt-sensitive versus salt-resistant patients, renal blood flow was found to decrease in the face of an increased filtration fraction (implying an increased P_{GC}) in salt-sensitive patients whereas the converse occurred in salt-resistant patients.[398] These observations are consistent with the notion that salt loading injures the glomerulus through glomerular capillary hypertension and that salt-sensitive individuals, and blacks in particular, are at added risk of this form of injury. The incidence of ESRD due to diabetic nephropathy is fourfold higher among African Americans than among white Americans.[458] It is notable that after controlling for the higher prevalence of diabetes and hypertension as well as age, socioeconomic status, and access to health care, the excess incidence of ESRD due to diabetes in blacks versus whites was confined to type 2 diabetics.[470] Among type 1 diabetics, blacks were not found to be at higher risk than whites. Indeed, the majority of blacks with diabetic ESRD (77%) had type 2 diabetes whereas the majority of whites with diabetic ESRD (58%) had type 1 diabetes.[471] Black race was also found to be associated with a threefold higher risk of early renal function decline (increase in serum creatinine of ≥0.4 mg/dl) among adults with diabetes.[472]

Several potential factors contributing to the different prevalence and severity of renal disease among population groups have been analyzed. Adjustment for socioeconomic factors reduces, but does not eliminate the increased risk of African Americans to develop ESRD.[458,461,472] African Americans have lower birth weights than their white counterparts and may therefore have programmed or genetically determined deficits in nephron number, rendering them more susceptible to hypertension and subsequent ESRD.[473,474] Finally, 40% of African-American patients with hypertensive ESRD and 35% with type 2 diabetes associated ESRD have first-, second-, or third-degree relatives with ESRD implying a strong familial susceptibility to ESRD and therefore a genetic predisposition.[475] Other ethnic groups including Asians,[406,476] Hispanics,[477] Native Americans,[478] Mexican Americans,[479] and Australian Aboriginals[480] have also been found to be at increased risk of developing CKD and ESRD.

Obesity and Metabolic Syndrome

Obesity may directly cause a glomerulopathy characterized by proteinuria and histological features of focal and segmental glomerulosclerosis[481] but it is likely that it also exacerbates progression of other forms of CKD. Micropuncture studies have confirmed that obesity is another cause of glomerular hypertension and hyperfiltration that may contribute to the progression of CKD.[482,483] Detailed investigation of adipocyte function has revealed that they are not merely storage cells but produce a variety of hormones and proinflammatory molecules that may contribute to progressive renal damage.[484] In humans severe obesity is associated with increased renal plasma flow, glomerular hyperfiltration, and albuminuria, abnormalities that are reversed by weight loss.[485] Several large population-based studies have identified obesity as a risk factor for developing CKD[403,486] and one study has found a progressive increase in relative risk of developing ESRD associated with increasing body mass index (BMI) (RR 3.57; CI 3.05–4.18 for BMI 30.0–34.9kg/m² versus BMI 18.5–24.9kg/m²) among 320,252 subjects with no evidence of CKD at initial screening.[487] The metabolic syndrome (insulin resistance) defined by the presence of abdominal obesity, dyslipidemia, hypertension, and fasting hyperglycemia is also associated with an increased risk of developing CKD. Analysis of the Third National Health and Nutrition Examination Survey (NHANES) data revealed a significantly increased risk of CKD and microalbuminuria in subjects with the metabolic syndrome as well as a progressive increase in risk associated with the number of components of the metabolic syndrome present.[488] Furthermore, a longitudinal study of 10,096 patients without diabetes or CKD at baseline identified metabolic syndrome as an independent risk factor for the development of CKD over 9 years (adjusted OR 1.43; 95%CI 1.18–1.73). Again there was a progressive increase in risk associated with the number of traits of the metabolic syndrome present (OR 1.13; 95%CI 0.89–1.45 for one trait versus OR 2.45; 95%CI 1.32–4.54 for five traits).[489] Patient hip-waist ratio, a marker insulin resistance, was independently associated with impaired renal function even in lean individuals (BMI < 25 kg/m²) among a population-based cohort of 7676 subjects.[490] The effect of obesity on progression in cohorts of patients with established CKD is less well documented. In one study increased BMI was an independent predictor CKD progression among 162 patients with IgA Nephropathy.[491] On the other hand, obesity may be less relevant to progression in more advanced stages of CKD as evidenced by the observation that BMI was unrelated to the risk of ESRD among a cohort of patients with CKD stage 4 and 5.[451]

Sympathetic Nervous System

Overactivity of the sympathetic nervous system has been observed in patients with CKD and several lines of evidence suggest that this may be another factor that contributes to progressive renal injury.[492] The kidneys are richly supplied with afferent sensory and efferent sympathetic innervation and may therefore act as both a source and target of sympathetic activation. That the former is true is suggested by a study that compared postganglionic sympathetic nerve activity (SNA) measured via microelectrodes in the peroneal nerve in normal individuals and hemodialysis patients subdivided into those who retained their native kidneys and those who had undergone bilateral nephrectomy.[493] SNA was 2.5 times higher in non-nephrectomized dialysis patients compared to both normals and nephrectomized patients, in whom SNA was similar. Furthermore, increased SNA was associated with increased vascular tone and mean arterial blood pressure in non-nephrectomized patients. SNA did not vary as a function of age, blood pressure, antihypertensive agents, or body fluid status. The authors speculated that intrarenal accumulation of uremic compounds stimulates renal afferent nerves via chemoreceptors, leading to reflex activation of efferent sympathetic nerves and increased SNA. Other studies, however, have observed increased SNA in the absence of uremia in patients with renovascular disease,[494] hypertensive ADPKD,[495] and non-diabetic CKD[496] or increased noradrenaline secretion in patients with nephrotic syndrome[497] and ADPKD.[495,498] Furthemore, correction of uremia by renal transplantation does not abrogate the increased SNA.[499] Interestingly, investigation of eight living kidney donors found no increase in SNA after donor nephrectomy, suggesting that the rise in SNA is related to renal damage rather than nephron loss.[496] Together, these findings suggest that a variety of forms of renal injury may provoke increased SNA and that uremia is not required for this response.

Evidence from experimental studies indicates that sympathetic overactivity resulting from renal disease may also accelerate renal injury. Ablation of afferent sensory signals from the kidneys by bilateral dorsal rhizotomy in 5/6 nephrectomized rats prevented the expected rise in systemic blood pressure, attenuated the rise in serum creatinine, and reduced the severity of glomerulosclerosis in the remnant kidneys when compared with sham rhizotomized controls.[500] To further investigate whether these benefits were solely attributable to the prevention of hypertension, 5/6 nephrectomized rats were treated with non-hypotensive doses of the sympatholytic drug moxonidine.[501] Despite the lack of effect on blood pressure, moxonidine treatment was associated with lower levels of proteinuria and less severe glomerulosclerosis than untreated rats. In a similar study, 5/6 nephrectomized rats were treated the α-blocker, phenoxybenzamine, the β-blocker, metoprolol, or a combination.[502] As in the previous study, the doses used did not lower blood pressure, but all three treatments significantly lowered albuminuria and almost normalized the reductions in capillary length density (an index of glomerular capillary obliteration) and podocyte number. Metoprolol and combination therapy significantly lowered the glomerulosclerosis index versus untreated controls. Taken together, these results indicate that increased SNA accelerates renal injury independent of its effect on blood pressure, and that the adverse effects are not mediated by sympathetic cotransmitters but by catecholamines. Furthermore, sympathetic nerve overactivity has been proposed to contribute to the development of tubulointerstitial injury by reducing of peritubular capillary perfusion to the extent that tubular and interstitial ischemia result.[503]

Preliminary evidence suggests that sympathetic overactivity may also be important in the progression of human CKD. Among patients with type 1 diabetes mellitus and proteinuria, evidence of parasympathetic dysfunction (that permits unopposed sympathetic tone) was associated with an increase in serum creatinine over the next 12 months.[504] Furthermore, among 15 normotensive type 1 diabetics, 3 weeks' treatment moxonidine significantly lowered albumin excretion rates without affecting blood pressure.[505] In other studies, chronic treatment with an ACEI or AT$_1$RA, of proven benefit in renoprotection, was associated with a reduction in sympathetic overactivity.[506,507] In contrast, treatment with amlodipine was associated with increased SNA. Because ACEIs and AT$_1$RAs do not readily enter the CNS, it is possible that RAS inhibition modulates neurotransmitter release in the kidney and reduces afferent signaling. Several questions remain to be answered regarding the role of increased SNA in CKD progression. Whereas the renoprotective effects of sympatholytic drugs appear to be independent of effects on systemic blood pressure, it is as yet unknown what effect they have on glomerular hemodynamics. Further studies are also required to determine the extent to which chronic inhibition of sympathetic overactivity may be beneficial in a variety of forms of human CKD and whether or not this benefit is additive to that derived from ACEI treatment.

Dyslipidemia

Moorhead and colleagues advanced the hypothesis that abnormalities in lipid metabolism may contribute to the progression of CKD.[508] Glomerular injury, accompanied by an alteration in basement membrane permeability, was envisaged as the initiator of a vicious cycle of hyperlipidemia and progressive glomerular injury. They proposed that urinary losses of albumin and lipoprotein lipase activators result in an increase in circulating low-density lipoproteins (LDL), which in turn bind to the glomerular basement membrane further impairing its permselectivity; filtered lipoproteins accumulate in the mesangium, stimulating extracellular matrix synthesis and mesangial cell proliferation; filtered LDL is taken up and metabolized by the tubules, leading to cell injury and interstitial disease. Notably, this hypothesis did not propose hyperlipidemia as an initiating factor in renal injury, but rather as a participant in a self-sustaining mechanism of disease progression.

Several lines of experimental evidence confirm the association between dyslipidemia and renal injury. Both intact and uninephrectomized rats with dietary-induced hypercholesterolemia developed more extensive glomerulosclerosis than their normocholesterolemic controls, and the severity of glomerulosclerosis correlated with serum cholesterol levels[509]; aging female Nagase analbuminemic rats (NAR) have endogenous hypertriglyceridemia and hypercholesterolemia and develop proteinuria and glomerulosclerosis by 9 and 18 months of age respectively whereas male NAR have lower lipid levels and have no glomerulosclerosis by 22 months of age.[442] Interestingly, ovariectomy in female NAR lowers triglyceride levels and reduces their renal injury. In seeming contradiction, however, young and aging male Sprague-Dawley rats developed more extensive glomerulosclerosis than age and sex matched NAR, despite increased cholesterol levels in the NAR.[510] Triglyceride levels, however, were lower in the NAR, again suggesting an independent role for triglycerides in lipid-mediated renal injury. Whereas data regarding the role of lipids in initiating renal disease are conflicting, several studies support the notion that dyslipidemia may promote renal damage. Cholesterol feeding has been shown to exacerbate glomerulosclerosis in uninephrectomized rats, pre-diabetic rabbits, rats with puromycin aminonucleoside nephropathy (PAN), and in the unclipped kidney of rats with two kidney, one clip (2-K,1C) hypertension. When hypertension and dyslipidemia are superimposed, a synergistic effect that dramatically accelerates renal functional deterioration is observed.[511,512]

In humans, the extent of the role of lipids in initiation and progression of renal disease remains unclear. At autopsy, a highly significant correlation was found between the presence of systemic atherosclerosis and the percentage of sclerotic glomeruli in normal individuals, fostering speculation that the development of glomerulosclerosis may be analogous to that of atherosclerosis.[513] A study designed to identify the clinical correlates of hypertensive ESRD found a strong association between atherosclerosis and hypertensive ESRD among older white patients.[514] Furthermore, dyslipidemia has been identified in several large studies as a risk factor for subsequent development of CKD in apparently healthy individuals.[403,515,516] The common forms of primary hypercholesterolemia are not associated with an increased incidence of renal disease in the general population but renal injury has been described in association with rare inherited disorders of lipoprotein metabolism.[517,518]

Whereas primary lipid-mediated renal injury is rare among patients with CKD, the latter is frequently accompanied by elevations in serum lipids, as a result of urinary loss of albumin and lipoprotein lipase activators, defective clearance of triglycerides, modification of LDL by advanced glycation end products, reduced plasma oncotic pressure, adverse effects of medication, and underlying systemic diseases.[519,520] Among a cohort of adult patients with CKD, the most frequent lipid abnormalities noted were hypertriglyceridemia, low high density lipoprotein (HDL), and increased apolipoprotein levels.[521] Furthermore, in a study of 631 routine renal biopsies, lipid deposits were detected in non-sclerotic glomeruli in 8.4% of kidneys and staining for apo B was positive in approximately one quarter of biopsies, suggesting that lipid deposition is not infrequent in diverse renal diseases.[368] Several epidemiological studies have found a strong association between CKD progression and dyslipidemia: in the MDRD study, low serum HDL cholesterol was found to be an independent predictor of more rapid rates of decline in GFR[522]; elevated total cholesterol, LDL-cholesterol, and apo B have been found to correlate strongly with GFR decline in CKD patients[523]; hypercholesterolemia was shown to be a predictor of loss of renal function in type 1 and type 2 diabetics[524,525]; among non-diabetic patients CKD advanced more rapidly in patients with hypercholesterolemia and hypertriglyceridemia, independent of blood pressure control[526]; among patients with IgA nephropathy hypertriglyceridemia was independently predictive of progression.[527] Not all studies confirm these findings, however: in the Multiple Risk Factor Intervention Trial (MRFIT), dyslipidemias were not associated with a decline in renal function[466]; in a retrospective analysis of patients with nephrotic syndrome, hypercholesterolemia at diagnosis was not found to be a predictor of renal disease progression.[528] In the latter study, however, both progressors and non-progressors had markedly elevated serum cholesterol levels that may have confounded the analysis. Interpretation of these data is complicated by the fact that in patients with renal insufficiency, dyslipidemias do not occur in isolation and are associated with other factors that also affect renal disease progression including hypertension, hyperglycemia, and proteinuria. Levels of serum cholesterol and triglycerides have been found to correlate with blood pressure and circulating AII levels in type 1 and type 2 diabetics with renal disease and to rise with increasing proteinuria in patients with nephrotic syndrome.[518]

The possible mechanisms whereby hyperlipidemia may contribute to renal injury have not been fully elucidated. Cholesterol feeding has been associated with an increase in mesangial lipid content,[509] glomerular macrophages, and TGF-β as well as fibronectin mRNA levels.[529,530] Furthermore, reduction of glomerular macrophages by whole-body X-irradiation in the setting of nephrotic syndrome, significantly reduced albuminuria without affecting serum lipids, indicating that macrophages play a central role in hyperlipidemic glomerular injury.[530] Mesangial cells express receptors for LDL and uptake is stimulated by vasoconstrictor and mitogenic peptides such as endothelin-1 and PDGF.[371] Metabolism of LDL by mesangial cells leads to increased synthesis of fibronectin and MCP-1, which may contribute to mesangial matrix expansion and recruitment of circulating macrophage/monocytes into the glomerulus.[372] Moreover, triglyceride-rich lipoproteins (very low density lipoprotein, VLDL, and intermediate density lipoprotein, IDL) induce mesangial cell proliferation and elaboration of IL-6, PDGF, and TGF-β in vitro.[531] Mesangial cells, macrophages, and renal tubule cells all have the capacity to oxidize LDL via formation of reactive oxygen species, a step that may be inhibited by antioxidants and HDL.[361,532,533] Oxidized LDL may induce dose-dependent mesangial cell proliferation or mesangial cell death as well as production of TNF-α, eicosanoids, monocyte chemotaxins, and glomerular vasoconstriction. These pathways, together with free radicals generated during LDL oxidation, may each contribute to renal inflammation and injury.[531,532] Hyperlipidemia is also associated with elevated P_{GC}, raising the possibility of a further pathway to glomerulosclerosis via hemodynamic injury.[509] The elevated P_{GC} appears to be mediated, in part, by an increase in renal vascular resistance that occurs in the context of increased plasma viscosity. In diabetic patients, circulating AII levels have been found to correlate with serum cholesterol[534] and both oxidized LDL and lipoprotein(a) have been shown to stimulate renin production by juxtaglomerular

cells in vitro.[533] Moreover, oxidized LDL has been found to reduce nitric oxide synthesis by endothelial cells[533] raising the possibility that alterations in activity of the renin angiotensin system and nitric oxide metabolism could also contribute to the increase in P_{GC} observed with hyperlipidemia.

It would follow that if hyperlipidemia exacerbates renal injury, interventions designed to lower serum lipids should ameliorate disease progression. Treatment with a 3-hydroxyl-3-methylglutaryl coenzyme A (HMG-CoA) reductase inhibitor or clofibric acid in the obese Zucker rat (a strain with endogenous hyperlipidemia and spontaneous glomerulosclerosis) and 5/6 nephrectomized rats (which develop hyperlipidemia secondary to renal insufficiency), resulted in lowering of serum lipid levels, reduction in albuminuria, reduction in mesangial cell DNA synthesis, and attenuation of glomerulosclerosis, despite a lack of effect on either systemic blood pressure or P_{GC}.[9,535] In rats in the nephrotic phase of PAN, HMG-CoA reductase inhibitor treatment resulted in reduction of albuminuria and serum cholesterol, reduction of MCP-1 mRNA expression, and a 77% reduction in glomerular macrophage accumulation.[536] The HMG-CoA reductase inhibitors may therefore exert beneficial effects on renal disease progression, not only by a reducing serum lipid levels, but also by inhibiting mesangial cell proliferation and mechanisms for the recruitment of macrophages due to decreased expression of chemotactic factors and cell adhesion molecules.[537] Cholesterol-fed rats with PAN treated with the antioxidants probucol or vitamin E showed significant reductions in proteinuria and glomerulosclerosis compared to untreated controls.[538] Furthermore, plasma VLDL and LDL from the treated animals were less susceptible to in vitro oxidation and less renal lipid peroxidation was evident, implying that lipid peroxidation plays an important role in renal injury associated with hyperlipidemia. In some clinical studies, dietary or pharmacological lowering of serum lipids has also been associated with a reduction in proteinuria and lower rates of decline in renal function but other studies have failed to demonstrate significant beneficial effects of lipid-lowering therapy on proteinuria or decline of renal function, despite adequate therapeutic reductions in serum lipids. A meta-analysis of 13 small studies that included both diabetic and non-diabetic renal disease found that lipid-lowering therapy significantly reduced the rate of decline in GFR (mean reduction of 1.9 ml/min/year).[539] The results of large clinical trials of lipid lowering therapies in patients with CKD are still awaited. Several secondary analyses of data from clinical trials suggest that lipid-lowering therapy may slow progression in human CKD but these data should be interpreted with caution. Secondary analysis of data from a randomized trial of pravastatin treatment for patients with a history of myocardial infarction found that pravastatin slowed the rate of GFR decline in patients with estimated GFR < 40 ml/min/1.73m², an effect that was also more pronounced in those with proteinuria.[540] Similarly, patients with previous cardiovascular disease or diabetes randomized to simvastatin treatment in the Heart Protection Study evidenced a smaller increase in serum creatinine than those who received placebo.[541] In a placebo-controlled open-label study, atorvastatin treatment in patients with CKD, proteinuria, and hypercholesterolemia was associated with preservation of creatinine clearance whereas those receiving placebo evidenced a significant decline.[542] Whereas these renoprotective effects were associated with cholesterol lowering it is possible that they may also be due to the direct pleiotropic effects of HMG-CoA reductase inhibitors. This notion is further supported by the observation that lipid lowering with fibrates was not associated with preservation of renal function,[543,544] although one study did show reduced progression to microalbuminuria among type 2 diabetics receiving fenofibrate.[545]

Calcium and Phosphate Metabolism

As is the case with many of the adaptations that follow nephron loss, evidence is accumulating that alterations in calcium and phosphate metabolism may also contribute to progressive renal damage. A retrospective analysis of 15 patients with non-progressing CKD (GFR 27–70 mL/min, observed for up to 17 years) revealed that the single feature common to all these patients was an enhanced capacity to excrete phosphate when compared to patients with similar GFR but progressive renal disease.[546] In all of the non-progressors, serum phosphate and calcium remained within normal limits without use of phosphate binders, calcium supplementation, or vitamin D. It is not yet clear which factor is most important but evidence suggests that hyperphosphatemia, renal calcium deposition, hyperparathyroidism, and activated vitamin D deficiency may each play a role.

Hyperphosphatemia

Uninephrectomized rats receiving a high phosphate diet (1%) developed renal calcium and phosphate deposition and tubulointerstitial injury within 5 weeks of nephrectomy.[171] Similar changes were observed in a proportion of intact rats fed a 2% phosphate diet. Phosphate excess, therefore, does appear to have some intrinsic nephrotoxicity that is enhanced in the setting of reduced nephron number. A high phosphate diet has also been associated with the development of parathyroid hyperplasia and hyperparathyroidism in remnant kidney rats.[547] Conversely, in both animals and humans with renal insufficiency, dietary phosphate restriction or treatment with oral phosphate binders has been associated with reductions in proteinuria and glomerulosclerosis and attenuation of disease progression as well as prevention of hyperparathyroidism.[548–551] Dietary phosphate restriction, however, almost inevitably also imposes dietary protein restriction. It is therefore not clear whether the benefit was derived directly from reduced phosphate intake or indirectly from protein restriction. One study in humans has reported additional renoprotection when phosphate restriction was superimposed on protein restriction.[552]

Renal Calcium Deposition

Calcium-phosphate deposition is a frequent histologic finding in end-stage kidney biopsies, irrespective of the underlying cause of renal failure.[175,553] Calcium levels in end-stage kidneys have been found to be approximately nine times greater than levels in control kidneys.[553] Histologically, deposits were seen in cortical tubule cells, basement membranes, and the interstitium.[553,554] Furthermore, the severity of renal parenchymal calcification has been found to correlate with the degree of renal dysfunction, implicating calcium-phosphate deposition in disease progression.[548,555] To determine whether the calcium deposits observed in end-stage kidneys precede or follow renal parenchymal fibrosis, rats with reduced renal mass were maintained on a high phosphate diet, thus ensuring a high calcium-phosphate product. A subgroup was treated with 3-phosphocitrate, an inhibitor of calcium-phosphate deposition.[555] Treatment with 3-phosphocitrate led to a significant reduction in renal injury compared to controls, indicating that calcium-phosphate deposition within the kidney occurs during the evolution of renal injury and may exacerbate nephron loss. Calcium deposition in the renal parenchyma is associated with ultrastructural evidence of mitochondrial disorganization and calcium accumulation[554] and may therefore contribute to renal injury via uncoupling of mitochondrial respiration and generation of reactive oxygen species.[556] Mitochondrial calcium deposition was reduced by dietary protein restriction or calcium channel blocker therapy.[554,556] Other potential roles for cellular calcium in renal disease progression include effects on vascular smooth muscle tone, mesangial cell contractility, cell growth and proliferation, extracellular matrix synthesis, and immune cell modulation.[557]

Hyperparathyroidism

Podocytes express a unique transcript of parathyroid hormone (PTH) receptor and PTH has been shown to have several effects on the kidney including decreasing SNGFR (without change in Q_A, P_{GC}, or ΔP), lowering K_f as well as stimulating renin production.[551] Furthermore, increased PTH levels may exacerbate renal damage through effects on blood pressure,[558] glucose intolerance, and lipid metabolism.[559,560] Two experimental studies have provided evidence that PTH may contribute to CKD progression. In the first parathyroidectomy was shown to improve survival, reduce the increased renal mass as well as renal calcium content, and attenuate the rise in serum creatinine observed in 5/6 nephrectomized rats fed high protein diet.[561] In the other, calcimimetic treatment and parathyroidectomy after 5/6 nephrectomy each abrogated tubulointerstitial fibrosis and glomerulosclerosis.[562] Interpretation of these data are, however, complicated by the observation in the latter study that both interventions also lowered blood pressure.

Activated Vitamin D Deficiency

It is perhaps not surprising that vitamin D, normally 1-hydroxylated in the kidney and therefore deficient in CKD, has several potentially beneficial effects on the kidney. In experimental studies 1,25 $(OH)_2D_3$ has been shown to inhibit proliferation of mesangial as well as tubule cells, inhibit renal hypertrophy after uninephrectomy,[563] and inhibit renin expression.[551] Several experiments have reported amelioration of renal damage in rats treated with 1,25 $(OH)_2D_3$ or vitamin D analogue after 5/6 nephrectomy.[564,565] Interestingly, a further study found that 1,25 $(OH)_2D_3$ treatment also preserved podocyte number, volume, and structure after 5/6 nephrectomy.[234] To date controlled trials examining the effect of 1,25 $(OH)_2D_3$ treatment on human CKD are not available.

Anemia

Anemia is a frequent consequence of CKD but may also influence its progression. Both acute and chronic anemias are associated with reversible increases in renal vascular resistance and a normal or reduced filtration fraction in animals and humans. Conversely, an increase in hematocrit is associated with an increase in filtration fraction. Thus hematocrit may influence renal hemodynamics and thereby affect the rate of progression of CKD. The effects of anemia on glomerular hemodynamics have been studied in rats subjected to 5/6 nephrectomy, DOCA-salt hypertension, and diabetes.[566–568] Irrespective of the model, anemia was associated with significant amelioration of glomerulosclerosis and consistently associated with reduction in P_{GC}. Reduced P_{GC} arose predominantly through reductions in efferent arteriolar resistance in rats with renal ablation, lowered systolic blood pressure in DOCA-salt rats and increased afferent arteriolar resistance in diabetic rats. Similarly, in the MWF/Ztm rat, which develops spontaneous glomerulosclerosis with age, anemia induced by dietary iron deficiency was associated with lower blood pressure, reduced urinary protein excretion and less extensive glomerulosclerosis compared with controls fed diet of normal iron content.[569] In contrast, however, prevention of anemia by administration of erythropoietin to remnant kidney rats in order to maintain a normal hematocrit, resulted in increased systemic and glomerular blood pressures and markedly increased glomerulosclerosis.[566]

Despite the apparently favorable hemodynamic effects of anemia in experimental models of CKD, humans studies suggest that anemia may in fact accelerate CKD progression. In patients with inherited hemoglobinopathies, chronic anemia is associated with glomerular hyperfiltration that eventuates in proteinuria, hypertension, and ESRD.[570,571] Furthermore, reduced hemoglobin was an independent predictor of increased risk of developing ESRD among patients with diabetic nephropathy in the RENAAL trial.[572] Several longitudinal studies of patients with other forms of CKD have identified lower hemoglobin as a risk factor for progression.[573,574] Further confirmation that anemia has an adverse effect of CKD progression is derived from two small randomized studies that have reported renoprotective benefit when anemia is corrected with erythropoietin. Among non-diabetic patients with serum creatinine 2 mg/dL to 6 mg/dL early treatment (started when hemoglobin <11.6 g/dL) with erythropoietin alpha was associated with a 60% reduction in the risk of doubling serum creatinine, ESRD, or death versus delayed treatment (started when hemoglobin <9.0 g/dL)[575] and in patients with serum creatinine 2 mg/dL to 4 mg/dL and hematocrit <30%, erythropoietin treatment was associated with significantly improved renal survival.[576] On the other hand, two other studies that had effect on left ventricular mass as their primary end point, found no effect of high versus low hemoglobin target on rate of decline in GFR[577,578] and one study reported a more rapid progression to ESRD among erythropoietin-treated patients randomized to a high (13.0–15.0 g/dL) versus a low (10.5–11.5 g/dL) hemoglobin target.[579]

The reasons for the apparent contradiction between the beneficial hemodynamic effects of anemia in experimental models and the identification of anemia as a risk factor for CKD progression in clinical studies, are unknown. It is possible that the benefit of the hemodynamic effects is outweighed by other factors such as increased renal hypoxia and ROS formation that may contribute to progressive renal damage. Issues related to the treatment of anemia in CKD are discussed further in Chapter 55.

Tobacco Smoking

Smoking produces acute sympathetic nervous system activation resulting in tachycardia and an increase in systolic blood pressure of up to 21 mm Hg.[580] Vasoconstriction occurs in several vascular beds, including the kidneys. Among healthy, non-smoking volunteers, acute exposure to cigarette smoke caused an 11% increase in renovascular resistance accompanied by a 15% reduction in GFR and an 18% decrease in filtration fraction. These effects appear to be mediated, at least in part, by nicotine because similar responses were observed after chewing nicotine gum.[581] Furthermore the renal hemodynamic effects of smoking can be blocked by pre-treatment with a β-blocker, indicating that β-adrenergic stimulation is also involved.[582] The effects of chronic smoking on the normal kidney are less well defined. Renal plasma flow but not GFR is reduced in chronic smokers and plasma endothelin levels are elevated. In one population-based study, chronic smoking was associated with a small increase in creatinine clearance, implying that smoking may cause glomerular hyperfiltration.[583] That these functional abnormalities may result in structural changes to blood vessels is suggested by the observation of abnormal intrarenal vasculature in smokers.[584,585] Moreover epidemiological studies have found smoking to be an important predictor of albuminuria in the general population.[583,586] In one study, heavy smoking (>20 cigarettes/day) was associated with a relative risk for albuminuria of 1.92.[586] Furthermore, in other epidemiological studies, smoking has been identified as a significant risk factor for renal impairment[403,587,588] and the development of ESRD.[402]

Whereas more studies are required to elucidate the effects of smoking on healthy kidneys, a growing body of evidence attests to the role smoking as an important risk factor for disease progression in a variety of forms of CKD. The first published studies focused on diabetic nephropathy. Among type 1 diabetics smoking has been found to be significant a risk factor for the development of microalbuminuria and overt nephropathy.[589,590] Furthermore, smoking was associated with more rapid progression from microalbuminuria to overt nephropathy[591] and with almost double the rate of decline in GFR in non-smokers.[592] Similar observations have been made among type 2 diabetics.[593–595] Several studies have also reported associations between smoking and accelerated CKD progression among non-diabetic forms of CKD. Among men with ADPKD or IgA nephropathy, a dose-dependent association between smoking and ESRD was observed, with an odds ratio of 5.8 for those with >15 pack years versus <5 pack years.[596] The median time to ESRD was almost halved in smokers versus non-smokers in patients with lupus nephritis.[597] Among 295 patients with a primary glomerulonephritis, those with a serum creatinine >1.7 mg/dl were significantly more likely to be smokers than those with normal creatinine.[598] Similarly, among 73 patients with primary renal disease, the rate of decline in GFR was doubled in heavy smokers versus non-smokers.[599] Finally, smoking was the most powerful predictor of a rise in serum creatinine among patients with severe essential hypertension.[600]

Mechanisms whereby cigarette smoking may result in renal injury include are the subject of ongoing research but are thought to include sympathetic nervous system activation, glomerular capillary hypertension, endothelial cell injury, and direct tubulotoxocity.[601] Among patients with CKD the hemodynamic effects were variable, but smoking was associated with a consistent increase in albumin/creatinine excretion.[581] Analysis of urine from both smokers and non-smokers has revealed significantly higher excretions of thromboxane- and prostacycline-derived products in smokers.[602] The authors suggest that increased synthesis of thromboxanes and prostacyclines may have pathologic importance for vascular injury given the biologic effects of these compounds on platelets and smooth muscle cells. An important role for sympathetic nervous system activation was suggested by a recent experimental study in which sympathetic denervation abrogated renal injury induced by exposure to cigarette smoke condensate.[603] A growing body of evidence thus supports the notion that the kidney is yet another organ that is adversely affected by smoking. Preliminary studies indicate that smoking cessation is therefore another intervention that may contribute to slowing the rate of progression of CKD.[604]

FUTURE DIRECTIONS

The development of pharmacological inhibitors of the RAS provided powerful and incisive tools to explore renal hemodynamic and other associated adaptations in the setting of progressive renal injury. These physiological insights paved the way for clinical studies that have now provided clear evidence for the use of ACEI and AT₁RA treatment as the mainstay of renoprotective strategies. Nevertheless, these studies have shown at best a halving of the rate of CKD progression. Ongoing research involving cell biology and molecular cloning as well as genomics and proteomics continues to yield novel insights into the mechanisms of progressive renal injury that promise to direct researchers to potential new molecular targets for renoprotective interventions. The development of the means to specifically inhibit molecular targets may provide new forms of therapy for those with CKD and enable physicians to realize the ultimate goal of achieving remission of progressive renal injury in the majority of patients and even regression of renal damage in some.

References

1. Kidney Disease Outcomes Quality Initiative: K/DOQI clinical practice guidelines for chronic kidney disease: evaluation, classification, and stratification. Am J Kidney Dis 39:S1–266, 2002.

2. Brenner BM: Retarding the progression of renal disease. Kidney Int 64:370–378, 2003.

3. Brenner BM, Meyer TW, Hostetter TH: Dietary protein intake and the progressive nature of kidney disease: The role of hemodynamically mediated glomerular injury in the pathogenesis of progressive glomerular sclerosis in aging, renal ablation and intrinsic renal disease. N Engl J Med 307:652–659, 1982.

4. Deen WM, Maddox DA, Robertson CR, et al: Dynamics of glomerular ultrafiltration in the rat. VII. Response to reduced renal mass. Am J Physiol 227:556–562, 1974.

5. Miller PL, Rennke HG, Meyer TW: Glomerular hypertrophy accelerates hypertensive glomerular injury in rats. Am J Physiol (Renal Fluid Electrolyte Physiol) 261:F459–F465, 1991.

6. Hostetter TH, Olson JL, Rennke HG, et al: Hyperfiltration in remnant nephrons: A potentially adverse response to renal ablation. J Am Soc Nephrol 12:1315–1325, 2001.

7. Griffin KA, Picken MM, Churchill M, et al: Functional and structural correlates of glomerulosclerosis after renal mass reduction in the rat. J Am Soc Nephrol 11:497–506, 2000.

8. Pelayo JC, Quan AH, Shanley PF: Angiotensin II control of the renal microcirculation in rats with reduced renal mass. Am J Physiol (Renal Fluid Electrolyte Physiol) 258:F414–F422, 1990.

9. Kasiske BL, O'Donnel MP, Garvis WJ, et al: Pharmacologic treatment of hyperlipidemia reduces injury in rat 5/6 nephrectomy model of chronic renal failure. Circ Res 62:367–374, 1988.

10. Buerkert J, Martin D, Prasad J, et al: Response of deep nephrons and the terminal collecting duct to a reduction in renal mass. Am J Physiol (Renal Fluid Electrolyte Physiol) 236:F454–F464, 1979.

11. Brown SA, Finco DR, Crowell WA, et al: Single-nephron adaptations to partial renal ablation in the dog. Am J Physiol (Renal Fluid Electrolyte Physiol) 258:F495–F503, 1990.

12. Kasiske BL, Ma JZ, Louis TA, et al: Long-term effects of reduced renal mass in humans. Kidney Int 48:814–819, 1995.

13. Blantz RC, Konnen KS, Tucker BJ: Angiotensin II effects upon the glomerular microcirculation and ultrafiltration coefficient of the rat. J Clin Invest 57:419–434, 1976.

14. Denton KM, Anderson WP, Sinniah R: Effects of angiotensin II on regional afferent and efferent arteriole dimensions and the glomerular pole. Am J Physiol Regul Integr Comp Physiol 279:R629–638, 2000.

15. Anderson S, Meyers TW, Rennke HG, et al: Control of glomerular hypertension limits glomerular injury in rats with reduced renal mass. J Clin Invest 76:612–619, 1985.

16. Anderson S, Rennke HG, Brenner BM: Therapeutic advantage of converting enzyme inhibitors in arresting progressive renal disease associated with systemic hypertension in the rat. J Clin Invest 77:1993–2000, 1986.

17. Lafayette RA, Mayer G, Park SK, et al: Angiotensin II receptor blockade limits glomerular injury in rats with reduced renal mass. J Clin Invest 90:766–771, 1992.

18. Mackenzie HS, Troy JL, Rennke HG, et al: TCV116 prevents progressive renal injury in rats with extensive renal mass ablation. J Hypertension 12 (suppl 9):S11–S16, 1994.

19. Rosenberg ME, Kren SM, Hostetter TH: Effect of dietary protein on the renin-angiotensin system in subtotally nephrectomized rats. Kidney Int 38:240–248, 1990.

20. Baboolal K, Meyer TW: The effect of acute angiotensin II blockade on renal function in rats with reduced renal mass. Kidney Int 46:980–985, 1994.

21. Mackie FE, Campbell DJ, Meyer TW: Intrarenal angiotensin and bradykinin peptide levels in the remnant kidney model of renal insufficiency. Kidney Int 59:1458–1465, 2001.

22. Correa-Rotter R, Hostetter TH, Manivel JC, et al: Renin expression in renal ablation. Hypertension 20:483–490, 1992.

23. Pupilli C, Chevalier RL, Carey RM, et al: Distribution and content of renin and renin mRNA in remnant kidney of adult rat. Am J Physiol (Renal Fluid Electrolyte Physiol) 263:F731–F738, 1992.

24. Rosenberg ME, Correa-Rotter R, Inagami T, et al: Glomerular renin synthesis and storage in the remnant kidney in the rat. Kidney Int 40:677–683, 1991.

25. Mackie FE, Meyer TW, Campbell DJ: Effects of antihypertensive therapy on intrarenal angiotensin and bradykinin levels in experimental renal insufficiency. Kidney Int 61:555–563, 2002.

26. Arima S, Kohagura K, Xu HL, et al: Nongenomic vascular action of aldosterone in the glomerular microcirculation. J Am Soc Nephrol 14:2255–2263, 2003.

27. Uhrenholt TR, Schjerning J, Hansen PB, et al: Rapid inhibition of vasoconstriction in renal afferent arterioles by aldosterone. Circ Res 93:1258–1266, 2003.

28. Uhrenholt TR, Schjerning J, Rasmussen LE, et al: Rapid non-genomic effects of aldosterone on rodent vascular function. Acta Physiol Scand 181:415–419, 2004.

29. Abassi Z, Francis B, Wessale J, et al: Effects of endothelin receptors ET(A) and ET(B) blockade on renal haemodynamics in normal rats and in rats with experimental congestive heart failure. Clin Sci (Lond) 103:245S-248S, 2002.

30. Granger JP: Endothelin. Am J Physiol Regul Integr Comp Physiol 285:R298–301, 2003.

31. Okada Y, Nakata M, Izumoto H, et al: Role of endothelin ETB receptor in partial ablation-induced chronic renal failure in rats. Eur J Pharmacol 494:63–71, 2004.

32. Benigni A, Perico N, Gaspari F, et al: Increased renal endothelin production in rats with reduced renal mass. Am J Physiol 260:F331–339, 1991.

33. Orisio S, Benigni A, Bruzzi I, et al: Renal endothelin gene expression is increased in remnant kidney and correlates with disease progression. Kidney Int 43:354–358, 1993.

34. Katoh T, Chang H, Uchida S, et al: Direct effects of endothelin in the rat kidney. Am J Physiol 258:F397–402, 1990.

35. Claria J, Jimenez W, La VG, et al: Effects of endothelin on renal haemodynamics and segmental sodium handling in conscious rats. Acta Physiol Scand 141:305–308, 1991.

36. Takabatake T, Ise T, Ohta K, et al: Effects of endothelin on renal hemodynamics and tubuloglomerular feedback. Am J Physiol 263:F103–108, 1992.

37. Martinez F, Deray G, Dubois M, et al: Chronic effects of endothelin-3 on blood pressure and renal haemodynamics in rats. Nephrol Dial Transplant 11:270–274, 1996.

38. Badr KF, Murray JJ, Breyer MD, et al: Mesangial cell, glomerular and renal vascular responses to endothelin in the rat kidney. J Clin Invest 83:336–342, 1989.

39. Kon V, Yoshioka T, Fogo A, et al: Glomerular actions of endothelin in vivo. J Clin Invest 83:1762–1767, 1989.

40. King AJ, Brenner BM, Anderson S: Endothelin: A potent renal and systemic vasoconstrictor peptide. Am J Physiol 256:F1051–1058, 1989.

41. Munger KA, Takahashi K, Awazu M, et al: Maintenance of endothelin-induced renal arteriolar constriction in rats is cyclooxygenase dependent. Am J Physiol 264:F637–644, 1993.

42. Qiu C, Samsell L, Baylis C: Actions of endogenous endothelin on glomerular hemodynamics in the rat. Am J Physiol 269:R469–473, 1995.

43. Sasser JM, Pollock JS, Pollock DM: Renal endothelin in chronic angiotensin II hypertension. Am J Physiol Regul Integr Comp Physiol 283:R243–248, 2002.

44. Hocher B, Schwarz A, Slowinski T, et al: In-vivo interaction of nitric oxide and endothelin. J Hypertension 22:111–119, 2004.

45. Ortola FV, Ballermann BJ, Brenner BM: Endogenous ANP augments fractional excretion of Pi, Ca, and Na in rats with reduced renal mass. Am J Physiol 255:F1091–1097, 1988.

46. Zhang PL, Mackenzie HS, Troy JL, et al: Effects of natriuretic peptide receptor inhibition on remnant kidney function in the rat. Kidney Int 46:414–420, 1994.

47. Dunn BR, Ichikawa I, Pfeffer JM, et al: Renal and systemic hemodynamic effects of synthetic atrial natriuretic peptide in the anesthetized rat. Circ Res 59:237–246, 1986.

48. de los Angeles Costa M, Elesgaray R, Loria A, et al: Atrial natriuretic peptide influence on nitric oxide system in kidney and heart. Regul Pept 118:151–157, 2004.

49. Nath KA, Chmielewski DH, Hostetter TH: Regulatory role of prostanoids in glomerular microcirculation of remnant nephrons. Am J Physiol 252:F829–837, 1987.

50. Pelayo JC, Shanley PF: Glomerular and tubular adaptive responses to acute nephron loss in the rat. Effect of prostaglandin synthesis inhibition. J Clin Invest 85:1761–1769, 1990.

51. Stahl RA, Kudelka S, Paravicini M, et al: Prostaglandin and thromboxane formation in glomeruli from rats with reduced renal mass. Nephron 42:252–257, 1986.

52. Jackson EK, Heidemann HT, Branch RA, et al: Low dose intrarenal infusions of PGE2, PGI2, and 6-keto-PGE1 vasodilate the in vivo rat kidney. Circ Res 51:67–72, 1982.

53. Fujihara CK, Antunes GR, Mattar AL, et al: Cyclooxygenase-2 (COX-2) inhibition limits abnormal COX-2 expression and progressive injury in the remnant kidney. Kidney Int 64:2172–2181, 2003.

54. Ren Y, Garvin JL, Falck JR, et al: Glomerular autacoids stimulated by bradykinin regulate efferent arteriole tone. Kidney Int 63:987–993, 2003.

55. De Nicola L, Blantz RC, Gabbai FB: Nitric oxide and angiotensin II. Glomerular and tubular interaction in the rat. J Clin Invest 89:1248–1256, 1992.

56. Griffin KA, Bidani AK, Ouyang J, et al: Role of endothelium-derived nitric oxide in hemodynamic adaptations after graded renal mass reduction. Am J Physiol 264:R1254–1259, 1993.

57. Aiello S, Noris M, Todeschini M, et al: Renal and systemic nitric oxide synthesis in rats with renal mass reduction. Kidney Int 52:171–181, 1997.

58. Fujihara CK, Mattar AL, Vieira JM, Jr, et al: Evidence for the existence of two distinct functions for the inducible NO synthase in the rat kidney: Effect of aminoguanidine in rats with 5/6 ablation. J Am Soc Nephrol 13:2278–2287, 2002.

59. Fujihara CK, De NG, Zatz R: Chronic nitric oxide synthase inhibition aggravates glomerular injury in rats with subtotal nephrectomy. J Am Soc Nephrol 5:1498–1507, 1995.

60. Valdivielso JM, Perez-Barriocanal F, Garcia-Estan J, et al: Role of nitric oxide in the early renal hemodynamic response after unilateral nephrectomy. Am J Physiol 276:R1718–1723, 1999.

61. Sigmon DH, Gonzalez-Feldman E, Cavasin MA, et al: Role of nitric oxide in the renal hemodynamic response to unilateral nephrectomy. J Am Soc Nephrol 15:1413–1420, 2004.

62. Granger JP, Hall JE: Acute and chronic actions of bradykinin on renal function and arterial pressure. Am J Physiol 248:F87–92, 1985.

63. Lortie M, Regoli D, Rhaleb NE, et al: The role of B1- and B2-kinin receptors in the renal tubular and hemodynamic response to bradykinin. Am J Physiol 262:R72–76, 1992.

64. Yu H, Carretero OA, Juncos LA, et al: Biphasic effect of bradykinin on rabbit afferent arterioles. Hypertension 32:287–292, 1998.

65. Ren Y, Garvin J, Carretero OA: Mechanism involved in bradykinin-induced efferent arteriole dilation. Kidney Int 62:544–549, 2002.

66. Bidani AK, Schwartz MM, Lewis EJ: Renal autoregulation and vulnerability to hypertensive injury in remnant kidney. Am J Physiol (Renal Fluid Electrolyte Physiol) 252:F1003–F1010, 1987.

67. Pelayo JC, Westcott JY: Impaired autoregulation of glomerular capillary hydrostatic pressure in the rat remnant nephron. J Clin Invest 88:101–105, 1991.

68. Loutzenhiser R, Bidani A, Chilton L: Renal myogenic response: Kinetic attributes and physiological role. Circ Res 90:1316–1324, 2002.

69. Salmond R, Seney FD: Reset tubuloglomerular feedback permits and sustains glomerular hyperfunction after extensive renal ablation. Am J Physiol (Renal Fluid Electrolyte Physiol) 260:F395–F401, 1991.

70. Braam B, Mitchell KD, Koomans HA, et al: Relevance of the tubuloglomerular feedback mechanism in pathophysiology. J Am Soc Nephrol 4:1257–1274, 1993.

71. Müller-Suur R, Norlén B-J, Persson EG: Resetting of tubuloglomerular feedback in rat kidneys after unilateral nephrectomy. Kidney Int 18:48–57, 1980.

72. Taal MW, Nenov VD, Wong W, et al: Vasopeptidase inhibition affords greater reno-protection than angiotensin-converting enzyme inhibition alone. J Am Soc Nephrol 12:2051–2059, 2001.

73. Biswas P, Roy A, Gong R, et al: Hepatocyte growth factor induces an endothelin-mediated decline in glomerular filtration rate. Am J Physiol Renal Physiol 288:F8–15, 2005.

74. Arima S, Ren Y, Juncos LA, et al: Platelet-activating factor dilates efferent arterioles through glomerulus-derived nitric oxide. J Am Soc Nephrol 7:90–96, 1996.

75. Ashton N: Renal and vascular actions of urotensin II. Kidney Int 70:624–629, 2006.

76. Fine L: The biology of renal hypertrophy. Kidney Int 29:619–634, 1986.

77. Wesson LG: Compensatory growth and other growth responses of the kidney. Nephron 51:149–184, 1989.

78. Hauser P, Kainz A, Perco P, et al: Transcriptional response in the unaffected kidney after contralateral hydronephrosis or nephrectomy. Kidney Int 68:2497–2507, 2005.

79. Liu B, Preisig PA: Compensatory renal hypertrophy is mediated by a cell cycle-dependent mechanism. Kidney Int 62:1650–1658, 2002.

80. Gomez AB, Carrero LV, Diaz GR: Image-directed color Doppler ultrasound evaluation of the single kidney after unilateral nephrectomy in adults. J Clin Ultrasound 25:29–35, 1997.

81. Prassopoulos P, Gourtsoyiannis N, Cavouras D, et al: CT evaluation of compensatory renal growth in relation to postnephrectomy time. Acta Radiol 33:566–568, 1992.

82. Prassopoulos P, Cavouras D, Gourtsoyiannis N: Pre- and post-nephrectomy kidney enlargement in patients with contralateral renal cancer. Eur Urol 24:58–61, 1993.

83. Seyer-Hansen K, Gundersen HJ, Osterby R: Stereology of the rat kidney during compensatory renal hypertrophy. Acta Pathol Microbiol Immunol Scand 93:9–12, 1985.

84. Nyengaard JR: Number and dimensions of rat glomerular capillaries in normal development and after nephrectomy. Kidney Int 43:1049–1057, 1993.

85. Schwartz MM, Churchill M, Bidani A, et al: Reversible compensatory hypertrophy in rat kidneys: Morphometric characterization. Kidney Int 43:610–614, 1993.

86. Lee GS, Nast CC, Peng SC, et al: Differential response of glomerular epithelial and mesangial cells after subtotal nephrectomy. Kidney Int 53:1389–1398, 1998.

87. Amann K, Irzyniec T, Mall G, et al: The effect of enalapril on glomerular growth and glomerular lesions after subtotal nephrectomy in the rat: A stereological analysis. J Hypertens 11:969–975, 1993.

88. Bidani AK, Mitchell KD, Schwartz MM, et al: Absence of glomerular injury or nephron loss in a normotensive rat remnant kidney model. Kidney Int 38:28–38, 1990.

89. Daniels BS, Hostetter TH: Adverse effects of growth in the glomerular microcirculation. Am J Physiol 258:F1409–F1416, 1990.

90. Schwartz MM, Evans J, Bidani AK: The mesangium in the long-term remnant kidney model. J Lab Clin Med 124:644–651, 1994.

91. Cortes P, Zhao X, Riser BL, et al: Regulation of glomerular volume in normal and partially nephrectomized rats. Am J Physiol 270:F356–370, 1996.

92. Miller PL, Meyer TW: Effects of tissue preparation on glomerular volume and capillary structure in the rat. Lab Invest 83:862–866, 1990.

93. Churchill M, Churchill PC, Schwartz M, et al: Reversible compensatory hypertrophy in transplanted brown Norway rat kidneys. Kidney Int 40:13–20, 1991.

94. Valentin JP, Sechi LA, Griffin CA, et al: The renin-angiotensin system and compensatory renal hypertrophy in the rat. Am J Hypertens 10:397–402, 1997.

95. Mulroney SE, Pesce C: Early hyperplastic renal growth after uninephrectomy in adult female rats. Endocrinology 141:932–937, 2000.

96. Haramati A, Lumpkin MD, Mulroney SE: Early increase in pulsatile growth hormone release after unilateral nephrectomy in adult rats. Am J Physiol 266:F628–632, 1994.

97. Flyvbjerg A, Bennett WF, Rasch R, et al: Compensatory renal growth in uninephrectomized adult mice is growth hormone dependent. Kidney Int 56:2048–2054, 1999.

98. Hammerman MR, O'Shea M, Miller SB: Role of growth factors in regulation of renal growth. Annu Rev Physiol 55:305–321, 1993.

99. Fine LG, Hammerman MR, Abboud HE: Evolving role of growth factors in the renal response to acute and chronic disease. J Am Soc Nephrol 2:1163–1170, 1992.

100. Shohat J, Davidowitz M, Erman A, et al: Serum and renal IGF-I levels after uninephrectomy in the rat. Scand J Clin Lab Invest 57:167–173, 1997.

101. Flyvbjerg A, Schrijvers BF, De Vriese AS, et al: Compensatory glomerular growth after unilateral nephrectomy is VEGF dependent. Am J Physiol Endocrinol Metab 283:E362–366, 2002.

102. Fervenza FC, Tsao T, Hsu F, et al: Intrarenal insulin-like growth factor-1 axis after unilateral nephrectomy in rat. J Am Soc Nephrol 10:43–50, 1999.

103. Gronboek H, Nielsen B, Flyvbjerg A, et al: Effect of graded renal ablation on kidney and serum insulin-like growth factor-I (IGF-I) and IGF binding proteins in rats: Relation to compensatory renal growth. Metabolism 46:29–35, 1997.

104. Stiles AD, Sosenko IR, D'Ercole AJ, et al: Relation of kidney tissue somatomedin-C/insulin-like growth factor I to postnephrectomy renal growth in the rat. Endocrinology 117:2397–2401, 1985.

105. El Nahas AM, Le Carpentier JE, Bassett AH: Compensatory renal growth: Role of growth hormone and insulin-like growth factor-I. Nephrol Dial Transplant 5:123–129, 1990.

106. Horiba N, Masuda S, Takeuchi A, et al: Gene expression variance based on random sequencing in rat remnant kidney. Kidney Int 66:29–45, 2004.

107. Smith LE, Shen W, Perruzzi C, et al: Regulation of vascular endothelial growth factor-dependent retinal neovascularization by insulin-like growth factor-1 receptor. Nature Med 5:1390–1395, 1999.

108. Kanda S, Saha PK, Nomata K, et al: Transient increase in renal epidermal growth factor content after unilateral nephrectomy in the mouse. Acta Endocrinol (Copenh) 124:188–193, 1991.

109. Miller SB, Rogers SA, Estes CE, et al: Increased distal nephron EGF content and altered distribution of peptide in compensatory renal hypertrophy. Am J Physiol 262:F1032–1038, 1992.

110. Rogers SA, Miller SB, Hammerman MR: Insulin-like growth factor I gene expression in isolated rat renal collecting duct is stimulated by epidermal growth factor. J Clin Invest 87:347–351, 1991.

111. Ishibashi K, Sasaki S, Sakamoto H, et al: Expressions of receptor gene for hepatocyte growth factor in kidney after unilateral nephrectomy and renal injury. Biochem Biophys Res Commun 187:1454–1459, 1992.

112. Nagaike M, Hirao S, Tajima H, et al: Renotropic functions of hepatocyte growth factor in renal regeneration after unilateral nephrectomy. J Biol Chem 266:22781–22784, 1991.

113. Joannidis M, Spokes K, Nakamura T, et al: Regional expression of hepatocyte growth factor/c-met in experimental renal hypertrophy and hyperplasia. Am J Physiol 267:F231–236, 1994.

114. Flyvbjerg A, Thorlacius UO, Naeraa R, et al: Kidney tissue somatomedin C and initial renal growth in diabetic and uninephrectomized rats. Diabetologia 31:310–314, 1988.

115. Hayslett JP, Kashgarian M, Epstein FH: Functional correlates of compensatory renal hypertrophy. J Clin Invest 47:774–782, 1968.

116. Hayslett JP, Kashgarian M, Epstein FH: Mechanism of change in the excretion of sodium per nephron when renal mass is reduced. J Clin Invest 48:1002, 1969.

117. Trizna W, Yanagawa N, Bar-Khayim Y, et al: Functional profile of the isolated uremic nephron. J Clin Invest 68:760–767, 1981.

118. Fine LG, Trizna W, Bourgoignie JJ, et al: Functional profile of the isolated uremic nephron. Role of compensatory hypertrophy in the control of fluid reabsorption by the proximal straight tubule. J Clin Invest 61:1508–1518, 1978.

119. Salehmoghaddam S, Bradley T, Mikhail N, et al: Hypertrophy of basolateral Na-K pump activity in the proximal tubule of the remnant kidney. Lab Invest 53:443–452, 1985.

120. Tabei K, Levenson DJ, Brenner BM: Early enhancement of fluid transport in rabbit proximal straight tubules after loss of contralateral renal excretory function. J Clin Invest 72:871–881, 1983.

121. Hwang S, Bohman R, Navas P, et al: Hypertrophy of renal mitochondria. J Am Soc Nephrol 1:822–827, 1990.

122. Hruska K, Klahr S, Hammerman MR: Decreased luminal membrane transport of phosphate in chronic renal failure. Am J Physiol 242:F17–F22, 1982.

123. Bouby N, Hassler C, Parvy P, et al: Renal synthesis of arginine in chronic renal failure: In vivo and in vitro studies in rats with 5/6 nephrectomy. Kidney Int 44:676–683, 1993.

124. Yanagawa N, Nissenson RA, Edwards B, et al: Functional profile of the isolated uremic nephron: Intrinsic adaptation of phosphate transport in the rabbit proximal tubule. Kidney Int 23:674–683, 1983.

125. Buerkert J, Martin D, Trigg D, et al: Effect of reduced renal mass on ammonium handling and net acid formation by the superficial and juxtamedullary nephron of the rat. Evidence for reentrapment rather than decreased production of ammonium in the acidosis of uremia. J Clin Invest 71:1661–1675, 1983.

126. Yamauchi A, Sugiura T, Kitamura H, et al: Effects of partial nephrectomy on the expression of osmolyte transporters. Kidney Int 51:1847–1854, 1997.

127. Fine LG, Yanagawa N, Schultze RG, et al: Functional profile of the isolated uremic nephron. Potassium adaptation in the rabbit cortical collecting tubule. J Clin Invest 64:1033–1043, 1979.

128. Zalups RK, Stanton BA, Wade JB, et al: Structural adaptation in initial collecting tubule following reduction in renal mass. Kidney Int 27:636–642, 1985.

129. Allison MEM, Wilson CB, Gottschalk CW: Pathophysiology of experimental glomerulonephritis in rats. J Clin Invest 53:1402–1423, 1974.

130. Kramp RA, MacDowell M, Gottschalk CW, et al: A study by microdissection and micropuncture of the structure and the function of the kidneys and the nephrons of rats with chronic renal damage. Kidney Int 5:147–176, 1974.

131. Brenner BM: Nephron adaptation to renal injury or ablation. Am J Physiol 249:F324–F337, 1985.

132. Pennell JP, Bourgoignie J: Adaptive changes of juxtaglomerular filtration in the remnant kidney. Pflugers Arch 389:131–135, 1981.

133. Ichikawa I, Hoyer JR, Seiler MW, et al: Mechanism of glomerulotubular balance in the setting of heterogeneous glomerular injury. J Clin Invest 69:185–198, 1982.

134. Marcussen N: Atubular glomeruli and the structural basis for chronic renal failure. Lab Invest 66:265–284, 1992.

135. Mitch WE, Wilcox CS: Disorders of body fluids, sodium and potassium in chronic renal failure. Am J Med 72:536–550, 1982.

136. Slatopolsky E, Elkan IO, Weerts C, et al: Studies on the characteristics of the control system governing sodium excretion in uremic man. J Clin Invest 47:521–530, 1968.

137. Weber H, Lin K-Y, Bricker NS: Effect of sodium intake on single nephron glomerular filtration rate and sodium reabsorption in experimental uremia. Kidney Int 8:14–20, 1975.

138. Bank N, Aynedjian HS: Individual nephron function in experimental bilateral pyelonephritis. I. Glomerular filtration rate and proximal tubular sodium, potassium, and water reabsorption. J Lab Clin Med 68:713–727, 1966.

139. Wilson DR, Sonnenberg H: Medullary collecting duct function in the remnant kidney before and after volume expansion. Kidney Int 15:487–501, 1979.

140. Hayslett JP: Functional adaptation to reduction in renal mass. Physiol Rev 59:137–164, 1979.

141. Woolf AS: Does atrial natriuretic factor contribute to the progression of renal disease? Med Hypoth 31:261–263, 1990.

142. Smith S, Anderson S, Ballerman BJ, et al: Role of atrial natriuretic peptide in adaptation of sodium excretion with reduced renal mass. J Clin Invest 77:1395–1398, 1986.

143. Zhang PL, Mackenzie HS, Troy JL, et al: Effects of natriuretic peptide receptor inhibition on remnant kidney function in rats. Kidney Int 46:414–420, 1993.

144. Guyton AC, Coleman TG, Young DB, et al: Salt balance and long-term blood pressure control. Ann Rev Med 31:15–27, 1980.

145. Langston JB, Guyton AC, Douglas BH, et al: Effect of changes in salt intake on arterial pressure and renal function in partially nephrectomized dogs. Circ Res XII:508–513, 1963.

146. Dormois JC, Young JL, Nies AS: Minoxidil in severe hypertension: Value when conventional drugs have failed. Am Heart J 90:360–368, 1975.

147. Gonick HC, Maxwell MH, Rubini ME, et al: Functional impairment in chronic renal disease. I. Studies on sodium-conserving ability. Nephron 3:137–152, 1966.

148. Bricker NS: Sodium homeostasis in chronic renal disease. Kidney Int 21:886–897, 1982.

149. Bricker NS, Dewey RR, Lubowitz H, et al: Observations on the concentrating and diluting mechanisms of the diseased kidney. J Clin Invest 38:516–523, 1959.

150. Mees EJD: Relation between maximal urine concentration, maximal water reabsorption capacity, and mannitol clearance in patients with renal disease. Br Med J 1:1159–1160, 1959.

151. Conte G, Dal Canton A, Fuiano G, et al: Mechanism of impaired urinary concentration in chronic primary glomerulonephritis. Kidney Int 27:792–798, 1985.

152. Duback UC, Rosner B, Muller A, et al: Relationship between regular intake of phenacitin-containing analgesics and laboratory evidence of uro-renal disease in a working female population of Switzerland. Lancet 1:539–543, 1975.

153. Hatch FE, Culberston JW: Nature of the renal concentrating defect in sickle cell disease. J Clin Invest 46:336–345, 1967.

154. Pennell JP, Bourgoignie JJ: Water reabsorption by papillary collecting ducts in the remnant kidney. Am J Physiol 242:F657–F663, 1982.

155. Klahr S, Schwab SJ, Stokes TJ: Metabolic adaptations of the nephron in renal disease. Kidney Int 29:80–89, 1986.

156. Milanes CL, Jamison RL: Effect of acute potassium load on reabsorption in Henle's loop in chronic renal failure in the rat. Kidney Int 27:919–927, 1985.

157. Bourgoignie JJ, Kaplan M, Pincus J, et al: Renal handling of potassium in dogs with chronic renal insufficiency. Kidney Int 20:482–490, 1981.

158. Bengele HH, Evan A, McNamara ER, et al: Tubular sites of potassium regulation in the normal and uninephrectomized rat. Am J Physiol 234:F146–F153, 1978.

159. Schon DA, Silva P, Hayslett JP: Mechanism of potassium excretion in renal insufficiency. Am J Pathol 227:1323–1330, 1974.

160. Palmer BF: Managing hyperkalemia caused by inhibitors of the renin-angiotensin-aldosterone system. N Engl J Med 351:585–592, 2004.

161. Gonick HC, Kleeman CR, Rubini ME, et al: Functional impairment in chronic renal disease. III. Studies of potassium excretion. Am J Med Sci 261:281–261, 1971.

162. Widmer B, Gerhardt RE, Harrington JT, et al: Serum electrolyte and acid base composition. The influence of graded degrees of chronic renal failure. Arch Intern Med 139:1099–1102, 1979.

163. Wong NL, Quamme GA, Dirks JH: Tubular handling of bicarbonate in dogs with experimental renal failure. Kidney Int 25:912–918, 1984.

164. Schwartz WB, Hall PW, Hays RM, et al: On the mechanism of acidosis in chronic renal disease. J Clin Invest 38:39–52, 1959.

165. Muldowney FP, Donohoe JF, Carrol DV, et al: Parathyroid acidosis in uremia. Q J Med 41:321–342, 1972.

166. Purkerson ML, Lubowitz H, White RW, et al: On the influence of extracellular fluid volume expansion on bicarbonate reabsorption in the rat. J Clin Invest 48:1754–1760, 1969.

167. Sastrasinh S, Tanen RL: Effect of plasma potassium on renal NH_3 production. Am J Physiol 244:F383 F391, 1083.

168. Wrong O, Davies HEF: Excretion of acid in renal disease. Q J Med 28:259, 1959.

169. Silver J, Levi R: Cellular and molecular mechanisms of secondary hyperparathyroidism. Clin Nephrol 63:119–126, 2005.

170. Slatopolsky E, Robson AM, Elkan I, et al: Control of phosphate excretion in uremic man. J Clin Invest 47:1865–1874, 1968.

171. Haut LL, Alfrey AC, Guggenheim S, et al: Renal toxicity of phosphate in rats. Kidney Int 17:722–731, 1980.

172. Brooks DP, Ali SM, Contino LC, et al: Phosphate excretion and phosphate transporter messenger RNA in uremic rats treated with phosphonoformic acid. J Pharmacol Exp Ther 281:1440–1445, 1997.

173. Kraus E, Briefel G, Cheng L, et al: Phosphate excretion in uremic rats: Effects of parathyroidectomy and phosphate restriction. Am J Physiol 248:F175–F182, 1985.

174. Campese VM: Neurogenic factors and hypertension in chronic renal failure. J Nephrol 10:184–187, 1997.

175. Hsu CH: Are we mismanaging calcium and phosphate metabolism in renal failure? Am J Kidney Dis 29:641–649, 1997.

176. Better OS, Kleeman CR, Gonick HC, et al: Renal handling of calcium, magnesium and inorganic phosphate in chronic renal failure. Isr J Med Sci 3:60–79, 1967.

177. Better OS, Kleeman CR, Maxwell MH, et al: The effect of induced hypercalcemia on renal handling of divalent ions in patients with renal disease. Isr J Med Sci 5:33–42, 1969.

178. Finkelstein FO, Kliger AS: Medullary structures in calcium reabsorption in rats with renal insufficiency. Am J Physiol 233:F197–200, 1977.

179. Zatz R, Dunn BR, Meyer TW, et al: Prevention of diabetic glomerulopathy by pharmacological amelioration of glomerular capillary hypertension. J Clin Invest 77:1925–1930, 1986.

180. Zatz R, Meyer TW, Rennke HG, et al: Predominance of hemodynamic rather than metabolic factors in the pathogenesis of diabetic glomerulopathy. Proc Natl Acad Sci U S A 82:5963–5967, 1985.

181. Dworkin LD, Hostetter TH, Rennke HG, et al: Hemodynamic basis for glomerular injury in rats with desoxycorticosterone-salt hypertension. J Clin Invest 73:1448–1461, 1984.

182. Steffes MW, Brown DM, Mauer SM: Diabetic glomerulopathy following unilateral nephrectomy in the rat. Diabetes 27:35–41, 1978.

183. Mauer SM, Steffes MW, Azar S, et al: The effects of Goldblatt hypertension on development of the glomerular lesions of diabetes mellitus in the rat. Diabetes 27:738–744, 1978.

184. Ots M, Troy JL, Mackenzie HS, et al: Isograft supplementation slows the progression of chronic experimental renal injury [abstract]. J Am Soc Nephrol 7:1861, 1996.

185. Mackenzie HS, Tullius SG, Heemann UW, et al: Nephron supply is a major determinant of long-term renal allograft outcome in rats. J Clin Invest 94:2148–2152, 1994.

186. Mackenzie HS, Azuma H, Troy JL, et al: Augmenting kidney mass at transplantation abrogates chronic renal allograft injury in rats. Proc Assoc Am Phys 108:127–133, 1996.

187. Novick AC, Gephardt G, Guz B, et al: Long-term follow-up after partial removal of a solitary kidney. N Engl J Med 325:1058–1062, 1991.

188. Remuzzi A, Mazerska M, Gephardt GN, et al: Three-dimensional analysis of glomerular morphology in patients with subtotal nephrectomy. Kidney Int 48:155–162, 1995.

189. Anderson S, Meyer TW, Rennke HG, et al: Control of glomerular hypertension limits glomerular injury in rats with reduced renal mass. J Clin Invest 76:612–619, 1985.

190. Taal MW, Chertow GM, Rennke HR, et al: Mechanisms underlying renoprotection during renin-angiotensin system blockade. Am J Physiol 280:F343–F355, 2001.

191. Anderson S, Rennke HG, Garcia DL, et al: Short and long term effects of antihypertensive therapy in the diabetic rat. Kidney Int 36:526–536, 1989.

192. Fujihara CK, Padilha RM, Zatz R: Glomerular abnormalities in long-term experimental diabetes. Role of hemodynamic and nonhemodynamic factors and effects of antihypertensive therapy. Diabetes 41:286–293, 1992.

193. Simons JL, Provoost AP, Anderson S, et al: Pathogenesis of glomerular injury in the fawn-hooded rat: Early glomerular capillary hypertension predicts glomerular sclerosis. J Am Soc Nephrol 3:1775–1782, 1993.

194. Ziai F, Ots M, Provoost AP, et al: The angiotensin receptor antagonist, irbesartan, reduces renal injury in experimental chronic renal failure. Kidney Int 50 (suppl 57): S-132-S-136, 1996.

195. Mackenzie HS, Ziai F, Nagano H, et al: Candesartan cilexetil reduces chronic renal allograft injury in Fisher to Lewis rats. J Hypertens 15 Suppl 4:S21–S25, 1997.

196. Ziai F, Nagano H, Kusaka M, et al: Renal allograft protection with losartan in Fisher–>Lewis rats: Hemodynamics, macrophages, and cytokines. Kidney Int 57:2618–2625, 2000.

197. Benediktsson H, Chea R, Davidoff A, et al: Antihypertensive drug treatment in chronic renal allograft rejection in the rat. Effect on structure and function. Transplantation 62:1634–1642, 1996.

198. Remuzzi A, Malanchini B, Battaglia C, et al: Comparison of the effects of angiotensin-converting enzyme inhibition and angiotensin II receptor blockade on the evolution of spontaneous glomerular injury in male MWF/Ztm rats. Exp Nephrol 4:19–25, 1996.

199. Anderson S, Rennke HG, Zatz R: Glomerular adaptations with normal aging and with long-term converting enzyme inhibition in rats. Am J Physiol 267:F35–F43, 1994.

200. Schmitz PG, O'Donnell MP, Kasiske BL, et al: Renal injury in obese Zucker rats: Glomerular hemodynamic alterations and effects of enalapril. Am J Physiol 263:F496–F502, 1992.

201. Anderson S, Diamond JR, Karnovsky MJ, et al: Mechanisms underlying transition from acute renal injury to late glomerular sclerosis in a rat model of nephrotic syndrome. J Clin Invest 82:1757–1768, 1988.

202. Lewis EJ, Hunsicker LG, Bain RP, et al: The effect of angiotensin-converting-enzyme inhibition on diabetic nephropathy. N Engl J Med 329:1456–1462, 1993.

203. Gruppo Italiano di Studi Epidemiologici in Nefrologia: Randomised placebo-controlled trial of effect of ramipril on decline in glomerular filtration rate and risk of terminal renal failure in proteinuric, non-diabetic nephropathy. Lancet 349:1857–1863, 1997.

204. Lewis EJ, Hunsicker LG, Clarke WR, et al: Renoprotective effect of the angiotensin-receptor antagonist irbesartan in patients with nephropathy due to type 2 diabetes. N Engl J Med 345:851–860, 2001.

205. Brenner BM, Cooper ME, de Zeeuw D, et al: Effects of losartan on renal and cardiovascular outcomes in patients with type 2 diabetes and nephropathy. N Engl J Med 345:861–869, 2001.

206. Hou FF, Zhang X, Zhang GH, et al: Efficacy and safety of benazepril for advanced chronic renal insufficiency. N Engl J Med 354:131–140, 2006.

207. Hostetter TH: Progression of renal disease and renal hypertrophy. Ann Rev Physiol 57:263–278, 1995.

208. Fujihara CK, Limongi DM, Falzone R, et al: Pathogenesis of glomerular sclerosis in subtotally nephrectomized analbuminemic rats. Am J Physiol 261:F256–264, 1991.

209. Rennke HG, Klein PS: Pathogenesis and significance of nonprimary focal and segmental glomerulosclerosis. Am J Kidney Dis 13:443–456, 1989.

210. Bohle A, Mackensen-Haen S, Wehrmann M: Significance of postglomerular capillaries in the pathogenesis of chronic renal failure. Kidney Blood Press Res 19:191–195, 1996.

211. Kang DH, Joly AH, Oh SW, et al: Impaired angiogenesis in the remnant kidney model: I. Potential role of vascular endothelial growth factor and thrombospondin-1. J Am Soc Nephrol 12:1434–1447, 2001.

212. Kang DH, Hughes J, Mazzali M, et al: Impaired angiogenesis in the remnant kidney model: II. Vascular endothelial growth factor administration reduces renal fibrosis and stabilizes renal function. J Am Soc Nephrol 12:1448–1457, 2001.

213. Brooks AR, Lelkes PI, Rubanyi GM: Gene expression profiling of vascular endothelial cells exposed to fluid mechanical forces: Relevance for focal susceptibility to atherosclerosis. Endothelium: J Endothelial Cell Res 11:45–57, 2004.

214. Nagel T, Resnick N, Atkinson WJ, et al: Shear stress selectively upregulates intercellular adhesion molecule-1 expression in cultured human vascular endothelial cells. J Clin Invest 94:885–891, 1994.

814

215. Shyy JYJ, Lin MC, Han JH, et al: The cis-acting phorbol ester 12-O-tetradecanoylp[horbol-13-acetate-responseive element is involved in shear stress-induced monocyte chemotactic protein—1 expression. Proc Natl Acad Sci U S A 92:8069–8073, 1995.

216. Gimbrone MA, Nagel T, Topper JN: Biomechanical activation: An emerging paradigm in endothelial adhesion biology. J Clin Invest 99:1809–1813, 1997.

217. Ingram AJ, Ly H, Thai K, et al: Activation of mesangial cell signaling cascades in response to mechanical strain. Kidney Int 55:476–485, 1999.

218. Riser BL, Cortes P, Zhao X, et al: Intraglomerular pressure and mesangial stretching stimulate extracellular matrix formation in the rat. J Clin Invest 90:1932–1943, 1992.

219. Harris RC, Haralson MA, Badr KF: Continuous stretch-relaxation in culture alters rat mesangial cell morphology, growth characteristics, and metabolic activity. Lab Invest 66:548–554, 1992.

220. Giunti S, Pinach S, Arnaldi L, et al: The MCP-1/CCR2 system has direct proinflammatory effects in human mesangial cells. Kidney Int 69:856–863, 2006.

221. Riser BL, Cortes P, Heilig C, et al: Cyclic stretching force selectively up-regulates transforming growth factor-beta isoforms in cultured rat mesangial cells. Am J Pathol 148:1915–1923, 1996.

222. Riser BL, Ladson-Wofford S, Sharba A, et al: TGF-beta receptor expression and binding in rat mesangial cells: modulation by glucose and cyclic mechanical strain. Kidney Int 56:428–439, 1999.

223. Riser BL, Denichilo M, Cortes P, et al: Regulation of connective tissue growth factor activity in cultured rat mesangial cells and its expression in experimental diabetic glomerulosclerosis. J Am Soc Nephrol 11:25–38, 2000.

224. Becker BN, Yasuda T, Kondo S, et al: Mechanical stretch/relaxation stimulates a cellular renin-angiotensin system in cultured rat mesangial cells. Exp Nephrol 6:57–66, 1998.

225. Kagami S, Border WA, Miller DE, et al: Angiotensin II stimulates extracellular matrix protein synthesis through induction of transforming growth factor-beta expression in rat glomerular mesangial cells. J Clin Invest 93:2431–2437, 1994.

226. Mattana J, Singhal PC: Applied pressure modulates mesangial cell proliferation and matrix synthesis. Am J Hypertens 8:1112–1120, 1995.

227. Kato H, Osajima A, Uezono Y, et al: Involvement of PDGF in pressure-induced mesangial cell proliferation through PKC and tyrosine kinase pathways. Am J Physiol 277:F105–F112, 1999.

228. Suda T, Osajima A, Tamura M, et al: Pressure-induced expression of monocyte chemoattractant protein-1 through activation of MAP kinase. Kidney Int 60:1705–1715, 2001.

229. Hamasaki K, Mimura T, Furuya H, et al: Stretching mesangial cells stimulates tyrosine phosphorylation of focal adhesion kinase pp125FAK. Biochem Biophys Res Commun 212:544–549, 1995.

230. Homma T, Akai Y, Burns KD, et al: Activation of S6 kinase by repeated cycles of stretching and relaxation in rat glomerular mesangial cells. Evidence for involvement of protein kinase C. J Biol Chem 267:23129–23135, 1992.

231. Durvasula RV, Shankland SJ: Podocyte injury and targeting therapy: An update. Curr Opin Nephrol Hypertens 15:1–7, 2006.

232. Nagata M, Kriz W: Glomerular damage after uninephrectomy in young rats. II. Mechanical stress on podocytes as a pathway to sclerosis. Kidney Int 42:148–160, 1992.

233. Yu D, Petermann A, Kunter U, et al: Urinary podocyte loss is a more specific marker of ongoing glomerular damage than proteinuria. J Am Soc Nephrol 16:1733–1741, 2005.

234. Kuhlmann A, Haas CS, Gross ML, et al: 1,25-Dihydroxyvitamin D3 decreases podocyte loss and podocyte hypertrophy in the subtotally nephrectomized rat. Am J Physiol Renal Physiol 286:F526–503, 2004.

235. Kriz W, LeHir M: Pathways to nephron loss starting from glomerular diseases-insights from animal models. Kidney Int 67:404–419, 2005.

236. Morton MJ, Hutchinson K, Mathieson PW, et al: Human podocytes possess a stretch-sensitive, Ca²⁺-activated K⁺ channel: Potential implications for the control of glomerular filtration. J Am Soc Nephrol 15:2981–2987, 2004.

237. Petermann AT, Hiromura K, Blonski M, et al: Mechanical stress reduces podocyte proliferation in vitro. Kidney Int 61:40–50, 2002.

238. Endlich N, Kress KR, Reiser J, et al: Podocytes respond to mechanical stress in vitro. J Am Soc Nephrol 12:413–422, 2001.

239. Martineau LC, McVeigh LI, Jasmin BJ, et al: p38 MAP kinase mediates mechanically induced COX-2 and PG EP4 receptor expression in podocytes: Implications for the actin cytoskeleton. Am J Physiol Renal Physiol 286:F693–701, 2004.

240. Petermann AT, Pippin J, Durvasula R, et al: Mechanical stretch induces podocyte hypertrophy in vitro. Kidney Int 67:157–166, 2005.

241. Durvasula RV, Petermann AT, Hiromura K, et al: Activation of a local tissue angiotensin system in podocytes by mechanical strain. Kidney Int 65:30–39, 2004.

242. vanGoor H, Fidler V, Weening JJ, et al: Determinants of focal and segmental glomerulosclerosis in the rat after renal ablation. Evidence for involvement of macrophages and lipids. Lab Invest 64:754–765, 1991.

243. Taal MW, Omer SA, Nadim MK, et al: Cellular and molecular mediators in common pathway mechanisms of chronic renal disease progression. Curr Opin Nephrol Hypertens 9:323–331, 2000.

244. Mai M, Geiger H, Hilgers KF, et al: Early interstitial changes in hypertension-induced renal injury. Hypertension 22:754–765, 1993.

245. Wolf G, Schneider A, Wenzel U, et al: Regulation of glomerular TGF-beta expression in the contralateral kidney of two-kidney, one-clip hypertensive rats. J Am Soc Nephrol 9:763–772, 1998.

246. Floege J, Burns MW, Alpers CE, et al: Glomerular cell proliferation and PDGF expression precede glomerulosclerosis in the remnant kidney model. Kidney Int 41:297–302, 1992.

247. Taal MW, Zandi-Nejad Z, Weening B, et al: Proinflammatory gene expression and macrophage recruitment in the rat remnant kidney. Kidney Int 58:1664–1676, 2000.

248. Wu LL, Cox A, Roe CJ, et al: Transforming growth factor beta 1 and renal injury following subtotal nephrectomy in the rat: role of the renin-angiotensin system. Kidney Int 51:1553–1567, 1997.

249. vanGoor H, vanderHorst ML, Fidler V, et al: Glomerular macrophage modulation affects mesangial expansion in the rat after renal ablation. Lab Invest 66:564–571, 1992.

250. Fujihara CK, Malheiros D, Zatz R, et al: Mycophenolate mofetil attenuates renal injury in the rat remnant kidney. Kidney Int 54:1510–1519, 1998.

251. Fujihara CK, De Lourdes Noronha I, Malheiros DM, et al: Combined mycophenolate mofetil and losartan therapy arrests established injury in the remnant kidney. J Am Soc Nephrol 11:283–290, 2000.

252. Remuzzi G, Zoja C, Gagliardini E, et al: Combining an antiproteinuric approach with mycophenolate mofetil fully suppresses progressive nephropathy of experimental animals. J Am Soc Nephrol 10:1542–1549, 1999.

253. Romero F, Rodriguez-Iturbe B, Parra G, et al: Mycophenolate mofetil prevents the progressive renal failure induced by 5/6 renal ablation in rats. Kidney Int 55:945–955, 1999.

254. Tapia E, Franco M, Sanchez-Lozada LG, et al: Mycophenolate mofetil prevents arteriolopathy and renal injury in subtotal ablation despite persistent hypertension. Kidney Int 63:994–1002, 2003.

255. Fujihara CK, Malheiros DM, Donato JL, et al: Nitroflurbiprofen, a new nonsteroidal anti-inflammatory, ameliorates structural injury in the remnant kidney. Am J Physiol 274:F573–579, 1998.

256. Jones SE, Kelly DJ, Cox AJ, et al: Mast cell infiltration and chemokine expression in progressive renal disease. Kidney Int 64:906–913, 2003.

257. Remuzzi G, Bertani T: Pathophysiology of progressive nephropathies. N Engl J Med 339:1448–1456, 1998.

258. Anders HJ, Ninichuk V, Schlondorff D: Progression of kidney disease: Blocking leukocyte recruitment with chemokine receptor CCR1 antagonists. Kidney Int 69:29–32, 2006.

259. Wada T, Furuichi K, Sakai N, et al: Gene therapy via blockade of monocyte chemoattractant protein-1 for renal fibrosis. J Am Soc Nephrol 15:940–948, 2004.

260. Mu W, Ouyang X, Agarwal A, et al: IL-10 suppresses chemokines, inflammation, and fibrosis in a model of chronic renal disease. J Am Soc Nephrol 16:3651–3660, 2005.

261. Ng YY, Huang TP, Yang WC, et al: Tubular epithelial-myofibroblast transdifferentiation in progressive tubulointerstitial fibrosis in 5/6 nephrectomized rats. Kidney Int 54:864–876, 1998.

262. Badid C, Vincent M, McGregor B, et al: Mycophenolate mofetil reduces myofibroblast infiltration and collagen III deposition in rat remnant kidney. Kidney Int 58:51–61, 2000.

263. Ma LJ, Marcantoni C, Linton MF, et al: Peroxisome proliferator-activated receptor-gamma agonist troglitazone protects against nondiabetic glomerulosclerosis in rats. Kidney Int 59:1899–1910, 2001.

264. Border WA, Noble NA: Fibrosis linked to TGF-beta in yet another disease. J Clin Invest 96:655–656, 1995.

265. Kato S, Luyckx VA, Ots M, et al: Renin-angiotensin blockade lowers MCP-1 expression in diabetic rats. Kidney Int 56:1037–1048, 1999.

266. Ketteler M, Noble NA, Border WA: Transforming growth factor-beta and angiotensin II: the missing link from glomerular hyperfiltration to glomerulosclerosis? Annu Rev Physiol 57:279–295, 1995.

267. Tamaki K, Okuda S, Ando T, et al: TGF-beta 1 in glomerulosclerosis and interstitial fibrosis of adriamycin nephropathy. Kidney Int 45:525–536, 1994.

268. Hancock WH, Whitley WD, Tullius SG, et al: Cytokines, adhesion molecules, and the pathogenesis of chronic rejection of rat renal allografts. Transplantation 56:643–650, 1993.

269. Niemir ZI, Stein H, Noronha IL, et al: PDGF and TGF-beta contribute to the natural course of human IgA glomerulonephritis. Kidney Int 48:1530–1541, 1995.

270. Yamamoto T, Noble NA, Cohen AH, et al: Expression of transforming growth factor-beta isoforms in human glomerular diseases. Kidney Int 49:461–469, 1996.

271. Yamamoto T, Noble NA, Miller DE, et al: Increased levels of transforming growth factor-beta in HIV-associated nephropathy. Kidney Int 55:579–592, 1999.

272. Yamamoto T, Nakamura T, Noble NA, et al: Expression of transforming growth factor beta is elevated in human and experimental diabetic nephropathy. Proc Natl Acad Sci U S A 90:1814–1818, 1993.

273. Shihab FS, Yamamoto T, Nast CC, et al: Transforming growth factor-beta and matrix protein expression in acute and chronic rejection of human renal allografts. J Am Soc Nephrol 6:286–294, 1995.

274. Isaka Y, Fujiwara Y, Ueda N, et al: Glomerulosclerosis induced by in vivo transfection of transforming growth factor-beta or platelet-derived growth factor gene into the rat kidney. J Clin Invest 92:2597–2601, 1993.

275. Isaka Y, Brees DK, Ikegaya K, et al: Gene therapy by skeletal muscle expression of decorin prevents fibrotic disease in rat kidney. Nat Med 2:418–423, 1996.

276. Dahly AJ, Hoagland KM, Flasch AK, et al: Antihypertensive effects of chronic anti-TGF-beta antibody therapy in Dahl S rats. Am J Physiol Regul Integr Comp Physiol 283:R757–767, 2002.

277. Kelly DJ, Zhang Y, Gow R, et al: Tranilast attenuates structural and functional aspects of renal injury in the remnant kidney model. J Am Soc Nephrol 15:2619–2629, 2004.

278. Hou CC, Wang W, Huang XR, et al: Ultrasound-microbubble-mediated gene transfer of inducible Smad7 blocks transforming growth factor-beta signaling and fibrosis in rat remnant kidney. Am J Pathol 166:761–771, 2005.

279. Matsuda H, Fukuda N, Ueno T, et al: Development of gene silencing pyrrole-imidazole polyamide targeting the TGF-beta1 promoter for treatment of progressive renal diseases. J Am Soc Nephrol 17:422–432, 2006.

280. Ito Y, Aten J, Bende RJ, et al: Expression of connective tissue growth factor in human renal fibrosis. Kidney Int 53:853–861, 1998.

CH 25

281. Murphy M, Godson C, Cannon S, et al: Suppression subtractive hybridization identifies high glucose levels as a stimulus for expression of connective tissue growth factor and other genes in human mesangial cells. J Biol Chem 274:5830–5834, 1999.
282. Igarashi A, Okochi H, Bradham DM, et al: Regulation of connective tissue growth factor gene expression in human skin fibroblasts and during wound repair. Mol Biol Cell 4:637–645, 1993.
283. Clarkson MR, Gupta S, Murphy M, et al: Connective tissue growth factor: A potential stimulus for glomerulosclerosis and tubulointerstitial fibrosis in progressive renal disease. Curr Opin Nephrol Hypertens 8:543–548, 1999.
284. Chan LY, Leung JC, Tang SC, et al: Tubular expression of angiotensin II receptors and their regulation in IgA nephropathy. J Am Soc Nephrol 16:2306–2317, 2005.
285. Lapinski R, Perico N, Remuzzi A, et al: Angiotensin II modulates glomerular capillary permselectivity in rat isolated perfused kidney. J Am Soc Nephrol 7:653–660, 1996.
286. Hoffmann S, Podlich D, Hahnel B, et al: Angiotensin II type 1 receptor overexpression in podocytes induces glomerulosclerosis in transgenic rats. J Am Soc Nephrol 15:1475–1487, 2004.
287. Arai M, Wada A, Isaka Y, et al: In vivo transfection of genes for renin and angiotensinogen into the glomerular cells induced phenotypic change of the mesangial cells and glomerular sclerosis. Biochem Biophys Res Commun 206:525–532, 1995.
288. van Leeuwen RT, Kol A, Andreotti F, et al: Angiotensin II increases plasminogen activator inhibitor type 1 and tissue-type plasminogen activator messenger RNA in cultured rat aortic smooth muscle cells. Circulation 90:362–368, 1994.
289. Vaughan DE, Lazos SA, Tong K: Angiotensin II regulates the expression of plasminogen activator inhibitor-1 in cultured endothelial cells. A potential link between the renin-angiotensin system and thrombosis. J Clin Invest 95:995–1001, 1995.
290. Feener EP, Northrup JM, Aiello LP, et al: Angiotensin II induces plasminogen activator inhibitor-1 and -2 expression in vascular endothelial and smooth muscle cells. J Clin Invest 95:1353–1362, 1995.
291. Ruiz-Ortega M, Bustos C, Hernandez-Presa MA, et al: Angiotensin II participates in mononuclear cell recruitment in experimental immune complex nephritis through nuclear factor-kappa B activation and monocyte chemoattractant protein-1 synthesis. J Immunol 161:430–439, 1998.
292. Gomez-Garre D, Largo R, Tejera N, et al: Activation of NF-kappaB in tubular epithelial cells of rats with intense proteinuria: role of angiotensin II and endothelin-1. Hypertension 37:1171–1178, 2001.
293. Rice EK, Tesch GH, Cao Z, et al: Induction of MIF synthesis and secretion by tubular epithelial cells: A novel action of angiotensin II. Kidney Int 63:1265–1275, 2003.
294. Hahn AW, Jonas U, Buhler FR, et al: Activation of human peripheral monocytes by angiotensin II. FEBS Lett 347:178–180, 1994.
295. Hernandez J, Astudillo H, Escalante B: Angiotensin II stimulates cyclooxygenase-2 mRNA expression in renal tissue from rats with kidney failure. Am J Physiol Renal Physiol 282:F592–598, 2002.
296. Goncalves AR, Fujihara CK, Mattar AL, et al: Renal expression of COX-2, ANG II, and AT1 receptor in remnant kidney: Strong renoprotection by therapy with losartan and a nonsteroidal anti-inflammatory. Am J Physiol Renal Physiol 286:F945–954, 2004.
297. Vazquez E, Coronel I, Bautista R, et al: Angiotensin II-dependent induction of AT(2) receptor expression after renal ablation. Am J Physiol Renal Physiol 288:F207–213, 2005.
298. Hashimoto N, Maeshima Y, Satoh M, et al: Overexpression of angiotensin type 2 receptor ameliorates glomerular injury in a mouse remnant kidney model. Am J Physiol Renal Physiol 286:F516–525, 2004.
299. Pitt B, Zannad F, Remme WJ, et al: The effect of spironolactone on morbidity and mortality in patients with severe heart failure. Randomized Aldactone Evaluation Study Investigators. N Engl J Med 341:709–717, 1999.
300. Greene EL, Kren S, Hostetter TH: Role of aldosterone in the remnant kidney model in the rat. J Clin Invest 98:1063–1068, 1996.
301. Quan ZY, Walser M, Hill GS: Adrenalectomy ameliorates ablative nephropathy in the rat independently of corticosterone maintenance level. Kidney Int 41:326–333, 1992.
302. Terada Y, Kobayashi T, Kuwana H, et al: Aldosterone stimulates proliferation of mesangial cells by activating mitogen-activated protein kinase 1/2, cyclin D1, and cyclin A. J Am Soc Nephrol 16:2296–2305, 2005.
303. Miyata K, Rahman M, Shokoji T, et al: Aldosterone stimulates reactive oxygen species production through activation of NADPH oxidase in rat mesangial cells. J Am Soc Nephrol 16:2906–2912, 2005.
304. Aldigier JC, Kanjanbuch T, Ma LJ, et al: Regression of existing glomerulosclerosis by inhibition of aldosterone. J Am Soc Nephrol 16:3306–3314, 2005.
305. Ma J, Weisberg A, Griffin JP, et al: Plasminogen activator inhibitor-1 deficiency protects against aldosterone-induced glomerular injury. Kidney Int 69:1064–1072, 2006.
306. Sun Y, Zhang J, Zhang JQ, et al: Local angiotensin II and transforming growth factor-beta1 in renal fibrosis of rats. Hypertension 35:1078–1084, 2000.
307. Han KH, Kang YS, Han SY, et al: Spironolactone ameliorates renal injury and connective tissue growth factor expression in type II diabetic rats. Kidney Int 70:111–120, 2006.
308. Ibrahim HN, Hostetter TH: Aldosterone in renal disease. Curr Opin Nephrol Hypertens 12:159–164, 2003.
309. Hostetter TH, Kren SM, Ibrahim HN: Mineralocorticoid receptor blockade in the remnant kidney model [abstract]. J Am Soc Nephrol 10:75, 1999.
310. Brown NJ, Nakamura S, Ma L, et al: Aldosterone modulates plasminogen activator inhibitor-1 and glomerulosclerosis in vivo. Kidney Int 58:1219–1227, 2000.
311. Rocha R, Chander PN, Khanna K, et al: Mineralocorticoid blockade reduces vascular injury in stroke-prone hypertensive rats. Hypertension 31:451–458, 1998.
312. Ponda MP, Hostetter TH: Aldosterone antagonism in chronic kidney disease. Clin J Am Soc Nephrol 1:668–677, 2006.
313. Epstein M, Buckaleaw V, Martinez F: Eplerenone reduces proteinuria in type 2 diabetes mellitus [abstract]. J Am Coll Cardiol 39:249A, 2002.
314. Miller SB, Martin DR, Kissane J, et al: Hepatocyte growth factor accelerates recovery from acute ischemic renal injury in rats. Am J Physiol 266:F129–134, 1994.
315. Liu Y, Tolbert EM, Lin L, et al: Up-regulation of hepatocyte growth factor receptor: an amplification and targeting mechanism for hepatocyte growth factor action in acute renal failure. Kidney Int 55:442–453, 1999.
316. Liu Y: Hepatocyte growth factor and the kidney. Curr Opin Nephrol Hypertens 11:23–30, 2002.
317. Liu Y, Rajur K, Tolbert E, et al: Endogenous hepatocyte growth factor ameliorates chronic renal injury by activating matrix degradation pathways. Kidney Int 58:2028–2043, 2000.
318. Matsumoto K, Morishita R, Moriguchi A, et al: Prevention of renal damage by angiotensin II blockade, accompanied by increased renal hepatocyte growth factor in experimental hypertensive rats. Hypertension 34:279–284, 1999.
319. Mizuno S, Matsumoto K, Kurosawa T, et al: Reciprocal balance of hepatocyte growth factor and transforming growth factor-beta 1 in renal fibrosis in mice. Kidney Int 57:937–948, 2000.
320. Azuma H, Takahara S, Matsumoto K, et al: Hepatocyte growth factor prevents the development of chronic allograft nephropathy in rats. J Am Soc Nephrol 12:1280–1292, 2001.
321. Yang J, Liu Y: Blockage of tubular epithelial to myofibroblast transition by hepatocyte growth factor prevents renal interstitial fibrosis. J Am Soc Nephrol 13:96–107, 2002.
322. Yang J, Dai C, Liu Y: Systemic administration of naked plasmid encoding hepatocyte growth factor ameliorates chronic renal fibrosis in mice. Gene Ther 8:1470–1479, 2001.
323. Tanaka T, Ichimaru N, Takahara S, et al: In vivo gene transfer of hepatocyte growth factor to skeletal muscle prevents changes in rat kidneys after 5/6 nephrectomy. Am J Transplant 2:828–836, 2002.
324. Inoue T, Okada H, Kobayashi T, et al: Hepatocyte growth factor counteracts transforming growth factor-beta1, through attenuation of connective tissue growth factor induction, and prevents renal fibrogenesis in 5/6 nephrectomized mice. FASEB J 17:268–270, 2003.
325. Takayama H, LaRochelle WJ, Sabnis SG, et al: Renal tubular hyperplasia, polycystic disease, and glomerulosclerosis in transgenic mice overexpressing hepatocyte growth factor/scatter factor. Lab Invest 77:131–138, 1997.
326. Laping NJ, Olson BA, Ho T, et al: Hepatocyte growth factor: a regulator of extracellular matrix genes in mouse mesangial cells. Biochem Pharmacol 59:847–853, 2000.
327. Almanzar MM, Frazier KS, Dube PH, et al: Osteogenic protein-1 mRNA expression is selectively modulated after acute ischemic renal injury. J Am Soc Nephrol 9:1456–1463, 1998.
328. Wang SN, Lapage J, Hirschberg R: Loss of tubular bone morphogenetic protein-7 in diabetic nephropathy. J Am Soc Nephrol 12:2392–2399, 2001.
329. Dube PH, Almanzar MM, Frazier KS, et al: Osteogenic Protein-1: Gene expression and treatment in rat remnant kidney model. Toxicol Pathol 32:384–392, 2004.
330. Hruska KA, Guo G, Wozniak M, et al: Osteogenic protein-1 prevents renal fibrogenesis associated with ureteral obstruction. Am J Physiol Renal Physiol 279:F130–143, 2000.
331. Wang S, Chen Q, Simon TC, et al: Bone morphogenic protein-7 (BMP-7), a novel therapy for diabetic nephropathy. Kidney Int 63:2037–2049, 2003.
332. Gould SE, Day M, Jones SS, et al: BMP-7 regulates chemokine, cytokine, and hemodynamic gene expression in proximal tubule cells. Kidney Int 61:51–60, 2002.
333. Zeisberg M, Kalluri R: The role of epithelial-to-mesenchymal transition in renal fibrosis. J Mol Med 82:175–181, 2004.
334. Wang S, Hirschberg R: BMP7 antagonizes TGF-beta -dependent fibrogenesis in mesangial cells. Am J Physiol Renal Physiol 284:F1006–1013, 2003.
335. Wang S, de Caestecker M, Kopp J, et al: Renal bone morphogenetic protein-7 protects against diabetic nephropathy. J Am Soc Nephrol 17:2504–2512, 2006.
336. Fogo A, Ichikawa I: Evidence for a pathogenic linkage between glomerular hypertrophy and sclerosis. Am J Kidney Dis 17:666–669, 1991.
337. Yoshida Y, Kawamura T, Ikoma M, et al: Effects of antihypertensive drugs on glomerular morphology. Kidney Int 36:626–635, 1989.
338. McGraw M, Poucell S, Sweet J, et al: The significance of focal segmental glomerulosclerosis in oligomeganephronia. Int J Pediatr Nephrol 5:67–72, 1984.
339. Fogo A, Hawkins EP, Berry PL, et al: Glomerular hypertrophy in minimal change disease predicts subsequent progression to focal glomerular sclerosis. Kidney Int 38:115–123, 1990.
340. Lax DS, Benstein JA, Tolbert E, et al: Effects of salt restriction on renal growth and glomerular injury in rats with remnant kidneys. Kidney Int 41:1527–1534, 1992.
341. Lafferty HM, Brenner BM: Are glomerular hypertension and "hypertrophy" independent risk factors for progression of renal disease? Semin Nephrol 10:294–304, 1990.
342. Griffin KA, Picken M, Giobbie-Hurder A, et al: Low protein diet mediated renoprotection in remnant kidneys: Renal autoregulatory versus hypertrophic mechanisms. Kidney Int 63:607–616, 2003.
343. Zatz R: Haemodynamically mediated glomerular injury: The end of a 15-year-old controversy? Curr Opin Nephrol Hypertens 5:468–475, 1996.
344. Olson JL, Hostetter TH, Rennke HG, et al: Altered glomerular permselectivity and progressive sclerosis following extreme ablation of renal mass. Kidney Int 22:112–126, 1982.
345. Bohrer MP, Deen WM, Robertson CR, et al: Mechanism of angiotensin II-induced proteinuria in the rat. Am J Physiol 233:F13–F21, 1977.
346. Abbate M, Zoja C, Remuzzi G: How does proteinuria cause progressive renal damage? J Am Soc Nephrol 17:2974–2984, 2006.
347. Eddy AA, Giachelli CM: Renal expression of genes that promote interstitial inflammation and fibrosis in rats with protein-overload proteinuria. Kidney Int 47:1546–1557, 1995.

348. Zoja C, Morigi M, Figliuzzi M, et al: Proximal tubular cell synthesis and secretion of endothelin-1 on challenge with albumin and other proteins. Am J Kidney Dis 26:934–941, 1995.
349. Wang Y, Chen J, Chen L, et al: Induction of monocyte chemoattractant protein-1 in proximal tubule cells by urinary protein. J Am Soc Nephrol 8:1537–1545, 1997.
350. Zoja C, Donadelli R, Colleoni S, et al: Protein overload stimulates RANTES production by proximal tubular cells depending on NF-kappa B activation. Kidney Int 53:1608–1615, 1998.
351. Tang S, Leung JC, Abe K, et al: Albumin stimulates interleukin-8 expression in proximal tubular epithelial cells in vitro and in vivo. J Clin Invest 111:515–527, 2003.
352. Donadelli R, Zanchi C, Morigi M, et al: Protein overload induces fractalkine upregulation in proximal tubular cells through nuclear factor kappaB- and p38 mitogen-activated protein kinase-dependent pathways. J Am Soc Nephrol 14:2436–2446, 2003.
353. Nakajima H, Takenaka M, Kaimori JY, et al: Activation of the signal transducer and activator of transcription signaling pathway in renal proximal tubular cells by albumin. J Am Soc Nephrol 15:276–285, 2004.
354. Erkan E, De Leon M, Devarajan P: Albumin overload induces apoptosis in LLC-PK(1) cells. Am J Physiol Renal Physiol 280:1107–1114, 2001.
355. Morais C, Westhuyzen J, Metharom P, et al: High molecular weight plasma proteins induce apoptosis and Fas/FasL expression in human proximal tubular cells. Nephrol Dial Transplant 20:50–58, 2005.
356. Zandi-Nejad K, Eddy AA, Glassock RJ, et al: Why is proteinuria an ominous biomarker of progressive kidney disease? Kidney Int Suppl 92:S76-S89, 2004.
357. Burton CJ, Combe C, Walls J, et al: Secretion of chemokines and cytokines by human tubular epithelial cells in response to proteins. Nephrol Dial Transplant 14:2628–2633, 1999.
358. Burton CJ, Harper SJ, Bailey E, et al: Turnover of human tubular cells exposed to proteins in vivo and in vitro. Kidney Int 59:507–514, 2001.
359. Kees-Folts D, Sadow JL, Schreiner GF: Tubular catabolism of albumin is associated with the release of an inflammatory lipid. Kidney Int 45:1697–1709, 1994.
360. Arici M, Chana R, Lewington A, et al: Stimulation of proximal tubular cell apoptosis by albumin-bound fatty acids mediated by peroxisome proliferator activated receptor-gamma. J Am Soc Nephrol 14:17–27, 2003.
361. Ong ACM, Moorhead JF: Tubular lipidosis: Epiphenomenon or pathogenetic lesion in human renal disease? Kidney Int 45:753–762, 1994.
362. Ong ACM, Jowett TP, Moorhead JF, et al: Human high density lipoproteins stimulate endothelin-1 release by cultured human renal proximal tubular cells. Kidney Int 46:1315–1321, 1994.
363. Hirschberg R: Bioactivity of glomerular ultrafiltrate during heavy proteinuria may contribute to renal tubulo-interstitial lesions: Evidence for a role for insulin-like growth factor I. J Clin Invest 98:116–124, 1996.
364. Hirschberg R, Wang S: Proteinuria and growth factors in the development of tubulointerstitial injury and scarring in kidney disease. Curr Opin Nephrol Hypertens 14:43–52, 2005.
365. Nomura A, Morita Y, Maruyama S, et al: Role of complement in acute tubulointerstitial injury of rats with aminonucleoside nephrosis. Am J Pathol 151:539–547, 1997.
366. He C, Imai M, Song H, et al: Complement inhibitors targeted to the proximal tubule prevent injury in experimental nephrotic syndrome and demonstrate a key role for C5b-9. J Immunol 174:5750–5757, 2005.
367. Perna A, Remuzzi G: Abnormal permeability to proteins and glomerular lesions: a meta-analysis of experimental and human studies. Am J Kidney Dis 27:34–41, 1996.
368. Lee HS, Lee JS, Koh HI, et al: Intraglomerular lipid deposition in routine biopsies. Clin Nephrol 36:67–75, 1991.
369. Sato H, Suzuki S, Ueno M, et al: Localization of apolipoprotein(a) and B-100 in various renal diseases. Kidney Int 43:430–435, 1993.
370. Wheeler DC, Persaud JW, Fernando R, et al: Effects of low-density lipoproteins on mesangial cell growth and viability in vitro. Nephrol Dial Transplant 5:185–191, 1990.
371. Grone EF, Abboud HE, Hohne M, et al: Actions of lipoproteins in cultured human mesangial cells: Modulation by mitogenic vasoconstrictors. Am J Physiol 263:F686–696, 1992.
372. Rovin BH, Tan LC: LDL stimulates mesangial fibronectin production and chemoattractant expression. Kidney Int 43:218–225, 1993.
373. Nakajima H, Takenaka M, Kaimori JY, et al: Gene expression profile of renal proximal tubules regulated by proteinuria. Kidney Int 61:1577–1587, 2002.
374. Thomas ME, Harris KP, Walls J, et al: Fatty acids exacerbate tubulointerstitial injury in protein-overload proteinuria. Am J Physiol Renal Physiol 283:F640–647, 2002.
375. van Timmeren MM, Bakker SJ, Stegeman CA, et al: Addition of oleic acid to delipidated bovine serum albumin aggravates renal damage in experimental protein-overload nephrosis. Nephrol Dial Transplant 20:2349–2357, 2005.
376. Abbate M, Zoja C, Corna D, et al: In progressive nephropathies, overload of tubular cells with filtered proteins translates glomerular permeability dysfunction into cellular signals of interstitial inflammation. J Am Soc Nephrol 9:1213–1224, 1998.
377. Abbate M, Zoja C, Rottoli D, et al: Proximal tubular cells promote fibrogenesis by TGF-beta1-mediated induction of peritubular myofibroblasts. Kidney Int 61:2066–2077, 2002.
378. Bonegio RG, Fuhro R, Wang Z, et al: Rapamycin ameliorates proteinuria-associated tubulointerstitial inflammation and fibrosis in experimental membranous nephropathy. J Am Soc Nephrol 16:2063–2072, 2005.
379. Gandhi M, Olson JL, Meyer TW: Contribution of tubular injury to loss of remnant kidney function. Kidney Int 54:1157–1165, 1998.
380. Eardley KS, Zehnder D, Quinkler M, et al: The relationship between albuminuria, MCP-1/CCL2, and interstitial macrophages in chronic kidney disease. Kidney Int 69:1189–1197, 2006.
381. Peterson JC, Adler S, Burkart JM, et al: Blood pressure control, proteinuria, and the progression of renal disease. The Modification of Diet in Renal Disease Study. Ann Intern Med 123:754–762, 1995.
382. de Zeeuw D, Remuzzi G, Parving HH, et al: Proteinuria, a target for renoprotection in patients with type 2 diabetic nephropathy: lessons from RENAAL. Kidney Int 65:2309–2320, 2004.
383. Ruggenenti P, Perna A, Remuzzi G: Retarding progression of chronic renal disease: The neglected issue of residual proteinuria. Kidney Int 63:2254–2261, 2003.
384. Jafar TH, Stark PC, Schmid CH, et al: Proteinuria as a modifiable risk factor for the progression of non-diabetic renal disease. Kidney Int 60:1131–1140, 2001.
385. The HOPE Study Investigators: Effects of ramipril on cardiovascular and microvascular outcomes in people with diabetes mellitus: results of the HOPE study and MICRO-HOPE substudy. Lancet 355:253–259, 2000.
386. Ruggenenti P, Perna A, Gherardi G, et al: Renoprotective properties of ACE-inhibition in non-diabetic nephropathies with non-nephrotic proteinuria. Lancet 354:359–364, 1999.
387. Wright JT, Jr., Bakris G, Greene T, et al: Effect of blood pressure lowering and antihypertensive drug class on progression of hypertensive kidney disease: Results from the AASK trial. JAMA 288:2421–2431, 2002.
388. Parving HH, Lehnert H, Brochner-Mortensen J, et al: The effect of irbesartan on the development of diabetic nephropathy in patients with type 2 diabetes. N Engl J Med 345:870–878, 2001.
389. Nakao N, Yoshimura A, Morita H, et al: Combination treatment of angiotensin-II receptor blocker and angiotensin-converting-enzyme inhibitor in non-diabetic renal disease (COOPERATE): A randomised controlled trial. Lancet 361:117–124, 2003.
390. Schmieder RE, Klingbeil AU, Fleischmann EH, et al: Additional antiproteinuric effect of ultrahigh dose candesartan: A double-blind, randomized, prospective study. J Am Soc Nephrol 16:3038–3045, 2005.
391. Casas JP, Chua W, Loukogeorgakis S, et al: Effect of inhibitors of the renin-angiotensin system and other antihypertensive drugs on renal outcomes: Systematic review and meta-analysis. Lancet 366:2026–2033, 2005.
392. The ALLHAT Investigators: Major outcomes in high-risk hypertensive patients randomized to angiotensin-converting enzyme inhibitor or calcium channel blocker vs diuretic: The Antihypertensive and Lipid-Lowering Treatment to Prevent Heart Attack Trial (ALLHAT). JAMA 288:2981–2997, 2002.
393. Rahman M, Pressel S, Davis BR, et al: Renal outcomes in high-risk hypertensive patients treated with an angiotensin-converting enzyme inhibitor or a calcium channel blocker vs a diuretic: a report from the Antihypertensive and Lipid-Lowering Treatment to Prevent Heart Attack Trial (ALLHAT). Arch Intern Med 165:936–946, 2005.
394. Mann JF, McClellan WM, Kunz R, et al: Progression of renal disease—can we forget about inhibition of the renin-angiotensin system? Nephrol Dial Transplant 2006:2348–2351, 2006.
395. Jafar TH, Schmid CH, Landa M, et al: Angiotensin-converting enzyme inhibitors and progression of nondiabetic renal disease. A meta-analysis of patient-level data. Ann Int Med 135:73–87, 2001.
396. Strippoli GFM, Craig M, Deeks JJ, et al: Effects of angiotensin converting enzyme inhibitors and angiotensin II receptor antagonists on mortality and renal outcomes in diabetic nephropathy: Systemic review. BMJ 329:828–831, 2004.
397. Li PK, Weening JJ, Dirks J, et al: A report with consensus statements of the International Society of Nephrology 2004 Consensus Workshop on Prevention of Progression of Renal Disease, Hong Kong, June 29, 2004. Kidney Int Suppl 94:S2-S7, 2005.
398. Campese VM, Karubian F: Salt sensitivity in hypertension: Implications for the kidney. J Am Soc Nephrol 2:S53–61, 1991.
399. Zucchelli P, Zuccala A: The diagnostic dilemma of hypertensive nephrosclerosis: The nephrologist's view. Am J Kidney Dis 21:87–91, 1993.
400. Iseki K, Iseki C, Ikemiya Y, et al: Risk of developing end-stage renal disease in a cohort of mass screening. Kidney Int 49:800–805, 1996.
401. Perry Jr HM, Miller P, Fornoff JR, et al: Early predictors of 15-year end-stage renal disease in hypertensive patients. Hypertension 25 [part 1]:587–594, 1995.
402. Haroun MK, Jaar BG, Hoffman SC, et al: Risk factors for chronic kidney disease: A prospective study of 23,534 men and women in Washington County, Maryland. J Am Soc Nephrol 14:2934–2941, 2003.
403. Fox CS, Larson MG, Leip EP, et al: Predictors of new-onset kidney disease in a community-based population. JAMA 291:844–850, 2004.
404. Klag MJ, Whelton PK, Randall BL, et al: Blood pressure and end-stage renal disease in men. N Engl J Med 334:13–18, 1996.
405. Hsu CY, McCulloch CE, Darbinian J, et al: Elevated blood pressure and risk of end-stage renal disease in subjects without baseline kidney disease. Arch Int Med 165:923–928, 2005.
406. Retnakaran R, Cull CA, Thorne KI, et al: Risk factors for renal dysfunction in type 2 diabetes: U.K. Prospective Diabetes Study 74. Diabetes 55:1832–1839, 2006.
407. Taal MW: Slowing the progression of adult chronic kidney disease: Therapeutic advances. Drugs 64:2273–2289, 2004.
408. Alkhunaizi AM, Chapman A: Renal artery stenosis and unilateral focal and segmental glomerulosclerosis. Am J Kidney Dis 29:936–941, 1997.
409. Berkman J, Rifkin H: Unilateral nodular diabetic glomerulosclerosis (Kimmelsteil-Wilson): Report of a case. Metabolism 22:715–722, 1973.
410. Klahr S, Levey AS, Beck GJ, et al: The effects of dietary protein restriction and blood-pressure control on the progression of chronic renal disease. Modification of Diet in Renal Disease Study Group. N Engl J Med 330:877–884, 1994.
411. Peterson JC, Adler S, Burkart JM, et al: Blood pressure control, proteinuria, and the progression of renal disease. Ann Intern Med 123:754–762, 1995.
412. Sarnak MJ, Greene T, Wang X, et al: The effect of a lower target blood pressure on the progression of kidney disease: Long-term follow-up of the modification of diet in renal disease study. Ann Intern Med 142:342–351, 2005.

413. Bidani AK, Griffin KA, Bakris G, et al: Lack of evidence of blood pressure-independent protection by renin-angiotensin system blockade after renal ablation. Kidney Int 57:1651–1661, 2000.

414. Lewis JB, Berl T, Bain RP, et al: Effect of intensive blood pressure control on the course of type 1 diabetic nephropathy. Am J Kidney Dis 34:809–817, 1999.

415. Schrier R, McFann K, Johnson A, et al: Cardiac and renal effects of standard versus rigorous blood pressure control in autosomal-dominant polycystic kidney disease: Results of a seven-year prospective randomized study. J Am Soc Nephrol 13:1733–1739, 2002.

416. Ruggenenti P, Perna A, Loriga G, et al: Blood-pressure control for renoprotection in patients with non-diabetic chronic renal disease (REIN-2): Multicentre, randomised controlled trial. Lancet 365:939–946, 2005.

417. Pohl MA, Blumenthal S, Cordonnier DJ, et al: Independent and additive impact of blood pressure control and angiotensin II receptor blockade on renal outcomes in the Irbesartan Diabetic Nephropathy Trial: Clinical implications and limitations. J Am Soc Nephrol 16:3027–3037, 2005.

418. Bosch JP, Lew S, Glabman S, et al: Renal hemodynamic changes in humans. Response to protein loading in normal and diseased kidneys. Am J Med 81:809–815, 1986.

419. Bosch JP, Lauer A, Glabman S: Short-term protein loading in assessment of patients with renal disease. Am J Med 77:873–879, 1984.

420. Krishna GG, Kapoor SC: Preservation of renal reserve in chronic renal disease. Am J Kidney Dis 17:18–24, 1991.

421. O'Connor WJ, Summerill RA: The excretion of urea by dogs following a meat meal. J Physiol 256:93–102, 1976.

422. O'Connor WJ, Summerill RA: Sulphate excretion by dogs following ingestion of ammonium sulphate or meat. J Physiol 260:597–607, 1976.

423. Wiseman MJ, Hunt R, Goodwin A, et al: Dietary composition and renal function in healthy subjects. Nephron 46:37–42, 1987.

424. Meyer TW, Ichikawa I, Zatz R, et al: The renal hemodynamic response to amino acid infusion in the rat. Trans Assoc Am Phys 96:76083, 1983.

425. Johannesen J, Lie M, Kiil F: Effect of glycine and glucagon on glomerular filtration and renal metabolic rates. Am J Physiol 233:F61-F66, 1977.

426. Maack T, Johnson V, Tate SS, et al: Effects of amino-acids (AA) on the function of the isolated perfused rat kidney [abstract]. Fed Proc 33:305, 1974.

427. Castellino P, Coda B, DeFronzo RA: The effect of intravenous amino acid infusion on renal hemodynamics in man [abstract]. Kidney Int 27:243, 1985.

428. King A: Nitric oxide and the renal hemodynamic response to proteins. Semin Nephrol 15:405–414, 1995.

429. Krishna GG, Newell G, Miller E, et al: Protein-induced glomerular hyperfiltration: Role of hormonal factors. Kidney Int 33:578–583, 1988.

430. Nakamura T, Fukui M, Ebihara I, et al: Effects of low-protein diet in glomerular endothelin family gene expression in experimental focal glomerular sclerosis. Clin Sci 88:29–37, 1995.

431. Benabe JE, Wang J, Wilcox JN, et al: Modulation of ANG II receptor and its mRNA in normal rat by low-protein feeding. Am J Physiol 265:F660–669, 1993.

432. Bertani T, Zoja C, Abbate M, et al: Age-related nephropathy and proteinuria in rats with intact kidneys exposed to diets with different protein content. Lab Invest 60:196–204, 1989.

433. Levey AS, Beck GJ, Bosch JP, et al: Short-term effects of protein intake, blood pressure, and antihypertensive therapy on glomerular filtration rate in the Modification of Diet in Renal Disease Study. J Am Soc Nephrol 7:2097–2109, 1996.

434. Pedrini MT, Levey AS, Lau J, et al: The effect of dietary protein restriction on the progression of diabetic and nondiabetic renal diseases: a meta-analysis. Ann Intern Med 124:627–632, 1996.

435. Fouque D, Wang P, Laville M, et al: Low protein diets delay end-stage renal disease in non-diabetic adults with chronic renal failure. Nephrol Dial Transplant 15:1986–1992, 2000.

436. Kasiske BL, Lakatua JD, Ma JZ, et al: A meta-analysis of the effects of dietary protein restriction on the rate of decline in renal function. Am J Kidney Dis 31:954–961, 1998.

437. Mitch WE, Remuzzi G: Diets for patients with chronic kidney disease, still worth prescribing. J Am Soc Nephrol 15:234–237, 2004.

438. Baylis C: Age-dependent glomerular damage in the rat. Dissociation between glomerular injury and both glomerular hypertension and hypertrophy. Male gender as a primary risk factor. J Clin Invest 94:1823–1829, 1994.

439. Baylis C, Corman B: The aging kidney: insights from experimental studies. J Am Soc Nephrol 9:699–709, 1998.

440. Sakemi T, Toyoshima H, Morito F: Testosterone eliminates the attenuating effect of castration on progressive glomerular injury in hypercholesterolemic male Imai rats. Nephron 67:469–476, 1994.

441. Sakemi T, Ohtsuka N, Yoshiyuki T, et al: Testosterone does not eliminate the attenuating effect of estrogen on progressive glomerular injury in estrogen-treated hypercholesterolemic male Imai rats. Kidney Blood Press Res 20:51–56, 1997.

442. Joles JA, van Goor H, van der Horst MLC, et al: High lipid levels in very low density lipoprotein and intermediate density lipoprotein may cause proteinuria and glomerulosclerosis in aging female analbuminemic rats. Lab Invest 73:912–921, 1995.

443. Lombet JR, Adler SG, Anderson PS, et al: Sex vulnerability in the subtotal nephrectomy model of glomerulosclerosis in the rat. J Lab Clin Med 114:66–74, 1989.

444. Reckelhoff JF, Baylis C: Glomerular metalloproteinase activity in the aging rat kidney: Inverse correlation with injury. J Am Soc Nephrol 3:1835–1838, 1993.

445. Neugarten J, Silbiger SR: Effects of sex hormones on mesangial cells. Am J Kidney Dis 26:147–151, 1995.

446. United States Renal Data System: Incidence and Prevalence. USRDS Annual Data Report:66–80, 2005.

447. Iseki K, Ikemiya Y, Fukiyama K: Risk factors of end-stage renal disease and serum creatinine in a community-based mass screening. Kidney Int 51:850–854, 1997.

448. Hannedouche T, Chauveau P, Kalou F, et al: Factors affecting progression in advanced chronic renal failure. Clin Nephrol 39:312–320, 1993.

449. Jungers P, Hannedouche T, Itakura Y, et al: Progression rate to end-stage renal failure in non-diabetic kidney diseases: A multivariate analysis of determinant factors. Nephrol Dial Transplant 10:1353–1360, 1995.

450. Eriksen BO, Ingebretsen OC: The progression of chronic kidney disease: A 10-year population-based study of the effects of gender and age. Kidney Int 69:375–382, 2006.

451. Evans M, Fryzek JP, Elinder CG, et al: The natural history of chronic renal failure: Results from an unselected, population-based, inception cohort in Sweden. Am J Kidney Dis 46:863–870, 2005.

452. Neugarten J, Acharya A, Silbiger SR: Effect of gender on the progression of nondiabetic renal disease: A meta-analysis. J Am Soc Nephrol 11:319–329, 2000.

453. Jafar TH, Schmid CH, Stark PC, et al: The rate of progression of renal disease may not be slower in women compared with men: A patient-level meta-analysis. Nephrol Dial Transplant 18:2047–2053, 2003.

454. Silbiger SR, Neugarten J: The impact of gender on the progression of chronic renal disease. Am J Kidney Dis 25:515–533, 1995.

455. Buckalew VM, Jr, Berg RL, Wang SR, et al: Prevalence of hypertension in 1,795 subjects with chronic renal disease: the modification of diet in renal disease study baseline cohort. Modification of Diet in Renal Disease Study Group. Am J Kidney Dis 28:811–821, 1996.

456. Luyckx VA, Brenner BM: Low birth weight, nephron number, and kidney disease. Kidney Int Suppl 97:S68-S77, 2005.

457. Nenov VD, Taal MW, Sakharova OV, et al: Multi-hit nature of chronic renal disease. Curr Opin Nephrol Hypertens 9:85–97, 2000.

458. Price DA, Owen WF Jr: African-Americans on maintenance dialysis: A review of racial differences in incidence, treatment and survival. Adv Ren Repl Therapy 4:3–12, 1997.

459. Striker GE: Kidney disease and hypertension in blacks. Am J Kidney Dis 20:673, 1992.

460. Klag MJ, Whelton PK, Randall BL, et al: End-stage renal disease in African-American and white men. 16-year MRFIT findings. JAMA 277:1293–1298, 1997.

461. Tarver-Carr ME, Powe NR, Eberhardt MS, et al: Excess risk of chronic kidney disease among African-American versus white subjects in the United States: A population-based study of potential explanatory factors. J Am Soc Nephrol 13:2363–2370, 2002.

462. McClellan W, Warnock DG, McClure L, et al: Racial differences in the prevalence of chronic kidney disease among participants in the Reasons for Geographic and Racial Differences in Stroke (REGARDS) Cohort Study. J Am Soc Nephrol 17:1710–1715, 2006.

463. Korbet SM, Genchi RM, Borok RZ, et al: The racial prevalence of glomerular lesion in nephrotic adults. Am J Kidney Dis 27:647–651, 1996.

464. Ingulli E, Tejani A: Racial differences in the incidence and renal outcome of idiopathic focal segmental glomerulosclerosis in children. Pediatr Nephrol 5:393–397, 1991.

465. Tierney WM, McDonald CJ, Luft FC: Renal disease in hypertensive adults: Effect of race and type II diabetes mellitus. Am J Kidney Dis 13:485–493, 1989.

466. Walker WG, Neaton JD, Cutler JA, et al: Renal function change in hypertensive members of the Multiple Risk Factor Intervention Trial. JAMA 268:3085–3091, 1992.

467. Hunsicker LG, Adler S, Caggiula A, et al: Predictors of the progression of renal disease in the Modification of Diet in Renal Disease Study. Kidney Int 51:1908–1919, 1997.

468. Whittle JC, Whelton PK, Seidler AJ, et al: Does racial variation in risk factors explain black-white differences in the incidence of hypertensive end-stage renal disease? Arch Intern Med 151:1359–1364, 1991.

469. Eisner GM: Hypertension: Racial differences. Am J Kidney Dis 16:35–40, 1990.

470. Brancati FL, Whittle JC, Whelton PK, et al: The excess incidence of diabetic end-stage renal disease among blacks. A population based study of potential explanatory factors. JAMA 268:3079–3084, 1992.

471. Cowie CC, Port FK, Wolfe RA, et al: Disparities in incidence of diabetic end-stage renal disease according to race and type of diabetes. N Engl J Med 321:1074–1079, 1989.

472. Krop JS, Coresh J, Chambless LE, et al: A community-based study of explanatory factors for the excess risk for early renal function decline in blacks vs whites with diabetes: The Atherosclerosis Risk in Communities study. Arch Int Med 159:1777–1783, 1999.

473. Lopes AAS, Port FK: The low birth weight hypothesis as a plausible explanation for the black/white differences in hypertension, non-insulin-dependent diabetes and end-stage renal disease. Am J Kidney Dis 25:350–356, 1995.

474. David RJ, Collins Jr JW: Differing birth weight among infants of U.S.-born blacks, African-born blacks and U.S.-born whites. N Engl J Med 337:1209–1214, 1997.

475. Freedman BI, Spray BJ, Tuttle AB, et al: The familial risk of end-stage renal disease in African Americans. Am J Kidney Dis 21:387–393, 1993.

476. Roderick PJ, Raleigh VS, Hallam L, et al: The need and demand for renal replacement therapy in ethnic minorities in England. J Epidemiol Comm Health 50:334–339, 1996.

477. de Zeeuw D, Ramjit D, Zhang Z, et al: Renal risk and renoprotection among ethnic groups with type 2 diabetic nephropathy: A post hoc analysis of RENAAL. Kidney Int 69:1675–1682., 2006.

478. Hoy WE, Megill DM, Hughson MD: Epidemic renal disease of unknown etiology in the Zuni Indians. Am J Kidney Dis 9:485–496, 1987.

479. Pugh JA, Stern MP, Haffner SM, et al: Excess incidence of treatment of end-stage renal disease in Mexican Americans. Am J Epidemiol 127:135–144, 1988.

480. Spencer JL, Silva DT, Snelling P, et al: An epidemic of renal failure among Australian Aboriginals. Med J Aust 168:537–541, 1998.

CH 25

481. Kambham N, Markowitz GS, Valeri AM, et al: Obesity-related glomerulopathy: An emerging epidemic. Kidney Int 59:1498–1509, 2001.
482. Schmitz PG, O'Donnell MP, Kasiske BL, et al: Renal injury in obese Zucker rats: Glomerular hemodynamic alterations and effects of enalapril. Am J Physiol 263:F496–502, 1992.
483. Park SK, Kang SK: Renal function and hemodynamic study in obese Zucker rats. Korean J Int Med 10:48–53, 1995.
484. Wolf G: After all those fat years: Renal consequences of obesity. Nephrol Dial Transplant 18:2471–2474, 2003.
485. Chagnac A, Weinstein T, Herman M, et al: The effects of weight loss on renal function in patients with severe obesity. J Am Soc Nephrol 14:1480–1486, 2003.
486. Gelber RP, Kurth T, Kausz AT, et al: Association between body mass index and CKD in apparently healthy men. Am J Kidney Dis 46:871–880, 2005.
487. Hsu CY, McCulloch CE, Iribarren C, et al: Body mass index and risk for end-stage renal disease. Ann Int Med 144:21–28, 2006.
488. Chen J, Muntner P, Hamm LL, et al: The metabolic syndrome and chronic kidney disease in U.S. adults. Ann Int Med 140:167–174, 2004.
489. Kurella M, Lo JC, Chertow GM: Metabolic syndrome and the risk for chronic kidney disease among nondiabetic adults. J Am Soc Nephrol 16:2134–2140, 2005.
490. Pinto-Sietsma SJ, Navis G, Janssen WM, et al: A central body fat distribution is related to renal function impairment, even in lean subjects. Am J Kidney Dis 41:733–741, 2003.
491. Bonnet F, Deprele C, Sassolas A, et al: Excessive body weight as a new independent risk factor for clinical and pathological progression in primary IgA nephritis. Am J Kidney Dis 37:720–727, 2001.
492. Rump LC, Amann K, Orth S, et al: Sympathetic overactivity in renal disease: a window to understand progression and cardiovascular complications of uraemia? Nephrol Dial Transplant 15:1735–1738, 2000.
493. Converse RL, Jr, Jacobsen TN, Toto RD, et al: Sympathetic overactivity in patients with chronic renal failure. N Engl J Med 327:1912–1918, 1992.
494. Johansson M, Elam M, Rundqvist B, et al: Increased sympathetic nerve activity in renovascular hypertension. Circulation 99:2537–2542, 1999.
495. Klein IH, Ligtenberg G, Oey PL, et al: Sympathetic activity is increased in polycystic kidney disease and is associated with hypertension. J Am Soc Nephrol 12:2427–2433, 2001.
496. Klein IH, Ligtenberg G, Neumann J, et al: Sympathetic nerve activity is inappropriately increased in chronic renal disease. J Am Soc Nephrol 14:3239–3244, 2003.
497. Rahman SN, Abraham WT, Van Putten VJ, et al: Increased norepinephrine secretion in patients with the nephrotic syndrome and normal glomerular filtration rates: Evidence for primary sympathetic activation. Am J Nephrol 13:266–270, 1993.
498. Cerasola G, Vecchi M, Mule G, et al: Sympathetic activity and blood pressure pattern in autosomal dominant polycystic kidney disease hypertensives. Am J Nephrol 18:391–398, 1998.
499. Kosch M, Barenbrock M, Kisters K, et al: Relationship between muscle sympathetic nerve activity and large artery mechanical vessel wall properties in renal transplant patients. J Hypertension 20:501–508, 2002.
500. Campese VM, Kogosov E, Koss M: Renal afferent denervation prevents the progression of renal disease in the renal ablation model of chronic renal failure in the rat. Am J Kidney Dis 26:861–865, 1995.
501. Amann K, Rump LC, Simonaviciene A, et al: Effects of low dose sympathetic inhibition on glomerulosclerosis and albuminuria in subtotally nephrectomized rats. J Am Soc Nephrol 11:1469–1478, 2000.
502. Amann K, Koch A, Hofstetter J, et al: Glomerulosclerosis and progression: Effect of subantihypertensive doses of alpha and beta blockers. Kidney Int 60:1309–1323, 2001.
503. Johnson RJ, Schreiner GF: Hypothesis: The role of acquired tubulointerstitial disease in the pathogenesis of salt-dependent hypertension. Kidney Int 52:1169–1179, 1997.
504. Weinrauch LA, Kennedy FP, Gleason RE, et al: Relationship between autonomic function and progression of renal disease in diabetic proteinuria: Clinical correlations and implications for blood pressure control. Am J Hypertension 11:302–308, 1998.
505. Strojek K, Grzeszczak W, Gorska J, et al: Lowering of microalbuminuria in diabetic patients by a sympathicoplegic agent: Novel approach to prevent progression of diabetic nephropathy? J Am Soc Nephrol 12:602–605, 2001.
506. Ligtenberg G, Blankestijn PJ, Oey PL, et al: Reduction of sympathetic hyperactivity by enalapril in patients with chronic renal failure. N Engl J Med 340:1321–1328, 1999.
507. Klein IH, Ligtenberg G, Oey PL, et al: Enalapril and losartan reduce sympathetic hyperactivity in patients with chronic renal failure. J Am Soc Nephrol 14:425–430, 2003.
508. Cases A, Coll E: Dyslipidemia and the progression of renal disease in chronic renal failure patients. Kidney Int Suppl 99:S87–S93, 2005.
509. Kasiske B, O'Donnell MP, Schmitz PG, et al: Renal injury of diet-induced hypercholesterolemia in rats. Kidney Int 37:880–891, 1990.
510. Fujihara CK, Limongi DMZP, De Oliveira HCF, et al: Absence of focal glomerulosclerosis in aging analbuminemic rats. Am J Physiol 262:R947–R954, 1992.
511. Grone HJ, Walli AK, Grone EF: Arterial hypertension and hyperlipidemia as determinants of glomerulosclerosis. Clin Invest 71:834–839, 1993.
512. Keane WF, Kasiske BL, O'Donnell MP, et al: Hypertension, hyperlipidemia and renal damage. Am J Kidney Dis 21:43–50, 1993.
513. Kasiske B: Relationship between vascular disease and age-associated changes in the human kidney. Kidney Int 31:1153–1159, 1987.
514. Bleyer AJ, Chen R, D'Agostino RB, Jr, et al: Clinical correlates of hypertensive end-stage renal disease. Am J Kidney Dis 31:28–34, 1998.
515. Muntner P, Coresh J, Smith JC, et al: Plasma lipids and risk of developing renal dysfunction: the atherosclerosis risk in communities study. Kidney Int 58:293–301, 2000.
516. Schaeffner ES, Kurth T, Curhan GC, et al: Cholesterol and the risk of renal dysfunction in apparently healthy men. J Am Soc Nephrol 14:2084–2091, 2003.
517. Shohat J, Boner G: Role of lipids in the progression of renal disease in chronic renal failure: Evidence from animal studies and pathogenesis. Isr J Med Sci 29:228–239, 1993.
518. Keane WF: Lipids and the kidney. Kidney Int 46:910–920, 1994.
519. Bucala R, Makita Z, Vega G, et al: Modification of low density lipoprotein by advanced glycation end products contributes to the dyslipidemia of diabetes and renal insufficiency. Proc Natl Acad Sci U S A 91:9441–9445, 1994.
520. Kasiske BL, Ma JZ, Kalil RSN, et al: Effects of antihypertensive therapy on serum lipids. Ann Intern Med 122:133–141, 1995.
521. Monzani G, Bergesio F, Ciuti R, et al: Lipoprotein abnormalities in chronic renal failure and dialysis patients. Blood Purif 14:262–272, 1996.
522. Hunsicker LG, Adler S, Caggiulia A, et al: Predictors of progression of renal disease in the Modification of Diet in Renal Disease Study. Kidney Int 51:1908–1919, 1997.
523. Samuelsson O, Mulec H, Knight-Gibson C, et al: Lipoprotein abnormalities are associated with increased rate of progression of human chronic renal insufficiency. Nephrol Dial Transplant 12:1908–1915, 1997.
524. Krolewski AS, Warram JH, Christlieb AR: Hypercholesterolemia- a determinant of renal function loss and deaths in IDDM patients with nephropathy. Kidney Int 45:S-125–S-131, 1994.
525. Ravid M, Brosh D, Ravid-Safran D, et al: Main risk factors for nephropathy in type 2 diabetes mellitus are plasma cholesterol levels, mean blood pressure, and hyperglycemia. Arch Intern Med 158:998–1004, 1998.
526. Maschio G, Oldrizzi L, Rugiu C, et al: Serum lipids in patients with chronic renal failure on long-term, protein-restricted diets. Am J Med 87:51N–54N, 1989.
527. Syrjanen J, Mustonen J, Pasternack A: Hypertriglyceridaemia and hyperuricaemia are risk factors for progression of IgA nephropathy. Nephrol Dial Transplant 15:34–42, 2000.
528. Radhakrishnan J, Appel AS, Valeri A, et al: The nephrotic syndrome, lipids, and risk factors for cardiovascular disease. Am J Kidney Dis 22:135–142, 1993.
529. Ding G, Pesek-Diamond I, Diamond JR: Cholesterol, macrophages, and gene expression of TGF-β1 and fibronectin during nephrosis. Am J Physiol 264:F577–F584, 1993.
530. Diamond JR, Ding G, Frye J, et al: Glomerular macrophages and the mesangial proliferative response in the experimental nephrotic syndrome. Am J Pathol 141:887–894, 1992.
531. Nishida Y, Yorioka N, Oda H, et al: Effect of lipoproteins on cultured human mesangial cells. Am J Kidney Dis 29:919–930, 1997.
532. Wheeler DC, Chana RS, Topley N, et al: Oxidation of low density lipoprotein by mesangial cells may promote glomerular injury. Kidney Int 45:1628–1636, 1994.
533. Wanner C, Greiber S, Kramer-Guth A, et al: Lipids and progression of renal disease: Role of modified low density lipoprotein and lipoprotein(a). Kidney Int 52:S-102–S-106, 1997.
534. Walker WG: Relation of lipid abnormalities to progression of renal damage in essential hypertension, insulin-dependent and non insulin-dependent diabetes mellitus. Miner Electrolyte Metab 19:137–143, 1993.
535. O'Donell MP, Kasiske BL, Kim Y, et al: Lovastatin retards the progression of established glomerular disease in obese Zucker rats. Am J Kidney Dis 22:83–89, 1993.
536. Park Y-S, Guijarro C, Kim Y, et al: Lovastatin reduces glomerular macrophage influx and monocyte chemoattractant protein-1 mRNA in nephrotic rats. Am J Kidney Dis 31:190–194, 1998.
537. Keane WF: Lipids and progressive renal failure. Wiener Klinische Wochenschrift 108:420–424, 1996.
538. Lee HS, Jeong JY, Kim BC, et al: Dietary antioxidant inhibits lipoprotein oxidation and renal injury in experimental focal segmental glomerulosclerosis. Kidney Int 51:1151–1159, 1997.
539. Fried LF, Orchard TJ, Kasiske BL: Effect of lipid reduction on the progression of renal disease: A meta-analysis. Kidney Int 59:260–269, 2001.
540. Tonelli M, Moye L, Sacks FM, et al: Effect of pravastatin on loss of renal function in people with moderate chronic renal insufficiency and cardiovascular disease. J Am Soc Nephrol 14:1605–1613, 2003.
541. Collins R, Armitage J, Parish S, et al: MRC/BHF Heart Protection Study of cholesterol-lowering with simvastatin in 5963 people with diabetes: A randomised placebo-controlled trial. Lancet 361:2005–2016, 2005.
542. Bianchi S, Bigazzi R, Caiazza A, et al: A controlled, prospective study of the effects of atorvastatin on proteinuria and progression of kidney disease. Am J Kidney Dis 41:565–570, 2003.
543. Manttari M, Tiula E, Alikoski T, et al: Effects of hypertension and dyslipidemia on the decline in renal function. Hypertension 26:670–675, 1995.
544. Tonelli M, Collins D, Robins S, et al: Effect of gemfibrozil on change in renal function in men with moderate chronic renal insufficiency and coronary disease. Am J Kidney Dis 44:832–839, 2004.
545. Ansquer JC, Foucher C, Rattier S, et al: Fenofibrate reduces progression to microalbuminuria over 3 years in a placebo-controlled study in type 2 diabetes: Results from the Diabetes Atherosclerosis Intervention Study (DAIS). Am J Kidney Dis 45:485–493, 2005.
546. Plante GE: Urinary phosphate excretion determines the progression of renal disease. Kidney Int 36:S-128-S-132, 1989.
547. Denda M, Finch J, Slatopolsky E: Phosphorus accelerates the development of parathyroid hyperplasia and secondary hyperparathyroidism in rats with renal failure. Am J Kidney Dis 28:596–602, 1996.
548. Alfrey AC, Zhu J-M: The role of hyperphosphatemia. Am J Kidney Dis 17:53–56, 1991.
549. Delmez JA, Slatopolsky E: Hyperphosphatemia: its consequences and treatment in patients with chronic renal disease. Am J Kidney Dis 19:303–317, 1992.

550. Shimamura T: Prevention of 11-deoxycorticosterone-salt-induced glomerular hypertrophy and glomerulosclerosis by dietary phosphate binder. Am J Pathol 136:549–556, 1990.

551. Ritz E, Gross ML, Dikow R: Role of calcium-phosphorous disorders in the progression of renal failure. Kidney Int Suppl 99:S66–S70, 2005.

552. Barsotti G, Giannoni A, Morelli E, et al: The decline of renal function slowed by very low phosphorus intake in chronic renal patients following a low nitrogen diet. Clin Nephrol 21:54–59, 1984.

553. Ibels LS, Alfrey AC, Huffer WE, et al: Calcification in end-stage kidneys. Am J Med 71:33–37, 1981.

554. Goligorsky MS, Chiamovitz C, Rapoport J, et al: Calcium metabolism in uremic nephrocalcinosis: preventive effect of verapamil. Kidney Int 27:774–779, 1985.

555. Lau K: Phosphate excess and progressive renal failure: The precipitation-calcification hypothesis. Kidney Int 36:918–937, 1989.

556. Schrier RW, Shapiro JI, Chan L, et al: Increased nephron oxygen consumption: Potential role in progression of chronic renal disease. Am J Kidney Dis 23:176–182, 1994.

557. Kramer HJ, Meyer-Lehnert H, Mohaupt M: Role of calcium in the progression of renal disease: Experimental evidence. Kidney Int 41:S-2–S-7, 1992.

558. Trachtman H, Chan JCM, Boyle R, et al: The relationship between calcium, phosphorus and sodium intake, race, and blood pressure in children with renal insufficiency: A report of the growth failure in children with renal diseases (GFRD) study. J Am Soc Nephrol 6:126–131, 1995.

559. Bro S, Olgaard K: Effects of excess PTH on nonclassical target organs. Am J Kidney Dis 30:606–620, 1997.

560. Akmal M, Kasim SE, Soliman AR, et al: Excess parathyroid hormone adversely affects lipid metabolism in chronic renal failure. Kidney Int 37:854–858, 1990.

561. Shigematsu T, Caverzasio J, Bonjour JP: Parathyroid removal prevents the progression of chronic renal failure induced by high protein diet. Kidney Int 44:173–181, 1993.

562. Ogata H, Ritz E, Odoni G, et al: Beneficial effects of calcimimetics on progression of renal failure and cardiovascular risk factors. J Am Soc Nephrol 14:959–967, 2003.

563. Matthias S, Busch R, Merke J, et al: Effects of 1,25(OH)2D3 on compensatory growth in the growing rat. Kidney Int 40:212–218, 1991.

564. Schwarz U, Amann K, Orth SR, et al: Effect of 1,25 (OH)2 vitamin D3 on glomerulosclerosis in subtotally nephrectomized rats. Kidney Int 53:1696–1705, 1998.

565. Hirata M, Makibayashi K, Katsumata K, et al: 22-Oxacalcitriol prevents progressive glomerulosclerosis without adversely affecting calcium and phosphorus metabolism in subtotally nephrectomized rats. Nephrol Dial Transplant 17:2132–2137, 2002.

566. Garcia DL, Anderson S, Rennke HG, et al: Anemia lessens and treatment with recombinant human erythropoietin worsens glomerular injury and hypertension in rats with reduced renal mass. Proc Natl Acad Sci U S A 85:6142–6146, 1988.

567. Lafferty HM, King AJ, Troy JL, et al: Normalization of the renal hemodynamic abnormalities of early anemia in the anemic rat [abstract]. Kidney Int 37:511, 1990.

568. Lafferty HM, Garcia DL, Rennke HG, et al: Anemia ameliorates progressive renal injury in experimental DOCA-Salt hypertension. J Am Soc Nephrol 1:1180–1185, 1991.

569. Puntorieri S, Brugnetti B, Remuzzi G, et al: Renoprotective effect of low iron diet and its consequence on glomerular hemodynamics [abstract]. J Am Soc Nephrol 1:693, 1990.

570. Ataga KI, Orringer EP: Renal abnormalities in sickle cell disease. Am J Hematol 63:205–211, 2000.

571. Scheinman JI: Sickle cell disease and the kidney. Semin Nephrol 23:66–76, 2003.

572. Mohanram A, Zhang Z, Shahinfar S, et al: Anemia and end-stage renal disease in patients with type 2 diabetes and nephropathy. Kidney Int 66:1131–1138, 2004.

573. Ravani P, Tripepi G, Malberti F, et al: Asymmetrical dimethylarginine predicts progression to dialysis and death in patients with chronic kidney disease: A competing risks modeling approach. J Am Soc Nephrol 16:2449–2455, 2005.

574. Kovedsy CP, Trivedi BK, Kalantar-Zadeh K, et al: Association of anemia with outcomes in men with moderate and severe chronic kidney disease. Kidney Int 69:560–564, 2006.

575. Gouva C, Nikolopoulos P, Ioannidis JP, et al: Treating anemia early in renal failure patients slows the decline of renal function: A randomized controlled trial. Kidney Int 66:753–760, 2004.

576. Kuriyama S, Tomonari H, Yoshida H, et al: Reversal of anemia by erythropoietin therapy retards the progression of chronic renal failure, especially in nondiabetic patients. Nephron 77:176–185, 1997.

577. Roger SD, McMahon LP, Clarkson A, et al: Effects of early and late intervention with epoetin alpha on left ventricular mass among patients with chronic kidney disease (stage 3 or 4): results of a randomized clinical trial. J Am Soc Nephrol 15:148–156, 2004.

578. Levin A, Djurdjev O, Thompson C, et al: Canadian randomized trial of hemoglobin maintenance to prevent or delay left ventricular mass growth in patients with CKD. Am J Kidney Dis 46:799–811, 2005.

579. Drüeke TB, Locatelli F, Clyne N, et al: Normalization of hemoglobin level in patients with chronic kidney disease and anemia, N Engl J Med 244:2071–2084, 2006.

580. Groppelli A, Giorgi DM, Omboni S, et al: Persistent blood pressure increase induced by heavy smoking. J Hypertension 10:495–499, 1992.

581. Ritz E, Benck U, Franek E, et al: Effects of smoking on renal hemodynamics in healthy volunteers and in patients with glomerular disease. J Am Soc Nephrol 9:1798–1804, 1998.

582. Benck U, Clorius JH, Zuna I, et al: Renal hemodynamic changes during smoking: effects of adrenoreceptor blockade. Eur J Clin Invest 29:1010–1018, 1999.

583. Halimi JM, Giraudeau B, Vol S, et al: Effects of current smoking and smoking discontinuation on renal function and proteinuria in the general population. Kidney Int 58:1285–1292, 2000.

584. Oberai B, Adams CW, High OB: Myocardial and renal arteriolar thickening in cigarette smokers. Atherosclerosis 52:185–190, 1984.

585. Lhotta K, Rumpelt HJ, Konig P, et al: Cigarette smoking and vascular pathology in renal biopsies. Kidney Int 61:648–654, 2002.

586. Pinto-Sietsma SJ, Mulder J, Janssen WM, et al: Smoking is related to albuminuria and abnormal renal function in nondiabetic persons. Ann Int Med 133:585–591, 2000.

587. Bleyer AJ, Shemanski LR, Burke GL, et al: Tobacco, hypertension, and vascular disease: risk factors for renal functional decline in an older population. Kidney Int 57:2072–2079, 2000.

588. Goetz FC, Jacobs DR, Jr, Chavers B, et al: Risk factors for kidney damage in the adult population of Wadena, Minnesota. A prospective study. Am J Epidemiol 145:91–102, 1997.

589. Chase HP, Garg SK, Marshall G, et al: Cigarette smoking increases the risk of albuminuria among subjects with type I diabetes. JAMA 265:614–617, 1991.

590. Muhlhauser I, Overmann H, Bender R, et al: Predictors of mortality and end-stage diabetic complications in patients with Type 1 diabetes mellitus on intensified insulin therapy. Diabet Med 17:727–734, 2000.

591. Stegmayr B, Lithner F: Tobacco and end stage diabetic nephropathy. Br Med J 295:581–582, 1987.

592. Biesenbach G, Janko O, Zazgornik J: Similar rate of progression in the predialysis phase in type I and type II diabetes mellitus. Nephrol Dial Transplant 9:1097–1102, 1994.

593. Mehler PS, Jeffers BW, Biggerstaff SL, et al: Smoking as a risk factor for nephropathy in non-insulin-dependent diabetics. J Gen Int Med 13:842–845, 1998.

594. Pijls LT, de Vries H, Kriegsman DM, et al: Determinants of albuminuria in people with Type 2 diabetes mellitus. Diabetes Res Clin Practice-Suppl 52:133–143, 2001.

595. Orth SR, Schroeder T, Ritz E, et al: Effects of smoking on renal function in patients with type 1 and type 2 diabetes. Nephrol Dial Transplant 20:2414–2419, 2005.

596. Orth SR, Stockmann A, Conradt C, et al: Smoking as a risk factor for end-stage renal failure in men with primary renal disease. Kidney Int 54:926–931, 1998.

597. Ward MM, Studenski S: Clinical prognostic factors in lupus nephritis. The importance of hypertension and smoking. Arch Intern Med 152:2082–2088, 1992.

598. Stengel B, Couchoud C, Cenee S, et al: Age, blood pressure and smoking effects on chronic renal failure in primary glomerular nephropathies. Kidney Int 57:2519–2526, 2000.

599. Samuelsson O, Attman PO: Is smoking a risk factor for progression of chronic renal failure? Kidney Int 58:2597, 2000.

600. Regalado M, Yang S, Wesson DE: Cigarette smoking is associated with augmented progression of renal insufficiency in severe essential hypertension. Am J Kidney Dis 35:687–694, 2000.

601. Orth SR, Ritz E: The renal risks of smoking: an update. Curr Opin Nephrol Hypertens 11:483–488, 2002.

602. Barrow SE, Ward PS, Sleightholm MA, et al: Cigarette smoking: Profiles of thromboxane- and prostacycline-derived products in human urine. Bioch Biophys Acta 993:121–127, 1989.

603. Odoni G, Ogata H, Viedt C, et al: Cigarette smoking condensate aggravates renal injury in the renal ablation model. Kidney Int 61:2090–2098, 2002.

604. Sawicki PT, Didjurgeit U, Muhlhauser I, et al: Smoking is associated with progression of diabetic nephropathy. Diabetes Care 17:126–131, 1994.

CHAPTER 26

Renal and Systemic Manifestations of Glomerular Disease

Sharon Anderson • Radko Komers • Barry M. Brenner

PROTEINURIA

Proteinuria characterizes most forms of glomerular injury and causes or contributes to all of the complications of the nephrotic syndrome. This section reviews the physiology and pathophysiology of glomerular proteinuria and the mechanisms by which proteinuria engenders systemic complications. Extensive discussion of the mechanisms of proteinuria may also be found in several reviews.[1-7]

Mechanisms of Proteinuria

Prerenal, Glomerular, and Tubular Proteinuria

The amount of protein excreted in the urine is a function of three factors: the amount of protein presented to the glomerulus (the filtered load); the permeability of the glomerular capillary wall (GCW); and the efficiency of proximal tubule reabsorption of filtered proteins. The major clinically relevant proteinuric syndromes, and the only ones that may lead to massive proteinuria, result from alterations in glomerular permeability to normally filtered proteins. Defense against proteinuria is dependent upon the structure and function of the GCW, characteristics of the protein molecule being presented to the glomerular barrier, and hemodynamic factors.

The Anatomic Barrier to Proteinuria: The Glomerular Capillary Wall

The classic view of the anatomic barrier to the filtration of protein has been extensively reviewed[1] and is briefly summarized here. As detailed later, recent years have seen a major advance in our insight into this process through the discovery of nephrin and associated studies of the molecular nature of the slit diaphragm.

The glomerular capillary barrier consists of multiple layers: the fenestrated endothelial cell surface layer (glycocalyx); the glomerular basement membrane (GBM); and the epithelial podocytes and intercalated slit diaphragms. Early studies concluded that the GBM was the component of the GCW that restricted passage of proteins.[8] Subsequent studies were consistent with this "single-barrier" hypothesis,[1] until studies with peroxidative tracers found that the slit diaphragm was an effective barrier to filtration.[9] Later studies led to the "double-barrier" hypothesis: that the GBM restricts the passage of larger macromolecules, whereas slit diaphragms regulate the passage of smaller ones.[10] However, this hypothesis failed to explain the findings that some relatively large tracers were restricted just beneath the slit diaphragm and some were completely restricted at the level of the inner layers of the GBM, so the potential contribution of charge needed to be addressed. Rennke and co-workers[11] used several ferritin fractions of similar size with varying isoelectric points (pIs). A stepwise

increase in the pI of ferritin resulted in a proportionate increase in its permeation into the GBM, with the more negatively charged particles penetrating furthest. Thus, these studies pointed to the existence of an intrinsic electrical charge in the GBM that was imparted by fixed anionic sites.[11]

These anionic sites have been localized to the surfaces of endothelial and epithelial cells, as well as GBM interposed between these cells.[1,12] The podocyte and its foot processes are covered with a surface coat of acidic glycoproteins (sialoproteins or glomerular polyanions) that are highly negatively charged. Stainable polyanion has been identified to be podocalyxin, a sialoprotein that carries most of the glomerular sialic acid.[13] The epithelial slit diaphragm also consists, in part, of glycosialoproteins,[14] as does the endothelial cell coat.

The biochemical composition of the GBM has been extensively studied.[1,15] The GBM consists of a nonpolar collagen-like component and a more polar noncollagen fraction of asparagine-linked polysaccharide units. Glomerular epithelial cells are capable of synthesizing all major GBM components. Integral components of the GBM include type IV collagen, laminin, entactin/nidogen, and various proteoglycans, including chondroitin sulfate proteoglycan and heparan sulfate proteoglycan (HS-PG). Of the latter, HS-PG has been shown to be particularly important in imparting charge selectivity to the GBM.[1,16] Normally, polyanions (particular HS-PG) act as "anticlogging" agents to prevent the adsorption of plasma protein so that ultrafiltration may proceed.[16] Many studies have indicated the importance of anionic sites and HS-PG specifically in the defense against proteinuria.[17,18] However, as discussed later, newer evidence points away from a predominant role of the GBM in filtration barrier function.

The role of glomerular cells in the defense against proteinuria has recently taken center stage, in view of innovative technologies and improvements in understanding of the molecular basis of the GCW. Daniels and colleagues[19,20] used confocal microscopy to examine diffusion of fluorescent macromolecules across individual glomerular capillaries in intact glomeruli. Studies in this system showed that protein (dextran) clearance in intact glomeruli is much less than that for the GBM alone; most of the selectivity of the GCW resides in the cells rather than in the GBM.[20] In further support of this concept, removal of perlecan, the principal proteoglycan of the GBM, does not produce proteinuria.[21]

Observations of changes in the structure of podocytes in various clinical proteinuric diseases prompted speculation that defects in that cell might be responsible for increased GCW permeability. In vivo studies have provided further confirmation of the importance of podocytes[22] and slit diaphragms[2,3,23] in the restrictive properties of the GCW. In 1998, Kestilä and associates[24] identified the gene mutation in congenital nephrotic syndrome of the Finnish type (CNF, NPHSI), which is characterized by congenital proteinuria and absence of the slit diaphragm. The disease gene was shown to encode the protein nephrin in the slit diaphragm.[25,26] Experimentally, nephrin-deficient mice were shown to develop massive proteinuria at birth, resulting in neonatal mortality.[26] Clinically, nephrin deficiency has been identified in a number of proteinuric renal diseases, including diabetic nephropathy.[27]

The structure and function of the slit diaphragm is an area of active investigation. Although the actual structure is not yet fully understood, there are a number of interacting components.[3,6] A hypothetical model of the slit diaphragm is depicted in Figure 26–1.[6] According to this model, the slit diaphragm components nephrin and Neph1 likely interact with each other and form the backbone of the slit diaphragm. The function of other included proteins, such as P-cadherin and FAT, are unresolved. Nephrin and Neph1 interact with the intracellular adapter molecules podocin, CD2AP and Zona Occludens-1 (ZO-1), which connect the slit diaphragm to the actin cytoskeleton of foot process. The adapter molecules also enhance the signaling function of nephrin and Neph1. Regulation of these molecules and their interactions is under active investigation.[3,6] Interestingly, it has recently been reported that angiotensin II induces reorganization of F-actin fibers and redistribution of ZO-1 that is physically associated with actin in murine podocytes and that the F-actin stabilizer jasplakinolide prevented both ZO-1 redistribution and albumin leakage.[28]

Several other candidate genes have been identified as potentially being associated with nephrotic syndromes; further details are available in Chapter 39 and several recent reviews.[3–6]

Whereas most attention has centered on the role of the podocyte, the role of the endothelial cell and its surface coat, the glycocalyx, is beginning to receive some attention.[5] The glycocalyx consists of highly negatively charged proteoglycans and glycosaminoglycans reinforced with plasma proteins such as orosomucoid (a protein produced by endothelial cells).[29] Synthesis of proteoglycans and glycosaminoglycans is down-regulated when endothelial cells are exposed to puromycin, a proteinuric toxin.[30] In an extrarenal system (the peritoneum), transvascular protein transport is markedly increased in mice lacking endothelial caveolae,[31] suggesting another mechanism by which the endothelial layer retards protein filtration.

Proximal Tubule Protein Reabsorption

"Tubular proteinuria" results from impairment in the normal proximal tubular degradation of filtered proteins. In the normal kidney, significant amounts of albumin are filtered, but the amount reaching the final urine is less than 30 mg/day. The degradation of filtered proteins occurs through lysosomal or endosomal activity; protein degradation consists of lysosomal protein uptake from the tubular fluid and subsequent exocytosis of peptide products back into the urine. It now appears that reabsorption of albumin is receptor-mediated (see reviews[32–35]). Luminal endocytosis is initiated by ligand binding to receptors localized in the clathrin-coated pits, followed by internalization, segregation of ligands and receptors in early and late endosomes, and directing of ligands to lysosomes for degradation, whereas the receptors are directed back to the apical plasma membrane via dense apical tubules.[7] Pathways of albumin handling in the kidney are schematized in Figure 26–2.[35] The initial recognition step by receptor-mediated endocytosis involves at least two proteins, megalin and cubilin, that appear to operate cooperatively.[32] Their importance is demonstrated in studies in mouse knockout models. In animals lacking CLC-5,[36] megalin,[37] or cubulin[38] proteinuria increases markedly.

Glomerular Permselectivity

Proteinuria has been further characterized by studies of permselectivity, the extent to which the GCW discriminates among molecules of different size, charge, and configuration. Classically, measurement of the Bowman space–to–plasma concentration ratio (the "sieving coefficient," θ) for various proteins has been determined by direct sampling via micropuncture techniques.[2] These studies indicate that small substances appear in the glomerular filtrate in concentrations similar to those in plasma, whereas the serum albumin is filtered to a much lesser extent (<0.1% that of inulin). The most extensively used method to quantify glomerular capillary permselectivity involves measurement of the fractional clearance of test macromolecules. If, like inulin, the test macromolecule is not reabsorbed or secreted, its fractional clearance will exactly equal its Bowman space–to–plasma concentration ratio, θ.[2] Proteins are not ideal test markers because of variations in size, charge, and shape, as well as tubule reabsorption of filtered protein. These difficulties may be circumvented with the use of a variety of exogenous nonprotein polymers, and much of the available permselectivity data relate to the use of dextran.[1] However, Ficoll has been evaluated and appears to be superior.[2,39]

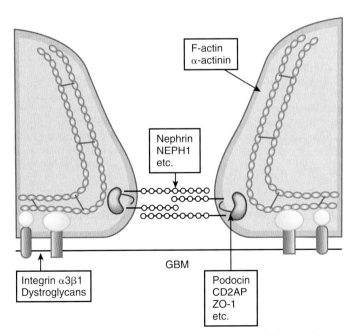

FIGURE 26–1 Hypothetical model of the podocyte slit diaphragm. See text for discussion. (Reproduced from Jalanko H: Pathogenesis of proteinuria: Lessons learned from nephrin and podocin. Pediatr Nephrol 18:487–491, 2003, with permission.)

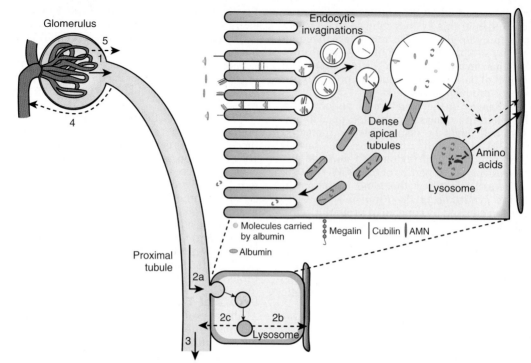

FIGURE 26–2 Pathways of albumin degradation in the proximal tubule. Albumin is filtered in the glomeruli (1) and reabsorbed by the proximal tubule cells by receptor-mediated endocytosis (2a). Internalization by endocytosis is followed by transport into lysosomes for degradation. Classically, this is considered to result in the formation of free amino acids released into the circulation (2b); however, it has been recently suggested that significant amounts of albumin fragments are excreted in the urine, possibly resulting from tubular degradation of filtered albumin (2c). Some intact albumin may escape tubular reabsorption (3), the amount being greater as the glomerular filtration fraction of albumin increases or tubular function is compromised. The *upper right* shows a schematic representation of the intracellular pathways following endocytic uptake of albumin and possible associated substances. Following binding to the receptors, cubilin or megalin, the receptor-albumin complex is directed into coated pits for endocytosis, a process that may also involve amnionless (AMN). The complex dissociates following vesicular acidification, most likely also leading to the release of any bound substances. Albumin is transferred to the lysosomal compartment for degradation. Some albumin may be degraded within a late endocytic compartment and recycled as fragments to be released at the luminal surface. Alternatively, albumin fragments may be recycled from the lysosomal compartment by a yet unknown route. Receptors recycle through dense apical tubules, whereas released substances carried by albumin may be released into the cytosol or transported across the tubular cell. An alternative high-capacity retrieval pathway for nondegraded albumin located immediately distal to glomerular basement membrane has been proposed (4), but yet not characterized. Misdirected filtration of albumin into the interstitium resulting from pathologic, glomerular changes has been proposed as a pathway for progression of renal disease (5). (From Birn H, Christensen EI: Renal albumin absorption in physiology and pathology. Kidney Int 69:440–449, 2006.)

Permselectivity Based on Molecular Size

The use of neutral dextran to analyze glomerular size selectivity is illustrated in the middle curve of Figure 26–3.[40–42] A value of 1.0 on the ordinate denotes a dextran clearance equal to that of inulin (e.g., no measurable resistance to the filtration of dextran). Measurable restriction to filtration of neutral dextran does not occur until the effective radius exceeds about 20 Å. As dextran size increases, fractional dextran clearance (θ_D) decreases progressively.

Theoretical Interpretation of Size Selectivity

ISOPOROUS MODELS. The most useful theoretical descriptions of macromolecular transport are based on the concept of hindered movement of solutes through water-filled pores. Dextran filtration data such as those in Figure 26–3 are predicted by models that envision transport as taking place through numerous, identical cylindrical pores with a radius of approximately 55 Å. Fluxes are hindered both by a partitioning phenomenon in which the macromolecule is partially excluded by virtue of its shape, size, or charge and by a hydrodynamic effect related to the nearby presence of the pore wall.[2] For relatively high fluid flow rates through the pore and for large solutes that diffuse poorly, solute movement is primarily via convection. For lower fluid flow rates or small solutes that diffuse rapidly, solute movement is governed primarily by diffusion. The rate of filtration of a solute depends on two independent glomerular membrane proper-

ties: K_f, the glomerular capillary ultrafiltration coefficient, and r_p, the apparent glomerular pore radius. A more complete discussion of the theories of partitioning and hindered particle motion has been recently reviewed.[2]

Application of this theoretical model to the data in Figure 26–3 results in calculated values of r_p that are relatively independent of molecular size. Presumably, all molecules "see" the same pores, so the finding that the "best-fit" value of r_p is independent of molecular size confirms that the theory successfully correlates most of the available data. Values of θ calculated with the use of the theory for neutral dextran are shown by the *middle solid curve* in Figure 26–3. In this case, a pore radius of 47 Å provides an excellent fit to the data presented, except for molecular radii smaller than 24 Å, for which the isoporous theory appears to underestimate dextran transport.

An additional parameter that may be derived from values of K_f and r_p is the ratio of total pore area to pore length. For pores of a given radius and length, this parameter is a measure of "pore density," the apparent number of pores per unit area of the GCW. Further calculations suggest that some 10% of the glomerular capillary surface area is perforated by pores.

HETEROPOROUS MODELS. Theoretical calculations indicate that the normal GCW behaves much as an isoporous filter with a pore radius of about 50 to 55 Å.[42] However, in some human diseases, experimental data are incompatible with the isoporous theory. In these proteinuric patients, θ_D was

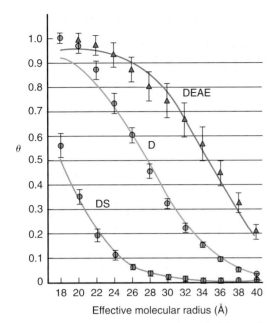

FIGURE 26-3 Filtrate-to-plasma concentration ratio (θ) as a function of molecular size for tritiated dextran sulfate (DS), neutral dextran (D), and diethylaminoethyl dextran (DEAE). Data points are means $\pm$ SE measured in the normal Munich-Wistar rat.[51,52] All three *solid curves* were calculated theoretically by using the membrane parameters $K_f = 4.8$ nL/(min $\cdot$ mm Hg), $r_p = 47$ Å, and $C_m = 165$ mEq/L. (From Deen WM, Satvat B, Jamieson JM: Theoretical model for glomerular filtration of charged solutes. Am J Physiol 238:F126, 1980.)

enhanced for the largest dextrans (>45 Å), but it was often decreased for the smallest dextrans.[43] These findings suggested that the selective increase in filtration of large dextrans could be explained by a second population of pores, fewer in number but with larger radii. Accordingly, Deen and co-workers[43] formulated a heteroporous model of glomerular size selectivity designed to account for the experimental observations. Data in nephrotic humans more closely fit a model of solute transport through a heteroporous membrane with a subpopulation of large pores. This model assumes that most of the GCW is perforated by cylindrical pores of radius r_o and that a smaller portion of the GCW is permeated by large, nondiscriminatory "shunt" pathways that do not exhibit size selectivity. The portion of the GCW permeated by shunt pores is denoted ω_o, a parameter that quantitates the magnitude of the size selectivity defect. The fractional area of the membrane occupied by this shunt pathway, though small, increases with each successive grade of barrier injury. This subpopulation of large pores is presumed to allow passage of immunoglobulin G (IgG) and probably most of the filtered albumin. Therefore, nonselective heavy proteinuria appears to result from loss of barrier size selectivity, which renders the glomerular membrane more porous to large plasma proteins.[43]

LOGNORMAL MODELS. In some cases, better results are obtained with a model assuming lognormal distribution of pore radii. Remuzzi and colleagues[44] used this model to define an index of the size of the largest pores in the GCW. By definition, 5% of the glomerular filtrate passes through pores with radii greater than r* (5%) and 1% passes through pores with radii greater than r* (1%).

Dextran, which has been used to obtain most of the available permselectivity data, appears to overestimate the true θ. Oliver and colleagues[39] proposed that Ficoll is a better probe of glomerular pore size; the use of Ficoll is now being extended to studies in rats, humans, and in vitro models.[19,45,46] For

Ficoll, a lognormal plus shunt pathway model was found to be the most effective.[39]

Interestingly, it has been reported that cultured podocytes are capable of establishing a size-selective barrier, regulated by specific signaling pathways,[47] opening up a new pathway for study of the function of the glomerular barrier.

Permselectivity Based on Molecular Charge

The charge-selective characteristics of the GCW have traditionally been evaluated with negatively charged markers such as dextran sulfate (DS). In a normal kidney, fractional DS clearance is lower than that for neutral dextran at any given molecular radius, whereas positively charged molecules pass through more freely (see Fig. 26-3).[48] However, the use of DS as an appropriate marker to assess charge selectivity has been challenged by observations that it is not as inert a tracer as once believed and that earlier studies probably overestimated the effects of charge.[2] For example, Guasch and co-workers[49] found that DS binds with plasma proteins. Furthermore, cellular uptake and intracellular desulfation of DS may affect the interpretation of fractional clearance data.[50] A detailed discussion of controversies in this field may be found in recent reviews.[2,5] Though not believed to invalidate the concept of charge selectivity, these observations indicate a need for further study in this area.

Permselectivity Based on Molecular Configuration

To compare sieving of molecules with different conformations, the effects of molecular shape or configuration must be taken into account. Bohrer and colleagues[51] compared the fractional clearance of neutral dextran with that of Ficoll, an uncharged cross-linked copolymer of sucrose and epichlorohydrin. At any given effective radius, the flexible coil dextran was filtered more readily than Ficoll, a nearly rigid sphere; the superior accuracy of Ficoll was subsequently confirmed.[39] More recently, available studies indicate that the shape and deformability of a protein are important and that polysaccharides may exhibit more physiologically appropriate shape characteristics.[52] Overall, these studies suggest that protein configuration also plays a role in filtration, although size and charge appear to be more important.[2,52]

Influence of Hemodynamic Factors on Filtration of Macromolecules

Hemodynamic factors influence the filtration of macromolecules (see review[53]). Often, θ varies inversely with the single-nephron glomerular filtration rate (SNGFR).[42] Thus, filtration of macromolecules is influenced not only by the intrinsic membrane properties of the GCW but also by other determinants of SNGFR: Q_A, the glomerular capillary plasma flow rate; ΔP, the glomerular transcapillary hydraulic pressure difference; and C_A, the afferent arteriolar plasma protein concentration. The absolute single-nephron clearance of a macromolecule is given by the product $\theta \times$ SNGFR.[42] Absolute clearance usually increases as Q_A is elevated, but less than in proportion to SNGFR; hence, θ decreases. Absolute macromolecular clearance rates also increase as ΔP rises. For neutral and anionic macromolecules, this increase is less than the increase in SNGFR, and as a result, θ decreases. For highly anionic molecules, this trend reverses at sufficiently high ΔP, and θ may increase. The opposite behavior is observed for positively charged molecules, with θ increasing with rising ΔP. The theoretical effects of C_A on θ are similar to those for inverse changes in ΔP because C_A and ΔP exert opposing effects on SNGFR. The actual effects of changes in C_A are likely to be more complicated because of parallel changes in K_f.[54] Hemodynamic factors may also influence rates of volume flux through the shunt pathway. Not surprisingly, interventions that alter glomerular hemodynamics also influence permselectivity, as has been best described using blockers of

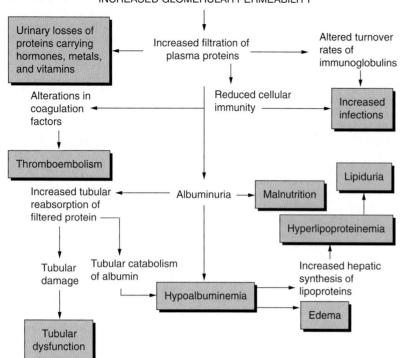

FIGURE 26–4 Pathophysiology of nephrotic syndrome. All abnormalities originate from increased glomerular permeability to plasma proteins; hypoalbuminemia initiates the major manifestations. (From Bernard DB: Extrarenal complications of the nephrotic syndrome. Kidney Int 33:1184, 1988.)

the renin-angiotensin system (RAS). For example, angiotensin-converting enzyme inhibitors (ACEIs) and angiotensin-receptor blockers (ARBs), which routinely reduce ΔP and proteinuria, have been shown to reduce the clearance of neutral dextrans of all sizes.[45,55]

Clinical Consequences of Proteinuria

Loss of albumin and other proteins into urine is the hallmark of nephrotic syndrome and a proximate or contributing cause to virtually all the systemic complications of this disorder. As depicted in Figure 26–4[56] and detailed later, increased filtration of plasma proteins contributes to hypoalbuminemia and its complications, to hyperlipidemia, to alterations in coagulation factors, and to alterations in cellular immunity, hormonal status, and mineral and electrolyte metabolism (see reviews[56–61]).

▌ HYPOALBUMINEMIA

Pathogenesis of Hypoalbuminemia

Nephrotic hypoalbuminemia results from multiple abnormalities in albumin homeostasis and is only partially explained by urinary albumin loss. Normal albumin metabolism is schematized in the *upper panel* of Figure 26–5.[59] The liver normally synthesizes 12 to 14 g/day of albumin, 90% of which is catabolized in extrarenal sites, primarily the vascular endothelium.[62] About 10% of the albumin synthesized daily is catabolized in the kidney, mainly by proximal tubule reabsorption of filtered albumin.[63] About 150 g of albumin (or 30%–50% of the total exchangeable pool) is located intravascularly, with the remainder in interstitial fluid, mostly skin and muscle.[64] The fractional catabolic rate, or the percentage of the plasma pool that is catabolized daily, is about 6% to 10%.[62,65] Thus, nephrotic hypoalbuminemia could result from some combination of urinary loss, decreased or insufficiently increased hepatic albumin synthesis, increased albumin catabolism, or altered albumin distribution.[66]

EXTRACORPOREAL LOSSES. The magnitude of hypoalbuminemia tends to increase with increasing proteinuria, but the relationship is inconsistent. Urinary losses alone should not lead to hypoalbuminemia because the liver can easily augment albumin synthesis and thus compensate for such losses. Evidence for enhanced intestinal albumin loss, or increased albumin catabolism, in the nephrotic syndrome is not strong.[66] As discussed later, renal albumin catabolism is increased, thereby contributing to the greater tendency to hypoalbuminemia.

HEPATIC ALBUMIN SYNTHESIS. Hepatic albumin synthesis is not impaired and, in fact, may be significantly increased in the nephrotic syndrome.[67,68] In nephrotic rats, hepatic release of albumin is enhanced, and the relative synthetic rate of albumin is markedly increased, with a comparable increase in albumin mRNA.[69,70] Oncotic pressure may play a role in albumin synthesis, as albumin gene expression varies inversely with oncotic pressure in experimental models.[71] That a transcriptional process is mainly responsible is suggested by findings that both steady-state levels and transcription rates of albumin mRNA are increased in the livers of nephrotic rats.[72] However, the increase in hepatic albumin synthesis is inadequate for the degree of hypoalbuminemia; thus, the albumin synthetic response rate is relatively impaired.

ALBUMIN CATABOLISM. In some hypoalbuminemic states, albumin catabolic rates are reduced.[73] In contrast, the possibility that hypoalbuminemia might be exacerbated by a maladaptive increase in albumin catabolism was suggested by Katz and associates,[74] who speculated that the increased urinary albumin load might up-regulate tubular albumin catabolism. In that case, most filtered albumin would be catabolized, and thus urinary albumin would represent only a small fraction of the filtered load. In confirmation of this notion, tubule albumin reabsorptive rates increase in nephrotic rats, though variably.[75] Additional support for the concept comes from evidence of a dual transport system for albumin uptake in the isolated perfused rabbit proximal tubule. This model exhibits both a low-capacity system that becomes saturated once the protein load exceeds physiologic

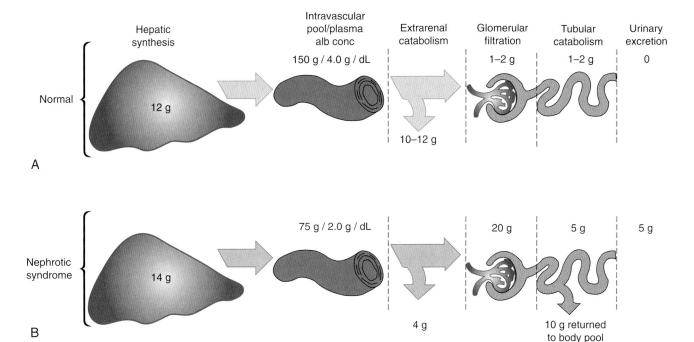

	Hepatic synthesis	Intravascular pool/plasma alb conc	Extrarenal catabolism	Glomerular filtration	Tubular catabolism	Urinary excretion

FIGURE 26–5 Daily albumin turnover in normal individuals **(A)** and in patients with nephrotic syndrome **(B)**. (Reproduced from Bernard DB: Metabolic complications in nephrotic syndrome: Pathophysiology and complications. *In* Brenner BM, Stein JH [eds]: The Nephrotic Syndrome, vol. 9. New York, Churchill Livingstone, 1982.)

levels and a high-capacity, low-affinity system that permits tubule albumin reabsorptive rates to rise as the filtered load increases.[76] Thus, an increase in the fractional catabolic rate may occur in the nephrotic syndrome. Regardless of whether fractional catabolism is normal or increased, total body albumin stores are markedly decreased. The net result is that absolute catabolic rates are normal or decreased.[66] Nutritional considerations affect this process. In nephrotic rats, absolute catabolic rates are decreased in rats fed adequate dietary protein but increased in rats receiving a low-protein diet.[77] Although decreased catabolism may serve to preserve total albumin stores, it is obviously insufficient to maintain albumin homeostasis.

ALBUMIN DISTRIBUTION. In nephrotic syndrome, the extravascular albumin pool is even more depleted than the intravascular pool.[78] Mobilization of extravascular albumin represents an early response to acute albumin loss, but this compensatory mechanism is clearly inadequate in the setting of continuing albumin loss, as in nephrotic syndrome.

Regulation of Albumin Metabolism in Nephrotic Syndrome

Several factors contribute to regulation of albumin metabolism and dysregulation in nephrotic syndrome.[66] The most widely studied factors regulating albumin synthesis are serum oncotic pressure and nutritional status. Albumin synthetic rates do not correspond to either serum albumin concentration or oncotic pressure in nephrotic patients.[67] It has been postulated that the hepatic albumin synthetic rate is more directly determined by changes in the hepatic extravascular interstitial albumin pool than by plasma characteristics and that this hepatic pool is not depleted in nephrotic syndrome and thus albumin synthesis is not stimulated.[79] More recently, it has been suggested that some serum factor or factors in hypo-oncotic states may stimulate albumin synthesis. In support of this hypothesis, incubation of rat hepatocytes with serum from nephrotic rats led to increased albumin and trans-

ferrin synthesis, even when oncotic pressure in the medium was normalized.[80]

Dietary factors also play a role. Albumin synthesis and serum albumin are not correlated in nephrotic rats fed a low-protein diet, but in the presence of high protein intake, albumin synthetic rates vary inversely with serum albumin.[72] Increasing dietary protein intake in nephrotic rats results in increased hepatic albumin mRNA content, as well as increased transcription, whereas decreased dietary protein intake limits hepatic albumin synthesis.[72,81] However, increasing dietary protein intake does not increase serum albumin or body albumin pools in nephrotic animals[77,81] or patients.[67] Feeding a high-protein diet stimulates hepatic albumin synthesis in nephrotic rats, but does not correct hypoalbuminemia, however, because dietary protein supplementation also increases urinary protein loss.[77,81] This unfortunate consequence of a high-protein diet also occurs in nephrotic patients; those eating a high-protein diet exhibit higher albumin synthetic rates, but also increased albuminuria, which results in no change in serum albumin levels.[67]

Factors contributing to enhanced proteinuria in the setting of a high-protein diet may include increased renal blood flow and glomerular filtration rate (GFR), with enhanced fractional renal clearance of albumin.[82] However, the net result is that, despite enhanced albumin synthesis, increased urinary losses predominate, so the serum albumin concentration and body albumin pools are further reduced.[82] Experimentally, blockade of the RAS in the setting of a high-protein diet allows increased hepatic synthesis but limits proteinuria, thereby allowing some amelioration of the hypoalbuminemia.[83] In nephrotic patients, both dietary protein restriction and ACEIs reduce proteinuria; however, protein restriction also reduces hepatic albumin synthesis, whereas albumin synthetic rates are maintained with angiotensin-converting enzyme (ACE) inhibition.[84]

Many hormones are needed for albumin synthesis,[66] but their relevance to nephrotic hypoalbuminemia is not well understood. Albumin synthesis is suppressed in the presence of inflammation,[85] and it is possible that elevated levels of lymphokines such as tumor necrosis factor[86] interfere with albumin synthesis in nephrotic syndrome.

In summary, nephrotic hypoalbuminemia is characterized by large urinary albumin losses and a marked reduction in the total exchangeable albumin pool. Mechanisms tending to counteract these forces are mobilization of extravascular pools, increases in albumin synthesis, and decreases in albumin catabolism. However, these compensatory mechanisms are insufficient to correct the hypoalbuminemia. Comparisons between normal and nephrotic albumin homeostasis are schematized in the *bottom panel* of Figure 26–5.[59] Normally, hepatic synthesis equals catabolism, with a yield of 1 to 2 g, which undergoes glomerular filtration and proximal tubular catabolism. In the nephrotic state, hepatic synthesis may be slightly increased, but the plasma albumin pool is smaller because catabolism is proportionally enhanced. Larger amounts are presented to the glomerulus, thereby resulting in both increased urinary loss and enhanced tubule catabolism.

Consequences of Hypoalbuminemia

Edema Formation and Blood Volume Homeostasis

Mechanisms of edema formation in the nephrotic syndrome are complex and have been recently reviewed.[87–90] Nephrotic edema does not result solely from hypoalbuminemia. The balance of Starling forces at the arteriolar end of the capillary favors net filtration of fluid into the interstitium. However, ongoing fluid transudation (edema accumulation) is normally limited by at least three protective mechanisms. First, lymphatics expand and proliferate so that increased lymphatic flow provides protection. Second, transudation of protein-free filtration into the interstitium reduces interstitial oncotic pressure, thus decreasing the oncotic pressure gradient and slowing ultrafiltration. Third, fluid flux tends to increase interstitial hydrostatic pressure, thereby reducing the transcapillary pressure gradient and further slowing filtration. Furthermore, the compliance characteristics of the interstitium resist fluid accumulation.[91] Thus, the appearance of edema in glomerulonephritis implies substantial disruption of the normal defenses against edema formation[88]; the role of primary sodium retention in this setting is discussed later.

RELATIONSHIP OF EDEMA FORMATION TO REDUCED PLASMA ONCOTIC PRESSURE. Hypoalbuminemia lowers the colloid oncotic pressure of blood, thereby favoring movement of water from the vascular to the interstitial space. However, continued edema formation would require disruption of normal defenses against edema, and evidence for such derangement is not clearly found. Patients studied during relapse and remission show almost equivalent changes in interstitial and plasma colloid osmotic pressure.[92] The reduction in interstitial oncotic pressure results in part from acceleration of lymphatic flow, which in turn returns interstitial protein to the intravascular space.[88] It has been suggested that this "wash-down" phenomenon is triggered by a slight increase in interstitial volume and hydraulic pressure induced by the initial loss of fluid into the interstitium. Body albumin pools are thus redistributed so that a greater fraction is located in the intravascular space.[78] These events thus serve to maintain blood volume and defend against edema formation.

Another mechanism related to nephrotic edema is the finding that capillary filtration capacity is higher in nephrotic patients.[90,93] Capillary hydraulic conductivity is determined by intercellular macromolecular complexes between endothelial cells, for example, tight junctions made of occludins, claudins, and ZO proteins, and adherens junctions made of cadherin, actinin, and catenins. These junctional complexes are closely related to the actin cytoskeleton.[94,95] Such a mech-

anism may increase capillary conductivity in nephrotic patients, under the influence of circulating permeability factors such as tumor necrosis factor-α.[86,96]

Taken together, it appears that substantial disruption of the renal mechanisms responsible for extracellular fluid homeostasis, rather than the level of hypoalbuminemia per se, is the primary determinant of the severity of edema formation. In assessing the relative contribution of hypoalbuminemia to edema formation, it is necessary to take into consideration the prevailing intravascular volume as well.

RELATIONSHIP OF EDEMA FORMATION TO THE PREVAILING INTRAVASCULAR VOLUME. One postulated scenario linking hypoalbuminemia to edema formation relates to the "underfill mechanism," as depicted in Figure 26–6.[97] According to this scenario, reductions in serum albumin and plasma oncotic pressure lead to edema formation, but also to hypovolemia. The reduced plasma volume (PV) then triggers compensatory mechanisms (e.g., nonosmotic vasopressin release, the RAS, and the sympathetic nervous system) that stimulate renal Na$^+$ and water retention. The latter serve to restore intravascular volume but also exacerbate hypoalbuminemia, so edema formation continues. However, some experimental observations are at odds with this hypothesis.[88,98,99] Moreover, the presence of hypovolemia is questionable; there has been inability to document hypovolemia by direct measurements, inability to consistently find changes in hormonal modulators compatible with hypovolemia, and failure of predicted changes to occur after remission or diuretic therapy. In nephrotic patients, PV and blood volume are not usually reduced; in fact, they are generally normal or even expanded.[100–102] Available studies note a range of PV in nephrotic patients, and methodologic issues may interfere with the interpretation of these studies.[97,102,103] Nonetheless, it should be possible to indirectly estimate blood volume by measurement of vasoactive hormones that are volume-responsive. Such functional evidence of hypovolemia is not

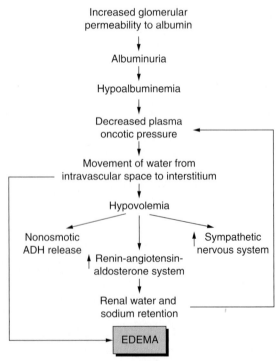

FIGURE 26–6 The "underfill" mechanism of edema formation. Hypovolemia (resulting from hypoalbuminemia and decreased plasma oncotic pressure) is viewed as the key event promoting Na$^+$ and water retention by the kidney. (From Perico N, Remuzzi G: Edema of the nephrotic syndrome: The role of the atrial peptide system. Am J Kidney Dis 22:355, 1993.)

consistently found in nephrotic syndrome.[59,97–99,101,102] Plasma renin activity (PRA) and aldosterone levels tend to be low and do not always correlate well with changes in PV.[102,104] Similarly, plasma levels of norepinephrine, arginine vasopressin (AVP), and atrial natriuretic peptide (ANP) tend to be normal or inconsistently changed.[105,106] Moreover, PV expansion by infusion of hyperoncotic plasma[107] or salt-poor albumin[108] and head-out water immersion[109] does not regularly result in diuresis or natriuresis. Nevertheless, some studies have found evidence consistent with hypovolemia and a natriuretic response to these maneuvers.[97,104,107]

Evidence from patients undergoing remission from nephrotic syndrome is also unclear. In responsive patients, steroid therapy leads to diuresis and natriuresis before any change in serum albumin. PRA and aldosterone levels are initially high and fall during natriuresis. After resolution of edema, PRA and aldosterone again rise to high levels, whereas plasma albumin and blood volume remain low; however, Na+ retention does not occur, and Na+ balance is maintained.[104] Taken together, these observations suggest a wide spectrum in prevailing PVs. These data have important therapeutic implications. The data suggest that edema is not necessary for maintenance of blood volume and, as a corollary, that vigorous treatment of edema with diuretics does not cause failure to maintain blood volume.[110]

ROLE OF INTRARENAL MECHANISMS. Most of the evidence implicates a primary intrarenal defect in the pathogenesis of nephrotic edema. This hypothesis, termed the "overfill theory," is schematized in Figure 26–7.[97] According to this hypothesis, a primary increase in renal Na+ retention leads to extracellular fluid volume expansion, altered Starling forces, and edema formation. Evidence in support of this mechanism comes from observations that Na+ retention occurs only in the ipsilateral kidney of rats with unilateral glomerulonephritis.[111] Moreover, the reduction in GFR that is often present would further limit Na+ excretion and contribute to renal sodium retention.

Micropuncture and other studies have localized the primary Na+ handling abnormality to the distal nephron.[111] Regarding mechanisms, considerable attention has focused on the role of ANP. Clinical[112] and experimental[113] studies have noted renal ANP resistance (i.e., blunted or absent natriuretic responses to ANP) in the nephrotic syndrome. ANP resistance is confined to the ipsilateral kidney in unilateral glomerulonephritis,[113] thus suggesting a role for this hormone in primary renal Na+ retention. Some evidence relates this finding of ANP resistance to heightened efferent sympathetic nervous activity.[114] At the level of the tubular cell, evidence suggests that the problem is accelerated breakdown of normally produced cyclic guanosine monophosphate.[115–117]

Recently, insight has been gained into the molecular mechanisms of renal sodium avidity. The hydrolytic and transport activities of sodium-potassium–adenosine triphosphatase (Na+,K+-ATPase) are increased in the cortical collecting duct in nephrotic rats. The proportional increases in Na+,K+-ATPase activity, cell surface expression, and total cellular content are associated with increased amounts of α- and β-subunit mRNA.[118] In principal cells from nephrotic rats, the epithelial sodium channel (ENaC) activity is increased in the absence of transcriptional induction of the mRNA encoding any of the ENaC subunits.[119] Though clearly invoked in some studies of the nephrotic syndrome,[119,120] ENaC activation and targeting may be secondary to hyperaldosteronism.[119,121] Overall, Na+ retention in the cortical collecting duct appears to be due, at least in part, to coordinated overactivity of the Na+,K+-ATPase and ENaC sodium transporters.[118] Finally, a role for the proximal tubule has been invoked with the observation that Na+ retention may also be associated with a shift of the cortical Na+/H+ exchanger NHE3 from an inactive to an active pool.[122] Indeed, it has recently been reported that NHE3 is activated in nephrotic rats,[122] and that NH3 is activated in vitro by albumin.[123]

A novel hypothesis regarding the interrelationship of sodium retention, interstitial inflammation, and nephrotic edema has recently been advanced by Rodríguez-Iturbe and co-workers.[124] The authors hypothesize that interstitial inflammation of the kidney induces primary sodium retention (Fig. 26–8). The generation of interstitial vasoconstrictors, driven by the inflammatory cell infiltrate, leads to reduction in K_f and SNGFR. As a consequence, there is a net increase in tubular Na+ reabsorption leading to primary sodium retention ("overfill"). The decrease in plasma oncotic pressure favors fluid extravasation from the intravascular compartment, thereby buffering changes in PV induced by sodium retention. If hypoalbuminemia is severe or the inflammatory infiltrate is absent, the reduction in plasma oncotic pressure may lead to "underfill" and secondary compensatory sodium retention. In support of this hypothesis are experimental observations that administration of mycophenolate mofetil prevents salt-sensitive hypertension after inflammation produced by infusion of angiotensin II[125]; the hypothesis has not yet been rigorously tested clinically.

Though less well studied, the mechanisms underlying abnormalities in water handling in experimental nephrotic syndrome have begun to be explored. These studies have noted reduced renal medullary water channel expression,[126] impaired aquaporin and urea transporter expression,[127] and decreased abundance of thick ascending limb Na+ transporters.[128]

Alterations in Renal Function

The Starling equation would predict that hypoalbuminemia and thus reduced plasma colloid oncotic pressure would reduce the forces opposing ultrafiltration, thereby increasing glomerular filtration. However, clinical[129] and experimental[130] studies indicate that such is not the case and that values of GFR are in fact reduced in conditions of reduced plasma protein levels. Baylis and colleagues[54] reported that the failure of SNGFR to rise resulted from a concomitant reduction in K_f. Reduced values of SNGFR, primarily caused by a reduction in K_f, have subsequently been observed in some,[130] but not all,[131] experimental nephrotic models; these differences in SNGFR derive, in part, from the presence or absence of compensatory elevations in ΔP. These observations suggest that serum albumin per se may not directly affect K_f, or that other factors may mitigate the effects of hypoalbuminemia on K_f. Innovative methods for estimating values of SNGFR and

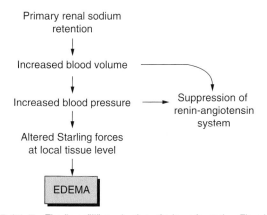

FIGURE 26–7 The "overfill" mechanism of edema formation. The abnormal renal Na+ retention is viewed as the primary event that through the increased plasma volume leads to alteration of the Starling forces at the local tissue level. (From Perico N, Remuzzi G: Edema of the nephrotic syndrome: The role of the atrial peptide system. Am J Kidney Dis 22:355, 1993.)

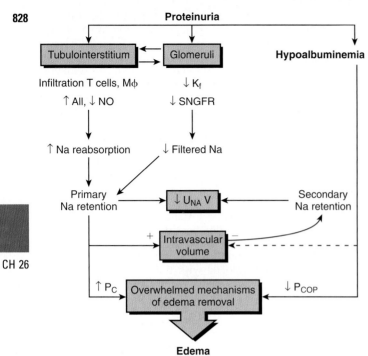

Proteinuria

Tubulointerstitium ⟷ Glomeruli   **Hypoalbuminemia**

Infiltration T cells, Mφ   ↓ K_f

↑ AII, ↓ NO   ↓ SNGFR

↑ Na reabsorption   ↓ Filtered Na

Primary Na retention → ↓ $U_{NA}V$ ← Secondary Na retention

\+ Intravascular volume −

↑ P_C Overwhelmed mechanisms of edema removal   ↓ P_{COP}

Edema

FIGURE 26–8 Pathophysiology of edema in the nephrotic syndrome. Proteinuria induces tubulointerstitial inflammation, with stimulation of vasoconstrictive mediators (angiotensin II, AII) and inhibition of vasodilatory mediators (e.g., nitric oxide [NO]). In the glomeruli, proteinuria causes a reduction in glomerular capillary untrafiltration coefficient (K_f) and single nephron glomerular filtration rate (SNGFR). Consequently, there is a net increase in tubular Na^+ reabsorption leading to primary Na^+ retention ("overfill") and increased capillary hydrostatic pressure (P_c). The decreased plasma oncotic pressure (P_{COP}) favors fluid movement outward, thereby buffering changes in PV induced by Na^+ retention. If hypoalbuminemia is severe and inflammation is minimal, the reduction in P_{COP} may cause "underfill" and secondary Na^+ retention. (From Rodríguez-Iturbe B, Herrera-Acosta J, Johnson RJ: Interstitial inflammation, sodium retention, and the pathogenesis of nephrotic edema: A unifying hypothesis. Kidney Int 62:1379–1384, 2002, with permission.)

its determinants in humans also suggest that a reduction in K_f commonly accompanies clinical glomerulonephritis as well. For example, this pattern has been observed in patients with minimal change disease[132] and membranous nephropathy.[133]

Alterations in Drug Pharmacokinetics

Kidney disease induces changes in all aspects of drug handling, including changes in bioavailability, the volume of distribution, renal drug metabolism, and renal excretion of drug and/or its metabolites.[134] Guidelines for modification of drug dosage in kidney disease are readily available[134–137] and are detailed in Chapter 57. The nephrotic syndrome poses special problems in drug handling. Hypoalbuminemia limits sites available for protein binding, thus increasing the amount of circulating free drug and potentially increasing first-pass hepatic drug removal. In addition, binding of organic bases and especially acids and bases is altered in hypoalbuminemia. In nephrotic patients, reduced protein binding results both from hypoalbuminemia and from a decrease in albumin's affinity for drugs. Accordingly, the unbound fraction of acidic drugs, including salicylate and phenytoin, may be markedly increased.[137] The clinical consequences of altered protein binding may be difficult to predict: Decreased binding allows for a higher concentration of free drug, but this effect may be counteracted by a larger volume of distribution and/or faster metabolism. Furthermore, protein binding may enhance tubule drug secretion;

the lesser protein binding in nephrotic syndrome may result in delayed renal excretion of some drugs.[134] Edema and ascites may increase the apparent volume of distribution of drugs that are highly water soluble or protein bound, thereby resulting in inadequate plasma levels, an effect particularly prominent with aminoglycoside antibiotics.[134]

The actions of diuretics are substantially altered in kidney disease and nephrotic syndrome, thereby contributing to the observed resistance to these drugs in these conditions.[138–140] The unbound fraction of furosemide increases markedly in severely hypoalbuminemic patients.[141] Nephrotic patients with a normal GFR deliver normal amounts of loop diuretics into the urine, but drug delivery is decreased in the setting of renal insufficiency.[142] When proteinuria is present, a substantial amount of furosemide may bind to urinary proteins, thereby reducing the amount of active, unbound drug in urine.[143] Tubule albumin blunts the inhibitory effects of furosemide on fractional loop Cl^- reabsorption,[144] whereas agents that block albumin-furosemide binding in the proximal tubule, such as warfarin and sulfisoxazole, partially restore diuretic responsiveness in experimental animals.[145] However, a careful study found that sulfisoxazole was ineffective in nephrotic patients.[146] Nephrotic patients also exhibit abnormal pharmacodynamic responses to furosemide,[143] so that the renal response to the drug is diminished even when adequate amounts of unbound, active drug reach the active site. Furthermore, animal studies indicate that furosemide is less potent in inhibiting Cl^- reabsorption in the loop in nephrotic rats.[147] Thus, both the pharmacodynamics and the pharmacokinetics of loop diuretics are altered in nephrotic syndrome. Single intravenous doses of 80 to 120 mg may be required to attain therapeutic levels of furosemide in urine, but doses above this range are unlikely to achieve any added therapeutic response.[138]

Studies in analbuminemic rats indicated that injection of furosemide bound to albumin resulted in natriuresis, with normalization of the plasma disappearance rate and increased urinary excretion of furosemide.[148] Thus, binding to plasma albumin appeared to be necessary for efficient delivery of drug into urine. These investigators then examined hypoalbuminemic patients with furosemide resistance and found that injecting furosemide as an admixture with equimolar albumin produced a diuresis, whereas giving either alone was without effect. Whether natriuresis occurred was not specifically mentioned. However, the available literature overall is conflicting as to the efficacy of combining albumin and furosemide in nephrotic patients.[149] Because administration of large amounts of albumin alone is both ineffective and expensive, this therapeutic combination will require clear validation before its routine use can be recommended. Other interventions, such as use of ultrafiltration[150] or combining furosemide with indapamide,[151] have been reported but also require further validation.

Therapy for glomerular disease or nephrotic syndrome may also be associated with drug interactions. For example, corticosteroids may inhibit hepatic microsomal enzymes, thereby altering the metabolism of other drugs. Clinically important drug interactions may be seen with other immunosuppressive drugs, including cyclosporine and azathioprine, as well as with diuretics and antihypertensive agents.[137]

Alterations in Platelet Function

Hypoalbuminemia may contribute to abnormal platelet function in nephrotic patients because conversion of arachidonic acid to metabolites that aggregate platelets is regulated by albumin.[152] In the presence of hypoalbuminemia, arachidonic acid may be metabolized to platelet-aggregating substances such as endoperoxides and thromboxane A_2.[153] In support of this notion, the degree of platelet dysfunction tends to correlate with the severity of hypoalbuminemia and proteinuria.[154]

Platelets from nephrotic patients are refractory to adenylate cyclase stimulation by prostaglandin E_1, further enhancing the tendency toward increased platelet aggregation.[155] However, a firm correlation between the plasma albumin concentration and platelet aggregability is not well established clinically.[155]

HYPERLIPIDEMIA

Hyperlipidemia is a frequent complication of nephrotic syndrome. Marked dysregulation of lipid metabolism occurs, with both quantitative and qualitative abnormalities in plasma lipids and lipoproteins. Although hyperlipidemia may be found in any kidney disease, it is most striking in nephrotic syndrome, in which such changes occur even when the GFR remains normal. The major lipid abnormalities are listed in Table 26–1 and described later.

Lipid Abnormalities in Nephrotic Syndrome

The nephrotic syndrome is characterized by abnormalities in virtually every aspect of lipid and lipoprotein metabolism.[156–158] Increased levels of the apolipoprotein B (apo B)–containing lipoproteins, very low density (VLDL), intermediate-density (IDL), and low-density (LDL) lipoproteins

TABLE 26–1	Mechanisms in the Pathophysiology of Lipid Abnormalities in Nephrotic Syndrome

Alterations in low-density lipoprotein and cholesterol metabolism
  Increased LDL generation
    Increased apo B synthesis
    Increased CETP activity
  Increased cholesterol synthesis
    Increased HMG-CoA reductase activity
    Decreased cholesterol 7α-hydroxylase
    Up-regulation of hepatic ACAT
  Defects in LDL clearance
    Reduction in hepatic LDL expression
    Reductions in apo B catabolism

Alterations in very low density lipoprotein metabolism
  Impaired VLDL clearance
    Reduced LPL and hepatic lipase activity
    Reduced VLDL receptor
    Impaired enrichment with apo E and apo C
  Increased hepatic production of fatty acids and triglycerides
    Elevated enzymatic activity of acyl-CoA carboxylase and fatty acid synthase
    Increased hepatic DGAT activity

Alterations in high-density lipoprotein
  Diminished LCAT activity
  Apo A-I enrichment of HDL*
  Reduced expression of HDL (SR-B1) receptor

Increased Lp(a) synthesis

*Observed in rats. Unlike experimental models, fractional catabolism of apo A-I in nephrotic patients is increased because of the increase in CETP, which is absent in rats. CETP mediates conversion of the larger HDL2 to the smaller HDL3, which has less affinity for apo A-I, and thus indirectly facilitates clearance of apo A-I.
ACAT, acetyl coenzyme A:cholesterol actytransferase; acyl-CoA, acyl coenzyme A; apo A-I, apolipoprotein A-I; apo B, apolipoprotein B; apo C, apolipoprotein C; apo E, apolipoprotein E; CETP, cholesterol ester transferase protein; DGAT, diacylglycerol acyltransferase; HDL, high-density lipoprotein; HMG-CoA, 3-hydroxy-3-methylglutaryl coenzyme A; LCAT, lecithin-cholesterol acyltransferase; LDL, low-density lipoprotein; Lp(a), lipoprotein (a); LPL, lipoprotein lipase; VLDL, very low density lipoprotein.

result in hypercholesterolemia, sometimes with hypertriglyceridemia. Cholesterol and phospholipid levels rise early in the disease course, whereas triglyceride (TG) elevations are more commonly found with more severe disease. Total high-density lipoprotein (HDL) levels are usually normal, but in severely proteinuric patients, HDL may be lost in the urine, with resultant reduced levels.[156–158] Subtype analysis demonstrates an abnormal distribution with significant reductions in the protective subtype HDL2.[159,160] Plasma concentrations of lipoprotein (a) (Lp[a]) are also elevated in nephrotic syndrome.[161–163] In addition, nephrotic patients show qualitative abnormalities in lipoprotein composition. The cholesterol-to-TG ratio is elevated in all classes of lipoproteins, which also tend to be enriched with cholesterol ester.[164] The highly atherogenic small LDL-III fraction is elevated as well.[165] The apolipoprotein content is also abnormal, with reduced apo C and E despite elevations in apo B, C-II, and E and an increased ratio of apo C-III to apo C-II.[158,166,167] Taken together, these abnormalities result in an increased atherogenic profile.[168]

Pathogenesis of Nephrotic Hyperlipidemia

Nephrotic hyperlipidemia results from both overproduction and impaired catabolism or composition of serum lipids and lipoproteins. A major issue is whether the lipid abnormalities in nephrotic syndrome arise as a consequence of hypoalbuminemia or proteinuria. In general, the severity of hyperlipidemia tends to correlate with the severity of hypoalbuminemia. In addition, remission of nephrotic syndrome is usually associated with a decrease in serum cholesterol as the albumin level rises, whereas albumin infusion acutely raises serum albumin and lowers serum cholesterol levels.[59,159,169] Because hepatic synthetic rates of albumin and lipoproteins react to similar stimuli and follow the same synthetic pathways, it has been hypothesized that increased lipoprotein synthesis was simply a side effect of increased albumin synthesis. However, although albumin synthesis is increased, no clear correlation has been found between hyperlipidemia and the rate of albumin synthesis in nephrotic patients. Kaysen and associates[170] showed that serum cholesterol levels in nephrotic patients were dependent only on the renal clearance of albumin and were totally independent of albumin synthetic rates, but that serum TG levels showed some dependence on albumin synthesis. Similarly, serum lipid levels in nephrotic rats correlated with proteinuria and not with albumin synthetic rates.[171] An alternative stimulus may be the reduction in plasma oncotic pressure. Infusion of either albumin or dextran into nephrotic patients and animals reduces serum lipid levels, thus suggesting that low plasma oncotic pressure may stimulate hepatic lipoprotein synthesis.[170,172,173] These findings correspond to in vitro observations demonstrating modulation of lipoprotein synthesis in hepatocytes cultured in media containing variable amounts of albumin.[69]

It is now apparent that reductions in plasma albumin levels or oncotic pressure, as well as the direct consequences of proteinuria, contribute to lipid alterations in nephrotic syndrome. As discussed later, these major factors operate on various levels of the lipid metabolic pathways. Metabolism of lipoproteins is closely linked. For purposes of this review, defects in the metabolism of individual fractions are discussed separately, with the understanding that one mechanism may alter the levels and composition of multiple lipoproteins.

Alterations in Low-Density Lipoprotein and Cholesterol Metabolism

Increases in LDL and total cholesterol in nephrotic syndrome are attributable to both increased synthesis and impaired catabolism. It has been shown that some nephrotic patients have increased absolute synthetic rates of apo B-100, the principal apoprotein constituent of LDL. Importantly, increased LDL apo B synthesis does not correlate with the synthetic rate of albumin.[174] Moreover, significant reductions in apo B catabolism have also been demonstrated.[175,176] Another line of evidence has suggested that plasma levels and the activity of cholesterol ester transfer protein (CETP) are enhanced in nephrotic syndrome.[177] This protein, which is present in humans but not in rats, mediates the transfer of esterified cholesterol from HDL to VLDL remnants to yield LDL.

Hepatic cholesterol synthesis is increased in experimental nephrotic syndrome. Complex studies by Vaziri and co-workers[178,179] have identified enzymatic defects in the liver of nephrotic rats that can collectively enhance hepatic cholesterol synthesis. These studies have shown increased hepatic activity of hydroxymethylglutaryl-coenzyme A (HMG-CoA) reductase, the rate-limiting enzyme for biosynthesis, in nephrotic rats. These changes are typical for the induction phase of proteinuria and are followed by a gradual decline to baseline levels.[178] This may explain why some other studies failed to find increases in this enzyme in nephrotic models.[180] In contrast to HMG-CoA reductase, hepatic expression of cholesterol 7α-hydroxylase, the rate-limiting enzyme responsible for conversion of cholesterol to bile acids, is reduced in nephrotic rats.[179,181]

More recently, the same group described marked up-regulation of hepatic acetyl coenzyme A:cholesterol acyltransferase (ACAT) in nephrotic rats.[182] This multifunctional enzyme is involved in the catalysis of intracellular cholesterol esterification and is responsible for lowering intracellular free cholesterol. By lowering hepatic free cholesterol, ACAT up-regulation may be responsible for the aforementioned defects in HMG-CoA reductase and 7α-hydroxylase activity and the enhanced cholesterol synthesis. Furthermore, enhanced ACAT activity leads to intracellular accumulation of cholesterol ester. Increases in hepatic cholesterol concentrations could contribute to hyperlipidemia both by increasing VLDL production and by down-regulating expression of LDL receptors, as discussed later.[180] In the vascular system, this phenomenon leads to foam cell formation and atherosclerosis.[183] Indeed, recent evidence has further suggested that ACAT plays a crucial role in complex alterations of lipid metabolism in nephrotic syndrome, at least experimentally.[180] Treatment of rats with puromycin nephrosis with an ACAT inhibitor resulted in reductions in plasma cholesterol and TGs, normalized the total cholesterol–to-HDL ratio, and lowered hepatic ACAT. This was accompanied by near normalization of plasma LCAT, hepatic SRB-1, and the LDL receptor (see later) and significant amelioration of proteinuria and hypoalbuminemia.[180]

Results of studies in humans are less clear. Turnover studies using radiolabeled glycerol and mevalonate have suggested increases in cholesterol synthesis.[164] In contrast, the serum lathosterol–to-cholesterol ratio, an index of cholesterol synthesis, is not elevated and does not change in response to antiproteinuric treatment.[184] Whether increased cholesterogenesis actually occurs in human nephrotic syndrome requires further clarification.

In addition to the defects discussed earlier, acquired defects in LDL clearance could also be responsible for LDL elevation in the nephrotic syndrome. Some earlier clinical studies have suggested reduced receptor-mediated LDL clearance with associated increases in LDL catabolism via alternative pathways.[176,177] Supporting this hypothesis, Vaziri and co-workers[179,185] described marked reduction in hepatic LDL receptor protein expression in nephrotic rats. These changes were present despite normal LDL receptor mRNA, suggesting inefficient LDL receptor translation or enhanced protein turnover in these rats. The authors hypothesized that, in addition

to reduced LDL clearance, an acquired hepatic LDL receptor defect could contribute to low hepatocellular cholesterol levels and consequent dysregulation of hepatic HMG-CoA reductase and 7α-hydroxylase, as discussed previously.[186] Another defect in nephrotic syndrome is the finding of marked up-regulation of hepatic LDL receptor–related protein expression, which is partly reversed with statin administration.[187]

Alterations in Very Low Density Lipoprotein Metabolism

The increased VLDL levels in nephrotic syndrome occur predominantly as a result of impaired VLDL clearance. Early studies demonstrated defective chylomicron clearance in nephrotic rats,[171] a phenomenon that correlated with proteinuria rather than with hypoalbuminemia. In addition, plasma TG levels are higher in nephrotic than in analbuminemic rats despite similar increases in hepatic TG production.[188] Defective VLDL clearance has also been documented in nephrotic patients.[174]

As a major determinant of chylomicron and VLDL clearance, the functional integrity of lipoprotein lipase (LPL) has been a logical focus for study in this area. Reduced LPL activity in nephrotic patients was proposed by Garber and colleagues.[189] Earlier reports suggested that decreased LPL activity may relate to the increased levels of circulating free fatty acids that result from hypoalbuminemia and the lowered protein-binding capacity of plasma. The increased free fatty acid level contributes by providing the lipid substrate for increased hepatic lipoprotein synthesis and by leading to decreased activity of LPL.[190,191]

LPL is attached to the endothelium by ionic bonding to a negatively charged matrix of glycosaminoglycans such as heparan sulfate.[190] This endothelium-bound LPL is an active, metabolically important pool, which is reduced in nephrotic rats.[171,191] Urinary excretion is markedly increased in nephrotic patients,[192] and circulating levels of heparan sulfate are reduced in nephrotic plasma and contribute to the decrease in LPL activity. In support of this concept, studies in nephrotic rats show that the markedly delayed plasma disappearance of radiolabeled chylomicrons may be completely normalized by injection of minute amounts of purified urinary heparan sulfate.[193] The heparan sulfate deficiency may also result from deficient hepatic synthesis of glycosaminoglycans. Nephrotic syndrome is characterized by excessive urinary losses of orosomucoid, a plasma glycoprotein synthesized by the liver. Urinary losses may lead to an increase in hepatic synthesis with a resultant excessive drain of key sugar intermediates from liver parenchymal cells, thus limiting the substrates available for heparan sulfate synthesis.[1] Because the endothelial pool of LPL in Nagase analbuminuric rats is reduced to the same extent as in nephrotic rats but TG levels are much higher in the latter model, it has been hypothesized that, in addition to defects in endothelial LPL, other important determinants of VLDL levels are present in nephrotic syndrome.

Indeed, more recent studies have revealed abnormalities in other determinants of VLDL clearance. In several models of nephrotic syndrome, Liang and Vaziri[194,195] demonstrated that elevated serum TG levels are in part attributable to reduced VLDL receptor and LPL expression. Reductions in VLDL receptor protein and mRNA were inversely related to plasma VLDL and TG concentrations. The same group implicated secondary hyperparathyroidism in the reduced LPL and hepatic lipase activity of proteinuric rats with progressive renal failure and suggested that, because of depletion of hepatic LPL in nephrotic rats, there is no liver compensation for the LPL defect.[196] Furthermore, defective receptor-mediated clearance and a metabolic defect in recognition and removal by the liver owing to hepatic lipase deficiency may underlie the elevated remnant particles in nephrotic syndrome.[197]

VLDL isolated from nephrotic rats hydrolyzes at a different rate in vitro than it does in control animals.[198] Shearer and associates[199] perfused hearts from normal, analbuminemic, and nephrotic rats with chylomicrons and found identical clearance of these particles in analbuminemic and nephrotic rats that was correctable with albumin. In contrast, binding of VLDL from nephrotic rats to cultured rat aortic endothelial cells was reduced as compared with binding in analbuminemic rats. These observations suggest that altered structure or composition of TG-rich lipoproteins must play a role in altered VLDL clearance. In both studies, the defects in lipolysis in nephrotic rats were corrected by normal HDL, thus suggesting that a component within HDL played a role in the genesis of these alterations. To facilitate VLDL receptor–mediated and LPL-mediated clearance, HDL supplies VLDL with most of the apo E and apo C. Alterations in these molecules in nephrotic syndrome have been described; apo E is reduced in the HDL of nephrotic rats and in the VLDL of nephrotic patients.[167] Apo C has been found to be markedly reduced per unit of VLDL in nephrotic patients[166,167] despite normal or even increased plasma levels. Reductions in VLDL apo C and apo E correlate with particle size.[167] The significance of alterations in apo E content in VLDL has more recently been further emphasized.[200] The authors have demonstrated normal binding of nascent VLDL from livers from nephrotic rats to endothelial cells. However, prior incubation of nascent VLDL with nephrotic HDL reduced binding in association with lower apo E content. The defect was corrected by reintroduction of apo E and suggests failure of nephrotic HDL to enrich VLDL with apo E. Thus, in addition to reduced LPL activity, VLDL clearance in nephrotic syndrome is delayed because of altered composition.

VLDL synthesis has been also evaluated. Increased hepatic production of fatty acids and TGs has been demonstrated in various nephrotic models.[188,201] Increased hepatic production of fatty acids in nephrotic rats has been shown to be caused by elevated enzymatic activity of acyl-CoA carboxylase and fatty acid synthase, the key enzymes in fatty acid biosynthesis.

More recently, the possible role of acyl CoA:diacylglycerol acyltransferase (DGAT) has been studied in this context. DGAT is a microsomal enzyme that joins acyl CoA to 1,2-diacylglycerol to form TG. Nephrotic rats demonstrated up regulation of hepatic DGAT-1 expression and activity, which could contribute to the associated hypertriglyceridemia by enhancing TG synthesis.[202] Although the reduced clearance of VLDL seems to play the principal role in hypertriglyceridemia, slightly increase or even normal TG synthesis in the face of reduced VLDL clearance, documented previously, could also contribute.

Alterations in High-Density Lipoprotein
Nephrotic syndrome is associated with specific abnormalities in enzymatic functions required for effective function of HDL. Diminished activity of the enzyme lecithin-cholesterol acyltransferase (LCAT) appears to contribute to the lipoprotein abnormalities in nephrotic syndrome.[203,204] LCAT is involved in catalyzing the esterification of cholesterol and its incorporation into HDL particles, as well as the conversion of HDL3 to HDL2. Low LCAT levels would impair this HDL maturation, in turn reducing the transfer of apo C-II to VLDL and thus inhibiting the catabolism of TG-rich lipoproteins.[164] Nephrotic patients have a distribution in HDL isoforms that corresponds to the LCAT defect; the higher-molecular-weight HDL2 is reduced and replaced by an increase in the lower-molecular-weight HDL3. The LCAT deficiency in nephrotic rats is due to urinary losses.[204] However, hypoalbuminemia may also play a role by increasing levels of free (unbound) lysolecithin, an inhibitor of LCAT.[205]

Increased hepatic production and elevated plasma CETP levels may contribute to HDL abnormalities in nephrotic

patients.[178] As a mediator of transfer of esterified cholesterol from HDL to VLDL, elevated CETP levels might contribute to cholesterol enrichment of TG-rich lipoproteins, as well as the observed reductions in HDL2.[178,206]

Elevated HDL in nephrotic rats is associated with apo A-I enrichment of HDL particles.[207,208] This abnormality has been linked to hypoalbuminemia and reduced oncotic pressure, and the accumulation of apo A-I–rich HDL is due to increased hepatic synthesis and reduced catabolism of HDL and apo A-I.[207,208] In addition, recent studies indicate that HDL is structurally altered by levels of albuminuria, associated with changes in concentrations of apo A-IV, apo E, apo A-II, apo C-II, and apo C-III.[209] Importantly, the relevance of these observations for human studies is unknown. Unlike experimental models, fractional catabolism of apo A-I in nephrotic patients is increased because of the increase in CETP that is absent in rats. CETP mediates conversion of the larger HDL2 to the smaller HDL3, which has less affinity for apo A-I, and thus indirectly facilitates clearance of apo A-I.[210]

Finally, the altered plasma HDL levels and composition in nephrotic rats are at least partly attributable to reduced protein expression of SR-B1.[211] This molecule has been identified as an HDL receptor responsible for the clearance of these particles. This situation closely resembles the defect in the LDL receptor in nephrotic rats, described previously.[175,185] Combined LDL and HDL receptor deficiency has been proposed as a crucial factor for development of hypercholesterolemia in the nephrotic syndrome.[186]

Lipoprotein (a)
Lp(a) is increased in nephrotic patients.[162,163,184] In view of the atherogenic potential of Lp(a), these findings are important. The principal mechanism leading to elevations in Lp(a) seems to be increased synthesis.[162] Lp(a) is related to apo B synthesis in nephrotic humans. As demonstrated by Noto and coworkers,[163] Lp(a) levels in nephrotic children inversely correlate with apo(a) isoform size and plasma albumin levels, but not with proteinuria.

Clinical Consequences of Nephrotic Hyperlipidemia

Many of the lipid abnormalities in nephrotic syndrome are significant risk factors for atherosclerotic cardiovascular (CV) disease in the general population, including increases in total cholesterol, LDL- and VLDL-cholesterol, apo B, and Lp(a) and reductions in HDL2 cholesterol. Furthermore, additional risk factors, such as hypertension, endothelial dysfunction, and hypercoagulability, may also contribute to the risk of atherosclerotic CV disease. A small study found elevated plasma homocysteine levels in nephrotic patients as well.[212] Nonetheless, evidence that CV risk is indeed increased in these patients remains controversial, and prospective long-term data are not available. Studies attempting to define CV risk in nephrotic patients have been flawed by inclusion of patients with minimal change disease, which typically remits; diabetes, which is inherently atherogenic; or failure to control for the presence of other risk factors. Indeed, the risk of CV disease in adults with a history of relapsing nephrotic syndrome during childhood is similar to that of the general population.[213] This observation agrees with early studies, which included relatively young patients, contained small numbers, and were retrospective in design, but also did not uniformly find an increased risk of CV events.[214–216] However, in a retrospective analysis of 142 currently nephrotic patients without diabetes, Ordonez and colleagues[217] found that, after correction for hypertension and smoking, the relative risk of myocardial infarction was increased 5.5-fold and that of coronary death was increased 2.8-fold in comparison to non-nephrotic controls. In addition, Falaschi and colleagues[218] evaluated the carotid intima–media wall thickness (IMT) in young patients with lupus as a marker of early atherosclerosis and CV risk. Patients with nephrotic-range proteinuria had a significantly higher IMT than did those without. The IMT did not correlate with the lupus activity score or other possible risk factors except for proteinuria, thus suggesting a higher risk of early atherosclerosis even in this young age group.[218]

Recent studies have focused on alterations in endothelial function associated with nephrotic syndrome. These complex changes with multifactorial etiology may be a common denominator of the clinical consequences of nephrotic syndrome, such as atherosclerosis, hypertension, and hyper-coagulability. Nephrotic patients may exhibit impaired endothelium-dependent relaxation[219,220] and decreased total plasma antioxidant potential.[221] Hyperlipidemia itself is also a risk factor for impaired endothelial function. Indeed, treatment with HMG-CoA reductase inhibitors resulting in significant reductions in hypercholesterolemia has been associated with substantial improvement in endothelium-dependent vasodilation in patients with nephrotic syndrome.[222] Altered lysophosphatidylcholine metabolism, linked to both hyperlipidemia and hypoalbuminemia, is another factor responsible for the endothelial dysfunction in nephrotic syndrome.[223]

Hyperlipidemia probably contributes to other adverse consequences of nephrotic syndrome. The increased platelet aggregation tends to correlate with the magnitude of hyper-lipidemia.[153] Hyperlipidemia may also contribute to the increased susceptibility of nephrotic patients to infection inasmuch as serum from nephrotic patients inhibits lymphocyte proliferation in response to specific and nonspecific antigen stimulation.[224] In addition to increasing the risk for CV disease, Lp(a), which may act to inhibit plasminogen, could contribute to hypercoagulability. Finally, the role of hyperlipidemia as a risk factor for progression of chronic kidney disease is discussed in detail in Chapters 47 and 48.

Therapy for Nephrotic Hyperlipidemia

In view of the magnitude of the CV risk in this population, further studies are needed to establish the need for aggressive hypolipidemic therapy.[168] Attempts to modify the lipoprotein profile may be worthwhile in patients with unremitting nephrotic syndrome, particularly if other CV risk factors are present. The principles of therapy are similar to those in other populations and include alterations in diet, the use of pharmacologic agents, and attention to other CV risk factors. Although few studies have systematically looked at the impact of standard dietary therapy in proteinuric patients, a moderate reduction in dietary cholesterol intake appears to be relatively ineffective.[225] Studies of vegetarian soy diets that are low in protein and rich in monounsaturated and polyunsaturated fatty acids have demonstrated improvements in serum cholesterol, LDL, and apo B in patients with proteinuria.[226] Supplementation of this diet with fish oil was of no additional benefit,[227] although it may provide some beneficial effect on TG levels.[164,226] Fibric acid derivatives have a more prominent effect on TG metabolism than on cholesterol. In one study of 11 patients treated with gemfibrozil, TG levels fell and HDL levels rose, with little change in total cholesterol or LDL-cholesterol levels.[228] Controlled prospective studies have indicated that colestipol and probucol may also have modest hypolipidemic effects.[229,230]

The preferred agents in nephrotic patients are HMG-CoA reductase inhibitors, which induce the greatest and most consistent hypolipidemic effect.[230] Experimentally, statins have been shown to ameliorate hepatic LDL receptor and HDL receptor deficiencies and to lower plasma total cholesterol, LDL, and the total cholesterol–to–HDL-cholesterol ratio.[231] Clinically, these drugs reduce total cholesterol, LDL, apo B-

100, and TG, and increase HDL.[232–235] Lp(a) levels may also be reduced by statins.[234,235] but the literature regarding Lp(a) is inconsistent. In the largest reported study, Olbricht and associates[236] conducted a prospective, randomized, placebo-controlled trial of 102 patients with glomerulonephritis and at least 3 g of proteinuria per day. With simvastatin, mean changes from baseline in total cholesterol, LDL-cholesterol, HDL-cholesterol, and serum TG were −39%, −47%, +1%, and −30%; serum Lp(a) was not affected. Another study demonstrated a possible benefit of combinations of statins with fibrates.[237] Other than lipid lowering, the beneficial effects of statins could be associated with their pleiotropic, non–lipid-lowering effects and may include a reduction in platelet aggregation and procoagulant factors, inhibition of mesangial cell proliferation and matrix accumulation, and anti-inflammatory effects.[238] Use of ezetimibe in nephrotic hyperlipidemia has not yet been reported.

In addition to standard hypolipidemic therapies, interventions that reduce proteinuria may also indirectly improve serum lipid profiles. Several studies of ACEI or ARB therapy have demonstrated improvement in lipid profiles, including reductions in Lp(a).[239–241] Finally, several reports have indicated beneficial effects of lipoprotein apheresis on severely hyperlipidemic nephrotic patients,[242,243] although evidence of long-term outcomes from this intervention are currently lacking.

HYPERTENSION

Hypertension frequently accompanies glomerular diseases. Hypertension in the absence of renal insufficiency is more likely to be present in primary glomerular diseases than in diseases of tubulointerstitial origin. The relationship between hypertension and glomerular disease has been the subject of many reviews[244,245] and is discussed in detail in Chapters 43 and 47. In nephrotic syndrome, hypertensive patients also appear to fall in the group with plasma volume expansion,[102] with blood pressures falling after remission or diuretic therapy.[246] Though not well studied, urinary loss of an anti-hypertensive substance is a possibility.

HEMATOLOGIC ABNORMALITIES
(see also Chapter 49)

Hypercoagulable State and Renal Vein Thrombosis

The nephrotic syndrome is frequently a hypercoagulable state, with increased risk of thromboembolic complications. The most common manifestation in adults is the development of renal vein thrombosis, most frequently associated with membranous glomerulonephritis. Prospective studies of the incidence of renal vein thrombosis in patients with membranous nephropathy indicated an average incidence of about 12%, with individual studies finding a range of 5% to 62%.[153,247,248] The incidence is lower in other forms of glomerulonephritis, for unknown reasons.

The incidence of thrombotic complications at other sites ranges from 8% to 44%, with an average of about 20%.[247–249] Of such complications, pulmonary embolism is the most frequent and serious. In a study of 204 children and 116 adults with nephrotic syndrome, children exhibited a lower incidence of events than adults did. However, the complications tended to be more severe in children, almost half of whom exhibited arterial thrombosis.[250] As mentioned earlier, the relative risk of coronary thrombotic events is increased in these patients,[217] and hypercoagulability could well contribute.

Pathogenesis of Hypercoagulability

The numerous abnormalities in the coagulation and hemostasis systems in the nephrotic syndrome have been extensively reviewed[56,57,153,247,251] and are briefly summarized here. These abnormalities include altered levels and activity of factors in the intrinsic and extrinsic coagulation cascades, levels of antithrombotic and fibrinolytic components of plasma, platelet counts and platelet function, blood viscosity, and other factors. A pathogenetic mechanism for these abnormalities is depicted in Figure 26–9,[153] and reported abnormalities are summarized in Table 26–2. As reviewed by Llach,[153] abnormalities of coagulation in the nephrotic syndrome may relate to each of the five major functional classes of coagulation components: (1) zymogens (factors II, V, VII, IX, X, XI, and XII), which are activated to enzymes, and cofactors (factors V and VIII), which accelerate the conversion of zymogens; (2) fibrinogen; (3) the fibrinolytic system; (4) clotting inhibitors; and (5) components of platelet reaction and thrombogenesis.

Alterations in Zymogens and Cofactors
Most studies have noted deficiencies in levels of factors IX, XI, and XII,[251,252] which are likely to relate to urinary loss of these low-molecular-weight proteins. Deficient factor XII levels are particularly important because this factor regulates coagulation activity as well as the fibrinolytic and kinin-kallikrein pathways.[253] Increased levels of factor II and combined factors VII and X have also been noted.[254] These zymogen abnormalities usually normalize with clinical remission of nephrotic syndrome.[252] The nephrotic syndrome is also characterized by increased levels of the cofactors V and VIII, which may correlate inversely with the serum albumin level.[254–256] The serum elevations appear to result from increased hepatic synthesis, perhaps in response to the decreased oncotic pressure and/or hypoalbuminemia. These abnormalities in zymogens and cofactors have not been clearly associated with thrombotic complications.[153]

Alterations in Fibrinogen Levels and the Fibrinolytic System
The nephrotic syndrome is associated with elevated plasma fibrinogen levels,[250,254–257] likely resulting from increased hepatic synthesis and normal catabolic rates.[258] Fibrinogen levels correlate directly with urinary protein and serum cholesterol levels and inversely with serum albumin levels.[254–257] Fibrinogen is an important determinant of plasma viscosity, and the increased levels may be important in the hypercoagulability of nephrotic syndrome. Indeed, by inducing fibrin deposition, hyperfibrinogenemia may be a major factor determining thrombotic risk.[258]

The data on fibrinolytic abnormalities in nephrotic syndrome are conflicting. Several studies noted deficient plasma levels of plasminogen, with the decrease correlating with the magnitude of hypoalbuminemia and proteinuria.[259,260] Other reported abnormalities include low antiplasmin activity (α_1-antitrypsin)[255] and increased antiplasmin activity (α_2-macroglobulin fraction, which is the primary plasmin inhibitor and may be the most reliable marker of renal vein thrombosis).[261]

Alterations in Coagulation Inhibitors
Nephrotic patients exhibit increased urinary losses and decreased plasma levels of antithrombin III (AT III), the most important inhibitor of coagulation and thrombin.[250,262] Deficient serum levels of AT III are sometimes,[262] though not always[263] present and correlated with thromboembolic phenomena in nephrotic patients. AT III deficiency is reversible with steroid therapy.[264]

Abnormalities in other coagulation inhibitors, including protein C and protein S, may also occur; congenital deficiencies of each are associated with recurrent venous thrombosis.[265,266] Both are found in the urine of nephrotic patients.[267,268] Levels of total protein S and protein C antigens are elevated, but the activity of protein S is reduced because of a significant reduction in free (active) protein S levels, a consequence of elevated urinary losses.[268] Protein C anticoagulant activity is elevated, although a marked reduction in specific activity has been noted.[268] Nephrotic patients may exhibit elevations in serum thrombin activatable fibrinolysis inhibitor (TAFI), as well as a deficiency in protein Z, two additional factors that may predispose to thrombosis.[269] A reduction in tissue factor

TABLE 26–2	Coagulation Abnormalities in Nephrotic Syndrome

Alterations in zymogens and cofactors
Deficiency in factors IX, XI, and XII
Increased levels of factor II and combined factors VII and X
Increased levels of factors V and VIII

Increased plasma fibrinogen levels
Alterations in the fibrinolytic system
Deficiency of plasma plasminogen
Low antiplasmin activity (α_1-antitrypsin)

Increased antiplasmin activity (α_2-macroglobulin fraction)
Increased α_1-antiplasmin

Alterations in coagulation inhibitors
Deficiency of antithrombin III
Deficiency of protein S
Deficiency of protein C (possible)

Alterations in platelet function
Enhanced platelet aggregability
Increased levels of β-thromboglobulin

Data modified from Llach F: Hypercoagulability, renal vein thrombosis, and other thrombotic complications of nephrotic syndrome. Kidney Int 28:429, 1985.

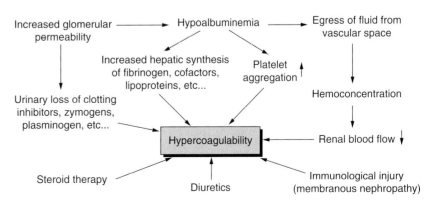

FIGURE 26–9 Schematic representation of pathogenetic factors leading to hypercoagulability, thromboembolic phenomena, and renal vein thrombosis in nephrotic syndrome. (From Llach F: Hypercoagulability, renal vein thrombosis, and other thrombotic complications of nephrotic syndrome. Kidney Int 28:429, 1985.)

pathway inhibitor (TFPI) has been postulated, but one study found that proteinuria was in fact associated with increased TFPI levels, so the thrombotic tendencies cannot be readily ascribed to TFPI deficiency.[270] Another study noted that many markers of endothelial cell injury (thrombomodulin, intracellular adhesion molecule-1, vascular cell adhesion molecule, TAFI, and vascular endothelial growth factor levels, but not protein Z) were elevated in nephrotic patients, but did not correlate with levels of proteinuria or serum albumin in general.[269] Finally, one study examined the incidence of genetic mutations in factor V Leiden. In 35 patients with nephrotic syndrome, 10 developed thrombotic events. Of these, 2 were heterozygous for a factor V gene mutation, 1 with thrombosis and 1 without.[271]

Alterations in Platelet Function

Platelet counts in nephrotic patients tend to be normal or elevated.[254,255] Platelet aggregability may be increased.[263,272] Potential contributions of hyperlipidemia and hypoalbuminemia to this abnormality were discussed earlier. Nephrotic patients may also exhibit elevations in β-thromboglobulin, a specific protein released by platelets on aggregation.[273,274]

In summary, numerous coagulation abnormalities are found in nephrotic syndrome. Furthermore, nephrotic syndrome may be characterized by increased blood viscosity,[274] as a result of both hyperlipidemia and increased fibrinogen. Steroid therapy may also exacerbate hypercoagulability in nephrotic patients.[275]

The specific role of each of these abnormalities in the pathogenesis of thromboembolic complications remains incompletely defined.[153] An increased tendency toward thrombotic events has been correlated with increased α_2-antiplasmin levels,[261] and the presence of factor XII and prekallikrein in subepithelial deposits has been noted in patients with membranous glomerulonephritis.[276] However, a prospective study of nephrotic adults monitored for an average of 21 months found significant increases in factor I, factor VIIIc, factor VIIIr:Ag, α_1-antitrypsin, and α_2-macroglobulin, as well as platelet hyperaggregability, in the group as a whole, but no correlation between these abnormalities and thromboembolic events. Low levels of AT III and severe hypoalbuminemia were of no predictive value for thromboembolic events.[263]

HORMONAL AND OTHER SYSTEMIC MANIFESTATIONS

Other systemic manifestations of glomerular disease, which are covered in detail elsewhere in this volume, include enhanced susceptibility to infection,[59,277] possibly as a result of urinary loss of components of the alternate complement pathway, including factor B, and loss of IgG.[277] IgG synthesis may also be impaired.[278]

Deficiencies of trace metals such as copper, zinc, and iron may occur.[279,280] Urinary losses of thyroxine-binding globulin, triiodothyronine, and thyroxine have been noted, although patients remain clinically euthyroid.[281] Urinary levels of corticosteroid-binding globulin[282] and insulin-like growth factor type I[283] are elevated, although the clinical consequences are unclear. Abnormalities in Ca^{2+} and vitamin D metabolism, such as hypocalcemia, hypocalciuria, and low serum levels of vitamin D, also characterize the nephrotic syndrome.[59,284,285] It is not clear that clinically significant hypovitaminosis D occurs in the majority of nephrotic patients,[57] but one study found an increased incidence of isolated osteomalacia and bone resorption in association with defective mineralization in patients with sustained nephrotic syndrome.[286] Urinary levels of erythropoietin are increased, and plasma levels fail to rise despite anemia[287]; erythropoietin deficiency can occur and cause anemia even in the setting of normal kidney function.[288,289] Transferrin synthesis is increased, but not sufficiently to replace urinary losses.[290,291] Finally, extrarenal protein loss in the presence of inadequate protein intake may be associated with negative nitrogen balance and protein malnutrition.[66]

References

1. Kanwar YS, Liu ZZ, Kashihara N, et al: Current status of the structural and functional basis of glomerular filtration and proteinuria. Semin Nephrol 4:390–413, 1991.
2. Deen WM, Lazzara MJ, Myers BD: Structural determinants of glomerular permeability. Am J Physiol 281:F579–F596, 2001.
3. Tryggvason K, Patrakka J, Wartiovaara J: Hereditary proteinuria syndromes and mechanisms of proteinuria. N Engl J Med 243:1387–1401, 2006.
4. Mathieson PW: The cellular basis of albuminuria. Clin Sci 107:533–538, 2004.
5. Haraldsson B, Sörensson J: Why do we not all have proteinuria? An update of our current understanding of the glomerular barrier. News Physiol Sci 19:7–10, 2004.
6. Jalanko H: Pathogenesis of proteinuria: Lessons learned from nephrin and podocin. Pediatr Nephrol 18:487–491, 2003.
7. D'Amico G, Bazzi C: Pathophysiology of proteinuria. Kidney Int 63:809–825, 2003.
8. Farquhar MG, Wissig SL, Palade GE: Glomerular permeability. I. Ferritin transfer across the normal glomerular capillary wall. J Exp Med 113:47–91, 1961.
9. Graham RC, Kellermeyer RW: Bovine lactoperoxidase as a cytochemical protein tracer for electron microscopy. J Histochem Cytochem 16:275–278, 1968.
10. Venkatachalam MA, Cotran RS, Karnovsky MJ: An ultrastructural study of glomerular permeability in aminonucleoside nephrosis using catalase as a tracer protein. J Exp Med 132:1168–1180, 1970.
11. Rennke HG, Cotran RS, Venkatachalam MA: Role of molecular charge in glomerular permeability: Tracer studies with cationized ferritins. J Cell Biol 67:638–646, 1975.
12. Venkatachalam MA, Rennke HG: The structural and molecular basis of glomerular filtration. Circ Res 43:337–347, 1978.
13. Kerjaschki D, Sharkey DJ, Farquhar MG: Identification and characterization of podocalyxin—The major sialoprotein of the renal glomerular epithelial cell. J Cell Biol 98:1591–1596, 1984.
14. Dekan G, Gabel CA, Farquhar MG: Sulfate contributes to the negative charge of podocalyxin—The major sialoglycoprotein of the filtration slits. Proc Natl Acad Sci U S A 88:5398–5402, 1991.
15. Miner JH: Renal basement membrane components. Kidney Int 56:2016–2024, 1999.
16. Kanwar YS, Rosenzweig LJ: Clogging of the glomerular basement membrane. J Cell Biol 93:489–494, 1982.
17. Kanwar YS, Jakubowski ML: Unaltered anionic sites of glomerular basement membrane in aminonucleoside nephrosis. Kidney Int 25:613–618, 1984.
18. Groggel GC, Stevenson J, Hovingh P, et al: Changes in heparan sulfate correlate with increased glomerular permeability. Kidney Int 33:517–523, 1988.
19. Bolton GR, Deen WM, Daniels BS: Assessment of the charge selectivity of glomerular basement membrane using Ficoll sulfate. Am J Physiol 274:F889–F896, 1998.
20. Daniels BS: Increased albumin permeability in vitro following alterations of glomerular charge is mediated by the cells of the filtration barrier. J Lab Clin Med 124:224–230, 1994.
21. Rossi M, Morita H, Sormunen R, et al: Heparan sulfate chains of perlecan are indispensable in the lens capsule but not in the kidney. EMBO J 22:236–245, 2003.
22. Laurens W, Battaglia C, Foglieni C, et al: Direct podocyte damage in the single nephron leads to albuminuria in vivo. Kidney Int 47:1078–1086, 1995.
23. Blantz RC, Gabbai FB, Peterson O, et al: Water and protein permeability is regulated by the glomerular epithelial slit diaphragm. J Am Soc Nephrol 4:1957–1964, 1994.
24. Kestilä M, Lenkkeri U, Männikko M, et al: Positionally cloned gene for a novel glomerular protein—Nephrin is mutated in congenital nephrotic syndrome. Mol Cell 1:575–582, 1998.
25. Ruitsalainen V, Ljungberg P, Wartiovaara J, et al: Nephrin is specifically located at the slit diaphragm of glomerular podocytes. Proc Natl Acad Sci U S A 96:7962–7967, 1999.
26. Putaala H, Souneninen R, Kilpelainen P, et al: The murine nephrin gene is specifically expressed in kidney, brain and pancreas: Inactivation of the gene leads to massive proteinuria and death. Hum Mol Genet 10:1–8, 2001.
27. Benigni A, Gagliardini E, Tomasoni S, et al: Selective impairment of gene expression and assembly of nephrin in human diabetic nephropathy. Kidney Int 65:2193–2200, 2004.
28. Macconi D, Abbate M, Morigi M, et al: Permselective dysfunction of podocyte-podocyte contact upon angiotension II unravels the molecular target for renoprotective intervention. Am J Pathol 168:1073–1085, 2006.
29. Sörensson J, Matejka GL, Ohlson M, Haraldsson B: Human endothelial cells produce orosomucoid, an important component of the capillary barrier. Am J Physiol 276:H530–H534, 1999.
30. Sörensson J, Björnson A, Ohlson M, et al: Synthesis of sulfated proteglycans by bovine glomerular endothelial cells in culture. Am J Physiol 2834:F373–F380, 2003.
31. Rosengren BI, Rippe A, Rippe C, et al: Transvascular protein transport in mice lacking endothelial caveolae. Am J Physiol Heart Circ Physiol 291:H1371–H1377, 2006.
32. Christensen EI, Bern H: Megalin and cubilin: Synergistic endocytic receptors in renal proximal tubule. Am J Physiol Heart Circ Physiol 280:F562–F573, 2001.
33. Gekle M: Renal tubule albumin transport. Annu Rev Physiol 67:573–592, 2005.

34. Christensen EI, Gburek J: Protein reabsorption in renal proximal tubule—Function and dysfunction in kidney pathophysiology. Pediatr Nephrol 19:714–721, 2004.

35. Birn H, Christensen EI: Renal albumin absorption in physiology and pathology. Kidney Int 69:440–449, 2006.

36. Christensen EI, Devuyst O, Dom G, et al: Loss of chloride channel ClC-5 impairs endocytosis by defective trafficking of megalin and cubilin in kidney proximal tubules. Proc Natl Acad Sci USA 100:8472–8477, 2003.

37. Leheste JR, Rolinski B, Vorum H, et al: Megalin knockout mice as an animal model of low molecular weight proteinuria. Am J Pathol 155:1361–1370, 1999.

38. Birn H, Fyfe JC, Jacobsen C, et al: Cubilin is an albumin binding protein important for renal tubular albumin reabsorption. J Clin Invest 105:1353–1361, 2000.

39. Oliver JD III, Anderson S, Troy JL, et al: Determination of glomerular size-selectivity in the normal rat with Ficoll. J Am Soc Nephrol 3:214–228, 1992.

40. Bohrer MP, Deen WM, Robertson CR, et al: Mechanism of angiotensin II–induced proteinuria in the rat. Am J Physiol 233:F13–F21, 1977.

41. Bohrer MP, Baylis C, Humes HD, et al: Permselectivity of the glomerular capillary wall. Facilitated filtration of circulating polycations. J Clin Invest 61:72–78, 1978.

42. Deen WM, Satvat B, Jamieson JM: Theoretical model for glomerular filtration of charged solutes. Am J Physiol 238:F126–F139, 1980.

43. Deen WM, Bridges CR, Brenner BM, et al: Heteroporous model of glomerular size selectivity: Application to normal and nephrotic humans. Am J Physiol 249:F374–F389, 1985.

44. Remuzzi A, Battaglia C, Rossa L, et al: Glomerular size selectivity in nephrotic rats exposed to diets with different protein contents. Am J Physiol 253:F318–F327, 1987.

45. Remuzzi A, Perico N, Amuchastegui CS, et al: Short- and long-term effect of angiotensin II receptor blockade in rats with experimental diabetes. J Am Soc Nephrol 4:40–49, 1993.

46. Blouch K, Deen WM, Fauvel J-P, et al: Molecular configuration and glomerular size selectivity in healthy and nephrotic humans. Am J Physiol 273:F430–F437, 1997.

47. Hunt JL, Pollak MR, Denker BM: Cultured podocytes establish a size-selective barrier regulated by specific signaling pathways and demonstrate synchronized barrier assembly in a calcium switch model of junction formation. J Am Soc Nephrol 16:1593–1602, 2005.

48. Brenner BM, Hostetter TH, Humes DH: Molecular basis of proteinuria of glomerular origin. N Engl J Med 298:826–833, 1978.

49. Guasch A, Deen WM, Myers BD: Charge selectivity of the glomerular filtration barrier in healthy and nephrotic humans. J Clin Invest 92:2274–2282, 1993.

50. Vyas SV, Parker JA, Comper WD: Uptake of dextran sulphate by glomerular intracellular vesicles during kidney ultrafiltration. Kidney Int 47:945–950, 1995.

51. Bohrer MP, Deen WM, Robertson CR, et al: Influence of molecular configuration on the passage of macromolecules across the glomerular capillary wall. J Gen Physiol 74:583–593, 1979.

52. Venturoli D, Rippe B: Ficoll and dextran vs. globular proteins as probes for testing glomerular permselectivity: Effects of molecular size, shape, charge, and deformability. Am J Physiol Renal Physiol 288:F605–F613, 2005.

53. Anderson S, Komers R, Brenner BM: Renal and systemic manifestations of glomerular disease. In Brenner BM (ed): The Kidney, 7th ed. Philadelphia: Saunders, 2004, pp 1927–1954.

54. Baylis C, Ichikawa I, Willis WT, et al: Dynamics of glomerular ultrafiltration. IX. Effects of plasma protein concentration. Am J Physiol 232:F58–F64, 1977.

55. Remuzzi A, Puntorieri S, Battaglia C, et al: Angiotensin converting enzyme inhibition ameliorates glomerular filtration of macromolecules and water and lessens glomerular injury in the rat. J Clin Invest 85:541–549, 1990.

56. Bernard DB: Extrarenal complications of the nephrotic syndrome. Kidney Int 33:1184–1202, 1988.

57. Harris RC, Ismail N: Extrarenal complications of the nephrotic syndrome. Am J Kidney Dis 23:477–497, 1994.

58. Orth SR, Ritz E: The nephrotic syndrome. N Engl J Med 338:1202–1211, 1998.

59. Bernard DB: Metabolic complications in nephrotic syndrome: Pathophysiology and complications. In Brenner BM, Stein JH (eds): The Nephrotic Syndrome. New York, Churchill Livingstone, 1982, pp 85–120.

60. Crew RJ, Radhakrishnan J, Appel G: Complications of the nephrotic syndrome and their treatment. Clin Nephrol 62:245–259, 2004.

61. Roth KS, Amaker BH, Chan JC: Nephrotic syndrome: pathogenesis and management. Pediatr Rev 23:237–248, 2002.

62. Rothschild MA, Oratz M, Schreiber SS: Albumin synthesis. N Engl J Med 286:748–757, 1972.

63. Sellers AL, Katz J, Bonorris G, et al: Determination of extravascular albumin in the rat. J Lab Clin Med 68:177–185, 1966.

64. Katz J, Bonorris G, Okuyama S, et al: Albumin synthesis in perfused liver of normal and nephrotic rats. Am J Physiol 212:1255–1260, 1967.

65. Katz J, Rosenfeld S, Sellers AL: Role of the kidney in plasma albumin catabolism. Am J Physiol 198:814–818, 1960.

66. Kaysen GA: Albumin metabolism in the nephrotic syndrome: The effect of dietary protein intake. Am J Kidney Dis 12:461–480, 1988.

67. Kaysen GA, Gambertoglio J, Jimenez I, et al: Effect of dietary protein intake on albumin homeostasis in nephrotic patients. Kidney Int 29:572–577, 1986.

68. Ballmer PE, Weber BK, Roy-Chaudhury P, et al: Elevation of albumin synthesis rates in nephrotic patients measured with [1-13C]leucine. Kidney Int 41:132–138, 1992.

69. Yamauchi A, Fukuhara Y, Yamamoto S, et al: Oncotic pressure regulates gene transcription of albumin and apolipoprotein B in cultured rat hepatoma cells. Am J Physiol 263:C397–C404, 1992.

70. Sun X, Martin V, Weiss RH, et al: Selective transcriptional augmentation of hepatic gene expression in the rat with Heymann nephritis. Am J Physiol 264:F441–F447, 1993.

71. Pietrangelo A, Panduro A, Chowdhury JR, et al: Albumin gene expression is down-regulated by albumin or macromolecule infusion in the rat. J Clin Invest 89:1755–1760, 1992.

72. Kaysen GA, Jones H Jr, Martin V, et al: A low protein diet restricts albumin synthesis in nephrotic rats. J Clin Invest 81:1623–1629, 1989.

73. Hoffenberg R, Gordon AH, Black EG, Louis LN: Plasma protein catabolism by the perfused rat liver: The effect of alteration of albumin concentration and dietary protein depletion. Biochem J 118:401–404, 1970.

74. Katz J, Bonorris G, Sellers AL: Albumin metabolism in aminonucleoside nephrotic rats. J Lab Clin Med 62:910–934, 1963.

75. Galaske RG, Baldamus CA, Stolte H: Plasma protein handling in the rat kidney: Micropuncture experiments in the acute heterologous phase of anti-GBM-nephritis. Pflugers Arch 375:269–277, 1978.

76. Park CH, Maack T: Albumin absorption and catabolism by isolated perfused proximal convoluted tubules of the rabbit. J Clin Invest 73:767–778, 1984.

77. Kaysen GA, Kirkpatrick WG, Couser WG: Albumin homeostasis in the nephrotic rat: Nutritional considerations. Am J Physiol 247:F192–F202, 1984.

78. Sellers AL, Katz J, Bonorris G: Albumin distribution in the nephrotic rat. J Lab Clin Med 71:511–516, 1968.

79. Rothschild MA, Oratz M, Evans CD, et al: Role of hepatic interstitial albumin in regulating albumin synthesis. Am J Physiol 210:57–62, 1966.

80. Sun X, Kaysen GA: Albumin and transferrin synthesis are increased in H4 cells by serum from analbuminemic or nephrotic rats. Kidney Int 45:1381–1387, 1994.

81. Kaysen GA, Jones H Jr, Hutchison FN: High protein diets stimulate albumin synthesis at the site of albumin mRNA transcription. Kidney Int 36(suppl 27):168–172, 1989.

82. Kaysen GA, Rosenthal C, Hutchison FN: GFR increases before renal mass or ODC activity increase in rats fed high protein diets. Kidney Int 36:441–446, 1989.

83. Hutchison FN, Schambelan M, Kaysen GA: Modulation of albuminuria by dietary protein and converting enzyme inhibition. Am J Physiol 253:F719–F727, 1987.

84. Don B, Kaysen GA, Hutchison F, et al: The effect of angiotensin converting enzyme inhibition and protein restriction in the treatment of proteinuria. Am J Kidney Dis 17:10–17, 1991.

85. Moshage HJ, Janssen JAM, Franssen JH, et al: Study of the molecular mechanism of decreased liver synthesis of albumin in inflammation. J Clin Invest 79:1635–1641, 1987.

86. Suranyi MG, Guasch A, Hall BM, et al: Elevated levels of tumor necrosis factor-alpha in the nephrotic syndrome in humans. Am J Kidney Dis 21:251–259, 1993.

87. Koomans HA: Pathophysiology of oedema in idiopathic nephrotic syndrome. Nephrol Dial Transplant 18(suppl 6):vi30–vi32, 2003.

88. Vande Walle JGJ, Donckerwolcke RA: Pathogenesis of edema in the nephrotic syndrome. Pediatr Nephrol 16:283–293, 2001.

89. Deschênes G, Feraille E, Doucet A: Mechanisms of oedema in nephrotic syndrome: Old theories and new ideas. Nephrol Dial Transplant 18:454–456, 2003.

90. Camici M: Molecular pathogenetic mechanisms of nephrotic edema: Progress in understanding. Biomed Pharmacother 59:214–223, 2005.

91. Aukland K, Nicolaysen G: Interstitial fluid volume: Local regulatory mechanisms. Physiol Rev 61:556–643, 1981.

92. Koomans HA, Kortlandt W, Geers AB, et al: Lowered protein content of tissue fluid in patients with the nephrotic syndrome: Observations during disease and recovery. Nephron 40:391–395, 1985.

93. Lewis DM, Tooke JE, Beaman M, et al: Peripheral microvascular parameters in the nephrotic syndrome. Kidney Int 54:1261–1266, 1998.

94. Schnittler HJ: Structural and functional aspects of intercellular junctions in vascular endothelium. Basic Res Cardiol 93:30–39, 1998.

95. Curry FR: Microvascular solute and water transport. Microcirculation 12:17–31, 2005.

96. Ferro T, Neumann P, Gertzberg N, et al: Protein kinase C-alpha mediates endothelial barrier dysfunction induced by TNF-alpha. Am J Physiol 278:L1107–L1117, 2000.

97. Schrier RW: Pathogenesis of sodium and water retention in high-output and low-output cardiac failure, nephrotic syndrome, cirrhosis, and pregnancy. N Engl J Med 319:1065–1076, 1988.

98. Perico N, Remuzzi G: Edema of the nephrotic syndrome: The role of the atrial peptide system. Am J Kidney Dis 22:355–366, 1993.

99. Humphreys MH: Mechanisms and management of nephrotic edema. Kidney Int 45:266–281, 1994.

100. Meltzer JL, Keim HJ, Laragh JH, et al: Nephrotic syndrome: Vasoconstriction and hypervolemic types indicated by renin-sodium profiling. Ann Intern Med 91:688–696, 1979.

101. Dorhout Mees EJ, Roos JC, Boer P, et al: Observations on edema formation in the nephrotic syndrome in adults with minimal lesions. Am J Med 67:378–384, 1979.

102. Dorhout Mees EJ, Geers AB, Koomans HA: Blood volume and sodium retention in the nephrotic syndrome: A controversial pathophysiological concept. Nephron 36:201–211, 1984.

103. Brown EA, Markandu N, Sagnella GA, et al: Sodium retention in nephrotic syndrome is due to an intrarenal defect: Evidence from steroid-induced remission. Nephron 39:290–295, 1985.

104. Schrier RW, Fassett RG: A critique of the overfill hypothesis of sodium and water retention in the nephrotic syndrome. Kidney Int 53:1111–1117, 1998.

105. Tulassay T, Rascher W, Lange RE, et al: Atrial natriuretic peptide and other vasoactive hormones in nephrotic syndrome. Kidney Int 31:1391–1395, 1987.

106. Usberti M, Federico S, Meccariello S, et al: Role of plasma vasopressin in the impairment of water excretion in nephrotic syndrome. Kidney Int 25:422–429, 1984.

107. Koomans HA, Geers AB, van der Meiracker AH, et al: Effects of plasma volume expansion on renal salt handling in patients with the nephrotic syndrome. Am J Nephrol 4:227–234, 1984.

Renal and Systemic Manifestations of Glomerular Disease

108. Brown EA, Markandu ND, Sagnella GA, et al: Evidence that some mechanism other than the renin system causes sodium retention in nephrotic syndrome. Lancet 2(8310):1237–1240, 1982.

109. Krishna GG, Danovitch GM: Effects of water immersion on renal function in the nephrotic syndrome. Kidney Int 21:395–401, 1982.

110. Koomans HA, Geers AB, Dourhout Mees EJ, et al: Lowered tissue-fluid oncotic pressure protects the blood volume in the nephrotic syndrome. Nephron 42:317–322, 1986.

111. Ichikawa I, Rennke HG, Hoyer JR, et al: Role for intrarenal mechanisms in the impaired salt excretion of experimental nephrotic syndrome. J Clin Invest 71:91–103, 1983.

112. Peterson C, Madsen B, Perlmann A, et al: Atrial natriuretic peptide and the renal response to hypervolemia in nephrotic humans. Kidney Int 34:825–831, 1988.

113. Perico N, Delaini F, Lupini C, et al: Blunted excretory response to atrial natriuretic peptide in experimental nephrosis. Kidney Int 36:57–64, 1989.

114. DiBona GF, Herman PJ, Sawin LL: Neural control of renal function in edema-forming states. Am J Physiol 254:R1017–R1024, 1988.

115. Valentin J-P, Qiu CQ, Muldowney WP, et al: Cellular basis for blunted volume expansion natriuresis in experimental nephrotic syndrome. J Clin Invest 90:1302–1312, 1992.

116. Valentin J-P, Ying W-Z, Sechi LA, et al: Phosphodiesterase inhibitors correct resistance to natriuretic peptides in rats with Heymann nephritis. J Am Soc Nephrol 7:582–593, 1996.

117. Valentin J-P, Ying W-Z, Couser WG, et al: Extrarenal resistance to atrial natriuretic peptide in rats with experimental nephrotic syndrome. Am J Physiol 274:F556–F563, 1998.

118. Deschênes G, Gonin S, Zolty E, et al: Increased synthesis and AVP unresponsiveness of Na,K-ATPase in collecting duct from nephrotic rats. J Am Soc Nephrol 12:2241–2252, 2001.

119. Lourdel S, Loffing J, Favre G, et al: Hyperaldosteronism and activation of the epithelial sodium channel are not required for sodium retention in puromycin-induced nephrosis. J Am Soc Nephrol 16:3642–3650, 2005.

120. Kim SW, Wang W, Nielsen J, et al: Increased expression and apical targeting of renal ENaC subunits in puromycin aminonucleoside-induced nephrotic syndrome in rats. Am J Physiol 286:F922–F935, 2004.

121. de Seigneux S, Kim SW, Hemmingsen SC, et al: Increased expression but not targeting of ENaC in adrenalectomized rats with PAN-induced nephrotic syndrome. Am J Physiol Renal Physiol 291:F208–F217, 2006.

122. Besse-Eschmann V, Klisic J, Nief V, et al: Regulation of the proximal tubular sodium/proton exchanger NHE3 in rats with puromycin aminonucleoside (PAN)-induced nephrotic syndrome. J Am Soc Nephrol 13:2199–2206, 2002.

123. Klisic J, Zhang J, Nief V, et al: Albumin regulates the Na$^+$/H$^+$ exchanger 3 in OKP cells. J Am Soc Nephrol 14:3008–3016, 2003.

124. Rodríguez-Iturbe B, Herrera-Acosta J, Johnson RJ: Interstitial inflammation, sodium retention, and the pathogenesis of nephrotic edema: A unifying hypothesis. Kidney Int 62:1379–1384, 2002.

125. Rodríguez-Iturbe B, Pons H, Quiroz Y, et al: Mycophenolate mofetil prevents salt-sensitive hypertension resulting from angiotensin II exposure. Kidney Int 59:2222–2232, 2001.

126. Apostol E, Ecelbarger CA, Terris T, et al: Reduced renal medullary water channel expression in puromycin aminonucleoside–induced nephrotic syndrome. J Am Soc Nephrol 8:15–24, 1997.

127. Fernández-Llama P, Andrews P, Nielsen S, et al: Impaired aquaporin and urea transporter expression in rats with Adriamycin-induced nephrotic syndrome. Kidney Int 53:1244–1253, 1998.

128. Fernández-Llama P, Andrews P, Ecelbarger CA, et al: Concentrating defect in experimental nephrotic syndrome: Altered expression of aquaporins and thick ascending limb Na$^+$ transporters. Kidney Int 54:170–179, 1998.

129. Klahr S, Alleyne GAO: Effects of chronic protein-calorie malnutrition on the kidney. Kidney Int 3:129–141, 1973.

130. Anderson S, Diamond JR, Karnovsky MJ, et al: Mechanisms underlying transition from acute glomerular injury to late glomerular sclerosis in a rat model of nephrotic syndrome. J Clin Invest 82:1757–1768, 1988.

131. Meyer TW, Rennke HG: Increased single-nephron protein excretion after renal ablation in nephrotic rats. Am J Physiol 255:F1243–F1248, 1988.

132. Guasch A, Myers BD: Determinants of glomerular hypofiltration in nephrotic patients with minimal change nephropathy. J Am Soc Nephrol 4:1571–1581, 1998.

133. Squarer A, Lemley KV, Ambalavanan S, et al: Mechanisms of progressive glomerular injury in membranous nephropathy. J Am Soc Nephrol 9:1389–1398, 1998.

134. Aronoff GR, Abel SR: Principles of administering drugs to patients with renal failure. In Bennett WM, McCarron DA, Brenner BM, Stein JH (eds): Pharmacotherapy of Renal Disease and Hypertension. New York, Churchill Livingstone, 1987, pp 1–20.

135. Aronoff GR, Berns JS, Brier ME, et al: Drug Prescribing in Renal Failure. Philadelphia, American College of Physicians, 1999.

136. The Renal Drug Book, Online Edition. www.kdp-baptist.louisville.edu/renalbook/

137. Morrison G, Audet PR, Singer I: Clinically important drug interactions for the nephrologist. In Bennett WM, McCarron DA, Brenner BM, Stein JH (eds): Pharmacotherapy of Renal Disease and Hypertension. New York, Churchill Livingstone, 1987, pp 49–98.

138. Brater DC: Diuretic therapy. N Engl J Med 339:387–395, 1998.

139. Ellison DH: Diuretic resistance: Physiology and therapeutics. Semin Nephrol 19:581–597, 1999.

140. Wilcox CS: New insights into diuretic use in patients with chronic renal disease. J Am Soc Nephrol 13:798–805, 2002.

141. Andreasen F: Determination of furosemide in blood plasma and its binding to proteins in normal plasma and in plasma from patients with acute renal failure. Acta Pharmacol Toxicol 32:417–423, 1973.

142. Keller E, Hoppe-Seyler G, Schollmeyer P: Disposition and diuretic effect of furosemide in the nephrotic syndrome. Clin Pharmacol Ther 32:442–449, 1982.

143. Voelker JR, Jameson DM, Brater DC: In vitro evidence that urine composition affects the fraction of active furosemide in the nephrotic syndrome. J Pharmacol Exp Ther 250:772–778, 1989.

144. Kirchner KA, Voelker JR, Brater DC: Intratubular albumin blunts the response to furosemide: A mechanism for diuretic resistance in nephrotic syndrome. J Pharmacol Exp Ther 252:1097–1101, 1990.

145. Kirchner KA, Voelker JR, Brater DC: Binding inhibitors restore furosemide potency in tubule fluid containing albumin. Kidney Int 40:418–424, 1991.

146. Agarwal A, Gorski JC, Sundblad K, Brater DC: Urinary protein binding does not affect response to furosemide in patients with nephrotic syndrome. J Am Soc Nephrol 11:1100–1105, 2000.

147. Kirchner KA, Voelker JR, Brater DC: Tubular resistance to furosemide contributes to the attenuated diuretic response in nephrotic rats. J Am Soc Nephrol 2:1201–1207, 1992.

148. Inoue M, Okajima K, Itoh K, et al: Mechanism of furosemide resistance in analbuminemic rats and hypoalbuminemic patients. Kidney Int 32:198–202, 1987.

149. Elwell RJ, Spencer AP, Eisele G: Combined furosemide and human albumin treatment for diuretic-resistant edema. Ann Pharmacother 37:695–700, 2003.

150. Davenport A: Ultrafiltration in diuretic-resistant volume overload in nephrotic syndrome and patients with ascites due to chronic liver disease. Cardiology 96:190–195, 2001.

151. Tanaka M, Oida E, Nomura K, et al: The Na$^+$-excreting efficacy of indapamide in combination with furosemide in massive edema. Clin Exp Nephrol 9:122–126, 2005.

152. Yoshida A, Aoki N: Release of arachidonic acid from human platelets: A key role for the potentiation of platelet aggregability in normal subjects as well as in those with the nephrotic syndrome. Blood 52:969–978, 1978.

153. Llach F: Hypercoagulability, renal vein thrombosis, and other thrombotic complications of nephrotic syndrome. Kidney Int 28:429–439, 1985.

154. Bang N, Tygstad C, Schroeder J, et al: Enhanced platelet function in glomerular renal disease. J Lab Clin Med 81:651–660, 1973.

155. Remuzzi G, Mecca G, Marchesi D, et al: Platelet hyperaggregability and the nephrotic syndrome. Thromb Res 16:345–354, 1979.

156. Kaysen GA: Hyperlipidemia of the nephrotic syndrome. Am J Kidney Dis 39(suppl 31):8–15, 1991.

157. Kaysen GA, de Sain-van der Velden MGM: New insights into lipid metabolism in the nephrotic syndrome. Kidney Int 55(suppl 71):S-18–S-21, 1999.

158. Joven J, Villabona C, Vilella E, et al: Abnormalities of lipoprotein metabolism in patients with the nephrotic syndrome. N Engl J Med 323:579–584, 1990.

159. Muls E, Rosseneu M, Daniels R, et al: Lipoprotein distribution and composition in the human nephrotic syndrome. Atherosclerosis 54:225–237, 1985.

160. Short CD, Durrington PN, Mallick NP, et al: Serum and urinary high density lipoproteins in glomerular disease with proteinuria. Kidney Int 29:1224–1228, 1986.

161. Wanner C, Rader D, Bartens W, et al: Elevated plasma lipoprotein(a) in patients with the nephrotic syndrome. Ann Intern Med 119:263–269, 1993.

162. de Sain-van der Velden MG, Reijngoud DJ, Kaysen GA, et al: Evidence for increased synthesis of lipoprotein(a) in the nephrotic syndrome. J Am Soc Nephrol 9:1474–1481, 1998.

163. Noto D, Barbagallo CM, Cascio AL, et al: Lipoprotein(a) levels in relation to albumin concentration in childhood nephrotic syndrome. Kidney Int 55:2433–2439, 1999.

164. Wheeler DC, Bernard DB: Lipid abnormalities in the nephrotic syndrome: Causes, consequences and treatment. Am J Kidney Dis 23:331–346, 1994.

165. Deighan CJ, Caslake MJ, McConnell M, et al: The atherogenic lipoprotein phenotype: Small dense LDL and lipoprotein remnants in nephrotic range proteinuria. Atherosclerosis 157:211–220, 2001.

166. Kashyap ML, Srivastava LS, Hynd BA, et al: Apolipoprotein CII and lipoprotein lipase in human nephrotic syndrome. Atherosclerosis 35:29–40, 1980.

167. Deighan CJ, Caslake MJ, McConnell M, et al: Patients with nephrotic-range proteinuria have apolipoprotein C and E deficient VLDL1. Kidney Int 58:1238–1246, 2000.

168. Radhakrishnan J, Appel AS, Valeri A, et al: The nephrotic syndrome, lipids, and risk factors for cardiovascular disease. Am J Kidney Dis 22:135–142, 1993.

169. Appel GB, Blum CB, Chien S, et al: The hyperlipidemia of the nephrotic syndrome: Relation to plasma albumin concentration, oncotic pressure, and viscosity. N Engl J Med 312:1544–1548, 1985.

170. Kaysen GA, Gambertoglio J, Felts J, et al: Albumin synthesis, albuminuria, and hyperlipemia in nephrotic patients. Kidney Int 31:1368–1376, 1987.

171. Davies RW, Staprans I, Hutchison FN, et al: Proteinuria, not altered albumin metabolism, affects hyperlipidemia in the nephrotic rat. J Clin Invest 86:600–605, 1990.

172. Allen JC, Baxter JH, Goodman HC: Effects of dextran, polyvinylpyrrolidone and gamma globulin on the hyperlipidemia of experimental nephrosis. J Clin Invest 40:499–508, 1961.

173. Heymann W, Nash G, Gilkey C, et al: Studies on the causal role of hypoalbuminemia in experimental nephrotic hyperlipemia. J Clin Invest 37:808–819, 1958.

174. de Sain-van der Velden MG, Kaysen GA, Barrett HA, et al: Increased VLDL in nephrotic patients results from a decreased catabolism while increased LDL results from increased synthesis. Kidney Int 53:994–1001, 1998.

175. Warwick GL, Packard CJ, Demant T, et al: Metabolism of apolipoprotein B–containing lipoproteins in subjects with nephrotic-range proteinuria. Kidney Int 40:129–138, 1991.

176. Warwick GL, Caslake MH, Boulton-Jones M, et al: Low-density lipoprotein metabolism in the nephrotic syndrome. Metabolism 39:187–192, 1990.

177. Braschi S, Masson D, Rostoker G, et al: Role of lipoprotein-bound NEFAs in enhancing the specific activity of plasma CETP in the nephrotic syndrome. Arterioscler Thromb Vasc Biol 17:2559–2567, 1997.

178. Vaziri ND, Liang KH: Hepatic HMG-CoA reductase gene expression during the course of puromycin-induced nephrosis. Kidney Int 48:1979–1985, 1995.

179. Vaziri ND, Sato T, Liang K: Molecular mechanisms of altered cholesterol metabolism in rats with spontaneous focal glomerulosclerosis. Kidney Int 63:1756–1763, 2003.

180. Vaziri ND, Liang KH: Acyl-coenzyme A:cholesterol acyltransferase inhibition ameliorates proteinuria, hyperlipidemia, lecithin-cholesterol acyltransferase, SRB-1, and low-density lipoprotein receptor deficiencies in nephrotic syndrome. Circulation 110:419–425, 2004.

181. Liang KH, Oveisi F, Vaziri ND: Gene expression of hepatic cholesterol 7 alpha-hydroxylase in the course of puromycin-induced nephrosis. Kidney Int 49:855–860, 1996.

182. Vaziri ND, Liang K: Up-regulation of acyl-coenzyme A:cholesterol acyltransferase (ACAT) in nephrotic syndrome. Kidney Int 61:1769–1775, 2002.

183. Bocan TM, Krause BR, Rosebury WS, et al: The combined effect of inhibiting both ACAT and HMG-CoA reductase may directly induce atherosclerotic lesion regression. Atherosclerosis 157:97–105, 2001.

184. Dullaart RP, Gansevoort RT, Sluiter WJ, et al: The serum lathosterol to cholesterol ratio, an index of cholesterol synthesis, is not elevated in patients with glomerular proteinuria and is not associated with improvement in hyperlipidemia in response to antiproteinuric treatment. Metabolism 45:723–730, 1996.

185. Vaziri ND, Liang K: Downregulation of hepatic LDL receptor expression in experimental nephrosis. Kidney Int 50:887–893, 1996.

186. Vaziri ND: Molecular mechanisms of lipid disorders in nephrotic syndrome. Kidney Int. 63:1964–1976, 2003.

187. Kim S, Kim CH, Vaziri ND: Upregulation of hepatic LDL receptor-related protein in nephrotic syndrome: Response to statin therapy. Am J Physiol Endocrinol Metab 288:E813–E817, 2004.

188. Joles JA, Bijleveld C, van Tol A, et al: Plasma triglyceride levels are higher in nephrotic than in analbuminemic rats despite a similar increase in hepatic triglyceride secretion. Kidney Int 47:566–572, 1995.

189. Garber DW, Gottlieb BA, Marsh JB, et al: Catabolism of very low density lipoproteins in experimental nephrosis. J Clin Invest 74:1375–1383, 1984.

190. Olivecrona T, Bengtsson G, Markland SE, et al: Heparin–lipoprotein lipase interactions. Fed Proc 36:60–65, 1977.

191. Kaysen GA, Pan XM, Couser WG, et al: Defective lipolysis persists in hearts of rats with Heymann nephritis in the absence of nephrotic plasma. Am J Kidney Dis 22:128–134, 1993.

192. Staprans I, Garon SJ, Hooper J, et al: Characterization of glycosaminoglycans in urine from patients with nephrotic syndrome and control subjects, and their effects on lipoprotein lipase. Biochim Biophys Acta 678:414–422, 1981.

193. Staprans I, Felts JM, Couser WG: Glycosaminoglycans and chylomicron metabolism in control and nephrotic rats. Metabolism 36:496–501, 1987.

194. Liang KH, Vaziri ND: Acquired VLDL receptor deficiency in experimental nephrosis. Kidney Int 51:1761–1765, 1997.

195. Sato T, Liang K, Vaziri ND: Down-regulation of lipoprotein lipase and VLDL receptor in rats with focal glomerulosclerosis. Kidney Int 61:157–162, 2002.

196. Vaziri ND, Wang XQ, Liang K: Secondary hyperparathyroidism downregulates lipoprotein lipase expression in chronic renal failure. Am J Physiol 273:F925–930, 1997.

197. Liang K, Vaziri ND: Down-regulation of hepatic lipase expression in experimental nephrotic syndrome. Kidney Int 51:1933–1937, 1997.

198. Furukawa S, Hirano T, Mamo JC, et al: Catabolic defect of triglyceride is associated with abnormal very-low-density lipoprotein in experimental nephrosis. Metab Clin Exp 39:101–107, 1990.

199. Shearer GC, Stevenson FT, Atkinson DN, et al: Hypoalbuminemia and proteinuria contribute separately to reduced lipoprotein catabolism in the nephrotic syndrome. Kidney Int 59:179–189, 2001.

200. Shearer GC, Couser WG, Kaysen GA: Nephrotic livers secrete normal VLDL that acquire structural and functional defects following interaction with HDL. Kidney Int 65:228–237, 2004.

201. Joles JA, Bijleveld C, van Tol A, et al: Estrogen replacement during hypoalbuminemia may enhance atherosclerotic risk. J Am Soc Nephrol 12:1870–1876, 1997.

202. Vaziri ND, Kim CH, Phan D, et al: Up-regulation of hepatic Acyl CoA:diacylglycerol acyltransferase-1 (DGAT-1) expression in nephrotic syndrome. Kidney Int 66:262–267, 2004.

203. Moorhead JF, El Nahas AM, Harry D, et al: Focal glomerulosclerosis and nephrotic syndrome with partial lecithin:cholesterol acetyltransferase deficiency and discoidal high density lipoprotein in plasma and urine. Lancet 1:936–938, 1983.

204. Vaziri ND, Liang K, Parks JS: Acquired lecithin-cholesterol acyltransferase deficiency in nephrotic syndrome. Am J Physiol 280:F823–F828, 2001.

205. Cohen SL, Cramp DG, Lewis AD, Tickner TR: The mechanism of hyperlipidaemia in nephrotic syndrome: Role of low albumin and the LCAT reaction. Clin Chim Acta 104:393–400, 1980.

206. Moulin P, Appel GB, Ginsberg HN, et al: Increased concentration of plasma cholesteryl transfer protein in nephrotic syndrome: Role in dyslipidemia. J Lipid Res 33:1817–1822, 1992.

207. Sun X, Jones H Jr, Joles JA, et al: Apolipoprotein gene expression in analbuminemic rats and in rats with Heymann nephritis. Am J Physiol 262:F755–F761, 1992.

208. Kaysen GA, Hoye E, Jones H Jr: Apolipoprotein AI levels are increased in part as a consequence of reduced catabolism in nephrotic rats. Am J Physiol 268:F532–F540, 1995.

209. Shearer GC, Newman JW, Hammock BD, Kaysen GA: Graded effects of proteinuria on HDL structure in nephrotic rats. J Am Soc Nephrol 16:1309–1319, 2005.

210. Tall AR: Plasma high density lipoproteins. Metabolism and relationship to atherogenesis. J Clin Invest 86:379–384, 1990.

211. Liang K, Vaziri ND: Down-regulation of hepatic high-density lipoprotein receptor, SR-B1, in nephrotic syndrome. Kidney Int 56:621–626, 1999.

212. Joven J, Arcelus R, Camps J, et al: Determinants of plasma homocyst(e)ine in patients with nephrotic syndrome. J Mol Med 78:147–154, 2000.

213. Lechner BL, Bockenhauer D, Iragorri S, et al: The risk of cardiovascular disease in adults who have had childhood nephrotic syndrome. Pediatr Nephrol 19:744–748, 2004.

214. Berlyne GM, Mallick NP: Ischaemic heart disease as a complication of nephrotic syndrome. Lancet 2:399–440, 1969.

215. Wass VJ, Jarrett RJ, Chilvers C, et al: Does the nephrotic syndrome increase the risk of cardiovascular disease? Lancet 2:664–667, 1979.

216. Wass V, Cameron JS: Cardiovascular disease and the nephrotic syndrome: The other side of the coin. Nephron 27:58–61, 1981.

217. Ordonez JD, Hiatt R, Killebrew EJ, et al: The increased risk of coronary heart disease associated with nephrotic syndrome. Kidney Int 44:638–642, 1993.

218. Falaschi F, Ravelli A, Martignoni A, et al: Nephrotic-range proteinuria, the major risk factor for early atherosclerosis in juvenile-onset systemic lupus erythematosus. Arthritis Rheum 43:1405–1409, 2000.

219. Stroes ESG, Joles JA, Chang P, et al: Impaired endothelial function in patients with nephrotic range proteinuria. Kidney Int 48:544–550, 1995.

220. Watts GF, Herrmann S, Dogra GK, et al: Vascular function of the peripheral circulation in patients with nephrosis. Kidney Int 60:182–189, 2001.

221. Dogra G, Ward N, Croft KD, et al: Oxidant stress in nephrotic syndrome: Comparison of F(2)-isoprostanes and plasma antioxidant potential. Nephrol Dial Transplant 16:1626–1630, 2001.

222. Dogra GK, Watts GF, Herrmann S, et al: Statin therapy improves brachial artery endothelial function in nephrotic syndrome. Kidney Int 62:550–557, 2002.

223. Vuong TD, de Kimpe S, de Roos R, et al: Albumin restores lysophosphatidylcholine-induced inhibition of vasodilation in rat aorta. Kidney Int 60:1088–1096, 2001.

224. Lenorsky C, Jordan SC, Ladisch S: Plasma inhibition of lymphocyte proliferation in nephrotic syndrome: Correlation with hyperlipidemia. J Clin Immunol 2:276–281, 1982.

225. D'Amico G, Gentile MG: Influence of diet on lipid abnormalities in human renal disease. Am J Kidney Dis 22:151–157, 1993.

226. Gentile MG, Fellin G, Cofano F, et al: Treatment of proteinuric patients with vegetarian soy diet and fish oil. Clin Nephrol 40:315–320, 1993.

227. Hall AV, Parbtani A, Clark WF, et al: Omega-3 fatty acid supplementation in primary nephrotic syndrome: Effects on plasma lipids and coagulopathy. J Am Soc Nephrol 3:1321–1329, 1992.

228. Groggel GC, Cheung AK, Ellis-Benigni K, et al: Treatment of the nephrotic hyperlipoproteinemia with gemfibrozil. Kidney Int 36:266–271, 1989.

229. Valeri A, Gelfand J, Blum C, et al: Treatment of the hyperlipidemia of the nephrotic syndrome: A controlled trial. Am J Kidney Dis 8:388–396, 1986.

230. Massy ZA, Ma JZ, Louis TA, et al: Lipid-lowering therapy in patients with renal disease. Kidney Int 48:188–198, 1995.

231. Vaziri ND, Liang K: Effects of HMG-CoA reductase inhibition on hepatic expression of key cholesterol-regulatory enzymes and receptors in nephrotic syndrome. Am J Nephrol 24:606–613, 2004.

232. Vega GL, Grundy SM: Lovastatin therapy in nephrotic hyperlipidemia: Effects on lipoprotein metabolism. Kidney Int 33:1160–1165, 1988.

233. Rabelink AJ, Hene RJ, Erkelens DW, et al: Effects of simvastatin and cholestyramine on lipoprotein profile in hyperlipidaemia of nephrotic syndrome. Lancet 2:1335–1338, 1988.

234. Brown CD, Azrolan N, Thomas L, et al: Reduction of lipoprotein(a) following treatment with lovastatin in patients with unremitting nephrotic syndrome. Am J Kidney Dis 26:170–177, 1995.

235. Wanner C, Boehler J, Eckardt HG, et al: Effects of simvastatin on lipoprotein(a) and lipoprotein composition in patients with nephrotic syndrome. Clin Nephrol 41:138–143, 1994.

236. Olbricht CJ, Wanner C, Thiery J, et al: Simvastatin in nephrotic syndrome. Kidney Int 56(suppl 71):113–116, 1999.

237. Deighan CJ, Caslake MJ, McConnell M, et al: Comparative effects of cerivastatin and fenofibrate on the atherogenic lipoprotein phenotype in proteinuric renal disease. J Am Soc Nephrol 12:341–348, 2001.

238. Buemi M, Nostro L, Crasci E, et al: Statins in nephrotic syndrome: A new weapon against tissue injury. Med Res Rev 25:587–609, 2005.

239. Keilani T, Schlueter WA, Levin ML, et al: Improvement of lipid abnormalities associated with proteinuria using fosinopril, an angiotensin converting enzyme inhibitor. Ann Intern Med 18:246–254, 1993.

240. Ruggenenti P, Mise N, Pisoni R, et al: Diverse effects of increasing lisinopril doses on lipid abnormalities in chronic nephropathies. Circulation 107:586–592, 2003.

241. de Zeeuw D, Gansevoort RT, Dullaart RPF, et al: Angiotensin II antagonism improves the lipoprotein profile in patients with nephrotic syndrome. J Hypertens 13(suppl):53–58, 1995.

242. Brunton C, Varghese Z, Moorhead JF: Lipopheresis in the nephrotic syndrome. Kidney Int 56(suppl 71):6–9, 1999.

243. Stenvinkel P, Alvestrand A, Angelin B, et al: LDL-apheresis in patients with nephrotic syndrome: Effects on serum albumin and urinary albumin excretion. Eur J Clin Invest 30:866–870, 2000.

244. Herrera Acosta J: Hypertension in chronic renal disease. Kidney Int 22:702–712, 1982.

245. Campese VM, Mitra N, Sandee D: Hypertension in renal parenchymal disease: Why is it so resistant to treatment? Kidney Int 69:967–973, 2006.

246. Küster S, Mehls O, Seidel C, et al: Blood pressure in minimal change and other types of nephrotic syndrome. Am J Nephrol 10(suppl 1):76–80, 1990.

247. Llach F: Hypercoagulability, renal vein thrombosis, and other thromboembolic complications. In Brenner BM, Stein JH (eds): The Nephrotic Syndrome. New York, Churchill Livingstone, 1982, pp 121–144.

CH 26

Renal and Systemic Manifestations of Glomerular Disease

248. Hoyer PF, Gonda S, Barthels M, et al: Thromboembolic complications in children with nephrotic syndrome. Acta Paediatr Scand 75:804–810, 1986.

249. Sullivan MJ III, Hough DR, Agodoa LCY: Peripheral arterial thrombosis due to the nephrotic syndrome: The clinical spectrum. South Med J 76:1011–1016, 1983.

250. Mehls O, Andrassy K, Koderisch J, et al: Hemostasis and thromboembolism in children with nephrotic syndrome: Differences from adults. J Pediatr 110:862–867, 1987.

251. Singhal R, Brimble KS: Thromboembolic complications in the nephrotic syndrome: pathophysiology and clinical management. Thromb Res 118:397–407, 2006.

252. Handley DA, Lawrence JR: Factor IX deficiency in the nephrotic syndrome. Lancet 1:1079–1081, 1967.

253. Vaziri ND, Ngo J-CT, Ibsen KH, et al: Deficiency and urinary loss of factor XII in adult nephrotic syndrome. Nephron 32:342–346, 1982.

254. Kendall AG, Lohmann RE, Dossetor JB: Nephrotic syndrome: A hypercoagulable state. Arch Intern Med 127:1021–1027, 1971.

255. Kanfer A, Kleinknecht D, Broyer M, et al: Coagulation studies in 45 cases of nephrotic syndrome without uremia. Thromb Diathes Haemorrh 24:562–571, 1970.

256. Thompson C, Forbes CD, Prentice CRM, et al: Changes in blood coagulation and fibrinolysis in the nephrotic syndrome. Q J Med 43:399–407, 1974.

257. Vaziri ND, Gonzales EC, Shayesthfar B, et al: Plasma levels and urinary excretion of fibrinolytic and protease inhibitory proteins in nephrotic syndrome. J Lab Clin Med 124:118–124, 1994.

258. Takeda Y, Chen A: Fibrinogen metabolism and distribution in patients with the nephrotic syndrome. J Lab Clin Med 70:678–685, 1967.

259. Wu KK, Koak JC: Urinary plasminogen and chronic glomerulonephritis. Am J Clin Pathol 60:915–919, 1973.

260. Lau SO, Tkachuk JY, Hasegawa DK, et al: Plasminogen and antithrombin III deficiencies in the childhood nephrotic syndrome associated with plasminogenuria and antithrombinuria. J Pediatr 96:390–392, 1980.

261. Du XH, Glas-Greenwalt P, Kant KS, et al: Nephrotic syndrome with renal vein thrombosis: Pathogenetic importance of a plasmin inhibitor (a2-antiplasmin). Clin Nephrol 24:186–191, 1985.

262. Kauffman RH, Veltkamp JJ, Van Tilburg NC, et al: Acquired antithrombin III deficiency and thrombosis in the nephrotic syndrome. Am J Med 65:607–613, 1978.

263. Robert A, Olmer M, Sampol J, et al: Clinical correlation between hypercoagulability and thrombo-embolic phenomena. Kidney Int 31:830–835, 1987.

264. Thaler E, Blazar E, Kopsa H, et al: Acquired anti-thrombin III deficiency in patients with glomerular proteinuria. Haemostasis 7:257–272, 1978.

265. Griffin JH, Evati B, Zimmerman TS, et al: Deficiency of protein C in congenital thrombotic disease. J Clin Invest 68:1370–1373, 1981.

266. Comp PC, Esmon DT: Recurrent venous thromboembolism in patients with a partial deficiency of protein S. N Engl J Med 311:1525–1528, 1984.

267. Mannucci PM, Valsecchi C, Bottaso B, et al: High plasma levels of protein C activity and antigen in the nephrotic syndrome. Thromb Haemost 55:31–33, 1986.

268. Vigano-D'Angelo S, D'Angelo A, Kaufman CE Jr, et al: Protein S deficiency occurs in the nephrotic syndrome. Ann Intern Med 107:42–47, 1987.

269. Malyszko J, Malyszko JS, Mysliwiec M: Markers of endothelial injury and thrombin activatable fibrinolysis inhibitor in nephrotic syndrome. Blood Coagul Fibrinolysis 13:615–621, 2002.

270. Ariens RA, Mioa M, Rivolta E, et al: High levels of tissue factor pathway inhibitor in patients with nephrotic proteinuria. Thromb Haemost 82:1020–1023, 1999.

271. Irish AB: The factor V Leiden mutation and the risk of thrombosis in patients with the nephrotic syndrome. Nephrol Dial Transplant 12:1680–1683, 1997.

272. Boneu B, Boissou F, Abbal M, et al: Comparison of progressive antithrombin activity and concentration of three thrombin inhibitors in nephrotic syndrome. Thromb Haemost 46:623–625, 1981.

273. Andrassy K, Depperman D, Walter E, et al: Is beta thromboglobulin a useful indicator of thrombosis nephrotic syndrome? Thromb Haemost 42:486, 1979.

274. McGinley E, Lowe GDO, Boulton-Jones M, et al: Blood viscosity and hemostasis in nephrotic syndrome. Thromb Haemost 49:155–157, 1983.

275. Mukherjee AP, Toh BH, Chan GL, et al: Vascular complications in nephrotic syndrome: Relationship of steroid therapy and accelerated thromboplastin generation. BMJ 4:273–276, 1970.

276. Berger J, Yaneva H: Hageman factor deposition in membranous nephropathy. Transplant Proc 3:472–473, 1982.

277. McLean RH, Forsgren A, Bjorksten B, et al: Decreased serum factor B concentration associated with decreased opsonization of *Escherichia coli* in idiopathic nephrotic syndrome. Pediatr Res 11:910–916, 1977.

278. Heslan JM, Lautie JP, Intrator L, et al: Impaired IgG synthesis in patients with the nephrotic syndrome. Clin Nephrol 18:144–147, 1982.

279. Pedraza-Chaverrí J, Torres-Rodríguez GA, Cruz C, et al: Copper and zinc metabolism in aminonucleoside-induced nephrotic syndrome. Nephron 66:87–92, 1994.

280. Perrone L, Gialanella G, Giordano V, et al: Impaired zinc metabolic status in children affected by idiopathic nephrotic syndrome. Eur J Pediatr 149:438–440, 1990.

281. Fonseca V, Thomas M, Sweny P: Can urinary thyroid hormone loss cause hypothyroidism? Lancet 338:475–476, 1991.

282. Musa BU, Seal US, Doe RP: Excretion of corticosteroid-binding globulin, thyroxine-binding globulin and total protein in adult males with nephrosis: Effect of sex hormones. J Clin Endocrinol 27:768–774, 1967.

283. Haffner D, Tönshoff B, Blum WF, et al: Insulin-like growth factors (IGFs) and IGF binding proteins, serum acid-labile subunit and growth hormone binding protein in nephrotic children. Kidney Int 52:802–810, 1997.

284. Khamiseh G, Vaziri N, Oveisi F, et al: Vitamin D absorption, plasma concentration and urinary excretion of 25(OH) vitamin D in nephrotic syndrome. Proc Soc Exp Biol Med 196:210–213, 1991.

285. Weng FL, Shults J, Herskovitz RM, et al: Vitamin D insufficiency in steroid-sensitive nephrotic syndrome in remission. Pediatr Nephrol 20:56–63, 2005.

286. Mittal SK, Dash SC, Tiwari SC, et al: Bone histology in patients with nephrotic syndrome and normal renal function. Kidney Int 55:1912–1919, 1999.

287. Vaziri ND, Kaupke CJ, Barton CH, et al: Plasma concentration and urinary excretion of erythropoietin in adult nephrotic syndrome. Am J Med 92:35–40, 1992.

288. Feinstein S, Becker-Cohen R, Algur N, et al: Erythropoietin deficiency causes anemia in nephrotic children with normal kidney function. Am J Kidney Dis 37:736–742, 2001.

290. Vaziri ND: Erythropoeitin and transferrin metabolism in nephrotic syndrome. Am J Kidney Dis 38:1–8, 2001.

291. Prinsen BHCMT, de Sain-Van der Velden MGM, Kaysen GA, et al. Transferrin synthesis is increased in nephrotic patients insufficiently to replace urinary losses. J Am Soc Nephrol 12:1017–1025, 2001.

CHAPTER 27

Diagnostic Kidney Imaging

William D. Boswell, Jr. • Hossein Jadvar • Suzanne L. Palmer

Imaging has evolved over the past 100 plus years, but the most changes have been seen in the past 20 years with marked changes in technology. In the beginning only anatomic information was available. Many different imaging examinations are now performed for the evaluation of the kidneys and the urinary tract providing not only anatomic, but also functional and metabolic information. X-ray studies include plain films, intravenous urography (IVU), antegrade and retrograde pyelograms, and computed tomography (CT). Most of these studies provide anatomic information, as does ultrasound, which employs high-frequency sound waves, not ionizing radiation. Magnetic resonance imaging (MRI) yields primarily anatomic information, but shows potential for functional evaluation as well. Nuclear medicine studies contribute primarily functional information with positron emission tomography (PET) yielding a means of metabolic assessment. Each modality has something to offer in the evaluation of the kidney as technical advances in all the areas have led to better means for renal evaluation. To properly evaluate the clinical question in patients, it is important to understand the benefits, the limitations, and the diagnostic yields of each modality.

PLAIN FILM OF THE ABDOMEN

The plain film of the abdomen has been used for years as the starting point or first step in the evaluation of the kidneys as well as the rest of the abdomen. This study may also be known as the KUB or radiograph of the kidneys, ureters, and bladder (Fig. 27–1). It is the scout film, first film, for many studies of the abdomen, including the IVU. The examination itself yields little significant information on its own. Renal size and contour may be estimated if the renal outlines can be seen, calcifications may be visualized, and other findings in the abdomen may be noted. If performed, it should be only the starting point in the evaluation of the kidneys. Intravenous iodinated contrast material is usually necessary for the opacification of the kidneys and urinary tract on radiograph examinations.

INTRAVENOUS UROGRAPHY

The intravenous urography (IVU) is still used by many as the primary means of investigation of the kidneys and urinary tract.[1,2] The IVU is also known as the intravenous pyelogram (IVP). The manner in which it is performed is best tailored to the clinical problem that is being studied. A scout film or plain film of the abdomen (KUB) is done before any contrast material is injected intravenously. This provides a starting point for the investigation of the urinary tract, but also serves as an overall assessment of the abdomen and pelvis in general. Subsequently, 25 grams to 40 grams of iodine in the form of iodinated contrast media (generally 75 cc to 150 cc) are injected intravenously for the study. The method of choice is a bolus injection, which leads to peak iodine concentrations in the plasma. Infusion techniques for contrast media injection have been used in the past but lead to a lower peak iodine concentration and poorer assessment overall. Timed sequential images of the kidneys and remainder of the genitourinary system are then obtained.[3,4]

As the iodinated contrast media is filtered by the glomerulus, the plasma iodine concentration determines the concentration of iodine in the glomerular filtrate. The higher the concentration of iodine injected, the greater the amount of iodine within the kidney and thus the better visualization of the kidney and subsequently the pelvocalyceal system.[5] The first film obtained in an IVU is taken immediately after the completion of the injection of the contrast media (generally within 30 to 60 seconds). It will demonstrate a nephrogram or image of the kidneys that reflects the iodine concentration within the tubular system of the kidneys (Fig. 27–2).[6] A higher plasma concentration of iodine leads to a higher iodine concentration in the glomerular filtrate. A higher iodine concentration in the tubular system results in a denser nephrogram or better depiction of the kidneys. This nephrogram may be used to evaluate the size, shape, and contour of the kidneys. The overall appearance and density of the kidneys should be symmetrical. The outlines of the kidneys are usually well seen contrasted by the lower or darker appearance of perirenal fat. The presence of renal

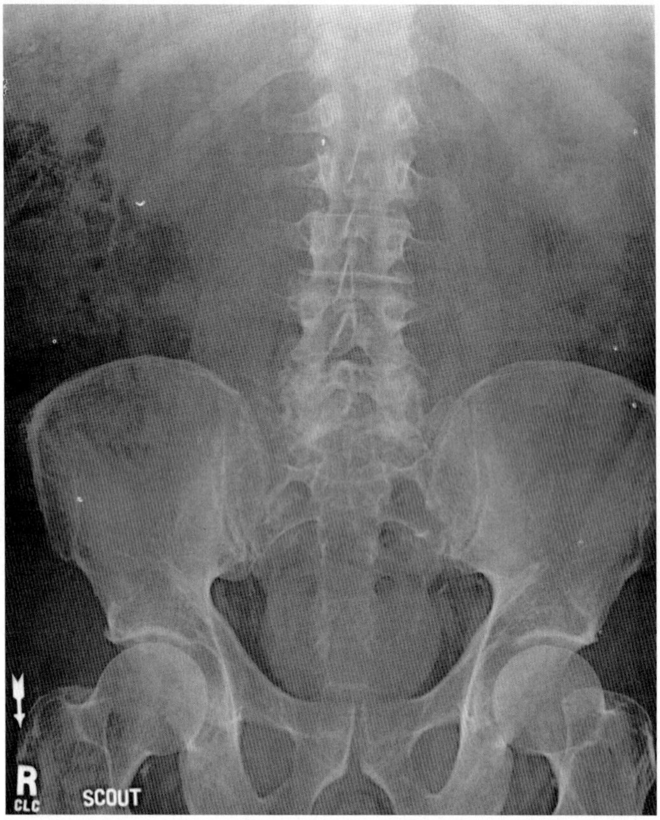

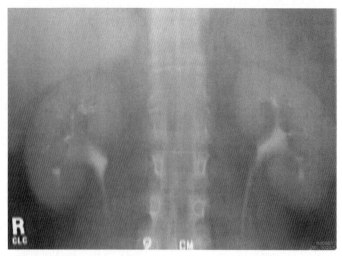

FIGURE 27–3 Intravenous urography—Nephrotomogram. This film is obtained between 5 to 7 minutes after the injection of contrast material. The overall outline of kidney is well seen with the calyces, renal pelvis, and proximal ureter opacified with the excreted contrast.

FIGURE 27–1 Plain film of the abdomen or KUB. The kidneys lie posteriorly in the retroperitoneum in the upper abdomen. They may be seen because they are surrounded by fat. The ribs overlie the kidney and bowel gas can be seen in the right upper quadrant. The psoas muscles are also well seen because retroperitoneal fat abuts them.

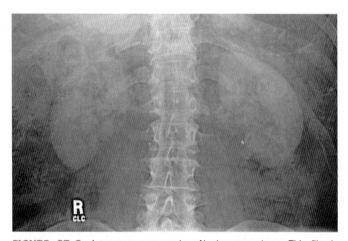

FIGURE 27–2 Intravenous urography—Nephrogram phase. This film is obtained within 60 seconds of the injection of contrast material. The kidneys are seen with smooth borders with the overlying bowel gas.

cortical scars and contour abnormalities caused by renal masses are usually well seen. The kidneys are usually homogenous in appearance throughout with a cyst or mass within the kidney causing an alteration to the overall density of the kidney.

By 3 to 5 minutes after the completion of the injection of contrast material, the iodinated contrast has reached the calyceal system. The excretion of the contrast media by the kidneys should always be symmetrical and the time of

appearance of contrast in the calyces similar. The anatomic depiction of the calyces, infundibula, and pelvis is best displayed by 5 to 10 minutes. Tomography may be performed, usually at 5 to 7 minutes, and it assists in the delineation of the renal contours, calyceal system, and renal pelvis (Fig. 27–3). The calyces have a well-formed cup shape with sharp fornices and end in a thin smooth infundibulum, which leads into the renal pelvis. The calyces may be compound or complex with several ending in one infundibulum. Abdominal compression may improve visualization of the renal elements early in the study with subsequent release allowing for the drainage of the contrast into the ureters and better visualization of the ureters. Imaging of the ureters is usually accomplished at 10 to 15 minutes. The drainage of the contrast material from the kidney and ureters allows for a global assessment of the urinary bladder (Fig. 27–4). The total number of images for the complete study is driven by the clinical question to be answered.[2–4]

IODINATED CONTRAST MEDIA

Over the years, many different intravascular contrast media have been employed.[7] All these contrast agents contain iodine in the form of a tri-iodinated benzoic acid ring in solution. Contrast agents are characterized as either ionic or nonionic and either monomers or dimmers. These agents are also known as high osmolar contrast media (HOCM), low osmolar contrast media (LOCM), and isotonic contrast media (IOCM) depending on their osmolality relative to plasma. HOCM has been used successfully for more than 50 years through the 1990's for most intravascular applications, including IVU, CT scanning, and angiographic applications. With the introduction of LOCM in the mid-1980's and IOCM in the 1990's, there has been a gradual shift to these agents. In the mid-2000's virtually all studies needing intravascular contrast injection are now performed with LOCM or IOCM.

All the HOCM agents are ionic. They are categorized as diatrizoates, iothalamates, and metrizoates. These compounds are all water-soluble salt solutions and all are hyperosmolar with relationship to plasma. The osmolality of these compounds is generally 5 to 8 times that of plasma (300 mOsm/liter). The anion is the iodine containing portion of the salt with the cation generally being either sodium or meglumine. Ionic media dissociate in water, whereas non-ionic media

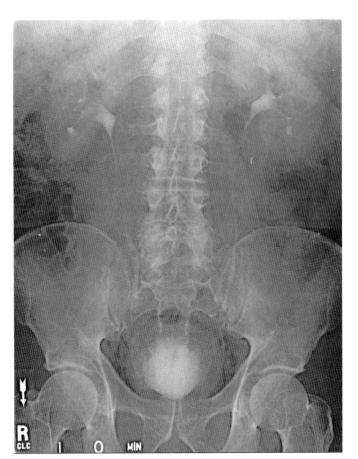

FIGURE 27–4 Intravenous urography—Excretory phase. This film is obtained 10 minutes after the injection of the contrast material. The kidneys are well visualized with contrast outlining the calyces, pelvis, ureters, and bladder.

remains in solution. Within the bloodstream, these agents are not bound to any plasma proteins and therefore filtered by the glomerulus directly. Virtually all of the contrast media injected is filtered by the glomerulus with no tubular reabsorption of excretion in the patient with normal renal function.[7] For patients experiencing renal failure, contrast media may be excreted by other routes including the biliary system or GI tract. All iodinated contrast agents are dialyzable.

Contrast material within the plasma has a half-life of 1 to 2 hours in the patient with normal renal function. Virtually all contrast will be excreted by the kidneys within 24 hours. The volume of contrast material injected, the concentration of contrast within the plasma, and the glomerular filtration rate (GFR) determine the amount of contrast material excreted into the collecting systems and subsequently the calyces, renal pelvis, and ureters. Thus, in patients with normal renal function the concentration of iodine in the plasma will ultimately determine the quality of the study. Other factors, most particularly the state of hydration, also come into play as well. Changes in the tubular reabsorption of water along the nephron will affect the concentration of iodine within the tubule and thus the subsequent iodine concentration in the urine, which is visualized in the calyces and renal pelvis on the radiograph studies.

Most LOCM agents are nonionic compounds, with the exception of Ioxaglate, which is an ionic dimer.[8] These compounds do not dissociate in solution. The LOCM are still hyperosmolar relative to plasma but to a much lesser degree compared with HOCM. LOCM are generally 2 to 3 times the osmolality of plasma. These agents are filtered by the glomerulus, just as HOCM, but have a higher concentration within the tubular system because there is less water reabsorption. The osmotic affect of LOCM is less than HOCM in the tubular system and with a higher overall concentration; therefore, within the urine, the quality of imaging studies are generally improved.[9] Iohexol, Iopamidol, and Ioversol make up the group of nonionic LOCM.

Isotonic contrast media (IOCM) are nonionic dimers: Iodixanol and Iotrol. These agents are isotonic relative to plasma. They are handled in the kidney, just as HOCM and LOCM, filtered by the glomerulus with no tubular reabsorption or excretion. These agents are generally not used for renal imaging. Their use is almost exclusively for cardiac catherizations. Cost is the major difference with IOCM being 2 to 4 times higher.

Reactions to the injection of any of the contrast agents may occur. These reactions are not "allergic" in the sense of an antigen-antibody reaction.[10] No antibodies to contrast media have ever been isolated. The reactions, however, have the appearance of an allergic reaction. Although the majority of these reactions are mild or minor, severe reactions and deaths do occur. With ionic HOCM the reaction rate for the general population is 5% to 6%.[11] In patients with a history of allergy, the reaction rate is 10% to 12% and in those who have had a previous reaction to IV contrast administration the rate is 15% to 20%. The rate of reactions with LOCM and IOCM is much lower.[12,13] Most reactions are mild consisting of flushing, nausea, and vomiting and do not require treatment. Mild dermal reactions, primarily urtica, do occur and may or may not require treatment. Moderate and severe reactions occur with considerably less frequency and include bronchospasm, laryngeal edema, seizures, arrhythmias, syncope shock, and cardiac arrest. All moderate and severe reactions require treatment. The risk of death has decreased from 1 in 8000 to 12,000 with HOCM and to 1 in 75,000 to 100,000 with LOCM and IOCM.[12]

As the reaction that occurs in patients after contrast injection is not antigen-antibody medicated, pretesting plays no role.[14] Neither the rate of injection nor dose of contrast material has been clearly established as a determinant in the occurrence of contrast-related reactions.[12,15] Premedication with antihistamines is used in some patients with prior minor reactions. The use of glucocorticoids plus H1 & H2 blockers is reserved for patients who need to be studied with iodinated contrast agents and have a history of prior contrast related reaction—usually moderate or severe in nature. There are few if any controlled studies available to critically evaluate this pretreatment regime.[16]

Contrast-related nephropathy occurs with a significant frequency, especially in the hospitalized patient base. Acute kidney injury (AKI/ARF) resulting from the administration of iodinated contrast agents is the third leading cause of hospital acquired AKI/ARF, after surgery and hypotension.[17–19] The etiology of contrast-related nephropathy is unknown but felt to be multifactorial.[19] Contrast-induced nephropathy is commonly defined as acute kidney injury occurring within 48 hours of the administration of intravascular iodinated contrast material and that no other causes are readily apparent. The definition is actually quite variable within the literature, but is most commonly associated with a rise of 0.5 mg/dL of serum creatinine above a baseline value.[20,21]

Most cases of contrast-related nephropathy present as an asymptomatic transient decrease in renal function and are nonoliguric. The rise in serum creatinine usually peaks at 3 to 5 days with a return to baseline within 10 to 14 days. Oliguric kidney injury occurs in a much smaller group with a peak creatinine elevation at 5 to 10 days and a return to baseline by 14 to 21 days. Rarely, oliguric kidney injury related to contrast media administration may require transient or long-term dialysis.

Risk factors for patients who may develop contrast-induced acute kidney injury are well known.[22] These include preexisting renal impairment, diabetes with renal insufficiency, dehydration, advancing age, congestive heart failure, ongoing treatment with nephrotoxic drugs, peripheral vascular disease, multiple myeloma, cirrhosis and liver failure, prior contrast load within 48 to 72 hours, and diuretic use, especially furosemide.[23,24] Contrast-related AKI/ARF rarely if ever occurs in individuals who are well hydrated and have normal renal function.[25,26] Although there is somewhat conflicting data, contrast-related nephropathy occurs with all types of contrast material.[20,27,28] Prevention of contrast-induced nephropathy is best done by recognizing the known risk factors.[29] Proper hydration is of paramount importance and must be performed beginning 12 hours before the contrast study.[30,31] Various methods of pretreatment have been tried with variable success. These include mannitol, diuretics, calcium channel blockers, adenosine antagonists (Theophylline), dopamine agonists, N-acetylcysteine, and sodium bicarbonate.[32–35] Again, with appropriate hydration and normal renal function, contrast-related nephropathy rarely occurs.

ULTRASOUND

Ultrasonography is a leading diagnostic examination used in the investigation of the kidneys and urinary tract.[36] It is non-invasive and requires little or no patient preparation. It is the first-line examination in the azotemic patient for assessing renal size and the presence or absence of hydronephrosis and obstruction. It is used to assess the vasculature of native and transplanted kidneys. Renal morphology and the characterization of renal masses are also done with ultrasound. As a guide for renal biopsy, ultrasound has helped to decrease morbidity and mortality.

Diagnostic ultrasonography is an outgrowth of SONAR (Sound Navigation and Ranging technology) used first during World War II for the detection of objects underwater. Medical ultrasound uses high-frequency sound waves to investigate diagnostic problems. In the abdomen and more particularly the kidney, 2.5 mHz to 4.0 mHz sound waves are generally employed.

The ultrasound unit consists of a transducer that sends and receives the sound waves, a microprocessor or computer that acquires and processes the returning signal, and an image display system or monitor that displays the processed images. The piezoelectric transducer converts electrical energy into high-frequency sound waves that are transmitted through the patient. It converts the returning reflected sound waves back into electrical energy that can be processed by the computer. Sound travels as a waveform through the tissues being imaged. The speed of the sound wave depends on the tissue through which it is traveling. In air, sound travels at 331 M/second and in the soft tissues of the body it travels at approximately 1540 M/second.

Different tissues and the interface between these tissues have different acoustic impedance. As the sound wave travels through different tissues, part of the wave is reflected back to the transducer. The depth of the tissue interface is measured by the time the sound wave takes to return to the transducer. A grey-scale image is produced by the measured reflected sound with the intensity of the pixels (picture elements) being proportional to the intensities of the reflected sound (Fig. 27–5). When the acoustic interfaces are quite large, strong echoes result. These are known as specular reflectors are a seen from the renal capsule and bladder wall. Non-specular reflectors generate lower amplitude echoes are seen in the renal parenchyma. Strong reflection of sound by bone and air results in little or no information from the tissues beneath; this is known as shadowing. Lack of acoustic impedance as seen in fluid-filled structures, such as the urinary bladder and renal cysts, allows the sound waves to penetrate further resulting in a relative increase in intensity distal to the structures; this is known as increased through transmission. Real-time ultrasound, which provides sequential images at a rapid frame rate, allows the demonstration of motion of organs and pulsation of vessels.

Doppler ultrasound, based on the Doppler frequency shift of the sound wave caused by moving objects, can be used to assess venous and arterial blood flow (Fig. 27–6).[37,38] Assessment of the waveforms can be used in diagnosis. The peripheral arterial resistance can be measured within the kidney. (Resistive Index RI = Peak Systolic velocity – lowest Diastolic velocity/Peak systolic velocity) (Fig. 27–7). Generally speaking, a normal RI is 0.70 or less. Native and transplanted kidneys can be evaluated. Increased RI is a nonspecific indicator of disease and a sign of increased peripheral vascular resistance.[39] With color Doppler ultrasound, the image is encoded with colors assigned to the pixels representing the direction, velocity, and volume of flow within vessels.[38] Power Doppler ultrasound uses the amplitude of the signal to produce a color map of the intrarenal vasculature and flow within the kidney (Fig. 27–8).[37]

Ultrasound—Normal Anatomy

The kidneys are located within Gerota's fascia and are surrounded by perinephric fat in the retroperteoneum. Sonographic images of the kidneys are generally obtained in the longitudinal and transverse planes. Parasagittal images are also obtained.[40] The perinephric fat has a variable appearance from slightly less echogenic to highly echogenic compared with the renal cortex. The renal capsule is seen as an echogenic line surrounding the kidney. The centrally located renal sinus or hilum, containing renal sinus fat, vessels, and the collecting system, is usually echogenic due to the presence of renal sinus fat (see Fig. 27–5). The amount of renal sinus fat generally increases with age. Tubular structures may be seen in the renal hilum corresponding to vessels and the collecting system. Color Doppler ultrasound may be used to differentiate the vessels from the collecting system.

Overall renal echogenicity is generally compared with the liver on the right and the spleen on the left (see Fig. 27–5). The normal renal cortex is less echogenic than the liver and spleen. Underlying liver disease may alter this picture. The medullary pyramids are hypoechoic and their triangular shape points to the renal hilum. The renal cortex lies peripherally and the separation from the medulla is usually demarcated by an echogenic focus due to the arcuate arteries along the corticomedullary junction. Columns of Bertin have the same echogenicity as the renal cortex and separate the renal pyramids. Occasionally a large column of Bertin may be seen and simulate a mass, a "pseudotumor." Even when large or prominent, a column of Bertin maintains similar echogenicity to the cortex and the vascular pattern seen on power Doppler image is also the same.

Renal size is easily measured sonographically. The normal longitudinal dimension of right kidney is 11 cm ± 1 cm and the left kidney is 11.5 cm ± 1 cm. The contours of the kidney are usually smooth although there may occasionally be some slight nodularity due to fetal lobulation. The renal arteries and veins may be seen extending from the renal hilum to the aorta and inferior vena cava. The veins lie anterior to the arteries. The renal arterial branching pattern within the kidneys may be seen with color Doppler sonography (see Fig. 27–6).[41] The resistive indices (RI) of the main, intralobar, and arcuate vessels may be calculated (see Fig. 27–7). With power Doppler imaging the intrarenal vasculature may be assessed demonstrating an overall increased pattern in the cortex relative to the medulla, corresponding to the normal arterial flow

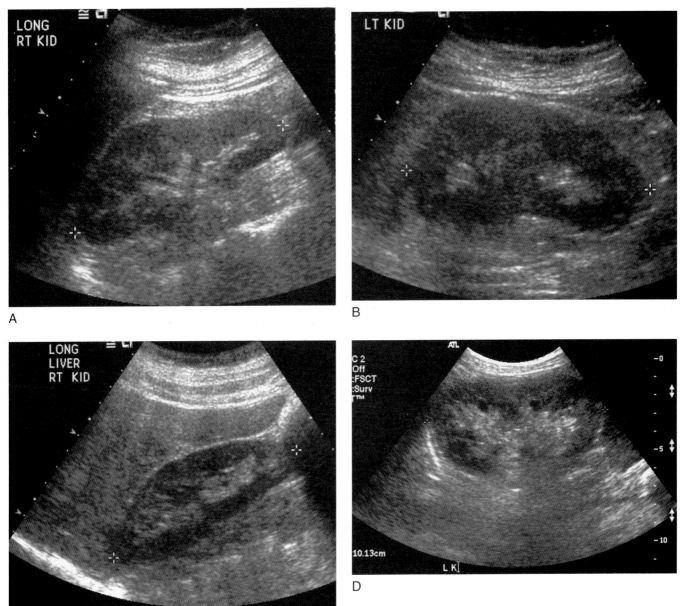

FIGURE 27–5 Normal renal ultrasounds. Normal right kidneys (**A, C**) and left kidneys (**B, D**) are shown. The central echogenic structure represents the vascular elements, calyces, and renal sinus fat. The peripheral cortex is noted to be smooth and regular. Renal pyramids are seen as hypoechoic structures between the central echo complex and the cortex in D.

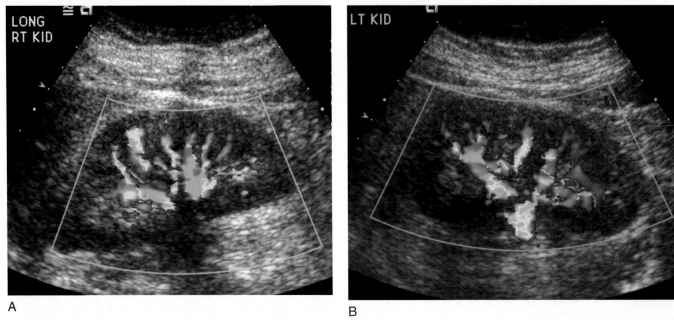

FIGURE 27-6 Normal color Doppler ultrasound. Normal right **(A)** and left **(B)** kidneys are seen. The red echogenic areas represent arterial flow (flow toward the transducer) and blue echogenic areas venous flow (flow away from the transducer).

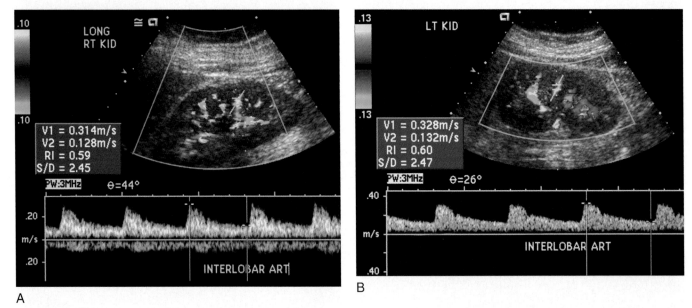

FIGURE 27-7 Normal power Doppler ultrasound. Normal right **(A)** and left **(B)** kidneys are seen. The color image represents a summation of all flow—arterial and venous—within the kidney.

to the kidney (see Fig. 27–8).[42,43] The renal calyces and collecting systems are not typically seen with ultrasound unless there is fullness or distension caused by a diuresis or obstruction. When seen the collecting systems are branching anechoic structures in the renal sinus fat connecting together to the renal pelvis. The urinary bladder is seen in the pelvis as a fluid-filled sonolucent structure. The entrance of the ureters into the bladder at the trigone may be visualized using color Doppler sonography. Ureteral jets should be seen bilaterally.

When a kidney is not identified in its normal location in the retroperitoneum, assessment of the remainder of the abdomen and pelvis should be undertaken. Ectopic kidneys may lie lower in the abdomen or within the pelvis and may also be located on the opposite side, even fused with the other kidney. Horseshoe kidneys tend to lie lower in the retroperitoneum and the axes of the kidneys may be different than the normal kidney.

The demonstration of increased echogenicity within the renal cortex may be useful in suggesting the presence of renal parenchymal (medical renal) disease.[43,44] The renal cortex may show increased echogenicity in patients with either acute or chronic kidney injury. This finding is nonspecific and does not correlate with the degree or severity of kidney injury. The finding is bilateral. The increased cortical echogenicity in patients with chronic kidney injury is generally related to interstitial fibrosis.[39] A patient with small, echogenic kidneys usually has end-stage renal disease (ESRD).

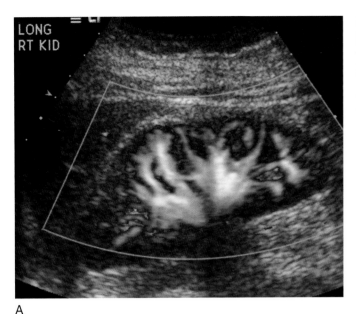

A

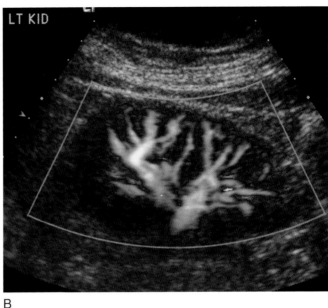

B

FIGURE 27–8 Normal duplex Doppler ultrasound. Normal right **(A)** and left **(B)** kidneys are seen. The waveforms within the interlobar arteries are visualized with the resistive indices calculated for each kidney.

Ultrasound has been very useful in directing renal biopsy for patients with either acute or chronic kidney injury. Renal identification and localization greatly facilitates the procedure. Its use has decreased the procedure time as well as decreased morbidity and mortality.

COMPUTED TOMOGRAPHY

Computed tomography (CT) has become an essential tool for diagnosis in virtually all areas of the body. In the genitourinary tract, it has supplanted the IVU, which had been the mainstay of diagnosis for years. Even in areas where ultrasound is employed, CT offers a complementary and sometimes superior means of imaging. CT is now the first examination to be performed in patients with renal colic, renal stone disease, renal trauma, renal infection and abscess, renal mass, hematuria, and finally, urothelial abnormalities.

Computed tomography has been heralded as the greatest improvement in diagnostic radiology since Roentgen discovered x-rays in 1895. Sir Godfrey Hounsfield developed the first CT scanner in 1970.[45] The first clinical applications in 1971 were in the head. The first body CT scanner was installed in Georgetown University Medical Center in 1974. The field has grown rapidly since that time with new technical innovations, image processing, and visualization methods. For his outstanding work in the field and for demonstrating the unique and remarkable clinical capabilities of CT, Sir Godfrey Hounsfield was awarded the Nobel Prize for Medicine in 1979.

Computer tomography is the computer reconstruction of an x-ray–generated image that typically depicts a slice through the area being studied in the body. The x-ray tube produces a highly collimated fan-bean and is mounted opposite an array of electronic detectors. This system rotates in tandem around the patient. The detector system collects hundreds of thousands of samples representing the x-ray attenuation along the line formed from the x-ray source to the detector as the rotation occurs. These data are transferred to a computer, which reconstructs the image. The image may then be displayed on a computer monitor or transferred to radiograph film for reviewing.

The CT image is actually made up of numerous pixels (picture elements) each corresponding to a CT number representing the amount of x-rays absorbed by the patient at a particular point in the cross-sectional image. These pixels represent a 2D display of a 3D object. Each pixel element actually has a third dimension—the slice thickness or depth. Thus, the CT number is actually the average x-ray attenuation of all the tissues within a specific volume element, voxel, which is used to create the individual image or slice.

Computed tomography numbers are the x-ray attenuation of each voxel relative to the attenuation of water (CT number = 0). Tissues that attenuate more x-rays than water have positive CT numbers and those with less attenuation have negative numbers. Bone may have a CT number greater than 1000, with air in the lungs having a CT number of ≈ −1000. Different shades of grey on a scale of white to black are assigned to the CT numbers (highest = white, lowest = black). The image of each slice is thus created on the monitor with image manipulation possible to accentuate the regions being imaged. The image data is constant but by varying the range of CT numbers, the appearance of the image may be changed, a key element of any digital image.

The initial CT scanners were relatively slow as the technology required a point and shoot process. One slice was obtained, the patient moved, and the next slice obtained. This initial generation of body CT scanner led to a scan of the abdomen that took up to 2 to 4 minutes or more to complete. In 1990, helical/spiral technology was introduced in which the x-ray tube and detector system continuously rotated around the patient and the patient moved continuously through the gantry. Scan time was reduced to 25 to 35 seconds through the abdomen. After helical/spiral CT, a two detector system was introduced that produced two slices for every 360° rotation of the x-ray tube and detector system. This was the first multi-detector CT scanner (MDCT). By 1998, four-detector systems were introduced by all manufactures. Today 10, 16, 32, 40, and 64 detector systems are available with more technological advances on the horizon. With MDCT, each 360° rotation of results in the number of slices equal to the number of detectors (i.e., 64 detector system = 64 slices in one 360° rotation). These technological advances have led to dramatic increase in the speed of scans (4 to 10 seconds), routine use of thin slices or collimation (1 mm to 2 mm), and marked improvement in spatial resolution (ability to resolve small objects).[46]

The faster scan times have led to improved utilization and optimization of intravenous contrast enhancement.[47] For example, the kidney can be scanned in the arterial, venous, nephrographic, and delay phases allowing for a more complete assessment. With a 16–64 detector scan, a single acquisition of CT data takes from 3 to 7 seconds with slice thickness being less than 1 mm. The images are normally displayed as transverse or axial images. As the slice thickness has been reduced to the point that the voxel has become a cube or near cube (isotropic voxel), sagittal, coronal, and oblique image may be displayed with no loss of resolution. The data acquisition may also be displayed as a 3D volumetric display with the regions of interest highlighted.[47] Scanning today is done with a single breath hold acquisitions leading to the elimination of virtually all motion artifacts, and the misregistration artifacts seen with breathing. In imaging the heart, ECG gated-acquisition to the cardiac cycle eliminates the motion of the heart resulting in clear assessment of the coronary arteries, valves, and related anatomy. The kidney is well suited for assessment with MDCT as sagittal, coronal, and 3D displays are additive to the information content of the study.[47–51]

Computed tomography urogram was introduced in 1999 to 2000 and is an outgrowth of the advances made with MDCT technology and state-of-the-art workstations with their added computer processing and display capabilities.[46,52] The CT urogram provides a complete examination of the kidney and the remainder of genitourinary tract. CT urography assesses the kidney as a whole (anatomic), the vascular tree (function and perfusion), and the excretory (urothelial) patterns. Noncontrast scans provide for assessment of renal calculi, high density cysts, and contour abnormalities.[53] Early phase scans (12–15 seconds) leads to arterial assessment. Scanning at 25 to 30 seconds yields a combined arterial-venous phase image with clear corticomedullary differentiation. With imaging done at 90 to 100 seconds, true nephrographic phase imaging of the kidneys is obtained.[47] Delayed imaging, typically at 3 to 7 minutes and up to 10 minutes, provides excretory phase images with evaluation of the urothelium—calyces, renal pelvis, ureters, and bladder.[54] Axial images, multiplanar reconstructions, maximum intensity projection (MIP) images, and 3D volumetric displays complement each other in the CT urogram.[52] Properly performed, the CT urogram has replaced the IVU in 2005.[55–58]

Computed Tomography Technique

Noncontrast images are obtained through the kidneys and the remainder of the GU tract to the pelvic floor if stone disease is the primary problem. In the case of vascular problems and renal masses, arterial-venous phase imaging is usually required and accomplished by a rapid bolus injection of iodinated contrast media, generally 4 to 5 cc/second and a volume of 100 to 120 cc, with scans in the arterial-venous phases at 25 to 30 seconds. When needed as in cases of suspected renal artery stenosis, true arterial phase imaging may be performed beginning at 12 to 15 seconds. Nephrographic imaging at 90 to 100 seconds is subsequently performed with excretory imaging to follow. Slice thickness is general 2 mm or less, which will allow for workstation reconstruction as necessary. The radiation dose for this technique is approximately 1.5 times that of the IVU, but the information content is exceedingly higher.

Computed Tomography Anatomy

The kidneys lie in the retroperitoneum, surrounded by Gerota's fascia in the perinephric space. Fat will generally

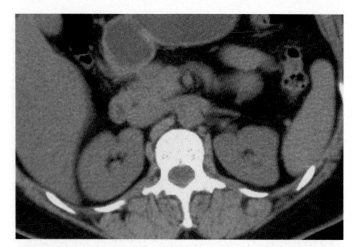

FIGURE 27–9 Normal noncontrast CT scan through the mid-portion of the kidneys. The kidneys lie in the retroperitoneum with the lumbar spine and psaos muscles more centrally. The liver is seen anterolateral to the right kidney and the spleen anterolateral to the left kidney.

outline the kidneys with the liver anterior-superior on the right, the spleen superior on the left, and the spine, aorta, and inferior vena cava (IVC) central to each kidney (Fig. 27–9). The abdominal contents lie anteriorly. This anatomy is easily seen with all phases of scanning. With arterial and venous phase scans, the renal arteries are easily seen, generally posterior to the venous structures (Fig. 27–10). The right renal artery is located behind the IVC (Fig. 27–11). The left renal vein courses anterior to the aorta before it enters the IVC and the right renal vein generally is seen obliquely entering the IVC. The adrenal glands are found in a location superior to the upper poles of the kidneys. In venous phase imaging, true separation of the renal cortex from the medulla is easily accomplished. Cortical thickness and medullary appearance may easily be assessed (see Fig. 27–10). The nephrographic phase should demonstrate the symmetrical enhancement for each of the kidneys (Fig. 27–12).[47] At 7 to 10 minutes in the excretory phase, the calyces should be well seen with sharp fornices, a cupped central section, and a narrow smooth infundibulum leading to the renal pelvis (Fig. 27–13).[54] Coronal images in a slab MIP format will display this to the best advantage. Three-dimensional volumetric reformations also may display the anatomic delay (Fig. 27–14).[57] The excretory phase images also delineate the ureters from the renal pelvis to the bladder. A curved reformatted series of images or 3D display will be needed to display the ureters in their entirety. Proper tailoring of the examination to the diagnostic problem will lead the correct imaging acquisition.[48,50,58]

MAGNETIC RESONANCE IMAGING

Like CT, magnetic resonance imaging (MRI) is a computer-based, multiplanar imaging modality. But instead of using ionizing radiation, MRI uses electromagnetic radiation. MRI is an alternative to contrast-enhanced CT, especially in patients with iodinated contrast allergy and renal insufficiency. MRI is also used when reduction of radiation exposure is desired, such as during pregnancy and in the pediatric population. MRI routinely allows detailed tissue characterization of the kidney and surrounding structures. The physics behind MRI is complex and will only be addressed briefly.

Clinical MRI is based on the interaction of hydrogen ions (protons) and radiofrequency waves in the presence of a

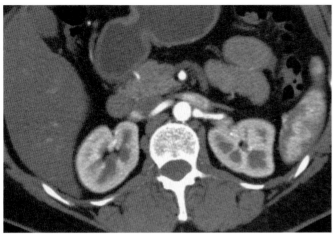
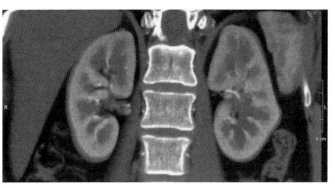

A

B

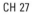

FIGURE 27-10 Normal corticomedullary phase CT scan. Axial CT slice **(A)** and coronal image **(B)** demonstrate the dense enhancement of the cortex relative to the medulla containing the renal pyramids.

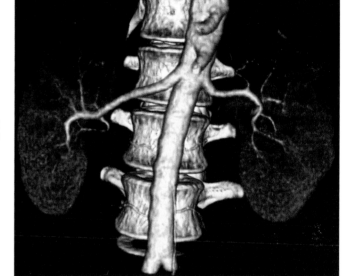

FIGURE 27-11 Normal renal CT angiogram. The aorta and the exiting renal arteries on the right and left are seen. The kidneys are seen peripherally with the branching renal arteries.

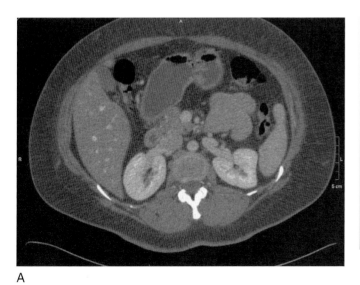
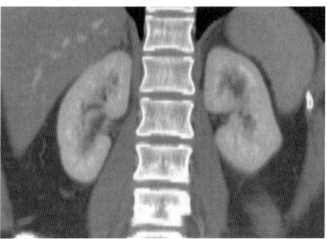

A

B

FIGURE 27-12 Normal nephrogram phase CT scan. The axial image **(A)** and the coronal image **(B)** demonstrate the homogenous appearance of the kidneys with the cortex and medulla no longer differentially enhanced. These images are typically obtained at 80 to 120 seconds after the injection of contrast material.

strong magnetic field.[59-61] The strong magnetic field, called the external magnetic field, is generated by a large bore, high field strength magnet. Most magnets in clinical use are superconducting magnets. The magnet strength is measured in Tesla (T) and can range from 0.2T to 3T for clinical imaging and up to 15T for animal research. Renal imaging is performed best on high field magnets (1.5T–3T) that allow for higher spatial resolution and faster imaging.

Images of the patient are obtained through a multistep process of energy transfer and signal transmission. When a patient is placed in the magnet, the mobile protons associated with fat and water molecules align longitudinal to the external magnetic field. No signal is obtained unless a resonant radiofrequency (RF) pulse is applied to the patient. The RF pulse causes the mobile protons within the patient to move from a lower, stable energy state to a higher, unstable energy state (excitation). When the RF pulse is removed, the protons return to the lower energy steady state while emitting frequency transmissions or signals (relaxation). In radiology lingo, an external RF pulse "excites" the protons causing them to "flip" to a higher energy state. When the RF pulse is removed, the protons "relax" with emission of a "radio signal". The signals produced during proton relaxation are separated from one another with applied magnetic field gradients. The emitted signals are captured by a receiving coil and reconstructed into images through a complex computerized algorithm: the Fourier Transform.[59-61]

Different tissues have different relaxation rates that lead to different levels of signal production or signal intensity. The signal intensity of each tissue is determined by three characteristics:

1. *Proton density of the tissue.* The greater the number of mobile protons, the greater the signal produced by the tissue. For example: a volume of urine has more mobile protons than the same volume of renal tissue, therefore urine will give more signal than the kidney. Stones have far fewer mobile protons per unit volume and therefore will produce little signal.
2. *T1 relaxation time.* How quickly a proton returns to the pre-excitation energy state. The shortest T1 times (rapid relaxation) produce the strongest signal.
3. *T2 relaxation time.* How quickly the proton signal decays due to non-uniformity of the magnetic field. A non-uniform field accelerates signal decay and leads to signal loss.[59-61]

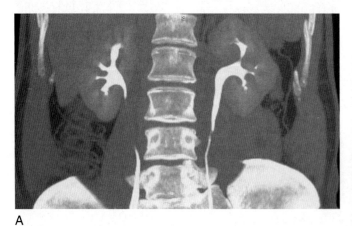

FIGURE 27–13 Normal excretory phase CT scan. The calyces and renal pelvis are now easily noted as they are opacified by the excreted contrast. This scan is obtained 5 to 10 minutes after the injection of contrast material.

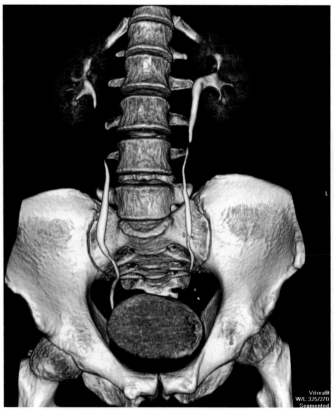

FIGURE 27–14 Normal CT urogram. The maximum-intensity projection (MIP) image **(A)** and volume rendered image **(B)** demonstrate the calyces, renal pelvis, ureters, and bladder. The MIP image is a slab—15 mm thick done in the coronal plane. The volume rendered image as the extraneous tissues adjacent to the kidneys removed and highlight the genitourinary track.

Magnetic resonance imaging involves the acquisition of multiple pulse sequences. A pulse sequence is a set of defined RF pulses and timing parameters used to acquire image data. These sequences include, but are not limited to, spin echo, gradient echo, inversion recovery, and steady-state precession. The data are acquired in volumes (voxels), reconstructed as 2D pixels, and displayed relative to tissue signal intensity variations (tissue contrast). Tissue contrast, like signal intensity, is determined by proton density and relaxation times. T1 weighting is related to the rate of T1 relaxation and the pulse repetition time (TR), also known as the time allowed for relaxation. T2 weighting is related to the rate of T2 relaxation and the time at which the "radio signal" is sampled by the receiver coil, also known as the time to echo (TE). TR and TE are programmable parameters that can be altered to accentuate T1 and T2 contrast weighting.[59-61] For the general observer, T1-weighted sequences have short TR and TE and show simple fluid as black. T2-weighted sequences have long TR and TE and show simple fluid as white (Fig. 27–15).

There are many programmable parameters, other than TR and TE, used to optimize imaging. These include, but are not limited to, choice of pulse sequence, coil types and gradients, slice orientation and thickness, field of view and matrix, gating to reduce motion, and use of intravenous (IV) contrast. Although there are many pulse sequences used in clinical MR imaging, ultrafast sequences are preferred for renal imaging. These fast sequences can be acquired in less than 30 seconds while the patients hold their breath. The benefits of rapid acquisition include improved image quality due to reduction of motion artifact, reduction of total scan time, and the ability to perform dynamic imaging.[62]

Use of IV contrast is routine in renal imaging due to the improved lesion detection and diagnostic accuracy provided by IV gadolinium-chelates (Gd-C). Gadolinium is a paramagnetic substance that shortens the T1 and T2 relaxation times, resulting in increased signal intensity on T1-weighted images and decreased signal intensity on T2-weighted sequences (Fig. 27–16). The pharmacokinetics and enhancement patterns of IV Gd-C agents are similar to iodinated contrast agents used for radiograph examinations. Unlike iodinated contrast agents, the dose response to Gd-C is non-linear; the signal intensity increases at low concentrations and then decreases at higher concentrations. Hence, the collecting systems, ureters, and bladder first brighten and then darken on T1-weighted sequences as the gadolinium concentration within the urine increases. Gd-C agents are well tolerated and can be used in patients with iodinated contrast allergies or who have renal insufficiency.[63] Severe contrast reactions to Gd-C agents are rare, as is nephrotoxicity.[64-66] There have been some reports of nephrotoxicity with IV Gd-C in high-risk populations: those with moderate to severe kidney injury.[67,68] Gd-C may interfere with serum calcium and magnesium measurements, especially in patients with renal insufficiency.[69] As with iodinated contrast, dialysis filters Gd-C effectively and dialysis is therefore recommended after contrast use in patients with kidney injury.[70]

Gd-C agents are not without risk, however. There have been recent reports of Gd-C associated development of nephrogenic systemic fibrosis (NSF), a rare fibrosing disease seen predominantly in dialysis dependent patients.[71-76] NSF was first described in 1997 and published in the literature in 2000[77]; but it was not until January 2006 that a possible causal relationship between Gd-C and NSF was presented in the literature. To date, over 215 cases have been reported to the International Center for Nephrogenic Fibrosing Dermopathy (ICNFD).[78] A cause and effect link between Gd-C and NSF has not been proven as of yet, but NSF has been strongly associated with high dose IV gadodiamide administration in the setting of high-risk patients. Gadodiamide is one of 5 U.S. Food and Drug Administration (FDA) approved Gd-C contrast agents for MRI. High-risk patients include patients with dialysis dependent chronic renal insufficiency, low glomerular filtration rate (GFR) of <30 mL/min/1.73 m^2 and acute hepatorenal syndrome. To date, no cases of NSF have been documented in patients with normal renal function.

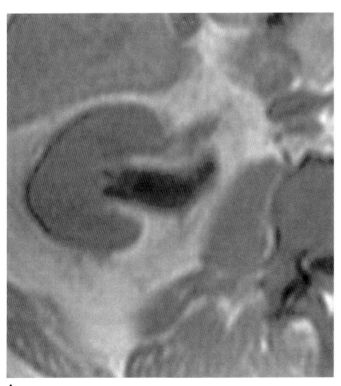

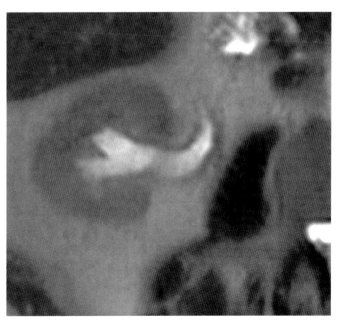

B

A

FIGURE 27–15 Normal MR signal characteristics of simple fluids. **A,** Urine is dark on T1-weighted sequences and **(B)** bright on T2-weighted sequences.

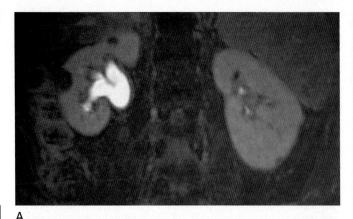

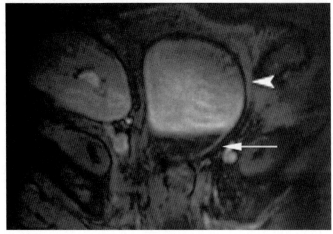

FIGURE 27-16 Paramagnetic effects of gadolinium on urine. **A,** Coronal T1-weighted image from an MR urogram demonstrates enhancement of the urine in the collection system. **B,** Coronal T2-weighted image from an MR urogram demonstrates low signal intensity urine in the collecting system secondary to effects of gadolinium. **C,** Axial T1-weighted, delayed post contrast image demonstrates layering of contrast. The denser, more concentrated gadolinium is dark (*arrow*). The less concentrated gadolinium is brighter and layers above (*arrowhead*).

Potential for NSF to occur in association with all the FDA approved Gd-C agents is suspected, but not proven. As more medical research is available, recommendations for the usage of Gd-C in patients with moderate to severe renal disease will be modified.[76,79] At the time of publication of this book, our approach to the use of Gd-C in high-risk patients is as follows: We do not administer gadodiamide to our patients. The Gd chelates that we use are at the FDA approved doses, or lower. If the patient is high-risk (dialysis dependent chronic renal insufficiency, GFR of <30 mL/min/1.73 m² or acute hepatorenal syndrome) we restrict the use of Gd-C agents to those patients who require contrast to make a diagnosis or direct therapy. We also recommend dialysis after exposure to Gd-C for dialysis dependent patients, although this has not been found to reduce the incidence of NSF. Suspected cases of NSF should be confirmed by skin biopsy and reported to ICNFD to help further our understanding of NSF and its association with Gd-C.

Contrast-enhanced MRI (CE-MRI) allows for dynamic evaluation of the kidney and surrounding structures. Serial acquisitions are obtained after bolus injection of gadolinium (0.1 mmol/kg–0.2 mmol/kg body weight) at 2 cc sec.[80,81] The injection should be administered by means of an automatic, MR-compatible power injector to assure accuracy of the timed bolus, including volume and rate of injection.[81,82] The corticomedullary/arterial phase (approximately 20 sec) best evaluates the arterial structures and corticomedullary differentiation. The nephrographic phase (70 to 90 sec) maximizes tumor detection and best demonstrates the renal veins and surrounding structures (Fig. 27–17). Imaging can be performed in any plane, but the coronal plane is the most frequently used for dynamic imaging as it allows imaging of the kidneys, ureters, vessels, and surrounding structures in the fewest number of images.

Magnetic resonance imaging is not indicated for every patient due to the presence of some implanted medical devices such as pacemakers, ferromagnetic CNS aneurysm clips, and ferromagnetic stapedial implants. Not all implants or devices are a problem, but knowledge of the type of device is critical to determine if the patient can safely enter the magnet.[83]

MAGNETIC RESONANCE IMAGING PROTOCOLS

Diagnostic Magnetic Resonance Imaging; Routine Renal Exam

Routine MRI evaluation of the kidneys includes axial and coronal T1-weighted and T2-weighted sequences. Both can be obtained with and without fat suppression. Dynamic contrast-enhanced T1-weighted sequences are also routinely obtained. In patients with normal renal function the renal cortex and medullary pyramids are easily differentiated due to the excellent tissue differentiation provided by MRI. On T1-weighted sequences the renal cortex is higher in signal intensity than the medullary pyramids. On T2-weighted

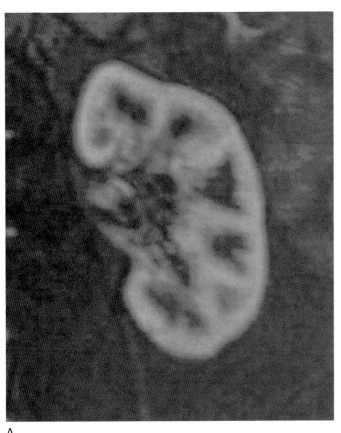

A

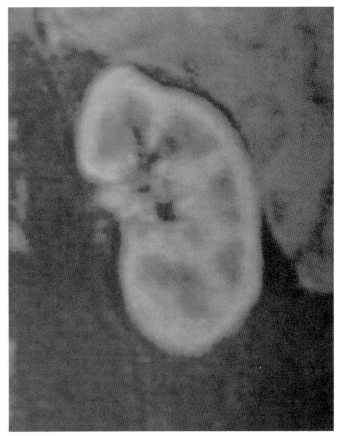

B

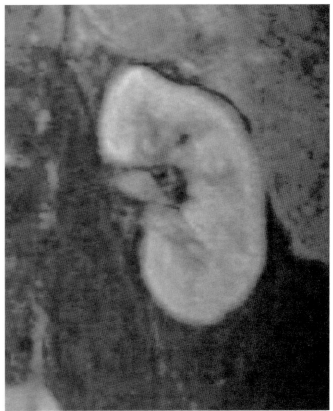

C

FIGURE 27–17 Magnetic resonance appearance of a normal kidney after bolus injection of gadolinium contrast material at **(A)** 20 seconds, **(B)** 50 seconds, and **(C)** 80 seconds after start of injection.

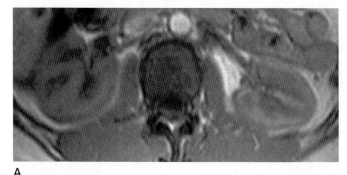
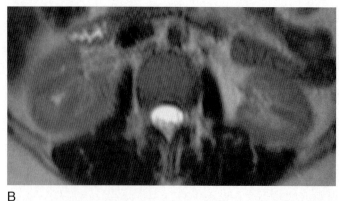

A

B

FIGURE 27–18 Normal MRI appearance of corticomedullary differentiation. **A,** Axial T1-weighted image demonstrates increased signal intensity of the renal cortex relative to the medullary pyramids. **B,** Axial T2-weighted image demonstrates decreased signal intensity of the renal cortex relative to the medullary pyramids.

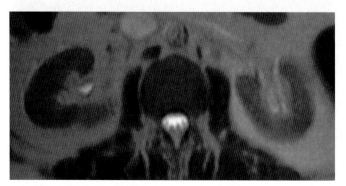

FIGURE 27–19 Axial T2-weighted image demonstrates loss of corticomedullary differentiation in patient with elevated creatinine.

sequences the renal cortex is lower in signal intensity than the medullary pyramids (Fig. 27–18). With kidney injury this corticomedullary differentiation disappears (Fig. 27–19).[84,85] Urine, like water, is normally black on T1-weighted and white on T2-weighted sequences (see Fig. 27–15). The parenchymal enhancement characteristics are similar to those seen on contrast-enhanced CT.

Renal Vascular Evaluation; Magnetic Resonance Angiography/Venography

On routine, precontrast imaging, the vessels can be variable in signal intensity, ranging from white to black due to many factors including, but not limited to, flow-related parameters, location and orientation of the imaged vessel, and choice of pulse sequence. Non contrast-enhanced pulse sequences can be used for angiography and venography, but these sequences take longer to acquire and their use is limited in abdominal imaging. These sequences are sometimes called "bright-blood" sequences and include time-of-flight MR angiography, which is based on flow-related enhancement, and phase contrast MR angiography, which is based on velocity and direction of flow. Phase contrast MR angiography can be used in conjunction with contrast-enhanced MR angiography (CE-MRA) to detect turbulent flow and high velocities associated with stenoses.

Unlike the "bright blood" sequences, CE-MRA minimizes flow-related enhancement and motion. CE-MRA depends on the T1 shortening properties of gadolinium, which allow for faster imaging, increased coverage, and improved resolution.[60,86] Accurate timing of the contrast bolus is critical for CE-MRA. The time at which the bolus arrives at the renal arteries may be determined with a bolus injection of 1 cc of gadolinium followed by a saline flush. A 3D T1-weighted

gradient-echo MR imaging pulse sequence is then acquired in the coronal plane during the injection of approximately 15 cc to 20 cc of gadolinium at 2 cc/sec, timed to capture the arterial phase.[80,81] Sequential 3D sequences are acquired to capture the venous phase (MR venography). The data sets can be post processed into multiple formats, improving ease and accuracy of interpretation (Fig. 27–20).[87–89]

Collecting System Evaluation: Magnetic Resonance Urography

Magnetic resonance urography (MRU) consists of protocols tailored to the evaluation of the renal collecting system and the pathology found there. MRU can be performed with heavily T2-weighted sequences, where urine gives the intrinsic contrast, or with contrast-enhanced T1-weighted sequences, which mimic conventional IV urography (IVU) and CT urography (CTU). Heavily T2-weighted sequences are most useful in patients with dilated collecting systems, where all water-filled structures are bright (Fig. 27–21), and in patients with impaired renal excretion, where contrast urography is most limited. Unfortunately, without adequate distention of the collecting system, T2-weighted evaluation is limited. Although a good morphologic examination, T2-weighted urography is ultimately limited by a lack of functional information. For example, T2-weighted urography cannot reliably differentiate between an obstructed system and an ectatic collecting system (Fig. 27–22).[90] Contrast-enhanced, excretory T1-weighted urography is superior to T2-weighted urography because both morphology and function can be evaluated.[90–92]

T2- and contrast-enhanced T1-weighted sequences are complementary and are frequently acquired together as part of a complete MRU examination. In non dilated systems, both techniques require hydration and furosemide for adequate distention of the renal collecting system.[90,93] A typical MRU will start with a coronal, heavily T2-weighted sequence where simple fluid (urine, CSF, ascites) is bright and all other tissues are dark (see Fig. 27–21). This rapid breath-hold sequence takes less than 5 seconds to acquire and is presented as a urographic-like image. The T2-weighted sequence is used as an initial survey of fluid within collecting system. Low-dose furosemide (0.1 mg/kg body weight, maximum dose 10 mg) is administered intravenously, 30 to 60 seconds before the intravenous administration of gadolinium (0.1 mmol/kg).[91,92] Furosemide is given to increase urine volume and dilute the gadolinium within the collecting system.[91,93] Coronal, post contrast, 3D T1-weighted sequences are acquired with the same technique as renal MRA, in the corticomedullary/arterial phase, nephrographic phase, and excretory phase (see Fig. 27–21).[92] Additional sequences may be acquired in any plane to better evaluate suspected pathology.

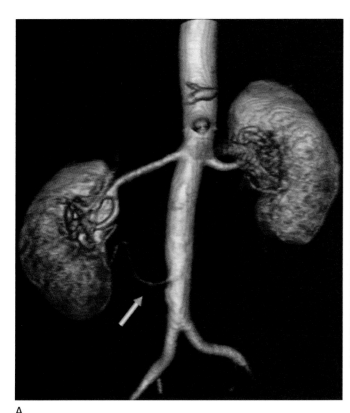
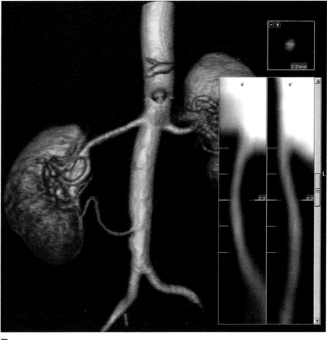

B

A

FIGURE 27-20 Magnetic resonance angiogram reconstructed with 3D software. **A,** Demonstrates excellent visualization of small accessory right renal artery (*arrow*). **B,** Presents the accessory artery in a way to make more accurate luminal measurements.

By combining renal MRI and MRU, a comprehensive morphologic and functional evaluation of urinary tract can be obtained. MRU gives accurate evaluation of the upper urinary tract, and is useful in the evaluation of anatomic anomalies including duplications, ureteropelvic obstruction, anomalous crossing vessels, and ureteroceles[93,94] (Fig. 27–23). Obstructive disease is well evaluated no matter whether the etiology is intrinsic or extrinsic to the collecting system.

NUCLEAR MEDICINE

Scintigraphy offers imaging-based diagnostic information on renal structure and function. Many single-photon radiotracers have long been in routine clinical use in renal scintigraphy, which are tailored to provide physiological information complementing the primarily anatomic and structural-based imaging modalities such as ultrasonography (US), computed tomography (CT), and magnetic resonance imaging (MRI). With the rapid expansion of positron emission tomography, and more recently hybrid structural-functional imaging systems such as PET-CT, additional unprecedented opportunities have developed for quantitative imaging evaluation of renal diseases in clinical medicine and in the research arena. In this section, we review the unique contribution of scintigraphy, including PET, in the imaging evaluation of renal structure and function. We first launch with a brief discussion of the common radiopharmaceuticals used in renal scintigraphy.

Radiopharmaceuticals

Technetium 99m diethylenetriaminepentaacetic Acid (Tc-99m DTPA)
Tc-99m DTPA is the common agent for assessing glomerular filtration rate (GFR). The ideal agent for measuring GFR is cleared only by glomerular filtration and is not secreted or reabsorbed. Tc-99m DTPA satisfies the first requirement but has variable degrees of protein binding, which deviates its kinetics from the ideal agent such as inulin. For a 20 mCi (740 MBq) dose, the radiation exposures to the kidneys and to the urinary bladder are 1.8 rads and 2.3 rads, respectively.[95]

Iodine-131 Orthoiodohippurate (I-131 OIH)
The mechanism of I-131 OIH renal clearance is about 20% by GFR and about 80% by tubular secretion. I-131 OIH is an acceptable alternative to para-aminohippuric acid (PAH) for determining renal plasma flow although its clearance is 15% lower than that of PAH. PAH is not entirely cleared by the kidneys with about 10% of arterial PAH remaining in the renal venous blood. Therefore, I-131 OIH measures *effective* renal plasma flow (ERPF). The tubular extraction efficiency of I-131 OIH is 90% and there is no hepatobiliary excretion. OIH may also be labeled with I-123 that not only provides equivalent urinary kinetics as that for I-131 label but also offers improved image quality due to typically larger administered dose in view of its more favorable radiation exposure. For a 300 uCi (11 MBq) dose of I-131 OIH, the radiation exposures to the kidneys and to the urinary bladder are 0.02 rads and 1.4 rads, respectively. Few drops of nonradioactive iodine (e.g., saturated solution of potassium iodide) orally minimize the thyroid uptake of free I-131.[95]

Technetium 99m Mercaptoacetyltriglycine (Tc-99m MAG3)
Tc-99m MAG3 has similar properties to OIH but has significant advantages of better image quality and less radiation exposure. The tubular extraction fraction of MAG3 is lower than OIH at about 60% to 70%. There is also about 3% hepatobiliary excretion, which increases with renal insufficiency. Despite these features, however, MAG3 is a common agent used in scintigraphic evaluation of renal function. For a 10 mCi (370 MBq) dose, the radiation exposures to the kidneys and to the urinary bladder are 0.15 rads and 4.4 rads, respectively.[95]

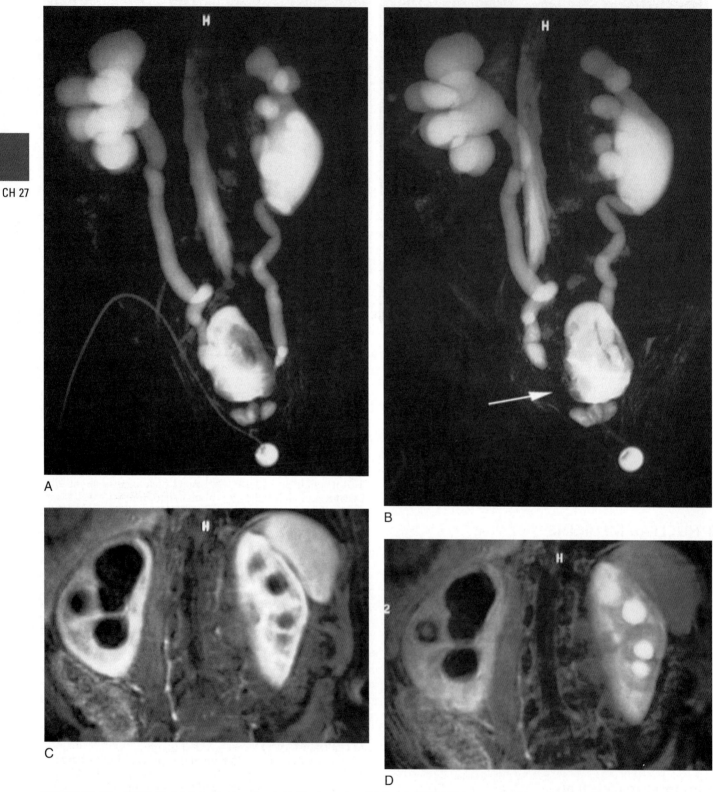

FIGURE 27–21 Bilateral hydronephrosis secondary to bladder tumor. **A and B,** Heavily T2W MRU demonstrate bilateral hydronephrosis and hydroureter due to bladder mass (arrow). **C,** Contrast-enhanced MRU nephrographic phase demonstrates asymmetric enhancement of the kidneys and **(D)** excretory phase demonstrates asymmetric excretion of gadolinium. There is no excretion on the right as demonstrated by unenhanced (dark) urine within the collecting system.

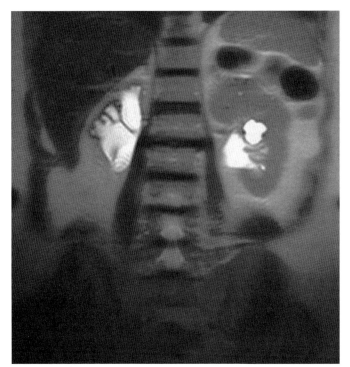
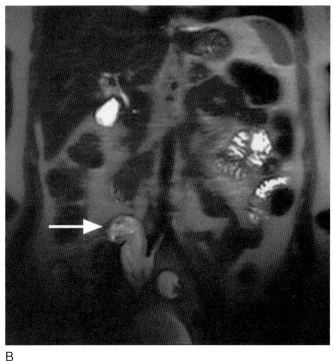

FIGURE 27–22 **A and B,** Coronal T2-weighed images demonstrate right renal atrophy and dilatation of the right collecting system in a patient after bladder resection and ilio-conduit reconstruction (*arrow*). On these static images it is difficult to differentiate between an obstructed and non obstructed system. This patient has pelvocaliectasis without obstruction, demonstrated on the contrast-enhanced portion of the examination.

Technetium 99m Dimercaptosuccinic Acid (Tc-99m DMSA)

Tc-99m DMSA localizes to renal cortex at high concentration and has slow urinary excretion rate. About 50% of the injected dose accumulates in the renal cortex at 1 hour. The tracer is bound to the renal proximal tubular cells. In view of the high retention of DMSA in the renal cortex, it has become useful for imaging of the renal parenchyma. For a 6 mCi (11 MBq) dose, the radiation exposures to the kidneys and to the urinary bladder are 3.78 rads and 0.42 rads, respectively.[95]

Fluorine-18 Fluorodeoxyglucose (FDG)

Fluorine-18 Fluorodeoxyglucose (FDG) is the most common positron-labeled radiotracer in positron emission tomography (PET). F-18 labeled deoxyglucose is a modified form of glucose in which the hydroxyl group in the 2-position is replaced by the F-18 positron emitter. FDG accumulates in cells in proportion to glucose metabolism. Cell membrane glucose transporters facilitate the transport of glucose and FDG across the cell membrane. Both glucose and FDG are phosphorylated in the 6-position by the hexokinase. The conversion of glucose-6-phosphate or FDG-6-phosphate back to glucose or FDG, respectively, is effected by the enzyme phosphatase. In most tissues, including cancer, there is little phosphatase activity. FDG-6-phosphate cannot undergo further conversions and is therefore trapped in the cell. FDG is excreted in the urine. The typical FDG dose is 0.144 mCi/kg (minimum 1 mCi, maximum 20 mCi). The urinary bladder wall receives the highest radiation dose from FDG.[96,97] The radiation dose depends on the excretion rate, the varying size of the bladder, the bladder volume at the time of FDG administration, and an estimated bladder time activity curve. For a typical 15 mCi FDG dose and voiding at 1 hour after tracer injection, the average estimated absorbed radiation dose to the adult bladder wall is 3.3 rads (0.22 rads/mCi).[98] The doses to other organs are between 0.75 and 1.28 rads (0.050–0.085 rads/mCi) for an average organ dose of 1.0 rad.[98]

NORMAL RENAL FUNCTION

Glomerular filtration rate and ERPF may be assessed using dynamic quantitative nuclear imaging techniques. The GFR quantifies the amount of filtrate formed per minute (normal: 125 mL/min in adults). Only 20% of renal plasma flow is filtered through the semipermeable membrane of the glomerulus. The filtrate is protein-free and nearly completely reabsorbed in the tubules. Filtration is maintained over a range of arterial pressures with autoregulation. The ideal agent for the determination of GFR is inulin, which is only filtered but is neither secreted nor reabsorbed.[95,99]

Tc-99m DTPA is often employed to demonstrate renal perfusion and assess glomerular filtration, although 5% to 10% of injected DTPA is protein-bound and 5% remains in the kidneys at 4 hours. A typical imaging protocol includes posterior 5-second flow images for 1 minute followed by 1-minute per frame images for 20 minutes. The GFR may be obtained using the Gates method that employs images of renal uptake during the second through third minute after DTPA administration. Regions of interest (ROIs) are drawn over the kidneys and background activity correction is applied. A standard dose is counted by the gamma camera for normalization. Depth photon attenuation correction is made based on a formula relating body weight and height. A split GFR can be obtained for each kidney, which is not possible with the creatinine clearance method.[95,99]

The ERPF (normal: 585 mL/min in adults) can be obtained by using OIH and MAG3 imaging.[100] However, OIH has been largely replaced by MAG3 because of MAG3's better imaging characteristics and dosimetry (due to radiolabeling with Tc-99m). Currently MAG3 is the renal imaging agent of choice primarily because of the combined renal clearance of MAG3 by both filtration and tubular extraction, which leads to the ability for obtaining relatively high-quality images even in patients with impaired renal function. The imaging protocol includes posterior 1-second images for 60 seconds (flow

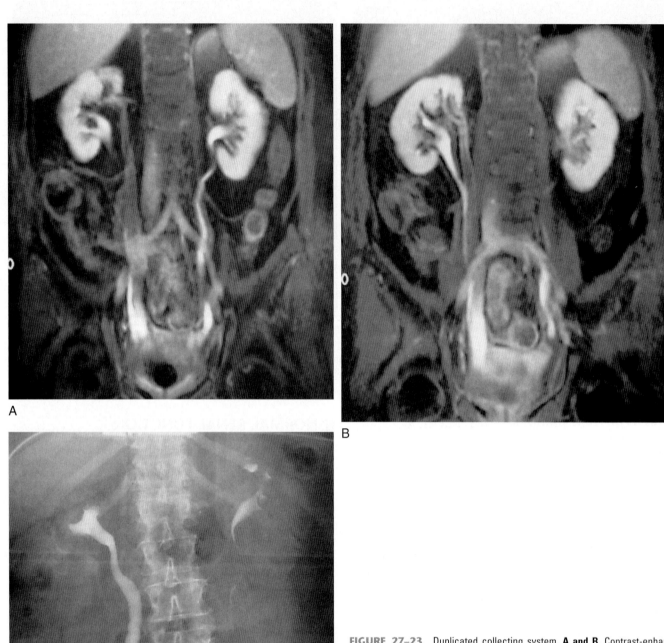

A

B

C

FIGURE 27–23 Duplicated collecting system. **A and B,** Contrast-enhanced MRU demonstrates a duplicated collecting system on the right with delayed excretion of the upper pole moiety. **C,** Obstruction of the upper pole moiety is confirmed on intravenous urogram.

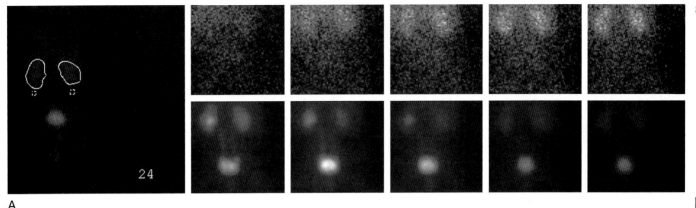

A

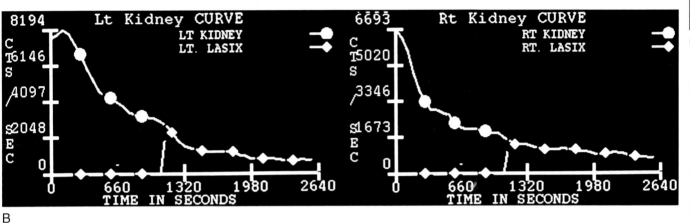

B

FIGURE 27–24 **A and B,** Normal Tc-99m MAG3 renogram.

study) followed by 1-minute images for 5 minutes and then 5-minute images to 30 minutes. The relative tubular function may be obtained by drawing renal ROIs corrected for background activity. A renogram is constructed to depict the renal tracer uptake over time. The first portion of the renogram has a sharp upslope occurring in about 6 seconds following peak aortic activity (phase I) representing perfusion followed by extension to the peak value representing both renal perfusion and early renal clearance (phase II). The next phase (phase III) is downsloping and represents excretion. Normal perfusion of the kidneys is symmetric (50% +/– 5%). The renogram peak occurs at about 2 to 3 minutes (versus 3 to 5 minutes with DTPA) in normal adults and by 30 minutes, more than 70% of tracer is cleared and present in the urinary bladder (Fig. 27–24).[95,99] Renal cortical structure can be imaged with DMSA, which correlates strongly with differential glomerular filtration and differential renal blood flow. Imaging is started 90 to 120 minutes after tracer administration, although images can be obtained at up to 4 hours. Planar images are obtained in the anterior, posterior, LAO/RAO, RPO/LPO projections. Single-photon computed tomography (SPECT) is also often obtained. A normal scan shows evenly distributed renal cortical uptake. Normal variations include dromedary hump (splenic impression on the left kidney), fetal lobulation, horseshoe kidney, crossed fused ectopia, and hypertrophied column of Bertin. The renal images also allow accurate assessment of the relative renal size, position, and axis.[95,99]

KIDNEY INJURY—ACUTE AND CHRONIC

Acute kidney injury (AKI/ARF) is characterized as pre-renal, renal, or post-renal in etiology. AKI/ARF is commonly encountered in the hospital setting. In these patients it is most frequently caused by hypotension, dehydration, nephrotoxic drugs, or hypoperfusion of the kidneys.[17] These pre-renal and renal causes account for more than 90% of all cases. The least common type of AKI/ARF, post-renal, is also the most potentially curable. Post-renal AKI/ARF is most often due to urinary tract obstruction or obstructive uropathy. Radiographic evaluation is done to exclude post-renal AKI/ARF in the form of obstructed kidneys. Once post-renal AKI/ARF is excluded, pre-renal and intrinsic causes of AKI/ARF can be managed medically.

Plain films offer little in the assessment of AKI/ARF. Only renal size and the presence or absence of renal stones can be assessed. The IVU plays no role in AKI/ARF as iodinated contrast is required for the study. Ultrasonography is the method of choice in evaluating patients with AKI/ARF. Renal size, echogenicity of the kidneys, cortical thickness, and the presence or absence of hydronephrosis are generally easily imaged.[101] A thin rim of decreased echogenicity may surround the kidneys in patients experiencing kidney injury.[102] For patients with AKI/ARF, the accuracy of ultrasound is greater than 95% in detecting hydronephrosis that is dilatation of the collecting systems and renal pelvis.[103,104] To make the diagnosis of a post-renal etiology for AKI/ARF, both kidneys should exhibit hydronephrosis.[105] The specific cause may not be elucidated with ultrasound and other methods must be employed, such as CT or MRI.

The principal ultrasonographic finding of hydronephrosis is the separation of the central renal sinus echo complex by a sonolucent fluid-filled renal pelvis, which directly connects to the dilated calyces and infundibula in the more peripheral aspects of the kidney. Hydronephrosis is generally graded by the extent of calyceal dilatation and the degree of cortical thinning.[103,106,107] Mild, or grade I, hydronephrosis is diag-

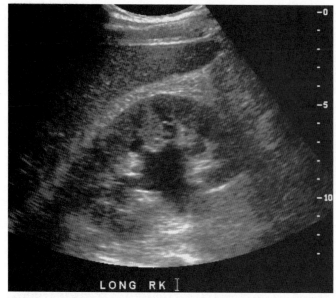

FIGURE 27–25 Mild hydronephrosis—ultrasound. The central echo complex is separated by the mildly distended calyces and renal pelvis. Notice the connection between the calyces and the renal pelvis. The cortex is preserved in thickness and the renal border remains smooth.

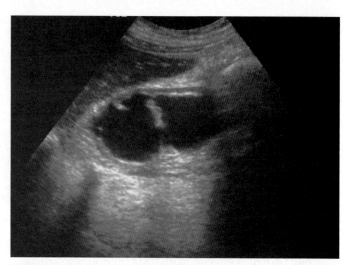

FIGURE 27–27 Marked hydronephrosis—ultrasound. Longitudinal image of the right kidney demonstrates a large fluid-filled sac with no normal remaining elements of the kidney visible. The cortex is almost gone but the outer border of the kidney remains smooth.

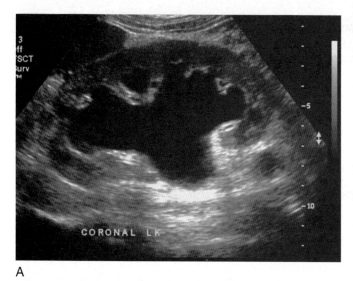

A

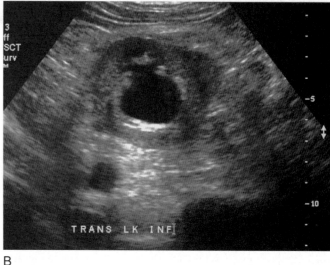

B

FIGURE 27–26 Moderate hydronephrosis—ultrasound. The dilated calyces are rounded and urine filled. The renal pelvis is dilated as well. Again note the connection between the calyces and the renal pelvis. The cortex is mildly thinned and the renal border is smooth. Longitudinal image (**A**) and transverse image (**B**).

nosed by noting the fluid-filled pelvicaliceal system causing slight separation of the central renal sinus fat (Fig. 27–25). The calyces are not distorted and the renal cortex appears of normal thickness. In grade II hydronephrosis the pelvicalyceal system appears more distended with greater separation of the central echo complex. The contour of the calyces becomes round, but the cortical thickness is unaltered (Fig. 27–26). With grade III hydronephrosis the calyces are more distended and cortical thinning is recognized. Severe, or grade IV, hydronephrosis exhibits marked dilation of the calyceal system (Fig. 27–27). The calyces appear as large ballooned fluid-filled structures with a dilated renal pelvis of variable size. Cortical loss is evident with the dilated calyces approaching or reaching the renal capsule. Generally speaking, the length and overall size of a hydronephrotic kidney is increased. Longstanding obstruction may, however, result in renal parenchymal atrophy and a somewhat small kidney with marked cortical thinning. The degree of hydronephrosis does not always correlate with the amount of obstruction.

Although hydronephrosis is usually easily diagnosed with ultrasound, it must not be confused with renal cystic disease. With hydronephrosis the dilated calyces have a direct visible communication with the renal pelvis, which is also dilated.[40] In cystic disease, the round fluid-filled cysts have walls with no direct communication evident between each and the renal pelvis. Peripelvic cysts frequently lead to a misdiagnosis of a dilated renal pelvis. Renal artery aneurysm may also be confused with a dilated renal pelvis, but the correct diagnosis can be made with added color Doppler ultrasound.

Nonobstructive hydronephrosis may present a confusing picture ultrasonographically.[108,109] Grade I hydronephrosis and possibly more severe grades may be seen in patients with no obstructive cause found. To some, mild dilatation of the pelvicalyceal system has been considered a normal variant. Nonobstructive causes of hydronephrosis include increased urine production and flow such as occurs with a diuresis from any cause, pregnancy, acute and chronic infection, vesicoureteral reflux, papillary necrosis, congenital megacalices,

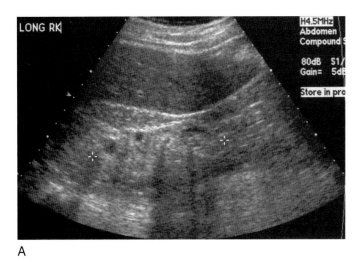
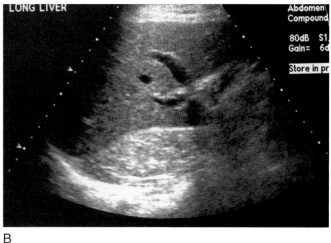

A   B

FIGURE 27-28 Chronic kidney injury—ultrasound. End–stage renal disease (ESRD) is noted **(A, B)** with the kidneys being high echogenic relative to the adjacent liver. There are no normal renal structures seen but the kidneys remain smooth in overall contour. Note the two small hypoechoic renal cysts in the surface in A.

over distended bladder, and post obstructive dilatation.[110] In patients with repeated episodes of intermittent or partial obstruction, the calyces become quite distensible or compliant leading to a variable picture of hydronephrosis depending on their state of hydration and urine production. Patients with vesicoureteral reflux also demonstrate distensible pelvicalyceal systems. Duplex Doppler ultrasound has been suggested as an additive means of differentiating obstructive from nonobstructive hydronephrosis.[111,112] The measurement of resistive indices has been investigated as a means of diagnosing acute renal obstruction.[113] The results have been variable leading to no consistent recommendation.[114,115]

The use of ultrasound also extends to patients with chronic kidney injury or medical renal disease. Increased cortical echogenicity may be seen in both acute and chronic renal parenchymal disease (Fig. 27–28).[116] The pattern should be bilateral. In chronic kidney injury, the degree of cortical echogenicity correlates with the severity of the interstitial fibrosis, global sclerosis, focal tubular atrophy, and number of hyaline casts per glomerulus.[39] Similar correlation is seen with decreasing renal size. These findings, however, remain nonspecific and renal biopsy is required for diagnosis. Loss of the normal corticomedullary function is seen with increasing cortical echogenicity.[44] Increased cortical echogenicity may also be seen in some patients with AKI/ARF such as glomerulonephritis and lupus nephritis. Sequential studies over time may be used to assess the progression of disease by monitoring the renal size and cortical echogenicity.

The key to the diagnosis of renal parenchymal disease is renal core biopsy and resulting histopathologic diagnosis.[116] Ultrasound facilitates the performance of renal biopsy by demonstrating the kidney and the proper location for biopsy. Ultrasound may also be used to evaluate for complications associated with renal biopsy such as perirenal hematoma.

Computed tomography scanning in AKI/ARF and CRF usually follows ultrasound evaluation that demonstrated bilateral hydronephrosis. Noncontrast CT easily demonstrates the dilated pelvocalyceal systems in the kidney. The parenchymal thickness relative to the dilated collecting systems can be visualized. The urine-filled calyces and pelvis are less dense than the surrounding parenchyma. The dilated ureters may be followed distally to establish the site of obstruction. The cause may be frequently seen, such as the case with pelvic tumors, distal ureteral stones, and retroperitoneal adenopathy or mass. If obstruction is not the cause, other potential etiologies such as cirrhosis and ascites with accompanying

hepatic failure may be evident. In CRF, CT scanning will usually demonstrate small contracted kidneys, which may also show evidence of adult acquired polycystic disease (Fig. 27–29). In general, the overall size and thickness of the renal parenchyma appears to decrease with age.[117] For patients with chronic longstanding obstruction as the cause of their kidney injury, CT will generally demonstrate large fluid-containing kidneys with little or no cortex remaining. Autosomal dominant polycystic disease may also be seen with CT (Fig. 27–30). The innumerable cysts are seen throughout the enlarged kidneys. Frequently, some of the cyst walls may contain thin rims of calcification. There may also be variation in the density of the internal contents of the cysts due to hemorrhage or proteinaceous debris. For patients undergoing regular dialysis, iodinated contrast may be given if necessary for CT scans as the material is dialyzable.

Magnetic resonance imaging is accurate in demonstrating pre-renal and post-renal causes of kidney injury, but unless the cause of injury is secondary to vascular occlusion or collection system obstruction, MRI becomes less specific. MRI is sensitive for the detection of renal parenchymal disease, but the renal parenchymal causes of injury have nonspecific findings and generally require biopsy (Figs. 27–31 and 27–32).[118]

Initial experience with diffusion weighted MR imaging has demonstrated reproducible information on renal function, with the possibility of determining the degree of dysfunction.[119] No large studies have been performed and further research is required before the usefulness of diffusion imaging is confirmed. Animal research is being performed with the hope of developing therapy for chronic nephropathy. MRI is being used in molecular imaging to follow the targeting of focal areas of glomerular damage by intravenously injected superparamagnetic iron oxide-labeled mesenchymal stem cells.[120]

In kidney injury, glomerular and tubular dysfunctions are reflected by abnormal renal scintigraphy and renograms. Renal uptake of MAG3 is prolonged with tubular tracer stasis and little or no excretion. It has been shown that in patients with acute kidney injury, the demonstration of MAG3 renal activity more than hepatic activity at 1 to 3 minutes indicates likely recovery whereas when renal uptake is less than the hepatic uptake, dialysis may be needed.[121] In chronic kidney injury, there is diminished renal perfusion, cortical tracer extraction, and excretion. However, this imaging pattern is nonspecific and will need to be interpreted in the clinical context.[95]

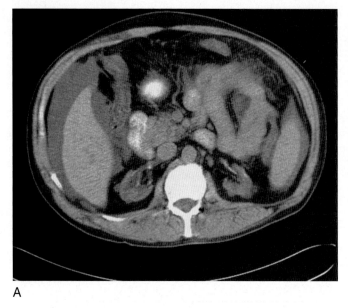

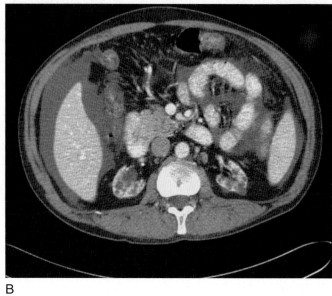

A

B

FIGURE 27–29 Adult acquired polycystic kidney disease—CT scan. Axial noncontrast **(A)** and post contrast **(B)** images. Small kidneys are seen bilaterally with multiple small 1-cm cysts primarily in the cortex.

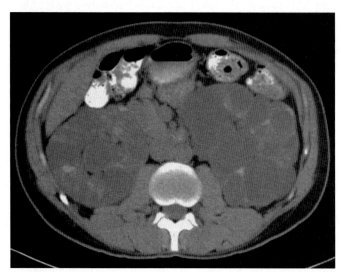

FIGURE 27–30 Autosomal dominant polycystic kidney disease—CT scan. This noncontrast CT images demonstrates the markedly enlarged kidney bilaterally with multiple low density cysts throughout both kidneys. The little remaining renal parenchyma is noted by the sparse higher density material squeezed by the cysts.

▌UNILATERAL OBSTRUCTION

Although ultrasound is frequently the first imaging method used to detect the obstructed kidney, it usually is unable to establish the cause of the obstruction. Contrast studies, primarily IVU and CT are the methods of choice for the patient with normal renal function. Antegrade or retrograde pyelograms are used as secondary means of assessment. Of these methodologies, CT is the most helpful in establishing the site and cause of unilateral obstruction.

The IVU has been used for years in evaluating the obstructed kidney.[3] The scout film may give a hint as to the cause (i.e., mass in the pelvis). The obstructed kidney is usually larger than the normal other side. The initial nephrogram and appearance of contrast material in the collecting system may be delayed. With time the nephrogram may be increased over that of the normal kidney.[3] Once the collecting system and

renal pelvis are opacified with the excreted contrast, they are dilated and distended. The ureters will fill late in relationship to the opposite normal kidney. Delayed images may be required with prone or upright views to identify the site of obstruction. With the IVU, the site of obstruction will be noted, but again the cause may only be inferred; this is also true with the antegrade and retrograde pyelograms.

Contrast-enhanced CT and more specifically, the CT urogram will be most useful in assessing the patient with unilateral obstruction.[51] The findings seen with the IVU are only amplified with the CT urogram. Small differences in the enhancement pattern of the kidney that are not notable on an IVU may be seen with CT (Fig. 27–33). Differential excretion differences are also more sensitively seen on CT.[50,51] The urine-filled or contrast-filled ureters point to the obstruction. The dilated ureters on the obstructed side may be followed in axial or coronal sections to the cause. The multiple causes of unilateral obstruction may be seen on CT—including both intra- and extra-ureteral cases (Fig. 27–34). MRI demonstrates similar findings although its sensitivity and specificity are only now being established.

Nuclear medicine assessment by means of diuretic renography may also be used to evaluate for obstructive uropathy. It is a noninvasive procedure and yields excellent results. In general, it is recommended that the patient be well hydrated. In children and in adults with noncompliant bladder, catheterization of the bladder may be used to ensure drainage and reduce back pressure in the urinary system. MAG3 scintigraphy is often employed. Furosemide (Lasix) is administered intravenously (1 mg/kg; higher dose in cases of renal insufficiency) when the renal pelvis and ureter are maximally distended.[122] This may occur in as early as 10 to 15 minutes and as late as 30 to 40 minutes after tracer administration. ROIs are drawn around each renal pelvis with the background regions as crescent shapes lateral to each kidney. Following furosemide administration, rapid emptying of the collecting system with a subsequent steep decline in the renogram curve is compatible with dilatation without obstruction. Obstruction can be excluded if the clearance half time (T1/2) of the renal pelvic emptying is less than 10 minutes. A curve that reaches a plateau or continues to rise after administration of furosemide is an obstructive pattern with a clearance T1/2 of greater than 20 minutes (Fig. 27–35). A slow downslope after

Text continued on p. 865

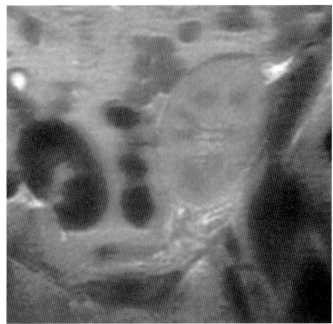

A

FIGURE 27–31 Renal transplant graft with acute tubular necrosis. **A,** Axial T2-weighted; **B,** axial T1-weighted; and **C,** gadolinium-enhanced T1-weighted images show reversal of the normal corticomedullary differentiation in this patient with biopsy-proven acute tubular necrosis.

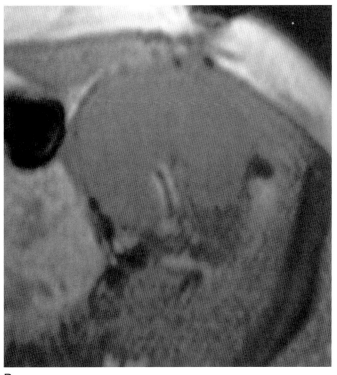

B

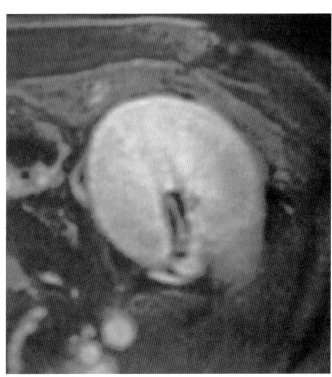

C

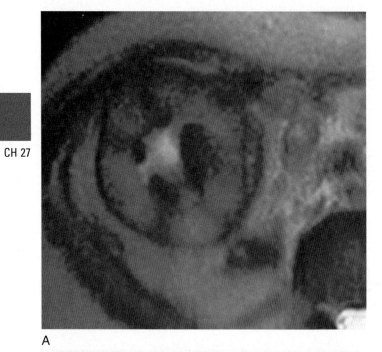

A

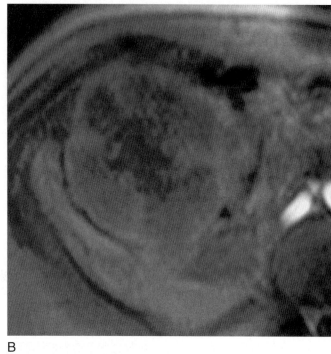

B

C

FIGURE 27–32 Renal transplant graft with chronic injury due to IgA nephropathy. **A**, Axial T2-weighted; **B**, axial T1-weighted; and **C**, gadolinium-enhanced T1-weighted image demonstrate accentuation of the corticomedullary differentiation.

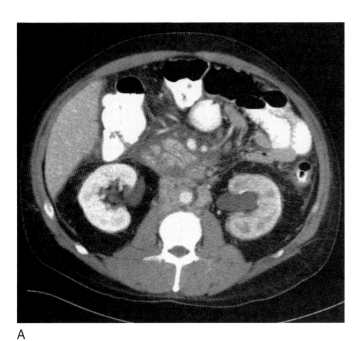

A

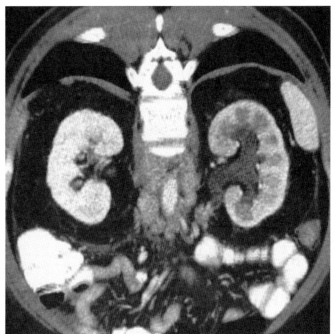

B

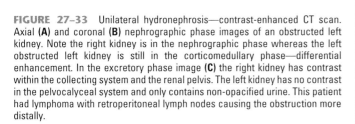

FIGURE 27–33 Unilateral hydronephrosis—contrast-enhanced CT scan. Axial (A) and coronal (B) nephrographic phase images of an obstructed left kidney. Note the right kidney is in the nephrographic phase whereas the left obstructed left kidney is still in the corticomedullary phase—differential enhancement. In the excretory phase image (C) the right kidney has contrast within the collecting system and the renal pelvis. The left kidney has no contrast in the pelvocalyceal system and only contains non-opacified urine. This patient had lymphoma with retroperitoneal lymph nodes causing the obstruction more distally.

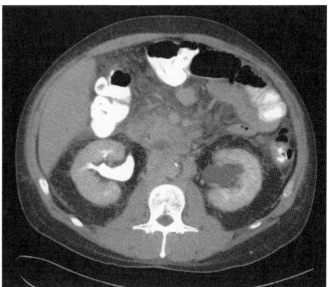

C

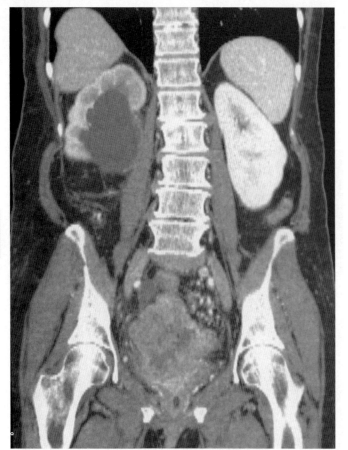

FIGURE 27-34 Unilateral obstruction—contrast-enhanced CT scan. The coronal image demonstrates the differential enhancement between the two kidneys with the moderately dilated renal pelvis and calyces on the right. The large heterogeneous pelvis mass is the source of the obstruction—recurrent rectal carcinoma.

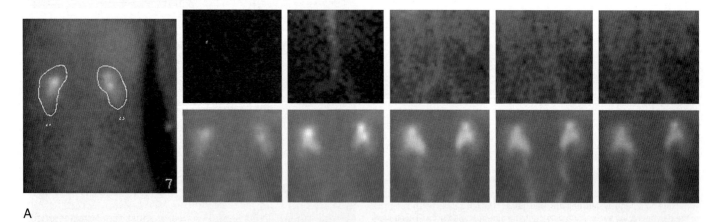

A

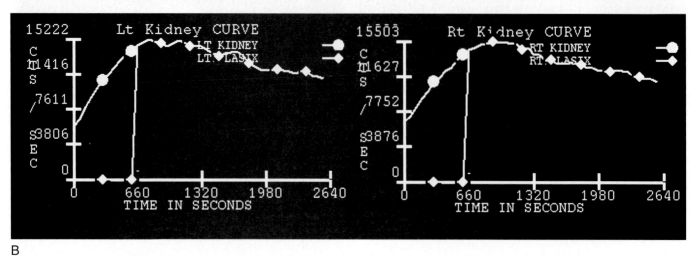

B

FIGURE 27-35 Abnormal Tc-99m MAG3 renogram demonstrating obstructive urinary kinetics with a poor response to furosemide. **A,** Static and timed images. **B,** Individual curves for each kidney.

furosemide may indicate partial obstruction. An apparent poor response to furosemide may also be seen in severe pelvic dilatation (reservoir effect). Other pitfalls include poor injection technique of either the diuretic or the radiotracer, impaired renal function, and dehydration in which delayed tracer transit and excretion may not be overcome by the effect of a diuretic. Kidneys in neonates (<1 month in age) may be too immature to respond to furosemide and are not suitable candidates for diuretic renal scintigraphy.[95,123]

RENAL CALCIFICATIONS AND RENAL STONE DISEASE

Calcifications may occur in many regions of the kidney.[124] Nephrolithiasis or renal calculi are the most common and occur in the pelvocalyceal system. Nephrocalcinosis refers to renal parenchymal calcification occurring in either the medulla or cortex. These calcifications are usually associated with diseases in which patients have hypercalcemia or hypercalcuria or in conditions with specific pathologic lesions in the cortex or medulla. Nephrocalcinosis may have diffuse or punctate calcifications and is usually bilateral. Some patients with nephrocalcinosis may also develop nephrolithiasis. Calcifications may also occur in vascular structures, particularly in patients with diabetes and advanced atherosclerotic disease. Rim-like calcifications may occur in simple renal cysts and polycystic disease. Renal carcinomas may exhibit variable calcifications as well. Sloughed papilla may also calcify within the calyx. All of these calcifications may be seen on plain films of the abdomen but will be seen to better advantage with noncontrast CT sans of the abdomen (Fig. 27–36).

Cortical calcification is most often associated with the results of acute cortical necrosis from any cause.[124] Dystrophic calcification develops in the damaged cortex after the episode of acute cortical necrosis. The calcifications tend to

be tram track-like and circumferential. Other entities in which cortical calcification are found include hyperoxaluria, Alport syndrome, and rarely, chronic glomerulonephritis. The stippled calcifications of hyperoxaluria may be found in both the cortex and medulla as well as other organs, such as the heart. With Alport syndrome only cortical calcifications are found.

Calcifications in the medulla are much more common than cortical calcifications.[124] The most common cause of medullary nephrocalcinosis is primary hyperparathyroidism. Intratubular deposition of calcium oxalate crystals occurs first with later deposits in the interstitial renal parenchyma. The distribution appears to be within the renal pyramid. The radiological picture may be focal or diffuse, and unilateral or bilateral. Nephrolithiasis also occurs in patients with primary hyperparathyroidism. Nephrocalcinosis occurs in other diseases in which hypercalcemia or hypercalciuria occur. These include hyperthyroidism, sarcoidosis, hypervitaminosis D, immobilization, multiple myeloma, and metastatic neoplasms to name a few. These calcifications are nonspecific and punctate in appearance and are usually medullary in location.

In 70% to 75% of cases of renal tubular acidosis (RTA) there is evidence of nephrocalcinosis. The calcifications tend to be uniform and distributed throughout the renal pyramids bilaterally. With medullary sponge kidney, renal tubular ectasia, small calculi form in the distal collecting tubules probably because of stasis. The appearance is varied from only a single calyx being involved to both kidneys throughout. The calcifications are small, round, and within the peak of the pyramid adjacent to the calyx. Medullary sponge kidney is also associated with nephrolithiasis, as the small calculi in the distal collecting tubules may pass into the collecting systems and ureters resulting in renal colic.[125]

The calcifications that occur in renal tuberculosis are typically medullary in location and may mimic other forms of nephrocalcinosis.[126] Renal tuberculosis begins in the renal cortex and progresses to the medulla. Invasion and erosion of the calyceal system subsequently occurs resulting in spread of the tuberculous infection down the ureters into the bladder. Calcification occurs in the pyramids as part of the healing process. With overwhelming involvement of the kidney, the entire kidney may be destroyed resulting in an autonephrectomy with diffuse, heavy calcification throughout the entire kidney, which is small and scarred. Medullary calcifications are also seen in patients with renal papillary necrosis. With necrosis of the papilla, the material is sloughed into the calyces. Retained tissue fragments may calcify and give the appearance of medullary nephrocalcinosis.

Nephrolithiasis is a common clinical entity. The lifetime risk of developing renal calculi is 12% with males being 2 to 3 times more at risk than females.[127] Most renal stones occur in individuals aged 30 to 60. Renal stone disease is a multifactorial problem with metabolic disorders and other factors, such as geography, diet, family history, diabetes, sedentary lifestyle, and dehydration, contributory to the disorder. Most urinary tract stones are composed of calcium salts of either oxalate or phosphate or a combination of the two.[128–131] This leads to the dense appearance on radiographs. Stasis contributes to the formation of stones in the urinary tract. Renal colic or flank pain is the most common presenting symptom. Most patients will also have hematuria although it may be absent if there is complete obstruction of the ureters by the obstructing stone. The pain that occurs with a passing renal stone is likely due to the distension of the tubular system and renal capsule of the kidney and the peristalsis associated with ureteral contractions as the stone moves distally.

Plain films of the abdomen require a stone that is densely calcified and of sufficient size to be visible (see Fig. 27–36). Frequently overlying bowel gas and feces may make visualization difficult. Costal cartilage calcifications in the upper

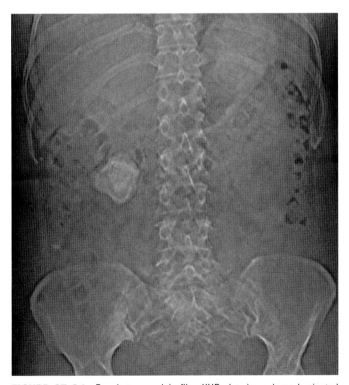

FIGURE 27-36 Renal stone—plain film. KUB showing a large laminated stone in the renal pelvis of the right kidney. The outline of the normal left kidney can be seen with no calcifications overlying it. The right kidney outline cannot be seen.

abdomen may be confused with renal calculi as may gallstones in the right upper quadrant. For years the IVU has been the method of choice for the assessment of the patient with renal colic.[132,133] After the injection of IV contrast media, there is an unequal nephrogram with a delayed appearance on the affected sides. Once the nephrogram appears, it may also be prolonged and increase in density with time, specifically with complete obstruction caused by a ureteric stone. The excretion of contrast into the collecting system is usually delayed and there is dilatation of the pelvocalyceal system. Delayed images up to 24 hours may occasionally be necessary to visualize the contrast-filled dilated collecting systems, pelvis, and ureter to the point of obstruction by the calculus. When the pelvocalyceal system is contrast filled and the ureter is not, upright or prone films may help fill the ureter with contrast. The injection of contrast, being a fluid load, may assist the stone in passage through the ureters into the bladder.

Most urinary calculi that are 4 mm or smaller will pass with conservative treatment.[134] The larger the stone the more likely other measures will be necessary in order to treat the stone and associated obstruction. Extracorporal shockwave lithotripsy (ESWL) is the method of choice for treating larger stones. Success rates are best for stones in the renal pelvis and kidney.[135]

Ultrasound assessment has also been used in the evaluation of renal colic.[136] This is quick and usually easily performed examination. One is looking for the effects of a passing renal stone, which is obstruction. Unilateral hydronephrosis may be seen although the examination may be normal early in the passage of a renal stone. Renal stones may be visualized within the kidney as hyperechoic foci with distal acoustic shadowing or reverberation artifacts (Fig. 27–37).[136] Ureteric stones are rarely seen due to overlying bowel gas and stone. Distal ureteral stones near the uretovesical junction may be visualized through the urine-filled bladder transabdominally. Transvaginal and transperineal ultrasound has also been suggested as a method for evaluating for distal ureteral stones. Ultrasound may demonstrate an absent ureteral jet in the bladder on the side in which a stone is being passed. Doppler ultrasound and assessment of the peripheral vasculature resistance may occasionally be helpful in pointing to the affected kidney, but the study results have been variable.[113]

Noncontrast CT scanning of the abdomen and pelvis has emerged as the standard for evaluation of patients with renal colic.[137–139] The sensitivities for CT of 96% to 100%, specificities of 95% to 100%, and accuracies of 96% to 98%, nonenhanced CT has supplanted the plain film, IVU, and US.[138,140–142] Comparing noncontrast CT and the IVU, CT performs much better with sensitivity of 94% to 100% and specificity of 92% to 100% versus the IVU with sensitivity of 64% to 97% and specificity of 92% to 94%.[138] Also, when noncontrast CT was used as the reference standard comparing US, a sensitivity of 24% and specificity of 90% was found for US.[143,144] As CT scanning uses x-ray radiation for the study, US examination should be reserved for the pediatric population and pregnant women. Alternative diagnosis is made in patients with "renal colic" in 9% to 29% of cases when noncontrast CT is used for evaluation.[145]

Nonenhanced CT scans are performed from the top of the kidneys to below the pubic symphysis. No preparation is needed. Intravenous contrast is rarely needed. The studies are performed using 3 mm collimation or less with the slices reconstructed contiguously or slightly overlapped.[146–148] The images should be viewed on a monitor as axial images with multiplanar reconstructions (MPR) used as an adjunct. Virtually all renal stones are denser than the adjacent soft tissues (Fig. 27–38)[149]; exceptions are renal stones associated with Indinavir, a protease inhibitor used in the management of AIDS, and very small uric acid stones (<1–2 mm).[150,151] As expected, calcium oxalate and calcium phosphate stones are the most dense.[129,130] Matrix stones, which are rare, may also be relatively low in density, but they usually contain calcium imparities that make them visible.[128,131]

Calculi appear as calcifications within the urinary tract. The most common locations for obstruction to occur are at the ureteropelvic junction, at the pelvic brim where the ureters cross over the iliac vessels, and at the uretovesical junction. The diagnosis is made on the CT scan by demonstrating the calcified stone within the urine-filled ureters (Fig. 27–39).[146] Secondary signs may be present to assist in the diagnosis.[140] Hydronephrosis and hydroureter to the point of the stone may be visible (see Fig. 27–39). Asymmetric perinephric and periureteral stranding may also be seen related to forniceal rupture and urine leak (Fig. 27–40).[152] The density of the involved kidney may be less than the opposite normal side due to increased interstitial fluid and edema.[153,154] The affected kidney may also be larger than the normal kidney. At the point of obstruction, the stone may be seen within the

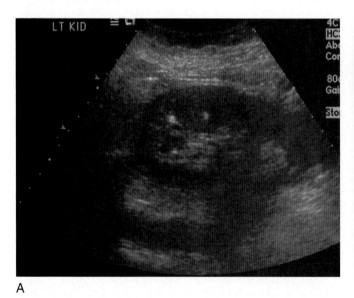

A

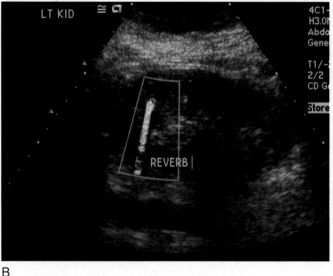

B

FIGURE 27–37 Renal stone—ultrasound. Longitudinal image **(A)** and color Doppler image **(B)** demonstrate an echogenic focus at the corticomedullary junction. Not all stones show shadowing but in this case reverberation artifact can be seen on the color Doppler image helping make the diagnosis.

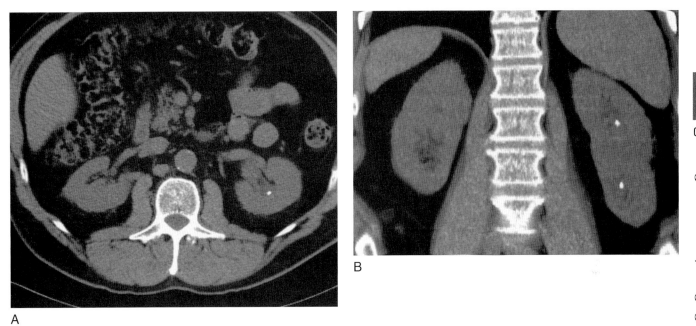

A

B

FIGURE 27-38 Renal stones—noncontrast CT scan. Axial image **(A)** and coronal image **(B)** demonstrate 4 mm to 5 mm stones in the upper and lower poles of the left kidney. There are no signs of obstruction.

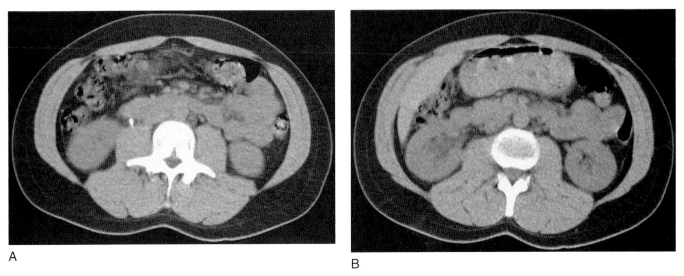

A

B

FIGURE 27-39 Ureteral stone—noncontrast CT scan. **(A)** A 5 mm to 6 mm right mid-ureteral stone is noted. **(B)** Axial images of the middle portion of the kidneys reveals the urine-filled right renal pelvis and a slightly less dense kidney when compared with the left. These are signs of obstruction.

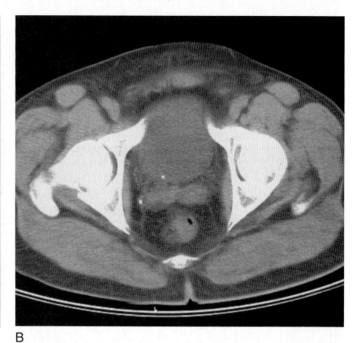

A   B

FIGURE 27–40 Ureteral stone—noncontrast CT scan. Axial images of the kidneys **(A)** show perinephric and peripelvic stranding and fluid on the right caused by forniceal rupture and leak of urine due to the distal obstructing stone at the right ureterovesical junction **(B)**. Note the phlebolith on the right posterior to the bladder and lateral to the seminal vesicle—a common pitfall.

ureter with soft tissue thickening of the ureteral wall at that level. This is likely due to edema and inflammation associated with the passage of the stone. Noncontrast CT has the advantage as well of assessing the overall stone burden of the patient, not just the passing stone. Also the size may be accurately measured allowing for treatment decisions to be made.[134,155,156] Distal ureteral stones may occasionally be confused with phleboliths, which are common in the pelvis (see Fig. 27–40). Multiplanar imaging coronal images of the ureters down to the level of the stone may be helpful. Also, close inspection of phleboliths frequently demonstrates a small soft tissue tag leading to the calcification—the comet tail sign.[157] Contrast material injection may occasionally be necessary in confusing or difficult cases. Also, it may be used in complicated cases in which the patient is febrile and pyelonephritis or pyohydronephrosis is suspected.

Computed tomography is more sensitive for the evaluation of renal and collecting system calcifications, especially in the absence of urinary tract obstruction. In the evaluation of acute stone disease, MRI is not the examination of first choice, but is a suitable alternative for selected patients.[158] Stones are difficult to identify in non-dilated systems, even in retrospect. When stones are seen on MRI they are seen as black foci on both T1- and T2-weighted sequences. Stones become more conspicuous in a dilated collecting system (Fig. 27–41); however, a non-enhancing filling defect is a nonspecific finding. Blood, air, or debris may have the same appearance. If stones or other calcifications are a concern, noncontrast CT is the examination of choice for improved conspicuity (Fig. 27–42).

When iodinated contrast is contraindicated or when reduction of radiation exposure is desired, MR urography (MRU) can be used to determine the etiology and location of an obstructing process (Fig. 27–43). MRU is highly accurate in demonstrating obstruction whether the process is acute or chronic.[158] Acute obstruction may be associated with perinephric fluid, which is well demonstrated on T2-weighted sequences.[158,159] However, perinephric fluid is a nonspecific finding and can be found associated with other renal pathology.

Although MRI is not the imaging modality of choice for acute renal trauma evaluation, MRI is useful in evaluating the patient who is recently post op for renal stone disease, especially in the patient with impaired renal function. MRI has been reported as being more accurate than CT in differentiating perirenal and intrarenal hematomas (Figs. 27–44 to 27–46).[160] With contrast, MRI can also demonstrate damage to the collecting system and areas of ischemia without the risk of nephrotoxicity.

RENAL INFECTION

Acute pyelonephritis is typically a clinical diagnosis based on signs and symptoms of flank pain, tenderness, and fever with accompanying laboratory findings of leukocytosis, pyuria, positive urine culture, and occasionally bacteremia and hematuria.[161] Most cases of acute pyelonephritis occur by the ascending route from the bladder.[161] Vesicoureteral reflux is viewed as the major cause. The gram negative bacteria are transported to the renal pelvis where intrarenal reflux occurs with the bacteria traversing the calyceal system to the ducts and tubules within the renal pyramid. With the bacteria within the tubules, there is a leukocyte response. Enzyme release results in destruction of tubular cells with subsequent bacterial invasion of the interstitum. The resultant inflammatory response involves both the interstitum and tubules. As the infection progresses it spreads throughout the pyramid and to the adjacent parenchyma. The inflammatory response leads to focal or more diffuse swelling of the kidney. Vasoconstriction of the involved arteries and arterioles is noted. Without adequate treatment there is necrosis of the involved regions and micro-abscess formation. These may coalesce into larger macro-abscesses, which tend to be surrounded by a rim of granulation tissue.[162] Perinephric abscess results from the rupture of an intrarenal abscess through the renal capsule or the leak from pyonephrosis, an infected and obstructed kidney. The overall distribution in the kidney is usually

Text continued on p. 873

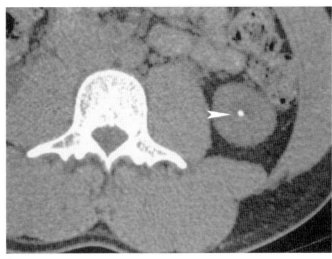

A

FIGURE 27–41   Renal stones. **(A)** Calcification well seen on CT (*arrowhead*) is **(B)** difficult to demonstrate on MRI (*arrow*), even in retrospect. **C,** A stone (*arrowhead*) is more conspicuous when it is located within a mildly dilated collection system.

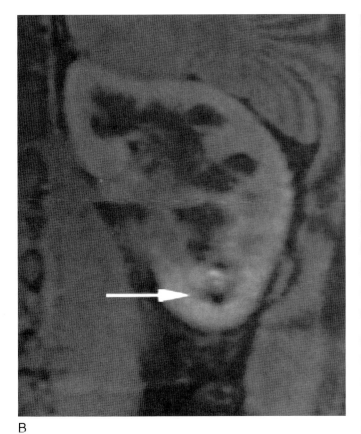

B

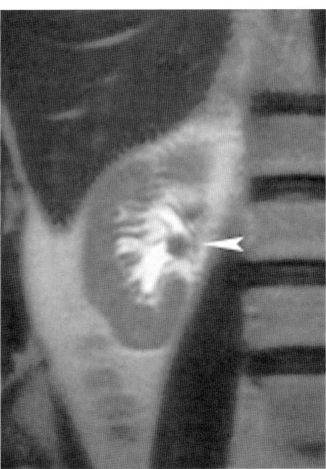

C

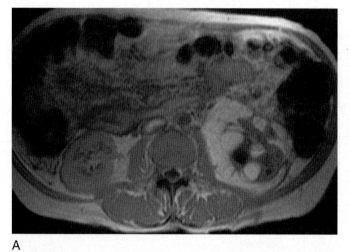

A

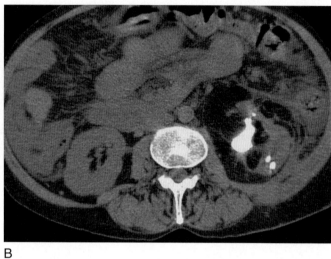

B

FIGURE 27–42 Staghorn calculus. **(A)** MRI and **(B)** CT demonstrating large pelvic calculus with associated left renal atrophy. Even large stones may be difficult to recognize on MRI. Calcifications are more conspicuous on CT.

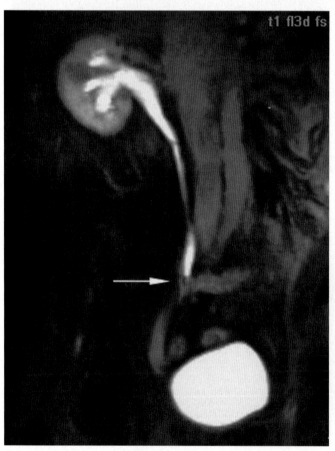

A

FIGURE 27–43 Magnetic resonance urogram reconstructions demonstrating a non occluding distal ureteral stone (*arrow*). **A-C,** 3D post processing techniques are used to mimic IV urography. **D,** Post contrast, axial imaging demonstrates a stone within the lumen of the distal ureters.

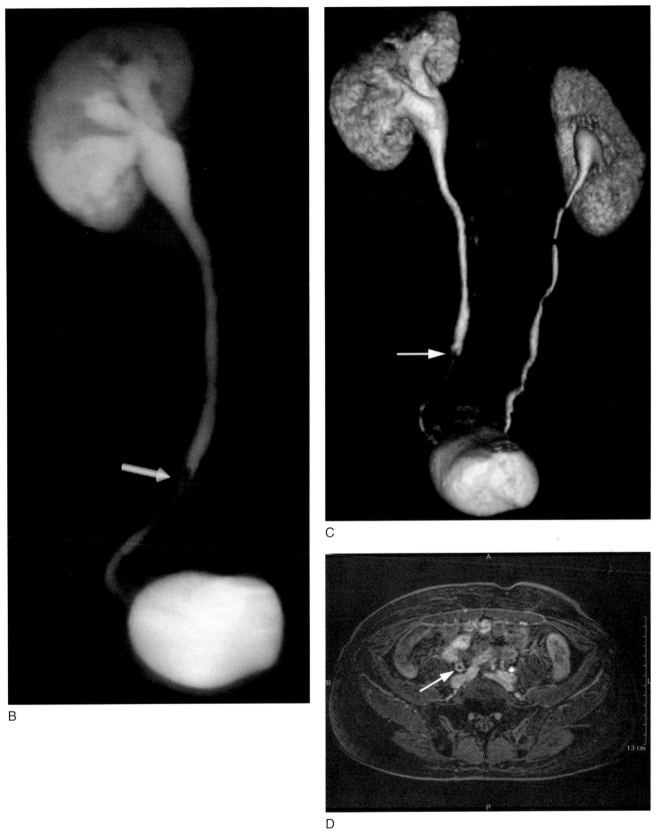

B

C

D

FIGURE 27–43—cont'd

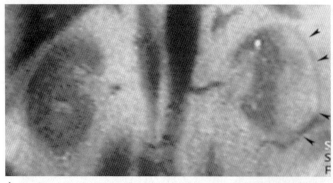

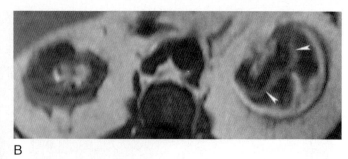

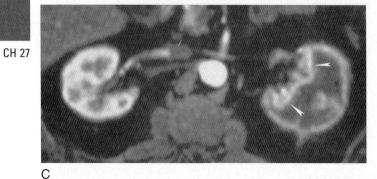

FIGURE 27–44 Subcapsular hematoma post lithotripsy. **A,** Coronal T2-weighted sequence demonstrating high-signal intensity blood contained by left renal capsule (*arrowheads*). **B,** Axial T1-weighted and **(C)** gadolinium-enhanced T1-weighted image show mass effect on left kidney (*arrowheads*) caused by a subcapsular hematoma. The signal intensity is consistent with intracellular methemoglobin.

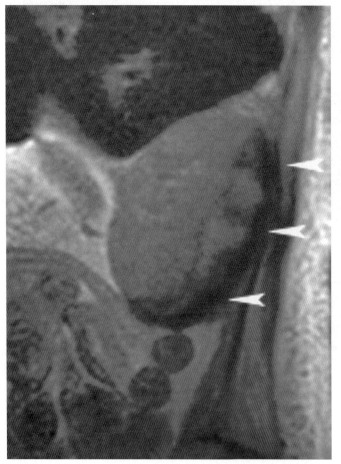

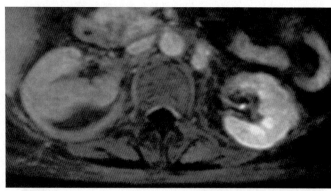

FIGURE 27–45 Post traumatic subcapsular hematoma. **A,** Sagittal T2-weighted and **(B)** post contrast T1-weighted images show a subcapsular hematoma (*arrowheads*) with signal intensity consistent with extracellular methemoglobin. This hematoma is older than the one shown in Figure 27–44.

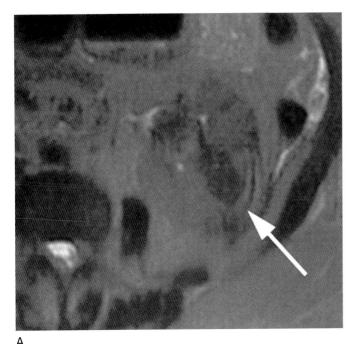

A

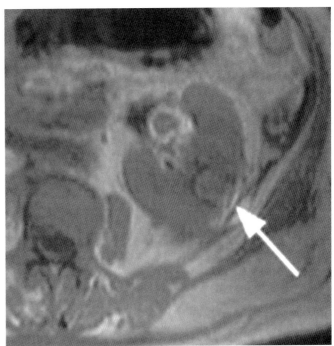

B

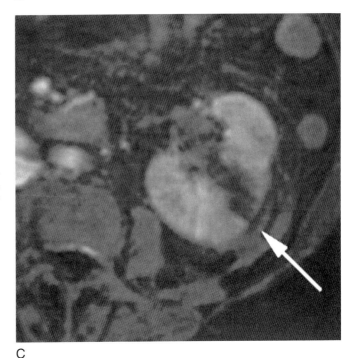

C

FIGURE 27-46 Hematoma status post surgical removal of staghorn calculus. **A,** T2-weighted, axial; **B,** T1-weighted, axial; and **C,** T1-weighted post contrast, axial images show an intrarenal hematoma (arrows) at the site of incision plane. This extends into the renal pelvis. No urine extravasation was demonstrated.

patchy or lobar although sometimes diffuse.[161] Subsequent scarring of the kidney after treatment reflects the magnitude of the infection and tissue destruction that occurred. Reflux is most common in childhood but may occur in adults with lower urinary tract infections or neurogenic bladders.

Hematogenous infection occurs initially in the cortex of the kidney. It eventually involves the medulla. It does not tend to be lobar or pyramidal in distribution. The areas of involvement are usually round, peripheral, and frequently multiple. These infections are usually caused by gram positive bacteria, such as staph aureus and streptococcus species. Bloodborne infection is less common than ascending infections and is usually seen in IV drug abusers, immunocompromised

patients, or patients with a source of infection outside the kidney such as heart valves or teeth.

In the patient with AIDS, urinary tract infections are quite common.[163] The infections are frequently hematogenous with unusual organisms such as pneumocystitis carinii, cytomegalovirus, and mycobacterium avium-intracellulare (MAI). The infections may also be seen in other abdominal organism—liver, spleen, and adrenals.[164,165]

Imaging is rarely used or needed in the uncomplicated case of acute pyelonephritis. It is reserved for the patient who is not responding to conventional antibiotic treatment, patients with an unclear diagnosis, patients with coexisting stone disease and possible obstruction, patients with diabetes and

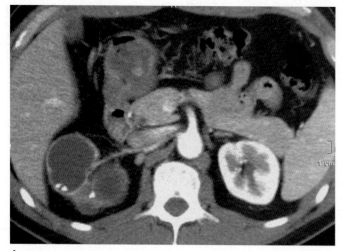

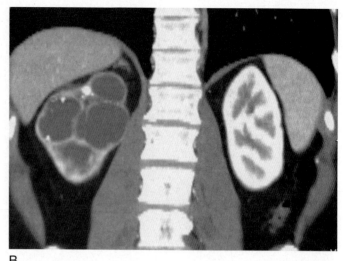

A   B

FIGURE 27–47 Renal tuberculosis—contrast-enhanced CT scan. Axial **(A)** and coronal **(B)** images show the destroyed right kidney due to renal tuberculosis. Parenchymal calcifications are present with dilated calyces due to the attenuated and truncated renal pelvis and ureter.

poor antibiotic response, and immunocompromised patients. Imaging is used to assist in confirming the diagnosis and determine the extent of the disease. It is also used in assessing complications of acute pyelonephritis including renal abscess, emphysematous pyelonephritis, and perinephric abscess.

Renal abscess formation is more common with hematogenous infection, although it does occur with ascending infection.[161] Emphysematous pyelonephritis is a severe necrotizing infection of the renal parenchyma usually caused by gram negative bacteria (E. coli, Klebsiella pneumoniae, Proteus Mirabilis).[166] Ninety percent of those with emphysematous pyelonephritis have un-contributed diabetes.[167] It is characterized by severe acute pyelonephritis, urosepsis, and hypotension. It is felt that the gas found in the renal parenchyma is formed due to the high levels of glucose in the tissue by fermentation with the production of CO_2. The gas may also be seen in the pelvocalyceal system or perinephric space (or both). Xanthogranulomatous pyelonephritis is a complication of longstanding obstruction and chronic infection, usually with Proteus or E. coli.[168] There is destruction of the renal parenchyma with replacement by vast amounts of lipid laden macrophages. Staghorn calculi are commonly encountered. The kidney is usually barely functional or nonfunctional. The destruction is typically global, but may involve only a portion of the kidney.

Renal tuberculosis occurs by hematogenous spread of pulmonary infections. The genitourinary track is the second most common site of involvement. Evidence of previous pulmonary tuberculosis is found in 70% to 75% of patients with genitourinary tuberculosis. Only 5% may have active tuberculosis. Renal involvement is bilateral with the findings being determined by the extent of the infection, stage of the infection, and host response. Calcified granuloma may be found within the cortex or medullar, papillary necrosis may be seen, and hydrocalyx with infundibular strictures may develop (Fig. 27–47). The kidney may become focally or globally scarred as the disease progresses. There may be areas of nonfunction with dystrophic calcifications. In its end stage, a small scarred kidney with bizarre calcifications may be found—the so-called autonephrectomy.[126,169]

In uncomplicated acute pyelonephritis the IVU may be normal in up to 75% of cases.[162,170] When present, the findings are usually unilateral and may be segmental. The findings include renal enlargement, altered nephrogram, decreased concentration of contrast material, and delayed appearance of contrast in the calyces. The calyces and renal pelvis may

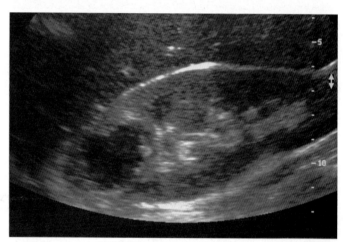

FIGURE 27–48 Acute pyelonephritis—renal ultrasound. The hypoechoic region in the upper pole represents an area affected by acute pyelonephritis. The surrounding parenchyma is somewhat distorted with loss of the normal corticomedullary junction.

be attenuated or mildly dilated as is the ureter. The kidney may be globally enlarged due to edema or may show a contour bulge with more focal involvement. The nephrogram may be diminished in intensity or even absent when compared to the opposite normal side. Delayed images may occasionally show a prolonged nephrogram on the affected side. The appearance time of the excreted contrast in the calyces may be delayed segmentally or globally and the overall density of the contrast may be diminished compared with the opposite side. The affected region will show attenuated calyces due to the edema although on occasion the calyces may be dilated. Dilatation of the pelvocalyceal system and ureter is due to atony or poor peristalsis with the system. This is a form of nonobstructive dilatation or hydronephrosis. The IVU usually will return to normal within 3 to 6 weeks of the occurrence of the episode of acute pyelonephritis.

Ultrasound is normal in the majority of patients with acute pyelonephritis. When the examination is abnormal, the findings are often nonspecific. Ultrasound is performed to look for a cause for acute pyelonephritis, such as obstruction or renal calculi, and to search for complications. Altered parenchymal echogenicity is the most frequent finding with loss of the normal corticomedullary differentiation. The echogenicity is usually decreased or heterogeneous in the affected area (Fig. 27–48). There may be focal or generalized swelling of the kidney. Power Doppler imaging may improve sensitivity in demonstrating focal hypoperfusion, but this is nonspecific. In patients with AIDS, renal nephropathy is found to have increased cortical echogenicity with loss of the corticomedullary differentiation (Fig. 27–49).[165] Renal size is also increased and this is generally a bilateral process.

Computed tomography is the most sensitive and specific means to image the patient with acute pyelonephritis.[170] Although the study may be normal in mild, uncomplicated pyelonephritis, it is still the most effective means of assisting in establishing the diagnosis, judging the extent, and evaluating for complications. Generally, noncontrast and post-contrast scans are used with the contrast-enhanced study being the most effective. The nephrographic phase of the CT scan is best for imaging the patient with acute pyelonephritis (Fig. 27–50). Wedge-shaped areas of decreased density extending from the renal pyramid to the cortex are most characteristic.[170] The nephrogram may be streaky or striated in a focal or global manner (Fig. 27–51).[171] There may be focal or diffuse swelling of the kidney.[172] The areas of involvement may appear almost mass-like (see Fig. 27–50). The changes in the nephrogram are related to decreased concentration of contrast media in the tubules with focal ischemia. There is also tubular destruction and obstruction with debris. There is usually a sharp demarcation with the normal parenchyma that continues to enhance normally in the nephrographic phase. There is soft tissue stranding and thickening of Gerota's fascia due to the adjacent inflammatory process (see Fig. 27–51).[162] There may be thickening of the walls of the renal pelvis and proximal ureter. Effacement of the calyces and renal pelvis may be seen. Mild dilation may also be occasionally noted. The kidney may have a single focal area of involvement or multiple areas with similar findings. With hematogenous-related pyelonephritis the early findings tend to be multiple, round cortical regions of hypodensity that become more confluent and involve the medulla with time.[172] These findings will persist for weeks despite successful treatment with antibiotics.

Complications of acute pyelonephritis include renal abscess, perinephric abscess, emphysematous pyelonephritis, and xanthogranulomatous pyelonephritis. All of these entities are imaged best with cross-sectional imaging

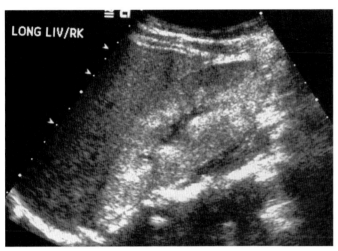

FIGURE 27–49 AIDS nephropathy—ultrasound. Longitudinal image of the right kidney. The kidney is of normal size to slightly increased size. The corticomedullary distinction is lost with diffuse increased cortical echogenicity.

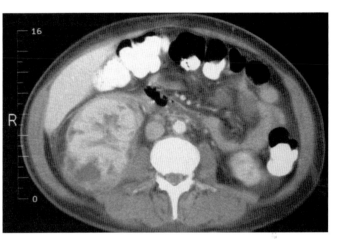

FIGURE 27–51 Acute pyelonephritis—contrast enhanced CT scan. The heterogeneous CT nephrogram shows the diffuse involvement of the right kidney. There is stranding and some fluid seen in the perinephritic space with thickening of Gerota's fascia.

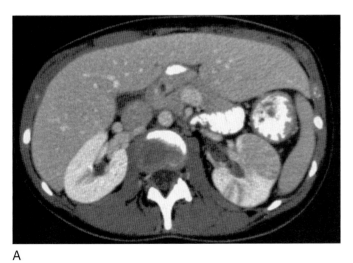

A

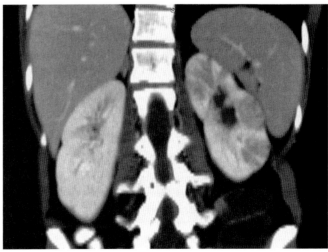

B

FIGURE 27–50 Acute pyelonephritis—contrast-enhanced CT scan. Axial (A) and coronal (B) images. The left kidney shows multiple areas of involvement. The hypodense region in the mid kidney appears almost mass-like (A, B). A striated nephrogram is seen in the region of involvement in the upper pole (B).

techniques, most specifically CT. Renal abscess results from severe pyelonephritis with coalescence of necrotic regions and microabcesses. They occur two to three times more frequently in diabetic patients.[167] The findings on IVU are nonspecific with renal mass being suggested by the contour bulge of the kidney and the hypodense region in the nephrogram. Adjacent calyces are not visualized due to edema or their destruction by the abscess cavity. Ultrasound assessment reveals an anechoic or hypoechoic mass with irregular walls. There is usually debris within the abscess leading to some low level echoes. There is usually poor through transmission. Highly echogenic foci within an abscess may represent microbubbles or gas. The wall may demonstrate increased vascular on color Doppler sonography. CT findings in renal abscess include a reasonably well-defined mass with a low density central region and a thick irregular wall or pseudocapsule (Fig. 27–52).[170] There is variable enhancement seen in the region adjacent to the abscess depending on the amount of inflammation. Mature abscesses may demonstrate a more sharply demarcated border with peripheral rim enhancement. Gas may be seen within the abscess.

Perinephric abscess formation is the result of renal abscesses rupturing through the renal capsule or emphysematous pyelonephritis extending through the capsule into the perinephric space.[172] The IVU may demonstrate on the nephrogram lucency around the kidney. The kidney is usually poorly functioning so complete assessment is difficult. Ultrasound assessment may show fluid or debris (or both) in a localized or generalized fashion around the kidney. With CT, the complete extent of perinephric involvement may be seen. Subcapsular extension may be separated from perinephric involvement. Generally, there is heterogeneous fluid density material seen in the perinephric space. It may contain gas as well. Extension within the retropertoneum is easily recognized into the psoas muscle and adjacent structures (see Fig. 27–52). With psoas involvement, it may extend into the pelvis and as far as the groin following the course of the iliopsoas muscle.

With emphysematous pyelonephritis, gas is seen within the renal parenchyma.[166] If the gas is extensive enough, it may be visible on plain films or KUB. The gas is usually mottled, bubbly, or streaky in appearance and may be seen in the areas over the kidneys. With gas in the pelvicalyceal system, it may be seen as the gas-filled outline of the renal pelvis and collecting systems. The IVU contributes little to the diagnosis as the involved kidney is usually nonfunctional. Nephrotomography may displace the gas within the kidney to better advantage. Ultrasound may suggest the diagnosis of emphysematous pyelonephritis by the demonstration of gas within the kidney.[173] With gas present there will be acoustic shadowing in the involved region with adjacent microbubbles causing ring down artifacts. CT is most specific in that the gas may be visualized and the extent of involvement determined.[174] There is generally extensive parenchymal destruction with streaks of gas or mottled collections of gas within the kidney (Fig. 27–53). There is little or no fluid seen. The gas is seen dissecting through the parenchyma in a linear focal or global manner. The gas usually radiates along the pyramid to the cortex. It may extend through into the perinephric space. Emphysematous pyelitis represents gas in the pelvocalyceal system only.[175] It is best diagnosed with CT where parenchymal gas is easily seen. The diagnosis distinction is important in that emphysematous pyelitis carries a less grave prognosis.

Xanthogranulomatous pyelonephritis is an end-stage condition resulting from chronic obstruction with longstanding infection.[168] The plain film or KUB will show a staghorn calculus or large calcification overlying the region of the kidney with a large mass filling the space. An enlarged kidney with loss of identifiable landmarks is seen with ultrasound. The renal sinus echoes are lost. There is usually a large calculus or staghorn calculus filling the space with adjacent debris-filled hypoechoic regions (Fig. 27–54). At times it appears as a large heterogeneous mass. CT defines the extent and adjacent organ involvement best in patients with xanthogranulomatous pyelonephritis. The CT findings include an enlarged but generally reniform mass filling the perinephric space.[168,176] Calcification, specifically calculi and staghorn calculi are found in 75% of cases. There is absent or markedly decreased excretion seen in 85% of cases and the involved region appears as a mass in more than 85% of cases.[168] In less than 15% of cases the process is focal with normally functioning area of the kidney remaining. The kidney appears enlarged and usually nonfunctional with multiple round

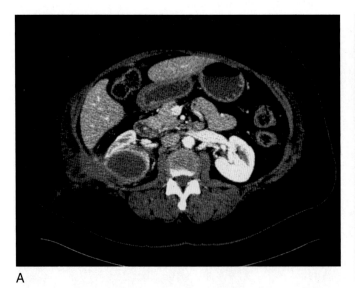

A

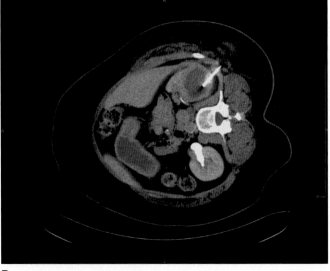

B

FIGURE 27–52 Renal abscess—contrast-enhanced CT scan. Axial image **(A)** demonstrates the hypodense abscess in the right kidney with extension into the perinephritic space and the right flank. Axial image **(B)** with the patient in the decubitus position reveals the method of diagnosis—needle aspiration. A drainage catheter was subsequently placed for treatment.

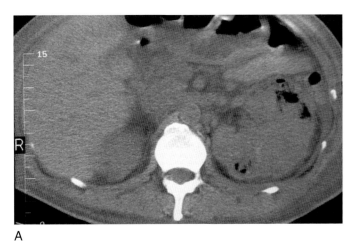

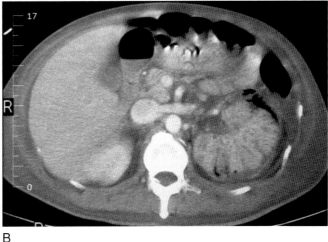

FIGURE 27–53 Emphysematous pyelonephritis—contrast-enhanced CT scan. A noncontrast image **(A)** and contrast-enhanced image **(B)** demonstrate gas in the renal parenchyma with extension into the perinephritic space. The nephrogram is striated throughout. Global involvement of the kidney is frequent.

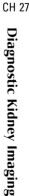

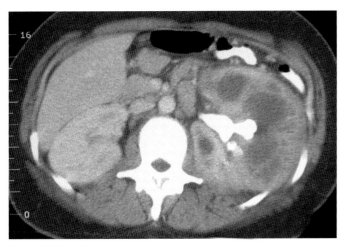

FIGURE 27–54 Xanthogranulomatous pyelonephritis—contrast-enhanced CT scan. A large staghorn calculus fills the renal pelvis and collecting systems in the left kidney. Much of the remainder of the kidney is replaced by hypodense material—the xanthogranulomatous infection—within the calyces and parenchyma with some minimal remaining enhancement of the cortex.

hypoattenuating regions with adjacent calcification. There is frequent perinephric extension. Fistulas may occur to adjacent structures with adenopathy noted in the retroperitoneum.

Chronic pyelonephritis is usually associated with vesicoureteral reflux occurring in childhood.[169] The kidney has focal scars that are associated with calyceal dilatation. The scarring is often separated by normal regions of the kidney and normal appearing calyces. When there is global involvement the kidney may be small. The IVU demonstrates dilated or ballooned calyces that extend to the cortical surface, which is thinned. The outline of the kidney will be distorted. One or both kidneys may be involved. With ultrasound the kidneys have irregular outlines with regions of cortical loss. Underlying dilated calyces may be visible. The regions of scarring may be echogenic compared with the adjacent normal kidney. CT scans will demonstrate abnormal architecture within the kidney.[172] Nephrographic phase images reveal the regions of cortical loss with the involved dilated calyces extending to the capsular surface. Variable dilatation of the calyces is seen. Again, the process may be unilateral or bilateral. Excretory

phase images will best delineate the extent of involvement especially when presented in a coronal format.

Magnetic resonance imaging is comparable to contrast-enhanced CT for the evaluation of pyelonephritis, abscess, and post infectious scarring.[177] Because CT is more sensitive for the evaluation of stones and gas, MRI is reserved for those patients with contraindications to iodinated contrast or radiation exposure (Fig. 27–55).

Acute pyelonephritis is associated with fever, flank pain, leukocytosis, and pyuria. Radiolabeled leukocyte (e.g., In-111 WBC) and gallium-67 citrate scans can be helpful in identifying acute pyelonephritis. However, these methods have the drawbacks of extended imaging time (more than 24 hours) and higher radiation exposure. Cortical imaging with DMSA has been shown to be highly sensitive for detecting acute pyelonephritis in the appropriate clinical setting.[178] Acute pyelonephritis demonstrates segmental regions of decreased tracer uptake in oval, round, or wedge pattern. There may also be diffuse generalized decrease in renal uptake, which in association with normal or slightly enlarged kidney is suspicious for an acute infectious process. The pathophysiologic basis for decline in DMSA cortical uptake in infection is related to diminished tracer delivery to the infected area and to direct infectious injury to the tubular cells compromising their function and tracer uptake. A wedge-shaped cortical defect with regional decrease in renal size is compatible with post-infectious scarring. Renal infarcts may also have similar appearance.[95,99]

RENAL MASS—CYSTS TO RENAL CELL CARCINOMA

Renal masses are quite common with simple renal cysts found in more than 50% of patients over the age of 50. The vast majority of renal masses are simple cysts with solid renal masses, such as renal cell carcinoma, in the minority. Renal masses produce variable findings in the kidney depending on their location. The contour of the kidney may be deformed, calyces displaced or splayed, density of the kidney altered, or the axis of the kidney changed. For years, the IVU was the method of choice for detection of renal masses. Studies have shown it is the low sensitivity for detection of renal masses especially those less than 3 cm in size.[179] A normal IVU does not exclude a renal mass. Using CT as the "gold standard", IVU detected 10% of masses less than 1 cm, 21% of masses

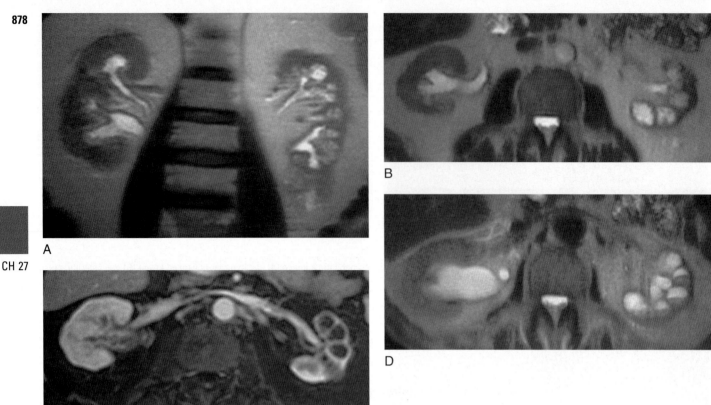

A

B

C

D

FIGURE 27–55 Renal tuberculosis. **A and B**, T2-weighted images demonstrate asymmetrical cortical thinning and focal areas of increased signal intensity in the distribution of the medullary pyramids. **C**, Post contrast T1-weighted image shows absence of enhancement consistent with granulomas with caseous necrosis. **D**, T2-weighed image after treatment shows distorted, dilated calyces containing debris. Right hydronephrosis is seen due to a distal ureteral stricture.

1 cm to 2 cm in size, 52% of those 2 cm to 3 cm in size and 85% of renal masses greater than 3 cm.[179] Ultrasound fared better but still detected only 26% of masses less than 1 cm, 60% of those 1 cm to 2 cm in size, 82% of masses 2 cm to 3 cm, and 85% of renal masses greater than 3 cm.[179] The findings on IVU are frequently nonspecific and further imaging is required to accurately characterize the renal mass. Ultrasound, CT, and MRI are needed to differentiate solid from cystic renal masses.

Simple renal cysts are commonly encountered with all imaging studies today. They are rarely seen in individuals under the age of 25, but are seen in with great frequency in individuals over the age of 50. Typically, renal cysts are asymptomatic, cortical in location, and may be single or multiple. The cause is unknown. The plain film (KUB) is rarely helpful unless the cyst is quite large. A thin peripheral curvilinear rim calcification may be seen in 1% to 2% of cases. The findings on IVU depend on the position in the kidney and associated deformity of the renal contour and splaying of the pelvocalyceal system. Nephrotomography will yield a well outlined, homogenous lesion that is less dense than the surrounding kidney (Fig. 27–56). The wall of the cyst will be paper thin with a sharp, clear-cut demarcation with the adjacent kidney. The interface with the kidney when a cyst lies on the surface will be beak-like. The calyces will be displaced or splayed.

Ultrasound is an excellent means of diagnosing a simple renal cyst if all imaging criteria are met.[40] The lesion in the kidney will be round or oval and must be anechoic (no echoes within) (Fig. 27–57). It must be well circumscribed with a smooth wall. There must be enhanced through transmission of the sound beyond the cyst with a sharp interface of the back wall with the renal parenchyma. Thin septa may be seen

within the cyst, but no nodules on the wall. If all criteria are met, the diagnosis is sound. If there is any deviation from the findings discussed earlier, further imaging with CT or MRI is necessary.

Computed tomography is the method of choice for characterizing and differentiating renal masses.[180–182] A simple renal cyst will appear as a well-circumscribed, round, water-dense lesion within the kidney (Fig. 27–58). The CT numbers of the cyst will be near zero. There will be no significant enhancement of the contents after the injection of contrast media. The CT numbers may vary slightly from water density, but no more than 10–15 Hounsfield units. The cyst must be uniform throughout with no measurable wall. The interface with the adjacent parenchyma must be sharp. The margins must be smooth with no perceptible nodules. Thin rim-like calcification may be seen. Occasionally, "high density" cysts may be encountered with CT numbers of 50 to 80 range. These are cysts containing hemorrhage or proteinaceous debris. They demonstrate no wall nodularity and again have no significant enhancement after contrast injection. They are common in polycystic kidneys.

Polycystic renal disease is classified as infantile, adult, or acquired. The infantile form is inherited as an autosomal recessive disorder.[183] It has a variable presentation with severe kidney injury being found with a neonatal presentation and congenital hepatic fibrosis and hepatic failure when presenting in older children. Organomegaly is common with bilateral symmetrical renal enlargement. The IVU yields poor visualization of the kidneys due to renal impairment with a prolonged, mottled nephrogram with a striated or streaky appearance. Ultrasound reveals enlarged, diffusely hyperechoic kidneys due to the abnormality involved, that of dilated, ectatic collecting tubules.[184] There is loss of the

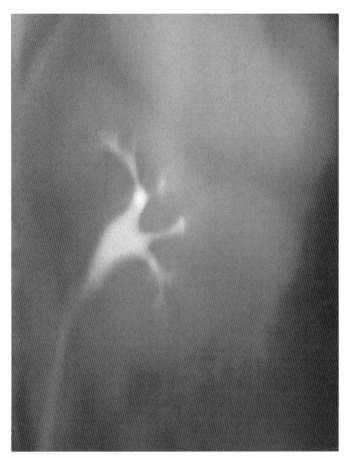

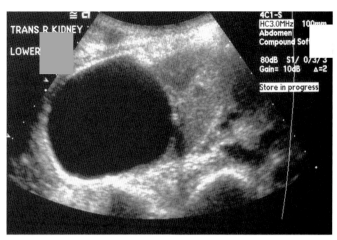

FIGURE 27–57 Renal cyst—ultrasound. A large anechoic renal mass is seen projecting off the lateral border of the right kidney. The cyst features include a well-circumscribed lesion with a sharp back wall and increased through transmission. There are no internal echoes or nodularity and the wall is smooth. There is a clear interface with the kidney.

FIGURE 27–56 Renal mass—nephrotomogram. The left kidney reveals a slightly hypodense mass projecting off the lateral border of the kidney. This proved to be a renal cyst with subsequent imaging.

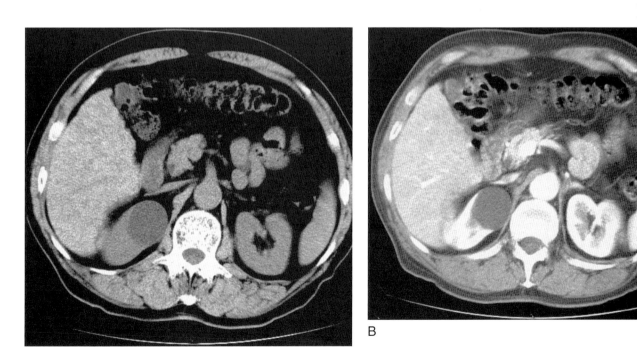

FIGURE 27–58 Renal cyst—CT scan. Axial noncontrast (A) and post contrast (B) images. The cyst is well circumscribed with no enhancement. It displays water density with CT numbers of 0–5. There is a sharp interface with the kidney and no perceptible wall. There are no nodules seen and it is uniform throughout.

corticomedullary differentiation as well. CT and MRI are rarely used as the diagnosis is made clinically with the associated ultrasound findings.

Autosomal dominant polycystic disease (ADPK) is the adult form.[185] The plain film will be normal early in the disease process, but as the cysts increase in size so does the overall renal size. When advanced, there will be large bilateral masses present with occasional curvilinear calcifications in the wall of some of the cysts. The IVU will demonstrate multiple lucencies throughout the kidneys, a Swiss-cheese appearance. When renal function is still normal there is extensive splaying and distortion of the pelvicalyceal system. Ultrasound reveals enlarged kidneys bilaterally, which are markedly lobulated containing multiple sonolucent areas of varying size throughout the kidneys.[186]

Computed tomography in ADPK yields enlarged, lobulated kidneys with a myriad of cysts of varying size throughout (Fig. 27–59). One kidney may be more involved than the other. The cysts may have calcifications with the wall. It is not uncommon to encounter cysts with varying density due to episodes of hemorrhage that occur within the cysts. A fluid level may be seen due to the presence of debris or hemorrhage within some of the cysts. In the excretory phase there is marked distortion of the calyces. The extent of renal involvement by ADPK is better appreciated in CT than US or IVU. Cysts may be found in the lever, spleen, and pancreas as well.

Adult acquired polycystic kidney disease (AAPKD) occurs in patients with kidney injury undergoing continuous peritoneal dialysis or hemodialysis.[187] The longer the patient has undergone dialysis, the higher the likelihood of AAPKD.[188] Most patients will have undergone dialysis for several years before it is discovered.[189] The cysts are generally quite small (0.5 cm to 2 cm in most). Calcification may occur in the wall. Plain films and IVU play no role due to impaired renal function. Ultrasound reveals small, shrunken kidneys with

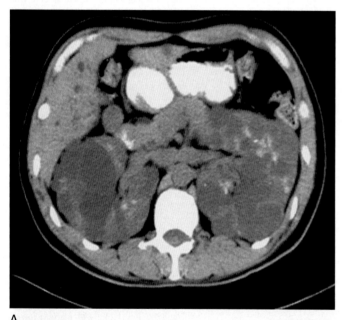

A

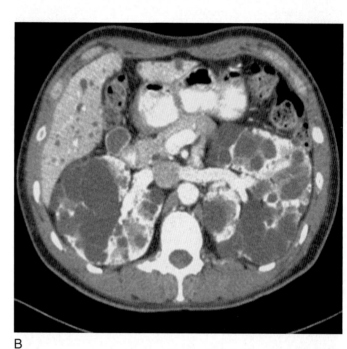

B

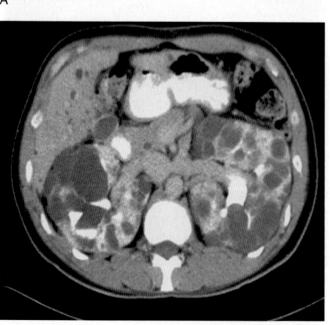

C

FIGURE 27–59 Autosomal dominant polycystic kidney disease—CT scan. Axial noncontrast **(A)**, nephrographic phase **(B)**, and excretory phase **(C)** images. The equally enlarged kidneys are seen bilaterally with the multiple varying sized cysts involving both kidneys. The calyces are splayed apart and distorted in the excretory phase image **(C)**. Note the multiple small cysts also present in the involved liver.

anechoic or hypoechoic regions representing the cysts. The findings are usually bilateral. CT or MRI will show the small bilateral kidneys with cysts of varying size but usually in the 1 cm to 2 cm range (see Fig. 27–29).[190,191] These cysts must be closely evaluated for solid components as carcinomas and adenomas occur with increased frequency in these patients. Solid lesions less than 3 cm in size may represent either adenomas or renal cell carcinomas, whereas most lesions greater than 3 cm are renal cell carcinomas.[192,193] Screening for AAPKD is usually done with ultrasound every 6 months, with CT or MRI reserved for patients with questionable or solid lesions.[194]

Medullary sponge kidney, or renal tubular ectasia is a non-hereditary developmental disorder with ectasia and cystic dilation of the distal collecting tubules. The cystic spaces predispose to stasis leading to stone formation and potential infection. Involvement is usually bilateral although not always symmetric with as few as one calyx involved. The kidneys are typically normal sized with a medullary nephrocalcinosis picture when the small stones are present.[125] The IVU reveals linear or round collections of contrast extending from the calyceal border forming parallel brush like striations. With more severe involvement the cystic dilatations may appear grape-like or bead-like. CT is an excellent method for demonstrating the calculi, although the striations or cystic dilatation may be difficult to visualize even with thin section excretory phase imaging.

Multicystic dysplastic kidney is an uncommon, congenital, non-hereditary condition. It is usually unilateral and affects the entire kidney. Rarely only a portion of the kidney is involved. The affected kidney is nonfunctional on IVU. Ultrasound reveals multiple anechoic cystic structures of varying size replacing the kidney with no normal parenchyma seen. Calcification in the wall of the cystic spaces may be seen. CT demonstrates multiple fluid-filled structures filling the renal fossa. Septa and some rim calcifications may be visible. The density of the fluid is usually that of water ($\approx$0) or slightly higher. There is no contrast enhancement seen with the injection of IV contrast. The renal artery to the affected size is not visible. It may be difficult to differentiate from severe hydronephrosis if no cyst walls or septa are visible.

Small cortical cysts may be seen in some hereditary syndromes (i.e., tuberous sclerosis). These cysts are typically multiple and very small (i.e., a few millimeters). They are seen best with MRI, but may also be seen on CT if the cysts are slightly larger. Pyelogenic cysts or calyceal diverticula are small cystic structures that connect with a portion of the pelvicalyceal system. On IVU, a calyceal diverticulum appears as a small round or oval collection of contrast connected to the fornix of the calyx. As stasis occurs within the diverticulum, renal stone formation may occur.

Para- and peripelvic cysts are extraparenchymal cysts that occur in the region of the renal pelvis. They may be single or multiple, unilateral or bilateral. With the increased use of cross-sectional imaging techniques, they are seen with increased frequency. They may result from lymphangiectasia from prior insult to the kidney. Depending on the size and number, IVU reveals compression of the renal pelvis and infundibula, but no calyceal dilatation. The condition may be confused with renal sinus lipomatosis. Ultrasound, CT, and MRI reveal the true nature of the process with the water-filled cystic structures in the renal sinus (Fig. 27–60).

All imaging modalities have been used to discover renal masses. The distinction between solid and cystic lesions is paramount as it guides differential diagnosis and subsequent treatment as needed. As discussed previously, these are significant limitations with both IVU and US in discovering renal masses less than 2 cm to 3 cm in size.[179] The IVU also is very limited in differentiating cystic from solid lesions and should not be used for that purpose. Although less accurate than CT, US provides a noninvasive means for differentiating solid from cystic renal masses. If all imaging criteria for a renal cyst are met with US, an accurate diagnosis can be made. CT is the imaging modality of choice for the characterization of all solid mass, suspected solid masses, or masses that do not meet US criteria for a true renal cyst.[195–197] The advantage of CT lies in the multiphase manner in which studies can be performed. Noncontrast, arterial, corticomedullary, nephrographic, and excretory phase imaging may all play a role in the accurate display and characterization of renal masses. MRI has sensitivities and specificities in line with CT but is generally reserved for a case in which the patient has impaired renal function or a contraindication to iodinated contrast medium. It is technically more demanding but may be helpful in cases of indeterminate CT assessed renal masses, those with venous involvement, and in distinguishing vessels from retroperitoneal lymph nodes. The findings of any and all studies must be linked to the clinical history, especially in the case of complex or complicated cystic renal masses.

Renal neoplasms may arise from either the renal parenchyma or the urotheliem of the pelvicalyceal system. Renal tumors have been reported during every decade of life, including the newborn.[198] Both benign and malignant tumors occur within the kidney. Benign tumors of any significant size are extremely uncommon. The diagnosis is typically made at autopsy as they rarely cause symptoms. With the increased use of cross-sectional imaging techniques, more are being discovered. The renal adenoma is the most common benign neoplasm. Arising from mature renal tubular cells, it almost always is less than 2 cm to 3 cm in size. There are no characteristic radiologic features that distinguish it from often solid tumors. Typically these lesions will be corticomedullary in location, solid on US, and demonstrate uniform enhancement on CT. Other benign lesions have been reported including hamartomas, oncocytomas, fibromas, myomas, lipomas, and hemangiomas, but uncommonly.

Hamartomas of the kidney, angiomyolipomas (AML), are one group of benign renal tumors that are distinguishable radiologically.[199] As the AML is composed of different tissues, including fat, muscle, vascular elements, and even cartilage, the fat in particular may be detected radiographically.[200] AML occur in two different groups of patients. A solitary unilateral form is most frequently found in women from the third to fifth decade. These are usually discovered due to pain associated with hemorrhage. Multiple bilateral AMLs are found in patients with tuberous sclerosis. With marked involvement of the kidneys, there are multiple masses found bilaterally with an appearance not unlike that of polycystic disease, except for the presence of fat in the masses. The solitary AML may be seen as a renal mass on conventional studies, KUB, and IVU, if of sufficient size. US will demonstrate the mass to be solid with increased echoes due to the presence of fat in the lesion.[201,202] CT is diagnostic in that fat will be seen with the mass (Fig. 27–61). Usually the CT numbers will be −20 or less. Most AML have a large amount of fat and the diagnosis can be made with ease. Uncommonly only a minimal amount of fat is present, and it must be searched for diligently on thin-section noncontrast CT scans.[203,204] All solid lesions in the kidney should be searched for fat; if it is present the diagnosis of AML is virtually assured.[205–207] Most AML 4 cm or less will be watched with surgery reserved for those of larger size, especially with hemorrhage.[208,209] Oncocytoma is another benign renal tumor that may occasionally be suggested pre-operatively in a patient with a solid renal mass.[210] This uncommon benign tumor originates in the epithelium of the proximal collecting tubule. Radiologically, it is usually found incidentally in asymptomatic adults. Its features include a solid mass with homogenous enhancement, a central stellate scar that may be seen with US, CT, or MRI,

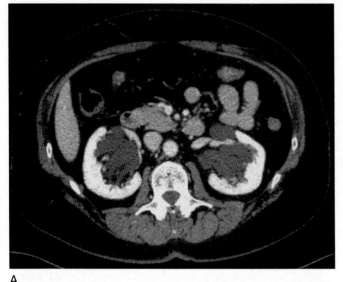

A

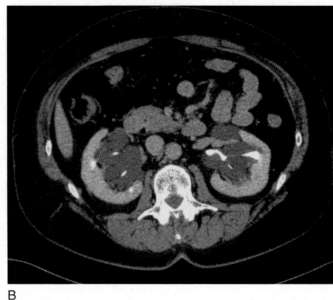

B

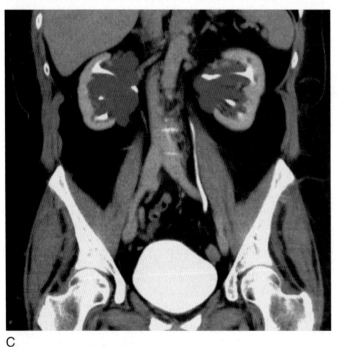

C

FIGURE 27–60 Peripelvic cysts—CT scan. Axial nephrographic phase (**A**) and excretory phase (**B**) images with a coronal excretory phase (**C**) image. Multiple bilateral water density cysts fill the renal hilum displacing and splaying the collecting system and renal pelvis (**B, C**). The cortex is preserved with no cysts visible in the cortex.

and on angiographic spoked wheel pattern.[211-213] These findings are nonspecific, however, and histologic confirmation is needed.[214,215] Oncocytic renal cell carcinomas also occur and surgery is generally needed for the correct diagnosis.

Renal cell carcinoma is the third most common tumor of the genitourinary tract after carcinoma of the prostate and bladder. This tumor constitutes 2% to 3% of all adult tumors and is the most common retroperitoneal tumor. Clear cell renal carcinoma is the most common subtype accounting for 70% of cases. Its average 5-year survival is 55% to 60%. Papillary renal carcinoma represents 15% to 20% of cases with a 5-year survival of 80% to 90%; 6% to 11% of renal cell carcinomas are of the chromophobe subtype with a 5-year survival of 90%. Collecting duct renal cell carcinomas are the rarest with 1% of cases and a 5-year survival of less than 5%. Chromophobe and papillary tumors tend to grow slower, are less aggressive, and more likely to contain calcification within.[216-218]

Imaging studies in renal cell carcinoma are used for initial detection, characterization, and staging. Accurate staging is

imperative as it drives the treatment decision. Surgery is the primary means of treatment with radical nephrectory, simple nephrectory, or nephron-sparing partial nephrectory being options.[219,220] More recently radiofrequency ablation or cryoablation have been used successfully in a limited population.[221-223] Recently, immunotherapy for metastatic renal cell carcinoma has been delivered by CT guidance.[224]

The classic presentation of a renal cell carcinoma in a patient with painless hematuria is that of a renal mass.[50,58] The plain film may reveal an enlarged kidney or mass in the region of the kidney; 10% to 20% of cases may demonstrate calcification on the KUB. Calcification may be seen however, in benign and malignant renal masses. Peripheral rim-like calcification on plain film does not exclude malignancy. Most often malignant lesions have central, punctuate, or mottled calcification.

Until recently the IVU has been the standard examination performed in patients suspected of having a mass lesion in the kidney.[179] Renal cell carcinoma will distort the kidney outline or cause renal enlargement.[50] The mass will have an

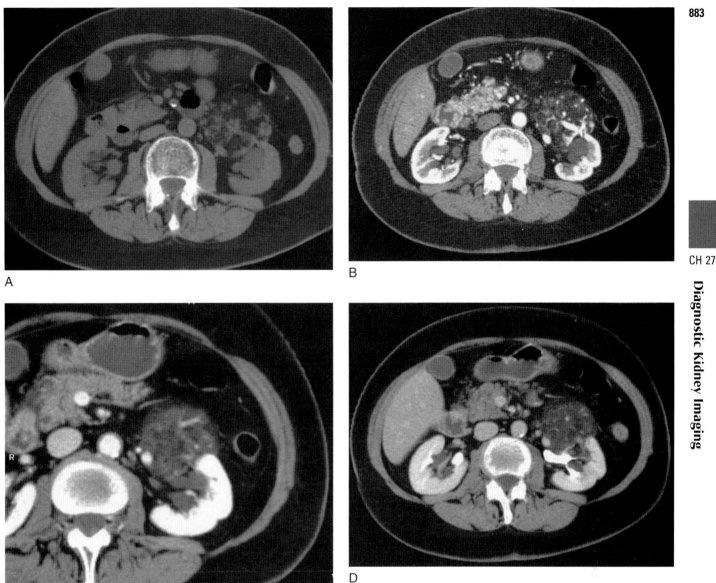

FIGURE 27–61 Angiomyolipoma—CT scan. Axial CT images—noncontrast **(A)**, corticomedullary phase **(B)**, nephrographic phase **(C)**, and excretory phase **(D)**. The fat-containing mass is seen projecting anteriorly from the left kidney. It has internal structure that demonstrates enhancement in this very vascular benign tumor.

irregular or indistinct junction with the normal renal paren-chyma. The calyces will be stretched, distorted, or obliterated by the tumor. When the neoplasm extends medially into the renal pelvis, it will narrow or obliterate the renal pelvis or cause an irregular filling defect that represents either tumor or blood clot within the pelvis. A nonfunctioning kidney may be seen with renal vein occlusion, replacement of the major-ity of the kidney by tumor, or complete involvement of the renal pelvis. A mass lesion in the kidney requires further evaluation with cross-sectional imaging techniques. The US findings in a renal cell carcinoma include a mass with vari-able complex internal echoes, impaired through transmission and poor definition of the back wall or distal aspect of the lesion (Fig. 27–62). Mural nodules may be seen in cystic lesions and the internal wall may be thickened and irregular. US is less accurate than CT for revealing small renal masses. Normal findings on US do not exclude a small renal mass. In one study of 205 lesions seen on CT, 79 were missed with US.[225] Thirty of these lesions were solid renal masses. Power

Doppler US, phase-inversion tissue harmonic imaging, and US contrast-enhanced harmonic imaging may improve the sensitivity of US for the detection and characterization of solid renal masses.[226–229]

Computed tomography is the modality of choice for imaging renal cell carcinoma as it has been proven effective in detection, diagnosis, characterization, and staging with accuracy exceeding 90%.[219,230] On noncontrast CT scans, renal cell carcinomas appear as an ill-defined, irregular area in the kidney with CT numbers close to that of renal parenchyma (Fig. 27–63). After the injection of intravenous iodinated contrast, the vast majority of RCC will show signifi-cant enhancement. The best phase for depiction of the mass is the nephrographic phase, although lesions are certainly detectable on the corticomedullary and excretory phases as well (Figs. 27–63 and 27–64).[231–233] In the corticomedullary phase, there is maximal enhancement of the arteries and veins that must be seen for accurate staging and preoperative planning (see Fig. 27–64).[234,235] The excretory phase is most

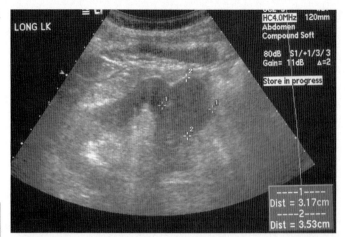

FIGURE 27–62 Renal cell carcinoma—ultrasound. Longitudinal image reveals a solid mass projecting from the left kidney. The mass contains internal echoes and does not have any of the features of a renal cyst. It has an ill-defined interface with the kidney and no increased through transmission.

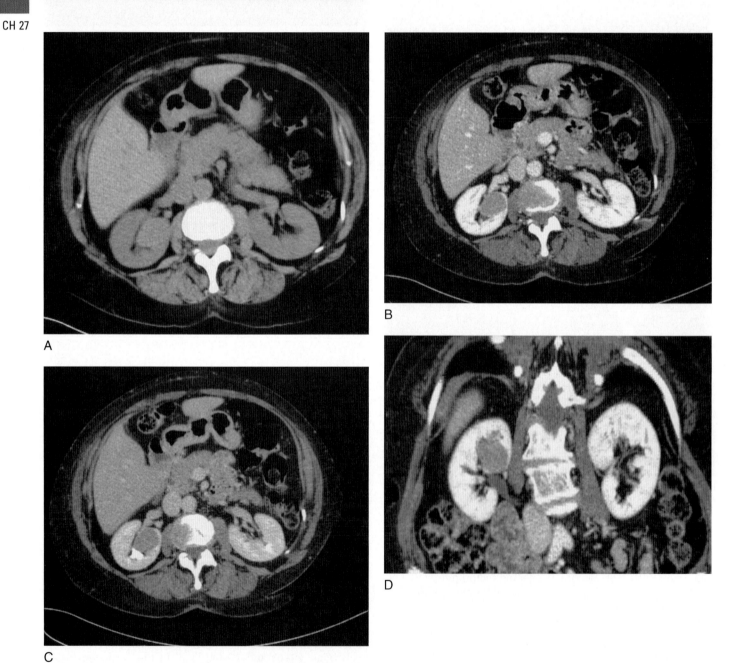

FIGURE 27–63 Renal cell carcinoma—CT scan. Axial noncontrast **(A)**, nephrographic phase **(B)**, and excretory phase **(C)** images combined with a coronal nephrographic phase image. On the noncontrast scan **(A)** the right renal mass is slightly hyperdense relative to the rest of the kidney. Contrast-enhanced scans **(B, C, D)** show the enhancing surrounded by the normal renal parenchyma. This proved to be a renal cell carcinoma—chromophobe type.

helpful for showing the relationship of the RCC to the pelvi-calyceal system and in preoperative planning for nephron-sparing partial nephrectomy (see Fig. 27–63).[236,237] Clear cell RCC will tend to have greater enhancement than the papillary or chromophobe RCC (see Figs. 27–63 and 27–64).[238,239] Enhancement patterns for clear cell and papillary RCC will appear more heterogeneous with the chromophobe RCC frequently showing a homogeneous enhancement pattern (see Fig. 27–63).[238] Chromophobe and papillary types will more often contain calcification than the clear cell type.[240]

The staging of RCC is important in predicting survival rates and planning the proper surgical approach to the mass. Both the WHO and Robson classifications are used in the staging of renal cell carcinoma.[219] With the Robson classification, in a stage I RCC, the tumor is confined to the renal parenchyma by the renal capsule (see Fig. 27–63). In stage II RCC, there is tumor extension through the renal capsule into the perinephric fat but still within Gerota's fascia (see Fig. 27–64). Stage III lesions are subdivided as IIIa—tumor extension into the renal vein or IVC; IIIb—tumor involvement of regional retroperitoneal lymph nodes; and IIIc—tumor involving the veins and nodes (Fig. 27–65). Stage IVa RCC will have progression of tumor outside Gerota's fascia with involvement of adjacent organs or muscles other than the ipsilateral adrenal gland. Stage IVb RCC represents tumor with distant

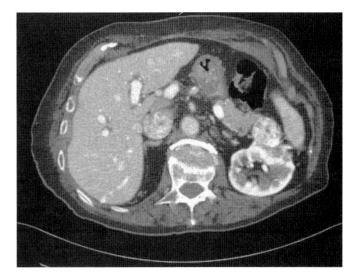

FIGURE 27–64 Renal cell carcinoma—CT scan. Axial contrast-enhanced corticomedullary phase image. Note the heterogeneously enhancing mass in the anterior aspect of the left kidney. This is a stage II RCC as it has extended through the renal capsule into Gerota's fascia. This proved to be a renal cell carcinoma—clear cell type.

FIGURE 27–65 Renal cell carcinoma—CT scan. Coronal contrast-enhanced (A), axial contrast-enhanced (B), and coronal contrast-enhanced (C) images. Stage IIIA RCC with mass in the right kidney shows a tumor thrombus extending into the right renal vein. In a different patient the right renal mass also has a tumor thrombus, but it has extended into the inferior vena cava (B, C). Both these RCCs proved to be of the clear cell type.

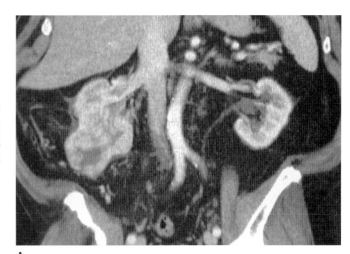

A

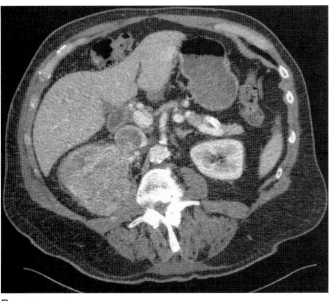

B

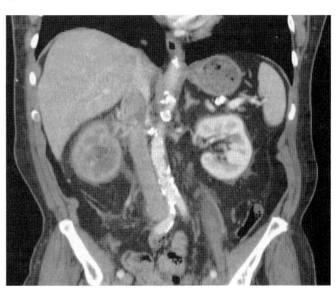

C

metastases, the most common sites being the lungs, mediastinum, liver, and bone.

Although RCC is the most common primary malignancy in the kidney, transitional cell carcinoma (TCC) also occurs within the kidney.[241] Most TCC involve the urothelium and project into the lumen of the renal pelvis or ureter. This leads to a picture of a filling defect within the renal pelvis or ureter that can be confused with a renal stone, blood clot, or debris (Fig. 27–66). Transitional cell carcinoma of the bladder is much more common than TCC of the kidney or ureter.[242] The

neoplasm may extend into the renal parenchyma and appears as a mass within the kidney. The imaging findings are similar to that of RCC except the lesions do not tend to enhance as much with contrast injection. Renal vein involvement is rare. Retrograde pyelograms with ureteroscopy are diagnostic.

Lymphoma may involve the kidney as part of multi-organ involvement, or rarely as a primary neoplasm.[243] Lymphoma presents with single or multiple masses within one or both kidneys. Perirenal extension may be seen as well. An infiltrative picture may also be seen with lymphomatous replacement of the kidney. This form usually has adjacent retroperitoneal adenopathy. The imaging findings will be representative of either the mass or infiltrative involvement. CT has usually been the imaging method of choice in these patients. Metastatic disease may also involve the kidney. Actually, it is quite often found at autopsy. With individuals living longer with cancer and the development of new drugs, we will probably see a rise in the number of cases of visible renal metastases. Metastases are most commonly hematogenous and result in usually multiple foci of involvement, although single lesions do occur (Fig. 27–67). They are most frequently seen with CT scanning, as CT is used for the regular follow-up of most cancer patients. Hypodense round masses usually in the periphery are the typical finding. When present as a single lesion, a metastasis cannot be differentiated from a primary renal neoplasm without biopsy.

Cystic renal masses present a vexing problem in that they are not all benign.[244] Cystic renal cell carcinomas occur, as do tumors within the wall of benign cysts. In 1986, Bosniak developed a classification system for cystic masses that has stood the test of time.[196,245,246] It is not a pathologic classification system, but actually an imaging and clinical management guide for handling the cystic renal mass. Category 1 represents simple benign cyst (see Fig. 27–58). Category 2 cysts are benign with thin septa, fine rim-like calcification, and/or uniform high-density cysts less than 3 cm that do not enhance with IV contrast injection on CT (Fig. 27–68). Category 2F was added to deal with a group of lesions falling between category 2 and 3 that need follow-up, usually at 6 to 12 months, to prove benignity (Fig. 27–69).[247] These cystic lesions may have multiple septa, an area of thick or nodular calcification, or a high-density cyst greater than 3 cm. Category 3 cystic lesions have thickened, irregular walls, which demonstrate some enhancement with contrast injection. Dense irregular calcification may also be seen. In these cases,

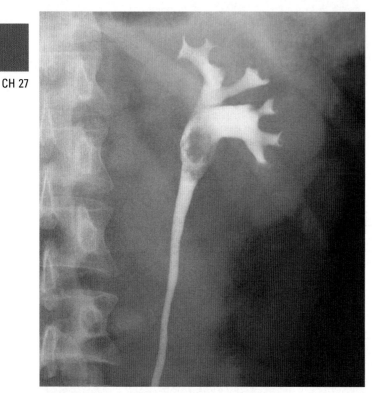

FIGURE 27–66 Transitional cell carcinoma—IVU. The irregular filling defect in the left renal pelvis represents a TCC. Note that there is no significant obstruction of the left kidney with normal appearing calyces.

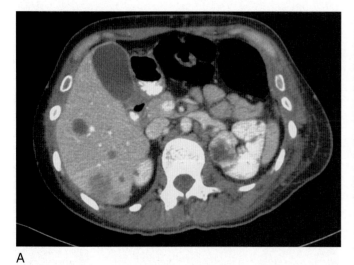

A

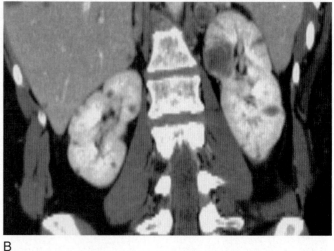

B

FIGURE 27–67 Metastases to the kidney—CT scan. Contrast-enhanced nephrographic phase axial (A) and coronal (B) images. Multiple heterogeneous, but hypodense lesions are seen in the kidneys bilaterally with the largest in the left upper pole. These appeared in a 2-month period in a patient with metastatic lung carcinoma. Note the metastases also present in the liver.

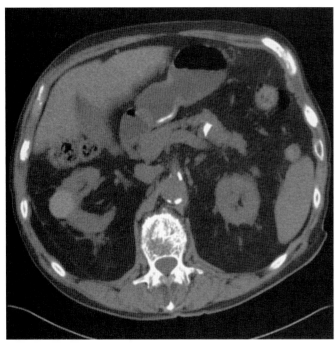

FIGURE 27–68 Hyperdense renal cyst—CT scan. Axial noncontrast CT image. A single well-circumscribed hyperdense mass is seen in the right kidney. This represents a Bosniak type II renal cyst. It is sharply defined, less than 3 cm, and demonstrated no enhancement on the contrast-enhanced scan.

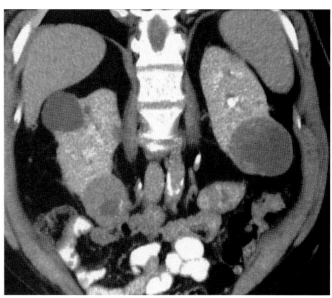

FIGURE 27–70 Bosniak type IV renal cyst—CT scan. Coronal nephrographic phase image. The left kidney shows a cystic mass with an internal solid component in the lower pole. In the lower pole of the right kidney there is a solid mass with central necrosis with represents a RCC. Note the Bosniak type I cysts in the upper pole of the right kidney. There is also a renal calculus in the mid portion of the left kidney. The left lower pole cystic lesion proved to be a RCC—papillary type.

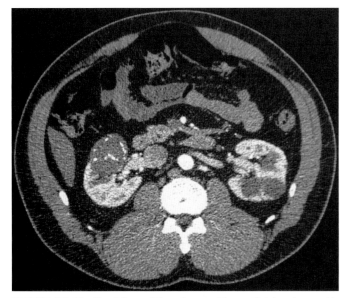

FIGURE 27–69 Bosniak type IIF renal cyst—CT scan. Axial nephrographic phase image. A cystic lesion in the right kidney also demonstrates large clumps of calcification on the outer wall and on internal septae. There was not change in the CT numbers between the noncontrast scan and the enhanced images. This requires follow-up. Note the Bosniak type I cysts in the left kidney.

clinical history may be helpful in pointing toward a renal abscess or infected cyst. Although many of these lesions will be benign, surgery may be necessary for diagnosis and treatment.[248] Biopsy has been advocated by some (see Fig. 27–52).[249–252] Category 4 cystic masses are clearly malignant and demonstrate distinct enhancing soft tissue masses or nodules within the cyst (Fig. 27–70). These lesions require nephrectomy, although if not larger than 5 cm to 6 cm and properly located, a nephron-sparing procedure may be performed.

Cysts are well demonstrated on MRI due to excellent soft tissue contrast. On MR imaging, simple cysts are well circumscribed, thin-walled structures containing fluid that is dark on T1-weighted sequences and bright on T2-weighted sequences (Fig. 27–71). Complex cysts are those that contain signal intensity material that is not characteristic for simple fluid. Complex cysts contain proteinaceous or hemorrhagic fluid and may have septations and calcification. The T1 signal intensity of the fluid is higher than expected for simple fluid, ranging from isointense to hyperintense. T2 signal intensity is lower than expected for simple fluid and may be black depending on the blood content. Cysts do not enhance. When compared to CT, MRI has been found to have a higher contrast resolution allowing for better visualization of septae.[253,254] MRI also better characterizes blood products. MRI is more sensitive to subtle enhancement, especially with subtraction techniques, allowing MRI to surpass CT in differentiating a complex cyst from a cystic neoplasm[253–255] (Figs. 27–72 and 27–73). As with CT, MRI easily demonstrated the cysts of ADPK, AAPKD, and the cysts seen in hereditary disorders, such as chronic kidney injury (Fig. 27–74), ADPCKD (Fig. 27–75), and von Hippel-Lindau (Fig. 27–76). MRI is a noninvasive way to confirm lithium toxicity by demonstrating characteristic parenchymal microcysts, in patients with chronic renal insufficiency who are on long-term lithium therapy.[256]

Differentiating benign masses from malignant masses is not always possible. Oncocytomas and lipid poor angiomyolipomas may have similar characteristics to renal cell cancer. In most cases MRI characteristics are similar to CT and except for AML, most benign lesions cannot be distinguished from malignant lesions. Because angiomyolipomas contain macroscopic fat, MR imaging with fat suppressed and opposed-phase chemical shift sequences can be used to make an accurate diagnosis.[257] Signal intensity of fat is high on both T1- and T2-weighted sequences. Macroscopic fat in AML will drop in signal intensity with fat suppression sequences. Opposed-phase chemical shift sequences causes an "India

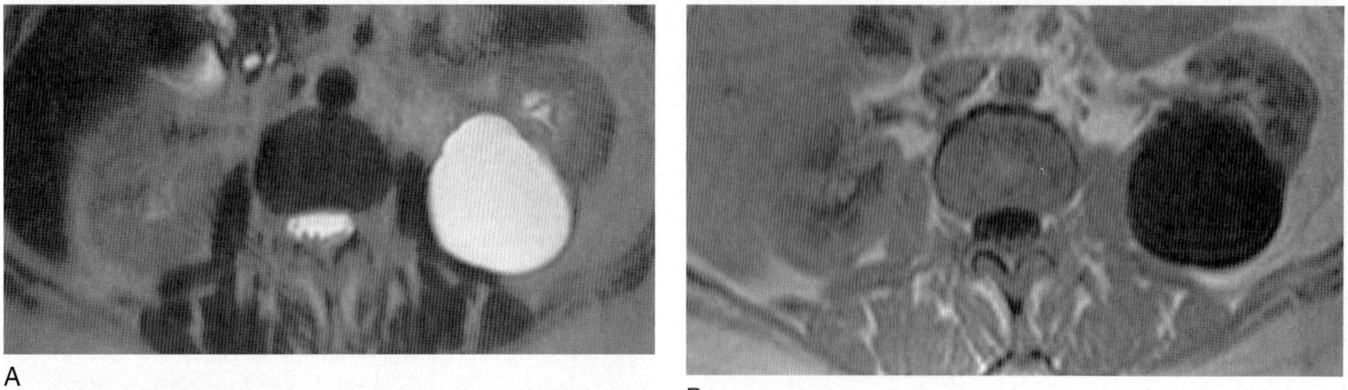

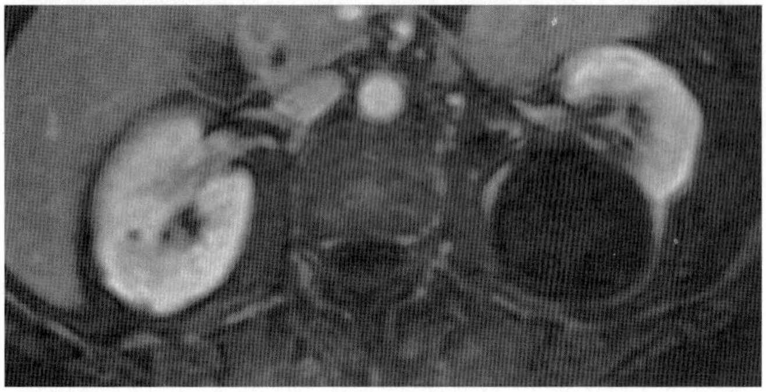

A

B

C

FIGURE 27–71 Simple cysts follow simple fluid signal intensity. **A,** On T2-weighted images cysts are bright and **(B)** on T1-weighted images cysts are dark. **C,** No enhancement is seen on gadolinium-enhanced T1-weighted images.

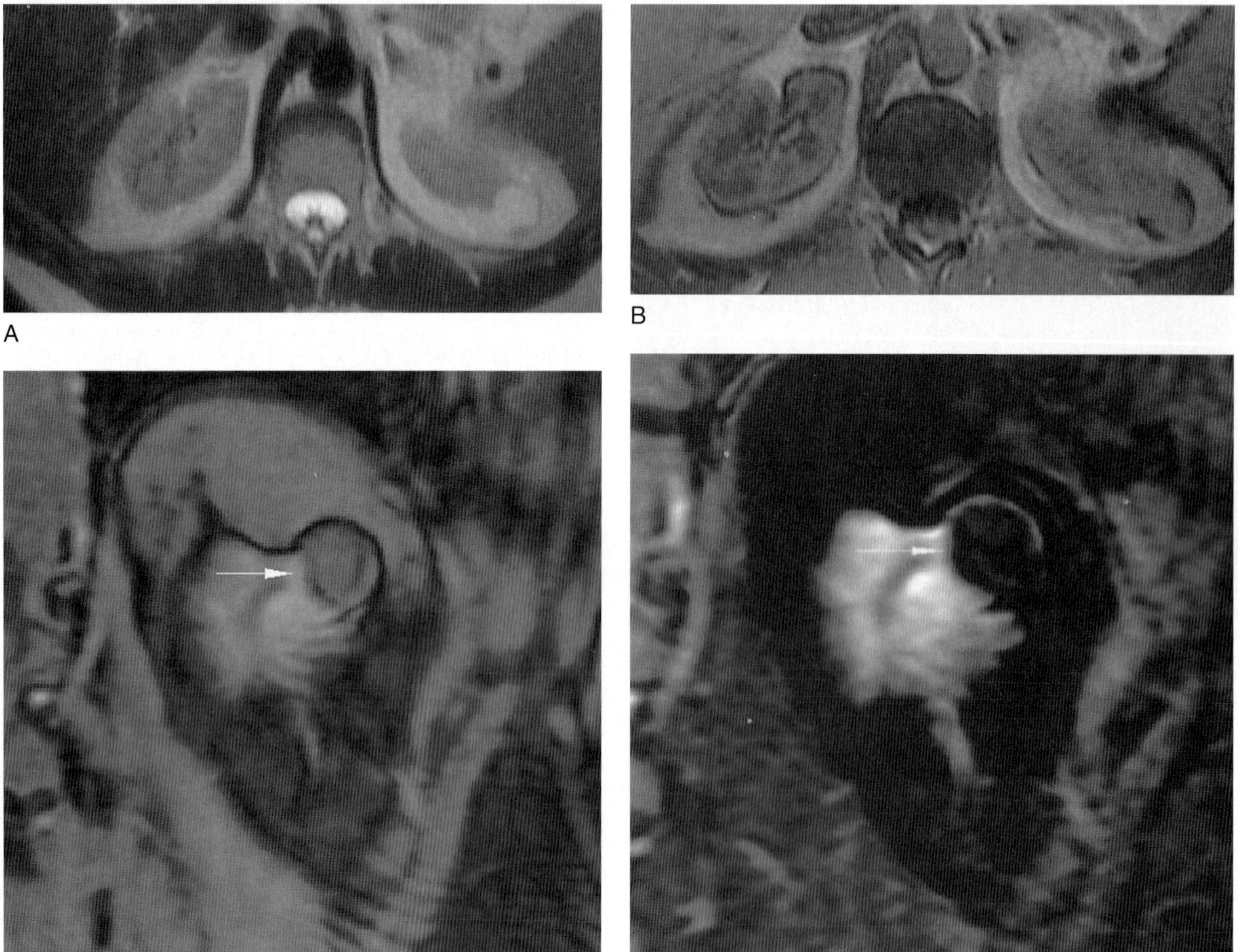

A

B

C

D

FIGURE 27–72 Complex cyst confirmed with image subtraction. **A,** T2-weighted axial image shows a bright left upper pole structure. **B,** T1-weighted axial image shows the same structure as intermediate in signal intensity. Because **(C)** post contrast T1 coronal shows higher signal intensity than expected for a cyst (*arrow*), **(D)** post contrast subtraction images are needed to confirm absence of enhancement (*arrow*).

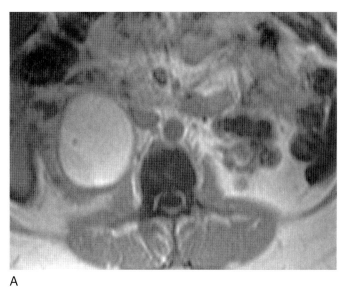

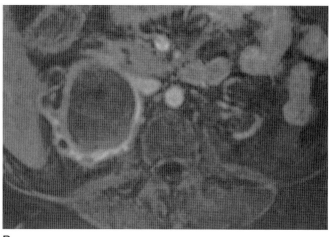

FIGURE 27–73 Complex hemorrhagic cyst. **A,** T1-weighted axial images show a complex right renal structure, bright on both sequences and with internal septations. **B,** There is no enhancement on gadolinium-enhanced T1-weighted images. This was diagnosed as a hemorrhagic cyst with fine needle aspiration.

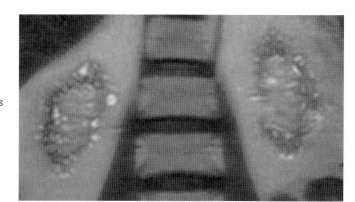

FIGURE 27–74 Chronic kidney injury. T2-weighted coronal image shows diffuse atrophy and multiple cysts in a patient on chronic dialysis.

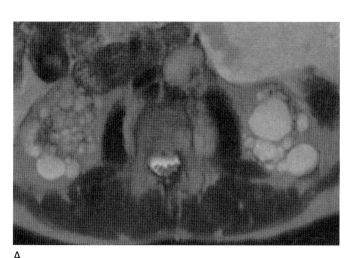

FIGURE 27–75 Autosomal dominant polycystic kidney disease. **A,** Axial and **(C)** coronal T2-weighted images showing bilateral renal cortical atrophy and multiple cysts, most of which are bright. **B,** Axial T1-weighted images with multiple dark structures. These structures do not enhance after gadolinium injection, **(D)** and are therefore consistent with cysts.

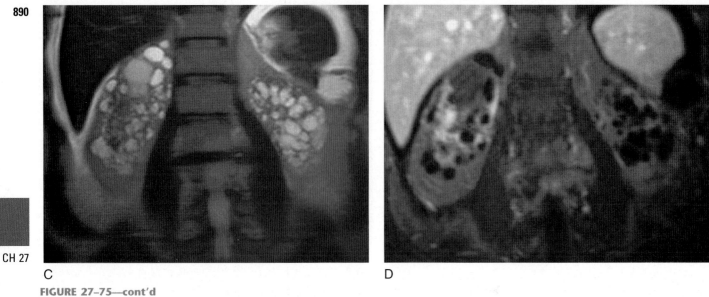

C   D

FIGURE 27–75—cont'd

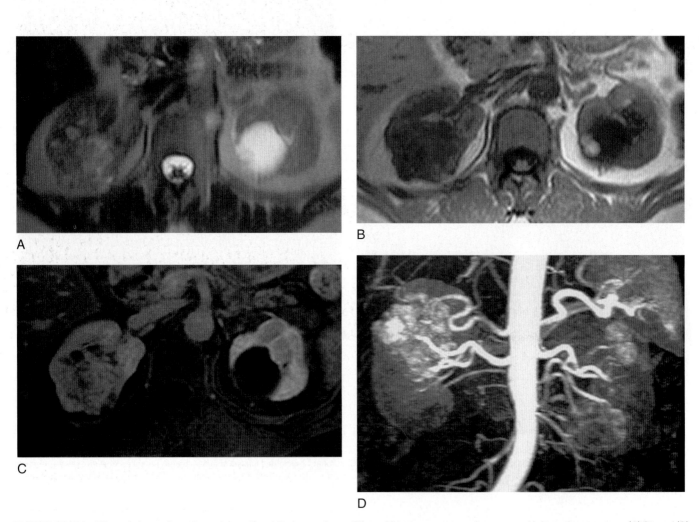

A   B

C   D

FIGURE 27–76 Bilateral clear cell carcinoma in von Hippel-Lindau syndrome. Bilateral heterogeneous renal masses and left renal cyst seen on **(A)** T2- and **(B)** T1-weighted images **(C)** demonstrates heterogeneous enhancement of the larger right renal mass and more homogeneous enhancement of two smaller left renal masses. **D,** Maximum intensity projection presents the multiple renal masses in angiogram format.

ink" outline of the tumor at its interface with normal renal parenchyma. The enhancement pattern of AML is variable and depends on the composition of the lesion.

The MR appearance of renal cell carcinoma (RCC) can be variable because RCC is a neoplasm with many histological types. These include clear cell, which tend to be larger with associated hemorrhage and necrosis (Figs. 27–77 and 27–78), papillary (Fig. 27–79), and chromophobe. RCC most commonly is heterogeneously hyperintense on T2-weighted sequences and hypointense to isointense on T1-weighted sequences (Fig. 27–80). RCC enhances less than normal renal cortex and may be quite heterogeneous. The heterogeneity increases with increasing size due to variable amounts of necrosis and intraluminal lipid. The intraluminal lipid may make areas of the mass drop in signal intensity on opposed phase T1-weighted sequences. Differentiating histological types is difficult due to overlap in their imaging appearance. The feasibility of RCC differentiation using advanced MR imaging techniques such as echoplanar is being evaluated but further research is required.[258]

Although MRI has been found to be highly accurate in staging RCC, the areas of greatest challenge remain the evaluation for local invasion of the perinephric fat and direct invasion of adjacent organs, especially with large tumors.[259] Presence of an intact pseudocapsule aids in excluding local invasion. A pseudocapsule is a hypointense rim around the tumor seen best on T2-weighted images (see Fig. 27–80). These are most frequently seen in association with small or slow-growing tumors. When the tumor extends beyond the confines of the kidney, the pseudocapsule is made of fibrous tissue, otherwise it is made up of compressed normal renal tissue.[260] If the pseudocapsule is intact, invasion of the perinephric fat is unlikely.[260]

CH 27

Diagnostic Kidney Imaging

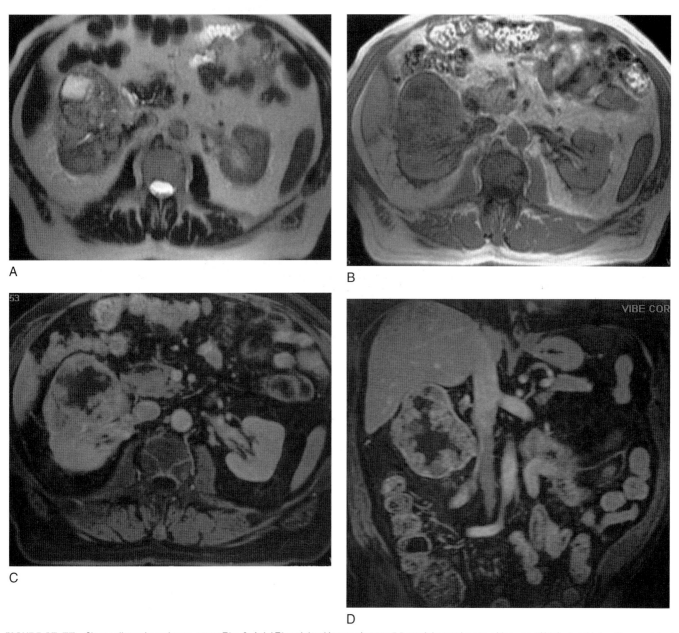

FIGURE 27–77 Clear cell renal carcinoma, stage T3a. **A**, Axial T2-weighted image shows a 7.5 cm right renal mass with areas of high signal intensity, consistent with necrosis and cystic degeneration. **B**, Axial T1-weighted image showing a heterogeneous isointense mass with increased perinephric fat stranding. **C and D**, Axial and coronal gadolinium-enhanced images confirm central areas of necrosis. No venous invasion is seen. Focal microinvasion of the perinephric fat was seen at surgery.

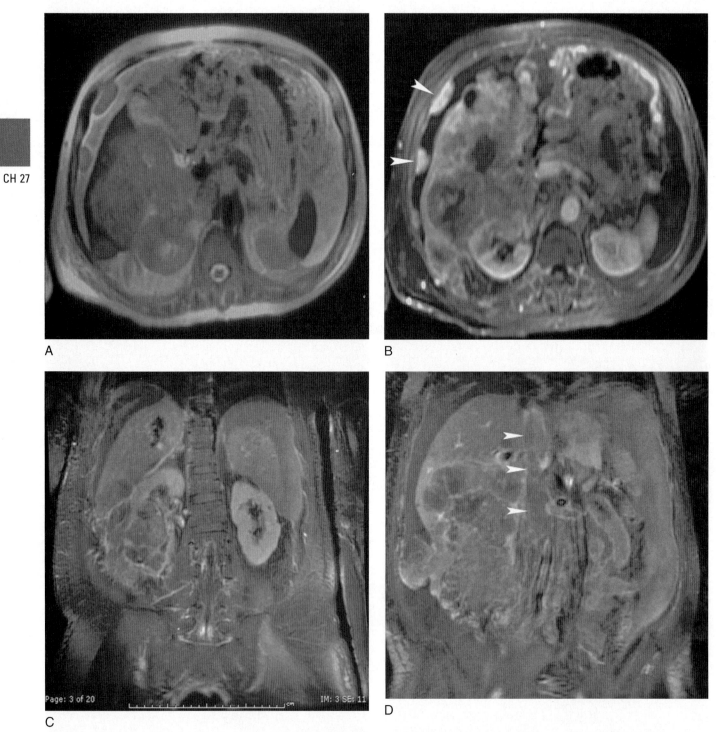

A

B

C

Page: 3 of 20   IM: 3 SE: 11

D

FIGURE 27–78 Metastatic renal cell carcinoma, stage T4N2M1. **A,** Axial T2 and **(B)** gadolinium-enhanced T1-weighted images show a large heterogeneous mass with invasion of the adjacent liver and peritoneal metastases (*arrowheads*). **C and D,** Coronal gadolinium-enhanced T1-weighted images show the large mass extending inferiorly and medially, with invasion of the inferior vena cava to the level of the hepatic veins (*arrowheads*).

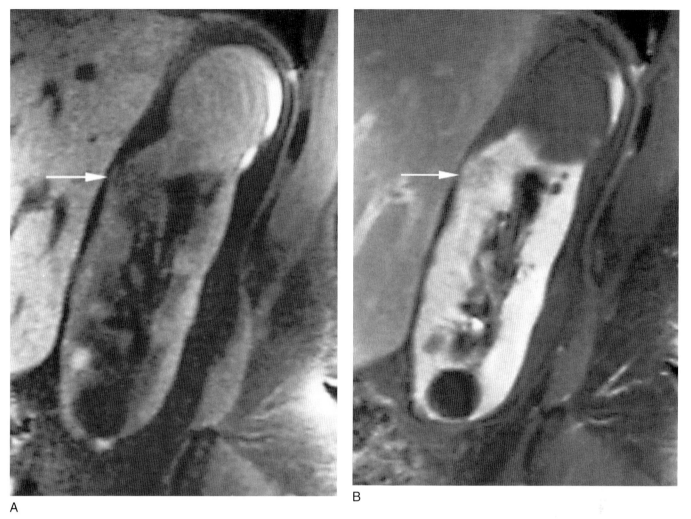

A

B

FIGURE 27-79 Papillary renal cell carcinoma, stage T1. Sagittal T1-weighted images **(A)** before and **(B)** after the administration of gadolinium show a subtle mass (*arrow*) in the anterior cortex and multiple nonenhancing cysts. No perinephric invasion was found at surgery.

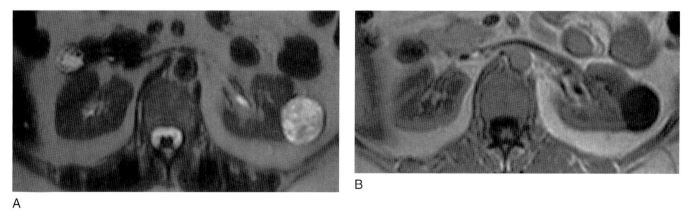

A

B

FIGURE 27-80 Renal cell carcinoma with pseudocapsule, Stage 1. **A,** T2-weighted image shows a heterogeneous, bright mass on the left with a well-defined pseudocapsule. **B,** T1-weighted image confirms a well-defined dark mass involving the left renal cortex.

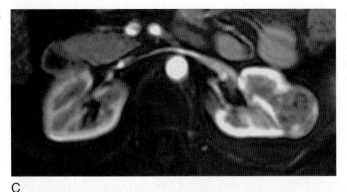

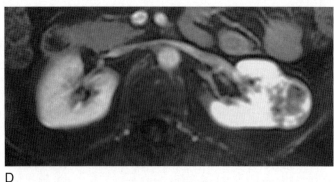

FIGURE 27–80—cont'd **C-E,** Axial gadolinium-enhanced T1-weighted images in the arterial, venous, and excretory phases demonstrate heterogeneous enhancement and no evidence of renal vein involvement. No perinephric invasion was found at surgery.

Detecting and assessing vascular thrombosis in patients with RCC is highly accurate and reliable with contrast-enhanced MR imaging.[259,261] Coronal imaging in the venous and delayed phases demonstrates the presence or absence of venous invasion, determines the extent of venous invasion, if present, and differentiates tumor thrombus, which enhances, from nonenhancing bland thrombus (Fig. 27–81). Accurate determination of renal vein, inferior vena cava, and right atrial involvement is important for deciding the surgical approach.[262]

Because findings of lymphoma are similar to CT, MRI likely will show no additional findings that would affect patient treatment. Lymphoma is typically hypointense on T1-weighted sequences and heterogeneous to slightly hypointense on T2-weighted sequences. Enhancement is minimal on post contrast sequences[263] (Fig. 27–82). Vessels are usually encased, are not invaded, and necrosis is usually not seen. Treated lymphoma may vary in signal intensity, likely secondary to effects of therapy.[263]

Computed tomography urography and MR urography likely will show similar findings. TCC in the upper collecting system can either be a focal, irregular enhancing mass within the collecting system (Fig. 27–83) or an ill-defined mass infiltrating the renal parenchyma. When small, they may be difficult to identify on both CT and MRI. Evaluation of the entire collecting system is required because synchronous lesions may be present. MRU is valuable for complete evaluation of the collecting system.

RENAL CANCER—POSITRON EMISSION TOMOGRAPHY AND POSITRON EMISSION TOMOGRAPHY-COMPUTED TOMOGRAPHY

Renal cell carcinoma (RCC) arises from the renal tubular epithelium and accounts for the majority of the adult kidney tumors. The tumor is angioinvasive and is associated with widespread hematogenous and lymphatic metastases especially to the lung, liver, lymph nodes, bone, and brain. Metastases are present in about 50% of patients at initial presentation. Radical nephrectomy is the main treatment for the early stages of disease, although palliative nephrectomy may also be performed in advanced disease with intractable bleeding. Solitary metastasis may also be resected. RCC responds poorly to chemotherapy. Radiation therapy for RCC is used for palliation of metastatic sites, specifically, bone and brain. Immunotherapy with biologic response modifiers such as interleukin-2 and interferon-α has the most impact on the treatment of metastatic disease. The 5-year survival may be as high as 80% to 90% for early stages of disease whereas advanced disease carries a poor prognosis.[264]

Preliminary studies of PET imaging of RCC have revealed a promising role in the evaluation of indeterminate renal masses, in preoperative staging and assessment of tumor burden, in detection of osseous and non-osseous metastases, in restaging after therapy, and in the determination of effect of imaging findings on clinical management.[265–270] However, other PET studies have demonstrated less enthusiastic results and no advantage over standard imaging methods.[271–273]

A relatively high false-negative rate of 23% has been reported with FDG PET in the preoperative staging of RCC when compared with histological analysis of surgical specimens. In one recent study, PET exhibited a sensitivity of 60% (versus 91.7% for CT) and specificity of 100% (versus 100% for CT) for primary RCC tumors. For retroperitoneal lymph node metastases and/or renal bed recurrence, PET was 75.0% sensitive (versus 92.6% for CT) and 100.0% specific (versus 98.1% for CT). PET had a sensitivity of 75.0% (versus 91.1% for chest CT) and a specificity of 97.1% (versus 73.1% for chest CT) for metastases to the lung parenchyma. PET had a sensitivity of 77.3% and specificity of 100.0% for bone metastases, compared with 93.8% and 87.2% for combined CT and bone scan.[274] For re-staging RCC, a sensitivity of 87% and a specificity of 100% have been reported.[275] A comparative

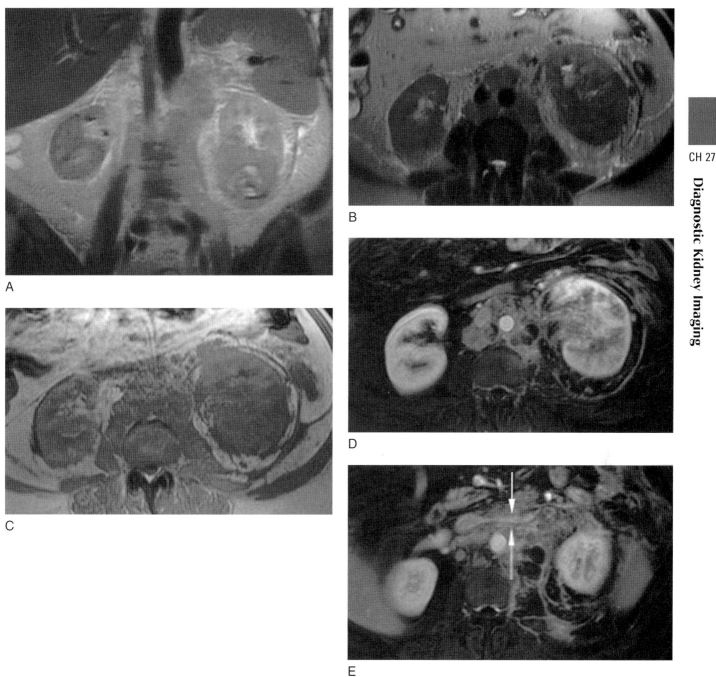

FIGURE 27–81 Poorly differentiated renal cell carcinoma, T4N2. **A and B,** Coronal and axial T2-weighted images show a heterogeneous mass in the lower pole of the left kidney with infiltration of the perinephric fat and extensive retroperitoneal lymphadenopathy. **C,** T1-weighted image shows the masses to be intermediate in signal intensity. **D and E,** axial gadolinium-enhanced T1-weighted images make the local invasion and adenopathy more conspicuous and show that the left renal vein is encased, not invaded (*arrows*).

896

CH 27

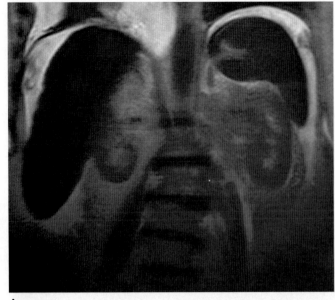

A

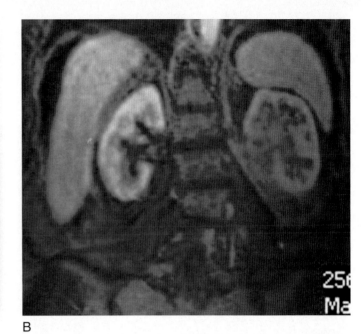

B

256
Ma

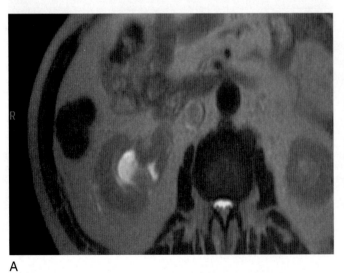

C

FIGURE 27–82 Lymphoma. **A,** Coronal T2-weighted image shows a large, infiltrating left renal mass extending into the perirenal fat. **B,** Coronal gadolinium-enhanced T1-weighted image better delineates the mass from the renal cortex. **C,** Axial gadolinium-enhanced T1-weighted image shows encasement of the left renal vein (*arrows*).

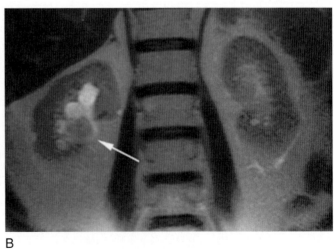

A

B

FIGURE 27–83 Transitional cell carcinoma. **(A)** Axial and **(B)** coronal T2-weighted images showing intermediate signal intensity masses (*arrow*) within the right renal pelvis associated with mild hydronephrosis.

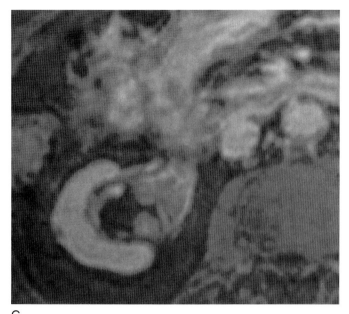

C

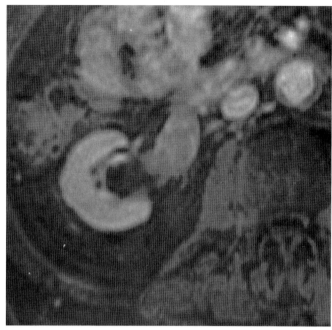

D

FIGURE 27–83—cont'd **C and D,** Axial gadolinium-enhanced T1-weighted images show heterogeneous enhancement and no evidence of invasion of the renal parenchyma.

investigation of bone scan and FDG PET for detecting osseous metastases in RCC revealed sensitivity and specificity of 77.5% and 59.6% for bone scan and 100% and 100% for PET, respectively.[270] Another report revealed a negative predictive value of 33% and positive predictive value of 94% for restaging RCC.[266] Other studies have reported high accuracy in characterizing indeterminate renal masses with a mean tumor-to-kidney uptake ratio of 3.0 for malignancy.[265]

These mixed observations are probably related to the heterogeneous expression of glucose transporter-1 (GLUT-1) in RCC, which may not correlate with the tumor grade or extent.[276,277] A negative study may not exclude disease whereas a positive study is highly suspicious for malignancy. If the tumor is FDG avid, then PET can be a reasonable imaging modality for follow-up after treatment and for surveillance (Fig. 27–84). In fact, it has been shown that FDG PET can alter clinical management in up to 40% of patients with suspicious locally recurrent and metastatic renal cancer.[268]

The diagnostic accuracy of FDG PET appears not to be improved by semi-quantitative image analysis, which is probably due to the fundamental variability of glucometabolism in RCC.[273] In one study, the maximum and average standardized uptake values (SUVs) for FDG-positive primary renal malignant tumors were 7.9 +/− 4.9 and 6.0 +/− 3.6, respectively. The maximum and average SUVs of metastatic renal masses were 6.1 +/− 3.4 and 4.7 +/− 2.8, respectively. There was no significant difference in maximum and average SUVs between primary and metastatic renal masses.[278] Because FDG is excreted in the urine, the intense urine activity may confound lesion detection in and near the renal bed. Intravenous administration of furosemide has been proposed to improve urine clearance from the renal collecting system although the exact benefit of such intervention in improving lesion detection remains undefined.

Other PET tracers (e.g., 11C-acetate, 18F-fluoromisonidazole) have been investigated in the imaging evaluation of patients with RCC but further studies are needed to establish the exact role of these and other non-FDG tracers in this clinical setting.[279,280] Moreover, many studies have now reported on the diagnostic synergism of the combined PET-CT imaging systems. The role of PET-CT in renal cancer imaging and its impact on both the short-term and the long-term clinical management and decision making will also need to be investigated.

RENAL VASCULAR DISEASE

Renal artery stenosis is a potential treatable cause of hypertension but is found in less than 5% of the hypertensive population.[281] When the expected signs and symptoms are present, the diagnosis may be made in 20% to 30% of patients.[282] RAS is usually defined as 50% or greater stenosis of the renal artery.[283] Atherosclerosis is the most common cause accounting for up to 70% of cases and is typically found in males over 50 years of age. The stenosis is caused by an atherosclerotic plaque with or without calcification located in the proximal renal artery at or near the ostia (Fig. 27–85).[284] It is bilateral in 30% of cases. Fibromuscular dysplasia is the second most common cause—approximately 25%.[285] Fibromuscular dysplasia is sub-classified by the location of the involvement within the vessel wall with medial fibroplasia being the most common. This form has the classic findings of the string of beads in the distal main renal artery and segmental branches caused by the alternating areas of stenosis and dilatation.

The IVU is of only historical note in the assessment of patients with renovascular hypertension. The hypertensive IVU was performed by obtaining a series of radiographs of the kidneys after the injection of contrast at 1-minute intervals looking for discrepancies in renal size, appearance of the nephrogram, prolongation of the nephrogram, and excretion patterns. This study is no longer performed because it has been supplanted by Doppler US, CT and MRI angiography, and captopril renography.[286,287]

Conventional US and Doppler US have been used to assess patients with renovascular hypertension.[288] Renal size and the presence or absence of medical renal disease may be evaluated with grey-scale ultrasound. Doppler ultrasound has been employed to assess the main renal arteries for renal

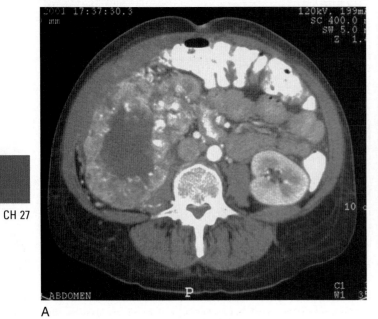

A

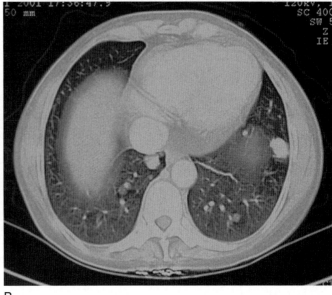

B

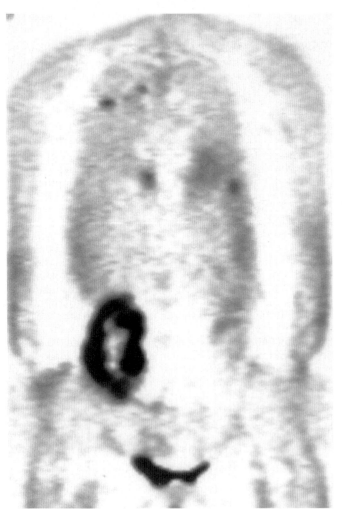

C

FIGURE 27–84 Renal cell carcinoma. CT shows a large necrotic renal mass **(A)** with several bilateral pulmonary nodules **(B)**. The PET scan **(C)** shows hypermetabolism at the periphery of the large renal mass and within the pulmonary nodules. The interior hypometabolism of the renal mass is compatible with central tumor necrosis.

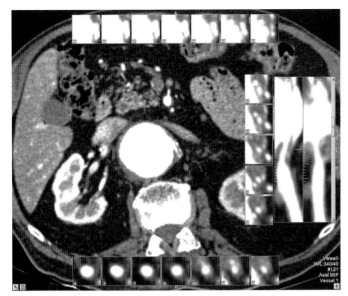

FIGURE 27-85   Renal artery stenosis—CT angiogram. Axial CT image with vessel analysis. The origin of the left renal artery is markedly narrowed by calcified and non-calcified atherosclerotic plaque. The vessel analysis demonstrates the renal artery in cross section for accurate calculation of the degree of stenosis—greater than 70% in this case.

artery stenosis and the intrarenal vasculature for secondary effects with variable success.[289,290] Doppler ultrasound is highly operator dependent and may be inadequate or incomplete due to overlying bowel gas, body habitus, or aortic pulsatility.[289] A stable Doppler signal may be difficult to reproduce in some patients. A complete examination has been possible in 50% to 90% of patients. Accessory renal arteries, which occur in 15% to 20% of patients may not be imaged.[291] The criteria used for evaluation of the main renal artery include an increase in the peak systolic velocity to greater than 185 cm/sec, a renal to aortic ratio of peak systolic velocity of greater than 3.0, and turbulent flow beyond the region of the stenosis.[292] Visualization of the main renal artery with no detectable Doppler signal would suggest renal artery occlusion. Intrarenal Doppler ultrasound vascular assessment has looked at the shape and character of the waveform. A dampened appearance to the waveform with a slowed systolic upstroke and delay to peak velocity, tardus-parvus effect, has shown variable results in renal artery stenosis.[293] A difference in the resistive indices of greater than 5% between the kidneys has also been suggestive of renal artery stenosis. Sensitivity and specificity for the techniques have generally been in the 50% to 70% range. Contrast-enhanced ultrasound has been suggested as a means to improve the accuracy of Doppler ultrasound.[294,295]

Computed tomography angiography performed with a multidetector CT (MDCT) scanner has sensitivity and specificity at or near 100% (see Fig. 27–85).[296–298] A normal result should rule out renal artery stenosis.[299] This study is performed with a contrast injection of 4 to 5 cc/sec, volume of contrast of 100 to 120 cc, and rapid scanning at 15 to 20 seconds for proper assessment of the renal arteries. The angiographic study takes less than 10 seconds to complete.[296] Computer processing of images is imperative with 3D volume renderings and maximum intensity projection (MIP) images required (Figs. 27–86 and 27–87).[299–301] Assessment of the axial images alone is insufficient. The main renal artery as well as its segmental braches can be viewed and evaluated. Accessory renal arteries down to 1 mm in diameter can be seen.[302] CTA may also demonstrate other findings in the patient with RAS including a smaller kidney with a smooth

contour, thinning of the cortex, a delayed or prolonged nephrogram—all on the affected side. Patients with renal artery stents can be successfully imaged with CTA (Fig. 27–88).[303,304] CTA and MRA are equivalent in the detection of hemodynamically significant renal artery stenosis.[305] Patients with impaired renal function or contrast allergy will need evaluation with MRA as a CTA with iodinated contrast cannot be done. Digital subtraction angiography should be reserved for those patients requiring an intervention, either angioplasty or angioplasty and stent placement. It is unnecessary for diagnosis today.

Ultrasound, CTA, and MRA have been shown to be accurate alternatives to conventional angiography.[306,307] Because CTA is sensitive, accurate, fast, and reproducible, MRA is reserved for patients for whom iodinated contrast is contraindicated. Renal insufficiency is not uncommon in the population clinically selected for high risk of renal artery stenosis. For this reason CE-MRA is widely accepted as a reliable and accurate examination for the evaluation of renal artery stenosis in this patient group.[88,305,308,309] Like CTA, MRA is noninvasive and provides excellent visualization of the aortoiliac and renal arteries.[305]

Contrast-enhanced–MRA has over 95% sensitivity for demonstrating the main renal arteries and has a high negative predictive value. A normal CE-MRA almost completely excludes a stenosis in the visualized vessels.[307] CE-MRA is a reliable examination but has been limited by incomplete visualization of segmental and small accessory vessels.[310] Whereas visualization of all accessory vessels is desired, Bude and colleagues[311] found isolated hemodynamically significant stenosis of an accessory artery in only 1.5% of their patients (1 of 68). The authors concluded that this limitation does not substantially reduce the rate of detection of renovascular hypertension by MRI. With the use of 3D reconstruction, studies have demonstrated no significant difference between CE-MRA and multidetector CTA in the detection of hemodynamically significant renal artery stenosis.[305] Volume rendering and multiplanar reformatting improve accuracy in depicting renal artery stenosis.[87] Volume rendering increases the positive predictive value of CE-MRA by reducing the overestimation of stenosis found with earlier reconstruction techniques (Fig. 27–89).[88,307] Volume rendering has better correlation with digital subtraction angiography and improves delineation of the renal arteries.[88]

Limitations of MRA are due in part to limitations in resolution and motion artifacts.[306,312] Advancements in MR gradient strengths and newer MRA techniques are resulting in continued improvement in image resolution and reduction in motion artifacts, while reducing imaging times.[312] Work with cardiac imaging has demonstrated that imaging at 3T can result in higher spatial and temporal resolution, when compared with imaging at 1.5T. This higher resolution was found to improve the evaluation of smaller structures of the heart.[313] Further evaluation is needed to determine how imaging at 3T will affect MRA of the renal arteries.[314]

Phase contrast MRA can be used to calculate blood flow through the renal artery.[315] Phase contrast flow curves can be generated and the severity of the hemodynamic abnormalities can be graded as normal, low-grade, moderate, and high-grade stenosis. This is similar to the Doppler ultrasound method. Grading can be used to evaluate the hemodynamic significance of a detected stenosis.[316] The significance of a stenosis on parenchymal function, however, is not currently evaluated by conventional MRA. Initial renal MR imaging perfusion studies are being performed to grade the effect of renal artery stenosis on parenchymal perfusion. Initial results show that MRI perfusion measurements with high spatial and temporal resolution reflect renal function as measured with serum creatinine.[317] Volumetric analysis of functional renal cortical tissue may also give clinically useful information in

A

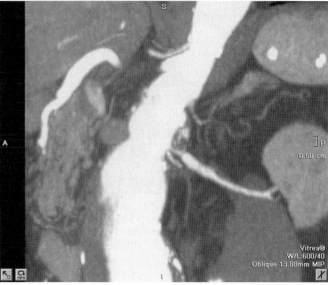

B

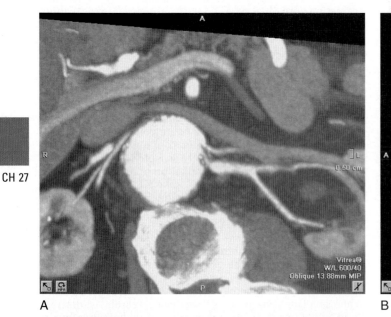

C

FIGURE 27–86 Renal artery stenosis—CT angiogram. Image processing applied to case in Figure 27–53. Axial **(A)** and coronal **(B)** slab MIP images demonstrate the atherosclerotic stenosis of the proximal renal artery. Note the accessory renal artery arising adjacent to the left main renal artery. Volume rendering of the CT angiogram **(C)** results in this 3D display, which may be rotated for best viewing and analysis.

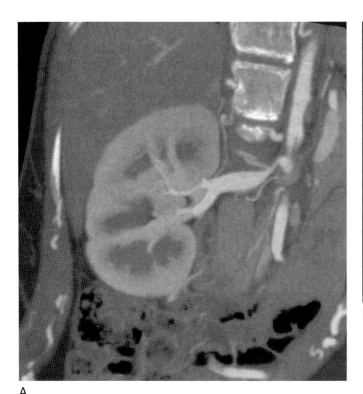

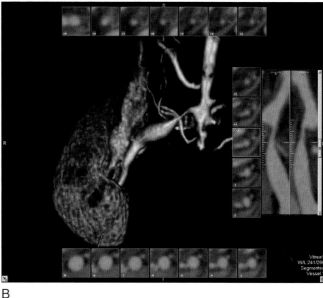

A

B

FIGURE 27–87   Renal artery stenosis—CT angiogram. Image progressing of abdominal CT angiogram. Coronal slab MIP (**A**) demonstrates the smooth narrowing of the proximal right renal artery in this patient with Takayasu arteritis. Note the markedly abnormal aorta with occlusion distal to the origin of the renal artery. Volume rendering (**B**) of the CT angiogram with vessel analysis reveals the 80% stenosis of the right renal artery. The left renal artery had been occluded previously and the kidney was supplied by collateral vessels.

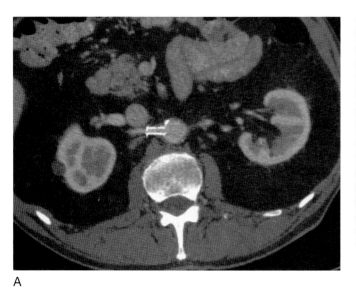

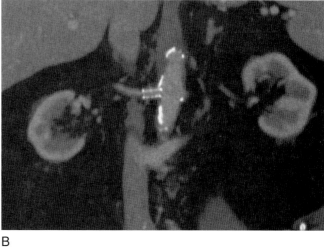

A

B

FIGURE 27–88   Renal artery stent—CT scan. Axial (**A**) and coronal (**B**) images of a contrast-enhanced CT scan in the corticomedullary phase. The metallic stent is seen at the origin of the right renal artery. It had been placed for treatment of renal artery stenosis due to atherosclerosis. Good flow through the stent is seen as contrast fills the lumen.

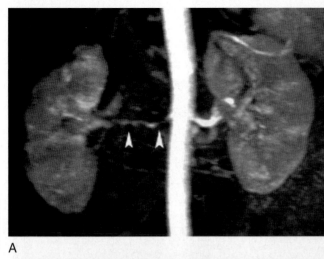

A

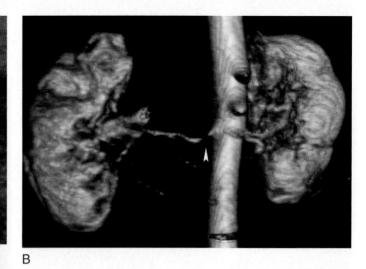

B

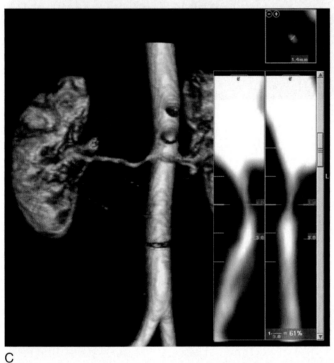

C

FIGURE 27–89 Renal artery stenosis. Advancements in post processing allow for more accurate evaluation of stenosis with MR angiography. **A,** Maximum intensity projection shows a high-grade stenosis near the renal artery origin with areas of apparent narrowing in the mid renal artery (*arrowheads*), mimicking fibromuscular dysplasia. **B,** Volume image show the proximal stenosis (*arrowhead*), but the mid artery is more normal in appearance. **C,** Image showing the artery in 2D allows measurement of the proximal stenosis and demonstrated a normal mid artery. This stenosis was confirmed with angiography.

patients with renal artery stenosis.[318] Further research is required before this will be known, however.

Magnetic resonance angiography is currently of limited value for the evaluation of restenosis in patients with renal artery stents. Although stent technology is rapidly changing, metal artifact still obscures the stent lumen to varying degrees due to susceptibility artifacts (Fig. 27–90). Phase-contrast MRA may be used to measure velocities proximal and distal to the stent, but this is an indirect approach to evaluating for stenosis. Work is being done to develop a metallic renal artery MR imaging stent that will allow for lumen visualization; however, this is not currently available clinically.[319]

Fibromuscular dysplasia (FMD) has a characteristic appearance of focal narrowing and dilatation ("string of beads") (Fig. 27–91). Because FMD frequently involves the mid to distal renal artery and segmental branches, resolution limits MRA evaluation. For this reason, MRA is not as reliable for diagnosis of FMD as it is for RAS. Renal infarctions are well demonstrated on MRA as wedge-shaped areas of decreased parenchymal enhancement. These are most conspicuous on the nephrographic phase. Evaluation of the arterial and venous structures may demonstrate the origin of the emboli or thrombosis (Fig. 27–92).

NUCLEAR IMAGING AND RENOVASCULAR DISEASE

Angiotensin converting enzyme (ACE) inhibition prevents conversion of angiotensin I to angiotensin II. In renal artery stenosis, angiotensin II constricts the efferent arterioles as a compensatory mechanism to maintain GFR despite diminished afferent renal blood flow. Therefore, ACE inhibition in renal artery stenosis reduces GFR by interfering with the compensatory mechanism. Captopril renography has been successful in evaluating patients with renal artery stenosis.

Before the study, the patient should be well hydrated. ACE inhibitors should be discontinued (captopril for 2 days; enalapril or lisinopril for 4 to 5 days) because otherwise

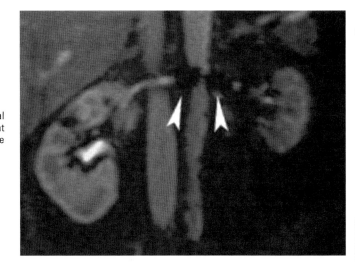

FIGURE 27–90 Magnetic resonance angiography in a patient with bilateral renal artery stents (*arrowheads*). The metal in the stent causes artifact that obscures the vessel lumen. Contrast is seen beyond the stent indicating that there is no complete occlusion.

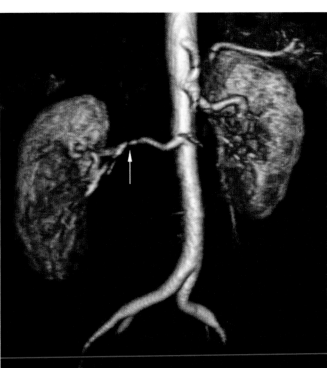

A

B

FIGURE 27–91 **A and B,** MR angiography with volume reconstruction demonstrates a subtle irregularity in the mid right renal artery (*arrow*). Fibromuscular dysplasia was confirmed with conventional angiography.

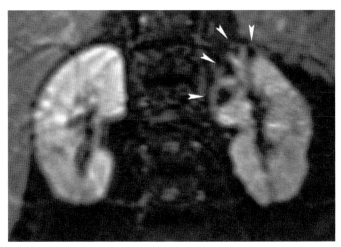

A

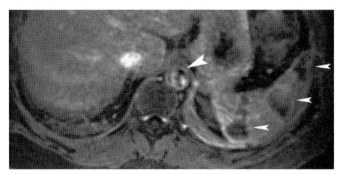

B

FIGURE 27–92 Renal infarcts due to embolic disease. **A,** Coronal gadolinium-enhanced T1-weighted image shows wedge-shaped cortical areas of absent enhancement (*arrowheads*). **B,** Axial gadolinium-enhanced T1-weighted image shows an irregular filling defect in the aorta (large arrowhead) consistent with thrombus, and three focal defects in the spleen (small arrowheads) consistent with splenic infarcts.

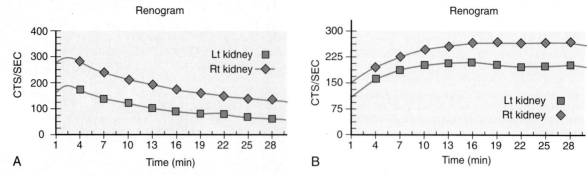

FIGURE 27–93 Tc-99m MAG3 renograms before (**A**) and after (**B**) ACE inhibition with captopril. Note the relatively normal renograms in **A** and the reduced initial slope, delayed time to peak activity, and plateau compatible with captopril-induced cortical tracer retention in **B**. These findings suggest a high probability for hemodynamically significant bilateral renal artery stenosis that is more severe on the left side (connected squares) than the right side (connected diamonds). Bilateral renal artery stenosis was later confirmed with angiography. (Adapted from Saremi F, Jadvar H, Siegel M: Pharmacologic interventions in nuclear radiology: Indications, imaging protocols, and clinical results. Radiographics 22:447–490, 2002.)

diagnostic sensitivity may be reduced. Diuretics should be discontinued preferably for 1 week. Dehydration resulting from diuretics may potentiate the effect of captopril and contribute to hypotension. Captopril (25 mg to 50 mg) crushed and dissolved in 250 mL water is administered orally followed by blood pressure monitoring every 15 minutes for 1 hour. Alternatively, enalaprilat (40 μg/kg up to 2.5 mg) is administered intravenously over 3 to 5 minutes. A baseline scan can be performed before captopril renography (1-day protocol) or the next day, only if captopril study is abnormal (2-day protocol).

The affected kidney in renovascular hypertension (RVH) often has a renogram curve with reduced initial slope, a delayed time to peak activity, prolonged cortical retention, and a slow downslope following peak (Fig. 27–93). These findings are due to slowed renal tracer transit owing to increased solute and water retention in response to ACE inhibition. Reduced urine flow causes delayed and decreased tracer washout into the collecting system in Tc-99m MAG3 and I-131 OIH studies. Tc-99m DTPA demonstrates reduced uptake on the affected side.[320]

Consensus reports regarding methods and interpretation of ACE renography elaborate on a scoring system of renogram curves.[321–323] It has been recommended that high (>90%), intermediate (10% to 90%), and low (<10%) probability categories be applied to captopril renography based on change of renogram curve score between baseline and post-captopril renograms. Among quantitative measurements, relative renal function, the time to peak activity, and the ratio of 20-minute renal activity to peak activity (20/peak) are used more commonly than other parameters. For MAG3 renal scintigraphy, a 10% change in relative renal function, peak activity increase of 2 minutes or more, and a parenchymal increase in 20/peak post captopril by 0.15 represent a high probability of renovascular hypertension.[324]

Captopril renography has a sensitivity of 80% to 95% and a specificity of 50%; the detection of stenosis by captopril-stimulated renography may be more complicated.[320] It is more the exception than the rule for bilateral renovascular stenosis to have symmetric findings on captopril renography. Studies in canine model with bilateral renal artery stenosis demonstrated that captopril produced striking changes in the time-activity curve of each kidney, which are more pronounced in the more severely stenotic kidney.[320]

RENAL VEIN THROMBOSIS

Renal vein thrombosis is usually clinically unsuspected. It is found in patients with a hypercoagulable state, underlying renal disease, or both.[325] The classic presentation of acute RVT with gross hematuria, flank pain, and decreasing renal function is uncommon.[326] Nephrotic syndrome is a common mode of presentation.[327] Two thirds of patient will present with minimal or no symptoms. In one study, 22% of patients with nephrotic syndrome were found to have RVT, usually chronic and asymptomatic; 60% of these patients had membranous glomemlonephritis.[327] Other etiologies include collagen vascular diseases, diabetic nephropathy, trauma, and tumor thrombus. Renal venography has been the definitive method of diagnosis in the past, but other methods of evaluation including Doppler US, CT, and MR have supplemented it.

The IVU is nonspecific in the diagnosis of RVT and is no longer employed. It may be normal in more than 25% of cases. With grey-scale and Doppler US the involved kidney appears enlarged and swollen with relative hypoechogenicity when compared with the normal size.[326] The finding of a filling defect in the renal vein is both sensitive and specific for diagnosis and is the only convincing sign of RVT. The lack of flow on Doppler US, however, is a nonspecific finding and is frequently due to a technically limited study. Absence or reversal of the diastolic waveform with Doppler US should not be used to suggest RVT.

A contrast-enhanced CT study is needed to properly assess the patient with suspected renal vein thrombosis. If there is renal function impairment MRI must be employed. CT findings include an enlarged renal vein with a low attenuating filling defect representing the clot within the renal vein.[328] There may be abnormal parenchymal enhancement with prolonged corticomedullary differentiation and a delay or persistent nephrogram. The kidney will appear to be enlarged with edema in the renal sinus. There may be stranding and thickening of Gerota's fascia. A striated nephrogram may occasionally be seen. Attenuation of the pelvicalyceal system may occur due to edema. Delayed appearance or absence of the pelvicalyceal system altogether may also be seen. Within chronic RVT, the RV may be attenuated or narrowed due to clot retraction and peri-capsular collateral veins may be noted. There is an increased risk of pulmonary emboli in these patients as well. With renal and rarely adrenal tumors, there may be thrombus that develops in the RV with extension to the IVC. Inhomogeneous enhancement of the thrombus suggests direct tumor involvement, not a bland thrombus.

The appearance of renal vein thrombosis on non contrast-enhanced MRI is variable. If the thrombosis is acute, the renal vein will be distended, no normal flow void is seen, and the affected kidney will be enlarged. Renal infarction may also be present. If the thrombosis is chronic, the renal vein will be small and difficult to see. The vein will contain a non-enhancing filling defect on contrast-enhanced MR venography consistent with thrombus. Enhancement of the thrombus is characteristic of tumor.

■ RENAL TRANSPLANTATION ASSESSMENT

The treatment of choice for patients with end-stage renal disease is renal transplantation. Although there has been significant improvement in continuous peritoneal dialysis and hemodialysis, patient survival is longer and overall quality of life is better after renal transplantation. Radiological evaluation is performed on the renal transplant donor and in the post-operative assessment of the transplant recipient. Although IVU and angiography were used in the past, US, CT, MRI, and renal scintigraphy are the current methods employed in these patients (Fig. 27–94).[329-331]

A comprehensive radiological assessment of the living renal transplant donor is crucial.[332] The anatomic information that is necessary is vascular, parenchymal, and pelvocalyceal. The renal artery must be visualized for number, length, location, and branching pattern. The parenchyma must be evaluated for scars, overall volume, renal masses, and calculi. The venous anatomy must be seen and the number of veins, anatomic variants, and significant systemic tributaries noted. The pelvocalyceal system must be scrutinized for anomalies such as duplication and papillary necrosis. As a choice exists for the type of nephrectomy, laparoscopic or open, complete and accurate information is necessary. The limited field of view with laparoscopic nephrectomy requires this information for a safe procedure.[333-336]

With the development of multidetector CT (MDCT) scanners, the complete evaluation of the living renal transplant donor is possible.[333,337,338] A non-contrast low-dose CT scan is performed just to search for renal stones, locate the kidneys, and identify renal masses (see Fig. 27–9). Arterial phase scanning is generally performed at 15 to 25 seconds to demonstrate the main renal artery, branching pattern of the artery, and abnormalities such as atherosclerotic plaques or fibromuscular dysplasia (see Fig. 27–11); 25% to 40% of patients have accessory renal arteries and 10% have early branching patterns in the main renal artery.[334,336] The transplant surgeon requires a main renal artery free of branching for the first 15 mm to 20 mm. Due to the rapid transit of contrast through the kidney, most renal veins are well seen in this phase also (see Fig. 27–10). Venous variants occur in 15% to 28% of patients with multiple renal veins being most common, especially in the right. On the left side 8% to 15% have a circumaortic renal vein and 1% to 3% a retroaortic vein.[336,339] Venous tributaries are also important to visualize including the gonadal, left adrenal, and lumbar veins. These are best seen on the nephrographic phase.[334,335] This phase is performed at 80 to 120 seconds after injection and is used to evaluate the cortex and medulla for scars and masses (see Fig. 27–12). Excretory phase imaging is performed with a CT scan, CT digital radiograph, or plain films to note the pelvocalyceal system for anomalies or abnormalities (see Figs. 27–13 and 27–14). CT has demonstrated accuracy of 91% to 97% for arterial phase imaging, 93% to 100% for the venous phase, and 99% for the pelvocalyceal system.[338,340,341] Similar results have been noted for MRI with the biggest discrepancy being found in imaging accessory renal arteries.[342,343] The lack of ionizing radiation and iodinated contrast will make MRI attractive in the future. Most centers today use CT in the evaluation of living renal transplant donors.

Magnetic resonance imaging, MRA, and MRU can be combined into one examination for the evaluation of the renal transplant donor.[344] MRI and CT are comparable for the evaluation of renal vasculature, morphology, and function. In order to avoid radiation exposure and nephrotoxicity, MRI may be chosen over CT for pre-operative evaluation.

Quantification of functional renal volume with MRA has been demonstrated to be feasible in healthy renal donors by determining the cortical volume.[345] The hypothesis supported by Van den Dool and colleagues was that glomerular filtration is an important component of renal function, and because the majority of glomeruli are in the cortex, there should be good correlation between renal function and cortical volume. Further research is required to confirm the authors' findings, however.

After surgically successful renal transplantation, radiological evaluation is frequently necessary. Conventional sonography, Doppler US, CT, MRI, and renal scintigraphy are used in various settings. Ultrasound assumes the primary role for assessing patients with changes in serum creatinine, urine output, pain, or hematuria.[346] It is also used to direct renal biopsy. Doppler US is used to evaluate renal perfusion, the patency of the renal artery and venous, and the integrity of the vascular anastomoses.[347] CT, MRI, and renal scintigraphy are adjunctive studies.

Conventional grey-scale ultrasound is essential to assess for transplant obstruction and peritransplant fluid collections.[331] Conventional sonography yields nonspecific findings in ATN and acute rejection including obliteration of the corticomedullary junction, prominent swollen pyramids, and loss of the renal sinus echoes.[330,332] All these findings indicate edema of the transplant, which leads to increased peripheral vascular resistance, decreased diastolic perfusion, and elevation of the resistive index (>0.80) (Fig. 27–95).[334] Chronic rejection

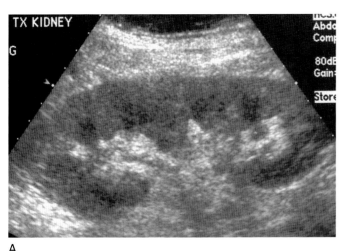

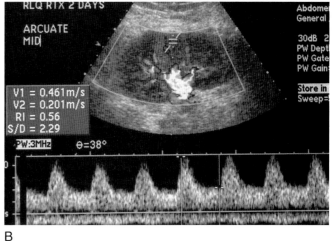

FIGURE 27–94   Normal renal transplant—ultrasound. Coronal image **(A)** of a recently transplanted kidney in the right lower quadrant. The central echo complex, medullary pyramids, and cortex are well seen. The duplex Doppler **(B)** image demonstrates normal flow to the transplant with a normal resistive index of 0.56.

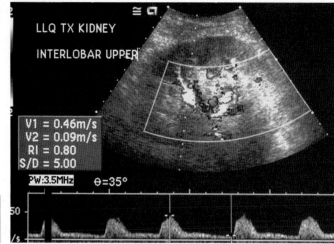

FIGURE 27–95 Renal transplant with ATN—ultrasound. Duplex Doppler image of the transplanted kidney shows a normal size and normal appearing kidney with a high resistive index of 0.80 in the interlobar artery. The patient recovered with return of normal renal function in 5 days.

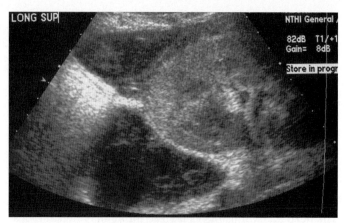

FIGURE 27–96 Renal transplant with hematoma—ultrasound. Longitudinal image of the upper aspect of the transplanted kidney shows two hypoechoic collections adjacent to the kidney. The heterogeneous hypoechoic nature of the collections suggests that they represent hematomas as opposed to urinomas or lymphoceles, which generally would be anechoic.

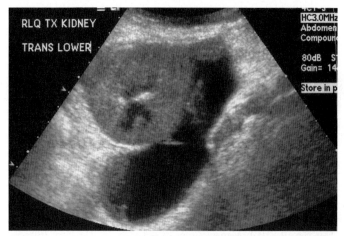

FIGURE 27–97 Renal transplant with urinoma—ultrasound. Transverse image through the lower aspect of the transplanted kidney reveals a normal appearing kidney with a large anechoic fluid collection adjacent to it. This was aspirated under ultrasound guidance leading to the diagnosis of urinoma. The patient was treated with catheter placement and drainage also performed with ultrasound guidance.

may lead to a kidney with diffusely increased echogenicity throughout.

Doppler US adds valuable information pertaining to the integrity of the vascular elements. Despite early enthusiasm with the ability of Doppler US to differentiate acute transplant rejection from acute tubular necrosis, it is now known that the findings are nonspecific and cannot obviate the need for renal biopsy in these cases.[348] Both ATN and acute rejection can cause increased peripheral vascular resistance.[349,350] A significant number of patients with acute rejection have a normal resistive index (<0.80). It is now known that vascular rejection is no more likely to cause increased peripheral vascular resistance than cellular rejection.[348] Neither the timing nor clinical symptoms of the renal dysfunction can be used to differentiate acute rejection from ATN.[348] Doppler US is most helpful in detecting acute arterial thrombosis where there is an absent signal in the artery or renal vein thrombosis where there is a plateau-like waveform and retrograde diastolic flow. An abnormal Doppler waveform in the allograft indicates a compromised transplant.[351] Sequential examinations may be used to show improvement or deterioration in the condition affecting the kidney and to note the progress of treatment.

Magnetic resonance imaging is useful in patients where the transplant is obscured by overlying bowel gas or in patients with large body habitus where ultrasound may be limited by the depth of the transplant. MRI is favored over contrast-enhanced CT due to lower risk of renal parenchymal injury associated with gadolinium. If any doubt exists after a thorough ultrasound evaluation, MR imaging may be performed to clarify or confirm the ultrasound findings.

Peri-transplant fluid collections are very common, occurring in up to 50% of cases.[346] These fluid collections may represent urinoma, hematoma, lymphocele, abscess, or seroma. The impact of the collection depends on the size and location. Urinomas and hematomas are found early, usually immediately after surgery. Lymphoceles generally are not found until 3 to 6 weeks after surgery. Abscesses are usually associated with transplant infection. On US evaluation, extra-renal or subcapsular hematomas usually have a complex echogenic appearance, which becomes less echogenic with time (Fig. 27–96).[346] CT will demonstrate a high attenuation fluid collection early. These are usually too complex to be drained successfully percutaneously. Urine leaks and the associated urinoma are also found in the immediate postop-

erative period (Fig. 27–97).[346] US will show an anechoic fluid collection with no septations. They may rapidly increase in size. Drainage may be performed by either US or CT guidance.[352] Antegrade pyelography via a percutaneous nephrostomy is needed to detect the site of leak, usually the ureteral anastomoses. Stent placement for treatment is necessary. Lymphoceles are recognized weeks to years after transplantation and occur in up to 20% of cases.[346] They form from the leakage of lymph from the interrupted lymphatics at surgery. Lymphoceles appear as anechoic fluid collections on US with septations. The size and effect on the kidney determine the need for treatment. As they are frequently located medial and inferior to the kidney, they are a common cause of obstruction to the kidney. US or CT guidance for drainage may be used. Sclerotherapy may be needed in a minority of cases to treat the lymphocele.[352] Peri-transplant abscess usually develops in association with renal infection or the infection of other fluid collections in the immunocompromised patient. Abscess on US examination appears as a complex fluid collection, possibly containing gas.[346] Fluid aspiration is usually necessary for the accurate characterization of fluid within a collection. Because blood products have characteristic signal intensities on T1- and T2-weighted sequences, MRI can provide specific diagnostic information that may help avoid an unnecessary interventional procedure, in cases of hematoma.

Renal obstruction or hydronephrosis may be seen in the transplanted kidney with renal dysfunction and is reversible. US is the best means for assessment.[347] In the immediate post-transplant period, mild caliectasis is common due to edema at the ureteric anastomosis site. Obstruction may also be caused by peritransplant fluid collections that may be seen also with US. Blood clots within the pelvicalyceal system may also yield hydronephrosis. Later strictures may occur primarily at the ureteral anastomosis site. Renal stones may also cause hydronephrosis during their passage to the bladder. A functional obstruction may be seen with an over distended bladder. US will demonstrate a resolution of the hydrone-phrosis with bladder emptying.

Hypertension with or without renal dysfunction may be seen in many post-transplant patients.[346] Vascular and non-vascular causes must be differentiated. Doppler US is the first line of evaluation. Renal artery stenosis may be found in up to 23% of patients.[353] The stenosis may occur before the anastomosis in the iliac artery, at the anastomosis site or more distally. More than half of the cases have the stenosis at the anastomotic site with it being more common in end to end anastomosis. CT or MR angiography is used to determine the site and the degree of stenosis (Fig. 27–98). Angioplasty is successful in managing most cases.[353]

Arteriovenous fistula occurs in transplant patients after renal biopsy. Most will close spontaneously within 4 to 6 weeks. Color and duplex Doppler imaging demonstrate high velocity and turbulent flow localized to a single segmental or interlobar artery and the adjacent vein. There is arterialized flow noted in the draining vein. Grey-scale images only dem-onstrate a simple or complex appearing cystic structure. If large and growing, embolization may become necessary.

Neoplasm occurs in transplant patients with increased frequency, up to 100 fold.[346] Neoplasms develop due to pro-longed immunosuppression. Skin cancers and lymphoma are the most common. There may be an increased risk of renal cell carcinoma in the transplanted kidney. Post-transplanta-tion lymphoproliferative disorder (PDLD) may occur in renal transplant patients.[354] Although the transplanted kidney may be involved, the most frequent sites are the brain, liver, lungs, and gastrointestinal tract. The appearance is similar to that found in conventional lymphomas with mass lesions in the organs with or without associated adenopathy.

The MRI findings of rejection are nonspecific (Figs. 27–31, 27–32, and 27–99). More recently, Sadowski and colleagues demonstrated the feasibility of using blood oxygen level-dependent MR imaging to evaluate the renal transplant oxygen status and presence of acute rejection.[355] The authors conclude that MR imaging may differentiate acute rejection from normal function and acute tubular necrosis, but further research is required. Animal research is being performed with the hope of using noninvasive diffusion MR imaging tech-niques as a tool for monitoring early renal graft rejection after transplantation.[356]

Nuclear medicine procedures are also employed in the renal transplant patient and play a role in the assessment of the complications associated with transplantation. These include vascular compromise (arterial or venous thrombosis), lympho-cele formation, urine extravasation, acute tubular necrosis, drug toxicity, and organ rejection. Scintigraphy provides important imaging information about these potential compli-cations, which can then prompt corrective intervention.[357]

An earliest complication may be hyperacute rejection, which is often apparent immediately after transplantation and is due to preformed cytotoxic antibodies. Other early

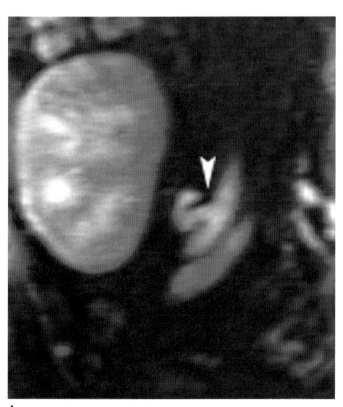
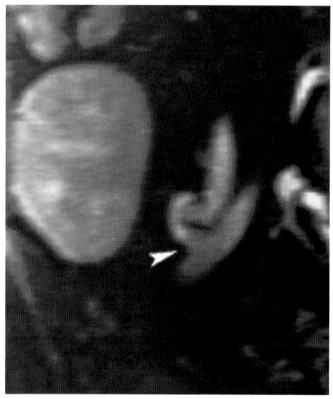

A
B

FIGURE 27–98 Renal transplant MR angiography showing **(A)** normal arterial and **(B)** normal venous anastomoses.

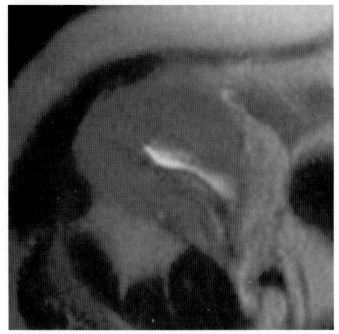

A

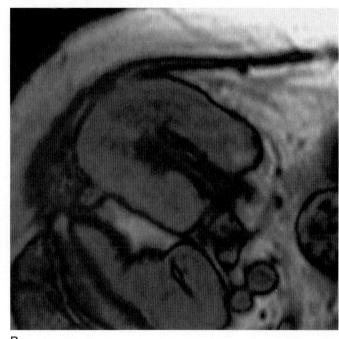

B

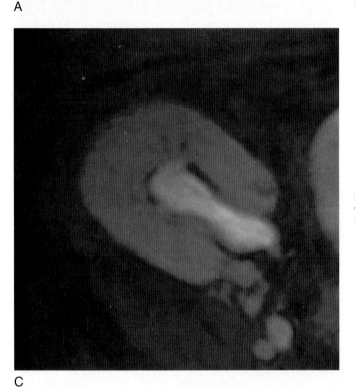

C

FIGURE 27–99 Renal transplant graft with normal function. **A,** Axial T2-weighted; **B,** axial T1-weighted; and **C,** axial gadolinium-enhanced T1-weighted images.

complications may include sudden urine output decline and acute urinary obstruction. Scintigraphy with DTPA or MAG3 shows absence of perfusion and function with complete renal artery or vein thrombosis. A sensitive but nonspecific finding for acute rejection occurs when there is greater than 20% decline in the ratio of renal activity to the aortic activity.[358]

Renal scintigraphy performed a few days after the transplantation often shows intact perfusion but delayed and decreased tracer excretion and some cortical tracer retention. This is typically due to acute tubular necrosis (ATN) and is more common with cadaveric grafts than with living-related grafts (Fig. 27–100). If both perfusion and function continue to decline, then rejection should be considered. However,

ATN, obstruction, drug (cyclosporine) toxicity, and rejection can have relatively similar scintigraphic appearance. The differential diagnosis should be considered in the clinical context and the interval since transplantation, although two or more of these conditions may coexist. In one report, a non-ascending second phase of MAG3 renogram curve was predictive of graft dysfunction. However, patients with ATN were not significantly more likely to have a non-ascending curve than those with acute rejection. An ascending curve was nonspecific and could be seen in both normally and poorly functioning grafts.[359]

Urine extravasation may be noted on the renal scans as collection of excreted radiotracer outside of the transplant

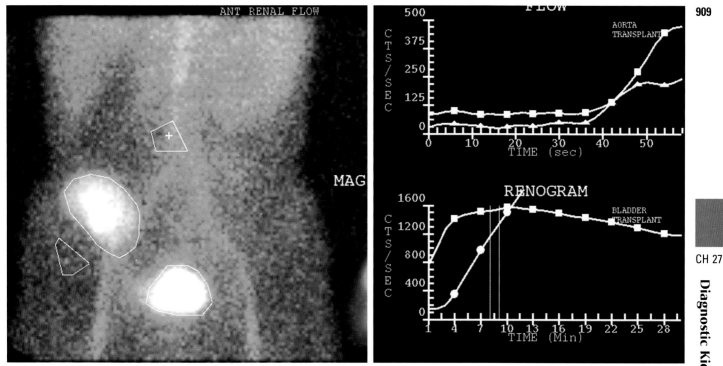

FIGURE 27–100 Abnormal Tc-99m MAG3 renogram demonstrating pattern compatible with acute tubular necrosis involving the right pelvic living-related renal transplant.

and the urinary bladder. Small urine leaks and impaired renal transplant function make the identification of a leak difficult on scintigraphy. However, a cold defect that becomes warmer with time on the sequential images usually represents an urinoma or a urinary leak. If the activity declines with voiding, then the finding is likely an urinoma. A chronic photopenic defect may represent a hematoma or a lymphocele (or both).[360] For assessing potential obstructive disease, scintigraphy with a diuretic may be considered as previously discussed.

References

1. Amis ES: Epitaph for the urogram (editorial). Radiology 213:639–640, 1999.
2. Pollack HM, Banner MP: Current status of excretory urography: A premature epitaph? Urol Clin North Am 12(4):585–601, 1985.
3. Dyer RB, Chen MYM, Zagoria RF: Intravenous urography: Technique and interpretation. RadioGraphics 21:799–824, 2001.
4. Hattery RR, Williamson B, Jr, Hartman GW, et al: Intravenous urographic technique. Radiology 167:593–599, 1988.
5. Saxton HM: Review article: Urography. Br J Radiol 42:321–346, 1969.
6. Fry IK, Cattell WR: The nephrographic pattern during excretion urography. Br Med Bull 28:227–232, 1972.
7. Katzberg RW: Urography into the 21st century: New contrast media, renal handling, imaging characteristics and nephrotoxicity. Radiology 204:297–312, 1997.
8. Almer T: Contrast agent design: Some aspects of synthesis of water-soluble contrast agents of low osmolality. J Theo Biol 24:216–226, 1969.
9. McClennan BL: Ionic and nonionic iodinated contrast media: Evolution and strategies for use. Am J Roentgenol 155:225–233, 1990.
10. Lasser EC: Etiology of anaphylactoid responses: The promise of nonionics. Invest Radiol 20:579–583, 1985.
11. Shehadi WH: Contrast media adverse reactions: Occurrence, recurrence, and distribution patterns. Radiology 143:11–17, 1982.
12. Katayama H, Yamaguchi K, Kozuka T, et al: Adverse reactions to ionic and nonionic contrast media: A report from the Japanese Committee on the Safety of Contrast Media. Radiology 175:621–628, 1990.
13. Jacobsson BF, Jorulf H, Kalantar MS, Narasimham DL: Nonionic versus ionic contrast media in intravenous urography: Clinical trial in 1000 consecutive patients. Radiology 167(3):601–605, 1988.
14. Brasch RC: Allergic reactions to contrast media: Accumulated evidence. Am J Roentgenol 134:797–801, 1980.
15. Lasser EC: Basic mechanisms of contrast media reactions: Theoretical and experimental considerations. Radiology 91:63–65, 1968.
16. Lasser EC, Berry CC, Talner LB, et al., and other Contrast Material Reaction Study participants: Pre-treatment with corticosteroids to alleviate reactions to intravenous contrast material. N Engl J Med 317(14):845–849, 1987.
17. Taliercio CP, Vietstra RE, Fisher LD, Burnett JC: Risks of renal dysfunction with cardiac angiography. Ann Intern Med 104:501–504, 1986.
18. Hou SS, Bushinsky DA, Wish JB, et al: Hospital-acquired renal insufficiency: A prospective study. Am J Med 74:243–248, 1983.
19. Tublin ME, Murphy ME, Tessler FN: Current concepts in contrast media-induced nephropathy. Am J Roentgenol 171:933–939, 1998.
20. Barrett BJ, Carlisle EJ: Metaanalysis of the relative nephrotoxicity of high-and low-osmolality iodinated contrast media. Radiology 188:171–178, 1993.
21. Aspelin P, Aubry P, Fransson S-G, et al: Nephrotoxic effects in high-risk patients undergoing angiography. N Engl J Med 348:491–499, 2003.
22. Gleeson TG, Bulugahapitiya S: Contrast-induced nephropathy. Am J Roentgenol 183:1673–1689, 2004.
23. Heinrich MC, Kuhlmann MK, Grgic A, et al: Cytotoxic effects of ionic high-osmolar, nonionic, monomeric, and nonionic iso-osmolar dimeric iodinated contrast media on renal tubular cells in vitro. Radiology 235:843–849, 2005.
24. Katzberg RW: Contrast medium-induced nephrotoxicity: Which pathway? Radiology 235:752–755, 2005.
25. Cohan RH, Dunnick NR: Intravascular contrast media: Adverse reactions. Am J Roentgenol 149:665–670, 1987.
26. Thomsen HS: Guidelines for contrast media from the European Society of Urogenital Radiology. Am J Roentgenol 181:1463–1471, 2003.
27. Bettmann MA, Heeren T, Greenfield A, Goudey C: Adverse events with radiographic contrast agents: Results of the SCVIR Contrast Agent Registry. Radiology 203:611–620, 1997.
28. Rudnick MR, Goldfarb S, Wexler L, et al., for the Iohexol Cooperative Study: Nephrotoxicity of ionic and nonionic contrast media in 1196 patients: A randomized trial. Kidney Int 47:254–261, 1995.
29. Ashley JB, Millward SF: Contrast agent-induced nephropathy: A simple way to identify patients with preexisting renal insufficiency. Am J Roentgenol 181:451–454, 2003.
30. American College of Radiology Committee on Drugs and Contrast Media. Manual on Contrast Media. 5th ed. Reston, VA, American College of Radiology, 2004.
31. Trivedi HS, Moore H, Nasr S, et al: A randomized prospective trial to assess the role of saline hydration on the development of contrast nephrotoxicity. Nephron Clin Pract 93(1):c29–c34, 2003.
32. Tepel M, Van Der Giet M, Schwarzfeld C, et al: Prevention of radiographic-contrast-agent-induced reductions in renal function by acetylcysteine. N Engl J Med 343:180–184, 2000.
33. Pannu N, Manns B, Lee H, Tonelli M: Systematic review of the impact of N-acetylcysteine on contrast nephropathy. Kidney Int 65:1366–1374, 2004.
34. Merten GJ, Burgess WP, Gray LV, et al: Prevention of contrast-induced nephropathy with sodium bicarbonate: A randomized controlled trial. JAMA 291(19):2328–2334, 2004.
35. Murphy SW, Barrett BJ, Parfrey PS: Contrast nephropathy. J Am Soc Nephrol 11:177–182, 2000.

36. Amis ES, Hartman DS: Renal ultrasonography 1984: A practical overview. Radiol Clin North Am 22(2):315–332, 1984.

37. Chen P, Maklad N, Redwine: Color and power Doppler imaging of the kidneys. World J Urol 16(1):41–45, 1998.

38. Jafri SZ, Madrazo BL, Miller JH: Color Doppler ultrasound of the genitourinary tract. Curr Opin Radiol 4(2):16–23, 1992.

39. Hricak H, Cruz C, Romanski R, et al: Renal parenchymal disease: Sonographic-histologic correlation. Radiology 144:141–147, 1982.

40. Coleman BG: Ultrasonography of the upper genitourinary tract. Urol Clin North Am 12(4):633–644, 1985.

41. Wells PNT: Doppler ultrasound in medical diagnosis. Br J Radiol 62:399–420, 1989.

42. Tublin ME, Bude RO, Platt JF: Review—The resistive index in renal Doppler sonography: Where do we stand? Am J Roentgenol 180:885–892, 2003.

43. Keogan MT, Kliewer MA, Hertzberg BS, et al: Renal resistive indexes: Variability in Doppler US measurements in a healthy population. Radiology 199:165–169, 1996.

44. Page JE, Morgan SH, Eastwood JB, et al: Ultrasound findings in renal parenchymal disease: Comparison with histological appearances. Clin Radiol 49(12):867–870, 1994.

45. Hounsfield GN: Computerized transverse axial scanning (tomography): Part I. Description of system. Br J Radiol 46:1016–1022, 1973.

46. Horton KM, Sheth S, Corl F, Fishman EK: Multidetector row CT: Principles and clinical applications. Crit Rev Comput Tomogr 43(2):143–181, 2002.

47. Saunders HS, Dyer RB, Shifrin RY, et al: The CT nephrogram: Implications for evaluation of urinary tract disease. RadioGraphics 15:1069–1085, 1995.

48. Perlman ES, Rosenfield AT, Wexler JS, Glockman MG: CT urography in the evaluation of urinary tract disease. J Comput Assist Tomogr 20(4):620–626, 1996.

49. Sudakoff GS, Dunn DP, Hellman RS, et al: Opacification of the genitourinary collecting system during MDCT urography with enhanced CT digital radiography: Nonsaline versus saline bolus. Am J Roentgenol 186:122–129, 2006.

50. Lang EK, MacChia RJ, Thomas R, et al: Improvided detection of renal pathologic features on multiphasic helical CT compared with IVU in patients presenting with microscopic hematuria. Urology 61:528–532, 2003.

51. Kawashima A, Glockner JF, King BF: CT urography and MR urography. Radiol Clin North Am 41:945–961, 2003.

52. McTavish JD, Jinzaki M, Zou KH, et al: Multi-detector row CT urography: Comparison of strategies for depicting the normal urinary collecting system. Radiology 225:783–790, 2002.

53. Engelstad BL, McClennan BL, Levitt RG, et al: The role of pre-contrast images in computed tomography of the kidney. Radiology 136:153–155, 1980.

54. McNicholas MM, Raptopoulos VD, Schwartz RK, et al: Excretory phase CT urography for opacification of the urinary collecting system. Am J Roentgenol 170:1261–1267, 1998.

55. Caoili EM: Imaging of the urinary tract using multidetector computed tomography urography. Semin Urol Oncol 20(3):174–179, 2002.

56. Kocakoc E, Bhatt S, Dogra VS: Renal multidetector row CT. Radiol Clin North Am 43(6):1021–1047, 2005.

57. Caoili EM, Cohan RH, Korobkin M, et al: Urinary tract abnormalities: Initial experience with multi-detector row CT urography. Radiology 222:353–360, 2002.

58. Joffe SA, Servaes S, Okon S, Horowitz M: Multi-detector row CT urography in the evaluation of hematuria. RadioGraphics 23:1441–1455, 2003.

59. Schild HH: MRI made easy. Wayne, NJ, Berlex Laboratories, Inc., 1999.

60. Hashemi RH, Bradley WG, Lisanti CJ: MRI: The Basics. 2nd ed. Philadelphia, Lippincott Williams & Wilkins, 2004.

61. Mitchell DG, Cohen MS: MRI Principles. 2nd ed. Philadelphia, Saunders, 2004.

62. Keogan MT, Edelman RR: Technologic advances in abdominal MR imaging. Radiology 220:310–320, 2001.

63. Nelson KL, Gifford LM, Lauber-Huber C, et al: Clinical safety of gadopentetate dimeglumine. Radiology 196:439–443, 1995.

64. Prince MR, Arnoldus C, Frisoli JK: Nephrotoxicity of high-dose gadolinium compared with iodinated contrast. J Magn Reson Imaging 6(1):162–166, 1996.

65. Rofsky NM, Weinreb JC, Bosniak MA, et al: Renal lesion characterization with gadolinium-enhanced MR imaging: Efficacy and safety in patients with renal insufficiency. Radiology 180:85–89, 1991.

66. Townsend RR, Cohen DL, Katholi R, et al: Safety of intravenous gadolinium (Gd-BOPTA) infusion in patients with renal insufficiency. Am J Kidney Dis 36(6):1207–1212, 2000.

67. Sam AD, Morasch MD, Collins J, et al: Safety of gadolinium contrast angiography in patients with chronic renal insufficiency. J Vasc Surg 38:313–318, 2003.

68. Ergün I, Keven K, Uruc I, et al: The safety of gadolinium in patients with stage 3 and 4 renal failure. Nephrol Dial Transpl 21(3):697–700, 2006.

69. Zhang HL, Ersoy H, Prince MR: Effects of gadopentetate dimeglumine and gadodiamide on serum calcium, magnesium, and creatinine measurements. J Magn Reson Imaging 23(3):383–387, 2006.

70. Choyke PL, Girton ME, Frank JA, et al: Clearance of gadolinium chelates by hemodialysis: An in vitro study. J Magn Reson Imaging 5(4):470–472, 2005.

71. Grobner T: Gadolinium: a specific trigger for the development of nephrogenic fibrosing dermopathy and nephrogenic systemic fibrosis? Nephrol Dial Transplant 21(4):1104–1108, 2006.

72. Marckmann P, Skov L, Rossen K, et al: Nephrogenic systemic fibrosis: suspected causative role of gadodiamide used for contrast-enhanced magnetic resonance imaging. J Am Soc Nephrol 17(9):2359–2362, 2006.

73. Maloo M, Abt P, Kashyap R, et al: Nephrogenic systemic fibrosis among liver transplant recipients: a single institution experience and topic update. Am J Transplant 6(9):2212–2217, 2006.

74. Sadowski EA, Bennett LK, Chan MR, et al: Nephrogenic systemic fibrosis: risk factors and incidence estimation. Radiology 243(1):148–157, 2007

75. Broome DR, Girguis MS, Baron PW, et al: Gadodiamide-associated nephrogenic systemic fibrosis: Why radiologists should be concerned. Am J Radiol 188:586–592, 2007.

76. Public health advisory: gadolinium-containing contrast agents for magnetic resonance imaging (MRI)—Omniscan, OptiMARK, Magnevist, ProHance, and MultiHance. U.S. Food and Drug Administration. Published June 8, 2006. Updated December 22, 2006.

77. Cowper SE, Robin HS, Steinberg HM, et al: Scleromyxedema-like cutaneous disease in renal-dialysis patients. Lancet 356:1000–1001, 2000.

78. Cowper SE: Nephrogenic fibrosing dermopathy (NFD/NSF) Web site, 2001–2007. Available at http://www.icnfdr.org. Last accessed May 25, 2007.

79. Thomsen HS: European Society of Urogenital Radiology guidelines on contrast media application. Curr Opin Urol 17(1):70–76, 2007.

80. Lee VS, Rofsky NM, Krinsky GA, et al: Single-dose breath-hold gadolinium-enhanced three-dimensional MR angiography of the renal arteries. Radiology 211:69–78, 1999.

81. Kopka L, Vosshenrich R, Rodenwaldt J, Grabbe E: Differences in injection rates on contrast-enhanced breath-hold-three-dimensional MR angiography. Am J Roentgenol 170:345–348, 1998.

82. Mitsuzaki K, Yamashita Y, Ogata I, et al: Optimal protocol for injection of contrast material at MR angiography: Study of healthy volunteers. Radiology 213:913–918, 1999.

83. Shellock FG: Reference manual for magnetic resonance safety, implants and devices. 2006 ed. Los Angeles, Biomedical Research Publishing Company, 2006.

84. Chung JJ, Semelka RC, Martin DR: Acute renal failure: Common occurrence of preservation of corticomedullary differentiation on MR images. Magn Reson Imaging 19(6):789–793, 2001.

85. Semelka RC, Corrigan K, Ascher SM, et al: Renal corticomedullary differentiation: Observation in patients with differing serum creatinine levels. Radiology 190:149–152, 1994.

86. Alley MT, Shifrin RY, Pelc NJ, Herfkens RJ: Ultrafast contrast-enhanced three-dimensional MR angiography: State of the art. RadioGraphics 18:273–285, 1998.

87. Baskaran V, Pereles FS, Nemcek AA, et al: Gadolinium-enhanced 3D MR angiography of renal artery stenosis: A pilot comparison of maximum intensity projection, multiplanar reformatting, and 3D Volume-rendering postprocessing algorithms. Acad Radiol 9(1):50–59, 2002.

88. Prince MR, Schoenberg SO, Ward JS, et al: Hemodynamically significant atherosclerotic renal artery stenosis: MR angiographic features. Radiology 205:128–136, 1997.

89. Willmann JK, Wildermuth S, Pfammatter T, et al: Aortoiliac and renal arteries: Prospective intraindividual comparison of contrast-enhanced three-dimensional MR angiography and multi-detector row CT angiography. Radiology 226:798–811, 2003.

90. Jara H, Barish MA, Yucel EK, et al: MR Hydrography: Theory and practice of static fluid imaging. Am J Roentgenol 170:873–882, 1998.

91. Nolte-Ernsting CCA, Bücker A, Adam GB, et al: Gadolinium-enhanced excretory MR urography after low-dose diuretic injection: Comparison with conventional excretory urography. Radiology 209:147–157, 1998.

92. Sudah M, Vanninen RL, Partanen K, et al: Patients with acute flank pain: Comparison of MR urography with unenhanced helical CT. Radiology 223:98–105, 2002.

93. Nolte-Ernsting CCA, Staatz G, Tacke J, Gunther RW: MR urography today. Abdom Imaging 28(2):191–209, 2003.

94. El-Diasty T, Mansour O, Farouk A: Diuretic contrast-enhanced magnetic resonance Urography versus intravenous urography for depiction of nondilated urinary tracts. Abdom Imaging 28(1):135–145, 2003.

95. Perlman SB, Bushnell DL, Barnes WE: Genitourinary System. In Wilson MA (ed): Textbook of Nuclear Medicine. Philadelphia, Lippincott-Raven Publishers, 1998, pp 117–136.

96. Mejia AA, Nakamura T, Masatoshi I, et al: Estimation of absorbed doses in humans due to intravenous administration of fluorine-18-fluorodeoxyglucose in PET studies. J Nucl Med 32:699–706, 1991.

97. Hays MT, Watson EE, Thomas SR, et al: MIRD dose estimate report No. 19: Radiation absorbed dose estimates from 18F-FDG. J Nucl Med 43:210–214, 2002.

98. Jones SC, Alavi A, Christman D, et al: The radiation dosimetry of 2[F-18]fluoro-2-deoxy-D-glucose in man. J Nucl Med 23(7):613–617, 1982.

99. Kuni C, duCret RP: Genitourinary system. In Manual of Nuclear Medicine Imaging, New York, Thieme Medical Publishers, 1997, pp 106–128.

100. Bagni B, Portaluppi F, Montanari L, et al: 99mTc-MAG3 versus 131I-orthoiodohippurate in the routine determination of effective renal plasma flow. J Nucl Med Allied Sci 34(2):67–70, 1990.

101. Ritchie WW, Vick CW, Glocheski SK, Cook DE: Evaluation of azotemic patients: Diagnostic yield of initial US examination. Radiology 167:245–247, 1988.

102. Yassa NA, Peng M, Ralls PW: Perirenal lucency ("kidney sweat"): A new sign of renal failure. AJR Am J Roentgenol 173:1075–1077, 1999.

103. Lee JKT, Baron RL, Melson GL, et al: Can real-time ultrasonography replace static B-scanning in the diagnosis of renal obstruction? Radiology 139:161–165, 1981.

104. Ellenbogen PH, Schieble FW, Talner LB, Leopold GR: Sensitivity of gray scale US in detecting urinary tract obstruction. Am J Roentgenol 130:731–733, 1978.

105. Stuck KJ, White GM, Granke DS, et al: Urinary obstruction in azotemic patients: Detection by sonography. Am J Roentgenol 149:1191–1193, 1987.

106. Platt JF: Advances in ultrasonography of urinary tract obstruction. Abdom Imaging 23:3–9, 1998.

107. Platt JF: Urinary obstruction. Radiol Clin North Am 34:1113–1129, 1996.

108. Kamholtz RG, Cronan JJ, Dorfman GS: Obstruction and the minimally dilated renal collecting system: US evaluation. Radiology 170:51–53, 1989.

109. Cronan JJ: Contemporary concepts in imaging urinary tract obstruction. Radiol Clin North Am 29(3):527–542, 1991.

110. Mallek R, Bankier AA, Etele-Hainz A, et al: Distinction between obstructive and nonobstructive hydronephrosis: Value of diuresis duplex Doppler sonography. Am J Roentgenol 166:113–117, 1996.

111. Scola FH, Cronan JJ, Schepps B: Grade I hydronephrosis: Pulsed Doppler US evaluation. Radiology 171:519–520, 1989.

112. Platt JF, Rubin JM, Ellis JH, DiPietro MA: Duplex Doppler US of the kidneys: Differentiation of obstructive from nonobstructive dilatation. Radiology 171:515–517, 1989.

113. Cronan JJ, Tublin ME: Role of the resistive index in the evaluation of acute renal obstruction. Am J Roentgenol 164:377–378, 1995.

114. Platt JF, Ellis JH, Rubin JM: Role of renal Doppler imaging in the evaluation of acute renal obstruction. Am J Roentgenol 164:379–380, 1995.

115. Platt JF: Looking for renal obstruction: The view from renal Doppler US. Radiology 193:610–612, 1994.

116. Platt JF, Rubin JM, Bowerman RA, Marn CS: The inability to detect kidney disease on the basis of echogenicity. Am J Roentgenol 151(2):317–319, 1988.

117. Gourtsoyiannis N, Prassopoulos P, Cavouras D, Pantelidis N: The thickness of the renal parenchyma decreases with age: A CT study of 360 patients. Am J Roentgenol 155:541–544, 1990.

118. Marotti M, Hricak H, Terrier F, et al: MR in renal disease: Importance of cortical-medullary distinction. Magn Reson Med 5:160–172, 1987.

119. Thoeny HC, De Keyzer F, Oyen RH, Peeters RR: Diffusion-weighted MR imaging of kidneys in healthy volunteers and patients with parenchymal diseases: Initial experience. Radiology 235:911–917, 2005.

120. Hauger O, Frost EE, van Heeswijk R, et al: MR Evaluation of the glomerular homing of magnetically labeled mesenchymal stem cells in a rat model of nephropathy. Radiology 238(1):200–210, 2006.

121. Lin EC, Gellens ME, Goodgold HM: Prognostic value of renal scintigraphy with Tc-99m MAG3 in patients with acute renal failure. J Nucl Med 36:232P-233P, 1995.

122. Saremi F, Jadvar H, Siegel M: Pharmacologic interventions in nuclear radiology: Indications, imaging protocols, and clinical results. Radiographics 22(3):477–490, 2002.

123. Kuni CC, duCret RP: Genitourinary system. In Manual of Nuclear Medicine Imaging. New York, Thieme Medical Publishers, 1997, pp 106–128.

124. Dyer RB, Chen MYM, Zagoria RJ: Abnormal calcifications in the urinary tract. RadioGraphics 18:1405–1424, 1998.

125. Ginalski JM, Portmann L, Jaeger PH: Does medullary sponge kidney cause nephrolithiasis? Am J Roentgenol 155:299–302, 1990.

126. Gibson MS, Puckett ML, Shelly ME: Renal tuberculosis. RadioGraphics 24:251–256, 2004.

127. Clark JY, Thompson IM, Optenberg SA: Economic impact of urolithiasis in the United States. J Urol 154:2020–2042, 1995.

128. Tublin ME, Murphy ME, Delong DM, et al: Conspicuity of renal calculi at unenhanced CT: Effects of calculus composition and size and CT technique. Radiology 225:91–96, 2002.

129. Newhouse JH, Prien EL, Amis ES, et al: Computed tomographic analysis of urinary calculi. Am J Roentgenol 142:545–548, 1984.

130. Hillman BJ, Drach GW, Tracey P, Gaines JA: Computed tomographic analysis of renal calculi. Am J Roentgenol 142:549–552, 1984.

131. Mostafavi MR, Ernst RD, Saltzman B: Accurate determination of chemical composition of urinary calculi by spiral computerized tomography. J Urol 159(3):673–675, 1998.

132. Smith RC, Rosenfield AT, Choe KA, et al: Acute flank pain: Comparison of non-contrast-enhanced CT and intravenous urography. Radiology 194:789–794, 1995.

133. Haddad MC, Sharif HS, Abomelha MS, et al: Management of renal colic: Redefining the role of the urogram. Radiology 184(1):35–36, 1992.

134. Coll DM, Varanelli MJ, Smith RC: Relationship of spontaneous passage of ureteral calculi to stone size and location as revealed by unenhanced helical CT. Am J Roentgenol 178:101–103, 2002.

135. Smith RC, Varanelli M: Diagnosis and management of acute ureterolithiasis. Am J Roentgenol 175:3–6, 2000.

136. Middleton WD, Dodds WJ, Lawson TL, Foley WD: Renal calculi: Sensitivity for detection with US. Radiology 167:239–244, 1988.

137. Gottlieb RH, La TC, Erturk EN, et al: CT in detecting urinary tract calculi: Influence on patient imaging and clinical outcomes. Radiology 225:441–449, 2002.

138. Sourtzis S, Thibeau JF, Damry N, et al: Radiologic investigation of renal colic: Unenhanced helical CT compared with excretory urography. Am J Roentgenol 172:1491–1494, 1999.

139. Boulay I, Holtz P, Foley WD, et al: Ureteral calculi: Diagnostic efficacy of helical CT and implications for treatment of patients. Am J Roentgenol 172:1485–1490, 1999.

140. Katz DS, Hines J, Rausch DR, et al: Unenhanced helical CT for suspected renal colic. Am J Roentgenol 173:425–430, 1999.

141. Haddad MC, Sharif HS, Shahed MS, et al: Renal colic: Diagnosis and outcome. Radiology 184:83–88, 1992.

142. Smith RC, Rosenfield AT, Choe KA, et al: Acute flank pain: Comparison of non-contrast-enhanced CT and intravenous urography. Radiology 194:789–794, 1995.

143. Flowler KAB, Locken JA, Duchesne JH, Williamson MR: US for detecting renal calculi with nonenhanced CT as a reference standard. Radiology 222:109–113, 2002.

144. Catalano O, Nunziata A, Altei F, Siani A: Suspected ureteral colic: Primary helical CT versus selective helical CT after unenhanced radiography and sonography. Am J Roentgenol 178:379–387, 2002.

145. Rucker CM, Menias CO, Bhalla S: Mimics of renal colic: Alternative diagnoses at unenhanced helical CT. RadioGraphics 24:S11-S33, 2004.

146. Tamm EP, Silverman PM, Shuman WP: Evaluation of the patient with flank pain and possible ureteral calculus. Radiology 228:319–329, 2003.

147. Diel J, Perlmutter S, Venkataramanan, et al: Unenhanced helical CT using increased pitch for suspected renal colic: An effective technique for radiation dose reduction? J Computer Assist Tomogr 24:795–801, 2000.

148. Katz DS, Venkataramanan, Napel S, Sommer FG: Can low-dose unenhanced multidetector CT be used for routine evaluation of suspected renal colic? Am J Roentgenol 180:313–315, 2003.

149. Saw KC, McAteer JA, Monga AG, et al: Helical CT of urinary calculi: Effect of stone composition, stone size, and scan collimation. Am J Roentgenol 175:329–332, 2000.

150. Nadler RB, Rubenstein JN, Eggener SE, et al: The etiology of urolithiasis in HIV infected patients. J Urol 169:475–477, 2003.

151. Blake SP, McNicholas MMJ, Raptopoulos V: Nonopaque crystal deposition causing ureteric obstruction in patients with HIV undergoing indinavir therapy. Am J Roentgenol 171:717–720, 1998.

152. Boridy IC, Kawashima A, Goldman SM, Sandler CM: Acute ureterolithiasis: Nonenhanced helical CT findings of perinephric edema for prediction of degree of ureteral obstruction. Radiology 213:663–667, 1999.

153. Georgiades CS, Moore CJ, Smith DP: Differences of renal parenchymal attenuation for acutely obstructed and unobstructed kidneys on unenhanced helical CT: A useful secondary sign? Am J Roentgenol 176:965–968, 2001.

154. Goldman SM, Faintuch S, Ajzen SA, et al: Diagnostic value of attenuation measurements of the kidney on unenhanced helical CT of obstructive ureterolithiasis. Am J Roentgenol 182:1251–1254, 2004.

155. Narepalem N, Sundaram CP, Boridy IC, et al: Comparison of helical computerized tomography and plain radiography for estimating urinary stone size. J Urol 167(3):1235–1238, 2002.

156. Takahashi N, Kawashima A, Ernst RD, et al: Ureterolithiasis: Can clinical outcome be predicted with unenhanced helical CT? Radiology 208:97–102, 1998.

157. Dalrymple NC, Casford B, Raiken DP, et al: Pearls and pitfalls in the diagnosis of ureterolithiasis with unenhanced helical CT. RadioGraphics 20:439–447, 2000.

158. Sudah M, Vanninen RL, Partanen K, et al: Patients with acute flank pain: Comparison of MR urography with unenhanced helical CT. Radiology 223:98–105, 2002.

159. Regan F, Bohlman ME, Khazan R, et al: MR urography using HASTE imaging in the assessment of ureteric obstruction. Am J Roentgenol 167:1115–1120, 1996.

160. Ku JH, Jeon YS, Kim ME, et al: Is there a role for magnetic resonance imaging in renal trauma? Int J Urol 8:261–267, 2001.

161. Talner LB, Davidson AJ, Lebowitz RL, et al: Acute pyelonephritis: Can we agree on terminology? Radiology 192:297–305, 1994.

162. Papanicolaou N, Pfister RC: Acute renal infections. Radiol Clin North Am 34(5):965–995, 1996.

163. Hamper UM, Goldblum LE, Hutchins GM, et al: Renal involvement in AIDS: Sonographic-pathologic correlation. Am J Roentgenol 150:1321–1325, 1988.

164. Koh, DM, Langroudi A, Padley SPG: Abdominal CT in patients with AIDS. Imaging. Br Inst Radiol (14);24–34, 2002.

165. Kay CJ: Renal diseases in patients with AIDS: Sonographic findings. Am J Roentgenol 159:551–554, 1992.

166. Grayson DE, Abbott RM, Levy AD, et al: Emphysematous infections of the abdomen and pelvis: A pictorial review. RadioGraphics 22:543–561, 2002.

167. Rodriguez-de-Velasquez A, Yoder IC, Velasquez PA, Papanicolaou N: Imaging the effects of diabetes on the genitourinary system. RadioGraphics 15:1051–1068, 1995.

168. Hayes WS, Hartman DS, Sesterbenn I: From the archives of the AFIP. Xanthogranulomatous pyelonephritis. RadioGraphics 11:485–498, 1991.

169. Kenney PJ: Imaging of chronic renal infections. Am J Roentgenol 155:485–494, 1990.

170. Soulen MC, Fishman EK, Goldman SM, Gatewood OMB: Bacterial renal infection: Role of CT. Radiology 171:703–707, 1989.

171. Sheth S, Fishman EK: Multi-detector row CT of the kidneys and urinary tract: Techniques and applications in the diagnosis of benign diseases. RadioGraphics 24:e20, 2004.

172. Kawashima A, Sandler CM, Goldman SM, et al: CT of renal inflammatory disease. RadioGraphics 17:851–866, 1997.

173. Gervais DA, Shitman GJ: Emphysematous pyelonephritis. Am J Roentgenol 162:348, 1994.

174. Wan Y-L, Lee T-Y, Bullard MJ, Tsai C-C: Acute gas-producing bacterial renal infection: Correlation between imaging findings and clinical outcome. Radiology 198:433–438, 1996.

175. Roy C, Pfleger DD, Tuchmann CM, et al: Emphysematous pyelitis: Findings in five patients. Radiology 218:647–650, 2001.

176. Fan CM, Whitman GJ, Chew FS: Xanthogranulomatous pyelonephritis. Am J Roentgenol 165:862, 1995.

177. Majd M, Blask ARN, Markle BM, et al: Acute pyelonephritis: Comparison of diagnosis with 99mTc-DMSA SPECT, spiral CT, MR imaging, and power Doppler US in an experimental pig model. Radiology 218:101–108, 2001.

178. Bjorgvinsson E, Majd M, Eggli KD: Diagnosis of acute pyelonephritis in children: Comparison of sonography and 99mTc-DMSA scintigraphy. Am J Roentgenol 157:539–543, 1991.

179. Warshauer DM, McCarthy SM, Street L, et al: Detection of renal masses: Sensitivities and specificities of excretory urography/linear tomography, US, and CT. Radiology 169:363–365, 1988.

180. Bosniak, Morton A: The use of the Bosniak classification system for renal cysts and cystic tumors. J Urol 157(5):1852–1853, 1997.

181. Jinzaki M, McTavish JD, Zou KH, et al: Evaluation of small (≤3 cm) renal masses with MDCT: Benefits of thin overlapping reconstructions. Am J Roentgenol 183:223–228, 2004.

182. Silverman SG, Lee BY, Seltzer SE, et al: Small (≤3 cm) renal masses: Correlation of spiral CT features and pathologic findings. Am J Roentgenol 163:597–605, 1994.

183. Hayden CK, Swischuk LE, Smith TH, Armstrong EA: Renal cystic disease in childhood. RadioGraphics 6(1):97–116, 1986.

184. Lonergan GF, Rice RR, Suarez ES: Autosomal recessive polycystic kidney disease: Radiologic-pathologic correlation. RadioGraphics 20:837–855, 2000.

185. Walker FC, Loney LC, Root ER, et al: Diagnostic evaluation of adult polycystic kidney disease in childhood. Am J Roentgenol 142:1273–1277, 1984.

186. Nicolau C, Torra R, Badenas C, et al: Autosomal dominant polycystic kidney disease types 1 and 2: Assessment of US sensitivity for diagnosis. Radiology 213:273–276, 1999.

912

187. Heinz-Peer G, Schoder M, Rand T, et al: Prevalence of acquired cystic kidney disease and tumors in native kidneys of renal transplant recipients: A prospective US study. Radiology 195:667–671, 1995.

188. Levine E: Acquired cystic kidney disease. Radiol Clin North Am 34(5):947–964, 1996.

189. Levine E, Slusher SL, Grantham JJ, Wetzel LH: Natural history of acquired renal cystic disease in dialysis patients: A prospective longitudinal CT study. Am J Roentgenol 156:501–506, 1991.

190. Takebayashi S, Hidai H, Chiba T, et al: Using helical CT to evaluate renal cell carcinoma in patients undergoing hemodialysis: Value of early enhanced images. Am J Roentgenol 172:429–433, 1999.

191. Taylor AJ, Cohen EP, Erickson SJ, et al: Renal imaging in long-term dialysis patients: A comparison of CT and sonography. Am J Roentgenol 153:765–767, 1989.

192. Takase K, Takahashi S, Tazawa S, et al: Renal cell carcinoma associated with chronic renal failure: Evaluation with sonographic angiography. Radiology 192:787–792, 1994.

193. Siegel SC, Sandler MA, Alpern MB, Pearlberg JL: CT of renal cell carcinoma in patients on chronic hemodialysis. Am J Roentgenol 150:583–585, 1988.

194. Matson MA, Cohen EP: Acquired cystic kidney disease: Occurrence, prevalence, and renal cancers. Medicine 69(4):217–226, 1990.

195. Choyke PL, Glenn GM, Walther MM, et al: Hereditary renal cancers. Radiology 226:33–46, 2003.

196. Bosniak MA: State of the Art. The current radiological approach to renal cysts. Radiology 158:1–10, 1986.

197. Zagoria RJ: Imaging of small renal masses: A medical success story. Am J Roentgenol 175:945–955, 2000.

198. Lowe LH, Isuani BH, Heller RM, et al: Pediatric renal masses: Wilms tumor and beyond. RadioGraphics 20:1585–1603, 2000.

199. Wagner BJ, Maj MC, Wong-You-Cheong JJ, Davis CJ: Adult renal hamartomas. Radio-Graphics 17:155–169, 1997.

200. Bosniak MA, Megibow AJ, Hulnick DH, et al: CT diagnosis of renal angiomyolipoma: The importance of detecting small amounts of fat. Am J Roentgenol 151:497–501, 1988.

201. Silverman SG, Pearson GDN, Seltzer SE, et al: Small (≤3 cm) hyperechoic renal masses: Comparison of helical and conventional CT for diagnosing angiomyolipoma. Am J Roentgenol 167:877–881, 1996.

202. Siegel CL, Middleton WD, Teefey SA, McClennan BL: Angiomyolipoma and renal cell carcinoma: US differentiation. Radiology 198:789–793, 1996.

203. Kim JK, Park SY, Shon JH, Cho KS: Angiomyolipoma with minimal fat: Differentiation from renal cell carcinoma at biphasic helical CT. Radiology 230:677–684, 2004.

204. Jinzaki M, Tanimoto A, Narimatsu Y, et al: Angiomyolipoma: Imaging findings in lesions with minimal fat. Radiology 205:497–502, 1997.

205. Lesavre A, Correas JM, Merran S, et al: CT of papillary renal cell carcinoma with cholesterol necrosis mimicking angiomyolipomas. Am J Roentgenol 181:143–145, 2003.

206. Israel GM, Bosniak MA, Slywotzky CM, Rosen RJ: CT differentiation of large exophytic renal angiomyolipomas and perirenal liposarcomas. Am J Roentgenol 179:769–773, 2002.

207. Bosniak M, Megibow AJ, Hulnick DH, et al: CT diagnosis of renal angiomyolipoma: The importance of detecting small amounts of fat. Am J Roentgenol 151:497–501, 1988.

208. Lemaitre L, Robert Y, Dubrulle F, et al: Renal angiomyolipoma: Growth followed up with CT and/or US. Radiology 197:598–602, 1995.

209. Yamakado K, Tanaka N, Nakagawa T, et al: Renal angiomyolipoma: Relationships between tumor size, aneurysm formation, and rupture. Radiology 225:78–82, 2002.

210. Palmer WE, Chew FS: Renal oncocytoma. Am J Roentgenol 156:1144, 1991.

211. Levine E, Huntrakoon M: Computed tomography of renal oncocytoma. Am J Roentgenol 141(4):741–746, 1983.

212. On the Am J Roentgenol Viewbox. Renal oncocytoma displaying intense activity on ^{18}F-FDG PET. Am J Roentgenol 186:269–271, 2006.

213. Neisius D, Braedel HU, Schindler E, et al: Computed tomographic and angiographic findings in renal oncocytoma. Br J Radiol 61(731):1019–1025, 1988.

214. Davidson AJ, Hayes WS, Hartman DS, et al: Renal oncocytoma and carcinoma: Failure of differentiation with CT. Radiology 186:693–696, 1993.

215. Curry NS, Schabel SI, Garvin AJ, Fish G: Case Report. Intratumoral fat in a renal oncocytoma mimicking angiomyolipoma. Am J Roentgenol 154:307–308, 1990.

216. Bostwick DG, Eble JN, Murphy GP: Conference summary. Diagnosis and prognosis of renal cell carcinoma: 1997 Workshop, Rochester, Minnesota, March 21–22, 1997. Cancer 80(5):975–976, 1997.

217. Bonsib SM: Risk and prognosis in renal neoplasms. A pathologist's prospective. Urol Clin North Am 26(3):643–660, 1999.

218. Russo P: Renal cell carcinoma: Presentation, staging, and surgical treatment. Semin Oncol 27(2):160–176, 2000.

219. Sheth S, Scatarige JC, Horton KM, et al: Current concepts in the diagnosis and management of renal cell carcinoma: Role of multidetector CT and three-dimensional CT. RadioGraphics 21:S237-S254, 2001.

220. Coll DM, Herts BR, Davros WJ, et al: Preoperative use of 3D volume rendering to demonstrate renal tumors and renal anatomy. RadioGraphics 20:431–438, 2000.

221. Gervais DA, McGovern FJ, Arellano RS, et al: Renal cell carcinoma: Clinical experience and technical success with radio-frequency ablation of 42 tumors. Radiology 226:417–424, 2003.

222. Mayo-Smith WW, Dupuy DE, Parikh PM, et al: Imaging-guided percutaneous radio-frequency ablation of solid renal masses: Techniques and outcomes of 38 treatment sessions in 32 consecutive patients. Am J Roentgenol 180:1503–1508, 2003.

223. Zagoria RF: Imaging-guided radio-frequency ablation of renal masses. RadioGraphics 24:S59-S71, 2004.

224. Suh RD, Goldin JG, Wallace AB, et al: Metastatic renal cell carcinoma: CT-guided immunotherapy as a technically feasible and safe approach to delivery of gene therapy for treatment. Radiology 231:359–364, 2004.

225. Jamis-Dow CA, Choyke PL, Jennings SB, et al: Small (<3-cm) renal masses: Detection with CT versus US and pathologic correlation. Radiology 198:785–788, 1996.

226. Jinzaki M, Ohkuma K, Tanimoto A, et al: Small solid renal lesions: Usefulness of power Doppler US. Radiology 209:543–550, 1998.

227. Forman HP, Middleton WD, Melson GL, McClennan BL: Hyperechoic renal cell carcinomas: Increase in detection at US. Radiology 188:431–434, 1993.

228. Ascenti G, Gaeta M, Magno C, et al: Contrast-enhanced second-harmonic sonography in the detection of pseudocapsule in renal cell carcinoma. Am J Roentgenol 182:1525–1530, 2004.

229. Schmidt T, Hohl C, Haage P, et al: Diagnostic accuracy of phase-inversion tissue harmonic imaging versus fundamental B-mode sonography in the evaluation of focal lesions of the kidney. Am J Roentgenol 180:1639–1647, 2003.

230. Davidson AJ, Hartman DS, Choyke PL, Wagner BJ: Radiologic assessment of renal masses: Implications for patient care. Radiology 202:297–305, 1997.

231. Yuh BI, Cohan RH: Different phases of renal enhancement: Role in detecting and characterizing renal masses during helical CT. Am J Roentgenol 173:747–755, 1999.

232. Cohan RH, Sherman LS, Korobkin M, et al: Renal masses: Assessment of corticome-dullary-phase and nephrographic-phase CT scans. Radiology 196:445–451, 1995.

233. Suh M, Coakley FV, Qayyum A, et al: Distinction of renal cell carcinomas from high-attenuation renal cysts at portal venous phase contrast-enhanced CT. Radiology 228:330–334, 2003.

234. Birnbaum BA, Jacobs JE, Ramchandani P: Multiphasic renal CT: Comparison of renal mass enhancement during the corticomedullary and nephrographic phases. Radiology 200:753–758, 1996.

235. Kopka L, Fischer U, Zoeller G, et al: Dual-phase helical CT of the kidney: Value of the corticomedullary and nephrographic phase for evaluation of renal lesions and preoperative staging of renal cell carcinoma. Am J Roentgenol 169:1573–1578, 1997.

236. Macari M, Bosniak MA: Delayed CT to evaluate renal masses incidentally discovered at contrast-enhanced CT: Demonstration of vascularity with deenhancement. Radiology 213:674–680, 1999.

237. Zeman RK, Zeiberg A, Hayes WS: Helical CT of renal masses: The value of delayed scans. Am J Roentgenol 177:771–776, 1996.

238. Benjaminov O, Atri M, O'Malley M, et al: Enhancing component on CT to predict malignancy in cystic renal masses and interobserver agreement of different CT features. Am J Roentgenol 186:665–672, 2006.

239. Ruppert-Kohlmayr AJ, Uggowitzer M, Meissnitzer T, Ruppert G: Differentiation of renal clear cell carcinoma and renal papillary carcinoma using quantitative CT enhancement parameters. Am J Roentgenol 183:1387–1391, 2004.

240. Kim JK, Kim TK, Ahn HJ, et al: Differentiation of subtypes of renal cell carcinoma on helical CT scans. Am J Roentgenol 178:1499–1506, 2002.

241. Browne RFJ, Meehan CP, Colville J, et al: Transitional cell carcinoma of the upper urinary tract: Spectrum of imaging findings. RadioGraphics 25:1609–1627, 2005.

242. Pickhardt PF, Lonergan GF, Davis CF, et al: From the archives of the AFIP. Infiltrative renal lesions: Radiologic-pathologic correlation. RadioGraphics 20:215–243, 2000.

243. Urban BA, Fishman EK: Renal lymphoma: CT patterns with emphasis on helical CT. RadioGraphics 20:197–212, 2000.

244. Hartman DS, Choyke PL, Hartman MS: From the RSNA refresher courses. A practical approach to the cystic renal mass. RadioGraphics 24:S101-S115, 2004.

245. Israel GM, Hindman N, Bosniak MA: Evaluation of cystic renal masses: Comparison of CT and MR imaging by using the Bosniak classification system. Radiology 231:365–371, 2004.

246. Siegel CL, McFarland EG, Brink JA, et al: CT of cystic renal masses: Analysis of diagnostic performance and interobserver variation. Am J Roentgenol 169:813–818, 1997.

247. Israel GM, Bosniak MA: Follow-up CT of moderately complex cystic lesions of the kidney (Bosniak Category IIF). Am J Roentgenol 181:627–633, 2003.

248. Curry NS, Cochran ST, Bissada NK: Cystic renal masses: Accurate Bosniak classification requires adequate renal CT. Am J Roentgenol 175:339–342, 2000.

249. Harisinghani MG, Maher MM, Gervais DA, et al: Incidence of malignancy in complex cystic renal masses (Bosniak Category III): Should imaging-guided biopsy precede surgery? Am J Roentgenol 180:755–758, 2003.

250. Dechet CB, Sebo T, Farrow G, et al: Prospective analysis of intraoperative frozen needle biopsy of solid renal masses in adults. J Urol 162:1282–1285, 1999.

251. Wood BJ, Khan MA, McGovern F, et al: Imaging guided biopsy of renal masses: Indications, accuracy and impact on clinical management. J Urol 161:1470–1474, 1999.

252. Rybicki FJ, Shu KM, Cibas ES, et al: Percutaneous biopsy of renal masses: Sensitivity and negative predictive value stratified by clinical setting and size of masses. Am J Roentgenol 180:1281–1287, 2003.

253. Israel GM, Hindman N, Bosniak MA: Evaluation of cystic renal masses: Comparison of CT and MR imaging by using the Bosniak classification system. Radiology 231:365–371, 2004.

254. Semelka RC, Shoenut JP, Kroeker MA, et al: Renal lesions: Controlled comparison between CT and 1.5-T MR imaging with nonenhanced and gadolinium-enhanced fat-suppressed spin-echo and breath-hold FLASH techniques. Radiology 182:425–430, 1992.

255. Hecht EM, Israel GM, Krinsky GA, et al: Renal masses: Quantitative analysis of enhancement with signal intensity measurements versus qualitative analysis of enhancement with image subtraction for diagnosing malignancy at MR imaging. Radiology 232:373–378, 2004.

256. Farres MT, Ronco P, Saadoun D, et al: Chronic lithium nephropathy: MR imaging for diagnosis. Radiology 229:570–574, 2003.

257. Israel GM, Hindman N, Hecht E, Krinsky G: The use of opposed-phase chemical shift MRI in the diagnosis of renal angiomylipomas. Am J Roentgenol 184:1868–1872, 2005.

CH 27

258. Yoshimitsu K, Kakihara D, Irie H, et al: Papillary renal carcinoma: Diagnostic approach by chemical shift gradient-echo and echo-planar MR imaging. J Magn Reson Imaging 23(3):339–344, 2006.

259. Ergen FB, Hussain HK, Caoili EM, et al: MRI for preoperative staging of renal cell carcinoma using the 1997 TNM classification: Comparison with surgical and pathologic staging. Am J Roentgenol 182:217–225, 2004.

260. Roy C, El Ghali S, Buy X, et al: Significance of the pseudocapsule on MRI of renal neoplasms and its potential application for local staging: A retrospective study. Am J Roentgenol 184:113–120, 2005.

261. Choyke PL, Walther MM, Wagner JR: Renal cancer: Preoperative evaluation with dual-phase three-dimensional MR angiography. Radiology 205:767–771, 1997.

262. El-Galley R: Surgical management of renal tumors. Radiol Clin North Am 41:1053–1065, 2003.

263. Semelka RC, Kelekis NL, Burdeny DA, et al: Renal lymphoma: Demonstration by MR imaging. Am J Roentgenol 166:823–827, 1996.

264. Frank IN, Graham Jr S, Nabors WL: Urologic and male genital cancers. In Holleb AI, Fink DJ, Murphy GP (eds): Clinical Oncology. American Cancer Society, 1991, pp 272–274.

265. Goldberg MA, Mayo-Smith WW, Papanicolaou N, et al: FDG PET characterization of renal masses: Preliminary experience. Clin Radiol 52:510–515, 1997.

266. Jadvar H, Kherbache HM, Pinski JK, Conti PS: Diagnostic role of [F-18]-FDG positron emission tomography in restaging renal cell carcinoma. Clin Nephrol 60:395–400, 2003.

267. Mankoff DA, Thompson JA, Gold P, et al: Identification of interleukin-2-induced complete response in metastatic renal cell carcinoma by FDG PET despite radiographic evidence suggesting persistent tumor. Am J Roentgenol 169:1049–1050, 1997.

268. Ramdave S, Thomas GW, Berlangieri SU, et al: Clinical role of F-18 fluorodeoxyglucose positron emission tomography for detection and management of renal cell carcinoma. J Urol 166:825–830, 2001.

269. Wahl RL, Harney J, Hutchins G, Grossman HB: Imaging of renal cancer using positron emission tomography with 2-deoxy-2-(18f)-fluoro-D-glucose: Pilot animal and human studies. J Urol 146(6):1470–1474, 1991.

270. Wu HC, Yen RF, Shen YY, et al: Comparing whole body 18F-2-deoxyglucose positron emission tomography and technetium-99m methylene diphosphate bone scan to detect bone metastases in patients with renal cell carcinomas—A preliminary report. J Cancer Res Clin Oncol 128:503–506, 2002.

271. Majhail NS, Urbain JL, Albani JM, et al: F-18 Fluorodeoxyglucose positron emission tomography in the evaluation of distant metastases from renal cell carcinoma. J Clin Oncol 21:3995–4000, 2003.

272. Seto E, Segall GM, Terris MK: Positron emission tomography detection of osseous metastases of renal cell carcinoma not identified on bone scan. Urology 55:286, 2000.

273. Zhuang H, Duarte PS, Pourdehand M, et al: Standardized uptake value as an unreliable index of renal disease on fluorodeoxyglucose PET imaging. Clin Nucl Med 25:358–360, 2000.

274. Kang DE, White RL Jr, Zuger JH, et al: Clinical use of fluorodeoxyglucose F 18 positron emission tomography for detection of renal cell carcinoma. J Urol 171(5):1806–1809, 2004.

275. Safaei A, Figlin R, Hoh CK, et al: The usefulness of F-18 deoxyglucose whole-body positron emission tomography (PET) for re-staging of renal cell cancer. Clin Nephrol 57:56–62, 2002.

276. Miyakita H, Tokunaga M, Onda H, et al: Significance of 18F-fluorodeoxyglucose positron emission tomography (FDG-PET) for detection of renal cell carcinoma and immunohistochemical glucose transporter 1 (GLUT-1) expression in the cancer. Int J Urol 9:15–18, 2002.

277. Nagase Y, Takata K, Moriyama N, et al: Immunohistochemical localization of glucose transporters in human renal cell carcinoma. J Urol 153(3 Pt 1):798–801, 1995.

278. Kumar R, Chauhan A, Lakhani P, et al: 2-Deoxy-2-[F-18]Fluoro-D-Glucose-Positron emission tomography in characterization of solid renal masses. Mol Imaging Biol 7(6):431–439, 2005.

279. Shreve P, Chiao PC, Humes HD, et al: Carbon-11-acetate PET imaging in renal disease. J Nucl Med 36:1595–1601, 1995.

280. Lawrentschuk N, Poon AM, Foo SS, et al: Assessing regional hypoxia in human renal tumors using 18F-Fluoromisonidazole positron emission tomography. BJU Int 96(4):540–546, 2005.

281. Hillman BJ: Imaging advances in the diagnosis of renovascular hypertension. Am J Roentgenol 153:5–14, 1989.

282. Albers FJ: Clinical characteristics of atherosclerotic renovascular disease. Am J Kidney Dis 24(4):636–41, 1994.

283. Ota H, Takase K, Rikimaru H, et al: Quantitative vascular measurements in arterial occlusive disease. RadioGraphics 25:1141–1158, 2005.

284. Siegel CL, Ellis JH, Korobkin M, Dunnick NR: CT-Detected renal arterial calcification: Correlation with renal artery stenosis on angiography. Am J Roentgenol 163:867–872, 1994.

285. Beregi JP, Louvegny S, Gautier C, et al: Fibromuscular dysplasia of the renal arteries: Comparison of helical CT angiography and arteriography. Am J Roentgenol 172:27–34, 1999.

286. Bolduc JP, Oliva VL, Therasse E, et al: Diagnosis and treatment of renovascular hypertension: A cost-benefit analysis. Am J Roentgenol 184:931–937, 2005.

287. Soulez G, Oliva VL, Turpin S, et al: Imaging of renovascular hypertension: Respective values of renal scintigraphy, renal Doppler US, and MR angiography. RadioGraphics 20:1355–1368, 2000.

288. Desberg AL, Paushter DM, Lammert GK, et al: Renal artery stenosis: Evaluation with color Doppler flow imaging. Radiology 177:749–753, 1990.

289. Hamper UM, DeJong MR, Caskey CI, Sheth S: Power Doppler imaging: Clinical experience and correlation with color Doppler US and other imaging modalities. RadioGraphics 17:499–513, 1977.

290. Helenon O, El Rody F, Correas JM, et al: Color Doppler US of renovascular disease in native kidneys. RadioGraphics 15:833–854, 1995.

291. Halpern EJ, Needleman L, Nack TL, East SA: Renal artery stenosis: Should we study the main renal artery or segmental vessels? Radiology 195:799–804, 1995.

292. House MK, Dowling RJ, King P, Gibson RN: Using Doppler sonography to reveal renal artery stenosis: An evaluation of optimal imaging parameters. Am J Roentgenol 173:761–765, 1999.

293. Kliewer MA, Tupler RH, Carroll BA, et al: Renal artery stenosis: Analysis of Doppler waveform parameters and Tardus-Parvus pattern. Radiology 189:779–787, 1993.

294. Melany ML, Grant EG, Duerinckx AJ, et al: Ability of a phase shift US contrast agent to improve imaging of the main renal arteries. Radiology 205:147–152, 1997.

295. Claudon M, Plouin PF, Baxter GM, et al: Renal arteries in patients at risk of renal arterial stenosis: Multicenter evaluation of the echo-enhancer SH U 508A at color and spectral Doppler US. Radiology 214:739–746, 2000.

296. Urban BA, Ratner LE, Fishman EK: Three-dimensional volume-rendered CT angiography of the renal arteries and veins: Normal anatomy, variants, and clinical applications. RadioGraphics 21:373–386, 2001.

297. Kaatee R, Beek FJA, DeLange EE, et al: Renal artery stenosis: Detection and quantification with spiral CT angiography versus optimized digital subtraction angiography. Radiology 205:121–127, 1997.

298. Beregi JP, Elkohen M, Deklunder G, et al: Helical CT angiography compared with arteriography in the detection of renal artery stenosis. Am J Roentgenol 167:495–501, 1996.

299. Kawashima A, Sandler CM, Ernst RD, et al: CT evaluation of renovascular disease. RadioGraphics 20:1321–1340, 2000.

300. Rubin GD, Dake MD, Napel S, et al: Spiral CT of renal artery stenosis: Comparison of three-dimensional rendering techniques. Radiology 190:181–189, 1994.

301. Brink JA, Lim JT, Wang G, et al: Technical optimization of spiral CT for depiction of renal artery stenosis: In vitro analysis. Radiology 194:157–163, 1995.

302. Bude RO, Forauer AR, Caoili EM, Nghiem HV: Is it necessary to study accessory arteries when screening the renal arteries for renovascular hypertension? Radiology 226:411–416, 2003.

303. Mallouhi A, Rieger M, Czermak B, et al: Volume-rendered multidetector CT angiography: Noninvasive follow-up of patients treated with renal artery stents. Am J Roentgenol 180:233–239, 2003.

304. Behar JV, Nelson RC, Zidar JP, et al: Thin-section multidetector CT angiography of renal artery stents. Am J Roentgenol 178:1155–1159, 2002.

305. Willmann J, Wildermuth S, Pfammatter T, et al: Aortoiliac and renal arteries: Prospective intraindividual comparison of contrast-enhanced three-dimensional MR angiography and multi-detector row CT angiography. Radiology 226:798–811, 2003.

306. Thornton MJ, Thornton F, O'Callaghan J, et al: Evaluation of dynamic gadolinium-enhanced breath-hold MR angiography in the diagnosis of renal artery stenosis. Am J Roentgenol 173:1279–1283, 1999.

307. Qanadli SD, Soulez G, Therasse E, et al: Detection of renal artery stenosis: Prospective comparison of captopril-enhanced Doppler sonography, captopril-enhanced scintigraphy, and MR angiography. Am J Roentgenol 177:1123–1129, 2001.

308. Mallouhi A, Schocke M, Judmaier W, et al: 3D MR angiography of renal arteries: Comparison of volume rendering and maximum intensity projection algorithms. Radiology 223:509–516, 2002.

309. Schoenberg SO, Knopp MV, Londy F, et al: Morphologic and functional magnetic resonance imaging of renal artery stenosis: A multireader tricenter study. J Am Soc Nephrol 13:158–169, 2002.

310. Soulez G, Olivia VL, Turpin S, et al: Imaging of renovascular hypertension: Respective values of renal scintigraphy, renal Doppler US and MR angiography. RadioGraphics 20:1355–1368, 2000.

311. Bude RO, Forauer AR, Caoili EM, Nghiem HV: Is it necessary to study accessory arteries when screening the renal arteries for renovascular hypertension? Radiology 226:411–416, 2003.

312. Wilson GJ, Hoogeveen RM, Willinek WA, et al: Parellel imaging in MR angiography. Top Magn Reson Imaging 15(3):169–185, 2004.

313. Gutberlet M, Noeske R, Schwinge K, et al: Comprehensive cardiac magnetic resonance imaging at 3.0 tesla: Feasibility and implications for clinical applications. Invest Radiol 41(2):154–167, 2006.

314. Chen Q, Quijano CV, Mai VM, et al: On improving temporal and spatial resolution of 3D contrast-enhanced body MR angiography with parallel imaging. Radiology 231:893–899, 2004.

315. de Haan MW, van Engelshoven JMA, Houben AJHM, et al: Phase-contrast magnetic resonance flow quantification in renal arteries comparison with 133 Xenon washout measurements. Hypertension 41:114–118, 2003.

316. Schoenberg SO, Knopp MV, Londy F, et al: Morphologic and functional magnetic resonance imaging of renal artery stenosis: A multireader tricenter study. J Am Soc Nephrol 13:158–169, 2002.

317. Michaely HJ, Schoenberg SO, Oesingmann N, et al: Renal artery stenosis: Functional assessment with dynamic MR perfusion measurements—feasibility study. Radiology 238(2):586–596, 2006.

318. van den Dool SW, Wasser MN, de Fijter JW, et al: Functional renal volume: Quantitative analysis at gadolinium-enhanced MR angiography—feasibility study in healthy potential kidney donors. Radiology 236:189–195, 2005.

319. Spuentrup E, Ruebben A, Stuber M, et al: Metallic renal artery MR imaging stent: Artifact-free lumen visualization with projection and standard renal MR angiography. Radiology 227:897–902, 2003.

320. Nally JV Jr, Black HR: State-of-the-art review: Captopril renography—Pathophysiological considerations and clinical observations. Semin Nucl Med 22:85–97, 1992.

321. Taylor A, Nally J, Aurell M, et al: Consensus report on ACE inhibitor renography for detecting renovascular hypertension. Radionuclides in Nephrourology Group. Consensus Group on ACEI Renography. J Nucl Med 37:1876–1882, 1996.

322. Taylor AT Jr, Fletcher JW, Nally JV Jr, et al: Procedure guideline for diagnosis of renovascular hypertension. Society of Nuclear Medicine. J Nucl Med 39:1297–1302, 1998.

323. Nally JV Jr, Chen C, Fine E, et al: Diagnostic criteria of renovascular hypertension with captopril renography: A consensus statement. Am J Hypertens 4:749S-752S, 1991.

324. Fine EJ: Interventions in renal scintigraphy. Semin Nucl Med 29:128–145, 1999.

325. Llach F, Papper S, Massey SG: The clinical spectrum of renal vein thrombosis: Acute and chronic. Am J Med 69(6):819–827, 1980.

326. Witz M, Kantarovsky A, Baruch M, Shifrin EG: Renal vein occlusion: A review. J Urol 155(4):1173–1179, 1996.

327. Llach F, Koffler A, Finck E, Massry SG: On the incidence of renal vein thrombosis in the nephrotic syndrome. Arch Intern Med 137(3): 333–336, 1977.

328. Gatewood OMB, Fishman EK, Burrow CR, et al: Renal vein thrombosis in patients with nephrotic syndrome: CT diagnosis. Radiology 159:117–122, 1986.

329. Sebastia C, Quiroga S, Boye R, et al: Helical CT in renal transplantation: Normal findings and early and late complications. RadioGraphics 21:1103–1117, 2001.

330. Brown ED, Chen MYM, Wolfman NT, et al: Complications of renal transplantation: Evaluation with US and radionuclide imaging. RadioGraphics 20:607–622, 2000.

331. Letourneau JG, Day DL, Ascher NL, Castaneda-Zuniga WR: Perspective. Imaging of renal transplants. Am J Roentgenol 150:833–838, 1988.

332. Kelcz F, Pazniak MA, Pirsch JD, Oberly TD: Pyramidal appearance and resistive index: Insensitive and nonspecific sonographic indicators of renal transplant rejection. Am J Roentgenol 155:531–535, 1990.

333. Smith PA, Ratner LE, Lynch FC, et al: Role of CT angiography in the preoperative evaluation for laparoscopic nephrectomy. RadioGraphics 18:589–601, 1998.

334. Holden A, Smith A, Dukes P, et al: Assessment of 100 live potential renal donors for laparoscopic nephrectomy with multi-detector row helical CT. Radiology 237:973–980, 2005.

335. Rydberg J, Kopecky KK, Tann M, et al: Evaluation of prospective living renal donors for laparoscopic nephrectomy with multisection CT: The marriage of minimally invasive imaging with minimally invasive surgery. RadioGraphics 21:S223-S236, 2001.

336. Kawamoto S, Montgomery R, Lawler LP, et al: Multi-detector row CT evaluation of living renal donors prior to laparoscopic nephrectomy. Radiographics 24:1513–1514, 2003.

337. Hofmann LV, Smith PA, Kuszyk BS, et al: Original report. Three-dimensional helical CT angiography in renal transplant recipients: A new problem-solving tool. Am J Roentgenol 173:1085–1089, 1999.

338. Pozniak MA, Balison DJ, Lee FT, et al: CT angiography of potential renal transplant donors. RadioGraphics 18:565–587, 1998.

339. Kawamoto S, Lawler LP, Fishman EK: Evaluation of the renal venous system on late arterial and venous phase images with MDCT angiography in potential living laparoscopic renal donors. Am J Roentgenol 184:539–545, 2005.

340. Sahani DV, Rastogi N, Greenfield AC, et al: Multi-detector row CT in evaluation of 94 living renal donors by readers with varied experience. Radiology 235:905–910, 2005.

341. Rubin GD: Invited commentary. Helical CT of potential living renal donors: Toward a greater understanding. RadioGraphics 18(3):601–604, 1998.

342. Hohenwalter MD, Skowlund CJ, Erickson SJ, et al: Renal transplant evaluation with MR angiography and MR imaging. RadioGraphics 21:1505–1517, 2001.

343. Hussain SM, Kock MCJM, Ifzermans JNM, et al: MR imaging: A "one-stop shop" modality for preoperative evaluation of potential living kidney donors. RadioGraphics 23:505–520, 2003.

344. Israel GM, Lee VS, Edye M, et al: Comprehensive MR imaging in the preoperative evaluation of living donor candidates for laparoscopic nephrectomy: Initial experience. Radiology 225:427–432, 2002.

345. Van den Dool SW, Wasser MN, de Fijter JW, et al: Functional renal volume: Quantitative analysis at gadolinium-enhanced MR angiography—feasibility study in healthy potential kidney donors. Radiology 236:189–195, 2005.

346. Akbar SA, Jafri ZH, Amendola MA, et al: Complications of renal transplantation. RadioGraphics 25:1335–1356, 2005.

347. Allen KS, Jorkasky DK, Arger PH, et al: Renal allografts: Prospective analysis of Doppler sonography. Radiology 169:371–376, 1998.

348. Grant EG, Perrella RR: Commentary. Wishing won't make it so: Duplex Doppler sonography in the evaluation of renal transplant dysfunction. Am J Roentgenol 155:538–539, 1990.

349. Reuther G, Wanjura D, Bauer H: Acute renal vein thrombosis in renal allografts: Detection with duplex Doppler US. Radiology 170:557–558, 1989.

350. Buckley AR, Cooperberg PL, Reeve CE, Magil AB: The distinction between acute renal transplant rejection and cyclosporine nephrotoxicity: Value of duplex sonography. Am J Roentgenol 149:521–525, 1987.

351. Kaveggia LP, Perrella RR, Grant EG, et al: Duplex Doppler sonography in renal allografts: The significance of reversed flow in diastole. Am J Roentgenol 155:295–298, 1990.

352. Voegeli DR, Crummy AB, McDermott JC, et al: Percutaneous management of the urological complications of renal transplantation. RadioGraphics 6(6):1007–1022, 1986.

353. Patel NH, Jindal RM, Wilkin T, et al: Renal arterial stenosis in renal allografts: Retrospective study of predisposing factors and outcome after percutaneous transluminal angioplasty. Radiology 219:663–667, 2001.

354. Vrachliotis TG, Vaswani KK, Davies EA, et al: Pictorial essay. CT findings in posttransplantation lymphoproliferative disorder of renal transplants. Am J Roentgenol 175:183–188, 2000.

355. Sadowski EA, Fain SB, Alford SK, et al: Assessment of acute renal transplant rejection with blood oxygen level-dependent MR imaging: Initial experience. Radiology 236:911–191, 2005.

356. Yang D, Ye Q, Williams DS, et al: Normal and transplanted rat kidneys: Diffusion MR imaging at 7 T. Radiology 231:702–709, 2004.

357. Dubovsky EV, Russell CD, Erbas B: Radionuclide evaluation of renal transplants. Semin Nucl Med 25(1):49–59, 1995.

358. Dunagin P, Alijani M, Atkins F, et al: Application of the kidney to aortic blood flow index to renal transplants. Clin Nucl Med 8:360–364, 1983.

359. Lin E, Alavi A: Significance of early tubular extraction in the first minute of Tc-99m MAG3 renal transplant scintigraphy. Clin Nucl Med 23(4):217–22, 1998.

360. Fortenbery EJ, Blue PW, Van Nostrand D, Anderson JH: Lymphocele: The spectrum of scintigraphic findings in lymphoceles associated with renal transplant. J Nucl Med 31:1627–1631, 1990.

CHAPTER 28

Interventional Nephrology

Ivan D. Maya • Michael Allon • Souheil Saddekni • David G. Warnock

OVERVIEW OF VASCULAR ACCESS FOR DIALYSIS

Most patients with end-stage renal disease undergo hemodialysis thrice weekly to optimize their survival, minimize medical complications, and enhance their quality of life. A reliable vascular access is a critical requirement for providing adequate hemodialysis. The ideal vascular access would be easy to place, be ready to use as soon as it is placed, deliver high blood flows indefinitely, and be free of complications. None of the existing types of vascular access achieves this ideal. Among the three types of vascular access currently available, native arteriovenous (AV) fistulas are superior to AV grafts, which, in turn, are superior to dialysis catheters. Recognizing the relative merits of the vascular access types, the Kidney Disease Outcomes Quality Initiative (K/DOQI) guidelines recommend placement of AV fistulas in at least 50% of hemodialysis patients, AV grafts in 40%, and dialysis catheters in no more than 10%.[1] The actual current distribution of vascular accesses among prevalent hemodialysis patients in the United States is 25% to 30% fistulas, 45% to 50% grafts, and 25% dialysis catheters.[2,3]

Vascular access procedures and their subsequent complications represent a major cause of morbidity, hospitalization, and cost for chronic hemodialysis patients.[4–8] Over 20% of hospitalizations in hemodialysis patients in the United States are access related, and the annual cost of access morbidity is close to $1 billion.[7] AV grafts are prone to recurrent stenosis and thrombosis and require multiple radiologic or surgical interventions to ensure their long-term patency for dialysis. Fistulas have a much lower incidence of stenosis and thrombosis than grafts do and require a much lower frequency of interventions to maintain their long-term patency for dialysis.[7–9] Conversely, fistulas have a higher primary failure rate (fistulas that never become usable for dialysis) than grafts do. Tunneled dialysis catheters have the highest frequency of infection and thrombosis but are a necessary evil, either as a bridge device in patients waiting for a fistula or graft or as an access of last resort in patients who have exhausted all options for a permanent vascular access.[10,11] Compared with patients who continue to dialyze with catheters, those who switch from a catheter to a fistula or graft have a substantially lower mortality risk.[12]

Even with aggressive efforts to follow the K/DOQI guideline on vascular access, it is likely that all three types of vascular access will remain in use for the foreseeable future. Much more clinical research is necessary to learn how to minimize the complications and optimize the outcomes of each type of vascular access.

RATIONALE FOR INTERVENTIONAL NEPHROLOGY

Patients with stage 4 chronic kidney disease are regularly seen by their nephrologists and referred to different subspecialists, including vascular surgeons and interventional radiologists, for access placement for hemodialysis or peritoneal dialysis. Once these patients start their dialysis treatments, vascular access becomes a very important aspect of their care. The patients undergo frequent placement of temporary or tunneled hemodialysis catheters, revision of a permanent access, surgical or percutaneous thrombectomies, and other related endovascular procedures. For a long time, nephrologists have taken a passive role in this very complicated but important area of dialysis care. However, nephrologists who were interested in improving the quality and timely provision of these services have developed a growing interest in having such procedures performed by appropriately trained nephrologists.[13]

During the last decade, some nephrologists have become directly motivated in providing access procedures for their patients. This initiative was pioneered by Gerald Beathard[14] and subsequently adopted by nephrologists at other medical centers.[15–20] It is not uncommon at present to find well-trained nephrologists getting actively involved in performing the various imaging and interventional dialysis procedures. Depending on the degree and depth of their training, interventional nephrologists can provide ultrasound and biopsy of kidneys, vascular mapping before access surgery, and continued involvement after surgery by providing procedures necessary for the maintenance of long-term patency of the vascular access. A decrease in hospitalizations for vascular access–related complications and missed outpatient hemodialysis sessions has been documented at one dialysis center when nephrologists performed interventional access procedures.[20]

In 2000, a group of physicians, including nephrologists and radiologists, formed the American Society of Diagnostic and Interventional Nephrology (ASDIN). This organization provides certification to interventional nephrologists as well as accreditation to the institutions involved in the practice and teaching of interventional procedures in the nephrology specialty.[18] Certification and accreditation are given for diagnostic ultrasound, peritoneal dialysis insertion, and endovascular procedures on AV fistulas, grafts, and chronic central venous catheters for dialysis. Comprehensive training is required to achieve dexterity and knowledge. Several academic centers in the United States already have interventional nephrology programs in place, either in a freestanding interventional facility or in a hospital-based radiology suite. A comprehensive list of procedures performed by interventional nephrologists is provided in Table 28–1.

A given interventional nephrology program may provide only a subset of these procedures, depending on the local needs and arrangements with other medical subspecialties. A solo nephrologist may decide to perform selected procedures necessary to provide an immediate dialysis access (such as insertion of dialysis catheters), thus eliminating delays resulting from scheduling difficulties. Conversely, a nephrology group practice may designate one or two nephrologists to be fully trained to perform a spectrum of interventional procedures.

At University of Alabama at Birmingham (UAB), a unique multidisciplinary model has been adopted to the patients' best advantage. This model consists of a joint interventional radiology/nephrology program, with interventional nephrologists and interventional radiologists sharing the same radiology suites, and working side by side to perform all dialysis access procedures. This program draws its success by using all existing technical, clinical, imaging, and surgical talents at the same institution.

A key element of any successful interventional program, whether it involves radiologists or nephrologists, is to have actively involved nephrology and dialysis program directors tracking the outcomes of the procedures and implementing timely quality improvement initiatives to improve outcomes. This can be best accomplished by having dedicated vascular access coordinators who maintain prospective, computerized records of all access procedures performed.[21]

RADIATION AND PERSONAL SAFETY

The understanding of basic radiation safety is very important to protect the patient, the physician, and the staff involved in the care of the patient. Unnecessary radiation exposure is harmful and can be easily prevented. The U.S. Food and Drug Administration (FDA) oversees the rules and regulations for use of x-ray equipment. The U.S. Occupational Safety and Health Administration (OSHA) regulates the radiation exposure of workers. Each state has its own regulatory office to ensure that workers do not exceed a predetermined radiation dose.

Exposure is the amount of ionizing radiation reaching a subject, and it is measured in units of Roentgen. The amount of energy absorbed by a material when it is exposed to ionizing radiation is measured in rads. The absorbed dose is always lower than the exposure, because the tissue does not absorb all the energy from the radiation. An absorbed dose equivalent is used to relate the amount of biologic damage and is measured in rem. The OSHA occupational dose limit for the whole body is 1.25 rem/quarter; for the extremities, it is 18.75 rem/quarter. A dosimeter must be worn at all times on the outside of the lead apron, and the absorbed dose measured monthly. To protect against radiation, the interventionist should minimize the time of exposure to radiation, minimize the use of magnification imaging, properly use collimators and field filters, maximize the distance between the source of radiation and the personnel involved with the procedure, minimize the use of cineangiography and continuous fluoroscopy, and use proper shielding, including lead aprons, thyroid collars, leaded glasses, and lead shields.

Knowledge of these facts and application of appropriate safeguards are particularly important in dialysis access procedures, especially those involving vascular access interventions in the upper extremity. The operators' proximity to the x-ray tube and difficulty in shielding increases their radiation exposure

PROCEDURES INVOLVING ARTERIOVENOUS GRAFTS

Surveillance for Graft Stenosis

About 80% of graft failures are due to thrombosis, whereas 20% are due to infection.[22,23] Thus, improving graft longevity requires implementing measures to reduce the frequency of graft thrombosis. When grafts are referred for thrombectomy, a significant underlying stenosis is observed, most commonly at the venous anastomosis, the draining vein, or the central veins.[24–26] This observation suggests that prophylactic angioplasty of hemodynamically significant graft stenosis may reduce the frequency of graft thrombosis, and thereby increase cumulative graft survival.

A seminal study by Schwab and co-workers[27] was the first to provide evidence supporting this approach. This group of investigators performed measurements of dynamic dialysis venous pressures during consecutive hemodialysis sessions under carefully standardized conditions. They discovered that a persistent elevation in the dialysis venous pressure measured at a low dialysis blood flow was predictive of

TABLE 28–1	Procedures Performed by Interventional Nephrologists
Diagnostic renal ultrasound	
Ultrasound guided percutaneous renal biopsy	
Placement of nontunneled and tunneled dialysis catheters	
Exchange of tunneled dialysis catheters	
Implantation of subcutaneous dialysis devices	
Preoperative vascular mapping	
Surveillance for stenosis	
Diagnostic fistulograms of arterio-venous grafts and fistulas	
Angioplasty of peripheral and central venous stenosis	
Deployment of endoluminal stents for peripheral and central venous stenosis	
Mechanical thrombectomy of arterio-venous grafts and fistulas	
Sonographic or angiographic assessment of immature fistulas	
Salvage procedures for immature fistulas	
Placement of peritoneal dialysis catheters	

hemodynamically significant stenosis. The investigators then instituted a program of clinical monitoring for graft stenosis, with referral for prophylactic angioplasty if there was a suspicion of graft stenosis. Compared with the historical control period, a regimen of stenosis monitoring and prophylactic angioplasty reduced the frequency of graft thrombosis by about two thirds, from 0.6 to 0.2 events per year. This landmark study stimulated a large volume of subsequent clinical research directed at two fundamental issues: (1) identifying a variety of noninvasive methods to screen for graft stenosis and (2) evaluating whether stenosis surveillance and prophylactic angioplasty improved graft outcomes.

A variety of methods have been validated for detection of hemodynamically significant graft *stenosis* (Table 28–2). Clinical monitoring consists of using information that is readily available from physical examination of the AV graft, abnormalities experienced during the dialysis sessions (difficult cannulation or prolonged bleeding from the needle puncture sites), or unexplained decreases in the dose of dialysis (Kt/V).[24,25,28] Graft surveillance uses noninvasive tests requiring specialized equipment or technician training that are not obtained as part of the routine dialysis treatment. These include measurement of static dialysis venous pressure (normalized for the systemic pressure),[29,30] measurement of the access blood flow,[31–34] or duplex ultrasound to evaluate directly for evidence of stenosis.[35–38] Each of these monitoring or surveillance tools has been reported to have a positive predictive value for graft stenosis between 70% and 100% (Table 28–3). The negative predictive value has not been studied systematically, as it would require obtaining routine fistulograms in patients whose screening test is negative. However, it can be inferred from the proportion of graft thromboses not preceded by abnormalities of graft surveillance (~25%).[34]

In contrast, the predictive value of these surveillance methods for graft *thrombosis* is much less impressive. Thus, when grafts with abnormal monitoring criteria suggestive of stenosis are observed without preemptive angioplasty, only about 40% of the grafts clot over the next 3 months.[39,40] In practice, this means that in any program of graft monitoring, about half of the preemptive angioplasties that are performed are superfluous. Unfortunately, there are no reliable tests to distinguish between the subset of grafts with stenosis that will progress to thrombosis from those that will remain patent without any intervention.

Several observational studies have documented that introduction of a monitoring or surveillance program for graft stenosis with preemptive angioplasty lowered the frequency of graft thrombosis by 40% to 80%, compared with the historical control period during which there was no monitoring program (Table 28–4).[21,27–29,41,42] The promising findings from multiple observational studies have led to the K/DOQI recommendations of implementing a program of graft surveillance and preemptive angioplasty in all dialysis centers in order to reduce the frequency of graft thrombosis.[1]

Only in the last few years has the value of graft stenosis surveillance been subjected to rigorous testing in randomized clinical trials. To date, there have been six such trials, evalu-

TABLE 28–2   Methods of Stenosis Monitoring

Clinical monitoring
Physical examination (abnormal bruit, absent thrill, distal edema)
Dialysis abnormalities (prolonged bleeding from needle sites, difficult cannulation)
Unexplained decrease in Kt/V

Surveillance
Static dialysis venous pressure (adjusted for systemic pressure)
Access blood flow
  Qa < 600 mL/min
  Qa decreased by > 25% from baseline
Doppler ultrasound

Kt/V, dialysis dose; Qa, access blood flow.

TABLE 28–3   Positive Predictive Value of Monitoring Methods for Graft Stenosis

Surveillance Method	Measurements (N)	Positive Predictive Value (%)
Clinical monitoring		
Cayco et al, 1998[41]	68	93
Robbin et al, 1998[37]	38	89
Safa et al, 1996[28]	106	92
Maya et al, 2004[25]	358	69
Robbin et al, 2006[38]	151	70
Static venous pressure		
Besarab et al, 1995[29]	87	92
Flow monitoring		
Schwab, 2001[48]	35	100
Moist et al, 2003[45]	53	87
Ultrasound		
Robbin et al, 2006[38]	122	80

TABLE 28–4   Effect of Surveillance on Graft Thrombosis: Observational Studies

Reference	Surveillance Method	Thrombosis Rate (Per Graft-Yr) Historical Control	Surveillance Period	Reduction (%)
Schwab et al, 1989[27]	Dynamic dialysis venous pressure	0.61	0.20	67
Besarab et al, 1995[29]	Static dialysis venous pressure	0.50	0.28	64
Safa et al, 1996[28]	Clinical monitoring	0.48	0.17	64
Allon et al, 1998[21]	Clinical monitoring	0.70	0.28	60
Cayco et al, 1998[41]	Clinical monitoring	0.49	0.29	41
McCarley et al, 2001[42]	Flow monitoring	0.71	0.16	77

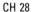

TABLE 28–5 Randomized Clinical Trials of Graft Surveillance

Reference	Surveillance Method	Subjects (N)		PTA/Yr		Thromb-free Survival at 1 Yr		Cum Survival at 1 Yr	
		Con	Surv	Con	Surv	Con	Surv	Con	Surv
Lumsden et al, 1997[173]	Doppler US	32	32	0	1.5	0.51	0.47	N/A	N/A
Ram et al, 2003[36]	Access flow	34	32	0.22	0.34	0.45	0.52	0.72	0.80
	Doppler US		35		0.65		0.70		0.80
Moist et al, 2003[45]	Access flow	53	59	0.61	0.93	0.74	0.67	0.83	0.83
Dember et al, 2004[43]	Static DVP	32	32	0.04	2.1	N/A	N/A	0.74	0.56
Malik et al, 2005[35]	Doppler US	92	97	N/A	N/A	N/A	N/A	0.73	0.93
Robbin et al, 2006[38]	Doppler US	61	65	0.64	1.06	0.57	0.63	0.83	0.85

Con, control; Cum, cumulative; DVP, dialysis venous pressure; N/A, not available; PTA, percutaneous transluminal angioplasty; Surv, surveillance; Thromb, thrombosis; US, ultrasound.

CH 28

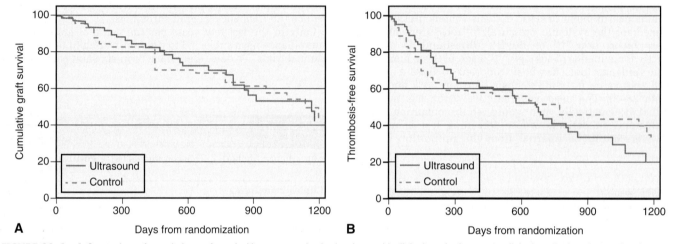

FIGURE 28–1 **A,** Comparison of cumulative graft survival between randomized patients with clinical monitoring versus clinical monitoring plus regular ultrasound surveillance of grafts. $P = .93$ by the log rank test. **B,** Comparison of thrombosis-free graft survival between randomized patients with clinical monitoring versus clinical monitoring plus regular ultrasound surveillance of grafts. $P = .33$ by the log rank test. (Reproduced from Robbin ML, Oser RF, Lee JY, et al: Randomized comparison of ultrasound surveillance and clinical monitoring on arteriovenous graft outcomes. Kidney Int 69:730–735, 2006.)

ating surveillance with access flow monitoring, static dialysis venous pressure, or ultrasound (Table 28–5). Only one of the six randomized trials has demonstrated a benefit of ultrasound graft surveillance[35]; the other five studies were negative, despite a substantial increase in the frequency of preemptive angioplasty in the surveillance group.[36,38,43–45] For example, one study randomized patients with grafts to standard clinical monitoring alone or to a combination of clinical monitoring and ultrasound surveillance for stenosis. The patients in the ultrasound group underwent a 66% higher frequency of preemptive angioplasty, yet there was no difference between the two randomized groups in terms of frequency of graft thrombosis, time to first thrombosis, or likelihood of graft failure (Fig. 28–1).[38] Because the randomized studies have been relatively small in size, it is possible they were inadequately powered to detect a modest benefit of graft surveillance. A large-scale, multicenter study would be required to provide a definitive answer to this controversial question. In the meantime, the value of surveillance of graft stenosis and preemptive angioplasty in improving graft outcomes remains controversial.[46,47]

If underlying graft stenosis is an important predictor of graft thrombosis, why is preemptive angioplasty not more successful in reducing graft thrombosis? The fundamental problem appears to be the short-lived efficacy of angioplasty to relieve graft stenosis. When serial access blood flows have been used as a surrogate marker of successful angioplasty, 20% of grafts have recurrent stenosis within 1 week of angioplasty and 40% within 1 month of angioplasty.[45,48] In another study, the mean access blood flow after angioplasty increased from 596 to 922 mL/min. However, 3 months later, the mean flow had decreased to 672 mL/min.[49] In addition, there is published evidence suggesting that the injury from balloon angioplasty can actually accelerate myointimal hyperplasia, thereby resulting in recurrent stenosis.[50] Not surprisingly, patients undergoing angioplasty for graft stenosis require frequent re-interventions owing to recurrent stenosis. The median intervention-free patency after graft stenosis is only about 6 months.[24,25]

The pathophysiology of graft stenosis involves proliferation of vascular smooth muscle cells (myointimal hyperplasia), with progressive encroachment of the lesion into the graft lumen.[51] To improve the patency of grafts after angioplasty, some investigators have attempted stent deployment. The rationale is that the rigid scaffold of the stent helps to keep the vascular lumen open. There has also been an ongoing

TABLE 28–6	Location of Stenosis in Patients with Grafts Undergoing Angioplasty				
Reference	All Stenotic Lesions (%)				
	VA	VO	CV	IG	AA
Beathard, 1992[26]	42	34	4	20	0
Lilly et al, 2001[24] Elective PTA	55	22	15	6	2.5
Lilly et al, 2001[24] Thrombectomy	60	14	9	10	7
Maya et al, 2004[25]	62	16	8	12	1.5

AA, arterial anastomosis; CV, central vein; IG, intragraft; PTA, percutaneous transluminal angioplasty; VA, venous anastomosis; VO, venous outflow.

TABLE 28–7	Primary Graft Patency After Elective Angioplasty			
Reference	Procedures (N)	Primary Patency At		
		3 Mo	6 Mo	12 Mo
Beathard, 1992[26]	536	79	61	38
Kanterman et al, 1995[174]	90		63	41
Safa et al, 1996[28]	90	70	47	16
Turmel-Rodrigues et al, 2000[92]	98	85	53	29
Lilly et al, 2001[24]	330	71	51	28
Maya et al, 2004[25]	155	79	52	31

CH 28

Interventional Nephrology

interest in pharmacologic approaches to prevention of myo-intimal hyperplasia. Two small, single-center, randomized clinical trials have documented a beneficial effect of dipyridamole and fish oil in preventing graft thrombosis.[52,53] A multi-center, randomized, double-blinded study compared clopidogrel plus aspirin with placebo for prevention of graft thrombosis. The study was terminated early owing to an excess of bleeding complications in the intervention group; there was no difference in the rate of graft thrombosis between the two randomized groups.[54] The Dialysis Access Consortium (sponsored by the National Institute of Diabetes and Digestive and Kidney Diseases [NIDDK]) is currently conducting a large, multicenter, randomized, double-blinded clinical trial to compare Aggrenox (long-acting dipyridamole + low-dose aspirin) with placebo in prevention of graft failure.[55] Details of pharmacologic approaches to prophylaxis of graft stenosis and thrombosis are beyond the scope of this chapter.

Angioplasty of Graft Stenosis

As described in the previous section, patients with patent grafts are frequently referred for elective angioplasty when hemodynamically significant stenosis is detected either by clinical monitoring or by one of several methods of graft surveillance. The goal of elective angioplasty is to correct the stenotic lesion that impairs optimal delivery of dialysis and, hopefully, delay graft thrombosis. The most common location of the stenosis by angiography is the venous anastomosis, followed by the peripheral draining vein, central vein, and intragraft (Table 28–6). Inflow (arterial anastomosis) stenosis has been rare (<5%) in most series. However, a recent study using retrograde angiography with manual occlusion of the venous limb documented an inflow stenosis in 29% of grafts referred for diagnostic angiography.[56]

A number of published series have documented the short-lived primary patency (time to next radiologic or surgical intervention) of grafts after elective angioplasty (Table 28–7), with only 50% to 60% patent at 6 months and 30% to 40% at 1 year. This means that, on average, each graft requires two angioplasties per year. The primary patency is shorter after angioplasty of central vein stenosis compared with other stenotic locations. In one study, the primary patency at 6 months was only 29% for central vein stenosis compared with 67% for stenosis at the venous anastomosis.[26] Most studies have documented progressively shorter patency after each consecutive angioplasty, although one investigator found comparable primary patency for the first and subsequent graft angioplasties.[26]

The primary patency of AV grafts after elective angioplasty is not affected by patient age, race, diabetes, or peripheral vascular diseases.[25] However, the patency is shorter in women than in men.[25] The primary patency after angioplasty is also not influenced by the location of the graft or the number of concurrent stenotic lesions found.[24]

The technical success of an angioplasty procedure may be assessed in several ways. The first is a visual inspection of the graft before and after the procedure to determine whether the magnitude (percent of stenosis relative to the normal vessel diameter) has been reduced. The degree of stenosis of each lesion can be quantified with calipers or graded semi-quantitatively using the following scale: grade 1, no (<10%) stenosis; grade 2, mild (10%–49%) stenosis; grade 3, moderate (50%–69%) stenosis; and grade 4, severe (70%–99%) stenosis.[24,25] A second approach is to measure the intragraft pressure before and after the procedure and normalize it for the systemic blood pressure. A third approach is to measure the change in access blood flow before and after the procedure. Each of these measures has been shown to be predictive of the primary patency of grafts after elective angioplasty. In one large series, after elective angioplasty, the median intervention-free survival of graft with no residual stenosis was 6.9 months compared with 4.6 months if there was any degree of residual stenosis.[24] Similarly, the median primary patency of grafts after angioplasty was inversely proportional to the intragraft-to–systemic pressure ratio, being 7.6, 6.9, and 5.6 months, when this ratio was less than 0.4, 0.4 to 0.6, and greater than 0.6, respectively.[24] Finally, a failure to significantly increase the access blood flow after angioplasty is observed in 20% of grafts at 1 week and in 40% by 1 month,[45,48] confirming the short-lived benefit of this intervention.

Technical Procedure: Percutaneous Graft Angioplasty

The AV graft is accessed with a micropuncture single needle at the arterial limb of the graft toward the venous outflow. The needle is exchanged for a 4-French catheter. Digitally subtracted antegrade angiograms are taken through the catheter to visualize the venous limb of the graft, the draining vein and central vessels. After applying pressure to the venous outflow, a retrograde angiogram is performed to visualize the arterial anastomosis. The presence or absence of stenotic lesions and their number and location, arterial anastomosis, intragraft, venous anastomosis, draining vein and central vein are recorded. The degree of stenosis of each lesion is quantified with calipers or graded semiquantitatively.[24,25] Lesions with at least 50% stenosis are considered to be hemodynamically significant and undergo angioplasty. If a stenotic lesion is encountered, then the 4-French catheter is exchanged for a 6-French sheath. An angioplasty balloon is introduced through the sheath. Balloon sizes (7–12 mm in diameter to 20–80 mm in length) vary depending on the

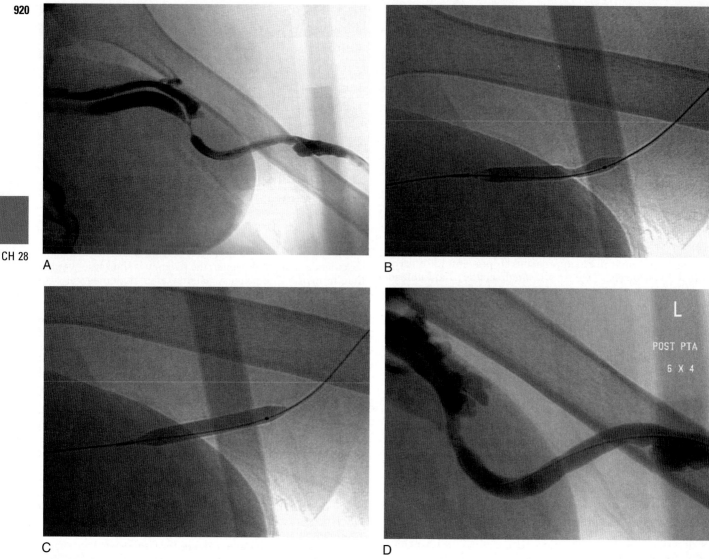

FIGURE 28–2 **A,** Left upper arm arteriovenous (AV) graft angiogram shows a severe (95%) stenotic lesion at the level of the venous anastomosis. **B,** Left upper arm AV graft stenotic lesion at the venous anastomosis with the angioplasty balloon partially inflated. **C,** Left upper arm AV graft stenotic lesion at the venous anastomosis with the angioplasty balloon fully inflated. **D,** Final postangioplasty left upper arm AV graft angiogram shows a treated lesion with minimal residual stenosis.

vessel to be treated; usually the balloon is selected to be 1 mm larger than the size of the graft or the vessel to be treated. The balloon is placed at the level of the stenotic lesion and inflated to its nominal pressure for 30 to 90 seconds (Figs. 28–2 and 28–3). The majority of anastomotic lesions require higher pressure than those required for peripheral arterial angioplasty. Therefore, high-pressure balloons with minimal burst pressure greater than 15 atm are routinely used.[57] If a residual (>30%) stenosis is found, prolonged angioplasty (5-min inflation), higher-pressure balloons (≤30 atm), and occasionally, stent deployment may be required to treat these lesions. At UAB, the patient's intragraft pressure and systemic pressure are measured before and immediately after the intervention. In addition to angiographic findings, we rely on a reduction of intragraft-to-systemic pressure ratio to confirm technical success and hemodynamic improvement. Other centers rely on different criteria, such as increases in access flow rate.

The major complications of this procedure are vessel extravasations and rupture of the vessel after the angioplasty treatment. Deploying a covered stent (endograft) can treat these complications. Surgical repair is indicated if the rupture is not corrected by stent placement.

Thrombectomy of Grafts

The majority of graft failures are due to thrombosis, which occurs most commonly in the context of underlying stenosis at the venous anastomosis.[23,24] For this reason, successful graft thrombectomy requires both resolution of the clot and correction of the underlying stenotic lesion. The primary patency of grafts after thrombectomy and angioplasty (Table 28–8) ranges from 30% to 63% at 3 months and 11% to 39% at 6 months. These outcomes are considerably worse than the primary patency observed after elective angioplasty (see Table 28–7), which is 71% to 85% at 3 months and 47% to 63% at 6 months. The primary graft patency is similar for mechanical thrombectomy and pharmacomechanical thrombectomy.[58] A large series comparing the outcomes of both types of radiologic procedures at one institution found that the primary patency was only 30% at 3 months for clotted grafts compared with 71% for patent grafts undergoing elective angioplasty (Fig. 28–4A).[24] The discrepancy was still apparent when the analysis was restricted to the subset of procedures in which there was no residual stenosis, with a median primary patency of 2.5 months after thrombectomy

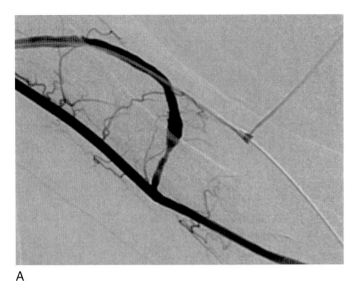

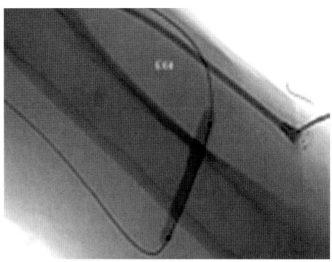

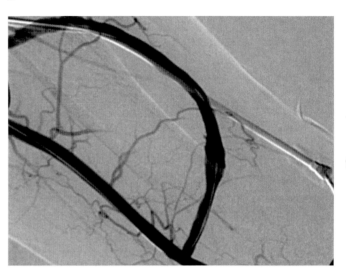

FIGURE 28–3 **A,** Digital subtraction angiography (DSA) of a left upper arm AV graft shows a moderate stenotic lesion at the level of the arterial limb of the graft. **B,** Spot film shows the stenotic lesion being angioplastied. **C,** Final postangioplasty DSA shows excellent results.

CH 28

Interventional Nephrology

TABLE 28–8	Primary Graft Patency After Thrombectomy		
		Primary Patency At	
Reference	Procedures (N)	3 Mo	6 Mo
Valji et al, 1991[175]	121	53	34
Trerotola et al, 1994[176]	34	45	19
Beathard, 1994[58]	55 mech / 48 pharm	37 / 46	
Cohen et al, 1994[177]	135	33	25
Sands et al, 1994[178]	71		11
Beathard, 1995[179]	425	50	33
Beathard et al, 1996[180]	1176	52	39
Trerotola et al, 1998[181]	112	40	25
Turmel-Rodrigues et al, 2000[92]	58	63	32
Lilly et al, 2001[24]	326	30	19

Mech, mechanical; pharm, pharmacomechanical.

compared with 6.9 months after elective angioplasty (see Fig. 28–4B).[24]

The duration of graft patency after thrombectomy does not differ between diabetic and nondiabetic patients. It is also not affected by the graft location or the number of concurrent graft stenoses found.[24] However, similar to the observations obtained after elective angioplasty, the primary patency of grafts after thrombectomy is inversely proportional to the magnitude of residual stenosis at the end of the procedure.[24]

Technical Procedure: Percutaneous Graft Thrombectomy

The AV graft is initially accessed with a single-wall needle at level of the arterial limb of the graft. A glidewire is passed up to the venous outlet and the needle exchanged for a 6-French catheter sheath. A catheter is placed beyond the clotted graft, and a venogram is performed of the venous outflow and central circulation. Extreme caution is exercised not to pressure-inject contrast into the graft, because it can dislodge clot and cause arterial emboli. Because greater than 60% of the stenotic lesions are located at the venous anastomosis, an angioplasty balloon, usually 8 by 40 mm, is placed at that site and inflated to its nominal pressure (15 atm). The

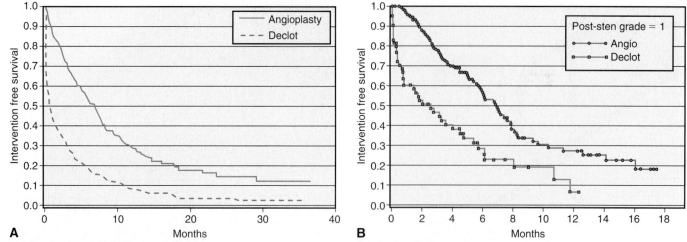

FIGURE 28–4 **A,** Intervention-free graft survival following elective angioplasty *(solid line)* or thrombectomy + angioplasty *(dotted line).* Graft survival was calculated from the date of the initial intervention to the date of the next intervention (angioplasty, declot, or surgical revision). *P* < .001 for the comparison between the two groups. **B,** Intervention-free graft survival following elective angioplasty *(circles)* or thrombectomy + angioplasty *(triangles)* in the subset of procedures with no residual stenosis. Graft survival was calculated from the date of the initial intervention to the date of the next intervention (angioplasty, declot, or surgical revision). *P* < .001 for the comparison between the two groups. (Reproduced from Lilly RZ, Carlton D, Barker J, et al: Clinical predictors of A-V graft patency following radiologic intervention in hemodialysis patients. Am J Kidney Dis 37:945–953, 2001.)

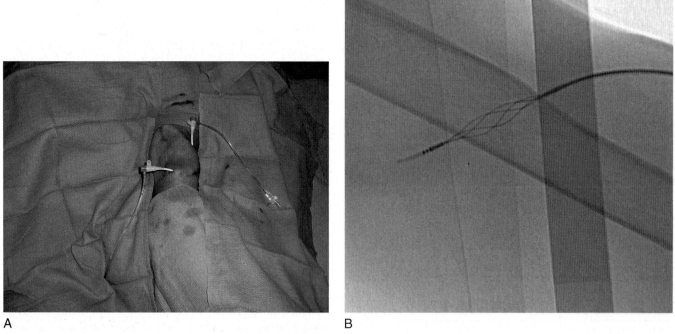

FIGURE 28–5 **A,** Percutaneous mechanical thrombectomy: A left upper arm AV graft site is prepped and two 6-French sheaths are in place. **B,** Percutaneous mechanical thrombectomy: Spot film shows the use of a percutaneous thrombectomy device (PTD). (Arrow-Trerotola-PTD.)

balloon is removed, and then a mechanical thrombectomy can be achieved by several methods including manual aspiration of the clots, infusion of a thrombolytic agent (tissue-type plasminogen activator [t-PA], urokinase), use of a clot-buster device (Angiojet, Arrow-Trerotola, Cragg thrombolytic brush, Hydrolyser, Prolumen, Amplatz thrombectomy device), or a combination of any of these (Fig. 28–5). Pure mechanical thrombectomy is sufficient, and thrombolysis rarely necessary. The graft is accessed for a second time with a single-wall needle at the venous limb of the graft. The needle is exchanged

over a wire for a 6-French catheter sheath. A glidewire is passed into the arterial circulation. A Fogarty balloon is passed beyond the arterial anastomosis and pulled back to dislodge the arterial plug. Aspiration of the clots through both sheaths is performed; the clot-bluster device is used again to clear all debris still in the graft. Once blood flow in the graft is restored, as assessed by physical examination, small amounts of contrast are injected to check for residual clots. Finally, antegrade and retrograde angiograms of the graft are performed to assess for patency and look for other stenotic lesions. Angioplasty of any residual hemodynamically significant stenotic lesion in the vascular access circuit is performed. Intra-access pressure and systemic pressure (measured inside the graft by occluding the venous outflow) are measured. The ratio is calculated to confirm acceptable angioplasty results. High intragraft pressures indicate residual venous anastomotic obstruction, whereas low pressures indicate obstruction at the arterial inflow.

Major complications of this procedure are vessel extravasations and rupture of the vein either because of wire manipulation or as a result of the angioplasty; stent deployment is the treatment of choice. Arterial emboli distal to the AV anastomosis may occur, and if encountered, either intervention or surgical embolectomy is required. One interventional method to treat this complication is back bleeding; which is simply an occlusion of the artery before its anastomosis to the graft, causing a retrograde blood flow that brings the clot into the graft. The use of a Fogarty balloon to remove the clot and the use of thrombolytics agents can also be performed to treat this complication.[59] Pulmonary embolism is common (~35%) in patients undergoing graft thrombectomy but is rarely of clinical significance.[60]

Deployment of Stents for Graft Stenosis/Thrombosis

As mentioned previously, the primary patency of grafts after angioplasty is short-lived, and there is evidence that the vascular injury from angioplasty may actually accelerate myointimal hyperplasia.[50] In view of these considerations, there has been considerable interest in technical modifications to improve the patency of grafts after angioplasty. Endoluminal stents work by forming a rigid scaffold preventing elastic recoil and helping to keep the vascular lumen open. Therefore, although myointimal hyperplasia recurs, it is less likely to narrow the vascular lumen. Stent placement has been attempted for the treatment for rapidly recurrent stenosis. A stenosis that is highly resistant to balloon angioplasty and cannot be expanded with a balloon is a contraindication for stent placement, because the stent will be as narrow as the original stenosis. On rare occasions, when trying to overcome such resistant stenoses with very high pressure, angioplasty may result in venous rupture and extravasation. Surgery is not necessary in these situations, as the complication can be converted to success by using stents or stent grafts (endograft).

Several small series have reported the outcomes after stent deployment for refractory vascular access stenosis.[61-67] Most of these studies have been limited by retrospective data collection, absence of a suitable control group, lumping together of patent and thrombosed accesses, and combining grafts with fistulas. A small randomized study comparing stents with conventional angioplasty found no difference in primary graft patency after the intervention.[62] However, this study enrolled a mixture of clotted and patent grafts, and the stenotic lesions were at a variety of locations, thus limiting the interpretation of the findings.

Because primary graft patency is particularly short-lived in clotted grafts undergoing thrombectomy, those grafts may experience better patency after stent deployment. One series reported the outcomes of 34 clotted grafts undergoing thrombectomy with stent placement at the venous anastomosis.[65] The primary patency after intervention in this homogeneous group of grafts was 63% at 6 months. Although there was no matched control group treated with angioplasty alone, the primary graft patency was much higher than that reported previously (11%–39% at 6 months) (see Table 28–8). A nonrandomized study comparing outcomes of clotted grafts treated with thrombectomy and stent placement at the venous anastomosis with matched control patients treated with only thrombectomy and angioplasty observed a significantly longer primary patency in grafts treated with a stent compared with those treated with angioplasty alone.[68] A definitive, randomized clinical trial is warranted to evaluate whether the patency of grafts after thrombectomy is enhanced by stent deployment.

A number of stent types are available, including covered and noncovered stents and either balloon or self-expandable. However, there are no published clinical trials comparing the outcomes between stent types. It is also possible that the administration of antiplatelet agents after stent placement or employment of drug-eluting stents (Sirolimus) may further improve the primary patency of grafts after thrombectomy, but again, there is no literature available at this time. Clopidrogel, an antiplatelet agent, is prescribed routinely after coronary stent placement to decrease early rethrombosis. It is not known whether administration of clopidogrel would prolong primary patency after AV graft stent placement.

Technical Procedure: Percutaneous Deployment of Stents

Percutaneous mechanical thrombectomy is achieved as described in the previous section. If a severe elastic recoil is seen on the final angiogram or a very significant residual stenosis (>30%) is seen at the level of the original stenotic lesion, then a stent could be deployed.[59] Stent sizes vary from 6 to 12 mm in diameter and 10 to 80 mm in length. The most commonly used stents are nitinol or nitinol covered with expanded polytetrafluoroethylene (e-PTFE). The appropriate size and length are determined by grading the stenotic lesion at the time of placement; usually, the stent is selected to be 1 mm larger than the size of the graft or the vessel to be treated and the length 5 mm longer than the stenotic lesion on each side. The stent comes already mounted in a device that is inserted through the sheath located at the arterial limb of the graft. A roadmap, contrast injection, of the stenotic lesion is performed. The stent is placed at the site of the stenotic lesion and deployed under fluoroscopic guidance (Fig. 28–6). A final angiogram is performed to assess for patency and proper placement of the stent.

Complications of stent deployment include those related to angioplasty. In addition, underestimation of the required stent size may result in stent migration to the systemic circulation. If the stent is placed at a site at which another vessel joins the main venous outlet, that vessel may be completely or partially occluded. Finally, a potential long-term complication is intrastent restenosis or thrombosis, which will require multiple frequent reinterventions.

PROCEDURES INVOLVING ARTERIOVENOUS FISTULAS

Preoperative Vascular Mapping

The need to increase placement of native AV fistulas has been highlighted by the K/DOQI guidelines[1] and by the Fistula First initiative (www.fistulafirst.org). There is widespread consensus among nephrologists and surgeons about the importance of maximizing fistula prevalence among hemodialysis patients. Achieving this goal, however, requires overcoming a number of hurdles, including timely referral of the patient with chronic kidney disease to the nephrologist and access surgeon, timely placement of an AV fistula, adequate maturation of new fistulas, and successful cannulation of the fistula for dialysis.[8] In the past, the surgeon's decision about the type and location of vascular access placed was determined by a physical examination of the extremity, with and without a tourniquet. This approach had the potential for

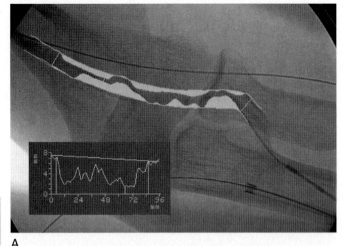

A

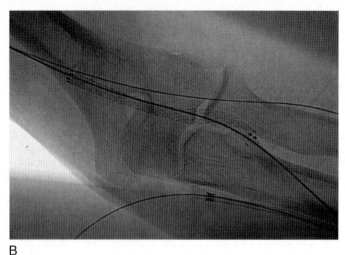

B

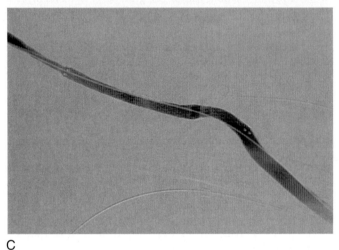

C

FIGURE 28–6 **A,** Angiogram demonstrates a severe stenotic lesion at the level of the venous anastomosis and the draining vein of a left forearm AV graft. The stenotic lesion has been graded before stent deployment. **B,** Spot film shows the stent fully deployed. **C,** DSA of the left forearm AV graft shows excellent results after stent deployment.

substantial errors. The surgeon may not be able to adequately visualize the veins in obese patients. As a result, the surgeon might place an AV graft when a fistula could have been feasible. In other patients, the surgeon may decide to place a radiocephalic fistula after visualizing a large diameter cephalic vein at the wrist. However, an unsuspected stenosis or thrombosis in a proximal portion of that vein would doom the success of this fistula.

The use of preoperative sonographic vascular mapping has been shown to substantially increase the proportion of patients receiving a fistula rather than a graft. A prospective pilot study at UAB compared the surgeon's decision about access placement in 70 consecutive chronic kidney disease patients, before and after the results of preoperative vascular mapping were provided to the surgeon.[69] In almost one third of the patients, the surgeon changed her or his mind about the intended access procedure after receiving the mapping results. In most of these cases, the surgeon decided to place a fistula rather than a graft, or changed her or his mind about the location of the fistula.[69] On the basis of these promising results, a program of routine preoperative vascular mapping was implemented. The results were dramatic: compared with the historical control period, the proportion of patients having a fistula placed increased from 34% to 64%. Moreover, the proportion of patients dialyzing with an AV fistula doubled from 16% to 34%.[70] Similar increases in fistula placement and fistula placement after introduction of preoperative vascular mapping have been documented by other investigators (Table 28–9), although a reduction in

primary fistula failure has not been a consistent finding in all studies.[70–73]

Although most centers have utilized sonographic vascular mapping, some have used venograms.[74] In patients with stage 4 chronic kidney disease who have not yet started dialysis, there is a theoretical concern of contrast nephropathy precipitating the need for initiation of dialysis. However, in a series of 25 patients with a mean glomerular filtration rate of 13 mL/min, none developed acute renal failure after undergoing angiography with 10 to 20 mL of low-osmolality contrast material.[75] Another potential risk is that venography of difficult-to-stick veins may injure veins required for future fistula creation. Venipuncture should be performed in the hand veins if at all possible, and the cephalic vein should be avoided at all costs.

Technical Procedure: Sonographic Preoperative Vascular Mapping

Vascular measurements are performed with the patient in a seated position, with the arm resting comfortably on a Mayo stand. All measurements are performed in the anteroposterior dimension in the transverse plane (Fig. 28–7). The minimum vein diameter for a native arteriovenous fistula is 2.5 mm. The minimum vein diameter for graft placement is 4.0 mm. The minimum arterial diameter for either fistula or graft placement is 2.0 mm. Veins are assessed for stenosis, thrombus, and sclerosis (thickened walls).

First, the radial artery diameter at the wrist is measured. A tourniquet is then placed at the mid to upper forearm.

TABLE 28–9	Effect of Preoperative Vascular Mapping on Vascular Access Outcomes					
Reference	**Fistulas Placed (%)**		**Primary Fistula Failure (%)**		**Prevalence of Fistula Use (%)**	
	Pre-VM	Post-VM	Pre-VM	Post-VM	Pre-VM	Post-VM
Silva et al, 1998[73]	14	63	36	8	8	64
Ascher et al, 2000[71]	0	100	N/A	18	5	68
Gibson et al, 2001[72]	11	95	18	25	N/A	N/A
Allon et al, 2001[70]	34	64	54	46	16	34
Sedlacek et al, 2001[182]	N/A	62	N/A	25	N/A	N/A
Mihmanli et al, 2001[183]			25	6		
Miller et al, 1997[184]	N/A	76				

N/A, not available; VM, preoperative vascular mapping.
Reproduced from Allon M, Robbin ML: Increasing arteriovenous fistulas in hemodialysis patients: Problems and solutions. Kidney Int 62:1109–1124, 2002.

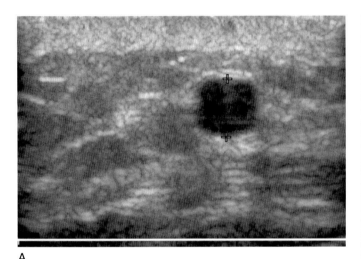
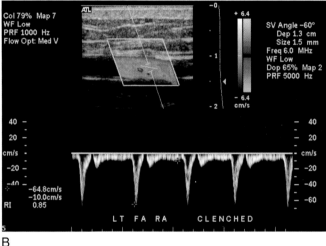

A   B

FIGURE 28–7   **A,** Venous mapping: Venous ultrasound shows a transverse section of a cephalic vein being measured (0.36 cm). **B,** Venous mapping: Doppler flow measurements and color Doppler ultrasound shows a longitudinal section of a left forearm radial artery that is 1.3 cm deep and 1.5 mm in diameter.

The veins above the wrist are percussed for 2 minutes, with special emphasis on the cephalic vein area. Sequential measurements are made of the cephalic vein at the wrist and mid and cranial forearm. Any other dorsal or volar veins at the wrist are also measured and followed up the arm, according to established diameter criteria. The tourniquet is sequentially moved up the arm, and cephalic, basilic, and brachial vein diameters are measured.

After the tourniquet is removed, the subclavian and jugular veins are assessed for stenosis and thrombus. Evidence of a more central stenosis is determined by analysis of the spectral Doppler waveform for respiratory phasicity and transmitted cardiac pulsatility. If there is a clinical or sonographic suspicion of central vein stenosis, a venogram or magnetic resonance venography (MRV) is obtained.

Measurements are recorded on a worksheet. The sonographic measurements are used by the surgeon to select the most appropriate vascular access, on the basis of the following list agreed upon by our nephrologists, radiologists, and vascular surgeons, from most desirable to least desirable:

1. Nondominant forearm cephalic vein fistula.
2. Dominant forearm cephalic vein fistula.
3. Nondominant or dominant upper arm cephalic vein fistula.

4. Nondominant or dominant upper arm basilic vein transposition fistula.
5. Forearm loop graft.
6. Upper arm straight graft.
7. Upper arm loop graft (axillary artery to axillary vein).
8. Thigh graft.

Salvage of Immature Fistulas

Compared with AV grafts, fistulas require a much lower frequency of intervention (angioplasty or thrombectomy) to maintain their long-term patency for dialysis. However, fistulas have a substantially higher primary failure rate (fistulas that are never usable for dialysis). The proportion of fistulas with primary failure has ranged from 20% to 50% in multiple recent series, even when routine preoperative vascular mapping has been employed.[8] Primary fistula failures fall into two major categories: early thrombosis and failure to mature.[76-78] *Early thrombosis* refers to fistulas that clot within 3 months of their creation, before they have been used for dialysis. *Failure to mature* refers to fistulas that never develop adequately to be cannulated reproducibly for dialysis.

Native fistulas are created by performing a direct anastomosis between a high-pressure artery and a low-pressure vein. Exposure of the vein to the high arterial pressure causes it to dilate and increase its blood flow. To be used reproducibly for dialysis, a fistula must have a large enough diameter to be safely cannulated with large-bore dialysis needles, and a sufficiently high access blood flow to permit a dialysis blood flow of 350 mL/min or higher. It also must be superficial enough for the landmarks to be easily appreciated by the dialysis staff performing the cannulation. The increases in blood flow and draining vein diameter occur fairly rapidly after fistula creation. Whereas the blood flow in a normal radial artery is only 20 to 40 mL/min, it increases more than 10-fold within a few weeks of fistula creation. In one study, the mean access blood flow in successful fistulas was 634 mL/min 2 weeks postoperatively[79]; in a second study, it was 650 mL/min 12 weeks after fistula creation.[80] Moreover, the mean access blood flows and fistula diameters are not significantly different in the 2nd, 3rd, and 4th months after fistula creation.[81] This implies that determination of whether a new fistula is likely to be used successfully for dialysis should be possible within 4 to 6 weeks of the initial surgery.

In some patients, maturation of the fistula can be assessed easily by clinical evaluation by the nephrologist, surgeon, or an experienced dialysis nurse. In less straightforward cases, duplex ultrasound may be useful in predicting whether a new fistula can be used successfully for dialysis. One pilot study used a combination of two simple sonographic criteria to assess fistula maturation: fistula diameter and access blood flow.[81] When the ultrasound documented a draining vein diameter 4 mm or more *and* an access blood flow of 500 mL/min or more, 95% of the fistulas were subsequently usable for dialysis. In contrast, when neither criterion was met, only 33% of the fistulas achieved adequacy for dialysis. The likelihood of fistula adequacy for dialysis was intermediate (~70%) when only one of the two criteria was met.

Failure of a fistula to mature can be caused by one of several anatomic defects, which can be identified by either sonography or angiography.[82] Stenosis at the anastomosis or in the draining vein is one such problem. Another possibility is that the draining vein has one or more large side branches. When this occurs, the arterial blood flow is distributed among two or more competing veins, thereby limiting the increase in blood flow in each. A third scenario may be observed in obese patients, in which the fistula has adequate caliber and blood flow but is simply too deep to be cannulated safely by the dialysis staff. In most patients, these anatomic lesions can be corrected by radiologic or surgical interventions. Stenotic lesions can be treated by angioplasty or surgical revision. Superficial side branches can be ligated by a suture through the skin; deeper branches can be embolized. Finally, the surgeon can superficialize fistulas that are too deep to be cannulated safely.

In immature fistulas with one or more of these anatomic lesions, specific interventions to correct the underlying lesion may promote subsequent fistula maturation. Several published series have evaluated the ability to salvage immature fistulas to ones that are subsequently usable for dialysis. A number of studies utilizing only radiographic procedures (angioplasty of stenotic lesions or obliteration of side branches) in immature fistulas have had a high success rate (Table 28–10).[74,83-86] An initial salvage (ability to use the fistula for dialysis) was accomplished in 80% to 90% of patients, with a subsequent 1-year primary patency of 39% to 75%. In another study utilizing a combination of radiologic and surgical salvage procedures in an unselected dialysis population, the salvage rate was more modest at 44%.[78] Of interest, the frequency of a salvage procedure for immature fistulas in that study was twice as high in women as in men.

Technical Procedure: Salvage of Immature Fistulas
Angioplasty of Stenotic Lesions
The stenosis at the juxta-arterial anastomosis can be treated with sequential balloon dilatations. This requires two to five treatments until the size of the anastomosis is appropriate. Long segments of stenotic lesions at the level of the most proximal part of the venous outlet near the anastomosis are amenable to balloon angioplasty and sometimes may require several follow-up interventions.

The AV fistula is initially accessed at its most proximal portion with a 21-gauge micropuncture needle. A cope-mandrel-wire is passed into the venous circulation, and then a 4-French catheter sheet is exchanged for the needle. Digital subtracted angiograms (DSAs) of the venous outlet and central circulation and a reflux retrograde arteriogram are performed. Once the lesion is identified, then the proper technique is selected.

If the lesion is at the juxta-arterial anastomosis, then a second access is achieved by inserting a micropuncture needle from the most distal portion of the fistula toward the AV anastomosis. The needle is exchanged for a 5-French catheter sheath and a wire (0.014–0.018 inch) is passed into the fistula and through the arterial anastomosis into the arterial circulation. An arteriogram of the AV anastomosis is performed, and the stenotic lesion is evaluated and graded. Depending on the severity of the stenosis, a balloon is selected from sizes between 2 and 6 mm in diameter and from 10 to 40 mm in length. The balloon is introduced into the stenotic

TABLE 28–10	Effect of Salvage Procedures on Immature Fistulas			
Reference	Pts (*N*)	Type of Intervention	Usable for Dialysis (%)	Primary Patency at 1 Yr (%)
Beathard et al, 1999[83]	63	PTA, vein ligation	82	75
Turmel-Rodrigues et al, 2001[85]	69	PTA, vein ligation	97	39
Miller et al, 2003[78]	41	PTA, vein ligation, surgical revision	44	N/A
Beathard et al, 2003[84]	100	PTA, vein ligation	92	68
Asif et al, 2005[74]	24	PTA, vein ligation	92	N/A
Nassar et al, 2006[86]	119	PTA, vein ligation	83	65

N/A, not available; PTA, percutaneous transluminal angioplasty.

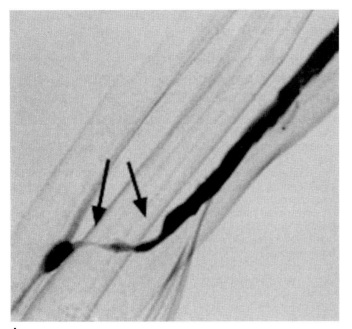

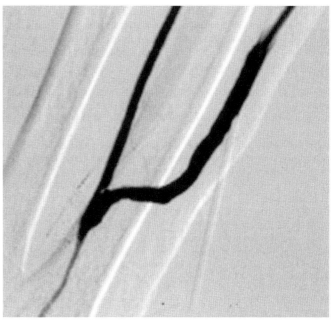

A   B

FIGURE 28–8 **A,** Fistula salvage: DSA of a radiocephalic AV fistula shows a severe stenotic lesion at the level of the juxta-arterial anastomosis. **B,** Fistula salvage: Postangioplasty DSA of a radiocephalic fistula shows radiologic improvement of the stenotic lesion at the level of the juxta-arterial anastomosis.

lesion and inflated carefully up to its nominal pressure. Subsequent angiograms are performed for a postangioplasty grading of the lesion (Fig. 28–8). Intrafistula and systemic pressures are taken before and after the angioplasty and the corresponding ratios calculated. Patients are brought back to the intervention suite 2 to 4 weeks later for a second-look angiogram of the fistula.

If the lesion is located in the proximal part of the fistula or at the central vessels, then the initial venous access is appropriate. The initial 4-French catheter is exchanged for a 4- to 6-French sheath and a glidewire passed into the central venous circulation. The balloon is selected depending on the severity of the lesion and also its location. Sizes can range from 4 to 8 mm in the peripheral venous circulation and up to 14 mm in the central circulation. Once the angioplasty is done, DSAs are performed for postangioplasty grading of the lesion. Intrafistula and systemic pressures are measured. Patients are followed at their local dialysis center and if the fistula does not mature or the nursing personnel are still having problems cannulating the fistula, then a second-look angiogram of the fistula is indicated.

Ligation of Accessory Veins
Accessory veins can be treated either by surgical ligation or by endovascular coil deployment. Treatment of these lesions requires a well-trained interventionist owing to the difficult technical approach to these lesions. Accessory veins are treated depending on size, location, and number (Fig. 28–9). Some interventionists advocate percutaneous ligation of superficial accessory veins at time of the initial angiogram of the fistula.[87] If the accessory vein is deep and has a good lumen size, then surgical ligation is indicated. If the accessory vein is deep but has a small lumen size, then a coil deployment should be considered.

The fistula is accessed and, depending on its size, an appropriate sheath is introduced. A selective catheter is introduced in each accessory vein, and an appropriate size coil is deployed. A final angiogram of the fistula is taken to ascertain proper coil deployment and occlusion of all collateral veins.

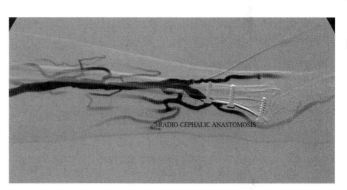

FIGURE 28–9 DSA of a left radiocephalic AV fistula showing multiple collaterals. There is a metallic plate from a prior open reduction and internal fixation of a radius bone fracture.

Angioplasty of Fistulas
Although the frequency of interventions is severalfold lower in fistulas than in grafts,[8] fistulas are also susceptible to developing stenosis and thrombosis. Most studies have documented a comparable primary patency of fistulas and grafts after elective angioplasty (Table 28–11), although one study observed a higher primary patency in fistulas.[88] As is the case with angioplasty of grafts, the primary patency of fistulas after angioplasty is inversely related to both the magnitude of postangioplasty stenosis and the magnitude of the postangioplasty intra-access–to–systemic pressure ratio.[25] Patient age, race, diabetic status, presence of peripheral vascular disease, access location, and number of stenotic sites have not been associated with the likelihood of vascular access patency after angioplasty.[25]

Technical Procedure: Angioplasty of Fistulas
The fistula is accessed at its most proximal portion with a 21-gauge micropuncture needle. A cope-mandrel-wire is passed into the venous circulation. The needle is exchanged for a 4-French catheter. Initial DSA of the fistula is performed,

including the venous outlet and central circulation. Lesions with more than 50% stenosis are considered to be hemodynamically significant and undergo angioplasty. Once the stenotic lesion has been identified and graded, then a glidewire is introduced to the central circulation and the catheter exchanged for a 6-French catheter sheath. An angioplasty balloon is introduced through the catheter sheath. Balloon sizes vary depending on the vessel to be treated. The balloon is placed at the level of the stenotic lesion and inflated to its nominal pressure for 30 to 90 seconds. High pressures (>20 atm) are frequently needed in fistulas.[57] A final DSA is performed to assess for residual stenosis and further treatment of the stenotic lesion (Fig. 28–10). The patient's intrafistula pressure and systemic pressure are measured before and immediately after the intervention, and a reduction intrafistula-to–systemic pressure ratio is used to confirm hemodynamic improvement.

The major complications of this procedure are vessel extravasations and rupture of the vessel after the angioplasty (Fig. 28–11). Deploying a covered stent can treat these com-

plications. Surgical repair is indicated if the rupture is not corrected by stent placement.

Percutaneous Mechanical Thrombectomy and Thrombolysis of Arteriovenous Fistulas

Dealing with thrombosed fistulas is one of the most challenging aspects in interventional nephrology.[89] Thrombectomy of aneurysmally dilated fistulas is the most difficult technically. The most common cause of fistula thrombosis is an underlying stenotic lesion in the venous outflow circulation (either peripherally or centrally). Less common causes include needle infiltration,[90] excessive manual pressure for hemostasis at the needle insertion site, or severe and prolonged hypotension. Successful restoration of patency in a thrombosed fistula requires expeditious thrombectomy. Several series have reported on the outcomes of radiologic thrombectomy of fistulas.[89,91–97] The immediate technical success has been fairly high, ranging from 73% to 93%. The primary patency of these fistulas after thrombectomy has ranged from 27% to 81% at 6 months and 18% to 70% at 1 year (Table 28–12). In one study, the primary patency after thrombectomy was lower in upper arm fistulas than in those in the forearm.[92] However, with additional interventions, the secondary patency of these fistulas has been 44% to 93% at 1 year. Considering that the alternative would be to abandon the thrombosed fistula and proceed with placement of a new fistula, concerted efforts to salvage thrombosed fistulas are extremely worthwhile.

Technical Procedure: Percutaneous Thrombectomy of Fistulas

Although more challenging than graft thrombectomy, AV fistulas can be declotted successfully. There are few contraindications, including concurrent infection, fistula immaturity, and very large aneurysms. The technical challenges include difficulty in the initial cannulation of a thrombosed fistula,

TABLE 28–11	Primary Patency After Elective Angioplasty: Fistulas Versus Grafts	
Reference	Primary Access Patency at 6 Mo	
	Grafts (%)	Fistulas (%)
Safa et al, 1996[28]	43	47
Turmel-Rodrigues et al, 2000[92]	53	67
McCarley et al, 2001[42]	37	34
Van der Linden et al, 2002[88]	25	50
Maya et al, 2004[25]	52	55

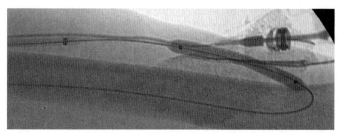

A

B

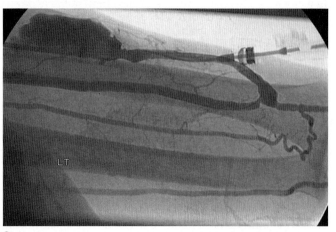

C

FIGURE 28–10 **A,** DSA of a left radiocephalic AV fistula shows a longs severe segment of stenosis distal to the arterial anastomosis followed by a pseudoaneurysm of the fistula. **B,** Spot film of a left radiocephalic AV fistula shows the segment of stenosis being angioplastied. **C,** Postangioplasty DSA shows a successful treatment; the pseudoaneurysm is unchanged.

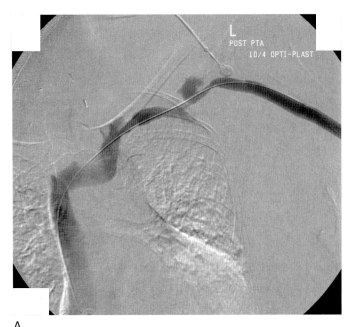

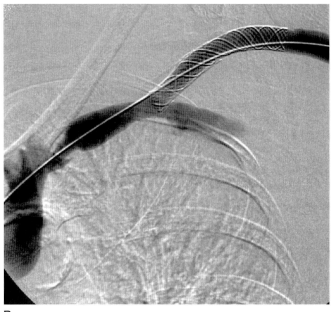

FIGURE 28–11 **A,** Angioplasty complication: DSA shows a rupture of the left cephalic vein after aggressive percutaneous transluminal angioplasty. There is a coexisting stenosis of the left subclavian. **B,** Angioplasty complication: DSA shows salvage and correction of the complication by deploying a covered stent.

TABLE 28–12	Primary Fistula Patency After Thrombectomy*		
Reference	Procedures (*N*)	Primary Patency At	
		6 Mo (%)	*12 Mo (%)*
Haage et al, 2000[91]	54	N/A	27
Turmel-Rodrigues et al, 2000[92]	54 FA 9 UA	74 27	47 27
Rajan et al, 2002[96]	30	28	24
Liang et al, 2002[95]	42	81	70
Shatsky et al, 2005[97]	44	38	18

*Series with fewer than 25 procedures not included.
FA, forearm; N/A, not available; UA, upper arm.

complete removal of large thrombi, and successful treatment of recalcitrant stenotic lesions.

The fistula is accessed at its most distal portion toward the arterial anastomosis with an 18-gauge needle, either blind or by guided ultrasonography. A glidewire is introduced and a catheter placed over the glidewire. A thrombolytic agent, 2 to 4 mg of Alteplase (t-PA), is infused and left in the fistula for 1 hour. The patient is taken back to the intervention suite, the glidewire is repositioned, and the catheter is replaced with a conventional 6-French sheath. A percutaneous thrombectomy over-the-wire device can be used, but the wire must be advanced into the arterial circulation. After a successful thrombolysis of the fistula, a Fogarty balloon is passed beyond the arterial anastomosis and pulled back to dislodge the plugging clot. Once the thrombus is cleared and blood flow reestablished, a DSA of the fistula is taken to evaluate for stenotic lesions along the venous outlet track or central circulation. If a lesion is encountered in the upstream or central circulation, then a second access is placed and the lesion angioplastied.

Manual aspiration without the use of thrombolytic agents is another approach. A sheath is placed to gain access to the venous outflow. A guide catheter with a large lumen is introduced through the sheath. The aspiration is performed with a 50-mL syringe connected to the guide catheter, while the catheter is removed with back-and-forth movements. The contents of the syringe are flushed, and the aspiration maneuver is repeated several times to remove all the thrombus. A second sheath is introduced toward the arterial anastomosis, and the same aspiration technique is performed to aspirate the rest of the thrombus located between the introducer and the anastomosis. A Fogarty balloon is passed beyond the arterial anastomosis and pulled back to dislodge the arterial plug clot. Digitally subtracted anterograde angiograms of the fistula are performed to assess for patency and look for stenotic lesions. Angioplasty of any hemodynamically stenotic lesion in the vascular access circuit is performed. A final DSA of the fistula is performed, and the patient's intra-access pressure and systemic pressure are measured before and immediately after the intervention. The pressure ratio is calculated to confirm improvement in blood flow.

The major complications of this procedure are vessel extravasations and rupture of the vessel after the angioplasty. Pulmonary embolism is of greater concern with fistula Thrombectomy than with graft thrombectomy, owing to the larger volume of thrombus. Finally, arterial emboli distal to the AV anastomosis may occur with greater frequency than for grafts.

NOVEL TECHNIQUES FOR TREATMENT OF SEVERE STENOTIC LESIONS

Cutting Balloon

Despite the use of angioplasty with high-pressure balloons and prolonged inflations, some lesions remain severely stenotic. The use of cutting balloons has been advocated as a tool to treat these lesions by creating a controlled rupture of the vessel wall. The cutting balloon catheter is a balloon with four blades arranged along the balloon. When the balloon is inflated, it exposes the blades to the offending lesion, creating a controlled rupture of the intima or hyperplastic fibrous tissue. A regular angioplasty balloon can be used afterward to shape the vessel and expand it to the desired diameter. It has been used in lesions at all levels from intragraft to central lesions. Preliminary reports suggested that cutting balloons may result in superior outcomes than those obtained with conventional angioplasty.[98,99] In one series of nine patients, grafts with high-grade venous anastomosis stenosis were treated with cutting balloon plus stent deployment.[98] The patients were followed up to 20 months with a functional graft. However, a randomized, multicenter clinical trial comparing use of the cutting balloon with conventional angioplasty for treatment of graft stenosis observed no advantage to the cutting balloon. The primary patency at 6 months was 48% in grafts treated with a cutting balloon versus 40% for grafts treated with angioplasty. Device-related complications occurred in 5% of the patients in the cutting balloon group (primarily vein rupture or dissection) compared with none of the patients whose grafts were treated with angioplasty alone.[100] The considerable additional cost of cutting balloons is substantial and precludes it ever being used routinely.

Cryoplasty Balloon

Cryotherapy with the cryoballoon is a novel therapy for patients with intractable stenoses at the venous anastomosis of AV grafts. This technique utilizes cold temperatures at the balloon site to cause apoptosis of the intima layer. Rifkin and co-workers[101] reported the outcomes of five patients with recurrent stenotic lesions at the venous anastomosis that were treated with the cryoballoon. The primary patency increased from 3 weeks after angioplasty alone to more than 16 weeks after cryoplasty. There are no published randomized studies comparing the outcomes of graft stenosis treated with cryoplasty versus with angioplasty alone.

█ CENTRAL VEIN STENOSIS

Central vein stenosis is a frequent occurrence in hemodialysis patients.[11] Acute or chronic trauma of the central vessels by either temporary or permanent dialysis catheters is the major cause.[102] Stenosis leads to impairment of venous return on the ipsilateral extremity and might, in turn, result in malfunction or thrombosis of the vascular access. Although it may be asymptomatic, patients with central vein stenosis most commonly present with ipsilateral upper extremity edema. In some patients, a previously unappreciated central vein stenosis becomes evident clinically after creation of an ipsilateral fistula or graft. The diagnosis can be confirmed by angiography, ultrasound, or MRV.

The most commonly encountered location of central vein stenosis is at the junction of the cephalic vein with the subclavian vein (not catheter injury related). Other central veins that may be affected include the subclavian vein, brachiocephalic vein, and superior vena cava (Fig. 28–12). In patients with tunneled femoral catheters, central vein stenosis may occur in the external iliac vein, common iliac vein, or inferior vena cava, resulting in ipsilateral lower extremity edema. The stenotic lesion is an aggressive myointimal proliferation or clot and fibrin sheath formation around indwelling dialysis catheters that is organized and incorporated into the vessel wall. These may progress over time to complete occlusion of the venous circulation. If left untreated, central vein stenosis may cause increased retrograde pressure and formation of venous collaterals. In some patients, the collaterals are sufficiently well developed to permit adequate venous drainage that prevents formation of edema.

The treatment of choice of central vein stenosis is percutaneous transluminal angioplasty (PTA) of the stenotic lesion.[44,103–109] Unfortunately, the long-term success is quite poor owing to a combination of elastic recoil and aggressive myointimal hyperplasia. In one study, the primary patency was substantially shorter after angioplasty of central vein

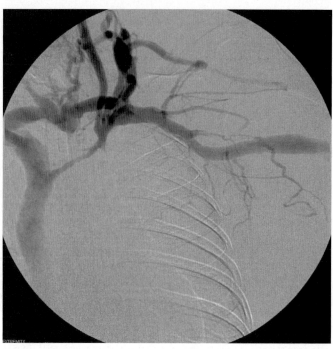

FIGURE 28–12 DSA shows a severe stenosis of the left innominate vein. There are multiple ipsilateral and across-the-neck collaterals draining into a normal right innominate vein.

stenosis compared with stenoses at more peripheral locations.[26] As a result, patients with central vein stenosis require frequent angioplasties to treat recurrent lesions.

Stent placement has been attempted in the management of refractory central vein stenosis owing to elastic recoil (Fig. 28–13). Several small series have reported the outcomes of stent placement for refractory central venous stenotic lesions. These studies have been limited by their retrospective study design, the small numbers of patients, and the absence of a control group. In two uncontrolled series, the primary patency after stent deployment for central vein stenosis was 42% to 50% at 6 months and only 14% to 17% at 1 year.[44,103] Although there are no published randomized studies comparing stent deployment with angioplasty of central vein stenosis, the primary patency in series utilizing stents has been no better than that achieved with angioplasty alone. In patients with ipsilateral vascular access and persistent upper extremity edema despite attempted angioplasty, the only recourse may be ligation of the vascular access.

█ INDWELLING HEMODIALYSIS CATHETERS

Nontunneled Temporary Hemodialysis Catheters

Temporary hemodialysis catheters are indicated for acute dialysis treatments. They are made of polyurethane, polyethylene, or polytetrafluoroethylene; they have a double lumen and are semirigid and easy to place in the internal jugular (preferably on the right side), femoral, and rarely, subclavian veins. Each site has its advantages and disadvantages, but if the catheters are placed in the femoral vein, the catheter should not stay longer than 72 hours, and the internal jugular vein catheters not longer than 1 week, owing to the high risk of bacteremia with longer dwell times.[110] The subclavian vein is usually used only if there is no other access available because there is an increased risk for stenosis and occlusion of the central vessels.[102] If the upper vessels are used, the

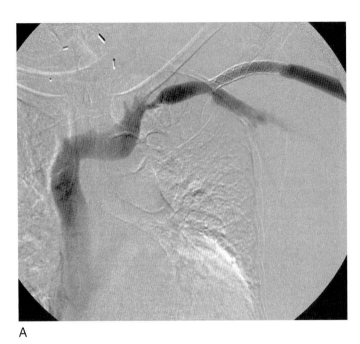

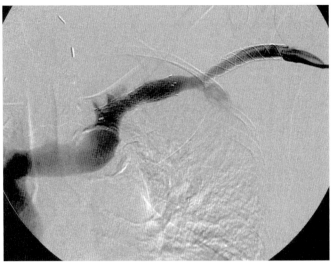

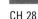

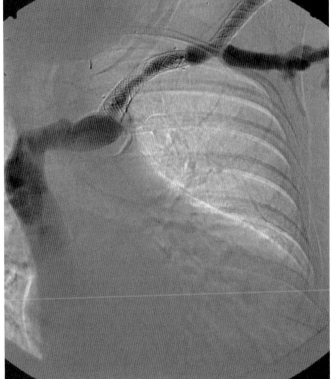

FIGURE 28–13 **A,** DSA shows a severe stenotic lesion of the left subclavian. There is also a stent at the left cephalic vein. **B,** DSA shows a stent deployed at the severe stenotic lesion of the left subclavian with excellent initial results. **C,** DSA taken 12 months after the initial placement of a stent at the left subclavian shows intrastent stenosis due to significant myointimal hyperplasia.

catheter should be long enough to have its tip at the junction of the right atrium and superior vena cava. If the femoral vein is used, the catheter's tip should be located in the inferior vena cava. If the patient is expected to remain catheter-dependent for a longer time period, a tunneled catheter should be placed. Temporary hemodialysis catheters can be placed blindly, by ultrasound or fluoroscopic guidance. A chest radiograph should always be obtained after placement of a central vein dialysis catheter in the chest; it is not needed after placement of a femoral dialysis catheter.

Technical Procedure: Insertion of Temporary Dialysis Catheters

The procedure is usually performed at patient's bedside, but occasionally, it is performed in the interventional suite. Strict sterile technique and use of local anesthesia are indicated. Access to the femoral or internal jugular vein may be done either blindly or by real-time ultrasound guidance. Real-time ultrasound is highly recommended, as it decreases the number of attempts at vein cannulation and minimizes the risk of inadvertent arterial cannulation. An 18-guage needle is used for access. Once the vein has been cannulated, a J-wire is introduced through the needle and advanced into the venous circulation. The needle is exchanged for a series of dilators, and then a temporary dialysis catheter (19–24 cm in length) is introduced and sutured in place. The lumens are flushed and filled with heparin.

Potential complications at time of placement at the upper vessels include pneumothorax, vein or arterial perforation; mediastinal or pericardial perforation with possibility of hemothorax and cardiac tamponade; air embolism; and local hematoma with possible extension into the soft subcutaneous tissue of the neck and possible external obstruction of the airways. The long-term complications include development of stenotic lesions along the trajectory of the catheter, which may preclude the use of the ipsilateral limb for future creation of a vascular access. If the patient already has a documented stenotic lesion of the central vessels, placement of an indwelling catheter may cause life-threatening acute central vessel occlusion. Exit site infections and catheter-related bacteremia (CRB) are frequent complications of temporary dialysis catheters. Development of CRB requires institution of systemic antibiotics and removal of the nontunneled dialysis catheter.

The complications at the femoral site are less dramatic, but vein or arterial perforation and formation of AV fistula are possible. Deep vein thrombosis, local hematomas, exit site infections, and bacteremia are not uncommon complications. There is also a possibility of causing stenosis of the femoral, iliac, or inferior vena cava.

Tunneled Hemodialysis Catheters

Tunneled hemodialysis catheters are used for temporary vascular access in patients waiting for a maturation of a permanent vascular AV fistula or graft. They are also required for long-term access in patients who have exhausted all options for placement of a permanent access in all four extremities. Tunneled dialysis catheters are usually placed in a central vein in the chest, most commonly in the internal jugular vein and, rarely, in the subclavian vein. They have the same characteristics as temporary catheters but are longer and have a Dacron cuff, which is tunneled in the subcutaneous tissue. An inflammatory response around the cuff results in scar tissue, creating a mechanical barrier that prevents introduction of infection from the exit site into the bloodstream. As a result, the frequency of CRB is lower with tunneled dialysis catheters than with acute catheters.[111,112]

Technical Procedure: Insertion of Tunneled Hemodialysis Catheters

Strict sterile technique, topical local anesthesia (1% lidocaine [Xylocaine]), and conscious sedation are used. Access to the internal jugular vein is guided by real-time ultrasound. A 21-guage micropuncture needle is used for access. Once the vein has been cannulated, a 0.018-inch guidewire is introduced through the needle and advanced under fluoroscopic guidance. The needle is removed and exchanged for a 4-French catheter. The guidewire and inner dilator are removed and a stiff 0.035-inch wire is passed through the catheter down into the inferior vena cava under fluoroscopic guidance. A skin pocket of about 1 cm is created at this location. The permanent indwelling hemodialysis catheter is attached to a tunneler device, and a tunnel is created lateral, down, and approximately 5 to 7 cm from the initial needle insertion. The catheter is buried under the skin. At this point, the tunneler device is discarded and a series of dilators are passed over the wire under fluoroscopic guidance, leaving a peel-away catheter sheath and inner dilator in place. The inner dilator and wire are removed, leaving the peel-away sheath behind. The tip of the catheter is introduced into the opening of the sheath and fed up to the junction of the superior vena cava and right atrium. The peel-away sheath is then removed. A final x-ray is taken to assess for kinks of the catheter and for placement (Fig. 28–14). Sutures are placed at the initial skin incision and also at the entry site of the catheter. The catheter lumens are filled with heparin. The catheters are 14.5 or 15 French with lengths from 24 cm for right internal jugular, 28 cm for left internal jugular, and from 36 to 42 cm for femoral veins.

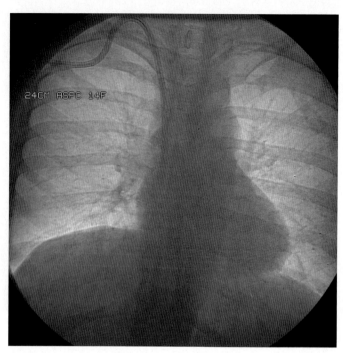

FIGURE 28–14 Spot film of an appropriate placement of a right internal jugular vein tunneled chronic dialysis catheter.

Complications at the time of placement are similar to those associated with temporary catheters. Internal jugular thrombosis develops in about 25% of tunneled catheters but is usually asymptomatic.[113] Other long-term complications include dysfunction due to intraluminal thrombosis or fibrin sheaths, exit site infections, tunnel infections, and CRB.[11]

Less Common Locations for Tunneled Hemodialysis Catheters

If prolonged use of upper extremity dialysis catheters leads to bilateral central vein occlusion, it becomes necessary to place a *tunneled catheter in the femoral vein*.[114,115] The procedure for placement of a tunneled femoral catheter is similar to that for a tunneled internal jugular vein catheter, except that a longer (36–42 cm) catheter is required, and the catheter tip is placed in either the proximal inferior vena cava or in the right atrium (Fig. 28–15).[114] The subcutaneous tunnel is created in the anterior upper thigh. The primary patency of tunneled femoral catheters is significantly worse than that of tunneled internal jugular catheters.[114] Presumably, some failures are due to kinking of the catheter in the groin when the thigh is flexed. However, the frequency of CRB is similar for patients with femoral and internal jugular dialysis catheters. The likelihood of CRB is proportional to the duration of catheter use.[116] There is high (~25%) frequency of symptomatic ipsilateral deep vein thrombosis after placement of a tunneled femoral catheter.[114] Fortunately, this complication can be treated with long-term anticoagulation; thereby permitting continued use of the catheter. In patients on hemodialysis in whom the central veins in the chest and groin have been exhausted, the placement of tunneled dialysis catheters at unconventional sites (translumbar and transhepatic) has been described. Catheters at these locations should be considered as last-resort options, as they are associated with a substantial risk for complications.

For *translumbar catheters*, the insertion site is located at the level of vertebra L3, the needle is directed toward the inferior vena cava under fluoroscopic guidance; once venous

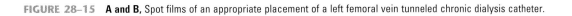

FIGURE 28–15 **A and B,** Spot films of an appropriate placement of a left femoral vein tunneled chronic dialysis catheter.

access is achieved, a glidewire is placed. A tunnel is created from initial needle insertion at the lower back and around the waist of the patient with the entry site located at lower part of the abdominal flank. The permanent hemodialysis catheter is advanced through the tunnel and the cuff is buried in the adjacent subcutaneous tissue (Fig. 28–16).[117,118] The risk of bleeding and retroperitoneal hematoma is considerably higher than that associated with tunneled femoral vein catheters. The most common complication of translumbar catheters in one series of 10 patients is partial dislodgment of the catheters.[118]

Interventional radiologists at some centers have placed *transhepatic catheters*. The right upper quadrant is propped and draped in the usual manner. A 21-gauge needle is placed halfway through the liver in a direction parallel to the right of the middle hepatic veins under fluoroscopic guidance. Contrast material is injected through the needle, and the needle is withdrawn until a hepatic vein is visualized. Once a suitable vein is accessed, a glidewire is placed and advanced to the right atrium. A subcutaneous tunnel is created inferiorly to the insertion site, and a dual-lumen, cuffed hemodialysis catheter is placed.[119–121] The major complications are bleeding and perihepatic hematoma. Stavropoulos and associates[120] reported a series of 36 transhepatic dialysis catheters placed in 12 patients. The mean survival of these catheters was only 24 days. The thrombosis rate was 2.40 per 100 catheter-days. The poor catheter patency rates were due to a high rate of late thrombosis.

Exchange of Tunneled Hemodialysis Catheters

There are two major indications for catheter exchange: dysfunction and infection. Catheter *dysfunction* is diagnosed when blood cannot be aspirated from the catheter lumen at the time of dialysis initiation, or more commonly, if it is not possible to consistently achieve a dialysis blood flow greater than 250 mL/min. In catheters that were previously

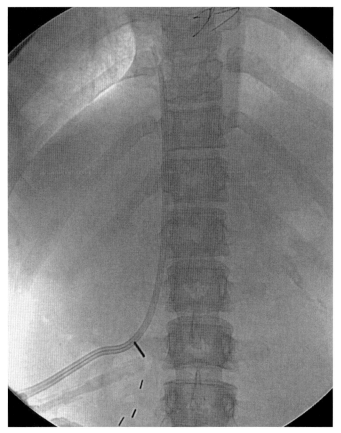

FIGURE 28–16 Spot film of an appropriate placement of a translumbar tunneled chronic dialysis catheter.

TABLE 28–13	Management Strategies for Catheter-Related Bacteremia
Systemic antibiotics alone	
Catheter removal with delayed placement of a new, tunneled catheter	
Catheter exchange over a guidewire	
Antibiotic lock	

delivering an adequate blood flow; intraluminal thrombus is the most common etiology for dysfunction, although a fibrin sheath may be the culprit in some patients. This problem is usually treated empirically in the dialysis unit by instilling t-PA into the catheter lumens.[122] t-PA instillation is successful in about 70% to 80% of catheters, but problems with poor flow frequently recur within 2 to 3 weeks. If the thrombolytic agent does not improve the catheter flow, the patient is referred for catheter exchange.

An exit site *infection* usually resolves with topical antimicrobial agents or oral antibiotics and is not usually an indication for catheter removal. However, if the patient has a tunnel track infection, catheter removal is mandatory. Finally, CRB is a common indication for catheter replacement.[10] In one series, the cumulative risk of CRB among catheter-dependent patients was 35% at 3 months and 48% at 6 months.[116] CRB is suspected when a catheter-dependent patient experiences fever or chills, and it is confirmed by blood cultures from the catheter and a peripheral vein growing the same organism.[10] When a single set of blood cultures is positive, CRB is still the most likely diagnosis in the absence of clinical evidence of an alternative source of infection.

The clinical management of CRB has evolved in the past few years (Table 28–13).[10] In the subset of patient whose fever persists after 48 to 72 hours of appropriate systemic antibiotics (~10%–15% of patients with CRB), removal of the infected catheter is mandatory. For the remaining patients, several management options are available. The first option is to continue systemic antibiotics without removal of the infected catheter. Unfortunately, the infection is infrequently eradicated with this approach; once the course of systemic antibiotics has been completed, bacteremia recurs in 63% to 78% of patients.[123–127] Moreover, delays in removing an infected catheter may result in metastasic infection, such as endocarditis, septic arthritis, or epidural abscess.[128] Prompt removal of the catheter removes the source of infection. However, in order to continue delivering dialysis to the patient, it is necessary to place a temporary (nontunneled) dialysis catheter. Once the bacteremia has resolved, a new tunneled catheter is placed. In an effort to reduce the number of required access procedures, a number of investigators have evaluated the strategy of exchanging the infected catheter for a new one over a guidewire. Several publications have documented the safety and efficacy of this approach.[126,129–132]

In the past few years, there has been a growing recognition of the central role of bacterial biofilms in causing CRB. Biofilms develop on the inner surface of the lumens of central vein catheters in as little as 24 hours and are relatively refractory to conventional plasma concentrations of antibiotics.[133–135] Instillation of a concentrated antibiotic solution into the catheter lumen after each dialysis session ("antibiotic lock") can frequently kill the bacteria in the biofilm. This approach can potentially remove the source of the infection (the biofilm) while permitting catheter salvage. The use of antibiotic locks, in conjunction with systemic antibiotics, has been shown to eradicate the infection, while salvaging the catheter, in about two thirds of the patients.[10,136–139] This strat-

egy is not associated with an increased risk of metastasic infections compared with prompt catheter removal or exchange of the infected catheter over a guidewire. At the authors' institution, implementation of an antibiotic lock protocol has dramatically reduced the frequency of catheter exchanges owing to infection.

Technical Procedure: Exchange of Tunneled Hemodialysis Catheters

Patients are brought to the interventional suite for exchange of permanent indwelling hemodialysis catheters. Strict sterile technique, topical local anesthesia (1% lidocaine), and conscious sedation are provided. Under fluoroscopic guidance, an extra-stiff 0.035-inch wire is passed through one of the lumens of the catheter and advanced to the inferior vena cava. The catheter cuff located near the exit site in the subcutaneous tissue is dissected, and the catheter is pulled out, leaving the wire behind. The exit site and the wire are cleaned and wiped with antibacterial soap. The operators' gloves are exchanged. A new permanent hemodialysis catheter is then prepped and advanced over the wire into place. The tip of the catheter is advanced to the inferior vena cava for the femoral vein or to the junction of the superior vena cava and right atrium for the internal jugular vein. Finally, the wire is removed, and the catheter is sutured in place. The lumens of the catheter are filled with heparin.

Subcutaneous Hemodialysis Ports

Implantable subcutaneous vascular access devices (e.g., LifeSite) have been available commercially for several years.[140] There is no clear indication for their use, except as a bridge device while waiting for maturation of a fistula. Theoretically, the risk of CRB should be lower with subcutaneous dialysis devices, as there is no portion protruding through the skin. However, a randomized clinical trial comparing a subcutaneous dialysis device with conventional tunneled dialysis catheters found no difference in the frequency of bacteremia, unless isopropyl alcohol was instilled into the subcutaneous device after each dialysis session.[141] Although these devices are no longer commercially available, some dialysis patients still have them in place.

Technical Procedure: Implantation of Subcutaneous Dialysis Ports

This access device has two titanium valves that are connected to two silicone catheters, which are placed individually into the central venous circulation with the same technique as the one described for tunneled catheters. The tip of one of the catheters is placed in the right atrium and the other tip in the superior vena cava. The most common placement site is the internal jugular vein, but external jugular and femoral veins can also be used. If the femoral vein is used, the tips of both catheters should be in the inferior vena cava, about 2 to 3 cm apart. Two different subcutaneous tissue pockets are created next to the tunneled catheters, and the titanium valve devices are implanted and connected to the catheters. The pockets are created in an area of easy access for cannulation by the dialysis nursing personnel. It is important to avoid creating the pockets in areas that will cause discomfort to the patient (i.e., above the clavicle or above the inguinal area). The device should not be deeper than 10 to 15 mm below the skin for easy access but not less than 10 mm because skin erosion and necrosis can occur. The medial titanium valve device is used for blood drawing, and the lateral is used for blood return during dialysis. To access the system and establish high blood flow rates, a standard 14-gauge needle is inserted through the skin into the device, and the needle opens the internal valve, allowing blood to flow.

Complications at time of placement are similar to those for tunneled catheters because the insertion technique of the indwelling catheters is similar. In addition, there is a risk for bleeding and hematoma formation at the site of the created subcutaneous tissue pocket. Late complications include malfunction of the valve devices, clotting and infection of the catheter lines, infection of the subcutaneous tissue pockets, and erosion and necrosis of the skin overlying the devices.

PERITONEAL DIALYSIS CATHETER PROCEDURES

Peritoneal dialysis (PD) is an alternative to hemodialysis in patients with end-stage renal disease. Although it is widely used in many countries, less than 10% of the U.S. dialysis population is treated by this modality.[142] PD catheters can be placed into the abdominal cavity by surgeons,[143-145] interventional radiologists,[146] or interventional nephrologists.[147] There are several techniques: blind (Seldinger) technique,[148] surgical placement,[143] peritoneoscopic,[149] laparoscopic,[150] Moncrief-Popovich technique,[151] and fluoroscopic insertion.[147] Incorporation of PD catheter placement in an established interventional nephrology program increases the utilization of this dialysis modality.[152]

Peritoneal catheters are made of either silicone rubber or polyurethane. The Tenckhoff catheter is still the most common type of PD catheter placed. The intraperitoneal portion of the catheter can be either straight, coiled, Ash (T-Flutted), or fitted with a silicone disk.[153] The extraperitoneal portion of the catheter may be straight or have a swan-neck design with single- or double inner cuffs, or a combination of a single cuff and a silicone disk. The most widely used PD catheter is the double-cuff, swan-neck, coiled Tenckhoff design. This design has been shown to decrease mechanical complications (i.e. inflow and outflow problems). It also decreases pain during infusion and has fewer propensities for migration. The swan-neck design was introduced to avoid cuff extrusions.[154] The intraperitoneal portion of the catheter should be placed between the visceral and the parietal peritoneum near the pouch of Douglas. The inner cuff should be inserted in the abdominal wall musculature (rectus muscle) to prevent leaks. The outer cuff should be located in the subcutaneous tissue to create a dead space between the two cuffs, which is believed to prevent migration of infections coming from the exit site. The subcutaneous tract and exit site should face downward and laterally to avoid exit site infection. The exit site should be determined and marked prior to the insertion while the patient is in the upright position. The belt-line, prior surgical sites, and the abdominal midline should be avoided. Postoperative catheter care is very important. The catheter should be covered with a nonocclusive dressing and should not to be used for 10 to 14 days. The catheter should be flushed at least two or three times per week with saline or dialysate solution until the patient is ready to start PD.[155] Usually, PD is started 2 to 3 weeks after placement of the catheter to allow for wound healing and avoid leaks. Low-volume PD may be attempted within 24 hours of catheter placement, if no other dialysis access is available.[156]

Two studies comparing swan-neck and straight Tenckhoff catheters have shown a similar risk for peritonitis and exit infection, but less cuff extrusion, with the swan-neck design. The lower incidence of cuff extrusion enhances the survival of the swan-neck catheters.[157-159] A technique that modifies the swan-neck catheter to a presternal exit site location has been reported by Twardowski and colleagues[160,161] and has shown an increase in access survival up to 95% at 2 years. It has shown a decrease in peritonitis, exit wound infection. The authors advocate the use of the catheter in obese patients, patients with ostomies, children with diapers and fecal incontinence. Gadallah and colleagues[162] demonstrated that placement of PD catheters by peritoneoscopic approach had a longer survival rate than those placed surgically, and the rates of exit infection and leak were lower. Moncrief and associates[151] described a technique in which the extraperitoneal portion of the catheter is buried in the abdominal subcutaneous tissue until the patient is ready for PD. It appears that it lowers the risk for initial infection of the tract.[151] A major complication during placement of the catheter is bowel perforation. It is infrequent with all techniques except for blind placement, but once identified, it requires bowel rest, intravenous antibiotic therapy, and rarely, surgical exploration.[143,152] Tip migration is a very common ($\leq 35\%$) late complication, which could cause problems with draining of the PD fluid. It can be fixed with either radiologic or surgical manipulation.[163,164] PD leaks around the catheter have been reported as much as 10%, but the use of double-cuff swan-neck catheters have decreased the incidence.[165] Perioperative infection and bleeding are very rare; prophylactic antibiotics are usually given.[164]

Technical Procedure: Insertion of Peritoneal Catheters by Fluoroscopic and Ultrasound Techniques

The abdomen is prepped and draped in a sterile fashion. Conscious sedation is administered with midazolam hydrochloride and fentanyl citrate. A registered nurse obtains vitals signs and administers the conscious sedation during the procedure. Insertion site is selected to be 2 cm to the left or right and below the umbilicus. An ultrasound machine with a properly sterilely covered 5-MHz transducer is used to guide a 21-gauge needle into the peritoneum. Under ultrasound guidance, the needle penetrates through the skin, the subcutaneous tissue, the outer fascia of rectus muscle, the muscle fibers, the inner fascia, and the parietal layer of peritoneum. Three to 5 mL of contrast is injected into the peritoneal cavity under fluoroscopy to ensure appropriate location; a radiologic pattern of bowel delineation is indicative of a good placement. A 0.018-inch cope-mandrel-wire is introduced through the needle. The needle is exchanged for a 6-French catheter sheath. A 2-cm incision is made on the skin, and the subcutaneous tissue is digitally dissected up to the rectus muscle. A series of dilators (8, 12, and 14 French) are passed over a stiff glidewire, and an 18-French peel-away sheath is placed. A double-cuff, swan-neck, Tenckhoff PD catheter is introduced over the stiff glidewire into the peritoneal cavity. The coiled intraperitoneal portion is placed in the lower intra-abdominal area. The inner cuff is pushed into the muscle before the peel-away sheath is removed. A tunnel is created with an exit site located distal, lateral, and below the initial incision with the outer cuff buried in the subcutaneous tissue. A final fluoroscopic imaging is performed to verify placement of the Tenckhoff catheter (Fig. 28–17). Inflow and outflow of the PD catheter is tested with 500 mL of normal saline. The PD catheter is flushed with 10 to 15 mL of heparin. The subcutaneous tissue and skin are sutured, and the site is dressed.

Technical Procedure: Insertion of Peritoneal Catheters by Peritoneoscopic Technique

Peritoneal catheters placed peritoneoscopically are implanted through the rectus muscle using a peritoneoscope device. It has the same initial preparation as for the fluoroscopic/ultrasound technique. With the patient under local anesthesia, a 2-cm skin incision is made. The subcutaneous tissue is dissected up to the rectus muscle. A catheter guide is inserted into the abdomen and the peritoneoscope is placed into the catheter to assess initial entry to the peritoneal cavity. The scope is removed, and 500 mL of air is infused into the cavity. The scope is again replaced and advanced to the pelvic area.

CH 28

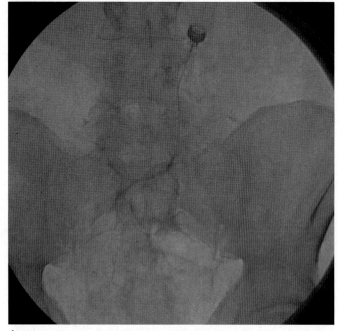

A

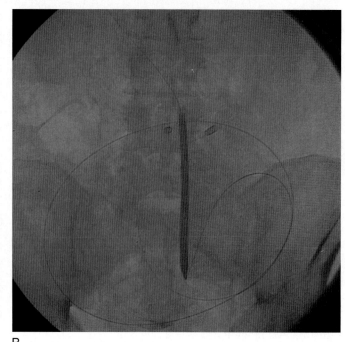

B

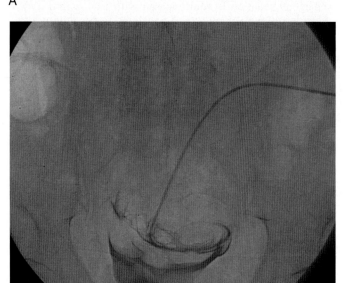

C

FIGURE 28–17 **A,** Spot film demonstrates free flow of contrast injection into the peritoneal cavity. **B,** Spot film shows a peel-away sheath in place during insertion of a Tenckhoff catheter. **C,** Spot film shows appropriate placement of a Tenckhoff catheter.

This area is inspected for adhesions and bowel loops. The scope is again removed, and the peritoneal catheter is introduced through the catheter with the help of a stainless steel stylette. The catheter is advanced to the pelvic area. The stylette is removed, and the inner cuff is buried into the musculature. The exit location is determined, and the catheter is tunneled to that location.

Technical Procedure: Insertion of Peritoneal Catheters by Pre-Sternal Catheter Placement

The PD catheter implantation technique is the same as the peritoneoscopic insertion, except that the PD catheter has a straight design instead of a swan neck. After the PD catheter is placed, then a second catheter is tunneled from the midabdomen up to the chest wall. The two catheters are connected by a titanium joint piece. The second catheter has the swan-neck design and two cuffs. The exit site is located lateral to the midsternal line.

▌PERCUTANEOUS RENAL BIOPSY

Percutaneous renal biopsy is an important procedure in the diagnosis of renal disease. The results of a renal biopsy are helpful in guiding medical therapy and providing a prognosis. The goal of a renal biopsy should be to maximize the yield of adequate renal tissue while minimizing the risk of complications. Percutaneous renal biopsies have evolved from a blind procedure to a real-time ultrasound-guided needle biopsy. Although some nephrologists still use the Franklin-Silverman needle and the Tru-Cut needle for blind biopsy, several authors have documented that the use of real-time ultrasonography along with the use of an automatic biopsy gun minimizes complications and provides a high yield of adequate tissue for pathologic diagnosis (Table 28–14). Cozens and co-workers[166] retrospectively compared a 15-gauge Tru-Cut renal biopsy with ultrasound localization and marking with an 18-gauge, spring-loaded gun renal biopsy under real-time ultrasound guidance. They reported

TABLE 28–14	Adequacy of Kidney Tissue Retrieval and Complications by Real-Time Ultrasound-Guided Percutaneous Renal Biopsy		
Reference	Biopsies (N)	Adequate Tissue (%)	Major Complications* (%)
Maya et al, 2007[185]	65	100	0
Doyle et al, 1994[186]	86	99	0.8
Hergesell et al, 1998[187]	1090	98.8	<0.5
Donovan et al, 1991[188]	192	97.8	<1
Burstein et al, 1993[168]	200	97.5	5.6
Cozens et al, 1992[166]		93	N/A
Marwah and Korbet, 1996[169]	394		6.6

*Definitions of major complications differed among studies.
N/A, not available.

a 79% yield of adequate renal tissue with the blind technique compared with 93% with real-time ultrasound guidance.[166] Similarly, two other comparative studies reported a higher mean number of glomeruli from biopsies obtained under real-time ultrasound compared with those performed blindly.[167,168]

Major complications of renal biopsies, including gross hematuria or retroperitoneal hematoma requiring blood transfusion, invasive procedure, or surgical intervention, have been reported in less than 1% of biopsies in some series and 5% to 6% by others (see Table 28–14). The likelihood of major complications was not associated with patient age, blood pressure, or serum creatinine in one large series.[167] Among those patients with major complications, the time interval from biopsy to diagnosis of the complication was 4 hours or less in 52%, 8 hours or less in 79%, and 12 hours or less in 100% of patients.[167] Thus, the minimal period of observation after a renal biopsy should be 12 hours. Minor complications, including transient gross hematuria or perinephric hematoma not requiring transfusion or intervention, occurred after 6.6% of biopsies in one series.[169] Either ultrasound or computed tomography can be used to diagnose perinephric hematomas.[170] Most hematomas resolve spontaneously within a few weeks with no significant sequelae. Major bleeding complications that do not resolve with conservative measures require further intervention. In the past, this entailed urgent surgical nephrectomy. However, selective renal arteriogram with embolization of the bleeding arteriole is often able to stop the bleeding in most cases. A review article reported only 0.3% major complications and less than 0.1% death rates in 9595 percutaneous renal biopsies performed over the last 50 years.

For patients at high risk of bleeding complications or liver disease with coagulopathy in whom a kidney biopsy is indicated, a transjugular kidney biopsy may be performed by an interventional radiologist or nephrologist. Thompson and colleagues[171] reported 91% adequate tissue retrieval with an average of 9 glomeruli for light microscopy in 23 patients undergoing transjugular renal biopsy. A capsular perforation was encountered in 17 patients, of whom 6 required coil embolization of the bleeding vessel. Two major complications were reported, 1 arteriocalyceal system fistula and 1 renal vein thrombosis 6 days after the biopsy.[171] Abbott and coworkers[172] reported a series of nine patients undergoing transjugular renal biopsy. Adequate tissue was obtained from all patients. Capsular perforation occurred in 90% of the patients, and two patients developed gross hematuria requiring transfusion.[172]

A bleeding disorder is an absolute contraindication to performing a percutaneous renal biopsy. However, if it can be

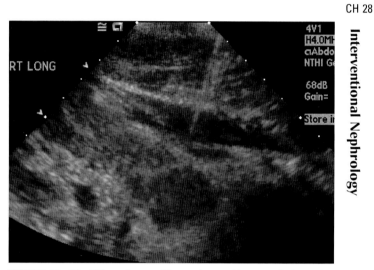

FIGURE 28–18 Kidney ultrasound image shows a biopsy needle located at the lower pole of the kidney.

corrected medically, and if the benefit of doing a biopsy outweighs the potential risk, the biopsy can still be performed. Some relative contraindications to renal biopsy include a solitary kidney, pyelonephritis, perinephric abscess, uncontrolled hypertension, hydronephrosis, polycystic kidney disease, severe anemia, pregnancy, renal masses, and renal artery aneurysms.

Technical Procedure: Percutaneous Renal Biopsy Under Real-Time Ultrasound Guidance

A complete blood count, prothrombin time, and partial thromboplastin time are checked before the procedure. The patient is taken to the ultrasound suite and placed in the prone position. An initial ultrasound examination is performed to confirm the presence of two kidneys. Sterile technique is observed and sterile cover placed over the ultrasound probe. The lower pole of the left kidney is preferred for right-handed operators. The skin and subcutaneous tissue are anesthetized with 1% lidocaine. A small incision is made with a scalpel at the site of needle insertion. Under real-time ultrasound guidance, a biopsy needle gun is advanced up to the capsule of the kidney (Fig. 28–18). The patient is asked to hold his or her breath, and the spring-loaded gun is activated. The gun is retrieved, and the specimen is placed in a container with media. There are different types of needle biopsy guns: full-core, half-core, or three quarters of a core. Sizes vary from 14-French to 18-French and lengths vary from 10

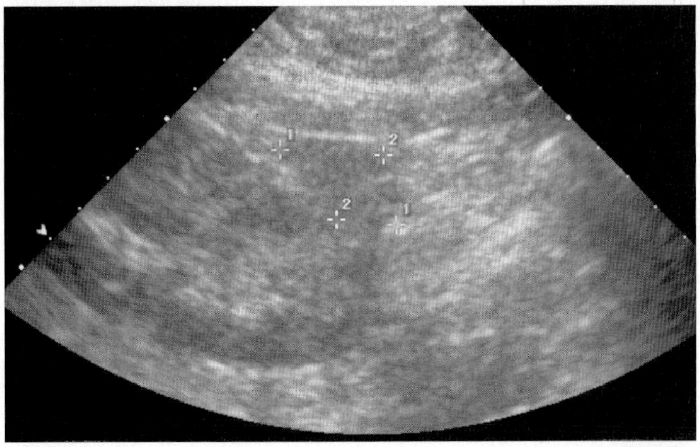

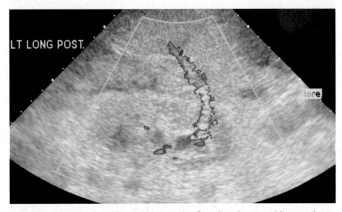

FIGURE 28–19 Postbiopsy kidney ultrasound image of a perinephric hematoma.

FIGURE 28–20 Postbiopsy kidney color Doppler ultrasound image shows active bleeding.

to 20 cm. Also, the throw (amount of tissue that the gun can obtained) of the device can be adjusted from 13 to 33 mm. Usually two or three biopsy pieces are taken in one setting to provide enough tissue for light microscopy, immunofluorescence, and electron microscopy studies. After the biopsy is completed, a second-look ultrasound examination is performed to assess for perinephric hematomas (Fig. 28–19). A color Doppler ultrasound postbiopsy surveillance imaging examination would also be helpful to localize any active bleeding (Fig. 28–20). Vital signs are obtained frequently in the 1st hour and then every 2 to 4 hours. Hematocrits are checked every 6 hours for the next 24 hours.

References

1. NKF-DOQI clinical practice guidelines for vascular access: Update 2000. Am J Kidney Dis 37(suppl 1):S137–S181, 2001.
2. Pisoni RL, Young EW, Dykstra DM, et al: Vascular access use in Europe and in the United States: Results from the DOPPS. Kidney Int 61:305–316, 2002.
3. Stehman-Breen CO, Sherrard DJ, Gillen D, Caps M: Determinants of type and timing of initial permanent hemodialysis vascular access. Kidney Int 57:639–645, 2000.
4. Fan PY, Schwab SJ: Vascular access: concepts for the 1990s. J Am Soc Nephrol 3:1–11, 1992.
5. Windus DW: Permanent vascular access: A nephrologist's view. Am J Kidney Dis 21:457–471, 1993.
6. Porile JL, Richter M: Preservation of vascular access. J Am Soc Nephrol 4:997–1003, 1993.
7. Feldman HI, Kobrin S, Wasserstein A: Hemodialysis vascular access morbidity. J Am Soc Nephrol 7:523–535, 1996.
8. Allon M, Robbin ML: Increasing arteriovenous fistulas in hemodialysis patients: Problems and solutions. Kidney Int 62:1109–1124, 2002.
9. Schwab SJ: Vascular access for hemodialysis. Kidney Int 55:2078–2090, 1999.
10. Allon M: Dialysis catheter-related bacteremia: Treatment and prophylaxis. Am J Kidney Dis 44:779–791, 2004.
11. Schwab SJ, Beathard GA: The hemodialysis catheter conundrum: Hate living with them, but can't live without them. Kidney Int 56:1–17, 1999.
12. Allon M, Daugirdas JT, Depner TA, et al: Effect of change in vascular access on patient mortality in hemodialysis patients. Am J Kidney Dis 47:469–477, 2006.
13. Allon M, Warnock DG: Interventional nephrology: Work in progress. Editorial. Am J Kidney Dis 42:388–391, 2003.
14. Beathard GA: What is the current and future status of interventional nephrology? Semin Dial 18:370–371, 2005.
15. Asif A, Byers P, Vieira CF, Roth D: Developing a comprehensive diagnostic and interventional nephrology program at an academic center. Am J Kidney Dis 42:229–233, 2003.
16. Work J: Hemodialysis catheters and ports. Semin Nephrol 22:211–220, 2002.
17. Rasmussen RL: Establishing an interventional nephrology suite. Semin Nephrol 22:237–241, 2002.
18. Saad TF: Training, certification, and reimbursement for nephrology procedures. Semin Nephrol 22:276–285, 2002.
19. O'Neill WC: Renal ultrasonography: A procedure for nephrologists. Am J Kidney Dis 30:579–585, 1997.
20. Mishler R, Sands JJ, Osfsthun NJ, et al: Dedicated outpatient vascular access center decreases hospitalization and missed outpatient dialysis treatments. Kidney Int 69:393–398, 2006.
21. Allon M, Bailey R, Ballard R, et al: A multidisciplinary approach to hemodialysis access: prospective evaluation. Kidney Int 53:473–479, 1998.
22. Miller PE, Carlton D, Deierhoi MH, et al: Natural history of arteriovenous grafts in hemodialysis patients. Am J Kidney Dis 36:68–74, 2000.
23. Miller CD, Robbin ML, Barker J, Allon M: Comparison of arteriovenous grafts in the thigh and upper extremities in hemodialysis patients. J Am Soc Nephrol 14:2942–2947, 2003.
24. Lilly RZ, Carlton D, Barker J, et al: Clinical predictors of A-V graft patency following radiologic intervention in hemodialysis patients. Am J Kidney Dis 37:945–953, 2001.
25. Maya ID, Oser R, Saddekni S, et al: Vascular access stenosis: Comparison of arteriovenous grafts and fistulas. Am J Kidney Dis 44:859–865, 2004.
26. Beathard GA: Percutaneous transvenous angioplasty in the treatment of vascular access stenosis. Kidney Int 42:1390–1397, 1992.
27. Schwab SJ, Raymond JR, Saeed M, et al: Prevention of hemodialysis fistula thrombosis. Early detection of venous stenosis. Kidney Int 36:707–711, 1989.
28. Safa AA, Valji K, Roberts AC, et al: Detection and treatment of dysfunctional hemodialysis access grafts: Effect of a surveillance program on graft patency and the incidence of thrombosis. Radiology 199:653–657, 1996.
29. Besarab A, Sullivan KL, Ross RP, Moritz MJ: Utility of intra-access pressure monitoring in detecting and correcting venous outlet stenoses prior to thrombosis. Kidney Int 47:1364–1373, 1995.
30. Besarab A, Frinak S, Sherman RA, et al: Simplified measurement of intra-access pressure. J Am Soc Nephrol 9:284–289, 1998.
31. Bosman PJ, Boereboom FTJ, Eikelboom BC, et al: Graft flow as a predictor of thrombosis in hemodialysis grafts. Kidney Int 54:1726–1730, 1998.
32. May RE, Himmelfarb J, Yenicesu M, et al: Predictive measures of vascular access thrombosis: A prospective study. Kidney Int 52:1656–1662, 1997.
33. Neyra NR, Ikizler TA, May RE, et al: Change in access blood flow over time predicts vascular access thrombosis. Kidney Int 54:1714–1719, 1998.
34. Smits JHM, Van der Linden J, Hagen EC, et al: Graft surveillance: Venous pressure, access flow, or the combination? Kidney Int 59:1551–1558, 2001.
35. Malik J, Slavikova M, Svobodova J, Tuka V: Regular ultrasound screening significantly prolongs patency of PTFE grafts. Kidney Int 67:1554–1558, 2005.
36. Ram SJ, Work J, Caldito GC, et al: A randomized controlled trial of blood flow and stenosis surveillance of hemodialysis grafts. Kidney Int 64:272–280, 2003.
37. Robbin ML, Oser RF, Allon M, et al: Hemodialysis access graft stenosis: US detection. Radiology 208:655–661, 1998.
38. Robbin ML, Oser RF, Lee JY, et al: Randomized comparison of ultrasound surveillance and clinical monitoring on arteriovenous graft outcomes. Kidney Int 69:730–735, 2006.
39. Dember LM, Holmberg EF, Kaufman JS: Value of static venous pressure for predicting arteriovenous graft thrombosis. Kidney Int 61:1899–1904, 2002.
40. McDougal G, Agarwal R: Clinical performance characteristics of hemodialysis graft monitoring. Kidney Int 60:762–766, 2001.
41. Cayco AV, Abu-Alfa AK, Mahnensmith RL, Perazella MA: Reduction in arteriovenous graft impairment: Results of a vascular access surveillance protocol. Am J Kidney Dis 32:302–308, 1998.
42. McCarley P, Wingard RL, Shyr Y, et al: Vascular access blood flow monitoring reduces access morbidity and costs. Kidney Int 60:1164–1172, 2001l
43. Dember LM, Holmberg EF, Kaufman JS: Randomized controlled trial of prophylactic repair of hemodialysis arteriovenous graft stenosis. Kidney Int 66:390–398, 2004.
44. Lumsden AB, MacDonald MJ, Isiklar H, et al: Central vein stenosis in the hemodialysis patient: Incidence and efficacy of endovascular treatment. Cardiovasc Surg 5:504–509, 1997.
45. Moist LM, Churchill DN, House AA, et al: Regular monitoring of access flow compared with monitoring of venous pressure fails to improve graft survival. J Am Soc Nephrol 14:2645–2653, 2003.
46. White JJ, Bander SJ, Schwab SJ: Is percutaneous transluminal angioplasty an effective intervention for arteriovenous graft stenosis? Semin Dial 18:190–202, 2005l
47. Besarab A: Access monitoring is worthwhile and valuable. Blood Purif 24:77–89, 2006.
48. Schwab SJ, Oliver MJ, Suhocki P, McCann R: Hemodialysis arteriovenous access: Detection of stenosis and response to treatment by vascular access blood flow. Kidney Int 59:358–362, 2001.

49. Murray BM, Rajczak S, Ali B, et al: Assessment of access blood flow after preemptive angioplasty. Am J Kidney Dis 37:1029–1038, 2001.
50. Chang CJ, Ko PJ, Hsu LA, et al: Highly increased cell proliferation activity in restenotic hemodialysis vascular access after percutaneous transluminal angioplasty: Implication in prevention of stenosis. Am J Kidney Dis 43:74–84, 2004.
51. Roy-Chaudhury P, Kelly BS, Miller MA, et al: Venous neointimal hyperplasia in polytetrafluoroethylene dialysis grafts. Kidney Int 59:2325–2334, 2001.
52. Schmitz PG, McCloud LK, Reikes ST, et al: Prophylaxis of hemodialysis graft thrombosis with fish oil: Double-blind, randomized, prospective trial. J Am Soc Nephrol 13:184–190, 2002.
53. Sreedhara R, Himmelfarb J, Lazarus JM, Hakim RM: Anti-platelet therapy in graft thrombosis: Results of a prospective, randomized, double-blind study. Kidney Int 45:1477–1483, 1994.
54. Kaufman JS, O'Connor TZ, Zhang JH, et al and the Veterans Affairs Cooperative Study Group on Hemodialysis Access Graft Thrombosis: Randomized controlled trial of clopidogrel plus aspirin to prevent hemodialysis access graft thrombosis. J Am Soc Nephrol 14:2313–2321, 2003.
55. Dixon BS, Beck GJ, Dember LM, et al for the DAC Study Group: Design of the Dialysis Access Consortium (DAC) Aggrenox prevention of access stenosis trial. Clin Trials 2:400–412, 2005.
56. Asif A, Gadalean FN, Merrill D, et al: Inflow stenosis in arteriovenous fistulas and grafts: A multicenter, prospective study. Kidney Int 67:1986–1992, 2005.
57. Trerotola SO, Kwak A, Clark TW, et al: Prospective study of balloon inflation pressures and other technical aspects of hemodialysis access angioplasty. J Vasc Interv Radiol 16:1613–1618, 2005.
58. Beathard GA: Mechanical versus pharmacomechanical thrombolysis for the treatment of thrombosed dialysis access grafts. Kidney Int 45:1401–1406, 1994.
59. Patel AA, Truite CM, Trerotola SO: Mechanical thrombectomy of hemodialysis fistulae and grafts. Cardiovasc Intervt Radiol 28:704–713, 2005.
60. Smits HF, Van Rijk PP, Van Isselt JW, et al: Pulmonary embolism after thrombolysis of hemodialysis grafts. J Am Soc Nephrol 8:1458–1461, 1997.
61. Beathard GA: Gianturco self-expanding stent in the treatment of stenosis in dialysis access grafts. Kidney Int 45:872–877, 1995.
62. Hoffer EK, Sultan S, Herskowitz MM, et al: Prospective randomized trial of metallic intravascular stent in hemodialysis graft maintenance. J Vasc Interv Radiol 8:965–973, 1997.
63. Hood DB, Yellin AE, Richman MF, et al: Hemodialysis graft salvage with endoluminal stents. Am Surg 60:733–737, 1994.
64. Patel RI, Peck SH, Cooper SG, et al: Patency of Wallstents placed across the venous anastomosis in hemodialysis grafts after percutaneous recanalization. Radiology 209:365–370, 1998.
65. Sreenarasimhaiah VP, Margassery SK, Martin KJ, Bander SJ: Salvage of thrombosed dialysis access grafts with venous anastomosis stents. Kidney Int 67:678–684, 2005.
66. Turmel-Rodrigues LA, Blanchard D, Pengloan J, et al: Wallstents and Craggstents in hemodialysis grafts and fistulas. Results for selective indications. J Vasc Interv Radiol 8:975–982, 1997.
67. Vogel PM, Parise C: SMART stent for salvage of hemodialysis access grafts. J Vasc Interv Radiol 15:1051–1060, 2004.
68. Maya ID, Allon M: Outcomes of thrombosed arteriovenous grafts: Comparison of stents versus angioplasty. Kidney Int 69:934–937, 2006.
69. Robbin ML, Gallichio ML, Deierhoi MH, et al: US vascular mapping before hemodialysis access placement. Radiology 217:83–88, 2000.
70. Allon M, Lockhart ME, Lilly RZ, et al: Effect of preoperative sonographic mapping on vascular access outcomes in hemodialysis patients. Kidney Int 60:2013–2020, 2001.
71. Ascher E, Gade P, Hingorani A, et al: Changes in the practice of angioaccess surgery: Impact of dialysis outcomes quality initiative recommendations. J Vasc Surg 31:84–92, 2000.
72. Gibson KD, Caps MT, Kohler TR, et al.: Assessment of a policy to reduce placement of prosthetic hemodialysis access. Kidney Int 59:2335–2345, 2001.
73. Silva MB, Hobson RW, Pappas PJ, et al: A strategy for increasing use of autogenous hemodialysis access procedures: Impact of preoperative noninvasive evaluation. J Vasc Surg 27:302–308, 1998.
74. Asif A, Cherla G, Merrill D, et al: Conversion of tunneled hemodialysis catheter–consigned patients to arteriovenous fistula. Kidney Int 67:2399–2406, 2005.
75. Asif A, Cherla G, Merrill D, et al: Venous mapping using venography and the risk of radio-contrast–induced nephropathy. Semin Dial 18:239–242, 2005.
76. Lockhart ME, Robbin ML, Allon M: Preoperative sonographic radial artery evaluation and correlation with subsequent radiocephalic fistula outcome. J Ultrasound Med 23:161–168, 2004.
77. Miller PE, Tolwani A, Luscy CP, et al: Predictors of adequacy of arteriovenous fistulas in hemodialysis patients. Kidney Int 56:275–280, 1999.
78. Miller CD, Robbin ML, Allon M: Gender differences in outcomes of arteriovenous fistulas in hemodialysis patients. Kidney Int 63:346–352, 2003.
79. Lin SL, Huang CH, Chen HS, et al: Effects of age and diabetes on blood flow rate and primary outcome of newly created hemodialysis arteriovenous fistulas. Am J Nephrol 18:96–100, 1998.
80. Wong V, Ward R, Taylor J, et al: Factors associated with early failure of arteriovenous fistulae for hemodialysis access. Eur J Vasc Endovasc Surg 12:207–213, 1996.
81. Robbin ML, Chamberlain NE, Lockhart ME, et al: Hemodialysis arteriovenous fistula maturity: US evaluation. Radiology 225:59–64, 2002.
82. Asif A, Roy-Chaudhury P, Beathard GA: Early arteriovenous fistula failure: A logical proposal for when and how to intervene. Clin J Am Soc Nephrol 1:332–339, 2006.
83. Beathard GA, Settle SM, Shields MW: Salvage of the nonfunctioning arteriovenous fistula. Am J Kidney Dis 33:910–916, 1999.
84. Beathard GA, Arnold P, Jackson J, Litchfield T, Physician Operators Forum of RMS Lifeline: Aggressive treatment of early fistula failure. Kidney Int 64:1487–1494, 2003.
85. Turmel-Rodrigues L, Mouton A, Birmele B, et al: Salvage of immature forearm fistulas for haemodialysis by interventional radiology. Nephrol Dial Transplant 16:2365–2371, 2001.
86. Nassar GM, Nguyen B, Rhee E, Achkar K: Endovascular treatment of the "failing to mature" arteriovenous fistula. Clin J Am Soc Nephrol 1:275–280, 2006.
87. Faiyaz R, Abreo K, Zaman F, et al: Salvage of poorly developed arteriovenous fistulae with percutaneous ligation of accessory veins. Am J Kidney Dis 39:824–827, 2002.
88. Van der Linden J, Smits JHM, Assink JH, et al: Short- and long-term functional effects of percutaneous transluminal angioplasty in hemodialysis vascular access. J Am Soc Nephrol 13:715–720, 2002.
89. Turmel-Rodrigues L, Pengloan J, Rodrigue H, et al: Treatment of failed native arteriovenous fistulae for hemodialysis by interventional radiology. Kidney Int 57:1124–1140, 2000.
90. Lee T, Barker J, Allon M: Needle infiltration of arteriovenous fistulas in hemodialysis: Risk factors and consequences. Am J Kidney Dis 47:1020–1026, 2006.
91. Haage P, Vorwerk D, Wilberger JE, et al: Percutaneous treatment of thrombosed primary arteriovenous hemodialysis access fistulae. Kidney Int 57:1169–1175, 2000.
92. Turmel-Rodrigues L, Pengloan J, Baudin S, et al: Treatment of stenosis and thrombosis in haemodialysis fistulas and grafts by interventional radiology. Nephrol Dial Transplant 15:2029–2036, 2000.
93. Zaleski GX, Funaki B, Kenney S, et al: Angioplasty and bolus urokinase infusion for the restoration of function in thrombosed Brescia-Cimino dialysis fistulas. J Vasc Interv Radiol 10:129–136, 1999.
94. Rocek M, Peregrin JH, Lasovickova J, et al: Mechanical thrombolysis of thrombosed hemodialysis native fistulas with use of the Arrow-Trerotola percutaneous thrombolytic device: Our preliminary experience. J Vasc Interv Radiol 11:1153–1158, 2000.
95. Liang HL, Pan HB, Chung HM, et al: Restoration of thrombosed Brescia-Cimino dialysis fistulas by using percutaneous transluminal angioplasty. Radiology 223:339–344, 2002.
96. Rajan DK, Clark TW, Simons ME, et al: Procedural success and patency after percutaneous treatment of thrombosed autogenous arteriovenous dialysis fistulas. J Vasc Interv Radiol 13:1211–1218, 2002.
97. Shatsky JB, Berns JS, Clark TW, et al: Single-center experience with the Arrow-Trerotola percutaneous thrombectomy device in the management of thrombosed native dialysis fistulas. J Vasc Interv Radiol 16:1605–1611, 2005.
98. Sreenarasimhaiah VP, Margassery SK, Martin KJ, Bander SJ: Cutting balloon angioplasty for resistant venous anastomotic stenoses. Semin Dial 17:523–527, 2004.
99. Ryan JM, Dumbleton SA, Smith TP: Using a cutting balloon to treat resistant high-grade dialysis graft stenosis. AJR Am J Roentgenol 180:1072–1074, 2003.
100. Vesely TM, Siegel JB: Use of the peripheral cutting balloon to treat hemodialysis-related stenoses. J Vasc Interv Radiol 16:1593–1603, 2005.
101. Rifkin BS, Brewster UC, Aruny JE, Perazella MA: Percutaneous balloon cryoplasty: A new therapy for rapidly recurrent anastomotic venous stenoses of hemodialysis grafts? Am J Kidney Dis 45:e27–e32, 2005.
102. Schillinger F, Schillinger D, Montagnac R, Milcent T: Post catheterisation vein stenosis in haemodialysis: Comparative angiographic study of 50 subclavian and 50 internal jugular acceses. Nephrol Dial Transplant 6:722–724, 1991.
103. Ayetkin C, Boyvat F, Yagmurdur MC, et al: Endovascular stent placement in the treatment of upper extremity central venous obstruction in hemodialysis patients. Eur J Radiol 49:81–85, 2004.
104. Buriankova E, Kocher M, Bachleda P, et al: Endovascular treatment of central vein stenoses in patients with dialysis shunts. Biomed Papers 147:203–206, 2003.
105. Kovalik EC, Newman GE, Suhocki PV, et al: Correction of central vein stenoses: Use of angioplasty and vascular Wallstents. Kidney Int 45:1177–1181, 1994.
106. Maskova J, Komarkova J, Kivanek J, et al: Endovascular treatment of central vein stenoses and/or occlusions in hemodialysis patients. Cardiovasc Interv Radiol 26:27–30, 2003.
107. Sprouse LR, Lesar CJ, Meier GH, et al: Percutaneous treatment of symptomatic central venous stenosis angioplasty. J Vasc Surg 39:578–582, 2004.
108. Surowiec SM, Fegley AJ, Tanski WJ, et al: Endovascular management of central venous stenoses in the hemodialysis patient: Results of percutaneous therapy. Vasc Endovasc Surg 38:349–354, 2004.
109. Vesely TM, Hovsepian DM, Pilgram TK, et al: Upper extremity ventral venous obstruction in hemodialysis patients: Treatment with Wallstents. Radiology 204:343–348, 1997.
110. Oliver MJ, Callery SM, Thorpe KE, et al: Risk of bacteremia from temporary hemodialysis catheters by site of insertion and duration of use: A prospective study. Kidney Int 58:2543–2545, 2000.
111. Stevenson KB, Hannah EL, Lowder CA, et al: Epidemiology of hemodialysis vascular access infections from longitudinal infection surveillance data: Predicting the impact of NKF-DOQI clinical practice guidelines for vascular access. Am J Kidney Dis 39:549–555, 2002.
112. Weijmer MC, Vervloet MG, ter Wee PM: Compared to tunnelled cuffed haemodialysis catheters, temporary untunnelled catheters are associated with more complications already within 2 weeks of use. Nephrol Dial Transplant 19:670–677, 2004.
113. Wilkin TD, Kraus MA, Lane KA, Trerotola SO: Internal jugular vein thrombosis associated with hemodialysis catheters. Radiology 228:697–700, 2003.
114. Maya ID, Allon M: Outcomes of tunneled femoral hemodialysis catheters: Comparison with internal jugular vein catheters. Kidney Int 68:2886–2889, 2005.
115. Zaleski GX, Funaki B, Lorenz JM, et al: Experience with tunneled femoral hemodialysis catheters. AJR Am J Roentgenol 172:493–496, 1999.
116. Lee T, Barker J, Allon M: Tunneled catheters in hemodialysis patients: Reasons and subsequent outcomes. Am J Kidney Dis 46:501–508, 2005.
117. Gupta A, Karak PK, Saddekni S: Translumbar inferior vena cava catheter for long-term hemodialysis. J Am Soc Nephrol 5:2094–2097, 1995.

118. Biswal R, Nosher JL, Siegel RL, Bodner LJ: Translumbar placement of paired hemodialysis catheters (Tesio catheters) and follow-up in 10 patients. Cardiovasc Interv Radiol 23:75–78, 2000.

119. Duncan KA, Karlin CA, Beezley M: Percutaneous transhepatic PermCath for hemodialysis vascular access. Am J Kidney Dis 25:973, 1995.

120. Stavropoulos SW, Pan JJ, Clark TWI, et al: Percutaneous transhepatic venous access for hemodialysis. J Vasc Interv Radiol 14:1187–1190, 2003.

121. Smith TP, Ryan JM, Reddan DN: Transhepatic catheter access for hemodialysis. Radiology 232:246–251, 2004.

122. Daeihagh P, Jordan J, Chen GJ, Rocco M: Efficacy of tissue plasminogen activator administration on patency of hemodialysis access catheters. Am J Kidney Dis 36:75–79, 2000.

123. Lund GB, Trerotola SO, Scheel PF, et al: Outcome of tunneled hemodialysis catheters placed by radiologists. Radiology 198:467–472, 1996.

124. Marr KA, Sexton DJ, Conlon PJ, et al: Catheter-related bacteremia and outcome of attempted catheter salvage in patients undergoing hemodialysis. Ann Intern Med 127:275–280, 1997.

125. Pourchez T, Moriniere P, Fournier A, Pietri J: Use of Permcath (Quinton) catheter in uremic patients in whom the creation of conventional vascular access for hemodialysis is difficult. Nephron 53:297–302, 1989.

126. Saad TF: Bacteremia associated with tunnneled, cuffed hemodialysis catheters. Am J Kidney Dis 34:1114–1124, 1999.

127. Swartz RD, Messana JM, Boyer CJ, et al: Successful use of cuffed central venous hemodialysis catheters inserted percutaneously. J Am Soc Nephrol 4:1719–1725, 1994,

128. Kovalik EC, Raymond JR, Albers FJ, et al: A clustering of epidural abscesses in chronic hemodialysis patients: Risks of salvaging access catheters in cases of infection. J Am Soc Nephrol 7:2264–2267, 1996.

129. Beathard GA: Management of bacteremia associated with tunneled-cuffed hemodialysis catheters. J Am Soc Nephrol 10:1045–1049, 1999.

130. Robinson D, Suhocki P, Schwab SJ: Treatment of infected tunneled venous access hemodialysis catheters with guidewire exchange. Kidney Int 53:1792–1794, 1998.

131. Shaffer D: Catheter-related sepsis complicating long-term, tunnelled central venous dialysis catheters: Management by guidewire exchange. Am J Kidney Dis 25:593–596, 1995.

132. Tanriover B, Carlton D, Saddekni S, et al: Bacteremia associated with tunneled dialysis catheters: Comparison of two treatment strategies. Kidney Int 57:2151–2155, 2000.

133. Costerton JW, Stewart PS, Greenberg EP: Bacterial biofilms: A common cause of persistent infections. Science 284:1318–1322, 1999.

134. Donlan RM: Biofilm formation: a clinically relevant microbiologic process. Clin Infect Dis 33:1387–1392, 2001.

135. Donlan RM: Biofilms: Microbial life on surfaces. Emerg Infect Dis 8:881–890, 2002.

136. Allon M: Saving infected catheters: Why and how. Blood Purif 23:23–28, 2005.

137. Krishnasami Z, Carlton D, Bimbo L, et al: Management of hemodialysis catheter related bacteremia with an adjunctive antibiotic lock solution. Kidney Int 61:1136–1142, 2002.

138. Poole CV, Carlton D, Bimbo L, Allon M: Treatment of catheter-related bacteremia with an antibiotic lock protocol: Effect of bacterial pathogen. Nephrol Dial Transplant 19:1237–1244, 2004.

139. Vardhan A, Davies J, Daryanani I, et al: Treatment of haemodialysis catheter–related infections. Nephrol Dial Transplant 17:1149–1150, 2002.

140. Beathard GA, Posen GA: Initial clinical results with the LifeSite Hemodialysis Access System. Kidney Int 58:2021–2027, 2000.

141. Schwab SJ, Weiss MA, Rushton F, et al: Multicenter clinical trial results with the Lifesite hemodialysis access system. Kidney Int 62:1026–1033, 2002.

142. Prichard S: Will peritoneal dialysis be left behind? Semin Dial 18:167–170, 2005.

143. Wang JY, Chen FM, Huang TJ, et al: Laparoscopic assisted placement of peritoneal dialysis catheters for selected patients with previous abdominal operation. J Invest Surg 18:59–62, 2005.

144. Comert M, Borazan A, Kulah E, Ucan BH: A new laparoscopic technique for placement of a permanent peritoneal dialysis catheter: The preperitoneal tunneling method. Surg Endosc 19:245–248, 2005.

145. Soontrapornchai P, Simapatanapong T: Comparison of open and laparoscopic secure placement of peritoneal dialysis catheters. Surg Endosc 19:137–139, 2005.

146. Degesys GE, Miller GA, Ford KK, Dunnick NR: Tenckhoff peritoneal dialysis catheters: The use of fluoroscopy in management. Radiology 154:819–820, 1985.

147. Zaman F, Pervez A, Atray NK, et al: Fluoroscopy-associated placement of peritoneal dialysis catheters by nephrologists. Semin Dial 18:247–251, 2005.

148. Zappacosta AR, Perras ST, Closkey GM: Seldinger technique for Tenckhoff catheter placement. ASAIO J 37:13–15, 1991.

149. Copley JB, Lindberg JS, Tapia NP, et al: Peritoneoscopic placement of swan neck peritoneal dialysis catheters. Perit Dial Int 14:295–296, 1994.

150. Tsimoyiannis EC, Siakas P, Glantzounis G, et al: Laparoscopic placement of the Tenckhoff catheter for peritoneal dialysis. Surg Laparosc Endosc Percutan Tech 10:218–221, 2000.

151. Moncrief JW, Popovich RP, Broadrick LJ, et al: The Moncrief-Popovich catheter: A new peritoneal access technique for patients on peritoneal dialysis. ASAIO J 39:62–65, 1993.

152. Asif A, Byers P, Vieira CE, et al: Peritoneoscopic placement of peritoneal dialysis catheter and bowel perforation: Experience of an interventional nephrology program. Am J Kidney Dis 42:1270–1274, 2003.

153. Gokal R: Peritoneal dialysis: Global update. Perit Dial Int 19(suppl 2):S11–S15, 1999.

154. Nebel M, Marczewski K, Finke K: Three years of experience with the swan-neck Tenckhoff catheter. Adv Perit Dial 7:208–213, 1991.

155. Lye WC, Giangg MM, van der Straaten JC, Lee EJ: Breaking-in after the insertion of Tenckhoff catheters: A comparison of two techniques. Adv Perit Dial 9:236–239, 1993.

156. Song JH, Kim GA, Lee SW, Kim MJ: Clinical outcomes of immediate full-volume exchange one year after peritoneal catheter implantation for CAPD. Perit Dial Int 2:194–199, 2000.

157. Eklund BH, Honkanen EO, Kala AR, Kyllonen LE: Catheter configuration and outcome in patients on continuous ambulatory peritoneal dialysis: A prospective comparison of two catheters. Perit Dial Int 14:70–74, 1994.

158. Eklund BH, Honkanen EO, Kala AR, Kyllonen LE: Peritoneal dialysis access: Prospective randomized comparison of the swan-neck and Tenckhoff catheters. Perit Dial Int 15:353–356, 1995.

159. Hwang TL, Huang CC: Comparison of swan-neck catheters with Tenckhoff catheters for CAPD. Adv Perit Dial 10:203–205, 1994.

160. Twardowski ZJ, Prowant BF, Nichols WK, et al: Six-year experience with swan-neck presternal peritoneal dialysis catheter. Perit Dial Int 18:598–602, 1998.

161. Twardowski ZJ: Presternal peritoneal catheter. Adv Ren Replace Ther 9:125–132, 2002.

162. Gadallah MF, Pervez A, el-Shahawy MA, et al: Peritoneoscopic versus surgical placement of peritoneal dialysis catheters: A prospective randomized study on outcome. Am J Kidney Dis 33:118–122, 1999.

163. Simons ME, Pron G, Voros M, et al: Fluoroscopically-guided manipulation of malfunctioning peritoneal dialysis catheters. Perit Dial Int 19:544–549, 1999.

164. Gadallah MF, Arora N, Arumugam R, Moles K: Role of Fogarty catheter manipulation in management of migrate, nonfunctional peritoneal dialysis catheters. Am J Kidney Dis 35:301–305, 2000.

165. Ash SR: Chronic peritoneal dialysis catheters: Overview of design, placement, and review procedures. Semin Dial 16:323–334, 2003.

166. Cozens NJ, Murchison JT, Allan PL, Winney RJ: Conventional 15 G needle technique for renal biopsy compared with ultrasound-guided spring-loaded 18 G needle biopsy. Br J Radiol 65:594–597, 1992.

167. Marwah DS, Korbet SM: Timing of complications in percutaneous renal biopsy: What is the optimal period of observation? Am J Kidney Dis 28:47–52, 1996.

168. Burstein DM, Korbet SM, Schwartz MM: The use of the automatic core biopsy system in percutaneous renal biopsies: A comparative study. Am J Kidney Dis 22:545–552, 1993.

169. Marwah DS, Korbet SM: Timing of complications in percutaneous renal biopsy: What is the optimal time of observation? Am J Kidney Dis 28:47–52, 1996.

170. Ginsburg JC, Fransman SL, Singer MA, et al: Use of computerized tomography to evaluate bleeding after renal biopsy. Nephron 26:240–243, 1980.

171. Thompson BC, Kingdon E, Johnston M, et al: Transjugular kidney biopsy. Am J Kidney Dis 43:651–662, 2004.

172. Abbott KC, Musio FM, Chung EM, et al: Transjugular renal biopsy in high-risk patients: An American case series. BMC Nephrol 3:5, 2002.

173. Lumsden AB, MacDonald MJ, Kikeri D, et al: Prophylactic balloon angioplasty fails to prolong the patency of expanded polytetrafluoroethylene arteriovenous grafts: Results of a prospective randomized study. J Vasc Surg 26:382–392, 1997.

174. Kanterman RY, Vesely TM, Pilgram TK, et al: Dialysis access grafts: anatomic location of venous stenosis and results of angioplsty. Radiology 195:153–159, 1995.

175. Valji K, Brookstein JJ, Roberts AC, Davis GB: Parmacomechanical thrombolysis and angioplasty in the management of clotted hemodialysis grafts: Early and late clinical results. Radiology 178:243–247, 1991.

176. Trerotola SO, Lund GB, Schell PJ, et al: Thrombosed dialysis access grafts: Percutaneous mechanical declotting without urokinase. Radiology 191:721–726, 1994.

177. Cohen MAH, Kumpe DA, Durham JD, Zwerdlinger SC: Improved treatment of thrombosed hemodialysis access sites with thrombolysis and angioplasty. Kidney Int 46:1375–1380, 1994.

178. Sands JJ, Patel S, Plaviak DJ, Miranda CL: Pharmacomechanical thrombolysis with urokinase for treatment of thrombosed hemodialysis access grafts: A comparison with surgical thrombectomy. ASAIO Trans 40:M886–M888, 1994.

179. Beathard GA: Thrombolysis versus surgery for the treatment of thrombosed dialysis access grafts. J Am Soc Nephrol 6:1619–1624, 1995.

180. Beathard GA, Welch BR, Maidment HJ: Mechanical thrombolysis for the treatment of thrombosed hemodialysis access grafts. Radiology 200:711–716, 1996.

181. Trerotola SO, Vesely TM, Lund GB, et al: Treatment of thrombosed hemodialysis access grafts: Arrow-Trerotola percutaneous thrombolytic device versus pulse-spray thrombolysis. Radiology 206:403–414, 1998.

182. Sedlacek M, Teodorescu V, Falk A, et al: Hemodialysis access placement with preoperative noninvasive vascular mapping: Comparison between patients with and without diabetes. Am J Kidney Dis 38:560–564, 2001.

183. Mihmanli I, Besirli K, Kurugoglu S, et al: Cephalic vein and hemodialysis fistula: Surgeon's observation versus color Doppler ultrasonographic findings. J Ultrasound Med 20:217–222, 2001.

184. Miller A, Holzenbein TJ, Gottlieb MN, et al: Strategies to increase the use of autogenous arteriovenous fistula in end-stage renal disease. Ann Vasc Surg 11:397–405, 1997.

185. Maya ID, Maddela P, Barker J, Allon M: Percutaneous renal biopsy: comparison of blind and real-time ultrasound-guided technique. Semin Dial 20:355–358, 2007.

186. Doyle AJ, Gregory MC, Terreros DA: Percutaneous native renal biopsy: Comparison of 1.2 mm spring-driven system with a traditional 2-mm hand-driven system. Am J Kidney Dis 23:498–503, 1994.

187. Hergessel O, Felten H, Andrassy K, et al: Safety of ultrasound-guided percutaneous renal biopsy—Retrospective analysis of 1090 consecutive vases. Nephrol Dial Transplant 13:975–977, 1998.

188. Donovan KL, Thomas DM, Wheeler DC, et al: Experience with a new method for percutaneous renal biopsy. Nephrol Dial Transplant 6:731–733, 1991.

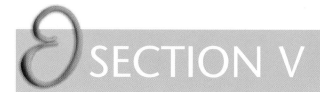

SECTION V

Disorders of Kidney Function

CHAPTER 29

Acute Kidney Injury

Michael R. Clarkson • John J. Friedewald • Joseph A. Eustace • Hamid Rabb

DEFINITION AND CLASSIFICATION

Acute kidney injury (AKI) is a protean syndrome of varied severity. It is characterized by a rapid (hours to weeks) decline in the glomerular filtration rate (GFR) and retention of nitrogenous waste products such as blood urea nitrogen (BUN) and creatinine.[1,2] In recent years, it has been recognized that the time-honored term acute renal failure (ARF) fails to adequately describe what is a dynamic process extending across initiation, maintenance, and recovery phases, each of which may be of variable duration and severity. The term acute renal *failure* suggests that the syndrome is dichotomous and places an undue emphasis on whether or not renal function has overtly failed. This belies the now well-established fact that even mild decrements in glomerular filtration may be associated with adverse clinical outcomes.[3-7] The alternative proposed term acute kidney injury has much to recommend it, perhaps better captures the diverse nature of this syndrome, and has entered into widespread clinical use. In this chapter, the two terms are used interchangeably. In clinical practice, acute tubular necrosis (ATN) has come to be used almost synonymously with AKI, although preferably, its use should be limited to a histologic context.

Historically, patients with AKI have been classified as being nonoliguric (urine output >400 mL/day), oliguric (urinary output <400 mL/day), or anuric (urinary output <100 mL/day).[8] Lower levels of urinary output typically reflect a more severe initial injury, have implications for volume overload and electrolyte disturbances, and are of prognostic importance. However, the therapeutic manipulation of the urine output does not ameliorate this prognostic association (vide infra).

For purposes of diagnosis and management, AKI has been divided into three categories (Table 29–1):

1. Diseases characterized by renal hypoperfusion in which the integrity of renal parenchymal tissue is preserved (prerenal states),
2. Diseases involving renal parenchymal tissue (intrarenal AKI or intrinsic AKI), and
3. Diseases associated with acute obstruction of the urinary tract (postrenal or obstructive AKI).

Most acute intrinsic AKI is caused by ischemia or nephrotoxins and is classically associated with ATN.

AKI may occur in someone either with previously normal renal function or as an acute and unanticipated deterioration in function in the setting of previously established chronic kidney disease. The etiology and outcome of AKI is heavily influenced by the circumstances in which it occurs, such as whether it develops in the community or in the hospital. It is similarly important to distinguish whether the kidney injury occurs as an isolated process, which is more common in community-acquired AKI, or if it occurs as part as a more extensive multiorgan syndrome. In the former context, management is often, at least initially, conservative and follows an expectant approach—deferring renal replacement therapy when possible while awaiting the spontaneous recovery of renal function. In the case of a critically ill patient with multiorgan failure, dialysis may be commenced much earlier, because the goal is not simply control of azotemia but rather one of renal support in an attempt to optimize the subject's physiologic parameters.[9]

More than 35 different definitions of AKI have been used in the recent literature.[10] These are typically based on either a fixed or relative increment in the serum creatinine level or reductions in urinary output. Most of these definitions are arbitrary and have not been validated with regard to their prognostic importance. Not surprisingly, this has limited the comparability of different studies and has hampered the translation of bench research into clinical practice.[11] Recently, a consensus conference sponsored by the Acute Dialysis Quality Improvement Initiative (ADQI) has proposed a new definition of ARF, that has been widely endorsed and is increasingly being used.[12] In keeping with the spectrum of changes seen in AKI, a diagnostic classification scheme was developed. This scheme is referred to by the acronym RIFLE, and includes three levels of renal dysfunction of increasing severity, namely, *R*isk of renal dysfunction, *I*njury to the kidney and *F*ailure of kidney function, and two outcome categories: *L*oss of function, and *E*nd stage kidney disease (Fig.

TABLE 29–1 **Classification and Major Disease Categories Causing Acute Kidney Injury**

Disease Category	Percentage of Patients with Acute Kidney Injury
Prerenal azotemia caused by acute renal hypoperfusion	55–60

Intrinsic renal azotemia caused by acute diseases of renal parenchyma
    Diseases involving large renal vessels
    Diseases of small renal vessels and glomeruli
    Acute injury to renal tubules mediated by ischemia or toxins*
    Acute diseases of the tubulointerstitium
	35–40

Postrenal azotemia caused by acute obstruction of urinary collecting system	<5

*Accounts for more than 90% of cases in the intrinsic renal azotemia category in most series.

CH 29

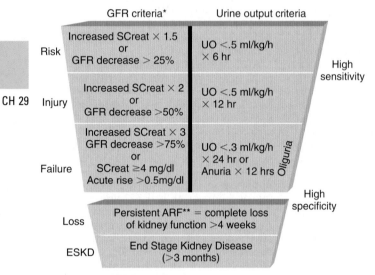

FIGURE 29–1 RIFLE classification scheme for acute renal failure. The classification system includes separate criteria for creatinine and urine output. A patient can fulfill the criteria through changes in serum creatinine (SCreat) or changes in urinary output, or both. The criteria that lead to the worst possible classification should be used. The shape of the figure denotes the fact that more patients (high sensitivity) will be included in the mild category, including some without actually having renal failure (less specificity). In contrast, at the bottom of the figure, the criteria are strict and therefore specific, but some patients will be missed. (From Bellomo R, Ronco C, Kellum JA, et al: Acute renal failure—definition, outcome measures, animal models, fluid therapy and information technology needs: the Second International Consensus Conference of the Acute Dialysis Quality Initiative (ADQI) Group. Crit Care 8:R204–R212, 2004.)

29–1). Renal dysfunction is defined in terms of either a rise in creatinine or a reduction in urine output, the more severe of the two criteria being selected. RIFLE-F (Failure) is present even if the rise in serum creatinine is less than threefold above baseline, provided that the new serum creatinine is greater than 4 mg/dL and has risen by at least 0.5 mg/dL. When the achieved designation results from urine output criteria a subscript "o" is added e.g. RIFLE-F$_o$. Similarly, a subscript "c" is used to denote the presence of preexisting chronic kidney disease. An inevitable limitation of any definition that uses relative changes in renal function is the problem of when the patient's baseline function is unknown and, therefore, can only be estimated. A worse RIFLE criteria score is associated with a progressively worse APACHE II score and higher mortality at both 1 and 6 months.[5,13] A more extensive classification system based on an multidimensional approach, as used in several other area of medicine such as with cirrhosis, has also recently been proposed for AKI.[14]

This includes 4 separate axis, namely (1) susceptibility—the prior level of renal function, (2) the nature and timing of the applied insult, (3) the response to this injury as measured by the RIFLE criteria and (4) the associated number of failed organs. This more complicated schema has the advantage of including not only the renal response but also of quantifying the clinical circumstances in which the injury occurs, factors that influence the clinical outcome and which therefore should equally be considered in estimating clinical risks and determining the optimal management.

A major challenge in the investigation and management of AKI is the timely recognition of the syndrome. It remains difficult to easily and reliably measure rapid changes in the GFR. Although the severity in decline in GFR correlates with the onset of oliguria, the latter is insensitive marker of the syndrome because many subjects with severe renal failure remain nonoliguric. In AKI, there is poor agreement between serum creatinine and GFR, at least until a serum creatinine steady state is reached, and even then, the absolute rise in serum creatinine must take into account differences in creatinine generation rates.[15] As a result, definitions of AKI that are based on a fixed increment in serum creatinine would be expected to be biased toward making an early diagnosis in well-muscled as compared with malnourished subjects or in men as compared with women. Creatinine clearances, especially when measured over a short time frame such as 2 to 4 hours, has some utility but may substantially overestimate GFR at low levels of renal function owing to a relatively high proportion of tubular secretion. Even the use of markers such as iothalamate to estimate GFR may be less precise in the acute as compared with the chronic setting owing to alterations in their volume of distribution as well as issues relating to tubular obstruction and backleak. The use of cystatin C or of other alternative makers of early AKI is an area of ongoing research.[16]

INCIDENCE

The incidence of in hospital AKI is difficult to estimate because no registry of its occurrence exists and because up until recently there was no standardized definition. From a variety of predominantly single center studies it is estimated that 3% to 7% of hospitalized patients develop AKI.[17–19] More detailed information is available regarding its development in the intensive care unit (ICU) environment, where approximately 25% to 30% of unselected patients develop some degree of AKI, although again estimates vary considerable depending on the definition used and the population casemix. Renal replacement therapy is typically required in 5% to 6% of the general ICU population or 8.8 to 13.4 cases per 100,000 population/year.[5,20–24] However, with the increasing prevalence of older subjects, higher degrees of comorbidity and preexisting chronic kidney disease in some centers, the proportion of patients requiring dialysis is substantially higher, two thirds of patients with AKI in one large multicenter study.[25] The occurrence of AKI and the need for renal replacement therapy may also be much higher in specific high-risk populations, such as those with haematologic malignancies, in whom in one study the requirement for renal replacement therapy was 22.5% as compared with 5.8% in those without haematological malignancies.[26]

A recent analysis of a random 5% sample of Medicare beneficiaries based on inpatient claims data from between 1992 and 2001 found an overall AKI incidence of 23.8 cases per 1000 hospital discharges. The rate per 1000 discharges progressively increased—by approximately 11% per year—over the decade from 14.6 in 1992 to 36.4 in 2001 and was consistently higher in older subjects, men, and blacks.[27] A similar incidence rate—9.2 cases per 1000 hospitalizations, equivalent to 1.9% of all hospital discharges—and similar demographic associations were observed using the 2001 National Hospital Discharge Survey, a national collected database based on a representative sample of nonfederal acute care hospitals.[28]

ETIOLOGY OF ACUTE KIDNEY INJURY

Prerenal Acute Kidney Injury

Prerenal AKI is the most common cause of AKI and is an appropriate physiologic response to renal hypoperfusion.[2,22,29] By definition, the integrity of renal parenchymal tissue is maintained and GFR is corrected rapidly with restoration of renal perfusion. Severe renal hypoperfusion may cause ischemic ATN. Thus, prerenal AKI and ischemic ATN are part of a spectrum of manifestations of renal hypoperfusion, and the clinical and biochemical features of prerenal ARF and ischemic ATN coexist in many patients.

Prerenal AKI can complicate any disease characterized by hypovolemia, low cardiac output, systemic vasodilatation, or intrarenal vasoconstriction (Table 29–2). True or "effective" hypovolemia leads to a fall in mean systemic arterial pressure, which, in turn, activates arterial (e.g., carotid sinus) and

cardiac baroreceptors and initiates a series of neural and humoral responses that include activation of the sympathetic nervous system and renin-angiotensin-aldosterone system and release of antidiuretic hormone (see Fig. 29–1).[30–32] Norepinephrine, angiotensin II, and antidiuretic hormone act in concert in an attempt to maintain blood pressure and preserve cardiac and cerebral perfusion by stimulating vasoconstriction in relatively "less important" vascular beds such as the musculocutaneous and splanchnic circulations, by inhibiting salt loss through sweat glands, by stimulating thirst and salt appetite, and by promoting renal salt and water retention. Glomerular perfusion, ultrafiltration pressure, and filtration rate are preserved during mild hypoperfusion through several compensatory mechanisms. Stretch receptors in the walls of afferent arterioles detect a reduction in perfusion pressure, triggering relaxation of afferent arteriolar smooth muscle cells and vasodilatation (autoregulation). Intrarenal biosynthesis of vasodilator prostaglandins (e.g., prostacyclin, prostaglandin E_2), kallikrein and kinins, and possibly nitric oxide (NO) is enhanced. Angiotensin II may induce preferential constriction of efferent arterioles, probably because most angiotensin II receptors are found at this location.[33] As a result, intraglomerular pressure is preserved, the fraction of renal plasma that is filtered by glomeruli (filtration fraction) is increased, and GFR is maintained.

These compensatory renal responses are overwhelmed during states of moderate to severe hypoperfusion, and ARF ensues. Autoregulatory dilatation of afferent arterioles is maximal at a mean systemic arterial blood pressure of about 70 to 80 mm Hg, and hypotension below this level is associated with a precipitous decline in glomerular ultrafiltration pressure and GFR.[34,35] Lesser degrees of hypotension may provoke prerenal AKI in the elderly, in patients with renovascular disease, and in patients with diseases affecting the integrity of afferent arterioles (e.g., hypertensive nephrosclerosis, diabetic nephropathy).[36] In addition, very high levels of angiotensin II, as are found in patients with marked circulatory failure, provoke constriction of both afferent and efferent arterioles, thus negating the relatively selective effect of low levels of this peptide on efferent arteriolar resistance.

Several classes of commonly used drugs impair renal adaptive responses and can convert compensated renal hypoper-

TABLE 29–2	Major Causes of Prerenal Azotemia

Intravascular volume depletion
Hemorrhage: traumatic, surgical, gastrointestinal, postpartum
Gastrointestinal losses: vomiting, nasogastric suction, diarrhea
Renal losses: drug-induced or osmotic diuresis, diabetes insipidus, adrenal insufficiency
Skin and mucous membrane losses: burns, hyperthermia, and other causes of increased
    insensible losses
"Third-space" losses: pancreatitis, crush syndrome, hypoalbuminemia

Decreased cardiac output
Diseases of myocardium, valves, pericardium, or conducting system
Pulmonary hypertension, pulmonary embolism, positive-pressure mechanical ventilation
Systemic vasodilatation
Drugs: antihypertensives, afterload reduction, anesthetics, drug overdoses
Sepsis, liver failure, anaphylaxis

Renal vasoconstriction
Norepinephrine, ergotamine, liver disease, sepsis, hypercalcemia

Pharmacologic agents that acutely impair autoregulation and glomerular filtration rate in specific settings
Angiotensin-converting enzyme inhibitors in renal artery stenosis or severe renal
    hypoperfusion
Inhibition of prostaglandin synthesis by nonsteroidal anti-inflammatory drugs during renal
    hypoperfusion

fusion to overt prerenal AKI or trigger progression of prerenal AKI to ischemic ATN.[37] Nonsteroidal anti-inflammatory drugs (NSAIDs), including cyclooxygenase II (COX-II) inhibitors, inhibit renal prostaglandin biosynthesis. They do not compromise GFR in normal individuals but may precipitate prerenal AKI in subjects with true hypovolemia or decreased effective arterial blood volume, or in patients with chronic renal insufficiency in whom GFR is maintained in part by prostaglandin-mediated hyperfiltration through remnant nephrons.[38–41] Similarly, inhibitors of angiotensin-converting enzyme (ACE) and angiotensin II receptor blockers (ARBs) may trigger prerenal AKI in individuals in whom intraglomerular pressure and GFR are dependent on angiotensin II. This complication is classically seen in patients with bilateral renal artery stenosis or unilateral stenosis in a solitary functioning kidney.[42–47] Here, angiotensin II preserves glomerular filtration pressure distal to renal arterial stenosis by increasing systemic arterial pressure and by triggering selective constriction of efferent arterioles. ACE inhibitors and ARBs blunt these compensatory responses and can precipitate reversible AKI in such patients. ACE inhibitors or ARBs, like NSAIDs, may also precipitate prerenal AKI in patients with compensated renal hypoperfusion of other causes, mandating close monitoring of the serum creatinine level when these drugs are administered to high-risk individuals.

The classic urinary and biochemical sequelae of prerenal AKI can be predicted from the stimulatory actions of norepinephrine, angiotensin II, antidiuretic hormone, and low urine flow rate on salt and water reabsorption from urine and include concentrated urine (specific gravity >1.018, osmolality >500 mOsm/kg H_2O, low urinary Na^+ concentration, and benign urine sediment. Nonoliguric prerenal ARF may be seen in patients with renal concentrating deficits (e.g., diabetes insipidus) and in the setting of large endogenous (glucose/urea) or exogenous (mannitol) solute loads.[48,49] Hypernatremia due to increased free water losses is a clue to the presence of a polyuric prerenal state.

Some vasoactive mediators, drugs, and diagnostic agents stimulate intense intrarenal vasoconstriction and induce glomerular hypoperfusion and AKI with many of the functional, clinical, and biochemical features of prerenal AKI. Examples include hypercalcemia, endotoxin, radiocontrast agents, calcineurin inhibitors (cyclosporin, FK506/tacrolimus), amphotericin B, cocaine, and norepinephrine (e.g., therapeutic administration, pheochromocytoma, brain damage).[50–52] Cyclosporine and tacrolimus precipitate ARF by inducing intrarenal vasoconstriction and hypoperfusion, and by stimulating mesangial cell contraction and a fall in glomerular filtration surface area.[53,54] Frank tubule necrosis is rare in this setting, although long-term calcineurin inhibition may lead to irreversible renal impairment, probably as a consequence of obliterative arteriopathy and chronic medullary ischemia.

Intrinsic Acute Kidney Injury

Ischemic ATN and toxic ATN account for about 80% to 90% of intrinsic AKI.[22,55,56] From a clinicopathologic viewpoint, it is helpful to categorize the causes of intrinsic ARF into the following categories (Table 29–3)
- Diseases involving large renal vessels,
- Diseases of the renal microvasculature and glomeruli,
- Ischemic and nephrotoxic ATN, and
- Other acute processes involving the tubulointerstitium.

Diseases of Large Renal Vessels, Microvasculature, and Tubulointerstitium

Occlusion of large renal vessels, either arteries or veins, is an uncommon cause of AKI. To affect BUN and serum creatinine, occlusion must be either bilateral or unilateral in patients with underlying chronic renal insufficiency or a solitary functioning kidney. Renal arteries may be occluded acutely by atheroemboli, thromboemboli, thrombosis, dissection of an aortic aneurysm, or, rarely, vasculitis. Atheroem-

---

TABLE 29–3 Major Causes of Acute Intrinsic Renal Azotemia

Diseases involving large renal vessels
Renal arteries*: thrombosis, atheroembolism, thromboembolism, dissection, vasculitis (e.g., Takayasu)
Renal veins*: thrombosis, compression

Diseases of glomeruli and the renal microvasculature (see Table 29–4)
Inflammatory: acute or rapidly progressive glomerulonephritis, vasculitis, allograft rejection, radiation
Vasospastic: malignant hypertension, toxemia of pregnancy, scleroderma, hypercalcemia, drugs, radiocontrast agents
Hematologic: hemolytic-uremic syndrome or thrombotic thrombocytopenic purpura, disseminated intravascular coagulation, hyperviscosity syndromes

Diseases characterized by prominent injury to renal tubules often with ATN†‡
Ischemia caused by renal hypoperfusion (see Table 29–2)
Exogenous toxins (e.g., antibiotics, anticancer agents, radiocontrast agents, poisons; see Table 29–6)
Endogenous toxins (e.g., myoglobin, hemoglobin, myeloma light chains, uric acid, tumor lysis; see Table 29–7)

Acute diseases of the tubulointerstitium (see Table 29–5)
Allergic interstitial nephritis (e.g., antibiotics, nonsteroidal anti-inflammatory drugs)
Infectious (viral, bacterial, fungal)
Acute cellular allograft rejection
Infiltration§ (e.g., lymphoma, leukemia, sarcoid)

*Acute renal failure (ARF) in this context usually implies bilateral disease or unilateral disease in a solitary functioning kidney.
†The majority of cases of acute intrinsic renal azotemia fall into this category.
‡Although frank necrosis of renal tubules is not invariably present, the term acute tubule necrosis (ATN) is used by convention to denote ARF related to tubule injury by either ischemia or nephrotoxins (see section on pathophysiology of ischemic ATN).
§Although infiltration of renal parenchyma is common, renal failure rarely occurs.

boli are the most common culprits and are usually dislodged from an atheromatous aorta during arteriography, angioplasty, or aortic surgery.[57] Cholesterol emboli lodge in medium or small renal arteries, where they incite an inflammatory reaction characterized classically by intimal proliferation, infiltration of vessel wall by macrophages and giant cells, fibrosis, and irreversible occlusion of the vessel lumen. Thromboemboli may originate in the heart in patients with atrial arrhythmias or mural thrombi and trigger acute infarction of renal tissue.[58,59] This may present with sudden flank pain and signs of a systemic inflammatory response. Renal artery thrombosis is usually superimposed on an atheromatous plaque but may also complicate traumatic intimal tears or the site of surgical anastomosis after renal transplantation. Outside of the immediate post-transplantation period, renal vein thrombosis is an exceedingly rare cause of AKI and is usually encountered as a complication of the nephrotic syndrome in adults or of severe dehydration in children.[60,61]

Virtually all diseases that compromise blood flow within the renal microvasculature may induce AKI.[62–64] These include inflammatory (e.g., glomerulonephritis or vasculitis) and noninflammatory (e.g., malignant hypertension) diseases of the vessel wall, thrombotic microangiopathies, and hyperviscosity syndromes (Table 29–4). Indeed, the decrement in renal perfusion in these settings may be severe enough to trigger superimposed ischemic ATN.[65] In general, these disorders can be distinguished from prerenal AKI and ischemic or nephrotoxic ATN by clinical or laboratory criteria; however, a renal biopsy may be required for definitive diagnosis (see later section on differential diagnosis). Disorders of the tubulointerstitium that induce AKI, other than ischemia or tubule cell toxins, include allergic interstitial nephritis, severe infections, allograft rejection, and, rarely, infiltrative disorders such as sarcoid, lymphoma, or leukemia (Table 29–5). A comprehensive discussion of these diseases is beyond the scope of this chapter and is presented elsewhere in this book.

Acute Tubule Necrosis

As discussed earlier, the pathologic term ATN and the clinical term ARF/AKI are often used interchangeably when referring to ischemic and nephrotoxic renal injury, evidence of frank necrosis of renal tubules is sparse or absent in most cases (vide infra).[66] Prerenal AKI and ischemic ATN are part of a spectrum of manifestations of renal hypoperfusion-prerenal AKI being a response to mild or moderate hypoperfusion and ischemic ATN being the result of more severe or prolonged hypoperfusion, often coexistent with other renal insults.[25] It is notable that extracellular fluid losses or transient renal hypoperfusion (e.g., cardiac arrest or aortic cross clamping) generally do not cause ATN in the absence of either preexisting renal impairment or the coincidence of another nephrotoxic insult (e.g., vasoactive drugs, sepsis, or rhabdomyolysis).[67] Prerenal AKI differs from ischemic ATN in that it is associated with injury to renal parenchyma and does not resolve immediately on restoration of renal perfusion. In its more extreme form, renal hypoperfusion may result in bilateral renal cortical necrosis and irreversible renal failure.

Ischemic ATN is observed most frequently in patients who have major surgery, trauma, severe hypovolemia, overwhelming sepsis, and burns.[55,68–72] The risk of ischemic ATN after cardiac surgery correlates directly with the duration of cardiopulmonary bypass and the degree of preoperative and postoperative cardiac impairment.[73–76] ATN most commonly complicates aortic surgery in patients undergoing emergency repair of ruptured abdominal aneurysms or after complicated elective procedures requiring prolonged (>60 minutes) clamping of the aorta above the origin of the renal arteries.[77,78] However, 50% of cases of postsurgical ATN occur in the absence of documented hypotension. ATN complicating

TABLE 29–4	Some Diseases of Glomeruli and the Renal Microvasculature Associated with Acute Intrinsic Renal Azotemia

Glomerulonephritis or vasculitis
Associated with antiglomerular basement membrane antibody (anti-GBM Ab)
  (Goodpasture syndrome if associated with lung hemorrhage)
Associated with antineutrophil cytoplasmic antibodies (ANCA)
  Wegener granulomatosis
  Microscopic or Churg-Strauss variant of polyarteritis nodosa
  Renal-limited crescentic glomerulonephritis
Associated with glomerular immune complexes and hypocomplementemia
  Acute diffuse proliferative glomerulonephritis (postinfectious)
  Membranoproliferative glomerulonephritis
  Subacute bacterial endocarditis
  Cryoglobulinemia
  Systemic lupus erythematosus (SLE)
Associated with absence of hypocomplementemia, ANCA, and anti-GBM Ab
  Immunoglobulin A nephropathy
  Schönlein-Henoch purpura
  Classic polyarteritis nodosa
  Radiation injury
Associated with collapsing glomerulopathy
  Infection (HIV)
  Pamidronate

Hyperviscosity syndromes
Multiple myeloma
Waldenström macroglobulinemia
Polycythemia

Hemolytic-uremic syndrome or thrombotic thrombocytopenic purpura
Infections
  Viral (e.g., enterovirus, coxsackievirus, influenza virus, hepatitis A virus, HIV)
  Bacterial (e.g., *Escherichia coli* O157:H7, *Shigella dysenteriae, Salmonella, Yersinia, Campylobacter*)
Radiotherapy
Disseminated malignancy (e.g., gastric adenocarcinoma)
Chemotherapeutic agents (mitomycin C, cisplatin, bleomycin, gemcytabine)
Calcineurin inhibitors, oral contraceptives, ticoldipine, clopidrogrel
Immunologic Diseases
SLE, rheumatoid arthritis, Sjögren, ankylosing spondylitis
Other
  Idiopathic, familial, pregnancy and puerperium

Miscellaneous
Atheroemboli
Accelerated hypertension
Scleroderma crisis
Toxemia of pregnancy
Drugs
  Calcineurin inhibitors
  Amphotericin B
  Cocaine
Radiocontrast agents

trauma is frequently multifactorial in origin and due to the combined effects of hypovolemia and myoglobin or other toxins released by damaged tissue. ATN occurs in 20% to 40% of patients who suffer burns involving more than 15% of their surface area and, again is frequently multifactorial and due to the combined effects of hypovolemia, rhabdomyolysis, sepsis, and nephrotoxic antibiotics.[79] Sepsis induces renal hypoperfusion by provoking a combination of systemic vasodilatation and intrarenal vasoconstriction.[17,69,71,80–85] In addition, endotoxin sensitizes renal tissue to the deleterious effects of ischemia.[85–87] The pathophysiology, pathology,

TABLE 29–5 Diseases of the Tubulointerstitium Associated with Acute Intrinsic Renal Azotemia

Drug-Induced Allergic Interstitial Nephritis

β-Lactams	Other Antibiotics	NSAIDs	Diuretics	Other	Infections	Miscellaneous
Ampicillin	Ethambutol	Aspirin	Chlorthalidone	α-Methyldopa	Bacterial	Systemic disease
Amoxicillin	p-Aminosalicylate	Celecoxib	Furosemide	Allopurinol	Acute pyelonephritis[†]	SLE
Carbenicillin	Rifampin	Fenoprofen	Bumetanide	Azathioprine	Leptospirosis	Sjögren syndrome
Methicillin	Sulfonamides	Ibuprofen	Thiazides	Carbamazepine	Scarlet fever	TINU
Nafcillin	Trimethoprim	Indomethacin		Cimetidine	Typhoid Fever	Cancer
Oxacillin	Ciprofloxacin	Mefenamic acid		Omeprazole	Legionaires Disease	Lymphoma
Penecillin G	Levofloxacin	Naproxen		Clofibrate	Viral	Leukemia
Cephalexin	Norfloxacxin	Phenazone		Clozapine	Cytomegalovirus	Myeloma
Cephatholin	Vancomycin	Phenylbutazone		Famotidine	Measles	Sarcoidosis
Cephradine		Tolmetin		Sulfinpyrazone	Infectious	
Cefotaxime				Phenobarbital	Mononucleosis	
					Rocky Mountain	
					spotted fever	
					Other	
					Candidiasis, other	
					fungi[‡]	
					Toxoplasmosis	

NSAIDS, nonsteroidal anti-inflammatory drugs; SLE, systemic lupus erythematosus; TINU, tubulointerstitial nephritis and uveitis syndrome.
[†]Rare to get AKI unless bilateral disease in diabetic patients.
[‡]May cause AKI by obstruction of tubules (fungus balls), in addition to causing acute interstitial nephritis.

management, and clinical course of ischemic ATN are discussed in detail later in this chapter.

Nephrotoxic ATN complicates the administration of many structurally diverse pharmacologic agents and poisons.[38,52,88–92] The proliferation in recent years of novel antimicrobial and anticancer agents has broadened the range of known therapeutic agents that cause nephrotoxic renal injury and has re-enforced the need for vigilance amongst clinicians (Table 29–6).[93–97] In addition, some endogenous compounds provoke AKI when present in the circulation at high concentrations.[70,98] In general, nephrotoxins cause renal injury by inducing a varying combination of intrarenal vasoconstriction, direct tubule toxicity, and intratubular obstruction.[88] The kidney is particularly vulnerable to nephrotoxic renal injury by virtue of its rich blood supply (25% of cardiac output) and its ability to concentrate toxins to high levels within the medullary interstitium (via the renal countercurrent mechanisms) and renal epithelial cells (via specific transporters). In addition, the kidney is an important site for xenobiotic metabolism and may transform relatively harmless parent compounds into toxic metabolites. The nephrotoxic potential of most agents is dramatically increased in the presence of borderline or overt renal ischemia, sepsis, or other renal insults. A detailed description of the pathophysiology and clinical features of drug-induced toxic nephropathies is presented in Chapter 63 and only a brief review of some common nephrotoxic syndromes is included here.

Tables 29–6 and 29–7 list the toxins that are most frequently associated with ATN. Acute intrarenal vasoconstriction is an important pathophysiologic event in AKI associated with radiocontrast agents (contrast nephropathy) and calcineurin inhibitors.[54,90,99–102] Contrast nephropathy typically presents as an acute decline in GFR within 24 to 48 hours of administration, a peak in serum creatinine value after 3 to 5 days, and return of the serum creatinine value to the "normal" range within 1 week.[99,100] The diagnosis is usually straightforward given the temporal correlation with contrast administration; however, consideration must be given to other potential diagnoses including atheroembolic renal disease, renal ischemia (e.g., aortic dissection) and other nephrotoxins. Individuals with chronic renal insufficiency (serum creatinine >2.0 mg/dL) are at the greatest risk of contrast-induced

TABLE 29–6 Some Exogenous Nephrotoxins That Are Common Causes of Acute Intrinsic Renal Azotemia with Acute Tubule Necrosis

Antibiotics	Chemotherapeutic agents
Acyclovir	Cisplatin
Cidofovir	Ifosfamide
Indinavir	Anti-inflammatory and immunosuppressive
Foscarnet	agents
Pentamidine	
Aminoglycosides	
Amphotericin B	NSAIDs (including COX-II inhibitors)
Organic solvents	Cyclosporin/tacrolimus
Ethylene glycol	Intravenous immune globulin
Toluene	Radiocontrast agents
Poisons	Bacterial toxins
Paraquat	
Snake bites	

renal injury.[99,103,104] Other risk factors include diabetic nephropathy, congestive heart failure, jaundice, volume depletion, multiple myeloma, the volume of contrast used, and the coincident use of ACE inhibitors or NSAIDs. Patients usually present with benign urine sediment, concentrated urine, and low fractional excretion of Na+ and, thus, have many features of prerenal AKI; however, in more severe cases, tubule cell injury may be evident.[105]

Postulated mechanisms of contrast agent–induced renal injury favor a combination of medullary ischemia and direct contrast-mediated tubular toxicity due to reactive oxygen species generation.[101,106–108] Contrast induces a biphasic hemodynamic response within the kidney; an initial transient vasodilation is followed by a period of sustained vasoconstriction. With regard to the latter, changes in the synthesis and release of NO, endothelin, and adenosine from endothelial cells combine to shunt blood flow away from the renal medulla, which has a high oxygen demand, to the renal cortex.[109–111] Although most patients recover renal function and the need for dialysis is unusual, contrast nephropathy is associated with a significant prolongation of hospital stay and increased patient mortality.[7]

TABLE 29–7 Some Sources of Endogenous Nephrotoxins That Cause Acute Intrinsic Renal Azotemia with Acute Tubule Necrosis*

Rhabdomyolysis with myoglobinuria†

Muscle injury	Trauma,‡ electric shock, hypothermia, hyperthermia (e.g., malignant hyperpyrexia)
Extreme muscular exertion	Seizures,‡ delirium tremens,‡ physical exercise
Muscle ischemia	Prolonged compression‡ (e.g., coma), compromise of major vessels (e.g., thromboembolism, dissection)
Metabolic disorders	Hypokalemia, hypophosphatemia, hypo- and hypernatremia, diabetic ketoacidosis, hyperosmolar states
Infections	Influenza, infectious mononucleosis, legionnaires' disease, tetanus
Toxins	Ethanol,‡ isopropyl alcohol, ethylene glycol, toluene, snake and insect bites
Drugs	Cocaine, HMG CoA reductase inhibitors, amphetamines, phencyclidine, lysergic acid diethylamide, heroin, methadone, salicylate overdose, succinylcholine
Immunologic diseases	Polymyositis, dermatomyositis
Inherited diseases	Myophosphorylase, phosphofructokinase, carnitine palmityltransferase, or myoadenylate deaminase deficiency

Hemolysis with hemoglobinuria†

Immunologic	Transfusion reactions‡
Infections and venoms	Malaria,‡ clostridia, spider bite (e.g., tarantula, brown recluse), snake bite‡ (e.g., rattlesnake, copperhead)
Drugs and chemicals	Aniline, arsine, benzene, cresol, fava beans, glycerol, hydralazine, phenol, quinidine, methydopa
Genetic diseases	Glucose 6-phosphate deficiency, paroxysmal nocturnal hemoglobinuria, march hemoglobinuria
Mechanical	Valvular prosthesis, extracorporeal circulation, microangiopathic hemolytic anemias, distilled water (intravenous dialysis, transurethral prostatectomy)

Increased uric acid production with hyperuricosuria

Primary increase in uric acid production	Hypoxanthine-guanine phosphoribosyltransferase Deficiency
Secondary increase in uric acid production	Treatment of malignancies‡ (especially lymphoproliferative or myeloproliferative)

Miscellaneous

	Myeloma light chains,‡ oxalate‡ (e.g., ethylene glycol toxicity), products of tumor lysis other than uric acid

*All of these diseases are sources of potential nephrotoxins, but not all have been definitively associated with acute renal failure (ARF).
†Hemoglobin and myoglobin cause little compromise of glomerular filtration when administered to experimental animals. Thus, it remains to be determined whether ARF in these settings is due to hemoglobin or myoglobin, metabolites of these compounds, or other toxic species released from red blood cells or muscle, or requires the coexistence of other renal insults (e.g., hypoperfusion).
‡Denotes most common causes of ARF. Renal failure is rare in other circumstances.

Intrarenal vasoconstriction is also a central component of AKI complicating hypercalcemia and, in addition, contributes to the nephrotoxicity of myoglobin and hemoglobin.[51,70,112–115] Interestingly, hemoglobin and myoglobin may promote vasoconstriction, at least in part by scavenging the vasodilator NO and thereby disrupting the balance between vasodilators and vasoconstrictors that is critical for maintenance of normal renal perfusion.[116–118]

Therapeutic agents that are directly toxic to renal tubule epithelium include antimicrobials such as aminoglycosides, amphotericin B, acyclovir, indinavir, cidofovir, pentamidine, and foscarnet, and chemotherapeutic agents such as cisplatin and ifosfamide (see Table 29–6). Nonoliguric ATN complicates 10% to 30% of courses of aminoglycoside antibiotics, even when blood levels are in the therapeutic range.[89,119–122] Aminoglycosides are polycations and are freely filtered across the glomerular filtration barrier and accumulated by proximal tubule cells by absorbtive endocytosis after interaction with negatively charged phospholipid residues on brush border membranes. Important risk factors for aminoglycoside nephrotoxicity include use of high or repeated doses or prolonged therapy, preexisting renal insufficiency, advanced age, volume depletion, and the coexistence of renal ischemia or other nephrotoxins.[120,121,123–126] Although the precise subcellular mechanisms by which aminoglycosides perturb renal function has not yet been fully elucidated, gentamicin has been demonstrated to bind to megalin, an endocytic receptor in the clathrin-coated pits of the apical cell membrane. When endocytosed, this complex may induce cellular injury by inhibiting endosomal fusion events.[127] Hypomagnesemia is a relatively common additional finding in patients with aminoglycoside-induced ATN and suggests coexistent injury to the thick ascending limb of the loop of Henle, the major site of Mg^{2+} reabsorption. AKI is usually detected during the second week of therapy, probably reflecting a requirement for accumulation within epithelial cells, but may be manifest earlier in the presence of ischemia or other nephrotoxins. ARF is almost invariable in patients receiving cumulative doses of amphotericin B of more than 1 g and is a common complication even with lower doses.[52,97,128] Amphotericin B induces direct renal vasoconstriction and exerts direct toxicity on a variety of tubular segments. The tubular dysfunction is manifested by an increase in tubuloglomerular feedback with resultant suppression of GFR, ATN, hypomagnesemia, hypophosphatemia, hypocalcemia, and a renal tubular acidosis due to backleakage of secreted H^+ in the distal cortical nephron. ATN due to amphotericin B is typically reversible, but chronic use can lead to nephrocalcinosis. High-dose intravenous acyclovir causes AKI within 24 to 48 hours in 10% to 30% of patients, particularly if they are volume depleted or if the drug is administered as a bolus.[129,130] ARF is usually nonoliguric; frequently associated with colic, nausea, and vomiting; and appears to be induced by intratubular precipitation of acyclovir crystals. A similar syndrome in now recognized in patients receiving the oral antiretroviral drug indinavir.[131] Asymptomatic crystalluria in seen in up to 10% of patients, with half this number presenting with loin pain and hematuria. A Fanconi-like syndrome is seen in up to 40% of patients receiving adefovir, a nucleoside reverse transcriptase inhibitor due to a direct toxic effect on tubular cell mitochondrial function.[132] A similar syndrome has also been decribed with tenofovir.[133] Cidofovir, a nucleotide analog used to treat cytomegaolvirus infections is also nephrotoxic.[134] Pentamidine induces AKI in 25% to 95% of patients, usually during the second week of therapy and frequently in association with hypomagnesemia, hypo- or hyperkalemia, and a distal renal tubular acidosis.[135–137] The mechanism of injury is unclear but may involve an immune process, because AKI does not appear to be dose dependent and is often associated with pyuria, hematuria, proteinuria, and casts. Foscarnet causes a distinct pattern of renal injury characterized by nonoliguric, often polyuric, ARF within 7 days, hyperphosphatemia, ATN, interstitial fibrosis, and a slow recovery that may take months.[138–140] ATN complicates up to 70% of courses of cisplatin and ifosfamide, two commonly used chemotherapeutic agents.[94,95,141–143] Cisplatin is accumulated by proximal tubule cells and induces mitochondrial injury, inhibition of ATPase activity and solute transport, and free radical–mediated injury to cell membranes.[2,95,142–147] In addition, cisplatin may cause severe hypomagnesemia, even in the absence of AKI, which may persist long after therapy has been stopped. Ifosfamide-induced ATN is being recognized increasingly and is often associated with the Fanconi syndrome, an unusual complication of proximal tubule injury by other agents.[141,148,149] The mechanism of proximal tubule injury in this setting is unknown. Methotrexate is primarily excreted unchanged in the urine. With the advent of high-dose intravenous methotrexate administration, typically in the setting of autologous bone marrow transplantation, AKI due to intratubular deposition of methotrexte is increasingly recognized.[94,150] Recently, there have been increasing reports of ATN associated with sucrose-containing intravenous immunoglobulin preparations.[151–153] The pathogenesis is believed to involve osmotic injury to the renal tubular epithelial cells by filtered sucrose.

Myoglobin, hemoglobin, uric acid, and myeloma light chains are the endogenous toxins that are most commonly associated with ATN. Renal dysfunction complicates approximately 30% of cases of rhabdomyolysis, the most common causes of which are listed in Table 29–7.[70,114,154–159] Hemoglobin-induced ATN is rare and is most commonly encountered after blood transfusion reactions (see Table 29–7).[117,160] The precise mechanisms by which rhabdomyolysis and hemolysis impair GFR are unclear, but intrarenal vasoconstriction, intratubular obstruction, and tubule injury have been well documented as contributory pathophysiologic events in experimental animals. Neither myoglobin nor hemoglobin is markedly nephrotoxic when injected *in vivo*. Both pigments induce intrarenal vasoconstriction, probably by scavenging the vasodilator NO in the renal microcirculation. At acid pH, myoglobin and hemoglobin are also sources of ferrihemate, a substance that is a potent inhibitor of tubule transport. In this regard, it is noteworthy that hypovolemia and acidosis predispose experimental animals and humans to pigment-induced ATN. Finally, both pigments, being ferrous iron compounds, may potentially induce tubule injury by stimulating local production of OH^-.[114,157,161–164]

Intratubular obstruction has been implicated as a central event in the pathophysiology of ATN induced by some other endogenous (e.g., myeloma light chains, uric acid) and exogenous (ethylene glycol) nephrotoxins. Casts, composed of filtered immunoglobulin light chains and other urinary proteins such as Tamm-Horsfall protein (THP), induce AKI in patients with multiple myeloma (myeloma-cast nephropathy).[98,112,165–169] High urinary salt concentrations and low urine pH promote this process. The correlation between cast formation and renal insufficiency is relatively weak, however, suggesting that light chains may be directly toxic to tubule epithelial cells. Acute uric acid nephropathy typically complicates treatment of lymphoproliferative or myeloprolif-

erative disorders and is usually associated with other biochemical evidence of tumor lysis such as hyperkalemia, hyperphosphatemia, and hypocalcemia.[170–173] Acute uric acid nephropathy is rare when plasma concentrations are less than 15 to 20 mg/dL but may be precipitated at relatively low levels by volume depletion or low urine pH. Both myeloma cast nephropathy and acute urate nephropathy are usually encountered in the setting of widespread malignancy and massive tumor destruction, and other potential contributory toxins in these clinical settings include hypercalcemia, hyperphosphatemia, and other products of tumor lysis (see later discussion of AKI in the cancer patient). Oxalate-induced AKI is usually encountered as a complication of ethylene glycol toxicity but occasionally complicates primary defects in oxalate metabolism (primary hyperoxaluria) or other secondary forms of hyperoxaluria (e.g., malabsorption, massive vitamin C ingestion, methoxyflurane anesthesia).[174–179]

Postrenal Acute Kidney Injury

Urinary tract obstruction accounts for less than 5% of cases of AKI. Because one kidney has sufficient clearance capacity to excrete the nitrogenous waste products generated daily, AKI resulting from obstruction requires either obstruction of urine flow between the external urethral meatus and bladder neck, bilateral ureteric obstruction, or unilateral ureteric obstruction in a patient with one functioning kidney or underlying chronic renal insufficiency (Table 29–8). Obstruction of the bladder neck is the most common cause of postrenal AKI and may complicate prostatic disease (e.g., hypertrophy, neoplasia, or infection), neurogenic bladder, or therapy with anticholinergic drugs. Less common causes of acute lower urinary tract obstruction include blood clots, calculi, and urethritis with spasm. Ureteric obstruction may result from intraluminal obstruction (e.g., calculi, blood clots, sloughed renal papillae), infiltration of the ureteric wall (e.g., neoplasia) or external compression (e.g., retroperitoneal fibrosis, neoplasia or abscess, inadvertent surgical ligature). During the early stages of obstruction (hours to days), continued glomerular filtration leads to increased intraluminal pressure upstream of the site of obstruction. This results in gradual distention of proximal ureter, renal pelvis, and calyces, and a fall in GFR. Although acute obstruction may lead to an initial modest increase in renal blood flow, arterial vasoconstriction soon supervenes, leading to a further decline in glomerular filtration. The pathophysiology and treatment of obstructive uropathy are discussed extensively in Chapter 36.

TABLE 29–8 Causes of Acute Postrenal Azotemia

Ureteric obstruction
Intraluminal: stones, blood clot, sloughed renal papillae, uric acid or sulfonamide crystals, fungus balls
Intramural: postoperative edema after ureteric surgery, BK virus–induced ureteric fibrosis in renal allograft
Extraureteric: iatrogenic (ligation during pelvic surgery)
Periureteric: hemorrhage, tumor, or fibrosis[†]

Bladder neck obstruction
Intraluminal: stones, blood clots, sloughed papillae
Intramural: bladder carcinoma, bladder infection with mural edema, neurogenic, drugs (e.g., tricyclic antidepressants, ganglion blockers)
Extramural: prostatic hypertrophy, prostatic carcinoma

Urethral obstruction
Phimosis, congenital valves, stricture, tumor

THE PATHOLOGY AND PATHOPHYSIOLOGY OF ACUTE TUBULE NECROSIS

Morphology of Acute Tubule Necrosis

Tubular injury is the hallmark of ATN and is most severe in the outer medulla of the kidney during injury from reduced blood flow with ischemia.[100] This damage involves the pars recta (S3 segments) of the proximal tubule and the medullary thick ascending limb (mTAL) of the distal nephron. Other areas of injury can be seen within the renal cortex, involving both proximal and distal segments of the nephron.[181-184] Although the term ATN is often used, synonymous with ARF/AKI, in fact, actual necrosis of tubular epithelial cells is a less common finding in ATN than cellular injury and dysfunction.[181,185] These forms of cell injury can include apoptosis, loss of cells forming gaps in the tubular architecture and denuded basement membrane, and cells sloughing into tubular lumens (Fig. 29–2).[181,185]

Damage to the brush border of the proximal tubules in the cortex is a common feature seen in ATN. The microvilli that make up the brush border are shortened or completely absent and can be found collecting in the tubular lumen.[66,181,185,186] Also frequently seen in ATN is the accumulation of tubular casts containing THP along with exfoliated tubular cells, remnants of shed brush border, and other cellular debris.[66,181,186,187]

Pathophysiology of Kidney Dysfunction in Acute Kidney Injury

The effect of renal injury, whether from ischemia or from other causes, is a profound decrease in the GFR. This large decrease in filtration capacity of the kidney often occurs in the absence overwhelmingly evident damage to the kidney as seen on light microscopy. There are at least three major classic proposed mechanisms for the fall in GFR, as determined by micropuncture studies on animals and indirect methods in humans. The first mechanism is a drop in the filtration pressure in the glomerulus. This drop in pressure is caused by afferent arteriolar vasoconstriction and proximal tubular obstruction.[188-192] This first mechanism leads to a direct fall in the GFR. Afferent arteriolar vasoconstriction is thought to be a result of endothelial cell injury.[193] This leads to an imbalance in vasoactive substances, with a predominance of vasoconstrictive activity. The second mechanism, tubular back-leakage, leads to a fall in the *effective* GFR. Glomerular filtrate that enters the tubular/urinary space is allowed to leak back into the renal interstitium and consequently be reabsorbed into the systemic circulation. Back-leakage of glomerular filtrate occurs in the setting of damage and loss of epithelial cells (denuded basement membranes) (Fig. 29–3) and loss of tight junctions between those cells that are critical to maintaining separation of tubular filtrate and the surrounding interstitium (see the section entitled The Epithelial Cell).[194] The role of tight junctions in normal solute trafficking is discussed later. Tight junctions are disrupted in the setting of adenosine triphosphate (ATP) depletion, allowing back-leakage of sodium and other solutes into the renal interstitium.[195,196] The third mechanism, tubular obstruction, is a result of cast formation from sloughed tubular epithelial cells as well as THP. THP tends to polymerize and form a gel that can further trap cells and tubular cell debris following AKI. The concentration of various molecules in the renal tubules in evolving ATN further promotes THP gel formation.[187]

Besides a fall in GFR, there is also a decreased ability of the kidney to concentrate urine following AKI. This is due in part to the loss of aquaporin water channel expression in different parts of the nephron including the collecting duct and the proximal tubules, as has been shown in animal models.[197] Blocking inflammation with alpha-melanocyte–stimulating hormone (α-MSH) infusion can partially normalize aquaporin expression and allow the kidney to retain concentrating ability. Moreover, the addition of erythropoietin (EPO) can either on its own, or in combination with α-MSH, be protective by maintaining aquaporin expression and concentrating ability.[198] Sodium and acid-base transporters are also dysregulated by kidney injury.[199]

Inflammation

Inflammation plays a central role in AKI. From initiation to extension through repair, inflammatory cells and soluble mediators are likely major determinants of the outcome from ARF. A number of different inflammatory cells and soluble mediators have been shown to be necessary for full renal damage and loss of glomerular filtration to occur.[200] Inflammatory pathways are attractive targets for therapy, and there has been great success with interventions in experimental models of AKI. The limitation of this approach seems to be that blocking inflammation after the renal insult has occurred affords much less protection to the kidney.

CH 29

Acute Kidney Injury

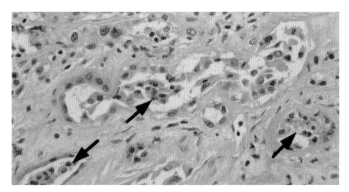

FIGURE 29–2 Cellular cast formation *(arrows)* in renal tubules of a human renal biopsy with acute tubular necrosis. (Courtesy of Dr. Yashpal Kanwar.)

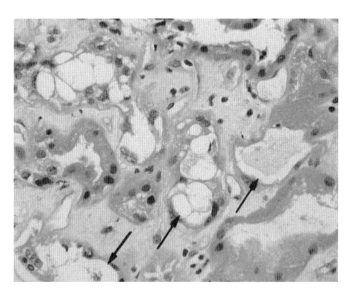

FIGURE 29–3 Cellular debris and cast formation in renal tubules of a human renal biopsy with acute tubular necrosis. (Courtesy of Dr. Yashpal Kanwar.)

Microvascular Inflammation

The proximal events leading to damage of renal tubular epithelial cells likely start in the microvasculature. The kidney receives 20% to 25% of cardiac output, and most of that blood flow is directed to the renal cortex.[201-203] Postglomerular vessels, branching from efferent arterioles, eventually become the vessels of the vasa recta. The low-flow state in the vasa recta is a critical aspect of the countercurrent multiplier, allowing for appropriate trafficking of water and solutes.[202] However, the low-flow state leaves the medulla relatively hypoxic when compared with other regions of the kidney. Unlike the renal cortex with a partial pressure of oxygen of about 50 mm Hg, the outer medulla has a partial pressure of oxygen in the 10 to 20 mm Hg range (Fig. 29–4).[204] Consequently, very slight decreases in the blood flow and oxygen delivery can lead to anoxic damage. Anoxic injury to local cells, including vascular smooth muscle cells and endothelial cells, leads to depletion of cellular energy stores and resultant disruption of their actin cytoskeleton.[205] The cellular deformities and hypoxia in and around the microvasculature leads to endothelial-erythrocyte interactions and promotes sludging of erythrocytes (RBCs) in a way that is analogous to a sickle cell vaso-occlusive crisis. Vascular congestion with RBC sludging has been described on renal biopsies.[206,207] Elegant video-microscopy has shed light on the kinetics of RBC sludging and blood flow.[208] These studies have demonstrated that peritubular capillaries had cessation of blood flow following an ischemic event as compared with glomerular capillaries that had diminished but never absent flow. Peritubular capillaries also took longer to recover normal blood flow when compared with other intrarenal vessels. The combination of hypoxic injury, changes in endothelial cell morphology, and heightened interactions between RBC and endothelium leads to the extension of the initial renal injury and contributes to our understanding of the regionalization of injury within the kidney. Hypoxia in the renal medulla can also predispose to other forms of renal injury, such as damage from aminoglycoside antibiotics.[209]

Leukocytes

Neutrophils have been extensively studied in ischemic reperfusion injury (IRI) models of AKI. Infiltrating neutrophils are infrequently seen on biopsies of human ATN but are known to infiltrate the kidney following an acute experimental ischemic insult.[210] Nonetheless, some experimental studies have demonstrated that decreased renal injury occurs when neutrophil migration and activity are blocked (see later), whereas others have not found a protective effect of neutrophil blockade or depletion on the course of ARF.[211,212]

Early inflammation is classically characterized by margination of neutrophils to vascular endothelium. Tethering interactions between selectins and their ligands initially slows neutrophils, allowing firmer adhesion and transmigration by integrins and their ligands. Platelet P-selectin was shown to be the main determinant of the P-selectin mediated renal injury.[213] Blockade of the shared ligand to all three selectins (E-, P-, and L-selectin) significantly protected rats from both renal IRI and associated mortality.[214] A key fucosyl sugar on

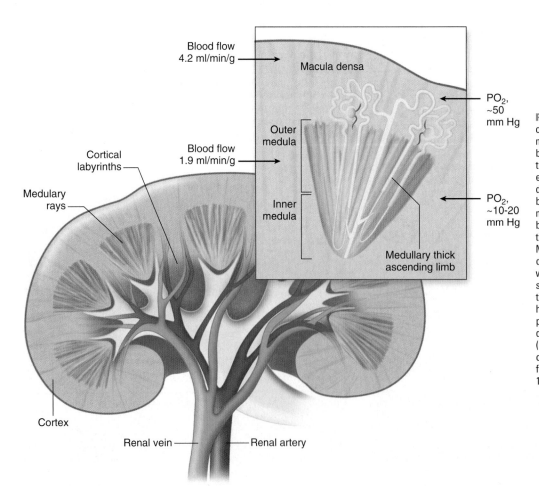

FIGURE 29–4 Anatomic and physiologic features of the renal cortex and medulla. The cortex, whose ample blood supply optimizes glomerular filtration, is generally well oxygenated, except for the medullary-ray areas devoid of glomeruli, which are supplied by venous blood ascending from the medulla. The medulla, whose meager blood supply optimizes the concentration of the urine, is poorly oxygenated. Medullary hypoxia results both from countercurrent exchange of oxygen within the vasa recta and from the consumption of oxygen by the medullary thick ascending limbs. Renal medullary hypoxia is an obligatory part of the process of urinary concentration. PO_2 denotes partial pressure of oxygen. (From Brezis M, Rosen S: Hypoxia of the renal medulla—its implications for disease. N Engl J Med 332:647–655, 1995.)

the selectin ligands appears to be the critical determinant of the renal injury after ischemia. Both in rats and mice, selectin ligand blockade, initially targeted to abrogate neutrophil infiltration, resulted in renal protection while neutrophils continued to infiltrate the post ischemic kidney.[215] Thus, it appears that modulation of the selectin pathway can alter outcome of ARF through neutrophil-independent ways. Owing to the promising nature of these experimental studies, a multicenter clinical trial is under way blocking selectin ligands to reduce ischemic kidney injury in deceased donor transplants.

After the slowing of leukocytes at the site of injury by selectins, firm adhesion occurs by the interactions of integrins with intercellular adhesion molecule-1 (ICAM-1). Blockade of the integrin CD11/CD18 protects from experimental IRI-induced ARF in rats; mice deficient in ICAM-1 were also found to have relative protection from renal ischemic injury.[212,216] Interestingly, neutrophil depletion in the rat model did not lead to protection, whereas it was protective in the mouse.[216,217] The importance of ICAM-1 interactions has also been studied in human renal transplant models. An initial study showed treatment with anti-ICAM-1 (or CD54) monoclonal antibodies protected human patients receiving a "high-risk" deceased donor renal allograft. Their rates of delayed graft function were lower than patients who received the sister organ but were not treated with the antibody.[218] However, a randomized controlled trial (RCT) of anti-ICAM-1 monoclonal antibody in recipients of deceased donor renal transplants showed that short-term induction with anti-ICAM-1 did not reduce the rate of delayed graft function or acute rejection.[219] A major logistic challenge for clinical use is that experimental studies demonstrate a dramatic protection by adhesion molecule blockade when given preischemia, whereas human studies had administered adhesion blockade after ischemia.

Mice and rats were treated with α-MSH, a known inhibitor of interleukin-8 (IL-8, a murine neutrophil chemokine) and ICAM-1 induction.[220] Significantly less renal damage was seen following IRI, both by measurements of serum creatinine and by renal histology. In a follow-up study, it was demonstrated that α-MSH inhibited renal injury in a neutrophil-depleted model, suggesting a more complex role for α-MSH, possibly by acting directly on renal tubular cells.[221] Other possible effects of α-MSH suggest a role in limiting apoptosis and down-regulating fas and fas ligand expression, as seen in animal models of AKI.[222] Other studies demonstrating a renal protection by an anti-inflammatory intervention have attributed the mechanism of protection to neutrophil blockade, only to later find the neutrophil was less important: A_{2A} adenosine receptor blockade lead to renoprotective effects in IRI models; however, recent data demonstrates that this is working primarily through CD4 T cells rather than neutrophils.[223,224] Blockage of platelet-activating factor (PAF), which is thought to play a mediating role in neutrophil adherence to endothelium, was protective in a rat cold ischemia reperfusion model.[225] Cumulative results suggest a real but only modest role for the neutrophil in ischemic AKI.

Although classic models of immunology or acute tissue injury do not predict a role for T cells in ischemic ARF, studies on human ARF had identified predominately mononuclear leukocytes, not neutrophils, in the vasa recta.[184] The production of T cell associated cytokines occurs in experimental IRI.[226] In addition, the same leukocyte adhesion molecules targeted for neutrophil blockade in renal IRI (e.g., selectins, CD11/CD18, and ICAM-1) also mediate T cell adhesion. Using special stains, T cells have been identified in the kidneys of rats and mice following IRI.[227,228] This led to studies that have now identified a modulatory role for T cells in experimental ARF. Double CD4/CD8 knockout mice had renal protection from IRI.[228] When T cell deficient (nu/nu) knockout mice were subjected to renal IRI, they also had less

depression of kidney function following IRI when compared with wild-type mice, primarily mediated by CD4 T cells. Adoptive transfer of T cells from wild type animals into the (nu/nu) mice restored ischemic injury, proving the role of the T cell in ischemic injury.[229] The CD4+ T cell effect was found to require interferon-γ (IFN-γ) and the B7-CD28 pathway. Wild-type mice depleted of T cells to very low levels, particularly of CD4+ cells, had significant protection from renal IRI, but simple CD4 depletion was not protective.[230,231] Alternative approaches using CTLA4Ig to block the B7-CD28 interaction significantly attenuated renal dysfunction in a rat renal IRI model.[232] It appears that B7-1 and not the B7-2 pathway is the important T cell co-stimulatory pathway in ARF.[233] An early, transient increase in T cells, a so-called hit-and-run hypothesis, might explain how T cells could play a role in the initiation of ARF. Recently, T cells have been shown to infiltrate postischemic kidney within 3 hours of reperfusion, which supports the hit-and-run model.[234]

The role for T cells in ARF is becoming increasingly complex, with the surprising finding that specific T cells can serve a protective function in ARF, which could be dependent one whether one examines early injury, extension, or repair. It appears that the Th1 phenotype of T cells is deleterious, and the Th2 phenotype is protective. These data, elicited with STAT6- and STAT4-deficient mice that have impaired Th2 and Th1 responses, respectively, is opposite to the asthma model of T cell engagement.[231] In addition, mice deficient in both T and B cells, are not protected from renal IRI.[235] This may be in part due to enhanced innate immunity in these mice, possibly from up-regulation of natural killer cells. Identification of the role of the T cell in renal IRI opens up the opportunity to evaluate well-characterized T cell reagents to prevent and treat ARF. Another mononuclear leukocyte that could be playing an important role in ARF is the macrophage.[224]

There are many other key inflammatory pathways that mediate the pathogenesis of AKI. Toll receptors (TLRs) likely play an important role. TLR2 has been shown to mediate experimental ischemic ARF, and TLR4 mediates ARF in a mouse endotoxemia (LPS) model.[236,237] TLR4 and MyD88 have been implicated in a mouse sepsis model.[238] Many of the cytokines and chemokines play a role in ARF, which is a rapidly advancing and promising area of investigation.

Apoptosis

Apoptosis, or programmed cell death, plays an important role in the pathophysiology of ARF. Apoptosis differs from cellular necrosis. Cellular necrosis is characterized by swelling of cells, loss of plasma membrane integrity, and eventually cell rupture with spillage of cellular contents into the extracellular space.[239] In apoptosis, the cell nucleus and cytoplasm condense and then split off into smaller apoptotic bodies.[239] Cytoplasmic organelles, including the mitochondria, are often intact and are phagocytized by macrophages or other cells, which leads to less spillage of cellular contents to cause inflammation.[239]

The effects of apoptosis on the host may change during the course of AKI, ranging from harmful to beneficial, depending on the phase of AKI. Initially, apoptosis may be deleterious to the kidney and overall renal function, whereas during the recovery phase, apoptosis may be an important mechanism to regulate cell number and morphology.[240] The signs of apoptosis in the kidney, initially heralded by DNA fragmentation in the cells of the thick ascending limb, can be seen within 15 minutes of a hypoxic insult in the rat kidney.[241] The same findings were seen following a radiocontrast nephropathy injury model in rats. These early findings of apoptosis often precede any discernable deterioration in renal function.[240] A second peak in the amount of apoptosis in renal tissue occurs days to weeks after the initial insult.[240] This peak often follows removal of necrotic tubular cells from the area, and may be a way to help regulate the number of newly generated cells.

Why some cells are destined for apoptosis and others for necrosis may have to do with the duration of ischemia as a surrogate for the extent of intracellular ATP depletion. Studies of cell culture found that the initial hypoxic injury triggers apoptotic pathways in some cells, but if the hypoxia is prolonged, then cells switch to primarily a necrosis pathway.[242,243] When human kidneys were examined at autopsy using 3' end labeling (TUNEL stain) to identify apoptotic cells following a hypoxic insult, apoptosis was found in most cases. Interestingly, findings of apoptosis did not correlate with renal function (as compared with a classic histologic finding such as fibrosis).[244]

Renal transplantation induces ischemic renal injury in the donor kidney. The duration and severity of that injury often correlates with the type of donor, deceased or living, and the cold ischemic time. Deceased donor kidneys were compared with living donor kidneys to determine if there were differences in rates of apoptosis.[245] Very little apoptosis was found in the kidneys of live donors. Apoptosis was seen in all deceased donor kidneys, with a direct correlation between the duration of cold ischemic time and the amount of apoptosis.[245,246] Also noted in the study of apoptosis in human renal allografts was the consistent activation of several proapoptotic factors from the mitochondrial pathway, mainly Bax and Bak. These are proapoptotic members of the Bcl-2 family can translocate from their normal cytosolic location to the mitochondria in response to ischemic stimuli. Once in the mitochondria, they cause release of cytochrome c and active caspase 9.[245,247,248]

Blocking apoptosis, using the active caspase inhibitor Z-Val-Ala-Asp(OMe)-CH2F (ZVAD-fmk) attenuated reperfusion-induced inflammation in a murine model of renal IRI.[249] Animals treated with the caspase inhibitor before renal IRI had significant protection from renal damage and loss of renal function, but that protection was lost if animals were treated following the onset of apoptosis. The expression of caspases in the cascade of events leading to apoptosis was found to be a critical step in the release of proinflammatory mediators, such as endothelial monocyte-activating polypeptide-II, which can further induce P- and E-selectins.[250]

Blocking caspase activity and apoptosis has been the target of other interventions, often successfully limiting renal damage in models of ischemic injury. Minocycline, the tetracycline antibiotic, was shown to block renal damage through reduction of apoptosis in a rat model of IRI.[251] Other studies have targeted different pathways of apoptosis. Death-associated protein kinase (DAPK) modulates cell death induced by IFN-γ, tumor necrosis factor-α (TNF-α), Fas, and detachment from the extracellular matrix.[252,253] DAPK has been also implicated in TGF-β–induced apoptosis in several cultured cell lines in which Smad proteins mediate transcriptional activation of DAPK.[254] DAPK-mutant mice had less apoptosis, and were protected from renal IRI when compared with wild-type mice.[253]

EPO administration can protect the kidney from the effects of IRI in experimental models. Many investigators have shown that EPO can decrease the number of apoptotic cells following an ischemic insult.[198,255-258] There have been several purported mechanisms, but an exact pathway has not been elucidated. Down-regulation of the proapoptotic intracellular molecule Bax, as well as down-regulation of NF-κβ and caspase-3, -8, and -9 has been shown.[256,257] Treatment with α-MSH, which was protective in animal models of ARF, was shown to decrease apoptosis in the rat kidney in an IRI model.[259]

Apoptosis has been shown to be an important pathway of injury in the kidney in other models as well. The use of cell cycle inhibitors that also effectively blocked caspase-3 were found to protect cultured renal tubular epithelial cells from an otherwise lethal dose of cisplatin.[260,261] Cisplatin is a highly nephrotoxic chemotherapeutic agent that damages cells in the S3 segment of the proximal tubule.[262]

The Endothelial Cell

The endothelial cell plays an important role in the development of ARF. When an initial insult damages the endothelium of the renal vessels, the result is an endothelial bed that is ineffective in regulating local blood flow and cell migration into tissues, and preventing coagulation.[263,264] This vascular dysregulation, as perpetuated by dysfunctional endothelial cells, leads to continued ischemic injury following the initial insult, the extension phase of AKI. The structural alterations that occur in the endothelial cell following an ischemic injury have been partially elucidated and help explain the functional changes that occur during this injury process. The baseline structure of the endothelial cell is maintained by a network of protein filaments that make up the cytoskeleton. Actin filament bundles, which have been shown to shrink in the setting of ATP depletion, form a supportive ring around the periphery of the endothelial cell.[265] The assembly and disassembly of actin filaments is regulated by a family of actin binding proteins. The actin depolymerizing factor/cofilin (ADF) family of proteins is known to regulate actin dynamics and play a role in the changes to the actin cytoskeleton during ischemia.[266] ADF/cofilin has a concentration-dependent effect on changes to the actin cytoskeleton under ATP-depleted conditions (such as ischemia).[267] Modulation of the ADF/cofilin-mediated changes to the actin cytoskeleton in ischemic endothelial cells has potentially important therapeutic implications for ischemic AKI, and may have applications in other organ systems as well.

Many of the endothelial changes in ARF are more functional rather than structural in origin. It was found that tubuloglomerular feedback is preserved in prolonged ischemic AKI, and that excessive NO as well as endothelium-derived hyperpolarizing factor antagonize autoregulation and cause endothelial dysfunction and a drop in GFR.[268] Further evidence for the role of endothelial cells in ARF comes from animal models of transplanted endothelial cells or surrogate cells expressing endothelial NO synthase. Animals subjected to renal ischemia had functional protection by the transplanted endothelial cells.[269] Interactions between endothelial cells and inflammatory cells also changes with an ischemic insult. Both P- and E-selectin are up-regulated on endothelial cells in the setting of ischemic damage as is ICAM-1.[200,270-272] Understanding the damage and dysfunction of renal endothelium in AKI opens the door to several potential therapeutic targets, some of which have been demonstrated in animal models of AKI.

The Renal Tubular Epithelial Cell

The renal tubular epithelial cells, which are visible on routine light microscopy as well as urine analysis, are the most obvious cell type injured in ARF. Injury and loss of epithelial cells, through necrosis or apoptosis can lead to loss of kidney function and apparent drop in GFR through processes of back-leakage of glomerular filtrate and tubular obstruction. The renal tubular cell has a remarkable ability to recover from an ischemic injury.[273] The tubular epithelial cell progresses through a series of morphologic changes that finally leads to restoration of normal structure and function. These steps include an initial loss of cell polarity and brush border, which contributes to altered solute trafficking.[274] Some cells die and are sloughed into the tubular lumen, and the remaining viable cells dedifferentiate and proliferate leading to final restoration of normal epithelium. The initial insult to the tubular epithelial cell depletes cellular ATP, which, in turn, leads to disruption of the apical actin cytoskeleton in a fashion that mirrors the changes in vascular endothelial cells in the kidney (see the section on endothelial cells earlier).[275] This structural change in the cell leads to the formation of membrane-bound vesicles or blebs that can either be internalized or shed into the tubular lumen as part of the cellular debris leading to cast formation and tubular obstruction.[276] Another important consequence of disruption of the apical cytoskeleton is the loss of tight junctions and adherens junctions.[194] The loss of these junctions contributes to the back-leakage of glomerular filtrate as a result of tubular obstruction.

Some elements of the basolateral cytoskeleton in epithelial cells are disrupted during AKI. The Na,K-ATPase that is found in the basolateral membrane as well as integrins that help tether cells to the basement membrane are both affected during IRI. The loss of the Na,K-ATPase decreases proximal tubular sodium reabsorption and increases the fractional excretion of sodium (FENa) contributing to tubuloglomerular feedback and drop in GFR.[276,277] The elevated FENa is a hallmark of intrinsic AKI (see previous section of this chapter). Loss of integrin polarity, particularly the β1 integrins, away from the basolateral membrane to the apical domain can lead to detachment of viable cells from the basement membrane and sloughing of cells into the tubular lumen.[276]

Stem Cells

A better understanding of the repair process and renal recovery holds great therapeutic promise for AKI. Whereas it is well known that renal tubular epithelial and other resident kidney cells repair and repopulate following AKI, the source of these cells has been unclear. If stem cells did play a role in renal recovery, are the cells found in the kidney? Do they migrate to the kidney from the bone marrow or other organs? Recently, some of these questions surrounding the role of stem cells in the repair of ARF have been answered.

Stem cells have been shown to have the ability to differentiate into a limited number of cell types. Hematopoietic stem cells (HSCs) and mesenchymal stem cells (MSCs) located in the adult bone marrow can differentiate into all types of blood cells, in the former case, or into adipocyte, chondrocyte or osteocyte lineages in the latter case.[278–280] Initial reports suggested that HSCs play a role in the recovery of ARF. An ischemic insult to the kidneys can mobilize bone marrow–derived HSCs, which can then differentiate into renal tubular cells. HSCs derived from the bone marrow were stained and shown to migrate to the postischemic kidney to repopulate and repair intrinsic kidney cells that were damaged.[281,282] In animal models, tracking transplanted exogenous HSCs showed their migration into the damaged kidney, particularly segments of the kidney that are known to be susceptible to ischemic damage such as the proximal tubule.[282] Ablation of the bone marrow in animal models led to increased renal damage and dysfunction following an ischemic renal injury, whereas reinfusion of HSCs conferred protection from renal IRI.[281] The evidence against HSCs as the major source of cells for renal recovery includes the absence of significant detection of these cells in the kidney during the recovery phase.

Other studies using animal models of IRI have demonstrated renoprotection by infusions of MSCs.[283,284] Infusions of MSCs at the time of, or up to 24 hours following an ischemic insult to the kidney, provided significant renal protection. Contrary to the initial thoughts, the renoprotective effects of MSCs are due more likely due to paracrine effects than to their differentiation into target kidney cells.[279,283] In fact, MSCs were not identified in the kidney, but local expression of inflammatory mediators had shifted to a predominantly anti-inflammatory milieu.[283,285] These anti-inflammatory substances include hepatocyte growth factor, vascular endothelial growth factor, and insulin-like growth factor 1 (IGF-1), which have all been shown to improve the course of experimental AKI.[276,286] MSC infusions can also lead to

improvement of AKI by providing endothelial progenitor cells to repair injured microvasculature.[287,288]

The most recent thinking about the role of stem cells in renal recovery favors the dedifferentiation of intrarenal cells and their eventual transformation to replace the loss of neighboring cells.[273] There is also new evidence of a resident pool of stem cells located within the renal papillae.[289,290]

Distant Organ Pathophysiology

ARF is a systemic disease, and with the availability of dialysis, most deaths during ARF are due to hypotension, cardiorespiratory failure, sepsis, and gastrointestinal bleeding. Organ cross-talk during ARF is being increasingly studied, and may help explain the excess morbidity and mortality associated with even mild degrees of acute kidney impairment (Fig. 29–5). There is a strong association between ARF and acute lung injury, and the mortality rate during ARF rises from 50% to 80% when both lung and kidney are involved.[291,292] Evidence for direct AKI-induced distant organ dysfunction was demonstrated when clamping of the renal artery in rats increased pulmonary vascular permeability with microvascular inflammation and both leukocyte and RBC sludging.[293] This effect occurred as early as 24 hours following IRI and peaks around 48 hours, with return to baseline near 96 hours. When rats were randomly treated with CNI-1493, which blocks the release of macrophage derived inflammatory products, the lung injury was blunted but the course of ARF was unchanged. In the same rat model, AKI led to pulmonary edema that was associated with a down regulation of pulmonary epithelial sodium channels, sodium/potassium ATP-ase (Na/K ATPase), and aquaporin-5 following IRI and ARF.[294] These changes likely impaired lung clearance of salt and water during ARF. In mice prone to sickle cell anemia, small amounts of kidney injury markedly increased lung and distant organ inflammation.[295]

Acute ischemic kidney injury can also produce cross-talk between the kidney and bone marrow, perhaps supporting or enhancing the inflammation that is seen during ARF. Mice that were subjected to renal ischemia through a clamp model were found to have increased levels of serum granulocyte colony–stimulating factor (G-CSF).[296] Increased levels of G-CSF mRNA and G-CSF protein were found in the kidneys of these animals. This production was localized to the epithelial cells of the mTAL. It was also demonstrated that cultured mTAL cells produce G-CSF mRNA and protein in response to stimulation with reactive oxygen species in vitro.

Cross-talk between the kidney and liver has also been demonstrated in the setting of AKI. The injured kidney produces IL-6, which exerts local proinflammatory and distant

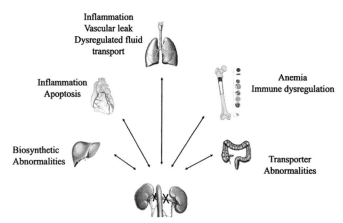

FIGURE 29–5 Organ cross-talk: Distant organ effects following ischemic acute kidney injury. Organ cross-talk can include the liver, heart, lungs, bone marrow, and gastrointestinal tract.

anti-inflammatory effects.[297,298] IL-6 is produced by several different cells in the body following injury (brain, muscle, gut). IL-6 can stimulate hepatic Kupffer cells to produce IL-10, which has been shown to be protective in animal models of AKI.[298] It was also recognized that ischemic renal injury leads to up-regulation of IL-10 receptors in the kidney. AKI in mice can also lead to cardiac apoptosis, which in part is cytokine mediated.[299] Cross-talk between kidney and heart has also been demonstrated, potentially involving apoptotic mechanisms and TNF. Studies to dissect mechanisms of kidney influence on distant organ dysfunction could elucidate key therapeutic targets that will reduce mortality during AKI.

New Experimental Models

Several new experimental models of ATN have been developed to allow better understanding of its underlying pathophysiology as well as to enable discovery of new therapeutics. Although there are several new models of AKI arising from a variety of causes, only a few new models are highlighted.[300] One of the most widely used classic small animal models involves a clamp applied to one or both kidneys. The length of injury as well as the site of injury (clamping one or both kidneys) can be controlled. Cold ischemia with warm reperfusion can also be achieved by removing a kidney, placing it on ice, and then re-implanting the kidney. This model mimics the situation commonly seen in renal transplantation.[300] However, the more an experimental model is distilled from what happens to humans in vivo, the less likely it is to encompass the complexity of the actual process. It is very rare in human native kidney that an isolated ischemic insult to the kidneys alone leads to AKI. In reality, a host of factors (concomitant medication use—NSAIDS, ACE-Inhibitors; sepsis; shock; congestive heart failure or hepatic failure) all set the stage for the ischemic insult. One cause of human renal IRI is sudden shock from hemorrhage or cardiac arrest. AKI develops in nearly a third of patients that survive an in-hospital cardiac arrest.[301] Whole-body IRI followed by resuscitation is also highly pertinent to the non-heart-beating deceased donor kidney, in which there is an opportunity to use more transplantable kidneys. To mimic this injury, a mouse cardiac arrest model was developed.[302] Cardiac arrest was induced by an infusion of potassium chloride and was allowed to persist for 10 minutes. Following this time, resuscitation was achieved by cardiac compressions, epinephrine, ventilation, and fluids, as is commonly done in cases of human cardiac arrest. This mouse model produced very similar findings to isolated renal artery clamp models. One significant difference was that only 10 minutes of ischemia was required with whole body ischemia, whereas with isolated clamp models, usually at least 30 minutes of warm ischemia is necessary to lead to significant renal injury. The reason for this difference was posited to be the effects of ischemia on distant organs and the release of inflammatory mediators. The implication of this finding to human IRI is that only brief episodes of systemic arterial hypotension may be sufficient to induce AKI.

A new model of AKI in sepsis has been developed in the mouse.[238,303] This model sought to expand upon a commonly used lipopolysaccharide (LPS) model that was in use. In the LPS model, the animal was injected with LPS to mimic the vascular collapse seen in septic shock. A newer model was developed and compared with the LPS model. The new model used a cecal ligation puncture (CLP) to induce polymicrobial sepsis, to more closely echo the events in humans leading to sepsis-related AKI. Mice were given a period of fluid resuscitation as well as antimicrobial therapy, which differentiates this model from the LPS model, and more closely mimics the events surrounding human sepsis and resultant ARF. The CLP model was applied to both young and old mice. It was noticed that the best fit of the model to human disease was found in the CLP model in older mice when compared with the LPS model. In the mouse CLP model, it was discovered that a single dose of ethyl pyruvate, which is known to scavenge free radicals and down-regulate inflammatory cytokines (IL-6 and TNF-α), provided significant protection from ARF.[303] The benefits of ethyl pyruvate therapy were found even when the drug was given up to 12 hours after the initiation of sepsis.

Another model of ATN has been developed in the zebrafish.[304] The advantage of the larval zebrafish model is the relative simplicity and visual accessibility of the kidney. With a primarily nephrotoxic model using the aminoglycoside gentamicin and the chemotherapeutic agent cisplatin, similar histologic changes in the zebrafish where found compared with changes caused by known nephrotoxic medications frequently implicated in human ARF. The possibility exists for genetic manipulation in the zebrafish to allow for knockout models to probe specific pathways in AKI.

Novel Biomarkers

New biomarkers hold the promise of allowing clinicians to detect kidney injury earlier, to guide future therapy, and to better prognosticate. The currently employed, traditional markers of AKI in the blood (creatinine and urea nitrogen) are insensitive, lagging indicators that are not specific for any given disease process.[305] The urinary sediment is made up of byproducts of cellular injury (i.e., casts) that are also lagging indicators of a previous and sometimes ongoing injury. There are several biomarkers currently under investigation, as detailed later (Table 29–9). Using known models of human ATN, such as deceased donor renal transplantation with delayed graft function, as well as animal models of IRI, investigators have found blood and urine proteins that may be effective biomarkers of AKI.

Keratinocyte-derived chemokine (KC) was shown to be upregulated very early in the course of IRI in a mouse model in the urine, blood and kidney. It was subsequently shown that the human analog of KC, Gro-α, is abundant in the urine of human deceased donor renal allograft recipients who have delayed graft function. The early elevation of urine Gro-α distinguished kidney transplants that had immediate function or a live donor kidney transplant from those with worse outcomes.[306] Elevations in KC/Gro-α in serum and urine were evident as early as 3 hours postischemia, well before the onset of histologic changes or rise in serum creatinine.

Neutrophil gelatinase-associated lipocalin (NGAL) is a promising early biomarker of AKI. NGAL is highly upregulated in the postischemic kidney of the human, mouse, and the rat, as well as in animal models of cisplatin nephrotoxicity.[307–309] NGAL is rapidly excreted in the urine to allow detection. Interestingly, NGAL is highly expressed in proliferating renal tubular cells, and NGAL has been used as a therapeutic agent in experimental models of AKI.[276]

Kidney injury molecule-1 (KIM-1) is a transmembrane protein that is expressed in high levels on dedifferentiated renal tubular epithelial cells in humans and rodents following ischemic or toxic injury.[305,310] Human KIM-1 ectodomain can be found in the urine, and elevations occur as early as 12 hours following IRI and persist until repair of the epithelium. KIM-1 is expressed at low levels in the noninjured kidney and so potentially represents a useful marker for AKI.

The sodium/hydrogen exchanged isoform 3 (NHE3) protein is an apical sodium transporter widely expressed in renal tubules and found primarily in the proximal tubule and thick ascending limb cells.[305,311] NHE3 is not detected in the urine of normal control subjects but is found in cases of prerenal

TABLE 29–9 Novel Biomarkers in Acute Renal Failure

Host	Reference	Marker	Substrate—Test	Comments
Rat	Zahedi et al[323]	SSAT	Rat kidney—RT-PCR and Northern blot	SSAT was able to distinguish ARF with tubular injury from ARF without ATN
Rat & Mouse	Muramatsu et al[319]	CYR61	Kidney and urine—Western blot	CYR61 is upregulated in kidneys with IRI—able to distinguish prerenal from intrarenal ARF
Human	Parikh et al[313]	IL-18	Urine—ELISA	IL-18 elevated in human kidney ATN (native and transplanted kidneys)
Human	du Cheyron et al[312]	NHE3	Urine—semiquantitative immunoblotting	NHE3 differentiated prerenal from intrarenal ischemic ATN from other intrarenal causes of ARF
Human	Nguyen et al[322]	Urine Proteome pattern	Urine—mass spectroscopy	Humans following cardiopulmonary bypass surgery—markers at 2 and 6 hours postoperative highly sensitive and highly predictive of AKI
Human	Han et al[310]	KIM-1	Urine, kidney—multiple methods	Specific for *ischemic* ARF/ATN when compared with other forms of kidney disease
Human, Mouse	Molls et al[306]	Gro-α, KC	Urine, blood—ELISA	Gro-α correlates well with renal recovery from AKI/DGF in transplant, early increase in urine and blood well before rise in serum creatinine in ARF models
Human	Mishra et al[307,308]	NGAL	Blood, urine—western blot and ELISA	NGAL sensitive, specific and predictive marker of ARF in blood and urine of patients after cardiopulmonary bypass
Human	Kwon et al[316]	Actin, IL-6 and IL-8	Urine—dot immunoblot and ELISA	All three markers predicted prolonged ARF following renal transplantation in humans

AKI, acute kidney injury; CYR61, cysteine-rich protein 61; DGF, delayed graft function; Gro-α, human growth-related oncogene-α; IL-6, interleukin-6; IL-8, interleukin-8; IL-18, interleukin-18; KC, keratinocyte-derived chemokine; KIM-1, kidney injury molecule 1; NGAL, neutrophil gelatinase–associated lipocalin; NHE3, Na$^+$/H$^+$ exchanger isoform 3; SSAT, spermidine/spermine N1-acetyltransferase.

CH 29

Acute Kidney Injury

AKI, postrenal AKI, and ATN. It was not detected in subjects with intrinsic causes of AKI such as glomerulonephritis, transplant rejection, or interstitial nephritis.[312] Levels of NHE3 in ATN and prerenal AKI were different, suggesting NHE3 as a possible marker to differentiate the two conditions.

Several urinary cytokines have been suggested as markers of AKI. IL-18 is a mediator of inflammation and ischemic tissue injury in a variety of organs. Quantification of urinary IL-18 levels in a series of patients showed different levels between normal controls, patients with ATN, prerenal ARF, urinary tract infection, and nephrotic syndrome. Importantly, levels were highest in patients with ATN, including recipients of deceased donor renal allografts with delayed graft function.[313] For this reason, IL-18 may be a good potential marker of ischemic AKI.[314] Other markers of inflammation, such as the macrophage chemoattractant protein-1, have been found in increased amounts in the urine of rats in experimental models of IRI.[315]

In studies of human renal transplantation, the urinary cytokines IL-6, IL-8, and the cytoskeletal protein actin were found to be markers of sustained AKI following transplant. These molecules were found in abundance in the urine samples of patients with prolonged delayed graft function when compared with those that had early recovery or immediate graft function.[316] In critically ill patients with ARF, plasma cytokine levels, particularly IL-6, IL-8, and IL-10, were associated with mortality.[317] Patients with high plasma levels of these three cytokines had a higher risk of death when compared with patients with lower levels. In another study of critically ill patients, plasma IL-6, IL-8, and IL-10 were up-regulated in patients with AKI, but the levels were not predictive of mortality in that cohort.[318]

Certain genomic markers, such as urinary mRNA, have been studied as early markers of AKI. mRNA for *cyr61*, a secreted growth factor–inducible immediate early gene in the proximal straight tubules, was up-regulated in the kidney 2 hours following an ischemic injury.[319] The *cyr61* protein levels peaked 6 to 9 hours postischemia, and they were not elevated in the setting of volume depletion, helping to differentiate intrinsic AKI from prerenal AKI. Another genomic biomarker for ischemic AKI is Zf9, a Kruppel-like transcription factor involved in the regulation of a number of downstream targets, such as transforming growth factor-β1 (TGF-β1).[320] Zf9 is expressed in stable kidneys at low levels in both proximal and distal tubular cells in a diffuse cytoplasmic distribution. Zf9 is highly up-regulated in the postischemic renal tubular cells in animal models as well as in cultured cells. Zf9 is also expressed in the developing kidney. Gene silencing of Zf9 abrogated TGF-β1 overexpression and mitigated the apoptotic response to ATP in vitro.[276,320] TGF-β has been shown in other models to be up-regulated following ischemic renal damage, and it undoubtedly plays an important role in either injury, repair, or both.[321] New techniques such as microarrays and advanced proteomic technology have generated many other new possible biomarkers for AKI.[322] Stathmin, spermidine acetyl transferase, and thrombospondin-1 are among the promising biomarkers for ARF that were discovered using microarray analysis in a rodent model of ARF.[323–325] As the fields of biomarker discovery and genomics advance, they will undoubtedly change the way we diagnose and treat AKI.

COURSE OF ACUTE TUBULE NECROSIS

As discussed earlier, the clinical course of ATN can be divided into three phases: the initiation, maintenance phase, and recovery phases. The initiation phase is the period when patients are exposed to the ischemia or toxins and parenchymal renal injury is evolving but not yet established. ATN is potentially preventable during this period, which may last hours to days. The initiation phase is followed by a maintenance phase, during which parenchymal injury is established and GFR stabilizes at a value of 5 to 10 mL/min.[326–328] Urine output is usually lowest during this period. The maintenance phase typically lasts 1 to 2 weeks but may be prolonged for 1 to 11 months before recovery. The recovery phase is the period, during which patients recover renal function through repair and regeneration of renal tissue. Its onset is typically heralded by a gradual increase in urine output and a fall in serum creatinine, although the latter may lag behind the onset of diuresis by several days. This post-ATN diuresis may reflect appropriate excretion of salt and water accumulated during the maintenance phase, osmotic diuresis induced by filtered urea and other retained solutes, and the actions of diuretics administered to hasten salt and water excretion.[329–331] Occasionally, diuresis may be inappropriate and excessive if recovery of tubule reabsorptive processes lags behind glomerular filtration, although this phenomenon is more common after relief of urinary tract obstruction.[332–335]

DIFFERENTIATION OF ACUTE TUBULE NECROSIS FROM OTHER CAUSES OF ACUTE KIDNEY INJURY

Clinical Features, Urinary Findings, and Confirmatory Tests

The assessment of patients with AKI requires a meticulous history, physical examination and urinalysis, in-depth review of previous records and recent drug history, judicious utilization of laboratory tests, renal imaging, assessment of response to fluid repletion, and occasionally renal biopsy (Table 29–10).[1,2,29,336] A graph of remote and recent serum creatinine levels versus time, incorporating drug therapy and interventions, is invaluable for differentiation of acute and chronic renal failure and the identification of the cause of AKI. An acute process is easily established if review of laboratory records reveals a recent rise in BUN and serum creatinine

TABLE 29–10	Clinical Approach to the Diagnosis of Acute Kidney Injury

History, physical examination (including fundoscopy and weight), detailed review of hospital chart, previous records, and drug history

Urinalysis including specific gravity, dipstick, sulfosalicylic acid, microscopy, and staining for eosinophils

Flowchart of serial blood pressures, weights, BUN, serum creatinine, major clinical events, interventions, and therapies

Routine blood chemistry assays (BUN, creatinine, Na^+, K^+, Ca^{2+}, HCO_3^-, Cl^-, PO_4^{3-}) and hematologic tests (complete blood count and differential white blood cell count)

Selected special investigations:
  Urine chemistry, eosinophils, and/or immunoelectrophoresis
  Serologic tests: antiglomerular basement membrane antibodies, antineutrophil cytoplasmic antibodies, complement, antinuclear antibodies, cryoglobulins, serum protein electrophoresis, anti–streptolysin O or anti-DNase titers
  Radiologic evaluation: plain abdominal film, renal ultrasonography, intravenous pyelography, renal angiography, magnetic resonance angiography.

Renal biopsy

BUN, blood urea nitrogen.

levels. Spurious causes of increased BUN or serum creatinine values should be excluded (see Fig. 29–1). When previous measurements are not available, anemia, hyperparathyroidism, neuropathy, band keratopathy, and radiologic evidence of renal osteodystrophy or small scarred kidneys are useful indicators of a chronic process. However, it should be noted that anemia may also complicate AKI, particularly if prolonged, and renal size can be normal or increased in a variety of chronic renal diseases (e.g., diabetic nephropathy, amyloid, polycystic kidney disease). Once a diagnosis of AKI is established, attention should focus on the differentiation between prerenal, intrinsic renal, and postrenal AKI, and the identification of the specific causative disease. Table 29–11 summarizes some clinical features, urinary findings, and confirmatory tests that are useful for diagnosis of the most common causes of AKI.

Clinical Assessment

Prerenal AKI should be suspected when the serum creatinine value rises after hemorrhage; excessive gastrointestinal, urinary, or insensible fluid losses; or extensive burns, particularly if access to fluids is restricted (e.g., comatose, sedated, or obtunded patients). Supportive findings on clinical assessment include symptoms of thirst or orthostatic dizziness and objective evidence of orthostatic hypotension (postural fall in diastolic pressure greater than 10 mm Hg) and tachycardia (postural increase of more than 10 beats/min), reduced jugular venous pressure, decreased skin turgor, dry mucous membranes, and reduced axillary sweating. However, florid symptoms or signs of hypovolemia are usually not manifest until extracellular fluid volume has fallen by 10% to 20%. Nursing and pharmacy records should be reviewed for evidence of a progressive fall in urine output and body weight and recent use of NSAIDs, ACE inhibitors or ARBs. Consideration should be given to the misuse of illicit drugs such as cocaine. Careful clinical examination may reveal stigmata of chronic liver disease and portal hypertension (e.g., palmar erythema, jaundice, telangiectasia, caput medusae, splenomegaly, ascites), advanced cardiac failure (e.g., peripheral edema, hepatic congestion, ascites, elevated jugular venous pressure, bibasilar lung crackles, pleural effusion, cardiomegaly, gallop rhythm, cold extremities), or other causes of reduced effective critical blood volume. Although clinical assessment provides a satisfactory index of cardiac output and tissue perfusion in most patients, invasive hemodynamic monitoring (central venous and Swan-Ganz catheterization) is often necessary in critically ill patients in whom edema can obscure the clinical examination and complicate the assessment of body weight and fluid balance.

Definitive diagnosis of prerenal AKI hinges on prompt resolution of AKI after restoration of renal perfusion. There is a high likelihood of ischemic ATN if AKI follows a period of severe renal hypoperfusion and persists despite restoration of renal perfusion.[34,37,71,337] It should be noted, however, that significant hypotension is recorded in the case notes of less than 50% of patients with postsurgical ATN. The diagnosis of nephrotoxic ATN requires scouring of clinical, pharmacy, nursing, and radiology records for evidence of recent administration of nephrotoxic medications or radiocontrast agents.[52,88,90,119,132,338,339] AKI after cancer chemotherapy suggests a diagnosis of tumor lysis syndrome and acute urate nephropathy, although other diagnoses must be considered (see later section on differential diagnosis in specific settings).[340–343] Pigment-induced ATN may be suspected if the clinical assessment reveals clues to rhabdomyolysis (e.g., seizures, excessive exercise, alcohol or drug abuse, muscle tenderness, limb ischemia) or hemolysis (e.g., recent transfusion).[68,70,114,344]

Although most AKI is either prerenal or due to ischemic and nephrotoxic ATN, patients should be assessed carefully

TABLE 29–11	Useful Clinical Features, Urinary Findings, and Confirmatory Tests in the Differential Diagnosis of Major Causes of Acute Azotemia		
Cause of Acute Kidney Injury	**Some Suggestive Clinical Features**	**Typical Urinalysis**	**Some Confirmatory Tests**
Prerenal azotemia	Evidence of true volume depletion (thirst, postural or absolute hypotension and tachycardia, low jugular vein pressure, dry mucous membranes and axillae, weight loss, fluid output > input) or decreased effective circulatory volume (e.g., heart failure, liver failure), treatment with NSAIDs or ACE inhibitor	Hyaline casts FENa < 1% UNa < 10 mEq/L SG > 1.018	Occasionally requires invasive hemodynamic monitoring; rapid resolution of AKI on restoration of renal perfusion
Intrinsic renal azotemia Diseases involving large renal vessels Renal artery thrombosis	History of atrial fibrillation or recent myocardial infarct, nausea, vomiting, flank or abdominal pain	Mild proteinuria Occasionally red cells	Elevated LDH with normal transaminases, renal arteriogram, MAG-3 renal scan, MRA
Atheroembolism	Usually > 50 y, recent manipulation of aorta, retinal plaques, subcutaneous nodules, palpable purpura, livedo reticularis, vasculopathy, hypertension	Often normal, eosinophiliuria Rarely casts.	Eosinophilia, hypocomplentemia, skin biopsy, renal biopsy
Renal vein thrombosis	Evidence of nephrotic syndrome or pulmonary embolism, flank pain	Proteinuria, hematuria	Inferior venocavogram, Doppler flow studies, MRV
Disease of the small vessels and glomeruli			
Glomerulonephritis or vasculitis	Compatible clinical history (e.g., recent infection) sinusitis, lung hemorrhage, rash or skin ulcers, arthralgias, hypertension, edema	Red blood cell or granular casts, red blood cells, white blood cells, proteinuria	Low C3, antineutrophil cytoplasmic antibodies, antiglomerular basement membrane antibodies. Anti–streptolysin O antibodies, anti-DNase, cryoglobulins, renal biopsy
HUS or TTP	Compatible clinical history (e.g., recent gastrointestinal infection, cyclosporine, anovulants), pallor, ecchymoses, neurologic abnormalities	May be normal, red blood cells, mild proteinuria, rarely red blood cell or granular casts	Anemia, thrombocytopenia, schistocytes on peripheral blood smear, low haptoglobin, increased LDH, renal biopsy
Malignant hypertension	Severe hypertension with headaches, cardiac failure retinopathy, neurological dysfunction papilledema	May be normal, red blood cells, mild proteinuria, rarely red blood cell casts	LVH by echocardiography or EKG Resolution of ARF with BP control
ARF mediated by ischemia or toxins (ATN)			
Ischemia	Recent hemorrhage, hypotension (e.g. cardiac arrest), surgery often in combination with vasoactive medication (e.g. ACE-inhibitor or NSAID) or chronic renal insufficiency	Muddy brown granular or tubule epithelial cell casts, FENa > 1%, UNa > 20 mEq/L, SG = 1.010	Clinical assessment and urinalysis usually sufficient for diagnosis
Exogenous toxin	Recent radiocontrast study, nephrotoxic antibiotic or chemotherapy often with coexistent volume depletion, sepsis or chronic renal insufficiency	Muddy brown granular or tubule epithelial cell casts, FENa > 1%, UNa > 20 mEq/L, SG = .010	Clinical assessment and urinalysis usually sufficient for diagnosis.
Endogenous toxin	History suggestive of rhabdomyolysis (coma, seizures, drug abuse, trauma)	Urine supernatant tests positive for heme in absence of red cells	Hyperkalemia, hyperphosphatemia, hypocalcemia, increased CK, MM, and myoglobin
	History suggestive of hemolysis (recent blood transfusion)	Urine supernatant pink and tests positive for hee in absence of red cells	Hyperkalemia, hyperphosphatemia, hypocalcemia, hyperuricemia and free circulating hemoglobin
	History suggestive of tumor lysis (recent chemotherapy), myeloma (bone pain), or ethylene glycol ingestion	Urate crystals, dipstick negative proteiuria, oxalate crystals respectively	Hyperuricemia, hyperkalemia, hyperphosphatemia (for tumor lysis); circulating or urinary monoclonal spike (for myeloma); toxicology screen, acidosis, osmolal gap (forethylene glycol)

CH 29

Acute Kidney Injury

Continued

TABLE 29-11	Useful Clinical Features, Urinary Findings, and Confirmatory Tests in the Differential Diagnosis of Major Causes of Acute Azotemia—cont'd		
Cause of Acute Kidney Injury	**Some Suggestive Clinical Features**	**Typical Urinalysis**	**Some Confirmatory Tests**
Acute diseases of the tubulointerstitium Allergic interstitial nephritis	Recent ingestion of drug and fever, rash, loin pain or arthralgia	White blood cellcasts, white blood cells (frequently eosinophiluria), red blood cells, rarely red blood cell casts, proteinuria (occasionally nephrotic)	Systemic eosinophilia, skin biopsy of rash area (leukocytoclastic vasculitis), renal biopsy
Acute bilateral pyelonephritis	Fever, flank pain and tenderness, toxic state	Leukocytes, occasionally white cell casts, red blood cells, bacteria	Urine and blood cultures
Post renal azotemia	Abdominal and flank pain, palpable bladder	Frequently normal, hematuria if stones, hemmorhage, prostatic hypertrophy	Plain film, renal ultrasonography, intravenous pyelography, computed tomography, retrograde or antegade pyelography

ACE, angiotensin-converting enzyme; ATN, acute tubular necrosis; ARF, acute renal failure; BP, blood pressure; CK, creatinine kinase; EKG, electrocardiogram; FENa, fractional excretion of sodium; HUS, hemolytic-uremic syndrome; LDH, lactate dehydropgenase; LVH, left ventricular hypertrophy; MM, multiple myeloma; MRA, magnetic resonance angiography; MRV, magnetic resonance venography; NSAID, nonsteroidal anti-inflammatory drug; SG, specific gravity; TTP, thrombotic thrombocytopenic purpura; UNa, urine Na+ concentration.

for evidence of other renal parenchymal diseases, because many of the latter are treatable and their diagnosis alters management and prognosis. Flank pain may be a prominent symptom of acute renal artery or vein occlusion, acute pyelonephritis, and occasionally necrotizing glomerulonephritis.[345–352] Interstitial edema leading to distention of the renal capsule and flank pain is seen in up to one third of patients with acute interstitial nephritis.[353] Close examination of the skin may reveal the subcutaneous nodules, livedo reticularis, digital ischemia, and palpable purpura of atheroembolism or vasculitis, the butterfly rash of systemic lupus erythematosus (SLE), impetigo in patients with postinfectious glomerulonephritis, a maculopapular rash suggestive of allergic interstitial nephritis, the yellow hue of liver disease or phenazopyridine (Pyridium) toxicity, telltale puncture marks of intravenous drug abuse, or the scarlatiniform eruption of staphylococcal toxic shock syndrome.[354–357] The eyes should be assessed for evidence of atheroembolism; hypertensive or diabetic retinopathy; the keratitis, scleritis, uveitis, and iritis of autoimmune vasculitides; icterus; and the rare but nevertheless pathognomonic band keratopathy of hypercalcemia and flecked retina of hyperoxalemia. Uveitis may also be an indicator of coexistent allergic interstitial nephritis, the tubulointerstitial nephritis and uveitis syndrome.[353,358,359] Examination of the ears, nose, and throat may reveal conductive deafness and mucosal inflammation or ulceration suggestive of Wegener granulomatosis or the neural deafness caused by aminoglycoside toxicity. Respiratory difficulty or the stigmata of chronic liver disease should immediately suggest a pulmonary-renal or hepatorenal syndrome (HRS), respectively. Cardiovascular assessment may be notable for marked elevation in systemic blood pressure and suggest malignant hypertension or scleroderma, or it may reveal a new arrhythmia or murmur that is a potential source of thromboemboli or subacute bacterial endocarditis (acute glomerulonephritis), respectively. Chest or abdominal pain and reduced pulses in the lower limbs should suggest aortic dissection or rarely Takayasu arteritis, and widespread atheromatous disease increases the likelihood of atheroembolic disease. Abdominal pain and nausea are frequent clinical correlates of atherombolic disease in a patient who has recently undergone an angiographic examination. Pallor and recent bruising are

important clues to the thrombotic microangiopathies, and the combination of bleeding and fever should raise the possibility of AKI in association with viral hemorrhagic fevers. A recent jejunoileal bypass may be a vital clue to a rare but reversible cause of AKI in obese patients.[178,360] Hyperreflexia and asterixis often portends the development of uremic encephalopathy, or may, in the presence of focal neurological signs, suggest a diagnosis of thrombotic thrombocytopenic purpura.

Postrenal AKI may be asymptomatic if obstruction develops relatively slowly. Alternatively, patients may present with suprapubic or flank pain if there is acute distention of the bladder or renal collecting system and capsule, respectively. Colicky flank pain radiating to the groin suggests acute ureteric obstruction. Prostatic disease should be suspected in patients with a history of nocturia, frequency, and hesitancy and an enlarged or indurated prostate gland on rectal examination. Similarly, a rectal or pelvic examination may reveal obstructing tumors in female patients. Neurogenic bladder is a likely diagnosis in patients receiving anticholinergic medications (e.g., tricyclic antidepressants) or with physical evidence of neurologic disease and autonomic insufficiency (e.g., paralysis, abnormal rectal sphincter tone, postvoid urine volume more than 200 to 300 mL). Bladder distention may be evident on abdominal percussion and palpation in patients with bladder neck or urethral obstruction. Definitive diagnosis of postrenal ARF usually relies on judicious use of radiologic investigations and rapid improvement in renal function after relief of obstruction.

Urinalysis

Assessment of the urine is a mandatory and inexpensive tool in the evaluation of AKI.[361–364] Urine volume is a relatively unhelpful parameter in differential diagnosis. Anuria suggests complete urinary tract obstruction but may be a complication of severe prerenal or intrinsic ARF (e.g., renal artery occlusion, severe proliferative glomerulonephritis or vasculitis, bilateral cortical necrosis). Wide fluctuations in urine output suggest intermittent obstruction. Patients with partial urinary tract obstruction may present with polyuria caused by secondary impairment of urine concentrating mechanisms. In contrast, analysis of the sediment and supernatant of a

TABLE 29-12	Urine Sediment in the Differential Diagnosis of Acute Kidney Injury

Normal or few red blood cells or white blood cells
Prerenal azotemia
Arterial thrombosis or embolism
Preglomerular vasculitis
HUS or TTP
Scleroderma crisis
Postrenal azotemia

Granular casts
ATN (muddy brown)
Glomerulonephritis or vasculitis
Interstitial nephritis

Red blood cell casts
Glomerulonephritis or vasculitis
Malignant hypertension
Rarely interstitial nephritis

White blood cell casts
Acute interstitial nephritis or exudative glomerulonephritis
Severe pyelonephritis
Marked leukemic or lymphomatous infiltration

Eosinophiluria (>5%)
Allergic interstitial nephritis (antibiotics > NSAIDs)
Atheroembolic disease

Crystalluria
Acute urate nephropathy
Calcium oxalate (ethylene glycol toxicity)
Acyclovir
Indinavir
Sulfonamides
Radiocontrast agents

ATN, acute tubular necrosis; HUS, hemolytic-uremic syndrome; NSAIDS, nonsteroidal anti-inflammatory drugs; TTP, thrombotic thrombocytopenic purpura.

centrifuged urine specimen is valuable for distinguishing between prerenal, intrinsic renal, and postrenal AKI and elucidating the precise etiology of intrinsic renal AKI (Table 29–12). Urine sediment should be inspected for the presence of cells, casts, and crystals. The sediment is typically acellular in prerenal AKI and may contain transparent hyaline casts ("bland," "benign," "inactive" urine sediment). Hyaline casts are formed in concentrated urine from normal constituents of urine, principally THP secreted by epithelial cells of the loop of Henle. Postrenal ARF may also present with a benign sediment, although hematuria and pyuria are common in patients with intraluminal obstruction (e.g., stones, sloughed papilla, blood clot) or prostatic disease. Pigmented "muddy brown" granular casts and tubule epithelial cell casts are characteristic of ischemic or nephrotoxic ATN. They are usually found in association with microscopic hematuria and mild "tubular" proteinuria (<1 g/d). Casts may be absent, however, in approximately 20% to 30% of patients with ischemic or nephrotoxic ATN and are not a requisite for diagnosis.[362,363] Indeed, there is generally a poor correlation between the severity of renal failure and the amount of debris in the urine sediment in these conditions (see section on pathology and pathophysiology of ischemic ATN). Red blood cell (RBC) casts almost always indicate acute glomerular injury but may also be observed, albeit rarely, in acute interstitial nephritis. Dysmorphic RBCs are a more common urinary finding in patients with glomerular injury but are a significantly less specific finding than RBC casts. Urine sediment abnormalities vary in diseases involving preglomerular blood vessels, such as hemolytic-uremic syndrome (HUS), thrombotic thrombocytopenic purpura (TTP), atheroembolic disease, and vasculitis involving medium-sized or large

vessels, and range from benign to frankly nephritic. White blood cell casts and nonpigmented granular casts suggest interstitial nephritis, and broad granular casts are characteristic of chronic renal disease and probably reflect interstitial fibrosis and dilatation of tubules. Eosinophiluria (between 1% and 50% of urine leukocytes) is a common finding (90%) in drug-induced allergic interstitial nephritis.[365,366] However, eosinophiluria is only 85% specific for allergic interstitial nephritis, and eosinophiluria of 1% to 5% can occur in a variety of other diseases including atheroembolization, ischemic and nephrotoxic ARF, proliferative glomerulonephritis, pyelonephritis, cystitis, and prostatitis. Uric acid crystals (pleomorphic) may be seen in urine in prerenal AKI but should raise the possibility of acute urate nephropathy if seen in abundance. Oxalate (envelope-shaped) and hippurate (needle-shaped) crystals suggest a diagnosis of ethylene glycol toxicity.[367,368]

Increased urinary protein excretion, characteristically less than 1 g/d, is a common finding in ischemic or nephrotoxic ARF and reflects both failure of injured proximal tubule cells to reabsorb normally filtered protein and excretion of cellular debris (tubule proteinuria). Proteinuria greater than 1 g/d suggests injury to the glomerular ultrafiltration barrier (glomerular proteinuria) or excretion of myeloma light chains.[98,112,369,370] The latter are not detected by conventional dipsticks (which detect albumin) and must be sought by other means (e.g., sulfosalicylic acid test, immunoelectrophoresis). Heavy proteinuria is also a frequent finding (80%) in patients with allergic interstitial nephritis triggered by NSAIDs. These patients have a glomerular lesion that is almost identical to minimal-change glomerulonephritis, in addition to acute interstitial inflammation.[371–373] A similar syndrome has been reported in patients receiving other agents such as ampicillin, rifampin, and interferon alfa.[374,375] Hemoglobinuria or myoglobinuria should be suspected if urine is strongly positive for hemoglobin by dipstick but contains few RBCs and if the supernatant of centrifuged urine is pink and also positive for free hemoglobin. Hemolysis and rhabdomyolysis can usually be differentiated by inspection of plasma. The latter is usually pink in hemolysis, but not in rhabdomyolysis, because free hemoglobin (65,000 daltons) is a larger molecule than myoglobin (17,000 daltons) that is heavily protein bound and filtered slowly by the kidney.

Confirmatory Tests

The pattern of change in serum creatinine value often provides clues to the cause of AKI. Prerenal AKI is typified by rapid fluctuations in creatinine that parallel changes in hemodynamic function and renal perfusion. The serum creatinine level begins to rise within 24 to 48 hours in patients with ARF after renal ischemia, atheroembolization, and radiocontrast exposure, three major diagnostic possibilities in patients undergoing emergency cardiac or aortic angiography and surgery. Creatinine levels, as already discussed, usually peak after 3 to 5 days in contrast nephropathy and return to the normal range within 5 to 7 days. In contrast, creatinine levels typically peak later (7 to 10 days) in ischemic ATN and atheroembolic disease. AKI usually resolves in the next 7 to 14 days in ischemic AKI, whereas AKI is frequently irreversible in atheroembolic disease. These rapid changes are in marked contrast to the delayed elevation in serum creatinine levels (7 to 10 days) that is characteristic of many tubule epithelial cell toxins (e.g., aminoglycosides, cisplatin).

Additional diagnostic clues can be gleaned from routine biochemical and hematologic tests. Hyperkalemia, hyperphosphatemia, hypocalcemia, and elevated serum uric acid and creatine kinase levels suggest a diagnosis of rhabdomyolysis.[114,155,157] A similar biochemical profile in association with AKI after cancer chemotherapy, but with higher levels of uric acid, a urine uric acid to creatinine ratio greater than

1.0, and normal or marginally elevated creatine kinase, is typical of acute urate nephropathy and tumor lysis syndrome.[340,343,376] Severe hypercalcemia of any cause can induce AKI. Widening of the serum anion ($Na^+ - [HCO_3^- + Cl^-]$) and osmolal (measured serum osmolality minus calculated osmolality) gaps is a clue to the diagnosis of ethylene glycol toxicity and should prompt a search for urine oxalate crystals.[367,377] Severe anemia in the absence of hemorrhage may reflect the presence of hemolysis, multiple myeloma, or thrombotic microangiopathy (e.g., HUS, TTP, toxemia, disseminated intravascular coagulation, accelerated hypertension, SLE, scleroderma, radiation injury). Other laboratory findings suggestive of thrombotic microangiopathy include thrombocytopenia, dysmorphic RBCs on a peripheral blood smear, a low circulating haptoglobin level, and elevated circulating levels of lactate dehydrogenase. Systemic eosinophilia suggests allergic interstitial nephritis but may also be a prominent feature in other diseases such as atheroembolic disease and polyarteritis nodosa, particularly the Churg-Strauss variant. Depressed complement levels and high titers of antiglomerular basement membrane antibodies, antineutrophil cytoplasmic antibodies, antinuclear antibodies, circulating immune complexes, or cryoglobulins are useful diagnostic tools in patients with suspected glomerulonephritis or vasculitis (see Table 29–4).

Imaging of the urinary tract by plain film of the abdomen, ultrasonography, computed tomography (CT), or magnetic resonance is recommended for most patients with ARF to distinguish between acute and chronic renal failure and exclude acute obstructive uropathy.[378–380] The plain film of the abdomen, with tomography if necessary, usually provides a reliable index of kidney size and may detect Ca^{2+}-containing kidney stones. However, the capacity of ultrasonography to determine cortical thickness, differences in cortical and medullary density, and the integrity of the collecting system, in addition to kidney size, makes it the screening modality of choice in most cases of AKI.[378,379,381–383] Although pelvicalyceal dilatation is usual in cases of urinary tract obstruction (98% sensitivity), dilatation may not be observed in the volume-depleted patient during the initial 1 to 3 days after obstruction when the collecting system is relatively noncompliant or in patients with obstruction caused by ureteric encasement or infiltration (e.g., retroperitoneal fibrosis, neoplasia).[384] CT scanning has largely replaced retrograde pyelography through cystography or percutaneous anterograde pyelography for definitive diagnosis when obstruction without dilatation is considered likely. The latter procedures remain useful for precise localization of the site of obstruction in selected cases and facilitate decompression of the urinary tract. Intravenous pyelography should be avoided in patients with AKI to avoid adding contrast nephropathy to already compromised renal function. Radionuclide scans have been touted as useful for assessing renal blood flow, glomerular filtration, tubule function, and infiltration by inflammatory cells in AKI; however, these tests generally lack specificity or yield conflicting or poor results in controlled studies and their use is largely restricted to the immediate postrenal transplantation period.[378,379,385] Magnetic resonance angiography (MRA) of the kidneys is extremely useful for detecting renal artery stenosis, and its role has been extended to the evaluation of acute renovascular crises.[378,380,386,387] MRA is a time-efficient and safe test when compared with conventional arteriography. Doppler ultrasonography and spiral CT are also useful in patients with suspected vascular obstruction; however, contrast angiography remains the gold standard for definitive diagnosis.

Renal biopsy is usually reserved for patients in whom prerenal and postrenal failure have been excluded and the cause of intrinsic AKI is unclear.[186] Renal biopsy is particularly useful when clinical assessment, urinalysis, and laboratory investigation suggest diagnoses other than ischemic or nephrotoxic injury that may respond to specific therapy. Examples include antiglomerular basement membrane disease and other forms of necrotizing glomerulonephritis, vasculitis, HUS and TTP, allergic interstitial nephritis, myeloma cast nephropathy, and acute allograft rejection.

Renal Failure Indices for Differentiation of Prerenal Acute Kidney Injury and Ischemic Acute Tubule Necrosis

Analysis of urine and blood biochemistry is useful for discriminating between the major categories of oliguric ARF, namely prerenal ARF and intrinsic ARF caused by ischemia or nephrotoxins (Table 29–13). The fractional excretion of Na^+

TABLE 29–13	Urine Indices Used in the Differential Diagnosis of Prerenal and Ischemic Intrinsic Renal Azotemia	
Diagnostic Index	Prerenal Azotemia	Ischemic Intrinsic Azotemia
Fractional excretion of Na+ (%),* $\dfrac{UNa \times Pcr}{PNa \times Ucr} \times 100$	<1	>1
Urinary Na+ concentration (mEq/L)	<10	>20
Urinary creatinine/plasma creatinine ratio	>40	<20
Urinary urea nitrogen/plasma urea nitrogen ratio	>8	<3
Urine specific gravity	>1.018	<1.012
Urine osmolality (mOsm/kg H2O)	>500	<250
Plasma BUN/creatinine ratio	>20	<10–15
Renal failure index,* UNa/Ucr/Pcr	<1	>1
Urine sediment	Hyaline casts	Muddy brown granular casts

BUN, blood urea nitrogen.
*Most sensitive indices. UNa, urine Na+ concentration; Ucr, urine creatinine concentration; PNa, plasma Na+ concentration; Pcr, plasma creatinine concentration.

(FENa) is the most sensitive index for this purpose.[388–391] The FENa relates Na⁺ clearance to creatinine clearance. Na⁺ is reabsorbed avidly from glomerular filtrate in patients with prerenal AKI as a consequence of suppression of atrial natriuretic peptide (ANP) secretion, activation of renal nerves and the renin-angiotensin-aldosterone axis, and local changes in peritubular hemodynamics. In contrast, Na⁺ reabsorption is inhibited in ATN as a result of tubule cell injury. Creatinine is reabsorbed to a much smaller extent than Na⁺ in both conditions. Consequently, oliguric patients with prerenal ARF typically have a FENa of less than 1.0% (frequently <0.01%), whereas the FENa is usually greater than 2.0% in patients with ischemic or nephrotoxic AKI. The renal failure index (see Table 29–13) provides comparable information, because clinical variations in serum Na⁺ concentration are relatively small. Urinary Na⁺ concentration is a less sensitive index for distinguishing prerenal AKI from ATN. Similarly, indices of urinary concentrating ability such as urine specific gravity, urine osmolality, urine/plasma creatinine or urea ratios, and serum urea nitrogen/creatinine ratio are of limited value in differential diagnosis. This is particularly true for elderly subjects, in whom urine concentrating mechanisms are frequently impaired while mechanisms for Na⁺ reabsorption are preserved.

Although beloved by textbooks and clinical teachers, the FENa is only of limited discriminatory value. The FENa is frequently greater than 1.0% in prerenal AKI in patients receiving diuretics or with bicarbonaturia (when HCO_3^- is excreted with Na⁺ to maintain electroneutrality), underlying chronic renal failure complicated by salt wasting, or adrenal insufficiency.[337,388,389,392–394] On the other hand, approximately 15% of patients with nonoliguric ischemic or nephrotoxic AKI have a FENa less than 1.0%, which probably reflects a milder form of renal injury (sometimes termed the intermediate syndrome). The latter has been described in patients with ATN of a variety of causes, including ischemia, radiocontrast agents, burns, sepsis, and HRS. Under these circumstances, epithelial cell damage is probably localized to the corticomedullary junction and outer medulla with relative preservation of function in other Na⁺-transporting segments. The apparent increase in frequency of the intermediate syndrome may reflect increasing attention by physicians to volume status and drug therapy in high-risk patients. It should be noted that the FENa is often less than 1.0% in AKI caused by urinary tract obstruction, glomerulonephritis, and diseases of the renal vasculature, and other parameters must be employed to distinguish these conditions from prerenal AKI.

Differential Diagnosis of Acute Kidney Injury in Specific Clinical Settings

The differential diagnosis of ARF in several common clinical situations warrants special mention (Table 29–14).

Acute Kidney Injury in a Patient with Cancer

Most AKI in patients with cancer is due to either prerenal AKI—often induced by vomiting and diarrhea in the presence of NSAIDs use—or hypercalcemia.[170,340,395–400] Intrinsic AKI can be triggered by chemotherapeutic agents or by the products of tumor lysis. Renal parenchymal invasion by solid and hematologic cancers occurs in 5% to 10% of autopsy studies but is rarely of clinical significance.[341,401] AKI consequent to leukemic infiltration of the kidney parenchyma typically presents with hematuria, proteinuria, and enlarged kidneys on ultrasound imaging. The diagnosis is an important one because the AKI may respond to chemotherapeutic intervention.

The tumor lysis syndrome is characterized by AKI associated with hyperuricemia, hyperphosphatemia and hypocalcemia.[402,403] It occurs most often following initiation of chemotherapy in patients with poorly differentiated lymphoproliferative malignancies, particularly the acute leukemias.[342,343,402–404] It occasionally occurs spontaneously, or in patients with solid organ tumors. AKI is triggered by direct tubular injury/obstruction by uric acid and calcium phosphate crystals. Less common causes of AKI include tumor-associated glomerulonephritis or a thrombotic microangiopathy (TMA) induced by drugs or irradiation.[96,405,406] In regard to the latter, chemotherapy-associated TMA is a well-recognized complication of several chemotherapeutic agents of which mitomycin C and gemcitabine are pre-eminent.[406–408]

AKI in association with multiple myeloma carries a wide differential diagnosis that includes in decreasing order of frequency hypovolemia, myeloma cast nephropathy, sepsis, hypercalcemia, ATN induced by drugs or tumor lysis during therapy, light chain deposition disease, cryoglobulinemia, hyperviscosity syndrome, plasma cell infiltration and vascular amyloidosis.[98,112,165,166,169,370,409,410]

Acute Kidney Injury in Pregnancy

The incidence of AKI requiring dialysis complicating pregnancy in industrialized countries is approximately 1 in 20,000 births.[411–418] The marked decline over the past 50 years is a result of improved prenatal care and obstetric practice. In early pregnancy, ATN induced by nephrotoxic abortifacients is still a relatively common cause of AKI in developing countries but is rarely seen in the developed world. Ischemic ATN, severe toxemia of pregnancy, and postpartum HUS and TTP are the most common causes later in pregnancy (see Table 29–14).[412,414,415,419] Ischemic ATN is usually provoked by postpartum hemorrhage or abruptio placentae and less commonly by amniotic fluid embolism or sepsis.[413,415,418] Glomerular filtration is usually normal in mild or moderate pre-eclampsia; however, AKI may complicate severe disease.[414,417,418,420] In this setting, AKI is typically transient and found in association with intrarenal vasospasm, marked hypertension and neurologic abnormalities. A variant of pre-eclampsia, the HELLP syndrome (Hemolysis, Elevated Liver enzymes, Low Platelets), is characterized by an initial benign course that can rapidly deteriorate with the development of a thrombotic microangiopathy characterized by hemolysis and derangement of coagulation, and hepatic and renal function.[416,420,421] Immediate delivery of the fetus is indicated in such cases. This presentation contrasts with that of postpartum thrombotic microangiopathy, which typically occurs against a background of normal pregnancy; is characterized by postpartum thrombocytopenia, microangiopathic anemia, and normal prothrombin and partial thromboplastin times; and frequently causes long-term impairment of renal function.[422–424] Acute fatty liver of pregnancy (AFLP) occurs in approximately 1 in 7000 pregnancies and induces acute renal impairment probably by triggering intrarenal vasoconstriction, as in other HRSs. Although the exact origin of AFLP is not known, the incidence is increased in women who carry a fetus with a defect in fatty acid oxidation, and who are themselves carriers of a genetic mutation that compromises intramitochondrial fatty acid oxidation.[421] Acute bilateral pyelonephritis may also precipitate AKI in pregnancy and should be obvious from clinical assessment (fever, flank pain) and routine urinalysis (bacteria, leukocytes) and laboratory tests (leukocytosis, increase in serum creatinine from basal levels).[414,416,425,426] The diagnosis of postrenal AKI is complicated in pregnancy by the fact that the collecting system undergoes a physiologic dilatation in the second and third trimesters, thus complicating the interpretation of ultrasonographic imaging.[427]

AKI in the cancer patient
Prerenal azotemia
   Hypovolemia (e.g., poor intake, vomiting, diarrhea)
Intrinsic renal azotemia
   Exogenous nephrotoxins: chemotherapy, antibiotics, radiocontrast agents
   Endogenous toxins: hyperuricemia, hypercalcemia, tumor lysis, light chains
   Other: radiation, HUS, TTP, glomerulonephritis, amyloid, infiltration
Postrenal azotemia
   Ureteric or bladder neck obstruction

AKI after cardiac surgery
Prerenal azotemia
   Hypovolemia (surgical losses, diuretics), cardiac failure, vasodilators
Intrinsic renal azotemia
   Ischemic renal failure with ATN (even in absence of documented hypotension)
   Atheroembolic renal disease after aortic manipulation/intra-aortic balloon pump
   Pre- or perioperative administration of radiocontrast agent
   Allergic interstitial nephritis induced by perioperative antibiotics
Postrenal azotemia
   Blocked urinary catheter

AKI in pregnancy
Intrinsic renal azotemia
   Pre-eclampsia or eclampsia
   Ischemia: postpartum hemorrhage, abruptio placentae, amniotic fluid embolus
   Direct toxicity of illegal abortifacients
   Postpartum HUS or TTP
   Acute fatty liver of pregnancy
Postrenal
   Obstruction with pyelonephritis

AKI after solid organ or bone marrow transplantation (BMT)
Prerenal azotemia
   Intravascular volume depletion (e.g., diuretic therapy)
   Vasoactive drugs (e.g., calcineurin inhibitors, amphotericin B)
   Hepatorenal syndrome, veno-occlusive disease of liver (BMT)
Intrinsic renal azotemia
   Post operative ischemic renal failure with ATN (even in absence of documented hypotension)
   Sepsis
   Exogenous nephrotoxins: aminoglycosides, amphoterincin B, radiocontrast
   Endogenous toxins: light chains
   HUS, TTP (e.g., cyclosporine or myeloablative radiotherapy-related)
   Allergic tubulointerstitial nephritis
Postrenal azotemia
   Blocked urinary catheter

AKI and pulmonary disease (pulmonary-renal syndrome)
Vasculitis: Goodpasture syndrome, Wegener syndrome, SLE, Churg-Strauss syndrome, or classic polyarteritis nodosa; cryoglobulinemia;
   right-sided endocarditis; lymphomatoid granulomatosis; sarcoidosis; scleroderma
Toxins: ingestion of paraquat or diquat
Infections: Legionnaire disease, *Mycoplasma* infection, tuberculosis, disseminated viral or fungal infection
Acute renal azotemia from any cause with hypervolemia and pulmonary edema
Prerenal azotemia caused by diminished cardiac output complicating pulmonary embolism, severe pulmonary hypertension, or positive-
   pressure mechanical ventilation
Lung cancer with hypercalcemia, tumor lysis, or glomerulonephritis

AKI and liver disease
Prerenal azotemia
   Primary liver disease with secondary renal failure caused by reduced effective (hypoalbuminemia, splanchnic vasodilatation) or true
     (gastrointestinal hemorrhage,diuretics) circulatory volume
   Right-sided heart failure with liver and renal failure
Intrinsic renal azotemia
   Ischemia (severe hypoperfusion—see above) or direct nephrotoxicity and hepatotoxicity of drugs or toxins (e.g., carbon tetrachloride,
     acetaminophen, tetracyclines, methoxyflurane)
   Tubulointerstitial nephritis + hepatitis caused by drugs (e.g., sulfonamides, rifampin, phenytoin, allopurinol, phenindione), infections
     (leptospirosis, brucellosis, Epstein-Barr virus infection, cytomegalovirus infection), malignant infiltration (lymphoma, leukemia), or
     sarcoidosis
   Glomerulonephritis or vasculitis (e.g., polyarteritis nodosa, Wegener syndrome, cryoglobulinemia, SLE, postinfections hepatitis or liver
     abscess)
   Occlusion of renal veins: tense ascites

AKI and nephrotic syndrome
Prerenal azotemia
  Intravascular volume depletion (diuretic therapy, hypoalbuminemia)
Intrinsic renal azotemia
  Manifestation of primary glomerular disease
  Collapsing glomerulopathy (e.g., HIV, pamidronate)
  Associated ATN (elderly hypertensive males)
  Associated interstitial nephritis (NSAIDs, rifampin, interferon alfa)
Myeloma cast nephropathy or light chain deposition disease
Renal vein thrombosis
Severe interstitial edema

ATN, acute tubular necrosis; HUS, hemolytic-uremic syndrome; SLE, systemic lupus erythematosus; TTP, thrombotic thrombocytopenic purpura.

Acute Kidney Injury after Cardiovascular Surgery

AKI requiring dialytic support is seen in 1% to 5% of patients undergoing coronary bypass grafting procedures.[4,74,428–430] Patients undergoing cardiac surgery are frequently predisposed to the development of postoperative AKI owing to the presence of preoperative hypertensive nephrosclerosis, diabetic nephropathy, and silent renal ischemia.[4,74] AKI in this setting can usually be attributed to prerenal AKI, ischemic ATN, atheroembolic disease, or the effects of radiocontrast material administered perioperatively (see Table 29–14).[57,74,431,432] The pattern of rise in serum creatinine may be extremely helpful in the differential diagnosis of ARF in this setting. As noted earlier, prerenal AKI is typified by rapid fluctuations in serum creatinine values that usually precede surgery and mirror changes in systemic hemodynamics and renal perfusion. Overzealous use of diuretics or afterload-reducing agents is a frequent cause of prerenal AKI postoperatively, particularly in elderly patients in whom renal autoregulation is frequently reduced secondary to hypertensive atherosclerotic or diabetic vasculopathy. The serum creatinine value characteristically rises for 3 to 4 days after the administration of contrast agent and returns rapidly to the normal range within 1 week. This pattern contrasts with those observed with ischemic ATN and atheroembolic disease, in which the serum creatinine value also rises progressively after surgery but typically takes 7 to 14 days before recovery begins (ATN) or fails to resolve (atheroemboli).[17,99,100] Rarer but nevertheless important causes include allergic tubulointerstitial nephritis induced by antibiotics administered perioperatively and obstruction of urine drainage. Independent preoperative risk factors for the development of AKI following cardiovascular surgery include advanced age, creatinine clearance less than 60 mL/min, peripheral vascular disease, cardiomegaly, and a left ventricular ejection fraction of less than 35%. Intraoperative risk factors include emergent surgery, bypass time greater than 100 minutes, intra-aortic balloon pump insertion, and combined valvular and coronary revascularization procedures.[74,431] Off-pump coronary artery bypass grafting surgery has been suggested to lessen the risk of postoperative renal failure in some but not all prospective studies.[433–435]

Acute Kidney Injury after a Solid Organ or Bone Marrow Transplant

Nonrenal solid organ transplant recipients have a notably high risk of developing AKI from cardiopulmonary, hepatic failure, sepsis, and the nephrotoxic effects of antimicrobials and immunosuppressive agents. The differential diagnosis of renal impairment following renal transplantation is discussed in detail in Chapter 36. In a large retrospective multicenter study, 25% of all nonrenal solid organ transplant recipients developed AKI, with 8% requiring renal replacement therapy. The development of dialysis-requiring AKI was associated with a 9- to 12-fold increase in patient mortality in this study.[436] AKI occurred in 35% of heart transplants and 15% of lung transplant recipients. Approximately 20% to 30% of liver transplantation patients will develop AKI, with a significant proportion of these having had, preoperative renal dysfunction.[437,438] There is conflicting evidence as to whether pretransplant renal dysfunction predicts outcome in patients undergoing orthotopic liver transplantation; however, patients with preoperative renal failure have significantly longer hospital and intensive care unit stays and an increased need for dialysis compared with patients with normal preoperative renal function.[439–441]

AKI is a recognized complication of myeloablative allogenic and, to a lesser extent, autologous hematopoetic cell transplantation (HCT).[400,442–444] The incidence of AKI following myeloablative HCT is as high as 50%, with 20% to 31% of patients requiring hemodialysis. The prognosis is grave, particularly for patients requiring dialysis (>80% mortality rate).[445–448] The incidence of AKI following autologous HCT is considerably lower.[448] A study of 232 patients following autologous HCT found reported an incidence of moderate to severe ARF of 21%, with an associated mortality of 18% in affected cases. Causes of AKI in this setting include hypovolemia, sepsis, tumor lysis syndrome, direct tubular toxicity from cytoreductive therapy, antibiotics, and calcineurin inhibitors. The most common cause of severe AKI complicating myeloablative HCT is the HRS complicating the development of veno-occulsive disease (VOD) of the liver.[448,449] VOD is most common in conditioning regimens that include total body irradiation and cyclophosphamide and or busulphan. The syndrome is characterized clinically by profound jaundice and avid salt retention with edema and ascites within the first month after engraftment. Oliguric AKI is common in moderate disease and certain in severe cases. The mortality rate approaches 100% for severe VOD.

Acute Kidney Injury in Association with Pulmonary Disease

The coexistence of AKI and pulmonary disease (pulmonary-renal syndrome) classically suggests a diagnosis of Goodpasture syndrome, Wegener granulomatosis, or other vasculitides.[450–455] The detection of circulating antineutrophil cytoplasmic antibodies, antiglomerular basement membrane antibodies, or hypocomplementemia can be useful in the differentiation of these diseases (see Tables 29–4 and 29–14), although the urgent need for definitive diagnosis and treatment may mandate a lung or renal biopsy. Several toxic ingestions and infections may also cause simultaneous pulmonary and renal injury that mimics a vasculitic process (see Table 29–14). Furthermore, intrinsic renal or postrenal AKI of any cause may be complicated by secondary hypervolemia and pulmonary edema, and severe lung diseases may compromise cardiac output and induce prerenal AKI (see Table 29–14).

Acute Kidney Injury in Association with Chronic Liver Disease

The differential diagnosis for AKI in association with liver disease is similarly large. In chronic liver disease, causes of AKI include volume depletion, gastrointestinal hemorrhage, sepsis, nephrotoxins (antibiotic radiocontrast), and the HRS. The term HRS is usually reserved for a syndrome of irreversible AKI that usually complicates advanced cirrhosis; however, this syndrome has been described in association with fulminant viral and alcoholic hepatitis.[456–462] The syndrome is characterized by renal failure and disturbed regulation of circulatory function. The latter is characterized by intense intrarenal vasoconstriction, whereas in the extrarenal circulation, arteriolar vasodilation triggers a reduction in total peripheral vascular resistance and a decrease in effective systemic circulatory volume despite an expanded total extracellular fluid volume.[456,459,460,463–466] Most patients have clinical evidence of advanced cirrhosis. HRS almost certainly represents the terminal stage of a hypoperfusion state that begins early in the course of chronic liver disease. The pathogenic mechanisms for the dramatic hemodynamic alterations are incompletely understood. In the early stages of HRS, arterial underfilling is thought to trigger activation of the renin-angiotensin and sympathetic nervous systems.[456,463,466,467] Renal perfusion is initially preserved by the local release of renal vasodilatory factors; however these compensatory mechanisms are eventually overwhelmed and progressive renal hypoperfusion ensues. The splanchnic circulation is protected from the effects of the vasoconstrictors such as angiotensin II owing to the local production of mediators such as NO, prostaglandins, and vasoactive peptides; a process that likely accentuates arterial underfilling in other vascular beds including the kidney. Mean arterial blood pressure is typically low, reflecting the reduction in peripheral vascular resistance.

Two subtypes of HRS have been described; type 1 is characterized by a rapid onset of renal failure with a doubling of serum creatinine to greater than 2.5 mg/dL or a 50% reduction in GFR to less than 20 mL/min over a 2-week period.[460,461,468] This subtype is characterized by a fulminant course with oliguria, encephalopathy, marked hyperbilirubinemia, and death usually within 1 month of presentation. Type II HRS is typified by a more indolent course with a stable reduction in GFR accompanying diuretic resistant ascites and avid sodium retention. The diagnosis of HRS is one of exclusion. Other diagnoses that must be entertained in the patient with AKI and liver disease include prerenal AKI due to gastrointestinal losses, drug toxicity, combined hepatitis and tubulointerstitial nephritis induced by drugs or infectious agents, and multiorgan involvement in vasculitides (e.g., hepatitis C–induced cryoglobulinemia; see Table 29–14). The BUN and serum creatinine values are characteristically deceptively low, despite marked impairment of GFR, because of impaired urea generation and coexisting muscle wasting.[469] The urinary findings include a benign sediment and a low FENa.[337] The most common precipitant of the HRS in patients with compensated cirrhosis is spontaneous bacterial peritonitis.[459,470] Other postulated trigger factors include vigorous diuresis or paracentesis, gastrointestinal bleeding, infections, minor surgery, or the use of NSAIDs and other drugs. However, caution must be exerted in these cases to exclude reversible causes of AKI. Adverse prognostic features include type I variant and the severity of the liver failure (Child-Pugh Class).[457,459,465,471] In the past, type I HRS was associated with a very bleak prognosis, with a median survival of less than a month. However, advances in the management of HRS discussed later suggest that in those patients who respond to therapy, there may be a trend toward better survival.

Acute Kidney Injury and the Nephrotic Syndrome

AKI in the context of the nephrotic syndrome presents a unique array of potential diagnoses. Epithelial cell injury, if severe, can trigger both nephrotic range proteinuria and acute or subacute renal failure.[472,473] This typically occurs as a manifestation of a primary glomerular disease such as collapsing glomerulopathy or crescentic membranous nephropathy. Less dramatic visceral epithelial cell injury, in combination with proximal tubular injury (e.g., panepithelial cell injury induced by NSAIDs or possibly undiagnosed viral illness) or interstitial nephritis (e.g., rifampicin induced) can also present as AKI complicating the nephrotic syndrome.[474–476] Massive excretion of light chain protein in patients with myeloma may present in a similar fashion.[98,477,478] ATN in association with the nephrotic syndrome is seen in a subpopulation of older patients with minimal change disease. These patients are more hypertensive and have heavier proteinuria than patients without AKI.[472] The higher incidence of arteriosclerosis in biopsy samples from these patients may point to preexisting hypertensive nephrosclerosis as a risk factor in the development of this complication. Renal vein thrombosis must always be considered in the differential diagnosis, particularly in the pediatric population; however, the commonest cause for ARF in the patient with the nephrotic syndrome is prerenal ARF complicating diuretic therapy for mobilization of edema.[60,61]

COMPLICATIONS OF ACUTE KIDNEY INJURY

AKI impairs renal excretion of Na^+, K^+, and water; divalent cation homeostasis; and urinary acidification mechanisms. As a result, AKI is frequently complicated by intravascular volume overload, hyperkalemia, hyponatremia, hyperphosphatemia, hypocalcemia, hypermagnesemia, and metabolic acidosis (Table 29–15). In addition, patients are unable to excrete nitrogenous waste products and may develop the uremic syndrome. In general, the severity of these complica-

TABLE 29–15	Common Complications of Acute Kidney Injury					
Metabolic	**Cardiovascular**	**Gastrointestinal**	**Neurologic**	**Hematologic**	**Infectious**	**Other**
Hyperkalemia	Pulmonary edema	Nausea	Neuromuscular irritability	Anemia	Pneumonia	Hiccups
Metabolic Acidosis	Arrhythmias	Vomiting	Asterixis	Bleeding	Septicemia	Elevated parathroid hormone
Hyponatremia	Pericardiitis	Malnutition	Seizures		Urinary tract infection	
Hypocalcemia	Pericardial effusion	GI hemorrhage	Mental status changes			Low total triiodothyronine and throxine
Hyperphosphatemia	Pulmonary Embolism					
Hypermagnesemia	Hypertension					Normal free throxine
Hyperuricemia	Myocardial Infarction					

GI, gastrointestinal.

tions mirrors the severity of renal injury and the catabolic state of the patient.[29,326,479] For example, the average daily increases in BUN and serum creatinine values in patients with nonoliguric, noncatabolic renal failure range from 10 to 20 mg/dL and 0.5 to 1.0 mg/dL, respectively. Comparable increments in BUN and creatinine levels in oliguric, catabolic patients typically range from 20 to 100 mg/dL and 2 to 3 mg/dL, respectively. Not surprisingly, therefore, the latter group is at significantly higher risk for life-threatening metabolic complications and has a worse prognosis[8] (see later).

Intravascular volume overload is an almost inevitable consequence of diminished salt and water excretion in AKI and may present clinically as mild hypertension, increased jugular venous pressure, bibasilar lung crackles, pleural effusions or ascites, peripheral edema, increased body weight, and life-threatening pulmonary edema. Hypervolemia may be particularly troublesome in patients receiving multiple intravenous medications, sodium bicarbonate for correction of acidosis, or enteral or parenteral nutrition. Moderate or severe hypertension is unusual in ATN and should suggest other diagnoses such as hypertensive nephrosclerosis, glomerulonephritis, renal artery stenosis, and other diseases of the renal vasculature.[62,414,452,480–482] Excessive water ingestion or administration of hypotonic saline or isotonic dextrose solutions can trigger hyponatremia, which, if severe, may cause cerebral edema, seizures, and other neurologic abnormalities.[483]

Hyperkalemia is a common and potentially life-threatening complication of AKI.[13,484–487] Serum K^+ typically rises by 0.5 mEq/L/day in oligoanuric patients and reflects impaired excretion of K^+ derived from diet, K^+-containing solutions, drugs administered as potassium salts (e.g., penicillin V), and K^+ released from injured tubule epithelium. Hyperkalemia may be compounded by coexistent metabolic acidosis that promotes K^+ efflux from cells. Severe hyperkalemia or hyperkalemia present at the time of diagnosis of AKI suggests massive tissue destruction such as rhabdomyolysis, hemolysis, or tumor lysis.[68,155,404,488] Mild hyperkalemia (<6.0 mEq/L) is usually asymptomatic. Higher levels are frequently associated with electrocardiographic abnormalities, typically peaked T waves, prolongation of the PR interval, flattening of P waves, widening of the QRS complex, and left axis deviation.[489–493] These changes may antecede the onset of life-threatening cardiac arrhythmias such as bradycardia, heart block, ventricular tachycardia or fibrillation, and asystole. In addition, hyperkalemia may induce neuromuscular abnormalities such as paresthesias, hyporeflexia, weakness, ascending flaccid paralysis, and respiratory failure. Hypokalemia is unusual in AKI but may complicate nonoliguric ATN caused by aminoglycosides, cisplatin, or amphotericin B, presumably by causing epithelial cell injury in the thick ascending limb of the loop of Henle, the last major site of K^+ reabsorption.[5,494–496]

Normal metabolism of dietary protein yields between 50 and 100 mmol/day of fixed nonvolatile acids (principally sulfuric and phosphoric acid), which must be excreted by the kidneys for preservation of acid-base homeostasis. Predictably, AKI is commonly complicated by metabolic acidosis, typically with a widening of the serum anion gap.[497] Acidosis may be severe (daily fall in plasma HCO_3^- >2 mEq/L) when the generation of H+ is increased by additional mechanisms (e.g., diabetic or fasting ketoacidosis; lactic acidosis complicating generalized tissue hypoperfusion, liver disease, or sepsis; metabolism of ethylene glycol).[176,368,459] In contrast, metabolic alkalosis is an infrequent finding but may complicate overzealous correction of acidosis with HCO_3^- or loss of gastric acid by vomiting or nasogastric aspiration.

Uric acid is cleared from blood by glomerular filtration and secretion by proximal tubule cells, and mild asymptomatic hyperuricemia (12 to 15 mg/dL) is typical in established AKI. Higher levels suggest increased production of uric acid and

should suggest a diagnosis of acute urate nephropathy.[170,498,499] In borderline cases, measurement of the urinary urate/creatinine ratio on a random specimen may help distinguish between hyperuricemia caused by overproduction and impaired excretion. This ratio is typically greater than 1.0 when uric acid production is increased and less than 0.75 in normal individuals and patients with renal failure.[173]

Mild hyperphosphatemia (5 to 10 mg/dL) is a common consequence of AKI, and hyperphosphatemia may be severe (10 to 20 mg/dL) in highly catabolic patients or when AKI is associated with rapid cell death as in rhabdomyolysis, hemolysis, or tumor lysis.[398,500–502] Metastatic deposition of calcium phosphate can lead to hypocalcemia, particularly when the product of serum Ca^{2+} (mg/dL) and PO_4^{3-} (mg/dL) concentrations exceeds 70.[484,503] Other factors that potentially contribute to hypocalcemia include skeletal resistance to the actions of parathyroid hormone, reduced levels of 1,25-dihydroxyvitamin D, and Ca^{2+} sequestration in injured tissues.[484,504,505] Hypocalcemia is usually asymptomatic, possibly because of the counterbalancing effects of acidosis on neuromuscular excitability. However, symptomatic hypocalcemia can occur in patients with rhabdomyolysis or acute pancreatitis or after treatment of acidosis with HCO_3^-.[484] Clinical manifestations of hypocalcemia include perioral paresthesias, muscle cramps, seizures, hallucinations and confusion, and prolongation of the QT interval, and nonspecific T-wave changes on an electrocardiogram. The Chvostek sign (contraction of facial muscles on tapping of the jaw over the facial nerve) and the Trousseau sign (carpopedal spasm after occlusion of arterial blood supply to the arm for 3 minutes with a blood pressure cuff) are useful indicators of latent tetany in high-risk patients. Mild asymptomatic hypermagnesemia is usual in oliguric AKI and reflects impaired excretion of ingested magnesium (dietary magnesium, magnesium-containing laxatives, or antacids).[506–508] Hypomagnesemia occasionally complicates nonoliguric ATN associated with cisplatin or amphotericin B and, as with hypokalemia, probably reflects injury to the thick ascending limb of loop of Henle, the principal site for Mg^{2+} reabsorption.[495,509,510] Hypomagnesemia is usually asymptomatic but may occasionally be manifest as neuromuscular instability, cramps, seizures, cardiac arrhythmias, or resistant hypokalemia or hypocalcemia.[506,508]

Anemia develops rapidly in AKI and is usually mild and multifactorial in origin. Contributing factors include inhibition of erythropoiesis, hemolysis, bleeding, hemodilution, and reduced RBC survival time.[511,512] Prolongation of the bleeding time and leukocytosis are also common.[513,514] Prolongation of the bleeding time may result from mild thrombocytopenia, platelet dysfunction, and clotting factor abnormalities (e.g., factor VIII dysfunction), and the complementary actions of administered drugs (e.g., penicillins), and leukocytosis usually reflects sepsis, stress response, and other concurrent illness.[513,515–517] Infection is the most common and serious complication of AKI, occurring in 50% to 90% of cases and accounting for up to 75% of deaths.[13,17–20,29,428,485,518] It is unclear whether this high incidence of infection is due to a defect in host immune responses or repeated breaches of mucocutaneous barriers (e.g., intravenous cannulae, mechanical ventilation, bladder catheterization).

Cardiac complications include arrhythmias, myocardial infarction, and pulmonary embolism. Although these events may reflect primary cardiac disease, abnormalities in myocardial contractility and excitability may be triggered or compounded by hypervolemia, acidosis, hyperkalemia, and other metabolic sequelae of AKI. The increased incidence of pulmonary embolism probably reflects protracted periods of immobilization. Mild gastrointestinal bleeding is common (10% to 30%) and is usually due to stress ulceration of gastric or small intestinal mucosa.[519,520] Alterations in neurologic function may reflect the onset of the uremic syndrome, metabolic complications of AKI, impaired excretion of prescribed neuropsychiatric medications, or primary neurologic disease including TTP.[521–524]

Malnutrition remains one of the most frustrating and troublesome complications of AKI. The majority of patients have net protein breakdown, which may exceed 200 g/day in catabolic subjects.[525,526] Malnutrition is usually multifactorial in origin and may reflect (1) inability to eat or loss of appetite; (2) the catabolic nature of the underlying medical disorder (e.g., sepsis, rhabdomyolysis, trauma); (3) nutrient losses in drainage fluids or dialysate; (4) increased breakdown and reduced synthesis of muscle protein and increased hepatic gluconeogenesis, probably through the actions of toxins, hormones (e.g., glucagon, parathyroid hormone), or other substances (e.g., proteases) that are accumulated in AKI; and (5) inadequate nutritional support.[527–531] Nutrition may also be compromised by the high incidence of acute gastrointestinal hemorrhage, which complicates up to 15% of cases of AKI.

Protracted periods of severe ARF or short periods of catabolic, anuric AKI often lead to the development of the uremic syndrome. Clinical manifestations of the uremic syndrome, in addition to those already listed, include pericarditis, pericardial effusion, and cardiac tamponade; gastrointestinal complications such as anorexia, nausea, vomiting, and ileus; and neuropsychiatric disturbances including lethargy, confusion, stupor, coma, agitation, psychosis, asterixis, myoclonus, hyperreflexia, restless leg syndrome, focal neurologic deficit, or seizures (see Table 29–15). The uremic toxin (or toxins) responsible for this syndrome has yet to be defined. Candidate molecules include (1) urea and its breakdown products, (2) other products of nitrogen metabolism such as guanidino compounds, (3) products of bacterial metabolism such as aromatic amines and skatoles, and (4) other compounds that are inappropriately retained in the circulation in AKI, or are underproduced, such as NO.[479]

A vigorous diuresis may complicate the recovery phase of AKI and precipitate intravascular volume depletion and a delay in recovery of renal function. This diuretic response probably reflects the combined effects of an osmotic diuresis induced by retained urea and other waste products and delayed recovery of tubule function relative to glomerular filtration.[330,331,333,334] Hypernatremia may also complicate this recovery phase if free water losses are not replenished or are inappropriately replaced by relatively hypertonic saline solutions. Hypokalemia, hypomagnesemia, hypophosphatemia, and hypocalcemia are rarer metabolic complications during recovery from AKI. Mild transient hypercalcemia is relatively frequent during recovery and appears to be a consequence of hyperparathyroidism. In addition, hypercalcemia may complicate recovery from rhabdomyolysis because of mobilization of sequestered Ca^{2+} from injured muscle.

MANAGEMENT OF ACUTE KIDNEY INJURY

The goals of management of AKI encompass the need to prevent death, ameliorate metabolic and extracellular volume complications, and preserve renal function so as to prevent the development of chronic kidney disease.

Prerenal Acute Kidney Injury

By definition, prerenal AKI is rapidly reversible on restoration of renal perfusion.[48] The composition of replacement fluids for treatment of hypovolemia varies depending on the source of fluid loss. Hypovolemia caused by hemorrhage is ideally corrected with packed RBCs if the patient is hemodynamically unstable or if the hematocrit is dangerously low. In the absence of active bleeding or hemodynamic instability,

isotonic saline may suffice. The choice of replacement for nonhemorrhagic renal, extrarenal, or third-space losses is controversial. Recent critical reviews of RCTs comparing crystalloid with colloid replacement for resuscitation in critically ill patients conclude that the routine use of colloids may be associated with an adverse outcome and is not justified.[532–538] A study comparing the use of hydroxyethylstarch or gelatin as a volume expander in patients with sepsis found that the use of hydroxyethylstarch was an independent risk factor for the development of AKI, and its routine use should be discouraged in the management of prerenal AKI and sepsis.[539] Thus, isotonic saline is the appropriate replacement fluid for plasma losses (e.g., burns, pancreatitis). The SAFE trial compared the use of either 4% albumin or normal saline for fluid resuscitation in ICU patients.[540] At 28 days, there was no significant difference noted between the two groups with respect to the primary outcome of death or secondary outcomes of organ failure, need for renal replacement therapy, or duration of hospitalisation. Colloid solutions should be used only sparingly, with regular monitoring of renal function and the risk of hyperoncotic renal failure minimized by the concomitant use of appropriate crystalloid solutions.[532] Urinary or gastrointestinal fluids vary greatly in composition but are usually hypotonic. Accordingly, initial replacement is best achieved with hypotonic solutions (e.g., 0.45% saline), and subsequent therapy should be based on measurements of the volume and ionic content of excreted or drained fluids. Serum K^+ and acid-base status should be monitored in all subjects. K^+ supplementation of replacement fluids is rarely required unless sodium bicarbonate induces hypokalemia during treatment of metabolic acidosis. Cardiac failure may require aggressive management with loop diuretics, antiarrhythmic drugs, positive inotropes, preload- and afterload-reducing agents, and mechanical aids such as an intra-aortic balloon pump. Invasive hemodynamic monitoring of the central venous pressure can be an important aid for guiding therapy in complicated patients in whom clinical assessment of cardiovascular function and intravascular volume may be difficult and unreliable. The routine use of pulmonary artery catheters is discouraged based on recent trial data.[541]

Fluid management may be particularly challenging in patients with AKI and cirrhosis.[457,458,462,463] Although these subjects typically have intense intrarenal vasoconstriction and expanded total plasma volume because of pooling of blood in the splanchnic circulation, true hypovolemia or reduced effective systemic arterial blood volume may be an important contributory factor to AKI. The relative contribution of hypovolemia to AKI in this setting can be determined only by administration of a fluid challenge. Fluids should be administered slowly, because nonresponders may suffer an increase in ascites formation and pulmonary edema. Spontaneous bacterial peritonitis is a common trigger factor for HRS in patients with advanced cirrhosis and ascites. The administration of albumin (1.5 g/kg on diagnosis and 1 g/kg on day 3) in combination with standard antibiotic therapy in this setting has been demonstrated to reduce the incidence of HRS and improve patient survival.[470] Paracentesis can be employed to remove large volumes of ascitic fluid. Albeit controversial, simultaneous administration of albumin intravenously is touted by some investigators to minimize the risk of prerenal AKI and full-blown HRS during large-volume paracentesis.[458,462,542] Indeed, large-volume paracentesis may occasionally improve GFR, possibly by lowering intra-abdominal pressure and promoting blood flow in renal veins. Shunting of ascitic fluid from the peritoneum to a central vein (transjugular portosystemic shunt, peritoneojugular shunt, LeVeen or Denver shunt) is an alternative approach in refractory cases.[457,543–546] These maneuvers can cause an improvement in GFR and Na^+ excretion, probably because the increase in central blood volume stimulates the release of ANP and inhibits aldosterone and norepinephrine secretion; however, definitive data on whether the improvement in renal function is associated with improved survival are lacking. Given that these procedures carry significant morbidity (e.g., hepatic encephalopathy); thus, their role needs to be determined by prospective controlled studies.

Vaospressin (V1) receptor agonists have shown promise in the reversal of established HRS.[547-549] The use of vaso-contrictors in patients with HRS is based on the premise that reversal of splanchnic vasodilatation will augment peripheral vascular resistance, suppress the generation of endogenous vasoconstrictors, and thus improve renal perfusion. In most studies, albumin is administered concomitantly to further aid renal perfusion. Several studies have suggested that intravenous terlipressin improves renal function in patients with HRS, especially when combined with intravenous albumin.[548-550] In a small randomized trial, terlipressin (1 mg IV twice daily) combined with albumin resuscitation (goal CVP 10–12 mm Hg) resulted in 5 of 12 patients surviving 15 days as opposed to none of the placebo group.[550] Predictors of nonresponse include older age and more severe liver failure (Child-Pugh score >13). Further large-scale RCTs are awaited with interest.

Intrinsic Acute Kidney Injury

Prevention

Optimization of cardiovascular function and intravascular volume is the single most important maneuver in the management of intrinsic AKI. There is compelling evidence that aggressive restoration of intravascular volume dramatically reduces the incidence of ATN after major surgery or trauma, burns, and cholera.[344,534,551-555] Sepsis-related AKI is a common clinical presentation and is associated with mortality rates as high as 80%.[17,20,556,557] Recent studies have emphasized two salient features of successful management of sepsis that may be of importance in the prevention of AKI. Early goal-directed resuscitation to defined hemodymanic targets (MAP >65 mm Hg, CVP 10–12, urine output >0.5 mL/kg per hour, ScvO2 >70%) using a combination of crystalloid solutions, red cell transfusion, and vasopressors results in a significant reduction in organ dysfunction and mortality in patients with the sepsis syndrome.[558] Although the therapeutic goals chosen in this study were to a degree arbitrary, this study emphasizes the imperative for early and aggressive volume resuscitation in the management of patients with the sepsis syndrome. In another study of critically ill patients, intensive insulin therapy to maintain a glucose level of 180 to 220 mg/dL resulted in a 41% decrease in AKI requiring renal replacement therapy.[559]

Volume depletion has been identified as a risk factor for nephrotoxic ATN induced by radiocontrast material, acyclovir, aminoglycosides, amphotericin B, cisplatin, acute urate nephropathy, rhabdomyolysis, hemolysis, multiple myeloma, hypercalcemia, and numerous other nephrotoxins.[98,112,402,404,499,555,560-564] Restoration of volume prevents the development of experimental and human ATN in many of these settings. The importance of maintaining euvolemia in high-risk clinical situations has been demonstrated most convincingly with contrast nephropathy, in which close attention to intravascular volume status ensures a low frequency of AKI.[565,566] Multiple studies have addressed this issue in an attempt to identify the optimal preventive strategy. Prophylactic infusion of half-normal saline (1 mL/kg for 12 hours before and after procedure) is more effective in preventing AKI than either mannitol and furosemide, both of which should be avoided in this setting.[567] In another large randomized trial, isotonic saline significantly reduced the incidence of contrast nephropathy following coronary angiography compared with half-normal saline with a

particular benefit noted in diabetic patients and those receiving large contrast loads.[568] In a smaller single trial, hydration with sodium bicarbonate before contrast exposure was more effective than hydration with isotonic saline for the prevention of contrast nephropathy.[569] In aggregate, the key message from these studies is that the avoidance of hypovolaemia is the key intervention in preventing contrast nephropathy. Definitive data regarding the optimal hydration regimen require additional confirmatory studies. In the interim, a hydration regimen of isotonic saline (~1 mL/kg per hour) starting the morning of the procedure and continuing for several hours afterward would appear most appropriate. The rate of administration must take into consideration the patient's cardiopulmonary status and may require adjustment in this regard.

N-acetylcysteine has been suggested as an ideal agent to prevent the nephrotoxicity of contrast mediums through antioxidant and vasodilatory effects.[570] Prophylactic oral administration of oral acetylcysteine (600 mg twice a day pre- and postprocedure), in combination with hydration, reduces the incidence of contrast nephropathy in patients with moderate renal insufficiency in several new trials.[570-576] The regimen is inexpensive and safe, and although definitive data are lacking, the use of prophylactic oral N-acetylcysteine should be considered in all patients with impaired renal function before receiving intravenous or intra-arterial iodinated contrast material. The use of low- or iso-osmolar contrast media has been suggested to reduce the incidence of contrast-induced AKI.[577] In a large randomized trial of patients undergoing coronary angiography, use of the low-osmolar contrast agent iohexol was associated with a reduction in the incidence of contrast nephropathy in patients with CKD and diabetes mellitus when compared with the standard high-osmolar diatrizoate.[578] In a second smaller study comparing the iso-osmolar agent iodixanol (~290 mOsm) with iohexol, the former reduced the risk of contrast nephropathy among diabetics with renal insufficiency when given with standard hydration regimens, albeit that the incidence of renal dysfunction in the iohexol group was remarkably high.[579] On balance, it would appear appropriate to use low-osmolar agents in patients with known diabetic nephropathy. However, definitive trial data is awaited regarding the generalizabilty of these findings to all patients with CKD. Other important interventions include spacing the timing of repeated contrast interventions as allowed by the patient's clinical need and considering alternate imaging techniques. The use of less nephrotoxic contrast agents (e.g., gadolinium or carbon dioxide) in combination with enhanced digital subtraction technology as an alternative to standard iodinated contrast administration is an evolving area of interest that offers the possibility of adequate imaging with significantly less renal injury.[580] Recent years have seen the wider application of MRA.[380,386,581] Its safety and accuracy make it a useful diagnostic tool for screening and diagnostic angiography of the abdominal aorta, renal, and visceral arteries in patients with renal impairment; however, interventional procedures (i.e., angioplasty and stenting) still require conventional digital subtraction angiography.

Diuretics, NSAIDs (including COX-II inhibitors), ACE inhibitors, and other vasodilators should be used with caution in patients with suspected true or effective hypovolemia or renovascular disease, because they may convert prerenal ARF to ischemic ATN and sensitize such patients to the actions of nephrotoxins. Careful monitoring of circulating drug levels appears to reduce the incidence of ARF associated with aminoglycoside antibiotics or calcineurin inhibitors.[89,121,582] Interestingly, the antimicrobial efficacy of aminoglycosides appears to persist in tissues even after the drug has been cleared from the circulation. Also, there is convincing evidence that once-daily dosing with these agents affords equal antimicrobial activity and less nephrotoxicity than conventional regimens.[123,125,582,583] The use of lipid-encapsulated formulations of amphotericin B may offer some protection against renal injury.[52,128] Several other agents are commonly employed to prevent AKI in specific clinical settings. Allopurinol (10 mg/kg/day in 3 divided doses, max 800 mg) is useful for limiting uric acid generation in patients at high risk for acute urate nephropathy; however, occasional patients receiving allopurinol still develop AKI, probably through the toxic actions of hypoxanthine crystals on tubule function.[170,395,402,404,499,584] In this setting, the use of recombinant urate oxidase (raburicase, 0.05–0.2 mg/kg) should be considered. Raburicase promotes the degradation of uric acid to allantoin and has been proven efficacy both as prophylaxis and treatment for acute uric acid–mediated tumor lysis syndrome.[404,584–587] In oligoanuric patients, prophylactic hemodialysis to remove excess uric acid may be of value.

Amifostine, an organic thiophosphate, has been demonstrated to ameliorate cisplatin nephrotoxicity in patients with solid organ or hematologic malignancies.[93,588–590] N-Acetylcysteine limits acetaminophen-induced renal injury if given within 24 hours of ingestion, and dimercaprol, a chelating agent, may prevent heavy metal nephrotoxicity.[591,592] Ethanol inhibits ethylene glycol metabolism to oxalic acid and other toxic metabolites but has been superceded by the introduction of fomepizole, an effective alcohol dehydrogenase inhibitor that decreases production of ethylene glycol metabolites and thence prevents the development of renal injury.[593–596]

Specific Therapies

During the past 2 decade there has been extensive investigation into the pathogenesis of AKI using experimental animal models and cultured cells. These studies have led to substantial advances in our understanding of the mechanisms that could potentially play a role in ATN in humans. This information has led to an exciting array of potentially novel targets for the treatment of this common and serious disease. However, a number of interventions shown to be effective in ameliorating AKI in animals have failed to be effective in humans with ATN. There are many possible reasons for lack of success in translating therapeutic successes for AKI from "bench to bedside." We lack adequate information regarding the pathology of ATN in humans in the current era, because there has been a lack of systematic studies in this area for many years. It is possible that human tissue, subjected to conventional histologic stains as well as more "state-of-the-art" approaches (such as gene array and proteomics) would facilitate the identification of those patients most likely to response to treatment.

Dopamine

Renal dose dopamine (1 to 3 mg/kg/min) has been widely advocated for the management of oliguric AKI.[597–599] In experimental animals and healthy human volunteers, renal dose dopamine increases renal blood flow and, albeit to a lesser extent, GFR. Renal dose dopamine has not been demonstrated to prevent or alter the course of ischemic or nephrotoxic ATN in prospective controlled clinical trials.[600–603] Indeed, the available evidence would suggest lack of efficacy. Furthermore, dopamine, even at low doses, is potentially toxic in critically ill patients and can induce tachyarrhythmias, myocardial ischemia, extravasation necrosis among other complications.[604] Thus, the routine administration of dopamine to patients with oliguric AKI is not justified based on the balance of experimental and clinical evidence.[605,606]

Fenoldopam

Fenoldopam is a selective postsynaptic dopamine agonist (D1-receptors) that mediates more potent renal vasodilatation and natriuresis than dopamine.[607] However, it also promotes hypotension by decreasing peripheral vasculature resistance.

Early positive results from small studies suggested a possible benefit renoprotective effect of fenoldopam in high-risk clinical situations.[608,609] However, a subsequent larger randomized trial comparing fenoldopam to standard hydration in patients undergoing invasive angiographic procedures found no benefit.[610] Moreover, in a large RCT, fenoldopam administration did not reduce mortality or the need for renal replacement therapy in ICU patients with early ATN.[611]

Natriuretic Peptides

ANP is a 28-amino acid polypeptide synthesized in cardiac atrial muscle.[598,612–614] ANP augments GFR by triggering afferent arteriolar vasodilatation and increasing Kf. In addition, ANP inhibits sodium transport and lowers oxygen requirements in several nephron segments. Synthetic analogs of ANP have shown promise in the management of ATN in the laboratory setting. To date, this promise has failed to translate into clinically apparent benefit and a large multicenter, prospective, randomized placebo controlled trial of anaritide, a synthetic analog of ANP, failed to show clinically significant improvement in dialysis-free survival or overall mortality in ATN.[615] Subgroup analysis suggested an improvement in dialysis-free survival in treated patients, but this was not confirmed in a subsequent prospective trial of patients with oliguric AKI. Ularitide (urodilantin) is a natriuretic pro-ANP fragment produced within the kidney. In a small randomized trial, ularitide did not reduce the need for dialysis in patients with AKI.[616]

Loop Diuretics

The administration of high-dose intravenous diuretics to individuals with oliguric AKI is commonly practiced.[617] Although this strategy may minimize fluid overload, there is no evidence that it alters mortality or dialysis-free survival. Some retrospective analyses have reported an increased risk of death and nonrecovery of renal function in patients treated in this manner.[618] In a recent large RCT, high-dose intravenous furosemide augmented urine output but did not alter the outcome of established AKI.[619] Given the risks of loop diuretics in AKI, including irreversible ototoxicity and exacerbation of prerenal AKI, their use should be restricted to the conservative management of volume overload (vide infra).[620,621]

Mannitol

No adequate data exist to support the routine administration of mannitol to oliguric patients. Moreover, when administered to severely oliguric or anuric patients, mannitol may trigger expansion of intravascular volume and pulmonary edema, and severe hyponatremia owing to an osmotic shift of water from the intracellular to the intravascular space.[555,567,617,622–626]

AKI caused by other intrinsic renal diseases such as acute glomerulonephritis or vasculitis may respond to corticosteroids, alkylating agents, and plasmapheresis, depending on the primary disease. Corticosteroids appear to hasten remission in some cases of allergic interstitial nephritis.[353,359,627,628] Plasma exchange is useful in treatment of sporadic TTP and possibly sporadic HUS in adults.[629,630] The role of plasmapheresis in the drug-induced thrombotic microangiopathies is less clear, and removal of the offending agent is the most important initial therapeutic maneuvre.[400,405,406] Postdiarrheal HUS in children is usually managed conservatively and evidence exists suggesting that early antibiotic therapy may actually promote the development of HUS.[631] Early studies suggested that plasmapheresis may be of benefit in ARF due to myeloma cast nephropathy.[167,564] Clearance of circulating light chains with concomitant chemotherapy to decrease the rate of production had been postulated to reverse renal injury in patients with circulating light chains, heavy Bence Jones proteinuria, and AKI. A recent relatively large

RCT compared plasma exchange and standard chemotherapy with chemotherapy alone. The study did not demonstrate improvement with plasma exchange with regard to the composite variable of death, dialysis dependence, or GFR less than 30 mL/min at 6 months, and its routine use in this setting can no longer be justified.[632]

Aggressive control of systemic arterial pressure is of paramount importance in limiting renal injury in malignant hypertensive nephrosclerosis, toxemia of pregnancy, and other vascular diseases. Hypertension and AKI associated with scleroderma may be exquisitely sensitive to treatment with ACE inhibitors.[633-635] The specifics of treatment strategies for these disorders are discussed in other chapters.

Management of Complications

Metabolic complications such as intravascular volume overload, hyperkalemia, hyperphosphatemia, and metabolic acidosis are almost invariable in oliguric AKI, and preventive measures should be taken from the time of diagnosis (Table 29–16). Prescription of nutrition should be designed to meet caloric requirements and minimize catabolism. In addition, doses of drugs excreted through the kidney must be adjusted for the degree of renal impairment.

After correction of intravascular volume deficits, salt and water intake should be adjusted to match losses (urinary, gastrointestinal, drainage sites, insensible losses). Intravascular volume overload can usually be managed by restriction of salt and water intake and by use of diuretics. Indeed, there is as yet no proven rationale for routine administration of diuretics to patients with AKI other than to treat this compli-cation. In the volume-overloaded patient, high doses of loop diuretics such as furosemide (bolus doses of up to 200 mg or up to 20 mg/hr as an IV infusion) or sequential thiazide and loop diuretic may be required if they fail to respond to conventional doses. Diuretic therapy should be discontinued in resistant patients to avoid complications such as ototoxicity. Caution should be exerted in the use of pharmacologic agents that require an obligate sodium and fluid load. Ultrafiltration or dialysis may be required for removal of volume when conservative measures fail. Hyponatremia associated with a fall in effective serum osmolality can usually be corrected by restriction of water intake. Conversely, hypernatremia is treated by administration of water, hypotonic saline solutions, or hypotonic dextrose-containing solutions (the latter are effectively hypotonic because dextrose is rapidly metabolized).

Mild hyperkalemia (<5.5 mEq/L) should be managed initially by restriction of dietary potassium intake and elimination of potassium supplements and potassium-sparing diuretics. Moderate hyperkalemia (5.5 to 6.5 mEq/L) in patients without clinical or electrocardiographic evidence of hyperkalemia can usually be controlled by administration of K+-binding ion exchange resins such as sodium polystyrene sulfonate (15 to 30 g every 3 or 4 hours) with sorbitol (50 to 100 mL of 20% solution) by mouth or as a retention enema. Loop diuretics also increase K+ excretion in diuretic-responsive patients. Emergency measures should be employed for patients with serum K+ values greater than 6.5 mEq/L and all patients with electrocardiographic abnormalities or clinical features of hyperkalemia. Intravenous insulin (5–10 U of

TABLE 29–16	Supportive Management of Intrinsic Acute Kidney Injury
Complication	**Treatment**
Intravascular Volume Overload	Restriction of salt (<1–1.5 g/day) and water (<1 L/day) Consider diuretics (usually loops +/– thiazide) Ultrafiltration
Hyponatremia	Restriction of oral and intravenous free water
Hyperkalemia	Restriction of dietary potassium Discontinue K+ supplements or K+-sparing diuretics K+-binding resin Loop diuretic Glucose (50 mls of 50%) + insulin (10–15 U regular) IV Sodium bicarbonate (50–100 meq IV) Calcium gluconate (10 mLs of 10% solution over 5 min) Dialysis/hemofiltration
Metabolic Acidosis	Restriction of dietary protein Sodium bicarbonate (if HCO_3^- <15 mEq/L) Dialysis/hemofiltration
Hyperphosphatemia	Restriction of dietary phosphate intake Phosphate binding agents (calcium carbonate, calcium acetate, sevalemer)
Hypocalcemia	Calcium carbonate (if symptomatic or sodium bicarbonate to be administered)
Hypermagnesemia	Discontinue magnesium containing antacids
Nutrition	Restriction of dietary protein (<0.8 g/kg/day up to 1.5 g/kg/day on CVVHD) 25–30 kcal/day Enteral route of nutrition preferred
Drug Dosage	Adjust all doses for GFR and renal replacement modality
Absolute Indications for RRT	Clinical evidence of uremia Intractable volume overload Hyperkalemia or severe acidosis resistant to conservative management

CVVHD, continuous venovenous hemodialysis; GFR, glomerular filtration rate; IV, intravenous; RRT, renal replacement therapy.

regular insulin) and glucose (50 mL of 50% dextrose) promote K^+ shift into cells within 30 to 60 minutes, a benefit that lasts for several hours. Sodium bicarbonate (1 ampule, 44.6 mEq intravenously over 5 minutes) also promotes rapid (onset less than 15 minutes, duration 1 to 2 hours) shift of K+ into the intracellular space as does nebulized (5–10 mg) albuterol. Sodium polysterene sulfonate and sodium bicarbonate have an obligatory sodium load; these compounds should be used judiciously for oliguric patients to avoid intravascular volume overload and life-threatening pulmonary edema. Calcium solutions such as calcium gluconate (10 mL of 10% solution intravenously over 5 minutes) antagonize the cardiac and neuromuscular effects of hyperkalemia and is a valuable emergency temporizing measure, whereas other agents reduce serum K^+ concentration. Dialysis is indicated if hyperkalemia is resistant to these measures.

Metabolic acidosis does not require treatment unless the serum HCO_3^- concentration falls below 15 mEq/L. More severe acidosis can be corrected by either oral or intravenous bicarbonate administration. Initial rates of replacement should be based on estimates of HCO_3^- deficit and adjusted thereafter according to serum levels. Patients should be monitored for complications of bicarbonate administration including metabolic alkalosis, hypocalcemia, hypokalemia, volume overload, and pulmonary edema. Hyperphosphatemia can usually be controlled by restriction of dietary phosphate intake and oral administration of agents (e.g., aluminum hydroxide, calcium carbonate or sevelamer) that reduce absorption of $PO4^{3-}$ from the gastrointestinal tract. Hypocalcemia does not usually require treatment unless it is severe, as may occur in patients with rhabdomyolysis or pancreatitis or after administration of bicarbonate. Hyperuricemia is usually mild in ARF (<15 mg/dL) and does not require specific intervention.

Nutritional management in patients with AKI requires close collaboration among physicians, nurses, and dietitians. Patients with ARF represent a heterogenous group and individualized nutritional management is required, especially in critically ill patients on renal replacement therapy in whom protein catabolic rates can exceed 1.5 g/kg body weight/day.[9,526–529,636] The objective of dietary modification in ARF is to provide sufficient calories to preserve lean body mass, avoid starvation ketoacidosis, and promote healing and tissue repair while minimizing production of nitrogenous waste. If the duration of renal insufficiency is likely to be short and the patient is not catabolic, then dietary protein should be restricted to <0.8 g/kg body weight/day. Catabolic patients, including those on continuous renal replacement therapy, may receive up to 1.4 mg/kg body weight/day. Total caloric intake should not exceed 35 kcal/kg body weight/day and will typically be in the range of 25 to 30 kcal/kg body weight/day.[526,528] The enteral route of nutrition is preferred, because it avoids the morbidity associated with parenteral nutrition while providing support to intestinal function. Management of nutrition is easier in nonoliguric patients and after institution of dialysis. Vigorous parenteral hyperalimentation has been claimed to improve prognosis in AKI; however, a consistent benefit has yet to be demonstrated in this regard. Water-soluble vitamin supplementation is advised with the exception of vitamin C, which can, in high doses (>200 mg/day), promote urinary oxalate excretion and stone formation.

Anemia may necessitate blood transfusion or administration of recombinant human erythropoietin if severe or if recovery is delayed. Uremic bleeding usually responds to desmopressin, correction of anemia, estrogens, or dialysis. Doses of drugs that are excreted by the kidney must be adjusted for the degree of renal impairment.[513] Gastric stress ulcer prophylaxis is not indicated unless the patient is intubated or has a concurrent coagulopathy. Febrile patients must be investigated aggressively for infection and may require treatment with broad-spectrum antibiotics while awaiting identification of specific organisms. Meticulous care of intravenous cannulas, Foley catheters, and other invasive devices is mandatory. Unfortunately, prophylactic antibiotics have not been shown to reduce the incidence of infection in these high-risk patients.

Indications and Modalities of Dialysis
General Comments
Dialysis does not hasten recovery from AKI. Initial studies suggesting that early dialysis therapy improved prognosis for patients with AKI have not been confirmed.[637–639] Similarly, there is no consensus on the optimal renal replacement therapy in AKI. The preferred mode of renal replacement therapy is an area of active research.[640,641] The claimed superiority of the continuous renal replacement techniques remains unproven. Neither are there evidenced-based guidelines on the initiation of dialysis in AKI.[12,642] Absolute indications for the commencement of renal replacement therapy include symptomatic uremia (asterixis, pericardial rub, encephalopathy) and acidosis, hyperkalemia, or volume overload that proves refractory to medical management. However, in clinical practice, most nephrologists initiate renal replacement therapy (RRT) before the onset of overt metabolic disarray when the need for renal support appears inevitable. The choice of dialysis modality (peritoneal dialysis, hemodialysis, or hemofiltration) is often guided by the resources of the health care institution, the technical expertise of the physician and the clinical status of the patient.

Peritoneal Dialysis
Peritoneal dialysis in AKI is effected through a temporary intraperitoneal catheter. With the development of intermittent hemodialysis, and more recently, the slow continuous blood purification therapies, there has been a decline in the use of peritoneal dialysis in the acute setting.[643–647] It is still used in the treatment of AKI in regions where access to acute intermittent or slow continuous hemodialysis is not possible. Peritoneal dialysis has the advantage of being relatively "low-tech" and portable, thus facilitating its use in remote or resource-constrained areas.[646] Systemic hypotension is typically avoided, and other benefits include the avoidance of systemic anticoagulation and need for angioaccess. Solute clearance and control of metabolic disarray in critically ill patients may be inferior to continuous veno-veno hemofiltration, and this has been associated with an adverse outcome in infection-associated AKI.[643] Other drawbacks include the risk of visceral injury during catheter placement and peritonitis subsequently.

Acute Intermittent Hemodialysis
Acute intermittent hemodialysis has been the mainstay of renal replacement therapy in AKI over the past 40 years.[638] Typically, patients undergo dialysis for 3 to 4 hours daily or on alternate days depending on their catabolic state. Vascular access for short-term hemodialysis or hemofiltration is usually achieved using a double-lumen catheter inserted into the internal jugular vein. Subclavian canulation offers an alternative but is associated with high rates of venous stenosis and is best avoided.[648] Femoral vein catheterization is technically easy and relatively free of complications. It is useful in patients who cannot tolerate the Trendelenburg position or who require only an abbreviated treatment course (e.g., removal of an exogenous toxin). Jugular lines are preferred for more prolonged treatment courses, but with careful nursing management, it is possible to maintain a femoral line in situ in the bedbound patient without incurring a significant excess infection risk.[649] The choice of membrane used during dialysis may have an effect on outcome.[650,651] Several,

although not all, RCTs indicate that the maintenance phase of ATN is significantly shorter with use of more biocompatible synthetic dialysis membranes (e.g., polysulphone, polyacrylonitrile) than with cuprophane membranes. However, systematic reviews of the literature have failed to convincingly demonstrate a benefit of synthetic over more modern substituted cellulose membranes.[652-657]

Anticoagulation with heparin is the standard method for preventing thrombosis of the extracorporeal circuit during acute intermittent dialysis.[658] Routine bedside measurement of the activated clotting time (ACT) allows heparin dosage adjustment as required to maintain a target ACT of baseline value plus 80%. Heparin-free dialysis can be performed in patients at high risk of hemorrhagic complications. This involves prerinsing the dialyzer with a heparinized solution (3000 U/L) and setting the blood flow rate at least 250 to 300 mL/min. A periodic saline rinse is then administered every 30 minutes to prevent the clotting in the extracorporeal circuit. If heparin-induced thrombocytopenia (HIT) is a concern then the heparin prerinse should be avoided. Other anticoagulation techniques include the administration of a single bolus of low-molecular-weight heparin at the start of dialysis.[659,660] Less used anticoagulant strategies include (1) regional heparinization with protamine infusion in the venous return line, (2) regional citrate anticoagulation, (3) continuous prostacyclin infusion, and (4) use of direct thrombin inhibitors: hirudin, argatroban, and lepirudin.[661-665]

The major complications of acute intermittent hemodialysis relate to rapid shifts in plasma volume and solute composition, the angioaccess procedure, and the necessity for anticoagulation.[486,524,645,666] Intradialytic hypotension is common in patients undergoing acute intermittent hemodialysis. Hypotension impairs solute clearance and the efficiency of dialysis. In addition, hypotension can further compromise renal perfusion and exacerbate tubular necrosis (see earlier). Intradialytic hypotension is typically triggered by excessive fluid removal during ultrafiltration.[667-671] The latter, in turn, may occur if the degree of hypervolemia is overestimated, if the fluid removed is not matched by flux of fluid into the intravascular space from interstitial and cellular compartments, if the volume of fluid removed is excessive, or if the patient's compensatory responses are impaired as a result of microvascular disease or vasodilatatory medications (e.g., nitrates, antihypertensive medication). Hypotension may be particularly problematic in critically ill patients with ATN and concurrent sepsis, hypoalbuminemia, malnutrition, or large third-space losses. Management of intradialytic hypotension requires careful assessment of intravascular volume, by invasive hemodynamic monitoring, if necessary; prescription of realistic ultrafiltration targets; and close observation for tachycardia or hypotension during dialysis. The immediate management of hypotension involves the discontinuation of hemofiltration, placing the patient in the Trendelenburg position, and the rapid infusion of 250 to 500 mL of normal saline.

The dialysis disequilibrium syndrome is a self-limited condition characterized by nausea, vomiting, headache, altered consciousness, and rarely, seizures or coma. It typically occurs after a first dialysis in patients with long-standing severe uremia.[524,638] The syndrome is triggered by rapid movement of water into brain cells following the development of transient plasma hypo-osmolality as solutes are rapidly cleared from the bloodstream during dialysis. The incidence of this complication has fallen in recent years, with the more gradual institution of dialysis, and the target reduction in BUN levels following the first dialysis treatment should not exceed 40%. The precise prescription of dialysis to achieve this outcome includes such variables as membrane size, blood flow rate, and duration of treatment. Typically, this will involve an initial treatment time of approximately 2 hours

with a blood flow rate of 200 to 250 mL/min. Isolated ultrafiltration can continue for a longer period if volume removal is the critical management issue.[672]

Once the patient is established on dialysis, the optimal dose of dialysis is controversial. The standards for dialysis adequacy using intermittent hemodialysis in ARF are not defined. Of note, the catabolic state observed in critically ill patients may justify large dialysis dose delivery.[12,642] In patients with AKI, the discrepancy between delivered versus prescribed hemodialysis dialysis dose may be significant owing to hemodynamic instability, filter clotting and inadequate vascular access, among other reasons. A randomized prospective trial of daily versus alternate-day hemodialysis suggested a significant mortality benefit in patients receiving daily dialysis.[486] In this study, daily hemodialysis afforded better uremic control while facilitating more intensive nutritional support without additional hemodynamic compromise and is now considered the standard of care.

The potential importance of dialysis membrane bioincompatibility as a determinant of outcome in ATN has been discussed earlier. Occasionally robust complement and leukocyte activation by cellulosic membranes is followed by leukocyte sequestration in the lungs, hypoxemia, dyspnea, and back pain; this is also called the first use syndrome.[654] More dramatic anaphylactoid reactions were occasionally seen in the past as a result of hypersensitivity to ethylene oxide used to sterilize the dialysis circuitry. These reactions are now uncommon as a result of changes in commercial sterilization techniques and the routine prerinsing of the dialysis circuit. Rarely, anaphylactoid reactions are observed in patients dialyzed on AN60 synthetic membranes who receive concomitant ACE inhibition. AN69 activates the kallikrein system and promotes bradykinin generation. The breakdown of bradykinin is inhibited by ACE inhibition so that in combination, ACE inhibitors and an AN69 membrane can dramatically augment circulating bradykinin levels.

Continuous Renal Replacement Therapy

Many patient with ATN are critically ill, hypercatabolic, and hemodynamically unstable. They frequently have large obligate fluid requirements, being on intravenous medication and parenteral alimentation. In this setting, ultrafiltration of large volumes of plasma over a relatively short period by acute intermittent hemodialysis may induce circulatory compromise. Even if tolerated hemodynamically, acute intermittent hemodialysis may not achieve adequate ultrafiltration or solute clearance to avoid life-threatening pulmonary edema or uremia, and continuous renal replacement therapy (CRRT) may be more appropriate. Hemofiltration was first described in 1977 for the management of refractory edema. Technical advances over the past 2 decades have yielded a variety of slow continuous dialytic therapies (Table 29-17) that are now well established in the management of AKI.[673,674] Whereas the various techniques differ slightly in their technical detail, they share several attractive features such as relative simplicity of operation, the ability to remove large volumes of fluid over a prolonged period with minimal hemodynamic compromise, and the capacity to control uremia and electrolyte and acid-base abnormalities with minimal perturbation of plasma osmolality.

Continuous venovenous hemodialysis (CVVHD), continuous venovenous hemofiltration (CVVH), or a combination thereof, called continuous venovenous hemodiafiltration (CVVHDF) are the techniques favored by most centers.[675] Angioaccess is achieved through a double-lumen venous catheter as described earlier. A roller pump ensures constant blood flow and generates hydraulic pressure for ultrafiltration. A variety of dialysates and filtrates are available and range from standard solutions used for peritoneal dialysis to solutions specifically tailored for CRRT. Importantly, all are

TABLE 29–17 Dialytic Modalities in Acute Kidney Injury

Modality	Dialyzer	Physical Principle	Urea Clearance (mL/min)	Middle Molecule Clearance
Hemodialysis				
Conventional	Hemodialyzer	Intermittent diffusive clearance and ultrafiltration (UF) concurrently	160	+
Sustained low efficiency dialysis (SLED)	Hemodialyzer	Intermittent, but prolonged diffusive clearance and ultrafiltration (UF) concurrently	40	+
Sequential ultrafiltration and clearance	Hemodialyzer	Intermittent (UF), followed by diffusive clearance	160	+
Continuous arteriovenous hemodialysis (CAVHD)	Hemofilter	Slow diffusive clearance and UF concurrently without a blood pump	17–21	+
Continuous venovenous hemodialysis (CVVHD)	Hemofilter	Slow diffusive clearance and UF concurrently with a blood pump	17–21	++
Hemofiltration				
Continuous arteriovenous hemofiltration (CAVHF)	Hemofilter	Continuous convective clearance without a blood pump	7–10	++
Continuous venovenous hemofitration (CVVHF)	Hemofilter	Continuous convective clearance with a blood pump	15–17	+++
Continuous venovenous hemodialysis plus hemofitration (CVVHDF)	Hemofilter	Continuous convective clearance plus diffusive clearance with a blood pump	25–26	+++
Ultrafiltration (UF)				
Isolated UF	Hemodialyzer	Intermittent UF alone	–	–
Slow continuous UF (SCUF)	Hemofilter	Continuous arteriovenous or venovenous hemofiltration UF alone without convective or diffusive clearance	1–3	
Peritoneal dialysis				
Continuous	Peritoneum	Continuous clearance and UF via exchanges performed at varying intervals	<15	+
Intermittent	Peritoneum	Intermittent clearance and UF via exchanges performed at varying intervals	<15	+

Adapted from Owen WF, Lazarus JM: Dialytic management of acute renal failure. *In* Lazarus JM, Brenner BM (eds): Acute Renal Failure, 3rd ed. New York, Churchill Livingstone, 1993.

isotonic and contain potassium well below the serum concentration. Standard solutions use lactate as their bicarbonate equivalent; however, tailored solutions may use bicarbonate or citrate as the base. Systemic heparinization is usually instituted; however, heparin requirements may be relatively low in patients with coagulopathy or thrombocytopenia, or in patients receiving replacement fluids into the dialysis circuitry before the dialysis filter (predilution fluid replacement). Regional citrate anticoagulation is an alternative anticoagulant strategy with several advantages in the critically ill patient.[676,677] Anticoagulation is achieved by infusion of trisodium citrate into the arterial blood inflow line, thus lowering the ionized calcium level and impairing the activity of calcium-dependent clotting factors. The process is reversed by a calcium infusion into the venous return line. This method provides highly effective local anticoagulation with prolonged filter life and is particularly useful in patients with HIT or in those at high risk of bleeding in whom systemic anticoagulation is contraindicated. Other anticoagulant options include prostacyclin or argatroban and lepirudin both direct thrombin inhibitors that have been used successfully for anticoagulant therapy in patients with HIT.[661,663,678]

Most modern units contain an air trap, air detector, venous pressure monitor, and automated control of the ultrafiltration rate. Clearance of low-molecular-weight solutes can be enhanced by an increase in the blood flow and dialysate rates, or by increasing the rate of hemofiltration if this technique is being used. On a milliliter-for-milliliter basis, increasing the

ultrafiltration rate is the most efficient way of improving clearance using the combined technique of CVVHDF. Some authorities have advocated prophylactic high-volume hemofiltration (>50 L/day) as an adjunctive therapy in sepsis with a view to removing septic mediators from the circulation.[679,680] No compelling prospective data exist at this time to recommend such an approach unless there is coexistent ARF requiring renal replacement therapy. As with hemodialysis, the optimal clearance targets in the slow continuous therapies is a matter of active debate. In patients undergoing continuous hemofiltration, an RCT has demonstrated that an ultrafiltration rate of 35/mL/kg/hr or above is associated with improved outcomes when compared to 20 mL/kg/hr suggesting a dose-response relationship in AKI.[681] However, further improvements in outcome from even higher ultrafiltration volumes have not been observed in randomized studies.[682]

The venovenous forms of CRRT have supplanted continuous arteriovenous techniques such as continuous arteriovenous hemodialysis and continuous arteriovenous hemodialysis plus hemofiltration (see Table 29–17) in the management of AKI. The latter techniques use arterial and venous cannulas, and rely on the patient's own blood pressure to provide the driving force for blood flow and ultrafiltration.[683,684] In the critically ill and often hemodynamically unstable patient, such methods afford less reliable blood flow rates, and the necessity for arterial cannulation incurs a risk of distal atheroembolic or artery-occlusive complications. Slow continuous ultrafiltration is a similar technique to the other slow continuous therapies described earlier except that the dialysis flow rate is set at zero and no replacement solution is administered.[685] This technique yields "pure" ultrafiltration and is typically used in the patient with marked volume overload as a result of obligate fluid intake and heart failure or capillary leak syndrome in the absence of overt uremic or metabolic indications for renal replacement.

The disadvantages of CRRT include its high cost and the need for specialized training of large numbers of nursing staff. Miscalculations in flow sheet computation can lead to significant errors in ultrafiltration rates and the continuous nature of the procedure restricts patient access to investigative procedures. Occasionally, lactate or citrate accumulation is a concern, especially in patients with severe hepatic dysfunction.[686–689] This usually manifests as a rise in total serum calcium combined with a fall in the ionized calcium level in the case of citrate accumulation. Hypophosphatemia can occur due to the higher clearance of phosphate as compared with conventional hemodialysis.

The persistent high mortality among patients with AKI requiring dialysis begs the question as to whether the continuous forms of renal replacement therapy offer any survival advantage over acute intermittent hemodialysis.[5,17,26,27,556] Several retrospective studies suggest an improvement in outcome in critically ill patients treated with CRRT; however, randomized prospective trials have failed to show a survival benefit and a more recent systematic review found no significant difference between continuous techniques and intermittent hemodialysis with regard to overall mortality.[9,690,691] However, the observed trend toward increasing use of slow continuous therapies will likely continue, especially in the hemodynamically unstable and catabolic patient.

An emerging alternative approach in the hemodynamically unstable patient is the use of slow, low-efficiency daily dialysis for prolonged periods of up to 12 hours a day.[670,692] The development of slow, low-efficiency daily dialysis is an attempt to harness the most attractive features of both intermittent hemodialysis (high efficiency, relative inexpensiveness, no requirement for presterilized fluids) and CRRT (hemodynamic stability, smooth metabolic control). This hybrid technique typically requires blood flows of less than 175 mL/min and dialysate flows less than 330 mL/min can achieve adequate solute and volume control in the critically ill patients with comparable hemodynamic stability to CRRT with less anticoagulation.[693]

Given the deficiencies of current renal replacement therapies several investigators have been investigating the potential of so-called bioartificial kidneys. These employ bioartificial tubule device using hollow fiber membranes lined with proximal tubular epithelial cells.[694–696] A small pilot study has been completed in human subjects with AKI and multiorgan failure. The renal assist device was demonstrated to possess metabolic activity with systemic effects and a randomized, controlled phase II clinical trial is under way to further assess the clinical safety and efficacy of this new therapeutic approach.[697]

Postrenal Acute Kidney Injury

Management of postrenal AKI usually involves a multidisciplinary approach and requires close collaboration among nephrologist, urologist, and radiologist. This topic is reviewed extensively in Chapter 36. Urethral or bladder neck obstruction is usually relieved temporarily by transurethral or suprapubic placement of a bladder catheter, thereby providing a window for identification and treatment of the obstructing lesion. Similarly, ureteric obstruction may be treated initially by percutaneous catheterization of the dilated ureteric pelvis or ureter. Indeed, obstructing lesions can often be removed percutaneously (e.g., calculus, sloughed papilla) or bypassed

by insertion of a ureteric stent (e.g., carcinoma). Most patients experience an appropriate diuresis for several days after relief of obstruction; however, approximately 5% develop a transient salt-wasting syndrome, because of delayed recovery of tubule function relative to GFR, that may require intravenous fluid replacement to maintain blood pressure.[332,334]

■ OUTCOME

The crude mortality rate among patients with intrinsic AKI approximates 50% and has changed little over the past 3 decades.[13,17,19–21,23,25,26,485,486,518,556,557,691,698–701] This lack of improvement in outcome, despite significant advances in supportive care, may be more apparent than real and reflect a reduction in the percentage of isolated AKI combined with an increase in AKI complicating the multiple-organ dysfunction syndrome.[25,556,702,703] When allied with the current trend for more aggressive surgical and medical intervention in the aging population, these factors probably mask an improvement in outcome. Mortality rates differ markedly depending on the cause of AKI: being approximately 15% in obstetric patients, 30% in toxin-related AKI, and 60% to 90% in patients with sepsis.[17,20,80,414,702,704] Although it was once widely held that the provision of effective renal replacement therapy largely corrected the prognostic import of an episode of AKI, more recent observations clearly demonstrate that this is not and probably never was the case, and that all too often, the development of AKI directly contributes to poor patient outcomes.[487] Factors associated with a poor prognosis include male sex, advanced age, oliguria (<400 mL/day), and a rise in the serum creatinine value of greater than 3 mg/dL, factors reflecting more severe renal injury and failure of other organ systems.

Even mild decreases in renal function are now recognized as being associated with worse patient outcomes. In a study of contrast nephropathy subjects whose serum creatinine rose by at least 25% to 2 mg/dL or over was associated with a greater than fivefold increase in mortality even after adjustment for potential confounders.[7] Although it is unclear with the use of dichotomized levels of renal function, to what extent the relationship is driven by the subjects with more extreme deteriorations in function. A study of 6000 general ICU patients found significant association between early degrees of AKI as assessed by RIFLE score and mortality.[705] Even with the use of renal replacement therapy, mortality remains elevated as compared with those with maintained independent renal function.[6,23,705]

In addition to its clinical consequences, ARF prolongs hospital stays and is associated with substantially increased medical expenditure.[5,485,706–708] The U.S. cost of treated AKI per Quality Adjusted Life Year (QALY) was estimated in 1999 to be $50,000 per QALY, a level that often raises concerns regarding the cost effectiveness of an intervention.[709] In a more recent analysis of long-term outcomes of ICU survivors who had recovered from renal failure quality adjusted survival was poor—15 QALYs per 100 patient-years in the first year postdischarge. However the subject's self-perceived health satisfaction was not significantly different from that of the general population.[710]

There are many problems with the design of most of the clinical studies that have examined the efficacy of several novel therapeutic interventions on the outcome of AKI. Measurement of the effect of treatment interventions in AKI is complicated by our inability to accurately define the onset and resolution of ARF. In addition, most clinical trials of AKI in humans have been limited because of an imbalance in the randomization of risk factors among control and experimental patients. This problem could be dealt with either by stratifying patients before randomization (using a score of severity of illness), or ideally, by studying numbers of patients large enough to ensure adequate randomization. Accurate scoring systems are needed to stratify patients enrolled in clinical trials and also to allow physicians to make informed treatment decisions including the withdrawal of medical care when the patient's condition make further intervention futile. The three most widely used general outcome mathematical models for critically ill patients are version II of the Acute Physiology and Chronic Health Evaluation (APACHE II), version II of the Acute Physiology Score and version II of the Mortality Probability Model at 24 hours.[13,525,711–713] These models were developed for critically ill patients with and without ARF, and although APACHE II may be superior in patients requiring renal replacement therapy, none are reliably predictive of outcome in the subgroup of patients with ARF. More recently, several ARF specific indices have been developed, but their generalizability outside the environment in which they were developed is uncertain.[714] In general, although several of these scoring systems are of interest from an epidemiology and research context, they remain poor discriminators of outcome in the individual patient. Finally, many human studies of AKI suffer from a lack of well-defined "end points."[12] Although the need for dialysis has been used as an end point in many trials of AKI, uniform criteria for the initiation and discontinuation of dialysis has have often not been set before the study. The necessary duration of follow-up to fully capture the sequelae of an episode of AKI is uncertain. Follow-up clearly needs to extend beyond ICU discharge and equally beyond hospital discharge, because there is some evidence that mortality rates start to stabilize after 2 months following hospital discharge.[715]

Most patients who survive an episode of AKI regain independent renal function. However, 50% have subclinical functional defects in glomerular filtration, tubule solute transport, H^+ secretion, and urinary concentrating mechanisms, and glomerular or tubulointerstitial scarring on renal biopsy (Table 29–18). AKI is irreversible in approximately 5% of patients, usually as a consequence of complete cortical necrosis, and requires long-term renal replacement therapy with dialysis or transplantation. An additional 5% of patients suffer progressive deterioration in renal function after an initial recovery phase, probably because of hyperfiltration and subsequent sclerosis of remnant glomeruli. Experimental animals and humans who experience one episode of AKI are at increased risk of additional episodes of AKI on subsequent exposure to ischemia or nephrotoxins. It is possible that the latter predisposition to acute and chronic renal failure may become increasingly relevant as human life expectancy increases.

References

1. Brady HR, Singer GG: Acute renal failure. Lancet 346:1533–1540, 1995.
2. Lameire N, Van Biesen W, Vanholder R: Acute renal failure. Lancet 365:417–430, 2005.
3. Lassnigg A, Schmidlin D, Mouhieddine M, et al: Minimal changes of serum creatinine predict prognosis in patients after cardiothoracic surgery: a prospective cohort study. J Am Soc Nephrol 15:1597–1605, 2004.
4. Thakar CV, Worley S, Arrigain S, et al: Influence of renal dysfunction on mortality after cardiac surgery: modifying effect of preoperative renal function. Kidney Int 67:1112–1119, 2005.
5. Hoste EA, Kellum JA: Acute renal failure in the critically ill: impact on morbidity and mortality. Contrib Nephrol 144:1–11, 2004.
6. Chertow GM, Levy EM, Hammermeister KE, et al: Independent association between acute renal failure and mortality following cardiac surgery. Am J Med 104:343–348, 1998.
7. Levy EM, Viscoli CM, Horwitz RI: The effect of acute renal failure on mortality. A cohort analysis. JAMA 275:1489–1494, 1996.
8. Klahr S, Miller SB: Acute oliguria. N Engl J Med 338:671–675, 1998.
9. Mehta RL, McDonald B, Gabbai FB, et al: A randomized clinical trial of continuous versus intermittent dialysis for acute renal failure. Kidney Int 60:1154–1163, 2001.
10. Kellum JA, Levin N, Bouman C, et al: Developing a consensus classification system for acute renal failure. Curr Opin Crit Care 8:509–514, 2002.
11. Bellomo R, Kellum J, Ronco C: Acute renal failure: time for consensus. Intensive Care Med 27:1685–1688, 2001.
12. Bellomo R, Ronco C, Kellum JA, et al: Acute renal failure—definition, outcome measures, animal models, fluid therapy and information technology needs: the Second International Consensus Conference of the Acute Dialysis Quality Initiative (ADQI) Group. Crit Care 8:R204–R212, 2004.
13. Abosaif NY, Tolba YA, Heap M, et al: The outcome of acute renal failure in the intensive care unit according to RIFLE: model application, sensitivity, and predictability. Am J Kidney Dis 46:1038–1048, 2005.
14. Mehta RL, Chertow GM: Acute renal failure definitions and classification: time for change? J Am Soc Nephrol 14:2178–2187, 2003.
15. Dagher PC, Herget-Rosenthal S, Ruehm SG, et al: Newly developed techniques to study and diagnose acute renal failure. J Am Soc Nephrol 14:2188–2198, 2003.
16. Herget-Rosenthal S, Marggraf G, Husing J, et al: Early detection of acute renal failure by serum cystatin C. Kidney Int 66:1115–1122, 2004.
17. Nash K, Hafeez A, Hou S: Hospital-acquired renal insufficiency. Am J Kidney Dis 39:930–936, 2002.
18. Metcalfe W, Simpson M, Khan IH, et al. Acute renal failure requiring renal replacement therapy: incidence and outcome. QJM 95:579–583, 2002.
19. Silvester W, Bellomo R, Cole L: Epidemiology, management, and outcome of severe acute renal failure of critical illness in Australia. Crit Care Med 29:1910–1915, 2001.
20. Soubrier S, Leroy O, Devos P, et al: Epidemiology and prognostic factors of critically ill patients treated with hemodiafiltration. J Crit Care 21:66–72, 2006.
21. Clermont G, Acker CG, Angus DC, et al: Renal failure in the ICU: comparison of the impact of acute renal failure and end-stage renal disease on ICU outcomes. Kidney Int 62:986–996, 2002.
22. Liano F, Pascual J: Epidemiology of acute renal failure: a prospective, multicenter, community-based study. Madrid Acute Renal Failure Study Group. Kidney Int 50:811–818, 1996.
23. Metnitz PG, Krenn CG, Steltzer H, et al: Effect of acute renal failure requiring renal replacement therapy on outcome in critically ill patients. Crit Care Med 30:2051–2058, 2002.
24. Guerin C, Girard R, Selli JM, et al: Initial versus delayed acute renal failure in the intensive care unit. A multicenter prospective epidemiological study. Rhone-Alpes Area Study Group on Acute Renal Failure. Am J Respir Crit Care Med 161:872–879, 2000.
25. Mehta RL, Pascual MT, Soroko S, et al: Spectrum of acute renal failure in the intensive care unit: the PICARD experience. Kidney Int 66:1613–1621, 2004.
26. Benoit DD, Hoste EA, Depuydt PO, et al: Outcome in critically ill medical patients treated with renal replacement therapy for acute renal failure: comparison between patients with and those without haematological malignancies. Nephrol Dial Transplant 20:552–558, 2005.
27. Xue JL, Daniels F, Star RA, et al: Incidence and mortality of acute renal failure in Medicare beneficiaries, 1992 to 2001. J Am Soc Nephrol 17:1135–1142, 2006.
28. Waikar SS, Wald R, Chertow GM, et al: Validity of international classification of diseases, ninth revision, clinical modification codes for acute renal failure. J Am Soc Nephrol 17:1688–1694, 2006.
29. Thadhani R, Pascual M, Bonventre JV: Acute renal failure. N Engl J Med 334:1448–1460, 1996.

TABLE 29–18	Residual Defects in Renal Structure and Function after Acute Kidney Injury (AKI)

Glomerular abnormalities

Thickening and/or splitting of the glomerular basement membrane
Glomerular hyalinosis
Decrease in GFR
Hyperfiltration in remnant nephrons
Increase in filtration fraction

Tubular abnormalities

Tubule atrophy
Interstitial fibrosis
Decrease in phenolsulfonphthalein excretion
Concentrating defects

Other

Proteinuria
Decrease in renal size
Predisposition to further episodes of ARF
Occasional progression to end-stage renal disease

GFR, glomerular filtration rate.
Adapted from Finn WF. Recovery from acute renal failure. *In* Lazarus JM, Brenner BM (eds): Acute Renal Failure, 3rd ed. New York: Churchill Livingstone, 1993.

30. Kon V, Yared A, Ichikawa I: Role of renal sympathetic nerves in mediating hypoperfusion of renal cortical microcirculation in experimental congestive heart failure and acute extracellular fluid volume depletion. J Clin Invest 76:1913–1920, 1985.

31. Blume A, Kaschina E, Unger T: Angiotensin II type 2 receptors: signalling and pathophysiological role. Curr Opin Nephrol Hypertens 10:239–246, 2001.

32. Aisenberry GA, Handleman WA, Arnold P, et al: Vascular effects of arginine vasopressin during fluid deprivation in the rat. J Clin Invest 67:961–968, 1981.

33. Kontogiannis J, Burns KD: Role of AT₁ angiotensin II receptors in renal ischemic injury. Am J Phtsiol 274:F79–F90, 1998.

34. Badr KF, Ichikawa I: Prerenal failure: a deleterious shift from renal compensation to decompensation. N Engl J Med 319:623–629, 1988.

35. Hall JE, Guyton AC, Jackson TE, et al: Control of glomerular filtration rate by renin-angiotensin system. Am J Physiol 233:F366–F372, 1977.

36. Lameire N, Nelde A, Hoeben H, et al: Acute renal failure in the elderly. Geriatr Nephrol Urol 9:153–165, 1999.

37. Fisch BJ, Linas LL: Prerenal acute renal failure. In Brady HR, Wilcox CS (eds): Therapy in Nephrology and Hypertension. Philadelphia, W.B. Saunders, 1998, pp 17–20.

38. Wali RK, Henrich WL: Recent developments in toxic nephropathy. Curr Opin Hyperten Nephrol 11:155–163, 2002.

39. Palmer BF: Clinical acute renal failure with non-steroidal anti-inflammatory drugs. Semin Nephrol 15:214–227, 1995.

40. Gutthann SP, Rodriguez LAG, Raiford DS, et al: Nonsteroidal anti-inflammatory drugs and the risk of hospitalization for acute renal failure. Arch Int Med 156:2433–2439, 1996.

41. Bennett WM, Henrich WL, Stoff JS: The renal effects of non-steroidal anti-inflammatory drugs: summary and recommendations. Am J Kidney Dis 29:356–362, 1996.

42. Textor SC: Renal failure related to angiotensin-converting enzyme inhibitors. Semin Nephrol 17:67–76, 1997.

43. Hays R, Aquino A, Lee BB, et al: Captopril-induced acute renal failure in a kidney transplant recipient. Clin Nephrol 19:320–321, 1983.

44. Kawamura J, Okada Y, Nishibuchi S, et al: Transient anuria following administration of angiotensin I-converting enzyme inhibitor (SQ 14225) in a patient with renal artery stenosis of the solitary kidney successfully treated with renal autotransplantation. J Urol 127:111–113, 1982.

45. Hricik DE, Browning PJ, Kopelman R, et al: Captopril-induced functional renal insufficiency in patients with bilateral renal-artery stenoses or renal-artery stenosis in a solitary kidney. N Engl J Med 308:373–376, 1983.

46. Mason JC, Hilton PJ: Reversible renal failure due to captopril in a patient with transplant artery stenosis. Case report. Hypertension 5:623–627, 1983.

47. Chrysant SG, Dunn M, Marples D, et al: Severe reversible azotemia from captopril therapy. Report of three cases and review of the literature. Arch Intern Med 143:437–441, 1983.

48. Blantz RC: Pathophysiology of pre-renal azotemia. Kidney Int 53:512–523, 1998.

49. Miller PD, Krebs RA, Neal BJ, et al: Polyuric prerenal failure. Arch Intern Med 140:907–909, 1980.

50. Singhal P, Horowitz B, Quinones MC, et al: Acute renal failure following cocaine abuse. Nephron 52:76–78, 1989.

51. Lins LE: Reversible renal failure caused by hypercalcemia. A retrospective study. Acta Med Scand 203:309–314, 1978.

52. Deray G: Amphotericin B nephrotoxicity. J Antimicrob Chemother 49(suppl 1):37–41, 2002.

53. Kon V, Awazu M: Endothelin and cyclosporine nephrotoxicity. Ren Fail 14:345–350, 1992.

54. Kunz J, Hall MN: Cyclosporin A, FK506 and rapamycin: more than just immunosuppression. Trends Biochem Sci 18:334–338, 1993.

55. Gill N, Nally JV Jr, Fatica RA: Renal failure secondary to acute tubular necrosis: epidemiology, diagnosis, and management. Chest 128:2847–2863, 2005.

56. Lieberthal W, Levinsky NG: Treatment of acute tubular necrosis. Semin Nephrol 10:571–583, 1990.

57. Thadhani RI, Camargo CA, Xavier RJ, et al: Atheroembolic renal failure after invasive procedures. Medicine 74:350–358, 1995.

58. Haimovici H: Arterial embolism, myoglobinuria, and renal tubular necrosis. Arch Surg 100:639–645, 1970.

59. Lessman RK, Johnson SF, Coburn JW, et al: Renal artery embolism: clinical features and long-term follow-up of 17 cases. Ann Intern Med 89:477–482, 1978.

60. Harrington JT, Kassirer JP: Renal vein thrombosis. Ann Rev Med 33:255–262, 1982.

61. Llach F: Hypercoagulability, renal vein thrombosis, and other thrombotic complications of nephrotic syndrome. Kidney Int 28:429–439, 1985.

62. Levine JS, Lieberthal W, Bernard DB, et al: Acute renal failure asscociated with renal vascular disease, vasculitis, glomerulonephritis and nephrotic syndrome. In Lazarus JM, Brenner BM (eds): Acute Renal Failure, 3rd ed. New York, Churchill Livingstone, 1993, pp 247–260.

63. Balow JE: Renal vasculitis. Kidney Int 27:954–964, 1985.

64. Serra A, Cameron JS, Turner DR, et al: Vasculitis affecting the kidney: Presentation, histopathology and long-term outcome. QJM LIII:181–207, 1984.

65. Kincaid-Smith P, Bennett WM, Dowling JP, et al: Acute renal failure and tubular necrosis associated with hematuria due to glomerulonephritis. Clin Nephrol 19:206–210, 1983.

66. Racusen LC: The morphologic basis of acute renal failure. In Molitorids BA, Finn WF, (eds): Acute Renal Failure. New York, W.B. Saunders Company, 2001, pp 1–12.

67. Domanovits H, Schillinger M, Mullner M, et al. Acute renal failure after successful cardiopulmonary resuscitation. Intensive Care Med 27:1194–1199, 2001.

68. Abernethy VE, Lieberthal W: Acute renal failure in the critically ill patient. Crit Care Clin 18:203–222, 2002.

69. Breen D, Bihari D: Acute renal failure as part of multi-organ failure: The slippery slope of critical illness. Kidney Int 53:S52–S33, 1998.

70. Abassi ZA, Hoffman A, Better OS: Acute renal failure complicating muscle crush injury. Semin Nephrol 18:558–565, 1998.

71. Bock HA: Pathophysiology in septic shock: From prerenal failure to renal failure. Kidney Int 53:S15–S19, 1998.

72. Brivet F, Kleinicht D, Loirat P, et al: Acute renal failure in intensive care units—causes, outcome and prognostic factors of hospital mortality: a prospective, multi-center study. Crit Care Med 24:192–198, 1996.

73. Chertow GM, Lazarus JM, Christiansen CL, et al: Preoperative renal risk stratification. Circulation 95:878–884, 1997.

74. Fortescue EB, Bates DW, Chertow GM: Predicting acute renal failure after coronary bypass surgery: cross-validation of two risk-stratification algorithms. Kidney Int 57:2594–2602, 2000.

75. Hilberman M, Myers BD, Carrie BJ, et al: Acute renal failure following cardiac surgery. J Thorac Cardiovasc Surg 77:880–888, 1979.

76. Bhat JG, Gluck MC, Lowenstein J, et al: Renal failure after open heart surgery. Ann Intern Med 84:677–682, 1976.

77. Gornick CC Jr, Kjellstrand CM: Acute renal failure complicating aortic aneurysm surgery. Nephron 35:145–157, 1983.

78. Chawla SK, Najafi H, Ing TS, et al: Acute renal failure complicating ruptured abdominal aortic aneurysm. Arch Surg 110:521–526, 1975.

79. Planas M, Wachtel T, Frank H, et al: Characterization of acute renal failure in the burned patient. Arch Intern Med 142:2087–2091, 1982.

80. Schrier RW, Wang W: Acute renal failure and sepsis. N Engl J Med 351:159–69, 2004.

81. Cole L, Bellomo R, Hart G, et al: A phase II randomized, controlled trial of continuous hemofiltration in sepsis. Crit Care Med 30:100–106, 2002.

82. Hotchkiss RS, Karl IE: The pathophysiology and treatment of sepsis. N Engl J Med 348:135–150, 2003.

83. Schor N: Acute renal failure and the sepsis syndrome. Kidney Int 61:764–776, 2002.

84. Thijs A, Thijs LG: Pathogenesis of renal failure in sepsis. Kidney Int Suppl 53:S34–S37, 1998.

85. Bone R: The pathogenesis of sepsis. Ann Intern Med 115:457–469, 1991.

86. Heyman SN, Darmon D, Goldfarb M, et al: Endotoxin-induced renal failure. I. A role for altered renal microcirculation. Exp Nephrol 8:266–274, 2000.

87. Zager RA: Endotoxemia, renal hypoperfusion and fever: interactive risk factors for aminoglycoside and sepsis-associated acute renal failure. Am J Kidney Dis 20:223–230, 1992.

88. Swan SK, Bennett WM: Nephrotoxic acute renal failure. In Lazarus JM, Brenner BM (eds): Acute Renal Failure, 3rd ed. New York, Churchill Livingstone, 1993, pp 357–370.

89. Appel GB: Aminoglycoside nephrotoxicity. Am J Med 18:558–565, 1990.

90. Berns AS: Nephrotoxicity of contrast media. Kidney Int 36:730–740, 1989.

91. Dillon JJ: Nephrotoxicity from antibacterial, antifungal and antiviral drugs. In Molitoris BA, Finn WF (eds): Acute Renal Failure. Philadelphia, W.B. Saunders, 2001, pp 349–364.

92. Andoh TF, Burdmann EA, Bennett WM: Nephrotoxicity of immunosuppressive drugs: experimental and clinical observations. Semin Nephrol 17:34–45, 1997.

93. Santini V: Amifostine: chemotherapeutic and radiotherapeutic protective effects. Expert Opin Pharmacother 2:479–489, 2001.

94. Koch Nogueira PC, Hadj-Aissa A, Schell M, et al. Long-term nephrotoxicity of cisplatin, ifosfamide, and methotrexate in osteosarcoma. Pediatr Nephrol 12:572–575, 1998.

95. Safirstein R, Winston J, Goldstein M, et al: Cisplatin nephrotoxicity. Am J Kidney Dis 8:356–367, 1986.

96. Jackson AM, Rose BD, Graff LG, et al: Thrombotic microangiopathy and renal failure associated with antineoplastic chemotherapy. Ann Intern Med 101:41–44, 1984.

97. Porter GA, Bennett WM: Nephrotoxic acute renal failure due to common drugs. Am J Physiol 241:F1–F8, 1981.

98. Winearls CG: Acute myeloma kidney. Kidney Int 48:1347–1361, 1995.

99. Murphy SA, Barrett BJ, Parfrey PS: Contrast nephropathy. J Am Soc Nephrol 11:177–182, 2000.

100. Solomon R: Radiocontrast-induced nephropathy. Semin Nephrol 18:551–557, 1998.

101. Solomon R: Contrast-medium-induced acute renal failure. Kidney Int 53:230–242, 1998.

102. Myers BD: Cyclosporine nephrotoxicity. Kidney Int 30:964–974, 1986.

103. Tepel M, Zidek W: Acetylcysteine and contrast media nephropathy. Curr Opin Nephrol Hypertens 11:503–506, 2002.

104. D'Elia JA, Gleason RE, Alday M, et al: Nephrotoxicity from angiographic contrast material. A prospective study. Am J Med 72:719–725, 1982.

105. Fang LST, Sirota RA, Ebert TH, et al: Low fractional excretion of sodium with contrast media-induced acute renal failure. Arch Intern Med 140:531–533, 1980.

106. Heyman SN, Reichman J, Brezis M: Pathophysiology of radiocontrast nephropathy: a role for medullary hypoxia. Invest Radiol 34:685–691, 1999.

107. Hizoh I, Strater J, Schick CS, et al: Radiocontrast-induced DNA fragmentation of renal tubular cells in vitro: role of hypertonicity. Nephrol Dial Transplant 13:911–918, 1998.

108. Brezis M, Epstein FH: A closer look at radiocontrast-induced nephropathy. N Engl J Med 320:179–181, 1989.

109. Heyman SN, Clark BA, Kaiser N, et al: Radiocontrast agents induce endothelin release in vivo and in vitro. J Am Soc Nephrol 3:58–65, 1992.

110. Oldroyd SD, Haylor JL, Morcos SK: Bosentan, an orally active endothelin antagonist: effect on the renal response to contrast media. Radiology 196:661–665, 1995.

111. Cantley L, Spokes K, Clark B, et al: Role of endothelin and prostaglandins in radiocontrast-induced renal artery constriction. Kidney Int 44:1217–1223, 1993.

112. Cohen DJ, Sherman WH, Osserman EF, et al: Acute renal failure in patients with multiple myeloma. Am J Med 76:247–256, 1984.

113. Benabe JE, Martinez-Maldonado M: Hypercalcemia nephropathy. Arch Intern Med 138:777–779, 1978.

114. Zager R: Rhabdomyolysis and myoglobinuric renal failure. Kidney Int 49:314–326, 1996.

115. Vetterlein R, Hoffman F, Pedina J, et al: Disturbances in the renal microcirculation induced by myoglobin and hemorrhagic hypotension in anesthetized rats. Am J Physiol 268:F839–F846, 1995.

116. Paller M: Hemoglobin- and myoglobin-induced acute renal failure in rats: role of iron in nephrotoxicity. Am J Physiol 255:F539–F544, 1988.

117. Flamenbaum W, Dubrow A: Acute renal failure associated with myoglobinuria and hemoglobinuria. In Lazarus JM, Brenner BM (eds): Acute Renal Failure, 2nd ed. New York, Churchill Livingston, 1988, pp 351–361.

118. Zager RA, Foerder CA: Effects of inorganic iron and myoglobin on in vitro proximal tubular lipid peroxidation and cytotoxicity. J Clin Invest 89:989–995, 1992.

119. Humes H: Aminoglycoside nephrotoxicity. Kidney Int 33:900–911, 1988.

120. Meyer RD: Risk factors and comparisons of clinical nephrotoxicity of aminoglycosides. Am J Med 80:119–125, 1986.

121. Moore RD, Smith CR, Lipsky JJ, et al: Risk factors for nephrotoxicity in patients treated with aminoglycosides. Ann Intern Med 100:352–357, 1984.

122. Matzke GR, Lucarotti RL, Shapiro HS: Controlled comparison of gentamicin and tobramycin nephrotoxicity. Am J Nephrol 3:11–17, 1983.

123. Hatala R, Dinh T, Cook DJ: Once-daily aminoglycoside dosing in immunocompetent adults: a meta- analysis. Ann Intern Med 124:717–725, 1996.

124. Prins JM, Buller HR, Kuijper EJ, et al: Once versus thrice daily gentamicin in patients with serious infections. Lancet 341:335–339, 1993.

125. Gilbert DN: Once-daily aminoglycoside therapy. Antimicrob Agents Chemother 35:399–405, 1991.

126. Moore RD, Smith CR, Lietman PS: Increased risk of renal dysfunction due to interaction of liver disease and aminoglycoside. Am J Med 80:1093–1097, 1986.

127. Moestrup SK, Cui S, Vorum H, et al: Evidence that epithelial glycoprotein 330/megalin mediates uptake of polybasic drugs. J Clin Invest 96:1404–1413, 1995.

128. Sorkine P, Nagar H, Weinbroum A, et al: Administration of amphotericin B in lipid emulsion decreases nephrotoxicity: results of a prospective, randomized, controlled study in critically ill patients. Crit Care Med 24:1311–1315, 1996.

129. Sawyer MH, Webb DE, Balow JE, et al: Acyclovir-induced renal failure. Clinical course and histology. Am J Med 84:1067–1071, 1988.

130. Spiegal DM, Lau K: Acute renal failure and coma secondary to acyclovir therapy. JAMA 255:1882–1883, 1986.

131. Flexner C: HIV-protease inhibitors. N Engl J Med 338:1281–1292, 1998.

132. Izzedine H, Launay-Vacher V, Deray G: Antiviral drug-induced nephrotoxicity. Am J Kidney Dis 45:804–817, 2005.

133. Malik A, Abraham P, Malik N: Acute renal failure and Fanconi syndrome in an AIDS patient on tenofovir treatment—case report and review of literature. J Infect 51:E61–E65, 2005.

134. Kay TD, Hogan PG, McLeod SE, et al: Severe irreversible proximal renal tubular acidosis and azotaemia secondary to cidofovir. Nephron 86:348–349, 2000.

135. Chapelon C, Raguin G, De Gennes C: Renal insufficiency with nebulised pentamidine. Lancet 2:1045–1046, 1989.

136. Miller RF, Delany S, Semple SJ: Acute renal failure after nebulised pentamidine. Lancet 1:1271–1272, 1989.

137. Lachaal M, Venuto RC: Nephrotoxicity and hyperkalemia in patients with acquired immunodeficiency syndrome treated with pentamidine. Am J Med 87:260–263, 1989.

138. Deray G, Martinez F, Katlama C, et al: Foscarnet nephrotoxicity: mechanism, incidence and prevention. Am J Nephrol 9:316–321, 1989.

139. Deray G, Katlama C, Dohin E: Prevention of foscarnet nephrotoxicity. Ann Intern Med 113:332, 1990.

140. Farese RV Jr, Schambelan M, Hollander H, et al: Nephrogenic diabetes insipidus associated with foscarnet treatment of cytomegalovirus retinitis. Ann Intern Med 112:955–956, 1990.

141. Skinner R, Pearson AD, Price L, et al: Nephrotoxicity after ifosfamide. Arch Dis Child 65:732–738, 1990.

142. Weiner M, Jacobs C: Mechanism of cisplatin nephrotoxicity. Federation Proc 42:2974–2978, 1983.

143. Goldstein R, Mayor G: The nephrotoxicity of cisplatin. Life Sci 32:685–690, 1983.

144. Humes HD, Weinberg JM, Knauss TC: Clinical and pathophysiologic aspects of aminoglycoside nephrotoxicity. Am J Kidney Dis 2:5–29, 1982.

145. Orrenius S: Apoptosis: molecular mechanisms and implications for human disease. J Int Med 237:529–536, 1995.

146. Lieberthal W, Triaca V, Levine J: Mechanisms of death induced by cisplatin in proximal tubular epithelial cells: apoptosis vs. necrosis. Am J Physiol 270:F700–F708, 1996.

147. Sanchez-Perez I, Perona R: Lack of c-Jun activity increases survival to cisplatin. FEBS Lett 453:151–158, 1999.

148. Smeitink J, Verreussel M, Schroder C, et al: Nephrotoxicity associated with ifosfamide. Eur J Pediatr 148:164–166, 1988.

149. Patterson WP, Khojasteh A: Ifosfamide-induced renal tubular defects. Cancer 63:649–651, 1989.

150. Abelson HT, Fosburg MT, Beardsley GP, et al: Methotrexate-induced renal impairment: clinical studies and rescue from systemic toxicity with high-dose leucovorin and thymidine. J Clin Oncol 1:208–216, 1983.

151. Chacko B, John GT, Balakrishnan N, et al: Osmotic nephropathy resulting from maltose-based intravenous immunoglobulin therapy. Ren Fail 28:193–195, 2006.

152. Shah S, Vervan M: Use of i.v. immune globulin and occurrence of associated acute renal failure and thrombosis. Am J Health Syst Pharm 62:720–725, 2005.

153. Chapman SA, Gilkerson KL, Davin TD, et al: Acute renal failure and intravenous immune globulin: occurs with sucrose-stabilized, but not with D-sorbitol-stabilized, formulation. Ann Pharmacother 38:2059–2067, 2004.

154. Sever M, Vanholder R, Lameire N: Management of crush-related injuries after disasters. N Engl J Med 354:1052–1063, 2006.

155. Vanholder R, Sever M, Erek E, et al: Rhabdomyolysis. J Am Soc Nephrol 11:1553–1561, 2000.

156. Ward M: Factors predictive of acute renal failure in rhabdomyolysis. Arch Intern Med 148:1553–1557, 1988.

157. Honda N, Kurokawa K: Acute renal failure and rhabdomyolysis. Kidney Int 23:888–898, 1983.

158. Knochel JP: Rhabdomyolysis and myoglobinuria. Annu Rev Med 33:435–443, 1982.

159. Gabow PA, Kaehny WD, Kelleher SP: The spectrum of rhabdomyolysis. Medicine (Baltimore) 61:141–152, 1982.

160. Dubrow A, Flamenbaum W: Acute renal failure associated with myoglobinuria and hemoglobinuria. In Brenner BM, Lazarus JM (eds): Acute Renal Failure, 2nd ed. New York, Churchill Livinstone, 1988, pp 279–293.

161. Nath KA, Bella G, Vercellotti GM, et al: Induction of heme oxygenase is a rapid, protective response in rhabdomyolysis in the rat. J Clin Inv 90:267–270, 1992.

162. Zager RA: Heme-protein induced tubular resistance: expression at the plasma membrane level. Kidney Int 47:1336–1345, 1995.

163. Karam H, Bruneval P, Clozel J-P, et al: Role of endothelin in acute renal falure due to rhabdomyolysis in rats. J Pharmacol Exp Ther 274:481–486, 1995.

164. Ron D, Taitelman U, Michaelson M, et al: Prevention of acute renal failure in traumatic rhabdomyolysis. Arch Intern Med 144:277–280, 1984.

165. Siami GA, Siami FS: Plasmapheresis and paraproteinemia: cryoprotein-induced diseases, monoclonal gammopathy, Waldenstrom's macroglobulinemia, hyperviscosity syndrome, multiple myeloma, light chain disease, and amyloidosis. Ther Apher 3:8–19, 1999.

166. Buxbaum JN, Chuba JV, Hellman GC, et al: Monoclonal immunoglobulin deposition disease: light chain and light and heavy chain deposition diseases and their relation to light chain amyloidosis. Clinical features, immunopathology, and molecular analysis. Ann Intern Med 112:455–464, 1990.

167. Zucchelli P, Pasquali S, Cagnoli L, et al: Controlled plasma exchange trial in acute renal failure due to multiple myeloma. Kidney Int 33:1175–1180, 1988.

168. Sanders PW, Booker BB: Pathobiology of cast nephropathy from human Bence Jones proteins. J Clin Invest 89:630–639, 1992.

169. Hill GS, Morel-Maroger L, Mery JP, et al: Renal lesions in multiple myeloma: Their relationship to associated protein abnormalities. Am J Kidney Dis II:423–438, 1983.

170. Conger JD: Acute uric acid nephropathy. Med Clin North Am 74:859–871, 1990.

171. Weinman EJ, Knight TF: Uric acid and the kidney. In Suki W, Ecknoyan G (eds): The Kidney in Systemic Disease. London, Suki and Eknoyan, 1981, pp 285–305.

172. Conger JD: Acute uric acid nephropathy. Semin Nephrol 1:69–74, 1981.

173. Tungsanga K, Boonwichit D, Lekhakula A, et al: Urine uric acid and urine creatine ratio in acute renal failure. Arch Intern Med 144:934–937, 1984.

174. Lawton JM, Conway LT, Crosson JT, et al: Acute oxalate nephropathy after massive ascorbic acid administration. Arch Intern Med 145:950–951, 1985.

175. Gilboa N, Largent JA, Urizar RE: Primary oxalosis presenting as anuric renal failure in infancy: diagnosis by x-ray diffraction of kidney tissue. J Pediatr 103:88–90, 1983.

176. Frommer JP, Ayus JC: Acute ethylene glycol intoxication. Am J Nephrol 2:1–5, 1982.

177. Mandell I, Krauss E, Millan JC: Oxalate-induced acute renal failure in Crohn's disease. Am J Med 69:628–632, 1980.

178. Ehlers SM, Posalaky Z, Strate RG, et al: Acute reversible renal failure following jejunoileal bypass for morbid obesity: a clinical and pathological (EM) study of a case. Surgery 82:629–634, 1977.

179. Merino GE, Buselmeier TJ, Kjellstrand CM: Postoperative chronic renal failure: a new syndrome? Ann Surg 182:37–44, 1975.

180. Olsen TS, Hansen HE: Ultrastructure of medullary tubules in ischemic acute tubular necrosis and acute interstitial nephritis in man. Apmis 98:1139–1148, 1990.

181. Racusen LC: Pathology of acute renal failure: structure/function correlations. Adv Renal Replacement Ther 4:3–16, 1997.

182. Venkatachalam MA, Bernard DB, Donohoe J, et al: Ischemic damage and repair in the rat proximal tubule. Differences among S1, S2 and S3 segments. Kidney Int 14:31–49, 1978.

183. Olsen S, Burdick JF, Keown PA, et al: Primary acute renal failure ('acute tubular necrosis') in the transplanted kidney: Morphology and pathogenesis. Medicine 68:173–187, 1989.

184. Solez K, Morel-Moroger L, Sraer JD: The morphology of "acute tubular necrosis" in man: analysis of 57 renal biopsies and a comparison with the glycerol modeL. Medicine 58:362–376, 1979.

185. Olsen TS, Hansen HE, Olsen HS: Tubular ultrastructure in acute renal failure: alterations of cellular surfaces (brush-border and basolateral infoldings). Virchows Arch A Pathol Anat Histopathol 406:91–104, 1985.

186. Solez K, Racusen LC: Role of the renal biopsy in acute renal failure. Contrib Nephrol 132:68–75, 2001.

187. Wangsiripaisan A, Gengaro PE, Edelstein CL, et al: Role of polymeric Tamm-Horsfall protein in cast formation: oligosaccharide and tubular fluid ions. Kidney Int 59:932–940, 2001.

188. Kwon O, Nelson WJ, Sibley R, et al: Backleak, tight junctions and cell-cell adhesion in postischemic injury to the renal allograft. J Clin Invest 101:2054–2064, 1998.

189. Alejandro V, Scandling JD Jr, Sibley RK, et al: Mechanisms of filtration failure during postischemic injury of the human kidney. A study of the reperfused renal allograft. J Clin Invest 95:820–831, 1995.

190. Burke TJ, Cronin RE, Duchin KL, et al: Ischemia and tubule obstruction during acute renal failure in dogs: mannitol in protection. Am J Physiol 238:F305–F314, 1980.

191. Tanner GA, Sophasan S: Kidney pressures after temporary artery occlusion in the rat. Am J Physiol 230:1173–1181, 1976.

192. Arendshorst WJ, Finn WF, Gottschalk CW, et al: Micropuncture study of acute renal failure following temporary renal ischemia in the rat. Kidney Int 10(suppl 6):S100–S105, 1976.

193. Sutton TA, Fisher CJ, Molitoris BA: Microvascular endothelial injury and dysfunction during ischemic acute renal failure. Kidney Int 62:1539–1549, 2002.

194. Lee DB, Huang E, Ward HJ: Tight junction biology and kidney dysfunction. Am J Physiol Renal Physiol 290:F20–F34, 2006.

195. Canfield PE, Geerdes AM, Molitoris BA: Effect of reversible ATP depletion on tight-junction integrity in LLC-PK1 cells. Am J Physiol 261:F1038–F1045, 1991.

196. Ye J, Tsukamoto T, Sun A, et al: A role for intracellular calcium in tight junction reassembly after ATP depletion-repletion. Am J Physiol 277:F524–F532, 1999.

197. Kwon TH, Frokiaer J, Fernandez-Llama P, et al: Reduced abundance of aquaporins in rats with bilateral ischemia-induced acute renal failure: prevention by alpha-MSH. Am J Physiol 277:F413–F427, 1999.

198. Gong H, Wang W, Kwon TH, et al: EPO and alpha-MSH prevent ischemia/reperfusion-induced down-regulation of AQPs and sodium transporters in rat kidney. Kidney Int 66:683–695, 2004.

199. Wang Z, Rabb H, Haq M, et al: A possible molecular basis of natriuresis during ischemic-reperfusion injury in the kidney. J Am Soc Nephrol 9:605–613, 1998.

200. Friedewald JJ, Rabb H: Inflammatory cells in ischemic acute renal failure. Kidney Int 66:486–491, 2004.

201. Chou SY, Porush JG, Faubert PF: Renal medullary circulation: hormonal control. Kidney Int 37:1–13, 1990.

202. Pallone TL, Turner MR, Edwards A, et al: Countercurrent exchange in the renal medulla. Am J Physiol Regul Integr Comp Physiol 284:R1153–R1175, 2003.

203. Pallone TL, Zhang Z, Rhinehart K: Physiology of the renal medullary microcirculation. Am J Physiol Renal Physiol 284:F253–F266, 2003.

204. Brezis M, Rosen S: Hypoxia of the renal medulla—its implications for disease. N Engl J Med 332:647–655, 1995.

205. Kwon O, Phillips CL, Molitoris BA: Ischemia induces alterations in actin filaments in renal vascular smooth muscle cells. Am J Physiol Renal Physiol 282:F1012–F1019, 2002.

206. Olof P, Hellberg A, Kallskog O, et al: Red cell trapping and post-ischemic renal blood flow. Differences between the cortex, outer and inner medulla. Kidney Int 40:625–631, 1991.

207. Mason J, Welsch J, Torhorst J: The contribution of vascular obstruction to the functional defect that follows renal ischemia. Kidney Int 31:65–71, 1987.

208. Yamamoto T, Tada T, Brodsky SV, et al: Intravital videomicroscopy of peritubular capillaries in renal ischemia. Am J Physiol Renal Physiol 282:F1150–F1155, 2002.

209. Spiegel DM, Shanley PF, Molitoris BA: Mild ischemia predisposes the S3 segment to gentamicin toxicity. Kidney Int 38:459–464, 1990.

210. Ysebaert DK, De Greef KE, Vercauteren SR, et al: Identification and kinetics of leukocytes after severe ischaemia/reperfusion renal injury. Nephrol Dial Transplant 15:1562–1574, 2000.

211. Paller MS: Effect of neutrophil depletion on ischemic renal injury in the rat. J Lab Clin Med 113:379–386, 1989.

212. Thornton MA, Winn R, Alpers CE, et al: An evaluation of the neutrophil as a mediator of in vivo renal ischemic-reperfusion injury. Am J Pathol 135:509–515, 1989.

213. Singbartl K, Forlow SB, Ley K: Platelet, but not endothelial, P-selectin is critical for neutrophil-mediated acute postischemic renal failure. FASEB J 15:2337–2344, 2001.

214. Nemoto T, Burne MJ, Daniels F, et al: Small molecule selectin ligand inhibition improves outcome in ischemic acute renal failure. Kidney Int 60:2205–2211, 2001.

215. Burne MJ, Rabb H: Pathophysiological contributions of fucosyltransferases in renal ischemia reperfusion injury. J Immunol 169:2648–2652, 2002.

216. Rabb H, Mediola C, Dietz J, et al: Role of CD11a and CD11b in ischemic acute renal failure in rats. Am J Physiol 267:F1052–F1058, 1994.

217. Kelly KJ, Williams WW, Colvin RB, et al: Intercellular adhesion molecule-1-deficient mice are protected against ischemic renal injury. J Clin Invest 97:1056–1063, 1996.

218. Haug C, Colvin R, Delmonico F, et al: Phase 1 trial of immunosuppression with anti-ICAM (CD54) mAb in renal allograft recipients. Transplantation (Baltimore) 55:766–773, 1993.

219. Salmela K, Wramner L, Ekberg H, et al: A randomized multicenter trial of the anti-ICAM-1 monoclonal antibody (enlimomab) for the prevention of acute rejection and delayed onset of graft function in cadaveric renal transplantation: a report of the European Anti-ICAM-1 Renal Transplant Study Group. Transplantation 67:729–736, 1999.

220. Chiao H, Kohda Y, McLeroy P, et al: Alpha-melanocyte-stimulating hormone protectes againts acute renal injury after ischemia in mice and rats. J Clin Invest 99:1165–1172, 1997.

221. Chiao H, Kohda Y, McLeroy P, et al: Alpha-melanocyte-stimulating hormone inhibits renal injury in the absence of neutrophils. Kidney Int 54:765–774, 1998.

222. Jo SK, Yun SY, Chang KH, et al: Alpha-MSH decreases apoptosis in ischaemic acute renal failure in rats: possible mechanism of this beneficial effect. Nephrol Dial Transplant 16:1583–1591, 2001.

223. Okusa MD, Linden J, Huang L, et al: A(2A) adenosine receptor-mediated inhibition of renal injury and neutrophil adhesion. Am J Physiol Renal Physiol 279:F809–F818, 2000.

224. Day YJ, Huang L, Ye H, et al: Renal ischemia-reperfusion injury and adenosine 2A receptor-mediated tissue protection: the role of CD4+ T cells and IFN-gamma. J Immunol 176:3108–3114, 2006.

225. Riera M, Torras J, Herrero I, et al: Neutrophils accentuate renal cold ischemia-reperfusion injury. Dose-dependent protective effect of a platelet-activating factor receptor antagonist. J Pharmacol Exp Ther 280:786–794, 1997.

226. Lemay S, Rabb H, Postler G, et al: Prominent and sustained up-regulation of gp130-signaling cytokines and the chemokine MIP-2 in murine renal ischemia-reperfusion injury. Transplantation 69:959–963, 2000.

227. Takada M, Nadeau KC, Shaw GD, et al: The cytokine-adhesion molecule cascade on ischemia/reperfusion injury of the rat kidney: inhibition by a soluble P-selectin ligand. J Clin Invest 99:2682–2690, 1997.

228. Rabb H, Daniels F, O'Donnell M, et al: Pathophysiological role of T lymphocytes in renal ischemia-reperfusion injury in mice. Am J Physiol Renal Physiol 279:F525–F531, 2000.

229. Burne MJ, Daniels F, El Ghandour A, et al: Identification of the CD4(+) T cell as a major pathogenic factor in ischemic acute renal failure. J Clin Invest 108:1283–1290, 2001.

230. Faubel S, Ljubanovic D, Poole B, et al: Peripheral CD4 T-cell depletion is not sufficient to prevent ischemic acute renal failure. Transplantation 80:643–649, 2005.

231. Yokota N, Daniels F, Crosson J, et al: Protective effect of T cell depletion in murine renal ischemia-reperfusion injury. Transplantation 74:759–763, 2002.

232. Takada M, Chandraker A, Nadeau KC, et al: The role of the B7 costimulatory pathway in experimental cold ischemia/reperfusion injury. J Clin Invest 100:1199–1203, 1997.

233. De Greef KE, Ysebaert DK, Dauwe S, et al: Anti-B7-1 blocks mononuclear cell adherence in vasa recta after ischemia. Kidney Int 60:1415–1427, 2001.

234. Ascon DB, Lopez-Briones S, Liu M, et al: Phenotypic and functional characterization of kidney-infiltrating lymphocytes in renal ischemia reperfusion injury. J Immunol 177:3380–3387, 2006.

235. Park P, Haas M, Cunningham PN, et al: Injury in renal ischemia-reperfusion is independent from immunoglobulins and T lymphocytes. Am J Physiol Renal Physiol 282:F352–F357, 2002.

236. Leemans JC, Stokman G, Claessen N, et al: Renal-associated TLR2 mediates ischemia/reperfusion injury in the kidney. J Clin Invest 115:2894–2903, 2005.

237. Cunningham PN, Wang Y, Guo R, et al: Role of Toll-like receptor 4 in endotoxin-induced acute renal failure. J Immunol 172:2629–2635, 2004.

238. Dear JW, Yasuda H, Hu X, et al: Sepsis-induced organ failure is mediated by different pathways in the kidney and liver: Acute renal failure is dependent on MyD88 but not renal cell apoptosis. Kidney Int 69:832–836, 2006.

239. Ueda N, Kaushal GP, Shah SV: Apoptotic mechanisms in acute renal failure. Am J Med 108:403–415, 2000.

240. Ortiz A: Nephrology forum: apoptotic regulatory proteins in renal injury. Kidney Int 58:467–485, 2000.

241. Beeri R, Symon Z, Brezis M, et al: Rapid DNA fragmentation from hypoxia along the thick ascending limb of rat kidneys. Kidney Int 47:1806–1810, 1995.

242. Allen J, Winterford C, Axelsen RA, et al: Effects of hypoxia on morphological and biochemical characteristics of renal epithelial cell and tubule cultures. Ren Fail 14:453–460, 1992.

243. Wiegele G, Brandis M, Zimmerhackl LB: Apoptosis and necrosis during ischaemia in renal tubular cells (LLC-PK1 and MDCK). Nephrol Dial Transplant 13:1158–1167, 1998.

244. Jaffe R, Ariel I, Beeri R, et al: Frequent apoptosis in human kidneys after acute renal hypoperfusion. Exp Nephrol 5:399–403, 1997.

245. Castaneda MP, Swiatecka-Urban A, Mitsnefes MM, et al: Activation of mitochondrial apoptotic pathways in human renal allografts after ischemiareperfusion injury. Transplantation 76:50–54, 2003.

246. Burns AT, Davies DR, McLaren AJ, et al: Apoptosis in ischemia/reperfusion injury of human renal allografts. Transplantation 66:872–876, 1998.

247. Adams JM, Cory S: The Bcl-2 protein family: arbiters of cell survival. Science 281:1322–1326, 1998.

248. Thornberry NA, Lazebnik Y: Caspases: enemies within. Science 281:1312–1316, 1998.

249. Daemen MA, van 't Veer C, Denecker G, et al: Inhibition of apoptosis induced by ischemia-reperfusion prevents inflammation. J Clin Invest 104:541–549, 1999.

250. Daemen MA, de Vries B, van't Veer C, et al: Apoptosis and chemokine induction after renal ischemia-reperfusion. Transplantation 71:1007–1011, 2001.

251. Kelly KJ, Sutton TA, Weathered N, et al: Minocycline inhibits apoptosis and inflammation in a rat model of ischemic renal injury. Am J Physiol Renal Physiol 287:F760–F66, 2004.

252. Cohen O, Inbal B, Kissil JL, et al: DAP-kinase participates in TNF-alpha- and Fas-induced apoptosis and its function requires the death domain. J Cell Biol 146:141–148, 1999.

253. Kishino M, Yukawa K, Hoshino K, et al: Deletion of the kinase domain in death-associated protein kinase attenuates tubular cell apoptosis in renal ischemia-reperfusion injury. J Am Soc Nephrol 15:1826–1834, 2004.

254. Wang WJ, Kuo JC, Yao CC, et al: DAP-kinase induces apoptosis by suppressing integrin activity and disrupting matrix survival signals. J Cell Biol 159:169–179, 2002.

255. Patel NS, Sharples EJ, Cuzzocrea S, et al: Pretreatment with EPO reduces the injury and dysfunction caused by ischemia/reperfusion in the mouse kidney in vivo. Kidney Int 66:983–989, 2004.

256. Sharples EJ, Patel N, Brown P, et al: Erythropoietin protects the kidney against the injury and dysfunction caused by ischemia-reperfusion. J Am Soc Nephrol 15:2115–2124, 2004.

257. Spandou E, Tsouchnikas I, Karkavelas G, et al: Erythropoietin attenuates renal injury in experimental acute renal failure ischaemic/reperfusion model. Nephrol Dial Transplant 21:330–336, 2006.

258. Vesey DA, Cheung C, Pat B, et al: Erythropoietin protects against ischaemic acute renal injury. Nephrol Dial Transplant 19:348–355, 2004.

259. Jo SK, Yun SY, Chang KH, et al: Alpha-MSH decreases apoptosis in ischaemic acute renal failure in rats: possible mechanism of this beneficial effect. Nephrol Dial Transplant 16:1583–1591, 2001.

260. Arany I, Megyesi JK, Kaneto H, et al: Cisplatin-induced cell death is EGFR/src/ERK signaling dependent in mouse proximal tubule cells. Am J Physiol Renal Physiol 287: F543–F549, 2004.

261. Price PM, Safirstein RL, Megyesi J: Protection of renal cells from cisplatin toxicity by cell cycle inhibitors. Am J Physiol Renal Physiol 286:F378–F384, 2004.

262. Pinzani V, Bressolle F, Haug IJ, et al: Cisplatin-induced renal toxicity and toxicity-modulating strategies: a review. Cancer Chemother Pharmacol 35:1–9, 1994.

263. Sutton TA, Fisher CJ, Molitoris BA: Microvascular endothelial injury and dysfunction during ischemic acute renal failure. Kidney Int 62:1539–1549, 2002.

264. Molitoris BA, Sutton TA: Endothelial injury and dysfunction: role in the extension phase of acute renal failure. Kidney Int 66:496–499, 2004.

265. Hinshaw DB, Burger JM, Miller MT, et al: ATP depletion induces an increase in the assembly of a labile pool of polymerized actin in endothelial cells. Am J Physiol 264: C1171–C1179, 1993.

266. Bamburg JR: Proteins of the ADF/cofilin family: essential regulators of actin dynamics. Annu Rev Cell Dev Biol 15:185–230, 1999.

267. Suurna MV, Ashworth SL, Hosford M, et al: Cofilin mediates ATP depletion-induced endothelial cell actin alterations. Am J Physiol Renal Physiol 290:F1398–F1407, 2006.

268. Guan Z, Gobe G, Willgoss D, et al: Renal endothelial dysfunction and impaired auto-regulation after ischemia-reperfusion injury result from excess nitric oxide. Am J Physiol Renal Physiol 291:619–628, 2006.

269. Brodsky SV, Yamamoto T, Tada T, et al: Endothelial dysfunction in ischemic acute renal failure: rescue by transplanted endothelial cells. Am J Physiol Renal Physiol 282:F1140–F1149, 2002.

270. Eppihimer MJ, Russell J, Anderson DC, et al: Modulation of P-selectin expression in the postischemic intestinal microvasculature. Am J Physiol 273:G1326–G1332, 1997.

271. Molitoris BA, Marrs J: The role of cell adhesion molecules in ischemic acute renal failure. Am J Med 106:583–592, 1999.

272. Singbartl K, Ley K: Leukocyte recruitment and acute renal failure. J Mol Med 82:91–101, 2004.

273. Bonventre JV: Dedifferentiation and proliferation of surviving epithelial cells in acute renal failure. J Am Soc Nephrol 14(suppl 1):S55–S61, 2003.

274. Molitoris BA, Dahl R, Geerdes A: Cytoskeleton disruption and apical redistribution of proximal tubule Na(+)-K(+)-ATPase during ischemia. Am J Physiol 263:F488–F495, 1992.

275. Molitoris BA: Actin cytoskeleton in ischemic acute renal failure. Kidney Int 66:871–883, 2004.

276. Devarajan P: Update on mechanisms of ischemic acute kidney injury. J Am Soc Nephrol 17:1503–1520, 2006.

277. Woroniecki R, Ferdinand JR, Morrow JS, et al: Dissociation of spectrin-ankyrin complex as a basis for loss of Na-K-ATPase polarity after ischemia. Am J Physiol Renal Physiol 284:F358–F364, 2003.

278. Mollura DJ, Hare JM, Rabb H: Stem-cell therapy for renal diseases. Am J Kidney Dis 42:891–905, 2003.

279. Lin F: Stem cells in kidney regeneration following acute renal injury. Pediatr Res 59:74R–78R, 2006.

280. Pittenger MF, Mackay AM, Beck SC, et al: Multilineage potential of adult human mesenchymal stem cells. Science 284:143–147, 1999.

281. Kale S, Karihaloo A, Clark PR, et al: Bone marrow stem cells contribute to repair of the ischemically injured renal tubule. J Clin Invest 112:42–49, 2003.

282. Lin F, Cordes K, Li L, et al: Hematopoietic stem cells contribute to the regeneration of renal tubules after renal ischemia-reperfusion injury in mice. J Am Soc Nephrol 14:1188–1199, 2003.

283. Lange C, Togel F, Ittrich H, et al: Administered mesenchymal stem cells enhance recovery from ischemia/reperfusion-induced acute renal failure in rats. Kidney Int 68:1613–1617, 2005.

284. Togel F, Hu Z, Weiss K, et al: Administered mesenchymal stem cells protect against ischemic acute renal failure through differentiation-independent mechanisms. Am J Physiol Renal Physiol 289:F31–F42, 2005.

285. Rabb H: Paracrine and differentiation mechanisms underlying stem cell therapy for the damaged kidney. Am J Physiol Renal Physiol 289:F29–F30, 2005.

286. Mizuno S, Nakamura T: Prevention of neutrophil extravasation by hepatocyte growth factor leads to attenuations of tubular apoptosis and renal dysfunction in mouse ischemic kidneys. Am J Pathol 166:1895–1905, 2005.

287. Patschan D, Plotkin M, Goligorsky MS: Therapeutic use of stem and endothelial progenitor cells in acute renal injury: ca ira. Curr Opin Pharmacol 6:176–183, 2006.

288. Patschan D, Krupincza K, Patschan S, et al: Dynamics of mobilization and homing of endothelial progenitor cells after acute renal ischemia: modulation by ischemic pre-conditioning. Am J Physiol Renal Physiol 1:176–185, 2006.

289. Al-Awqati Q, Oliver JA: Stem cells in the kidney. Kidney Int 61:387–395, 2002.

290. Oliver JA, Maarouf O, Cheema FH, et al: The renal papilla is a niche for adult kidney stem cells. J Clin Invest 114:795–804, 2004.

291. Moore FA, Moore EE: Evolving concepts in the pathogenesis of postinjury multiple organ failure. Surg Clin North Am 75:257–277, 1995.

292. Rabb H, Chamoun F, Hotchkiss J: Molecular mechanisms underlying combined kidney-lung dysfunction during acute renal failure. Contrib Nephrol 132:41–52, 2001.

293. Kramer AA, Postler G, Salhab KF, et al: Renal ischemia/reperfusion leads to macro-phage-mediated increase in pulmonary vascular permeability. Kidney Int 55:2362–2367, 1999.

294. Rabb H, Wang Z, Nemoto T, et al: Acute renal failure leads to dysregulation of lung salt and water channels. Kidney Int 63:600–606, 2003.

295. Nath KA, Grande JP, Croatt AJ, et al: Transgenic sickle mice are markedly sensitive to renal ischemia-reperfusion injury. Am J Pathol 166:963–972, 2005.

296. Zhang Y, Woodward VK, Shelton JM, et al: Ischemia-reperfusion induces G-CSF gene expression by renal medullary thick ascending limb cells in vivo and in vitro. Am J Physiol Renal Physiol 286:F1193–F1201, 2004.

297. Kielar ML, John R, Bennett M, et al: Maladaptive role of IL-6 in ischemic acute renal failure. J Am Soc Nephrol 16:3315–3325, 2005.

298. Kielar ML, Rohan Jeyarajah D, Lu CY: The regulation of ischemic acute renal failure by extrarenal organs. Curr Opin Nephrol Hypertens 11:451–457, 2002.

299. Kelly KJ: Distant effects of experimental renal ischemia/reperfusion injury. J Am Soc Nephrol 14:1549–1558, 2003.

300. Heyman SN, Lieberthal W, Rogiers P, et al: Animal models of acute tubular necrosis. Curr Opin Crit Care 8:526–534, 2002.

301. Mattana J, Singhal PC: Prevalence and determinants of acute renal failure following cardiopulmonary resuscitation. Arch Intern Med 153:235–239, 1993.

302. Burne-Taney MJ, Kofler J, Yokota N, et al: Acute renal failure after whole body ischemia is characterized by inflammation and T cell–mediated injury. Am J Physiol Renal Physiol 285:F87–F94, 2003.

303. Miyaji T, Hu X, Yuen PS, et al: Ethyl pyruvate decreases sepsis-induced acute renal failure and multiple organ damage in aged mice. Kidney Int 64:1620–1631, 2003.

304. Hentschel DM, Park KM, Cilenti L, et al: Acute renal failure in zebrafish: a novel system to study a complex disease. Am J Physiol Renal Physiol 288:F923–F929, 2005.

305. Han WK, Bonventre JV: Biologic markers for the early detection of acute kidney injury. Curr Opin Crit Care 10:476–482, 2004.

306. Molls RR, Savransky V, Liu M, et al: Keratinocyte-derived chemokine is an early bio-marker of ischemic acute kidney injury. Am J Physiol Renal Physiol 290:F1187–F1193, 2006.

307. Mishra J, Ma Q, Prada A, et al: Identification of neutrophil gelatinase-associated lipocalin as a novel early urinary biomarker for ischemic renal injury. J Am Soc Nephrol 14:2534–2543, 2003.

308. Mishra J, Mori K, Ma Q, et al: Neutrophil gelatinase-associated lipocalin: a novel early urinary biomarker for cisplatin nephrotoxicity. Am J Nephrol 24:307–315, 2004.

309. Mishra J, Ma Q, Kelly C, et al: Kidney NGAL is a novel early marker of acute injury following transplantation. Pediatr Nephrol 21:856–863, 2006.

310. Han WK, Bailly V, Abichandani R, et al: Kidney Injury Molecule-1 (KIM-1): a novel biomarker for human renal proximal tubule injury. Kidney Int 62:237–244, 2002.

311. Attmane-Elakeb A, Chambrey R, Tsimaratos M, et al: Isolation and characterization of luminal and basolateral plasma membrane vesicles from the medullary thick ascending loop of Henle. Kidney Int 50:1051–1057, 1996.

312. du Cheyron D, Daubin C, Poggioli J, et al: Urinary measurement of Na+/H+ exchanger isoform 3 (NHE3) protein as new marker of tubule injury in critically ill patients with ARF. Am J Kidney Dis 42:497–506, 2003.

313. Parikh CR, Jani A, Melnikov VY, et al: Urinary interleukin-18 is a marker of human acute tubular necrosis. Am J Kidney Dis 43:405–414, 2004.

314. Hropot M, Juretschke HP, Langer KH, et al: S3226, a novel NHE3 inhibitor, attenuates ischemia-induced acute renal failure in rats. Kidney Int 60:2283–2289, 2001.

315. Rice JC, Spence JS, Yetman DL, et al: Monocyte chemoattractant protein-1 expression correlates with monocyte infiltration in the post-ischemic kidney. Ren Fail 24:703–723, 2002.

316. Kwon O, Molitoris BA, Pescovitz M, et al: Urinary actin, interleukin-6, and interleukin-8 may predict sustained ARF after ischemic injury in renal allografts. Am J Kidney Dis 41:1074–1087, 2003.

317. Simmons EM, Himmelfarb J, Sezer MT, et al: Plasma cytokine levels predict mortality in patients with acute renal failure. Kidney Int 65:1357–1365, 2004.

318. Ahlstrom A, Hynninen M, Tallgren M, et al: Predictive value of interleukins 6, 8 and 10, and low HLA-DR expression in acute renal failure. Clin Nephrol 61:103–110, 2004.

319. Muramatsu Y, Tsujie M, Kohda Y, et al: Early detection of cysteine rich protein 61 (CYR61, CCN1) in urine following renal ischemic reperfusion injury. Kidney Int 62:1601–1610, 2002.

320. Tarabishi R, Zahedi K, Mishra J, et al: Induction of Zf9 in the kidney following early ischemia/reperfusion. Kidney Int 68:1511–1519, 2005.

321. Spurgeon KR, Donohoe DL, Basile DP: Transforming growth factor-beta in acute renal failure: receptor expression, effects on proliferation, cellularity, and vascularization after recovery from injury. Am J Physiol Renal Physiol 288:F568–F577, 2005.

322. Nguyen MT, Ross GF, Dent CL, et al: Early prediction of acute renal injury using urinary proteomics. Am J Nephrol 25:318–326, 2005.

323. Zahedi K, Wang Z, Barone S, et al: Expression of SSAT, a novel biomarker of tubular cell damage, increases in kidney ischemia-reperfusion injury. Am J Physiol Renal Physiol 284:F1046–F1055, 2003.

324. Zahedi K, Wang Z, Barone S, et al. Identification of stathmin as a novel marker of cell proliferation in the recovery phase of acute ischemic renal failure. Am J Physiol Cell Physiol 286:C1203–C1211, 2004.

325. Thakar CV, Zahedi K, Revelo MP, et al: Identification of thrombospondin 1 (TSP-1) as a novel mediator of cell injury in kidney ischemia. J Clin Invest 115:3451–3459, 2005.

326. Brady HR, Lieberthal W: Acute renal failure. In Brenner B (ed): The Kidney, 6th ed. Philadelphia, WB Saunders, 1999.

327. Ward EE, Richards P, Wrong OM: Urine concentration after acute renal failure. Nephron 3:289–294, 1966.

328. Belizon IJ, Chou S, Porush JG, et al: Recovery without a diuresis after protracted acute tubular necrosis. Arch Intern Med 140:133–134, 1980.

329. Liano F, Gallego A, Pascual J, et al: Prognosis of acute tubular necrosis: an extended prospectively contrasted study. Nephron 63:21–31, 1993.

330. Finn WF: Diagnosis and management of acute tubular necrosis. Med Clin North Am 74:873–891, 1990.

331. Belizon IJ, Chou S, Porush JG, et al: Recovery without a diuresis after protracted acute tubular necrosis. Arch Intern Med 140:133–134, 1980.

CH 29

332. Coar D: Obstructive nephropathy. Del Med J 63:743–749, 1991.

333. Jones BF, Nanra RS: Post-obstructive diuresis. Aust N Z J Med 13:519–521, 1983.

334. Wahlberg J: The renal response to ureteral obstruction. Scand J Urol Nephrol Suppl 73:1–30, 1983.

335. Boone TB, Allen TD: Unilateral post-obstructive diuresis in the neonate. J Urol 147:430–432, 1992.

336. Faber MD, Kupin WL, Krishna GG, et al: The differential diagnosis of acute renmal failure. *In* Lazarus JM, Brenner BM (eds): Acute Renal Failure. New York, Churchill Livingstone, 1993, pp 133–192.

337. Nanji AI: Increased fractional excretion of sodium in prerenal azotemia: need for careful interpretation. Clin Chem 27:1314–1315, 1981.

338. Rudnick MR, Berns JS, Cohen RM, et al: Contrast media associated nephrotoxicity. Curr Opinion Nephrol Hypert 5:127–133, 1996.

339. Fillastre JP, Viotte G, Morin JP, et al: Nephrotoxicity of antitumoral agents. Adv Nephrol 17:175–218 L33, 1988.

340. Boles JM, Dutel JL, Briere J, et al: Acute renal failure caused by extreme hyperphosphatemia after chemotherapy of an acute lymphoblastic leukemia. Cancer 53:2425–2429, 1984.

341. Lundberg WB, Cadman ED, Finch SC, et al: Renal failure secondary to leukemic infiltration of the kidneys. Am J Med 62:636–642, 1977.

342. Cohen LF, Balow JE, Magrath IT, et al: Acute tumor lysis syndrome. A review of 37 patients with Burkitt's lymphoma. Am J Med 68:486–491, 1980.

343. Razis E, Arlin ZA, Ahmed T, et al: Incidence and treatment of tumor lysis syndrome in patients with acute leukemia. Acta Haematol 91:171–174, 1994.

344. Sever MS, Vanholder R, Lameire N: Management of crush-related injuries after disasters. N Engl J Med 354:1052–1063, 2006.

345. Pontremoli R, Rampoldi V, Morbidelli A, et al: Acute renal failure due to acute bilateral renal artery thrombosis: successful surgical revascularization after prolonged anuria. Nephron 56:322–324, 1990.

346. Delans RJ, Ramirez Z, Farber MS, et al: Renal artery thrombosis: a cause of reversible acute renal failure. J Urol 128:1287–1289, 1982.

347. Fogel RI, Endreny RG, Cronan JJ, et al: Acute renal failure with anuria caused by aortic thrombosis and bilateral renal artery occlusion. A report of two cases. R I Med J 70:501–504, 1987.

348. Nahar A, Akom M, Hanes D, et al: Pyelonephritis and acute renal failure. Am J Med Sci 328:121–123, 2004.

349. Turner ME, Weinstein J, Kher K: Acute renal failure secondary to pyelonephritis. Pediatrics 97:742–743, 1996.

350. Jones BF, Nanra RS, White KH: Acute renal failure due to acute pyelonephritis. Am J Nephrol 11:257–259, 1991.

351. Nunez JE, Perez E, Gunasekaran S, et al: Acute renal failure secondary to acute bacterial pyelonephritis. Nephron 62:240–241, 1992.

352. Lorentz WB, Iskandar S, Browning MC, et al: Acute renal failure due to pyelonephritis. Nephron 54:256–258, 1990.

353. Clarkson MR, Giblin L, O'Connell FP, et al: Acute interstitial nephritis: clinical features and response to corticosteroid therapy. Nephrol Dial Transplant 19:2778–2783, 2004.

354. Roth S, Andrassy K, Schmidt KH, et al: Febrile lady with acute renal failure and desquamating erythema. Am J Kidney Dis 34:150–154, 1999.

355. Bachhuber R, Parker RA, Bennett WM: Acute renal failure in toxic shock syndrome owing to rhabdomyolysis. Ann Clin Lab Sci 13:25–26, 1983.

356. Raper RF, Ibels LS: Toxic-shock syndrome in a male complicated by oliguric acute renal failure. Aust N Z J Med 12:60–62, 1982.

357. Alano FA Jr, Webster GD Jr: Acute renal failure and pigmentation due to phenazopyridine (Pyridium). Ann Intern Med 72:80–91, 1970.

358. Sessa A, Meroni M, Battini G, et al: Acute renal failure due to idiopathic tubulointestinal nephritis and uveitis: "TINU syndrome." Case report and review of the literature. J Nephrol 13:377–380, 2000.

359. Vanhaesebrouck P, Carton D, De Bel C, et al: Acute tubulo-interstitial nephritis and uveitis syndrome (TINU syndrome). Nephron 40:418–422, 1985.

360. Zsigmond GL, Verrier E, Way LW: Sudden reversal of renal failure after take-down of a jejunoileal bypass. Report of a case involving hemorrhagic proctocolitis, and renal and hepatic failure late after jejunoileal bypass for obesity. Am J Gastroenterol 77:216–219, 1982.

361. da Silva Magro MC, de Fatima Fernandes Vattimo M: Does urinalysis predict acute renal failure after heart surgery? Ren Fail 26:385–392, 2004.

362. Tsai JJ, Yeun JY, Kumar VA, et al: Comparison and interpretation of urinalysis performed by a nephrologist versus a hospital-based clinical laboratory. Am J Kidney Dis 46:820–829, 2005.

363. Szwed JJ: Urinalysis and clinical renal disease. J Am Med Technol 46:720–725, 1980.

364. Marcussen N, Schumann J, Campbell P, et al: Cytodiagnostic urinalysis is very useful in the differential diagnosis of acute renal failure and can predict the severity. Ren Fail 17:721–729, 1995.

365. Nolan CR 3rd, Anger MS, Kelleher SP: Eosinophiluria—a new method of detection and definition of the clinical spectrum. N Engl J Med 315:1516–1519, 1986.

366. Corwin HL, Korbet SM, Schwartz MM: Clinical correlates of eosinophiluria. Arch Intern Med 145:1097–1099, 1985.

367. Tadokoro M, Ozono Y, Hara K, et al: A case of acute renal failure due to ethylene glycol intoxication. Nippon Jinzo Gakkai Shi 37:353–356, 1995.

368. Meier M, Nitschke M, Perras B, et al: Ethylene glycol intoxication and xylitol infusion—metabolic steps of oxalate-induced acute renal failure. Clin Nephrol 63:225–228, 2005.

369. Smolens P, Venkatachalam M, Stein JH: Myeloma kidney cast nephropathy in a rat model of multiple myeloma. Kidney Int 24:192–204, 1983.

370. McCarthy CS, Becker JA: Multiple myeloma and contrast media. Radiology 183:519–521, 1992.

371. Revai T, Harmos G: Nephrotic syndrome and acute interstitial nephritis associated with the use of diclofenac. Wien Klin Wochenschr 111:523–524, 1999.

372. Nortier J, Depierreux M, Bourgeois V, et al: Progression of a naproxen and amoxicillin induced acute interstitial nephritis with nephrotic syndrome: case report. Clin Nephrol 35:187–189, 1991.

373. Lofgren RP, Nelson AE, Ehlers SM: Fenoprofen-induced acute interstitial nephritis presenting with nephrotic syndrome. Minn Med 64:287–290, 1981.

374. Averbuch SD, Austin HA 3rd, Sherwin SA, et al: Acute interstitial nephritis with the nephrotic syndrome following recombinant leukocyte a interferon therapy for mycosis fungoides. N Engl J Med 310:32–35, 1984.

375. Neugarten J, Gallo GR, Baldwin DS: Rifampin-induced nephrotic syndrome and acute interstitial nephritis. Am J Nephrol 3:38–42, 1983.

376. Schelling JR, Ghandour FZ, Strickland TJ, et al: Management of tumor lysis syndrome with standard continuous arteriovenous hemodialysis: case report and a review of the literature. Ren Fail 20:635–644, 1998.

377. Baud FJ, Galliot M, Astier A, et al: Treatment of ethylene glycol poisoning with intravenous 4-methylpyrazole. N Engl J Med 319:97–100, 1988.

378. Pozzi Mucelli R, Bertolotto M, Quaia E: Imaging techniques in acute renal failure. Contrib Nephrol 132:76–91, 2001.

379. Mucelli RP, Bertolotto M: Imaging techniques in acute renal failure. Kidney Int Suppl 66:S102–S105, 1998.

380. Marcos WJ, Choyke PL: Magnetic resonance angiography of the kidney. Semin Nephrol 20:450–455, 2000.

381. Webb JA: Ultrasonography in the diagnosis of urinary tract obstruction. Brit Med J 301:994–988, 1990.

382. Rascoff JH, Golden RA, Spinowitz BS, et al: Nondilated obstructive nephropathy. Arch Intern Med 143:696–698, 1983.

383. Ellenbogen PH, Scheible FW, Talner LB, et al: Sensitivity of gray scale ultrasound in detecting urinary tract obstruction. AJR Am J Roentgenol 130:731–733, 1978.

384. Bhandari S: The patient with acute renal failure and non-dilated urinary tract. Nephrol Dial Transplant 13:1888, 1998.

385. Sherman RA, Byun KJ: Nuclear medicine in acute and chronic renal failure. Semin Nucl Med 12:265–279, 1982.

386. Weise WJ, Jaffrey JB: Review: CT angiography and magnetic resonance imaging are the best less-invasive tests for renal artery stenosis. ACP J Club 136:69, 2002.

387. Schoenberg SO, Essig M, Hallscheidt P, et al: Multiphase magnetic resonance angiography of the abdominal and pelvic arteries: results of a bicenter multireader analysis. Invest Radiol 37:20–28, 2002.

388. Zarich S, Fang LST, Diamond JR: Fractional excretion of sodium. Exceptions to its diagnostic value. Arch Intern Med 145:108–112, 1985.

389. Vaz AJ: Low fractional excretion of urine sodium in acute renal failure due to sepsis. Arch Intern Med 143:738–739, 1983.

390. Fang LS, Sirota RA, Ebert TH, et al: Low fractional excretion of sodium with contrast media-induced acute renal failure. Arch Intern Med 140:531–533, 1980.

391. Espinel CH: The FENa test. Use in the differential diagnosis of acute renal failure. JAMA 236:579–581, 1976.

392. Corwin HL, Schreiber MJ, Fang LS: Low fractional excretion of sodium. Occurrence with hemoglobinuric- and myoglobinuric-induced acute renal failure. Arch Intern Med 144:981–982, 1984.

393. Steiner RW: Low fractional excretion of sodium in myoglobinuric renal failure. Arch Intern Med 142:1216–1217, 1982.

394. Diamond JR, Yoburn DC: Nonoliguric acute renal failure associated with a low fractional excretion of sodium. Ann Intern Med 96:597–600, 1982.

395. Andreoli SP, Clark JH, McGuire WA, et al: Purine excretion during tumor lysis in children with acute lymphocytic leukemia receiving allopurinol: relationship to acute renal failure. J Pediatr 109:292–298, 1986.

396. Boles JM, Dutel JL, Briere J, et al: Acute renal failure caused by extreme hyperphosphatemia after chemotherapy of an acute lymphoblastic leukemia. Cancer 53:2425–2429, 1984.

397. Gilboa N, Lum GM, Urizar RE: Early renal involvement in acute lymphoblastic leukemia and non-Hodgkin's lymphoma in children. J Urol 129:364–367, 1983.

398. Kaplan BS, Hebert D, Morrell RE: Acute renal failure induced by hyperphosphatemia in acute lymphoblastic leukemia. Can Med Assoc J 124:429–431, 1981.

399. Eckman LN, Lynch EC: Acute renal failure in patients with acute leukemia. South Med J 71:382–385, 1978.

400. Humphreys BD, Soiffer RJ, Magee CC: Renal failure associated with cancer and its treatment: an update. J Am Soc Nephrol 16:151–161, 2005.

401. Srinivasa NS, McGovern CH, Solez K, et al: Progressive renal failure due to renal invasion and parenchymal destruction by adult T-cell lymphoma. Am J Kidney Dis 16:70–72, 1990.

402. Cairo MS, Bishop M: Tumour lysis syndrome: new therapeutic strategies and classification. Br J Haematol 127:3–11, 2004.

403. Lotfi M, Brandwein JM: Spontaneous acute tumor lysis syndrome in acute myeloid leukemia? A single case report with discussion of the literature. Leuk Lymphoma 29:625–628, 1998.

404. Del Toro G, Morris E, Cairo MS: Tumor lysis syndrome: pathophysiology, definition, and alternative treatment approaches. Clin Adv Hematol Oncol 3:54–61, 2005.

405. Humphreys BD, Sharman JP, Henderson JM, et al: Gemcitabine-associated thrombotic microangiopathy. Cancer 100:2664–2670, 2004.

406. Magee CC: Renal thrombotic microangiopathy induced by interferon-alpha. Nephrol Dial Transplant 16:2111–2112, 2001.

407. Giroux L, Bettez P, Giroux L: Mitomycin-C nephrotoxicity: A clinico-pathologic study of 17 cases. Am J Kidney Dis VI:28–39, 1985.

408. Medina PJ, Sipols JM, George JN: Drug-associated thrombotic thrombocytopenic purpura-hemolytic uremic syndrome. Curr Opin Hematol 8:286–293, 2001.

409. Bernstein SP, Humes HD: Reversible renal insufficiency in multiple myeloma. Arch Intern Med 142:2083–2086, 1982.

410. Defronzo RA, Humphrey RL, Wright JR, et al: Acute renal failure in multiple myeloma. Medicine 54:209–223, 1975.

411. Prakash J, Kumar H, Sinha DK, et al: Acute renal failure in pregnancy in a developing country: twenty years of experience. Ren Fail 28:309–313, 2006.

412. Gammill HS, Jeyabalan A: Acute renal failure in pregnancy. Crit Care Med 33:S372–S384, 2005.

413. Selcuk NY, Tonbul HZ, San A, et al: Changes in frequency and etiology of acute renal failure in pregnancy (1980–1997). Ren Fail 20:513–517, 1998.

414. Ventura JE, Villa M, Mizraji R, et al: Acute renal failure in pregnancy. Ren Fail 19:217–220, 1997.

415. Stratta P, Besso L, Canavese C, et al: Is pregnancy-related acute renal failure a disappearing clinical entity? Ren Fail 18:575–584, 1996.

416. Pertuiset N, Grunfeld JP: Acute renal failure in pregnancy. Baillieres Clin Obstet Gynaecol 8:333–351, 1994.

417. Alexopoulos E, Tambakoudis P, Bili H, et al: Acute renal failure in pregnancy. Ren Fail 15:609–613, 1993.

418. Stratta P, Canavese C, Dogliani M, et al: Pregnancy-related acute renal failure. Clin Nephrol 32:14–20, 1989.

419. Hayslett JP: Current concepts. Postpartum renal failure. N Engl J Med 312:1556–1559, 1985.

420. Sibai BM, Kustermann L, Velasco J: Current understanding of severe preeclampsia, pregnancy-associated hemolytic uremic syndrome, thrombotic thrombocytopenic purpura, hemolysis, elevated liver enzymes, and low platelet syndrome, and postpartum acute renal failure: different clinical syndromes or just different names? Curr Opin Nephrol Hypertens 3:436–445, 1994.

421. Treem WR: Mitochondrial fatty acid oxidation and acute fatty liver of pregnancy. Semin Gastrointest Dis 13:55–66, 2002.

422. Weiner CP: Thrombotic microangiopathy in pregnancy and the postpartum period. Semin Hematol 24:119–129, 1987.

423. Lampinen K, Peltonen S, Pettila V, et al: Treatment of postpartum thrombotic microangiopathy with plasma exchange using cryosupernatant as replacement. Acta Obstet Gynecol Scand 83:175–179, 2004.

424. Bauwens M, Hauet T, Malin F, et al: Postpartum thrombotic microangiopathy with plasma exchange dependence. Ann Med Interne (Paris) 143(Suppl 1):37, 1992.

425. Grunfeld JP, Ganeval D, Bournerias F: Acute renal failure in pregnancy. Kidney Int 18:179–191, 1980.

426. Davies MH, Wilkinson SP, Hanid MA, et al: Acute liver disease with encephalopathy and renal failure in late pregnancy and the early puerperium—a study of fourteen patients. Br J Obstet Gynaecol 87:1005, 1980.

427. D'Elia FL, Brennan RE, Brownstein PK: Acute renal failure secondary to ureteral obstruction by a gravid uterus. J Urol 128:803–804, 1982.

428. Bahar I, Akgul A, Ozatik MA, et al: Acute renal failure following open heart surgery: risk factors and prognosis. Perfusion 20:317–322, 2005.

429. Mangos GJ, Brown MA, Chan WY, et al: Acute renal failure following cardiac surgery: incidence, outcomes and risk factors. Aust N Z J Med 25:284–289, 1995.

430. Conlon PJ, Stafford-Smith M, White WD, et al: Acute renal failure following cardiac surgery. Nephrol Dial Transplant 14:1158–1162, 1999.

431. Corwin HL, Sprague SM, DeLaria GA, et al: Acute renal failure associated with cardiac operations. A case-control study. J Thorac Cardiovasc Surg 98:1107–1112, 1989.

432. Davis RF, Lappas DG, Kirklin JK, et al: Acute oliguria after cardiopulmonary bypass: renal functional improvement with low-dose dopamine infusion. Crit Care Med 10:852–856, 1982.

433. Chukwuemeka A, Weisel A, Maganti M, et al: Renal dysfunction in high-risk patients after on-pump and off-pump coronary artery bypass surgery: a propensity score analysis. Ann Thorac Surg 80:2148–2153, 2005.

434. Ascione R, Lloyd CT, Underwood MJ, et al: On-pump versus off-pump coronary revascularization: evaluation of renal function. Ann Thorac Surg 68:493–498, 1999.

435. Stallwood MI, Grayson AD, Mills K, et al: Acute renal failure in coronary artery bypass surgery: independent effect of cardiopulmonary bypass. Ann Thorac Surg 77:968–972, 2004.

436. Wyatt CM, Arons RR: The burden of acute renal failure in nonrenal solid organ transplantation. Transplantation 78:1351–1355, 2004.

437. Bilbao I, Charco R, Balsells J, et al: Risk factors for acute renal failure requiring dialysis after liver transplantation. Clin Transplant 12:123–129, 1998.

438. Brown RS, Jr, Lombardero M, Lake JR: Outcome of patients with renal insufficiency undergoing liver or liver- kidney transplantation. Transplantation 62:1788–1793, 1996.

439. Nair S, Verma S, Thuluvath PJ: Pretransplant renal function predicts survival in patients undergoing orthotopic liver transplantation. Hepatology 35:1179–1185, 2002.

440. Lafayette RA, Pare G, Schmid CH, et al: Pretransplant renal dysfunction predicts poorer outcome in liver transplantation. Clin Nephrol 48:159–164, 1997.

441. Gonwa TA, Klintmalm GB, Levy M, et al: Impact of pretransplant renal function on survival after liver transplantation. Transplantation 59:361–365, 1995.

442. Zager RA: Acute renal failure syndromes after bone marrow transplantation. Adv Nephrol Necker Hosp 27:263–280, 1997.

443. Gruss E, Bernis C, Tomas JF, et al: Acute renal failure in patients following bone marrow transplantation: prevalence, risk factors and outcome. Am J Nephrol 15:473–479, 1995.

444. Zager R: Acute renal failure in the setting of bone marrow transplantation. Kidney Int 14:341–344, 1994.

445. Parikh CR, McSweeney PA, Korular D, et al: Renal dysfunction in allogeneic hematopoietic cell transplantation. Kidney Int 62:566–573, 2002.

446. Parikh CR, McSweeney P, Schrier RW: Acute renal failure independently predicts mortality after myeloablative allogeneic hematopoietic cell transplant. Kidney Int 67:1999–2005, 2005.

447. Parikh CR, Sandmaier BM, Storb RF, et al: Acute renal failure after nonmyeloablative hematopoietic cell transplantation. J Am Soc Nephrol 15:1868–1876, 2004.

448. Parikh CR, Schrier RW, Storer B, et al: Comparison of ARF after myeloablative and nonmyeloablative hematopoietic cell transplantation. Am J Kidney Dis 45:502–509, 2005.

449. Jones RJ, Lee KS, Beschorner WE, et al: Venoocclusive disease of the liver following bone marrow transplantation. Transplantation 44:778–783, 1987.

450. Dalpiaz G, Nassetti C, Stasi G: Diffuse alveolar haemorrhage from a rare primary renal-pulmonary syndrome: micropolyangiitis. Case report and differential diagnosis. Radiol Med (Torino) 106:114–119, 2003.

451. Gallagher H, Kwan JT, Jayne DR. Pulmonary renal syndrome: a 4-year, single-center experience. Am J Kidney Dis 39:42–47, 2002.

452. Sanchez M, Bosch X, Martinez C, et al: Idiopathic pulmonary-renal syndrome with antiproteinase 3 antibodies. Respiration 61:295–299, 1994.

453. Koss MN, Antonovych T, Hochholzer L: Allergic granulomatosis (Churg-Strauss syndrome): pulmonary and renal morphologic findings. Am J Surg Pathol 5:21–28, 1981.

454. Bonsib SM, Walker WP: Pulmonary-renal syndrome: clinical similarity amidst etiologic diversity. Mod Pathol 2:129–37, 1989.

455. Herman PG, Balikian JP, Seltzer SE, et al: The pulmonary-renal syndrome. AJR Am J Roentgenol 130:1141–1148, 1978.

456. Ruiz-del-Arbol L, Monescillo A, Arocena C, et al: Circulatory function and hepatorenal syndrome in cirrhosis. Hepatology 42:439–447, 2005.

457. Guevara M, Gines P: Hepatorenal syndrome. Dig Dis 23:47–55, 2005.

458. Gines P, Cardenas A, Arroyo V, et al: Management of cirrhosis and ascites. N Engl J Med 350:1646–1654, 2004.

459. Gines P, Guevara M, Arroyo V, et al: Hepatorenal syndrome. Lancet 362:1819–1827, 2003.

460. Gines P, Arroyo V: Heopatorenal syndrome. J Am Soc Nephrol 10:1833–1839, 1999.

461. Epstein M: Hepatorenal syndrome. In Brady HR, Wilcox CS (eds): Therapy in Nephrology and Hypertension. Philadelphia, W.B. Saunders, 1998, pp 45–52.

462. Bataller R, Sort P, Gines P, et al: Hepatorenal syndrome: definition, pathophysiology, clinical features and management. Kidney Int Suppl 66:S47–S53, 1998.

463. Gines P, Sort P: Pathophysiology of renal dysfunction in cirrhosis. Digestion 59(suppl 2):11–15, 1998.

464. Attucha N, Garcia-Estan J: Intrarenal alterations in experimental liver cirrhosis. News Physiol Sci 11:48–52, 1996.

465. Epstein M: Hepatorenal syndrome: emerging perspectives of pathophysiology and therapy. J Am Soc Nephrol 4:1735–1753, 1994.

466. Schrier R, Arroyo V, Bernardi M, et al: Peripheral arterial vasodilatation hypothesis: a proposal for the initiation of renal sodium and water retention in cirrhosis. Hepatology 8:1151–1157, 1988.

467. Weigert AL, Martin P-Y, Schrier RW: Vascular hyporesponsiveness in cirrhotic rats; role of different nitrix oxide isoforms. Kidney Int 52:S41–S44, 1997.

468. Arroyo V, Gines P, Gerbes AL, et al: Definition and diagnostic criteria of refractory ascites and hepatorenal syndrome in cirrhosis. International Ascites Club. Hepatology 23:164–176, 1996.

469. Papadakis MA, Arieff AI: Unpredictability of clinical evaluation of renal function in cirrhosis. Prospective study. Am J Med 82:945–952, 1987.

470. Sort P, Navasa M, Arroyo V, et al: Effect of intravenous albumin on renal impairment and mortality in patients with cirrhosis and spontaneous bacterial peritonitis. N Engl J Med 341:403–409, 1999.

471. Alessandria C, Ozdogan O, Guevara M, et al: MELD score and clinical type predict prognosis in hepatorenal syndrome: relevance to liver transplantation. Hepatology 41:1282–1289, 2005.

472. Loghman-Adham M, Siegler RL, Pysher TJ: Acute renal failure in idiopathic nephrotic syndrome. Clin Nephrol 47:76–80, 1997.

473. James SH, Lien YH, Ruffenach SJ, et al: Acute renal failure in membranous glomerulonephropathy: a result of superimposed crescentic glomerulonephritis. J Am Soc Nephrol 6:1541–1546, 1995.

474. Blackshear JL, Davidman M, Stillman MT: Identification of risk for renal insufficiency from nonsteroidal anti-inflammatory drugs. Arch Intern Med 143:1130–1134, 1983.

475. Clive DM, Stoff JS: Renal syndromes associated with nonsteroidal antiinflammatory drugs. N Engl J Med 310:563–572, 1984.

476. Brezin JH, Katz SM, Schwartz AB, et al: Reversible renal failure and nephrotic syndrome associated with nonsteroidal anti-inflammatory drugs. N Engl J Med 301:1271–1273, 1979.

477. Booth LJ, Minielly JA, Smith EK: Acute renal failure in multiple myeloma. Can Med Assoc J 111:334–335, 1974.

478. Kjeldsberg CR, Holman RE: Acute renal failure in multiple myeloma. J Urol 105:21–23, 1971.

479. Yu A, Brenner BM, Yu ASL: Uremic syndrome revisited: A pathogenetic role for retained endogenous inhibitors of nitric oxide synthesis. Curr Opin Hyperten Nephrol 1:3–7, 1992.

480. Mattern WD, Sommers SC, Kassirer JP: Oliguric acute renal failure in malignant hypertension. Am J Med 52:187–197, 1972.

481. Rasmussen HH, Ibels LS: Acute renal failure. Multivariate analysis of causes and risk factors. Am J Med 73:211–218, 1982.

482. Salant DJ, Adler S, Bernard DB, et al: Acute renal failure associated with renal vascular disease, vasculitis, glomerulonephritis and nephrotic syndrome. In Brenner, BM, Lazarus JM (eds): Acute Renal Failure, 2nd ed. New York, Churchill Livinstone, 1988, pp 371–490.

483. Anderson RJ, Chung HM, Kluge R, et al: Hyponatremia: a prospective analysis of its epidemiology and the pathogenetic role of vasopressin. Ann Intern Med 102:164–168, 1985.

484. May RC, Stivelman JC, Maroni BJ: Metabolic and electrolyte disturbances in acute renal failure. *In* Lazarus JM, Brenner BM (eds): Acute Renal Failure, 3rd ed. New York, Churchill Livingston, 1993, pp 107–117.

485. Chertow GM, Burdick E, Honour M, et al: Acute kidney injury, mortality, length of stay, and costs in hospitalized patients. J Am Soc Nephrol 16:3365–3370, 2005.

486. Schiffl H, Lang SM, Fischer R: Daily hemodialysis and the outcome of acute renal failure. N Engl J Med 346:305–310, 2002.

487. Kellum JA, Angus DC: Patients are dying of acute renal failure. Crit Care Med 30:2156–2157, 2002.

488. Akmal M, Bishop JE, Telfer N, et al: Hypocalcemia and hypercalcemia in patients with rhabdomyolysis with and without acute renal failure. J Clin Endo Metabol 63:137–142, 1986.

489. Kahloon MU, Aslam AK, Aslam AF, et al: Hyperkalemia induced failure of atrial and ventricular pacemaker capture. Int J Cardiol 105:224–226, 2005.

490. Esposito C, Bellotti N, Fasoli G, et al: Hyperkalemia-induced ECG abnormalities in patients with reduced renal function. Clin Nephrol 62:465–468, 2004.

491. Mattu A, Brady WJ, Robinson DA: Electrocardiographic manifestations of hyperkalemia. Am J Emerg Med 18:721–729, 2000.

492. Acker CG, Johnson JP, Palevsky PM, et al: Hyperkalemia in hospitalized patients: causes, adequacy of treatment, and results of an attempt to improve physician compliance with published therapy guidelines. Arch Intern Med 158:917–924, 1998.

493. Arnsdorf MF: Electrocardiogram in hyperkalemia: electrocardiographic pattern of anteroseptal myocardial infarction mimicked by hyperkalemia-induced disturbance of impulse conduction. Arch Intern Med 136:Unknown, 1976.

494. Cronin RE, Bulger RE, Southern P, et al: Natural history of aminoglycoside nephrotoxicity in the dog. J Lab Clin Med 95:463–474, 1980.

495. Patel R, Savage A: Symptomatic hypomagnesemia associated with gentamicin therapy. Nephron 23:50–52, 1979.

496. Eknoyan G, Roberts AD: Nephrotoxicity of amphotericin B: Observations on the mechanism of hypokalemia. Antimicrob Agents Chemother 2:497–501, 1962.

497. Miltenyi M, Tulassay T, Korner A, et al: Tubular dysfunction in metabolic acidosis. First step to acute renal failure. Contrib Nephrol 67:58–66, 1988.

498. Conger JD, Falk SA: Intrarenal dynamics in the pathogenesis and prevention of acute urate nephropathy. J Clin Invest 59:786–793, 1977.

499. Cairo MS: Prevention and treatment of hyperuricemia in hematological malignancies. Clin Lymphoma 3(Suppl 1):S26–S31, 2002.

500. Singhal P, Kumar A, Desroches L, et al: Prevalence and predictors of rhabdomyolysis in patients with hyperphosphatemia. Am J Med 92:458–464, 1992.

501. Tsokos GC, Balow JE, Spiegel RJ, et al: Renal and metabolic complications of undifferentiated and lymphoblastic lymphomas. Medicine (Baltimore) 60:218–229, 1981.

502. Ettinger D, Harker WG, Gerry HW, et al: Hyperphosphatemia, hypocalcemia and transient renal failure: Results of cytotoxic treatment of acute lymphoblastic leukemia. JAMA 239:2472–2480, 1978.

503. Massry SG, Arieff AI, Coburn JW, et al: Divalent ion metabolism in patients with acute renal failure: studies on the mechanism of hypocalcemia. Kidney Int 5:437–445, 1974.

504. Pietrek J, Kokot F, Kuska J: Serum 25-hydroxyvitamin D and parathyroid hormone in patients with acute renal failure. Kidney Int 13:178–185, 1978.

505. Arieff AI, Massry SG: Calcium metabolism of brain in acute renal failure. Effects of uremia, hemodialysis, and parathyroid hormone. J Clin Invest 53:387–392, 1974.

506. Zaman F, Abreo K: Severe hypermagnesemia as a result of laxative use in renal insufficiency. South Med J 96:102–103, 2003.

507. Massry SG, Seelig MS: Hypomagnesemia and hypermagnesemia. Clin Nephrol 7:147–153, 1977.

508. Schelling JR: Fatal hypermagnesemia. Clin Nephrol 53:61–65, 2000.

509. Schilsky RL, Anderson T: Hypomagnesemia and renal magnesium wasting in patients receiving cisplatin. Ann Intern Med 90:929–931, 1979.

510. Blachley J, Hill J: Renal and electrolyte disturbances associated with cisplatin. Ann Intern Med 95:628–632, 1981.

511. du Cheyron D, Parienti JJ, Fekih-Hassen M, et al: Impact of anemia on outcome in critically ill patients with severe acute renal failure. Intensive Care Med 31:1529–1536, 2005.

512. Radtke HW, Claussner A, Erbes PM, et al: Serum erythropoietin concentration in chronic renal failure: relationship to degree of anemia and excretory renal function. Blood 54:877–884, 1979.

513. Mannucci PM, Remuzzi G, Pusineri F, et al: Deamino-8-D-arginine vasopressin shortens the bleeding time in uremia. N Engl J Med 308:8–12, 1983.

514. Brown CH 3rd, Bradshaw MJ, Natelson EA, et al: Defective platelet function following the administration of penicillin compounds. Blood 47:949–956, 1976.

515. Andrassy K, Ritz E, Hasper B, et al: Penicillin-induced coagulation disorder. Lancet 2:1039–1041, 1976.

516. Deykin D: Uremic bleeding. Kidney Int 24:698–705,1983.

517. Janson PA, Jubelirer SJ, Weinstein MJ, et al: Treatment of the bleeding tendency in uremia with cryoprecipitate. N Engl J Med 303:1318–1321, 1980.

518. Ympa YP, Sakr Y, Reinhart K, et al: Has mortality from acute renal failure decreased? A systematic review of the literature. Am J Med 118:827–832, 2005.

519. Priebe HJ, Skillman JJ, Bushnell LS, et al: Antacid versus cimetidine in preventing acute gastrointestinal bleeding. A randomized trial in 75 critically ill patients. N Engl J Med 302:426–430, 1980.

520. Fiaccadori E, Maggiore U, Clima B, et al: Incidence, risk factors, and prognosis of gastrointestinal hemorrhage complicating acute renal failure. Kidney Int 59:1510–1519, 2001.

521. Pimentel JL Jr, Brusilow SW, Mitch WE: Unexpected encephalopathy in chronic renal failure: hyperammonemia complicating acute peritonitis. J Am Soc Nephrol 5:1066–1073, 1994.

522. Hyneck ML: Current concepts in clinical therapeutics: drug therapy in acute renal failure. Clin Pharm 5:892–910, 1986.

523. Hogg JE: Neurologic complications of acute and chronic renal failure. Adv Neurol 19:637–46, 1978.

524. Bagshaw SM, Peets AD, Hameed M, et al: Dialysis disequilibrium syndrome: brain death following hemodialysis for metabolic acidosis and acute renal failure—a case report. BMC Nephrol 5:9, 2004.

525. Fiaccadori E, Lombardi M, Leonardi S, et al: Prevalence and clinical outcome associated with preexisting malnutrition in acute renal failure: a prospective cohort study. J Am Soc Nephrol 10:581–593, 1999.

526. Druml W: Nutritional management of acute renal failure. Am J Kidney Dis 37:S89–S94, 2001.

527. Riella MC: Nutrition in acute renal failure. Ren Fail 19:237–252, 1997.

528. Fiaccadori E, Maggiore U, Giacosa R, et al: Enteral nutrition in patients with acute renal failure. Kidney Int 65:999–1008, 2004.

529. Chima CS, Meyer L, Hummell AC, et al: Protein catabolic rate in patients with acute renal failure on continuous arteriovenous hemofiltration and total parenteral nutrition. J Am Soc Nephrol 3:1516–1521, 1993.

530. Sponsel H, Conger JD: Is parenteral nutrition therapy of value in acute renal failure patients? Am J Kidney Dis 25:96–102, 1995.

531. Mitch WE: Mechanisms causing loss of muscle in acute uremia. Ren Fail 18:389–394, 1996.

532. Ragaller MJ, Theilen H, Koch T: Volume replacement in critically ill patients with acute renal failure. J Am Soc Nephrol 12(Suppl 17):S33–S39, 2001.

533. Waiker SS, Chertow GM: Crystalloids versus colloids for resuscitation in shock. Curr Opin Nephrol Hypertens 9:501–504, 2000.

534. Alderson P, Schierhout G, Roberts I, et al: Colloids versus crystalloids for fluid resuscitation in critically ill patients. Cochrane Database Syst Rev 2, 2000.

535. Choi PT-L, Yip G, Quionez LG, et al: Crystalloids vs. colloids in fluid resusitation. A critical review. Crit Care Med 27:200–210, 1999.

536. Schierhout G, Roberts I: Fluid resuscitation with colloid or crystalloid solutions in critically ill patients: a systematic review of randomized trials. BMJ 316:961–964, 1998.

537. Roberts JS, Bratton SL: Colloid volume expanders. Problems, pitfalls and possibilities. Drugs 55:621–630, 1998.

538. Davidson IJ: Renal impact of fluid management with colloids: a comparative review. Eur J Anaesthesiol 23:721–738, 2006.

539. Schortgen F, Lacherade JC, Bruneel F, et al: Effects of hydroxyethylstarch and gelatin on renal function in severe sepsis: a multicentre randomised study. Lancet 357:911–916, 2001.

540. Finfer S, Bellomo R, Boyce N, et al: A comparison of albumin and saline for fluid resuscitation in the intensive care unit. N Engl J Med 350:2247–2256, 2004.

541. Wheeler AP, Bernard GR, Thompson BT, et al: Pulmonary-artery versus central venous catheter to guide treatment of acute lung injury. N Engl J Med 354:2213–2224, 2006.

542. Kellerman P: Large volume paracentesis in treatment of ascites. Ann Intern Med 112:889–891, 1990.

543. Levinsky NG, Bernard DB: The LeVeen shunt. *In* Isselbacher KJ, Braunwald E, Wilson JD (eds): Update II, Harrison's Principles of Internal Medicine. New York, McGraw Hill, 1982, pp 147–148.

544. Smadja C, Franco D: The LeVeen shunt in the elective treatment of intractable ascites in cirrhosis. A prospective study on 140 patients. Ann Surg 201:488–493, 1985.

545. Lake J, Ring E, LaBerge J, et al: Transjugular intrahepatic portocaval stent in patients with renal insufficiency. Transplant Proc 25:1766–1767, 1992.

546. Guevara M, Gines P, Bandi JC, et al: Transjugular intrahepatic portosystemic shunt in hepatorenal syndrome: effects on renal function and vasoactive systems. Hepatology 1998;28:416–22.

547. Moreau R, Lebrec D: The use of vasoconstrictors in patients with cirrhosis: type 1 HRS and beyond. Hepatology 43:385–394, 2006.

548. Ortega R, Gines P, Uriz J, et al: Terlipressin therapy with and without albumin for patients with hepatorenal syndrome: results of a prospective, nonrandomized study. Hepatology 36:941–948, 2002.

549. Uriz J, Gines P, Cardenas A, et al: Terlipressin plus albumin infusion: an effective and safe therapy of hepatorenal syndrome. J Hepatol 33:43–48, 2000.

550. Solanki P, Chawla A, Garg R, et al: Beneficial effects of terlipressin in hepatorenal syndrome: a prospective, randomized placebo-controlled clinical trial. J Gastroenterol Hepatol 18:152–156, 2003.

551. Carpenter CC, Mitra PP, Sack RB, et al: Clinical studies in Asiatic cholera I. Preliminary observations. Bull Johns Hopkins Hosp 118:165–173, 1966.

552. Carpenter CC, Mitra PP, Sack RB, et al: Clinical studies in Asiatic cholera II. Development of a 2:1 saline:lactate regimen. Comparison of this regimen with traditional methods of treatment. Bull Johns Hopkins Hosp 118:174–196, 1966.

553. Carpenter CC, Mitra PP, Sack RB, et al: Clinical studies in Asiatic cholera III. Physiological studies during treatment of the acute cholera patient: Comparison of lactate and bicarbonate in correction of acidosis; effects of potassium depletion. Bull Johns Hopkins Hosp 118:197–207, 1966.

554. Bunn F, Lefebvre C, Li Wan Po A, et al: Human albumin solution for resuscitation and volume expansion in critically ill patients. The Albumin Reviewers. Cochrane Database Syst Rev 2, 2000.

555. Gunal AI, Celiker H, Dogukan A, et al: Early and vigorous fluid resuscitation prevents acute renal failure in the crush victims of catastrophic earthquakes. J Am Soc Nephrol 15:1862–1867, 2004.

556. Uchino S, Kellum JA, Bellomo R, et al: Acute renal failure in critically ill patients: a multinational, multicenter study. JAMA 294:813–818, 2005.

557. Brivet FG, Kleinknecht DJ, Loirat P, et al: Acute renal failure in intensive care units—causes, outcome, and prognostic factors of hospital mortality; a prospective, multicenter study. French Study Group on Acute Renal Failure. Crit Care Med 24:192–198, 1996.

558. Rivers E, Nguyen B, Havstad S, et al: Early goal-directed therapy in the treatment of severe sepsis and septic shock. N Engl J Med 345:1368–1377, 2001.

559. van den Berghe G, Wouters P, Weekers F, et al: Intensive insulin therapy in the critically ill patients. N Engl J Med 345:1359–1367, 2001.

560. Ozols RF, Corden BJ, Jacob J, et al: High-dose cisplatin in hypertonic saline. Ann Intern Med 100:19–24, 1984.

561. Ozols R, Corden B, Jacob J, et al: High-dose cisplatin in hypertonic saline. Ann Intern Med 100:19–24, 1984.

562. Heyman SN, Reuss S, Silva P, et al: Protective action of glycine in cisplatin nephrotoxicity. Kidney Int 40:273–279, 1991.

563. Bush HL Jr, Huse JB, Johnson WC, et al: Prevention of renal insufficiency after abdominal aortic aneurysm resection by optimal volume loading. Arch Surg 116:1517–1524, 1981.

564. Johnson WJ, Kyle RA, Pineda AA, et al: Treatment of renal failure associated with multiple myeloma. Plasmapheresis, hemodialysis, and chemotherapy. Arch Intern Med 150:863–869, 1990.

565. Barrett BJ, Parfrey PS: Clinical practice. Preventing nephropathy induced by contrast medium. N Engl J Med 354:379–386, 2006.

566. Parfrey P: The clinical epidemiology of contrast-induced nephropathy. Cardiovasc Intervent Radiol 28(Suppl 2):S3–S11, 2005.

567. Solomon R, Werner C, Mann D, et al: Effects of saline, mannitol, and furosemide to prevent acute decreases in renal function induced by radiocontrast agents. N Engl J Med 331:1416–1420, 1994.

568. Mueller C, Buerkle G, Buettner HJ, et al: Prevention of contrast media–associated nephropathy: randomized comparison of 2 hydration regimens in 1620 patients undergoing coronary angioplasty. Arch Intern Med 162:329–336, 2002.

569. Merten GJ, Burgess WP, Gray LV, et al: Prevention of contrast-induced nephropathy with sodium bicarbonate: a randomized controlled trial. JAMA 291:2328–2334, 2004.

570. Fishbane S, Durham JH, Marzo K, et al: N-acetylcysteine in the prevention of radiocontrast-induced nephropathy. J Am Soc Nephrol 15:251–260, 2004.

571. Tepel M, van der Giet M, Schwarzfeld C, et al: Prevention of radiographic-contrast-agent-induced reductions in renal function by acetylcysteine. N Engl J Med 343:180–184, 2000.

572. Shyu KG, Cheng JJ, Kuan P: Acetylcysteine protects against acute renal damage in patients with abnormal renal function undergoing a coronary procedure. J Am Coll Cardiol 40:1383–1388, 2002.

573. Kay J, Chow WH, Chan T, et al. Acetylcysteine for prevention of acute deterioration of renal function following elective coronary angiography and intervention: a randomized controlled trial. JAMA 289:553–558, 2003.

574. Marenzi G, Assanelli E, Marana I, et al: N-acetylcysteine and contrast-induced nephropathy in primary angioplasty. N Engl J Med 354:2773–2782, 2006.

575. Zagler A, Azadpour M, Mercado C, et al: N-acetylcysteine and contrast-induced nephropathy: a meta-analysis of 13 randomized trials. Am Heart J 151:140–145, 2006.

576. Kshirsagar AV, Poole C, Mottl A, et al: N-acetylcysteine for the prevention of radiocontrast induced nephropathy: a meta-analysis of prospective controlled trials. J Am Soc Nephrol 15:761–769, 2004.

577. Barrett BJ, Carlisle EJ: Metaanalysis of the relative nephrotoxicity of high- and low-osmolality iodinated contrast media. Radiology 188:171–178, 1993.

578. Rudnick MR, Goldfarb S, Wexler L, et al: Nephrotoxicity of ionic and nonionic contrast media in 1196 patients: a randomized trial. The Iohexol Cooperative Study. Kidney Int 47:254–261, 1995.

579. Aspelin P, Aubry P, Fransson SG, et al: Nephrotoxic effects in high-risk patients undergoing angiography. N Engl J Med 348:491–499, 2003.

580. Rieger J, Sitter T, Toepfer M, et al: Gadolinium as an alternative contrast agent for diagnostic and interventional angiographic procedures in patients with impaired renal function. Nephrol Dial Transplant 17:824–828, 2002.

581. Pereles FS, Baskaran V: Abdominal magnetic resonance angiography: principles and practical applications. Top Magn Reson Imaging 12:317–326, 2001.

582. Blaser J, Konig C: Once-daily dosing of aminoglycosides. Eur J Clin Microbiol Infect Dis 14:1029–1038, 1995.

583. Craig WA: Once-daily versus multiple-daily dosing of aminoglycosides. J Chemother 7(Suppl 2):47–52, 1995.

584. Goldman SC, Holcenberg JS, Finklestein JZ, et al: A randomized comparison between rasburicase and allopurinol in children with lymphoma or leukemia at high risk for tumor lysis. Blood 97:2998–3003, 2001.

585. Bessmertny O, Robitaille LM, Cairo MS: Rasburicase: a new approach for preventing and/or treating tumor lysis syndrome. Curr Pharm Des 11:4177–4185, 2005.

586. Navolanic PM, Pui CH, Larson RA, et al: Elitek-rasburicase: an effective means to prevent and treat hyperuricemia associated with tumor lysis syndrome, a Meeting Report, Dallas, Texas, January 2002. Leukemia 17:499–514, 2003.

587. Cairo MS: Recombinant urate oxidase (rasburicase): a new targeted therapy for prophylaxis and treatment of patients with hematologic malignancies at risk of tumor lysis syndrome. Clin Lymphoma 3:233–234, 2003.

588. Hartmann JT, von Vangerow A, Fels LM, et al: A randomized trial of amifostine in patients with high-dose VIC chemotherapy plus autologous blood stem cell transplantation. Br J Cancer 84:313–320, 2001.

589. Koukourakis MI: Amifostine in clinical oncology: current use and future applications. Anticancer Drugs 13:181–209, 2002.

590. Vaira M, Barone R, Aghemo B, et al: [Renal protection with amifostine during intraoperative peritoneal chemohyperthermia (IPCH) with cisplatin (CDDP) for peritoneal carcinosis. Phase 1 study]. Minerva Med 92:207–211, 2001.

591. Morgan JM: Chelation therapy in lead nephropathy. South Med J 68:1001–1006, 1975.

592. Murray KM, Hedgepeth JC: Intravenous self-administration of elemental mercury: efficacy of dimercaprol therapy. Drug Intell Clin Pharm 22:972–975, 1988.

593. Brent J, McMartin K, Phillips S, et al: Fomepizole for the treatment of ethylene glycol poisoning. Methylpyrazole for Toxic Alcohols Study Group. N Engl J Med 340:832–838, 1999.

594. Goldfarb DS: Fomepizole for ethylene-glycol poisoning. Lancet 354:1646, 1999.

595. Najafi CC, Hertko LJ, Leikin JB, et al: Fomepizole in ethylene glycol intoxication. Ann Emerg Med 37:358–359, 2001.

596. Battistella M: Fomepizole as an antidote for ethylene glycol poisoning. Ann Pharmacother 36:1085–1089, 2002.

597. Graziani G, Cantaluppi A, Casati S, et al: Dopamine and frusemide in oliguric acute renal failure. Nephron 37:39–42, 1984.

598. Conger JD, Falk SA, Hammond WS: Atrial natriuretic peptide and dopamine in established acute renal failure in the rat. Kidney Int 40:21–28, 1991.

599. Parker S, Carlon GC, Isaacs M, et al: Dopamine administration in oliguria and oliguric renal failure. Crit Care Med 9:630–632, 1981.

600. Kellum JA, M Decker J: Use of dopamine in acute renal failure: a meta-analysis. Crit Care Med 29:1526–1531, 2001.

601. Denton MD, Chertow GM, Brady HR: "Renal-dose" dopamine for the treatment of acute renal failure: scientific rationale, experimental studies and clinical trials. Kidney Int 50:4–14, 1996.

602. Marik PE, Iglesias J: Low-dose dopamine does not prevent acute renal failure in patients with septic shock and oliguria. NORASEPT II Study Investigators. Am J Med 107:387–390, 1999.

603. Bellomo R, Chapman M, Finfer S, et al: Low-dose dopamine in patients with early renal dysfunction: a placebo-controlled randomised trial. Australian and New Zealand Intensive Care Society (ANZICS) Clinical Trials Group. Lancet 356:2139–2143, 2000.

604. Lauschke A, Teichgraber UK, Frei U, et al: "Low-dose" dopamine worsens renal perfusion in patients with acute renal failure. Kidney Int 69:1669–1674, 2006.

605. Jones D, Bellomo R: Renal-dose dopamine: from hypothesis to paradigm to dogma to myth and, finally, superstition? J Intensive Care Med 20:199–211, 2005.

606. Bellomo R: Has renal-dose dopamine finally been relegated to join the long list of medical myths? Crit Care Resusc 3:7–10, 2001.

607. Singer I, Epstein M: Potential of dopamine A-1 agonists in the management of acute renal failure. Am J Kidney Dis 31:743–755, 1998.

608. Tumlin JA, Wang A, Murray PT, et al: Fenoldopam mesylate blocks reductions in renal plasma flow after radiocontrast dye infusion: a pilot trial in the prevention of contrast nephropathy. Am Heart J 143:894–903, 2002.

609. Caimmi PP, Pagani L, Micalizzi E, et al: Fenoldopam for renal protection in patients undergoing cardiopulmonary bypass. J Cardiothorac Vasc Anesth 17:491–494, 2003.

610. Stone GW, McCullough PA, Tumlin JA, et al: Fenoldopam mesylate for the prevention of contrast-induced nephropathy: a randomized controlled trial. JAMA 290:2284–2291, 2003.

611. Tumlin JA, Finkel KW, Murray PT, et al: Fenoldopam mesylate in early acute tubular necrosis: a randomized, double-blind, placebo-controlled clinical trial. Am J Kidney Dis 46:26–34, 2005.

612. Kurnik BRC, Kurnik PB, Cuttler I, et al: Protective effect of atrial natriuretic peptide (ANP) in patients with chronic renal failure (CRF) receiving contrast. Kidney Int 35:411–417, 1989.

613. Conger JD, Falk SA, Yuan BH, et al: Atrial natriuretic peptide and dopamine in a rat model of ischemic acute renal failure. Kidney Int 35:1126–1132, 1989.

614. Nakamoto M, Shapiro JI, Shanley PF, et al: In vitro and in vivo protective effect of atriopeptin III on ischemic acute renal failure. J Clin Invest 80:698–705, 1987.

615. Lewis J, Salem MM, Chertow GM, et al: Atrial natriuretic factor in oliguric acute renal failure. Anaritide Acute Renal Failure Study Group. Am J Kidney Dis 36:767–774, 2000.

616. Meyer M, Pfarr E, Schirmer G, et al: Therapeutic use of the natriuretic peptide ularitide in acute renal failure. Ren Fail 21:85–100, 1999.

617. Levinsky NG, Bernard DB: Mannitol and loop diuretics in acute renal failure. In Brenner BM, Lazarus JM (eds): Acute Renal Failure, 2nd ed. New York, W.B. Saunders; 1988, pp 841–856.

618. Mehta RL, Pascual MT, Soroko S, et al: Diuretics, mortality, and nonrecovery of renal function in acute renal failure. JAMA 288:2547–2553, 2002.

619. Cantarovich F, Rangoonwala B, Lorenz H, et al: High-dose furosemide for established ARF: a prospective, randomized, double-blind, placebo-controlled, multicenter trial. Am J Kidney Dis 44:402–409, 2004.

620. Rybak LP, Whitworth C, Scott V: Comparative acute ototoxicity of loop diuretic compounds. Eur Arch Otorhinolaryngol 248:353–357, 1991.

621. Ikeda K, Oshima T, Hidaka H, et al: Molecular and clinical implications of loop diuretic ototoxicity. Hear Res 107:1–8, 1997.

622. Hanley MJ, Davidson K: Prior mannitol and furosemide infusion in a model of ischemic acute renal failure. Am J Physiol 241:F556–F564, 1981.

623. Vanholder R, Leusen I, Lameire N: Comparison between mannitol and saline infusion in HgCl$_2$-induced acute renal failure. Nephron 38:193–201, 1984.

624. Grino JM, Miravitlles R, Castelao AM, et al: Flush solution with mannitol in the prevention of post-transplant renal failure. Transplant Proc 19:4140–4142, 1987.

625. Zager RA, Mahan J, Merola AJ: Effects of mannitol on the postischemic kidney: Biochemical, functional and morphologic assessments. Lab Invest 53:433–442, 1985.

626. van Valenberg PL, Hoitsma AJ, Tiggeler RG, et al: Mannitol as an indispensable constituent of an intraoperative hydration protocol for the prevention of acute renal failure after renal cadaveric transplantation. Transplantation 44:784–788, 1987.

627. Pusey CD, Saltissi D, Bloodworth L, et al: Drug associated acute interstitial nephritis: Clinical and pathological features and the response to high dose steroid therapy. Q J Med 52:194–211, 1983.

628. Bender WL, Whelton A, Beschorner WE, et al: Interstitial nephritis, proteinuria, and renal failure caused by nonsteroidal anti-inflammatory drugs. Immunologic characterization of the inflammatory infiltrate. Am J Med 76:1006–1012, 1984.

629. von Baeyer H: Plasmapheresis in thrombotic microangiopathy-associated syndromes: review of outcome data derived from clinical trials and open studies. Ther Apher 6:320–328, 2002.

630. Madore F, Lazarus JM, Brady HR: Therapeutic plasma exchange in renal diseases. J Am Soc Nephrol 7:367–386, 1996.

631. Wong CS, Jelacic S, Habeeb RL, et al: The risk of the hemolytic-uremic syndrome after antibiotic treatment of Escherichia coli O157:H7 infections. N Engl J Med 342:1930–1936, 2000.

632. Clark WF, Stewart AK, Rock GA, et al: Plasma exchange when myeloma presents as acute renal failure: a randomized, controlled trial. Ann Intern Med 143:777–784, 2005.

633. Beckett VL, Donadio JVJ, Brennan LAJ, et al: Use of captopril as early therapy for renal scleroderma: A prospective study. Mayo Clin Proc 60:763–771, 1985.

634. Lopez-Ovejero JA, Saal SD, D'Angelo WA, et al: Reversal of vascular and renal crises of scleroderma by oral angiotensin-converting enzyme blockade. N Engl J Med 300:11417–1419, 1979.

635. Traub YM, Shapiro AP, Rodnan GP, et al: Hypertension and renal failure (scleroderma renal crisis) in progressive systemic sclerosis. Review of a 25 year experience with 68 cases. Medicine 62:335–352, 1983.

636. Wolfson M, Kopple JD: Nutritional management of acute renal failure. In Lazarus JM, Brenner BM (eds): Acute Renal Failure, 3rd ed. New York, Churchill Livingstone, 1993, pp 267–270.

637. Teschan PE, Baxter CR, O'Brien TF, et al: Early dialysis in the treatment of acute renal failure. Ann Intern Med 53:992–1016, 1960.

638. Owen WF, Lazarus JM: Dialytic management of acute renal failure. In Lazarus JM, Brenner BM (eds): Acute Renal Failure, 3rd ed. New York, Churchill Livingstone, 1993, p 487.

639. Fischer RP, Griffen WO Jr, Reiser M, et al: Early dialysis in the treatment of acute renal failure. Surg Gynecol Obstet 123:1019–1023, 1966.

640. Mehta RL: Outcomes research in acute renal failure. Semin Nephrol 23:283–294, 2003.

641. Kellum JA, Ronco C, Mehta R, et al: Consensus development in acute renal failure: The Acute Dialysis Quality Initiative. Curr Opin Crit Care 11:527–532, 2005.

642. Kellum JA, Mehta RL, Angus DC, et al: The first international consensus conference on continuous renal replacement therapy. Kidney Int 62:1855–1863, 2002.

643. Phu NH, Hien TT, Mai NT, et al: Hemofiltration and peritoneal dialysis in infection-associated acute renal failure in Vietnam. N Engl J Med 347:895–902, 2002.

644. Ash SR: Peritoneal dialysis in acute renal failure of adults: the safe, effective, and low-cost modality. Contrib Nephrol 132:210–221, 2001.

645. Eustace J, Heffernan A, Watson A: Acute hemodialysis and acute peritoneal dialysis. In Brady HR, Wolcox CS (eds): Therapy in Nephrology and Hypertension. Philadelphia, W.B. Saunders, 1999, pp 53–69.

646. Ash SR, Bever SL: Peritoneal dialysis for acute renal failure: the safe, effective, and low-cost modality. Adv Ren Replace Ther 2:160–163, 1995.

647. Holley HL, Pirano BM: Complications of peritoneal dialysis: Diagnosis and management. Semin Nephrol 3:245–255, 1990.

648. Cimochowski GE, Worley E, Rutherford WE, et al: Superiority of the internal jugular over the subclavian access for temporary dialysis. Nephron 54:154–61, 1990.

649. Kirkpatrick WG, Culpepper RM, Sirmon MD: Frequency of complications with prolonged femoral vein catheterization for hemodialysis access. Nephron 73:58–62, 1996.

650. Cheung A, Hohnholt M, Gilson J: Adherence of neutrophils to hemodialysis membranes: role of complement receptors. Kidney Int 40:1123–1133, 1991.

651. Hakim RM: Clinical implications of hemodialysis membrane biocompatibility. Kidney Int 44:484–494, 1993.

652. Tonelli M, Pannu N, Manns B: Influence of dialysis membranes on outcomes in acute renal failure. Kidney Int 63:1957–1958; author reply 1958, 2003.

653. Hakim R, Wingard R, Parker R: Effect of the dialysis membrane in the treatment of patients with acute renal failure. N Engl J Med 331:1338–1342, 1994.

654. Schiffl H, Lang SM, Konig A, et al: Biocompatible membranes in acute renal failure: prospective case-controlled study. Lancet 344:570–572, 1994.

655. Himmelfarb J, Tolkoff Rubin N, Chandran P, et al: A multicenter comparison of dialysis membranes in the treatment of acute renal failure requiring dialysis. J Am Soc Nephrol 9:257–66, 1998.

656. Parker RA, Himmelfarb J, Tolkoff-Rubin N, et al: Prognosis of patients with acute renal failure requiring dialysis: results of a multicenter study. Am J Kidney Dis 32:432–443, 1998.

657. Subramanian S, Venkataraman R, Kellum JA: Influence of dialysis membranes on outcomes in acute renal failure: a meta-analysis. Kidney Int 62:1819–1823, 2002.

658. Caruana RJ, Keep DM: Anticoagulation. In Duagirdas JT, Ing TS (eds): Handbook of dialysis. Boston, Little, Brown and Company, 1994, pp 121–136.

659. Leu JG, Chiang SS, Lin SM, et al: Low molecular weight heparin in hemodialysis patients with a bleeding tendency. Nephron 86:499–501, 2000.

660. Ward DM: Anticoagulation in patients on dialysis. In Nissenson AR, Fine RN, Gentile DE (eds): Clinical Dialysis, 3rd ed. East Norwalk, CT, Appelton and Lange, 1995, pp 127–152.

661. Abramson S, Niles JL: Anticoagulation in continuous renal replacement therapy. Curr Opin Nephrol Hypertens 8:701–707, 1999.

662. Davenport A: Management of heparin-induced thrombocytopenia during continuous renal replacement therapy. Am J Kidney Dis 32:E3, 1998.

663. Tang IY, Cox DS, Patel K, et al: Argatroban and renal replacement therapy in patients with heparin-induced thrombocytopenia. Ann Pharmacother 39:231–236, 2005.

664. Dager WE, White RH: Argatroban for heparin-induced thrombocytopenia in hepatorenal failure and CVVHD. Ann Pharmacother 37:1232–1236, 2003.

665. Vargas Hein O, von Heymann C, Lipps M, et al: Hirudin versus heparin for anticoagulation in continuous renal replacement therapy. Intensive Care Med 27:673–679, 2001.

666. Lien J, Chan V: Risk factors influencing survival in acute renal failure treated by hemodialysis. Arch Intern Med 145:2067–2069, 1985.

667. Doshi M, Murray PT: Approach to intradialytic hypotension in intensive care unit patients with acute renal failure. Artif Organs 27:772–780, 2003.

668. Schreiber MJ Jr: Clinical case-based approach to understanding intradialytic hypotension. Am J Kidney Dis 38:S37–S47, 2001.

669. Ifudu O, Miles AM, Friedman EA: Hemodialysis immediately after acute myocardial infarction. Nephron 74:104–109, 1996.

670. Marshall MR, Ma T, Galler D, et al: Sustained low-efficiency daily diafiltration (SLEDD-f) for critically ill patients requiring renal replacement therapy: towards an adequate therapy. Nephrol Dial Transplant 19:877–884, 2004.

671. Al-Hilali N, Al-Humoud HM, Ninan VT, et al: Profiled hemodialysis reduces intradialytic symptoms. Transplant Proc 36:1827–1828, 2004.

672. Po CL, Afolabi M, Raja RM: The role of sequential ultrafiltration and varying dialysate sodium on vascular stability during hemodialysis. Asaio J 39:M798–M800, 1993.

673. Forni LG, Hilton PJ: Continuous hemofiltration in the treatment of acute renal failure. N Engl J Med 336:1303–1309, 1997.

674. Ronco C, Brendolan A, Bellomo R: Continuous renal replacement techniques. Contrib Nephrol 132:236–251, 2001.

675. Ronco C, Zanella M, Brendolan A, et al: Management of severe acute renal failure in critically ill patients: an international survey in 345 centres. Nephrol Dial Transplant 16:230–237, 2001.

676. Palsson R, Niles JL: Regional citrate anticoagulation in continuous venovenous hemofiltration in critically ill patients with a high risk of bleeding. Kidney Int 55:1991–1997, 1999.

677. Flanigan MJ, Pillsbury L, Sadewasser G, et al: Regional hemodialysis anticoagulation: hypertonic tri-sodium citrate or anticoagulant citrate dextrose-A. Am J Kidney Dis 27:519–524, 1996.

678. Chen JL: Argatroban: a direct thrombin inhibitor for heparin-induced thrombocytopenia and other clinical applications. Heart Dis 3:189–198, 2001.

679. Bellomo R, Baldwin I, Cole L, et al: Preliminary experience with high-volume hemofiltration in human septic shock. Kidney Int Suppl 66:S182–S185, 1998.

680. Cornejo R, Downey P, Castro R, et al: High-volume hemofiltration as salvage therapy in severe hyperdynamic septic shock. Intensive Care Med 32:713–722, 2006.

681. Ronco C, Bellomo R, Homel P, et al: Effects of different doses in continuous venovenous haemofiltration on outcomes of acute renal failure: a prospective randomised trial. Lancet 356:26–30, 2000.

682. Bouman CS, Oudemans-Van Straaten HM, Tijssen JG, et al: Effects of early high-volume continuous venovenous hemofiltration on survival and recovery of renal function in intensive care patients with acute renal failure: a prospective, randomized trial. Crit Care Med 30:2205–2211, 2002.

683. Mault JR, Dechert RE, Lees P, et al: Continuous arteriovenous filtration: an effective treatment for surgical acute renal failure. Surgery 101:478–484, 1987.

684. Stevens PE, Davies SP, Brown EA, et al: Continuous arteriovenous haemodialysis in critically ill patients. The Lancet 1:150–152, 1988.

685. Ronco C, Bellomo R, Ricci Z: Hemodynamic response to fluid withdrawal in overhydrated patients treated with intermittent ultrafiltration and slow continuous ultrafiltration: role of blood volume monitoring. Cardiology 96:196–201,2001.

686. Levraut J, Ciebiera JP, Jambou P, et al: Effect of continuous venovenous hemofiltration with dialysis on lactate clearance in critically ill patients. Crit Care Med 25:58–62, 1997.

687. Bohler J: Treatment of acute renal failure in intensive care patients. Int J Artif Organs 19:108–110, 1996.

688. Bohm R, Gladziwa U, Clasen W, et al: Which bicarbonate concentration is adequate to lactate-buffered substitution fluids in maintenance hemofiltration? Clin Nephrol 42:257–262, 1994.

689. Clasen M, Bohm R, Riehl J, et al: Lactate or bicarbonate for intermittent hemofiltration? Contrib Nephrol 93:152–155, 1991.

690. Uehlinger DE, Jakob SM, Ferrari P, et al: Comparison of continuous and intermittent renal replacement therapy for acute renal failure. Nephrol Dial Transplant 20:1630–1637, 2005.

691. Tonelli M, Manns B, Feller-Kopman D: Acute renal failure in the intensive care unit: a systematic review of the impact of dialytic modality on mortality and renal recovery. Am J Kidney Dis 40:875–885, 2002.

692. Marshall MR, Golper TA, Shaver MJ, et al: Sustained low-efficiency dialysis for critically ill patients requiring renal replacement therapy. Kidney Int 60:777–785, 2001.

693. Marshall MR, Golper TA, Shaver MJ, et al: Urea kinetics during sustained low-efficiency dialysis in critically ill patients requiring renal replacement therapy. Am J Kidney Dis 39:556–570, 2002.

694. Humes HD, Fissell WH, Weitzel WF: The bioartificial kidney in the treatment of acute renal failure. Kidney Int Suppl 80:121–125, 2002.

695. Fissell WH, Kimball J, MacKay SM, et al: The role of a bioengineered artificial kidney in renal failure. Ann N Y Acad Sci 944:284–295, 2001.

696. Woods JD, Humes HD: Prospects for a bioartificial kidney. Semin Nephrol 17:381–386, 1997.

697. Humes HD, Weitzel WF, Bartlett RH, et al: Initial clinical results of the bioartificial kidney containing human cells in ICU patients with acute renal failure. Kidney Int 66:1578–1588, 2004.

698. Palevsky PM, Metnitz PG, Piccinni P, et al: Selection of endpoints for clinical trials of acute renal failure in critically ill patients. Curr Opin Crit Care 8:515–518, 2002.

699. Chertow GM, Lazarus JM, Paganini EP, et al: Predictors of mortality and the provision of dialysis in patients with acute tubular necrosis. The Auriculin Anaritide Acute Renal Failure Study Group. J Am Soc Nephrol 9:692–698, 1998.

700. Rasmussen HH, Pitt EA, Ibels LS, et al: Prediction of outcome in acute renal failure by discriminant analysis of clinical variables. Arch Intern Med 145:2015–2018, 1985.

986

701. Wilkins RG, Faragher EB: Acute renal failure in an intensive care unit: incidence, prediction and outcome. Anaesthesia 38:628–634, 1983.

702. Turney JH, Marshall DH, Brownjohn AM, et al: The evolution of acute renal failure, 1956–1988. Q J Med 74:83–104, 1990.

703. Biesenbach G, Zazgornik J, Kaiser W, et al: Improvement in prognosis of patients with acute renal failure over a period of 15 years: an analysis of 710 patients in a dialysis center. Am J Nephrol 12:319–325, 1992.

704. Frankel MC, Weinstein AM, Stenzel KH: Prognostic patterns in acute renal failure: the New York Hospital, 1981–1982. Clin Exp Dial Apheresis 7:145–167, 1983.

705. Hoste EA, Clermont G, Kersten A, et al: RIFLE criteria for acute kidney injury are associated with hospital mortality in critically ill patients: a cohort analysis. Crit Care 10:R73–R83, 2006.

706. Manns B, Doig CJ, Lee H, et al. Cost of acute renal failure requiring dialysis in the intensive care unit: clinical and resource implications of renal recovery. Crit Care Med 31:449–455, 2003.

707. Bates DW, Su L, Yu DT, et al: Mortality and costs of acute renal failure associated with amphotericin B therapy. Clin Infect Dis 32:686–693, 2001.

708. Fischer MJ, Brimhall BB, Lezotte DC, et al: Uncomplicated acute renal failure and hospital resource utilization: a retrospective multicenter analysis. Am J Kidney Dis 46:1049–1057, 2005.

709. Hamel MB, Phillips RS, Davis RB, et al: Outcomes and cost-effectiveness of initiating dialysis and continuing aggressive care in seriously ill hospitalized adults. SUPPORT Investigators. Study to Understand Prognoses and Preferences for Outcomes and Risks of Treatments. Ann Intern Med 127:195–202, 1997.

710. Ahlstrom A, Tallgren M, Peltonen S, et al: Survival and quality of life of patients requiring acute renal replacement therapy. Intensive Care Med 31:1222–1228, 2005.

711. Fiaccadori E, Maggiore U, Lombardi M, et al: Predicting patient outcome from acute renal failure comparing three general severity of illness scoring systems. Kidney Int 58:283–292, 2000.

712. Halstenberg WK, Goormastic M, Paganini EP: Validity of four models for predicting outcome in critically ill acute renal failure patients. Clin Nephrol 47:81–86, 1997.

713. van Bommel EF, Bouvy ND, Hop WC, et al: Use of APACHE II classification to evaluate outcome and response to therapy in acute renal failure patients in a surgical intensive care unit. Ren Fail 17:731–742, 1995.

714. Mehta RL, Pascual MT, Gruta CG, et al: Refining predictive models in critically ill patients with acute renal failure. J Am Soc Nephrol 13:1350–1357, 2002.

715. Bell M, Liljestam E, Granath F, et al: Optimal follow-up time after continuous renal replacement therapy in actual renal failure patients stratified with the RIFLE criteria. Nephrol Dial Transplant 20:354–360, 2005.

CHAPTER 30

Primary Glomerular Disease

Patrick H. Nachman • J. Charles Jennette • Ronald J. Falk

The underlying cause of most glomerular diseases remains an enigma. Infectious agents, autoimmunity, drugs, inherited disorders, and environmental agents have been implicated as causes of certain glomerular diseases. Until the precise etiology and pathogenesis of glomerular disorders is unraveled, we continue in the tradition of Richard Bright—studying the relationship of clinical, pathological, and laboratory signs and symptoms of disease, and basing our diagnostic categorization on these features rather than on etiology.

Glomerular diseases may be categorized into those that primarily involve the kidney (primary glomerular diseases), and those in which kidney involvement is part of a systemic disorder (secondary glomerular diseases). This chapter will focus on primary glomerular diseases. This separation of glomerular disease into primary versus secondary is somewhat problematic, because in some instances, what are considered primary glomerular diseases is similar, if not identical, to secondary glomerular diseases. For example, IgA nephropathy, pauci-immune necrotizing and crescentic glomerulonephritis, anti-GBM glomerulonephritis, membranous glomerulopathy, and type I membranoproliferative glomerulonephritis can occur as primary renal diseases or as components of systemic diseases (i.e., Henoch-Schönlein purpura, pauci-immune small-vessel vasculitis, Goodpasture syndrome, systemic lupus erythematosus, and cryoglobulinemic vasculitis, respectively). This chapter will focus on the diagnosis and management of glomerular diseases that do not appear to be a component of a systemic disease.

When a patient presents with glomerular disease, clinicians must evaluate the clinical signs and symptoms of renal disease, and must also be vigilant for evidence of a systemic disease that could be causing the renal disease. Clinical evaluation includes assessment of proteinuria, hematuria, the presence or absence of renal insufficiency, and the presence or absence of hypertension. Some glomerular diseases cause isolated proteinuria or isolated hematuria with no other signs or symptoms of disease. More severe glomerular disease often results in the nephrotic syndrome or nephritic (glomerulonephritic) syndrome. Glomerular disease may have an indolent course or begin abruptly, leading to acute or rapidly progressive glomerulonephritis. Whereas some glomerular disorders consistently cause a specific syndrome (e.g., minimal change glomerulopathy resulting in the nephrotic syndrome), most disorders are capable of causing features of both nephrosis and nephritis (Table 30–1). This sharing and variability of clinical manifestations among different glomerular diseases confounds determination of an accurate diagnosis based on clinical features alone. Therefore, renal biopsy has an important role in the evaluation of many patients with glomerular disease.

This chapter will focus initially on the clinical syndromes caused by glomerular diseases, including isolated proteinuria, isolated hematuria, the nephrotic syndrome, and nephritic syndrome. Then, specific forms of primary glomerular disease that cause these syndromes will be considered in detail, beginning with glomerular diseases that cause predominantly the nephrotic syndrome, and concluding with glomerular diseases that cause predominantly the nephritic syndrome.

GENERAL DESCRIPTION OF GLOMERULAR SYNDROMES

Isolated Proteinuria

Proteinuria can be caused by systemic overproduction (e.g., multiple myeloma with Bence Jones proteinuria), tubular dysfunction (e.g., Fanconi syndrome), or glomerular dysfunction. It is important to identify patients in whom proteinuria is a manifestation of substantial glomerular disease as opposed to those patients who have benign functional, transient, postural (orthostatic), or intermittent proteinuria.

Plasma proteins larger than 70 kD cross the basement membrane in a manner normally restricted by both size-selective and charge-selective barriers.[1,2] The functional characteristics of the glomerular capillary filter have been extensively studied by the evaluation of the fractional clearance of molecules of different size and charge.[3] The size-selective barrier is most likely a consequence of functional pores within the glomerular basement membrane that restrict the filtration of plasma proteins of more than 150 kD. There is also a shape restriction of molecules that allows elongated molecules to cross the glomerular capillary wall more readily than molecules of the same molecular weight, and there is a charge-selective nature of the barrier largely a consequence of glycosaminoglycans arranged along the capillary wall. Loss of charge selectivity may be the defect in minimal change glomerulopathy, whereas a loss of size selectivity may be the cause of proteinuria in, for instance, membranous glomerulopathy.[2]

A number of factors have proven to be important in the disruption of the glomerular capillary wall as a consequence of tissue-degrading enzymes, complement components that assemble upon it, and oxygen radicals that target both the glomerular basement membrane and the slit

TABLE 30–1	Manifestations of Nephrotic and Nephritic Features by Glomerular Disease	
	Nephrotic Features	Nephritic Features
Minimal change glomerulopathy	++++	–
Membranous glomerulopathy	++++	+
Focal segmental glomerulosclerosis	+++	++
Fibrillary glomerulonephritis	+++	++
Mesangioproliferative glomerulopathy*	++	++
Membranoproliferative glomerulonephritis[†]	++	+++
Proliferative glomerulonephritis*	++	+++
Acute diffuse proliferative glomerulonephritis[‡]	+	++++
Crescentic glomerulonephritis[¶]	+	++++

*Mesangioproliferative and proliferative glomerulonephritis (focal or diffuse) are structural manifestations of a number of glomerulonephritides, including IgA nephropathy and lupus nephritis.
[†]Both type I (mesangiocapillary) and type II (dense deposit disease).
[‡]Often a structural manifestation of acute post-streptococcal glomerulonephritis.
[¶]Can be immune complex mediated, anti-glomerular basement membrane antibody mediated, or associated with anti-neutrophil cytoplasmic autoantibodies.
Modified from Jennette JC, Mandal AK: The nephrotic syndrome. *In* Mandel SR, Jennette JC (eds): Diagnosis and Management of Renal Disease and Hypertension, 2nd ed. Durham, Carolina Academic Press, 1994, pp 235–272.

diaphragm. Heparinase and hyaluronidase alterations in the amino glycan content of the glomerular capillary wall may play a role in increased protein excretion.[4,5] Genetic studies have provided exciting clues to the specific components of the glomerular capillary wall, including mutations in the podocyte or proteins in the slit diaphragm, which result in proteinuria (recently reviewed by Tryggvason and colleagues[6]).

Another major mechanism resulting in proteinuria is impaired reabsorption of plasma proteins by proximal tubular epithelial cells. A number of low-molecular-weight proteins, including β1, β2, and α1 microglobulins, are filtered by the glomerulus and absorbed by tubular epithelial cells. When tubular epithelial cells are damaged, these proteins are excreted. The qualitative nature of proteinuria forms the basis for the observation that excretion of high-molecular-weight proteins (e.g., fractional excretion of IgG) is indicative of glomerular damage, whereas excretion of low-molecular-weight proteins (e.g., fractional excretion of alpha1 microglobulin) is more likely when there is tubular epithelial damage. This separation of high- from low-molecular-weight proteinuria has been suggested to be a predictor of clinical outcome in a number of glomerular diseases.[7] The uptake of filtered proteins, including albumin by tubular cells, may produce a reaction that results in tubular atrophy and interstitial fibrosis. This is a controversial area, however, in that a number of studies suggest that exposure of tubular epithelium to albumin or other proteins may not be a phlogistic event.[8–11]

The term "isolated proteinuria" is used in several conditions, including mild transient proteinuria of less than one gram that typically accompanies physiologically stressful conditions such as fever in hospitalized patients, exercise, and congestive heart failure.[12] In other patients, transient proteinuria is a consequence of the overflow of proteins of low molecular weight due to over-production of light chains, heavy chains, or other fragments of immunoglobulins. The differential diagnosis of overproduction of proteinuria includes multiple myeloma, Bence Jones proteinuria, β2 microglobulinuria, and hemoglobinuria.

The term "orthostatic proteinuria" is defined by the absence of proteinuria while the patient is in a recumbent posture and its appearance during upright posture, especially during ambulation or exercise.[13] The total amount of protein excretion in a 24-hour period is generally less than 1.0 gram, but may be as much as 2 grams. Orthostatic proteinuria is more common in adolescents and is uncommon in individuals over the age of 30.[13,14] Two to five percent of adolescents have orthostatic proteinuria. Renal biopsy of patients with orthostatic proteinuria reveals that 47% have normal glomeruli by light microscopy, 45% have minimal to moderate glomerular abnormalities of nonspecific nature, and the remainder have evidence of a primary glomerular disease.[15] Why is proteinuria increased during upright posture in individuals with normal glomeruli by light microscopy? Although the answer to this question remains an enigma, there are several likely possibilities. Orthostatic proteinuria may occur as a consequence of alterations in glomerular hemodynamics. It is possible that even in histologically "normal" glomeruli, where there are no specific lesions, there are subtle glomerular abnormalities, including abnormal basement membranes, or focal changes of the mesangium.[16] Alternatively, orthostatic proteinuria has been demonstrated with entrapment of the left renal vein by the aorta and superior mesenteric artery. Thirteen of 15 children with orthostatic proteinuria had venous entrapment compared with 9 of 80 with normal protein excretion.[17] In addition, the observation that surgical correction of a kink in an allograft renal vein resulted in the disappearance of orthostatic proteinuria gives credence to venous entrapment as a cause for orthostatic proteinuria.[16]

There are several approaches to the diagnosis of orthostatic proteinuria. These include comparison of protein excretion in two 12-hour urine collections, one recumbent and one during ambulation. Another approach is to compare protein in a split collection of 16 hours during ambulation and 8 hours of overnight collection. Importantly, patients should be recumbent for at least 2 hours before their ambulatory collection is completed to avoid the possibility of contamination of the "recumbent" collection by urine formed during ambulation. The diagnosis of orthostatic proteinuria requires that protein excretion during recumbency is less than 50 mg during those 8 hours. Little convincing data exists on the usefulness of urinary protein-to-creatinine ratio measurements during recumbency versus ambulation as a diagnostic test for orthostatic proteinuria.

Long-term follow-up of orthostatic proteinuria for 20 years suggests a benign long-term course.[14] Orthostatic proteinuria resolves in most patients. It is present in one half of patients after 10 years and only 17% of patients after 20 years.[14] In the absence of a kidney biopsy, an underlying glomerulopathy cannot be completely excluded, and an orthostatic component of proteinuria may be found in early glomerular disease. Thus, it is important to reassess patients after an interval of about 1 year to be certain that the degree or pattern of proteinuria has not changed.

Fixed proteinuria is present whether the patient is upright or recumbent. The proteinuria disappears in some patients whereas others will have a more ominous glomerular lesion that portends an adverse long-term outcome. The prognosis depends on the persistence and severity of the proteinuria. If proteinuria disappears, it is less likely that the patient will develop hypertension or reduced glomerular filtration rate. These patients must be evaluated periodically for as long as proteinuria persists.

RECURRENT OR PERSISTENT HEMATURIA

Hematuria is the presence of an excessive number of red blood cells in the urine and is categorized as either microscopic (visible only with the aid of a microscope) or macroscopic (urine that is tea-colored or cola-colored, pink, or even red). Hematuria can result from injury to the kidney or to another site in the urinary tract.

Healthy individuals may excrete as many as 10^5 red cells in the urine in a 12-hour period. An acceptable definition of hematuria is more than two red cells per high-power field in centrifuged urine.[18] However, the approach to processing urine varies from laboratory to laboratory, thus the number of red cells per high-power field that is an accurate indicator of hematuria may vary slightly among different laboratories. The urinary dipstick detects one to two red cells per high power field and results in a very sensitive test. A negative dipstick examination virtually excludes hematuria.[19]

Hematuria is present in about 5% to 6% of the general population[20] and 4% of school children. In the majority of children, follow-up urinalyses are normal.[21] In most people, the hematuria emanates from the lower urinary tract, especially in the conditions affecting the urethra, bladder, and prostate. Less than 10% of hematuria is caused by glomerular bleeding.[18] Persistent hematuria, especially in older individuals, should raise the possibility of malignancy. The incidence of malignancy, especially from the bladder, ranges from 5% in individuals with persistent microscopic hematuria to over 20% in individuals with gross hematuria.[22] Other causes of non-glomerular hematuria include neoplasms, trauma, metabolic defects such as hypercalciuria, vascular diseases including renal infarctions and renal vein thrombosis, cystic diseases of the kidney including polycystic kidney disease, medullary cystic disease and medullary sponge kidney, and interstitial kidney disease such as papillary necrosis, hydronephrosis, and drug-induced interstitial nephritis. In children with asymptomatic hematuria, hypercalciuria is the cause in 15% of cases, and 10% to 15% will have IgA nephropathy. Up to 80% of children and 15% to 20% of adults with hematuria will have no identifiable cause.[23]

Transient hematuria has been found in a number of settings. Transient hematuria is present in 13% of postmenopausal women.[24] Episodic hematuria in a cyclical pattern during a menstrual cycle is most likely a consequence of the invasion of the urinary tract by endometrial implants.[25] In 1000 males between the ages of 18 and 33, hematuria was present at least once in 39%, and on two or more occasions in 16%. Patients with isolated, asymptomatic hematuria without proteinuria or renal insufficiency have resolution of

their hematuria in 20% of cases; however, even in these cases, some will develop hypertension and proteinuria.[26] In older individuals, transient hematuria should raise a concern of malignancy.[18,27,28] In some individuals, transient hematuria may be a consequence of exercise.

Glomerular hematuria, in contrast to hematuria caused by injury elsewhere in the urinary tract, is characterized by misshapen red cells that have been distorted by osmotic and chemical stress to red blood cells as they passed through the nephron. Dysmorphic hematuria, especially cells that have membrane blebs producing the picture of acanthocyturia, is strong evidence for glomerular bleeding.[22] The findings of proteinuria (especially >2 grams per day), hemoglobin, or red cell casts enhance the possibility that hematuria is of glomerular origin. Although the presence of brown or cola-colored urine is most commonly associated with glomerular hematuria, its absence does not exclude glomerular disease. Interestingly, the presence of clots in the urine does not occur with glomerular bleeding.

The differential pathologic diagnosis of glomerular hematuria without proteinuria, renal insufficiency, or red blood cell casts is IgA nephropathy, thin basement membrane nephropathy, hereditary nephritis, or histologically normal glomeruli.[29] In a study by Tiebosch,[30] 80 normotensive adults underwent renal biopsy to evaluate recurrent macroscopic hematuria or persistent microscopic hematuria. Twenty-seven individuals had IgA nephropathy, 42 had normal renal tissue by light microscopy, of which electron microscopy revealed thin basement membrane nephropathy in 18 patients, and normal glomerular basement membrane thickness in 24 patients. Hematuria disappeared in 13 of these latter patients. The remaining 11 patients had mesangioproliferative glomerulonephritis, interstitial nephritis, or focal glomerulosclerosis. Importantly, of the 54 patients who presented with microscopic hematuria, 31% had thin basement membrane nephropathy, illustrating the importance of this disease as a cause for asymptomatic glomerular hematuria.

Table 30-2 provides data from an analysis of native kidney biopsy specimens of patients from the University of North Carolina Nephropathology Laboratory, all of whom had hematuria. Patients with systemic lupus erythematosus were excluded from the study. The patients were selected based on a serum creatinine of less than 1.5 mg/dL or greater than 3 mg/dL. The patients with a serum creatinine of less than 1.5 mg/dL were further divided into those with proteinuria less than 1 gram per day, versus those with proteinuria of 1 gram to 3 grams per day. The data showed that patients with relatively normal serum creatinine, hematuria, and less than 1 gram per day of proteinuria were most likely to have thin basement membrane nephropathy, IgA nephropathy, or no identifiable renal lesion. When hematuria is accompanied by 1 gram to 3 grams per day of proteinuria, but no significant renal insufficiency, IgA nephropathy was the most likely specific cause. Patients with hematuria and a serum creatinine of greater than 3 mg/dL most often have aggressive glomerulonephritis with crescents.

Despite these overall tendencies, it is not possible to definitively determine the cause of asymptomatic hematuria without renal biopsy, and even renal biopsy evaluation fails to reveal a cause in a minority of patients. Certain rules generally apply to the clinical prediction of the most likely cause. Gross hematuria is most commonly found in IgA nephropathy or hereditary nephritis. Patients with thin basement membrane nephropathy typically do not have substantial proteinuria.

Potential benefits of renal biopsy in patients with isolated hematuria include reduction of patient and physician uncertainty by confirming a specific diagnosis. Nonetheless, the role of renal biopsy in the evaluation of individuals with asymptomatic hematuria without proteinuria, hypertension,

TABLE 30–2	Renal Disease in Patients with Hematuria Undergoing Renal Biopsy		
	Hematuria Proteinuria <1 Creatinine <1.5	Hematuria Proteinuria 1–3 Creatinine <1.5	Hematuria Creatinine >3
No abnormality	30%	2%	0%
Thin basement nephropathy	26%	4%	0%
IgA nephropathy	28%	24%	8%
Glomerulonephritis without crescents*	9%	26%	23%
Glomerulonephritis with crescents*	2%	24%	44%
Other renal disease†	5%	20%	25%
Total	100% n = 43	100% n = 123	100% n = 255

Units: proteinuria, g/24 h; serum creatinine, mg/dl.
*Proliferative or necrotizing glomerulonephritis other than IgA nephropathy or lupus nephritis.
†Includes causes for the nephrotic syndrome, such as membranous glomerulopathy and focal segmental glomerulosclerosis.
An analysis of renal biopsy specimens evaluated at by the University of North Carolina Nephropathology Laboratory. Patients with systemic lupus erythematosus were excluded from the analysis.
Derived from Caldas MLR, Jennette JC, Falk RJ, Wilkman AS, NC Glomerular Disease Collaborative Network Lab Invest 62:15A, 1990.

or kidney insufficiency remains unclear. In biopsy series from patients in whom asymptomatic hematuria is accompanied by low-grade proteinuria, specific glomerular diseases including IgA nephropathy and membranoproliferative glomerular disease may be discovered when there is no proteinuria, and IgA nephropathy and thin basement membrane disease or non-diagnostic minor changes remain the most common findings.[31,32] Confirmation of a glomerular cause eliminates repeated unnecessary urologic studies and determination of a more accurate long-term prognosis can be made (e.g., thin basement membrane nephropathy is less likely to progress than IgA nephropathy). However, isolated glomerular hematuria without proteinuria or renal insufficiency may not warrant a renal biopsy because the findings often will not affect management. In one study of patients with isolated hematuria, the biopsy results altered patient management in only 1 of 36 patients.[33]

Nephrotic Syndrome

The nephrotic syndrome results from greater than 3.5 grams per day of proteinuria and is characterized by edema, hyperlipidemia, hypoproteinemia, and other metabolic disorders (described in detail below). In addition to primary (idiopathic) glomerular diseases, the nephrotic syndrome may be secondary to a large number of identifiable disease states (Table 30–3, *modified from previous edition*). Despite the differences in these causes, the loss of substantial amounts of protein in the urine results in a shared set of abnormalities that comprise the nephrotic syndrome.

Edema

Edema is the most common presenting symptom of patients with the nephrotic syndrome. Various theories for the cause of nephrotic edema have been proposed. Hypovolemia as a consequence of reduced plasma oncotic pressure has long been considered the proximal cause of salt and water retention by the kidney. Enhanced tubular sodium reabsorption is thought to be a function of multiple mediator systems responding to the "perceived volume depletion" with activation of the renin-angiotensin aldosterone, sympathetic nervous, and vasopressor systems.[34]

Although there is evidence to support the "underfilling" hypothesis of edema formation,[35] other investigators have suggested that a primary disorder of the kidney results in

increased intravascular volume and subsequent suppression of renin angiotensin aldosterone access and elevated natriuretic peptide levels.[36] The literature is unclear whether plasma volume is low or high. These issues are of more than academic interest, in that fluid assessment in a patient with the nephrotic syndrome may require substantial alterations in diuretic use.[35]

It is reasonable to assert that hypoproteinemia results in a fall in the plasma oncotic pressure and the movement of fluid into the interstitial space. Several factors mitigate this phenomenon. Normally, the transcapillary oncotic pressure gradient (plasma oncotic pressure minus the interstitial oncotic pressure) acts synergistically to retain fluid within the vascular space. In normal patients, colloid osmotic pressure in the plasma is approximately 26 mm Hg. The interstitial oncotic pressure may be as high as 10 mm Hg to 15 mm Hg because of the filtration of albumin across the capillary wall. In nephrotic patients, the interstitial oncotic pressure may fall to as low as 2.6 mm Hg in the lower extremity. The fall in the interstitial oncotic pressure functions as a protecting factor in hypoproteinemic patients.[37] There may be a consequent parallel decline in interstitial oncotic pressure matching the fall in the plasma oncotic pressure and minimizing the change in the transcapillary gradient. Thus, there would be a smaller change in the transcapillary gradient and a reduced drive of fluid shifting from the vascular compartment into the interstitium. Other factors limiting the amount of fluid movement into the interstitium include compliance of the interstitium in most tissues and increased lymphatic fluid flow. Marked dietary salt ingestion or the administration of saline to patients who are hypoproteinemic may result in a rapid fall in the transcapillary oncotic pressure gradient and subsequent substantial edema.

What factors are responsible for sodium retention in the nephrotic state? Does the propensity for avid sodium retention derive entirely from hypovolemia due to loss of fluid into the interstitium? Most likely in some patients, hypovolemia plays an important role in the retention of salt and water by the kidney.[38] However, there have been several challenges to the concept that sodium retention and edema formation are the consequence of hypovolemia. These arguments suggest that in adult patients with the nephrotic syndrome, there may be normal or even increased plasma volume.[39] High blood pressure argues against hypovolemia and, in fact, suggests hypervolemia.[40]

Idiopathic Nephrotic Syndrome due to Primary Glomerular Disease

Nephrotic Syndrome Associated with Specific Etiologic Events or in Which Glomerular Disease Arises as a Complication of Other Diseases:

1. Medications
   Organic, inorganic, elemental mercury*
   Organic gold
   Penicillamine, bucillamine
   "Street" heroin
   Probenecid
   Captopril
   NSAIDs
   Lithium
   Interferon alfa
   Chlorpropamide
   Rifampin
   Pamidronate
   Paramethadione (Paradione), trimethadione (Tridione)
   Mephenytoin (Mesantoin)
   Tolbutamide[†]
   Phenindione[†]
   Warfarin
   Clonidine[†]
   Perchlorate[†]
   Bismuth[†]
   Trichloroethylene[†]
   Silver[†]
   Insect repellent[†]
   Contrast media
2. Allergens, venoms, immunizations
   Bee sting
   Pollens
   Poison ivy and poison oak
   Antitoxins (serum sickness)
   Snake venom
   Diphtheria, pertussis, tetanus toxoid
   Vaccines
3. Infections
   a. Bacterial-PSGN, infective endocarditis, "shunt nephritis," leprosy, syphilis (congenital and secondary), Mycoplasma infection, tuberculosis, [†]chronic bacterial pyelonephritis with vesicoureteral reflux.
   b. Viral-hepatitis B, hepatitis C, cytomegalovirus, infectious mononucleosis (Epstein-Barr virus), herpes zoster, vaccinia, human immunodeficiency virus type I
   c. Protozoal-malaria (especially quartan malaria), toxoplasmosis
   d. Helminthic-schistosomiasis, trypanosomiasis, filariasis
4. Neoplastic
   a. Solid tumors (carcinoma and sarcoma): lung, colon, stomach, breast, cervix, kidney, thyroid, ovary, melanoma, pheochromocytoma, adrenal, oropharynx, carotid body, [†]Wilms tumor, prostate, mesothelioma, oncocytoma
   b. Leukemia and lymphoma: Hodgkin disease, chronic lymphatic leukemia, multiple myeloma (amyloidosis), Waldenström macroglobulinemia, lymphoma.
   c. Graft versus host disease after bone marrow transplantation
5. Multisystem disease[‡]
   Systemic lupus erythematosus
   Mixed connective tissue disease
   Dermatomyositis
   Rheumatoid arthritis
   Goodpasture disease
   Schönlein-Henoch purpura (see also IgA nephropathy, Berger disease)

Systemic vasculitis (including Wegener granulomatosis)
Takayasu arteritis
Mixed cryoglobulinemia
Light and heavy chain disease (Randall-type)
Partial lipodystrophy
Sjögren syndrome
Toxic epidermolysis
Dermatitis herpetiformis
Sarcoidosis
Ulcerative colitis
Amyloidosis (primary and secondary)
6. Heredofamilial and metabolic disease[‡]
   Diabetes mellitus
   Hypothyroidism (myxedema)
   Graves disease
   Amyloidosis (familial Mediterranean fever and other hereditary forms, Muckle-Wells syndrome)
   Alport syndrome
   Fabry disease
   Nail-patella syndrome
   Lipoprotein glomerulopathy
   Sickle cell disease
   α_1-Antitrypsin deficiency
   Asphyxiating thoracic dystrophy (Jeune syndrome)
   Von Gierke disease
   Podocyte/Slit diaphragm
      Nephrin
      FAT2
      Podocin
      CD2AP
      Denys-Drash syndrome (WT1)
      ACTN4
   Charcot-Marie-Tooth syndrome
   Congenital nephrotic syndrome (Finnish-type)
   Cystinosis (adult)
   Galloway-Mowat syndrome
   Hurler syndrome
   Familial dysautonomia
7. Miscellaneous[‡]
   Pregnancy-associated (preeclampsia, recurrent, transient)
   Chronic renal allograft failure
   Accelerated or malignant nephrosclerosis
   Unilateral renal arterial hypertension
   Intestinal lymphangiectasia
   Chronic jejunoileitis[†]
   Spherocytosis[†]
   Renal artery stenosis
   Congenital heart disease[†] (cyanotic)
   Severe congestive heart failure[†]
   Constrictive pericarditis[†]
   Tricuspid insufficiency[†]
   Massive obesity
   Vesicoureteric reflux nephropathy
   Papillary necrosis
   Gardner-Diamond syndrome
   Castleman disease
   Kartagener syndrome
   Buckley syndrome
   Kimura disease
   Silica exposure

*Diseases and other agents in italics are the more commonly encountered causes of nephrotic syndrome.
[†]Single case reports or small series in which cause-and-effect relationship cannot be established. Other factors (e.g., mercurial diuretics in heart failure) may have been true inciting event.
[‡]See Chapter 31 for detailed discussion of the secondary forms of nephrotic syndrome.

The resolution of edema due to normalization of plasma oncotic pressure, for example by administration of albumin, supports the argument that hypoalbuminemia is important in the generation of edema. In some patients, however, the administration of albumin does not result in amelioration of edema, nor does maintenance of a normal serum albumin level in any given patient necessarily prevent the development of edema over the course of time. There are normal levels of serum albumin in some edematous patients. This may be due to contraction of the blood volume, or of homeostatic increase in other proteins that may rise to varying degrees. Thus, the serum albumin may not be indicative of the plasma oncotic pressure. Some of the most convincing data that hypovolemia may not necessarily play a role in the development of edema stems from studies in children with relapse of minimal change glomerulopathy. Vande Walle and colleagues investigated the cause of sodium retention in the nephrotic syndrome in children with early relapse of minimal change glomerulopathy.[41] In this study, children presented with severe hypoproteinemia and the nephrotic syndrome with or without clinical symptoms or laboratory signs of hypovolemia. Sodium retention preceded the reduction in serum protein concentrations in some patients, and natriuresis developed before proteinuria had resolved in others.

The levels of atrial natriuretic factor (ANF) and plasma renin activity (PRA) in patients with acute glomerulonephritis have been compared to patients with the nephrotic syndrome and to normal individuals.[42] The amount of edema was similar in the two groups of patients with glomerular disease, and they had similar urinary sodium excretion. Interestingly, patients with acute glomerulonephritis had five times higher levels of ANF and six times lower PRA when compared to patients with the nephrotic syndrome. In fact, the degree of edema correlated with the ANF levels found with acute glomerulonephritis, but not in those patients with the nephrotic syndrome. There was a strong negative correlation between the level of ANF and the PRA. At the same level of sodium excretion, nephrotic patients had ANF and PRA levels equivalent to normal subjects ingesting a usual amount of sodium in their diet. These results suggest that renal sodium retention in nephrosis is probably a consequence of primary renal sodium retention rather than a consequence of plasma hormone effects on the kidney. It is reasonably certain that sodium retention in nephrotic states is not dependent on changes in activity in the renin-angiotensin-aldosterone system.[43-46] Whether the inability of angiotensin converting enzyme inhibitors to result in natriuresis is a function of over-activity of this system that cannot be inhibited, or this system is not causing sodium retention has not been elucidated. On the other side of the controversy, capillary filtration capacity at the calf, a noninvasive measure of capillary pressure, demonstrated that patients with the nephrotic syndrome had no evidence of capillary hypertension or evidence to support the overflow hypothesis of edema formation. In fact, there was no difference in capillary pressure between nephrotic subjects and controls.[47]

Recently, a hypothesis has been advanced that sodium and water retention in the nephrotic syndrome is due to over-excretion of vasopressin as a consequence of either volume or osmotic stimuli. This vasopressin-dependent process results in fluid retention.[48] The availability of selective antagonists of vasopressin's action with respect to vascular and tubular effects should make it possible to explore this hypothesis more fully.

There are certain important issues to consider when making decisions about management of edema in the nephrotic syndrome. In some patients, the edema is only of minimal discomfort whereas in others the edema causes substantial morbidity. The goal should be to have a slow resolution of edema. In all instances, the institution of rapid diuresis,

resulting in hypovolemia and even hypotension, must be avoided. Dietary restriction of sodium intake has been the mainstay of therapy in the management of nephrotic edema. Patients with nephrosis have sodium avidity and therefore the amount of sodium in the urine may be as low as 10 mmol/day.[49] Consequently, it is virtually impossible to lower the sodium intake to these levels. It is more important to suggest mild sodium restriction. Mild diuretics, including thiazide diuretics, may be sufficient in many patients with mild edema. Potassium sparing diuretics, such as triamterene, amiloride, or spironolactone, are useful in those patients in whom hypokalemia becomes a clinical problem, but their use is limited in those patients with renal insufficiency. Furosemide and other loop diuretics are typically used for moderate to severe nephrotic edema. Although the high protein content of tubular fluid was once thought to inhibit furosemide and other loop diuretics by binding to them, data now suggests that urinary protein binding does not effect the response to furosemide.[50,51] Metolazone may be effective when used by itself or in combination with loop diuretics (i.e., furosemide) in patients with refractory nephrotic edema. In patients treated with diuretics, episodes of profound volume depletion may occur. The resultant peripheral vasoconstriction, tachycardia, orthostatic hypotension and, at times, oliguria and renal insufficiency are usually amenable to cessation of the diuretic and rehydration. Albumin infusions transiently increase plasma volume and are most useful in patients with profound volume depletion.[52,53] Unfortunately, because of the rapid excretion of the infused albumin within 48 hours,[54] the utility of this approach is short-lived and may result in transient development of pulmonary edema. In extreme cases of marked edema, and especially pulmonary edema typically in the setting of reduced glomerular filtration rate, filtration using either intermittent or continuous extracorporeal dialysis is useful.

Hyperlipidemia

Hyperlipidemia is one of the sentinel features of the nephrotic syndrome. Patients develop numerous alterations in lipid profiles including hypercholesterolemia and hypertriglyceridemia with elevations in low-density lipoprotein (LDL), very low-density lipoprotein (VLDL), intermediate-density lipoprotein (IDL), and lipoprotein(a) [LP(a)]. Reduced or unchanged high-density lipoprotein (HDL) concentrations result in an increase in the adverse cardiovascular risk ratio of LDL/HDL cholesterol.[55-59] Hyperlipidemia is thought to be the consequence of both increased synthesis and decreased catabolism of individual lipid fractions. In part, hypercholesterolemia is due to the overproduction by the liver of lipoproteins that contain both cholesterol and lipoprotein B.[55,57] It has been hypothesized that this overproduction by the liver is a consequence of a fall in the oncotic pressure. Oncotic pressure may play a role in the regulation of the transcription of albumin and apolipoprotein B genes.[60] Data now suggest that hyperlipidemia in nephrotic patients is driven by a complex interplay of relative elevation or diminution of a number of enzymes that are important in cholesterol synthesis. In a number of studies, Vaziri and colleagues have shown that there is a relative elevation of hepatic 3-hydroxy-3-methylglutaryl-coenzyme A (HMG-CoA) reductase, the rate-limiting enzyme in cholesterol biosynthesis, and a reduction in hepatic cholesterol (Ch) 7α-hydroxylase. The expression of Ch 7α-hydroxylase is rate-limiting in the catabolism of cholesterol. In addition, LDL receptor deficiency limits hepatic cholesterol uptake and is complemented by the upregulation of the liver-specific enzyme acylcoenzyme A: cholesterol acyltransferase-2 (ACAT-2) that lowers liver-free cholesterol concentrations.[61] In the nephrotic syndrome, abnormalities in HDL may be a consequence of urinary loss of the critical enzyme lecithin:cholesterol acyltransferase

(LCAT), which decreases HDL-mediated uptake of surplus cholesterol from tissues outside of the liver. Accompanying the loss of LCAT is the down-regulation of hepatic HDL receptor-limiting cholesterol and triglyceride removal by the liver. Hypertriglyceridemia seen in the nephrotic syndrome is most likely a consequence of a number of factors, including the down-regulation of lipoprotein lipase, the down-regulation of the VLDL receptor, and the impairment of hepatic triglyceride lipase (reviewed by Vaziri[61]).

Finally, LP(a) is an independent risk factor for atherosclerotic disease.[62] In patients with the nephrotic syndrome, plasma LP(a) increases significantly as a consequence of an increased rate of synthesis with a normal fractional catabolic rate.[63] LP(a) binds to apolipoprotein(a) [Apo(a)] with a disulfide bond. Apo(a) has a high degree of homology with plasminogen,[64] and Apo(a) interferes with plasminogen-mediated fibrinolysis; thus, an elevation of LP(a) produces a prothrombotic event.

There are many clinical benefits of lipid-lowering therapy. In the landmark study of the Lipid Research Clinics Program coronary primary prevention trial, cholestyramine demonstrated a reduction of serum cholesterol that could reduce the rate of adverse coronary events.[65,66] Numerous subsequent studies have further elucidated the relationship of coronary artery disease with hypercholesterolemia.[67-72] Premature coronary atherosclerosis and increased incidence of myocardial infarction have been reported in patients with the nephrotic syndrome.[73] Hyperlipidemia of the nephrotic syndrome is likely a separate risk factor for atherosclerotic cardiovascular disease.[56,58] In a case-controlled study, individuals with nephrotic syndrome were at a substantially increased risk of coronary artery disease with a relative risk when compared to controls of 5.5 for myocardial infarction and a relative risk of 2.8 for coronary death in general.[73] Most studies, however, have not confirmed a predisposition for accelerated atherosclerosis in nephrotic patients.[74] This may be due to the relatively small number of younger patients studied and the relatively short duration that patients have been examined.

Sensitive measures of endothelial dysfunction suggest that in patients with the nephrotic syndrome, endothelial function is altered. Postischemic flow-mediated dilatation (FMD) of the brachial artery was significantly lower in nephrotic patients and primary hyperlipidemia patients when compared with control patients.[75] Using an HMG-CoA reductase inhibitor, brachial artery endothelial function improved.[76]

In addition to the cardiovascular risk, there is a risk of the hyperlipidemia promoting progression of renal disease. These data largely stem from animal studies suggesting that hyperlipidemia enhances the rate of progressive glomerular injury.[77] The potentially atherogenic apo-B containing lipoproteins may be associated with glomerular and interstitial lesions. How these lipoproteins cause renal disease is not clear, although there is non-receptor-mediated uptake of lipoproteins by mesangial cells that accelerate both sclerotic processes and proliferative ones. Most importantly, increased concentrations of APO-B containing lipoproteins are associated with more rapid progression of renal injury in both diabetic nephropathy and primary glomerular diseases.[78] In some patients, hyperlipidemia may persist well after clinical remission has occurred.

The management of hyperlipidemia in the nephrotic syndrome is difficult. Remission of the nephrotic syndrome leads to optimum resolution of hypercholesterolemia and hypertriglyceridemia. Dietary therapy provides very little benefit.[79] However, Gentile and colleagues evaluated the effect of a soy vegetable diet rich in mono- and polyunsaturated fatty acids.[80] Using this approach, a 25% to 30% reduction in lipid levels was observed that could not be improved by the addition of fish oils to the diet. This approach must be confirmed by larger trials.

Virtually all forms of lipid-lowering drugs have been used to treat patients with the nephrotic syndrome.[79,81-86] The most useful agents to lower lipid levels in patients with nephrosis are the HMG-CoA reductase inhibitors and agents that sequester bile acids, including cholestyramine and colestipol. The bile acid sequestrants lower total cholesterol levels by up to 30% when used alone[81] and when used with HMG-CoA reductase inhibitors, they have an additive benefit. The HMG-CoA reductase inhibitors lower total and LDL cholesterol levels by between 10% and 45%, coupled with a reduction in triglyceride levels.[56,79,82] The use of these agents in patients with unremitting nephrotic syndrome resulted in a moderate decline in Lp(a) in patients with an elevated Lp(a).[84] Although the fibric acid derivatives including gemfibrozil and clofibrate lower cholesterol by only 10% to 30%, they also lower plasma triglycerides and may raise HDL level. Unfortunately, they are associated with increased risk of myopathy. Nicotinic acid may have a positive effect on hyperlipidemia, but the side effects of headaches and flushing usually limit its usefulness. At present, treatment of HMG-CoA reductase inhibitors appears to be the treatment of choice.

Functional Consequence of Urinary Loss of Plasma Proteins

In addition to the urinary losses of albumin in the nephrotic syndrome, glomerular permeability causes the loss of proteins of similar molecular weight (Table 30-4). Not all proteins are lost in the urine, especially larger proteins such as IgM, fibrinogen, alpha-1 and alpha-2 macroglobulin, and larger lipoproteins that never traverse the glomerular

TABLE 30-4	Alterations of Plasma Protein in the Nephrotic Syndrome[114,115,1280-1293]

- Immunoglobulins
  Decreased IgG
  Normal or increased IgA, IgM, or IgE
  Increased alpha$_2$k and beta globulins
  Decreased alpha$_1$ globulin
- Metal-binding proteins
  Loss of metal binding proteins
    Iron
    Copper
    Zinc
- Loss of erythropoietin
- Depletion of transferrin
- Transcortin deficiency

- Complement deficiency
  Decreased factor B
  Decreased C3
  Decreased C1q, C2, C8, Ci
  Increased C3, C4bp
  Normal C1s, C4, and C1 inhibitor
- Coagulation components
  Decreased factors XI, XII, kallikrein inhibitor
  Decreased factors IX, XII
  Decreased anti-plasmin, alpha$_1$ antitrypsin
    Plasminogen activator, endothelial
    prostacyclin stimulating factor
  Decreased anti-thrombin III
  Elevated beta thromboglobulin
  Procoagulant

capillary wall and thus are of normal or increased concentration in the plasma.[87]

Hormone-binding proteins are typically lost in the urine resulting in several endocrine or metabolic abnormalities. The urinary loss of thyroid binding globulins and thyroxine results in a low T4, both free and bound, in about one half of all patients with the nephrotic syndrome and a normal glomerular filtration rate.[88–90] Additionally, total T3 levels are reduced probably because of decreased binding to thyroid binding globulins.[90] Total reversed T3 levels tend to be normal in the nephrotic syndrome, but the free reverse T3 level is elevated.[90] Despite these abnormalities, most patients remain clinically euthyroid. In some patients, loss of thyroid proteins in the urine has been associated with hypothyroidism in patients with the nephrotic syndrome,[91] with hypothyroidism resolving coincident with remission of the nephrotic syndrome. Moreover, treatment of the nephrotic syndrome with corticosteroid therapy may reduce TSH levels and, in some patients, inhibit the conversion of T4 to T3,[92] As a practical matter, free T4 levels or the level of the TSH are the best markers of the clinical status of the thyroid.

Calcium and vitamin D levels are typically altered in the nephrotic syndrome. Vitamin D binding protein is a relatively small protein of 59 kD that is filtered as readily as albumin.[93] 25-hydroxyvitamin D, the precursor of Calcitriol, is bound to vitamin D binding proteins and is lost in the urine with the nephrotic syndrome.[94,95] Similarly, there may be low serum concentrations of total 1,25-dihydroxyvitamin D.[96] With the loss of vitamin D binding protein, it is important to measure free 1,25-dihydroxyvitamin D levels to accurately assess the status of this factor in these patients. Further, hypoalbuminemia results in low total serum calcium concentration. Coupled with alterations in vitamin D binding proteins, of issue is which patients with true hypocalcemia are at risk for osteopenia. Bone biopsies in patients with normal serum PTH levels, relatively normal levels of 1,25-hydroxyvitamin D3, and low to normal range normal vitamin D binding proteins usually have no evidence of osteomalacia or hyperparathyroidism on bone biopsy.[97] Because osteomalacia and hyperparathyroidism have been reported to occur with low levels of 25-hydroxyvitamin D in other situations, this report provides comfort that preservation of bone occurs in this group of patients. Thus, in patients with nephrotic syndrome, normal renal function, and abnormalities in circulating vitamin D and calcium, there is little data to suggest that there are alterations in bone mineralization. The concomitant use of corticosteroid therapy or the development of renal insufficiency or other mitigating factors will induce osteoporosis. Therefore, replacement of either calcium or vitamin D in patients with the nephrotic syndrome is not recommended except in prolonged courses of nephrosis or when patients receive corticosteroid therapy. Careful evaluation of bone mineralization with bone densitometry scanning and early administration of vitamin D and other agents may prevent loss of bone mineralization.

Because of the urinary loss of immunoglobulins and defects in the complement cascade, nephrotic patients have an increased susceptibility of infection, particularly peritonitis. Peritonitis caused by either gram-negative or gram-positive organisms remains a serious complication of the nephrotic syndrome.[98–100] Children of African American descent appear to be at greater risk for peritonitis.[100,101] The etiology of the susceptibility to bacterial infections, especially by encapsulated organisms, is not entirely clear. Acquired IgG deficiency due to urinary losses is certainly a cause of enhanced infection. The deficiency of both factor B and D urinary protein loss results in impaired opsonization of these microorganisms. Controversy regarding the presence of functional splenic abnormalities is a matter of debate.[102,103] Treatment protocols include intravenous antibiotics with broad-spectrum coverage of both gram-positive and gram-negative organisms until appropriate culture results are available. Although pneumococcal vaccination is recommended with the nephrotic syndrome,[104] there are reports of patients who develop peritonitis despite vaccination. Whether this results from poor immunoglobulin response to the vaccine or exposure to other serotypes of pneumococcus is uncertain.[98]

Hypoalbuminemia is a cardinal feature of the nephrotic syndrome. Serum albumin levels are depressed not only as a consequence of loss in the urine, but also because of an increased albumin catabolism.[105] Hepatic albumin synthesis is increased from 145 ± 9 mg/kg/day to 213 ± 17 mg/kg/day in nephrotic patients.[106] The transcriptional regulation of human albumin synthesis is not correlated with plasma oncotic pressure or serum albumin concentration, but rather with a urinary albumin excretion.[107] In fact, a fall in plasma oncotic pressure may not be a stimulus to albumin synthesis by the liver at all.[105] Although there is a correlation between the amount of proteinuria and the degree of hypoalbuminemia, there are individuals who have normal, or near normal levels of serum albumin despite severe proteinuria.[108–110] Prolonged and massive proteinuria may lead to malnutrition.

There are several abnormalities of the coagulation system in the nephrotic syndrome (Table 30–5). The thrombotic abnormalities in the nephrotic syndrome are a consequence of hyperfibrinogemia, increased *in vitro* platelet hyperaggregability, increased fibrinogen to fibrin transition, decreased levels of antithrombin III, and decreased fibrinolysis. These abnormalities may result in venous and arterial thrombi. Prevalence of coagulation disorders in series of adult nephrotic patients varies substantially, but averages 26% in an accumulated study of eight series.[111] The incidence of thromboembolic problems in children is substantially less, and is approximately 1.8%. Deep venous thrombosis may occur in virtually any venous bed, whereas arterial thromboses occur less frequently in almost any vessel.[112,113] The cause of hypercoagulability is uncertain, but there are numerous possibilities.[114–117] Studies on the plasma levels of fibrinopeptide, anti-thrombin III complex, products of thrombin activation in 21 patients with the nephrotic syndrome compared with 16 controls suggest that the low anti-thrombin III level in nephrotic patients may not only be due to urinary loss, but

TABLE 30–5	Coagulation Factors in the Nephrotic Syndrome[116,529,1292,1294–1307]
Increased blood viscosity	
Hemoconcentration	
Increased plasma fibrinogen	
Increased intravascular fibrin formation	
Increased α-2 macroglobulins	
Increased tissue type plasminogen activator	
Increased factors II, V, VII, VIII, X, XIII	
Decreased factors IX, XI, XII	
Decreased α-antitrypsin	
Decreased fibrinolytic activity	
Decreased plasma plasminogen	
Decreased antithrombin III	
Decreased protein S	
Thrombocytosis	
Increased platelet aggregability	

also to intravascular consumption.[118] Steroid administration alters the level of certain clotting factors and may provide yet another stimulus for procoagulant activity.[114] Many patients with the nephrotic syndrome are anemic as a consequence of decreased renal function and decreased erythropoietin levels. The increase in hepatic synthesis of transferrin does not match urinary losses of transferrin. There are urinary losses of erythropoietin as well.[119,120]

GLOMERULAR DISEASES THAT CAUSE NEPHROTIC SYNDROME

Minimal Change Glomerulopathy

Epidemiology

Minimal change glomerulopathy, also known as minimal change disease, was first described in 1913 by Monk who called it "lipoid nephrosis" because of the lipid in the tubular epithelial cells and urine.[121] Minimal change glomerulopathy is most common in children, accounting for 70% to 90% of nephrotic syndrome in children under age 10 and 50% in older children. Minimal change glomerulopathy also causes 10% to 15% of primary nephrotic syndrome in adults (Fig. 30–1).

The incidence of minimal change glomerulopathy has geographic variations. Minimal change glomerulopathy is more common in Asia than in North America or Europe.[122] This may be a consequence of differences in renal biopsy practices, or of differences in environmental or genetic influences. The disease may also affect elderly patients in whom there is a higher propensity for the clinical syndrome of minimal change glomerulopathy and acute renal failure (discussed later). There appears to be a male preponderance of this process in some series, especially in children in whom male-to-female ratio is 2 to 3:1,[123] however, our own data do not support this (Table 30–6).

Pathology

Light Microscopy

Minimal change glomerulopathy has no glomerular lesions by light microscopy (Fig. 30–2), or only minimal focal segmental mesangial prominence.[124] This mesangial prominence should have no more than three or four cells embedded in the matrix of a segment, and the matrix should not be expanded to the extent that capillary lumens are compromised. Capillary walls should be thin and capillary lumens patent.

The most consistent tubular lesion is increased protein and lipid resorption droplets in tubular epithelial cells. These droplets are periodic acid-Schiff positive. Conspicuous resorbed lipid in epithelial cells prompted the designation lipoid nephrosis for this disease prior to the recognition of the ultrastructural glomerular lesion. Interstitial edema is rare, even in patients with severe nephrotic syndrome and anasarca. Focal proximal tubular epithelial flattening (simplification), which is histologically identical to that seen with ischemic acute renal failure, occurs in patients who have the syndrome of minimal change glomerulopathy with acute renal failure.[125]

Focal areas of interstitial fibrosis and tubular atrophy in a specimen that otherwise looks like minimal change glomerulopathy, especially in a young person, should raise the possibility of focal segmental glomerulosclerosis that was not

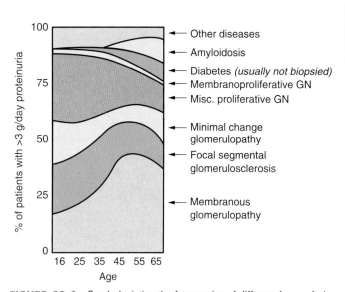

FIGURE 30–1 Graph depicting the frequencies of different forms of glomerular disease identified in renal biopsy specimens from patients with proteinuria of greater than 3 g/day evaluated in the University of North Carolina Nephropathology Laboratory. Some diseases that cause proteinuria are underrepresented because they are not always evaluated by renal biopsy. For example, many patients with steroid-responsive proteinuria may be given a presumptive diagnosis of minimal change glomerulopathy and are not subjected to biopsy, and most patients with diabetes and proteinuria are presumed to have diabetic glomerulosclerosis and are not biopsied.

TABLE 30–6 Diseases that Cause the Nephrotic Syndrome*			
Glomerular Lesion	**N**	**Male:Female Ratio**	**White:Black Ratio**
Minimal change glomerulopathy	522	1.1:1.0	1.9:1.0
Focal segmental glomerulosclerosis (FSGS) (typical)	1103	1.4:1.0	1.0:1.0
Collapsing glomerulopathy FSGS	135	1.2:1.0	1.0:7.8
Glomerular tip lesion FSGS	94	1.0:1.0	4.7:1.0
Membranous glomerulopathy	1120	1.4:1.0	1.9:1.0
C1q nephropathy	114	1.0:1.0	1.0:4.8
Fibrillary glomerulonephritis	76	1.0:1.2	14.3:1.0

*Information in this table is from 9605 native kidney biopsies from the UNC Nephropathology Laboratory. This laboratory evaluates kidney biopsies from a base population of approximately 10 million throughout the southeastern United States and centered in North Carolina. The expected white-to-black ratio in this renal biopsy population is approximately 2:1.

sampled in the biopsy specimen. Examination of additional levels of section may reveal a sclerotic glomerulus.

Immunofluorescence Microscopy

Glomeruli usually show no staining with antisera specific for IgG, IgA, IgM, C3, C4, or C1q. The most frequent positive finding is low-level mesangial staining for IgM, sometimes accompanied by low-level staining for C3. If the IgM staining is not accompanied by mesangial electron dense deposits by electron microscopy, it is consistent with a diagnosis of minimal change glomerulopathy. Patients with mesangial IgM by immunofluorescence microscopy (in the absence of dense deposits by electron microscopy) do not have a worse prognosis than those without IgM.[126,127] The presence of mesangial dense deposits identified by electron microscopy worsens the prognosis and thus justifies altering the diagnosis, for example to IgM mesangial nephropathy.[128] Anything more than trace staining for IgG or IgA casts substantial doubt

on a diagnosis of minimal change glomerulopathy. Even when no sclerotic glomerular lesions are seen by light microscopy, well-defined irregular focal segmental staining for C3 and IgM should raise the possibility of focal segmental glomerulosclerosis because sclerotic lesions usually trap C3 and IgM. Glomerular and tubular epithelial cell cytoplasmic droplets and tubular casts may stain positively for immunoglobulins and other plasma proteins when there is substantial proteinuria.

Electron Microscopy

The pathologic *sine qua non* of minimal change glomerulopathy is effacement of visceral epithelial cell foot processes observed by electron microscopy (Figs. 30–3 and 30–4). However, this is not a specific feature, because it occurs in the glomeruli of patients with severe proteinuria of any cause. During active nephrosis, the effacement often is very extensive, with only a few scattered intact foot processes. As the patient enters remission, the extent of foot process effacement diminishes. The effacement usually is accompanied by microvillous transformation, which is the development of numerous villous projections from the epithelial surface into the urinary space. The effacement also is accompanied by increased density of the cytoskeleton, including actin filaments, in clumps near the basement membrane surface of the visceral epithelial cells. These intracytoplasmic densities should not be confused with subepithelial immune complex dense deposits. Glomerular and proximal tubular epithelial cells have increased clear and dense cytoplasmic droplets.

All of these ultrastructural glomerular changes occur in other glomerular disease when there is nephrotic-range proteinuria. Therefore, minimal change glomerulopathy is a diagnosis by exclusion that is made only when there is no evidence by light, immunofluorescence, and electron microscopy for any other glomerular disease.

Pathogenesis

Although the pathogenesis of minimal change glomerulopathy remains unclear, this disorder is most likely a consequence of abnormal regulation of T-cell subset[129–133] and pathologic elaboration of circulating permeability factor. Specifically, corticosteroids and alkylating drugs cause a remission of minimal change glomerulopathy, there is an association of minimal change glomerulopathy with Hodgkin disease,[134,135]

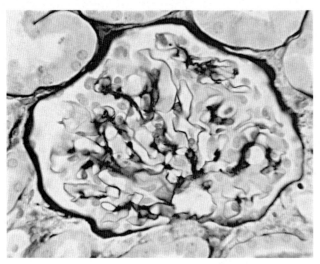

FIGURE 30–2 Unremarkable light microscopic appearance of minimal change glomerulopathy. Glomerular basement membranes are thin, and there is no glomerular hypercellularity or mesangial matrix expansion. (Jones methenamine silver, ×300.)

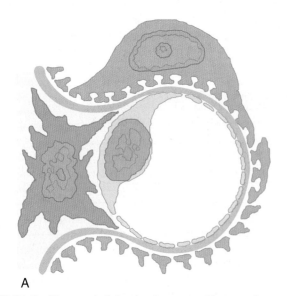

A

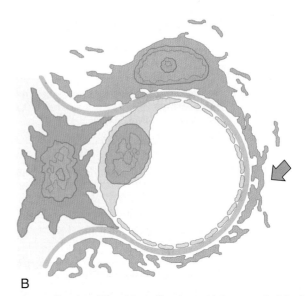

B

FIGURE 30–3 Diagrams depicting the ultrastructural features of a normal glomerular capillary loop (**A**) and a capillary loop with features of minimal change glomerulopathy (**B**). The latter has effacement of epithelial foot processes (arrow) and microvillous projections of epithelial cytoplasm. (Used with permission from J.C. Jennette.)

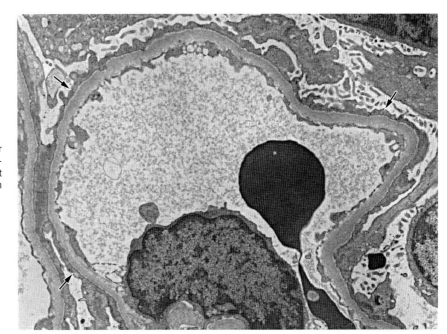

FIGURE 30-4 Electron micrograph of a glomerular capillary wall from a patient with minimal change glomerulopathy showing extensive foot process effacement (arrows) and microvillous transformation (magnification ×5000).

and remissions are associated with depression of cell-mediated immunity during viral infections such as measles. Specific evidence stems from the finding that a glomerular permeability factor is produced by human T cell hybridomas obtained from a patient with minimal change nephrosis. When this factor was injected into rodents, proteinuria occurred with partial fusion of glomerular epithelial cell foot processes.[136] Although there are no observable abnormalities in T or B cell populations in patients with relapsing or quiescent minimal change glomerulopathy,[137-140] lymphocytes have depressed reactivity when challenged with mitogens.[141-149] T cells apparently produce a product, most likely a lymphokine, which increases glomerular permeability to protein. When the glomerular permeability factor is removed from the kidney, it functions normally. This is supported by the intriguing observation that transplantation of a kidney from a patient with refractory minimal change glomerulopathy resulted in rapid disappearance of proteinuria.[150]

This factor my have specificity for glomerular epithelial cells that results in loss of the charge selective barrier of the glomerular basement membrane. The loss of charge selectivity has been assessed by dextran studies.[151,152] In these studies, there is less evidence for a defect in the size selective barrier and more of an alteration of the basement membrane electrostatic charge. The glomerular negative charge is reduced in relapse.[153]

There are other potential pathogenic mechanisms for the pathological changes described as minimal change glomerulopathy. Circulating immune complexes have been found in patients who have been presumed to have minimal change glomerulopathy,[154,155] the level of which fell during remission. Moreover, there have been studies of the presence of an IgM rheumatoid factor in patients with minimal change glomerulopathy. The significance of these observations is questionable given the lack of immune complex deposition within glomeruli.

Clinical Features and Natural History

The cardinal clinical feature of minimal change glomerulopathy in children is the relatively abrupt onset of proteinuria and development of the nephrotic syndrome with heavy proteinuria, hypoalbuminemia, and hyperlipidemia.[124] The edematous picture is typically what prompts the parents of

TABLE 30–7	Common Disease Associations with Minimal Change Glomerulopathy[159,160,194-196,877,1308-1315]
Infections	**Tumors**
• Viral	• Hodgkin disease
• Parasitic	• Lymphoma/leukemia
Pharmaceutical agents	• Solid tumors
• Non-steroidal anti-inflammatory drugs	**Allergies**
• Gold	• Food
• Lithium	• Dust
• Interferon	• Bee stings
• Ampicillin	• Pollen
• Rifampin	• Poison ivy and poison oak
• Trimethadione	• Dermatitis herpetiformis
• Tiopronin	

children to seek medical attention. Hematuria is distinctly unusual, and in children, hypertension is uncommon. In the International Study of Kidney Disease in Children (ISKDC) series, diastolic hypertension was found in 13% of patients.[156] The clinical features of adults with minimal change glomerulopathy tend to be somewhat different. In a group of 89 adults over the age of 60, hypertension, sometimes severe, as well as renal insufficiency, was more common.[157] Because individuals over the age of 60 account for almost one-quarter of adult patients with minimal change glomerulopathy, this presentation must be considered.

Minimal change glomerulopathy has been associated with several other conditions, including viral infections, pharmaceutical agents, malignancy, and allergy (Table 30–7). In some patients, there is a history of a drug reaction before the onset of minimal change glomerulopathy. The use of non-steroidal anti-inflammatory drugs and, in particular, fenoprofen has been associated with, and may cause minimal change glomerulopathy.[158] In this setting, most patients have not only proteinuria, but also pyuria and renal insufficiency as a consequence of the simultaneous development of acute tubulointerstitial nephritis. This same process has also been described with other compounds, including interferon,[159] penicillins, and rifampin. In most of these patients, discontinuation of the offending drug leads to resolution of the proteinuria, but it may take weeks to months for complete amelioration of pyuria and renal insufficiency.

Rarely, minimal change glomerulopathy is associated with a lymphoid malignancy, usually Hodgkin disease.[160] Minimal change glomerulopathy may also occur with solid tumors as an apparent paraneoplastic phenomenon.

There is also an association of minimal change glomerulopathy with food allergy. This is an important association in that, in some patients, removal of the allergen has resulted in the resolution of the proteinuria. In 42 patients of non-biopsied idiopathic nephrotic syndrome, 16 of 42 had positive skin tests for food allergy. In 13 of 42 an oligo-antigenic diet was prescribed resulting in a significant reduction in proteinuria.[161] Thus, it is important to ask patients about potential allergens, especially those found with food.

A syndrome of minimal change glomerulopathy accompanied by a reversible acute renal failure has a higher incidence in adults than in children.[157,162,163] This syndrome of adult minimal change glomerulopathy with acute renal failure was studied in 21 patients who, on presentation, had a serum creatinine greater than 177 mmol/L, and were compared with 50 adult patients with minimal change glomerulopathy and a serum creatinine of less than 133 mmol/L. Patients who presented with acute renal failure were older (59 years versus 40 years), had a higher systolic blood pressure (158 mm Hg versus 138 mm Hg), and had more proteinuria (13.5 versus 7.9 grams/24 hours). Importantly, renal biopsy demonstrated evidence of atherosclerosis and focal tubular epithelial simplification compatible with ischemic acute renal failure. Of the 18 patients with renal failure for whom follow-up data were available, all had recovery of renal function, but some only after substantial dialytic support.[125]

A review of 79 patients in the literature since 1966 revealed a similar finding in an older population with high urinary protein excretion, a low serum albumin, and the persistence of acute renal failure for up to 77 weeks. The presence of histopathological findings of acute tubular necrosis was found in 60% of these patients.[162] When treating older patients, it is important to recognize that acute renal failure may be present in the setting of minimal change glomerulopathy, and that dialytic therapy may be necessary to tide the patient over while corticosteroid treatment induces a response.

Laboratory Findings

The ubiquitous laboratory feature of minimal change glomerulopathy is severe proteinuria.[124] Microscopic hematuria is seen in less than 15% of patients, with only rare episodes of macroscopic hematuria. The rapidity of the development of proteinuria in some patients is associated with evidence of volume contraction with increased hematocrit and hemoglobin. The erythrocyte sedimentation rate is increased as a consequence of the hyperfibrinogenemia as well as hypoalbuminemia. The serum albumin concentration is usually depressed, whereas the total cholesterol, LDL, and triglyceride levels are increased. Total serum protein concentration is usually reduced to between 4.5 g/dL and 5.5 g/dL with a serum albumin concentration of generally less than 2 g/dL and, in more severe cases, less than 1 g/dL. Pseudohyponatremia has been observed in the setting of marked hyperlipidemia. Serum calcium may be low largely due to hypoproteinemia.

Several abnormalities that promote thrombosis are frequent in patients with severe nephrosis, including increased plasma viscosity, increased red cell aggregation, low plasminogen, and low anti-thrombin III.[164] Renal function is usually normal, although the serum creatinine may be slightly increased at the time of presentation. A minority of patients (usually older

adults) has substantial acute renal failure as discussed earlier.

The loss of albumin into the urine is largely a function of a loss of charge-selective permselectivity.[151,152,165,166] Consequently, the fractional excretion of albumin is proportionately greater than the fractional excretion of IgG. IgG levels, however, may be profoundly decreased—a factor that occurs most notably during episodes of relapse. This low level of immunoglobulin may result in susceptibility to infections. IgM levels may be elevated after a remission.[167] Mean serum IgA levels may be substantially elevated in patients with minimal change glomerulopathy compared to those with other renal disease 168 and are also elevated in association with relapse in children.[169] Among adult patients with minimal change glomerulopathy, over half have elevated levels of serum IgE and two thirds of patients have evidence of some allergic symptoms.[170] Elevation of IgE suggests a relationship between minimal change glomerulopathy and allergy. Complement levels are typically normal in patients with minimal change glomerulopathy.

Treatment

The general approach to treatment of patients with minimal change glomerulopathy has been to institute corticosteroid therapy. For children, the dose of prednisone is 60 mg/M^2/day. For adults, the dose of prednisone is 1 mg/kg of body weight, not to exceed 80 mg/day. In children, this form of therapy results in a complete remission with disappearance of proteinuria in over 90% of patients within 4 to 6 weeks of therapy. A response to prednisone therapy has occurred if the patient has had no proteinuria by dipstick analysis for at least three days. It should be noted that the serum albumin and serum lipid levels might not return to normal for prolonged periods of time following resolution of proteinuria.[171]

Treatment is generally continued for 6 weeks after there is complete remission of proteinuria. During those 6 weeks, the dose should be changed to alternate-day prednisone or to a step-wise reduction in the daily dose of prednisone. If the dose is changed to alternate-day when remission has occurred, the dose may be decreased in children from 60 mg/M^2/day to 40 mg/M^2/day.[133,172–176] In adult patients with minimal change glomerulopathy, a response to corticosteroid treatment may take up to 15 weeks.[157] In a study of 89 adult patients given prednisolone, 60% were in remission after 8 weeks, 76% after 16 weeks, and 81% over the course of the study. Of the 58 treated patients who responded, 24% never relapsed, 56% relapsed on a single occasion or infrequently, and only 21% were frequent relapsers. Of these 89 patients, only four remained nephrotic, and two of these presented with acute renal failure. Cyclophosphamide therapy was administered in 36 of the 89 patients, with 66% of these patients being in remission at 5 years.

One of the most controversial issues with respect to treatment pertains to the regimen for tapering the prednisone after the initial response. Sudden withdrawal of corticosteroids, or a rapid taper of prednisone immediately following complete remission, may prompt a relapse. Whether this is a consequence of adrenal insufficiency or depression of the pituitary adrenal access has been a matter of debate.[176–178] At least in children, likelihood of relapse is decreased with prolonged use of corticosteroids over a 10- to 12-week period.[174,179,180] Once remission has been obtained, an alternate-day schedule should begin within at least 4 weeks of the response in order to decrease the steroid-induced side effects.

In children who have not been biopsied prior to treatment, a renal biopsy is usually appropriate when there is failure to respond to a 4- to 6-week course of prednisone, particularly if there have been changes in the clinical course during this period of time, suggestive of another glomerular disease. Many pediatricians advocate a biopsy at the onset of the

TABLE 30–8	Patterns of Response of Minimal Change Glomerulopathy to Corticosteroid Treatment[156,174,175,191]

Primary responder, no relapse

Primary responder with only one relapse in the first 6 months after an initial response

Initial steroid response with two or more relapses within 6 months (frequent relapse)

Initial steroid-induced remission with relapses during tapering of corticosteroid, or within 2 weeks after their withdrawal (steroid dependent)

Steroid-induced remission, but no response to a subsequent relapse

No response to treatment (steroid resistant)

disease if there are clinical features suggesting a diagnosis other than minimal change glomerulopathy (e.g., hypertension, red blood cell casts in the urine, or hypocomplementemia), or if the nephrotic syndrome begins in the first year of life or after 6 years of age.

After the clinical response to initial treatment, as few as 25% have a long-term remission,[163] 25% to 30% have infrequent relapses (no more than one per year), and the remainder have frequent relapses, steroid-dependence or steroid-resistance (Table 30–8). The treatment of frequently relapsing or steroid-dependent nephrotic patients requires additional forms of therapy. The treatment is aimed at minimizing the complications of corticosteroid therapy. In general, induction of a remission with prednisone therapy followed by the institution of cyclophosphamide results in higher urine flow rates and reduced risk of hemorrhagic cystitis. When cyclophosphamide has been used in doses of 2 mg/kg for 8 to 12 weeks, 75% of patients remain free of proteinuria for at least 2 years.[157,181–183] The response to cyclophosphamide may be predicted from the response to corticosteroids. Patients who have had an immediate relapse after the cessation of corticosteroids will have a greater chance of relapsing immediately after the cessation of cyclophosphamide. Those who have had longer remissions after corticosteroid therapy will have a decreased risk of relapse after cyclophosphamide.[184] In those patients who are steroid-dependent, the response to cyclophosphamide has been improved by increasing the duration of therapy to up to 12 weeks.[181] In at least one other study, the 12-week course of cyclophosphamide has not been proven efficacious.[185]

Chlorambucil has many of the same toxicities as cyclophosphamide, and in children, may be associated with a higher incidence of malignancy.[186,187] However, the use of chlorambucil at a dose of 0.1 mg/kg/day to 0.2 mg/kg/day in an 8-week course may produce more stable remission than cyclophosphamide,[188,189] and has been reported to be effective even in some cyclophosphamide-resistant children.[190] Both cyclophosphamide and chlorambucil have profound side effects that include life-threatening infection, gonadal dysfunction, hemorrhagic cystitis, bone marrow suppression, and potential mutagenic event. The disadvantage of chlorambucil is the inherent higher risk of leukemia than with cyclophosphamide.[160]

In individuals who do not respond to an alkylating agent, yet have a predictable response to corticosteroid therapy, the challenge becomes how best to decrease the major complications associated with prolonged and repetitive bouts of corticosteroid therapy. In addition to the development of life-threatening infections, prolonged corticosteroid therapy may

lead to osteoporosis, diabetes mellitus, and accelerated atherosclerosis. Many patients have profound mental status changes, especially emotional lability with intermittent corticosteroid treatment. Thus, in those patients not responding to alkylating therapy, the question is whether other forms of therapy are indicated. Notably, end-stage renal failure is an extremely unusual event in minimal change glomerulopathy. In light of these considerations, additional forms of therapy must be considered carefully with respect to the cumulative addition of other immunosuppressive drugs.

Steroid-Resistant Minimal Change Glomerulopathy

Approximately 5% of children with minimal change glomerulopathy appear to be steroid-resistant. In those patients who never had a renal biopsy, resistance to corticosteroid therapy is an indication for renal biopsy. Often, the renal biopsy evaluation will demonstrate focal segmental glomerulosclerosis or other forms of glomerular injury other than minimal change glomerulopathy.[191]

If the diagnosis remains minimal change glomerulopathy after renal biopsy evaluation, there may be several reasons for steroid resistance. Some patients, especially those for whom corticosteroid therapy is overly toxic, may skip doses or not fully comply with therapy. In other patients, especially some adults, alternate-day therapy may not provide sufficient amounts of corticosteroid to induce clinical remission. In very edematous patients, oral corticosteroid therapy may not be well absorbed, and a dose of intravenous methylprednisolone may provide a more reliable route of administration. Available data suggest that pulse methylprednisolone may induce remission in some corticosteroid-resistant children. In one study, five of eight corticosteroid-resistant children had a remission with pulse methylprednisolone,[192] although this experience is not universal.[193]

Cyclosporine can be administered at a dose of approximately 5 mg/kg. Up to 90% of patients may have either a partial or complete remission with cyclosporine.[169,174,194–196] Unfortunately, there are only rare patients who experience long-term remission once cyclosporine is discontinued.[175] Two trials examined the use of cyclosporine in steroid-resistant nephrosis. The French Society of Pediatric Nephrology used cyclosporine with prednisone at a dose of 30 mg/M²/day for the first month, and then alternate-day prednisone for 5 months. Cyclosporine was administered at a dose of 150 to 200 mg/M²/day.[197] In this study, 48% of patients with minimal change glomerulopathy had complete remission, some within the first month of therapy. A minority of the responders became steroid-sensitive when they later relapsed. In a study by Ponticelli,[198] 13 of 45 patients had minimal change glomerulopathy and were treated with cyclosporine. In those patients with minimal change glomerulopathy, partial or complete remission occurred within 2 months of beginning therapy. Unfortunately, the early positive results of this study were associated with relapses in all patients after cyclosporine was stopped.

In a summary of nine studies,[199] only 20% of children had complete remission with cyclosporine, and many, if not most, relapsed with cessation of therapy. Moreover, cyclosporine and cyclophosphamide appear to have a similar degree of efficacy with respect to controlling the nephrotic syndrome, but cyclophosphamide-treated patients have a more stable long-term remission.[200] In this study, the likelihood of a long-term remission in patients treated with cyclophosphamide was 63%, and was only 25% in those treated with cyclosporine.

To counteract the usual relapse of nephrosis when cyclosporine has been used for 6 months, an alternative approach to cyclosporine treatment relies on a long-term course of this drug, using gradually lower doses in order to maintain the patient in remission. In one study,[201] patients in complete remission for more than 1 year on cyclosporine remained in remission if the cyclosporine was gradually tapered and then stopped. Repeat biopsies in patients treated for as long as 20 months showed no overt sign of nephrotoxicity.

Levamisole is an anti-helminthic drug that also has an immunostimulating role.[197,202] A typical dose is 2.5 mg/kg of body weight given orally on alternate days or three times per week. In one study, 61 children were given a 3- to 4-month course of placebo or levamisole after remission of proteinuria was induced by corticosteroids. In that study, 14 of 31 patients using levamisole were able to discontinue steroid use and remain in remission, compared with only 4 of 30 control subjects.[202] Moreover, when levamisole was administered to patients after a steroid-induced remission, relapse was substantially decreased from 5.2 episodes to less than 0.7 episodes per year during 24 months of treatment.[203] The side effects of this drug, at least in children, include transient cytopenia in two thirds of patients. More profound complications have been reported in treatment with levamisole.[112] Levamisole is not currently available in the United States.

Focal Segmental Glomerulosclerosis

Focal segmental glomerulosclerosis (FSGS) is not a single disease but rather is a diagnostic term for a clinical-pathological syndrome that has multiple etiologies and pathogenic mechanisms.[204,205] The ubiquitous clinical feature of the syndrome is proteinuria, which may be nephrotic or non-nephrotic, and the ubiquitous pathologic feature is focal segmental glomerular consolidation or scarring, which my have several distinctive patterns (Fig. 30–5). These patterns can be classified as collapsing FSGS, tip lesion FSGS, cellular FSGS, perihilar FSGS and FSGS not otherwise specified (NOS).[204,205] The collapsing variant of FSGS is a clinically aggressive variant that is much more common in African American than Caucasian populations, and is characterized pathologically by segmental collapse of capillaries accompanied by hypertrophy and hyperplasia of epithelial cells. The glomerular tip lesion variant of FSGS, which typically presents with marked nephrosis but often has a good outcome, is characterized by consolidation and sclerosis in the glomerular segment that is adjacent to the origin of the proximal tubule.[205] The term cellular FSGS has been used in a number of ways in the literature. For example, this term has been used to describe the collapsing variant and the tip lesion variant of FSGS. Thus care must be taken when reading the literature to determine if this term is being used as defined by D'Agati and colleagues or in some other way.[204] As defined by D'Agati, the cellular variant is relatively uncommon.[205] The perihilar variant of FSGS is characterized pathologically by sclerosis at the hilum of the glomerulus that typically contains foci of hyalinosis.[204] As shown in Table 30–9, FSGS may appear to be a primary renal disease, or it may be associated with, and possibly caused by, a variety of other conditions. When FSGS is secondary to obesity or reduced numbers of nephrons, it often has a perihilar pattern and is accompanied by glomerular enlargement. FSGS that is associated with HIV infection has a collapsing pattern.

Epidemiology

Over the past two decades, there has been an increased incidence of focal segmental glomerulosclerosis (FSGS). Whether this is a true increase in incidence or whether the condition has been better defined and more readily diagnosed by nephropathologists is debatable. Nonetheless, for the past 20 years, the yearly incidence of primary FSGS has risen from less than 10% to approximately 25% of adult nephropathies.[206–210] A substantial portion of this increase may be attributable to an increase in the collapsing glomerulopathy variant of FSGS[210,211] and obesity.[212]

Moreover, there appears to be an emerging racial difference in the prevalence of FSGS in that there are progressively more African-American patients with FSGS than there are white

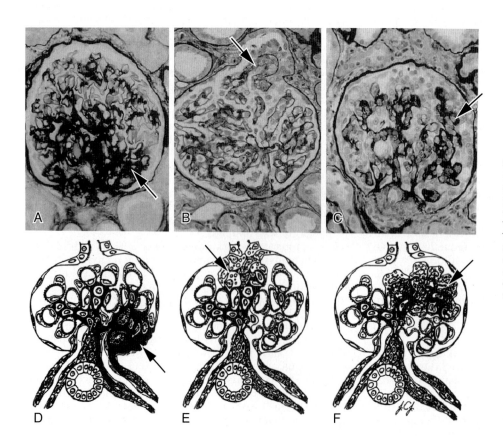

FIGURE 30–5 Light micrographs and diagrams depicting patterns of focal segmental glomerulosclerosis. One pattern (**A and D**) has a predilection for sclerosis in the perihilar regions of the glomeruli. The glomerular tip lesion variant has segmental consolidation confined to the segment adjacent to the origin of the proximal tubule (**B and E**). The collapsing glomerulopathy variant has segmental collapse of capillaries with hypertrophy and hyperplasia of overlying epithelial cells (**C and F**). (Jones methenamine silver, ×100.)

TABLE 30–9	Focal Segmental Glomerulosclerosis

Primary (idiopathic) FSGS
  FSGS not otherwise specified (NOS)
  Glomerular tip lesion variant of FSGS
  Collapsing variant of FSGS
  Perihilar variant of FSGS
  Cellular variant of FSGS

Secondary FSGS
  With HIV disease
  With IV drug abuse
  With other drugs (e.g., pamidronate, interferon)
  With identified genetic abnormalities (e.g., in podocin, alpha-actinin-4, TRPC6)
  With glomerulomegaly
    Morbid obesity
    Sickle cell disease
    Cyanotic congenital heart disease
    Hypoxic pulmonary disease
  With reduced nephron numbers
    Unilateral renal agenesis
    Oligomeganephronia
    Reflux-interstitial nephritis
    Post-focal cortical necrosis
    Post nephrectomy

patients.[209,213,214] The data in these studies are similar to the cases seen in the UNC Nephropathology Laboratory, which demonstrates that the proportional prevalence of typical FSGS and collapsing FSGS in African-American patients is substantially higher than in whites, although the glomerular tip lesion variant of FSGS has a predilection for whites (see Table 30–6).[214] Although the ratio of African Americans to whites is equivalent in FSGS, the proportion of African American patients in our biopsy population is approximately 30%. Thus, the relative incidence of FSGS is higher for African American than Caucasian patients.

Pathology
Light Microscopy
Focal segmental glomerulosclerosis is characterized by focal and segmental glomerular sclerosis.[204,205] The sclerosis may begin as segmental consolidation caused by insudation of plasma proteins causing hyalinosis, by accumulation of foam cells, by swelling of epithelial cells, and by collapse of capillaries resulting in obliteration of capillary lumens. These events are accompanied by increase in collagenous matrix material that ultimately produces a genuinely sclerosis component to the lesion.

Focal segmental glomerulosclerosis is, by definition, a focal process and the limited number of glomeruli in a renal biopsy specimen may not include any of segmentally sclerotic glomeruli that are present in the kidney. In this instance, focal tubulointerstitial injury or glomerular enlargement, which often accompanies focal segmental glomerulosclerosis, can be used as surrogate markers. For example, focal segmental glomerulosclerosis should be considered in renal biopsy specimens of patients with the nephrotic syndrome when there is relatively well-circumscribed focal tubular atrophy and interstitial fibrosis with slight chronic inflammation, even when there are no light microscopic glomerular lesions, no immune deposits, and no ultrastructural changes other than foot process effacement. Diagnostic segmental sclerosis that is adequate for diagnosis may be present only in the tissue examined by immunofluorescence or electron microscopy.

The focal segmental glomerular scarring is not specific. Many injurious processes can cause focal glomerular scarring and must be ruled out before making a diagnosis of focal segmental glomerulosclerosis. For example, hereditary nephritis causes progressive glomerular scarring that can mimic focal segmental glomerulosclerosis. This is revealed by identification of the ultrastructural changes that are characteristic for hereditary nephritis. Focal segmental glomerulonephritis, for example caused by IgA nephropathy, lupus nephritis, anti-neutrophil cytoplasmic antibody-(ANCA) associated glomerulonephritis, can result in focal segmental glomerular scarring that is histologically indistinguishable from that caused by focal segmental glomerulosclerosis. Findings by immunofluorescence and electron microscopy, and by serology, can reveal a glomerulonephritic basis for focal glomerular scarring.

Based on the character and glomerular distribution of lesions, five major structural variants of focal segmental glomerulosclerosis can be recognized that correlate to a degree with the outcome (prognoses) and may be caused by different etiologies and pathogenic mechanisms.[204,205] The five pathologic variants are collapsing FSGS, tip lesion FSGS, cellular FSGS, perihilar FSGS, and FSGS not otherwise specified (NOS).[204,205]

The collapsing variant of FSGS has segmental to global collapse of capillaries with obliteration of lumens. The characteristic feature is focal segmental or global collapse of glomerular capillaries with obliteration of capillary lumens. Visceral epithelial cells overlying collapsed segments are usually enlarged and contain conspicuous resorption droplets. Hyperplasia of visceral epithelial cells raises the possibility of crescentic glomerulonephritis. The convention among most renal pathologists is not to refer to the epithelial hyperplasia of collapsing glomerulopathy as crescent formation. The degree of adhesion formation relative to the extent of glomerular sclerosis is much less in collapsing glomerulopathy than in typical focal segmental glomerulosclerosis. This may result in contracted (collapsed) tuft basement membranes and sclerotic matrix separated from Bowman capsule by hypertrophied and hyperplastic epithelial cells. The collapsing glomerulopathy variant of focal segmental glomerulosclerosis is the major pathologic expression of HIV nephropathy,[124,215–217] and also occurs with intravenous drug abuse and as an idiopathic process.[210,211] In renal transplants, this phenotype of FSGS occurs as both recurrent and *de novo* disease.[218,219]

Relative to the extent of glomerular sclerosis, tubulointerstitial injury is more severe in collapsing glomerulopathy than in typical focal segmental glomerulosclerosis. Tubular epithelial cells have larger resorption droplets, extensive proteinaceous casts, and marked focal dilation of lumens (microcystic change). There also is more extensive interstitial infiltration by mononuclear leukocytes. Immunofluorescence microscopy findings are similar to those observed in typical focal segmental glomerulosclerosis except for the usual finding of larger resorption droplets in glomerular visceral epithelial cells and tubular epithelial cells. Electron microscopy reveals the same structural changes seen by light microscopy. In a specimen with the collapsing glomerulopathy variant of focal segmental glomerulosclerosis, the most important ultrastructural assessment is for the presence or absence of endothelial tubuloreticular inclusions. Endothelial tubuloreticular inclusions are identified in over 90% of patients with HIV infection and collapsing glomerulopathy, but in less than 10% of patients with idiopathic collapsing glomerulopathy or collapsing glomerulopathy associated with intravenous drug abuse. The only other settings in which endothelial tubuloreticular inclusions are numerous are in patients with systemic lupus erythematosus and in patients treated with alpha-interferon.

The tip lesion variant of FSGS has consolidation of segments contiguous with the proximal tubule. These lesions may be sclerotic or cellular. However, the increased cellularity is predominantly within the tuft unlike the extracapillary hypercellularity of collapsing FSGS. Foam cells often contribute to this endocapillary hypercellularity.

The glomerular tip lesion variant of FSGS was first described by Howie and is characterized by consolidation of the glomerular segment that is adjacent to the origin of the proximal tubule, and thus opposite the hilum (Figs. 30–5B and Fig. 30–5E).[220–225] The initial consolidation usually has obliteration of capillary lumens by foam cells, swollen endothelial cells, and increase in collagenous matrix material (sclerosis). Hyalinosis is seen less often than with typical focal segmental glomerulosclerosis. Visceral epithelial cells adjacent to the consolidated segment are enlarged and contain clear vacuoles and hyaline droplets. These altered visceral epithelial cells often are contiguous to, if not attached to, adjacent parietal epithelial cells and tubular epithelial cells at the origin of the proximal tubule, which also have irregular enlargement and vacuolation. The tip lesion may project into the lumen of the proximal tubule. Some lesions are less cellular with a predominance of matrix and collagenous adhesions to Bowman capsule at the origin of the proximal tubule.

The cellular variant of FSGS as defined by D'Agati and colleagues has lesions that resemble the cellular lesion for the tip variant, but they are distributed throughout the glomerular tuft.[204] Perihilar FSGS is characterized by the perihilar predilection of lesions and the presence of hyalinosis. The NOS FSGS category is a nonspecific category that is used when the lesions do not have the distinctive features of any of the other four distinctive variants.

As will be discussed later, different pathologic variants of FSGS have distinctive clinical presentations and outcomes.

Immunofluorescence Microscopy

In all of the histologic variants, non-sclerotic glomeruli and segments usually have no staining for immunoglobulins or complement. As in patients with minimal change glomerulopathy, as well as individuals with no renal dysfunction, a minority of patients with focal segmental glomerulosclerosis will have low-level mesangial staining for IgM in non-sclerotic glomeruli. Low-level mesangial C3 staining is less frequent and low-level IgG and IgA is rare. The presence of substantial staining of non-sclerotic glomeruli for immunoglobulins, especially if immune complex-type electron dense deposits are present, points toward the sclerotic phase of a focal immune complex glomerulonephritis rather than focal segmental glomerulosclerosis.

Sclerotic segments typically have irregular staining for C3, C1q, and IgM (Fig. 30–6). Other plasma constituents are less frequently identified in the sclerotic areas. Epithelial resorption droplets stain for plasma proteins.

Electron Microscopy

The ultrastructural features of focal segmental glomerulosclerosis are nonspecific. Electron microscopy plays an important role in the diagnosis of focal segmental glomerulosclerosis by helping to identify other causes for glomerular scarring that can be mistaken for focal segmental glomerulosclerosis by light microscopy alone.

Foot process effacement in focal segmental glomerulosclerosis affects sclerotic and non-sclerotic glomeruli, and usually is more focal than in minimal change glomerulopathy. Foot process effacement is less extensive in some forms of secondary FSGS than in idiopathic FSGS. Occasionally, glomerular capillaries have focal denudation of foot processes. Non-sclerotic glomeruli and segments should have no immune complex-type electron dense deposits. One must be careful not to confuse electron dense insudative lesions with immune complex deposits. These lesions equate with the hyalinosis seen by light microscopy and result from the accumulation of plasma proteins within sclerotic areas. Thus, if the electron dense material is present in sclerotic but not in non-sclerotic

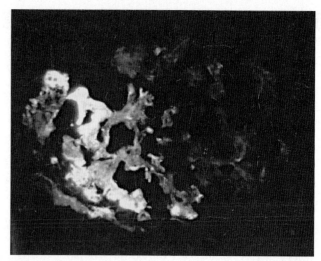

FIGURE 30–6 Immunofluorescence micrograph showing irregular segmental staining for C3 corresponding to a site of segmental sclerosis. (Fluorescein isothiocyanate [FITC] anti-C3, ×3000.)

glomerular segments, it should not be considered to be evidence for immune complex mediated glomerular disease. On the other hand, well-defined mesangial or capillary wall electron dense deposits in non-sclerotic segments indicate immune complex-mediated glomerulonephritis with secondary scarring, which should be confirmed and further characterized by immunofluorescence microscopy.

Pathogenesis

The pathogenesis of FSGS remains poorly understood. The advanced segmental lesions are essentially segmental scars composed predominantly of collagen. The pathogenesis must involve an injurious factor (the etiology) that initiates a sequence of events that ultimately causes the segmental glomerular scarring. As with many patterns of glomerular injury, it is likely that multiple different etiologies can initiate shared pathogenic pathways that can ultimately result in segmental glomerular sclerosis. In addition, different sets of etiologic factors may initiate the different pathogenic pathways that lead to the different structural variants of FSGS.

Some of the same pathogenic events that cause segmental scarring secondary to focal glomerular injury caused by a proliferative or necrotizing glomerulonephritis are probably operative in producing the sclerosis of FSGS. In this regard, the overproduction of TGF-β1 in glomeruli due to acute inflammatory lesions may cause glomerular sclerosis.[226] In experimental models of glomerular inflammation, the administration of antibodies to TGF-β or other inhibitors to TGF-β results in a decrease in matrix accumulation and a reduction in the severity of glomerular scarring.[227] Whether these events occur in human disease is yet to be proven, although there is increased expression of TGF-β in many different types of renal disease, including FSGS.[228] Several mechanisms are associated with the fibrosis of renal disease. Extracellular matrix, and proteoglycans such as decorin and biglycan, may have a pathogenic role in fibrosing diseases by regulation of transforming growth factor beta.[229]

Focal segmental glomerulosclerosis also results from the loss of nephrons, which causes compensatory intraglomerular hypertension and hypertrophy in the remaining glomeruli. The compensatory glomerular hypertension results in both epithelial and endothelial cell injury, as well as mesangial alterations that lead to progressive focal and segmental sclerosis.[230–237] This process, at least in experimental animals, is made worse by increased dietary protein intake and is ameliorated by both protein restriction and antihypertensive therapy. Several other abnormalities also may play a role in the pathogenesis of FSGS, including disorders of lipid metabolism, such as the urinary loss of lecithin-cholesterol acyltransferase,[238–241] abnormalities of the coagulation pathway, and alterations in T cell function.[242] The role of growth factors in addition to TGF-β and platelet-derived growth factor certainly may participate in these lesions.

Whether the loss of nephron number leads to glomerular sclerosis in humans remains controversial. There are well-documented examples of patients who have had either congenital absence or surgical removal of a kidney prior to the development of FSGS.[243] As expected, patients with a greater loss of renal mass have a greater incidence of secondary FSGS. However, data from long-term studies of individuals donating a kidney for renal transplantation have not demonstrated an increased incidence of hematuria or proteinuria when compared to siblings.[244,245] Long-term studies of men who have had a unilateral nephrectomy due to trauma indicate that there is only a small increase in mild proteinuria and systolic hypertension when compared to age-matched controls.[246,247]

Glomerular enlargement accompanied by the development of FSGS occurs in the setting of hypoxemia, for example in patients with sickle cell anemia, congenital pulmonary disease, or cyanotic congenital heart disease. Obesity appears to predispose to FSGS.[248,249] Weight loss and the administration of an ACE inhibitor decreased protein excretion by 80% to 85%.[250] Patients with sleep apnea may have proteinuria that is more functional in nature, but with little or no evidence of glomerular scarring or epithelial injury observed on biopsy.[251,252] The association between sleep apnea and proteinuria is questioned by an analysis of 148 patients referred for polysomnography who were not diabetic and had not been treated previously for obstructive sleep apnea.[253] In this patient population, clinically significant proteinuria was uncommon, was associated with older age, hypertension, coronary artery disease, and arousal index by univariate analysis, and only with age and hypertension in multiple regression analysis. Body mass index and apnea hypopnea index were not associated with urine protein-creatinine ratio. The authors concluded that nephrotic-range proteinuria should not be ascribed to sleep apnea and deserves a thorough renal evaluation.

A permeability factor has been described in some patients with FSGS. In a seminal study, 33 patients with recurrent FSGS after transplantation had a higher mean permeability to albumin value than normal subjects.[254] After plasmapheresis, the permeability factor in six patients was reduced and proteinuria significantly decreased. This circulating factor bound to protein A and had an apparent molecular weight of about 50,000 D.[255,256] In a minority of patients with steroid-resistant FSGS in the native kidneys, plasmapheresis may diminish proteinuria and stabilize renal function. In most patients, however, there is no improvement in proteinuria despite loss of the permeability factor after plasmapheresis.[257] An exact description of this permeability factor in the pathogenesis of FSGS remains unknown despite attempts at elucidating its origin.

The past decade has witnessed an explosion of interest in the role of the podocyte in FSGS (see Chapter 39). Podocytes are highly differentiated postmitotic cells whose function is based on their architecture. Several proteins have now been detected on the podocyte, and their role in various diseases is becoming clear. Thus, in collapsing forms of focal sclerosis, podocytes undergo irreversible ultrastructural changes. This is in contrast to minimal change disease and membranous nephropathy where mature podocyte markers are retained at normal levels. In collapsing FSGS and HIV nephropathy, all of the podocyte markers disappear, suggesting a dysregulated podocyte phenotype in these diseases.[258–260] In fact, podocyte proliferation is seen in some examples of FSGS, which may be a consequence of the decrease in cyclin-dependent kinase inhibitors P27 and P57.[261] The effacement of foot processes may be a consequence of the overproduction of oxygen radicals and accumulation of lipid peroxidase.[262] In theory, the loss of visceral epithelial cells could result in focal areas of glomerular basement membrane denudation with diminished barrier function. The concept that podocyte dropout is a major factor in the development of glomerulosclerosis in general, and specifically in the development of collapsing FSGS, has been highly touted.[263–266] In fact, collapsing FSGS is prototypical of the concept that podocytes become dysregulated and proliferate[267]; however, there have been challenges to the concept. In a mouse model of focal sclerosis, parietal epithelial and not visceral epithelial cells were involved in the proliferative event.[268] In a single patient, it was found that parietal epithelial cells, not the podocyte, were responsible for FSGS, including collapsing FSGS. Which cell(s) are to be the real culprit remains to be determined. It is well established that there are familial forms of FSGS.[269] In a study of 18 families with 45 biopsy-proven cases of FSGS, the disorder appeared to be transmitted in an autosomal dominant pattern. It was associated with HLA alleles, including HLA DR4, HLA-B12, HLA-DRW8, and HLA-DRW5.[270] Even nonfamilial FSGS is associated with specific HLA types. In children of Hispanic origin, FSGS has been linked to HLA DRW8,[271,272] and B8 is associated with DR3 and DR7 in children of Germanic origin.[273] In adults, FSGS is found with an increased incidence of HLA DR4[274] and HLA BW53 in some patients with FSGS associated with heroin.[275]

Recent genetic case studies of familial FSGS have led to the identification of podocyte proteins and have highlighted the important role of podocyte proteins in the glomerular filtration barrier. For instance, positional cloning has led to the identification of a gene that encodes a podocyte actin-binding protein called α-actin 4 as the cause of autosomal-dominant FSGS.[276] The same strategy has been used to clone two other genes, NPHS1 (encoding the protein nephrin) and NPHS2 (encoding the protein podocin). Mutations in the nephrin gene are responsible for autosomal-recessive congenital nephrotic syndrome of the Finnish type.[277] Earlier familial studies on mutations in NPHS2 described the early childhood onset of proteinuria, rapid progression to end-stage renal disease, and no recurrence after renal transplantation.[278] Further studies have shown that mutations in NPHS2 resulting in familial autosomal recessive FSGS are due to nonsense, missense, frame shift, or premature stop codons.[279] The frequency of podocin mutation varies depending on the population studied.[280–282] Mutations in podocin are found in familial autosomal recessive FSGS in European children and adolescents with steroid-resistant nephrotic syndrome. One study suggested that children with familial or sporadic FSGS had NPHS2 mutations in 21% of 152 patients. In another study of 338 patients with autosomal-recessive or sporadic steroid-resistant nephrotic syndrome, a number of NPHS2 mutations were found, including 43% in the familial autosomal-recessive group and 10% in the sporadic group. Mutations in α-actinin-4 (ACTN-4) have been described in patients with autosomal-dominant FSGS as well. There are now a total of 5 ACTN-4 genes believed to cause disease 6,[283] and may account for about 4% of familial FSGS. A cautionary note must be made in that most studies of genetic mutations in FSGS have been examined in children. In an adult study[284] of patients with FSGS from 33 sporadic cases in Italy, disease-associated podocin mutation was present but there were no disease-causative ACTN4 genes. Interestingly, the genotype does not necessarily correlate with the phenotype. Some patients appear to be steroid-sensitive, others steroid-resistant, and yet others sensitive to cyclosporine therapy.[285]

Two very interesting studies describe the TRPC6 cation channel family in FSGS. In one study,[286] a large family with hereditary FSGS with a missense mutation to the TRPC6 gene caused mutation from an amino acid from proline to glutamine, which enhanced the TRPC6 calcium signal in response to a number of stimuli. Another study[287] found TRPC6 abnormalities in patients with FSGS in 5 families with autosomal-dominant FSGS. How this calcium channel regulates podocyte structure and function remains to be fully elucidated, but it is possible that TRPC6 channel activity in the slit diaphragm is important for podocyte structure. There are a number of other mutations that may be associated with FSGS, including genes for proteins, such as WT-1.[6]

A number of infections cause FSGS. HIV-associated FSGS is pathologically identical to idiopathic collapsing FSGS, except for the presence of endothelial tubuloreticular inclusions in the former but not the latter. This close association of HIV infection with collapsing FSGS, as well as experimental evidence of focal glomerular sclerosis in mice transgenic for HIV type I genes,[209,215,226,228,243,288–290] raise the possibility that the HIV virus can be an etiologic agent of FSGS. Whether other viral diseases, including parvovirus B19, cause the idiopathic collapsing variant of FSGS remains to be elucidated.[291,292] Parvovirus B19 has been found with greater frequency in patients with idiopathic and collapsing FSGS compared with patients with other diagnoses.[292] The polyomavirus SV40 may also play a role.[293] Focal sclerosis is associated with a number of malignant conditions that have been associated with lymphoproliferative disease. In a recent study,[294] there was an association of FSGS in monoclonal gammopathies of undetermined significance (MGUS) that responded in MGUS or multiple myeloma. When the lymphoproliferative disease was treated, the renal lesion improved.

Clinical Features and Natural History

In all forms of primary FSGS, proteinuria of varying degrees is the hallmark feature. The degree of proteinuria varies from non-nephrotic (1 to 2 grams) to massive proteinuria (over 10 grams) associated with all of the morbid features of the nephrotic syndrome. Hematuria occurs in over half of FSGS patients and approximately one third of patients present with some degree of renal insufficiency. Gross hematuria is more commonly seen in FSGS than in minimal change glomerulopathy.[295] Hypertension is found as a presenting feature in one third of patients. There are differences in the presentation of FSGS in adults and children.[206,296–298] Children tend to present with more proteinuria, while hypertension is more common in adults.

Differences in clinical manifestations correlate with different pathologic phenotypes of FSGS.[214] For example, patients with perihilar FSGS accompanied by glomerular hypertrophy more commonly have non-nephrotic-range proteinuria than FSGS patients who do not have glomerular hypertrophy. Additionally there are differences in the clinical presentation of the collapsing variant of FSGS and the glomerular tip lesion variant of FSGS. For example, the collapsing variant often has more severe proteinuria and renal insufficiency but less hypertension than the typical variant, and the glomerular tip lesion variant often presents with rapid onset of edema similar to minimal change glomerulopathy.

Weiss[299] first reported six patients with a collapsing variant of FSGS, and larger series of such patients have subsequently been studied.[210,211] Patients with collapsing FSGS have substantially more proteinuria, a lower serum albumin, and higher serum creatinine than patients with either perihilar FSGS. The development of proteinuria, edema, or hypoalbuminemia may occur rapidly over the course of days to weeks, in contrast to the more insidious development of proteinuria

in most patients with typical FSGS. Moreover, patients with collapsing FSGS more frequently have extrarenal manifestations of disease a few weeks prior to onset of the nephrosis, such as episodes of diarrhea, upper respiratory tract infections, or pneumonic-like symptoms that are usually ascribed to viral or other infectious process. However, the systemic symptoms of fever, malaise, and anorexia occur in less than 20% of patients at the time of onset of nephrosis.

Pamidronate, a bisphosphonate that prevents bone disease in myeloma and metastatic tumors, has been reported to be associated with collapsing FSGS in a number of series.[268,300] With discontinuation of the drug, kidney function stabilized in all patients except those with collapsing FSGS.

The clinical presentation of glomerular tip lesion differs from that of both perihilar FSGS and the collapsing FSGS.[214] Patients with glomerular tip lesion tend to be older white males, in sharp contrast to the younger black male prevalence in collapsing FSGS. The proteinuria in these patients usually is severe and the onset is abrupt with sudden development of edema and hypoalbuminemia. The rapidity of onset of the disease process is similar to the clinical presentation of minimal change glomerulopathy.[223,301,302] Glomerular tip lesion patients may develop reversible acute renal failure, especially at the time of initial presentation when the degree of proteinuria, edema, and hypoalbuminemia are at their peak. This also is similar to minimal change glomerulopathy but rarely occurs with other variants of FSGS.

It is difficult to ascribe a survival by year for the aggregate group of patients with FSGS. In general, patients with perihilar FSGS have a better long-term outcome than those with collapsing FSGS. Because a greater number of patients with glomerular tip lesion respond to corticosteroid therapy, the long-term outcome for patients with this histological variant may be better than that for patients with typical FSGS.[214] Some authorities do not believe there is an association between the pathological variants of FSGS and the long-term course.[303]

The degree of proteinuria is a predictor for the long-term clinical outcome. Non-nephrotic-range proteinuria correlates with a more favorable renal survival of over 80% after 10 years of follow-up.[304,305] In contrast, patients who have more than 10 grams of proteinuria per day have a very poor long-term renal survival with the majority of patients reaching end-stage renal disease within 3 years.[306,307] This rapid decline in renal function has been termed "malignant FSGS" due to the morbid nature of the nephrosis and the rapidity of the deterioration in renal function.[305] Patients with FSGS and protein excretion that measures between non-nephrotic range and massive proteinuria have a variable long-term renal outcome. In general, these have a relatively poor outcome, with half of these patients reaching end-stage renal disease by 10 years.[206,298,308]

One of the most useful prognostic indicators for patients with FSGS is whether they attain a remission of their nephrotic syndrome.[297] Patients who have a remission of nephrosis have a substantially greater renal survival than those who do not.[297,304,305,309,310] According to Korbet,[206,298] less than 15% of patients with complete or partial remission progress to end-stage renal disease within 5 years of follow-up. Up to 50% of patients not attaining remission progress to end-stage disease within 6 years of follow-up.

As in other forms of glomerular injury, entry serum creatinine is associated with a poor long-term renal survival.[304,306,311,312] Patients with a serum creatinine of over 1.3 mg/dL have a poorer renal survival than those with lower serum creatinine, irrespective of the level of proteinuria (10-year renal survival of 27% versus 100%).[206] Entry serum creatinine by multivariate analysis may be more important than proteinuria as a predictor of progression to end-stage renal disease.[304,305,307,308,311,312]

Controversy abounds regarding whether there is a poorer long-term prognosis in black patients compared to white patients. In children, Inguli and Tejani noted that within 8.5 years of follow-up, 78% of black patients but only 33% of white patients progressed to end-stage renal disease.[312,322] The racial predilection for poor long-term prognosis has not been corroborated in adult patients with nephrosis.[304,305]

Some pathological discriminators correlate with long-term clinical outcome. Neither the degree of scarring within the glomerulus nor the number of glomeruli that are totally obsolescent is predictive of long-term renal outcome.[301,303,312,313] As in most forms of glomerular disease, interstitial fibrosis and tubular atrophy correlate with poor prognosis. Substantial controversy has surrounded the prognostic value of discriminating between different types of focal segmental glomerulosclerosis. Most investigators agree that there is a much more rapid deterioration in renal function with collapsing FSGS than typical FSGS.[207,210,314]

Another controversial issue is the prognostic significance of the location of the sclerosis within the glomerular tuft. The original descriptions of the glomerular tip lesion by Howie[222-224] suggested that this variant of FSGS has a better response to corticosteroid therapy and a more benign clinical course than typical FSGS. Other investigations have not confirmed an improved long-term renal survival with glomerular tip lesion. These latter studies, however, included very few patients with glomerular tip lesions in the cohort of patients who were studied.[225,301,303] Thomas and colleagues observed that tip lesion FSGS had a higher rate of remission and a better 3-year renal survival that other pathologic variants of FSGS.[205]

The prognostic significance of mesangial hypercellularity associated with FSGS also is controversial. Some studies have identified a correlation between mesangial hypercellularity and poor outcomes, such as poor response to steroids,[315,316] more frequent relapses, and more progression of renal insufficiency.[317] However, other studies have not confirmed the more rapid loss of renal function.[225,301,303]

Laboratory Findings

Hypoproteinemia is common in patients with FSGS, with total serum protein reduced to varying extents. The serum albumin concentration may fall to below 2 g/dL, especially in patients with the collapsing and glomerular tip variants of FSGS. As in other forms of the nephrotic syndrome, levels of immunoglobulins are typically depressed; and levels of lipids are increased, especially serum cholesterol. Serum complement components are generally in normal range in FSGS. Circulating immune complexes have been detected in patients with FSGS,[154,318] although their pathogenic significance has not been determined. Serologic testing for HIV infection should be obtained for patients with FSGS, especially those with the collapsing pattern.

Treatment

Other than the study by the ISKD, there have been no prospective randomized treatment trials for focal segmental glomerulosclerosis. Thus, available data are based entirely on anecdotal series using different treatment protocols, different definitions of remission, response, relapse, and resistance, and different lengths of therapy.[297,304,309,319] One review of studies suggested that only 15% of patients with FSGS responded to treatment, in sharp contrast to those with minimal change glomerulopathy.[320] More optimistic reports have been obtained by groups in Toronto and Chicago[297,298] that suggest that 30% to 40% of adult patients may attain some form of remission with corticosteroid treatment. A compilation of these studies by Korbet and co-workers[206] suggests that of 177 patients who received a variety of different forms of therapy, 45% attained complete remission, 10% attained partial remission, and 45% had no response.[297,304,309,319,321]

In children, the initial treatment of focal segmental glomerulosclerosis is similar to that of minimal change glomerulopathy, because so many pediatricians treat patients without having histological confirmation of the disease process. Thus, the International Study of Kidney Diseases in Children recommended using an initial course of prednisone of 60 mg/day/M², up to 80 mg/day for 4 weeks. This should be followed with 40 mg/day/M², up to 60 mg/day, administered in divided doses for 3 consecutive days of 7, for 4 weeks, and then tapered off for 4 more weeks. Similar to the adult patients with minimal change glomerulopathy, a longer course of therapy at higher doses of prednisone may be necessary to induce remission. Thus, in those series where there is an increased remission rate,[198,297,304,309,319,322,323] prednisone treatment was continued for 16 weeks in order to achieve remission. In adult patients, median time for complete remission was 3 to 4 months.[201]

Among patients with a positive response to corticosteroid treatment, a portion will relapse. Guidelines for re-treatment of this group of patients are similar to those of relapsing minimal change glomerulopathy. In patients whose remission prior to relapse was prolonged (over 6 months), a repeat course of corticosteroid therapy may again induce a remission. In steroid-dependent patients who develop frequent relapses, repeated high-dose corticosteroid therapy results in unacceptable cumulative toxicity. Thus, alternative strategies such as the addition of cyclophosphamide or cyclosporine may be useful. In some individuals, reestablishment of remission may result when cyclophosphamide is administered for 8 to 12 weeks at a dose of 2 mg/kg/day.[298] In patients with the glomerular tip lesion variant of FSGS, a trial of corticosteroids is appropriate because many patients have a decline in protein excretion.[221,302,303]

The practice of using higher doses of corticosteroids in order to reach remission has resulted in alternative therapeutic approaches in patients who are resistant to oral prednisone. In these forms of therapy, prednisone-resistant FSGS has been treated with methylprednisolone boluses of 30 mg/kg/day to a maximum of 1 gram given every other day for 6 doses, followed by this same dose on a weekly basis for 10 weeks; subsequently, similar doses are given on a tapering schedule. In addition to these large doses of methylprednisolone, oral prednisone is given.[324,325] Some patients are also given alkylating agents. With this treatment protocol, 12 of 23 children entered remission, and six had decreased urinary protein losses.

These very high doses of corticosteroids in children, and the duration of daily prednisone for up to 6 to 9 months in adults is not without enormous short- and long-term side effects. In studies in which long-term, high-dose corticosteroids are administered, few analyses have been undertaken of the development of osteoporosis, short- and long-term risk of infection, and the development of cataract, diabetes, or other long-term sequelae. Thus, the available data do not allow for careful understanding of risk-benefit ratios. Until the use of very large dose of Solu-Medrol is subject to controlled clinical trials, the utility of this potential yet dangerous approach must be viewed with caution. There are some authorities who feel that most treatment of FSGS with corticosteroids is hazardous.[326]

Attempts at alternate-day steroid therapy have not been successful except in elderly populations. The Toronto group[327] demonstrated that patients over the age of 60 achieved a 40% remission rate using up to 100 mg of prednisone on alternate days for 3 to 5 months. This therapy was well tolerated in this population without obvious side effects during the study period. Alternate-day prednisone most likely works in this population because of an increased susceptibility to the immunosuppressive effects of corticosteroids and altered glucocorticoid kinetics in the elderly.

Several studies have failed to document the effectiveness of cytotoxic drugs in the treatment of FSGS.[309,328] In one review, only 23% of 247 children with FSGS were steroid-responsive, and 70 patients were treated with cytotoxic drugs. Of these, 30% responded. In the final analysis, less than 20% of the 247 children were in remission. The use of cytotoxic drugs has been evaluated in only one series of adults.[309] Although their use correlated with longer remissions and fewer relapses, no other study has corroborated these results.

The International Study of Kidney Diseases in Children carefully examined the role of cyclophosphamide in the treatment of children with FSGS. For 3 months, cyclophosphamide was used in combination with a 12-month course of every-other-day prednisone therapy. When this regimen was compared to prednisone alone, there was no improvement in response between patients treated with cyclophosphamide compared to those receiving prednisone alone.[329]

Patients resistant to prednisone may be induced into remission with cyclosporine. A randomized trial demonstrates the utility of cyclosporine in patients with steroid resistance, resulting in remission in the majority of patients.[330] This study compared 46 cyclosporine-treated steroid-resistant FSGS patients to 45 control patients. Of the 46 patients, nine achieved complete remission whereas none of the controls did. Partial remissions were observed in 40% to 70% of the cyclosporine-treated patients, and in 17% to 33% of the control patients. These results are statistically significant when both complete and partial remissions are considered. Withdrawal of treatment results in relapse in over 75% of patients.[320]

How long should patients be treated with cyclosporine? In a study by Meyrier,[201] when patients remained in remission for over 12 months, cyclosporine was slowly tapered and eventually removed without subsequent relapse.[201] Unfortunately, long-term treatment with cyclosporine was associated with increases in tubular atrophy and interstitial fibrosis.[201] The degree of tubulointerstitial disease was positively correlated with the initial serum creatinine, the number of segmental scars on initial biopsy, and on a cyclosporine dose of more than 5.5 mg/kg/day. Thus, there is a clear trade-off in the use of cyclosporine over the long term in the well-established development of interstitial fibrosis and tubular atrophy.

Angiotensin-converting enzyme (ACE) inhibitors angiotensin receptor blockers (ARB) have been evaluated in the treatment of FSGS. ACE inhibitors have been shown to decrease proteinuria and the rate of progression to end-stage renal disease.[331–334] These results have been obtained not only in the presence of diabetes, but also in cases of non-diabetic renal disease. In patients with sickle cell disease, glomerulomegaly, and FSGS, ACE inhibitors decreased proteinuria acutely while maintaining glomerular filtration rate and renal plasma flow.[335] In general, these studies suggest that angiotensin-converting enzyme inhibitors, and perhaps angiotensin II receptor antagonists would provide a substantial ameliorative effect in nephrotic symptoms of FSGS. In fact, in patients with glomerulomegaly and resultant non-nephrotic-range proteinuria, an ACE inhibitor or angiotensin II receptor antagonist sufficiently decreases proteinuria and potentially decreases hyperlipidemia, edema, and other manifestations of persistent loss of protein in the urine in this population with excellent long-term prognosis. Regardless of other forms of anti-inflammatory or immunosuppressive therapy employed, the beneficial effects of these agents indicates that they should be added, despite the well-known side effects of hyperkalemia and reduction in glomerular filtration rate, especially in patients with serum creatinines of over 3 mg/dL.

Other forms of treatment have been used. Plasmapheresis or protein absorption strategies to remove circulating factors responsible for FSGS have led to remission of recurrent FSGS, but it does not appear to be beneficial in the primary disease.[257,336] Anecdotal cases suggest that mycophenolate mofetil may be useful in some patients as well.

In summary, patients with primary FSGS remain frustrating patients to treat. Enthusiasm for the use of high-dose, prolonged corticosteroid therapy in adults and children has prompted the use of this therapy in many FSGS patients. Only a prospective randomized trial that carefully evaluates this approach will determine its precise effectiveness. In patients who have protein excretion of less than 3 grams/day or with glomerulomegaly found on biopsy (or both), a trial of angiotensin converting enzyme inhibitors or angiotensin II receptor antagonist is warranted. In those patients who have nephrotic-range proteinuria, careful supportive care and consideration of a trial of oral corticosteroids in adult patients may be an acceptable approach after the patient is carefully informed about the risks and potential benefits of 12 to 16 weeks of daily corticosteroid therapy. Alternating a trial of cyclosporine may be warranted at a dose of 5 mg/kg/day for less than 12 months. In all of these patients, an angiotensin converting enzyme inhibitor may provide a substantial reduction in proteinuria and a potential long-term benefit that may be equal to or greater than that of the immunosuppressive therapy.

C1q Nephropathy

C1q nephropathy is a relatively rare cause for proteinuria and nephrotic syndrome that can mimic FSGS clinically and histologically.[337,338] The diagnosis is based on the presence of mesangial immune complex deposits that have conspicuous staining for C1q. The C1q staining usually is accompanied by staining for IgG, IgM, and C3. Electron microscopy demonstrates well-defined mesangial immune complex type dense deposits. Light microscopic findings vary from no lesion (mimicking minimal change glomerulopathy), to focal glomerular hypercellularity, to focal segmental sclerosing lesions that may be indistinguishable histologically from FSGS. The findings by immunofluorescence microscopy and electron microscopy, however, readily differentiate C1q nephropathy from minimal change glomerulopathy and FSGS. The pathologic features suggest an immune complex pathogenesis, but the details of the pathogenic mechanism and the etiology are unknown.

Patients with C1q nephropathy are predominantly black and male, with a black to white ratio of 4.7:1 and a male to female ratio of 1.8:1. Patients are usually between the ages of 15 and 30 when diagnosed, and all of them have proteinuria. Almost half have edema, 40% have hypertension, and 30% have hematuria. Interestingly, many patients are relatively asymptomatic, and proteinuria is first detected at the time of a "sports physical" or induction into the armed forces. These patients, by definition, have no clinical or serological evidence of systemic lupus erythematosus, despite the presence of C1q in the renal biopsy. C1q nephropathy may have a spontaneous improvement.[339]

Ninety percent of C1q nephropathy patients followed by the Glomerular Disease Collaborative Network continue to have proteinuria at 2.5 years of follow-up. Whether corticosteroids have a role in the treatment of patients with this disease process is not certain. Life table analysis demonstrates that renal survival at 3 years is 84%, and treatment with corticosteroids had no statistical improvement in proteinuria or preservation of renal function. Yet, there are reports of some patients who have had complete remission with corticosteroids.[340]

Membranous Glomerulopathy

Epidemiology

Idiopathic membranous glomerulopathy is the most common cause for nephrotic syndrome in adults.[211,221-225,230-237,239-242,256,295,297,299,302,305,306,309,324,341-391] Membranous glomerulopathy occurs as an idiopathic (primary) or secondary disease. Secondary membranous glomerulopathy is caused by autoimmune diseases (e.g., lupus erythematosus, autoimmune thyroiditis), infection (e.g., hepatitis B, hepatitis C), drugs (e.g., penicillamine, gold), and malignancies (e.g., colon cancer, lung cancer). Secondary membranous glomerulopathy, especially that caused by hepatitis B[380,381,392-397] and lupus, is more frequent in children than adults. In patients over the age of 60, membranous glomerulopathy is associated with a malignancy in from 20% to 30% of patients.[375]

Membranous glomerulopathy is the cause for nephrotic syndrome in approximately 25% of adults.[398-407] A study of patients with more than 1 gram of proteinuria in the United Kingdom by the Medical Research Council from 1978 to 1990 determined that 20% had membranous glomerulopathy. Membranous glomerulopathy is uncommon in children. The peak incidence of membranous glomerulopathy is in the fourth or fifth decade of life.[401,408-412] Membranous glomerulopathy is most common in middle-aged males. In a pooled analysis of patients with idiopathic membranous glomerulopathy derived from articles in North America, Europe, Australia, Asia, and Japan, there was a 2:1 predominance of males (1190 males and 598).[400-403,406,409-411,413-433] The adult-to-child ratio was 26:1 (1734 adults and 67 children), however, this low incidence of membranous glomerulopathy in children was biased by the exclusion of children from some of the studies that were pooled. Membranous glomerulopathy affects all races.

Although most patients with membranous glomerulopathy present with the nephrotic syndrome, there may be 10% to 20% of patients who have proteinuria that remains less than 2 g/day.[434] Thus, it is likely that the frequency of membranous glomerulopathy in the general population is underestimated because of individuals who have membranous glomerulopathy that is causing subclinical proteinuria that never prompts renal biopsy.

There are geographic variations in the clinical manifestations of membranous glomerulopathy. Patients in studies from Australia or Japan have lower percentages of the nephrotic syndrome at entry when compared to patients from Europe or North America. The geographic differences may be caused by different frequencies and causes of secondary membranous glomerulopathy in different geographical locations, such as different frequencies of membranous glomerulopathy caused by hepatitis B, malaria, and other infections.[381,395]

Pathology
Electron Microscopy

The pathologic *sine qua non* of membranous glomerulopathy is the presence of subepithelial immune complex deposits, or their structural consequences.[435] Electron microscopy provides the most definitive diagnosis of membranous glomerulopathy, although a relatively confident diagnosis can be made based on typical light microscopic and immunofluorescence microscopic findings.

Figure 30-7 depicts the four ultrastructural stages of membranous glomerulopathy as described by Ehrenreich and Churg.[436] The earliest ultrastructural manifestation, stage I, is the presence of scattered or more regularly distributed small immune complex-type electron dense deposits in the subepithelial zone between the basement membrane and the epithelial cell. Epithelial foot process effacement and microvillous transformation occur in all stages of membranous

glomerulopathy when there is substantial proteinuria. Stage II is characterized by projections of basement membrane material around the subepithelial deposits. In three dimensions, these projections surround the sides of the deposits, but when observed in cross sections, they appear as spikes extending between the deposits (Figs. 30-7 and 30-8). In stage III, the new basement membrane material surrounds the deposits and thus in cross-sections there is basement membrane material between the deposits and the epithelial cytoplasm. At this point the deposits are in essence intramembranous rather than subepithelial; however, the ultrastructural appearance allows the inference that they once were subepithelial and thus indicative of membranous glomerulopathy. Stage IV is characterized by loss of the electron density of the deposits, often resulting in irregular electron lucent zones within an irregularly thickened basement membrane. Although not described by Ehrenreich and Churg, some nephropathologists recognize stage V, which is characterized by a repaired outer basement membrane zone with the only residual basement membrane disturbance in the inner aspect of the basement membrane. At the time of renal biopsy, most patients in the United States have stage I or II disease (Table 30-10).

Mesangial dense deposits are rare in idiopathic membranous glomerulopathy but are frequent in secondary membranous glomerulopathy (see Table 30-10). This suggests, but does not prove, that idiopathic membranous glomerulopathy is caused by subepithelial *in situ* immune complex formation with antibodies from the circulation complexing with antigens derived from the capillary wall. Immune complexes formed only at this site could not go against the direction of filtration to reach the mesangium. Secondary forms of membranous glomerulopathy usually are caused by immune complexes that contain antigens that are in the circulation, such as antigens derived from infections (e.g., hepatitis B), tumor antigens (e.g., colon cancer), or autoantigens (e.g., thyroglobulin). With both the antigens and antibodies in the systemic circulation, it is likely that some immune complexes wold form that would localize not only in the subepithelial zone but also in the mesangium or subendothelial zone. This is demonstrated in the secondary form of membranous glomerulopathy that occurs in patients with systemic lupus erythematosus. Over 90% of lupus membranous glomerulopathy specimens have mesangial dense deposits identified by electron microscopy.[437] Therefore, the presence of mesangial dense deposits should raise the index of suspicion for secondary rather than primary membranous glomerulopathy.

Immunofluorescence Microscopy

The characteristic immunofluorescence microscopy finding in membranous glomerulopathy is diffuse global granular capillary wall staining for immunoglobulin and complement (Fig. 30-9).[435] IgG is the most frequent and usually the most intensely staining immunoglobulin, although less staining for IgA and IgM is common (see Table 30-10). C3 staining is present over 95% of the time but typically is relatively low intensity. C1q staining is uncommon and of low intensity in idiopathic membranous glomerulopathy but is frequent and of high intensity in lupus membranous glomerulopathy.[437] Although not usually evaluated in routine diagnostic preparations, there is very intense staining of capillary walls for terminal complement components (i.e., components of the membrane attack complex). In the rare patients who have concurrent anti-GBM glomerulonephritis and membranous glomerulopathy, linear staining for IgG can be discerned just below the granular staining.[438]

Tubular basement membrane staining for immunoglobulins or complement is rare in idiopathic membranous glomerulopathy, but is common in secondary membranous glomerulopathy, especially lupus membranous glomerulopathy.[437]

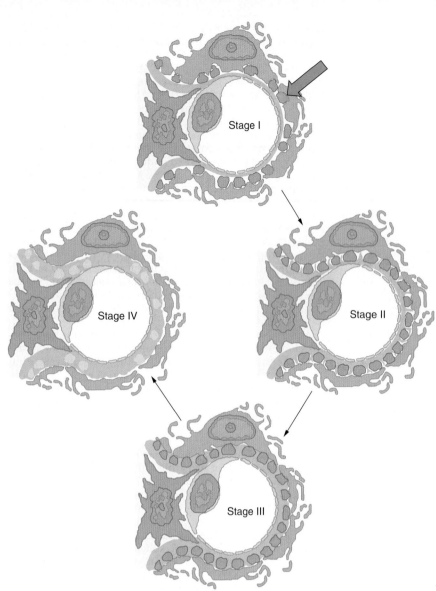

FIGURE 30–7 Diagram depicting the four ultrastructural stages of membranous glomerulopathy. Stage I has subepithelial dense deposits (arrow) without adjacent basement membrane reaction. Stage II has projections of basement membrane adjacent to deposits. Stage III has deposits surrounded by basement membrane. Stage IV has thickened basement membrane with irregular lucent zones. (Reproduced with permission of J.C. Jennette.)

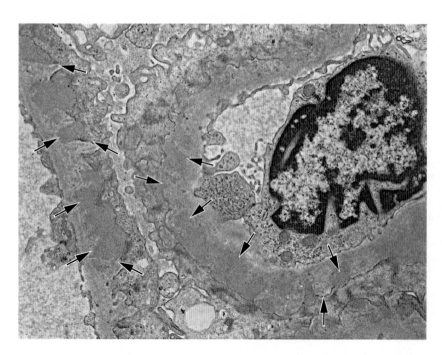

FIGURE 30–8 Electron micrograph of stage II membranous glomerulopathy with numerous subepithelial dense deposits (straight arrows) and adjacent projections of basement membrane material (curved arrows) (magnification ×100).

<table>
<tr><td colspan="2">TABLE 30–10 Pathologic Features of 350 Consecutive Non-Lupus Membranous Glomerulopathy Renal Biopsy Specimens Evaluated by the UNC Nephropathology Laboratory</td></tr>
</table>

	% Positive and Mean Intensity when Positive
Immunofluorescence microscopy	
IgG	99% (3.5+)
IgM	95% (1.2+)
IgA	84% (1.1+)
C3	97% (1.6+)
C1q	34% (1.1+)
Kappa	98% (3.1+)
Lambda	98% (2.8+)
Electron microscopy	**% with**
Subepithelial electron dense deposits	99%
Mesangial electron dense deposits	16%
Subendothelial electron dense deposits	7%
Endothelial tubuloreticular inclusions	3%
Stage I	38%
Stage II	32%
Stage III	6%
Stage IV	5%
Stage V	1%
Mixed stage	20%

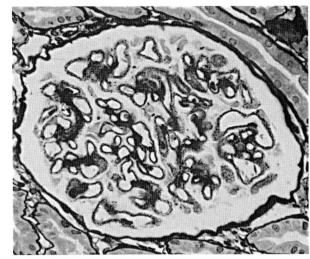

FIGURE 30–10 Light micrograph of a glomerulus with stage II membranous glomerulopathy demonstrating spikes along the outer aspects of the glomerular basement membrane (cf. Fig. 30–2). These correspond to the projections of basement membrane material between the immune deposits. (Jones methenamine silver, ×300.)

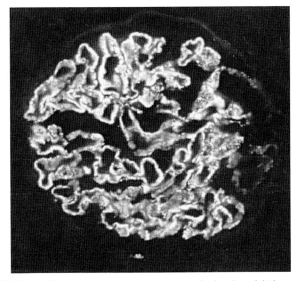

FIGURE 30–9 Immunofluorescence micrograph showing global granular capillary wall staining for IgG in a glomerulus with membranous glomerulopathy. (FITC anti-IgG, ×300.)

Light Microscopy

The characteristic histologic abnormality is diffuse global capillary wall thickening in the absence of significant glomerular hypercellularity.[439] The light microscopic features of membranous glomerulopathy, however, vary with the stage of the disease and with the degree of secondary chronic sclerosing glomerular and tubulointerstitial injury. Mild stage I lesions may not be discernible by light microscopy, especially using only a hematoxylin and eosin stain. Stage II, III, and IV lesions usually have readily discernible thickening of capillary walls.

Masson trichrome stains may demonstrate the subepithelial immune complex deposits as tiny fuchsinophilic (red) grains along the outer aspect of the glomerular basement membranes. However, this is not a sensitive, specific, or technically reliable method for detecting glomerular immune complex deposits. Special stains that accentuate basement membrane material, such as the Jones' silver methenamine stain, may reveal the basement membrane changes that are induced by the subepithelial immune deposits. Spikes along the outer aspect of the glomerular basement membrane usually are seen in stage II lesions (Fig. 30–10). Stage III and IV lesions have irregularly thickened and trabeculated basement membranes, which resemble changes that occur with membranoproliferative glomerulonephritis and chronic thrombotic microangiopathy.

Overt mesangial hypercellularity is uncommon in idiopathic membranous glomerulopathy, although it is more frequent in secondary membranous glomerulopathy.[437] Crescent formation is rare unless there is concurrent anti-GBM disease or ANCA disease.[440–446]

With disease progression, chronic sclerosing glomerular and tubulointerstitial lesions develop. Glomeruli become segmentally and globally sclerotic, and develop adhesions to Bowman capsule. Worsening tubular atrophy, interstitial fibrosis, and interstitial infiltration by mononuclear leukocyte parallels progressive loss of renal function.[447]

Pathogenesis

Membranous glomerulopathy is caused by immune complex localization in the subepithelial zone of glomerular capillaries. The pathogenetic mechanisms that lead to this immune complex localization and the subsequent development of a proteinuria remain incompletely understood. The nature of the antigen involved in the immune complex deposits of membranous glomerulopathy and its source remain unknown. In fact, it is apparent that may different antigen-antibody combinations cause membranous glomerulopathy. The nephritogenic antigens can be endogenous to the glomerulus itself or can be exogenous. In the latter case, the antigen may be deposited in the subepithelial zone as part of preformed, circulating, immune complexes, or could be produced in or planted in the subepithelial zone as free antigen to which antibodies bind to form immune complexes *in situ.*

In rat Heymann nephritis, which closely resembles human idiopathic membranous glomerulopathy, there is convincing evidence that the subepithelial immune deposits form *in situ* as a result of the binding of antibodies to glycoproteins produced by visceral epithelial cells followed by accumulation of masses of the immune complexes in the subepithelial zone.[448-450]

If the nephritogenic antigens in human membranous glomerulopathy are intrinsic to the glomerulus, one could postulate that they should be distributed along the lamina rara externa or at the base of the visceral epithelial cells.[451,452] Antibodies reactive *in vitro* with normal glomerular capillary walls have only rarely been described in human membranous glomerulopathy.[453-455] Antibodies to endothelin I and III were unexpectedly found to stain immune deposits in kidneys with idiopathic membranous glomerulonephritis, but not other primary glomerular diseases. As endothelin mRNA was not expressed in renal tissues of patients with membranous glomerulopathy, it was implied that the endothelin found in immune deposits waste of non-renal origin.[456] Identifying the target antigen(s) associated with membranous nephropathy is a key question. A number of antigens have been detected in human membranous nephropathy associated with either infectious disease or cancers. To date, the most convincing identification of a target antigen intrinsic to the normal podocyte membrane comes from the identification of antibodies to neutral endopeptidase in four cases of antenatal membranous nephropathy.[457] Mothers who lack this neural endopeptidase (NEP) and become pregnant with a normal fetus were described to form antibodies to this protein (also expressed on syncytiotrophoblastic cells), which can then cross the placenta and induce typical membranous nephropathy in the fetus.[458] NEP has not been found in the subendothelial immune deposits of patients with idiopathic membranous nephropathy.[459] Nevertheless, these cases of membranous nephropathy caused by alloimmunization to a protein intrinsic to the podocyte foot process raises the possibility that a similar mechanism could be involved in the pathogenesis of adult idiopathic disease.[457]

Regardless of the nature of the immune complex deposits in membranous glomerulopathy, the mechanisms leading to the proteinuric and nephrotic state are somewhat more completely understood. The current understanding of these mechanisms is largely based on data emerging from studies of passive Heyman nephritis.[450,451] In this model, immune complex formation in the subepithelial zone leads to the activation of the complement pathway leading to the formation of the C5b-C9 membrane attack complex. This results in complement-mediated injury to the epithelial cells.[460-462] The characteristic findings of a predominance of IgG4 with less IgG3 and no IgG1 in subepithelial deposits,[463,464] and the paucity of C1q and C4 in these deposits,[465] argues against a predominant role for the classical pathway of complement activation in membranous nephropathy, but rather points to a role of the alternative pathway.[466] The fact that the alternative pathway is spontaneously active in turn points to the likely importance of the complement regulatory proteins. Podocytes primarily rely on membrane complement receptor 1 (CR1) (Crry in rodents), decay accelerating factor (DAF) and have the capability to make their own factor H. The importance of complement-mediated injury (at least in passive Heymann nephritis) comes from the evidence that nephritogenic serum contains antibodies to membrane complement regulatory proteins [Crry].[467,468] In a model of active Heymann nephritis, immunization with Fx1A lacking Crry leads to the formation of anti-Fx1A antibodies and subepithelial immune complex deposits, but no complement activation or the development of proteinuria.[469] Conversely, the over-expression of Crry or treatment with exogenous Crry has a salutatory effect on immune complex-mediated glomerulonephritis.[470,471] Subsequent injury to the epithelial cell membrane and to the glomerular basement membrane is hypothesized to be mediated at least in part by the production of reactive oxygen species and lipid peroxidation of cell membrane proteins and of type IV collagen.[472] Complement activation seems to be involved in the tubular injury as well, which eventually leads to tubulointerstitial atrophy and fibrosis.[473,474]

The alteration in the glomerular extracellular matrix seen in membranous glomerulopathy may not be mediated entirely by complement activation and formation of the membrane attack complex. This is evidenced by GBM thickening in the autologous immune complex nephritis model but not in passive Heymann nephritis.[472] Recent studies suggest that the thickening of the basement membrane seen in membranous glomerulopathy may be caused at least in part by a decrease in fibrinolytic activity, due to the stabilization of active plasminogen activator inhibitor I (PAI I) in conjunction with vitronectin in the subepithelial deposits.[475]

The human leukocyte antigen (HLA) class II DR3 has been associated with membranous glomerulopathy.[476-488] In fact, there may be a relative risk of 12 for developing membranous glomerulopathy if HLA DR3 is inherited.[476] In a Japanese population, there is an increased incidence of HLA DR2[479,480] and Dqw1.[481] It is possible that a haplotype containing DR3 and specific HLA Class I antigens may be common in these patients as well.[476] For instance, HLA-B18 and HLA DR3 haplotype may confer an even greater risk for the development of membranous glomerulopathy.[482] C4 null alleles are more frequently found in patients with membranous glomerulopathy, especially in Caucasian populations.[483] Whether or not these immunogenetic markers confer at worsening prognosis has been controversial.[393] Despite the relative risk associated with some of these immunogenetic markers, there are relatively few examples of familial membranous glomerulopathy.[484-488]

Clinical Features and Natural History

Patients with membranous glomerulopathy usually have the nephrotic syndrome with hypoalbuminemia, hyperlipidemia, peripheral edema, and lipiduria. This presentation occurs in 70% to 80% of patients with membranous glomerulopathy.[374,405,410,423,427,489-496] The onset of this nephrotic process is usually not associated with any prodromal disease process or other antecedent infections. Hypertension may be absent at the outset of disease.[401,403] In most series, the incidence of hypertension at onset varies from 13% to 55%.[400-403,406,409-411] Most patients present with normal or slightly decreased renal function.

If progressive renal insufficiency develops, it is usually relatively indolent. An abrupt change to more acute renal insufficiency should prompt investigation of a superimposed condition. For instance, crescentic glomerulonephritis has been observed in some patients with membranous glomerulopathy.[497] Most of these patients have an idiopathic cause for the crescentic transformation. One third of these patients have anti-glomerular basement membrane antibodies, and some may have anti-neutrophil cytoplasmic autoantibodies.

Other causes for sudden deterioration of renal function include acute bilateral renal vein thrombosis, and hypovolemia in the setting of massive nephrosis. The incidence of renal vein thrombosis in the setting of membranous glomerulopathy[498] varies from 4% to 52%.[115] The diagnosis of renal vein thrombosis may be clinically apparent based on the sudden development of macroscopic hematuria, flank pain, and reduction in renal function. It is more persistent, and insidious development of renal vein thrombosis is not uncommon.[167,499] Although ultrasonography with Doppler studies may demonstrate the renal thrombus, intravenous venography with contrast remains the gold standard. Magnetic resonance imaging with gadolinium allows for visualization of clots involving arterial and venous systems and may prove to be a useful diagnostic test.

Drug-induced renal injury is another reason for the sudden deterioration in renal function in a patient with membranous glomerulopathy. The use of non-steroidal anti-inflammatory drugs, diuretics, and anti-microbials is linked with the occurrence of acute interstitial nephritis or acute tubular necrosis.

An estimate of renal survival in patients with membranous glomerulopathy can be obtained from a pooled analysis of outcomes in clinical studies.[500] In this analysis of 1189 pooled patients,[400-403,406,409-411,413-433,501-503] the probability of renal survival was 46% in 5 years, 65% in 10 years, and 59% years at 15 years. Although 35% of patients may progress to renal disease at 10 years, 25% may have a complete spontaneous remission of proteinuria within 5 years.[430] In a study from Italy of 100 untreated patients with membranous glomerulopathy who were observed for 10 years, 30% had progressive renal impairment after 8 years of follow-up. On the other hand, of the 62% who presented with nephrotic-range proteinuria, 50% underwent spontaneous remission in 5 years.[426] When pooling data from many studies on membranous glomerulopathy,[500] 10% of non-treated patients are in complete remission at 12 months, 16% at 24 months, and 22% at 36 months. Spontaneous remission may take 36 to 48 months to develop.

Although population studies provide an estimate of the prognosis in patient populations, sequential examination of any given patient over time provides a much stronger predictor of the long-term renal outcome in that individual. Thus, several studies have attempted to estimate the prognosis of patients with membranous glomerulopathy. Patients with overtly declining renal function are at higher risk for progressive renal deterioration.[430] In addition to declining renal function, Pei and colleagues[504] have reported that persistent proteinuria is more predictive of renal insufficiency than proteinuria at a single time point. Thus, persistent proteinuria of ≥8 grams per day for ≥6 months was associated with a 66% probability of progression to chronic renal failure. Patients with at least 6 grams of protein per day for 9 or more months had a 55% probability of developing chronic renal insufficiency. Even moderate levels of persistent proteinuria (≥4 grams/day) for over 18 months were associated with increased risk of chronic renal insufficiency. Although the data of Pei and colleagues described the persistence of proteinuria as a poor long-term prognostic factor, the amount of proteinuria at the time of presentation may also confer some degree of long-term prognostic information. Adults who present with non-nephrotic proteinuria have a more favorable 10-year survival rate than those with advanced proteinuria.[426] In contrast, patients with ≥10 grams or proteinuria per day at the onset of disease have a 60% probability of developing end-stage renal disease during 8 years of follow-up.[432] Despite these assertions, it should be noted that some patients with non-nephrotic proteinuria may develop a more progressive course,[432] and others with massive proteinuria at the time of presentation may have spontaneous remission.

In addition to renal insufficiency and proteinuria, other factors may be associated with an increased risk of progressive renal failure. These include male gender, advanced age (over age 50 years), poorly controlled hypertension, and reduced glomerular filtration rate at the outset of presentation.[409,424,126,130,132,494,504-506] In addition to the clinical prognostic features, the presence of advanced membranous glomerulopathy on renal biopsy (stage III or IV), tubular atrophy, and interstitial fibrosis can also be associated with increased risk. In fact, chronic interstitial fibrosis and tubular atrophy are shown to be independent predictors of progressive renal failure in idiopathic membranous glomerulopathy.[428,502,507-509] The presence of crescents on renal biopsy may also portend a poor long-term prognosis.

There is considerable controversy regarding the predictive value of the stage of glomerular lesions detected by electron microscopy. Some studies[493,510,511] suggest that a poor prognosis is associated with stage III or IV lesions. Other studies[400,418,424,428,432,502,512] refute this observation. The presence of frequent mononuclear cells in the interstitium may carry an increased risk of progressive renal failure.[513]

Focal segmental glomerulosclerosis superimposed on membranous has a worse long-term renal prognosis than membranous glomerulopathy without sclerosis.[514,515] In one study, renal insufficiency in patients with concurrent FSGS and membranous glomerulopathy occurred at a rate of 52% at 5 years compared to 12% at 5 years in patients with membranous glomerulopathy alone.[514]

In summary, strong indicators of progressive disease are persistent moderate proteinuria, impaired renal function, severe proteinuria at presentation, and the presence of substantial interstitial infiltrates on biopsy. Patients with superimposed crescentic glomerulonephritis or segmental sclerosis fare poorly.

Laboratory Findings

Proteinuria is the hallmark of patients with membranous glomerulopathy. Well over 80% have more than 3 grams of protein per 24 hours. In some patients, the amount of proteinuria may exceed 20 grams/day. The MRC study reported 30% of patients had more than 10 grams per day at the time of presentation.[434] Microscopic hematuria is present in 30% to 50% of patients at the time of presentation.[410,495,516] Macroscopic hematuria on the other hand, is distinctly uncommon and occurs in less than 4% of adult patients[517,518] although it may be common in children.[519] Most patients present with either normal or only slightly decreased renal function. In fact, impaired renal function is found in less than 10% of patients at the time of presentation.[423,495]

In patients with severe nephrosis, hypoalbuminemia is common, as well as the loss of other serum proteins, including IgG. Serum lipoproteins are characteristically elevated, as they are in other forms of the nephrotic syndrome. Elevated LDL and VLDL are common in membranous glomerulopathy. In one study, elevated levels of lipoprotein (A) normalized in those patients who are in remission.[520]

Complement component levels, C3 and C4, are typically normal in patients with membranous glomerulopathy. The complex of terminal complement components known as C5b-9 is found in the urine in some patients with active membranous glomerulopathy. There is increased excretion of this complex in patients with active immune complex formation. The excretion may decrease during disease inactivity.[460-462,521-526]

To exclude common causes of secondary membranous glomerulopathy, one should obtain serologic tests for nephritogenic infections such as hepatitis B, hepatitis C, and syphilis, and tests for immunological disorders such as lupus, mixed connective tissue disease, and cryoglobulinemia. Membranous nephropathy has been associated with graft versus host disease following allogenic stem cell transplant, and this should be considered as well.[527]

Although patients with nephrosis in general appear to be hypercoagulable, this tendency may be enhanced in patients with membranous glomerulopathy.[115,498,528] Thus, patients with membranous glomerulopathy have hyperfibrinogenemia with increased circulating pro-coagulants and decreased anti-coagulant factors such as anti-thrombin 3.[529] The thrombotic tendency may be increased by the erythrocytosis that occurs in some patients, as well as by the effect of lipoprotein (a) to retard thrombolysis. Consequently, renal vein thrombosis is reported more frequently in patients with membranous glomerulopathy than in other causes of nephrotic syndrome.[498,530-533] The prevalence of renal vein thrombosis in patients with membranous glomerulopathy ranges from approximately 5% to 63%, with an averaged of less than 15%. The prevalence of all forms of deep vein thrombosis in patients with membranous glomerulopathy in general ranges from 9% to 44%. Renal vein thrombosis secondary to membranous glomerulopathy is often silent, pulmonary embolism is typically the phenomenon that presents the first clinical evidence of an underlying thrombotic tendency. It is the concern for the morbidity and, at times, mortality associated with pulmonary embolism that has led to the use of prophylactic anticoagulation for patients of severe nephrotic syndrome and membranous glomerulopathy. A decision analysis suggests the risk of life-threatening complications of pulmonary embolism outweigh the risks associated with anticoagulation.[534]

Treatment

Corticosteroids

Of all glomerular diseases, the management of membranous nephropathy has been most intensively studied, yet remains greatly controversial. The difficulty in the management of membranous glomerulopathy is a consequence of the chronic nature of the disease, the tendency for spontaneous remission and relapse, the variability of clinical severity, and the lack of efficacy of existing treatment protocols. The role of corticosteroids and alkylating agents in the treatment of this disease has been debated for decades. The common therapeutic approaches for new-onset disease include (1) no specific treatment, that is, placebo or supportive care, (2) corticosteroids (usually prednisone or methylprednisolone), and (3) alkylating agents, such as chlorambucil or cyclophosphamide, with or without concurrent corticosteroid treatment. Numerous studies using corticosteroid treatment have demonstrated different outcomes.[400–403,406,409–411,413–433,501–503] In a pooled analysis of these studies, corticosteroid therapy resulted in no better probability of renal survival than no treatment.[500]

There have been three large, prospective, randomized trials examining the efficacy of oral corticosteroid therapy in adult patients.[414,415,535] These prospective studies have differed in outcome. The US Collaborative Study[405] suggested that 8 weeks of 100 mg to 150 mg of prednisone given on alternate days resulted in a transient decrease in proteinuria to less than 2 grams when compared to placebo. In this trial, prednisone was discontinued after 3 months unless a relapse of proteinuria occurred after either a partial or complete remission. Relapses were treated by reinstitution of high-dose prednisone for 1 month, and then prednisone was tapered. Interestingly, the results of this study suggested that patients who were treated with prednisone were less likely to double their entry serum creatinine, were more likely to experience a transient decrease in proteinuria to less than 2 grams a day, and that even a partial remission of proteinuria was associated with well-preserved, long-term renal function. This seminal study guided treatment for more than a decade, but was criticized because the placebo group faired substantially worse than non-treated patients in several other studies.

The US Collaborative Study prompted other similar prednisone-treatment protocols. For instance, the protocol of Cameron and co-workers[414] for the British Medical Research Council, was similar in a number of ways, except that prednisolone was discontinued after 8 weeks without tapering and without treatment of the relapse of proteinuria. Moreover, patients with lower creatinine clearance (≤30 ml/min) were included in the study. Three to nine months after study entry, there was no improvement in renal function, and the urine protein excretion and albumin level improved only transiently. A third corticosteroid treatment protocol was reported by Cattran.[415] The entry criteria included patients with relatively small amounts of proteinuria (≤0.3 g/day). The prednisone treatment included alternate-day dosage of 45 mg/

M[2] of body surface area. In this prospective study, prednisone had no effect on either proteinuria or renal function.

Meta-analysis of the US Collaborative study and the studies by Cameron, Cattran, and Kobayashi[400,414–416] compared glucocorticoid-treated patients to those not receiving treatment.[500] There was a tendency for patients to achieve complete remission at 24 to 36 months, but this result did not reach statistical significance. A pooled analysis of randomized trials and prospective studies using adjusted values from logistic regression analysis again demonstrated a lack of benefit of corticosteroid therapy in inducing a remission of the nephrotic syndrome. There was no benefit of corticosteroids on renal survival in general.

The issue, then, is whether prednisone has any role in the treatment of patients with idiopathic membranous glomerulopathy. The three studies described above employed relatively short courses of prednisone, anticipating long-term effects. It has been argued by several investigators that higher doses (60 to 200 mg QOD) of prednisone and longer courses of therapy (up to 1 year) are essential for treatment in these patients.[399,494] The studies of these investigators suffer from the fact that they are retrospective and contain reasonably small numbers of patients. Moreover, the side effects of extended courses of very high dose corticosteroids do not favor the risk/benefit ratio of this form of therapy.[535,536]

An alternative to oral glucocorticoid therapy has been treatment with pulse methylprednisolone. This approach has been largely aimed at patients with membranous glomerulopathy who have deteriorating renal function. Short and colleagues[537] treated patients with membranous glomerulopathy and renal insufficiency using pulse methylprednisolone at 1 gram/day for 5 days followed by oral prednisone. Improvement in renal function was sustained for 6 months, and there was reduction in proteinuria. Yet, long-term outcomes were discouraging in almost half of these patients, including renal failure in one third and myocardial infarction with renal dysfunction in 13%. A similar study[538] combined pulse methylprednisolone with azathioprine or cyclophosphamide. Although there may have been some improvement in proteinuria and renal function in a minority of patients, substantial side effects afflicted almost the entire study population.

The evidence to date does not support the use of oral corticoids for the treatment of idiopathic membranous glomerulopathy. This said, it should be noted that there is an uncommon group of patients with membranous glomerulopathy who are highly steroid-responsive and have a natural history of response and relapse in a fashion very reminiscent of minimal change glomerulopathy.[172,173,539] These patients are rare with respect to the entire spectrum of patients with idiopathic membranous glomerulopathy.[172,173,539]

Interestingly, emerging data suggest that ACTH may have a different effect on the nephritic syndrome of membranous nephropathy than high-dose oral glucocorticoids.[540] In a recently published randomized controlled trial which compared treatment with methylprednisolone alternated with a cytotoxic drug every other month for 6 months to intramuscular synthetic adrenocorticotropic hormone administered twice a week for 1 year, the two forms of therapy led to significant and comparable reductions of proteinuria in most patients.[541]

Use of Cyclophosphamide

Cytotoxic drugs, including cyclophosphamide and chlorambucil have been used for the treatment of idiopathic membranous glomerulopathy. In a number of studies, Ponticelli demonstrated that chlorambucil has a salutary effect in the treatment of membranous glomerulopathy.[418,502,510,512] In these studies, patients with idiopathic membranous glomerulopathy were treated initially with intravenous pulse methylprednisolone at 1 gram per day for the first 3 days of each month, with daily oral glucocorticoid (methylprednisolone at 0.4 mg/kg/day or prednisone 0.5 mg/kg/day) therapy, given on an alternating monthly schedule with chlorambucil at a dose of 0.2 mg/kg/day. Patients randomized to the treatment group had their nephrotic syndrome for a significantly shorter duration of nephrotic syndrome and had a complete or partial remission of proteinuria in 83% of patients compared with 38% of control patients.[512] The slope of the mean reciprocal plasma creatinine remained stable in the treatment group, but declined in the untreated patients beginning at 12 months. At follow-up at 10 years, the probability of a functioning kidney was 92% in the treated patients and 60% in controls. Only 10% of patients were withdrawn from therapy as a consequence of side effects. When compared to treatment with glucocorticoids alone, treatment with a combination of chlorambucil and methylprednisolone was associated with an earlier remission of the nephrotic syndrome, and a greater stability of complete or partial remission of proteinuria.[418] Interestingly, the overall decline in renal function was not different in the two treatment groups. Unfortunately, this difference persisted for the first 3 years of follow-up but was no longer statistically significantly different by 4 years (62% versus 42%, p = 0.102). In a study comparing cyclophosphamide with chlorambucil, cyclophosphamide was found to be at least as effective as chlorambucil when used in a similar dosing protocol, and appeared to have somewhat fewer side effects.[542]

Despite these reported benefits, the salutary effects of alkylating agents combined with prednisone or other agents have not been confirmed in other trials.[417,429,433,503] These conflicting results prompted two meta-analyses of controlled trials of either cyclophosphamide or chlorambucil treatment of membranous glomerulopathy.[500,543] Both meta-analyses suggested that cytotoxic agents improve the chance of a complete remission of proteinuria by four- to five-fold, but have no long-term protective effect on renal survival. In a recent study comparing patients treated with prednisone tapered over 6 months plus chlorambucil, when compared to conservative treatment of historical controls, patients treated with combined glucocorticoid and chlorambucil regimen did much better over the long term.[544]

Some patients with membranous glomerulopathy present with progressive deterioration of renal function. Several rescue therapies with alkylating agents have been tried.[545–552] These studies suggest that oral cyclophosphamide or chlorambucil may stabilize renal function and induce a remission of the nephrotic syndrome. Intravenous cyclophosphamide has been shown to be ineffective.[548,549] These regimens have used large doses of prednisone (60 mg to 100 mg QOD for a year)[547] and oral cyclophosphamide from 1 to 4.5 years. In general, complete or partial remission of proteinuria can be obtained in up to 50% of patients, and stability of renal function in approximately the same number. The risk-to-benefit ratio of these aggressive treatment protocols must be acceptable to the patient. As a consequence, these treatments result in substantial side effects during the study follow up. Recent long-term follow up using prolonged oral cyclophosphamide in patients with Wegener granulomatosis[553] suggests that 15% of patients will develop transitional cell carcinoma of the bladder with a substantial increase in the incidence of lymphomas. The development of bladder cancer may become apparent up to seven years after the cyclophosphamide has been given. Thus, these aggressive salvage strategies for membranous glomerulopathy must be balanced against the immediate and long-term consequences of alkylating agents.

Cyclosporine
There has been substantial interest in the use of cyclosporine that has resulted in improvement in proteinuria and stability of renal function in many patients.[554–556] In most studies

however, protein excretion increased in the majority of patients soon after the cessation of cyclosporine therapy. Yet, in one series,[557] improvement in renal function and proteinuria was sustained in 75% of patients for 20 months after cyclosporine was discontinued. Cyclosporine treatment may play a role in patients with steroid-resistant membranous nephropathy. In a randomized, controlled trial comparing 26 weeks of cyclosporine treatment plus low-dose prednisone to placebo plus prednisone, 75% of the treatment group versus 22% of the control group (P < 0.001) had a partial or complete remission of their proteinuria by 26 weeks. Relapse occurred in about 40% of patients achieving remission in either treatment group. The fraction of patients in sustained remission then remained significantly different between the groups until the end of the study (cyclosporine 39%, placebo 13%, P = 0.007). Renal function was unchanged and equal in the two groups over the test medication period.[558] It is interesting to consider how cyclosporine induces a remission of membranous glomerulopathy while the drug is administered, and the repeated observation of relapse after the drug is withdrawn. Some understanding of this issue was obtained examining the effect of three months of cyclosporine and three months of enalapril in a randomized cross-over study.[559] Cyclosporine did improve proteinuria without alterations in glomerular filtration or plasma flow (dextran analysis revealed that cyclosporine improved the size-selective and charge-selective properties of the glomerular capillary wall). These results were not obtained by use of enalapril. However, 75% of these study patients relapsed in the month after stopping cyclosporine. Repeat biopsy of a subset of these patients revealed persistent deposition of immunoglobulin and complement, suggesting that the disease process was ongoing.

Other Forms of Immunosuppressive Therapy
Other forms of therapy have been tried in idiopathic membranous glomerulopathy, with varying results. These include the use of azathioprine,[419,420] which demonstrated no positive effect of prednisone and azathioprine combinations. Pooled intravenous immunoglobulin[560] was tested in nine patients with resultant decline in proteinuria and stabilization of renal function with minimal side effects. This small case series must be evaluated in a larger prospective trial. In a retrospective analysis of 86 patients with primary MN, 30 patients were non-randomly treated with one to three courses of intravenous immune globulin, (100–150 mg/kg/day) for 6 consecutive days. There was no difference in the initial demographic or clinicopathological states between the two treatment groups. Among patients with homogeneous ("synchronous") immune complex deposits, treatment with IVIg was associated with earlier remission as compared to patients treated with corticosteroid ± cyclophosphamide alone (57 versus 10% remission at 6 months respectively, P = 0.006). No benefit was demonstrated among patients with heterogeneous immune complex deposits or in the final outcome for all groups.[561]

Mycophenolate mofetil has been tried in the management of membranous nephropathy. In general, patients have been treated with this drug after they have failed ACE inhibitors, ARBs, glucocorticoids, alkylating agents, and even cyclosporine. In a pilot open label study of 16 patients treated for 6 to 16 months, 6 patients had a decrease in proteinuria of >50%, within a period of 6 months.[562] The role (if any) of mycophenolate mofetil in the therapy of membranous nephropathy remains to be elucidated.[562–566]

The recent years have seen great interest in the use of the anti-CD20 monoclonal antibody rituximab for the management of a number of antibody mediated autoimmune diseases, including membranous nephropathy. In an initial report of eight patients, treatment with rituximab (4 weekly doses of 375 mg/M² body surface area) was associated with prompt and sustained reduction in proteinuria.[567,568] There has since been followed an additional open-label study from the same group,[569] but no controlled trial of this agent has been undertaken yet, and its effects on long-term renal outcome are unproven.

Based on the greater appreciation of the role of complement activation and especially that of complement regulatory proteins, in the pathogenesis of membranous nephropathy, a great deal of interest exists in targeting this pathway for therapy. Several compounds are under development. To date human trials were conducted only for eculizumab, a monoclonal antibody directed against the fifth component of complement (C5). In a randomized trial of patients with *de novo* membranous nephropathy, treatment with eculizumab was not associated with a statistically significant improvement in proteinuria or preservation of renal function. These disappointing results were likely due to insufficient dosing, as only a minority of patients attained consistent inhibition of complement inhibition.[570] Nevertheless, this general approach is thought to hold a great deal of promise based on early animal studies.

In the absence of full understanding of the pathogenesis of membranous glomerulopathy, and thus an effective targeted therapy, the current approach to the treatment of membranous glomerulopathy must rely on risk stratification. The indolent disease process that results in spontaneous remissions in one quarter of patients, coupled with the known adverse consequences of long-term oral glucocorticoids and alkylating agents, should prompt a careful analysis of the risk-benefit ratio in treatment of any given patient. All patients should receive excellent supportive care, including the use of angiotensin converting enzyme inhibitors[331,571–574] or angiotensin receptor blockers, therapy using lipid-lowering agents described previously, and perhaps the use of a prophylactic anticoagulant. The usefulness of lipid-lowering therapy in membranous nephropathy may be more than just the diminution of plasma cholesterol. In fact, certain agents, especially probucol, may inhibit the lipid peroxidation, which may alter the composition of the glomerular basement membrane.[575]

Several predictors of a progressive loss of GFR have been described in patients with membranous nephropathy. Both age and gender have been identified as predictors of outcome, with men having a worse prognosis than women.[576] Although older age is associated with a poorer renal outcome, it appears that the rate of decline in renal function is comparable in older and younger patients, however, older patients have a lower creatinine clearance at presentation.[577] Important predictors of progression are the rate of decline in GFR over the an observation period of 6 months[577] and the degree and duration of proteinuria. Patients presenting with non-nephrotic proteinuria have an improved 10-year renal survival rate; whereas those with more than grams of proteinuria have a 60% probability of ESRD at 8 years. In addition, several histologic features on renal biopsy have been associated with a poor outcome, including the severity of tubulointerstitial damage, and vascular sclerosis, the amount of complement deposition on immunofluorescence, the presence of the lesion of focal and segmental glomerulosclerosis and the findings of heterogeneous versus homogeneous (synchronous) morphology of the subepithelial electron-dense deposits. In a recent analysis of renal biopsies of 389 adult patients with membranous nephropathy, associations were tested between these variables and the rate of decline of renal function decline, renal survival, remission in proteinuria, and response to immunosuppression.[578] Although these histologic features were associated with a reduced renal survival, they did not predict this outcome independently of the baseline clinical variables nor did they correlate with the rate of decline in

function or with baseline proteinuria. Furthermore, the severity of tubulointerstitial and vascular lesions did not preclude a remission in proteinuria in treated patients. The amount of complement deposition did not predict renal survival, remissions in proteinuria, or response to immunosuppressive drugs, but did correlate with a faster rate of renal function decline.[578] Additional predictors of outcome include the degree of IgG and α(1)microglobulin excretions as reflecting the alteration of permselectivity in the glomerular capillary wall and the reabsorption impairment of low-molecular-weight proteins respectively. Remission was reported in 100% versus 20% in patients with IgG excretion <110 mg/g Cr versus >110 mg/g Cr (P = 0.0001) and 77% versus 17% in patients with α(1)microglobulin excretion <33.5 mg/g Cr versus >33.5 mg/g Cr (P = 0.0009).[579] Similarly urinary β-2-microglobulin has also been found to predict progressive loss of renal function.[580]

Most patients should be observed for the development of adverse prognostic factors or the development of spontaneous remissions. In adult patients with good prognostic features, with less than 4 grams or proteinuria per day and normal renal function should be managed conservatively without the use of glucocorticoid or cytotoxic agents, but with an ACE inhibitor and or an angiotensin receptor blocker. These patients should receive excellent supportive care. Patients at moderate risk (persistent proteinuria between 4 and 6 grams per day after 6 months of conservative therapy and normal renal function) or high risk of progression (persistent proteinuria greater than 8 grams per day with or without renal insufficiency) should be considered for immunosuppressive therapy with either the combination of glucocorticoids and cyclophosphamide (or chlorambucil) in alternating monthly pulses ("Ponticelli protocol"); or a regimen consisting of cyclosporine with low-dose glucocorticoids. A current recommendation gives preference for the use a cytotoxic treatment approach in patients with moderate risk of progression, and for the use of cyclosporine in patients at high risk of progression.[581] This decision must be individualized to each patient's comorbidities and assessment of the risk associated with each kind of therapy. Whenever cyclosporine is used, close attention must be given to the consistent use of a same formulation over time, and initiating therapy at a low- to moderate dose (e.g., starting at 2 mg/day to 2.5 mg/day in divided dose of the microemulsion formulation), followed by a dose adjustment with careful evaluation of changes in blood pressure and creatinine clearance. Individuals who have advanced chronic renal failure and in whom serum creatinine exceeds 3 mg/dL to 4 mg/dL are best treated by supportive care awaiting dialysis and renal transplantation. Acute renal insufficiency in this population should prompt evaluation of interstitial nephritis, crescentic nephritis, or renal vein thrombosis.

Membranoproliferative Glomerulonephritis (Mesangial Capillary Glomerulonephritis)

Epidemiology

The majority of patients with membranoproliferative glomerulonephritis (MPGN) are children between the ages of 8 and 16 years.[582] In pediatric populations, 90% of type I MPGN and 70% of type II are found in individuals between the ages of 8 and 16 years. There is nearly an equal proportion of males to females in both type I and type II disease.[583–593] There was a male to female ratio of 1.2 to 1.0 in the last 248 examples of type I MPGN diagnosed in the UNC Nephropathology Laboratory. MPGN is identified in approximately 10% of renal biopsy specimens.[583,585] MPGN appears to be decreasing in frequency.[594]

Type I Membranoproliferative Glomerulonephritis

Light Microscopy

The most common histologic features of type I MPGN are diffuse global capillary wall thickening and endocapillary hypercellularity.[584,595] Infiltrating mononuclear leukocytes and neutrophils also contribute to the glomerular hypercellularity. The consolidation of glomerular segments that results from these changes often causes an accentuation of the segmentation referred to as "hypersegmentation" or lobulation. As a consequence, an earlier name for this phenotype of glomerular injury was "lobular glomerulonephritis." Markedly expanded mesangial regions may develop a nodular appearance with a central zone of sclerosis that may resemble diabetic glomerulosclerosis or light chain deposition disease. However, the integration of light, immunofluorescence, and electron microscopy findings readily differentiates type I MPGN from other diseases that can mimic it by light microscopy.

A distinctive but not completely specific feature of type I MPGN is doubling or more complex replication of glomerular basement membranes that can be seen with stains that highlight basement membranes, such as Jones' silver methenamine stain or periodic acid-Schiff stain (Fig. 30–11). This change is caused by the production of basement membrane material between and around projections of mesangial cytoplasm that extend into an expanded subendothelial zone, probably in response to the presence of subendothelial immune complex deposits (Fig. 30–12). The presence of "hyaline thrombi" within capillary lumens should raise the possibility of cryoglobulinemia or lupus as the cause for the MPGN. Hyaline thrombi are not true thrombi but rather are aggregates of immune complexes filling capillary lumens. A minority of patients with type I MPGN have crescents, but these rarely involve more than 50% of glomeruli.[596,597] As with other types of glomerulonephritis, substantial crescent formation correlates with a more rapid progression of disease.[595]

Immunofluorescence Microscopy

The characteristic pattern of staining is peripheral granular to band-like staining for complement, especially C3, and usually immunoglobulins (Fig. 30–13). This corresponds to the prominent subendothelial immune complex localization seen by electron microscopy. The staining pattern is less granular and less symmetrical than that usually seen with membranous glomerulopathy. Mesangial granular staining may be conspicuous or inconspicuous. The hypersegmentation or lobulation that is seen by light microscopy often can be discerned by immunofluorescence microscopy. A minority of patients with type I MPGN have staining of immune complexes along tubular basement membranes or in extraglomerular vessels or both.

The composition of the immune deposits is variable, which probably reflects the many different causes of type I MPGN. Most specimens have more intense staining for C3 than for any immunoglobulin, but some specimens have more intense staining for IgG or IgM. Rare specimens have a predominance of IgA and can be considered a MPGN expression of IgA nephropathy. Even when C3 is the most intensely staining immune determinant, most specimens have clear cut staining

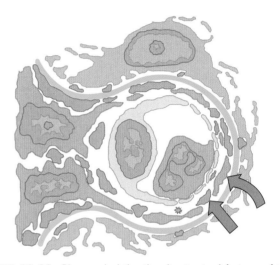

FIGURE 30–12 Diagram depicting the ultrastructural features of type I MPGN. Note the subendothelial dense deposits (straight arrow), subendothelial mesangial cytoplasm interposition (curved arrow), and production of new basement material (asterisk). (Reproduced with permission of J.C. Jennette.)

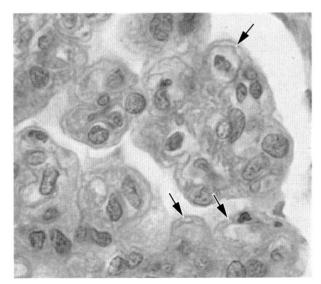

FIGURE 30–11 Light micrograph of a glomerular segment from a patient with type I membranoproliferative glomerulonephritis (MPGN) demonstrating doubling (arrows) and more complex replication of glomerular basement membranes. (Periodic acid–Schiff [PAS], ×1000.)

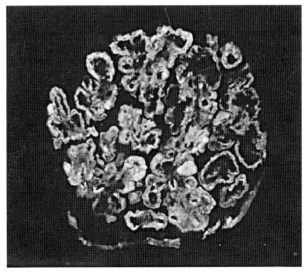

FIGURE 30–13 Immunofluorescence micrograph of a glomerulus with type I MPGN showing global bandlike capillary wall staining for C3, as well as irregular mesangial staining. (FITC anti-C3, ×300.)

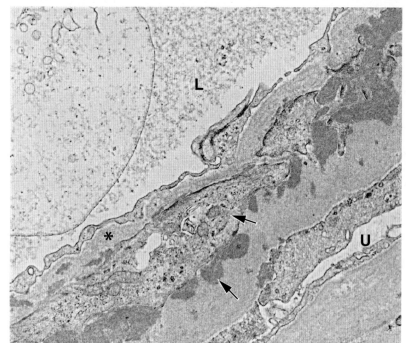

FIGURE 30–14 Electron micrograph of a capillary wall from a glomerulus with type I MPGN. The capillary lumen (L) is in the upper left and the urinary space is in the lower right (U). In the subendothelial zone are dense deposits (straight arrow), extensions of mesangial cytoplasm (curved arrow), and new basement membrane material (cf. Fig. 30–12) (magnification ×10,000).

for IgG or IgM or both. The presence of intracapillary globular structures that stain intensely for immunoglobulin and complement corresponds to the hyaline thrombi seen by light microscopy raise the possibility of MPGN caused by lupus or cryoglobulinemia.

Electron Microscopy

The ultrastructural hallmark of type I MPGN is mesangial interposition into and expanded subendothelial zone that contains electron dense immune complex deposits (Figs. 30–12 and 30–14). This distinct pattern of mesangial and capillary involvement has prompted a synonym for type I MPGN, "mesangiocapillary glomerulonephritis." New basement membrane material is formed around the subendothelial deposits and around the projections of mesangial cytoplasm, which is the basis for the basement membrane replication seen by light microscopy (see Fig. 30–11). Scattered mesangial dense deposits are usually found in association with mesangial hypercellularity and mesangial matrix expansion. Variable numbers of subepithelial electron dense deposits occur. When they are numerous enough to resemble membranous glomerulopathy, some nephropathologists apply the diagnosis "mixed membranous and proliferative glomerulonephritis" or "type III MPGN" as proposed by Burkholder.[598] The term type III MPGN also has been applied to a very rare pattern of glomerular injury that resembles type I MPGN by light microscopy and immunofluorescence microscopy, but is characterized ultrastructurally by irregularly thickened glomerular basement membranes with numerous intramembranous deposits of variable density.[589,599]

The hyaline thrombi seen by light microscopy appear as intraluminal spherical densities. When these structures, or any of the other electron dense deposits, have a microtubular substructure, the possibility of cryoglobulinemic glomerulonephritis or immunotactoid glomerulopathy should be considered.

Type II Membranoproliferative Glomerulonephritis

An alternative term for type II MPGN is dense deposit disease.[595] This term emphasizes the pathognomonic feature of type II MPGN, which is the development of discontinuous

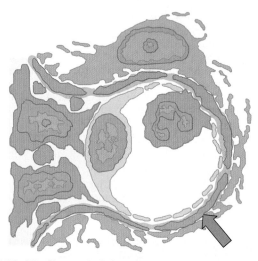

FIGURE 30–15 Diagram depicting a glomerular capillary loop with features of type II MPGN (dense deposit disease) with bandlike intramembranous dense deposits (arrow) and spherical mesangial dense deposits. (Reproduced with permission of J.C. Jennette.)

electron dense bands within glomerular basement membranes (Figs. 30–15 and 30–16). These are accompanied by spherical to irregular mesangial dense deposits, and occasional subendothelial and subepithelial deposits, some of which may resemble the "humps" of postinfectious glomerulonephritis.

Immunofluorescence microscopy demonstrates intense capillary wall linear to band-like staining for C3 (Fig. 30–17), with little or no staining for immunoglobulin.[600,601] The capillary wall staining may have a fine double contour with outlining of the outer and inner aspects of the dense deposits. The mesangial deposits usually appear as scattered spherules or rings, with the latter resulting from staining of the outer surface but not the interior of the spherical deposits.

The light microscopic appearance of type II MPGN is much more variable than that of type I MPGN, and does not always have a membranoproliferative appearance. This has prompted

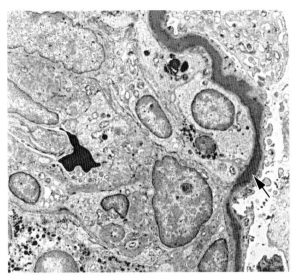

FIGURE 30–16 Electron micrograph of a glomerular capillary from a patient with type II MPGN showing a bandlike intramembranous dense deposit that has essentially replaced the normal glomerular basement membrane. Also note the endocapillary hypercellularity (magnification ×5000).

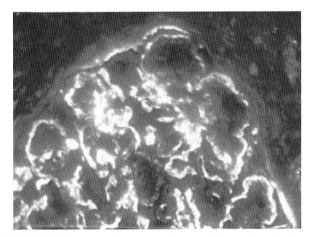

FIGURE 30–17 Immunofluorescence micrograph of a portion of a glomerulus with type II MPGN demonstrating discontinuous bandlike capillary wall staining and granular mesangial staining for C3. (FITC anti-C3, ×600.)

some nephropathologists to prefer the term dense deposit disease rather than type II MPGN.[601] The histologic appearance can be a typical membranoproliferative pattern with thickened capillary walls and marked lobular hypercellularity that closely resembles type I MPGN. However, some specimens have predominantly capillary wall thickening with focal or absent hypercellularity, and some specimens have focal or diffuse hypercellularity without substantial capillary wall thickening. A minority of patients will have crescent formation. Therefore, the histologic appearance of type II MPGN (dense deposit disease) can mimic many other categories of glomerulonephritis and the findings by immunofluorescence and especially electron microscopy are required for accurate diagnosis.

Pathogenesis

Although the pathologic findings indicate that type I MPGN is an immune complex disease, the identity of the nephritogenic antigen is unknown in most patients. In the minority of patients in whom the nature of the antigen is identified, the sources have included infections, neoplasms, hereditary

TABLE 30–11	Classification of Membranoproliferative Glomerulonephritis[612,1019,1316–1323]

Idiopathic
  Type I
  Type II
  Type III

Secondary
  Infections
    Hepatitis C and B
    Visceral abscesses
    Infective endocarditis
    Shunt nephritis
    Quartan malaria
    Schistosoma nephropathy
    Mycoplasmin infection
  Rheumatologic diseases
    Systemic lupus erythematosus
    Scleroderma
    Sjögren syndrome
    Sarcoidosis
    Mixed essential cryoglobulinemia with or without hepatitis C infection
    Anti-smooth muscle syndrome
  Malignancy
    Carcinoma
    Lymphoma
    Leukemia
  Inherited
    Alpha1 antitrypsin deficiency
    Complement deficiency (C2 or C3), with or without partial lipodystrophy

diseases, and autoimmune diseases (Table 30–11). The pathological finding of intense immune complex deposition with hypercellularity suggests that the inflammation caused by the immune complexes has resulted in both proliferation of mesangial and endothelial cells, and the recruitment of inflammatory cells, including neutrophils and monocytes. These leukocytes are attracted to the glomerulus by activation of multiple mediator systems, including the complement system, cytokines, and chemokines.

Type II MPGN is characterized by deposits of dense material within the basement membranes of glomeruli, Bowman capsule, and tubules. Interestingly, these deposits do not appear to contain immunoglobulins, but seem to activate the alternate pathway of complement. A porcine model of MPGN (porcine-dense deposit disease) suggests that there is massive deposition of C3 and the terminal C5b-9 complement complex (the membrane attack complex). In the circulation, there is extensive complement activation with very low C3 and high circulating terminal complement components. No immune complex deposits were detected in renal tissue. At least in this animal model of type II MPGN, the pathogenetic mechanism does not appear to involve immune complexes, but rather utilizes some other mechanism for the activation of complement and the trapping of activating complement components within the glomerular basement membrane.[602]

Hypocomplementemia is a characteristic feature of all types of MPGN. Complement activation in MPGN type I occurs through the classical pathway initiated by immune complex formation. The hypocomplementemia in MPGN type II is more than likely a consequence of alternate pathway activation. C3 nephritic factor is an antibody that prolongs the half-life of C3 convertase. It does so in one of two ways—by either binding to C3bBb, or IgG-C3b-C3bBb of the assembled convertase. The stabilization of this complex results in perpetual C3 breakdown. It is tempting to impugn this factor as central to the pathogenesis of MPGN. C3 nephritic factor does not always correlate with disease activity and, more importantly, progressive renal damage still occurs in patients who have normal levels of complement.[603-605] Normal protective, or regulatory, mechanisms control C3bBb levels and complement deposition, of which Factor H is one of the most important. Factor H is a soluble glycoprotein that regulates complement in the fluid phase and on cell surfaces by binding to C3b.[606] Some mutations in Factor H result in MPGN-like diseases.[607,608]

Clinical Features and Natural History

The clinical features of all forms of membranoproliferative glomerulonephritis are usually that of the nephrotic syndrome. At least half of patients present with all of the components of the nephrotic syndrome, and one quarter of patients present with a combination of asymptomatic hematuria and asymptomatic proteinuria. Finally, one quarter to one third of patients present with the acute nephritic syndrome associated with red cells, red call casts, hypertension, and renal insufficiency.[584,585,609,610] Hypertension is typically mild, although in some cases, especially those with MPGN type II, severe hypertension can occur. Renal dysfunction occurs in at least half of cases. When present at the outset of disease, renal dysfunction portends a poor prognosis. There is an association of respiratory tract infections that may precede cases of MPGN in half of patients.

Membranoproliferative glomerular diseases are also associated with a number of other disease processes (see Table 30–11). A wide variety of infectious and autoimmune conditions are associated with MPGN suggesting that, in addition to the known association of hepatitis, infections in and by themselves may present with a pathological presentation of MPGN.

Of note are those patients who have either deficiency of the second or third component of complement with or without partial lipodystrophy.[605,611-615] This disease process may have an X-linked transmission and is associated with the systemic manifestations of this disease process.[615] In addition to partial lipodystrophy, congenital complement deficiency states, and deficiency in alpha-1 anti-trypsin also predispose to MPGN type I.

The prognosis for MPGN type I has been reviewed and described in several studies.[584,585,616] D'Amico and Ferrario in Italy[585] found a 10-year renal survival of less than 65%. Cameron in the United Kingdom found a 10-year survival of 40% in patients with MPGN type I and persistent nephrosis.[584] Non-nephrotic patients had a 10-year survival of 85%.

The prognosis for type II disease is worse than that for type I. The worsened prognosis is probably because dense deposit disease is frequently associated with crescentic glomerulonephritis and chronic tubulointerstitial nephritis at the time of biopsy.[617-619] In type II MPGN, clinical remissions are rare,[584,586] with a clinical remission rate less than 5% in children. Patients generally enter renal failure between years 8 through 12 of their disease. The parameters suggestive of poor prognosis in idiopathic MPGN type I include hypertension,[593,619] impaired glomerular filtration rate,[593,619-621] nephrotic rather than non-nephrotic,[584,619,620,622] and cellular crescents on biopsy.[584,621,623]

What differentiates MPGN type I from type II? Do they represent different diseases, or are they a continuum? The argument that they are different diseases is based on the distinct morphologic, histopathologic, and immunopathologic changes differentiating the two types.[586,592,624-626] Type II MPGN tends to present with nephritis whereas MPGN type I presents with more nephrotic features. Type II disease is associated with persistently low serum C3 concentrations.[584,586,592,593,620,626,627] Type II MPGN occurs in individuals who are usually less than 20 years old, although there are

occasional exceptions. Type II MPGN recurs in the transplanted kidney much more regularly than type I.[586,628-630]

Type III MPGN occurs in a very small number of children and young adults. Regardless of the pathological distinctions of MPGN type III of Burkholder[598] or of Strife,[599] there are few clinical parameters noted on these patients. These patients may have clinical features of disease quite similar to that of MPGN type I, and the long-term, clinical course is quite similar as well. Patients with MPGN described by Strife[589] have low C3 levels in the absence of C3 nephritic factor. Patients with non-nephrotic proteinuria do better patients presenting with nephrotic syndrome. In our own experience, progression to end-stage renal disease is quite variable, but it appears that some patients stabilize or even improve with long-term renal survival.

Laboratory Findings

Hematuria is the hallmark of presentation. Hematuria may be microscopic or macroscopic in nature. Proteinuria can be mild and asymptomatic in 30% of patients, but half of patients may have the nephrotic syndrome. Renal insufficiency occurs in a variable number of cases, but it becomes the most ominous feature of the acute nephritic syndrome. Decreasing glomerular filtration rate associated with retention of salt and water results in hypertension that can occasionally be severe.

Type I MGPN often is secondary to recognizable causes, such as cryoglobulinemia, hepatitis C, hepatitis B, osteomyelitis, subacute bacterial endocarditis, or infected ventriculoatrial shunt. Serologic and clinical evidence of these processes should be sought. The observation that upper respiratory tract infections precede the onset of what is considered idiopathic MPGN in as many as one half of patients[582] raises the possibility that infectious agents contribute to the pathogenesis of many examples of idiopathic type I MPGN.

One of the hallmarks of the laboratory abnormalities in types I and II MPGN is alteration in the complement cascade (Table 30–12). C3 is persistently depressed in approximately 75% of MPGN patients.[584,585,609,610,631] This is in contrast to post-streptococcal glomerulonephritis in which depressed C3 levels typically return to normal levels within 2 months.[632-634] The persistent depression of C3 and the nephritic syndrome should suggest type I MPGN. The depression of C3 is a consequence of both the activation of the alternate complement pathway and low synthetic levels. Activation of the alternate pathway is suggested by the observation that in type I MPGN, C3 levels are depressed, whereas classical pathway activator C1q and C4 usually are normal. However, when MPGN is caused by cryoglobulinemia there may be more depression of C4 than C3.[635] In type II MPGN, C3 depression occurs in 80% to 90% of patients and, if anything, C3 levels persist longer in type II disease[432] associated with decrements in terminal complement components C5b-9.

Complement activation is enhanced by C3 nephritic factor (C3 NeF) an autoantibody that reacts with convertase of C3 (C3b Bb).[636-639] The autoantibody results in the stabilization of C3 convertase resulting in persistent enzyme activity. Thus, C3 cleavage occurs unabated due to the inability of usual inhibitory proteins to degrade the alternative pathway convertase. C3 nephritic factor occurs in over 60% of patients with MPGN type II and may be responsible for the persistently low levels of C3 in these patients. C3 nephritic factor or its analogues are not only found in type II MPGN, but may be found in other glomerular diseases as well, usually those associated with nephritis.[631,640] Other factors capable of cleaving C3 are not clear, but are found in patients with other acute glomerulonephritis and especially lupus.[632]

Some proportion of type I MPGN is attributable to hepatitis C with or without cryoglobulinemia. The precise percentage of patients with MPGN due to hepatitis C may vary according

Disease	C4	C3	ASO, ADNase B	Cryo Ig	aGBM	ANCA
TABLE 30–12 Selected Serologic Findings in Patients with Primary Glomerular Disease						
Minimal change glomerulopathy	N	N	—	—	—	—
Focal glomerulosclerosis	N	N	—	—	—	—
Membranous GN	N	N	—	—	—	—
Membranoproliferative GN						
Type I	N or ↓↓	↓↓	+	++	—	—
Type II	N	↓↓↓	+	—	—	—
Fibrillary GN	N	N	—	—	—	—
IgA nephropathy	N	N	—	—	—	—
Acute poststreptococcal GN	N or ↓	↓↓	+++	++	—	—
Crescentic GN						
Anti-GBM	N	N	—	—	+++	±
Immune complex	N or ↓	N or ↓↓	—	N/++	—	±
ANCA-SVV	N	N	—	—	±	+++

ADNase B, antideoxyribonuclease B; ANCA, antineutrophil cytoplasmic antibodies; aGBM, anti–glomerular basement membrane antibodies; ASO, antistreptolysin-O; Cryo, cryoglobulins; GN, glomerulonephritis; Ig, immunoglobulins.

CH 30

Primary Glomerular Disease

to geographic area and cultural factors. Consequently, the overall percentage of patients with MPGN type I with hepatitis C across the globe is still unknown. When MPGN is secondary to other disease processes such as malignancy or a rheumatic condition, the laboratory features associated with the systemic disease (for instance SLE) are positive (e.g., antibodies to double-stranded DNA).

Treatment

In general, one third of patients with type I MPGN will have a spontaneous remission, one third will have progressive disease, and one third will have a disease process that will wax and wane but never completely disappear.[585]

The management of type I MPGN is based on the underlying cause of the disease process. Thus, the therapy for MPGN associated with cryoglobulinemia and hepatitis C should be aimed at treating hepatitis C virus infection; whereas, the management of MPGN associated with lupus or with scleroderma should be based on the principles of care of those rheumatological conditions. Most recommendations for the treatment of type I MPGN are limited to studies in children.[641-648] West and colleagues touted the benefits of prednisone therapy provided on a continuous basis for improved renal survival.[643] Whether the benefit of low-dose prednisone therapy is only seen in children, or whether similar effects are achieved in adults has never been subject to a prospective randomized trial. However, low-dose, alternate-day prednisone may have a salutary effect on improving renal function.[646,647]

In addition to glucocorticoids, a host of other forms of immunosuppressive and anti-coagulant treatment has been used in the management of type I MPGN. Studies with dipyridamole, aspirin, and warfarin with and without cyclophosphamide have been tried in both controlled and uncontrolled studies.[417,583,648-653] A retrospective study of patients treated with warfarin, dipyridamole, and cyclophosphamide[648] touted a long-term survival of 82% compared to historical untreated controls in which there were no survivors. The reason for the extremely adverse outcome of the historical untreated controls is not clear, and a controlled trial in Canada using this approach[415] did not demonstrate a benefit.

Initial reports of a positive response in renal survival were associated with treatment with aspirin and dipyridamole.[583] This approach was widely accepted; however, statistical design flaws resulted in re-analysis of the data revealing no difference in the treatment and control groups with respect to long-term outcome.[609] A subsequent study using acetylsalicylic acid with dipyridamole demonstrated a slight decrease in urine protein excretion by 3 years without differences in renal function.[652]

Type I MPGN is significantly ameliorated by the use of cyclosporine in the very rare condition known as Buckley syndrome.[172,173,654] Cyclosporine does seem to have an effect on the long-term outcome of this process.

Unfortunately, there is not a good form of therapy for MPGN type II. This is compounded by the fact that MPGN type II recurs almost invariably in renal transplant patients, especially if crescentic disease is present in the native kidney biopsy.[584,593,604,610,630,655-657] MPGN type I may also recur after transplantation, albeit less frequently.

Glomerulonephritis

The syndrome of glomerulonephritis is characterized by hematuria, red blood cell casts, proteinuria, hypertension, and renal insufficiency. The clinical presentation varies from asymptomatic hematuria or proteinuria (or both) to acute nephritis to rapidly progressive nephritis to chronic nephritis. These varied clinical manifestations are the result of different expressions of inflammatory glomerular injury that ranges from structurally imperceptible abnormalities, to pure mesangial hypercellularity, to endocapillary proliferative glomerulonephritis, to crescentic glomerulonephritis, or to chronic sclerosing glomerulonephritis (Fig. 30–18). These structural categories of glomerulonephritis are not specific diseases, but rather are patterns of glomerular injury that can be caused by many different etiologies and pathogenic mechanisms.[657]

Acute Post-Streptococcal Glomerulonephritis (PSGN)

Epidemiology

Acute PSGN is a disease that affects primarily children with the peak incidence being between ages of 2 and 6 years. Children younger than age 2 years and adults older than age 40 account for only about 15% of patients affects with acute PSGN. Subclinical, microscopic hematuria may be four times more common as overt acute PSGN, as documented in studies of family members of affected patients.[658-660] Only rarely do

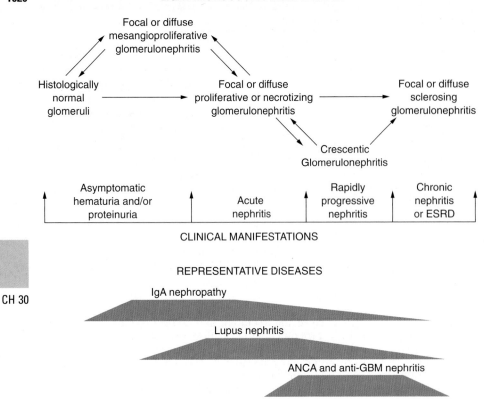

CH 30

CLINICAL MANIFESTATIONS

REPRESENTATIVE DISEASES

IgA nephropathy

Lupus nephritis

ANCA and anti-GBM nephritis

FIGURE 30–18 Diagram depicting the continuum of structural changes that can be caused by glomerular inflammation (top), the usual clinical syndromes that are caused by each expression of glomerular injury (middle), and the portion of the continuum that is most often attained by several specific categories of glomerular disease (bottom). (From Ferrario F, Kourilsky O, Morel-Maroger L: Acute endocapillary glomerulonephritis in adults: A histologic and clinical comparison between patients with and without initial acute renal failure. Clin Nephrol 19:17–23, 1983, with permission.)

PSGN and rheumatic fever occur concomitantly.[661] Males are more likely than females to have overt nephritis.

Acute PSGN may occur as part of an epidemic or sporadic disease. During epidemic infections of streptococci of proven nephrogenicity, the clinical attack rate appears to be about 12%,[662–664] but may be as high as 25%.[665] Indeed, the attack rate may be as high as 38% in certain affected families.[660]

Differences in attack rates among different families are used to argue the existence of host factors affecting susceptibility to overt nephritis.[666] An association was found between HLA-DRW4 and acute PSGN in a study of 18 families involving 67 siblings in Venezuela. More recently, Mori and colleagues reported an increased incidence of HLA-DP5 antigen in 58 Japanese patients when compared to 317 healthy unrelated controls.[667] These authors report a statistically significant increase in frequency of HLA-DPA*02-022 and DPB1*05-01; whereas, HLA-DPA*01 and DPA*0201 were significantly decreased when compared to controls.

The attack rate of acute PSGN after sporadic infections with group A streptococci of potentially nephritogenic types is quite variable,[668,669] again pointing to ill-defined host factors. The minority of streptococcal infections lead to the nephritic syndrome, arguing for the presence of certain nephritogenic "characteristics of the offending agent." Indeed, Rammelkamp and co-workers identified in the 1950s[668,669] certain strains of streptococci within the Lancefield group A in particular, type XII that are capable of leading to an acute glomerulonephritis. Other nephritogenic serotypes include M types 1, 2, 3, 4, 18, 25, 49, 55, 57, 59, and 60. Other potential nephritogenic types include types 31, 52, 56, 59, and 61. There are differences among these serotypes in their propensity to be associated with nephritis depending on the site of infection. Certain strains, such as type 2, 49, 55, 57 and 60, are usually associated with nephritis after a pyoderma,[670,671] whereas M type 49 can lead to nephritis after either a pharyngitis or pyoderma. Besides the group A beta hemolytic streptococci, acute PSGN

has also been described after infection with group C streptococci and possibly group G streptococci.[672,673]

Acute PSGN is on the decline in developed countries, whereas it continues to occur in developing communities.[674] Epidemic PSGN is frequently associated with skin infections as opposed to pharyngitides associated with sporadic PSGN in developed countries. Overt glomerulonephritis is found in about 10% of children at risk, but when one includes subclinical disease as evidenced by microscopic hematuria, about 25% of children at risk are affected.[675,676] In some developing countries, acute PSGN remains the most common form of acute nephritic syndrome among children. The "attack rate" appears to follow a cyclical pattern every ten years or so.[677] Based on 11 published population-based studies, a recent study estimated the median incidence of post-streptococcal glomerulonephritis in children from less developed country studies or those that included substantial minority populations in more developed countries at 24 cases per 100,000 person-years, whereas the incidence in adults was conservatively estimated at 2 cases per 100,000 person-years in less developed countries and 0·3 cases per 100,000 person-years in more developed countries.[678] These authors estimated that over 470,000 cases of acute post-streptococcal glomerulonephritis occur annually, with approximately 5000 deaths (1% of total cases), 97% of which are in less developed countries.

Pathology
Light Microscopy
The pathologic appearance of acute PSGN varies during the course of the disease. The acute histologic change is influx of neutrophils that results in diffuse global hypercellularity (Fig. 30–19).[679–683] Endocapillary proliferation of mesangial cells and endothelial cells also contributes to the hypercellularity. The hypercellularity often is very marked and results in enlarged consolidated glomeruli. The descriptive designa-

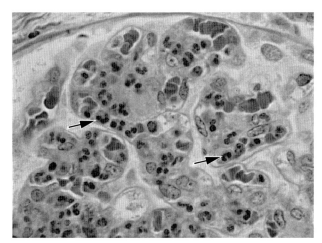

FIGURE 30–19 Light micrograph of a glomerulus with acute poststreptococcal glomerulonephritis demonstrating marked influx of neutrophils (arrows). (Masson trichrome, ×700.)

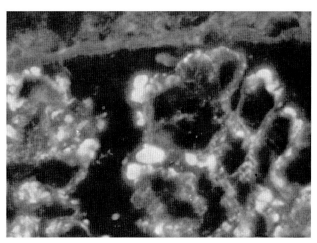

FIGURE 30–20 Immunofluorescence micrograph of a glomerular segment from a patient with acute poststreptococcal glomerulonephritis (PSGN) showing coarsely granular capillary wall staining for C3. Compare this to the finely granular capillary wall staining of membranous glomerulopathy in Figure 30–9. (FITC anti-C3, ×800.)

tion acute diffuse proliferative glomerulonephritis often is used as a pathologic designation for this stage of acute PSGN. A minority of patients has crescent formation that usually affects only a small proportion of glomeruli.[684] Extensive crescent formation is rare.[685,686] Special stains that have differential reactions with immune deposits may demonstrate subepithelial deposits. For example, the subepithelial deposits may stain red (fuchsinophilic) with Masson trichrome stain.

Interstitial edema and interstitial infiltration of predominantly mononuclear leukocytes usually is present and occasionally is pronounced, especially with unusually severe disease with crescents. Focal tubular epithelial cell simplification (flattening) also may accompany severe disease. Arteries and arterioles typically have no acute changes, although there may be preexisting sclerotic changes in older patients.

During the resolving phase of self-limited PSGN, which usually begins within several weeks of onset, the infiltrating neutrophils disappear and endothelial hypercellularity resolves leaving behind only mesangial hypercellularity.[679,687] This mesangioproliferative stage often is present in patients with APSG who have had resolution of nephritis but have persistent isolated proteinuria, and may persist for several months in patients who have complete clinical resolution. There may be focal segmental glomerular scarring as sequelae of particularly injurious inflammation, but this is rarely extensive except in the rare patients with crescentic APGN. Ultimately, the pathologic changes of APGN can resolve completely.[687,688]

Immunofluorescence Microscopy

Immunofluorescence microscopy demonstrates immune glomerular immune complex deposits in PSGN.[680,682,683,689] The pattern and composition of deposits change during the course of PSGN. During the acute diffuse proliferative phase of the disease there is diffuse global coarsely granular capillary wall and mesangial staining that usually is very intense for C3 and of varying degrees for IgG from intense to absent (Fig. 30–20). Staining for IgM and IgA is less frequent and usually less intense. In self-limited disease, biopsy should be performed later in the disease course as it is more likely that the staining will be predominantly or exclusively for C3 with little or no immunoglobulin staining. Because most patients with uncomplicated new onset acute PSGN undergo renal biopsy, most biopsy specimens are obtained later in the course when there is diagnostic uncertainty because of equivocal serologic con-

firmation, or unusually aggressive or persistent clinical features. At this time, the immunofluorescence microscopy staining is usually predominantly for C3. This may reflect termination of nephritogenic immune complex localization in the kidney with masking of residual complexes by complement. The continued presence of intense staining for IgG a month or more into the course of what otherwise looks like pathologically typical PSGN is cause for concern that the process will not be self-limited.

Several patterns of immune staining have been described but are of limited prognostic value.[680,683,690] The garland pattern has numerous large closely apposed granular deposits along the capillary walls. Patients with this pattern usually have nephrotic range proteinuria as a component of their disease. The starry sky pattern has more scattered granular staining, which corresponds somewhat to less severe disease. The mesangial pattern, especially when it is predominantly C3 staining, corresponds to the resolving phase with a mesangioproliferative light microscopic appearance.

Electron Microscopy

The hallmark ultrastructural feature of PSGN is the subepithelial hump-like dense deposits (Figs. 30–21 and 30–22).[682,687–689,691] However, small subendothelial and mesangial dense deposits can usually be identified when carefully observed and theoretically may be more important in the pathogenesis of the disease, especially the neutrophilic influx and endocapillary proliferative response, than the subepithelial humps. The subepithelial humps are covered by effaced epithelial foot processes, which usually contain condensed cytoskeletal filaments (including actin) that form a corona around the immune deposits (see Fig. 30–22). During the acute phase, capillary lumens often contain marginated neutrophils, some of which are in direct contact with glomerular basement membranes (see Fig. 30–22). Lesser numbers of monocytes and macrophages contribute to the leukocyte influx. Mesangial regions are expanded by increased numbers of mesangial cells and leukocytes as well as increased matrix material and varying amounts of electron dense material.

During the resolution phase, usually 6 to 8 weeks into the course, the subepithelial humps disappear, leaving behind only mesangial and sometimes a few scattered subendothelial and intramembranous dense deposits. The subepithelial first become electron lucent and then disappear completely. The humps in peripheral capillary loops disappear before the

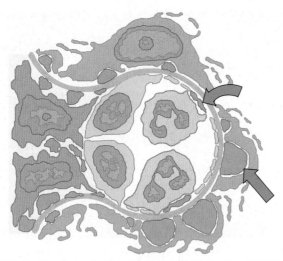

FIGURE 30–21 Diagram of the ultrastructural features of acute PSGN. Note the subepithelial humplike dense deposits (straight arrow), subendothelial deposits (curved arrow), and mesangial deposits. There is endocapillary hypercellularity caused by neutrophil infiltration, and endothelial and mesangial proliferation. (Reproduced with permission of J.C. Jennette.)

CH 30

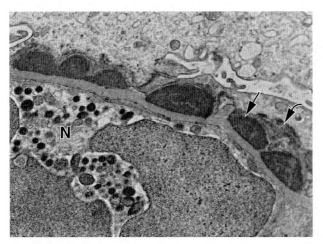

FIGURE 30–22 Electron micrograph of a portion of a glomerular capillary from a patient with acute PSGN showing subepithelial dense deposits (straight arrow), condensation of cytoskeleton in adjacent epithelial cytoplasm (small curved arrow), and a neutrophil (N) marginated against the basement membrane with no intervening endothelial cytoplasm (magnification ×5000).

humps in the subepithelial zone adjacent to the perimesangial basement membrane.

Pathogenesis

Acute post-streptococcal glomerulonephritis is the prototype disease of an acute glomerulonephritis associated with an infectious etiology. The first description of this link dates back to the early 18th century after Scarlet Fever epidemics in Florence and Vienna. Richard Bright first described the association in 1836, reporting that Scarlet Fever was sometimes followed by hematuria and kidney disease.[692] In 1907, Schick described an asymptomatic interval of 12 days to 7 weeks between the onset of streptococcal infection and that of nephritis.[693] In the early 1950s, Rammelkamp and Weaver further refined the association of post-streptococcal glomerulonephritis with specific serotypes of streptococci.[668,694]

Despite the early recognition of an association between streptococcal infection and an acute glomerulonephritis, the pathogenic mechanism of disease remains incompletely

understood. Conceptually, acute post-streptococcal glomerulonephritis (PSGN) could be secondary to either a direct toxic effect on the glomerulus of a streptococcal protein, or the streptococcal product could induce an immune-complex-mediated injury. This could occur by a number of different mechanisms: (1) by introducing an antigen to the glomerulus (planted antigen), (2) by the deposition of circulating immune complexes, (3) by altering a normal renal antigen, causing it to become a self antigen, (4) by inducing an autoimmune response to a self antigen by way of antigenic mimicry. It is conceivable that more than one streptococcal antigen may be involved in the pathogenesis of acute PSGN, and more than one pathogenic mechanism may be at play simultaneously.

Several streptococcal proteins have been implicated in the pathogenesis of acute PSGN.[695] M protein molecules protruding from the surface of group A streptococci contain epitopes which cross-react with glomerular antigens. Shared sequences of M protein types V, VI, and XIX have been shown to elicit antibodies that react with several myocardial and skeletal muscle proteins.[696] Conversely, monoclonal antibodies raised against human renal cortex have been shown to cross-react with types VI and XII M proteins, bringing evidence that certain M proteins may share antigenic determinants between all glomeruli.[697] The renal glomerular cross-reactivity of the amino terminal region of type I M protein was further localized to a tetra peptide sequence at position 23–26.[698] Antibodies raised against amino terminal of type I M protein was shown to cross-react with the cytoskeletal protein of glomerular mesangial cells, namely, the filament protein vimentin.[696]

Currently, the spectrum of infectious agents associated with a post-infectious glomerulonephritis or a peri-infectious glomerulonephritis includes many more bacterial pathogens than streptococci. These include staphylococci, gram negative rods, and intracellular bacteria.[699] Likewise, the population at risk for peri-infectious glomerulonephritis has changed to include alcoholics, intravenous drug users, and patients with ventricular atrial shunts. However, post-streptococcal glomerulonephritis remains the infectious glomerulonephritis, which is the most extensively studied and documented.

Clinical Features and Natural History

Classically, the syndrome of acute PSGN presents abruptly with hematuria, proteinuria, hypertension, and azotemia. This syndrome can present with an entire spectrum of severity from asymptomatic to oliguric acute renal failure.[700] A latent period is present from the onset of pharyngitis to that of nephritis. In post-pharyngitic cases, the latent period averages 10 days after pharyngitis with a range from 7 to 21 days. The latent period may be longer after a skin infection (from 14 to 21 days), although this period is harder to define after impetigo.[701] The latency period can exceed 3 weeks.[702] Conversely, short latency periods of less than one week are suggestive of a "synpharyngitic syndrome" corresponding typically to exacerbation of an underlying IgA nephropathy.

The hematuria is microscopic in more than two-thirds of cases, but may be macroscopic on occasions. Patients commonly report gross hematuria and transient oliguria. Anuria, however, is infrequent and, if persistent, may indicate the development of crescentic glomerulonephritis.

Mild to moderate hypertension occurs in more than 75% of patients that is most evident at the onset of nephritis and typically subsides promptly after diuresis.[661] Antihypertensive treatment is necessary in only about one half of patients. Signs and symptoms of congestive heart failure may occur and, indeed, dominate the clinical picture. These include jugular venous distention, the presence of an S3 gallop, dyspnea, and signs of pulmonary congestion.[702–705] Frank heart failure may be a complication in as many of 40% of elderly patients with PSGN.

Edema may be the presenting symptom in two thirds of patients, and is present in as many as 90% of patients.[658] The presence of edema is based on primary renal sodium and fluid retention. The edema typically presents in the face and upper extremities. Ascites and anasarca may occur in children.

Encephalopathy presenting as confusion, headache, somnolence, or even convulsion, is not frequent, and may affect children more frequently than adults. This encephalopathy is not always attributable to severe hypertension, but may be the result of CNS vasculitis instead.[702,704–706]

The clinical manifestations of acute PSGN typically resolve in 1 to 2 weeks as the edema and hypertension disappear after diuresis, the patient remains typically asymptomatic. Both the hematuria and proteinuria may persist for several months, but are usually resolved within a year. However, proteinuria may persist in those patients who initially presented with nephrotic syndrome.[658] The long-term persistence of proteinuria and, especially albuminuria, may be an indication of persistence of proliferative glomerulonephritis.[664]

Differential diagnosis of acute PSGN includes (1) IgA nephropathy[707] and Henoch-Schönlein purpura, (especially when the acute nephritic syndrome is associated with gross or rusty hematuria), (2) MPGN, or (3) acute crescentic glomerulonephritis (RPGN immune complex mediated, anti-GBM-mediated, or pauci-immune). The occurrence of an acute nephritis in the setting of persistent fever should raise the suspicion of a peri-infectious GN especially with a persistence of an infection such as an occult abscess or infective endocarditis.

Although rheumatic fever and post-streptococcal glomerulonephritis rarely occur concomitantly, their concurrence has recently been described.[708]

Laboratory Findings

Hematuria, microscopic or gross, is nearly always present in acute PSGN. There are, however, rare cases of documented acute PSGN with no associated hematuria.[660,709] Microscopic examination of urine typically reveals the presence of dysmorphic red blood cells[710] or red blood cell casts. Other findings on microscopy are those of leukocytes, renal tubule epithelial cells, as well as hyaline and granular casts.[661] When the hematuria is macroscopic, the urine typically has a rusty or tea-color.

Proteinuria is nearly always present but typically in the sub-nephrotic range. In half of patients, it may be less than 500 mg per day.[711,712] Nephrotic-range proteinuria may occur in as many as 20% of patients and is more frequent in the adults than in children.[658] The proteinuria may often contain large amounts of fibrin degradation products, and fibrinopeptides.[709,713]

A pronounced decline in urine glomerular filtration rate (GFR) is common in the elderly population with acute PSGN affecting nearly 60% of patients 55 years of age and older.[704] This profound decrease in GFR is uncommon in children to middle-aged adults. Indeed, because of the accompanying fluid retention and increase in circulatory volumes, a mild decrease in GFR may not be accompanied by an increase in serum creatinine concentration above laboratory limits of normal. Renal plasma flow, tubular reabsorptive capacity, and concentrating ability are typically not affected. On the other hand, urinary sodium excretion and calcium excretion are greatly reduced.[714]

A transient hyporeninemic hypoaldosteronism may lead to mild to moderate hyperkalemia. This may be exacerbated by a concomitant decrease in GFR and a reduced distal delivery of solute. This type IV renal tubular acidosis may resolve with the resolution of nephritis in the event of diuresis, but may be persistent beyond that point in some patients.[715] The suppressed plasma renin activity may be a consequence of the volume expansion present in those patients.[716]

Throat or skin cultures frequently reveal group A streptococci.[661,717] The sensitivity and specificity of these tests are likely affected by the methodology of obtaining a throat culture and the test used.[718] Such cultures may be less satisfactory than serologic studies to evaluate the presence of recent streptococcal infection in patients suspected of having PSGN.[665] The antibodies most commonly studied for the detection of a recent streptococcal infection are anti-streptolysin-O (ASO), anti-streptokinase, anti-hyaluronidase, anti-deoxyribonuclease-B, and anti-nicotinamide adenine dinucleotidase.[719] Of these, the most commonly used test is the ASO. An elevated ASO titer above 200 units may be found in 90% of patients with pharyngeal infection.[661] In the diagnosis of an acute post-streptococcal glomerulonephritis however, a rise in titer is more specific than the absolute level of a titer. The latter is likely affected by the geographic and socioeconomic prevalence of pharyngeal infections with group A streptococci. Increased ASO titers may be present in about two-thirds of patients with upper respiratory tract infection, but in only about one-third of patients following streptococcal impetigo.[658] Serial ASO titer measurements with a two-fold or greater rise in titer are highly indicative of a recent infection.[658,661]

The streptozyme test combines several anti-streptococcal antibody assays and may be a useful screening test.[720] Because certain strains of type XII group A streptococci do not produce streptolysin S or O and in patients in whom impetigo-associated PSGN is suspected, testing for anti-deoxyribonuclease B and anti-hyaluronidase titers is a useful procedure.[670] Antibodies to other streptococcal cell wall glycoproteins may also increase, including those for endostreptosin.[661,721–724] On occasion, autoantibodies to collagen and laminin may be detected.[661,725] Positive throat cultures or skin cultures may be present in a few as one fourth of patients.

The serial estimation of complement components is important in the diagnosis of PSGN. Early in the acute phase, the levels of hemolytic complement activity (CH-50 and C3) are reduced. These levels return to normal usually within 8 weeks.[661,702,726–731] The reduction in serum C3 levels is especially marked in patients with C3 nephritic factor, which is capable of cleaving native C3.[632–634] The finding of low properdin and C3 levels, and the concomitant normal to modestly reduced levels of C1q, C2, and C4[726,727,732] all point to the importance of the activation of the alternate pathway of the complement activation cascade.[726] There is some evidence as well for activation via the classic pathway.[733] Other complement level abnormalities include a mild depression of C5 levels, whereas C6 and C7 are most often normal.[632,661,732] Plasma level of soluble terminal complement components (C5b-9) rises acutely and then falls to normal.[727] As complement levels typically return to normal within eight weeks, the presence of persistent depression of C3 levels may be indicative of another diagnosis, such as MPGN, endocarditis, occult sepsis, SLE, atheromatous emboli, or congenital chronic state of complement deficiency.[726]

Circulating cryoglobulins,[734,735] as well as circulating immune complexes[736–739] may be detected in some patients with PSGN. The pathophysiologic importance of these circulating immune complexes as to the development of acute nephritis is unclear.[738–740]

Abnormalities in blood coagulation systems may be detected in acute PSGN, thus thrombocytopenia may be seen.[741] Elevated levels of fibrinogen, factor VIII, plasmin activity, and circulating high molecular weight fibrinogen complexes may be seen and correlate with disease activity, and unfavorable prognosis.[742–746]

Although complement studies suggest that the alternative pathways are primarily involved in acute PSGN, there is some evidence also for activation via the classic pathway.[733]

Treatment

Treatment of acute post-streptococcal glomerulonephritis is largely that of supportive care. Children almost invariably recover from the initial episode.[489,665,747] Of concern to clinicians are those patients who present with acute renal failure. An initial episode of acute renal failure is not necessarily associated with a bad prognosis.[700] In a study of 20 adult patients with diffuse proliferative glomerulonephritis, 11 had acute renal failure and 9 had normal or mild renal insufficiency. There were no differences in the clinical, immunological, or histological features between the groups. After 18 months of follow-up, outcome was similar in the two groups. Thus, there is little evidence to suggest the need for any form of immunosuppressive therapy. Because of the profound salt and water retention observed in these patients, and, in some, pulmonary congestion, it is important to use loop diuretics such as furosemide to avoid volume expansion and hypertension. When volume expansion does occur, antihypertensive agents are frequently useful to ameliorate the hypertension. Interestingly, plasma renin levels are reduced; yet, captopril has been shown to lower blood pressure and improve glomerular filtration rate in patients with post-streptococcal glomerulonephritis.[748]

Some patients with substantial volume expansion and marked pulmonary congestion do not respond to diuretics. In those individuals, dialytic support is appropriate, either hemodialysis or continuous venovenous hemofiltration in adults or peritoneal dialysis in children. Some patients develop substantial hyperkalemia. In those patients, exchange resins or dialysis may be useful. Importantly, so-called potassium sparing agents, including triamterene, spironolactone, and amiloride, should not be used in this disease state. Usually, patients undergo a spontaneous diuresis within 7 to 10 days after the onset of their illness and no longer require supportive care.[700,749] There is no evidence to date that early treatment of streptococcal disease, either pharyngitic or cellulitic, will alter the risk of post-streptococcal glomerulonephritis. It has long been speculated whether penicillin can control the spread of outbreaks of epidemic poststreptococcal glomerulonephritis. In studies from aboriginal communities in Australia, the use of benzathine penicillin prevented new cases of poststreptococcal glomerulonephritis, especially in children with skin sores and household contacts with affected cases.[750]

The long-term prognosis of patients with post-streptococcal glomerulonephritis is not as benign as previously considered. Widespread crescentic glomerulonephritis results in an increased number of obsolescent glomeruli associated with tubulointerstitial disease that results in progressive reduction of the renal mass over time.[751] A proportion of patients with streptococcal glomerulonephritis develop hypertension, proteinuria and renal insufficiency from 10 to 40 years after the illness.[751–753] Nonetheless, it is most common that the long-term disease process is marked only by mild hypertension.

In some patients, there is evidence to suggest that the original diagnosis of post-streptococcal glomerulonephritis may have been in error. This is especially true for those individuals in whom a renal biopsy was never performed. For instance, a patient who has an upper respiratory tract infection and then develops a glomerulonephritis may be considered to have post-streptococcal glomerulonephritis, when in fact they have another proliferative form of glomerulonephritis. In these patients, lack of resolution of their renal disease should prompt a renal biopsy to elucidate the underlying cause of the glomerular injury.

IgA Nephropathy

Epidemiology

IgA nephropathy remains one of, if not the most common glomerular lesion of all of the forms of glomerulonephritis. Initially described in the late 1960s by Berger and Hinglais,[754,755] patients were described based on the finding of predominant IgA deposition (and, to a lesser extent other immunoglobulins) in the mesangium with a mesangial proliferation, and with clinical features that span the spectrum from asymptomatic hematuria to rapidly progressive glomerulonephritis. The disease process was initially considered a benign form of hematuria. However, over the past decades, it has become clear that up to 40% of patients may progress to end-stage kidney disease. Moreover, it has become recognized that, in addition to an idiopathic form of disease, IgA nephropathy is also associated with a variety of disease processes (Table 30–13).

IgA nephropathy occurs in individuals of all ages, but it is still most common in the second and third decade of life, and it is much more common in males than females (Table 30–14). IgA nephropathy is uncommon in children under 10 years of age. In fact, 80% of patients are between the ages of 16 and 35 at the time of renal biopsy.[756–761] The male-to-female ratio has been described anywhere from 2 : 1 to 6 : 1.[756–761]

The distribution of IgA nephropathy varies in different geographic regions throughout the world.[762] It is the most common form of primary glomerular disease in Asia, accounting for up to 30% to 40% of all biopsies, 20% in Europe, and 10% of all biopsies performed for glomerular disease in North America.[762] The reason for this wide variance in incidence is partly attributable to indications for renal biopsy in Asia compared to those in North America. In Asia, urinalyses are performed routinely on children of school age, and renal biopsies of this population with asymptomatic hematuria may lead to an increased number of patients who have the diagnosis of IgA nephropathy. Genetic issues may also be important in the geographic difference. IgA nephropathy is

TABLE 30–13	IgA Nephropathy: The Syndrome[795,810,822,906,907,976,1324–1350]

Primary IgA nephropathy

Secondary IgA nephropathy
  Henoch-Schönlein purpura
  HIV infection
  Toxoplasmosis
  Seronegative spondyloarthropathy
  Celiac disease
  Dermatitis herpetiformis
  Crohn disease
  Liver disease
  Alcoholic cirrhosis
  Ankylosing spondylitis
  Reiter syndrome
  Neoplasia
    Mycosis fungoides
    Lung CA
    Mucin-secreting CA
  Cyclic neutropenia
  Immunothrombocytopenia
  Gluten sensitive enteropathy
  Scleritis
  Sicca syndrome
  Mastitis
  Pulmonary hemosiderosis
  Berger's
  Leprosy

Familial IgA nephropathy

TABLE 30-14	Diseases that Cause Glomerulonephritis*		
Glomerular Lesion	N	Male:Female Ratio	White:Black Ratio
IgA nephropathy	693	2.0:1.0	14.0:1.0
MPGN I	248	1.2:1.0	3.3:1.0
Anti-GBM	82	1.1:1.0	7.9:1.0
ANCA-GN	257	1.0:1.0	6.7:1.0
Fibrillary glomerulonephritis	76	1.0:1.2	14.3:1.0

*Information in this table is from 9605 native kidney biopsies from the UNC Nephropathology Laboratory. This laboratory evaluates kidney biopsies from a base population of approximately 10 million throughout the southeastern United States and centered in North Carolina. The expected white to black ratio in this renal biopsy population is approximately 2:1.

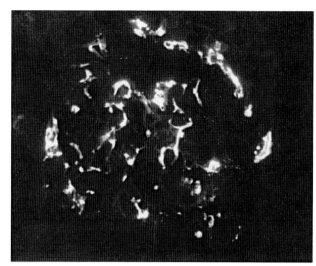

FIGURE 30-23 Immunofluorescence micrograph of a glomerulus with IgA nephropathy showing intense mesangial staining for IgA. (FITC anti-IgA, ×300.)

rare in African Americans (see Table 30-14)[763,764] and quite common in Native Americans of the Zuni and Navajo tribes.[765] The prevalence of IgA in the general population has been estimated to be between 25 and 50 cases per 100,000,[762,766] although notably, almost 5% of all biopsied patients have at least some IgA deposits in their glomeruli.[767] Population studies in Germany and in France calculated an incidence of 2 cases per 10,000,[768-771] although autopsy studies performed in Singapore[772] suggested that 2% to 4.8% of the population had IgA deposition in their glomeruli.

Genetics

IgA nephropathy is a histological diagnosis that is unlikely to be due to a single genetic locus. In fact, the genetics of IgA nephropathy likely results from interaction of multiple susceptibility and progression genes in combination with environmental factors.[773] A number of studies suggest that there are genes that render an individual susceptible to IgA nephropathy and genes that portend a more rapid progression of IgA nephropathy. Polymorphism occurs in a number of genes, including the angiotensin converting enzyme, angiotensinogen, angiotensin II receptor, major histocompatibility loci, T cell receptor, interleukin-1 and -6, and interleukin receptor antagonist, transforming growth factor, mannose binding lectin, uteroglobin, nitric oxide synthesis, and tumor necrosis factor.[774-780] There have been a number of studies examining in the angiotensin converting enzyme (ACE) gene in IgA nephropathy with or without progressive disease.[781-783] Data obtained[784] in a group of 168 white patients with IgA nephropathy suggest that the angiotensinogen gene and the insertion-deletion polymorphism of the angiotensin converting enzyme were important markers for predicting progression to chronic renal failure.[784] Studies in this arena have been relative small and, as a consequence, definitive statements about these genes in IgA nephropathy are difficult to make.

A familial form of IgA nephropathy has also been described.[785-789] IgA has been described in siblings and in twins. In some kindred, it may be associated with deafness. Familial IgA nephropathy must be differentiated from Alport syndrome. In Italy, the familial IgA nephropathy was linked in 60% of case to 6q22-23 locus and was associated with poor prognosis. The 20-year renal survival in these families was only 41% versus the 20-year renal survival in sporadic cases of 94%.[790] Ghavari[791] studied 30 kindred with IgA nephropathy and found a strong linkage on chromosome 6q22-23 with a load score of 5.6. This was not linked to a major histocompatibility locus, uteroglobin, the IgA Fc receptor, or galactosyl transferase. Uteroglobin is an antiinflammatory protein that binds to IgA fibronectin complexes, thereby reducing their inflammatory potential. Interestingly, uteroglobin knockout mice develop IgA nephropathy. Some Japanese patients with IgA nephropathy are homozygous for mutations of uteroglobin and have low uteroglobin plasma levels.[777] Italian patients with IgA nephropathy have an increased amount of uteroglobin bound to IgA fibronectin complexes.[792]

The prevailing hypothesis pertaining to the pathogenesis of IgA nephropathy pertains to defects in protein glycosylation, particularly in B cells secreting IgA1. It has been difficult, however, to demonstrate consistent defects in the β-1,3-galactosyltransferase enzyme that places galactose on O-linked carbohydrate side chains of the IgA1 molecule. Recently, the gene responsible for protein glycosylation of the Tn antigen on red blood cells in patients with the autoimmune disease known as Tn syndrome has been discovered.[793] This gene, known as Cosmc, is located on the X chromosome and is a molecular chaperone for an enzyme T-synthase that glycosylates the Tn antigen on defective red blood cells in the Tn syndrome. This defect was similarly found in B cells from IgA nephropathy.[794] The defect in IgA nephropathy may be due to an improper folding of the β-1,3-galactosyltransferase enzyme, reducing its activity in B cells in patients with IgA nephropathy.

Pathology
Immunofluorescence Microscopy

IgA nephropathy can only be definitively diagnosed by the immunohistologic demonstration of glomerular immune deposits that stain dominantly or co-dominantly for IgA compared to staining for IgG and IgM (Fig. 30-23).[795-798] The staining is usually exclusively or predominantly mesangial, although a minority of specimens, especially from patients with severe disease, will have substantial capillary wall staining. By definition, 100% of IgA nephropathy specimens stain for IgA. On a scale of 0 to 4+, the mean intensity of IgA staining is approximately 3+.[797] IgM staining is observed in 84% of specimens with a mean intensity (when present) of only approximately 1+. IgG staining is observed in 62% of specimens, also with a mean intensity (when present) of approximately 1+. Early studies of IgA nephropathy described more frequent and more intense IgG staining than is seen today, but this probably was caused by less specific antibodies that cross reacted between IgA and IgG. Almost all IgA nephropathy specimens have substantial staining for C3 but staining for C1q is rare and weak when present. If there is intense staining in a specimen that has substantial IgA and IgG, the possibility of lupus nephritis rather than IgA nephropathy should be considered.[797] An additional relatively distinctive feature of IgA nephropathy is that, unlike any other glomerular immune complex disease, the immune deposits usually have more intense staining for lambda light chains than kappa light chains.[795,797]

Electron Microscopy

The ubiquitous ultrastructural finding is mesangial electron dense deposits that correspond to the immune deposits seen by immunohistology (Figs. 30–24 and 30–25).[796] The mesangial deposits often are immediately beneath the perimesangial basement membrane. They are accompanied by varying degrees of mesangial matrix expansion and hypercellularity. Most specimens do not have capillary wall deposits, but a minority, especially from patients with more severe disease, will have scattered subendothelial dense deposits or subepithelial dense deposits or both. The extent of endocapillary

proliferation and leukocyte infiltration parallel the pattern of injury observed by light microscopy. Epithelial foot process effacement is observed in those patients with substantial proteinuria.

Light Microscopy

IgA nephropathy can cause any of the light microscopic phenotypes of proliferative glomerulonephritis (Fig. 30–26) or may cause no discernible histologic changes.[796–803] As depicted in Figure 30–18, this spectrum of glomerular inflammatory responses is shared by a variety of glomerulonephritides that have different etiologies but induce similar or identical light microscopic alterations in glomeruli. Figure 30–18 also depicts the most frequent clinical manifestations of the different histologic phenotypes of glomerulonephritis, all of which can be caused by IgA nephropathy. At the time of biopsy, IgA nephropathy usually manifests as a

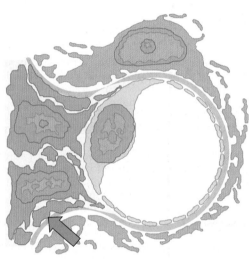

FIGURE 30–24 Diagram depicting the ultrastructural features of IgA nephropathy. Note the mesangial dense deposits (straight arrow) and mesangial hypercellularity. (Reproduced with permission of J.C. Jennette.)

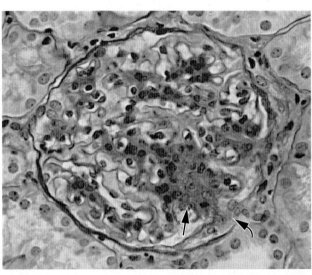

FIGURE 30–26 Light micrograph of a glomerulus with IgA nephropathy showing segmental mesangial matrix expansion and hypercellularity (straight arrow), and an adhesion to the Bowman capsule (curved arrow). (PAS, ×300.)

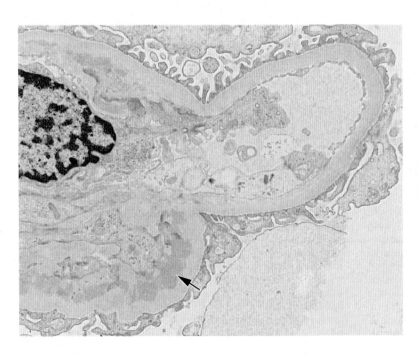

FIGURE 30–25 Electron micrograph of a capillary and adjacent mesangium from a patient with IgA nephropathy showing mesangial dense deposits immediately beneath the paramesangial basement membrane (magnification ×7000).

focal or diffuse, mesangioproliferative or proliferative glomerulonephritis, although a few patients will have no lesion by light microscopy, a few patients will have aggressive disease with crescents, and occasional patients will already have chronic sclerosing disease. Different criteria for renal biopsy result in different frequencies of the various phenotypes of IgA nephropathy among different series of patients. If nephrologists who are contributing patients to series have liberal criteria, for example performing biopsies on patients with hematuria, normal renal function and little or no proteinuria, the phenotypes of IgA nephropathy will be skewed to the left of the diagram in Figure 30–18. Alternatively, if the contributing nephrologists reserve biopsy only for patients with some degree of renal insufficiency or substantial proteinuria, the IgA nephropathy phenotypes will be skewed to the right. Of 668 consecutive native kidney IgA nephropathy specimens diagnosed in the UNC Nephropathology Laboratory, 4% had no lesion by light microscopy, 13% had exclusively mesangioproliferative glomerulonephritis, 37% had focal proliferative glomerulonephritis (25% of these had <50% crescents), 28% had diffuse proliferative glomerulonephritis (45% of these had <50% crescents), 4% had crescentic glomerulonephritis (50% or more crescents), 6% had focal sclerosing glomerulonephritis without residual proliferative activity, 6% had diffuse chronic sclerosing glomerulonephritis, and 2% had lesions that did not fall within this categorization.

The mildest light microscopic expression of IgA nephropathy, other than no discernible lesion, is focal or diffuse mesangial hypercellularity without more complex endocapillary hypercellularity, such as endothelial proliferation or influx of leukocytes. This is analogous to class II lupus nephritis. More severe inflammatory injury causes focal (involving less than 50% of glomeruli) or diffuse proliferative glomerulonephritis as the pathologic expression of IgA nephropathy, which is pathologically analogous to class III and class IV lupus nephritis. The lesions are characterized by not only mesangial hypercellularity but also some degree of endothelial proliferation or leukocyte infiltration that distorts or obliterates some capillary lumens. Extensive necrosis is rare in IgA nephropathy, although slight focal segmental necrosis with karyorrhexis often occurs in severely inflamed glomeruli. With time, destructive glomerular inflammatory lesions progress to sclerotic lesions that may form adhesions to Bowman capsule. Occasional patients with IgA nephropathy will have focal glomerular sclerosis by light microscopy that is indistinguishable from focal segmental glomerulosclerosis until the immunofluorescence microscopy is taken into consideration. Because of the episodic nature of IgA nephropathy, many patients will have combinations of focal sclerotic lesions and focal active proliferative lesions. Patients with the most severe IgA nephropathy have crescent formation because of extensive disruption of capillaries.[803] Advanced chronic disease is characterized by extensive glomerular sclerosis associated with marked tubular atrophy, interstitial fibrosis, and interstitial infiltration by mononuclear leukocytes.

Pathogenesis

Thirty years after the first description of IgA nephropathy, the pathogenesis of this disease is becoming clearer.[661,804] The characteristic pathologic finding by immunofluorescence microscopy of granular deposits of IgA and C3 in the glomerular mesangium, and in the case of Henoch-Schönlein purpura, in dermal capillaries suggests that this disease is the result of the deposition of circulating immune complexes leading to the activation of the complement cascade via the alternate pathway. The deposited IgA is predominantly polymeric IgA-1.[805–808] The fact that polymeric IgA-1 is usually derived mainly from the mucosal immune system, and the

association of some cases of IgA nephropathy with syndromes that affect the respiratory tract or gastrointestinal tract, has led to the suggestion that IgA nephropathy is a disease of the mucosal immune system.[809] This concept was supported by the finding in some patients with IgA nephropathy of Ig antibodies to dietary antigens or various infectious agents, both viral and bacterial.[810–823] This concept is also supported by the clinical observations that in some patients with IgA nephropathy, the hematuria increases acutely at the time of upper respiratory tract or gastrointestinal infections. However, it has now been determined that the increased polymeric IgA-1 antibody synthesis is reduced from the mucosa but is increased after systemic immunization.[806,824,825] In addition, increase in IgA secreting B cells was documented both from the peripheral blood of patients[826] and in the bone marrow.[827] It is unlikely that the pathogenesis of IgA nephropathy is related to a quantitative increase in serum levels of polymeric IgA-1, as those are only modestly increased,[806,828] and the occurrence of IgA nephropathy in patients with IgA myeloma or AIDS is decreased despite very high levels of circulating IgA in these diseases.[828] In addition, the inability to identify a consistent antigen associated with IgA deposition in IgAN argues against the concept that this disease is primarily due to the deposition of circulating immune complexes. Alternatively, the deposition of IgA in IgAN may occur by mechanisms other than classical antigen antibody interactions.[806]

It has been suggested that rather than a quantitative abnormality in IgA antibodies in this disease, the anomaly may be in the IgA molecule itself, namely in its glycosylation.[829] In humans, the heavy chain of IgA-1, but not IgA-2, contains a hinge region which includes five serine residues. To these serine residues, are O-linked mono- or oligosaccharides consisting of N-acetylgalactosamine (GalNac). This GalNac is usually substituted with a terminal galactose.[830] It has been demonstrated by lectin-binding studies and by carbohydrate composition that the IgA-1 in patients with IgA nephropathy contains less terminal galactose than that of healthy controls.[806,831] As IgA-1 is normally cleared from the circulation by the liver via the asialoglycoprotein receptor (ASGPR),[832–834] it is thought that the defective galactosylation of the hinge region in IgA-1 may lead to decreased clearance of IgA-1 molecule in patients with IgA nephropathy.[835,836] This altered galactosylation also leads to an increased binding of polymeric IgA-1 in the kidney.[829,836,837] This defect in IgA-1 glycosylation is thought to be synthetic rather than degradative.[838] It has now been demonstrated that there is a reduced activity of the beta-1,3 galactosyl transferase (beta-1, 3GT), (the specific enzyme responsible for galactosylation of olein sugars), in B cells of patients with IgA nephropathy. However, the activity of that enzyme in other cells is maintained intact compared to normal controls.[806,839]

The pathogenesis of IgA nephropathy is most likely a consequence of defective mucosal immunity.[840] As a consequence of this abnormality, there is exposure to any number of environmental antigens that may stimulate IgA-1 B cells. Defective beta-1,3 galactosyltransferase in these B cells results in exaggerated synthesis of galactose deficient IgA-1 molecules in the circulation.[831,839,841] Autoantibody response to galactose deficient IgA-1 molecule results in circulating immune complexes that are poorly removed by the reticuloendothelial system.[842] Galactose-deficient IgA-1 molecules also deposit in the mesangium where they induce a variety of phlogistic mediators including cytokines, chemokines, and growth factors.[843–845] A mesangial receptor for IgA immune complexes has now been identified.[846] In addition, IgA1-containing immune complexes alter the proliferation of mesangial cells as well.[847]

The existence, nature, and role of other autoantibodies in IgA nephropathy is also a hypothesis under investigation. A number of autoantibodies to various putative autoantigens have been described in IgA nephropathy and have recently been reviewed.[848] Such autoantigens include a mesangial cell membrane antigen,[849] endothelial cells (human umbilical vein endothelial cells),[811,848] single-stranded DNA,[811] cardiolipin,[811,850] and antibodies to galactose deficient IgA-1 models. Most of these autoantibodies were found in a subset of patients rarely exceeding 3% of patients with IgA nephropathy and may sometimes be the result of high circulating levels of IgA in these patients.[850] The presence of IgG antineutrophil cytoplasmic autoantibodies has been described to occur in a minority of patients with IgA nephropathy.[851] In addition, IgA ANCA have been rarely associated with a systemic vasculitis of the Henoch-Schönlein purpura type.[852–854] In the setting of IgA ANCA, the autoantigen seems to be different from the major ANCA autoantigens, namely myeloperoxidase (MPO) and proteinase 3 (PR3). Circulating IgA-fibronectin complexes have also been described in the circulation of patients with IgA nephropathy and HIV infection.[855] The fibronectin in these complexes may then mediate binding to collagen. However, these complexes may not be true immune complexes and once again may be directly related to increased IgA levels in patients with IgA nephropathy.[856] Lastly, IgA rheumatoid factor has been described in about 50% of patients with IgA nephropathy[857,858] and may have a functional role in the impaired solubilization of antigen antibody complexes.[859]

An alternative hypothesis as to the increased levels of serum IgA in patients with IgAN is that of increased production of IgA antibodies rather than a decrease in the hepatic clearance due to abnormal glycosylation. Previous studies have suggested increases in circulating IgA-bearing cells in peripheral blood[860] as well as an increase in the *in vitro* production of IgA by peripheral blood lymphocytes.[861–863] More recent data suggests that polymorphisms in the regulatory region of the I alpha-1 gene may account for the hypersynthesis of IgA in patients with IgA nephropathy.[864,865]

Regardless of the mechanism leading to the increased deposition of IgA or IgA-containing immune complexes in the glomeruli, the mechanisms responsible for the glomerular injury remains poorly understood, especially when one keeps in mind the poor phlogistic nature of IgA and its inability to activate complement. Despite the demonstration of a specific IgA receptor on mesangial cells[866] and in the glomerulus of patients with IgA nephropathy,[867] studies of the expression of Fc-alpha R on peripheral blood mononuclear cells and granulocytes led to conflicting results.[867,868] IgAN may be linked to the expression of an IgAN-specific variant of Fc alpha R receptor on monocytes.[869] The role, if any, of Fc alpha R in the pathogenesis of IgA nephropathy remains to be elucidated. Alternatively, IgA-IgG immune aggregates have been hypothesized to activate C3 by the IgG contained in those aggregates.[870]

Clinical Features and Natural History

Approximately 40% to 50% of patients present with macroscopic hematuria at the time of their initial presentation. The episodes tend to occur with a close temporal relationship to upper respiratory infection, including tonsillitis or pharyngitis. This synchronous association of pharyngitis and macroscopic hematuria has been give the name "synpharyngitic" nephritis. Much less commonly, episodes of macroscopic hematuria may follow infections that involve the urinary tract or gastroenteritis. Macroscopic hematuria may be entirely asymptomatic, but more often is associated with dysuria that may prompt the treating physician to consider bacterial cystitis. Systemic symptoms are frequently found, including nonspecific symptoms such as malaise, fatigue, muscle aches and pains, and fever. Some patients present with abdominal or flank pain.[871,872] In a minority of patients (<5%), malignant hypertension may be an associated presenting feature.[873] In

the most severe cases (less than 10%), acute glomerulonephritis results in acute renal insufficiency and failure.[874,875] Recovery typically occurs with resolution of symptoms, even in those patients who have been temporarily dialysis dependent.[875]

Macroscopic hematuria due to IgA nephropathy occurs more often in children than young adults. When it occurs in older individuals, it should raise the possibility of the more common causes of urinary tract bleeding, such as stones or malignancy.

The second most common presentation is that of microscopic hematuria, occurring in 30% to 40% of patients. Patients with IgA nephropathy present for evaluation of asymptomatic hematuria with or without the presence of proteinuria. In addition to glomerulonephritis, these patients may commonly have hypertension. In fact, in white patients with hypertension and hematuria, IgA nephropathy is the most common form of hematuria.[876] Intermittent macroscopic hematuria occurs in 25% of these patients. Microscopic hematuria and proteinuria persist between episodes of macroscopic hematuria.

Approximately one third of patients with IgA nephropathy present with macroscopic hematuria, one third present with microscopic hematuria (with or without proteinuria) and the final one third of patients have a variety of presentations, including the nephrotic syndrome or chronic glomerular disease.

Patients presenting with the nephrotic syndrome may have a widespread proliferative glomerulonephritis, or coexisting of IgA nephropathy and minimal change glomerulopathy.[877] Finally, some patients with IgA nephropathy have reached end-stage renal disease at the time of their first presentation. These individuals typically have had asymptomatic microscopic hematuria and proteinuria that has remained undetected.[874]

In addition to idiopathic IgA nephropathy, IgA nephropathy may be the glomerular expression of a systemic disease (see Table 30–13). For example, patients with Henoch-Schönlein purpura have abdominal pain, arthritis, a vasculitic rash, and a glomerulonephritis that is indistinguishable from primary IgA nephropathy. This condition is discussed more fully in the next chapter.

Although IgA nephropathy was thought to carry a relatively benign prognosis, it is estimated that 1% to 2% of all patients with IgA nephropathy will develop end-stage renal failure each year from the time of diagnosis. In a study of 1900 patients derived from 11 separate series, the long-term renal survival was estimated to be 78% to 87% within a decade of the presentation.[878] Similarly, European studies have suggested that renal insufficiency may occur in 20% to 30% of patients within two decades of the original presentation.[760] In a study from Hong Kong, patients with mild IgA nephropathy were followed prospectively. Significant proteinuria or renal insufficiency was found in a number of patients, suggesting that, even in patients presenting with milder forms of disease, there is a significant risk of progression.

Nonetheless, there are patients in whom there is no tendency toward progressive disease, whereas other patients have a fulminate course resulting in a rapid progression to end-stage renal disease.[879] Several studies have assessed features that predict a poor prognosis. Sustained hypertension, persistent proteinuria (especially proteinuria over 1 gram), impaired renal function, and the nephrotic syndrome, constitute poor prognostic markers.[798,880–882] Male gender and an older age at the onset of disease may also connote a poor prognosis.[881,883–887] Controversy persists with respect to the issue of recurring bouts of macroscopic hematuria.[888] It is possible that macroscopic hematuria is an overt manifestation of disease and, therefore, identifies patients earlier in the course of their disease. Alternatively, macroscopic hematuria may represent an episodic process that results in self-limited inflammation, in contrast to persistent hematuria that represents ongoing, low-grade inflammation. In general, persistent microscopic hematuria is associated with a poor prognosis.[889] It is important to note that acute renal failure associated with macroscopic hematuria does not affect long-term prognosis. The fact that acute renal failure does occur during gross episodes of hematuria has been confirmed.[890–892] In these patients, the acute renal failure is most likely associated with acute tubular damage and not too crescentic disease. After the episodes of gross hematuria, renal function typically returns to baseline and the long-term prognosis is good. The degree of proteinuria is more than likely an additional marker of glomerular disease. Whether this is a consequence of the relationship between proteinuria and tubular dysfunction found in many forms of glomerular disease or specific to IgA nephropathy is not clear. In a study by Chen,[893] mice that had been proteinuric by various methods had enhanced deposition of administered IgA immune complexes. This suggests that these complexes might be more easily deposited in proteinuric states. More importantly, the amount of protein excretion one year after diagnosis was highly predictive of the development of end-stage renal disease within 7 years of subsequent follow-up. Individuals with less than 500 mg/dL per 24 hours had no renal failure within 7 years whereas those with over 3 g had approximately 60% chance of end-stage renal disease.[894]

Histological features that are associated with progression to end-stage renal disease include interstitial fibrosis, tubular atrophy, and glomerular scarring. Presence or absence of immune deposits in capillary loops and the mesangium, and crescent formation have also been correlated with disease. Whether crescents found on renal biopsy constitute a poor prognostic factor has also been a controversial issue. Crescentic glomerulonephritis is most likely to occur in patients who have macroscopic hematuria. Thus, it is not clear whether the presence of crescentic disease can be separately associated with a poor prognosis. However, in IgA as in other forms of glomerular disease, the severity of tubulointerstitial nephritis appears to correlate more closely with the risk of progression than with glomerular damage.

Women with IgA tolerate pregnancy well. Only those women with uncontrolled hypertension, a glomerular filtration rate less than 70 ml/min, or severe arteriolar or interstitial damage on renal biopsy are at risk for renal dysfunction.[895,896] Pregnant women with creatinine levels greater than 1.4 mg/dL have a higher propensity for hypertension and a progressive increase in creatinine during the course or pregnancy, and pregnancy-related loss of maternal renal function occurs in 43% of patients. The infant survival rate was 93% in this study, and pre-term delivery occurred in almost two thirds, and growth retardation in one third of infants.[897]

Laboratory Findings

To date, there are no specific serologic/laboratory tests diagnostic of IgA nephropathy or Henoch-Schönlein purpura. Although the serum IgA levels are elevated in up to 50% of patients, the presence of elevated IgA in the circulation is not specific for IgA nephropathy. The detection of IgA-fibronectin complexes was initially thought to be a marker in patients with IgA nephropathy.[898–900] This was not proven a clinically significant test. In our own experience, some patients with IgA nephropathy have elevated IgA-fibronectin levels that are maintained throughout the course of their disease, whereas in other patients, IgA fibronectin levels are never discovered. Polymeric IgA also appears to be found in some patients with IgA nephropathy.[805,901–905] The polymeric IgA itself appears to be that of the IgA1 subclass. IgA may also be contained in circulating immune complexes that are non-complement binding. Similar immune complexes have been described in

Henoch-Schönlein purpura.[906–923] The level of circulating immune complexes wax and wane and may sometimes correlate with episodes of macroscopic hematuria. In one interesting study, the level of circulating immune complexes was increased after patients drank cow's milk. This phenomenon occurred in 10% to 15% of patients, possibly suggesting sensitivity to bovine serum albumin. Unfortunately, none of these findings is pathognomonic of IgA nephropathy.

Some patients with IgA nephropathy have antibodies to the glomerular basement membrane,[924] the mesangium,[925,926] glomerular endothelial cells,[810] and IgA rheumatoid factor.[857,858] The IgA rheumatoid factor has been found and may participate in the pathogenetic process.[857,858] Others have found antibodies to anti-neutrophil cytoplasmic constituents,[812,813] although it is possible that the IgA ANCA are a laboratory artifact.[858] Antibodies to infectious agents such as herpes, Haemophilus parainfluenza, and normal pathogens found in both the respiratory tract as well as in the gut have been described, as well as antibodies to both bovine serum proteins and soy proteins.[815–822,927,928] Until studies demonstrate that certain patients have sensitivity to a particular pathogen or food allergen, it is difficult to know whether to obtain antibody testing to eliminate certain foods from the patient's diet. None of these antibody tests has been standardized well enough in large patient populations to make their study in all patients with IgA nephropathy meaningful.

Complement levels such as C3 and C4 are typically normal and, in some patients, even elevated,[929] as are complement components C1q, C2-C9.[758,906,907,929,930] The fact that these complement levels are normal may belie the fact that either the alternate or the classical pathway of complement may be activated. In this regard, C3 fragments are increased in 50% to 75% of patients,[931,932] as well as C4 binding protein concentrations.[930]

A typical finding is microscopic hematuria on urinalysis that may persist, even at very low levels of macroscopic hematuria. The finding of dysmorphic erythrocytes in the urine is typical.[933] Proteinuria is found in many patients with IgA nephropathy, although the majority of them have less than one gram of protein per day. Patients who have a more persistent course or a more aggressive diffuse proliferative glomerulonephritis may have a greater amount of proteinuria. Other factors found in the urine of patients with IgA nephropathy include platelet-derived growth factor and interleukin-6. The initial interest in elevated urinary interleukin-6 is tempered by the fact that this same protein is found in association with urinary tract infections.[934–936]

A frequently asked question is whether skin biopsy provides any diagnostic utility in patients with IgA nephropathy. In one study, the sensitivity of finding dermal capillary IgA deposits in the skin of patients with IgA nephropathy was found to be 75% with a specificity of 88%.[937] When the IgA is present along the dermal capillaries, it is also accompanied by C3, properdin, and fibrin deposits.[937–940] In these biopsies, it is important to note that IgG or IgM should not be found in the dermal vasculature. If they are, other diagnoses, such as systemic lupus erythematosus, should be considered. The value of skin biopsy in recurrent episodes of macroscopic hematuria has not gained widespread acceptance, largely because of the substantial variation in sensitivity and specificity of skin biopsies in finding IgA in patients with nephropathy.[940]

Treatment

Without a clear understanding of the pathogenesis of IgA nephropathy, it is difficult to describe precise treatment for this condition. As in any form of chronic renal insufficiency, antihypertensive therapy may ameliorate a possibility of secondary glomerular damage. The angiotensin converting enzyme inhibitors have been demonstrated to be beneficial in IgA in reducing proteinuria, even in normotensive patients with IgAN nephropathy.[941] A report by Woo suggests that in patients with normal renal function and mild proteinuria (<500 mg/day), blood pressure should be controlled with an ACE inhibitors or angiotensin receptor blockers.[942] These agents may also improve proteinuria due to altering glomerular size selectivity.[943] In a retrospective analysis, ACE inhibitors were compared to other anti-hypertensive medicines. The ACE-inhibitor treated group experienced a slower loss of renal function and a higher percentage of remission of proteinuria than the no treatment group.[944] These agents have been similarly demonstrated to decrease the deterioration in renal function when compared to beta blockers.[945] In the ACE gene DD genotype, anti-proteinuric effects of the ACE inhibitor were more profound in patients with the DD genotype than in other patients with IgA nephropathy.[781] The combined effects of ACE-inhibitors and angiotensin receptor blocker (ARB) was assessed in a large controlled trial in which 263 patients with non-diabetic kidney disease were randomized to trandolapril alone, losartan alone or both drugs.[946] Fifty percent of enrolled patients had IgA nephropathy. All patients received other antihypertensive medications to maintain a target blood pressure <130/80 mm Hg. Compared to either agent alone, the combination of trandolapril and losartan resulted in a significantly greater reduction in proteinuria and decreased likelihood of reaching the combined primary endpoint of time to doubling of serum creatinine or reaching end stage kidney disease. The combination therapy was not associated with a higher frequency of side effects (including hyperkalemia).

Therapy with glucocorticoids for IgA nephropathy has generated substantial controversy. While prednisone was initially considered to be without effect,[947] some cohort studies suggest that corticosteroids may have an important effect.[948,949] Recently, a randomized trial demonstrated that glucocorticoids may be useful in patients with IgA nephropathy and well-preserved renal function (serum creatinine <1.5 mg/dL and proteinuria between 1 and 3.5 gm/day).[950] Patients were treated with IV methylprednisolone for three consecutive days in months 1, 3, and 5 and oral prednisone given at a dose of 0.5 mg/kg qod for months 1 to 6, compared to standard therapy. After a 5-year follow-up, the risk of a doubling in plasma creatinine was significantly lower in the corticosteroid-treated patients, who also showed a significant decrease in mean urinary protein excretion after 1 year that persisted throughout the follow-up.[950] This beneficial effect was maintained after 10 years of follow up as reflected by a renal survival (failure to double the serum creatinine) of 97% in the treated group as compared to 53% (log rank test $P = 0.0003$) in the placebo group.[951] On the other hand, in the multicenter, randomized controlled trial conducted by the Southwest Pediatric Nephrology Study Group,[952] there was no statistically significant improvement in the rate of renal failure (defined as a 60% decrease in GFR) among patients who were treated with an alternate day regime of high dose prednisone (60 mg/M² every other day for 3 months, then 40 mg/M² every other day for 9 months, then 30 mg/M² every other day for 12 months) when compared to placebo. This negative result is however mitigated by the fact that patients in the placebo group had a statistically significantly lower degree of proteinuria at baseline. The potential role of corticosteroids in the management of IgA nephropathy was also evaluated in a metaanalysis of six randomized trials in which various regimen were compared to placebo or dipyridamole and encompassing a total of 181 patients.[953] This analysis did not include the study by the Southwest Pediatric Nephrology Study Group.[952] Based on this analysis, the use of corticosteroids was associated with a decreased risk of doubling serum creatinine (RR 0.45; 95% CI 0.29, 0.69) or reaching ESKD (RR 0.44; 95% CI 0.25, 0.80).

Another circumstance in which prednisone has a demonstrated substantial beneficial effect is in the treatment of patients with IgA nephropathy and concurrent minimal change glomerulopathy. These patients have nephrotic-range proteinuria and diffuse foot process fusion. They respond to prednisone in a manner very similar to that of patients with minimal change glomerulopathy.[194,877,954] However, the nephrotic syndrome might also be a consequence of advanced glomerular scarring or diffuse proliferative glomerulonephritis. In these patients, resolution of the nephrotic syndrome by corticosteroids is not as forthcoming.

More aggressive treatment may be appropriate in patients with progressive IgA nephropathy. In a randomized, controlled trial, patients with a serum creatinine >1.5 mg/dL and a GFR declining at a rate >15% per year received either no immunosuppression or were treated with oral prednisolone (initially at 40 mg/day) and cyclophosphamide (at 1.5 mg/kg/day) for 3 months followed by 2 years of azathioprine (1.5 mg/kg/day).[955] Over a follow-up of 2 to 6 years, treated patients had 72% 5-year renal survival, versus only 6% in untreated patients.[955] This approach of prednisone coupled with oral azathioprine for 2 years in patients with over 2.5 g of proteinuria was also observed in a retrospective survey by Goumenos.[956,957]

In patients who have rapidly progressive glomerulonephritis with widespread crescentic transformation, there are reports on the use of pulse methylprednisolone, oral prednisone, and/or cyclophosphamide.[958–960] It is reasonable to treat crescentic disease in IgA nephropathy in a manner similar to other forms of crescentic glomerulonephritis (e.g., ANCA glomerulonephritis). Of concern, however, was the finding in 12 patients of the persistence of crescents on repeat biopsy, despite the early and aggressive treatment with pulse methylprednisolone and oral prednisone, and a short-term reversal of the acute crescentic glomerulonephritis.[960] This study suggests that there was only a diminution in the rate of progression to end-stage renal disease.

Other Modalities

It is reasonably clear that treatment with the combination of oral cyclophosphamide, dipyridamole, and low-dose warfarin[961] has very little long-term benefit in patients with IgA nephropathy. At 8 years, there was no difference between placebo and control patients, and 25% to 30% of patients in both groups had progressed to end-stage renal disease.

Whether mycophenolate mofetil is useful in the treatment of IgA nephropathy has not been established. Four randomized trials of MMF have been published with conflicting results.[962–965] The studies based in China and Hong Kong report a beneficial effect of MMF on proteinuria and hyperlipidemia[962,963] without an effect on renal function.[962] On the other hand the two placebo controlled studies of MMF in white populations of 32 and 34 patients failed to demonstrate a benefit of MMF on proteinuria or the preservation of renal function.[964,965] It is noteworthy however that in one study,[964] patients had relatively advanced renal insufficiency (mean serum creatinine of 2.4 mg/dL). Collectively, these underpowered studies fail to establish a role for MMF in IgA nephropathy and raise the question as to whether certain ethnic groups (Asians) may be more responsive to this form of therapy. MMF is currently the focus of a large randomized placebo-controlled trial in the United States.[966]

Intravenous immunoglobulins have been used in at least one study for IgA nephropathy.[967] Treatment of 9 patients with IgA nephropathy produced some favorable results, including a reduction in proteinuria, hematuria, and leukocyturia. There was a decrease in the progressive decline in renal function. The conclusions of these studies must be tempered by the relatively small numbers of patients enrolled in any of them, and the absence of appropriate control populations.

There has been much discussion in the literature about the use of tonsillectomy in IgA nephropathy. The results of the retrospective trials are inconsistent.[968–970] Based on a retrospective multivariate analysis 969 of large cohort of patients (329 patients) from Japan, treatment with tonsillectomy and pulse glucocorticoid therapy (methylprednisolone [0.5 g/day for 3 days for three courses] followed by oral prednisolone at an initial dose of 0.6 mg/kg on alternate days, with a decrease of 0.1 mg/kg every 2 months) was associated with clinical remission. Similarly, a multivariate analysis[971] of the focusing on the subgroup of patients 70 patients from the same cohort with a baseline serum creatinine >1.5 mg/dL, treatment with the combination of tonsillectomy and pulse glucocorticoids was associated with improved long-term renal survival. Another retrospective analysis[968] however, showed no benefit of tonsillectomy on the clinical course of IgA nephropathy. No study has yet demonstrated a superiority of tonsillectomy alone, or superiority over similar course of pulse glucocorticoids, and no randomized controlled trials assessing the value of tonsillectomy has been performed. At this point, there is therefore no convincing evidence in support for tonsillectomy in the treatment of IgA nephropathy. Such measure could however be beneficial in patients with recurrent tonsillitis.

Fish Oil

The advent of treatment of IgA nephropathy with fish oil has led to substantial difficulties in treatment of the individual patient with IgA nephropathy. Because of the widespread publicity of the potential beneficial effect of omega-3 fatty acids and IgA nephropathy,[972–974] it has been difficult to avoid this form of treatment in patients who have learned about it either from the news media or the Internet. A study by the Mayo Clinic[973] randomized 106 patients to either 12 grams of fish oil containing N-3 fatty acids or olive oil for 2 years. Only 6% of patients treated with fish oil had a doubling of their plasma creatinine concentration when compared to 33% of those treated with olive oil. In the fish oil-treated patients, only 14% excreted over 3.5 grams of protein per day, in contrast to 65% of those treated with olive oil. Impressively, the incidence of death or end-stage renal disease by 4 years of follow-up was 10% in the fish oil group and 40% in the olive oil-treated group. There was no difference between the two groups with respect to blood pressure control. The fish oil was apparently well tolerated. The enthusiasm for this approach must be tempered by two other much smaller trials that showed absolutely no benefit of fish oil therapy.[972,975] A meta-analysis of the available trials suggested that some of the differences in the positive versus negative trials were a consequence of differences in follow-up time.[974] When all studies were combined, there was not a statistically significant benefit of fish oil therapy, although there was at least a minor beneficial effect. If any effect was to be observed with fish oil therapy, it was found in those individuals who had more proteinuria. In the multicenter, randomized controlled trial conducted by the Southwest Pediatric Nephrology Study Group,[952] treatment with Omacor 4 gm/day for 2 years was not associated with a statistically significant improvement in the rate of renal failure (defined as a 60% decrease in GFR) when compared to placebo. This negative result is however mitigated by the fact that patients in the placebo group had a statistically significantly lower degree of proteinuria at baseline.

Dietary Modification

If IgA nephropathy is a consequence of the mucosal immune reaction to certain dietary products, then a diet avoiding these products may have a salutary effect. In a study from Italy, a low antigen diet was used to treat 51 patients with IgA nephropathy. In these patients, a diet was selected to avoid most meats, all dairy products, eggs, and gluten. In this group of 21 patients, proteinuria fell in 12 whose baseline protein excretion was greater than 1 gram/day. A subsequent post-treatment biopsy suggested that there was a reduction in mesangial immunoglobulin deposition, C5 deposition, and fibrin. Similar results were described in an uncontrolled study of a gluten-free diet. These dietary modification studies must be subjected to a longer clinical trial.

There have been reports on a variety of potential mechanisms to decrease the level of IgA or to alter dietary antigen exposure. These include tonsillectomy,[976] antibiotics,[977] sodium cromoglycate,[978] or dietary manipulation.[979,980] Attempts at decreasing IgA production have been explored by using phenytoin.[981,982] None of these approaches has been widely tested, nor are they considered approved treatment modalities.

In summary, patients with IgA nephropathy should be treated with an ACE inhibitor or angiotensin receptor blocker.[983] The use of the combination of an angiotensin receptor blocker and ACE inhibitor should be attempted especially in hypertensive patients who have substantial proteinuria.[946,984,985] This may occur without further decline in blood pressure.[986,987] Patients with significant proteinuria and microscopic hematuria that persists over time should be considered for treatment with alternate month intravenous methylprednisolone and alternate-day corticosteroids. In those patients with progressive renal insufficiency, the use of prednisone and cyclophosphamide followed by azathioprine should be considered.[955] High-dose corticosteroids and/or cyclophosphamide should also be considered for patients with widespread crescentic glomerulonephritis, whereas patients with acute renal failure associated with tubular necrosis and little glomerular damage should be treated conservatively, as these individuals have an excellent long-term response. Although there is still no conclusive evidence of efficacy, the relatively benign side effect profile of omega-3 fatty acids warrants its use in patients who have an unfavorable prognosis. Those patients with the nephrotic syndrome and minimal change glomerulopathy may benefit from oral glucocorticoids. If there is a clear sensitivity to certain types of dietary products, it is useful to attempt an antigen-free diet.

Other Glomerular Diseases that Cause Hematuria

The clinical designation of benign familial hematuria often refers to thin basement membrane nephropathy. The prevalence of thin basement membrane nephropathy in the general population has been estimated from morphometry studies in transplant and allografts to be approximately 5.2% to 9.2%.[988] Similarly, of over 1078 native kidney biopsies, thin basement membrane nephropathy was found in 5% of patients.

Males and females are equally effected patients and are typically found to have microscopic hematuria when they are adolescents or young adults. The majority of patients have microscopic hematuria at presentation. Many have had previous urological examinations in search of a lower urinary tract source of bleeding, including cystoscopy and IVP or ultrasound. The presence of dysmorphic red cells or red cell casts may make the diagnosis of thin basement membrane nephropathy more readily apparent. Unlike IgA nephropathy, however, macroscopic hematuria is uncommon.[747,989] Similarly, unlike many patients with IgA nephropathy, most have no proteinuria, although some may have mild to moderate proteinuria, usually less than 1 to 2 grams.[30,990,991] The pattern of hematuria is sometimes familial, and assessing the urine of family members can further complement a diagnosis. In some patients, there is no obvious pattern of inheritance.[30,989,992–994] In a search for hematuria in first-degree relatives, approximately one half of those undiagnosed patients may have hematuria.[993,995] Father-to-son transmission, not found in X-linked hereditary nephritis, may be found in thin basement membrane nephropathy. It has long been known that Alport syndrome is a consequence of molecular defect in the COL-413/4 genes. Mutations within the COL-4A3 gene have been described in patients with familial hematuria.[996]

The long-term course of patients with thin basement membrane nephropathy is thought to be excellent.[30,990,997] In a study of 19 normotensive adults with normal renal function and hematuria, all patients had thin basement membrane nephropathy on biopsy. These patients were followed for a mean of 12 years. The incidence of hypertension in this population was 35% and was statistically more common than in healthy controls. Although thin basement membrane nephropathy has been thought to be of long-term benign prognosis, it is important to note that in this population, some patients have premature glomerular obsolescence, increased incidence of hypertension, and potential late onset of renal insufficiency. In this same study,[998] 6 of 89 first-degree elderly relatives had renal failure compared to only 1 of 129 relatives with IgA nephropathy. At the end of 12 years of follow-up, 3 of 7 subjects over the age of 50 had a slight decline in glomerular filtration rate.

Persistent isolated hematuria is also present in hereditary nephritis associated with Alport syndrome.[29,999,1000] By examining the urine of asymptomatic family members, it may be possible to elicit a hereditary cause. By history, hereditary nephritis is usually associated with an x-linked dominant form of inheritance[1001] and is associated with hearing loss and ocular abnormalities in many cases. It may be possible to differentiate thin basement membrane nephropathy from Alport disease by skin biopsy using an antibody to the alpha-5 chain of type IV collagen. In males with hereditary nephritis, there was no staining with this antibody along the epidermal basement membrane and, interestingly, there was discontinuous staining in female carriers who had no urinary abnormalities. In contrast, there was normal staining of this antibody in control patients.[1002]

The syndrome of loin pain hematuria is another condition causing hematuria. This uncommon syndrome occurs primarily in young women.[1003–1005] Oral contraceptives have been associated with this condition.[1003–1006] The clinical picture is reminiscent of that of IgA nephropathy. There are recurrent episodes of gross hematuria, usually with flank pain that is typically described as dull or aching. Patients sometimes have fever, malaise, and anorexia. Hypertension and proteinuria are uncommon. It has been suggested that the cause of the pain is due to small vessel thrombi resulting in infarction of the kidney. Thus, arteriograms have been performed which occasionally reveal narrowing of intrarenal vessels.[1005] In the few renal biopsies that have been performed, normal glomeruli have been demonstrated,[640,1006,1007] although C3 and IgM deposits have been found. Some patients have a substantial psychological overlay. Continued pain may lead to narcotics addiction.[1006] The treatment of loin pain hematuria usually begins with cessation of the oral contraceptives,[640,1003–1006] or treatment with anticoagulant drugs. There have been reports of a renal denervation by autotransplantation of the kidney,[1008] but 30% of these patients have recurrence of their symptoms. In a study by Lucas,[1009] 15 patients with loin pain hematuria were compared to 10 with nephrolithiasis and flank pain. Patients with loin pain hematuria syndrome tended to have somatic symptoms, adverse psychological events, and a history of analgesic ingestion to a greater degree than those patients with nephrolithiasis.[1005]

Fibrillary Glomerulonephritis and Immunotactoid Glomerulopathy

Nomenclature

Fibrillary glomerulonephritis and immunotactoid glomerulopathy are glomerular diseases that are characterized by patterned deposits seen by electron microscopy (Figs. 30–27 and 30–28).[1010–1017] There is controversy over how to categorize these diseases. Most renal pathologists prefer to distinguish fibrillary glomerulonephritis from immunotactoid glomerulopathy based on the presence of fibrils of approximately 20 nm diameter in the former and larger 30 nm to 40 nm diameter microtubular structures in the latter[1010,1012–1015] (see Figs. 30–27 and 30–28). A minority of pathologists,

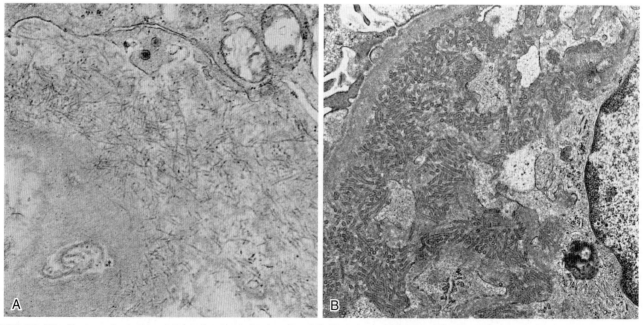

FIGURE 30–27 Electron micrographs showing the glomerular deposits of fibrillary glomerulonephritis (**A**) and immunotactoid glomerulopathy (**B**). Note the random orientation of the former, and the microtubular appearance and greater organization of the latter (magnification ×20,000).

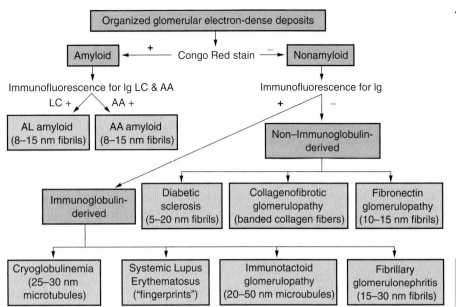

FIGURE 30-28 Algorithm for the pathologic categorization of glomerular diseases with patterned or organized deposits. The first dichotomy is into amyloid versus nonamyloid disease, and the second is into diseases caused by immunoglobulin molecule deposition versus those that are not. By the approach illustrated, fibrillary glomerulonephritis is distinguished from immunotactoid glomerulopathy based on the ultrastructural characteristics of the deposits.

however, advocate grouping glomerular diseases with either fibrillary deposits or microtubular deposits under the term immunotactoid glomerulopathy.[1014,1017]

Pathology

Electron Microscopy

The diagnosis of fibrillary glomerulonephritis requires the identification by electron microscopy of irregular accumulation of randomly arranged non-branching fibrils of approximately 20 nm diameter in glomerular mesangium or capillary walls or both[1010–1016,1018] (Fig. 30–27A). In capillary walls, the fibrillary deposits can be subepithelial, subendothelial, or intramembranous. The fibrillary deposits often contain blotchy electron dense material, but only rarely have associated well-defined electron dense deposits. The fibrils are distinctly larger than the actin filaments in adjacent cells, which is a useful observation that helps distinguish the fibrils of fibrillary glomerulonephritis from those of amyloidosis, which are only slightly larger than actin. The fibrils of fibrillary glomerulonephritis are not as large as the microtubular deposits of immunotactoid glomerulopathy or cryoglobulinemia, and they do not have the "fingerprint" configuration occasionally observed in lupus nephritis dense deposits. Most patients with fibrillary glomerulonephritis have substantial proteinuria and therefore there usually is extensive effacement of visceral epithelial foot processes.

The tubular substructure of the deposits of immunotactoid glomerulopathy is readily discerned at 5000 to 10,000 magnification (Fig. 30–27B). At this magnification, the deposits of fibrillary glomerulonephritis have no tubular structure. The microtubules of immunotactoid glomerulopathy also have a greater tendency to align in parallel arrays whereas the fibrils of fibrillary glomerulonephritis always are randomly distributed.[1018] The ultrastructural deposits of immunotactoid glomerulopathy resemble those seen with cryoglobulinemic glomerulonephritis, and thus the latter must be ruled out before making a diagnosis of immunotactoid glomerulopathy.

Light Microscopy

In fibrillary glomerulonephritis, extensive localization of fibrils in capillary walls causes capillary wall thickening. Mesangial localization causes increased mesangial matrix and usually stimulates mesangial hypercellularity. Varying distributions of the fibrillary deposits causes the light micro-scopic appearance of fibrillary glomerulonephritis to be extremely variable.[1010–1016] Therefore, fibrillary glomerulonephritis can mimic the light microscopic appearance of membranoproliferative glomerulonephritis, proliferative glomerulonephritis, or membranous glomerulopathy. Crescents occur in the most aggressive phenotypes. Of 74 sequential fibrillary glomerulonephritis specimens evaluated at UNC, 28% had crescents with an average involvement of 29% of glomeruli (range 5% to 80%). The fibrillary deposits typically have a moth-eaten appearance when stained with a Jones silver methenamine stain. They are negative with Congo red staining, which distinguishes them from amyloid deposits. Immunotactoid glomerulopathy also has a varied light microscopic appearance. Combined capillary wall thickening and mesangial expansion is most common, often giving a membranoproliferative appearance.

Immunofluorescence Microscopy

The deposits of fibrillary glomerulonephritis almost always stain more intensely for IgG than for IgM or IgA, and many specimens have little of no staining for IgM and IgA.[1010–1016] IgG4 is the dominant subclass. Only rare specimens have staining for only one light chain type. C3 staining usually is intense. The immunofluorescence staining pattern of fibrillary glomerulonephritis is relatively distinctive (Fig. 30–29). It is not granular or linear, but rather has an irregular band-like appearance in capillary walls and an irregular shaggy appearance in the mesangium.

The deposits of immunotactoid glomerulopathy usually are IgG dominant with staining for both kappa and lambda light chains. Some investigators conclude that the immunoglobulin in the deposits of immunotactoid glomerulopathy more often is monoclonal than in fibrillary glomerulonephritis.[1012]

Pathogenesis

The etiology and pathogenesis of fibrillary glomerulonephritis and immunotactoid glomerulopathy are not known. Fibrillary glomerulonephritis and immunotactoid glomerulonephritis have been associated with lymphoproliferative disease (for instance with chronic lymphocytic leukemia or B-cell lymphomas).[1012,1018,1019] In fact, the treatment of some patients with chemotherapy has caused improvement in renal function and reduction in proteinuria. The possible oligoclonal character of the deposits of fibrillary glomerulonephritis may facilitate self-association and fibrillar

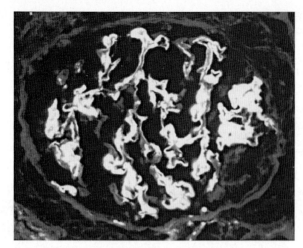

FIGURE 30–29 Immunofluorescence micrograph of a glomerulus with fibrillary glomerulonephritis showing mesangial and bandlike capillary wall staining for IgG. (FITC anti-IgG, ×300.)

organization in an analogous fashion to the monoclonal light chains of AL amyloidosis.[1015] The resemblance of immunotactoid deposits to those of cryoglobulinemia, which often contain a monoclonal component, also raises the possibility that the presence of some type of uniformity of the immunoglobulin in the deposits may be causing the patterned organization in immunotactoid glomerulopathy.

Epidemiology and Clinical Features

An analysis of 9085 consecutive native kidney biopsies evaluated in the UNC Nephropathology laboratory reveals a frequency of fibrillary glomerulonephritis of 0.8%, compared to 14.5% for membranous glomerulopathy, 7.5% for IgA nephropathy, 2.6% for type I MPGN I, 1.5% for amyloidosis, 0.8% for anti-GBM glomerulonephritis, 0.2% for type II, and 0.1% for immunotactoid glomerulonephritis. Thus, fibrillary glomerulonephritis is about as common as anti-GBM glomerulonephritis and much more frequent than immunotactoid glomerulopathy.

Patients with fibrillary glomerulonephritis present with a mixture of the nephrotic and nephritic syndrome features.[1013,1015,1018] Patients may have microscopic or macroscopic hematuria, renal insufficiency (including RPGN in a few patients), hypertension, and proteinuria, which may be nephrotic range. In a series of 28 patients with fibrillary glomerulonephritis, the mean age was 49 years, with a range of 21 to 75. The ratio of males to females was 1:1.8, and the ratio of whites to blacks was 8.3:1, suggesting a predilection for whites over blacks.[1015] The mean amount of proteinuria was 6 grams/day. Unfortunately, after 24 months of follow-up, renal survival was only 48%.[1015] Renal insufficiency is common at the time of presentation, as are hematuria and hypertension. Patients with these disorders must not have cryoglobulinemia, lupus, or paraproteinemia. Some controversy exists as to whether patients with immunotactoid glomerular disease should be separate from those with fibrillary glomerulopathy. Fibrillary glomerulopathy have microfibrils less than 30 nm, whereas those with immunotactoid have microfibrils greater than 30 nm. Most investigators suggest there is a difference, in that patients with immunotactoid glomerular disease are more likely to have a lymphoproliferative disorder. Such patients have progressive renal failure in less than 5 years, although long-term patient survival is greater than 80% at 5 years.[1020,1021]

In a group of six patients with immunotactoid glomerulopathy, the mean age was 62, suggesting that patients with immunotactoid glomerulopathy may be significantly older than those with fibrillary glomerulonephritis.[1013] On clinical presentation, these patients look very much like those with fibrillary glomerulonephritis with proteinuria, hematuria and renal insufficiency. Importantly, those patients with immunotactoid glomerular disease are more likely to have an associated hematopoietic process and poor long-term survival.[1013] In a review study of patients presenting with fibrillary glomerulopathy or immunotactoid glomerulopathy, 161 patients were observed. Those who had fibrillary glomerulopathy, all patients had proteinuria and three quarters of both types of presentations had the nephrotic syndrome. Hematuria occurred in approximately two-thirds of patients and hypertension in half to two thirds. Renal insufficiency was discovered in half the patient population. There were no real statistical differences in the clinical presentation of either the fibrillary glomerular disease group or those with immunotactoid glomerulopathy. The patients who had a more rapid progression to end-stage renal disease had a higher incidence of nephrosis and hypertension than those with milder disease. Four patients eventually received transplants and recurrent disease was found in three of five allografts, although there was a slower rate of deterioration of renal function in the allograft.[1022] In fibronectin glomerulonephritis, patients present with proteinuria in adolescence and the clinical course is characterized by proteinuria with hematuria in one half of these patients. The few patients that have been reported either have stable renal function, yet some have persistent decline in renal function.[1023]

In one report of extrarenal manifestations of fibrillary glomerulonephritis, there was evidence of pulmonary hemorrhage[1024] and in one patient with immunotactoid glomerulopathy, there were extrarenal deposits in both the liver and bone.[1025]

Treatment

At this time, there is no convincingly effective form of treatment for patients with either fibrillary glomerulonephritis or immunotactoid glomerulopathy.[1018] The dismal prognosis in patients with either of these diseases prompts physicians to search for some immunosuppressive form of treatment. Fully 40% to 50% of patients with these diseases develop end-stage renal disease within 6 years of presentation.[1010,1011,1013,1015] Efforts for treatment with either glucocorticoids or alkylating agents such as cyclophosphamide have typically shown either no response or, at best, some amelioration of proteinuria.[1026] In our own experience, prednisone therapy alone has had no benefit at all. Efforts at treatment with colchicine therapy in a fashion analogous to treatment of systemic amyloidosis have also not provided any substantial beneficial effect. Nonetheless, in fibrillary glomerulonephritis or other forms of glomerulonephritis associated with chronic lymphocytic leukemia or other forms of lymphocytic lymphoma, there is a report of improvement in a minority of patients treated with chlorambucil. Thus, it is possible that the treatment of the underlying malignancy if one is detected may make the glomerulonephritis better.[1019]

There is only one report in the literature[1022] that describes the predictors of disease progression in transplantation in fibrillary glomerulopathy. Four patients received five renal allografts followed for four to eleven years. Recurrence of fibrillary glomerulonephritis was documented in three of these allografts, although the rate of deterioration in the allograft was slower.

Rapidly Progressive Glomerulonephritis and Crescentic Glomerulonephritis

Nomenclature and Categorization

The term rapidly progressive glomerulonephritis (RPGN) refers to a clinical syndrome characterized by a rapid loss of renal function, often accompanied by oliguria or anuria, and with features of glomerulonephritis, including dysmorphic erythrocyturia, erythrocyte cylindruria, and glomerular proteinuria.[1027] Aggressive glomerulonephritis that causes RPGN usually has extensive crescent formation.[1028] For this reason, the clinical term RPGN is sometimes used interchangeably with pathologic term crescentic glomerulonephritis. Crescentic glomerulonephritis is the most aggressive structural phenotype in the continuum of injury that results from glomerular inflammation (see Fig. 30–18). The crescent formation results from disruption of glomerular capillaries that allows inflammatory mediators and leukocytes to enter Bowman space where they induce epithelial cell proliferation and macrophage maturation that together produce cellular crescents (Fig. 30–30).[1029–1031] Therefore, a ubiquitous pathologic feature of crescentic glomerulonephritis is focal rupture of glomerular capillary walls that can be seen by light microscopy and electron microscopy.[1028,1032,1033]

Renal diseases other than crescentic glomerulonephritis can cause the sign and symptoms of RPGN. Two examples are acute thrombotic microangiopathy and atheroembolic renal disease. Although acute tubular necrosis and acute tubulointerstitial nephritis may cause rapid loss renal function and oliguria, these processes typically do not cause dysmorphic erythrocyturia, erythrocyte cylindruria, or substantial proteinuria.

A small minority of all patients with glomerulonephritis develops RPGN. The incidence of the clinical syndrome has been estimated to be as low as seven cases per million population per year.[661,1034] The three major immunopathologic categories of crescentic glomerulonephritis have different frequencies in different age groups (Table 30–15).[1027,1028,1032,1035] In a patient who has RPGN clinically and crescentic glomerulonephritis identified light microscopy of a renal biopsy specimen, the precise diagnostic categorization of the disease requires integration of clinical, serologic, immunohistologic, and electron microscopic data (Fig. 30–31).

Immune complex crescentic glomerulonephritis is caused by immune complex localization within glomeruli. It is the most common cause for RPGN in children (Table 30–16).[1028] The major clinical differential diagnosis in children is hemolytic uremic syndrome, which also can cause rapid loss of renal function, hypertension, hematuria, and proteinuria. The presence of microangiopathic hemolytic anemia and thrombocytopenia are indicators that the rapid loss of renal function is more likely caused by hemolytic uremic syndrome than crescentic glomerulonephritis. Pauci-immune crescentic glomerulonephritis, which has no evidence for immune complex or anti-GBM localization in glomeruli and is usually associated with ANCA, is the most common cause for RPGN and crescentic glomerulonephritis in adults, especially older adults (Tables 30–16 and 30–17).[1027,1035,1036] In most patients, pauci-immune crescentic glomerulonephritis is a component of a systemic small-vessel vasculitis, such as Wegener granulomatosis or microscopic polyangiitis, however, some patients have renal-limited (primary) disease.[1028,1037–1039] This entity will be more fully discussed in Chapter 33. Anti-GBM disease is the least frequent cause for crescentic glomerulonephritis (see Tables 30–16 and 30–17).[1027,1028,1035,1036] It is most frequent in young males and older females, but is not common in any setting.

Immune Complex-Mediated Crescentic Glomerulonephritis

Epidemiology

Most patients with immune complex crescentic glomerulonephritis have clinical or pathologic evidence for a specific category of primary glomerulonephritis, such as IgA nephropathy, post-infectious glomerulonephritis, or membranoproliferative glomerulonephritis, or they have glomerulonephritis that is a component of a systemic immune complex disease, such as systemic lupus erythematosus, cryoglobulinemia, or Henoch-Schönlein purpura. A minority of patients with immune complex crescentic glomerulonephritis, however, do

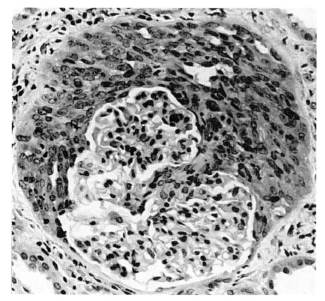

FIGURE 30–30 Light micrograph showing a large cellular crescent (magnification ×500).

TABLE 30–15	Frequency of Immunopathologic Categories of Glomerulonephritis in over 3000 Consecutive Non-Transplant Renal Biopsies Evaluated by Immunofluorescence Microscopy in the University of North Carolina Nephropathology Laboratory			
Immunohistology	**All Proliferative GN (n = 1093)**	**Any Crescents (n = 540)**	**>50% Crescents (n = 195)**	**Arteritis in Biopsy (n = 37)**
Pauci-immune (<2+ Ig)	45% (496/1093)	51% (227/540)	61% (118/195)*	84% (31/37)
Immune Complex (≥2+ Ig)	52% (570/1093)	44% (238/540)	29% (56/195)	14% (5/37)‡
Anti-GBM	3% (27/1093)	5% (25/540)†	11% (21/195)	3% (1/37)¶

*70 of 77 patients tested for ANCA were positive (91%) (44 P-ANCA and 26 C-ANCA).
†3 of 19 patients tested for ANCA were positive (16%) (2 P-ANCA and 1 C-ANCA).
‡4 patients had lupus and 1 post-streptococcal glomerulonephritis.
¶This patient also had a P-ANCA (MPO-ANCA).
Derived from Jennette JC, Falk RJ: The pathology of vasculitis involving the kidney. Am J Kidney Dis 24:130–141, 1994.

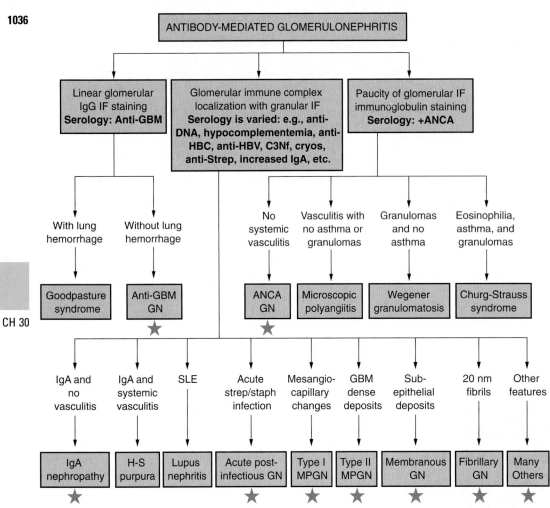

FIGURE 30–31 Algorithm for categorizing glomerulonephritis that is known or suspected of being mediated by antibodies. This categorization applies to glomerulonephritis with crescents as well as to glomerulonephritis without crescents. The diseases with stars beneath them can be considered primary glomerular diseases, whereas those without stars are secondary to (components of) systemic diseases.

TABLE 30–16	Relative Frequency of Immunopathologic Categories of Crescentic Glomerulonephritis in Different Age Groups*			
Categories of CGN	**Age in Years**			
	1–100 (n = 632)	1–20 (n = 73)	21–60 (n = 303)	>60(n = 256)
Anti-GBM CGN	15%	12%	15%	15%
Immune complex CGN	24%	45%	35%	6%
Pauci-immune CGN[†]	60%	42%	48%	79%
Other	1%	0%	3%	0%

ANCA, antineutrophil cytoplasmic antibodies; CGN, crescentic glomerulonephritis.

*CGN is defined as >50% of glomeruli with crescents.

[†]Approximately 90% associated with ANCA. Frequency is determined with respect to age in patients whose renal biopsies were evaluated in the University of North Carolina Nephropathology Laboratory. Notice the very high frequency of pauci-immune (usually ANCA-associated) disease in the elderly.

Derived from Jennette JC, Nickeleit V: Anti-glomerular basement membrane glomerulonephritis and Goodpasture's syndrome. *In* Jennette JC, Olson JL, Schwartz MM, Silva FG (eds): Heptinstall's Pathology of the Kidney, 6th ed. Philadelphia, Lippincott Williams & Wilkins, 2006, pp 613–642.

not have patterns of immune complex localization that readily fit into the specific categories of immune complex glomerulonephritis.[1040] This category is sometimes called idiopathic crescentic immune complex glomerulonephritis.

Immune complex crescentic GN accounts for the majority of crescentic glomerulonephritides in children, but accounts for only a minority of crescentic glomerulonephritis in the elderly (see Table 30–16). The higher frequency in children

reflects the general trend for many types of immune complex glomerulonephritis to be more frequent in younger individuals, for example, IgA nephropathy, poststreptococcal glomerulonephritis, membranoproliferative glomerulonephritis type I and II, and lupus nephritis.

Data in Table 30–17 demonstrate that immune complex glomerulonephritis less often has crescent formation, and, when crescents are present, they involve a smaller proportion

TABLE 30–17	Patients with Various Glomerular Diseases who Have Crescent Formation Based on Analysis of over 6000 Native Kidney Biopsies*			
Disease		**Pts. with Crescents (%)**	**Pts. with ≥50% Crescents**	**Avg. % of Glomeruli with Crescents**
Anti-GBM antibody-mediated glomerulonephritis		97	85	77
ANCA-associated glomerulonephritis		90	50	49
Immune complex-mediated glomerulonephritis				
Lupus glomerulonephritis (classes III and IV)		56	13	27
Henoch-Schönlein purpura glomerulonephritis[+]		61	10	27
IgA nephropathy[+]		32	4	21
Acute postinfectious glomerulonephritis[+]		33	3	19
Fibrillary glomerulonephritis		23	5	26
Type I membranoproliferative glomerulonephritis		24	5	25
Membranous lupus glomerulonephritis (class V)		12	1	17
Membranous glomerulonephritis (non-lupus)		3	0	15

*Evaluated in the University of North Carolina Nephropathology Laboratory. In general, diseases that most often have crescents also have the largest percentage of glomeruli involved by crescents when they are present.

[+]Because more severe examples of IgA nephropathy and postinfectious glomerulonephritis are more often evaluated by renal biopsy, the extent of crescent formation in the biopsied patients shown in this table is higher than in all patients with these diseases.

Derived from Jennette JC: Rapidly progressive crescentic glomerulonephritis. Kidney Int 63:1164–1177, 2003.

of glomeruli than is the case with anti-GBM glomerulonephritis or ANCA glomerulonephritis. The data in Table 30–17 overestimate the extent of crescent formation in immune complex glomerulonephritis because patients with severe disease are more likely to undergo renal biopsy than patients with less severe disease. For example the frequency of glomerular crescents in all patients with post-streptococcal glomerulonephritis or IgA nephropathy is likely much lower than the frequency shown in Table 30–17 because of the bias in the patients selected for renal biopsy. Nevertheless, the data show the much greater propensity for crescent formation in anti-GBM and ANCA glomerulonephritis compared with immune complex glomerulonephritis.

Pathology
Light Microscopy
The light microscopic appearance of crescentic immune complex glomerulonephritis depends upon the underlying category of glomerulonephritis, for example, in their most aggressive expressions, membranoproliferative glomerulonephritis, membranous glomerulopathy, acute postinfectious glomerulonephritis, or proliferative glomerulonephritis, including IgA nephropathy, can all have crescent formation.[440–445,596,697,680,685,686,708,800,802,803,960,1034,1041–1052] This underlying phenotype of immune complex glomerulonephritis is recognized best in the intact glomeruli or glomerular segments. There usually are varying combinations of capillary wall thickening and endocapillary hypercellularity in the intact glomeruli. This is in contrast to anti-GBM glomerulonephritis and ANCA-glomerulonephritis, which tend to have surprisingly little alteration in intact glomeruli and segments in spite of the severe necrotizing injury in involved glomeruli and segments. In glomerular segments adjacent to crescents in immune complex glomerulonephritis, there usually is some degree of necrosis with karyorrhexis; however, the necrosis rarely is as extensive as that typically seen with anti-GBM or ANCA-glomerulonephritis. In addition, there is less destruction of Bowman capsule associated with crescents in immune complex glomerulonephritis, as well as less pronounced periglomerular tubulointerstitial inflammation. Crescents in immune complex glomerulonephritis have a higher proportion of epithelial cells to macrophages than crescents in anti-GBM or ANCA glomerulonephritis, which may be related to the less severe disruption of Bowman capsule and thus less opportunity for macrophages to migrate in from the interstitium.[1040]

Immunofluorescence Microscopy
Immunofluorescence microscopy, as well as electron microscopy, provides the evidence that crescentic glomerulonephritis is immune complex mediated versus anti-GBM antibody mediated versus likely to be ANCA-associated. The pattern and composition of immunoglobulin and complement staining depends on the underlying category of immune complex glomerulonephritis that has induced crescent formation.[441,619,623,684,685,800,1027,1044,1046,1052–1054] For example, crescentic glomerulonephritis with predominantly mesangial IgA-dominant deposits is indicative of crescentic IgA nephropathy, C3-dominant deposits with peripheral band-like configurations suggest crescentic membranoproliferative glomerulonephritis, coarsely granular capillary wall deposits raise the possibility of crescentic post-infectious glomerulonephritis, and finely granular IgG-dominant capillary wall deposits suggest crescentic membranous glomerulopathy. The latter may be a result of concurrent anti-GBM disease, which will also cause linear GBM staining beneath the granular staining, or concurrent ANCA disease, which can be documented serologically. About a quarter of all patients with crescentic immune complex glomerulonephritis are ANCA-positive, whereas less than 5% of patients with non-crescentic immune complex glomerulonephritis are ANCA-positive. This suggests that the presence of ACA in patients with immune complex glomerulonephritis may predispose to disease that is more aggressive.

Electron Microscopy
As with the immunofluorescence microscopy, the findings by electron microscopy in patients with crescentic immune complex glomerulonephritis are dependent upon the type of immune complex disease that has induced crescent formation. The hallmark ultrastructural finding is immune complex-type electron dense deposits. These can be mesangial, subendothelial, intramembranous, subepithelial, or any combinations of these. The pattern and distribution of deposits may indicate a particular phenotype of primary crescentic immune complex glomerulonephritis, such as postinfectious, membranous, or membranoproliferative type I or II.[441,685,1052] Ultrastructural findings also may suggest that the disease is secondary to some unrecognized systemic process. For example, endothelial tubuloreticular inclusions suggest lupus nephritis, and microtubular configurations in immune deposits suggest cryoglobulinemia.

As with all types of crescentic glomerulonephritis, breaks in glomerular basement membranes usually can be identified if looked for carefully, especially in glomerular segments adjacent to crescents. Dense fibrin tactoids occur in thrombosed capillaries, in sites of fibrinoid necrosis, and in the interstices between the cells in crescents. In general, the extent of fibrin tactoid formation in areas of fibrinoid necrosis is less conspicuous in crescentic immune complex glomerulonephritis than in crescentic anti-GBM or ANCA glomerulonephritis.

Pathogenesis

Crescentic glomerulonephritis is the result of a final common pathway of glomerular injury that results in crescent formation. Multiple etiologies and pathogenic mechanisms can lead to the final common pathway, including many types of immune complex disease. The general dogma is that immune complex localization in glomerular capillary walls and mesangium, by either deposition or in situ formation or both, activates multiple inflammatory mediator systems.[237,1027,1028] This includes humoral mediator systems, such as the coagulation system, kinin system, and complement system, as well as phlogogenic cells, such as neutrophils, monocytes/macrophages, platelets, lymphocytes, endothelial cells, and mesangial cells. The activated cells also release soluble mediators, such as cytokines and chemokines. If the resultant inflammation is contained within the glomerular basement membrane, a proliferative or membranoproliferative phenotype of injury ensues with only endocapillary hypercellularity. However, if the inflammation breaks through capillary walls into Bowman space, extracapillary hypercellularity (crescent formation) results.

Complement activation has often been considered a major mediator of injury in immune complex glomerulonephritis, however, experimental data indicate the importance of Fc receptors in immune complex mediated injury.[1055,1056] For example, mice deficient for the Fc gamma R1 and Fc gamma R3 receptors have a markedly reduced capacity to develop immune complex glomerulonephritis.[1057,1058]

Treatment

The therapy for crescentic immune complex glomerulonephritis is influenced by the nature of the underlying category of immune complex glomerulonephritis. For example, acute post-streptococcal glomerulonephritis with 50% crescents might not prompt the same therapy as IgA nephropathy with 50% crescents. However, there are inadequate controlled prospective studies to guide therapy for most forms of crescentic immune complex glomerulonephritis. Some nephrologists extrapolate from the lupus nephritis experience and choose to treat patients with crescentic immune complex disease with immunosuppressive drugs which they would not use if the glomerular lesions appeared less aggressive. For example, there are advocates for treating crescentic IgA nephropathy with immunosuppressive drugs and even plasmapheresis who would not recommend such treatment for patients without crescents.[960] For the minority of patients who have idiopathic immune complex crescentic glomerulonephritis, the most common treatment is immunosuppressive therapy with pulse methylprednisolone followed by prednisone at a dose of 1 mg/kg daily, and then tapered over the second to third month to an alternate-day regimen until completely discontinued.[661,1059-1061] In patients with a rapid decline in renal function, cytotoxic agents in addition to corticosteroids may be considered. As with anti-GBM and ANCA disease, institution of immunotherapy should occur as early as possible during the course of crescentic immune complex glomerulonephritis to reduce the likelihood of reaching the irreversible stage of advanced scarring. There is evidence, however, that crescentic glomerulonephritis with an underlying immune complex proliferative glomerulonephritis is less responsive to aggressive immuno-suppressive therapy than is anti-GBM or ANCA crescentic glomerulonephritis.[960,1040]

Anti-Glomerular Basement Membrane Glomerulonephritis

Epidemiology

Anti-GBM disease accounts for about 10% to 20% of crescentic glomerulonephritides.[661,1038] This disease is characterized by circulating antibodies to the glomerular basement membrane (anti-GBM) and deposition of IgG or rarely IgA along glomerular basement membranes.[661,1040,1062-1074] Anti-GBM antibodies may be eluted from renal tissue samples from patients with anti-GBM disease, thus allowing verification that the antibodies are specific to the glomerular basement membrane.[661,1068,1072] The antibodies eluted from renal tissue bind to the same epitope of type IV collagen as the circulating anti-GBM antibodies from the same patient.[1075]

Anti-GBM disease occurs as a renal-limited disease (anti-GBM glomerulonephritis) and as a pulmonary-renal vasculitic syndrome (Goodpasture syndrome).[661,1040,1062-1074,1076] The incidence of anti-GBM disease has two peaks with respect to age. The first peak is in the second and third decade of life and the second peak is in the sixth and seventh decade. The first peak has a male preponderance and higher frequency of pulmonary hemorrhage (Goodpasture syndrome), whereas the second peak has a predominance of women who more often have renal-limited disease.

Genetic susceptibility to anti-GBM disease is associated with HLA DR2 specificity.[1077] Further analysis of the association with HLA DR2 reveals an association with the DRB1 alleles, DRB1*1501 and DQB*0602.[1078-1081] Further refinement of this association showed that polymorphic residues in the second peptide-binding region of the HLA class II antigen segregated with disease, supporting the hypothesis that the HLA association in GBM disease reflects the ability of certain class II molecules to bind and present anti-GBM peptides to T helper cells.[1078] This concept is further supported by mouse models of anti-GBM disease in which crescentic glomerulonephritis and lung hemorrhage are restricted to only certain MHC haplotypes, despite the ability of mice of all haplotypes to produce anti-alpha 3 NC1 antibodies.[1082]

Pathology

Immunofluorescence Microscopy

The pathologic finding of linear staining of the glomerular basement membranes for immunoglobulin is indicative of anti-GBM glomerulonephritis (Fig. 30–32).[1069,1072,1073,1083-1086] This is predominantly IgG, however, rare patients with IgA-dominant anti-GBM glomerulonephritis have also been reported.[1070,1087] Linear staining for both kappa and lambda light chains typically accompanies the staining for gamma heavy chains. Linear staining for gamma heavy chains alone indicates gamma heavy chain deposition disease. Most specimens with anti-GBM glomerulonephritis have discontinuous linear to granular capillary wall staining for C3, but a minority has little or no C3 staining. Linear staining for IgG may also occur along tubular basement membranes.[1073]

The linear IgG staining of glomerular basement membranes frequently seen in patients with diabetic glomerulosclerosis and the less intense linear staining seen in older patients with hypertensive vascular disease must not be confused with anti-GBM disease. The clinical data and light microscopic findings should help make this distinction. Serologic confirmation should always be obtained to substantiate the diagnosis of anti-GBM disease.

Serologic testing for ANCA should be ordered simultaneously because a quarter to a third of patients with anti-GBM disease are also ANCA-positive, and this may modify the

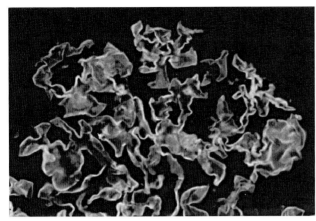

FIGURE 30–32 Immunofluorescence micrograph of a portion of a glomerulus with anti-GBM glomerulonephritis showing linear staining of glomerular basement membranes for IgG. (FITC anti-IgG, ×600.) (Modified from Ferrario F, Kourilsky O, Morel-Maroger L: Acute endocapillary glomerulonephritis in adults: A histologic and clinical comparison between patients with and without initial acute renal failure. Clin Nephrol 19:17–23, 1983, with permission.)

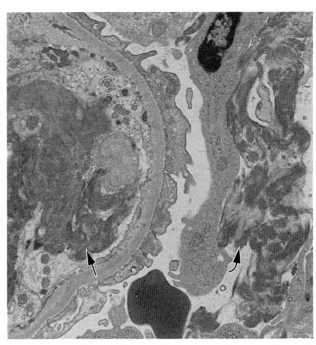

FIGURE 30–33 Electron micrograph of a portion of a glomerular capillary wall and adjacent urinary space from a patient with anti-GBM glomerulonephritis. Note the fibrin tactoids within a capillary thrombus (straight arrow) and in the Bowman space (curved arrow) between the cells of a crescent. Also note the absence of immune complex–type electron dense deposits in the capillary wall (magnification ×6000).

prognosis and the likelihood of systemic small-vessel vasculitis.[1038,1088]

Light Microscopy

At the time of biopsy, 95% of patients have some degree of crescent formation and 81% have crescents in 50% or more of glomeruli (see Table 30–17).[1028,1083] On average, 77% of glomeruli have crescents. Glomeruli with crescents typically have fibrinoid necrosis in adjacent glomerular segments. Non-necrotic segments may look entirely normal by light microscopy, or may have slight infiltration by neutrophils or mononuclear leukocytes. This differs from crescentic immune complex glomerulonephritis, which typically has capillary wall thickening and endocapillary hypercellularity in the intact glomeruli. Special stains that outline basement membranes, such a Jones silver methenamine or periodic acid-Schiff stains, often demonstrate focal breaks in glomerular basement membranes in areas of necrosis, and also show focal breaks in Bowman capsule. The most severely injured glomeruli have global glomerular necrosis, circumferential cellular crescents, and extensive disruption of Bowman capsule.

The acute necrotizing glomerular lesions and the cellular crescents evolve into glomerular sclerosis and fibrotic crescents, respectively.[1083] If the renal biopsy specimen is obtained several weeks into the course of anti-GBM disease, the only lesions may be these chronic sclerotic lesions. There may be a mixture of acute and chronic lesions; however, the glomerular lesions of anti-GBM glomerulonephritis tend to be more in synchrony than those of ANCA-glomerulonephritis, which more often show admixtures of acute and chronic injury.

Tubulointerstitial changers are commensurate with the degree of glomerular injury. Glomeruli with extensive necrosis and disruption of Bowman capsule typically have intense periglomerular inflammation, including occasional multinucleated giant cells. There also is focal tubular epithelial acute simplification or atrophy, focal interstitial edema and fibrosis, and focal interstitial infiltration of predominantly mononuclear leukocytes. There are no specific changes in arteries or arterioles. If necrotizing inflammation is observed in arteries or arterioles, the possibility of concurrent anti-GBM and ANCA disease should be considered.

Electron Microscopy

The findings by electron microscopy reflect those seen by light microscopy.[1083,1089] In acute disease, there is focal glomerular necrosis with disruption of capillary walls. Bowman capsule also may have focal gaps. Leukocytes, including neutrophils and monocytes, often are present at sites of necrosis, but are uncommon in intact glomerular segments. Fibrin tactoids, which are electron dense curvilinear accumulations of polymerized fibrin, accumulate at sites of coagulation system activation, including sites capillary thrombosis, fibrinoid necrosis and fibrin formation in Bowman space (Fig. 30–33). Cellular crescents contain cells with ultrastructural features of macrophages and epithelial cells. An important negative observation is the absence of immune complex type electron dense deposits. These occur only in anti-GBM disease patients who have concurrent immune complex disease. Glomerular segments that do not have necrosis may appear remarkably normal, with only focal effacement of visceral epithelial foot processes. There may be slight lucent expansion of the lamina rara interna, but this is an inconstant and nonspecific feature. In chronic lesions, amorphous and banded collagen deposition distorts or replaces the normal architecture.

Pathogenesis

The landmark studies opening the way to the understanding of the pathogenesis of anti-GBM disease were those of Lerner, Glassock and Dixon.[1068] In these studies, antibodies eluted from nephritic kidneys of patients with Goodpasture syndrome and injected in monkeys led to the induction of fulminant glomerulonephritis, proteinuria, renal failure, and pulmonary hemorrhage along with intense staining of the glomerular basement membrane for human IgG.

The antigen to which anti-GBM antibodies react was initially found to be in the collagenase-resistant part of type IV collagen, the "non-collagenous domain," or NC1 domain.[1090–1093] The antigenic epitopes found in the NC1 domain is in a cryptic form as evidenced by the fact that little reactivity is found against the native hexameric structure of the NC1 domain. However, when the hexameric NC1 domain is denatured and dissociates into dimers and monomers, the reactivity of antibodies increases 15-fold.[1093] On the other hand, if the antigen is reduced and alkylated, antibody binding to such denatured NC1 domain almost disappears.[1094] About 90% of anti-type IV collagen antibodies are directed against the alpha-3 chain of type IV collagen.[1060,1095] Furthermore, the majority of patients express antibody to two major conformational epitopes (EA and EB) located within the carboxyterminal non-collagenous (NC1) domain of the alpha-3 chain of type IV collagen.[1096,1097] This is further supported by inhibition assays using the monoclonal antibody to an antigenic epitope on alpha-3 (IV collagen),[1098] or with the use of a polyclonal anti-idiotype to anti-alpha-3 IV NC1 antibodies.[1099] The Goodpasture epitopes in the native autoantigen are sequestered within the NC1 hexamers of the $\alpha3\alpha4\alpha5$(IV) collagen network. The crypticity of the target epitopes is a feature of the quaternary structure of two distinct subsets of $\alpha3\alpha4\alpha5$(IV) NC1 hexamers. Goodpasture antibodies only breach the quaternary structure of hexamers containing only monomer subunits, whereas hexamers composed of both dimer and monomer subunits (D-hexamers) are resistant to autoantibodies under native conditions. The epitopes of D-hexamers are structurally sequestered by dimer reinforcement of the quaternary complex.[1100] It is presumed that environmental factors, such as exposure to hydrocarbons,[1101] tobacco smoke,[1102] and endogenous oxidants[1103] can also expose the cryptic Goodpasture epitopes. In patients with anti-GBM disease who do not have antibodies to the classic epitope on the alpha 3 chain, antibodies to entactin have been detected.[1104] A small percentage of patients with anti-GBM disease may additionally have limited reactivity with the NC1 domains of the alpha-1 or alpha-4 chains of type IV collagen. These additional reactivities seem to be more frequent in patients with anti-GBM mediated glomerulonephritis alone.[1105] Up to one third of patients with anti-GBM disease have circulating ANCA.[1045,1088,1098,1105,1106] Both anti-myeloperoxidase specific P-ANCA and anti-proteinase 3 specific C-ANCA can occur in patients with anti-GBM disease. Interestingly, no differences in the antigenic specificity of anti-GBM antibodies were detected between sera with or without concurrent expression of ANCA.[1098] Coexistence of ANCA in patients with anti-GBM antibodies is associated with small-vessel vasculitis in organs in addition to lung and kidney. In experimental models, antibodies to myeloperoxidase (MPO) aggravate experimental anti-GBM disease.[1088,1107] In a recent study comparing patients with anti-GBM, MPO-ANCA and both, patients with both anti-GBM and anti-MPO autoantibodies had a similar renal outcome as patients with anti-GBM alone, and both groups had a significantly worse renal survival than patients with MPO-ANCA alone.[1108] Patient survival at one year was best among patients with MPO-ANCA alone, although the differences did not reach statistical significance.

A number of animal models of anti-GBM disease have been developed over the years. These have been based on the immunization of animals with heterologous or homologous glomerular basement membrane as exemplified in the Steblay nephritis model.[1109] Alternatively, anti-GBM antibody induced injury has been experimentally induced passively by the intravenous injection of heterologous anti-GBM antibodies. This leads to two phases of injury. The first, or so-called heterologous phase, occurs in the first 24 hours and is mediated by the direct deposition of the heterologous antibodies on the glomerular basement membrane with subsequent recruitment of neutrophils. This is usually followed by an autologous phase, depending on the host's immune response to the heterologous immunoglobulin bound to the GBM.[1109] The rat model induced by injection of heterologous anti-GBM has permitted the study of the roles of various inflammatory mediators in the development of anti-GBM disease.[1110–1113] The more recent development of analogous murine models

of anti-GBM disease opens the way for more specific evaluations of the inflammatory processes with the use of strains of mice with specific gene "knockouts".[1082] For example, this approach has been used to assess the role of T cells in the development of anti-GBM disease. When mice of eight different strains representing the major histocompatibility complex haplotypes were immunized with purified bovine alpha-3 (IV) NC1 dimers, this led to the production of anti-alpha-3 IV NC1 antibodies in all strains of mice. However, only a subset of strains developed nephritis and lung hemorrhage. The novelty of this new murine model is that it is derived by direct immunization of mice with bovine alpha-3 chain of type IV collagen as opposed to being induced by the passive transfer of heterologous anti-GBM antibodies from other animal species or strains.

A role for T cells in the initiation or pathogenesis of anti-GBM disease is suggested by the increased susceptibility to the disease in the setting of the HLA class II antigens of the DR2 family, and more specifically, with the DRB1 alleles mentioned earlier.[1078] Further evidence of the involvement of T cell activation in the development of the autoimmune response to the NC1 domain of the alpha-3 chain of type IV collagen comes from studies of T cell proliferation in response to other monomeric components of the glomerular basement membrane[1114] and synthetic oligopeptides.[1115] Only the mouse strains capable of mounting a Th1 type response developed nephritis.[1082] The role of T cells in this model was further documented by the fact that passive transfer of lymphocytes or antibodies from nephritogenic strains to syngenetic recipients led to the development of nephritis, whereas the passive transfer of antigen antibodies to T cell receptor deficient mice failed to do so. In fact, special T cell repertoires capable of generating nephritogenic lymphocytes are critical in the development of anti-glomerular basement membrane disease.[1082]

Both TH2 and TH1 responses may occur, depending upon the host response. In TH2 prone animals, glomerular injury results because of antibody deposition, complement activation and neutrophil infiltration, whereas immune responses to the same antigen in TH1 prone mice result in a delayed hypersensitivity reaction.[1116]

The study of the role of complement activation in anti-GBM disease is largely from studies of passive injection of heterologous antibodies to GBM. This model suggests that the terminal components of the complement system are not involved in the pathogenesis of this model.[1117] Further studies in rabbits that are congenitally deficient in the sixth component of complement also suggested that the terminal components of complement do not play a major part in the pathogenesis of the disease except in leucocyte-depleted animals.[1118,1119] The role of complement cascade activation in a murine model of heterologous anti-GBM has previously led to conflicting results as to the role of complement activation in this model.[1120] More recent data using the same model in mice rendered completely deficient of complement components C3 or C4 revealed a protective effect of C3 deficiency more than that of C4 deficiency. Both the protective effects could be overcome if the dose of nephritogenic antibodies was increased.[1121] The role of complement activation in the human disease is poorly understood although it is usually along with the immunoglobulin deposits along the basement membrane.

The role of the Fc receptor in mediating glomerulonephritis has been debated. There are various Fc gamma receptors, some of which appear injurious and others protective. For instance, the Fc gamma receptor 2b is the central regulatory receptor for immunoglobulin antibody expression and function. Mice that are deficient in this receptor develop massive pulmonary hemorrhage when immunized with anti-glomerular basement membrane antibodies.[1122] In others,

Fc gamma receptors give mice anti-glomerular basement membrane disease.[1123,1124]

The role of nitric oxide radicals has been investigated in many glomerular diseases, especially anti-GBM disease. Nitrous oxide radicals generated by endothelial nitric oxide synthetase are involved in the regulation of vascular tone and inhibition of platelet aggregation and leukocyte adhesion to the endothelium. Consequently, they have an anti-inflammatory effect. In animals deficient in eNOS, glomerulonephritis is more severe, especially with capillary thrombosis and neutrophil accumulation.[1125]

In the model of heterologous transfer of anti-GBM disease, the role of macrophage infiltration in anti-GBM disease seems to be species dependent.[1126–1128] Finally, many drugs that influence T cell mediated autoimmune responses have been tried in animal models of anti-GBM disease.[1129] Nonetheless, macrophage infiltration occurs in many types of progressive renal diseases. Macrophages produce interleukin-1 beta, TNF alpha, and, in appropriate conditions, transforming growth factor beta TGF beta. Coordinated upregulation of several molecules results in additional macrophage recruitment and activation.[1130] In contrast, interleukin-10 inhibits macrophage induced glomerular injury that may attenuate macrophage-mediated glomerular disease.[1131]

Conclusions about the pathogenesis of human anti-GBM disease that are drawn from these animal models must be tempered by the realization that the animal models may not be exact replicas of the human disease.

Clinical Features and Natural History

The onset of renal anti-GBM disease is typically characterized by an abrupt, acute glomerulonephritis with severe oliguria or anuria. There is a high risk of progression to end stage renal disease if appropriate therapy is not instituted promptly. Prompt treatment with plasmapheresis, corticosteroids, and cyclophosphamide results in patient survival of approximately 85% and renal survival of approximately 60%.[1059,1132–1136]

Rarely, patients have a more insidious onset that remains essentially asymptomatic until the development of uremic symptoms and fluid retention.[661,1076,1086,1137] The onset of disease may be associated with arthralgias, fever, myalgias, and abdominal pain; however, gastrointestinal complaints or neurologic disturbances are rare.

Goodpasture syndrome is characterized by the presence of pulmonary hemorrhage concurrent with glomerulonephritis. In some patients, the pulmonary involvement may be, however, the usual pulmonary manifestation is sever pulmonary hemorrhage that may be life threatening. Pulmonary bleeding can be demonstrated early in the course of disease by the finding of unexplained anemia, careful inspection of high-quality radiographs, observation of expectorated sputum looking for the presence of hemosiderin-laden macrophages, and the serial measurement of the alveolar arterial oxygen gradient.[661,1069] In patients with anti-GBM disease, the occurrence of pulmonary hemorrhage is far more common in smokers than non-smokers.[1138] Pulmonary hemorrhage may be associated with environmental exposures to hydrocarbons[1138–1141] or other exposures, such as cocaine or upper respiratory tract infections.[1142] Occupational exposure to petroleum-based mineral oils is a risk factor for the development of anti-GBM antibodies per se.[1143] The association of pulmonary hemorrhage with environmental exposures and infection raises the theoretical possibility of exposure of the cryptic antigen in the alveolar basement membrane thus allowing for recognition by circulating anti-basement membrane antibodies.

Laboratory Findings

Renal involvement by anti-GBM disease typically causes an acute nephritic syndrome with hematuria including dysmorphic erythrocyturia and red blood cells casts. Although nephrotic-range proteinuria may occur, a full nephrotic syndrome is rarely seen.[1073,1076,1083,1086,1137]

The diagnostic laboratory finding in anti-GBM disease is detection of circulating antibodies to glomerular basement membrane, and specifically to the alpha-3 chain of type IV collagen. These antibodies are detected by radioimmunoassay or enzyme immunoassay in approximately 90% of patients. Indirect immunofluorescence microscopy assays are not sensitive enough to be adequate serologic tests for anti-GBM antibodies. The anti-GBM antibodies are most often of the IgG1 subclass, but may also be of IgG4 subclass, the latter being more often seen in females.[1144]

Treatment

The standard treatment for anti-GBM disease includes intensive plasmapheresis combined with corticosteroids and cyclophosphamide or azathioprine.[1059,1133,1145–1148] Plasmapheresis consists of removal of two to four liters of plasma with replacement with a 5% albumin solution continued on a daily basis until circulating antibody levels become undetectable. In those patients with pulmonary hemorrhage, clotting factors should be replaced by administering fresh-frozen plasma at the end of each treatment. Prednisone should be administered at a dose of 1 mg/kg of body weight for at least the first month and then tapered to alternate-day therapy during the second and third months of treatment. Cyclophosphamide is administered either orally (at a dose of 2 mg/kg/day) or intravenous cyclophosphamide is used at a starting dose of 0.5 grams/M^2 of body surface area. The dose of cyclophosphamide must be adjusted with consideration for the degree of impairment of renal function and the white blood cell count. Cytotoxic therapy is usually continued for about six to twelve months with the possibility of switching cyclophosphamide to azathioprine after three to four months in selected patients. The role of high-dose intravenous methylprednisolone pulses remains unproven in the treatment of anti-GBM disease.[1149–1153] Nonetheless, the urgent nature of the clinical process prompts some nephrologists to administer methylprednisolone as part of induction therapy in this and other forms of crescentic glomerulonephritis. A dose of 7 mg/kg of methylprednisolone given on a daily basis for three consecutive days is usually sufficient.

Using the regimen of aggressive plasmapheresis with corticosteroids and cyclophosphamide, patient survival is approximately 85% with 40% progression to end-stage renal disease.[1059,1132–1137] These results are better than those before the introduction of plasmapheresis are when patient survival was less than 50% with a near 90% rate of end-stage renal disease. In a recent study from the Hammersmith Hospital in the United Kingdom, Pusey and colleagues have demonstrated that aggressive plasmapheresis, even in patients with severe renal insufficiency, may have an ameliorative effect, and provide improved long-term patient and renal survival.[1154] In that cohort, patients who presented with a creatinine concentration of 500 mmol/L or more (>5.7 mg/dL) but did not require immediate dialysis, patient and renal survival were 83% and 82% at 1 year and 62% and 69% at last follow-up. The renal prognosis of patients who presented with dialysis-dependent renal failure was however very poor at only 8% at 1 year. All patients who required immediate dialysis and had 100% crescents on renal biopsy remained dialysis dependent.[1155]

The major prognostic marker for the progression to end-stage renal disease is the serum creatinine at the time of initiation of treatment. Patients with a serum creatinine above 7 mg/dL are unlikely to recover sufficient renal function to discontinue renal replacement therapy.[1071] At issue is whether and for how long aggressive immunosuppression should persist in dialysis-dependent patients. Aggressive immunosuppression and plasmapheresis are warranted in patients with pulmonary hemorrhage. Aggressive immunosuppression should be withheld in patients with disease limited to the kidney who present with widespread glomerular and interstitial scarring on renal biopsy and a serum creatinine greater than 7 mg/dL. In such patients, the risks of therapy outweigh the potential benefits. In those patients in whom the serum creatinine is elevated, yet on biopsy there is active crescentic glomerulonephritis, aggressive treatment should continue for at least 4 weeks. If there is no restoration of renal function by 4 to 8 weeks, and in the absence of pulmonary bleeding, immunosuppression should be discontinued.

In patients who have both circulating anti-GBM and ANCA, the chance of recovery of renal function may be better than that of patients with anti-GBM alone. In these patients, immunosuppressive therapy should not be withheld, even with serum creatinine levels above 7 mg/dL, as the concomitant presence of ANCA was associated with a more favorable renal outcome in some[1153,1156] but not all studies.[1108]

The adjunctive use of anti-coagulant therapy in addition to corticosteroids and cytotoxic agents has been considered, in part because of the pathologic finding of fibrin in the glomerular lesions. There are currently no proven benefits of such treatment. In fact, the use of heparin or warfarin may be associated with increased of pulmonary hemorrhage and its inherent morbidity and mortality.

Once remission of anti-GBM disease is achieved with immunosuppressive therapy, recurrent disease occurs only rarely.[1157–1160] Similarly, the recurrence of anti-GBM disease after renal transplantation is also rare, especially when transplantation is delayed until after disappearance or substantial diminution of anti-GBM antibody in the circulation.[1161]

Pauci-Immune Crescentic Glomerulonephritis

Epidemiology

The characteristic feature of the glomerular lesion in this category of disease is focal necrotizing and crescentic glomerulonephritis with little or no glomerular staining for immunoglobulin by immunofluorescence microscopy.[1028,1063,1146,1148,1162] Pauci-immune crescentic glomerulonephritis usually is a component of a systemic small-vessel vasculitis, however, some patients have renal-limited (primary) pauci-immune crescentic glomerulonephritis.[1028,1037,1038,1163] ANCA-associated small-vessel vasculitis is discussed in more detail in Chapter 33. Pauci-immune crescentic glomerulonephritis, including that accompanying small-vessel vasculitis, is the most common category of RPGN in adults (see Table 30–15), especially older adults (see Table 30–16). There is a predilection for whites compared to blacks (see Table 30–14). There is no sex preference (see Table 30–14).

Pathology
Light Microscopy

The light microscopic appearance of ANCA-associated pauci-immune crescentic glomerulonephritis is indistinguishable from that of anti-GBM crescentic glomerulonephritis.[441,684,1032,1039,1040,1163–1165] Renal-limited (primary) pauci-immune crescentic glomerulonephritis also is indistinguishable from pauci-immune crescentic glomerulonephritis that occurs as a component of a systemic small-vessel vasculitis, such as Wegener granulomatosis, microscopic polyangiitis, or Churg-Strauss syndrome. As illustrated in Figure 30–18, ANCA glomerulonephritis and anti-GBM glomerulonephritis most often manifest as crescentic glomerulonephritis.

At the time of biopsy, approximately 90% of renal biopsy specimens with ANCA-associated pauci-immune glomerulo-

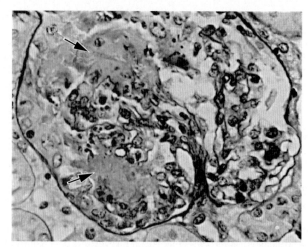

FIGURE 30–34 Light micrograph showing segmental fibrinoid necrosis in a glomerulus from a patient with antineutrophil cytoplasmic antibody–associated pauci-immune crescentic glomerulonephritis. (PAS, ×300.)

nephritis have some degree of crescent formation, and approximately half of the specimens have crescents involving 50% or more of glomeruli (see Table 30–18). Over 90% of specimens have focal segmental to global fibrinoid necrosis (Fig. 30–34). As with anti-GBM disease, the intact glomerular segments often have no light microscopic abnormalities. The most severely injured glomeruli have not only extensive necrosis of glomerular tufts but also extensive lysis of Bowman capsule with resultant periglomerular inflammation. The periglomerular inflammation contains varying mixtures of neutrophils, eosinophils, lymphocytes, monocytes and macrophages, including occasional multinucleated giant cells. This periglomerular inflammation may have a granulomatous appearance, especially when the glomerulus that was the nidus of inflammation has been destroyed or is not in the plane of section. This granulomatous appearance is a result of the periglomerular reaction to extensive glomerular necrosis and is not specific for a particular category of necrotizing glomerulonephritis. This pattern of injury can be seen with anti-GBM glomerulonephritis, renal-limited pauci-immune crescentic glomerulonephritis, and crescentic glomerulonephritis secondary to microscopic polyangiitis, Wegener granulomatosis, and Churg-Strauss syndrome. Necrotizing granulomatous inflammation that is not centered on a glomerulus, but rather is in the interstitium or centered on an artery raises the possibility of Wegener granulomatosis or Churg-Strauss syndrome. The presence of arteritis in a biopsy specimen that has pauci-immune crescentic glomerulonephritis indicates that the glomerulonephritis is a component of a more widespread vasculitis, such as microscopic polyangiitis, Wegener granulomatosis, or Churg-Strauss syndrome.

The acute necrotizing glomerular lesions evolve into sclerotic lesions. During completely quiescent phases, a renal biopsy specimen may have only focal sclerotic lesions that may mimic focal segmental glomerulosclerosis. ANCA-associated glomerulonephritis often has many recurrent bouts of exacerbation. Therefore, combinations of active acute necrotizing glomerular lesions and chronic sclerotic lesions often occur in the same renal biopsy specimen.

Immunofluorescence Microscopy

By definition, the distinguishing pathologic difference between pauci-immune crescentic glomerulonephritis and anti-GBM and immune complex crescentic glomerulonephritis is the absence or paucity of glomerular staining for immunoglobulins. How pauci-immune is pauci-immune crescentic glomerulonephritis? One basis for the categorization as pauci-immune crescentic glomerulonephritis is to identify patients who are likely to be ANCA-positive, which increases the likelihood of certain systemic small-vessel vasculitides.[446,1037,1038,1163] The likelihood of a positive ANCA is inversely proportional to the intensity of glomerular immunoglobulin staining by immunofluorescence microscopy in a specimen with crescentic glomerulonephritis.[1165] The likelihood of a positive ANCA serologic assay is approximately 90% if there is no staining for immunoglobulin, approximately 80% if there is trace to 1+ staining (on a scale of 0 to 4+), approximately 50% if there is 2+ staining, approximately 30% if there is 3+ staining, and less than 10% if there is 4+ staining. Therefore, even patients with definite evidence for immune complex glomerulonephritis have a higher than expected frequency of ANCA, but the highest frequency is in those patients with little or no evidence for immune complex or anti-GBM mediated disease. The presence of ANCA at higher than expected frequency in immune complex disease is intriguing, and raises the possibility that ANCA is contributing to the pathogenesis of not only pauci-immune crescentic glomerulonephritis but also the most severe examples of immune complex disease.[446] Looking at this issue from a different perspective, approximately 25% of patients with idiopathic immune complex crescentic glomerulonephritis (i.e., immune complex glomerulonephritis that does not fit well into one of the categories of primary or secondary immune complex disease) are ANCA positive, compared to less than 5% of patients who have idiopathic immune complex glomerulonephritis with no crescents.[446]

Glomerular capillary wall or mesangial staining usually accompanies immunoglobulin staining and is present in occasional specimens that do not have immunoglobulin staining. There is irregular staining for fibrin at sites of intraglomerular fibrinoid necrosis and capillary thrombosis, and in the interstices of crescents. Foci of glomerular necrosis and sclerosis also may have irregular staining for C3 and IgM.

Electron Microscopy

The findings by electron microscopy are indistinguishable from those described earlier for anti-GBM glomerulonephritis.[1089] Specimens with pure pauci-immune crescentic glomerulonephritis have no immune complex type electron dense deposits. Foci of glomerular necrosis have leukocyte influx, breaks in glomerular basement membranes, and fibrin tactoids in capillary thrombi and sites of fibrinoid necrosis. Sclerotic areas have effacement by amorphous of banded collagen.

Pathogenesis

The pathogenesis of pauci-immune crescentic glomerulonephritis is currently not fully understood.[1166,1167] In the absence or paucity of immune complex deposition within glomeruli or other vessels, it is difficult to implicate classic mechanisms of immune complex mediated damage in the pathogenesis of pauci-immune crescentic glomerulonephritis. On the other hand, the substantial accumulation of polymorphonuclear leukocytes at the sites of vascular necrosis has led to the study of the role of neutrophil activation in this disease. There is now convincing evidence that ANCA are directly involved in the pathogenesis of pauci-immune small-vessel vasculitis or glomerulonephritis. Substantial *in vitro* data implicates a pathogenic role for ANCA based on the demonstration that these autoantibodies activate normal human polymorphonuclear leukocytes.[1165,1166,1168] In order for anti-MPO, anti-PR3, or autoantibodies to other neutrophil antigens contained within the azurophilic granules[1169] to interact with their corresponding antigens, the antibodies have either to penetrate the cell or alternatively those antigens must translocate to the cell surface. Indeed, small amounts of cytokine (e.g., TNF and interleukin-1) at concentrations too low to cause full neutrophil activation, are capable of inducing such a translocation of ANCA antigens to the cell surface.[1170] This translocation of ANCA antigens to the cell surface has been demonstrated *in vivo* on the neutrophils of patients with Wegener granulomatosis or in patients with sepsis.[1171-1173] In the presence of circulating ANCA, the interaction of the autoantibody with their externalized antigen results in full activation of the neutrophil leading to the respiratory burst and degranulation of primary and secondary granule constituents.[1173,1174] The current hypothesis stipulates that ANCA induce a premature degranulation and activation of neutrophil at the time of their margination and diapedesis, leading to the release of lytic enzymes and toxic oxygen metabolites at the site of the vessel wall, thus producing a necrotizing inflammatory injury. This paradigm is supported by *in vitro* studies demonstrating that neutrophils activated by ANCA lead to the damage and destruction of human umbilical vein endothelial cells in culture.[1175,1176]

In addition to direct damage of the endothelium by neutrophil degranulation, ANCA antigens released from neutrophils and monocytes enter endothelial cells and cause cell damage. PR3 can enter the endothelial cells by a receptor-mediated process[1177-1179] and result in the production of IL-8 production[1180] and chemoattractant protein-1. PR3 also induces an apoptotic event from both proteolytic and non-proteolytic mechanisms.[1181,1182] Similarly, MPO enters endothelial cells by an energy-dependent process,[1183] and transcytoses intact endothelium to localize within the extracellular matrix. There, in the presence of the substrates H_2O_2 and NO_2-, MPO catalyzes nitration of tyrosine residues on extracellular matrix proteins,[1184] resulting in the fragmentation of extracellular matrix protein.[1185] However, a recent study suggests that endothelial cells inhibit superoxide generation by ANCA-activated neutrophils, and that serine proteases may play a more important role than reactive oxygen species as mediators of endothelial injury during ANCA-associated systemic vasculitis.[1186]

Neutrophil activation by ANCA is likely mediated by both the antigen binding portion of the autoantibodies (F(ab')2) and by the engagement of their Fc fraction to Fc gamma receptors on the surface of neutrophils.[1169,1176,1187,1188] Human neutrophils constitutively express the IgG receptors Fc gamma RIIa and Fc gamma RIIIb.[1189] Engagement of the Fc receptors results in a number of neutrophil-activation events, including respiratory burst, degranulation, phagocytosis, cytokine production, and upregulation of adhesion molecules. ANCA have been shown to engage both types of receptors.[1176,1190] In particular, FcgammaRIIa engagement by ANCA appears to increase neutrophil actin polymerization leading to distortion in their shape and possibly decreasing their ability to pass through capillaries (the primary site of injury in ANCA vasculitis).[1191] Furthermore, polymorphisms of the Fc gamma RIIIb receptors[1192,1193] (but not of Fc gammaRII[1194,1195]) appear to influence the severity of ANCA-vasculitis. In addition to the Fc receptor–mediated mechanism, substantial data supports a role for the F(ab')$_2$ portion of the antibody molecule in leukocyte activation. ANCA F(ab')$_2$ induce oxygen radical production[1188] and the transcription of cytokine genes in normal human neutrophils and monocytes. Microarray gene chip analysis showed that ANCA IgG and ANCA-F(ab')2 stimulate transcription of a distinct subset of genes, some unique to whole IgG, some unique to F(ab')2 fragments, and some common to both.[1196] It is most likely that F(ab')$_2$ portions of ANCA are capable of low-level neutrophil and monocyte activation.[1188] The Fc portion of the molecule almost certainly causes leukocyte activation once the F(ab')$_2$ portion of the immunoglobulin has interacted with the antigen, either on the cell surface or in the microenvironment.[1176] Recently, the signal transduction pathways of F(ab')2 and Fc receptor activation through a specific p21ras (Kristen-ras) pathway were elucidated.[1197]

The role of T cells in the pathogenesis of pauci-immune necrotizing small-vessel vasculitis or glomerulonephritis, although suspected,[1198,1199] is less well-defined. This role is suggested by the presence of CD4 positive T cells in the granulomatous[1200] and active vasculitic lesions,[1201-1205] and by some correlation of soluble markers of T cell activation with disease activity,[1200,1206] specifically, soluble interleukin-2 receptor and sCD3.[1207,1208] Also, leukocytes isolated from patients with Wegener granulomatosis and anti-PR3 antibodies have been shown to proliferate in response to crude neutrophil extracts that contain PR3 or to purified PR3,[1208-1212] whereas T cells from patients with MPO-ANCA did not have a similar proliferative response to MPO.[1213]

Further establishment of a pathogenetic role between ANCA and the development of pauci-immune necrotizing glomerulonephritis and small-vessel vasculitis greatly benefited from the development of animal models of this disease.

Early models of disease were based on the finding of circulating anti-MPO antibodies in 20% of female MRL/lpr/lpr mice,[1214] and in an inbred strain of mice, SCG/Kj, derived from the MRL/lpr mice and BXSB strains that develop a severe form of crescentic glomerulonephritis and a systemic necrotizing vasculitis.[1215] Anti-MPO antibodies have been isolated from these strains of mice. Treatment of rats with mercuric chloride led to the development of widespread inflammation, including necrotizing vasculitis in the presence of anti-MPO antibodies and anti-GBM antibodies.[1216] A more convincing model implicates a pathogenetic role for ANCA. Aggravation of a mild anti-glomerular basement membrane mediated glomerulonephritis in the rat when the animals were previously immunized with myeloperoxidase[1107] suggests that minor pro-inflammatory events could be driven to severe necrotizing processes in the presence of ANCA.

Compelling models for ANCA small-vessel vasculitis were recently described. Myeloperoxidase knockout mice were immunized with murine myeloperoxidase. Splenocytes from these mice were transferred to immunoincompetent Rag'2 resulting in the development of anti-MPO antibodies, a severe necrotizing and crescentic glomerulonephritis and, in some animals, vasculitis in the lung and other organ systems. In a separate but similar set of experiments, anti-MPO antibodies alone (not splenocytes) were transferred into Rag'2–/– mice. These mice developed a pauci-immune necrotizing and crescentic glomerulonephritis.[1217] These studies indicate that anti-MPO antibodies cause pauci-immune necrotizing disease. This disease process occurred without antigen-driven T cells.[1218] The glomerulonephritis induced by anti-MPO antibodies is aggravated by the administration of LPS into recipient mice.[1219] Conversely, the disease was abrogated when the neutrophils of anti-MPO recipient mice were depleted by a selective anti-neutrophil monoclonal antibody (NIMP-R14).[1220] In experiments to assess the role of T cells using this animal model, the transfer of T cell enriched splenocytes (>99% T cells) did not cause glomerular crescent formation or vascular necrosis. These data do not support a pathogenic role for anti-MPO T cells in the induction of acute injury.[1221]

The pathogenic role of anti-MPO antibodies is also documented in a second animal model whereby rats immunized with human MPO developed anti-rat-MPO antibodies and a necrotizing and crescentic glomerulonephritis, as well as pulmonary capillaritis.[1222] These two animal models document that anti-MPO antibodies are capable of causing a necrotizing and crescentic glomerulonephritis and a widespread systemic vasculitis. A model of anti-PR3-induced vascular injury was developed in proteinase 3/neutrophil elastase-deficient mice

whereby the passive transfer of murine anti-mouse PR3 was associated with a stronger localized cutaneous inflammation and perivascular infiltrates were observed around cutaneous vessels at the sites of intradermal injection of tumor necrosis factor alpha.[1221,1223] In summary, these animal studies document that both anti-MPO and proteinase-3 antibodies are capable of causing disease.

As is true for most autoimmune responses, the inciting events in the breakdown of tolerance and the generation of anti-MPO or anti-PR3 antibodies are not known. Although genetic predispositions,[1224] environmental exposure to foreign pathogens,[1225] and notably to silica[1226,1227] have been implicated, no direct link between these exposure and the formation of ANCA has been established. A serendipitous finding in ANCA vasculitis has spawned a theory of autoantigen complementarity.[1228,1229] This theory rests on evidence that proteins transcribed and translated from the sense strand of DNA bind to proteins that are transcribed and translated from the anti-sense strand of DNA. It has been recently demonstrated that some patients with PR3-ANCA harbor antibodies to an antigen complementary to the middle portion of PR3. These anti-complementary PR3 antibodies form an anti-idiotypic pair with PR3-ANCA. Moreover, cloned complementary PR3 proteins bind to PR3 and function as a serine proteinase inhibitor. Preliminary data suggest that the complementary PR3 antigens are found on a variety of microbes, some of which have been associated with ANCA vasculitis and also found in the genome of some patients with both PR3- and MPO-ANCA.[1229] While these studies need to be confirmed and expanded to determine the source of the complementary PR3 antigen and their role (if any) in inducing vasculitis, these observations may provide a promising avenue for the detection of the proximate cause of the ANCA autoimmune response.

Clinical Features and Natural History

The majority of patients with pauci-immune necrotizing crescentic glomerulonephritis and ANCA have glomerular disease as part of a systemic small-vessel vasculitis. The disease is clinically limited to the kidney in about one-third of patients.[1230] When both renal-limited and vasculitis-associated pauci-immune crescentic glomerulonephritis are considered, this category of crescentic glomerulonephritis is the most common cause of rapidly progressive glomerulonephritis in adults.[1028,1034,1038,1230,1231] When part of a systemic vasculitis, patients may present with a pulmonary-renal, dermal-renal, or a multisystem disease. Frequent sites of involvement include the lungs, upper airways, sinuses, ears, eyes, gastrointestinal tract, skin, peripheral nerves, joints, and central nervous system. The three major ANCA-associated syndromes are microscopic polyangiitis, Wegener granulomatosis, and the Churg-Strauss syndrome.[1039,1050,1232] Even when the patients have no clinical evidence of extra renal manifestation of active vasculitis, systemic symptoms consisting of fever, fatigue, myalgias and arthralgias are common.

Although most patients with ANCA-associated pauci-immune necrotizing glomerulonephritis have RPGN with rapid loss of renal function associated with hematuria, proteinuria, and hypertension, some patients follow a more indolent course of slow decline in function and less active urine sediment. In the latter group of patients, episodes of focal necrosis and hematuria resolve with focal glomerular scarring. Subsequent relapses result in cumulative damage to glomeruli.

It is important to note that patients presenting with pauci-immune crescentic glomerulonephritis alone may later develop signs and symptoms of systemic disease with involvement of extra renal organ systems.[1233] An autopsy study was conducted in patients with ANCA-associated vasculitis. This study revealed the widespread presence of glomerulonephritis, but also demonstrated the finding of clinically silent extrarenal vasculitis. Eight percent of patients died either from septic infections or from progressive recurrent vasculitis.[1233]

No studies currently available specifically examine the prognostic factors of pauci-immune crescentic glomerulonephritis in the absence of extra-renal manifestations of disease. In studies addressing the question of prognosis of patients with ANCA small-vessel vasculitis in general,[1037,1233,1234] the presence of pulmonary hemorrhage was the most important determinant of patient survival. With respect to the risk of end-stage renal disease, the most important predictor of outcome is the entry serum creatinine at the time of initiation of treatment.[1234] This parameter remained the most important predictive factor of renal outcome in a multivariate analysis correcting for such variables as the presence or absence of extra-renal disease. Treatment resistance and progression to end-stage kidney disease is also predicted by the presence of greater disease chronicity and vascular sclerosis on renal biopsy (presence of glomerular sclerosis, interstitial infiltrates, tubular necrosis, and atrophy,[1235] and clinical markers of chronic disease including cumulative organ damage (measured by the Vasculitis Damage Index).[1236] Vascular sclerosis on biopsy was also found to be an independent predictor of treatment resistance[1237] and may be a reflection of chronic renal damage due to hypertension or other atherosclerotic processes, with ANCA-associated nephritis inducing an additional insult. The impact of renal damage as a predictor of resistance emphasizes the importance of early diagnosis and prompt institution of therapy. It is important to note that while the entry serum creatinine is the most important predictor of renal outcome, there is no threshold of renal dysfunction for which treatment is deemed futile, as more than half the patients presenting with a GFR less than 10 ml/min may reach a remission and have a substantial improvement in renal function. Therefore, aggressive immunosuppressive therapy in all newly diagnosed patients is warranted.[1237] However, the risk of progression to ESKD is also determined by the change in GFR within the first 4 months of treatment. In the absence of other disease manifestations, the decision to continue immunosuppressive therapy among patients with sharply declining GFR should be weighed against the diminishing chance of renal recovery.[1237]

Relapses of ANCA small-vessel vasculitis occurs in up to 40% of patients. Based on a large cohort study of patients, the risk of relapse appears to be predicted by the presence of PR3-ANCA (as opposed to MPO-ANCA) and the presence of upper-respiratory tract or lung involvement.[1237] Patients with glomerulonephritis alone, who predominantly have an MPO-ANCA would therefore belong to the subgroup of patients with a relatively low risk of relapse—with a rate of relapse around 25% in a median of 62 months.

Pauci-immune necrotizing glomerulonephritis and small-vessel vasculitis may recur after renal transplantation.[1238,1239] The rate of recurrence for ANCA small-vessel vasculitis in general, including pauci-immune necrotizing glomerulonephritis alone, is about 20%.[1240] The rate of recurrence in the subset of patients who have pauci-immune necrotizing glomerulonephritis alone without systemic vasculitis is unknown, but may be lower than 20%. A positive ANCA test at the time of transplantation does not seem to be associated with an increased risk of recurrent disease.

Laboratory Findings
Approximately 80% to 90% of patients with pauci-immune necrotizing and crescentic glomerulonephritis will have circulating ANCA.[446,1037,1050,1167,1241–1243] By indirect immunofluorescence microscopy on alcohol fixed neutrophils, ANCA cause two patterns of staining; perinuclear (P-ANCA) and cytoplasmic (C-ANCA).[1167,1243] The two major antigen specificities for ANCA are myeloperoxidase (MPO) and proteinase 3 (PR3).[1163,1243–1247] Both proteins are found in the primary granules of neutrophils and the lysosomes of monocytes. With rare exceptions, anti-MPO antibodies produce a P-ANCA pattern of staining on indirect immunofluorescence microscopy, whereas anti-PR3 antibodies cause a C-ANCA pattern of staining. About two-thirds of patients with pauci-immune necrotizing crescentic glomerulonephritis without clinical evidence of systemic vasculitis will have MPO-ANCA or P-ANCA, and approximately 30% will have PR3-ANCA or C-ANCA.[1039,1248] The relative frequency of MPO-ANCA to PR3-ANCA is higher in patients with renal-limited disease than in patients with microscopic polyangiitis or Wegener granulomatosis.[1039] As mentioned previously, about one third of patients with anti-GBM disease and approximately a quarter of patients with idiopathic immune complex crescent glomerulonephritis are ANCA positive, therefore, ANCA-positivity is not completely specific for pauci-immune crescentic glomerulonephritis.[446] Maximal sensitivity and specificity with ANCA testing is best performed when both immunofluorescence and antigen-specific assays are performed. Antigen-specific assays may be either an ELISA or radioimmune assay. A variety of commercial tests are now available, and their diagnostic specificity ranges from 70% to 90%, and sensitivity from 81% to 91%.[446,1249] Tests still do not provide the necessary sensitivity/specificity and predictive power to use them as the basis for initiating or altering cytotoxic therapy.

The positive predictive value (PPV) of a positive ANCA result (i.e., the percent of positive patients who have pauci-immune crescentic glomerulonephritis) depends on the signs and symptoms of disease in the patient who is tested. The signs and symptoms indicate the pretest likelihood of pauci-immune crescentic glomerulonephritis (predicted prevalence), which greatly influences predictive value. The PPV of a positive ANCA result in a patient with classic features of RPGN is 95%.[446] In patients with hematuria and proteinuria, the PPV of a positive ANCA result is 84% if the serum creatinine is >3 mg/dL, 60% if the serum creatinine is 1.5 to 3.0 mg/dL, and only 29% if the serum creatinine is less than 1 mg/dL.[1250] Although the PPV is not good in this last setting, the negative predictive value is greater than 95% and thus a negative result can allay any concerns that the patient has early or mild pauci-immune necrotizing glomerulonephritis.

Urinalysis findings in pauci-immune crescentic glomerulonephritis include hematuria with dysmorphic red blood cells, with or without red cell casts, and proteinuria. The proteinuria ranges from 1 gram/24 hours to as much as 16 grams/24 hours.[1233,1251] Serum creatinine usually is elevated at the time of diagnosis and rising, although a minority of patients will have relatively indolent disease. ESR and C-reactive protein are elevated during active disease. Serum complement component levels are typically within normal limits.

Whether a renal biopsy is essential for the management of ANCA-associated pauci-immune glomerulonephritis depends on a number of factors, including the diagnostic accuracy of ANCA testing, the pre-test probability of finding pauci-immune glomerulonephritis, the value of knowing the activity and chronicity of the renal lesions, and the risk associated with immunotherapy of ANCA pauci-immune necrotizing glomerulonephritis. Based on a study of 1000 patients with proliferative and/or necrotizing glomerulonephritis and a positive test for either PR3-ANCA or MPO-ANCA, the positive predictive value of ANCA testing was found to be 86% with a false positive rate of 14% and a false negative rate of 16%. Considering the serious risks inherent to treatment with high-dose corticosteroids and cytotoxic agents, it is prudent to confirm the diagnosis and characterize the activity and chronicity of ANCA-associated pauci-immune crescentic glomerulonephritis by renal biopsy unless the patient is too ill to tolerate the procedure.[1250]

Treatment

The treatment of pauci-immune crescentic glomerulonephritis remains varying regimens of corticosteroids and cyclophosphamide.[1234,1252,1253] In view of the potential explosive and fulminant nature of this disease, induction therapy should be instituted using pulse methylprednisolone at a dose of 7 mg/kg/day for three consecutive days in an attempt to halt the aggressive, destructive, inflammatory process. This is followed by the institution of daily oral prednisone, as well as cyclophosphamide, either orally or intravenously. Prednisone is usually started at a dose of 1 mg/kg/day for the first month, then tapered to an alternate-day regimen, and then discontinued by the end of the third to fourth month of treatment. When a regimen of monthly intravenous doses of cyclophosphamide is used, the starting dose should be about 0.5 grams/M^2 and adjusted upward to 1 gram/M^2 based on the two-week leukocyte count nadir.[1216,1253] A regimen based on daily oral cyclophosphamide should begin at a dose of 2 mg/kg/day[1252] and is adjusted downward as needed to keep a nadir leukocyte count above 3000 cells/mm³.

The optimal length of therapy with cyclophosphamide remains to be determined. Typically, patients are treated for 6 to 12 months, at which time it is reasonable to discontinue the cyclophosphamide in patients who are in remission. For patients who have not achieved the remission by that time, continuing a longer duration is a reasonable approach. In some patients, the monthly intravenous regimen is not sufficiently immunosuppressive necessitating daily oral cyclophosphamide treatment (which results in a higher cumulative dosage). For patients who attain an early complete remission with cyclophosphamide, it is possible to switch therapy after three months to Azathioprine, 2 mg/kg/day for an additional eighteen months.[1110] This approach appears as effective as 12 months of oral cyclophosphamide followed by 12 months of azathioprine based on renal function, and the frequency of relapse.

In three randomized control trials addressing the role of plasmapheresis in the treatment of ANCA-associated small-vessel vasculitis and glomerulonephritis,[1254–1256] plasmapheresis was not found to provide any added benefit over immunosuppressive treatment alone in patients with renal limited disease or in patients with mild to moderate renal dysfunction. However, the use of plasmapheresis in addition to immunosuppressive therapy appears to be beneficial in the subset of patients who require dialysis at the time of presentation.[1256,1257] In a study performed by a European vasculitis study group, the use of pulse plasma exchange was found to be superior to pulse methylprednisolone in recovery of renal function among patients with severe renal dysfunction at the time of entry into study (serum creatinine >500 micromols [5.7 mg/dl]).[1258] Patients who eventually come off dialysis usually do so within twelve weeks of initiation of therapy.[1216] For this reason, continuing immunosuppressive therapy beyond twelve weeks in a patient who is still on dialysis is unlikely to be of added benefit (unless they continue to have extra-renal manifestations of vasculitis). Because of the clinically observed increased risk of severe bone marrow suppression with the use of cyclophosphamide in patients on dialysis, such treatment should be pursued with extreme caution.

Although high-dose intravenous pooled immunoglobulin has been used in the treatment of systemic vasculitis resistant to usual immunosuppressive treatment,[1259–1264] there are no published reports of its use in patients with pauci-immune crescentic glomerulonephritis alone without systemic involvement.

Trimethoprim sulfamethoxazole has been suggested to be of benefit in the treatment of patients with Wegener granulomatosis.[1265,1266] Such beneficial effects, if any, seem to be limited to the upper respiratory tract and this antibiotic are unlikely to have a role in the treatment of pauci-immune crescentic glomerulonephritis alone. Methotrexate has been used in the treatment of patients with Wegener granulomatosis who did not have immediately life-threatening pulmonary or renal disease.[1267,1268] The dose of methotrexate must be reduced in patients whose creatinine clearance is less than 80 ml/min, and its use is contraindicated when creatinine clearances are less than 10 ml/min. Moreover, in our experience there are patients on methotrexate who have progressive glomerulonephritis. Methotrexate is, therefore, unlikely to have any role in the treatment of pauci-immune crescentic glomerulonephritis alone.

Recently, other agents including rituximab,[1269–1272] alemtuzumab (Campath H1),[1273] and infliximab[1274–1277] have been evaluated in small studies for the management of patients resistant to conventional therapy with glucocorticoids and cyclophosphamide. These studies were performed among patients with Wegener granulomatosis or microscopic polyangiitis rather than patients with isolated pauci-immune necrotizing glomerulonephritis alone. Whether the use of such agents is indicated or beneficial among patients with glomerulonephritis is currently unknown. Similarly, the studies pertaining to maintenance immunosuppression for the prevention of relapse are primarily geared to patients with Wegener granulomatosis or microscopic polyangiitis. Current data suggest that patients with pauci-immune glomerulonephritis alone and MPO-ANCA are at a relatively low risk of relapse. The value of prolonged maintenance immunosuppression in this group of patients is unknown, and any benefit in preventing a relapse would have to be weighed against the potential toxicity and risks associated with immunosuppressive agents.

The diagnosis and management of ANCA-associated small-vessel vasculitis is discussed in more detail in Chapter 31.

References

1. Brenner BM, Hostetter TH, Humes HD: Glomerular permselectivity: Barrier function based on discrimination of molecular size and charge. Am J Physiol 234:F455–F460, 1978.
2. Shemesh O, Deen WM, Brenner BM, et al: Effect of colloid volume expansion on glomerular barrier size-selectivity in humans. Kidney Int 29:916–923, 1986.
3. Brenner BM, Bohrer MP, Baylis C, Deen WM: Determinants of glomerular permselectivity: Insights derived from observations in vivo. Kidney Int 12:229–237, 1977.
4. Levidiotis V, Freeman C, Tikellis C, et al: Heparanase is involved in the pathogenesis of proteinuria as a result of glomerulonephritis. J Am Soc Nephrol 15:68–78, 2004.
5. Jeansson M, Haraldsson B: Glomerular size and charge selectivity in the mouse after exposure to glucosaminoglycan-degrading enzymes. J Am Soc Nephrol 14:1756–1765, 2003.
6. Tryggvason K, Patrakka J, Wartiovaara J: Hereditary proteinuria syndromes and mechanisms of proteinuria. N Engl J Med 354:1387–1401, 2006.
7. Bazzi C, Petrini C, Rizza V, et al: A modern approach to selectivity of proteinuria and tubulointerstitial damage in nephrotic syndrome. Kidney Int 58:1732–1741, 2000.
8. Rippe B: What is the role of albumin in proteinuric glomerulopathies? Nephrol Dial Transplant 19:1–5, 2004.
9. Brunskill NJ: Albumin signals the coming of age of proteinuric nephropathy. J Am Soc Nephrol 15:504–505, 2004.
10. Bakoush O, Torffvit O, Rippe B, Tencer J: Renal function in proteinuric glomerular diseases correlates with the changes in urine IgM excretion but not to the changes in the degree of albuminuria. Clin Nephrol 59:345–352, 2003.
11. Osicka TM, Strong KJ, Nikolic-Paterson DJ, et al: Renal processing of serum proteins in an albumin-deficient environment: An in vivo study of glomerulonephritis in the Nagase analbuminaemic rat. Nephrol Dial Transplant 19:320–328, 2004.
12. Albright R, Brensilver J, Cortell S: Proteinuria in congestive heart failure. Am J Nephrol 3:272–275, 1983.
13. Wingo CS, Clapp WL: Proteinuria: Potential causes and approach to evaluation. Am J Med Sci 320:188–194, 2000.
14. Springberg PD, Garrett LE, Jr, Thompson AL, Jr, et al: Fixed and reproducible orthostatic proteinuria: Results of a 20-year follow-up study. Ann Intern Med 97:516–519, 1982.

15. Robinson RR, Ashworth CT, Glover SN, et al: Fixed and reproducible orthostatic proteinuria. II. Electron microscopy of renal biopsy specimens from five cases. Am J Pathol 39:405–417, 1961.

16. Devarajan P: Mechanisms of orthostatic proteinuria: Lessons from a transplant donor. J Am Soc Nephrol 4:36–39, 1993.

17. Shintaku N, Takahashi Y, Akaishi K, et al: Entrapment of left renal vein in children with orthostatic proteinuria. Pediatr Nephrol 4:324–327, 1990.

18. Mariani AJ, Mariani MC, Macchioni C, et al: The significance of adult hematuria: 1000 hematuria evaluations including a risk-benefit and cost-effectiveness analysis. J Urol 141:350–355, 1989.

19. Schroder FH: Microscopic haematuria. BMJ 309:70–72, 1994.

20. Kincaid-Smith P, Fairley K: The investigation of hematuria. Semin Nephrol 25:127–135, 2005.

21. Meyers KE: Evaluation of hematuria in children. Urol Clin North Am 31:559–573, 2004.

22. Schramek P, Schuster FX, Georgopoulos M, et al: Value of urinary erythrocyte morphology in assessment of symptomless microhaematuria. Lancet 2:1316–1319, 1989.

23. Mazhari R, Kimmel PL: Hematuria: An algorithmic approach to finding the cause. Cleve Clin J Med 69:870, 872–874, 876, 2002.

24. Mohr DN, Offord KP, Owen RA, Melton LJ, III: Asymptomatic microhematuria and urologic disease. A population-based study. JAMA 256:224–229, 1986.

25. Case records of the Massachusetts General Hospital. Weekly clinicopathological exercises. Case 33–1992. A 34-year-old woman with endometriosis and bilateral hydronephrosis. N Engl J Med 327:481–485, 1992.

26. Chow KM, Kwan BC, Li PK, Szeto CC: Asymptomatic isolated microscopic haematuria: Long-term follow-up. Q J Med 97:739–745, 2004.

27. Murakami S, Igarashi T, Hara S, Shimazaki J: Strategies for asymptomatic microscopic hematuria: A prospective study of 1034 patients. J Urol 144:99–101, 1990.

28. Britton JP, Dowell AC, Whelan P: Dipstick haematuria and bladder cancer in men over 60: Results of a community study. BMJ 299:1010–1012, 1989.

29. Topham PS, Harper SJ, Furness PN, et al: Glomerular disease as a cause of isolated microscopic haematuria. Q J Med 87:329–335, 1994.

30. Tiebosch AT, Frederik PM, Breda Vriesman PJ, et al: Thin-basement-membrane nephropathy in adults with persistent hematuria. N Engl J Med 320:14–18, 1989.

31. Assadi FK: Value of urinary excretion of microalbumin in predicting glomerular lesions in children with isolated microscopic hematuria. Pediatr Nephrol 20:1131–1135, 2005.

32. Eardley KS, Ferreira MA, Howie AJ, et al: Urinary albumin excretion: A predictor of glomerular findings in adults with microscopic haematuria. Q J Med 97:297–301, 2004.

33. Richards NT, Darby S, Howie AJ, et al: Knowledge of renal histology alters patient management in over 40% of cases. Nephrol Dial Transplant 9:1255–1259, 1994.

34. Vande Walle JG, Donckerwolcke RA, van Isselt JW, et al: Volume regulation in children with early relapse of minimal-change nephrosis with or without hypovolaemic symptoms. Lancet 346:148–152, 1995.

35. Schrier RW, Fassett RG: A critique of the overfill hypothesis of sodium and water retention in the nephrotic syndrome. Kidney Int 53:1111–1117, 1998.

36. Plum J, Mirzaian Y, Grabensee B: Atrial natriuretic peptide, sodium retention, and proteinuria in nephrotic syndrome. Nephrol Dial Transplant 11:1034–1042, 1996.

37. Noddeland H, Riisnes SM, Fadnes HO: Interstitial fluid colloid osmotic and hydrostatic pressures in subcutaneous tissue of patients with nephrotic syndrome. Scand J Clin Lab Invest 42:139–146, 1982.

38. Joles JA, Rabelink TJ, Braam B, Koomans HA: Plasma volume regulation: Defences against edema formation (with special emphasis on hypoproteinemia). Am J Nephrol 13:399–412, 1993.

39. Geers AB, Koomans HA, Roos JC, et al: Functional relationships in the nephrotic syndrome. Kidney Int 26:324–330, 1984.

40. Kuster S, Mehls O, Seidel C, Ritz E: Blood pressure in minimal change and other types of nephrotic syndrome. Am J Nephrol 10 Suppl 1:76–80, 1990.

41. Vande W, Donckerwolcke RA, van I, et al: Volume regulation in children with early relapse of minimal-change nephrosis with or without hypovolaemic symptoms. Lancet 346:148–152, 1995.

42. Rodriguez-Iturbe B, Colic D, Parra G, Gutkowska J: Atrial natriuretic factor in the acute nephritic and nephrotic syndromes. Kidney Int 38:512–517, 1990.

43. Brown EA, Markandu ND, Sagnella GA, et al: Lack of effect of captopril on the sodium retention of the nephrotic syndrome. Nephron 37:43–48, 1984.

44. Brown EA, Markandu ND, Roulston JE, et al: Is the renin-angiotensin-aldosterone system involved in the sodium retention in the nephrotic syndrome? Nephron 32:102–107, 1982.

45. Brown EA, Markandu ND, Sagnella GA, et al: Evidence that some mechanism other than the renin system causes sodium retention in nephrotic syndrome. Lancet 2:1237–1240, 1982.

46. Dusing R, Vetter H, Kramer HJ: The renin-angiotensin-aldosterone system in patients with nephrotic syndrome: Effects of 1-sar-8-ala-angiotensin II. Nephron 25:187–192, 1980.

47. Lewis DM, Tooke JE, Beaman M, et al: Peripheral microvascular parameters in the nephrotic syndrome. Kidney Int 54:1261–1266, 1998.

48. Crew RJ, Radhakrishnan J, Appel G: Complications of the nephrotic syndrome and their treatment. Clin Nephrol 62:245–259, 2004.

49. Vande W, Donckerwolcke RA, van I, et al: Volume regulation in children with early relapse of minimal-change nephrosis with or without hypovolaemic symptoms. Lancet 346:148–152, 1995.

50. Kirchner KA, Voelker JR, Brater DC: Binding inhibitors restore furosemide potency in tubule fluid containing albumin. Kidney Int 40:418–424, 1991.

51. Agarwal R, Gorski JC, Sundblad K, Brater DC: Urinary protein binding does not affect response to furosemide in patients with nephrotic syndrome. J Am Soc Nephrol 11:1100–1105, 2000.

52. Davison AM, Lambie AT, Verth AH, Cash JD: Salt-poor human albumin in management of nephrotic syndrome. Br Med J 1:481–484, 1974.

53. Haws RM, Baum M: Efficacy of albumin and diuretic therapy in children with nephrotic syndrome. Pediatrics 91:1142–1146, 1993.

54. Churg J, Strauss L: Allergic granulomatosis, allergic angiitis and periarteritis nodosa. Am J Pathol 27:277–301, 1951.

55. Joven J, Villabona C, Vilella E, et al: Abnormalities of lipoprotein metabolism in patients with the nephrotic syndrome. N Engl J Med 323:579–584, 1990.

56. Wheeler DC, Bernard DB: Lipid abnormalities in the nephrotic syndrome: causes, consequences, and treatment. Am J Kidney Dis 23:331–346, 1994.

57. Appel G: Lipid abnormalities in renal disease. Kidney Int 39:169–183, 1991.

58. Radhakrishnan J, Appel AS, Valeri A, Appel GB: The nephrotic syndrome, lipids, and risk factors for cardiovascular disease. Am J Kidney Dis 22:135–142, 1993.

59. Stenvinkel P, Berglund L, Heimburger O, et al: Lipoprotein(a) in nephrotic syndrome. Kidney Int 44:1116–1123, 1993.

60. Yamauchi A, Fukuhara Y, Yamamoto S, et al: Oncotic pressure regulates gene transcriptions of albumin and apolipoprotein B in cultured rat hepatoma cells. Am J Physiol 263:C397–C404, 1992.

61. Vaziri ND: Molecular mechanisms of lipid disorders in nephrotic syndrome. Kidney Int 63:1964–1976, 2003.

62. Liu AC, Lawn RM: Vascular interactions of lipoprotein (a). Curr Opin Lipidol 5:269–273, 1994.

63. De Sain-Van Der Velden MG, Reijngoud DJ, Kaysen GA, et al: Evidence for increased synthesis of lipoprotein(a) in the nephrotic syndrome. J Am Soc Nephrol 9:1474–1481, 1998.

64. McLean JW, Tomlinson JE, Kuang WJ, et al: cDNA sequence of human apolipoprotein(a) is homologous to plasminogen. Nature 330:132–137, 1987.

65. The Lipid Research Clinics Coronary Primary Prevention Trial results. I. Reduction in incidence of coronary heart disease. JAMA 251:351–364, 1984.

66. The Lipid Research Clinics Coronary Primary Prevention Trial results. II. The relationship of reduction in incidence of coronary heart disease to cholesterol lowering. JAMA 251:365–374, 1984.

67. Shepherd J, Cobbe SM, Ford I, et al: Prevention of coronary heart disease with pravastatin in men with hypercholesterolemia. West of Scotland Coronary Prevention Study Group. N Engl J Med 333:1301–1307, 1995.

68. Randomised trial of cholesterol lowering in 4444 patients with coronary heart disease: The Scandinavian Simvastatin Survival Study (4S). Lancet 344:1383–1389, 1994.

69. Sacks FM, Pfeffer MA, Moye LA, et al: The effect of pravastatin on coronary events after myocardial infarction in patients with average cholesterol levels. Cholesterol and Recurrent Events Trial investigators. N Engl J Med 335:1001–1009, 1996.

70. Summary of the second report of the National Cholesterol Education Program (NCEP) Expert Panel on Detection, Evaluation, and Treatment of High Blood Cholesterol in Adults (Adult Treatment Panel II). JAMA 269:3015–3023, 1993.

71. Law MR, Wald NJ, Thompson SG: By how much and how quickly does reduction in serum cholesterol concentration lower risk of ischaemic heart disease? BMJ 308:367–372, 1994.

72. Holme I: Relationship between total mortality and cholesterol reduction as found by meta-regression analysis of randomized cholesterol-lowering trials. Control Clin Trials 17:13–22, 1996.

73. Ordonez JD, Hiatt RA, Killebrew EJ, Fireman BH: The increased risk of coronary heart disease associated with nephrotic syndrome. Kidney Int 44:638–642, 1993.

74. Habib R: Nephrotic syndrome in the 1st year of life. Pediatr Nephrol 7:347–353, 1993.

75. Watts GF, Herrmann S, Dogra GK, et al: Vascular function of the peripheral circulation in patients with nephrosis. Kidney Int 60:182–189, 2001.

76. Dogra GK, Watts GF, Herrmann S, et al: Statin therapy improves brachial artery endothelial function in nephrotic syndrome. Kidney Int 62:550–557, 2002.

77. Hayslett JP, Krassner LS, Bensch KG, et al: Progression of "lipoid nephrosis" to renal insufficiency. N Engl J Med 281:181–187, 1969.

78. Attman PO, Samuelsson O, Alaupovic P: Progression of renal failure: Role of apolipoprotein B-containing lipoproteins. Kidney Int Suppl 63:S98–101, 1997.

79. Massy ZA, Ma JZ, Louis TA, Kasiske BL: Lipid-lowering therapy in patients with renal disease. Kidney Int 48:188–198, 1995.

80. Gentile MG, Fellin G, Cofano F, et al: Treatment of proteinuric patients with a vegetarian soy diet and fish oil. Clin Nephrol 40:315–320, 1993.

81. Valeri A, Gelfand J, Blum C, Appel GB: Treatment of the hyperlipidemia of the nephrotic syndrome: A controlled trial. Am J Kidney Dis 8:388 396, 1986.

82. Rabelink AJ, Hene RJ, Erkelens DW, et al: Effects of simvastatin and cholestyramine on lipoprotein profile in hyperlipidaemia of nephrotic syndrome. Lancet 2:1335–1338, 1988.

83. Thomas ME, Harris KP, Ramaswamy C, et al: Simvastatin therapy for hypercholesterolemic patients with nephrotic syndrome or significant proteinuria. Kidney Int 44:1124–1129, 1993.

84. Brown CD, Azrolan N, Thomas L, et al: Reduction of lipoprotein(a) following treatment with lovastatin in patients with unremitting nephrotic syndrome. Am J Kidney Dis 26:170–177, 1995.

85. Keilani T, Schlueter WA, Levin ML, Batlle DC: Improvement of lipid abnormalities associated with proteinuria using fosinopril, an angiotensin-converting enzyme inhibitor. Ann Intern Med 118:246–254, 1993.

86. Olbricht CJ, Wanner C, Thiery J, Basten A: Simvastatin in nephrotic syndrome. Simvastatin in Nephrotic Syndrome Study Group. Kidney Int Suppl 71:S113–S116, 1999.

87. de Sain van der Velden MG, Kaysen GA, de Meer K, et al: Proportionate increase of fibrinogen and albumin synthesis in nephrotic patients: Measurements with stable isotopes. Kidney Int 53:181–188, 1998.

88. Afrasiabi MA, Vaziri ND, Gwinup G, et al: Thyroid function studies in the nephrotic syndrome. Ann Intern Med 90:335–338, 1979.

89. Gavin LA, McMahon FA, Castle JN, Cavalieri RR: Alterations in serum thyroid hormones and thyroxine-binding globulin in patients with nephrosis. J Clin Endocrinol Metab 46:125–130, 1978.

90. Feinstein EI, Kaptein EM, Nicoloff JT, Massry SG: Thyroid function in patients with nephrotic syndrome and normal renal function. Am J Nephrol 2:70–76, 1982.

91. Fonseca V, Thomas M, Katrak A, et al: Can urinary thyroid hormone loss cause hypothyroidism? Lancet 338:475–476, 1991.

92. Chopra IJ, Williams DE, Orgiazzi J, Solomon DH: Opposite effects of dexamethasone on serum concentrations of 3,3′,5′-triiodothyronine (reverse T3) and 3,3′5-triiodothyronine (T3). J Clin Endocrinol Metab 41:911–920, 1975.

93. Alon U, Chan JC: Calcium and vitamin D homeostasis in the nephrotic syndrome: Current status. Nephron 36:1–4, 1984.

94. Sato KA, Gray RW, Lemann J: Urinary excretion of 25-hydroxyvitamin D in health and the nephrotic syndrome. J Lab Clin Med 99:325–330, 1982.

95. Barragry JM, France MW, Carter ND, et al: Vitamin-D metabolism in nephrotic syndrome. Lancet 2:629–632, 1977.

96. Koenig KG, Lindberg JS, Zerwekh JE, et al: Free and total 1,25-dihydroxyvitamin D levels in subjects with renal disease. Kidney Int 41:161–165, 1992.

97. Korkor A, Schwartz J, Bergfeld M, et al: Absence of metabolic bone disease in adult patients with the nephrotic syndrome and normal renal function. J Clin Endocrinol Metab 56:496–500, 1983.

98. Gorensek MJ, Lebel MH, Nelson JD: Peritonitis in children with nephrotic syndrome. Pediatrics 81:849–856, 1988.

99. Feinstein EI, Chesney RW, Zelikovic I: Peritonitis in childhood renal disease. Am J Nephrol 8:147–165, 1988.

100. Krensky AM, Ingelfinger JR, Grupe WE: Peritonitis in childhood nephrotic syndrome: 1970–1980. Am J Dis Child 136:732–736, 1982.

101. Rubin HM, Blau EB, Michaels RH: Hemophilus and pneumococcal peritonitis in children with the nephrotic syndrome. Pediatrics 56:598–601, 1975.

102. Berns JS, Pearson HA, Gaudio KM, et al: Normal splenic function in children with the nephrotic syndrome. Pediatr Nephrol 2:244–246, 1988.

103. McVicar MI, Chandra M, Margouleff D, Zanzi I: Splenic hypofunction in the nephrotic syndrome of childhood. Am J Kidney Dis 7:395–401, 1986.

104. Pneumococcal polysaccharide vaccine. Recommendation of the Immunization Practices Advisory Committee. Ann Intern Med 96:203–205, 1982.

105. Kaysen GA: Plasma composition in the nephrotic syndrome. Am J Nephrol 13:347–359, 1993.

106. Ballmer PE, Weber BK, Roy C, et al: Elevation of albumin synthesis rates in nephrotic patients measured with [1–13C]leucine. Kidney Int 41:132–138, 1992.

107. Pedraza C, Huberman A: Actinomycin D blocks the hepatic functional albumin mRNA increase in aminonucleoside-nephrotic rats. Nephron 59:648–650, 1991.

108. Glassock RJ: Proteinuria. In Massry SG, Glassock RJ (eds): Textbook of Nephrology, 3rd ed. Baltimore, Williams and Wilkins, 1995, pp 600–604.

109. Praga M, Borstein B, Andres A, et al: Nephrotic proteinuria without hypoalbuminemia: Clinical characteristics and response to angiotensin-converting enzyme inhibition. Am J Kidney Dis 17:330–338, 1991.

110. Bernard DB: Metabolic abnormalities in the nephrotic syndrome. In Brenner BM, Stein JH (eds): Pathophysiology and Complications in Nephrotic Syndrome. New York, Churchill Livingstone, 1982, p 86.

111. Mohos SC, Skoza L: Glomerular sialoprotein. Science 164:1519–1521, 1969.

112. Palcoux JB, Niaudet P, Goumy P: Side effects of levamisole in children with nephrosis. Pediatr Nephrol 8:263–264, 1994.

113. Bohrer MP, Deen WM, Robertson CR, Brenner BM: Mechanism of angiotensin II-induced proteinuria in the rat. Am J Physiol 233:F13–F21, 1977.

114. Cameron JS: Coagulation and thromboembolic complications in the nephrotic syndrome. Adv Nephrol Necker Hosp 13:75–114, 1984.

115. Llach F: Hypercoagulability, renal vein thrombosis, and other thrombotic complications of nephrotic syndrome. Kidney Int 28:429–439, 1985.

116. Kanfer A: Coagulation factors in nephrotic syndrome. Am J Nephrol 10 Suppl 1:63–68, 1990.

117. Wygledowska G: Haemostasis in nephrotic syndrome. Med Wieku Rozwoj 5:389–396, 2001.

118. Chen TY, Huang CC, Tsao CJ: Hemostatic molecular markers in nephrotic syndrome. Am J Hematol 44:276–279, 1993.

119. Shibasaki T, Misawa T, Matsumoto H, et al: Characteristics of anemia in patients with nephrotic syndrome. Nippon Jinzo Gakkai Shi 36:896–901, 1994.

120. Vaziri ND: Erythropoietin and transferrin metabolism in nephrotic syndrome. Am J Kidney Dis 38:1–8, 2001.

121. Munk F: Die nephrosen. Med Klin 12:1019, 1946.

122. Sharples PM, Poulton J, White RH: Steroid responsive nephrotic syndrome is more common in Asians. Arch Dis Child 60:1014–1017, 1985.

123. Wyatt RJ, Marx MB, Kazee M, Holland NH: Current estimates of the incidence of steroid responsive idiopathic nephrosis in Kentucky children 1–9 years of age. Int J Pediatr Nephrol 3:63–65, 1982.

124. Olson JL: The nephrotic syndrome and minimal change disease. In Jennette JC, Olson JL, Schwartz MM, Silva FG (eds): Heptinstall's Pathology of the Kidney, 6th ed. Philadelphia, Lippincott Williams & Wilkins, 2006.

125. Jennette JC, Falk RJ: Adult minimal change glomerulopathy with acute renal failure. Am J Kidney Dis 16:432–437, 1990.

126. Murphy MJ, Bailey RR, McGiven AR: Is there an IgM nephropathy? Aust N Z J Med 13:35–38, 1983.

127. Pardo V, Riesgo I, Zilleruelo G, Strauss J: The clinical significance of mesangial IgM deposits and mesangial hypercellularity in minimal change nephrotic syndrome. Am J Kidney Dis 3:264–269, 1984.

128. Cohen AH, Border WA, Glassock RJ: Nehprotic syndrome with glomerular mesangial IgM deposits. Lab Invest 38:610–619, 1978.

129. Shalhoub RJ: Pathogenesis of lipoid nephrosis: A disorder of T-cell function. Lancet 2:556–560, 1974.

130. Schnaper HW, Aune TM: Identification of the lymphokine soluble immune response suppressor in urine of nephrotic children. J Clin Invest 76:341–349, 1985.

131. Mallick NP: The pathogenesis of minimal change nephropathy. Clin Nephrol 7:87–95, 1977.

132. Fujimoto S, Yamamoto Y, Hisanaga S, et al: Minimal change nephrotic syndrome in adults: Response to corticosteroid therapy and frequency of relapse. Am J Kidney Dis 17:687–692, 1991.

133. Mendoza SA, Tune BM: Treatment of childhood nephrotic syndrome. J Am Soc Nephrol 3:889–894, 1992.

134. Branten AJ, Wetzels JF: Immunosuppressive treatment of patients with a nephrotic syndrome due to minimal change glomerulopathy. Ned Tijdschr Geneeskd 142:2832–2838, 1998.

135. Walker F, Neill S, Carmody M, Dwyer WF: Nephrotic syndrome in Hodgkins disease. Int J Pediatr Nephrol 4:39–41, 1983.

136. Koyama A, Fujisaki M, Kobayashi M, et al: A glomerular permeability factor produced by human T cell hybridomas. Kidney Int 40:453–460, 1991.

137. Kobayashi K, Yoshikawa N, Nakamura H: T-cell subpopulations in childhood nephrotic syndrome. Clin Nephrol 41:253–258, 1994.

138. Fiser RT, Arnold WC, Charlton RK, et al: T-lymphocyte subsets in nephrotic syndrome. Kidney Int 40:913–916, 1991.

139. Sasdelli M, Rovinetti C, Cagnoli L, et al: Lymphocyte subpopulations in minimal-change nephropathy. Nephron 25:72–76, 1980.

140. Kerpen HO, Bhat JG, Kantor R, et al: Lymphocyte subpopulations in minimal change nephrotic syndrome. Clin Immunol Immunopathol 14:130–136, 1979.

141. Lagrue G, Branellec A, Blanc C, et al: A vascular permeability factor in lymphocyte culture supernants from patients with nephrotic syndrome. II. Pharmacological and physicochemical properties. Biomedicine 23:73–75, 1975.

142. Savin VJ: Mechanisms of proteinuria in noninflammatory glomerular diseases. Am J Kidney Dis 21:347–362, 1993.

143. Boulton J, Tulloch I, Dore B, McLay A: Changes in the glomerular capillary wall induced by lymphocyte products and serum of nephrotic patients. Clin Nephrol 20:72–77, 1983.

144. Sewell RF, Short CD: Minimal-change nephropathy: how does the immune system affect the glomerulus? Nephrol Dial Transplant 8:108–112, 1993.

145. Bakker WW, van Luijk WH, Hene RJ, et al: Loss of glomerular polyanion in vitro induced by mononuclear blood cells from patients with minimal-change nephrotic syndrome. Am J Nephrol 6:107–111, 1986.

146. Maruyama K, Tomizawa S, Seki Y, et al: Inhibition of vascular permeability factor production by ciclosporin in minimal change nephrotic syndrome. Nephron 62:27–30, 1992.

147. Tomizawa S, Maruyama K, Nagasawa N, et al: Studies of vascular permeability factor derived from T lymphocytes and inhibitory effect of plasma on its production in minimal change nephrotic syndrome. Nephron 41:157–160, 1985.

148. Trompeter RS, Barratt TM, Layward L: Vascular permeability factor and nephrotic syndrome. Lancet 2:900, 1978.

149. Lagrue G, Xheneumont S, Branellec A, et al: A vascular permeability factor elaborated from lymphocytes. I. Demonstration in patients with nephrotic syndrome. Biomedicine 23:37–40, 1975.

150. Pru C, Kjellstrand CM, Cohn RA, Vernier RL: Late recurrence of minimal lesion nephrotic syndrome. Ann Intern Med 100:69–72, 1984.

151. Winetz JA, Robertson CR, Golbetz HV, et al: The nature of the glomerular injury in minimal change and focal sclerosing glomerulopathies. Am J Kidney Dis 1:91–98, 1981.

152. Carrie BJ, Salyer WR, Myers BD: Minimal change nephropathy: An electrochemical disorder of the glomerular membrane. Am J Med 70:262–268, 1981.

153. Kitano Y, Yoshikawa N, Nakamura H: Glomerular anionic sites in minimal change nephrotic syndrome and focal segmental glomerulosclerosis. Clin Nephrol 40:199–204, 1993.

154. Levinsky RJ, Malleson PN, Barratt TM, Soothill JF: Circulating immune complexes in steroid-responsive nephrotic syndrome. N Engl J Med 298:126–129, 1978.

155. Cairns SA, London A, Mallick NP: Immune complexes in minimal-change glomerulopathy. N Engl J Med 302:1033, 1980.

156. The primary nephrotic syndrome in children. Identification of patients with minimal change nephrotic syndrome from initial response to prednisone. A report of the International Study of Kidney Disease in Children. J Pediatr 98:561–564, 1981.

157. Nolasco F, Cameron JS, Heywood EF, et al: Adult-onset minimal change nephrotic syndrome: A long-term follow-up. Kidney Int 29:1215–1223, 1986.

158. Artinano M, Etheridge WB, Stroehlein KB, Barcenas CG: Progression of minimal-change glomerulopathy to focal glomerulosclerosis in a patient with fenoprofen nephropathy. Am J Nephrol 6:353–357, 1986.

159. Averbuch SD, Austin HA, Sherwin SA, et al: Acute interstitial nephritis with the nephrotic syndrome following recombinant leukocyte a interferon therapy for mycosis fungoides. N Engl J Med 310:32–35, 1984.

160. Kaldor JM, Day NE, Pettersson F, et al: Leukemia following chemotherapy for ovarian cancer. N Engl J Med 322:1–6, 1990.

161. Laurent J, Rostoker G, Robeva R, et al: Is adult idiopathic nephrotic syndrome food allergy? Value of oligoantigenic diets. Nephron 47:7–11, 1987.

162. Smith JD, Hayslett JP: Reversible renal failure in the nephrotic syndrome. Am J Kidney Dis 19:201–213, 1992.

163. Grupe WE: Childhood nephrotic syndrome: Clinical associations and response to therapy. Postgrad Med 65:229–6, 1979.

164. Ueda N: Effect of corticosteroids on some hemostatic parameters in children with minimal change nephrotic syndrome. Nephron 56:374–378, 1990.

165. Bridges CR, Myers BD, Brenner BM, Deen WM: Glomerular charge alterations in human minimal change nephropathy. Kidney Int 22:677–684, 1982.

166. Ghiggeri GM, Candiano G, Ginevri F, et al: Renal selectivity properties towards endogenous albumin in minimal change nephropathy. Kidney Int 32:69–77, 1987.

167. Giangiacomo J, Cleary TG, Cole BR, et al: Serum immunoglobulins in the nephrotic syndrome. A possible cause of minimal-change nephrotic syndrome. N Engl J Med 293:8–12, 1975.

168. Groshong T, Mendelson L, Mendoza S, et al: Serum IgE in patients with minimal-change nephrotic syndrome. J Pediatr 83:767–771, 1973.

169. Meadow SR, Sarsfield JK: Steroid-responsive and nephrotic syndrome and allergy: clinical studies. Arch Dis Child 56:509–516, 1981.

170. Lagrue G, Laurent J, Hirbec G, et al: Serum IgE in primary glomerular diseases. Nephron 36:5–9, 1984.

171. Zilleruelo G, Hsia SL, Freundlich M, et al: Persistence of serum lipid abnormalities in children with idiopathic nephrotic syndrome. J Pediatr 104:61–64, 1984.

172. Glassock RJ: Therapy of idiopathic nephrotic syndrome in adults. A conservative or aggressive therapeutic approach? Am J Nephrol 13:422–428, 1993.

173. Ponticelli C, Passerini P: Treatment of the nephrotic syndrome associated with primary glomerulonephritis. Kidney Int 46:595–604, 1994.

174. Nephrotic syndrome in children: A randomized trial comparing two prednisone regimens in steroid-responsive patients who relapse early. Report of the international study of kidney disease in children. J Pediatr 95:239–243, 1979.

175. Alternate-day versus intermittent prednisone in frequently relapsing nephrotic syndrome. A report of "Arbetsgemeinschaft fur Padiatrische Nephrologie". Lancet 1:401–403, 1979.

176. Leisti S, Hallman N, Koskimies O, et al: Association of postmedication hypocortisolism with early first relapse of idiopathic nephrotic syndrome. Lancet 2:795–796, 1977.

177. Leisti S, Koskimies O, Perheentupa J, et al: Idiopathic nephrotic syndrome: Prevention of early relapse. Br Med J 1:892, 1978.

178. Leisti S, Koskimies O: Risk of relapse in steroid-sensitive nephrotic syndrome: Effect of stage of post-prednisone adrenocortical suppression. J Pediatr 103:553–557, 1983.

179. Ehrich JH, Brodehl J: Long versus standard prednisone therapy for initial treatment of idiopathic nephrotic syndrome in children. Arbeitsgemeinschaft fur Pediatrische Nephrologie. Eur J Pediatr 152:357–361, 1993.

180. Short versus standard prednisone therapy for initial treatment of idiopathic nephrotic syndrome in children. Arbeitsgemeinschaft for Pediatrische Nephrologie. Lancet 1:380–383, 1988.

181. Cyclophosphamide treatment of steroid dependent nephrotic syndrome: Comparison of eight week with 12 week course. Report of Arbeitsgemeinschaft fur Pediatrische Nephrologie. Arch Dis Child 62:1102–1106, 1987.

182. Berns JS, Gaudio KM, Krassner LS, et al: Steroid-responsive nephrotic syndrome of childhood: A long-term study of clinical course, histopathology, efficacy of cyclophosphamide therapy, and effects on growth. Am J Kidney Dis 9:108–114, 1987.

183. Schulman SL, Kaiser BA, Polinsky MS, et al: Predicting the response to cytotoxic therapy for childhood nephrotic syndrome: Superiority of response to corticosteroid therapy over histopathologic patterns. J Pediatr 113:996–1001, 1988.

184. Effect of cytotoxic drugs in frequently relapsing nephrotic syndrome with and without steroid dependence. N Engl J Med 306:451–454, 1982.

185. Ueda N, Kuno K, Ito S: Eight and 12 week courses of cyclophosphamide in nephrotic syndrome. Arch Dis Child 65:1147–1150, 1990.

186. Muller W, Brandis M: Acute leukemia after cytotoxic treatment for nonmalignant disease in childhood. A case report and review of the literature. Eur J Pediatr 136:105–108, 1981.

187. Kleinknecht C, Guesry P, Lenoir G, Broyer M: High-cost benefit of chlorambucil in frequent relapsing nephrosis. N Engl J Med 296:48–49, 1977.

188. Grupe WE, Makker SP, Ingelfinger JR: Chlorambucil treatment of frequently relapsing nephrotic syndrome. N Engl J Med 295:746–749, 1976.

189. Williams SA, Makker SP, Ingelfinger JR, Grupe WE: Long-term evaluation of chlorambucil plus prednisone in the idiopathic nephrotic syndrome of childhood. N Engl J Med 302:929–933, 1980.

190. Elzouki AY, Jaiswal OP: Evaluation of chlorambucil therapy in steroid-dependent and cyclophosphamide-resistant children with nephrosis. Pediatr Nephrol 4:459–462, 1990.

191. Primary nephrotic syndrome in children: Clinical significance of histopathologic variants of minimal change and of diffuse mesangial hypercellularity. A Report of the International Study of Kidney Disease in Children. Kidney Int 20:765–771, 1981.

192. Murnaghan K, Vasmant D, Bensman A: Pulse methylprednisolone therapy in severe idiopathic childhood nephrotic syndrome. Acta Paediatr Scand 73:733–739, 1984.

193. Rose GM, Cole BR, Robson AM: The treatment of severe glomerulopathies in children using high dose intravenous methylprednisolone pulses. Am J Kidney Dis 1:148–156, 1981.

194. Cheng IK, Chan KW, Chan MK: Mesangial IgA nephropathy with steroid-responsive nephrotic syndrome: Disappearance of mesangial IgA deposits following steroid-induced remission. Am J Kidney Dis 14:361–364, 1989.

195. Lagrue G, Laurent J: Allergy and lipoid nephrosis. Adv Nephrol Necker Hosp 12:151–175, 1983.

196. Lagrue G, Laurent J: Is lipoid nephrosis an "allergic" disease? Transplant Proc 14:485–488, 1982.

197. Niaudet P, Drachman R, Gagnadoux MF, Broyer M: Treatment of idiopathic nephrotic syndrome with levamisole. Acta Paediatr Scand 73:637–641, 1984.

198. Ponticelli C, Rizzoni G, Edefonti A, et al: A randomized trial of cyclosporine in steroid-resistant idiopathic nephrotic syndrome. Kidney Int 43:1377–1384, 1993.

199. Niaudet P, Habib R: Cyclosporine in the treatment of idiopathic nephrosis. J Am Soc Nephrol 5:1049–1056, 1994.

200. Ponticelli C, Edefonti A, Ghio L, et al: Cyclosporin versus cyclophosphamide for patients with steroid-dependent and frequently relapsing idiopathic nephrotic syndrome: A multicentre randomized controlled trial. Nephrol Dial Transplant 8:1326–1332, 1993.

201. Meyrier A, Noel LH, Auriche P, Callard P: Long-term renal tolerance of cyclosporin A treatment in adult idiopathic nephrotic syndrome. Collaborative Group of the Societe de Nephrologie. Kidney Int 45:1446–1456, 1994.

202. Levamisole for corticosteroid-dependent nephrotic syndrome in childhood. British Association for Paediatric Nephrology. Lancet 337:1555–1557, 1991.

203. Ginevri F, Trivelli A, Ciardi MR, et al: Protracted levamisole in children with frequent-relapse nephrotic syndrome. Pediatr Nephrol 10:550, 1996.

204. D'Agati VD, Fogo AB, Bruijn JA, Jennette JC: Pathologic classification of focal segmental glomerulosclerosis: A working proposal. Am J Kidney Dis 43:368–382, 2004.

205. Thomas DB, Franceschini N, Hogan SL, et al: Clinical and pathologic characteristics of focal segmental glomerulosclerosis pathologic variants. Kidney Int 69:920–926, 2006.

206. Korbet SM: Primary focal segmental glomerulosclerosis. J Am Soc Nephrol 9:1333–1340, 1998.

207. Haas M, Spargo BH, Coventry S: Increasing incidence of focal-segmental glomerulosclerosis among adult nephropathies: A 20-year renal biopsy study. Am J Kidney Dis 26:740–750, 1995.

208. Cameron JS: The enigma of focal segmental glomerulosclerosis. Kidney Int Suppl 57:S119–S131, 1996.

209. Haas M, Meehan SM, Karrison TG, Spargo BH: Changing etiologies of unexplained adult nephrotic syndrome: A comparison of renal biopsy findings from 1976–1979 and 1995–1997. Am J Kidney Dis 30:621–631, 1997.

210. Valeri A, Barisoni L, Appel GB, et al: Idiopathic collapsing focal segmental glomerulosclerosis. Kidney Int 50:1734–1746, 1996.

211. Detwiler RK, Falk RJ, Hogan SL, Jennette JC: Collapsing glomerulopathy: A clinically and pathologically distinct variant of focal segmental glomerulosclerosis. Kidney Int 45:1416–1424, 1994.

212. Kambham N, Markowitz GS, Valeri AM, et al: Obesity-related glomerulopathy: An emerging epidemic. Kidney Int 59:1498–1509, 2001.

213. Pontier PJ, Patel TG: Racial differences in the prevalence and presentation of glomerular disease in adults. Clin Nephrol 42:79–84, 1994.

214. Korbet SM, Genchi RM, Borok RZ, Schwartz MM: The racial prevalence of glomerular lesions in nephrotic adults. Am J Kidney Dis 27:647–651, 1996.

215. D'Agati V: The many masks of focal segmental glomerulosclerosis. Kidney Int 46:1223–1241, 1994.

216. Cohen AH, Nast CC: HIV-associated nephropathy. A unique combined glomerular, tubular, and interstitial lesion. Mod Pathol 1:87–97, 1988.

217. D'Agati V, Suh JI, Carbone L, et al: Pathology of HIV-associated nephropathy: A detailed morphologic and comparative study. Kidney Int 35:1358–1370, 1989.

218. Clarkson MR, Meara YM, Murphy B, et al: Collapsing glomerulopathy—recurrence in a renal allograft. Nephrol Dial Transplant 13:503–506, 1998.

219. Meehan SM, Pascual M, Williams WW, et al: De novo collapsing glomerulopathy in renal allografts. Transplantation 65:1192–1197, 1998.

220. Howie AJ, Lee SJ, Green NJ, et al: Different clinicopathological types of segmental sclerosing glomerular lesions in adults. Nephrol Dial Transplant 8:590–599, 1993.

221. Beaman M, Howie AJ, Hardwicke J, et al: The glomerular tip lesion: A steroid responsive nephrotic syndrome. Clin Nephrol 27:217–221, 1987.

222. Howie AJ: Changes at the glomerular tip: A feature of membranous nephropathy and other disorders associated with proteinuria. J Pathol 150:13–20, 1986.

223. Howie AJ, Brewer DB: The glomerular tip lesion: A previously undescribed type of segmental glomerular abnormality. J Pathol 142:205–220, 1984.

224. Howie AJ, Brewer DB: Further studies on the glomerular tip lesion: Early and late stages and life table analysis. J Pathol 147:245–255, 1985.

225. Yoshikawa N, Ito H, Akamatsu R, et al: Focal segmental glomerulosclerosis with and without nephrotic syndrome in children. J Pediatr 109:65–70, 1986.

226. Sharma K, Ziyadeh FN: The emerging role of transforming growth factor-beta in kidney diseases. Am J Physiol 266:F829–F842, 1994.

227. Border WA, Okuda S, Languino LR, et al: Suppression of experimental glomerulonephritis by antiserum against transforming growth factor beta 1. Nature 346:371–374, 1990.

228. Yoshioka K, Takemura T, Murakami K, et al: Transforming growth factor-beta protein and mRNA in glomeruli in normal and diseased human kidneys. Lab Invest 68:154–163, 1993.

229. Stokes MB, Holler S, Cui Y, et al: Expression of decorin, biglycan, and collagen type I in human renal fibrosing disease. Kidney Int 57:487–498, 2000.

230. Eagen JW: Glomerulopathies of neoplasia. Kidney Int 11:297–303, 1977.

231. Olson JL, Hostetter TH, Rennke HG, et al: Altered glomerular permselectivity and progressive sclerosis following extreme ablation of renal mass. Kidney Int 22:112–126, 1982.

232. Brenner BM, Meyer TW, Hostetter TH: Dietary protein intake and the progressive nature of kidney disease: The role of hemodynamically mediated glomerular injury in the pathogenesis of progressive glomerular sclerosis in aging, renal ablation, and intrinsic renal disease. N Engl J Med 307:652–659, 1982.

233. Brenner BM: Hemodynamically mediated glomerular injury and the progressive nature of kidney disease. Kidney Int 23:647–655, 1983.

234. el Nahas AM: Glomerulosclerosis: Insights into pathogenesis and treatment. Nephrol Dial Transplant 4:843–853, 1989.

235. Simons JL, Provoost AP, Anderson S, et al: Modulation of glomerular hypertension defines susceptibility to progressive glomerular injury. Kidney Int 46:396–404, 1994.

236. Johnson RJ: The glomerular response to injury: progression or resolution? Kidney Int 45:1769–1782, 1994.

237. Couser WG: Mechanisms of glomerular injury: An overview. Semin Nephrol 11:254–258, 1991.

238. Keane WF: Lipids and the kidney. Kidney Int 46:910–920, 1994.

239. Moorhead JF, el Nahas M, Harry D, et al: Focal glomerular sclerosis and nephrotic syndrome with partial lecithin:cholesterol acetyltransferase deficiency and discoidal high density lipoprotein in plasma and urine. Lancet 1:936–937, 1983.

240. Moorhead JF, Chan MK, el Nahas M, Varghese Z: Lipid nephrotoxicity in chronic progressive glomerular and tubulo-interstitial disease. Lancet 2:1309–1311, 1982.

241. Diamond JR, Karnovsky MJ: Focal and segmental glomerulosclerosis: Analogies to atherosclerosis. Kidney Int 33:917–924, 1988.

242. Matsumoto K, Osakabe K, Katayama H, Hatano M: Concanavalin A-induced suppressor cell activity in focal glomerular sclerosis. Nephron 31:27–30, 1982.

243. Novick AC, Gephardt G, Guz B, et al: Long-term follow-up after partial removal of a solitary kidney. N Engl J Med 325:1058–1062, 1991.

244. Najarian JS, Chavers BM, McHugh LE, Matas AJ: 20 years or more of follow-up of living kidney donors. Lancet 340:807–810, 1992.

245. Saran R, Marshall SM, Madsen R, et al: Long-term follow-up of kidney donors: A longitudinal study. Nephrol Dial Transplant 12:1615–1621, 1997.

246. Narkun B, Nolan CR, Norman JE, et al: Forty-five year follow-up after uninephrectomy. Kidney Int 43:1110–1115, 1993.

247. Kasiske BL, Ma JZ, Louis TA, Swan SK: Long-term effects of reduced renal mass in humans. Kidney Int 48:814–819, 1995.

248. Verani RR: Obesity-associated focal segmental glomerulosclerosis: Pathological features of the lesion and relationship with cardiomegaly and hyperlipidemia. Am J Kidney Dis 20:629–634, 1992.

249. Kambham N, Markowitz GS, Valeri AM, et al: Obesity-related glomerulopathy: An emerging epidemic. Kidney Int 59:1498–1509, 2001.

250. Praga M, Hernandez E, Andres A, et al: Effects of body-weight loss and captopril treatment on proteinuria associated with obesity. Nephron 70:35–41, 1995.

251. Chaudhary BA, Sklar AH, Chaudhary TK, et al: Sleep apnea, proteinuria, and nephrotic syndrome. Sleep 11:69–74, 1988.

252. Sklar AH, Chaudhary BA: Reversible proteinuria in obstructive sleep apnea syndrome. Arch Intern Med 148:87–89, 1988.

253. Casserly LF, Chow N, Ali S, et al: Proteinuria in obstructive sleep apnea. Kidney Int 60:1484–1489, 2001.

254. Savin VJ, Sharma R, Sharma M, et al: Circulating factor associated with increased glomerular permeability to albumin in recurrent focal segmental glomerulosclerosis. N Engl J Med 334:878–883, 1996.

255. Dantal J, Bigot E, Bogers W, et al: Effect of plasma protein adsorption on protein excretion in kidney-transplant recipients with recurrent nephrotic syndrome. N Engl J Med 330:7–14, 1994.

256. Artero ML, Sharma R, Savin VJ, Vincenti F: Plasmapheresis reduces proteinuria and serum capacity to injure glomeruli in patients with recurrent focal glomerulosclerosis. Am J Kidney Dis 23:574–581, 1994.

257. Feld SM, Figueroa P, Savin V, et al: Plasmapheresis in the treatment of steroid-resistant focal segmental glomerulosclerosis in native kidneys. Am J Kidney Dis 32:230–237, 1998.

258. Yang Y, Gubler MC, Beaufils H: Dysregulation of podocyte phenotype in idiopathic collapsing glomerulopathy and HIV-associated nephropathy. Nephron 91:416–423, 2002.

259. Schmid H, Henger A, Cohen CD, et al: Gene expression profiles of podocyte-associated molecules as diagnostic markers in acquired proteinuric diseases. J Am Soc Nephrol 14:2958–2966, 2003.

260. Ohtaka A, Ootaka T, Sato H, Ito S: Phenotypic change of glomerular podocytes in primary focal segmental glomerulosclerosis: Developmental paradigm? Nephrol Dial Transplant 17 Suppl 9:11–15, 2002.

261. Shankland SJ, Eitner F, Hudkins KL, et al: Differential expression of cyclin-dependent kinase inhibitors in human glomerular disease: Role in podocyte proliferation and maturation. Kidney Int 58:674–683, 2000.

262. Binder CJ, Weiher H, Exner M, Kerjaschki D: Glomerular overproduction of oxygen radicals in Mpv17 gene-inactivated mice causes podocyte foot process flattening and proteinuria: A model of steroid-resistant nephrosis sensitive to radical scavenger therapy. Am J Pathol 154:1067–1075, 1999.

263. Kretzler M: Role of podocytes in focal sclerosis: Defining the point of no return. J Am Soc Nephrol 16:2830–2832, 2005.

264. Johnstone DB, Holzman LB: Clinical impact of research on the podocyte slit diaphragm. Nature Clin Pract Nephrol 2:271–282, 2006.

265. Kriz W, LeHir M: Pathways to nephron loss starting from glomerular diseases-insights from animal models. Kidney Int 67:404–419, 2005.

266. Barisoni L, Kopp JB: Update in podocyte biology: Putting one's best foot forward. Curr Opin Nephrol Hypertens 12:251–258, 2003.

267. Wiggins JE, Goyal M, Sanden SK, et al: Podocyte hypertrophy, "adaptation," and "decompensation" associated with glomerular enlargement and glomerulosclerosis in the aging rat: Prevention by calorie restriction. J Am Soc Nephrol 16:2953–2966, 2005.

268. Dijkman H, Smeets B, van der Laak J, et al: The parietal epithelial cell is crucially involved in human idiopathic focal segmental glomerulosclerosis. Kidney Int 68:1562–1572, 2005.

269. Winn MP, Conlon PJ, Lynn KL, et al: Clinical and genetic heterogeneity in familial focal segmental glomerulosclerosis. International Collaborative Group for the Study of Familial Focal Segmental Glomerulosclerosis. Kidney Int 55:1241–1246, 1999.

270. Faubert PF, Porush JG: Familial focal segmental glomerulosclerosis: Nine cases in four families and review of the literature. Am J Kidney Dis 30:265–270, 1997.

271. Tejani A, Nicastri A, Phadke K, et al: Familial focal segmental glomerulosclerosis. Int J Pediatr Nephrol 4:231–234, 1983.

272. McCurdy FA, Butera PJ, Wilson R: The familial occurrence of focal segmental glomerular sclerosis. Am J Kidney Dis 10:467–469, 1987.

273. Ruder H, Scharer K, Opelz G, et al: Human leucocyte antigens in idiopathic nephrotic syndrome in children. Pediatr Nephrol 4:478–481, 1990.

274. Dennis VW, Robinson RR: Proteinuria. In Edelman CM (ed): Pediatric Kidney Disease. Boston, Little, Brown, 1978, p 306.

275. Haskell LP, Glicklich D, Senitzer D: HLA associations in heroin-associated nephropathy. Am J Kidney Dis 12:45–50, 1988.

276. Kaplan JM, Kim SH, North KN, et al: Mutations in ACTN4, encoding alpha-actinin-4, cause familial focal segmental glomerulosclerosis. Nat Genet 24:251–256, 2000.

277. Gigante M, Monno F, Roberto R, et al: Congenital nephrotic syndrome of the finnish type in Italy: a molecular approach. J Nephrol 15:696–702, 2002.

278. Boute N, Gribouval O, Roselli S, et al: NPHS2, encoding the glomerular protein podocin, is mutated in autosomal recessive steroid-resistant nephrotic syndrome. Nat Genet 24:349–354, 2000.

279. Tsukaguchi H, Sudhakar A, Le TC, et al: NPHS2 mutations in late-onset focal segmental glomerulosclerosis: R229Q is a common disease-associated allele. J Clin Invest 110:1659–1666, 2002.

280. Caridi G, Bertelli R, Carrea A, et al: Prevalence, genetics, and clinical features of patients carrying podocin mutations in steroid-resistant nonfamilial focal segmental glomerulosclerosis. J Am Soc Nephrol 12:2742–2746, 2001.

281. Frishberg Y, Rinat C, Megged O, et al: Mutations in NPHS2 encoding podocin are a prevalent cause of steroid-resistant nephrotic syndrome among Israeli-Arab children. J Am Soc Nephrol 13:400–405, 2002.

282. Karle SM, Uetz B, Ronner V, et al: Novel mutations in NPHS2 detected in both familial and sporadic steroid-resistant nephrotic syndrome. J Am Soc Nephrol 13:388–393, 2002.

283. Weins A, Kenlan P, Herbert S, et al: Mutational and biological analysis of alpha-actinin-4 in focal segmental glomerulosclerosis. J Am Soc Nephrol 16:3694–3701, 2005.

284. Aucella F, De Bonis P, Gatta G, et al: Molecular analysis of NPHS2 and ACTN4 genes in a series of 33 Italian patients affected by adult-onset nonfamilial focal segmental glomerulosclerosis. Nephron Clin Pract 99:c31–c36, 2005.

285. Antignac C: Genetic models: Clues for understanding the pathogenesis of idiopathic nephrotic syndrome. J Clin Invest 109:447–449, 2002.

286. Winn MP, Conlon PJ, Lynn KL, et al: A mutation in the TRPC6 cation channel causes familial focal segmental glomerulosclerosis. Science 308:1801–1804, 2005.

287. Reiser J, Polu KR, Moller CC, et al: TRPC6 is a glomerular slit diaphragm-associated channel required for normal renal function. Nat Genet 37:739–744, 2005.

288. Rennke HG, Klein PS: Pathogenesis and significance of nonprimary focal and segmental glomerulosclerosis. Am J Kidney Dis 13:443–456, 1989.

289. Fogo A, Glick AD, Horn SL, Horn RG: Is focal segmental glomerulosclerosis really focal? Distribution of lesions in adults and children. Kidney Int 47:1690–1696, 1995.

290. Border WA, Noble NA, Yamamoto T, et al: Natural inhibitor of transforming growth factor-beta protects against scarring in experimental kidney disease. Nature 360:361–364, 1992.

291. Moudgil A, Nast CC, Bagga A, et al: Association of parvovirus B19 infection with idiopathic collapsing glomerulopathy. Kidney Int 59:2126–2133, 2001.

292. Tanawattanacharoen S, Falk RJ, Jennette JC, Kopp JB: Parvovirus B19 DNA in kidney tissue of patients with focal segmental glomerulosclerosis. Am J Kidney Dis 35:1166–1174, 2000.

293. Li RM, Branton MH, Tanawattanacharoen S, et al: Molecular identification of SV40 infection in human subjects and possible association with kidney disease. J Am Soc Nephrol 13:2320–2330, 2002.

294. Dingli D, Larson DR, Plevak MF, et al: Focal and segmental glomerulosclerosis and plasma cell proliferative disorders. Am J Kidney Dis 46:278–282, 2005.

295. Focal segmental glomerulosclerosis in children with idiopathic nephrotic syndrome. A report of the Southwest Pediatric Nephrology Study Group. Kidney Int 27:442–449, 1985.

296. Newman WJ, Tisher CC, McCoy RC, et al: Focal glomerular sclerosis: Contrasting clinical patterns in children and adults. Medicine (Baltimore) 55:67–87, 1976.

297. Pei Y, Cattran D, Delmore T, et al: Evidence suggesting under-treatment in adults with idiopathic focal segmental glomerulosclerosis. Regional Glomerulonephritis Registry Study. Am J Med 82:938–944, 1987.

298. Korbet SM, Schwartz MM, Lewis EJ: Primary focal segmental glomerulosclerosis: Clinical course and response to therapy. Am J Kidney Dis 23:773–783, 1994.

299. Weiss MA, Daquioag E, Margolin EG, Pollak VE: Nephrotic syndrome, progressive irreversible renal failure, and glomerular "collapse": A new clinicopathologic entity? Am J Kidney Dis 7:20–28, 1986.

300. Barri YM, Munshi NC, Sukumalchantra S, et al: Podocyte injury associated glomerulopathies induced by pamidronate. Kidney Int 65:634–641, 2004.

301. Schwartz MM, Korbet SM: Primary focal segmental glomerulosclerosis: Pathology, histological variants, and pathogenesis. Am J Kidney Dis 22:874–883, 1993.

302. Ito H, Yoshikawa N, Aozai F, et al: Twenty-seven children with focal segmental glomerulosclerosis: correlation between the segmental location of the glomerular lesions and prognosis. Clin Nephrol 22:9–14, 1984.

303. Schwartz MM, Korbet SM, Rydell J, et al: Primary focal segmental glomerular sclerosis in adults: Prognostic value of histologic variants. Am J Kidney Dis 25:845–852, 1995.

304. Rydel JJ, Korbet SM, Borok RZ, Schwartz MM: Focal segmental glomerular sclerosis in adults: Presentation, course, and response to treatment. Am J Kidney Dis 25:534–542, 1995.

305. Korbet SM, Schwartz MM, Lewis EJ: The prognosis of focal segmental glomerular sclerosis of adulthood. Medicine (Baltimore) 65:304–311, 1986.

306. Velosa JA, Holley KE, Torres VE, Offord KP: Significance of proteinuria on the outcome of renal function in patients with focal segmental glomerulosclerosis. Mayo Clin Proc 58:568–577, 1983.

307. Brown CB, Cameron JS, Turner DR, et al: Focal segmental glomerulosclerosis with rapid decline in renal function ("malignant FSGS"). Clin Nephrol 10:51–61, 1978.

308. Korbet SM: Clinical picture and outcome of primary focal segmental glomerulosclerosis. Nephrol Dial Transplant 14 Suppl 3:68–73, 1999.

309. Banfi G, Moriggi M, Sabadini E, et al: The impact of prolonged immunosuppression on the outcome of idiopathic focal-segmental glomerulosclerosis with nephrotic syndrome in adults. A collaborative retrospective study. Clin Nephrol 36:53–59, 1991.

310. Arbus GS, Poucell S, Bacheyie GS, Baumal R: Focal segmental glomerulosclerosis with idiopathic nephrotic syndrome: Three types of clinical response. J Pediatr 101:40–45, 1982.

311. Wehrmann M, Bohle A, Held H, et al: Long-term prognosis of focal sclerosing glomerulonephritis. An analysis of 250 cases with particular regard to tubulointerstitial changes. Clin Nephrol 33:115–122, 1990.

312. Ingulli E, Tejani A: Racial differences in the incidence and renal outcome of idiopathic focal segmental glomerulosclerosis in children. Pediatr Nephrol 5:393–397, 1991.

313. Mongeau JG, Robitaille PO, Clermont MJ, et al: Focal segmental glomerulosclerosis (FSG) 20 years later. From toddler to grown up. Clin Nephrol 40:1–6, 1993.

314. Lewis EJ: Management of the nephrotic syndrome in adults. In Cameron J, Glassock R (eds): The Nephrotic Syndrome. New York, Marcel Dekker, 1988, pp 461–521.

315. Garin EH, Donnelly WH, Geary D, Richard GA: Nephrotic syndrome and diffuse mesangial proliferative glomerulonephritis in children. Am J Dis Child 137:109–113, 1983.

316. Allen WR, Travis LB, Cavallo T, et al: Immune deposits and mesangial hypercellularity in minimal change nephrotic syndrome: Clinical relevance. J Pediatr 100:188–191, 1982.

317. Schoeneman MJ, Bennett B, Greifer I: The natural history of focal segmental glomerulosclerosis with and without mesangial hypercellularity in children. Clin Nephrol 9:45–54, 1978.

318. Cairns SA, London RA, Mallick NP: Circulating immune complexes in idiopathic glomerular disease. Kidney Int 21:507–512, 1982.

319. Agarwal SK, Dash SC, Tiwari SC, Bhuyan UN: Idiopathic adult focal segmental glomerulosclerosis: A clinicopathological study and response to steroid. Nephron 63:168–171, 1993.

320. Meyrier A, Simon P: Treatment of corticoresistant idiopathic nephrotic syndrome in the adult: Minimal change disease and focal segmental glomerulosclerosis. Adv Nephrol Necker Hosp 17:127–150, 1988.

321. Miyata J, Takebayashi S, Taguchi T, et al: Evaluation and correlation of clinical and histological features of focal segmental glomerulosclerosis. Nephron 44:115–120, 1986.

322. Schwartz MM, Evans J, Bain R, Korbet SM: Focal segmental glomerulosclerosis: Prognostic implications of the cellular lesion. J Am Soc Nephrol 10:1900–1907, 1999.

323. Ponticelli C, Villa M, Banfi G, et al: Can prolonged treatment improve the prognosis in adults with focal segmental glomerulosclerosis? Am J Kidney Dis 34:618–625, 1999.

324. Griswold WR, Tune BM, Reznik VM, et al: Treatment of childhood prednisone-resistant nephrotic syndrome and focal segmental glomerulosclerosis with intravenous methylprednisolone and oral alkylating agents. Nephron 46:73–77, 1987.

325. Mendoza SA, Reznik VM, Griswold WR, et al: Treatment of steroid-resistant focal segmental glomerulosclerosis with pulse methylprednisolone and alkylating agents. Pediatr Nephrol 4:303–307, 1990.

326. Meyrier A: Focal segmental glomerulosclerosis: To treat or not to treat? 2. Focal and segmental glomerulosclerosis is not a disease, but an untreatable lesion of unknown pathophysiology. Its treatment must not be uselessly hazardous. Nephrol Dial Transplant 10:2355–2359, 1995.

327. Nagai R, Cattran DC, Pei Y: Steroid therapy and prognosis of focal segmental glomerulosclerosis in the elderly. Clin Nephrol 42:18–21, 1994.

328. Melvin T, Bennett W: Management of nephrotic syndrome in childhood. Drugs 42:30–51, 1991.

329. Tarshish P, Tobin JN, Bernstein J, Edelmann CM: Cyclophosphamide does not benefit patients with focal segmental glomerulosclerosis. A report of the International Study of Kidney Disease in Children. Pediatr Nephrol 10:590–593, 1996.

330. Cattran DC, Appel GB, Hebert LA, et al: A randomized trial of cyclosporine in patients with steroid-resistant focal segmental glomerulosclerosis. North America Nephrotic Syndrome Study Group. Kidney Int 56:2220–2226, 1999.

331. Praga M, Hernandez E, Montoyo C, et al: Long-term beneficial effects of angiotensin-converting enzyme inhibition in patients with nephrotic proteinuria. Am J Kidney Dis 20:240–248, 1992.

332. Huissoon AP, Meehan S, Keogh JA: Reduction of proteinuria with captopril therapy in patients with focal segmental glomerulosclerosis and IgA nephropathy. Ir J Med Sci 160:319–321, 1991.

333. Bedogna V, Valvo E, Casagrande P, et al: Effects of ACE inhibition in normotensive patients with chronic glomerular disease and normal renal function. Kidney Int 38:101–107, 1990.

334. Maschio G, Alberti D, Janin G, et al: Effect of the angiotensin-converting-enzyme inhibitor benazepril on the progression of chronic renal insufficiency. The Angio-tensin-Converting-Enzyme Inhibition in Progressive Renal Insufficiency Study Group. N Engl J Med 334:939–945, 1996.

335. Falk RJ, Scheinman J, Phillips G, et al: Prevalence and pathologic features of sickle cell nephropathy and response to inhibition of angiotensin-converting enzyme. N Engl J Med 326:910–915, 1992.

336. Haas M, Godfrin Y, Oberbauer R, et al: Plasma immunadsorption treatment in patients with primary focal and segmental glomerulosclerosis. Nephrol Dial Transplant 13:2013–2016, 1998.

337. Jennette JC, Hipp CG: C1q nephropathy: A distinct pathologic entity usually causing nephrotic syndrome. Am J Kidney Dis 6:103–110, 1985.

338. Jennette JC, Falk RJ: C1q nephropathy. In Massry S, Glassock R (eds): Textbook of Nephrology, 3rd ed. Baltimore, Williams and Wilkins, 1995, pp 749–752.

339. Nishida L, Kawakatsu H, Komatsu H, et al: Spontaneous improvement in a case of C1q nephropathy. Am J Kidney Dis 35:E22, 2000.

340. Iskandar SS, Browning MC, Lorentz WB: C1q nephropathy: A pediatric clinicopathologic study. Am J Kidney Dis 18:459–465, 1991.

341. Yamamoto T, Noble NA, Miller DE, Border WA: Sustained expression of TGF-beta 1 underlies development of progressive kidney fibrosis. Kidney Int 45:916–927, 1994.

342. Thomsen OF, Ladefoged J: Glomerular tip lesions in renal biopsies with focal segmental IgM. APMIS 99:836–843, 1991.

343. Gephardt GN, Tubbs RR, Popowniak KL, McMahon JT: Focal and segmental glomerulosclerosis. Immunohistologic study of 20 renal biopsy specimens. Arch Pathol Lab Med 110:902–905, 1986.

344. Markovic L, Muller CA, Risler T, et al: Mononuclear leukocytes, expression of HLA class II antigens and intercellular adhesion molecule 1 in focal segmental glomerulosclerosis. Nephron 59:286–293, 1991.

345. Glasser RJ, Velosa JA, Michael AF: Experimental model of focal sclerosis. I. Relationship to protein excretion in aminonucleoside nephrosis. Lab Invest 36:519–526, 1977.

346. Velosa JA, Glasser RJ, Nevins TE, Michael AF: Experimental model of focal sclerosis. II. Correlation with immunopathologic changes, macromolecular kinetics, and polyanion loss. Lab Invest 36:527–534, 1977.

347. Bolton WK, Westervelt FB, Sturgill BC: Nephrotic syndrome and focal glomerular sclerosis in aging man. Nephron 20:307–315, 1978.

348. Marks MI, Drummond KN: Nephropathy and persistent proteinuria after albumin administration in the rat. Lab Invest 23:416–420, 1970.

349. Kreisberg JI, Karnovsky MJ: Focal glomerular sclerosis in the fawn-hooded rat. Am J Pathol 92:637–652, 1978.

350. Remuzzi G, Bertani T: Is glomerulosclerosis a consequence of altered glomerular permeability to macromolecules? Kidney Int 38:384–394, 1990.

351. Thomas ME, Schreiner GF: Contribution of proteinuria to progressive renal injury: Consequences of tubular uptake of fatty acid bearing albumin. Am J Nephrol 13:385–398, 1993.

352. Agarwal A, Nath KA: Effect of proteinuria on renal interstitium: Effect of products of nitrogen metabolism. Am J Nephrol 13:376–384, 1993.

353. Ueda Y, Ono Y, Sagiya A, et al: Mesangial anionic sites are decreased in human focal glomerular sclerosis. Clin Nephrol 37:280–284, 1992.

354. Hoyer JR, Vernier RL, Najarian JS, et al: Recurrence of idiopathic nephrotic syndrome after renal transplantation. Lancet 2:343–348, 1972.

355. Leumann EP, Briner J, Donckerwolcke RA, et al: Recurrence of focal segmental glomerulosclerosis in the transplanted kidney. Nephron 25:65–71, 1980.

356. Axelsen RA, Seymour AE, Mathew TH, et al: Recurrent focal glomerulosclerosis in renal transplants. Clin Nephrol 21:110–114, 1984.

357. Artero M, Biava C, Amend W, et al: Recurrent focal glomerulosclerosis: Natural history and response to therapy. Am J Med 92:375–383, 1992.

358. Kim EM, Striegel J, Kim Y, et al: Recurrence of steroid-resistant nephrotic syndrome in kidney transplants is associated with increased acute renal failure and acute rejection. Kidney Int 45:1440–1445, 1994.

359. Dantal J, Baatard R, Hourmant M, et al: Recurrent nephrotic syndrome following renal transplantation in patients with focal glomerulosclerosis. A one-center study of plasma exchange effects. Transplantation 52:827–831, 1991.

360. Li PK, Lai FM, Leung CB, et al: Plasma exchange in the treatment of early recurrent focal glomerulosclerosis after renal transplantation. Report and review. Am J Nephrol 13:289–292, 1993.

361. Futrakul P, Poshyachinda M, Mitrakul C: Focal sclerosing glomerulonephritis: A kinetic evaluation of hemostasis and the effect of anticoagulant therapy: A controlled study. Clin Nephrol 10:180–186, 1978.

362. Purkerson ML, Joist JH, Yates J, et al: Inhibition of thromboxane synthesis ameliorates the progressive kidney disease of rats with subtotal renal ablation. Proc Natl Acad Sci U S A 82:193–197, 1985.

363. Border WA, Okuda S, Languino LR, Ruoslahti E: Transforming growth factor-beta regulates production of proteoglycans by mesangial cells. Kidney Int 37:689–695, 1990.

364. Mongeau JG, Corneille L, Robitaille P, et al: Primary nephrosis in childhood associated with focal glomerular sclerosis: Is long-term prognosis that severe? Kidney Int 20:743–746, 1981.

365. Ramirez F, Travis LB, Cunningham RJ, et al: Focal segmental glomerulosclerosis, crescent, and rapidly progressive renal failure. Int J Pediatr Nephrol 3:175–178, 1982.

366. Packham DK, North RA, Fairley KF, et al: Pregnancy in women with primary focal and segmental hyalinosis and sclerosis. Clin Nephrol 29:185–192, 1988.

367. Geary DF, Farine M, Thorner P, Baumal R: Response to cyclophosphamide in steroid-resistant focal segmental glomerulosclerosis: A reappraisal. Clin Nephrol 22:109–113, 1984.

368. Tejani AT, Butt K, Trachtman H, et al: Cyclosporine A induced remission of relapsing nephrotic syndrome in children. Kidney Int 33:729–734, 1988.

369. Okada S, Kurata N, Ota Z, Ofuji T: Effect of dipyridamole on proteinuria of nephrotic syndrome. Lancet 1:719–720, 1981.

370. Velosa JA, Torres VE, Donadio JV, et al: Treatment of severe nephrotic syndrome with meclofenamate: An uncontrolled pilot study. Mayo Clin Proc 60:586–592, 1985.

371. Kooijmans-Coutinho MF, Tegzess AM, Bruijn JA, et al: Indomethacin treatment of recurrent nephrotic syndrome and focal segmental glomerulosclerosis after renal transplantation. Nephrol Dial Transplant 8:469–473, 1993.

372. Velosa JA, Torres VE: Benefits and risks of nonsteroidal antiinflammatory drugs in steroid-resistant nephrotic syndrome. Am J Kidney Dis 8:345–350, 1986.

373. Muso E, Yashiro M, Matsushima M, et al: Does LDL-apheresis in steroid-resistant nephrotic syndrome affect prognosis? Nephrol Dial Transplant 9:257–264, 1994.

374. Coggins CH: Is membranous nephropathy treatable? Am J Nephrol 1:219–221, 1981.

375. Glassock RJ: Secondary membranous glomerulonephritis. Nephrol Dial Transplant 7 Suppl 1:64–71, 1992.

376. Cahen R, Francois B, Trolliet P, et al: Aetiology of membranous glomerulonephritis: A prospective study of 82 adult patients. Nephrol Dial Transplant 4:172–180, 1989.

377. Warms PC, Rosenbaum BJ, Michelis MF, Haas JE: Idiopathic membranous glomerulonephritis occurring with diabetes mellitus. Arch Intern Med 132:735–738, 1973.

378. Shearn MA, Hopper J, Biava CG: Membranous lupus nephropathy initially seen as idiopathic membranous nephropathy. Possible diagnostic value of tubular reticular structures. Arch Intern Med 140:1521–1523, 1980.

379. Adu D, Williams DG, Taube D, et al: Late onset systemic lupus erythematosus and lupus-like disease in patients with apparent idiopathic glomerulonephritis. Q J Med 52:471–487.

380. Kleinknecht C, Levy M, Gagnadoux MF, Habib R: Membranous glomerulonephritis with extra-renal disorders in children. Medicine (Baltimore) 58:219–228, 1979.

381. Takekoshi Y, Tanaka M, Shida N, et al: Strong association between membranous nephropathy and hepatitis-B surface antigenaemia in Japanese children. Lancet 2:1065–1068, 1978.

382. Samuels B, Lee JC, Engleman EP, Hopper J: Membranous nephropathy in patients with rheumatoid arthritis: Relationship to gold therapy. Medicine (Baltimore) 57:319–327, 1978.

383. Schwartzberg M, Burnstein SL, Calabro JJ, Jacobs JB: The development of membranous glomerulonephritis in a patient with rheumatoid arthritis and Sjgren's syndrome. J Rheumatol 6:65–70.

384. Yamada A, Mitsuhashi K, Miyakawa Y, et al: Membranous glomerulonephritis associated with eosinophilic lymphfolliculosis of the skin (Kimura's disease): Report of a case and review of the literature. Clin Nephrol 18:211–215, 1982.

385. Dupont AG, Verbeelen DL, Six RO: Weber-Christian panniculitis with membranous glomerulonephritis. Am J Med 75:527–528, 1983.

386. Taylor RG, Fisher C, Hoffbrand BI: Sarcoidosis and membranous glomerulonephritis: A significant association. Br Med J (Clin Res Ed) 284:1297–1298, 1982.

387. Weetman AP, Pinching AJ, Pussel BA, et al: Membranous glomerulonephritis and autoimmune thyroid disease. Clin Nephrol 15:50–51, 1981.

388. Kobayashi K, Harada A, Onoyama K, et al: Idiopathic membranous glomerulonephritis associated with diabetes mellitus: Light, immunofluorescence and electron microscopic study. Nephron 28:163–168, 1981.

389. Sanchez I, Sobrini B, Guisantes J, et al: Membranous glomerulonephritis secondary to hydatid disease. Am J Med 70:311–315, 1981.

390. Brueggemeyer CD, Ramirez G: Membranous nephropathy: A concern for malignancy. Am J Kidney Dis 9:23–26, 1987.

391. Burstein DM, Korbet SM, Schwartz MM: Membranous glomerulonephritis and malignancy. Am J Kidney Dis 22:5–10, 1993.

392. Del Vecchio B, Polito C, Caporaso N, et al: Membranous glomerulopathy and hepatitis B virus (HBV) infection in children. Int J Pediatr Nephrol 4:235–238, 1983.

393. Hsu HC, Lin GH, Chang MH, Chen CH: Association of hepatitis B surface (HBs) antigenemia and membranous nephropathy in children in Taiwan. Clin Nephrol 20:121–129, 1983.

394. Kirdpon S, Vuttivirojana A, Kovitangkoon K, Poolsawat SS: The primary nephrotic syndrome in children and histopathologic study. J Med Assoc Thai 72 Suppl 1:26–31, 1989.

395. Yoshikawa N, Ito H, Yamada Y, et al: Membranous glomerulonephritis associated with hepatitis B antigen in children: A comparison with idiopathic membranous glomerulonephritis. Clin Nephrol 23:28–34, 1985.

396. Del Vecchio B, Polito C, Caporaso N, et al: Membranous glomerulopathy and hepatitis B virus (HBV) infection in children. Int J Pediatr Nephrol 4:235–238, 1983.

397. Slusarczyk J, Michalak T, Nazarewicz D, et al: Membranous glomerulopathy associated with hepatitis B core antigen immune complexes in children. Am J Pathol 98:29–43, 1980.

398. Black DA, Rose G, Brewer DB: Controlled trial of prednisone in adult patients with the nephrotic syndrome. Br Med J 3:421–426, 1970.

399. Bolton WK, Atuk NO, Sturgill BC, Westervelt FB: Therapy of the idiopathic nephrotic syndrome with alternate day steroids. Am J Med 62:60–70, 1977.

400. A controlled study of short-term prednisone treatment in adults with membranous nephropathy. Collaborative Study of the Adult Idiopathic Nephrotic Syndrome. N Engl J Med 301:1301–1306, 1979.

401. Forland M, Spargo BH: Clinicopathological correlations in idiopathic nephrotic syndrome with membranous nephropathy. Nephron 6:498–525, 1969.

402. Hayslett JP, Kashgarian M, Bensch KG, et al: Clinicopathological correlations in the nephrotic syndrome due to primary renal disease. Medicine (Baltimore) 52:93–120, 1973.

403. Miller RB, Harrington JT, Ramos CP, et al: Long-term results of steroid therapy in adults with idiopathic nephrotic syndrome. Am J Med 46:919–929, 1969.

404. Nyberg M, Petterson E, Tallqvist G, Pasternack A: Survival in idiopathic glomerulonephritis. Acta Pathol Microbiol Scand [A] 88:319–325, 1980.

405. Comparison of idiopathic and systemic lupus erythematosus-associated membranous glomerulonephropathy in children. The Southwest Pediatric Nephrology Study Group. Am J Kidney Dis 7:115–124, 1986.

406. Pierides AM, Malasit P, Morley AR, et al: Idiopathic membranous nephropathy. Q J Med 46:163–177, 1977.

407. Medawar W, Green A, Campbell E, et al: Clinical and histopathologic findings in adults with the nephrotic syndrome. Ir J Med Sci 159:137–140, 1990.

408. Churg J, Ehrenreich T: Membranous nephropathy. Perspect Nephrol Hypertens 1 Pt 1:443–448, 1973.

409. Hopper J, Trew PA, Biava CG: Membranous nephropathy: Its relative benignity in women. Nephron 29:18–24, 1981.

410. Noel LH, Zanetti M, Droz D, Barbanel C: Long-term prognosis of idiopathic membranous glomerulonephritis. Study of 116 untreated patients. Am J Med 66:82–90, 1979.

411. Ehrenreich T, Porush JG, Churg J, et al: Treatment of idiopathic membranous nephropathy. N Engl J Med 295:741–746, 1976.

412. Honkanen E, Tornroth T, Gronhagen R: Natural history, clinical course and morphological evolution of membranous nephropathy. Nephrol Dial Transplant 7 Suppl 1:35–41, 1992.

413. Row PG, Cameron JS, Turner DR, et al: Membranous nephropathy. Long-term follow-up and association with neoplasia. Q J Med 44:207–239, 1975.

414. Cameron JS, Healy MJ, Adu D: The Medical Research Council trial of short-term high-dose alternate day prednisolone in idiopathic membranous nephropathy with nephrotic syndrome in adults. The MRC Glomerulonephritis Working Party. Q J Med 74:133–156, 1990.

415. Cattran DC, Delmore T, Roscoe J, et al: A randomized controlled trial of prednisone in patients with idiopathic membranous nephropathy. N Engl J Med 320:210–215, 1989.

416. Kobayashi Y, Tateno S, Shigematsu H, Hiki Y: Prednisone treatment of non-nephrotic patients with idiopathic membranous nephropathy. A prospective study. Nephron 30:210–219, 1982.

417. Donadio JV, Holley KE, Anderson CF, Taylor WF: Controlled trial of cyclophosphamide in idiopathic membranous nephropathy. Kidney Int 6:431–439, 1974.

418. Ponticelli C, Zucchelli P, Passerini P, Cesana B: Methylprednisolone plus chlorambucil as compared with methylprednisolone alone for the treatment of idiopathic membranous nephropathy. The Italian Idiopathic Membranous Nephropathy Treatment Study Group. N Engl J Med 327:599–603, 1992.

419. Controlled trial of azathioprine and prednisone in chronic renal disease. Report by Medical Research Council Working Party. Br Med J 2:239–241, 1971.

420. Controlled trial of azathioprine in the nephrotic syndrome secondary to idiopathic membranous glomerulonephritis. Can Med Assoc J 115:1209–1210, 1976.

421. Olbing H, Greifer I, Bennett BP, et al: Idiopathic membranous nephropathy in children. Kidney Int 3:381–390, 1973.

422. Erwin DT, Donadio JV, Holley KE: The clinical course of idiopathic membranous nephropathy. Mayo Clin Proc 48:697–712, 1973.

423. Honkanen E: Survival in idiopathic membranous glomerulonephritis. Clin Nephrol 25:122–128, 1986.

424. MacTier R, Boulton J, Payton CD, McLay A: The natural history of membranous nephropathy in the West of Scotland. Q J Med 60:793–802, 1986.

425. Shearman JD, Yin ZG, Aarons I, et al: The effect of treatment with prednisolone or cyclophosphamide-warfarin-dipyridamole combination on the outcome of patients with membranous nephropathy. Clin Nephrol 30:320–329, 1988.

426. Schieppati A, Mosconi L, Perna A, et al: Prognosis of untreated patients with idiopathic membranous nephropathy. N Engl J Med 329:85–89, 1993.

427. Franklin WA, Jennings RB, Earle DP: Membranous glomerulonephritis: Long-term serial observations on clinical course and morphology. Kidney Int 4:36–56, 1973.

428. Ramzy MH, Cameron JS, Turner DR, et al: The long-term outcome of idiopathic membranous nephropathy. Clin Nephrol 16:13–19, 1981.

429. Suki WN, Chavez A: Membranous nephropathy: Response to steroids and immuno-suppression. Am J Nephrol 1:11–16, 1981.

430. Davison AM, Cameron JS, Kerr DN, et al: The natural history of renal function in untreated idiopathic membranous glomerulonephritis in adults. Clin Nephrol 22:61–67, 1984.

431. Harrison DJ, Thomson D, MacDonald MK: Membranous glomerulonephritis. J Clin Pathol 39:167, 1986.

432. Donadio JV, Torres VE, Velosa JA, et al: Idiopathic membranous nephropathy: The natural history of untreated patients. Kidney Int 33:708–715, 1988.

433. Alexopoulos E, Sakellariou G, Memmos D, et al: Cyclophosphamide provides no additional benefit to steroid therapy in the treatment of idiopathic membranous nephropathy. Am J Kidney Dis 21:497–503, 1993.

434. Mallick NP, Short CD, Manos J: Clinical membranous nephropathy. Nephron 34:209–219, 1983.

435. Schwartz MM: Membranous glomerulonephritis. In Jennette JC, Olson JL, Schwartz MM, Silva FG (eds): Heptinstall's Pathology of the Kidney, 6th ed. Philadelphia, Lippincott Williams & Wilkins, 2006, pp 205–252.

436. Magori A, Sonkodi S, Szabo E, Ormos J: Clinical pathology of membranous nephropathy based on kidney biopsy studies. Orv Hetil 118:2013–2020, 1977.

437. Jennette JC, Iskandar SS, Dalldorf FG: Pathologic differentiation between lupus and nonlupus membranous glomerulopathy. Kidney Int 24:377–385, 1983.

438. Jennette JC, Lamanna RW, Burnette JP, et al: Concurrent antiglomerular basement membrane antibody and immune complex mediated glomerulonephritis. Am J Clin Pathol 78:381–386, 1982.

439. Silva FG: Membranoproliferative glomerulonephritis. In Jennette JC, Olson JL, Schwartz MM, Silva FG (eds): Heptinstall's Pathology of the Kidney. Philadelphia, Lipincott-Raven, 1998, pp 309–368.

440. Abreo K, Abreo F, Mitchell B, Schloemer G: Idiopathic crescentic membranous glomerulonephritis. Am J Kidney Dis 8:257–261, 1986.

441. Jennette JC, Falk RJ: Nephritic syndrome and glomerulonephritis. In Silva FG, D'Agati VD, Nadasdy R (eds): Renal Biopsy Interpretation. New York, Churchill Livingstone, 1996, pp 71–114.

442. Klassen J, Elwood C, Grossberg AL, et al: Evolution of membranous nephropathy into anti-glomerular-basement-membrane glomerulonephritis. N Engl J Med 290: 1340–1344, 1974.

443. Kurki P, Helve T, von Bonsdorff M, et al: Transformation of membranous glomerulonephritis into crescentic glomerulonephritis with glomerular basement membrane antibodies. Serial determinations of anti-GBM before the transformation. Nephron 38:134–137, 1984.

444. Mathieson PW, Peat DS, Short A, Watts RA: Coexistent membranous nephropathy and ANCA-positive crescentic glomerulonephritis in association with penicillamine. Nephrol Dial Transplant 11:863–866, 1996.

445. Mitas JA, Frank LR, Swerdlin AR, et al: Crescentic glomerulonephritis complicating idiopathic membranous glomerulonephropathy. South Med J 76:664–667, 1983.

446. Lim LC, Taylor JG, III, Schmitz JL, et al: Diagnostic usefulness of antineutrophil cytoplasmic autoantibody serology. Comparative evaluation of commercial indirect fluorescent antibody kits and enzyme immunoassay kits. Am J Clin Pathol 111:363–369, 1999.

447. Schwartz MM: Membranous glomerulonephritis. In Jennette JC, Olson JL, Schwartz MM, Silva FG (eds): Heptinstall's Pathology of the Kidney, 5th ed. Philadelphia, Lippincott-Raven, 1998, pp 259–308.

448. Camussi G, Noble B, Van Liew J, et al: Pathogenesis of passive Heymann glomerulonephritis: Chlorpromazine inhibits antibody-mediated redistribution of cell surface antigens and prevents development of the disease. J Immunol 136:2127–2135, 1986.

449. Kerjaschki D, Farquhar MG: Immunocytochemical localization of the Heymann nephritis antigen (GP330) in glomerular epithelial cells of normal Lewis rats. J Exp Med 157:667–686, 1983.

450. Cavallo T: Membranous nephropathy. Insights from Heymann nephritis. Am J Pathol 144:651–658, 1994.

451. Kerjaschki D: Molecular pathogenesis of membranous nephropathy. Kidney Int 41:1090–1105, 1992.

452. Eddy AA, Fritz IB: Localization of clusterin in the epimembranous deposits of passive Heymann nephritis. Kidney Int 39:247–252, 1991.

453. Zager RA, Couser WG, Andrews BS, et al: Membranous nephropathy: A radioimmunologic search for anti-renal tubular epithelial antibodies and circulating immune complexes. Nephron 24:10–16, 1979.

454. Douglas MF, Rabideau DP, Schwartz MM, Lewis EJ: Evidence of autologous immune-complex nephritis. N Engl J Med 305:1326–1329, 1981.

455. Zanetti M, Mandet C, Dubost A, et al: Demonstration of a passive Heymann nephritis-like mechanism in a human kidney transplant. Clin Nephrol 15:272–277, 1981.

456. Honkanen E, Tikkanen I, Tornroth T: [Pathogenesis of glomerulonephritis]. Duodecim 111:1426–1434, 1995.

457. Ronco P, Debiec H: New insights into the pathogenesis of membranous glomerulonephritis. Curr Opin Nephrol Hypertens 15:258–263, 2006.

458. Debiec H, Guigonis V, Mougenot B, et al: Antenatal membranous glomerulonephritis due to anti-neutral endopeptidase antibodies. N Engl J Med 346:2053–2060, 2002.

459. Ronco P, Debiec H: Molecular pathomechanisms of membranous nephropathy: From Heymann nephritis to alloimmunization. J Am Soc Nephrol 16:1205–1213, 2005.

460. Cybulsky AV, Rennke HG, Feintzeig ID, Salant DJ: Complement-induced glomerular epithelial cell injury. Role of the membrane attack complex in rat membranous nephropathy. J Clin Invest 77:1096–1107, 1986.

461. Couser WG, Schulze M, Pruchno CJ: Role of C5b-9 in experimental membranous nephropathy. Nephrol Dial Transplant 7 Suppl 1:25–31, 1992.

462. Coupes B, Brenchley PE, Short CD, Mallick NP: Clinical aspects of C3dg and C5b-9 in human membranous nephropathy. Nephrol Dial Transplant 7 Suppl 1:32–34, 1992.

463. Doi T, Mayumi M, Kanatsu K, et al: Distribution of IgG subclasses in membranous nephropathy. Clin Exp Immunol 58:57–62, 1984.

464. Haas M: IgG subclass deposits in glomeruli of lupus and nonlupus membranous nephropathies. Am J Kidney Dis 23:358–364, 1994.

465. Doi T, Kanatsu K, Nagai H, et al: Demonstration of C3d deposits in membranous nephropathy. Nephron 37:232–235, 1984.

466. Cunningham PN, Quigg RJ: Contrasting roles of complement activation and its regulation in membranous nephropathy. J Am Soc Nephrol 16:1214–1222, 2005.

467. Quigg RJ, Holers VM, Morgan BP, Sneed AE: Crry and CD59 regulate complement in rat glomerular epithelial cells and are inhibited by the nephritogenic antibody of passive Heymann nephritis. J Immunol 154:3437–3443, 1995.

468. Salant DJ, Belok S, Madaio MP, Couser WG: A new role for complement in experimental membranous nephropathy in rats. J Clin Invest 66:1339–1350, 1980.

469. Schiller B, He C, Salant DJ, et al: Inhibition of complement regulation is key to the pathogenesis of active Heymann nephritis. J Exp Med 188:1353–1358, 1998.

470. Nangaku M, Quigg RJ, Shankland SJ, et al: Overexpression of Crry protects mesangial cells from complement-mediated injury. J Am Soc Nephrol 8:223–233, 1997.

471. Quigg RJ, Kozono Y, Berthiaume D, et al: Blockade of antibody-induced glomerulonephritis with Crry-Ig, a soluble murine complement inhibitor. J Immunol 160:4553–4560, 1998.

472. Neale TJ, Ojha PP, Exner M, et al: Proteinuria in passive Heymann nephritis is associated with lipid peroxidation and formation of adducts on type IV collagen. J Clin Invest 94:1577–1584, 1994.

473. Hsu SI, Couser WG: Chronic progression of tubulointerstitial damage in proteinuric renal disease is mediated by complement activation: A therapeutic role for complement inhibitors? J Am Soc Nephrol 14:S186–S191, 2003.

474. Tang S, Lai KN, Sacks SH: Role of complement in tubulointerstitial injury from proteinuria. Kidney Blood Press Res 25:120–126, 2002.

475. Nakamura T, Tanaka N, Higuma N, et al: The localization of plasminogen activator inhibitor-1 in glomerular subepithelial deposits in membranous nephropathy. J Am Soc Nephrol 7:2434–2444, 1996.

476. Klouda PT, Manos J, Acheson EJ, et al: Strong association between idiopathic membranous nephropathy and HLA-DRW3. Lancet 2:770–771, 1979.

477. Laurent B, Berthoux FC, le Petit JC, et al: Immunogenetics and immunopathology of human idiopathic membranous glomerulonephritis. Proc Eur Dial Transplant Assoc 19:629–634, 1983.

478. lePetit JC, Laurent B, Berthoux FC: HLA-DR3 and idiopathic membranous nephritis (IMN) association. Tissue Antigens 20:227–228, 1982.

479. Hiki Y, Kobayashi Y, Itoh I, Kashiwagi N: Strong association of HLA-DR2 and MT1 with idiopathic membranous nephropathy in Japan. Kidney Int 25:953–957, 1984.

480. Tomura S, Kashiwabara H, Tuchida H, et al: Strong association of idiopathic membranous nephropathy with HLA-DR2 and MT1 in Japanese. Nephron 36:242–245, 1984.

481. Ogahara S, Naito S, Abe K, et al: Analysis of HLA class II genes in Japanese patients with idiopathic membranous glomerulonephritis. Kidney Int 41:175–182, 1992.

482. Dyer PA, Klouda PT, Harris R, Mallick NP: Properdin factor B alleles in patients with idiopathic membranous nephropathy. Tissue Antigens 15:505–507, 1980.

483. Sacks SH, Nomura S, Warner C, et al: Analysis of complement C4 loci in Caucasoids and Japanese with idiopathic membranous nephropathy. Kidney Int 42:882–887, 1992.

484. Short CD, Feehally J, Gokal R, Mallick NP: Familial membranous nephropathy. Br Med J (Clin Res Ed) 289:1500, 1984.

485. Sato K, Oguchi H, Hora K, et al: Idiopathic membranous nephropathy in two brothers. Nephron 46:174–178, 1987.

486. Dumas R, Dumas ML, Baldet P, Bascoul S: [Membranous glomerulonephritis in two brothers associated in one with tubulo-interstitial disease, Fanconi syndrome and anti-TBM antibodies (author's transl)]. Arch Fr Pediatr 39:75–78, 1982.

487. Elshihabi I, Kaye CI, Brzowski A: Membranous nephropathy in two human leukocyte antigen-identical brothers. J Pediatr 123:940–942, 1993.

488. Vangelista A, Tazzari R, Bonomini V: Idiopathic membranous nephropathy in 2 twin brothers. Nephron 50:79–80, 1988.

489. Lewy JE, Salinas M, Herdson PB, et al: Clinico-pathologic correlations in acute poststreptococcal glomerulonephritis. A correlation between renal functions, morphologic damage and clinical course of 46 children with acute poststreptococcal glomerulonephritis. Medicine (Baltimore) 50:453–501, 1971.

490. Pollak VE, Pirani CL, Dujovne I, Dillard MG: The clinical course of lupus nephritis: relationship to the renal histologic findings. Perspect Nephrol Hypertens 1 Pt 2:1167–1181, 1973.

491. Beregi E, Varga I: Analysis of 260 cases of membranous glomerulonephritis in renal biopsy material. Clin Nephrol 2:215–221.

492. Kida H, Asamoto T, Yokoyama H, et al: Long-term prognosis of membranous nephropathy. Clin Nephrol 25:64–69, 1986.

493. Abe S, Amagasaki Y, Konishi K, et al: Idiopathic membranous glomerulonephritis: Aspects of geographical differences. J Clin Pathol 39:1193–1198, 1986.

494. Tu WH, Petitti DB, Biava CG, et al: Membranous nephropathy: predictors of terminal renal failure. Nephron 36:118–124, 1984.

495. Murphy BF, Fairley KF, Kincaid S: Idiopathic membranous glomerulonephritis: long-term follow-up in 139 cases. Clin Nephrol 30:175–181, 1988.

496. Sherman RA, Dodelson R, Gary NE, Eisinger RP: Membranous nephropathy. J Med Soc N J 77:649–652, 1980.

497. James SH, Lien YH, Ruffenach SJ, Wilcox GE: Acute renal failure in membranous glomerulonephropathy: A result of superimposed crescentic glomerulonephritis. J Am Soc Nephrol 6:1541–1546, 1995.

498. Wagoner RD, Stanson AW, Holley KE, Winter CS: Renal vein thrombosis in idiopathic membranous glomerulopathy and nephrotic syndrome: Incidence and significance. Kidney Int 23:368–374, 1983.

499. Kanwar YS, Farquhar MG: Anionic sites in the glomerular basement membrane. In vivo and in vitro localization to the laminae rarae by cationic probes. J Cell Biol 81:137–153, 1979.

500. Hogan SL, Muller KE, Jennette JC, Falk RJ: A review of therapeutic studies of idiopathic membranous glomerulopathy. Am J Kidney Dis 25:862–875, 1995.

501. Pollak VE, Rosen S, Pirani CL, et al: Natural history of lipoid nephrosis and of membranous glomerulonephritis. Ann Intern Med 69:1171–1196, 1968.

502. Ponticelli C, Zucchelli P, Passerini P, et al: A randomized trial of methylprednisolone and chlorambucil in idiopathic membranous nephropathy. N Engl J Med 320:8–13, 1989.

503. Murphy BF, McDonald I, Fairley KF, Kincaid S: Randomized controlled trial of cyclophosphamide, warfarin and dipyridamole in idiopathic membranous glomerulonephritis. Clin Nephrol 37:229–234, 1992.

504. Pei Y, Cattran D, Greenwood C: Predicting chronic renal insufficiency in idiopathic membranous glomerulonephritis. Kidney Int 42:960–966, 1992.

505. Cattran DC, Pei Y, Greenwood C: Predicting progression in membranous glomerulonephritis. Nephrol Dial Transplant 7 Suppl 1:48–52, 1992.

506. Honkanen E, Tornroth T, Gronhagen R, Sankila R: Long-term survival in idiopathic membranous glomerulonephritis: Can the course be clinically predicted? Clin Nephrol 41:127–134, 1994.

507. Wehrmann M, Bohle A, Bogenschutz O, et al: Long-term prognosis of chronic idiopathic membranous glomerulonephritis. An analysis of 334 cases with particular regard to tubulo-interstitial changes. Clin Nephrol 31:67–76, 1989.

508. Austin HA, Boumpas DT, Vaughan EM, Balow JE: High-risk features of lupus nephritis: Importance of race and clinical and histological factors in 166 patients. Nephrol Dial Transplant 10:1620–1628, 1995.

509. D'Amico G: Influence of clinical and histological features on actuarial renal survival in adult patients with idiopathic IgA nephropathy, membranous nephropathy, and

membranoproliferative glomerulonephritis: Survey of the recent literature. Am J Kidney Dis 20:315–323, 1992.

510. Ponticelli C, Zucchelli P, Imbasciati E, et al: Controlled trial of methylprednisolone and chlorambucil in idiopathic membranous nephropathy. N Engl J Med 310:946–950, 1984.

511. Zucchelli P, Cagnoli L, Pasquali S, et al: Clinical and morphologic evolution of idiopathic membranous nephropathy. Clin Nephrol 25:282–288, 1986.

512. Ponticelli C, Zucchelli P, Passerini P, et al: A 10-year follow-up of a randomized study with methylprednisolone and chlorambucil in membranous nephropathy. Kidney Int 48:1600–1604, 1995.

513. Alexopoulos E, Seron D, Hartley RB, et al: Immune mechanisms in idiopathic membranous nephropathy: The role of the interstitial infiltrates. Am J Kidney Dis 13:404–412, 1989.

514. Wakai S, Magil AB: Focal glomerulosclerosis in idiopathic membranous glomerulonephritis. Kidney Int 41:428–434, 1992.

515. Lee HS, Koh HI: Nature of progressive glomerulosclerosis in human membranous nephropathy. Clin Nephrol 39:7–16, 1993.

516. Zucchelli P, Pasquali S: Membranous nephropathy. In Cameron JS (ed): Oxford Textbook of Clinical Nephrology. Oxford, Oxford University Press, 1992.

517. Pruchno CJ, Burns MW, Schulze M, et al: Urinary excretion of C5b-9 reflects disease activity in passive Heymann nephritis. Kidney Int 36:65–71, 1989.

518. Rosen S, Tornroth T, Bernard DB: Membranous glomerulonephritis. In Tischer CC, Brenner BM (eds): Renal Pathology. Philadelphia, Lippincott, 1989.

519. Habib R, Kleinknecht C, Gubler MC: Extramembranous glomerulonephritis in children: report of 50 cases. J Pediatr 82:754–766, 1973.

520. Short CD, Durrington PN, Mallick NP, et al: Serum lipoprotein (a) in men with proteinuria due to idiopathic membranous nephropathy. Nephrol Dial Transplant 7 Suppl 1:109–113, 1992.

521. Schulze M, Donadio JV, Pruchno CJ, et al: Elevated urinary excretion of the C5b-9 complex in membranous nephropathy. Kidney Int 40:533–538, 1991.

522. Ogrodowski JL, Hebert LA, Sedmak D, et al: Measurement of SC5b-9 in urine in patients with the nephrotic syndrome. Kidney Int 40:1141–1147, 1991.

523. Brenchley PE, Coupes B, Short CD, et al: Urinary C3dg and C5b-9 indicate active immune disease in human membranous nephropathy. Kidney Int 41:933–937, 1992.

524. Coupes BM, Kon SP, Brenchley PE, et al: The temporal relationship between urinary C5b-9 and C3dg and clinical parameters in human membranous nephropathy. Nephrol Dial Transplant 8:397–401, 1993.

525. Savin VJ, Johnson RJ, Couser WG: C5b-9 increases albumin permeability of isolated glomeruli in vitro. Kidney Int 46:382–387, 1994.

526. Kusunoki Y, Akutsu Y, Itami N, et al: Urinary excretion of terminal complement complexes in glomerular disease. Nephron 59:27–32, 1991.

527. Lin J, Markowitz GS, Nicolaides M, et al: Membranous glomerulopathy associated with graft-versus-host disease following allogeneic stem cell transplantation. Report of 2 cases and review of the literature. Am J Nephrol 21:351–356, 2001.

528. Llach F: Thromboembolic complications in nephrotic syndrome. Coagulation abnormalities, renal vein thrombosis, and other conditions. Postgrad Med 76:111–8, 121, 1984.

529. Kauffmann RH, Veltkamp JJ, Van Tilburg NH, Van Es LA: Acquired antithrombin III deficiency and thrombosis in the nephrotic syndrome. Am J Med 65:607–613, 1978.

530. Velasquez F, Garcia P, Ruiz M: Idiopathic nephrotic syndrome of the adult with asymptomatic thrombosis of the renal vein. Am J Nephrol 8:457–462, 1988.

531. Llach F, Koffler A, Finck E, Massry SG: On the incidence of renal vein thrombosis in the nephrotic syndrome. Arch Intern Med 137:333–336, 1977.

532. Llach F, Arieff AI, Massry SG: Renal vein thrombosis and nephrotic syndrome. A prospective study of 36 adult patients. Ann Intern Med 83:8–14, 1975.

533. Trew PA, Biava CG, Jacobs RP, Hopper J: Renal vein thrombosis in membranous glomerulonephropathy: Incidence and association. Medicine (Baltimore) 57:69–82, 1978.

534. Sarasin FP, Schifferli JA: Prophylactic oral anticoagulation in nephrotic patients with idiopathic membranous nephropathy. Kidney Int 45:578–585, 1994.

535. Saag KG, Koehnke R, Caldwell JR, et al: Low dose long-term corticosteroid therapy in rheumatoid arthritis: An analysis of serious adverse events. Am J Med 96:115–123, 1994.

536. Stuck AE, Minder CE, Frey FJ: Risk of infectious complications in patients taking glucocorticosteroids. Rev Infect Dis 11:954–963.

537. Short CD, Solomon LR, Gokal R, Mallick NP: Methylprednisolone in patients with membranous nephropathy and declining renal function. Q J Med 65:929–940, 1987.

538. Williams PS, Bone JM: Immunosuppression can arrest progressive renal failure due to idiopathic membranous glomerulonephritis. Nephrol Dial Transplant 4:181–186, 1989.

539. Manos J, Short CD, Acheson EJ, et al: Relapsing idiopathic membranous nephropathy. Clin Nephrol 18:286–290, 1982.

540. Berg AL, Nilsson-Ehle P, Arnadottir M: Beneficial effects of ACTH on the serum lipoprotein profile and glomerular function in patients with membranous nephropathy. Kidney Int 56:1534–1543, 1999.

541. Ponticelli C, Passerini P, Salvadori M, et al: A randomized pilot trial comparing methylprednisolone plus a cytotoxic agent versus synthetic adrenocorticotropic hormone in idiopathic membranous nephropathy. Am J Kidney Dis 47:233–240, 2006.

542. Branten AJ, Reichert LJ, Koene RA, Wetzels JF: Oral cyclophosphamide versus chlorambucil in the treatment of patients with membranous nephropathy and renal insufficiency. Q J Med 91:359–366, 1998.

543. Imperiale TF, Goldfarb S, Berns JS: Are cytotoxic agents beneficial in idiopathic membranous nephropathy? A meta-analysis of the controlled trials. J Am Soc Nephrol 5:1553–1558, 1995.

544. Torres A, Dominguez-Gil B, Carreno A, et al: Conservative versus immunosuppressive treatment of patients with idiopathic membranous nephropathy. Kidney Int 61:219–227, 2002.

545. West ML, Jindal KK, Bear RA, Goldstein MB: A controlled trial of cyclophosphamide in patients with membranous glomerulonephritis. Kidney Int 32:579–584, 1987.

546. Jindal K, West M, Bear R, Goldstein M: Long-term benefits of therapy with cyclophosphamide and prednisone in patients with membranous glomerulonephritis and impaired renal function. Am J Kidney Dis 19:61–67, 1992.

547. Bruns FJ, Adler S, Fraley DS, Segel DP: Sustained remission of membranous glomerulonephritis after cyclophosphamide and prednisone. Ann Intern Med 114:725–730, 1991.

548. Falk RJ, Hogan SL, Muller KE, Jennette JC: Treatment of progressive membranous glomerulopathy. A randomized trial comparing cyclophosphamide and corticosteroids with corticosteroids alone. The Glomerular Disease Collaborative Network [see comments]. Ann Intern Med 116:438–445, 1992.

549. Reichert LJ, Huysmans FT, Assmann K, et al: Preserving renal function in patients with membranous nephropathy: Daily oral chlorambucil compared with intermittent monthly pulses of cyclophosphamide. Ann Intern Med 121:328–333, 1994.

550. Mathieson PW, Turner AN, Maidment CG, et al: Prednisolone and chlorambucil treatment in idiopathic membranous nephropathy with deteriorating renal function. Lancet 2:869–872, 1988.

551. Warwick GL, Geddes CG, Boulton-Jones JM: Prednisolone and chlorambucil therapy for idiopathic membranous nephropathy with progressive renal failure. Q J Med 87:223–229, 1994.

552. Brunkhorst R, Wrenger E, Koch KM: Low-dose prednisolone/chlorambucil therapy in patients with severe membranous glomerulonephritis. Clin Invest 72:277–282, 1994.

553. Tarlar-Williams C, Hijazi Y, Walther M: Cyclophosphamide-induced cystitis and bladder cancer in patients with Wegener's granulomatosis. Ann Intern Med 124:477–484, 1996.

554. Meyrier A: Treatment of idiopathic nephrotic syndrome with cyclosporine A. J Nephrol 10:14–24.

555. Guasch A, Suranyi M, Newton L, et al: Short-term responsiveness of membranous glomerulopathy to cyclosporine. Am J Kidney Dis 20:472–481, 1992.

556. Rostoker G, Belghiti D, Ben M, et al: Long-term cyclosporin A therapy for severe idiopathic membranous nephropathy. Nephron 63:335–341, 1993.

557. Cattran DC, Greenwood C, Ritchie S, et al: A controlled trial of cyclosporine in patients with progressive membranous nephropathy. Canadian Glomerulonephritis Study Group. Kidney Int 47:1130–1135, 1995.

558. Cattran DC, Appel GB, Hebert LA, et al: Cyclosporine in patients with steroid-resistant membranous nephropathy: A randomized trial. Kidney Int 59:1484–1490, 2001.

559. Ambalavanan S, Fauvel JP, Sibley RK, Myers BD: Mechanism of the antiproteinuric effect of cyclosporine in membranous nephropathy. J Am Soc Nephrol 7:290–298, 1996.

560. Palla R, Cirami C, Panichi V, et al: Intravenous immunoglobulin therapy of membranous nephropathy: Efficacy and safety. Clin Nephrol 35:98–104, 1991.

561. Yokoyama H, Goshima S, Wada T, et al: The short- and long-term outcomes of membranous nephropathy treated with intravenous immune globulin therapy. Kanazawa Study Group for Renal Diseases and Hypertension. Nephrol Dial Transplant 14:2379–2386, 1999.

562. Miller G, Zimmerman R, Radhakrishnan J, Appel G: Use of mycophenolate mofetil in resistant membranous nephropathy. Am J Kidney Dis 36:250–256, 2000.

563. Briggs WA, Choi MJ, Scheel Jr, PJ: Successful mycophenolate mofetil treatment of glomerular disease. Am J Kidney Dis 31:213–217, 1998.

564. Choi MJ, Eustace JA, Gimenez LF, et al: Mycophenolate mofetil treatment for primary glomerular diseases. Kidney Int 61:1098–1114, 2002.

565. Nowack R, Birck R, van der Woude FJ: Mycophenolate mofetil for systemic vasculitis and IgA nephropathy. Lancet 349:774, 1997.

566. Zhao M, Chen X, Chen Y, et al: [Mycophenolate mofetil in the treatment of primary nephrotic syndrome]. Zhonghua Yi Xue Za Zhi 81:528–531, 2001.

567. Remuzzi G, Chiurchiu C, Abbate M, et al: Rituximab for idiopathic membranous nephropathy. Lancet 360:923–924, 2002.

568. Ruggenenti P, Chiurchiu C, Brusegan V, et al: Rituximab in idiopathic membranous nephropathy: A one-year prospective study. J Am Soc Nephrol 14:1851–1857, 2003.

569. Ruggenenti P, Chiurchiu C, Abbate M, et al: Rituximab for idiopathic membranous nephropathy: Who can benefit? Clin J Am Soc Nephrol 1:738–748, 2006.

570. Appel GB, Nachman PH, Hogan SL, et al: Eculizumab (c5 complement inhibitor) in the treatment of idiopathic membranous nephropathy [Abstract]. J Am Soc Nephrol 13: 2002.

571. Rostoker G, Ben M, Remy P, et al: Low-dose angiotensin-converting-enzyme inhibitor captopril to reduce proteinuria in adult idiopathic membranous nephropathy: A prospective study of long-term treatment. Nephrol Dial Transplant 10:25–29, 1995.

572. Thomas DM, Hillis AN, Coles GA, et al: Enalapril can treat the proteinuria of membranous glomerulonephritis without detriment to systemic or renal hemodynamics. Am J Kidney Dis 18:38–43, 1991.

573. Gansevoort RT, Heeg JE, Vriesendorp R, et al: Antiproteinuric drugs in patients with idiopathic membranous glomerulopathy. Nephrol Dial Transplant 7 Suppl 1:91–96, 1992.

574. Ruilope LM, Casal MC, Praga M, et al: Additive antiproteinuric effect of converting enzyme inhibition and a low protein intake. J Am Soc Nephrol 3:1307–1311, 1992.

575. Haas M, Kerjaschki D, Mayer G: Lipid-lowering therapy in membranous nephropathy. Kidney Int Suppl 71:S110–S112, 1999.

576. Neugarten J, Acharya A, Silbiger SR: Effect of gender on the progression of nondiabetic renal disease: A meta-analysis. J Am Soc Nephrol 11:319–329, 2000.

577. Zent R, Nagai R, Cattran DC: Idiopathic membranous nephropathy in the elderly: a comparative study. Am J Kidney Dis 29:200–206, 1997.

578. Troyanov S, Roasio L, Pandes M, et al: Renal pathology in idiopathic membranous nephropathy: A new perspective. Kidney Int 69:1641–1648, 2006.

579. Bazzi C, Petrini C, Rizza V, et al: Urinary excretion of IgG and alpha(1)-microglobulin predicts clinical course better than extent of proteinuria in membranous nephropathy. Am J Kidney Dis 38:240–248, 2001.

580. Branten AJ, du Buf-Vereijken PW, Klasen IS, et al: Urinary excretion of {beta}2-microglobulin and IgG predict prognosis in idiopathic membranous nephropathy: A validation study. J Am Soc Nephrol 16:169–174, 2005.

581. Cattran D: Management of membranous nephropathy: When and what for treatment. J Am Soc Nephrol 15:1188–1194, 2005.

582. Levy M, Gubler MC, Habib R: New concepts in membranoproliferative glomerulonephritis. In Kincaid-Smith P, d'Apice AJF, Atkins RC (eds): Progress in Glomerulonephritis. New York, John Wiley and Sons, 1979, p 177.

583. Donadio JV, Jr, Anderson CF, Mitchell JC, III, et al: Membranoproliferative glomerulonephritis. A prospective clinical trial of platelet-inhibitor therapy. N Engl J Med 310:1421–1426, 1984.

584. Cameron JS, Turner DR, Heaton J, et al: Idiopathic mesangiocapillary glomerulonephritis. Comparison of types I and II in children and adults and long-term prognosis. Am J Med 74:175–192, 1983.

585. D'Amico G, Ferrario F: Mesangiocapillary glomerulonephritis. J Am Soc Nephrol 2:S159–S166, 1992.

586. Habib R, Gubler MC, Loirat C, et al: Dense deposit disease: A variant of membranoproliferative glomerulonephritis. Kidney Int 7:204–215, 1975.

587. Davis AE, Schneeberger EE, McCluskey RT, Grupe WE: Mesangial proliferative glomerulonephritis with irregular intramembranous deposits. Another variant of hypocomplementemic nephritis. Am J Med 63:481–487, 1977.

588. King JT, Valenzuela R, McCormack LJ, Osborne DG: Granular dense deposit disease. Lab Invest 39:591–596, 1978.

589. Strife CF, Jackson EC, McAdams AJ: Type III membranoproliferative glomerulonephritis: Long-term clinical and morphologic evaluation. Clin Nephrol 21:323–334, 1984.

590. Klein M, Poucell S, Arbus GS, et al: Characteristics of a benign subtype of dense deposit disease: Comparison with the progressive form of this disease. Clin Nephrol 20:163–171, 1983.

591. Sasdelli M, Santoro A, Cagnoli L, et al: [Membranoproliferative glomerulonephritis. Clinical, biological and histological study of 31 cases]. Minerva Nefrol 22:229–238.

592. Vargas R, Thomson KJ, Wilson D, et al: Mesangiocapillary glomerulonephritis with dense "deposits" in the basement membranes of the kidney. Clin Nephrol 5:73–82, 1976.

593. Donadio JV, Jr, Slack TK, Holley KE, Ilstrup DM: Idiopathic membranoproliferative (mesangiocapillary) glomerulonephritis: A clinicopathologic study. Mayo Clin Proc 54:141–150, 1979.

594. Barbiano D, Baroni M, Pagliari B, et al: Is membranoproliferative glomerulonephritis really decreasing? A multicentre study of 1548 cases of primary glomerulonephritis. Nephron 40:380–381, 1985.

595. Zhou XJ, Silva FG: Membranoproliferative glomerulonephritis. In Jennette JC, Olson JL, Schwartz MM, Silva FG (eds): Heptinstall's Pathology of the Kidney 6h ed. Philadelphia, Lippincott Williams & Wilkins, 2006, pp 253–320.

596. Korzets Z, Bernheim J, Bernheim J: Rapidly progressive glomerulonephritis (crescentic glomerulonephritis) in the course of type I idiopathic membranoproliferative glomerulonephritis. Am J Kidney Dis 10:56–61, 1987.

597. McCoy R, Clapp J, Seigler HF: Membranoproliferative glomerulonephritis. Progression from the pure form to the crescentic form with recurrence after transplantation. Am J Med 59:288–292, 1975.

598. Burkholder PM, Marchand A, Krueger RP: Mixed membranous and proliferative glomerulonephritis. A correlative light, immunofluorescence, and electron microscopic study. Lab Invest 23:459–479, 1970.

599. Strife CF, McEnery PT, McAdams AJ, West CD: Membranoproliferative glomerulonephritis with disruption of the glomerular basement membrane. Clin Nephrol 7:65–72, 1977.

600. Jennette JC: Immunohistology of renal disease. In Jennette JC (ed): Immunohistopathology in Diagnostic Pathology. Boca Raton, CRC Press, 1989, pp 29–84.

601. Sibley RK, Kim Y: Dense intramembranous deposit disease: New pathologic features. Kidney Int 25:660–670, 1984.

602. Jansen JH, Hogasen K, Mollnes TE: Extensive complement activation in hereditary porcine membranoproliferative glomerulonephritis type II (porcine dense deposit disease). Am J Pathol 143:1356–1365, 1993.

603. Mathieson PW, Peters K: Are nephritic factors nephritogenic? Am J Kidney Dis 24:964–966, 1994.

604. Droz D, Nabarra B, Noel LH, et al: Recurrence of dense deposits in transplanted kidneys: I. Sequential survey of the lesions. Kidney Int 15:386–395, 1979.

605. Eisinger AJ, Shortland JR, Moorhead PJ: Renal disease in partial lipodystrophy. Q J Med 41:343–354, 1972.

606. Appel GB, Cook HT, Hageman G, et al: Membranoproliferative glomerulonephritis type II (dense deposit disease): An update. J Am Soc Nephrol 16:1392–1403, 2005.

607. Dragon-Durey MA, Fremeaux-Bacchi V, Loirat C, et al: Heterozygous and homozygous factor h deficiencies associated with hemolytic uremic syndrome or membranoproliferative glomerulonephritis: Report and genetic analysis of 16 cases. J Am Soc Nephrol 15:787–795, 2004.

608. Ault BH, Schmidt BZ, Fowler NL, et al: Human factor H deficiency. Mutations in framework cysteine residues and block in H protein secretion and intracellular catabolism. J Biol Chem 272:25168–25175, 1997.

609. Donadio JV, Jr, Offord KP: Reassessment of treatment results in membranoproliferative glomerulonephritis, with emphasis on life-table analysis. Am J Kidney Dis 14:445–451, 1989.

610. Holley KE, Donadio JV: Mesangioproliferative glomerulonephritis. In Tisher CC, Brenner BM (eds): Renal Pathology: With Clinical and Functional Correlations. Philadelphia, Lippincott, 1994, pp 294–329.

611. Peters DK, Charlesworth JA, Sissons JG, et al: Mesangiocapillary nephritis, partial lipodystrophy, and hypocomplementaemia. Lancet 2:535–538, 1973.

612. Sissons JG, West RJ, Fallows J, et al: The complement abnormalities of lipodystrophy. N Engl J Med 294:461–465, 1976.

613. Bennett WM, Bardana EJ, Wuepper K, et al: Partial lipodystrophy, C3 nephritic factor and clinically inapparent mesangiocapillary glomerulonephritis. Am J Med 62:757–760, 1977.

614. Ipp MM, Minta JO, Gelfand EW: Disorders of the complement system in lipodystrophy. Clin Immunol Immunopath 7:281–287, 1977.

615. Stutchfield PR, White RH, Cameron AH, et al: X-linked mesangiocapillary glomerulonephritis. Clin Nephrol 26:150–156, 1986.

616. Schmitt H, Bohle A, Reineke T, et al: Long-term prognosis of membranoproliferative glomerulonephritis type I. Significance of clinical and morphological parameters: An investigation of 220 cases. Nephron 55:242–250, 1990.

617. Kashtan CE, Burke B, Burch G, et al: Dense intramembranous deposit disease: A clinical comparison of histological subtypes. Clin Nephrol 33:1–6, 1990.

618. Dense deposit disease in children: Prognostic value of clinical and pathologic indicators. The Southwest Pediatric Nephrology Study Group. Am J Kidney Dis 6:161–169, 1985.

619. di Belgiojoso B, Tarantino A, Colasanti G, et al: The prognostic value of some clinical and histological parameters in membranoproliferative glomerulonephritis (MPGN): Report of 112 cases. Nephron 19:250–258, 1977.

620. Habib R, Kleinknecht C, Gubler MC, Levy M: Idiopathic membranoproliferative glomerulonephritis in children. Report of 105 cases. Clin Nephrol 1:194–214, 1973.

621. Swainson CP, Robson JS, Thomson D, MacDonald MK: Mesangiocapillary glomerulonephritis: A long-term study of 40 cases. J Pathol 141:449–468, 1983.

622. Antoine B, Faye C: The clinical course associated with dense deposits in the kidney basement membranes. Kidney Int 1:420–427, 1972.

623. Miller MN, Baumal R, Poucell S, Steele BT: Incidence and prognostic importance of glomerular crescents in renal diseases of childhood. Am J Nephrol 4:244–247, 1984.

624. Droz D, Zanetti M, Noel LH, Leibowitch J: Dense deposits disease. Nephron 19:1–11, 1977.

625. Hume DM, Bryant CP: The development of recurrent glomerulonephritis. Transplant Proc 4:673–677, 1972.

626. Lamb V, Tisher CC, McCoy RC, Robinson RR: Membranoproliferative glomerulonephritis with dense intramembranous alterations. A clinicopathologic study. Lab Invest 36:607–617, 1977.

627. Davis AE, Schneeberger EE, Grupe WE, McCluskey RT: Membranoproliferative glomerulonephritis (MPGN type I) and dense deposit disease (DDD) in children. Clin Nephrol 9:184–193, 1978.

628. Cameron JS: Glomerulonephritis in renal transplants. Transplantation 34:237–245, 1982.

629. Cameron JS, Turner DR: Recurrent glomerulonephritis in allografted kidneys. Clin Nephrol 7:47–54, 1977.

630. Curtis JJ, Wyatt RJ, Bhathena D, et al: Renal transplantation for patients with type I and type II membranoproliferative glomerulonephritis: Serial complement and nephritic factor measurements and the problem of recurrence of disease. Am J Med 66:216–225, 1979.

631. Varade WS, Forristal J, West CD: Patterns of complement activation in idiopathic membranoproliferative glomerulonephritis, types I, II, and III. Am J Kidney Dis 16:196–206, 1990.

632. Williams DG, Peters DK, Fallows J, et al: Studies of serum complement in the hypocomplementaemic nephritides. Clin Exp Immunol 18:391–405, 1974.

633. Pickering RJ, Gewurz H, Good RA: Complement inactivation by serum from patients with acute and hypocomplementemic chronic glomerulonephritis. J Lab Clin Med 72:298–307, 1968.

634. Halbwachs L, Leveille M, Lesavre P, et al: Nephritic factor of the classical pathway of complement: Immunoglobulin G autoantibody directed against the classical pathway C3 convetase enzyme. J Clin Invest 65:1249–1256, 1980.

635. Misiani R, Bellavita P, Fenili D, et al: Hepatitis C virus infection in patients with essential mixed cryoglobulinemia. Ann Intern Med 117:573–577, 1992.

636. Daha MR, Austen KF, Fearon DT: Heterogeneity, polypeptide chain composition and antigenic reactivity of C3 nephritic factor. J Immunol 120:1389–1394, 1978.

637. Spitzer RE, Vallota EH, Forristal J, et al: Serum C'3 lytic system in patients with glomerulonephritis. Science 164:436–437, 1969.

638. Schreiber RD, Gotze O, Muller-Eberhard HJ: Nephritic factor: Its structure and function and its relationship to initiating factor of the alternative pathway. Scand J Immunol 5:705–713, 1976.

639. Williams DG, Bartlett A, Duffus P: Identification of nephritic factor as an immunoglobulin. Clin Exp Immunol 33:425–429, 1978.

640. Siegler RL, Brewer ED, Hammond E: Platelet activation and prostacyclin supporting capacity in the loin pain hematuria syndrome. Am J Kidney Dis 12:156–160, 1988.

641. McAdams AJ, McEnery PT, West CD: Mesangiocapillary glomerulonephritis: Changes in glomerular morphology with long-term alternate-day prednisone therapy. J Pediatr 86:23–31, 1975.

642. McEnery PT, McAdams AJ, West CD: Membranoproliferative glomerulonephritis: Improved survival with alternate day prednisone therapy. Clin Nephrol 13:117–124, 1978.

643. West CD: Childhood membranoproliferative glomerulonephritis: An approach to management. Kidney Int 29:1077–1093, 1986.

644. McEnery PT, McAdams AJ, West CD: The effect of prednisone in a high-dose, alternate-day regimen on the natural history of idiopathic membranoproliferative glomerulonephritis. Medicine (Baltimore) 64:401–424, 1985.

645. McEnery PT, McAdams AJ: Regression of membranoproliferative glomerulonephritis type II (dense deposit disease): Observations in six children. Am J Kidney Dis 12:138–146, 1988.

646. Ford DM, Briscoe DM, Shanley PF, Lum GM: Childhood membranoproliferative glomerulonephritis type I: Limited steroid therapy. Kidney Int 41:1606–1612, 1992.

647. Warady BA, Guggenheim SJ, Sedman A, Lum GM: Prednisone therapy of membranoproliferative glomerulonephritis in children. J Pediatr 107:702–707, 1985.

648. Kincaid-Smith P: The natural history and treatment of mesangiocapillary glomerulonephritis. Perspect Nephrol Hypertens 1 Pt 1:591–609, 1973.

649. Kher KK, Makker SP, Aikawa M, Kirson IJ: Regression of dense deposits in Type II membranoproliferative glomerulonephritis: Case report of clinical course in a child. Clin Nephrol 17:100–103, 1982.

650. Chapman SJ, Cameron JS, Chantler C, Turner D: Treatment of mesangiocapillary glomerulonephritis in children with combined immunosuppression and anticoagulation. Arch Dis Child 55:446–451, 1980.

651. Zimmerman SW, Moorthy AV, Dreher WH, et al: Prospective trial of warfarin and dipyridamole in patients with membranoproliferative glomerulonephritis. Am J Med 75:920–927, 1983.

652. Zauner I, Bohler J, Braun N, et al: Effect of aspirin and dipyridamole on proteinuria in idiopathic membranoproliferative glomerulonephritis: A multicentre prospective clinical trial. Collaborative Glomerulonephritis Therapy Study Group (CGTS). Nephrol Dial Transplant 9:619–622, 1994.

653. Cattran DC, Cardella CJ, Roscoe JM, et al: Results of a controlled drug trial in membranoproliferative glomerulonephritis. Kidney Int 27:436–441, 1985.

654. Glassock RJ: Role of cyclosporine in glomerular diseases. Cleve Clin J Med 61:363–369, 1994.

655. Leibowitch J, Halbwachs L, Wattel S, et al: Recurrence of dense deposits in transplanted kidney: II. Serum complement and nephritic factor profiles. Kidney Int 15:396–403, 1979.

656. Glicklich D, Matas AJ, Sablay LB, et al: Recurrent membranoproliferative glomerulonephritis type 1 in successive renal transplants. Am J Nephrol 7:143–149, 1987.

657. Jennette JC, Falk RJ: Diagnosis and management of glomerular diseases. Med Clin North Am 81:653–677, 1997.

658. Rodriguez-Iturbe B: Poststreptococcal glomerulonephritis. In Glassock RJ (ed): Current Therapy in Nephrology and Hypertension, 4th ed. St. Louis, Mosby-Year Book, Inc., 1998, pp 141–145.

659. Ginsburg BE, Wasserman J, Huldt G, Bergstrand A: Case of glomerulonephritis associated with acute toxoplasmosis. Br Med J 3:664–665, 1974.

660. Rodriguez-Iturbe B, Rubio L, Garcia R: Attack rate of poststreptococcal nephritis in families. A prospective study. Lancet 1:401–403, 1981.

661. Glassock RJ, Adler SG, Ward HJ, Cohen AH: Primary glomerular diseases. In Brenner BM, Rector FC Jr (eds): The Kidney, 4th ed. Philadelphia, WB Saunders, 1991, pp 1182–1279.

662. Mota-Hernandez F, Briseno-Mondragon E, Gordillo-Paniagua G: Glomerular lesions and final outcome in children with glomerulonephritis of acute onset. Nephron 16:272–281, 1976.

663. Popovic-Rolovic M, Kostic M, Antic-Peco A, et al: Medium- and long-term prognosis of patients with acute poststreptococcal glomerulonephritis. Nephron 58:393–399, 1991.

664. Buzio C, Allegri L, Mutti A, et al: Significance of albuminuria in the follow-up of acute poststreptococcal glomerulonephritis. Clin Nephrol 41:259–264, 1994.

665. Tejani A, Ingulli E: Poststreptococcal glomerulonephritis. Current clinical and pathologic concepts. Nephron 55:1–5, 1990.

666. Layrisse Z, Rodriguez-Iturbe B, Garcia-Ramirez R, et al: Family studies of the HLA system in acute post-streptococcal glomerulonephritis. Hum Immunol 7:177–185, 1983.

667. Mori K, Sasazuki T, Kimura A, Ito Y: HLA-DP antigens and post-streptococcal acute glomerulonephritis. Acta Paediatr 85:916–918, 1996.

668. Rammelkamp CH, Weaver RS: Acute glomerulonephritis. The significance of the variations in the incidence of the disease. J Clin Invest 32:345–358, 1953.

669. Stetson CA, Rammelkamp CH, Krause RM: Epidemic acute nephritis: Studies on etiology, natural history, and prevention. Medicine 34:431, 1955.

670. Dillon HC, Jr: The treatment of streptococcal skin infections. J Pediatr 76:676–684, 1970.

671. Dillon HC, Jr, Reeves MS: Streptococcal immune responses in nephritis after skin infections. Am J Med 56:333–346, 1974.

672. Reid HF, Bassett DC, Poon-King T, et al: Group G streptococci in healthy schoolchildren and in patients with glomerulonephritis in Trinidad. J Hyg (Lond) 94:61–68, 1985.

673. Svartman M, Finklea JF, Earle DP, et al: Epidemic scabies and acute glomerulonephritis in Trinidad. Lancet 1:249–251, 1972.

674. Oner A, Demircin G, Bulbul M: Post-streptococcal acute glomerulonephritis in Turkey. Acta Paediatr 84:817–819, 1995.

675. Streeton CL, Hanna JN, Messer RD, Merianos A: An epidemic of acute poststreptococcal glomerulonephritis among aboriginal children. J Paediatr Child Health 31:245–248, 1995.

676. Thomson PD: Renal problems in black South African children. Pediatr Nephrol 11:508–512, 1997.

677. Zoric D, Kelmendi M, Shehu B, et al: Acute poststreptococcal glomerulonephritis in children. Adv Exp Med Biol 418:125–127, 1997.

678. Carapetis JR, Steer AC, Mulholland EK, Weber M: The global burden of group A streptococcal diseases. Lancet Infect Dis 5:685–694, 2005.

679. Rosenberg HG, Vial SU, Pomeroy J, et al: Acute glomerulonephritis in children. An evolutive morphologic and immunologic study of the glomerular inflammation. Pathol Res Pract 180:633–643, 1985.

680. Edelstein CL, Bates WD: Subtypes of acute postinfectious glomerulonephritis: A clinico-pathological correlation. Clin Nephrol 38:311–317, 1992.

681. Feldman JD, Mardiney MR, Shuler SE: Immunology and morphology of acute post-streptococcal glomerulonephritis. Lab Invest 15:283–301, 1966.

682. Fish AJ, Herdman RC, Michael AF, et al: Epidemic acute glomerulonephritis associated with type 49 streptococcal pyoderma. II. Correlative study of light, immunofluorescent and electron microscopic findings. Am J Med 48:28–39, 1970.

683. Nadasdy T, Silva FG: Acute postinfectious glomerulonephritis. In Jennette JC, Olson JL, Schwartz MM, Silva FG (eds): Heptinstall's Pathology of the Kidney, 6th ed. Philadelphia, Lippincott Williams & Wilkins, 2006, pp 321–396.

684. Jennette JC, Thomas DB: Crescentic glomerulonephritis. Nephrol Dial Transplant 16 Suppl 6:80–82, 2001.

685. Modai D, Pik A, Behar M, et al: Biopsy proven evolution of post streptococcal glomerulonephritis to rapidly progressive glomerulonephritis of a post infectious type. Clin Nephrol 23:198–202, 1985.

686. Montseny JJ, Kleinknecht D, Meyrier A: [Rapidly progressive glomerulonephritis of infectious origin]. Ann Med Interne (Paris) 144:308–310, 1993.

687. Velhote V, Saldanha LB, Malheiro PS, et al: Acute glomerulonephritis: Three episodes demonstrated by light and electron microscopy, and immunofluorescence studies—a case report. Clin Nephrol 26:307–310, 1986.

688. Rosenberg HG, Donoso PL, Vial SU, et al: Clinical and morphological recovery between two episodes of acute glomerulonephritis: A light and electron microscopic study with immunofluorescence. Clin Nephrol 21:350–354, 1984.

689. Michael AF, Jr., Drummond KN, Good RA, Vernier RL: Acute poststreptococcal glomerulonephritis: Immune deposit disease. J Clin Invest 45:237–248, 1966.

690. Sorger K, Gessler M, Hubner FK, et al: Follow-up studies of three subtypes of acute postinfectious glomerulonephritis ascertained by renal biopsy. Clin Nephrol 27:111–124, 1987.

691. Jennings RB, Earle DP: Poststreptococcal glomerulonephritis: Histopathologic and clinical studies on the acute, subsiding acute and early chronic latent phases. J Clin Invest 40:1525, 1961.

692. Bright R: Cases and observations, illustrative of renal disease accompanied with the secretion of albuminous urine. Guy's Hospital Reports 1:338–400, 1836.

693. Schick B: Die nachkrankheiten des scharlachs. Jahrb Kinderheilkd 65 (supplement):132–173, 1907.

694. Rammelkamp CH, Weaver RS, Dingle JH: Significance of the epidemiological differences between acute nephritis and acute rheumatic fever. Trans Assoc Am Physicians 65:168, 1952.

695. Holm SE: The pathogenesis of acute post-streptococcal glomerulonephritis in new lights. Review article. APMIS 96:189–193, 1988.

696. Kraus W, Ohyama K, Snyder DS, Beachey EH: Autoimmune sequence of streptococcal M protein shared with the intermediate filament protein, vimentin. J Exp Med 169:481–492, 1989.

697. Goroncy-Bermes P, Dale JB, Beachey EH, Opferkuch W: Monoclonal antibody to human renal glomeruli cross-reacts with streptococcal M protein. Infect Immun 55:2416–2419, 1987.

698. Kraus W, Beachey EH: Renal autoimmune epitope of group A streptococci specified by M protein tetrapeptide Ile-Arg-Leu-Arg. Proc Natl Acad Sci U S A 85:4516–4520, 1988.

699. Montseny JJ, Meyrier A, Kleinknecht D, Callard P: The current spectrum of infectious glomerulonephritis. Experience with 76 patients and review of the literature. Medicine (Baltimore) 74:63–73, 1995.

700. Ferrario F, Kourilsky O, Morel-Maroger L: Acute endocapillary glomerulonephritis in adults: A histologic and clinical comparison between patients with and without initial acute renal failure. Clin Nephrol 19:17–23, 1983.

701. Richards J: Acute post-streptococcal glomerulonephritis. W V Med J 87:61–65, 1991.

702. Madaio MP, Harrington JT: Current concepts. The diagnosis of acute glomerulonephritis. N Engl J Med 309:1299–1302, 1983.

703. Lee HA, Stirling G, Sharpstone P: Acute glomerulonephritis in middle-aged and elderly patients. Br Med J 2:1361–1363, 1966.

704. Washio M, Oh Y, Okuda S, et al: Clinicopathological study of poststreptococcal glomerulonephritis in the elderly. Clin Nephrol 41:265–270, 1994.

705. Rovang RD, Zawada ET, Jr, Santella RN, et al: Cerebral vasculitis associated with acute post-streptococcal glomerulonephritis. Am J Nephrol 17:89–92, 1997.

706. Kaplan RA, Zwick DL, Hellerstein S, et al: Cerebral vasculitis in acute post-streptococcal glomerulonephritis. Pediatr Nephrol 7:194–195, 1993.

707. Okada K, Saitoh S, Sakaguchi Z, et al: IgA nephropathy presenting clinicopathological features of acute post-streptococcal glomerulonephritis. Eur J Pediatr 155:327–330, 1996.

708. Akasheh MS, al-Lozi M, Affarah HB, et al: Rapidly progressive glomerulonephritis complicating acute rheumatic fever. Postgrad Med J 71:553–554, 1995.

709. Dodge WF, Spargo BH, Travis LB, et al: Poststreptococcal glomerulonephritis. A prospective study in children. N Engl J Med 286:273–278, 1972.

710. Fairley KF, Birch DF: Hematuria: A simple method for identifying glomerular bleeding. Kidney Int 21:105–108, 1982.

711. Baldwin DS, Gluck MC, Schacht RG, Gallo G: The long-term course of poststreptococcal glomerulonephritis. Ann Intern Med 80:342–358, 1974.

712. Hinglais N, Garcia T, Kleinknecht D: Long-term prognosis in acute glomerulonephritis. The predictive value of early clinical and pathological features observed in 65 patients. Am J Med 56:52–60, 1974.

713. Cortes P, Potter EV, Kwaan HC: Characterization and significance of urinary fibrin degradation products. J Lab Clin Med 82:377–389, 1973.

714. Wilson RJ: Renal excretion of calcium and sodium in acute nephritis. Br Med J 4:713–715, 1969.

715. Don BR, Schambelan M: Hyperkalemia in acute glomerulonephritis due to transient hyporeninemic hypoaldosteronism. Kidney Int 38:1159–1163, 1990.

716. Martin DR: Rheumatogenic and nephritogenic group A streptococci. Myth or reality? An opening lecture. Adv Exp Med Biol 418:21–27, 1997.

717. Rodriguez I: Epidemic poststreptococcal glomerulonephritis. Kidney Int 25:129–136, 1984.

718. Tanz RR, Gerber MA, Shulman ST: What is a throat culture? Adv Exp Med Biol 418:29–33, 1997.

719. Peter G, Smith AL: Group A streptococcal infections of the skin and pharynx (first of two parts). N Engl J Med 297:311–317, 1977.

720. Bergner R, Fleiderman S, Ferne M, et al: The new streptozyme test for streptococcal antibodies. Studies in the value of this multiple antigen test in glomerulonephritis, acute pharyngitis, and acute rheumatic fever. Clin Pediatr (Phila) 14:804–809, 1975.

721. Lange K, Seligson G, Cronin W: Evidence for the in situ origin of poststreptococcal glomerulonephritis: Glomerular localization of endostreptosin and the clinical significance of the subsequent antibody response. Clin Nephrol 19:3–10, 1983.

722. Lange K, Ahmed U, Kleinberger H, Treser G: A hitherto unknown streptococcal antigen and its probable relation to acute poststreptococcal glomerulonephritis. Clin Nephrol 5:207–215, 1976.

723. Cronin WJ, Lange K: Immunologic evidence for the in situ deposition of a cytoplasmic streptococcal antigen (endostreptosin) on the glomerular basement membrane in rats. Clin Nephrol 34:143–146, 1990.

724. Yoshimoto M, Hosoi S, Fujisawa S, et al: High levels of antibodies to streptococcal cell membrane antigens specifically bound to monoclonal antibodies in acute poststreptococcal glomerulonephritis. J Clin Microbiol 25:680–684, 1987.

725. Kefalides NA, Pegg MT, Ohno N, et al: Antibodies to basement membrane collagen and to laminin are present in sera from patients with poststreptococcal glomerulonephritis. J Exp Med 163:588–602, 1986.

726. Hebert LA, Cosio FG, Neff JC: Diagnostic significance of hypocomplementemia. Kidney Int 39:811–821, 1991.

727. Matsell DG, Roy S, Tamerius JD, et al: Plasma terminal complement complexes in acute poststreptococcal glomerulonephritis. Am J Kidney Dis 17:311–316, 1991.

728. McLean RH, Schrager MA, Rothfield NF, Berman MA: Normal complement in early poststreptococcal glomerulonephritis. Br Med J 1:1326, 1977.

729. Lewis EJ, Carpenter CB, Schur PH: Serum complement component levels in human glomerulonephritis. Ann Intern Med 75:555–560, 1971.

730. Cameron JS, Vick RM, Ogg CS, et al: Plasma C3 and C4 concentrations in management of glomerulonephritis. Br Med J 3:668–672, 1973.

731. Sjoholm AG: Complement components and complement activation in acute poststreptococcal glomerulonephritis. Int Arch Allergy Appl Immunol 58:274–284, 1979.

732. Schreiber RD, Muller-Eberhard HJ: Complement and renal disease. In Wilson CB, Brenner BM, Stein JH (eds): Contemporary Issues in Nephrology. New York, Churchill Livingstone, 1979, p 67.

733. Wyatt RJ, Forristal J, West CD, et al: Complement profiles in acute post-streptococcal glomerulonephritis. Pediatr Nephrol 2:219–223, 1988.

734. McIntosh RM, Kulvinskas C, Kaufman DB: Cryoglobulins. II. The biological and chemical properties of cryoproteins in acute post-streptococcal glomerulonephritis. Int Arch Allergy Appl Immunol 41:700–715, 1971.

735. McIntosh RM, Griswold WR, Chernack WB, et al: Cryoglobulins. III. Further studies on the nature, incidence, clinical, diagnostic, prognostic, and immunopathologic significance of cryoproteins in renal disease. Q J Med 44:285–307, 1975.

736. Rodriguez-Iturbe B, Carr RI, Garcia R, et al: Circulating immune complexes and serum immunoglobulins in acute poststreptococcal glomerulonephritis. Clin Nephrol 13:1–4, 1980.

737. Yoshizawa N, Treser G, McClung JA, et al: Circulating immune complexes in patients with uncomplicated group A streptococcal pharyngitis and patients with acute poststreptococcal glomerulonephritis. Am J Nephrol 3:23–29.

738. Mezzano S, Olavarria F, Ardiles L, Lopez MI: Incidence of circulating immune complexes in patients with acute poststreptococcal glomerulonephritis and in patients with streptococcal impetigo. Clin Nephrol 26:61–65, 1986.

739. Sesso RC, Ramos OL, Pereira AB: Detection of IgG-rheumatoid factor in sera of patients with acute poststreptococcal glomerulonephritis and its relationship with circulating immunecomplexes. Clin Nephrol 26:55–60, 1986.

740. Villarreal H, Jr., Fischetti VA, van de Rijn I, Zabriskie JB: The occurrence of a protein in the extracellular products of streptococci isolated from patients with acute glomerulonephritis. J Exp Med 149:459–472, 1979.

741. Kaplan BS, Esseltine D: Thrombocytopenia in patients with acute post-streptococcal glomerulonephritis. J Pediatr 93:974–976, 1978.

742. Ekert H, Powell H, Muntz R: Hypercoagulability in acute glomerulonephritis. Lancet 1:965–966, 1972.

743. Ekberg M, Nilsson IM: Factor VIII and glomerulonephritis. Lancet 1:1111–1113, 1975.

744. Alkjaersig NK, Fletcher AP, Lewis ML, et al: Pathophysiological response of the blood coagulation system in acute glomerulonephritis. Kidney Int 10:319–328, 1976.

745. Adhikari M, Coovadia HM, Greig HB, Christensen S: Factor VIII procoagulant activity in children with nephrotic syndrome and post-streptococcal glomerulonephritis. Nephron 22:301–305, 1978.

746. Mezzano S, Kunick M, Olavarria F, et al: Detection of platelet-activating factor in plasma of patients with streptococcal nephritis. J Am Soc Nephrol 4:235–242, 1993.

747. Potter EV, Lipschultz SA, Abidh S, et al: Twelve to seventeen-year follow-up of patients with poststreptococcal acute glomerulonephritis in Trinidad. N Engl J Med 307:725–729, 1982.

748. Parra G, Rodriguez-Iturbe B, Colina-Chourio J, Garcia R: Short-term treatment with captopril in hypertension due to acute glomerulonephritis. Clin Nephrol 29:58–62, 1988.

749. Leonard CD, Nagle RB, Striker GE, et al: Acute glomerulonephritis with prolonged oliguria. An analysis of 29 cases. Ann Intern Med 73:703–711, 1970.

750. Johnston F, Carapetis J, Patel MS, et al: Evaluating the use of penicillin to control outbreaks of acute poststreptococcal glomerulonephritis. Pediatr Infect Dis J 18:327–332, 1999.

751. Baldwin DS: Chronic glomerulonephritis: Nonimmunologic mechanisms of progressive glomerular damage. Kidney Int 21:109–120, 1982.

752. Baldwin DS: Poststreptococcal glomerulonephritis. A progressive disease? Am J Med 62:1–11, 1977.

753. Lien JW, Mathew TH, Meadows R: Acute post-streptococcal glomerulonephritis in adults: a long-term study. Q J Med 48:99–111, 1979.

754. Berger J: IgA glomerular deposits in renal disease. Transplant Proc 1:939–944, 1969.

755. Berger J, Hinglais N: Intercapillary deposits of IgA-IgG. J Urol Nephrol (Paris) 74:694–695, 1968.

756. Niaudet P, Murcia I, Beaufils H, et al: Primary IgA nephropathies in children: Prognosis and treatment. Adv Nephrol Necker Hosp 22:121–140, 1993.

757. Schena FP: A retrospective analysis of the natural history of primary IgA nephropathy worldwide. Am J Med 89:209–215, 1990.

758. Clarkson AR, Seymour AE, Thompson AJ, et al: IgA nephropathy: A syndrome of uniform morphology, diverse clinical features and uncertain prognosis. Clin Nephrol 8:459–471, 1977.

759. Colasanti G, Banfi G, di Belgiojoso GB, et al: Idiopathic IgA mesangial nephropathy: clinical features. Contrib Nephrol 40:147–155, 1984.

760. Clarkson AR, Woodroffe AJ, Bannister KM, et al: The syndrome of IgA nephropathy. Clin Nephrol 21:7–14, 1984.

761. Schena FP, Gesualdo L, Montinaro V: Immunopathological aspects of immunoglobulin A nephropathy and other mesangial proliferative glomerulonephritides. J Am Soc Nephrol 2:S167–S172, 1992.

762. D'Amico G: The commonest glomerulonephritis in the world: IgA nephropathy. Q J Med 64:709–727, 1987.

763. Crowley-Nowick PA, Julian BA, Wyatt RJ, et al: IgA nephropathy in blacks: Studies of IgA2 allotypes and clinical course. Kidney Int 39:1218–1224, 1991.

764. Jennette JC, Wall SD, Wilkman AS: Low incidence of IgA nephropathy in blacks. Kidney Int 28:944–950, 1985.

765. Hoy WE, Hughson MD, Smith SM, Megill DM: Mesangial proliferative glomerulonephritis in southwestern American Indians. Am J Kidney Dis 21:486–496, 1993.

766. Power DA, Muirhead N, Simpson JG, et al: IgA nephropathy is not a rare disease in the United Kingdom. Nephron 40:180–184, 1985.

767. Waldherr R, Rambausek M, Duncker WD, Ritz E: Frequency of mesangial IgA deposits in a non-selected autopsy series. Nephrol Dial Transplant 4:943–946, 1989.

768. Rambausek M, Rauterberg EW, Waldherr R, et al: Evolution of IgA glomerulonephritis: Relation to morphology, immunogenetics, and BP. Semin Nephrol 7:370–373, 1987.

769. Simon P, Ang KS, Bavay P, et al: Immunoglobulin A glomerulonephritis. Epidemiology in a population of 250 000 inhabitants. Presse Med 13:257–260, 1984.

770. Simon P, Ramee MP, Ang KS, Cam G: Course of the annual incidence of primary glomerulopathies in a population of 400,000 inhabitants over a 10-year period (1976–1985). Nephrologie 7: 1986.

771. Simon P, Ramee MP, Autuly V, et al: Epidemiology of primary glomerular diseases in a French region. Variations according to period and age. Kidney Int 46:1192–1198, 1994.

772. Levy M, Berger J: Worldwide perspective of IgA nephropathy. Am J Kidney Dis 12:340–347, 1988.

773. Frimat L, Kessler M: Controversies concerning the importance of genetic polymorphism in IgA nephropathy. Nephrol Dial Transplant 17:542–545, 2002.

774. Frimat L, Philippe C, Maghakian MN, et al: Polymorphism of angiotensin converting enzyme, angiotensinogen, and angiotensin II type 1 receptor genes and end-stage renal failure in IgA nephropathy: IGARAS—a study of 274 Men. J Am Soc Nephrol 11:2062–2067, 2000.

775. Gong R, Liu Z, Li L: Mannose-binding lectin gene polymorphism associated with the patterns of glomerular immune deposition in IgA nephropathy. Scand J Urol Nephrol 35:228–232, 2001.

776. Kim W, Kang SK, Lee DY, et al: Endothelial nitric oxide synthase gene polymorphism in patients with IgA nephropathy. Nephron 86:232–233, 2000.

777. Matsunaga A, Numakura C, Kawakami T, et al: Association of the uteroglobin gene polymorphism with IgA nephropathy. Am J Kidney Dis 39:36–41, 2002.

778. Lee EY, Yang DH, Hwang KY, Hong SY: Is tumor necrosis factor genotype (TNFA2/TNFA2)a genetic prognostic factor of an unfavorable outcome in IgA nephropathy? J Korean Med Sci 16:751–755, 2001.

779. Schroeder HW, Jr: Genetics of IgA deficiency and common variable immunodeficiency. Clin Rev Allergy Immunol 17:127–140, 2000.

780. Niemir ZI, Stein H, Noronha IL, et al: PDGF and TGF-beta contribute to the natural course of human IgA glomerulonephritis. Kidney Int 48:1530–1541, 1995.

781. Yoshida H, Mitarai T, Kawamura T, et al: Role of the deletion of polymorphism of the angiotensin converting enzyme gene in the progression and therapeutic responsiveness of IgA nephropathy. J Clin Invest 96:2162–2169, 1995.

782. Harden PN, Geddes C, Rowe PA, et al: Polymorphisms in angiotensin-converting-enzyme gene and progression of IgA nephropathy. Lancet 345:1540–1542, 1995.

783. Hunley TE, Julian BA, Phillips JA, III, et al: Angiotensin converting enzyme gene polymorphism: Potential silencer motif and impact on progression in IgA nephropathy. Kidney Int 49:571–577, 1996.

CH 30

Primary Glomerular Disease

784. Pei Y, Scholey J, Thai K, et al: Association of angiotensinogen gene T235 variant with progression of immunoglobin A nephropathy in Caucasian patients. J Clin Invest 100:814–820, 1997.

785. Julian BA, Quiggins PA, Thompson JS, et al: Familial IgA nephropathy. Evidence of an inherited mechanism of disease. N Engl J Med 312:202–208, 1985.

786. Montoliu J, Darnell A, Torras A, et al: Familial IgA nephropathy: Report of two cases and brief review of the literature. Arch Intern Med 140:1374–1375, 1980.

787. Tolkoff-Rubin NE, Cosimi AB, Fuller T, et al: IGA nephropathy in HLA-identical siblings. Transplantation 26:430–433, 1978.

788. Chahin J, Ortiz A, Mendez L, et al: Familial IgA nephropathy associated with bilateral sensorineural deafness. Am J Kidney Dis 19:592–596, 1992.

789. Levy M, Lesavre P: Genetic factors in IgA nephropathy (Berger's disease). Adv Nephrol Necker Hosp 21:23–51, 1992.

790. Schena FP, Cerullo G, Rossini M, et al: Increased risk of end-stage renal disease in familial IgA nephropathy. J Am Soc Nephrol 13:453–460, 2002.

791. Gharavi AG, Yan Y, Scolari F, et al: IgA nephropathy, the most common cause of glomerulonephritis, is linked to 6q22–23. Nat Genet 26:354–357, 2000.

792. Coppo R, Chiesa M, Cirina P, et al: In human IgA nephropathy uteroglobin does not play the role inferred from transgenic mice. Am J Kidney Dis 40:495–503, 2002.

793. Ju T, Cummings RD: Protein glycosylation: Chaperone mutation in Tn syndrome. Nature 437:1252, 2005.

794. Qin W, Zhou Q, Yang LC, et al: Peripheral B lymphocyte beta1,3-galactosyltransferase and chaperone expression in immunoglobulin A nephropathy. J Intern Med 258:467–477, 2005.

795. Lai KN, Chan KW, Mac-Moune F, et al: The immunochemical characterization of the light chains in the mesangial IgA deposits in IgA nephropathy. Am J Clin Pathol 85:548–551, 1986.

796. Emancipator SN: IgA nephropathy and Henoch-Schonlein purpura. In Jennette JC, Olson JL, Schwartz MM, Silva FG (eds): Heptinstall's Pathology of the Kidney, 5th ed. Philadelphia, Lippincott-Raven, 1998, pp 479–450.

797. Jennette JC: The immunohistology of IgA nephropathy. Am J Kidney Dis 12:348–352, 1988.

798. Haas M: Histologic subclassification of IgA nephropathy: A clinicopathologic study of 244 cases. Am J Kidney Dis 29:829–842, 1997.

799. Lee SM, Rao VM, Franklin WA, et al: IgA nephropathy: Morphologic predictors of progressive renal disease. Hum Pathol 13:314–322, 1982.

800. Abuelo JG, Esparza AR, Matarese RA, et al: Crescentic IgA nephropathy. Medicine (Baltimore) 63:396–406, 1984.

801. Hogg RJ, Silva FG, Wyatt RJ, et al: Prognostic indicators in children with IgA nephropathy—report of the Southwest Pediatric Nephrology Study Group. Pediatr Nephrol 8:15–20, 1994.

802. Croker BP, Dawson DV, Sanfilippo F: IgA nephropathy. Correlation of clinical and histologic features. Lab Invest 48:19–24, 1983.

803. Streather CP, Scoble JE: Recurrent IgA nephropathy in a renal allograft presenting as crescentic glomerulonephritis. Nephron 66:113–114, 1994.

804. Barratt J, Feehally J: IgA nephropathy. J Am Soc Nephrol 16:2088–2097, 2005.

805. Egido J, Sancho J, Blasco R, et al: Immunopathogenetic aspects of IgA nephropathy. Adv Nephrol Necker Hosp 12:103–137, 1983.

806. Allen A, Feehally J: IgA glycosylation in IgA nephropathy. Adv Exp Med Biol 435:175–183, 1998.

807. Feehally J: Immune mechanisms in glomerular IgA deposition. Nephrol Dial Transplant 3:361–378, 1988.

808. Conley ME, Cooper MD, Michael AF: Selective deposition of immunoglobulin A1 in immunoglobulin A nephropathy, anaphylactoid purpura nephritis, and systemic lupus erythematosus. J Clin Invest 66:1432–1436, 1980.

809. Bene MC, Hurault DL, Kessler M, Faure GC: Confirmation of tonsillar anomalies in IgA nephropathy: A multicenter study. Nephron 58:425–428, 1991.

810. Wang MX, Walker RG, Kincaid-Smith P: Endothelial cell antigens recognized by IgA autoantibodies in patients with IgA nephropathy: Partial characterization. Nephrol Dial Transplant 7:805–810, 1992.

811. Frampton G, Walker RG, Perry GJ, et al: IgA affinity to ssDNA or endothelial cells and its deposition in glomerular capillary walls in IgA nephropathy. Nephrol Dial Transplant 5:841–846, 1990.

812. Saulsbury FT, Kirkpatrick PR, Bolton WK: IgA antineutrophil cytoplasmic antibody in Henoch-Schonlein purpura. Am J Nephrol 11:295–300, 1991.

813. Savige JA, Gallicchio M: IgA antimyeloperoxidase antibodies associated with crescentic IgA glomerulonephritis. Nephrol Dial Transplant 7:952–955, 1992.

814. O'Donoghue DJ, Feehally J: Autoantibodies in IgA nephropathy. Contrib Nephrol 111:93–103, 1995.

815. Fornasieri A, Sinico RA, Maldifassi P, et al: IgA-antigliadin antibodies in IgA mesangial nephropathy (Berger's disease). Br Med J (Clin Res Ed) 295:78–80, 1987.

816. Laurent J, Branellec A, Heslan JM, et al: An increase in circulating IgA antibodies to gliadin in IgA mesangial glomerulonephritis. Am J Nephrol 7:178–183, 1987.

817. Yagame M, Tomino Y, Eguchi K, et al: Levels of circulating IgA immune complexes after gluten-rich diet in patients with IgA nephropathy. Nephron 49:104–106, 1988.

818. Nagy J, Scott H, Brandtzaeg P: Antibodies to dietary antigens in IgA nephropathy. Clin Nephrol 29:275–279, 1988.

819. Rostoker G, Andre C, Branellec A, et al: Lack of antireticulin and IgA antiendomysium antibodies in sera of patients with primary IgA nephropathy associated with circulating IgA antibodies to gliadin. Nephron 48:81, 1988.

820. Davin JC, Malaise M, Foidart J, Mahieu P: Anti-alpha-galactosyl antibodies and immune complexes in children with Henoch-Schonlein purpura or IgA nephropathy. Kidney Int 31:1132–1139, 1987.

821. Yap HK, Sakai RS, Woo KT, et al: Detection of bovine serum albumin in the circulating IgA immune complexes of patients with IgA nephropathy. Clin Immunol Immunopathol 43:395–402, 1987.

822. Suzuki S, Nakatomi Y, Sato H, et al: Haemophilus parainfluenzae antigen and antibody in renal biopsy samples and serum of patients with IgA nephropathy. Lancet 343:12–16, 1994.

823. Drew PA, Nieuwhof WN, Clarkson AR, Woodroffe AJ: Increased concentration of serum IgA antibody to pneumococcal polysaccharides in patients with IgA nephropathy. Clin Exp Immunol 67:124–129, 1987.

824. Layward L, Allen AC, Hattersley JM, et al: Elevation of IgA in IgA nephropathy is localized in the serum and not saliva and is restricted to the IgA1 subclass. Nephrol Dial Transplant 8:25–28, 1993.

825. Layward L, Allen AC, Harper SJ, et al: Increased and prolonged production of specific polymeric IgA after systemic immunization with tetanus toxoid in IgA nephropathy. Clin Exp Immunol 88:394–398, 1992.

826. Schena FP, Mastrolitti G, Fracasso AR, et al: Increased immunoglobulin-secreting cells in the blood of patients with active idiopathic IgA nephropathy. Clin Nephrol 26:163–168, 1986.

827. Harper SJ, Allen AC, Pringle JH, Feehally J: Increased dimeric IgA producing B cells in the bone marrow in IgA nephropathy determined by in situ hybridisation for J chain mRNA. J Clin Pathol 49:38–42, 1996.

828. Emancipator SN, Lamm ME: IgA nephropathy: pathogenesis of the most common form of glomerulonephritis. Lab Invest 60:168–183, 1989.

829. Mestecky J, Hashim OH, Tomana M: Alterations in the IgA carbohydrate chains influence the cellular distribution of IgA1. Contrib Nephrol 111:66–71, 1995.

830. Baenziger J, Kornfeld S: Structure of the carbohydrate units of IgA1 immunoglobulin. II. Structure of the O-glycosidically linked oligosaccharide units. J Biol Chem 249:7270–7281, 1974.

831. Mestecky J, Tomana M, Crowley-Nowick PA, et al: Defective galactosylation and clearance of IgA1 molecules as a possible etiopathogenic factor in IgA nephropathy. Contrib Nephrol 104:172–182, 1993.

832. Stockert RJ, Kressner MS, Collins JC, et al: IgA interaction with the asialoglycoprotein receptor. Proc Natl Acad Sci U S A 79:6229–6231, 1982.

833. Moldoveanu Z, Moro I, Radl J, et al: Site of catabolism of autologous and heterologous IgA in non-human primates. Scand J Immunol 32:577–583, 1990.

834. Tomana M, Kulhavy R, Mestecky J: Receptor-mediated binding and uptake of immunoglobulin A by human liver. Gastroenterology 94:762–770, 1988.

835. Andre PM, Le Pogamp P, Chevet D: Impairment of jacalin binding to serum IgA in IgA nephropathy. J Clin Lab Anal 4:115–119, 1990.

836. Hiki Y, Iwase H, Saitoh M, et al: Reactivity of glomerular and serum IgA1 to jacalin in IgA nephropathy. Nephron 72:429–435, 1996.

837. Tomana M, Matousovic K, Julian BA, et al: Galactose-deficient IgA1 in sera of IgA nephropathy patients is present in complexes with IgG. Kidney Int 52:509–516, 1997.

838. Allen AC, Harper SJ, Feehally J: Galactosylation of N- and O-linked carbohydrate moieties of IgA1 and IgG in IgA nephropathy. Clin Exp Immunol 100:470–474, 1995.

839. Allen AC, Topham PS, Harper SJ, Feehally J: Leucocyte beta 1,3 galactosyltransferase activity in IgA nephropathy. Nephrol Dial Transplant 12:701–706, 1997.

840. de Fijter JW, Eijgenraam JW, Braam CA, et al: Deficient IgA1 immune response to nasal cholera toxin subunit B in primary IgA nephropathy. Kidney Int 50:952–961, 1996.

841. Hiki Y, Kokubo T, Iwase H, et al: Underglycosylation of IgA1 hinge plays a certain role for its glomerular deposition in IgA nephropathy. J Am Soc Nephrol 10:760–769, 1999.

842. Tomana M, Novak J, Julian BA, et al: Circulating immune complexes in IgA nephropathy consist of IgA1 with galactose-deficient hinge region and antiglycan antibodies. J Clin Invest 104:73–81, 1999.

843. Kokubo T, Hashizume K, Iwase H, et al: Humoral immunity against the proline-rich peptide epitope of the IgA1 hinge region in IgA nephropathy. Nephrol Dial Transplant 15:28–33, 2000.

844. Hiki Y, Odani H, Takahashi M, et al: Mass spectrometry proves under-O-glycosylation of glomerular IgA1 in IgA nephropathy. Kidney Int 59:1077–1085, 2001.

845. Leung JC, Tang SC, Lam MF, et al: Charge-dependent binding of polymeric IgA1 to human mesangial cells in IgA nephropathy. Kidney Int 59:277–285, 2001.

846. Novak J, Vu HL, Novak L, et al: Interactions of human mesangial cells with IgA and IgA-containing immune complexes. Kidney Int 62:465–475, 2002.

847. Novak J, Tomana M, Matousovic K, et al: IgA1-containing immune complexes in IgA nephropathy differentially affect proliferation of mesangial cells. Kidney Int 67:504–513, 2005.

848. O'Donoghue DJ, Darvill A, Ballardie FW: Mesangial cell autoantigens in immunoglobulin A nephropathy and Henoch-Schonlein purpura. J Clin Invest 88:1522–1530, 1991.

849. Ballardie FW, Brenchley PE, Williams S, O'Donoghue DJ: Autoimmunity in IgA nephropathy. Lancet 2:588–592, 1988.

850. Goshen E, Livne A, Nagy J, et al: Antinuclear autoantibodies in sera of patients with IgA nephropathy. Nephron 55:33–36, 1990.

851. O'Donoghue DJ, Nusbaum P, Noel LH, et al: Antineutrophil cytoplasmic antibodies in IgA nephropathy and Henoch-Schonlein purpura. Nephrol Dial Transplant 7:534–538, 1992.

852. Esnault VL, Ronda N, Jayne DR, Lockwood CM: Association of ANCA isotype and affinity with disease expression. J Autoimmunol 6:197–205, 1993.

853. Ramirez SB, Rosen S, Niles S, Somers MJ: IgG antineutrophil cytoplasmic antibodies in IgA nephropathy: A clinical variant? Am J Kidney Dis 31:341–344, 1998.

854. Martin SJ, Audrain MA, Baranger T, et al: Recurrence of immunoglobulin A nephropathy with immunoglobulin A antineutrophil cytoplasmic antibodies following renal transplantation. Am J Kidney Dis 29:125–131, 1997.

855. van den Wall Bake AW, Kirk KA, Gay RE, et al: Binding of serum immunoglobulins to collagens in IgA nephropathy and HIV infection. Kidney Int 42:374–382, 1992.

856. Eitner F, Schulze M, Brunkhorst R, et al: On the specificity of assays to detect circulating immunoglobulin A-fibronectin complexes: Implications for the study of serologic phenomena in patients with immunoglobulin A nephropathy. J Am Soc Nephrol 5:1400–1406, 1994.

857. Czerkinsky C, Koopman WJ, Jackson S, et al: Circulating immune complexes and immunoglobulin A rheumatoid factor in patients with mesangial immunoglobulin A nephropathies. J Clin Invest 77:1931–1938, 1986.

858. Sinico RA, Fornasieri A, Oreni N, et al: Polymeric IgA rheumatoid factor in idiopathic IgA mesangial nephropathy (Berger's disease). J Immunol 137:536–541, 1986.

859. Schena PF, Pastore A, Sinico RA, et al: Polymeric IgA and IgA rheumatoid factor decrease the capacity of serum to solubilize circulating immune complexes in patients with primary IgA nephropathy. J Immunol 141:125–130, 1988.

860. Nomoto Y, Sakai H, Arimori S: Increase of IgA-bearing lymphocytes in peripheral blood from patients with IgA nephropathy. Am J Clin Pathol 71:158–160, 1979.

861. Hale GM, McIntosh SL, Hiki Y, et al: Evidence for IgA-specific B cell hyperactivity in patients with IgA nephropathy. Kidney Int 29:718–724, 1986.

862. Waldo FB, Beischel L, West CD: IgA synthesis by lymphocytes from patients with IgA nephropathy and their relatives. Kidney Int 29:1229–1233, 1986.

863. Yano N, Asakura K, Endoh M, et al: Polymorphism in the Ialpha1 germ-line transcript regulatory region and IgA productivity in patients with IgA nephropathy. J Immunol 160:4936–4942, 1998.

864. Yano N, Endoh M, Miyazaki M, et al: Altered production of IgE and IgA induced by IL-4 in peripheral blood mononuclear cells from patients with IgA nephropathy. Clin Exp Immunol 88:295–300, 1992.

865. Demaine AG, Rambausek M, Knight JF, et al: Relation of mesangial IgA glomerulonephritis to polymorphism of immunoglobulin heavy chain switch region. J Clin Invest 81:611–614, 1988.

866. Gomez-Guerrero C, Gonzalez E, Egido J: Evidence for a specific IgA receptor in rat and human mesangial cells. J Immunol 151:7172–7181, 1993.

867. Kashem A, Endoh M, Yano N, et al: Glomerular Fc alphaR expression and disease activity in IgA nephropathy. Am J Kidney Dis 30:389–396, 1997.

868. Grossetete B, Launay P, Lehuen A, et al: Down-regulation of Fc alpha receptors on blood cells of IgA nephropathy patients: Evidence for a negative regulatory role of serum IgA. Kidney Int 53:1321–1335, 1998.

869. Toyabe S, Kuwano Y, Takeda K, et al: IgA nephropathy-specific expression of the IgA Fc receptors (CD89) on blood phagocytic cells. Clin Exp Immunol 110:226–232, 1997.

870. Waldo FB, Cochran AM: Mixed IgA-IgG aggregates as a model of immune complexes in IgA nephropathy. J Immunol 142:3841–3846, 1989.

871. Walshe JJ, Brentjens JR, Costa GG, et al: Abdominal pain associated with IgA nephropathy. Possible mechanism. Am J Med 77:765–767, 1984.

872. MacDonald IM, Fairley KF, Hobbs JB, Kincaid-Smith P: Loin pain as a presenting symptom in idiopathic glomerulonephritis. Clin Nephrol 3:129–133, 1975.

873. Perez-Fontan M, Miguel JL, Picazo ML, et al: Idiopathic IgA nephropathy presenting as malignant hypertension. Am J Nephrol 6:482–486, 1986.

874. Kincaid-Smith P, Bennett WM, Dowling JP, Ryan GB: Acute renal failure and tubular necrosis associated with hematuria due to glomerulonephritis. Clin Nephrol 19:206–210, 1983.

875. Delclaux C, Jacquot C, Callard P, Kleinknecht D: Acute reversible renal failure with macroscopic haematuria in IgA nephropathy. Nephrol Dial Transplant 8:195–199, 1993.

876. Kapoor A, Mowbray JF, Porter KA, Peart WS: Significance of haematuria in hypertensive patients. Lancet 1:231–232, 1984.

877. Mustonen J, Pasternack A, Rantala I: The nephrotic syndrome in IgA glomerulonephritis: Response to corticosteroid therapy. Clin Nephrol 20:172–176, 1983.

878. D'Amico G: Influence of clinical and histological features on actuarial renal survival in adult patients with idiopathic IgA nephropathy, membranous nephropathy, and membranoproliferative glomerulonephritis: Survey of the recent literature. Am J Kidney Dis 20:315–323, 1992.

879. Nicholls K, Walker RG, Dowling JP, Kincaid-Smith P: "Malignant" IgA nephropathy. Am J Kidney Dis 5:42–46, 1985.

880. D'Amico G: Influence of clinical and histological features on actuarial renal survival in adult patients with idiopathic IgA nephropathy, membranous nephropathy, and membranoproliferative glomerulonephritis: Survey of the recent literature. Am J Kidney Dis 20:315–323, 1992.

881. Alamartine E, Sabatier JC, Guerin C, et al: Prognostic factors in mesangial IgA glomerulonephritis: An extensive study with univariate and multivariate analyses. Am J Kidney Dis 18:12–19, 1991.

882. Johnston PA, Brown JS, Braumholtz DA, Davison AM: Clinico-pathological correlations and long-term follow-up of 253 United Kingdom patients with IgA nephropathy. A report from the MRC Glomerulonephritis Registry. Q J Med 84:619–627, 1992.

883. D'Amico G: Influence of clinical and histological features on actuarial renal survival in adult patients with idiopathic IgA nephropathy, membranous nephropathy, and membranoproliferative glomerulonephritis: Survey of the recent literature. Am J Kidney Dis 20:315–323, 1992.

884. Bogenschutz O, Bohle A, Batz C, et al: IgA nephritis: On the importance of morphological and clinical parameters in the long-term prognosis of 239 patients. Am J Nephrol 10:137–147, 1990.

885. Donadio JV, Bergstralh EJ, Offord KP, et al: Clinical and histopathologic associations with impaired renal function in IgA nephropathy. Mayo Nephrology Collaborative Group. Clin Nephrol 41:65–71, 1994.

886. Katafuchi R, Oh Y, Hori K, et al: An important role of glomerular segmental lesions on progression of IgA nephropathy: a multivariate analysis. Clin Nephrol 41:191–198, 1994.

887. Clarkson AR, Woodroffe AJ: Therapeutic perspectives in mesangial IgA nephropathy. Contrib Nephrol 40:187–194, 1984.

888. Bennett WM, Kincaid-Smith P: Macroscopic hematuria in mesangial IgA nephropathy: Correlation with glomerular crescents and renal dysfunction. Kidney Int 23:393–400, 1983.

889. Bradford WD, Croker BP, Tisher CC: Kidney lesions in Rocky Mountain spotted fever: a light-, immunofluorescence-, and electron-microscopic study. Am J Pathol 97:381–392, 1979.

890. Packham DK, Hewitson TD, Yan HD, et al: Acute renal failure in IgA nephropathy. Clin Nephrol 42:349–353, 1994.

891. Praga M, Gutierrez-Millet V, Navas JJ, et al: Acute worsening of renal function during episodes of macroscopic hematuria in IgA nephropathy. Kidney Int 28:69–74, 1985.

892. Fogazzi GB, Imbasciati E, Moroni G, et al: Reversible acute renal failure from gross haematuria due to glomerulonephritis: Not only in IgA nephropathy and not associated with intratubular obstruction. Nephrol Dial Transplant 10:624–629, 1995.

893. Chen A, Ding SL, Sheu LF, et al: Experimental IgA nephropathy. Enhanced deposition of glomerular IgA immune complex in proteinuric states. Lab Invest 70:639–647, 1994.

894. Donadio JV, Bergstralh EJ, Grande JP, Rademcher DM: Proteinuria patterns and their association with subsequent end-stage renal disease in IgA nephropathy. Nephrol Dial Transplant 17:1197–1203, 2002.

895. Abe S: Pregnancy in IgA nephropathy. Kidney Int 40:1098–1102, 1991.

896. Abe S: The influence of pregnancy on the long-term renal prognosis of IgA nephropathy. Clin Nephrol 41:61–64, 1994.

897. Jones DC, Hayslett JP: Outcome of pregnancy in women with moderate or severe renal insufficiency. N Engl J Med 335:226–232, 1996.

898. Cederholm B, Wieslander J, Bygren P, Heinegard D: Circulating complexes containing IgA and fibronectin in patients with primary IgA nephropathy. Proc Natl Acad Sci U S A 85:4865–4868, 1988.

899. Davin JC, Li VM, Nagy J, et al: Evidence that the interaction between circulating IgA and fibronectin is a normal process enhanced in primary IgA nephropathy. J Clin Immunol 11:78–94, 1991.

900. Baldree LA, Wyatt RJ, Julian BA, et al: Immunoglobulin A-fibronectin aggregate levels in children and adults with immunoglobulin A nephropathy. Am J Kidney Dis 22:1–4, 1993.

901. Jones CL, Powell HR, Kincaid-Smith P, Roberton DM: Polymeric IgA and immune complex concentrations in IgA-related renal disease. Kidney Int 38:323–331, 1990.

902. Cosio FG, Lam S, Folami AO, et al: Immune regulation of immunoglobulin production in IgA-nephropathy. Clin Immunol Immunopathol 23:430–436, 1982.

903. Trascasa ML, Egido J, Sancho J, Hernando L: Evidence of high polymeric IgA levels in serum of patients with Berger's disease and its modification with phenytoin treatment. Proc Eur Dial Transplant Assoc 16:513–519, 1979.

904. Newkirk MM, Klein MH, Katz A, et al: Estimation of polymeric IgA in human serum: an assay based on binding of radiolabeled human secretory component with applications in the study of IgA nephropathy, IgA monoclonal gammopathy, and liver disease. J Immunol 130:1176–1181, 1983.

905. Sancho J, Egido J, Sanchez-Crespo M, Blasco R: Detection of monomeric and polymeric IgA containing immuno complexes in serum and kidney from patients with alcoholic liver disease. Clin Exp Immunol 47:327–335, 1982.

906. Evans DJ, Williams DG, Peters DK, et al: Glomerular deposition of properdin in Henoch-Schonlein syndrome and idiopathic focal nephritis. Br Med J 3:326–328, 1973.

907. Gluckman JC, Jacob N, Beaufils H, et al: Clinical significance of circulating immune complexes detection in chronic glomerulonephritis. Nephron 22:138–145, 1978.

908. Coppo R, Basolo B, Martina G, et al: Circulating immune complexes containing IgA, IgG and IgM in patients with primary IgA nephropathy and with Henoch-Schoenlein nephritis. Correlation with clinical and histologic signs of activity. Clin Nephrol 18:230–239, 1982.

909. Danielsen H, Eriksen EF, Johansen A, Solling J: Serum immunoglobulin sedimentation patterns and circulating immune complexes in IgA glomerulonephritis and Schonlein-Henoch nephritis. Acta Med Scand 215:435–441, 1984.

910. Doi T, Kanatsu K, Sekita K, et al: Detection of IgA class circulating immune complexes bound to anti-C3d antibody in patients with IgA nephropathy. J Immunol Methods 69:95–104, 1984.

911. Hall RP, Stachura I, Cason J, et al: IgA-containing circulating immune complexes in patients with igA nephropathy. Am J Med 74:56–63, 1983.

912. Lesavre P, Digeon M, Bach JF: Analysis of circulating IgA and detection of immune complexes in primary IgA nephropathy. Clin Exp Immunol 48:61–69, 1982.

913. Mustonen J, Pasternack A, Helin II, et al: Circulating immune complexes, the concentration of serum IgA and the distribution of HLA antigens in IgA nephropathy. Nephron 29:170–175, 1981.

914. Sancho J, Egido J, Rivera F, Hernando L: Immune complexes in IgA nephropathy: presence of antibodies against diet antigens and delayed clearance of specific polymeric IgA immune complexes. Clin Exp Immunol 54:194–202, 1983.

915. Tomino Y, Miura M, Suga T, et al: Detection of IgA1-dominant immune complexes in peripheral blood polymorphonuclear leukocytes by double immunofluorescence in patients with IgA nephropathy. Nephron 37:137–139, 1984.

916. Tomino Y, Sakai H, Endoh M, et al: Detection of immune complexes in polymorphonuclear leukocytes by double immunofluorescence in patients with IgA nephropathy. Clin Immunol Immunopathol 24:63–71, 1982.

917. Woodroffe AJ, Gormly AA, McKenzie PE, et al: Immunologic studies in IgA nephropathy. Kidney Int 18:366–374, 1980.

918. Doi T, Kanatsu K, Sekita K, et al: Circulating immune complexes of IgG, IgA, and IgM classes in various glomerular diseases. Nephron 32:335–341, 1982.

919. Nagy J, Fust G, Ambrus M, et al: Circulating immune complexes in patients with IgA glomerulonephritis. Acta Med Acad Sci Hung 39:211–218, 1982.

920. Ooi YM, Ooi BS, Pollak VE: Relationship of levels of circulating immune complexes to histologic patterns of nephritis: a comparative study of membranous glomerulonephropathy and diffuse proliferative glomerulonephritis. J Lab Clin Med 90:891–898, 1977.

921. Valentijn RM, Kauffmann RH, de la Riviere GB, et al: Presence of circulating macromolecular IgA in patients with hematuria due to primary IgA nephropathy. Am J Med 74:375–381, 1983.

922. Kauffmann RH, Herrmann WA, Meyer CJ, et al: Circulating IgA-immune complexes in Henoch-Schonlein purpura. A longitudinal study of their relationship to disease activity and vascular deposition of IgA. Am J Med 69:859–866, 1980.

923. Levinsky RJ, Barratt TM: IgA immune complexes in Henoch-Schonlein purpura. Lancet 2:1100–1103, 1979.

924. Cederholm B, Wieslander J, Bygren P, Heinegard D: Patients with IgA nephropathy have circulating anti-basement membrane antibodies reacting with structures common to collagen I, II, and IV. Proc Natl Acad Sci U S A 83:6151–6155, 1986.

925. Tomino Y, Sakai H, Endoh M, et al: Cross-reactivity of eluted antibodies from renal tissues of patients with henoch-Schonlein purpura nephritis and IgA nephropathy. Am J Nephrol 3:315–318, 1983.

926. Tomino Y, Sakai H, Miura M, et al: Specific binding of circulating IgA antibodies in patients with IgA nephropathy. Am J Kidney Dis 6:149–153, 1985.

927. Nagy J, Uj M, Szucs G, et al: Herpes virus antigens and antibodies in kidney biopsies and sera of IgA glomerulonephritic patients. Clin Nephrol 21:259–262, 1984.

928. Tomino Y, Yagame M, Omata F, et al: A case of IgA nephropathy associated with adeno- and herpes simplex viruses. Nephron 47:258–261, 1987.

929. Julian BA, Wyatt RJ, McMorrow RG, Galla JH: Serum complement proteins in IgA nephropathy. Clin Nephrol 20:251–258, 1983.

930. Miyazaki R, Kuroda M, Akiyama T, et al: Glomerular deposition and serum levels of complement control proteins in patients with IgA nephropathy. Clin Nephrol 21:335–340, 1984.

931. Geiger H, Good RA, Day NK: A study of complement components C3, C5, C6, C7, C8 and C9 in chronic membranoproliferative glomerulonephritis, systemic lupus erythematosus, poststreptococcal nephritis, idiopathic nephrotic syndrome and anaphylactoid purpura. Z Kinderheilkd 119:269–278, 1975.

932. Wyatt RJ, Kanayama Y, Julian BA, et al: Complement activation in IgA nephropathy. Kidney Int 31:1019–1023, 1987.

933. Birch DF, Fairley KF, Whitworth JA, et al: Urinary erythrocyte morphology in the diagnosis of glomerular hematuria. Clin Nephrol 20:78–84, 1983.

934. Ohta K, Takano N, Seno A, et al: Detection and clinical usefulness of urinary interleukin-6 in the diseases of the kidney and the urinary tract. Clin Nephrol 38:185–189, 1992.

935. Tomino Y, Funabiki K, Ohmuro H, et al: Urinary levels of interleukin-6 and disease activity in patients with IgA nephropathy. Am J Nephrol 11:459–464, 1991.

936. Taira K, Hewitson TD, Kincaid-Smith P: Urinary platelet factor four (Pf4) levels in mesangial IgA glomerulonephritis and thin basement membrane disease. Clin Nephrol 37:8–13, 1992.

937. Hene RJ, Velthuis P, van de Wiel A, et al: The relevance of IgA deposits in vessel walls of clinically normal skin. A prospective study. Arch Intern Med 146:745–749, 1986.

938. de la Faille-Kuyper EH, de la Faille H, van der Meer JB: Letter: An immunohistochemical study of the skin of healthy individuals. Acta Derm Venereol 56:317–318, 1976.

939. Faille-Kuyper EH, Kater L, Kuijten RH, et al: Occurrence of vascular IgA deposits in clinically normal skin of patients with renal disease. Kidney Int 9:424–429, 1976.

940. Hasbargen JA, Copley JB: Utility of skin biopsy in the diagnosis of IgA nephropathy. Am J Kidney Dis 6:100–102, 1985.

941. Maschio G, Cagnoli L, Claroni F, et al: ACE inhibition reduces proteinuria in normotensive patients with IgA nephropathy: A multicentre, randomized, placebo-controlled study. Nephrol Dial Transplant 9:265–269, 1994.

942. Woo KT, Lau YK: Proteinuria: Clinical signficance and basis for therapy. Singapore Med J 42:385–389, 2001.

943. Remuzzi A, Perticucci E, Ruggenenti P, et al: Angiotensin converting enzyme inhibition improves glomerular size-selectivity in IgA nephropathy. Kidney Int 39:1267–1273, 1991.

944. Cattran DC, Greenwood C, Ritchie S: Long-term benefits of angiotensin-converting enzyme inhibitor therapy in patients with severe immunoglobulin a nephropathy: A comparison to patients receiving treatment with other antihypertensive agents and to patients receiving no therapy. Am J Kidney Dis 23:247–254, 1994.

945. Rekola S, Bergstrand A, Bucht H: Deterioration rate in hypertensive IgA nephropathy: Comparison of a converting enzyme inhibitor and beta-blocking agents. Nephron 59:57–60, 1991.

946. Nakao N, Yoshimura A, Morita H, et al: Combination treatment of angiotensin-II receptor blocker and angiotensin-converting-enzyme inhibitor in non-diabetic renal disease (COOPERATE): A randomised controlled trial. Lancet 361:117–124, 2003.

947. D'Amico G: Influence of clinical and histological features on actuarial renal survival in adult patients with idiopathic IgA nephropathy, membranous nephropathy, and membranoproliferative glomerulonephritis: survey of the recent literature. Am J Kidney Dis 20:315–323, 1992.

948. Galla JH: IgA nephropathy. Kidney Int 47:377–387, 1995.

949. Kobayashi Y, Hiki Y, Fujii K, et al: Moderately proteinuric IgA nephropathy: Prognostic prediction of individual clinical courses and steroid therapy in progressive cases. Nephron 53:250–256, 1989.

950. Pozzi C, Bolasco PG, Fogazzi GB, et al: Corticosteroids in IgA nephropathy: A randomised controlled trial. Lancet 353:883–887, 1999.

951. Pozzi C, Andrulli S, Del VL, et al: Corticosteroid effectiveness in IgA nephropathy: Long-term results of a randomized, controlled trial. J Am Soc Nephrol 15:157–163, 2004.

952. Hogg RJ, Lee J, Nardelli N, et al: Clinical trial to evaluate omega-3 fatty acids and alternate day prednisone in patients with IgA nephropathy: Report from the Southwest Pediatric Nephrology Study Group. Clin J Am Soc Nephrol 1:467–474, 2006.

953. Samuels JA, Strippoli GF, Craig JC, et al: Immunosuppressive treatments for immunoglobulin A nephropathy: A meta-analysis of randomized controlled trials. Nephrology (Carlton) 9:177–185, 2004.

954. Lai KN, Lai FM, Ho CP, Chan KW: Corticosteroid therapy in IgA nephropathy with nephrotic syndrome: A long-term controlled trial. Clin Nephrol 26:174–180, 1986.

955. Ballardie FW, Roberts IS: Controlled prospective trial of prednisolone and cytotoxics in progressive IgA nephropathy. J Am Soc Nephrol 13:142–148, 2002.

956. Goumenos D, Ahuja M, Shortland JR, Brown CB: Can immunosuppressive drugs slow the progression of IgA nephropathy? Nephrol Dial Transplant 10:1173–1181, 1995.

957. Ahuja M, Goumenos D, Shortland JR, et al: Does immunosuppression with prednisolone and azathioprine alter the progression of idiopathic membranous nephropathy? Am J Kidney Dis 34:521–529, 1999.

958. Welch TR, McAdams AJ, Berry A: Rapidly progressive IgA nephropathy. Am J Dis Child 142:789–793, 1988.

959. Lai KN, Lai FM, Leung AC, et al: Plasma exchange in patients with rapidly progressive idiopathic IgA nephropathy: A report of two cases and review of literature. Am J Kidney Dis 10:66–70, 1987.

960. Roccatello D, Ferro M, Coppo R, et al: Report on intensive treatment of extracapillary glomerulonephritis with focus on crescentic IgA nephropathy. Nephrol Dial Transplant 10:2054–2059, 1995.

961. Woo KT, Lee GS, Lau YK, et al: Effects of triple therapy in IgA nephritis: A follow-up study 5 years later. Clin Nephrol 36:60–66, 1991.

962. Tang S, Leung JC, Chan LY, et al: Mycophenolate mofetil alleviates persistent proteinuria in IgA nephropathy. Kidney Int 68:802–812, 2005.

963. Chen X, Chen P, Cai G, et al: A randomized control trial of mycophenolate mofeil treatment in severe IgA nephropathy. Zhonghua Yi Xue Za Zhi 82:796–801, 2002.

964. Frisch G, Lin J, Rosenstock J, et al: Mycophenolate mofetil (MMF) vs placebo in patients with moderately advanced IgA nephropathy: A double-blind randomized controlled trial. Nephrol Dial Transplant 20:2139–2145, 2005.

965. Maes BD, Oyen R, Claes K, et al: Mycophenolate mofetil in IgA nephropathy: results of a 3-year prospective placebo-controlled randomized study. Kidney Int 65:1842–1849, 2004.

966. Hogg RJ, Wyatt RJ: A randomized controlled trial of mycophenolate mofetil in patients with IgA nephropathy [ISRCTN62557616]. BMC Nephrol 5:3, 2004.

967. Rostoker G, Desvaux-Belghiti D, Pilatte Y, et al: High-dose immunoglobulin therapy for severe IgA nephropathy and Henoch-Schonlein purpura. Ann Intern Med 120:476–484, 1994.

968. Rasche FM, Schwarz A, Keller F: Tonsillectomy does not prevent a progressive course in IgA nephropathy. Clin Nephrol 51:147–152, 1999.

969. Hotta O, Miyazaki M, Furuta T, et al: Tonsillectomy and steroid pulse therapy significantly impact on clinical remission in patients with IgA nephropathy. Am J Kidney Dis 38:736–743, 2001.

970. Xie Y, Nishi S, Ueno M, et al: The efficacy of tonsillectomy on long-term renal survival in patients with IgA nephropathy. Kidney Int 63:1861–1867, 2003.

971. Sato M, Hotta O, Tomioka S, et al: Cohort study of advanced IgA nephropathy: Efficacy and limitations of corticosteroids with tonsillectomy. Nephron Clin Pract 93:c137–c145, 2003.

972. Pettersson EE, Rekola S, Berglund L, et al: Treatment of IgA nephropathy with omega-3-polyunsaturated fatty acids: A prospective, double-blind, randomized study. Clin Nephrol 41:183–190, 1994.

973. Donadio JV, Jr, Bergstralh EJ, Offord KP, et al: A controlled trial of fish oil in IgA nephropathy. Mayo Nephrology Collaborative Group. N Engl J Med 331:1194–1199, 1994.

974. Dillon JJ: Fish oil therapy for IgA nephropathy: Efficacy and interstudy variability. J Am Soc Nephrol 8:1739–1744, 1997.

975. Bennett WM, Walker RG, Kincaid-Smith P: Treatment of IgA nephropathy with eicosapentanoic acid (EPA): A two-year prospective trial. Clin Nephrol 31:128–131, 1989.

976. Lagrue G, Sadreux T, Laurent J, Hirbec G: Is there a treatment of mesangial IgA glomerulonephritis? Clin Nephrol 16:161, 1981.

977. Kincaid-Smith P, Nicholls K: Mesangial IgA nephropathy. Am J Kidney Dis 3:90–102, 1983.

978. Sato M, Takayama K, Kojima H, et al: Sodium cromoglycate therapy in IgA nephropathy: A preliminary short-term trial. Am J Kidney Dis 15:141–146, 1990.

979. Coppo R, Basolo B, Rollino C, et al: Mediterranean diet and primary IgA nephropathy. Clin Nephrol 26:72–82, 1986.

980. Coppo R, Roccatello D, Amore A, et al: Effects of a gluten-free diet in primary IgA nephropathy. Clin Nephrol 33:72–86, 1990.

981. Clarkson AR, Seymour AE, Woodroffe AJ, et al: Controlled trial of phenytoin therapy in IgA nephropathy. Clin Nephrol 13:215–218, 1980.

982. Coppo R, Basolo B, Bulzomi MR, Piccoli G: Ineffectiveness of phenytoin treatment on IgA-containing circulating immune complexes in IgA nephropathy. Nephron 36:275–276, 1984.

983. Nolin L, Courteau M: Management of IgA nephropathy: Evidence-based recommendations. Kidney Int Suppl 70:S56–S62, 1999.

984. Kincaid-Smith P, Fairley K, Packham D: Randomized controlled crossover study of the effect on proteinuria and blood pressure of adding an angiotensin II receptor antagonist to an angiotensin converting enzyme inhibitor in normotensive patients with chronic renal disease and proteinuria. Nephrol Dial Transplant 17:597–601, 2002.

985. Laverman GD, Navis G, Henning RH, et al: Dual renin-angiotensin system blockade at optimal doses for proteinuria. Kidney Int 62:1020–1025, 2002.

986. Pisoni R, Ruggenenti P, Sangalli F, et al: Effect of high dose ramipril with or without indomethacin on glomerular selectivity. Kidney Int 62:1010–1019, 2002.

987. Haas M, Leko-Mohr Z, Erler C, Mayer G: Antiproteinuric versus antihypertensive effects of high-dose ACE inhibitor therapy. Am J Kidney Dis 40:458–463, 2002.

988. Dische FE, Anderson VE, Keane SJ, et al: Incidence of thin membrane nephropathy: Morphometric investigation of a population sample. J Clin Pathol 43:457–460, 1990.

989. Dische FE, Weston MJ, Parsons V: Abnormally thin glomerular basement membranes associated with hematuria, proteinuria or renal failure in adults. Am J Nephrol 5:103–109, 1985.

990. Aarons I, Smith PS, Davies RA, et al: Thin membrane nephropathy: A clinico-pathological study. Clin Nephrol 32:151–158, 1989.

991. Thin-membrane nephropathy—how thin is thin? Lancet 336:469–470, 1990.

992. Rogers PW, Kurtzman NA, Bunn SM, Jr, White MG: Familial benign essential hematuria. Arch Intern Med 131:257–262, 1973.

993. Cosio FG, Falkenhain ME, Sedmak DD: Association of thin glomerular basement membrane with other glomerulopathies. Kidney Int 46:471–474, 1994.

994. McLay AL, Jackson R, Meyboom F, Jones JM: Glomerular basement membrane thinning in adults: Clinicopathological correlations of a new diagnostic approach. Nephrol Dial Transplant 7:191–199, 1992.

995. Blumenthal SS, Fritsche C, Lemann J, Jr: Establishing the diagnosis of benign familial hematuria. The importance of examining the urine sediment of family members. JAMA 259:2263–2266, 1988.

996. Badenas C, Praga M, Tazon B, et al: Mutations in theCOL4A4 and COL4A3 Genes Cause Familial Benign Hematuria. J Am Soc Nephrol 13:1248–1254, 2002.

997. Chrysostomou A, Walker RG, Russ GR, et al: Diltiazem in renal allograft recipients receiving cyclosporine. Transplantation 55:300–304, 1993.

998. Nieuwhof CM, de Heer F, de Leeuw P, et al: Thin GBM nephropathy: Premature glomerular obsolescence is associated with hypertension and late onset renal failure. Kidney Int 51:1596–1601, 1997.

999. Tiebosch AT, Wolters J, Frederik PF, et al: Epidemiology of idiopathic glomerular disease: A prospective study. Kidney Int 32:112–116, 1987.

1000. Trachtman H, Weiss RA, Bennett B, Greifer I: Isolated hematuria in children: Indications for a renal biopsy. Kidney Int 25:94–99, 1984.

1001. Hebert LA, Betts JA, Sedmak DD: Loin pain-hematuria syndrome associated with thin glomerular basement membrane disease and hemorrhage into renal tubules. Kidney Int 49:168–173, 1996.

1002. Yoshioka K, Hino S, Takemura T, et al: Type IV collagen alpha 5 chain. Normal distribution and abnormalities in X-linked Alport syndrome revealed by monoclonal antibody. Am J Pathol 144:986–996, 1994.

1003. Little PJ, Sloper JS, De Wardener HE: A syndrome of loin pain and haematuria associated with disease of peripheral renal arteries. Q J Med 36:253–259, 1967.

1004. Burden RP, Dathan JR, Etherington MD, et al: The loin-pain/haematuria syndrome. Lancet 1:897–900, 1979.

1005. Weisberg LS, Bloom PB, Simmons RL, Viner ED: Loin pain hematuria syndrome. Am J Nephrol 13:229–237, 1993.

1006. Boyd WN, Burden RP, Aber GM: Intrarenal vascular changes in patients receiving oestrogen-containing compounds—a clinical, histological and angiographic study. Q J Med 44:415–431, 1975.

1007. Fletcher P, Al Khader AA, Parsons V, Aber GM: The pathology of intrarenal vascular lesions associated with the loin-pain-haematuria syndrome. Nephron 24:150–154, 1979.

1008. Dimski DS, Hebert LA, Sedmak D, et al: Renal autotransplantation in the loin pain-hematuria syndrome: A cautionary note. Am J Kidney Dis 20:180–184, 1992.

1009. Lucas PA, Leaker BR, Murphy M, Neild GH: Loin pain and haematuria syndrome: a somatoform disorder. Q J Med 88:703–709, 1995.

1010. Alpers CE, Rennke HG, Hopper J, Jr, Biava CG: Fibrillary glomerulonephritis: An entity with unusual immunofluorescence features. Kidney Int 31:781–789, 1987.

1011. Korbet SM, Schwartz MM, Lewis EJ: Immunotactoid glomerulopathy. Am J Kidney Dis 17:247–257, 1991.

1012. Alpers CE: Immunotactoid (microtubular) glomerulopathy: An entity distinct from fibrillary glomerulonephritis? Am J Kidney Dis 19:185–191, 1992.

1013. Fogo A, Qureshi N, Horn RG: Morphologic and clinical features of fibrillary glomerulonephritis versus immunotactoid glomerulopathy. Am J Kidney Dis 22:367–377, 1993.

1014. Korbet SM, Schwartz MM, Lewis EJ: The fibrillary glomerulopathies. Am J Kidney Dis 23:751–765, 1994.

1015. Iskandar SS, Falk RJ, Jennette JC: Clinical and pathologic features of fibrillary glomerulonephritis. Kidney Int 42:1401–1407, 1992.

1016. Jennette JC, Falk RJ: Fibrillary glomerulonephritis. In Tisher CC, Brenner BM (eds): Renal Pathology with Clinical and Functional Correlations. Philadelphia, Lippincott, 1994, pp 553–563.

1017. D'Agati V, Jennette JC, Silva FG: Non-neoplastic renal disease. In American Registry of Pathology. Washington DC, 2005, pp 199–238.

1018. Schwartz MM: Glomerular diseases with organized deposits. In Jennette JC, Olson JL, Schwartz MM, Silva FG (eds): Heptinstall's Pathology of the Kidney 5th ed. Philadelphia, Lippincott-Raven, 1998, pp 369–388.

1019. Moulin B, Ronco PM, Mougenot B, et al: Glomerulonephritis in chronic lymphocytic leukemia and related B-cell lymphomas. Kidney Int 42:127–135, 1992.

1020. Bridoux F, Hugue V, Coldefy O, et al: Fibrillary glomerulonephritis and immunotactoid (microtubular) glomerulopathy are associated with distinct immunologic features. Kidney Int 62:1764–1775, 2002.

1021. Schwartz MM, Korbet SM, Lewis EJ: Immunotactoid glomerulopathy. J Am Soc Nephrol 13:1390–1397, 2002.

1022. Pronovost PH, Brady HR, Gunning ME, et al: Clinical features, predictors of disease progression and results of renal transplantation in fibrillary/immunotactoid glomerulopathy. Nephrol Dial Transplant 11:837–842, 1996.

1023. Fujigaki Y, Kimura M, Yamashita F, et al: An isolated case with predominant glomerular fibronectin deposition associated with fibril formation. Nephrol Dial Transplant 12:2717–2722, 1997.

1024. Masson RG, Rennke HG, Gottlieb MN: Pulmonary hemorrhage in a patient with fibrillary glomerulonephritis. N Engl J Med 326:36–39, 1992.

1025. Wallner M, Prischl FC, Hobling W, et al: Immunotactoid glomerulopathy with extra-renal deposits in the bone, and chronic cholestatic liver disease. Nephrol Dial Transplant 11:1619–1624, 1996.

1026. D'Agati V, Sacchi G, Truong L: Fibrillary glomerulopathy: Defining the disease spectrum [Abstract]. J Am Soc Nephrol 2:591, 1991.

1027. Couser WG: Rapidly progressive glomerulonephritis: Classification, pathogenetic mechanisms, and therapy. Am J Kidney Dis 11:449–464, 1988.

1028. Jennette JC: Rapidly progressive crescentic glomerulonephritis. Kidney Int 63:1164–1177, 2003.

1029. Jennette JC, Hipp CG: The epithelial antigen phenotype of glomerular crescent cells. Am J Clin Pathol 86:274–280, 1986.

1030. Hancock WW, Atkins RC: Cellular composition of crescents in human rapidly progressive glomerulonephritis identified using monoclonal antibodies. Am J Nephrol 4:177–181, 1984.

1031. Guettier C, Nochy D, Jacquot C, et al: Immunohistochemical demonstration of parietal epithelial cells and macrophages in human proliferative extra-capillary lesions. Virchows Arch A Pathol Anat Histopathol 409:739–748, 1986.

1032. Jennette JC: Crescentic glomerulonephritis. In Jennette JC, Olson JL, Schwartz MM, Silva FG (eds): Heptinstall's Pathology of the Kidney, 5th ed. Philadelphia, Lippincott-Raven, 1998, pp 625–656.

1033. Bonsib SM: Glomerular basement membrane necrosis and crescent organization. Kidney Int 33:966–974, 1988.

1034. Andrassy K, Kuster S, Waldherr R, Ritz E: Rapidly progressive glomerulonephritis: analysis of prevalence and clinical course. Nephron 59:206–212, 1991.

1035. Stilmant MM, Bolton WK, Sturgill BC, et al: Crescentic glomerulonephritis without immune deposits: Clinicopathologic features. Kidney Int 15:184–195, 1979.

1036. Prasad AN, Kapoor KK, Katarya S, Mehta S: Periarteritis nodosa in a child. Indian Pediatr 20:57–61, 1983.

1037. Jennette JC, Falk RJ: Antineutrophil cytoplasmic autoantibodies and associated diseases: A review. Am J Kidney Dis 15:517–529, 1990.

1038. Jennette JC, Falk RJ, Milling DM: Pathogenesis of vasculitis. Semin Neurol 14:291–299, 1994.

1039. Jennette JC, Wilkman AS, Falk RJ: Anti-neutrophil cytoplasmic autoantibody-associated glomerulonephritis and vasculitis. Am J Pathol 135:921–930, 1989.

1040. Ferrario F, Tadros MT, Napodano P, et al: Critical re-evaluation of 41 cases of "idiopathic" crescentic glomerulonephritis. Clin Nephrol 41:1–9, 1994.

1041. Yeung CK, Wong KL, Wong WS, et al: Crescentic lupus glomerulonephritis. Clin Nephrol 21:251–258, 1984.

1042. Weber M, Kohler H, Fries J, et al: Rapidly progressive glomerulonephritis in IgA/IgG cryoglobulinemia. Nephron 41:258–261, 1985.

1043. Chugh KS, Gupta VK, Singhal PC, Sehgal S: Case report: Poststreptococcal crescentic glomerulonephritis and pulmonary hemorrhage simulating Goodpasture's syndrome. Ann Allergy 47:104–106, 1981.

1044. Connolly CE, Gallagher B: Acute crescentic glomerulonephritis as a complication of a Staphylococcus aureus abscess of hip joint prosthesis. J Clin Pathol 40:1486, 1987.

1045. Kalluri R, Meyers K, Mogyorosi A, et al: Goodpasture syndrome involving overlap with Wegener's granulomatosis and anti-glomerular basement membrane disease. J Am Soc Nephrol 8:1795–1800, 1997.

1046. Gao GW, Lin SH, Lin YF, et al: Infective endocarditis complicated with rapidly progressive glomerulonephritis: A case report. Zhonghua Yi Xue Za Zhi (Taipei) 57:438–442, 1996.

1047. Grcevska L, Polenakovic M: Crescentic glomerulonephritis as renal cause of acute renal failure. Ren Fail 17:595–604, 1995.

1048. Toth T: Crescentic involved glomerulonephritis in infective endocarditis. Int Urol Nephrol 22:77–88, 1990.

1049. Wu MJ, Osanloo EO, Molnar ZV, et al: Poststreptococcal crescentic glomerulonephritis in a patient with preexisting membranous glomerulonephropathy. Nephron 35:62–65, 1983.

1050. Lai FM, Li PK, Suen MW, et al: Crescentic glomerulonephritis related to hepatitis B virus. Mod Pathol 5:262–267, 1992.

1051. Squier MK, Sehnert AJ, Cohen JJ: Apoptosis in leukocytes. J Leukoc Biol 57:2–10, 1995.

1052. Moorthy AV, Zimmerman SW, Burkholder PM, Harrington AR: Association of crescentic glomerulonephritis with membranous glomerulonephropathy: a report of three cases. Clin Nephrol 6:319–325, 1976.

1053. Bacani RA, Velasquez F, Kanter A, et al: Rapidly progressive (nonstreptococcal) glomerulonephritis. Ann Intern Med 69:463–485, 1968.

1054. Jardim HM, Leake J, Risdon RA, et al: Crescentic glomerulonephritis in children. Pediatr Nephrol 6:231–235, 1992.

1055. Hazenbos WL, Gessner JE, Hofhuis FM, et al: Impaired IgG-dependent anaphylaxis and Arthus reaction in Fc gamma RIII (CD16) deficient mice. Immunity 5:181–188, 1996.

1056. Sylvestre DL, Ravetch JV: Fc receptors initiate the Arthus reaction: Redefining the inflammatory cascade. Science 265:1095–1098, 1994.

1057. Clynes R, Dumitru C, Ravetch JV: Uncoupling of immune complex formation and kidney damage in autoimmune glomerulonephritis. Science 279:1052–1054, 1998.

1058. Park SY, Ueda S, Ohno H, et al: Resistance of Fc receptor-deficient mice to fatal glomerulonephritis. J Clin Invest 102:1229–1238, 1998.

1059. Lockwood CM, Rees AJ, Pearson TA, et al: Immunosuppression and plasma-exchange in the treatment of Goodpasture's syndrome. Lancet 1:711–715, 1976.

1060. Hellmark T, Johansson C, Wieslander J: Characterization of anti-GBM antibodies involved in Goodpasture's syndrome. Kidney Int 46:823–829, 1994.

1061. O'Neill WM, Jr., Etheridge WB, Bloomer HA: High-dose corticosteroids: their use in treating idiopathic rapidly progressive glomerulonephritis. Arch Intern Med 139:514–518, 1979.

1062. Salant DJ: Immunopathogenesis of crescentic glomerulonephritis and lung purpura. Kidney Int 32:408–425, 1987.

1063. Glassock RJ: A clinical and immunopathologic dissection of rapidly progressive glomerulonephritis. Nephron 22:253–264, 1978.

1064. Angangco R, Thiru S, Esnault VL, et al: Does truly "idiopathic" crescentic glomerulonephritis exist? Nephrol Dial Transplant 9:630–636, 1994.

1065. Couser WG: Idiopathic rapidly progressive glomerulonephritis. Am J Nephrol 2:57–69, 1982.

1066. Beirne GJ, Wagnild JP, Zimmerman SW, et al: Idiopathic crescentic glomerulonephritis. Medicine (Baltimore) 56:349–381, 1977.

1067. Neild GH, Cameron JS, Ogg CS, et al: Rapidly progressive glomerulonephritis with extensive glomerular crescent formation. Q J Med 52:395–416, 1983.

1068. Lerner RA, Glassock RJ, Dixon FJ: The role of anti-glomerular basement membrane antibody in the pathogenesis of human glomerulonephritis. J Exp Med 126:989–1004, 1967.

1069. Briggs WA, Johnson JP, Teichman S, et al: Antiglomerular basement membrane antibody-mediated glomerulonephritis and Goodpasture's syndrome. Medicine (Baltimore) 58:348–361, 1979.

1070. Border WA, Baehler RW, Bhathena D, Glassock RJ: IgA antibasement membrane nephritis with pulmonary hemorrhage. Ann Intern Med 91:21–25, 1979.

1071. Savage CO, Pusey CD, Bowman C, et al: Antiglomerular basement membrane antibody mediated disease in the British Isles 1980–4. Br Med J (Clin Res Ed) 292:301–304, 1986.

1072. Senekjian HO, Knight TF, Weinman EJ: The spectrum of renal diseases associated with anti-basement membrane antibodies. Arch Intern Med 140:79–81, 1980.

1073. Conlon PJ, Jr, Walshe JJ, Daly C, et al: Antiglomerular basement membrane disease: the long-term pulmonary outcome. Am J Kidney Dis 23:794–796, 1994.

1074. Savige JA, Kincaid-Smith P: Antiglomerular basement membrane (GBM) antibody-mediated disease. Am J Kidney Dis 13:355–361, 1989.

1075. Kalluri R, Melendez E, Rumpf KW, et al: Specificity of circulating and tissue-bound autoantibodies in Goodpasture syndrome. Proc Assoc Am Physicians 108:134–139, 1996.

1076. Kelly PT, Haponik EF: Goodpasture syndrome: Molecular and clinical advances. Medicine (Baltimore) 73:171–185, 1994.

1077. Rees AJ, Peters DK, Compston DA, Batchelor JR: Strong association between HLA-DRW2 and antibody-mediated Goodpasture's syndrome. Lancet 1:966–968, 1978.

1078. Fisher M, Pusey CD, Vaughan RW, Rees AJ: Susceptibility to anti-glomerular basement membrane disease is strongly associated with HLA-DRB1 genes. Kidney Int 51:222–229, 1997.

1079. Huey B, McCormick K, Capper J, et al: Associations of HLA-DR and HLA-DQ types with anti-GBM nephritis by sequence-specific oligonucleotide probe hybridization. Kidney Int 44:307–312, 1993.

1080. Dunckley H, Chapman JR, Burke J, et al: HLA-DR and -DQ genotyping in anti-GBM disease. Dis Markers 9:249–256, 1991.

1081. Burns AP, Fisher M, Li P, et al: Molecular analysis of HLA class II genes in Goodpasture's disease. Q J Med 88:93–100, 1995.

1082. Kalluri R, Danoff TM, Okada H, Neilson EG: Susceptibility to anti-glomerular basement membrane disease and Goodpasture syndrome is linked to MHC class II genes and the emergence of T cell-mediated immunity in mice. J Clin Invest 100:2263–2275, 1997.

1083. Jennette JC, Nickeleit V: Anti-glomerular basement membrane glomerulonephritis and Goodpasture's syndrome. In Jennette JC, Olson JL, Schwartz MM, Silva FG (eds): Heptinstall's Pathology of the Kidney, 6th ed. Philadelphia, Lippincott Williams & Wilkins, 2006, pp 613–642.

1084. Germuth FG, Jr, Choi IJ, Taylor JJ, Rodriguez E: Antibasement membrane disease. I. The glomerular lesions of Goodpasture's disease and experimental disease in sheep. Johns Hopkins Med J 131:367–384, 1972.

1085. McPhaul JJ, Jr, Mullins JD: Glomerulonephritis mediated by antibody to glomerular basement membrane. Immunological, clinical, and histopathological characteristics. J Clin Invest 57:351–361, 1976.

1086. Walker RG, Scheinkestel C, Becker GJ, et al: Clinical and morphological aspects of the management of crescentic anti-glomerular basement membrane antibody (anti-GBM) nephritis/Goodpasture's syndrome. Q J Med 54:75–89, 1985.

1087. Fivush B, Melvin T, Solez K, McLean RH: Idiopathic linear glomerular IgA deposition. Arch Pathol Lab Med 110:1189–1191, 1986.

1088. Short AK, Esnault VL, Lockwood CM: Anti-neutrophil cytoplasm antibodies and anti-glomerular basement membrane antibodies: Two coexisting distinct autoreactivities detectable in patients with rapidly progressive glomerulonephritis. Am J Kidney Dis 26:439–445, 1995.

1089. Poskitt TR: Immunologic and electron microscopic studies in Goodpasture's syndrome. Am J Med 49:250–257, 1970.

1090. Wieslander J, Barr JF, Butkowski RJ, et al: Goodpasture antigen of the glomerular basement membrane: localization to noncollagenous regions of type IV collagen. Proc Natl Acad Sci U S A 81:3838–3842, 1984.

1091. Wieslander J, Bygren P, Heinegard D: Isolation of the specific glomerular basement membrane antigen involved in Goodpasture syndrome. Proc Natl Acad Sci U S A 81:1544–1548, 1984.

1092. Wieslander J, Langeveld J, Butkowski R, et al: Physical and immunochemical studies of the globular domain of type IV collagen. Cryptic properties of the Goodpasture antigen. J Biol Chem 260:8564–8570, 1985.

1093. Hellmark T, Segelmark M, Wieslander J: Anti-GBM antibodies in Goodpasture syndrome; anatomy of an epitope. Nephrol Dial Transplant 12:646–648, 1997.

1094. Hellmark T, Brunmark C, Trojnar J, Wieslander J: Epitope mapping of anti-glomerular basement membrane (GBM) antibodies with synthetic peptides. Clin Exp Immunol 105:504–510, 1996.

1095. Kalluri R, Sun MJ, Hudson BG, Neilson EG: The Goodpasture autoantigen. Structural delineation of two immunologically privileged epitopes on alpha3(IV) chain of type IV collagen. J Biol Chem 271:9062–9068, 1996.

1096. Netzer KO, Leinonen A, Boutaud A, et al: The goodpasture autoantigen. Mapping the major conformational epitope(s) of alpha3(IV) collagen to residues 17–31 and 127–141 of the NC1 domain. J Biol Chem 274:11267–11274, 1999.

1097. Hellmark T, Segelmark M, Unger C, et al: Identification of a clinically relevant immunodominant region of collagen IV in Goodpasture disease. Kidney Int 55:936–944, 1999.

1098. Hellmark T, Niles JL, Collins AB, et al: Comparison of anti-GBM antibodies in sera with or without ANCA. J Am Soc Nephrol 8:376–385, 1997.

1099. Meyers KE, Kinniry PA, Kalluri R, et al: Human Goodpasture anti-alpha3(IV)NC1 autoantibodies share structural determinants. Kidney Int 53:402–407, 1998.

1100. Borza DB, Bondar O, Colon S, et al: Goodpasture autoantibodies unmask cryptic epitopes by selectively dissociating autoantigen complexes lacking structural reinforcement: novel mechanisms for immune privilege and autoimmune pathogenesis. J Biol Chem 280:27147–27154, 2005.

1101. Stevenson A, Yaqoob M, Mason H, et al: Biochemical markers of basement membrane disturbances and occupational exposure to hydrocarbons and mixed solvents. QJM 88:23–28, 1995.

1102. Donaghy M, Rees AJ: Cigarette smoking and lung haemorrhage in glomerulonephritis caused by autoantibodies to glomerular basement membrane. Lancet 2:1390–1393, 1983.

1103. Kalluri R, Cantley LG, Kerjaschki D, Neilson EG: Reactive oxygen species expose cryptic epitopes associated with autoimmune goodpasture syndrome. J Biol Chem 275:20027–20032, 2000.

1104. Saxena R, Bygren P, Butkowski R, Wieslander J: Entactin: A possible auto-antigen in the pathogenesis of non-Goodpasture anti-GBM nephritis. Kidney Int 38:263–272, 1990.

1105. Kalluri R, Danoff T, Neilson EG: Murine anti-alpha3(IV) collagen disease: A model of human Goodpasture syndrome and anti-GBM nephritis. J Am Soc Nephrol 6:833, 1995.

1106. Savage CO, Lockwood CM: Antineutrophil antibodies in vasculitis. Adv Nephrol Necker Hosp 19:225–236, 1990.

1107. Heeringa P, Brouwer E, Klok PA, et al: Autoantibodies to myeloperoxidase aggravate mild anti-glomerular-basement-membrane-mediated glomerular injury in the rat. Am J Pathol 149:1695–1706, 1996.

1108. Rutgers A, Slot M, van Paassen P, et al: Coexistence of anti-glomerular basement membrane antibodies and myeloperoxidase-ANCAs in crescentic glomerulonephritis. Am J Kidney Dis 46:253–262, 2005.

1109. Wilson CB: Immunologic aspects of renal diseases. JAMA 268:2904–2909, 1992.

1110. Gaskin G, Savage CO, Ryan JJ, et al: Anti-neutrophil cytoplasmic antibodies and disease activity during long-term follow-up of 70 patients with systemic vasculitis. Nephrol Dial Transplant 6:689–694, 1991.

1111. Sado Y, Naito I: Experimental autoimmune glomerulonephritis in rats by soluble isologous or homologous antigens from glomerular and tubular basement membranes. Br J Exp Pathol 68:695–704, 1987.

1112. Sado Y, Naito I, Okigaki T: Transfer of anti-glomerular basement membrane antibody-induced glomerulonephritis in inbred rats with isologous antibodies from the urine of nephritic rats. J Pathol 158:325–332, 1989.

1113. Bolton WK, May WJ, Sturgill BC: Proliferative autoimmune glomerulonephritis in rats: A model for autoimmune glomerulonephritis in humans. Kidney Int 44:294–306, 1993.

1114. Derry CJ, Ross CN, Lombardi G, et al: Analysis of T cell responses to the autoantigen in Goodpasture's disease. Clin Exp Immunol 100:262–268, 1995.

1115. Steblay RW, Rudofsky U: Experimental glomerulonephritis induced in sheep by injections of human lung and Freund's adjuvant. Science 160:204–206, 1968.

1116. Huang XR, Holdsworth SR, Tipping PG: Th2 responses induce humorally mediated injury in experimental anti-glomerular basement membrane glomerulonephritis. J Am Soc Nephrol 8:1101–1108, 1997.

1117. Adler S, Baker PJ, Pritzl P, Couser WG: Detection of terminal complement components in experimental immune glomerular injury. Kidney Int 26:830–837, 1984.

1118. Groggel GC, Salant DJ, Darby C, et al: Role of terminal complement pathway in the heterologous phase of antiglomerular basement membrane nephritis. Kidney Int 27:643–651, 1985.

1119. Tipping PG, Boyce NW, Holdsworth SR: Relative contributions of chemo-attractant and terminal components of complement to anti-glomerular basement membrane (GBM) glomerulonephritis. Clin Exp Immunol 78:444–448, 1989.

1120. Schrijver G, Assmann KJ, Bogman MJ, et al: Antiglomerular basement membrane nephritis in the mouse. Study on the role of complement in the heterologous phase. Lab Invest 59:484–491, 1988.

1121. Sheerin NS, Springall T, Carroll MC, et al: Protection against anti-glomerular basement membrane (GBM)-mediated nephritis in C3- and C4-deficient mice. Clin Exp Immunol 110:403–409, 1997.

1122. Nakamura A, Yuasa T, Ujike A, et al: Fcgamma receptor IIB-deficient mice develop Goodpasture's syndrome upon immunization with type IV collagen: A novel murine model for autoimmune glomerular basement membrane disease. J Exp Med 191:899–906, 2000.

1123. Wakayama H, Hasegawa Y, Kawabe T, et al: Abolition of anti-glomerular basement membrane antibody-mediated glomerulonephritis in FcRgamma-deficient mice. Eur J Immunol 30:1182–1190, 2000.

1124. Suzuki Y, Shirato I, Okumura K, et al: Distinct contribution of Fc receptors and angiotensin II-dependent pathways in anti-GBM glomerulonephritis. Kidney Int 54:1166–1174, 1998.

1125. Heeringa P, van Goor H, Itoh-Lindstrom Y, et al: Lack of endothelial nitric oxide synthase aggravates murine accelerated anti-glomerular basement membrane glomerulonephritis. Am J Pathol 156:879–888, 2000.

1126. Neugarten J, Feith GW, Assmann KJ, et al: Role of macrophages and colony-stimulating factor-1 in murine antiglomerular basement membrane glomerulonephritis. J Am Soc Nephrol 5:1903–1909, 1995.

1127. Lan HY, Bacher M, Yang N, et al: The pathogenic role of macrophage migration inhibitory factor in immunologically induced kidney disease in the rat. J Exp Med 185:1455–1465, 1997.

1128. Tang T, Rosenkranz A, Assmann KJ, et al: A role for Mac-1 (CDIIb/CD18) in immune complex-stimulated neutrophil function in vivo: Mac-1 deficiency abrogates sustained Fcgamma receptor-dependent neutrophil adhesion and complement-dependent proteinuria in acute glomerulonephritis. J Exp Med 186:1853–1863, 1997.

1129. Luca ME, Paul LC, Der Wal AM, et al: Treatment with mycophenolate mofetil attenuates the development of Heymann nephritis. Exp Nephrol 8:77–83, 2000.

1130. Taal MW, Zandi N, Weening B, et al: Proinflammatory gene expression and macrophage recruitment in the rat remnant kidney. Kidney Int 58:1664–1676, 2000.

1131. Huang XR, Kitching AR, Tipping PG, Holdsworth SR: Interleukin-10 inhibits macrophage-induced glomerular injury. J Am Soc Nephrol 11:262–269, 2000.

1132. Lockwood CM, Boulton-Jones JM, Lowenthal RM, et al: Recovery from Goodpasture's syndrome after immunosuppressive treatment and plasmapheresis. Br Med J 2:252–254, 1975.

1133. Pusey CD: Plasma exchange in immunological disease. Prog Clin Biol Res 337:419–424, 1990.

1134. Peters DK, Rees AJ, Lockwood CM, Pusey CD: Treatment and prognosis in antibasement membrane antibody-mediated nephritis. Transplant Proc 14:513–521, 1982.

1135. Pusey CD, Lockwood CM, Peters DK: Plasma exchange and immunosuppressive drugs in the treatment of glomerulonephritis due to antibodies to the glomerular basement membrane. Int J Artif Organs 6 Suppl 1:15–18, 1983.

1136. Madore F, Lazarus JM, Brady HR: Therapeutic plasma exchange in renal diseases. J Am Soc Nephrol 7:367–386, 1996.

1137. Wilson CB, Dixon FJ: Anti-glomerular basement membrane antibody-induced glomerulonephritis. Kidney Int 3:74–89, 1973.

1138. Zimmerman SW, Groehler K, Beirne GJ: Hydrocarbon exposure and chronic glomerulonephritis. Lancet 2:199–201, 1975.

1139. Churchill DN, Fine A, Gault MH: Association between hydrocarbon exposure and glomerulonephritis. An appraisal of the evidence. Nephron 33:169–172, 1983.

1140. Ravnskov U, Lundstrom S, Norden A: Hydrocarbon exposure and glomerulonephritis: Evidence from patients' occupations. Lancet 2:1214–1216, 1983.

1141. Daniell WE, Couser WG, Rosenstock L: Occupational solvent exposure and glomerulonephritis. A case report and review of the literature. JAMA 259:2280–2283, 1988.

1142. Rees AJ, Lockwood CM, Peters DK: Enhanced allergic tissue injury in Goodpasture's syndrome by intercurrent bacterial infection. Br Med J 2:723–726, 1977.

1143. Merkel F, Kalluri R, Marx M, et al: Autoreactive T-cells in Goodpasture's syndrome recognize the N-terminal NC1 domain on alpha 3 type IV collagen. Kidney Int 49:1127–1133, 1996.

1144. Segelmark M, Butkowski R, Wieslander J: Antigen restriction and IgG subclasses among anti-GBM autoantibodies. Nephrol Dial Transplant 5:991–996, 1990.

1145. Strauch BS, Charney A, Doctorouff S, Kashgarian M: Goodpasture syndrome with recovery after renal failure. JAMA 229:444, 1974.

1146. Lang CH, Brown DC, Staley N, et al: Goodpasture syndrome treated with immunosuppression and plasma exchange. Arch Intern Med 137:1076–1078, 1977.

1147. Johnson JP, Whitman W, Briggs WA, Wilson CB: Plasmapheresis and immunosuppressive agents in antibasement membrane antibody-induced Goodpasture's syndrome. Am J Med 64:354–359, 1978.

1148. Smith PK, d'Apice JF: Plasmapheresis in rapidly progressive glomerulonephritis. Am J Med 65:564–566, 1978.

1149. Thysell H, Bygren P, Bengtsson U, et al: Immunosuppression and the additive effect of plasma exchange in treatment of rapidly progressive glomerulonephritis. Acta Med Scand 212:107–114, 1982.

1150. Glassock RJ: The role of high-dose steroids in nephritic syndromes: The case for a conservative approach. In Narins R (ed): Controversies in Nephrology and Hypertension. New York, Churchill Livingstone, 1984, p 421.

1151. Bolton WK: The role of high-dose steroids in nephritic syndromes: the case for aggressive use. In Narins R (ed): Controversies in Nephrology and Hypertension. New York, Churchill Livingstone, 1984, p 421.

1152. Adler S, Bruns FJ, Fraley DS, Segel DP: Rapid progressive glomerulonephritis: Relapse after prolonged remission. Arch Intern Med 141:852–854, 1981.

1153. Jayne DR, Marshall PD, Jones SJ, Lockwood CM: Autoantibodies to GBM and neutrophil cytoplasm in rapidly progressive glomerulonephritis. Kidney Int 37:965–970, 1990.

1154. Gaskin G, Pusey CD: Plasmapheresis in antineutrophil cytoplasmic antibody-associated systemic vasculitis. Ther Apher 5:176–181, 2001.

1155. Levy JB, Turner AN, Rees AJ, Pusey CD: Long-term outcome of anti-glomerular basement membrane antibody disease treated with plasma exchange and immunosuppression. Ann Intern Med 134:1033–1042, 2001.

1156. O'Donoghue DJ, Short CD, Brenchley PE, et al: Sequential development of systemic vasculitis with anti-neutrophil cytoplasmic antibodies complicating anti-glomerular basement membrane disease. Clin Nephrol 32:251–255, 1989.

1157. Dahlberg PJ, Kurtz SB, Donadio JV, et al: Recurrent Goodpasture's syndrome. Mayo Clin Proc 53:533–537, 1978.

1158. Klasa RJ, Abboud RT, Ballon HS, Grossman L: Goodpasture's syndrome: Recurrence after a five-year remission. Case report and review of the literature. Am J Med 84:751–755, 1988.

1159. Wu MJ, Moorthy AV, Beirne GJ: Relapse in anti glomerular basement membrane antibody mediated crescentic glomerulonephritis. Clin Nephrol 13:97–102, 1980.

1160. Hind CR, Bowman C, Winearls CG, Lockwood CM: Recurrence of circulating anti-glomerular basement membrane antibody three years after immunosuppressive treatment and plasma exchange. Clin Nephrol 21:244–246, 1984.

1161. Almkuist RD, Buckalew VM, Jr, Hirszel P, et al: Recurrence of anti-glomerular basement membrane antibody mediated glomerulonephritis in an isograft. Clin Immunol Immunopathol 18:54–60, 1981.

1162. Jennette JC, Thomas DB: Pauci-immune and antineutrophil cytoplasmic autoantibody glomerulonephritis and vasculitis. In Jennette JC, Olson JL, Schwartz MM, Silva FG (eds): Heptinstall's Pathology of the Kidney, 6th ed. Philadelphia, Lippincott Williams & Wilkins, 2006, pp 643–674.

1163. Jennette JC, Falk RJ: Anti-neutrophil cytoplasmic autoantibodies: Discovery, specificity, disease associations and pathogenic potential. Adv Pathol Lab Med 363–377, 1995.

1164. Jennette JC: Antineutrophil cytoplasmic autoantibody-associated diseases: A pathologist's perspective. Am J Kidney Dis 18:164–170, 1991.

1165. Harris AA, Falk RJ, Jennette JC: Crescentic glomerulonephritis with a paucity of glomerular immunoglobulin localization. Am J Kidney Dis 32:179–184, 1998.

1166. Jennette JC, Falk RJ: Pathogenic potential of anti-neutrophil cytoplasmic autoantibodies. Adv Exp Med Biol 336:7–15, 1993.

1167. Kallenberg CG, Brouwer E, Weening JJ, Tervaert JW: Anti-neutrophil cytoplasmic antibodies: Current diagnostic and pathophysiological potential. Kidney Int 46:1–15, 1994.

1168. Keogan MT, Esnault VL, Green AJ, et al: Activation of normal neutrophils by anti-neutrophil cytoplasm antibodies. Clin Exp Immunol 90:228–234, 1992.

1169. Falk RJ, Terrell RS, Charles LA, Jennette JC: Anti-neutrophil cytoplasmic autoantibodies induce neutrophils to degranulate and produce oxygen radicals in vitro. Proc Natl Acad Sci U S A 87:4115–4119, 1990.

1170. Charles LA, Caldas ML, Falk RJ, et al: Antibodies against granule proteins activate neutrophils in vitro. J Leukoc Biol 50:539–546, 1991.

1171. Braun MG, Csernok E, Muller-Hermelink HK, Gross WL: Distribution pattern of proteinase 3 in Wegener's granulomatosis and other vasculitic diseases. Immun Infekt 19:23–24, 1991.

1172. Brouwer E, Huitema MG, Mulder AH, et al: Neutrophil activation in vitro and in vivo in Wegener's granulomatosis. Kidney Int 45:1120–1131, 1994.

1173. Ewert BH, Jennette JC: Anti-myeloperoxidase antibodies (aMPO) stimulate neutrophils to adhere to cultured human endothelial cells utilizing the beta-2-integrin CD11/18. [Abstract]. J Am Soc Nephrol 3:585, 1992.

1174. Braun MG, Csernok E, Gross WL, Muller-Hermelink HK: Proteinase 3, the target antigen of anticytoplasmic antibodies circulating in Wegener's granulomatosis. Immunolocalization in normal and pathologic tissues. Am J Pathol 139:831–838, 1991.

1175. Savage CO, Pottinger BE, Gaskin G, et al: Autoantibodies developing to myeloperoxidase and proteinase 3 in systemic vasculitis stimulate neutrophil cytotoxicity toward cultured endothelial cells. Am J Pathol 141:335–342, 1992.

1176. Porges AJ, Redecha PB, Kimberly WT, et al: Anti-neutrophil cytoplasmic antibodies engage and activate human neutrophils via Fc gamma RIIa. J Immunol 153:1271–1280, 1994.

1177. Taekema-Roelvink ME, van Kooten C, Heemskerk E, et al: Proteinase 3 interacts with a 111-kD membrane molecule of human umbilical vein endothelial cells. J Am Soc Nephrol 11:640–648, 2000.

1178. Kurosawa S, Esmon CT, Stearns-Kurosawa DJ: The soluble endothelial protein C receptor binds to activated neutrophils: Involvement of proteinase-3 and CD11b/CD18. J Immunol 165:4697–703, 2000.

1179. Esmon CT: Structure and functions of the endothelial cell protein C receptor. Crit Care Med 32:S298–S301, 2004.

1180. Ballieux BE, Hiemstra PS, Klar-Mohamad N, et al: Detachment and cytolysis of human endothelial cells by proteinase 3. Eur J Immunol 24:3211–3215, 1994.

1181. Yang JJ, Kettritz R, Falk RJ, et al: Apoptosis of endothelial cells induced by the neutrophil serine proteases proteinase 3 and elastase. Am J Pathol 149:1617–1626, 1996.

1182. Taekema-Roelvink ME, van Kooten C, Janssens MC, et al: Effect of anti-neutrophil cytoplasmic antibodies on proteinase 3-induced apoptosis of human endothelial cells. Scand J Immunol 48:37–43, 1998.

1183. Baldus S, Eiserich JP, Mani A, et al: Endothelial transcytosis of myeloperoxidase confers specificity to vascular ECM proteins as targets of tyrosine nitration. J Clin Invest 108:1759–1770, 2001.

1184. Brennan ML, Wu W, Fu X, et al: A tale of two controversies: Defining both the role of peroxidases in nitrotyrosine formation in vivo using eosinophil peroxidase and myeloperoxidase-deficient mice, and the nature of peroxidase-generated reactive nitrogen species. J Biol Chem 277:17415–17427, 2002.

1185. Woods AA, Linton SM, Davies MJ: Detection of HOCl-mediated protein oxidation products in the extracellular matrix of human atherosclerotic plaques. Biochem J 370:729–735, 2003.

1186. Lu X, Garfield A, Rainger GE, et al: Mediation of endothelial cell damage by serine proteases, but not superoxide, released from antineutrophil cytoplasmic antibody-stimulated neutrophils. Arthritis Rheum 54:1619–1628, 2006.

1187. Mulder AH, Broekroelofs J, Horst G, et al: Anti-neutrophil cytoplasmic antibodies (ANCA) in inflammatory bowel disease: Characterization and clinical correlates. Clin Exp Immunol 95:490–497, 1994.

1188. Kettritz R, Jennette JC, Falk RJ: Crosslinking of ANCA-antigens stimulates superoxide release by human neutrophils. J Am Soc Nephrol 8:386–394, 1997.

1189. Kimberly RP: Fcgamma receptors and neutrophil activation. Clin Exp Immunol 120 (Suppl 1):18–19, 2000.

1190. Kocher M, Edberg JC, Fleit HB, Kimberly RP: Antineutrophil cytoplasmic antibodies preferentially engage Fc gammaRIIIb on human neutrophils. J Immunol 161:6909–6914, 1998.

1191. Tse WY, Nash GB, Hewins P, et al: ANCA-induced neutrophil F-actin polymerization: Implications for microvascular inflammation. Kidney Int 67:130–139, 2005.

1192. Wainstein E, Edberg J, Csernok E, et al: FcgammaRIIIb alleles predict renal dysfunction in Wegener's granulomatosis (WG). Arthritis Rheum 39:210, 1995.

1193. Dijstelbloem HM, Scheepers RH, Oost WW, et al: Fcgamma receptor polymorphisms in Wegener's granulomatosis: Risk factors for disease relapse. Arthritis Rheum 42:1823–1827, 1999.

1194. Edberg JC, Wainstein E, Wu J, et al: Analysis of FcgammaRII gene polymorphisms in Wegener's granulomatosis. Exp Clin Immunogenet 14:183–195, 1997.

1195. Tse WY, Abadeh S, McTiernan A, et al: No association between neutrophil FcgammaRIIa allelic polymorphism and anti-neutrophil cytoplasmic antibody (ANCA)-positive systemic vasculitis. Clin Exp Immunol 117:198–205, 1999.

1196. Yang JJ, Alcorta DA, Preston GA, et al: Genes activated by ANCA IgG amd ANCA F(ab')2 fragments [Abstract]. J Am Soc Nephrol 11:485A, 2000.

1197. Williams JM, Savage COS: Characterization of the regulation and functional consequences of p21ras activation in neutrophils by antineutrophil cytoplasm antibodies. J Am Soc Nephrol 16:90–96, 2005.

1198. Franssen CF, Stegeman CA, Kallenberg CG, et al: Antiproteinase 3- and antimyeloperoxidase-associated vasculitis. Kidney Int 57:2195–2206, 2000.

1199. Harper L, Savage CO: Pathogenesis of ANCA-associated systemic vasculitis. J Pathol 190:349–359, 2000.

1200. Schmitt WH, Heesen C, Csernok E, et al: Elevated serum levels of soluble interleukin-2 receptor in patients with Wegener's granulomatosis. Association with disease activity. Arthritis Rheum 35:1088–1096, 1992.

1201. Bolton WK, Innes DJ, Jr, Sturgill BC, Kaiser DL: T-cells and macrophages in rapidly progressive glomerulonephritis: Clinicopathologic correlations. Kidney Int 32:869–876, 1987.

1202. Csernok E, Trabandt A, Muller A, et al: Cytokine profiles in Wegener's granulomatosis: predominance of type 1 (Th1) in the granulomatous inflammation. Arthritis Rheum 42:742–750, 1999.

1203. Balding CE, Howie AJ, Drake-Lee AB, Savage CO: Th2 dominance in nasal mucosa in patients with Wegener's granulomatosis. Clin Exp Immunol 151:332–339, 2001.

1204. Komocsi A, Lamprecht P, Csernok E, et al: Peripheral blood and granuloma CD4(+)CD28(−) T cells are a major source of interferon-gamma and tumor necrosis factor-alpha in Wegener's granulomatosis. Am J Pathol 160:1717–1724, 2002.

1205. Cunningham MA, Huang XR, Dowling JP, et al: Prominence of cell-mediated immunity effectors in "pauci-immune" glomerulonephritis [see comments]. J Am Soc Nephrol 10:499–506, 1999.

1206. Wang G, Hansen H, Tatsis E, et al: High plasma levels of the soluble form of CD30 activation molecule reflect disease activity in patients with Wegener's granulomatosis. Am J Med 102:517–523, 1997.

1207. Stegeman CA, Tervaert JW, Huitema MG, Kallenberg CG: Serum markers of T cell activation in relapses of Wegener's granulomatosis. Clin Exp Immunol 91:415–420, 1993.

1208. Van Der Woude FJ, van Es LA, Daha MR: The role of the c-ANCA antigen in the pathogenesis of Wegener's granulomatosis. A hypothesis based on both humoral and cellular mechanisms. Neth J Med 36:169–171, 1990.

1209. Ballieux BE, van der Burg SH, Hagen EC, et al: Cell-mediated autoimmunity in patients with Wegener's granulomatosis (WG) [see comments]. Clin Exp Immunol 100:186–193, 1995.

1210. Brouwer E, Stegeman CA, Huitema MG, et al: T cell reactivity to proteinase 3 and myeloperoxidase in patients with Wegener's granulomatosis (WG). Clin Exp Immunol 98:448–453, 1994.

1211. King WJ, Brooks CJ, Holder R, et al: T lymphocyte responses to anti-neutrophil cytoplasmic autoantibody (ANCA) antigens are present in patients with ANCA-associated systemic vasculitis and persist during disease remission. Clin Exp Immunol 112:539–546, 1998.

1212. Griffith ME, Coulthart A, Pusey CD: T cell responses to myeloperoxidase (MPO) and proteinase 3 (PR3) in patients with systemic vasculitis. Clin Exp Immunol 103:253–258, 1996.

1213. Monaghan P, Robertson D, Amos TA, et al: Ultrastructural localization of bcl-2 protein. J Histochem Cytochem 40:1819–1825, 1992.

1214. Esnault VL, Mathieson PW, Thiru S, et al: Autoantibodies to myeloperoxidase in brown Norway rats treated with mercuric chloride. Lab Invest 67:114–120, 1992.

1215. Harper MC, Milstein C, Cooke A: Pathogenic anti-MPO antibody in MRL/lpr mice [Abstract]. Clin Exp Immunol 101:54, 1995.

1216. Nachman PH, Hogan SL, Jennette JC, Falk RJ: Treatment response and relapse in antineutrophil cytoplasmic autoantibody-associated microscopic polyangiitis and glomerulonephritis. J Am Soc Nephrol 7:33–39, 1996.

1217. Xiao H, Heeringa P, Hu P, et al: Antineutrophil cytoplasmic autoantibodies specific for myeloperoxidase cause glomerulonephritis and vasculitis in mice. J Clin Invest 110:955–963, 2002.

1218. Falk RJ, Jennette JC: ANCA are pathogenic—oh yes they are! J Am Soc Nephrol 13:1977–1979, 2002.

1219. Huugen D, Xiao H, van Esch A, et al: Aggravation of anti-myeloperoxidase antibody-induced glomerulonephritis by bacterial lipopolysaccharide: Role of tumor necrosis factor-alpha. Am J Pathol 167:47–58, 2005.

1220. Xiao H, Heeringa P, Liu Z, et al: The role of neutrophils in the induction of glomerulonephritis by anti-myeloperoxidase antibodies. Am J Pathol 167:39–45, 2005.

1221. Jennette JC, Xiao H, Falk RJ: Pathogenesis of vascular inflammation by anti-neutrophil cytoplasmic antibodies. J Am Soc Nephrol 17:1235–1242, 2006.

1222. Little MA, Smyth CL, Yadav R, et al: Antineutrophil cytoplasm antibodies directed against myeloperoxidase augment leukocyte-microvascular interactions in vivo. Blood 106:2050–2058, 2005.

1223. Pfister H, Ollert M, Froehlich LF, et al: Anti-neutrophil cytoplasmic autoantibodies (ANCA) against the murine homolog of proteinase 3 (Wegener's autoantigen) are pathogenic in vivo. Blood 101:1411–1418, 2004.

1224. Spencer SJ, Burns A, Gaskin G, et al: HLA class II specificities in vasculitis with antibodies to neutrophil cytoplasmic antigens. Kidney Int 41:1059–1063, 1992.

1225. Stegeman CA, Tervaert JW, Sluiter WJ, et al: Association of chronic nasal carriage of Staphylococcus aureus and higher relapse rates in Wegener granulomatosis [see comments]. Ann Intern Med 120:12–17, 1994.

1226. Gregorini G, Ferioli A, Donato F, et al: Association between silica exposure and necrotizing crescentic glomerulonephritis with p-ANCA and anti-MPO antibodies: A hospital-based case-control study. Adv Exp Med Biol 336:435–440, 1993.

1227. Hogan SL, Satterly KK, Dooley MA, et al: Silica exposure in anti-neutrophil cytoplasmic autoantibody-associated glomerulonephritis and lupus nephritis. J Am Soc Nephrol 12:134–142, 2001.

1228. Pendergraft WF, III, Pressler BM, Jennette JC, et al: Autoantigen complementarity: A new theory implicating complementary proteins as initiators of autoimmune disease. J Mol Med 83:12–25, 2005.

1229. Pendergraft WF, Preston GA, Shah RR, et al: Autoimmunity is triggered by cPR-3(105–201), a protein complementary to human autoantigen proteinase-3. Nat Med 10:72–79, 2004.

1230. Bonsib SM, Walker WP: Pulmonary-renal syndrome: Clinical similarity amidst etiologic diversity. Mod Pathol 2:129–137, 1989.

1231. Niles JL, Bottinger EP, Saurina GR, et al: The syndrome of lung hemorrhage and nephritis is usually an ANCA-associated condition. Arch Intern Med 156:440–445, 1996.

1232. Jennette JC, Falk RJ, Andrassy K, et al: Nomenclature of systemic vasculitides. Proposal of an international consensus conference. Arthritis Rheum 37:187–192, 1994.

1233. Savage CO, Winearls CG, Evans DJ, et al: Microscopic polyarteritis: Presentation, pathology and prognosis. Q J Med 56:467–483, 1985.

1234. Hogan SL, Nachman PH, Wilkman AS, et al: Prognostic markers in patients with antineutrophil cytoplasmic autoantibody-associated microscopic polyangiitis and glomerulonephritis. J Am Soc Nephrol 7:23–32, 1996.

1235. Bajema IM, Hagen EC, Hermans J, et al: Kidney biopsy as a predictor for renal outcome in ANCA-associated necrotizing glomerulonephritis. Kidney Int 56:1751–1758, 1999.

1236. Koldingsnes W, Nossent JC: Baseline features and initial treatment as predictors of remission and relapse in Wegener's granulomatosis. J Rheumatol 30:80–88, 2003.

1237. Hogan SL, Falk RJ, Chin H, et al: Predictors of relapse and treatment resistance in antineutrophil cytoplasmic antibody-associated small-vessel vasculitis. Ann Intern Med 143:621–631, 2005.

1238. Frasca GM, Neri L, Martello M, et al: Renal transplantation in patients with microscopic polyarteritis and antimyeloperoxidase antibodies: Report of three cases. Nephron 72:82–85, 1996.

1239. Rosenstein ED, Ribot S, Ventresca E, Kramer N: Recurrence of Wegener's granulomatosis following renal transplantation. Br J Rheumatol 33:869–871, 1994.

1240. Nachman PH, Segelmark M, Westman K, et al: Recurrent ANCA-associated small vessel vasculitis after transplantation: A pooled analysis. Kidney Int 56:1544–1550, 1999.

1241. Geffriaud-Ricouard C, Noel LH, Chauveau D, et al: Clinical spectrum associated with ANCA of defined antigen specificities in 98 selected patients. Clin Nephrol 39:125–136, 1993.

1242. Kallenberg CG, Mulder AH, Tervaert JW: Antineutrophil cytoplasmic antibodies: A still-growing class of autoantibodies in inflammatory disorders. Am J Med 93:675–682, 1992.

1243. Falk RJ, Jennette JC: Anti-neutrophil cytoplasmic autoantibodies with specificity for myeloperoxidase in patients with systemic vasculitis and idiopathic necrotizing and crescentic glomerulonephritis. N Engl J Med 318:1651–1657, 1988.

1244. Ludemann J, Utecht B, Gross WL: Anti-neutrophil cytoplasm antibodies in Wegener's granulomatosis recognize an elastinolytic enzyme. J Exp Med 171:357–362, 1990.

1245. Goldschmeding R, van der Schoot CE, ten Bokkel HD, et al: Wegener's granulomatosis autoantibodies identify a novel diisopropylfluorophosphate-binding protein in the lysosomes of normal human neutrophils. J Clin Invest 84:1577–1587, 1989.

1246. Jennette JC, Hoidal JR, Falk RJ: Specificity of anti-neutrophil cytoplasmic autoantibodies for proteinase 3. Blood 75:2263–2264, 1990.

1247. Niles JL, McCluskey RT, Ahmad MF, Arnaout MA: Wegener's granulomatosis autoantigen is a novel neutrophil serine proteinase. Blood 74:1888–1893, 1989.

1248. Bosch X, Mirapeix E, Font J, et al: Anti-myeloperoxidase autoantibodies in patients with necrotizing glomerular and alveolar capillaritis. Am J Kidney Dis 20:231–239, 1992.

1249. Choi HK, Liu S, Merkel PA, et al: Diagnostic performance of antineutrophil cytoplasmic antibody tests for idiopathic vasculitides: Metaanalysis with a focus on antimyeloperoxidase antibodies. J Rheumatol 28:1584–1590, 2001.

1250. Falk RJ, Moore DT, Hogan SL, Jennette JC: A renal biopsy is essential for the management of ANCA-positive patients with glomerulonephritis. Sarcoidosis Vasc Diffuse Lung Dis 13:230–231, 1996.

1251. Savage CO, Harper L, Adu D: Primary systemic vasculitis. Lancet 349:553–558, 1997.

1252. Fauci AS, Katz P, Haynes BF, Wolff SM: Cyclophosphamide therapy of severe systemic necrotizing vasculitis. N Engl J Med 301:235–238, 1979.

1253. Falk RJ, Hogan S, Carey TS, Jennette JC: Clinical course of anti-neutrophil cytoplasmic autoantibody-associated glomerulonephritis and systemic vasculitis. The Glomerular Disease Collaborative Network. Ann Intern Med 113:656–663, 1990.

1254. Glockner WM, Sieberth HG, Wichmann HE, et al: Plasma exchange and immunosuppression in rapidly progressive glomerulonephritis: A controlled, multi-center study. Clin Nephrol 29:1–8, 1988.

1255. Cole E, Cattran D, Magil A, et al: A prospective randomized trial of plasma exchange as additive therapy in idiopathic crescentic glomerulonephritis. The Canadian Apheresis Study Group. Am J Kidney Dis 20:261–269, 1992.

1256. Pusey CD, Rees AJ, Evans DJ, et al: Plasma exchange in focal necrotizing glomerulonephritis without anti-GBM antibodies. Kidney Int 40:757–763, 1991.

1257. Levy JB, Pusey CD: Still a role for plasma exchange in rapidly progressive glomeru-lonephritis? J Nephrol 10:7–13, 1997.

1258. Gaskin G, Jayne DR, European Vasculitis Study Group: Adjunctive plasma exchange is superior to methylprednisolone in acute renal failure due to ANCA-associated glomerulonephritis. J Am Soc Nephrol 13:2A-3A, 2002.

1259. Jayne DR, Davies MJ, Fox CJ, et al: Treatment of systemic vasculitis with pooled intravenous immunoglobulin. Lancet 337:1137–1139, 1991.

1260. Tuso P, Moudgil A, Hay J, et al: Treatment of antineutrophil cytoplasmic autoanti-body-positive systemic vasculitis and glomerulonephritis with pooled intravenous gammaglobulin. Am J Kidney Dis 20:504–508, 1992.

1261. Jayne DR, Lockwood CM: Pooled intravenous immunoglobulin in the management of systemic vasculitis. Adv Exp Med Biol 336:469–472, 1993.

1262. Richter C, Schnabel A, Csernok E, et al: Treatment of anti-neutrophil cytoplasmic antibody (ANCA)-associated systemic vasculitis with high-dose intravenous immu-noglobulin. Clin Exp Immunol 101:2–7, 1995.

1263. Richter C, Schnabel A, Csernok E, et al: Treatment of Wegener's granulomatosis with intravenous immunoglobulin. Adv Exp Med Biol 336:487–489, 1993.

1264. Jayne DR, Chapel H, Adu D, et al: Intravenous immunoglobulin for ANCA-associated systemic vasculitis with persistent disease activity. Q J Med 93:433–439, 2000.

1265. DeRemee RA, McDonald TJ, Weiland LH: Wegener's granulomatosis: Observations on treatment with antimicrobial agents. Mayo Clin Proc 60:27–32, 1985.

1266. Stegeman CA, Tervaert JW, De Jong PE, Kallenberg CG: Trimethoprim-sulfamethoxa-zole (co-trimoxazole) for the prevention of relapses of Wegener's granulomatosis. Dutch Co-Trimoxazole Wegener Study Group. N Engl J Med 335:16–20, 1996.

1267. Hoffman GS, Leavitt RY, Kerr GS, Fauci AS: The treatment of Wegener's granuloma-tosis with glucocorticoids and methotrexate. Arthritis Rheum 35:1322–1329, 1992.

1268. Sneller MC, Hoffman GS, Talar-Williams C, et al: An analysis of forty-two Wegener's granulomatosis patients treated with methotrexate and prednisone. Arthritis Rheum 38:608–613, 1995.

1269. Keogh KA, Ytterberg SR, Fervenza FC, et al: Rituximab for refractory Wegener's granulomatosis: report of a prospective, open-label pilot trial. Am J Respir Crit Care Med 173:180–187, 2006.

1270. Eriksson P: Nine patients with anti-neutrophil cytoplasmic antibody-positive vascu-litis successfully treated with rituximab. J Intern Med 257:540–548, 2005.

1271. Stasi R, Stipa E, Poeta GD, et al: Long-term observation of patients with anti-neutrophil cytoplasmic antibody-associated vasculitis treated with rituximab. Rheumatology (Oxford) 45:1432–1436, 2006.

1272. Aries PM, Lamprecht P, Gross WL: Rituximab in refractory Wegener's granulomato-sis: Favorable or not? Am J Respir Crit Care Med 173:815a–8816, 2006.

1273. Jayne DR: Campath-1H (anti-CD52) for refractory vasculitis: Retrospective Cam-bridge experience 1989–1999. Cleve Clin J Med 69:SII-129, 2002.

1274. Lamprecht P, Voswinkel J, Lilienthal T, et al: Effectiveness of TNF-alpha blockade with infliximab in refractory Wegener's granulomatosis. Rheumatology (Oxford) 41:1303–1307, 2002.

1275. Bartolucci P, Ramanoelina J, Cohen P, et al: Efficacy of the anti-TNF-alpha antibody infliximab against refractory systemic vasculitides: An open pilot study on 10 patients. Rheumatology (Oxford) 41:1126–1132, 2002.

1276. Booth A, Harper L, Hammad T, et al: Prospective study of TNFalpha blockade with infliximab in anti-neutrophil cytoplasmic antibody-associated systemic vasculitis. J Am Soc Nephrol 15:717–721, 2004.

1277. Booth AD, Jefferson HJ, Ayliffe W, et al: Safety and efficacy of TNFalpha blockade in relapsing vasculitis. Ann Rheum Dis 61:559, 2002.

1278. Jennette JC, Mandal AK: The nephrotic syndrome. In Mandel SR, Jennette JC (eds): Diagnosis and Management of Renal Disease and Hypertension, 2 ed. Durham, Caro-lina Academic Press, 1994, pp 235–272.

1279. Caldas ML, Charles LA, Falk RJ, Jennette JC: Immunoelectron microscopic documen-tation of the translocation of proteins reactive with ANCA to neutrophil cell surfaces during neutrophil activation. [Abstract]. Third International Workshop on ANCA 1990.

1280. Ellis D: Anemia in the course of the nephrotic syndrome secondary to transferrin depletion. J Pediatr 90:953–955, 1977.

1281. Harris RC, Ismail N: Extrarenal complications of the nephrotic syndrome. Am J Kidney Dis 23:477–497, 1994.

1282. Howard RL, Buddington B, Alfrey AC: Urinary albumin, transferrin and iron excre-tion in diabetic patients. Kidney Int 40:923–926, 1991.

1283. Cartwright GE, Gubler CJ, Wintrobe MM: Studies on copper metabolism. XI. Copper and iron metabolism in the nephrotic syndrome. J Clin Invest 33:685, 1954.

1284. Pedraza C, Torres R, Cruz C, et al: Copper and zinc metabolism in aminonucleoside-induced nephrotic syndrome. Nephron 66:87–92, 1994.

1285. Freeman RM, Richards CJ, Rames LK: Zinc metabolism in aminonucleoside-induced nephrosis. Am J Clin Nutr 28:699–703, 1975.

1286. Hancock DE, Onstad JW, Wolf PL: Transferrin loss into the urine with hypochromic, microcytic anemia. Am J Clin Pathol 65:73–78, 1976.

1287. Bergrem H: Pharmacokinetics and protein binding of prednisolone in patients with nephrotic syndrome and patients undergoing hemodialysis. Kidney Int 23:876–881, 1983.

1288. Frey FJ, Frey BM: Altered prednisolone kinetics in patients with the nephrotic syn-drome. Nephron 32:45–48, 1982.

1289. Strife CF, Jackson EC, Forristal J, West CD: Effect of the nephrotic syndrome on the concentration of serum complement components. Am J Kidney Dis 8:37–42, 1986.

1290. Kaysen GA, Gambertoglio J, Jimenez I, et al: Effect of dietary protein intake on albumin homeostasis in nephrotic patients. Kidney Int 29:572–577, 1986.

1291. Panicucci F, Sagripanti A, Vispi M, et al: Comprehensive study of haemostasis in nephrotic syndrome. Nephron 33:9–13, 1983.

1292. Adler AJ, Lundin AP, Feinroth MV, et al: Beta-thromboglobulin levels in the nephro-tic syndrome. Am J Med 69:551–554, 1980.

1293. Kuhlmann U, Steurer J, Rhyner K, et al: Platelet aggregation and beta-thromboglo-bulin levels in nephrotic patients with and without thrombosis. Clin Nephrol 15:229–235, 1981.

1294. Alkjaersig N, Fletcher AP, Narayanan M, Robson AM: Course and resolution of the coagulopathy in nephrotic children. Kidney Int 31:772–780, 1987.

1295. Kendall AG, Lohmann RC, Dossetor JB: Nephrotic syndrome. A hypercoagulable state. Arch Intern Med 127:1021–1027, 1971.

1296. Coppola R, Guerra L, Ruggeri ZM, et al: Factor VIII/von Willebrand factor in glo-merular nephropathies. Clin Nephrol 16:217–222, 1981.

1297. Thomson C, Forbes CD, Prentice CR, Kennedy AC: Changes in blood coagulation and fibrinolysis in the nephrotic syndrome. Q J Med 43:399–407, 1974.

1298. Vaziri ND, Ngo JL, Ibsen KH, et al: Deficiency and urinary losses of factor XII in adult nephrotic syndrome. Nephron 32:342–346, 1982.

1299. Lau SO, Tkachuck JY, Hasegawa DK, Edson JR: Plasminogen and antithrombin III deficiencies in the childhood nephrotic syndrome associated with plasminogenuria and antithrombinuria. J Pediatr 96:390–392, 1980.

1300. Shimamatsu K, Onoyama K, Maeda T, et al: Massive pulmonary embolism occurring with corticosteroid and diuretics therapy in a minimal-change nephrotic patient. Nephron 32:78–79, 1982.

1301. Vaziri ND, Gonzales EC, Shayestehfar B, Barton CH: Plasma levels and urinary excre-tion of fibrinolytic and protease inhibitory proteins in nephrotic syndrome. J Lab Clin Med 124:118–124, 1994.

1302. Ozanne P, Francis RB, Meiselman HJ: Red blood cell aggregation in nephrotic syn-drome. Kidney Int 23:519–525, 1983.

1303. Boneu B, Bouissou F, Abbal M, et al: Comparison of progressive antithrombin activ-ity and the concentration of three thrombin inhibitors in nephrotic syndrome. Thromb Haemost 46:623–625, 1981.

1304. Jorgensen KA, Stoffersen E: Antithrombin III and the nephrotic syndrome. Scand J Haematol 22:442–448, 1979.

1305. Thaler E, Balzar E, Kopsa H, Pinggera WF: Acquired antithrombin III deficiency in patients with glomerular proteinuria. Haemostasis 7:257–272, 1978.

1306. Vigano D, Angelo A, Kaufman CE, et al: Protein S deficiency occurs in the nephrotic syndrome. Ann Intern Med 107:42–47, 1987.

1307. Mehls O, Andrassy K, Koderisch J, et al: Hemostasis and thromboembolism in chil-dren with nephrotic syndrome: Differences from adults. J Pediatr 110:862–867, 1987.

1308. Warren GV, Korbet SM, Schwartz MM, Lewis EJ: Minimal change glomerulopathy associated with nonsteroidal antiinflammatory drugs. Am J Kidney Dis 13:127–130, 1989.

1309. Tornroth T, Skrifvars B: The development and resolution of glomerular basement membrane changes associated with subepithelial immune deposits. Am J Pathol 79:219–236, 1975.

1310. Criteria for diagnosis of Behcet's disease. International Study Group for Behcet's Disease. Lancet 335:1078–1080, 1990.

1311. Korzets Z, Golan E, Manor Y, et al: Spontaneously remitting minimal change nephropathy preceding a relapse of Hodgkin's disease by 19 months. Clin Nephrol 38:125–127, 1992.

1312. Dabbs DJ, Striker LM, Mignon F, Striker G: Glomerular lesions in lymphomas and leukemias. Am J Med 80:63–70, 1986.

1313. Alpers CE, Cotran RS: Neoplasia and glomerular injury. Kidney Int 30:465–473, 1986.

1314. Meyrier A, Delahousse M, Callard P, Rainfray M: Minimal change nephrotic syn-drome revealing solid tumors. Nephron 61:220–223, 1992.

1315. Lagrue G, Laurent J, Rostoker G: Food allergy and idiopathic nephrotic syndrome. Kidney Int Suppl 27:S147–S151, 1989.

1316. Rennke HG: Secondary membranoproliferative glomerulonephritis. Kidney Int 47:643–656, 1995.

1317. Beaufils M, Morel-Maroger L, Sraer JD, et al: Acute renal failure of glomerular origin during visceral abscesses. N Engl J Med 295:185–189, 1976.

1318. Martinelli R, Noblat AC, Brito E, Rocha H: Schistosoma mansoni-induced mesangio-capillary glomerulonephritis: Influence of therapy. Kidney Int 35:1227–1233, 1989.

1319. Molle D, Baumelou A, Beaufils H, et al: Membranoproliferative glomerulonephritis associated with pulmonary sarcoidosis. Am J Nephrol 6:386–387, 1986.

1320. Zell SC, Duxbury G, Shankel SW: Alveolar hemorrhage associated with a membra-noproliferative glomerulonephritis and smooth muscle antibody. Am J Med 82:1073–1076, 1987.

1321. Strife CF, Hug G, Chuck G, et al: Membranoproliferative glomerulonephritis and alpha 1-antitrypsin deficiency in children. Pediatrics 71:88–92, 1983.

1322. Lagrue G, Laurent J, Dubertret L, Branellec A: Buckley's syndrome and membrano-proliferative glomerulonephritis. Nephron 31:279–280, 1982.

1323. Swarbrick ET, Fairclough PD, Campbell PJ, et al: Coeliac disease, chronic active hepatiti, and mesangiocapillary glomerulonephritis in the same patient. Lancet 2:1084–1085, 1980.

1324. Katz A, Dyck RF, Bear RA: Celiac disease associated with immune complex glomeru-lonephritis. Clin Nephrol 11:39–44, 1979.

1325. Pasternack A, Collin P, Mustonen J, et al: Glomerular IgA deposits in patients with celiac disease. Clin Nephrol 34:56–60, 1990.

1326. Jennette JC, Ferguson AL, Moore MA, Freeman DG: IgA nephropathy associated with seronegative spondylarthropathies. Arthritis Rheum 25:144–149, 1982.

1327. Woodroffe AJ: IgA, glomerulonephritis and liver disease. Aust N Z J Med 11:109–111, 1981.

1328. Hirsch DJ, Jindal KK, Trillo A, Cohen AD: Acute renal failure in Crohn's disease due to IgA nephropathy. Am J Kidney Dis 20:189–190, 1992.

1329. Kalsi J, Delacroix DL, Hodgson HJ: IgA in alcoholic cirrhosis. Clin Exp Immunol 52:499–504, 1983.

1330. Ramirez G, Stinson JB, Zawada ET, Moatamed F: IgA nephritis associated with mycosis fungoides. Report of two cases. Arch Intern Med 141:1287–1291, 1981.

1066

1331. Sinniah R: Mucin secreting cancer with mesangial IgA deposits. Pathology 14:303–308, 1982.

1332. Monteiro GE, Lillicrap CA: Case of mumps nephritis. Br Med J 4:721–722, 1967.

1333. Spichtin HP, Truniger B, Mihatsch MJ, et al: Immunothrombocytopenia and IgA nephritis. Clin Nephrol 14:304–308, 1980.

1334. Woodrow G, Innes A, Boyd SM, Burden RP: A case of IgA nephropathy with coeliac disease responding to a gluten-free diet. Nephrol Dial Transplant 8:1382–1383, 1993.

1335. Nomoto Y, Sakai H, Endoh M, Tomino Y: Scleritis and IgA nephropathy. Arch Intern Med 140:783–785, 1980.

1336. Andrassy K, Lichtenberg G, Rambausek M: Sicca syndrome in mesangial IgA glomerulonephritis. Clin Nephrol 24:60–62, 1985.

1337. Thomas M, Ibels LS, Abbot N: IgA nephropathy associated with mastitis and haematuria. Br Med J (Clin Res Ed) 291:867–868, 1985.

1338. Yum MN, Lampton LM, Bloom PM, Edwards JL: Asymptomatic IgA nephropathy associated with pulmonary hemosiderosis. Am J Med 64:1056–1060, 1978.

1339. Remy P, Jacquot C, Nochy D, et al: Buerger's disease associated with IgA nephropathy: Report of two cases. Br Med J (Clin Res Ed) 296:683–684, 1988.

1340. Kimmel PL, Phillips TM, Ferreira-Centeno A, et al: Brief report: Idiotypic IgA nephropathy in patients with human immunodeficiency virus infection. N Engl J Med 327:702–706, 1992.

1341. Newell GC: Cirrhotic glomerulonephritis: Incidence, morphology, clinical features, and pathogenesis. Am J Kidney Dis 9:183–190, 1987.

1342. Beaufils H, Jouanneau C, Katlama C, et al: HIV-associated IgA nephropathy—a post-mortem study. Nephrol Dial Transplant 10:35–38, 1995.

1343. van de Wiel A, Valentijn RM, Schuurman HJ, et al: Circulating IgA immune complexes and skin IgA deposits in liver disease. Relation to liver histopathology. Dig Dis Sci 33:679–684, 1988.

1344. Druet P, Bariety J, Bernard D, Lagrue G: [Primary glomerulopathy with IgA and IgG mesangial deposits. Clinical and morphological study of 52 cases]. Presse Med 78:583–587, 1970.

1345. Garcia-Fuentes M, Martin A, Chantler C, Williams DG: Serum complement components in Henoch-Schonlein purpura. Arch Dis Child 53:417–419, 1978.

1346. Gartner HV, Honlein F, Traub U, Bohle A: IgA-nephropathy (IgA-IgG-nephropathy/IgA-nephritis)—a disease entity? Virchows Arch A Pathol Anat Histol 385:1–27, 1979.

1347. Frasca GM, Vangelista A, Biagini G, Bonomini V: Immunological tubulo-interstitial deposits in IgA nephropathy. Kidney Int 22:184–191, 1982.

1348. Gutierrez M, Navas P, Ortega R, et al: Familial and hereditary mesangial glomerulonephritis with IgA deposits (author's transl). Med Clin (Barc) 76:1–7, 1981.

1349. Garcia-Fuentes M, Chantler C, Williams DG: Cryoglobulinaemia in Henoch-Schonlein purpura. Br Med J 2:163–165, 1977.

1350. Galla JH, Kohaut EC, Alexander R, Mestecky J: Racial difference in the prevalence of IgA-associated nephropathies. Lancet 2:522, 1984.

1351. Jennette JC, Falk RJ: The pathology of vasculitis involving the kidney. Am J Kidney Dis 24:130–141, 1994.

CH 30

Secondary Glomerular Disease

Gerald B. Appel • Jai Radhakrishnan • Vivette D'Agati

SYSTEMIC LUPUS ERYTHEMATOSUS

Lupus nephritis (LN) is a frequent and potentially serious complication of systemic lupus erythematosus (SLE).[1-6] Serious kidney disease influences morbidity and mortality both directly and indirectly through complications of therapy. Recent studies have more clearly defined the spectrum of clinical, prognostic and renal histopathologic findings in SLE. Treatment trials have focused on the benefits of a variety of immunosuppressive regimens both in severe proliferative LN and membranous lupus. The new histopathologic, epidemiologic, and clinical data have led to further large controlled randomized trials to define the optimal treatment for LN.

Epidemiology

The incidence and prevalence of SLE depend on the population studied and the diagnostic criteria for defining SLE. Females greatly outnumber males by 8–13 : 1.[3,7,8] However, males with SLE have the same incidence of renal disease as do females.[7,8] Younger adults outnumber older individuals with over 85% of patients younger than 55 years of age. SLE is more likely to be associated with severe nephritis in children, and is less likely in the elderly.[2-4,8] SLE appears to be more common and certainly is associated with more severe renal involvement in the African American population although the precise roles of biologic–genetic versus socioeconomic factors have not been clearly defined.[7-12] Thus, the overall incidence of SLE ranges from 1.8 to 7.6 cases per 100,000 with a prevalence of from 4 to 250 cases per 100,000.[7,8,13] The incidence of renal involvement is even more variable depending on the populations studied as well as the diagnostic criteria for kidney disease and whether involvement is defined by renal biopsy or clinical findings. Approximately 25% to 50% of unselected lupus patients will have clinical renal disease at onset whereas as many as 60% of adults with SLE will develop renal disease during their course.[3-5,7,8]

Although the etiology of SLE remains unknown, certain genetic, hormonal, and environmental factors clearly influence the course and severity of disease expression. A genetic predisposition for the development of SLE is supported by a high concordance rate in monozygotic twins, the significant percentage of relatives of patients with the disease who develop SLE (5%–12%), the higher frequency of certain HLA genotypes (e.g., HLA-B8, DR2, DR3, and DQW1), and the higher frequency of SLE in populations with deficiencies of certain complement components (e.g., C1q, C2, and C4 deficiency).[8] Inherited abnormalities of Fc receptors may also influence the incidence and severity of renal disease in SLE.[14] A multiplicity of genes appears to be involved in the abnormalities related to SLE. Evidence for a predisposing role for hormonal factors includes the strong predominance of females in the childbearing age and the increased incidence of SLE in postmenopausal females given estrogen.[14] There is also more severe and earlier disease in female murine models of SLE (F1 NZB/NZW), which is ameliorated by oophorectomy or androgen therapy. Environmental factors other than estrogens may also affect the occurrence and expression of SLE. Although alterations of the immune system induced by viral or bacterial antigens have been proposed, their role in SLE induction remains far from clear.[15] However, exposure to sunlight, UV radiation, and certain medications can all predispose to the development of SLE.

The diagnosis of SLE is often clinically established by the presence of certain clinical and laboratory features defined by the 1997 modified American Rheumatism Association criteria.[16] Development of 4 of the 11 criteria over a lifetime gives a 96% sensitivity and specificity for SLE. The criteria include malar rash, discoid lupus, dermal disease, photosensitivity, oral or nasal ulcerations, non-deforming arthritis, serositis including pleuritis and pericarditis, and central nervous system disease such as seizures or psychoses. Hematologic involvement is manifested by anemia, leukopenia, lymphopenia or thrombocytopenia, and immunologic markers of disease including a positive anti-DNA antibody, anti-Sm antibody, and test for antiphospholipid antibodies or by a positive ANA. The last remaining criterion is renal involvement defined for these purposes as persistent proteinuria exceeding 500 mg daily (or 3+ on the dipstick) or the presence of cellular casts (consisting of erythrocyte, hemoglobin, granular, tubular, or mixed casts). Although the criteria were not designed for diagnosis in individual patients, they are useful to follow the evolution and treatment response of patients with SLE. Because some patients, especially those with mesangial or membranous glomerular lesions, will present with clinical renal disease before they have fulfilled 4 of the 11 ARA criteria for SLE, the diagnosis of SLE remains a clinical diagnosis with histopathologic findings supporting or confirming the presumed diagnosis.[17]

Pathogenesis

Although numerous immunologic abnormalities have been noted in patients with SLE, it is unclear which factors are directly related to the pathogenesis of the disease itself and which factors are epiphenomena.[15] SLE is a disease in which abnormalities of immune regulation lead to a loss of self-tolerance and subsequent autoimmune responses.[15,18-20] SLE has been associated with a decreased number of cytotoxic and suppressor T cells, increased helper (CD4+) T cells, polyclonal activation of B cells, defective B cell tolerance, dysfunctional T cell signaling, and abnormal Th1 and Th2 cytokine production.[8,21-23] Some of these abnormalities contribute to the activation and clonal expansion of CD4+ T cells, which via cytokine release cause activation of autoreactive B cells leading to their proliferation and differentiation into cells that produce an excess of antibodies against nuclear antigens.[8,15] Ultimately unique idiotypic autoantibodies are produced by clones of B cells leading to high levels of antibodies directed against nuclear antigens such as ANA, DNA, Sm, RNA, Ro, La, and other nuclear antigens.[15,24,25] The formation of circulating immune complexes and their deposition with complement activation is important for certain patterns of glomerular damage. Immune complexes are also detectable in the skin at the dermal–epidermal junction, in the choroid plexus, pericardium, and pleural spaces. The propensity of these immune complexes to cause disease depends not only on size and charge, but also on the rate of clearance by Fc receptors in the liver and spleen.

Glomerular involvement in SLE has often been considered a human prototype of classic chronic immune complex-induced glomerulonephritis as defined in experimental models.[26] The chronic deposition of circulating immune complexes plays a major role in the mesangial and the proliferative patterns of LN. Size, charge, and avidity of the immune complexes influence their localization within the glomerulus. The clearing ability of the mesangium and local hemodynamic factors may also play a role.[27] In diffuse proliferative LN the deposited complexes consist of nuclear antigens (e.g., DNA) and high affinity complement fixing IgG antibodies.[8,26] Cationic histones bind to glomerular basement membrane (GBM) as well and may facilitate antinuclear antibody localization.[8,26] Once deposited, the complement cascade is activated leading to complement mediated damage, activation of procoagulant factors, leukocyte infiltration, release of proteolytic enzymes, and various cytokines regulating glomerular cellular proliferation and matrix synthesis. Other patients may have a different mechanism of immune complex mediated damage. The initiating event may be the local binding of nuclear or other antigens to glomerular sites particularly the subepithelial regions of the GBM, followed by in situ immune complex formation. Glomerular and vascular damage may be potentiated by hypertension and coagulation abnormalities. The presence of anti-phospholipid antibodies, directed against a phospholipid-beta$_2$ glycoprotein complex, and their attendant alterations in endothelial and platelet function, including reduced production of prostacyclin and

other endothelial anticoagulant factors, activation of plasminogen, inhibition of protein C or S, and enhanced platelet aggregation, can also potentiate glomerular and vascular lesions.

Pathology of Lupus Nephritis

The histopathology of LN is extremely pleomorphic.[1-5,8] This diversity of disease expression is evident when comparing adjacent glomeruli in a single biopsy or comparing biopsy findings among different patients. Moreover, the lesions have the capacity to transform from one pattern to another spontaneously or with therapy. Initial attempts to classify biopsies were hindered by the variable expression of the disease, its ability to transform, and the lack of well-defined clinical–pathologic correlation. Early classifications of LN divided glomerular changes into mild and severe forms.[2,26] The World Health Organization Classification (WHO), used for almost 30 years,[28] combined light microscopic (LM) findings with the immunofluorescence (IF) and electron microscopic (EM) findings to present an accurate and precise classification system. Although it greatly advanced the study of clinical pathologic correlations, provided valuable prognostic information, and has also allowed the development of controlled collaborative clinical trials of LN, it still had limitations. In 2003 a new classification schema of LN, the International Society of Nephrology/Renal Pathology Society (ISN/RPS) classification, addressed these limitations.[29,30] This classification is now widely used by nephrologists, pathologists, and rheumatologists (Table 31–1). Although it still divides the biopsies of SLE patients into six classes akin to the older WHO classification, it should provide better data from clinical pathologic correlations and more prognostic information to the clinician.

International Society of Nephrology (ISN) Class I denotes normal glomeruli by light microscopy but with mesangial immune deposits by IF and EM. Even patients without clinical renal disease often have mesangial immune deposits when studied carefully by the more sensitive techniques of IF and EM.[2,17]

TABLE 31–1	International Society of Nephrology/Renal Pathology Society (2003) Classification of Lupus Nephritis
Class I	Minimal mesangial LN
Class II	Mesangial proliferative LN
Class III	Focal LN* (<50% of glomeruli) III (A): Active lesions III (A/C): Active and chronic lesions III (C): Chronic lesions
Class IV	Diffuse LN* (≥50% of glomeruli) Diffuse segmental (IV-S) or global (IV-G) LN IV (A): Active lesions IV (A/C): Active and chronic lesions IV (C): Chronic lesions
Class V†	Membranous LN
Class VI	Advanced sclerosing LN (≥90% globally sclerosed glomeruli without residual activity)

LN, lupus nephritis.
†Class V may occur in combination with III or IV in which case both will be diagnosed.

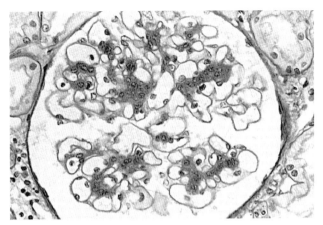

FIGURE 31–1 Lupus nephritis class II: There is mild global mesangial hyper-cellularity (Periodic acid-Schiff, ×400).

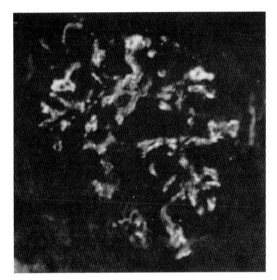

FIGURE 31–2 Lupus nephritis class II: Immunofluorescence photomicrograph showing deposits of C3 restricted to the glomerular mesangium (×400).

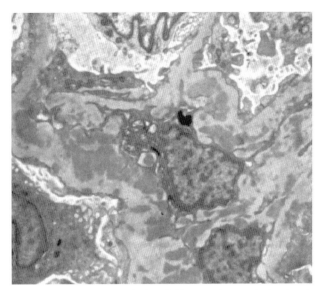

FIGURE 31–3 Lupus nephritis class II: Electron micrograph showing abundant mesangial electron-dense deposits (×12,000).

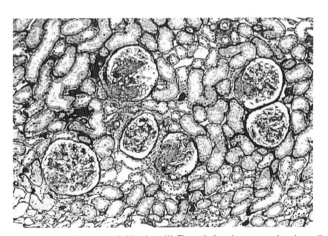

FIGURE 31–4 Lupus nephritis class III: There is focal segmental endocapillary proliferation (Jones methenamine silver, ×100).

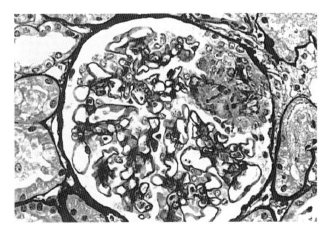

FIGURE 31–5 Lupus nephritis class III: The glomerular endocapillary proliferation is discretely segmental with necrotizing features and an early cellular crescent (Jones methenamine silver, ×400).

International Society of Nephrology Class II is defined on LM by pure mesangial hypercellularity, with mesangial immune deposits on IF and EM (Figs. 31–1, 31–2, and 31–3).[2,8,31,32] Mesangial hypercellularity is defined as greater than three cells in mesangial regions distant from the vascular pole in 3 μm-thick sections. There may be rare minute subendothelial or subepithelial deposits visible by IF or EM, but not by LM.

International Society of Nephrology Class III, focal lupus nephritis, is defined as focal segmental and/or global endocapillary and/or extracapillary glomerulonephritis affecting less than 50% of the total glomeruli sampled. There is usually focal segmental endocapillary proliferation including mesangial cells and endothelial cells, with infiltrating mononuclear and polymorphonuclear leukocytes (Figs. 31–4, 31–5, and 31–6).[2,8,33] Class III biopsies may have active (proliferative), inactive (sclerosing), or active and inactive lesions subclassified as A, C, or A/C respectively. Active lesions may display fibrinoid necrosis, nuclear pyknosis or karyorrhexis, and rupture of the glomerular basement membrane (GBM). Hematoxylin bodies, consisting of swollen basophilic nuclear material acted upon by anti-nuclear antibodies, are occasionally found in association with necrotizing lesions. Subendo-thelial immune deposits may be visible by LM as "wire loop" thickenings of the glomerular capillary walls or large intralu-minal masses, so-called "hyaline thrombi". Segmental scar-ring involving less than 50% of the glomeruli qualifies for an ISN Class III C lesion. In Class III biopsies, some glomeruli adjacent to those with severe histologic changes may show only mesangial changes or no abnormality by LM. In Class III, diffuse mesangial and focal and segmental subendothelial immune deposits are typically identified by IF and EM. The segmental subendothelial deposits are usually present in the distribution of the segmental endocapillary proliferative lesions.

International Society of Nephrology Class IV, diffuse pro-liferative LN, have glomeruli with qualitatively similar endo-capillary glomerular proliferation as in Class III biopsies, but the proliferation involves more than 50% of the glomeruli (Figs. 31–7, 31–8, and 31–9).[2–4,8,17,26,32,34,35] The ISN Classi-

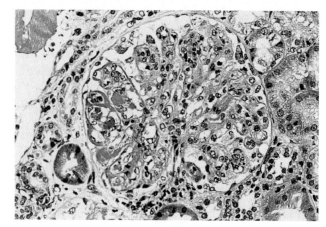

FIGURE 31–7 Lupus nephritis class IV: There is global endocapillary proliferation with infiltrating neutrophils and segmental wire loop deposits (Hematoxylin-eosin, ×320).

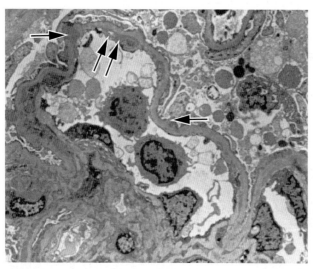

FIGURE 31–6 Lupus nephritis class III: Electron micrograph showing deposits in the mesangium as well as involving the peripheral capillary wall in subendothelial (double arrow) and subepithelial (single arrow) locations (×4900).

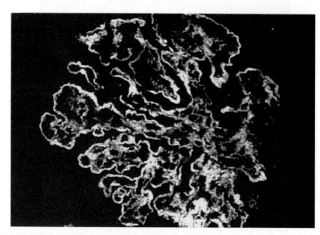

FIGURE 31–8 Lupus nephritis class IV: Immunofluorescence photomicro-graph showing global deposits of IgG in the mesangial regions and outlining the subendothelial aspect of the peripheral glomerular capillary walls (×600).

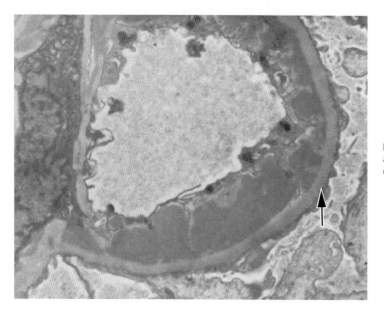

FIGURE 31–9 Lupus nephritis class IV: Electron micrograph showing a large subendothelial electron-dense deposit as well as a few small sub-epithelial deposits (arrow) (×1200).

fication subdivides lupus nephritis Class IV into diffuse segmental versus diffuse global proliferation to facilitate future studies addressing possible differences in outcome and pathogenesis between these subgroups. Class IV-S is used if more than 50% of affected glomeruli have segmental lesions, whereas Class IV-G is used if more than 50% of affected glomeruli have global lesions. All the active features described earlier for Class III (including fibrinoid necrosis, leukocyte infiltration, wire loop deposits, hyaline thrombi, and hematoxylin bodies) may be encountered in Class IV lupus nephritis. In general, there is more extensive peripheral capillary wall subendothelial immune deposition in Class IV biopsies and extracapillary proliferation in the form of crescents is not uncommon. Some patients with ISN Class IV lesions have features similar to idiopathic membranoproliferative (mesangiocapillary glomerulonephritis) with mesangial interposition along the peripheral capillary walls and double contours of the GBMs.

International Society of Nephrology Class V is defined by regular subepithelial immune deposits producing a membranous pattern (Figs. 31–10, 31–11, and 31–12).[2,8,26,32,36–38] The co-existence of mesangial immune deposits and mesangial hypercellularity in most cases helps to distinguish membranous LN from idiopathic membranous glomerulopathy.[39] Early membranous lupus nephropathy Class V may have no identifiable abnormalities by LM. In well-developed membranous glomerulonephritis, there is typically thickening of the glomerular capillary walls and "spike" formation. When the membranous alterations are accompanied by additional focal or diffuse proliferative lesions and subendothelial immune complex deposition they are classified as V + III and V + IV. Because sparse subepithelial deposits may also be encountered in other classes (III or IV) of LN, a diagnosis of pure lupus membranous LN should be reserved only for those cases in which the membranous pattern predominates.

International Society of Nephrology Class VI is advanced sclerosing lupus nephritis or end-stage LN and is reserved for those biopsies with over 90% of the glomeruli sclerotic. There are no active lesions and it may be difficult in such biopsies to even establish the diagnosis of LN without the identification of residual glomerular immune deposits by IF and EM.

CH 31

Secondary Glomerular Disease

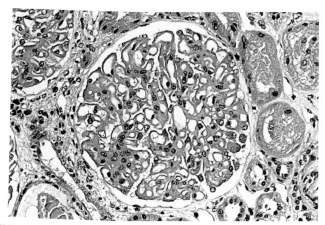

FIGURE 31–10 Lupus nephritis class V: There is diffuse uniform thickening of glomerular basement membranes accompanied by mild segmental mesangial hypercellularity (Hematoxylin-eosin, ×320).

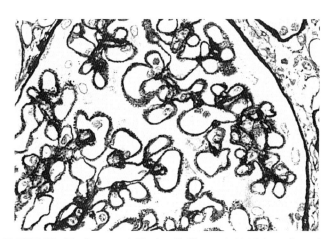

FIGURE 31–11 Lupus nephritis class V: Silver stain highlights uniform glomerular basement membrane spikes projecting from the glomerular basement membranes (Jones methenamine silver, ×800).

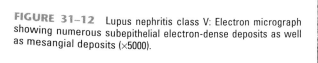

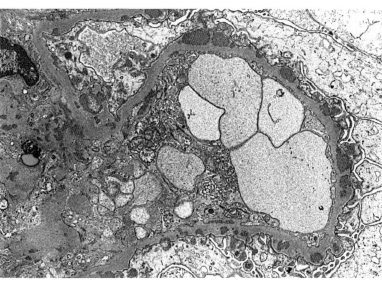

FIGURE 31–12 Lupus nephritis class V: Electron micrograph showing numerous subepithelial electron-dense deposits as well as mesangial deposits (×5000).

In LN immune deposits can be found in all renal compartments, the glomeruli, tubules, interstitium, and blood vessels.[2,8,26,38] IgG is almost universally present, with co-deposits of IgM and IgA in most specimens. Both C3 and C1q are commonly identified.[2,8,26] The presence of all three immunoglobulins, IgG, IgA, and IgM, along with the two complement components,C1q and C3, is known as "full house" staining (after the poker hand!) and is highly suggestive of lupus nephritis, as is strong C1q staining.

Staining for fibrin-fibrinogen is common in the distribution of crescents and segmental necrotizing lesions. In biopsies of patients with lupus the "tissue ANA,"[39] nuclear staining of renal epithelial cells in sections stained with fluoresceinated antisera to human IgG is a frequent finding in all classes. It results from the binding of patient's own ANA to nuclei that have been exposed in the course of cryostat sectioning.

Electron Microscopy

The distribution of glomerular, tubulointerstitial, and vascular deposits seen by EM correlates closely with the pattern observed by IF.[2-6,8,26] Deposits are typically electron-dense and granular. Some deposits exhibit a fingerprint substructure composed of curvilinear parallel arrays measuring 10 nm to 15 nm in diameter.[2,4,26] Tubulo-reticular inclusions (TRIs), intracellular branching tubular structures measuring 24 nm in diameter located within dilated cisternae of the endoplasmic reticulum of glomerular and vascular endothelial cells, are commonly observed in SLE biopsies.[2,4,26] TRI's are inducible upon exposure to α-interferon (so-called "interferon footprints") and are also present in biopsies of HIV-infected patients and those with other viral infections.[40]

Other Histopathologic Features

Some investigators have also found it useful to grade biopsies for features of activity (potentially reversible lesions) and chronicity (irreversible lesions).[41] The system of activity and chronicity indices developed at the NIH is widely used. For activity index, the biopsy is graded on a scale of 0 to 3+ for each of six histologic features including endocapillary proliferation, glomerular leukocyte infiltration, wire loop deposits, fibrinoid necrosis and karyorrhexis, cellular crescents, and interstitial inflammation. The severe lesions of crescents and fibrinoid necrosis are assigned double weight. The sum of the individual components yields a total histologic activity index score of from 0 to 24. Likewise, a Chronicity Index of 0 to 12 is derived from the sum of glomerulosclerosis, fibrous crescents, tubular atrophy, and interstitial fibrosis, each graded on a scale of 0 to 3+. Studies at the NIH correlated with both a high Activity Index (>12) and especially a high Chronicity Index (>4) with a poor 10-year renal survival.[2,8,27,41] However, in several other large studies neither the activity Index nor the Chronicity Index correlated well with long-term prognosis.[17,42,43] These studies have included both patients with all WHO classes as well as those with predominantly severe Class IV patients. Other studies from the NIH have shown that a combination of elevated Activity Index (>7) and Chronicity Index (>3) adds prognostic information about the long-term outcome of the patients.[41] Moreover, in these studies the combination of cellular crescents and interstitial fibrosis also predicted a poor outcome. A major beneficial value of calculating an Activity and Chronicity Index is in the comparison of sequential biopsies in individual patients. This provides useful information about the efficacy of therapy and the relative degree of reversible versus irreversible lesions.[44,45]

Some patients with SLE have major changes in the tubulointerstitial compartment.[46-50] Active tubulointerstitial lesions include edema and inflammatory infiltrates including T lymphocytes (both CD4 and CD8 positive cells), monocytes, and plasma cells.[50] Tubulointerstitial immune deposits of immunoglobulin or complement (or both) may be present along the basement membranes of tubules and interstitial capillaries. Severe acute interstitial changes and tubulo-interstitial immune deposits are most commonly found in patients with active proliferative Class III and IV LN. The degree of interstitial inflammation does not correlate well with the presence or quantity of tubulo-interstitial immune deposits.[46,48] Interstitial fibrosis or tubular atrophy (or both) are commonly encountered in the more chronic phases of LN. A recent study of over 150 LN patients documents a strong inverse correlation between the degree of tubular damage and renal survival. In addition renal survival was higher for patients with less expression on their renal biopsy of the adhesion molecule ICAM-I.[47,49]

Vascular lesions are not included in the formulation of either the ISN classification or the NIH Activity or Chronicity Indices despite their frequent occurrence and clinical significance.[51-53] The most frequent vascular lesion is simple vascular immune deposition, most common in patients with active Class III and IV biopsies. The vessels may show no abnormalities by LM, but by IF and EM there are granular immune deposits in the media and intima of small arteries and arterioles. Non-inflammatory necrotizing vasculopathy, most common in arterioles in active Class IV LN, is a fibrinoid necrotizing lesion without leukocyte infiltration that severely narrows or occludes the arteriolar lumen. True inflammatory vasculitis resembling polyangiitis is extremely rare in biopsies from SLE patients. It may be limited to the kidney or be part of a more generalized systemic vasculitis.[52,53] Thrombotic microangiopathy involving vessels and glomeruli may be associated with anticardiolipin/anti-phospholipid antibody or hemolytic uremic syndrome-thrombocytopenic purpura (HUS-TTP)-like syndrome due to autoantibody to the Von Willebrand factor cleaving protease.[52,53]

A number of other renal diseases have been documented on biopsy in SLE patients including minimal change disease, focal glomerulosclerosis, and HIV-associated–like lesions.[54-56] In some, the relationship between SLE and the second disease suggests this is not a coincidental occurrence but related to the interaction of the disease processes.

Clinical Manifestations

Although SLE predominantly affects young females, the clinical manifestations are similar in both sexes and in adults and children.[3,7,8] SLE is a pleomorphic multisystem disease that can affect virtually any organ system. Organ systems commonly involved include the kidneys, joints, serosal surfaces including pleura and pericardium, central nervous system, and skin. In addition, involvement of other organ systems including cardiac, hepatic, pulmonary, hematopoietic, and gastrointestinal is not infrequent.

The clinical manifestations of kidney involvement in SLE are as varied as the extrarenal manifestations of the disease. Renal involvement often develops concurrently or shortly following the onset of SLE and may follow a protracted course with periods of remissions and exacerbations. Clinical renal involvement usually correlates well with the degree of glomerular involvement in SLE. However, some patients may have severe vascular or tubulointerstitial disease leading to major clinical manifestations despite a benign pattern of glomerular involvement.[46,52,53] Although the clinical features of renal involvement in relation to the histologic findings on renal biopsy have not clearly been defined for the new ISN/

RPS classification, they are very likely to be similar to the correlations of the older WHO classification.

Patients with Class I biopsies often have no, or at most mild, evidence of clinical renal disease. Likewise, most patients with disease confined to the mesangial regions of the glomeruli (Class II) have mild or minimal clinical renal findings.[1–6,31,32] They may have a high anti-DNA antibody titer and low serum complement, but urinary sediment is inactive, hypertension is infrequent, proteinuria is usually less than 1 g daily, and the serum creatinine and GFR are usually normal. Nephrotic range proteinuria is extremely rare and may represent a concurrence of minimal change disease with LN when present.[55]

Class III, focal proliferative LN, is often associated with active lupus serologies, although the degree of serologic activity does not necessarily correlate with the severity or extent of the histologic damage.[17,31,33] Hypertension and active urinary sediment are commonly present. Proteinuria is often more than 1 g daily, and as many as one quarter to one third of patients with focal LN will have the nephrotic syndrome at presentation. Many patients will have an elevated serum creatinine at presentation. Patients with less extensive glomerular involvement by the focal proliferative process and those with fewer necrotizing features and those without crescents are more likely to be normotensive and have preserved renal function.

Most treatment trials deal largely with patients with ISN Class IV, diffuse proliferative disease, which typically presents with the most active and severe clinical features. These patients often have high anti-DNA antibody titers, low serum complement levels, and very active urinary sediment, with erythrocytes, red cell, and other casts on urinalysis.[1–6,8,17,31,34,35] Virtually all have proteinuria and as many as half of the patients will have the nephrotic syndrome. Likewise, hypertension and renal dysfunction are typical, and even when the serum creatinine appears normal, the GFR is usually depressed.

Patients with lupus membranous nephropathy, ISN Class V, typically present with proteinuria, edema, and other manifestations of the nephrotic syndrome.[1,3,4,8,17,36–38] However, as many as 40% will have less than 3 g proteinuria daily, and 16% to 20% less than 1 g of proteinuria at biopsy. Up to 60% of membranous patients will have a low serum complement and an elevated anti-DNA antibody titer.[17] Likewise, active urine sediment, hypertension, and renal dysfunction may all occur in patients with pure membranous lupus without superimposed proliferative lesions. Patients with lupus membranous nephropathy may present with heavy proteinuria or what appears to be idiopathic nephrotic syndrome before developing other clinical and laboratory manifestations of SLE.[8,17,34] As with idiopathic membranous nephropathy, patients with lupus membranous nephropathy are predisposed to developing thrombotic complications such as renal vein thrombosis and pulmonary emboli.[52,53] Patients with mixed membranous and proliferative patterns on biopsy have clinical features that reflect both components of their renal disease.

End-stage LN, ISN Class VI, is usually the result of "burnt out" LN of long duration.[1–6,8,26] It is often the end result of years of lupus flares alternating with periods of inactivity. Much of the renal histologic damage may represent non-immunologic progression of disease in remaining glomeruli as a result of reduced number of functioning nephrons. Although the lesions are sclerosing and fibrotic without activity on biopsy, patients may still have microhematuria and proteinuria. Virtually all such patients have both hypertension and a decreased GFR. Levels of anti-DNA antibodies and serum complement levels have usually normalized by the time these patients reach stage VI lesions.

"Silent LN"[8,57] has been described in patients without clinical evidence of renal involvement despite the presence of proliferative LN on renal biopsy. Some investigators consider a patient to have "silent lupus nephritis" if there are active biopsy lesions without active urinary sediment, proteinuria, or a depressed GFR, whereas others require negative lupus serologies as well. Although silent LN is well described in some studies, others have been unable to find even isolated examples.[8,17,26] Thus, "silent LN" certainly appears to be a rare phenomenon. Moreover, it is highly likely that even patients with true "silent disease" will manifest clinical renal involvement shortly into their course.

Serologic Tests

Abnormal autoantibody production is the hallmark of SLE. The presence of antibodies directed against nuclear antigens (ANA) and especially against DNA (anti-DNA) antibodies are included in the ARA's diagnostic criteria for SLE, and are commonly used to monitor the course of patients with SLE. Autoantibodies may have wide range of cross-reactivity and autoantibodies of unrelated SLE patients may share idiotypes.[8,24,58] ANA's are a highly sensitive screen for SLE, being found in more than 90% of untreated patients, but they are not specific for SLE and occur in many other rheumatologic diseases as well as a variety of infectious diseases including HIV infection.[8,24] It is unclear how well a particular pattern of ANA fluorescence (e.g., homogeneous, speckled, nucleolar, rim) correlates with any specific rheumatologic disease or with the presence of renal disease. In FANA-negative patients antibodies against nuclear antigens can often be detected by other techniques such as radioimmunoassay. The titer of the ANA does not correlate well with the presence of the severity of renal involvement in SLE.[3,8,24]

Autoantibodies directed against double stranded DNA (ant-dsDNA) are a more specific but less sensitive marker of SLE and are found an almost three fourths of untreated patients with active SLE.[24] These antibodies may be detected by a number of techniques including the Farr radioimmunoassay, and an immunofluorescence test directed against the DNA in the kinetoplast of the single celled organism Crithidia luciliae, and by ELISA.[24] Anti-ds DNA IgG antibodies of high avidity that fix complement have correlated best with the presence of renal disease[3,8,27] and such anti-dsDNA antibodies have been found in the immune glomerular deposits of animal models and humans with LN.[27,59] High anti-dsDNA antibody titers correlate well with clinical activity. Anti-single stranded DNA antibodies (anti-ssDNA) are commonly found in patients with SLE as well as in many other collagen-vascular diseases and do not correlate well with clinical lupus activity.

A variety of other autoantibodies directed against ribonucleic antigens are commonly present in lupus patients. These include anti-Sm and anti-nRNP against extracted nuclear antigen (ENA).[24] Anti-Sm antibodies, although very specific for SLE are found in only about 25% of lupus patients. The prognostic value of anti-Sm antibodies is not clear. In some studies, patients who are anti-Sm-positive have had a greater incidence of renal and CNS disease or more cutaneous vasculitis, cardiopulmonary disease, and a worse prognosis. Anti-nRNP antibodies, found in over one third of SLE patients, are also present in many rheumatologic diseases other than SLE, particularly mixed connective tissue disease (MCTD).[24,60] AntiRo/SAA antibodies are directed against the protein complex of a cytoplasmic RNA and are present in 25% to 30% of SLE patients. Anti-La/SSB autoantibodies are directed against a nuclear RNP antigen distinct from ENA and are present in from 5% to 15% of lupus patients. Neither are specific for SLE and both are found in other collagen disease especially Sjögren syndrome. Maternal anti-Ro antibodies are related to lupus in the newborn with its associated cardiac conduction abnormalities.[61] Anti-Ro antibodies are also associated with a unique dermal form of lupus with psoriaform features, with SLE patients who are homozygous C2 deficient, and with a vasculitic disease associated with CNS involvement and cutaneous ulcers.[62] In addition, lupus patients may develop antibodies directed against histones, endothelial cells, antiphospholipids, and neutrophil cytoplasmic antigens (ANCA).[64-67]

Levels of total hemolytic complement (CH50) and complement components are usually decreased during active SLE and especially active renal disease.[3,4,8] Levels of C4 and C3 often decline before a clinical flare of active lupus.[8,58] Serial monitoring of complement levels, with a decline in levels predicting a flare, is considered more useful clinically than an isolated depressed C3 or C4 value.[3,8] Likewise, normalization of depressed serum complement levels is often associated with improved renal outcome.[68] Levels of total complement and C3 levels may be decreased in the absence of active clinical or renal disease in patients with extensive dermatologic involvement by SLE. Isolated complement deficiency states (including C1r, C1s, C2, C4, C5, and C8) have been associated with SLE and such patients may have depressed total complement levels despite inactive disease.[69]

Other immunologic tests commonly found in lupus patients include elevated levels of circulating immune complexes (CIC), a positive lupus band test, and the presence of cryoglobulins. None of these tests has been shown to clearly correlate with lupus activity and in specific LN.[8,70] In patients with both SLE and isolated discoid lupus, immune complex deposits containing IgG antibody and complement are found along the dermal epidermal junction of involved skin lesions.[3,8,71] In clinically uninvolved skin the presence of granular deposits in this location has been found only in systemic disease. However, the specificity and sensitivity of this test is debated, it requires immunofluorescence of the dermal biopsy, and its correlation with clinical lupus activity or renal disease is unproven.[8] Mixed IgG-IgM cryoglobulins containing anti-DNA antibodies, DNA, and fibronectin may be found in patients with SLE and active renal disease. Patients with SLE commonly have a false positive VDRL due to the presence of antiphospholipid antibodies.[72]

Monitoring Clinical Disease

It is important in the treatment of patients with lupus to be able to predict clinical and renal relapses and prevent their occurrence through the judicious use of immunosuppressive agents. Serial measurements of many serologic tests for clinical activity (including complement components, autoantibodies, sedimentation rate, C-reactive protein, circulating immune complexes, and recently levels of cytokines and interleukins) have been used to predict flares of lupus activity. Although there is controversy regarding the value of a declining C3 and C4 level and a rising anti-DNA antibody titer in predicting a clinical flare of SLE or active renal disease,[3,8,67] clearly these are the most widely used serologic tests to monitor SLE activity. Serum levels of anti-ds DNA typically rise and serum complement levels typically fall as the clinical activity of SLE increases and usually before clinical renal deterioration. In patients with active renal involvement the urinalysis frequently reveals dysmorphic erythrocytes, rbc casts, and other formed elements. An increase in proteinuria from levels of less than 1 g daily to over this amount and certainly from low levels to nephrotic levels is a clear indication of either increased activity or a change in renal histologic class.[8,17]

Drug-Induced Lupus

A variety of medications may induce a lupus-like syndrome or exacerbate an underlying predisposition to SLE. Although a number of drugs have produced this entity, those metabolized by acetylation such as procainamide and hydralazine are common causes.[73,74] This occurs more commonly in patients with a genetic decrease in hepatic N-acyltransferase who are slow acetylators.[75] Procainamide-induced SLE may be mediated by its metabolite procainamide hydroxylamine as opposed to the active metabolite N-acetylprocainamide, which does not produce an SLE-like syndrome.[73-75] Diltiazem, minocycline, penicillamine, isoniazid, methyldopa, chlorpromazine, and practolol are other drugs that have all clearly produced a drug-related lupus syndrome.[73,74,76,77] A number of other drugs that are possibly but not conclusively associated with this syndrome include phenytoin, quinidine, antithyroid drugs, sulfonamides, lithium, β blockers, nitrofurantoin, PAS, captopril, glyburide, hydrochlorothiazide, alfa interferon, carbamazepine, sulfasalazine, and rifampin.[78,79] Clinical manifestations of drug-induced lupus include fever, rash, myalgias, arthralgias and arthritis, and serositis. CNS and renal involvement are relatively uncommon in drug-induced disease.[80,81] Although elevated anti-DNA antibodies and depressed serum complement levels are unusual in drug-induced lupus, antihistone autoantibodies are present in more than 95% of patients.[73] These are usually formed against a complex of the histone dimer H2A-H2B and DNA and other histone components.[73,82] Antihistone antibodies are also present in the vast majority of idiopathic, non-drug–related SLE patients, but they are directed primarily against different histone antigens (H1 and H2B).[73] The diagnosis of drug-related SLE depends on documenting the offending agent and achieving a remission with withdrawal of the drug. The presence of antihistone antibodies in the absence of anti-DNA antibodies and other serologic markers for SLE is also indicative of drug-induced disease.[73] The primary treatment consists of discontinuing the offending drug, although NSAIDs and corticosteroids may be effective in suppressing the serositis and constitutional symptoms of the disease.

Pregnancy and Systemic Lupus Erythematosus

Because SLE occurs so commonly in women of childbearing age, the issue of pregnancy arises often in the care of this population. Independent but related issues are the fate of the mother both in terms of flares of lupus activity and progression of renal disease and the fate of the fetus. It is unclear whether flares of lupus activity occur more commonly during pregnancy or shortly after delivery.[83-86] Some controlled studies found no increased in lupus flares in pregnant patients over non pregnant controls.[83-86] Patients who were clinically inactive at the time of pregnancy were especially unlikely to experience an exacerbation of SLE. However, in two retrospective studies, in 37 and 68 patients, flares of lupus activity including renal involvement occurred in over 50% of the pregnancies.[85,86] This was significantly increased over the rate after delivery and in non pregnant lupus patients. Because the numbers of patients studied are small, it is unclear whether there is an increased risk of exacerbation of SLE during pregnancy. Women with quiescent disease, however, will fare the best.[83]

Pregnancy in patients with LN has also been associated with worsening of renal function.[87,88] This is less likely to occur in patients who have been in remission for at least 6 months. Patients with hypertension are likely to have higher levels and those who have proteinuria are likely to have increased levels during pregnancy. Patients with elevated serum creatinines are most likely to suffer worsening of renal function and to be at highest risk for fetal loss. Both high-dose corticosteroids and azathioprine have been used in pregnant lupus patients, but cyclophosphamide is contraindicated due to its teratogenicity and newer agents such as mycophenolate and rituximab are not recommended, making the treatment of severe LN more difficult.

The rate of fetal loss in all SLE patients in most series is 20% to 40% and may approach 50% in some series.[84,86,88-90] Although fetal mortality is increased in SLE patients with renal disease, it may be decreasing in the modern treatment era.[84,85,87,88] Patients with anticardiolipin antibodies, hypertension, or heavy proteinuria are at higher risk for fetal loss.[84] One review of 10 studies in over 550 women with SLE found fetal death in between 38% and 59% of all pregnant SLE patients with antiphospholipid antibodies as opposed to 16% to 20% of those without antibodies.[91]

Dialysis and Transplantation

The percentage of patients with severe LN who progress to end-stage renal disease (ESRD) varies from 5% to 50% depending on the population studied, the length of follow-up, and the response to therapy.[8,17,44,57,92-95] Many with progressive renal failure have a resolution of their extrarenal manifestations of disease and serologic activity.[96-98] With duration of dialysis the incidence of clinically active patients declines further, decreasing in one study from 55% at the onset of dialysis to less than 10% at the fifth year and 0% by the tenth year of dialysis.[97] Although ESRD has been described as an immunosuppressed state it is unclear precisely what mechanisms underlie this immune suppression of dialysis and ESRD. Patients with ESRD due to LN have increased mortality during the early months of dialysis due to infectious complications as a result of their immunosuppressive treatment.[96,98,99] Long-term survival for SLE patients on chronic hemodialysis or continuous ambulatory peritoneal dialysis is similar to other patients with ESRD with most common cause of long-term death being cardiovascular.[97-99]

In general, most renal transplant programs allow patients with active SLE to undergo a period of dialysis for from 3 to 12 months to allow clinical and serologic disease activity to become quiescent.[97] Allograft survival rates in patients with ESRD due to LN are comparable to the rest of the ESRD population.[8,98-102] The rate of recurrent SLE in the allograft has been low in most series (<4%)[96,97,100] although in several recent reports a higher recurrence rate has been noted.[102] The low recurrence rate is in part due to the immune suppressant action of ESRD prior to transplantation and in part the immunosuppressive regimens used to prevent allograft rejection. Lupus patients with an antiphospholipid antibody may benefit from anticoagulation therapy during the post transplant period.[103,104]

Course and Prognosis of Lupus Nephritis

The course of patients with LN is extremely varied with from less than 5% to over 60% of patients developing progressive renal failure.[1,5,8,17,33,44,92-95,105] This course is defined by the initial pattern and severity of renal involvement as modified by therapy, exacerbations of the disease, and complications of treatment. The prognosis has clearly improved in recent decades with wider and more judicious use of new immunosuppressives. Most studies have found additional prognostic value of renal biopsy over clinical data in SLE populations.[106-108]

Patients with lesions limited to the renal mesangium generally have an excellent course and prognosis.[1-6,8] Those who do not transform into other patterns are unlikely to develop progressive renal failure and mortality is generally due to extrarenal manifestations and complications of therapy. It is unknown why some patients will progress to more serious renal disease whereas others do not over a lifetime. Patients with focal proliferative disease have an extremely varied course. Those with mild proliferation in a small percentage of glomeruli respond well to therapy and less than 5% progress to renal failure over 5 years of follow-up.[1-6,8,17,109,110] Patients with more proliferation, those with necrotizing features, and those with crescent formation have a prognosis more akin to patients with Class IV diffuse proliferative disease. Some Class III patients will transform or evolve to Class IV over time. In one study, patients with "severe" Class III lesions actually had a lower remission rate and renal survival than patients with Class IV lesions.[111] This emphasizes the different patterns within the designation focal proliferative lupus nephritis among investigators in the older WHO classification. Clearly patients with very active segmental proliferative and necrotizing lesions fare worse than those with global milder proliferative lesions in only some of the glomeruli.

Patients with diffuse proliferative disease have the least favorable prognosis in most series.[1-6,8,17] Nevertheless, the prognosis for this group has markedly improved. Five-year renal survival rates, commonly less than 50% in the past are now over 90% in some series of patients treated with modern immunosuppressive agents.[8,35,110,112] In recent trials from NIH the risk of doubling the serum creatinine, a surrogate marker for progressive renal disease, at 5 years in diffuse proliferative lupus treated with cyclophosphamide containing regimens ranged from 35% to less than 5%.[93,94,112] Groups with a better prognosis received more intensive regimens of therapy. In an Italian study of diffuse proliferative disease survival was 77% at 10 years and over 90% if extrarenal deaths were excluded.[35] In a recent U.S. study of 89 patients with diffuse proliferative disease, renal survival was 89% at 1 year and 71% at 5 years.[10] It is unclear whether the improved survival in these recent series is largely due to improved therapy with immunosuppressive medications, or better supportive care and clinical use of these medications.

In the past some studies have found age, gender, and race to be as important prognostic variables as clinical features in patient and renal survival in SLE[1,4,6,8,16,108,113-115]; however, a consistent finding is that African Americans have a greater frequency of LN and a worse renal and overall prognosis.[1,4,8,16,110,113,116] This worse prognosis appears to relate to both biologic/genetic factors and to socioeconomic ones.[9,10,16] In a study from NIH of 65 patients with severe LN, clinical features at study entry associated with progressive renal failure included age, black race, hematocrit less than 26%, and serum creatinine greater than 2.4 mg/dl.[41] Patients with combined severe activity and chronicity (Activity Index >7 plus Chronicity Index >3 on renal biopsy) as well as those with the combination of cellular crescents and interstitial fibrosis also had a worse prognosis. In another U.S. study of 89 patients with diffuse proliferative LN, none of the following features impacted on renal survival: age, gender, SLE duration, uncontrolled hypertension, or any individual histologic variable.[10] Entry serum creatinine over 3.0 mg/dl, combined activity and chronicity on the biopsy, and black race did predict a poor outcome. Renal survival for the white patients was 95% at 5 years but only 58% for the black patients at 5 years. In a study of over 125 LN patients with WHO Class III or IV from New York both racial and socioeconomic factors influenced the poor outcome in African Americans.[116] African Americans and Hispanics had a worse renal prognosis. In the Hispanics this was entirely related to socioeconomic factors whereas in the blacks both socioeconomic and genetic biologic factors appeared to be involved in the adverse outcome.[116] An evaluation of 203 patients from the Miami area confirms a worse renal outcome in both African Americans and Hispanics related to both biologic factors and more aggressive disease as well as economic factors.[117]

A more rapid renal remission and more complete remission have been related to improved long-term prognosis.[118,119] Renal flares during the course of SLE also may predict a poor renal outcome.[105,120,121] Relapses of severe LN occur in up to 50% of patients over 5 to 10 years of follow-up and usually respond less well and more slowly to repeated course of cytotoxics.[8,105,122–124] A retrospective analysis of 70 Italian patients in which over half had diffuse proliferative disease found excellent patient survival (100% at 10 years and 86% at 20 years) as well as preserved renal function with probability of not doubling the serum creatinine at 10 years to be 85% and at 20 years to be 72%.[105] Most patients in this study were white and this may be associated with the excellent long-term prognosis. Multivariate analysis in the Italian study showed males, those more anemic, and especially those with flare ups of disease to have a worse outcome. Patients with renal flares of any type had 6.8 times the risk of renal failure, and those with flares with rapid rises in the creatinine had 27 times the chance of doubling their serum creatinine. Another Italian study of 91 patients with diffuse proliferative lupus nephritis showed over 50% having a renal flare that correlated with a younger age at biopsy (<30 years old), higher activity index, and karyorrhexis on biopsy.[120] The number of flares, nephritic flares, and flares with increased proteinuria correlated with a doubling of the serum creatinine. The role of relapses in predicting progressive disease has been documented by others as well, although relapse does not invariably predict a bad outcome.[125]

Although an elevated anti-DNA antibody titer and low serum complement levels have in some studies predicted progressive renal disease, they may normalize with therapy and in most prognostic studies they have not correlated with long-term prognosis.[8,10,17,92,105] In several studies anemia has been a poor prognostic finding regardless of the underlying etiology.[41,105] Severe hypertension has also been related to renal prognosis in some studies, but not others.[17] Renal dysfunction as noted by an elevated serum creatinine or decreased GFR or by heavy proteinuria and the nephrotic syndrome are indicative of a poor renal prognosis in the vast majority of series.[1–8,116] Not all studies have found an elevation of the initial serum creatinine to predict a poor prognosis long-term and in some the initial serum creatinine only predicted short-term renal survival over years, not long-term renal prognosis.[10] Other renal features such as duration of nephritis and rate of decline of GFR may also predict prognosis.[92,110]

Finally, histologic features such as class, the degree of activity and chronicity, and the severity of tubulointerstitial damage on biopsy have also been predictive of prognosis. In a number of studies the pattern of renal involvement, especially when using the ISN or older WHO classification, has been a useful guide to prognosis.[1–6,8,17,30,55] In early clinical trials at the NIH, patients with severe proliferative LN who had higher Activity Index or Chronicity Index were more likely to have a progressive course to renal failure.[110] Other studies with different referral populations could not confirm that an elevated activity or chronicity index predicted a poor prognosis.[2,4,8,17,26,42,92] Although there is disagreement about the role of individual indices, the contribution of chronic scarring to a poor long-term outcome has been confirmed by many studies.[49,92,120,125,126] Some studies have found the initial renal biopsy to have little predicative value in terms of long-term outcome, but features on a repeat biopsy at 6 months to be a strong predictor of doubling the serum creatinine or progression to ESRD.[47,127] These features at 6 months include ongoing inflammation with cellular crescents and macrophages in the tubular lumens, persistent immune deposits (especially C3) on IF, and persistent subendothelial and mesangial deposits. More recent studies by this group suggest that reversal of interstitial fibrosis and glomerular segmental scarring along with remission of initial inflammation and immune deposition is an important favorable prognostic finding on the 6-month biopsy.[125] Thus, chronic changes on biopsy are not always cumulative and immutable and their reversal may be crucial in preventing ESRD when new acute lesions develop.

The natural history of membranous lupus is unclear. In early studies with short follow-up, the course of membranous lupus appeared far better than that of patients with active proliferative lesions.[32] Subsequent studies with longer follow-up suggested a worse outcome for some patients especially those with persistent nephrotic syndrome.[17] Recent retrospective studies with long-term follow-up show 5-year renal survival rates largely depend on whether patients have true pure membranous lesions (pure Class V) or superimposed proliferative lesions either in a focal segmental (Class III + V) or diffuse distribution (IV + V).[37,38] One U.S. study found the 10-year survival rate was 72% for patients with pure membranous lesions but only 20% to 48% for those with superimposed proliferative lesions.[37] Black race, elevated serum creatinine, higher degrees of proteinuria, hypertension, and transformation to another WHO pattern all portended a worse outcome.[1,4] The poor survival in blacks with membranous lupus nephropathy may explain the excellent results in retrospective Italian studies, which are largely white. One such Italian study found the 10-year survival of membranous patients to be 93%.[38] Even in this Italian population survival was far better than in patients with superimposed proliferative lesions (Classes III + V or IV + V). Thus, at least in part the variability of prognosis in older studies can be explained by the differences in racial background, underlying histology of the membranous lesions, as well as differences in therapy.

Management of Lupus Nephritis

The treatment of many patients with severe LN remains controversial.[1,3,6–8] Although recent controlled randomized studies have better defined the course and therapy for these patients, the most effective and least toxic regimen for any given patient is often less clear cut. Although some newer therapies may offer clear short-term benefits, it is unclear whether they prevent chronic renal failure at 5 and 10 years later. Moreover, as patient survival improves it is crucial to find regimens that have equivalent efficacy but less side effects and toxicity.

Patients with Class I and Class II biopsies have an excellent renal prognosis and need no therapy directed at the kidney. Transformation to another histologic class is usually heralded by increasing proteinuria and urinary sediment activity.[30] At this point repeat renal biopsy may serve as a guide to therapy.[8] There is no general consensus on the treatment of patients with focal proliferative LN, Class III lesions. This is, in part, due to the spectrum of disease that occurs in Class III. Patients with only mild or moderate proliferative lesions involving a few glomeruli, with no necrotizing features and no crescent formation, have a good prognosis and will often respond to a short course of high-dose corticosteroid therapy. Patients with severe segmental lesions and with necrotizing features and crescent formation usually require more vigorous therapy similar to patients with diffuse proliferative LN.

Patients with diffuse proliferative disease, Class IV lesions, require aggressive treatment to avoid irreversible renal damage and progression to ESRD.[1–6,8] The precise form of immunosuppressive regimen is still debated and may include high-dose daily or alternate day corticosteroids, azathioprine, intravenous pulse methylprednisolone, oral or intravenous cyclophosphamide, cyclosporine, mycophenolate mofetil, and rituximab. There is also data in the literature on other less well-studied therapies such as ancrod treatment, total lymphoid irradiation, thromboxane inhibitors, intravenous gamma-globulin, tolerance-inducing molecules (e.g., LJP 394), blockers of lymphocyte co-stimulation, and total marrow ablation with stem cell rescue therapy. Only a few of the latter therapies have been examined in well-designed long-term studies. No current regimen of immunosuppressives is without major potential side effects and no agent is universally effective. Thus, newer therapeutic agents are being developed, not only to manage active disease or to prevent flare ups of LN, but also to minimize the side effects of current regimens. The concept of more vigorous initial treatment, an induction phase, followed by more prolonged lower dose therapy, a maintenance phase of treatment, is widely accepted.[8]

Prednisone has been used for almost 50 years to treat LN. Despite the lack of controlled trials, higher doses of corticosteroids appeared more effective than low-dose therapy (<30 mg Prednisone daily) in retrospective studies.[1,3–6,8] Even the high-dose corticosteroids given in early studies were in doses far lower than in modern regimens. Initial use of high-dose corticosteroid treatment for severe LN, reserving other immunosuppressives agents only for those patients who fail to respond to several months of therapy or who have evidence of rapid clinical progression of disease, is still utilized by some clinicians especially for limited focal proliferative disease. However, for severe proliferative LN, either Class III or Class IV, most clinicians institute corticosteroids along with other immunosuppressives.[8] Some have utilized regimens of 1 mg/kg/day of prednisone converting to 2 mg/kg/day on alternate days after 4 to 6 weeks of treatment. Others prefer to start with pulses of IV Solu-Medrol (see later).

Controlled randomized trials at the NIH and elsewhere have helped clarify the role of cyclophosphamide in the management of severe LN.[44,93,94,112,128,129] In one trial, patients were randomly assigned to treatment regimens of high-dose corticosteroids for 6 months, or oral cyclophosphamide, oral azathioprine, combined oral azathioprine plus cyclophosphamide, or every third month intravenous cyclophosphamide all given with low-dose corticosteroids.[112] Evaluation at 120 months of follow-up showed a significant improvement in renal survival in the intravenous cyclophosphamide group versus the steroid group. At longer follow-up to 200 months, the renal survival of the azathioprine group was now statistically no better than that of the corticosteroid group.[112] Thus, the cyclophosphamide groups seemed most successful in preventing renal failure. Because side effects appeared least severe in the intravenous cyclophosphamide group, subsequent protocols at NIH have utilized regimens of the drug intravenously. Recent trials use monthly pulses of intravenous cyclophosphamide for 6 consecutive months as opposed to every third monthly regimens.[9,44,93,94,122,128,129]

There have been few randomized trials using pulse methyl prednisolone therapy for severe LN.[93,94] Initial trials of pulse methylprednisolone in patients with diffuse proliferative disease and a rising serum creatinine showed favorable results utilizing a regimen of three consecutive daily one gram pulses.[1,8] Subsequent reports and uncontrolled trials used a variety of immunosuppressive regimens with the pulse steroids with favorable results. Two NIH trials have found pulse corticosteroids to be less effective than intravenous cyclophosphamide in preventing progressive renal failure.[93,94,130] In one diffuse proliferative LN patients were randomized to receive either monthly pulse methylpredniso-

lone (1 g/m²) or one of two cyclophosphamide regimens.[94] At 60 months, 48% of the pulse steroid treated patients doubled their serum creatinine in comparison to only 25% of the cyclophosphamide groups.

A number of other groups have confirmed the benefits and response rate of intravenous cyclophosphamide regimens in severe LN.[44,122,128,129,159] In a meta-analysis of 19 prospective controlled trials in 440 patients with severe LN treated with oral prednisone, azathioprine, oral cyclophosphamide, or intravenous cyclophosphamide, other immunosuppressive agents were more effective than prednisone for reducing both total mortality and ESRD.[131] In most patients treated with intravenous cyclophosphamide side effects such as hemorrhagic cystitis, alopecia, and so far tumors have been infrequent.[1,3–6,8] Exceptions are menstrual irregularities and premature menopause, which is most common in women over 25 years of age who have received IV cyclophosphamide for over 6 months treatment.[132] The dose of IV cyclophosphamide must be reduced in patients with significant renal impairment and adjusted for some removal by hemodialysis in ESRD patients. MESNA therapy has been beneficial in reducing bladder complications from the toxic metabolite of cyclophosphamide, acrolein.[133] Not all investigators feel the promising results obtained with intravenous cyclophosphamide can be attributed to the immunosuppression alone, but rather to improved medical management of hypertension, and the metabolic and infectious complications of SLE as well.[134]

A controlled randomized trial at NIH of 1 year of monthly doses of intravenous methylprednisolone versus monthly intravenous cyclophosphamide for 6 months and then every third month doses, versus the combination of both therapies found the remission rate was highest with the combined treatment regimen (85%) as opposed to cyclophosphamide alone (62%) and methylprednisolone alone (29%).[93] Mortality was low and similar in all groups. Although the combined regimen was the most effective, it also appeared to have the greatest incidence of short-term adverse side effects. Longer follow-up of this same population indicates that over time drug toxicity was not different between the cytotoxic group and the combined cytotoxic-methylprednisolone group.[130] Side effects included premature menopause (56% cyclophosphamide versus 56% combined), aseptic necrosis (28% cyclophosphamide versus 30% combined), Herpes zoster (28% cyclophosphamide versus 25% combined), and major infections (33% cyclophosphamide versus 45% combined). It is likely through higher sustained remissions and fewer long-term relapses less patients required repeated treatments in the combined cyclophosphamide steroid treated group. Moreover, the long-term efficacy was greatest for the combination therapy group especially in terms of renal outcomes. Thus, for many patients combined Solu-Medrol pulses and intravenous cyclophosphamide pulses together became a standard therapy for severe LN despite problems with side effects.

Mycophenolate mofetil (MMF) has proven to be an effective immunosuppressive in transplant patients and has replaced azathioprine in many transplant centers. It is a reversible inhibitor of inosine monophosphate dehydrogenase and blocks B and T cell proliferation, inhibits antibody formation, and decreases expression of adhesion molecules among other effects. MMF has been effective in treating animal models of LN.[135–137] Initially evaluated in small non-randomized trials in LN patients either intolerant or resistant to intravenous cyclophosphamide therapy, MMF has now been shown to have benefits in efficacy and in reduction of complications of therapy when compared to standard treatment regimens in a number of well-performed randomized trials.[138–149] In one 6-month Chinese trial of over 40 patients randomized to either MMF or IV pulse cyclophosphamide for induction therapy of severe LN,[141] proteinuria and microhematuria decreased more in the MMF patients than in the cytotoxic group, with renal impairment pre and post therapy, activity index on biopsy pre and post therapy, and serologic improvement equivalent. MMF was better tolerated with fewer gastrointestinal side effects and fewer infections. In another randomized controlled trial of 42 LN patients given either prednisone plus oral MMF or a regimen of prednisone plus cyclophosphamide orally for 6 months followed by oral azathioprine for another 6 months both drugs proved to be similar in efficacy.[142] Of the MMF group 81% achieved complete remission and 14% partial remission versus 76% complete and 14% partial remission for the cyclophosphamide-azathioprine group. Treatment failures, relapses post therapy, discontinuations of therapy, mortality, and time to remission were similar. Although these results were very promising the initial study was short term and in a Chinese populations with unclear applicability to the U.S. population and especially to African Americans.[143] Longer follow-up of these patients with the addition of 22 more patients showed the MMF to have comparable efficacy to the cyclophosphamide with no significant difference in complete or partial remissions, doubling of baseline creatinine, or relapses. Significantly fewer MMF patients developed severe infections, leukopenia, or amenorrhea, and all deaths and ESRD were in the cyclophosphamide group.[144] Thus, in this population, at long-term follow-up induction treatment of severe LN with MMF was as effective as oral cyclophosphamide but with fewer side effects.

A recent U.S. study compared MMF to IV cyclophosphamide for induction therapy for 140 patients with severe Class III and IV LN.[145] The LN patients, including over 50% blacks, had heavy proteinuria and active urinary sediment. They were randomized to either receive standard monthly pulses of IV cyclophosphamide $0.5-1\,g/m^2$ for 6 months or oral MMF 2 to 3 g/day. Although this was designed as an equivalency study to test the hypothesis of equal efficacy between treatments but superior toxicity profile, the MMF proved superior in an intention-to-treat analysis in both complete and complete and partial remissions. Side effect profile also appeared better with MMF. At 3-year follow-up there was a trend to less renal failure and mortality favoring the MMF. Thus, in a patient population at high risk for poor renal outcomes, MMF proved superior to IV cyclophosphamide. It should be stressed that the mean entry serum creatinine of both arms of this study was only slightly greater than 1 mg/dl and it is unknown whether patients with severe depressions of the GFR or with severe histologic damage on biopsy will respond as well. An ongoing international multicenter randomized controlled trial will compare MMF to IV cyclophosphamide for induction therapy in over 370 enrolled LN patients (The Aspreva Lupus Management Trial/ALMS trial).[146]

Although these trials focused on the induction of remission in severe LN patients, other trials have looked at maintenance of remission and prevention of activation of disease. The Euro Lupus Nephritis Trial, a multicenter prospective trial of 90 patients with severe LN compared low-dose versus "conventional" high-dose IV cyclophosphamide for both induction and remission.[147] Patients were randomized to either a standard high dose regimen of 6 monthly IV pulses of 0.5 to $1\,g/m^2$ cyclophosphamide followed by 2 quarterly pulses or only 500 mg IV every 2 weeks for a total of 6 doses both followed by oral azathioprine (AZA) as maintenance therapy. At long-term follow-up (over 40 months) there were no statistically significant differences in treatment failures, renal remissions, or renal flares, but twice as many infections occurred in the high-dose group. Although this trial may have included some patients with milder renal disease (mean creatinine 1–1.3 mg/dl; mean proteinuria 2.5–

3.5 g/day for both groups), and may be applicable only to a white population, nevertheless, it supports the use of shorter duration and lower total dose cyclophosphamide for induction therapy for some patients and confirms the benefit of azathioprine maintenance. Longer follow-up of the same population to 73 months confirms these data and suggests that early response to therapy is predictive of a good long-term outcome.[148]

A randomized controlled trial from Miami examined LN patients who had successfully completed induction of remission with 4 to 7 monthly pulses of IV cyclophosphamide and were then randomized to either continued every third month IV cyclophosphamide, oral azathioprine, or oral MMF.[5,149] The 54 LN patients randomized were largely composed of blacks and Hispanics (50% black) and included many patients with the nephrotic syndrome (64%), renal dysfunction, and severe proliferative LN on biopsy (81% Class IV); 87% achieved remission following cyclophosphamide therapy. Fewer patients in the azathioprine and the mycophenolate group reached the primary end points of death and chronic renal failure compared to the cyclophosphamide group. The cumulative probability of remaining relapse free was higher with MMF (78%) and azathioprine (58%) compared with cyclophosphamide (43%), and there was increased mortality in patients given continued IV cyclophosphamide. Complications of therapy were all reduced in the MMF and azathioprine groups including days of hospitalization, amenorrhea, and infections. Thus, maintenance therapy with either MMF or azathioprine was superior to IV cyclophosphamide with less toxicity. An ongoing trial by the European Working Party on SLE compares MMF to azathioprine as remission maintaining treatment for severe LN (MAINTAIN Nephritis Trial).

A number of other commonly used immunosuppressive agents have been used in small studies in LN patients. Low dose cyclosporine (4–6 mg/kg/day) has been used usually in combination with other immunosuppressive agents in over 100 SLE patients.[150] One uncontrolled trial of SLE patients with disease resistant to other therapies described 26 patients with LN who received 2 years of cyclosporine plus tapering corticosteroids.[151] The patients experienced improvement in lupus serology, clinical activity, proteinuria, and renal histology without any increase in serum creatinine over the 2 years of treatment. Others have found that cyclosporine along with low-dose corticosteroids is not satisfactory therapy for severe proliferative disease with decreases in the dose of cyclosporine (e.g., for rises in the serum creatinine) leading to flares of disease activity.[150] Tacrolimus, widely used in solid organ transplantation, has been compared successfully to standard cyclophosphamide therapy in a number of small trials in LN patients. In one study of 48 severe LN patients, 59% of tacrolimus-treated patients experienced a complete remission versus 32% of IV cyclophosphamide-treated patients.[152]

Rituximab, a chimeric monoclonal antibody directed against the B7 antigen on B lymphocytes, depletes CD20 B cells through multiple mechanisms including complement-dependent cell lysis, FcRγ dependent antibody dependent cell mediated cytotoxicity, and induction of apoptosis. Rituximab has been utilized with varying success in many immunologic and autoimmune diseases including a variety of primary glomerular diseases. In LN it has been used in over 100 patients mostly in case reports and open-labeled uncontrolled trials.[153,154] Although it is difficult to draw conclusions based on these studies, it clearly has been successful in some patients with both severe and refractory LN. A typical trial included 10 patients with focal or diffuse proliferative LN who received 4 weekly infusions of rituximab ($375\,mg/m^2$) with oral prednisolone.[153] Eight patients achieved a partial remission and five patients subsequently developed complete remissions of their LN. Complete remission was sustained in four of five patients at 12 months. Rituximab has been used with repeated administration up to three cycles in some patients with severe LN.[155] Of the initial 15 resistant LN patients treated by the Columbia Nephrology group with IV rituximab for resistant disease, half had a beneficial response in terms of reductions of proteinuria and improvement in GFR. A current multicenter prospective randomized placebo controlled trial compares the combination of rituximab and MMF to MMF alone for induction and maintenance therapy in 140 patients with severe LN.[156]

Other therapies used in LN include plasmapheresis, total lymphoid irradiation, ancrod, thromboxane antagonists, tolerance molecules, marrow ablation with stem cell rescue, use of blockers of co-stimulatory molecules, and IV gammaglobulin. All are still experimental since none has of yet undergone large successful controlled clinical trials.

There are isolated cases or small series of LN patients who have experienced improvement of severe clinical and histologic renal disease with plasmapheresis in combination with a number of other treatments. A large multicenter controlled trial of 86 patients with severe LN randomized to standard therapy or standard therapy plus plasmapheresis found no benefit in the plasmapheresis group beyond a more rapid lowering of anti-DNA antibody titers.[157] There was no difference in clinical remission, progression to renal failure, or patient survival. Likewise, plasmapheresis synchronized to IV cyclophosphamide pulse therapy has not proven effective.[158] At present plasmapheresis is not standard therapy and should be reserved for only certain patients with LN as those with severe pulmonary hemorrhage failing other therapy, patients with a TTP-like syndrome, patients with anticardiolipin antibodies and a clotting episode who cannot be anticoagulated due to hemorrhage, etc.[159]

Intravenous immune globulin has been used successfully in a number of immunologic disease, including a number of SLE patients to treat thrombocytopenia as well as LN.[160,161] In one series of nine patients with LN resistant to standard therapy, IVIG therapy resulted in clinical and histologic improvement.[161] However, other studies have not found success with IVIG and its role remains unclear. The one controlled trial included only 14 patients but did show stabilization of the plasma creatinine, creatinine clearance, and proteinuria when IVGG was used as maintenance therapy after successful induction of remission with IV cyclophosphamide.[162]

T lymphocytes activation requires two signals.[163] The first occurs when the antigen is presented to the T cell receptor (TCR) in the context of MHC class II molecules on antigen presenting cells and the second by the interaction of costimulatory molecules on T lymphocytes and antigen presenting cells. Disruption of costimulatory signals interrupts the (auto)immune response. In murine lupus models an important role for CD40:CD40L and CD28:B7 costimulatory molecules has been established. However, two clinical trials using different humanized antiCD40L monoclonal antibodies (BG9588 and IDEC-131) in LN patients have not been successful.[164-166] A study using BG9588 (riplizumab) showed improved renal function and lupus serology, but was terminated prematurely due to thromboembolic complications. A second trial with IDEC-131, although showing no major safety concerns, did not show clinical efficacy in human SLE. Another costimulatory pathway is mediated through the interaction of CD28-CD80/86. CTLA4 antagonizes CD28 dependent costimulation.[1] CTLA-4 Ig, a fusion molecule that combines the extracellular domain of human CTLA4 with the constant region (Fc) of the human IgG$_1$ heavy chain, interrupts the CD28-CD80/86 interaction. Two preparations, Abatacept and Belatacept (LEA29Y), are being evaluated. However, clinical trials using these monoclonal antibodies in lupus are only in an early stage.

One new agent that has been evaluated in large multicenter blinded trials is a designer molecule directed at inducing tolerance and preventing anti-DNA antibody formation.[167,168] LJP 340 (Riquent, Abetimus sodium) has been developed as a tolerogen to block B cell antibody formation by binding to immunoglobulin receptors on B cells. In animal models it decreases antiDNA antibody titers, lupus renal histopathologic manifestations, proteinuria, and renal dysfunction in lupus prone animals.[167] In an initial trial of over 230 patients treated for over 76 weeks it did not prove more effective than placebo in preventing flares of the disease and decreasing ant-ds DNA anti body levels. However, in the subgroup of 189 patients whose anti-DNA antibodies had a high affinity to the molecule it significantly reduced renal flares, the concurrent need for high-dose corticosteroid use, and major clinical SLE flares.[168] In a subsequent randomized trial the drug failed to reduce flares at a rate greater than placebo. It is of interest that the renal flare rate was much lower both in the treatment and placebo groups showing the benefits of modern maintenance background therapy.

Total lymphoid irradiation, similar to that used in management of Hodgkin disease, has been used in one series of LN patients.[169] The long-term results of therapy do not appear advantageous enough to warrant such potentially aggressive regimen. Because there may be evidence of microthromboses of the glomerular capillaries in severe LN, ancrod or pit-viper venom has been used in one series of patients with severe LN.[170] Again, the results in terms of preventing progressive disease were not impressive. In a short-term trial in a small group of patients with lupus, an intravenous thromboxane antagonist led to an improvement in GFR and renal blood flow.[171] However, it is doubtful that oral therapy will produce complete enough blockade of thromboxane synthesis to sustain improved function in patients clinically. Other agents under preliminary investigation that have successfully been used in lupus prone animal models include an antibody directed against the fifth component of complement to block the membrane attack complex (antiC5 antibody), and blockers of inflammatory mediators such as gamma interferon.[172,173] Immunoablative therapy with high-dose cyclophosphamide with and without stem cell transplantation has been used successfully in a limited number of SLE patients with only a short period of follow-up.[174-176]

For patients with Class V, membranous lupus nephropathy, there have been conflicting data regarding the course, prognosis, and response to treatment.[1,8] The degree of superimposed proliferative lesions greatly influences outcome in Class V patients, and it is unclear if older trials really only included true membranous patients. Some patients with pure membranous lupus nephropathy will have a prolonged course of asymptomatic proteinuria or the nephrotic syndrome yet little progression to renal failure over time. Others with active serology, severe nephrotic syndrome, and a progressive course will more clearly benefit from therapy. Early trials reported low response rates and inconsistent response rates with oral corticosteroids.[36] Excellent long-term results with intensive immunosuppressive regimens from Italian studies and others raise questions of whether the results are related to the therapeutic intervention or to the population studied and better supportive treatments.[38] A retrospective Italian trial found better remission with a regimen of chlorambucil and methylprednisolone over that with corticosteroids alone.[177] In a small nonrandomized trial of cyclosporine in membranous lupus there was an excellent remission rate of the nephrotic syndrome with mean proteinuria decreasing from 6 to 1 g to 2 g daily by 6 months.[45] At long-term follow-up and re biopsy there was no evidence of cyclosporine-induced renal damage, but two patients had developed superimposed proliferative lesions over time. An NIH trial of 42 patients with membranous lupus nephropathy and the nephrotic syndrome comparing cyclosporine, prednisone, and intravenous cyclophosphamide found superior remission rates for the cyclosporine and cyclophosphamide regimens but a trend toward more relapses when the cyclosporine was withdrawn.[178] A study of 38 patients with pure membranous LN evaluated long-term treatment with prednisone plus azathioprine.[179] At 12 months 67% of the patients had experienced a complete remission and 22% a partial remission. At 3 years only 12% had relapsed, at 5 years only 16%, and at 90 months only 19% relapsed. At the end of follow-up no patients had doubled their serum creatinine. Clearly in this population a regimen of steroids plus azathioprine was highly effective.

The response of patients with membranous LN to MMF has been varied. In one series of 18 patients with different classes of LN treated with MMF, all four treatment failures were in those with membranous LN.[180] Others in small trials have reported more favorable results.[181–183] In the randomized multicenter study of 140 LN patients, 27 had pure membranous lupus nephropathy. Analysis of all membranous patients who completed the study showed no difference in rates of partial or complete remission, changes in SCr, serum albumin, urinary protein excretion, or serologies between the MMF and IV cyclophosphamide groups at follow-up.[184] Based on this limited data management of MLN should be based on severity of disease. Patients with pure MLN and a good renal prognosis (subnephrotic levels of proteinuria and preserved GFR) may benefit from a short course of cyclosporine with low-dose corticosteroids along with inhibitors of the renin-angiotensin system and statins. For those at higher risk of progressive disease (e.g., blacks, those who are fully nephrotic) options include cyclosporine, monthly IV pulses of cyclophosphamide, MMF, or azathioprine plus corticosteroids. Patients with mixed membranous nephropathy and proliferative disease are treated in the same way as those with proliferative disease alone.

As effective and safer therapies for LN have evolved, greater attention has been directed at other causes of morbidity and mortality in this population. Lupus patients have accelerated atherogenesis and a disproportionate rate of coronary vascular disease leading to a high mortality many years after the onset of their LN.[185] The high cardiovascular risk rate has been attributed to concurrent hypertension, hyperlipidemia, nephrotic syndrome, prolonged corticosteroid use, antiphospholipid antibody syndrome, and in some, the added vascular risks of CKD.[186,187] Despite limited data on therapeutic interventions in this population, aggressive management of modifiable cardiovascular risk factors may alter the morbidity and mortality of this population. Extrapolating from other CKD populations, closely monitored BP control (<130/80), the use of ACEI and/or ARBs, and correction of dyslipidemia with statins are reasonable in all LN patients. In addition, use of calcium, vitamin D supplements, and bisphosphonates to prevent glucocorticoid-induced osteoporosis may be useful.

Some form of antiphospholipid antibodies are present in 25% to 75% of lupus patients. Because most do not experience thrombotic complications, it is clear most require no special attention directed to the prevention of large vessel and microvascular thromboses.[188–190] In SLE patients with evidence of a clinical thrombotic event most investigators use chronic anticoagulation with Coumadin as long as the antibody remains present in high titer. Although the standard practice has been not to anticoagulate other patients, in one recent series of over 100 SLE patients over one fourth had antiphospholipid antibodies, of whom almost 80% had a thrombotic event. The antibody positive patients also had a greater incidence of chronic renal failure than the antibody negative patients.[91] (See Anticardiolipin antibodies and glomerulonephritis in following section.)

ANTIPHOSPHOLIPID ANTIBODY SYNDROME

The presence of antiphospholipid (APL) antibodies may be associated with glomerular disease, large vessel renal involvement, as well as coagulation problems in dialysis and renal transplant patients.[188–190,192] Patients with the antiphospholipid syndrome have arterial and venous thromboses and an increased risk of fetal loss associated with a variety of antibodies directed against plasma proteins bound to phospholipids including anticardiolipin antibodies, antibodies causing a false positive VDRL, the lupus anticoagulant, and antibodies directed against beta$_2$ glycoprotein 1.[193] Specific criteria for a definitive diagnosis of APL antibody syndrome have recently been developed and include at least one of the following clinical features and at least one of the following laboratory findings. Clinical criteria include either one or more episodes of venous, arterial, or small vessel thrombosis and/or morbidity with pregnancy, whereas laboratory criteria include the presence of aPL (on two or more occasions at least 12 weeks apart and no more than 5 years prior to clinical manifestations) as demonstrated by one or more of the following: IgG and/or IgM anticardiolipin antibody in moderate or high titer, antibodies to β2-glycoprotein 1 of IgG or IgM isotype at high titer, or lupus anticoagulant activity.[194,195] In some studies the presence of specific beta$_2$ glycoprotein 1 antibodies has been correlated with the presence of anticardiolipin antibodies and an increased risk of thrombotic events in patients with antiphospholipid syndrome.[196,197] Catastrophic APL syndrome occurs when there is rapid thromboses in multiple organ systems.[198,199] Antiphospholipid antibodies have been associated with increased endothelial production of adhesion molecules such as VCAM 1, and may contribute to atherosclerosis by binding to oxidized LDL.[200] The pathogenesis of the thrombotic tendency in patients with antiphospholipid antibodies remains to be elucidated, but may involve a combination of dysregulation of coagulation, platelet activation, and endothelial injury.[188,190,192]

Thirty percent to 50% of patients with APL antibodies have the primary APL syndrome in which there is no associated autoimmune disease.[188,190,192] A number of commonly used tests are available to confirm the suspicion of APL syndrome including the "lupus anticoagulant", anticardiolipin antibodies, or broader APL antibodies (against cardiolipin, phosphatidylserine, and other phospholipids) by an ELISA assay. APL antibodies have also been found in from 25% to 75% of SLE patients, although most of these patients never experience the clinical features of the APL syndrome.[188,190,192] In an analysis of 29 published series comprising over 1000 SLE patients, 34% were positive for the lupus anticoagulant and 44% for anticardiolipin antibodies.[201] Although some studies have not found a high incidence of thrombotic events in SLE patients positive for antiphospholipid antibodies, others with longer follow-up generally have correlated their presence with a higher thrombotic event rate.[202,203] A recent European study of almost 575 patients with SLE found the prevalence of IgG anticardiolipin antibodies to be 23% and for IgM 14%.[204] Patients with IgG antibodies had a clear association with thrombocytopenia and thromboses. A recent multicenter European analysis of 1000 SLE patients found thromboses in 7% of patients over 5 years. Patients with IgG anticardiolipin antibodies again had a higher incidence of thromboses, as did those with a lupus anticoagulant.[205] APL antibodies are also found in up to 2% of normal individuals and in those with a variety of infections and drug reactions, but these are not usually associated with the clinical spectrum of the APL syndrome.[206] HIV-infected patients and those infected with hepatitis C have much higher frequencies of anticardiolipin

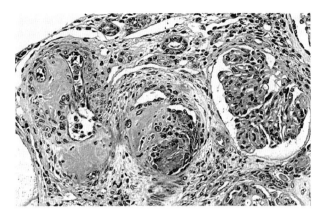

FIGURE 31-13 Anti-phospholipid antibody syndrome: Organizing recanalized thrombi narrow the lumens of two interlobular arteries. The adjacent glomerulus displays ischemic retraction of its tuft (Hematoxylin-eosin, ×200).

antibodies but no antibodies to beta$_2$-glycoprotein 1, and usually do not have manifestations of the antiphospholipid syndrome.[207–209]

The clinical features of the APL syndrome relate to thrombotic events and consequent ischemia. In one series of 1000 APL syndrome patients the most common features were deep vein thrombosis 32%, thrombocytopenia 22%, livedo reticularis 20%, stroke 13%, pulmonary embolism 9%, and fetal loss 9%.[210] Patients may also experience pulmonary hypertension, memory impairment and other neurologic manifestations and fever, malaise, and constitutional symptoms.[188–192]

Renal involvement occurs in as many as 25% of patients with primary APL syndrome.[188–192] The renal pathology of APL syndrome is characterized by thrombosis of blood vessels ranging from the glomerular capillaries to the main renal artery and vein.[188–190,210,211] Lesions involving the arteries and arterioles often have both a thrombotic component and a reactive or proliferative one with intimal mucoid thickening, subendothelial fibrosis, and medial hyperplasia (Fig. 31–13).[210,211] Inflammatory vasculitis has been identified rarely. Interstitial fibrosis and cortical atrophy may occur due to tissue ischemia.[211] Glomerular lesions include glomerular capillary thrombosis with associated mesangiolysis, mesangial interposition and duplication of glomerular basement membrane, and electron lucent, fluffy, subendothelial deposits resembling other forms of glomerular thrombotic microangiopathy such as HUS-TTP.

A recent study retrospectively evaluated renal biopsies from 81 patients with aPL.[212] APL syndrome nephropathy existed in almost 40% of APL-positive patients versus only 4% of patients without aPL and was associated with both lupus anticoagulant and anticardiolipin antibodies. Among APL-positive SLE patients, APS nephropathy was found in two thirds of those with APL syndrome and in one third of those without APL syndrome. Although patients with APL nephropathy had a higher frequency of hypertension and elevated serum creatinine levels at biopsy in this series, they did not have a higher frequency of renal insufficiency, end-stage renal disease, or death at follow-up.[212] This is in contrast to another recent series of over 100 lupus patients that found the presence of APL antibodies to be associated with both thrombotic events and a greater progression to renal failure.[191] Some renal biopsies have been misclassified as focal segmental glomerulosclerosis, membranous nephropathy, and membranoproliferative GN when they truly display a thrombotic microangiopathy.[213] However, a recent study reports patients

with a number of glomerular histologic patterns on light microscopic including membranous nephropathy, minimal change/focal sclerosis, mesangial proliferative GN, and pauci immune rapidly progressive GN to have classic APL syndrome.[214]

The most frequent clinical renal features are proteinuria, at times in the nephrotic range, active urinary sediment, hypertension, and progressive renal dysfunction.[188,190,210] Some patients present with acute deterioration of renal function.[213] With major renal arterial involvement there may be renal infarction, and renal vein thrombosis may be silent or present with sudden flank pain and a decrease in renal function. Renal artery stenosis has been reported with and without malignant hypertension in both SLE patients and others with antiphospholipid antibody syndrome.[215–218] In SLE, APL antibodies have been associated with a history of systemic thromboses, neurologic disorders, and thrombocytopenia.[188,190,192,201] Although only about 10% of biopsied lupus patients have glomerular microthromboses as their major histopathologic finding, nevertheless, therapy of this glomerular lesion clearly differs from that of immune complex mediated glomerulonephritis.[52] One study of 114 biopsied SLE patients found vaso-occlusive lesions in one third of biopsies, which both correlated with hypertension and an increased serum creatinine level.[219] In SLE features that correlate well with high titers of IgG APL antibodies are thrombocytopenia, the presence of a false positive VDRL for syphilis (FTA negative), and a prolonged APTT.[188–190,192,219] Neither the titer of anti-DNA antibodies nor the serum complement levels correlate well with the APL antibody levels. In SLE, in general, high titers of IgG ACL antibody correlate well with risk of thromboses. However, not all studies have been able to correlate the presence of anticardiolipin or specific APL antibodies with thrombotic events in SLE patients. For example, in one study of 114 biopsied patients renal thrombi were related to anti lupus antibodies but not anticardiolipin antibodies.[219] The clinical features of APL syndrome in SLE patients are identical to the in primary APL syndrome. One recent study documents the prevalence of APL antibodies in 26% of 111 LN patients observed a mean of 173 months. Of the APL antibody positive patients 79% developed a thrombotic event or fetal loss and the presence of antibodies was strongly correlated with the developed of progressive chronic kidney disease.[191] Studies in ESRD patients have shown a high prevalence of APL antibodies in patients on hemodialysis (10%–30%).[220,221] Studies in patients with renal insufficiency and patients on peritoneal dialysis have shown a much lower incidence of APL antibodies.[188] Studies have found antiphospholipid antibodies to be present in 31% of hemodialysis patients with a varying prevalence of the lupus anticoagulant and anticardiolipin antibodies.[220,221] In general, there has been no association with age, gender, or duration of the dialysis. One cross-sectional study of hemodialysis patients found 22% of 74 patients with arteriovenous grafts had a raised titer of IgG anticardiolipin antibody versus only 6% of 17 patients with arteriovenous fistulas.[221] There was a significant increase in the odds of having two or more episodes of AV graft thrombosis in patients with raised ACLP titer. Whether AV grafts induce ACLN antibodies or whether patients with ACLN antibodies require AV grafts remains unclear.[222] In a study of 230 hemodialyzed patients titers of IgG anticardiolipin antibodies were elevated in 26% of the patients as opposed to elevated titers of IgM antibodies in only 4%, and elevated titers of both antibodies in 3%.[223] The mean time to AV graft failure was significantly shorter in the group with elevated IgG antibodies but there was no difference in AV fistula clotting between those with and without high IgG antibody titers. The use of Coumadin increased graft survival in patients with elevated IgG anticardiolipin levels.

The presence of APL antibodies may also damage the renal allograft. In several studies 20% to 60% of SLE patients with APL antibodies who received renal transplants had evidence of related problems with venous thromboses, pulmonary emboli, or persistent thrombocytopenia.[224-227] In one large study of non-SLE patients 28% of 178 transplant patients had antiphospholipid antibodies that were associated with a threefold to fourfold increased risk of arterial and venous thromboses.[225] However, a recent study of 337 renal transplant recipients found the 18% who were IgG or IgM ACL antibody positive (even after correction for the effects of anticoagulation) had no greater allograft loss or reduction in GFR over time than did patients who were ACL antibody negative.[228] Although most hepatitis C virus positive patients with antiphospholipid antibodies do not have evidence of increased thromboses and the antiphospholipid syndrome, HCV-positive renal transplant patients with anticardiolipin antibodies appear to have a higher risk of thrombotic microangiopathy in the allograft.[229] In many of these transplant studies treatment with anticoagulation has proven successful in preventing recurrent thromboses and graft loss.[224,226,227]

Treatment

The optimal treatment of patients with APL antibodies or the APL syndrome (or both) remains to be defined.[188-190] Many patients with SLE with APL antibodies do not experience thrombotic events and do not require anticoagulation or other special therapy. Higher titers of IgG APL antibody have been related to a greater incidence of thrombotic events.[204,205] In patients without evidence of the APL syndrome, and no thrombotic events, some are treated only with daily aspirin therapy. In patients with the full APL syndrome either primary or secondary to SLE high-dose anticoagulation has proven more effective than either no therapy, aspirin, or low-dose anticoagulation in preventing recurrent thromboses.[188,192,230] A retrospective analysis of 147 patients with the APL syndrome and documented prior thromboses (62 primary disease and 66 SLE and 19 lupus-like syndrome) recorded 186 recurrent thrombotic events in 69% of the patients.[230] The median time between the initial thrombosis and the first recurrence was 12 months but with a huge range (0.5 to 144 months). Treatment with warfarin to produce an INR >3 was significantly more effective than treatment with low-dose warfarin (INR <3) or treatment with aspirin alone. The highest rate of thrombosis (1.3 per patient-year) occurred in patients in the 6 months after discontinuing anticoagulation with Coumadin. Bleeding complications occurred in 29 of the 147 patients but were severe in only 7 patients. The role of immunosuppressive agents has been uncertain in treating this syndrome.[188,192,206,231] Thus, in SLE patients the anti-DNA antibody titer and the serum complement may normalize in response to immunosuppressive medication without a significant change in a high titer of IgG APL antibody.[231] In pregnant patients with antiphospholipid syndrome heparin and low-dose aspirin have been successful in several studies but prednisone use has not.[232-234] In rare patients who cannot tolerate anticoagulation due to recent bleeding, who have thromboembolic events despite adequate anticoagulation, or who are pregnant, plasmapheresis with corticosteroids and other immunosuppressives have been used with some success.[235,236] Use of other treatments such as intravenous gammaglobulin and hydroxychloroquine remains anecdotal.[237,238]

MIXED CONNECTIVE TISSUE DISEASE

Mixed connective tissue disease (MCTD), first described in 1972, is defined by a combination of clinical and serologic features.[239-241] Patients with MCTD share many overlapping features with patients with SLE, scleroderma, and polymyositis.[240-244] They also typically have distinct serologic findings with a very high ANA titer, often with a speckled pattern, and antibodies directed against a specific ribonuclease sensitive extractable nuclear antigen (ENA), U1 RNP.[240-244] MCTD is far more common in females than males with a 16:1 sex ratio. Genetic predisposition to MCTD has been linked to HLA-DR4 and DR 2 genotypes.[245] Not all patients with clinical features of the syndrome have a positive ENA, and not all patients with a positive ENA have the clinical features of MCTD.[242,244] Moreover, because some patients fulfill diagnostic criteria for other connective tissue diseases, investigators have questioned whether MCTD is a distinct syndrome. The term "undifferentiated autoimmune rheumatic and connective tissue disorder" or overlap syndrome is sometimes used because many patients with features of MCTD will eventually develop into SLE, scleroderma, or rheumatoid arthritis.[242-246]

In the early stages of MCTD patients do not usually manifest overlapping features of other connective tissue disorders, but rather nonspecific symptoms such as malaise, fatigue, myalgias, arthralgias, and low-grade fever. Over time systemic clinical features of MCTD similar to those found in each of the various rheumatologic connective tissue disease often appear. These include arthralgias and in some deforming arthritis, myalgias and myositis, Raynaud phenomenon, swollen hands and fingers, restrictive pulmonary disease and pulmonary hypertension, esophageal dysmotility, pericarditis and myocarditis, serositis, oral and nasal ulcers, digital ulcers and gangrene, discoid lupus-like lesions, malar rash, alopecia, photosensitivity, and lymphadenopathy.[241-244,246-249] However, patients with MCTD and especially those documented to have anti-U1RNP antibodies, infrequently have major CNS disease or severe proliferative glomerulonephritis.[241-244,246-249] Low-grade anemia, lymphocytopenia, and hypergammaglobulinemia are all common in MCTD.

The most widely used serologic test to confirm a diagnosis of MCTD is the ENA with anti-U1RNP antibodies.[242-244,250] The diagnosis of MCTD is even firmer in those patients with IgG antibodies against an antigenic component of U1RNP, the 68 kD protein.[250,251] Antibodies to other nuclear antigens have been found in MCTD and some correlate better with some clinical features of specific rheumatologic diseases.[241-244,246] Thus antibodies to Ku and anti-Jo-1 correlate with individual clinical spectrums of overlapping rheumatologic disease. Antibodies against dsDNA, Sm antigen, and Ro are infrequently positive in MCTD, but up to 70% of patients will have a positive rheumatoid factor.[242] Antiphospholipid antibodies are found less frequently than in SLE.

In initial studies of patients with MCTD renal disease was infrequent.[242-244] In subsequent studies the incidence of involvement has varied from 10% to 26% of adults and from 33% to 50% of children with MCTD.[242-244,246,248] Many patients may have mild or minimal clinical manifestations with only microhematuria and less than 500 mg proteinuria daily. However, heavier proteinuria and the nephrotic syndrome occur.[248,252] Other patients will have severe hypertension and acute renal failure reminiscent of "scleroderma renal crisis".[248,253] Although the titer of anti-RNP does not correlate with renal involvement, the presence of serologic markers typical of active SLE, high anti-dsDNA antibody titers, anti-Sm antibody are more common with renal disease.[242-244] Low serum complement levels have not always correlated with the presence of renal involvement.[248] Children with MCTD more often have glomerular involvement even though many will not have clinical or urinary findings suggestive of renal involvement.[254] Hypocomplementemia in these children is often associated with a membranous or mixed pattern of GN.

The pathology of MCTD is pleomorphic with the glomerular lesions resembling the spectrum found in SLE and vascular lesions resembling those found in scleroderma. Glomerular disease is most common and is usually superimposed on a background of mesangial deposits and mesangial hypercellularity as in SLE.[248,252,254–258] As many as 30% of cases have mesangial deposits of IgG and C3. Other patients have focal proliferative glomerulonephritis with both mesangial and subendothelial deposits, but glomerular fibrinoid necrosis and crescent formation is rare. The most common pattern of glomerular involvement is that of membranous nephropathy reported in up to 35% of cases[248,252,254–257] with typical granular capillary wall staining for IgG, C3, and at times IgA and IgM. Some patients, especially children, will have a mixed pattern of membranous plus mesangial proliferative GN.[254] Patients may evolve or transform from one pattern of glomerular involvement to another in a fashion similar to SLE patients. By ultrastructural analysis findings similar to those in SLE have been reported including endothelial tubuloreticular inclusions, deposits with "fingerprint" substructure, and tubular basement membrane deposits.[248,257] In one review of 100 biopsied patients with MCTD 12% had normal biopsies, 35% mesangial lesions, 10% proliferative lesions, and 36% membranous nephropathy.[257] In addition 15% to 25% of patients had interstitial disease and vascular lesions. In autopsy series in which two thirds of patients had clinical renal disease a similar distribution of glomerular lesions with a predominance of membranous features was found.[258] Other renal pathology findings in MCTD include secondary renal amyloidosis,[259] vascular sclerosis ranging from intimal sclerosis to medial hyperplasia,[248] and vascular lesions resembling those in scleroderma kidney with involvement of the interlobular arteries by intimal mucoid edema and fibrous sclerosis.

Therapy of MCTD with corticosteroid is effective in treating the inflammatory features of joint disease and serositis.[242–244,248] There are no controlled treatment trials in patients with MCTD. Steroids are less effective in treating scleradermatous features such as cutaneous disease, esophageal involvement, Raynaud phenomenon, and especially pulmonary hypertension, which has been treated with CCB's, ACE inhibitors, prolonged immunosuppression, or IV prostacyclin.[260] IV immunoglobulin has been used as in SLE patients with decreased platelets, hemolytic anemia, and erythema skin disease.[261] Glomerular involvement can vary as in SLE and treatment is generally directed at the glomerular lesion in a similar fashion to treating active LN.

Originally MCTD was felt to have a good prognosis with little mortality and few patients developing clear cut other connective tissue disorders. The longer patients with MCTD are observed the greater percentage who evolve more clearly into a specific connective tissue disorder.[242–244,246] In some series almost half of the patients with a short duration of follow-up were still felt to have true MCTD, but in those with longer follow-up the percentage had dropped to 15% or less.[242–244,246,248] Most patients evolve toward a picture of either SLE or systemic sclerosis, but some develop prominent features of rheumatoid arthritis.[248] Mortality rates have been found to range from 15% to 30% at 10 to 12 years with patients with more clinical features of scleroderma and polymyositis having a worse prognosis.[242–244,248] The leading causes of mortality in MCTD are pulmonary hypertension, myocarditis, and renovascular hypertension with cerebral hemorrhage.[242–244] Patients with IgG anticardiolipin antibodies may be at greater risk. Other causes include vascular lesions of the coronary and other vessels, hypertensive scleroderma crisis, and chronic renal failure. Clearly the view of MCTD as a benign disorder is incorrect, and it is a disease with significant morbidity and mortality.

Wegener granulomatosis is usually classified together with a number of other small vessel vasculitides including microscopic polyangiitis and Churg-Strauss syndrome.[262] There is often considerable overlap in the clinical, histologic, and laboratory features of these entities, all may by associated with anti-neutrophil cytoplasmic antibodies (ANCA), and the treatment for all is often similar involving potent immunosuppressives. Wegener granulomatosis has been traditionally defined by the triad of systemic vasculitis associated with necrotizing, granulomatous inflammation of the upper and lower respiratory tracts, and glomerulonephritis.[263] Subsequent descriptions of "limited" upper respiratory tract disease, of multiorgan system involvement, and of the nature and potential pathogenesis of the serologic marker of ANCA have enhanced our understanding of this disease.[264–268] Even in the pre-ANCA era these criteria yielded a sensitivity of 88% and a specificity of 92%. Clearly adding ANCA to the diagnostic criteria increases these percentages.[269–271]

Wegener granulomatosis has a slight male predominance and although it may occur at any age of life has a peak incidence in the fourth to sixth decade of life.[263,267,272,273] Pauciimmune rapidly progressive glomerulonephritis (including Wegener and microscopic polyangiitis) are the most common forms of crescentic glomerulonephritis at all ages, and especially in the elderly.[274] Most reported patients have been white, although with use of newer serologic tests such as the ANCA patients of all races are being diagnosed.[275] The occurrence of Wegener granulomatosis in more than one family member has rarely been noted.[276] Although certain HLA frequencies such as HLA DR2, HLA B7, and HLA DR1 and DR1-DQW1 have been reported more commonly in Wegener patients, the data is far from conclusive about a genetic profile of the disease.[277]

Pathology

The classic histopathologic finding in Wegener granulomatosis is a focal segmental necrotizing and crescentic glomerulonephritis (Fig. 31–14).[267,278] Although the percentage of affected glomeruli can vary widely, the necrotizing changes are usually segmental in nature.[267,278,279] Unaffected glomeruli typically appear normal. Global proliferation and necrotizing glomerular tuft involvement may be more common in more severe disease when greater numbers

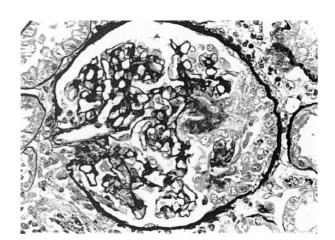

FIGURE 31–14 Wegener granulomatosis: A typical glomerulus displays segmental fibrinoid necrosis with rupture of glomerular basement membrane, fibrin extravasation into the urinary space, and an overlying segmental cellular crescent (Jones methenamine silver, ×500).

1084

of glomeruli are affected. "Intracapillary thrombosis" with deposition of eosinophilic "fibrinoid" material is common in early lesions together with endothelial cell swelling, infiltration by polymorphonuclear leukocytes, and pyknosis or karyorrhexis (nuclear dust).[267,278,279] In areas of active necrotizing glomerular lesions "gaps" may be present in the GBM and crescents typically overlie the segmental lesions. Crescents vary from segmental to circumferential. They may be associated with destruction of Bowman capsule.[280] Granulomatous crescents containing epithelioid histiocytes and giant cells may involve from less than 15% to over 50% of cases; the finding of large numbers of them is more typical of Wegener granulomatosis and C-ANCA positive patients than other vasculitides. Chronic segmental or global glomerulosclerosis with fibrous crescents often occur side by side with more active glomerular lesions in the same biopsy. Although there is much overlap in the histologic findings in patients who have microscopic polyangiitis and Wegener granulomatosis, some differences have been noted. Patients with microscopic polyangiitis are more likely to have a greater degree and severity of glomerulosclerosis, interstitial fibrosis, and tubular atrophy on initial biopsy.[281] Likewise, these findings are all more extensive in patients who are myeloperoxidase-ANCA positive (MPO) rather than anti-proteinase 3 (PR3) ANCA positive.[281]

CH 31

The vasculitis in Wegener granulomatosis may affect small and medium sized renal arteries, veins, and capillaries[267,278,279] The vasculitis, which is focal in nature, has been reported in 5% to 10% of biopsies of Wegener patients.[263,266,267,282] It is more commonly found at autopsy with larger tissue samples and where serial sectioning and a directed search for the lesions have been performed. The necrotizing arteritis consists of endothelial cell swelling and denudation, intimal fibrin deposition, and mononuclear and polymorphonuclear leukocytes infiltration of the vessel wall with mural necrosis (Fig. 31–15). The vasculitis may be associated with granuloma formation. Tubules show areas of focal tubular degenerative and regenerative changes, and cortical infarcts may be found.[262,267] Interstitial inflammatory infiltrates of lymphocytes, monocytes, plasma cells, and polymorphonuclear leukocytes associated with edema are common. Granulomas with giant cells have been noted in interstitium of the cortex and medulla in from 3% to 20% of cases.[272] Papillary necrosis, which is usually bilateral and affects most papillae, has been reported is as many as one-fifth of Wegener patients and may be related to impaired papillary blood supply due to medullary capillaritis.[283] Biopsy of extrarenal tissue may

show necrotizing and granulomatous inflammation or evidence of vasculitis.[266–278]

Immunopathologic Features

There is no glomerular immune staining in most cases of Wegener granulomatosis. Although some reports have described the localization of various immunoglobulins and complement components in the glomerular tuft and vasculature, this likely represents non-immunologic trapping in areas of necrosis and sclerosis. Most reports describe only focal low intensity IF staining, a pattern referred to as "pauci-immune".[263–267,278] Positivity for fibrin/fibrinogen is common in the distribution of the necrotizing glomerular lesions, crescents, and vasculitic lesions. Reports of immunofluorescent staining in pulmonary vasculature, sinus tissue, and alveolar tissue have all been inconsistent.

Electron Microscopy

By electron microscopy glomeruli affected by necrotizing lesions often show areas of intraluminal and subendothelial fibrin deposition associated with endothelial necrosis and gaps in the GBM through which fibrin and leukocytes extravasate into Bowman space.[263–267,278] There may be subendothelial accumulation of electron lucent "fluffy" material associated with intravascular coagulation. True electron-dense immune type deposits are not usually identified and when present are sparse and ill defined.[263–267,278] Thus, Wegener granulomatosis like polyarteritis fits into the category of "pauci-immune" glomerulonephritides. Electron microscopy of the vessels in Wegener granulomatosis may show swelling and denudation of endothelial cells, and subendothelial accumulation of fibrin, platelets, and amorphous electron-dense material, but no typical immune-type electron-dense deposits.

Pathogenesis

Although the pathogenesis of Wegener granulomatosis remains unknown, abnormalities of both humoral and cell mediated immunity have been noted.[266,267] The disease shares many morphologic features of the type IV hypersensitivity reaction, an immunologic response resulting from interaction of sensitized lymphocytes with specific antigens leading to the release of lymphokines, macrophage accumulation, and activation and transformation to epithelioid histiocytes and giant cells. Vasculitis in other systems (such as the cutaneous necrotizing vasculitis) suggests additional mechanisms of vessel injury mediated by polymorphonuclear leukocytes or ANCA-induced neutrophil degranulation, an Arthus reaction (type II reaction) or immune complex injury similar to the model of acute serum sickness (type III reaction).

Recent in vitro and animal experiments strongly support a role for ANCA in the pathogenesis of the disease.[284,285] In RAG-2 mice, transfer of anti-MPO IgG causes glomerulonephritis with necrosis and crescent formation that appears identical to human ANCA-associated glomerulonephritis by LM and IF.[286] This can occur in the absence of antigen-specific T lymphocytes strongly suggesting a pathogenetic role for the antibodies themselves. In humans, neonatal microscopic polyangiitis with pulmonary hemorrhage and renal disease has occurred secondary to the transfer of maternal MPO-ANCA.[287] However, there is still support for cell mediated mechanisms of tissue injury with a predominance of CD 4-positive T lymphocytes and monocytes in the inflammatory respiratory tract infiltrates, defects in delayed hypersensitivity, a rise in soluble markers of T cell activation as soluble

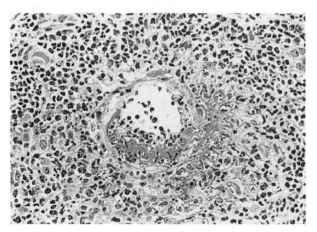

FIGURE 31–15 Wegener granulomatosis: An interlobular artery displays necrotizing vasculitis with intimal fibrin deposition and transmural inflammation by neutrophils and lymphocytes (Hematoxylin-eosin, ×375).

interleukin-2 receptor and CD 30, impaired lymphocyte blastogenesis, and T cell response to protease 3.[268,288–291]

With prominent respiratory tract involvement it is logical to envision an inhaled pathogen or environmental allergen as the initiator of the disease process. Nevertheless, no specific microbes or antigenic substances has been identified. Again ANCA antibodies have been proposed as promoters of the vasculitic process rather than just markers of the disease process. The expression of granule proteins on the surface of neutrophils and monocytes allows for the interaction with ANCA leading to a respiratory burst in the cell, degranulation and local release of damaging and chemoattractant products, and neutrophil apoptosis.[266–268,292,293] Chemoattractant products and the activated cells result in damage to the endothelium. In the presence of ANCA, neutrophils exhibit exaggerated adhesion and transmigration through endothelium.[294] A spectrum of glomerular and vascular disease reaction is seen depending on antigen expression, host leukocyte activation, circulating and local cytokines and chemokines, the condition of the endothelium, and the nature of T and B cell interactions.[266–268,292] The membranes of leukocytes from Wegener patients may be primed with PR 3 molecules on their surfaces ripe for activation of the disease process.[268,293,295,296] This might explain the exacerbations of disease activity associated with respiratory infections causing the cytokine release that leads to neutrophil and monocyte priming, as well as the potential benefits of therapy with trimethoprim sulfamethoxazole.[297,298]

Clinical and Laboratory Features

Patients with Wegener granulomatosis may present with an indolent slowly progressive involvement of the respiratory tract and mild renal findings or with fulminant acute glomerulonephritis leading to the necessity for dialysis. In the past there was often a several month period between onset of symptoms and the establishment of the diagnosis.[263,272] Despite greater awareness of disease symptoms, the more rapid use of renal biopsy and the use of ANCA assays, diagnosis is still often delayed. Most patients will have constitutional symptoms including fever, weakness, and malaise at presentation.[263–267,272,299] From 70% to 80% of patients will have upper respiratory findings at presentation and even more will develop this over time.[263–267,272,299] There may be rhinitis, purulent or bloody nasal discharge and crusting, and sinusitis.[263–267,272] Sinus involvement demonstrated by radiographs or by CT scanning typically involves the maxillary sinus and less commonly the sphenoid, ethmoid, and frontal sinuses.[263,272] There may be opacification, air fluid levels, mass lesion, or rarely bony erosions. Upper respiratory tract involvement can also be manifest by tinnitus and hearing loss, otic discharge and earache, and perforation of the tympanic membrane, hoarseness and throat pain.[263–267,272] Chronic sequelae of the upper respiratory disease include deafness, chronic sinusitis with repeated secondary infections and nasal septal collapse with saddle nose deformity.

Lower respiratory tract disease, found at presentation in up to 75% of patients eventually develops in most patients.[263–267,272] Symptoms include cough often with sputum production, dyspnea on exertion and shortness of breath, alveolar hemorrhage and hemoptysis, and pleuritic pain.[300,301] Chest radiographs and CT scans may reveal single or multiple nodules some with areas of cavitation, alveolar infiltrates and interstitial changes, and less commonly small pleural effusions and atelectatic areas. Chest radiograph or CT scan may document lower respiratory tract disease in the absence of pulmonary symptoms or clinical findings.[272] Airflow obstruction and a reduced carbon monoxide diffusing capacity are typically present.[302]

Wegener granulomatosis is a multisystem disease with many organs involved by the vasculitic process and its sequelae.[263–267,272] Cutaneous involvement, present in 15% to over 50% of patients, may occur with a variety of macular lesions, papules, nodules, or purpura usually on the lower extremities. Patients may also present with rheumatologic involvement with arthralgias of large and small joints as well as non-deforming arthritis of the knees and ankles or more rarely a myopathy or myositis. Up to 65% of patients have ophthalmologic disease manifested by conjunctivitis, episcleritis and uveitis, optic nerve vasculitis, or proptosis due to retro-orbital inflammation. Nervous system involvement is most typically manifested as a mononeuritis multiplex, but may involve cranial nerves or the central nervous system. Other organs involved include the liver, parotids, thyroid, gall bladder, and the heart.[263–267,272]

Abnormal laboratory tests in Wegener granulomatosis include a normochromic, normocytic anemia, a mild leukocytosis, and a mild thrombocytosis.[263,267,272] Eosinophilia is uncommon and there have been no abnormalities of circulating lymphocytes subsets in the disease.[273] Non-specific markers of an inflammatory disease process such as an elevated sedimentation rate, C-reactive protein levels, and rheumatoid factor tests are often positive and correlate with the general disease activity. Other serologic tests including those for ANA, serum complement levels, and cryoglobulins are normal or negative.[263] CIC are found in a variable percentage of patients, but relation to disease activity is debated. Likewise elevated levels of IgA or IgE have been reported but are of unclear significance.[264–267,272]

The vast majority of patients with active Wegener granulomatosis will be positive for ANCA by a variety of assays. ANCA has been detected in from 88% to 96% of these patients.[264–269] In general patients with granulomatous lesions are more likely to be C-ANCA positive with antibody directed against a serine proteinase of the neutrophilic granules. Protease 3 is a 228 amino acid serine proteinase found in azurophilic granules of neutrophils and the lysosomes of monocytes.[264–269] However, many patients fitting the clinical and histologic definition of Wegener granulomatosis will be P-ANCA positive with antibodies directed against myeloperoxidase, a highly cationic 140 kD dimer located in a similar distribution to proteinases.[264–269] In a recent study of 89 patients from China who fulfilled clinical and histopathologic criteria for Wegener granulomatosus according to the Chapel Hill Consensus Conference, 61% were -MPO ANCA positive and only 38% PR3 ANCA positive.[275] Although the specificity of C-ANCA for Wegener granulomatosis has been as high as 98% to 99% by different assays, the sensitivity may be low in certain populations with inactive disease or limited disease.[264–269,303] False positive C-ANCA tests have been reported in patients with certain infections (e.g., HIV, tuberculosis, subacute bacterial endocarditis), neoplastic disease, and drug-induced conditions.[304,305] Although there has been debate whether the ANCA levels parallel the clinical and histologic activity of the disease, many patients will normalize their ANCA titer during periods of quiescence.[264–268,306] Nevertheless approximately 40% of patients in remission will have positive tests for C-ANCA.[306,307] A subsequent rise in ANCA titer from low titer has been suggested as predictive of renal and systemic flares.[264–268,306,308–310]

Renal Findings

Renal findings in Wegener granulomatosis are extremely variable and usually occur along with other systemic manifestations.[263–268,272,299] Most patients have evidence of clinical renal disease at presentation, and from 50% to 95% of patients with Wegener granulomatosis will eventually develop clinical evidence of renal involvement. There is typically mild proteinuria and urinary sediment findings often with microscopic hematuria, and red cell casts present. Patients with more severe glomerular involvement often have a decrease in GFR and greater levels of proteinuria, but the nephrotic syndrome is uncommon. The level of proteinuria may be high in those without severe renal insufficiency and may actually increase during therapy as the GFR improves.[272–299] The degree of renal failure and serum creatinine do not always correlate well with the percent of glomerular necrotizing lesions, the percent of glomerular crescent formation, or the presence of interstitial granulomas or vasculitis. The incidence of both acute oliguric renal failure and significant hypertension varies among reports but is higher in reports from renal centers. Intravenous pyelograms are typically normal, and by angiography aneurysms are not usually present.[263–268]

In addition to glomerular and vascular lesions, other renal conditions associated with Wegener granulomatosis have included pyelonephritis and hydronephrosis due to vasculitis causing ureteral stenosis, papillary necrosis, perirenal hematoma from arterial aneurysm rupture, and lymphoreticular malignancies with neoplastic infiltration of the renal parenchyma in patients treated with immunosuppression.[311]

Course and Treatment

The course of the active glomerulonephritis is typical of rapidly progressive glomerulonephritis with progression to renal failure over days to months.[263–268,272] Patients with severe necrotizing granulomatous glomerulonephritis are more likely to develop renal failure, and patients with more global glomerulosclerosis are more likely to develop ESRD.[312] One study found greater glomerulosclerosis and interstitial fibrosis to predict a poor renal outcome, but greater numbers of active crescents actually predicted a better outcome.[313] Even with immunosuppressive therapy, a significant number of patients will eventually progress over the long term to renal failure.[313]

The introduction of effective cytotoxic immunosuppressive therapy has dramatically changed the course of Wegener granulomatosis. Initial studies of untreated patients and even those utilizing corticosteroids alone documented survivals of 20% to 60% at 1 year.[263] Although corticosteroids lead to some clinical improvement there has been documentation of the progression of both renal and extrarenal lesions during corticosteroid therapy.[263–268] Although other immunosuppressive agents have been used, and despite few controlled trials, cyclophosphamide has become the treatment of choice for Wegener granulomatosis.[263–268,314] Long-term survival with cyclophosphamide-based regimens range from 87% at 8 years to 64% at 10 years in different series.[263–268,315] Using a regimen of combined cyclophosphamide (1.5–2 mg/kg/day) and corticosteroids investigators at the NIH achieved remissions in 85% to 90% of 133 Wegener patients.[263] Most patients were converted to every other day steroid usage in several months and were able to discontinue steroid use by 1 year. Although one half of the patients eventually relapsed many patients remained in long-term remission off immunosuppressives. Similar results have been found by other investigators using cyclophosphamide-based regimens.[265–268,305,314,315] Complete remissions of renal and extrarenal symptoms including severe pulmonary disease, and renal failure requiring dialysis have been well described.[265–268,314–317] Over 50% of dialysis-dependent patients will be able to discontinue dialysis and remain stable for periods up to a number of years. Although resistance to therapy is well documented, some patients are documented as treatment failures due to non-compliance, intercurrent infection requiring decreased treatment, or inadequate duration of therapy. Other immunosuppressives

appear less effective in inducing an initial remission in Wegener granulomatosis and cyclophosphamide has been effective in patients who have failed treatment with azathioprine or chlorambucil.

Because there are few randomized controlled trials the optimal dose, duration of treatment, route of administration, and concomitant therapy to be given with cyclophosphamide remain unclear. Although cyclophosphamide is usually administered with corticosteroids initially as the patient responds to treatment the dose of the steroids are often tapered or changed to alternate day therapy.[263] Some regimens have included administration of intravenous high-dose "pulse" corticosteroids initially and others have used plasmapheresis as well in critically ill patients.[316–319] A typical regimen for induction therapy for severe Wegener granulomatosis might include IV pulse methylprednisolone 7 mg/kg for 3 days followed by daily oral prednisone 1 mg/kg for the first month with subsequent tapering of the dose along with either IV or oral cyclophosphamide given for approximately 6 months. Doses can be adjusted for leucopenia and other side effects as well for treatment response. Several studies have evaluated the role of pulse IV cyclophosphamide versus oral cyclophosphamide in ANCA positive small vessel vasculitis.[264,320–322] In one study of 50 patients with Wegener granulomatosis randomly assigned to either 2 years of IV or oral cyclophosphamide, remissions at 6 months occurred in 89% of the IV group versus 78% of the oral group.[322] At the end of the study remissions occurred in 67% of the IV group and 57% of the oral group, but relapses were more common in the IV group (60% versus 13%). In a meta-analysis of 11 nonrandomized studies including over 200 ANCA-associated vasculitis patients, complete remissions occurred in over 60% of patients and partial remissions in another 15%.[323] IV pulse cyclophosphamide was more likely to induce remission and less likely to cause infection than oral cyclophosphamide. The rate of relapse, although not statistically significant, was greater in the IV pulse group. It is unclear how frequent the initial intravenous "pulses" of cyclophosphamide should be given, with some investigators using monthly doses and others starting with smaller doses every 2 to 3 weeks. Despite these uncertainties, it is clear that early application of an intensive immunosuppressive regimen can prevent long-term morbidity and end organ damage. Because the total dose of the cyclophosphamide is far less in patients receiving pulsed IV therapy, many prefer to use it as a less toxic regimen and try to enhance maintenance therapy to avoid relapse.

In several studies the addition of plasmapheresis to cyclophosphamide-based regimens did not improve outcome.[313,316–319] However, there appears to be a role for plasmapheresis in certain patients with severe renal failure, those with pulmonary hemorrhage, those with coexistent anti-GBM antibodies, and those failing all other therapeutic agents.[313,316–319] In one study of 20 ANCA positive small vessel vasculitis patients with massive pulmonary hemorrhage treated with methylprednisolone, IV cyclophosphamide, and plasmapheresis all 20 patients had resolution of their pulmonary hemorrhage with this regimen.[326] Likewise a review of 88 patients with ANCA-positive renal vasculitis in seven series in the literature showed a benefit in renal survival with plasmapheresis added (67%) over standard steroid and cyclophosphamide therapy (40%).[327] Unpublished preliminary results of a trial of over 150 patients with ANCA-positive glomerulonephritis with a marked elevation of the serum creatinine treated with either induction therapy with plasma exchange plus oral prednisone plus oral cyclophosphamide versus pulsed methylprednisolone plus oral steroids plus oral cyclophosphamide showed an advantage for the plasma exchange group.[327] The addition of etanercept to a standard induction regimen for Wegener granulomatosis was evaluated in 174 patients and provided no additional benefit in terms of sustained remissions, or time to achieve remission.[328] Disease flares and adverse events were common in both treatment groups and solid tumors developed in six patients in the etanercept group. A small number of uncontrolled trials have evaluated rituximab, a chimeric monoclonal antibody directed against CD-19 and CD20 B cells, with sustained remissions in most of the patients studied.[329] Likewise, a study of Alemtuzumab, an anti-CD52 monoclonal antibody, in 70 patients gave a remission rate of 83% but this was associated with a high rate of relapse, infection, and mortality.[327] The use of infliximab a TNF-α blocker in four uncontrolled trials was associated with an 80% remission rate but a high rate of infectious complications.[330] Relapse rates from 20% to 50% have been reported often when infectious complications have led to a discontinuation of immunosuppressive therapy.[305,309,314,331] Predictors of relapse in a cohort of 350 patients with ANCA-positive vasculitis included C-ANCA or PR 3 positivity, lung involvement, upper respiratory involvement as opposed to factors not predicting relapse such as age, gender, race, and a clinical diagnosis of Wegener granulomatosis rather than microscopic polyangiitis or renal limited vasculitis.[332] Most relapses respond to another course of cyclophosphamide therapy.[314] In patients whose ANCA level has declined during remission, a major rise in titer may predict a relapse although ANCA levels and clinical disease activity do not always correlate well. Although some studies have found unacceptably high relapse rates with intravenous cyclophosphamide, others have found patients to respond equally well to this regimen as to oral cyclophosphamide.[268,314,323-325] Clearly IV cyclophosphamide appears to have fewer side effects than oral cyclophosphamide but a higher risk of relapses.

Because of the potential for multiple severe complications with cyclophosphamide therapy (e.g., infections, infertility, hemorrhagic cystitis, and an increased risk of long-term malignancy once an initial remission has been achieved) some patients have been switched to less toxic immunosuppressives such as azathioprine, low-dose methotrexate, or mycophenolate mofetil.[333-335] A recent study of 155 patients with ANCA-positive vasculitis treated patients with cyclophosphamide and steroids to induce a remission and then randomized patients to either oral azathioprine or continued cyclophosphamide therapy.[336] Of the 155 patients 144 entered remission and were randomized. There was no difference in the relapse rate of 10 vs. 11 patients in the two groups or in the adverse event rate. Relapse rates were lower in patients with microscopic polyangiitis than in the Wegener group. Cyclosporine has also been used in small numbers of patients successfully.[336,337] Infections of the respiratory tract may be associated with flares of disease activity in patients with Wegener granulomatosis. Prophylactic use of trimethoprim-sulfamethoxazole may reduce the incidence of respiratory infections and in some studies prevent activation of the disease process.[338] Methotrexate has been evaluated in an uncontrolled trial of over 40 patients with remission in 80% of patients and reasonable evidence of real improvement or stabilization long term.[339,340] Other agents being evaluated in Wegener granulomatosis include IV gammaglobulin, the chemotherapeutic agent etoposide, and humanized monoclonal antibodies directed at T cells.[341-346] Supportive measures such as sinus drainage procedures, hearing aids, and corrective surgery for nasal septal collapse may be helpful in individuals with chronic sequelae of upper respiratory involvement.[263-267]

Dialysis and transplantation have been performed in increasing numbers of Wegener patients.[336,347-354] Some patients' disease activity diminishes with onset of renal failure, but others still require intensive immunosuppression and relapses have been reported after onset of ESRD. Fatality rates may be high in the ESRD population due to slow

recognition of relapses of the vasculitic process in the presence of dialysis. Most patients receiving allografts have been maintained on prednisone and cyclosporine or tacrolimus with or without mycophenolate.[336,347-352] Recurrent active glomerulonephritis in the allograft occurs in 15% to 20% of patients[345] and may respond to cyclophosphamide therapy.[336,348-350] There is no evidence that regimens including mycophenolate mofetil or tacrolimus have advantages over older immunosuppressive regimens in preventing recurrences of Wegener activity. There is only limited experience with sirolimus.[354]

MICROSCOPIC POLYANGIITIS AND POLYARTERITIS NODOSA

Polyarteritis was first described by Rokitansky in 1852 and the term "periarteritis nodosa" was first used by Kussmaul and Maier in 1866.[355] The disease has been divided into a "classic" pattern with a systemic necrotizing vasculitis primarily affecting muscular arteries, often at branch points, producing lesions of varying ages with focal aneurysm formation and a "microscopic" polyangiitis with a necrotizing inflammation of small arteries, veins, and capillaries involving multiple viscera, including lung and dermis and producing lesions of similar age, usually without aneurysms. There are some patients with overlapping features of both patterns.[356] Moreover, many patients with both presentations of polyarteritis may have anti-neutrophil cytoplasmic antibodies along with pauci-immune segmental necrotizing and crescentic glomerulonephritis similar to patients with isolated pauci-immune idiopathic rapidly progressive glomerulonephritis and Wegener granulomatosis.[357] At present ANCA-positive microscopic polyangiitis should be considered as part of the spectrum of ANCA-associated vasculitides ranging from renal-limited idiopathic RPGN, to multisystem diseases including Wegener granulomatosis, Churg-Strauss syndrome, and other vasculitides.[357-359]

The incidence of renal disease associated with vasculitis has been increasing in a number of series.[360] While in part this may be due to wider use of serologic tests such as the ANCA and wider use of renal biopsy in older individuals, many investigators feel the absolute incidence has increased. In one large series ANCA-associated crescentic glomerulonephritis made up almost 10% of all glomerular diseases diagnosed by renal biopsy in a 2-year period.[361] Polyarteritis is more common in males than females (sex ratio 2.5:1) and occurs most often in the fifth and sixth decades of life although it has been reported in all age groups. There are rare reports of familial incidence of necrotizing vasculitis, and an increased frequency of certain HLA haplotypes (e.g., All, B35) has been reported.[362]

Clinically, the prevalence of renal disease in polyangiitis varies from 64% to 76% in unselected series and virtually 100% in nephrology-based series.[363-365] Moreover, the prevalence of pathologic renal involvement may exceed that of clinically evident renal disease. Although a number of diseases have been associated with glomerular disease and a systemic and/or renal vasculitis, true idiopathic polyarteritis is a primary vasculitis. "Secondary" vasculitis associated with cryoglobulinemia, systemic lupus, and Henoch-Schönlein purpura is usually readily distinguished. Likewise, vasculitis and glomerulonephritis similar to that seen in microscopic polyangiitis have been noted in relapsing polychondritis.[366,367] ANCA-positive polyangiitis has been associated with use of oral anti-thyroid medication propylthiouracil.[368] Classic polyarteritis has been associated with drug abuse with amphetamines and other illicit drugs, but it is unclear how many of these patients had associated viral infectious hepatitis.[369] Patients with both anti-GBM

1088

antibodies and ANCA have been described,[370–372] some of whom have a prominent systemic vasculitis. (See section on Goodpasture syndrome.) The most common associated illness to be found in patients with classic polyarteritis is hepatitis B infection. The incidence ranges from 0% to 30% to 55% of different series but is probably less than 10% of all cases.[373] It is unclear how many of these patients have had concomitant hepatitis C infection. Hairy cell leukemia has also been reported in association with polyarteritis.[374]

Pathology

Classic (Macroscopic) Polyangiitis

In classic polyarteritis the glomeruli are usually unaffected. Some glomeruli may show ischemic collapse of the tuft and sclerosis of Bowman capsule. Some patients with large vessel vasculitis may also have a focal necrotizing glomerulonephritis with or without crescents identical to that seen in microscopic polyarteritis and idiopathic pauci-immune RPGN.[311,375] Whether these represent overlap with microscopic polyangiitis awaits further clarification about pathogenesis. The vasculitis in classic polyarteritis affects the medium size to large arteries (i.e., those of subarcuate, arcuate, and interlobar caliber) in a segmental distribution often producing lesions of different ages, including acute, healing, and chronic lesions.[361,375] There are areas of involvement interspersed with normal areas of the vessel and even in the involved portions the vessel wall has eccentric inflammation in only some parts of its circumference. In areas of active vasculitis there is an inflammation of the vessel wall involving the intima alone, the intima and media, or all three layers of the vessel wall. Inflammatory infiltrates are composed of lymphocytes, polymorphonuclear leukocytes, monocytes, and occasionally eosinophils. Lesions are often necrotizing with mural fibrin deposition and rupture of the elastic membranes. These areas of necrosis may lead to aneurysm formation particularly in larger arteries (i.e., arcuate, interlobar), which can be associated with rupture and hemorrhage into the renal parenchyma. Superimposed thrombosis with luminal occlusion is not uncommon. In the healing phase, the vascular inflammation subsides and the vessel wall is thickened by concentric cellular proliferation of myointimal cells separated by a loose ground substance. Localized destruction of elastic lamellae is demonstrable with elastic stains. Eventually the media is replaced by areas of broad fibrous scars. There may be almost total occlusion of the vessel lumen by intimal fibroplasia with areas of concentric reduplication and discontinuity of the internal elastic membrane. Wedge-shaped, macroscopic cortical infarcts are common in "classic" polyarteritis and are usually caused by thrombotic occlusion of vasculitic lesions.[361] In more chronic biopsies there is tubular atrophy and interstitial fibrosis.

Microscopic Polyangiitis

Patients with microscopic polyangiitis infrequently have true arteritis identified on renal biopsy. The frequency ranges from 11% to 22% with predominant involvement of interlobular arteries and arterioles rather than larger vessels as in "classic" polyarteritis.[361] Involvement is circumferential, lesions are of the same age, and aneurysm formation is rare. The acute vasculitis may resemble that of the classic form histologically or it may be granulomatous with the vessel media expanded by infiltrating mononuclear and polymorphonuclear leukocytes, epithelioid cells, and focal giant cells. In the same vessel features of granulomatous and necrotizing vasculitis may co-exist. In later stages of the disease there may be narrowing of the lumens of small arteries due to concentric intimal fibroplasia and elastic reduplication, but medial scarring is less frequent and severe than in the classic form of

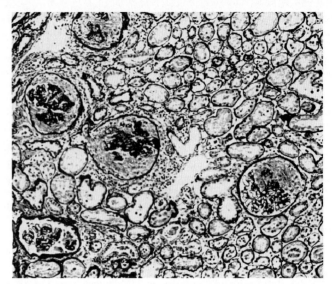

FIGURE 31–16 Microscopic polyarteritis (polyangiitis): There are diffuse crescents with focal segmental necrosis of the glomerular tuft (Jones methenamine silver, ×125).

periarteritis. In microscopic polyangiitis there is often a diffuse interstitial inflammatory cell infiltrate with plasma cells, lymphocytes, and polymorphonuclear leukocytes especially around glomeruli and vessels. In some biopsies this contains large numbers of eosinophils, in others inflammatory cells penetrate the tubular basement membrane causing tubulitis.[376] In more chronic stages there is patchy tubular atrophy and interstitial fibrosis that parallels the glomerular and vascular damage.

In microscopic polyangiitis the most prominent histologic finding is typically a focal segmental necrotizing glomerulonephritis with crescents affecting from few to many glomeruli (Fig. 31–16).[361,376] There is focal destruction of the glomerular basement membrane associated with polymorphonuclear infiltration, karyorrhexis, and deposition of fibrin within the tuft and adjacent Bowman space. The tuft may show a variable degree of hypercellularity. Crescents characteristically overlie areas of segmental tuft necrosis and may be segmental or circumferential. Both cellular and fibrous crescents often appear in the same biopsy. Some crescents are voluminous with a "sunburst" appearance due to massive circumferential destruction of Bowman capsule. In the chronic or healing phase of the disease there is segmental and global glomerulosclerosis with focal fibrous crescents. A recent study documents differences between biopsies of patients with microscopic polyangiitis and Wegener granulomatosis. Biopsies from patients with polyangiitis are more likely to show glomerulosclerosis, interstitial fibrosis, and tubular atrophy. This is also true of P(MPO)-ANCA–positive patients. This suggests a more prolonged, less fulminant course of these patients' renal disease than in patients with Wegener granulomatosis.

Immunofluorescent and Electron Microscopic Findings

In most cases the glomeruli show no or only weak immune staining by IF consistent with the designation "pauci-immune" glomerulonephritis.[361,376] A review of a number of large series reported positivity for one or another immunoglobulin in from 3% to 35% of cases with great heterogeneity and variability of intensity.[361] Fibrinogen was most commonly present in glomeruli, followed by C3 and then by IgG and Clq.[376] The pattern is felt to be consistent with "nonspecific trapping" in areas of glomerular necrosis and sclerosis rather than immune complex deposition. Vascular staining is similar.

By electron microscopy the glomeruli in most patients with either macroscopic or microscopic polyarteritis have no electron-dense deposits.[365,376,377] Patients may have sparse irregular deposits in various glomerular locations. Glomeruli may show endothelial swelling, subendothelial accumulation of "fluffy" electron lucent material, and subendothelial and intracapillary fibrin deposition and occasional fibrin-platelet thrombi. Through gaps in the GBM, fibrin tactoids and neutrophils may exude into Bowman space associated with epithelial crescents. In the chronic phase glomeruli develop segmental or global glomerulosclerosis with fibrous crescents. Vascular changes have included swelling and focal degeneration of the endothelium, separation of the endothelium from its basement membrane with subendothelial fibrin deposition, and with severe damage intraluminal fibrin, platelet thrombi, erythrocyte sludging, severe subendothelial fibrin deposition, edema and inflammatory infiltration of the intima and media by leukocytes.[361,376,377] As in the glomeruli, no electron-dense deposits are found in the vessels. In biopsies with chronic changes there may be expansion of the vessel intima by concentric layers of elastic tissue, fibrillar collagen and non fibrillar basement membrane material, and scarring of the media.

Pathology of Extrarenal Systemic Disease

Autopsy studies in polyarteritis describe the kidneys as being the most commonly affected organ (65%) followed by the liver (54%), peri adrenal tissue (41%), pancreas (39%), and less commonly muscle and brain.[361,376,378] It is unclear what percent of patients with microscopic polyangiitis have pulmonary involvement due to overlap in classification with Wegener granulomatosis and Churg-Strauss syndrome. When biopsied other tissues giving high yields for diagnosing the vasculitis of polyarteritis include the testes, the sural nerve, skin, rectum, and skeletal muscle.

Pathogenesis

The vasculitis of polyarteritis may be mediated by a number of diverse pathogenetic factors including humoral vascular immune deposits, cellular immunity, endothelial cytopathic factors, and anti-neutrophilic cytoplasmic antibody. An immune complex (IC) pathogenesis of vasculitis is suggested by experiments of acute serum sickness in which an acute glomerulonephritis is produced along with a systemic vasculitis resembling polyarteritis.[361] The vasculitis can be largely prevented by complement or neutrophile depletion. The experimental Arthus reaction can also induce a vasculitis resulting from in situ vascular immune complex formation with vessel injury preventable by neutrophil or complement depletion.[379] MRL-1 mice develop an immune complex glomerulonephritis with necrotizing vasculitis similar to polyarteritis nodosa[380] in association with high levels of circulating immune complexes, predominantly autoantibodies containing anti-DNA. Viral infection of the muscle cells of the vessel media by murine leukemia virus is also associated with a necrotizing vasculitis and lupus-like syndrome with vascular deposits of immunoglobulin and complement.[381] However, glomerular and vascular immune deposits are rarely found in human polyarteritis despite significant levels of CIC's.

Two models of cell mediated vasculitis have been produced experimentally in mice.[382] There is no evidence in these models for vascular immune deposits and some have a granulomatous form of vasculitis similar to that of polyarteritis in multiple organs. In Kawasaki vasculitis IgM anti-endothelial antibodies directed against endothelial surface antigens inducible by cytokines have been found.[383] Likewise, several viral infections in humans are capable of inducing direct cytopathic injury to arterial endothelium.[361]

ANCA may play a pathogenetic role in ANCA-associated microscopic polyangiitis and glomerulonephritis in a manner similar to Wegener granulomatosis (see section on Wegener granulomatosis). There may be initial priming of the neutrophil with cytokines and other mediators of inflammation, perhaps in response to infection, leading to expression of ANCA antigens on cell surfaces. These antigens can then react with circulating ANCAs. Myeloperoxidase is expressed on neutrophil cell surfaces following neutrophil priming with tumor necrosis factor and ANCAs have been demonstrated to stimulate a respiratory burst, with release of reactive oxygen species by primed neutrophils and monocytes, as well as degranulation of activated neutrophils and monocytes. Prior infection may set in motion the priming mechanisms that eventuate in vasculitis and in vitro evidence supports injury to endothelial cells by primed neutrophils exposed to ANCA. The induction of ANCA-positive microscopic polyangiitis associated with use of the antithyroid drug propylthiouracil suggests a pathogenetic role for ANCA as well.[368,384] Although ANCA develop in relation to many different antigens in these patients (e.g., elastase, cathepsin G, lactoferrin), it is those patients with high titers of specific anti-MPO antibodies characteristics (e.g., high avidity and complement binding) who develop the disease.

Clinical Features

The clinical features of polyarteritis are quite variable depending on the population studied and the diagnostic criteria used for the disease. Because both the classic and microscopic forms of the disease share many clinical findings they are often included together despite the marked differences in pathology. Many patients with ANCA-positive idiopathic pauci-immune rapidly progressive glomerulonephritis will have evidence of extrarenal symptoms. If these patients are included in the spectrum of polyarteritis the clinical presentation and features will also differ from older series.[385]

The most common clinical findings relate to constitutional symptoms of fever, weight loss, and malaise.[386] Gastrointestinal involvement may include nausea, vomiting, abdominal pain, gastrointestinal bleeding, bowel infarcts, and perforations.[361,387,388] Liver involvement may be associated with hepatitis B or C, and vasculitis of the mesenteric vessels, hepatic arteries, and of the gall bladder leading to cholecystitis have all been found.[361,387,388] Patients may develop heart failure, coronary artery ischemia with angina or myocardial infarction, and less commonly pericarditis and conduction abnormalities.[361] Disease of the nervous system may be central, with seizures and cerebro-vascular accidents, or related to peripheral nerves, with mononeuritis multiple and peripheral neuropathies.[361,389,391] Patients may develop muscle weakness, myalgias or myositis, and arthralgias but frank arthritis is less common.[361,392] Clinical findings also may relate to disease in the gonads, salivary glands, pancreas, adrenal, ureter, breast, and eyes.[361,393] In general, with the exception of liver manifestations and arthralgias, there is little difference between the clinical findings of patients who are hepatitis B positive or negative. Patients with cutaneous disease may present with "palpable purpura" with a leukocytoclastic angiitis on biopsy, or with petechiae, nodules, papules, livedo reticularis, and skin ulcerations.[361,394] The extent of pulmonary involvement is variable depending on the criteria for classification of polyarteritis versus other vasculitic disease such as Wegener granulomatosis and Churg-Strauss syndrome.[361]

There are a number of differences in the presentation of patients with the classic pattern and the microscopic form of polyarteritis.[361] In the classic form patients typically have findings related to visceral organ infarction and ischemia, and abdominal, cardiac, and neurologic findings are prominent. In the microscopic form cutaneous disease and pulmonary findings are more frequent. Patients with idiopathic focal segmental necrotizing glomerulonephritis and ANCA-positive rapidly progressive glomerulonephritis have similar clinical findings and presentations regardless of whether vasculitis has been documented on renal biopsy.[386] Likewise the extrarenal findings in patients with ANCA positive rapidly progressive glomerulonephritis have been similar whether the patients are P-ANCA or C-ANCA positive.[386]

Laboratory Tests

Laboratory tests in patients with polyarteritis include an elevated erythrocyte sedimentation rate in almost all patients and anemia, leukocytosis, and thrombocytosis present in over two thirds.[361,385] Eosinophilia is found in from 10% to 40%, being higher in patients with the microscopic form of PAN and in those overlapping with Churg-Strauss syndrome. Most patients have negative tests for anti-nuclear antibodies and normal serum complement values. Tests for circulating immune complexes and rheumatoid factor are often positive.[395] Although cryoglobulins have often been reported to be positive in many patients it is unclear what percent have had associated hepatitis infection.[361] The incidence of hepatitis B antigenemia has been variable ranging from 0% to as many as 40% in some series weighted heavily for classic polyarteritis. It is usually positive in less than 10% of unselected patients.[361,395]

The widespread use of accurate assays for ANCA have facilitated the clinical diagnosis of polyangiitis. There is considerable clinical overlap between patients with polyarteritis, Wegener granulomatosis, and Churg-Strauss, and all have high rates of ANCA positivity. Although C-ANCA positive patients are more likely to have biopsy proven necrotizing vasculitis or granulomatous inflammation of the sinuses or lower respiratory tract there is a large overlap in the clinical manifestations between C-ANCA positive and P-ANCA positive patients. Patients with classic polyarteritis are usually ANCA negative. ANCA titers vary considerable among patients with similar clinical manifestation and the role of the titre in predicting flares of the disease is not fully defined. Some patients will retain high ANCA levels despite clinical remission and some patients are positive for anti-GBM antibodies as well as ANCA (see section on Wegener granulomatosis).

Renal Findings

Although the kidney is typically the organ most commonly involved in polyarteritis, the pattern may vary considerably.[361,396] In the microscopic form of the disease vasculitis and glomerulonephritis relate to the clinical findings, whereas in the classic pattern renal ischemia and infarction due to larger vessel disease predominate. Hypertension is common in polyarteritis and is found initially in up to one half of patients.[361] Hypertension may be mild or severe, and if not present initially can develop at any time during the course of the disease.[397] Presenting symptoms related to kidney disease

are uncommon in "classic" polyarteritis with the exception of hypertension but may include hemorrhage from a renal artery aneurysm, flank pain, and gross hematuria. Oliguric acute renal failure is uncommon as are symptoms related to the nephrotic syndrome.[397]

Most patients will have laboratory evidence of their renal involvement at presentation. The majority of cases of microscopic polyangiitis and some of classic polyarteritis have urinary sediment changes with microscopic hematuria and often red blood cell casts.[361] Proteinuria is found in most patients but the nephrotic syndrome is rarely present. A decreased GFR is present in up to half of the patients in unselected series, and more in those selected for renal involvement. Severe renal insufficiency may be found at presentation in some patients. These renal findings are similar to those found in patients with ANCA-positive idiopathic RPGN, whether or not associated with systemic involvement.[385] In microscopic polyarteritis the severity of the clinical renal findings generally correlates with the degree of glomerular involvement akin to patients with Wegener granulomatosis. Patients with normal serum creatinines or creatinine clearances are likely to have normal glomeruli on biopsy or only ischemic glomerular changes, whereas patients with reduced or deteriorating renal function are more likely to exhibit severe segmental necrotizing glomerulonephritis or diffuse proliferative features.[361,365,398] Extensive crescent formation correlates with oliguria, severe renal failure, and a residual decrease in GFR after therapy.[361,376]

Angiographic examination of the vasculature for evidence of polyarteritis is far more likely to be positive in patients with the classic pattern. Angiograms reveal multiple rounded, saccular aneurysms of medium-sized vessels in about 70% of cases as well as thromboses, stenoses, and other luminal irregularities.[361,387,398] Aneurysms most commonly involve the hepatic, splanchnic, and renal vessels, are usually bilateral, multiple, and vary in size from 1 mm to 12 mm.[398] There is no way to clinically predict the presence of aneurysms.[398] Vasculitic changes and even aneurysms can heal with time as documented by angiography usually in correlation with the clinical response of the patient.[387,398] Similar aneurysms have been documented in Wegener granulomatosis, SLE, TTP, bacterial endocarditis, and Churg-Strauss syndrome.

Prognosis and Treatment

In retrospective studies of untreated patients with polyarteritis survival has been dismal with 5-year survival less than 15%.[361] Many patients had a fulminant course with a high early mortality due to the acute vasculitic process. A poor prognosis has been found in the elderly, those with a delay in diagnosis, with gastrointestinal tract catastrophes such as bowel infarction and hemorrhage, and with severe renal disease. Hypertension has been variably found to adversely affect the prognosis or have no effect on it. Renal prognosis has been reported to be adversely affected by increased activity on the biopsy, more crescents, severity of endocapillary proliferation, and glomerulosclerosis.[361] Early mortality in polyarteritis relates to the active vasculitis leading to renal failure, gastrointestinal hemorrhage or acute cardiovascular events whereas late mortality has been attributed to chronic vascular changes with chronic renal failure, and heart disease with congestive heart failure.[363] Survival has not been different in a series of over 150 patients with focal segmental necrotizing glomerulonephritis either alone or with associated arteritis.[396]

Corticosteroid use improved the survival of polyarteritis patients significantly with 5-year survivals of approximately 50%.[361] Nevertheless some patients achieve only partial remissions of the disease with continued activity leading to long-term morbidity and mortality. The addition of cytotoxic immunosuppressives to corticosteroid regimens has greatly improved the survival with 5-year survival rate increased to well over 80%. Although a number of immunosuppressives including azathioprine, busulfan, methotrexate, 6-mercaptopurine, and antithymocyte globulin have all been used successfully, many feel cyclophosphamide is the most effective agent.[399] Initial therapy of polyarteritis usually consists of high doses of cyclophosphamide (e.g., 1–2 mg/kg/day), adjusted to avoid leukopenia, commonly given along with high doses of corticosteroids (e.g., 60 mg Prednisone/day). The steroid dose is then tapered over time. Successful treatment can lead to complete inactivity of the vasculitic process and reversal of even severe renal failure requiring dialytic support. Other regimens have used various combinations of pulse methylprednisolone, plasma exchange, and intravenous cyclophosphamide with good short-term results. These regimens are discussed extensively in the section on Wegener granulomatosis because many treatment studies included all ANCA-positive vasculitis patients together. One trial of intravenous versus oral cyclophosphamide along with corticosteroids in ANCA-positive patients with microscopic polyarteritis nodosa or Wegener granulomatosis found equivalent efficacy and less side effects with the intravenous regimen. ANCA-positive patients with rapidly progressive glomerulonephritis many of which fit the definition of microscopic polyangiitis have responded well to regimens of oral corticosteroids and bolus intravenous methylprednisolone, with either bolus intravenous cyclophosphamide, or oral cyclophosphamide. The frequency of administration of the intravenous cyclophosphamide has varied from monthly to every 2 to 3 weeks at doses ranging from 0.5 to 1 g/m², whereas pulse methylprednisolone has been given at daily doses of 500 mg or up to 7 mg/kg body weight for several days. Although the benefits of oral versus IV cyclophosphamide have been debated, they are discussed under Wegener granulomatosus. A recent large multicenter prospective randomized trial comparing oral to IV cyclophosphamide in 144 ANCA-positive polyangiitis patients for induction therapy found no difference in efficacy, BVAS score, or serum creatinine between the two regimens. Even patients with dialysis requiring renal failure may respond to these regimens. Although controlled trials have shown ambiguous results regarding the benefit of adding plasmapheresis to standard regimens in ANCA-positive polyangiitis, it may benefit a subset of patients with severe glomerulonephritis requiring dialysis, or those with pulmonary hemorrhage. Even patients with a good response to therapy may suffer residual glomerular damage and progress long term to end-stage renal disease. Thus, aggressive, vigorous early therapy to turn off the disease process is felt to be crucial in preventing residual organ damage.[401–403] Therapeutic intervention in addition to immunosuppressive therapy includes control of hypertension, and measures to prevent non-immunologic glomerular disease progression such as use of anti-hypertensives that blockade the renin-angiotensin system, and use of low protein diets in some patients. Alpha interferon and other anti-viral agents have been used in the management of polyarteritis associated with hepatitis B infection and Hairy cell leukemia.[404,405]

For patients with ESRD, immunosuppressive therapy should be continued for 6 months to 1 year after the disease appears inactive. Although transplantation has been performed in only a limited number of patients with polyarteritis, by extrapolation of results from populations with ANCA positive rapidly progressive glomerulonephritis and Wegener granulomatosis, most patients should do well on standard immunosuppressive regimens; the risk of recurrence remains in the 15% to 20% range.

CHURG-STRAUSS SYNDROME (ALLERGIC GRANULOMATOSIS)

Churg-Strauss syndrome, or allergic granulomatosis and angiitis, is a rare systemic disease characterized by vasculitis, asthma, organ infiltration by eosinophils, and peripheral eosinophilia.[406,407] Churg and Strauss first fully described the syndrome in 1951.[361] Although there may be some overlap with other vasculitic and allergic processes such as polyarteritis nodosa, Wegener granulomatosis and microscopic polyangiitis, Loeffler syndrome, and chronic eosinophilic pneumonitis, the clinical and pathologic features of "Churg-Strauss syndrome" are distinct.[409,410]

Churg-Strauss syndrome is an uncommon disease with only several hundred cases reported in the literature. In a review of almost 185,000 asthmatic patients taking medications only 21 cases of Churg-Strauss syndrome were identified.[411] The low incidence may reflect under recognition and there might also be a higher disease incidence if a looser definition of the disease was applied with only some clinical and histopathologic features required for defining the diagnosis. A more inclusive definition includes (1) asthma, (2) peripheral blood eosinophilia, and (3) systemic vasculitis involving two or more extrapulmonary organs. Using this definition, many cases described as other vasculitic syndromes in asthmatics would fit the definition of Churg-Strauss syndrome.

There is no gender predominance in Churg-Strauss syndrome, and although the disease has been reported at all ages, the mean age of diagnosis is about 50 years old.[406–410] The clinical renal involvement in Churg-Strauss syndrome is clearly less prevalent than morphological renal involvement. However, a recent series from one center reports a high incidence of clinical renal disease.[413] In autopsy series, the kidney is affected in over one half of patients, whereas clinical renal disease has been described in from 25% to over 90% of patients.[406–410,413]

A number of studies document the rare occurrence of Churg-Strauss syndrome in steroid-dependent asthmatics taking leukotriene receptor antagonists (montelukast, zafirlukast, pranlukast).[414–420] This may represent unmasking of the vasculitic syndrome as the leukotriene receptor antagonist permits steroid withdrawal because similar cases have been reported in "asthmatics" with a change from oral to inhaled steroids.[418,419] Rarely, substitution of a leukotriene receptor antagonist for inhaled steroids has led to Churg-Strauss syndrome.[420] Other investigators have not been able to find evidence to support a pathogenic role for leukotriene receptor antagonists in the development of the disease.[421]

Pathology

Renal biopsies in Churg-Strauss syndrome vary from normal kidney tissue to severe glomerulonephritis, vasculitis, and interstitial inflammation.[361,406–408,412,413,422,423] There may be a focal segmental necrotizing glomerulonephritis sometimes with small crescents. In most cases the glomerulonephritis is mild, affects only several glomeruli, and involves the tuft segmentally. The glomerulonephritis may, however, be diffuse and global with severe necrotizing features and crescents. Rarely there is only mesangial hypercellularity without endocapillary proliferation or necrosis. In autopsy studies vasculitis was found in the kidney in over one half of the original cases studied by Churg and Strauss and it has been noted on renal biopsy as well.[361] It may involve any size artery from arterioles to arcuates and histologically may vary from fibrinoid necrotizing to granulomatous. Although resembling other forms of vasculitis, the arteritis is characterized by eosinophilic granulocytes within the arterial wall and in the

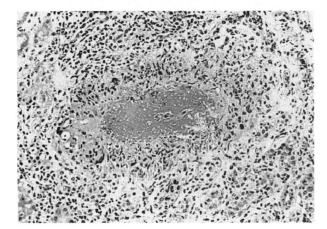

FIGURE 31–17 Churg-Strauss syndrome: Granulomatous vasculitis involves an arcuate artery. There is granulomatous transmural inflammation with focal giant cells and superimposed luminal thrombosis (Hematoxylin-eosin, ×125).

surrounding connective tissue (Fig. 31–17). Destruction of elastic membrane, aneurysms, and luminal thrombosis with recanalization may occur as may epithelioid cells and multinucleated giant cells in the media, adventitia, and perivascular connective tissue. Active and healed lesions may co-exist. Less commonly, venules and small veins of interlobular size may be affected, often with granulomatous features and in close association with adjacent interstitial granulomatous inflammation. The tubulointerstitial region is involved by an inflammatory infiltrate containing eosinophils and some lymphocytes, plasma cells, and polymorphonuclear leukocytes in association with interstitial edema.[361,413] In some cases there are interstitial granulomas composed of a core of eosinophilic or basophilic necrotic material surrounded by a rim of radially oriented macrophages, giant cells of the Langhans type, and numerous eosinophils. Interstitial nephritis may be present without glomerular pathology.

By IF areas of segmental necrosis in the glomeruli may contain IgM, C_3, and fibrinogen.[361,412,413] A single report describes IgA staining in the glomerulus.[412] Several investigators have described complement in arteries in Churg-Strauss syndrome. The presence of IgE in renal or other tissues has not been adequately investigated.[424] EM of the glomeruli, pulmonary granulomas, venules, and capillaries reveals no electron-dense deposits.[361,406–408]

Pathogenesis

Although the pathogenesis of Churg-Strauss syndrome remains unclear, allergic or hypersensitivity mechanisms are supported by the presence of asthma, hypereosinophilia, and elevated plasma levels of IgE.[406–408,412,424,425] Eosinophils in patients with Churg-Strauss syndrome have prolonged survival due to inhibition of CD95 mediated apoptosis; T cell secretion of eosinophil activating cytokines may play a role as well.[425] Human eosinophil cationic proteins, which are capable of tissue destruction in a variety of hypereosinophilic syndromes, have been found in granulomatous tissue from patients with Churg-Strauss syndrome.[426,427] Higher serum levels of eosinophil cationic protein (ECP), soluble interleukin-2 receptor (sIl-2R) and soluble thrombomodulin levels have been associated with active disease in Churg-Strauss syndrome.[427] Although a pathogenetic role for immune complex deposition has been suggested, hypocomplementemia and CIC's have rarely been observed and the negative IF and EM findings do not support an immune complex pattern

of injury. Cell mediated immunity may be involved in the pathogenesis of the lesions and high helper/suppressor ratios in the peripheral blood during the acute phase of the disease are reported as well as a preponderance of helper T cells in the granulomas of skin biopsies.[361] It is likely that ANCA may play a role akin to that in Wegener granulomatosis and microscopic polyarteritis.

Clinical and Laboratory Features

Patients may have initial constitutional symptoms such as weight loss, fatigue, malaise, and fever.[361,406–408] Characteristic extrarenal features include asthma (present in over 95% of cases), an allergic diathesis, allergic rhinitis, and peripheral eosinophilia.[406,410,412] Asthmatic disease typically precedes the onset of the vasculitis by years, but it may occur simultaneously. The severity of the asthma does not necessarily parallel the severity of the vasculitis. Many patients subsequently develop eosinophilia in the blood along with eosinophilic infiltrates in multiple organs. This is followed by vasculitis of organs in some patients. This multisystem disease often involves the heart with pericarditis, heart failure, and/or ischemic disease, the gastrointestinal tract with abdominal pain, ulceration, diarrhea, or bowel perforation, and the skin with subcutaneous nodules, petechiae, and/or purpuric lesions.[406–410,412,428–430] A peripheral neuropathy with mononeuritis multiplex is common, but migrating polyarthralgia or arthritis (or both) occur less frequently.[431] The eye, prostate, and genitourinary tract may be involved. Some patients with Churg-Strauss syndrome have overlapping features with polyarteritis or other vasculitides.[406–410]

Laboratory evaluation typically reveals anemia, leukocytosis, and an elevated erythrocyte sedimentation rate.[361,406–410] Eosinophilia is universally present and may reach 50% of the total peripheral leukocyte count. The degree of eosinophilia and the erythrocyte sedimentation rate may correlate with disease activity as may the level of eosinophilic cationic protein, soluble interleukin-2 receptor, and soluble thrombomodulin levels.[427] Rheumatoid factor is often positive and C-reactive protein levels are increased, whereas serum complement, hepatitis markers, CIC's, ANA, and cryoglobulins are usually negative.[361,406–410] Elevated serum IgE levels and IgE-containing CIC's are frequently found.[406–410,412,424] Chest radiograph may show patchy infiltrates, nodules, diffuse interstitial disease, and pleural effusion.[406–410,431,432] Pleural effusions my be exudative and contain large numbers of eosinophils.[433] On angiography visceral aneurysms may be present in patients with both polyarteritis overlap syndromes and classic Churg-Strauss syndrome.

ANCA levels have been elevated in 40% to 80% of Churg-Strauss patients.[421,428,434,435] Most patients are P-ANCA positive with antibody directed against myeloperoxidase, but some are positive for C-ANCA. In one recent analysis of almost 100 patients 35% were ANCA positive by immunofluorescence with a perinuclear pattern and antimyeloperoxidase specificity in about three quarters.[435] Some investigators have found a good correlation between ANCA positivity and ANCA titers and clinical activity whereas others have not.[421,428,435] Clearly in some, ANCA titers may remain positive despite clinical remissions. In Churg-Strauss patients ANCA positivity has been correlated variably with renal involvement, pulmonary disease, peripheral neuropathy, and the presence of vasculitis.[434,435]

Although the clinical renal findings in Churg-Strauss syndrome are diverse, as opposed to other vasculitides, renal involvement rarely predominates.[361,406–410] Microscopic hematuria and mild proteinuria are common, but nephrotic range proteinuria is infrequent. Hypertension is found in up to 75% of patients. In pure Churg-Strauss syndrome, renal failure has been uncommon although it occurs in patients with overlap syndromes. Recent reports, however, suggest a higher incidence of renal involvement and renal failure.[409,410,413,422]

Prognosis, Course, and Treatment

Patients may have several phases of the syndrome over many years.[406-410] There may be a prodromal phase of asthma or allergic rhinitis followed by a phase of peripheral blood and tissue eosinophilia remitting and relapsing over months to years before development of systemic vasculitis. A shorter duration of asthma prior to onset of vasculitis has been associated with a worse prognosis.[412] The correlation between ANCA levels with the disease activity in Churg-Strauss syndrome has been variable. In general, renal disease is mild with only 7% of one large literature review having renal failure as a cause of death even in untreated patients.[361,412,413] Most patients surviving the initial insult usually fare well with survival rates in treated patients approximately 90% at 1 year and 70% at 5 years.[406-410,428] Patients with significant cardiac, CNS, gastrointestinal involvement, and those with greater degrees of renal damage have a poor long-term survival.[428] However, cases progressing to severe renal failure and dialysis have certainly been reported.[410,413,422]

Corticosteroid therapy is successful in most patients with Churg-Strauss syndrome.[406-410] Patients respond rapidly to high daily oral prednisone therapy and even relapses respond to retreatment. Extra renal disease often responds as well. Resistant cases may benefit from treatment with other immunosuppressive agents such as azathioprine, methotrexate, cyclophosphamide, or plasma exchange although one meta-analysis could find no benefit from the addition of plasma exchange to other treatments.[406-410,435,436] Pulse intravenous cyclophosphamide has also been used successfully.[437] IV immune globulin has been used successfully in some small groups of patients resistant to other forms of therapy.[438,439] TNF blocking agents such as infliximab and etanercept have also been useful in some such patients.[434] Alpha interferon has been used to treat successfully several patients resistant to corticosteroids and cyclophosphamide.[440] Although recovery is usually complete, some patients relapse and others have chronic sequelae such as peripheral neuropathy, chronic pulmonary changes, and hypertension.[406,428]

GLOMERULAR INVOLVEMENT IN OTHER VASCULITIDES (TEMPORAL ARTERITIS, TAKAYASU DISEASE, LYMPHOMATOID ARTERITIS)

Temporal Arteritis

Temporal arteritis or giant cell arteritis is a systemic vasculitis with a characteristic giant cell vasculitis of medium size and large arteries.[441-444] The disease is slightly more prevalent in females than in males and is the most common form of arteritis in western countries.[441-446] Temporal arteritis is primarily a disease of the elderly, the average age of onset of symptoms being 72 years, with over 95% of patients exceeding 50 years of age.[445,446] Extra cranial vascular involvement occurs in from 10% to 15% of patients with giant cell arteritis.[441,444,447] Renal manifestations are rare and generally mild, consisting of mild hematuria and proteinuria, without renal functional impairment.[441-444] Renal failure occurring in patients with temporal arteritis is exceedingly unusual.

There are several reports of a polyarteritis nodosa-like renal involvement occurring in association with temporal arteritis or polymyalgia rheumatica.[448] Some patients are P-ANCA positive and less commonly patients have been C-ANCA positive.[449] The renal pathology has been described as a focal segmental necrotizing glomerulonephritis with focal crescents and vasculitis of the PAN type, primarily affecting small arteries and arterioles. Rarely visceral aneurysms have been demonstrable angiographically. Whether these cases represent true manifestations of temporal arteritis or forms of "overlap" with polyarteritis nodosa is not clear. There is also single report of probable LN occurring in a patient with temporal arteritis.[450] In a report of membranous glomerulopathy occurring in a patient with temporal arteritis, it was not clear whether the association was fortuitous or pathogenetically linked because both the proteinuria and systemic symptoms responded to steroid therapy.[451] Renal amyloidosis has also rarely been noted in patients with temporal arteritis.

The most common renal manifestations of mild proteinuria and microhematuria are present in less than 10% of patients.[442-444,447] Erythrocyte casts have been found on urinalysis in some patients and especially those with extracranial large vessel involvement. Renal excretory function is usually unaffected and renal insufficiency is uncommon. Rare cases of renal insufficiency or renal failure (or both) have been attributed to renal arteritis affecting the main renal artery or its intraparenchymal branches.[448,449] In some cases the pathology has been inadequate to diagnose the precise etiology of the renal failure. The nephrotic syndrome has been reported in a patient with temporal arteritis and membranous glomerulopathy.[451] In this case steroid therapy produced a partial response with reduction in proteinuria from 6.8 to 1.3 grams/day. Hypertension is infrequent and most often mild to moderate when present.

The vasculitis seen in temporal arteritis is characterized by segmental transmural inflammation of medium size and large elastic arteries by a mixed infiltrate of lymphocytes, monocytes, polymorphonuclear leukocytes, scattered eosinophils, and giant cells.[441-444] Giant cells are quite variable in number and are usually most prominent in the region of the internal and external elastic membrane, with associated gaps in the elastica. Necrosis of the intima and media may occur in the acute phases. In the chronic phase, exuberant intimal fibroplasia may lead to marked narrowing of the arterial lumen.

The management of temporal arteritis with corticosteroids causes rapid and dramatic improvement in general well being, specific symptomatology, and laboratory abnormalities.[441-444] A number of corticosteroid sparing and secondary immunosuppressives have been used successfully in temporal arteritis.[452,453] Abnormal urinary sediment changes disappear, and there is resolution of extracranial large vessel involvement.[451-453] However, once established, visual loss is often permanent, despite resolution of the active disease process. Exacerbation of systemic vasculitis may occur if corticosteroids are tapered too rapidly.

Takayasu Arteritis

Takayasu arteritis is a rare vasculitic disease of unknown pathogenesis characterized by inflammation and stenosis of medium and large arteries, with a predilection for the aortic arch and its branches.[454-457] The disease most commonly affects young women between the ages of 10 and 40, and Asians are much more commonly affected.[454-457] Although findings are typically confined to the aortic arch, the subclavian, carotid, and pulmonary arteries, in some cases the abdominal aorta and its branches are affected.[454] The histopathologic findings of the vessels include arteritis with transmural infiltration by lymphocytes, monocytes, polymorphonuclear leukocytes, and in some cases Langhans giant cells. In the chronic phase of the disease, intimal fibroplasia and medial scarring may result in severe vascular stenoses or total luminal obliteration.

Although in the past renal disease was believed to be uncommon, renal involvement is now reported more frequently.[457–462] This is usually due to an obliterative arteritis of the main renal artery or narrowing of the renal ostia by abdominal aortitis leading to renovascular hypertension. Arteriography is usually used to make the diagnosis of Takayasu arteritis although computerized tomography, MR, and PET scan imaging have been used as well.[454,463,464] Laboratory abnormalities reveal mild anemia, elevated erythrocyte sedimentation rate, increased levels of C-reactive protein, and elevated gammaglobulin levels but other serologic tests such as ANA, latex fixation, VDRL, ASLO, and serum complement levels are normal. Some patients have antiendothelial cell antibodies.[465] Hypertension, which may be severe occurs in 40% to 60% of patients and has been attributed to decreased elasticity of the aorta, increased renin secretion due to stenosis of major renal arteries, and other mechanisms.[459,461,466,467] Although mild proteinuria and hematuria are found in some patients, nephrotic range proteinuria is uncommon and should suggest the possibility of secondary renal amyloidosis.[468] The serum creatinine is usually normal, but may be mildly elevated or associated with a high BUN to creatinine ratio suggestive of "pre-renal" azotemia. Progressive renal failure is uncommon.[455,456,459]

A mild mesangial proliferative glomerulonephritis may occur in patients with Takayasu arteritis.[458,460,468] Mesangial deposits of IgG, IgM, IgA, C_3, and C_4 have been reported and mesangial electron-dense deposits are found on EM. Most patients have normal renal function and only mild hematuria and proteinuria. Elevated serum levels of IgA have been noted, and some patients have had glomerular involvement typical of IgA nephropathy.[460,468] Whether this is coincidental or part of the disease process is unclear. One series of patients with Takayasu arteritis had unusual glomerular histopathology with mesangial sclerosis and nodules, as well as mesangiolysis and glomerular microaneurysms resembling diabetic nephropathy.[458] None of these patients had diabetic nephropathy. IF and EM in these cases of "centrolobular mesangiopathy" did not support an immune pathogenesis. There are also rare reports of renal amyloidosis occurring in association with Takayasu arteritis[468] and cases of membranoproliferative glomerulonephritis, crescentic glomerulonephritis, and proliferative glomerulonephritis.[469]

Treatment

In the majority of patients, corticosteroids are effective therapy for the vasculitis and systemic symptoms and further vascular deterioration is suppressed.[454–456] Other medications including azathioprine, methotrexate, cyclophosphamide, mycophenolate, and anti-TNF therapy have also been used successfully in individuals as have anticoagulants, vasodilators, and acetyl salicylic acid.[470–474] Residual morbidity and mortality may result from the progressive fibrosis and stenosis of previously inflamed arteries.[475]

Lymphomatoid Granulomatosis

Lymphomatoid granulomatosis is a rare disease that may encompass a spectrum from premalignant disease to frank neoplastic lymphoproliferative disorder.[476] Many cases are now felt to be associated with EB virus B cell lymphomas. Although in a recent review of over 150 cases renal involvement was found on histopathology in almost one third of

cases at autopsy, glomerular involvement is unusual. Histologically, there is focal infiltration of the renal interstitium by a polymorphous infiltrate of mature lymphocytes, plasma cells, histiocytes, immunoblasts, and atypical lymphoid cells whereas the glomeruli are spared. Lymphomatoid granulomatosis may cause diagnostic confusion with true vasculitides such as Wegener granulomatosis, allergic granulomatosis, and polyarteritis nodosa.

◼ HENOCH-SCHÖNLEIN PURPURA

Henoch-Schönlein purpura (HSP) is a systemic vasculitic syndrome with involvement of the skin and gastrointestinal tract and joints in association with a characteristic glomerulonephritis.[477–480] In HSP IgA containing immune complexes deposit in the skin, kidney, and other organs in association with an inflammatory reaction of the vessels. In the skin this leads to a leukocytoclastic angiitis with petechiae and purpura. In gastrointestinal tract involvement there may be ulcerations, pain, and bleeding, and in the kidney an immune complex glomerulonephritis is found.[477–480]

Males are slightly more commonly affected than females, and children are far more frequently affected than adults although the disease can occur at any age.[477,481–485] The peak age of patients with HSP is approximately 5 years old as opposed to IgA nephropathy, which has a peak age of 15 to 30 years old.[477–484] HSP may account for up to 15% of all glomerulonephritis in young children.[477–484] More severe renal disease occurs in older children and adults.[485] HSP is uncommon in blacks.[487] Familial occurrence has rarely been reported and the frequency of HLA-Bw35 has been reported to be increased in some but not all patients with HSP.[489,490] About one fourth of patients will have a history of allergy but exacerbations related to a specific allergen are rare. In some cases relapses of the syndrome have occurred after exposure to allergens or the cold and seasonal variations show peak occurrence in the winter months.

Although HSP with classic organ system involvement is readily diagnosed, the syndrome may be confused with other systemic illnesses such as SLE and polyarteritis nodosa, with infectious agents such as meningococcemia, gonococcemia, and Yersinia enterocolitis. Likewise, certain medications and vaccination-related hypersensitivity reactions may mimic this disease as can post-infectious glomerulonephritis, which may have at times systemic manifestations. Although an upper respiratory infection precedes HSP in 30% to 50% of patients, serologic evidence of streptococcal infection is lacking. Abdominal pains may be mistaken for appendicitis, cholecystitis, or another surgical emergency and lead to exploratory laparotomy.

Clinical Findings

The classic tetrad of findings in HSP includes dermal involvement, gastrointestinal disease, joint involvement, and glomerulonephritis, but not all patients will have all organ systems clinically involved.[477–480] Constitutional symptoms such as fever, malaise, and fatigue and weakness may be associated with active isolated dermal involvement or full-blown systemic diseases. Skin lesions are almost universal in both children and adults with HSP and are commonly found on the lower and upper extremities but may also be on the buttocks or elsewhere.[477,479,491] They are characterized by urticarial macular and papular reddish-violaceous lesions that do not blanch. Lesions may be discrete or may coalesce into palpable purpuric lesions associated with lower extremity edema even in the absence of the nephrotic syndrome. New crops of lesions may recur over weeks or months. On skin biopsy there is a leukocytoclastic angiitis with evidence of IgA containing immune complexes along with IgG, C3, properidine but not C4 or C1q.[808] Gastrointestinal manifestations are present in from 25% to 90% of patients and may include colicky pain, nausea and vomiting, melena, and hematochezia.[477–480,492–495] One recent study of over 260 patients found that 58% had abdominal pain and 18% evidence of GI bleeding.[496] In patients with gastrointestinal involvement, endoscopy may reveal purpuric lesions, and rarely patients may develop areas of intussusception or perforation. Rheumatologic involvement is most common in the ankles and knees and less commonly in elbows and wrists, and may consist of arthralgias or frank arthritis with painful, tender effusions.[477–480] Patients do not develop joint deformities or erosive arthritis. Rarely patients will have evidence of other organ involvement with pulmonary, central nervous system, or ureteritis.[477–480,497]

Renal involvement varies from 20% to 100% of patients with HSP depending on the method of detection of renal disease and referral source of the patients.[477–480,484–486,491] In one recent series of over 260 patients 20% developed renal disease.[498] In studies routinely examining the urine, renal involvement ranges from 40% to 60% of patients.[499] In a series of 250 adults with HSP 32% had renal insufficiency usually with proteinuria (97%) and hematuria (93%).[491] The onset of active renal disease usually follows the onset of the systemic manifestations by days to weeks and is characterized by microscopic hematuria, active urinary sediment, and proteinuria.[477,479,487,491] Gross hematuria is uncommon. Even in children without clinical evidence of renal disease excessive excretion of erythrocytes in the urine has been documented. Some patients with clinical renal involvement will develop the nephrotic syndrome and some will have a nephritic picture. There is no relationship between the severity of extra renal organ involvement and the severity of the renal lesions.

Laboratory Features

In HSP platelet counts and serum complement levels are all usually normal.[477–480] Rarely slightly low CH50 and properidine levels or evidence of alternate pathway activation of complement is observed. Serum IgA levels are elevated in up to one half of patients especially during active phases of the illness, but do not correlate well with the severity of clinical manifestations or course of the disease.[477–480,483] A number of abnormal IgA antibodies have been noted including IgA rheumatoid factor, CIC's with IgA and IgG, IgA anticardiolipin antibodies, IgA fibronectin aggregates, IgA anti-alpha-galactosyl antibodies, and IgA ANCA.[502–510] The relationship of these to active renal or systemic disease remains to be confirmed although concentrations of IgA and IgG immune complexes, IgA rheumatoid factor, and IgA anti-galactosyl antibodies have been correlated with clinical renal disease manifestations.[503–505,509] Some patients have cryoglobulins.

Pathology

Although by LM the renal biopsy findings of HSP resemble those of IgA nephropathy, there are some histopathologic differences. The typical glomerular pathology of HSP is a mesangio-proliferative glomerulonephritis with variable crescent formation.[477–481,484,485,491,501,511] The mesangial changes include both increased mesangial cellularity and matrix expansion that may be focal or diffuse (Fig. 31–18). In severe cases, polymorphonuclear cells and mononuclear cells may also infiltrate the glomerular tufts and there may be necrotizing features. By monoclonal antibody staining increased numbers of monocyte/macrophages and CD4 and CD8 T cells are found.[512,513] Some cases have a well-developed membranoproliferative pattern with double contours of the GBM. Crescents vary from segmental to circumferential and are initially cellular but later fibrotic in nature (Fig. 31–19).

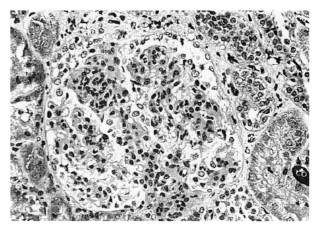

FIGURE 31–18 Henoch-Schönlein purpura nephritis: An example with global mesangial proliferation and focal infiltrating neutrophils (Hematoxylin-eosin, ×500).

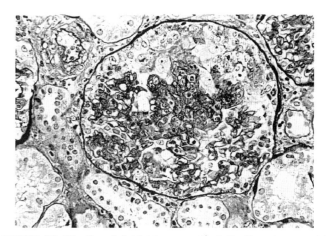

FIGURE 31–19 Henoch-Schönlein purpura nephritis: There is segmental endocapillary proliferation with an overlying segmental cellular crescent (Periodic acid Schiff, ×475).

Tubulointerstitial changes of atrophy and interstitial fibrosis are consistent with the degree of glomerular damage. In general, endocapillary and extracapillary proliferation as well as glomerular fibrin deposition are more frequent and severe in HSP than in IgA nephropathy.[481] The histopathologic classification system proposed by the International Study of Kidney Disease of Childhood correlates the glomerular lesions with clinical manifestations as well as prognosis.[484,501] These categories include Class I with minimal glomerular alterations; Class II with mesangial proliferation only; Class III with either focal (a) or diffuse (b) mesangial proliferation but less than 50% of glomeruli containing crescents or segmental lesions of thrombosis, necrosis, or sclerosis; Class IV with similar mesangial proliferation as IIIa and IIIb but 50% to 75% of glomeruli with crescents; Class V with similar changes and over 75% crescents; and Class VI a "pseudo" membranoproliferative pattern. Although hematuria is common to all groups, and proteinuria of some degree may be found in all, the nephrotic syndrome is present in only 25% of groups I, II, and III. Likewise, groups IIIb, IV, and V tend to have a progressive course toward renal failure.[515] Even by LM deposits may be seen in the mesangial regions and rarely along the capillary walls as well. It is unusual to find the presence of a vasculitis on renal biopsy.

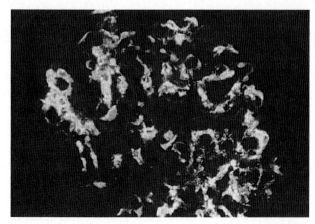

FIGURE 31-20 Henoch-Schönlein purpura nephritis: Immunofluorescence photomicrograph showing intense deposits of IgA distributed throughout the mesangium and also extending into a few peripheral glomerular capillary walls (×600).

Immunofluorescence and Electron Microscopy

By IF, IgA is the dominant or co-dominant immunoglobulin. Co-deposits of IgG and IgM, C3, and properidine are common. Deposits are typically found in the mesangium, especially involving the paramesangial regions, and may extend into the subendothelial areas (Fig. 31-20).[477-481] Early classical complement components of C1q and C4 are rarely present. These findings contrast with LN in which IgG usually predominates and C1q is almost always present. The deposited IgA is usually IgA1 subclass and may have the J chain indicating its polymeric nature, but secretory piece is not found.[477-481,516,517] Fibrin-related antigens are also commonly present.[515] IgA may be deposited along with C3 and C5 in both involved and uninvolved skin in the small vessels similar to the findings in IgA nephropathy.[518,519] IgA is also found in vasculitic lesions in the intestinal tract.[493-495] Similar IgA deposits may also occur in the skin in dermatitis herpetiformis (at the tips of the dermal papillae) and in SLE along with early and late complement components (at the dermal epidermal junction).

By EM characteristic immune type electron-dense deposits are found predominantly in the mesangial regions, accompanied by increase in mesangial cellularity and matrix.[477-481,514] In some capillaries, the deposits extend subendothelially from the adjacent mesangial regions. Occasionally, subepithelial deposits are also present and may resemble the humps of post-streptococcal disease.[515] Immunoelectron microscopy has confirmed the predominance of IgA in association with some C3 and IgG in the deposits.[511] Evidence of coagulation with fibrin and platelets thrombi may be found in capillary lumina. In cases with severe crescent involvement there may be disruption or rupture of the capillary walls.

Pathogenesis

The pathogenesis of HSP remains unknown. It is clearly a systemic immune complex disease with IgA-containing CIC's that are associated with a small vessel vasculitis and capillary damage.[477-480] The complexes contain polymeric IgA of the IgA1 subclass and late-acting complement components. This composition together with the presence of terminal complement components suggests alternate pathway complement activation. Whether IgA immune complexes trigger this com-

plement activation and the ultimate role of complement participation in the glomerular disease process are unclear. The presence of circulating polymeric IgA complexes, the deposition of IgA in the kidney as well as the skin, intestines and other organs, and recurrence of disease in the allograft all point to the systemic nature of the disease process.[520-522] Again the precise role of the IgA containing complexes or various IgA containing antibodies in the disease process is unclear because IgA is deposited in some diseases (e.g., celiac disease and chronic liver disease) without major clinical glomerular damage.[523] Complement activation, platelet activation and coagulation, and vasoactive prostanoids, cytokines, and growth factors may all play a role here. Impaired T cell activity has also been implicated in the pathogenesis of HSP.[524] HSP has also been reported in a patient with an IgA monoclonal gammopathy.[525] The relationship of HSP to IgA nephropathy is obscure with some investigators considering the disease separate entities and others describing them as different ends of the same pathogenetic spectrum.[477-480] Similar renal histologic findings and similar immunologic abnormalities such as circulating IgA levels, IgA fibronectin aggregates, and anti-mesangial cell antibodies suggest a common mechanism of renal injury.[527,528] IgG autoantibodies against mesangial cells parallel the course of the renal disease. Both IgA nephropathy and HSP have occurred in different members of the same families and in monozygotic twins after adenovirus infection.[488,526,529] Infectious agents associated with the occurrence of HSP have included varicella, measles, adenovirus, hepatitis A and/or B, Yersinia, Shigella, mycoplasma, HIV infection, and staphylococci including methicillin resistant organisms, but none has been proven as the etiology of the vasculitic disease.[478,479,526,530-532] Likewise, HSP has been reported to occur in association with vaccinations, insect bites, cold exposure, and trauma, although an etiologic relation is unproven.[533]

Course, Prognosis, and Treatment

In most patients HSP is a self-limited disease with a good long-term outcome.[477-480] Patients may have recurrences of the rash, joint symptoms, and gastrointestinal symptoms for months or years, but most patients have a benign short-term and long-term renal course. In general there is a good correlation between the clinical renal presentation and the ultimate prognosis.[477-480,484,491,501,515] Patients with focal mesangial involvement and only hematuria and mild proteinuria tend to have an excellent prognosis. In one recent large pediatric study renal survival was 100%.[498] In another series of 150 patients with 50% renal involvement only two patients had residual hematuria and no patient abnormal renal function at 2.5 years.[477] In most series by several years from presentation over half of the patients had no renal abnormalities, less than one fourth sediment abnormalities or proteinuria, only 10% decreased GFR, and less than 10% patients with severe clinical renal involvement at onset had persistent hypertension or declining GFR over a long period of time. A review of over 50 patients observed over 24 years after childhood onset HSP found 7 of 20 with severe HSP at onset with residual renal impairment as adults as opposed to only 2 of 27 patients with mild initial renal disease.[534] In a large series unselected for renal involvement only 2% to 5% of patients will develop ESRD. Long-term renal function may not be as good in adults with HSP.[491,535,536] In a series of over 250 adults with HSP observed almost 15 years, 11% developed ESRD, 13% severe renal impairment with a clearance less than 30 ml/min, and 15% moderate renal insufficiency.[491] A poor renal prognosis is predicted by an acute nephritic presentation, older age, and especially by larger amounts of proteinuria and more severe nephrotic syndrome.[535,537]

On renal biopsy, a poor prognosis is predicted by IgA deposits extending from the mesangium out along the peripheral capillary walls, increased interstitial fibrosis, glomerular fibrinoid necrosis, and especially the presence of greater percentage of crescents on renal biopsy.[491,537,538] In one large study of over 150 children with HSP those with greater than 50% glomeruli with crescents had at last follow-up over one third of patients with ESRD and another 18% with chronic renal insufficiency.

Repeat biopsies in patients with HSP who have clinically improved show decreased mesangial deposits and hypercellularity. Although complete clinical recovery occurs in 95% of affected children and most adults with HSP over one third of HSP patients who become pregnant have associated hypertension or proteinuria.[501] Mortality in HSP is less than 10% at 10 years.

There is no proven therapy for HSP.[477–480] Most patients fare well in the short term regardless of lack of any immunosuppressive intervention. Although steroids have been associated with decreased abdominal and rheumatological symptoms they have not been proven to ameliorate the renal lesions in any controlled fashion.[539–543] One study did find improved long-term renal findings in patients who received a trial of corticosteroids, and pulse intravenous methylprednisolone followed by high-dose corticosteroids has been successful in some studies leading to a low progression to renal failure despite the presence of poor prognostic findings.[539,543] However, other studies have not found long-term benefit from pulse steroids or oral corticosteroids. Patients with more severe clinical features and especially those with more crescents on biopsy have also been treated with anticoagulants, azathioprine, cyclophosphamide, chlorambucil and other immunosuppressives, and even plasma exchange.[543–550] Although these reports have shown anecdotal success in reversing the renal progression, controlled trials have not yet shown benefits of using cytotoxic immunosuppressive therapy.[537,538] IV immune globulin has been used in several patients with the nephrotic syndrome and decreased GFR in an uncontrolled non-randomized but apparently successful fashion.[548]

Clinical renal disease due to HSP has only rarely been reported to recur in the renal allograft.[520–522,551] However, as in IgA nephropathy, histologic recurrence is more common than clinical recurrence. Rarely recurrent disease in the allograft occurs along with extrarenal involvement and leads to loss of the allograft.[520–522] This may be more common in patients who are transplanted either with living related donors or while still active clinically within the first few years of developing ESRD.

ANTI-GLOMERULAR BASEMENT MEMBRANE DISEASE AND GOODPASTURE SYNDROME

Anti-GBM disease is caused by circulating antibodies directed against an antigenic site on type 4 collagen in the GBM.[552–555] In 1919 Goodpasture described the case of an 18-year-old male who died with an influenza-like illness characterized by pulmonary hemorrhage and a proliferative glomerulonephritis. However, pulmonary hemorrhage can occur in many diseases associated with glomerulonephritis aside from true Goodpasture syndrome including SLE, ANCA positive vasculitides, HSP, MCTD, and with renal vein thrombosis in the nephrotic syndrome.[556–559] True Goodpasture syndrome should consist of the triad of (1) proliferative, usually crescentic, glomerulonephritis, (2) pulmonary hemorrhage, (3) and the presence of anti-GBM antibodies.[552–555] In

anti-GBM disease the pulmonary hemorrhage may precede, occur concurrently with, or follow the glomerular involvement.[552–555,560,561] Some patients with anti-GBM antibodies and glomerulonephritis and hence "anti-GBM" disease never experience pulmonary involvement and thus do not have true "Goodpasture" syndrome.[554,555,560] Documentation of anti-GBM antibody-induced disease may be via renal biopsy,[561–563] or by establishing the presence of circulating anti-GBM antibodies. Indirect IF although insensitive is specific for the presence of anti-GBM antibodies, and it is positive in more than three fourths of patients.[562] Radioimmunoassay, enzyme-linked immunoabsorbent assay, and immunoblotting for the antibodies are highly specific and sensitive.[554,555]

Pathogenesis

Anti-GBM autoantibodies react with epitopes on the noncollagenous domain of type IV collagen.[552,553,564–567] This is encoded for by genes in the q35-37 region of chromosome 2. In many cases the primary antigenic site is between amino acids 198 and 237 of the terminal region of the alpha 3 chain of the type IV collagen.[552–554] This epitope is found in GBM, the basement membrane of alveoli, and several other locations in the body. The structure of the epitope is identical in the glomeruli and the alveolar basement membranes and may require partial denaturation for full exposure to antibody. The alpha 3 chain of type IV collagen is found predominantly in the GBM and alveolar capillary basement membranes, perhaps explaining the limited distribution of disease involvement in Goodpasture syndrome.[554] Eluates of antibody from lung and kidney of patients with Goodpasture syndrome cross react with GBM and the alveolar basement membrane and can produce disease in animal models.[568] Most anti-GBM antibodies belong to the IgG1 subclass and not all fix complement.[569] Antibody reacting with its antigen(s) and perhaps via autoreactive T cells leads to an inflammatory response, the formation of a proliferative glomerulonephritis, breaks in the GBM, and the subsequent extracapillary proliferation or crescent formation.[554,555] A role for T cells in Goodpasture syndrome is supported by the T cell infiltrates on biopsy, patient T cell proliferation in response to alpha 3 (IV) NC1 domain, the correlation of autoreactive T cells with disease activity, and the role of CD4+CD25+ regulatory cells controlling the autoreactive T cell response.[554,570,571] When the anti-GBM antibodies cross react with and cause damage to the basement membrane of pulmonary capillaries the patient will develop pulmonary hemorrhage and hemoptysis. An initial insult to the pulmonary vascular integrity may be required because alveolar capillaries are not normally permeable to passage of anti-GBM antibodies.[572] Exacerbations of disease and especially pulmonary disease with hemoptysis have been related to hydrocarbon fume exposure, cigarette smoking, hair dyes, exposure to metallic dust, D-penicillamine, and cocaine inhalation.[572–579] Although smokers with anti-GBM disease have a higher incidence of pulmonary hemorrhage, circulating anti-GBM antibody levels are no higher than in patients with disease who are non-smokers.[572,573] Goodpasture syndrome has occasionally been reported in more than one family member and has rarely occurred in clusters of unrelated patients occasionally at a particular season of the year.[554,560] Certain HLA types, HLA-DRw15 and DR4 and DRw2 may predispose to the syndrome and perhaps more severe disease.[580,581] Influenza A2 infection has also been associated with Goodpasture syndrome. Anti-GBM disease can also occur in patients with typical membranous nephropathy and in 5% to 10% of patients receiving allografts for ESRD secondary to Alport hereditary nephritis.[582,583]

Clinical Features

Glomerulonephritis mediated by anti-GBM antibodies, although reported in hundreds of patients in the literature and well studied immunopathogenetically, is an infrequent pattern of glomerular injury.[552–555,560] Although some studies suggested estimates as high as 3% to 5% of all glomerular diseases, most studies reduce this estimate to 1% to 2%. The disease has two peaks of occurrence, the first in younger males and the second in elderly females, but it can occur at any age and in either sex.[552–555,560,573,584–587] Anti-GBM disease limited to the kidney may be more common in older patients. Goodpasture syndrome is less common in blacks perhaps due to less frequent occurrence of certain predisposing HLA antigens in this population.[552–555,560,573,584–587] An upper respiratory infection precedes the onset of disease in 20% to 60% of cases.[552–555,573]

The most common extrarenal findings are by far related to pulmonary involvement. Patients may have cough, dyspnea, and shortness of breath, and hemoptysis may vary from trivial amounts to life-threatening massive amounts associated with exsanguination and suffocation.[554–556,573,585] In almost three fourths of cases pulmonary hemorrhage precedes or is coincident with the glomerular disease.[552–555] Although some patients have constitutional symptoms with weakness, fatigue, weight loss, chills, and fevers, this is less prominent than in systemic vasculitides; others may have skin rash, hepatosplenomegaly, nausea and vomiting, and arthralgias or arthritic complaints at onset.[554]

The clinical renal presentation may be with an acute nephritic picture with hypertension, edema, hematuria and active urinary sediment, and reduced renal function; however, only 20% of patients are hypertensive at onset.[552–555,585] Renal function is usually already reduced at presentation and may deteriorate from normal to dialysis requiring levels in a matter of days to weeks.[552–555,585] However, one recent study found over one third of patients to have a normal GFR.[587] There is a good correlation between the serum creatinine level and the percentage of glomeruli involved by severe crescent formation.

Laboratory Findings

Laboratory evaluation in patients with Goodpasture syndrome typically shows active urinary sediment with red cells and red cell casts.[554,555,585] Proteinuria although commonly present is usually not in the nephrotic range perhaps secondary to the reduction in GFR commonly present. Serologic tests such as ASLO, ANA, serum complement levels, rheumatoid factor, cryoglobulins, and CIC's are all either negative or normal.[554,555,585–587] Circulating anti-GBM antibodies are present in over 90% of patients although the antibody titer does not always correlate well with the manifestations or course of either the pulmonary or renal disease.[552,554,555,588] Most patients have a decrease in serum antibody titer with time. From 10% to 38% of patients will have both positive anti-GBM antibodies and ANCA tests usually directed against myeloperoxidase but occasionally against serine proteinase.[554,586,589–592] The anti-GBM antibodies in patients who are ANCA positive have the same antigenic specificity as in patients who are ANCA negative.[592] The ANCA titers are also similar in patients with and without coexistent anti-GBM antibodies. Some studies suggest that the course of patients double positive for anti-GBM antibodies and ANCA parallels that of patients with anti-GBM antibody disease with a much poorer renal prognosis for patients with severe renal failure than ANCA-positive patients.[593] Some patients have a clinical systemic vasculitis with purpura and arthralgias and arthritis—findings rarely seen in isolated Goodpasture syndrome without coexistent ANCA.[586,589,590] In Goodpasture syndrome

a microcytic, hypochromic anemia is common even without overt pulmonary hemorrhage. Other patients may have a leukocytosis. Iron deposition in the lungs may be documented by either Fe59 scanning or by pulmonary lavage or expectorated sputum showing hemosiderin laden macrophages. In patients with pulmonary involvement chest radiograph is abnormal in over 75% and typically shows infiltrates corresponding to areas of pulmonary hemorrhage, but it may also demonstrate atelectasis, pulmonary edema, and areas of coexistent pneumonia.[552–555] Hypoxemia and an increased arterial alveolar gradient is present in severe cases.

Pathology

By LM patients with mild clinical involvement often have a focal, segmental proliferative glomerulonephritis.[552,554,555,588] This is typically associated with areas of segmental necrosis and overlying small crescents.[588] However, the most common biopsy picture is diffuse crescentic glomerulonephritis involving over 50% of glomeruli, with exuberant circumferential crescents (Fig. 31–21).[554,594] The underlying tuft is compressed but displays focal necrotizing features. Disruption and destruction of portions of the GBM and the basement membrane of Bowman capsule may be seen on silver stain.[594] Early crescents are formed by proliferating epithelial cells and infiltrating T lymphocytes, monocytes, and polymorphonuclear leukocytes, whereas older ones are composed predominantly of spindled fibroblast-like cells, with few if any infiltrating leukocytes.[594,595] An associated tubulointerstitial nephritis with inflammatory cell infiltration and edema is commonly found. Multinucleated giant cells may be present in the crescents or tubulointerstitial regions. Some patients have necrotizing vasculitis of small arteries and arterioles. This is particularly common in those with associated ANCA seropositivity. In biopsies taken later in the course of the glomerulonephritis there is progressive global and segmental sclerosis and interstitial fibrosis. Pulmonary histology reveals intra-alveolar hemorrhage with widening and disruption of the alveolar septa and hemosiderin laden macrophages.[552–555]

The IF findings define the disease process in Goodpasture syndrome and differentiate it from pauci-immune and immune complex-mediated forms of crescentic glomerulonephritis that may have similar light microscopic features. The diagnostic finding is an intense and diffuse linear staining for IgG, especially IgG1 and IgG4, involving GBM's (Fig. 31–22).[569,596,597] Rarely have IgM or IgA been identified in a linear

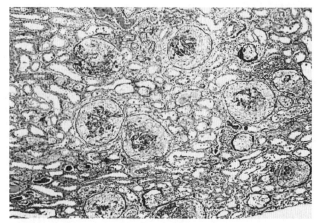

FIGURE 31–21   Goodpasture disease: There is diffuse crescentic glomerulonephritis with large circumferential cellular crescents and severe compression of the glomerular tuft (Periodic acid Schiff, ×80).

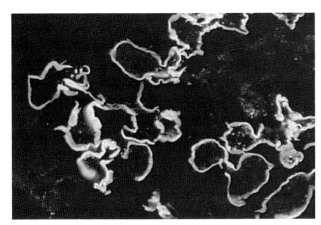

FIGURE 31–22 Goodpasture disease: Immunofluorescence photomicrograph showing linear glomerular basement membrane deposits of IgG. Some of the glomerular basement membranes are discontinuous, indicating sites of rupture (×800).

distribution.[595] C3 deposits are found in a more finely granular GBM distribution in many patients. C1q is typically absent. Linear IF staining with IgG may also be found along the tubular basement membranes in some but not all cases. Fibrin-related antigens are commonly present within the crescents and segmental necrotizing lesions. In the lungs, similar linear deposition of IgG occurs along the alveolar capillary walls.[554]

Electron microscopic analysis of glomeruli in patients with Goodpasture syndrome typically does not reveal any immune type electron-dense deposits. Some rare reports of such deposits may represent partially degraded products of coagulation.[597] There may be widening of the subendothelial space by a semi lucent zone containing fibrin-like material, and gaps in the GBM and in Bowman capsule are commonly present.[595] Rare patients have co-existent membranous glomerulopathy with typical findings by light microscopy, IF, and EM.[582] EM of pulmonary tissue may demonstrate hyperplasia of pneumocytes and alveolar basement membrane thickening.

Course, Treatment, and Prognosis

The course of untreated Goodpasture syndrome is one of progressive renal dysfunction leading to uremia.[552–555,585] Early studies reported almost all patients with the disease dying from either pulmonary hemorrhage or progressive renal failure. Recent studies have shown a marked decrease in mortality to less than 10% probably related to improved supportive care and more rapid diagnosis and treatment.[554,597,598] Some patients have one or more relapses of the pulmonary disease.[599,600] Spontaneous remission of the renal involvement is rare although with therapy many patients will have a stable course and some dramatic improvement of their renal function.[552–555,597,598] If treatment is started early in the course of the disease patients may regain considerable kidney function. The plasma creatinine correlates fairly well with the degree of crescentic involvement of the glomeruli, and if the plasma creatinine is markedly elevated and the patient requires dialysis, most go on to develop ESRD.[554,555,597] A recent study from China in over 100 patients with anti-GBM antibodies noted a poorer prognosis in patients with creatinines over 600 μmol/L, oligo-anuria at presentation, over 85% crescents on biopsy, and renal involvement before pulmonary hemorrhage.

Anti-GBM disease is an uncommon disease with no large randomized studies defining the benefits of any given therapy.

Pulmonary hemorrhage and clinical lung involvement has abated with high-dose oral or intravenous corticosteroid therapy.[552–555,598] Frequently with resolution of pulmonary disease, patients are left with few clinical sequelae or respiratory symptoms. Renal involvement appears less responsive to corticosteroid alone. Plasmapheresis may have a dramatic effect in reversing pulmonary hemorrhage and renal disease when used early in the course in combination with immunosuppressants.[554,597,601–603] Plasmapheresis removes the circulating anti-GBM antibodies whereas immunosuppressive therapy prevents new antibody formation and controls the ongoing inflammatory response. One review of uncontrolled trials found that 40% of patients had stabilized or improved renal function with plasmapheresis.[603] Patients with severe renal failure who are already on dialysis or who have serum creatinines greater than 8 mg/dl are less likely to respond to therapy, but some have recovered.[554,597,602,603] One recent series of patients who were positive for both anti-GBM antibodies and ANCA behaved similar to those with anti-GBM antibodies alone with a 1-year renal survival of 73% in those with a plasma creatinine less than 500 mmoles/L and 0% in those on dialysis.[593] In other series dialysis-dependent patients who are both anti-GBM antibody and ANCA positive are still more likely to recover than patients who are dialysis dependent with only anti-GBM antibody positivity.[586,589–591] One therapy for Goodpasture syndrome includes a combination of prednisone (1 mg/kg/day) or IV pulse methylprednisolone (30 mg/kg/day or 1000 mg/day) for several days followed by high-dose oral therapy along with plasmapheresis and cyclophosphamide (2 mg/kg/day). Although daily plasmapheresis is usually maintained for weeks, its frequency can be determined by the rapidity of clinical response. Exacerbations of disease may occur with intercurrent infections.[600] Immunosuppressive therapy is usually continued for 6 to 12 months with a tapering regimen to allow spontaneous cessation of autoantibody production. Some patients with early disappearance of circulating anti-GBM antibodies may respond to shorter therapy or tolerate change to less toxic immunosuppressives such as azathioprine.[554,555,585] There is limited data on other immunosuppressive regimens such as cyclosporine, and experimental protocols such as using blockade of CD28-B7 T cell costimulatory pathways in Goodpasture syndrome.[604,605] Immunoadsorption has also been used to remove the anti-GBM antibodies in Goodpasture syndrome.[606] Even in patients with initial improvement of renal function, some with severe crescentic glomerular involvement will progress to renal failure over time perhaps related to non-immunologic progression of disease. The incidence of ESRD in patients with significant glomerular involvement is over 50% and the renal outcome is usually progressively downhill unless vigorous prompt therapy is instituted.

Anti-GBM mediated renal disease may recur in the renal allograft.[607–610] As with a number of other forms of glomerulonephritis evidence of histologic recurrence (i.e., linear staining for IgG along GBM's) is far higher than clinical involvement and may be as high as 50%. The low recurrence rate reported in transplants recently probably reflects a combination of waiting sufficient time to document the absence of anti-GBM antibodies, the use of immunosuppressives and plasmapheresis to remove current antibody, and the "one-shot" nature of the disease.[611,612] Patients with recurrence typically have hematuria and proteinuria. Graft loss secondary to recurrent disease is rare. Patients should not be transplanted during the acute phase of their illness when autoantibody levels are high, and prophylactic pretransplant immunosuppression has been recommended for those receiving allografts from living related donors. Although patients with resolving pulmonary disease may have residual diminished gas exchange, most pulmonary function tests return to normal and do not limit the renal transplant process.[613]

Sjögren syndrome is characterized by a chronic inflammatory cell infiltration of the exocrine salivary and lacrimal glands and is associated with the "sicca complex" of xerostomia and xerophthalmia.[614–617] Although this may occur as isolated exocrine gland involvement, patients may have involvement by a systemic inflammatory disease of the kidneys, lungs, esophagus, thyroid, stomach, and pancreas.[614–617] Other patients have manifestations of a collagen vascular disease most commonly rheumatoid arthritis, and less frequently SLE, scleroderma, polymyositis, or MCTD. Still other patients will have different immunologic disorders such as chronic active hepatitis, primary biliary cirrhosis, Crohn disease, and fibrosing alveolitis or develop lymphoma or Waldenström macroglobulinemia. Serologic abnormalities are common in Sjögren syndrome and include hypergammaglobulinemia, rheumatoid factor, cryoglobulins, a homogeneous or speckled pattern ANA, anti-Ro/SSA and anti-La/SSB, but serum complement levels are generally normal unless the patient has associated SLE.[614–617]

The major clinical renal manifestations of patients with Sjögren syndrome usually relate to tubulointerstitial involvement of the kidneys with tubular defects such as a distal RTA, impaired concentrating ability, hypercalciuria, and less frequently proximal tubular defects.[614–621] Most patients do not have clinical evidence of glomerular disease and have relatively negative urinalysis with only mild elevations of the serum creatinine. In one recent analysis of over 470 patients with primary Sjögren syndrome observed for a mean of 10 years only 20 patients (4%) developed overt renal disease.[618] Ten patients had interstitial nephritis on biopsy, eight patients glomerular lesions, and two both lesions. In those infrequent patients with glomerular lesions, hematuria, proteinuria, and renal insufficiency are found. Some patients will develop the full nephrotic syndrome whereas others may develop renal vasculitis with prominent hypertension and renal insufficiency.

In most cases the renal pathology shows prominent tubulointerstitial nephritis with sparing of the glomeruli.[614–618,621] There is a chronic active interstitial inflammation by a predominantly lymphocytic infiltrate occasionally with granuloma formation and with variable interstitial fibrosis and tubular atrophy. By IF, there may be no detectable deposits. However, in some cases tubular basement membrane deposits of IgG and C3 have been described. A nonspecific glomerulosclerosis with mesangial sclerosis, GBM thickening and wrinkling is found in those with chronic and severe tubulointerstitial damage. Infrequently patients will have an immune complex mediated glomerular involvement.[615,616,621–627] In one recent series of biopsied patients with primary Sjögren syndrome, patients had either mesangial proliferative glomerulonephritis or membranoproliferative glomerulonephritis, usually associated with cryoglobulins, on biopsy.[618] In other series patients may have associated features of SLE. As in SLE, the spectrum of glomerular involvement ranges from mesangial proliferative[625] to focal proliferative,[621] diffuse proliferative,[625,626] and membranous nephropathy. A membranoproliferative pattern of proliferative glomerulonephritis has been reported in patients with associated cryoglobulinemia.[624,627] By IF and EM, immune deposits have been localized in the various patterns to the mesangial region or the subendothelial or subepithelial aspect of the GBM as in SLE. Some patients with Sjögren syndrome have a necrotizing arteritis of the kidney occasionally with extra renal involvement.[628] Most patients with severe tubulointerstitial disease and Sjögren syndrome respond to treatment with corticosteroids.[615,629] Patients with immune complex glomerulonephritis and Sjögren syndrome are generally treated in a similar fashion to those with SLE, and those with vasculitis generally receive cytotoxic therapy similar to other necrotizing vasculitides.[615]

SARCOIDOSIS

Most manifestations of sarcoidosis are not related to the kidney.[630] The most common renal findings are interstitial nephritis (typically granulomatous), nephrolithiasis, and tubular functional abnormalities.[631,632] Glomerular disease is infrequent and may be the coincidental expression of two unrelated disease processes in one individual rather than secondary to the sarcoidosis itself. A variety of glomerular lesions have been described in patients with sarcoidosis including minimal change disease, focal segmental glomerulosclerosis, membranous nephropathy, IgA nephropathy, membranoproliferative glomerulonephritis, and proliferative and crescentic glomerulonephritis.[631–642] ANCA-positive crescentic glomerulonephritis has also been reported.[643] The IF and EM features conform to the various histologic patterns. Some patients have granulomatous renal interstitial nephritis in addition to the glomerular lesions, whereas others have only extrarenal histologic documentation of the sarcoidosis. The clinical presentation of glomerular disease in sarcoidosis is usually that of proteinuria, active urinary sediment at times, and most commonly the nephrotic syndrome. Patients have been treated with various forms of immunosuppression including steroids depending on their glomerular lesions.[633–643]

AMYLOIDOSIS

Amyloidosis comprises a diverse group of systemic and local diseases characterized by the extracellular deposition of fibrils in various organs.[644–646] Although the precursor proteins vary, all share an antiparallel beta pleated sheet configuration on X-ray diffraction leading to their amyloidogenic properties and unique staining characteristics.[644–646] All amyloid fibrils bind Congo red (leading to characteristic apple green birefringence under polarized light) and thioflavin T, and have a characteristic ultrastructural appearance. All types of amyloid contain a 25 Kd glycoprotein, serum amyloid P component (SAP), a member of the pentraxin family that includes C-reactive protein. Amyloid deposits may also contain restricted subsets of heparin and dermatan sulfated glycosaminoglycans (GAGS) and proteoglycans non covalently linked to the amyloid fibrils.[647] Amyloid fibrils may be composed of many different proteins, but only some proteins produce deposition in the kidney. In AL amyloidosis, the deposited fibrils are derived from the variable portion of immunoglobulin light chains produced by a clonal population of plasma cells.[644–646] AA amyloid is due to the deposition of serum amyloid A protein in chronic inflammatory states.[644] Forms of hereditary amyloid involving the kidney include mutations in transthyretin, fibrinogen A chain, apolipoprotein A1, lysozyme, apolipoprotein AII, cyclostatin C, and gelosin.[646,648–650] These include two predominantly neuropathic forms and forms related to deposition of a fibrinogen fragment or a fragment of an apolipoprotein variant.[650]

The pathogenesis of amyloidosis remains unclear.[651–655] Because diverse proteins may produce amyloid, co-factors such as amyloid P component may have an important role in the pathogenesis of tissue deposition. These may act by promoting fibrillogenesis, stabilization of the fibrils, binding to matrix proteins, or affect the metabolism and proteolysis of formed fibrils. It is also possible that cofactors are deposited after fibrillogenesis.[646,650–655] It is unclear what factors allow some proteins to aggregate into amyloid fibrils. Amyloid fibrils generally resist biodegradation and accumulate in the tissues resulting in organ dysfunction. However, amyloid deposits have been shown to exist in a dynamic state and have been shown to regress by radiolabeled SAP scintigraphy.[656] Patients with secondary amyloidosis have levels of circulating SAA protein no greater than those patients with inflammatory diseases who do not have amyloid deposition. Therefore, some additional unknown stimulus is required for amyloid fibrils to form and precipitate. In AL amyloid biochemical characteristics of the light chain, such as an aberrant amino acid composition at certain sites, appear important in determining amyloid formation.[654,655] This may account for the reproducibility of a given form of renal disease (cast nephropathy versus amyloid) in animal models infused with monoclonal light chains from affected patients.[657] Certain light chains may also form high molecular weight aggregates in vitro.[658] Macrophage dependent generation of pre amyloid fragments with chemical properties allowing aggregation may also play a role.[658] Amyloid P component may prevent degradation of amyloid fibrils once formed.[659,660]

AL and AA Amyloidosis

In AL amyloidosis, fibrils are composed of the N terminal amino acid residues of the variable region of an immunoglobulin light chain. Lambda light chains predominate over kappa in AL amyloidosis, and there is an increased incidence of monoclonal lambda type VI.[661] Although the diagnosis of AL amyloidosis may be suspected on clinical grounds, confirmation requires biopsy documentation. Organ involvement is quite variable, and the absence of other organ involvement does not exclude amyloidosis as a cause of major renal disease.[644,645] The kidneys are the most common major organ involved by AL amyloid and most patients will eventually have renal amyloid on autopsy.[662] In patients over the age of 60 years old as many as 10% to 20% of patients with presumed idiopathic nephrotic syndrome will have amyloidosis on renal biopsy.[663] Multiple myeloma occurs in up to 20% of primary amyloidosis cases. Amyloidosis should be suspected in all patients with circulating serum monoclonal M proteins, and approximately 90% of primary amyloid patients will have a paraprotein spike in the serum or urine by immunofixation.

The incidence of AL amyloid is about 8 per million annually but varies greatly in different locations.[664] Most patients with AL amyloidosis are over 50 years old (median age 59–63) and less than 1% are under 40 years old. Men are affected twice as often as women.[644,645,662] Presenting symptoms include weight loss, fatigue, light-headedness, shortness of breath, peripheral edema, pain due to peripheral neuropathy, and purpura. Patients may have hepatosplenomegaly, macroglossia, or rarely enlarged lymph nodes. Multisystem organ involvement is typical with most commonly affected organs being the kidney (50%), heart (40%), and peripheral nerves (up to 25%).[644,645,662]

Amyloidosis due to the deposition of AA protein occurs in chronic inflammatory diseases. AA amyloid is composed of the amino terminal end of the acute phase reactant serum amyloid A protein (SAA).[644–647,653,665] SAA is produced in the liver and circulates in association with high density lipoprotein (HDL). AA amyloid is commonly found in rheumatoid arthritis, inflammatory bowel disease, familial Mediterranean fever, quadriplegics with chronic urinary infections and decubitus ulcers, chronic heroin addicts who inject drugs subcutaneously, bronchiectasis, and occasionally in poorly treated osteomyelitis.[644,653,666–669] In an autopsy study of 150 addicts 14% of subcutaneous and 26% of those with chronic suppurative infections had renal amyloidosis.[669] This form of amyloid typically occurs in older addicts with a long history

of substance abuse who have exhausted sites of intravenous access and resorted to skin popping.

The diagnosis of amyloid is usually established by tissue biopsy of an affected organ.[644–648,670] Liver and kidney biopsy are positive in as many as 90% of clinically affected cases. A diagnosis may be made with less invasive techniques with fat pad aspirate (60%–90%), rectal biopsy (50%–80%), bone marrow aspirate (30%–50%), gingival biopsy (60%), or dermal biopsy (50%) in selected series.[670–673] Serum amyloid P whole body scintigraphy, following injection of radiolabeled SAP, may allow the noninvasive diagnosis of amyloidosis as well as allowing quantification of the extent of organ system involvement and non-invasive assessment of the therapeutic response to treatment.[674] This test may be positive even when tissue biopsy has been negative and may be more accurate in AA than in AL amyloidosis. In AL amyloidosis detection of an abnormal ratio of free kappa to lambda light chains in the serum is a new technique to detect plasma cell dyscrasias, which has a higher sensitivity than either serum or urinary electrophoretic techniques.[675] This technique also allows assessment of response to therapy by following the level of abnormal free light chain in the serum.[676] Patients with hereditary amyloidosis due to deposition of abnormal transthyretin, apolipoproteins, lysozyme, and other protein may present in a fashion similar to AL amyloid. In one series 10% of 350 cases of hereditary amyloidosis were misdiagnosed as having AL amyloid.[650,677] Hereditary amyloidosis may present at any age from the second to eighth decade. Although the course is often more prolonged and benign than that of AL amyloid its presentation can be identical. Establishing the correct diagnosis is crucial because the management of hereditary amyloid may include liver transplantation rather than chemotherapy and stem cell transplantation as in AL amyloid.

Clinical manifestations of renal disease depend on the location and extent of amyloid deposition. Renal involvement predominates in AL amyloidosis with one third to one half of patients having renal manifestations at presentation.[644–646] Most patients have proteinuria, approximately 25% have the nephrotic syndrome at diagnosis, and others present with varying degrees of azotemia.[644–646,662] Over time as many as 40% will develop the nephrotic syndrome whereas others have lesser degrees of proteinuria or azotemia. Urinalysis is typically bland but micro hematuria and cellular casts have been reported. Proteinuria is typically nonselective and almost 90% of patients with greater than 1 gram/day urinary protein will have a monoclonal protein in the urine. Hypercholesterolemia is less common than in other forms of the nephrotic syndrome. The amount of glomerular amyloid deposition does not correlate well with the degree of renal dysfunction.[644,645] Despite the literature suggestion of enlarged kidneys in AL amyloid, by ultrasonography most patients have normal-sized kidneys.[644] Hypertension is found in from 20% to 50% of patients, but many will have orthostatic hypotension either due to peripheral neuropathy, autonomic neuropathy, and/or the nephrotic syndrome. Patients with predominantly vascular involvement may have little proteinuria but renal insufficiency due to decreased renal blood flow. Infrequently patients will have predominantly tubular deposition of amyloid with tubular defects such as distal RTA and nephrogenic diabetes insipidus.[644–646,662]

Pathology

In patients with clinical renal disease, the sensitivity of renal biopsy with adequate tissue sampling approaches 100%.[645,678–681] Renal biopsy is useful to distinguish primary AL amyloid from AA amyloid, and to rule out involvement by other renal disease in patients with known amyloidosis of other organ systems.

By LM there is a glomerular deposition of amorphous hyaline material that usually begins in the mesangium and extends into the peripheral capillary walls (Fig. 31–23). This material is eosinophilic, weakly PAS positive, and non argyrophilic. In trichrome-stained sections it may appear lavender or grey-blue. Affected glomeruli appear hypocellular and may have a nodular aspect. In the peripheral GBM, amyloid deposits form spicular hair-like projections that resemble the spikes of membranous glomerulopathy (Fig. 31–24). Congo red stain gives an orange staining reaction and the diagnostic apple green birefringence under polarized light (Fig. 31–25). Amyloid deposits stain metachromatically with crystal or methyl violet and fluoresce under ultraviolet light following thioflavin T staining. Amyloid deposition may be confined to the glomeruli or involve other renal components including tubular basement membranes, interstitium, and blood vessels. IF in AL amyloidosis gives strong staining with antisera to the pathogenic light chain, usually lambda (Fig. 31–26). In AA amyloidosis, immunostaining for immunoglobulins and complement components is generally negative, whereas for SAA protein there is strong reactivity by IF or immunoperoxidase staining (Fig. 31–27). Hereditary amyloidoses should stain neither selectively with a single light chain nor for AA protein. Under EM, typical non branching 8 nm to 12 nm wide fibrils are randomly distributed in the mesangium and along

the GBM in the subepithelial, intramembranous, and subendothelial locations (Fig. 31–28). Mild cases may have deposition limited to the mesangium. More severe cases usually have more extensive deposition in the peripheral capillary walls. By EM glomerular capillary wall deposits may form

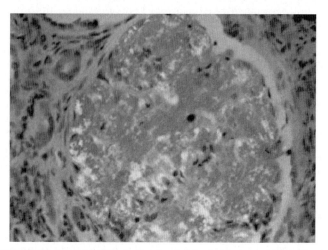

FIGURE 31–25 Amyloidosis: Congo red stain of a glomerulus that is largely replaced by amyloid demonstrates the characteristic birefringence under polarized light (×450).

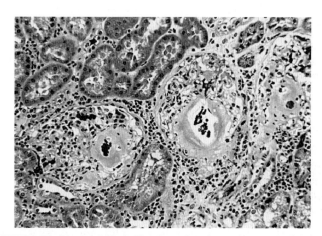

FIGURE 31–23 Amyloidosis: The glomerular tuft contains segmental deposits of amorphous eosinophilic hyaline material involving the vascular pole and some mesangial regions (Hematoxylin-eosin, ×375).

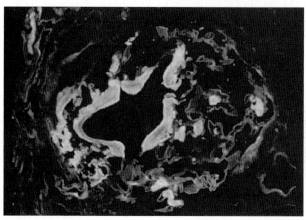

FIGURE 31–26 Amyloidosis: Immunofluorescence photomicrograph showing glomerular staining for lambda light chain in the distribution of the glomerular amyloid deposits in a patient with AL amyloidosis and plasma cell dyscrasia (×600).

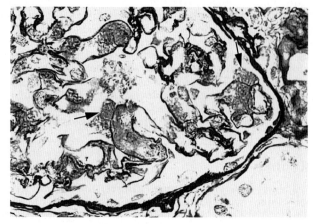

FIGURE 31–24 Amyloidosis: The amyloid deposits expand the mesangium and form focal spicular projections through the glomerular capillary walls, resembling spikes (arrows) (Jones methenamine silver, ×800).

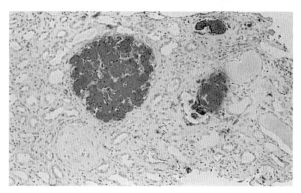

FIGURE 31–27 Amyloidosis: Immunoperoxidase staining for SAA protein outlines the glomeruli and arteries of a patient with secondary AA amyloidosis (×125).

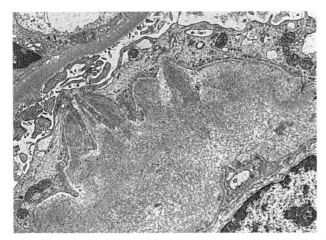

FIGURE 31–28 Amyloidosis: Electron micrograph showing extensive infiltration of the glomerular basement membrane by 10-nm fibrils that project toward the urinary space (×8000).

characteristic spike-like projections along the subepithelial aspect of the glomerular capillary wall.

Course, Prognosis, and Treatment

The prognosis of patients with AL amyloidosis in the past has been poor with some series having a median survival of less than 2 years.[644,645] The baseline serum creatinine at diagnosis and the degree of proteinuria are predictive of the progression to ESRD. The median time from diagnosis to onset dialysis is 14 months, and from dialysis to death only 8 months in some series.[645,662] Recent data suggests improved survival in at least some amyloid patients. Factors associated with decreased patient survival include evidence of cardiac involvement, lambda versus kappa proteinuria, renal dysfunction with an elevated serum creatinine, and interstitial fibrosis on renal biopsy.[662,682] Cardiac involvement with associated heart failure and arrhythmias is the primary cause of death in amyloidosis followed by renal disease.[683,684]

The optimal treatment for AL amyloid differs dependent on age, organ systems involved, and overall health of the patient.[644–647] A number of treatment strategies focus on methods to decrease the production of monoclonal light chains akin to myeloma therapy using chemotherapeutic drugs such as melphalan and prednisone, cyclophosphamide, or VAD therapy. In some patients there has been evidence of resolution of proteinuria, stabilization of renal function, improvement of symptoms, and occasionally evidence of decreased organ involvement such as decreased hepatosplenomegaly.[685] In a review of 153 AL amyloid patients treated with melphalan and prednisone only 18% of the patients had a regression of organ manifestations of amyloidosis with responders having a 5-year survival of 78% versus only 7% in the non-responders.[686] Patients with renal amyloidosis fared best with 25% having a 50% resolution in nephrotic range proteinuria and stable or improved GFR. Colchicine was used to manage AL amyloidosis in the past.[687] Most trials have demonstrated a clear benefit of chemotherapeutic options over colchicine, and even the addition of colchicine to these regimens provided only a small benefit.[688,689] A study compared therapy with melphalan, prednisone, and colchicine therapy to colchicine alone in 100 consecutive patients seen between 1987 and 1992.[688] The group receiving combined chemotherapy plus colchicine had less long-term mortality than the colchicine group.

Another study of 220 AL amyloid patients randomized to colchicine, melphalan plus prednisone, or all three drugs found a median survival of 8.5 months for the colchicine

group as opposed to 17 to 18 months for the other groups.[689] Eighteen percent of the chemotherapy groups had a 50% decrease in proteinuria as opposed to 6% of the colchicine group. However, renal failure developed in a similar percentage, 14% to 21% of each of the three groups. Thus, current therapy focuses on chemotherapy. A recent prospective trial in over 100 patients compared an intensive regimen with five agents (vincristine, BCNU, melphalan, cyclophosphamide, and prednisone) to melphalan and prednisone alone. This showed no survival advantage for the intensive treatment group over the standard therapy.[690]

Other therapies for primary amyloid used experimentally to treat small numbers of patients include dimethyl sulfoxide, 4′-iodo-4′-deoxydoxorubicin, fludarabine, vitamin E, and interferon alpha-2.[644,691–694] None has proven efficacy at this time. High-dose dexamethasone therapy has been suggested to have benefits in isolated patients, but in a trial of 25 patients it yielded only a 12% response rate and a 14-month mean survival time.[695] Recent reports using high-dose melphalan followed by allogeneic bone marrow transplant or stem cell transplant have given promising results.[696–700]

The use of high-dose chemotherapy followed by peripheral blood stem cell transplantation has led to resolution of the nephrotic syndrome and biopsy proven improvement of amyloid organ involvement in isolated cases.[697–701] Although there was a high mortality in early reports (20% in the first 3 months), 60% of the survivors had a complete hematologic response and at 2 years over two thirds of the patients were alive.[697] Of those patients with renal involvement all survived and two thirds had a 50% decrease in proteinuria without a worsening of GFR. One retrospective study analyzed 65 AL amyloid patients with over 1 g daily proteinuria treated with dose-intensive ablative chemotherapy followed by autologous blood stem-cell transplantation.[702] Three fourths of the patients survived the first year and among those a good renal response was found in 36% at 1 year and 52% at 2 years. Patients with a complete hematologic response were more likely to have a good renal response and patient survival was superior in patients with less than three organ systems involved, younger patients, and those able to tolerate higher doses of the ablative therapy. Toxicities included mucositis, edema, elevated liver function tests, pulmonary edema, gastrointestinal bleeding, and in 23% transient acute renal failure. Thus, for younger patients with predominantly renal involvement stem cell transplantation is currently a reasonable alternative therapy for AL amyloid. Subsequent studies from other centers have supported stem cell transplantation as a beneficial therapy for some patients with AL amyloid.[703] Even patients with ESRD due to amyloidosis may undergo this form of therapy with results no different from non-ESRD patients with AL amyloidosis.[704]

Regardless of whether chemotherapy or marrow transplant is used, the treatment of amyloid patients with nephrotic syndrome involves supportive care. This may include judicious use of diuretics and salt restriction in those with edema, treatment of orthostatic hypotension with compression stockings, fludrocortisone, and in some midodrine, an oral alpha adrenergic agonist.[644,705]

The management of AA amyloid focuses on the management of the underlying inflammatory disease process. This has included surgical debridement of inflammatory tissue, antibiotic therapy of infectious processes, and anti-inflammatory medications and immunosuppressive agents in rheumatoid arthritis and inflammatory bowel disease. Therapy may lead to stabilization of renal function, reduction in proteinuria, and partial resolution of amyloid deposits. Prognosis may be good if the underlying disease can be controlled and there is not already extensive amyloid deposition. Alkylating agents have been used to control AA amyloidosis secondary to rheumatologic diseases in a number of studies with evidence of increased GFR and decreased proteinuria, with prolonged renal survival.[706,707] Similar results have been achieved with other immunosuppressive agents with improvement in proteinuria, prolonged survival compared with controls, and in several cases regression of amyloid deposits on repeat biopsy.[644]

In familial Mediterranean fever, an autosomal recessive disease primarily found in Sephardic Jews, Turks, Armenians, and Arabs, there are recurrent attacks of fever and serositis associated with the development of AA amyloidosis in up to 90% of untreated patients.[708] Colchicine has long been used successfully to prevent the febrile attacks and was effective in preventing the development of proteinuria and stabilizing proteinuria in other patients.[708] However, renal function did deteriorate in all patients with the nephrotic syndrome at presentation. A retrospective analysis of FMF patients with milder renal clinical involvement and at least 5 years' follow-up concluded that high doses of colchicine were more effective in preventing renal dysfunction, and that patients with lower levels of serum creatinine at presentation responded better to therapy.[708] Once the serum creatinine level was elevated, however, increasing the dose of colchicine did not seem to prevent progression to ESRD. Secondary amyloidosis seen in drug abusers with suppurative skin lesions secondary to subcutaneous injection of drugs has occasionally responded to colchicine therapy, although most investigators feel the key to improvement appears to be management of the underlying infections and cessation of skin popping.[669,709]

A recent multicenter randomized controlled trial compared a GAG mimetic, used to inhibit the binding between heparin sulfate, perlecan, and the amyloid fibril protein and thus block fibrillogenesis, to placebo in 183 patients with AA amyloid. Although the specified end point of the study was not achieved, the GAG mimetic did reduce the risk of doubling the serum creatinine by 54% and halved the risk of a 50% decrease in creatinine clearance.[710] This study clearly shows the need for newer therapies for amyloidosis and the value of controlled trials in studying these agents.[710] Several promising experimental therapies for managing amyloid include using anti-amyloid antibodies, and the use of an inhibitor of the binding of amyloid P component to amyloid fibrils.[647]

End-Stage Renal Disease in Amyloidosis

In most series the median survival of amyloid patients with ESRD is less than 1 year with the primary cause of death being complications of cardiac amyloid.[711,712] However, for patients who survive the first month of ESRD replacement therapy the survival rate is over 50% at 2 years and 30% at 5 years.[712] This is still 20% lower than an age-matched general ESRD population. There appears to be no survival advantage to the use of a specific dialytic technique such as peritoneal dialysis or hemodialysis.[712] Experience with renal transplantation is largely in patients with AA amyloid and is limited in AL amyloid.[713,714] One series on transplantation in amyloid included 45 patients (with 42 with AA amyloid) and found an overall low patient survival, particularly in the early posttransplant period in older patients due to infectious and cardiovascular complications.[713] Graft survival, however, was not decreased despite rates of recurrence of amyloidosis in the allograft as high as 20% to 33%.[713–715]

Fibrillary Glomerulonephritis and Immunotactoid Glomerulonephritis

Patients with glomerular lesions may have fibrillar deposition differing in size from that of amyloid and without the typical staining properties of amyloid.[644,716–720] In the past similar patients were reported as having Congo red-negative amyloid, amyloid-like glomerulopathy, and non-amyloidotic fibrillary glomerulopathy. Many investigators have subdivided these patients into two major groups depending on clinical associations and fibril size. In fibrillary GN the fibrils are approximately 16 nm to 24 nm (mean 20 nm) in diameter and in immunotactoid GN there are larger microtubules of 30 nm to 50 nm in diameter. It has been suggested that the fibrils represent a slow-acting cryoprecipitate of polyclonal or monoclonal immunoglobulin.[721] A third rare form of fibrillary renal disease is fibronectin glomerulopathy in which the glomeruli are involved with massive deposition of fibronectin.[722–724]

Although some would choose to classify both fibrillary GN and immunotactoid GN as a single disease entity, most clinicians and nephropathologists would divide them into distinct disorders.[644,716–720] Almost 90% of cases have the smaller 20 nM fibrils of fibrillary glomerulopathy.[716–720] Fibrillary GN occurs mostly in adults, in both sexes, in all age groups, and most commonly in whites. It is usually an isolated renal entity. Patients with immunotactoid GN tend to be older, may have a less rapidly progressive course, and in all series are more likely to have an associated lymphoproliferative disease often with a circulating paraprotein.[716–720] Patients with both disease usually have proteinuria, and most have hypertension and hematuria. About 70% have the nephrotic syndrome at biopsy, but this may represent a bias in biopsy selection. At presentation renal insufficiency is common and most patients progress to ESRD. The course to ESRD appears to be more rapid than in patients with renal amyloidosis, particularly in older patients, those with an elevated serum creatinine, and those with crescentic lesions on biopsy. Fibronectin GN is a familial disease with probable autosomal dominant inheritance that presents with proteinuria and hematuria usually in adolescents and eventually progresses to the nephrotic syndrome and slow deteriorating renal function.[722–724]

The diagnosis of all of these fibrillary diseases is made solely on renal biopsy.[716–720,725] LM findings in fibrillary glomerulonephritis are highly variable and include mesangial proliferation, mesangial expansion by amorphous amyloidlike material, membranous, membranoproliferative, and crescentic glomerulonephritis (Fig. 31–29). In immunotactoid glomerulonephritis, glomerular lesions are often nodular and sclerosing whereas others are proliferative or membranous (Fig. 31–30). The pathognomonic findings are seen on EM and consist of non branching fibrils of 16 nm to 24 nm in diameter in fibrillary glomerulopathy (as opposed to 8 nm–12 nm for amyloid) (Fig. 31–31) and hollow microtubules of 30 nm to 50 nm in immunotactoid glomerulonephritis (Fig. 31–32). In fibrillary glomerulonephritis, fibrils are arranged randomly in the mesangial matrix and GBMs. By contrast the microtubules of immunotactoid glomerulopathy are often arranged in parallel stacks. The fibrils and microtubules do not stain with Congo red or thioflavin T. In fibrillary GN, IF is almost always positive for IgG (Fig. 31–33) (especially subclass IgG4), C3, and both kappa and lambda chains.[716–720,725] Staining for IgM, IgA, and C1 has been reported in a minority of cases. In immunotactoid glomerulonephritis, the immunoglobulin deposits are often monoclonal. In both diseases the fibril-related deposits are usually limited to the glomerulus. In fibronectin GN the fibrils may be admixed with more granular glomerular electron-dense deposits.[722–724] Rare patients with fibrillary glomerulopathy have been reported to have extrarenal deposits involving alveolar capillaries, and in the case of immunotactoid GN, the bone marrow.[726,727]

No proven therapy for fibrillary GN is known. Some clinicians choose to treat the LM pattern observed on renal biopsy

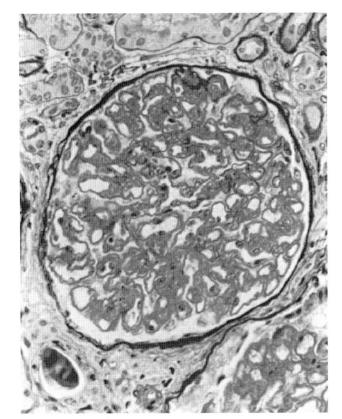

FIGURE 31-29 Fibrillary glomerulonephritis: The mesangium is mildly expanded and the capillary basement membranes appear thickened with segmental double contours (Periodic acid Schiff, ×300).

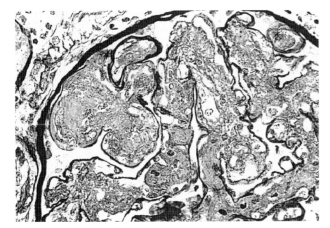

FIGURE 31-30 Immunotactoid glomerulopathy: There is lobular expansion of the glomerular tuft by abundant mesangial deposits of silver-negative material. Segmental extension of deposits into the subendothelial aspect of some glomerular capillaries is also seen (Jones methenamine silver, ×500).

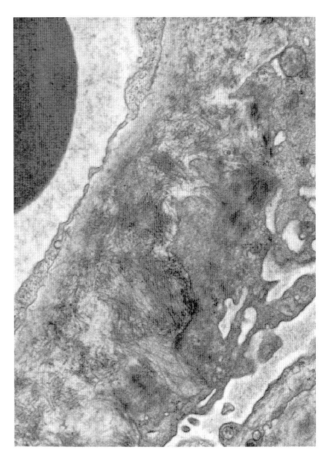

FIGURE 31-31 Fibrillary glomerulonephritis: Electron micrograph showing the characteristic randomly oriented fibrils, measuring 16–20 nm within the glomerular basement membrane. The foot processes are effaced (×8,000).

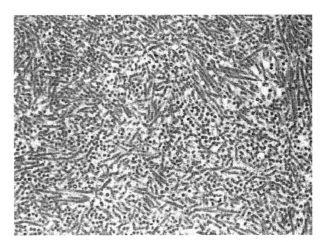

FIGURE 31-32 Immunotactoid glomerulopathy: Electron micrograph showing abundant mesangial deposits of tubulo-fibrillar structures measuring approximately 35 nm in diameter (×10,000).

FIGURE 31-33 Fibrillary glomerulonephritis: Immunofluorescence photomicrograph showing smudgy deposits of IgG throughout the mesangium, with segmental extension into the peripheral glomerular capillary walls (×800).

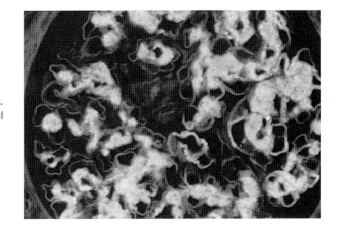

CH 31

Secondary Glomerular Disease

(e.g., membranous, crescentic GN) and ignore the presence of the precipitated fibrils.[644,716] Prednisone, cyclophosphamide, and colchicine have not led to consistent benefit in most patients.[644,716,717] However, in some patients with crescentic GN, cyclophosphamide and corticosteroid therapy has led to a dramatic improvement of GFR and proteinuria with some patients being able to discontinue dialytic support. Cyclosporine has also been used successfully in some patients with fibrillary GN and a membranous pattern on light microscopy.[644] In patients with associated with CLL, treatment with chemotherapy has been associated with improved renal function and decreased proteinuria.[644,716] Dialysis and transplantation have been performed in fibrillary GN but there is a recurrence of disease in one half of patients.[716,728–730]

Monoclonal Immunoglobulin Deposition Disease

Monoclonal immunoglobulin deposition disease (MIDD), which includes light chain deposition disease (LCDD), light and heavy chain deposition disease (LCDD/HCDD), and heavy chain deposition disease (HCDD), is a systemic disease caused by the overproduction and extracellular deposition of a monoclonal immunoglobulin protein.[731–735] LCDD is by far the most common pattern. As opposed to amyloidosis, in LCDD the deposits in approximately 80% of cases are composed of kappa rather than lambda light chains.[731–738] The deposits are also granular in nature, do not form fibrils or beta pleated sheets, do not bind Congo red stain or thioflavine-T, and are not associated with amyloid P protein.[731–738] In amyloid the fibrils are usually derived from the variable region of the light chains, whereas in LCDD it is usually the constant region of the immunoglobulin light chain that is deposited. This may explain the far brighter IF staining for light chains found in LCDD as opposed to amyloidosis. The pathogenesis of the glomerulosclerosis in LCDD is not entirely clear but mesangial cells from patients with LCDD produce transforming growth factor-β, which acting as an autacoid in turn promotes these cells to produce matrix proteins such as type IV collagen, laminin, and fibronectin.[739]

Patients with LCDD are generally over 45 years old.[731–739] Many such patients develop frank myeloma and others clearly have a lymphoplasmacytic B cell disease such as lymphoma or Waldenström macroglobulinemia.[734–737] Even in such patients without an overt plasma cell dyscrasia, it is excessive production of abnormal monoclonal light chains that produce the disease. As in amyloidosis, the clinical features vary with the location and extent of organ deposition of the monoclonal protein. Patients typically have cardiac, neural, hepatic, and renal involvement, but other organs such as the skin, spleen, thyroid, adrenal, and gastrointestinal tract may be involved.[731–739] Patients with renal involvement usually have significant glomerular involvement and thus present with proteinuria, with the nephrotic syndrome in up to one half. This is often accompanied by hypertension and renal insufficiency. Some patients may have greater tubulointerstitial involvement and less proteinuria along with renal insufficiency.[737]

The glomerular pattern by LM is usually nodular sclerosing with mesangial nodules of acellular eosinophilic material resembling the nodular glomerulosclerosis seen in diabetic glomerulosclerosis (Fig. 31–34).[731–740] Glomerular capillary microaneurysms may also be found.[741] Some glomeruli have associated membranoproliferative features. In LCDD the nodules are more strongly PAS positive and less argyrophilic than in diabetes.[731,742] Unlike diabetic glomerulosclerosis the GBMs in LCDD are not usually thickened by LM. Other glomeruli may be entirely normal or have only mild mesangial

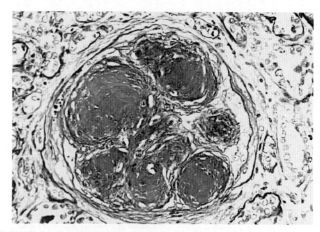

FIGURE 31–34 Light chain deposition disease: There is nodular glomerulosclerosis with marked global expansion of the mesangium by intensely PAS-positive material, but without appreciable thickening of the glomerular capillary walls (Periodic acid Schiff, ×375).

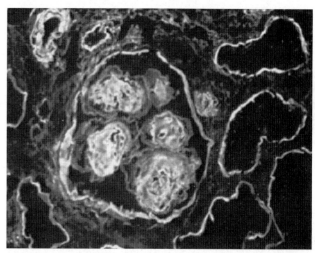

FIGURE 31–35 Light chain deposition disease: Immunofluorescence photomicrograph showing linear staining for kappa light chain involving glomerular and tubular basement membranes, the mesangial nodules, Bowman capsule, and vessel walls (×250).

sclerosis. IF is usually diagnostic with a monoclonal light chain (kappa in 80%) staining in a diffuse linear pattern along the GBMs, in the nodules, and along the tubular basement membranes and vessel walls (Fig. 31–35).[731–738] Staining for complement components is usually negative. By EM deposition of a finely granular punctate electron-dense material occurs along the lamina rara interna of the GBM in the mesangium and along tubular and vascular basement membranes.[731–738,742]

The prognosis for patients with LCDD is uncertain and appears to be better than that for AL amyloidosis. As in amyloidosis death is often attributed to cardiac disease and heart failure or infectious complications.[731–738,740] In one recent large series of 63 patients 65% of patients developed myeloma.[735] Of the total 63 patients 36 developed uremia and 37 died. Predictors of worse renal outcome included increased age and elevated serum creatinine at presentation. Predictors of worse patient survival included increased age, occurrence of frank myeloma, and extrarenal deposition of light chains. Treatment with melphalan and prednisone, as in amyloid, has led to stabilized or improved renal function in LCDD. However, this therapy is not successful in patients with

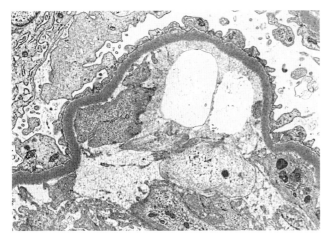

FIGURE 31-36 Heavy chain deposition disease: Electron micrograph showing band-like finely granular electron-dense deposits involving the glomerular basement membrane, with greatest intensity along the inner aspect (×5000).

significant renal dysfunction and a plasma creatinine above 4 mg/dl at initiation of treatment.[740] Patient survival is about 90% at 1 year and 70% at 5 years, with renal survival 67% and 37% at 1 and 5 years.[740] Patients with LCDD and associated cast nephropathy have a worse renal and patient survival. Marrow or stem cell transplantation may be the optimal treatment for many patients with LCDD in the future.[731,735] Although there is little data on dialysis and transplantation in LCDD, patients appear to fare as well as those with amyloidosis. Recurrences in the renal transplant have been reported [731,737,740,743–745] and one recent trial of seven patients with LCDD who received renal transplants found recurrences in five of seven in a mean time of less than 1 year.[746] Thus, suppression of the abnormal paraprotein producing cel clone is crucial prior to renal transplantation.

In some patients with a plasma cell dyscrasia either both light and heavy immunoglobulin chains (LCDD/HCDD) or truncated heavy chains alone (HCDD) are deposited in the tissue (Fig. 31–36).[731,732,736,747,748] The clinical features are similar to those of LCDD and amyloidosis.[731,748] Most patients are middle age or older although at least one patient has been 35 years of age. They present with renal insufficiency, proteinuria, hypertension, and often the nephrotic syndrome. In most patients a monoclonal protein is detected in the serum or urine. In contrast to amyloid and LCDD, HCDD often manifests hypocomplementemia.[748] All patients with HCDD have a deletion of the CH1 domain of the heavy chain, which causes it to be secreted prematurely from the plasma cell.[748–751] The characteristic light microscopic finding in HCDD is a nodular sclerosing glomerulopathy at times with crescents.[731,748] The diagnosis is made by IF with linear positivity for the heavy chain of immunoglobulin (usually gamma) and negativity for both kappa and lambda light chains.[748] The distribution is diffuse involving glomerular, tubular, and vascular basement membranes. Treatment has been similar to LCDD, and most patients have progressed to renal failure. Recurrence in the renal transplant has been documented with eventual loss of the allograft.[731]

Glomerular Disease in Myeloma and Benign Gammopathies

Patients with plasma cell dyscrasia may develop pathology in the tubulo-interstitial, glomerular, and vascular compartments.[752] Glomerular and vascular lesions are usually restricted to those patients with associated AL amyloidosis or monoclonal light or heavy chain deposition disease (or both)(see Amyloid and MIDD). In myeloma cast nephropathy, there are severe tubulo-interstitial lesions. The glomeruli are usually spared and appear normal by LM or have only mild GBM thickening or minor amounts of mesangial matrix deposition without mesangial hypercellularity. Recently patients with a proliferative glomerulonephritis resembling immune complex glomerulonephritis have been described in patients with plasma cell disorders.[753] These patients presented with renal insufficiency and proteinuria with many having the nephrotic syndrome, but no evidence of cryoglobulinemia. On biopsy all had granular electron-dense deposits in the mesangial, subendothelial, and subepithelial sites, but by IF these were restricted to a single monoclonal gamma subclass and light chain isotype (e.g., IgG1kappa or IgG2lambda). No patient developed overt myeloma or lymphoma during the follow-up period. In rare cases intracellular glomerular crystals within the podocytes have been noted, sometimes in association with tubular epithelial crystalline deposits.[754,755] Pamidronate-associated focal sclerosis has been noted in myeloma[756] as have crescentic glomerulonephritis and membranoproliferative glomerulonephritis have been reported rarely, particularly in patients with associated cryoglobulinemia.

Monoclonal gammopathies of undetermined significance (MGUS), also known as benign gammopathies, are premalignant plasma cell disorders that occur in 3.2% of the population over 50 years of age.[757] The prevalence of MGUS increases with age from 5% of those over 70 years old to 7.5% of those 85 years of age or older. Patients with benign monoclonal gammopathies have an abnormal circulating immunoglobulin and abnormal clonal proliferation of plasma cells producing this protein without evidence of myeloma, amyloidosis, Waldenström macroglobulinemia, or other dysproteinemia.[757] Only a small percentage of these patients will progress to myeloma or other clinically relevant plasma cell dyscrasia. Clinical renal disease is uncommon in patients with true benign monoclonal gammopathy and only some patients will have mild proteinuria or hematuria.[752]

The literature on the pathology of this disorder is complicated by the fact that not all patients have had IF or EM evaluation making it possible that some actually had amyloidosis, light chain deposition disease, or cryoglobulinemia. By LM most patients with benign monoclonal gammopathies have had mild or focal proliferative glomerular lesions.[752] Some patients have a more severe and diffuse proliferative glomerulonephritis with invading polymorphonuclear cells and macrophages whereas others have been reported to have membranoproliferative picture, membranous or minimal change pattern. Few biopsies have been examined by IF but those studied with a proliferative glomerulonephritis have glomerular immunoglobulin deposits corresponding to the circulating monoclonal immunoglobulin. Other patients have had deposits of IgG, and IgM and C3. By EM patients with minimal change and membranous nephropathy have had findings similar to patients without a monoclonal paraproteinemia. Other patients have had fibrillar deposits along the GBM or crystalline deposits in endothelial cells. Some have a rapidly progressive glomerulonephritis.[758,759] Again it is unclear if these patients have had a coexistent cryoglobulinemia or other disorder.

WALDENSTRÖM MACROGLOBULINEMIA

Waldenström macroglobulinemia is a syndrome in which patients have an abnormal circulating monoclonal IgM protein

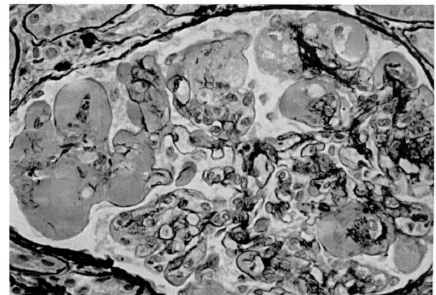

FIGURE 31-37 Waldenström macroglobulinemia: Large Aprotein thrombi corresponding to the monoclonal IgM deposits fill the glomerular capillary lumina, with minimal associated glomerular hypercellularity (Jones methenamine silver, ×600).

in association with a B cell lymphoproliferative disorder involving small lymphocytes.[760-763] This slowly progressive disorder occurs in older patients (median age 60 with a slight male predominance) who present with fatigue, weight loss, bleeding, visual disturbances, peripheral neuropathy, and with hepatosplenomegaly, lymphadenopathy, anemia, and often hyperviscosity syndrome.[760-763] Renal involvement is uncommon, but glomerular lesions are found in some patients.[764,765] Renal involvement is usually manifested by microscopic hematuria and proteinuria, which may be nephrotic or at lower levels. In some cases it is due to excreted light chains. Patients may have enlarged kidneys. The pathology seen in Waldenström macroglobulinemia is varied.[764,765] Some patients will have invasion of the renal parenchyma by neoplastic lymphoplasmacytic cells. Acute renal failure associated with intraglomerular occlusive thrombi of the IgM paraprotein has also been reported. These cases have large eosinophilic, amorphous, PAS positive, deposits occluding the glomerular capillary loops with little or no glomerular hypercellularity (Fig. 31–37). By IF these glomerular "thrombi" stain for IgM and a single light chain, consistent with monoclonal IgM deposits, but complement components are usually negative. By EM the deposits contain non-amyloid fibrillar or amorphous electron-dense material.[766] Some patients develop membranoproliferative glomerulonephritis with an associated Type 1 or Type 2 cryoglobulinemia (Fig. 31–38). Cases of LCDD have also been reported. At times intratubular casts similar to those of myeloma cast nephropathy may be present. Amyloid has been found in a number of patients with Waldenström macroglobulinemia. Management of Waldenström macroglobulinemia is directed against the lymphoproliferative disease with alkylating agents, melphalan, and prednisone, and at times plasmapheresis for hyperviscosity signs and symptoms as well as newer therapies including fludarabine, cladribine, α-interferon, and Rituximab, and marrow transplantation.[767-769]

MIXED CRYOGLOBULINEMIA

Cryoglobulinemia refers to a pathologic condition caused by the production of circulating immunoglobulins that precipitate upon cooling and resolubilize on warming.[770-773] Cryoglobulinemia is associated with a variety of infections, especially hepatitis C virus (see later) as well as collagen-

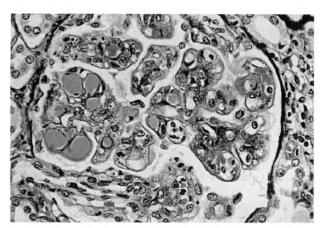

FIGURE 31-38 Waldenström macroglobulinemia: An example with cryoglobulinemic glomerulonephritis showing the characteristic intraluminal deposits, infiltrating leukocytes, and double contoured glomerular basement membranes (Jones methenamine silver, ×600).

vascular disease, and lymphoproliferative diseases. Cryoglobulins have been divided into three major groups based on the nature of the circulating immunoglobulins.[770-772] In type I cryoglobulinemia the cryoglobulin is a single monoclonal immunoglobulin often found associated with Waldenström macroglobulinemia or myeloma.[773] Both Type II and Type III cryoglobulinemia are defined as mixed cryoglobulins, containing a least two immunoglobulins. In Type II a monoclonal immunoglobulin (IgM kappa in over 90%) is directed against polyclonal IgG and has rheumatoid factor activity.[774] In Type III the antiglobulin is polyclonal in nature with both polyclonal IgG and IgM in most cases. The majority of patients with Type II and III mixed cryoglobulins have now been clearly shown to have HCVirus infection.[775,776] To establish a diagnosis of cryoglobulinemia, the offending cryoglobulins or the characteristic renal tissue involvement must be demonstrated. Hypocomplementemia, especially of the early components C1q-C4, is a characteristic and often helpful finding.

In the past in 30% of all mixed cryoglobulinemias there was no clear etiology and the name essential mixed cryoglobulinemia was appropriate.[770,771,776-778] The disease was uncommon but not rare, and it occurred predominantly in adult females. Systemic manifestation of mixed cryoglobulinemia included weakness, malaise, Raynaud phenomena, arthralgias-arthritis, hepato-splenomegaly with abnormal liver function tests in two thirds to three quarters of patients, peripheral neuropathy, and purpuric-vasculitic skin lesions.[770-774,776,777] Low levels of total complement and especially C4 levels are common.

Renal disease occurs at presentation in less than one fourth of patients, but develops in as many as 50% over time.[770-772,775-777] In up to one quarter to one third of patients an acute nephritic picture with hematuria, hypertension, proteinuria, and acute renal insufficiency develops. An oliguric rapidly progressive GN picture is present only rarely. About 20% of patients present with the nephrotic syndrome. The majority of patients with renal disease have a slow indolent renal course characterized by proteinuria, hypertension, hematuria, and renal insufficiency.

Many studies of Type II cryoglobulinemia have shown evidence of hepatitis B infection or other viral infections (e.g., Epstein-Barr virus).[779,780] However, recent studies have clearly documented HCV as a major cause of cryoglobulin production in most patients previously felt to have essential mixed cryoglobulinemia.[775,781-783] Antibodies to HCV antigens have been documented in the serum and HCV RNA and anti-HCV antibodies are enriched in the cryoglobulins of these patients.[775,781-785] This is true even for patients with normal levels of aminotransferases and no clinical evidence of hepatitis. HCV antigens have also been localized by immunohistochemistry in the glomerular deposits.[783]

In cryoglobulinemia immunoglobulin complexes deposit in the glomeruli and small and medium-sized arteries binding complement and inciting a proliferative response.[775,777] The serum cryoglobulin has been clearly shown to participate in the formation of the glomerular immune complex. In vitro studies have shown that IgM kappa rheumatoid factor from patients with Type II cryoglobulinemia are much more likely to bind to cellular fibronectin (a component of the glomerular mesangium) than IgM from patients with Waldenström's, normal controls, or IgM containing rheumatoid factor from rheumatoid arthritis patients.[786] The particular physicochemical characteristics of the variable region of the immunoglobulin cryoglobulin may be important in the localization of the renal deposits.

Although by LM the glomerular lesions of cryoglobulinemia may show a variety of proliferative and sclerosing features (Fig. 31–39), certain features help to distinguish the

proliferative GN of essential mixed cryoglobulinemia from other proliferative glomerulonephritides.[770,773,774,782] These include massive exudation of monocytes and to a lesser degree polymorphonuclear leukocytes; amorphous eosinophilic PAS positive, Congo red negative deposits on the inner side of the glomerular capillary wall and sometimes filling the lumens; membranoproliferative features with double contoured GBMs and interposition of deposits, mesangial cells, and monocytes; and the rarity of extracapillary proliferation despite the intense intracapillary proliferation. The glomerular lesions may be accompanied by an acute vasculitis of small- or medium-sized vessels. The monocytes of patients with active cryoglobulinemia and associated nephritis have been shown to phagocytose cryoglobulins but to be unable to catabolize them. By IF (Fig. 31–40), the glomeruli in Type II or Type III cryoglobulinemia contain deposits of both IgM as well as IgG with C3 and frequently C1q in the distribution of subendothelial and mesangial deposits and the intracapillary "thrombi". By EM (Fig. 31–41), deposits present in the subendothelial position or filling the capillary lumens, often appear as either amorphous electron-dense deposits or organized deposits of curvilinear parallel fibrils that appear tubular in cross section and have a diameter of 20 nM to 35 nM.[770,772,786,787]

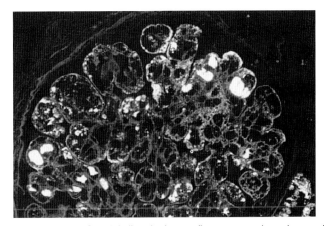

FIGURE 31–40 Cryoglobulinemia: Immunofluorescence photomicrograph showing deposits of IgM corresponding to the large glomerular intracapillary deposits, with more finely granular subendothelial deposits outlining the glomerular capillary walls (×900).

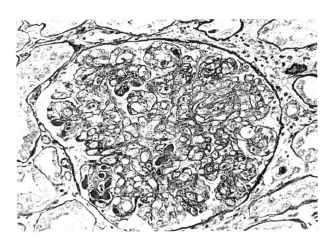

FIGURE 31–39 Cryoglobulinemia: There is global endocapillary proliferative glomerulonephritis with membranoproliferative features and focal intraluminal cryoglobulin deposits, forming Athrombi (Periodic acid Schiff, ×375).

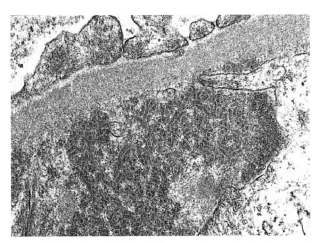

FIGURE 31–41 Cryoglobulinemia: Electron micrograph showing organized subendothelial deposits with an annular-tubular substructure. These curvilinear tubular structures measure approximately 30 nm in diameter (×30,000).

Some patients with mixed cryoglobulinemia will have a partial or total remission of their disease whereas most have episodic exacerbations of their systemic and renal disease.[770,782] Before the association of mixed cryoglobulinemia and HCV was discovered, many patients were treated successfully with prednisone and cytotoxic agents such as cyclophosphamide and chlorambucil.[770,772] None was used in a controlled fashion. In patients with severe renal disease, in those with digital necrosis from the cryoglobulins, and in those with life-threatening organ involvement, plasmapheresis has also been used in combination with steroids and cytotoxics.[778,789,782] Currently most patients with HCV-associated cryoglobulinemia are treated with antiviral agents.[790,791] (See section on Hepatitis C Virus.) Aggressive immunosuppressive therapy carries the risk of promoting HCV replication in HCV-infected patients and of lymphoma in others. Most patients with cryoglobulinemia in the past did not die of renal disease, but rather of cardiac or other systemic disease and infectious complications.[789] Rituximab has recently been used successfully for management of Type II mixed cryoglobulinemia in patients with and without evidence of HCV infection.[792] Dialysis and transplantation in cryoglobulinemia have been used, but recurrences in the allograft have been reported.[793-795]

HEREDITARY NEPHRITIS INCLUDING ALPORT SYNDROME

Alport syndrome is an inherited (usually X-linked) disorder with characteristic glomerular pathology, frequently associated with hearing loss and ocular abnormalities. Guthrie first reported a family with recurrent hematuria.[796] Alport reported additional observations on this family, the occurrence of deafness associated with hematuria, and the observation that affected males died of uremia whereas affected females lived to an old age.[797] Since then, several hundred unrelated kindreds exhibiting hereditary nephritis, with and without deafness, have been described, representing a wide variety of geographic and ethnic groups.[798-804] Alport syndrome accounts for 2.5% of children and 0.3% of adults with end-stage renal disease in the United States.[805]

Clinical Features

The disease usually manifests in children or young adults.[802,803,806] Males have persistent microscopic hematuria, with episodic gross hematuria, which may be exacerbated by respiratory infections or exercise. There may be flank pain or abdominal discomfort accompanying these episodes. Proteinuria is usually mild at first and increases progressively with age. The nephrotic syndrome has also been described.[807] Hypertension is a late manifestation. Slowly progressive renal failure is common in males. End-stage renal disease usually occurs in males between the ages of 16 and 35. In some kindred, the course may be more delayed with renal failure occurring between 45 and 65 years of age. In most females, the disease is mild and only partially expressed, however, some females have experienced renal failure.[808] In the European Community Alport Syndrome Concerted Action (ECASCA) cohort, hematuria was observed in 95% of carriers and consistently absent in the others. Proteinuria, hearing loss, and ocular defects developed in 75%, 28%, and 15%, respectively.[809] This variability in disease severity in females can be explained by the degree of random inactivation of the mutated versus wild-type X chromosome due to Lyonization.

High-frequency sensorineural deafness occurs in 30% to 50% of patients. Hearing impairment is always accompanied by renal involvement. The severity of hearing loss is variable

and there is no relation between the severity of hearing loss and of the renal disease. Based on brain stem auditory evoked responses, the site of the aural lesion is in the cochlea.[810,811] Families with hereditary nephritis, but without sensorineural hearing loss have been described.[811,812]

Ocular abnormalities occur in 15% to 30% of patients.[813] Anterior lenticonus, which is the protrusion of the central portion of the lens into the anterior capsule, is virtually pathognomonic of Alport syndrome. Other ocular abnormalities include keratoconus, spherophakia, myopia, retinal flecks, cataracts, retinitis pigmentosa, and amaurosis.[802,803,814] Other variants of Alport syndrome, now known to be distinct entities, include the association of hereditary nephritis with thrombocytopathia (mega thrombocytopenia), so-called Epstein syndrome,[815,816] diffuse leiomyomatosis,[817] ichthyosis and hyperprolinuria,[818] and Fechtner syndrome (nephritis, macrothrombocytopenia, Döhle-like leukocyte inclusions, deafness, and cataract).[819]

Pathology

The LM appearance of biopsies is non-specific.[820] The diagnosis rests on the EM findings. By LM most biopsies have glomerular and tubulointerstitial lesions. In the early stages (<5 years of age), the kidney biopsy may be normal or nearly normal.[821] The only abnormality may be the presence of superficially located fetal glomeruli involving 5% to 30% of the glomeruli or interstitial foam cells.[822,823] In the older child (5–10 years of age), mesangial and capillary wall lesions may be visible. These consist of segmental to diffuse mesangial cell proliferation, matrix increase, and thickening of the glomerular capillary wall.[824] Special stains such as Jones methenamine silver or periodic acid Schiff may reveal thickening and lamellation of the GBM. Segmentally or globally sclerosed glomeruli may be present. Tubulointerstitial changes may include interstitial fibrosis, tubular atrophy, focal tubular basement membrane thickening, and interstitial foam cells. The glomerular and tubular lesions progress over time. A pattern of focal segmental and global glomerulosclerosis with hyalinosis is common in advanced cases, especially those with nephrotic-range proteinuria. Tubulointerstitial lesions progress from focal to diffuse involvement.[822,825]

By IF many specimens are negative[822,826] but some may have nonspecific granular deposits of C3 and IgM within the mesangium and vascular pole and along the glomerular capillary wall in a segmental or global distribution.[803,811] The finding in rare cases of nonspecifically trapped immune deposits within the lamellated glomerular basement membranes may lead to an erroneous diagnosis of immune complex GN.[827] With segmental sclerosis, subendothelial deposits of IgM, C3, properdin, and C4 are found.[803,822] The GBM of males with Alport syndrome frequently lacks reactivity with sera from patients with anti-GBM antibody disease, or with monoclonal antibodies directed against the Goodpasture epitope.[828,829] This abnormality can help in diagnosing equivocal cases where the electron microscopic findings are not specific.[820]

In the mature kidney, collagen IV is composed of heterotrimers made up of six possible alpha chains. Chains composed of $\alpha 1$, $\alpha 1$, $\alpha 2$ are distributed in all renal basement membranes. Collagen IV chains composed of $\alpha 3$, $\alpha 4$, $\alpha 5$ are present in mature GBM and some distal TBM. Chains of $\alpha 5$, $\alpha 5$, $\alpha 6$ are distributed in Bowman capsule and collecting duct TBM, as well as in epidermal basement membrane. Commercially available antisera to the subunits of collagen IV reveal preservation of the α_1 and α_2 subunits but loss of immunoreactivity for the α_3, α_4 and α_5-subunits from the GBM of affected males with X-linked disease. In addition, there is loss of α_5 staining from Bowman capsule, distal tubular basement membranes and skin in affected males with X-linked disease.

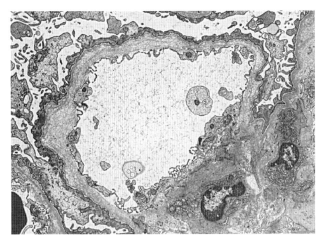

FIGURE 31–42 Alport disease: Electron micrograph showing a thickened, lamellated glomerular basement membrane with the characteristic split and splintered appearance (×4000).

Females are chimeras with segmental loss of α_5 in glomerular and epidermal basement membranes due to random inactivation of the mutated X chromosome in podocytes and basal keratinocytes. Patients with autosomal recessive forms of Alport disease typically lack the α_3, α_4, and α_5 subunits in GBM but retain α_5 immunoreactivity in Bowman capsule, collecting ducts, and skin (where $\alpha5$ forms a heterotrimer with $\alpha6$). Thus, absence of α_5 staining in skin biopsies is highly specific for the diagnosis of X-linked Alport syndrome.[830]

On EM the earliest change is thinning of the GBM (which is not specific for hereditary nephritis and can occur in thin basement membrane disease).[831] The cardinal ultrastructural abnormality is the variable thickening, thinning, basket weaving, and lamellation of the GBM (Fig. 31–42). These abnormalities may also be seen in some patients without a family history of nephritis[832]; these patients may be offspring of asymptomatic carriers, or may represent new mutations. The endothelial cells are intact, and foot process effacement may be seen overlying the altered capillary walls. The mesangium may be normal in early cases, but with time, matrix and cells increase and mesangial interposition into the capillary wall may be observed.[803,826] In males, the number of glomeruli showing lamellation increases from about 30% by age 10 to over 90% by age 30. In females with mild disease, less than 30% of the glomeruli may be affected.[833]

The specificity of the GBM findings has been questioned.[834] Foci of lamina densa lamellation and splitting have been seen in 6% to 15% of unselected renal biopsies. These changes also may be seen focally in other glomerulopathies. Thus clinical correlation and immunofluorescence examination are essential when the ultrastructural features suggest Alport syndrome. Although diffuse thickening and splitting of the GBM strongly suggests Alport syndrome, not all Alport kindreds show these characteristic features. Thick, thin, normal, and nonspecific changes have also been described.

Pathogenesis and Genetics of Hereditary Nephritis

There are three genetic forms of hereditary nephritis. In the majority of cases, the disease is transmitted via an X-linked inheritance (i.e., father-to-son transmission does not occur, and women tend to be carriers because of Lyonization). Autosomal dominant and recessive inheritance have also been described, as has sporadic occurrence.[800,802,835] The frequency

of the Alport gene has been estimated to be 1:5000 in Utah[836] and 1:10,000 in the United States.[837]

Hereditary nephritis is caused by defects in type IV collagen. Six genes for type IV collagen have been characterized. Mutations in the COL4A5 gene (encoding the α-5 subunit of collagen type IV) on the X chromosome are responsible for the more frequent X-linked form of hereditary nephritis.[838] The identified mutations include deletions, insertions, substitutions, and duplications.[838–842] However, there are other abnormalities that are not encoded by the COL4A5 gene. Other Type IV collagen peptides are abnormally distributed. The α_1 and α_2 peptides that are normally confined to the mesangial and subendothelial regions, become distributed throughout the full thickness of the GBM in hereditary nephritis. With progressive glomerular obsolescence, these peptide chains disappear, with an increase in collagen V and VI.[843] Moreover, the basement membranes of these patients do not react with anti-GBM antibodies. This implies that the NC1 domain of the α_3 subunit of type IV collagen is not incorporated normally into the GBM, probably because the α_5 subunit is required for normal assembly of the minor alpha chains of collagen IV into heterotrimers.[844] Cationic antigenic components are also absent.[845] The reason why these GBM abnormalities occur is not known, but may be due to alteration in the incorporation of other collagens into the GBM.[846]

Genetic screening is difficult because of the large number of mutations and the lack of hot spots on the genomic sequence involved.[847] Autosomal recessive and autosomal dominant hereditary nephritis have been shown to involve the α-3 or α-4 chains. The genes for these proteins are encoded on chromosome 2. An abnormality of any of these chains could impair the integrity of the basement membranes in the glomerulus and cochlea, leading to similar clinical findings.

Recently, the minor causes of familial hematuria, the Fechtner and Epstein syndromes, along with two other genetic conditions featuring macrothrombocytes (Sebastian syndrome and May-Hegglin anomaly), were shown to result from heterozygous mutations in the gene *MYH9,* which encodes nonmuscle myosin heavy chain IIA (NMMHC-IIA).[848]

Course and Treatment

Recurrent hematuria and proteinuria may be present for many years followed by the insidious onset of renal failure. Virtually all affected males reach ESRD but there is considerable interkindred variability in the rate of progression. The rate of progression within male members of an affected family is usually but not always relatively constant.[803,849,850] The presence of gross hematuria in childhood, nephrotic syndrome, sensorineural deafness, anterior lenticonus, and diffuse GBM thickening are indicative of an unfavorable outcome in females.[808] A European Community Alport Syndrome Concerted Action (ECASCA) has been established to define the AS phenotype and to determine genotype–phenotype correlations. A report on 401 male patients belonging to the 195 families with COL4A5 mutation showed a 90% probability rate of progression to end-stage renal failure by age 30 years in patients with large deletions, nonsense mutations, or frameshift mutations. The same risk was of 50% and 70%, respectively, in patients with missense or splice site mutations. The risk of developing hearing loss before 30 years of age was approximately 60% in patients with missense mutations, compared with 90% for the other types of mutations.[804] Female carriers with the COL4A5 mutation generally have less severe disease. In the ECASCA cohort described earlier, the probability of developing ESRD before the age of 40 years was 12%, in females versus 90%, in males. The risk of progression to end-stage renal disease appears to increase after the age of 60 years in women. Risk factors for renal failure in women included the development and progressive increase in proteinuria, and the occurrence of a hearing defect.

There is no proven therapy for Alport syndrome. Proteinuria-reduction strategies, such as aggressive control of hypertension and use of angiotensin-converting enzyme inhibitors (ACEI) might slow the rate of progression in patients with hereditary nephritis.[851] A small number of patients showed apparent stabilization when treated long term with cyclosporine.[852] However, the potential for calcineurin inhibitor toxicity exists.

Renal replacement therapy (either dialysis or transplantation) may be performed in patients with hereditary nephritis. Allograft and patient survival were comparable to survival rates in the UNOS database.[853] In approximately 2% to 4% of male patients receiving a renal transplant, anti-GBM antibody disease may develop.[854] These antibodies are directed against the Goodpasture antigen in the α-3 chain. This antigen, which presumably does not exist in the kidney in patients with hereditary nephritis, is present in normal kidneys and is thus recognized as foreign.[855,856] A profile of these patients has been compiled.[820] The patients are usually male, always deaf, and likely to have reached end-stage renal disease before the age of 30. There is a suggestion that certain mutations in the COL4A5 gene, such as deletions (which account for 11%–12% of Alport cases), may predispose patients to the development of allograft anti-GBM nephritis.[856] In 75% of cases, the onset of anti-GBM nephritis occurs within the first year after transplantation, and 76% of the allografts were lost.

THIN BASEMENT MEMBRANE NEPHROPATHY

Thin basement membrane nephropathy (TBMN) (also known as benign familial hematuria and thin GBM nephropathy) describes a condition that differs from Alport disease in its generally benign course and lack of progression. The typical finding on renal pathology is diffuse thinning of the glomerular basement membranes (GBM). However, thin GBM may be found in other conditions as well (including early Alport disease and IgA nephropathy).[857] The true incidence of TBMN disease is unknown; reports evaluating patients with isolated hematuria suggest that 20% to 25% of such patients have thin GBM disease.[858–860]

Clinical Features

Patients usually present in childhood with microhematuria. Hematuria is usually persistent but may be intermittent in some patients. Episodic gross hematuria may occur particularly with upper respiratory infections.[861,862] Patients do not typically have overt proteinuria, but when present, this may suggest progression of disease.[858,863]

Pathology

Renal biopsies typically show no histologic abnormalities with the exception of focal erythrocyte casts. By IF, no glomerular deposits of immunoglobulins or complement are found. By EM, there is diffuse and relatively uniform thinning of the GBM (Fig. 31–43). The normal thickness of the GBM is age and gender dependent. Vogler and colleagues[864] have defined normal ranges for children: at birth 169 ± 30 nm, at 2 years of age 245 ± 49 nm, at 11 years 285 ± 39 nm. Steffes and associates[865] have defined normal ranges for adults 373 ± 42 (males) 326 ± 45 nm (females). Each laboratory should attempt to establish its own normals for GBM thickness. A cutoff value of 250 nm has been reported by some authors,[866–868] whereas other groups have used a cutoff

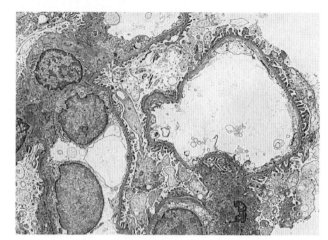

FIGURE 31–43 Thin basement membrane disease: By electron microscopy, the glomerular basement membranes are diffusely and uniformly thinned, measuring less than 200 nm in thickness (×2500).

of 330 nm.[863] There is often accentuation of the lamina rara interna and externa. Focal GBM gaps may be identified ultrastructurally. Immunostaining for the alpha subunits of collagen IV reveal a normal distribution in the GBM.

Pathogenesis

About 40% of TBMN disease has been linked to mutations of the COL4A3 and COL4A4 genes.[869] In most kindreds with TBMN, the disorder appears to be transmitted in an autosomal dominant pattern. In a few families with several affected children and apparently unaffected parents suggests a recessive mode of inheritance or that one parent was an asymptomatic carrier.[860,861,870] There appears to be a reduction or loss of the subepithelial portion of the basement membrane, which apparently contains normal amounts of type IV collagen.[871]

Differential Diagnosis of Familial Hematurias

Type IV collagen defects can cause both TBMN and Alport syndrome. Patients with TBMN can be considered carriers of autosomal recessive Alport syndrome.[872,873] With advances in molecular biology and immunopathology, hereditary forms of hematuria have been better characterized. Table 31–2 shows a summary of the clinical, pathologic, and genetic aspects of the various forms of hereditary nephritis.[874] Because GBM thinning may be seen in early cases of Alport syndrome, immunohistochemical analysis of α_3, α_4, and α_5-subunits should be undertaken (because genetic tests are not practical). Table 31–3 shows the typical immunostaining patterns in the kidney and skin basement membranes.

NAIL-PATELLA SYNDROME (HEREDITARY OSTEO-ONYCHODYSPLASIA)

Nail-patella syndrome (NPS) is an autosomal dominant condition affecting tissues of both ectodermal and mesodermal origin, manifested as symmetrical nail, skeletal, ocular, and renal anomalies.

Clinical Features

The classical tetrad of anomalies of the nails, elbows and knees, and iliac horns was described by Mino and colleagues

TABLE 31–2	Classification of Familial Hematurias					
	Locus	**Progressive Nephropathy**	**Deafness**	**Ocular Changes**	**GBM Changes**	**Hematologic Features**
Type IV collagen disorders						
Alport syndrome						
X-linked	COL4A5	+	+	+	Thickening	No
X-linked + diffuse leiomyomatosis	COL4A5 + COL4A6	+	+	No	Thickening	No
Autosomal recessive	COL4A3 or COL4A4	+	+	+	Thickening	No
Autosomal dominant	COL4A3 or COL4A4	+	+	No	Thickening	No
Thin basement membrane nephropathy*	COL4A3 or COL4A4	No	No	No	Thinning	No
Non-collagen disorders						
Fechtner syndrome	MYH9	+	+	+	Thickening	Thrombocytopenia May-Hegglin
Epstein syndrome	MYH9	+	+	+	Thickening	Thrombocytopenia

*Some families with thin basement membrane disease have mutations at loci other than the type IV collagen genes.
From Kashtan CE: Familial hematurias: What we know and what we don't. Pediatr Nephrol 20(8):1027–1035, 2005.

TABLE 31–3	Immunostaining Patterns for α_5 in Kidney and Epidermal Basement Membranes		
	Glomerular Basement Membrane	**Bowman Capsule**	**Epidermal Basement Membrane**
Normal	Present/Normal	Present/Normal	Present/Normal
X-linked Alport Males	Absent	Absent	Absent
X-linked Alport Female carriers	Present/Mosaic	Present/Mosaic	Present/Mosaic
Autosomal recessive Alport	Absent	Present/Normal	Present/Normal
Thin Basement Membrane Disease	Present/Normal	Present/Normal	Present/Normal

in 1948.[875] Nail dysplasia and patellar aplasia or hypoplasia are essential features for the diagnosis of NPS. The presence of triangular nail lunulae is a pathognomonic sign for NPS. Other skeletal abnormalities include dysplasia of the elbow joints, posterior iliac horns, and foot deformities. Various ocular anomalies have sporadically been found in NPS patients, including microcornea, sclerocornea, congenital cataract, iris processes, pigmentation of the inner margin of the iris, and congenital glaucoma.[876]

Renal involvement is variable, being present in up to 38% of patients. Renal manifestations first appear in children and young adults and may include proteinuria, hematuria, hypertension, or edema. The nephrotic syndrome and progressive renal failure may occasionally occur. The course is generally benign with renal failure being a late feature.[877,878] Congenital malformations of the urinary tract and nephrolithiasis are also more frequent in these patients.

Pathology

The findings on LM are nonspecific and include focal and segmental glomerular sclerosis, segmental thickening of the glomerular capillary wall, and mild mesangial hypercellular-

ity.[879] IF microscopy is nonspecific and IgM and C3 have been observed in sclerosed segments. Ultrastructural studies show a thickened basement membrane that contains irregular lucencies, imparting a "moth-eaten" appearance (Fig. 31–44A). The presence of intramembranous fibrils with the periodicity of collagen is revealed by phosphotungstic acid stains in electron microscopic sections, corresponding to the distribution of the intramembranous lucencies (Fig. 31–44B). These must be distinguished from the occasional collagen fibrils that can accumulate nonspecifically in the sclerotic mesangium in a variety of sclerosing glomerular conditions.[879]

Pathogenesis

The genetic locus for this syndrome appears to be on chromosome 9, in linkage with ABO and the locus for adenylate kinase.[880,881] Features reminiscent of nail patella syndrome have been produced in mice with targeted disruption of the LIM-homeodomain protein Lmx1b. Lmx1b plays a central role in dorso-ventral patterning of the vertebrate limb. The authors also showed that LMX1B mapped to the NPS locus and that three NPS patients carried de novo heterozygous

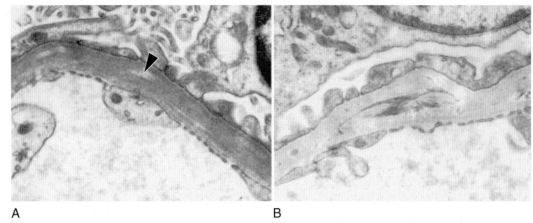

A   B

FIGURE 31–44   Nail-Patella syndrome. **A,** Routine electron micrograph showing thickening of a glomerular basement membrane with focal irregular internal lucencies (×15,000). **B,** Phosphotungstic acid-stained electron micrograph demonstrating the characteristic banded collagen fibrils within the rarefied segments of glomerular basement membrane (×15,000).

mutations in this gene.[882] This finding has been confirmed in other kindreds with NPS.[883]

Treatment

There is no treatment for this condition; occasional patients with renal failure have been successfully transplanted.[884]

FABRY DISEASE (ANGIOKERATOMA CORPORIS DIFFUSUM UNIVERSALE)

Fabry disease[885] is an X-linked inborn error of glycosphingolipid metabolism involving a lysosomal enzyme, α-galactosidase A (also known as ceramide trihexosidase). The enzyme deficiency leads to the accumulation of globotriaosylceramide (ceramide trihexoside) and related neutral glycosphingolipids leading to multisystem involvement and dysfunction. Clinical guidelines for the diagnosis and treatment of Fabry disease have recently been published.[886]

Clinical Features

Fabry disease has been reported in all ethnic groups, and the estimated incidence in males is 1 in 40,000 to 1 in 60,000. In male hemizygotes, the initial clinical presentation usually begins in childhood with episodic pain in the extremities and acroparesthesias. Renal involvement is common in male hemizygotes and is occasional in female heterozygotes. The disease presents with hematuria and proteinuria, which often progresses to nephrotic levels. In men, progressive renal failure generally develops by the fifth decade. In the United States, Fabry disease accounted for 0.02% of patients who began renal replacement therapy between 1995 and 1998.[887]

The skin is commonly involved with reddish-purple macules (angiokeratomas) typically found on the abdomen, buttocks, hips, genitalia, and upper thighs. Other findings include palmar erythema, conjunctival and oral mucous membrane telangiectasia, and subungual splinter hemorrhages. The nervous system is involved with peripheral and autonomic neuropathy. Premature arterial disease of coronary vessels leads to myocardial ischemia and arrhythmias at a young age. Similarly, cerebrovascular involvement leads to early onset of strokes. In the heart, valvular disease and hypertrophic cardiomyopathy have also been reported. Corneal opacities are seen in virtually all hemizygotes and most heterozygotes. Posterior capsular cataracts, edema of

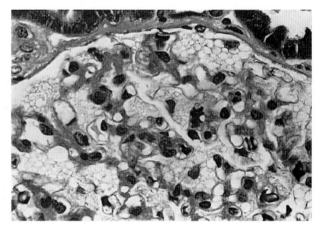

FIGURE 31–45   Fabry disease: By light microscopy, the visceral epithelial cells are markedly enlarged with foamy-appearing cytoplasm (Trichrome, ×800).

retina and eyelids, tortuous retinal and conjunctival vessels may also been seen in the eye. Generalized lymphadenopathy, hepatosplenomegaly, aseptic necrosis of femoral and humeral heads, myopathy, hypoalbuminemia, and hypogammaglobulinemia have been reported.

In carrier females, clinical manifestations may range from asymptomatic to severe disease similar to male hemizygotes. Up to one third of female carriers have been reported to have significant disease manifestations.[888]

Pathology

Glycosphingolipid accumulation begins early in life[889] and the major renal site of accumulation is the podocyte (visceral epithelial cells). By LM, these cells are enlarged with numerous clear, uniform vacuoles in the cytoplasm causing a foamy appearance (Fig. 31–45). These vacuoles can be shown to contain lipids when fat stains (such as Oil Red-O) are used, or when viewed under the polarizing microscope where they exhibit a double refractile appearance before being processed with lipid solvents. All renal cells may accumulate the lipid. These include (in addition to podocytes) parietal epithelial cells, glomerular endothelial cells, mesangial cells, interstitial capillary endothelial cells, distal convoluted tubule cells, and to a lesser extent, cells of the loops of Henle, and proximal tubular cells. Indeed, vascular endothelial cells are

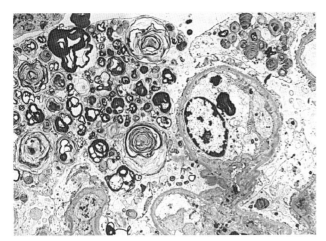

FIGURE 31–46 Fabry disease: Electron micrograph showing abundant whorled myelin figures within the cytoplasm of the podocytes. A few similar inclusions are also identified within the glomerular endothelial cells (×2000).

involved in virtually every organ and tissue.[890] In the kidney, the myocytes and endothelial cells of arteries are commonly involved. In heterozygotes, similar changes are present but with less severity.[891] Characteristic findings are noted on EM (Fig. 31–46). The major finding is large numbers of "myelin figures" or "zebra bodies" within the cytoplasm of the podocytes, and to a variable extent, in other renal cell types. These intracytoplasmic vacuoles consist of single membrane-bound dense bodies with a concentric whorled or multilamellar appearance. Glomerular podocytes exhibit variable foot process effacement. The GBMs are initially normal, but with progression of disease, there may be thickening and collapse of the GBM, focal and segmental glomerular sclerosis, with accompanying tubular atrophy and interstitial fibrosis.[892] Findings on IF microscopy are usually negative except in areas of segmental sclerosis, where IgM and complement may be demonstrated. Orange autofluorescence corresponding to the lipid inclusions may be found in podocytes and other renal cells.

Pathogenesis

The entire gene for α-galactosidase has been sequenced.[893] Specific molecular defects vary from family to family, and include rearrangements, deletions, and point mutations.[894] Deficiency of the enzyme leads to accumulation of globotriaosylceramide especially in the vascular endothelium, with subsequent ischemic organ dysfunction. Patients with blood groups B and AB have earlier and more severe symptoms, likely related to accumulation of the terminal α-galactose substance occurring during the synthesis of the B antigen on red blood cell membranes.[895] Globosyltriaosylceramide accumulation in podocytes may lead to proteinuria and renal dysfunction, but functional abnormalities are not always noted, especially in female heterozygotes. A gene-knockout mouse model of Fabry disease has been produced, which shows the characteristic changes.[896]

Diagnosis

The diagnosis in affected males can be established by measuring levels of α-galactosidase-A in plasma or peripheral blood leukocytes. Hemizygotes have almost no measurable enzyme activity. Female carriers may have enzyme levels in the low to normal range; to diagnose female carriers, the specific mutation in the family must be demonstrated.[886] The measurement of urinary ceramide digalactoside and trihexoside levels may also be of use to identify the carrier state. Prenatal diagnosis can be made by measuring amniocyte enzyme levels in amniotic fluid.

Treatment

Two randomized, controlled trials have shown that recombinant human α-galactosidase-A replacement therapy is safe and can improved clinical parameters. In one short-term study α-galactosidase-A treatment was associated with improved neuropathic pain, decreased mesangial widening, and improved creatinine clearance.[897] In the second study, repeat renal biopsies showed decreased microvascular endothelial deposits of globotriaosylceramide.[890,898,898a,898b] Clinical guidelines for the management of Fabry disease have recently been published: enzyme replacement therapy should be administered as early as possible in all males with Fabry disease (including those with end-stage renal disease) and female carriers with substantial disease manifestations.[886]

The European Renal Association-European Dialysis and Transplant Association (ERA-EDTA) Registry has reported outcomes on patients with Fabry disease. Since 1985, 4 to 13 new patients per year have commenced renal replacement therapy in Europe. Patient survival on dialysis was 41% at 5 years; cardiovascular complications (48%) and cachexia (17%) were the main causes of death. Graft survival at 3 years in 33 patients was not inferior to that of other nephropathies (72% versus 69%), and patient survival after transplantation was comparable to that of patients under 55 years of age.[899] In the U.S. population, survival of Fabry patients was lower than non-diabetic renal failure patients.[887]

Long-term allograft function in patients with Fabry disease has been reported. Glycosphingolipid deposits do recur in allografts, but have not been reported to cause graft failure.[900] It is likely that enzyme therapy will benefit patients on dialysis and those who have been transplanted.

◼ SICKLE CELL NEPHROPATHY

Renal disease associated with sickle cell disease includes gross hematuria, papillary necrosis, nephrotic syndrome, renal infarction, inability to concentrate urine, renal medullary carcinoma, and pyelonephritis.[901,902] Microscopic or gross hematuria is likely the result of microinfarcts in the renal medulla. Glomerular lesions however, are less commonly encountered and may be seen in patients with HbSS, HbSC, and sickle cell-thalessemia.[903]

Clinical Features

In one study, the prevalence of proteinuria (>1+ on a dipstick) in SS disease was 26%.[903] The majority of proteinuric patients had less than 3g/d and an elevated serum creatinine levels was present in 7% of patients. In another study, 4.2% with SS disease, and 2.4% with sickle C disease developed renal failure. The median age of disease onset for these patients was 23.1 and 49.9 years, respectively. Survival time for patients with SS anemia after the diagnosis of renal failure, despite dialysis, was 4 years, and the median age at the time of death was 27 years. The risk for renal failure was increased in patients with the Central African Republic beta s-gene cluster haplotype, hypertension, proteinuria, and severe anemia.[904] The course of SS renal disease is progressive; in one series, 18% of patients with SS disease progressed to ESRD.[905]

Two patterns of glomerular lesions may be seen in patients with SS-associated glomerulopathy. Immune-mediated glomerulonephritis with a membranoproliferative pattern exhibits mesangial proliferation with mild to moderate capillary wall thickening due to GBM reduplication and mesangial interposition (Fig. 31–47). Some of these patients also exhibit features of chronic thrombotic microangiopathy, with narrow double contours of the GBM and mesangiolysis. A pattern of membranous glomerulonephritis has also been described. On IF microscopy, irregular granular deposits of IgG and C3 have been reported in association with membranous or mesangiocapillary findings on LM.[906] Ultrastructural studies show granular dense deposits in the mesangial and subepithelial area. Some cases have no detectable deposits, but subendothelial accumulation of electron lucent "fluff" resembling the changes in chronic thrombotic microangiopathies may be seen. Mild mesangial proliferation and peripheral mesangial interposition is frequently seen. Sickled erythrocytes containing para crystalline inclusions may be identified within glomerular capillaries.[906–910]

In the second form of sickle glomerulopathy, focal and segmental glomerulosclerosis is seen associated with glomerulomegaly (Fig. 31–48). Two patterns of FSGS may be observed: a "collapsing" pattern and an "expansive" pattern.[901,903,911–913] On IF nonspecific IgM and C3 are seen in sclerosed segments. In all these forms, there may be prominent intracapillary erythrocyte sickling and congestion.

Pathogenesis

The mechanism(s) for glomerular abnormalities in SS patients is not fully understood. One theory proposes that mesangial cells are activated by the presence of fragmented RBCs in glomerular capillaries. This activation of mesangial cells promotes synthesis of matrix proteins and GBM reduplication.[914] In another study, renal tubular epithelial antigens and complement components were detected in a granular pattern along the GBM; the authors hypothesized that glomerulonephritis was mediated by glomerular deposition of immune complexes containing renal tubular epithelial antigen and antibody to renal tubular epithelial antigen (the antigen possibly released after tubular damage secondary to decreased oxygenation and hemodynamic alterations related to SS disease).[906]

In patients with the FSGS pattern, it is proposed that the collapsing pattern represents an initial but progressive obliteration of the glomerular capillary bed by red blood cell sickling, which cannot be compensated by further glomerular hypertrophy. Hemodynamic glomerular injury then supervenes from the sustained or increasing hyperfiltration in a diminishing capillary bed, manifesting morphologically as the expansive pattern of sclerosis.[903,911] The role of reactive oxygen species in producing chronic vascular endothelial injury has also been suggested.[915]

Treatment

The management of renal disease has generally not been satisfactory. Treatment of patients with SS nephropathy with angiotensin-converting enzyme inhibitors reduces the degree of proteinuria.[903,916] However, their effectiveness in preserving renal function remains to be established.

SS nephropathy accounts for 0.1% of ESRD patients in the United States.[917] Renal transplantation has been performed in SS patients. One-year graft survival in SS patients was similar to other transplanted patients; however, long-term renal outcome was worse, as was short-term and long-term mortality.[918] Transplanted sickle patients commonly experience SS crises.[919,920] Recurrent SS nephropathy has been reported in the transplanted kidney.[912,921]

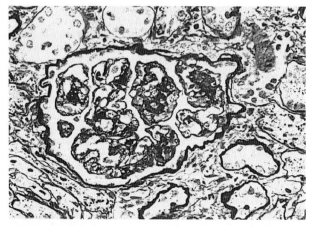

FIGURE 31–47 Sickle cell disease: An example of sickle cell glomerulopathy with membranoproliferative features. There are double contours of the glomerular basement membrane associated with segmental mesangiolysis (Jones methenamine silver, ×500).

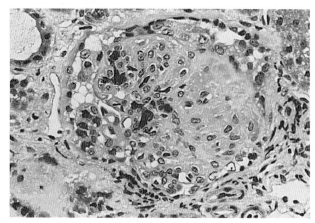

FIGURE 31–48 Sickle cell disease: An example with focal segmental glomerulosclerosis. The nonsclerotic glomerular capillaries are congested with sickled erythrocytes (Hematoxylin-eosin, ×500).

▌ LIPODYSTROPHY

Lipodystrophies are rare diseases in which there is loss of fat, which may be localized to the upper part of the body in partial lipodystrophy (PLD) or more diffuse in generalized lipodystrophy (GLD).[922,923] PLD is commonly associated with Type II mesangiocapillary (membranoproliferative glomerulonephritis).

Partial lipodystrophy most often presents in girls between ages 5 and 15 years. In addition to the loss of fat, the lipodystrophies are associated with a wide variety of metabolic and systemic abnormalities. Hyperinsulinism, insulin resistance, and diabetes are common. Other metabolic abnormalities include hyperlipidemia, hyperproteinemia, and euthyroid hypermetabolism. Clinical findings may include tall stature, muscular hypertrophy, hirsutism, macroglossia, abdominal distension, subcutaneous nodules, acanthosis nigricans, hepatomegaly, cirrhosis, clitoral or penile enlargement, febrile adenopathy, cerebral atrophy, cerebral ventricular dilatation, hemiplegia, mental retardation, and cardiomegaly.[922,923] Renal disease occurs in 20% to 50% of patients with PLD,[922,923] and

PLD occurs in 10% of patients with membranoproliferative glomerulonephritis (MPGN) Type II.[924,925] Patients are noted to have asymptomatic proteinuria and microhematuria, but the nephrotic syndrome is occasionally present.[926,927] Diminished C3 levels in association with the C3 nephritic (C3NeF) is the most prominent serologic abnormality. The course of glomerular disease is fairly rapid progression to ESRD and the prognosis of PLD is determined mainly by renal disease.[923]

In GLD, the nephrotic syndrome, non-nephrotic proteinuria, and hypertension have been reported.[922] In a recent report, 88% of these patients had albumin excretion greater than 30 mg/24 h, 60% had albuminuria (>300 mg/24 h), and 20% had nephrotic-range proteinuria greater than 3500 mg/24 h.[928]

Pathology

Partial lipodystrophy is frequently associated with mesangiocapillary (membranoproliferative) glomerulonephritis Type II or dense deposit disease.[926,927,929,930] Patients with type III MPGN[931] and minimal change disease[932] have also been reported. Focal and segmental glomerulosclerosis, membranoproliferative glomerulonephritis, and diabetic glomerulosclerosis have been reported in patients with GLD.[928]

Pathogenesis and Treatment

The pathogenesis of PLD and GLD is poorly understood. It is unlikely that one unifying link will be found given the differences in epidemiology, genetics, and clinical features. Acquired forms of lipodystrophy are believed to be autoimmune disorders. Most patients with PLD possess an IgG autoantibody, C3 nephritic factor (C3NeF), which binds to and stabilizes the alternate pathway convertase, C3 convertase-C3bBb. In the presence of C3NeF, C3bBb becomes resistant to its regulatory proteins H and I. Although the majority of patients with partial dystrophy have low serum C3, not all patients will exhibit nephritis.[930] Recombinant leptin appears to decrease the proteinuria in some patients with GLD.[928] There is no effective therapy for PLD, and although renal transplantation is the treatment of choice when ESRD ensues, recurrence in transplants has been reported.[923,929,933]

LECITHIN-CHOLESTEROL ACYLTRANSFERASE (LCAT) DEFICIENCY

Gjone and Norum reported a familial disorder characterized by proteinuria, anemia, hyperlipidemia, and corneal opacity.[934,935] Most of the initial patients were of Scandinavian origin; subsequent reports have been from other countries.[936,937]

Clinical Features

The triad of anemia, nephrotic syndrome, and corneal opacities suggests this disorder. Renal disease is a universal finding with albuminuria noted early in life. Proteinuria increases in severity during the fourth and fifth decades, often with development of the nephrotic syndrome. The latter is accompanied by hypertension and progressive renal failure. Most patients are mildly anemic with target cells and poikilocytes on the peripheral smear. There is evidence of low-grade hemolysis. During childhood, corneal opacities appear as grayish spots over the cornea accompanied by a lipoid arcus. Visual acuity is unimpaired. Atherosclerotic events are accelerated in these patients.[934,938–941]

Pathology

Abnormalities are found mainly in the glomeruli, but arteries and arterioles may also be affected.[934,935,940,942] By light microscopy (Fig. 31–49), the glomerular capillary walls are thickened and there is mesangial expansion. Basement membranes are irregular and often appear to contain vacuoles, resembling stage 3 membranous alterations. Double contouring of capillary walls is occasionally present. Similar vacuoles in the mesangium impart a honeycomb appearance. There is no associated glomerular hypercellularity. By immunofluorescence microscopy, there is typically negative staining for all immunoglobulin and complement components. On electron microscopy (Fig. 31–50), the vacuolated areas seen by light microscopy correspond to extracellular irregular lucent zones (lacunae) in the mesangial matrix and GBM containing lipid inclusions. These inclusions contain rounded, small, dense structures, either solid or with a lamellar substructure.

Pathogenesis

The disorder is inherited in an autosomal recessive pattern. Patients have little or no LCAT activity in their blood

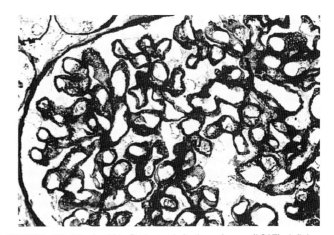

FIGURE 31–49 Lecithin-Cholesterol Acyltransferase (LCAT) deficiency: The glomerular basement membranes and mesangium have a vacuolated appearance, resembling stage 3 membranous glomerulopathy (Jones methenamine silver, ×800).

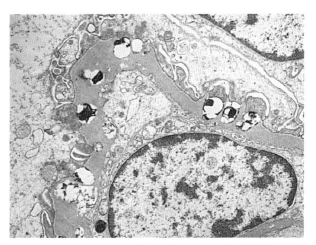

FIGURE 31–50 Lecithin-Cholesterol Acyltransferase (LCAT) deficiency: Electron micrograph showing intramembranous lacunae with rounded structures containing an electron-dense membranous core and electron lucent periphery (×5000).

circulation because of mutations in the *LCAT* gene.[943,944] LCAT is an enzyme that circulates in the blood primarily bound to high-density lipoprotein and catalyzes the formation of cholesteryl esters via the hydrolysis and transfer of the sn-2 fatty acid from phosphatidylcholine to the 3-hydroxyl group of cholesterol. Thus patients with LCAT deficiency have high levels of phosphatidylcholine and unesterified cholesterol, with corresponding low levels of lysophosphatidylcholine and cholesteryl ester in the blood. An abnormal lipoprotein, lipoprotein-X (Lp-X) is present in patients' plasma. Lp-X is thought to arise from the surface of chylomicron remnants that are not further metabolized due to the absence of active LCAT. Accumulation of lipid component occurs in both intra- and extracellular sites. Damage to the GBM occurs from these lipids resulting in proteinuria. Endothelial damage and resulting vascular insufficiency may contribute to renal insufficiency. It has been proposed that Lp-X stimulates mesangial cells, leading to the production of MCP-1 (monocyte chemoattractant protein-1), promoting monocyte infiltration, foam cell formation, and progressive glomerulosclerosis in a manner similar to atherosclerosis.[945]

Diagnosis

In patients suspected of having LCAT deficiency, measurements of plasma enzyme should be performed. The enzyme levels and activity vary among kindreds[939]; thus enzyme measurements should include activity as well as mass. Other abnormalities of lipids frequently accompany LCAT deficiency. The plasma is turbid, total cholesterol varies, triglycerides are increased, HDL is reduced, and all fractions contain higher amounts of cholesterol.

Treatment

A low lipid diet or lipid lowering drugs have not shown to be of benefit.[940] Plasma infusions may provide reversal of erythrocytic abnormalities, but long-term benefits have yet to be demonstrated.[946] The lesions may recur in the allograft but renal function is adequately preserved.[947]

LIPOPROTEIN GLOMERULOPATHY

Lipoprotein glomerulopathy (LPG) is a newly recognized glomerular characterized by dysbetalipoproteinemia, lipid deposition in the kidney leading to glomerulosclerosis and renal failure. The majority of patients have been from Japan.[948,949]

The histologic hallmark of LPG is the presence of laminated thrombi consisting of lipids within the lumina of dilated glomerular capillaries. The pathogenesis of LGP is unknown, but the presence of thrombi consisting of lipoproteins raised the possibility that LPG might be related to a primary abnormality in lipid metabolism.[950] Indeed Type III hyperlipidemia (elevated LDL and high apo-E levels) have been reported in Japanese patients, associated with apo-E variants.[949,951–955] Furthermore, LPG-like deposits were detected in apo-E deficient mice transfected with apo-E (Sendai), one of the apo-E variants associated with LPG. Abnormal apo-E has not been found in the single European patient with this disease.[956]

There is no uniformly effective therapy for LPG; however, intensive lipid-lowering therapy has been reported to be effective in one patient with LPG.[957] Recurrence of lesions of LPG have occurred in renal allografts.[958,959]

GLOMERULAR INVOLVEMENT WITH BACTERIAL INFECTIONS

Infectious Endocarditis

The natural history of endocarditis-associated glomerulonephritis has changed significantly in parallel with the changing epidemiology of infectious endocarditis (IE) and the advent of antibiotics. In the pre-antibiotic era, *Streptococcus viridans* was the most common organism and glomerulonephritis occurred in between 50% to 80% of cases.[960] During that era, glomerulonephritis was less common in association with acute endocarditis.[961,962] With the use of prophylactic antibiotics in patients with valvular heart disease, and an increase in intravenous drug use, *Staphylococcus aureus* has replaced *S. viridans* as the primary pathogen. Glomerulonephritis in these patients with acute IE occurs as commonly as in subacute endocarditis.[960,963–965] The incidence of glomerulonephritis with endocarditis with *S. aureus* ranges from 22% to 78%[963,966] being higher in those series consisting predominantly of intravenous drug users.[966,967]

Clinical Features

Renal complications of IE include infarcts, abscesses, and glomerulonephritis (all of which may coexist). In focal glomerulonephritis, mild asymptomatic urinary abnormalities including hematuria, pyuria, and albuminuria may be noted. Infrequently, with severe focal glomerulonephritis, renal insufficiency or uremia may be present. Renal dysfunction, micro or gross hematuria and the nephrotic-range proteinuria may be present with diffuse glomerulonephritis.[960,963,968] Rapidly progressive renal failure with crescents has been reported.[960,969] Rarely, patients may present with vasculitic features (including purpura).[970] Although hypocomplementemia is frequent, it is neither invariable (occurring in 60% to 90% of patients with glomerulonephritis), nor specific for renal involvement.[965,966] The majority of patients demonstrate activation of the classical pathway.[966,971] Alternate pathway activation has been described in some cases of *S. aureus* endocarditis.[966] The degree of complement activation correlates with the severity of renal impairment[966] and the complement levels normalize with successful therapy of the infection. Circulating immune complexes have been found in the serum in up to 90% of patients.[971,972] Mixed cryoglobulins and rheumatoid factor may also be present in the serum of patients.[965,973] ANCA positivity has been occasionally reported in biopsy-proven immune complex glomerulonephritis associated with IE.[974] Anti-GBM antibody in eluates from diseased glomeruli has been reported.[975]

Pathology

On light microscopy, focal and segmental endocapillary proliferative glomerulonephritis with focal crescents is the most typical finding. Some patients may exhibit a more diffuse proliferative glomerulonephritis lesion with or without crescents.[960,961,963,976,977] IF reveals granular capillary and mesangial deposits of IgG, IgM, and C3.[960,963,976] EM shows electron-dense deposits in mesangial, subendothelial, and occasionally subepithelial locations, with varying degrees of mesangial and endocapillary proliferation.[960,963,976]

Pathogenesis

The diffuse deposition of immunoglobulin, the depression of complement and electron-dense deposits supports an immune complex mechanism for the production of this form of glomerulonephritis. The demonstration of specific antibody in kidney eluates and the detection of bacterial antigen in the deposits further supported this view. Both *S. aureus*[978] and hemolytic *Streptococcus*[979] antigens have been identified.

Treatment

With the initiation of antibiotic therapy, the manifestations of glomerulonephritis begin to subside. Rarely, microhematuria and proteinuria may persist for years.[960] Plasmapheresis and corticosteroids have been reported to promote renal recovery in some patients with renal failure.[969,980] However, this approach should be taken cautiously because of the risk of promoting infectious aspects of the disease while ameliorating the immunologic manifestations.

Shunt Nephritis

Ventriculovascular (ventriculoatrial, ventriculojugular) shunts use for the management of hydrocephalus used to be colonized commonly with microorganisms, particularly *Staph. albus* (75%).[981] Less often, other bacteria (e.g., *Propionibacterium acnes*) have been implicated.[982] Ventriculoperitoneal shunts are more resistant to infection. However, glomerulonephritis has been reported with these shunts as well.[983] Infected peritoneovenous (LeVeen) shunts also have been associated occasionally with glomerulonephritis.[984]

Patients commonly present with fever. Anemia, hepatosplenomegaly, purpura, arthralgias, and lymphadenopathy are found on examination. Renal manifestations include hematuria (microscopic or gross), proteinuria (nephrotic syndrome in 30% of patients), azotemia, and hypertension. Laboratory abnormalities include presence of rheumatoid factor, cryoimmunoglobulins, elevated sedimentation rate and C-reactive protein levels, hypocomplementemia, and presence of circulating immune complexes.[985,986] Shunt nephritis usually presents within a few months of shunt placement, but delayed manifestations, as late as 17 years have been reported.[987] By LM, glomeruli exhibit mesangial proliferation or membranoproliferative changes. IF reveals diffuse granular deposits of IgG, IgM, and C3. Electron-dense mesangial and subendothelial deposits are found by EM.[988]

Antibiotic therapy and prompt removal of the infected catheter usually leads to remission of the glomerulonephritis.[989] However, cases progressing to chronic renal failure have been reported.[990] Rarely, patients have elevated proteinase-3-specific ANCA titers, which also improved after removal of the infected shunt, with or without corticosteroid therapy.[991]

Visceral Infection

Visceral infections in the form of abdominal, pulmonary, and retroperitoneal abscesses are known to be associated with glomerulonephritis.[992] The clinical and pathological syndrome resembles infective endocarditis. Beaufils and colleagues reported on 11 patients who had visceral abscesses and in whom acute renal failure developed. Circulating cryoglobulins, decreased serum complement levels, and circulating immune complexes were found in some of these patients. All renal biopsies showed a diffuse proliferative and crescentic glomerulonephritis. The evolution of the glomerulonephritis, documented by serial biopsies, closely paralleled the course of the infection. A complete recovery of renal function occurred in those cases in which a rapid and complete cure of the infection was obtained. For those patients in whom the infection was not cured or in whom therapy was delayed, chronic renal failure also developed.[993]

Other Bacterial Infections and Fungal Infections

Congenital, secondary, and latent forms of syphilis rarely may be complicated by glomerular involvement. Patients are typically nephrotic and proteinuria usually responds to penicillin therapy.[994–998] Membranous nephropathy with varying degrees of proliferation and with granular IgG and C3 deposits is the commonest finding on biopsies. Treponemal antigen and antibody have been eluted from deposits. Rarely minimal change lesions[999] and crescentic glomerulonephritis[1000] or amyloidosis may be seen.

Renal involvement including azotemia, proteinuria, nephrotic syndrome, renal tubular defects, and hematuria is not uncommon in leprosy, especially with the lepra reaction.[1001–1006] Rarely, presentation with RPGN can occur[1007] and ESRD.[1008] Mesangial proliferation, diffuse proliferative glomerulonephritis, crescentic glomerulonephritis, membranous nephropathy, membranoproliferative glomerulonephritis, microscopic angiitis, and amyloidosis may all be seen in kidney biopsies. Organisms consistent with *M. Leprae* have been found in glomeruli.

Aspergillosis has been associated with immune complex-mediated glomerulonephritis.[1009] Membranous nephropathy, membranoproliferative glomerulonephritis, crescentic glomerulonephritis, and amyloidosis have been associated with *M. tuberculosis*.[1010–1013] *Mycoplasma* has been reported to be associated with nephrotic syndrome and rapidly progressive glomerulonephritis. Antibiotics do not seem to alter the course of the disease. Mycoplasmal antigen has been reported to be present in glomerular lesions.[1014–1018] Acute glomerulonephritis with hypocomplementemia has been reported with pneumococcal infections. Proliferative glomerulonephritis with deposition of IgG, IgM, complements C1q, C3, C4, and pneumococcal antigens have been observed in renal biopsies.[1019,1020] Nocardiosis has been associated with mesangiocapillary glomerulonephritis.[1021] In infections with *Brucella,* patients may present with hematuria, proteinuria (usually nephrotic), and varying degrees of renal functional impairment. There usually is improvement after antibiotics, but histologic abnormalities, proteinuria, and hypertension may persist. Glomerular mesangial proliferation, focal and segmental endocapillary proliferation, diffuse proliferation, and crescents may be found in renal biopsies. IF may show no deposits, IgG, or occasionally IgA.[1022–1026] Asymptomatic urinary abnormalities may be seen in up to 80% of patients infected with *Leptospira.* Patients usually present with acute renal failure due to tubulointerstitial nephritis. Rarely, mesangial or diffuse proliferative glomerulonephritis may be seen.[1027,1028] From 1% to 4% of patients with typhoid fever secondary to *Salmonella* experience glomerulonephritis. Asymptomatic urinary abnormalities may be more frequent. Renal manifestations are usually transient and resolve within 2 to 3 weeks. Serum C3 may be depressed. Mesangial proliferation with deposits of IgG, C3, and C4 is the most common finding. IgA nephropathy has also been reported.[1029–1031]

GLOMERULAR INVOLVEMENT WITH PARASITIC DISEASES

Malaria

Four strains of malaria parasite cause human disease: Plasmodium vivax, P. falciparum, P. malariae (causing quartan malaria), and P. ovale. Of these, renal involvement has been extensively documented and studied in P. malariae and falciparum. In falciparum malaria, clinically overt glomerular disease is uncommon. Asymptomatic urinary abnormalities may occur with sub-nephrotic proteinuria and hematuria or pyuria. Renal function is usually normal. Renal biopsies show mesangial proliferation or membranoproliferative lesions.[1032] Severe malaria may be manifest with hemoglobinuric acute renal failure.[1033] In quartan malaria with renal involvement, proteinuria is the cardinal manifestation, ranging from mild and transient to florid nephrotic syndrome. Significant hematuria is unusual. Serum complement may be depressed in early stages of the disease. There is progression to end-stage renal failure within 3 to 5 years. Spontaneous remissions may occur, but are rare. Antimalarial treatment fails to improve the renal outcome, and response to steroids is disappointing.[1034] Renal biopsies in Ugandan adults and children with quartan malaria show some form of proliferative glomerulonephritis (diffuse, focal, lobular, or minimal). Membranous nephropathy has also been described in these patients.[1035] However, in Nigerian children, the most common lesion was a localized or diffuse thickening of glomerular capillary walls with focal or generalized double-contouring and segmental sclerosis of the tuft.[1036] IF examination revealed deposits of IgG, IgM, C3, and P. malariae antigen in the glomeruli. By EM electron-dense material has been observed within the irregularly thickened GBM.[1037] Immune complex deposition is thought to mediate quartan malarial nephropathy through deposition of malarial antigens and antibody within the glomerulus. An experimental model in mice using P. berghei supports this hypothesis.[1038] However, late in the course of the disease, these antigens cannot be detected and possibly, non-immune mechanisms lead to persistence of disease.

Schistosomiasis is a visceral parasitic disease caused by the blood flukes of the genus Schistosoma. S. mansoni and S. japonicum cause cirrhosis of the liver and S. hematobium causes cystitis. Glomerular involvement in S. Mansoni includes mesangial proliferation, focal sclerosis, membranoproliferative lesions, crescentic changes, membranous nephropathy, amyloidosis, and eventually end-stage kidneys.[1039-1041] Schistosomal antigens have been demonstrated in renal biopsies in such patients.[1042] Treatment with antiparasitic agents does not appear to influence progression of renal disease.[1043] S. hematobium is occasionally associated with the nephrotic syndrome, which may respond to treatment of the parasite.[1039] In some patients with schistosomiasis, renal involvement may be related to concomitant Salmonella infection.[1044]

Leishmaniasis also known as Kala-Azar is caused by Leishmania donovani. Renal involvement in Kala-Azar appears to be mild and reverts with anti-leishmanial treatment. Renal biopsies show glomerular mesangial proliferation or focal endocapillary proliferation. IgG, IgM, C3 may be observed in areas of proliferation. Amyloidosis may also complicate Kala-Azar.[1045,1046] In Trypanosomiasis, Trypanosome brucei, T. gambiense, and T. rhodesiense cause African sleeping sickness and have rarely been associated with proteinuria.[1047] Filariasis caused by organisms in the genus Onchocerca, Brugia, Loa loa, and Wuchereria. Hematuria, proteinuria (including nephrotic syndrome) has been described. Renal manifestations may appear with management of infection. Renal biopsy findings have included mesangial proliferative glomerulonephritis with C3 deposition, diffuse proliferative glomerulonephritis, and collapsing glomerulopathy with loiasis.[1048-1053] Trichinosis is caused by Trichinella spiralis and may be associated with proteinuria and hematuria, which abated after specific treatment. Renal biopsies in patients with trichinosis have shown mesangial proliferative glomerulonephritis with C3 deposition.[1054,1055] Echinococcus granulosus and E. multilocularis cause hydatid disease or echinococcosis in humans. Mesangiocapillary glomerulonephritis and membranous nephropathy have occasionally been associated with hepatic hydatid cysts.[1056,1057] Toxoplasmosis may be associated with nephrotic syndrome in infants and rarely, in adults. Mesangial and endothelial proliferation may be found, with deposition of IgG, IgA, IgM, C3, and fibrinogen in areas of proliferation.[1058-1060]

GLOMERULAR INVOLVEMENT WITH VIRAL INFECTIONS

Viruses have been postulated to cause glomerular injury by various mechanisms including direct cytopathic effects, the deposition of immune complexes, or by initiation of autoimmune mechanisms.

In a study of previously healthy people with non-streptococcal upper respiratory infections, 4% had erythrocyte casts and glomerulonephritis on biopsy. A reduction in serum complement and serologic evidence of infection with adenovirus, influenza A, or influenza B were observed in some. Initial renal biopsy showed either focal or diffuse mesangial proliferation in all nine, with mesangial C3 deposits in six specimens. Sequential creatinine clearances were reduced in about half these patients during follow-up.[1061]

The nephrotic syndrome has been described with Epstein-Barr virus (EBV) infections.[1062] Renal biopsies in patients with urinary abnormalities have included immune complex-mediated glomerulonephritis with tubulointerstitial nephritis,[1063] minimal glomerular lesions with IgM deposition,[1064] and widespread glomerular mesangiolysis sometimes admixed with segmental mesangial sclerosis.[1065] In addition, the presence of EBV DNA in the glomerulus is thought to worsen glomerular damage in chronic glomerulopathies.[1066] Other viruses have rarely been associated with glomerulonephritis including herpes zoster, mumps, adenovirus, echovirus, Coxsackie virus, and influenza A and B.[1067]

HIV-Related Glomerulopathies

Over 42 million people have been infected with the human immunodeficiency virus (HIV) worldwide, with an estimated 5 million new infections each year.[1068] A variety of glomerular lesions and in particular, a unique form of glomerular damage, HIV-associated nephropathy (HIVAN), have emerged as significant forms of renal disease in HIV-infected patients.[1069,1070]

HIV-Associated Nephropathy

Clinical Features

In 1984, the first detailed report of a new pattern of sclerosing glomerulopathy in HIV-infected patients was reported.[1071] Subsequent studies mainly from large urban centers confirmed the occurrence and described the features of HIVAN.[1071-1081] In these largely urban eastcoast centers, the prevalence of HIVAN approached 90% in nephrotic HIV-positive patients in contrast to a prevalence of only 2% in San Francisco where most seropositive patients were white homosexuals.[1082-1084]

There is a strong predilection for HIVAN among HIV-infected patients of African Heritage. The black:white ratio among patients with HIVAN is 12:1.[1085] HIVAN is the third leading cause of ESRD among African Americans aged 20 to 64, following only diabetes and hypertension.[1078,1086] Of HIV-infected adults, who do not use intravenous drugs, with glomerular lesions, 17% of whites had very mild FSGS, 75% diffuse mesangial hyperplasia (DMH), and none severe FSGS in contrast to blacks in whom only 27% had DMH but in whom 55% had severe FSGS. Blacks were also more likely to have more severe clinical renal disease with heavier proteinuria, a higher incidence of the nephrotic syndrome, and greater renal insufficiency. A similar presentation has been found in Los Angeles and Europe.[1087,1088] Racial factors are important in mutations of HIV receptors, which may in part explain some differences in the racial predisposition to HIV infection and HIVAN.[1089-1091] Although intravenous drug use has been the most common risk factor for the HIVAN, the disease has been seen in all groups at risk for AIDS including homosexuals, perinatally acquired disease, heterosexual transmission, and exposure to contaminated blood products.[1069] HIVAN usually occurs in patients with a low CD4 count, but full-blown AIDS is certainly not a prerequisite for the disease. In one New York study the onset of HIVAN was most common in otherwise asymptomatic HIV-infected patients (i.e., 12 of 26 were asymptomatic patients).[1071,1075] There is no relationship between the development of HIVAN and patient age and duration of HIV infection, or types of opportunistic infections or malignancies.[1069] The prevalence of HIVAN in patients who test positive for HIV is reported to be 3.5% in patients screened in the clinic setting[1092]; the same group reported that HIVAN was found in 6.9% of autopsies in HIV-infected patients.[1093]

The clinical features of HIVAN include presenting features of proteinuria, typically in the nephrotic range (and often massive), and renal insufficiency. Other manifestation of the nephrotic syndrome including edema, hypoalbuminemia, and hypercholesterolemia have been common in some series but less so in others despite the heavy proteinuria.[1069,1071,1074,1075,1079,1081,1094] Likewise, the incidence of hypertension has been variable even in patients with severe renal failure. Some patients, however, present with subnephrotic range proteinuria, and urinary sediment findings of microhematuria and sterile pyuria.[1095] The renal ultrasound in HIVAN show echogenic kidneys with preserved or enlarged size with an average of over 12 cm in spite of the severe renal insufficiency.[1075,1079] Echogenicity may correlate with the histopathologic tubulo-interstitial changes better than the glomerular changes.[1079]

Pathology

The term HIVAN is reserved for the characteristic LM pattern of focal segmental glomerulosclerosis and related mesangiopathies.[1070] The focal sclerosing features are typically collapsing with retraction of the glomerular capillary walls and luminal occlusion either in a segmental or global distribution (Fig. 31–51).[1070,1073,1096] In the acute phase, this occurs without a substantial increase in matrix or hyalinosis. There is striking hypertrophy and hyperplasia of the visceral epithelial cells, which form a cellular crown over the collapsed glomerular lobules (Fig. 31–52). In one study analyzing the expression pattern of podocyte differentiation and proliferation markers, there was disappearance of all podocyte differentiation markers from collapsed glomeruli, associated with cell proliferation suggesting that the podocyte phenotype is

dysregulated.[1097] Patients with HIVAN have a higher percentage of glomerular collapse, less hyalinosis, and greater visceral cell swelling than patients with classic idiopathic FSGS or heroin nephropathy even when matched for serum creatinine and degree of proteinuria.[1073] The tubulointerstitial disease is also more severe in HIVAN with tubular degenerative changes and regenerative features, interstitial edema, fibrosis, and inflammation.[1070,1073] Tubules are often greatly dilated into microcysts containing proteinaceous casts (see Fig. 31–51). By IF, IgM and C3 are present; however, by EM, immune deposits are not detected (Fig. 31–53). In almost all biopsies of HIVAN there are numerous tubulo-reticular inclusions (TRI) within the glomerular and vascular endothelial cells (Fig. 31–54).[1069,1070,1073,1096] These 24-nm interanastomosing tubular structures are found within the dilated cisternae of the endoplasmic reticulum.

Pathogenesis

Recent evidence strongly supports a role for direct HIV-1 infection of renal parenchymal cells. By in-situ hybridization, HIV-1 RNA was detected in renal tubular epithelial cells, glomerular epithelial cells (visceral and parietal), and interstitial leukocytes.[1098] Renal epithelial cells may be an

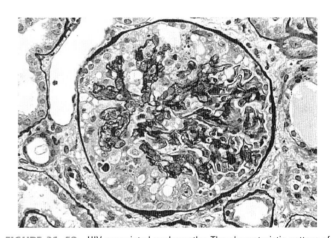

FIGURE 31–52 HIV-associated nephropathy: The characteristic pattern of collapsing glomerular sclerosis is depicted. Glomerular capillary lumina are occluded by wrinkling and retraction of the glomerular capillary walls associated with marked hypertrophy and hyperplasia of the podocytes, forming a pseudocrescent (Periodic acid-Schiff, ×325).

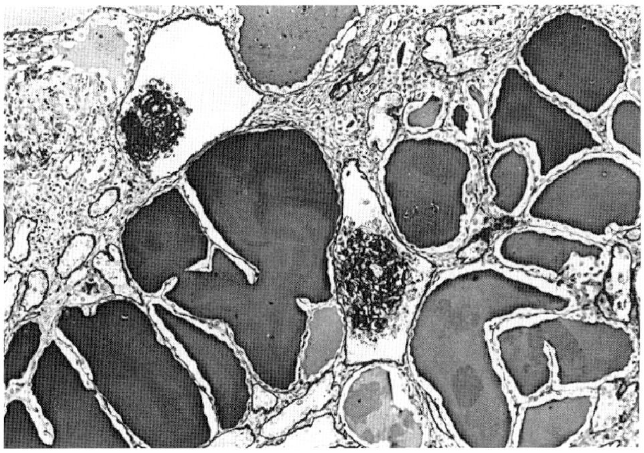

FIGURE 31–51 HIV-associated nephropathy: Glomeruli have collapsed tufts with capping of the overlying podocytes and dilatation of the urinary space. The tubules are dilated forming microcysts with abundant proteinaceous casts (Periodic acid Schiff, ×125).

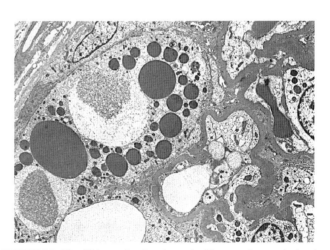

FIGURE 31–53 HIV-associated nephropathy: Electron micrograph showing wrinkling of glomerular basement membranes with marked podocyte hypertrophy, complete foot process effacement, and numerous intracytoplasmic protein resorption droplets (×2500).

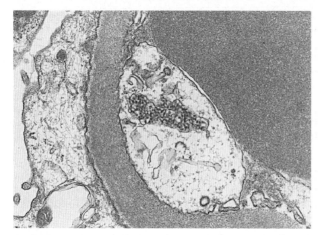

FIGURE 31–54 HIV-associated nephropathy: Electron micrograph showing a typical tubuloreticular inclusion within the endoplasmic reticulum of a glomerular endothelial cell (×6000).

important reservoir for HIV because HIV RNA was found in the kidney of patients with undetectable viral loads in peripheral blood.[1098] Moreover, HIV-infected tubular epithelium can support viral replication, as evidenced by the detection of HIV quasispecies separate from those found in peripheral blood of the same patient.[1099]

A replicative-deficient transgenic mouse model of HIVAN has been developed with lesions identical to HIV nephropathy.[1100–1102] It was subsequently demonstrated that the HIV transgene expression is required for development of the HIVAN phenotype.[1103] Thus, viral replication may not be necessary for the development of the disease and it is likely that a viral gene product with direct effects on renal cells is operative.

The lesions of collapsing glomerulopathy are associated with podocyte proliferation and de-differentiation.[1097,1104] The specific gene(s) responsible for producing these changes are being investigated. The nef gene (which is thought to act by activation of tyrosine kinases) was found to be essential in producing HIV-induced changes in podocyte cultures[1105] and in one murine model of HIVAN.[1106] Recent evidence supports a synergistic role for nef and vpr on podocyte dysfunction and progressive glomerulosclerosis.[1107] Host genes may also play a role in the pathogenesis of HIVAN. The expression of two cyclin-dependent kinase inhibitors (which regulate cell cycle), p27 and p57, were decreased in podocytes from HIVAN biopsies whereas expression of another CDK inhibitor, p21, was increased.[1108]

Course and Treatment

The natural history of HIVAN during the early part of the AIDS epidemic was characterized by rapid progression to end-stage renal disease (ESRD). Case series from the United States that were published during the years that HIVAN was first described demonstrated an almost universal requirement for dialysis within less than 1 year of diagnosis.[1071,1074,1075] There are no randomized controlled trials to define the optimal treatment of HIVAN. There are several early case reports and retrospective analyses in which patients with biopsy-documented or presumed HIVAN have experienced either remissions of the nephrotic syndrome or improvement in GFR when treated with AZT or AZT with acyclovir.[1109–1112] Recently, the role of combined antiviral therapies and the use of newer agents in the management of HIVAN have been investigated in small numbers of patients with apparent beneficial effects.[1113–1115] Corresponding to the introduction of highly active anti-retroviral therapy (HAART) the rise in new cases of ESRD due to HIVAN slowed markedly.[1116]

There have been a few studies using corticosteroids in HIVAN. In an early study, prednisone was not associated with improvement in children with HIVAN.[1117,1118] Remissions in HIV-infected children with the minimal change pattern on biopsy treated with steroids have been noted, but not in children with sclerosing or collapsing lesions.[1069] In adults, however, several retrospective studies have shown short-term improvement in clinical parameters.[1119–1121]

Three pediatric patients with HIVAN on biopsy had sustained remissions of the nephrotic syndrome when treated with cyclosporine.[1117] They eventually developed opportunistic infections requiring the cyclosporine to be discontinued and subsequently experienced relapses of the nephrotic proteinuria and renal failure.

In isolated patients and in several small trials use of ACE inhibitors has been shown to decrease proteinuria in HIVAN and to slow the progression to renal failure.[1122–1124] Serum ACE levels are elevated in HIV patients and ACE inhibitors may prevent proteinuria and glomerulosclerosis by either hemodynamic mechanisms or through modulation of matrix production and mesangial cell proliferation or even by affecting HIV protease activity.[1122–1124] Although some of these studies used control groups of untreated HIV patients of similar age, sex, race, and degree of renal insufficiency and proteinuria the studies were not randomized, blinded trials. Nevertheless in each study the ACE-treated group had less proteinuria, less rise in serum creatinine, and less progression to ESRD.

At present the therapy of HIVAN should include use of multiple anti-viral agents as in HIV infected patients without nephropathy. Use of ACE inhibitors or perhaps angiotensin II receptor blockers, with careful attention to hyperkalemia and acute rises in the serum creatinine, may be beneficial. Immunosuppressive therapy with steroids or cyclosporine should be used only in certain patients where the potential benefits of therapy outweigh the risks of further immunocompromise and opportunistic infections.

Several studies have documented favorable outcomes in HIVAN patients who received renal transplants.[1125,1126] The current consensus is that renal transplantation is no longer a contraindication in HIV-positive patients, and the British HIV Association have published guidelines on this topic.[1127]

Other Glomerular Lesions in Patients with HIV Infection

Although HIVAN is the most common form of glomerulopathy found in HIV-infected patients, other lesions have been reported as well. In one series of over 100 biopsies for glomerular disease in HIV-positive patients, 73% were classic HIVAN, but other lesions included MPGN in 10%, minimal change disease in 6%, amyloid in 3%, lupus-like nephritis in 3%, acute postinfectious glomerulonephritis in 2%, membranous nephropathy 2%, and 1% each of focal and segmental necrotizing glomerulonephritis, thrombotic microangiopathy, IgA nephropathy, and immunotactoid nephropathy.[1070] Collapsing FSGS is most common in urban centers with large black populations, whereas higher rates of immune complex glomerulonephritis are found in other cities and especially European white populations.[1087,1088] In a study from Paris, immune complex GN was found in over 50% of the white HIV seropositive patients but only 21% of the blacks.[1087,1088] Likewise in a study from northern Italy of 26 biopsies on HIV-infected patients most cases were of immune complex GN but none of classic HIVAN.[1128]

IgA nephropathy has been reported in a number of series of HIV-infected patients.[1129–1133] This has occurred in both whites and blacks despite the rarity of typical IgA nephropathy in black populations. The clinical features usually include hematuria, proteinuria, and some renal insufficiency. Cases with leukocytoclastic angiitis of the skin (consistent with Henoch-Schönlein purpura) have also been noted. The histology shows a variety of changes from mesangial proliferative glomerulonephritis to collapsing glomerulosclerosis with mesangial IgA deposits. IgA anti-HIV immune complexes have been eluted from the kidneys of several such patients, and several patients have had circulating immune complexes containing IgA idiotypic antibodies directed against viral proteins, either anti-HIV p24 or HIV gp41.[1132]

Membranoproliferative glomerulonephritis may be the most common pattern of immune complex-mediated glomerulonephritis seen in HIV-infected patients. Two series document a high occurrence in intravenous drug abusers co-infected with HIV and hepatitis C.[1134,1135] Most patients have had microscopic hematuria, nephrotic-range proteinuria, and renal insufficiency at biopsy. Cryoglobulins are commonly positive, as is hypocomplementemia, and some have had both hepatitis B and hepatitis C infection. The pathology of the glomerulopathy may be similar to idiopathic MPGN Type 1 or Type 3 although some patients also have features of segmental membranous or mesangioproliferative features.

A lupus-like immune complex glomerulonephritis has been reported in a number of patients.[1078,1136–1138] Most of these patients have had positive serology for SLE with positive ANA, anti-DNA, and low complement levels. This contrasts with a low incidence of ANA positivity and almost no anti-DNA positivity in the general HIV-infected population.[1139]

A not-infrequent association in both white and black HIV-infected patients has been thrombotic thrombocytopenic purpura (TTP). Most have been in an advanced stage of HIV infection and had renal involvement with hematuria, proteinuria, and variable renal insufficiency. Other typical findings of TTP such as fever, neurologic symptoms, thrombocytopenia, and microangiopathic hemolytic anemia are often present. There is no known association with *E.coli* O157:H7 or other agents implicated in the epidemic forms of hemolytic uremic syndrome. Mortality is high even if treated with vigorous therapy (e.g., plasmapheresis, fresh frozen plasma infusion, and corticosteroids).[1140]

Glomerular Manifestations of Liver Disease

Hepatitis B

Hepatitis B antigenemia has been associated with glomerulonephritis for over 30 years. Hepatitis B has a worldwide distribution. In countries where the virus is endemic (sub-Saharan Africa, Southeast Asia, and Eastern Europe) there is vertical transmission from mother to infant and horizontal transmission between siblings. Hepatitis B-associated nephropathy occurs in these children with a 4:1 male preponderance.[1141–1143] In the United States and Western Europe where hepatitis B is acquired by parenteral routes or sexually, the nephropathy affects mainly adults and has a different clinical course from the endemic form.[1144–1146] However, hepatitis B-associated nephropathy is rare in hepatitis B carriers.[1147] Polyarteritis nodosa has also been associated with hepatitis B.[1148]

Clinical Features

Most patients present with proteinuria or the nephrotic syndrome. In endemic areas, there may not be a preceding history of hepatitis. The majority of patients have normal renal function at time of presentation. There may be urinary erythrocytes but the majority have a bland sediment. Liver disease may be absent (carrier state) or chronic, and clinically mild. Serum aminotransferases may be normal or modestly elevated (between 100–200 IU/L). Liver biopsies in these patients

often show chronic active hepatitis. Some patients ultimately develop cirrhosis in their biopsies. There is often spontaneous resolution of the carrier state with resolution of renal abnormalities. Spontaneous resolution of HBV-associated nephropathy is particularly common in children from endemic areas. The probability of a spontaneous remission may be as high as 80% after 10 years.[1149,1150]

Pathology

Most cases of hepatitis B-associated nephropathy manifest membranous nephropathy, although mesangial proliferation and sclerosis have also been reported.[1141,1142,1144–1146,1151,1152] A few patients with membranoproliferative glomerulonephritis have also been described, with mesangial cell interposition, reduplication of the GBM, and subendothelial glomerular deposits.[1144,1146,1151] In a few series Type III MPGN have been reported in which there are electron-dense subepithelial deposits in addition to the changes seen in Type I MPGN.[1146] Crescentic glomerulonephritis in association with membranous changes and primary crescentic glomerulonephritis have also been described.[1153,1154] The glomerular lesions appear to be immune complex-mediated. HBsAg, HBcAg, and HBeAg[1155] have all been demonstrated in glomerular lesions, as has HBV DNA.[1143,1156]

Treatment

In children with mild endemic form of hepatitis B-associated nephropathy, no treatment other than supportive care is advocated. In patients with progressive renal dysfunction, interferon has been used with mixed results.[1157–1160] Steroids do not significantly improve proteinuria and may potentially enhance viral replication.[1161,1162] Adenine arabinoside and thymic extract (Thymostimuline) for 6 months have shown to be of some benefit in these cases.[1163] Nucleoside analogs including lamivudine (3TC), adefovir, and lobucavir have also demonstrated clinical utility in treating hepatitis B infection; Lamivudine was shown to reduce proteinuria and lead to a lesser incidence of ESRD in 10 patients with hepatitis B-associated nephropathy.[1164] Preemptive lamivudine therapy in renal transplant recipients has shown improved survival compared to historical controls.[1165,1166]

Hepatitis C

Renal disease associated with hepatitis C virus (HCV) infection includes membranoproliferative glomerulonephritis with or without associated mixed cryoglobulinemia and membranous glomerulopathy. The membranoproliferative glomerulonephritis is most often type 1, with fewer cases of type 3.[1167–1169] Rare cases of diffuse proliferative and exudative glomerulonephritis, polyarteritis, and fibrillary and immunotactoid glomerulopathy have also been described in association with HCV.[1170] Most patients have evidence of liver disease as reflected by elevated plasma transaminase levels. However, transaminase levels are normal in some cases and a history of acute hepatitis is often absent.

Pathogenesis

The pathogenesis of HCV-related nephropathies is immune complex-mediated. HCV-specific proteins have been isolated from glomerular lesions.[1171] The disappearance of viremia in response to interferon (see later) is associated with a diminution of proteinuria; a relapse of viremia is accompanied by rising proteinuria.

Clinical and Pathologic Features

Mixed cryoglobulinemia is associated with hepatitis C virus and may cause a systemic vasculitis; patients may exhibit constitutional systemic symptoms, palpable purpura, peripheral neuropathy, and hypocomplementemia. The renal manifestations include hematuria, proteinuria (often in the nephrotic range), and renal insufficiency. The histologic findings resemble those in idiopathic MPGN type 1 or type 3

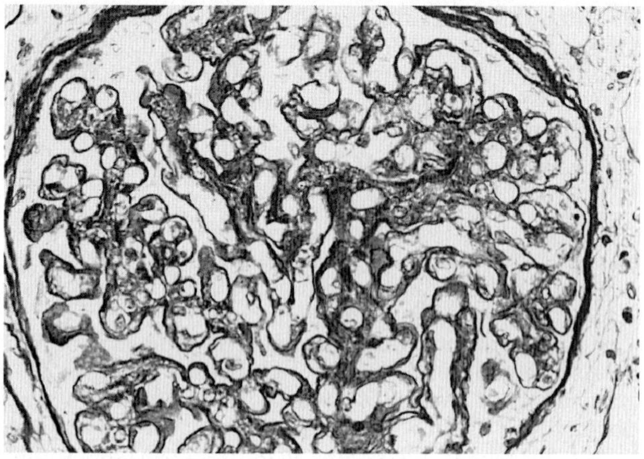

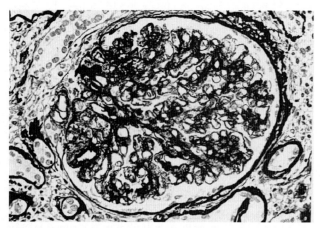

FIGURE 31–55 Hepatitis C-associated membranoproliferative glomerulonephritis type 1: The mesangium is expanded by global mesangial hypercellularity associated with numerous double contours of the glomerular basement membranes (Periodic acid Schiff, ×500).

FIGURE 31–56 Hepatitis C-associated membranoproliferative glomerulonephritis type 3: There are mixed features of membranoproliferative glomerulonephritis type 1 (with mesangial proliferation and duplication of glomerular basement membrane) and membranous glomerulopathy (with basement membrane spikes) (Jones methenamine silver, ×325).

(Figs. 31–55 and 31–56) except for intraluminal protein "thrombi" on light microscopy and the organized annular-tubular substructure of the electron-dense deposits on electron microscopy. Prior to the advent of hepatitis C serological tests, mixed cryoglobulinemia had been considered an idiopathic disease ("essential" mixed cryoglobulinemia). Up to 95% of these patients show signs of HCV infection.[1172] Few patients with thrombotic microangiopathy associated with cryoglobulinemia have been described.[1173] Membranoproliferative glomerulonephritis without associated cryoglobulinemia may occur, but is much less common.[1168]

Rarely, membranous nephropathy may be associated with HCV infection. Patients present with the nephrotic syndrome or proteinuria. Complement levels tend to normal and neither cryoglobulins nor rheumatoid factors are present in HCV-associated membranous nephropathy.[1174]

Both Type I MPGN (with and without cryoglobulinemia) and membranous nephropathy may recur in the allograft after renal transplantation, sometimes leading to graft loss.[1175–1178] Similar lesions have occurred in native kidneys after liver transplantation in HCV-positive patients.[1179,1180]

Treatment

A number of reports demonstrating a beneficial response to α-interferon therapy in patients with HCV-induced renal disease.[1174,1181,1182] Vasculitic symptoms, viral titers, proteinuria, and in some studies, plasma creatinine improved in 50% to 60% of patients receiving α-interferon for periods up to 1 year. Cessation of interferon therapy, however, was associated with recurrence of viremia and cryoglobulinemia in a majority of patients in these studies. Longer periods of treatment (18 months) show some additional benefit in liver disease, but has not been evaluated in the HCV-induced renal disease.[1183] Interferon therapy may paradoxically exacerbate proteinuria and hematuria that appears to be unrelated to viral antigenic effects.[1184]

Combination therapy with ribavirin and interferon has shown better response rates as initial therapy, and in α-interferon relapses in patients with HCV liver disease.[1185–1187] Combination therapy appeared to improve biochemical parameters of renal dysfunction in 20 HCV-GN patients, which was not accompanied by a significant virological response.[1188] Another report on 18 patients showed sustained virologic responses in two thirds of patients which was associated with improvement in renal parameters.[1189] Combination therapy (especially ribavirin) may not be well tolerated in the presence of significant renal dysfunction. Interferon-α treatment of renal transplant patients with HCV has been associated with acute renal failure[1190] and acute humoral rejection.[1191]

Cyclophosphamide treatment has been used successfully in HCV-glomerulonephritis,[1192] even if interferon-resistant.[1193] Cyclophosphamide treatment may be associated with a temporary, reversible increase in viral load and a change of quasispecies.[1194] Fludarabine has been reported to decrease proteinuria in HCV-associated cryoglobulinemic MPGN.[1195] Recently, there have been reports of rituximab-induced remissions of proteinuria in HCV-GN.[1196] In renal transplant patients with HCV-GN, similar improvement in renal parameters have been reported, albeit with a higher incidence of infectious complications.[1197]

Autoimmune Chronic Active Hepatitis

Autoimmune chronic hepatitis is a distinctive progressive necrotic and fibrotic disorder of the liver with clinical or serologic evidence (or both) of a generalized autoimmune disorder.[1198] Two distinct clinical lesions have been associated with this disorder: glomerulonephritis and interstitial nephritis. Patients with the glomerular lesion present with nephrotic syndrome or renal insufficiency. On renal biopsy they have membranous or membranoproliferative glomerulonephritis. In two patients with membranous nephropathy, circulating immune complexes containing U1-RNP (ribonucleoprotein) and IgG have been reported. Eluates from the kidney tissue revealed higher concentrations of anti U1-RNP antibody. It is not known whether immunosuppressive therapy ameliorates the renal disorder.[1198] It is unclear if coexistent hepatitis C infection had been present in many of these patients.

Liver Cirrhosis

Glomerulonephritis is a rare manifestation of liver cirrhosis. Glomerular morphologic abnormalities with IgA deposition have been noted in more than 50% of patients with cirrhosis at both necropsy and biopsy[1199,1200] although this has also been found in some autopsies of non-cirrhotic kidneys.[1201] Clinically, there may be mild proteinuria or hematuria (or both). There are two patterns on histology: a mesangial sclerosis ("cirrhotic glomerular sclerosis") or membranoproliferative glomerulonephritis. The latter may be associated with more severe renal symptoms and a depression of serum complement C3 levels.[1202] Again, it is unclear if some patients had co-existent hepatitis C infection. Rarely, HSP with rapidly progressive glomerulonephritis has been described in association with cirrhosis.[1203]

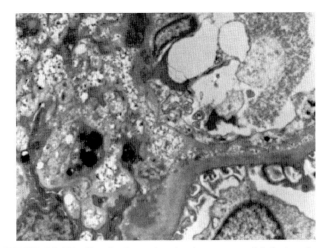

FIGURE 31–57 Hepatic glomerulopathy: A paramesangial electron-dense deposit corresponding to IgA is present. In addition, there are irregular lucencies containing dense granular and rounded membranous structures within the mesangial matrix and extending into the subendothelial space (×6000).

Renal biopsies of patients with cirrhosis on light microscopy show an increase in mesangial matrix with little on no increase in mesangial cellularity, a lesion known as "hepatic glomerulopathy". Less commonly, the distinctive pathologic findings consist of mesangial proliferative glomerulonephritis with mesangial IgA deposits usually accompanied by complement deposition and less intense IgG and/or IgM.[1199,1204,1205] By electron microscopy, the mesangium and subendothelial regions contain lucencies with dense granular and rounded membranous structures consistent with lipid inclusions (Fig. 31–57). Increased serum IgA levels are found in over 90% of cirrhotic patients with glomerular IgA deposition. Other authors have reported IgM as the dominant immunoglobulin.[1200] Cirrhotic glomerulonephritis is usually a clinically silent disease; however, the diagnosis can be suspected by finding proteinuria, or abnormalities of the urine sediment. The pathogenesis may relate to defective hepatic clearance of IgA as well as altered processing or portacaval shunting (or both) of circulating immune complexes.[1206] This theory is bolstered by the finding of increased deposits of IgA in skin and hepatic sinusoids in cirrhotic patients.[1207] Moreover, in patients with non-cirrhotic portal fibrosis who underwent portal-systemic bypass procedures there was an increase in the incidence of clinically overt glomerulonephritis (from 78% to 32%) associated with deposition of IgA after the procedure. In the latter group, there was also a significant incidence of renal failure (50% after 5 years).[1208] Similar findings were noted in children with end-stage liver disease from α-1 antitrypsin deficiency or biliary atresia, which resolved after liver transplantation.[1209]

Glomerular Lesions Associated with Neoplasia

The occurrence of glomerular syndromes, both nephrotic and nephritic, may be associated with malignancy, but is rare (<1%). Glomerular disease may be seen with a wide variety of malignancies. Carcinomas of the lung, stomach, breast, and colon are most frequently associated with glomerular lesions. Membranous nephropathy is the most common lesion associated with carcinoma.[1210–1212] Patients over the age of 50 presenting with nephrotic syndrome should be reviewed for the presence of a malignancy.[1213,1214]

Clinical and Pathologic Features

Clinically, the glomerulopathy of neoplasia may be manifested by proteinuria or the nephrotic syndrome, an active urine sediment, and/or diminished glomerular filtration. Sig-

nificant renal impairment is uncommon, and is usually associated with the proliferative forms of glomerulonephritis. In evaluating an erythrocyte sedimentation rate (ESR) in patients with nephrotic syndrome, it should be noted that most such patients have an ESR above 60 mm/h, with roughly 20% being above 100 mm/h. As a result, an elevated ESR alone in a patient with the nephrotic syndrome (or with end-stage renal disease) is not an indication to evaluate the patient for an occult malignancy or underlying inflammatory disease.[1215,1216]

Membranous Nephropathy

Membranous nephropathy may be associated with malignancies in 10% to 40% of cases.[1214,1217] These include carcinoma of bronchus,[1218] breast,[1219] colon,[1220,1221] stomach, ovary,[1222] kidney,[1223] pancreas,[1224] and prostate,[1225,1226] as well as testicular seminoma,[1227] parotid adenolymphoma, carcinoid tumor,[1228,1229] and Hodgkin disease and carotid body tumor.[1230] In some cases of membranous nephropathy associated with malignancy, tumor antigens have been detected within the glomeruli. It is postulated that tumor antigen deposition in the glomerulus is followed by antibody deposition, causing "in situ" immune complex formation, and subsequent complement activation.[1231,1232] Immune complexes and complement have been found in cancer patients without overt renal disease.[1231] Removal of the tumor may lead to remission of the nephrotic syndrome, which may then recur, following the development of metastasis. In many instances successful treatment of the neoplasm has induced a partial or complete remission of the associated glomerulopathy.

Minimal Change Disease or Focal Glomerulosclerosis

Minimal change disease or focal glomerulosclerosis may occur in association with Hodgkin disease,[1233–1235] and, less often, non-Hodgkin lymphoma or leukemia,[1234] and rarely thymoma,[1236] mycosis fungoides,[1237] renal cell carcinoma,[1238] and other solid tumors.[1239–1241] Secretion of a lymphokine by abnormal T cells may underlie glomerular injury in these disorders.[1242,1243]

Secondary amyloidosis has been described with a number of malignancies, particularly renal cell carcinoma, Hodgkin disease, and chronic lymphocytic leukemia.[1,2,4] In Hodgkin disease, for example, renal amyloidosis is generally a late event resulting from a chronic inflammatory state; by comparison, minimal change disease most often occurs at the time of initial presentation.[5]

Proliferative Glomerulonephritides and Vasculitides

Both membranoproliferative and rapidly progressive glomerulonephritis have been described in patients with solid tumors and lymphomas, although the etiologic relationship between these conditions is not proven.[1241,1244] The association is probably strongest for membranoproliferative glomerulonephritis and chronic lymphocytic leukemia and may be associated with circulating cryoglobulins.[1245,1246] Mesangial proliferation with IgA deposition has been associated with mucosa-associated lymphoid tissue (MALT) lymphoma, which resolved following management of the malignancy with chlorambucil.[1247] Although the association between crescentic glomerulonephritis and vasculitis with tumors may be coincidental, it has been suggested that the malignancy may act as a trigger for the vasculitis.[1248–1250] In contrast to the nephrotic states described earlier in which renal function is generally well preserved at presentation and the urine sediment is usually benign, patients with proliferative glomerulonephritis often have an acute decline in renal function and an active urine sediment.

Thrombotic Microangiopathy

Both the hemolytic-uremic syndrome (HUS) and the related disorder thrombotic thrombocytopenic purpura (TTP) can occur in patients with malignancy. An underlying carcinoma of the stomach, pancreas, or prostate may be associated with HUS. More commonly, however, anti-tumor therapy is implicated: mitomycin, the combination of bleomycin and cisplatin, and radiation plus high-dose cyclophosphamide prior to bone marrow transplantation all can lead to the HUS, which may first become apparent months after therapy has been discontinued.[1251] This topic is reviewed elsewhere in this book.

GLOMERULAR DISEASE ASSOCIATED WITH DRUGS

Heroin Nephropathy

In the 1970's, reports began to appear linking heroin abuse to the nephrotic syndrome and renal biopsy findings of focal and segmental glomerulosclerosis. This syndrome was referred to as heroin-associated nephropathy (HAN).[1252-1257] Similar lesions were seen in users of intravenous pentazocine (Talwin), and tripelennamine (pyribenzamine) so-called T's and Blues.[1258] This syndrome occurred almost exclusively in blacks; it has been suggested that blacks may have a genetic predisposition for developing HAN.[1259,1260] The mean age was less than 30 years old with 90% of the patients being males. The duration of drug abuse varied from 6 months to 30 years (mean 6 years) prior to the onset of renal disease. Most patients presented with the nephrotic syndrome. The course of HAN was relentless progression to ESRD over many years in those addicts who continued to use heroin, whereas a regression of abnormalities was seen in patients that were able to stop using the drug. Kidney biopsies of these patients showed lesions of focal segmental and global sclerosis. Nonspecific trapping leads to the deposition of IgM and C3 in areas of sclerosis. There was usually significant interstitial inflammation associated with the glomerular lesion. The pathogenesis of HAN is unknown. Abnormalities of cellular and humoral immunity have been well described in heroin addicts.[1261] It has been suggested that morphine itself could act as an antigen and that contaminants used to "cut" the heroin could contribute to the pathogenesis. Morphine (the active metabolite of heroin) has been shown to stimulate proliferation and sclerosis of mesangial cells and fibroblasts.[1262,1263] The syndrome of HAN has almost disappeared among drug addicts presenting with renal failure; for example, there has been a sharp decline in incident cases of HAN and there have been no reported cases of HAN-associated ESRD from Brooklyn, New York during the period of 1991 to 1993.[1264,1265] In part this trend coincides with the rise of HIV infection and HIVAN.

Nonsteroidal Anti-Inflammatory Drugs (NSAID)-Induced Nephropathy

Nonsteroidal anti-inflammatory drugs are being used by approximately 50 million of the general public in the United States at any point in time. Approximately 1% to 3% of patients exposed to NSAIDs will manifest one of the renal abnormalities associated with its use: fluid and electrolyte disturbances, acute renal failure, and nephrotic syndrome with interstitial nephritis and papillary necrosis.[1266] The combination of acute interstitial nephritis and nephrotic syndrome is characteristic of this group of compounds. Essentially all NSAIDS can cause this type of renal disease,[1267-1269] including the cyclooxygenase-2 inhibitors.[1270,1271]

Clinical and Pathologic Features
Minimal-Change Disease with Interstitial Nephritis
The onset of NSAID-induced nephrotic syndrome is usually delayed, with a mean time of onset of 5.4 months (range 2

weeks to 18 months). Patients may present with edema and oliguria. Systemic signs of allergic interstitial nephritis are usually absent. The urine exhibits microhematuria and pyuria. Proteinuria is usually in the nephrotic range. The extent of renal dysfunction may be mild to severe. On LM the findings consist of minimal-change disease with interstitial nephritis. A focal of diffuse interstitial infiltrate consists predominantly of cytotoxic T lymphocytes (also other T cell subsets, B cells, and plasma cells).[1272,1273] The syndrome usually reverses after discontinuing therapy, and the time to recovery may be between 1 month to 1 year.[1269] Complete remission is usually seen.[1274] Relapse of proteinuria has been reported.[1275] Treatment of the nephrotic syndrome is usually unnecessary because the disorder is self-limiting. However, a short course of corticosteroids may be beneficial in patients in whom no response is seen after several weeks of discontinuation of the drug.[1276] Plasma exchange was reported with being associated with rapid recovery of renal function in two patients.[1277]

Other Patterns
Minimal-change nephrotic syndrome without interstitial disease has been occasionally reported.[1278] Granulomatous interstitial disease without glomerular changes has also been described.[1279] Membranous nephropathy has also been reported in association with NSAID use,[1280] including the newer COX-2 inhibitors.[1271] As in minimal change nephrotic syndrome, there is rapid recovery after drug withdrawal in NSAID-induced membranous nephropathy.

Pathogenesis
The mechanism of NSAID-induced nephrotic syndrome has not been defined. It has been proposed that inhibition of cyclooxygenase by NSAID inhibits prostaglandin synthesis and shunts arachidonic acid pathways towards the production of leukotrienes. These byproducts of arachidonic acid metabolism may promote T lymphocyte activation and enhanced vascular permeability, leading to minimal change disease.[1267-1269]

Anti Rheumatoid Arthritis Therapy-Induced Glomerulopathy

Gold Salts and D-Penicillamine
Proteinuria and nephrotic syndrome have been reported to occur in association with both oral and parenteral gold.[1281,1282] Dermatitis may occur concurrently. Membranous nephropathy, and rarely minimal-change disease have been reported.[1283] A higher incidence of nephropathy has been reported in patients with HLA B8/DR3.[1284,1285]

Proteinuria in association with membranous nephropathy is the most common lesion reported. Less commonly, minimal-change disease and mesangial proliferative lesions have been reported.[1285] Goodpasture-like syndrome,[1286] minimal-change nephrotic syndrome,[1287] and membranous nephropathy concurrently with vasculitis[1288] have been described rarely. HLA B8/DR3 haplotypes are also associated with penicillamine nephropathy.[1289] Tiopronin and bucillamine (a penicillamine-like compound) have also been associated with the same renal lesions described for penicillamine.[1290,1291] The onset of proteinuria with gold or penicillamine therapy is usually between 6 to 12 months after starting therapy. Proteinuria usually resolves after withdrawing the offending agent; persistent renal dysfunction is uncommon.[1285,1289,1292] Under close supervision, gold and penicillamine has been continued in patients with nephropathy with no obvious adverse effect on renal function.[1293] Anti-TNF alpha agents have been reported to promote the development of lupus-like nephritis and ANCA-associated glomerulonephritis in patients with rheumatoid arthritis.[1294]

Other Medications

Organic mercurial exposure can occur with diuretics, skin lightening creams, gold refining, and industrial exposure. Proteinuria and nephrotic syndrome have been reported.[1295–1297] Renal biopsy in such patients has shown membranous nephropathy[1298,1299] or minimal-change disease.[1300] The nephrotic syndrome has been associated with the anticonvulsants ethosuccimide,[1301] trimethadione,[1302] and paradione.[1303] Diffuse proliferative glomerulonephritis may be seen with mesantoin (mephenytoin).[1304] ANCA-associated vasculitis as well as a lupus-like nephritis has been reported with propylthiouracil.[1305–1308] Captopril has been associated with the development of proteinuria and the nephrotic syndrome due to membranous nephropathy.[1309] Substituting enalapril for captopril has been reported to ameliorate the nephrotic syndrome.[1310] Interferon-α has been associated with interstitial nephritis, minimal-change disease, focal and segmental glomerulosclerosis and acute renal failure,[1311,1312] thrombotic microangiopathy,[1313,1314] and crescentic glomerulonephritis.[1315] Mercapto propionyl glycine(2-MPG) used in the management of cystinuria has been associated with membranous glomerulopathy.[1316] Lithium use has been associated with minimal change disease,[1317,1318] membranous nephropathy,[1319] and focal and segmental glomerulosclerosis.[1320,1321] The use of high-dose pamidronate in patients with malignancies has been associated with HIV-negative collapsing focal and segmental glomerulosclerosis.[1322]

Miscellaneous Diseases Associated with Glomerular Lesions

Well-documented cases exist of nephrotic syndrome associated with unilateral renal artery stenosis, which improved after correction of the stenosis. The mechanism of proteinuria presumably relates to high levels of angiotensin-II.[1323–1325]

Acute silicosis has been associated with a proliferative glomerulonephritis with IgM and C3 deposits, leading to renal failure.[1326] A patient with dense lamellar inclusions in swollen glomerular epithelial cells, similar to those seen in Fabry disease has also been described.[1327]

Membranous nephropathy and membranoproliferative glomerulonephritis[1328] have been described in association with ulcerative colitis.[1329]

Kimura disease and angiolymphoid hyperplasia with eosinophilia (ALHE) produce skin lesions that appear as single or multiple red-brown papules or as subcutaneous nodules with a predilection for the head and neck region. Other associated features include eosinophilia and elevated IgE levels. Both Kimura disease and the similar ALHE are frequently associated with glomerular disease. Mesangial proliferative glomerulonephritis[1330] and minimal change disease[1331] have been described.

Renal complications of Castleman disease (angiofollicular lymph node hyperplasia) are uncommon. The reported cases are very heterogeneous and their renal pathology includes minimal-change disease, mesangial proliferative glomerulonephritis,[1332] membranous nephropathy,[1333] membranoproliferative glomerulonephritis,[1334] crescentic glomerulonephritis,[1335] fibrillary glomerulonephritis,[1336] and amyloidosis.[1337] Serum Il-6 levels appear to be elevated and declines with corticosteroid therapy.[1332] Removal of tumor mass, or management with steroids appears to ameliorate the renal manifestations in some cases.

Angioimmunoblastic lymphadenopathy has been associated with diffuse proliferative glomerulonephritis with necrotizing arteritis, and minimal-change disease.[1234,1338]

Acknowledgment

The authors thank Dr. Alice Appel for excellent editorial assistance in the completion of this chapter.

References

1. Waldman M, Appel GB: Update on the treatment of lupus nephritis. Kidney Int 70:1403–1412, 2006.
2. Appel GB, D'Agati VD: Lupus nephritis—pathology and pathogenesis. Chapter 55. In Wallace DJ, Hahn BH (eds): Dubois' Lupus Erythematosus. 7th ed. Philadelphia, Lippincott Williams and Wilkins, 2006, pp 1094–1112.
3. Cameron JS. Lupus nephritis. J Am Soc Nephrol 10:413–424, 1999.
4. Appel GB, D'Agati V: Renal involvement in systemic lupus erythematosus. Chapter 44. In Massary S, Glassock R (eds): Text of Kidney Disease. Philadelphia, Williams and Wilkins, 2000, pp. 787–797.
5. Contreras G, Roth D, Pardo V, et al: Lupus nephritis: A clinical review for the practicing nephrologist. Clin Nephrol 57:95–107, 2002.
6. Berden JHM: Lupus nephritis. Kidney Int 52:538–558, 1997.
7. Wallace DJ, Dubois EL: Definition, classification, and epidemiology of systemic lupus erythematosus. In Wallace DJ, Dubois EL (eds): Lupus Erythematosus, 3rd ed. Philadelphia, Lea and Febiger, 1987.
8. Appel GB, Cameron JS: Lupus nephritis. In Johnson RJ, Feehaly J, Floege J (eds): Comprehensive Clinical Nephrology, 3rd ed. St. Louis, Mosby, 2007, pp 291–305.
8a. Rothfield N: Clinical features of systemic lupus erythematosus. In Kelley WN, Harris ED, Ruddy S, Sledge CB (eds): Textbook of Rheumatology. Philadelphia, WB Saunders, 1981.
9. Appel GB: Cyclophosphamide therapy of severe lupus nephritis. Am J Kidney Dis 30:872–878, 1997.
10. Dooly MA, Hogan S, Jenette C, Falk R, for the Glomerulonephritis Disease Collaborative Network: Cyclophosphamide therapy for lupus nephritis: Poor survival in black Americans. Kidney Int 51:1188–1195, 1997.
11. Barr RG, Seliger S, Appel GB, et al: Prognosis in proliferative lupus nephritis: Role of socioeconomic status and race/ethnicity. Nephrol Dial Transplant 18:2039–2046, 2003.
12. Contreras G, Lenz O, Pardo V, et al: Outcome in African Americans and Hispanics with lupus nephritis. Kidney Int 69:1846–1851, 2006.
13. Hess EV, Farhey Y: Epidemiology, genetics, etiology, and environment relationships of systemic lupus erythematosus. Curr Opin Rheumatol 6:474, 1994.
14. Salmon J, Millard S, Schacter L, et al. FcgammaRIIA alleles are heritable risk factors for lupus nephritis in African-Americans. J Clin Invest 97:1348–1354, 1996.
15. Waldman M, Madaio MP: Pathogenic autoantibodies in lupus nephritis. Lupus 14:19–24, 2005.
16. Hochberg MC: Updating the American College of Rheumatology revised criteria for the classification of SLE. Arthritis Rheum 40:1725, 1997.
17. Appel GB, Cohen DJ, Pirani CL, et al: Long term follow-up of lupus nephritis: A study based on the WHO classification. Am J Med 83:877, 1987.
18. Kotzin BL: Systemic lupus erythematosus. Cell 85:303, 1996.
19. Theofilopoulos AN: The basis of autoimmunity. 1. Mechanisms of aberrant self recognition. Immunol Today 16:90, 1995.
20. Klimnan DM, Steinberg AD: Inquiry into murine and human lupus. Immunol Rev 144:157, 1995.
21. Stohl W: Impaired polyclonal T cell cytolytic activity. A possible risk factor for SLE. Arthritis Rheum 38:506, 1995.
22. Tsokos GC: Lymphocytes, cytokines, inflammation, and immune trafficking. Curr Opin Rheumatol 7:376, 1995.
23. Mo C, Datta SK: Lupus: Key pathogenic mechanisms and contributing factors. Clin Immunol Immunopathol 77:209, 1995.
24. Hahn BH: Antibodies to DNA. N Engl J Med 338:1359–1368, 1998.
25. Chabre H, Amoura Z, Piette J-C, et al: Presence of nucleosome-restricted antibodies in patients with SLE. Arthritis Rheum 38:1485, 1995.
26. D'Agati VD: Renal disease in systemic lupus erythematosus, mixed connective tissue disease, Sjögren's syndrome, and rheumatoid arthritis. In Jennette CJ, Olson L, Schwartz MM, Silva F (eds): Pathology of the Kidney, 5th ed. Philadelphia, Lippincott-Raven, 1998, pp. 541–624.
27. D'Andrea DK, Coupaye-Gerard B, Kleyman TR, et al: Lupus autoantibodies interact directly with distinct glomerular and vascular cell surface antigens. Kidney Int 49:1214, 1996.
28. Churg J, Bernstein J, Glassock R: Renal Disease: Classification and Atlas of Glomerular Diseases. 2nd ed. New York, Igaku-Shoin, 1995, p 152.
29. Weening JJ, D'Agati VD, Appel GB, et al: The classification of glomerulonephritis in systemic lupus nephritis revisited. Kidney Int 65:521–530, 2004.
30. Weening JJ, D'Agati VD, Appel GB, et al: The classification of glomerulonephritis in systemic lupus nephritis revisited. J Am Soc Nephrol 15:241–250, 2004.
31. Baldwin DS: Clinical usefulness of the morphological classification of lupus nephritis. Am J Kidney Dis II:142–149, 1982.
32. Appel GB, Silva FG, Pirani CL, et al: Renal involvement in systemic lupus erythematosus: A study involving 56 patients emphasizing histologic classification. Medicine 57:371–410, 1978.
33. Magil AB, Ballon HS, Rae A: Focal proliferative lupus nephritis: A clinicopathologic study using the WHO classification. Am J Med 72:620–630, 1982.
34. Magil AB, Puterman ML, Ballon HS, et al: Prognostic factors in diffuse proliferative lupus glomerulonephritis. Kidney Int 34:511–517, 1988.
35. Ponticelli C, Zucchelli P, Moroni G, et al: Long-term prognosis of diffuse lupus nephritis. Clin Nephrol 28:263, 1987.

36. Donadio JV Jr, Burgess JK, Holley KE: Membranous lupus nephropathy: A clinico-pathologic study. Medicine 56:527, 1977.

37. Sloane RP, Schwartz MM, Korbet SM, et al: Long-term outcome in systemic lupus erythematosus membranous glomerulonephritis. J Am Soc Nephrol 7:299–305, 1996.

38. Pasquali S, Banfi G, Zucchelli A, et al: Lupus membranous nephropathy: Long-term outcome. Clin Nephrol 39:175–182, 1993.

39. Jennette JC, Iskander SS, Dalldorf FG: Pathologic differentiation between lupus and nonlupus membranous glomerulopathy. Kidney Int 24:377, 1983.

40. D'Agati VD, Appel GB: Renal pathology of HIV infection. Semin Nephrol 18:406–421, 1998.

41. Austin HA, Boumpas DT, Vaughan EM, Balow JE: Predicting renal outcomes in severe lupus nephritis: Contributions of clinical and histologic data. Kidney Int 43:544–550, 1994.

42. Schwartz M, Berstein J, Hill GS, et al: Predictive value of renal pathology in diffuse proliferative lupus glomerulonephritis. Kidney Int 36:891–896, 1989.

43. Schwartz MM: The Holy Grail: Pathological indices in LN. Kidney Int 58:1354–1355, 2000.

44. Valeri A, Rhadhakrishnan J, D'Agati V, et al: IV Pulse Cytoxan treatment of severe lupus nephritis. Clin Nephrol 42:71–78, 1994.

45. Radharkrishnan J, Kunis CL, D'Agati V, Appel GB: Cyclosporin treatment of membranous lupus nephropathy. Clin Nephrol 42:147–154, 1994.

46. Park MH, D'Agati VD, Appel GB, Pirani CL: Tubulointerstitial disease in lupus nephritis: Relationship to immune deposits, interstitial inflammation, glomerular changes, renal function, and prognosis. Nephron 44:309–319, 1986.

47. Hill G, Delahousse M, Nochy D, et al: A new index for evaluation of renal biopsies in lupus nephritis. Kidney Int 58:11600–1173, 2000.

48. Hill GS, Delahousse M, Nochy D, et al: Proteinuria and tubulointerstitial lesions in LN. Kidney Int 60:1893–1903, 2001.

49. Daniel L, Sichez H, Giorgi R, et al: Tubular lesions and tubular cell adhesion molecules for the prognosis of lupus nephritis. Kidney Int 60:2215–2221, 2001.

50. D'Agati V, Appel GB, Knowles D, et al: Monoclonal antibody identification of mononuclear cells in renal biopsies of lupus nephritis. Kidney Int 30:573, 1986.

51. Banfi G, Bertani T, Boeri V, et al: Renal vascular lesions as a marker of a poor prognosis in patients with lupus nephritis. Am J Kidney Dis 18:240, 1991.

52. Appel GB, Pirani CL, D'Agati VD: Renal vascular complications of systemic lupus erythematosus. J Am Soc Nephrol 4:1499, 1994.

53. Appel GB: Renal vascular involvement in SLE. In Lewis EJ, Schwartz M, Korbet SM (eds): Lupus Nephritis. Oxford, Oxford Press, 1999, pp. 241–262.

54. Hertig A, Droz D, Lesavre P, et al: SLE and idiopathic nephrotic syndrome: Coincidence or not? Am J Kidney Dis 40:1179–1184, 2002.

55. Dube GK, Markowitz GS, Radhakrishnan J, et al: Minimal change disease in SLE. Clin Nephrol 57:120–126, 2002.

56. Chang BG, Markowitz GS, Seshan SV, et al: Renal manifestations of concurrent SLE and HIV infection. Am J Kidney Dis 33:441–449, 1999.

57. Font J, Torras A, Cervera R, et al: Silent renal disease in systemic lupus erythematosus. Clin Nephrol 27:283–288, 1987.

58. Isenberg DA, Collins C: Detection of cross-reactive anti-DNA antibody idiotypes on renal tissue-bound immunoglobulins from lupus patients. J Clin Invest 76:287, 1985.

59. Foster MH, Cizman B, Madaio MP: Nephritogenic autoantibodies in systemic lupus erythematosus: Immunochemical properties, mechanisms of immune deposition, and genetic origins. Lab Invest 69:494, 1993.

60. Sharp GC, Irvin WS, Tan EJ, et al: Mixed connective tissue disease: An apparently distinct rheumatic disease syndrome associated with a specific antibody to an extractable nuclear antigen (ENA). Am J Med 52:148, 1972.

61. Franco HL, Weston WL, Peebles C, et al: Autoantibodies directed against sicca syndrome antigens in the neonatal lupus syndrome. J Acad Dermatol 4:67, 1981.

62. Reichlin M: Clinical and immunologic significance of antibodies to Ro and La in systemic lupus erythematosus. Arthritis Rheum 25:767, 1982.

63. Termaat RM, Assmann KJM, Dijkman HBPM, et al: Anti-DNA antibodies can bind to the glomerulus via two distinct mechanisms. Kidney Int 43:1363, 1992.

64. Morioka T, Woitas R, Fujigaki Y, et al: Histone mediates glomerular deposition of small size DNA anti-DNA complex. Kidney Int 45:991, 1994.

65. D'Cruz DP, Houssiau FA, Ramirez G, et al: Antibodies to endothelial cells in systemic lupus erythematosus: A potential marker for nephritis and vasculitis. Clin Exp Immunol 85:254, 1991.

66. Hughson MD, Nadasdy T, McCarty GA, et al: Renal thrombotic microangiopathy in patients with systemic lupus erythematosus and the antiphospholipid syndrome. Am J Kidney Dis 20:150, 1992.

67. Frampton G, Hicks J, Cameron JS: Significance of anti-phospholipid antibodies in patients with lupus nephritis. Kidney Int 39:1225, 1991.

68. Laitman RS, Glicklich D, Sablay L, et al: Effect of long-term normalization of serum complement levels on the course of lupus nephritis. Am J Med 87:132, 1989.

69. Walport MJ: Complement. N Engl J Med 344:1058–1060, 1140–1144, 2001.

70. Greisman SG, Redecha PB, Kimberly RP, Christian CL: Differences among immune complexes: Association of C1q in SLE immune complexes with renal disease. J Immunol 138:739, 1987.

71. Noel L-H, Droz D, Rothfield NF: Clinical and serologic significance of cutaneous deposits of immunoglobulins, C3 and C1q, in SLE patients with nephritis. Clin Immunol Immunopathol 10:318, 1978.

72. Joseph R, Radlakrishnan J, Appel GB: Anticardiolipin antibodies and renal disease. Curr Opin Nephrol Hypertens 10:175, 2001.

73. Yung, RL, Johnson, KJ, Richardson, BC: New concepts in the pathogenesis of drug-induced lupus. Lab Invest 73:746, 1995.

74. Fritzler MJ: Drugs recently associated with lupus syndromes. Lupus 3:455, 1994.

75. Reidenberg, MM, Drayer, DE, Lorenzo, B, et al: Acetylation phenotypes and environmental chemical exposure of people with idiopathic systemic lupus erythematosus. Arthritis Rheum 36:971–973, 1992.

76. Crowson AN, Magro CM: Diltiazem and subacute cutaneous lupus erythematosus-like lesions (letter). N Engl J Med 333:1429, 1995.

77. Gough A, Chapman S, Wagstaff K, et al: Minocycline induced autoimmune hepatitis and systemic lupus erythematosus-like syndrome. BMJ 312:169, 1996.

78. Laversuch CJ, Collins DA, Charles PJ, Bourke BE: Sulphasalazine-induced autoimmune abnormalities in patients with rheumatic disease. Br J Rheumatol 34:435, 1995.

79. Beming SE, Iseman MD: Rifamycin-induced lupus syndrome. Lancet 349:1521, 1997.

80. Shapiro KS, Pinn VW, Harrington JT, Levey AS: Immune complex glomerulonephritis in hydralazine-induced SLE. Am J Kidney Dis 3:270, 1984.

81. Short AK, Lockwood CM: Antigen specificity in hydralazine associated ANCA positive vasculitis. Q J Med 88:775, 1995.

82. Burlingame RW, Rubin RL: Drug-induced anti-histone autoantibodies display two patterns of reactivity with substructures of chromatin. J Clin Invest 88:680, 1991.

83. Urowitz MIB, Gladman DD, Farewell VT, et al: Lupus and pregnancy studies. Arthritis Rheum 36:1392, 1993.

84. Moroni G, Quaglini S, Banfi G, et al: Pregnancy in LN. Am J Kidney Dis 40:713–720, 2002.

85. Ruiz-Irastorza G, Lima F, Alves J, et al: Increased rate of lupus flare during pregnancy and the puerperium; a prospective study of 78 pregnancies. Br J Rheumatol 35:133, 1996.

86. Petri K, Howard D, Repke J: Frequency of lupus flare in pregnancy: The Hopkins lupus pregnancy center experience. Arthritis Rheum 34:1358, 1991.

87. Hayslett JP: Maternal and fetal complications in pregnant women with systemic lupus erythematosus. Am J Kidney Dis 17:123, 1991.

88. Julkunen K, Kaaja R, Palosuo T, et al: Pregnancy in lupus nephropathy. Acta Obstet Gynecol Scand 72:258, 1993.

89. Julkunen EL, Jouhaikainen T, Kaaja R, et al: Fetal outcome in lupus pregnancy: A retrospective case-control study of 242 pregnancies in 112 patients. Lupus 2:125, 1993.

90. Petri M, Albritton J: Fetal outcome of lupus pregnancy: A retrospective case-control study of the Hopkins lupus cohort. J Rheumatol 20:650, 1993.

91. McNeil HP, Chesterman CN, Krilis SA: Immunology and clinical importance of antiphospholipid antibodies. Adv Immunol 49:193, 1991.

92. Conlon PJ, Fischer CA, Levesqu MC, et al: Clinical, biochemical, and pathological predictors of poor response to IV cyclophosphamide in DPLN. Clin Nephrol 46:170–175, 1996.

93. Gourley MF, Austin HA, Scott D, et al: Methylprednisolone and cyclophosphamide, alone or in combination, in patients with lupus nephritis. Ann Intern Med 125:549–557, 1996.

94. Boumpas DT, Austin HA, Vaughn EM, et al: Controlled trial of pulse methylprednisolone versus two regimens of cyclophosphamide in severe lupus nephritis. Lancet 340:741–745, 1992.

95. Chagnac A, Kiberd BA, Farinas MC, et al: Outcome of the acute glomerular injury in porliferative lupus nephritis. J Clin Invest 84:922–930, 1989.

96. Mojcik CF, Klippel, JH: End-stage renal disease and SLE. Am J Med 101:100–107, 1996.

97. Cheigh JS, Stenzel KH: End-stage renal disease in SLE. Am J Kidney Dis 21:2, 1993.

98. Nissenson AR, Port FK: Outcome of ESRD in patients with rare causes of kidney failure. Q J Med 273:63–74, 1996.

99. Ward MM: Cardiovascular and cerebrovascular morbidity and mortality among women with ESRD attributed to LN. Am J Kidney Dis 36:516–525, 2000.

100. Ward MM: Outcomes of renal transplantation among patients with end-stage renal disease caused by lupus nephritis. Kidney Int 57:2136–2143, 2000.

101. Lochhead KM, Pirsch JD, D'Alessandro AK et al: Risk factors for renal allograft loss in patients with systemic lupus erythematosus. Kidney Int 49:512, 1996.

102. Stone JII, Millwood CL, Olson JL, et al: Frequency of recurrent lupus nephritis among 97 renal transplant patients during the cyclophosphamide era. Arthritis Rheum 41:678–686, 1998.

103. Radhakrishnan J, Williams GS, Appel GB, Cohen DJC: Renal transplantation in anticardiolipin positive lupus erythematosus patients. Am J Kidney Dis 23:286, 1994.

104. Stone JH, Amend WJ, Criswell LA: Antiphospholipid antibody syndrome in renal transplantation: Occurrence of clinical events in 96 consecutive patients with systemic lupus erythematosus. Am J Kidney Dis 34:1040, 1999.

105. Moroni G, Qualini S, Maccario M, et al: "Nephritic flares" are predictors of bad long-term renal outcome in lupus nephritis. Kidney Int 50:2047–2053, 1996.

106. Magil AB, Puterman ML, Ballon HS, et al: Prognostic factors in diffuse proliferative lupus glomerulonephritis. Kidney Int 34:511, 1988.

107. Nossent HC, Henzen-Logmans SC, Vroom TM, et al: Contribution of renal biopsy data in predicting outcome in lupus nephritis. Analysis of 116 patients. Arthritis Rheum 33:970, 1990.

108. Esdaile JM, Federgreen W, Quintal H, et al: Predictors of one year out-come in lupus nephritis: The importance of renal biopsy. Q J Med 81:907, 1991.

109. Schwartz MM, Lan S-P, Bernstain J, et al: Role of pathology indices in the management of severe lupus glomerulonephritis. Kidney Int 42:743–748, 1992.

110. Balow JE, Boumpas DT, Fessler BJ, Austin HA III: Management of lupus nephritis. Kidney Int 49 Suppl:S88–92, 1996.

111. Najafi CC, Korbet SM, Lewis EJ, et al: Significance of histologic patterns of glomerular injury upon long-term prognosis in severe lupus glomerulonephritis. Kidney Int 59:2156–2163, 2001.

112. Steinberg AD, Steinberg SC: Long-term preservation of renal function in patients with lupus nephritis receiving treatment that includes cyclophosphamide versus those treated with prednisone only. Arthritis Rheum 34:945–950, 1991.

113. Bakir AA, Levy PS, Dunea G: The prognosis of lupus nephritis in African-Americans: A retrospective Analysis. Am J Kidney Dis 24:159, 1994.

114. Tejani A, Nicastri AD, Chen C-K et al: Lupus nephritis in Black and Hispanic children. Am J Dis Child 137:481–483, 1983.

115. Austin HA, Boumpas DT, Vaughan EM, Balow JE: Predicting renal outcomes in severe lupus nephritis: Contributions of clinical and histologic data. Kidney Int 43:544–550, 1994.

116. Seliger S, Barr RG, Appel GB, et al: Prognosis in proliferative lupus nephritis: The role of socioeconomic status and race/ethnicity. Nephrol Dial Transplant 18:2039–2046, 2003.

117. Contreras G, Lenz O, Pardo V, et al: Outcome in African Americans and Hispanics with lupus nephritis. Kidney Int 69:1846–1851, 2006.

118. Houssieau FA, Vasconcelos C, D'Cruz D, et al: Early response to immunosuppressive therapy predicts good renal outcome in lupus nephritis: Lessons from long-term follow of patients in the Euro-Lupus Nephritis Trial. Arthritis Rheum 50:3934–3940, 2004.

119. Korbet SM, Lewsi EJ, Schwartz MM, et al: Factors predictive of outcome in severe lupus nephritis. Am J Kidney Dis 35:904–914, 2000.

120. Mosca M, Bencivelli W, Neri R, et al: Renal flares in 91 SLE patients with diffuse proliferative glomerulonephritis. Kidney Int 61:1502–1509, 2002.

121. Ponticelli C, Moroni G: Flares in lupus nephritis: Incidence, impact on renal survival and management. Lupus 7:635–638, 1998.

122. Ioannidis JPA, Boki KA, Katsorida ME, et al: Remission, relapse, and re-remission of LN treated with cyclophosphamide. Kidney Int 57:258–264, 2000.

123. Pablos JL, Gutierrez-Millet V, Gomez-Reino JJ: Remission of LN with cyclophosphamide and late relapse following therapy withdrawal. Scand J Rheumatol 23:142–144, 1994.

124. Ciruelo E, DelaCruz J, Lopez I, Gomez-Reino JJ: Cumulative rate of relapse of LN after successful treatment with cyclophosphamide. Arthritis Rheum 12:2028–2034, 1996.

125. Hill GS, Delahousse M, Nochy D, et al: Outcome of relapse in lupus nephritis: Roles of reverse of renal fibrosis and response of inflammation therapy. Kidney Int 61:2176–2186, 2002.

126. Martins L, Rocha G, Rodriguez A, et al: LN: A retrospective review of 78 cases from a single center. Clin Nephrol 57:114–119, 2002.

127. Hill GS, Delahousse M, Nochy D, et al: Predictive power of the second renal biopsy in lupus nephritis: Significance of macrophages. Kidney Int 59:304–316, 2001.

128. McCune WJ, Golbus J, Zeldes W, et al: Clinical and immunologic effects of monthly administration of intravenous cyclophosphamide in severe lupus erythematosus. N Engl J Med 318:1423–1431, 1988.

129. Lehman TJA, Sherry DD, Wagner-Weiner L, et al: Intermittent intravenous cyclophosphamide therapy for lupus nephritis. J Pediatr 114:1055–1060, 1989.

130. Illei GG, Austin HA, Crane M, et al: Combination therapy with pulse cyclophosphamide plus pulse methylprednisolone improves long-term renal outcome without adding toxicity in patients with LN. Ann Int Med 21:248–257, 2001.

131. Bansal VK, Beto JA: Treatment of lupus nephritis: A meta-analysis of clinical trials. Am J Kidney Dis 29:193–199, 1997.

132. Boumpas DT, Austin HA, Vaughn EM, et al: Risk for sustained amenorrhea in patients with SLE receiving intermittent pulse cyclophosphamide therapy. Ann Intern Med 119:366–369, 1993.

133. Kleta R: Cyclophosphamide and mercaptoethane sulfonate (MESNA) therapy for minimal lesion glomerulonephritis. Kidney Int 56:2312–2313, 1999.

134. Donadio JV, Glassock RJ: Immunosuppressive drug therapy in lupus nephritis. Am J Kidney Dis 21:239–250, 1993.

135. Corna D, Moriji M, Facchinetti D, et al: MMF limits renal damage and prolongs life in murine lupus autoimmune disease. Kidney Int 51:1583–1589, 1997.

136. Van Bruggen MCJ, Walgreen B, Rijko TPM, Berden JHM: Attenuation of murine LN by MMF. J Am Soc Nephrol 9:1407–1415, 1998.

137. Zoja C, Begnini R, Noris M, et al: MMF combined with a cyclooxygenase-2 inhibitor ameliorates murine LN. Kidney Int 60:653–663, 2001.

138. Dooley MA, Cosio FG, Nachman PH, et al: MMF therapy in LN: Clinical observations. J. Am Soc Nephrol 10:833–839, 1999.

139. Kingdon EJ, McLean AG, Psimerrou E, et al: The safety and efficacy of MMF in lupus nephritis: A pilot study. Lupus 10:606–611, 2001.

140. Mok CC, Lai KN: Mycophenolate mofetil in lupus glomerulonephritis. Am J Kidney Dis 40:447–457, 2002.

141. Li LS, Hu WX, Chen HP, Liu ZH: Comparison of MMF versus cyclophosphamide pulse therapy in the induction treatment of severe diffuse proliferative LN in Chinese population. J Am J Nephrol 11:486A, 2000.

142. Chan TM, Li FK, Tang CS, et al: Efficacy of mycophenolate mofetil in patients with diffuse proliferative LN. N Engl J Med 343:1156–1162, 2000.

143. Falk R (ed): Treatment of LN—a work in progress. N Engl J Med 343:1182–1183, 2000.

144. Chan TM, Tse KC, Tang CS, et al: Hong Kong Nephrology Study Group. Long-term study of mycophenolate mofetil as continuous induction and maintenance treatment of diffuse proliferative lupus nephritis. J Am Soc Nephrol 16:1076–1084, 2005.

145. Ginzler E, Dooley MA, Aranow C, et al: Mycophenolate mofetil or intravenous cyclophosphamide for lupus nephritis. N Engl J Med 353:2219–2228, 2005.

146. Sinclair A, Appel GB, Dooley MA, et al: Protocol for the Aspreva Lupus Management Study. J Am Soc Nephrol 16:528A, 2005.

147. Houssieau FA, Vasconcelos C, D'Cruz D, et al: Euro-Lupus Trial. Arthritis Rheum 46:2121–2131, 2002.

148. Houssieau FA, Vasconcelos C, D'Cruz D, et al: Early response to immunosuppressive therapy predicts good renal outcome in lupus nephritis: Lessons from long-term follow of patients in the Euro-Lupus Nephritis Trial. Arthritis Rheum 50:3934–3940, 2004.

149. Contreras G, Pardo V, Leclercq B, et al: Sequential therapies for proliferative lupus nephritis. N Engl J Med 350:971–980, 2004.

150. Radhakrishnan J, Valeri A, Kunis C, Appel GB: Use of cyclosporin in systemic lupus. Contrib Nephrol 114:59–72, 1995.

151. Favre H, Miescher PA, Huang YP, et al: Cyclosporin in the treatment of lupus nephritis. Am J Nephrol 9S:57–60, 1989.

152. Lei-Shi L, Hai-Tao Z, Shu-Quiong S, et al: Controlled trial of tecrolimus versus intravenous cyclophosphamide as induction therapy for severe lupus nephritis. J Am Soc Nephrol 16: 556A, 2005.

153. Sfikakis PP, Boletis JN, Tsokos GC: Rituximab anti-B cell therapy in systemic lupus erythematosus: Pointing to the future. Curr Opin Rheumatol 17:550–557, 2005.

154. Leandro MJ, Cambridge G, Edwards JC, et al: B cell depletion in the treatment of patients with SLE: A longitudinal analysis of 24 patients. Rheumatology 44:1542–1545, 2005.

155. Ng KP, Leandro MJ, Edwards JC, et al: Repeated B cell depletion in treatment of refractory SLE. Ann Rheum Dis 65:942–945, 2006.

156. Appel GB, Looney RJ, Eisenberg RA: Protocol for the Lupus Nephritis Assessment with Rituximab (LUNAR) study. J Am Soc Nephrol 17:573A, 2006.

157. Lewis EJ, Hunsicker LG, Lau SP, et al: For the Lupus Collaboration Study Group. A Controlled Trial of Plasmapheresis in Severe Lupus Nephritis. N Engl J Med 326:1373–1379, 1992.

158. Euler HH, Schroeder JO, Marten P, et al: Treatment free remission in severe SLE following synchronization of plasmapheresis with subsequent pulse cyclophosphamide. Arthritis Rheum 37:1784–1794, 1994.

159. Gelfand J, Truong L, Stern L, et al: Thrombotic thrombocytopenic purpura syndrome in SLE: Treatment with plasma infusion. Am J Kidney Dis 6:154–160, 1985.

160. Jordan SC: Intravenous gamma-globulin in SLE and immune complex disease. Clin Immunol Immunopathol 53:S164–169, 1989.

161. Lin C-Y, Hsu H-C, Chiang H: Improvement of histological and immunological change in steroid and immunosuppressive drug-resistant lupus nephritis by high-dose intravenous gamma globulin. Nephron 53:303–310, 1989.

162. Boletis JN, Ioannidis JPA, Boki KA, Moutsopoulos HM: Intravenous immunoglobulin compared with cyclophosphamide for proliferative LN. Lancet 354:569, 1999.

163. Sharpe AH, Abbas AK: T-Cell costimulation-biology, therapeutic potential, and challenges. N Engl J Med 355:973–975, 2006.

164. Kato K, Santana-Sahagun E, Rassenti LZ, et al: The soluble CD40 ligands CD154 in SLE. J Clin Invest 104:949–955, 1999.

165. Davis J, Totoritis M, Rosenberg J, et al: Phase I Clinical Trial of AntiCD40 Ligand (IDEC 131) in patients with SLE. J Rheum 28:95–101, 2001.

166. Kawai T, Andrews D, Colvin RB et al: Thromboembolitic complications after treatment with AntiCD40 ligand. Nature Med 6:114, 2000.

167. Weisman MH, Bluesteuin HG, Berne CM, et al: Reduction in circulating dsDNA antibody titer after administration of LJ394. J Rheumatol 24:314–318, 1997.

168. Alarcon-Segovia D, Tumlin JA, Furie RA, et al: LJP 394 for the prevention of renal flare in patients with SLE. Arthritis Rheum 48:442–454, 2003.

169. Chagnac A, Kiberd BA, Farinas MC, et al: Outcome of the acute glomerular injury in porliferative lupus nephritis. J Clin Invest 84:922–930, 1989.

170. Hariharan S, Pollak VE, Kant KS, et al: Diffuse proliferative lupus nephritis: Long-term observation in patients treated with ancrod. Clin Nephrol 34:61–69, 1990.

171. Pierucci A, Simonetti BM, Pecci G, et al: Improvement of renal function with selective thromboxane antagonism in lupus nephritis. N Engl J Med 320:421–425, 1989.

172. Wang Y, Hu Q, Madri JA, et al: Amelioration of lupus-like autoimmune disease in NZB/NZW F1 mice after treatment with a blocking monoclonal antibody specific for complement component 5. Proc Natl Acad Sci 93:8563–8568, 1996.

173. Lawson, Prud'homme GJ, Chang Y, et al: Treatment of murine lupus with cDNA encoding IFN gamma receptor/Fc. J Clin Invest 106:207, 2000.

174. Brodsky R, Petri M, Smith D, et al: Immunoablative high dose cyclophosphamide without stem cell rescue for refractory severe autoimmune disease. Ann Intern Med 129:1031–1035, 1998.

175. Burt RK, Traynor AE, Pope R, et al: Treatment of autoimmune disease by intense immunosuppressive conditioning and autologous hematopoietic stem cell transplantation. Blood 92:3505–3514, 1998.

176. Traynor AE, Schroeder J, Rosa RM, et al: Stem cell transplantation for resistant lupus. Arthritis Rheum 42:5170, 1999.

177. Moroni G, Moccario M, Banfi G, et al: Treatment of membranous lupus nephritis. Am J Kidney Dis 31:681–686, 1998.

178. Austin HA, Vaugham EK Boumpas DT, et al: Lupus membranous nephropathy: Controlled trial of prednisone, pulse cyclophosphamide, and cyclosporine (abstract). J Am Soc Nephrol 2004.

179. Mok CC, Ying KY, Lau CS et al: Treatment of membranous lupus with azathioprine and prednisone. Am J Kidney Dis 43: 269, 2004.

180. Kapitsinou PP, Boletis JN, Skopoul FN, et al: Lupus nephritis treatment with mycophenolate. Rheumatology (Oxford) 43:377–380, 2000.

181. Spetie DN, Tang Y, Rovin BH, et al: Mycophenolate mofetil therapy of SLE membranous nephropathy. Kidney Int 66: 2411–2415, 2004.

182. Kanda H, Kubo K, Tateishi S, et al: Antiproteinuric effect of ARB in lupus nephritis patients with persistent proteinuria despite immunosuppressive therapy. Lupus 14:288–292, 2005.

183. Kavim MY, Pisoni CN, Ferro L, et al: Reduction of proteinuria with mycophenolate mofetil in predominantly membranous lupus nephropathy. Rheumatology (Oxford) 44:1317–1321, 2005.

184. Radhakrishnan J, Ginzler E, Appel GB: Mycophenolate vs IV cyclophosphamide for membranous lupus nephropathy. J Am Soc Nephrol 16:8A, 2005.

185. Uramoto KM, Michet CJ, Jr, Thumboo J, et al: Trends in the incidence and mortality of systemic lupus erythematosus, 1950–1992. Arthritis Rheum 42(1):46–50, 1999.

186. Roman MJ, Shanker BA, Davis A, et al: Prevalence and correlates of accelerated atherosclerosis in systemic lupus erythematosus. N Engl J Med 349:2399–406, 2003.

187. Bruce IN, Urowitz MB, Gladman DD, et al: Risk factors for coronary heart disease in women with systemic lupus erythematosus: The Toronto Risk Factor Study. Arthritis Rheum 48:3159–3167, 2003.

188. Joseph RE, Radhakrishnan J, Appel GB: Antiphospholipid antibody syndrome and renal disease. Curr Opin Nephrol Hypertens 10:175–181, 2001.

189. Singh AK: Lupus nephritis and the anti-phospholipid antibody syndrome in pregnancy. Kidney Int 58:2240–2254, 2000.

190. Nzerue CM, Hewann-Lowe K, Pierangeli S, Harris EN: "Black Swan in the Kidney." Renal involvement in the antiphospholipid antibody syndrome. Kidney Int 62:733–734, 2002.

191. Moroni G, Ventura D, Riva P, Panzeri P: Antiphospholipid antibodies are associated with an increased risk for chronic renal insufficiency in patients with lupus nephritis. Am J Kidney Dis 43:28, 2004.

192. Levine JS, Brauch DW, Rauch J: The Antiphospholipid Syndrome. N Engl J Med 346:752–763, 2002.

193. Avcin T, Cimaz R, Meroni PL: Recent advances in antiphospholipid antibodies and antiphospholipid syndromes in pediatric populations. Lupus 11:4, 2002.

194. Miyakis S, Lockshin MD, Atsumi T, et al: International consensus statement on an update of the classification criteria for definite antiphospholipid syndrome (APS). J Thromb Haemost 4:295, 2006.

195. Reber G, Tincani A, Sanmarco M, et al: Proposals for the measurement of anti-beta2-glycoprotein I antibodies. Standardization group of the European Forum on Antiphospholipid Antibodies. J Thromb Haemost 2:1860, 2004.

196. Tsutsumi A, Matsuura E, Ichikawa K, et al: Antibodies to beta2-glycoprotein I and clinical manifestations in patients with systemic lupus erythematosus. Arthritis Rheum 39:1466–1474, 1996.

197. Detkova D, Gil-Aguado A, Lavilla P, et al: Do antibodies to beta2-glycoprotein I contribute to the better characterization of the antiphospholipid syndrome? Lupus 6:430–436, 1999.

198. Asherson RA, Espinosa G, Cervera R, et al: Disseminated intravascular coagulation in catastrophic antiphospholipid syndrome: Clinical and haematological characteristics of 23 patients. Ann Rheum Dis 64:943, 2005.

199. Cervera R, Font J, Gomez-Puerta JA, et al: Validation of the preliminary criteria for the classification of catastrophic antiphospholipid syndrome. Ann Rheum Dis 64:1205, 2005.

200. Kaplanski G, Cacoub P, Farnarier C, et al: Increased soluble vascular cell adhesion molecule 1 concentrations in patients with primary or systemic lupus erythematosus-related antiphospholipid syndrome. Correlations with severity of thrombosis. Arthritis Rheum 43:55–64, 2000.

201. Love PE, Santoro SA: Antiphospholipid antibodies: Anticardiolipin and the lupus anticoagulant in SLE and in SLE disorders. Ann Intern Med 112:682–698, 1990.

202. de Bandt M, Benali K, Guillevin L, et al: Longitudinal determination of antiphospholipid antibodies in lupus patients without previous manifestations of antiphospholipid syndrome. A prospective study. J Rheumatol 26:91–96, 1999.

203. Shah NM, Khamashta MA, Alsumi T, et al: Outcome of patients with anticardiolipin antibodies: A 10 year follow-up of 52 patients. Lupus 7:3–6, 1998.

204. Sebastiani GD, Galeazzi M, Tincani A, et al: Anticardiolipin and antibetaGP1 antibodies in a large series of European patients with systemic lupus erythematosus. Prevalence and clinical associations. Scand J Rheumatol 28:344–351, 1999.

205. Cervera R, Khamashta MA, Font J, et al: Morbidity and mortality in systemic lupus erythematosus during a 5-year period. A multicenter prospective study of 1000 patients. European Working Party on Systemic Lupus Erythematosus. Medicine 78:167–175, 1999.

206. Lockshin MD: Answers to the Antiphospholipid Antibody Syndrome. N Engl J Med 332:1025–1027, 1995.

207. Harada M, Fujisawa Y, Sakisaka S, et al: High prevalence of anticardiolipin antibodies in hepatitis C virus infection: Lack of effects on thrombocytopenia and thrombotic complications. J Gastroenterol 35:272–277, 2000.

208. Ordi-Ros J, Villarreal J, Monegal F, et al: Anticardiolipin antibodies in patients with hepatitis C virus infection: Characterization in relation to antiphospholipid syndrome. Clin Diagn Lab Immunol 7:241–244, 2000.

209. Ankri A, Bonmarchand M, Coutellier A, et al: Antiphospholipid antibodies are an epiphenomenon in HIV-infected patients [letter]. AIDS 13:1282–1283, 1999.

210. Venkataseshan S, Barisoni L, Smith S, et al: Renal disease in antiphospholipid antibody syndrome (a study of 26 biopsied patients). J Am Soc Nephrol 7:1343, 1996.

211. Nochy D, Daugas E, Droz D, et al: The intrarenal vascular lesions associated with primary antiphospholipid syndrome. J Am Soc Nephrol 10:507–518, 1999.

212. Tektonidou MG, Sotsiou F, Nakopoulou L, et al: Antiphospholipid syndrome nephropathy in patients with systemic lupus erythematosus and antiphospholipid antibodies: Prevalence, clinical associations, and long-term outcome. Arthritis Rheum 50:2569, 2004.

213. Saracino A, Ramunni A, Pannarale G, Coratelli P: Kidney disease associated with primary antiphospholipid syndrome: Clinical signs and histopathological features in an case experience of five cases. Clin Nephrol 63:471, 2005.

214. Fakhouri F, Noel LH, Zuber J, Beaufils H: The expanding spectrum of renal diseases associated with antiphospholipid syndrome. Am J Kidney Dis 41:1205, 2003.

215. Godfrey T, Khamsahta MA, Hughes GRV: Antiphospholipid syndrome and renal artery stenosis. Q J Med 93:127–129, 2000.

216. Remondino GI, Mysler E, Pissano MN, et al: A reversible bilateral renal artery stenosis in association with the antiphospholipid syndrome. Lupus 9:65–67, 2000.

217. Riccialdelli L, Arnaldi G, Giacchetti G, et al: Hypertension due to renal artery occlusion in a patient with the antiphospholipid syndrome. Am J Hypertens 14:62–65, 2001.

218. Sirvent AE, Euriquez R, Antholin A, et al: Malignant hypertension in antiphospholipid syndrome. Nephron 73:368–369, 1996.

219. Daugas E, Nochy D, Huong DL, et al: Anti-phospholipid syndrome nephropathy in SLE. J Am Soc Nephrol 13:42, 2002.

220. Prakash R, Miller CC, Suki WN: Anticardiolipin antibody in patients on maintenance hemodialysis and its association with recurrent AV graft thrombosis. Am J Kidney Dis 26:347–352, 1995.

221. Brunet P, Aillaud MF, SanMarco M, et al: Antiphospholipids in hemodialysis patients relationships between lupus anticoagulant and thrombosis. Kidney Int 48:794–800, 1995.

222. Joseph RE, Radhakrishnan J, Appel GB, et al: Relationship of anticardiolipin antibodies to oxidative stress in hemodialysis. J Am Soc Nephrol 9:254, 1998.

223. Valeri A, Radhakrishnan J: Anti-cardiolipin antibodies (ACLA) in hemodialysis patients: A prospective study of 230 patients. J Am Soc Nephrol 7:1423, 1996.

224. Radhakrishnan J, Williams G, Appel GB, Cohen D: Renal transplantation in anticardiolipin antibody-positive lupus erythematosus patients. Am J Kidney Dis 23:286–289, 1994.

225. Ducloux D, Pellet E, Fournier V, et al: Prevalence and clinical significance of antiphospholipid antibodies in renal transplant recipients. Transplantation 67:90–93, 1999.

226. Stone JH, Amend WJ, Criswell LA: Antiphospholipid antibody syndrome in renal transplantation: Occurrence of clinical events in 96 consecutive patients with systemic lupus erythematosus. Am J Kidney Dis 34:1040, 1999.

227. Friedman GS, Meier-Kriesche HU, Kaplan B, et al: Hypercoaguable states in renal transplant candidates: Impact of anticoagulation upon incidence of renal allograft thrombosis. Transplantation 72:1073, 2001.

228. Forman JP, Lin J, Pascual M, et al: Significance of anticardiolipin antibodies on short and long-term allograft survival and function following kidney transplantation. Am J Transplant 11:1786–1791, 2004.

229. Baid S, Pascual M, Williams WW Jr, et al: Renal thrombotic microangiopathy associated with anticardiolipin antibodies in hepatitis C-positive renal allograft recipients. J Am Soc Nephrol 10:146–153, 1999.

230. Khamashta MA, Cuadrado MJ, Mujic F, et al: The management of thrombosis in the antiphospholipid-antibody syndrome. N Engl J Med 332:993–997, 1995.

231. Joseph RE, Valeri A, Radhakrishnan J, et al: Anticardiolipin antibody levels in lupus nephritis: Effects of immunosuppression. J Am Soc Nephrol 8:89, 1997.

232. Ginsberg JS, Greer I, Hirsh J: Use of antithrombotic agents during pregnancy. Chest 119S:1225–1315, 2001.

233. Kutteh WH: Antiphospholipid antibody-associated recurrent pregnancy: Treatment with heparin and low dose aspirin is superior to low dose aspirin alone. Am J Obstet Gynecol 174:1584–1589, 1996.

234. Kobayashi S, Tamura N, Tsuda H, et al: Immunoadsorbant plasmapheresis for a patient with antiphospholipid syndrome during pregnancy. Ann Rheum Dis 51(3):399–401, 1992.

235. Faria MS, Mota C, Barbot J, et al: Haemolytic uraemic syndrome, cardiomyopathy, cutaneous vasculopathy and anti-phospholipid activity. Nephrol Dial Transpl 15:1891–1892, 2000.

236. Takeshita Y, Turumi Y, Touma S, Takagi N: Successful delivery in a pregnant woman with lupus anticoagulant positive systemic lupus erythematosus treated with double plasmapheresis. Ther Apher 5:22–24, 2001.

237. Piette JC, Le Tiu Huong D, Wechsler B: Therapeutic use of intravenous immunoglobulins in the antiphospholipid syndrome. Ann Med Intern 151(Suppl 1):1551–1554, 2000.

238. Nasai R, Janicinova V, Petrikova M: Chloroquine inhibits stimulated platelets at the arachidonic acid pathway. Thromb Res 77:531–542, 1995.

239. Sharp GC, Irvin WS, Tan EM, et al: Mixed connective tissue disease: An apparently distinct rheumatic disease associated with a specific antibody to an extractable nuclear antigen (ENA). Am J Med 52:148, 1972.

240. Alarcon-Segovia D, Cardiel MH: Comparison between 3 diagnostic criteria for mixed connective tissue disease. Study of 593 patients. J Rheumatol 16:328, 1989.

241. Doria A, Ghirardello A, de Zambiasi P, et al: Japanese diagnostic criteria for mixed connective tissue disease in Caucasian patients. J Rheumatol 19:529, 1992.

242. Farhey Y, Hess EV: Mixed connective tissue disease. Arthritis Cure Res 10:333, 1997.

243. Kasukawa R: Mixed connective tissue disease. Intern Med 38:386, 1999.

244. Hoffman RW, Greidinger EL: Mixed connective tissue disease. Curr Opin Rheumatol 12:386, 2000.

245. Gendi NS, Welsh KI, van Venrooij WJ, et al: HLA type as a predictor of MCTD differentiation. Ten year clinical and immunogenetic follow-up of 46 patients. Arthritis Rheum 38:259, 1995.

246. Burdt MA, Hoffman RW, Deutscher SL, et al: Long-term outcome in MCTD. Longitudinal clinical and serologic findings. Arthritis Rheum 42:899, 1999.

247. Piirainen HI, Kurki PT: Clinical and serologic follow-up of patients with polyarthritis, Raynaud's phenomenon, and circulating RNP antibodies. Scand J Rheumatol 19:51, 1990.

248. Kitridou RC, Akmal M, Turkel SB, et al: Renal involvement in MCTD a longitudinal clinicopathologic study. Semin Arthritis Rheum 16:135, 1986.

249. Bennett RM: Scleroderma overlap syndromes. Rheum Dis Clin North Am 16:185, 1990.

250. Hoffman RW, Cassidy JT, Takeda Y, et al: U1–70kd autoantibody positive MCTD in children. A longitudinal clinical and serologic analysis. Arthritis Rheum 36:1599, 1993.

251. Appelboom T, Kahn MF, Mairesse N: Antibodies to small ribonucleoprotein and to 73 KD heat shock protein: Two distinct markers of MCTD. Clin Exp Immunol 100:486, 1995.

252. Fuller TJ, Richman AV, Auerbach D, et al: Immune complex glomerulonephritis in a patient with MCTD. Am J Med 62:761, 1977.

253. Satoh K, Imai H, Yasuda T, et al: Sclerodermatous renal crisis in a patients with MCTD. Am J Kidney Dis 24:215, 1994.

254. Ito S, Nakamura T, Kurosawa R, et al: Glomerulonephritis in children with mixed connective tissue disease. Clin Nephrol 66:160–165, 2006.

255. Pelferman TG, McIntosh CS, Kershaw M: MCTD associated with glomerulonephritis and hypocomplementemia. Postgrad Med J 56:177, 1980.

256. Kobayashi S, Nagase M, Kimura M, et al: Renal invovlement in MCTD. Am J Nephrol 5:282, 1985.

257. Bennett RM: MCTD. *In* Grishman E, Churg J, Needle MA, Venkataseshan VS (eds): The Kidney in Collagen Vascular Diseases. New York, Raven Press, 1993, p 167.

258. Sawait, Murakami K, Kurasano Y: Morphometric analysis of the kidney lesions in MCTD. Tohoku J Exp Med 174:141, 1994.

259. Kessler E, Halpern M, Chagnac A, et al: Unusual renal deposits in MCTD. Arch Pathol Lab Med 116:261, 1992.

260. McLaughlin VV, Genthner DE, Pannella MM, et al: Compassionate use of continuous prostacyclin in the management of secondary pulmonary hypertension: A case series. Ann Intern Med 130:740, 1999.

261. Ulmer A, Kotter I, Pfaff A, Fierlbech G: Efficacy of pulsed IV immunoglobulin therapy in MCTD. J Am Acad Dermatol 46:123, 2002.

262. Jennette JC, Falk RJ, Andrassy K, et al: Nomenclature of systemic vasculitides: Proposal of an international consensus conference. Arthritis Rheum 37:187–192, 1994.

263. Hoffman GS, Kerr GS, Leavitt RY, et al: Wegener's granulomatosis: An analysis of 158 patients. Ann Intern Med 116:488–498, 1992.

264. Falk RJ, Nachman PH, Hogan SL, Jennette JC: ANCA glomerulonephritis and vasculitis: A Chapel Hill Perspective. Semin Nephrol 20:233–242, 2000.

265. Savage J, Davies D, Falk RJ, et al: Antineutrophil cytoplasmic antibodies and associated diseases: A review of the clinical and laboratory features. Kidney Int 57:846, 2000.

266. Savage CO: ANCA-associated renal vasculitis—Nephrology Forum. Kidney Int 60:1614–1627, 2001.

267. Jennette JC, Falk RJ: Small-vessel vasculitis. N Engl J Med 337:1512–1523, 1997.

268. Franssen CF, Stegman CA, Kellenberg CGM, et al: Antiproteinase 3 and antimyeloperoxidase associated vasculitis. Kidney Int 57:2195–2206, 2000.

269. Hagen EC, Daha MR, Hermans J, et al: for the EC/BCR project for ANCA assay standardization. Diagnostic value of standardized assays for anti-neutrophil cytoplasmic antibodies in idiopathic systemic vasculitis. Kidney Int 53:754–761, 1998.

270. Kallenberg CG, Brouwer E, Weening JJ, Cohen Tervaert JW: Anti-neutrophil cytoplasmic antibodies: Current diagnostic and pathophysiological potential. Kidney Int 46:1, 1994.

271. Rao JK, Weinberger M, Oddone EZ, et al: The role of antineutrophil cytoplasmic antibody (c-ANCA) testing in the diagnosis of Wegener's granulomatosis. A literature review and meta-analysis. Ann Intern Med 123:925, 1995.

272. Appel GB, Gee B, Kashgarian M, Hayslett JP: Wegener's granulomatosis clinical-pathologic correlations and longterm course. Am J Kidney Dis 1:27–37, 1981.

273. ten Berge IJM, Wilmink JM, Meyer CJLM, et al: Clinical and immunological follow-up of patients with severe renal disease in Wegener's granulomatosis. Am J Nephrol 5:21–29, 1985.

274. Jennette JC: Rapidly progressive and crescentic glomerulonephritis. Kidney Int 63:1164–1172, 2003.

275. Chen M, Yu F, Zhang Y, et al: Characteristics of Chinese patients with Wegener's granulomatosis with anti MPO antibodies. Kidney Int 68:2225–2229, 2005.

276. Muniain MA, Moreno JC, Gonzalez Campora R: Wegener's granulomatosis in two sictoro. J Rheum Dis 45:417–421, 1986.

277. Papiha SS, Murty GE, Ad Hia A, et al: Association of Wegener's granulomatosis with HLA antigens and other genetic markers. Ann Rheum Dis 51:246–248, 1992.

278. Jennette, JC, Falk, RJ: The pathology of vasculitis involving the kidney. Am J Kidney Dis 24:130, 1994

279. Ronco P, Mougenot B, Bindi P, et al: Clinicohistological features and long-term outcome of Wegener's granulomatosis. Renal involvement in systemic vasculitis. Contrib Nephrol 94:47–57, 1991.

280. Boucher A, Droz D, Adafer E, Noel L-H: Relationship between the integrity of Bowman's capsule and the composition of cellular crescents in human crescentic glomerulonephritis. Lab Invest 56:526–533, 1987.

281. Hauer HA, Bajema IM, Van Houwelingen HC, et al: for the European Vasculitis Study Group (EUVAS). Renal histology in ANCA-associated vasculitis: Differences between diagnosis and serologic subgroups. Kidney Int 61:80–89, 2002.

282. Grotz W, Wanner C, Keller E, et al: Crescentic glomerulonephritis in Wegener's granulomatosis: Morphology, therapy, and outcome. Clin Nephrol 35:243–251, 1991.

283. Watanabe T, Nagafuchi Y, Yoshikawa Y, Toyoshima H: Renal papillary necrosis associated with Wegener's granulomatosis. Human Pathol 14:551–557, 1983.

284. Jennette JC: Rapidly progressive and crescentic glomerulonephritis. Kidney Int 63:1164–1172, 2003.

285. Jennette JC, Xiao H, Falk RJ: The pathogenesis of vascular inflammation by antineutrophil cytoplasmic antibodies. J Am Soc Nephrol 17:1236–1242, 2006.

286. Xiao H, Heeringa P, Hu P, et al: Antineutrophil cytoplastic autoantibodies specific for myeloperoxidase causes glomerulonephritis and vasculitis in mice. J Clin Invest 110:955–963, 2002.

287. Schlieben DJ, Korbet SM, Kimura RE, et al: Pulmonary-renal syndrome in a newborn with placental transmission of ANCAs. Am J Kidney Dis 45:758–761, 2003.

288. Wong J, Csernok E, Gross WL: High plasma levels of the soluble form of CD 30 activation molecule reflect disease activity in patients with Wegener's granulomatosis. Am J Med 102:517–523, 1997.

289. Stagman CA, Cohen Tervaot JW, Huitema MG, Kallenberg CGM: Serum markers of T cell activation in relapses of Wegener's granulomatosis. Clin Exp Immunol 91:415–420, 1993.

290. King WJ, Brooks CJ, Holder R, et al: T lymphocytes response to ANCA antigens are present in patients with ANCA-associated systemic vasculitis. Clin Exp Immunol 112:539–546, 1998.

291. Griffith ME, Coulhart A, Pusey CD: T cell responses to myeloperoxidase and proteinase 3 in patients with systemic vasculitis. Clin Exp Immunol 103:253–258, 1996.

292. Preston GA, Falk RJ: ANCA signaling is not just a matter of respiratory burst. Kidney Int 59:1981–1982, 2001.

293. Harper L, Crockwell P, Dwoma A, Savage C: Neutrophil priming and apoptosis in ANCA-associated vasculitis. Kidney Int 59:1729–1738, 2001.

294. Little MA, Pusey CD: Glomerulonephritis due to ANCA- associated vasculitis: An update on approaches to management. Nephrology 10:368–376, 2005.

295. Witko-Sarsat V, Lesavre P, Lopez S, et al: A large subset of neutrophils expressing membrane proteinase 3 is a risk factor for vasculitis and rheumatoid arthritis. J Am Soc Nephrol 10:1224–1233, 1995.

296. Franseen CF, Huitema MG, Kobold AC, et al: In vitro neutrophil activation by antibodies to proteinase 3 and myeloperoxidase from patients with crescentic glomerulonephritis. J Am Soc Nephrol 10:1506–1515, 1999.

297. Rarok AA, Stegman CA, Limburg PG, Kallenberg CGM: Neutrophil membrane expression of proteinase 3 is related to relapse in PR3-ANCA-Associated Vasculitis. J Am Soc Nephrol 13:2232–2238, 2002.

298. West B, Todd JR, King JW: Wegener's granulomatosis and Trimethoprim sulfamethoxazole. Ann Intern Med 106: 840–842, 1987.

299. Andrassy K, Erb A, Koderisch J, et al: Wegener's granulomatosis with renal involvement: Patient survival and correlations between initial renal function, renal histology, therapy, and renal outcome. Clin Nephrol 35:139–147, 1991.

300. Cordier JF, Valeyre D, Guillevin L, et al: Pulmonary Wegener's granulomatosis. A clinical and imaging study of 77 cases. Chest 97:906–912, 1990.

301. Gaudin PB, Askin FB, Falk RJ, Jennette JC: The pathologic spectrum of pulmonary lesions in patients with anti-neutrophil cytoplasmic autoantibodies specific for anti-proteinase 3 and anti-myeloperoxidase. Am J Clin Pathol 104:7, 1995.

302. Rosenberg DM, Weinberger SE, Fuhner JD, et al: Functional correlates of lung involvement in Wegener's granulomatosis. Use of pulmonary function tests in staging and follow-up. Am J Med 69:387, 1980.

303. Rao JK, Allen NB, Feussner JR, Weinberger M: A prospective study of c-ANCA and clinical criteria in diagnosing Wegener's granulomatosis. Lancet 346:926, 1995.

304. Rao JK, Weinberger M, Oddone EZ, et al: The role of antineutrophil cytoplasmic antibody (c-ANCA) testing in the diagnosis of Wegener granulomatosis. A literature review and meta-analysis. Ann Intern Med 123:925, 1995.

305. Geffiaud-Ricouard C, No'l LK, Chauveau D, et al: Clinical spectrum associated with antineutrophil cytoplasmic antibodies of defined antigen specificities in 98 selected patients. Clin Nephrol 39:125, 1993.

306. Pettersson E, Heigl Z: Antineutrophil cytoplasmic antibody (CANCA and PANCA) titers in relation to disease activity in patients with necrotizing vasculitis. A longitudinal study. Clin Nephrol 37:219, 1992.

307. Kerr GS, Fleisher TA, Hallahan CW, et al: Limited prognostic value of changes in antineutrophil cytoplasmic antibody titer in patients with Wegener's granulomatosis. Arthritis Rheum 36:365, 1993.

308. Cohen Tervaert JW, Huitema MG, Hene RJ, et al: Prevention of relapses in Wegener's granulomatosis by treatment based on antineutrophil cytoplasmic antibody titre. Lancet 336.709, 1990.

309. Jayne DR, Gaskin G, Pusey CD, Lockwood CM: ANCA and predicting relapse in systemic vasculitis. Q J Med 88:127, 1995.

310. Kyndt X, Renmanx D, Bridoux F, et al: Serial measurements of ANCA in patients with systemic vasculitis. Am J Med 106:527, 1999.

311. Rich LM, Piering WF: Ureteral stenosis due to recurrent Wegener's granulomatosis after kidney transplantation. J Am Soc Nephrol 4:1516, 1994.

312. Jennette JC, Hogan SL, Wilkman AS, et al: Pathologic features of antineutrophil cytoplasmic autoantibody-associated renal disease as predictors of long-term loss of renal function. Modern Pathol 5:102A, 1992.

313. Zauner I, Bach D, Braun N, et al: Predictive value of initial histology and effect of plasmapheresis on long-term prognosis of rapidly progressive glomerulonephritis. Am J Kidney Dis 39:28–35, 2002.

314. Nachman PH, Hogan SL, Jennette JC, Falk RJ: Treatment response and relapse in antineutrophil cytoplasmic antibody-associated microscopic polyangiitis and glomerulonephritis. J Am Soc Nephrol 7:33, 1996.

315. Matteson EL, Gold KN, Bloch DA, Hunder GG: Long-term survival of patients with Wegener's granulomatosis from the American College of Rheumatology Wegener's Granutomatosis Classification Criteria Cohort. Am J Med 101:129, 1996.

316. Cole E, Cattran D, Magil A, et al: A prospective randomized trial of plasma exchange as additive therapy in idiopathic crescentic glomerulonephritis. Am J Kidney Dis 20:261–265, 1992.

317. Glassock RJ: Intensive plasma exchange in crescentic glomerulonephritis: Help or no help? Am J Kidney Dis 20:270, 1992.

318. Gallagher H, Kwan JT, Jayne DR: Pulmonary Renal Syndrome: A 4 year single center experience. Am J Kidney Dis 39:42–47, 2002.

319. Pusey CD, Rees AJ, Evans DJ, et al: Plasma exchange in focal necrotizing glomerulonephritis without anti-GBM antibodies. Kidney Int 40:757, 1991.

320. Hoffman GS, Leavitt RY, Fleisher TA, et al: Treatment of Wegener's granulomatosis with intermittent high-dose intravenous cyclophosphamide. Am J Med 89:403–410, 1990.

321. Kunis CL, Kiss B, Williams G, et al: Intravenous "pulse" cyclophosphamide therapy of crescentic glomerulonephritis. Clin Nephrol 37:1–7, 1992.

322. Guillevin L, Cordier J-F, Lhote F, et al: A prospective multicenter randomized trial comparing steroids and pulse cyclophosphamide versus steroids and oral cyclophosphamide in the treatment of generalized Wegener's granulomatosis. Arthritis Rheum 40:2187, 1997.

323. de Groot K, Adu D, Savage CO: The value of pulse cyclophosphamide in ANCA-associated vasculitis: Meta-analysis and critical review. Nephrol Dial Transplant 16:2018, 2001.

324. Haubitz M, Schellang S, Gobel U, et al: Intravenous pulse administration of cyclophosphamide versus daily oral treatments in patients with ANCA-associated vasculitis and renal involvement in a prospective randomized study. Arthritis Rheum 41:1835, 1998.

325. Adu D, Pall A, Luqmani RA, et al: Controlled trial of pulse versus continuous prednisone and cyclophosphamide in the treatment of systemic vasculitis. Q J Med 90:401, 1997.

326. Klemmer PJ, Chalermskulrat W, Reif MS, et al: Plasmapheresis therapy for diffuse alveolar hemorrhage in patients with small-vessel vasculitis. Am J Kidney Dis 42:1149–1153, 2003.

327. Jayne D: Conventional treatment and outcome of Wegener's granulomatosus and microscopic polyangiitis. Cleve Clin J Med 69 S2:110–116, 2002.

328. Etanercept plus standard therapy for Wegener's granulomatosis. N Engl J Med 352: 351–361, 2005.

329. Keogh KA, Wylam ME, Stone JH, Specks U: Induction of remission by B lymphocyte depletion in eleven patients with antineutrophil cytoplasmic antibody associated vasculitis. Arthritis Rheum 52:262–268, 2005.

330. Booth AD, Almond MK, Burns A, et al: Outcome of ANCA-associated renal vasculitis. Am J Kidney Dis 41:776, 2003.

331. Westman KW, Bygren PG, Olsson H, et al: Relapse rate, renal survival, and cancer morbidity in patients with Wegener's granulomatosis or microscopic polyangiitis with renal involvement. J Am Soc Nephrol 9:842, 1998.

332. Hogan SL, Falk RJ, Chin H, et al: Predictors of relapse and treatment resistance in antineutrophil cytoplasmic antibody associated small vessel vasculitis. Ann Intern Med 143:621–631, 2005.

333. de Groot K, Reinhold-Keller E, Tatsis E, et al: Therapy for the maintenance of remission in 65 patients with generalized Wegener's granulomatosis. Arthritis Rheum 39:2052, 1996.

334. Langford CA, Talar-Williams C, Barron KS, et al: Use of a cyclophosphamide induction—methotrexate maintenance regimen for the treatment of Wegener's granulomatosis. Arthritis Rheum 44:271, 2001.

335. Luqmani R, Jayne D: EUVAS. European Vasculitis Study Group: A multicenter randomized trial of cyclophosphamide versus azathioprine during remission in ANCA-associated vasculitis. Arthritis Rheum 42:225, 1995.

336. Jayne D, Rasmussen N, Andrassy K, et al: A randomized trial for maintenance therapy for vasculitis associated with antineutrophil cytoplasmic antibodies. N Engl J Med 349:36–44, 2003.

337. Haubitz M, Koch KM, Brunkhorst R: Cyclosporin for the prevention of disease reactivation in relapsing ANCA-associated vasculitis. Nephrol Dial Transplant 13:2074, 1998.

338. Stegman CA, Cohen Tervaert JW, de Jong PE, et al: Trimethoprim-sulfamethoxazole (co-trimoxazole) for the prevention of relapses of Wegener's granulomatosis. N Engl J Med 335:16, 1996.

339. Sneller MC, Hoffinan GS, Tular-Williams C, et al: An analysis of 42 Wegener's granulomatosis patients treated with methotrexate and prednisone. Arthritis Rheum 38:608, 1995.

340. Langford CA, Tular-Williams C, Sneller MC: Use of methotrexate and glucocorticoids in the treatment of Wegener's granulomatosis. Long-term renal outcome in patients with glomerulonephritis. Arthritis Rheum 43:1836, 2000.

341. Jayne DR, Davies MJ, Fox CJ, et al: Treatment of systemic vasculitis with pooled intravenous immunoglobulin. Lancet 337:1137, 1991.

342. Tuso P, Moudgil A, Hay J, et al: Treatment of antineutrophil cytoplasmic autoantibody positive systemic vasculitis and glomerulonephritis with pooled intravenous gammaglobulin. Am J Kidney Dis 20:504, 1992.

343. Richter C, Schnabel A, Csemok E, et al: Treatment of antineutrophil cytoplasmic antibody (ANCA)-associated systemic vasculitis with high dose intravenous immunoglobulin. Clin Exp Immunol 101:2, 1995.

344. Pedersen RS, Bistrup C: Etoposide: More effective and less bone-marrow toxic than standard immunosuppressive therapy in systemic vasculitis. Nephrol Dial Transplant 11:1121, 1996.

345. Lockwood CM, Thiru S, Isaacs JD, et al: Long-term remission of intractable systemic vasculitis with monoclonal antibody therapy. Lancet 341:1620, 1993.

346. Hagen EC, de Keizer RJ, Andrassy K, et al: Compassionate treatment of Wegener's granulomatosis with rabbit anti-thymocyte globulin. Clin Nephrol 43:351, 1995.

347. Mekhail TM, Hoffman GS: Long-term outcome of Wegener's granulomatosis in patients with renal disease requiring dialysis. J Rheumatol 27:1237, 2000.

348. Nachman PH, Segelmark M, Westman K, et al: Recurrent ANCA associated small vessel vasculitis after transplantation. A pooled analysis. Kidney Int 56:1544, 1999.

349. Haubitz M, Koch KM, Brunkhorst R: Survival and vasculitis activity in patients with end-stage renal disease due to Wegener's granulomatosis. Nephrol Dial Transplant 13:1713, 1998.

350. Allen A, Pusey C, Gaskin G: Outcome of renal replacement therapy in ANCA associated systemic vasculitis. J Am Soc Nephrol 9:1258, 1998.

351. Haubitz M, de Groot T: Tolerance of mycophenolate mofetil in ESRD patients with ANCA associated vasculitis. Clin Nephrol 57:421, 2002.

352. Rostaing L, Modesto A, Oksman F, et al: Outcome of patients with antineutrophil cytoplasmic autoantibody-associated vasculitis following cadaveric kidney transplantation. Am J Kidney Dis 29:96, 1997.

353. Haubitz M, Kliem V, Koch KM, et al: Renal transplantation for patients with autoimmune diseases: Single-center experience with 42 patients. Transplantation 63:1251, 1997.

354. Constantinescu A, Liang M, Laskow DA: Sirolimus lowers myeloperoxidase and p-ANCA titers in a pediatric patient before kidney transplantation. Am J Kidney Dis 40:407–410, 2002.

355. Churg J: Nomenclature of vasculitic syndrome: A historical perspective. Am J Kidney Dis 18:148–153, 1991.

356. Deshazo RD, Levinson AI, Lawless OJ, Weisbaum G: Systemic vasculitis with coexistent large and small vessel involvement. A classification dilemma. JAMA 238:1940–1942, 1977.

357. Kallenberg CG, Brouwer E, Weening JJ, Cohen Tervaert JW: Anti-neutrophil cytoplasmic antibodies: Current diagnostic and pathophysiological potential. Kidney Int 46:1, 1994.

358. Gross WL, Schmitt WH, Csernok E: Antineutrophil cytoplasmic autoantibody-associated diseases: A rheumatologist's perspective. Am J Kidney Dis 18:175–179, 1991.

359. Cohen Tervaert JW, Goldschmeding R, Elema JD, et al: Association of autoantibodies to myeloperoxidase with different forms of vasculitis. Arthritis Rheum 33:1264–1272, 1990.

360. Woodrow G, Cook JA, Brownjohn AM, Turney JH: Is renal vasculitis increasing in incidence. Lancet 336: 1583, 1990.

361. D'Agati V, Appel GB: Polyarteritis, Wegener's granulomatosis, Churg-Strauss syndrome. In Brenner B, Tischer C (eds): Renal Pathology. 2nd ed. Philadelphia, JB Lippincott, 1994, pp. 1087–1154.

362. Barbiano di Belgiojoso G, Genderini A, Sinico RA, et al: Acute renal failure due to microscopic polyarteritis nodosa with the same histological and clinical patterns in a father and son in renal involvement in systemic vasculitis. Contrib Nephrol 94:107–114, 1991.

363. Leib SS, Restivo C, Paulus HE: Immunosuppressive and corticosteroid therapy of polyarteritis nodosa. Am J Med 67:941–947, 1979.

364. Scott DGI, Bacon PA, Elliott PJ, et al: Systemic vasculitis in a district general hospital, 1972–1980: Clinical and laboratory features, classification and prognosis of 80 cases. Q J Med 51 (203):292–311, 1982.

365. Serra A, Cameron JS, Turner DR, et al: Vasculitis affecting the kidney: Presentation, histopathology and long-term outcome. Q J Med 53:181–208, 1984.

366. Chang-Miller A, Okamura M, Torres VE, et al: Renal involvement in relapsing polychondritis. Medicine 66:202–217, 1987.

367. Espinoza LR, Richman A, Bocanegra T, et al: Immune complex-mediated renal involvement in relapsing polychondritis. Am J Med 71:181–183, 1983.

368. Zhao MH, Chen M, Gao Y, Wang H-Y: Propylthiouracil-induced ANCA-associated vasculitis. Kidney Int 69:1477–1481, 2006 .

369. Citron BP, Halpern M, McCarron M, et al: Necrotizing angiitis associated with drug abuse. N Engl J Med 283:1003–1011, 1970.

370. Jayne DRW, Marshall PD, Jones Si, Lockwood CM: Autoantibodies to GBM and neutrophil cytoplasm in rapidly progressive glomerulonephritis. Kidney Intern 37:965–970, 1990.

371. Komadina KH, Houk RW, Vicks SL, et al: Goodpasture's syndrome associated with pulmonary eosinophilic vasculitis. J Rheumatol 15:1298–1301, 1988.

372. O'Donoghue DJ, Short CD, Brenchley PEC, et al: Sequential development of systemic vasculitis with antineutrophil cytoplasmic antibodies complicating antiglomerular basement membrane disease. Clin Nephrol 32: 251–255, 1989.

373. Guillevin L, Lhote F, Cohen P, et al: Polyarteritis nodosa related hepatitis B virus. A prospective study with long-term observation of 41 patients. Medicine (Baltimore) 74:238, 1995.

374. Carpenter MT, West SG: Polyarteritis nodosa in hairy cell leukemia: Treatment with interferon-alpha. J Rheumatol 21:1150, 1994.

375. Jennette JC, Falk RJ: The pathology of vasculitis involving the kidney. Am J Kidney Dis 24:130, 1994.

376. D'Agati V, Chander P, Nash M, Mancilla-Jimenez R: Idiopathic microscopic polyarteritis nodosa: Ultrastructural observations on the renal vascular and glomerular lesions. Am J Kidney Dis 7:95–110, 1986.

377. Meroni M, Sessa A, Tarelu LT, et al: Renal ultrastructural features in primary systemic vasculitis in renal involvement in systemic vasculitis. Contrib Nephrol 94:123–132, 1991.

378. Cameron JS: Renal vasculitis: Microscopic polyarteritis and Wegener's granuloma in renal involvement in systemic vasculitis. Contrib Nephrol 94:38–46, 1991.

379. Crawford JP, Movat HZ, Ranadive NS, Hay JB: Pathways to inflammation induced by immune complexes: Development of the Arthus reaction. Fed Proc 41:2583–2587, 1982.

380. Berden JHM, Hang L, McConahey PJ, Dixon FJ: Analysis of vascular lesions in murine SLE. I. Association with serologic abnormalities. J Immunol 130:1699–1705, 1983.

381. Yoshiki T, Hayasaka T, Fukatso R, et al: The structural proteins of murine leukemia virus and the pathogenesis of necrotizing arteritis and glomerulonephritis in SL/Ni mice. J Immunol 122:1812–1820, 1979.

382. Hart MN, Tassell SK, Sadewasser KL, et al: Autoimmune vasculitis resulting from in vitro immunization of lymphocytes to smooth muscle. Am J Pathol 119:448–455, 1985.

383. Leung DYM, Geha RS, Newberger JW, et al: Two monokines, interlukin-1 and tumor necrosis factor, render cultured vascular endothelial cells susceptible to lysis by antibodies circulating during Kawasaki syndrome. J Exp Med 164:1958–1972, 1988.

384. Schwartz RA, Churg J: Churg-Strauss syndrome. Br J Dermatol 127:199, 1992.

385. Serra A, Cameron JS: Clinical and pathologic aspects of renal vasculitis. Semin Nephrol 5:15–33, 1985.

386. Falk RJ, Hogan S, Carey TS, Jennette JC, and The Glomerular Disease Collaborative Network: Clinical course of anti-neutrophil cytoplasmic autoantibody-associated glomerulonephritis and systemic vasculitis. Ann Intern Med 113:656–663, 1990.

387. Travers RL, Allison DJ, Brettle RP, Hughes GRV: Polyarteritis nodosa: A clinical and angiographic analysis of 17 cases. Semin Arthritis Rheum 8:184–199, 1979.

388. Guillevin L, Lhote L, Gallais V, et al: Gastrointestinal involvement in periarteritis nodosa and Churg-Strauss syndrome. Ann Med Intern 146:260, 1995.

389. Ohkoshi N, Mgusama K, Oguni E, Shoji S: Sural nerve biopsy in vasculitic neuropathies: Morphometric analysis of the caliber of involved vessels. J Med 27:153, 1996.

390. Cohen Tervaret JW, Kallenberg C: Neurologic manifestations of systemic vasculitides. Rheum Dis Clin North Am 19:913, 1993.

391. Moore PM: Neurologic manifestations of vasculitis: Update on immunopathogenic mechanisms and clinical features. Ann Neurol 37(Suppl 1): S131, 1995.

392. Plumley SG, Rubio R, Alasfar S, Jasin HE: Polyarteritis nodosa presenting as polymyositis. Semin Arthritis Rheum 31:377, 2002.

393. Ng WF, Chow LT, Lam PW: Localized polyarteritis of the breast: Report of two cases and a review of the literature. Histopathology 23:535, 1993.

394. Gibson LE, Su WP : Cutaneous vasculitis. Rheum Dis Clin North Am 21:1097, 1995.

395. Guillevin L, Ronco P, Verroust P: Circulating immune complexes in systemic necrotizing vasculitis of the polyarteritis nodosa group. Comparison of HBV-related polyarteritis nodosa and Churg-Strauss angiitis. J Autoimmunity 3:789–792, 1990.

396. Wilkowski MJ, Velosa JA, Holley KE, et al: Risk factors in idiopathic renal vasculitis and glomerulonephritis. Kidney Intern 36:1133–1141, 1989.

397. O'Connell MT, Kubrusly DB, Fournier AM: Systemic necrotizing vasculitis seen initially as hypertensive crisis. Arch Intern Med 145:265–267, 1985.

398. Vazquez JJ, San Martin P, Barbado FJ, et al: Angiographic findings in systemic necrotizing vasculitis. Angiology 32:773–779, 1981.

399. Fauci A, Doppman JL, Wolff SM: Cyclophosphamide-induced remissions in advanced polyarteritis nodosa. Am J Med 64: 890–894, 1978.

400. De Groot K, Jayne D, Tesar V, et al: European Multicenter Randomized Controlled Trial of daily oral vs. pulse cyclophosphamide for induction of remission in AWCA-associated systemic vasculitis. J Asoc Nephrol 16:7A, 2005.

401. Gayraud M, Guillevin L, Le Toumelin P, et al: Long-term follow up of polyarteritis nodosa, microscopic polyangiitis, and Churg-Strauss syndrome. Arthritis Rheum 44:666, 2001.

402. Guillevin L: Treatment of classic polyarteritis nodosa in 1999. Nephrol Dial. Transplant 14:2077, 1999.

403. Guillevin L, L'hoto F, Gayraud M, et al: Prognostic factors in polyarteritis nodosa and Churg-Strauss syndrome. A prospective study in 342 patients. Medicine 75:17, 1996.

404. Kruger, K Boker KK, Zeidler K, et al: Treatment of hepatitis B-related polyarteritis nodosa with famciclovir and interferon alfa-2b. J Hepatol 26:935, 1997.

405. Guillevin L, Lhote F, Cohen P, et al: Polyarteritis nodosa related hepatitis B virus. A prospective study with long-term observation of 41 patients. Medicine (Baltimore) 74:238, 1995.

406. Hellmich B, Ehlers S, Csernok E, Gross WL: Update on the pathognesis of Churg-Strauss syndrome. Clin Exp Rheumatol 21:S69–77, 2003.

407. Abril A, Calamia KT, Cohen MD: The Churg Strauss syndrome (allergic granulomatous angiitis): Review and update. Semin Arthritis Rheum 33:106–114, 2003.

408. Lhote F, Guillevin L: Polyarteritis nodosa, microscopic polyangiitis, and Churg-Strauss syndrome. Clinical aspects and treatment. Rheum Dis Clin North Am 21:911, 1995.

409. Reid AJC, Harrison BDW, Watts RH, et al: Churg-Strauss syndrome in a district hospital. Q J Med 91:219, 1998.

410. Guillevin L, Cohen P, Gayraud M, et al: Churg-Strauss syndrome. Clinical study and long-term follow-up of 96 patients. Medicine 78:26, 1999.

411. Harold LR, Andrade SE, Go AS, et al: The incidence of Churg Strauss syndrome in asthma drug users: A population-based prospective. J Rheumatol 32:1076–1080, 2005.

412. Cooper HJ, Bacal E, Patterson R: Allergic angiitis and granulomatosis. Arch Intern Med 138:367, 1978

413. Clutterbuck EJ, Evans DJ, Pusey CD: Renal involvement in Churg-Strauss Syndrome. Nephrol Dial Transplant 5:161–167, 1990.

414. Wechsler ME, Garpestad E, Flier SF, et al: Pulmonary infiltrates, eosinophilia, and cardiomyopathy following corticosteroid withdrawal in ptients with asthma receiving zafirlukast. JAMA 279:455, 1998.

415. Green RI, Vayonis AG: Churg-Strauss syndrome after zafirlukast in two patients not receiving systemic steroid treatment. Lancet 353:725, 1999.

416. Kinoshita M. Shiraishi T, Koga T, et al: Churg-Strauss syndrome after corticosteroid withdrawal in an asthmatic patient treated with pranlikast. J Allergy Clin Immunol 103:534, 1999.

417. Martin RM, Wilton LV, Mann RD: Prevalence of Churg-Strauss syndrome, vasculitis, eosinophilia and associated condition: Retrospective analysis of 58 prescription-event monitoring cohort studies. Pharmacoepidemiol Drug Safety 8:179, 1999.

418. Wechsler M, Finn D, Gunawardena D, et al: Churg-Strauss syndrome in patients receiving montelukast as treatment for asthma. Chest 117:708, 2000.

419. Le Gall C, Pham S, Vignes S, et al: Inhaled coticosteroids and Churg-Strauss syndrome: A report of five cases. Eur Respir J 15:978, 2000.

420. Tuggey JM, Hosker HS: Churg-Strauss syndrome associatd with montelukast therapy. Thorax 55:805, 2000.

421. Keogh KA, Specks U: Churg-Strauss syndrome: Clinical presentation, antineutrophil cytoplasmic antibodies, and leukotriene receptor antagonists. Am J Med 115:284–290, 2003.

422. Gaskin G, Clutterbuck EJ, Pusey CD: Renal disease in the Churg-Strauss Syndrome in renal involvement in systemic vasculitis. Contrib Nephrol 94:58–65, 1991.

423. Antiga G, Volpi A, Battini G, et al: Acute renal failure in a patient affected with Churg and Strauss Syndrome. Nephron 57:113–114, 1991.

424. Manger BJ, Krapf FE, Gramatzi M, et al: IgE-containing circulating immune complexes in Churg-Strauss vasculitis. Scand J Immunol 21:369, 1985.

425. Hellmich B, Ehlers S, Csernok K, Gross WL: Update on the pathogenesis of Churg-Strauss syndrome. Clin Exp Rheumatol 21:S69, 2003.

426. Tai PC, Kolt ME, Denny P, et al: Deposition of eosinophil cationic protein in granulomas in allergic granulomatosis and vasculitis: The Churg-Strauss syndrome. Br Med J 289:400, 1984.

427. Schmitt WH, Csernock E, Kobayashi S: Churg-Strauss syndrome markers of lymphocyte activation and endothelial damage. Arthritis Rheum 41:445, 1998.

428. Solans R, Bosch JA, Perez-Bocanegra C, et al: Churg-Strauss syndrome: Outcome and long-term follow-up of 32 patients. Rheumatology 40:763–771, 2001.

429. Hasley PB, Follansbee WP, Coulehan JL: Cardiac manifestations of Churg-Straus syndrome: Report of a case and review of the literature. Am Heart J 120:996, 1990.

430. Hattori N, Ichimura M, Nagamatsu M, et al: Clinicopathological features of Churg-Strauss syndrome-associated neuropathy. Brain 122:427, 1999.

431. Choi YH, Im JG, Han BK, et al: Thoracic manifestation of Churg-Strauss Syndrome: Radiologic and clinical findings. Chest 117:117, 2000.

432. Buschman DL, Waldron JA, King TE Jr: Churg-Strauss pulmonary vasculitis. High resoution CT scanning and pathologic findings. Am Rev Respir Dis 142:458, 1990.

433. Erzurum SC, Underwood GA, Hamilos DL, Waldron JA: Pleural effusion in Churg-Strauss syndrome. Chest 95:1357, 1989.

434. Hellmich B, Goss WL: Recent progress in thepharmacotherapy of Churg-Strauss syndrome. Expert Opin Pharmacother 5:25–35, 2004.

435. Sinico RA, DiToma L, Maggiore U, et al: Prevalence and clinical significance of anitneutrophil cytoplasmic antibodies in Churg-Strauss syndrome. Arthritis Rheum 52: 2926–2935, 2005.

436. Sable-Fourtassou R, Cohen P, Mahr A, et al: Antineutrophil cytoplasmic antibodies and the Churg-Strauss syndrome. Ann Intern Med 143:632–638, 2005.

437. Chow C-C, Li EKM, MacMoune Lai F: Allergic granulomatosis and angiitis (Churg Strauss Syndrome): Response to "pulse" intavenous cyclophosphamide. Ann Rheum Dis 48:605, 1989.

438. Tsurikisawa N, Taniguchi M, Saito H, et al: Treatment of Churg-Strauss syndrome with high dose intravenous immunoglobulin. Ann Allergy Asthma Immunol 92: 80–87, 2004.

439. Danielli MG, Cappelli M, Malcangi G, et al: Long term effectiveness of intravenous immunoglobulin in Churg-Strauss syndrome. Ann Rheum Dis 63:1649–1654, 2004.

440. Tatsis E, Schnabel A, Gross WL: Interferon-alpha treatment of four pattients with the Churg-Strauss syndrome. Ann Intern Med 129:370, 1998.

441. Gonzalez-Gay MA, Barros S, Lopez-Diaz MJ, et al: Giant cell arteritis: Disease patterns of clinical presentation in a series of 240 patients. Medicine 84:269–276, 2005.

442. Gonalez-Gay MA, Lopez-Diaz MJ, Barros S, et al: Giant cell arteritis: Laboratory tests at the time of diagnosis in a series of 240 patients. Medicine 84:277–290, 2005.

443. Hunder GG: Giant cell arteritis and polymyalgia rheumatica. Med Clin N Am 81:195–219, 1997.

444. Levine SM, Hellmann DB: Giant cell arteritis. Curr Opin Rheumatol 14:3–10, 2002.

445. Lawrence RC, Helmick CG, Arnett FC, et al: Estimates of the prevalence of arthritis and selected musculo-skeletal disorders in the US. Arthritis Rheum 41:778–799, 1998.

446. Solvarani C, Gabriel SE, Fallon WM, Hunder GG: The incidence of giant cell arteritis in Olmstead County Minnesota. Ann Intern Med 123:192–194, 1995.

447. Lie JT: Aortic and extracranial large vessel giant cell arteritis: A review of 72 cases with histopathologic documentation. Semin Arthritis Rheum 24:422–431, 1995.

448. Highton J, Anderson KR: Concurrent polyarteritis nodosa and temporal arteritis. N Z Med J 14:766, 1984.

449. Bosch X, Mirapeix E, Font J, et al: antimyeloperoxidase autoantibodies in patients with necrotizing glomerular and alveolar capillaritis. Am J Kidney Dis 20:231–239, 1992.

450. Fauchald P, Rygvold O, Oystese B: Temporal arteritis and polymyalgia rheumatica. Ann Intern Med 77:845, 1972.

451. Truong L, Kopelman RG, Williams GS, Pirani CL: Temporal arteritis and renal disease. Am J Med 78:171, 1985.

452. Jover JA, Hernandez-Garcia C, Murado IC, et al: Combined treatment of giant cell arteritis with methotrexate and prednisone. Ann Intern Med 134:106–114, 2001.

453. Wilke WS, Hoffman GS: Treatment of corticosteroid resistant giant cell arteritis. Rheum Dis Clin N Am 21:59–71, 1995.

454. Hata A, Noda M, Moriwaki R, Numaro F: Angiographic findings of Takayasu arteritis: New classification. Int J Cardiol 54 (Suppl):155, 1997.

455. Hall S, Barr W, Lie JT, et al: Takayasu arteritis. A study of 32 North American patients. Medicine 64:89, 1985.

456. Cid MC, Font C, Coll-Vincent B, Grau JM: Large vessel vasculitides. Curr Opin Rheumatol 10:18, 1998.

457. Sharma BK, Jain S, Sagar S: Systemic manifestations of Takayasu arteritis: The expanding spectrum. Int J Cardiol 54 (Suppl):149, 1997.

458. Yoshimura M, Kida H, Saito Y, et al: Peculiar glomerular lesions in Takayasu's arteritis. Clin Nephrol 24:120, 1985.

459. Weiss RA, Jodorkovsky R, Weiner S, et al: Chronic renal failure due to Takayasu's arteritis: Recovery of renal function after nine months of dialysis. Clin Nephrol 17:104, 1982.

460. Takagi M, Ikeda T, Kimura K, et al: Renal histological studies in patients with Takayasu's arteritis. Nephron 36:68, 1984.

461. Lagneau P, Michel JB: Renovascular hypertension and Takayasu's disease. J Urol 134:876, 1985.

462. Greene NB, Baughman RP, Kim CK: Takayasu's arteritis associated with interstitial lung disease and glomerulonephritis. Chest 89:605, 1986.

463. Andrews J, Al-Nahhas A, Pennell DJ, et al: Non-invasive imaging in the diagnosis and managemtn of Takayasu's arteritis. Ann Rheum Dis 63:995–1000, 2004.

464. Kissin EY, Merkel PA: Diagnostic imaging in Takayasu's arteritis. Curr Opin Rheumatol 16:31–37, 2004.

465. Eichorn J, Sima D, Thiele B, et al: Anti-endothelial cell antibodies in Takayasu's arteritis. Circulation 94:2396, 1996.

466. Simon D, Ledonx F, Lagneau P, et al: Takayasu's aortitis with renovascular hypertension. Successful complex vascularization. J Urol 125:91, 1981.

467. Yoneda S, Nukada T, Imaizumi M, et al: Hemodynamic and volume characteristics and peripheral plasma renin activity in Takayasu's arteritis. Jpn Circ J 44:951, 1980.

468. Graham AN, Delahunt B, Renouf JJ, Austad WI: Takayasu's disease assoociated with generalized amyloidosis. Aus N Z J Med 15:343, 1985.

469. Yoshikawa Y, Truong LD, Mattioli CA, Lederer E: Membranoproliferative Glomerulonephritis in Takayasuls Arteritis. Am J Nephrol 8:240–244, 1988.

470. Hoffman GS, Leavitt RY, Kerr GS, et al: Treatment of glucocorticoid resistant or relapsing Takayasu arteritis with methotrexate. Arthritis Rheum 37:578, 1994.

471. Mevavash D, Leibnitz G, Brezis M, Raz E: Induction of remission on a patient with Takayasu's arteritis by low dose pulse methotrexate. Ann Rheum Dis 51:904, 1992.

472. Daino E, Schieppati A, Remuzzi G: Mycophenolate mofetil for the treatment of Takayasu's arteritis: report of three cases. Ann Intern Med 130:422, 1999.

473. Valsakumar AK, Valappil UC, Jorapur V, et al: Role of immunosuppressive therapy on clinical, immunological, and angiographic outcome in active Takayasu's arteritis. J Rheumatol 30:1793–1798, 2003.

474. Hoffman GS, Merkel PA, Brasington RD, et al: Anti-tumor necrosis factor therapy in patients with difficult to treat Takayasu's arteritis. Arthritis Rheum 50:2296–2304, 2004.

475. Ishikawa K, Martani S: Long-term outcome for 120 Japanses patients with Takayasu's Disease. Circulation 90:1853, 1994.

476. Myers JL: Editorial. Lymphomatoid granulomatosis: Past, present . . . future. Mayo Clin Proc 65: 274–278, 1990.

477. Trapani S, Micheli A, Grisolia F, et al: Henoch Schonlein purpura in childhood: epidemiological and clinical analysis of 150 cases over a 5 year period and review of the literature. Semin Arthritis Rheum 35:143–153, 2005.

478. Rai A, Nast C, Adler S: Henoch-Schonlein purpura nephritis. J Am Soc Nephrol 10:2637, 1999.

479. Saulsbury FT: Henoch-Schoenlein Purpura in children. Report of 100 patients and review of the literature. Medicine 78:395, 1999.

480. Tizard EJ: Henoch-Schoenlein purpura. Arch Dis Child 80:380, 1999.

481. Yang YH, Hung CF, Hsu CR, et al: A nationwide survey on epideliologic characterisitics of childhood HSP in Taiwan. Rheumatology 44:618–622, 2005.

482. Gardner-Medwin JM, Dolezalova P, Cummins C, Southwood TR: Incidence of Henoch-Schonlein purpura, Kawasaki disease, and rare vasculitides in children of different ethnic origins. Lancet 360:1197–1202, 2002.

483. Davin JC, Ten Berge IJ, Weening JJ: What is the difference between IgA nephropathy and Henoch-Schonlein purpura nephritis? Kidney Int 59:823–834, 2001.

484. Yoshikawa N, Ito H, Yoshiya K, et al: Henoch-Schonlein nephritis and IgA nephropathy in children: A comparison clinical course. Clin Nephrol 27:233, 1987.

485. Fogazzi GB, Pasquali S, Moriggi M, et al: Long-term outcome of Schonlein Henoch nephritis in the adult. Clin Nephrol 31:60, 1989.

486. Blanco, R, Martinez-Taboada, VK Rodriguez-Valverde, V, et al: Henoch-Schonlein purpura in adulthood and childhood: Two dffferent expressions of the same syndrome. Arthritis Rheum 40:859, 1997.

487. Kurihara S, Fukuda Y, Saito Y, et al: Three cases of "IgA nephritis" associated with other disease. J Kanazawa Med Univ 7:51, 1982.

488. Levy M: Do genetic factors play a role in Berger's disease. Pediatr Nephrol 1:447, 1987.

489. Ostergaard JR, Storm K, Lamm LU: Lack of association between HLA and Schonlein-Henoch purpura. Tissue Antigens 35:234, 1990.

490. Farley TA, Gillespie S, Rasoulpour M, et al: Epidemiology of a cluster of Henoch-Schonlein purpura. Am J Dis Child 143:798, 1989.

491. Pillebout E, Thervet E, Hill G, et al: Henoch-Schonlein Purpura in adults: Outcome and prognostic factors. J Am Soc Nephrol 13:1271–1278, 2002.

492. Nathan K, Gunasekaran TS, Berman JH: Recurrent gastrointestinal Henoch-Schonlein purpura. J Clin Gastroenterol 29:86, 1999.

493. Nakasone H, Hokama A, Fukuch J, et al: Colonoscopic findings in an adult patient with HSP. Gastrointest Endosc 52:392, 2000.

494. Cappell MS, Gupta AM: Colonic lesions associated with Henoch-Schonlein purpura. Am J Gasterenterol 85:1186, 1990.

495. Yoshikawa N, Vamamuro F, Akita Y: Gastrointestinal lesions in an adult patient with HSP. Hepatogastroenterol 46:2823, 1999.

496. Chang WL, Yang YH, Lin YT, Chiang BL: Gastrointestinal manifestations in Hencoh-Schonlein purpura: A review of 261 patients. Acta Paediatr 93:142–1431, 2004.

497. Payton CD, Allison MEM, Boulton-Jones JM: Henoch-Schonlein purpura presenting with pulmonary hemorrhage. Scott Med J 32:26, 1987.

498. Chang WL, Yang YH, Wang LC, et al: Renal manifestations of Henoch-Schonlein purpura: A 10 year clinical study. Pediatr Nephrol 20:1269–1272, 2005.

499. Martini A, Ravelli A, Beluffi G: Urinary microscopy in the diagnosis of hematuria in Henoch-Schonlein purpura. Eur J Pediatr 144:591, 1986.

500. Zurowski AM, Wrzolkowa T, Uszycka KM: Henoch-Schönlein nephritis in children: A clinicopathological study. Int J Pediatr Nephrol 6:183, 1985.

501. Goldstein AR, White RK Akuse R, Chantler C: Long-term follow-up of childhood Henoch-Schonlein nephritis. Lancet 339:280, 1992.

502. Saulsbury FT: IgA rheumatoid factor in Henoch-Schönlein purpura. J Pediatr 108:71, 1986.

503. Coppo R, Basolo B, Martina G, et al: Circulating immune complexes containing IgA, IgM, and IgG in patients with primary IgA nephropathy and Henoch-Schönlein nephritis; correlation with clinical and histologic signs of activity. Clin Nephrol 18:230, 1982.

504. Shaw G, Ronda N, Bevan JS, et al: ANCA of IgA class correlate with disease activity in adult Henoch-Schönlein purpura. Nephrol Dial Transplant 7:1238, 1992.

505. Darvin J-C, Malaise M, Foidart J, Mahieu P: Anti-alpha- galactosyl antibodies and immune complexes in children with Henoch-Schönlein purpura or IgA nephropathy. Kidney Int 31:1132, 1987.

506. Saulsbury FT, Kirkpatrick PR, Bolton WK: IgA antineutrophil cytoplasmic antibody in Henoch-Schönlein purpura. Am J Nephrol 11:295, 1991.

507. Ronda N, Esnault Vl, Layward L, et al: ANCA of IgA isotype in adult Henoch-Schönlein purpura. Clin Exp Immunol 95:49, 1994.

508. Blanco QA, Blanco C, Alvarez J, et al: Antiimmunoglobulin antibodies in children with Schönlein-Henoch syndrome: Absence of serum IgA antibodies. Eur J Pediatr 153:103, 1994.

509. Burden A, Gibson I, Roger R, Tillman D: IgA anticardiolipin antibodies associated with Henoch-Schönlein purpura. Am Acad Dermatol 31:857–860, 1994.

510. Jennette JC, Wieslander J, Tuttle R, Falk RJ: Serum IgA fibronectin aggregates in patients with IgA nephropathy and Henoch-Schönlein purpura. Am J Kidney Dis 18:466, 1991.

511. Yoshiara S, Yoshikawa N, Matsuo T: Immunoelectronmicroscopic study of childhood IgA nephropathy and Henoch-Schönlein nephritis. Virchow Arch 412:95, 1987.

512. Nolasco F, Cameron J, Hartley B: Intraglomerular T cells and monocytes in nephritis: Study with monoclonal antibodies. Kidney Int 31:1160, 1987.

513. Yoshioka K, Takemura T, Aya N, et al: Monocyte infiltration and cross-linked fibrin deposition in IgA nephritis and Henoch-Schonlein purpura nephritis. Clin Nephrol 32:107, 1989.

514. Yoshikawa N, White RK, Cameron AH: Prognostic significance of the glomerular changes in Henoch-Schonlein nephritis. Clin Nephrol 16:223, 1981.

515. Niaudet P, Murcia I, Beaufils H, et al: Primary IgA nephropathies in children: Prognosis and treatment. Adv Nephrol 22:121–140, 1993.

516. Rajaraman S, Goldblum RM, Cavallo T: IgA-associated glomerulonephritides: A study with monoclonal antibodies. Clin Immunol Immunopathol 39:514, 1986.

517. Russel MW, Mestecky J, Julian BA, Gallo JH: IgA-associated renal diseases: Antibodies to environmental antigens in sera and deposition of immunoglobulins and antigens in glomeruli. J Clin Immunol 6:74, 1986.

518. Hene RJ, Velthuis P, van de Wiel A, et al: The relevance of IgA deposits in vessel walls of clinically normal skin. Arch Intern Med 146:745, 1986.

519. Kawana S, Nishiyama S: Serum SC5–9 (terminal complement complex), a sensitive indicator of disease activity in patients with Henoch-Schönlein purpura . Dermatology 184: 171, 1992.

520. Nast CC, Ward FU, Koyle MA, Cohen AH: Recurrent Henoch-Schönlein purpura following renal transplantation. Am J Kidney Dis 9:39, 1987.

521. Hasegawa A, Kawamura T, Ito FL, et al: Fate of renal grafts with recurrent Henoch-Schönlein purpura nephritis in children. Transplant Proc 21:2130, 1989.

522. Meulders Q, Pirson Y, Cosyns JP, et al: Course of Henoch-Schönlein nephritis after renal transplantation. Report of ten patients and review of the literature. Transplantation 58:1179, 1994.

523. Pasternack A, Collin P, Mustonen J, et al: Glomerular IgA deposits in patients with celiac disease. Clin Nephrol 34:56, 1990.

524. Cassaneuva B, Rodriguez VV, Farinas MC, et al: Autologous mixed lymphocyte reaction and T-cell suppressor activity in patients with Henoch-Schönlein purpura and IgA nephropathy. Nephron 54:224, 1990.

525. Dosa S, Cairns SA, Mallick NP, et al: Relapsing Henoch-Schönlein syndrome with renal involvement in a patient with an IgA monoclonal gammopathy: A study of the result of immunosuppressant and cytotoxic therapy. Nephron 26:145, 1980.

526. Meadow SR, Scott DG: Berger disease: Henoch-Schönlein syndrome without the rash. J Pediatr 106:27, 1985.

527. O'Donoghue DJ, Darvill A, Ballardie FW: Mesangial cell autoantigens in immunoglobulin A nephropathy and Henoch-Schönlein purpura. J Clin Invest 88:1522, 1991.

528. O'Donoghue DJ, Jewkes F, Postlethwaite RJ, Ballardie FW: Autoimmunity to glomerular antigens in Henoch Schönlein nephritis. Clin Sci 83:281, 1992.

529. Montoliu J, Lens XM, Torra A, Revert L: Henoch-Schönlein purpura and IgA nephropathy in a father and son. Nephron 54:77, 1990.

530. Garty BZ, Danon YL, Nitzan M: Schönlein-Henoch purpura associated with hepatitis A infection. Am J Dis Child 139:632, 1985.

531. Maggiore G, Martini A, Grifeo S, et al: Hepatitis B infection and Henoch-Schönlein purpura. Am J Dis Child 138:681, 1984.

532. Eftychiou C, Samarkos M, Golfinopoulou S, et al: Henoch-Schönlein purpura associated with methicillin-resistant Staphylococcus aureus infection. Am J Med 119:85–86, 2006.

533. Patel U, Bradley JR, Hamilton DV: Henoch-Schönlein purpura after influenza vaccination. Br Med J Clin Res Educ 296:1800, 1988.

534. Ronkainen J, Nuutinen M, Koskimies O: The adult kidney 24 years after childhood Henoch-Schönlein purpura: A retrospective cohort study. Lancet 360:666–670, 2002.

535. Rauta V, Tonroth T, Gronhagen-Riska C: Henoch-Schönlein nephritis in adults—clinical features and outcomes in Finnish patients. Clin Nephrol 58:1–8, 2002.

536. Shrestha S, Sumingan N, Tan J, et al: Henoch Schönlein purpura with nephritis in adults: Adverse prognostic indicators in a UK population. Q J Med 99:253–265, 2006.

537. Tarshish P, Bernstein J, Edelman CM Jr: Henoch-Schönlein purpura nephritis: Course of disease and efficacy of cyclophosphamide. Pediatr Nephrol 19: 51–56, 2004.

538. Shrestha S, Sumingan N, Tan J, et al: Henoch Schönlein purpura with nephritis in adults: Adverse factors in a UK population. Q J Med 99:253–265, 2006.

539. Mollica F, Li Volti S, Garozzo R, Russo G: Effectiveness of early prednisone treatment in preventing the development of nephropathy in anaphylactoid purpura. Eur J Pediatr 151:40, 1992.

540. Niaudet P, Levy M, Broyer M, Habib R: Clinicopathologic correlations in severe forms of Henoch-Schönlein purpura nephritis based on repeat biopsies. Contrib Nephrol 40:250, 1984.

541. Rosenblum ND, Winter HS: Steroid effects on the course of abdominal pain in children with Henoch-Schönlein purpura. Pediatrics 79:1018, 1987.

542. Saulsbury FT: Corticosteroid therapy does not prevent nephritis in Henoch-Schönlein purpura. Pediatr Nephrol 7:69, 1993.

543. Niaudet P, Habib R: Methylprednisolone pulse therapy in the treatment of severe forms of Schönlein-Henoch purpura nephritis. Pediatr Nephrol 12:238, 1998.

544. Bergstein J, Leiser J, Andreoli SP: Response of crescentic Henoch-Schönlein purpura nephritis to corticosteroid and azathioprine therapy. Clin Nephrol 49:9, 1998.

545. Kauffman RK, Honwert DA: Plasmapheresis in rapidly progressive Henoch-Schönlein glomerulonephritis and the effect on circulating IgA immune complexes. Clin Nephrol 16:155, 1981.

546. Kunis CL, Kiss B, Williams G, et al: Treatment of rapidly progressive glomerulonephritis with IV pulse cyclophosphamide. Clin Nephrol 37:1, 1992.

547. Coppo R, Basolo B, Roccatello D, Piccoli G: Plasma exchange in primary IgA nephropathy and Henoch-Schönlein syndrome nephritis. Plasma Ther 6:705, 1985.

548. Rostoker G, Desvaux-Belghiti D, Pilatte Y, et al: High dose immunoglobulin therapy for severe IgA nephropathy and Henoch-Schönlein purpura. Ann Intern Med 120:476, 1994.

549. Iijima K, Ito-Kariya S, Nakamura H, Yoshikawa N: Multiple combined therapy for severe Henoch-Schoenlein nephritis in children. Pediatr Nephrol 12:244, 1998.

550. Shin JI, Park JM, Kim JH, et al: Factors affecting histological regression of crescentic Henoch-Schönlein nephritis in children. Pedatr Nephrol 20:2005.

551. Bachman V, Biava C, Amend W, et al: The clinical course of IgA nephropathy and Henoch-Schönlein purpura following renal transplantation. Transplantation 42:511–515, 1986.

552. Hudson BG: The molecular basis of Goodpasture and Alport's syndromes: Beacon for the discovery of the collagen IV family. J Am Soc Nephrol 15:2514–2527, 2004.

553. Wang: J Am Soc Nephrol 2005.

554. Pusey C: Anti-glomerular basement membrane disease. Kidney Int 64:1535–1550, 2003.

555. Kluth DC, Rees AJ: Anti-glomerular basement membrane disease. J Am Soc Nephrol 10:2446, 1999.

556. Boyce NW, Holdsworth SR: Pulmonary manifestations of the clinical syndrome of acute glomerulonephritis and lung hemorrhage. Am J Kidney Dis 8:31, 1986.

557. Niles JL, Bottinger EP, Saurina GR, et al: The syndrome of lung hemorrhage and nephritis is usually an ANCA-associated condition. Arch Intern Med 156:440, 1996.

558. Markus HS, Clark JV: Pulmonary hemorrhage in Henoch-Schoenlein purpura. Thorax 44:525, 1989.

559. Esnault VL, Soleimani B, Keogan MT, et al: Association of IgM with IgG ANCA in patients presenting with pulmonary hemorrhage. Kidney Int 41:1304, 1992.

560. Kelly PT, Haponick EF: Goodpasture's syndrome: Molecular and clinical advances. Medicine 73:171, 1994.

561. Salama AD, Dougan T, Levy JB, et al: Goodpasture's disease in the absence of circulating anti-GBM antibodies as detected by standard techniques. Am J Kidney Dis 39:1162, 2002.

562. Lamriben L, Kourilsky O, Mougenot B, et al: Goodpasture's syndrome with asymptomatic renal involvement. Disappearance of anti-GBM antibodies and deposits after treatment. Nephrol Dial Transplant 8:1267–1269, 1993.

563. Knoll G, Rabin E, Burns BF: Anti-GBM mediated glomerulonephritis with normal pulmonary and renal function. A case report and review of the literature. Am J Nephrol 13:494, 1993.

564. Kalluri R, Wilson CB, Weber K, et al: Identification of the alpha-3 chain of type IV collagen as the common autoantigen in antibasement membrane disease and Goodpasture syndrome. J Am Soc Nephrol 6:1178, 1995.

565. Levy JB, Coulthart A, Pusey CD: Mapping B cell epitopes in Goodpasture's disease. J Am Soc Nephrol 8:1698, 1997.

566. Merkel F, Kalluri R, Marx M, et al: Autoreactive T-cells in Goodpasture's syndrome recognize the N-terminal NC I domain on a 3 type IV collagen. Kidney Int 49:1127, 1996.

567. Leinonen A, Netzer KO, Bontaud A, et al: Goodpasture antigen: Expression of the full-length alpha 3 (IV) chain of collagen IV and localization of epitopes exclusively to the noncollagenous domain. Kidney Int 55:926, 1999.

568. Rutgers A, Meyers KE, Canziani G, et al: High affinity of anti-GBM antibodies from Goodpasture and transplanted Alport patients to alpha3 (IV) NC I collagen. Kidney Int 58:115, 2000.

569. Weber M, Lohse A, Manus M, et al: IgG subclass distribution of autoantibodies to GBM in Goodpasture's syndrome compared to other autoantibodies. Nephron 49:54, 1988.

570. Salama AD, Chandhry AN, Molthaus KA, et al: Regulation of CD25+ lymphocytes of autoantigen-specific T-cell responses in Goodpasture's. Kidney Int 64:1685, 2003.

571. Pusey CD. Anti-glomerular basement membrane–antiGBM-disease. Kidney Int 64:1535–1550, 2003.

572. Stevenson A, Yaqoob M, Mason H, et al: Biochemical markers of basement membrane disturbances and occupational exposure to hydrocarbons and mixed solvents. Q J Med 88:23, 1995.

573. Herody M, Bobrie G, Gouarin C, et al: Anti-GBM disease: Predictive value of clinical, histological, and serological data. Clin Nephrol 40:249, 1993.

574. Donaghy K, Rees AJ: Cigarette smoking and lung hemorrhage in glomerulonephritis caused by antibodies to glomerular basement membrane. Lancet 2:1390, 1983.

575. Bombassei GJ, Kaplan AA: The association between hydrocarbon exposure and antiglomerular basement membrane antibody-mediated disease (Goodpasture's syndrome). Am J Ind Med 21:141, 1992.

576. Bernis P, Hamels J, Quoidbach A, et al: Remission of Goodpasture's syndrome after withdrawal of an unusual toxin. Clin Nephrol 23:312, 1985.

577. Ravnskov V: Possible mechanisms of hydrocarbon associated glomerulonephritis. Clin Nephrol 23:294, 1985.

578. Lechleitner P, DeFregger M, Lhotta K, et al: Goodpasture's syndrome. Unusual presentation after exposure to hard metal dust. Chest 103:956, 1993.

579. Siebels M, Andrassy K, Ritz E: Provocation of pulmonary hemorrhage in Goodpasture's syndrome by chlorine gas. Nephrol Dial Transplant 8:189, 1993.

580. Phelp RG, Rees AJ: The HLA complex in Goodpasture's Disease: A model for analyzing susceptibility to autoimmunity. Kidney Int 86:1638, 1999.

581. Burns AP, Fisher M, Li P, et al: Molecular analysis of HLA class II genes in Goodpasture's disease. Q J Med 88:93, 1995.

582. Petterson E, Tonroth T, Miettinen A: Simultaneous anti-GBM and membranous glomerulonephritis: Case report and literature review. Clin Immunol Immunopathol 31:171, 1984.

583. Kalluri R, Weber M, Netzer KO, et al: COL4A5 gene deletion and production of posttransplant anti-a3(IV) collagen alloantibodies in Alport syndrome. Kidney Int 45:721, 1994.

584. Yankowitz J, Kuller JA, Thomas RL: Pregnancy complicated by Goodpasture's syndrome. Obstet Gynecol 79:806, 1992.

585. Holdsworth S, Boyce N, Thomson N, Atkins R: The clinical spectrum of glomerulonephritis and lung hemorrhage (Goodpasture's syndrome). Q J Med 55:75, 1985.

586. Jayne DR, Marshall PD, Jones SJ, Lockwood CM: Autoantibodies to GBM and neutrophil cytoplasm in rapidly progressive glomerulonephritis. Kidney Int 37:965, 1990.

587. Ang C, Savige J, Dawborn J, et al: Antiglomerular basement membrane antibody mediated disease with normal renal function. Nephrol Dial Transplant 13:935, 1998.

588. Merkel R, Pullin O, Marx M, et al: Course and prognosis of anti-basement membrane antibody-mediated disease: Report of 35 cases. Nephrol Dial Transplant 9:372, 1994.

589. O'Donoghue DJ, Short CD, Brenchley PE, et al: Sequential development of systemic vasculitis with anti-neutrophil cytoplasmic antibodies complicating anti-glomerular basement membrane disease. Clin Nephrol 32:251, 1989.

590. Weber NE, Andrassy K, Pullig O, et al: Antineutrophil-cytoplasmic antibodies and antiglomerular basement membrane antibodies in Goodpasture's syndrome and in Wegener's granulomatosis. J Am Soc Nephrol 2:1227, 1992.

591. Kalluri R, Meyers KM, Mogyorosi H, et al: Goodpasture's Syndrome involving overlap with Wegener's granulomatosis and anti-GBM disease. J Am Soc Nephrol 8:1795, 1997.

592. Hellmark T, Niles JL, Collins AB, et al: A comparison of anti-GBM antibodies in sera with and without ANCA. J Am Soc Nephrol 8:376, 1997.

593. Levy JB, Hammad T, Coulhart A, et al: Clinical features and outcomes of patients with both ANCA and anti-GBM antibodies. Kidney Int 66:1535–1540, 2004.

594. Boucher A, Droz D, Adafer E, Noel L-H: Relationship between the integrity of Bowman's capsule and the composition of cellular crescents in human crescentic glomerulonephritis. Lab Invest 56:526, 1987.

595. Bonsib SM: Glomerular basement membrane discontinuities. Am J Pathol 119:357, 1985.

596. Segelmark M, Butkowski R, Wieslander J: Antigen restrictions and IgG subclasses among anti-GBM antibodies. Nephrol Dial Transplant 5:991, 1990.

597. Savage JA, Dowling J, Kincaid-Smith P: Superimposed glomerular immune complexes in anti-GBM disease. Am J Kidney Dis 14:145, 1989.

598. Jindal KK: Management of idiopathic crescentic and diffuse proliferative glomerulonephritis: Evidence-based recommendations. Kidney Int Suppl 70:533, 1999.

599. Mehler PS, Brunvand MW, Hutt AP, Anderson RJ: Chronic recurrent Goodpasture's syndrome. Am J Med 82:833, 1987.

600. Wu MJ, Moorthy AV, Beirne GJ: Relapse in anti-GBM mediated crescentic glomerulonephritis. Clin Nephrol 13:9, 1980.

601. Maxwell AD, Nelson WE, Hill CM: Reversal of renal failure in nephritis associated with antibodies to glomerular basement membrane. BMJ 297:333, 1988.

602. Cui Z, Zhao MH, Xin G, Wang HY: Characteristics and prognosis of Chinese patients with anti-glomerular basement membrane disease. Nephron Clin Pract 99:c49–55, 2005.

603. Levy JB, Turner AN, Rees AJ, Pusey CD: Long term outcome of anti-GBM antibody disease treated with plasma exchange and immunosuppression. Ann Intern Med 134:1033–1042, 2001.

604. Querin S, Schurch W, Beaulieu R: Cyclosporin in Goodpasture's syndrome. Nephron 60:355, 1992.

605. Reynolds J, Tam FW, Chandraker A, et al: CD28-B7 blockade prevents the development of experimental autoimmune glomerulonephritis. J Clin Invest 105:643, 2000.

606. Laczika K, Knapp S, Derflerk K, et al: Immunoadsorption in Goodpasture's syndrome. Am J Kidney Dis 36:392, 2000.

607. Bergrem H, Jervell J, Brodwall EK, et al: Goodpasture's syndrome: A report of seven patients including long-term follow-up of three who received a kidney transplant. Am J Med 68:54, 1980.

608. Kotanko P, Pusey CD, Levy JB: Recurrent glomerulonephritis following renal transplantation. Transplantation 63:2045, 1997.

609. Denton MD, Singh AK: Recurrent and de novo glomerulonephritis in the renal allograft. Seminars Nephrol 20:164, 2000.

610. Netzer KO, Merkel F, Weber M: Goodpasture's Syndrome and ESRD—to transplant or not to transplant? Nephrol Dial Transpl 13:1346, 1998.

611. Floege J: Recurrent glomerulonephritis following renal transplantation: An update. Nephrol Dial Transplant 18:1260–1263, 2003.

612. Knoll G, Cockfield S, Blydt-Hansen T, et al: Canadian Society of Transplantation consensus guidelines on eligibility for kidney transplantation. Can Med Assoc J 173:1181–1190, 2005.

613. Conlon PJ Jr, Walshe JJ, Daly C, et al: Anti-GBM disease: The long-term pulmonary outcome. Am J Kidney Dis 23:794, 1994.

614. Ramos-Casals M, Tzioufas AG, Font J: Primary Sjogren's syndrome: New clinical and therapeutic concepts. Ann Rheum Dis 64:347–354, 2005.

615. Goulos A, Masouridi S, Tzionfas AG, et al: Clinically significant and biopsy documented renal involvement in primary Sjögren syndrome. Medicine 79:241, 2000.

616. Bossini N, Savoldi S, Franceschin F, et al: Clinical and morphological features of kidney involvement in primary Sjogren's syndrome. Nephrol Dial Transplant 16:2328, 2001.

617. Pertovaarc M, Korpels M, Pasternack A: Factors predictive of renal involvement in patients with primary Sjogren's syndrome. Clin Nephrol 56:10, 2001.

618. Goules A, Masouridi S, Tzioufas AG, et al: Clinically significant and biopsy-documented renal involvement in primary Sjögren syndrome. Medicine 79: 241–249, 2000.

619. Bossini N, Savoldi S, Franceschini F, et al: Clinical and morphological features of kidney involvement in primary Sjogren's syndrome. Nephrol Dial Transplant 16:2328–2336, 2001.

620. Wrong OM, Feest TG, MacIlver AG: Immune related potassium losing interstitial nephritis: A comparison with distal RTA. Q J Med 86:513, 1993.

621. Rayaburg J, Koch AE: Renal insufficiency from interstitial nephritis in primary Sjogren's syndrome. J Rheumatol 17:1714, 1990.

622. Font J, Cervera R, Lopez-Soto A, et al: Mixed membranous and proliferative glomerulonephritis in primary Sjogren's syndrome. Br J Rheumatol 28:548, 1989.

623. Khan MA, Akhtar M, Taher SM: Membranoproliferative glomerulonephritis in a patient with primary Sjogren's syndrome. Am J Nephrol 8:235, 1988.

624. Palcoux JB, Janin-Mercier A, Campagne D, et al: Sjogren's syndrome and lupus erythematosus nephritis. Arch Dis Child 59:175, 1984.

625. Pokorny G, Sonkodi S, Ivanyi B, et al: Renal involvement in patients with primary Sjogren's syndrome. Scand J Rheumatol 18:231, 1989.

626. Schlesinger I, Carlson TS, Nelson D: Type III membranoproliferative glomerulonephritis in primary Sjogren's syndrome. Conn Med J 53:629, 1989.

627. Cortez MS, Sturgil BC, Bolton WK: Membranoproliferative glomerulonephritis with primary Sjogren's syndrome. Am J Kidney Dis 25:632, 1995.

628. Molina R, Provost TT, Alexander EL: Two types of inflammatory vascular disease in Sjogren's syndrome. Arthritis Rheum 28:1251, 1985.

629. Rosenberg AM, Dyck RF, George GH: Intravenous pulse methylprednisolone for the treatment of a child with Sjogren's nephropathy. J Rheumatol 17;391, 1990.

630. Baughman RP, Lowere EE, du Bois RM: Sarcoidosis. Lancet 361:1111–1118, 2003.

631. Gobel U, Kettritz R, Schneider W, Luft FC: The Protean face of renal sarcoidosis. J Am Soc Nephrol 12:616–623, 2001.

632. Brause M, Magnusson K, Degenhardt S, et al: Renal involvement in sarcoidosis—a report of 6 cases. Clin Nephrol 57:142–148, 2002.

633. Mundlein E, Greter T, Ritz E: Grave's disease, sarcoidosis in a patient with minimal change disease. Nephrol Dial Transplant 11:860–862, 1996.

634. Parry RG, Falk C: Minimal Change Disease in association with sarcoidosis. Nephrol Dial Transplant 12:2159–2160, 1997.

635. Veronese FS, Henn L, Faccin C, et al: Pulmonary sarcoidosis and focal segmental glomerulosclerosis: Case report and renal transplant follow up. Nephrol Dial Transplant 13:493–495, 1998.

636. Jones B, Fowler J: Membranous nephropathy associated with sarcoidosis. Response prednisolone. Nephron 52:101, 1989.

637. Toda T, Kimoto S, Nishio Y, et al: Sarcoidosis with membranous nephropathy and granulomatous nephritis. Intern Med 38:882–886, 1999.

638. Dimitriades C, Shetty AK, Vehaskari M, et al: Membranous nephropathy associated with childhood sarcoid. Pediatr Nephrol 13:444–447, 1999.

639. Paydas S, Abayli B, Kocabas A, et al: Membranoproliferative glomerulonephritis associated pulmonary sarcoidosis. Nephrol Dial Transplant 13:228–229, 1998.

640. Taylor JE, Ansell ID: Steroid sensitive nephrotic syndrome and renal impairment in a patient with sarcoidosis. Nephrol Dial Transplant 11:355–356, 1996.

641. Nishiki M, Murakami Y, Yamane Y, Kato Y: Steroid sensitive nephrotic syndrome, sarcoidosis, and thyroiditis. Nephrol Dial Transplant 14:2008–2010, 1999.

642. van Uum SH, Coorman MP, Assman WJ, Wetzels JF: A 58 year old man with sarcoidosis complicated by focal crescentic glomerulonephritis. Nephrol Dial Transplant 12:2703, 1997.

643. Auinger M, Irsigler K, Breiteneder S, Ulrich W: Normocalcemic hepatorenal sarcoidosis with crescentic glomerulonephritis. Nephrol Dial Transplant 12:1474, 1997.

644. Schwimmer JA, Joseph RE, Appel GB: Amyloid, fibrillary, and the glomerular deposition diseases in therapy. In Wilcox CS, Brady HR (eds): Nephrology and Hypertension. Philadelphia, Saunders, 2003, pp. 253–261.

645. Gertz MA, Lacy MQ, Dispenzier A: Immunoglobulin light chain amyloidosis and the kidney. Kidney Int 61:1–9, 2002.

646. Falk R, Skinner M: The systemic amyloidosis: an overview. Adv Intern Med 45:107–131, 2000.

647. Gillmore JD, Hawkins PN: Drug insight: Emerging therapies for amyloidosis. Nature Clinical Practice Nephrology 2:263–270, 2006.

648. Benson MD, Uemichi T: Transthyretin amyloidosis. J Exp Clin Invest 3:44–51, 1996.

649. Valleix S, Drunat S, Philit J-B, et al: Hereditary renal amyloidosis caused by a new variant lysozyme WG4R in a French family. Kidney Int 61:907–912, 2002.

650. Hawkins PM: Hereditary systemic amyloidosis with renal involvement. J Nephrol 16:443, 2003.

651. Gallo G, Wisiewski T, Choi-Miura NH, et al: Potential role of apolipoprotein E in fibrillogenesis. Am J Pathol 145:526, 1994.

652. Husby G, Stenstad T, Magnus JH, et al: Interaction between circulating amyloid fibril protein precursors and extracellular matrix components in the pathogenesis of systemic amyloidosis. Clin Immunol Immunopathol 70:2, 1994.

653. Cunnane G: Amyloid proteins in the pathogenesis of AA amyloidosis. Lancet 358:4–5, 2001.

654. Hurle M, Helms LR, Li L, et al: A role for destabilizing amino acid replacements in light-chain amyloidosis. Proc Natl Acad Sci U S A 91:5446, 1994.

655. Alim MA, Yamaki S, Hussein MS, et al: Structural relationship of kappa-type light chains with AL amyloid. Clin Exp Immunol 118:334–348, 1999.

656. Gilmore JD, Lovat LB, Persey MR, et al: Amyloid load and clinical outcome in AA amyloidosis in relation to circulating concentration of serum amyloid A protein. Lancet 358: 24–29, 2001.

657. Solomon A, Weiss DT, Kattine AA: Nephrotoxic potential of Bence Jones proteins. N Engl J Med 324:1845, 1991.

658. Myat EA, Westholm FA, Weiss, DT, et al: Pathogenic potential of human monoclonal immunoglobulin fight chains: Relationship between in vitro aggregation and in vivo organ deposition. Proc Natl Acad Sci U S A 91:3034, 1994.

659. Pepys MB: Amyloidosis. Ann Rev Med 57:223, 2006.

660. Pepys MB, Herbert J, Hutchinson WL, et al: Targeted pharmacological depletion of serum amyloid P component for treatment of human amyloidosis. Nature 417:254–259, 2002.

661. Harris AA, Wilkman AS, Hogan SL, et al: Amyloidosis and light chain deposition disease in renal biopsy specimen. Pathology, laboratory data, demographics and frequency (abstract). J Am Soc Nephrol 8:537A, 1997.

662. Kyle RA, Gertz MA: Primary systemic amyloidosis: Clinical and laboratory features in 474 cases. Semin Hematol 32:45–59, 1995.

663. Kunis CL, Teng SN: Treatment of glomerulonephritis in the elderly. Semin Nephrol 20:256–264, 2000.

664. Kyle RA, Linos A, Beard CM, et al: Incidence and natural history of primary systemic amyloidosis in Olmstead County Minnesota. Blood 79:1817–1822, 1992.

665. Gillmore J, Lovat L, Pearsey M, et al: Amyloid load and clinical outcome in AA amyloidosis in relation to circulating concentrations of serum amyloid A protein. Lancet 358:24–29, 2001.

666. Gertz M, Kyle RA: Secondary systemic amyloidosis. Response and survival in 64 patients. Medicine(Baltimore) 70:246, 1991.

667. Said R, Hamzeh Y, Said S, et al: Spectrum of renal involvement in familial Mediterranean fever. Kidney Int 41: 414, 1992.

668. Agha I, Mahoney R, Beardslee M, et al: Systemic amyloidosis associated with pleomorphic sarcoma of the spleen and remission of nephrotic syndrome after removal. Am J Kidney Dis 40:411–415, 2002.

669. Kunis CL, Ward H, Appel GB: Renal diseases associated with drugs of abuse. In Porter G, Verpooten GA, Debroe M, Bennett WM (eds): Nephrotoxicity in Clinical Medicine: Renal Injury from Drugs and Chemicals. Dordrecht, The Netherlands, Kluwer Academic Press, 2003.

670. Westermark P: Diagnosing amyloidosis. Scand J Rheumatol 24:327–329, 1995.

671. Masouye I: Diagnostic screening of systemic amyloidosis by abdominal fat pad aspiration. An analysis of 100 cases. Am J Dermatopathol 19:41–45, 1997.

672. Delgado WA, Arana-Chavez VE: Amyloid deposits in labial, salivary glands identified by electron microscopy. J Oral Pathol Med 26:51–52, 1997.

673. Gertz MA, Li CY, Shirahama T, Kyle RA: Utility of subcutaneous fat aspiration for the diagnosis of systemic amyloidosis (immunoglobulin light chain). Arch Int Med 148:929–933, 1988.

674. Hawkins PN, Lavender JP, Pepys MB: Evaluation of systemic amyloid by scintography with I^{123}-labeled serum amyloid P component. N Engl J Med 323:508–513, 1990.

675. Drayson M, Tang LX, Drew R, et al: Serum free light chain measurements for identifying and monitoring patients with nonsecretory multiple myeloma. Blood 97: 2900–2902, 2001.

676. Lachman HJ, Gallimore R, Gillmore JD, et al: Outcome in systemic AL amyloidosis in relationship to changing serum concentrations of circulating free immunoglobulin light chains following chemotherapy. Br J Hematol 122:78–84, 2003.

677. Lachmann HJ, Booth DR, Booth SE, et al: Misdiagnosis or hereditary amyloidosis as primary AL amyloidosis. N Engl J Med 346:1786–1781, 2002.

678. Piken MM, Pelton K, Frangione B, Gallo G: Primary amyloidosis A: Immunohistochemical and biochemical characterization. Am J Pathol 129:536, 1987.

679. Herrera G: Renal disease associated with plasma cell dyscrasias, amyloidosis, Waldenström's macroglobulinemia, and cryoglobulinemia. In Jennette JC, Olson JL, Schwartz MM (eds): Heptinstall's Pathology of the Kidney. 6th ed. pp. 853–910, 2006.

680. Picken MM: The changing concepts of amyloid. Arch Pathol Lab Med 25:38–46, 2001.

681. Markowitz GS: Dysproteinemias and the kidney. Adv Anatomic Pathol 11:49–63, 2004.

682. Getz MA, Kyle RA, Grieppe PR: Response rates and survival in primary systemic amyloidosis. Blood. 77:257, 1991.

683. Mathew V, Olsson LJ, Gertz MA, Hayes DL: Symptomatic conduction system disease in cardiac amyloidosis. Am J Cardiol 80:1491–1492, 1997.

684. Dubrey SW, Cha K, Anderson J, et al: The clinical features of immunoglobulin light-chain (AL) amyloidosis with heart involvement. Q J Med 91:141–157, 1998.

685. Kyle RA, Wagoner RD, Holley KE: Primary systemic amyloidosis, resolution of the nephrotic syndrome with melphalan and prednisone. Arch Intern Med 142:1445, 1982.

686. Gertz MA, Kyle RA, Greipp PR: Response rates and survival in primary systemic amyloidosis. Blood 77(2):257, 1991.

687. Cohen AS, Rubinow A, Anderson JJ, et al: Survival of patients with primary amyloidosis. Colchicine treated cases from 1976 to 1983 compared with cases seen in previous years (1961–1973). Am J Med 82:1182, 1987.

688. Skinner M, Anderson J, Simms R, et al: Treatment of 100 patients with primary amyloidosis: A randomized trial of melphalan, prednisone, and colchicine versus colchicine only. Am J Med 100:290, 1996.

689. Kyle RA, Gertz MA, Greipp PR, et al: A trial of those three regimens for primary amyloidosis: Colchicine alone, melphalan and prednisone, and melphalan, prednisone and colchicine. N Engl J Med 336:1202–1207, 1997.

690. Gertz MA, Lacy MQ, Lust JA, et al: Prospective randomized trial of melphalan and prednisone versus vincristine, carmustine, melphalan, cyclophosphamide, and prednisone in the treatment of primary amyloidosis. J Clin Oncol 17:262–267, 1999.

691. Wang WJ, Lin CD, Wong CK, et al: Response of systemic amyloidosis to dimethyl sulfoxide. J Am Acad Dermatol 15:402, 1986.

692. Merlini G, Anesi E, Garini P, et al: Treatment of AL amyloidosis with 4′-iodo-4′deoxydoxyrubicin: An update. Blood 93:1112–1113, 1999.

693. Gertz MA, Kyle RA: Phase II trial of alpha-tocopherol (vitamin E) in the treatment of primary systemic amyloidosis. Am J Hematol 34:55, 1990.

694. Gertz MA, Kyle RA: Phase II trial of recombinant interferon alfa-2 in the treatment of primary systemic amyloidosis. Am J Hematol 44:125, 1993.

695. Gertz MA, Lacy MQ, Lust JA, et al: Phase II trial of high dose dexamethasone for untreated patients with primary systemic amyloidosis. Am J Hematol 61:115–119, 1999.

696. Van Buren M, Hene RJ, Verdonck LF, et al: Clinical remission after syngeneic bone marrow transplantation in a patient with AL amyloidosis. Ann Intern Med 122:508, 1995.

697. Comenzo RI, Vosburgh E, Falk RH, et al: Dose-intensive melphalan with blood stem-cell support for the treatment of AL (amyloid light-chain) amyloidosis: Survival and responses in 25 patients. Blood 91:3662–3670, 1998.

698. Gertz MA, Lacy MQ, Dispenzieri A: Myeloablative chemotherapy with stem cell rescue for the treatment of primary systemic amyloidosis: A status report. Bone Marrow Transplant 25:465–470, 2000.

699. Comenzo RL: Hematopoietic cell transplantation for primary systemic amyloidosis: What have we learned? Leuk Lymphoma 37:245–258, 2000.

700. Gertz MA, Lacy MQ, Gastineau DA, et al: Blood stem cell transplantation as therapy for primary systemic amyloidosis (AL). Bone Marrow Transplant 26:963–969, 2000.

701. Moreau P, Leblond V, Bourquelot P, et al: Prognostic factors for survival and response after high-dose therapy and autologous stem cell transplantation in systemic AL amyloidosis: A report on 21 patients. Br J Haematol 101:766–769, 1998.

702. Dember LM, Sanchorawala V, Seldin DC, et al: Effect of dose-intensive intravenous melphalan and autologous blood stem-cell transplantation on AL amyloidosis-associated renal disease. Ann Intern Med 134:746–753, 2001.

703. Leung N, Dispenzieri A, Fervenza F, et al: Renal response after high dose melphalan and stem cell transplantation is a favorable marker in patients with primary systemic amyloid. Am J Kidney Dis 46:270–277, 2005.

704. Casserly LF, Fadia A, Sanchorawala V, et al: High dose intravenous melphalan with autologous stem cell transplantation in AL amyloid associated end stage renal disease. Kidney Int 63:11051–1057, 2003.

705. Blowey DL, Balfe JW, Gupta I, et al: Midodrine efficacy and pharmacokinetics in a patient with recurrent intradialytic hypotension. Am J Kidney Dis 28:132, 1996.

706. Berglund K, Thysell H, Keller C: Results principles and pitfalls in the management of renal AA amyloidosis; a 10–21 year follow-up of 16 patients with rheumatic disease treated with alkylating cytostatics. J Rheumatol 20:2051, 1993.

707. Chevrel G, Jenvrin C, McGregoe B, et al: Renal type AA amyloidosis associated with rheumatoid arthritis: A cohort study showing improved survival on treatment with pulse cyclophosphamide. Rheumatology (Oxford) 40:821–825, 2001.

708. Livneh A, Zemer D, Langevitz P, et al: Colchicine in the treatment of AA amyloidosis of familial mediterranean fever. Arthritis Rheum 37(12):1804, 1994.

709. Neugarten J, Gallo G, Buxbaum J, et al: Amyloidosis in subcutaneous heroin abusers. Am J Med 81:635–641, 1986.

710. Dember LM, Hawkins PN, Hazenberg BPC, et al: Eprodisate for the treatment of renal disease in AA amyloid. N Engl J Med 356:2349, 2007.

711. Gertz MA, Kyle RA, O'Fallon WM: Dialysis support of patients with primary systemic amyloidosis, a study of 211 patients. Arch Intern Med 152: 2245, 1992.

712. Moroni G, Banfi G, Montoli A, et al: Chronic dialysis in patients with systemic amyloidosis: The experience in Northern Italy. Clin Nephrol 38(2):81, 1992.

713. Pasternack A, Ahonen J, Kuhlback B: Renal transplantation in 45 patients with amyloidosis. Transplantation 42(6):598, 1986.

714. Sobh K, Refaie A, Moustafa F, et al: Study of live donor kidney transplantation outcome in recipients with renal amyloidosis. Nephrol Dial Transplant 9:704, 1994.

715. Tan AU Jr, Cohen AK, Levine BS: Renal amyloidosis in a drug abuser. J Am Soc Nephrol 5:1653, 1995.

716. Rosenstock J, Valeri A, Appel GB, et al: Fibrillary glomerulonephritis. Defining the disease spectrum. Kidney Int 63:1450–1462, 2003.

717. Brady HR: Fibrillary glomerulopathy. Kidney Int 53:1421–1429, 1998.

718. Schwartz MM, Korbet SM, Lewis EJ: Immunotactoid Glomerulopathy. J Am Soc Nephrol 13:1390–1397, 2002.

719. Iskandar SS, Falk RJ, Jennette JC: Clinical and pathological features of fibrillary glomerulonephritis. Kidney Int 42:1401, 1992.

720. Fogo A, Nauman Q, Horn RG: Morphological and clinical features of fibrillary glomerulonephritis versus immunotactoid glomerulopathy. Am J Kidney Dis 22(3):367, 1993.

721. Rostagno A, Vidal R, Kumar A, et al: Fibrillary glomerulonephritis related to serum fibrillar immunoglobulin-fibronectin complexes. Am J Kidney Dis 28:676, 1996.

722. Strom EH, Banfi G, Krapf R, et al: Glomerulopathy associated with predominant fibronectin deposits: A newly recognized hereditary disease. Kidney Int 48:163, 1995.

723. Assmann KJ, Koene RA, Wetzels JF: Familial glomerulonephritis characterized by massive deposits of fibronectin. Am J Kidney Dis 25:781, 1995.

724. Fujigaki Y, Kimura M, Yamashita F, et al: An isolated case with predominant glomerular fibronectin deposition associated with fibril formation. Nephrol Dial Transplant 12:2717, 1997.

725. Alpers CE: Immunotactoid (microtubular) glomerulopathy: An entity distinct from fibrillary glomerulonephritis. Am J Kidney Dis 19:185, 1992.

726. Masson RG, Rennke HG, Gottlieb MN: Pulmonary hemorrhage in a patient with fibrillary glomerulonephritis. N Engl J Med 326:36, 1992.

727. Wallner K, Prischl, FC, Hobling W, et al: Immunotactoid glomerulopathy with extra-renal deposits in the bone, and chronic cholestatic liver disease. Nephrol Dial Transplant 11:1619, 1996.

728. Samaniego M, Nadasdy GM, Laszik Z, et al: Outcome of renal transplantation in fibrillary glomerulonephritis. Clin Nephrol 55:159–166, 2001.

729. Korbet S, Rosenberg BF, Schwartz NM, Lewis EJ: Course of renal transplantation in immunotactoid glomerulopathy. Am J Med 89:91, 1990.

730. Pronovost PK, Brady HR, Gunning ME, et al: Clinical features, predictors of disease progression and results of renal transplantation in fibrillary/immunotactoid glomerulopathy. Nephrol Dial Transplant 11:837, 1996.

731. Lin J, Markowitz GS, Valeri AM, et al: Renal monoclonal immunoglobulin deposition disease: The disease spectrum. Am J Soc Nephrol 12:1482–1492, 2001.

732. Buxbaum J, Gallo G: Nonamyloidotic monoclonal immunoglobulin deposition disease. Light-chain, heavy-chain, and light- and heavy-chain deposition diseases. Hematol Oncol Clin North Am 13:1235–1248, 1999.

733. Sanders PW, Herrera GA: Monoclonal immunoglobulin light chain-related renal disease. Semin Nephrol 13:324–341, 1993.

734. Alpers CE: Glomerulopathies of dysproteinurias, abnormal immunoglobulin deposition, and lymphoproliferative disorders. Curr Opin Nephrol Hypertens 3:349–355, 1994.

735. Pozzi C, D'Amico M, Fogazzi GB, et al: Light chain deposition disease with renal involvement: clinical characteristics and prognostic factors. Am J Kidney Dis 42:1154–1163, 2003.

736. Preud'Homme JL, Aucouterier P, Touchard G, et al: Monoclonal immunoglobulin deposition disease (Randall type). Relationship with structural abnormalities of immunoglobulin chains. Kidney Int 46:965–972, 1994.

737. Buxbaum JN, Chuba JV, Hellman GC, et al: Monoclonal immunoglobulin deposition disease: Light chain and light and heavy chain deposition diseases and their relation to light chain amyloidosis. Ann Intern Med 12:455–464, 1990.

738. Ronco PM, Mougenot B, Touchard G, et al: Renal involvement in hematologic disorders: Monoclonal immunoglobulins and nephropathy. Curr Opin Nephrol Hypertens 4:130–138, 1995.

739. Zhu L, Herrera GA, Murphy-Ullrich JE, et al: Pathogenesis of glomerulosclerosis in LCDD: Role of TGF-beta. Am J Pathol 147:375–385, 1995.

740. Heilman RI, Velosa JA, Holley KE, et al: Long-term follow-up and response to chemotherapy in patients with LCDD. Am J Kidney Dis 20:34–41, 1992.

741. Sinniah R, Cohen AH: Glomerular capillary aneurysms in light chain nephropathy: An ultrastructural proposal of morphogenesis. Am J Pathol 118:298, 1985.

742. Noel LH, Droz D, Ganeval D, Grunfeld JP: Renal granular monoclonal light chain deposits: Morphological aspects in 11 cases. Clin Nephrol 21:263, 1984.

743. Lin JJ, Miller F, Waltzer W, et al: Recurrence of immunoglobulin A-kappa crystalline deposition disease after kidney transplantation. Am J Kidney Dis 25:75–78, 1995.

744. Gerlag PG, Koene RA, Berden HM: Renal transplantation in light chain nephropathy: A case report and review of the literature. Clin Nephrol 25:101–104, 1986.

745. Alpers CE, Marchioro TRL, Johnson RJ: Monoglobulin immunoglobulin deposition disease in a renal allograft: Probable recurrent disease in a patient without myeloma. Am J Kidney Dis 13:418–423, 1989.

746. Leung N, Lager DJ, Gertz MA, et al: Long-term outcome of renal transplantation in light-chain deposition disease. Am J Kidney Dis 43:147–153, 2004.

747. Aucouturier P, Khamlichi AA, Touchard G, et al: Brief report: Heavy chain deposition disease. N Engl J Med 329:1389, 1993.

748. Kambham N, Markowitz GS, Appel GB, et al: Heavy chain deposition disease: The disease spectrum. Am J Kidney Dis 33:954–962, 1999.

749. Cheng IKP, Ho SKN, Chan DMT, et al: Crescenteric nodular glomerulosclerosis secondary to truncated immunoglobulin a heavy chain deposition. Am J Kidney Dis 28:283–288, 1996.

750. Khamlichi AA, Aucouturier P, Preud'homme JL, Cogne M: Structure of abnormal heavy chains in human heavy-chain deposition disease. Eur J Biochem 229:54–60, 1995.

751. Preud'homme JL, Aucouturier P, Touchard G, et al: Monoclonal immunoglobulin deposition disease: A review of immunoglobulin chain alteratons. Int J Immunopharmacol 16:425–431, 1994.

752. Pirani CL, Silva F, D'Agati V, et al: Renal lesions in plasma cell dyscrasias: Ultrastructural observation. Am J Kidney Dis 10:208–221, 1987.

753. Nasr SH, Markowitz GS, Stokes B, et al: Proliferative glomerulonephritis with monoclonal IgG deposits: A distinct entity mimicking immune-complex glomerulonephritis. Kidney Int 65:85–96, 2004.

754. Nasr SH, Preddie DC, Markowitz GS, et al: Multiple myeloma, nephritic syndrome and crystalloid inclusions in podocytes. Kidney Int 69:616–620, 2006.

755. Tomioka M, Ueki K, Nakahashi H, et al: Widespread crystalline inclusions affecting podocytes, tubular cells, and interstitial histiocytes in the myeloma kidney. Clin Nephrol 62:229–233, 2004.

756. Markowitz G, Appel GB, Fine P, et al: Collapsing FSGS following treatment with high dose pamidronate. J Am Soc Nephrol 12:1164–1172, 2001.

757. Kyle RA, Therneau TM, Rajkumar SV, et al: Prevalence of monoclonal gammopathy of undetermined significance. N Engl J Med 354:1362–1369, 2006.

758. Kebler R, Kithier K, McDonald FD, Cadnapaphorncha P: Rapidly progressive glomerulonephritis and monoclonal gammopathy. Am J Med 78:133, 1985.

759. Meyrier A, Simon EC, Migan F, et al: Rapidly progressive glomerulonephritis and monoclonal gammopathies. Nephron 38:156, 1984.

760. Owen RG, Treon SP, Al-Katib A, et al: Clinicopathological definition of Waldenström's macroglobulinemia: Consensus panel recommendations for the Second International Workshop on Waldenström's Macroglobulinemia. Semin Oncol 30:110–115, 2003.

761. Groves FD, Travis LB, Devesa SS, et al: Waldenström's macroglobulinemia: Incidence patterns in the US 1988–1994. Cancer 82:1078, 1998.

762. Garcia Suz R, Mantoto S, Torrequebrada A, et al: Waldenström's macroglobulinemia: Presenting features and outcomes in a series with 217 cases. Br J Haematol 115:575, 2001.

763. Dimopoulos MA, Panayiotidis P, Moupoulos LA, et al: Waldenström's ulinemia: Clinical features, complications and management. J Clin Oncol 18:214, 2000.

764. Veltman GA, Van Veen S, Kluin-Nelemaus JC, et al: Renal disease in Waldenström's macroglobulinemia. Nephrol Dial Transplant 12:1256, 1997.

765. Tsuji M, Ochiai S, Taka T, et al: Non-amyloidogenic nephrotic syndrome in Waldenström's macroglobulinemia. Nephron 54:176, 1990.

766. Gallo GR, Feiner HE, Buxbaum JN: The kidney in lymphoplasmacytic disorders. Pathol Ann 17:291, 1982.

767. Treon SP, Gertz MA, Dimopouols M, et al: Update on treatment recommendations from the Third International Workshop on Waldenström's macroglobulinemia. Blood 107:3442–3446, 2006.

768. Annibali O, Petrucci MT, Martini V, et al: Treatment of 72 newly diagnosed Waldenström macroglobulinemia cases with oral melphalan, cyclophosphamide, and prednisone: Results and cost analysis. Cancer 103:582–587, 2005.

769. Gertz MA, Rue M, Blood E, et al: Multicenter phase 2 trial of Rituximab for Waldenström macroglobulinemia. Leuk Lymphoma 45:2047–2055, 2004.

770. D'Amico G, Colasanti G, Ferrario F, Sinico RA: Renal involvement in essential mixed cryoglobulinemia. Kidney Int 35:1004, 1989.

771. Tarantino A, de Vecchi A, Montaguino G, et al: Renal disease in essential mixed cryoglobulinemia: Long-term follow-up of 44 patients. Q J Med 50:1, 1981.

772. D'Amico G, Colasanti G, Ferrario F, et al: Renal involvement in essential mixed cryoglobulinemia: A peculiar type of immune complex mediated disease. Adv Nephrol 17:219, 1988.

773. Zago-Novaretti M, Khuri F, Miller KB, et al: Waldenstrom's macroglobulinemia with an IgM protein that is both a cold agglutinin and a cryoglobulin and has a suppressor effect of progenitor cell growth. Transfusion 34:910, 1994.

774. Frankel AK, Singer DR, Winearls CG, et al: Type 11 essential mixed cryoglobulinemia: Presentation, treatment and outcome in 13 patients. Q J Med 82:101, 1992.

775. Agnello V, Chung RT, Kaplan LM: A Role for Hepatitis C virus infection in type II cryoglobulinemia. N Engl J Med 327:1490–1495, 1992.

776. Cordonnier D, Vialfel P, Renversy J, et al: Renal disease in 18 patients with mixed type II IgM-IgG cryoglobulinemia: Monoclonal lymphoid infiltration and membranoproliferative glomerulonephritis (14 cases). Adv Nephrol 12:177, 1983.

777. Appel GB: Immune-Complex glomerulonephritis—Deposits plus interest. N Engl J Med 328:505–506, 1993.

778. Marti G, Galli K, Invemizzi F, et al: Cryoglobulinemias: A multi-centre study of the early clinical and laboratory manifestations of primary and secondary disease. Q J Med 88:115, 1995.

779. Galli M, Monti G, Invernizzi F, et al: Hepatitis B virus-related markers in secondary and essential mixed cryoglobulinemias: A multicenter study of 596 cases. Ann Ital Med Intern 7:209–214, 1992.

780. Agnello V: Case records of the Massachusetts General Hospital. N Engl J Med 323:1756, 1990.

781. Misiani R, Bellavita P, Fenili D, et al: Hepatitis C virus infection in patients with essential mixed cryoglobulinemia. Ann Intern Med 117:573, 1992.

782. D'Amico G, Ferrario F: Cryoglobulinemic glomerulonephritis: A MPGN induced by hepatitis C virus. Am J Kidney Dis 25:361–369, 1995.

783. Sansonno D, Gesualdo L, Manno C, et al: Hepatitis C virus-related proteins in kidney tissue from hepatitis C virus-infected patients with cryoglobulinemic membranoproliferative glomerulonephritis. Hepatology 25:1237, 1997.

784. Bichard P, Ounanian A, Girard M, et al: High prevalence of HCV RNA in the supernatant and the cryoprecipitate of patients with essential and secondary type II mixed cryoglobulinemia. J Hepatol 21:58–63, 1994.

785. Johnson RJ, Willson R, Yamabe K, et al: Renal manifestations of hepatitis C virus infection. Kidney Int 46:1255, 1994.

786. Fornasieri A, Armelloni S, Bernasconi P, et al: High binding of IgMk rheumatoid factor from type II cryoglobulins to cellular fibronectin. Am J Kidney Dis 27: 476–483, 1996.

787. Sinico RA, Winearls CG, Sabadini E, et al: Identification of glomerular immune complexes in cryoglobulinemia glomerulonephritis. Kidney Int 34:109, 1988.

788. Madore F, Lazarus JK, Brady HR: Therapeutic plasma exchange in renal diseases. J Am Soc Nephrol 7:367, 1996.

789. Tarantino A, Carnpise K, Banfi G, et al: Long-term predictors of survival in essential mixed cryoglobulinemic glomerulonephritis. Kidney Int 47:618, 1995.

790. Misiani R, Bellavita P, Baio P, et al: Successful treatment of HCV associated cryoglobulinemic glomerulonephritis with a combination of interferon and ribavirin. Nephrol Dial Transplant 14:1558, 1999.

791. Poynard T, Bedossa P, Chevalher K, et al: A comparison of three interferon alfa-2b regimens for the long-term treatment of chronic non-A, non-B hepatitis. N Engl J Med 332:1457, 1995.

792. Zaja F, De Vita S, Mazzaro C, et al: Efficacy and safety of rituximab in type II mixed cryoglobulinemia. Blood 101:3827–3834, 2003.

793. Tarantino A, Moroni G, Banfi G, et al: Renal replacement therapy in cryoglobulinemic nephritis. Nephrol Dial Transplant 9:1426, 1994.

794. Hiesse C, Bastuji-Garin G, Moulin B, et al: Recurrent essential mixed cryoglobulinemia in renal allografts. Report of two cases and review of the literature. Am J Nephrol 9:150, 1989.

795. Zuckerman E, Kerren D, Slobodin G, et al: Treatment of refractory, symptomatic, Hepatitis C virus related mixed cryoglobulinemia with ribavirin and interferon alpha. J Rheumatol 27:2172, 2000.

796. Guthrie LB: Idiopathic or congenital hereditary and family hematuria. Lancet 1:1243–1246, 1902.

797. Alport AC: Hereditary familial congenital hemorrhagic nephritis. Br Med J 1:504–506, 1927.

798. Kendall G, Hertz AF: Hereditary familial congenital hemorrhagic nephritis. Guys Hosp Rep 66:137, 1912.

799. Crawfurd MD, Toghill PJ: Alport's syndrome of hereditary chronic nephritis and deafness. Q J Med 37:563–576, 1968.

800. Gubler M-C, Antignac C, Deschenes G: Genetic, clinical and morphologic heterogeneity in Alport's syndrome. Adv Nephrol 22:15–35, 1993.

801. Chazan JA, Zacks J, Cohen JJ, Garella S: Hereditary nephritis: Clinical spectrum and mode of inheritance in five new kindreds. Am J Med 50:764–771, 1971.

802. Chugh KS, Sakhuja V, Agarwal A: Hereditary nephritis (Alport's syndrome)-clinical profile and inheritance in 28 kindreds. Nephrol Dial Transplant 8:690–695, 1993.

803. Gubler M, Levy M, Broyer M, et al: Alport's syndrome: A report of 58 cases and a review of the literature. Am J Med 70:493–505, 1981.

804. Jais JP, Knebelmann B, Giatras I, et al: X-linked Alport syndrome: Natural history in 195 families and genotype-phenotype correlations in males. J Am Soc Nephrol 11:649–657, 2000.

805. Excerpts from United States Renal Data System 1997 Annual Report. Incidence and prevalence of ESRD. Am J Kidney Dis 30:S40-S53, 1997.

806. O'Neill WM, Atkin CL, Bloomer HA: Hereditary nephritis: A re-examination of its clinical and genetic features. Ann Intern Med 88:176–182, 1978.

807. Knepshield JH, Roberts PL, Davis CJ, Moser RH: Hereditary chronic nephritis complicated by nephrotic syndrome. Arch Intern Med 122:156–158, 1968.

808. Grunfeld J-P, Noel LH, Hafex S, Droz D: Renal prognosis in women with hereditary nephritis. Clin Nephrol 23:267–271, 1985.

809. Jais JP, Knebelmann B, Giatras I, et al: X-linked Alport syndrome: Natural history and genotype-phenotype correlations in girls and women belonging to 195 families: A "European community Alport syndrome concerted action" study. J Am Soc Nephrol 14:2603–2610, 2003.

810. Gleeson MJ: Alport's syndrome: Audiological manifestations and implications. J Laryngol Otol 98:449–465, 1984.

811. Yoshikawa N, White RHR, Cameron AH: Familial hematuria: Clinicopathological correlations. Clin Nephrol 17:172–182, 1982.

812. Grunfeld J-P, Bois EP, Hinglais N: Progressive and non-progressive hereditary nephritis. Kidney Int 4:216–228, 1973.

813. Chance JK, Stanley JA: Alport's syndrome: Case report and review of ocular manifestations. Ann Ophthalmol 9:1527–1530, 1977.

814. Thompson SM, Deady JP, Willshaw HR, White RHR: Ocular signs in Alport's syndrome. Eye 1:146–153, 1987.

815. Epstein CJ, Sahud MA, Piel CF, et al: Hereditary macrothombocytopenia, nephritis and deafness. Am J Med 52:299–310, 1972.

816. Parsa KP, Lee DBN, Zamboni L, Glassock RJ: Hereditary nephritis, deafness and abnormal thrombopoiesis: Study of a new kindred. Am J Med 60:665–671, 1976.

817. Antignac C, Zhou J, Sanak M, et al: Alport syndrome and diffuse leiomyomatosis: Deletions in the 5' end of the COL4A5 collagen gene. Kidney Int 42:1178–1183, 1992.

818. Goyer RA, Reynolds J Jr, Burke J, Burkholder P: Hereditary renal disease with neurosensory hearing loss, prolinuria and ichthyosis. Am J Med Sci 256:166–179, 1968.

819. Ghiggeri GM, Caridi G, Magrini U, et al: Genetics, clinical and pathological features of glomerulonephritis associated with mutations of nonmuscle myosin IIA (Fechtner syndrome). Am J Kidney Dis 41:95–104, 2003.

820. Kashtan CE, Michael AF, Sibley RK, Vernier RL: Hereditary nephritis: Alport syndrome and thin glomerular basement membrane disease. In Craig Tisher C, Brenner BM (eds): Renal Pathology: With Clinical and Functional Correlation. 2nd ed. Philadelphia, JB Lippincott, 1994, pp 1239–1266.

821. Rumpelt HJ: Hereditary nephropathy (Alport's syndrome): Spectrum and development of glomerular lesions. In Rosen S (ed): Pathology of Glomerular Disease. New York, Churchill Livingstone, 1983, p. 225.

822. Gaboardi R, Edefonti A, Imbasciati E, et al: Alport's syndrome (progressive hereditary nephritis). Clin Nephrol 2:143–156, 1974.

823. Langer KH, Theones W: Alport syndrom: Licht und electronen-mikroskopische nierenefund im fruhstadium. Verh D Dtsch Ges Pathol 55:497–502, 1971.

824. Krickstein HI, Gloor FJ, Balogh K: Renal pathology in hereditary nephritis with nerve deafness. Arch Pathol 82:506–517, 1966.

825. Habib R, Gubler M-C, Hinglais N, et al: Alport's syndrome: Experience at Hopital Necker. Kidney Int 21:S20-S28, 1982.

826. Hinglais N, Grunfeld J-P, Bois LE: Characteristic ultrastructural lesion of the glomerular basement membrane in progressive hereditary nephritis (Alport's syndrome). Lab Invest 27:473–487, 1972.

827. Nasr SH, Markowitz GS, Goldstein CS, et al: Hereditary nephritis mimicking immune complex-mediated glomerulonephritis. Hum Pathol 37:547–554, 2006.

828. Olson FL, Anand SK, Landing BH, et al: Diagnosis of hereditary nephritis by failure of glomeruli to bind anti-glomerular basement membrane antibodies. J Pediatr 96:697–699, 1980.

829. Savage COS, Kershaw M, Pusey CD, et al: Use of a monoclonal antibody in differential diagnosis of children with hematuria and hereditary nephritis. Lancet 1:1459–1461, 1986.

830. Grunfeld JP: Contemporary diagnostic approach in Alport's syndrome. Renal Failure 22:759–763, 2000.

831. Kashtan CE, Michael AF: Alport syndrome. Kidney Int 2750:1445–1463, 1996.

832. Reznick VM, Griswold WR, Vazquez MD, et al: Glomerulonephritis with absent glomerular basement membrane antigens. Am J Nephrol 4:296–298, 1984.

833. Rumpelt HJ: Hereditary nephropathy (Alport's syndrome): Correlation of clinical data with glomerular basement membrane alterations. Clin Nephrol 13:203–207, 1980.

834. Hill GS, Jenis EH, Goodloe SG: The nonspecificity of the ultrastructural alterations in hereditary nephritis. Lab Invest 31:516–532, 1974.

835. Tryggvason K, Zhou J, Hostikka SL, Shows TB: Molecular genetics of Alport syndrome. Kidney Int 43:38–44, 1993.

836. Hasstedt SJ, Atkin CL: X-linked inheritance of Alport syndrome: Family P revisited. Am J Hum Gen 35:1241–1251, 1983.

837. Shaw RF, Kallen RJ: Population genetics of Alport's syndrome: Hypothesis of abnormal segregation and the necessary existence of mutation. Nephron 16:427–432, 1976.

838. Barker DF, Hostikka SL, Zhou J: Identification of mutations in the COL4A5 collagen gene in Alport syndrome. Science 248:1224–1227, 1990.

839. Kleppel MM, Kashtan C, Santi PA: Distribution of familial nephritis antigen in normal tissue and renal basement membranes of patients with homozygous and heterozygous Alport familial nephritis: Relationships of familial nephritis and Goodpasture antigens to novel collagen chains and type IV collagen. Lab Invest 61:278–289, 1989.

840. Hostikka SL, Eddy RL, Byers MG: Identification of a distinct type IV collagen α chain with restricted kidney distribution and assignment of its gene to the locus of X-chromosome-linked Alport syndrome. Proc Natl Acad Sci U S A 87:1606–1610, 1990.

841. Knebelman B, Antignac C, Gubler M-C, Grunfeld J-P: Molecular genetics of Alport's syndrome: The clinical consequences. Nephrol Dial Transplant 8:677–679, 1993.

842. Netzer KO, Renders L, Zhou J: Deletions of the COL4A5 gene in patients with Alport syndrome. Kidney Int 42:1336–1344, 1992.

843. Kashtan C, Kim Y: Distribution of the α1 and α2 chains of collagen IV and of collagens V and VI in Alport syndrome. Kidney Int 42:115–126, 1992.

844. Kalluri R, Weber M, Netzer K: COL4A5 gene deletion and production of posttransplant anti-α3(IV) collagen alloantibodies in Alport syndrome. Kidney Int 45:721–726, 1994.

845. Van den Heuvel LPWJ, Savage COS, Wong M: The glomerular basement membrane defect in Alport-type hereditary nephritis: Absence of cationic antigenic components. Nephrol Dial Transplant 4:770–775, 1989.

846. Nakanishi K, Yolhikawa N, Iijima K, Nakamura H: Expression of type IV collagen alpha-3 and alpha-4 chain mRNA in X-linked Alport syndrome. J Am Soc Nephrol 7:938–945, 1996.

847. Kashtan CE, Michael AF: Alport syndrome: From bedside to genome to bedside. Am J Kidney Dis 22:627–640, 1993.

848. Seri M, Pecci A, Di Bari F, et al: MYH9-related disease—May-Hegglin anomaly, Sebastian syndrome, Fechtner syndrome, and Epstein syndrome are not distinct entities but represent a variable expression of a single illness. Medicine 82:203–215, 2003.

849. Tishler PV, Rosner B: The genetics of the Alport syndrome. Birth Defects 10: 93–99, 1979.

850. Hasstedt SJ, Atkin CL, San Juan AC: Genetic heterogeneity among kindreds with Alport syndrome. Am J Hum Genet 38:940–953, 1986.

851. Cohen EP, Lemann J Jr: In hereditary nephritis, angiotensin converting enzyme inhibition decreases proteinuria and may slow the rate of progression. Am J Kidney Dis 27:199–203, 1996.

852. Callis L, Vila A, Carrera M, Nieto J: Long-term effects of cyclosporine A in Alport's syndrome. Kidney Int 55:1051–1056, 1999.

853. Byrne MC, Budisavljevic MN, Fan Z, et al: Renal transplant in patients with Alport's syndrome. Am J Kidney Dis 39:769–775, 2002.

854. Goldman M, Depierreux M, De Pauw L, et al: Failure of two subsequent renal grafts by anti-GBM glomerulonephritis in Alport's syndrome: Case report and review of literature. Transplant Int 3:82–85, 1990.

855. Hudson BG, Kalluri R, Gunwar S, et al: The pathogenesis of Alport syndrome involves type IV collagen molecules containing the α3(IV) chain: Evidence from anti-GBM nephritis after renal transplantation. Kidney Int 42:179–187, 1992.

856. Ding J, Zhou J, Tryggvason K, Kashtan CE: COL4A5 deletions in three patients with Alport syndrome and posttransplant antiglomerular basement membrane nephritis. J Am Soc Nephrol 5:161–168, 1994.

857. Cosio FG, Falkenhain ME, Sedmak DD: Association of thin glomerular basement membrane with other glomerulopathies. Kidney Int 46:471–474, 1994.

858. Perry GJ, George CRP, Field MJ, et al: Thin-membrane nephropathy: A common cause of glomerular haematuria. Med J Aust 151:638–642, 1989.

859. Lang S, Stevenson B, Risdon RA: Thin basement membrane nephropathy as a cause for recurrent haematuria in childhood. Histopathology 16:331–337, 1990.

860. Schroder CH, Bontemps CM, Assman KJM, et al: Renal biopsy and family studies in 65 children with isolated hematuria. Acta Pediatr Scand 79:630–636, 1990.

861. McConville JM, West CD, McAdams AJ: Familial and nonfamilial benign hematuria. J Pediatr 69:207–214, 1966.

862. Pardo V, Berian MG, Levi DF, Strauss J: Benign primary hematuria: Clinicopathologic study of 65 patients. Am J Med 67:817–822, 1979.

863. Dische FE, Anderson VER, Keane SJ, et al: Incidence of thin membrane nephropathy: Morphometric investigation o a population sample. J Clin Pathol 43:457–460, 1990.

864. Vogler C, McAdams AJ, Homan SM: Glomerular basement membrane and lamina densa in infants and children: An ultrastructural evaluation. Pediatr Pathol 7:527–534, 1987.

865. Steffes MW, Barbosa J, Basgen JM, et al: Quantitative glomerular morphology of the normal human kidney. Lab Invest 49:82–86, 1983.

866. Tiebosch ATMG, Frederik PM, van Breda Vriesman PJC, et al: Thin-basement-membrane nephropathy in adults with persistent hematuria. N Engl J Med 320:14–18, 1989.

867. Basta-Jovanovic G, Venkataseshan VS, Gil J, et al: Morphometric analysis of glomerular basement membranes (GBM) in thin basement membrane disease (TBMD). Clin Nephrol 33:110–114, 1990.

868. Abe S, Amagasaki Y, Iyori S, et al: Thin basement membrane syndrome in adults. J Clin Pathol 40:318–322, 1987.

869. Badenas C, Praga M, Tazon B, et al: Mutations in the COL4A4 and COL4A3 genes cause familial benign hematuria. J Am Soc Nephrol 13:1248–1254, 2002.

870. Eisenstein B, Stark H, Goodman RM: Benign familial hematuria in children from Jewish communities. J Med Genet 16:369–372, 1979.

871. Aarons I, Smith PS, Davies RA, et al: Thin membrane nephropathy: A clinicopathological study. Clin Nephrol 32:151–158, 1989.

872. Lemmink HH, Nillesen WN, Mochizuki T, et al: Benign familial hematuria due to mutation of the type IV collagen alpha4 gene. J Clin Invest 98:1114–1118, 1996.

873. Longo I, Porcedda P, Mari F, et al: COL4A3/COL4A4 mutations: From familial hematuria to autosomal-dominant or recessive Alport syndrome. Kidney Int 61:1947–1956, 2002.

874. Kashtan CE: Familial hematurias: What we know and what we don't. Pediatr Nephrol 20:1027–1035, 2005.

875. Mino RA, Mino VH, Livingstone RG: Osseous dysplasia and dystrophy of the nail: Review of literature and report of a case. Am J Roentgenol 60:633–641, 1948.

876. Bongers EM, Gubler MC, Knoers NV: Nail-patella syndrome. Overview on clinical and molecular findings. Pediatr Nephrol 17:703–712, 2002.

877. Hoyer JR, Michael AF, Vernier RL, Sisson S: Renal disease in nail-patella syndrome: Clinical and morphologic studies. Kidney Int 2:231, 1972.

878. Bennett WM, Musgrave JE, Campbell RA, et al: The nephropathy of the nail-patella syndrome: Clinicopathologic analysis of 11 kindreds. Am J Med 54:304, 1973.

879. Morita T, Laughlin LO, Kawano K, et al: Nail-patella syndrome: Light and electron microscopic studies of the kidney. Arch Intern Med 131:217, 1973.

880. Renwick JH, Lawler SD: Genetical linkage between the ABO and the nail patella loci. Ann Hum Genet 19:312–331, 1955.

881. Schleutermann DA, Bias WB, Murdock JL, McCusick VA: Linkate of the loci for the nail patella syndrome and adenylate kinase. Am J Hum Genet 21:606–630, 1969.

882. Dreyer SD, Zhou G, Baldini A, et al: Mutations in LMX1B cause abnormal skeletal patterning and renal dysplasia in nail patella syndrome. Nat Genet 19:47–50, 1998.

883. Vollrath D, Jaramillo-Babb VL, Clough MV, et al: Loss-of-function mutations in the LIM-homeodomain gene, LMX1B, in nail-patella syndrome. Hum Mol Genet 7:1091–1098, 1998.

884. Chan PCK, Chan KW, Cheng KP, Chan MK: Living related renal transplantation in a patient with nail-patella syndrome. Nephron 50:164–166, 1988.

885. Fabry J: Ein beitrag zur kenntnis der purpura hemorrhagica nodularis (purpura papulosa hemorrhagica hebrae). Arch Derm 43:187, 1898.

886. Eng CM, Germain DP, Banikazemi M, et al: Fabry disease: Guidelines for the evaluation and management of multi-system involvement. Genet Med 8:539, 2006.

887. Obrador GT, Ojo A, Thadhani R: End-stage renal disease in patients with Fabry disease. J Am Soc Nephrol 13 Suppl 2;S144-S146, 2002.

888. Whybra C, Kampmann C, Willers I, et al: Anderson-Fabry disease: Clinical manifestations of disease in female heterozygotes. J Inherit Metab Dis 24:715–724, 2001.

889. Gubler MC, Lenoir G, Grunfeld J-P, et al: Early renal changes in homozygous and heterozygous patients with Fabry's disease. Kidney Int 13:223, 1978.

890. Thurberg BL, Rennke H, Colvin RB, et al: Globotriaosylceramide accumulation in the Fabry kidney is cleared from multiple cell types after enzyme replacement therapy. Kidney Int 62:1933–1946, 2002.

891. Farge D, Nadler S, Wolfe LS: Diagnostic value of kidney biopsy in heterozygous Fabry's disease. Arch Pathol Lab Med 109:85, 1985.

892. Ferraggiana T, Churg J, Grishman E, et al: Light- and electron-microscopic histochemistry of Fabry's disease. Am J Pathol 103: 247, 1981.

893. Kornreich R, Desnic RJ, Bishop DF: Nucleotide sequences of the human alpha-galactosidase A gene. Nucleic Acids Res 17:3301, 1989.

894. Bernstein HS, Bishop DF, Astrin KH, et al: Fabry disease: Six gene rearrangements and an exonic point mutation in the alpha galactosidase gene. J Clin Invest 83:1390, 1989.

895. Wherret JR, Hakomori S: Characterization of blood group B glycolipid, accumulating in the pancreas of a patient with Fabry's disease. J Biol Chem 218:3046, 1973.

896. Ohshima T, Murray GJ, Swaim WD, et al: Alpha-galactosidase A deficient mice: A model of Fabry disease. Proc Natl Acad Sci U S A 94:2540–2544, 1997.

897. Schiffmann R, Kopp JB, Austin HA, III, et al: Enzyme replacement therapy in Fabry disease: A randomized controlled trial. JAMA 285:2743–2749, 2001.

898. Eng CM, Guffon N, Wilcox WR, et al: Safety and efficacy of recombinant human alpha-galactosidase A—replacement therapy in Fabry's disease. N Engl J Med 345:9–16, 2001.

898a. Banikazemi M, Bultas J, Waldek S, et al: Agalsidase-Beta therapy for advanced Fabry disease. Ann Int Med 146:77, 2007.

898b. Germain DP, Waldek S, Banikazemi M, et al: Sustained long-term renal stabilization after 54 months of agalsidase? Therapy in patients with Fabry disease. J Am Soc Nephrol 18:1547, 2007.

899. Tsakiris D, Simpson HK, Jones EH, et al: Report on management of renal failure in Europe, XXVI, 1995. Rare diseases in renal replacement therapy in the ERA-EDTA registry. Nephrol Dial Transplant 11 (suppl 7): 4–20, 1996.

900. Helin I: Fabry's disease: A brief review in connection with a Scandinavian survey. Scand J Urol Nephrol 13:335, 1979.

901. Falk RJ, Jennette JC: Sickle cell nephropathy. Adv Nephrol 23:133–147, 1994.

902. Davis CJ Jr, Mostofi FK, Sesterhenn IA: Renal medullary carcinoma. The seventh sickle cell nephropathy. Am J Surg Pathol 19:1–11, 1995.

903. Falk RJ, Scheinman J, Phillips G, et al: Prevalence and pathologic features of sickle cell nephropathy and response to inhibition of angiotensin-converting enzyme. N Engl J Med 326:910–915, 1992.

904. Powars DR, Elliott-Mills DD, Chan L, et al: Chronic renal failure in sickle cell disease: Risk factors, clinical course, and mortality. Ann Intern Med 115:614–620, 1991.

905. Thomas AN, Pattison C, Serjeant GR: Causes of death in sickle-cell disease in Jamaica. Br Med J 285:633–635, 1982.

906. Pardo V, Strauss J, Kramer H, et al: Nephropathy associated with sickle cell anemia: An autologous immune complex nephritis. II. Clinicopathologic study of seven patients. Am J Med 59:650–659, 1975.

907. Ozawa T, Mass M, Guggenheim S, et al: Autologous immune complex nephritis associated with sickle cell trait: Diagnosis of the hemoglobinopathy after renal structural and immunological studies. Br Med J 1:369–371, 1976.

908. Effenbeing IB, Patchefsky A, Schwartz W, Weinstein AG: Pathology of the glomerulus in sickle cell anemia with and without nephrotic syndrome. Am J Pathol 77:357, 1974.

909. McCoy RC. Ultrastructural alterations in the kidney of patients with sickle cell disease and the nephrotic syndrome. Lab Invest 21: 85, 1969.

910. Walker BR, Alexander F, Birdsall TR, Warren RL: Glomerular lesions in sickle cell nephropathy. JAMA 215:437–440, 1971.

911. Bhatena DB, Sondheimer JH: The glomerulopathy of homozygous sickle hemoglobin (SS) disease: Morphology and pathogenesis. J Am Soc Nephrol 1:1241–1252, 1991.

912. Tejani A, Phadke K, Adamson O, et al: Renal lesions in sickle cell nephropathy in children. Nephron 39:352–355, 1985.

913. Nasr SH, Markowitz GS, Sentman RL, D'Agati VD: Sickle cell disease, nephrotic syndrome, and renal failure. Kidney Int 69:1276–1280, 2006.

914. Elfenbein IB, Patchefsky A, Schwartz W, Weinstein AG: Pathology of glomerulus in sickle-cell anemia with and without nephrotic syndrome. Am J Pathol 77:357–374, 1974.

915. Wesson DE: The initiation and progression of sickle cell nephropathy. Kidney Int 61:2277–2286, 2002.

916. Foucan L, Bourhis V, Bangou J, et al: A randomized trial of captopril for microalbuminuria in normotensive adults with sickle cell anemia. Am J Med 104:339–342, 1998.

917. Abbott KC, Hypolite IO, Agodoa LY: Sickle cell nephropathy at end-stage renal disease in the United States: Patient characteristics and survival. Clin Nephrol 58:9–15, 2002.

918. Ojo AO, Govaerts TC, Schmouder RL, et al: Renal transplantation in end-stage sickle cell nephropathy. Transplantation 67:291–295, 1999.

919. Chatterjee SN: National study on natural history of renal allografts in sickle cell disease or trait. Nephron 25:199–201, 1980.

920. Chatterjee SN: National study in natural history of renal allografts in sickle cell disease or trait: A second report. Transplant Proc 19(2 Suppl 2): 33–35, 1987.

921. Miner DJ, Jorkasky DK, Perloff LJ, et al: Recurrent sickle cell nephropathy in a transplanted kidney. Am J Kidney Dis 10:306–313, 1987.

922. Senior B, Gellis SS: The syndromes of total lipodystrophy and partial lipodystrophy. Pediatrics 33:593–612, 1964.

923. Misra A, Peethambaram A, Garg A: Clinical features and metabolic and autoimmune derangements in acquired partial lipodystrophy—Report of 35 cases and review of the literature. Medicine 83:18–34, 2004.

924. Habib R, Gubler MC, Loirat C, et al: Dense deposit disease: A variant of membranoproliferative glomerulonephritis. Kidney Int 7:204–215, 1975.

925. Vargas RA, Thomson KJ, Wilson D, et al: Mesangiocapillary glomerulonephritis with "dense deposits" in the basement membranes of the kidney. Clin Nephrol 5:73–82, 1976.

926. Eisinger AJ, Shortland JR, Moorhead PJ: Renal disease in partial lipodystrophy. Q J Med 41:343–354, 1972.

927. Peters DK, Williams DG, Charlesworth JA, et al: Mesangiocapillary nephritis, partial lipodystrophy and hypocomplementaemia. Lancet 2:535–538, 1973.

928. Javor ED, Moran SA, Young JR, et al: Proteinuric nephropathy in acquired and congenital generalized lipodystrophy: Baseline characteristics and course during recombinant leptin therapy. J Clin Endocrinol Metab 89:3199–3207, 2004.

929. Cahill J, Waldron S, O'Neill G, Duffy BS: Partial lipodystrophy and renal disease. Ir J Med Sci 152:451–453, 1983.

930. Sissons JGP, West RJ, Fallows J, et al: The complement abnormalities of lipodystrophy. N Engl J Med 294:461–465, 1976.

931. Chartier S, Buzzanga JB, Paquin F: Partial lipodystrophy associated with a type 3 form of membranoproliferative glomerulonephritis. J Am Acad Dermatol 16:201–205, 1987.

932. Jacob DK, Date A, Shastry JCM: Minimal change disease with partial lipodystrophy. Child Nephrol Urol 9:116–117, 1988.

933. Schmidt P, Kerjaschki D, Syre G, et al: Recurrence of intramembranous glomerulonephritis in 2 consecutive kidney transplantations. Schweiz Med Wochenschr 108:781–788, 1998.

934. Norum KR, Gjone E: Familial plasma lecithin-cholesterol acyltransferase defciency: Biochemical study of a new inborn error of metabolism. Scand J Clin Lab Invest 20: 231–243, 1967.

935. Gjone E, Norum KR: Familial serum cholesterol ester deficiency: Clinical study of a patient with a new syndrome. Acta Med Scand 183:107–112, 1968.

936. Albers JJ, Chan C-H, Adolphson J, et al: Familial lecithin-cholesterol acyltransferase deficiency in a Japanese family: Evidence for functionally defective enzyme in homozygotes and obligate heterozygotes. Hum Genet 62:82–85, 1982.

937. Vergani C, Cataparo AL, Roma P, Giuduci G: A new case of familial LCAT deficiency. Acta Med Scand 214:173–176, 1983.

938. Gjone E: Familial lecithin-cholesterol acyltransferase deficiency. Birth Defects 18:423–432, 1982.

939. Borysiewicz LK, Soutar AK, Evans DJ, et al: Renal failure in lecithin-cholesterol acyltransferase deficiency. Q J Med 51:411–426, 1982.

940. Gjone E: Familial lecithin-cholesterol acyl transferase deficiency: A new metabolic disease with renal involvement. Adv Nephrol 10:167–185, 1981.

941. Vrabec MP, Shapiro MB, Koller E, et al: Lecithin-cholesterol acyltransferase deficiency: Ultrastructural examination of sequential renal biopsies. Arch Ophthalmol 106:225–229, 1988.

942. Magil A, Chase W, Frohlich J: Unusual renal biopsy findings in a patient with lecithin-cholesterol acyltransferase deficiency. Hum Pathol 13:283–285, 1982.

943. McLean G, Wion K, Drayna D, et al: Human lecithin-cholesterol acyltransferase gene: Complete gene sequence and sites of expression. Nucleic Acids Res 14:9397–9406, 1986.

944. McLean J, Fielding C, Drayna D, et al: Cloning and expression of human lecithin-cholesterol acyltransferase cDNA. Proc Natl Acad Sci U S A 83:2335–2339, 1986.

945. Lynn EG, Siow YL, Frohlich J, Cheung GT: Lipoprotein-X stimulates monocyte chemoattractant protein-1 expression in mesangial cells via nuclear factor-kappa B. Kidney Int 60:520–532, 2001.

946. Murayama N, Asano Y, Kato K, et al: Effects of plasma infusion on plasma lipids, apoproteins and plasma enxyme activities in familial lecithin-cholesterol acyltransferase deficiency. Eur J Clin Invest 12:122–129, 1984.

947. Flatmark A, Hovig T, Mythre E, Gjone E: Renal transplantation in patients with familial lecithin-cholesterol acyltransferase deficiency. Transplant Proc 9:1665–1671, 1977.

948. Saito T, Sato H, Kudo K, et al: Lipoprotein glomerulopathy: Glomerular lipoprotein thrombi in a patient with hyperlipoproteinemia. Am J Kidney Dis 13:148–153, 1989.

949. Saito T, Oikawa S, Sato H, Sasaki J: Lipoprotein glomerulopathy: Renal lipidosis induced by novel apolipoprotein E variants. Nephron 83:193–201, 1999.

950. Karet FE, Lifton RP: Lipoprotein glomerulopathy: A new role for apolipoprotein E? J Am Soc Nephrol 8:840–842, 1997.

951. Oikawa S, Matsunaga A, Saito T, et al: Apolipoprotein E Sendai (arginine 145–> proline): A new variant associated with lipoprotein glomerulopathy. J Am Soc Nephrol 8:820–823, 1997.

952. Konishi K, Saruta T, Kuramochi S, et al: Association of a novel 3-amino acid deletion mutation of apolipoprotein E (Apo E Tokyo) with lipoprotein glomerulopathy. Nephron 83:214–218, 1999.

953. Matsunaga A, Sasaki J, Komatsu T, et al: A novel apolipoprotein E mutation, E2 (Arg25Cys), in lipoprotein glomerulopathy. Kidney Int 56:421–427, 1999.

954. Ando M, Sasaki J, Hua H, et al: A novel 18-amino acid deletion in apolipoprotein E associated with lipoprotein glomerulopathy. Kidney Int 56:1317–1323, 1999.

955. Ogawa T, Maruyama K, Hattori H, et al: A new variant of apolipoprotein E (apo E Maebashi) in lipoprotein glomerulopathy. Pediatr Nephrol 14:149–151, 2000.

956. Meyrier A, Dairou F, Callard P, Mougenot B. Lipoprotein glomerulopathy: First case in a white European. Nephrol Dial Transplant 10:546–549, 1995.

957. Ieiri N, Hotta O, Taguma Y: Resolution of typical lipoprotein glomerulopathy by intensive lipid-lowering therapy. Am J Kidney Dis 41:244–249, 2003.

958. Andrews PA: Lipoprotein glomerulopathy: a new cause of nephrotic syndrome after renal transplantation. Implications for renal transplantation. Nephrol Dial Transplant 14: 239–240, 1999.

959. Miyata T, Sugiyama S, Nangaku M, et al: Apolipoprotein E2/E5 variants in lipoprotein glomerulopathy recurred in transplanted kidney. J Am Soc Nephrol 10:1590–1595, 1999.

960. Neugarten J, Baldwin DS: Glomerulonephritis in bacterial endocarditis. Am J Med 77: 297–304, 1984.

961. Baehr G: Glomerular lesions of subacute bacterial endocarditis. J Exp Med 15: 330–347, 1912.

962. Libman E: Characterization of the various forms of endocarditis. JAMA 80:813–818, 1923.

963. Neugarten J, Gallo GR, Baldwin DS: Glomerulonephritis in bacterial endocarditis. Am J Kidney Dis 3(5):371–379, 1984.

964. Garvey GJ, Neu HC: Infective endocarditis-and evolving disease. A review of endocarditis at the Columbia-Presbyterian Medical Center. Medicine(Baltimore) 57:105–127, 1978.

965. Pelletier LL Jr, Petersdorf RG: Infective endocarditis: A review of 125 cases from the Univeriy of Washington Hospitals, 1962–1972. Medicine(Baltimore) 56:287–313, 1977.

966. O'Connor DT, Weisman MH, Fierer J: Activation of the alternate complement pathway in Staph. aureus infective endocarditis and its relationship to thrombocytopenia, coagulation abnormalities, and acute glomerulonephritis. Clin Exp Immunol 19:131–141, 1978.

967. Levine DP, Cushing RD, Jui J, Brown WJ: Community-acquired methicillin-resistant Staphylococcus aureus endocarditis in the Detroit Medical Center. Ann Intern Med 97:330–338, 1982.

968. Gutman RA, Striker GE, Gilliland BC, Cutler RE: The immune complex glomerulonephritis of bacterial endocarditis. Medicine(Baltimore) 51:1–25, 1972.

969. Daimon S, Mizuno Y, Fujii S, et al: Infective endocarditis-induced crescentic glomerulonephritis dramatically improved by plasmapheresis. Am J Kidney Dis 32:309–313, 1998.

970. Kodo K, Hida M, Omori S, et al: Vasculitis associated with septicemia: Case report and review of the literature. Pediatr Nephrol 16:1089–1092, 2001.

971. Kauffman RH, Thompson J, Valentjin RM, et al: The clinical implications and the pathogenetic significance of circulating immune complexes in infective endocarditis. Am J Med 71:17–25, 1981.

972. Cabane J, Godeau P, Herreman G, et al: Fate of circulating immune complexes in infective endocarditis. Am J Med 66:277–282, 1979.

973. Hurwitz D, Quismorio FP, Friou GJ: Cryoglobulinemia in patients with infectious endocarditis. Clin Exp Immunol 19:131–141, 1975.

974. Subra JJ, Michelet C, Laporte J, et al: The presence of cytoplasmic antineutrophil cytoplasmic antibodies (C-ANCA) in the course of subacute bacterial endocarditis with glomerular involvement, coincidence or association? Clin Nephrol 49:15–18, 1998.

975. Levy RL, Hong R: The immune nature of subacute bacterial endocarditis (SBE) nephritis. Am J Med 54:645–652, 1973.

976. Morel-Maroger L, Sraer JD, Herreman G, Godeau P: Kidney in subacute endocarditis: Pathological and immunofluorescent findings. Arch Pathol 94:205–213, 1972.

977. Boulton JM, Sissons JG, Evans DJ, Peters DK: Renal lesions in subacute bacterial endocarditis. Br Med J 2:11–14, 1974.

978. Yum M, Wheat LJ, Maxwell D, Edwards JL: Immunofluuorescent localization of Staphylococcus aureus antigen in acute bacterial endocarditis nephritis. Am J Clin Pathol 70:832–835, 1978.

979. Perez GO, Rothfield N, Williams RC Jr: Immune-complex nephritis in baterial endocarditis. Arch Intern Med 136:334–336, 1976.

980. McKinsey DS, McMurray TI, Flynn JM: Immunosuppressive therapy and plasmapheresis in rapidly progressive glomerulonephritis associated with glomerulonephritis. Rev Infect Dis 12:125–127, 1990.

981. Schoenbaum SC, Gardner P, Shillito J: Infections of cerebrospinal fluid shunts: Epidemiology, clinical manifestations, and therapy. J Infect Dis 131:543–552, 1975.

982. Balogun RA, Palmisano J, Kaplan AA, et al: Shunt nephritis from Propionibacterium acnes in a solitary kidney. Am J Kidney Dis 38:E18, 2001.

983. Rifkinson-Mann S, Rifkinson N, Leong T: Shunt nephritis. Case report. J Neurosurg 74:656–659, 1991.

984. Salcedo JR, Sorkin L: Nephritis associated with an infected peritoneovenous LeVeen shunt. J Pediatr Gastroenterol Nutr 4:842–844, 1985.

985. Black JA, Challacombe DN, Ockenden BG: Nephrotic syndrome associated with bacteraemia after shunt operations for hydrocephalus. Lancet 2:921–924, 1965.

986. Stickler GB, Shin MH, Burke EC, et al: Diffuse glomerulonephritis associated with infected ventriculoatrial shunt. N Engl J Med 279:1077–1082, 1968.

987. Kubota M, Sakata Y, Saeki N, et al: A case of shunt nephritis diagnosed 17 years after ventriculoatrial shunt implantation. Clin Neurol Neurosurg 103:245–246, 2001.

988. McKenzie SA, Hayden K: Two cases of "shunt nephritis". Pediatrics 54:806–808, 1974.

989. Vella J, Carmody M, Campbell E, et al: Glomerulonephritis after ventriculo-atrial shunt. Q J Med 88:911–918, 1995.

990. Schoeneman M, Bennett B, Greifer I: Shunt nephritis progressing to chronic renal failure. Am J Kidney Dis 2:375–377, 1982.

991. Iwata Y, Ohta S, Kawai K, et al: Shunt nephritis with positive titers for ANCA specific for proteinase 3. Am J Kidney Dis 43e11–16, 2004.

992. Danovitch GM, Nord EP, Barki Y, Krugliak L: Staphylococcal lung abscess and acute glomerulonephritis. Isr J Med Sci 15:840–843, 1979.

993. Beaufils M, Morel-Maroger L, Sraer JD, et al: Acute renal failure of glomerular origin during visceral abscesses. N Engl J Med 295:185–189, 1976.

994. Yuceoglu AM, Sagel I, Tresser G, et al: The glomerulopathy of congenital syphilis. A curable immune- deposit disease. JAMA 229:1085–1089, 1974.

995. Hunte W, al-Ghraoui F, Cohen RJ: Secondary syphilis and the nephrotic syndrome. J Am Soc Nephrol 3:1351–1355, 1993.

996. Sanchez-Bayle M, Ecija JL, Estepa R, et al: Incidence of glomerulonephritis in congenital syphilis. Clin Nephrol 20:27–31, 1983.

997. Hruby Z, Kuzniar J, Rabczynski J, et al: The variety of clinical and histopathologic presentations of glomerulonephritis associated with latent syphilis. Int Urol Nephrol 24:541–547, 1992.

998. Gamble CN, Reardan JB: Immunopathogenesis of syphilitic glomerulonephritis. Elution of antitreponemal antibody from glomerular immune-complex deposits. N Engl J Med 292:449–454, 1975.

999. Krane NK, Espenan P, Walker PD, et al: Renal disease and syphilis: A report of nephrotic syndrome with minimal change disease. Am J Kidney Dis 9:176–179, 1987.

1000. Walker PD, Deeves EC, Sahba G, et al: Rapidly progressive glomerulonephritis in a patient with syphilis. Identification of antitreponemal antibody and treponemal antigen in renal tissue. Am J Med 76:1106–1112, 1984.

1001. Ponce P, Ramos A, Ferreira ML, et al: Renal involvement in leprosy. Nephrol Dial Transplant 4: 81–84, 1989.

1002. Ahsan N, Wheeler DE, Palmer BF: Leprosy-associated renal disease: Case report and review of the literature. J Am Soc Nephrol 5:1546–1552, 1995.

1003. Matsuo E, Furuno Y, Komatsu A, et al: Hansen's disease and nephropathy as its sequence. Nihon Hansenbyo Gakkai Zasshi 66:103–108, 1997.

1004. Chugh KS, Damle PB, Kaur S, et al: Renal lesions in leprosy amongst north Indian patients. Postgrad Med J 59:707–711, 1983.

1005. Grover S, Bobhate SK, Chaubey BS: Renal abnormality in leprosy. Lepr India 55:286–291, 1983.

1006. Nakayama EE, Ura S, Fleury RN, Soares V: Renal lesions in leprosy: A retrospective study of 199 autopsies. Am J Kidney Dis 38:26–30, 2001.

1007. Nigam P, Pant KC, Mukhija RD, et al: Rapidly progressive (crescentric) glomerulonephritis in erythema nodosum leprosum: case report. Hansenol Int 11:1–6, 1986.

1008. Chugh KS, Sakhuja V: End stage renal disease in leprosy. Int J Artif Organs 9:9–10, 1986.

1009. Slater DN, Brown CB, Ward AM, et al: Immune complex crescentic glomerulonephritis associated with pulmonary aspergillosis. Histopathology 7:957–966, 1983.

1010. Pecchini F, Bufano G, Ghiringhelli P: Membranoproliferative glomerulonephritis secondary to tuberculosis. Clin Nephrol 47:63–64, 1997.

1011. O'Brien AA, Kelly P, Gaffney EF, et al: Immune complex glomerulonephritis secondary to tuberculosis. Ir J Med Sci 159:187, 1990.

1012. Rodriguez-Garcia JL, Fraile G, Mampaso F, Teruel JL: Pulmonary tuberculosis associated with membranous nephropathy. Nephron 55:218–219, 1990.

1013. Somvanshi PP, Patni PD, Khan MA: Renal involvement in chronic pulmonary tuberculosis. Ind J Med Sci 43:55–58, 1989.

1014. Campbell JH, Warwick G, Boulton-Jones M, et al: Rapidly progressive glomerulonephritis and nephrotic syndrome associated with Mycoplasma pneumoniae pneumonia. Nephrol Dial Transplant 6:518–520, 1991.

1015. Cochat P, Colon S, Bosshard S, et al: Membranoproliferative glomerulonephritis and Mycoplasma pneumoniae infection. Arch Fr Pediatr 42:29–31, 1985.

1016. Von Bonsdorff M, Ponka A, Tornroth T: Mycoplasmal pneumonia associated with mesangiocapillary glomerulonephritis type II (dense deposit disease). Acta Med Scand 216:427–429, 1984.

1017. Vitullo BB, O'Regan S, de Chadarevian JP, Kaplan BS: Mycoplasma pneumonia associated with acute glomerulonephritis. Nephron 21:284–288, 1978.

1018. Said MH, Layani MP, Colon S, et al: Mycoplasma pneumoniae-associated nephritis in children. Pediatr Nephrol 13:39–44, 1999.

1019. Kaehny WD, Ozawa T, Schwarz MI, et al: Acute nephritis and pulmonary alveolitis following pneumococcal pneumonia. Arch Intern Med 138:806–808, 1978.

1020. Schachter J, Pomeranz A, Berger I, Wolach B: Acute glomerulonephritis secondary to lobar pneumonia. Int J Pediatr Nephrol 8:211–214, 1987.

1021. Jose MD, Bannister KM, Clarkson AR, et al: Mesangiocapillary glomerulonephritis in a patient with Nocardia pneumonia. Nephrol Dial Transplant 13:2628–2629, 1998.

1022. Dunea G, Kark RM, Lannigan R, et al: Brucella nephritis. Ann Intern Med 70:783–790, 1969.

1023. Volpi A, Doregatti C, Tarelli T, et al: Acute glomerulonephritis in human brucellosis. Report of a case. Pathologica 77:519–524, 1985.

1024. Elzouki AY, Akthar M, Mirza K: Brucella endocarditis associated with glomerulonephritis and renal vasculitis. Pediatr Nephrol 10:748–751, 1996.

1025. Siegelmann N, Abraham AS, Rudensky B, Shemesh O: Brucellosis with nephrotic syndrome, nephritis and IgA nephropathy. Postgrad Med J 68:834–836, 1992.

1026. Nunan TO, Eykyn SJ, Jones NF: Brucellosis with mesangial IgA nephropathy: successful treatment with doxycycline and rifampicin. Br Med J (Clin Res Ed) 288:1802, 1984.

1027. Sitprija V, Pipatanagul V, Mertowidjojo K, et al: Pathogenesis of renal disease in leptospirosis: Clinical and experimental studies. Kidney Int 17:827–836, 1980.

1028. Lai KN, Aarons I, Woodroffe AJ, Clarkson AR: Renal lesions in leptospirosis. Aust N Z J Med 12: 276–279, 1982.

1029. Sitprija V, Pipatanagul V, Boonpucknavig V, Boonpucknavig S: Glomerulitis in typhoid fever. Ann Intern Med 81:210–213, 1974.

1030. Lambertucci JR, Godoy P, Neves J, et al: Glomerulonephritis in Salmonella-Schistosoma mansoni association. Am J Trop Med Hyg 38:97–102, 1988.

1031. Indraprasit S, Boonpucknavig V, Boonpucknavig S: IgA nephropathy associated with enteric fever. Nephron 40:219–222, 1985.

1032. Bhamarapravati N, Boonpucknavig S, Boonpucknavig V, Yaemboonruang C: Glomerular changes in acute plasmodium falciparum infection. An immunopathologic study. Arch Pathol 96:289–293, 1973.

1033. Eiam-Ong S, Sitprija V: Falciparum malaria and the kidney: A model of inflammation. Am J Kidney Dis 32:361–375, 1998.

1034. Hendrickse RG, Adeniyi A: Quartan malarial nephrotic syndrome in children. Kidney Int 16:64–74, 1979.

1035. Kibukamusoke JW, Hutt MS: Histological features of the nephrotic syndrome associated with quartan malaria. J Clin Pathol 20:117–123, 1967.

1036. Hendrickse RG, Adeniyi A, Edington GM, et al: Quartan malarial nephrotic syndrome. Collaborative clinicopathological study in Nigerian children. Lancet 1:1143–1149, 1972.

1037. Houba V: Immunopathology of nephropathies associated with malaria. Bull World Health Organ 52:199–207, 1975.

1038. Boonpucknavig V, Boonpucknavig S, Bhamarapravati N: Plasmodium berghei-infected mice. Focal glomerulonephritis in hyperimmune state. Arch Pathol Lab Med 103:567–572, 1979.

1039. Greenham R, Cameron AH: Schistosoma haematobium and the nephrotic syndrome. Trans R Soc Trop Med Hyg 74:609–613, 1980.

1040. Rocha H, Cruz T, Brito E, Susin M: Renal involvement in patients with hepatosplenic Schistosomiasis mansoni. Am J Trop Med Hyg 25:108–115, 1976.

1041. Barsoum RS: Schistosomiasis and the kidney. Semin Nephrol 23:34–41, 2003.

1042. Sobh MA, Moustafa FE, Sally SM, et al: Characterisation of kidney lesions in early schistosomal-specific nephropathy. Nephrol Dial Transplant 3:392–398, 1988.

1043. Martinelli R, Noblat AC, Brito E, Rocha H: Schistosoma mansoni-induced mesangiocapillary glomerulonephritis: Influence of therapy. Kidney Int 35:1227–1233, 1989.

1044. Barsoum RS. Schistosomal glomerulopathy: Selection factors. Nephrol Dial Transplant 2: 488–497, 1987.

1045. Dutra M, Martinelli R, de Carvalho EM, et al: Renal involvement in visceral leishmaniasis. Am J Kidney Dis 6:22–27, 1985.

1046. De Brito T, Hoshino-Shimizu S, Neto VA, et al: Glomerular involvement in human kala-azar. A light, immunofluorescent, and electron microscopic study based on kidney biopsies. Am J Trop Med Hyg 24:9–18, 1975.

1047. Basson W, Page ML, Myburgh DP: Human trypanosomiasis in Southern Africa. S Afr Med J 51:453–457, 1977.

1048. Greene BM, Taylor HR, Brown EJ, et al: Ocular and systemic complications of diethylcarbamazine therapy for onchocerciasis: Association with circulating immune complexes. J Infect Dis 147:890–897, 1983.

1049. Cruel T, Arborio M, Schill H, et al: Nephropathy and filariasis from Loa loa. Apropos of 1 case of adverse reaction to a dose of ivermectin. Bull Soc Pathol Exot 90:179–181, 1997.

1050. Pakasa NM, Nseka NM, Nyimi LM: Secondary collapsing glomerulopathy associated with Loa loa filariasis. Am J Kidney Dis 30:836–839, 1997.

1051. Yap HK, Woo KT, Yeo PP, et al: The nephrotic syndrome associated with filariasis. Ann Acad Med Singapore 11:60–63, 1982.

1052. Date A, Gunasekaran V, Kirubakaran MG, Shastry JC: Acute eosinophilic glomerulonephritis with Bancroftian filariasis. Postgrad Med J 55:905–907, 1979.

1053. Chugh KS, Sakhuja V: Glomerular diseases in the tropics editorial. Am J Nephrol 10:437–450, 1990.

1054. Sitprija V, Keoplung M, Boonpucknavig V, Boonpucknavig S: Renal involvement in human trichinosis. Arch Intern Med 140:544–546, 1980.

1055. Trandafirescu V, Georgescu L, Schwarzkopf A, et al: Trichinous nephropathy. Morphol Embryol (Bucur) 25:133–137, 1979.

1056. Covic A, Mititiuc I, Caruntu L, Goldsmith DJ: Reversible nephrotic syndrome due to mesangiocapillary glomerulonephritis secondary to hepatic hydatid disease. Nephrol Dial Transplant 11:2074–2076, 1996.

1057. Vialtel P, Chenais F, Desgeorges P, et al: Membranous nephropathy associated with hydatid disease. N Engl J Med 304:610–611, 1981.

1058. Oseroff A: Toxoplasmosis associated with nephrotic syndrome in an adult. South Med J 81:95–96, 1988.

1059. Wickbom B, Winberg J: Coincidence of congenital toxoplasmosis and acute nephritis with nephrotic syndrome. Acta Paediatr Scand 61:470–472, 1972.

1060. Ginsburg BE, Wasserman J, Huldt G, Bergstrand A: Case of glomerulonephritis associated with acute toxoplasmosis. Br Med J 3:664–665, 1974.

1061. Smith MC, Cooke JH, Zimmerman DM, et al: Asymptomatic glomerulonephritis after nonstreptococcal upper respiratory infections. Ann Intern Med 91:697–702, 1979.

1062. Blowey DL: Nephrotic syndrome associated with an Epstein-Barr virus infection. Pediatr Nephrol 10:507–508, 1996.

1063. Joh K, Kanetsuna Y, Ishikawa Y, et al: Epstein-Barr virus genome-positive tubulointerstitial nephritis associated with immune complex-mediated glomerulonephritis in chronic active EB virus infection. Virchows Arch 432:567–573, 1998.

1064. Gilboa N, Wong W, Largent JA, Urizar RE: Association of infectious mononucleosis with nephrotic syndrome. Arch Pathol Lab Med 105:259–262, 1981.

1065. Nadasdy T, Park CS, Peiper SC, et al: Epstein-Barr virus infection-associated renal disease: Diagnostic use of molecular hybridization technology in patients with negative serology. J Am Soc Nephrol 2:1734–1742, 1992.

1066. Iwama H, Horikoshi S, Shirato I, Tomino Y: Epstein-Barr virus detection in kidney biopsy specimens correlates with glomerular mesangial injury. Am J Kidney Dis 32:785–793, 1998.

1067. Gallo G, Neugarten J, Baldwin DS: Glomerulonephritis associated with systemic bacterial and viral infections. In Tisher CC, Brenner BM (eds): Renal Pathology: With Clinical and Functional Correlations, 2nd ed. Philadelphia, JB Lippincott, 1994, pp. 564–595.

1068. AIDS epidemic update. UNAIDS/WHO. 2002.

1069. D'Agati V, Appel GB: HIV infection and the kidney. J Am Soc Nephrol 8:138–152, 1997.

1070. D'Agati V, Appel GB: Renal pathology of human immunodeficiency virus infection. Semin Nephrol 18:406–421, 1998.

1071. Rao TK, Filippone EJ, Nicastri AD, et al: Associated focal and segmental glomerulosclerosis in the acquired immunodeficiency syndrome. N Engl J Med 310:669–673, 1984.

1072. Gardenswartz MH, Lerner CW, Seligson GR, et al: Renal disease in patients with AIDS: a clinicopathologic study. Clin Nephrol 21:197–204, 1984.

1073. D'Agati V, Suh JI, Carbone L, et al: Pathology of HIV-associated nephropathy: A detailed morphologic and comparative study. Kidney Int 35:1358–1370, 1989.

1074. Rao TK, Friedman EA, Nicastri AD: The types of renal disease in the acquired immunodeficiency syndrome. N Engl J Med 316:1062–1068, 1987.

1075. Carbone L, D'Agati V, Cheng JT, Appel GB: Course and prognosis of human immunodeficiency virus-associated nephropathy. Am J Med 87:389–395, 1989.

1076. Langs C, Gallo GR, Schacht RG, et al: Rapid renal failure in AIDS-associated focal glomerulosclerosis. Arch Intern Med 150:287–292, 1990.

1077. Pardo V, Meneses R, Ossa L, et al: AIDS-related glomerulopathy: Occurrence in specific risk groups. Kidney Int 31:1167–1173, 1987.

1078. Strauss J, Abitbol C, Zilleruelo G, et al: Renal disease in children with the acquired immunodeficiency syndrome. N Engl J Med 321:625–630, 1989.

1079. Bourgoignie JJ, Meneses R, Ortiz C, et al: The clinical spectrum of renal disease associated with human immunodeficiency virus. Am J Kidney Dis 12:131–137, 1988.

1080. Seney FDJ, Burns DK, Silva FG: Acquired immunodeficiency syndrome and the kidney. Am J Kidney Dis 16:1–13, 1990.

1081. Glassock RJ, Cohen AH, Danovitch G, Parsa KP: Human immunodeficiency virus (HIV) infection and the kidney. Ann Intern Med 112:35–49, 1990.

1082. Humphreys MH: Human immunodeficiency virus-associated glomerulosclerosis. Kidney Int 48:311–320, 1995.

1083. Mazbar SA, Schoenfeld PY, Humphreys MH: Renal involvement in patients infected with HIV: Experience at San Francisco General Hospital. Kidney Int 37:1325–1332, 1990.

1084. Ross MJ, Klotman PE: Recent progress in HIV-associated nephropathy. J Am Soc Nephrol 13:2997–3004, 2002.

1085. Bourgoignie JJ, Ortiz-Interian C, Green DF: The human immunodeficiency virus epidemic and HIV associated nephropathy. In Hatano M (ed): Nephrology, 1st ed. Tokyo, Springer Verlag, 1990, pp. 484–492.

1086. Winston JA, Burns GC, Klotman PE: The human immunodeficiency virus (HIV) epidemic and HIV-associated nephropathy. Semin Nephrol 18: 373–377, 1998.

1087. Nochy D, Glotz D, Dosquet P, et al: Renal disease associated with HIV infection: A multicentric study of 60 patients from Paris hospitals. Nephrol Dial Transplant 8:11–19, 1993.

1088. Nochy D, Glotz D, Dosquet P, et al: Renal lesions associated with human immunodeficiency virus infection: North American vs. European experience. Adv Nephrol Necker Hosp 22:269–286, 1993.

1089. Liu R, Paxton WA, Choe S, et al: Homozygous defect in HIV-1 coreceptor accounts for resistance of some multiply-exposed individuals to HIV-1 infection. Cell 86:367–377, 1996.

1090. Smith MW, Dean M, Carrington M, et al: Contrasting genetic influence of CCR2 and CCR5 variants on HIV-1 infection and disease progression. Hemophilia Growth and Development Study (HGDS), Multicenter AIDS Cohort Study (MACS), Multicenter Hemophilia Cohort Study (MHCS), San Francisco City Cohort (SFCC), ALIVE Study. Science 277:959–965, 1997.

1091. Winkler C, Modi W, Smith MW, et al: Genetic restriction of AIDS pathogenesis by an SDF-1 chemokine gene variant. ALIVE Study, Hemophilia Growth and Development Study (HGDS), Multicenter AIDS Cohort Study (MACS), Multicenter Hemophilia Cohort Study (MHCS), San Francisco City Cohort (SFCC). Science 279:389–393, 1998.

1092. Ahuja TS, Borucki M, Funtanilla M, et al: Is the prevalence of HIV-associated nephropathy decreasing? Am J Nephrol 19:655–659, 1999.

1093. Shahinian V, Rajaraman S, Borucki M, et al: Prevalence of HIV-associated nephropathy in autopsies of HIV-infected patients. Am J Kidney Dis 35:884–888, 2000.

1094. Bourgoignie JJ: Renal complications of human immunodeficiency virus type 1. Kidney Int 37:1571–1584, 1990.

1095. Valeri A, Neusy AJ: Acute and chronic renal disease in hospitalized AIDS patients. Clin Nephrol 35:110–118, 1991.

1096. Chander P, Soni A, Suri A, et al: Renal ultrastructural markers in AIDS-associated nephropathy. Am J Pathol 126:513–526, 1987.

1097. Barisoni L, Kriz W, Mundel P, D'Agati V: The dysregulated podocyte phenotype: A novel concept in the pathogenesis of collapsing idiopathic focal segmental glomerulosclerosis and HIV-associated nephropathy. J Am Soc Nephrol 10:51–61, 1999.

1098. Bruggeman LA, Ross MD, Tanji N, et al: Renal epithelium is a previously unrecognized site of HIV-1 infection. J Am Soc Nephrol 11:2079–2087, 2000.

1099. Marras D, Bruggeman LA, Gao F, et al: Replication and compartmentalization of HIV-1 in kidney epithelium of patients with HIV-associated nephropathy. Nature Med 8:522–526, 2002.

1100. Dickie P, Felser J, Eckhaus M, et al: HIV-associated nephropathy in transgenic mice expressing HIV-1 genes. Virology 185:109–119, 1991.

1101. Kopp JB, Klotman ME, Adler SH, et al: Progressive glomerulosclerosis and enhanced renal accumulation of basement membrane components in mice transgenic for human immunodeficiency virus type 1 genes. Proc Natl Acad Sci U S A 89:1577–1581, 1992.

1102. Kopp JB, Ray PE, Adler SH, et al: Nephropathy in HIV-transgenic mice. Contrib Nephrol 107:194–204, 1994.

1103. Bruggeman LA, Dikman S, Meng C, et al: Nephropathy in human immunodeficiency virus-1 transgenic mice is due to renal transgene expression. J Clin Invest 100:84–92, 1997.

1104. Barisoni L, Bruggeman LA, Mundel P, et al: HIV-1 induces renal epithelial dedifferentiation in a transgenic model of HIV-associated nephropathy. Kidney Int 58:173–181, 2000.

1105. Husain M, Gusella GL, Klotman ME, et al: HIV-1 nef induces proliferation and anchorage-independent growth in podocytes. J Am Soc Nephrol 13:1806–1815, 2002.

1106. Hanna Z, Weng XD, Kay DG, et al: The pathogenicity of human immunodeficiency virus (HIV) type 1 Nef in CD4C/HIV transgenic mice is abolished by mutation of its SH3-binding domain, and disease development is delayed in the absence of Hck. J Virol 75:9378–9392, 2001.

1107. Zuo Y, Matsusaka T, Zhong J, et al: HIV-1 genes vpr and nef synergistically damage podocytes, leading to glomerulosclerosis. J Am Soc Nephrol 17:2832–2843, 2006.

1108. Shankland SJ, Eitner F, Hudkins KL, et al: Differential expression of cyclin-dependent kinase inhibitors in human glomerular disease: Role in podocyte proliferation and maturation. Kidney Int 58:674–683, 2000.

1109. Babut-Gay ML, Echard M, Kleinknecht D, Meyrier A: Zidovudine and nephropathy with human immunodeficiency virus (HIV) infection. Ann Intern Med 111:856–857, 1989.

1110. Harrer T, Hunzelmann N, Stoll R, et al: Therapy for HIV-1-related nephritis with zidovudine. AIDS 4:815–817, 1990.

1111. Lam M, Park MC: HIV-associated nephropathy—beneficial effect of zidovudine therapy. N Engl J Med 323:1775–1776, 1990.

1112. Ifudu O, Rao TK, Tan CC, et al: Zidovudine is beneficial in human immunodeficiency virus associated nephropathy. Am J Nephrol 15:217–221, 1995.

1113. Wali RK, Drachenberg CI, Papadimitriou JC, et al: HIV-1-associated nephropathy and response to highly-active antiretroviral therapy. Lancet 352:783–784, 1998.

1114. Kirchner JT: Resolution of renal failure after initiation of HAART: 3 cases and a discussion of the literature. AIDS Read 12:103–112, 2002.

1115. Atta MG, Gallant JE, Rahman MH, et al: Antiretroviral therapy in the treatment of HIV-associated nephropathy. Nephrol Dial Transplant 21:2809–2813, 2006.

1116. USRDS 2002. US Renal Data System: USRDS 2002 Annual Data Report. Bethesda, MD, National Institutes of Health, National Institute of Diabetes and Digestive and Kidney Diseases, Division of Kidney, Urologic, and Hematologic Diseases; 2002.

1117. Ingulli E, Tejani A, Fikrig S, et al: Nephrotic syndrome associated with acquired immunodeficiency syndrome in children. J Pediatr 119:710–716, 1991.

1118. Strauss J, Zilleruelo G, Abitbol C, et al: Human immunodeficiency virus nephropathy. Pediatr Nephrol 7:220–225, 1993.

1119. Smith MC, Pawar R, Carey JT, et al: Effect of corticosteroid therapy on human immunodeficiency virus- associated nephropathy. Am J Med 97:145–151, 1994.

1120. Smith MC, Austen JL, Carey JT, et al: Prednisone improves renal function and proteinuria in human immunodeficiency virus-associated nephropathy. Am J Med 101:41–48, 1996.

1121. Eustace JA, Nuermberger E, Choi M, et al: Cohort study of the treatment of severe HIV-associated nephropathy with corticosteroids. Kidney Int 58:1253–1260, 2000.
1122. Klotman PE: Early treatment with ACE inhibition may benefit HIV-associated nephropathy patients. Am J Kidney Dis 31:719–720, 1998.
1123. Burns GC, Paul SK, Toth IR, Sivak SL: Effect of angiotensin-converting enzyme inhibition in HIV-associated nephropathy. J Am Soc Nephrol 8:1140–1146, 1997.
1124. Ouellette DR, Kelly JW, Anders GT: Serum angiotensin-converting enzyme level is elevated in patients with human immunodeficiency virus infection. Arch Intern Med 152:321–324, 1992.
1125. Kumar MSA, Sierka DR, Damask AM, et al: Safety and success of kidney transplantation and concomitant immunosuppression in HIV-positive patients. Kidney Int 67:1622–1629, 2005.
1126. Long-term patient and graft survival after kidney transplantation in hiv positive patients. Transplantation 82:121–122, 2006.
1127. Bhagani S, Sweny P, Brook G: Guidelines for kidney transplantation in patients with HIV disease. HIV Med 7:133–139, 2006.
1128. Casanova S, Mazzucco G, Barbiano DB, et al: Pattern of glomerular involvement in human immunodeficiency virus- infected patients: An Italian study. Am J Kidney Dis 26:446–453, 1995.
1129. Kimmel PL, Phillips TM, Ferreira-Centeno A, et al: HIV-associated immune-mediated renal disease. Kidney Int 44:1327–1340, 1993.
1130. Beaufils H, Jouanneau C, Katlama C, et al: HIV-associated IgA nephropathy–a post-mortem study. Nephrol Dial Transplant 10:35–38, 1995.
1131. Kenouch S, Delahousse M, Mery JP, Nochy D: Mesangial IgA deposits in two patients with AIDS-related complex. Nephron 54:338–340, 1990.
1132. Kimmel PL, Phillips TM, Ferreira-Centeno A, et al: Brief report: Idiotypic IgA nephropathy in patients with human immunodeficiency virus infection. N Engl J Med 327:702–706, 1992.
1133. Katz A, Bargman JM, Miller DC, et al: IgA nephritis in HIV-positive patients: A new HIV-associated nephropathy? Clin Nephrol 38:61–68, 1992.
1134. Stokes MB, Chawla H, Brody RI, et al: Immune complex glomerulonephritis in patients coinfected with human immunodeficiency virus and hepatitis C virus. Am J Kidney Dis 29:514–525, 1997.
1135. Cheng JT, Anderson HL, Markowitz GS, et al: Hepatitis C virus-associated glomerular disease in patients with HIV co-infection. J Am Soc Nephrol 10:1566–1574, 1999.
1136. D'Agati V, Seigle R: Coexistence of AIDS and lupus nephritis: A case report. Am J Nephrol 10:243–247, 1990.
1137. Contreras G, Green DF, Pardo V, et al: Systemic lupus erythematosus in two adults with human immunodeficiency virus infection. Am J Kidney Dis 28:292–295, 1996.
1138. Faubert PF, Porush JG, Venkataseshan VS: Lupus like syndromes. *In* Grishman E, Churg J, Needleman P, Venkataseshan VS (eds): The Kidneys in Collagen Vascular Disease, 1st ed. New York, Raven Press, 1993, pp. 96–98.
1139. Kopelman RG, Zolla-Pazner S: Association of human immunodeficiency virus infection and autoimmune phenomena. Am J Med 84:82–88, 1988.
1140. Rarick MU, Espina B, Mocharnuk R, et al: Thrombotic thrombocytopenic purpura in patients with human immunodeficiency virus infection: A report of three cases and review of the literature. Am J Hematol 40:103–109, 1992.
1141. Kleinknecht C, Levy M, Peix A, et al: Membranous glomerulonephritis and hepatitis B surface antigen in children. J Pediatr 95: 946–952, 1979.
1142. Hsu HC, Wu CY, Lin CY, et al: Membranous nephropathy in 52 hepatitis B surface antigen (HBsAg) carrier children in Taiwan. Kidney Int 36:1103–1107, 1989.
1143. Wrzolkowa T, Zurowska A, Uszycka-Karcz M, Picken MM: Hepatitis B virus-associated glomerulonephritis: Electron microscopic studies in 98 children. Am J Kidney Dis 18:306–312, 1991.
1144. Venkataseshan VS, Lieberman K, Kim DU, et al: Hepatitis B-associated glomerulonephritis. Pathology, pathogenesis, and clinical course. Medicine (Baltimore) 69:200–216, 1990.
1145. Lai KN, Li PK, Lui SF, et al: Membranous nephropathy related to hepatitis B virus in adults. N Engl J Med 324:1457–1463, 1991.
1146. Johnson RJ, Couser WG: Hepatitis B infection and renal disease: Clinical, immunopathogenetic and therapeutic considerations. Kidney Int 37:663–676, 1990.
1147. McMahon BJ, Alberts SR, Wainwright RB, et al: Hepatitis B-related sequelae. Prospective study in 1400 hepatitis B surface antigen-positive Alaska native carriers. Arch Intern Med 150:1051–1054, 1990.
1148. Guillevin L, Lhote F, Cohen P, et al: Polyarteritis nodosa related to hepatitis B virus. A prospective study with long-term observation of 41 patients. Medicine (Baltimore) 74:238–253, 1995.
1149. Gilbert RD, Wiggelinkhuizen J: The clinical course of hepatitis B virus-associated nephropathy. Pediatr Nephrol 8:11–14, 1994.
1150. Levy M, Gagnadoux MF: Membranous nephropathy following perinatal transmission of hepatitis B virus infection—long-term follow-up study. Pediatr Nephrol 10:76–78, 1996.
1151. Ozdamar SO, Gucer S, Tinaztepe K: Hepatitis-B virus associated nephropathies: A clinicopathological study in 14 children. Pediatr Nephrol 18:23–28, 2003.
1152. Combes B, Shorey J, Barrera A, et al: Glomerulonephritis with deposition of Australia antigen-antibody complexes in glomerular basement membrane. Lancet 2:234–237, 1971.
1153. Lai FM, Li PK, Suen MW, et al: Crescentic glomerulonephritis related to hepatitis B virus. Mod Pathol 5:262–267, 1992.
1154. Li PK, Lai FM, Ho SS, et al: Acute renal failure in hepatitis B virus-related membranous nephropathy with mesangiocapillary transition and crescentic transformation. Am J Kidney Dis 19:76–80, 1992.
1155. Ohba S, Kimura K, Mise N, et al: Differential localization of s and e antigens in hepatitis B virus- associated glomerulonephritis. Clin Nephrol 48:44–47, 1997.
1156. Lai KN, Ho RT, Tam JS, Lai FM: Detection of hepatitis B virus DNA and RNA in kidneys of HBV related glomerulonephritis. Kidney Int 50:1965–1977, 1996.
1157. Conjeevaram HS, Hoofnagle JH, Austin HA, et al: Long-term outcome of hepatitis B virus-related glomerulonephritis after therapy with interferon alfa. Gastroenterology 109:540–546, 1995.
1158. Lin CY: Treatment of hepatitis B virus-associated membranous nephropathy with recombinant alpha-interferon. Kidney Int 47:225–230, 1995.
1159. Lisker-Melman M, Webb D, Di Bisceglie AM, et al: Glomerulonephritis caused by chronic hepatitis B virus infection: Treatment with recombinant human alpha-interferon. Ann Intern Med 111:479–483, 1989.
1160. Bhimma R, Coovadia HM, Kramvis A, et al: Treatment of hepatitis B virus-associated nephropathy in black children. Pediatr Nephrol 17:393–399, 2002.
1161. Lin CY: Clinical features and natural course of HBV-related glomerulopathy in children. Kidney Int Suppl 35:S46-S53, 1991.
1162. Lai KN, Tam JS, Lin HJ, Lai FM: The therapeutic dilemma of the usage of corticosteroid in patients with membranous nephropathy and persistent hepatitis B virus surface antigenaemia. Nephron 54:12–17, 1990.
1163. Lin CY, Lo SC: Treatment of hepatitis B virus-associated membranous nephropathy with adenine arabinoside and thymic extract. Kidney Int 39:301–306, 1991.
1164. Tang S, Lai FMM, Lui YH, et al: Lamivudine in hepatitis B-associated membranous nephropathy. Kidney Int 68:1750–1758, 2005.
1165. Chan TM, Fang GX, Tang CS, et al: Preemptive lamivudine therapy based on HBV DNA level in HBsAg-positive kidney allograft recipients. Hepatology 36:1246–1252, 2002.
1166. Lee WC, Wu MJ, Cheng CH, et al: Lamivudine is effective for the treatment of reactivation of hepatitis B virus and fulminant hepatic failure in renal transplant recipients. Am J Kidney Dis 38:1074–1081, 2001.
1167. Johnson RJ, Willson R, Yamabe H, et al: Renal manifestations of hepatitis C virus infection. Kidney Int 46:1255–1263, 1994.
1168. Johnson RJ, Gretch DR, Yamabe H, et al: Membranoproliferative glomerulonephritis associated with hepatitis C virus infection. N Engl J Med 328:465–470, 1993.
1169. D'Amico G: Renal involvement in hepatitis C infection: Cryoglobulinemic glomerulonephritis. Kidney Int 54:650–671, 1998.
1170. Markowitz GS, Cheng JT, Colvin RB, et al: Hepatitis C viral infection is associated with fibrillary glomerulonephritis and immunotactoid glomerulopathy. J Am Soc Nephrol 9:2244–2252, 1998.
1171. Sansonno D, Gesualdo L, Manno C, et al: Hepatitis C virus-related proteins in kidney tissue from hepatitis C virus-infected patients with cryoglobulinemic membranoproliferative glomerulonephritis. Hepatology 25:1237–1244, 1997.
1172. Agnello V, Chung RT, Kaplan LM: A role for hepatitis C virus infection in type II cryoglobulinemia. N Engl J Med 327:1490–1495, 1992.
1173. Herzenberg AM, Telford JJ, De Luca LG, et al: Thrombotic microangiopathy associated with cryoglobulinemic membranoproliferative glomerulonephritis and hepatitis C. Am J Kidney Dis 31:521–526, 1998.
1174. Stehman-Breen C, Alpers CE, Couser WG, et al: Hepatitis C virus associated membranous glomerulonephritis. Clin Nephrol 44:141–147, 1995.
1175. Hammoud H, Haem J, Laurent B, et al: Glomerular disease during HCV infection in renal transplantation. Nephrol Dial Transplant 11 Suppl 4:54–55, 1996.
1176. Morales JM, Campistol JM, Andres A, Rodicio JL: Glomerular diseases in patients with hepatitis C virus infection after renal transplantation. Curr Opin Nephrol Hypertens 6:511–515, 1997.
1177. Morales JM, Pascual-Capdevila J, Campistol JM, et al: Membranous glomerulonephritis associated with hepatitis C virus infection in renal transplant patients. Transplantation 63:1634–1649, 1997.
1178. Cruzado JM, Gil-Vernet S, Ercilla G, et al: Hepatitis C virus-associated membranoproliferative glomerulonephritis in renal allografts. J Am Soc Nephrol 7:2469–2475, 1996.
1179. Davis CL, Gretch DR, Perkins JD, et al: Hepatitis C-associated glomerular disease in liver transplant recipients. Liver Transpl Surg 1:166–175, 1995.
1180. Kendrick EA, McVicar JP, Kowdley KV, et al: Renal disease in hepatitis C-positive liver transplant recipients. Transplantation 63:1287–1293, 1997.
1181. Misiani R, Bellavita P, Fenili D, et al: Interferon alfa-2a therapy in cryoglobulinemia associated with hepatitis C virus. N Engl J Med 330:751–756, 1994.
1182. Johnson RJ, Gretch DR, Couser WG, et al: Hepatitis C virus-associated glomerulonephritis. Effect of alpha-interferon therapy. Kidney Int 46:1700–1704, 1994.
1183. Takano S, Satomura Y, Omata M. Effects of interferon beta on non-A, non-B acute hepatitis: A prospective, randomized, controlled-dose study. Japan Acute Hepatitis Cooperative Study Group. Gastroenterology 107:805–811, 1994.
1184. Ohta S, Yokoyama H, Wada T, et al: Exacerbation of glomerulonephritis in subjects with chronic hepatitis C virus infection after interferon therapy. Am J Kidney Dis 33:1040–1048, 1999.
1185. Davis GL, Esteban-Mur R, Rustgi V, et al: Interferon alfa-2b alone or in combination with ribavirin for the treatment of relapse of chronic hepatitis C. International Hepatitis Interventional Therapy Group. N Engl J Med 339:1493–1499, 1998.
1186. McHutchison JG, Gordon SC, Schiff ER, et al: Interferon alfa-2b alone or in combination with ribavirin as initial treatment for chronic hepatitis C. Hepatitis Interventional Therapy Group. N Engl J Med 339:1485–1492, 1998.
1187. Reichard O, Norkrans G, Fryden A, et al: Randomised, double-blind, placebo-controlled trial of interferon alpha-2b with and without ribavirin for chronic hepatitis C. The Swedish Study Group. Lancet 351:83–87, 1998.
1188. Sabry AA, Sobh MA, Sheaashaa HA, et al: Effect of combination therapy (ribavirin and interferon) in HCV-related glomerulopathy. Nephrol Dial Transplant 17:1924–1930, 2002.
1189. Alric L, Plaisier E, Theault S, et al: Influence of antiviral therapy in hepatitis C virus-associated cryoglobulinemic MPGN. Am J Kidney Dis 43:617–623, 2004.
1190. Rostaing L, Modesto A, Baron E, et al: Acute renal failure in kidney transplant patients treated with interferon alpha 2b for chronic hepatitis C. Nephron 74:512–516, 1996.

1191. Baid S, Tolkoff-Rubin N, Saidman S, et al: Acute humoral rejection in hepatitis C-infected renal transplant recipients receiving antiviral therapy. Am J Transplant 3:74–78, 2003.

1192. Quigg RJ, Brathwaite M, Gardner DF, et al: Successful cyclophosphamide treatment of cryoglobulinemic membranoproliferative glomerulonephritis associated with hepatitis C virus infection. Am J Kidney Dis 25:798–800, 1995.

1193. Beddhu S, Bastacky S, Johnson JP: The clinical and morphologic spectrum of renal cryoglobulinemia. Medicine (Baltimore) 81:398–409, 2002.

1194. Thiel J, Peters T, Mas MA, et al: Kinetics of hepatitis C (HCV) viraemia and quasispecies during treatment of HCV associated cryoglobulinaemia with pulse cyclophosphamide. Ann Rheum Dis 61:838–841, 2002.

1195. Rosenstock JL, Stern L, Sherman WH, et al: Fludarabine treatment of cryoglobulinemic glomerulonephritis. Am J Kidney Dis 40:644–648, 2002.

1196. Quartuccio L, Soardo G, Romano G, et al: Treatment of glomerulonephritis in type II mixed cryoglobulinemia with rituximab. Arthritis Rheum 50:S235, 2004.

1197. Basse G, Ribes D, Kamar N, et al: Rituximab therapy for de novo mixed cryoglobulinemia in renal transplant patients. Transplantation 80:1560–1564, 2005.

1198. Penner E: Nature of immune complexes in autoimmune chronic active hepatitis. Gastroenterology 92:304–308, 1987.

1199. Axelsen RA, Crawford DH, Endre ZH, et al: Renal glomerular lesions in unselected patients with cirrhosis undergoing orthotopic liver transplantation. Pathology 27:237–246, 1995.

1200. Kawaguchi K, Koike M: Glomerular lesions associated with liver cirrhosis: An immunohistochemical and clinicopathologic analysis. Hum Pathol 17:1137–1143, 1986.

1201. Bene MC, De Korwin JD, de Ligny BH, et al: IgA nephropathy and alcoholic liver cirrhosis. A prospective necropsy study. Am J Clin Pathol 89:769–773, 1988.

1202. Nochy D, Callard P, Bellon B, et al: Association of overt glomerulonephritis and liver disease: a study of 34 patients. Clin Nephrol 6:422–427, 1976.

1203. Aggarwal M, Manske CL, Lynch PJ, Paller MS: Henoch-Schonlein vasculitis as a manifestation of IgA-associated disease in cirrhosis. Am J Kidney Dis 20:400–402, 1992.

1204. Berger J, Yaneva H, Nabarra B: Glomerular changes in patients with cirrhosis of the liver. Adv Nephrol Necker Hosp 7:3–14, 1977.

1205. Callard P, Feldmann G, Prandi D, et al: Immune complex type glomerulonephritis in cirrhosis of the liver. Am J Pathol 80:329–340, 1975.

1206. Newell GC: Cirrhotic glomerulonephritis: Incidence, morphology, clinical features, and pathogenesis. Am J Kidney Dis 9:183–190, 1987.

1207. van de Wiel A, Valentijn RM, Schuurman HJ, et al: Circulating IgA immune complexes and skin IgA deposits in liver disease. Relation to liver histopathology. Dig Dis Sci 33:679–684, 1988.

1208. Dash SC, Bhuyan UN, Dinda AK, et al: Increased incidence of glomerulonephritis following spleno-renal shunt surgery in non-cirrhotic portal fibrosis. Kidney Int 52:482–505, 1997.

1209. Noble-Jamieson G, Thiru S, Johnston P, et al: Glomerulonephritis with end-stage liver disease in childhood. Lancet 339:706–707, 1992.

1210. Alpers CE, Cotran RS: Neoplasia and glomerular injury. Kidney Int 30:465–473, 1986.

1211. Norris SH: Paraneoplastic glomerulopathies. Semin Nephrol 13:258–272, 1993.

1212. Morel-Maroger Striker L, Striker GE: Glomerular lesions in malignancies. Contrib Nephrol 48:111–124, 1985.

1213. Brueggemeyer CD, Ramirez G: Membranous nephropathy: A concern for malignancy. Am J Kidney Dis 9:23–26, 1987.

1214. Zech P, Colon S, Pointet P, et al: The nephrotic syndrome in adults aged over 60: etiology, evolution and treatment of 76 cases. Clin Nephrol 17:232–236, 1982.

1215. Liverman PC, Tucker FL, Bolton WK: Erythrocyte sedimentation rate in glomerular disease: Association with urinary protein. Am J Nephrol 8:363–367, 1988.

1216. Bathon J, Graves J, Jens P, et al: The erythrocyte sedimentation rate in end-stage renal failure. Am J Kidney Dis 10:34–40, 1987.

1217. Burstein DM, Korbet SM, Schwartz MM: Membranous glomerulonephritis and malignancy. Am J Kidney Dis 22:5–10, 1993.

1218. da Costa CR, Dupont E, Hamers R, et al: Nephrotic syndrome in bronchogenic carcinoma: Report of two cases with immunochemical studies. Clin Nephrol 2:245–251, 1974.

1219. Barton CH, Vaziri ND, Spear GS: Nephrotic syndrome associated with adenocarcinoma of the breast. Am J Med 68:308–312, 1980.

1220. Couser WG, Wagonfeld JB, Spargo BH, Lewis EJ: Glomerular deposition of tumor antigen in membranous nephropathy associated with colonic carcinoma. Am J Med 57:962–970, 1974.

1221. Wakashin M, Wakashin Y, Iesato K, et al: Association of gastric cancer and nephrotic syndrome. An immunologic study in three patients. Gastroenterology 78:749–756, 1980.

1222. Beauvais P, Vaudour G, Boccon Gibod L, Levy M: Membranous nephropathy associated with ovarian tumour in a young girl: Recovery after removal. Eur J Pediatr 148:624–625, 1989.

1223. Nishibara G, Sukemi T, Ikeda Y, Tomiyoshi Y: Nephrotic syndrome due to membranous nephropathy associated with renal cell carcinoma. Clin Nephrol 45:424, 1996.

1224. Helin K, Honkanen E, Metsaniitty J, Tornroth T: A case of membranous glomerulonephritis associated with adenocarcinoma of pancreas. Nephrol Dial Transplant 13:1049–1050, 1998.

1225. Stuart K, Fallon BG, Cardi MA: Development of the nephrotic syndrome in a patient with prostatic carcinoma. Am J Med 80:295–298, 1986.

1226. Kon SP, Fan SL, Kwan JT, et al: Membranous nephropathy complicating adenolymphoma of the parotid (Warthin's tumour). Nephron 73:692–694, 1996.

1227. Schneider BF, Glass WF, Brooks CH, Koenig KG: Membranous glomerulonephritis associated with testicular seminoma. J Intern Med 237:599–602, 1995.

1228. Becker BN, Goldin G, Santos R, et al: Carcinoid tumor and the nephrotic syndrome: A novel association between neoplasia and glomerular disease. South Med J 89:240–242, 1996.

1229. Hotta O, Taguma Y, Kurosawa K, et al: Membranous nephropathy associated with nodular sclerosing Hodgkin's disease. Nephron 63:347–350, 1993.

1230. Lumeng J, Moran JF: Carotid body tumor associated with mild membranous glomerulonephritis. Ann Intern Med 65:1266–1270, 1966.

1231. Pascal RR, Iannaccone PM, Rollwagen FM, et al: Electron microscopy and immunofluorescence of glomerular immune complex deposits in cancer patients. Cancer Res 36:43–47, 1976.

1232. Helin H, Pasternack A, Hakala T, et al: Glomerular electron-dense deposits and circulating immune complexes in patients with malignant tumours. Clin Nephrol 14:23–30, 1980.

1233. Sherman RL, Susin M, Weksler ME, Becker EL: Lipoid nephrosis in Hodgkin's disease. Am J Med 52:699–706, 1972.

1234. Dabbs DJ, Striker LM, Mignon F, Striker G: Glomerular lesions in lymphomas and leukemias. Am J Med 80:63–70, 1986.

1235. Watson A, Stachura I, Fragola J, Bourke E: Focal segmental glomerulosclerosis in Hodgkin's disease. Am J Nephrol 3:228–232, 1983.

1236. Ishida I, Hirakata H, Kanai H, et al: Steroid-resistant nephrotic syndrome associated with malignant thymoma. Clin Nephrol 46:340–346, 1996.

1237. Cather JC, Jackow C, Yegge J, et al: Mycosis fungoides with focal segmental glomerular sclerosis and nephrotic syndrome. J Am Acad Dermatol 38:301–305, 1998.

1238. Auguet T, Lorenzo A, Colomer E, et al: Recovery of minimal change nephrotic syndrome and acute renal failure in a patient with renal cell carcinoma. Am J Nephrol 18:433–435, 1998.

1239. Gandini E, Allaria P, Castiglioni A, et al: Minimal change nephrotic syndrome with cecum adenocarcinoma. Clin Nephrol 45:268–270, 1996.

1240. Singer CR, Boulton-Jones JM: Minimal change nephropathy associated with anaplastic carcinoma of bronchus. Postgrad Med J 62:213–217, 1986.

1241. Thorner P, McGraw M, Weitzman S, et al: Wilms' tumor and glomerular disease. Occurrence with features of membranoproliferative glomerulonephritis and secondary focal, segmental glomerulosclerosis. Arch Pathol Lab Med 108:141–146, 1984.

1242. Moorthy AV, Zimmerman SW, Burkholder PM: Nephrotic syndrome in Hodgkin's disease. Evidence for pathogenesis alternative to immune complex deposition. Am J Med 61:471–477, 1976.

1243. Shalhoub RJ: Pathogenesis of lipoid nephrosis: A disorder of T cell function. Lancet ii: 556–560, 1974.

1244. Walker JF, O'Neil S, Campbell E, et al: Carcinoma of the oesophagus associated with membrano- proliferative glomerulonephritis. Postgrad Med J 57:592–596, 1981.

1245. Moulin B, Ronco PM, Mougenot B, et al: Glomerulonephritis in chronic lymphocytic leukemia and related B- cell lymphomas. Kidney Int 42:127–135, 1992.

1246. Feehally J, Hutchinson RM, Mackay EH, Walls J: Recurrent proteinuria in chronic lymphocytic leukemia. Clin Nephrol 16:51–54, 1981.

1247. Mak SK, Wong PN, Lo KY, Wong AK: Successful treatment of IgA nephropathy in association with low-grade B-cell lymphoma of the mucosa-associated lymphoid tissue type. Am J Kidney Dis 31:713–718, 1998.

1248. Edgar JD, Rooney DP, McNamee P, McNeill TA: An association between ANCA positive renal disease and malignancy. Clin Nephrol 40:22–25, 1993.

1249. Hruby Z, Bronowicz A, Rabczynski J, et al: A case of severe anti-neutrophil cytoplasmic antibody (ANCA)- positive crescentic glomerulonephritis and asymptomatic gastric cancer. Int Urol Nephrol 26:579–586, 1994.

1250. Biava CG, Gonwa TA, Naughton JL, Hopper J, Jr: Crescentic glomerulonephritis associated with nonrenal malignancies. Am J Nephrol 4:208–214, 1984.

1251. Gordon LI, Kwaan HC: Cancer- and drug-associated thrombotic thrombocytopenic purpura and hemolytic uremic syndrome. Semin Hematol 34:140–147, 1997.

1252. Kilcoyne MM, Gocke DJ, Meltzer JI, et al: Nephrotic syndrome in heroin addicts. Lancet 1:17–20, 1972.

1253. Rao TK, Nicastri AD, Friedman EA: Natural history of heroin-associated nephropathy. N Engl J Med 290:19–23, 1974.

1254. Cunningham EE, Brentjens JR, Zielezny MA, et al: Heroin nephropathy. A clinicopathologic and epidemiologic study. Am J Med 68:47–53, 1980.

1255. Llach F, Descoeudres C, Massry SG: Heroin associated nephropathy: Clinical and histological studies in 19 patients. Clin Nephrol 11:7–12, 1979.

1256. Treser G, Cherubin C, Longergan ET, et al: Renal lesions in narcotic addicts. Am J Med 57:687–694, 1974.

1257. Eknoyan G, Gyorkey F, Dichoso C, et al: Renal involvement in drug abuse. Arch Intern Med 132:801–806, 1973.

1258. May DC, Helderman JH, Eigenbrodt EH, Silva FG: Chronic sclerosing glomerulopathy (heroin-associated nephropathy) in intravenous T's and Blues abusers. Am J Kidney Dis 8: 404–409, 1986.

1259. Friedman EA, Rao TK: Why does uremia in heroin abusers occur predominantly among blacks? JAMA 250:2965–2966, 1983.

1260. Haskell LP, Glicklich D, Senitzer D: HLA associations in heroin-associated nephropathy. Am J Kidney Dis 12:45–50, 1988.

1261. Brown SM, Stimmel B, Taub RN, et al: Immunologic dysfunction in heroin addicts. Arch Intern Med 134:1001–1006, 1974.

1262. Singhal PC, Sharma P, Sanwal V, et al: Morphine modulates proliferation of kidney fibroblasts. Kidney Int 53:350–357, 1998.

1263. Singhal PC, Gibbons N, Abramovici M: Long term effects of morphine on mesangial cell proliferation and matrix synthesis. Kidney Int 41:1560–1570, 1992.

1264. Friedman EA, Rao TK: Disappearance of uremia due to heroin-associated nephropathy. Am J Kidney Dis 25:689–693, 1995.

1265. D'Agati V: The many masks of focal segmental glomerulosclerosis. Kidney Int 46:1223–1241, 1994.

1266. Whelton A, Watson AJ: Nonsteroidal anti-inflammatory drugs: Effects on kidney function. In DeBroe ME, Porter GA, Bennett WM, Verpoooten GA (eds): Clinical Nephrotoxins. Renal Injury from Drugs and Chemicals, 1st ed. Dordrecht, The Netherlands, Kluwer, 1998, pp. 203–216.

1267. Clive DM, Stoff JS: Renal syndromes associated with nonsteroidal anti-inflammatory drugs. N Engl J Med 310:563–572, 1984.

1268. Abraham PA, Keane WF: Glomerular and interstitial disease induced by nonsteroidal anti- inflammatory drugs. Am J Nephrol 4:1–6, 1984.

1269. Levin ML: Patterns of tubulo-interstitial damage associated with nonsteroidal anti-inflammatory drugs. Semin Nephrol 8:55–61, 1988.

1270. Alper AB, Jr, Meleg-Smith S, Krane NK: Nephrotic syndrome and interstitial nephritis associated with celecoxib. Am J Kidney Dis 40:1086–1090, 2002.

1271. Markowitz GS, Falkowitz DC, Isom R, et al: Membranous glomerulopathy and acute interstitial nephritis following treatment with celecoxib. Clin Nephrol 59:137–142, 2003.

1272. Stachura I, Jayakumar S, Bourke E: T and B lymphocyte subsets in fenoprofen nephropathy. Am J Med 75:9–16, 1983.

1273. Bender WL, Whelton A, Beschorner WE, et al: Interstitial nephritis, proteinuria, and renal failure caused by nonsteroidal anti-inflammatory drugs. Immunologic characterization of the inflammatory infiltrate. Am J Med 76:1006–1012, 1984.

1274. Warren GV, Korbet SM, Schwartz MM, Lewis EJ: Minimal change glomerulopathy associated with nonsteroidal antiinflammatory drugs. Am J Kidney Dis 13:127–130, 1989.

1275. Schwartzman M, D'Agati V: Spontaneous relapse of naproxen-related nephrotic syndrome. Am J Med 82:329–332, 1987.

1276. Neilson EG: Pathogenesis and therapy of interstitial nephritis. Kidney Int 35:1257–1270, 1989.

1277. Thysell H, Brun C, Larsen S, Norlin M: Plasma exchange in two cases of minimal change nephrotic syndrome with acute renal failure. Int J Artif Organs 6 Suppl 1:75–78, 1983.

1278. Bander SJ. Reversible renal failure and nephrotic syndrome without interstitial nephritis from zomepirac. Am J Kidney Dis 6:233–236, 1985.

1279. Schwarz A, Krause PH, Keller F, et al: Granulomatous interstitial nephritis after nonsteroidal anti-inflammatory drugs. Am J Nephrol 8:410–416, 1988.

1280. Radford MG, Jr, Holley KE, Grande JP, et al: Reversible membranous nephropathy associated with the use of nonsteroidal anti-inflammatory drugs. JAMA 276:466–469, 1996.

1281. Antonovych TT: Gold nephropathy. Ann Clin Lab Sci 11:386–391, 1981.

1282. Wilkinson R, Eccleston DW: Nephrotic syndrome induced by gold therapy. Br Med J 2:772, 1970.

1283. Francis KL, Jenis EH, Jensen GE, Calcagno PL: Gold-associated nephropathy. Arch Pathol Lab Med 108:234–238, 1984.

1284. Speerstra F, Reekers P, van de Putte LB, et al: HLA-DR antigens and proteinuria induced by aurothioglucose and D-penicillamine in patients with rheumatoid arthritis. J Rheumatol 10:948–953, 1983.

1285. Hall CL: The natural course of gold and penicillamine nephropathy: A longterm study of 54 patients. Adv Exp Med Biol 252:247–256, 1989.

1286. Matloff DS, Kaplan MM: D-Penicillamine-induced Goodpasture's-like syndrome in primary biliary cirrhosis—successful treatment with plasmapheresis and immunosuppressives. Gastroenterology 78:1046–1049, 1980.

1287. Falck HM, Tornroth T, Kock B, Wegelius O: Fatal renal vasculitis and minimal change glomerulonephritis complicating treatment with penicillamine. Report on two cases. Acta Med Scand 205:133–138, 1979.

1288. Mathieson PW, Peat DS, Short A, Watts RA: Coexistent membranous nephropathy and ANCA-positive crescentic glomerulonephritis in association with penicillamine. Nephrol Dial Transplant 11:863–866, 1996.

1289. Moens HJ, Ament BJ, Feltkamp BW, van der Korst JK: Longterm followup of treatment with D-penicillamine for rheumatoid arthritis: Effectivity and toxicity in relation to HLA antigens. J Rheumatol 14:1115–1119, 1987.

1290. Ferraccioli GF, Peri F, Nervetti A, et al: Tiopronin-nephropathy: Clinical, pathological, immunological and immunogenetic characteristics. Clin Exp Rheumatol 4:9–15, 1986.

1291. Yoshida A, Morozumi K, Suganuma T, et al: Clinicopathological findings of bucillamine-induced nephrotic syndrome in patients with rheumatoid arthritis. Am J Nephrol 11:284–288, 1991.

1292. Hall CL, Jawad S, Harrison PR, et al: Natural course of penicillamine nephropathy: A long term study of 33 patients. Br Med J (Clin Res Ed) 296:1083–1086, 1988.

1293. Hall CL, Tighe R: The effect of continuing penicillamine and gold treatment on the course of penicillamine and gold nephropathy. Br J Rheumatol 28:53–57, 1989.

1294. Stokes MB, Foster K, Markowitz GS, et al: Development of glomerulonephritis during anti-TNF-alpha therapy for rheumatoid arthritis. Nephrol Dial Transplant 20:1400–1406, 2005.

1295. Oliveira DB, Foster G, Savill J, et al: Membranous nephropathy caused by mercury-containing skin lightening cream. Postgrad Med J 63:303–304, 1987.

1296. Meeks A, Keith PR, Tanner MS: Nephrotic syndrome in two members of a family with mercury poisoning. J Trace Elem Electrolytes Health Dis 4:237–239, 1990.

1297. Hill GS: Drug-associated glomerulopathies. Toxicol Pathol 14:37–44, 1986.

1298. Kibukamusoke JW, Davies DR, Hutt MS: Membranous nephropathy due to skin-lightening cream. Br Med J 2:646–647, 1974.

1299. Tubbs RR, Gephardt GN, McMahon JT, et al: Membranous glomerulonephritis associated with industrial mercury exposure. Study of pathogenetic mechanisms. Am J Clin Pathol 77:409–413, 1982.

1300. Belghiti D, Patey O, Berry JP, et al: Lipoid nephrosis of toxic origin. 2 cases. Presse Med 15:1953–1955, 1986.

1301. Silverman SH, Gribetz D, Rausen AR. Nephrotic syndrome associated with ethosuccimide. Am J Dis Child 132:99, 1978.

1302. Bar-Khayim Y, Teplitz C, Garella S, Chazan JA: Trimethadione (Tridione)-induced nephrotic syndrome. A report of a case with unique ultrastructural renal pathology. Am J Med 54:272–280, 1973.

1303. Heymann W: Nephrotic syndrome after use of trimethadione and paramethadione in petit mal. JAMA 202:893–894, 1967.

1304. Snead C, Siegel N, Hayslett J: Generalized lymphadenopathy and nephrotic syndrome as a manifestation of mephenytoin (mesantoin) toxicity. Pediatrics 57:98–101, 1976.

1305. Yuasa S, Hashimoto M, Yura T, et al: Antineutrophil cytoplasmic antibodies (ANCA)-associated crescentic glomerulonephritis and propylthiouracil therapy. Nephron 73:701–703, 1996.

1306. Dolman KM, Gans RO, Vervaat TJ, et al: Vasculitis and antineutrophil cytoplasmic autoantibodies associated with propylthiouracil therapy. Lancet 342:651–652, 1993.

1307. Vogt BA, Kim Y, Jennette JC, et al: Antineutrophil cytoplasmic autoantibody-positive crescentic glomerulonephritis as a complication of treatment with propylthiouracil in children. J Pediatr 124:986–988, 1994.

1308. Prasad GV, Bastacky S, Johnson JP: Propylthiouracil-induced diffuse proliferative lupus nephritis: Review of immunological complications. J Am Soc Nephrol 8:1205–1210, 1997.

1309. Hoorntje SJ, Kallenberg CG, Weening JJ, et al: Immune-complex glomerulopathy in patients treated with captopril. Lancet 1:1212–1215, 1980.

1310. Webb DJ, Atkinson AB: Enalapril following captopril-induced nephrotic syndrome. Scott Med J 31:30–32, 1986.

1311. Coroneos E, Petrusevska G, Varghese F, Truong LD: Focal segmental glomerulosclerosis with acute renal failure associated with alpha-interferon therapy. Am J Kidney Dis 28:888–892, 1996.

1312. Shah M, Jenis EH, Mookerjee BK, et al: Interferon-alpha-associated focal segmental glomerulosclerosis with massive proteinuria in patients with chronic myeloid leukemia following high dose chemotherapy. Cancer 83:1938–1946, 1998.

1313. Honda K, Ando A, Endo M, et al: Thrombotic microangiopathy associated with alpha-interferon therapy for chronic myelocytic leukemia. Am J Kidney Dis 30:123–130, 1997.

1314. Ohashi N, Yonemura K, Sugiura T, et al: Withdrawal of interferon-alpha results in prompt resolution of thrombocytopenia and hemolysis but not renal failure in hemolytic uremic syndrome caused by interferon-alpha. Am J Kidney Dis 41:E10, 2003.

1315. Parker MG, Atkins MB, Ucci AA, Levey AS: Rapidly progressive glomerulonephritis after immunotherapy for cancer. J Am Soc Nephrol 5:1740–1744, 1995.

1316. Lindell A, Denneberg T, Enestrom S, et al: Membranous glomerulonephritis induced by 2-mercaptopropionylglycine (2-MPG). Clin Nephrol 34:108–115, 1990.

1317. Richman AV, Masco HL, Rifkin SI, Acharya MK: Minimal-change disease and the nephrotic syndrome associated with lithium therapy. Ann Intern Med 92:70–72, 1980.

1318. Tam VK, Green J, Schwieger J, Cohen AH: Nephrotic syndrome and renal insufficiency associated with lithium therapy. Am J Kidney Dis 27:715–720, 1996.

1319. Phan L, Coulomb F, Boudon M, et al: Extramembranous glomerulonephritis induced by lithium. Nephrologie 12:185–187, 1991.

1320. Santella RN, Rimmer JM, MacPherson BR: Focal segmental glomerulosclerosis in patients receiving lithium carbonate. Am J Med 84:951–954, 1988.

1321. Markowitz GS, Radhakrishnan J, Kambham N, et al: Lithium nephrotoxicity: A progressive combined glomerular and tubulointerstitial nephropathy. J Am Soc Nephrol 11:1439–1448, 2000.

1322. Markowitz GS, Appel GB, Fine PL, et al: Collapsing focal segmental glomerulosclerosis following treatment with high-dose pamidronate. J Am Soc Nephrol 12:1164–1172, 2001.

1323. Ie EH, Karschner JK, Shapiro AP: Reversible nephrotic syndrome due to high renin state in renovascular hypertension. Neth J Med 46:136–141, 1995.

1324. Chen R, Novick AC, Pohl M: Reversible renin mediated massive proteinuria successfully treated by nephrectomy. J Urol 153:133–134, 1995.

1325. Jardine DL, Pidgeon GB, Bailey RR: Renal artery stenosis as a cause of heavy albuminuria. N Z Med J 106:30–31, 1993.

1326. Giles RD, Sturgill BC, Suratt PM, Bolton WK: Massive proteinuria and acute renal failure in a patient with acute silicoproteinosis. Am J Med 64:336–342, 1978.

1327. Banks DE, Milutinovic J, Desnick RJ, et al: Silicon nephropathy mimicking Fabry's disease. Am J Nephrol 3:279–284, 1983.

1328. Moayyedi P, Fletcher S, Harnden P, et al: Mesangiocapillary glomerulonephritis associated with ulcerative colitis: Case reports of two patients. Nephrol Dial Transplant 10:1923–1924, 1995.

1329. Dhiman RK, Poddar U, Sharma BC, et al: Membranous glomerulonephritis in association with ulcerative colitis. Indian J Gastroenterol 17:62, 1998.

1330. Whelan TV, Maher JF, Kragel P, et al: Nephrotic syndrome associated with Kimura's disease. Am J Kidney Dis 11:353–356, 1988.

1331. Sud K, Saha T, Das A, et al: Kimura's disease and minimal-change nephrotic syndrome. Nephrol Dial Transplant 11:1349–1351, 1996.

1332. Lui SL, Chan KW, Li FK, et al: Castleman's disease and mesangial proliferative glomerulonephritis: The role of interleukin-6. Nephron 78:323–327, 1998.

1333. Ruggieri G, Barsotti P, Coppola G, et al: Membranous nephropathy associated with giant lymph node hyperplasia. A case report with histological and ultrastructural studies. Am J Nephrol 10:323–328, 1990.

1146

1334. Said R, Tarawneh M: Membranoproliferative glomerulonephritis associated with multicentric angiofollicular lymph node hyperplasia. Case report and review of the literature. Am J Nephrol 12:466–470, 1992.

1335. Tsukamoto Y, Hanada N, Nomura Y, et al: Rapidly progressive renal failure associated with angiofollicular lymph node hyperplasia. Am J Nephrol 11:430–436, 1991.

1336. Miadonna A, Salmaso C, Palazzi P, et al: Fibrillary glomerulonephritis in Castleman's disease. Leuk Lymphoma 28:429–435, 1998.

1337. Ikeda S, Chisuwa H, Kawasaki S, et al: Systemic reactive amyloidosis associated with Castleman's disease: Serial changes of the concentrations of acute phase serum amyloid A and interleukin 6 in serum. J Clin Pathol 50:965–967, 1997.

1338. Wood WG, Harkins MM: Nephropathy in angioimmunoblastic lymphadenopathy. Am J Clin Pathol 71:58–63, 1979.

CH 31

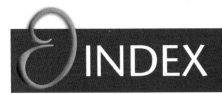

Note: Page numbers followed by the letter f refer to figures; those followed by the letter t refer to tables.

Amphotericin B
  for peritonitis, in CAPD patients, 2026t
  hypomagnesemia from, 597–598
Ampicillin, for peritonitis, in CAPD
  patients, 2026t
Amplatz thrombectomy device, for renal
  vein thrombosis, 1169
Amputation, in diabetic hemodialysis
  patient, 1288
Amrinone, for cardiogenic shock, 2051
Amyloidosis
  AL amyloid, 1101
  Alcoholics Anonymous amyloid in,
    1101
  end-stage renal disease in, 1104
  in familial Mediterranean fever, 1104
  pathology of, 1101–1103, 1102f, 1103f
  prognosis of, 1103
  treatment of, 1103–1104
Analgesics
  dosage considerations for, 1937
  for pain, in autosomal dominant
    polycystic kidney disease, 1441
  nephropathy due to, 1186–1188, 1215
    clinical features of, 1188
    diagnosis of, 1188, 1189f
    pathogenesis and pathology of, 1186–
      1188, 1187f
    treatment of, 1188
Anaphylactoid reactions
  ACE inhibitors causing, 1601
  to hemodialysis, 1997–1998
  to iron dextran, 1888, 1988
Anaritide, 355
ANAs. See Antinuclear antibodies (ANAs).
ANCAs. See Antineutrophil cytoplasmic
  antibodies (ANCAs).
Anemia
  and progressive renal injury, 809–810
  hemolytic, and rHuEPO resistance, 1892
  in acute kidney injury, 709–710, 967
    management of, 972
  in diabetic patients, with renal failure,
    1286
  in hemodialysis patient, 1986–1988
  in uremic platelet disorder, 1738
  renal, 647, 719–720, 1711, 1719–1720,
    1728–1738
    adverse effects of, 1730
    as contraindication to transplantation,
      2129–2130
    cardiac health and, 1735–1736, 1735f
    consequences of, 1733–1737
    definition of, 1728
    erythropoiesis in, 1729–1732, 1732f
    mortality risk with, 1734–1735
    pathobiology of, 1732–1733, 1733f
    prevalence of, 1728–1729, 1729f,
      1730f
    quality of life with, 1733–1734
    treatment of
      iron in, 1887–1889
      rHuEPO in, 1884–1887
  sickle cell, 1159. See also Sickle cell
    disease.
    genetic studies of, 1162
Anergy, T cell, 2172, 2173–2174, 2173f,
  2174f, 2174t
Aneurysm(s)
  after renal biopsy, 751
  intracranial, in autosomal dominant
    polycystic kidney disease,
    1440–1441
    management of, 1442
  renal artery. See Renal artery aneurysm.

Angina, in hemodialysis patient, 1997
Angioedema, as complication of ACE
  inhibitors, 1601
Angiogenesis, 6–7
  imbalance in, preeclampsia and, 1577–
    1578, 1577f, 1578f
  molecular genetics of, 16–18, 16f–18f
Angiography
  computed tomography. See Computed
    tomography angiography (CTA).
  coronary, in chronic kidney disease
    patient, 1713–1714
  digital subtraction. See Digital
    subtraction angiography (DSA).
  magnetic resonance. See Magnetic
    resonance angiography (MRA).
  of acute kidney injury, 711
Angioinfarction, for renal cell carcinoma,
  1360
Angiokeratoma, in Fabry disease, 1114
Angiokeratoma corporis diffusum
  universale, 1114–1115, 1114f
Angiolymphoblastic lymphadenopathy,
  glomerular lesions in, 1127
Angiolymphoid hyperplasia with
  eosinophilia, glomerular lesions in,
  1127
Angiomyolipoma
  computed tomography of, 881–882,
    883f
  in tuberous sclerosis, 1446
Angioplasty. See also Percutaneous
    transluminal renal angioplasty (PTRA).
  coronary, in chronic kidney disease
    patient, 1716
  for arteriovenous fistula
    stenotic lesions in, 926–927, 927f
    technique of, 927–928, 928f, 929f
  for arteriovenous graft stenosis, 919–920,
    919t
    technique of, 919–920, 920f, 921f
  for fibromuscular disease, 1559
Angiopoietin 1, in vasculogenesis, 17–18
Angiotensin(s), 338
Angiotensin I receptor(s), in preeclampsia,
  1576–1577
Angiotensin I receptor blockers,
  renoprotective effects of, 1858–1860
Angiotensin II
  and distal nephron acidification,
    265–266
  and proximal tubule acidification, 257
  biologic actions of, 407
  effects of
    on kidney, 344
    on proximal tubular Na+-Cl-
      absorption, 163–164, 163f
    on renal autoregulatory mechanisms,
      342
    on renal hemodynamics, 341–342
    on tubular transport, 342–343
  in aging kidney, 682–683
  in hypertension, 1483–1484
    smooth muscle stimulation by, 1482
  in ischemic nephropathy, 1536
  in nephrogenesis, 668
  in pregnant patient, 1569, 1569f
  in renal injury, after nephron loss, 797,
    798f
  in renal microcirculation, 103–104, 103f
  in tubuloglomerular feedback, 107–108
  removal of
    by aminopeptidases, 338
    by endopeptidases, 338
  renal effect of, 408

Angiotensin II receptor(s), 338–340
  AT$_1$, 339, 344
  AT$_2$, 339–340, 344
  AT$_4$, 340
Angiotensin II receptor blockers,
  1603–1606
  efficacy and safety of, 1606
  fixed-dose combination therapy with,
    1628t
  hyperkalemia from, 572–573, 572f
  mechanism of action of, 1603
  pharmacodynamic properties of, 1604t
  pharmacokinetic properties of, 1604t
  renal effects of, 1605–1606
  types of, 1603, 1604t
Angiotensin II Receptors Antagonist
  Losartan (RENAAL) study, 643
Angiotensin III, 1166–1167
Angiotensinases, 338
Angiotensin-converting enzyme (ACE),
  336–338, 338f
  neural endopeptidase and, dual
    inhibition of, 356. See also
    Vasopeptidase inhibitors.
  polymorphism of, 1864
  somatic, 337
  testicular, 337
Angiotensin-converting enzyme (ACE)
  genotype, 337, 1864
  in diabetic nephropathy progression,
    1278–1279
  in IgA nephropathy, 1025
Angiotensin-converting enzyme (ACE)
  inhibitors, 1596–1597
  and hyponatremia, 491
  complications due to, in plasmapheresis
    patients, 2074
  dosage considerations for, 1949–1950
  dose modifications of, 1601, 1602t
  efficacy and safety of, 1600–1601, 1602t,
    1603
  fixed-dose combination therapy with,
    1628t
  for cardiac disease and chronic kidney
    disease, 1716
  for congestive heart failure, 426, 426t
  for diabetes mellitus, 1278–1279, 1280–
    1284, 1281f, 1283f, 1204f
  for focal segmental glomerulosclerosis,
    1006
  for HIV-associated nephropathy, 1122
  for hypertension
    in autosomal dominant polycystic
      kidney disease, 1441
    in pre-dialysis patient, 1718
  for hypertension in pregnancy,
    1583–1584
  for hypertensive emergencies, 1634t,
    1635–1636, 1636t
  for IgA nephropathy, 1030
  for pheochromocytoma, 1491
  for radiation nephritis, 1157
  for renal artery stenosis, 1551–1553
  for systemic sclerosis, 1155
  hyperkalemia from, 572–573, 572f
  in aging kidney, 682–683, 683f
  indications for and contraindications to,
    1601
  mechanism of action of, 1596, 1597t
  pharmacodynamic properties of, 1597t
  pharmacogenetics of, 1864
  pharmacokinetic properties of, 1598t
  prerenal azotemia from, 945t, 946
  prophylactic, for vascular access
    dysfunction, 1965

Inflammation *(Continued)*
in peritoneal dialysis patient, 2023
interstitial, 1180–1182
effector cells in, 1180–1181
regulatory cells in, 1181–1182
rHuEPO resistance due to, 1892
Inflammatory bowel disease,
hypomagnesemia in, 597
Infliximab, for Wegener's granulomatosis,
1087
Influenza, glomerular involvement in,
1120
Infundibuloneurohypophysitis,
lymphocytic, 471
Inguinal hernia, in peritoneal dialysis
patient, 2027–2028
Inheritance pattern, of nephrolithiasis,
1301
Insulin
and phosphate transport, 201t, 203
and potassium transport, 548–549
for diabetic ketoacidosis, 536
in glomerular filtration and renal
circulation regulation, 115
in stimulation of endothelin, 347
with glucose, for hyperkalemia, 575
Insulin resistance
in dialysis patient, 1749–1750
in patient with chronic kidney disease
not on dialysis, 1750, 1750t
in patient with chronic kidney disease
on thiazolidinediones, 1750–1751
in transplant patient, 1750
Insulin-like growth factor (IGF)
in glomerular filtration and renal
circulation regulation, 115
serum, in assessment of protein stores in
renal failure, 1831
Insulin-like growth factor (IGF)-1
in chronic kidney disease, 1751
in hypertrophic response to nephron
loss, 789
in tubulointerstitial injury, 1176–1177
recombinant, use of, in dialysis patients,
1753
Insulin-like growth factor (IGF) binding
proteins, in chronic kidney disease,
1751
Integrin(s)
in glomerulogenesis, 19–20
in nephrogenesis, 14
Intensive care unit (ICU), 2037–2062
acute respiratory failure in, 2037–2038
adult respiratory distress syndrome in,
2038–2041
cardiogenic shock in, 2050–2053
fulminant hepatic failure in, 2053–2062
hypovolemic shock in, 2041–2045
renal replacement therapy in, 2056–2059
sepsis in, 2045–2050
Intercalated cell(s)
in connecting tubule, 62
in cortical collecting duct, 63, 64f–67f,
65–68
Interferon(s), for renal cell carcinoma,
1362–1363
Interferon-α
for HCV-induced renal disease, 1124
with interleukin-2, for renal cell
carcinoma, 1364, 1364t
Interferon-γ, in systemic sclerosis, 1155
Interleukin(s)
in systemic sclerosis, 1155
response of, to urinary tract infection,
1211

Interleukin-1, in sepsis, 2046, 2047f
Interleukin-2, for renal cell carcinoma,
1363–1365
alternative IL-2-based regimens and,
1363
high-dose, 1363
influence of subtype in, 1365
predictors of response and survival with,
1365, 1365t
toxicity-reduction strategies in,
1363–1364
with interferon-alpha, 1364, 1364t
Interleukin-4, for renal cell carcinoma,
1365
Interleukin-6
as biomarker, for acute kidney injury,
957
for renal cell carcinoma, 1365
in sepsis, 2046, 2047f
Interleukin-8
as biomarker, for acute kidney injury,
957
in sepsis, 2046
Interleukin-10
as biomarker, for acute kidney injury,
957
in sepsis, 2046
Interleukin-12, recombinant, for renal cell
carcinoma, 1365–1366
Interleukin-13, in sepsis, 2046
Interleukin-18, as biomarker, for acute
kidney injury, 957, 957t
Interlobular artery(ies)
anatomy of, 91–92, 92f
constriction of, norepinephrine in, 113
dilation of, atrial natriuretic peptide in,
116
relaxation response of, 104, 104f
International Cystinuria Consortium (ICC),
235, 236t
International Reflux Study Committee
classification, of vesicoureteral reflux,
1208, 1208f
International Society of Nephrology/Renal
Pathology Society classification, of
lupus nephritis, 1068–1071, 1068t,
1069f–1071f
Interstitial cell(s)
cortical, 77, 78f
medullary, 77–78, 79f
Interstitial fibrosis
in chronic kidney disease, 1701–
1702
in tubulointerstitial disease, 1182
tubular epithelial cell recovery from,
1257–1258
Interstitial fluid, accumulation of. *See also*
Edema.
local mechanisms in, 420
Interstitial inflammation, 1180–1182
effector cells in, 1180–1181
regulatory cells in, 1181–1182
Interstitial nephritis. *See also*
Tubulointerstitial disease(s).
acute, 1174, 1183–1186
clinical manifestations of, 1185
diagnosis of, 1185
drug-induced, 1183–1184, 1183t
etiology of, 1183–1184, 1183t
idiopathic, 1183t, 1184
infection-induced, 1183t, 1184
pathology of, 1184–1185
plasmapheresis for, 1186
prognosis of, 1185
treatment of, 1185–1186

Interstitial nephritis *(Continued)*
allergic
drug-induced, 948t
in allograft recipient, 2149
chronic, 1186–1197
5-aminosalicylic acid–induced, 1188–
1190, 1189t, 1190f
analgesic nephropathy and, 1186–
1188, 1189f, 1189t
aristolochic nephropathy and, 1189t,
1190–1192, 1191f
Balkan endemic nephropathy and,
1189t, 1195–1196, 1196f
cadmium nephropathy and, 1194–1195
causes of, 1186t
differential diagnosis of, 1189t
hyperuricemia and, 1196
hyperuricosuria and, 1196
hypokalemic nephropathy and,
1196–1197
lead nephropathy and, 1193–1194
lithium nephropathy and, 1192–1193,
1192f
NSAID-induced, 1188
sarcoidosis and, 1197
urate nephropathy and, 1196
hereditary cystic diseases with,
1448–1450
historical aspects of, 1174
NSAID-induced, 371, 1126
Interstitial pressure, sodium excretion and,
405–407, 406f
Interstitium, 77–80
cortical, 77, 78f
medullary, 77–80, 79f
Interventional nephrology, 915–946
in vascular access dysfunction, 1965
procedures performed in, 916t. *See
under specific procedure for
details.*
involving arteriovenous fistulas,
923–929
involving arteriovenous grafts,
916–923
involving indwelling hemodialysis
catheters, 930–943
involving peritoneal dialysis catheters,
943–944
Involving stenotic lesions, 929–930
renal biopsy as, 944–946
radiation and personal safety in, 916
rationale for, 915–916
Intestinal transport defects, in cystinuria,
1401
Intra-aortic balloon pumping, to improve
diastolic blood pressure, in
cardiogenic shock, 2052
Intracellular compartment
aquaporin-2 localization in, during
recycling, 291–293
composition and size of, 459–460, 460f
Intracranial aneurysm, in autosomal
dominant polycystic kidney disease,
1440–1441
management of, 1442
Intradialytic hemolysis, in hemodialysis
patient, 1998
Intrahepatic hypertension, and cirrhosis
with ascites, 438
Intramembranous particle aggregates
orthogonal arrays of, 288
water-permeable, 287–288
Intrarenal physical factor(s), in
extracellular fluid volume control,
402–407